NEUROTRAUMA

NOTICE

NEUROTRAUMA

Editors

RAJ K. NARAYAN, M.D., F.A.C.S.

Professor and Chairman
Department of Neurosurgery
Temple University School of Medicine
Philadelphia, Pennsylvania

JACK E. WILBERGER, JR., M.D., F.A.C.S.

Professor and Director
Division of Neurosurgery
Allegheny General Hospital
Pittsburgh, Pennsylvania

JOHN T. POVLISHOCK, Ph.D.

Professor and Chairman
Department of Anatomy
Medical College of Virginia
Virginia Commonwealth University
Richmond, Virginia

McGRAW-HILL
HEALTH PROFESSIONS DIVISION

New York St. Louis San Francisco
Auckland Bogotá Caracas Lisbon London Madrid
Mexico City Milan Montreal New Delhi San Juan
Singapore Sydney Tokyo Toronto

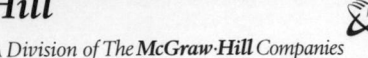

1234567890 QPK QPK 9876

ISBN 0-07-045662-3

This book was set in Times Roman by Bi-Comp, Inc.
The editors were Martin Wonsiewicz and Pamela Touboul; the production supervisor was Richard Ruzycka; the cover designers were Marsha Cohen and Dr. Carole Christman.
Quebecor/Kingsport was printer and binder.
This book is printed on acid-free paper.

Library of Congress Cataloging-in-Publication Data
Neurotrauma / editors, Raj K. Narayan, Jack E. Wilberger, Jr., John T. Povlishock.
p. cm.
Includes bibliographical references and index.
ISBN 0-07-045662-3 (hardcover)
1. Brain—Wounds and injuries. 2. Spinal cord—Wounds and injuries. I. Narayan, Raj K. II. Wilberger, Jack E. III. Povlishock, John T.
[DNLM: 1. Brain Injuries. 2. Spinal Cord Injuries. WL 354 N49448 1995]
RD593.N47 1995
617.4′8044—dc20
DNLM/DLC
for Library of Congress 95-40277

To our parents, wives, and children
without whose support, encouragement, and tolerance this book
would not have been possible
Brij and Rathna Narayan
Tina, Tara, Neil, and Gita Narayan
James and Florence Wilberger
Mary Ellen, Matthew, Adam, and Melanie Wilberger
Theodore and Mary Povlishock
Deborah, Alexandra, and Marisa Povlishock
and to
J. Douglas Miller, M.D., Ph.D.
1937–1995
Professor of Neurosurgery
University of Edinburgh
Neurosurgeon, scholar, gentleman and friend

CONTENTS

Imaging Techniques

Operating Room Management

Management of Associated Injuries

CONTRIBUTORS

Numbers in brackets refer to the contributors' chapters.

WAYNE M. ALVES, Ph.D.
Executive Director, Neuroclinical Trials Center, University of Virginia Health Sciences Center, Charlottesville, Virginia. **[63, 65]**

BRUCE J. ANDERSEN, M.D., Ph.D.
Chairman, Department of Neurosurgery, The Brooklyn Hospital Center; Assistant Professor of Neurosurgery, New York University, New York, New York. **[81]**

DOUGLAS K. ANDERSON, Ph.D.
C.M. & K.E. Overstreet Professor, Departments of Neuroscience and Neurological Surgery, University of Florida, College of Medicine, Gainesville, Florida. **[111]**

THOMAS E. ANDERSON, Ph.D.
Senior Staff Research Scientist, Research Technology Partnership, Biomedical Science Department, GM R and D Center, Warren, Michigan. **[100]**

BRIAN T. ANDREWS, M.D., F.A.C.S.
Attending Neurosurgeon, San Francisco General Hospital. Department of Neurosurgery, University of California at San Francisco. Attending Neurosurgeon, The California Pacific Medical Center. Attending Neurosurgeon, St. Mary's Hospital Medical Center, San Francisco, California. **[24]**

ROBERT L. ATMAR, M.D.
Assistant Professor of Infectious Disease, Department of Medicine and Department of Microbiology and Immunology, Baylor College of Medicine. The Medicine Service, Ben Taub General Hospital, Houston, Texas. **[48]**

THOMAS Y. BARNES
Program Analyst, Department of Biostatistics, Medical College of Virginia, Virginia Commonwealth University, Richmond, Virginia. **[53]**

DONALD P. BECKER, M.D.
Professor and Chief, Division of Neurosurgery, UCLA School of Medicine, Los Angeles, California. **[6]**

EDWARD C. BENZEL, M.D., F.A.C.S.
University of New Mexico, School of Medicine; Professor and Chief, Division of Neurosurgery, Albuquerque, New Mexico. **[78]**

ANDREW R. BLIGHT, Ph.D.
Professor and Director of Research Laboratory, Division of Neurosurgery, University of North Carolina, Chapel Hill, North Carolina. **[101]**

CORWIN BOAKE, M.D.
Assistant Professor, Department of Physical Medicine and Rehabilitation, University of Texas-Houston Medical School and the Institute for Rehabilitation and Research, Houston, Texas. **[58]**

CATHERINE F. BONTKE, M.D.
System Medical Director for Rehabilitation Services, The Rehabilitation Hospital of Connecticut, Hartford, Connecticut. **[58]**

DARREL C. BOONE, M.D.
Trauma/Critical Care Fellow, University of Pittsburgh Medical Center, Pittsburgh, Pennsylvania. **[21]**

ADAM P. BROWN, M.D.
Department of Neurological Surgery, Washington University School of Medicine, St. Louis, Missouri. **[45]**

ROSS BULLOCK, M.D., Ph.D.
Lind Laurence Associate Professor, Department of Surgery, Division of Neurosurgery, Medical College of Virginia, Virginia Commonwealth University, Richmond, Virginia. **[27]**

DAVID W. CAHILL, M.D.
Professor and Director, Division of Neurosurgery, University of South Florida, Tampa, Florida. **[88]**

ROBERT CANTU
Medical Student, Tufts University School of Medicine. **[95]**

ROBERT C. CANTU, M.D.
Chief, Neurosurgical Services, and Director, Service of Sports Medicine, Emerson Hospital, Concord, Massachusetts; Medical Director, National Center for Catastrophic Sports Injury Research, Chapel Hill, North Carolina. **[95]**

MICHAEL E. CAREY, M.D.
Professor, Department of Neurosurgery, Louisiana State University, New Orleans, Louisiana. **[99]**

MICHAEL CARON, M.D.
Associate Medical Director, CINN, Joliet, Illinois. **[11]**

DAVID A. CARRIER, M.D.
Chief of Neuroradiology, Wilford Hall Medical Center, Lackland AFB, Texas. **[9]**

R. EDWARD CARTER, M.D.
Professor of Clinical Physical Medicine and Rehabilitation, Baylor College of Medicine, Houston, Texas. **[93]**

L. PHILIP CARTER, M.D.
Professor and Chief, Department of Neurosurgery, University of Oklahoma Health Sciences Center, Oklahoma City, Oklahoma. **[35]**

CAMILLE CASH
Medical Student, Baylor College of Medicine, Houston, Texas. **[19]**

BRITTON CHANCE, Ph.D.
Professor Emeritus, University of Pennsylvania School of Medicine, Department of Biochemistry and Biophysics, Philadelphia, Pennsylvania. **[12]**

RANDALL CHESNUT, M.D.
Assistant Professor, Dept. of Neurosurgery, University of California at San Francisco; Chief, Neurosurgical Services, San Francisco General Hospital, San Francisco, California. **[32, 79]**

WEN-TA CHIU, M.D.
Department of Neurosurgery, Taipei Medical College, Taipei, Taiwan. **[62]**

SUNG C. CHOI, Ph.D.
Professor, Department of Biostatistics and Neurosurgery, Medical College of Virginia, Virginia Commonwealth University, Richmond, Virginia. **[53]**

SOPHIA CHUNG, M.D.
Assistant Professor, Department of Ophthalmology, Saint Louis University School of Medicine. Sec. Appointment, Assistant Professor, Department of Neurology, St. Louis University School of Medicine, St. Louis, Missouri. **[43]**

GUY L. CLIFTON, M.D.
Professor and Chairman, Department of Neurosurgery, University of Texas Health Sciences Center, Houston, Texas. **[29]**

MICHAEL COBURN, M.D.
Assistant Professor of Urology, Baylor College of Medicine. Deputy Chief of Urology, Ben Taub General Hospital, Houston, Texas. **[22]**

TIMOTHY I. COHEN, M.D.
Chief Resident, Division of Neurosurgery, University of North Carolina at Chapel Hill, Chapel Hill, North Carolina. **[47]**

NEWTON W. COKER, M.D.
Professor, Department of Otorhinolaryngology and Communicative Sciences, Baylor College of Medicine, Houston, Texas. **[17]**

WILLIAM COLLINS, M.D.
Chairman, Department of Surgery, Yale University, School of Medicine, New Haven, Connecticut. **[73]**

CHARLES F. CONTANT, JR. Ph.D.
Assistant Professor, Department of Neurosurgery, Baylor College of Medicine, Houston, Texas. **[64]**

PAUL COOPER, M.D.
Professor, Department of Neurological Surgery, NYU Medical Center, New York, New York. **[44]**

MICHAEL K. COPASS, M.D.
Director of Emergency Services, Professor Medicine/Neurology, University of Washington/Harborview Medical Center, Seattle, Washington. **[7]**

LEWIS COVELER, M.D.
Professor of Clinical Anesthesiology, Baylor College of Medicine, Chief of Anesthesiology, Ben Taub General Hospital, Houston, Texas. **[13]**

RALPH G. DACEY, JR., M.D.
Professor and Chairman, Department of Neurology and Neurological Surgery, Washington University School of Medicine at Washington University Medical Center, St. Louis, Missouri. **[45]**

PEDRO J. DIAZ-MARCHAN, M.D.
Assistant Professor, Department of Radiology, Baylor College of Medicine, Houston, Texas. Chief of Neuroradiology, Ben Taub General Hospital. **[9]**

CURTIS A. DICKMAN, M.D.
Director of Spinal Research, Associate Chief, Spine Section, Division of Neurosurgery, Barrow Neurological Institute, Phoenix, Arizona. **[80]**

W. DALTON DIETRICH, Ph.D.
Professor of Neurology & Anatomy & Cell Biology, University of Miami, School of Medicine, Miami, Florida. **[110]**

TUE DINH, M.D.
Fellow in Microsurgery, Division of Plastic Surgery, Baylor College of Medicine, Houston, Texas. **[15]**

JOHN F. DITUNNO, M.D.
Michie Professor and Chairman, Department of Rehabilitation Medicine, Thomas Jefferson University, Philadelphia, Pennsylvania. **[91]**

ED DIXON, Ph.D.
Visiting Associate Professor, Department of Neurosurgery, University of Pittsburgh Medical Center, Presbyterian University Hospital, Pittsburgh, Pennsylvania. **[98]**

CURTIS DOBERSTEIN, M.D.
Head, Section of Vascular Neurosurgery, Rhode Island Hospital. Assistant Professor, Department of Neurosurgery, Brown University School of Medicine, Providence, Rhode Island. **[6, 37]**

DAVID DOEZEMA, M.D.
University of New Mexico, School of Medicine, and Associate Professor, Department of Emergency Medicine, Albuquerque, New Mexico. **[78]**

WILLIAM H. DONOVAN, M.D.
Vice President of Medical Affairs, The Institute for Rehabilitation and Research, Houston, Texas; Professor and Chairman, Department of Physical Medicine and Rehabilitation, University of Texas, Health Science Center, Houston, Texas. **[96]**

S. KATHLEEN DOSTER, M.D., Ph.D.
Fellow, Neuromuscular Disease Program, Department of Neurology, Washington University, St. Louis, Missouri. **[106]**

JOSHUA L. DOWLING, M.D.
Resident, Department of Neurological Surgery, Washington University School of Medicine, St. Louis, Missouri. **[45]**

ANN-CHRISTINE DUHAIME, M.D.
Associate Neurosurgeon, Children's Hospital of Philadelphia, University of Pennsylvania, Philadelphia, Pennsylvania. **[26]**

A. BRENT EASTMAN, M.D.
Director of Trauma Services, Scripps Memorial Hospital Trauma Center. Associate Clinical Professor of Surgery, University of California at San Diego, La Jolla, California. **[67]**

HOWARD EISENBERG, M.D.
Professor and Head, Division of Neurosurgery, University of Maryland, Baltimore, Maryland. **[65]**

RANDOLPH W. EVANS, M.D.
Clinical Assistant Professor, University of Texas at Houston Medical School. Baylor College of Medicine, Chief of Neurology Section. Park Plaza Hospital, Houston, Texas. **[41]**

ALAN I. FADEN, M.D.
Dean of Research and Graduate Education, Professor of Neurology and Pharmacology, Georgetown University Medical Center, Washington, D.C. **[109]**

DAVID J. FELDMAN, M.D.
Postdoctoral Fellow of Neuroradiology, Department of Radiology, Baylor College of Medicine, Houston, Texas. **[9]**

ZEEV FELDMAN, M.D.
Department of Neurosurgery, Baylor College of Medicine, Houston, Texas. **[55]**

GLEN A. FENTON, M.D.
Associate Professor, Department of Neurology, St. Louis University School of Medicine, St. Louis, Missouri. **[43]**

RICHARD G. FESSLER, M.D., Ph.D.
Associate Professor, University of Florida, Department of Neurosurgery, Gainesville, Florida. **[77]**

PAUL C. FRANCEL, M.D., Ph.D.
Resident, Department of Neurosurgery, University of Virginia, Charlottesville, Virginia. **[54]**

JAMSHID B. GHAJAR, M.D., Ph.D.
Associate Professor of Neurosurgery, Aitken Institute, Cornell University Medical Center, New York, New York. **[70]**

RYAN S. GLASSER, M.D.
University of Florida, School of Medicine, Gainesville, Florida. **[77]**

J. CLAY GOODMAN, M.D.
Associate Professor, Departments of Pathology, Neurosurgery and Neurology, Baylor College of Medicine, Houston, Texas. **[40]**

SHANKAR P. GOPINATH, M.D.
Research Associate, Department of Neurosurgery, Baylor College of Medicine, Houston, Texas. **[12]**

DAVID IAN GRAHAM, MBBCH, Ph.D., FRCPATH.
University of Glasgow, Head, Department of Neuropathology, Institute of Neurological Sciences Southern General Hospital, Glasgow, Scotland. **[4]**

DANIEL E. GRAVES, B.S.
Instructor, Physical Medicine and Rehabilitation Department, Baylor College of Medicine, Houston, Texas. **[93]**

STEPHEN B. GREENBERG, M.D.
Professor and Vice-Chairman, Department of Medicine, Professor, Department of Microbiology and Immunology, Baylor College of Medicine. Chief of the Medical Service, Ben Taub General Hospital, Houston, Texas. **[48]**

STEVEN K. GUDEMAN, M.D.
Professor and Chief, Division of Neurosurgery, University of North Carolina at Chapel Hill, Chapel Hill, North Carolina. **[47]**

WILLIAM GRAHAM GUERRIERO, M.D.
Professor of Urology, Baylor College of Medicine. Director of the Abdominal Transplantation Program for The Methodist Hospital, Houston, Texas. **[57]**

G. GURURAJ, M.D.
Department of Epidemiology, National Institute of Mental Health and Neuroscience, India. **[62]**

MICHAEL HAGLUND, M.D., Ph.D.
Assistant Professor, Department of Neurological Surgery, Duke University, Durham, North Carolina. **[42]**

REGIS HAID, M.D.
Associate Professor, Department of Neurosurgery, Emory University, Atlanta, Georgia. **[85]**

EDWARD D. HALL, Ph.D.
Senior Scientist, CNS Diseases Research Unit, Upjohn Laboratories, Kalamazoo, Missouri. **[104]**

M. BOWES HAMILL, M.D.
Associate Professor of Clinical Ophthalmology, Cullen Eye Institute, Baylor College of Medicine, Houston, Texas. **[16]**

LINDA HANKINS, M.D.
Assistant Professor of Neuroradiology, Department of Radiology, University of Texas Houston Medical School, Houston, Texas. **[10]**

H. JULIA HANNAY, Ph.D.
Professor and Director of Clinical Neuropsychology Program, University of Houston. Adjunct Professor of Neurosurgery and Neurology, Baylor College of Medicine. Adjunct Professor of Psychiatry, University of Texas Medical Center, Houston, Texas. **[49]**

RONALD L. HAYES, Ph.D.
Professor, Department of Neurosurgery, University of Texas Health Sciences Center, Houston, Texas. **[29, 98]**

L. ANNE HAYMAN, M.D.
Professor, Department of Radiology, Director of Herbert J. Frensley Center for Imaging Research. Baylor College of Medicine, Houston, Texas. **[9, 10]**

EDWARD K. HERES, M.D.
Department of Anesthesiology, Allegheny General Hospital, Pittsburgh, Pennsylvania. **[82]**

W. KEITH HOOTS, M.D.
Associate Professor of Pediatrics and Internal Medicine, University of Texas-Houston Health Sciences Center. Associate Pediatrician and Associate Professor, Department of Pediatrics, University of Texas M.D. Anderson Cancer Center. Medical Director of the Gulf State Hemophilia Center, Houston, Texas. **[46]**

PHILIP J. HORNER, Ph.D.
Postdoctoral Research Associate, Salk Institute, Laboratory of Genetics, San Diego, California. **[103]**

DAVID A. HOVDA
Associate Professor, Division of Neurosurgery, UCLA School of Medicine, Los Angeles, California. **[108]**

DENA R. HOWLAND, Ph.D.
Research Scientist, Department of Neuroscience, University of Florida, College of Medicine, Gainesville, Florida. **[111]**

CHUNG Y. HSU, M.D., Ph.D.
Professor and Head, Cerebrovascular Disease Section, Department of Neurology, Washington University, St. Louis, Missouri. **[106]**

ZHONG Y. HU, M.D., Ph.D.
Research Associate, Cerebrovascular Disease Section, Department of Neurology, Washington University, St. Louis, Missouri. **[106]**

JOHN A. JANE, M.D., Ph.D.
Professor and Chairman, Department of Neurosurgery, University of Virginia, Charlottesville, Virginia. **[54]**

MADHANGI JAYARAMAN, MPH
Researcher, Southern California Injury Prevention Research Center, UCLA School of Public Health, Los Angeles, California. **[2]**

BRYAN JENNETT, CBE, M.D., F.R.C.S.
Emeritus Professor of Neurosurgery, Institute of Neurological Sciences, University of Glasgow, Glasgow, Scotland. **[1]**

IAIN H. KALFAS, M.D., F.A.C.S
Head, Section of Spinal Surgery, Department of Neurosurgery, Cleveland Clinic Foundation, Cleveland, Ohio. **[83]**

HOWARD H. KAUFMAN, M.D.
Professor and Chairman, Department of Neurosurgery, West Virginia School of Medicine, Morgantown, West Virginia. **[56]**

DIANA KELKER
Executive Director, THINK FIRST Program, Cinicinnati, Ohio. **[72]**

DANIEL F. KELLY, M.D.
Assistant Professor, Division of Neurosurgery-UCLA and Harbor UCLA Medical Center, Los Angeles, California. **[6]**

JOHN J. KNIGHTLY, LCDR, MC, USNR
Department of Neurosurgery, Naval Medical San Diego, San Diego, California. **[61]**

GLENN W. KNOX, M.D.
Assistant Professor, Department of Otorhinolaryngology, Director of Balance Center, University of Pennsylvania Hospital, Philadelphia, Pennsylvania. **[17]**

JESS F. KRAUSE, MPH, Ph.D.
Professor of Department of Epidemiology, Director of Southern California Injury Prevention Research Center, UCLA, Los Angeles, California. **[2]**

JOHN A. KUSSKE, M.D.
Clinical Professor, Department of Neurological Surgery, University of California, Irvine, Irvine, California. **[69]**

RONALD E. LAPORTE, M.D.
Department of Epidemiology, University of Pittsburgh, Pittsburgh, Pennsylvania. **[62]**

HARVEY S. LEVIN, Ph.D.
Professor and Director of Research, Department of Physical Medicine and Rehabilitation, Baylor College of Medicine, Houston, Texas. **[50]**

JAMES W. LIGHTHALL, Ph.D.
Staff Scientist, Field Performance Analysis, GMC, Detroit, Michigan. **[100]**

RONALD W. LINDSAY, M.D.
Associate Professor, Department of Orthopedic Surgery, Baylor College of Medicine, Houston, Texas. **[19]**

PAUL A. LOBAUGH, Ph.D.
Vice President, Allegheny Neuromonitoring, Inc., Pittsburgh, Pennsylvania. **[86]**

JEFFREY M. LOBOSKY, M.D.
Clinical Instructor, Department of Neurosurgery, University of California at San Francisco, University of California at Davis; Director, Neurosurgical Intensive Care Unit, N.T. Enlow Memorial Hospital, Chico, California. **[74]**

PAUL G. LOUBSER, M.D., C.H.B.
Assistant Professor, Department of Anesthesia, Baylor College of Medicine, Houston, Texas. **[90, 96]**

DONALD W. MARION, M.D.
Associate Professor of Neurological Surgery, Director, The Brain Trauma Research Center, University of Pittsburgh, Pittsburgh, Pennsylvania. **[33, 52]**

ANTHONY MARMAROU, Ph.D.
Professor and Vice-Chairman, Director of Research, Division of Neurosurgery, Medical College of Virginia, Virginia Commonwealth University, Richmond, Virginia. **[30]**

NEIL A. MARTIN, M.D.
Division of Neurosurgery, UCLA School of Medicine, Los Angeles, California. **[37]**

KENNETH L. MATTOX, M.D.
Professor of Surgery, Baylor College of Medicine, Chief of Staff, Ben Taub General Hospital, Houston, Texas. **[20]**

DAVID L. McARTHUR, Ph.D., MPH
Epidemiologist, Southern California Injury Prevention Research Center, UCLA School of Public Health, Los Angeles, California. **[2]**

BRUCE McCORMACK, M.D.
Assistant Professor, Department of Neurosurgery, UCSF Medical Center, San Francisco, California. **[44]**

TRACY K. McINTOSH, Ph.D.
Professor of Neurosurgery, Bioengineering and Pharmacology, Director, Head Injury Center, University of Pennsylvania, Philadelphia, Pennsylvania. **[107]**

GUY M. McKHANN II, M.D.
Resident, Department of Neurological Surgery, University of Washington, Seattle, Washington. **[7]**

ARNOLD H. MENEZES, M.D.
Professor and Vice Chairman, Division of Neurosurgery, University of Iowa, Iowa City, Iowa. **[92]**

MARY ELLEN MICHEL, Ph.D.
Health Scientist Administrator, Division of Stroke and Trauma, National Institute of Neurological Disorders and Stroke, National Institutes of Health, Bethesda, Maryland. **[66]**

J. DOUGLAS MILLER, M.D., Ph.D. (Deceased)
Professor of Surgical Neurology, Department of Clinical Neurosciences, University of Edinburgh, Edinburgh, United Kingdom. **[5, 31]**

J. PAUL MUIZELLAR, M.D., Ph.D.
Professor, Wayne State University. Director, Neurotrauma Institute of Wayne State University at Detroit Receiving Hospital, Detroit, Michigan. **[38]**

RAJ K. NARAYAN, M.D.
Professor and Chairman, Department of Neurosurgery, Temple University School of Medicine, Philadelphia, Pennsylvania. **[8, 14, 23, 60, 94]**

PAULINE T. NEWLON, Ph.D.
Assistant Professor, Department of Neurosurgery and Neurobiology, Eastern Virginia Medical School, Norfolk, Virginia. **[39]**

WALTER D. OBRIST, Ph.D.
Professor Emeritus of Neurosurgery, Department of Neurological Surgery, University of Pittsburgh, Pittsburgh, Pennsylvania. **[33]**

JOSE A. OROZCO, M.D.
Research Associate, Section of Neurosurgery, University of Arizona Medical Center, Tucson, Arizona. **[35]**

LINDA OTT, M.S.
Research Consultant, University of Kentucky Medical Center, Lexington, Kentucky. **[25]**

ANDREW B. PEITZMAN, M.D.
Director, Trauma and Surgical Critical Care, Associate Professor of Surgery, University of Pittsburgh Medical Center, Pittsburgh, Pennsylvania. **[21]**

JOSEPH M. PIEPMEIER, M.D.
Professor, Department of Neurosurgery, Yale University, New Haven, Connecticut. **[89]**

JOHN G. PIPER, M.D.
Division of Neurosurgery, University of Iowa, Iowa City, Iowa. **[92]**

IAN R. PIPER, BSC, Ph.D.
Research Fellow, Department of Clinical Neurosciences, University of Edinburgh, Edinburgh, Scotland. **[31]**

JOHN T. POVLISHOCK, Ph.D.
Professor and Chair of Anatomy, Director of Commonwealth Center for the Study of Brain Injury, Co-Director, MCV/VCU Neuroscience Center, Medical College of Virginia, Virginia Commonwealth University, Richmond, Virginia. **[97]**

MORRIS W. PULLIAM, CAPT, MC, USN
Chairman, Department of Neurosurgery, National Naval Medical Center. Professor and Chief, Division of Neurosurgery, Uniform Services University of The Health Sciences, Bethesda, Maryland. Clinical Professor, Department of Neurosurgery, George Washington School of Medicine, Washington, D.C. **[61]**

SALLY RATY, M.D.
Assistant Professor of Anesthesiology, Baylor College of Medicine, Staff Anesthesiologist, Ben Taub General Hospital, Houston, Texas. **[13]**

GLENN R. RECHTINE, M.D.
Florida Orthopaedic Institute, Tampa, Florida. **[88]**

PAUL J. REIER, Ph.D.
Mark F. Overstreet Professor, Department of Neurological Surgery & Neuroscience, University of Florida, College of Medicine, Gainesville, Florida. **[111]**

MICHAEL RHODES, M.D., FACS
Chief of Trauma, Lehigh Valley Hospital, Allentown, Pennsylvania. **[68]**

CLAUDIA S. ROBERTSON, M.D.
Professor, Department of Neurosurgery Baylor College of Medicine, Houston, Texas, Director, NICU, Ben Taub General Hospital, Houston, Texas. **[12, 34, 36]**

DANIEL P. ROBERTSON, M.D.
Chief Resident, Dept. of Neurosurgery, Baylor College of Medicine, Houston, Texas. **[94]**

GAYLAN L. ROCKSWOLD, M.D.
Chief of Neurosurgery, Hennepin County Medical Center. Professor of Neurosurgery, University of Minnesota, Minneapolis, Minnesota. **[28]**

GERALD S. RODTS JR., M.D.
Assistant Professor, Department of Neurosurgery, Emory University, Atlanta, Georgia. **[85]**

JOSEPH ROMANO, ESQUIRE
Attorney at Law, Rosenstein and Romano, PC, Norristown, Pennsylvania. **[71]**

THOMAS G. SAUL, M.D.
Medical Director, THINK FIRST Program, Cincinnati, Ohio. **[72]**

JOHN G. SCHMIDT, M.D.
Instructor, Department of Neurology, St. Louis University School of Medicine, St. Louis, Missouri. **[43]**

GARY W. SCHURMAN, M.S.
President, Allegheny Neuromonitoring, Inc., Pittsburgh, Pennsylvania. **[86]**

JOHN B. SELHORST, M.D.
Professor and Chairman, Department of Neurology, St. Louis University School of Medicine. Sec. Appointment, Professor, Department of Ophthalmology, St. Louis, Missouri. **[43]**

SALEH M. SHENAQ, M.D.
Professor, Division of Plastic Surgery, Baylor College of Medicine, Houston, Texas. **[15]**

MARK SHERER, Ph.D.
Director of Neuropsychology, The Institute for Rehabilitation and Research. Clinical Assistant Professor of Physical Medicine and Rehabilitation, Baylor College of Medicine. Adjunct Clinical Assistant Professor of Psychology, University of Houston, Houston, Texas. **[49]**

RICHARD K. SIMPSON, JR., M.D.
Associate Professor of Neurosurgery, Assistant Professor of Anesthesiology, Assistant Professor of Physical Medicine and Rehabilitation, Baylor College of Medicine; Chief of Neurosurgery, V.A. Medical Center, Houston, Texas. **[40, 94]**

PANAYIOTIS J. SIOUTOS, M.D.
Section of Neurosurgery, University of Arizona, Tucson, Arizona. [35]

DOUGLAS H. SMITH, M.D.
Assistant Professor, Division of Neurosurgery, University of Pennsylvania, Pennsylvania. [107]

PATRICK F. X. STATHAM, MB, BS, FRCS (ED), FRCS (ENG), FRCS (SN)
Consultant Neurosurgeon, Department of Clinical Neurosciences, University of Edinburgh, Edinburgh, Scotland. [31]

SHERMAN STEIN, M.D.
Professor, Division of Neurosurgery, Cooper Hospital/University Medical Center, University of Medicine and Dentistry of New Jersey, Robert Wood Johnson Medical School at Camden, Camden, New Jersey. [3, 51]

BRADFORD T. STOKES, Ph.D.
Associate Dean of Research & Graduate Education, Director, Spinal Cord Injury Research Center, Professor of Departments of Physiology and Surgery, Ohio State University, Columbus, Ohio. [103]

WARREN A. STRINGER, M.D.
Assistant Professor of Neuroradiology, University of Arkansas for Medical Sciences, Little Rock, Arkansas. [81]

MARIAELAINA SUMAS, M.D.
Chief Resident, Department of Neurosurgery, Temple University School of Medicine, Philadelphia, Pennsylvania. [23]

KATHERINE H. TABER, Ph.D.
Assistant Professor, Department of Radiology and Herbert J. Frensley Center for Imaging Research, Baylor College of Medicine, Houston, Texas. [10]

CHARLES H. TATOR, M.D., M.A., Ph.D., F.R.C.S.(C)
Professor and Chairman, Dept. of Neurosurgery, University of Toronto, Toronto Hospital, Toronto, Ontario, Canada. [18, 75]

EDWARD TEEPLE JR., M.D.
Associate Professor, Dept. of Anesthesiology, Medical College of Pennsylvania, Hahnemann University, Allegheny Campus, Allegheny General Hospital, Pittsburgh, Pennsylvania. [82]

NANCY T. TEMKIN, Ph.D.
Associate Professor of Neurological Surgery and Biostatistics, University of Washington, Seattle, Washington. [42]

TODD TRASK, M.D.
Assistant Professor, Department of Neurosurgery, Baylor College of Medicine, Houston, Texas. [60]

ALEX B. VALADKA, M.D
Assistanst Professor, Department of Neurosurgery, Baylor College of Medicine. Chief of Neurosurgery, Ben Taub General Hospital, Houston, Texas. [8, 14]

MATTHEW J. WALL, JR., M.D.
Assistant Professor of Surgery, Baylor College of Medicine, Chief of General Surgery, Ben Taub General Hospital, Houston, Texas. [20]

JON C. WALSH, M.D.
Associate Director of Trauma Services, Scripps Memorial Hospital Trauma Center, La Jolla, California. [67]

JOHN D. WARD, M.D.
Professor and Executive Vice-Chairman, Division of Neurosurgery, Chief of Pediatric Neurosurgery, Director of Neurosciences ICU, Medical College of Virginia, Richmond, Virginia. [59]

JACK E. WILBERGER, JR., M.D.
Professor and Director of Neurosurgery, Medical College of Pennsylvania, Hahnemann University, Allegheny Campus, Allegheny General Hospital, Pittsburgh, Pennsylvania. [86, 87, 95]

H. RICHARD WINN, M.D.
Professor and Chairman, Department of Neurological Surgery, University of Washington/Harborview Medical Center, Seattle, Washington. [7, 42]

TROY WOODMAN, B.S.
Research Assistant, Department of Neurosurgery, Baylor College of Medicine, Houston, Texas. [36]

JEAN R. WRATHALL, Ph.D.
Associate Professor, Department of Cell Biology, Georgetown University Medical Center, Washington, D.C. [102]

JOEL YEAKLEY, M.D.
Professor and Chief of Neuroradiology, Section and Professor of Neuroradiology, Department of Radiology, University of Texas Houston Medical School, Houston, Texas. [10]

BYRON YOUNG, M.D.
Chair of Surgery, Johnston-Wright. Professor and Chief of Neurosurgery, University of Kentucky Medical Center, Lexington, Kentucky. [25]

WISE YOUNG, M.D., Ph.D.
Professor of Neurosurgery, Physiology & Biophysics, Director of Neurosurgery Research Laboratory, New York University Medical Center, New York, New York. [76, 105]

NATHAN ZASLER, M.D.
CEO and Executive Medical Director, National NeuroRehabilitation Consortium, Inc. Medical Director, Concussion Care Centers of America, Inc., Richmond, Virginia. [58]

WILLIAM ZERICK, M.D.
Division of Neurosurgery, Barrow Neurological Institute, Phoenix, Arizona. [80]

PREFACE

The field of neurotrauma has made remarkable strides over the past two decades. From its beginning as an unpopular backwater subspecialty field pursued only by the most masochistic neurosurgeons, the study of head and spinal cord injury has come to draw the interest of a wide spectrum of physicians and scientists. Not long ago, when a patient suffered a central nervous system (CNS) injury, it was regarded as a condition for which little if anything could be done. Since all the damage was thought to occur at the moment of impact, any interventions were felt to be futile. However, it has become apparent that although much irreversible CNS damage occurs immediately, evolving destructive processes over the ensuing hours and days clearly worsen the ultimate outcome.

Much progress has been made in understanding these secondary insults at the clinical level as well as at the biochemical level. As a result, the management of these patients is continually being refined and several neuroprotective agents are being tested clinically. Although nationwide statistics are hard to come by, experience at many centers seems to demonstrate a clear trend toward improved outcomes from head and spinal cord injuries. As the field of neurotrauma has matured, the initial quasiscientific bean-counting and fishing expeditions have led to new insights. The clinicians who initially generated interest in this area have become much better educated in the scientific process, and basic scientists who would otherwise have hesitated to enter a "dirty" clinical arena have done so in large numbers. The resulting cross-fertilization between these disciplines has generated tremendous excitement and has propelled the field forward. This book attempts to capture this excitement and to provide the reader with a comprehensive guide to CNS injury from both a clinical and a basic research viewpoint.

Neurotrauma is primarily a clinical textbook. The section on basic research has been intentionally kept shorter than the first two clinical sections to maintain this emphasis. It is hoped that this book will serve as a ready reference for the wide spectrum of physicians and scientists who have become involved with this field. It is presented in a manner that should be easily digestible by a relative newcomer but is comprehensive enought to be useful to the more seasoned student. It is the largest single source of data on this subject ever published.

When the authors undertook this project two years ago, we recognized that it was going to be a challenge to bring this book to completion within a reasonable period. The field is advancing rapidly, and information can easily become dated, especially in the area of basic research. Virtually all the lead authors are acknowledged authorities, and such people tend to be chronically overcommitted. We therefore greatly appreciate their considerable efforts in producing such excellent chapters and trust that they will forgive our gentle harassment and nitpicking. The end, we hope, justifies the means.

We would like to acknowledge the critical roles several individuals played in bringing this project to fruition: Jane Pennington, who was then working for McGraw-Hill, first approached us with a proposal for this book and wouldn't take no for an answer. Roberta Abbott's editorial assistance and organization helped us through most of the initial process. Marty Wonsiewicz at McGraw-Hill inherited this project from Dr. Pennington and was most persuasive in getting the job done in a timely fashion with the help of James Morgan. Pamela Touboul, also of McGraw-Hill, did an excellent job of keeping the manuscripts, figures, and galleys flowing. Finally, Dr. Carole Christman produced the cover illustration in her usual inimitable fashion. To these individuals and to our colleagues who tolerated our preoccupation with this project, we are truly grateful.

Raj K. Narayan, M.D., F.A.C.S.
Jack E. Wilberger, M.D., F.A.C.S.
John T. Povlishock, Jr., Ph.D.

NEUROTRAUMA

PART I

HEAD INJURY

Overview

CHAPTER 1

HISTORICAL PERSPECTIVE ON HEAD INJURY*

Bryan Jennett

EDITORIAL COMMENT

While no one would disagree with Jennett's recommendation that more attention should be paid to mild and moderate head injuries, few neurosurgeons actively involved in research on head injuries are likely to share his pessimism about severe head injury. This constitutes an enormous challenge, and a certain proportion of head-injured patients will be unsalvageable despite all interventions; however, it has become obvious that not all brain injuries occur at the moment of impact and that ongoing destructive processes and secondary insults occur well after the initial injury. These processes can potentially be inhibited, and the secondary insults can be detected earlier and/or avoided. Recent basic and clinical research is yielding new drugs and monitoring techniques that will almost certainly favorably affect the outcome of head injury. The mortality from severe head injury is being reduced with better prehospital care, quicker neurosurgical intervention, and better monitoring and treatment in dedicated neurosurgical intensive care units.

The Traumatic Coma Data Bank (TCDB), which consisted of four U.S. centers reporting on 746 severe closed head injury patients treated between 1984 and 1987, reported a mortality rate of 36 percent. This was a clear improvement over the 50 percent mortality rate reported from three countries by Jennett and coworkers in 1977.[23] *Jennett describes this as being due to "differing selection criteria for entry," although the series were very similar in terms of the usual predictors of outcome, such as age, pupillary reaction, and percentage of mass lesions. Experience at the Baylor College of Medicine over the past 4 years with 214 patients sustaining severe head injury has shown a 30 percent mortality rate despite the fact that the series included a very large proportion of patients with surgically evacuated mass lesions (57 percent compared to 37 percent in the TCDB and 54 percent, 28 percent, and 56 percent in the three centers reported by Jennett in 1979). Several other centers are reporting a similar decline in mortality in recent years, probably as a result of a combination of interventions.*

In this chapter Jennett throws down the gauntlet: Does the hope for improving the mortality and morbidity from head injury lie in the development of newer therapies and interventions, or are prevention and organization the key? The rest of this book suggests that both strategies are worthwhile.

R.K.N.

Neurosurgery began with the treatment of head injuries. Compound depressed fractures caused by arrows have been preserved from ancient Chinese dynasties, and trephine openings for the evacuation of traumatic clots with evidence of healing, and therefore of survival, have been found in remains from the Incas onward. Hippocrates classified head injuries and recommended trephining for some; he also coined the aphorism that no head injury is too trivial to ignore or so serious that it should be cause for despair. More than a millennium later, Macewen of Glasgow pioneered elective intracranial surgery on the basis of deductions from recent knowledge of cerebral localization.[1] This occurred in the 1870s, years before x-rays were discovered and at a time when Harvey Cushing was still a schoolboy. Macewen worked for a time as a casualty surgeon for the Central Police Division in Glasgow, one of the roughest Victorian cities. An article from this period discussed the distinction between traumatic and alcoholic pupillary

* This is an updated version of an essay published in *Craniospinal Trauma*, Pits LH, Wagner FC (eds), New York: Thieme, 1990, with permission of editors and publishers.

abnormalities. Another article reported how the observation of focal epilepsy led to the detection and localization of complications distant from the site of trauma to the head. Macewen described first an abscess and then a subdural hematoma; the hematoma was successfully removed. A link between his era and the current period is provided by a patient who more than half a century after being operated on by Macewen came to the author's clinic at the Institute in Glasgow, where a computed tomography (CT) scan showed the bone defect resulting from Macewen's surgery.

LESSONS FROM TWENTIETH-CENTURY WARS

War provides an opportunity for surgeons to learn about trauma. When Cushing went to Europe during World War I, he found that no less than 60 percent of deaths after dural penetration were due to sepsis. He maintained that many of those deaths would be avoidable if delay in debridement could be reduced, and by the end of that conflict he had reduced mortality from 54 percent to 29 percent.[2] Neurosurgical services for the British Army in World War II were organized by Cairns, who had been a resident with Cushing. To minimize the delays Cushing had warned about, Cairns set up mobile neurosurgical units, each staffed by a neurosurgeon, a neurologist, and an anaesthetist.[3] He was fortunate to have the opportunity to perform the first tests with penicillin; this marked the beginning of a new era in the treatment of war wounds.

Many soldier-surgeons later became academics, but Cairns was a professor of surgery at Oxford before he became a brigadier. He imposed on his medical officers the academic discipline of careful note taking from the time of the first medical contact in the field. This provided data not only for accurate correlation of the severity and type of injury with the immediate outcome but also for research on the sequelae of head injury that continued for 20 years or more. The base hospital he set up in Oxford admitted injured men a few days after their surgery near the front, thanks to the development of air evacuation, and continued to operate until the mid-1950s.

The Korean conflict saw the further development of mobile army surgical hospitals (MASH) near the front and early helicopter evacuation to base hospitals. However, the same lesson had to be learned again: delays led to high infection rates even when antibiotics had been given prophylactically. Early in that campaign the infection rate had been 41 percent, but it fell to 1 percent by the end.[4]

The Vietnam war saw even more rapid evacuation of casualties to surgical facilities, which were often reached within an hour or less and were almost always reached within 6 h. One consequence was that the hospital mortality rate increased as casualties who in previous wars would have died on the battlefield reached a hospital. However, most of these patients were irrecoverable, and triage determined that many of them died without surgery. Such deaths accounted for 20 percent of admissions, whereas among 1455 wounded soldiers who were operated on, only 9 percent died in the hospital; the rate for those who were not in coma was only 3 percent.[5] Several of these lessons of war have had to be learned again by surgeons dealing with head injuries in civilian life, in particular, the importance of organization in minimizing delay before injured patients reach a specialist and the importance of triage.

THE LAST 30 YEARS IN CIVILIAN LIFE

Since World War II there have been two major developments in the management of head injuries. In 1958, a neurosurgeon, an otolaryngologist, and an anesthesiologist from Newcastle in the United Kingdom reported improved survival after severe injuries as a result of what later came to be known as intensive care. Their regimen involved frequent use of tracheostomy and drugs that reduced spasticity and facilitated the control of increased body temperature.[6] Since then, there has been a mushrooming of intensive care units, from almost none to 50,000 in the United States between 1960 and 1980. The main impetus was provided by the fact that mechanical ventilators became available in more hospitals, and this brought anesthesiologists on the scene as major actors in the management of severe head injuries. In collaboration with neurosurgeons, they developed regimens of intensive medical therapy for severe head injuries. It became clear that only a small minority of patients with head injuries, whether mild or severe, ever need surgery. Consequently, most head injuries, especially less severe ones, are now looked after by practitioners of disciplines other than neurosurgery. In the United States, however, there are a large number of neurosurgeons and they manage most head traumas.

The other dramatic advance has been CT scanning. When CT became available in the mid-1970s, it did away with amateur angiograms in the middle of the night and ended the woodpecker surgery of exploratory burr holes for patients suspected of harboring a life-threatening hematoma. As scanning became more widely used, it was realized that significant hematomas could be detected in patients who had not yet developed the clinical features of cerebral compression; thus, earlier intervention became possible. Scanning has also taught neurosurgeons much about the nature of the lesions associated with less severe injuries that seldom come to autopsy. Magnetic resonance imaging (MRI) is extending that knowledge further by revealing lesions that are not shown on CT scans. In particular, MRI demonstrates how extensive brain damage can be in patients who by clinical standards have been only mildly injured.

The wide availability of CT scanning in the United States changed attitudes concerning the investigation and management of head injuries, both severe and mild. This has led to interest in the hospitalwide organization of care for head-injured patients as distinct from what occurs only in neurosurgical and intensive care units. Hence, radiologists, trauma surgeons, and emergency room doctors have become involved in the management of head injury patients. The demand for scanners to deal with head injuries in the acute stage was one factor that showed the need for information about the scale of occurrence of these injuries, leading epidemiologists on both sides of the Atlantic to recognize that head injury presents a major public health problem. At the same time, there has been an unprecedented period of interest on the part of a small group of pathologists and neurosurgeons in exploring human lesions at autopsy and developing experimental models for head injury.

HUMAN AND EXPERIMENTAL PATHOLOGY

The autopsy has traditionally been the source of knowledge about the damage sustained by the brain during and after head injury. Although new imaging techniques have provided fresh insights, the interpretation of some of the radiological findings has depended on recognizing lesions during life that had previously been known only after death. For many years, however, the literature on the pathological aspects of head injury had been dominated by forensic pathologists whose accounts included many data from the injured who had died at the scene of an accident. These data account for only about half of all head injury deaths, and the lesions found after such overwhelming injuries are often different in kind from those found in patients who survive even 24 to 48 h. However, attempts to undertake a detailed neuropathologic examination of the brain after death in the hospital have been frustrated by the belief that the demand for an immediate report for legal purposes necessitates the slicing of the unfixed brain. Special arrangements with the legal authorities in Glasgow have allowed academic neuropathologists to receive uncut brains for prolonged fixation, an essential condition for carrying out detailed dissection and quantitative histological examination. This procedure has been carried out on more than 600 brains by Adams and Graham,[7] who have mapped the pattern of primary and secondary damage.

These studies showed that obvious cortical contusions were a much less important component of primary damage than was diffuse axonal injury (DAI) in the white matter, a lesion seldom detected without microscopy. It also became evident that the brainstem was not the main or only site of damage, although for years clinicians had been referring to comatose patients with extensor responses as having "brainstem injury." These studies also showed the frequency of secondary brain damage. Widespread hypoxic or ischemic lesions were found in over 40 percent of hospital deaths, with evidence of increased intracranial pressure (ICP) in 70 percent or more. The cause of the hypoxic brain damage was considered to be intracranial hypertension combined with systemic arterial hypotension and/or a reduced oxygen content of the blood. These systemic abnormalities commonly result from blood loss and respiratory insufficiency, usually as a consequence of the major extracranial injuries found in about a third of patients with severe head injuries. Another contribution of these clinicopathologic studies in Glasgow has been to identify how frequently patients "talk and die."[8] With this came the concept of avoidable factors that contribute to death after head injury; the most common factor is delayed evacuation of an intracranial hematoma.[9]

Experimental primate studies by Gennarelli and colleagues[10] over the last 20 years have confirmed and extended the work of Russell and Denny-Brown at Oxford in the first years of World War II, who showed that brain damage was more extensive when the head of a monkey was free to move when it was struck.[11] The findings of Gennarelli and coworkers also confirmed the predictions of the Oxford physicist Holbourn, who in the 1940s experimented with gelatin models of the brain and simulated the shearing lesion of white matter that is now called DAI. This was first described in detail by Strich,[12,13] who dissected the brains of patients who had survived long periods with severe disability.

As a result of collaborative research by teams in Philadelphia and Glasgow, it appears that all the lesions found in humans can be reproduced experimentally by varying the degree, duration, and direction of applied acceleration and deceleration forces.[10,14] There now is no doubt that shearing forces acting on nerve fibers and blood vessels are the main mechanism for producing impact or primary damage. These experiments have also shown that axonal damage in continuity can occur; whether this progresses to a permanent lesion may depend on factors that could be influenced by pharmacological interventions. This has altered the philosophy of impact brain damage, which had been based on the assumption that damage is maximal at onset and is irreversible.

CLINICAL RESPONSE TO PATHOLOGICAL DATA

The finding that many patients who died had suffered hypoxic or ischemic brain damage and increased ICP seemed to explain the benefit resulting from intensive respiratory care and other medical measures. There followed several years of efforts to control ICP by means of steroid drugs, osmotic agents, and hyperventilation[15] and to reduce the metabolic rate of the brain by inducing general body hypothermia and through the use of depressant drugs.[16] At the same time, there had been an abundance of experimental work on intracranial pressure and cerebral blood flow, using a number of models that were one step removed from trauma, with lesions that were usually induced by ischemia or cold. Means of measuring ICP and cerebral blood flow were also used in intensive care units at academic centers.[17] Many of the data were confusing, however, with no consistent correlation between pressure, blood flow, and clinical outcome except at the extremes of normality and abnormality. However, it has become clear that episodes of arterial hypotension and elevated ICP are common even after a patient is receiving neurosurgical care.[18] These episodes, combined with episodes occurring in the early stages after injury, explain why secondary ischemic brain damage is so common. Monitoring systems are now used to detect and correct such insults as soon as possible.[19]

It also came to be appreciated that most monitoring and therapeutic interventions involve hazards and that it was uncertain whether an improved outcome could justify some of the components of modern intensive care (often labeled "aggressive management"). It was tempting to assume that most severely injured patients who survived after such treatment would have died without it. In 1978, Langfitt[20] concluded that there was little evidence of a large decrease in mortality from head injury over the previous 50 years. The validity of comparisons between series was, however, limited by the lack of an accepted measure of the severity of injury. It had long been recognized that deeper and more long-lasting coma, along with injury in older patients, produced higher mortality rates. However, the course followed by individual patients often seemed capricious: Some patients who initially looked hopeless not only survived but sometimes even made a reasonable recovery, whereas others whose impact injury was less serious sometimes deteriorated and died.

It was this dilemma, in the context of the limited availability of intensive care, that led Glasgow neurosurgeons to begin prospective data collection in severely injured patients in 1968. The specific intention was to develop prognostic criteria that might help with decision making in the acute stage. This led to the development of both the Glasgow Coma Scale, a simple descriptive and numerical means of classifying the responsiveness of patients with impaired consciousness,[21] and the Glasgow Outcome Scale.[22] Data collection was later extended to include two centers in the Netherlands and one in Los Angeles. This international trauma data bank defined "coma" as not opening the eyes, not obeying commands, and not uttering understandable words. It also defined a head injury as severe only if coma lasted for at least 6 h. Analysis of the first 700 severely head injured patients revealed that the nature of intensive therapy differed considerably in the three countries (e.g., the use of steroids, osmotics, controlled ventilation, and tracheostomy). Despite this, the mortality and degree of recovery in survivors were strikingly similar.[23] The mortality was about 50 percent, similar to that found in Langfitt's review of previously published series,[20] although severity of injury was less well defined in these earlier studies. It seemed that in many cases the outcome depended more on the degree of brain damage and the patient's age than on the details of treatment, and in 1976 Jennett and associates reported that a confident prediction of outcome at 6 months could be made within a few days of injury in about half these patients.[24]

These conclusions were confirmed by an analysis of 1250 cases from the data bank[25] and again by a comparison of more than 700 recent cases from Glasgow with more than 400 cases from San Francisco.[26,27] Several reports from other places challenged these findings and claimed that the results could be improved through the use of various intensive therapeutic regimens.[15–17,28] A critique of these conflicting reports has drawn attention to the pitfalls inherent in the evaluation of therapy for life-threatening conditions such as severe head injury.[29] Many variations in outcome can be explained by differing selection criteria for entry, often reflecting local factors in the organization of care and methods of triage for severe injuries. When age and severity of injury are carefully accounted for, it is possible to predict with considerable accuracy what the outcome will be.[24–27,30] This was later reported by Knaus and coworkers for patients in general intensive care units in different parts of the United States[31] and was also found to be the case when patients in the United States were compared with those in France, where fewer interventions were undertaken.[32] The message of the international head injury study was sometimes misrepresented as indicating that treatment was of no value. In fact, all the patients in that study had been treated in specialist intensive care units and had had the benefit of first-class neurosurgical care, in particular the early detection and removal of intracranial hematomas.

Since then, several other large series of severe head injuries have been reported: the American Traumatic Coma Data Bank,[33] the British-Finnish trial of nimodipine,[34] the four-center study in the United Kingdom,[35] and the European nimodipine trial.[36] These studies have all recorded lower mortality rates than those in the original international study but included some less severely injured patients. More trials are under way to test several new drugs that are designed to control various aspects of the chemical cascade of events that follow brain injury or protect the brain from the effects of those events.

MANAGEMENT OF INTRACRANIAL HEMATOMA

None of these activities in the last 30 years has altered the importance of ensuring that acute intracranial hematomas are detected and dealt with expeditiously. Policies directed toward this end should result in fewer patients developing avoidable secondary brain damage leading to death or permanent disability.[37] More than half of a large series of patients with operated intracranial hematomas had talked between the time of injury and the operation, and hematomas were found much more often in patients who had talked and deteriorated than in those who were in coma from the outset.[37] Hopes ran high that CT scanning would improve the outcome of patients with an acute hematoma because it so effectively diagnosed this complication. However, three neurosurgical centers in Great Britain reported no improvement in the outcome of head injury during the first 3 to 4 years after scanning became available. It was clear from the Glasgow study that the potential for benefit depended on organizational changes that would ensure that more patients at high risk of developing this complication as well as those suspected of already having developed it were transferred early to centers that could provide not only scanning but skilled surgical intervention as well.

Both CT scanners and neurosurgeons are much scarcer in Europe than in the United States, making the issue of triage for scanning and neurosurgical consultation important. Intracranial hematoma is an infrequent complication (1 in 6000 attenders at emergency departments in the United States and 1 in 900 of those admitted in Britain). Therefore, it is vital to determine as soon as possible which patients are at risk of developing this complication, particularly among those who are awake and talking, and not be suspected of being at risk and in need of further observation and investigation. A study of several thousand of these patients in accident departments and general surgical wards in Scotland has shown that a fracture of the skull is a much more powerful predictor of hematoma than is altered consciousness. Patients who have recovered from briefly impaired consciousness and have no fracture are extremely unlikely to develop a clot.[39] On this basis, guidelines were agreed upon nationally by neurosurgeons in Great Britain, for x-raying the skull in accident departments, for admission for further observation, and for CT scanning and neurosurgical consultation.[40] These guidelines were originally applied to adults only; however, data on children were subsequently published (Table 1-1).[41]

As a result of the establishment of these guidelines, many more patients were referred to the neurosurgical units for scanning and arrived there sooner; moreover, more hematomas were detected, fewer patients were in coma by the time of surgery, and the mortality among operated patients was progressively reduced (Table 1-2).[42] In general hospitals the admission rate for mild

TABLE 1-1 Risk* of Acute Hematoma in Emergency Department Attenders after Head Injury

		Children	Adults
No skull fracture	Fully conscious	12,559	7,866
	Impaired	580	180
	Coma	65	27
With fracture	Fully conscious	157	45
	Impaired	25	5
	Coma	12	4
All cases		2,100	348

* Risk is equal to one in the number quoted.

SOURCE: Teasdale et al.[41]

TABLE 1-2 Effect of Transfer Policy on Mortality after an Operation for Acute Traumatic Hematoma

		Extradural		*Intradural*	
		n	% **Dead**	*n*	% **Dead**
1974–1977	Usually referred when deteriorating	119	25	186	47
1978–1984	Local criteria for early referral	233	18	426	36
1985–1988	After national guidelines	77	9	145	31

SOURCE: Teasdale et al.[42]

injuries with low risk of complications was reduced. A similar approach has been successful in Italy.[43,44] The widespread availability of CT scanners in the United States has reduced the need for skull radiography,[45,46] and this may also occur in Europe as more scanners are placed in general hospitals.

RECOVERY AFTER HEAD INJURY: REHABILITATION

When the Newcastle team reported improved survival rates for severe head injuries in 1958, it stated that most survivors made a good physical and mental recovery and predicted that most would be fit to return to productive work.[6] Ten years later, reports appeared showing that less than half of those patients were working at all several years after injury; many of those working were doing jobs of lower status compared with their jobs before the injury.

An English orthopedic surgeon reported in 1967 that 40 percent of 230 patients he treated were left disabled and coined the term "lamebrain."[47] An editorial asked whether survival might sometimes be more tragic than death and stressed the paucity of prognostic criteria to inform decision making involving patients in the acute stage.[48] Noting the tendency to use overly optimistic terms to describe the recovery associated with disability (satisfactory, practical, useful, worthwhile), Jennett and Bond[22] introduced the Glasgow Outcome Scale with categories of good, moderately disabled, severely disabled, vegetative, and dead. This scale showed that 6 months after severe head injury, only 40 percent of survivors in the International Data Bank had made a good recovery, 30 percent were moderately disabled, 25 percent were severely disabled, and 5 percent were vegetative.[23] Since the average age of disabled survivors was about 27 years, many of these patients faced 40 years of disability. The features of disability have been studied extensively in the last decade, and it is clear that the physical or neurological sequelae are much less disabling than the mental sequelae, which include disorders of memory, behavior, cognitive function, and emotional control.[49] Relatives report serious personality change in most injured survivors, and the burden of caring for them commonly results in family disruption. Psychologists have studied the nature of deficits that can be measured with tests and have helped set up numerous rehabilitation facilities, especially in the United States. There is some confusion between interventional treatment and the provision of continuing support, and considerable controversy remains about the impact of different forms of therapy on the rate of recovery and the achieved level of function.[50] Most patients reach their final category on the Glasgow Outcome Scale within 6 to 12 months,[49] although improvement continues for much longer within one category.

EPIDEMIOLOGY, PREVENTION, AND ORGANIZATION OF CARE

Accidents are now the leading cause of death among individuals under age 45 years in western countries. Head injuries account for 70 percent of accidental deaths and for most of the persisting disability after trauma; they are 10 to 40 times more common than spinal cord injury. Routinely collected statistics provide limited data that are most reliable about deaths. However, the last decade has seen large-scale surveys of patients in Scotland, several areas of the United States, and two Australian states.[51–54] Death rates from head injury per 100,000 population vary from 9 for Great Britain, to 25 for the United States, to 28 for Australia. Ten times as many patients are admitted as die in the United States, but in Britain the ratio is 30:1; attenders at accident departments outnumber admissions by 5 to 1 in Great Britain, where they account for 10 percent of all patients coming to those departments.[52] When disabled survivors with an expectation of a long life and the much larger number of patients who have symptoms for a few weeks after mild injuries are taken into account, the scale and scope of the problem posed by head injuries become obvious. Less than 10 percent of patients admitted to the hospital have serious impairment of consciousness, yet about half of all the patients who eventually need neurosurgery and half of those who stay in the hospital for more than a month come from the large number whose initial injuries were mild or moderate.[55] This fact, together with the recognition that paying so much attention to the most severe injuries has yielded only modest gains, is leading to increasing interest in milder injuries.

With regard to causation and prevention, researchers may overstate the importance of road accidents and the risk to vehicle occupants. Although road accidents are the most common single cause of severe and fatal injuries, they account for only 50 to 60 percent of these injuries and for a much smaller proportion of milder injuries.[54] Many accidents involve pedestrians, especially among the young and the elderly, in whom falls are also common. Alcohol is an important element not only in road accidents (including drivers and pedestrians) but also in assaults and falls. Preventive measures include control of drinking, improvements in vehicles and road engineering, and the use of seat belts and protective helmets.

Perhaps the main challenge for the health care system is to organize the management of the large number of patients with mild head injuries who come to a hospital in such a way that the minority who are at risk from complications are identified and dealt with appropriately. In Great Britain, many of these mild injuries are managed both in the emergency room and in the ward of first admission by doctors without training in neurosurgery. In the United States, most patients hospitalized after head injury are cared for by neurosurgeons or surgeons with trauma training. A variety of disciplines are involved in the care of head-injured patients in accordance with local arrangements, including emergency physicians; general, orthopedic, and trauma surgeons; pediatricians; neurologists; and radiologists. The role of the neurosurgeon may be different in the United States than in Europe because of the large differences in the availability not only of neurosurgeons but also of specialized diagnostic and therapeutic facilities. Seven times as many neurosurgeons are available in the United States, along with 10 times as many CT scanners and intensive care beds.

Although neurosurgeons outside the United States deal with only a small minority of the head-injured patients who are admitted to a hospital, they need to provide national and local leadership in devising policies for collaboration with other disciplines for the management of milder injuries.[56,57] These guidelines should include clear indications for investigations, admission to the hospital, and referral to specialist units such as those developed in Great Britain.[40,41] In the United States, there is a strong trend toward more regional organization of facilities for trauma in general as well as for head injuries.[58,59] Services provided for head injuries in a community should be monitored by audits that record the number of cases attending, admitted, investigated, and treated in various ways, with the catchment population as the denominator. The number of patients who talk and die and the number of hematomas detected per year, together with the proportion of survivors who make a reasonable recovery, can provide useful indicators of the quality of that service. It is increasingly being recognized that improved care for less severely injured or low-risk patients, directed toward minimizing secondary brain damage from complications, is likely to have more of an impact on avoidable mortality and morbidity from head injury than is more intensive treatment of those who are already severely brain damaged.[38,42,43,60] The most telling data in support of this claim come from the study of nearly 8000 head injuries in 41 U.S. hospitals.[60] These hospitals ranged from best (mortality only half that expected) to worst (almost twice that expected). Almost 70 percent of patients were not severe (expected mortality <10 percent). For these patients, the mortality in the best hospital was 9 times lower than expected and that in the worst hospital was 8 times greater than expected. For severe injuries, the mortality was only 1.2 times greater in the worst than in the best hospitals.

The specialty of neurosurgery will prosper in the competitive field of health care only if it is seen to deal effectively with the major problems of the community within its area of expertise.[56] Therefore, neurosurgery seems likely to need head injuries for its future welfare as much as head-injured patients need neurosurgeons for their best chance of survival and recovery.

References

1. Jennett B: Sir William Macewen 1848–1924: Pioneer Scottish neurosurgeon. *Surg Neurol* 6:57, 1976.
2. Cushing H: A study of a series of wounds involving the brain and its enveloping structures. *Br J Surg* 5:558, 1918.
3. Cairns H: Neurosurgery in the British Army 1939–1945. *Br J Surg* [*War Surg Suppl*] 1:9–26, 1947.
4. Meirowsky AM: *Neurological Surgery of Trauma.* U.S. Government Printing Office, 1965.
5. Hammon WM: Analysis of 2187 consecutive penetrating wounds of the brain from Vietnam. *J Neurosurg* 34:127, 1971.
6. MacIver IN, Frew JC, Matheson JG: The role of respiratory insufficiency in the mortality of severe head injuries. *Lancet* 1:390, 1958.

7. Adams JH, Graham DI: *An Introduction to Neuropathology.* Edinburgh: Churchill Livingstone, 1988.
8. Reilly PL, Graham DI, Adams H, et al: Patients with head injury who talk and die. *Lancet* 2:375, 1975.
9. Rose J, Valtonen S, Jennett B: Avoidable factors contributing to death after head injury. *Br Med J* 2:615, 1977.
10. Gennarelli TA, Thiebault LE, Adams JH, et al: Diffuse axonal injury and traumatic coma in the primate. *Ann Neurol* 12:564, 1982.
11. Denny-Brown D, Russell WR: Experimental cerebral concussion. *Brain* 64:93, 1941.
12. Strich SJ: Diffuse degeneration of cerebral white matter in severe dementia following head injury. *J Neurol Neurosurg Psychiatry* 19:163–185, 1956.
13. Strich SJ: Shearing of nerve fibres as a cause of brain damage due to head injury. *Lancet* 2:444–448, 1961.
14. Adams JH, Doyle D, Ford I, et al: Diffuse axonal injury in head injury: Definition, diagnosis and grading. *Histopathology* 15:49–59, 1989.
15. Becker DP, Miller JD, Ward JD, et al: The outcome from severe head injury with early diagnosis and intensive management. *J Neurosurg* 47:491–502, 1977.
16. Marshall LF, Smith RW, Shapiro HM: The outcome with aggressive treatment in severe head injuries: II. Acute and chronic barbiturate administration in the management of head injury. *Neurosurgery* 50:26–30, 1979.
17. Marshall LF, Smith RW, Shapiro HM: The outcome with aggressive treatment in severe head injuries: I. The significance of intracranial pressure monitoring. *Neurosurgery* 50:20–25, 1979.
18. Andrews PJD, Piper IR, Dearden NM, et al: Secondary insults during intrahospital transport of head injured patients. *Lancet* 335:327–330, 1990.
19. Gopinath SP, Robertson CS, Contant CF, et al: Jugular venous desaturation and outcome after head injury. *J Neurol Neurosurg Psychiatry* 57:717–723, 1994.
20. Langfitt TW: Measuring the outcome from head injuries. *J Neurosurg* 48:673–678, 1978.
21. Teasdale G, Jennett B: Assessment of coma and impaired consciousness: A practical scale. *Lancet* 2:81–84, 1974.
22. Jennett B, Bond M: Assessment of outcome after severe brain damage: A practical scale. *Lancet* 1:480–484, 1975.
23. Jennett B, Teasdale G, Galbraith S, et al: Severe head injuries in three countries. *J Neurol Neurosurg Psychiatry* 40:291, 1977.
24. Jennett B, Teasdale G, Braakman R, et al: Predicting outcome in individual patients after severe head injury. *Lancet* 1:1031, 1976.
25. Jennett B, Teasdale G, Fry J, et al: Treatment for severe head injury. *J Neurol Neurosurg Psychiatry* 43:289, 1980.
26. Jennett B: Outcome of intensive therapy for severe head injuries: An inter-centre comparison, in Parillo JE, Ayres SM (eds): *Major Issues in Critical Care Medicine.* Baltimore: Williams & Wilkins, 207–213, 1984.
27. Murray GD: Use of an international data bank to compare outcome following severe head injury in different centres. *Stat Med* 5:103, 1986.
28. Miller JD, Butterworth JF, Gudeman SK, et al: Further experience in the management of severe head injury. *J Neurosurg* 54:289, 1981.
29. Miller JD, Teasdale GM: Clinical trials for assessing treatment for severe head injury, in Becker DP, Povlishock JT (eds): *Central Nervous System Status Report.* Bethesda, MD: National Institutes of Health, 1985.
30. Murray GD, Murray LS, Barlow P, et al: Assessing the performance and clinical impact of a computerised prognostic system in severe head injury. *Stat Med* 6:403, 1986.
31. Knaus WA, Draper EA, Wagner DP, et al: Evaluation outcome from intensive care: A preliminary multihospital comparison. *Crit Care Med* 10:491, 1982.
32. Knaus WA, Wagner DP, Loirat P, et al: A comparison of intensive care in the USA and France. *Lancet* 2:642, 1982.
33. Varia: Report on the Trauma Coma Data Bank. *J Neurosurg* 75(Suppl):1–66, 1993.
34. Bailey I, Bell A, Gray J, et al: A trial of the effect of nimodipine on outcome after head injury. *Acta Neurochir (Wien)* 110:97–105, 1991.
35. Murray LS, Teasdale GM, Murray GD, et al: Does prediction of outcome alter potential management? *Lancet* 341:1487–1491, 1993.
36. European Study Group: A multicenter trial on the efficacy of mimodipine on severe head injury. *J Neurosurg* 80:797–804, 1994.
37. Marshall LF, Toole BM, Bowers SA: The National Traumatic Coma Data Bank: II. Patients who talk and deteriorate: Implications for treatment. *J Neurosurg* 59:285, 1983.
38. Jennett B: Epidemiology of severe head injury: Socioeconomic consequences of avoidable mortality and morbidity. *Proceedings 2nd International Symposium on Nimodipine 1990.* Berlin: Springer-Verlag, 1991.
39. Mendelow AD, Teasdale G, Jennett B, et al: Risks of intracranial haematoma in head injured adults. *Br Med J* 287:1173, 1983.
40. Guidelines for initial management after head injury in adults. *Br Med J* 288:983, 1984.
41. Teasdale G, Murray G, Anderson E, et al: Risks of acute traumatic intracranial haematoma in children and adults: Implications for managing head injuries. *Br Med J* 300:363–367, 1990.
42. Teasdale GM, Murray L, Murray G, et al: Guidelines for decision making to improve outcome after head injury. *J Neurotrauma* 10(Suppl):S101, 1993.
43. Tomei G, Taggi F, and Co-operative Study Group: Low risk head injuries: Definition and management strategies. *J Neurotrauma* 10(Suppl):S103, 1993.
44. Servadei F, Nasi MT, Vergoni G, et al: Extradural haematomas: How many deaths can be avoided with a clear protocol and prevention of deterioration in minor injuries? *J Neurotrauma* 10(Suppl):S194, 1993.
45. Masters SJ, McClean PM, Arcarese JS, et al: Skull X-ray examinations after head trauma: Recommendations by a multidisciplinary panel and validation study. *N Engl J Med* 316:84, 1987.
46. Thornbury JR, Masters SJ, Campbell JA: Imaging recommendations for head trauma: A new comprehensive strategy. *AJR* 149:781, 1987.
47. London PS: Some observations on the course of events after severe injury of the head. *Ann R Coll Surg Engl* 41:460, 1967.

48. Severe head injuries. *Lancet* 1:514, 1968.
49. Jennett B, Snoek J, Bond MR, et al: Disability after severe head injury. *J Neurol Neurosurg Psychiatry* 44:285, 1981.
50. Rosenthal M, Griffiths ER, Bond MR, et al (eds): *Rehabilitation of the Adult and Child with Traumatic Brain Injury* (2d ed). Philadelphia: FA Davis, 1989.
51. Frankowski RF, Annegers JF, Whitman S: The descriptive epidemiology of head trauma in US, in Becker DP, Povlishock JT (eds): *Central Nervous System Status Report.* Bethesda, MD: National Institutes of Health, 33–43, 1985.
52. Jennett B, MacMillan R: Epidemiology of head injury. *Br Med J* 282:101, 1981.
53. Trauma Subcommittee of the Neurosurgical Society of Australasia: Neurotrauma in Australia (report on surveys). *Aust N Z J Surg* 56: (Suppl) 1986.
54. Jennett B, Frankowski RF: The epidemiology of head injury, in Vinken PJ, Bruyn GW (eds): *Handbook of Clinical Neurology.* Amsterdam: Elsevier Science, 1990: vol 13, pp 1–16.
55. Miller JD, Jones PA: The work of a regional head injury service. *Lancet* 1:1141, 1985.
56. Jennett B: The future role of neurosurgery in the care of head injuries. *Neurosurg Rev* 9:129, 1986.
57. Jennett B, Teasdale G: *Management of Head Injuries.* Philadelphia: FA Davis, 1981.
58. California Association of Neurological Surgeons' Emergency Services Committee Report: Guidelines for Establishment of Trauma Centers. *J Neurosurg* 65:569, 1986.
59. Planning neurotrauma care: Appendix I to the Hospital Resources Document. *Bull Am Coll Surg* 71:22, 1986.
60. Klauber MR, Marshall LF, Luerssen TG, et al: Determinants of head injury mortality: Importance of the low risk patient. *Neurosurgery* 24:31–36, 1989.

CHAPTER 2

EPIDEMIOLOGY OF BRAIN INJURY*

Jess F. Kraus
David L. McArthur
Terry A. Silverman
Madhangi Jayaraman

SYNOPSIS

This chapter explores the recent English-language literature on the incidence, severity, and outcome of brain injury. Across studies, great variation is found in estimates of the numbers of persons suffering a brain injury as a result of substantial differences in definitions of terms, inclusion and exclusion criteria, and specific details of the research designs. The first half of the chapter presents estimates of the annual U.S. incidence rate for brain injury and describes the characteristics of high-risk groups and high-risk exposures. Recent findings from work conducted outside the United States provide important points for comparison. The second half examines recent literature dealing with relationships between demographic factors and severity, relationships between indexes of severity and outcome, and the general topic of epidemiological prognosis.

This chapter synthesizes a variety of published research papers that describe the incidence, severity, and outcome of brain injury and the possible relationships among those factors. Comparison of results between papers requires a level of uniformity among term definitions, variables, and measurement techniques that is rarely present. Therefore, while it is possible to report study findings and draw an overall picture of brain injury in the United States, such a portrayal is not without limitations.

The term "brain injury" is often defined quite differently in different papers (Table 2-1). While most authors clearly wish to study assaults to the nervous system, some use the term "head injury."[1,2] This practice allows for the inclusion of patients with physical injuries to the skull, facial fractures, or soft tissue damage to the face or head without neurological consequences.

Case inclusion criteria vary from study to study as well. Research populations may consist of patients referred to neurological intensive care units[3–5] or patients treated in emergency departments and released for outpatient observation.[6,7] In several studies, those experiencing immediate death or death on arrival at the emergency department are excluded.[8]

ESTIMATES OF OCCURRENCE OF BRAIN INJURY

Brain Injury and Death Rates

In 1990, almost 148,500 persons died of acute traumatic injury, accounting for about 8 percent of all deaths in the United States. The exact percentage of deaths involving significant brain injury is not known, but mortality estimates from Minnesota[1] and California[9] suggest that about 50 percent are due to brain trauma. National Center for Health Statistics data on multiple causes of death indicate that 28 percent of all deaths from injury involve significant brain trauma.[10] However, this value may be an underestimate by as much as 44 percent, since the case-finding process relied on a stringent and therefore exclusive list of injury diagnoses.

The reported mortality rate for brain injury varies from 14 to 30 per 100,000 population per year. This

* This work was supported by the Southern California Injury Prevention Research Center under Grant No. R49-CCR903622 from the Centers for Disease Control.

TABLE 2-1 Case Identification and Brain Injury Severity Criteria and Scoring: Selected U.S. Incidence Studies

Study Location (Reference)	Study Years	Case Definition	Severity Criteria/Scoring
Olmsted County, Minnesota (Annegers et al.[1])	1965–1974	Head injury with evidence of presumed brain involvement, i.e., concussion with loss of consciousness (LOC), posttraumatic amnesia (PTA), or neurological signs of brain injury, skull fracture	1. Fatal (<28 days) 2. Severe: intracranial hematoma, contusion, or LOC > 24 h or PTA > 24 h 3. Moderate: LOC or PTA 30 min–24 h, skull fracture, or both 4. LOC or PTA < 30 min without skull fracture
San Diego County, California, (Klauber et al.[33])	1978	ICD codes 800, 801, 804, 806, 850–854 with hospital admission diagnosis or cause of death with skull fracture, LOC, PTA, neurological deficit or seizure, no gunshot wounds	Glasgow Coma Scale (GCS) (categories formed from scores of 3, 4–5, 6–7, 8–15)
San Diego County, California (Kraus et al.[9])	1981	Physician diagnosed physical damage from acute mechanical energy exchange resulting in concussion, hemorrhage, contusion, or laceration of brain	Modified GCS (severe = ≤ 8; moderate = 9–15 and hospital stay of 4–8 h and brain surgery, or abnormal CAT or GCS = 9–12; mild = all others, GCS 13–15)
Maryland (MacKenzie et al.[12])	1986	ICD codes 800, 801, 803, 804, 850–854	ICDMAP—converts ICD codes to Abbreviated Injury Severity Scores
Central Virginia (Rimel et al.[5])	Oct. 1977–June 1979	CNS referral patients with significant head injury admitted to neurosurgical service	GCS (severe = ≤8, moderate = 9–12, mild = 13–15)
Chicago area (Whitman et al.[2])	1979–1980	Any hospital discharge diagnosis of ICD codes 800–804, 830, 850–854, 873, 920, 959.0; injury within 7 days prior to hospital visit and blow to head/face with LOC or laceration of scalp/forehead	1. Fatal 2. Severe = intracranial hematoma, contusion, LOC/PTA > 24 h 3. Moderate = LOC/PTA 30 min to ≤ 24 h 4. Mild LOC/PTA < 30 min 5. Trivial = remainder

range of rates probably reflects a lack of specificity of diagnosis on some death certificates (Fig. 2-1).

The only national estimate of nonfatal brain injury for the United States was derived from the National Health Interview Survey (NHIS) for 1985–1987, extrapolated to the 1990 U.S. Census population of about 249 million residents.[10] The NHIS reports that about 1,975,000 head injuries occur per year. Unfortunately, this estimate includes head injuries in which no brain injury has occurred. The extent of the diagnosis and treatment of brain injury in and outside emergency rooms is not known, but Fife,[11] on reexamining the NHIS database, concluded that only 16 percent of all head injuries resulted in admission to a hospital. Therefore, only one of six persons with a head (not necessarily brain) injury is in serious enough condition to be admitted to a hospital for medical treatment. Because the number of individuals who seek medical care that does not involve emergency room facilities is unknown, the NHIS figure of 1.975 million injuries remains an uncertain estimate of the true incidence in the population.

Data summarized in Fig. 2-2 show occurrence rates for brain injury that range from a low of 132 per 100,000 in Maryland[12] to a high of 367 per 100,000 in the Chicago

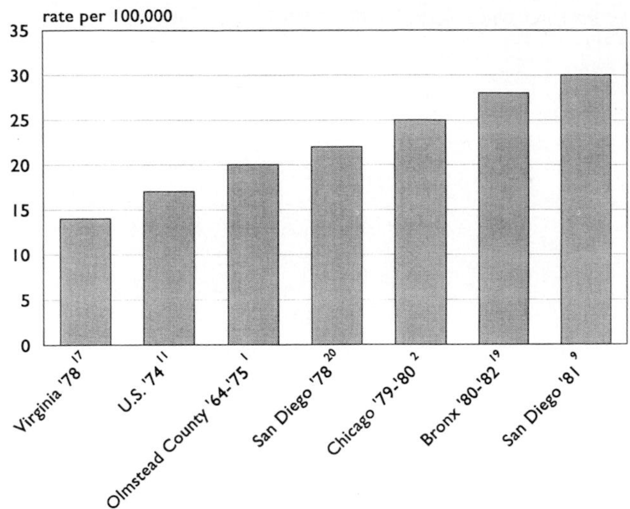

Figure 2-1. Brain injury mortality rates in the United States: selected studies.

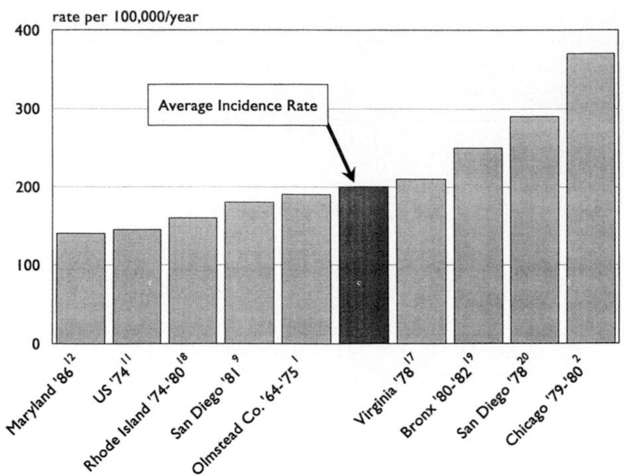

Figure 2-2. Brain injury incidence rates in the United States: selected studies.

area.[2] Despite several important differences that limit comparison between the two studies, it is possible to estimate an average rate of fatal plus nonfatal hospitalized brain injury reported in all U.S. studies of about 237 per 100,000 persons per year. If the highest and lowest estimates in Fig. 2-2 are excluded from consideration, the estimated rate is about 220 per 100,000 per year. A conservative rate used in this chapter for purposes of disability estimation is 200 per 100,000 per year.

An estimate derived from published national sources and summarized in Fig. 2-3 suggests that about 373,000 persons were discharged from a hospital in 1990 in the United States with a diagnosis of brain injury, for a hospital admission rate of about 150 per 100,000 population per year. The hospital discharge rate is useful in estimating the annual rate of disability from injury. The difference between estimates using average incidence values in aggregate U.S. studies and those using data from hospital discharges or visits is due to definitional variation. The actual U.S. incidence rate is therefore presumed to be between 180 and 220 per 100,000 persons per year.

A different perspective on brain injury rates is provided by Table 2-2, in which brain injury is compared with other leading diagnoses involving the head. The most frequently used first-listed diagnoses upon discharge (implying the primary reason for admission) from the NHIS data are presented in two ways: population rates and relative rates per 100 discharges in which

TABLE 2-2 Discharge Rates for Selected First-Listed Diagnoses per 100,000 Population and per 100 Diagnoses of Brain Injury

Diagnosis	ICD Codes	Rate per 100,000 Population	Rate Ratio per 100 Diagnoses of Brain Injury
Brain injury*	800–804, 850–854, 905, 907	149.6	(100.0)
Occlusion of cerebral arteries	434	96.5	64.3
Schizophrenic disorders	295	85.2	56.8
Other cerebrovascular disease	436, 437	83.6	55.8
Epilepsy	345	37.0	24.7
Intracerebral and intracranial hemorrhage	431, 432	29.8	19.8
Migraine	346	20.1	13.4
Multiple sclerosis	340	12.9	8.6
Malignant neoplasm of brain	191	12.1	8.0
Cerebral degeneration (nonchildhood)	331	8.0	5.4
Subarachnoid hemorrhage	430	8.0	5.4

* Not limited to first-listed diagnoses; may not include all admissions with brain injury.

SOURCE: Collins.[10]

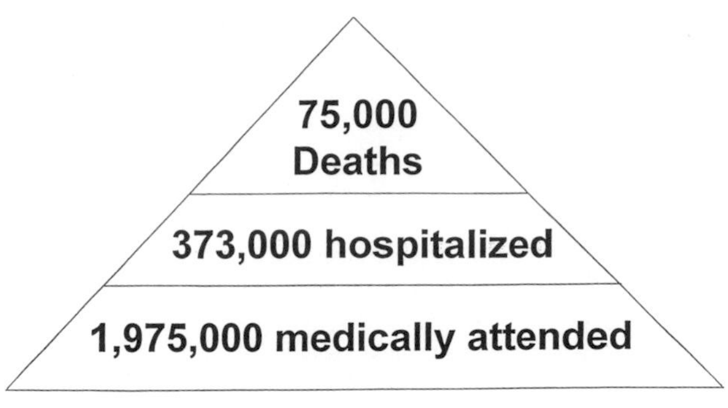

Figure 2-3. Annual brain injury frequency, 1990 U.S. estimates.

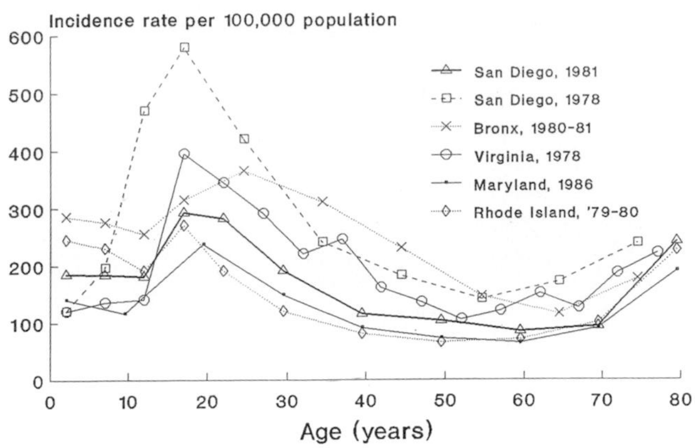

Figure 2-4. Age-specific brain injury incidence rates per 100,000 population: selected U.S. studies. (Used with permission from Kraus JF: Epidemiology of Head Injury, in Cooper PR (ed): *Head Injury* (3d ed) Baltimore: Williams & Wilkins, 1993.)

brain injury was one of the diagnoses. With few exceptions, many of the leading causes of hospitalization occur at no more than one-fifth the rate for brain injury. Occlusion of cerebral arteries occurs at two-thirds the rate for brain injury. Schizophrenic disorders and cerebrovascular diseases that are not separately categorized occur at a rate less than three-fifths the rate for brain injury. While these rates are not totally independent and are subject to the usual range of problems involving diagnostic bias, they illustrate the relative magnitudes of the various injuries and illnesses affecting the head. Accurate information on occurrence rates for brain injury allows monitoring of changes in incidence in the population, evaluation of the effects of specific countermeasures or treatments, and identification of risk groups or exposure circumstances.

Characteristics of High-Risk Groups

Age

All studies of the occurrence of brain injury in the United States show that persons 15 to 24 years old are at the highest risk. Patterns in age-specific rates (as shown in Fig. 2-4) illustrate high rates under the age of 10 in all studies and even higher rates under age 5 in some studies. The rates generally peak after age 15, decline after age 24, and continue to decline in the middle years. The rates increase again in the age range of 60 to 65 years.

Sex

All incidence reports agree that brain injuries are far more frequent for males than for females, with a rate ratio varying from approximately 2.0 to 2.8 (Fig. 2-5). Although variations in rate ratios exist, the differences may reflect different exposure levels.

Race and Ethnicity

Although some studies show a higher brain injury incidence in nonwhites compared with whites, there is justifiable concern over the quality of the data used to derive these rates. Hospital reporting practices vary widely in recording ethnicity or race in medical records; thus, racial and ethnic differences in brain injury rates have not been determined accurately.

Socioeconomic Status

As was shown above, age, gender, and race and ethnicity are risk markers for certain populations with a high

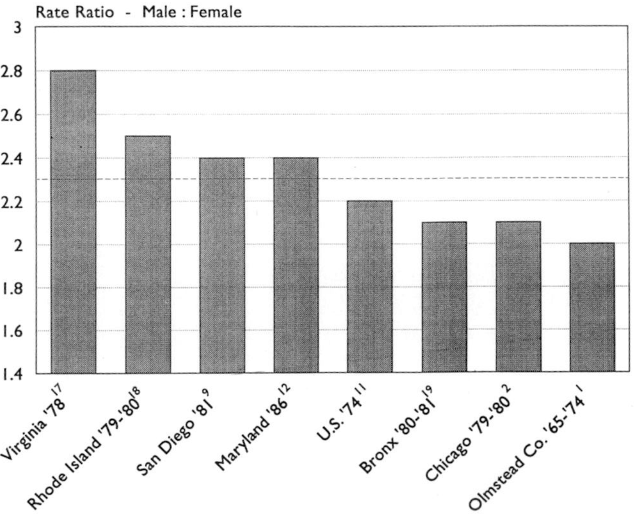

Figure 2-5. Rate ratio of brain injuries by gender: selected studies.

incidence of brain injury. Another risk marker is socioeconomic status, as measured by a number of indicators. The NHIS for 1985–1987 shows that the estimated average annual number of injuries and the rates per 100 persons per year are highest in families with the lowest income levels.[10] This finding was also observed by Kraus and colleagues[13] in their study in San Diego County and by Whitman and associates[2] in two socioeconomically different Chicago communities. In the report by Kraus et al.,[13] the surrogate for individual socioeconomic status was median family income per census tract. The findings did not change when race or ethnicity was taken into consideration. Multivariate analysis suggested that using race and/or ethnicity as a proxy for socioeconomic status may be inappropriate; other aspects of exposure nested within the "socioeconomic environment" should be explored.

CHARACTERISTICS OF EXPOSURES TO THE RISK OF BRAIN INJURY

Alcohol

The positive association between blood alcohol concentration (BAC) and risk of injury is well established for almost every type of external cause of injuries, including motor vehicle crashes, general aviation crashes, drownings, and violence.[14] Although animal studies demonstrate a variety of physiological effects of alcohol on CNS injuries, human data are equivocal. Less studied has been the role of alcohol and the outcome of specific kinds or anatomic locations of injuries such as CNS trauma or burns in humans. Kraus et al.[15] found that 56 percent of adults with a diagnosis of brain injury who were tested for BAC had a positive result. The prevalence of a positive BAC varied by severity of brain injury; the highest prevalence of BAC occurred among those with mild brain injury compared with moderate or severe brain injury (71 percent versus 49 percent, respectively). However, selection bias may occur in emergency department BAC testing of injured persons because of different severities, types of injuries, inherent sociodemographic differences, or differing external causes of injuries. For example, blood testing was less frequent for males, young adults, persons with mild brain injuries, and those injured from falls. Despite this potential bias, Kraus and colleagues[15] found that the BAC level was positively associated with physician-diagnosed neurological impairment and with length of hospitalization. Gurney et al.[16] found that brain-injured adults who were intoxicated at the time of injury were more likely to develop respiratory distress and/or pneumonia than were brain-injured adults who were not intoxicated at the time of injury. While the prevalence of pneumonia among intoxicated patients could not be assessed before their hospitalization, decreased immune function resulting from ethanol exposure may impair respiratory function sufficiently to lead to pneumonia after hospitalization.

Transport

The available data[1,2,9,11,12,17–20] suggest that the exposure most frequently associated with fatal and nonfatal brain injury is transportation (Fig. 2-6). This category embraces automobiles, trucks, bicycles, motorcycles, pedestrians, aircraft, watercraft, and farm equipment. Transportation causes of brain injury are followed in number by falls, usually among the elderly and patients with assault-related brain injury. In addition, sports and recreation are a significant factor for brain injury.

The dominant form of transportation exposure is motor vehicle crashes or impacts (Fig. 2-7). This form can be subdivided into three broad groups: vehicle occupants, riders on motorcycles, and pedestrians and bicyclists. As a result of classification difficulties across studies, it is not possible to characterize occupant location in the vehicle (e.g., driver versus passenger), but vehicle occupants as a whole are the most frequently brain-injured group. Exposure risk within different types of transportation appears to differ dramatically across re-

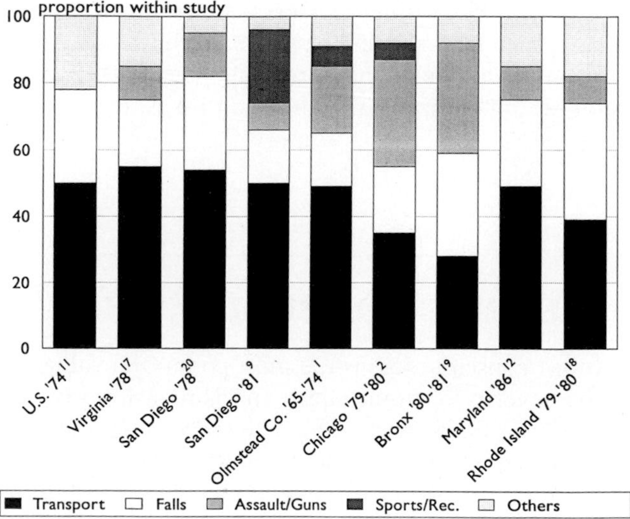

Figure 2-6. Distribution of brain injuries by external cause, selected studies.

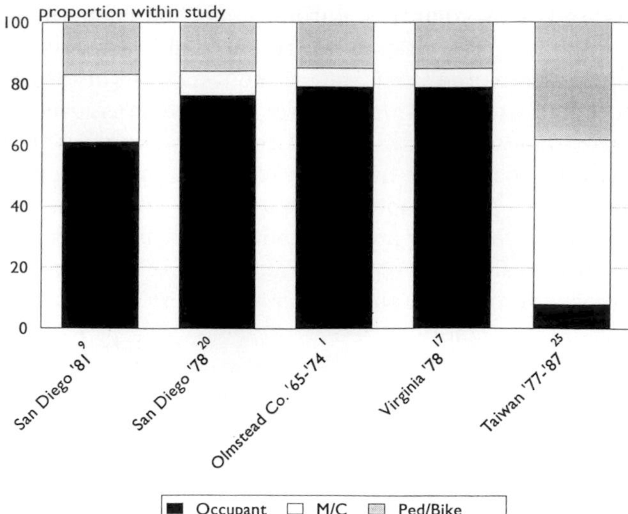

Figure 2-7. Distribution of motor-vehicle-related brain injuries by vehicle type.

Eye Opening	
Spontaneous	E4
To speech	3
To pain	2
Nil	1
Best Motor Response	
Obeys	M6
Localizes	5
Withdraws	4
Abnormal flexion	3
Extensor response	2
Nil	1
Verbal Response	
Oriented	V5
Confused conversation	4
Inappropriate words	3
Incomprehensible sounds	2
Nil	1

Coma Score (E + M + V) = 3 to 15
(From Teasdale and Jennett[39])

Figure 2-8. Scoring system of the Glasgow Coma Scale. (From Teasdale and Jennett.[39])

ports and is currently the subject of intense study (e.g., the contribution of seat belt use and motorcycle helmet use to the prevention of head injuries and fatalities).

Other Premorbid Exposures

A number of authors have taken up the issue of antecedent risk factors, asking whether various conditions predispose children to exposures that result in brain injury. Goldstein and Levin[21] reported that children with premorbid factors such as behavioral problems exhibit a greater tendency to have brain injuries. However, Klonoff[22] could not show any relationship between factors such as lower income and crowded housing and injury repetition. Though they possess no treatment implications, if such factors could be proved to have conclusive relationships, they might alert public health authorities to target populations for prevention measures.

SEVERITY OF BRAIN INJURY

Level of consciousness is the most common evaluation of the severity of brain injury and is measured by the Glasgow Coma Scale (GCS). The GCS scoring system is described in Fig. 2-8. The distribution of the severity of brain injury as assessed by the GCS is shown in Fig. 2-9. The majority of brain injuries in all studies are classified as "mild" (i.e., GCS of 13 to 15). However, "mild" connotes an imprecise description of brain trauma and is differentially conceived by various researchers (Fig. 2-10). Among those admitted to a hospital alive, 80 percent are mild (GCS 13 to 15), 10 percent are moderate (GCS 9 to 12), and 10 percent are severe (GCS $\leq$ 8). Only one study found a higher proportion of moderate and severe cases,[17] possibly because the study hospital was a referral institution to which serious injuries were more likely to be sent from the surrounding catchment area.

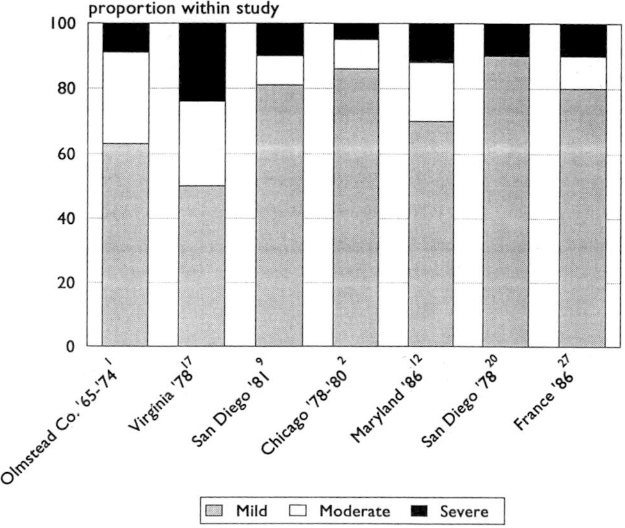

Figure 2-9. Distribution of brain injury severity: selected studies.

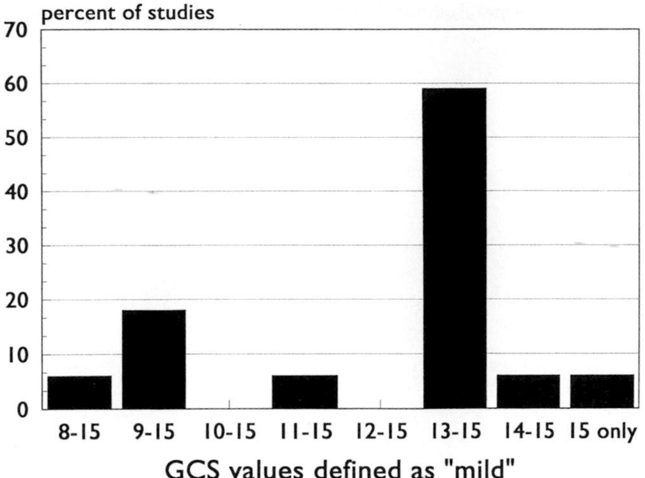

Figure 2-10. Percentage of studies reporting use of the Glasgow Coma Scale for mild brain injury by interval of scale employed.

HOSPITAL ADMISSIONS AND DIAGNOSES

Information on persons admitted to short care nonfederal hospitals in the United States in 1990 is available through the National Hospital Discharge Survey (NHDS).[23] This data source provides information on *any* listed diagnosis of brain injury coded to the International Classification of Diseases, 9th revision, Clinical Modification (ICD-9 CM), and in this regard brain injury may be the least severe of all injuries observed in the clinical assessment.[24] The rate for those admitted with a brain injury of any severity at short stay hospitals during 1990 is about 150 per 100,000 population. The hospital discharge rate is approximately twice as high for males as for females.

Rates are highest for those below 15 years old. Unfortunately, the only national data on hospital discharges are grouped into four generally heterogeneous groups. Thus, rates are not available for smaller age ranges. Most persons discharged from a hospital with a brain injury were diagnosed as having a concussion without fracture of the skull, which is consistent with the severity distribution from more focused studies. Approximately 30 percent of the discharges involve "other intracranial injury" without a skull fracture; intracranial injury with fracture represents less than 13 percent of all hospital discharges.

The age-specific injury incidence rates reported earlier in this chapter are considerably higher than the age-specific discharge rates from the NHDS. A possible explanation for the high brain injury rate among hospital discharges for infants is "birth trauma," a diagnosis excluded from most brain injury databases. Those who died at the scene, during emergency transportation, or in the emergency facility are not included in the NHDS estimates. In evaluating these data, the reader should be aware that the NHDS figures are based on *discharges* from short stay hospitals or on the same hospital on multiple occasions for the same injury. Therefore, the discharge does not represent an exclusive occurrence. Independent information from the authors' studies suggests that multiple hospital admissions to the same hospital or a different hospital for treatment of the same injury are a relatively common occurrence.

Types of Brain Lesions

Although the literature is replete with reports describing brain trauma, few epidemiological studies have addressed the question of the nature and severity of brain lesions. In the San Diego County cohort study,[9] however, clinical information was uniformly recorded and coded from the physician's notes in the medical record. The data are population-based, as they refer to a single period from all hospitals in the region and refer only to patients age 15 and older.

Figure 2-11 shows the distribution of brain injury lesions according to fracture status and type. Slightly less than half of all hospital-admitted brain injuries are concussions *without* a concurrent fracture. Nearly 11 percent of those with a laceration and/or contusion of the brain do not have a concurrent fracture. Similarly, among those diagnosed with a brain hemorrhage, one-

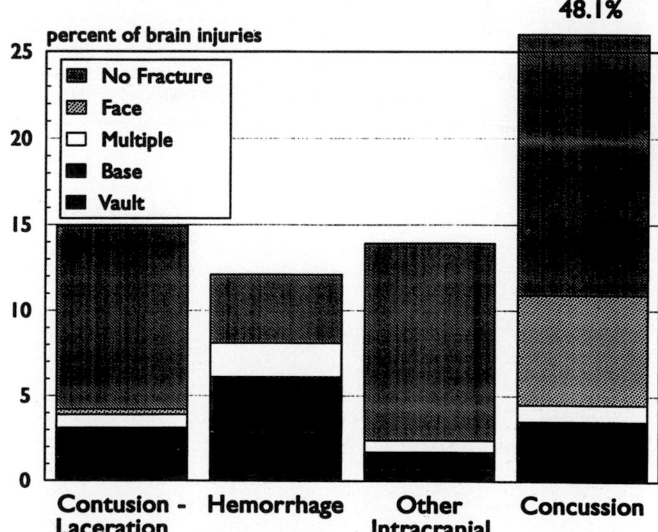

Figure 2-11. Distribution of injury diagnosis and fracture status: selected studies.

half do not have a concurrent skull fracture. In all four major brain lesion categories, at least one-half of the patients do not have a concurrent fracture of the skull. Fracture is much less common among patients with a diagnosis of concussion or another cranial injury than among patients with a diagnosis of contusion, laceration, or hemorrhage.

Case Fatality Rates

While the general fatality rate (or mortality rate) provides an idea of the level or magnitude of the most severe brain injuries in the general population, the case fatality rate after hospital admission measures the immediate gross consequences of the trauma and has been used to assess secondary prevention countermeasures.

Case fatality data are available from six U.S. population-based incidence studies (Fig. 2-12). Case fatality rates range from approximately 3 per 100 patients in Rhode Island[18] to about 8 per 100 hospitalized cases in the Bronx, New York.[19] While it is tempting to compare across these studies, it would not be appropriate, as they were not adjusted for hospital admission severity. One case fatality report from Taiwan[25] shows a high rate, but again, as cases are mixed by injury severity, comparison across study centers would not yield any meaningful information.

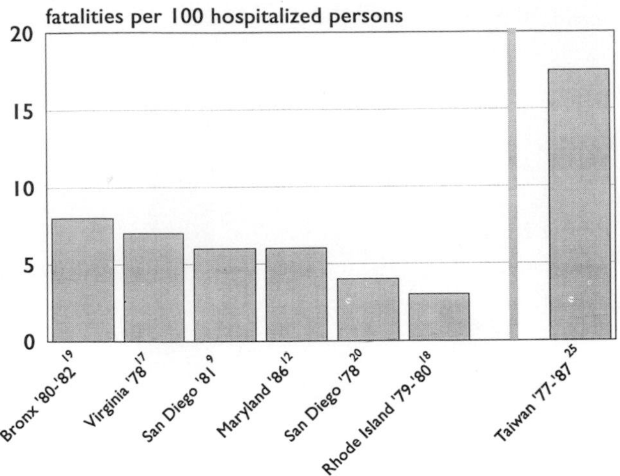

Figure 2-12. Case fatality rates of persons hospitalized for brain injury: selected studies.

International Studies

The epidemiology of brain injury is not independent of social and cultural factors, a fact which becomes clear when brain injury statistics in North America are compared with those in other parts of the world (Table 2-3). Studies from Cantabria, Spain,[26] and Aquitaine, France,[27] reveal that the incidence and causes of head injury are only slightly different from those in the United States. By contrast, data from Johannesburg, South Africa,[28] contrast sharply with other papers, reflecting the social and political instability in that nation.

The studies from France and Spain include all head injuries, not brain injury alone, and therefore cannot provide entirely comparable brain injury statistics. Nevertheless, broad generalizations are possible. While estimates of the incidence of head trauma in Aquitaine are

TABLE 2-3 Incidence Rate Characteristics: Selected International Studies

Study Location (Reference)	Study Years	No. Cases	Incidence Rate per 100,000	Age at Highest Risk	Male/ Female Ratio	Case Fatality Rate per 100	External Causes
Cantabria, Spain (Vasquez-Barquero et al.[26])	1988	477	91	15–24	2.7:1	0.020	Vehicle: 60%; falls: 24%; work-related: 8%; recreation: 4%
Aquitaine, France (Tiret et al.[27])	1986	8940	281	15–24	2.1:1	0.022	Traffic: 60%; falls: 32%; struck by object: 6%
Johannesburg, South Africa (Nell and Brown[28])	1987	6409	316	25–44	African: 4.4:1 White: 40.1:1	African: 0.088 White: 0.054 Colored: 0.045	Percentage of all causes by race and gender: African: vehicles: 27% (males), 24% (females); interpersonal: 51% (males), 52% (females) White: vehicles: 73% (males), 62% (females); interpersonal: 10% (males), 10% (females)

similar to those in the United States (280 in 100,000), the incidence in Cantabria is astonishingly lower (91 in 100,000). Since these studies included all head injuries, the actual incidence rates for brain injury are underestimated. The male-female incidence ratio is similar to the U.S. findings described in this chapter: 2.7 in Cantabria and 2.1 in Aquitaine. Also, the peak age of injury is 15 to 24 for males and females in both studies. In both Aquitaine and Cantabria, vehicle-related crashes accounted for 60 percent of the injuries. Falls accounted for 24 percent of the injuries in Spain and 32.5 percent of the injuries in France. Head injury from assault seems to be lower in Cantabria than in most cities in the United States. Case fatality in Aquitaine (0.022 in 100), though not severity-adjusted, is similar to that in U.S. studies. Further, 9 percent of survivors suffer severe injury. In Spain, the case fatality rate (0.020 in 100) is considerably lower than it is in the United States. It appears that severe brain injury is much less common in Cantabria than it is in the United States. Only 1 percent of patients have severe disability or are in a persistent vegetative state.

In Johannesburg, the picture is radically different. For all races, the age-adjusted incidence of brain injury is 316 in 100,000, much higher than the incidence rate in the United States. By race, the rate for age-adjusted nonfatal brain injury incidence for Africans is 355 in 100,000; for whites, 109 in 100,000; and for Coloreds, 298 in 100,000. Further, the male-female ratio among Africans is 4.4, while among whites it soars to 40.1. Despite this discrepancy, African females and males have considerably higher age-adjusted nonfatal incidence rates (133 in 100,000 and 582 in 100,000, respectively) than do their white counterparts (6 in 100,000 for females and 224 in 100,000 for males). While the age peak in nonfatal incidence rates is 15 to 24 years for white males (419 in 100,000), African males and females peak at ages 25 to 44 (763 in 100,000 and 200 in 100,000, respectively). Also, although the age peak is in the range of 25 to 44, the African male incidence at ages 15 to 24 (634 in 100,000) is higher than the white male incidence in this range, a phenomenon which the authors do not fully explain. Clearly, South Africans in general and Africans in particular have lived in a more violent society than the United States, France, or Spain, a fact which is borne out by the description of the causes of injury. For all Africans and Colored males, interpersonal violence accounts for the majority of nonfatal brain injuries, while vehicle-related causes account for more brain injuries among whites and other race-sex groups. Fatal brain injury, however, is primarily the result of vehicle crashes in all race-sex groups, with interpersonal violence running a close second among African males. Africans in vehicular crashes are generally pedestrians, while whites in such crashes are usually vehicle occupants, reflecting an economic disparity between the races. Among whites, the second highest cause of fatal brain injury is suicide for both males and females. According to the authors, this is due to social stress indirectly caused by apartheid.[28] Ironically, only 2.8 percent of all brain injuries among Africans are severe, while 18.2 percent of brain injuries among whites fall in that classification. According to the authors, vehicular crashes generally produce injuries of greater severity than does interpersonal violence.

INTERRELATIONSHIPS ACROSS DOMAINS

The interaction of incidence, severity, and outcome of brain injury has been considered by a variety of researchers in the past two decades. Some investigators have attempted to isolate optimal predictors of outcome by using longitudinal data sets. In other studies, the relations found between variables in one data set and variables in another data set are reported only cursorily, having emerged from the analyses as a perhaps unintended bonus of the original study. The deliberate search for links between early and late events, markers, behaviors, and outcomes shows itself in three broad types of reports in the professional literature. The largest group consists of treatment studies that seek to determine whether different interventions applied shortly after the trauma event might result in consistent (positive) differences in patient outcome.

A second group of contributions to this literature is driven by policy and planning considerations and searches for effective methods of patient triage and prognosis that provide in effect a "postdiction" of current results such that future patients' progress might be predicted both accurately and parsimoniously. A third group of results has been propelled by analytic considerations, in which increasingly powerful multivariate statistical methods are applied to admittedly subtle data to tease apart complex interrelationships between sets of variables. Just how far this third group can go has yet to be seen.

Analyzing the impact of sets of variables on outcome produces predictive models that are more accurate than an individual clinician's past experience.[29] Further, when clinical teams are provided with computer-generated predictions based on clinical data, they tend to diminish their use of certain types of intensive management. Apparently, this action does not produce an adverse effect on outcome, and neurosurgeons do not necessarily limit treatment when predictions are available.[29]

The following sections report briefly on successes and failures in the search for setwise relationships reported in recent studies. In most instances, the particular combinations of variables, measurement instruments, and clinical characteristics chosen by the researchers are unique to the individual study and have not been subjected to independent replication. When research teams share variables, frequently neither the patient populations nor the periods under consideration are comparable; the latter is important because of changes over time in diagnostic or treatment sophistication. Even the same authors reporting their work over time have had cause to vary their approaches between projects. Only through multicenter collaborative studies have sufficient sample sizes and common databases become available. The efforts involved in such large-scale investigations as Becker et al.[30] and others during the 1970s and of the Trauma Coma Data Bank investigators during the 1980s are to be commended. However, the overwhelming bulk of the professional literature has not been able to utilize these data-intensive methods. For all these reasons, the authors have not attempted a formal metaanalysis of the literature. However, in the material that follows, the authors attempt to provide logical underpinnings to unite a highly diverse group of reports. This section concludes with a brief look at selected current prediction models for head injury.

Relationships between Demographic Factors or Other Antecedents and Outcome

The relationship between age and severity, though well studied and often reported to be "firmly established," has not been confirmed in its entirety (Table 2-4). In some reports, severity is considerably lower at younger ages than at older ages.[30] Alternatively, various investigators have suggested a higher mortality rate in children under age 5 and adults over age 60, but there is no clear trend. Levi et al.[31] presented data in which the rates of severe disability or death show a positive trend with respect to age (from newborns to age 16 years). However, their confidence intervals are quite wide, and the regression equation is not significant.

In a review by Vollmer,[32] age is second only to injury severity indicators in predicting outcome. In general, mortality rates seem to increase with age.[33,34] Waxman et al.,[35] however, found that under 5 years of age, children either died or had a good recovery. Few recovered with disability. Children over 5, however, showed no relation between outcome and age. Patients older than 60, by contrast, were likely to die or have a recovery with disability. Levin et al.[36] found that the inverse relationship between age and mortality held in children 4 years old and older but not in younger children. Kraus[37]

TABLE 2-4 Relationships between Age and Outcome: Selected Studies

Study Location (Reference)	Year of Study	Sample Size	Study Type	Ages with Good Outcome	Ages with Poor Outcome	Comment
Virginia (Alberico et al.[40])	1976–1984	330	Case series	0–20 (5–9 among pediatric group)	61–80 (15–19 among pediatric group)	Outcome assessed by Glasgow Outcome Score (GOS)
Virginia (Becker et al.[30])	1972–1976	160	Case series	0–20	61–80	Outcome assessed by GOS
Israel (Groswasser et al.[38])	5 years prior to 1990	328	Case series	16–29	16–29	Good recovery = return to school or workplace
Israel (Levi et al.[31])	1984–1988	653	Case series	0–2	13–14	Outcome assessed by Injury Severity Score (ISS)
Trauma Coma Data Bank (USA) (Levin et al.[36])	1983–1988	103	Case series	5–10	0–4	Outcome assessed by mortality
State of Washington (Michaud et al.[41])	1985–1986	75	Case series	15–16	<2	Outcome assessed by GOS
Scotland and the Netherlands (Teasdale and Jennett[39])	5 years prior to 1976	326	Case series	5–29	>60	Recovery defined by GOS
California (Waxman et al.[35])	1985–1987	306	Case series	21–30	71–90	No patient over 60 survived with good recovery

has shown the difficulties inherent in attempting to relate age to outcome. Groswasser et al.,[38] using binary outcome scoring, could not show any connection between outcome and age. Nevertheless, several authors[39,40] have established that younger age groups have a better outcome as measured by the Glasgow Outcome Score (GOS), a relatively crude indicator of neurological complications or residual effects. In contrast, Michaud et al.[41] were able to show that functional recovery actually improves with increasing age.

Few demographic factors have conclusively been shown to affect severity. Gender and severity do not have a distinct correlation. MacKenzie et al.[12] were able to establish that males have a higher severity than do females, while Klauber et al.[42] showed no such relationship.

Relationships between Severity and Outcome

Numerous authors have researched the effect of the severity of a brain injury on an individual's outcome. The time after injury when outcome is observed differs considerably between papers, generally ranging from 3 months to 1 year. Kaufman et al.[43] warned that the course of outcome, specifically coma type, varies considerably over the first year and that predictions for outcome earlier than 1 year are not valid beyond the follow-up period. They suggested grouping patients into categories by GCS or Karnofsky score for functional abilities and then recording neurological function or complications such as infection at regular intervals. Jennett[44] used coma depth and duration as markers of outcome and in this way increased the comparability of samples from Los Angeles, Glasgow, and the Netherlands. In general, however, as authors frequently use unique severity and outcome measures, comparing results between papers is difficult. Nevertheless, compiling the impact of severity on outcome measures is vital for clinical prediction and management. Though several severity and outcome couplings are limited to one or two studies, a few relationships between specific severity and outcome classifications have been well studied.

Early GCS scores, along with numerous other direct measures of severity, have been exhaustively studied in relation to outcome (Table 2-5). While Vollmer[32] describes significant limitations of the GCS, several authors have successfully utilized the GCS for various outcome measures. GCS at admission appears to be a more than adequate predictor for the GOS.[31,36,39,45–49] Even more impressive, the relationship stands whether the GOS is taken at 1 year,[46,50] 6 months,[48,51] 3 months,[39] or 1 week.[49] Several authors assert that GCS after admission is a more accurate predictor of outcome. GCS scores obtained 6 h after admission accurately predicted GOS at death or discharge from the hospital, while GCS at admission correlated poorly with outcome.[36] When Young et al.[52] combined GCS scores after 48 h and computed tomography (CT) scan data, they were much better able to predict outcome as measured by GOS than they were with admission GCS alone. Similarly, Michaud et al.[41] found that the GCS motor score at 72 h and the level of oxygenation were the best predictors of disability outcome. Wagstyl et al.[50] found that the GCS trend over a 24-h period was useful in predicting outcome in children. Finally, Karzmark et al.[53] were able to show that long-term reading ability is also accurately predicted by GCS.

GOS, though widely used, is not necessarily the most viable outcome measure. GCS scores correlate well with various neuropsychiatric measures. The severity of GCS has a direct relationship to neurobehavioral outcome,[46] learning and memory,[54] general performance,[55] and the Halstead Impairment Index.[56] Pupillary reactivity, like the GCS, seems to be a good predictor for a wide variety of outcomes and is coupled with the GCS in numerous studies. It has been shown to accurately predict GOS as well as various neuropsychological outcome measures. Michaud et al.[41] found that pupillary reactivity and the Injury Severity Score[57] were excellent predictors of survival.

Another widely used measure of severity is the duration of posttraumatic amnesia (PTA). According to Bishara et al.,[45] PTA correlates well with GOS taken at 6 months and again at 1 year. Fearnside et al.[58] have shown a strong relationship between PTA and mortality. Mandelberg[59] asserted that PTA duration accurately predicts verbal and performance IQ at both 3 and 6 months as measured by the Weschler Adult Intelligence Scale. Brooks and Aughton[60] and Bond[61] agree that PTA adequately predicts recall ability. Further, Bond[61] and Brown et al.[62] found that PTA also predicts the results of psychiatric disorders. While investigators seem to find cognition outcome well accounted for by PTA, general cognitive functions are less clearly related to PTA. While Bennett-Levi[63] showed a relationship between PTA and general cognitive function, Gronwall and Wrightson[64] showed only a mild correlation and the study by Barth et al.[65] produced no correlation at all. VanZomeren and VanDenBurg[66] found that PTA duration is well correlated with an individual's ability to return to work.

Mortality after brain injury is not as commonly described as the GOS, but several studies have shown that various severity measures can predict mortality. In addition to PTA,[58] coma type,[67,68] duration of unconsciousness,[69] CT findings,[70] and various postoperative signs[71] can be used to predict the probability of death.

A variety of assessments made during the acute stage of an injury, while not constituting direct evaluations of

TABLE 2-5 Severity Measures Obtained in Acute Stage Predictive of Outcome: Selected Studies

Reference	Predictor Measure	Outcome Measure
Barth et al.[65]	Specific cerebral trauma	Neuropsychological testing
Bennett-Levy[63]	Posttraumatic amnesia (PTA)	Cognitive abilities
Berger et al.[51]	Glasgow Coma Scale (GCS)	Glasgow Outcome Score (GOS)
Bishara et al.[45]	PTA	GOS at 6 months, 1 year
Bond[61]	PTA	Social, mental, physical disability
Brooks and Aughton[60]	Duration of unconsciousness	Intelligence, memory, language
Brown et al.[62]	PTA	Cognitive abilities
Fearnside et al.[58]	PTA duration	Mortality
Filley et al.[67]	Duration of coma, CT findings	GOS, social behaviors
Gensemer et al.[56]	GCS	Halstead Impairment Index (cognitive dysfunction and behavioral outcomes)
Gronwall and Wrightson[64]	PTA	Information processing
Karzmark[53]	GCS	Long-term reading ability
Levi et al.[31]	GCS, Injury Severity Score (ISS)	GOS
Levin et al.[36]	GCS 6 h after admission	GOS at death or discharge
Levin et al.,[46] (see also Wagstyl et al.[50])	GCS	GOS at 1 year
Levin et al.[54]	GCS	GCS and cognitive abilities at 1 year
Lokkeberg and Grimes[47]	GCS	GOS
Mandelberg[59]	PTA duration	Verbal and performance IQ
Marmarou et al.[48] (see also Berger et al.[51])	GCS	GOS at 6 months
Michaud et al.[41]	GCS motor score at 72 h, oxygenization level	Disability
Pagni[68]	Duration of unconsciousness, type of skull fracture, intracranial hematoma	Epilepsy
Pazzaglia et al.[69]	Level of coma, intracranial lesions	Death or level of social integration
Pfenninger[70]	GCS and intracranial pressure (ICP), CT findings	Mortality
Richards and Hoff[71]	Intracranial damage	Mortality
Teasdale and Jennett[39]	GCS at admission	GOS at 3 months
VanZomeran and VanDenBerg[66]	PTA duration	Return to work, memory impairment
Wagstyl et al.[50]	GCS trend over 24 h	GOS (in children)
Wassertheil-Smoller et al.[49]	GCS at admission	GOS at 1 week
Winogran et al.[55]	GCS, duration of altered consciousness	Psychological test scores
Young et al.[52]	GCS, CT data	GOS

injury severity (they require transformations or decision processes before being interpreted as indexes of severity), are reliable indicators of long-term outcome (Table 2-6). One of the most widely used predictive measures is intracranial pressure (ICP). Like GCS and PTA, ICP is strongly correlated with early GOS[51] and GOS at 6 months.[48] Alberico et al.[40] were also able to show this correlation but added that age may confound the relationship. Cerebral blood flow also has a strong relationship with GOS.[72] Miller et al.[73] found that heightened ICP increases mortality. However, ICP is not as good a predictor of neuropsychiatric outcomes.[46,55]

Computed tomography findings seem to predict GOS scores well,[36,74] although Waxman et al.[35] showed only a weak correlation. Consistent with these findings, Waxman's group also found a much stronger correlation between extracranial complications such as elevated systolic blood pressure and GOS than did Piek et al.,[75] who concurred that intracranial complications have a weaker predictive power in that they showed no significant asso-

TABLE 2-6 Measures Other Than Severity Obtained in Acute Stage Predictive of Outcome: Selected Studies

Reference	Predictor Measure	Outcome Measure
Alberico et al.[40]	Infracranial pressure (ICP), diffuse vs. mass lesion	Glasgow Outcome Score (GOS)
Berger et al.[51]	ICP, neurological status	GOS
Bowers and Marshall[76]	Hematoma, multiple injuries	GOS
Kraus et al.[13]	Hemorrhage, skull fracture	Death, GOS, neurological deficit
Levin et al.[36]	ICP	GOS at 6 months
Levin et al.[46]	GOS at discharge	Neuropsychological performance at 6, 12, 24 months
Levin et al.[78] (see also Alexandre et al.[80])	Oculovestibular deficits	Cognitive outcome
Lokkeberg and Grimes[47]	Time to ER, time to intubation, mode of transport, type of injury	GOS
Marmarou et al.[48]	Computed tomography (CT) findings	GOS
Miller et al.[73]	Mass vs. diffuse lesion, ICP	GOS
Piek et al.[75]	Hypotension, pneumonia, coagulopathy, septicemia	GOS
Rimel et al.[74]	Glasgow Coma Scale (GCS) at discharge	GOS
Robertson et al.[72]	Cerebral blood flow	GOS
Teasdale and Jennett[39]	Age, pupillary response	GOS
Waxman et al.[35] (see also Piek et al.[75])	Extracranial complications	GOS
Winogran et al.[55]	Duration of unconsciousness	Psychological test scores

ciations with outcome. Similarly, Bowers and Marshall[76] and Lokkeberg and Grimes[47] showed that the specific type of treatment in the hospital significantly affects the outcome, legitimizing Piek's claim that extracranial complications deserve at least as much management attention as do those occurring intracranially.

Among intracranial complications that are strong predictors of outcome, oculovestibular reflex deficits[39] and the size of mass lesions[40,51,72] individually are good predictors of outcome as measured by GOS. Intracranial and extracranial complications certainly need not be mutually exclusive. Kraus et al.,[13] testing various predictor factors for brain injury in San Diego County, found that hemorrhage and fracture are important predictors for death, an unfavorable GOS score, or the presence of any neurological deficit. GCS and the Maximum Abbreviated Injury Score[57] are other factors which independently predict an unfavorable outcome. Although the San Diego findings may not apply to all brain-injured populations, along with similar clinical reports they assist in identifying important factors that require increased clinical attention to affect current diagnostic outcomes for brain injury.

Endless varieties of measures of cognitive function have been put forward to assess impaired function after brain injury. Because investigators frequently use different tests to measure abilities, comparison is difficult though not impossible. For example, duration of unconsciousness has been used repeatedly to predict cognitive function. Apparently, this measure can be used to predict outcomes involving intelligence, memory, language,[77] facial recognition,[78] personality changes,[55] ability to return to work, and motor function.[79] However, since such relationships have not been reported independently, the strength of the claim is somewhat weakened. Indeed, Barth et al.[65] found no relationship between duration of unconsciousness and general cognitive function.

Various authors have identified other predictors for cognitive outcome, such as oculovestibular deficits.[54,80] Hematoma does not appear, however, to predict general cognitive function.[54] Similarly, the laterality of the injury lesion has little or no impact on intelligence, memory, or language.[77] Stein et al.[81] explored the issue of delayed injury, the phenomenon in which lesions appear on CT scans or the patient worsens considerably after the initial admission diagnosis. The presence of delayed cerebral insults is strongly associated with the severity of the initial injury, cardiopulmonary resuscitation performed in the field, coagulopathy at admission, and an initial CT diagnosis of subdural hematoma. Delayed injury in turn is predictive of higher mortality, slowed recovery, and a significantly poorer outcome at 6 months.

Studies exploring the relationships between severity and outcome, then, vary considerably in variables used, intent, methods, and the like. Nevertheless, a summary of the literature illuminates the fact that some relationships, such as that between GCS and GOS, are well established and need only be refined for use as a predictor measure in a clinical setting. Cognitive sequelae, in contrast, have not been uniformly studied and require further research.

Predictor Factors and the Clinical Setting

Thatcher et al.[82] point out the need for a multivariate prognostic index in the prediction of the long-term outcome of head injury, since many more trauma patients are now surviving rather than dying of their injuries. Narayan et al.[83] noted the importance of objective prognostication for allocating services, matching in clinical trials, and developing comparisons across study locations. A number of investigators have pursued the question of predictor modeling (Table 2-7). While all agree that certain predictors are more accurate than others, none share common variables, even when the same or a similar outcome is used. This dissonance does not reflect disagreement among researchers; rather, it is a product of the unique focus of each paper.

For example, Narayan et al.,[83] Thatcher et al.,[82] and Wärme et al.[84] used GOS at 1 year as the outcome but explored different predictor variables. Narayan et al. dichotomized the outcome measure as good versus poor and, using logistic regression, evaluated the prognostic capability of six clinical variables and three physiological variables singly and in combination. The most successful combination was found to be all six clinical indicators (age, GCS score, pupillary reaction, surgical mass lesion, eye movements, and motor posturing) together with the results from multimodality evoked potential studies (89 percent correct prediction). In a multivariate analysis, Thatcher et al.[82] found that EEG and GCS account for over 95 percent of the variance if outcome is measured as a good outcome or death. However, EEG and GCS account for only 75 percent of the variance if the outcome was in an intermediate range of disability, perhaps indicating that discrete predictors can be used for extreme outcomes but are less useful in gauging the future degree of disability. Wärme et al.[84] were primarily concerned with hospital management. Using a multivariate analysis, they reported that GCS motor score, systemic hypotension, and duration of hyperventilation were the best predictors of good recovery as determined by GOS.

Choi et al.[85] predicted outcome in terms of four categories similar to the GOS. Unlike Thatcher, Choi established that the GCS motor score alone is as powerful a predictor of outcome as the entire GCS is. These researchers constructed three simple graphs by using age, best motor response, and pupillary response for a clinical estimation of the probability of outcome in severe head injury. The graphs were easy to read and were useful for triage determinations. Stewart et al.[86] used four prognostic discharge categories as outcome. Age and pattern of unconsciousness, ranging from limited contusion through lucid intervals to death, were found to be the best predictors.

A few authors attempted to predict cognitive functioning or disability. Tompkins et al.[87] selected cognitive performance in language, memory, and visuomotor speed as outcome. The severity of the injury as measured by GCS and a history of psychological, physical, or cognitive disorders before the injury were the best predictive measures. Lewin et al.[88] measured cognitive disability as changes in sensory, motor, and verbal skills (central nervous disability) and changes in behavior (mental disability). Age, posttraumatic amnesia, and the worst neurological response score were among the best predictors of cognitive outcome 10 to 24 years after an injury.

A number of authors have discussed the possibility of using CT scans to predict outcome. Gerber et al.[89] created an outcome prediction model for subarachnoid hemorrhage. When the best predictors for outcome appeared to be neurological grade and CT scan, Gerber et al. summed these variables and were able to describe the outcome 3 months after the injury. Outcomes measured by CT scans are not quite as easy to predict. Of 712 patients admitted with a GCS score of 15, Jeret et al.[90] found that 67 had acute traumatic lesions as displayed by CT. The CT abnormality was associated with older patients, whites, basilar skull fracture, injury by assault, and pedestrians hit by a motor vehicle. However, Jeret et al. were not able to find any single variable or group of variables that would correctly classify mildly head injured patients by normal or abnormal CT scans. The fact that the abnormality was found among elderly white patients may be due to selection bias, as less severely injured white patients might not have sought treatment at the city hospital.

While most of the predictor and outcome measures Michaud et al.[41] utilized are similar to those discussed in other papers, their model is unusual. The outcome measures were survival, quality of survival (or severity of disability), and morbidity. All outcomes were measured as values of GOS. Brain injury severity, extracranial injury severity, Injury Severity Score, and pupillary response in the emergency room were predictive of survival. However, GCS at 72 h after injury, brain injury severity, and extracranial injury severity were predictive of disability. Chest injuries and oxygenation level were predictive of increased mortality and morbidity among brain-injured patients. Disability predictors are particularly important for advising and counselling purposes.

TABLE 2-7 Models of Predictors and Clinical Outcome: Selected Studies

Reference	Predictors	Outcomes	Comments
Choi et al.[85]	Motor score and age and pupillary response	Four outcome categories	Motor score predicted 78% of outcomes; as powerful as Glasgow Coma Scale (GCS)
Gerber et al.[89]	Neurological grade (scored 1–6) and computed tomography (CT) scan (scored 0–3) at admission	Outcome 3 months after injury (scored 1–3)	Highly significant predictions of outcome
Jeret et al.[90]	Age and injury due to assault	CT abnormality	No single variable could predict normal vs. abnormal scans
Lewin et al.[88]	Age and posttraumatic amnesia (PTA) and worst neurological responsiveness	CNS deficiency, mental impairment 10–24 y after injury	Outcome determined at time of initial hemorrhage
Michaud et al.[41]	Injury Severity Scale (ISS) and pupillary response in emergency department (ED)	Mortality	Odds ratios (ORs) for fatality: ISS >40 compared to ISS $< 25 = 53.6$; abnormal pupillary response compared to normal = 18.4
	GCS motor score 72 h after injury *and* arterial P_{O_2} in ED	Disability at discharge from acute care hospital	ORs for good recovery or moderate disability: GCS motor score >4 compared to $\leq 4 = 36.5$; P_{O_2} ≥ 350 mmHg compared to ≤ 105 mmHg = 3.4
Narayan et al.[83]	Age and GCS score and pupillary reaction and surgical decompression and eye movements and motor posturing and multimodality evoked potential (MEP)	Outcome up to 12 months after injury (scored good, poor)	MEP data predicted 91% correctly with 25% of predictions >90% confidence; combination of variables predicted 89% correctly with 64% of predictions >90% confidence
Stewart et al.[86]	Age and pattern of consciousness	Outcome categories based on mortality and length of hospital stay	63% of patients' outcomes predicted
Thatcher et al.[82]	EEG and GCS	Glasgow Outcome Score (GOS) at 1 year; good outcome or death	EEG and GCS predicted 95% of variance
		Intermediate range of disability	EEG and GCS predicted 75% of variance
Tompkins et al.[87]	GCS and history of psychological, physical, cognitive disorders	Cognitive performance in language, memory, visuomotor speed	Severity is best predictor, improved by considering preinjury physical and psychological status
Wärme et al.[84]	GCS motor score and systemic hypotension and duration of hyperventilation and epilepsy	GOS	Improvements in diagnostic and therapeutic protocols resulted in improved outcomes

Interrelationships Across Domains

Brain injury research is difficult; for the most part, the researcher can only infer what the patient's prior brain function must have been before the traumatic injury event. Brain-injured survivors are generally poor at providing first-person accounts, and friends and relatives can give only surrogate impressions. Thus, the issue of psychosocial or behavioral changes or deficits caused by injury and the evolution of outcome from any given point in the recovery process to any given point further along must be interpreted cautiously.

In the absence of perfect reliability, perfect sensitivity, and specificity of factors, there will be, by definition, some degree of reduced credibility for a given measurement. This increases the inherent ambiguity of cross-group relationships over extended follow-up periods, since there are few inexpensive ways to counterbalance the inadequacy of the measurement. Moreover, such deficits in research design may confound one another in the multivariate context, with the unintended statistical consequence being a diminished ability to isolate subtle results from finite samples. In research aimed at unraveling the subtle combinations of "hard" and "soft" signs and symptoms of brain injury, particularly over time and across diverse patient populations, the deficits embedded in the measurement tools make it difficult to conduct definitive studies.

Despite these caveats, the relationships between demographic factors, incidence, severity, and outcome can be examined in a variety of meaningful ways and pursued by creative research designs. However, it is difficult to select a stringent set of predictive variables. An excellent example of a stringent modeling approach is that of Choi et al.,[85] who isolated only the three factors of age, motor score, and pupillary response as "a compact but highly predictive model" for the prediction of GOS scores among severely head injured patients at follow-ups as long as 12 months after injury. Further, the choice of variables should be neither overly broad nor overly narrow in scope (e.g., related cohesively to previous advancements in the field). An improved prognosis is unlikely unless the set of measurements is both demonstrably related to progress made to date and generalizable across a variety of brain injuries.

The epidemiological research challenge in prognosis is clear: The task is to devise optimal strategies to secure large, linkable data sets from trauma and rehabilitation services, the behavioral and social sciences, and both retrospective and prospective epidemiological assessments and then to sift through and interpret mountains of sometimes overlapping, often competing, and always demanding information to arrive at best estimates of risk. Epidemiological findings are the primary source of probabilistic models of causation, which themselves must be linked to specific clinical data to appropriately predict individual outcomes. Clinicians and researchers can also join forces effectively in validating predictions of individual outcome in an epidemiological sense.

References

1. Annegers JF, Grabow JD, Groover RV, et al: Seizures after head trauma: A population study. *Neurology* 30:683, 1980.
2. Whitman S, Coonley-Hoganson R, Desai BT: Comparative head trauma experiences in two socioeconomically different Chicago-area communities: A population study. *Am J Epidemiol* 119:570, 1984.
3. Auer LM, Gell G, Richling B, et al: Predicting lethal outcome after severe head injury: A computer-assisted analysis of neurological symptoms and laboratory values. *Acta Neurochir (Wien)* 52:225, 1980.
4. Bruce DA, Schut L, Bruno L, et al: Outcome following severe head injuries in children. *J Neurosurg* 48:679, 1978.
5. Rimel RW, Giordani B, Barth JT, et al: Disability caused by minor head injury. *Neurosurgery* 9:221, 1981.
6. Gronwall SL, Wrightson P: Delayed recovery of intellectual function after minor head injury. *Lancet* 2:605, 1974.
7. Plaut MR, Gifford RRM: Trivial head trauma and its consequences in a perspective of regional health care. *Milit Med* 141:244, 1976.
8. Jennett B, Murray A, Carlin J, et al: Head injuries in three Scottish neurosurgical units. *Br Med J* 2:955, 1979.
9. Kraus JF, Black MA, Hessol N, et al: The incidence of acute brain injury and serious impairment in a defined population. *Am J Epidemiol* 119:186, 1984.
10. Collins JG: Types of injuries by selected characteristics: United States, 1985–1987. *Vital Health Stat* 10:175, 1990.
11. Fife D: Head injury with and without hospital admission: Comparisons of incidence and shortterm disability. *Am J Public Health* 77:810, 1987.
12. MacKenzie EJ, Edelstein SL, Flynn JP: Hospitalized head-injured patients in Maryland: Incidence and severity of injuries. *Maryland Med J* 38:725, 1989.
13. Kraus JF, Fife D, Ramstein K, et al: The relationship of family income to the incidence, external causes, and outcomes of serious brain injury, San Diego County, California. *Am J Public Health* 76:1345, 1986.
14. Smith G, Kraus J: Alcohol and residential, recreational, and occupational injuries: A review of the epidemiologic evidence. *Annu Rev Public Health* 9:99, 1988.
15. Kraus J, Fife D, Conroy C, Nourjah P: Alcohol and brain injuries: Persons blood-tested, prevalence of alcohol involvement, and early outcome following injury. *Am J Public Health* 79:294, 1989.
16. Gurney JG, Rivara FP, Mueller BA, et al: The effects of alcohol intoxication on the initial treatment and hospital course of patients with acute brain injury. *J Trauma* 33:709, 1992.
17. Jagger J, Levine J, Jane J, et al: Epidemiologic features of head injury in a predominantly rural population. *J Trauma* 24:40, 1984.
18. Fife D, Faich G, Hollenshead W, Boynton W: Incidence and outcome of hospital-treated head injury in Rhode Island. *Am J Public Health* 76:773, 1986.
19. Cooper JD, Tabaddor K, Hauser WA: The epidemiology of head injury in the Bronx. *Neuroepidemiology* 2:70, 1983.
20. Klauber MR, Barrett-Connor E, Marshall LF, Bowers SA: The epidemiology of head injury: A prospective study of an entire community—San Diego County, California, 1978. *Am J Epidemiol* 113:500, 1981.
21. Goldstein FC, Levin HS: Epidemiology of pediatric

closed head injury: Incidence, clinical characteristics, and risk factors. *J Learning Disabil* 20:518, 1987.
22. Klonoff H: Head injuries in children: Predisposing factors, accident conditions, accident proneness and sequelae. *Am J Public Health* 61:2405, 1971.
23. Graves E: Detailed diagnoses and procedures, National Hospital Discharge Survey, 1990. *Vital Health Stat* 13:113, 1992.
24. Commission on Professional and Hospital Activities: *The International Classification of Diseases, 9th Revision, Clinical Modification* (*ICD.9.CM*). Ann Arbor: Commission on Professional and Hospital Activities, 1986.
25. Lee S, Lui T, Chang C, et al: Features of head injury in a developing country—Taiwan (1977–1987). *J Trauma* 30:194, 1990.
26. Vasquez-Barquero A, Vasquez-Barquero JL, Austin O, et al: The epidemiology of head injury in Cantabria. *Eur J Epidemiol* 8:832, 1992.
27. Tiret L, Hausherr E, Thicoipe M, et al: The epidemiology of head trauma in Aquitaine (France), 1986: A community-based study of hospital admissions and deaths. *Int J Epidemiol* 19:133, 1990.
28. Nell V, Brown SOD: Epidemiology of traumatic brain injury in Johannesburg: II. Morbidity, mortality and etiology. *Soc Sci Med* 33:289, 1991.
29. Braakman R: Early prediction of outcome in severe head injury. *Acta Neurochir* (*Wien*) 116:161, 1992.
30. Becker DP, Miller DJ, Ward JD, et al: The outcome from severe head injury with early diagnosis and intensive management. *J Neurosurg* 47:491, 1977.
31. Levi L, Guilburd JN, Linn S, Feinsod M: The association between skull fracture, intracranial pathology and outcome in pediatric head injury. *Br J Neurosurg* 5:617, 1991.
32. Vollmer DG: Prognosis and outcome of severe head injury, in Cooper PR (ed): *Head Injury* (3d ed). Baltimore: Williams & Wilkins, 1993: 553–581.
33. Klauber MR, Marshall LF, Luersson TG, et al: Determinants of head injury mortality: Importance of the low risk patient. *Neurosurgery* 24:31, 1989.
34. Luerssen TG, Klauber MR, Marshall LF: Outcome from head injury related to patient's age: A longitudinal prospective study of adult and pediatric head injury. *J Neurosurg* 68:409, 1988.
35. Waxman K, Sundine MJ, Young RF: Is early prediction of outcome in severe head injury possible? *Arch Surg* 126:1237, 1991.
36. Levin HS, Aldrich EF, Saydjari C, et al: Severe head injury in children: Experience of the Traumatic Coma Data Bank. *Neurosurgery* 31:435, 1992.
37. Kraus JF: Epidemiologic features of head and spinal cord injury. *Adv Neurol* 19:261, 1978.
38. Groswasser Z, Cohen M, Blankstein E: Polytrauma associated with traumatic brain injury: Incidence, nature and impact on rehabilitation outcome. *Brain Injury* 4:161, 1990.
39. Teasdale G, Jennett B: Assessment and prognosis of coma after head injury. *Acta Neurochir* (*Wien*) 34:45, 1976.
40. Alberico AM, Ward JD, Choi SC, et al: Outcome after severe head injury: Relationship to mass lesions, diffuse injury, and ICP course in pediatric and adult patients. *J Neurosurg* 67:648, 1987.
41. Michaud LJ, Rivara FP, Grady MS, Reay DT: Predictors of survival and severity of disability after severe brain injury in children. *Neurosurgery* 31:254, 1992.
42. Klauber MR, Marshall LF, Barrett-Connor E, Bowers SA: Prospective study of patients hospitalized with head injury in San Diego County, 1978. *Neurosurgery* 9:236, 1981.
43. Kaufman HH, Bretaudierre J-P, Rowlands BJ, et al: Head injury: Variability of course and presence of confounding factors. *Int J Technol Assessment Health Care* 5:631, 1989.
44. Jennett B: Some international comparisons, in Levin HS, Eisenberg HM, Benton AL (eds): *Mild Head Injury*. New York: Oxford University Press, 1989:23–34.
45. Bishara SN, Partridge FM, Godfrey HPD, Knight RG: Post-traumatic amnesia and Glasgow Coma Scale related to outcome in survivors in a consecutive series of patients with severe closed-head injury. *Brain Injury* 6:373, 1992.
46. Levin HS, Gary HE, Eisenberg HM, et al: Neurobehavioral outcome one year after severe head injury: Experience of the Traumatic Coma Data Bank. *J Neurosurg* 73:699, 1990.
47. Lokkeberg AR, Grimes RM: Assessing the influence of non-treatment variables in a study of outcome from severe head injuries. *J Neurosurg* 61:254, 1984.
48. Marmarou A, Anderson RL, Ward JD, et al: Impact of ICP instability and hypotension on outcome in patients with severe head trauma. *J Neurosurg* 75:S59, 1991.
49. Wassertheil-Smoller S, Tabaddor K, Feiner C, Shulman K: Factors affecting short-term outcome of head trauma patients. *Neuroepidemiology* 1:154, 1982.
50. Wagstyl J, Sutcliffe AJ, Alpar EK: Early prediction of outcome following head injury in children. *J Pediatr Surg* 22:127, 1987.
51. Berger MS, Pitts LH, Lovely M, et al: Outcome from severe head injury in children and adolescents. *J Neurosurg* 62:194, 1985.
52. Young B, Rapp RP, Pharm D, et al: Early prediction of outcome in head-injured patients. *J Neurosurg* 54:300, 1981.
53. Karzmark P: Prediction of long-term cognitive outcome of brain injury with neuropsychological, severity of injury, and demographic data. *Brain Injury* 6:213, 1992.
54. Levin HS, Grossman RG, Rose JE, Teasdale G: Long-term neuropsychological outcome of closed head injury. *J Neurosurg* 50:412, 1979.
55. Winogron HW, Knights RM, Bawden HN: Neuropsychological deficits following head injury in children. *J Clin Neuropsychol* 6:269, 1984.
56. Gensemer IB, Smith JL, Walker JC, et al: Psychological consequences of blunt head trauma and relation to other indices of severity of injury. *Ann Emerg Med* 18:29, 1989.
57. Association for the Advancement of Automotive Medicine: *The Abbreviated Injury Scale*, 1990 revision. Des Plaines: Association for the Advancement of Automotive Medicine, 1990.

58. Fearnside MR, Cook RJ, McDougall P, McNeil RJ: The Westmead Head Injury Project, outcome to severe head injury: A comparative analysis of pre-hospital, clinical and CT variables. *Br J Neurosurg* 7:267, 1993.
59. Mandelberg IA: Cognitive recovery after severe head injury. *J Neurol Neurosurg Psychiatry* 39:1001, 1976.
60. Brooks DN, Aughton ME: Cognitive recovery during the first year after severe blunt head injury. *Int Rehabil Med* 1:166, 1979.
61. Bond MR: Assessment of the psychosocial outcome of severe head injury. *Acta Neurochir (Wien)* 34:57, 1976.
62. Brown G, Chadwick O, Shaffer D, et al: A prospective study of children with head injuries: III. Psychiatric sequelae. *Psychol Med* 11:63, 1981.
63. Bennett-Levy JM: Long-term effects of severe closed head injury on memory: Evidence from a consecutive series of young adults. *Acta Neurol Scand* 70:285, 1984.
64. Gronwall D, Wrightson P: Memory and information processing capacity after closed head injury. *J Neurol Neurosurg Psychiatry* 44:889, 1981.
65. Barth JT, Macciocchi SN, Giordani B, et al: Neuropsychological sequelae of minor head injury. *Neurosurgery* 13:529, 1983.
66. VanZomeren AH, VanDenBurg W: Residual complaints of patients two years after severe head injury. *J Neurol Neurosurg Psychiatry* 48:21, 1985.
67. Filley CM, Cranberg LD, Alexander MP, Hart EJ: Neurobehavioral outcome after closed head injury in childhood and adolescence. *Arch Neurol* 44:194, 1987.
68. Pagni CA: The prognosis of head-injured patients in a state of coma with decerebrated posture: Analysis of 471 cases. *J Neurol Sci* 17:289, 1973.
69. Pazzaglia P, Frank G, Frank F, Gaist G: Clinical course and prognosis of acute post-traumatic coma. *J Neurol Neurosurg Psychiatry* 38:149, 1975.
70. Pfenninger J: Early prediction of outcome after severe head injury in children. *Z Kinderchir* 39:223, 1984.
71. Richards T, Hoff J: Factors affecting survival from acute subdural hematoma. *Surgery* 75:253, 1974.
72. Robertson CS, Contant CF, Gokaslan ZL, et al: Cerebral blood flow, arteriovenous oxygen difference, and outcome in head injured patients. *J Neurol Neurosurg Psychiatry* 55:594, 1992.
73. Miller JD, Becker DP, Ward JD, et al: Significance of intracranial hypertension in severe head injury. *J Neurosurg* 47:503, 1977.
74. Rimel RW, Giordani B, Barth JT, Jane JA: Moderate head injury: Completing the clinical spectrum of brain trauma. *Neurosurgery* 11:344, 1982.
75. Piek J, Chesnut RM, Marshall LF, et al: Extracranial complications of severe head injury. *J Neurosurg* 77:901, 1992.
76. Bowers SA, Marshall LF: Outcome in 200 consecutive cases of severe head injury treated in San Diego County: A prospective analysis. *Neurosurgery* 6:237, 1980.
77. Brooks DN: Wechsler Memory Scale Performance and its relationship to brain damage after severe closed head injury. *J Neurol Neurosurg Psychiatry* 39:593, 1976.
78. Levin HS, Grossman RG, Kelly PJ: Impairment of facial recognition after closed head injuries of varying severity. *Cortex* 13:119, 1977.
79. Brink JD, Imbus C, Woo-Sam J: Physical recovery after severe closed head trauma in children and adolescents. *J Pediatr* 97:721, 1980.
80. Alexandre A, Colombo F, Nertempi P, Benedetti A: Cognitive outcome and early indices of severity of head injury. *J Neurosurg* 59:751, 1983.
81. Stein SC, Spettell C, Young G, Ross SE: Delayed and progressive brain injury in closed-head trauma: Radiological demonstration. *Neurosurgery* 32:25, 1993.
82. Thatcher RW, Cantor DS, McAlaster R, et al: Comprehensive predictions of outcome in closed head-injured patients. *Ann NY Acad Sci* 620:82, 1991.
83. Narayan RK, Greenberg RP, Miller JD, et al: Improved confidence of outcome prediction in severe head injury: A comparative analysis of the clinical examination, multimodality evoked potentials, CT scanning, and intracranial pressure. *J Neurosurg* 54:751, 1981.
84. Wärme PE, Bergström R, Persson L: Neurosurgical intensive care improves outcome after severe head injury. *Acta Neurochirur (Wien)* 110:57, 1991.
85. Choi SC, Narayan RK, Anderson RL, Ward JD: Enhanced specificity of prognosis in severe head injury. *J Neurosurg* 69:381, 1988.
86. Stewart WA, Litten SP, Sheehe PR: A prognostic model for head injury. *Acta Neurochir (Wien)* 45:199, 1979.
87. Tompkins CA, Holland AL, Ratcliff G, et al: Predicting cognitive recovery from closed head-injury in children and adolescents. *Brain Cogn* 13:86, 1990.
88. Lewin W, Marshall TFD, Roberts AH: Long-term outcome after severe head injury. *Br Med J* 15:1533, 1979.
89. Gerber CJ, Lang DA, Neil-Dwyer G, Smith PWF: A simple scoring system for accurate prediction of outcome within four days of a subarachnoid hemorrhage. *Acta Neurochir (Wien)* 122:11, 1993.
90. Jeret JS, Mandell M, Anziska B, et al: Clinical predictors of abnormality disclosed by computed tomography after mild head trauma. *Neurosurgery* 32:9, 1993.

CHAPTER 3

CLASSIFICATION OF HEAD INJURY

Sherman C. Stein

"Order and simplicity are the first steps toward the mastery of a subject. . . ." Thomas Mann

SYNOPSIS

This chapter examines the purposes and elements of classification systems for closed head injury (CHI). It discusses existing systems, their applications and goals. None of the systems completely meets these goals, and limitations are discussed in detail. The advantages of a multidimensional classification scheme are stressed, and several such systems are introduced. An expanded severity scale, based primarily on the Glasgow Coma Scale, is proposed as one part of a multi-dimensional system.

INTRODUCTION

At present, there is no system of classifying head injury that is universally accepted and used. So many classification schemes have been proposed that the choice is bewildering. At the mild end of the head injury spectrum alone, there are so many systems that their creators cannot even agree on a common name (Table 3-1).

There are several reasons to impose a classification system upon the CHI population. Epidemiologic and demographic analyses provide insight into public health, prevention and resource allocation. Tabulation of the mechanisms of injury and their pathologic expression provides understanding about the pathophysiology of head injury. Radiological, clinical, and outcome groupings are all relevant to patient care. The severity of the initial brian injury and the potential to develop more severe damage are both of great importance. Outcome prediction in trauma could play a role in determining health care policy.[1]

In patients with mild head injury, the ideal classification method would identify those patients who, despite having relatively normal neurological exams, are harboring dangerous intracranial hematomas. There is also a need to identify patients with nonsurgical intracranial lesions, who are nevertheless likely to develop long-term neurobehavioral sequelae.[2]

Among patients with more serious injuries, a system is needed to identify the ones most likely to develop progression of their intracranial lesions. At the most severe end of the head injury spectrum, there is a need to determine the extent of cerebral damage beyond which therapeutic efforts are futile (i.e. define the limits of salvageability).

Standardization of the classification of head injury can provide guidance in patient care. Ghajar[3] and associates have shown a remarkable lack of consistency among neurosurgeons in the treatment of severe head injury. Advanced Trauma Life Support[4] courses, based in part on systematic classification of injuries, have allowed a more organized approach to general trauma. This approach has proven to be useful in both education and outcome.[5] It is hoped that improved classification of CHI will promote more uniform and improved neurosurgical care.

The ideal classification routine should have the flexibility to reliably predict who needs cranial CT scanning, who must be admitted for observation, who will require emergency surgery, who will develop dangerous intracranial hypertension, and so on. Needless to say, no clinical classification can be expected to be uniformly accurate in making such predictions. However, the need for a reasonable classification is apparent.

Several agents which show promise in limiting delayed neuronal injury are currently being developed for clinical use (see Chapter 27, Experimental Drug Therapies for Head Injury and Chapter 65, Head Injury Trials—Past and Present). An appropriate codification system may help delineate patients most suited for par-

TABLE 3-1 Definitions of Minor Head Injury

		*Allowable Symptoms**					*Allowable Signs**				
Author(s)	**Mildest Category**	**Loss of Consciousness**	**Headache**	**Nausea**	**Vomiting**	**Dizziness**	**Disorientation**	**Impaired Alertness**	**Memory Loss**	**Focal Deficit**	**Inability to Follow Commands**
Becker et al. 1990 (112)	Grade 1	transient	yes	yes	yes		no	no	no	no	no
Committee on Trauma, ACS 1993 (4)	Minor	<15 min	yes	yes	no	yes	no	no	no	no	no
Feuerman et al. 1988 (113)	Minor	yes					no	no	no	no	no
Fischer et al. 1981 (114)	Class 1	yes					yes	no		yes	no
Klauber et al. 1989 (115)	Low risk	yes					yes	yes			yes
LaHaye et al. 1988 (116)	Grade 1	transient	yes	yes	yes		no	no	no	no	no
Levin et al. 1987 (117)	Minor	<20 min					yes	yes	yes	no	yes
Mendelow et al. 1982 (118)	Mild	brief	no	no	no		no	no		no	no
Miller et al. 1990 (119)	Minor	yes	yes	yes	yes		no		yes	no	no
Narayan 1989 (120)	Grade 1	transient	yes	yes	yes		no	no	no	no	no
Rimel et al. 1981 (111)	Minor	<20 min					yes	yes	yes	yes	yes
Thornbury et al. 1987 (121)	Low risk	yes	no	no	no	no	no	no		no	no

* If no, the presence of this symptom or sign places the patient in a more serious category.
If blank, not addressed by author(s) and presumably allowable.

ticular clinical trials. It is likely that head-injured patients will need to be classified by a combination of clinical, radiographic, and laboratory parameters. Other systems may be useful in providing constantly updated outcome predictions and audits of treatment effectiveness, in guiding rehabilitation treatment, in assessing economic damages and in comparing the results of various treatment regimens.

Elements of a Classification System

The components of a particular classification system must suit the purposes to which that system is intended; a single system cannot possibly address every potential use. Enough individual parameters must be available to guide therapy or to make predictions. However, a system that employs too many parameters is unwieldy and rarely useful in practice. Input variables must therefore be few in number, easily obtained and subject to minimal inter-observer disagreement. Any worthwhile codification should be subject to statistical validation.

Information that may be relevant to classification includes the history of the accident, the severity of the impact to the head, the degree of neurologic dysfunction, its temporal course, the nature of the prehospital care, associated injuries, as well as the type, location,

TABLE 3-2 Elements Potentially Important in Classifying Head Injury

A. *History:*
   1. Premorbid medical, neurological and social history
   2. Type of accident
   3. Severity of impact
   4. Pre-hospital care
   5. Clinical course since accident
B. *Physical Findings*
   1. Neurological examination
      a. function involved
      b. severity
      c. course (serial exams)
   2. Associated injuries and findings
C. *Neurodiagnostic Studies*
   1. Radiological
      a. lesions (pathology, location)
      b. CT scan
      c. MRI scan
      d. skull radiography
   2. Physiological
      a. intracranial pressure
      b. cerebral blood flow and metabolism
   3. Electrodiagnostic
      a. sensory evoked potentials
      b. motor evoked response
      c. electroencephalography
D. *Other Laboratory Studies*
   1. Coagulation and other systemic markers
   2. Biochemical monitoring of brain and CSF
E. *Treatment*
   1. Medical
      a. general support
      b. drug therapy
   2. Surgical
      a. neurosurgery
      b. for non-neurological surgery
   3. Experimental
F. *Clinical Course and Complications*
G. *Miscellaneous Elements*
   1. Injury category
   2. Impact site, superficial injuries
   3. Population statistics
   4. Economic factors

and size of intracranial abnormalities. Furthermore, the patient's therapy, hospital courses and rehabilitation may all influence outcome. These potential elements of various CHI classification systems are shown in Table 3-2. This list is loosely based on factors considered important in the Traumatic Coma Data Bank.[6]

Existing Classification Systems

Most commonly used classification schemes are based on the severity of the CHI or the anatomy of the intracranial lesions. The list that follows is not exhaustive and deals with the more commonly used classification systems. One can divide such systems into those which separate CHI into anatomical or severity categories, those (algebraic scales) in which the total severity of a given head injury is determined by the sum of the scores of individual components, those classification systems with special purposes (neuroradiological, pediatric, outcome, etc.) and those which combine the variables of several scales.

Categorical systems

International Classification of Disease (ICD). This system is primarily anatomical and is based on the type and location of various parenchymal and extraparenchymal lesions.[7]

Abbreviated Injury Scale (AIS). This primarily anatomical system is also scored for severity, based on the relative seriousness of the lesion and the effect on consciousness.[8] Each anatomical lesion of the brain, cerebral vasculature, skull or scalp is documented by clinical examination, neuroimaging studies, surgical or autopsy findings. A seven digit code number is assigned which reflects the lesion location, size and severity. The final digit of each individual lesion AIS code is related to severity and is scored on a scale of 1 to 6 (Table 3-3). The severity code is precisely defined, the number reflecting the lesion location, size and expected consequences. For patients in whom serious anatomical lesions are lacking or not documented, the head AIS is scored on duration of unconsciousness, or on the level of consciousness at the scene or on hospital admission. If there are multiple lesions, the AIS code is the highest.

Reaction Level Scale (RLS 85). This system is a modification of the Glasgow Coma Scale (v.i.), which omits eye opening and verbal response in comatose patients, while grading responsiveness in more alert patients.[9]

Loss of Consciousness Grading Systems. A number of classification schemes divide traumatic unconsciousness into several grades, based on the depth of coma.

TABLE 3-3 Abbreviated Injury Scale (AIS)

AIS Code	Severity
1	Minor
2	Moderate
3	Serious
4	Severe
5	Critical
6	Maximum

These include the Grady Coma Scale[10] and scales introduced by Ranshoff and Fleischer[11] and Becker.[12]
CONCUSSION SCALES. There are several systems introduced to classify concussion, usually in the context of sports injuries.[13–15]

ALGEBRAIC SCALES

GLASGOW COMA SCALE (GCS). Introduced by Teasdale and Jennett,[16] this system is widely used in scoring mental status following head injury. The score is the sum of three components, eye opening, best verbal response, and best motor response (Table 3-4). In recent years, the GCS has become widely accepted in grading head injuries and other neurological causes of impaired consciousness.[17] Although the GCS can be assessed at any point after trauma, the score following resuscitation[18] is commonly used to signify status on hospital admission.
HEAD INJURY WATCH SHEET. This represents an expansion of the GCS to include stimulus to awaken, quality of consciousness, ability to move and pupillary reaction.[19]
MARYLAND COMA SCALE. An expansion of the GCS to include brainstem function, this scale was introduced to help calculate the rate of recovery from traumatic coma.[20]
GLASGOW-LIEGE SCALE. Introduced by Born,[21] it adds scores for the presence or absence of several brainstem reflexes.
LEEDS COMA SCALE. This system grades the severity of a head injury by adding a number of historical, clinical, and diagnostic scores. The scores are weighted according to the degree of abnormality. It was developed in an attempt to determine survivability in severe head injury.[22]

TABLE 3-4 Glasgow Coma Scale

Eye-Opening (E):	
Spontaneous	4
To Voice	3
To Pain	2
No Response	1
Best Motor Response (M):	
Obeys Commands	6
Localizes	5
Withdraws (Flexion)	4
Abnormal Flexion (Posturing)	3
Extension (Posturing)	2
No Response	1
Verbal Response (V):	
Oriented Conversation	5
Confused, Disoriented	4
Inappropriate Words	3
Incomprehensible Sounds	2
No Response	1
Score = E + M + V	

TABLE 3-5 Injury Severity Scale (ISS)

Body Region
1. Head or neck
2. Face
3. Chest
4. Abdominal or pelvic contents
5. Extremities or pelvic girdle
6. External

Other algebraic scales related to the GCS include the Comprehensive Level of Consciousness Scale (CLOCS),[23] the Clinical Neurological Assessment Tool (CNA),[24] the Coma Recovery Scale (CRS),[25] the Glasgow Pittsburgh Coma Scoring System,[26] and the Innsbruck Coma Scale (ICS).[27]
INJURY SEVERITY SCALE (ISS). This system was introduced to quantify the severity of multiple system injuries of which the CHI is a component.[28] The Abbreviated Injury Scale (AIS) is described above for head injury, as is the assignment of the severity code for each lesion (Table 3-3). An AIS code is assigned to each of the six body regions (Table 3-5). The total score is reached by determining the AIS codes of the three most seriously injured organ systems, squaring each individual system score, and summing the squares. The magnitude of the ISS is related to the overall severity of the injury.

SPECIAL PURPOSE GROUPINGS

NEURORADIOLOGY. These systems grade the extent of an injury by scoring the severity of lesions ascertained by neurodiagnostic studies.[29–32]
PEDIATRICS. Systems have been introduced to score the mental status examination in infants and young children to overcome the shortcomings of the GCS in this group of patients.[33–39]
MINOR CHI. A number of systems have been introduced to classify relatively minor head injuries. Only a few have been shown to have predictive power.[2,40]
OUTCOME SCALES. The Glasgow Outcome Scale[41] is a simple five point scale to grade outcome from good recovery to death. The Disability Rating Scale[42] is an expansion of the GOS with five additional outcome categories. The Cognitive Function or Rancho Scale[43] is a detailed assessment of one's level of functioning within a given environment. The Functional Assessment Measure was introduced to combine the strengths of these scales.[44] The International Classification of Impairments, Disability, and Handicaps[45] is more a listing of individual impairments than a functional scoring system.

Penetrating Cerebral Injury. Although this chapter is devoted to closed head injury, the interested reader is referred to an excellent classification system proposed by Shaffrey and associates.[46]

Treatment Intensity Scores. A number of therapy intensity scores have been adapted from the Intensive Care literature to apply to head injury. These are generally algebraic scales. They include the Therapeutic Intervention Scoring System (TISS),[47] Acute Physiologic and Chronic Health Evaluation (APACHE),[48] a simplified APACHE system,[49] the APACHE II[50] and APACHE III[51] systems.

Intracranial Therapeutic Intensity Level (TIL). This system was introduced to measure the degree of therapeutic effort expended in order to maintain the intracranial pressure within an acceptable range.[52,53]

Metabolic Scales. One system which scores head injury severity using a number of metabolic and general hematological variables was introduced by Stanbrook and associates.[54]

Combinations of Variables

Gennarelli and associates pointed out the futility of using a single variable (head injury severity) to predict outcome in CHI; they suggested improving prediction power by combining severity scores with the lesions diagnosed by CT scan.[55] A number of scoring systems have been introduced which combine clinical, radiological, and other laboratory variables. These include the system suggested by Karnaze et al.[56] which combines clinical and sensory evoked responses. The suggestion by Lindgren[57] of combining the anatomic specificity of the ICD scale with a suitable scale for head injury severity advances this concept. Changaris[58] combined the GCS with the cerebral perfusion pressure to form an algebraic severity scale, and Yamaura and associates[59] proposed a scale employing age and CT scan findings.

Stein and Spettell have introduced the Head Injury Severity Scale (HISS) to address the need for a multidimensional classification system.[60] The HISS is flexible and combines a standard clinical severity grade with a second measure, historical, physical or radiographic, appropriate to the severity of the injury.

APPLICATIONS OF EXISTING SYSTEMS

General Applications

Important applications of classification systems include guidance in resuscitation and acute patient care,[61] hospital resource allocation and length of stay estimation,[62] following the rate and completeness of recovery among individuals and groups of patients,[63] predicting and comparing outcome,[64] statistical comparison and research[65] and education.[61]

For any of these applications, a particular classification system must be precise, reliable, simple, and subject to minimal interobserver disagreement. Foulkes and associates[66] discuss the objectives, design, and collection of databases for head injury.

Comparison of Various Systems

As one would expect, many comparisons have shown strengths and weakness of various systems, depending on the purpose for which they are used.[50,67] A system designed to grade minor head injury would be of little value in predicting the needs or outcome for a severe or critical CHI patient. Conversely, a system that scores intensity of treatment in an intensive care unit would be unlikely to help an emergency room physician evaluate a minor head injury patient. An anatomic system such as the ICD[7] provides information valuable for epidemiological studies and might be valuable for seatbelt and drunk driving legislation. However, it is of little value in patient management or prediction.[68]

The Glasgow Coma Scale (GCS) is almost universally used as a system of grading severity, even if that was not its original intent.[16] As such, it is applied to patient management, comparison among various groups and outcome prediction. The Injury Severity Scale (ISS) has been successfully applied in guiding resuscitation, resource allocation and education.[61,62] Various outcome scales have been reviewed and their utility to research in CHI compared.[44] Assessment of outcome from head injury is reviewed by Hannay in this text (Chap. 49).

Prediction

Perhaps the most valuable function of a classification system is in its organization of patients into groups which can be compared for prediction purposes. Prediction may include which patients with minor head injury harbor intracranial lesions requiring CT scanning and hospital admission. It may be prediction of the need for neurosurgical intervention or critical care for moderate CHI. There is a role for predicting survival and recovery in severe head injury as well. Predictability is necessary for resource allocation, education, drafting relevant legislation, etc.

It is not the purpose of this chapter to review outcome prediction as there are some excellent reviews on the subject[68–70] (Chap. 53, Predicting Outcome in the Head-Injured Patient). However, a classification system must contain all of the elements necessary for a particular prediction scheme.

Accurate prediction systems can be constructed for guiding individual patient decisions[71] and can improve outcome over treatment decisions based on subjective approaches.[72] The group in Glasgow has shown that the concept of computer-based prediction systems for head injury is well accepted in the medical community[73] and has actually influenced therapeutic decisions when introduced into clinical practice.[74] This is not to say that accurate prediction statistics will necessarily lead to lockstep application of treatment decisions or cookbook medicine. Interpretation of information, therapeutic philosophy and local resources play a major role in determining management recommendations. One need only look at three disparate approaches to the treatment of minor head injury, all based on essentially the same predictive data![75–77]

LIMITATIONS OF EXISTING CLASSIFICATION SYSTEMS

Limitations Common to All Classification Systems

Oversimplification

Most common classification systems rely on a small number of elements. Although it is obvious that the ability to predict is rather severely restricted by this limitation, comparisons must utilize a small number of simple categories or they lose statistical power.

Prime examples are systems based on the severity of brain injury, the single most important factor in survival according to some authorities.[78] Scoring of brain injury severity by any system is usually done at a single point in time, dubbed a "snapshot" by Price.[79] The severity of the head injury alone is probably too limited to allow accurate prediction of outcome, and other factors are probably needed to strengthen its predictive ability.[55,80,81] The severity of the brain injury depends on a number of factors, the most important being the total global insult to the brain, both immediate and delayed, and compensation to this insult.[79] One must also consider the effect of interventions, of the underlying health status, etc.

Failure to account for complications

The predictive power of any system is always confounded by adverse events (both neurological and systemic), and no system can account for these complications. When they occur, they generally make outcome worse than predicted.[82]

Lack of flexibility

Most existing systems employ a set of criteria rigidly applied to all CHI patients. It makes sense that different criteria will be needed to answer different questions. Michaud et al.[83] have suggested the need to use different elements of information collected at different times to predict both survival and quality of life following CHI. Furthermore, there is a continual search for new approaches to improve outcome in head injury. Hence, as outcome improves, the value of various prediction schemes must necessarily change. Unless a classification system has the flexibility to adapt to therapeutic advances and their effect on outcome, it may soon be rendered obsolete as a tool for prediction.

Limitations Common to Algebraic Scales

Algebraic scales in common use for CHI are not parametric, in that they do not represent precise measurements of discrete quantities. Nor are they linear. The degree of functional loss, increased severity, or decreased therapeutic intensity associated with a two point drop in score is rarely twice the change incurred by a one point decrease. They are not even interval scales; a drop of two points in one component of an algebraic scale may not represent the same degree of change as does a two point decrease in another component. Almost all such scales are ordinal, i.e., the numbers used represent the "order" or position in a spectrum of function.

Performing mathematical manipulations on such scales, such as summing components or taking mean values, is not justified. There is no a priori reason to believe a sum score of 9 formed by three 3's is equivalent to a 9 reached by adding components of 6, 2, and 1. As Price[79] points out, "Mathematical addition of nonparametric data is however renowned for generating misleading results."

Severity scales

Severity scales have been shown to have serious limitations in predicting deterioration and death among "low-risk" patients[84,85] and an inability to predict recovery from prolonged coma.[68,86]

SPECIFIC LIMITATIONS OF EXISTING SYSTEMS

GLASGOW COMA SCALE

The GCS shares the limitations of all severity systems. In addition, intubation and orbital swelling interfere with accurate scoring when present. The former precludes any verbal response, and the latter may prevent eye opening. Since it is a common practice for emergency personnel to sedate and intubate combative patients in the field, and since many of these patients arrive at the hospital pharmacologically unresponsive due to sedation and neuromuscular blockade ("Chemical 3s"), there is a serious scoring problem. Post-resuscitation scoring must await metabolism of these pharmacologic agents. In one study, such complications interfered with direct assessment of at least one component of the GCS in 38 percent of patients; the GCS could not be confidently assigned in almost half that number.[87]

At the low end of the scale, the motor component is much more important than the other two elements of the GCS.[88] At the upper end of the scale, a wide range of patients exhibit a GCS of 15,[9] and the scale fails to account for the amount of stimulation needed to obtain an appropriate and oriented verbal response. The greatest number of scoring errors occurs in the middle range of scores.[89–91] Education is necessary in the proper application of the GCS,[92] as inexperienced users tend to make serious and consistent errors.[90] Statistical studies have cast doubt on the value of the sum score,[93] and psychometric analysis has questioned the reliability and the validity of the GCS compared to other scales.[94] The predictive value of the GCS, even when applied after the initial period, is still somewhat limited. Low scores do not necessarily predict bad outcome.[95] Since GCS scores do not follow a normal distribution, studies employing mean GCS values and standard statistical analysis are misleading.[96] Eisenberg[97] provides an excellent critique of the Glasgow Coma Scale. Investigators in Scandinavia have reported replacing the GCS in clinical practice.[98] However, despite these limitations, the GCS continues to be widely used.

OTHER SYSTEMS

Even the Leeds Scale, designed only to predict survival, is not infallible.[99] The ICD system is cumbersome to apply[57,79] and often requires several entries for each head-injured patient. Many injuries must be coded "unspecified," and ICD rubrics often combine injuries of very different severity.[100,101] The Injury Severity Scale was shown to underscore the severity of CHI.[102] Neurodiagnostic classification systems also have limited predictive value,[80] especially if applied early in the course of CHI.[103,104] There is considerable interobserver disagreement in the application of the Glasgow Outcome Scale.[105,106] However, as additional outcome categories are added to the five in the GOS, the confusion is only compounded.[107]

HEAD INJURY SEVERITY SCALE

BACKGROUND

A mutually agreed-upon clinical severity scale is necessary for communicating about individual CHI patients and patient groups. However, severity alone is ineffective in describing such groups. Each severity category, no matter how chosen, contains an enormously divergent patient population. Criteria such as age, presence or absence of intracranial lesions and intensity of treatment may influence decisions regarding care and prognosis. Langfitt has pointed out this shortcoming by a reminder that no patient ever died of a "mild head injury."[108] The unwritten assumption is that the unfortunate patient's injury was only "apparently" mild and that complications supervened.

Teasdale[109] has emphasized the need for a multidimensional classification system for head injury, thus providing varied dimensions for different purposes. Such a system can only be built on the foundation of a reliable clinical system to grade CHI severity.

SEVERITY CATEGORIES

The traditional scale of mild, moderate, and severe[110,111] has the advantage of providing a few, fairly distinct categories. Unfortunately, the range of severity encompassed by the mild and severe categories may be excessive,[91] and only a small percentage of patients fit into the moderate group. In the expanded scale presented here, minor and serious CHIs are divided into five categories, based primarily on the GCS score (Table 3-6). The limitations of the GCS notwithstanding, this is the most logical severity scale available. It is simple to apply, there is minimal interobserver disagreement, and it can be accurately used by a broad spectrum of health care workers. Furthermore, the GCS is presently ingrained in most head injury centers as a measure of severity. It is generally conceded that additional historical information is needed to supplement the GCS in minor CHI.

TABLE 3-6 Proposed Head Injury Severity Scale

Severity Category	GCS Interval
Minimal	15 no loss of consciousness (LOC) or amnesia
Mild	14; or 15 plus amnesia, or brief (<5 min) LOC, or impaired alertness or memory
Moderate	9–13 or LOC ≥ 5 min, or focal neurologic deficit
Severe	5–8
Critical	3–4

Loss of consciousness, amnesia, post-traumatic seizures, open, depressed skull fractures and focal neurological deficit are all incorporated in the definitions of various minor CHI categories.

A "critical" category has been added to the "serious" group because of the obvious differences in intensity of treatment, survival, and other outcome parameters seen in patients with GCS of 3 or 4, as compared to those with higher scores below 9. The time at which the severity is scored is flexible, but must be defined for a given application.

Applications

The utility of a scale depends on its desired application. One system may be valuable in collecting demographic data, but quite another may be needed to guide patient care. One scale may help determine which patients with minor CHI require neurodiagnostic testing but be unable to predict survivability in critical CHI patients. Experience has shown that no one-dimensional scale can meet all these goals. The challenge for the future is to devise flexible, multi-dimensional classification schemes for CHI, which meet the needs of clinical personnel, researchers and health care planners.

References

1. Medeloff JM, Cayten CG: Trauma systems and public policy. *Annu Rev Pub Health* 1991; 12:401–424.
2. Williams DH, Levin HS, Eisenberg HM: Mild head injury classification. *Neurosurgery* 1990; 27:422–428.
3. Ghajar J, Hariri RJ, Narayan RK, et al: Survey of critical care management of comatose, head-injured patients in the United States. *Crit Care Med* 1995; 23:560–567.
4. Committee on Trauma, American College of Surgeons: Advanced Trauma Life Support, Program for Physicians. Chicago: American College of Surgeons, 1993.
5. Townsend RN, Clark R, Ramenofsky ML, et al: ATLS-based videotape trauma resuscitation review: Education and outcome. *J Trauma* 1993; 34:133–138.
6. Foulkes MA: Neurosurgical data bases. *J Neurosurg* 1991; 75:S1–S7.
7. World Health Organization: Diseases of the Nervous System and Sense Organs. In: International Classification of Diseases, 9th revision, Clinical Modification (ICD-9-CM), 1993 edition. Los Angeles, Practice Management Information Corp., 1993, pp. 77–103, 213–248.
8. Association for the Advancement of Automotive Medicine: The Abbreviated Injury Scale, 1990 Revision. Des Plaines, IL: Association for the Advancement of Automotive Medicine, 1990: 15–24.
9. Starmark J-E, Stalhamar D, Holmgren E, et al: A comparison of the Glasgow Coma Scale and the Reaction Level Scale (RLS85) *J Neurosurg* 1988; 69:699–706.
10. Barrow DL, Wood J: Cerebral resuscitation, in Chernow B, Lake CR (eds): *The Pharmacological Approach to the Critically Ill Patient.* Baltimore: Williams & Wilkins, 1983: 76–84.
11. Ransohoff J, Fleischer A: Head Injuries. *JAMA* 1975; 234:861–864.
12. Becker DP, Miller JD, Young HF, et al: Diagnosis and treatment of head injury in adults, in Youmans JR (ed): *Neurological Surgery*, 2d ed. Philadelphia: WB Saunders, 1982: vol 4, 1938.
13. Torg JS: *Athletic Injuries to the Head, Neck and Face.* Philadelphia: JB Lippincott, 1982.
14. Kulund DN: *The Injured Athlete.* Philadelphia: JB Lippincott, 1982.
15. Nelson WE, Jane JA, Gieck JH: Minor head injury in sports: A new system of classification and management. *Physician Sports Med* 1984; 12:103.
16. Teasdale G, Jennett B: Assessment of coma and impaired consciousness. *Lancet* 1974; 1:81–83.
17. Bastos P, Sun X, Wagner DP, et al: Glasgow Coma Scale score in the evaluation of outcome in the intensive care unit: Findings from the Acute Physiology and Chronic Health Evaluation III study. *Crit Care Med* 1993; 21:1459–1465.
18. Marshall LF, Becker DP, Bowers SA, et al: The national traumatic coma data bank. Part I: Design, purpose, goals and results. *J Neurosurg* 1983; 59:276–284.
19. Yen JK, Bourke RS, Nelson LR, et al: Numerical grading of clinical neurological status after serious head injury. *J Neurol Neurosurg Psychiatry* 1978; 41:1125–1130.
20. Salcman M, Schepp RS, Ducker TB: Calculated recovery rates in severe head trauma. *Neurosurgery* 1981; 8:301–308.
21. Born JD: The Glasgow-Liege Scale. *Acta Neurochir* 1988; 91:1–11.
22. Gibson RM, Stephenson GC: Aggressive management of severe closed-head trauma: Time for a reappraisal. *Lancet* 1989; 2:369–371.
23. Stanczak DE, White VG, Gouview WD, et al: Assessment of level of consciousness following severe neurological insult. *J Neurosurg* 1984; 60:955–960.
24. Crosby L, Parsons LC: Clinical neurologic assessment tool: Development and testing of an instrument to index neurological status. *Heart Lung* 1989; 18:121–129.

25. Giacino JT, Kezmarksy MA, DeLuca J, Cicerone KD: Monitoring rate of recovery to predict outcome in minimally responsive patients. *Arch Phys Med Rehabil* 1991; 72:897–901.
26. Safar P: Resuscitation after brain ischemia. Grenvik A, Safar P (eds): *Brain Failure and Resuscitation.* New York: Churchill-Livingstone, 1981: 155–184.
27. Benzer A, Mittschiffthaker G, Marosi M, et al: Prediction of nonsurvival after trauma: Innsbruck coma scale. *Lancet* 1991; 338:977–978.
28. American Association of Automotive Medicine: Rating the severity of tissue damage: I. The Abbreviated Injury Scale. *JAMA* 1977; 215:277–280.
29. Marshall LF, Marshall SB, Klauber MR, et al: A new classification of head injury based on computerized tomography. *J Neurosurg* 1991; 75:S14–S20.
30. Marshall LF, Marshall SB, Klauber MR, et al: The diagnosis of head injury requires a classification based on computed axial tomography. *J Neurotrauma* 1992; 9 (Suppl 1):S287–S292.
31. Teasdale G, Teasdale E, Hadley D: Computed tomographic and magnetic resonance imaging classification of head injury. *J Neurotrauma* 1992; 9(Suppl 1):S249–S257.
32. Tomei G, Sganzerla E, Spugnoli D, et al: Posttraumatic diffuse cerebral lesions. Relationship between clinical course, CT findings and ICP. *J Neurosurg Sci* 1991; 35:61–75.
33. Seshia SS, Seshia MMK, Sachdeva RK: Coma in childhood. *Dev Med Child Neurol* 1977; 19:614–628.
34. Hahn YS, Chyung C, Barthel MJ, et al: Head injuries in children under 36 months of age: Demography and outcome. *Childs Nerv Syst* 1988;4:34–40.
35. Duncan CC, Ment LR, Smith B, et al: A scale for the assessment of neonatal neurologic status. *Childs Brain* 1981; 3:299–306.
36. Morray JP, Tyler DC, Jones TK, et al: Coma scale for use in brain-injured children. *Crit Care Med* 1984; 12:1018–1023.
37. Raimondi AJ, Hirschauer J: Head injury in the infant and toddler. Coma scoring and outcome scale. *Childs Brain* 1984; 11:12–35.
38. Yager JV, Johnston BM, Seshia SS: Coma scales in pediatric practice. *Am J Dis Child* 1990; 144:1088–1091.
39. Simpson DA, Cockington RA, Hanieh A, et al: Head injuries in infants and young children: The value of the Paediatric Coma Scale. *Childs Nerv Syst* 1991; 7:183–190.
40. Sano K, Manaka S, Kitamuru K, et al: Statistical studies on evaluation of mild disturbance of consciousness—study of a simpler scale for clinical use. *J Neurosurg* 1983; 58:223–230.
41. Jennett B, Snoek J, Bond MR, et al: Disability after severe head injury: Observation on the use of the Glasgow Outcome Scale. *J Neurol Neurosurg Psychiatry* 1981; 44:285–293.
42. Hall K, Cope DN, Rappaport M: Glasgow Outcome Scale and Disability Rating Scale: Comparative usefulness in following recovery in traumatic brain injury. *Arch Phys Med Rehab* 1985; 66:35–37.
43. Gouvier WD, Blanton PD, Laporte KK, et al: Reliability and validity of the Disability Rating Scale and the levels of Cognitive Functioning Scale in monitoring recovery from severe head injury. *Arch Phys Med Rehab* 1987; 68:94–97.
44. Ditunno JF Jr: Functional assessment measures in CNS trauma. *J Neurotrauma* 1992; 9(Suppl 1):S301–S305.
45. World Health Organization: *International Classification of Impairments, Disabilities and Handicaps: A Manual of Classification Relating to the Consequences of Disease.* Geneva, World Health Organization, 1980.
46. Shaffrey ME, Polin RS, Phillips CD, et al: Classification of civilian craniocerebral gunshot wounds: A multivariate analysis predictive of mortality. *J Neurotrauma* 9 (Suppl 1):S279–S285.
47. Cullen DJ, Civetta JM, Briggs BA, et al: Therapeutic Intervention Scoring System. A method for quantitative comparison of patient care. *Crit Care Med* 1974; 2:57–60.
48. Knaus WA, Zimmerman JE, Wagner DP, et al: Acute Physiology and Chronic Health Evaluation: A physiologically based classification system. *Crit Care Med* 1981; 9:591–597.
49. LeGall JR, Loirat P, Alperovitch A, et al: A simplified acute physiology score for ICU patients. *Crit Care Med* 1984; 12:975–977.
50. Gensemer IB, Smith JL, Walker JC, et al: Psychological consequences of blunt head trauma and relation to other indices of severity of injury. *Ann Emerg Med* 1989; 18:9–12.
51. Zimmerman JE (ed): The APACHE III study design: Analytic plan for evaluation of severity and outcome. *Crit Care Med* 1989; 17(Suppl):S169–S221.
52. Marmarou A, Anderson RL, Ward JD, et al: NINDS Traumatic Coma Data Bank intracranial pressure monitoring methodology. *J Neurosurg* 1991; 75:S21–S28.
53. Maset AL, Marmarou A, Ward JD, et al: Pressure-volume index in head injury. *J Neurosurgery* 1987; 67:832–840.
54. Stambrook M, Moore AD, Kowalchuk S, et al: Early metabolic and neurologic predictors of long-term quality of life after closed head injury. *Canad J Surg* 1990; 33:115–118.
55. Gennarelli TA, Spielman GM, Langfitt TW, et al: Influence of the type of intracranial lesion on outcome from severe head injury. *J Neurosurg* 1982; 56:25–32.
56. Karnaze DS, Weiner JM, Marshall LF: Auditory evoked potentials in coma after closed head injury: A clinical-neurophysiologic coma scale for predicting outcome. *Neurology* 1985; 35:1122–1126.
57. Lindgren S: Diagnostic terminology of head injuries—related to severity. *Acta Neurochir* 1986; (Suppl 36):70–80.
58. Changaris DG, McGraw P, Richardson JD, et al: Corre-

lation of cerebral perfusion pressure and Glasgow Coma Scale to outcome. *J Trauma* 1987; 27:1007–1013.

59. Yamaura A, Ono J, Watanabe Y, et al: CT findings and outcome in head injuries—effects of aging. *Neurosurg Rev* 1989; 12(Suppl 1):178–183.
60. Stein SC, Spettell C: The Head Injury Severity Scale (HISS): A practical classification of head injury. *Brain Injury* 1995; 5:437–444.
61. Trunkey D: Initial treatment of patients with extensive trauma. *N Engl J Med* 1991; 324:1259–1263.
62. Anderson J, Shaskey W, Schwartz ML, et al. Injury Severity Score, head injury and patient wait days: Contributions to extended trauma patient length of stay. *J Trauma* 1992; 33:219–220.
63. Lobato RD, Sarabia R, Rivas JJ: Normal computerized tomography scans in severe head injury. Prognostic and clinical management implications. *J Neurosurg* 1986; 65:784–789.
64. Rappaport M, Herrero-Backe C, Rappaport ML: Head injury outcome up to ten years later. *Arch Phys Med Rehabil* 1989; 70:885–892.
65. Titterington DM, Murray GD, Murray LS, et al: Comparison of discrimination techniques applied to a complex data set of head injured patients. *JR Statist Soc A* 1981; 144:145–175.
66. Foulkes MA, Eisenberg HM, Jane JA, et al: The Traumatic Coma Data Bank: Design, methods and baseline characteristics. *J Neurosurg* 1991; 75:S8–S13.
67. Rocca B, Martin C, Viviand X, et al: Comparison of severity scores in patients with head trauma. *J Trauma* 1989; 29:299–305.
68. Contant CF and Narayan RK: Prognosis after head injury, in Neurological Surgery, Youmans JR (Ed), 4th Ed, WB Saunders. 1996, p 1792–1812.
69. Deaton AV: Predicting outcomes: The slippery slope. *Brain Inj* 1993; 7:99–100.
70. Ruff RM, Marshall LF, Crouch J, et al: Predictors of outcome following severe head trauma: Follow-up data from the Traumatic Coma Data Bank. *Brain Inj* 1993; 7:101–111.
71. Murray GD, Murray LS, Barlow P, et al: Assessing the performance and clinical impact of a computerized prognostic system in severe head injury. *Statist Med* 1986; 5:403–410.
72. Kaufmann MA, Buchmann B, Scheidegger D, et al: Severe head injury: Should expected outcome influence resuscitation and first-day decisions? *Resuscitation* 1992; 23:199–206.
73. Barlow P, Teasdale G: Prediction of outcome and the management of severe head injuries: The attitudes of neurosurgeons. *Neurosurgery* 1986; 19:989–991.
74. Murray LS, Teasdale GM, Murray GD, et al: Does prediction of outcome alter patient management? *Lancet* 1993; 341:1487–1491.
75. Servadei F, Vergoni G, Nasi MT, et al: Management of low-risk head injuries in an entire area: Results of an 18-month survey. *Surg Neurol* 1993; 39:269–275.
76. Stein SC, Ross SE: Minor head injury: A proposed strategy for emergency management. *Ann Emerg Med* 1993; 22:1193–1196.
77. Reinus WR, Wippold FJ II, Erickson KK: Practical selection criteria for noncontrast cranial computed tomography in patients with head trauma. *Ann Emerg Med* 1993; 22:1148–1155.
78. Conroy C, Kraus JF: Survival after brain injury. *Neuroepidemiology* 1988; 7:13–22.
79. Price DJ: Is diagnostic severity grading for head injuries possible? *Acta Neurochir* 1986; (Suppl 36):67–69.
80. Van Dongen KJ, Braakman R, Gelpke GJ: The prognostic value of computerized tomography in comatose head-injured patients. *J Neurosurg* 1983; 59:951–957.
81. Williams JM, Gomes F, Drudge OW, et al: Predicting outcome from closed head injury by early assessment of trauma severity. *J Neurosurg* 1984; 61:581–585.
82. Jennett B, Teasdale G, Braakman R, et al: Predicting outcome in individual patients after severe head injury. *Lancet* 1976; 1:1031–1034.
83. Michaud LJ, Rivara FP, Grady MS, et al: Predictors of survival and severity of disability after severe brain injury in children. *Neurosurgery* 1992; 31:254–264.
84. Klauber MR, Marshall LF, Toole BM, et al: Cause of decline in head-injury mortality rate in San Diego County, California. *J Neurosurg* 1985; 62:528–531.
85. Dacey RG, Wayne AM, Rimel RW, et al: Neurosurgical complication after apparently minor head injury: Assessment of risk in a series of 160 patients. *J Neurosurg* 1986; 65:203–210.
86. Levin HS, Savdjari C, Eisenberg HM, et al: Vegetative state after closed head injury. A traumatic coma. Data Bank Report. *Arch Neurol* 1991; 48:580–585.
87. Gale JL, Dikmen S, Wyler A, et al: Head Injury in the Pacific Northwest. *Neurosurgery* 1983; 12:487–491.
88. Jagger J, Jane JA, Rimel R: The Glasgow Coma Scale: To sum or not to sum? *Lancet* 1983; 2:97.
89. Starmark J-E, Holmgren E, Stalhammar D: Current reporting of responsiveness in acute cerebral disorders: A survey of the neurosurgical literature. *J Neurosurg* 1988; 69:692–698.
90. Rowley G, Fielding K: Reliability and accuracy of the Glasgow Coma Scale with experienced and inexperienced users. *Lancet* 1991; 337:535–538.
91. Holmgren E, Lindgren S, Stalhammer D: Multiple or single scales in observation at bedside. *Acta Neurochir (Wien)* 1981; 56:141–142.
92. Teasdale G, Kril-Jones R, van der Sande J: Observer variability in assessing impaired consciousness and coma. *J Neurol Neurosurg Psychiatry* 1978; 41:603–610.
93. Koziol JA, Hacke W: Multivariate data reduction by principal components with application to neurological scoring instruments. *J Neurol* 1990; 237:461–464.
94. Segatore M, Way C: The Glasgow Coma Scale: Time for change. *Heart Lung* 1992; 21:548–557.
95. Waxman K, Sundine MJ, Young RF: Is early prediction of outcome in severe head injury possible? *Arch Surg* 1991; 126:1237–1242.
96. Gaddis GM, Gaddis ML: Non-normality of distribution

of Glasgow Coma Scores and Revised Trauma Scores. *Ann Emerg Med* 1994; 1994; 23:75–80.
97. Eisenberg H: Outcome after head injury: Part I: General considerations, in Becker DP, Povlishock JT (eds): *Central Nervous System Trauma Status Report, 1985.* Washington, DC: U.S. Government Printing Office, 1988:271–280.
98. Starmark J-E, Holmgren E, Stalhammar D, et al: Reliability and accuracy of the Glasgow Coma Scale. *Lancet* 1991; 337:1042–1043.
99. Feldman Z, Contant CF, Robertson CS, et al: Evaluation of the Leeds prognostic score for severe head injury. *Lancet* 1991; 337:1451–1453.
100. Langley J: The International Classification of Disease's codes for describing injuries and the circumstances surrounding injuries. *Accid Anal Prev* 1982; 14:195–197.
101. Garthe EA: Compatibility of ICD-9-CM with AIS-80. *AAAM The Quarterly/Journal* 1982; 4:42–46.
102. Gennarelli TA, Champion HR, Sacco WJ, et al: Mortality of patients with head injury and extracranial injury treated in trauma centers. *J Trauma* 1989; 29:1193–1202.
103. Cohadon R, Richer E, Reglade C, et al: Recovery of motor function after severe traumatic coma. *Scand J Rehab Med* 1988; (Suppl 17):75–85.
104. Wilson JTL, Wiedmann KD, Hadley DM, et al: Early and late magnetic resonance imaging and neurophsychological outcome after head injury. *J Neurol Neurosurg Psychiatry* 1988; 51:391–396.
105. Dodwell D: The heterogeneity of social outcome following head injury. *J Neurol Neurosurg Psychiatr* 1988; 51:833–838.
106. Tate RL, Lulham JM, Broe GA, et al: Psychosocial outcome for the survivors of severe blunt head injury: The results from a consecutive series of 100 patients. *J Neurol Neurosurg Psychiatry* 1989; 52:1128–1134.
107. Maas AIR, Braakman R, Schouten HJA, et al: Agreement between physicians on assessment of outcome following severe head injury. *J Neurosurg* 1983; 58:321–325.
108. Langfitt T: Concluding remarks, in Hoff JT, Anderson TE, Cole TM (eds): *Mild to Moderate Head Injury.* Boston: Blackwell Scientific, 1989:235–238.
109. Teasdale G: Workshop Consensus: Clinical Management of Mild to Moderate Head Injury, in Hoff JT, Anderson TE, Cole TM (eds): *Mild to Moderate Head Injury.* Boston: Blackwell Scientific, 1989:227–229.
110. Rimel RW, Giordani B, Barth JT, et al: Moderate head injury: Completing the clinical spectrum of brain trauma. *Neurosurgery* 1982; 11:344–351.
111. Rimel RW, Giordani B, Barth JT, et al: Disability caused by minor head injury. *Neurosurgery* 1981; 9:221–228.
112. Becker DP, Gade GF, Young HF, et al: Diagnosis and treatment of head injury in adults, in Youmans Jr (ed): *Neurological Surgery.* 3d ed. Philadelphia: WB Saunders, 1990:2017–2048.
113. Feuerman T, Wackym PA, Gade GF, et al: Value of skull radiography, head computed tomographic scanning and admission for observation in cases of minor head injury. *Neurosurgery* 1988; 22:449–453.
114. Fischer RP, Carlson J, Perry JF: Post-concussion hospital observation of alert patients in a primary trauma center. *J Trauma* 1981; 21:920–924.
115. Klauber MR, Marshall LF, Luerssen TG, et al: Determinants of head injury mortality: Importance of the low risk patient. *Neurosurgery* 1989; 24:31–36.
116. La Haye PA, Gade GF, Becker DP: Injury to the cranium, in Mattox KL, Moore EE, Feliciano DV (eds): *Trauma.* Norwalk, CT: Appleton & Lange, 1988: 237–249.
117. Levin HS, Mattiss, Ruff RM, et al: Neurobehavioral outcome following minor head injury: A three center study. *J Neurosurg* 1987; 66:234–243.
118. Mendelow AD, Campbell DA, Jeffrey RR, et al: Admission after mild head injury: Benefits and costs. *Brit Med J* 1982; 285:1530–1532.
119. Miller JD, Murray LS, Teasdale GM: Development of a traumatic intracranial hematoma after a "minor" head injury. *Neurosurgery* 1990; 27:669–673.
120. Narayan RK: Emergency room management of the head-injured patient, in Becker DP, Gudeman SK (eds): *Textbook of Head Injury.* Philadelphia: WB Saunders, 1989:23–66.
121. Thornbury JR, Masters SJ, Campbell JA: Imaging recommendations for head trauma: A new comprehensive strategy. *AJR* 1987; 149:781–783.

CHAPTER 4

NEUROPATHOLOGY OF HEAD INJURY

David Ian Graham

SYNOPSIS

The most important factor governing the outcome in a patient with a head injury is the damage sustained by the brain. Furthermore, it is well recognized that in many patients, not all the brain damage occurs at the time of injury. There is now considerable insight into the underlying mechanisms of traumatic coma as a result of advances in both the definition and, to some extent, the quantification of various types of brain damage. Although there is a trend toward classifying brain damage after head injury as focal or diffuse, there are basically two main stages in the development of brain damage after head injury: (1) primary damage, which occurs at the moment of injury and can include lacerations of the scalp, fracture of the skull, contusions and lacerations, diffuse axonal injury, intracranial hemorrhage, and other types of brain damage, and (2) secondary damage, which results from complicating processes that are initiated at the moment of injury but may not present clinically for a period of time afterward, including hypoxia/ischemia, swelling, infection, and brain damage due to elevated intracranial pressure. This chapter discusses in depth the pathology of both primary and secondary damage after trauma to the head.

The classification of brain damage after head injury has to be informed by two extremes: the patient who remains in a coma from the moment of injury until death and the patient who is apparently normal after the initial injury but who, as a result of a complication, lapses into a fatal coma. There is little doubt that traumatic coma may be attributed to many different types of brain damage.

There have been many studies on the classification of brain damage in patients who die from a head injury.[1–7] In the past, the existence of primary and secondary damage was emphasized in an attempt to provide clinicopathologic correlation. This approach has helped identify potentially preventable complications in patients with a head injury who "talk and die"[8] or "talk and deteriorate,"[9] since it is well recognized that an apparently trivial head injury can set in motion a progressive sequence of events leading to secondary brain damage with a fatal outcome or severe persistent disability.[10,11]

From a neuropathological point of view, it has been suggested that there are two main stages in the development of brain damage following injury to the head. Primary damage occurs at the moment of injury and takes the form of lacerations of the scalp, fractures of skull, contusions and lacerations, diffuse axonal injury, and intracranial hemorrhage. Secondary damage is produced by complicating processes that are initiated at the moment of injury but may not present clinically for a period of time after the injury. This includes brain damage due to raised intracranial pressure (ICP), hypoxia/ischemia, swelling, and infection.

In the last decade computed tomography (CT) has played a very important role in the diagnostic evaluation of head-injured patients. More recently magnetic resonance imaging (MRI) has been found to be particularly useful in the later diagnosis and classification of traumatic lesions in a closed head injury.[12–14] In an unconscious patient without any evidence of intracranial hematoma, it is usually concluded that the patient has sustained diffuse brain damage. However, even with improved CT scanning and MRI, the precise type of damage may not be identifiable during life. Furthermore, it may be difficult to define post mortem unless the brain is properly fixed before dissection and the appropriate histological studies are undertaken. This applies both to nonmissile injuries, which are generally most common in civilian practice, and to missile injuries.

Careful clinical and laboratory studies[15,16] have shown that the principal mechanisms of head injury are contact and acceleration/deceleration. Lesions due to contact result from an object striking the head or vice versa and include local effects such as laceration of the scalp, fracture of the skull, extradural hematoma, surface contusion, and intracerebral hemorrhage. In contrast, acceleration/deceleration results from head movement in the instant after injury and leads to intracranial and intracerebral pressure gradients as well as shear, tensile, and compressive strains. Such inertial (nonimpact) lesions are responsible for two of the most important types of damage encountered in nonmissile head injury: acute subdural hematoma resulting from the tearing of subdural bridging veins and diffuse axonal injury (DAI).

GLASGOW DATABASE

With the cooperation of the appropriate legal authorities and the forensic pathologists in the west of Scotland, a comprehensive database of brain damage in fatal head injuries was established. In the 25-year period between 1968 and 1982, it consisted of a consecutive series of 635 fatal nonmissile head injuries (Table 4-1).

In all cases, the brains were suspended in 10% Formol (Formaldehyde) saline for at least 3 weeks before being dissected in the standard fashion: The cerebral hemispheres were sliced in the coronal plane, the cerebellum at right angles to the folia, and the brainstem horizontally. Comprehensive histological studies were undertaken in the majority of cases.

TABLE 4-1 Data from a Consecutive Series of 635 Fatal Nonmissile Head Injuries over a 25-Year Period (1968–1982)

Factor	Percent
Sex	
Males	78
Females	22
Type of injury	
Road traffic accident	53
Falls	35
Assaults	5
Other	7
Incidence of	
Fracture of skull	75
Surface contusions	94: mild in 6%, moderate in 78%, severe in 10%
Diffuse axonal injury	29
Intracranial hematoma	60: EDH in 10%, SDH in 18%, intracerebral in 16%, "burst" lobe in 23%
Elevated intracranial pressure	75
Ischemic brain damage	55
Brain swelling	51: unilateral in 34%, bilateral in 17%
Intracranial infection	4

EDH = Extradural (epidurm) Hematoma
SDH = Subdural Hematoma

PATHOLOGICAL STUDIES

The role of the pathologist in the study of brain damage from head injury has been questioned when he or she is restricted to an examination of fatal cases only. However, experience has shown that in most cases the pathologist is able to define the sequence of events leading to the fatal outcome; thus, the clinicopathologic assessment can help identify at least potentially preventable factors, providing an audit of and quality assurance for the management of head-injured patients.[17] Furthermore, it is only through a study of fatal head injuries that insight can be gained into the types of brain damage present in patients who remain permanently disabled after a head injury.

PRIMARY DAMAGE

Lacerations of the Scalp

Not only do scalp lacerations indicate the site of injury, they may bleed profusely. Furthermore, if there is an associated open depressed fracture of the skull, a laceration may be a potential route for intracranial infection.

Fracture of the Skull

In general, the more severe the injury, the greater the frequency of fractures. This frequency is 3 percent in accident/emergency attenders, 65 percent in patients admitted to a neurosurgical unit, and 80 percent in fatal cases.[17] Patients with a fracture have a much higher incidence of intracranial hematoma than do those without a fracture.[18,19]

Linear fractures of the vault occur in 62 percent of patients with severe head injury and extend into the base of the skull in 17 percent. Fractures limited to the base of the skull are present in only 4 percent of cases. A fracture is said to be depressed if the fragments of the inner table of the skull are depressed by at least the thickness of the diploë, and such lesions are found in 11 percent of patients. A depressed fracture is said to be compound if there is an associated laceration of the skull and penetrating if there is also a tear in the dura. Both are potential routes for intracranial infection. Depressed fractures are also associated with an increased incidence of posttraumatic epilepsy. Fractures in the base of the skull may be complicated by intracranial infection as organisms spread from the air sinuses or the middle ear; this explains the clinical importance of CSF rhinorrhea, otorrhea, and traumatic pneumocephalus. If injury has been particularly severe, there may be a hinged fracture extending across the base of the skull, usually in the region of the posterior part of the pituitary fossa and the adjacent squamous part of the temporal bones. A fall on the occiput may be associated with a contrecoup fracture of the orbital ridges and ethmoid plates; particularly in childhood, a growing fracture may develop if brain tissue protrudes into the fracture.

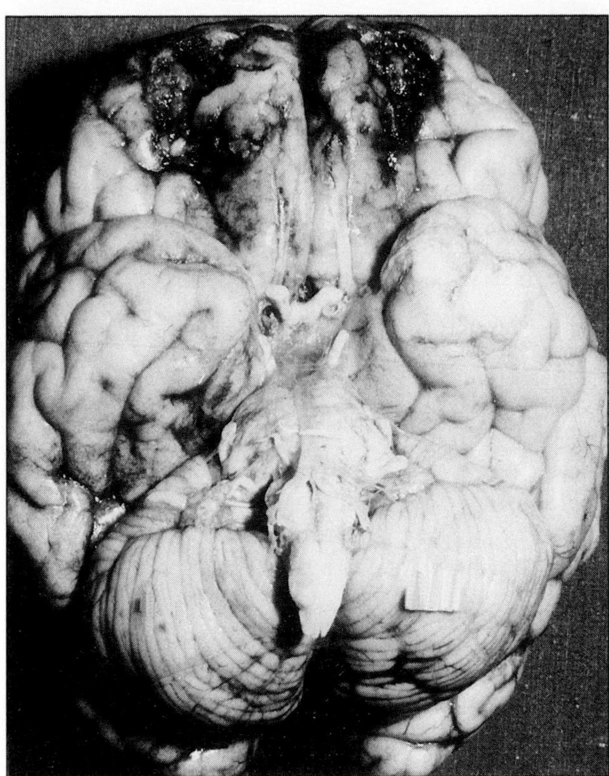

Figure 4-1. Surface contusions. There are recent hemorrhagic contusions affecting the poles and the underaspects of the frontal lobes.

Contusions and Lacerations of the Brain

A contusion is a type of focal brain damage caused mainly by contact between the surface of the brain and the bony protuberances of the base of the skull. By definition, the pia-arachnoid is intact over surface contusions but is torn in lacerations. Considered to be the hallmark of brain damage due to head injury, they have a very characteristic distribution affecting the frontal poles, the orbital gyri (Fig. 4-1), the cortex above and below the sylvian fissures, the temporal poles, and the lateral and inferior aspects of the temporal lobes. Less frequently, the inferior surfaces of the cerebellar hemispheres are affected. They are most severe on the crests of gyri and may extend to involve digitate white matter. In the early stages, they are hemorrhagic and swollen; when healed, they present as golden-brown shrunken scars. Healed contusions have been reported as incidental findings in 2.5 percent of autopsies in general hospitals. Typical surface contusions are rare in young infants, with the typical features of nonmissile head injury in this age group being contusional tears in the subcortical white matter and the outer layers of the cortex.

Various types of contusion have been defined. Fracture contusions occur at the site of a fracture and are particularly severe in the frontal lobes and in association with fractures of the anterior fossae; coup contusions occur at the site of impact in the absence of a fracture; contrecoup contusions occur in the brain diametrically opposite the point of impact; herniation contusions occur in areas where the medial parts of the temporal lobe make contact with the free edge of the tentorium or the cerebellar tonsils make contact at the foramen magnum at the time of injury; and intermediary coup contusions are single or multiple lesions in the deepest structures of the brain, including the corpus callosum, the basal ganglia, the hypothalamus, and the brainstem. Gliding contusions are focal hemorrhages in the cortex and the adjacent white matter of the superior margins of the cerebral hemispheres and are due to rotation, unlike the contusions listed above, which result from contact of the brain surface with bony protuberances. These types of contusions are often asymmetrical and are usually part of the spectrum of diffuse injuries that embraces both acute vascular injury and diffuse axonal injury.

A contusion index has been developed which allows the depth and extent of contusions in various parts of the brain to be expressed quantitatively.[20] Not surprisingly, contusions in the frontal and temporal lobes have been found to be (1) more severe in patients with a fracture of the skull than in those without a fracture, (2) significantly less severe in patients with diffuse axonal injury (see next section) than in those without this type of brain damage, and (3) more severe in patients who do not experience a lucid interval than in those who do. The use of a contusion index has also shed doubt on the concept that contrecoup contusions are the most severe. In patients who receive frontal or occipital injuries, contusions are always more severe in the frontal lobes. More recently Scott et al.[21] derived a hemorrhagic lesion score which provides finer discrimination of the distribution and severity of injury by including lesions involving the corpus callosum, deep white matter, and deep gray matter.

Lacerations of the frontal and temporal lobes are often associated with acute subdural and intracerebral hemorrhage. The terms "burst" frontal lobe and "burst" temporal lobe are then appropriate.

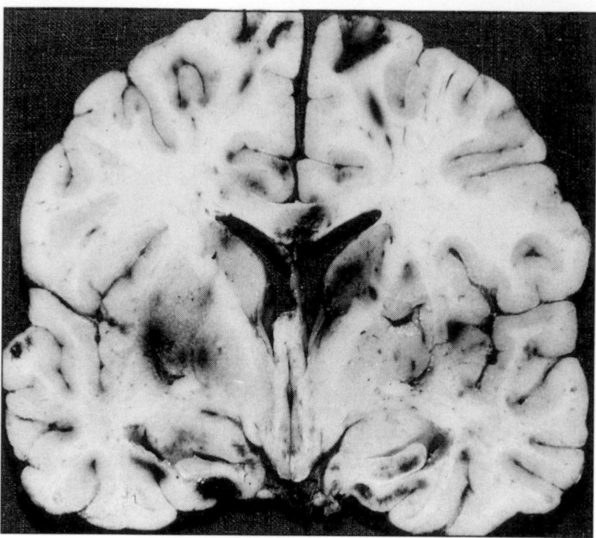

Figure 4-2. Diffuse axonal injury. Note the bilateral parasagittal "gliding" contusions, a hemorrhagic lesion in the corpus callosum and interventricular septum, small hematomas in the body of the right caudate nucleus and the left lentiform nucleus, and small hemorrhages in the anteromedial portions of each medial lobe.

Diffuse Axonal Injury

Severe DAI not accompanied by an intracranial mass lesion occurs in almost 50 percent of patients with a severe head injury, causes 35 percent of all deaths after head injury, and is the most common cause of the vegetative state and severe disability until death.[22] This type of brain damage was first called "diffuse degeneration of white matter."[23] A variety of descriptive terms have since been used, including "shearing injury,"[24,25] diffuse damage of immediate impact type,"[26] "diffuse white matter shearing injury,"[27] "inner cerebral trauma,"[28] and, most recently, "diffuse axonal injury."[29] From the outset, Strich[23] attributed the degeneration of white matter to a shearing injury that affects nerve fibers at the time of injury. However, the concept of DAI as a form of primary brain damage has not gone unchallenged. Some workers have suggested that the damage to white matter is often due to hypoxia/ischemia or edema or is secondary to brainstem damage after an intracranial expanding lesion.[30,31] The situation has now been clarified in favor of Strich's views. Structural abnormalities identical to those seen in humans have been produced in a variety of species subjected to either fluid percussion[32–34] or nonimpact controlled angular acceleration of the head without any concomitant increase in intracranial pressure or hypoxia/ischemia.[35]

Severe cases of DAI have three distinctive features:

1. A focal lesion in the corpus callosum which usually extends over an anteroposterior distance of several centimeters lies to one side of the midline, often involving the interventricular septum, and is associated with intraventricular hemorrhage (Fig. 4-2).
2. Focal lesions of various sizes in the dorsolateral quadrants of the rostral brainstem adjacent to the superior cerebellar peduncles.
3. Microscopic evidence of widespread damage to axons.

The first two abnormalities can often be seen macroscopically in properly fixed and dissected brains, although the appearance of individual lesions depends on the length of survival after injury. For example, if the patient survives for only a few days, the lesions in the corpus callosum and brainstem are usually hemorrhagic; however, with the passage of time, they become soft and granular and ultimately are represented by shrunken, often cystic scars. The third component—diffuse injury to axons—can be seen only microscopically, with the histological appearance depending on the length of survival. If survival is short (days), numerous axonal swellings may be seen as eosinophilic masses on nerve fibers in sections stained by hematoxylin and eosin or as argyrophilic swellings in silver-stained preparations (Fig. 4-3). These swellings can also be demonstrated by immunohistochemistry.[36,37] They occur especially in the parasagittal white matter, the corpus callosum, the internal capsule, deep gray matter, and various tracts in the brainstem, including the medial lemnisci, the medial longitudinal bundles, the central tegmental tracts, and the corticospinal tracts.

In patients with intermediate survival (weeks), there are large numbers of small clusters of microglia throughout the white matter of the cerebral and cerebellar hemispheres and the brainstem; these clusters are associated with astrocytosis and lipid-filled macrophages. If the patient survives for several months or longer, the break-

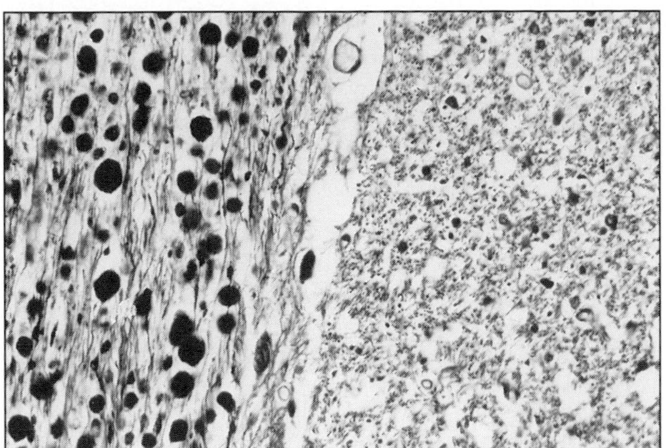

Figure 4-3. Diffuse axonal injury: axonal bulbs. There are axonal swellings in the brainstem, all on axons running in the same direction. Palmgren ×360.

down products of myelin can be detected by using the Marchi technique in the white matter of the cerebral and cerebellar hemispheres and the ascending and descending fiber tracts of the brainstem and spinal cord. A significant number of head-injured patients survive for long periods in a vegetative or severely disabled state. In these patients external abnormalities may be limited to small healed surface contusions at autopsy. On coronal section, the ventricles may be enlarged because of reduction in the white matter (Fig. 4-4). In some cases small cystic lesions may be seen in the corpus callosum and in or adjacent to one or both superior cerebellar peduncles. In microscopic DAI, microscopic abnormalities may be so difficult to identify that pathologists unaware of the syndrome may not establish the

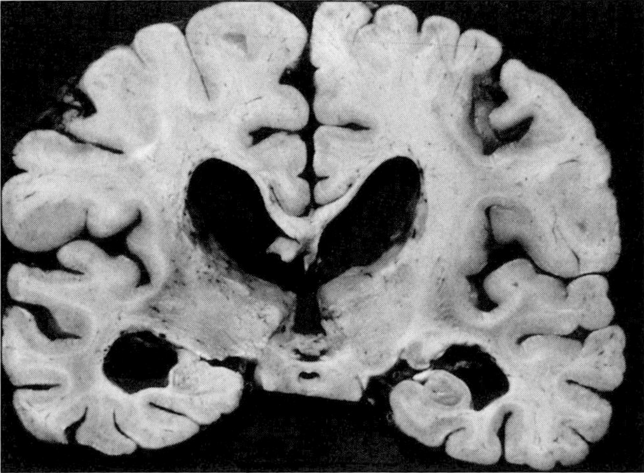

Figure 4-4. Diffuse axonal injury. There is generalized enlargement of the ventricles caused largely by loss of the centrum semiovale in a patient who survived for almost 2 years after a road traffic accident.

true nature of the condition unless the appropriate histological studies are undertaken.[38]

It is now apparent that patients with DAI form a distinct clinicopathologic group which at the severe end of the spectrum is characterized by a statistically significant lower incidence of lucid intervals, fractures of the skull, surface contusions, intracerebral hematomas, and evidence of a high ICP compared with patients who do not have this type of brain damage.[29] Gliding contusions[39] are often present, as are hematomas in the basal ganglia[40] and the hippocampi. Such lesions are particularly associated with road traffic accidents[29] but have also been described after an assault.[41,42] A small number of patients have suffered DAI from a fall from a height greater than their own.[43]

Grading of Diffuse Axonal Injury

The hypothesis that DAI may not represent an "all or nothing" phenomenon but may be part of a continuum of diffuse brain injury that ranges clinically from concussion up to and including persistent posttraumatic coma[44] has received support from the identification of less severe degrees of DAI in both humans and experimental animals. Pilz[45] described the occurrence of axonal swellings in human head injuries of varying severity, and as early as 1968 Oppenheimer[46] showed that occasional clusters of microglia can be found in patients dying from an unrelated cause soon after a minor head injury. Clark[47] also drew attention to the frequent occurrence of such clusters in the white matter in patients dying as a result of a head injury.

Strong support for this hypothesis has been provided by morphological studies after fluid percussion-induced head injury[32,33] and more recently in a model of axonal injury in the optic nerve.[48] In these studies, the earliest signs of axonal damage took the form of nodal blebs and varicosities which were thought to represent damage to axons at the node of Ranvier or to the cytoskeletons of axons at the time of injury with inhibition of axonal transport, thus leading to swellings at the point of injury.[34,49]

Support for the hypothesis has also been provided by a review of 122 cases of DAI in the Glasgow database.[50] In 10 cases there was microscopic evidence of axonal damage throughout the white matter of the brain; there was no focal accentuation in either the corpus callosum or the brainstem. These cases were referred to as grade 1 DAI. In 29 cases there was a focal lesion in the corpus callosum in addition to widely distributed axonal injury; the focal lesions were identified microscopically in only 11 of these cases. These cases were designated DAI grade 2. Eighty-three cases revealed focal lesions in both the corpus callosum and the dorsolateral quadrants of the rostral brainstem in addition to histological evidence of widely distributed axonal damage. These cases represent the most severe end of the spectrum and are referred to as grade 3 DAI. Thus, the severity of the DAI could be defined only by histological assessment in 24 of the 122 cases. Blumbergs et al.[51] also described a spectrum of axonal injury in fatal nonmissile head injuries in which they found that the hallmark of the more severe grades were lesions that could be seen macroscopically in the corpus callosum and the rostral brainstem. With the understanding that varying degrees of DAI may occur, it has been recognized that lesser degrees of axonal injury may be associated with either a completely or a partially lucid interval.[50] Among the 122 cases reviewed by Adams et al.,[50] there were 2 patients with grade 1 injuries who each had a completely lucid interval and 15 with grade 2 injuries who each experienced a partially lucid interval. None of the patients with grade 3 DAI talked, and all the patients who did talk after injury and subsequently died succumbed to the development of secondary complications.

Since it takes between 18 and 24 h for classic axonal bulbs to appear in the human brain, it is likely that the incidence of DAI is probably higher than the published figures suggest. This is being revealed by immunohistochemistry, which has demonstrated the presence of axonal swellings between 3[52] and 12 h[53] after an injury. However, caution must be exercised since axonal swellings and/or varicosities as demonstrated by conventional silver impregnation techniques can be induced artificially by handling unfixed tissue post mortem.[54] It has not been agreed that variation in axonal diameter without bulb formation but associated with an astrocytosis soon after head injury is diagnostic of DAI.[54,55] Although the definitive diagnosis of DAI cannot be made in patients who survive for only a short time after an injury, it may nevertheless be strongly suspected, particularly if there are focal lesions in the corpus callosum and in appropriate areas of the brainstem. The likelihood is even greater if there are gliding contusions and/or hematomas in the basal ganglia.

Concept of nondisruptive axotomy

Earlier studies in humans indicated that axons are torn at the time of injury, resulting in the extrusion of a ball of axoplasm into the extracellular space of the brain. However, immediate disruption of axons has not been identified by electron microscopy in experimental models of head injury[33] or in stretch preparations of the optic nerve of the guinea pig.[48,49] All these studies, however, have suggested that there is a process of delayed axonotomy in which actual disruption of some axons does not occur until hours after the original injury. Thus, the clinical severity and outcome depend not only on the total number of damaged axons but also on the proportion of disrupted to nondisrupted axons. This proportion obviously can change if secondary axonal damage occurs in nondisrupted axons, causing them to become disrupted (Fig. 4-5). This observation is important because if a means can be found to arrest this process, it may pave the way for the development of specific therapeutic interventions aimed at promoting axonal repair and eliminating secondary axonotomy to improve the outcome of DAI.

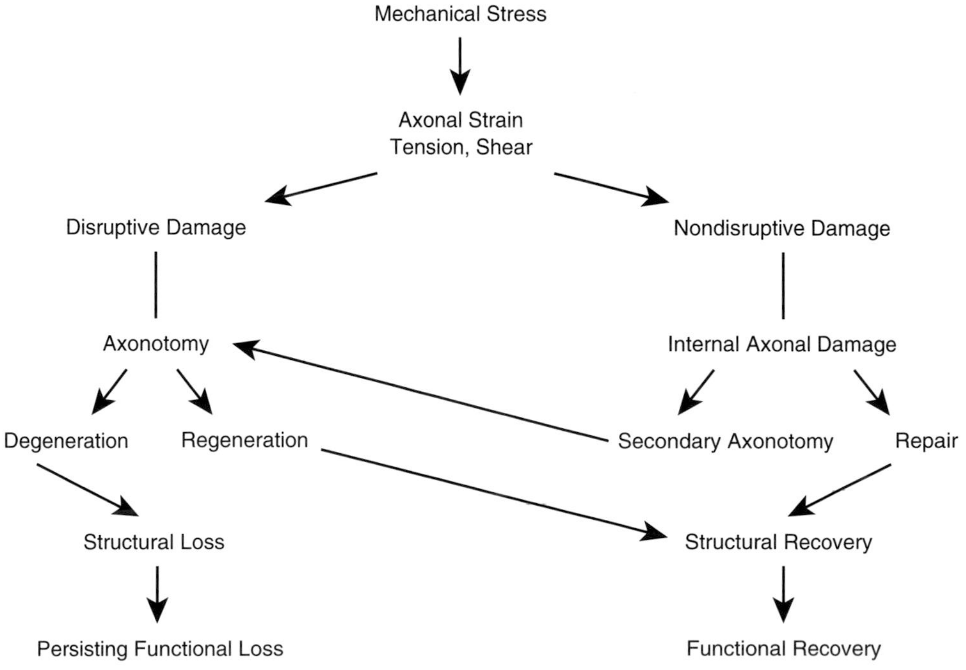

Figure 4-5. Schematic concept of diffuse axonal injury. From: Gennarelli TA, Adams JH, Graham DI: Diffuse axonal injury—a new conceptual approach to an old problem, in Baethmann A, Go KG, Unterberg A (eds): *Mechanisms of Secondary Brain Damage.* New York: Plenum Press, 1986: 15–28.

Vascular Lesions

In patients who die within minutes of a head injury, there are often multiple petechial hemorrhages throughout the cerebral hemispheres, particularly in the white matter of the frontal and temporal lobes and in the brainstem. This type of primary damage is now referred to as diffuse vascular injury.[7,56] The lesions are small and perivascular in distribution, with the source of bleeding being arterial, venous, or capillary. Many are identifiable macroscopically, but others can be recognized only by means of microscopy. Tomlinson[56] has suggested that such hemorrhages are not necessarily responsible for the death of the patient but are indicative of a type of damage that is incompatible with life. Under these circumstances, hemorrhages into the rostral brainstem are usually more numerous and severe than those in the medulla, although the latter may be severely affected in cases of traumatic hyperextension of the head or in patients with fracture dislocations of the atlanto-occipital joint.[57]

An occasional complication of an injury to the neck is traumatic thrombosis of a cervical artery.[58] The pathogenesis of the thrombosis is not always clear, but one precipitating mechanism is dissection in the wall of the blood vessel. It has been suggested that this may be caused by stretching of the artery when the neck is hyperextended at the time of injury. Subsequent thrombosis may lead to a massive cerebral infarction.

After injury to the neck, death may ensue rapidly as a result of massive subarachnoid hemorrhage due to traumatic rupture of a vertebral artery.[59] There is a variable bruise or laceration both below and behind one ear, and in some cases there is a fracture of the transverse process of the first cervical vertebra. The precise mechanism of the hemorrhage is not understood, but it appears that the vertebral artery in relation to the transverse process of the first cervical vertebra ruptures and that this is followed by massive subarachnoid hemorrhage. Most patients die very soon after injury; the striking post mortem feature is a severe and extensive subarachnoid hemorrhage in the posterior fossa. Caroticocavernous fistula is another uncommon sequel of head injury.

Primary Damage to the Brainstem

The term "primary damage to the brainstem" is often used by clinicians in referring to patients who are in coma from the moment of injury and do not have an intracranial expanding lesion. The term implies that the condition of the patient is due to focal primary damage to the brainstem. Although a number of cases have been described that suggest that this indeed is the case, in the author's experience it is a rare occurrence and the primary damage to the brainstem does not occur in isolation but is part of the clinicopathologic entity of DAI.

One type of primary damage to the brainstem consists of a tear at the junction between the pons and the medulla—the pontomedullary rent. In some instances there may be complete avulsion of the medulla from the pons, and there is often an associated ring fracture of the base of the skull with dislocation and/or fracture of the first or second cervical vertebra. Severe hyperextension of the head may be the pathogenetic factor in such cases.[60]

In a series of 988 autopsied fatalities caused by road accidents, Simpson et al.[61] found evidence of gross primary injury to the brainstem in 36 (3.6 percent). These cases fell into three groups: (1) 8 cases of pontomedullary tearing without other gross brain injury in 7 of which there were associated atlanto-occipital dislocations and/or high cervical fracture dislocations, (2) 17 cases of pontomedullary tearing associated with other brainstem lacerations and/or major damage elsewhere in the brain and a fracture of the base of the skull, and (3) 11 cases of brainstem lacerations in sites other than the pontomedullary junction, often with fracture of the skull thought to be induced by torsion of the calvaria.

Not all pontomedullary rents are immediately fatal. A number of patients have survived with clinical features suggestive of primary damage to the brainstem which were confirmed after death.[62–64]

Cranial Nerves

The most common deficit is loss of the sense of smell. This is not surprising in view of the relative severity of contusions that affect the undersurfaces of the frontal lobes and the frequency of fractures in the anterior fossae. Fractures of the orbit and anterior cranial fossae may be associated with damage to the optic nerves, and fractures that involve the petrous part of the temporal bone may damage the seventh and eighth cranial nerves[65] (see also Chap. 43).

Hypothalamus

There may be damage to the hypothalamus and pituitary gland. Occasionally, the pituitary stalk may be torn at the time of injury, resulting in massive infarction in the anterior lobe of the pituitary gland. However, it seems likely that most of the damage identified in the hypothalamus is secondary to elevated ICP, shift, and distortion in the brain[66] and to compression of the hypothalamo-hypophyseal portal vessels in the pituitary gland as a result of similar mechanisms.

Corpus Callosum

Lesions in the corpus callosum occur frequently.[67,68] It is not clear how many patients with these lesions also have DAI. In the author's experience, lesions within the corpus callosum are multifactorial in nature and include acute vascular injury, cerebral fat embolism, and infarction in the territory supplied by the pericallosal arteries, usually secondary to a supracallosal hernia.

Intracranial Hemorrhage

Intracranial hemorrhage is a common complication of a head injury, particularly in patients with a fracture of the skull, and is the most common cause of clinical deterioration and death in patients who experience a lucid interval after injury.[8,69–71] Traumatic intracranial hemorrhage is classified as follows:

1. Extradural (epidural) hematoma
2. Intradural hematoma
   a. Subdural hematoma
   b. Discrete intracerebral or intracerebellar hematoma not in continuity with the surface of the brain
   c. "Burst" lobe: an intracerebral or intracerebellar hematoma in continuity with the related subdural hematoma

Some degree of subarachnoid hemorrhage is invariably present in any serious head injury as a result of surface contusions. If the amount of hemorrhage is large, it may be a causative factor in the induction of the vasospasm that is frequently seen in the angiograms of patients with an acute head injury.[72] Large amounts of traumatically induced subarachnoid hemorrhage may cause an acute hydrocephalus, but in any patient in whom recovery is slower than expected, a delayed posttraumatic hydrocephalus should be ruled out.

CT scanning has shown that intracranial hematomas are often present long before they produce clinical deterioration; although some hematomas undoubtedly enlarge, the main effects of an intracranial hematoma are delayed because it is the associated swelling of the brain that is largely responsible for the subsequent events. The importance of intracranial hematomas as a source of secondary brain damage is emphasized by a study of patients who died although they had been able to talk after their head injuries.[9–11] The fact that they talked shows that these patients did not have severe diffuse primary brain damage, only to deteriorate and become unconscious later as a result of an expanding intracranial mass. This sequence of events is particularly characteristic of extradural hematomas, although some patients with acute subdural hematomas also have a similar clinical course.

CT scanning has made it possible to distinguish delayed hematomas from the development of a clot at the site of previous surgery. Thus, a delayed hematoma is usually defined as a lesion of increased attenuation developing in part of the brain or an intracranial cavity that the admission CT scan suggested was normal, even though in retrospect some abnormality is often recognized on the first CT scan. Such hematomas have been reported to occur in 1.5 to 7 percent of patients with a severe head injury.[73–75]

Some degree of intraventricular hemorrhage is a frequent occurrence, particularly in patients with DAI (see Diffuse Axonal Injury, above).

Extradural (Epidural) Hematoma

Extradural (epidural) hematoma occurs in approximately 2 percent of all types of injury.[4] In fatal head injuries, an epidural hematoma is found in between 5 percent[3] and 15 percent[2] of patients. It was present in 10 percent of the cases in the Glasgow database. A concomitant fracture of the skull is present in 85 percent of adult patients, but it is well recognized that epidural hematomas can occur in children in the absence of a fracture.

Epidural hematoma occurs most commonly in the temporal region; however, in 20 to 30 percent of cases it occurs elsewhere,[19,71] such as in the frontal and parietal regions or within the posterior fossa. Occasionally these hematomas are multiple. This type of hemorrhage results from torn meningeal blood vessels, and as the hematoma enlarges, it gradually strips the dura from the skull to form a circumscribed ovoid mass and progressively indents and flattens the adjacent brain (Fig. 4-6). Many extradural hematomas are associated with only

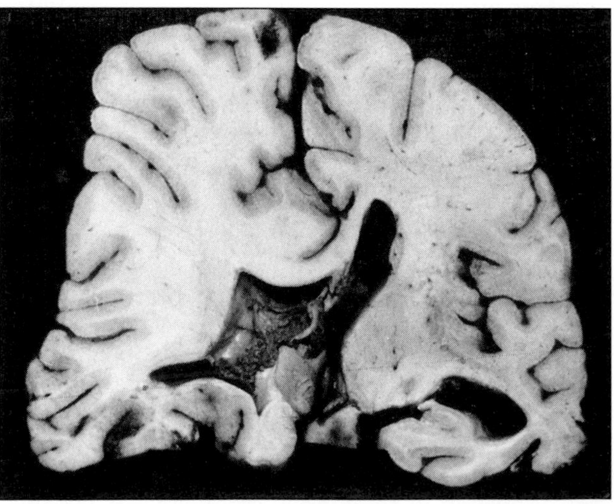

Figure 4-6. Extradural hematoma. Note the distortion and displacement of the brain produced by the hematoma.

minimal evidence of other types of brain damage if they are recognized and evacuated early.

With time, small hematomas become completely organized, but large hematomas may undergo partial organization, with their centers remaining cystic and filled with dark viscous fluid.[71] Studies have shown that the size of an extradural hematoma may increase by up to 50 percent during the first 10 to 14 days after injury; this is associated with liquefaction of the clot. After the second week, these hematomas become smaller and in the majority of patients are completely resolved by the fourth to sixth week after the injury.

In fire-related deaths where the head has been exposed to intense heat, there may be fissure fractures of the skull and heat hematomas in the extradural space. These artifactual hematomas have a pink spongy appearance which is said to be characteristic of thermal injury and may differ from the dark red appearance of the blood in an ordinary extradural hematoma. The pathogenesis of this type of hematoma is uncertain, although it has been assumed that the victim must have been alive in order for it to develop. The combination of extradural hematoma and fracture of the skull in fire victims may therefore cause difficulties in interpretation.

Intradural Hematoma

Subdural Hematomas

These hematomas are usually caused by rupture of the veins that bridge the subdural space where they connect the superior surfaces of the cerebral hemispheres to the sagittal sinus. Thin bilateral films of blood in the subdural space are common in acute fatal head injury, and in about 13 percent of cases the hematoma is pure with very little evidence of other brain damage. Because blood can spread freely throughout the subdural space, subdural hematomas tend to cover the entire hemisphere and are more extensive than extradural hematomas. Some subdural hematomas are arterial in origin, with the hemorrhage stemming from a cortical artery.[71]

Subdural hematomas thought to be large enough to act as significant mass lesions have been reported in 26 percent[3] and 63 percent[2] of nonmissile head injuries. In 8 percent of the cases in the Glasgow database, the hematoma was pure, acting in many respects like an extradural hematoma; however, most cases are associated with considerable brain damage, and therefore the mortality and morbidity are greater in subdural than in extradural hematomas (Fig. 4-7). A "burst" lobe was present in 23 percent of the Glasgow cases.

Subdural hematoma is the most common type of intracranial injury found in infants subjected to nonaccidental injury.[76] They are often associated with skeletal injuries. The hematoma may contain some blood clot consisting of encapsulated xanthochromic fluid. This is sometimes referred to as a subdural hygroma.

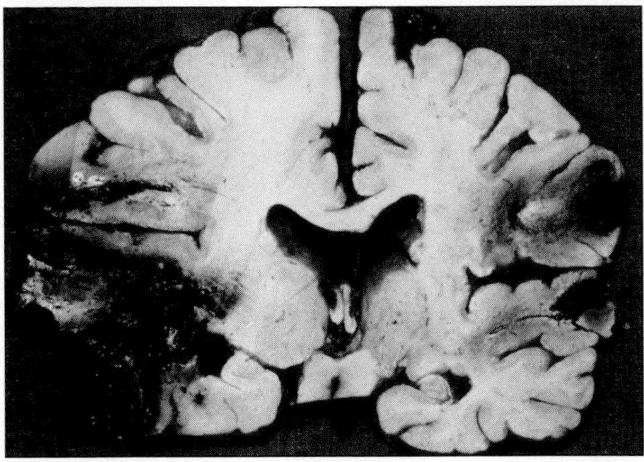

Figure 4-7. Intradural hematoma: "burst" lobe. The hematoma in the left temporal lobe was in continuity with an acute subdural hematoma. In addition, there are contusions over the lateral aspect of the right cerebral hemisphere.

Subdural hematomas have long been defined as acute, subacute, or chronic. There is no uniformity of nomenclature.[17,71] Attempts to age hematomas on the basis of histological studies have not proved satisfactory. Current opinion is moving toward classifying a subdural hematoma as acute when the hematoma is composed of clot and blood (usually within the first 48 h after an injury), subacute when there is a mixture of clotted and fluid blood (developing between 2 and 14 days after the injury), and chronic when the hematoma is fluid (developing more than 14 days after the injury).[17,71]

The blood remains clotted for at least 48 h and sometimes several days; thereafter, there is a mixture of blood clot and fluid blood. After about 3 weeks no clot remains. The characteristic neuropathologic observation is that despite the presence of an acute or subacute subdural hematoma and distortion of the brain, the gyral and sulcal pattern on the side of the hematoma is preserved; that is, there is no convolutional flattening, although there is marked flattening of the convolutions of the contralateral hemisphere. This occurs because the subdural blood is in contact with both gyri and sulci and therefore exerts uniform compression on the subjacent brain, preventing flattening of its surface. In about 25 percent of patients who undergo evacuation of an acute subdural hematoma, acute brain swelling occurs in the hemisphere beneath the clot and carries a bad prognosis.[77]

In a study of pure acute subdural hematoma, Gennarelli and Thibault[78] found that in 72 percent of patients the head injury was produced by a fall or an assault; in only 24 percent was the cause a road traffic accident. These figures are in marked contrast to patients without mass lesions who had been in coma for more than 24 h—i.e., patients with diffuse brain damage—90 percent of whom were injured in road traffic accidents and only 10 percent of whom suffered falls or assaults.

Chronic subdural hematomas typically present weeks or months after what may appear to have been a trivial head injury. The hematoma, which ultimately becomes encapsulated in a membrane, increases in size slowly, probably as a result of repeated small hemorrhages into it. It eventually becomes large enough to produce distortion and herniation of the brain. Chronic subdural hematoma is particularly common in older individuals in whom there is already some cerebral atrophy. As the hematoma slowly expands, the period of spatial compensation may be long enough to cause considerable distortion of the brain before there is a significant rise in ICP.

Intracerebral Hematomas

These hematomas are present in 16 percent of the cases in the Glasgow database. They are often multiple but occur most commonly in the frontal and temporal lobes,[71] although they may also occur deep within the hemispheres. They are found less commonly in the cerebellum. Their pathogenesis is not clear, but it seems likely that they are caused by the direct rupture of intracerebral vessels at the time of injury. Sometimes traumatic intracerebral hematomas develop several days after the injury, and the recognition of this possibility may have important medicolegal implications if the patient dies.

As a result of CT scanning, there is greater recognition of relatively small hematomas deeply seated in the brain. Patients with this type of hematoma have an increased incidence of gliding contusions and DAI (see Diffuse Axonal Injury, above), so that patients found to have a basal ganglia hematoma on CT shortly after a head injury are likely to have sustained diffuse brain damage at the time of injury. However, there are other cases of this pattern of deep hematoma formation in which evidence of DAI cannot be found.

If a solitary hematoma is found in the brain of a patient who has suffered a head injury, the possibility that it is due to either a hypertensive bleed or the rupture of a saccular aneurysm which resulted in the head injury should be considered. Interpretation of the findings post mortem can be difficult or even impossible, and much depends on the site of the hematoma. However, if the hemorrhage is in the subfrontal or temporal region, it is more likely to be traumatic than spontaneous.[79] Even when all the possibilities have been taken into consideration, it may be difficult to reach a final conclusion with regard to the primary event.

"Burst" Lobe

The term "burst" lobe describes an intracerebral or intracerebellar hematoma in continuity with a subdural hematoma. It is presumed to be due to hemorrhage from superficial cortical vessels. It was present in 23 percent of the cases in the Glasgow database and occurred most commonly in the frontal and temporal lobes.

SECONDARY DAMAGE

Secondary damage is most often associated with brain swelling, ischemia, and elevated intracranial pressure.

Brain Swelling

Brain swelling occurs frequently in association with head injury. It may be localized or generalized and may occur either alone or in combination with other pathological conditions. Furthermore, it may contribute to an elevation of ICP and death from secondary damage to the brainstem. The cause of the swelling is not always clear, but in general it is due to an increase in the cerebral blood volume (congestive brain swelling) or in the water content of the brain tissue (cerebral edema). There are three principal types of brain swelling: (1) swelling adjacent to contusions, (2) diffuse swelling of one cerebral hemisphere, and (3) diffuse swelling of both cerebral hemispheres.

Swelling of the Brain Adjacent to Contusions, Lacerations, or an Intracerebral Hematoma

In these contusions swelling of the brain is common and is due to physical disruption of the tissue. As a result of damage to the blood-brain barrier, water, electrolytes, and macromolecules leak into brain tissue and spread into the adjacent white matter to form vasogenic edema.[80] This edema can be detected by CT or MRI within 24 to 48 h of injury in many cases and appears to be maximal between days 4 and 8 after a head injury (Fig. 4-8). According to Wahl et al.,[81] for vasogenic brain edema to develop to the point where it causes mass effect, three conditions must be fulfilled: (1) increased capillary permeability, (2) a continuous force driving fluid out from the vessels into the interstitial space of the brain, and (3) retention of the fluid in the interstitial space. When there is actual physical disruption of blood

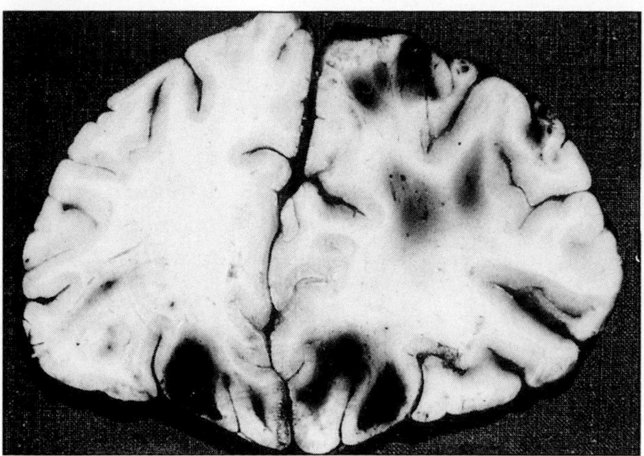

Figure 4-8. Brain swelling. There is considerable swelling of the right frontal lobe in association with contusions.

vessels, it is easy to envisage how this type of edema may develop, but there are many instances in which capillary permeability is increased in the absence of a known physical disruption. Under these circumstances, other mechanisms operate, including the opening of the tight junctions between endothelial cells and increased pinocytosis.[82]

Hydrostatic and osmotic forces are also responsible for driving fluid from the vascular bed into the interstitial space.[83] The rate at which fluid accumulates is determined by a combination of tissue compliance and the amount of protein that accumulates in the fluid.

Diffuse Swelling of One Cerebral Hemisphere

Swelling of one hemisphere is most often seen in association with an ipsilateral acute subdural hematoma.[6,77] When the hematoma is evacuated, the brain expands to fill the space. Situations similar to this have been seen in experimental studies and have been attributed to engorgement of a nonreactive vascular bed secondary to cerebral ischemia produced by high ICP.[84] However, the pathogenesis of this entity has not been fully ascertained.

Diffuse Swelling of Both Cerebral Hemispheres

Diffuse swelling of both hemispheres tends to appear particularly among young patients.[6,85] The pathogenesis of this type of brain swelling is not clear, but it seems possible that loss of vasomotor tone and consequent vasodilatation contributes to the swelling.[86,87] As was described previously, if vasodilatation persists, the blood-brain barrier may become defective, leading to true vasogenic edema. However, widespread cerebral edema has not been demonstrated consistently on MRI.[88–90]

After death, the brain is swollen diffusely and the ventricles are small and symmetrical.[91] In a detailed neuropathologic study of 63 children after head injury in the Glasgow database, diffuse brain swelling was found in 17 percent of cases.[92] In a few cases, swelling was associated with widespread ischemic brain damage secondary to posttraumatic status epilepticus or cardiorespiratory arrest. However, it is not clear from this study whether the swelling is due to the associated structural damage or simply adds further insult to an already damaged brain.

Ischemic Brain Damage

Ischemic brain damage is common in patients dying as a result of a nonmissile head injury. Just how common it is was not appreciated until a detailed study of 151 cases reported in 1978 revealed an incidence of 91 percent.[93] In this study, ischemic damage was assessed as being severe in 27 percent of patients, moderately severe in 43 percent, and mild in 30 percent. The highest incidence of ischemic damage was seen in the hippocampus (80 percent),[94] the basal ganglia (79 percent), and the cerebellum (44 percent). Ischemic damage was seen in the cerebral cortex in 46 percent of cases, either centered on or accentuated in the boundary zones, particularly between the anterior and middle cerebral arterial territories, or widespread throughout the neocortical ribbon.

A subsequent study published in 1989 established the fact that ischemic brain damage is still common in fatal nonmissile head injuries.[85] Although there was no statistical difference in the incidence of moderate to severe ischemic brain damage between the two reports, in the second study there was an increase in the number of patients with diffuse ischemic brain damage. Overall, the findings suggested that there had been an improvement in the early management of head injury, with less of the type of damage caused by systemic hypotension. There is increasing evidence that this type of brain damage occurs soon after injury.[95] Also, if an infarct is found in the brain of a head-injured patient, the possibility that this is the primary and hence precipitating injury has to be considered.

The pathogenesis of ischemic brain damage is not fully understood. According to Graham et al.,[93] it was more common in patients who sustained a known clinical episode of hypoxia [defined as systolic blood pressure less than 80 mmHg for 15 min or a Pa_{O_2} of 6.7 kPa (50 mmHg)] at some time after the injury than in those who did not. It was also more common in patients who experienced high ICP.[96] However, ischemic brain damage may occur without the ICP being high.[97] There is also a statistically significant correlation between ischemic brain damage and the presence of cerebral arterial spasm.[72] Postmortem studies have shown that an insufficient supply of oxygen to the brain is not uncommon in patients who have sustained a fatal head injury. Indeed, it may be the principal pathological finding in patients who remain vegetative or severely disabled after a head injury.[98] There is an awareness that at least some of the ischemic damage is avoidable, including factors such as obstruction of the airway, poorly controlled epilepsy, hypertension, and delay in the treatment of intracranial hematomas. Recent findings of silent episodes of cerebral ischemia as determined by jugular oxygen desaturation tie in nicely with these pathological data and begin to explain the frequency with which ischemic changes are seen in the brains of head-injured patients (see Chap. 36). Every effort must be made to reduce this potentially preventable complication of head injury.

Brain Damage Secondary to Elevated Intracranial Pressure

Brain damage secondary to elevated ICP is a common complication in patients who sustain a nonmissile head injury. There is deformation of brain tissue and a reduction in the volume of CSF within the skull as the mass enlarges. Shift and distortion in the brain occur, and herniation may eventually result in the intact skull. A space-occupying lesion in one cerebral hemisphere may result in herniation of the cingulate gyrus under the free edge of the falx or herniation of the parahippocampal gyrus of the medial part of the temporal lobe through the opening of the tentorium cerebelli. Space-occupying lesions in the cerebellum may result in herniation of the cerebellar tonsil through the foramen magnum. As herniation occurs, the cisterns are obliterated and pressure gradients develop between the various intracranial compartments. In addition, vascular lesions such as hemorrhage and ischemic necrosis of the brain are significant secondary complications. Using the previously defined structural criterion of pressure necrosis in one or both parahippocampal gyri,[99] which allows the pathologist to state with a reasonable degree of certainty whether ICP had been high during life, Graham et al. established that the ICP had been high in 75 percent (324 of 434) of patients with a fatal head injury.[96] The usual causes were intracranial hematoma and brain swelling, and the most common postmortem findings were secondary damage in the brainstem in the form of midline hemorrhages and/or infarction, followed by variable degrees of ischemic damage within particular arterial territories.

Principal among the infarcts were those within the distribution of one or both posterior cerebral arteries. This would typically result in cortical blindness and, in certain cases, Anton's syndrome (cortical blindness with denial of the deficit). Less commonly, infarctions were also seen within the distribution of the anterior cerebral, anterior choroidal, and superior cerebellar arteries. In 45 percent of cases, there was evidence of infarction in the anterior lobe of the pituitary gland.

In a series of 36 patients who survived more than 4 weeks after injury, neuropathologic studies found that there was not one case in which the clinical state could be attributed solely to secondary damage to the brainstem.[100] The two most common findings were DAI and diffuse ischemic damage. This study suggests that patients with secondary damage to the brainstem rarely survive for more than a few weeks. Among the cases in the Glasgow database without evidence of a high ICP, the most common types of brain damage were again DAI and ischemic brain damage.[97] However, such brain damage may not be easy to identify unless the specimen has been properly fixed before dissection and the appropriate histological studies have been undertaken.

Infection

Meningitis is a well-recognized complication after head injury and is usually associated with a basal fracture of the skull. If there is also a dural tear, CSF rhinorrhea or otorrhea may develop. In such cases, meningitis is not necessarily restricted to the early posttraumatic period but may be delayed many months or even years. A small traumatic fistula may also cause recurrent episodes of meningitis. Subdural or intracerebral abscesses are uncommon complications of nonmissile head injuries but are more common after penetrating injuries.

Fat Embolism

Extremity fractures are frequently present in patients who sustain a severe head injury, placing them at risk of developing a systemic fat embolism. Fat emboli can be demonstrated in the lungs of 90 to 100 percent of patients with fractures. Intravascular fat embolism is common, but clinically significant fat embolism is rare. At the site of fracture, fat from the marrow enters damaged veins in the form of small globules. If these fat globules are sufficiently numerous, some will not be trapped in the pulmonary circulation and will enter the systemic circulation as a potential source of cerebral embolism.[101]

The neuropathology of cerebral fat embolism has been reviewed.[102] In cases of fulminating fat embolism, the brain of a patient who has died within a day or two of injury may appear entirely normal macroscopically. However, in patients surviving 3 or 4 days, the white matter of the brain may be diffusely studded with petechial hemorrhages, although the majority of histological fat emboli are seen in gray matter because of its extensive vascular network. Fewer emboli are seen in white matter, where damage is greatest because many of the vessels are end arteries with poor collateral circulation. Histologically, there may be foci of myelin pallor or perivascular infarcts infiltrated by polymorphonuclear leukocytes. After survival for several days, changes may be found in the gray matter. In a case where the patient survived for a week,[103] there were multiple foci of necrosis chiefly in the deeper layers of the cortex and the cerebellum. Fat globules were present in the capillaries of both altered and normal brain. In a patient who survived for 12 days, Winkelman[104] found small infarcts in the deeper layers of the cortex in the white matter (especially in the frontal lobes) and the brainstem (especially the pons). In a case where the patient survived for 34 days, there was edema, multiple small hemorrhagic infarcts, and gliosis.[105] In patients who survived from 3 months to 7 years, there was gross atrophy of the cerebral white matter.[106–108] Therefore, in patients who die of multiple injuries, the brain should be screened routinely for fat embolism.

Progressive Neurological Disease

Diseases in which the possibility of a connection with head injury has been reported include Pick's disease,[109] Parkinsons's disease,[110] motor neuron disease, and Creutzfeldt-Jakob disease.[111] However, there is no convincing evidence that there is a direct correlation between any of these diseases and a previous head injury.

It is well recognized, however, that persons subjected to large numbers of concussive or subconcussive blows, such as boxers, sometimes develop neurological signs and progressive dementia.[112–114] This condition is often referred to as the "punch-drunk" syndrome (dementia pugilistica) and may not develop until years after the last injury. It usually develops in boxers with long careers who have been dazed or knocked out on many occasions. The pathogenesis of the brain damage is not understood, but it is characterized by defects in the interventricular septum, thinning of the corpus callosum, enlargement of the lateral ventricles, degeneration of the substantia nigra, and the presence of many neurofibrillary tangles throughout the cerebral cortex and the brainstem.[115] Recently, the cases originally reported by Corsellis et al.[115] have been reexamined by immunohistochemical methods, using an antibody to the beta amyloid protein present in neuritic plaques.[116] This revealed the presence of extensive beta amyloid protein immunoreactive deposits in the form of diffuse plaques; these deposits were not identified with Congo Red or standard silver stains. Thus, in addition to the neurofibrillary tangles identifiable by standard histological techniques, substantial deposition of beta amyloid protein has been found in the brains of patients with the punch-drunk syndrome. It is conceivable that this syndrome and the dementia of Alzheimer's disease share common pathogenetic mechanisms that lead to the formation of tangles and plaques.[117,118]

Hydrocephalus

A further complication of nonmissile head injury is posttraumatic hydrocephalus. In the acute phase, this is likely to be due to large amounts of blood within the subarachnoid space, whereas with survival, the ventricular enlargement is probably secondary to fibrosis and hemosiderosis of the meninges. In either case, the basic problem is an impairment of CSF absorption via the arachnoid granulations into the superior sagittal sinus. However, in patients who survive a nonmissile head injury, ventricular enlargement, whether symmetrical or asymmetrical, is likely to be due to a number of other pathological conditions. For example, in patients with DAI or severe ischemic brain damage, the ventricles enlarge as a result of loss of brain tissue. Thus, pathologically, as is the case clinically, the distinction between posttraumatic hydrocephalus and ex vacuo ventriculomegaly is not always clear.

THE AUTOPSY

From the above account, it should be apparent that there are various types of brain damage in nonmissile head injury, many of which are subtle. Too often, death is certified as being due to a fracture of the skull and cerebral contusions even though neither may be the reason for the patient being in coma. The great majority of patients with a fracture of the skull and even patients with severe cerebral contusions may make an excellent recovery if no other type of brain damage is present.

Pathologists must be present when the skull is opened so that the location and size of an intracranial hematoma can be accurately noted. The volume of the hematoma should be measured, since hematomas smaller than about 35 ml are unlikely to have caused a significant mass effect unless there was associated brain swelling. Pathologists should also assess the tightness of the dura, since this is a useful method of determining whether ICP was high during life.

In many severe head injuries, the cause of the fatal outcome may be immediately apparent, for example, if there is an intracranial hematoma, evidence of brain swelling, and secondary hemorrhage in the brainstem. Even in these patients there may be other types of brain damage. However, the pathologist may find a brain of almost entirely normal appearance while the clinical history clearly indicates that the patient died from a nonmissile head injury. The worst thing to do in such circumstances is to slice the unfixed brain, as it may be difficult to identify focal lesions of the corpus callosum or rostral brainstem and evidence suggestive of ischemic damage. Furthermore, ventricular size and displacement caused, for example, by swelling are almost impossible to assess. Even if the brain is sliced unfixed, it must be screened for diffuse axonal injury, ischemic brain damage, and fat embolism. The presence or absence of a fat embolism may easily be established by taking two or three blocks for frozen sections. To establish the presence of DAI or ischemic brain damage, tissue from the arterial boundary zones, the parasagittal white matter, the corpus callosum, the hippocampi, the cerebellum, and several levels of the brainstem must be examined histologically.

If a patient has survived in coma or is vegetative for weeks or months after a head injury, the most likely causes of brain damage are DAI and ischemic brain damage, since most patients who sustain secondary damage in the brainstem rarely survive for more than a few weeks. The situation should be clarified by a histological survey; however, if the patient has survived for more than 2 months after the injury, the need for identifying long tract degeneration in Marchi preparations has to be emphasized.

References

1. Lindenberg R, Freytag E: A mechanism of cerebral contusions: A pathologic-anatomic study. *Arch Pathol* 69:440, 1960.
2. Freytag E: Autopsy findings in head injuries from blunt forces. *Arch Pathol* 75:402, 1963.
3. Maloney AJF, Whatmore WJ: Clinical and pathological observations in fatal head injuries—a 5-year study of 172 cases. *Br J Surg* 56:23, 1969.
4. Lindenberg R: Trauma of meninges and brain, in Minckler J (ed): *Pathology of the Nervous System,* vol 2. New York: McGraw-Hill, 1971:1705–1765.
5. Hardman JM: The pathology of traumatic brain injuries, in Thompson RA, Green JR (eds): *Advances in Neurology,* vol 22: *Complications of Nervous System Trauma.* New York: Raven Press, 1979:15–50.
6. Adams JH, Graham DI, Scott G, et al: Brain damage in non-missile head injury. *J Clin Pathol* 33:1132, 1980.
7. Adams JH: Brain damage in fatal non-missile head injury in man, in Brakkman R (ed): *Handbook of Clinical Neurology,* vol 13: *Head Injury.* Amsterdam: Elsevier, 1990:43–63.
8. Reilly PL, Graham DI, Adams JH, Jennett B: Patients with head injury who talk and die. *Lancet* 2:375, 1975.
9. Marshall LF, Toole BM, Bowers SA: The national coma data bank: Patients who talk and deteriorate: Implications for treatment. *J Neurosurg* 59:285, 1983.
10. Rose J, Valtonen S, Jennett B: Avoidable factors contributing to death after head injury. *Br Med J* 2:615, 1977.
11. Dacey RG, Alves WM, Jane JA: Neurosurgical complications after apparently minor head injury: Assessment of risk in a series of 610 patients. *J Neurosurg* 65:203, 1986.
12. Gentry LR, Godersky JC, Thompson B: MR imaging of head trauma: Review of the distribution and radiopathologic features of traumatic lesions. *Am J Neuroradiol* 9:101, 1988.
13. Teasdale G, Teasdale E, Hadley D: Computed tomographic and magnetic resonance imaging classification of head injury, in Jane JA, Anderson DK, Torner JC, Young W (eds): Central nervous system trauma status report 1991. *J Neurotrauma* 9(Suppl 1):S249, 1992.
14. Marshall LF, Marshall SB, Klauber MR, et al: The diagnosis of head injury requires a classification based on computed axial tomography. *J Neurotrauma* 9(Suppl 1):S287, 1992.
15. Genneralli TA, Thibault LE: Biological models of head injury, in Becker JP, Povlishock JT (eds): *Central Nervous System Trauma Status Report.* Bethesda, MD: NINCDS, 1985:391–404.
16. Graham DI, Adams JH, Gennarelli TA: Mechanisms of nonpenetrating head injury, in Bond RF (ed): *Perspectives in Shock Research. Progress in Clinical and Biological Research,* vol 264. New York: Liss, 1988:159–168.
17. Jennett B, Teasdale G: *Management of Head Injuries.* Philadelphia: Davis, 1981.
18. Mendelow AD, Teasdale G, Jennett B: Risks of intracranial hematoma in head injured adults. *Br Med J* 287:1173, 1983.
19. Cooper PR: Post traumatic intracranial mass lesions, in Cooper PR (ed): *Head Injury* (3d ed). Philadelphia: Williams & Wilkins, 1993:275–329.
20. Adams JH, Doyle D, Graham DI, et al: The contusion index: A reappraisal in human and experimental nonmissile head injury. *Neuropathol Appl Neurobiol* 11:299, 1985.
21. Simpson DA, Ryan EA, Paix BR et al: Brain injuries in car occupants: A correlation of impact data with neuropathological findings. In: Proceedings of International Conference on the Biomechanics of Impact. Bron: International Research Council on Biomechanics on Impact. 1991, pp 89–100.
22. McLellan DR, Adams JH, Graham DI: The structural basis of the vegetative state and prolonged coma after

non-missile head injury, in Papo I, Cohadon F, Massarotti M (eds): *Le Coma Traumatique.* Padova: Liviana Editrice, 1986:165.
23. Strich SJ: Diffuse degeneration of the cerebral white matter in severe dementia following head injury. *J Neurol Neurosurg Psychiatry* 19:163, 1956.
24. Peerless SJ, Rewcastle NB: Shear injuries of the brain. *Can Med Assoc J* 96:577, 1967.
25. Strich SJ: Shearing of nerve fibres as a cause of brain damage due to head injury. *Lancet* 2:443, 1961.
26. Adams JH, Mitchell DE, Graham DI, Doyle D: Diffuse brain damage of immediate impact type. *Brain* 100:489, 1977.
27. Zimmerman RA, Larissa T, Bilaniuk LT, Gennarelli TA: Computed tomography of shearing injuries of the cerebral white matter. *Radiology* 127:393, 1978.
28. Grcevic N: The concept of inner cerebral trauma. *Scand J Rehabil Med* 25(Suppl 17):25, 1988.
29. Adams JH, Graham DI, Murray LS, Scott G: Diffuse axonal injury due to non-missile head injury in humans: An analysis of 45 cases. *Ann Neurol* 12:557, 1982.
30. Jellinger K, Seitelberger F: Protraced post-traumatic encephalopathy: Pathology, pathogenesis and clinical implications. *J Neurol Sci* 10:51, 1970.
31. Peters G, Rothemund E: Neuropathology of the traumatic apallic syndrome, in Ore GD, Gerstenbrand F, Lucking CH, et al (eds): *The Apallic Syndrome.* Berlin: Springer-Verlag, 1977:78–87.
32. Povlishock JT, Becker DP, Cheng CLY, Vavehan CW: Axonal change in minor head injury. *J Neuropathol Exp Neurol* 42:225, 1983.
33. Erb DE, Povlishock JT: Axonal damage in severe traumatic brain injury: An experimental study in the cat. *Acta Neuropathol* (*Berl*) 76:347, 1988.
34. Povlishock JT: Traumatically induced axonal injury: Pathogenesis and pathobiological implications. *Brain Pathol* 2:1, 1992.
35. Gennarelli TA, Thibault LE, Adams JH, et al: Diffuse axonal injury and traumatic coma in the primate. *Ann Neurol* 12:564, 1982.
36. Grady MS, McLaughlin MR, Christman CW, et al: The use of antibodies targeted against the neurofilament subunits for the detection of diffuse axonal injury in humans. *J Neuropathol Exp Neurol* 52:143, 1993.
37. Gentleman SM, Nash MJ, Sweeting CJ, et al: Beta amyloid precursor protein (BAPP) as a marker for axonal injury after head injury. *Neurosci Lett* 160:139, 1993.
38. Adams JH, Doyle D, Graham DI, et al: Microscopic diffuse axonal injury in cases of head injury. *Med Sci Law* 25:265, 1985.
39. Adams JH, Doyle D, Graham DI, et al: Gliding contusions in non-missile head injury in humans. *Arch Pathol Lab Med* 110:485, 1986.
40. Adams JH, Doyle D, Graham DI, et al: Deep intracerebral (basal ganglia) hematomas in fatal non-missile head injury in man. *J Neurol Neurosurg Psychiatry* 49:1039, 1986.
41. Imajo T, Challener RC, Roessman U: Diffuse axonal injury by assault. *Am J Forensic Med Pathol* 8:217, 1987.
42. Graham DI, Clark JC, Adams JH, Gennarelli TA: Diffuse axonal injury caused by assault. *J Clin Pathol* 45:840, 1992.
43. Adams JH, Doyle D, Graham DI, et al: Diffuse axonal injury in head injuries caused by a fall. *Lancet* 2:1420, 1984.
44. Gennarelli TA: Cerebral concussion and diffuse brain injuries, in Cooper PR (ed): *Head Injury* (3d ed). Philadelphia: Williams & Wilkins, 1993:137–158.
45. Pilz P: Axonal Injury in head injury. *Acta Neurochir* (*Wien*) [*Suppl*] 32:119, 1983.
46. Oppenheimer DR: Microscopic lesions in the brain following head injury. *J Neurol Neurosurg Psychiatry* 31:299, 1968.
47. Clark JM: Distribution of microglial clusters in the brain after head injury. *J Neurol Neurosurg Psychiatry* 37:463, 1974.
48. Gennarelli TA, Thibault LE, Tipperman R, et al: Axonal injury in the optic nerve: A model simulating diffuse axonal injury in the brain. *J Neurosurg* 71:244, 1989.
49. Maxwell WL, Irvine A, Graham D, et al: Focal axonal injury: The early axonal response to stretch. *J Neurocytol* 20:157, 1991.
50. Adams JH, Doyle D, Ford I, et al: Diffuse axonal injury in head injury: Definition, diagnosis and grading. *Histopathology* 15:49, 1989.
51. Blumbergs PC, Jones NR, North JB: Diffuse axonal injury in head trauma. *J Neurol Neurosurg Psychiatry* 52:838, 1989.
52. Sherriff FE, Bridges LR, Sivaloganathan S: Early detection of axonal injury after human head trauma using immunocytochemistry for beta amyloid precursor protein. *Acta Neuropathol* 88:433, 1994 (*Berl*) 88:433, 1994.
53. Yaghamai A, Povlishock JT: Traumatically induced reactive change as visualized through the use of monoclonal antibodies targeted to neurofilament subunits. *J Neuropathol Exp Neurol* 51:158, 1992.
54. Crooks DA: The pathological concept of diffuse axonal injury: Its pathogenesis and the assessment of severity. *J Pathol* 165:5, 1991.
55. Vanezis P, Chan KK, Scholtz CL: White matter damage following acute head injury. *Forensic Sci Int* 35:1, 1987.
56. Tomlinson BE: Brain stem lesions after head injury, in Sevitt S, Stoner HB (eds): *The Pathology of Trauma. J Clin Pathol* 23(Suppl):154, 1970.
57. Lindenberg R, Freytag E: Brainstem lesions characteristic of traumatic hyperextension of the head. *Arch Pathol* 90:509, 1970.
58. Batjer HH, Giller CA, Kopitnik TA, Purdy PD: Intracranial and cervical vascular injuries, in Cooper PR (ed): *Head Injury* (3d ed). Philadelphia: Williams & Wilkins, 1993:373–403.
59. Harland WA, Pitts JF, Watson AA: Subarachnoid hemorrhage due to upper cervical trauma. *J Clin Pathol* 36:1335, 1983.
60. Kakulas BA, Taylor JR: Pathology of injuries of the vertebral column and spinal cord, in Frankel HL (ed): *Handbook of Clinical Neurology,* vol 17: *Spinal Cord Trauma.* Amsterdam: Elsevier, 1992:21–51.
61. Simpson DA, Blumbergs PC, Cooter RD, et al: Pon-

tomedullary tears and other gross brainstem injuries after vehicular accidents. *J Trauma* 29:1519, 1989.
62. Britt RH, Herrick MK, Mason RT, Dorfman LJ: Traumatic lesions of the pontomedullary junction. *Neurosurgery* 6:623, 1980.
63. Pilz P: Survival after traumatic lesions of the pontomedullary junction: Report of 4 cases. *Acta Neurochir (Wien)* 32(Suppl):77, 1983.
64. Zampella EJ, Duvall ER, Langford KH: Computed tomography and magnetic resonance imaging in traumatic locked-in syndrome. *Neurosurgery* 22:591, 1988.
65. Rovit RL, Murali R: Injuries of the cranial nerves, in Cooper PR (ed): *Head Injury* (3d ed). Philadelphia: Williams & Wilkins, 1993:183–202.
66. Harper CG, Doyle D, Adams JH, Graham DI: Analysis of abnormalities in the pituitary gland in non-missile head injury. *J Clin Pathol* 39:769, 1986.
67. Lindenberg R, Fisher R, Durlacher SH, et al: Lesions of the corpus callosum following blunt mechanical trauma to the head. *Am J Pathol* 31:297, 1955.
68. Komatsu S, Sato T, Kagawa S, et al: Traumatic lesions of the corpus callosum. *Neurosurgery* 5:32, 1979.
69. Rockswold GL, Leonard PR, Nagib ME: Analysis of management in thirty-three closed injury patients who "talked and deteriorated." *Neurosurgery* 21:51, 1987.
70. Klauber MR, Marshall LF, Luerssen TG, et al: Determinants of head injury mortality: Importance of the low risk patient. *Neurosurgery* 24:31, 1989.
71. Bullock R, Teasdale G: Surgical management of traumatic intracranial hematomas, in Braackman R (ed): *Handbook of Clinical Neurology,* vol 15: *Head Injury.* Amsterdam: Elsevier, 1990:249–298.
72. Macpherson P, Graham DI: Correlation between angiographic findings and the ischemia of head injury. *J Neurol Neurosurg Psychiatry* 41:122, 1978.
73. Baratham G, Dennyson WG: Delayed traumatic intracranial hemorrhage. *J Neurol Neurosurg Psychiatry* 25:698, 1985.
74. Gentleman D, Nath F, MacPherson P: Diagnosis and management of delayed traumatic intracerebral hematoma. *Br J Neurosurg* 3:367, 1985.
75. Gudeman SK, Kishore PR, Miller JD, et al: The genesis and significance of delayed traumatic intracerebral hematoma. *Neurosurgery* 5:304, 1979.
76. Leestma JE: Neuropathology of child abuse, in Leestma JE, Kirpatrick JB (eds): *Forensic Neuropathology.* New York: Raven Press, 1988:333–356.
77. Lobato RD, Sarabia R, Cordobes F, et al: Post-traumatic cerebral hemispheric swelling: Analysis of 55 cases studied with computerized tomography. *J Neurosurg* 68:417, 1988.
78. Gennarelli TA, Thibault LE: Biomechanics of acute subdural hematoma. *J Trauma* 22:680, 1982.
79. Galbraith S: Misdiagnosis and delayed diagnosis in traumatic intracranial hematoma. *Br Med J* 1:1438, 1976.
80. Klatzo I: Cerebral oedema and ischemia, in Smith WT, Cavanagh JB (eds): *Recent Advances in Neuropathology.* New York: Churchill Livingstone, 1979:27–39.
81. Wahl M, Unterberg A, Baethmann A, Schilling L: Mediators of blood-brain barrier dysfunction and formation of vasogenic brain edema. *J Cereb Blood Flow Metab* 8:621, 1988.
82. Povlishock JT, Becker DP, Sullivan HG, Miller JD: Vascular permeability alterations to horseradish peroxidase in experimental brain injury. *Brain Res* 153:223, 1978.
83. Miller JD: Traumatic brain swelling and edema, in Cooper PR (ed): *Head Injury* (3d ed). Baltimore: Williams & Wilkins, 1993:331–354.
84. Langfitt TW, Weinstein JD, Kassell NF: Cerebral vasomotor paralysis produced by intracranial hypertension. *Neurology* 15:622, 1965.
85. Graham DI, Ford I, Adams JH, et al: Ischemic brain damage is still common in fatal non-missile head injury. *J Neurol Neurosurg Psychiatry* 52:346, 1989.
86. Bruce DA, Alavi A, Bilaniuk L, et al: Diffuse cerebral swelling following head injuries in children: The syndrome of "malignant brain edema." *J Neurosurg* 54:170, 1981.
87. Muizelaar JP, Marmarou A, De Salles AAF, et al: Cerebral blood flow and metabolism in severely head-injured children. *J Neurosurg* 71:63, 1989.
88. Bullock R, Smith R, Favier J, et al: Part 1: Relationship with GCS score, outcome, ICP, and PVI: Brain specific gravity and CT scan density measurements after human head injury. *J Neurosurg* 63:64, 1985.
89. Gomori JM, Grossman RI, Goldberg HI, et al: Intracranial hematomas: Imaging by high field MR. *Radiology* 157:87, 1985.
90. Jenkins A, Teasdale G, Hadley MDM, et al: Brain lesions detected by magnetic resonance imaging in mild and severe head injuries. *Lancet* 2:445, 1986.
91. Snoek J, Jennett B, Adams JH, et al: Computerized tomography after recent severe head injury in patients without acute intracranial hematoma. *J Neurol Neurosurg Psychiatry* 42:215, 1979.
92. Graham DI, Ford I, Adams JH, et al: Fatal head injury in children. *J Clin Pathol* 42:18, 1989.
93. Graham DI, Adams JH, Doyle D: Ischemic brain damage in fatal non-missile head injuries. *J Neurol Sci* 39:213, 1978.
94. Kotapka MJ, Graham DI, Adams JH, Gennarelli TA: Hippocampal damage in fatal non-missile human head injury: Frequency and distribution. *Acta Neuropathol (Berl)* 83:530, 1992.
95. Bouma GJ, Muizelaar JP, Stringer WA, et al: Ultra-early evaluation of regional cerebral blood flow in severely head-injured patients using xenon-enhanced computerized tomography. *J Neurosurg* 77:360, 1992.
96. Graham DI, Lawrence AE, Adams JH, et al: Brain damage in non-missile head injury secondary to high intracranial pressure. *Neuropathol Appl Neurobiol* 13:209, 1987.
97. Graham DI, Lawrence AE, Adams JH, et al: Brain damage in fatal non-missile head injury without high intracranial pressure. *J Clin Pathol* 41:34, 1988.
98. McLellan DR, Adams JH, Graham DI, et al: The structural basis of the vegetative state and prolonged coma

after non-missile head injury, in Papo I, Cohadon F, Massarotti M (eds): *Le Coma Traumatique.* Padova: Liviana Editrice, 1986:165–185.

99. Adams JH, Graham DI: The relationship between ventricular fluid pressure and neuropathology of raised intracranial pressure. *Neuropathol Appl Neurobiol* 2:323, 1976.
100. Graham DI, MacLellan D, Adams JH, et al: The neuropathology of severe disability after head injury. *Acta Neurochir.* [*Suppl*] (*Wien*) 32:65–67, 1983.
101. Watson AJ: Genesis of fat emboli. *Clin Pathol* 23(Suppl 4):132, 1970.
102. Kamenar E, Burger PC: Cerebral fat embolism: A neuropathological study of a micro-embolic state. *Stroke* 11:477, 1980.
103. Neuburger KT: Ueber cerebrale Fett und Luftembolie. *Z Gesamte Neurol Psychiat* 95:278, 1925.
104. Winkleman NW: Cerebral fat embolism: Clinico-pathologic study of 2 cases. *Arch Neurol Psychiatry* 47:57, 1942.
105. Koenig PA: Beitrag zur Protrahierten Fettembolie. *Monatsschr Unfallheilkunde* 59:289, 1956.
106. Brandenburg W: Spatfolgen der Luftembolie des Gehirns und ihr Pathologisch-anatomisches. *Bildgebung Verhandlung Deutschen Gesell Pathologie* 41:236, 1958.
107. Von Hochstetter AR, Friede RL: Residual lesions of cerebral fat embolism. *Neurology* 216:227, 1977.
108. McTaggart DM, Neubuerger KT: Cerebral fat embolism: Pathologic changes in the brain after survival of 7 years. *Acta Neuropathol* (*Berl*) 15:183, 1970.
109. McMenemey WH, Grant HC, Behrman S: Two examples of "presenile dementia" (Pick's disease and Stern-Garcin syndrome) with a history of trauma. *Arch Psychiat Nervenkrank* 208:162, 1965.
110. Grimberg L: Paralysis agitans and trauma. *Nerv Ment Dis* 79:14, 1934.
111. Behrman S, Mandybur T, McMenemey WH: Un cas de maladie Creutzfeld-Jakob a la suite d'un traumatisme cerebrale. *Rev Neurol,* (*Paris*) 107:453, 1962.
112. Critchley M: Medical aspects of boxing particularly from a neurological standpoint. *Br Med* 1:357, 1957.
113. Mawdsley C, Ferguson FR: Neurological disease in boxers. *Lancet* 2:795, 1963.
114. Corsellis JAN: Boxing and the brain. *Br Med* 298:105, 1989.
115. Corsellis JAN, Brunton CJ, Freeman-Browne D: The aftermath of boxing. *Psychol Med* 3:270, 1973.
116. Roberts GW, Allsop D, Bruton C: The occult aftermath of boxing. *J Neurol Neurosurg Psychiatry* 53:373, 1990.
117. Roberts GW, Gentleman SM, Lynch A, Graham DI: BA4 amyloid protein deposition in brain after head trauma. *Lancet* 338:1422, 1991.
118. Gentleman SM, Graham DI, Roberts EW: Molecular pathology of head trauma: Altered BAPP metabolism and the aetiology of Alzheimer's disease, in Kogure K, Hossmann KA, Siesjo BK (eds): *Progress in Brain Research,* vol 96. Amsterdam: Elsevier, 1993:237–246.

CHAPTER 5

PATHOPHYSIOLOGY OF HEAD INJURY

J. Douglas Miller
Ian R. Piper
Patricia A. Jones

SYNOPSIS

The evolution of knowledge about the pathophysiology of primary and secondary posttraumatic brain injury has improved management and is opening new therapeutic opportunities for treatments. Important secondary processes include brain herniation and cerebral ischemia, with the ischemia resulting from the superimposition of a secondary insult at a time when the normal regulatory mechanisms are in abeyance as a result of the injury. Raised intracranial pressure plays a major role in both processes, while arterial hypotension is important in brain ischemia. Such secondary insults occur much more frequently than has been recognized and have a major adverse effect on outcome even when other prognostic factors are taken into account. Some other secondary insults, notably pyrexia, were underemphasized in the past. Improved patient monitoring systems now offer an opportunity to study the incidence and interrelationships of secondary insults in greater detail, but valuable information also continues to emerge from the experimental laboratory, where better control of individual variables surrounding head injury can be obtained.

INTRODUCTION

For many years the pathophysiology of traumatic brain injury was divided into primary injury and secondary injury. It was assumed the damage caused by the physical forces associated with an injury occur more or less instantly and are nonreversible for the most part. While the contusions and lacerations that occur on the brain surface, especially at the temporal poles and the orbital surface of the frontal lobes, constitute obvious signs of injury,[1] it has been recognized for more than 30 years that diffuse axonal injury in the subcortical white matter is the primary basis for the prolonged loss of consciousness, impairment of motor response, and incomplete recovery that mark patients with a severe traumatic brain injury.[2] Recent work by Gennarelli and associates,[3] Maxwell and coworkers,[4] and Povlishock[5] has suggested that the process underlying at least some forms of diffuse axonal injury takes several hours to complete, during which time there is infolding of the axolemma, interruption of axoplasmic flow, formation of a localized swelling of the axon, and eventually separation of the axon to form a true retraction ball.

It is known from eyewitness reports of head injury and experimental studies that immediately after impact, there are alterations in arterial blood pressure (elevation in some cases and reduction in others) and an interruption of normal respiration, sometimes with a prolonged period of apnea, immediately after the impact.[6] Thus, traumatic brain injury seldom occurs in isolation but is accompanied in most cases by some disturbance of the physiological variables that are important in ensuring a continuous blood supply to and oxygenation of the brain. Head injuries are often accompanied by other injuries (more than 50 percent in the case of severe head injury). These other injuries also may contribute to secondary insults and secondary brain damage.[7]

In the days after a head injury, there are many occasions and opportunities for secondary damage to occur. In this chapter, the processes of secondary brain insult and injury will be described, along with recent data on their frequency, pathogenesis, and effect on outcome (Table 5-1).

TABLE 5-1 Processes and Factors Leading to Secondary Posttraumatic Brain Damage

Mass lesion, brain shift, and herniation
- Intracranial hematoma (EDH/SDH/ICH)
- Focal brain swelling/edema

Cerebral ischemia
- Reduced cerebral perfusion pressure
- Decreased arterial hypotension
  - intracranial hypertension
- Pyrexia
- Hypoxemia/anemia
- Cerebral vasospasm
- Epilepsy
- Infection
- Hyponatremia

INTRACRANIAL HEMATOMA

The occurrence of hemorrhage inside the cranial cavity and the formation of a hematoma after a head injury constitute the most important avoidable cause of death and disability after head injuries of all degrees of severity. Because of the exponential nature of the intracranial volume-pressure curve, the clinical manifestations of hematoma often occur relatively late in the evolution but then progress with startling rapidity. A preemptive diagnostic approach based on knowledge of risk factors that favor the development of hematoma and the early application of brain imaging in such cases is the recommended approach to diagnosis. The most important risk factor by far is the presence of a skull fracture (Table 5-2).[8,9] The outcome of intracranial hematoma is related to the level of consciousness of the patient at the time of detection of the hematoma [the lower the Glasgow Coma Scale (GCS) score, the worse the prognosis], the time lapse between onset of coma and first evacuation of the hematoma, the state of the pupillary responses, and the age of the patient.

EXTRADURAL HEMATOMA

Bleeding between the outer surface of the dura mater and the inner surface of the skull is nearly always caused by and located close to a skull fracture. Extradural hematomas (Fig. 5-1) may occur in patients who have never been unconscious after the injury, have been briefly comatose and recovered, or have been continuously comatose since the injury. More than half of extradural hematomas occur over the convexity of cerebral hemisphere, in the territory of the middle meningeal artery and its branches, since these are the vessels most commonly damaged by a skull fracture and are the source of the bleeding. It must be remembered, however, that approximately 10 percent of extradural hematomas occur in the extreme frontal area or the posterior fossa. Hematomas in the posterior fossa are extremely important, since patients with this problem may remain conscious until a late stage in the evolution of the hematoma and then simultaneously lose consciousness and become apneic, with death only minutes away. Probably the majority of posterior fossa epidural hematomas extend upward into the supratentorial compartment and in doing so strip off the dura overlying the transverse sinus, which may be a troublesome and diffcult source of hemorrhage. Because the hematoma consists of solid clotted blood in all cases, a craniotomy is necessary to remove the hematoma. In these combined lesions, it is important to leave intact the bridge of bone that overlies the lateral sinus so that homeostasis can be obtained by

TABLE 5-2 Relationship between Presence of Skull Fracture and Intracranial Hematoma in Patients with Severe, Moderate, and Minor Head Injury: Patients Managed in Edinburgh in 3 Years

Severity	Hematoma on CT	No Hematoma	Total
Severe (GCS 8)			
Fracture present	74 (44%)	94 (56%)	168
No fracture	43 (32%)*	91 (68%)	134
Moderate (GCS 9–12)			
Fracture present	49 (29%)	118 (71%)	167
No fracture	25 (8%)†	299 (92%)	324
Minor (GCS 13–15)			
Fracture	42 (10%)	391 (90%)	433
No fracture	27 (1%)‡	2549 (99%)	2576
Totals	260	3542	3802

* $p < 0.05$.
† $p < 0.001$.
‡ $p < 0.0001$.

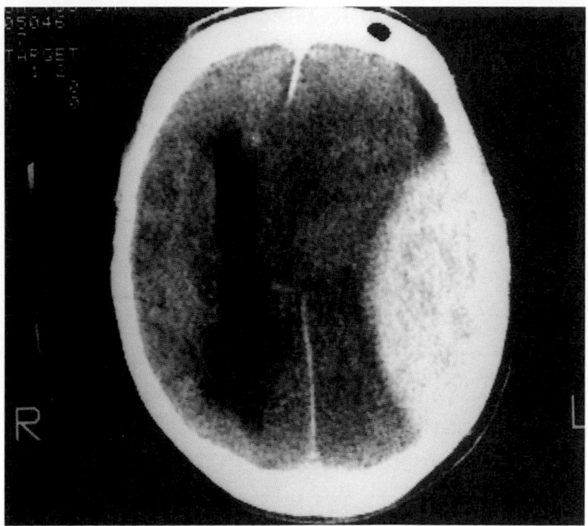

Figure 5-1. Large extradural hematoma with midline shift and dilatation of the contralateral ventricle.

overlaying a muscle graft on the dura and hitching it to the bony bridge.

Acute Subdural Hematoma

Acute subdural hematomas (Fig. 5-2) are lesions that are related to movement of the brain; although they are, like all hematomas, more common in the presence of a skull fracture, the skull fracture may be on the opposite side of the head from the subdural hematoma. The source of the hemorrhage may be a laceration of the brain, most commonly at the temporal pole, the so-called burst temporal lobe. It may be due to tearing of a vein bridging the brain surface and the inner surface of the dura or to damage to a small artery on the brain surface. The evolution of these hematomas can be extremely rapid, but in the case of a so-called hyperacute subdural hematoma, computed tomography (CT) imaging shows lucent areas within the hematoma that represent liquid blood that has not had time to clot.

A chronic subdural hematoma is quite different. Occurring mainly in the elderly, the very young, and those with prior brain atrophy and evolving over a period of weeks, the hematoma consists of liquid blood. While in some cases a relatively minor head injury that occurred some weeks previously is noted, in many cases no history of head injury can be obtained.

Subdural hygromas are collections of clear CSF or sometimes thin serous fluid over the surface of the brain. In most cases, they represent an evolution in patients with craniocerebral disproportion, but in some cases in which there is brain shift, a strong argument can be put forward that these lesions contribute to neurological impairment and that the collection should be evacuated.

Intracerebral Hematoma

The formation of a sizable blood clot within the substance of the brain may be a complication of a brain laceration resulting from a blunt acceleration/deceleration head injury, when the hematoma tends to form in the inferior frontal lobe or in the temporal lobes or occurs in the track of a penetrating head wound, in which case the location of the hematoma is dependent on the location and direction of brain penetration and its proximity to major vessels (Fig. 5-3).

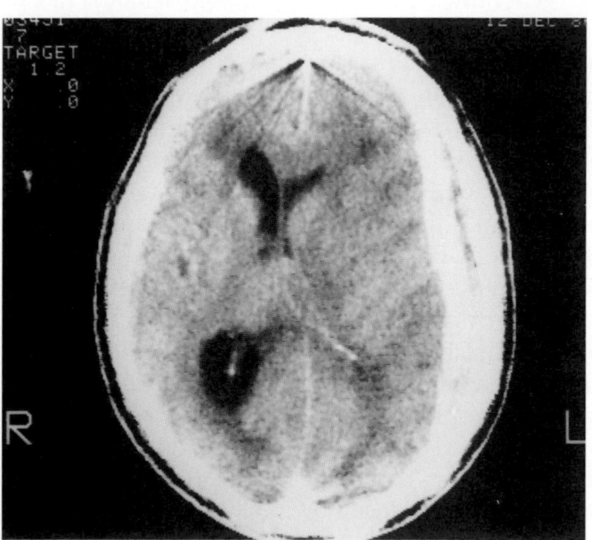

Figure 5-2. Acute subdural hematoma with midline shift, compression of the ipsilateral ventricle, and dilatation of the contralateral ventricle.

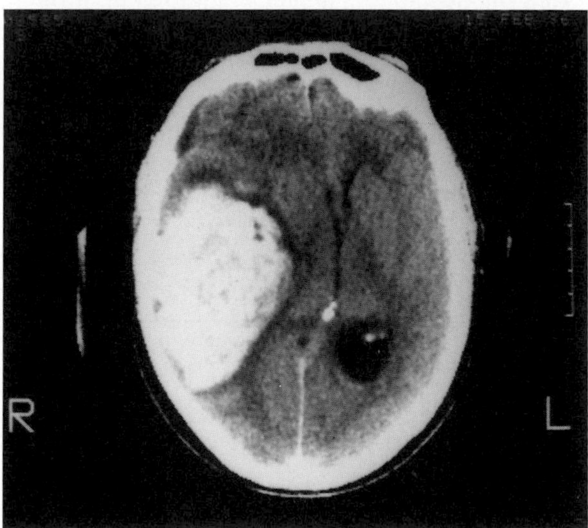

Figure 5-3. Large posttraumatic intracerebral hematoma in right temporal lobe.

Moderate-sized intracerebral hemorrhagic contusions may be seen in the basal ganglia in patients with particularly severe diffuse axonal injuries. This is the prime significance of such lesions, which, less significantly, also represents a problem resulting from mass effect.[1]

BRAIN SHIFT AND HERNIATION

With progressive enlargement of the hematoma or focal swelling of adjacent tissue, brain is shifted away from the mass, and structures that normally lie in the midline, such as the interventricular septum and the third ventricle, can be seen displaced away from the midline on CT imaging. Because the falx remains in the midline, the cingulate gyrus may herniate under the free edge of the falx and may cause compression or distortion of the pericallosal arteries.[10] Because the foramen of Monro becomes occluded in this process of midline shift, the contralateral ventricle may become dilated while the ventricle ipsilateral to the mass is compressed. This is a reliable indication that intracranial pressure is increased.[11] With hematomas compressing the supratentorial compartment, brain herniation eventually will also occur at the tentorial hiatus, usually laterally with compression of the posterior cerebral artery and the oculomotor nerve ipsilateral to the mass. In the case of bilateral or frontal lesions, the herniation may be posterior, with compression of the tectal plate resulting in bilateral pupil abnormalities and failure of upward gaze.[12] With infratentorial masses or further progression of a supratentorial mass, tonsillar herniation eventually occurs, with downward displacement of the cerebellar tonsils through the foramen magnum, compression of the medulla, and apnea followed by circulatory arrest.

An intracranial mass lesion sets the stage for brain herniation. The actual driving force behind the process is the development of a pressure gradient between the intracranial compartments that tends to displace brain from the compartment with the higher pressure toward that with the lower pressure.[13,14]

CEREBRAL PERFUSION PRESSURE, AUTOREGULATION, AND CEREBRAL BLOOD FLOW

Cerebral perfusion pressure (CPP), the difference between mean arterial pressure and intracranial pressure (ICP), may be reduced after a head injury by an increase in ICP or a decrease in arterial pressure[15] (Table 5-3).

TABLE 5-3 Causes of Reduced Cerebral Perfusion Pressure

Arterial hypotension
- Hypovolemia
- Cardiodepressant drugs
- Sepsis

Intracranial hypertension
- Mass lesion (hematoma)
- Vascular engorgement
- Cerebral edema
- Acute hydrocephalus

The extent to which a reduction in CPP leads to a fall in cerebral blood flow (CBF) may be a measure of autoregulation or at least the lower autoregulatory threshold, the CPP level below which CBF cannot be maintained. Ischemic brain damage is extremely common as a postmortem finding in patients with fatal head injuries.[16] Abnormally low levels of CBF are seldom found unless the first measurements are made within a few hours of a head injury.[17] Reduction in middle cerebral artery flow velocity was found consistently at the first recording in a study of 50 severely head injured patients by Chan and colleagues.[18] Certainly, a reduction in jugular venous oxygen saturation to 50% and below is not uncommon as a transient phenomenon.[19,20] In a number of studies, induced or spontaneous changes in CPP have been associated with pressure-passive changes in CBF. This has been interpreted as indicating that autoregulation is impaired, in keeping with the widely accepted concept that autoregulation is impaired or absent after a head injury of any severity. In contrast, the cerebrovascular response to a change in arterial P_{CO_2} generally is preserved until the patient is in extremis. If autoregulation is a protective homeostatic mechanism, it seems surprising that it should be so easily lost after a trauma. An alternative explanation for the pressure-passive changes in flow that accompany changes in CPP is that the entire autoregulatory curve has been shifted to the right so that the lower threshold level becomes higher in terms of the minimum acceptable level of CPP. In severely head injured patients, the Doppler pulsatility index increases progressively from the normal value of 0.7 to 0.9 to 3.0 or 4.0 as CPP falls, with the threshold CPP value being 70 mmHg.[20] There is a similar relationship between CPP and jugular venous oxygen saturation: with normal values as long as CPP is over 70 mmHg and a progressive fall in Sjv_{O_2} after CPP falls below 70 mmHg. The relationship is the same whether CPP is reduced by a fall in arterial pressure or a rise in ICP. It is also the same whether the CPP changes are spontaneous or change because of treatment.[21] It appears that the threshold level of CPP may vary in individual patients and over time, but as a general rule,

TABLE 5-4 Risk Factors for Ischemia in Traumatic Subarachnoid Hemorrhage

Reduced cerebral perfusion pressure
Upward shift of autoregulatory threshold
Cerebral vasospasm
Increased metabolic demand
Substrate lack

CPP needs to be higher than normal to ensure adequate cerebral perfusion in a severely head injured patient. This phenomenon also is seen in patients with long-standing arterial hypertension.[22] Presumably, it may result from generalized cerebral vasoconstriction from any cause. Possible mechanisms include the moderate hyperventilation that commonly accompanies head injury and is commonly employed in patients who are artificially ventilated after a head injury. A tempting alternative explanation is the liberation of vasoconstrictor substances such as an endothelin after a head injury. A similar phenomenon can be observed after subarachnoid hemorrhage, and it must not be forgotten that subarachnoid hemorrhage frequently accompanies traumatic brain injury (Table 5-4). In the generation of ischemic infarction after a head injury, it appears that a combination of the cerebral vasoconstriction and reduction in CPP is required to produce ischemia sufficient for infarction to follow.[23]

Raised Intracranial Pressure

Apart from the formation of an intracranial hematoma, which almost invariably raises ICP, there are three main causes of this common sequel to moderate and severe head injury. The first is cerebrovascular congestion with an increase in cerebral blood volume. This may be associated with cerebral hyperemia, an absolute or relative increase in CBF as related to the cerebral metabolic rate, which produces jugular venous saturation levels over 75% and a high oxygen content in the cerebral venous blood. Often, however, the cerebrovascular resistance is transferred to the venous end of the system and cerebral blood flow is normal or low. In the case of hyperemia, inducing cerebral vasoconstriction and reducing CBF by depressing metabolism may be suitable strategies, but these strategies are entirely unsuitable when blood flow is not increased and may simply make the ischemia worse.[24]

The second main contributor to raised ICP after a head injury is the formation of brain edema, an increase in brain volume that is due to an increase in the tissue water content. For some years it was considered that edema following a head injury, particularly perifocal edema around brain contusions, is mainly vasogenic. That is, protein-rich edema fluid crosses a defective blood-brain barrier to raise the levels of water and sodium in brain tissue and cause tissue expansion.[25] A variant of this type of edema is hydrostatic edema, a condition that follows flooding of the cerebrovascular bed with blood under high pressure because of a failure of cerebrovascular resistance, followed by accumulation of water in the extracellular space.[26] It now appears that most of the water in the areas of brain contusion is intracellular and represents cytotoxic edema caused by membrane pump failure that results from ischemia in which CBF falls to levels insufficient to maintain ionic homeostasis.[27]

Whatever its cause and nature, posttraumatic cerebral edema may be recognized eventually on CT imaging by a lucent area in white matter or on magnetic resonance imaging (MRI) by an increase in T_2 signal. Increased extracellular water content is most visible in white matter because, as a result of the arrangement of fibers, this tissue is more compliant and distensible than is gray matter, in which the increased density of cellular structures makes it more resistant to visible tissue expansion even though there is a significant increase in intracellular water. Formation of brain edema is favored by an elevation in body temperature[28] and a reduction in serum sodium, with both conditions occurring frequently after a head injury.[29]

The third and least common cause of raised ICP after a head injury is the development of acute hydrocephalus. Although enlargement of the lateral ventricles is common after a severe head injury, in nearly all instances this is an enlargement ex vacuo caused by the loss of white matter substance and is not associated with raised ICP. Acute hydrocephalus is most likely to occur when there has been a heavy posttraumatic subarachnoid hemorrhage or when infection in the CSF spaces has complicated the head injury.

Arterial Hypotension

Episodes of arterial hypotension may occur at any time after a head injury.[30] Hypotension in the first 72 h after an injury is most likely to be due to hypovolemia that may result from inadequate replacement of blood loss. Agonal hypotension occurs in patients with overwhelmingly severe head injury who have already suffered one or more waves of paroxysmal intracranial hypertension and elevation of the blood pressure, the Cushing vasopressor response. Inadequate fluid replacement, particularly after osmotically induced diuresis, also may produce a degree of hypovolemia, and this, when coupled with the cardiodepressant effect of sedative drugs such as barbiturates and propofol, may produce arterial hypotension. In young children, overventilation under high pressure may produce sufficient cardiac tamponade to lower blood pressure. In patients in whom there are a number of long indwelling lines, such as Swan-Ganz catheters or long central lines for parenteral feeding, there is always a risk of septicemia, and this may produce arterial hypotension as part of the clinical picture.

PYREXIA AFTER HEAD INJURY

Elevation of body temperature occurs very frequently after head injury and has a number of adverse consequences. It increases the metabolic demand of the brain at a time when CBF may be marginally inadequate. It favors increased brain congestion and an increased rate of formation of brain edema and is therefore associated with raised ICP.[28] The reasons for the elevation in body temperature are not entirely clear. Pyrexia cannot be explained simply on the basis of infection, since in the majority of cases, at least in the early stages, there is no evidence of infection but there is elevated body temperature. It has been suggested that cytokine release after injury plays a role.

HYPOXEMIA AND ANEMIA

One of the strong arguments in favor of the institution of artificial ventilation in all patients with severe head injury is the prevention of hypoxemia resulting from inadequate respiratory depth and rhythm, but despite that, there remain a number of potential sources of hypoxemia in head-injured patients. These include pulmonary infection, atelectasis, edema, and acute respiratory distress syndrome (ARDS). Reductions in hematocrit are also common in head-injured patients and have become more common because of increasing reluctance to replace lost blood with whole-blood transfusions. While it is claimed that a certain amount of reduction of the hematocrit may optimize perfusion of the cerebrovascular bed, the reduced oxygen carriage may be critical when there is a limited capacity for CBF to show a compensatory increase because of superimposed vasoconstrictory factors.

THE FREQUENCY OF SECONDARY INSULTS TO THE INJURED BRAIN AND THEIR SIGNIFICANCE FOR OUTCOME

In Edinburgh over the past 5 years, a system has been developed for the detection and quantification of secondary insults. This system, which uses a personal computer, has the capability of recording minute by minute up to 15 physiological variables.[31] The data from the patient's monitors are directed via serial links after analogue-to-digital conversion if required to a bedside computer that displays a subset of the information and stores all data on disk. Monitored variables include heart rate measured from the electrocardiogram (ECG), systolic and mean arterial blood pressure measured invasively, ICP recorded from a Camino pressure monitor, arterial oxygen saturation recorded from a pulse oximeter, peripheral and core temperatures, and in certain patients jugular venous oxygen saturation. From these variables, CPP is derived from the difference between mean arterial pressure and ICP and cerebral arteriovenous oxygen content difference is derived from the hemoglobin level, which is entered daily, and the oxygen saturation values.

The computer detects when a channel is not working and compares valid data with upper and lower rejection limits, which have been specified for each channel. Values falling outside these limits are considered nonphysiological and are rejected. The system also permits comments to be inserted by nurses and doctors, including the time of day of a comment.

At the outset of the study, abnormal levels of physiological variables were defined, beyond which an insult was considered to have occurred, provided that it lasted for 5 min or longer (or, in the case of pyrexia, 1 h or longer). Three ranges of abnormal values were defined to produce three grades of insult. These values, which are described as Edinburgh University Secondary Insult Grades (EUSIG), are listed in Table 5-5.

The study group consisted of 124 patients age 14 years or more who met the following criteria: The post-resuscitation GCS was 12 or less or was 13, 14, or 15, but the patient also had other major injuries sufficient to reach an Injury Severity Score of 16 points or more; there needed to be clinical indications for monitoring

TABLE 5-5 Grading of Secondary Insults

Variable	Grade 1	Grade 2	Grade 3
Raised ICP (mm/Hg)	≥20	≥30	≥40
CPP (mm/Hg)	≤60	≤50	≤40
Hypotension (mm/Hg)			
Systolic	≤90	≤70	≤50
Mean	≤70	≤55	≤40
Hypertension (mm/Hg)			
Systolic	≥160	≥190	≥220
Mean	≥110	≥130	≥150
Hypoxemia, Sa_{O_2} (%)	≤90	≤85	≤80
Cerebral oligemia, Sv_{O_2} (%)	≤54	≤49	≤45
Cerebral hyperemia, Sv_{O_2} (%)	≥75	≥85	≥95
Pyrexia (°C)	≥38	≥39	≥40
Tachycardia (bpm)	≥120	≥135	≥150
Bradycardia (bpm)	≤50	≤40	≤30

TABLE 5-6 Number of Patients Who Suffered One or More Secondary Insults

	Severe	Moderate	Minor	Total
Insult(s) found	67	29	17	113
No insults	1	7	3	11
Total	68	36	20	124

the patient in an intensive care unit (ICU); and the data collection process had to be started within 24 h of admission.[32]

Physiological parameters of raised ICP, arterial hypotension and hypertension, reduced CPP, hypoxemia, pyrexia, bradycardia, and tachycardia were studied in this group of 124 adult patients. Not all patients had all parameters measured; for example, ICP monitoring was seldom employed in patients with moderate or minor head injury. Of the 124 patients, a subgroup of 71 had full minute-by-minute monitoring of all eight of these parameters.[33]

Among the entire patient group, more than 90 percent were found to have one or more insults and 50 percent sustained at least one insult at the highest grade. Insults were frequent in all age groups and at all severities of head injury (Table 5-6 through 5-8).

The high frequency of secondary insults recorded in the ICU was at first surprising. In patients studied during transportation within the hospital, we had recorded a frequency of secondary insult of approximately 50 percent, although in that study we had noted that patients who sustained secondary insults during transportation were likely to have even more and more severe insults upon returning to the ICU.[34] The high incidence of episodes of intracranial hypertension seems to be consistent with previous studies in which the more intensively the patient is monitored and the data are recorded, the higher is the observed frequency of intracranial hypertension in 44 percent and 53 percent, respectively, in two series of severely head injured patients.[35,36] Marmarou and colleagues recorded intracranial hypertension in 72 percent of the more intensively studied patients in the Traumatic Coma Databank.[37] One of the important conclusions from the present study was that even patients with entirely normal admission CT images could subsequently develop intracranial hypertension. This has led us to widen our criteria for the use of ICP monitoring to all patients scoring 8 or less on the GCS regardless of admission CT findings.[38]

We have looked in particular detail at reduction in CPP to determine the time after injury when this becomes a particular problem, and at each time epoch we have examined the data to determine whether the reduction in CPP is due primarily to arterial hypotension, intracranial hypertension, or a combination of the two.[25] Data were available from 74 patients who had CPP monitored for periods of up to 14 days; of these 74 patients, 81 percent were found to have one or more CPP insult, with the peak for insult duration occurring on the sixth postinjury day. When examined day by day, arterial hypotension was a prominent cause of reduced CPP on the first and second postinjury days; raised ICP predominated on days 4, 5, and 6; and arterial hypotension became prominent again on days 9, 10, and 11.[30]

All the surviving patients in this prospective study have had a rigorous and objective assessment of outcome at 6, 12, and 24 months after injury. The 5-point Glasgow Outcome Score was used, with the outcome score determined after a patient assessment that employed a neuropsychometric test battery and a relatives' questionnaire; the scorer was unaware of the secondary insult data, and 12-month outcome data have been used for this part of the study.

Among the insult data that were obtained, five factors were found to be consistently important for outcome: arterial hypotension, reduced CPP, raised ICP, hypoxemia, and pyrexia. Using the Mann-Whitney U-test, the total duration of arterial hypotension at grade 1 insult level was found to be significantly and adversely related to outcome not only in terms of survival but also in terms of distinguishing between groups making a moderate recovery and groups that remained severely disabled. These differences were also apparent at more severe levels of arterial hypotension and with grade 2 and grade 3 CPP insults. Raised ICP considered in isolation was found to be significant only between patients who died and those who made a good recovery at grade 2 (over 30 mmHg) insult level.[33]

TABLE 5-7 Secondary Insults in 124 Head-Injured Patients

			Duration in min × 10^3	
Variable	**No. mon**	**No. Insult (%)**	**Grade 1 (%)**	**Total**
High ICP	77	65 (84%)	172 (78%)	221
Low blood pressure	112	82 (73%)	44 (90%)	49
Low CPP	75	61 (81%)	47 (72%)	65
Pyrexia	106	90 (85%)	254 (90%)	282
Hypoxemia	113	45 (40%)	2 (66%)	3

TABLE 5-8 Secondary Insults in Severe, Moderate, and Minor Head Injury

		Severe	*Moderate*	*Minor*
Variable	**No. mon**	***n* (%)***	***n* (%)**	***n* (%)**
High ICP	77	54 (89%)	18 (72%)	5 (80%)
Low BP	112	66 (80%)	31 (58%)	15 (73%)
Low CPP	75	54 (87%)	18 (72%)	3 (33%)
Pyrexia	106	64 (86%)	27 (89%)	15 (73%)
Hypoxemia	113	64 (47%)	33 (33%)	16 (25%)

* % refers to the proportion of patients in that category with one or more insults.

Secondary insults do not occur in isolation but appear in series of complex patterns and sequences. Furthermore, many other factors, including age, severity of initial head injury, pupillary light responses, and presence of other injuries, are known to have an effect on the outcome from head injury. Using logistic regression analysis, including the total duration in minutes of each of the eight monitored physiological variables and the four demographic factors of age, pupillary response, severity of injury, and other injuries, and comparing good or moderate outcome with poor outcome (dead, vegetative, or severely disabled), it was found that the total duration of arterial hypotension and pupillary response on admission were significant predictors of outcome. If outcome was considered as survival versus death, the total duration of the three insult variables of arterial hypotension, hypoxemia, and pyrexia was found to be significant.

Experimental Studies of Head Injury

Clinical studies of head injury have confirmed the fact that secondary insults occur frequently and carry an adverse significance for outcome. Further light can be shed on this influence by studying an experimental model of head injury followed by controlled secondary insults. Using the Marmarou weight drop model of closed head injury, anesthetized rats were instrumented with microdialysis probes and a ventricular catheter for ICP monitoring. After a period of 2 h elapsed after the injury, secondary insults of arterial hypotension and pyrexia were applied. Although others have shown outpouring of glutamate into the extracellular space immediately after trauma,[39] measurements at 2 h after injury did not show increased levels of any of the excitatory or inhibitory amino acids. Within minutes of the application of the secondary insults seen to be most harmful in patients—hypotension and pyrexia—steep rises were recorded in the extracellular fluid concentrations of glutamate, aspartate, gamma-aminobuytric acid, and taurine.[40] Some years earlier, Jenkins and colleagues had shown that an ischemic brain insult after a fluid percussion brain injury produced a disproportionately greater amount of ischemic brain damage than occurred when either insult was delivered on its own.[41] The data suggest that trauma in some way preconditions the brain to respond adversely to any superimposed secondary physiological insult.

All the evidence from our studies to date points toward the fact that the long-term outcome after head injuries, whether severe, moderate, or minor, can be influenced adversely by secondary pathophysiological insults, a number of which are both common and theoretically avoidable.

References

1. Adams JH: Head injury, in Adams SH, Duchen LW (eds): *Greenfield's Neuropathology,* 5th ed. London: Arnold, 1992:106–152.
2. Strich SJ: Shearing of nerve fibres as a cause of brain damage due to head injury. *Lancet* 2:443–448, 1961.
3. Gennarelli TA, Thibault LE, Tipperman R, et al: Axonal injury in the optic nerve: A model simulating diffuse axonal injury in the brain. *J Neurosurg* 71:244–253, 1989.
4. Maxwell WL, Graham DI, Adams JH, et al: Focal axonal injury: The early axonal response to stretch. *J Neurocytol* 20:157–164, 1991.
5. Povlishock JT: Traumatically induced axonal injury: Pathogenesis and pathobiological implications. *Brain Pathol* 2:1–12, 1992.
6. Sullivan HG, Martinez AJ, Becker DP, et al: Fluid percussion model of mechanical brain injury in the cat. *J Neurosurg* 45:520–534, 1976.
7. Miller JD, Jones PA, Dearden NM, Tocher JL: Progress in the management of head injury. *Br J Surg* 79:60–64, 1992.
8. Teasdale GM, Murray G, Anderson E, et al: Risks of acute traumatic intracranial haematoma in children and adults: Implications for managing head injuries. *Br Med J* 300:363–367, 1990.
9. Miller JD: Minor, moderate and severe head injury. *Neurosurg Rev* 9:135–139, 1986.
10. Miller JD, Adams JH: The pathophysiology of raised intracranial pressure, in Adams JH, Duchen E (eds): *Greenfield's Neuropathology,* 5th ed. London: Arnold, 1992:69–105.

11. Teasdale E, Cardoso E, Galbraith S, Teasdale G: CT scan in severe diffuse head injury: Physiological and clinical correlations. *J Neurol Neurosurg Psychiatry* 47:600–603, 1984.
12. Johnson RT, Yates PO: Clinical pathological aspects of pressure changes at the tentorium. *Acta Radiol* 46:241–249, 1956.
13. Langfitt TW, Weinstein JD, Kassell NF, Simeone FA: Transmission of increased intracranial pressure: I. Within the craniospinal axis. *J Neurosurg* 21:989–997, 1964.
14. Takizawa H, Gabra-Sanders T, Miller JD: Analysis of changes in intracranial pressure and pressure volume index at different locations in the craniospinal axis during supratentorial epidural balloon inflation. *Neurosurgery* 19:1–8, 1986.
15. Miller JD, Stanek AE, Langfitt TW: Concepts of cerebral perfusion pressure and vascular compression during intracranial hypertension, in Meyer JS, Schade J (eds): *Progress in Brain Research,* vol. 35: *Cerebral Blood Flow.* Amsterdam: Elsevier, 1972:411–432.
16. Graham DI, Ford I, Hume-Adams J, et al: Ischaemic brain damage is still common in fatal non-missile head injury. *J Neurol Neurosurg Psychiatry* 52:346–350, 1989.
17. Bouma GJ, Muizelaar JP, Choi SC, et al: Cerebral circulation and metabolism after severe traumatic brain injury: The elusive role of ischaemia. *J Neurosurg* 75:685–693, 1991.
18. Chan KH, Miller JD, Dearden NM: Intracranial blood flow velocity after head injury: Relationship to severity of injury, time, neurological status and outcome. *J Neurol Neurosurg Psychiatry* 55:787–791, 1992.
19. Sheinberg M, Kanter MJ, Robertson CS, et al: Continuous monitoring of jugular venous oxygen saturation in head injured patients. *J Neurosurg* 76:212–217, 1992.
20. Chan KH, Miller JD, Dearden NM, et al: Effect of changes in cerebral perfusion pressure upon middle cerebral artery blood flow velocity and jugular bulb venous oxygen saturation after severe head injury. *J Neurosurg* 77:55–61, 1992.
21. Chan KH, Dearden NM, Miller JD, et al: Multimodality monitoring as a guide to treatment of intracranial hypertension after severe brain injury. *Neurosurgery* 32:547–553, 1993.
22. Strandgaard S: Autoregulation of cerebral blood flow in hypertensive patients: The modifying influence of prolonged antihypertensive treatment on the tolerance to acute, drug induced hypotension. *Circulation* 53:720–727, 1976.
23. Chan KH, Dearden NM, Miller JD: The significance of post-traumatic increase in cerebral blood flow velocity: A transcranial Doppler ultrasound study. *Neurosurgery* 30:697–700, 1992.
24. Miller JD: Vasoconstriction as head injury treatment—right or wrong? *Intensive Care Med* 20:249–250, 1994.
25. Klatzo I: Neuropathological aspects of brain oedema. *J Neuropathol Exp Neurol* 26:1–14, 1967.
26. Schutta HS, Kassell NF, Langfitt TW: Brain swelling produced by injury and aggravated by arterial hypertension—a light and electron microscopic study. *Brain* 9:281–294, 1968.
27. Bullock R, Maxwell WL, Graham DI, et al: Glial swelling following human cerebral contusion: An ultrastructural study. *J Neurol Neurosurg Psychiatry* 54:427–434, 1991.
28. Clasen RA, Pandolfi S, Laing I, Casey D: Experimental study of relation of fever to cerebral oedema. *J Neurosurg* 41:476–581, 1974.
29. Arieff AI: Hyponatraemia associated with permanent brain damage. *Adv Intern Med* 32:325–344, 1987.
30. Cortbus F, Jones PA, Miller JD, et al: Cause, distribution and significance of episodes of reduced cerebral perfusion pressure following head injury. *Acta Neurochir (Wien)* 130:117–124, 1994.
31. Piper IR, Lawson A, Dearden NM, Miller JD: Computerised data collection: A microcomputer data collection system in head injury intensive care. *Br J Intensive Care* 1:73–78, 1991.
32. Corrie J, Piper IR, Housley A, et al: Microcomputer based data recording improves identification of secondary insults during intensive care management of head injured patients. *Br J Intensive Care* 3:225–233, 1993.
33. Jones PA, Andrews PJD, Midgley S, et al: Measuring the burden of secondary insults in head injured patients during intensive care. *J Neurosurg Anesth* 6:4–14, 1994.
34. Andrews PJD, Piper IR, Dearden NM, Miller JD: Secondary insults during intrahospital transport of head injured patients. *Lancet* 1:327–330, 1990.
35. Miller JD, Becker DP, Ward JD, et al: Significance of intracranial hypertension in severe head injury. *J Neurosurg* 47:503–516, 1977.
36. Miller JD, Butterworth JF, Gudeman SK, et al: Further experience in the management of severe head injury. *J Neurosurg* 54:289–299, 1981.
37. Marmarou A, Anderson RL, Ward JD, et al: NINDS Traumatic Coma Databank: Intracranial pressure monitoring methodology. *J Neurosurg* 75(Suppl):S21–S27, 1991.
38. O'Sullivan MG, Statham PFX, Jones PA, et al: Role of intracranial pressure monitoring in severely head injured patients without signs of intracranial hypertension of initial computerised tomography. *J Neurosurg* 80:46–50, 1994.
39. Katayama Y, Becker DP, Tamura T, Hovda DA: Massive increases in extracellular potassium and the indiscriminate use of glutamate following concussive brain injury. *J Neurosurg* 73:889–900, 1990.
40. Piper IR, Thomson D, Weir D, Miller JD: Post-traumatic pyrexia coupled with hypotenison increases hippocampal amino acids in a rodent model of impact acceleration head injury. *J Neurotrauma* 12:470, 1995.
41. Jenkins LW, Moszyski K, Lyeth BG, et al: increased vulnerability of the mildly traumatised rat brain to cerebral ischaemia: The use of a controlled second insult as a research tool. *Brain Res* 477:211–244, 1989.

CHAPTER 6

GENERAL PRINCIPLES OF HEAD INJURY MANAGEMENT

Daniel F. Kelly
Curtis Doberstein
Donald P. Becker

SYNOPSIS

This chapter provides an overview of current management of the craniocerebral trauma victim. The essential principles of care, established in the 1970s, include emergent evacuation of intracranial hematomas, prevention or treatment of intracranial hypertension and cerebral ischemia, and avoidance of other postinjury secondary insults. In recent years this basic approach has evolved substantially. The most important modifications of traditional management include a greater emphasis on maintaining an adequate cerebral perfusion pressure as a means of averting cerebral ischemia, and the recognition that aggressive hyperventilation to control intracranial hypertension may promote ischemia. Specifically, it is recommended that cerebral perfusion pressure be maintained at 70 mmHg or greater and that only mild hyperventilation to achieve a Pa_{CO_2} *of 30 to 35 mmHg be utilized in the treatment of severe head injury patients. Recommendations for emergent resuscitation of the head injury victim are also provided, including techniques of airway management, fluid resuscitation, initial treatment of intracranial hypertension, and criteria for evacuation of intracranial mass lesions. Critical care of the patient with severe head injury also is addressed, including methods of hemodynamic monitoring of cerebral physiology, and treatment of intracranial hypertension. The recently documented benefits of early enteral nutrition also are stressed, and the management of commonly encountered posttraumatic intracranial and extracranial complications is reviewed. Overall, these therapeutic modifications and advances in critical care appear to be impacting favorably on long-term neurological recovery. It is hoped that the addition of novel pharmacological neuroprotective therapies and the use of moderate hypothermia, currently being evaluated in clinical trials, will further reduce the substantial morbidity and mortality associated with traumatic brain injury*

INTRODUCTION

Traumatic brain injury continues to pose a serious health care challenge throughout the world. In the United States, trauma is the leading cause of death in individuals under 45 years of age and is a major cause of death and disability in older age groups as well. Brain injury results in more trauma deaths than do injuries to any other specific body region.[1] Half of the 150,000 injury-related deaths that occur annually in the United States involve a serious brain injury that is primarily responsible for the patient's demise.[2] Overall, approximately 500,000 head injuries per year in the United States are serious enough to require admission to a hospital. Despite intensive intervention, long-term disability or death occurs in the majority of severely head injured patients.[3–5] Significant neuropsychological sequelae and physical disabilities also are common in patients sustaining milder injuries.[3,6,7]

Meaningful recovery of function after head injury is possible if patients are rapidly and effectively resuscitated, if surgical mass lesions are emergently evacuated, and if secondary insults are prevented or minimized. A key factor in recovery is the heightened vulnerability of the brain millieu following injury.[8,9] After focal or diffuse insults, many neuronal, glial, and endothelial cell populations are functionally impaired. If conditions are favorable, these cells will recover with time. However, if such events as hypotension, hypoxia, or intracranial hypertension go unchecked, many vulnerable cells will succumb. Optimizing conditions for cellular recovery by maintaining adequate cerebral perfusion, normalizing intracranial pressure (ICP), and averting additional secondary insults is essential in the overall treatment strategy for the head-injured patient. Improvements in resuscitation, diagnosis, and surgical treatment may be reaching a plateau as means of further reducing morbidity and mortality. However, refinements in critical care continue to offer new avenues for enhancing outcome. Monitoring cerebral blood flow and metabolism for detection and prevention of ischemia, as well as new neuroprotective pharmacological therapies hold the greatest promise for achieving further meaningful recovery after head injury. This chapter will provide an overview of the essential principles involved in optimizing outcome after traumatic brain injury, including aspects of prehospital and emergency room care, operative and perioperative strategies, and intensive care monitoring and intervention.

PREVENTION

Clearly, the most effective means of addressing central nervous system trauma is through prevention. In the United States, Canada, and elsewhere, public education initiatives on brain and spinal cord injury, such as the Think First program, and enactment of safety legislation have begun to help. From 1982 to 1992, seat-belt use among drivers and passengers in the United States increased from approximately 11 to 66 percent; legislation now mandates their use in 46 of 50 states.[10] Since 1990, all new cars manufactured in the United States are equipped with automatic seat belts and/or a driver's side air bag. In 1992, air bags were estimated to have saved over 550 lives and prevented approximately 40,000 serious injuries. Motorcycle helmet laws also have been implemented in 47 of 50 states. Fatalities from motorcycle use have fallen from over 4600 in 1982 to approximately 2400 in 1992. Given that head injury is the primary cause of death in most motorcycle fatalities, these laws appear to be having a beneficial effect on reducing mortality. Similarly, infant restraint seats are now mandatory in automobiles throughout the United States. Increasing use of these devices from 1982 to 1992 was estimated to have saved over 2000 infant lives. The pervasive problem of alcohol-related traffic accidents is also starting to diminish owing to broad educational efforts and strict enforcement of drunk driving laws. The legal drinking age is now 21 throughout the United States. Between 1982 and 1992, alcohol-related traffic deaths fell by over 30 percent despite a rising number of vehicles on the road. Overall, these efforts have reduced the incidence of certain types of head injury, but further progress can still be made from broader implementation of such preemptive strategies.

SECONDARY BRAIN INJURY AND CELLULAR VULNERABILITY

Functional recovery after traumatic brain injury is determined by the severity of the initial trauma and by the occurrence of secondary insults. By definition, primary injury occurs immediately on impact and may lead to irreversible damage as a result of direct mechanical cell disruption. Secondary insults are physiological events that can occur within minutes, hours, or days after the primary injury and can lead to further damage of nervous tissue, prolonging and/or contributing to permanent neurological dysfunction. Following the initial injury, many cells are functionally compromised, but can recover if provided an optimal environment. Such cells, however, are particularly vulnerable to the physiological challenges imposed by secondary insults.[8] This state of vulnerability was illustrated by Jenkins and coworkers in a series of animal experiments in which a fluid percussion brain injury was followed 1 h later by a brief period of global ischemia.[9] Each insult alone produced no morphological cell death. However, in animals sustaining concussion followed by transient ischemia, extensive hippocampal neuronal cell death occurred. Such ischemic insults following human head injury appear to occur relatively frequently.[11–14] Bouma and colleagues documented regional or global ischemia, defined as a cerebral blood flow of 18 ml/100 g/min or less, by the xenon-133 method or by stable xenon-CT in approximately one-third of severe head injury patients evaluated within 6 to 8 h of injury.[11,12] Early ischemia correlated significantly with early mortality. Hypotension and/or hypoxia was documented in 57 percent of the severe head injury patients in the Traumatic Coma Data Bank (TCDB) cohort.[13] A single episode of hypotension was associated with an 85 percent increase in mortality.

The importance of secondary injury has been recognized for almost two decades. Graham and associates in 1978 documented ischemic brain damage in 92 percent of 151 head injury victims at autopsy, illustrating the ultimate consequences of postinjury hypotension, hypoxia, and intracranial hypertension.[15] Contemporaneous work by Jennett and Carlin suggested that further improvements in outcome after head injury would hinge largely on reversing or preventing such insults.[16] The concept of "early diagnosis and intensive management" to pre-empt secondary insults and thus improve outcome after severe head injury was emphasized by Becker and colleagues in 1977.[17] This aggressive medical and surgical approach, stressing maintenance of normothermia, optimizing hemodynamic function, treatment of hypoxia, cerebral ischemia, and intracranial hypertension, and emergent evacuation of intracranial hematomas, remains the basic therapeutic strategy for the 1990s.

RECENT THERAPEUTIC MODIFICATIONS

Although the essential treatment approach for head injury developed in the 1970s endures, the understanding of injury pathophysiology and the resultant therapeutic concepts have evolved substantially over the last decade. These modifications appear to affect long-term neurological recovery favorably. The most important changes are a greater emphasis on maintaining an adequate cerebral perfusion pressure in relation to ICP as a means of averting cerebral ischemia, and the recognition that aggressive hyperventilation to control ICP may promote cerebral ischemia. Recent investigations have delineated other causes of secondary brain injury, including excitatory amino acid release, coagulopathy, hyperthermia, hyperglycemia, and electrolyte disturbances.[18–27] Such insights have resulted in an intensified effort to prevent or minimize the impact of these insults (Fig. 6-1). The following discussion on cerebral perfusion pressure, ICP, cerebral blood flow, autoregulation, and the use of hyperventilation will provide the background and rationale for current management strategies in the patient with traumatic brain injury.

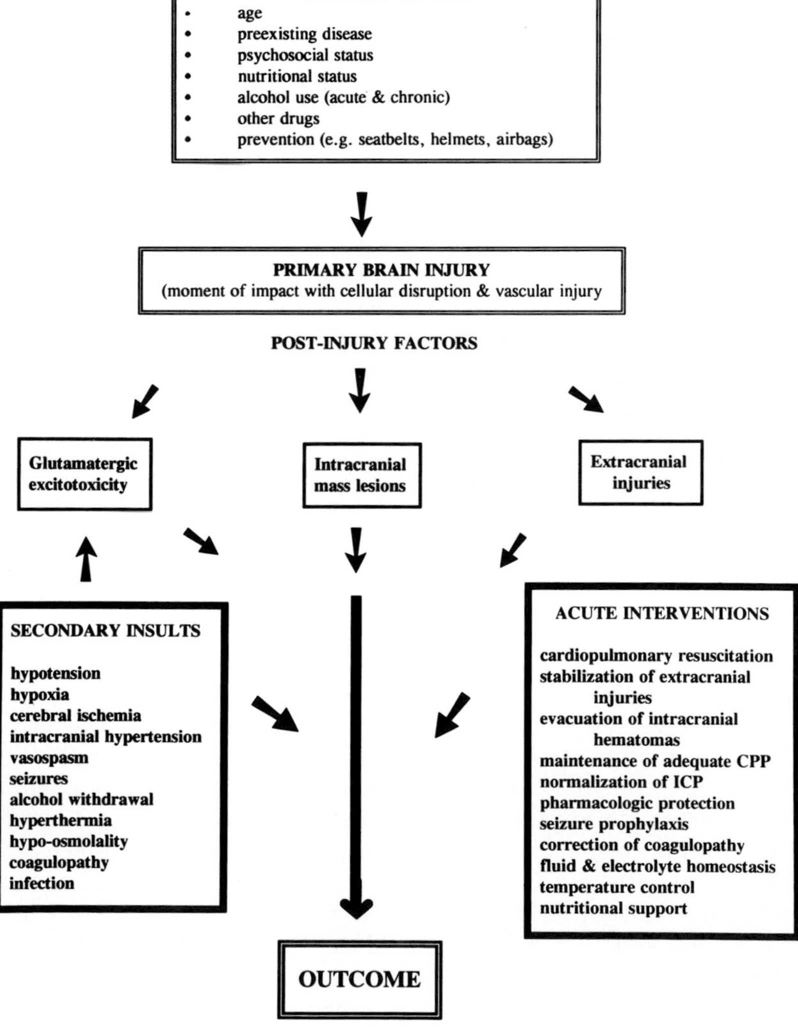

Figure 6-1. Schematic representation of factors and interventions that influence outcome before and after traumatic brain injury. (CPP = cerebral perfusion pressure.) (From Vollmer.[95])

TABLE 6-1 Outcome after Severe Closed Head Injury (GCS 7 or less) Comparing Cerebral Perfusion Pressure Therapy with Minimal Hyperventilation (*) to Traditional Management (TCDB cohort)

	Favorable (%)	Unfavorable (%)	Mortality (%)
Rosner et al*[(31)]	59	41	(29)
Marion et al*[(30)]	51	49	(20)
TCDB[(4)]	37	63	(40)

(outcome as defined by Glasgow Outcome Scale: favorable outcome includes good recovery and moderate disability; unfavorable outcome includes severe disability, vegetative, and dead; TCDB - Traumatic Coma Data Bank)

Outcome in Relation to Cerebral Perfusion Pressure (CPP)

Randomized trials have not been performed in patients with severe head injury by using different perfusion pressure goals. A retrospective report by McGraw of over 180 closed head injury patients demonstrated significantly better outcome and lower mortality when CPP was above 80 mmHg rather than below 80 mmHg during the first 48 h after injury.[28] In 116 severe head injury patients, Gopinath and coworkers demonstrated that mean and lowest recorded CPP correlated significantly with outcome.[27] The same investigators demonstrated in 163 severe head injury patients that a CPP of 60 mmHg was the critical level below which outcome was significantly worsened.[29]

Rosner and Rosner and Marion and colleagues studied outcome after severe closed head injury (Glasgow Coma Scale 7 or less) when perfusion pressure was maintained at 70 mmHg or greater and Pa_{CO_2} was kept in the range of 35 mmHg.[30,31] Rosner reported a favorable outcome (good recovery or moderate disability) in 59 percent of 158 patients and a mortality rate of 29 percent. Marion and colleagues documented favorable outcome in 51 percent of 84 patients at 6 months postinjury, with 20 percent mortality. These two reports compare favorably with the TCDB cohort in which a specific CPP goal was not established and hyperventilation to a Pa_{CO_2} below 30 mmHg was typically employed (Table 6-1).[4] In patients with an initial GCS of 7 or less analyzed by the TCDB, outcome was favorable in 37 percent, while mortality was 40 percent. Even more significant is a comparison of results in patients with traumatic hematomas requiring surgery who were treated by these two different management strategies. In the series by Rosner and Rosner, favorable outcome was achieved in 59 percent of operated patients; in the TCDB patients, a favorable outcome was seen in 23 percent of operated patients.

Autoregulation, Cerebral Perfusion Pressure, and ICP

Understanding the relationship between CPP and autoregulation is of fundamental importance in managing the head-injured patient. Autoregulation of cerebral blood flow is defined as the mechanism by which a constant flow is delivered to the brain over a wide range of systemic blood pressures or CPP.[32] CPP is the difference between the mean arterial pressure and the mean ICP. In normal subjects, mean arterial pressure ranges from 80 to 100 mmHg, ICP is 5 to 10 mmHg, and CPP ranges from 70 to 95 mmHg. Cerebral pressure autoregulation normally has a lower perfusion pressure limit of approximately 50 mmHg and an upper limit of approximately 140 mmHg. Below a perfusion pressure of 50 mmHg, compensatory cerebral arteriole vasodilation is exhausted, vessel collapse may occur, and cerebral ischemia ensues (Fig. 6-2). Above a perfusion pressure of 140 mmHg, cerebral vasoconstriction is overcome, and cerebral blood flow increases passively with perfusion pressure, resulting in blood brain barrier damage and brain edema.[33–35]

After traumatic brain injury, pressure autoregulation is often disturbed, yet there is considerable debate concerning the nature of this derangement. Recent studies by Bouma and Muizelaar indicate that one-third to one-half of severely head injured individuals will have some degree of autoregulatory impairment.[36–38] The most clinically relevant aspect of this derangement appears to be an elevation of the lower limit of perfusion pressure at which autoregulation will function.[39–41] Earlier studies suggested that a CPP of 50 mmHg to 60 mmHg was sufficient to achieve this autoregulatory threshold.[42–44] More recent investigations, however, indicate that most severe head injury patients require a perfusion pressure of at least 60 mmHg to 70 mmHg to achieve autoregulatory function and to reduce ischemic insults.[28–30,45,46] When perfusion pressure is maintained above this level, cerebral blood flow does not correlate

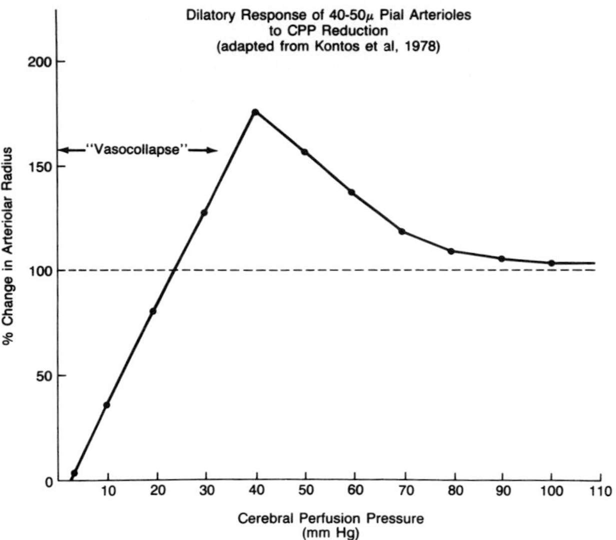

Figure 6-2. Diagram demonstrating autoregulatory arteriole vasodilation as cerebral perfusion pressure (CPP) is decreased. As the lower threshold for autoregulation is reached, cerebral blood flow falls passively with further decrements in perfusion pressure, and a state of "vasocollapse" is reached. (From Rosner.[48])

with CPP (Fig. 6-3).[47] Only when perfusion pressure falls below the lower autoregulatory threshold will cerebral blood flow become directly linked to perfusion pressure.[33,41,48]

A concern in maintaining relatively high CPP has been the exacerbation of intracranial hypertension through passive increases in cerebral blood flow in patients with impaired autoregulation.[49,50] In earlier studies, an association between "hyperemia" and intracranial hypertension was demonstrated in both adults and children after severe head injury.[50,51] However, more recent reports suggest that blood pressure elevations do not worsen intracranial hypertension in most head injury victims and that maintaining higher CPP may, in fact, facilitate ICP control.[36,37,46,52–54]

In a series of 66 head-injured adults, Kelly and coworkers documented hyperemia (cerebral blood flow > 55 ml/100 g/min) in 37 of 213 (17.4 percent) blood flow studies in 21 of 66 patients (31 percent).[54] Simultaneous intracranial hypertension occurred in 21.6 percent of the studies with hyperemia compared to 11.9 percent of the studies in which blood flow was below hyperemic levels. Although the incidence of intracranial hypertension was greater with simultaneous hyperemia, in approximately 80 percent raised ICP occurred in the setting of normal or low cerebral blood flow. This study suggests that hyperemia may be one of several causes of intracranial hypertension, but in the majority of head-injured patients high cerebral blood flow is not associated with high ICP. Investigations by Muizelaar and colleagues and Robertson and coworkers have also demonstrated a lack of correlation between elevated blood flow and intracranial hypertension.[52,53] In 158 severe head injury patients, Rosner and Rosner also found no positive correlation between CPP and intracranial

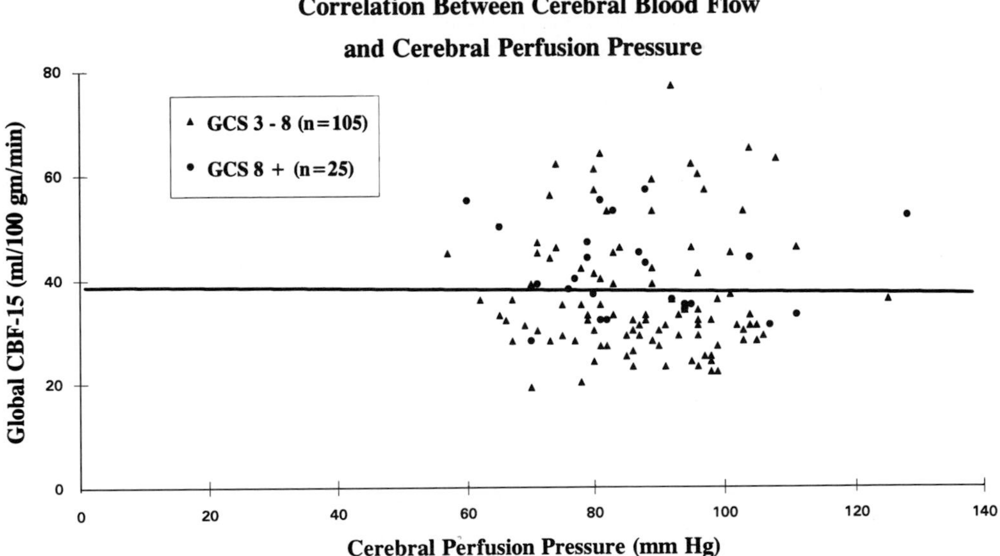

Figure 6-3. Lack of correlation between cerebral blood flow (CBF) and cerebral perfusion pressure in 130 measurements in 52 closed head injury patients. In 93 percent of the measurements, cerebral perfusion pressure was above 70 mmHg at the time of cerebral blood flow determination. (From Shalmon et al.[47])

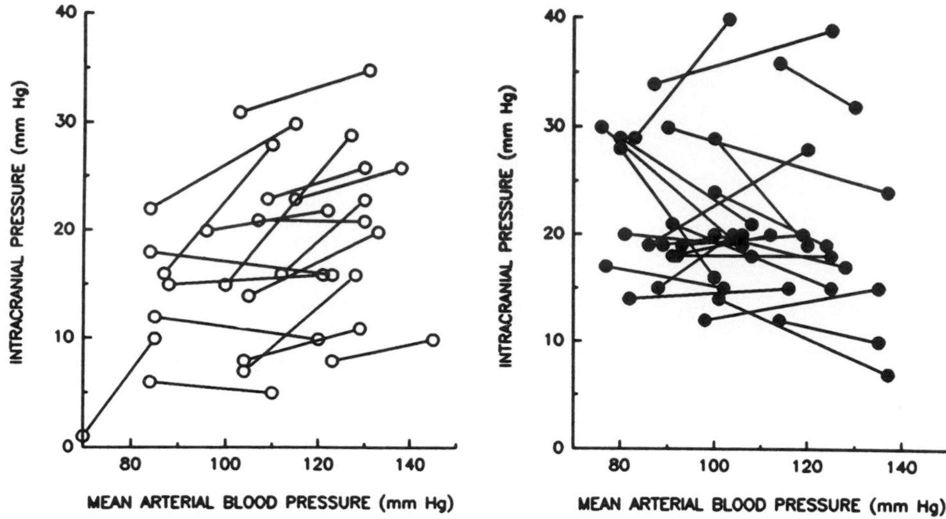

Figure 6-4. Graphs showing the relationship between changes in mean arterial blood pressure and ICP in severe head injury patients with defective (*left*) and intact (*right*) autoregulation. Note that in the majority of patients with defective autoregulation, a marked rise in ICP does not occur with blood pressure elevation. (From Bouma et al.[36])

hypertension.[46] On average, ICP decreased after CPP reached 72 mmHg and continued to decrease up to a perfusion pressure of 112 mmHg. In individual patients, however, this critical level of CPP above which ICP began to decline ranged widely from 43 to 130 mmHg.

In two reports of severe head injury patients by Bouma and associates autoregulation was directly tested and changes in cerebral blood flow and ICP were assessed in response to induced hypertension or hypotension[36,37] (Fig 6-4 and Table 6-2). These two studies demonstrated that, for the majority of patients with impaired autoregulation, induced hypertension will result in an increase in cerebral blood flow with a relatively low risk of significant intracranial hypertension. When individuals with impaired autoregulation were subjected to induced hypotension, a reduction in ICP and cerebral

TABLE 6-2 Physiological Parameters in Head-Injured Patients before and after Blood Pressure Manipulations

	Trimethaphan Group		*Phenylephrine Group*	
	Before	**After**	**Before**	**After**
Autoregulation intact				
MABP	120 ± 13	91 ± 10	93 ± 11	119 ± 11
ICP	20 ± 3	30 ± 2*	20 ± 6	20 ± 8
PVI	22 ± 5	22 ± 6	19 ± 6	21 ± 7
CBF	38 ± 6	35 ± 4	35 ± 10	37 ± 11
CMR_{O_2}	1.01 ± 0.29	0.99 ± 0.41	1.71 ± 0.62	1.60 ± 0.52
Autoregulation defective				
MABP	112 ± 19	90 ± 17	99 ± 12	126 ± 9
ICP	16 ± 5	11 ± 7*	16 ± 7	20 ± 9*
PVI	21 ± 9	24 ± 2**	22 ± 5	18 ± 4**
CBF	79 ± 38	37 ± 10	34 ± 6	50 ± 14
CMR_{O_2}	2.07 ± 0.29	1.86 ± 0.49	1.32 ± 0.39	1.50 ± 0.65

Values are means ± standard deviations, measured before and after administration of blood pressure regulatory agents. Autoregulation was intact in 40 patients and defective in 18 patients. (MABP = mean arterial blood pressure in mmHg; ICP = intracranial pressure; PVI = pressure-volume index (ml); CBF = cerebral blood flow; CMR_{O_2} = cerebral metabolic rate of oxygen in mL/100 g/min; statistical significance: * = $p < 0.01$, paired *t*-test, ** = $p < 0.05$).

SOURCE: From Bouma et al.[36] with permission.

blood flow occurred. Equally important was the finding that, in patients with intact autoregulation, induced hypertension did not cause changes in cerebral blood flow or ICP; however, a reduction of blood pressure resulted in a significant rise in ICP.

These investigations have important therapeutic implications. When autoregulation is intact, maintenance of an adequate perfusion pressure will help prevent intracranial hypertension. A fall in blood pressure generally will result in an increase in ICP because of reflex vasodilation and an increase in cerebral blood volume. An increase in blood pressure or perfusion pressure will cause a decrease or at least a stabilization of ICP due to reflex vasoconstriction.[33] The vasodilatory and vasoconstriction cascade models described by Rosner are helpful in understanding this process (Fig. 6-5).[55] Cyclic ICP waves originally defined by Lundberg, can be understood on the basis of these models (Fig. 6-6).[56,57] Both Lundberg A waves (plateau waves) and the shorter duration B waves appear to be initiated by decrements in systemic arterial pressure. When such pressure waves occur, efforts to rapidly improve perfusion pressure should be made by ICP reduction, blood pressure elevation, or both.

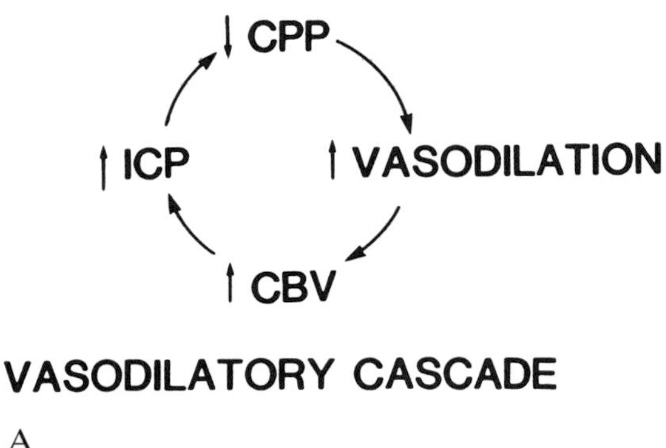

A

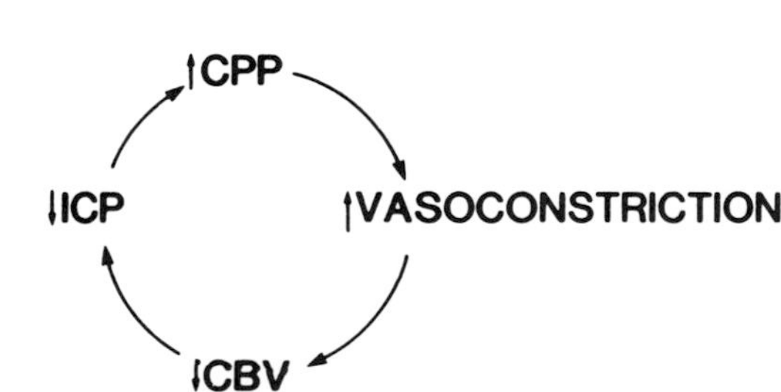

B

Figure 6-5. The vasodilatory and vasoconstriction cascades assume pressure autoregulatory mechanisms are intact. *A.* The vasodilatory cascade model illustrates how a decrease in cerebral perfusion pressure can result in cerebral vasodilation with an increase in cerebral blood volume and a rise in ICP. A drop in systemic arterial pressure is probably the most common cause of initiating the cascade. If blood pressure is not increased, perfusion pressure will continue to fall and ICP will continue to increase until vasodilation is maximal. *B.* The vasoconstriction cascade demonstrates the therapeutic effect on ICP of maintaining a higher cerebral perfusion pressure. Elevations of blood pressure with volume expansion, blood transfusion, bolus mannitol administration, and vasopressor therapy can all help initiate the cascade. (From Rosner.[55])

The vasoconstriction and vasodilation models do not apply when perfusion pressure falls below the lower autoregulatory threshold or exceeds the upper autoregulatory limit. In the latter situation, an increase in CPP may cause a significant rise in cerebral blood flow. The effect on ICP, however, is less dramatic, in that a significant exacerbation of intracranial hypertension does not commonly occur. The fact that ICP changed minimally with induced hypertension in the majority of patients with "impaired autoregulation" in the studies by Bouma and associates may indicate that a degree of autoregulatory control was achieved when higher perfusion pressures were reached.[36,37]

While the lower perfusion pressure autoregulatory limit appears to be in the range of 70 mmHg in most severe head injury patients, the upper limit is not well defined. Perfusion pressures in the range of 105 mmHg appear to have been well tolerated for relatively brief periods in the patients studied by Bouma and associates[36,37] Whether perfusion pressures of this level are ultimately beneficial when sustained for hours or days remains to be determined. Persistent induced hypertension to maintain perfusion pressures at this level may promote cerebral edema through a damaged blood-brain barrier and ultimately may prolong the period of intracranial hypertension. Additionally, systemic complications may result from prolonged vasopressor therapy utilized to maintain high perfusion pressure. In patients with significant autoregulatory impairment, induced hypertension may exacerbate intracranial hypertension through passive blood flow increases, although, as described above, this appears to be uncommon. High cerebral blood flow seen in the early injury period may also be partially attributable to transient glucose hypermetabolism, which could in turn exacerbate intracranial hypertension.[58,59] These forms of hyperemia-associated intracranial hypertension, although uncommon, are probably optimally treated by suppression of the cerebral metabolic rate using high-dose pentobarbital or propofol, while still maintaining an adequate CPP. If cerebral blood flow measurements are available, this modality can help determine if hyperemia is in fact contributing to elevated ICP.

In summary, maintaining CPP at or above 70 mmHg after severe head injury is recommended because it appears to reduce the risk of cerebral ischemia, facilitates ICP control in the majority of patients, and substantially

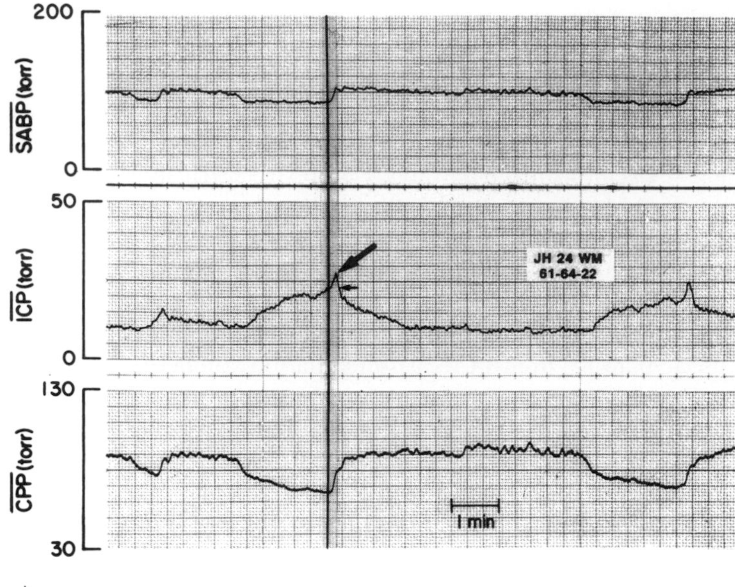

A

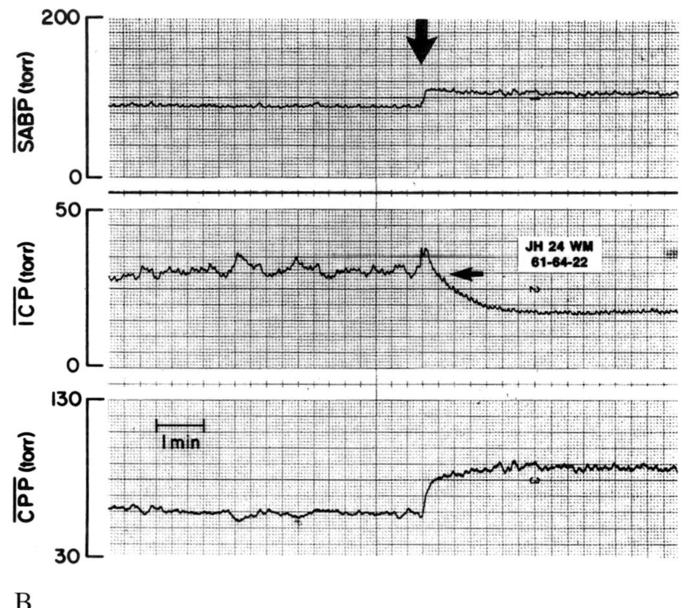

B

Figure 6-6. *A*. Two strong ICP waves are demonstrated in this patient. The first wave is initiated by a drop in systolic arterial blood pressure (SABP) of approximately 10 mmHg, beginning 2 minutes before the heavy black line. The ICP gradually increases over the next 2 minutes and then is arrested by a termination spike, marked by the *large arrow*. The second ICP wave is very similar in appearance and also is initiated by a decrement in systolic blood pressure. *B*. This patient demonstrates the effect of a spontaneous increase in mean systolic blood pressure from approximately 90 to 110 mmHg, which results in a rise in cerebral perfusion pressure from approximately 60 to 85 mmHg (*heavy black arrow*). At this point, there is an ICP termination spike from approximately 30 to 37 mmHg, lasting about 10 seconds, and then a sustained decrease in ICP to a level of approximately 18 mmHg. The cascade model explains this decrease in ICP based on restoration of an optimal perfusion pressure with resultant vasoconstriction and a decreased blood volume. (CPP = cerebral perfusion pressure) (From Rosner.[48])

improves long-term outcome compared with historical controls. This threshold, however, appears to have a rather wide range from patient to patient and has a variable time course. Some patients will maintain cerebral blood flow well above ischemic thresholds at a perfusion pressure below 70 mmHg; others may require perfusion pressures in the range of 80 to 100 mmHg. Although the upper safe range for perfusion pressure remains ill-defined, sustained levels of 90 to 100 mmHg appear to be well tolerated and may be beneficial in some patients for achieving autoregulatory function and control of ICP. When ICP and CPP cannot be maintained at normal levels (i.e., ICP below 20 mmHg and perfusion pressure above 70 mmHg), maintenance of an adequate perfusion pressure should still be aggressively pursued. With an adequate CPP, modest intracranial hypertension appears to be well tolerated if clinical status and CT findings do not suggest imprending herniation from a surgically amenable mass lesion.[31,60] The precise level and duration of raised ICP that does not adversely affect outcome, however, remains to be defined. Given the strong correlation between elevated ICP and poor outcome, an aggressive attempt to maintain ICP below 20 mmHg should still be made.[61–63]

Hyperventilation

Despite the effectiveness of hypocapnia in reducing cerebral blood volume and ICP, its use has recently been curtailed in severe head injury patients. This change is based on evidence that maintaining Pa_{CO_2} in the range of 25 to 30 mmHg can result in significant cerebral vasoconstriction and marked reductions in blood flow.[64,65] In a randomized trial by Muizelaar and coworkers of severe head injury patients maintained at an average Pa_{CO_2} of either 25 or 35 mmHg, the patients treated with normocapnia had a significantly better outcome at 3 and 6 months postinjury.[64] This difference in outcome, however, was seen only in patients with Glasgow motor scores of 4 or 5 and was not present 1 year after injury.

Gopinath and colleagues studied the effects of hypocapnia in 116 severe head injury patients with continuous jugular venous oxygen saturation (Sjv_{O_2}) monitoring.[27] In patients with episodes of oxygen desaturation, the cause was attributed to a Pa_{CO_2} of less than 29 mmHg in 27 percent. Single or multiple episodes of desaturation to an Sjv_{O_2} of less than 50 percent strongly correlated with poor outcome. The good outcome in severe head injury patients reported by Rosner and Rosner and Marion and coworkers with perfusion pressure management and maintenance of normocapnia, also suggests that hyperventilation is not essential for achieving a high rate of functional survivors.[30,31]

Hyperventilation probably has its most deleterious effect during the first 24 h after severe head injury, when cerebral blood flow is typically at its lowest.[12,66] It is therefore recommended that Pa_{CO_2} be maintained at approximately 35 mmHg within the first 24 h after injury, and in the range of 30 to 35 mmHg after that time if ICP control is problematic. Although hyperventilation is effective in lowering ICP at least transiently, it is generally not essential if other standard methods are utilized. Dissemination of this information to emergency room physicians and paramedics is warranted, given that significant hyperventilation is still commonly practiced in the initial management of the comatose head-injured patient.

INITIAL MANAGEMENT

Prehospital and Emergency Room Care

Assessment and stabilization of the head injury victim begins at the injury scene by emergency medical personnel. Their tasks include securing the patient's airway, initiating fluid resuscitation, stabilizing the cervical and thoracolumbar spine, identifying and stabilizing extracranial injuries, and assessing the patient's level of consciousness. Obtaining information on the mechanism of injury and providing rapid transport to a qualified medical facility are also critical components of initial management.

Once the victim is in the hospital, care should progress in a rapid and systematic manner, with diagnostic and therapeutic maneuvers proceeding simultaneously. This approach is best facilitated by a designated trauma team, which has become the standard of care for acute management of the trauma victim. As in the prehospital setting, the most immediate concerns are establishing a secure airway, providing adequate ventilation, and correcting or preventing hypoxia and hypotension. Adequate venous access with a minimum of two large-bore peripheral intravenous lines (16-gauge or larger) is essential in managing the hypotensive, hypovolemic trauma patient. Simultaneously, a general survey is performed to assess for major extracranial injuries. Life-threatening insults such as tension pneumothorax, cardiac tamponade, or major vascular injuries with hypovolemic shock take precedence over neurological injury and are addressed immediately. Initial radiological studies in the trauma patient include a three-view cervical spine series plus chest and pelvic films. An indwelling catheter to monitor urine output and an oro- or nasogastric tube are placed. Contraindications to nasogastric tube insertion include suspected anterior cranial base or midface fractures. Initial laboratory studies should include a type and cross-match for possible blood transfusion, complete blood count, serum electrolytes, glucose, creatinine, arterial blood gas, prothrombin time and parital thromboplastin time, and urinalysis. A blood alcohol level and a urine toxicology screen for narcotics, benzodiazepines, amphetamines, cocaine, and phencyclidine (PCP) are also useful.

Hypoxia and airway management

Hypoxia during resuscitation was documented in 46 percent of patients in the TCDB cohort and was significantly associated with poor outcome.[13] Transient or prolonged apnea after concussive brain injury is a well-recognized phenomenon and a major contributor to postinjury hypoxia.[67] Associated injuries such as flail chest, hemothorax or pneumothorax, upper airway trauma, and cervical spinal cord injury will also impair ventilation and oxygenation. Intoxication from alcohol or other sedative-hypnotics will diminish respiratory drive and protective airway reflexes as well.

In patients with poor airway protection or inadequate

ventilatory effort, prompt endotracheal intubation is required. In recent years, as emergency medical technicians have become more highly trained, endotracheal intubation at the injury scene has become commonly practiced. Specific indications for intubation in the head-injured patient include inability to maintain adequate ventilation, impending airway loss from a neck or pharyngeal injury, poor airway protection associated with depressed level of consciousness, or potential for neurological deterioration when being transported out of the emergency room. All patients who are not verbalizing and who cannot follow commands should be intubated promptly. In general, this means that all patients with GCS of 8 or less require intubation and assisted ventilation.

The vast majority of head injury victims can be safely intubated via the orotracheal route with in-line stabilization of the cervical spine, even prior to obtaining radiographs of the cervical spine. This method of intubation, with strict maintenance of a neutral head position and slight to no axial traction, causes minimal movement of the potentially unstable cervical spine and has not been associated with new neurological deficit in three clinical series.[68–70] The nasotracheal route of intubation is contraindicated in patients with possible fractures of the anterior cranial base and/or midface, requires considerably more experience and time, and has a lower success rate and a higher complication rate than does oral intubation.[71] In patients with major facial or upper airway trauma, a surgical airway by cricothyroidotomy may be required, although the complication rate in the emergency setting may be as high as 32 percent.[71]

Orotracheal intubation in the head-injured patient is best facilitated by rapid sequence induction utilizing thiopental, 3 to 5 mg/kg, and succinylcholine, 1 to 2 mg/kg.[70] In recent years, as an alternative to thiopental, the ultra-short-acting hypnotic anesthetic agent etomidate appears to be safe and effective for rapid sequence induction.[72,73] Once intubated, adequate sedation and paralysis are essential to help prevent dangerous spikes in ICP caused by "bucking" on the endotracheal tube or excessive motor activity. Narcotic sedation with morphine or fentanyl is effective, and neuromuscular blockade with vecuronium or pancuronium can be added if excessive motor activity persists.

Hypotension and Fluid Resuscitation

Hypotension was documented in almost 35 percent of the severe head injury patients in the TCDB cohort and was an even more ominous predictor of poor outcome than was hypoxia.[13] Klauber and colleagues documented a mortality of 35 percent in head-injured patients admitted with a systolic blood pressure of less than 85 mmHg compared with a mortality of only 6 percent in patients presenting with higher systolic blood pressures.[74] Hypotension or hypoxia also have been shown to correlate with diffuse brain swelling on CT.[75]

Most head injury victims with hypotension and multisystem trauma have sustained significant volume loss and require rapid fluid resuscitation. Volume replacement can significantly improve cerebral perfusion and often results in a dramatic improvement in neurological status.[76] The optimal method of fluid resuscitation in the hypotensive, hypovolemic brain-injured patient remains controversial. Isotonic saline (0.9% NaCl) is the most commonly used and least expensive preparation for volume resuscitation. A concern when using isotonic saline has been the development of brain edema. Experimental and clinical studies suggest that the risk of aggravating brain edema with isotonic crystalloid fluid resuscitation is minimal provided hypo-osmolality does not develop.[77,78] However, infusion of even mildly hypotonic saline for fluid resuscitation has been associated with increased brain edema in experimental studies.[79] Because commercially available Ringer's lactate solution is significantly more hypo-osmolar than its calculated osmolality of 273 mOsm/kg, use of 0.9% normal saline with an osmolality of 308 mOsm/kg is recommended.[78–80]

Recently, hypertonic saline or colloid infusions have been used in the acute resuscitative phase after head injury. Such solutions are potent volume expanders and may help prevent development of brain edema and intracranial hypertension by creating a favorable gradient for the movement of free water from the extravascular to the intravascular compartment.[81,82] Both experimental and clinical studies suggest that hypertonic saline may prove to be an effective form of early volume expansion in the head-injured patient.[83,84] The use of colloid for acute volume expansion is appealing because compounds such as albumin or 6% hetastarch have a high molecular weight and a relatively low vascular permeability. With longer intravascular retention time their effect on volume expansion is more sustained compared to isotonic crystalloid, and theoretically the risk of aggravating brain edema is diminished. However, reviews of randomized trials comparing crystalloid versus albumin for fluid resuscitation have shown no difference in survival and a significantly greater cost when using albumin.[85,86]

Currently, neither hypertonic saline nor colloid preparations appear to have a distinct advantage over isotonic crystalloid as a means of achieving prompt volume expansion in the head-injured hypovolemic patient. Rapid infusion of 1 to 2 liters of 0.9% NaCl generally is effective in hemodynamically stabilizing most trauma victims.[80] If hypotension is not reversed after 1 to 2 liters of crystalloid and/or colloid, a central venous line should be inserted, and transfusion of packed red blood cells is indicated. Despite their widespread use, no studies have demonstrated an improved survival with the use of military antishock trousers (MAST) in the multiple trauma patient.[87]

Neurological Evaluation

The Glasgow Coma Scale

One of the most important factors in early treatment decisions and in long-term outcome after head injury is the patient's initial level of consciousness.[4,6,7] Although many methods of defining level of consciousness exist, the most widely used measure is the Glasgow Coma Scale (GCS) first presented by Teasdale and Jennett in 1974 (Fig. 6-7).[88,89] The utility of this scaling system is in its objectivity, reproducibility, and simplicity. It provides paramedics, nurses, and physicians with a rapid measure of level of consciousness, obviating ambiguous terminology such as "lethargic," "stuporous," and "obtunded." Because the level of consciousness can be lowered independent of head injury by several factors, including shock, hypoxia, hypothermia, alcohol intoxication, the postictal state, and administration of sedatives or narcotics, the postresuscitation GCS is generally considered more reliable in providing an initial assessment of injury severity.[90,91] Although not consistently defined, this score generally refers to the best GCS obtained within the first 6 to 8 h of injury following nonsurgical resuscitation.[4,91,93–95] Injury severity is generally categorized into three levels based on the postresuscitation GCS. Minor or mild head injury includes patients whose initial GCS is 13 to 15; moderate injury includes patients with a GCS of 9 to 12; severe injury refers to a GCS of 3 to 8 or a subsequent deterioration to a GCS of 8 or less (Table 6-2).[6,7,88,93] These categorizations, although arbitrary, have helped to define the spectrum of traumatic brain injury and are useful in guiding therapy and providing important prognostic information.

Glasgow Coma Scale

EYE OPENING
- 4 = Spontaneously
- 3 = To voice
- 2 = To pain
- 1 = None

VERBAL RESPONSE
- 5 = Oriented
- 4 = Confused
- 3 = Inappropriate words
- 2 = Incomprehensible sounds
- 1 = None

MOTOR RESPONSE
- 6 = Follows commands
- 5 = Localizes to pain
- 4 = Withdrawal to pain
- 3 = Abnormal flexion
- 2 = Abnormal extension
- 1 = None

Figure 6-7. Introduced by Teasdale and Jennett in 1974, the Glasgow Coma Scale provides an objective, rapidly performed assessment of the level of consciousness.[88] The postresuscitation GCS is one of the strongest predictors of long-term outcome following craniocerebral trauma.

Neurological Examination

In the acutely head injured patient, the neurological examination is necessarily abbreviated and should focus on the level of consciousness, the pupillary light reflexes, extraocular eye movements, the motor examination, and lower brainstem reflexes for patients in deep coma. As part of this initial survey, the head should be carefully palpated to detect bony step-offs, and all scalp lacerations should be gently probed to assess for depressed fractures and foreign bodies. Signs of a basal skull fracture also should be sought, including hemotympanum, cerebrospinal fluid otorrhea or rhinorrhea, and retromastoid or periorbital ecchymosis and tenderness. This initial assessment, along with inspection of the neck and thoracolumbar spine, should take no longer than 5 to 10 min. Before leaving the emergency department for CT, the cervical spine should be evaluated with a lateral view x-ray, which includes the cervicothoracic junction. If time permits, anteroposterior and open mouth views should also be obtained before leaving the emergency department.

The triad of a deteriorating level of consciousness, pupillary dilation, and an associated hemiparesis has long been recognized as highly suggestive of a hemispheric mass lesion causing transtentorial herniation.[104] However, any one of these findings in a patient after head injury may be a manifestation of a traumatic hematoma and when noted should heighten the urgency of evaluation. Such signs also may be absent, falsely localizing, or may occur in patients with diffuse brain injuries.[105] Other etiologies of diminished consciousness also should be considered in the patient who appears to have sustained a head injury, including seizure activity, the postictal state, alcohol intoxication, drug over-

CT Scanning Criteria Following Craniocerebral Trauma

GCS 14 or less

GCS 15 with:

- **documented loss of consciousness**
- **amnesia for injury**
- **focal neurologic deficit**
- **signs of basal or calvarial skull fracture**

Figure 6-8. Given the significant risk of rapid deterioration in the mildly head injured patient, the threshold for obtaining a timely CT scan should be low.

dose, and severe hypoglycemia. Because the neurological examination is frequently unreliable in accurately predicting intracranial pathology, radiological evaluation, preferably with CT, is always indicated in the acutely head injured patient.

A CT is indicated in all head-injured patients with a depressed level of consciousness, including those who are heavily inebriated. Too frequently, alcohol-intoxicated patients are initially observed in the emergency room and CT is prompted by neurological deterioration. A timely CT is also indicated in all patients with a GCS of 15 who sustained a loss of consciousness, are amnestic to the injury, have a focal neurological deficit, or have signs of a basilar or calvarial skull fracture (Fig. 6-8). An axial CT without contrast rapidly defines intracranial lesions and determines whether urgent neurosurgical intervention is required. Obtaining both brain and bone "windows" will help determine the etiology and the significance of focal neurological findings and whether a skull fracture is present. When CT is available, skull x-rays are obviated.[102,103] When CT is of limited availability or nonexistent, skull x-rays still have a role, as demonstrated by the study of Miller and coworkers.[101] If a skull fracture is seen, and if the patient is stable, further close observation is indicated; or, preferably, the patient can be transferred to a facility where CT is available. In patients who are comatose or deteriorating, if a neurosurgeon is present, further diagnostic evaluation with cerebral angiography, contrast or air ventriculography, or exploratory burr holes is indicated.

The deteriorating patient

Despite the strong predictive value of the GCS, a significant portion of patients with seemingly minor injuries, based on their initial level of consciousness, will have sustained a serious intracranial insult. Klauber and associates analyzing over 7900 head trauma victims from 41 hospitals, concluded that the excessive mortality noted in some of the hospitals was likely due to inadequate observation of the less severely injured patients.[74] Stein and Ross specifically addressed individuals with a postresuscitation GCS of 13.[96,97] In 658 patients with an initial GCS of 13 to 15, 18 percent had abnormalities on CT scan and 5 percent required surgery. Of the 62 patients with a GCS of 13, 40 percent had CT abnormalities and 10 percent required surgery. They concluded that such patients should be considered to have sustained a moderate head injury and that their initial management should be more rigorous and vigilant than is customary for indivuduals with a GCS of 14 or 15.

Several reports have addressed the problem of patients who initially are conscious after injury but then worsen to a GCS of 8 or less. Such patients who "talk and deteriorate" have comprised 10 to 32 percent of severe head injury victims.[98–100] Lobato and colleagues noted that 25 percent of 838 severely head injured patients talked at some point prior to lapsing into coma.[99] Almost 36 percent of these patients were fully oriented during their lucid interval. Most notably, 80 percent had a focal mass lesion, requiring evacuation in the majority of cases. Over a 10-year period, Miller and coworkers documented 183 patients with closed head injury, an initial GCS of 15, and who subsequently required evacuation of a traumatic hematoma.[101] This cohort represented 17 percent of all patients requiring craniotomy for acute traumatic hematoma during the study period. Approximately 40 percent of patients reported no loss of consciousness, posttraumatic amnesia, headache, or vomiting when first evaluated. However, 33 percent had a focal neurological deficit despite being fully conscious, 19 percent had signs of a basal skull fracture, and 60 percent had a skull fracture on skull x-ray. These studies provide strong rationale for closely monitoring the conscious head-injured patient, including frequent neurological assessments and an early CT.

Early management of intracranial hypertension

Measures to control intracranial hypertension should begin prior to obtaining a CT in individuals who arrive in coma, have a precipitous decline in level of consciousness, or develop pupillary asymmetry or hemiparesis, given the likelihood that a traumatic mass lesion is responsible for the patient's deterioration. Such interventions include intubation and assisted ventilation, sedation, bolus mannitol therapy, and administration of prophylactic phenytoin. Prevention of hypotension by establishing euvolemia and in some cases vasopressor therapy also is critical to maintain adequate CPP and to help control ICP.[36,48] This aggressive approach will result in overtreatment of some patients, but may be a

Emergent Management of Intracranial Hypertension

- **Intubation**
- **Controlled ventilation to $PaCO_2$ 35 mmHg**
- **Volume resuscitation**
- **Establishment of normotension**
- **Narcotic sedation / neuromuscular blockade**
- **Bolus mannitol 1 gram/kg**
- **Phenytoin 18 mg/kg**

Figure 6-9. When head-injured patients arrive in coma (GCS 8 or less), precipitously deteriorate in level of consciousness, or have pupillary dilation or obvious hemiparesis, such interventions are urgently indicated prior to obtaining a head CT.

deciding factor in others whose precarious neurological state is greatly improved by such interventions. Rapid implementation of these maneuvers will generally "buy time" and allow for a precise CT diagnosis to be made (Fig. 6-9).

Once a secure airway is established, narcotic sedation with morphine or fentanyl should be achieved; a neuromuscular blocking agent such as vecuronium or pancuronium can be added when agitation or abnormal posturing persist. Mild hyperventilation to achieve a Pa_{CO_2} of 35 mmHg should be instituted and a 0.5 to 1.0 g/kg intravenous bolus of mannitol administered. The risk of inducing hypotension in the hypovolemic patient by mannitol administration is low, provided adequate fluid replacement with normal saline and/or colloid administration is occurring simultaneously. Mannitol used in this manner is highly effective in treating both intracranial hypertension and hypovolemia and will improve CPP.[48,106] Prophylactic anticonvulsant therapy with phenytoin (18 mg/kg intravenous loading dose) should be administered as an additional preemptive measure against intracranial hypertension given that generalized seizures in a patient with an intracranial mass lesion can have devastating consequences.

Special concerns in the multiple trauma patient

Extracranial trauma complicates 30 to 70 percent of head injuries; approximately 5 percent of head injury victims sustain a cervical spine injury.[98,107–109] In the TCDB cohort, multiple trauma occurred in 70 percent of patients but was not a major determinant of mortality in any age group.[109] Only when severe extracranial injuries accompany mild or moderate head injury is mortality significantly influenced by associated injuries.[170] Because of the aggressive prehospital and emergency care common today, many critically ill trauma patients are intubated, sedated, and pharmacologically paralyzed before being seen by a neurosurgeon. Close cooperation and communication with the trauma or emergency physicians is essential in order to obtain information on the patient's initial neurological status and to plan a coherent sequence of diagnostic and therapuetic procedures. If the neurosurgeon is not present during the initial moments of evaluation, the emergency or trauma physicians must be able to perform an adequate neurological examination and be adept at making appropriate early management decisions regarding the patient's neurological status. For example, patients should not be detained in the emergency room to undergo diagnostic peritoneal lavage or other lengthy investigative studies prior to a head CT if they are hemodynamically stable and have no findings to suggest a serious intraabdominal or thoracic injury. Adherence to this principle is especially important in all moderate and severe head injury patients and in those who have a focal neurological deficit or evidence of a calvarial or skull base fracture. On occasion, however, a patient will be so hemodynamically unstable as to require emergency thoracotomy or laparotomy prior to obtaining a head CT. In this situation, the initial neurological assessment should determine whether ICP monitoring or exploratory burr holes are required while the patient is under general anesthesia. In patients with localizing signs such as significant pupillary asymmetry or marked hemiparesis, or in those with abnormal posturing, exploratory burr holes are warranted. In patients with a GCS of 13 or less without localizing signs, intraoperative ICP monitoring is recommended, given that most of these patients will have significant intracranial injuries. Any patient with a GCS of 14 or 15 who has extensive external craniocervical trauma also should be considered for monitoring. For patients with a GCS of 8 or less, a ventriculostomy with the ability to drain cerebrospinal fluid is indicated, given the high likelihood of raised ICP in such patients.[63,110,118] For those with a GCS of 9 or greater, a less invasive monitoring technique such as parenchymal fiber-optic probe may be more prudent and fraught with fewer complications than "blind" ventriculostomy placement.

Because hypotension can significantly depress the level of consciousness independent of head injury, a significant number of patients who undergo intraoperative pressure monitoring as outlined by this algorithm ultimately will not have needed it. The consequences, however, of undiagnosed and untreated intracranial hypertension argue against a less invasive approach. When these patients leave the operating room after their emergency procedure, they should be taken directly for head CT. The noninvasive technique of transcranial near-infrared spectroscopy has recently been demonstrated by Gopinath and coworkers to be highly accurate in diagnosing traumatic intracranial hematomas.[111] This technique may have its most useful application in hemodynamically unstable multiple trauma patients who must be taken emergently to the operating room prior to CT.

Monitoring after initial resuscitation

Less than half of severe head injury victims and significantly fewer sustaining a moderate closed head injury will require evacuation of a traumatic intracranial hematoma. Whether surgery is required or not, the intensity of monitoring and medical intervention will be determined largely by the patient's level of consciousness and CT findings. Given the significant risk of neurological deterioration following closed or penetrating injuries of even moderate severity, all such individuals warrant careful and frequent observation, preferably in an intensive care unit. In nonintubated moderate head injury patients, minimal monitoring should include continuous electrocardiogram recording and pulse oximetry; neurological assessments should be performed every 30 min for at least the first 6 h after injury and then on an hourly basis until the patient's condition has clearly stabilized or is improving. A loss of two points or more on the GCS, new pupillary asymmetry, or hemiparesis warrant an urgent repeat CT. Worsening headache, persisent vomiting, or seizure activity also should prompt an urgent reevaluation by CT. Monitoring of severe head injury patients is deferred to the discussion of critical care in traumatic brain injury.

Early repeat CT and coagulopathy

When potential surgical lesions are seen on the initial CT, a repeat scan within 4 to 8 h of the first scan should be part of routine monitoring. Based on a review of 154 consecutive closed head injury patients requiring surgical intervention, McBride and colleagues found that 47.5 percent of patients who had initial nonoperative lesions on CT required surgical intervention based on the findings of the follow-up CT.[112] In a recent study by Stein and associates, 44.5 percent of 337 consecutive patients sustaining a closed head injury developed delayed or progressive lesions seen on a follow-up CT scan.[23] Factors that were significantly associated with the development of delayed cerebral insults included increasing severity of the initial head injury as defined by GCS, the need for cardiopulmonary resuscitation at the accident site, the presence of a subdural hematoma on the first CT scan, and the presence of coagulopathy upon admission. Further addressing coagulopathy after closed head injury, the same investigators found elevated prothrombin time, partial thromboplastin time, or low platelet count in 37.5 percent of 253 patients upon admission.[24] In those patients who developed delayed brain injury as defined above, 55 percent had an abnormal prothrombin time, partial thromboplastin time, or platelet count; in those whose follow-up CT scans did not worsen, only 9 percent had abnormal coagulation studies. The risk of developing a delayed insult on CT was 85 percent in those with at least one abnormal clotting study and only 31 percent for those without such abnormalities. When coagulopathy is present upon admission, Stein and associates advocate early repeat CT scanning. This concept of timely follow-up evaluation is particularly relevant in many of today's trauma centers, where patients are routinely scanned within 1 to 2 h of injury, when the hemorrhagic process may still be evolving.

Indications for Surgery

The most critical factors in deciding whether to proceed with surgical evacuation of an intracranial hematoma are the patient's neurological status, the imaging findings, and the extent of extracranial injury. There is little debate that surgical intervention is indicated in a rapidly deteriorating patient who harbors an expanding intracranial hematoma causing significant mass effect. In general, all acute traumatic extraaxial hematomas 1 cm or greater in thickness warrant urgent evacuation. For less obvious situations controversy persists, but several reasonable statements can be made. Generally, a subdural hematoma or epidural hematoma of over 5 mm in thickness with an equivalent midline shift in a comatose patient (GCS 8 or less) should be evacuated urgently. On the other hand, surgical decompression of a thin-rim subdural hematoma of 3 mm or less, associated with marked hemispheric swelling and a large midline shift, is unlikely to improve the patient's condition or reduce ICP.[60,113,114] Such patients are best managed medically. A CT should be repeated, especially if the first scan is obtained within a few hours of injury or if there are other associated lesions, such as contusions that may have progressed in the interim.

Another somewhat controversial group of patients are those with an acute epidural or subdural hematoma 5 to 10 mm thick who have a GCS of 9 to 13. An urgent operative course is warranted in all patients with a deteriorating level of consciousness, pupillary abnormalities, hemiparesis, or when CT reveals effacement of the basilar cisterns or a hematoma in the middle fossa causing mass effect. Patients that can be managed in an intensive care setting with frequent neurological examinations include those with a stable or improving level of consciousness, no focal deficits, and normal basilar cisterns on CT with no appreciable midline shift. Often such patients are older and have some degree of cortical atrophy. Any deterioration warrants a repeat CT or in some cases a direct trip to the operating room. Another group of patients who warrant initial conservative management are those with an interhemispheric subdural hematoma without neurological deficit, given the risks of operating along the sagittal sinus.

Perhaps the most controversy exists over when to evacuate intracerebral hematomas and hemorrhagic contusions, and whether such removal is helpful in controlling ICP and improving outcome.[60] Miller and coworkers in their experience with over 200 severely head injured patients found that despite removing such lesions, patients with contusions or intracerebral hematomas had the highest incidence of intracranial hypertension of all subgroups in the study.[108] Consequently, they recommend an initial nonoperative course in most cases, resorting to surgery if medical management of intracranial hypertension has failed. Others, such as Cooper, believe that early surgical removal of larger intracerebral hematomas and cerebral contusions provides early control of ICP and helps prevent the cascade of secondary events leading to later intracranial hypertension.[114]

Despite such debate, there is general agreement that the decision to remove an intracerebral hematoma or cerebral contusion should be based on several key factors, including the size of the lesion, its depth and exact location from the cortical surface, the presence of associated lesions, and the patient's neurological status and ICP.[60,114] Cortical contusions over 2 cm in diameter generally should be removed if there is significant mass effect and ICP is difficult to control medically. Frontal pole and temporal lobe hematomas or contusions 2 cm in diameter or more with significant mass effect, basilar cistern impingement, and midline shift of over 5 mm also should be removed if ICP management is problematic. An initial conservative approach is warranted, however, when eloquent cortex is involved, such as dominant temporal lobe lesions or lesions near the central sulcus. An expectant course is also indicated in comatose but neurologically stable patients with small lesions associated with less than 5 mm midline shift and open basilar cisterns on CT. Similarly, lesions confined to the deep white matter or basal ganglia are best managed without surgery. ICP should be carefully monitored and controlled by medical means. If such measures fail, the patient can be reconsidered for surgery. In patients with a GCS of 9 to 13, a conservative course in an intensive care setting is reasonable in individuals with cerebral contusions or an intracerebral hematoma, provided they have a stable or improving level of consciousness, midline shift of 3 mm or less, and no significant basilar cistern effacement is seen on CT.

Finally, there are situations where the dismal clinical status of the patient warrants a nonoperative course despite the presence of a radiographic surgical lesion. Such cases include the adult patient who after resuscitation remains flaccid with a GCS of 3, nonreactive and dilated pupils, and without spontaneous respirations. Similarly, in patients over the age of 75 with a GCS of 5 or less, a nonoperative course generally should be taken given their almost uniformly poor outcome with or without surgery.[109,115] All other patients with surgical mass lesions, even those with a postresuscitation GCS of 3, but at least one reactive pupil, warrant emergent operative intervention. A significant, albeit small, portion of such patients will make a satisfactory recovery. Additionally, in some patients a low GCS may in part be due to intoxication or the postictal state.[91]

CRITICAL CARE IN TRAUMATIC BRAIN INJURY

Intensive care of the patient with traumatic brain injury has two primary and interrelated goals: maintenance or reestablishment of neurological and systemic homeostasis and early detection of neurological deterioration. Of principal importance is achieving adequate CPP and normalizing ICP as well as minimizing or preventing additional secondary insults resulting from hypotension, hypoxia, seizures, hyperthermia, electrolyte disturbances, coagulopathy, and infection. Although the following guidelines pertain largely to patients sustaining severe head injuries, the discussion also is highly relevant to those with moderate injuries. In individuals with less severe injuries secondary insults may have the greatest impact.

Essential Monitoring

Monitoring equipment for the severe head injury patient should include an ICP monitor, central venous pressure line, an arterial pressure line, and continuous pulse oximetry. An end-tidal CO_2 monitor is also useful to allow timely adjustments of the ventilatory rate when spontaneous Pa_{CO_2} changes occur.

Hemodynamic Monitoring

Hemodynamic monitoring and support is a critical component in the overall management strategy of severe head injury patients. The goals of monitoring include optimizing volume status and cardiac function, maximizing tissue perfusion, and averting complications of fluid management and pharmacological hemodynamic therapy. A central venous pressure line or a pulmonary artery (Swan-Ganz) catheter is recommended for management of all severely injured patients. In most young healthy adults, central venous or right atrial pressures tend to reflect volume status and left ventricular function, especially when used in conjunction with other clinical parameters such as blood pressure, pulse rate, and urine output. However, in older or critically ill patients, this correlation often fails. Consequently, a pulmonary artery catheter is recommended for patients over the age of 50 to 60 years, for individuals with preexisting hypertension, cardiac or pulmonary disease, and for those with major extracranial trauma, particularly spinal cord, chest, or abdominal injuries, or when vasopressor or high-dose barbiturates are used. Hypovolemic or cardiogenic shock, respiratory failure, sepsis, or multisystem organ failure also are indications for Swan-Ganz catheterization. In critically ill patients, intracardiac monitoring with measurement of the pulmonary artery wedge pressure gives a more accurate estimation of left ventricular function and left ventricular preload than does the central venous pressure.[116] Other parameters such as mixed venous oxygen saturation and systemic vascular resistance also can be determined to further guide hemodynamic therapy.

Monitoring Cerebral Physiology

Intracranial pressure

Numerous reports demonstrate a significant correlation between intracranial hypertension and poor outcome following traumatic brain injury.[61–63,108,110,118] All patients with an initial postresuscitation GCS of 8 or less warrant ICP monitoring. Intracranial pressure monitoring also should be considered in patients with a postresuscitation GCS of 9 to 13 who have intracranial hematomas or cerebral contusions causing mass effect that initially do not warrant surgical evacuation. This statement is not meant to advocate an indiscriminate use of ICP monitoring; instead, it accepts the reality that a significant number of patients may subsequently deteriorate as their intracranial injuries evolve. Monitoring of ICP in these patients provides an early warning system for herniation or decreased cerebral perfusion.

The preferred method of monitoring is an intraventricular catheter, given the therapeutic benefit of cerebrospinal fluid drainage for ICP control. Even with diffuse cerebral swelling, most lateral ventricles can be cannulated after one or two attempts. If, however, a ventriculostomy is not placed within three passes, a parenchymal fiber-optic probe is an acceptable alternative. Repeated passes of a ventricular catheter have been associated with increased risk of intracerebral hematoma, especially in patients with coagulopathy.[119]

The criteria for how long to monitor ICP are not firmly established. Posttraumatic swelling, edema, and progression of hemorrhagic lesions typically are maximal within 48 to 96 h of injury. However, delayed rises in ICP are not uncommon. In a recent series of 53 severe head injury patients, 15 (31 percent) developed a secondary rise in ICP occurring 3 to 10 days after injury.[120] In 6 of the 15 patients, the delayed rise in ICP was uncontrollable, resulting in death; only 2 patients had a good outcome. The most frequent initial diagnoses in these 15 patients were multiple contusions and acute subdural hematoma.

Discontinuation of ICP monitoring is reasonable in patients who maintain normal ICP without specific therapy or with only minimal sedation for at least 24 h. Such patients should also show significant and steady clinical improvement to a GCS of 9 or greater (unless a primary brainstem or diffuse axonal injury is evident), and demonstrate resolving lesions on follow-up CT scans, including visible cisterns. Even if these criteria are met, a longer period of observation may be warranted when the initial diagnosis is acute subdural hematoma or multiple contusions, in patients with significant vasospasm, and in those patients with major systemic derangements. Intraoperative ICP monitoring is also generally recommended in moderate or severe head injury patients undergoing general anesthesia within 7 to 10 days of injury for an extracranial operation injury that cannot otherwise be delayed.

Cerebral blood flow

As the detrimental effects of cerebral ischemia have become more apparent, greater emphasis has been placed on assessing regional and global cerebral blood flow and metabolism.[14,15,60] Measurements of cerebral blood flow with xenon-133, stable xenon CT, or the nitrous oxide saturation method are established techniques and are becoming frequently utilized in the neurosurgical critical care setting.[11,12,30,36,50,53,66,123,124] Of the three methods cited, the largest experience has been with the xenon-133 method, starting in the mid-1970s with investigations by Obrist and colleagues.[124] The major advantage of this technique is that it can be performed at the patient's bedside and repeated as needed. Its major drawback is that it essentially provides a hemispheric cortical blood flow measurement, predominantly of the middle cerebral artery distribution. Local areas of critically low blood flow may not be detected. Stable xenon CT does have significantly higher resolution and can provide regional cortical, basal ganglia, and brainstem blood flow measures along with a simultaneous CT anatomic image.[123,125] The major problem with this technique is that it requires patient transport.

Regardless of the method used to measure cerebral blood flow, such assessments are ideally started within the first 24 h after severe head injury when ischemia is most likely to occur and then on a serial basis over the next several days. The patients most likely to benefit from regular blood flow measurements are those with problematic intracranial hypertension and marginal CPP. In such patients, blood flow assessment can help guide therapeutic maneuvers such as CPP management and use of hyperventilation.

Jugular Venous Oxygen Saturation

Indirect assessment of global cerebral blood flow and metabolism by measurement of jugular venous oxygen saturation is becoming more commonly employed in severely head injured patients.[45,53,121,122,127] Placement of a fiberoptic catheter into the jugular bulb allows continuous recording of jugular venous oxygen saturation (Sjv_{O_2}), determination of arteriojugular venous oxygen difference (AVD_{O_2}) and, in conjunction with cerebral blood flow measurement, determination of the cerebral metabolic rate for oxygen (CMR_{O_2}).[53,126] Jugular venous oxygen saturation monitoring appears to be an effective means of detecting episodes of global cerebral ischemia.[27,45,60,122] Normal Sjv_{O_2} is approximately 65 percent; an Sjv_{O_2} below 50 to 55 percent is considered indicative of global ischemia warranting treatment.[122,127] Because over one-half of recorded desaturations may be due to poor catheter position or calibration, an algorithm for diagnosing the cause of desaturation is necessary.[122] Once this process has been performed and a true episode of desaturation has been documented, appropriate intervention is warranted. In the majority of cases, reduction of ICP, elevation of the Pa_{CO_2} to normocarbic levels, or elevation of the systemic blood pressure will be required to correct the desaturation.[27]

Gopinath and colleagues have recently documented their experience with 116 severe head-injured patients undergoing continuous jugular venous oxygen saturation monitoring during the first five days after injury.[27] One or more confirmed episodes of desaturation to an Sjv_{O_2} of less than 50 percent occurred in 40 percent of patients and was significantly associated with poor outcome; 90 percent of patients sustaining multiple episodes of desaturation had a poor outcome compared to 55 percent of patients without episodes of desaturation. The most frequent causes of oxygen desaturation included intracranial hypertension (44 percent), hypocarbia to a Pa_{CO_2} of less than 28 mmHg (27 percent), systemic hypotension (10 percent), and hypoxia (8 percent).

Transcranial Doppler and Traumatic Vasospasm

Traumatic arterial spasm has been variably defined as a middle cerebral artery flow velocity greater than 100 or 120 cm/sec or a middle cerebral artery/internal carotid artery ratio (Lindegaard ratio) of greater than 3.[128–131] In patients with a GCS of 3 to 12, the incidence of traumatic vasospasm has ranged from 7 to 40 percent, with the highest incidence in patients with severe head injury.[128–131] Onset of increased flow velocity occurs between days 1 to 6 after injury, typically on day 2 or 3, with maximal velocities seen between days 5 to 13.[128,129] The development of spasm has been correlated with CT evidence of subarachnoid blood in several studies.[130–132] In a study by Martin and coworkers, all three patients with severe vasospasm (middle cerebral flow velocity >200 cm/s) had subarachnoid blood on CT.[129]

The incidence of cerebral infarction attributable to traumatic vasospasm appears to be relatively low. In four transcranial Doppler investigations, the incidence of spasm-related cerebral infarction ranged from 0 to 5 percent.[128–131] Combining these four studies, 6 of 226 patients (2.7 percent) developed infarction; all 6 had sustained a severe head injury and had subarachnoid blood on CT. In four patients who developed infarction in a study by Chan and associates, all had episodes of CPP less than 60 mmHg requiring treatment.[128] Martin and coworkers demonstrated a significant correlation between the highest mean middle cerebral artery flow velocity and the lowest hemispheric cerebral blood flow as measured by the xenon-133 method.[129]

In the TCDB cohort of 753 patients, a 39 percent incidence of CT-diagnosed subarachnoid hemorrhage was reported, which correlated with a twofold increase in mortality.[75] It is likely that this increased risk of dying in patients with traumatic subarachnoid hemorrhage was at least partially attributable to vasospasm. Although most studies have demonstrated an association between the presence of traumatic subarachnoid hemorrhage and transcranial Doppler diagnosed vasospasm, the presence of spasm has not been shown to be an independent predictor of outcome.[128–131] The favorable results associated with maintenance of an adequate CPP may be due in part to an amelioration of the hemodynamic effects of arterial narrowing.

Because transcranial Doppler is a noninvasive study that can be done at the patient's bedside, it is an attractive monitoring technique for the head-injured patient. Given that patients sustaining severe head injury with subarachnoid hemorrhage on CT are the most prone to develop clinically significant vasospasm, such patients are especially appropriate for frequent Doppler studies.

Hemodynamic Support and CPP Management

The first step in establishing adequate CPP is vascular volume expansion. If perfusion pressure remains insufficient after volume therapy and after treatment to reduce ICP, the use of induced hypertension or inotropic support is indicated. In patients with precipitous drops in blood pressure or perfusion pressure, urgent and simultaneous use of volume expansion and vasopressor therapy is often required. A search for the underlying cause of hemomdynamic instability should also be undertaken.

Volume Expansion

To establish euvolemia, administration of full maintenance intravenous fluids should be given at a rate of 1.5 ml/kg/h of half-normal or normal saline with 5% dextrose and potassium supplementation. If serum sodium is less than 140 mmol/L, the use of normal saline (D5 0.9% NaCl with KCl 20 mEq/L) as the maintenance fluid is indicated to prevent the development of a hypo-osmolar state. If the hematocrit falls below 30 percent, transfusion of packed red blood cells is generally indicated to optimize blood rheology and cerebral oxygen delivery, particularly in individuals with problematic ICP or marginal perfusion pressure.

If a central venous pressure line is being used, the central venous pressure should be maintained from 5 to 10 mmHg. If a pulmonary artery catheter is in place, the wedge pressure should be maintained between 10 and 14 mmHg. This range of wedge pressure is associated with maximal cardiac performance in most adults; raising wedge pressure above 14 mmHg typically will not improve cardiac or stroke volume indices but will increase the risk of pulmonary edema.[133] The need for higher intracardiac pressures can be determined by administering further volume and plotting a Starling curve with serial determinations of cardiac output and wedge pressure.

If central venous pressure falls below 5 mmHg or the wedge pressure is less than 10 mmHg, additional fluids should be given as needed in the form of cystalloid or colloid. Volume expansion with either crystalloid or colloid preparations in the brain-injured patient is acceptable, with care being taken not to induce a hypo-osmolar state with hypo-osmolar fluids or to incite coagulopathy with large doses of hetastarch.[134] When the CPP goal of 70 mmHg is not being met while the central venous pressure or the wedge pressure are in the desired range, additional volume expansion is indicated. Once central venous pressure is over 10 mmHg or wedge pressure is over 14 mmHg and perfusion pressure or blood pressure are still inadequate, induced hypertension or inotropic support generally is indicated.

Pharmacological Therapy

Use of vasopressor or inotropic support should be dictated by hemodynamic parameters, most important of which are the cardiac output (or cardiac index) and the systemic vascular resistance. Renal function is also an important consideration, given that vasopressors at higher doses can result in extracranial end-organ ischemia. Three vasopressors, dopamine (Intropin), norepinephrine (Levophed), and phenylephrine (Neo-Synephrine), and the inotropic agent, dobutamine (Dobutrex) are employed most commonly in the critical care setting (Tables 6-3 and 6-4). All are sympathomimetic amines with varying degrees of alpha and beta adrenergic activity. All should be administered with continuous arterial pressure monitoring and preferably with a pulmonary artery catheter in place.

Choice of Agent

For most young, previously healthy trauma patients, norepinephrine is an excellent first choice to achieve a significant increase in arterial blood pressure. Because it is a peripheral vasoconstrictor and an inotropic agent, both blood pressure and cardiac output usually are improved. Since it does not increase urine output like

TABLE 6-3 Sympathomimetics for the Maintenance of Cerebral Perfusion Pressure

	Sites of Action						
	Heart		*Peripheral Vasculature*		*Hemodynamic Response*		
	Contractility (inotropic) β_1	**Heart rate[1] (chronotropic)** β_1	**Vasoconstriction** α	**Vasodilatation** β_2	**Cardiac output**	**Systemic vascular resistance**	**Blood pressure**
Dopamine	+++	+	0 to +++[2]	0[3]	↑	↓[2] or ↑	0 to ↑
Norepinephrine	++	++	+++	0	↑ or 0	↑	↑
Phenylephrine	0	0[1]	+++	0	↓	↑	↑
Dobutamine	+++	0 to +	0 to +	0 to +	↑	↓	0 to ↑

(1 = decreased heart rate may result from reflex mechanisms; 2 = effects are dose dependent; 3 = dilates renal and splanchnic beds via dopaminergic effect at doses < 10 mg/kg/min).

SOURCE: Lyerly HK: Shock, in Lyerly HK (ed): *The Handbook of Surgical Intensive Care: Practices of the Surgery Residents at the Duke University Medical Center*, 2d ed. Chicago: Year Book Medical Publishers, 1989:15, with permission.

TABLE 6-4 Recommended Dosage Range of Sympathomimetics (μg/kg/min)

Agent	Low	Medium	High
Dopamine	2.00	10.00	20.00
Norepinephrine	0.02	0.10	0.20
Phenylephrine	1.00	2.50	5.00
Dobutamine	5.00	10.00	10.00

SOURCE: Damiano RJ: Cardiovascular system, in Lyerly HK (ed): *The Handbook of Surgical Intensive Care: Practices of the Surgery Residents at the Duke University Medical Center*, 2d ed. Chicago: Year Book Medical Publishers, 1989:79, with permission.

low- or moderate-dose dopamine, fluid replacement is typically simplified. The norepinephrine infusion generally should not exceed 0.20 mg/kg/min. If urine output falls below 0.5 ml/kg/h, or if a metabolic acidosis develops, renal dose dopamine should be started and the hemodynamic indices reassessed. When the cardiac index is less than 3.0 L/min/m^2, the cardiac inotropic agent dobutamine is an effective first agent in improving perfusion pressure.[135] Some patients occasionally will require more than one agent to achieve adequate cerebral perfusion. However, in most cases after reassessing the hemodynamic profile, it is apparent that further volume expansion is indicated.

Following traumatic brain injury with acute intraparenchymal blood on CT, an upper limit for systolic blood pressure of 180 to 200 mmHg is prudent, given the risk of worsening such hemorrhage with excessive hypertension. Chronic hypertensive patients, however, are likely to tolerate—and in fact require—higher arterial pressures to maintain adequate cerebral perfusion.[48]

Complications of Hemodynamic Therapy

Complications associated with central venous access, including pneumothorax, arterial injury, or local hematoma formation, occur at a rate of 1 to 2 percent.[116] With the use of strict sterile technique, catheter-related sepsis occurs in less than 1 percent of cases, but the risk does increase if lines are left in place over 72 to 96 h. In general, central venous lines and pulmonary artery catheters should be removed as soon as their clinical utility is exhausted. The benefits from intracardiac monitoring with a Swan-Ganz catheter probably are negligible in patients who have pulmonary artery wedge or pulmonary artery diastolic pressures that correlate well with central venous pressures. After 48 to 72 h of monitoring such patients, the Swan-Ganz catheter often can be removed and hemodynamic therapy can be based on central venous pressure, systemic blood pressure, and other clinical parameters. With aggressive volume expansion, however, the risk of pulmonary edema is significant. Central venous or wedge pressures should be carefully maintained within reasonable physiological ranges as described earlier. Regular physical examinations and daily chest x-rays are mandatory, especially in elderly patients and in those with multiple injuries. Strict and frequent monitoring of total fluid intake and output is essential in maintaining a euvolemic state. Negative fluid balance should be corrected by replacement of the fluid deficit at frequent intervals.

With the use of high-dose vasopressors, the risk of extracranial end-organ ischemia is significant. Arterial blood gases should be checked at least twice daily and serum lactate determinations obtained if a metabolic acidosis develops. The upper dosage limits of pressor agents should be strictly followed. In patients receiving other potentially nephrotoxic drugs such as aminoglycoside antibiotics and mannitol, pressor therapy carries an even higher risk. Renal dose dopamine is helpful in preserving kidney function in critically ill patients who require high dose vasopressor. Close monitoring of urine output, blood urea nitrogen, and creatinine also is important. If renal function does deteriorate, pharmacological therapy should be modified accordingly. Daily mannitol doses are ideally kept at 200 g per day or less, and significantly lower doses are recommended if renal insufficiency develops.[136]

Treatment of Intracranial Hypertension

Intracranial hypertension is variably defined as an ICP of over 10 to 15 mmHg; an ICP of over 20 mmHg sustained for more than 5 min warrants treatment. In patients with temporal lobe or deep frontal lobe lesions where the risk of uncal herniation is greater, an ICP treatment threshold of 15 mmHg may be indicated.[13] With progressive intracranial hypertension or increasing intensity of ICP treatment, the possibility of a new or a reaccumulating intracranial hematoma should be investigated by a repeat CT scan.

Treatment of intracranial hypertension should proceed in a stepwise manner (Fig. 6-10). Routine preemptive measures exercised in all severe head injury patients include maintenance of normothermia, head elevation to 30 degrees, and mild hyperventilation to a Pa_{CO_2} of approximately 35 mmHg.[138] Prophylactic anticonvulsants should also be utilized for at least the first week after injury.[139] When acute and sustained rises in ICP occur, rapid manual hyperventilation of the patient should be avoided because the Pa_{CO_2} may drop dramatically, resulting in critical cerebral vasoconstriction and ischemia. Instead the maneuvers outlined below should be followed in an expedient and, if necessary, simultaneous manner.

Medical Management of Intracranial Hypertension

Preemptive Measures
- head elevation to 30°, neutral alignment
- mild hyperventilation ($PaCO_2$ 30 - 35 mmHg)
- maintenance of euvolemia
- maintenance of CPP 70 mmHg or higher
- maintenance of normothremia (< 37.5° C)
- seizure prophylaxis (phenytoin)

Primary Therapy
- ventricular CSF drainage
- sedation (narcotics, benzodiazepines)
- neuromuscular blockade

Secondary Therapy
- bolus mannitol administration
- elevation of cerebral perfusion pressure

Tertiary Therapy
- metabolic suppressive therapy with high-dose barbiturates or propofol

Figure 6-10. Medical management of intracranial hypertension. (CSF = cerebrospinal fluid)

In patients whose ICP is easily controlled over the first 24 to 48 h after injury, suspension of sedation and neuromuscular blocking agents can be done early to permit clinical evaluation. However, in patients with problematic ICP, little is to be gained by early reversal of such therapy.[60] In fact, a significant spike in ICP may occur. During this period, neurological assessment may necessarily be limited to evaluation of pupillary responses.

Sedation and neuromuscular blocking agents

Sedation can be initiated with a 5 to 10 mg bolus of IV morphine, which may be repeated once. If it is effective in lowering ICP, a continuous morphine infusion starting at 5 mg/h should be instituted. The rate can be increased up to 20 mg/h, as needed for agitation or excess motor activity. When intracranial hypertension persists despite narcotic sedation, and if the patient is agitated, has increased motor tone, is shivering or resisting the ventilator, neuromuscular blockade should be added to help control ICP. These agents are effective in maintaining relaxation and can be given as needed or by a continuous infusion. Agitation secondary to alcohol withdrawal also may contribute to intracranial hypertension and is typically poorly controlled with narcotics. If withdrawal is suspected, a benzodiazepine such as lorazepam (Ativan) 2 to 5 mg IV every 6 h, can be administered empirically for 48 to 72 h. Alternatively, the shorter acting benzodiazepine, midazolam (Versed) can be used as a continuous infusion.

Ventricular drainage

When these initial measures are inadequate to control ICP, ventricular drainage should be utilized. In patients who exhibit no signs of agitation or increased motor tone, ventricular drainage should be used as the initial treatment to reduce ICP. The ventriculostomy chamber can be placed at 5 cm above the level of the lateral ventricle with the pressure monitored continuously. The ventriculostomy is opened when ICP exceeds the treatment threshold. Continuous ventricular drainage is not recommended because significant ICP spikes may be missed when the ICP is monitored only intermittently. Additionally, catheter occlusion secondary to ventricular collapse around the catheter is more likely to occur when continuous drainage is utilized.

Mannitol

Mannitol is an excellent volume expander, thereby improving perfusion pressure. As an osmotic diuretic, it also removes extravascular water from the brain. Additionally, blood viscosity is reduced with mannitol administration, and this improves cerebral blood flow.[37,48] Because boluses of 0.25 g/kg have been shown to be equally effective in lowering ICP as have larger doses, it is recommended that lower doses be used initially.[140] For most adults, a 25-g bolus is effective for lowering ICP and improving CPP and can be repeated as necessary. Serum osmolality should not be allowed to rise above 310 mOsm/kg. If total input and output are regularly matched, a hyperosmolar state will rarely develop. Given that excessive mannitol use can result in acute oliguric renal failure, total daily doses of mannitol ideally should not exceed 200 g; in patients with renal insufficiency, lower daily doses are recommended.[136]

Perfusion pressure manipulation

When ICP remains elevated and CPP is 70 mmHg or less, despite the above maneuvers, an attempt to raise perfusion pressure further to 80 to 100 mmHg can be made before resorting to barbiturate therapy. As discussed earlier in this chapter, many patients may require a perfusion pressure considerably above 70 mmHg before adequate ICP control is achieved.[48]

High-dose barbiturate therapy

The mechanism of ICP control with high-dose barbiturates is thought to be largely through a reduction in cerebral metabolism with a coupled decrease in cerebral blood flow and blood volume.[141,142] The response rate (i.e., control of ICP) has ranged from 30 to 80 percent in five different series reported from 1978 to 1988.[43,137,143–145] Of those patients who responded, mortality was 21 to 33 percent; in nonresponders, mortality ranged from 64 to 89 percent. In a prospective randomized study by Eisenberg and coworkers, only 30 percent of patients responded to high-dose pentobarbital therapy.[143] However, barbiturate treatment conferred a 2 : 1 benefit over conventional therapy, and this advantage rose to a 4 : 1 benefit if patients with prerandomization cardiac complications were excluded. These investigations indicate that high-dose barbiturate therapy for intractable intracranial hypertension is efficacious in some patients, although predicting which patients are likely to respond is not easy. Indications for initiating pentobarbital treatment have not been consistently defined. When all previously outlined measures fail to control ICP, barbiturate therapy can be considered.[13,60,143] For therapy to be effective in improving outcome it should be instituted before irreversible brainstem injury has occurred. If barbiturates are started too late, ICP may be controlled but the patient is likely to remain neurologically devastated. Reasonable indications to begin high-dose pentobarbital therapy include 30 min of ICP over 30 mmHg with CPP less than 70 mmHg, or ICP over 40 mmHg despite a CPP of 70 mmHg.

Given the high rate of complications with barbiturate therapy, extreme vigilance must be practiced. The patient should be in a normovolemic state prior to onset of therapy and a pulmonary artery catheter inserted. Electroencephalography is essential for monitoring the depth of barbiturate therapy. It is desirable to maintain a burst suppression pattern of isoelectric intervals with bursts of activity at 8 to 12 Hz.[146] However, if electroencephalography is not immediately available, instituting pentobarbital therapy should not be delayed. Pentobarbital administration should begin with a 10 mg/kg loading dose over 30 min followed by 5 mg/kg/h over the next 3 h. If systolic blood pressure drops, the loading dose infusion should be slowed. A maintenance infusion of 1 to 3 mg/kg/h generally will maintain burst suppression and control ICP. Serum pentobarbital levels should be followed; ICP control typically is achieved with serum levels of 30 to 50 mg/100 ml.[13] The lowest effective dose to control ICP should be utilized. An adverse hemodynamic response is most likely to occur in older patients and in those with preexisting cardiac instability. In such patients, initiating therapy with lower doses is prudent. Ideally, CPP should still be maintained above 70 mmHg. Loss of pupillary reactivity is common with high-dose pentobarbital therapy and should not be interpreted as treatment failure with irreversible loss of brainstem function. Gradual withdrawal of barbiturate therapy over several days can begin after ICP control has been achieved for 24 to 48 h. Patients in barbiturate coma are at increased risk for pneumonia and sepsis and should be carefully monitored for such infections.[13]

Temperature Regulation

Hyperthermia has been associated with worse outcome following servere head injury.[20,27] Conversely, the use of mild systemic hypothermia to 30 to 34°C in the treatment of severe head injury has yielded promising results in five preliminary clinical studies, and a randomized multicenter study is underway.[147–151] Therefore, maintenance of systemic normothermia (core temperature less than 37.5°C) appears warranted in moderate and severely head injured patients. A regimen utilizing a combination of acetaminophen, cooling blankets, and ice water lavage is generally effective. If shivering is noted, a neuromuscular blocking agent should be added. Given that brain temperatures are consistently higher than body temperatures, optimal temperature management in head-injured patients may best be served by monitoring brain temperature directly.[151,152]

Steroids

Failure of high-dose corticosteroid therapy to control ICP or improve outcome in patients with traumatic brain injury has been shown in numerous clinical trials. Additionally, associated complications, including blunted immune response, masking of infection, gastrointestinal hemorrhage, poor wound healing, and elevation in serum glucose levels, make high-dose glucocorticoids unsuitable for the head-injured patient.[153–157]

INTRACRANIAL COMPLICATIONS

Posttraumatic Seizures

Prevention of seizures is an important goal in patients following traumatic brain injury, particularly in individuals with problematic intracranial hypertension, those with significant cerebral swelling on CT, and in patients at risk for progession of hemorrhagic intracranial lesions.[158] Factors that lower the seizure threshold must be carefully monitored and addressed, including a low anticonvulsant level, electrolyte derangements (particularly low serum sodium, magnesium, or calcium levels), hypoglycemia, hypoxemia, alcohol withdrawal, or meningitis. An intracranial hematoma, brain swelling, or pneumocephalus may also incite seizure activity. Thus, an urgent CT scan is always indicated following an initial posttraumatic seizure.

Early posttraumatic seizures, occurring in the first week after injury, are seen in approximately 25 percent of patients with traumatic intracranial hematomas.[159] Temkin and colleagues in a prospective randomized study of head injury patients with intracranial injury on CT or a GCS of 10 or less demonstrated a 73 percent reduction in posttraumatic seizures during the first week after injury.[139] Use of phenytoin with maintenance of high therapeutic serum levels is thus recommended during the acute injury period. No randomized studies, however, have shown a clear effect from prophylactic anticonvulsant therapy in controlling onset of late seizures.[139,160,161]

Ventriculostomy-related Complications

Complications related to ventriculostomy placement include parenchymal injury, hemorrhage, and infection. The incidence of ventriculostomy-related hemorrhage was 1.4 percent in the series by Narayan and coworkers and was associated with coagulopathy and the number of passes made during catheter placement.[119] In patients with clotting abnormalities, placement of an ICP monitor should be deferred until such deficiencies are at least temporarily corrected.

Ventriculitis in association with ventricular catheter placement is a relatively frequent problem, being seen in 11 percent of general neurosurgical patients in the series of Mayhall and associates.[162] From this study the risk of infection was thought to be related largely to the length of time the catheter was in place. Only 6 percent of patients developed ventriculitis if the catheter was removed within 5 days, but 18 percent developed this complication when the catheter was in place longer. In a more recent series of 205 neurosurgical patients, including 76 with head injuries, no relationship was seen between duration of ICP monitoring and the average daily incidence of infection with up to 2 weeks of monitoring.[163] The overall infection rate was 7 percent, with an average monitoring time of 7 days. From these data and a review of the literature, Winfield and colleagues concluded that the duration of monitoring should be dictated by the clinical need to follow ICP, not the concern of infection. Additionally, the need for prophylactic antibiotics and for minimal manipulation and irrigation of the catheter system was stressed. Based on these data, it appears reasonable to leave a ventriculostomy in place for up to 2 weeks, provided prophylactic antibiotics are used, the catheter is tunneled several centimeters away from the insertion site, and cerebrospinal fluid surveillance samples are taken every 2 or 3 days. If ventriculitis does develop, removal of or changing the catheter to another site is mandatory and antibiotic coverage should be modified accordingly.

NUTRITIONAL SUPPORT

Moderate or severe head injury results in a generalized hypermetabolic and hypercatabolic state.[164–167] Robertson and coworkers estimated that the metabolic rate increases on average by 40 percent in the acute phase following severe head injury.[168] Multisystem trauma without head injury also increases overall energy expenditure by 30 to 50 percent.[169] In the absence of adequate nutritional support, the resultant hypercatabolic state causes endogenous protein breakdown to amino acids, which fuels the Kreb's cycle. If this rapid protein turnover is not mitigated, not only will skeletal muscle proteolysis occur, but eventually visceral and circulating proteins will be catabolized. Ultimately, this form of acute protein malnutrition results in multiorgan dysfunction and an immunocompromised state that can seriously hinder recovery. Gut function, cardiovascular function, ventilatory response, wound healing, and infection rate are all adversely affected if significant protein malnutrition is allowed to develop.[171–173] Conversely, when the accelerated metabolic needs are adequately met, wound healing is improved, infection and sepsis rates are diminished, intensive care unit stays are shortened, and mortality is reduced.[174–178] Currently, a consensus is emerging in support of early enteral feeding in the great majority of trauma victims, including those sustaining serious head injury.[169,179–182]

Jejunal feedings in head-injured patients appear to be superior to the gastric route. The ileus that occurs after moderate or severe head injury is predominantly restricted to the stomach and may persist for 4 or 5 days. Consequently, early gastric feeding will typically be inadequate to provide total nutritional needs and places patients at increased risk for aspiration.[173,182,183] In the moderate or severe head injury patient, full enteral feedings should begin ideally within 24 to 48 h of injury. Jejunal access can be established by nasojejunal tube (placed fluoroscopically or endoscopically), by a percutaneous gastrojejunostomy, by percutaneous endoscopic jejunostomy, or at the time of laparotomy if abdominal exploration is required.[182,184] Full-strength feedings usually can begin at 50 ml/h and increased over the next 24 to 36 h to a maximal rate of approximately 125 ml/h. Most critically ill neurosurgical patients will expend 25 to 35 kcal/kg/day, while protein requirements generally range from 1.5 to 2.0 g/kg/day. Actual energy requirements are best predicted by the Harris-Benedict formula or by indirect calorimetry and with consultations to the dietary department of the hospital.[183] Hyperglycemia is seen commonly after both experimental and human traumatic brain injury and is a significant predictor of poor outcome.[25] It is thought that high glucose levels enhance ischemia-mediated cell damage, probably through lactate accumulation.[25,26] Insulin should be administered as needed to maintain serum glucose below 150 to 200 mg/dl. If jejunal feedings cannot be initiated or tolerated within 36 to 48 h of injury, parenteral nutrition should begin instead.[169]

SYSTEMIC OR EXTRACRANIAL COMPLICATIONS

Electrolyte Derangements

Hyponatremia

Hyponatremia lowers the seizure threshold and can exacerbate cerebral edema.[19,22] Low serum sodium is relatively common after head injury, occurring in 8 percent of patients with moderate or severe injuries in one study.[19] The etiology of hyponatremia in head-injured patients is unclear. Cerebral salt-wasting and the syndrome of inappropriate antidiuretic hormone are both characterized by low serum sodium and serum osmolality and inappropriately high urine sodium and urine osmolality in a setting of normal renal, adrenal, and thyroid function. The major distinction among these entities is the volume status of the patient.[22,185,186] Patients with the syndrome of inappropriate antidiuretic hormone generally are responsive to fluid restriction; those with cerebral salt-wasting respond to volume and sodium administration.[186] For hyponatremia below 130 mmol/L, intravenous urea is safe and rapidly effective in correcting this problem, whether it is attributed to the syndrome of inappropriate antidiuretic hormone or to cerebral salt-wasting.[22,187] Urea is effective because it is a potent osmotic diuretic and significantly increases sodium reabsorption at the kidney. Forty g of urea in 150 ml of normal saline can be given over 2 h and repeated every 8 h. A significant rise in serum sodium typically is seen after two or three doses. On average the serum sodium will rise 6 and 10 mmol/L 24 and 48 h after initiating therapy. Central pontine myelinolysis from overly rapid correction of hyponatremia has not been reported with the use of urea.[22, 187] Infusion of hypertonic saline is also an effective method of correcting significant hyponatremia but generally takes longer and requires closer monitoring of urine electrolytes than when using urea. Marked fluid restriction to correct hyponatremia should be avoided given the importance of maintaining normovolemia in the head-injured patient.

Hypomagnesemia

Magnesium levels should be carefully followed in moderate and severe brain-injured patients because low serum and low brain magnesium levels frequently are seen after traumatic brain injury.[188] Hypomagnesemia lowers the seizure threshold, frequently complicates alcohol withdrawal, and in experimental traumatic brain injury hinders neurological recovery.[21] Postinjury administration of intravenous magnesium in an experimental head injury model was shown to improve motor function significantly.[21] Presently, it appears reasonable and safe to maintain serum magnesium levels in the upper range of normal (1.8–2.2 mEq/L), with intravenous supplementation, provided renal function is normal.

Pneumonia

Pneumonia is a frequent and often serious complication following severe head injury, occurring in 41 percent of the TCDB patients.[189] Aspiration at the scene of injury, impaired airway reflexes, prolonged intubation, and treatment with barbiturates make the traumatic brain injury victim highly predisposed to develop pneumonia. In febrile patients who develop new infiltrates on chest x-ray, an evolving leukocytosis, and sputum analysis showing copious white blood cells, empirical antibiotic treatment is indicated. Chest physiotherapy and frequent positional changes are important adjuncts to antimicrobial therapy.

An important contributing factor in the development of pneumonia in intubated neurosurgical patients appears to be the use of antacids or histamine type 2 (H2) antagonists (cimetidine or ranitidine) for stress ulcer prophylaxis. In three recent randomized trials comprised of over 250 ventilator-dependent intensive care unit patients, including neurosurgical patients, the incidence of pneumonia averaged 31 percent in the patients treated with antacids and/or H2 blockers; in patients treated with sucralfate, the incidence of pneumonia averaged 10 percent.[190–192] The frequency of clinically significant gastrointestinal hemorrhage by either method of ulcer prophylaxis was low in both groups, approximately 1 percent for the antacid/H2 antagonist-treated patients and 2 percent for those treated with sucralfate. The higher rate of pneumonia in the H2 antagonist/antacid-treated patients is thought to be related to a higher gastric pH, which allows gastric colonization of aerobic gram-negative bacilli and subsequent oropharyngeal and tracheal colonization. Sucralfate is thus recommended as the initial ulcer prophylactic agent in the intubated brain-injured patient. When using sucralfate, however, absorption of enterally administered medications may be impaired. In particular, this problem has been noted with anticonvulsants; consequently, the intravenous route of administration for such medications is recommended.

Thromboembolic Events

Deep vein thrombosis and pulmonary embolism are relatively frequent and often devastating complications in head-injured patients. The incidence of these complications is reduced by the use of pneumatic compression boots. In a study of both neurology and neurosurgical patients treated with compression boots, the incidence of clinically evident deep vein thrombosis was 2.3 percent and for pulmonary embolus was 1.8 percent.[193] More recently, Frim and associates administered low-dose subcutaneous heparin to 138 consecutive neurosurgical patients requiring operation, including 58 patients with head injuries.[194] The patients were treated with a regimen of perioperative compression stockings and with subcutaneous heparin, 5000 units twice daily, starting on postoperative day 1. In these patients, there were no thromboembolic events and no postoperative hemorrhages. In the control group of 473 patients treated with only intraoperative and postoperative compression stockings, 3.2 percent developed thromboembolic complications, including 8 with deep vein thrombosis and 7 with pulmonary embolus. From this study, low-dose subcutaneous heparin in conjunction with compression stockings appears safe and effective against thromboembolic events in the head injury victim. In a recent review of thromboembolic disease in patients with neurological illness, Hamilton and coworkers also recommended a regimen of pneumatic compression stockings and subcutaneous heparin in those at significant risk, including patients with head injuries.[195] Beginning low-dose subcutaneous heparin on the first postinjury or postoperative day appears reasonable in moderate and severe head injury patients, provided initial coagulation parameters are normal and hemorrhagic lesions seen on CT have stabilized.

A high degree of suspicion for deep vein thrombosis and pulmonary embolus must be maintained in the severe head injury victim. When a deep vein thrombosis is suspected by calf or thigh tenderness or lower extremity swelling, venous impedance plethysmography or contrast venography are urgently indicated. If a pulmonary embolus is suspected because of new-onset tachypnea, tachycardia, or a decrease in arterial oxygen saturation, a radionucleotide ventilation/perfusion (V/Q) scan should be obtained. In patients with indeterminate scans in whom the clinical suspicion of pulmonary embolus is high, a pulmonary angiogram is indicated. If an embolus is detected by a high-probability ventilation/perfusion scan or by angiography, an inferior vena cava filter should be placed without delay. A deep vein thrombosis occurring above the level of the knee also warrants filter placement.[196] The unacceptable risk of intracranial hemorrhage with full anticoagulation precludes such treatment in the acutely head injured patient for at least 7 to 14 days after injury. The ideal timing for safe anticoagulation after head injury remains unclear.[195,196]

Gastrointestinal Hemorrhage

Erosive gastrointestinal lesions are common after severe head injury. In one endoscopic study, 91 percent of such patients had gastritis within 24 h of injury.[197] Significant gastrointestinal bleeding requiring transfusion or other intervention has been reported in 2 to 11 percent of severely head injured patients.[198,199] Routine ulcer prophylaxis in all severe head injury patients is warranted. Use of sucralfate is recommended because of the significantly lower incidence of associated pnemonia and equivalent ulcer prophylaxis when compared to H2 antagonists or antacids.[190–192]

FUTURE EFFORTS

Further meaningful recovery after head injury will be forthcoming with greater understanding of secondary injury phenomena, more refined physiological and metabolic monitoring, and an even greater reduction of postinjury cerebral ischemia. Numerous neuroprotective agents are currently being investigated which may also significantly enhance outcome. These new compounds include the antioxidant 21-aminosteroids, which inhibit lipid peroxidation and stabilize cell membranes.[200] The preliminary results of a European/Australian efficacy study in patients with aneurysmal subarachnoid hemorrhage indicate a significant reduction in mortality with the use of the 21-aminosteroid, tirilazad mesylate. A similar trial of this agent in patients with moderate or severe closed head injury is nearing completion. Another free radical scavenger, superoxide dismutase (PEG-SOD) is also currently being investigated in a multicenter study in moderate and severe head injury patients.[201] The calcium channel antagonist, nimodipine, in a European multicenter trial was recently shown to modestly but significantly improve outcome in severe closed head injury victims who had subarachnoid hemorrhage on initial CT. Further investigations with nimodipine are underway.[202] The buffereing agent, tromethamine (THAM) has also been shown to ameliorate intracranial hypertension and shorten the length of stay in the intensive care unit; additional investigations of this agent are in progress.[64,203] Blunting of the excitatory amino acid secondary injury cascade with *N*-methyl-D-aspartate (NMDA) antagonists appears to be a promising area of neuroprotection.[204] A multicenter trial of the competitive NMDA antagonist, CGS 19755, is underway in severe closed head injury patients in North America. The use of mild hypothermia in severe head injury patients is also being further investigated in a multicenter trial, given that several pilot studies have demonstrated efficacy with its use.[147–151] Magnesium supplementation in the head-injured patient has also shown promise as a neuroprotective agent and is currently being studied in the clinical setting as well.[21,188] It is hoped that ongoing and future investigations will further reduce the devastating personal and societal impact of traumatic brain injury.

Portions of this chapter have appeared in previous chapters written by the authors, including: "Surgical Management of Severe Closed Head Injury in Adults" by Kelly DF, McBride DQ, and Becker DP, in *Operative Neurosurgical Techniques,* 3d ed, Philadelphia: WB Saunders, 1985; and "Diagnosis and Treatment of Moderate and Severe Head Injury in Adults" by Kelly DF, Nikas DL, and Becker DP, in *Neurological Surgery,* 4th ed, Philadelphia: WB Saunders, 1995.

References

1. Baker SP, O'Neill B, Ginsburg MJ, et al: Injuries in relation to other health problems, in *The Injury Fact Book* (2d ed). New York: Oxford University Press, 1992: 8–16.
2. Kraus JF: Epidemiology of head injury, in Cooper PR (ed): *Head Injury* (3d ed). Baltimore: Williams & Wilkins, 1993: 1–25.
3. Levin HS: Neurobehavioral sequelae of closed head injury, in Cooper PR (ed): *Head Injury* (3d ed). Baltimore: Williams & Wilkins, 1993: 525–551.
4. Marshall LF, Gautille T, Klauber MR, et al: The outcome of severe closed head injury. *J Neurosurg* 1991; 75(suppl):S28–36.
5. Van Zomeren AH, Van Den Burg W: Residual complaints of patients two years after severe head injury. *J Neurol Neurosurg Psychiatry* 1985; 48:21–28.
6. Rimel RW, Giordani B, Barth JT, et al: Disability caused by minor head injury. *Neurosurgery* 1981; 9:221–228.
7. Rimel RW, Giordani B, Barth JT: Moderate head injury: Completing the clinical spectrum of brain trauma. *Neurosurgery* 1982; 11:344–351.
8. Hovda DA, Becker DP, Katayama Y: Secondary injury and acidosis. *J Neurotrauma* 1990; 9:S47–60.
9. Jenkins LW, Moszynski K, Lyeth BG, et al: Increased vulnerability of the mildly traumatized rat brain to cerebral ischemia: The use of controlled secondary ischemia as a research tool to identify common mechanisms contributing to mechanical and ischemic brain injury. *Brain Res* 1989; 477:211–224.
10. U.S. Department of Transportation, National Highway Traffic Safety Administration: 1994 *Occupant Protection Idea Sampler.* Washington: U.S. Dept of Transportation, 1994.
11. Bouma CJ, Muizelaar JP, Choi SC, et al: Cerebral circulation and metabolism after severe traumatic brain injury: The elusive role of ischemia. *J Neurosurg* 1991; 75:685–693.
12. Bouma GJ, Muizelaar JP, Stringer WA, et al: Ultra-early evaluation of regional cerebral blood flow in severely head-injured patients using xenon-enhanced computerized tomography. *J Neurosurg* 1992; 77:17, 360–368.
13. Chesnut RM, Marshall LF, Marshall SB: Medical management of intracranial pressure, in Cooper PR (ed): *Head Injury* (3d ed). Baltimore: Williams & Wilkins, 1993: 225–246.
14. Graham DI, Ford I, Adams JH, et al: Ischaemic brain damage is still common in fatal non-missile head injury. *J Neurol Neurosurg Psychiatry* 1989; 52:346–350.
15. Graham DI, Adams JH, Doyle D: Ischaemic brain damage in fatal non-missile head injuries. *J Neurol Sci* 1978; 39:213–234.
16. Jennett B, Carlin J: Preventable mortality and morbidity after head injury. *Injury* 1978; 10:31–39.
17. Becker DP, Miller JD, Ward JD, et al: The outcome from severe head injury with early diagnosis and intensive management. *J Neurosurg* 1977; 47:491–502.
18. Katayama Y, Becker DP, Tamura T, et al: Massive increase in extracellular potassium and the indiscriminate release of glutamate following concussive brain injury. *J Neurosurg* 1990; 73:889–900.
19. Doczi T, Tarjanyi J, Huszka E, et al: Syndrome of inappropriate secretion of antidiuretic hormone (SIADH) after head injury. *Neurosurgery* 1982; 10:685–688.
20. Jones PA, Piper IR, Corrie J, et al: Microcomputer based detection of secondary insults and 12 month outcome after head injury. Abstract, 2nd International Neurotrauma Symposium, Glasgow, July 1993.
21. McIntosh TK: Pharmacologic strategies in the treatment of experimental brain injury. *J Neurotrauma* 1992; 9(suppl 1):S201–209.
22. Reeder RF, Harbaugh RE: Administration of intravenous urea and normal saline for treatment of hyponatremia in neurosurgical patients. *J Neurosurg* 1989; 70:201–206.
23. Stein SC, Spettell C, Young G, et al: Delayed and progressive brain injury in closed-head trauma: radiological demonstration. *Neurosurgery* 1993; 32:25–31.
24. Stein SC, Young GS, Talucci RC, et al: Delayed brain injury after head trauma: Significance of coagulopathy. *Neurosurgery* 1992; 30:160–165.
25. Young B, Ott L, Dempsey R, et al: Relationship between admission hyperglycemia and neurological outcome of severely brain-injured patients. *Ann Surg* 1989; 210:466–473.
26. Young B, Ott L, Yingling B, et al: Nutrition and brain injury. *J Neurotrauma* 1992; 9(suppl 1):S375–383.
27. Gopinath SP, Robertson CS, Contant CF, et al: Jugular

venous desaturation and outcome after head injury. *J Psychiatry Neurosci* 1994; 57:717–723.
28. McGraw CP: A cerebral perfusion pressure greater than 80 mmHg is more beneficial, in Hoff JT, Betz AL (eds): *Intracranial Pressure VII.* Berlin: Springer-Verlag, 1989: 839–841.
29. Contant CF, Robertson CF, Gopinath SP, et al: Determination of clinically important thresholds in continuously monitored patients with head injury. Abstract, 2d International Neurotrauma Symposium, Glasgow, July, 1993.
30. Marion DW, Obrist WD, Penrod LE, et al: Treatment of cerebral ischemia improves outcome following severe traumatic brain injury. Abstract, The 61st Annual Meeting of the American Association of Neurological Surgeons, Boston, April 1993; and personal communication.
31. Rosner MJ, Rosner SD: CPP management: I. Results. Presented at Ninth International Symposium on Intracranial Pressure, Nagoya, Japan, 1994.
32. Lassen NA: Cerebral blood flow and oxygen consumption in man. *Physiol Rev* 1959; 39:183–238.
33. Paulson OB, Strandgaard S, Edvinsson L: Cerebral autoregulation. *Cerebrovasc Brain Metab Rev* 1990; 2:161–192.
34. Sokad TE, Kalimio H, Olsson Y, et al: Transient hypertensive opening of the blood-brain barrier can lead to brain damage. *Acta Neuropathol* 1988; 75:557–565.
35. Kontos HA, Wei EP, Navari RM, et al: Responses of cerebral arteries and arterioles to acute hypotension and hypertension. *Am J Physiol* 1978; 234:H371–H383.
36. Bouma GJ, Muizelaar JP, Bandoh K, et al: Blood pressure and intracranial pressure-volume dynamics in severe head injury relationship with cerebral blood flow. *J Neurosurg* 1992; 77:15–19.
37. Bouma GJ, Muizelaar JP: Relationship between cardiac output and cerebral blood flow in patients with intact and with impaired autoregulation. *J Neurosurg* 1990; 73:368–374.
38. Muizelaar JP, Ward JD, Marmarou A, et al: Cerebral blood flow and metabolism in severely head-injured children: II. Autoregulation. *J Neurosurg* 1989; 71:72–76.
39. Gray WJ, Rosner MJ: Pressure-volume index as a function of cerebral perfusion pressure: II. The effects of low cerebral perfusion pressure and autoregulation. *J Neurosurg* 1987; 67:377–380.
40. El-Adawy Y, Rosner MJ: Cerebral perfusion pressure, autoregulation and the PVI reflection point: Pathological ICP, in Hoff JT, Betz AL (eds): *Intracranial Pressure VII.* Berlin: Springer-Verlag, 1989: 829–833.
41. Lewelt W, Jenkins LW, Miller JD: Autoregulation of cerebral blood flow after experimental fluid percussion injury of the brain. *J Neurosurg* 1980; 53:500–511.
42. Miller JD: Head injury and brain ischemia. *Br J Anaesth* 1985; 57:120–129.
43. Nordstrom CH, Messeter K, Sundbarg G, et al: Cerebral blood flow, vasoreactivity, and oxygen consumption during barbiturate therapy in severe traumatic brain lesions. *J. Neurosurg* 1988; 68:424–431.
44. Tsutsumi H, Ide K, Mizutani T, et al: The relationship between intracranial pressure, cerebral perfusion pressure and outcome in head injured patients: The critical level of cerebral perfusion pressure, in Miller JD, Teasdale GM, Rowan JO, et al (eds): *Intracranial Pressure VI.* Berlin: Springer-Verlag, 1986: 661–666.
45. Chan K, Dearden NM, Miller JD, et al: Multimodality monitoring as a guide to treatment of intracranial hypertension after severe brain injury. *Neurosurgery* 1993; 32:547–553.
46. Rosner MJ, Rosner SD: CPP management: II. Optimization of CPP or vasoparalysis does not exist in the living brain. Presented at Ninth International Symposium on Intracranial Pressure, Nagoya, Japan, 1994.
47. Shalmon E, Caron MJ, Martin NA, et al: Cerebral perfusion pressure and cerebral blood flow: lack of correlation. *Intracranial Pressure IX*, section XVII:348–352, 1994.
48. Rosner MJ: Pathophysiology and management of increased intracranial pressure, in Andrews BT (ed): *Neurosurgical Intensive Care.* New York: McGraw-Hill, 1993: 57–112.
49. Fieschi C, Battistini N, Beduschi A, et al: Regional cerebral blood flow and intraventricular pressure in acute head injuries. *J Neurol Neurosurg Psychiatry* 1974; 37:1378–1388.
50. Obrist WD, Langfitt TW, Jaggi JI, et al: Cerebral blood flow and metabolism in comatose patients with acute head injury. Relationship to intracranial hypertension. *J Neurosurg* 1984; 61:241–253.
51. Bruce DA, Alavi A, Bilaniuk L, et al: Diffuse cerebral swelling following head injuries in children: The syndrome of "malignant brain edema." *J Neurosurg* 1981; 54:170–178.
52. Muizelaar JP, Marmarou A, DeSalles AAF, et al: Cerebral blood flow and metabolism in severely head-injured children: Part 1. Relationship with GCS score, outcome, ICP, and PVI. *J Neurosurg* 1989; 71:63–71.
53. Robertson CS, Contant CF, Gokasian ZL, et al: Cerebral blood flow, arteriovenous oxygen difference, and outcome in head injured patients. *J Neurol Neurosurg Psychiatry* 1992; 5:594–603.
54. Kelly DF, Dordestani RK, Shalmon E: Hyperemia-associated intracranial hypertension following human traumatic brain injury is uncommon. To be presented at: Third International Neurotrauma Symposium, Toronto, 1995.
55. Rosner MJ, Daughton S: Cerebral perfusion pressure management in head injury. *J Trauma* 1990; 30:933–941.
56. Lundberg N: Continuous recording and control of ventricular fluid pressure in neurosurgical practice. *Acta Psychiatr Neurol Scnad* 1960; 36(suppl 149):1–193.
57. Rosner MJ, Becker DP: Origin and evolution of plateau waves: Experimental observations and a theoretical model. *J Neurosurg* 1984; 60:312–324.
58. Kuroda Y, Inglis FM, Miller JD, et al: Transient glucose hypermetabolism after acute subdural hematoma in the rat. *J Neurosurg* 1992; 76:471–477.
59. Bergsneider M, Kelly DF, Shalmon E, et al: Early hyperglycolysis following severe human traumatic brain in-

jury: A positron emission tomography study. To be presented at Third International Neurotrauma Symposium, Toronto, July, 1995.

60. Miller JD: Evaluation and treatment of head injury in adults. *Neurosurg Q* 1992; 2:28–43.
61. Alberico AM, Ward JD, Choi SC, et al: Outcome after severe head injury, relationship to mass lesions, diffuse injury, and ICP course in pediatric and adult patients. *J Neurosurg* 1987; 67:648–656.
62. Marmarou A, Anderson RL, Ward JD, et al: NINDS Traumatic Coma Data Bank: Intracranial pressure monitoring methodology. *J Neurosurg* 1991; 75:S21–27.
63. Marmarou A, Anderson RL, Ward JD, et al: Impact of ICP instability and hypotension on outcome in patients with severe head trauma. *J Neurosurg* 1991; 75:S59–66.
64. Muizelaar JP, Marmarou A, Ward JD, et al: Adverse effects of prolonged hyperventilation in patients with severe head injury: A randomized clinical trial. *J Neurosurg* 1991; 75:731–739.
65. Van Helden A, Schneider GH, Unterberg A, et al: Monitoring of jugular venous oxygen saturation as a guide to therapy of severe head injury. Abstract. 2d International Neurotrauma Symposium, Glasgow, July 1993.
66. Obrist WD, Marion DW, Aggarwal S: Time course of cerebral blood flow and metabolic changes following severe head injury. Abstract, 61st Annual Meeting of the American Association of Neurological Surgeons, Boston, April 1993.
67. Ommaya AK, Gennarelli TA: Experimental head injury, in Vinken PJ, Bruyn GW (eds): *Handbook of Clinical Neurology*, vol 23. Amsterdam: Elsevier-North Holland, 1975: 67–90.
68. Majernick TG, Bieniek R, Houston JB, et al: Cervical spine movement during orotracheal intubation. *Ann Emerg Med* 1986; 15:417–420.
69. Rhee KJ, Green W, Holcroft JW, et al: Oral intubation in the multiply injured patient: The risk of exacerbating spinal cord damage. *Ann Emerg Med* 1990; 19:511–514.
70. Talucci RC, Shaikh KA, Schwab CW: Rapid sequence induction with oral endotracheal intubation in the multiply injured patient. *Am Surg* 1988; 54:185–187.
71. Delaney KA, Goldfrank LR: Initial management of the multiply injured or intoxicated patient, in Cooper PR (ed): *Head Injury*, (3d ed). Baltimore: Williams & Wilkins, 1993: 43–63.
72. Ghoneim MM, Yamada T: Etomidate: A clinical and electroencephalographic comparison with thiopental. *Anesth Analg* 1977; 56:479–485.
73. Milde LM, Milde JH, Michenfelder JD: Cerebral functional, metabolic, and hemodynamic effects of etomidate in dogs. *Anesthesiology* 1985; 63:371–377.
74. Klauber MR, Marshall LF, Luerssen TG, et al: Determinants of head injury mortality: Importance of the low risk patient. *Neurosurgery* 1989; 24:31–36.
75. Eisenberg HM, Gary HE, Aldrich EF, et al: Initial CT findings in 753 patients with severe head injury: A report from the NIH Traumatic Coma Data Bank. *J Neurosurg* 1990; 73:688–698.
76. Wilberger JE: Emergency care and initial evaluation, in Cooper PR (ed): *Head Injury*, (3d ed). Baltimore: Williams & Wilkins, 1993: 27–41.
77. Scalea T, Maltz S, Duncan A, et al: Fluid resuscitation in head injury. *American Association for the Surgery of Trauma Abstract Book*. New York: American Association for the Surgery of Trauma, September, 1989.
78. Kaieda R, Todd MM, Cook LN, et al: Acute effects of changing plasma osmolality and colloid oncotic pressure on the formation of brain edema after cryogenic injury. *Neurosurgery* 1989; 24:671–678.
79. Tommasino C, Moore S, Todd MM: Cerebral effects of isovolemic hemodilution with crystalloid or colloid solutions. *Crit Care Med* 1988; 16:862–868.
80. Sutin KM, Ruskin KJ, Kaufman BS: Intravenous fluid therapy in neurologic injury. *Crit Care Clin* 1992; 8(2):367–408.
81. Zornow MH, Scheller MS, Shackford SR: Effect of hypertonic lactated Ringer's solution on intracranial pressure and cerebral water content in a model of traumatic brain injury. *J Trauma* 1989; 29:484–488.
82. Worthley LIG, Cooper DJ, Jones N: Treatment of resistant intracranial hypertension with hypertonic saline. *J Neurosurg* 1988; 68:478.
83. Gunnar WD, Merlotti GJ, Jonasson O, et al: Resuscitation from hemorrhagic shock: Alterations of the intracranial pressure after normal saline, 3% saline and dextran-40. *Ann Surg* 1986; 204: 686–692.
84. Vassar MJ, Perry CA, Gannaway WL, et al: 7.5% sodium chloride/dextran for resuscitation of trauma patients undergoing helicopter transport. *Arch Surg* 1991; 126:1065–1072.
85. Velanovich V: Crystalloid versus colloid fluid resuscitation: A meta-analysis of mortality. *Surgery* 1989; 105:65–71.
86. Bisonni RS, Holtgrave DR, Lawler F. et al: Colloids versus crystalloids in fluid resuscitation: An analysis of randomized controlled trials. *J Fam Pract* 1991; 32:387–390.
87. Weigelt JA: Resuscitation and initial management. *Crit Care Clin* 1993; 9:657–671.
88. Teasdale G, Jennett B: Assessment of coma and impaired consciousness: A practical scale. *Lancet* 1974; 2:81–84.
89. Starmark JE, Holmgren E, Stalhammar D: Current reporting of responsiveness in acute cerebral disorders: A survey of the neurosurgical literature. *J Neurosurg* 1988; 69:692–698.
90. Galbraith S, Murray WR, Patel AR, et al: The relationship between alcohol and head injury and its effect on the conscious level. *Br J Surg* 1976; 63:128–130.
91. Jagger J, Fife D, Venberg K, et al: Effect of alcohol intoxication on the diagnosis and apparent severity of brain injury. *Neurosurgery* 1984; 15:303–306.
92. Sivakumar V, Rajshekhar V, Chandy MJ: Management of neurosurgical patients with hyponatremia and natriuresis. *Neurosurgery* 1993; 34:269–274.
93. Foulkes MA, Eisenberg HM, Jane JA, et al: The traumatic coma data bank: Design, methods, and baseline characteristics. *J Neurosurg* 1991; 75(suppl):S8–13.

94. Pal J, Brown R, Fleiszer D: The value of the Glasgow Coma Scale and Injury Severity Score: Predicting outcome in multiple trauma patients with head injury. *J Trauma* 1989; 29:746–748.
95. Vollmer DG: Prognosis and outcome of severe head injury, in Cooper PR (ed): *Head Injury*, (3d ed). Baltimore: Williams & Wilkins, 1993: 533–581.
96. Stein SC, Ross SE: Moderate head injury: A guide to initial management. *J Neurosurg* 1992; 77:562–564.
97. Stein SC, Ross SE: The value of computed tomographic scans in patients with low-risk head injuries. *Neurosurgery* 1990; 26:638–640.
98. Jennett B, Teasdale G, Galbraith S, et al: Severe head injury in three countries. *J Neurol Neurosurg Psychiatry* 1977; 40:291–298.
99. Lobato RD, Rivas JJ, Gomez PA, et al: Head-injured patients who talk and deteriorate into coma: Analysis of 211 cases studied with computerized tomography. *J Neurosurg* 1991; 75:256–261.
100. Marshall LF, Toole BM, Bowers SA: The National Traumatic Coma Data Bank: II. Patients who talk and deteriorate: Implications for treatment. *J Neurosurg* 1983; 59:285–288.
101. Miller JD, Murray LS, Teasdale GM: Development of a traumatic intracranial hematoma after a "minor" head injury. *Neurosurgery* 1990; 27:669–673.
102. Feuerman T, Wackym PA, Gade GF, et al: Value of skull radiography, head computed tomographic scanning, and admission for observation in cases of minor head injury. *Neurosurgery* 1988; 22:449–453.
103. Masters ST, McClean PM, Arcarese JS, et al: Skull x-ray examinations after head trauma: Recommendations by a multi-disciplinary panel and validation study. *N Engl J Med* 1987; 316:84–91.
104. Meyer A: Herniation of the brain. *Arch Neurol Psychiatr* 1920; 4:387–400.
105. Wilberger JE, Rothfus WE, Tabas J, et al: Acute tissue tear hemorrhages of the brain: Computed tomography and clinicopathological correlations. *Neurosurgery* 1990; 27:208–213.
106. Brown FD, Johns L, Jafar JJ, et al: Detailed monitoring of the effects of mannitol following experimental head injury. *J Neurosurg* 1979; 50:423–432.
107. Gentleman D, Teasdale G, Murray L: Cause of severe head injury and risk of complications. *Br Med J* 1986; 292:449.
108. Miller JD, Butterworth JF, Gudeman SK, et al: Further experience in the management of severe head injury. *J Neurosurg* 1981; 54:289–299.
109. Vollmer DG, Torner JC, Jane JA, et al: Age and outcome following traumatic coma: why do older patients fare worse. *J Neurosurg* 75:S37–S49, 1991.
110. Miller JD, Becker DP, Ward JD, et al: Significance of intracranial hypertension in severe head injury. *J Neurosurg* 1977; 47:503–516.
111. Gopinath SP, Robertson CS, Grossman RG, et al: Near-infrared spectroscopic localization of intracranial hematomas. *J Neurosurg* 1993; 79:43–47.
112. McBride DQ, Patel AB, Caron M: Early repeat CT scan: Importance in detecting surgical lesions after closed head injury. Abstract. 2d International Neurotrauma Symposium, Glagow, July 1993.
113. Aldrich EF, Eisenberg HM: Acute subdural hematoma, in Apuzzo MLJ (ed): *Brain Surgery Complications: Avoidance and Management*. New York: Churchill Livingstone, 1993: 1283–1298.
114. Cooper PR: Post-traumatic intracranial mass lesions, in Cooper PR (ed): *Head Injury*, (3d ed). Baltimore: Williams & Wilkins, 1993: 275–329.
115. Howard MA, Gross AS, Dacey RG, et al: Acute subdural hematomas: An age-dependent clinical entity. *J Neurosurg* 1989; 71:858–863.
116. Voyce SJ, Urbach D, Rippe JM: Pulmonary artery catheters, in Rippe JM, Irwin RS, Alpert JS, et al (eds): *Intensive Care Medicine*, (2d ed). Boston: Little, Brown, 1991: 48–72.
117. Waxman K, Sundine MJ, Young RF: Is early prediction of outcome in severe head injury possible? *Arch Surg* 1991; 126:1237–1242.
118. Marshall LF, Smith RW, Shapiro HM: The outcome with aggressive treatment in severe head injuries: I. The significance of intracranial pressure monitoring. *J Neurosurg* 1979; 50:20–25.
119. Narayan RK, Kishore PRS, Becker DP, et al: Intracranial pressure: To monitor or not to monitor? A review of our experience with severe head injury. *J Neurosurg* 1982; 56:650–659.
120. Unterberg A, Kiening K, Schmiedek P, et al: Long-term observations of intracranial pressure after severe head injury: The phenomenon of secondary rise of intracranial pressure. *Neurosurgery* 1993; 32:17–24.
121. Chan K, Miller JD, Dearden NM, et al: The effect of changes in cerebral perfusion pressure upon middle cerebral artery blood flow velocity and jugular bulb venous oxygen saturation after severe brain injury. *J Neurosurg* 1992; 77:55–61.
122. Sheinberg M, Kanter MJ, Robertson CS, et al: Continuous monitoring of jugular venous oxygen saturation in head-injured patients. *J Neurosurg* 1992; 76:212–217.
123. Marion DW, Darby J, Yonas H: Acute regional blood flow changes caused by severe head injuries. *J Neurosurg* 1991; 74:407–414.
124. Obrist WD, Thompson HK Jr, Wang HS et al: Regional cerebral blood flow estimated by xenon-133 inhalation. *Stroke* 1975; 6:245–256.
125. Yonas H (ed): *Cerebral Blood Flow Measurement with Stable Xenon-Enhanced Computed Tomography*. New York: Raven Press, 1992.
126. Jaggi JL, Obrist WD, Gennarelli TA, et al: Relationship of early cerebral blood flow and metabolism to outcome in acute head injury. *J Neurosurg* 1990; 72:176–182.
127. Gibbs EL, Leenox WG, Nims LF, et al: Arterial and cerebral venous blood: Arterial-venous differences in man. *J Biol Chem* 1942; 144:325–332.
128. Chan K, Dearden NM, Miller JD: The significance of posttraumatic increase in cerebral blood flow velocity: A transcranial Doppler ultrasound study. *Neurosurgery* 1992; 30:697–700.
129. Martin NA, Doberstein C, Zane C, et al: Posttraumatic cerebral arterial spasm: Transcranial Doppler ultra-

sound, cerebral blood flow, and angiographic findings. *J Neurosurg* 1992; 77:575–583.

130. Steiger HJ, Aaslid R, Stooss et al: Transcranial Doppler monitoring in head injury: Relations between type of injury, flow velocities, vasoreactivity, and outcome. *Neurosurgery* 1994; 34:79–86.

131. Weber M, Grolimund P, Seiler RW: Evaluation of posttraumatic cerebral blood flow velocities by transcranial Doppler ultrasonography. *Neurosurgery* 1990; 27:106–112.

132. Martin NA, Doberstein C, Khanna R, et al: Posttraumatic cerebral arterial spasm. Abstract, 2d International Neurotrauma Symposium, Glasgow, July 1993.

133. Levy ML, Giannotta SL: Cardiac performance indices during hypervolemic therapy for cerebral vasospasm. *J Neurosurg* 1991; 75:27–31.

134. *Physicians Desk Reference 48.* Montvale, NJ: Medical Economics, 1994: 896–897.

135. Levy ML, Rabb CH, Zelman V, et al: Cardiac performance enhancement from dobutamine in patients refractory to hypervolemic therapy for cerebral vasospasm. *J Neurosurg* 1993; 79:494–499.

136. Dorman HR, Sondheimer JH, Cadnapaphornchai P: Mannitol-induced acute renal failure. *Medicine* 1990; 69:153–159.

137. Marshall LF, Smith RW, Shapiro HM: The outcome with aggressive treatment in severe head injuries: II. Acute and chronic barbiturate administration in the management of head injury. *J Neurosurg* 1979; 50:26–30.

138. Feldman Z, Kanter MJ, Robertson CS, et al: Effect of head elevation on intracranial pressure, cerebral perfusion pressure, and cerebral blood flow in head-injured patients. *J Neurosurg* 1992; 76:207–211.

139. Temkin NR, Dikmen SS, Wilensky AJ, et al: A randomized, double-blind study of phenytoin for the prevention of post-traumatic seizures. *N Engl J Med* 1990; 323:497–502.

140. Marshall LF, Smith R, Rauscher L, et al: Mannitol dose requirements in brain-injured patients. *J Neurosurg* 1978; 48:169–172.

141. Shapiro HM: Barbiturates in brain ischemia. *Br J Anesth* 1985; 57:82–95.

142. Miller JD: Barbiturates and raised intracranial pressure. *Ann Neurol* 1979; 6:189–193.

143. Eisenberg HM, Frankowski RF, Contant CF, et al: High-dose barbiturate control of elevated intracranial pressure in patients with severe head injury. *J Neurosurg* 1988; 69:15–23.

144. Rea GL, Rockswold GL: Barbiturate therapy in uncontrolled intracranial hypertension. *Neurosurgery* 1983; 12:401–404.

145. Rockoff MA, Marshall LF, Shapiro HM: High-dose barbiturate therapy in humans: A clinical review of 60 patients. *Ann Neurol* 1979; 6:194–199.

146. Donegan JH: The electroencephalogram, in Blitt CD (ed): *Monitoring in Anesthesia and Critical Care Medicine.* New York: Churchill Livingstone, 1985: 323–343.

147. Clifton GL, Steven A, Plenger PM, et al: A phase II study of systemic hypothermia in severe brain injury. Abstract, 61st Annual Meeting of the American Association of Neurological Surgeons, Boston, April 1993.

148. Marion DW, Obrist WD, Carlier PM, et al: The use of moderate therapeutic hypothermia for patients with severe head injuries: A preliminary report. *J Neurosurg* 1993; 79:354–362.

149. Shiozaki T, Sugimoto H, Taneda M, et al: Effect of mild hypothermia on uncontrollable intracranial hypertension after severe head injury. *J Neurosurg* 1993; 79:363–368.

150. Vice MV: A metabolic approach to the management of neurological trauma: Hypothermic hypokalemic coma. Abstract, 61st Annual Meeting of the American Association of Neurological Surgeons, Boston, April 1993.

151. Hayashi N, Hirayama T, Udagawa A, et al: Systemic management of cerebral edema based on a new concept in severe head injury patients. *Acta Neurochir* 1994; 60(suppl):541–543.

152. Mellergard P: Changes in human intracerebral temperature in response to different methods of brain cooling. *Neurosurgery* 1992; 31:671–677.

153. Cooper PR, Moody S, Clark WK, et al: Dexamethasone and severe head injury: A prospective double-blind study. *J Neurosurg* 1979; 51:307–316.

154. Dearden NM, Gibson JS, McDowall DG, et al: Effect of high-dose dexamethasone on outcome from severe head injury. *J Neurosurg* 1986; 64:81–88.

155. Gudeman S, Miller J, Becker D: Failure of high-dose steroid therapy to influence intracranial pressure in patients with severe head injury. *J Neurosurg* 1979; 51:301–306.

156. Marshall L, King J, Langfitt T: The complications of high-dose corticosteroid therapy in neurosurgical patients: A prospective study. *Ann Neurol* 1977; 1:201–203.

157. Saul T, Ducker T, Salman M, et al: Steroids in severe head injury: A prospective, randomized clinical trial. *J Neurosurg* 1981; 54:596–600.

158. Deutschman CS, Haines SJ: Anticonvulsant prophylaxis in neurological surgery. *Neurosurgery* 1985; 17:510–517.

159. Jennett B: *Epilepsy after Nonmissle Injuries,* (2d ed.) Chicago: Year Book, 1975.

160. Salazar AM, Jabbari B, Vance SC, et al: Epilepsy after penetrating head injury: I. Clinical correlates: A report of the Vietnam Head Injury Study. *Neurology* 1985; 35:1406–1414.

161. Young B, Rapp RP, Norton JA, et al: Failure of prophylactically administered phenytoin to prevent late posttraumatic seizures. *J Neurosurg* 1983; 58:236–241.

162. Mayhall CG, Archer NH, Lamb VA, et al: Ventriculostomy-related infection: A prospective epidemiologic study. *N Engl J Med* 1984; 310:553–559.

163. Winfield JA, Rosenthal P, Kanter RK, et al: Duration of intracranial pressure monitoring does not predict daily risk of infectious complications. *Neurosurgery* 1993; 33:424–431.

164. Clifton GL, Robertson CS, Choi SC: Assessment of nutritional requirements of head-injured patients. *J Neurosurg* 1986; 64:895–901.

165. Deutschman CS, Konstantinides FN, Raup S, et al:

Physiological and metabolic response to isolated closed-head injury: I. Basal metabolic state: Correlations of metabolic and physiologic parameters with fasting and stressed controls. *J Neurosurg* 1986; 64:89–98.

166. Hadley MN, Grahm TW, Harrington T, et al: Nutritional support and neurotrauma: A critical review of early nutrition in forty-five acute head injury patients. *Neurosurgery* 1986; 19:367–373.
167. Young B, Ott L, Twyman D, et al: The effect of nutritional support on outcome from severe head injury. *J Neurosurg* 1987; 67:668–676.
168. Robertson CS, Clifton GL, Grossman RG: Oxygen utilization and cardiovascular function in head-injured patients. *Neurosurgery* 1984; 15:307–314.
169. Moore FA, Moore EE: Trauma, in Zaloga GP (ed): *Nutrition in Critical Care.* St. Louis: Mosby, 1994: 571–586.
170. Gennarelli TA, Champion HR, Sacco WJ, et al: Mortality of patients with head injury and extracranial injury treated in trauma centers. *J Trauma* 1989; 29:1193–1202.
171. Abel RM, Grimes JB, Alonso D, et al: Adverse hemodynamic and ultrastructural changes in dog hearts subjected to protein-calorie malnutrition. *Am Heart J* 1979; 97:733–744.
172. Law DK, Dudrick SJ, Abdou NI: Immunocompetence of patients with protein-calorie malnutrition: The effects of nutritional repletion. *Ann Intern Med* 1973; 79:545–550.
173. Grahm TW, Zadrozny DB, Harrington T: The benefits of early jejunal hyperalimentation in the head-injured patient. *Neurosurgery* 1989; 25:729–735.
174. Haydock DA, Hill GL: Impaired wound healing in surgical patients with varying degrees of malnutrition. *J Parenter Enteral Nutr* 1986; 10:550–554.
175. Moore EE, Jones TN: Benefits of immediate jejunostomy feeding after major abdominal trauma—a prospective, randomized study. *J Trauma* 1986; 26:874–881.
176. Rapp RP, Young B, Twyman D, et al: The favorable effect of early parenteral feeding on survival in head-injured patients. *J Neurosurg* 1983; 58:906–912.
177. Zaloga GP, Bortenschlager L, Black KW, et al: Immediate postoperative enteral feeding decreases weight loss and improves wound healing after abdominal surgery in rats. *Crit Care Med* 1992; 20:115–118.
178. Deitch EA, Ma W, Ma L, et al: Protein malnutrition predisposes to inflammatory-induced gut-origin septic states. *Ann Surg* 1990; 211:560–568.
179. Inoune S, Lukes S, Alexander JW, et al: Increased gut blood flow with early enteral feeding in burned guinea pigs. *J Burn Care Rehab* 1989; 10:300–308.
180. Kudsk JF, Croce MA, Fabian TC, et al: Enteral versus parenteral feeding: Effects on septic morbidity after blunt and penetrating abdominal trauma. *Ann Surg* 1992; 215:503–513.
181. Zaloga GP: Timing and route of nutritional support, in Zaloga GP (ed): *Nutrition in Critical Care*. St. Louis: Mosby, 1994: 297–330.
182. Kudsk KA, Minard G: Enteral nutrition, in Zaloga GP (ed): *Nutrition in Critical Care.* St. Louis: Mosby, 1994:331–360.
183. Bowers DF: The initiation and progression of tube feedings, Brown FD, Johns L, Jafar JJ, et al: Detailed monitoring of the effects of mannitol following experimental head injury. *J Neurosurg* 1979; 50:423–432.
184. Kirby DF, Clifton GL, Turner H, et al: Early enteral nutrition after braininjury by percutaneous endoscopic gastrojejunostomy. *J Parenter Enteral Nutr* 1991; 15:298–302.
185. Bartter FC, Schwartz WB: The syndrome of inappropriate secretion of antidiuretic hormone. *Am J Med* 1967; 42:790–804.
186. Lolin Y, Jackowski A: Hyponatremia in neurosurgical patients: Diagnosis using derived parameter of sodium and water homeostasis. *Br J Neurosurg* 1992; 6:457–466.
187. Kelly DF, Laws ER, Fossett DT: Delayed hyponatremia after transphenoidal surgery for pituitary adenoma. *J Neurosurgery* 1995, August (in press).
188. Gennarelli TA: Personal communication, 1993.
189. Piek J, Chesnut RM, Marshall LF, et al: Extracranial complications of severe head injury. *J Neurosurg* 1992; 77:901–907.
190. Driks MR, Craven DE, Celli BR, et al: Nosocomial pneumonia in intubated patients given sucralfate as compared with antacids or histamine type 2 blockers: The role of gastric colonization. *N Engl J Med* 1987; 317:1376–1382.
191. Eddleston JM, Vohra A, Scott P, et al: A comparison of the frequency of stress ulceration and secondary pneumonia in sucralfate- or ranitidine-treated intensive care unit patients. *Crit Care Med* 1991; 19:1491–1496.
192. Tryba M: Risk of acute stress bleeding and nosocomial pneumonia in ventilated intensive care unit patients: Sucralfate versus antacids. *Am J Med* 1987; 83(suppl 3B):117–124.
193. Black PMcL, Baker MF, Snook CP: Experience with external pneumatic calf compression in neurology and neurosurgery. *Neurosurgery* 1986; 18:440–444.
194. Frim DM, Barker FG, Poletti CE: Postoperative low-dose heparin decreases thromboembolic complications in neurosurgical patients. *Neurosurgery* 1992; 30:830–833.
195. Hamilton MG, Hull RD, Pineo GF: Venous thromboembolism in neurosurgery and neurology patients: A review. *Neurosurgery* 1994; 34:280–296.
196. Chesnut RM: Medical complications of the head-injured patient, in Cooper RP (ed): *Head Injury*, (3d ed). Baltimore: Williams & Wilkins, 1993: 459–501.
197. Brown TH, Davidson PF, Larson GM: Acute gastritis occurring within 24 hours of severe head injury. *Gastrointest Endosc* 1989; 35:37–40.
198. Epstein FM, Ward JD, Becker DP: Medical complications of head injury, in Cooper PR (ed): *Head Injury*, (2d ed). Baltimore: Williams & Wilkins, 1987: 390–421.
199. Halloran LG, Zfass AM, Gayle WE, et al: Prevention of acute gastrointestinal complications after severe head injury: A controlled trial of cimetidine prophylaxis. *Am J Surg* 1980; 139:44–48.
200. Hall ED, Braughler JM, McCall JM: Antioxidant effects

in brain and spinal cord injury. *J Neurotrauma* 1992; 9(suppl 1):S165–172.

201. Muizelaar JP, Marmarou A, Young HF, et al: Improving the outcome of severe head injury with the oxygen radical scavenger polyethylene glycol-conjugated superoxide dismutase: A Phase II trial. *J Neurosur* 1993; 78:375–382.
202. European Study Group on Nimodipine in Severe Head Injury: A multicenter trial of the efficacy of nimodipine on outcome after severe head injury. *J Neurosurg* 1994; 80:797–804.
203. Rosner MJ, Rosner SD: THAM therapy and traumatic brain injury: A double-blind, randomized study. Presented at Ninth International Symposium on Intracranial Pressure, Nagoya, Japan, 1994.
204. Kuroda Y, Fujisawa H, Strebel S, et al: Effect of neuroprotective *N*-methyl-D-aspartate antagonist on increased intracranial pressure: Studies in the rat acute subdural hematoma model. *Neurosurgery* 1994; 35:106–112.

Early Care

CHAPTER 7

PREHOSPITAL CARE OF THE HEAD-INJURED PATIENT

Guy M. McKhann II
Michael K. Copass
H. Richard Winn

SYNOPSIS

Trauma accounts for approximately 1 in 12 deaths in the United States[1] *and is the leading cause of mortality in the age group from 1 to 34 years old.*[2] *Head injury is responsible for about 25 to 50 percent of those fatalities.*[3–6] *The mortality of trauma patients is nearly three times higher when head injury is present regardless of the mechanism of injury.*[6] *Prehospital care is an important component in the treatment of head-injured patients. Improved medical care at the scene of the injury, appropriate rapid triage to a facility with integrated trauma services, attention to airway management, prevention and treatment of hypotension and hypoxia, and early management of increased intracranial pressure have all contributed to improved prehospital care of patients with a head injury.*[7–9] *Despite advances in prehospital care, neurosurgeons have paid limited attention to this important phase of head injury. Prehospital care represents the initial intervention in the continuum of head injury assessment and treatment, and advances in therapy in this setting may have a profound impact on the ultimate outcome.*

DEVELOPMENT OF PREHOSPITAL CARE

The American College of Surgeons first directed attention toward the study of trauma when it formed the predecessor to the Committee on Trauma, the Committee on Treatment of Fractures, in 1922.[10] Except in the military setting, little progress was made over the next several decades, as evidenced by the 1966 report by the National Academy of Science terming accidental injury "the neglected disease of modern society."[11] This report stimulated new funding for emergency medical technician and paramedic training programs and for the development of systematized regional trauma care centers.[12,13]

The concept of preventable death was identified by Van Wagoner in 1961.[14] He determined that one-sixth of noncombat military deaths resulted from injuries from which recovery could be expected and another one-sixth resulted from suboptimal treatment. Jennett and Carlin, specifically referring to head injuries, stated that most preventable deaths from head injury were due to "inappropriate management of patients who reached hospitals alive."[15] Bruser estimated that 25 of 119 automobile deaths in Canada were potentially preventable and suggested that patients be triaged to medical facilities that meet minimum care standards.[16] Various studies of trauma death revealed that approximately one-third of trauma deaths in nondesignated hospitals were preventable.[17]

The American College of Surgeons subsequently developed criteria for the establishment of trauma center categorization and trauma system regionalization.[18] The Joint Section of Trauma of the American Association of Neurological Surgeons and the Congress of Neurological Surgeons supported these criteria and endorsed the establishment of regional neurotrauma centers.[19] Studies have subsequently shown a marked reduction in the percentage of preventable deaths from trauma in regions that have implemented a systemized approach to trauma care.[20,21] Appropriate triage and the development of regional trauma centers with rapid application of surgical care have contributed to improved survival and outcome.

TRANSPORTATION

A crucial component of regionalized trauma system care is the rapid transportation of medical services to the scene of an accident and the subsequent stabilization of the patient. Such an approach to on-site care is called in-the-field treatment. Another important component of regionalized trauma care is transportation of the patient to an appropriate trauma center. The importance of reducing the time between injury and definitive medical care was introduced by Napoleon's surgeon, D. J. Larrey. Larrey was a surgeon in the Army of the Rhine in 1792, a time when regulations required that army ambulances be stationed more than 2 miles from the battlefront. The wounded were left on the battlefield until the battle was over, often more than 24 h. Larrey realized that lives were being lost during this time period and developed the *ambulance volente,* or flying ambulance, to bring aid to the wounded on the battlefield and rapidly retrieve them (Figure 7-1*A* and *B*).[22] The modern extension of Larrey's concept is the rapid-response trauma transportation unit, either ambulance or aircraft, with advanced medical treatment crews. Whether ground or air transportation is the better method depends on the regional geography and travel times.[23]

Helicopters were first used for medical purposes in the Korean war. In the civilian setting, they were initially applied to patient care in Europe in the 1960s. Similar utilization occurred in the United States in the 1970s. Helicopters allow rapid delivery of medical expertise to the site of injury and subsequent retrieval of the patient to the trauma center. Aeromedical transportation of a small subset of severely injured patients has been shown to decrease predicted mortality by 52 percent.[12] The utility of helicopters compared with ground transport is related to the ability of rotocraft transport to conserve time. The maximum efficient distance for helicopter transportation between a rural accident scene and a tertiary care trauma center has been estimated to be 112 to 160 km (70 to 96 miles).[23] Helicopter transport has also been effective in urban areas where traffic congestion can greatly increase ground transportation times.[24] For greater distances, fixed-wing aircraft may be utilized.

The importance of shortening the time to treatment has been demonstrated by Seelig et al.[25] in patients with severe closed head injury and acute subdural hematoma. Patients with a hematoma that was evacuated within 4 h had a 30 percent mortality rate and a 65 percent functional outcome rate, whereas patients who were operated on after more than 4 h after an injury had a 90 percent mortality rate and less than a 10 percent

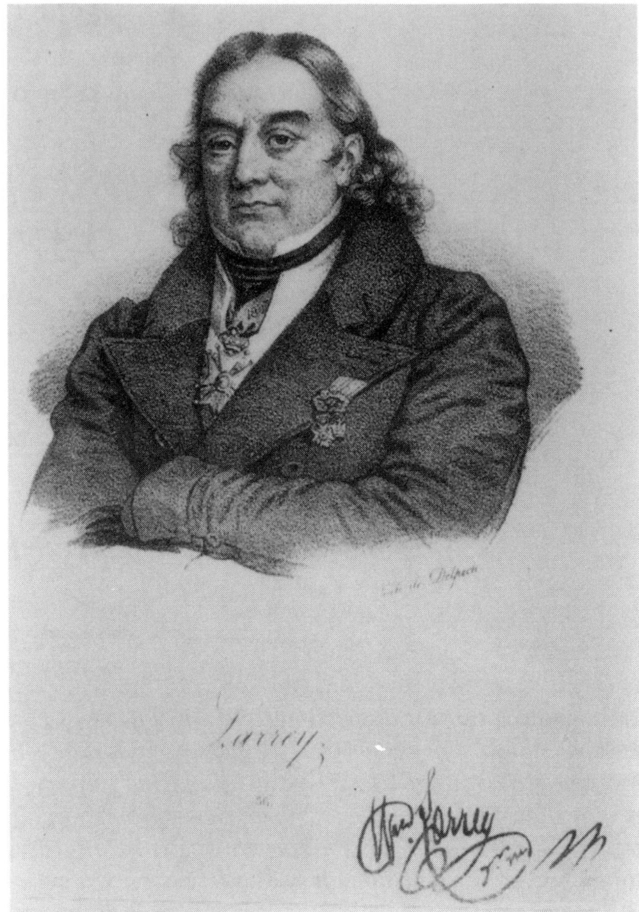

A

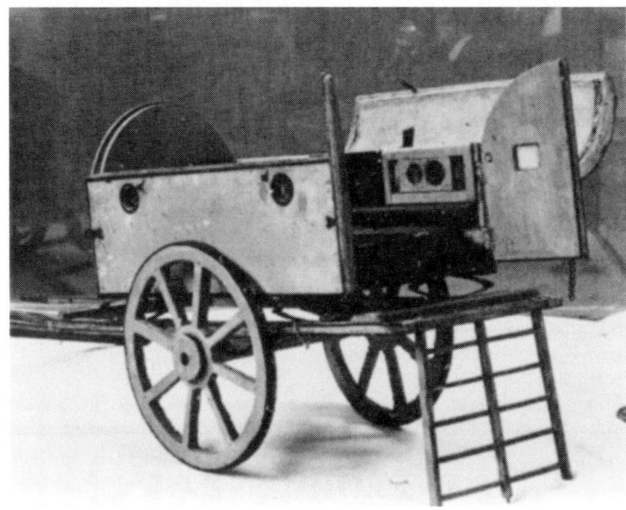

B

Figure 7-1. *A.* Napoleon's surgeon, D. J. Larrey. *B.* Larrey's *ambulance volente.* (Reproduced with permission from Dible.[22])

functional outcome rate.[25] Although further studies have not reproduced this degree of success, Wilberger et al. found a clear trend toward improved functional recovery in patients operated on within 4 h.[26] Considering that up to one-fourth of comatose head-injured patients admitted to hospitals have an acute subdural hematoma,[25] the benefits of rapid transportation are apparent.

PERSONNEL

Properly trained professionals, whether emergency medical technicians, paramedics, nurses, or physicians, are needed for the initial treatment of airway, respiratory, and circulatory problems as well as for the assessment of neurological function. Whether the level of training of the aeromedical personnel makes a difference in outcome is unclear, but some evidence suggests that it may. Schmidt et al.[27] compared prehospital care in Hanover, Germany, with that in Knoxville, Tennessee. They found an improved outcome in helicopter-transported multitrauma patients in Germany, which they attributed to more aggressive prehospital care provided by a trauma surgeon in the field. In a more recent study from the Royal London Hospital, Wilden et al.[24] suggested that an improved good recovery in head-injured patients (Traumatic Data Coma Bank Diffuse Injury II and Diffuse Injury III) may be related to the presence of a surgeon or anesthesiologist in the helicopter. Additionally, Sefrin reviewed prehospital care in Wurzberg, Germany, and estimated that 10 percent of accident victims who die could be saved if the "preclinical first aid system were exploited to the full by the appropriate emergency-medical qualifications of the doctors."[28]

PREVENTION OF SECONDARY INJURY

Aggressive treatment of head-injured patients reduces overall mortality and increases the number of patients who have a good recovery or moderate disability, while the number of severely disabled patients remains constant.[29] A major component of this care is the prevention of secondary insults to the brain after the primary brain injury. An acutely injured brain has been shown experimentally to be susceptible to secondary insults, including ischemia and hypoxia.[30] Hypoxia and hypercarbia induce vasodilation of intracerebral blood vessels, resulting in increased cerebral blood volume, increased intracranial pressure, and, potentially, cerebral herniation.[31,32] Cerebral autoregulation is impaired after a head injury,[33,34] resulting in cerebral hypoperfusion when systemic hypotension is present. Evidence of secondary brain injury has been found at autopsy in 66 to 92 percent of fatally head injured patients.[35–37] Prevention of these insults through proper airway management and maintenance, and the reestablishment of normal oxygenation and perfusion is critical in preventing worsening of the initial injury and death.

The importance of preventing hypoxia in head-injured patients was recognized in 1958 by MacIver et al., who stated that "anoxia is the main cause of death in patients who survive the accident but die at a later stage."[38] These authors went on to hypothesize that with proper management, "the onset of a secondary anoxic oedema can be prevented, and even severe intracerebral damage can be overcome; and damaged neurones, if receiving an adequate oxygen supply, can in many cases recover normal function." In support of this theory, they documented a lowering of mortality in severely head injured patients from 90 percent to 40 percent when proper attention was paid to respiratory insufficiency.[38]

Miller et al.[39] subsequently found that on initial presentation to a major trauma center, 30 percent of severely head injured patients were hypoxic (arterial P_{O_2} less than 65 mmHg), 13 percent were hypotensive (arterial pressure less than 95 mmHg systolic), and 12 percent were anemic (hematocrit below 30 percent). All but one of the hypotensive or anemic patients had multiple injuries, while 67 percent of the hypoxic patients had multiple injuries.[39] Early Traumatic Coma Data Bank (TCDB) analysis in 1983 found that 28 percent and 35 percent of severely head injured patients were hypoxic and hypotensive (systolic blood pressure <90 mmHg), respectively.[40] Subsequent analysis of TCDB data from the time of injury to the time of arrival at the emergency room revealed that hypoxia occurred in 46 percent of severely head injured patients and hypotension occurred in 35 percent.[41] More recently, Wald et al.[42] reported that 26 percent of severely head injured patients were hypotensive, hypoxic, or both on admission. Study of CT scans from head-injured patients in the TCDB revealed an association between hypoxia and diffuse cerebral swelling.[43]

The significance of secondary injury on the outcome of head-injured patients has been well documented.[15,39–42,44–50] Several studies, including Miller and Becker,[44] the TCDB 1983 analysis,[40] and Wald et al.,[42] have shown at least a doubling of mortality in the presence of hypoxia or hypotension. Rose et al.[45] found that

86 of 116 head-injured patients who talked before dying had an "avoidable factor" and that 55 of those patients had either airway obstruction or hypotension. In a prospective analysis of 200 consecutive head-injured patients, Bowers and Marshall[46] reported that only 4 of 17 patients with hypoxia or hypotension on arrival at the trauma center made a good recovery.

More recent studies have stressed the prognostic significance of hypotension. The 1993 TCDB review of 717 patients from four trauma centers revealed that only 33 percent of severely head injured patients with hypotension and 20 percent of patients with both hypoxia and hypotension had a good or moderate outcome, while 54 percent of patients with neither secondary insult had a good or moderate outcome. The presence of hypotension doubled the mortality in this cohort of patients. Hypoxia occurred more frequently than hypotension in the early posttraumatic period in these patients but increased overall mortality only minimally.[41]

Siegal et al.[47] reviewed 1709 patients admitted to a single institution with blunt head trauma and found that mortality was nearly double when brain injury was accompanied by systemic injury. The effect of visceral or lower extremity injury on mortality was found to result from hypovolemic hypoperfusion. Stratifying head injury by the Glasgow Coma Scale (GCS), the authors found that at each GCS level, mortality increased in relation to the amount of blood volume replacement required in the first 24 h after the injury. As blood replacement increased from 0 to ≥6 liters in the first 24 h after injury, mortality increased from 22 to 85 percent in severely head injured patients (GCS 4 to 6). In the moderately head injured GCS 9 to 12 group, mortality increased nearly 25 times as blood replacement increased from 0 to ≥6 liters/24 h.

In summary, hypoxia and hypotension adversely affect the outcome in head-injured patients. Prehospital management should be directed toward aggressively diagnosing and treating these abnormalities.

Airway Management

The first priority in prehospital resuscitation is the establishment and maintenance of a proper airway. The indications for airway management are altered consciousness, including agitation, combativeness, or obtundation; facial or neck trauma with potential or existent airway compromise; and the potential for neurological deterioration during transportation. The goals of airway management are to provide adequate ventilation and oxygen delivery with concomitant avoidance of hypoxia and hypercarbia and to protect the airway from aspiration. Airway compromise may be subtle but progressive and recurrent.[51] The causes of hypoxia and hypercarbia in head-injured patients are manifold. Drugs or alcohol, which can be detected in up to 83 percent of trauma patients,[52] can result in poor ventilatory effort. The head injury itself may result in significant apnea. Upper airway obstruction by the tongue, teeth, dentures, or vomitus is common. Mandibular fractures may result in hypopharyngeal tongue obstruction because of loss of masticatory muscle support, while other facial fractures may result in hemorrhage or secretions that obstruct the upper airway. Expanding neck lesions or direct laryngeal trauma may also affect the airway. In patients with multiple injuries, pulmonary contusion, flail chest, diaphragmatic injuries, pneumothorax, aspiration, and adult respiratory distress syndrome can all result in hypoxia and/or hypercarbia.[31] Neurogenic pulmonary edema occurs rarely.[53]

As taught in the Advanced Trauma Life Support (ATLS) course, initial airway management consists of (1) looking for agitation, cyanosis, or obtundation, which may indicate hypoxia, hypoxemia, or hypercarbia, respectively, (2) listening for upper airway gurgling sounds consistent with pharyngeal obstruction or hoarseness present with laryngeal obstruction, and (3) feeling for expiratory air movement and a midline trachea. Airway management techniques can then be applied to secure, protect, or provide an airway.[51] Initial airway maneuvers to clear and establish the upper airway include the chin lift and the jaw thrust. An oral or nasal airway can then be inserted to maintain the airway. It is essential during these maneuvers and during endotracheal intubation to avoid neck hyperextension, since as many as 1.8 to 15 percent of head-injured patients have a coexistent spine or spinal cord injury.[54–56] Whether the frequency of cervical spine injury in association with head injury is as high as was previously reported has been questioned. A recent review of 8285 blunt trauma victims at a single institution found that 7.3 percent of all head-injured patients who were intubated or had an admission GCS of 8 or less had a cervical spine fracture.[56] Cervical spine fracture should be assumed and the neck should be protected until such an injury is ruled out by roentgenographic and clinical examination.

If an oral airway is unable to achieve adequate oxygenation or if ventilation is precluded by one of the factors discussed above, endotracheal intubation should be performed expeditiously. The outcome of severely head injured patients is correlated significantly with their time to intubation.[57] In the emergent setting of an apneic or obstructed patient, orotracheal intubation with in-line manual cervical immobilization is the route of choice. In contrast to axial traction, which may distract or sublux an injured cervical spine,[58] in-line immobilization avoids movement of the cervical spine.[59] Oral intubation performed properly by experienced personnel has been demonstrated to be safe and effective, without significant risk of exacerbating a cervical cord injury.[60,61] Nasotracheal intubation is preferred in a spontaneously breathing patient, allowing the patient to continue breathing during intubation. However, it is a blind procedure that may require fiber-optic techniques and has variable success rates. Nasotracheal intubation is associated with a significant risk of hemorrhage or retropharyngeal perforation[62,63] and is less appropriate in the prehospital setting.

Tracheal intubation should be performed if possible despite facial injury (Fig. 7-2). If the trachea cannot be intubated, a needle or surgical cricothyrotomy can be performed. Surgical cricothyrotomy involves a skin incision extending through the cricothyroid membrane. Because of the time required for the procedure and the potential complications, including vocal cord paralysis, hemorrhage, incorrect endotracheal tube placement, and subglottic stenosis,[64] needle cricothyrotomy is preferred in the emergency prehospital setting. Because the risk of subglottic stenosis is particularly high in children, surgical cricothyrotomy is not recommended for children under age 12 years.[65] If oxygen at 15 liters/min (40 to 50 psi) is available in the transport vehicle, jet insufflation can be used to ventilate for 30 to 45 min but has the disadvantage of hypercarbia from inadequate exhalation in the head-injured setting. However, jet insufflation has the advantage of potentially expelling a glottic-level obstruction into the hypopharynx.[51]

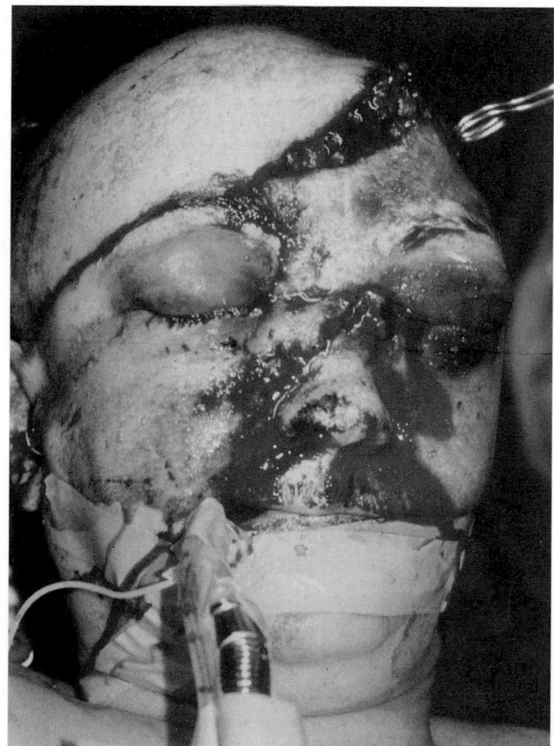

Figure 7-2. Despite the massive craniofacial injuries, including midface fractures, present in this patient, orotracheal intubation is the preferred method for airway control. (Photograph courtesy Joseph Gruss, M.D.)

It is imperative that a hypoxic or apneic patient be ventilated and oxygenated before intubation is attempted and between attempts at endotracheal or surgical intubation. Once an adequate airway is maintained, positive-pressure ventilation with 100% oxygen should be instituted. If intubation is not required, a tight-fitting face mask with 10 to 12 liters/min of high-flow oxygen can deliver an FI_{O_2} of .85. Pulse oxymetry is a valuable tool for monitoring oxygenation in the prehospital setting.[66]

Various pharmacological agents can be used to facilitate the intubation procedure. Vecuronium bromide (0.15 to 0.30 mg/kg IV), a nondepolarizing neuromuscular blocking agent, and succinylcholine (1.0 to 2.0 mg/kg IV), a depolarizing cholinergic motor endplate receptor binding agent, both provide chemical paralysis effectively. The use of succinylcholine and the stimulation of tracheal reflexes during intubation can result in rises in blood pressure, heart rate, and intracranial pressure with a potential concomitant risk for neurological deterioration.[67–69] Premedication with lidocaine (1.5 mg/kg IV) can help minimize reflex cardiovascular and intracranial pressure effects.[70,71] Etomidate (0.3 mg/kg IV), a short-acting hypnotic agent that has beneficial effects on intracranial pressure (ICP),[72] can be used in combination with lidocaine as an alternative to paralysis for intubation.[73] A neurological examination should be documented before intubation. Cricoid pressure should be applied during intubation to decrease the risk of aspiration.[74]

The importance of establishing a proper airway after head injury was prospectively documented in Singbartl's study of 147 neurotraumatized accident victims in Germany.[75] Singbartl found that 46.3 percent of patients who were not initially intubated developed aspiration and that 72.2 percent of the unintubated patients subsequently suffered from respiratory insufficiency. In contrast, 9.3 percent of intubated head-injured patients developed aspiration, while 35.5 percent of these patients had respiratory insufficiency.

Intravascular Volume Management

After the establishment of an appropriate airway in a head-injured patient, systemic perfusion must be optimized. Hypotension only rarely results from primary brain injury. If hypotension is present, it should be assumed to be the result of volume loss. After the placement of large-bore intravenous lines, fluid resuscitation should begin with isotonic normal saline or lactated Ringer's solution.[51] If a rapid response to bolus resuscitation with 1 to 2 liters of isotonic fluid (20 ml/kg in the pediatric population) is not achieved, group O Rh-negative blood can be used in the prehospital setting for further volume replacement. The restoration of systemic perfusion takes priority over concerns about the possible promotion or exacerbation of cerebral edema.[51] Many of the etiologies of significant blood loss in multitraumatized head-injured patients are occult[76] and thus cannot be rapidly diagnosed or treated in the field. However, bleeding from lacerations should be tamponaded and fractures should be splinted.

ATLS teaching recommends fluid resuscitation with isotonic fluids.[51] However, there is continuing debate over the potential benefits of hypertonic saline as an alternative resuscitant. Hypertonic saline (2400 mOsm/liter) infused at 5 ml/kg has been shown to increase systemic blood pressure and cardiac output,[77–80] presumably by osmotically redistributing fluid from the extravascular to the intravascular compartment.[81,82] An additional proposed mechanism of action of hypertonic solution is stimulation of a neurogenic reflex, resulting in peripheral vasodilation, venoconstriction, and increased myocardial contractility.[83,84] In comparison with isotonic fluids, hypertonic fluids have been shown in several experimental models to decrease ICP relatively during fluid resuscitation after head injury through dehydration of uninjured brain areas that have an intact blood-brain barrier.[85,86] In contrast, brain water content in injured areas of brain with a disrupted blood-brain barrier is increased to a similar degree with either hypertonic or isotonic fluid resuscitation.[87–90] Although case reports document improved ICP control in patients treated with hypertonic saline after a severe head injury,[91,92] a randomized clinical trial has not been performed.

Military antishock trousers (MASTs) are frequently used to provide external counterpressure for the treatment of traumatic hypovolemia caused by intraperitoneal, extraperitoneal, or pelvic hemorrhage. The concept of external counterpressure therapy was introduced by Crile[93] in 1903 and independently reapplied by Gardner and Dohn in 1956 in seated operative neurosurgical patients.[94] MASTs have subsequently become a standard component of prehospital care in many centers. They act by decreasing blood loss from intraabdominal, retroperitoneal, or pelvic sources while maintaining myocardial and cerebral perfusion.[95,96]

Both the favorable hemodynamic effects[97] and the clinical benefit of MAST[98,99] relative to mortality and cost have been questioned. In addition, significant complications associated with MAST treatment include the development of lactic acidosis, pulmonary complications, and lower extremity complications.[100] The effects of MAST on ICP in patients with severe head injury were investigated by Gardner et al.,[101] who found a small incremental increase in ICP during sequential MAST inflation that was compensated for by improved hemodynamic stability and elevated mean arterial blood pressure and cerebral perfusion pressure. All 12 patients in this study had an initial ICP below 20 mmHg. The effects of MAST on ICP in severely head injured patients with elevated ICP has not been studied.

The combination of hypertonic saline volume resuscitation and MAST external counterpressure has been studied in an experimental hemorrhagic shock model.[100] Hypertonic saline and MAST therapy resulted in improved hemodynamic parameters, including mean arterial pressure, cardiac index, and systemic vascular resistance, and prolonged the favorable effect of hypertonic saline on mean arterial pressure. The effects of this combined therapy on ICP management and outcome in experimental and clinical severe head injury deserve investigation.

Multitraumatized head-injured patients should be kept normovolemic in the prehospital setting to maximize systemic and cerebral perfusion. As was stated previously, volume resuscitation takes precedence over the potential effects of fluid resuscitation on ICP and cerebral edema.[51] Additionally, recent studies have questioned the belief that increased total fluid resuscitation alters ICP management or outcome. Schmoker et al.[102] retrospectively studied 40 adult trauma patients with severe head injuries and measured their total fluid balance from the time of injury to 72 h after the injury. They found no significant correlation between total fluid balance and either ICP or outcome. They concluded that "maintenance of normovolemia does not predispose the patient to uncontrolled ICP."[102] Similarly, in a rabbit cryogenic insult model, James and Schneider[103] found that an isotonic fluid load resulted in increased water content in the white matter in the region of the cryogenic injury but that ICP was not significantly elevated in comparison with controls. Whether the same results apply to a fluid challenge in the setting of a diffuse head injury was not addressed. Rosner and Daughton[104] documented an improved outcome in severely head injured patients who were treated with optimization of cerebral perfusion pressure in combination with control of increased ICP.

The deleterious effects of hyperglycemia on a head-injured patient should be considered during fluid resuscitation. Severe head injury results in a stress response with acute hypothalamic-adrenal activation. This in turn results in an increase in circulating catecholamines and elevated blood glucose levels. The levels of circulating catecholamines[105] and the degree of hyperglycemia[106,107] are both directly related to the severity of the head injury. Hyperglycemia has been shown to worsen the prognosis after cerebral ischemia from cardiac arrest or stroke.[108–110] Additionally, hyperglycemic severely head injured patients have a worse neurological outcome independent of the GCS score.[107]

The hypothesized mechanism by which hyperglycemia worsens outcome is that under ischemic conditions, when anaerobic metabolism is ongoing, increased glucose substrate results in increased production of lactate and hydrogen ions. Intracellular lactic acidosis triggers a cascade of events that results in secondary neuronal damage.[111,112] Whether controlling hyperglycemia in head-injured patients will improve the outcome has not been studied. However, in a dog cardiac arrest model, D'Alecy et al.[113] showed that infusion with 5% dextrose in lactated Ringer's solution resulted in significantly increased neurological deficits in comparison with control lactated Ringer's–infused animals. Until the effects of glucose control on the outcome of head injury are prospectively studied, minimization of supplemental glucose during fluid resuscitation in the prehospital phase is advisable.

NEUROLOGICAL ASSESSMENT AND TRIAGE

A rapid neurological assessment should be performed in the field to establish a neurological baseline that can be followed over time and allows the identification of lateralizing signs, including pupillary dilation and focal motor weakness. Although the ATLS course recommends a simple AVPU (alert, responds to verbal stimuli, responds to painful stimuli, unresponsive) neurological examination,[50] this system lacks the detail to allow serial monitoring of neurological function. The GCS developed by Jennett and Teasdale defines comatose patients as those who cannot open their eyes, speak words, or follow commands[114] (Table 7-1). The GCS is reliable and reproducible whether used in the field by paramedics, in the emergency room by physicians, or longitudinally by neurosurgeons.[114,115]

TABLE 7-1 Glasgow Coma Scale

Eye opening (E)	
Spontaneous	4
To voice	3
To pain	2
None	1
Motor response (M)	
Obeys commands	6
Localizes pain	5
Normal flexion (withdrew)	4
Abnormal flexion (decorticate)	3
Extension (decerebrate)	2
None (flaccid)	1
Verbal response (V)	
Oriented	5
Confused conversation	4
Inappropriate words	3
Incomprehensible sounds	2
None	1

GCS score = E + M + V. Best possible score = 15; worst possible score = 3.

The GCS allows stratification of patients into mild (GCS 13 to 15), moderate (GCS 9 to 12), and severe (GCS $\leq$ 8) head-injured groups. The initial GCS correlates well with the final outcome.[116] When combined with pupillary size and reactivity and with the mechanism of injury (vehicular versus nonvehicular), the GCS can be used to predict the likelihood of the need for intracranial surgery after a closed head injury.[117] It must be remembered that hypoxia, hypotension, other severe metabolic disturbances, and intoxication can all dramatically affect the neurological examination.

More detailed trauma scores have been designed to assist with in-the-field triage decisions and allow comparison of outcomes in patient groups while controlling for case mix severity. Trauma patient populations can be compared between institutions or in one institution over time. Early classification systems include the Injury Severity Score (ISS) and the Trauma Score (TS). The ISS scores body regions on the basis of severity of injury,[118] while the TS assesses circulatory, respiratory, and neurological function.[119] Both have been shown to correctly predict the probability of survival and to have high interrater reliability.[120] A third scale, the TRISS, combines the anatomic classification of the ISS, the physiological assessment of the TS, and the important prognostic factor of age in a logistic regression model.[119] Retrospective analysis of 262 multiply injured patients in Cologne, Germany, found the TRISS to be a more accurate predictor of survival than the GCS, TS, or ISS.[121]

The TS, ISS, and TRISS all potentially underestimate the severity of head-injured patients, a problem recognized by the Major Trauma Outcome Study of the American College of Surgeons. A Revised Trauma Score (RTS) was thus designed, appropriately weighing and incorporating the GCS, systolic blood pressure, and respiratory rate in logistic regression fashion. A triage form (T-RTS) of the RTS uses a 0 to 12 score that can easily be calculated in the prehospital setting. (Table 7-2). Patients with a T-RTS below 12 should be triaged to a trauma center. The RTS more accurately incorporates head injury and is more reliable than the TS.[122]

High-risk patients with a normal RTS score of 12 must also be identified in the prehospital setting. Included in this group are GCS 13 to 15 patients with a significant mechanism of injury who should be triaged to a trauma facility. The American College of Surgeons has proposed a three-stage triage decision algorithm that incorporates abnormal patient physiology, the mechanism of injury, and a combination of age, surroundings, and suspected total trauma.[123] When this algorithm is used, patients can be appropriately triaged and rapidly transported to a trauma center.

TABLE 7-2 Triage Revised Trauma Score

Glasgow Coma Scale (GCS)	Systolic Blood Pressure (SBP)	Respiratory Rate (RR)	Coded Value (C)
13–15	>89	10–29	4
9–12	76–89	>29	3
6–8	50–75	6–9	2
4–5	1–49	1–5	1
3	0	0	0

Triage RTS score = GCS + SBP + RR. Best possible score = 12; worst possible score = 0.

ICP MANAGEMENT

Intracranial hypertension has clearly been shown to be associated with a poor prognosis after a traumatic brain injury.[29,104,116,124–130] A recent analysis of TCDB records of 190 potential descriptors of outcome as defined by the Glasgow Outcome Score (GOS) found that in addition to age, admission motor score, and admission pupillary response, the factor most highly correlated with outcome was the proportion of ICP measurements greater than 20 mmHg. When logistic regression analysis was used, age, admission motor score, and admission pupillary response correctly explained 46 percent of observed patient outcomes. When the proportion of ICP measurements greater than 20 mmHg and the proportion of blood pressure measurements below 80 mmHg were factored in, 53 percent of observed outcomes were correctly explained. Unlike most other studies relating ICP management to prognosis, this report attempted to isolate the contribution of increased ICP to outcome from the contribution of other factors.[131]

If evidence of intracranial hypertension is present in the field, initial measures of treatment should be instituted. Pupillary asymmetry or lateralizing extremity weakness in the setting of an appropriate mechanism of injury indicates transtentorial herniation.[132] The presence of a focal intracranial mass lesion cannot be readily determined because localizing signs may be present in one-quarter of patients with diffuse axonal injury[133] or absent in up to one-half of patients with an epidural or subdural hematoma.[134–137] Initial strategies for the management of increased ICP in the prehospital setting include the establishment of an adequate airway with supplemental oxygenation and ventilation to prevent hypoxia or hypercarbia and the prevention or treatment of hypotension to optimize cerebral perfusion pressure. Both hypoxia and hypotension can stimulate intracranial vasodilation, with resultant increased ICP.[104] Further intracranial vasoconstriction and concomitant decreased ICP can be achieved by means of hyperventilation. Although hyperventilation, because of its transient beneficial effects,[138] is frequently reserved in the hospital setting for refractory increased ICP or increased ICP associated with hyperemia,[139] it is a useful way to lower ICP rapidly in the prehospital setting until further treatment measures are established. However, in the setting of hypotension or reduced cerebral blood flow early after severe head injury, hyperventilation can potentially exacerbate cerebral ischemia via vasoconstriction.[140]

Mannitol and furosemide (Lasix) can be used to further lower ICP. Hyperosmotic agents such as mannitol have been thought to act by osmotic withdrawal of water from cerebral tissue.[141,142] Although this mechanism probably explains some of the ICP-lowering properties of mannitol, after the administration of hyperosmolar solution the ICP falls significantly faster than the change in white matter water content.[142–144] Additionally, the blood-brain osmotic gradient has been shown not to correlate with ICP reduction or the duration of mannitol's effect.[145] Other, possibly more important mechanisms of the ICP-lowering effect of mannitol all act through cerebral vasoconstriction. These mechanisms include volume expansion with resultant increased systemic blood pressure and cerebral perfusion pressure,[146,147] hemodilution with concomitant decreased blood viscosity,[148,149] and increased deformity of red blood cells.[148] All these actions can increase oxygen delivery to the brain, resulting in cerebral vasoconstriction and lowering of ICP.[146,150] Mannitol should be administered as a 1 g/kg rapid 15- to 30-min infusion. Bolus infusion should be avoided, as it may result in a rapid, short-lived decrease in systemic blood pressure and an increase in ICP, possibly mediated by the release of atrial natriuretic peptide in response to acute volume expansion.[146,151]

Furosemide, a loop diuretic, can be used in synergy with mannitol to lower ICP. Osmotic diuresis induced by mannitol is enhanced by furosemide 0.5 to 1 mg/kg.[152,153] However, the ICP-lowering effects of furosemide may be lost in the setting of volume depletion or hemoconcentration.[153–155] As with mannitol, the hemodynamic and rheologic effects of furosemide may be important in lowering ICP in addition to the osmotic movement of water out of the brain and diuresis. Furosemide has also been shown to decrease CSF production.[156]

In the past, corticosteroids were used after a head injury as part of ICP management pharmacotherapy and in the hope of improving the outcome. Despite early studies suggesting decreased mortality in severely head injured patients who received large doses of corticosteroids,[157,158] there is now considerable evidence that corticosteroids do not improve ICP control or outcome.[159–163] A prospective multicenter randomized double-blind study of high-dose dexamethasone administered in the field is ongoing in Germany.[27] Lazaroids (21-aminosteroids) offer potentially beneficial effects in the treatment of head-injured patients without causing many of the adverse effects of glucocorticoids and are being investigated.

EFFICACY OF PREHOSPITAL CARE

The importance of prehospital care of head-injured patients is clear. The combination of rapid triage and transportation by appropriate medical personnel to a neurotrauma center, early recognition and prevention of secondary injury, and management of increased ICP all contribute to improved prehospital management. Klauber et al.[8] studied head injury mortality in San Diego County and found that mortality decreased from 21.3 in 100,000 in 1976 to 17.5 in 100,000 in 1982 with the institution of paramedical services and the initiation of a helicopter transportation service. Additionally, the number of individuals dead on arrival at hospitals declined by 68 percent between 1979 and 1981. The authors concluded that the improved mortality was due to the introduction of ground and air transportation services and rapid treatment of acute respiratory failure and hypotension.

Head injury mortality was compared in two centers with different emergency medical services—Charlottesville, Virginia, and New Delhi, India—over a 20-month period from 1977 to 1979.[7] Adjusting for differences in the distribution of motor scores, the mortality was found to be significantly higher in New Delhi. In particular, moderately injured patients (GCS motor score of 5) had 2½ times greater mortality in New Delhi. Most of the patients in New Delhi were transported to the hospital by nonmedical personnel and received no prehospital care. The majority of these patients arrived at the hospital over 2 h after injury. The authors felt that delays in transportation and lack of prehospital care might have contributed to the mortality difference between the two groups. Interestingly, the mortality for severely head injured patients (GCS motor score 1 to 4) was similar in the two centers.

In Germany, the cost-effectiveness of a rapid transportation system of prehospital care has been studied. A mathematic benefit of DM 5.30 (approximately $3) was calculated to result from each deutsche mask invested in the rescue service in north Bavaria.[164] A further review of prehospital care in Germany revealed that significantly more patients who received prehospital care survived craniocerebral trauma.[7]

FUTURE DIRECTIONS

Despite gains to date in the prehospital care of head injury, there is room for improvement. Remaining questions include the following:

1. What is the optimal fluid for initial resuscitation?
2. Will preventing hyperglycemia after head injury improve the outcome?
3. Should doctors be present in the field during the initial resuscitive phase?
4. Will further improvements in preventing secondary insults improve patient outcome?

Significant attention has been focused on the last of these questions. Jennett et al.[165] compared early characteristics and late outcome of head injury in Scotland, the Netherlands, and the United States. These authors found that despite significant differences in the organization of care and the details of management, mortality was the same. In comparison with the other two countries, patients in Scotland were referred secondarily to a neurosurgical unit, resulting in a significant delay between the time of injury and specialist care. On the basis of their findings, these authors speculated that "once a patient has sustained a certain degree of brain damage, the outcome depends largely upon the extent of this—whether it be damage due only from primary impact or includes that from secondary complications also."[165]

More recently, Wald et al.[42] compared the effects of hypoxia and hypotension after severe head injury in a rural area without a trauma system to the effects reported from TCDB data. Despite more than twice the average time from injury to arrival at the trauma center in the Vermont cohort, the TCDB group had a higher rate of secondary insults. Mortality was at least doubled in association with secondary insults in both groups. The authors suggested that because the outcomes of comparably grouped patients in a rural area and in the TCDB trauma centers were similar, rapid prehospital care may not be able to correct the deleterious effects of secondary insults. Data from their own laboratory support this conclusion in that cerebral ischemia remained after the restoration of systemic blood pressure in a hypotensive head injury model.[166] By contrast, Siegal et al.[47] demonstrated that mortality and the need for rehabilitation in survivors increased significantly in GCS-stratified groups of head-injured patients in relation to the amount of blood volume resuscitation that was required in the first 24 h after an injury. TCDB analysis revealed that hypotension is prognostically much more important than hypoxia in determining head injury outcome.[41]

On the basis of these studies, it is likely that more rapid prehospital correction of hypotension and, to a lesser degree, hypoxia can improve the outcome from traumatic head injury. However, a subset of patients probably exists whose secondary injury cascade is too far advanced to be reversed by correction of hypoxia or hypotension. In these patients, new clinical agents are required that can block or reverse cell injury. A myriad of potential agents are being investigated and will be discussed elsewhere in this book. Two compounds have already been tested on the clinical level: tromethamine (THAM) and polyethyleneglycol–conjugated superoxide dismutase (PEG-SOD).

Tromethamine, which reduces brain edema and cerebral acidosis and ICP through unclear mechanisms, has been shown in randomized prospective fashion to be beneficial in controlling ICP in patients with persistent elevation.[167] Outcome was not improved, but the drug dosage and timing of administration might have been suboptimal. PEG-SOD, a superoxide oxygen radical scavenger, has been tested in a phase II clinical trial in severely head injured patients.[168] Oxygen radicals have been implicated in head injury by several mechanisms, including direct neuronal injury, cerebral ischemia-reperfusion injury, and vasoconstriction. At 6 months of follow-up, 21 percent of patients receiving 10,000 U/kg PEG-SOD were vegetative or had died, while 36 percent of control patients were in those outcome categories.[168] The potentially beneficial effects of earlier dosing and higher doses of PEG-SOD are being studied.

Many more compounds are being investigated and developed, including growth factors, calcium channel blockers, antioxidants, excitatory neurotransmitter receptor antagonists, vasoactive agents, cytoprotective agents, opiate antagonists, and ICP-lowering agents. As these agents are demonstrated to have a clinically beneficial effect, they can be integrated into the prehospital care of patients with a head injury. As methylprednisolone can now be given in the field after spinal cord injury, cocktails of agents could potentially be given in the future to ameliorate the secondary effects of closed head injury.

Further standardization of prehospital criteria is important in comparing future studies. Although head-injured patients with significant extracranial trauma have higher morbidity and mortality, their worse outcome results from the severity of the head injury and the hypotension and hypoxia associated with extracranial trauma.[7,42,47] Future studies need to incorporate prehospital neurological status, injury severity, mechanism of injury, and measures of systemic perfusion and oxygenation to allow appropriate comparisons.

References

1. National Center for Health Statistics: Births, marriages, divorces, and deaths for 1990. *Monthly Vital Statistics Report,* vol 39, no 12. Hyattsville, MD: Public Health Services, 1991.
2. *Accident Facts.* Chicago: National Research Council, 1984.
3. Annegers JF, Grabow JD, Kurland LT, et al: The incidence, causes, and secular trends in head injury in Olmstead County, Minnesota, 1935–1974. *Neurology* 30:912–919, 1980.
4. Kraus JF, Black MA, Hessol N, et al: The incidence of acute brain injury and serious impairment in a defined population. *Am J Epidemiol* 119:186–201, 1984.
5. Sosin DM, Sacks JJ, Smith SM: Head injury-associated deaths in the United States from 1979 to 1986. *JAMA* 262:2251–2255, 1989.
6. Gennarelli TA, Champion HR, Sacco WJ, et al: Mortality of patients with head injury and extracranial injury treated in trauma centers. *J Trauma* 29:1193–1202, 1989.
7. Colohan ART, Alves WM, Gross CR, et al: Head injury mortality in two centers with different emergency medical services and intensive care. *J Neurosurg* 71:202–207, 1989.
8. Klauber MR, Marshall LF, Toole BM, et al: Cause of decline in head injury mortality rate in San Diego County, California. *J Neurosurg* 62:528–531, 1985.
9. West JG, Williams MJ, Trunkey DD, et al: Trauma systems: Current status—future challenges. *JAMA* 259:3597–3600, 1988.
10. Hampton OP Jr: The Committee on Trauma of the American College of Surgeons. *Bull Am Coll Surg* 57:7–13, 1972.
11. National Committee of Trauma and Committee of Shock: *Accidental Death and Disability: The Neglected Disease of Modern Society.* Washington, DC: National Academy of Sciences/National Research Council, 1966.
12. Baxt WG, Moody P: The impact of a rotocraft aeromedical emergency care service on trauma mortality. *JAMA* 249:3047–3051, 1983.
13. Committee on Trauma Research: *Injury in America.* Washington, DC: National Research Council, National Academy Press, 1985.
14. Van Wagoner FH: Died in hospital: A three-year study of deaths following trauma. *J Trauma* 1:401–408, 1961.

15. Jennett B, Carlin J: Preventable mortality and morbidity after head injury. *Injury* 10:31–39, 1978.
16. Bruser DM: Emergency care of auto crash victims, in Keeney AH (ed): *Proceedings of the 11th Annual Meeting of the American Association for Automotive Medicine.* Springfield, IL: Charles C Thomas, 1970: 232–239.
17. Cales RH, Trunkey DD: Preventable trauma deaths: A review of trauma care systems development. *JAMA* 254:1059–1063, 1985.
18. Committee on Trauma: Hospital and prehospital resources for the care of the injured patient. *Bull Am Coll Surg* 71:4–12, 1986.
19. Pitts LH, Ojemann RG, Quest DO: Neurotrauma care and the neurosurgeon: A statement from the Joint Section of Trauma of the AANS and CNS. *J Neurosurg* 67:783–785, 1987.
20. West JG, Cales RH, Grazzaniga AB: Impact of regionalization: The Orange County experience. *Arch Surg* 118:740–744, 1983.
21. Shackford SR, Hollingworth-Fridlund P, Cooper GF, et al: The effect of regionalization upon the quality of trauma care as assessed by concurrent audit before and after institution of a trauma system. *J Trauma* 26:812–820, 1986.
22. Dible JH: *Napoleon's Surgeon.* London: William Heinemann, 1970.
23. Champion HR: Helicopters in emergency trauma care. *JAMA* 249:3074–3075, 1983.
24. Wilden HN, Sutcliffe JC, McAvinchey R, et al: The effect of early management of head injuries on outcome. Congress of Neurological Surgeons 43rd Annual Meeting: 67, 1993.
25. Seelig JM, Becker DP, Miller JD, et al: Traumatic acute subdural hematoma: Major mortality reduction in comatose patients treated within four hours. *N Engl J Med* 304:1511–1518, 1981.
26. Wilberger JE, Harris M, Diamond D: Acute subdural hematoma: Morbidity and mortality related to timing of operative intervention. *J Trauma* 30:733–736, 1990.
27. Schmidt U, Herlich M, Frame SB, et al: On-scene helicopter transport of the multitrauma patient—comparison of a German and an American system. *J Trauma* 31:1038, 1991.
28. Sefrin P: Current level of prehospital care in severe head injury—potential for improvement. *Acta Neurochir* (*Wien*) S57:141–144, 1993.
29. Miller JD, Butterworth JF, Gudeman SK, et al: Further experience in the management of severe head injury. *J Neurosurg* 54:289–299, 1981.
30. Jenkins LW, Moszynski K, Lyeth BF, et al: Increased vulnerability of the mildly traumatized rat brain to cerebral ischemia: The use of controlled secondary ischemia as a research tool to identify common or different mechanisms contributing to mechanical and ischemic brain injury. *Brain Res* 477:211–224, 1989.
31. Lassen HA: Control of cerebral circulation in health and disease. *Circ Res* 34:749–760, 1967.
32. Klatzo I: Presidential address: Neuropathological aspects of brain edema. *J Neuropathol Exp Neurol* 26:1–14, 1967.
33. Bruce DA, Langfit TA, Miller JD, et al: Regional cerebral blood flow, intracranial pressure, and brain metabolism in comatose patients. *J Neurosurg* 38:131–144, 1973.
34. Enevoldson E: CBF in head injury. *Acta Neurochir* (*Wien*) S36:133–136, 1986.
35. Shackford SR, MacKersie RC, Davis JW, et al: Epidemiology and pathology of traumatic deaths occurring at a level I trauma center in a regionalized system: The importance of secondary brain injury. *J Trauma* 29:1392–1397, 1989.
36. Graham DI, Ford I, Adams JH, et al: Ischemic brain damage is still common in fatal non-missile head injury. *J Neurol Neurosurg Psychiatry* 52:346–350, 1989.
37. Graham DI, Adams JH, Doyle D, et al: Quantification of primary and secondary lesions in severe head injury. *Acta Neurochir* (*Wien*) S57:41–48, 1993.
38. MacIver IN, Frew IJC, Matheson JG: The role of respiratory insufficiency in the mortality of severe head injuries. *Lancet* 1:390–393, 1958.
39. Miller JD, Sweet RC, Narayan RK, et al: Early insult to the injured brain. *JAMA* 240:439–442, 1978.
40. Marshall LF, Becker DP, Bowers SA, et al: The National Traumatic Coma Data Bank: 1: Design, purpose, goals, and results. *J Neurosurg* 59:276–284, 1983.
41. Chesnut RM, Marshall LF, Klauber MR, et al: The role of secondary brain injury in determining outcome from severe head injury. *J Trauma* 34:216–222, 1993.
42. Wald SL, Shackford SR, Fenwick J: The effect of secondary insults on mortality and long-term disability after severe head injury in a rural region without a trauma system. *J Trauma* 34:377–381, 1993.
43. Eisenberg HM, Gary HE, Aldrich EF: Initial CT findings in 753 patients with severe head injury: A report from the NIH Traumatic Coma Data Bank. *J Neurosurg* 73:688–698, 1990.
44. Miller JD, Becker DP: Secondary insults to the injured brain. *J R Coll Surg Edinb* 27:292–298, 1982.
45. Rose J, Valtonen S, Jennett B: Avoidable factors contributing to death after head injury. *Br Med J* 21:615–618, 1977.
46. Bowers SA, Marshall LF: Outcome in 200 consecutive cases of severe head injury in San Diego County: A prospective analysis. *Neurosurgery* 6:237–242, 1980.
47. Siegal JH, Gens DR, Marmentov T, et al: Effect of associated injuries and blood volume replacement on death, rehabilitation needs, and disability in blunt traumatic brain injury. *Crit Care Med* 19:1252–1265, 1991.
48. Price DJE, Murray A: Influence of hypoxia and hypotension on recovery from head injury. *Injury* 3:218–224, 1972.
49. Klauber MR, Marshall LF, Luerssen TG, et al: Determinants of head injury mortality: Importance of the low risk patient. *Neurosurgery* 24:31–36, 1989.
50. Newfield P, Pitts L, Kaktis J, et al: The influence of shock on mortality after head trauma. *Crit Care Med* 8:254, 1980.
51. Advanced Trauma Life Support Course. Chicago: American College of Surgeons, 1989.
52. Sloan EP, Zalenski RJ, Smith RF, et al: Toxicology

screening in urban trauma patients: Drug prevalence and its relationship to trauma severity and management. *J Trauma* 29:1647–1653, 1989.
53. Frost EAM: The physiology of respiration in neurosurgical patients. *J Neurosurg* 50:699–714, 1979.
54. O'Malley KJ, Ross SE: The incidence of injury to the cervical spine in patients with craniocerebral injury. *J Trauma* 28:1476–1478, 1988.
55. Gbaanader G, Fruin A, Taylon C: Role of emergency cervical radiography in head trauma. *Am J Surg* 152:643–647, 1986.
56. Hills MW, Deane SA: Head injury and facial injury: Is there an increased risk of cervical spine injury? *J Trauma* 34:549–554, 1993.
57. Gildenberg PL, Makela M: The effect of early intubation and ventilation on outcome following head trauma, in Dacey RG, Winn HR, et al (eds): *Trauma of the Central Nervous System.* New York: Raven Press, 1985:79–90.
58. Bivins HG, Ford S, Bezmalinovic Z, et al: The effect of axial traction during orotracheal intubation of the trauma victim with an unstable cervical spine. *Ann Emerg Med* 17:53–57, 1988.
59. Majernick TG, Bienick R, Houston JB, et al: Cervical spine movement during orotracheal intubation. *Ann Emerg Med* 15:417–420, 1986.
60. Rhee KJ, Green W, Holcroft JW, et al: Oral intubation in the multiply injured patient: The risk of exacerbating spinal cord damage. *Ann Emerg Med* 19:45–48, 1990.
61. Talucci RC, Shaikh KA, Schwab CW: Rapid sequence induction with oral endotracheal intubation in the multiply injured patient. *Am Surg* 54:185–187, 1988.
62. Danzyl D, Thomas DM: Nasotracheal intubation in the emergency department. *Crit Care Med* 8:677–682, 1980.
63. Tintinelli JE, Claffey J: Complications of nasotracheal intubation. *Ann Emerg Med* 10:142–144, 1981.
64. McGill J, Clinton JE, Ruiz E: Cricothyrotomy in the emergency department. *Ann Emerg Med* 11:361–364, 1982.
65. Esses BA, Jafek BW: Cricothyroidotomy: A decade of experience in Denver. *Ann Otol Rhinol Laryngol* 96:519–524, 1987.
66. Silverston P: Pulse oxymetry at the roadside: A study of pulse oxymetry in immediate care. *Br Med J* 298:711–713, 1989.
67. Forbes AM, Dally FG: Acute hypertension during induction of anesthesia and endotracheal intubation in normotensive man. *Br J Anaesth* 42:618–624, 1970.
68. Fox EJ, Sklar GS, Hill CH, et al: Complications related to the pressor response to endotracheal intubation. *Anesthesiology* 47:524–525, 1977.
69. Halldin M, Wahlin A: Effects of succinylcholine on the intraspinal fluid pressure. *Acta Anesthesiol Scand* 3:155–161, 1959.
70. Donegan MF, Bedford RF: Intravenously administered lidocaine prevents intracranial hypertension during endotracheal suctioning. *Anesthesiology* 52:516–518, 1980.
71. Steinhaus JE, Gaskin L: A study of intravenous lidocaine as a suppressant of cough reflex. *Anesthesiology* 24:285–290, 1963.
72. Artru AA: Intracranial volume-pressure relationship following thiopental or etomidate. *Anesthesiology* 71:763–768, 1989.
73. Delaney KA, Goldfrank LR: Initial management of the multiply injured or intoxicated patient, in Cooper RR (ed): *Head Injury* (3d ed). Baltimore: Williams & Wilkins, 1993:46.
74. Sellick BA: Cricoid pressure to control regurgitation of stomach during induction of anesthesia. *Lancet* 2:404, 1961.
75. Singbartl G: Die Bedeutung der präklinischen Notfallversorgung für die Prognose von Patienten mit schwerem Schädel-Hirn-Trauma. *Anaesth Intensivther Notfallmed* 20:251–260, 1985.
76. Narayan RK: Emergency room management of the head-injured patient, in Becker DP, Gudeman SK (eds): *Textbook of Head Injury.* Philadelphia: Saunders, 1989:30.
77. Valesco IT, Pontieri Y, Rocha-e-Silva M, et al: Hypertonic NaCl and severe hemorrhagic shock. *Am J Physiol* 239:H664–H673, 1980.
78. Nakayama S, Sibley L, Gunther RA, et al: Small volume resuscitation with hypertonic saline (2400 mOsm/liter) during hemorrhagic shock. *Circ Shock* 13:149–159, 1984.
79. Rocha-e-Silva M, Negraes GA, Soares AM, et al: Hypertonic resuscitation from severe hemorrhagic shock: Patterns of regional circulation. *Circ Shock* 19:165–175, 1986.
80. Meningas PA, Mattox KL, Pepe PE, et al: Hypertonic saline-dextran solutions for the prehospital management of traumatic hypotension. *Am J Surg* 157:528–534, 1989.
81. Nakayama S, Kramer GC, Carlsen RC, et al: Infusion of very hypertonic saline to bled rats: Membrane potentials and fluid shifts. *J Surg Res* 38:180–186, 1985.
82. Auler JOC, Pereira MCH, Gioniele-Amaral RF, et al: Hemodynamic effects of hypertonic NaCl during surgical treatment of aortic aneurysms. *Surgery* 101:594–601, 1987.
83. Wildenthal K, Mierzwiak DS, Mitchell, JH: Acute effects of increased serum osmolality on left ventricular performance. *Am J Physiol* 216:898–904, 1969.
84. Wolf MB: Plasma volume dynamics after hypertonic fluid infusion in nephrectomized dogs. *Ma J Physiol* 221:1392–1395, 1971.
85. Gunnar W, Jonasson O, Merlotti G, et al: Head injury and hemorrhagic shock: Studies of the blood, brain, and intracranial pressure after resuscitation with normal saline solution, 3% saline solution, and dextran-40. *Surgery* 103:398–407, 1988.
86. Ducey JP, Mosirgo DW, Lamiell JM, et al: A comparison of the cerebral and cardiovascular effects of complete resuscitation with isotonic and hypertonic saline, hetastarch, and whole blood following hemorrhage. *J Trauma* 29:1510–1518, 1989.
87. Zornow MH, Scheller MS, Shackford SR: Effect of a hypertonic lactated Ringer's solution of intracranial pressure and cerebral water content in a model of traumatic brain injury. *J Trauma* 29:484–488, 1989.

88. Wisner DH, Schuster L, Gunn C: Hypertonic saline resuscitation of head injury: Effects on cerebral water content. *J Trauma* 30:75–78, 1990.
89. Battistella FD, Wisner DH: Combined hemorrhagic shock and head injury: Effects of hypertonic saline (7.5%) resuscitation. *J Trauma* 31:182–188, 1991.
90. Fulton RL, Flynn WJ, Mancino M, et al: Brain injury causes loss of cardiovascular response to hemorrhagic shock. *J Invest Surg* 6:117–131, 1993.
91. Worthey LG, Cooper DJ, Jones N: Treatment of resistant intracranial hypertension with hypertonic saline. *J Neurosurg* 68:478–481, 1988.
92. Holcroft JW, Vassar MJ, Turner JE, et al: Three percent NaCl and 7.5% NaCl-dextran in the resuscitation of severely head injured patients. *Ann Surg* 206:279–288, 1987.
93. Crile GW: *Blood Pressure in Surgery.* Philadelphia: Lippincott, 1903:289–291.
94. Gardner JW, Dohn DF: The antigravity suit (G suit) in surgery. *JAMA* 126:274–276, 1956.
95. Caplan BC, Civeta JM, Nagel EL: The military antishock trousers in civilian prehospital emergency care. *J Trauma* 13:843–848, 1973.
96. Pelligra R, Sandberg EC: Control of intractable abdominal bleeding by external counterpressure. *JAMA* 241:708–713, 1979.
97. McSwain NE: Pneumatic anti-shock garment: State of the art 1988. *Ann Emerg Med* 17:506–525, 1988.
98. MacKensie RC, Christensen JM, Lewis FR: The prehospital use of external counterpressure: Does MAST make a difference? *J Trauma* 24:882–888, 1984.
99. Pepe PE, Bass RR, Mattox KL: Clinical trials of the pneumatic antishock garment in the urban prehospital setting. *Ann Emerg Med* 15:1407–1410, 1986.
100. Landau EH, Gross D, Assalia A, et al: Hypertonic saline infusion in hemorrhagic shock treated by military antishock trousers (MAST) in awake sheep. *Crit Care Med* 21:1554–1562, 1993.
101. Gardner SR, Maull KI, Swensson EE, et al: The effects of the pneumatic antishock garment on intracranial pressure in man: A prospective study of 12 patients with severe head injury. *J Trauma* 24:896–900, 1984.
102. Schmoker JD, Shackford SR, Wald SL, et al: An analysis of the relationship between fluid and sodium administration and intracranial pressure after head injury. *J Trauma* 33:476–481, 1992.
103. James HE, Schneider S: Effects of acute isotonic saline administration on serum osmolality, serum electrolytes, brain water content, and intracranial pressure. *Acta Neurochir* (*Wien*) S57:89–93, 1993.
104. Rosner MJ, Daughton S: Cerebral perfusion pressure management in head injury. *J Trauma* 30:933–941, 1990.
105. Clifton GL, Zieglar MG, Grossman RG: Circulatory catecholamines and sympathetic activity after head injury. *Neurosurgery* 8:10–13, 1981.
106. Young B, Oh L, Dempsey R, et al: Relationship between admission hyperglycemia and neurologic outcome of severely brain-injured patients. *Ann Surg* 210:466–473, 1989.
107. Lam AM, Winn HR, Cullen BF, et al: Hyperglycemia and neurologic outcome in patients with head injury. *J Neurosurg* 75:545–551, 1991.
108. Combs DJ, Revland DS, Martin DB, et al: Glycolytic inhibition by 2-deoxyglucose reduces hyperglycemia-associated mortality and morbidity in the ischemic rat. *Stroke* 17:989–994, 1986.
109. Siesjo BK: Cell damage in the brain: A speculative synthesis. *J Cereb Blood Flow Metab* 1:155–185, 1981.
110. Longstreth WT, Inui TS: High blood glucose level on hospital admission and poor neurological recovery after cardiac arrest. *Ann Neurol* 15:59–63, 1984.
111. Hoffman WE, Braucher E, Palligrino DA, et al: Brain lactate and neurologic outcome following incomplete ischemia in fasted, nonfasted, and glucose loaded rats. *Anesthesiology* 72:1045–1050, 1990.
112. Pulsinelli WA, Waldman S, Rawlinson D, et al: Moderate hyperglycemia augments ischemic brain damage: A neuropathologic study in the rat. *Neurology* 11:1239–1246, 1982.
113. D'Alecy LG, Lindy EF, Barton KJ, et al: Dextrose containing intravenous fluid impairs outcome and increases death after eight minutes of cardiac arrest and resuscitation in dogs. *Surgery* 100:505–511, 1986.
114. Teasdale G, Jennett B: Assessment of coma and impaired consciousness. *Lancet* 2:81–84, 1974.
115. Menegazzi JJ, Davis EA, Sucov AH, et al: Reliability of the Glasgow Coma Scale when used by emergency physicians and paramedics. *J Trauma* 34:46–48, 1993.
116. Narayan RK, Greenberg RP, Miller DJ, et al: Improved confidence of outcome prediction in severe head injury: A comparative analysis of the clinical examination, multimodality evoked potentials, CT scanning, and intracranial pressure. *J Neurosurg* 54:751–762, 1981.
117. Gennarelli TA: Initial assessment and management of head injury, in Pitts LH, Wagner FC (eds): *Craniospinal Trauma.* New York: Thieme, 1990:20.
118. Baker ST, O'Neill B, Hadeon W, et al: The Injury Severity Score: A method for describing patients with multiple injuries and evaluation emergency care. *J Trauma* 14:187–196, 1974.
119. Champion HR, Sacco WJ, Carnazzo AJ, et al: The Trauma Score. *Crit Care Med* 9:672–676, 1981.
120. Champion HR, Sacco WJ: *Trauma Risk Assessment: Review of Severity Scales.* New York: Appleton-Centry-Crofts, 1983.
121. Bouillon B, Schweins M, Lechleuthrer A, et al: Assessment of emergency care in trauma patients. *Acta Neurochir* (*Wien*) 557:137–140, 1993.
122. Champion HR, Sacco WJ, Copes WS, et al: A revision of the Trauma Score. *J Trauma* 29:623–629, 1989.
123. American College of Surgeons Committee on Trauma: Appendix F to hospital resources documents: Field categorization of trauma patients (field triage), in *Hospital and Prehospital Resources for Optimal Care of the Injured Patient and Appendices A through J.* Chicago:1987.
124. Becker DP, Miller JD, Ward JD, et al: The outcome from severe head injury with early diagnosis and intensive management. *J Neurosurg* 47:491–502, 1977.
125. Eisenberg HM, Cayard C, Papanicolaou, et al: The ef-

fects of three potentially preventable complications on outcome after severe closed head injury, in Ishii S, Nagai H, Brock M (eds): *Intracranial Pressure V.* Berlin: Springer-Verlag, 1983:549–553.

126. Marshall LF, Smith RW, Shapiro HM: The outcome with aggressive treatment in severe head injuries: I. The significance of intracranial pressure monitoring. *J Neurosurg* 50:20–25, 1979.
127. Miller JD, Becker DP, Ward JD, et al: Significance of intracranial hypertension in severe head injury. *J Neurosurg* 47:503–516, 1977.
128. Nordby HK, Gunnerod N: Epidural monitoring of the intracranial pressure in severe head injury characterized by non-localizing motor response. *Acta Neurochir (Wien)* 74:21–26, 1985.
129. Saul TG, Ducker TB: Effect of intracranial pressure monitoring and aggressive treatment on mortality in severe head injury. *J Neurosurg* 56:498–503, 1982.
130. Pitts LH, Kaktis JV, Juster R, et al: ICP and outcome in patients with severe head injury, in Shulman K, Marmarou A, Miller JE, et al (eds): *Intracranial Pressure IV.* Berlin: Springer-Verlag, 1980:5–9.
131. Marmarou A, Anderson RL, Ward JD, et al: Impact of ICP instability and hypotension on outcome in patients with severe head trauma. *J Neurosurg* 75:559–566, 1991.
132. Meyer A: Herniation of the brain. *Arch Neurol Psychiat* 4:387–400, 1920.
133. Wilberger JE, Rothfus WF, Tabis J: Acute tissue tear hemorrhages of the brain: Computerized tomographic and clinicopathological correlations. *Neurosurgery* 27:561–569, 1990.
134. Kluge D: Cranial trephination for diagnosis and therapy of closed injuries to the head. *Am J Surg* 99:707–712, 1960.
135. Rand BO, Ward AA, White LE: The use of twist drill to evaluate head trauma. *J Neurosurg* 25:410–415, 1966.
136. Andrews BT, Pitts LH, Lovely MP, et al: Is computed tomographic scanning necessary in patients with transtentorial herniation? Results of immediate surgical exploration without computed tomography in 100 patients. *Neurosurgery* 19:408–414, 1986.
137. Mahoney BD, Rockswold GL, Ruiz E, et al: Emergency twist drill trephination. *Neurosurgery* 8:551–554, 1981.
138. van der Poel H: Cerebral vasoconstriction is not maintained with prolonged hyperventilation, in Hoff JT, Betz AL (eds): *Intracranial Pressure VII.* Berlin: Springer-Verlag, 1989:899–903.
139. Miner ME, in comments to Chan K-H, Dearden NM, Miller JD, et al: Multimodality monitoring as a guide to treatment of intracranial hypertension after severe brain injury. *Neurosurgery* 32:552, 1993.
140. Bouma GJ, Muizelaar JP, Choi SC, et al: Cerebral circulation and metabolism after severe traumatic brain injury: The elusive role of ischemia. *J Neurosurg* 75:685–693, 1991.
141. Hartwell RC, Sutton LN: Mannitol, intracranial pressure, and vasogenic edema. *Neurosurgery* 32:444–450, 1993.
142. Clasen RA, Cooke PN, Pandolf S, et al: Hypertonic urea in experimental cerebral edema. *Arch Neurol* 12:424–434, 1965.
143. Reed DJ, Woodbury DM: Effect of hypertonic urea on cerebrospinal fluid pressure and brain volume. *J Physiol (Lond)* 164:252–264, 1962.
144. Harbough RD, James HE, Marshall LF, et al: Acute therapeutic modalities for experimental vasogenic edema. *Neurosurgery* 5:656–665, 1979.
145. Pollay M, Fullenwider CH, Roberts PA, et al: The effect of mannitol and furosemide on the blood-brain barrier osmotic gradient and intracranial pressure. *J Neurosurg* 59:945–950, 1983.
146. Rosner MJ, Coley I: Cerebral perfusion pressure: A hemodynamic mechanism of mannitol and the postmannitol hemogram. *Neurosurgery* 21:147–156, 1987.
147. Wise BL, Chater ML: The value of hypertonic mannitol solution in decreasing brain mass and lowering cerebrospinal-fluid pressure. *J Neurosurg* 19:1038–1043, 1962.
148. Burke AM, Quest DO, Chien S, et al: The effects of mannitol on blood viscosity. *J Neurosurg* 55:550–553, 1981.
149. Muizelaar JP, Wei EP, Kontos HA, et al: Mannitol causes compensatory cerebral vasoconstriction and vasodilation in response to blood viscosity changes. *J Neurosurg* 59:822–828, 1983.
150. Kontos HA: Regulation of the cerebral circulation. *Annu Rev Physiol* 43:397–407, 1981.
151. Rosner MJ, in comments to Hartwell RC, Sutton LN: Mannitol, intracranial pressure and vasogenic edema. *Neurosurgery* 32:450, 1993.
152. Schettini A, Stahurski B, Young HF: Osmotic and osmotic-loop diuresis in brain surgery. *J Neurosurg* 56:679–684, 1982.
153. Wilkinson HA, Rosenfield S: Furosemide and mannitol in the treatment of acute experimental intracranial hypertension. *Neurosurgery* 12:405–410, 1983.
154. Gaab M, Knoblich OE, Schupp J, et al: Effect of furosemide (lasix) on acute severe experimental cerebral edema. *J Neurol* 220:185–197, 1979.
155. Tornheim PA, McLaurin RL, Sawaya R: Effect of furosemide on experimental traumatic cerebral edema. *Neurosurgery* 4:48–52, 1979.
156. Sahar A, Tsipstein E: Effects of mannitol and furosemide on the rate of formation of cerebrospinal fluid. *Exp Neurol* 60:584–591, 1978.
157. Faupel G, Ruelen HJ, Muller D, et al: Double blind studying of the effects of steroids on severe closed head injury, in Pappius HM, Feindel W (eds): *Dynamics of Brain Edema.* Berlin: Springer-Verlag, 1976:337–343.
158. Gobiet W, Bock WJ, Liesegang J, et al: Treatment of acute cerebral edema with high dose dexamethasone, in Beks JWF, Bosch DA, Brock M (eds): *Intracranial Pressure III.* Berlin: Springer-Verlag, 1976:232–235.
159. Braakman R, Schouten HJA, Dishoeck MB, et al: Megadose steroids in severe head injury: Results of a prospective double-blind clinical trial. *J Neurosurg* 58:326–330, 1983.
160. Cooper P, Moody S, Clark W, et al: Dexamethasone and severe head injury: A prospective double blind study. *J Neurosurg* 51:307–316, 1979.

161. Deardon NM, Gibson JS, McDowall DG, et al: Effect of high dose dexamethasone on outcome from severe head injury. *J Neurosurg* 64:81–88, 1986.
162. Gudeman S, Miller J, Becker D: Failure of high dose steroid therapy to influence intracranial pressure in patients with severe head injury. *J Neurosurg* 51:301–306, 1979.
163. Saul T, Ducker T, Salcman M, et al: Steroids in severe head injury: A prospective randomized clinical trial. *J Neurosurg* 54:596–600, 1981.
164. Deutscher Verkehrssicherheitsrat Bayer: Staatsministerium des Inneren Notfallrettung Unterfranken, Dokumentation Band II. Zur Wirksamkeit und Wirtschaft des Rettungsdienstes, 1985.
165. Jennett B, Teasdale G, Galbraith S, et al: Severe head injury in three countries. *J Neurol Neurosurg Psychiatry* 40:291–298, 1977.
166. Schmoker J, Zhuang J, Shackford SR: Hemorrhagic hypotension after brain injury causes an early and sustained decrease in oxygen delivery despite normalization of systemic oxygen delivery. *J Trauma* 31:1038, 1991.
167. Wolf AL, Levi L, Marmarou A, et al: Effect of THAM upon outcome in severe head injury: A randomized prospective clinical trial. *J Neurosurg* 78:54–59, 1993.
168. Muizelaar JP, Marmarou A, Young HF, et al: Improving the outcome of severe head injury with the oxygen radical scavenger polyethylene glycol-conjugated superoxide dismutase: A Phase II trial. *J Neurosurg* 78:375–382, 1993.

CHAPTER 8

EMERGENCY ROOM MANAGEMENT OF THE HEAD-INJURED PATIENT

Alex B. Valadka
Raj K. Narayan

SYNOPSIS

Emergency room management of head-injured patients is challenging because of the complexity of the associated problems and the unpredictable course of the intracranial processes. This chapter details current thinking on the management of mild, moderate, and severe head injuries and deals with some of the controversial issues relevant to these patients.

INTRODUCTION

The authors of this chapter attempt to summarize the current thinking related to the initial evaluation and treatment of head-injured patients. To some extent, the information contained here is a synthesis of the principles discussed in other chapters in this text, although it is conveyed with a more practical approach.

No universally accepted guidelines exist for the management of head injury. However, early efforts have been made to synthesize current knowledge in this field into a reasonable protocol.[1] The following material is evolving and will change as understanding of the pathophysiology of head injury improves. While the support systems and facilities to manage head-injured patients in this fashion are not available in much of the world, the information in this chapter represents what is considered optimal treatment at the present time.

CLASSIFICATION

Head injuries can be classified in several ways. For practical purposes, three descriptions are useful: (1) mechanism, (2) severity, and (3) morphology (Table 8-1).

Mechanism of Injury

Head injury may be classified broadly as blunt or penetrating. For practical purposes, the term "blunt head injury" usually is associated with automobile collisions, falls, and blunt assaults. Penetrating head injury usually results from gunshot and stab wounds. The distinction between the two depends on the presence of dural penetration.

Severity of Injury

The Glasgow Coma Scale (GCS) score is used to quantify neurological findings and has brought a degree of uniformity of description and discipline for patients with head injury.[2–4] The GCS score has even been adopted for the description of patients with altered levels of consciousness from other causes.

Coma is defined as the inability to obey commands, utter words, and open the eyes. Patients who open their eyes spontaneously, obey commands, and are oriented score a total of 15 points on the GCS, whereas flaccid patients who do not open their eyes or vocalize score the minimum of 3 points (Table 8-2). No single score within the range of 3 to 15 points forms a cutoff point for coma. However, 90 percent of all patients with a score of 8 or less and none of those with a score of 9 or more are found to be in coma according to the preceding definition. Therefore, a GCS score of 8 or less has become the generally accepted definition of coma. The distinction between patients with severe head injury and those with mild to moderate head injury is therefore fairly clear. However, distinguishing between mild and moderate head injuries is more of a problem. Somewhat arbitrarily, head-injured patients with a GCS sum score of 9 to 12 have been categorized as "moderate" and those with a score of 13 to 15 have been designated as "mild." Patients with a GCS score of 13 to 15 who also

TABLE 8-1 Classifications of Head Injury

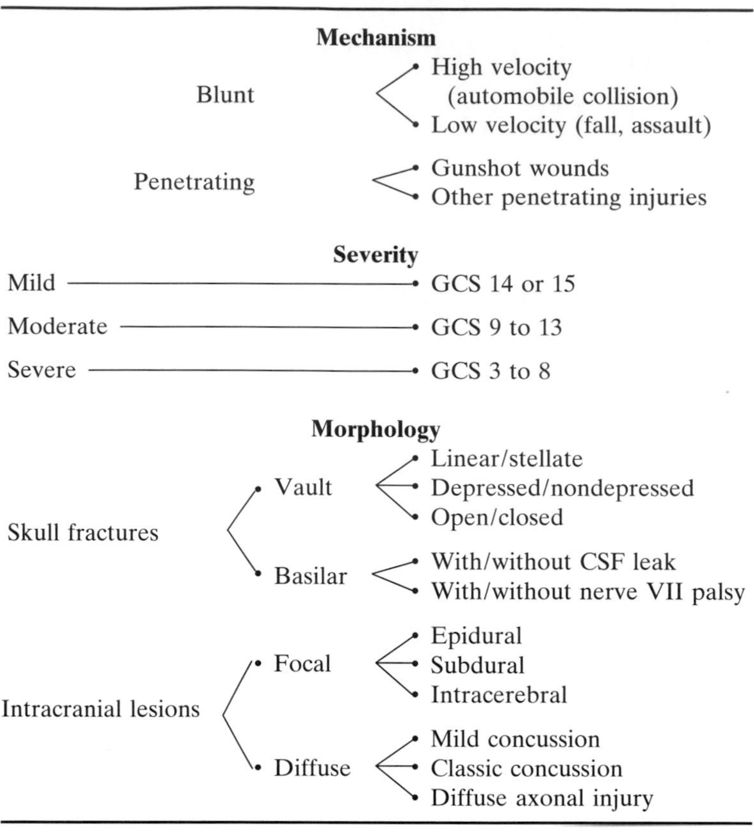

Mechanism		
Blunt		High velocity (automobile collision)
		Low velocity (fall, assault)
Penetrating		Gunshot wounds
		Other penetrating injuries
Severity		
Mild		GCS 14 or 15
Moderate		GCS 9 to 13
Severe		GCS 3 to 8
Morphology		
Skull fractures	Vault	Linear/stellate
		Depressed/nondepressed
		Open/closed
	Basilar	With/without CSF leak
		With/without nerve VII palsy
Intracranial lesions	Focal	Epidural
		Subdural
		Intracerebral
	Diffuse	Mild concussion
		Classic concussion
		Diffuse axonal injury

have computed tomography (CT) scan abnormalities have been shown to do significantly worse than those whose CT scans are normal. Note that in assessing the GCS, it is important to use the best motor response in calculating the score. However, one must record the response on both sides.

The increasing frequency of endotracheal intubation of comatose patients by paramedical personnel at the scene of the accident has raised some questions about the proper assessment of their GCS scores upon the arrival of these patients in the emergency room. One method is to designate the verbal score by the letter "T" (for "intubated"), which is recorded next to the sum of the motor and eye scores. Another problem arises when an occasional patient has such severe periorbital injury or edema that the eye score cannot be assessed properly. In cases in which only an incomplete assessment is possible, it becomes all the more important to ensure accuracy in recording the little information that is available. In particular, for predicting prognosis after a severe head injury, the combination of motor score and other important data, such as age and pupillary response, is as reliable as the complete GCS combined with the same information.[5] Hence, it becomes especially important to record the motor response after

TABLE 8-2 Glasgow Coma Scale

Assessment Area	Score
Eye opening (E)	
Spontaneous	4
To speech	3
To pain	2
None	1
Best motor response (M)	
Obeys commands	6
Localizes pain	5
Normal flexion (withdrawal)	4
Abnormal flexion (decorticate)	3
Extension (decerebrate)	2
None (flaccid)	1
Verbal Response (V)	
Oriented	5
Confused conversation	4
Inappropriate words	3
Incomprehensible sounds	2
None	1

GCS score = (E + M + V); best possible score = 15; worst possible score = 3.

resuscitation. However, considerable variability in the assessment of the GCS has been reported.[6]

Morphology of Injury

CT scanning has revolutionized the classification and management of head injury. Although patients who are deteriorating rapidly, neurologically or hemodynamically, may be taken to surgery without a CT scan, the vast majority should have a CT scan before surgical intervention. Furthermore, frequent follow-up CT scans are essential because the morphological picture in head injury often undergoes a remarkable evolution over the first few hours, days, and even weeks after an injury. Morphologically, head injuries may be broadly considered under two headings: (1) skull fractures and (2) intracranial lesions.

Skull fractures

Skull fractures may be seen in the cranial vault or skull base, may be linear or stellate, and may be depressed or nondepressed. Basal skull fractures usually require CT scanning with bone window settings for identification. The presence of the clinical signs of a basal skull fracture should increase the index of suspicion and help in their identification. These signs include periorbital ecchymosis (raccoon eyes), retroauricular ecchymosis (Battle's sign), CSF leaks, and seventh nerve palsy.

As a general guideline, fragments depressed more than the thickness of the skull require surgical elevation. Open or compound skull fractures have a direct communication between the scalp laceration and the cerebral surface because the dura is torn. These fractures require early surgical repair.

The significance of a skull fracture should not be underestimated, since it takes considerable force to fracture the skull. A linear vault fracture increases the likelihood of the presence of an intracranial hematoma by a factor of about 400 in a conscious patient and a factor of 20 in a comatose patient.[7] Basilar skull fractures are sometimes associated with a CSF leak from the nose (rhinorrhea) or the ear (otorrhea). They also may be associated with a seventh nerve palsy, which may occur immediately or a few days after the initial injury. Generally, the prognosis for the recovery of seventh nerve function is better in the delayed-onset variety.

Intracranial lesions

Intracranial lesions may be classified as focal or diffuse, although the two forms frequently coexist. Focal lesions include epidural hematomas, subdural hematomas, and contusions (intracerebral hematomas). Diffuse brain injuries in general show normal CT scans but demonstrate an altered sensorium or even deep coma. Based on the depth and duration of coma, diffuse injuries can be classified as mild concussion, classic concussion, or diffuse axonal injury.

Epidural Hematomas

Epidural hematomas are located outside the dura but within the skull and are typically biconvex or lenticular in shape. They are most often located in the temporal or temporoparietal region and often result from laceration of the middle meningeal artery caused by a fracture. While these clots usually are thought to be arterial in origin, they also may be due to venous bleeding associated with skull fractures in at least a third of cases. Occasionally, an epidural hematoma may result from torn venous sinuses, particularly in the parieto-occipital region or posterior fossa. Although epidural hematomas are relatively uncommon (less than 1 percent of all head-injured patients and less than 10 percent of those who are comatose),[8] they should always be considered in the diagnostic process. If they are treated early, the prognosis usually is excellent because the damage to the underlying brain will be limited. Outcome is directly related to the neurological status of the patient before surgery. Patients with epidural hematomas can present with the classical "lucid interval" and "talk and die." The decision to perform an operation is a difficult judgment that should be made by a neurosurgeon.

Subdural Hematomas

Subdural hematomas are much more common than are epidural hematomas, occurring in approximately 30 percent of severe head injuries. They result most frequently from the tearing of a bridging vein between the cerebral cortex and a draining venous sinus. However, they also can be associated with lacerations of the brain surface. Subdural hematomas normally cover the entire surface of the hemisphere. Furthermore, the brain damage underlying an acute subdural hematoma is usually much more severe and the prognosis is much worse than is the case with epidural hematomas. The high mortality rate associated with subdural hematomas can be lowered by very rapid surgical intervention and aggressive medical management.

Contusions and Intracerebral Hematomas

Pure cerebral contusions are fairly common. Their frequency has become much more apparent as the quality and number of CT scanners have increased. Furthermore, contusions of the brain are almost always seen in association with subdural hematomas. Although the vast majority of contusions occur in the frontal and temporal lobes, they can occur in any part of the brain, including the cerebellum and brainstem. The distinction between a contusion and a traumatic intracerebral hematoma remains ill defined. Contusions can, in a period of hours or days, evolve or coalesce to form an intracerebral hematoma.

Diffuse Injuries

Diffuse brain injuries form a continuum of brain damage caused by increasing amounts of acceleration-deceleration injury to the brain. Diffuse brain injury is the most common type of head injury.

A mild concussion is an injury in which consciousness is preserved but there is a noticeable degree of temporary neurological dysfunction. These injuries are exceedingly common and, because of their mild degree, often are not brought to medical attention. The mildest form of concussion results in confusion and disorientation without amnesia (loss of memory). This syndrome is completely reversible and is not associated with any major sequelae. A slightly greater injury causes confusion with both retrograde and anterograde amnesia (amnesia for events before and after the injury).

A classical cerebral concussion is an injury that results in loss of consciousness. This condition always is accompanied by some degree of posttraumatic amnesia, and the length of amnesia is a good measure of the severity of the injury. The loss of consciousness is transient and reversible. In a somewhat arbitrary definition, the patient has returned to full consciousness by 6 h, although this usually occurs much sooner. While many patients with a classical cerebral concussion have no sequelae other than amnesia for the events relating to the injury, some patients may have more long-lasting neurological deficits, including memory difficulties, dizziness, nausea, anosmia, and depression. This is referred to as a postconcussion syndrome and can be quite disabling.

Diffuse axonal injury (DAI) is the term used to explain prolonged posttraumatic coma that is not due to a mass lesion or ischemic insult. These patients are rendered deeply comatose and remain so for prolonged periods. They often demonstrate evidence of decortication or decerebration (motor posturing) and often remain severely disabled if they survive. They often exhibit autonomic dysfunction, such as hypertension, hyperhidrosis, and hyperpyrexia, and were previously thought to have a primary brainstem injury. Distinguishing between DAI and hypoxic brain injury is not easy in the clinical setting, and the two may coexist.

MANAGEMENT OF MILD HEAD INJURY (GCS 14 OR 15)

Approximately 80 percent of patients presenting to the emergency room with a head injury fall under the category of mild head injury (Algorithm 8-1). These patients are awake but may be amnesic for the events surrounding the injury. There may be a history of a brief loss of consciousness, which usually is difficult to confirm. The issue often is confounded by alcohol or other intoxicants.

Most patients with a mild head injury make uneventful recoveries, although with subtle neurological sequelae. However, about 3 percent of these patients deteriorate unexpectedly and can become neurologically devastated if the decline in mental status is not noticed early. How can a doctor avoid such an occurrence? The classic struggle between "cost-effective" management and the "best possible" management is clearly evident here.

Ideally, a CT scan should be obtained in all head-injured patients, especially if there is a history of more than a momentary loss of consciousness, amnesia, or severe headaches after the injury. However, if a CT scan is not immediately available and if the patient is asymptomatic, fully awake, and alert, she or he may alternatively be kept under observation in the hospital for 12 to 24 h. In a study of almost 700 patients with mild head injury (GCS score of 14 or 15) who experienced a brief loss of consciousness or amnesia, 18 percent had abnormalities on the initial CT and 5 percent required surgery.[9] The same investigators reported that 40 percent of patients with a GCS of 13 had abnormal CT scans,[10] prompting the authors to suggest that these patients should be classified as having moderate head injuries rather than being placed in the mild head injury group.[11] None of their patients with normal CT scans on admission showed subsequent deterioration or required surgery. Nevertheless, it is possible for a few isolated patients with normal early scans to develop mass lesions a few hours later.

At present, skull x-rays are recommended only in penetrating head injury or when CT scanning is not immediately available. If a skull x-ray is obtained, one must look for the following features: (1) linear or depressed skull fractures, (2) midline position of the pineal gland (if calcified), (3) air-fluid levels in the sinuses, (4) pneumocephalus, (5) facial fractures, and (6) foreign bodies.

How often does one find a skull fracture? This figure varies with the severity of injury, from 3 percent of patients with mild head injuries (those not admitted) to

ALGORITHM 8-1 Management of Mild Head Injury

Definition: Patient is awake and may be oriented (GCS 14 or 15)

History

- Name, age, sex, race, occupation
- Mechanism of injury
- Time of injury
- Loss of consciousness immediately after injury
- Subsequent level of alertness
- Amnesia: retrograde, anterograde
- Headache: mild, moderate, severe
- Seizures

General examination to exclude systemic injuries

Limited neurological examination

Cervical spine and other radiographs as indicated

Blood alcohol level and urine toxic screen

CT scan of the head in all patients except completely asymptomatic and neurologically normal patients is ideal

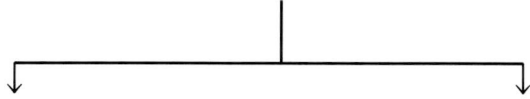

Observe in/admit to hospital
- No CT scanner available
- Abnormal CT scan
- All penetrating head injuries
- History of loss of consciousness
- Deteriorating level of consciousness
- Moderate to severe headache
- Significant alcoholic/drug intoxication
- Skull fracture
- CSF leak rhinorrhea or otorrhea
- Significant associated injuries
- No reliable companion at home
- Unable to return promptly
- Amnesia
- History of loss of consciousness

Discharge from hospital
- Patient does not meet any of the criteria for admission
- Discuss need to return if any problems develop and issue a "warning sheet"
- Schedule follow-up clinic visit, usually within 1 week

65 percent of those with severe head injuries. The vault is involved three times as often as the base is. Basal fractures often are not visualized on initial skull films, and clinical signs such as periorbital ecchymosis, CSF rhinorrhea or otorrhea, hemotympanum, and Battle's sign must be taken as presumptive evidence of a basal fracture and warrant admission for observation.

X-rays of the cervical spine and other parts must be obtained if there is any pain or tenderness. Nonnarcotic analgesics such as acetaminophen are preferred, although codeine may be used if there is an associated painful injury. Tetanus toxoid must be administered if there are any associated open wounds. Routine blood tests usually are not necessary if there are no systemic injuries. A blood alcohol level and urine toxic screen can be useful both for diagnostic and for medicolegal purposes. A mildly head injured patient with a normal CT scan who can be promptly brought back to the hospital may be discharged from the emergency department to the care of a reliable companion. The companion is instructed on a warning sheet to keep the patient under close observation for at least 12 h and bring the patient back if any adverse features develop (Table 8-3). If no reliable companion is available or if a CT scan cannot

TABLE 8-3 Head Injury Warning Discharge Instructions*

We have found no evidence to indicate that your head injury was serious. However, new symptoms and unexpected complications can develop hours or even days after the injury. The first 24 hours are the most crucial, and you should remain with a reliable companion at least during this period. If any of the following signs develop, call your doctor or come back to the hospital:

1. Drowsiness or increasing difficulty in awakening patient (awaken patient every 2 hours during period of sleep)
2. Nausea or vomiting
3. Convulsions or fits
4. Bleeding or watery drainage from the nose or ear
5. Severe headaches
6. Weakness or loss of feeling in the arm or leg
7. Confusion or strange behavior
8. One pupil (black part of the eye) much larger than the other, peculiar movements of the eyes, double vision, or other visual disturbances
9. A very slow, or very rapid, pulse or an unusual breathing pattern

If there is swelling at the site of injury, apply an ice pack, making sure that there is a cloth or towel between the ice pack and the skin. If swelling increases markedly in spite of the ice pack application, call us or come back to the hospital.

You may eat and drink as usual if you desire. However, you should *not* drink alcoholic beverages for at least 3 days after your injury.

Do not take any sedatives or any pain relievers stronger than Tylenol, at least for the first 24 hours. Do not use aspirin-containing medicines.

If you have any further questions, or in case of an emergency, we can be reached at (telephone number). ____________________.

Doctor's name: ____________________

* If a significant lesion is noted on CT scan, the patient must be admitted to the care of a neurosurgeon and managed according to his or her neurological progress over the next few days. A follow-up CT scan is usually obtained before discharge or sooner in the case of neurological deterioration.

be obtained, the patient may be kept in the hospital for several hours with frequent neurological checks and then discharged if she or he appears normal.

MANAGEMENT OF MODERATE HEAD INJURY (GCS 9 TO 13)

Patients with a moderate head injury constitute approximately 10 percent of head injury patients seen in the emergency department (Algorithm 8-2). They still are able to follow simple commands but usually are confused or somnolent and may have focal neurological deficits such as hemiparesis. Approximately 10 to 20 percent of these patients deteriorate and lapse into coma. Therefore, they should be managed in the same way as severely head injured patients, although they are not routinely intubated. However, every precaution should be taken to protect the airway.

On admission to the emergency department, a brief history is obtained and cardiopulmonary stability is ensured before a neurological assessment is performed. A CT scan of the head is obtained in all moderately head injured patients. In a review of 341 patients with a GCS of 9 to 12, 40 percent of the patients had an abnormal initial CT scan and 8 percent of those with a GCS of 9 to 13 required neurosurgical intervention.[10] These patients are admitted for observation even if the CT scan is normal. If the patient improves neurologically and a follow-up CT scan of the head shows no surgical mass lesion, the patient may be discharged from the hospital

ALGORITHM 8-2 Management of Moderate Head Injury

Definition: Patient may be confused or somnolent but is still able to follow simple commands (GCS 9 to 13)

Initial workup
- Same as for mild head injury, plus baseline blood work
- CT scan of the head obtained in all cases
- Admission for observation

After admission
- Frequent neurological checks
- Follow-up CT scan if condition deteriorates or preferably before discharge

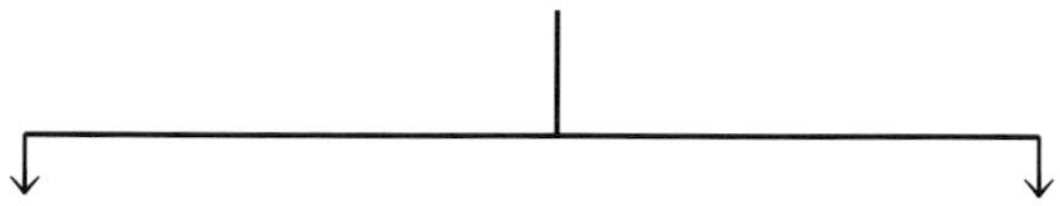

If patient improves (90%)
- Discharge when appropriate
- Follow-up in clinic

If patient deteriorates (10%)
- If the patient stops following simple commands, repeat CT scan and manage per severe head injury protocol.

over the next few days. However, if the patient lapses into coma, the management principles described for severe head injury are adopted.

MANAGEMENT OF SEVERE HEAD INJURY (GCS 3 TO 8)

Patients who have sustained a severe head injury are unable to follow simple commands even after cardiopulmonary stabilization (Algorithm 8-3). Although this definition includes a wide spectrum of brain injury, it identifies patients who are at the greatest risk of suffering significant morbidity and mortality. A "wait and see" approach in such patients can be disastrous, and prompt diagnosis and treatment are of the utmost importance.

Primary Survey and Resuscitation

Brain injury often is adversely affected by secondary insults. In a study of 100 consecutive patients with severe brain injury evaluated on arrival in the emergency department, 30 percent were hypoxemic (P_{O_2} <65 mmHg), 13 percent were hypotensive (systolic blood pressure <95 mmHg), and 12 percent were anemic (hematocrit <30 percent).[12] Hypotension on admission in patients with a severe head injury is associated with more than double the mortality seen in patients with no hypotension (60 versus 27 percent). The presence of hypoxia in addition to hypotension is associated with a mortality of approximately 75 percent. Therefore, it is imperative that cardiopulmonary stabilization be achieved rapidly in patients with severe head injury.

Airway and Breathing

A frequent concomitant of head injury is transient respiratory arrest. Prolonged apnea often may be the cause of "immediate" death at the injury scene. The most important aspect of immediately managing these patients is early endotracheal intubation. The patient is ventilated with 100% oxygen until blood gases can be obtained and appropriate adjustments can be made to the concentration of inspired oxygen.

Hyperventilation should be used cautiously in patients with severe head injury. While this may be used temporarily to correct acidosis and quickly bring down the increased intracranial pressure (ICP) in a patient with dilated pupils, it is a double-edged sword. (See "Hyperventilation," later in this chapter.) Hyperventilation may be used cautiously in patients who demonstrate a worsening GCS or pupillary dilatation. The P_{CO_2} should be kept between 25 and 35 mmHg.

Circulation

As was outlined previously, hypotension and hypoxia are the principal enemies of a head-injured patient. If

ALGORITHM 8-3 Initial Management of Severe Head Injury

Definition: Patient is unable to follow even simple commands because of impaired consciousness. (GCS 3 to 8)

Assessment and management
- ABC
- Primary survey and AMPLE history

Neurological reevaluation
- Eye opening
- Motor response
- Verbal response
- Pupillary light reaction
- Oculocephalics (doll's eyes) ±
- Oculovestibulars (caloric) ±

Therapeutic agents
- Mannitol
- Moderate hyperventilation
- Anticonvulsant

Diagnostic tests (in descending order of preference)
- CT scan, all patients
- Air ventriculogram
- Angiogram

(Air ventriculogram and Angiogram: Consider only if CT is not available)

Note: "AMPLE" history is mnemonic for *a*llergies, *m*edications currently taken, *p*ast illnesses, *l*ast meal, and *e*vents/environment related to the injury.

the patient is hypotensive, it is vital to restore normal blood volume as soon as possible. Hypotension usually is not due to the brain injury itself, except in the terminal stages, when medullary failure supervenes.

Far more commonly, hypotension is a marker of severe blood loss, which may be overt, occult, or both (Table 8-4). One also must consider associated spinal cord injury (quadriplegia or paraplegia), cardiac contusion or tamponade, and tension pneumothorax as possible causes.

While efforts are being made to determine the cause of hypotension, volume replacement should be initiated. Diagnostic peritoneal lavage (DPL) is used routinely in comatose patients because a clinical examination for abdominal tenderness is not possible in those patients. Establishing the priority of DPL versus CT scan of the head can sometimes create conflicts between trauma surgeons and neurosurgeons. A policy that helps clarify the decision-making process is useful (Algorithm 8-4). If necessary, the patient can be transported to the CT scanner while the DPL is still in progress. It must be emphasized that a patient's neurological examination is meaningless as long as the patient is hypotensive. Hypotensive patients who are unresponsive to any form of stimulation may revert to a nearly normal neurological examination soon after normal blood pressure is restored.

TABLE 8-4 Common Sites of Blood Loss in a Multiple Trauma Patient

Overt	Occult
1. Scalp lacerations	1. Intraperitoneal or retroperitoneal
2. Maxillofacial injuries	2. Hemothorax
3. Open fractures	3. Pelvic hematoma
4. Other soft tissue injuries	4. Bleeding into extremities at site of long bone fractures
	5. Subgaleal or extradural hematoma in an infant
	6. Traumatic aortic rupture

Secondary Survey

Patients with severe head injury often have multiple trauma. In a series of severely head injured patients, more than 50 percent had additional major systemic injuries requiring care by other specialists (Table 8-5).[12] In this chapter, the authors wish to emphasize only a few points: (1) The physicians participating in the initial assessment of these patients must have a high index of

TABLE 8-5 Systemic Injuries in 100 Patients with Severe Head Injury

Type of Injury	Incidence, %
Long bone or pelvic fracture	32
Maxillary or mandibular fracture	22
Major chest injury	23
Abdominal visceral injury	7
Spinal injury	2

SOURCE: Adapted with permission from Miller JD, Sweet RC, Narayan RK, et al: Early insults to the injured brain. *JAMA* 240:439–442, 1978.

ALGORITHM 8-4 DPL versus Scan in Head-Injured Patients

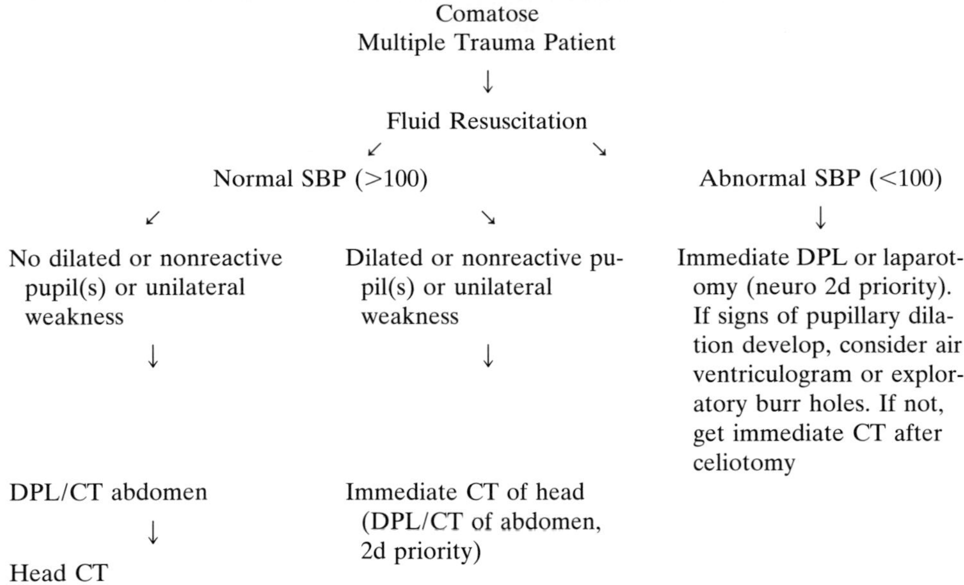

In borderline cases, i.e., when the systolic blood pressure (SBP) can be temporarily corrected but tends to slowly decrease, every effort should be made to get a head CT before taking the patient to the OR for laparotomy. Such cases call for great clinical judgment and cooperation between the trauma surgeon and the neurosurgeon.

Notes: 1. All comatose head injury patients will undergo resuscitation (ABCs) on arrival in the emergency room.
2. As soon as the BP is normalized, a minineurological exam is performed (GCS and pupillary reaction). If the BP cannot be normalized, the neurological exam is still performed and the hypotension is recorded.
3. If the patient's SBP cannot be brought up to over 100 mmHg despite aggressive fluid resuscitation, the priority is to establish the cause of the hypotension, with the neurosurgical evaluation taking second priority. In such cases the patient undergoes a DPL in the ER and may need to go directly to the OR for a laparotomy. The trauma surgeon takes primary responsibility for such patients. CT of the head is obtained after the laparotomy. If there is clinical evidence of an intracranial mass, an air ventriculogram, exploratory burr holes, or craniotomy may be undertaken in the OR while the laparotomy is being performed.
4. If the patient's SBP is >100 mmHg after resuscitation and the patient has clinical evidence of a possible intracranial mass (unequal pupils, asymmetrical motor exam), the first priority is to obtain a CT head scan. A DPL may be performed in the ER, CT area, or OR, but the patient's neurological evaluation or treatment should not be delayed. An abdominal CT may be used instead of the DPL at the discretion of the trauma surgeon.

suspicion for subtle or occult injuries, (2) expert consultation should be sought whenever such additional injuries are suspected or identified, and (3) it is acceptable to "miss" minor or noncritical injuries in the acute resuscitative phase. Once the patient's condition has stabilized, however, every effort should be made to identify such occult injuries.

Blood should be obtained and sent for electrolytes, complete blood count, platelet count, coagulation profile, typing and cross-matching, arterial blood gas, hepatic enzymes, amylase, and in females a pregnancy test. A urinalysis also should be obtained. Because they often take time to be completed and interpreted, radiographs of the cervical spine, chest, and pelvis should be called for immediately. Similarly, any other obvious or suspected injuries to bones or joints require radiographs of the involved area. Complete evaluation of all suspected injuries may require more complex radiographic procedures, such as arch aortograms, which can be performed only in the radiology department.

Neurological Examination

As soon as the patient's cardiopulmonary status has been stabilized, a rapid and directed neurological examination is performed. This consists primarily of the GCS score and pupillary light response. Doll's-eye movements (oculocephalics), calorics (oculovestibulars), and corneal responses may be deferred until a neurosurgeon becomes available. Although various factors may confound an accurate evaluation of the patient's neurological status, such as hypotension, hypoxia, and intoxication, valuable data can be obtained.

It is extremely important to obtain a reliable minineurological examination before sedating or paralyzing the patient. Because the patient's clinical condition can be extremely important in determining subsequent treatment, it is important not to use long-acting paralytic agents in patients with a head injury. For this reason, succinylcholine, vercuronium, or very small doses of pancuronium are recommended. Small repeated doses of intravenous morphine (4 to 6 mg) are useful in providing analgesia and sedation that is reversible.

MOTOR RESPONSE

In a comatose patient, motor responses can be elicited by nailbed or nipple pressure. If a patient demonstrates variable responses to stimulation or if the response on each side is different, the best motor response elicited is a more accurate prognostic indicator than is the worst response. However, to follow trends in a patient's progress, it is better to report both the best and the worst responses. In other words, the right-side and left-side motor responses should be recorded separately. Serial examinations should be performed because of the variability in responses over time. This also allows the examiner to get a better sense of the patient's stability and allows the detection of deterioration as early as possible. In addition to the GCS score, pupillary responses should be recorded. Furthermore, advanced age, hypotension, and hypoxia all adversely affect outcome. Indeed, there is considerable interplay among all these factors in determining the ultimate outcome in a severely head injured patient.

PUPILLARY REACTIVITY AND EXTRAOCULAR MOVEMENTS

Careful notation of pupillary size and response to light is very important during the initial examination of a head-injured patient (Table 8-6). A well-known early sign of temporal lobe herniation is mild dilatation of the pupil and a sluggish pupillary light response. With worsening of herniation, there is wide dilatation of the pupils, followed by ptosis and paresis of the medial rectus and other ocular muscles innervated by the third nerve. This results in the classical "down and out" position of the eye that is diagnostic of a third nerve palsy.

Bilaterally dilated and nonreactive pupils can be due to inadequate brain perfusion or, less commonly, to bilateral third nerve palsies. Reestablishment of adequate cerebral perfusion can result in normalization of this finding. A pupil that does not react directly to light but reacts to light in the opposite eye (Marcus Gunn pupil) is a classical indication of an optic nerve injury. Bilaterally small pupils suggest that the patient has used certain drugs, particularly opiates, or has one of several metabolic encephalopathies or a destructive lesion of the pons. In these conditions, pupillary light responses usually can be seen with the +20 diopter lens on a standard ophthalmoscope.

Traumatic third palsy is the diagnosis in patients with a history of a dilated pupil from the onset of injury, an improving level of consciousness, and appropriate ocular muscle weakness. A widely dilated pupil occurs occasionally with direct trauma to the globe of the eye. This traumatic mydriasis usually is unilateral and is not accompanied by ocular muscle paresis. In a sixth nerve palsy, which paralyzes the lateral rectus, the eye is deviated medially and cannot be made to go laterally with doll's-eye or caloric stimulation. Fourth nerve palsies ordinarily cannot be identified in a comatose patient because of the subtle action of the fourth nerve.

OCULOCEPHALIC TESTING

Other essential components of the initial neurological survey include assessment and documentation of oculocephalic and oculovestibular responses. By testing the function of areas such as the paramedian pontine reticular formation and the medial longitudinal fasciculus, these maneuvers provide valuable information about the functional integrity of the brainstem reticular formation and its rostral connections.[13] Oculocephalic or "doll's-eyes" testing requires the prior exclusion of cervical spine fractures. With the neck flexed 30 degrees from the horizontal, the head is rotated briskly from side to side. In an awake patient, cortical control can maintain the direction of gaze in whichever direction the patient chooses (i.e., doll's suppressed). In a comatose patient, the eyes move opposite to the direction of rotation; that is, they continue to stare upward at the ceiling. If brainstem connections and ocular cranial nerves are intact, the response is "full." If the test is performed properly, an impaired response suggests either a palsy of cranial nerve III or VI, or dysfunction of the brainstem or of the structures that detect and transmit afferent impulses to the eyes, such as the semicircular canals and the cervical proprioceptive neurons and their ascending connections.

OCULOVESTIBULAR TESTING

Ideally, oculovestibular testing is performed with a supine patient's head flexed 30 degrees. However, because oculovestibular testing can be performed without ma-

TABLE 8-6 Interpretation of Pupillary Findings in Head-Injured Patients

Pupil Size	Light Response	Interpretation
Unilaterally dilated	Sluggish or fixed	Nerve III compression secondary to tentorial herniation
Bilaterally dilated	Sluggish or fixed	Inadequate brain perfusion Bilateral nerve III palsy
Unilaterally dilated or equal	Cross-reactive (Marcus Gunn)	Optic nerve injury
Bilaterally constricted	May be difficult to determine	Drugs (opiates) Metabolic encephalopathy Pontine lesion
Unilaterally constricted	Preserved	Injured sympathetic pathway, e.g., carotid sheath injury

nipulating the patient's neck, it is not contraindicated in the presence of a cervical spine fracture. This test is more reliable and accurate than is oculocephalic testing.[14] Oculovestibular testing is performed by irrigating the external auditory canal with at least 20 ml of ice water after the integrity of the tympanic membrane has been verified. The subsequent movement of endolymph within the horizontal semicircular canal causes slow tonic deviation of the eyes ipsilaterally, provided that the regions in the pontomedullary reticular system that control ocular movement are intact. The compensatory rapid movement of the eyes in the contralateral direction creates the impression of a nystagmus in a direction opposite to the cold water irrigation.[13] This phenomenon, which is described by the nmemonic "cold opposite, warm same" or "cows," is not seen in the comatose patient. The absence of both oculovestibular and oculocephalic responses portends a grim prognosis.

RADIOLOGIC STUDIES

Plain Skull Radiography

Perhaps the most contentious debate about radiographic assessment of head-injured patients centers on the value of skull radiographs, especially in patients with minor head injuries. Before the advent of modern neuroimaging techniques, radiographs of the skull were for many years one of the few diagnostic tools available for the emergency room assessment of patients with head injuries. More recently, it has been said that the diagnostic yield of routine skull radiographs in patients with minor head injuries is too low to justify their continued use, especially since a CT scan of the head is often obtained whenever such a patient demonstrates even the slightest suggestion of a neurological abnormality after a blow to the head. This argument was strengthened by the findings of a large prospective multicenter trial.[15]

The cost of obtaining and having a radiologist formally interpret a CT scan of the head has dropped dramatically, whereas the cost of skull radiographs has continued to rise. Nevertheless, CT scans of the head remain four to five times more expensive than plain films of the skull. The authors justify their very liberal use of CT scanning with the knowledge that detecting an otherwise missed intracranial lesion more than makes up for this difference in cost.

It should be emphasized that the debate over the value of plain radiographs should not be interpreted to mean that the finding of a skull fracture is inconsequential. Because the likelihood of significant intracranial pathology increases 400-fold in the presence of a skull fracture,[7] a CT scan of the head should always be considered when plain films reveal a skull fracture.

CT Scanning

The single most important radiological study in a patient with a severe head injury is a CT scan of the head.[16] This is almost always done without contrast in order to identify acute intracranial hemorrhage, bony fractures, and abnormalities of the brain parenchyma. Also, special circumstances may require diagnostic studies to supplement the CT scan. For example, skull radiographs may be useful for penetrating injuries and depressed fractures.

Extra caution should be used in evaluating patients suspected of intoxication with alcohol or other drugs. All too often, an obtunded state in such patients is automatically attributed to the abused substance, when in fact the intoxication may be masking an expanding intracranial mass lesion. Thus, instead of arguing against the need to obtain a CT scan of the head, the combination of drug intoxication and minor head injury should encourage one to scan the patient.

Angiography and Magnetic Resonance Imaging

Cerebral angiography is seldom performed in the setting of acute head injury. Previously, an important indication for angiography was to facilitate the identification of an isodense subdural hematoma not seen on CT. However, this question can now be answered more effectively by the newer CT scanners or by magnetic resonance imaging (MRI). MRI, however, is not widely used to image acute head injuries because of the time involved, the need to place the patient's entire body into the bore of the magnet, and the potential difficulties posed by the ferromagnetic monitoring and resuscitative equipment used in emergency rooms. However, in cases of mild or moderate injury or after a severely head injured patient has passed the initial posttraumatic period, MRI may provide diagnostic and prognostic information that may not be detected by even the most sensitive CT scanners.[17–19]

Ultrasonography and Transcranial Doppler

Although ultrasonography is used routinely for elective imaging of the intracranial contents of neonates with patent fontanelles, the quality of the image produced is too low to suggest that ultrasonography will replace CT scanning for evaluating trauma in infants. In adults, the utility of ultrasound is restricted to the intraoperative setting, only after an opening has been made in the calvarium. Another application of ultrasound technology is in transcranial Doppler (TCD) studies, which can be employed in the intensive care unit to provide useful information about blood flow velocity and vasospasm in branches of the major cerebral arteries.[20] However, TCD does not play a useful role in the initial assessment and management of patients in the emergency room.

Air Ventriculography

A radiographic technique that currently is used only rarely but may be helpful in emergent situations is air ventriculography.[21] This is most commonly performed in patients whose hemodynamic instability makes a CT scan impractical or whose high probability of harboring an aortic dissection mandates that an aortogram be done before a CT scan of the head. While the patient is on the operating or angiographic table, a frontal ventriculostomy is performed, using the sterile technique described elsewhere in this text. After 10 ml of CSF is withdrawn and replaced with a similar volume of air, a portable anteroposterior x-ray of the skull is obtained to identify any displacements of the ventricular system, which are assumed to result from traumatic hematomas until proved otherwise. Any shift of the midline of 5 mm or more is considered an indication for surgical decompression. Depending on whether the patient is in the emergency room, the angiography suite, or the operating room, the exact type of emergent decompression may range from a few burr holes and dural incisions to a complete craniotomy and evacuation of a clot. Every attempt must be made to preserve a sterile field, and hemostasis and closure must be performed in as meticulous a fashion as circumstances allow. Needless to say, performing any such procedure outside the operating room is not desirable but may sometimes be mandated by the need for rapid decompression.

Other Technologies

Near-infrared spectroscopy represents an exciting new development for the rapid detection of intracranial hematomas.[22] Such studies can be performed at the bedside, either in the emergency room or in the intensive care unit. However, PET and SPECT studies play no role acutely, but during the patient's recovery they may help elucidate the metabolic status of various regions of the brain and thus may assist in prognostication.[23] At present, however, they must be regarded primarily as research tools.

COMMON CONFOUNDING FACTORS

Intoxication

Several confusing and potentially dangerous situations arise regularly in the emergency room assessment of severely head injured patients. Perhaps the most common is the presence of intoxicating levels of ethanol and/or other sedating drugs in a patient's blood. Especially when these levels are high and a history of head trauma is not available, a patient's coma or depressed mental status may prematurely be assumed to be due to those drugs. Such patients may then be left undisturbed while the drug in question is given time to become metabolized. If the alteration in consciousness is due not to the abused drug but rather to an intracranial mass lesion, the results of the delay can be disastrous. Such lesions are discovered only when a head CT is finally obtained because the patient fails to wake up after many hours or because the patient is eventually found to have a fixed and dilated pupil or other evidence of herniation. By this time, the patient's chances of making a meaningful recovery are markedly diminished. The painful lesson learned from these cases is that one's index of suspicion for significant intracranial pathology should be dramatically raised by the combination of head injury and sedating drugs.

Nontraumatic Coma

Another important but less common scenario concerns a comatose patient who has been assumed to have suffered a head injury but who later is found to have another etiology for his or her coma. The main pitfall in these cases is the delay in initiating the appropriate treatment for the patient's underlying condition. In most cases, however, the blood chemistry determinations obtained as part of the standard evaluation of a severely head injured patient uncover the common metabolic causes of coma, whereas the head CT will provide assurance that the patient does not harbor a structural lesion requiring emergent surgery. A few of the more common causes of metabolic coma are hypoglycemia, hyponatremia, anoxia, hypothermia, and hepatic encephalopathy.[24] Accidental or intentional overdosage of various drugs occurs commonly and must be considered.

Pharmacological Paralysis

An avoidable complicating factor in the assessment of many of these patients is premature and excessive administration of neuromuscular blocking agents such as pancuronium and vecuronium. A patient must be able to cooperate fully with his or her examiner to properly gauge the severity of the injury. Obviously, this is not possible if the patient has been pharmacologically paralyzed. Thus, the neurosurgeon is frequently confronted with a patient in whom the physical examination is confined to the pupillary response to light but one whose CT scan reveals a mass lesion that may or may not warrant surgical removal, depending on the patient's neurological condition. Furthermore, the neurological examination as reported by outside physicians or paramedics may be sketchy, and the large dose of paralyzing agents administered makes complete pharmacological reversal difficult. Waiting for these agents to wear off may subject the patient to a potentially harmful delay in treatment, but proceeding with an emergency craniotomy or even a ventriculostomy is also not without risk. No one would argue with the necessity of paralyzing a patient whose uncontrolled thrashing about might jeopardize himself or herself and the flight crew of an aeromedical transport helicopter. However, unnecessarily paralyzing a patient could subject that patient to some risk by eliminating potentially valuable clinical information. If paralysis is deemed necessary, short-acting agents such as succinylcholine and vecuronium are preferred. If longer-acting agents such as pancuronium are used, small doses (e.g., 2 mg) are recommended.

Spinal Cord Injury

The importance of prompt recognition of concomitant spinal column fractures is obvious. Such patients are at risk of developing neurological deficits even after admission to the hospital.[25] The authors have seen cervical spine fractures in less than 5 percent of patients with severe head injury, which corresponds to the incidence reported in the recent literature.[26–28] It has been shown that treatment within 8 h of injury with high doses of methylprednisolone can produce a slight but definite improvement in neurological outcome, but such treatment initiated more than 8 h after injury provides no benefit and may be harmful.[29] This underscores the importance of early diagnosis and treatment.

RELATED ISSUES AND CONTROVERSIES

There is no therapy that can reverse the neurological damage caused by a head injury. Instead, the goals of all therapeutic efforts are twofold: maintaining homeostasis so that the injured brain has an optimal internal milieu in which to conduct its own reparative processes and preventing any subsequent secondary insults to an already sensitized brain.[30] A variety of interventions are available to approach these goals simultaneously from many different directions. The many chapters that discuss them in detail constitute a significant portion of this textbook. A few specific topics are addressed below.

Transfusions

Most clinicians caring for head-injured patients are familiar with blood component therapy, the details of which will not be discussed here. However, one area often overlooked by trauma surgeons and emergency medicine personnel is the follow-up that may be needed to detect iatrogenic transmission of disease via blood component transfusion. Although the risk of AIDS is uppermost in public consciousness, viral hepatitis is a much more common threat. Estimates of the risk of HIV infection from transfusion of blood or blood components range from 1 in 40,000 (0.0025 percent) to 1 in 250,000 (0.0004 percent),[31] with perhaps the best estimate being 1 in 153,000 per unit transfused.[32] Former estimates of a 6 to 10 percent likelihood of acquiring non-A, non-B hepatitis[33] have currently been revised to 2 to 3 percent per transfusion episode (CM Leveque, personal communication). The reason for the progressive decrease in risk is the increasing number and sensitivity of available screening tests for the various forms of hepatitis.

After exposure to hepatitis A or B, passive immunization via the administration of gamma globulin is recommended by the Centers for Disease Control (CDC).[34] Guidelines are less clear in cases of non-A, non-B hepatitis because the efficacy of treatment in these cases is controversial. There are some reports describing a reduction in the incidence of non-A, non-B hepatitis or of hepatitis C after the administration of immune globulin in certain situations, including blood transfusions.[35,36] Thus, although hard data are not available, it seems reasonable to use immune globulin as soon as possible after percutaneous exposure to non-A, non-B hepatitis.[37] Chronic hepatitis is routinely treated with interferon,[38] but the value of this drug in acute cases remains controversial. Some patients at the authors' institution have shown some improvement, but their long-term outcome remains unknown. A randomized controlled trial of interferon-alpha in acute posttransfusion hepatitis C suggested that this treatment may mitigate the severity and duration of the acute symptoms, but the incidence of chronic cases was not decreased.[39]

Early treatment of documented seroconversion to a positive HIV test was initially hoped to slow the development of AIDS and prolong life span, but this conclusion was not borne out by the results of the Concorde trial.[40] However, documentation of seroconversion does permit the early institution of measures to prevent and treat various complications, which may be quite important. In a recent report, the initiation of these measures to control *Pneumocystis carinii* pneumonia was suggested to be more important than antiretroviral therapy in prolonging survival time.[41] In an accompanying editorial, Phair reviewed this and several other recent studies and concluded that zidovudine (AZT) has a limited but measurable benefit in the treatment of HIV infection and that prophylaxis of *P. carinii* pneumonia has significantly affected both AIDS-free time and overall survival of HIV-infected patients.[42]

More important, early detection of HIV infection provides an opportunity for early counseling of patients and their families. As a public health measure, identifying the donor of any suspected infectious blood product permits that donor to be contacted and also permits his or her exclusion from further donation. This is quite important, because the major reason for the safety of the blood supply in this country is the screening of donors and the exclusion of blood from those known or likely to be infected with transmissible diseases.[43] Most cases of HIV infection caused by transfusions occur because the donor was infected too recently to mount an antibody response to the HIV virus.[32,44]

At the authors' institution, the decision to perform posttransfusion testing is made on an individualized basis. Indications vary from suspected acute hepatitis to severe anxiety on the part of the patient. Such testing is carried out 6 months after the transfusion and includes screening for the HIV virus as well as for hepatitis. Unfortunately, such follow-up may be overlooked because of other priorities or perhaps because the personnel who administered the blood transfusion are often not the individuals who follow the patient in the hospital or after discharge.

Timing of Surgery

A significant percentage of head-injured patients harbor traumatic intracranial hematomas that require surgical evacuation. These patients must be taken to surgery without delay. A study of Seelig and colleagues concluded that outcome was significantly improved in patients in whom evacuation of an acute subdural hematoma could be accomplished within 4 h of injury.[45] A subsequent report by Wilberger and coworkers was unable to confirm the strong link between prompt evacuation of hematomas and better outcomes, but a trend was evident.[46] Anecdotal reports have demonstrated that prompt evacuation of acute subdural hematomas can immediately and dramatically improve cerebral blood flow.[47] Thus, although the emergency room evaluation of trauma patients must always be done expeditiously, this is even more true when localizing signs suggest the presence of an intracranial mass lesion. Unfortunately, even with prompt surgical intervention, some patients still have a poor outcome. In these cases, underlying diffuse axonal injury, ischemia, or other pathological processes are probably present in conjunction with the mass lesion.

CT Scanning versus Trephination

Because of the vital importance of rapid detection and decompression of traumatic hematomas and because of their frequency in severely head injured patients who display signs of tentorial herniation, some authors have advocated that some of these patients immediately receive exploratory burr holes in the emergency room.[48,49] Although this procedure may occasionally play a role in some cases, the authors overwhelmingly prefer prompt CT scanning after rapid assessment and stabilization in the emergency room. If refractory hypotension mandates that a CT scan be deferred until after a lifesaving laparotomy or thoracotomy, the authors may perform an air ventriculogram in the operating room, while the other procedure is in progress. This is less invasive than numerous burr holes, and furthermore, the drainage of even small amounts of CSF can significantly lower ICP. If the ventriculogram suggests the presence of a mass lesion, decompression can be performed. However, this is not a convenient or particularly reliable undertaking, and it may be preferable to wait until the surgery is completed and obtain a CT scan at that time. Features that may push the authors toward obtaining an air ventriculogram include dilated pupils in the face of an anticipated long operative time. The universal trend toward situating CT scanners near emergency departments should make rapid CT scanning even more feasible, especially with the development of spiral CT scanners.[50,51] Also, the refinement of near-infrared spectroscopy and other new technologies may facilitate the rapid and reliable diagnosis of intracranial hematomas by noninvasive means.[22]

Organ Donation

Despite the accelerating growth of knowledge about the pathophysiology of traumatic brain injury, over a third of patients with severe head injury ultimately expire.[52] Although frustration and a sense of failure are inevitable after the death of a patient, one must not miss the opportunity to develop something positive from such a tragedy by initiating consideration of organ donation by the family. As transplantation medicine continues to achieve increasing success with a greater variety of organ systems, the need for organ donors increases. Neurosurgeons are uniquely positioned to assume an active role in helping to meet this need.

Hyperventilation

Hyperventilation is recommended as a temporizing measure for patients with focal signs or acutely elevated ICP.[53] Such patients are hyperventilated only until the underlying abnormality can be treated. Prophylactically and aggressively hyperventilating all severely head injured patients has been shown to adversely affect outcome in some patients without improving outcome in any group of patients.[54] Excessive hyperventilation can cause cerebrovascular constriction of such severity that cerebral ischemia may develop.[55] Moreover, within 24 h, cerebral vessels become less responsive to continuously lowered carbon dioxide and may even return to baseline caliber.[56] The authors' current policy is to use hyperventilation judiciously, as needed. The authors aim to keep the P_{CO_2} at approximately 30 mmHg and restore normocapnia as soon as ICP and cerebral perfusion pressure (CPP) are normalized. Prophylactic hyperventilation is not used. Monitoring of jugular venous oxygen saturation may be a useful method of determining the degree of hypocapnia a particular patient can safely tolerate.

Mannitol and Hypertonic Fluids

Management of intravenous fluids in trauma patients has always been a contentious topic. Controversy still surrounds the issue of whether mannitol should be administered routinely or only when focal findings are present. Recent reports in the trauma literature suggest that resuscitation of trauma patients with small volumes of hypertonic fluid improves outcomes, including those of patients with head injuries.[57–61] Clearly, if a comatose patient has a dilated pupil and unilateral weakness, the decision to give mannitol is easy. On the other end of the spectrum, one would not give mannitol to a conscious patient without focal deficits. Patients between these two extremes are more problematic.

Fluid Resuscitation

Conventional wisdom states that hypotension in a trauma patient should be corrected immediately and aggressively. This is particularly true in patients with head injury.[12,62,63] However, recent reports in patients treated in an urban setting for penetrating thoracic and abdominal injuries suggest that such aggressive correction of hypotension may in fact worsen outcomes by aggravating blood loss.[64–66] The basic premise of this strategy equates hypotension with the body's attempt to minimize hemorrhage; iatrogenic hypertension via vigorous fluid resuscitation provides the patient with little additional benefit at the expense of promoting exsanguination. However, as was detailed previously, hypotension in head-injured patients is associated with dramatically worse outcomes.[62,63] Thus, the wisdom of following this strategy in patients with head injury is dubious.

Implicit in this discussion are the different perspectives and priorities of the various members of the trauma team. Although neurosurgeons, general surgeons, and orthopedic surgeons all tend to place their organ systems at the top of the priority list, each must recognize that the patient's overall care can be optimized only by communication and cooperation in the emergency room.

Steroids

The routine administration of steroids after a severe head injury is now discouraged.[67] Clear proof of benefit has not been shown in head-injured patients, and some studies have attributed deleterious effects to steroids.[68–71] In spinal cord injuries, however, prompt administration of large doses of methylprednisolone has been shown to have a slight beneficial effect.[29]

CONCLUSION

This chapter can give only a brief overview of the enormously difficult and complex task of caring for an acutely head injured patient in the emergency room. In concluding this chapter, the authors wish to emphasize the importance of a few major points. These include early intubation and ventilation, avoiding hypotension at all costs, avoiding prolonged pharmacological paralysis if at all possible, and prompt CT scanning. Adherence to these simple but important principles will significantly increase a patient's chances of achieving a good outcome.

REFERENCES

1. Narayan RK, Saul TG, Eisenberg HM, Pitts LH: Neurotrauma care, in Committee on Trauma of the American College of Surgeons (ed): *Resources for Optimal Care of the Injured Patient: 1993.* Chicago: American College of Surgeons, 1993: 41–45.
2. Teasdale G, Jennett B: Assessment of coma and impaired consciousness. *Lancet* 2:81–84, 1974.
3. Jennett B, Teasdale G: Aspects of coma after severe head injury. *Lancet* 1:878–881, 1977.
4. Rimel RW, Jane JA, Edlich RF: An injury severity scale for the comprehensive management of central nervous system trauma. *JACEP* 8:64–67, 1979.
5. Choi SC, Narayan RK, Anderson RL, Ward JD: Enhanced specificity of prognosis in severe head injury. *J Neurosurg* 69:381–385, 1988.
6. Marion DW, Carlier PM: Problems with initial Glasgow Coma Scale assessment caused by prehospital treatment of patients with head injury: Results of a national survey. *J Trauma* 36:89–95, 1994.
7. Jennett B, Teasdale G: *Management of head injuries.* Philadelphia: Davis, 1981.
8. Miller JD, Becker DP: General principles and pathophysiology of head injury, in Youmans JR (ed): *Neurological Surgery.* Philadelphia: Saunders, 1982: 1896–1937.
9. Stein SC, Spettell C, Young G, Ross SE: Limitations of neurological assessment in mild head injury. *Brain Injury* 7:425–430, 1993.
10. Stein SC, Ross SE: Moderate head injury: A guide to initial management. *J Neurosurg* 77:562–564, 1992.
11. Stein SC, Ross SE: Minor head injury: A proposed strategy for emergency management. *Ann Emerg Med* 22:1193–1196, 1993.
12. Miller JD, Sweet RC, Narayan R, Becker DP: Early insults to the injured brain. *JAMA* 240:439–442, 1978.
13. Bajandas FJ, Kline LB: *Neuro-Ophthalmology Review Manual,* 3d ed. Thorofare, N.J.: SLACK, 1988.
14. Narayan RK: Head injury, in Grossman RG (ed): *Principles of Neurosurgery.* New York: Raven Press, 1991: 235–291.
15. Masters SJ, McClean PM, Arcarese JS, et al: Skull x-ray examinations after trauma: Recommendations by a multidisciplinary panel and validation study. *N Engl J Med* 316:84–91, 1987.
16. Johnson MH, Lee SH: Computed tomography of acute cerebral trauma. *Radiol Clin North Am* 30:325–352, 1992.
17. Levin HS, Amparo E, Eisenberg HM, et al: Magnetic resonance imaging and computerized tomography in relation to the neurobehavioral sequelae of mild and moderate head injuries. *J Neurosurg* 66:706–713, 1987.
18. Levin HS, Williams D, Crofford MJ, et al: Relationship of depth of brain lesions to consciousness and outcome after closed head injury. *J Neurosurg* 69:861–866, 1988.
19. Levin HS, Williams DH, Valastro M, et al: Corpus callosal atrophy following closed head injury: Detection with magnetic resonance imaging. *J Neurosurg* 73:77–81, 1990.
20. Aaslid R, Markwalder TM, Nornes H: Noninvasive transcranial Doppler ultrasound recording of flow velocity in basal cerebral arteries. *J Neurosurg* 57:769–774, 1982.
21. Narayan RK: Emergency room management of the head-injured patient, in Becker DP, Gudeman SK (eds): *Textbook of Head Injury.* Philadelphia: Saunders, 1989: 23–66.
22. Gopinath SP, Robertson CS, Grossman RG, Chance B: Near-infrared spectroscopic localization of intracranial hematomas. *J Neurosurg* 79:43–47, 1993.
23. Valadka AB, Ward JD, Smoker WRK: Brain imaging in neurologic emergencies, in Society of Critical Care Medicine (ed): *Critical Care: State of the Art,* vol 14. Anaheim, Calif.: Society of Critical Care Medicine, 1993: 1–60.
24. Plum F, Posner JB: *The Diagnosis of Stupor and Coma,* 3d ed. Philadelphia: Davis, 1980.
25. Marshall LF, Knowlton S, Garfin SR, et al: Deterioration following spinal cord injury: A multicenter study. *J Neurosurg* 66:400–404, 1987.
26. Michael DB, Guyot DR, Darmody WR: Coincidence of head and cervical spine injury. *J Neurotrauma* 6:177–189, 1989.
27. O'Malley KF, Ross SE: The incidence of injury to the cervical spine in patients with craniocerebral injury. *J Trauma* 28:1476–1478, 1988.
28. Soicher E, Demetriades D: Cervical spine injuries in patients with head injuries. *Br J Surg* 78:1013–1014, 1991.
29. Bracken MB, Shepard MJ, Collins WF, et al: A randomized, controlled trial of methylprednisolone or naloxone in the treatment of acute spinal-cord injury. *N Engl J Med* 322:1405–1411, 1990.
30. Becker DP, Gardner S: Intensive management of head injury, in Wilkins RH, Rengachary SS (eds): *Neurosurgery.* New York: McGraw-Hill, 1985: 1593–1600.
31. Gerst PH, Fildes JJ, Rosario PG, Schorr JB: Risks of human immunodeficiency virus infection to patients and healthcare personnel. *Crit Care Med* 18:1440–1448, 1990.
32. Cumming PD, Wallace EL, Schorr JB, Dodd RY: Exposure of patients to human immunodeficiency virus through the transfusion of blood components that test antibody-negative. *N Engl J Med* 321:941–946, 1989.
33. Bove JR: Transfusion-associated hepatitis and AIDS: What is the risk? *N Engl J Med* 317:242, 1987.
34. Centers for Disease Control: Protection against viral hepatitis: Recommendations of the immunization practices advisory committee (ACIP). *MMWR* 39:1–26, 1990.

35. Sanchez-Quijano A, Pineda JA, Lissen E, et al: Prevention of post-transfusion non-A non-B hepatitis by nonspecific immunoglobulin in heart surgery patients. *Lancet* 4:1245–1249, 1988.
36. Conrad ME, Lemon SM: Prevention of endemic icteric viral hepatitis by administration of immune serum globulin. *J Infect Dis* 156:56–63, 1987.
37. Carey WD, Patel G: Viral hepatitis in the 1990s: III. Hepatitis C, hepatitis E, and other viruses. *Cleve Clin J Med* 59:595–601, 1992.
38. Bonino F: Chronic viral hepatitis: From clinical trials to the therapeutic decision in the individual patient. *J Hepatol* 13(Suppl 1):S27–S30, 1991.
39. Viladomiu L, Genesca J, Estaban JI, et al: Interferon alpha in acute posttransfusion hepatitis C: A randomized controlled trial. *Hepatology* 15:767–769, 1992.
40. Aboulker JP, Swart A: A preliminary analysis of the Concorde trial. *Lancet* 341:889–890, 1993.
41. Osmond D, Charlebois E, Lang W, et al: Changes in AIDS survival time in two San Francisco cohorts of homosexual men, 1983 to 1993. *JAMA* 271:1083–1087, 1994.
42. Phair JP: Effectiveness of zidovudine treatment of advanced HIV infection. *JAMA* 271:1121–1122, 1994.
43. Menitove JE: The decreasing risk of transfusion-associated AIDS. *N Engl J Med* 321:966–968, 1989.
44. Zuck TF: Transfusion-transmitted AIDS reassessed. *N Engl J Med* 318:511–512, 1988.
45. Seelig JM, Becker DP, Miller JD, et al: Traumatic acute subdural hematoma: Major mortality reduction in patients treated within four hours. *N Engl J Med* 304:1511–1518, 1981.
46. Wilberger JE Jr, Harris M, Diamond DL: Acute subdural hematoma: Morbidity and mortality related to timing of operative intervention. *J Trauma* 30:733–736, 1990.
47. Schroder ML, Muizelaar JP, Kuta AJ: Documented reversal of global ischemia immediately after removal of an acute subdural hematoma: Report of two cases. *J Neurosurg* 80:324–327, 1994.
48. Andrews BT, Pitts LH, Lovely MP, Bartkowski H: Is computed tomographic scanning necessary in patients with tentorial herniation? *Neurosurgery* 19:408–414, 1986.
49. Mahoney BD, Rockswold GL, Ruiz E, Clinton JE: Emergency twist drill trephination. *Neurosurgery* 8:551–554, 1981.
50. Heiken JP, Brink JA, Vannier MW: Spiral (helical) CT. *Radiology* 189:647–656, 1993.
51. Zimmerman RA, Gusnard DA, Bilaniuk LT: Pediatric craniocervical spiral CT. *Neuroradiology* 34:112–116, 1992.
52. Marshall LF, Gautille T, Klauber MR, et al: The outcome of severe closed head injury. *J Neurosurg* 75(Suppl):S28–S36, 1991.
53. Ward JD, Choi S, Marmarou A, et al: Effect of prophylactic hyperventilation on outcome in patients with severe head injury, in Hoff JT, Betz AL (eds): *Intracranial Pressure VII.* Berlin: Springer-Verlag, 1989: 630–633.
54. Muizelaar JP, Marmarou A, Ward JD, et al: Adverse effects of prolonged hyperventilation in patients with severe head injury: A randomized clinical trial. *J Neurosurg* 75:731–739, 1991.
55. Bouma GJ, Muizelaar JP: Cerebral blood flow, cerebral blood volume, and cerebrovascular reactivity after severe head injury. *J Neurotrauma* 9(Suppl 1):S333–S348, 1992.
56. Muizelaar JP, van der Poel H, Li Z, et al: Pial arteriolar vessel diameter and CO2 reactivity during prolonged hyperventilation in the rabbit. *J Neurosurg* 69:923–927, 1988.
57. Mattox KL, Maningas PA, Moore EE, et al: Prehospital hypertonic saline/dextran infusion for posttraumatic hypotension. *Ann Surg* 213:482–491, 1991.
58. Vassar MJ, Perry CA, Gannaway WL, Holcroft JW: 7.5% sodium chloride/dextran for resuscitation of trauma patients undergoing helicopter transport. *Arch Surg* 126:1065–1072, 1991.
59. Israel RS, Marx JA, Moore EE, Lowenstein SR: Hemodynamic effect of mannitol in a canine model of concomitant increased intracranial pressure and hemorrhagic shock. *Ann Emerg Med* 17:560–566, 1988.
60. Walsh JC, Zhuang J, Shackford SR: A comparison of hypertonic to isotonic fluid in the resuscitation of brain injury and hemorrhagic shock. *J Surg Res* 50:284–292, 1991.
61. Prough DS, Whitley JM, Taylor CL, et al: Regional cerebral blood flow following resuscitation from hemorrhagic shock with hypertonic saline. *Anesthesiology* 75:319–327, 1991.
62. Chesnut RM, Marshall LF, Klauber MR, et al: The role of secondary brain injury in determining outcome from severe head injury. *J Trauma* 34:216–222, 1993.
63. Marmarou A, Anderson RL, Ward JD, et al: Impact of ICP instability and hypotension on outcome in patients with severe head trauma. *J Neurosurg* 75(Suppl):S59–S66, 1991.
64. Martin RR, Bickwell WH, Pepe PE, et al: Prospective evaluation of preoperative fluid resuscitation in hypotensive patients with penetrating truncal injury: A preliminary report. *J Trauma* 33:354–361, 1992.
65. Bickwell WH, Shaftan GW, Mattox KL: Intravenous fluid administration and uncontrolled hemorrhage. *J Trauma* 29:409, 1989.
66. Bickwell WH, Wall MJ Jr, Pepe PE, et al: Immediate versus delayed fluid resuscitation for hypotensive patients with penetrating torso injuries. *N Engl J Med* 331:1105–1109, 1994.
67. Clifton GL: Controversies in medical management of head injury. *Clin Neurosurg* 34:587–603, 1988.
68. Fanconi S, Kloti J, Meuli M, et al: Dexamethasone therapy and endogenous cortisol production in severe pediatric head injury. *Intensive Care Med* 14:163–166, 1988.
69. Fast A, Alon M, Weiss S, Zer-Aviv FR: Avascular necrosis of bone following short-term dexamethasone therapy for brain edema. *J Neurosurg* 61:983–985, 1984.
70. Braakman R, Schouten HJA, Blaauw-van Dishoeck M, Minderhoud JM: Megadose steroids in severe head injury: Results of a prospective double-blind clinical trial. *J Neurosurg* 58:326–330, 1983.
71. Giannotta SL, Weiss MH, Apuzzo MLJ, Martin E: High-dose glucocorticoids in the management of severe head injury. *Neurosurgery* 15:497–501, 1984.

Imaging Techniques

CHAPTER 9

COMPUTED TOMOGRAPHY OF CLOSED HEAD INJURY

Pedro J. Diaz-Marchan
L. Anne Hayman
David A. Carrier
David J. Feldman

SYNOPSIS

Computed tomography (CT) is the imaging modality of choice for acute head-injured patients. It correlates with patient morbidity and even identifies patients with initially benign clinical scores who are at risk of developing serious complications. It is superior to magnetic resonance imaging (MRI) in the acute setting because it is widely available, is rapid, and allows continuous monitoring of the patient during the procedure. It is inferior to MRI in detecting diffuse nonhemorrhagic parenchymal injuries; however, these lesions do not require acute neurosurgical intervention.

The ability of CT to detect small density differences between brain and blood allows it to depict bleeding into the parenchyma and the extraaxial and/or CSF spaces. Large density differences between brain and normal CSF are exploited to detect compression of the CSF-filled ventricles and sulci caused by masses or brain swelling. This chapter illustrates these capabilities. In addition, it describes the pathophysiology underlying four types of closed head injuries: (1) primary parenchymal injury, (2) extraaxial collections, (3) hemorrhage into the CSF spaces, and (4) secondary effects of intracranial trauma (brain herniation, diffuse swelling, and posttraumatic CSF fistula).

Despite the introduction of magnetic resonance imaging (MRI), computed tomography (CT) remains the primary method for evaluating closed head injuries. The advantages of CT include widespread availability, rapid imaging time, low cost, and safety. The absolute head immobility and sedation often required for MRI are less crucial in obtaining adequate CT images. In addition, the appearance of the initial CT scan has been shown to correlate with mortality.[1] CT can be used to identify patients at increased risk despite an initially benign clinical evaluation.

Thus, CT has virtually replaced skull radiography as the primary imaging tool in head injury because it provides imaging of the brain and other soft tissues. Skull fractures are rarely detected by radiographs in patients with minor head trauma, and in patients with major trauma, prompt neurosurgical consultation and a brain CT scan are required.[2–6]

Attention to the technical aspects of a CT scan maximizes its usefulness. At the authors' institution we obtain 3-mm-thick axial slices from the foramen magnum through the sella, followed by 10-mm-thick slices through the supratentorial region, including the vertex. All slices are angled parallel to the orbitomeatal line. Slices which show motion artifact are repeated. The CT images are reconstructed in soft tissue, blood, and bone window algorithms (window widths of 80, 150, and 2000 to 4000; levels 40, 60, and 500, respectively). Improper windowing can obscure the vital density differential between blood and brain. These densities are measured in Hounsfield units (HU). The normal range for gray matter is 36 to 60 HU, the white matter measures 24 to 36 HU (average range for brain is 24 to 46 HU), and depending on the hematocrit, blood can measure 40 to 80 HU for hematocrits of 30 to 90, respectively.[7–9]

The infusion of intravenous contrast CT scan is not usually necessary, and an enhanced study may be contraindicated in the acute setting because foci of enhancement can obscure underlying areas of contusion. However, contrast enhancement sometimes is helpful in identifying isodense subacute or chronic extraaxial hematomas.[10,11]

This chapter discusses the CT appearance of the most common intracranial injuries, including primary parenchymal injuries, extraaxial collections, and hemorrhages into the CSF spaces. A brief review of the secondary effects of intracranial trauma with an emphasis on brain herniations is also included.

PRIMARY PARENCHYMAL INJURIES

All parenchymal injuries result from shear-strain forces caused by marked rotational acceleration of the head.[12–21] They can result in intraparenchymal hematomas of varying sizes. For clinical purposes, parenchymal injuries are usually categorized by the presence or size of the hematoma (Table 9-1). In this chapter, brain injuries are classified into four anatomic categories: (1) diffuse axonal injury (DAI), (2) cortical contusions, (3) subcortical gray matter injury, and (4) brainstem injury.[22–24]

TABLE 9-1 Classification of Diffuse Head Injury Based on Computed Tomography

Category	Initial CT Findings
Diffuse Injury I	No visible pathology
Diffuse Injury II	Cisterns are present; midline shift < 5 mm and/or lesion densities present, no high- or mixed-density lesion > 25 ml, may include bone fragments and foreign bodies
Diffuse Injury III (swelling)	Cisterns are compressed or absent; midline shift is 0–5 mm; no high- or mixed-density lesion > 25 ml
Diffuse Injury IV (shift)	Midline shift > 5 mm, no high- or mixed-density lesion > 25 ml
Evacuated mass	Any lesion surgically evacuated
Nonevacuated mass	High- or mixed density lesion > 25 ml, not surgically evacuated

SOURCE: Marshall et al.[1] Used with permission.

Diffuse Axonal Injury

DAI is caused by differential movement of brain regions with different densities. Shear-strain forces that develop during rotational acceleration/deceleration of the head are the forces most likely to produce DAI.[12,17,18,20] Most injuries occur in the lobar white matter, particularly at the corticomedullary junction of the frontal and temporal lobes.[16,17,23] DAI may also occur in the corpus callosum and the dorsolateral aspect of the brainstem in cases of severe trauma. Injuries in the corpus callosum or brainstem rarely occur without associated lesions in the lobar white matter. About 75 percent of callosal injuries occur in the posterior body and splenium of the corpus callosum because the posterior falx prevents lateral displacement of the hemispheres during rotational acceleration of the head.[23] This creates tensile forces across the posterior corpus callosum.[20] Clinically, severe DAI is usually associated with impairment of consciousness which begins at the moment of impact.[13,18,20]

Since most of the damage in DAI is microscopic, only 10 percent of patients with DAI demonstrate abnormalities on CT scan. These abnormalities are either confluent areas of damage or hemorrhage (Fig. 9-1*A* and *B*). Hemorrhagic lesions more than a few millimeters in size can be seen on CT. When they are large, they tend to be oval, with the long axis parallel to the involved axons.[23,24] Nonhemorrhagic lesions cannot be detected on CT unless they are large enough to demonstrate a focus of subtle hypodensity, possibly representing edema. Since this edema takes time to develop, these lesions are usually seen only on follow-up CT scans. Other delayed findings include a subtle halo of hypodense edema around hemorrhages and new foci of hemorrhage in previously bland areas. After the edema resolves and the blood is resorbed, the CT scan may appear "normal" even though the patient has significant clinical cognitive and behavioral abnormalities.[25] In other cases the follow-up CT scan may show only generalized atrophy.

Cortical Contusions

A cortical contusion is a contact injury that results from a gyrus striking the skull. It can result from a direct blow, leading to linear acceleration/deceleration forces, or from shear-strain forces produced by rotational acceleration.[12,16,17,21] The areas of the brain most vulnerable to this type of injury are those adjacent to the floor of the anterior and middle cranial fossae: the sphenoid wings and petrous ridges. Therefore, the frontal and temporal poles and the undersurfaces of the temporal lobes are most commonly involved. Less frequently, the inferior surface of the cerebellum is contused.[12,21,23,26]

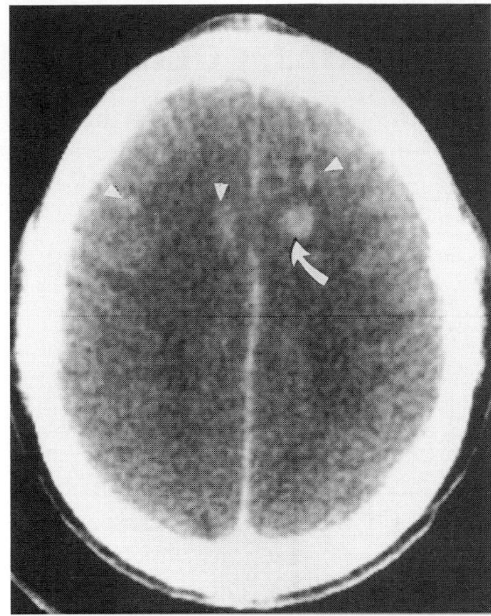

A

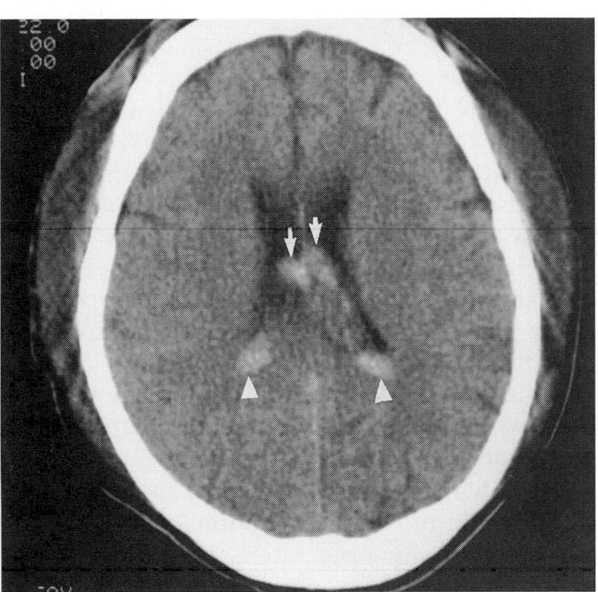

B

Figure 9-1. *A.* Noncontrast CT shows bifrontal hemorrhagic shearing injuries involving the gray–white matter junction (small arrowheads) and the left frontal lobar white matter (arrow). *B.* Noncontrast CT reveals a hemorrhagic shearing injury involving the body of the corpus callosum (arrows). Also note the acute blood within the ventricles which usually accompanies DAI (arrowheads).

These lesions are usually multiple and bilateral, but they often appear to be unrelated to the point of impact.[21,23,27]

On CT, contusions are seen as focal cortical hyperdensities associated with surrounding hypodense edema (Fig. 9-2). Local mass effect may be present, as manifested by effaced sulci and/or ventricles as well as by

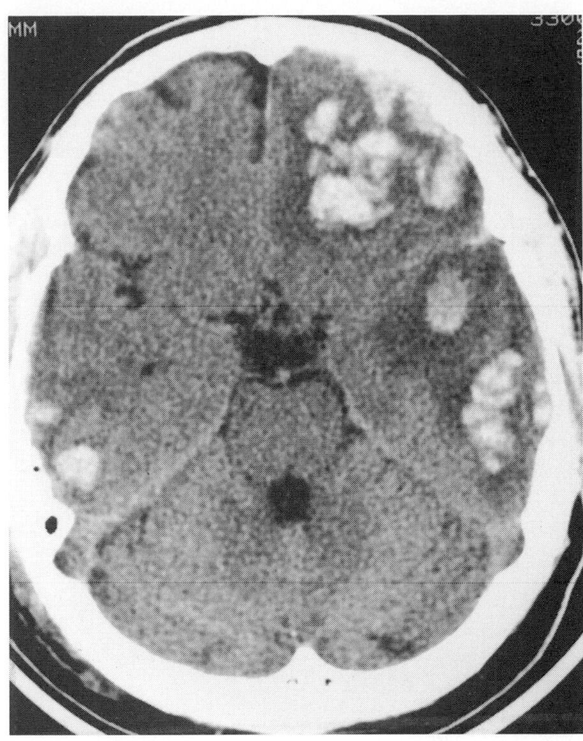

Figure 9-2. Noncontrast CT showing left frontal and bitemporal hemorrhagic contusions.

brain herniations. These lesions become isodense by the end of the first week and appear hypodense thereafter. In the chronic phase, local volume loss leads to nonspecific encephalomalacic changes.[22,26,28] Contusions can be seen on CT even if they are nonhemorrhagic. These lesions are identified as focal cortical hypodensities which may enlarge and become more conspicuous as edema develops during the first week. Delayed hemorrhage may occur in these areas.

Subcortical Gray Matter Injury

Injury to the subcortical gray matter is characterized by small focal hemorrhages in the basal ganglia and thalami (Fig. 9-3). The postulated mechanism is disruption of small penetrating arterioles at the base of the brain secondary to shear-strain forces.[13,29] This is a relatively uncommon finding which is seen in about 3 to 4.5 percent of severely head injured patients. It usually occurs in association with other primary injuries, such as DAI, and thus has a poor prognosis.[24]

Brainstem Injury

The most common location for acute posttraumatic brainstem injury is the dorsolateral aspect of the upper midbrain (Fig. 9-4). This injury occurs as the brainstem strikes the edge of the tentorium. Only 10 percent of

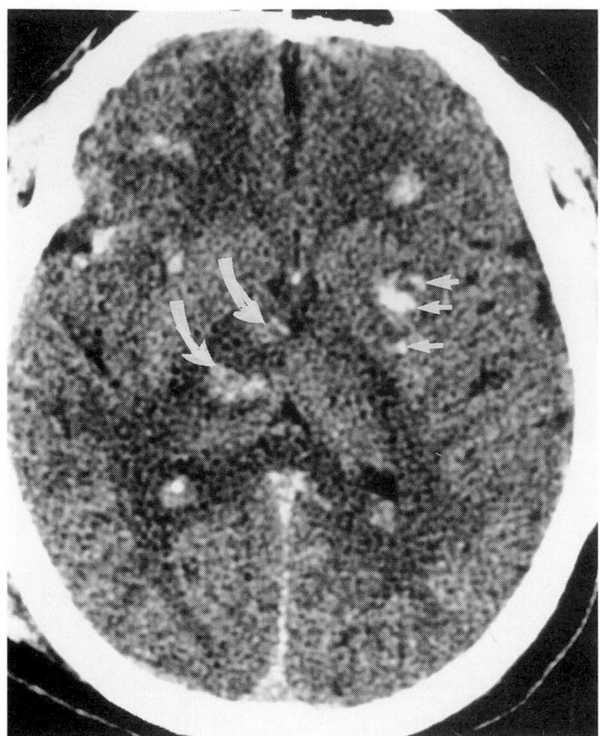

Figure 9-3. Noncontrast CT shows deep hemorrhages in the right thalamus (large arrows) and left putamen (small arrows). Bifrontal gray–white matter junction shearing injuries are also seen.

brainstem injuries are clearly detected on CT, and they are usually associated with DAI. These lesions may be confused with Duret's hemorrhages, which are caused by prolonged transtentorial herniation. However, Duret's hemorrhages are usually located in the midline in the midbrain and pontine tegmentum.[30,31]

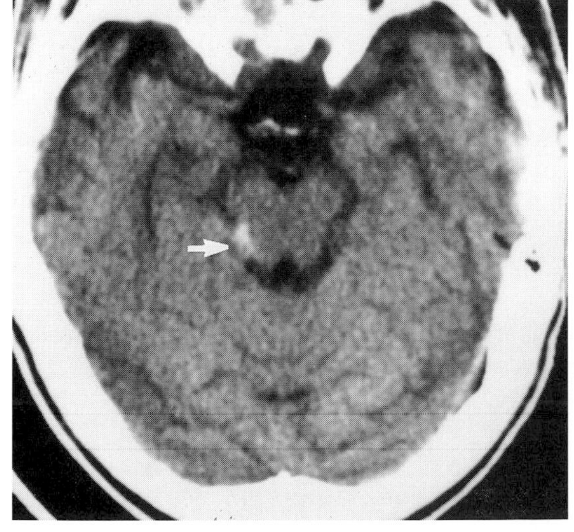

Figure 9-4. Noncontrast CT shows a focal hemorrhage involving the dorsolateral aspect of the brainstem (arrow).

EXTRAAXIAL COLLECTIONS

Blood or air may accumulate between the brain and the inner table of the skull. The pressure exerted by such collections can cause further injury to the brain. This section discusses the important imaging features of subdural and epidural hematomas and pneumocephalus.

SUBDURAL HEMATOMAS

Posttraumatic subdural hematomas (SDHs) most commonly result from tearing of the bridging veins by rapid acceleration/deceleration of the head. They are easily recognized on CT as extraaxial, crescentic, homogeneously hyperdense collections which conform to the cerebral surface (Fig. 9-5). Their mass effect is gauged by the degree of sulcal effacement, inward buckling of the gray–white matter interface, and midline shift. Although SDHs extend across suture lines, they do not cross the midline because they are fixed by sites of dural attachment (falx and tentorium).[32,33]

SDHs over 5 mm wide are usually clearly identified on CT. Smaller collections and occasionally larger ones occurring at the vertex may be missed because of partial volume effects. Occasionally, an acute SDH has a biconvex inner margin, mimicking the appearance of an epidural hematoma. This is usually seen during the first 6 h after an injury. It is thought to be caused by continued bleeding which for unknown reasons cannot spread farther in the subdural space.[34]

The density of an acute SDH is directly related to its hemoglobin content. Clot retraction contributes little to the progressive increase in density that occurs during the first 72 h after trauma. A gradual loss of the serum trapped within the mesh of a normal clot is the most likely basis for this observation. Over time, there is lysis of erythrocytes, protein removal, and progressive osmotic dilution; this results in a progressive loss of density on CT images. Thus, the SDH becomes progressively isodense (with respect to gray matter) over the first 2 to 3 weeks. By the fourth week, the SDH is generally hypodense compared with the gray matter. However, isodense SDH collections have been seen up to 10 weeks after trauma.[33] Thus, absolute reliance on CT density alone can lead to an inaccurate estimation of the age of an SDH. Several other pitfalls are associated with determining the age of an SDH by CT density criteria. An acute SDH can appear isodense to gray matter if the hemoglobin concentration does not increase the density to a level greater than that of the adjacent gray matter. This occurs if the SDH is formed from blood with a hemoglobin concentration below 10 to 11 g/dl, an arachnoidal tear allows CSF to dilute the

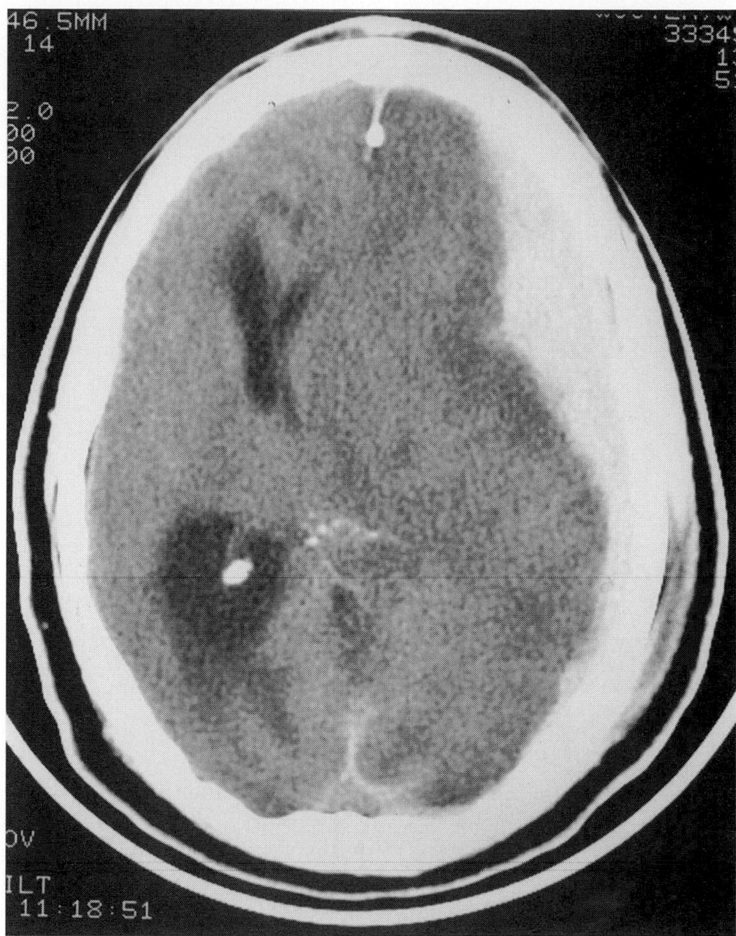

Figure 9-5. Noncontrast CT shows a left-sided homogeneously hyperdense subdural hematoma. Note the remarkable right-to-left shift of the midline structures caused by transfalcine herniation of the brain.

hematoma, or acute rebleeding into a chronic (hypodense) subdural collection takes place.[32,35,36]

An isodense SDH can be difficult to detect, especially on earlier-generation CT scanners. Careful evaluation of the cerebral convexities for evidence of extraaxial mass effect is necessary. Effaced sulci, distortion of the ipsilateral ventricle, and inward displacement of the white matter are all useful signs which should alert one to the presence of an SDH (Fig. 9-6).

Mixed-density acute subdural hematomas (MDSDHs) can also occur. In one study, this type of SDH was present in more than 30 percent of patients with an SDH. MDSDHs show associated focal, well-defined zones which are isodense to gray matter in marginal, irregular, or laminar patterns within the hyperdense hematoma[32] (Fig. 9-7). MDSDHs tend to be larger than hyperdense SDHs and are associated with a greater degree of midline shift and a higher mortality rate. Several theories have been proposed as possible explanations for this radiographic appearance.[32] Serum extrusion during the early phase of clot retraction and an associated arachnoidal tear are the most likely explanations. Acute rebleeding into a chronic subdural collection can mimic an MDSDH, but the presence of an ill-defined interface between the chronic and acute portions of the collection usually helps distinguish between the two.[32]

A sedimentation level may form in the dependent portion of an SDH if the patient is confined to bed in a brow-up position. The administration of contrast medium before CT may help define the lateral extent of the hypodense SDH by visualizing the displaced brain surfaces adjacent to the SDH.[10,11] The membrane of the SDH lies adjacent to the inner table of the skull and over the cortical surface (Fig. 9-8).

The incidence of delayed SDH varies from 0.2 to 10 percent.[37,38] This complication can be seen even in the absence of clinical deterioration or changes in intracranial pressure. It may occur after decompressive surgery or any other alteration of the intracranial equilibrium. Thus, a repeat CT scan within 24 h after admission for a closed head injury or decompressive surgery is often useful.[37,38]

Epidural Hematomas

Epidural hematomas (EDHs) are relatively less common. They usually result from a lacerated meningeal

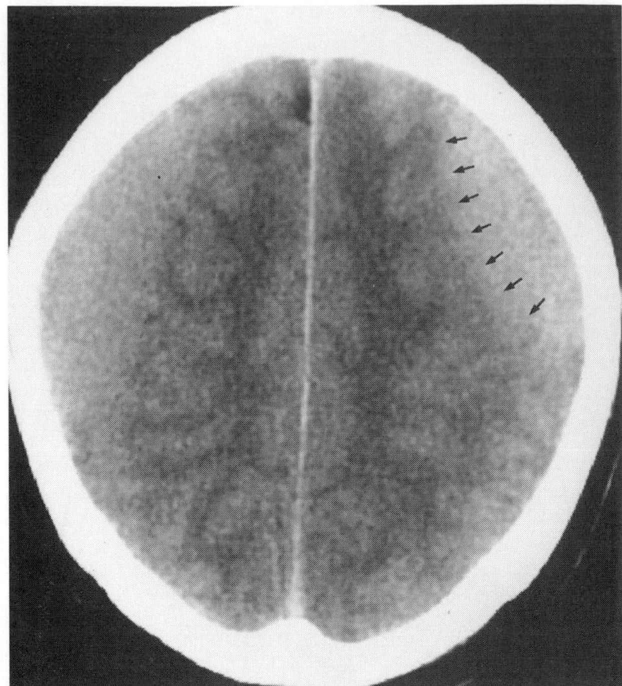

Figure 9-6. Noncontrast CT shows a bilateral isodense subdural collection at the anterior aspect of the vertex. Note the inward buckling of the cortex with preservation of the gray–white matter junction region. The surface of the displaced left cerebral hemisphere has been marked with arrows.

vessel or dural sinus but may result from bleeding from a fracture alone. An associated fracture is found in more than 95 percent of cases. However, in young children, because of calvarial plasticity, EDH can occur in the absence of a fracture. Blood accumulates in the epidural space and strips the dura away from the inner table of the skull.

EDHs are localized to the temporoparietal region in 60 to 80 percent of patients as a result of damage to the anterior or posterior branches of the middle meningeal artery as they run across the squamosal portion of the temporal bone. Frontal and parieto-occipital EDHs are less common. In the posterior fossa, 85 percent of EDHs result from a torn dural sinus. When an EDH occurs at the vertex, the superior sagittal sinus is usually involved.[33,39]

On CT, EDH forms an extraaxial lentiform, or biconvex, hyperdense collection which can cross the midline but is limited by bony sutures (Fig. 9-9*A* and *B*). The density of an EDH on CT depends on the factors previously described for an SDH. The CT appearance also depends on the source of the bleeding (arterial or venous), the time interval between the injury and CT, the severity of the hemorrhage, and the degree of clot organization or breakdown. Although an EDH is usually homogeneously hyperdense, visualization of focal isodensity or hypodensity zones within the hematoma usually indicates the presence of active bleeding or a coagulopathy (Fig. 9-10). An irregular hypodense "swirl" correlates with active bleeding in the majority of cases.[39] An isodense delayed EDH after surgery is a rare occurrence.[38,40,41]

EDHs are usually stable lesions that attain their maximum size within minutes after the initial injury. However, exceptions can occur during the first 24 h, presumably secondary to rebleeding or continuous oozing of blood (Fig. 9-11*A* and *B*). Enlarging EDHs have been reported as late as 2 weeks after head trauma. This subacute increase in size is probably related to osmotic factors rather than rebleeding since there is always an associated decrease in CT density within the EDH. Air collections within an EDH usually indicate the presence of either a skull or a mastoid air cell fracture. The presence of large quantities of air can contribute to the development of a delayed mass effect.

Although CT has lowered the morbidity and mortality from EDH by facilitating diagnosis and treatment, many small asymptomatic EDHs are being detected. Nonsurgical management of these lesions is appropriate when they are relatively small, have minimal associated mass effect, and are discovered several hours or days after an injury. However, they require careful observation and frequent follow-up CT scans to rule out a progressive increase in the size of the lesions.[42,43]

PNEUMOCEPHALUS

Posttraumatic pneumocephalus occurs most commonly in the subdural or subarachnoid spaces but may be found in the epidural or intraparenchymal compartments as well. Its significance derives from its association with fractures of the adjacent paranasal sinuses or mastoid air cells which can lead to CSF fistulas. Pneumocephalus can be seen in up to 13 percent of patients with a closed head injury.[44] Posttraumatic pneumatoceles and tension pneumocephalus have been described.[45] Because of its extremely low attenuation value, as little as 0.5 ml of intracranial air can be detected.[46]

HEMORRHAGE INTO THE CEREBROSPINAL SPACES

When an acute subarachnoid hemorrhage (SAH) or intraventricular hemorrhage (IVH) occurs in the setting

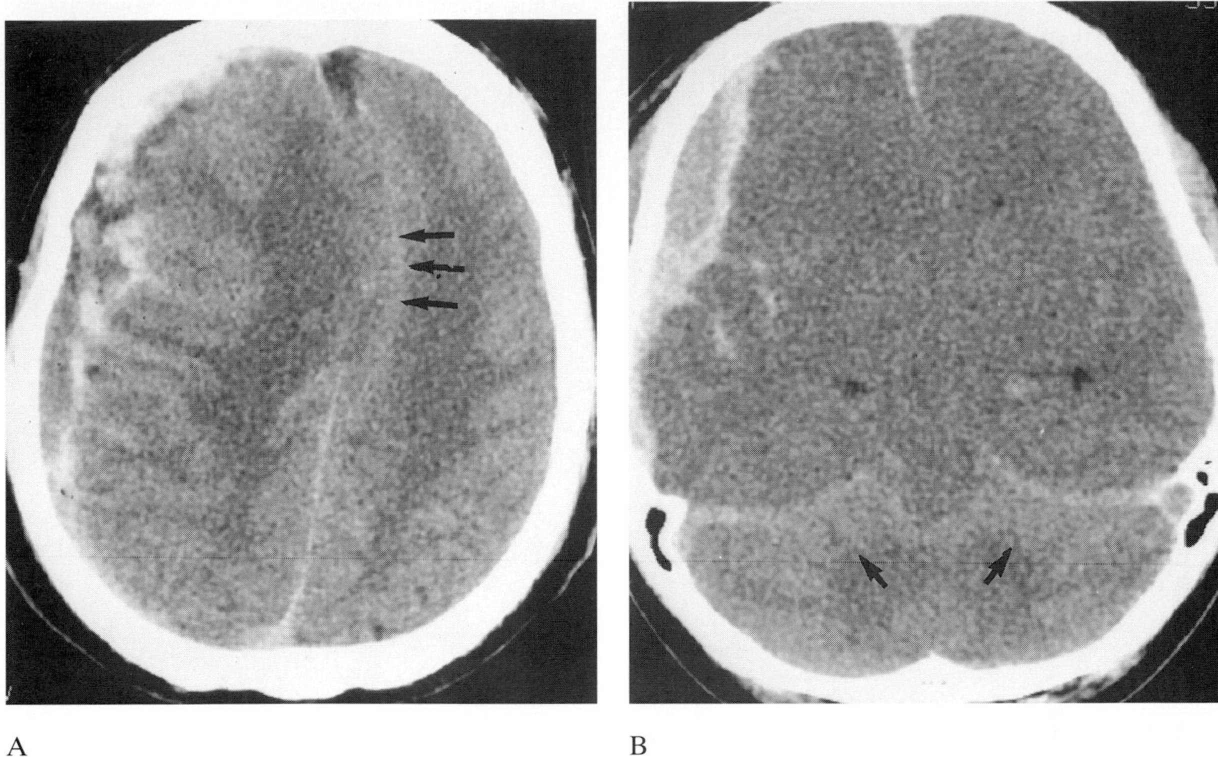

Figure 9-7. *A.* Noncontrast CT of a mixed-density right subdural hematoma. Mass effect has resulted in subfalcine herniation and midline shift. Arrows mark the surface of the displaced right cingulate gyrus. Note the absence of the normally CSF-filled convexity sulci as a result of the mass effect and cerebral swelling. *B.* Right frontal MDSDH with diffuse supratentorial brain swelling. Note both the diffuse hypodensity and the loss of discrimination of the gray–white matter junction in the cerebral hemispheres. The normal gray–white matter junction in the cerebellum is marked for comparison. Also note the absence of the CSF suprasellar and perimesencephalic cisterns. Figure 9-2 shows their normal appearance at a slightly higher level.

of trauma, it is usually associated with another intracranial pathological condition. SAH is identified as loss of the normal CSF hypodensity in the sulci or cisterns. Patients with mild SAH may show only an isodense obliteration of the basal cisterns. This may mimic cerebral swelling by simulating sulcal or cisternal effacement.[22–24] Areas of increased attenuation in the sulci, basal cisterns, or sylvian and interhemispheric fissures may be seen in cases of more severe SAH (Fig. 9-12).

The CT findings of SAH persist for only a few days because blood is rapidly cleared from the subarachnoid space. If the history of trauma is not clear, angiography is frequently necessary to exclude the presence of a ruptured aneurysm.[33]

As many as 25 percent of patients with severe head injury have IVH (Fig. 9-12). Focal and diffuse areas of high attenuation are identified within the ventricles in these cases. Blood tends to settle in the dependent portions of the ventricles (i.e., the occipital horns) where a CSF-blood level forms. In the absence of rebleeding, this clears rapidly, and IVH is rarely seen after about 1 week.

SECONDARY EFFECTS OF INTRACRANIAL TRAUMA

The secondary effects of a closed head injury occur when a space-occupying intracerebral and/or extraaxial mass rapidly forms within the closed confines of the skull. Cerebral herniation, posttraumatic cerebral infarction, and/or pressure necrosis of the brain can result. CSF fistulas, pneumocephalus, and posttraumatic encephaloceles are secondary events which occur if there is a skull fracture with an associated dural laceration.

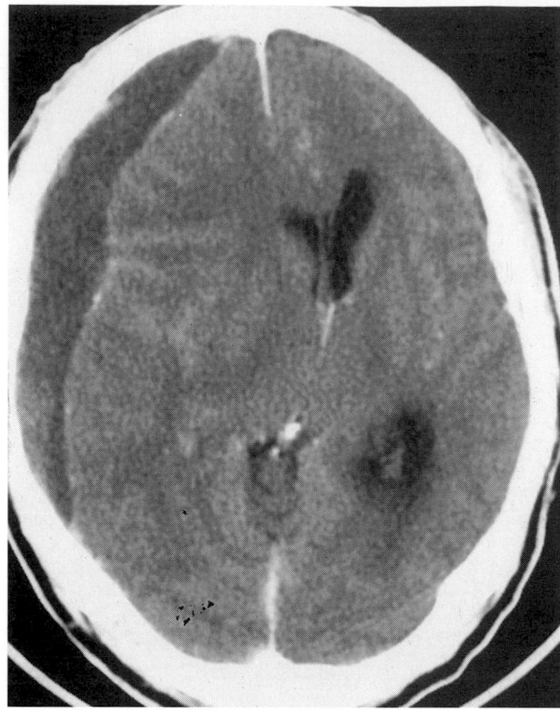

Figure 9-8. Contrast-enhanced CT of a right frontotemporal chronic subdural hematoma. Note the smooth enhancement along the inner margins of the collection and the large right-to-left shift.

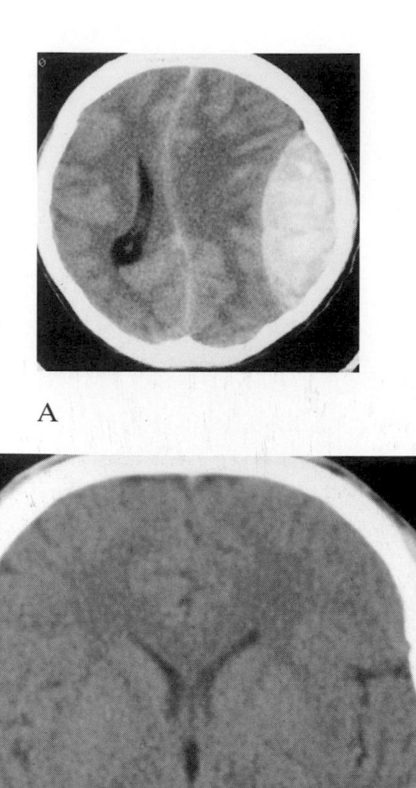

Figure 9-9. *A.* Noncontrast CT of an acute epidural hematoma resulting in mass effect and obliteration of the body of the left lateral ventricle. The anteroposterior extension of the hematoma is limited by the coronal suture (anteriorly) and the lambdoid suture (posteriorly). *B.* Noncontrast CT of a posterior fossa epidural hematoma (arrows). An underlying left occipital skull fracture was identified on the bone windows (not shown).

BRAIN HERNIATIONS

Cerebral herniation occurs when a space-occupying lesion displaces normal brain. There are five types of displacements: subfalcine, descending transtentorial, ascending transtentorial, transalar, and tonsillar herniations. All these displacements of brain cause compression or distortion of adjacent blood vessels which can result in specific patterns of ischemic brain injury.[47–52]

SUBFALCINE HERNIATION

Subfalcine herniation describes a midline shift which displaces the cingulate gyrus beneath the falx (Fig. 9-13). Midline shift is usually determined by drawing a line from the crista galli to the internal occipital protuberance and measuring the distance between the midline structures (usually the septum pellucidum and/or the pineal gland) and this landmark. This measurement is compared to the scale on the scan image to obtain the true degree of shift. A midline shift of 5 mm or more is considered significant from a surgical standpoint. A lesion causing such shift is classified as a category IV lesion and is associated with a 50 percent mortality rate (Table 9-1).[1]

Initially, there is compression of the ipsilateral lateral ventricle by the subfalcine herniation. As the mass effect increases, the *contralateral* ventricle may dilate because of mechanical obstruction of the foramen of Monro. Unilateral or bilateral infarction in the distribution of the anterior cerebral artery (ACA) may occur as it is pushed across the midline and/or compressed against the free margin of the falx. Individual anatomic varia-

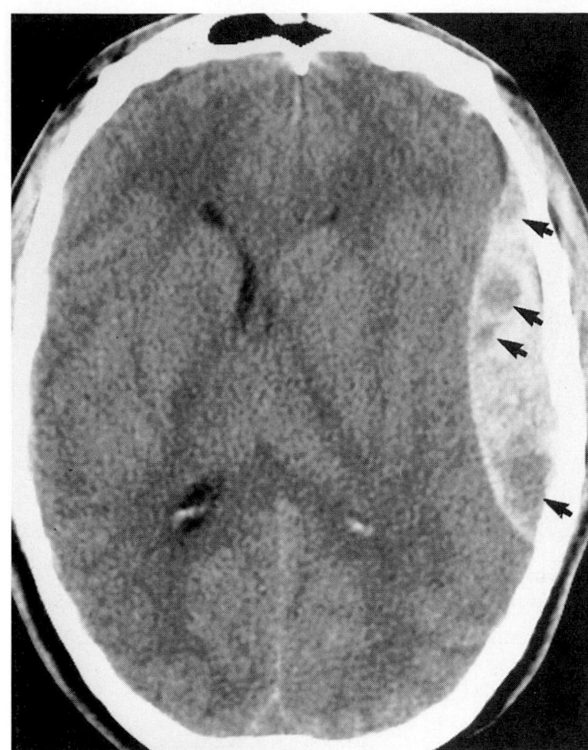

Figure 9-10. Noncontrast CT shows a large nonhomogeneous acute left epidural hematoma. Focal hypodensities within the hematoma (arrows) represent unclotted blood. Note the effacement of the left lateral ventricle and the shift from left to right.

tions in the relationship of the falx to the pericallosal or callosomarginal arteries determine the exact site of vascular injury.[47–50]

Descending Transtentorial Herniation

Descending transtentorial herniation or uncal herniation occurs as a result of medial and inferior displacement of the uncus and the parahippocampal gyrus of the temporal lobe through the tentorial notch. It is seen on CT as an encroachment on the lateral aspect of the ipsilateral suprasellar cistern. In severe cases, the brainstem is displaced and the contralateral cerebral peduncle is compressed against the adjacent tentorial incisura, resulting in the Kernohan's notch syndrome. Rotation of the brainstem and widening of the ipsilateral perimesencephalic cistern allow the medial temporal lobe to descend into the cerebellopontine angle cistern. Complete uncal herniation results in obliteration of the suprasellar and perimesencephalic cisterns[51,52] (Fig. 9-13).

Again, individual anatomic variations in the incisura and its relationship to the midbrain and the adjacent

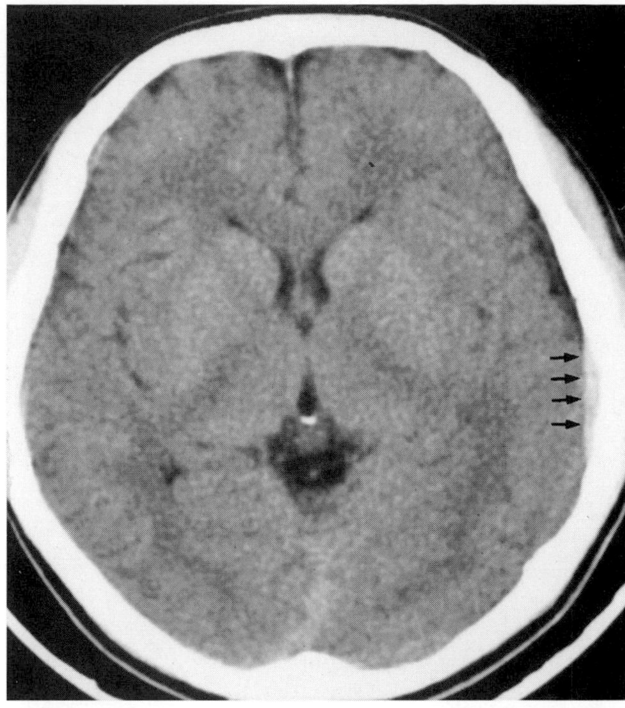

A

B

Figure 9-11. *A.* Noncontrast CT on admission shows a small extraaxial hematoma along the left temporal convexity (arrows). The associated fracture is not shown. *B.* Follow-up noncontrast CT of the same patient 10 h later shows a large epidural hematoma with midline shift. Note that the collection is limited by the coronal and lambdoid sutures.

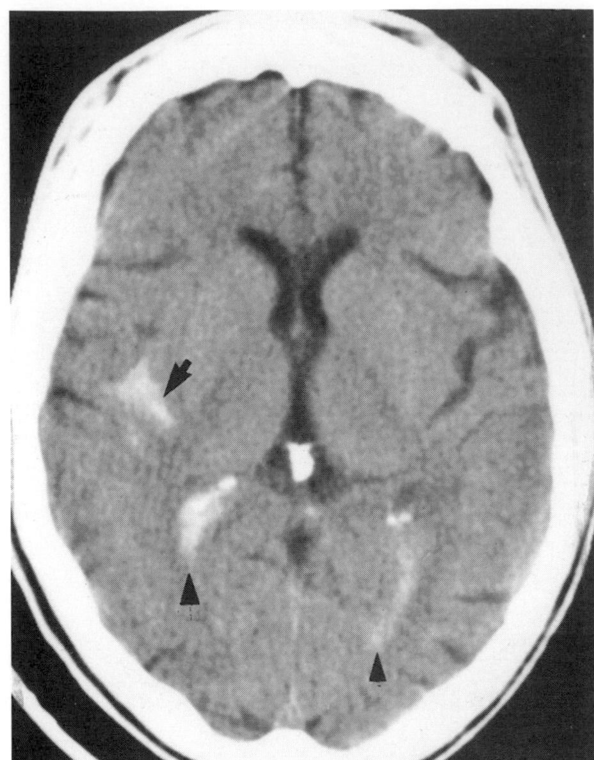

Figure 9-12. Nonenhanced CT shows a subarachnoid hemorrhage in the right sylvian fissure (arrow) and blood within the occipital horns of the lateral ventricles (arrowheads).

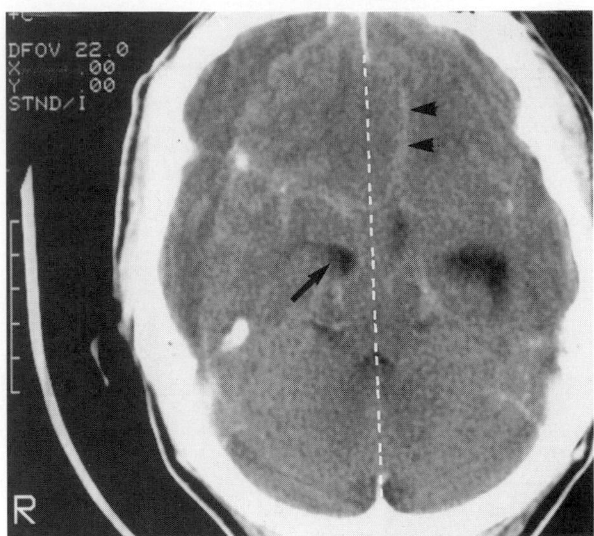

Figure 9-13. Contrast-enhanced CT of a right frontotemporal chronic SDH resulting in uncal herniation. The right temporal horn is displaced medially (arrow). Effacement of the suprasellar cistern is evident. Subfalcine herniation from right to left is also present (see arrowheads on interhemispheric fissure). Note that a line has been drawn from the anterior falx (just above its attachment to the crista galli) and the internal occipital protuberance. The distance between this landmark and the displaced interhemispheric fissure (arrowheads) can be measured and compared to the 1-cm scale marker on the left side of this image. In this case, there is a 1-cm transfalcine herniation.

vasculature determine the pattern of occlusive vascular compromise. The most commonly recognized ischemic injury is in the distribution of the posterior cerebral arteries (PCAs). Ipsilateral or contralateral occipital lobe infarctions result from direct compression by the herniating mass or compression of the PCA against the tentorial incisura, respectively. This can result in cortical blindness and Anton's syndrome. If the ipsilateral anterior choroidal artery is compressed, ischemic injury to the posterior limb of the internal capsule occurs. However, compression of the adjacent oculomotor (third) nerve usually leads to ipsilateral pupillary dilatation.[47,52]

Ascending Transtentorial Herniation

Ascending transtentorial herniation is much less common than the descending variety but may occur in two clinical situations. It can be the direct effect of a posterior fossa mass or may occur after rapid decompression of a supratentorial space-occupying lesion. In the first case, the vermis ascends to obliterate the quadrigeminal plate and/or superior cerebellar cisterns. CT detects flattening or distortion of the posterior aspect of the quadrigeminal plate cistern (Fig. 9-14). Eventually, the cistern develops an anterior rather than a posterior convexity. Finally, compression of the cerebral aqueduct causes hydrocephalus of the third and lateral ventricles.

Transalar Herniation

Transalar herniation refers to brain shifts across the sphenoid wing (ala). These shifts may be caused by anterior cranial fossa masses (descending) or middle cranial fossa masses (ascending). Anterior or posterior bowing of the ipsilateral, horizontal portion of the sylvian fissure which contains the horizontal (M1) segments of the middle cerebral artery (MCA) may be seen. This finding is visualized on CT if there is acute perisylvian subarachnoid blood or if the horizontal (M1) segment of the MCA is identified after contrast enhancement. Infarctions in the distribution of both anterior and middle cerebral artery branches have been described in cases of severe transalar herniation.[47,53]

Tonsillar Herniation

Tonsillar herniation results from an enlarging posterior fossa mass or as a late sequela of supratentorial cerebral

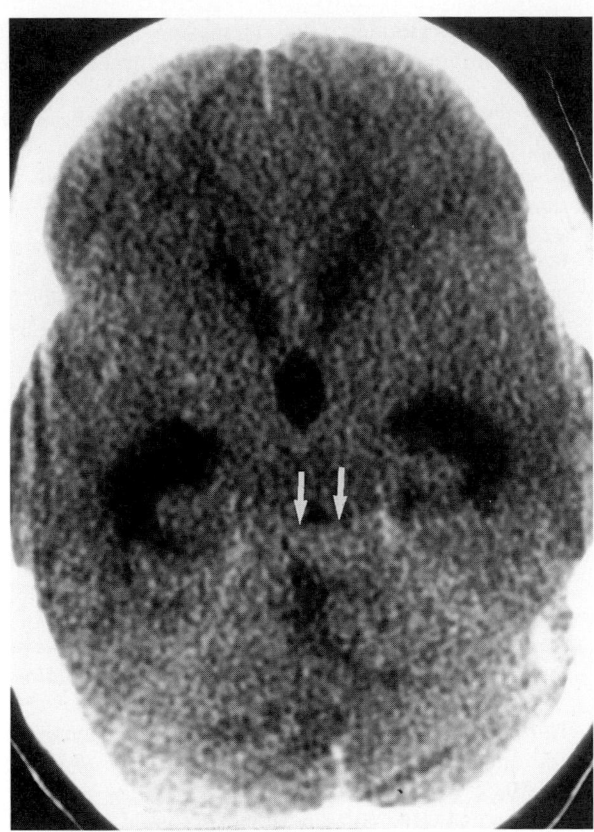

Figure 9-14. Nonenhanced CT of a patient with upward transtentorial herniation caused by a posterior fossa mass (not shown). There is effacement of the quadrigeminal plate cistern by the ascending vermis (arrows).

swelling. CT scans demonstrate crowding of the cisterna magna by the downward displacement of the cerebellar tonsils. This results in obliteration of the CSF cisterns around the medulla. Obstructive hydrocephalus caused by obstruction of the fourth ventricle may occur. The ultimate result of tonsillar herniation is cardiopulmonary arrest due to brainstem compression.

Diffuse Cerebral Swelling

The diffuse cerebral swelling commonly seen in association with closed head injury is well visualized by CT. In this condition, the cerebral sulci are effaced, the gray–white matter interface is lost, and the basal cisterns are obliterated (Fig. 9-7). On normal soft tissue window settings, the cerebellum, the cerebral vasculature, and the dural surfaces (falx and tentorium) appear hyperdense against the background of diffusely swollen edematous hypodense brain. Descending transtentorial herniation is commonly present. As one would expect, patients with these findings have a high mortality rate.

Posttraumatic CSF Fistula

Posttraumatic cerebrospinal fistulas occur in up to 9 percent of patients with head injury. Spontaneous closure of these fistulas occurs in over 80 percent of cases. A persistent CSF leak is significant, however, because it may result in meningitis.

CT cisternography is the best available diagnostic procedure with which to identify the site of the leak. In this procedure, approximately 8 to 10 ml of concentrated water-soluble nonionic contrast medium is injected into the lumbar subarachnoid space and is directed by gravity to the region of interest in the skull. Thin coronal and axial CT sections are then performed as necessary with the patient in the position which causes maximum CSF leakage. New techniques such as digital subtraction cisternography and MRI-modified RARE (rapid acquisition and relaxation enhancement) imaging using heavy T_2 weighting may eventually replace CT cisternography as the imaging procedure of choice.[54–58]

References

1. Marshall LF, Marshall SB, Klauber MR, et al: A new classification of head injury based on computerized tomography. *J Neurosurg* 75:S14–S20, 1991.
2. Hackney DB: Skull radiography in the evaluation of acute head trauma: A survey of current practice. *Radiology* 181:711–714, 1991.
3. Thornbury JR, Campbell JA, Masters SJ, et al: Skull fracture and the low risk of intracranial sequelae in minor head trauma. *AJR* 143:661–664, 1984.
4. Feuerman T, Wackym PA, Gade GF, et al: Value of skull radiography, head computed tomographic scanning and admission for observation in cases of minor head injury. *Neurosurgery* 22:449–453, 1988.
5. Thornbury JR, Masters SJ, Campbell JA: Imaging recommendations for head trauma: A new comprehensive strategy. *AJR* 149:781–783, 1987.
6. Masters SJ, McClean PM, Argarese JS, et al: Skull x-ray examinations after head trauma. *N Engl J Med* 316:84–91, 1987.
7. Norman D, Price D, Boyd D, et al: Quantitative aspects of computed tomography of the blood and cerebrospinal fluid. *Radiology* 123:335–338, 1977.
8. New PFJ, Scott WR, Schnur JA, et al: Computerized axial tomography with the EMI scanner. *Radiology* 110:109–123, 1974.
9. New PFJ, Aronow S: Attenuation measurements of whole blood and blood fractions in computed tomography. *Radiology* 212:635–640, 1976.
10. Mauser HW, vanNieuwenhuizen O: Is contrast-enhanced CT indicated in acute head injury? *Neuroradiology* 26:31–32, 1984.
11. Boyko OB, Cooper DF, Grossman CB: Contrast-enhanced CT of acute isodense subdural hematoma. *AJNR* 12:341–343, 1991.

12. Holbourn AHS: Mechanics of head injuries. *Lancet* 2:438–441, 1943.
13. Adams JH, Mitchell DE, Graham DI, et al: Diffuse brain damage of immediate impact type: Its relationship to primary brainstem damage in head injury. *Brain* 100:489–502, 1977.
14. Adams JH, Doyle D, Graham DI, et al: Microscopic diffuse axonal injury in cases of head injury. *Med Sci Law* 25:265, 1985.
15. Adams JH, Doyle D, Graham DI, et al: Deep intracerebral basal ganglia haematomas in fatal non-missile head injury in man. *J Neurol Neurosurg Psychiatry* 49:1039, 1966.
16. Adams JH, Graham DI: *An Introduction to Neuropathology.* Edinburgh: Churchill Livingstone, 1988.
17. Adams JH, Graham DI, Gennarelli TA: Contemporary neuropathological considerations regarding brain damage in head injury, in Becker DP, Porlischeck JT (eds): *Central Nervous System Trauma Status Report.* NINCDS, 1985: 65.
18. Adams JH, Graham DI, Murray LS, et al: Diffuse axonal injury due to nonmissile head injury in humans: An analysis of 45 cases. *Ann Neurol* 12:557–563, 1982.
19. Blumbergs PC, Jones NR, North JB: Diffuse axonal injury in head trauma. *J Neurol Neurosurg Psychiatry* 5:838, 1989.
20. Gennarelli TA, Thebault LE, Adams JH, et al: Diffuse axonal injury and traumatic coma in the primate. *Ann Neurol* 12:564, 1982.
21. Adams JH: Pathology of nonmissile head injury, in Gentry LR (ed): *Neuroimaging Clinics of North America,* vol 1, no 2. Philadelphia: Saunders, 1991: 397–410.
22. Gentry LR: Primary neuronal injuries, in Gentry LR (ed): *Neuroimaging Clinics of North America,* vol 1, no 2. Philadelphia: Saunders, 1991: 411–432.
23. Gentry LR, Godersky JC, Thompson B: MR imaging of head trauma: Review of the distribution and radiopathologic features of traumatic lesions. *AJNR* 9:101–110, 1988.
24. Gentry LR, Godersky JC, Thompson B, et al: Prospective comparative study of intermediate-field MR and CT in the evaluation of closed head trauma. *AJNR* 9:91–100, 1988.
25. Groswasser Z, Reider-Groswasser I, Soroker N, et al: Magnetic resonance imaging in head injured patients with normal late computed tomography scans. *Surg Neurol* 27:331–337, 1987.
26. Hesselink JR, Dowd CF, Healy ME, et al: MR imaging of brain contusions: A comparative study with CT. *AJR* 150:1133–1142, 1988.
27. Macpherson M, Macpherson P, Jennett B: Evidence of intracranial contusion and haematoma in relation to the presence, site and type of skull fracture. *Clin Radiol* 42:321–326, 1990.
28. Zimmerman RA, Bilaniuk LT, Dolinskes AC, et al: Computed tomography of acute intracerebral hemorrhagic contusion. *Comput Tomogr* 1:271–288, 1977.
29. Macpherson P, Teasdale E, Dhaker S, et al: The significance of traumatic haematomas in the region of the basal ganglia. *J Neurol Neurosurg Psychiatry* 49:29–34, 1989.
30. Gentry LR, Godersky JC, Thompson BH: Traumatic brainstem injury: MR imaging. *Radiology* 171:177–187, 1987.
31. Tsai FY, Teal JS, Quinn MF, et al: CT of brainstem injury. *AJR* 134:717–723, 1980.
32. Reed D, Robertson WD, Graeb DA, et al: Acute subdural hematomas: Atypical CT findings. *AJNR* 7:417–421, 1986.
33. Cornelius RS, Gaskill MF, Lukin RR: Traumatic intracranial hemorrhage, in Gentry LR (ed): *Neuroimaging Clinics of North America,* vol 1, no 2. Philadelphia: Saunders, 1991: 433–441.
34. Braun J, Borovich B, Guilburd JN, et al: Acute subdural hematoma mimicking epidural hematoma on CT. *AJNR* 8:171–173, 1987.
35. Smith WP, Batnitzky S, Rengachary SS: Acute isodense subdural hematomas: A problem in anemic patients. *AJR* 136:543–546, 1981.
36. Kaufman HH, Singer JM, Sadhu VK, et al: Isodense acute subdural hematoma. *J Comput Assist Tomogr* 4:557–559, 1980.
37. Lesoin F, Viaud C, Pruvo J, et al: Traumatic and alternating delayed intracranial hematomas. *Neuroradiology* 26:515–516, 1984.
38. Borovich B, Braun J, Guilburd N, et al: Delayed onset of traumatic extradural hematoma. *J Neurosurg* 63:30–34, 1985.
39. Zimmerman RA, Bilaniuk LT: Computed tomographic staging of traumatic epidural bleeding. *Radiology* 144:809–812, 1982.
40. Thibodeau M, Melanson D, Ethier R: Acute epidural hematoma following decompressive surgery of a subdural hematoma. *J Can Assoc Radiol* 38:52–53, 1987.
41. DiRocco A, Ellis SJ, Landes C: Delayed epidural hematoma. *Neuroradiology* 33:253–254, 1991.
42. Hamilton M, Wallace C: Nonoperative management of acute epidural hematoma diagnosed by CT: The neuroradiologist's role. *AJNR* 13:853–859, 1992.
43. Saghert O, Ribas GC, Jane JA: Nonoperative management of acute epidural hematoma diagnosed by CT: The neuroradiologist's role. *AJNR* 13:860–862, 1992.
44. Jacobs JB, Persky MS: Traumatic pneumocephalus. *Laryngoscope* 90:515–521, 1980.
45. Briggs M: Traumatic pneumocephalus. *Br J Surg* 61:307–312, 1974.
46. Osborn AG, Daines JH, Wing SD, et al: Intracranial air on computerized tomography. *J Neurosurg* 48:355–359, 1978.
47. Osborn AG: Secondary effects of intracranial trauma, in Gentry LR (ed): *Neuroimaging Clinics of North America,* vol 1, no 2. Philadelphia: Saunders, 1991:
48. Sohn D, Levine S: Frontal lobe infarcts caused by brain herniation. *Arch Pathol* 84:509–512, 1967.
49. Rothfus WE, Goldberg AL, Tabaas JH, et al: Callosomarginal infarction secondary to transfalcial herniation. *AJNR* 8:1073–1076, 1987.
50. Galligioni F, Bernardi R, Mingrino S: Anatomic variation of the height of the falx cerebri: Its relationship to displacement of the anterior cerebral artery in frontal space-occupying lesion. *AJR* 106:273–278, 1969.

51. Zimmerman RD, Yurberg E, Russell EJ, et al: Falx and interhemispheric fissure on axial CT: I. Normal anatomy. *AJNR* 189:899–904, 1982.
52. Osborn AG: Diagnosis of descending transtentorial herniation by cranial computed tomography. *Radiology* 123:93–96, 1977.
53. Lindenberg R: Compression of brain arteries as pathogenic factor for tissue necrosis and their areas of predilection. *J Neuropathol Exp Neurol* 14:223–243, 1955.
54. Wakhloo AK, vanVelthoven V, Schumacher M, et al: Evaluation of MR imaging, digital subtraction cisternography, and CT cisternography in diagnosing CSF fistula. *Acta Neurochir* (*Wien*) 111:119–127, 1991.
55. Byrne JV, Ingram CE, MacVicar C, et al: Digital subtraction cisternography: A new approach to fistula localisation in cerebrospinal fluid rhinorrhoea. *J Neurol Neurosurg Psychiatry* 53:1072–1075, 1990.
56. Ozgen T, Tekkok IH, Cila A, et al: CT cisternography in evaluation of cerebrospinal fluid rhinorrhea. *Neuroradiology* 32:481–484, 1990.
57. Rothfus WE, Deeb ZL, Daffner RH, et al: Head-hanging CT: An alternative method for evaluating traumatic CSF rhinorrhea. *AJNR* 8:155–156, 1987.
58. Prere J, Puech JL, Derover N, et al: *J Neuroradiol* 13:278–285, 1986.

CHAPTER 10

MAGNETIC RESONANCE IMAGING IN HEAD INJURY

Linda Hankins
Katherine H. Taber
Joel Yeakley
L. Anne Hayman

SYNOPSIS

Magnetic resonance (MR) imaging is more sensitive than computed tomography (CT) in evaluating the overall extent of brain damage, especially nonhemorrhagic diffuse axonal injuries (DAI) and small extraaxial hematomas. This feature may help in assessing the prognosis and rehabilitation potential of head-injured patients.[1–4] *It has not replaced CT in the evaluation of acute head injuries because: (1) CT detects all surgically significant lesions; (2) high-field MR units (greater than 0.5T) require special monitoring equipment to assess vital signs; and (3) MR is more motion-sensitive and takes longer than a CT scan. Nevertheless, MR can be helpful in assessing and monitoring brain injuries undetected by CT. Currently, MR has a role in patients with prolonged unconsciousness or focal neurological deficits that are not explained by their CT images. The optimal MR imaging techniques for evaluating these patients are discussed.*

INTRODUCTION

Magnetic resonance (MR) is more sensitive than computed tomography (CT) for the detection of acute abnormalities and delayed sequelae of head trauma.[1–14] If there is a focal neurological deficit not explained by CT, or if there is a prolonged period of unconsciousness, MR examination should be performed.

In the acute setting, CT remains the most frequently used imaging exam for several reasons. It detects almost all surgically significant lesions, costs less than MR, and it is widely available. In addition, CT is currently safer because it usually can be performed within 5 to 10 min while a brain MR takes approximately 30 min with conventional T1-weighted (T1W) and T2-weighted (T2W) spin echo (SE) scanning techniques. Other factors limiting the use of MR in acute trauma include the need for specialized life-support equipment and monitoring devices that can function in a high magnetic field without distorting the MR images. Also, the MR scanner frequently is some distance from the emergency room, and transportation of acutely injured patients is often undesirable.

The limited visualization of acute blood products on MR compared to CT has been cited as an additional reason for obtaining a CT in acutely traumatized patients. The biochemical/physical basis for the MR signal intensities observed in hemorrhage has been the subject of much speculation. The current theory implicates the presence of "deoxyhemoglobin" within intact red blood cells (RBCs) as the cause of the distinctive low signal seen on standard T2W SE images.[15–17] Other contributing factors such as dehydration of the RBCs[18,19] have been proposed.[20] The loss of RBC integrity and the formation of methemoglobin is thought to cause the bright signal commonly seen on both T1W and T2W SE MR images of subacute hemorrhage. The accumulation of hemosiderin at the site of chronic hemorrhage is easily detected as low signal on T2W SE images.

This perceived limitation of MR in detecting acute hematomas is largely overcome by using indirect signs, such as local edema and mass effect, to facilitate the diagnosis of brain injury. The optimal MR techniques for evaluating head trauma are discussed in the following section.

Technical Considerations in MR Imaging

Spin echo (SE) vs. fast spin echo (FSE)

A major disadvantage of MR compared with CT is the lengthy examination time. The newer, fast spin echo (FSE) MR techniques have decreased scan times from 15 to 20 min to 3 to 5 min for the T2W images. However, FSE MR techniques may be less sensitive to acute blood than is conventional SE, and thus less useful in the acute setting. A recent study comparing the contrast/noise on conventional SE and FSE companion images concluded that they were similar for lesions with a high signal intensity, but that the FSE was inferior to conventional SE for detection of small, low-intensity lesions (i.e., acute blood).[22] These lesions lacked surrounding edema to provide a contrasting background. Another study concludes that SE and FSE are comparable for imaging of blood, but this conclusion was based on signal-to-noise measurements and on clinical reading of the images.[23] The absolute signal intensities were almost identical in the "deoxyhemoglobin" of blood and white matter. Thus, the "hypointense" hemorrhage was identified on FSE by its contrast with the surrounding bright signal (edema and/or methemoglobin), rather than with brain.

Gradient echo (GE)

An alternative method for rapidly obtaining MR images is to use gradient echo (GE) images. These techniques are quite sensitive to magnetic susceptibility variations. Based on this sensitivity, it has been suggested that GE MR images should allow reliable visualization of blood.[24] In animal studies, hematomas were hypointense to brain and easily identified from the earliest timepoints on GE sequences.[25,26] This finding has also been reported in clinical studies.[24,27–29] However, hematomas are occasionally of intermediate or high signal intensity on GE images.[27] In addition, artifacts resulting from susceptibility gradients at interfaces between brain and surrounding structures (i.e., skull base) can cause lesions to be missed with this technique.

Low vs. high magnetic field strength

It is commonly accepted that hematomas are more reliably visualized at high (1.5T) than low (≤0.5T) magnetic field strength. Two major factors allow better delinea-

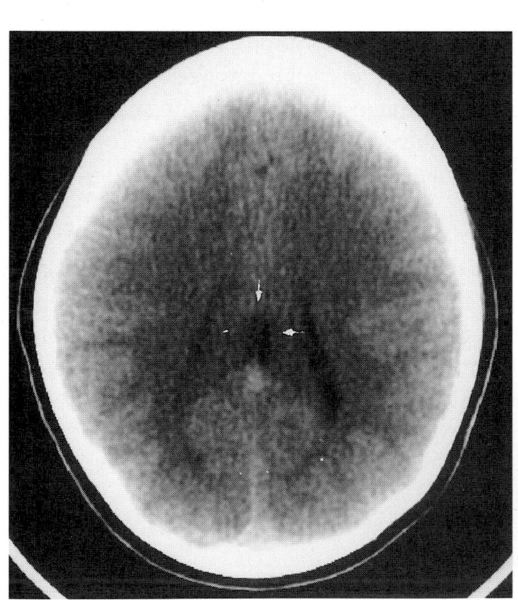

A

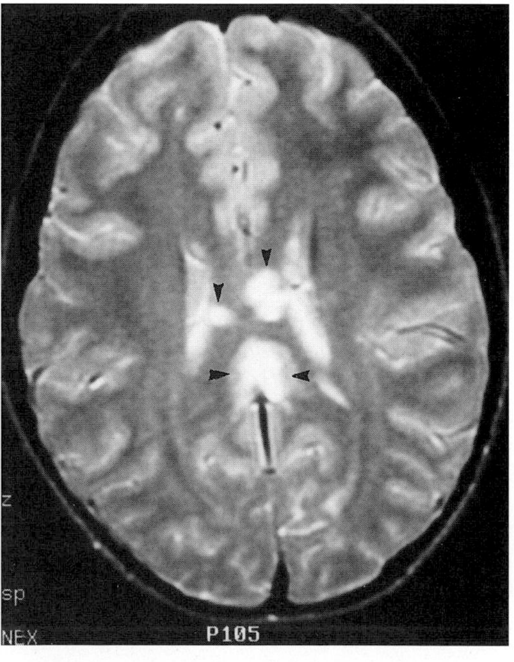

B

Figure 10-1*A*,*B*. Acute nonhemorrhagic shearing injury. Axial CT scans (*A*) show a subtle zone of hypodensity (*arrow*) in the corpus callosum secondary to a nonhemorrhagic shearing injury. Note the absence of intraventricular blood. Companion axial T2W SE MR scan (*B*) clearly shows edema at the site of shearing injury in the corpus callosum (*arrowheads*).

tion of lesions at higher magnetic field strength. One important factor is image resolution. The signal-to-noise increases with increasing magnetic field strength. As a result, images acquired at high magnetic field strength have higher resolution and, therefore, can theoretically identify smaller hematomas. Not all studies support the position that pathology will be missed on lower field strength images.[30]

Increasing the magnetic field strength also increases the effect of paramagnetic species (intracellular deoxyhemoglobin and methemoglobin) on the MR signal intensity. As a result, the effect of deoxyhemoglobin within a hematoma will be greater at 1.5T than at 0.5T. The differences in lesion appearance across field strength have been attributed primarily to this effect. Several reports indicate that a hematoma can have a hypointense appearance even at quite low magnetic field strength (0.064T), so the issue of whether the presence of intracellular deoxyhemoglobin is needed for detection cannot be considered completely resolved.[30,31]

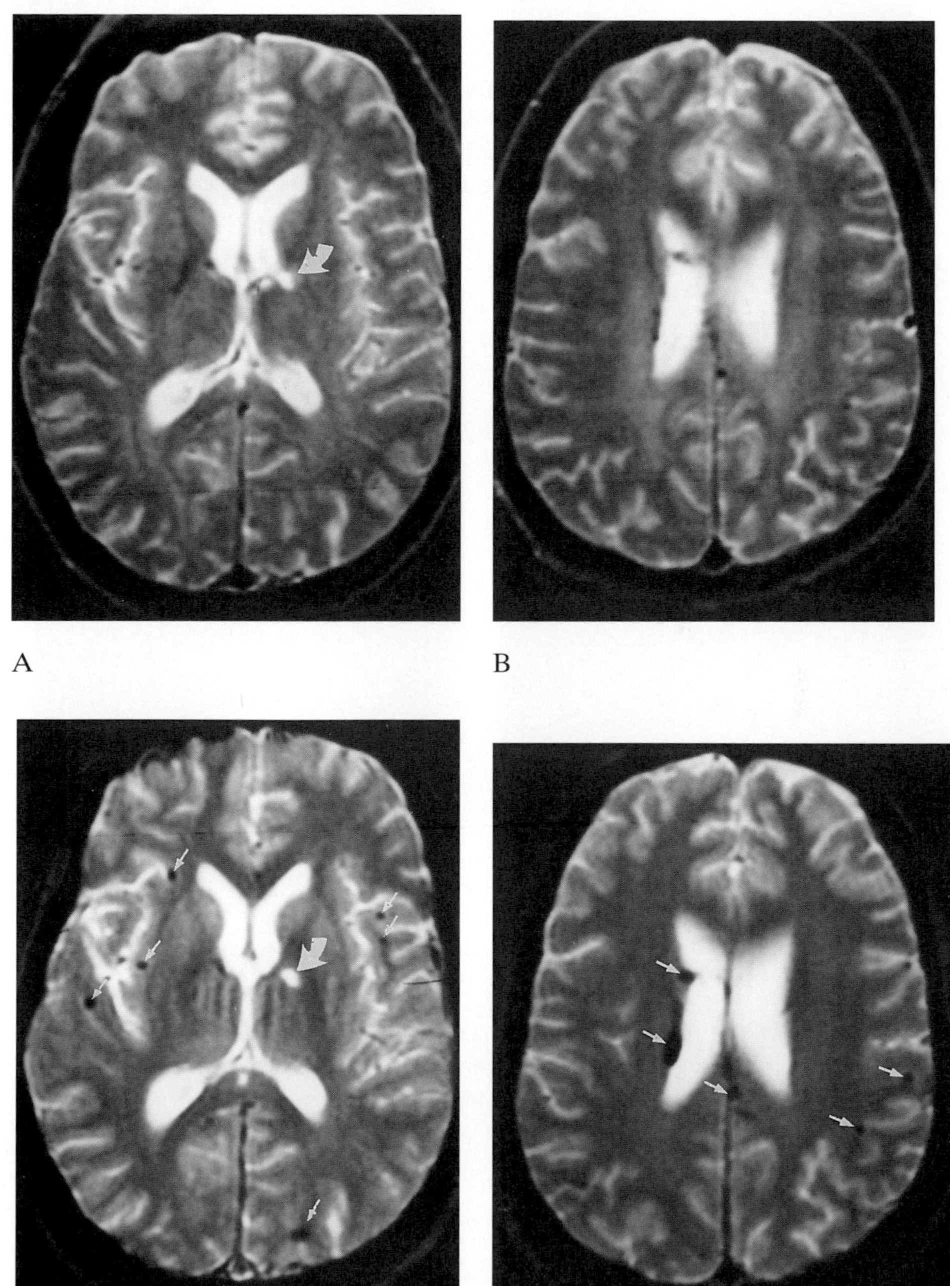

Figure 10-2*A–D*. Numerous acute small hemorrhagic injuries and a single nonhemorrhagic shearing injury. Axial T2W MR scans (*A*,*B*) show hemorrhagic shearing injuries less well than the companion GE sequences (*C*,*D*) (*arrows*). The nonhemorrhagic shearing injury in the genu of the right internal capsule is marked by a *curved arrow* in (*A*) and (*C*).

Optimal clinical MR examination

At our institutions MR scans are performed by obtaining the following sequences on a 1.5T MR unit (Signa, General Electric Company). A localizing sagittal T1W SE image is performed. This is followed by an axial double echo spin density (SD) and T2W SE image set. The latter image is needed to detect the hypointensity characteristic of acute blood products. If a coronal view is needed, it is obtained by using a T2W FSE image. Finally, an axial GE scan is done to detect small regions of blood.

Clinical Considerations

In this chapter, the MR appearance of the most common types of head injuries will be discussed. These include: (1) primary neuronal injuries; (2) extraaxial collections; (3) hemorrhage into the cerebrospinal fluid (CSF) spaces; and (4) primary vascular injuries. The pathophysiology of the first three of these conditions and details concerning their CT appearance were described in the preceding chapter, "Computed Tomography of Closed Head Injury." Therefore, these features will not be covered here.

PRIMARY NEURONAL INJURY

Marked rotation or acceleration of the head can cause one of two types of neuronal injury. These can be categorized as: (1) diffuse axonal injury (DAI) in the subcortical gray matter and brainstem injury; (2) cortical contusions.

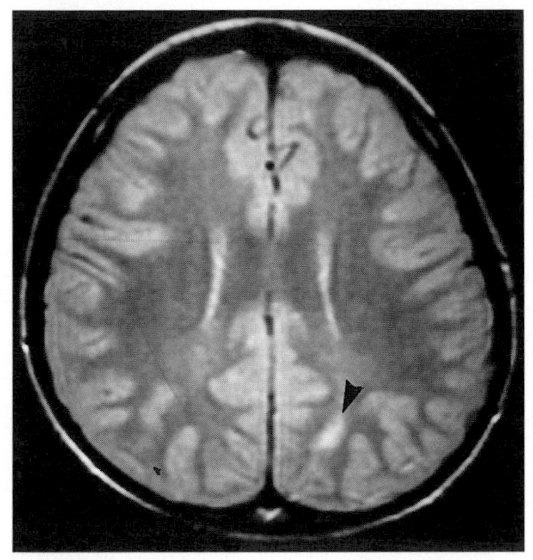

A

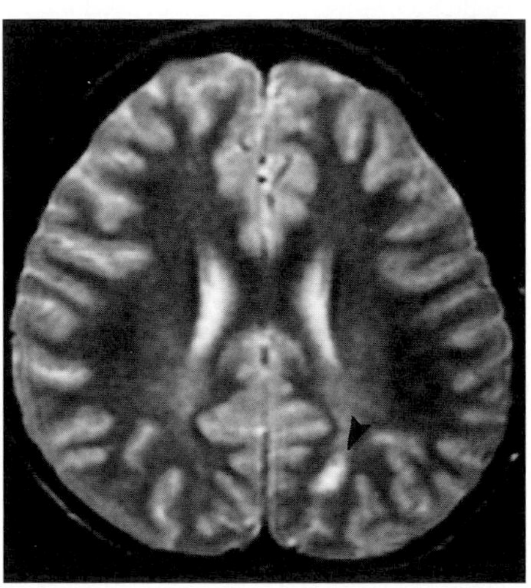

B

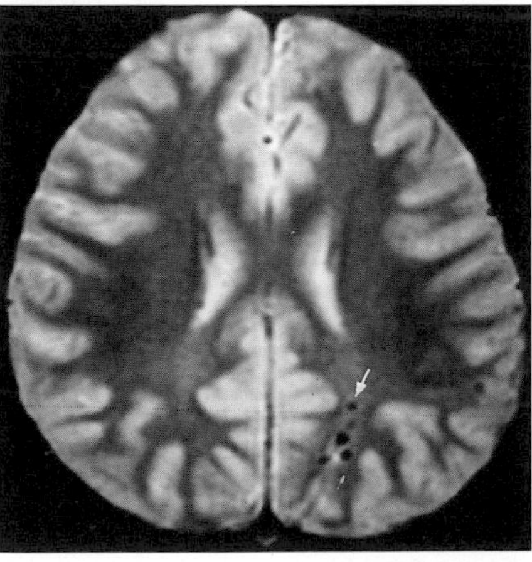

C

Figure 10-3*A–C*. Hemorrhagic acute shearing injury. Axial MR scans using standard SD (2000/30) (*A*) and T2W (2000/80) (*B*) techniques show a small hyperintense focus in the subcortical white matter of the left occipital lobe (*arrowheads*). (*C*) The compansion axial GE (750/33) MR scan shows numerous small hypointense foci of hemorrhage at this site (*arrows*).

Diffuse Axonal Injury in the Subcortical Regions and Brainstem

MR is superior to CT scanning in the detection of DAI. These lesions typically are located at the gray-white matter interface and are characterized by multiple, small, focal areas of damage.[21,32,33] Most are nonhemorrhagic, but up to 20 percent may contain a small amount of hemorrhage.[8,34] They occur in four primary locations: (1) lobar white matter; (2) corpus callosum; (3) dorsolateral aspect of the upper brainstem; and (4) internal capsule.[8,21,32,33,35–37]

In the acute phase (1–4 days), the nonhemorrhagic lesions are seen as small oval or round areas of hyperintensity, relative to brain parenchyma, on both T2W SD and SE images (Fig. 10-1). Acute hemorrhagic shear injuries may have a central hypointensity within them on the T2W and GE scans (Figs. 10-2, 10-3).[34–36] Chronic hemorrhagic shear injuries are visualized on T2W SE scans as foci of very low signal intensity because they contain hemosiderin. Shearing injuries are often associated with brainstem injury and long tract interruptions. Hence, they have a poor prognosis.[38,39]

MR is also sensitive to the gliotic areas that occur at the site of an old shearing injury. They may not be well seen on T1W images unless there is associated encephalomalecia. These areas are seen as increased signal on SD and T2W images.

Cortical Contusions

MR is extremely sensitive in the detection of hemorrhagic and nonhemorrhagic cortical contusions.[6–14] An acute clot produces low signal intensity on T2W SE and GE images. It is typically isointense to brain parenchyma on T1W SE images. In addition, MR can detect hemoglobin degradation products (i.e., hemosiderin) for months to years following the trauma.[14,15,24,28]

These lesions involve the superficial gray matter of the brain, most frequently in the inferior, lateral, and anterior aspects of the frontal and temporal lobes. Multiple series have demonstrated the superiority of T2W SE images over CT or T1W SE images in the detection of nonhemorrhagic contusions. The MR signal changes are likely related to abnormally increased water content within foci of edema.[3,7–10,12]

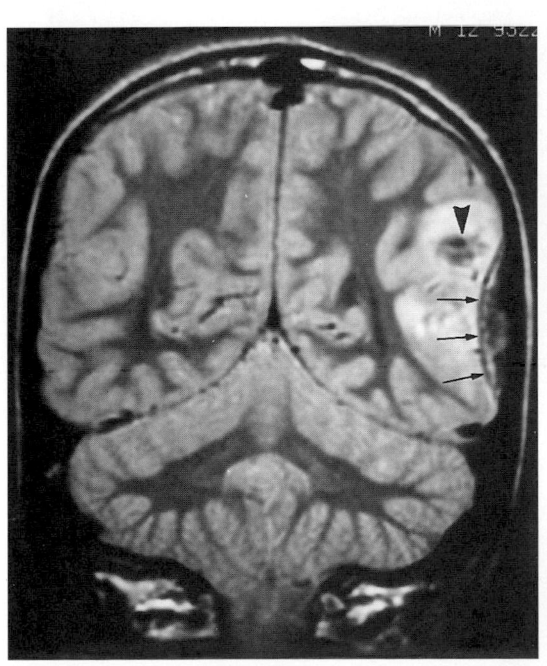

A

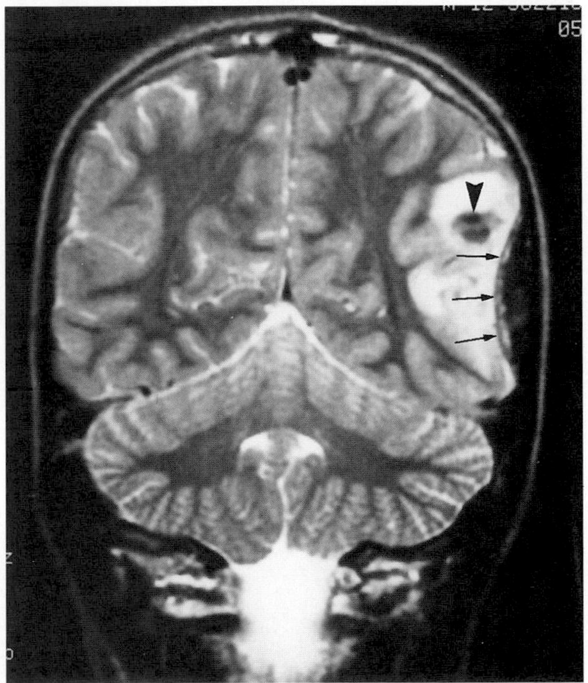

B

Figure 10-4*A*,*B*. Contusion and acute epidural hematoma. Coronal MR scans using double echo FSE SD (*A*) and FSE T2W (*B*) techniques show a large hypointense extraaxial collection displacing the edematous underlying brain which contains an associated hemorrhagic contusion (*arrowhead*). The thin dural line (*arrows*) correctly identifies this collection as an epidural hematoma.

EXTRAAXIAL COLLECTIONS

MR is superior to CT in detecting acute and subacute subdural hematomas. In one series, CT detected 53 percent of lesions compared with detection rates of 70 and 95 percent noted on T1 and T2W SE MR images.[9] In the chronic phase, MR can visualize subdural collections that have become isointense on CT scan. The MR imaging features of acute, subacute, and chronic extraaxial collections are described in the following discussion.

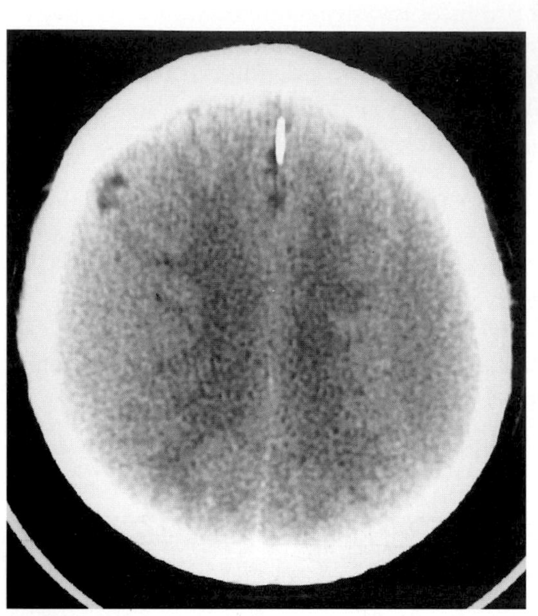

A

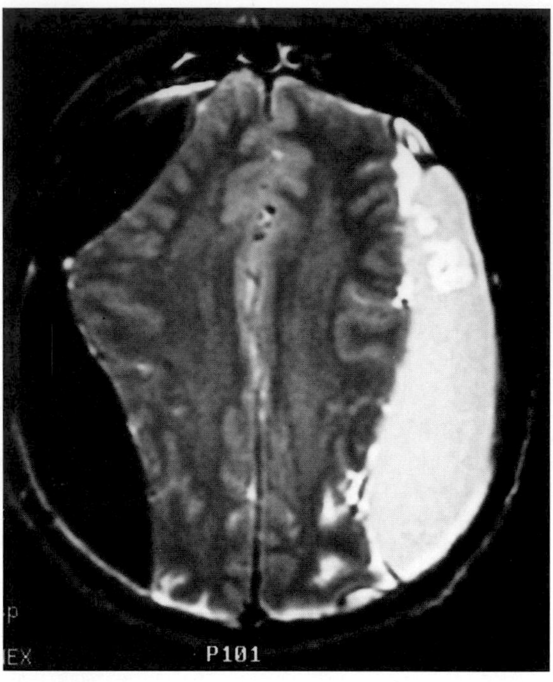

B

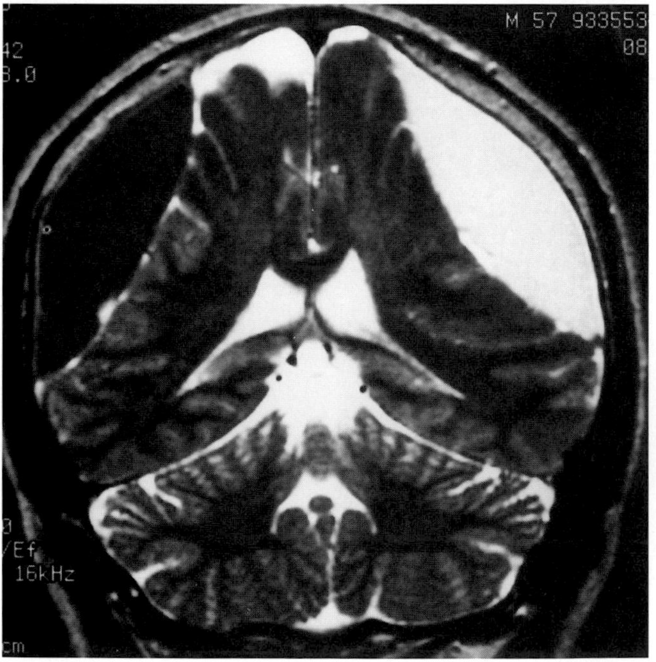

C

Figure 10-5*A–C*. Chronic subdural hematomas. Axial CT (*A*) shows bilateral isodense extraaxial collections which are identified primarily due to inward buckling of the white matter in the centrum ovale. Companion FSE T2W MR scans in axial (*B*) and coronal (*C*) projections show hypointense blood products ("deoxyhemoglobin") in the right-sided subdural and CSF signal intensities ("methemoglobin") within the left-sided subdural collection. Note the lentiform shape typical of a chronic subdural collection.

Acute Extraaxial Blood

The prompt identification of acute extracerebral hematomas is of critical importance because surgical intervention may be necessary. Although acute subdural or epidural hematomas of significant size can be recognized on MR, hematomas less than 3 mm could be missed because they are isointense to brain or skull on MR sequences. In clinical practice, this is usually not a problem because the signal intensities in the blood rapidly

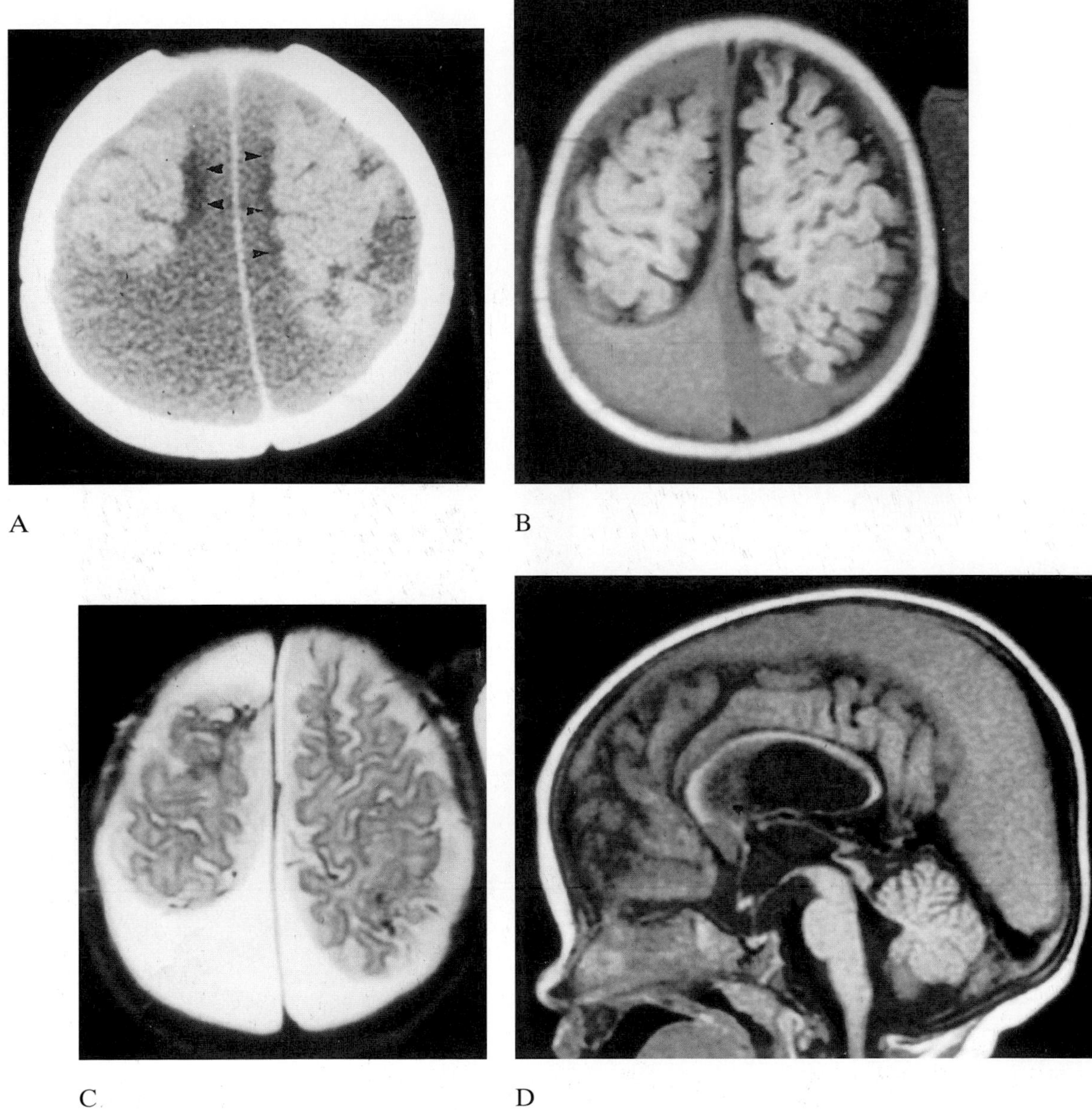

Figure 10-6*A–D*. Chronic bilateral subdural hematomas in an infant with nonaccidental trauma and the misleading history of "acute" trauma. Axial CT (*A*) shows the extensive subdural fluid surrounding the cerebral hemispheres. Note that the subarachnoid space (*arrowheads*) has reconstituted below these collections. It is seen as a hypodense rim surrounding the atrophic underlying brain. Axial T1W SE MR image (*B*) shows the resolving biconvexity and falx subdural collections. Again note the hypointense cerebrospinal fluid in the subarachnoid space surrounding the cerebral hemispheres. Axial T2W image (*C*) shows hyperintense signal in the arachnoid cerebrospinal fluid and subdural collections. Sagittal T1W MR (*D*) shows the full extent of the falx subdural hematoma in interhemispheric fissure.

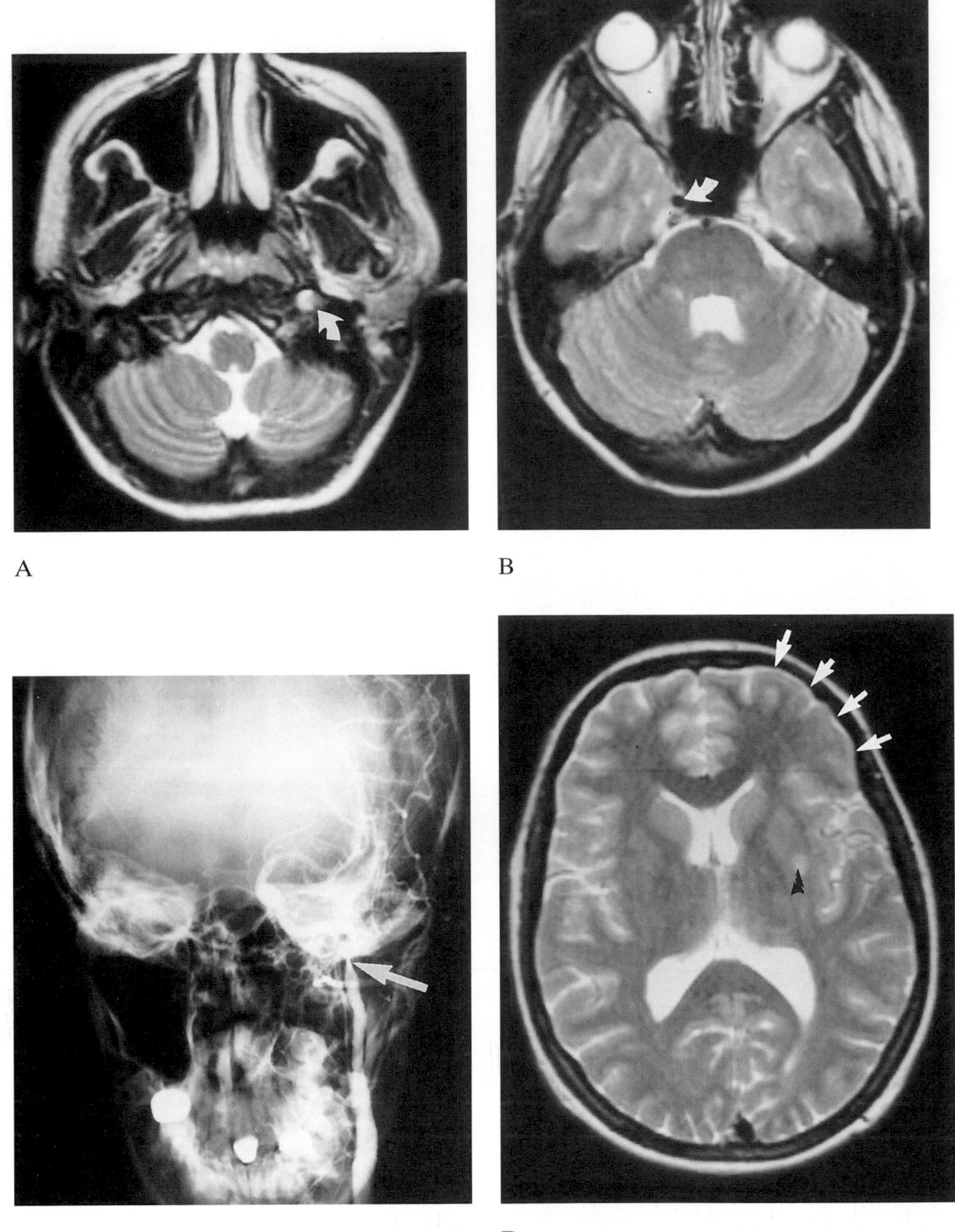

Figure 10-7*A–E*. Acute carotid dissection with secondary cerebral infarction and a shearing injury in the left putamen. Axial T2W (*A*,*B*) MR scans show hyperintense clot in the wall and lumen of the left carotid artery (*arrow*) as it enters the skull base. Note absence of the normal flow void in the left cavernous carotid segment (normal right side marked for comparison). Cerebral right arteriogram (*C*) done after the MR shows narrowing at the previously occluded site of dissection at the skull base (*arrow*). Axial T2W MR scans (*D*,*E*) show loss of the normal cortical signal intensity in the frontal cortex (*arrows*) due to embolic infarction from the thrombosed left carotid. Also noted abnormal hyperintense signal in the left putamen (*arrowhead*) due to vascular shearing injury of a lateral lenticulostriate vessel. Note that the edema is hyperintense at level (*D*) and that hypointense hemorrhage is present at level (*E*).

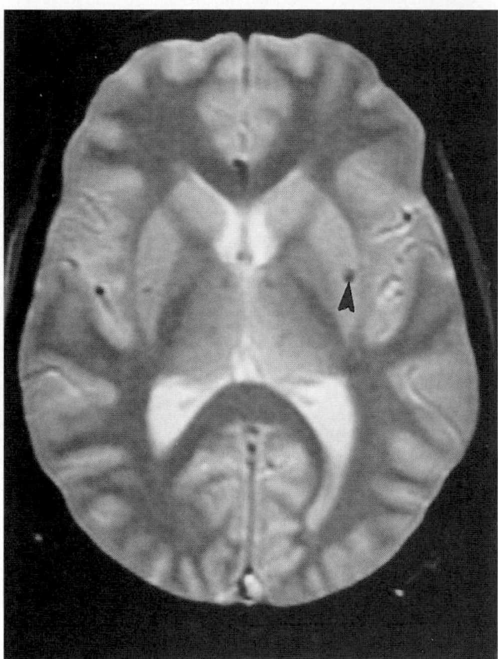

E

Figure 10-7 *Continued.*

develop characteristics that effectively separate it from the surrounding structures. These zones become hyperintense on T1W sequences. Convexity hematomas, which are sometimes missed by CT, can best be seen on coronal MR scan sequences.[40]

MR can be used to distinguish small epidural hematomas (which require careful follow-up) from incidental subdural collections (which require no additional images or therapy).[7–9,14,21] On MR, the displaced dura is seen as a line of low signal intensity between the brain and the extraaxial hematomas in these cases (Fig. 10-4). However, the skull fractures which are associated with epidural hematomas in 85 to 95 percent of cases are better seen with CT. MR scans can detect a skull fracture only when there is fluid or hemorrhage in the fracture site.[21]

Subacute Extraaxial Blood

Small, subacute extracerebral hematomas are easily detected with MR mainly because of the presence of methemoglobin, which is easily seen as a hyperintense region on the T1W images (Fig. 10-5).[7–9,12,14] This is partly because it offers better visualization of posterior fossa structures than CT, owing to its relative lack of artifact.[7,8,14] In addition, small extraaxial collections in the subfrontal, subtemporal, or clival regions are better seen on MR.[14] These collections are not, however, significant surgical lesions.

Chronic Extraaxial Blood

MR has also been shown to be superior to CT in detection of chronic subdural hematomas.[8] The MR signal characteristics of these collections vary with their age and the specific pulse sequences utilized (Fig. 10-6).[15,24,28,41,42] The presence of chronic subdural collections in children, elderly, or handicapped patients with acute trauma suggests nonaccidental injury (Fig. 10-7).[43]

Approximately 10 to 25 percent of chronic subdural hematomas are isodense relative to underlying brain parenchyma on CT scans.[13,44–47] These collections may be difficult to detect on axial CT imaging, especially if there is cortical atrophy and there are bilateral collections.[13,44,46] Thus, a CT diagnosis often depends on indirect signs (i.e., cortical effacement and separation of sulci from the inner table of the skull, unexplained midline shift, or buckling of white matter).[13,40,44–47] For these reasons, MR is superior to CT in detecting this phase of a subdural hematoma.

HEMORRHAGE INTO THE CEREBROSPINAL SPACE

Acute subarachnoid hemorrhage (SAH) is best seen on noncontrast CT scans.[40,48,49] In a prospective study, Gentry and coworkers found that detection of acute SAH by MR was limited unless there was a large clot within the subarachnoid space.[8] As SAH progresses to the subacute stage, it may become more visible on MR as an abnormally high signal intensity on T1W images.[49] In the late or chronic phase, MR may show hypointensity in the subarachnoid spaces secondary to hemosiderin deposition (i.e., "pial siderosis").

PRIMARY VASCULAR INJURIES

MR is uniquely able to detect acute occlusions of the major cerebral arteries and venous sinuses.[50–52] An acute clot within the carotid or vertebral arteries is seen as an absence of the normal hypointense flow void (Fig. 10-7). On T1W images the clot in the wall or lumen can be identified as a hyperintense focus in the expected location of the vessel flow void. Zones of cerebral infarction that occur secondary to total occlusion or emboli from this vessel also can be detected by MR scans (Fig. 10-7*D*,*E*).

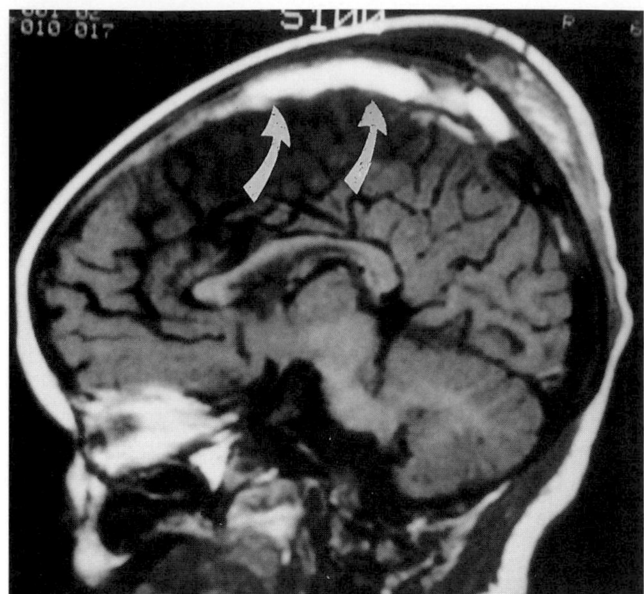

A

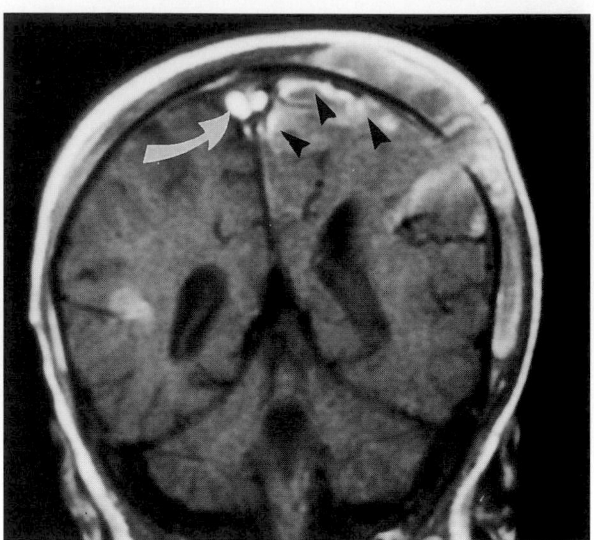

B

Figure 10-8*A*,*B*. Acute posttraumatic superior sagittal sinus thrombosis. T1W SE MR scans in sagittal (*A*) and coronal proportions (*B*) show hyperintense thrombus in the superior sagittal sinus (*arrows*). Note hemorrhagic hyperintense signal in the cortex which has suffered venous infarction (*arrowheads*) in (*B*). An incidental contusion is also present in the right sylvian cortex and a large subgaleal left hematoma is present in the right scalp.

Occlusion of the venous sinuses occurs as a result of local trauma to the superior sagittal or lateral sinus regions. It can be detected by MR as absence of the flow void. The hyperintense (bright) appearance of the intraluminal clot on T1W images should not be confused with the normally hyperintense signal from slow venous flow. When there is a doubt, a venous phase contrast MR angiogram can be performed. In severe cases, the MR can detect hemorrhagic venous infarction of the brain (Fig. 10-8).

References

1. Groswasser Z, Reider-Groswasser I, Soroker N, et al: Magnetic resonance imaging in head injured patients with normal late computed tomography scans. *Surg Neurol* 1987; 27:331–337.
2. Doezema D, King JN, Tandberg D, et al: Magnetic resonance imaging in minor head injury. *Ann Emerg Med* 1991; 20:1281–1285.
3. Yokota H, Kurokawa A, Otsuka T, et al: Significance of magnetic resonance imaging in acute head injury. *J Trauma* 1991; 31:351–357.
4. Tanaka T, Sakai T, Uemura K, et al: MR imaging as predictor of delayed posttraumatic cerebral hemorrhage. *J Neurosurg* 1988; 69:203–209.
5. Brant-Zawadzki M, Davis PL, Crooks LE, et al: NMR demonstration of cerebral abnormalities: Comparison with CT. *AJNR* 1983; 4:117–124.
6. Jenkins A, Hadley MDM, Teasdale G, et al: Brain lesions detected by magnetic resonance imaging in mild and severe head injuries. *Lancet* 1986; 2:445–446.
7. Snow RB, Zimmerman RD, Gandy SE, et al: Comparison of magnetic resonance imaging and computed tomography in the evaluation of head injury. *Neurosurgery* 1986; 18:45–51.
8. Gentry LR, Godersky JC, Thompson B, et al: Prospective comparative study of intermediate-field MR and CT in the evaluation of closed head trauma. *AJNR* 1988; 9:91–100.
9. Han JS, Kaufman B, Alfidi RJ, et al: Head trauma evaluated by magnetic resonance and computed tomography: A comparison. *Radiology* 1984; 150:71–77.
10. Hesselink JR, Dowd CF, Healy ME, et al: MR imaging of brain contusions: A comparative study with CT. *AJNR* 1988; 9:269–278.
11. Hadley DM, Teasdale GM, Jenkins A, et al: Magnetic resonance imaging in acute head injury. *Clin Radiol* 1988; 39:131–139.
12. Kelly AB, Zimmerman RD, Snow RB, et al: Head trauma: Comparison of MR and CT—Experience in 100 patients. *AJNR* 1988; 9:699–708.
13. Forbes GS, Sheedy PF, Piepgras DG, et al: Computed tomography in the evaluation of subdural hematomas. *Radiology* 1978; 126:143–148.

14. Yeakley JW, Pan G, Kulkarni MV: The role of magnetic resonance imaging in head trauma, in Miner ME, Wagner KA (eds): *Neurotrauma—Treatment, Rehabilitation and Related Issues,* 3d ed. Boston: Butterworths, 1989: 37–50.
15. Gomori JM, Grossman RI, Goldberg HI, et al: Intracranial hematomas: Imaging by high-field MR. *Radiology* 1985; 157:87–93.
16. Gomori JM, Grossman RI, Yu IPC, et al: NMR relaxation times of blood: Dependence on field strength, oxidation state and cell integrity. *J Comput Assist Tomogr* 1987; 11(4):684–690.
17. Gomori JM, Grossman RI: Mechanisms responsible for the MR appearance and evolution of intracranial hemorrhage. *Radiographics* 1988; 8:427–440.
18. Chin HY, Taber KH, Hayman LA, et al: Temporal changes in red blood cell hydration: Application to MRI of hemorrhage. *Neuroradiology* 1991; 33(suppl):79–81.
19. Taber KH, Ford JJ, Jensen RS, et al: Change in red blood cell relaxation with hydration: Application to MR imaging of hemorrhage. *JMRI* 1992; 2:203–208.
20. Hayman LA, Taber KH, Ford JJ, et al: Mechanisms of MR signal alteration by acute intracerebral blood: Old concepts and new theories. *AJNR* 1991; 12:899–907.
21. Gentry LR: Head trauma, in Atlas SW (ed): *Magnetic Resonance Imaging of the Brain and Spine.* New York: Raven Press, 1991: 439–466.
22. Norbash AM, Glover GH, Enzmann DR: Intracerebral lesion contrast with spin-echo and fast spin-echo pulse sequences. *Radiology* 1992; 185:661–665.
23. Jones KM, Maulkern RV, Mantello MT, et al: Brain hemorrhage: Evaluation with fast spin-echo and conventional dual spin-echo images. *Radiology* 1992; 182:53–58.
24. Edelman RR, Johnson K, Buxton R, et al: MR of hemorrhage: A new approach. *AJNR* 1986; 7:751–756.
25. Weingarten K, Zimmerman RD, Deo-Narine V, et al: MR imaging of acute intracranial hemorrhage: Findings on sequential spin-echo and gradient-echo images in a dog model. *AJNR* 1991; 12:457–467.
26. Hayman LA, McArdle CB, Taber KH, et al: MR imaging of hyperacute intracranial hemorrhage in the cat. *AJNR* 1989; 10:681–686.
27. Zyed A, Hayman LA, Bryan RN: MR imaging of intracerebral blood: Diversity in the temporal pattern at 0.5 and 1.0 T. *AJNR* 1991; 12:469–474.
28. Atlas SW, Mark AS, Grossman RI, et al: Intracranial hemorrhage: Gradient-echo MR imaging at 1.5 T. *Radiology* 1988; 168:803–807.
29. Seidenwurm D, Meng T, Kowalski H, et al: Intracranial hemorrhagic lesions: Evaluation with spin-echo and gradient-refocused MR imaging at 0.5 and 1.5 T. *Radiology* 1989; 172:189–194.
30. Orrison WW, Stimac GK, Stevens EA, et al: Comparison of CT, ultra-low field and high-field MRI. Presented at ASNR 30th Annual Meeting, 1992:144–145.
31. Chaney RK, Taber KH, Orrison WW, et al: Magnetic resonance imaging of intracerebral hemorrhage at different field strengths: A review of reported intraparenchymal signal intensities. *Neuroimag Clin North Am* 1992; 2(1):25–51.
32. Adams JH: Pathology of nonmissile head injury. *Neuroimag Clin North Am* 1991; 1:397–410.
33. Gentry LR: Primary neuronal injuries. *Neuroimag Clin North Am* 1991; 1:411–432.
34. Gentry LR, Godersky JC, Thompson B: MR imaging of head trauma: Review of the distribution and radiopathologic features of traumatic lesions. *AJNR* 1988; 9: 101–110.
35. Gentry LR, Godersky JC, Thompson BH: Traumatic brain stem injury: MR imaging. *Radiology* 1989; 171:177–187.
36. Gentry LR, Thompson B, Godersky JC: Trauma to the corpus callosum: MR features. *AJNR* 1988; 9:1129–1138.
37. Zimmerman RA, Bilaniuk LT, Genneralli T: Computed tomography of shearing injuries of the cerebral white matter. *Radiology* 1978; 127:393–396.
38. Adams JH, Graham DI, Murray LS, et al: Diffuse axonal injury due to nonmissile head injury in humans: An analysis of 45 cases. *Ann Neurol* 1982; 12:557–563.
39. Gennarelli TA, Spielman GM, Langfitt TW, et al: Influence of the type of intracranial lesion on outcome from severe head injury. *J Neurosurg* 1982; 56:26–32.
40. Cornelius RS, Gaskill MF, Lukin RR: Traumatic intracranial hemorrhage. *Neuroimag Clin North Am* 1991; 1: 433–441.
41. Sipponen JT, Sipponen RE, Sivula A: Chronic subdural hematoma: Demonstration by magnetic resonance. *Radiology* 1984; 150:79–85.
42. Unger EC, Cohen MS, Brown TR: Gradient-echo imaging of hemorrhage at 1.5 tesla. *Magn Reson Imaging* 1989; 7:163–172.
43. Sato Y, Yuh WTC, Smith WL, et al: Head injury in child abuse: Evaluation with MR imaging. *Radiology* 1989; 173:653–657.
44. Kim KS, Hemmati M, Weinberg PE: Computed tomography in isodense subdural hematoma. *Radiology* 1978; 128:71–74.
45. Moller A, Ericson K: Computed tomography of isoattenuating subdural hematomas. *Radiology* 1979; 130: 149–152.
46. Moon KL, Brant-Zawadzki M, Pitts LH, et al: Nuclear magnetic resonance imaging of CT-isodense subdural hematomas. *AJNR* 1984; 5:319–322.
47. Wilms G, Marchal G, Geusens E, et al: Isodense subdural haematomas on CT: MR findings. *Neuroradiology* 1992; 34:497–499.
48. Chakeres DW, Bryan RN: Acute subarachnoid hemorrhage: In vitro comparison of magnetic resonance and computed tomography. *AJNR* 1986; 7:223–228.
49. Bradley WG, Schmidt PG: Effect of methemoglobin formation on the MR appearance of subarachnoid hemorrhage. *Radiology* 1985; 156:99–103.
50. Zimmerman RA: Vascular injuries of the head and neck. *Neuroimag Clin North Am* 1991; 1:443–459.
51. Davis JM, Zimmerman RA: Injury of the carotid and vertebral arteries. *Neuroradiology* 1983; 25:55–69.
52. Goldberg HI, Grossman RI, Gomori JM, et al: Cervical internal carotid artery dissecting hemorrhage: Diagnosis using MR. *Radiology* 1986; 158:157–161.

CHAPTER 11

PET/SPECT IMAGING IN HEAD INJURY

Michael J. Caron

SYNOPSIS

Positron emission tomography (PET) and single photon emission computed tomography (SPECT) have been used to a limited degree in the clinical evaluation of the head-injured patient. Some of the advantages of these investigations include a more regionalized and quantitative assessment of cerebral blood flow and metabolism, and the correlation of these data with morphological studies. Applications under development include the determination of the biodistribution of neurotransmitters and drugs in the injured brain. Correlation of metabolic information with neuropsychological data may yield new insights into the functional organization of the brain. While currently these studies are primarily of research interest, it is conceivable that as their relevance is better understood, they may become routinely used in the clinical management of head injury patients.

INTRODUCTION

Throughout the history of modern medicine, imaging studies of the brain have been responsible for major advances in the treatment of all neurological disorders. In traumatic brain injury (TBI), imaging has been integral in development of current management strategies. Advances in neuroimaging have been rapidly incorporated into the acute treatment of TBI victims in an effort to reduce mortality and improve the quality of outcomes for individuals unfortunate to have suffered a traumatic cerebral insult.

The discovery of x-ray imaging by Roentgen in 1895 allowed for the first skull films.[1] Skull films allowed the early diagnosis of traumatic skull fractures and thus a clue for operative localization of intracranial hematomas. Angiography was added by Monitz in 1923.[2] The technique of direct bilateral carotid puncture and angiography provided the location of intracranial hematomas and the extent of midline shift to further refine early operative management of craniocerebral trauma. Ventriculopathy and pneumoencephalography contributed to advances in localization of intracranial lesions, allowed measurement of intracranial pressure, and led to the drainage of cerebrospinal fluid for treatment of raised intracranial pressure.

The single most important imaging advancement in modern management of traumatic brain injury was the introduction of computed axial tomography (CT) in 1972 by Godfrey Hounsfield. Along with the establishment of modern emergency transport of patients and the rapid identification and operative decompression of intracranial hematomas, CT dramatically helped improve the outcome of severe head injury.[3–5]

Future advances in the treatment of head injury will rely on development of new drugs for the protection and repair of the injured central nervous system (CNS) as well as further elucidation of the pathophysiological processes responsible for secondary brain injury.[6] Both of these approaches will rely upon the ever improving ability to image cerebral physiological events through the use of biochemical imaging. This chapter will briefly review the current capabilities of positron emission tomography (PET) and single photon emission computed tomography (SPECT) for imaging cerebral physiology. Studies conducted to date in TBI will be summarized, and the future potential of these techniques for the study of brain injury pathophysiology and clinical care will be discussed.

History of Biochemical Imaging

The universal radiation detector, the Anger gamma camera, was first introduced in 1958. The camera consists of a collimator, a sodium iodide scintillation crystal, and an array of photomultiplier tubes. The collimator is a lead baffle which ensures emitted electromagnetic radiation striking the crystal is travelling parallel to the collimator and thus coming from the target being studied. The emitted radiation strikes the sodium iodide crystals and is stopped. The energy of this impact releases a photon and the photomultipliers convert this photon into an electronic signal which is registered by the scanner for electronic image reconstruction. The discovery of technetium-99m (^{99m}Tc) by Harper in 1962 heralded the birth of modern nuclear medicine. This element is the photon emitting isotope used to label 90 percent of all radiopharmaceuticals employed in single photon emission computed tomography (SPECT) of the brain. The addition of CT technology was an essential element in the development of modern radiopharmaceutical imaging. In the late 1970s the addition of tomographic image processing to existing single photon techniques greatly improved the anatomic resolution of isotope imaging. Modern SPECT imaging with brain-dedicated tomographic units can provide fairly high-resolution three-dimensional reconstruction of a variety of cerebral physiological events.

The in vivo autoradiographic techniques developed by Sokoloff and coworkers[7] for measurement of cerebral metabolic rate of glucose utilization in animals provided the foundation for the development of clinical PET. In parallel with the development of quantitative autoradiography, tomographic PET scanning units and cyclotron-generated isotopes for labeling biologically active compounds were developed[8] and applied to the non-invasive quantification of glucose metabolism in the humans.[9,10] Along with the development of labeled compounds to study other biological processes, these advances in imaging technology have greatly expanded our ability to image cerebral physiological events.

BIOCHEMICAL IMAGING

All activity in the brain is biochemical in nature. The energy required to build cellular membranes, organelles, and to maintain cellular resting membrane potentials is biochemical. The production, release, and reuptake of neurotransmitters is biochemical. The autoregulation of cerebral blood flow is mediated by biochemical metabolites and tissue pH. It is for this reason that imaging of physiological events with biochemical radiopharmaceutical tracers and emission tomography is ideally suited to provide information not available with conventional CT transmission scanning or magnetic resonance imaging (MRI). Biochemical imaging utilizes tracer kinetic modeling and tomographic image reconstruction to both visually display the anatomic location of the biochemical pathway under examination and provide quantitative rates of the process. Selection of the appropriate biochemical tracer defines the biochemical pathway or physiological process which is imaged. Conventional CT and MR imaging in traumatic brain injury provide only anatomic information on location of intracranial blood, edema, and shifts of normal structures. Functional MR imaging sequences, which are currently under development, are approaching clinical and research utility. However, the new MRI techniques do not yet provide the quantitative biochemical measurements available with radiopharmaceutical emission imaging.

Tracer kinetic modeling employs the administration of a radiolabeled biologically active compound (tracer) and a mathematical model of the kinetics of the biological process which that tracer participates in. A dose of tracer with known radioactivity is administered and distributed throughout the body. The radioactivity emitted from the organ under examination is quantified by external counters in a tomographic fashion for reconstruction of three-dimensional images of the radioactive counts. For qualitative (clinical) studies, the raw images of counts can be displayed as anatomic representations of the location and intensity of the biodistribution of the tracer. Quantification of the biological processes, for research, is then calculated from the counts of the tracer in blood collected from the systemic circulation, application of the kinetic model of biochemical reactions or compartments which the tracer must pass through before it is counted, and the actual counts emitted from the organ under investigation.

Current PET and SPECT imaging can provide information about cerebral glucose metabolism, cerebral blood flow, cerebral blood volume, cerebral neurotransmitters, and protein synthesis. Recent studies have described labeling CNS-active drugs for the studies of biodistribution in the brain. Resolution refers to the smallest structure which, under ideal conditions, can be discriminated from an adjacent structure in a reconstructed brain image. The physics of tracer selection, image reconstruction, scanner construction, and tracer kinetic modeling are beyond the scope of this chapter. However, a gross simplification of image acquisition in both PET and SPECT is presented.

An energy-emitting isotope is created, the isotope is chemically incorporated into a biologically active compound, the compound is administered to the patient, and the distribution of the radioactivity emitted from the target organ is counted. The difference in PET and SPECT isotopes is in the type of energy emitted. Positron emission tomography isotopes are shorter lived, and when they decay a positron (positively charged electron) is released. The positron collides with an electron, and the two particles annihilate each other. The mass of the two particles is converted to two equal 511-keV photons. These two photons travel out of the body in exactly opposite (180 degrees) directions. The PET scanners electronically paired counting devices are positioned 180° from each other. A photon is not accepted as a count of tracer activity originating from the area being scanned unless its paired (coincident) detector is struck by a photon at the same instant. This coincident detection of paired photons provides more accurate localization in space of the origin of the tracer radioactivity than do the SPECT isotopes. In SPECT imaging the isotopes emit a single photon to an array of individual detectors configured circumferentially around the target organ.

The difference in physical characteristics of tracers utilized for PET and SPECT imaging impart advantages and disadvantages to each method. Single photon emission computed tomography isotopes, ^{99m}Tc HMPAO in particular, have the advantage of a volume of distribution in the brain which closely parallels CBF and it also has a long half-life. Once administered the radiopharmaceutical is stable enough that scanning within several hours provides the same physiological information as if imaging were performed immediately. The ability for absolute quantification is lost, but tracer can be administered at the time of a clinical event (seizure or administration of a drug, for example) and scanning can proceed within several hours instead of immediately as is necessary for most PET studies. Current resolution of brain structures is 8 to 9 mm for brain-dedicated SPECT systems[11] utilizing ^{99m}Tc-labeled compounds and 10 to 14 mm for ^{133}Xe compounds. PET resolution is approximately 2 mm for ^{18}F, and 5 mm for ^{15}O compounds.[12–14]

The technical challenges in biochemical imaging for traumatic brain injury utilizing both PET and SPECT are primarily that of providing accurate quantitative data on regional blood flow and metabolism for research studies. The difficulty with accuracy of quantitative studies originates in the breakdown in the tracer kinetic models due to tissue edema, dynamic changes in blood-brain barrier function, instability of cerebral blood flow and autoregulation, and the heterogeneous changes in mechanically disrupted brain. Despite these limitations the quantitative data collected is unique information which is unavailable by any other imaging modality. The practical aspect of utilizing these techniques for making clinical decisions regarding patient care and prognosis does not require the absolute quantitative data for interpretation. The images generated by the tomographic collection of the emitted radioactive counts can be presented in axial, coronal, sagittal, or three-dimensional surface renderings in either gray scale or color. "Imaging is an extremely efficient process (for screening the entire brain) because data are presented in pictorial form to the most efficient human sensory system for search, identification, and interpretation—the visual system."[14] Visual inspection of an image of the symmetry and intensity of regional changes in a given physiological process by an experienced observer knowledgeable in the anatomy and physiology of the brain along with a clinical examination of the patient provides an invaluable amount of information.

As stated previously, the selection of the appropriate tracer is the key to investigation of cerebral physiological events. The range of imaging sequences available with PET and SPECT are described below.

Cerebral Oxygen and Glucose Utilization

Only PET can provide a quantitative measurement of regional variations in brain oxygen utilization. The local cerebral metabolic rate of oxygen utilization ($LCMRO_2$) is a calculated value. Three methods of calculating $LCMRO_2$ have been utilized and the technique, advantages, and disadvantages of each are reviewed elsewhere.[15]

Cerebral Blood Flow (CBF) Studies

Cerebral blood flow (CBF) studies utilizing PET are performed by three different techniques. The tissue clearance, continuous inhalation of short half-life tracers (equilibrium), and tissue-trapping techniques have all been utilized.[14] Both methods employ $H_2{}^{15}O$ as the freely diffusible tracer necessary to meet the modeling criteria for quantitative studies. Because ^{15}O has a 2-min half-life, this method of quantitative CBF measurement requires a cyclotron for isotope generation in immediate proximity to the scanner. Simply stated, the clearance technique counts the inflow and outflow of the labeled water which is administered as an intravenous bolus. Alternatively a bolus of $C^{15}O_2$ is inhaled and immediately converted to labeled water by carbonic anhydrase in the lung. The equilibrium technique utilizes an infusion of $H_2{}^{15}O$ to reach equilibrium in the brain tissue. The blood flow is calculated from the difference in counts between arterial delivery of labeled water, the removal by venous outflow, and tracer decay. The PET resolution for studies of local CBF is $7 \times 6 \times 6$ mm^3.

This resolution is contrasted to resolution with other techniques for measurement of cerebral perfusion such as external ^{133}Xe washout (2 cm), stable xenon CT ($1.5 \times 1.5 \times 0.8$ cm^3), and HMPAO (1.0 cm^3).[12,13] New functional MR imaging sequences are under development and resolution for CBF imaging approaches $6 \times 6 \times 8$ mm^3.

Single photon emission computed tomography studies of cerebral perfusion are performed with two different tracers; ^{133}Xe and ^{99m}Tc-labeled HMPAO. The major advantage of ^{133}Xe is the ability to perform dynamic scanning during the uptake, distribution, and washout of this highly diffusible and inert gas from the brain. The dynamic scanning allows absolute quantitative measurement of CBF. The disadvantage of ^{133}Xe dynamic cerebral SPECT studies is much lower spatial resolution than other technniques and less accurate imaging of deep structures in the brain because of scattering of the low energy photons (81 keV) emitted by ^{133}Xe.[16] The second agent available for imaging cerebral perfusion is ^{99m}Tc HMPAO. This tracer is lipophilic and readily crosses the intact blood-brain barrier by passive diffusion. Through mechanisms not yet fully elucidated, HMPAO breaks down into a hydrophilic compound which cannot diffuse back across the blood-brain barrier for clearance from the brain.

Cerebral Blood Volume (CBV) Studies

Positron emission tomography utilizes ^{11}CO or $C^{15}O_2$ bound to red blood cells or tracers which remain in the vasculature such as ^{11}C-methyl-albumin, ^{68}Ga-EDTA, and ^{68}Ga-transferrin to quantitatively determine cerebral blood volume. Single photon emission computed tomography utilizes ^{99m}Tc-labeled red cells or albumin for quantitative microvascular hematocrit and qualitative cerebral blood volume studies, respectively.[17]

The average whole brain CBV value determined by Phelps and coworkers was 4.3 $\pm$ 0.4 ml/100 g.[18] As determined by Grubb and colleagues, this can vary depending on the presence or absence of large arterial or venous structures in the scanning plane.[19]

Image Registration

One of the difficulties in interpretation of PET and SPECT images has been the inability to clearly recognize anatomic landmarks routinely used in visual interpretation of conventional CT and MR images. Clinicians who do not routinely study emission-generated images often feel uncomfortable placing the anatomic location of an area of abnormal flow or metabolism seen on these studies. Recent advances in registration of PET and SPECT images with conventional CT and MR images allows superimposition of either line drawings of normal anatomic landmarks or the actual CT and MR images, onto the metabolic images.[20]

PET AND SPECT STUDIES IN HEAD INJURY

Relatively few studies utilizing PET in head-injured patients have been published. Langfitt and Alavi at the University of Pennsylvania were the first to report on glucose metabolism.[21,22] They compared CT, MRI, xenon CBF, and PET-FDG studies in three patients. Flouro deoxyglucose (FDG) studies were obtained at 4, 15, and 17 days postinjury, respectively, in the three cases studied. Two patients had repeat imaging batteries at 6 months postinjury. Correlation of glucose metabolism and CBF was inconsistent probably due to the lack of a xenon detector directly over the most anterior tip of the temporal lobes, a consistent site of decreased metabolism on PET. The analysis was semiquantitative, utilizing a ratio of regional to whole brain glucose metabolism within an individual subject. Absolute rates of whole brain or regional glucose metabolism were not reported. The degree of global depression of glucose metabolism correlated with the Glasgow Coma Scale (GCS) score of the patient at the time of the PET study.[23] The neuropsychological battery did not consistently correlate with the reported areas of decreased glucose metabolism. The important observation made in these early studies was that with the exception of a few punctate hemorrhages seen on MRI only, all areas of abnormality visualized on CT and MRI were demonstrated by PET. Additionally, the PET studies detected regions of abnormal metabolism which appeared normal on CT or MRI.

In an effort to define the quantitative thresholds for recovery of function on a neuroanatomic and neuropsychological basis, Caron and colleagues[24] initiated a comprehensive study of glucose metabolism and cerebral blood flow, utilizing PET, as one of the projects within the UCLA Brain Injury Research Center. Quantitative FDG analysis of regional cerebral glucose metabolism in combination with conventional CT, CT xenon blood flow studies, and a comprehensive neuropsychological battery in both the acute and one year follow-up of severely and moderately head injured patients, is in progress. This study has taken advantage of the greatly improved image resolution of the current generation of PET scanners. From the preliminary reports it is evident that the goal of obtaining a true regional evaluation of the changes in cerebral glucose metabolism in the entire brain will be realized.

The first report confirmed the observation of Langfitt regarding the ability of PET-FDG studies to visualize more lesions than CT in six moderately and severely injured patients.[25] The size of the PET abnormalities were larger than the corresponding CT lesion when both were detectable. The difference in size between the structural and metabolic lesions diminished during recovery and several chronic CT lesions were larger than the area of altered glucose metabolism seen on PET. Caron was the first to report absolute rates of local cerebral glucose metabolism in head-injured humans.[26] In three severely injured patients LCMRGlc was measured in the motor cortex, cerebellar hemispheres, within the center of unoperated contusions, in the resection cavity of operted contusions, and in brain adjacent to both the operated and unoperated contusions. The following observations were evident. Within an individual subject (1) LCMRGlc was higher in cortex adjacent to operatively decompressed versus unoperated intracerebral contusions, (2) crossed cerebellar hypometabolism was seen in a pattern similar to that seen in cerebral infarction,[15] and (3) unlike CT which loses resolution of viable versus nonviable cortex in the low attenuation areas of edema surrounding contusions, PET was sensitive enough to resolve areas with absent cortical metabolism from areas of low but still anatomically intact cortical ribbons.[26,27]

Imaging and outcome studies have been carried out for CT, MR, PET, and SPECT. Several excellent reviews summarize the results of neuropsychological evaluations in relationship to imaging studies.[16] Computed tomography scanning is useful for identification of acute intracranial hematomas and both ventricular enlargement and late cortical atrophy during long-term follow-up. The presence of any of these abnormalities is associated with poor neuropsychological outcomes. In either the acute or late stages of brain injury CT does not correlate well with specific localization of brain regions responsible for neurological deficits. Magnetic resonance imaging provides a better overall assessment of the diffuse nature of cerebral trauma than CT. While MRI has provided better correlation between site of lesions and neuropsychological outcome, the relationships are not consistent across studies. Magnetic resonance imaging often reveals multiple small frontal, temporal, and deep lesions not evident on CT. This diffuse pattern of injury may be responsible for the inability of neuropsychological testing to localize the exact anatomic correlate of specific functional deficits.

Positron emission tomography studies of long-term neuropsychological outcome in adults have yielded mixed results. The three patients reported by Langfitt demonstrated clear abnormalities of glucose metabolism in all areas suggested as damaged on the neuropsychological battery. Although sensitive, qualitative PET studies were not specific, PET visualized deficient glucose metabolism in areas not related to the neuropsychological abnormalities.[21] This underscores the need for regional quantitative measurement of glucose metabolism in association with neuropsychological testing as proposed by Caron and under investigation at the UCLA Brain Injury Research Center.[24] In a preliminary report Kelly describes an association between late decreased temporal and orbitofrontal glucose metabolism with abnormalities in memory and executive function, respectively.[28] Results from a large population of patients with a variety of lesion locations should be useful in correlating specific regional abnormalities in metabolism with the results of neuropsychological testing.[29,30]

CONCLUSIONS

Advances in radiopharmaceutical technology and imaging instrumentation have now placed PET and SPECT in a position to become extremely valuable tools for both routine clinical management and research studies of the metabolic consequences of traumatic brain injury. In combination with newly developing MR functional imaging sequences, the complex interplay between injury-mediated biochemical cascades, neuronal defense and repair mechanisms, cerebral blood flow and the mechanism of action of investigational drugs under development should be unraveled. Ultraearly PET and SPECT metabolic studies (FDG and HMPAO) may define salvageability and guide operative decompression of intracerebral lesions. Structural and blood flow information will likely be provided by MRI. Positron emission tomography and SPECT will provide regional metabolic information and characterize the biodistribution of drugs and neurotransmitters. Both PET and MRI are capable of providing functional activation studies which in combination with neuropsychological studies will provide insight into cerebral mechanisms of repair and reorganization. Positron emission tomography protein synthesis studies may predict both repair and memory function. Practitioners involved in all aspects of care for patients suffering from traumatic brain injury are encouraged to become familiar with the capability of the various biochemical imaging studies available and to take an active role in development of these capabilities at their institutions.

ACKNOWLEDGMENT

This work was supported in part by the UCLA Brain Injury Research Center grant from the National Institutes of Health (NINDS Grant NS30308), the Research and Education Institute at the Harbor-UCLA Medical Center, and the Chicago Institute of Neurosurgery and Neuroresearch.

References

1. Roentgen W: Ueber eine neue Art von Strahlen (Vorlaufige Mitteilung). *Sitzungs-Berichte der Physikalisch-medicineschen Gesellschaftzu Wurzburg* 1895; 9:132.

2. Monitz E: Diagnostic des tumeurs cerebrales et eprueve de L'encephalagraphie arterielle. Paris: Masson & Cie, 1931.
3. Becker DP, Miller JD, Ward JD: The outcome from severe head injury with early diagnosis and intensive management. *J Neurosurg* 1977; 47:491–502.
4. Bowers SA, Marshall LF: Outcome in 200 consecutive cases of severe injury treated in San Diego County: A prospective analysis. *Neurosurgery* 1980; 6:237–242.
5. Seelig JM, Becker DP, Miller JD, et al: Traumatic acute subdural hematoma: Major mortality reduction in comatose patients treated within four hours. *N Engl J Med* 1981; 304:1511–1512.
6. Caron MJ, Hovda DA, Becker DP: Changes in the treatment of head injuries, in Aldrich F, Eisenberg HM (eds): *Neurosurg Clin North Am* 1991; 2:483–491.
7. Sokoloff L, Reivich M, Kennedy C, et al: The (^{14}C)-deoxy glucose method for the measurement of local cerebral glucose utilization: Theory, procedure and normal values in the conscious and anesthetized albino rat. *J Neurochem* 1977; 28:897–916.
8. Phelps ME, Hoffman EJ, Mullani NA, Ter-Pogossian MM: Application of annihilation coincidence to transaxial reconstruction tomography. *J Nucl Med* 1975; 16:210–224.
9. Reivich M, Kuhl D, Wolf A, et al: The (^{18}F)fluoro-deoxyglucose method for the measurement of local cerebral glucose utilization in man. *Circ Res* 1979; 44:127–137.
10. Phelps ME, Huang SC, Hoffman EJ, et al: Tomographic measurement of local glucose metabolic rate in humans with (F-18) 2-fluoro-2-deoxy-D-glucose: Validation of method. *Ann Neurol* 1979; 6:371–388.
11. Lassen NA, Holm S: Single photon emission computed tomography (SPECT), in Mazziotta JC, Gilman S, (eds): *Clinical Brain Imaging: Principles and Applications, Contemporary Neurology Series.* Philadelphia: F.A. Davis Company, 1992: Chap 4, 108–134.
12. Brooks DJ, Frackowiak RSJ: Cerebrovascular disease, in Mazziotta JC, Gilman S (eds): *Clinical Brain Imaging: Principles and Applications, Contemporary Neurology Series.* Philadelphia: F. A. Davis Company, 1992: 217–243.
13. Frackowiac RSJ, Lenzi GL, Jones T, Heather JD: Quantitative measurement of regional cerebral blood flow and oxygen metabolism in man using ^{15}O and positron emission tomography: Theory, procedure, and normal values. *J Comput Assist Tomogr* 1980; 4:727–736.
14. Phelps ME: Positron emission tomography (PET), in Mazziotta JC, Gilman S (eds): *Clinical Brain Imaging: Principles and Applications, Contemporary Neurology Series*, Philadelphia: F.A. Davis Company, 1992: Chap 3, 71–107.
15. Baron JC, Frackowiak RSJ, Herholz K, et al: Use of PET methods for measurement of cerebral energy metabolism in hemodynamics in cerebral vascular disease: Review. *J Cereb Blood Flow Metab.* 1989; 9:723–742.
16. Van Heertum RL, Miller SH, Mosesson RE: SPECT brain imaging in neurologic disease. *Radiol Clin of North Am* 1993; 31(4):881–907.
17. Loutfi I, Frackowiak RSJ, Myers MJ, Lavender JP: Regional brain hematocrit in stroke by single photon emission computed tomography imaging. *Am J Physiol Imag* 1987; 2:10–16.
18. Phelps ME, Huang SC, Hoffman EJ, et al: Validation of tomographic measurement of cerebral blood volume with ^{11}C-labeled carboxyhemoglobin. *J Nuc Med* 1979; 20:328–334.
19. Grubb RL, Raichle ME, Higgins CS, et al: Measurement of regional cerebral blood volume by emission tomography. *Ann Neurol* 1978; 4:322–328.
20. Holman *J Nucl Med* 1991; 32:1478–1484.
21. Langfitt TW, Obrist WD, Alavi A, et al: Computerized tomography, magnetic resonance imaging, and positron emission tomography in the study of brain trauma. *J Neurosurg* 1986; 64:760–767.
22. Alavi A, Langfitt T, Fazekas F, et al: Correlation studies of head trauma with PET, MRI, and XCT. *J Nuc Med* 1986; 27:919.
23. Alavi A, Fazekas F, Alves W, et al: Positron emission tomography in the evaluation of head injury. *J Cereb Blood Flow Metab* 1987; 7(suppl):S646.
24. Caron MJ, Mazziotta JC, Hovda DA, et al: *Vulnerability in Brain Injury: Thresholds for Recovery.* Project No. 3, UCLA Brain Injury Research Center Grant, National Institute Health (NS 30308), Funded 1992–1995, submitted 1991.
25. Caron MJ, Mazziotta J, Woods R, et al: Comparison of positron emission tomography and computerized axial tomography in lesion identification in brain injured humans. *J Neurotrauma* 1992; 9(4):382.
26. Caron MJ, Mazziotta JC, Hovda DA, Becker DP: Quantification of Cerebral Glucose Metabolism in Brain Injured Humans Utilizing Positron Emission Tomography, *J Cereb Blood Flow Metab* 1993; 13(Suppl 1):S379.
27. Caron MJ, Hovda DA, Mazziotta JC, et al: The structural and metabolic anatomy of traumatic brain injury in humans: A computerized tomography and positron emission tomography analysis. *J Neurotrauma* 1993; 10(suppl 1):S58.
28. Kelly DF, Bergsneider M, Shalmon E, et al: Following traumatic brain injury, longterm neuropsychologic deficits are associated with regionally specific local depression of cerebral glucose utilization as measured by positron emission tomography. 3rd International Neurotrauma Symposium, Toronto, 1995.
29. Bergsneider M, Kelly DF, Shalmon E, et al: Early hyperglycolysis following severe human traumatic brain injury: A positron emission tomography study. 3rd International Neurotrauma Symposium, Toronto, 1995.
30. Shalmon E, Kelly DF, Bergsneider M, et al: Regional association between cerebral blood flow and glucose metabolism following human brain injury: A positron emission tomographic study. 3rd International Neurotrauma Symposium, Toronto, 1995.

CHAPTER 12

NEAR-INFRARED SPECTROSCOPY IN HEAD INJURY

Shankar P. Gopinath
Britton Chance
Claudia S. Robertson

SYNOPSIS

Traumatic intracranial hematoma, which can present acutely or in a delayed fashion, constitutes a common and treatable source of morbidity and mortality in patients who sustain head injuries. Early detection of an intracranial hematoma remains the cornerstone for successful therapy. Although CT scan is the diagnostic procedure of choice for detection, there can be difficulties in obtaining a timely CT scan while the patient is either in the emergency room or in the intensive care unit (ICU). Transcranial near-infrared spectroscopy is a simple, noninvasive, portable, and rapid method of detecting the intracranial hematoma and adds to the diagnostic armamentarium of the clinician. Near-infrared (NIR) light penetrates the skull and brain to a depth of several centimeters and is absorbed by the hemoglobin. Since the concentration of hemoglobin is greater in an acute hematoma than in normal brain tissue, less NIR light is reflected back on the side of the hematoma. This can be recorded as a difference in optical density (ΔOD) between the two sides of the head. Generally, an extracerebral hematoma has a ΔOD value of greater than 0.6, while the value is less than 0.4 in intracerebral hematomas. Future studies could explore the potential uses of NIR spectroscopy in the field or in the ICU.

INTRODUCTION

One of the major causes of death and disability in patients with head trauma is the development of an intracranial hematoma. With the advent of the CT scan and its use as the principal investigative method in patients with severe head injury, a high incidence of intracranial hematomas has been documented in this population. It is estimated that an intracranial hematoma, which may be acute or delayed, occurs in approximately 40 to 50 percent of patients with severe head injury.[1–3] The incidence of traumatic intracranial hematomas in patients over 50 years old is reported to be three to four times higher than in those under 30 years. A substantial incidence (29 percent) of operable mass lesions is seen even in patients presenting with a GCS score of 13 to 15 when associated with risk factors such as injury from a fall and age over 40 years.[4] Patients with mass lesions carry a higher mortality and morbidity than those with diffuse brain injury.

The role of delayed or secondary brain injury results in the eventual recovery of patients has been well documented.[5,6] Intracranial hematomas remain one of the most important causes of secondary brain insults, making it critical to detect them early. In a recent study, the occurrence of delayed cerebral injury, defined as the development of new or worsening intracranial lesions as compared with the admission CTs, was found to be approximately 45 percent. The presence of delayed cerebral injury was associated with a more serious outcome.[7] Intracranial hematoma is the cause of deterioration in approximately 75 percent of patients who "talk and deteriorate" after head injury.[8,9]

TYPES OF INTRACRANIAL HEMATOMAS

Acute subdural hematoma is the most common type of traumatic intracranial hematoma requiring neurosurgical intervention. It is seen in 24 percent of patients with severe closed head injuries.[3] Hemorrhage into the subdural space may be caused by cortical contusion, by laceration of meninges, or most commonly, by the tearing of a vein bridging the subdural space. Most of the patients are immediately symptomatic and are frequently unconscious when they reach the emergency room. Acute subdural hematoma is usually seen on a CT scan as a homogeneous high-density crescent conforming to the shape of the calvarium laterally and to the cerebral cortex medially. In patients who are comatose at the time of initial examination, the mortality rate may approach 100 percent without surgery, whereas it decreases to below 50 percent if surgical intervention occurs within 3 to 4 h of injury.[10] Increasing age, delay in the evacuation of the hematoma, and increasing size of the hematoma are factors associated with a poor prognosis.

Epidural hematoma occurs in fewer than 10 percent of patients with head trauma. Epidural hematoma is caused by bleeding between the inner table of the skull and the dura. Epidural hematoma develops commonly from an injury to the anterior or posterior branch of the middle meningeal artery resulting from a fracture of the squamous portion of the temporal bone. A skull fracture is seen in approximately 85 percent of the patients with epidural hematoma.[11] As the dura is firmly attached to the skull at the suture, an epidural hematoma rarely crosses the suture line, thus assuming a lenticular shape. The typical CT scan feature of epidural hematoma is a focal, smoothly marginated, biconvex high-density mass intimately related to the inner table of the skull. Epidural hematomas, are usually thought of as acute, but may be delayed in 9 percent of affected patients.[12] In approximately 7 percent, a small epidural hematoma will expand rapidly following evacuation of a contralateral hematoma.[13]

Intracerebral hematoma can be present on admission to the hospital or can be delayed, although usually appearing during the first 48 h after injury (delayed traumatic intracerebral hematomas, or DTICH).[14] Intracerebral hematomas are irregular, poorly marginated homogeneous collections of blood located in the white matter, predominantly in either frontal or temporal lobes.[15,16] Four percent of traumatic intracerebral hematomas occur in the basal ganglia.[17] In the Traumatic Coma Data Bank series, intracerebral hematoma was found as the primary lesion in 10 percent of the patients with severe closed head injury.[3]

Delayed intracerebral hematomas are highly unpredictable and can occur in any age group, in patients who are fully conscious on admission, and in patients with a normal CT scan, with or without associated fracture. The incidence of delayed intracerebral hematoma varies. In one series, it was seen in 3 to 8 percent of severely head injured patients.[8–20] In another series, 19 percent of the patients with a severe head injury who deteriorated neurologically after admission to the hospital had a large delayed intracerebral hematoma.[21] The occurrence of a delayed intracerebral hematoma also has been observed following evacuation of an acute epidural or subdural hematoma.

Most delayed intracerebral hematomas occur in the first 3 days after injury. In one study, 35 percent of intracerebral hematomas were found to develop within the first 24 h, 46 percent were detected 24 to 72 h after injury, and 20 percent 72 h after injury.[14] The general prognosis for functional recovery is poorer in patients who develop delayed intracerebral hematomas.

Studies have shown that early detection and treatment of intracranial hematomas reduces morbidity and/or mortality.[10,22,23] Available techniques for diagnosing intracranial hematomas include air ventriculogram, cerebral arteriogram, CT scan, and MRI scan. At the present time, the unenhanced CT scan is the procedure of choice in the acute evaluation of head-injured patients. However, since hematomas can develop after the initial evaluation, none of the currently available imaging techniques is ideal for early detection. Patients, often critically ill, must be taken out of the ICU for most of these diagnostic studies. A noninvasive method of detecting the development of an intracranial hematoma, even if the precise location can not be identified, would be very useful.

NEAR-INFRARED SPECTROSCOPY

Characteristics of Near-Infrared Light

The spectrum of light used in clinical investigations include gamma rays, x-rays, UV light, visible light, and infrared rays (Fig. 12-1). Although light in the visible part of the spectrum has been used for examining tissues and organs for more than 100 years, in vivo biochemical measurement using light was not realized practically until the twentieth century. The principles of spectrophotometry using ultraviolet, visible, and infrared wavelengths were largely developed and applied for in vitro chemical analysis. The technique of dual wavelength near infrared principles was first utilized in medical applications by Millikan, who developed a simple ear oximeter.[24] While optical methods were improved for the study of rapid reactions,[25] the clinical application of near-infrared spectroscopy (NIRS) in humans began with the work of Jobsis-Vandervliet in the adult head.[26]

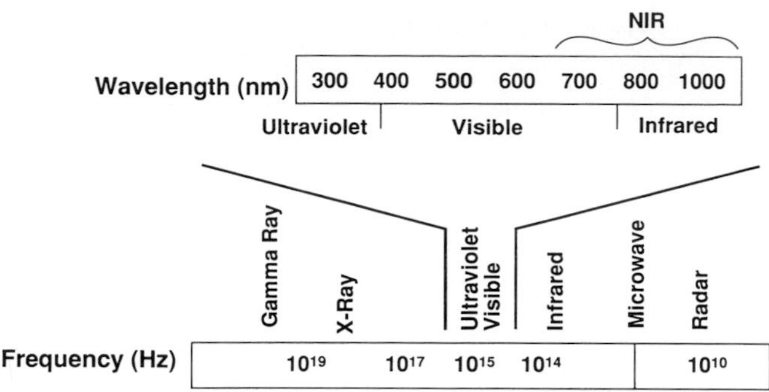

Figure 12-1. Spectrum of light showing the NIR range.

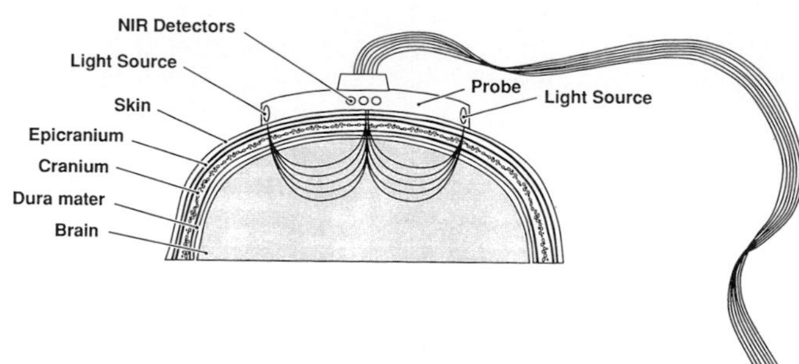

Figure 12-2. Diagram of NIRS probe on the scalp. The *curved lines* illustrate the area traversed by most of the photons entering at the light source and exiting at the light sensor.

Identification of intracranial hematomas with NIRS is a new application of an existing technology that provides information about changes in cerebral oxygen saturation, cerebral blood flow and volume, and oxygen utilization in the brain. The method is based on the fact that light in the near-infrared range (700–950 nm) can pass through biological tissues far more readily than does the light of visible or far-infrared spectrum. Light in the near-infrared range can penetrate scalp, skull, and brain to a depth of several centimeters.

Types of Spectroscopy

Two modes of spectroscopy have been used for monitoring the brain:

1. Transcranial or transillumination mode spectroscopy (forwardscattering of photons). NIR light is delivered to one hemisphere and collected over the opposite hemisphere. Clinical applications of this type are suitable only in neonates. In adults, the transillumination mode is not used because of the diameter of the head and consequent degree of light attenuation across it.
2. Reflection mode spectroscopy (backscattering of photons). In this arrangement of diffuse transmission spectroscopy, light propagates along a high probability course into the tissue of interaction and then back to the surface.[27] This process has the advantage of depth resolution, which allows cerebral hemoglobin to be measured independently of scalp and skull hemoglobin.[28]

Interaction of NIR Light with Biological Tissues

When NIR light enters tissues, it is both scattered and absorbed. The amount of scattering and absorption depends on the wavelength of the light and the tissue type.[29] Some photons migrate through the tissue and eventually exit at the site of the photosensor. Other photons follow paths that never interact with the sensor. The paths followed by most of the photons that eventually exist at the sensor site fall within a crescent-shaped area between the light source and the sensor (Fig. 12-2). The depth of this area is dependent on the distance between the light source and the sensor and can be increased by making this separation greater.

Attenuation due to light absorption is caused by chromophores, which in the brain include oxyhemoglobin, deoxyhemoglobin, and oxidized cytochrome aa_3.[30] Figure 12-3 shows the absorbance curves for the three chromophores at varying wavelengths of NIR light.[31] Oxyhemoglobin has an absorbance peak at 850 nm, while deoxyhemoglobin has an absorbance peak at 760 nm. The contribution from cytochrome aa_3 is relatively small. Therefore, for detecting changes in oxyhemoglobin, the difference in absorbance at 760 and 850 nm is recorded. For detecting changes in hemoglobin (or

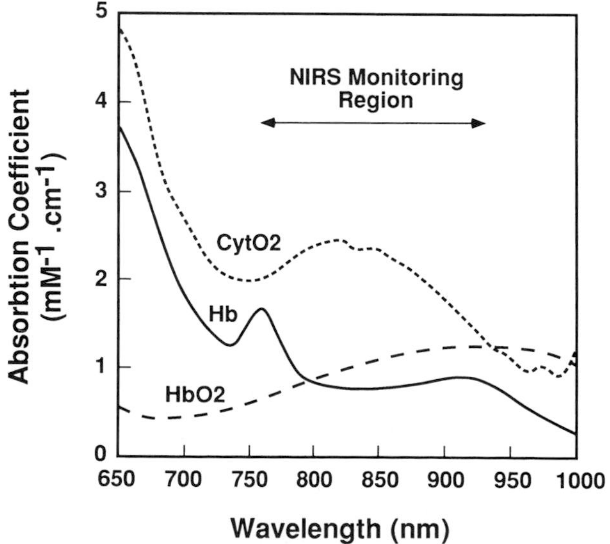

Figure 12-3. Graph of the absorbance of oxyhemoglobin, deoxyhemoglobin, and cytochrome aa_3 at varying wavelengths. [From Elwell et al.[31]]

blood) volume, the sum of the absorbances at 760 and 850 nm is recorded.

NIRS Monitoring of Cerebral Metabolism

Near-infrared spectroscopy has now been widely employed in neonates to monitor cerebral tissue oxygenation in a variety of clinical situations. Using qualitative NIR instrumentation, Kurth and associates[32] monitored changes in oxygenated hemoglobin during cooling and warming on cardiopulmonary bypass and circulatory arrest. They noted a progressive desaturation of hemoglobin in the brain vasculature during circulatory arrest that recovered during rewarming. Similarly, using NIRS, episodes of desaturation of brain vasculature hemoglobin have been observed in premature infants during endotracheal suctioning[33,34] and crying.[35] Several investigators have found the NIRS to be very useful in measuring cerebral blood volume in neonates.[35–37] Recently, the application of NIRS has been utilized even in the fetus to measure changes in fetal cerebral oxygenation during labor and childbirth.[38,39]

In normal adult volunteers, the changes in brain vasculature hemoglobin saturation to varying concentrations of inspired oxygen from 7 to 21 percent have been studied by McCormick and associates.[40] In this study, the transcranial saturation of 63.9 percent found during inspired oxygen of 21 percent fell to 35.2 percent on 7 percent inspired oxygen. In addition, a correlation was found between the onset of EEG slowing and cerebral hemoglobin desaturation as measured by NIRS. In another study involving patients requiring profound hypothermia and cardiac arrest for repair of cerebral aneurysm, NIRS has been used to track changes in cerebral vascular hemoglobin saturation.[40]

Early studies reported the use of NIRS in assessing

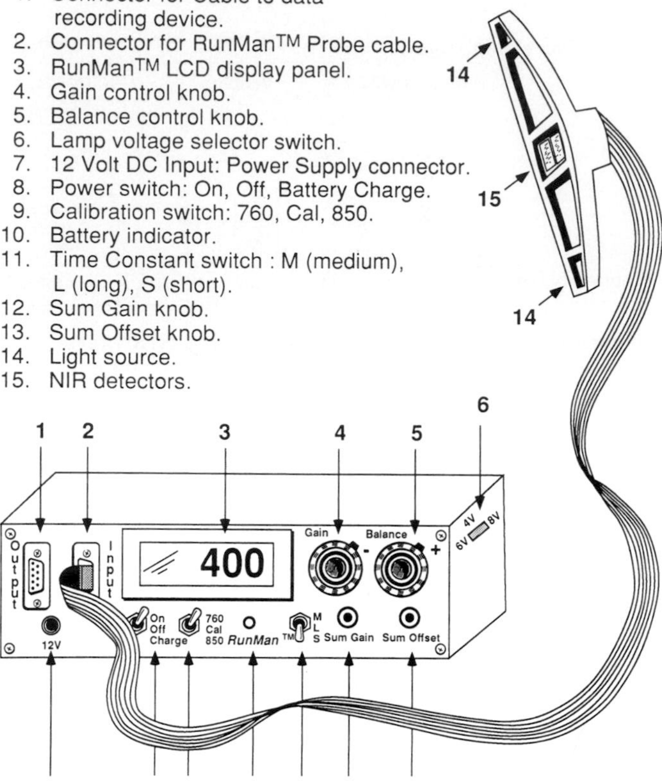

Figure 12-4. Diagram of NIRS monitor identifying all of the switches and knobs described in the text.

the qualitative changes in cerebral oxygen saturation and cerebral blood volume.[36,41,42] However, quantitative measurement of cerebral blood flow and cerebral blood volume and its response to changes in carbon dioxide has been made possible by recent technological and methodological developments.[43–46]

TABLE 12-1 To Determine ΔOD, Locate in the "Monitor" Column of the Chart the Reflected Light Value from the Hematoma Side (Assuming that the Normal Side Was Adjusted to 400). The ΔOD Is Opposite the Reflected Light Value.

Monitor	ΔOD	Monitor	ΔOD	Monitor	ΔOD	Monitor	ΔOD
10	1.60	110	0.56	210	0.27	310	0.11
20	1.30	120	0.52	220	0.26	320	0.09
30	1.12	130	0.49	230	0.24	330	0.08
40	1.00	140	0.45	240	0.22	340	0.07
50	0.90	150	0.42	250	0.20	350	0.05
60	0.82	160	0.39	260	0.18	360	0.04
70	0.75	170	0.37	270	0.17	370	0.03
80	0.69	180	0.34	280	0.15	380	0.02
90	0.64	190	0.32	290	0.14	390	0.01
100	0.60	200	0.30	300	0.12	400	0

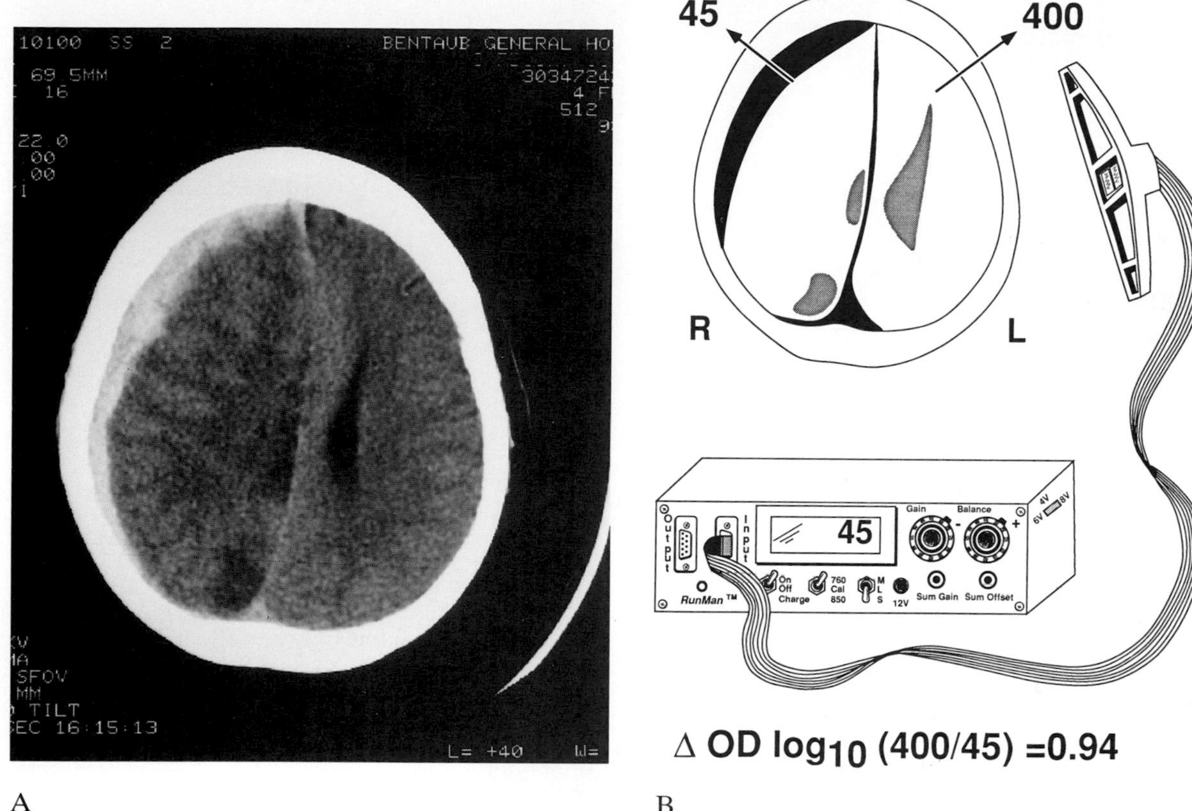

A

B

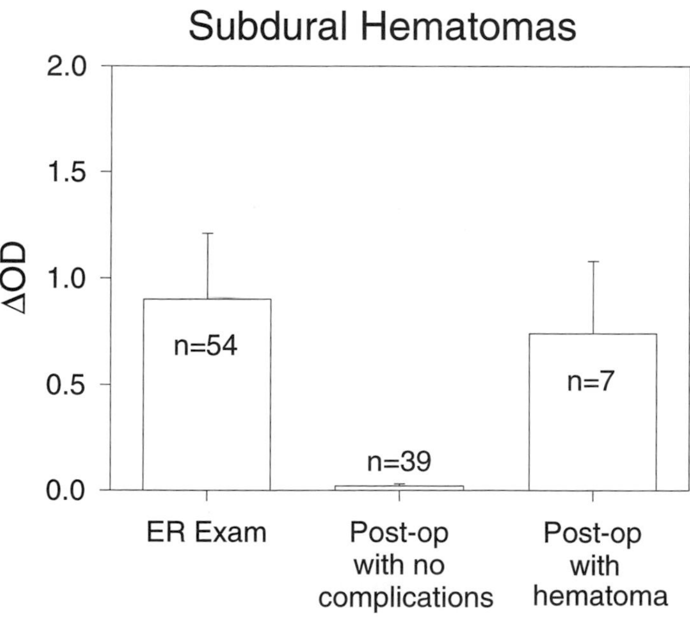

C

Figure 12-5. A typical CT scan (*A*) and the corresponding NIRS examination (*B*) of a patient with a subdural hematoma. The bar graph (*C*) shows the average ΔOD on the initial scan in all 54 patients, the average ΔOD postoperatively in the 39 patients with uncomplicated courses, and the average ΔOD in the 7 patients who developed some type of intracranial hematoma postoperatively. The scatterplot (*D*) shows the relationship ($n = 54$, $r = 0.64$, $p < .001$) between the thickness of the subdural hematoma on the initial CT scan and the ΔOD in the emergency room.

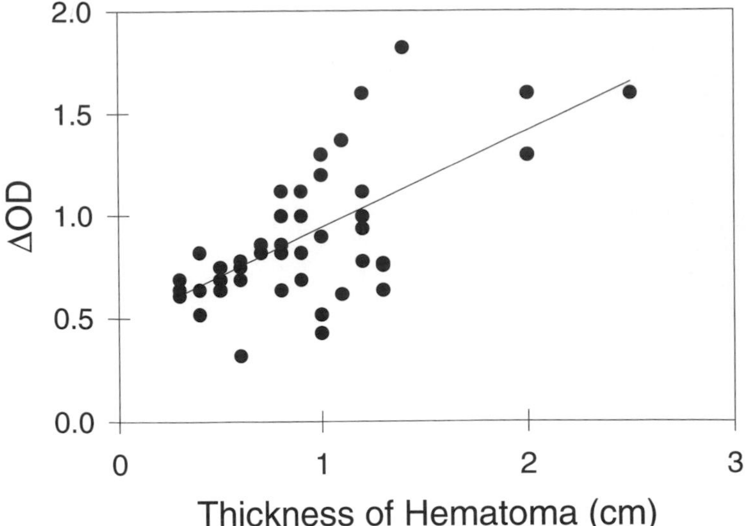

D

Figure 12-5. *Continued.*

The NIRS Examination for Localization of Intracranial Hematomas

Time-resolved studies using NIRS have been carried out on breast tissue samples in vitro for possible detection of breast cancer. Preliminary results suggest that the location of the tumor could be observed in breast tissue.[47] However, to our knowledge, no studies have been performed on brain using NIRS for imaging purposes.

The principle used in identifying intracranial hematomas with NIRS is that extravascular blood absorbs more NIR light than intravascular blood because there is a greater concentration of hemoglobin in the acute hematoma than in the brain tissue, where blood is contained within vessels. Therefore, the absorbance of NIR light is greater and the reflected light less on the side of the brain containing a hematoma than on the uninjured side.

For the studies described in this chapter, a dual-wavelength reflectance spectrometer was used (RunMan, NIM, Inc., Philadelphia). This monitor is small (6.5 in. × 4.5 in. × 2 in.), battery-operated, and can be easily transported into the ER or ICU. Figure 12-4 identifies the various switches and knobs that are described below. The LCD panel displays the intensity of the reflected light at 760 and 850 nm when the calibration switch is in the 760 and 850 position, respectively. The panel also displays the difference in reflected light at 760 and 850 nm when the calibration switch is in the "cal" position. The probe consists of two small incandescent bulbs placed 3.5 cm on either side of a 760- and 850-nm photodetector. The 3.5-cm separation of light source and detector allows measurement of NIR absorbance in a volume of tissue approximately 2 cm wide by 2 to 3 cm deep. Leakage of the light is minimized by the presence of rubber dams between the light emitter and detectors and around the circumference of the probe.

The procedure for a NIRS examination is simple and takes less than 10 min. The following steps are performed in sequence:

1. The NIRS probe is connected to the battery-operated, portable monitor. The unit is turned on and allowed to warm up for 10 min.
2. The light intensity switch is adjusted to either 4, 6, or 8 V. For adults with light skin color and for children, 4 V may be sufficient; for adults with dark skin color, 8 V should be selected.
3. The time constant switch is set to the "S" position.
4. The "gain" knob is adjusted to midposition.
5. The calibration switch is at the "cal" position.
6. The probe is placed on the frontal region of the suspected uninjured cerebral hemisphere, making certain that the rubber dams make a light seal against the scalp. If the patient has a subgaleal hematoma, avoid the area of subgaleal hematoma.

TABLE 12-2 Values of ΔOD in Patients without Intracranial Hematomas

Patient Group	ΔOD (right-left)
No head injury (n = 10)	0.02 ± 0.01
DBI (n = 30)	0.03 ± 0.01
Postop SDH (n = 39)	0.03 ± 0.01
Postop EDH (n = 19)	0.02 ± 0.01
Postop ICH (n = 10)	0.04 ± 0.01
Average of All Groups	0.03 ± 0.01

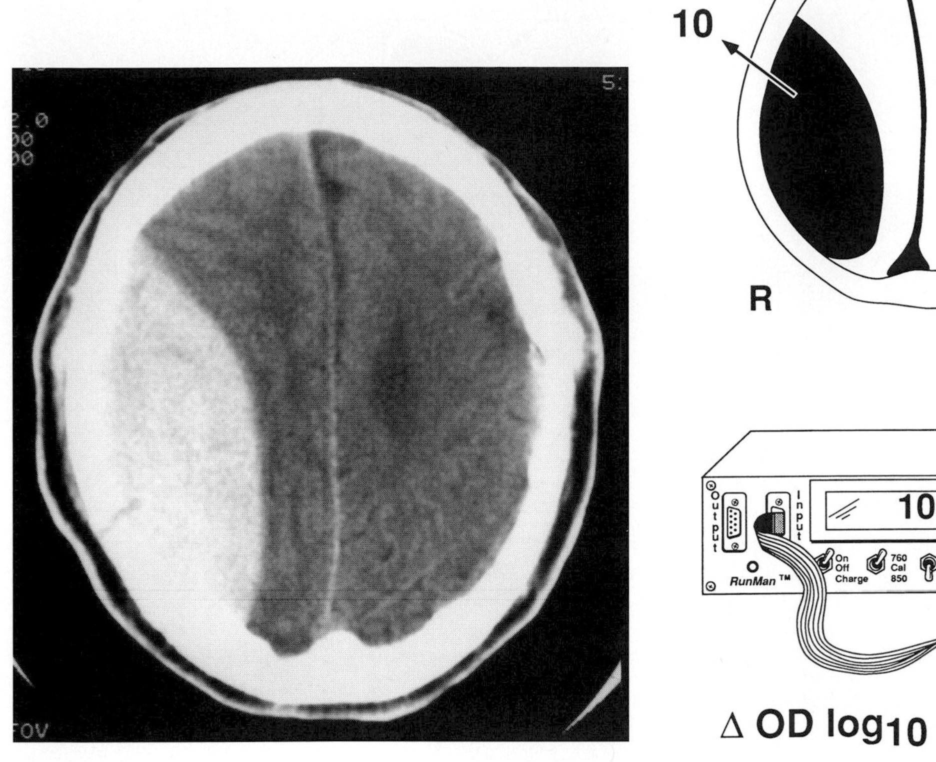

A

B

C

Figure 12-6. A typical CT scan (*A*) and the corresponding NIRS examination (*B*) of a patient with an epidural hematoma. The bar graph (*C*) shows the average ΔOD on the initial scan in all 28 patients, the average ΔOD postoperatively in the 19 patients with uncomplicated postoperative courses, and the average ΔOD in the 3 patients who developed some type of intracranial hematoma postoperatively. The scatterplot (*D*) shows the relationship ($n = 28$, $r = 0.73$, $p < .001$) between the thickness of the epidural hematoma on the initial CT scan and the ΔOD in the emergency room.

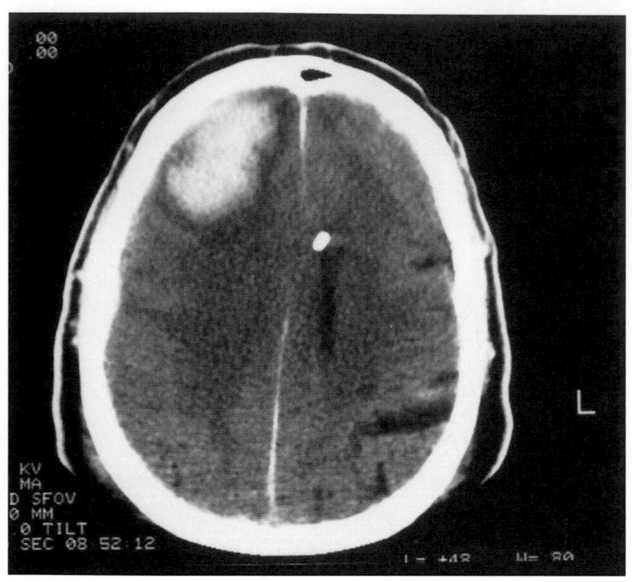

A

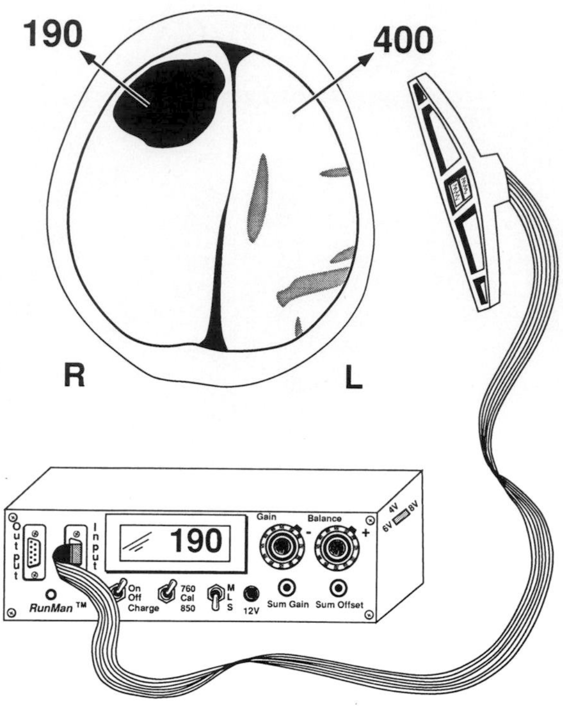

B

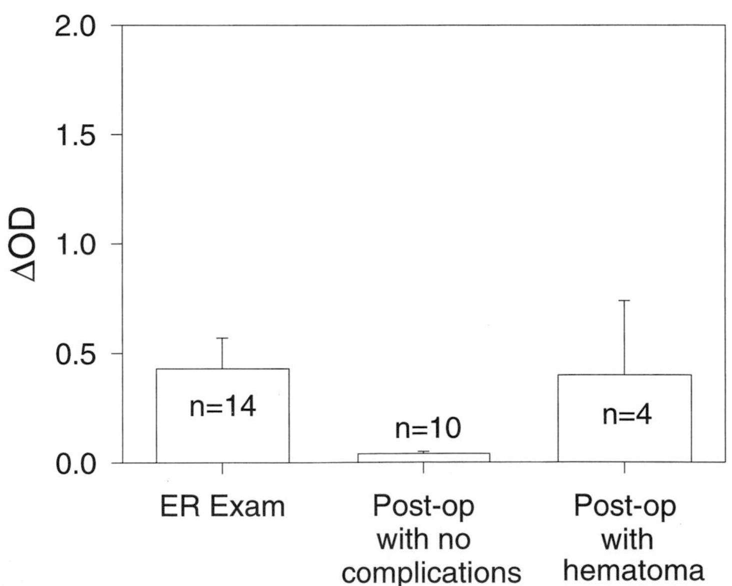

C

Figure 12-7. A typical CT scan (*A*) and the corresponding NIRS examination (*B*) of a patient with an intracerebral hematoma. The bar graph (*C*) shows the average ΔOD on the initial scan in all 14 patients, the average ΔOD postoperatively in the 10 patients who had uncomplicated postoperative courses, and the average ΔOD in the 4 patients who developed some type of intracranial hematoma postoperatively.

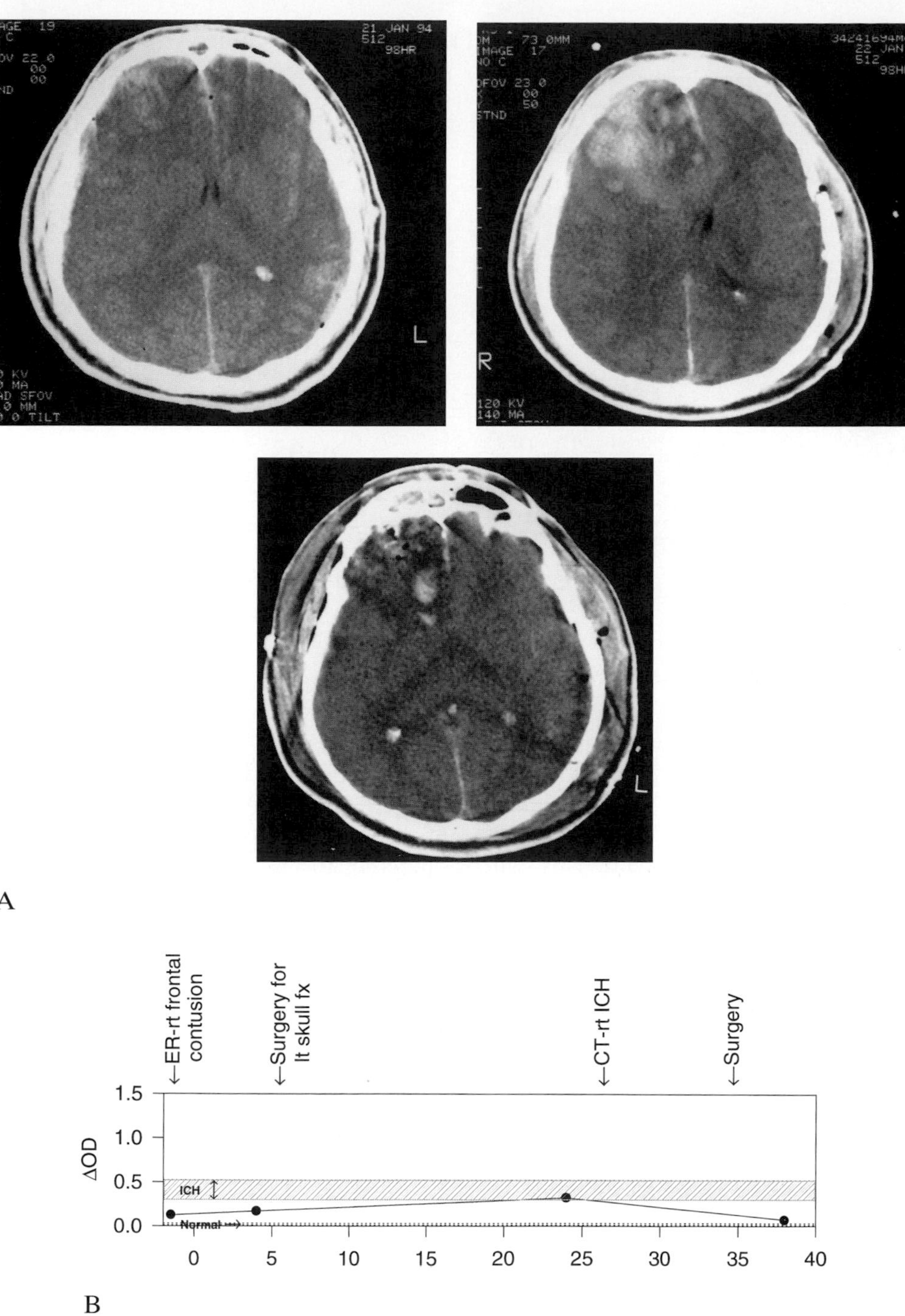

Figure 12-8. Typical series of CT scans (*A*) in a patient who developed a delayed intracerebral hematoma, (*B*) and the serial measurements of ΔOD corresponding to the CT scans. The bar graph (*C*) shows the average ΔOD on the initial CT scan; the follow-up CT scans show the delayed traumatic intracerebral hematoma, and postoperatively in the three patients who developed a delayed intracerebral hematoma.

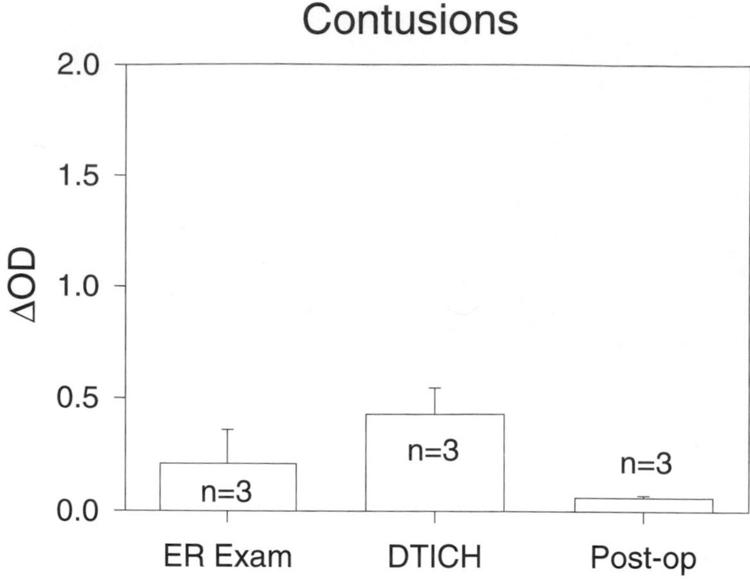

C

Figure 12-8. *Continued.*

7. The balance knob is adjusted until the LCD panel reads zero.
8. The calibration switch is flipped to the 760 nm position, and the gain knob is adjusted until the LCD panel reads 400. If the gain must be increased to greater than 9.5 to obtain a reading of 400 on the LCD panel, the light intensity switch is increased to a higher voltage setting, and steps 4 to 8 are repeated. If a reading of 400 cannot be obtained on the LCD panel with a light intensity of 8 V, an underlying hematoma is suggested. The probe is placed on the opposite cerebral hemisphere and steps 4 to 8 are repeated.
9. The NIRS probe is placed on the frontal region of the opposite cerebral hemisphere, making certain again that the rubber dams make a light seal against the scalp. The light intensity displayed on the LCD panel is recorded. This value will be close to 400 in patients without intracranial blood and considerably less than 400 in patients with an acute intracranial hematoma underlying the probe.
10. Steps 5 to 9 are repeated for the temporal, parietal, and occipital areas of the brain, comparing the values for the reflected light intensity for the right and left sides of each region.
11. The difference in optical density (ΔOD) is calculated from the following formula:

$$\Delta OD = \log_{10} \frac{I_N}{I_H},$$

where I_N = the intensity of reflected light on the normal side

I_H = the intensity of reflected light on the hematoma side

The difference in optical density can also be obtained by looking up the light intensity on the hematoma side from Table 12-1, if the light intensity on the normal side has been adjusted to 400.

CLINICAL EXPERIENCE

We have compared NIRS examinations to CT scans in a total of 131 head-injured patients. A NIRS examination was obtained in the ER at the time of the admission CT scan and then serial measurements were obtained during the hospital course, along with follow-up CT scans. The first 47 of these patients are described in detail in a publication.[48] In addition, a total of 10 patients with no head injuries but with other diagnoses were studied as a control group.

Table 12-2 lists the mean and standard deviations of the ΔOD values in all of the patients who have been studied to date without intracranial hematomas. This group includes the patients without head injury, the patients with diffuse brain injury, and postoperative head-injured patients whose intracranial hematomas were successfully evacuated. The average value was similar in all the patient groups, averaging 0.03 ± 0.01. The maximal value in all of the patients was 0.05.

Types of Intracranial Hematomas that Can Be Identified with NIRS

Subdural hematomas

A total of 54 patients with a subdural hematoma on initial CT scan were studied. Figure 12-5 shows a typical CT scan (*A*) and the corresponding NIRS examination (*B*) for one of these patients. Forty-six of the 54 patients had surgical evacuation of the subdural hematoma on admission to the hospital; 8 patients were not treated surgically because the hematoma was small. The bar graph (*C*) shows the average ΔOD on the initial scan in all 54 patients, the average ΔOD postoperatively in the 39 patients with uncomplicated courses, and the average ΔOD in the 7 patients who developed some type of intracranial hematoma postoperatively. These postoperative complications included four patients with reoccurrence of the subdural hematoma and three patients with epidural hematoma at the operative site. The scatterplot (*D*) shows the relationship ($n = 54$, $r = 0.64$, $p < .001$) between the thickness of the subdural hematoma on the initial CT scan and the ΔOD in the ER.

Epidural hematomas

A total of 28 patients with an epidural hematoma on the initial CT scan have been studied. Figure 12-6 shows a typical CT scan (*A*) and the corresponding NIRS examination (*B*) for one of these patients. Twenty-two of the patients had surgical evacuation of the hematoma on admission to the hospital; six patients were treated medically because the hematoma was small and localized. The bar graph (*C*) shows the average ΔOD on the initial scan in all 28 patients, the average ΔOD postoperatively in the 19 patients with uncomplicated postoperative courses, and the average ΔOD in the three patients who developed some type of intracranial hematoma postoperatively. These postoperative complications included one patient with reoccurrence of the epidural hematoma and two patients with delayed development of epidural hematoma on the opposite side. The scatterplot (*D*) shows the relationship ($n = 28$, $r = 0.73$, $p < .001$) between the thickness of the epidural hematoma on the initial CT scan and the ΔOD in the ER. The relationship is similar to that seen with the subdural hematoma, suggesting that the reason that the average ΔOD of the epidural hematoma group is greater than that of the subdural hematoma group is that the epidural hematoma tended to be thicker (1.3 ± 0.5 cm compared to 0.9 ± 0.4 cm, respectively).

Intracerebral hematomas

A total of 16 patients with an intracerebral hematoma on the initial CT scan have been studied. Fourteen of

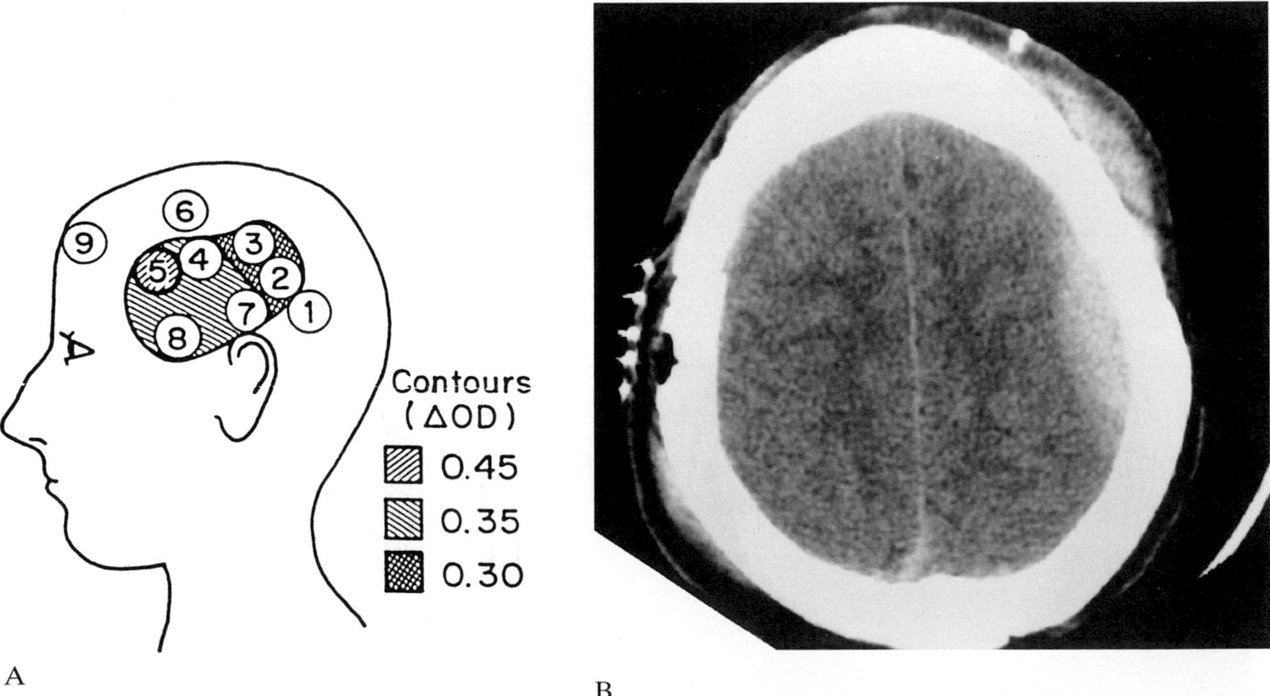

Figure 12-9. Example of a contour map for ΔOD (*A*) which outlines the epidural hematoma seen on the CT scan (*B*).

TABLE 12-3 NIRS Examinations Obtained in Patients with Chronic SDH

	Light Intensity		ΔOD
Patient	Ipsilateral	Contralateral	(Ipsicontralateral)
G.J	550	400	−0.14
L.A.	500	400	−0.10
S.E.	400	530	0.12

the patients had surgical evacuation of the hematoma on admission to the hospital; two were treated medically. Figure 12-7 shows a typical CT scan (*A*) and the corresponding NIRS examination (*B*) for one of these patients. The bar graph (*C*) shows the average ΔOD on the initial scan in all 16 patients, the average ΔOD postoperatively in the 10 patients who had uncomplicated postoperative courses, and the average ΔOD in the 4 patients who developed some type of intracranial hematoma postoperatively. These postoperative complications included three patients with reoccurrence of the intracerebral hematoma and one patient with epidural hematoma at the operative site.

Three patients were studied who each had a contusion present on the initial CT scan, followed by coalescence of the contusion into an intracerebral hematoma on a subsequent CT scan. Figure 12-8 shows an example of the CT scans in one of these patients (*A*), along with the serial measurements of ΔOD corresponding to the serial CT scans. The bar graph (*C*) shows the average ΔOD on the initial CT scan; at the time of the follow-up and postoperatively, CT scans showed the delayed traumatic intracerebral hematoma.

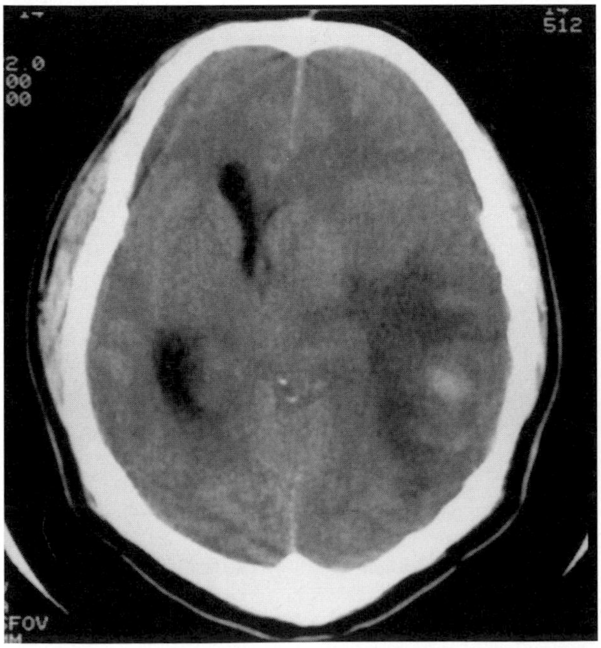

Figure 12-10. Example of a small temporal contusion which did not significantly affect the ΔOD.

LOCATION AND MAPPING OF HEMATOMAS

The ΔOD is partly determined by the thickness of the hematoma, and a contour map of ΔOD can outline a localized collection of blood, such as an epidural hematoma. Figure 12-9 illustrates a case that shows a localization and mapping of an epidural hematoma by obtaining different ΔOD within the hematoma. The correspond-

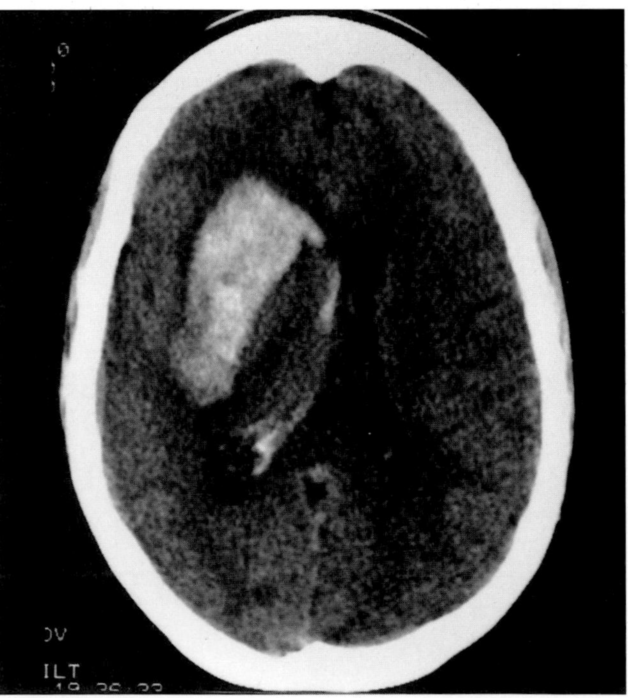

Figure 12-11. Example of a nontraumatic intracranial hematoma lying more than 2 cm beneath the surface of the brain, which was not detectable with the probe used for these studies.

ing CT confirms the location and extent of a clot as plotted by the NIRS method.

Types of Intracranial Hematomas that Cannot Be Identified with NIRS

Chronic subdural hematomas

Because the method relies on the characteristic absorbance of light by hemoglobin at 760 nm, it has not been possible to identify reliably chronic subdural hematoma in which the hemoglobin has been metabolized to varying degrees. As shown in Table 12-3, the light absorbance can be increased, decreased, or not changed on the side of a chronic subdural hematoma.

Hematomas that are small or deep

With the probe configuration that was used in these studies, the depth of brain examined is probably not more than 2.5 cm. This has been adequate to identify all the traumatic hematomas in the present series that were sufficiently large as to require surgery. Figure 12-10 shows a small temporal contusion that did not significantly affect the ΔOD. This contusion did not require surgery and was resolved with medical management; the contusion illustrates the size resolution of the NIRS examination. Figure 12-11 shows a type of intracranial hematoma lying more than 2 cm beneath the surface of the brain; this was not detectable with the probe used for these studies. While this was not a traumatic hematoma, it does illustrate another limitation of the NIRS examination. This is not an inherent limitation of the technique but rather of the probe configuration. The separation of the probe and the light source could be widened to increase the depth of the brain examined.

Comparison of Information Obtained with NIRS Examination and CT Scan

Table 12-4 gives a brief comparison of the information that can be obtained with NIRS and CT. The NIRS in its present form cannot replace the CT scan, but because

TABLE 12-4 Comparison of NIRS Examination and CT Scan

	NIRS Examination	CT Scan
Cost per examination	none	Approx. $1000
Time to perform	10 minutes	15–20 minutes
Special personnel required	none	technician, radiologist
Place of examination	monitor is taken to patient	patient must be taken to scanner
Type of information that can be obtained:	1. Single examination can determine if there is an intracranial hematoma in the area of the brain examined by the probe.	1. Detailed information about the location and size of the hematoma can be obtained. Usually it can be determined if a hematoma is subdural, epidural, or intracerebral.
	2. Serial examinations can determine if a hematoma is enlarging or resolving.	2. Associated information, such as the amount of midline shift, and compression of ventricles and basal cisterns can be determined.
Limitations:		
Extracerebral hematomas	SDH and EDH as small as 0.3 cm thick have been identified. Possibility of missing bilateral acute extracerebral collections exist.	At times, it is difficult to distinguish bone artifacts from thin collection of blood, especially in temporal region.
Intracerebral hematomas	Small hematomas and hematomas that are deep cannot be identified	

of its portability and low cost may give valuable information about which patients need to have a CT scan. Its applications may include the following: (1) In the field, a NIRS examination might help triage a patient with a head injury to a hospital with neurosurgical support. (2) In the mild head injury patient, a NIRS examination might help decide which patients require observation or a CT scan. (3) In the ICU, a NIRS examination might help decide when a patient requires a repeat CT scan to look for a postoperative or delayed intracranial hematoma. Further studies are needed to explore these potential uses of existing NIRS technology. Furthermore, future development of NIRS technology may help improve the resolution and localization of the information obtained.

References

1. Becker DP, Miller JD, Ward JD, et al. The outcome from severe head injury with early diagnosis and intensive management. *J Neurosurg* 1977; 47:491.
2. Jennett B, Teasdale G, Braakman R, et al: Prognosis of patients with severe head injury. *Neurosurgery* 1979; 4:283.
3. Foulkes M, Eisenberg HM, Jane JA, et al: The traumatic coma data bank: Design, methods, and baseline characteristics. *J Neurosurg* 1991; 75(suppl):S8–13.
4. Gutman MB, Moulton RJ, Sullivan I, et al: Risk factors predicting operable intracranial hematomas in head injury. *J Neurosurg* 1992; 77:9–14.
5. Miller JD, Sweet RC, Narayan R, Becker DP: Early insults to the injured brain. 1978; 240:439–442.
6. Miller JD: Head injury and brain ischemia: Implications for therapy. *Br J Anaesth* 1985; 57:120–129.
7. Stein SC, Spettell C, Young G, Ros RE: Delayed and progressive brain injury in closed-head trauma: Radiological demonstration. *Neurosurgery* 1993; 32:25–30.
8. Jennett B: Diagnosis and management of head trauma. *J Neurotrauma* 1991; 8(suppl 1):S15–S19.
9. Rockswold GL, Pheley PJ: Patients who talk and deteriorate. *Ann Emerg Med* 1993; 22:1004–1007.
10. Seelig JM, Becker DP, Miller JD, et al: Traumatic subdural hematoma: Major mortality reduction in comatose patients treated within four hours. *N Engl J Med* 1981; 304:1511–1518.
11. Kvarnes TL, Trumpy JH: Extradural hematomas: Report of 132 cases. *Acta Neurochir* 1978; 41:223–231.
12. Borovich B, Braun J, Guilburd JN, et al: Delayed onset of traumatic extradural hematomas. *J Neurosurg* 1985; 63:30–34.
13. Ban M, Agawa M, Fukami T: Delayed evolution of posttraumatic contralateral extracerebral hematoma after evacuation of initial hematoma. *Neurol Med Chir (Tokyo)* 1991; 31:927–930.
14. Soloniuk D, Pitts LH, Lovely M, Bartowski H: Traumatic intracerebral hematomas: Timing of appearance and indications for operative removal. *J Trauma* 1986; 26:787–794.
15. Rivano C, Barzonic M, Carta F, et al: Traumatic intracerebral hematoma: Seventy-two cases surgically treated. *J Neurol Sci* 1980; 24:77–84.
16. Jamieson KG, Yelland JDN: Traumatic intracerebral hematoma: Report of 63 surgically treated cases. *J Neurosurg* 1972; 37:528–532.
17. MacPherson P, Teasdale G, Khaker S, et al: The significance of traumatic intracranial hematoma in the region of basal ganglia. *J Neurol Neurosurg Psychiatry* 1986; 49:29–34.
18. Lipper MH, Kishore PR, Girevendulis AK, et al: Delayed intracranial hematoma in patients with head injury. *Neuroradiology* 1979; 133:645–649.
19. Gudeman SK, Kishore PRS, Miller JD, et al: The genesis and significance of delayed traumatic intracerebral hematoma. *Neurosurgery* 1979; 5:309–313.
20. Andrews BT: Management of delayed post-traumatic intracerebral hemorrhage. *Contemp Neurosurg* 1980; 2:8.
21. Clifton GL, Grossman RG, Makela ME, et al: Neurological course and correlated computerized tomography findings after severe closed head injury. *J Neurosurg* 1980; 52:611–624.
22. Mendelow AD, Karmi MZ, Paul KS, et al: Extradural hematomas: Effect of delayed treatment. *Br Med J* 1979; 1:1240–1242.
23. Moulton RJ: Traumatic intracranial mass lesions: How soon for evacuation? *Can J Surg* 1992; 35:35–37.
24. Millikan GA: The oxymeter, an instrument for measuring continuously the oxygen saturation of arterial blood in man. *Rev Sci Instrum* 1942; 13:434.
25. Chance B: Rapid and sensitive spectrophotometry: III. A double beam apparatus. *Rev Sci Instrum* 1951; 22:634–638.
26. Jobsis-Vandervliet FF: Noninvasive, infrared monitoring of cerebral and myocardial oxygen sufficiency and circulatory parameters. *Science* 1977; 198:1264–1267.
27. Patterson MS, Chance B, Wilson BC: Time resolved reflectance and transmittance for the non-invasive measurement of tissue optical properties. *Appl Optics* 1989; 28:2331–2336.
28. Chance B, Leigh JS, Miyake H, et al: Comparison of time-resolved and -unresolved measurements of deoxyhemoglobin in brain. *Proc Natl Acad Sci USA* 1988; 85:4971–4975.
29. Cheong WF, Prahl SC, Welch AJ: A review of the optical properties of biological tissues. *IEEE J Quant Electron* 26:2166–2185.
30. Nioka S, Chance B, Smith DS, et al: Cerebral energy metabolism and oxygen state during hypoxia in neonate and adult dogs. *Ped Res* 1990; 28:54–62.
31. Elwell CE, Owen-Reece H, Cope M, et al: Measurement of adult cerebral hemodynamics using near infrared spectroscopy. *Acta Neurochir* 1993; (Suppl) 59:74–80.
32. Kurth CD, Steven JM, Nicolson SC, et al: Kinetics of cerebral deoxygenation during deep hypothermic circulatory arrest in neonates. *Anesthesiology* 1992; 77:656–661.

33. Shah AR, Kurth CD, Gwiazdowski SG, et al: Fluctuations in cerebral oxygenation and blood volume during endotracheal suctioning in premature infants. *J Pediatr* 1992; 126:769–774.
34. Brazy JE, Lewis DV, Mitnick MH, Jobsis-Vandervliet FF: Non-invasive monitoring of cerebral oxygenation in preterm infants: Preliminary observations. *Pediatrics* 1985; 75:217–225.
35. Brazy JE: Effects of crying on cerebral blood volume and cytochrome aa_3. *J Pediatr* 1988; 112:457–461.
36. Ferrari M, De Marchis C, Giannini I, et al: Cerebral blood volume and hemoglobin oxygen saturation monitoring in neonatal brain by near IR spectroscopy. *Adv Exp Med Biol* 1986; 200:203–211.
37. Wyatt JS, Cope M, Delpy DT, et al: Quantitation of cerebral blood volume in newborn infants by near infrared spectroscopy. *J Appl Physiol* 1990; 68:1086–1091.
38. Peebles DM, Edwards AD, Wyatt JS, et al: Effect of oxytocin on fetal brain oxygenation during labour. *Lancet* 1991; 338:254–255.
39. Peebles DM, Edwards AD, Wyatt JS, et al: Changes in human fetal cerebral hemoglobin concentration and oxygenation during labour measured by near infrared spectroscopy. *Am J Obstet Gynecol* 1992; 166:1369–1373.
40. McCormick PW, Stewart M, Goetting MG, et al: Regional cerebrovascular oxygen saturation measured by optical spectroscopy in humans. *Stroke* 1991; 22:596–602.
41. Chance B, Smith DS, Nioka S, et al: Photon migration in muscle and brain, in Chance B (ed): *Photon Migration in Tissues.* New York: Plenum Press, 1989: 121–135.
42. Brazy JE, Lewis DV: Changes in cerebral blood volume and cytochrome aa_3 during hypertensive peaks in preterm infants. *Pediatrics* 1986; 108:983–987.
43. Skov L, Pryds O, Greisen G: Estimating cerebral blood flow in newborn infants: Comparison of near infrared spectroscopy and ^{133}Xenon clearance. *Paediatr Res* 1991; 30:570–573.
44. Livera LN, Spencer SA, Thorniley MS, et al: Effects of hypoxaemia and bradycardia on neonatal cerebral hemodynamics. *Arch Dis Child* 1991; 66:376–380.
45. Edwards AD, Reynolds EOR, Richardson CE, Wyatt JS: Estimation of blood flow in man using near infrared spectroscopy (NIRS). *J Physiol* 1988; 410:50P.
46. Pryds O, Greisen G, Skov LL, Fris-Hansen B: Carbon dioxide related changes in cerebral blood volume and cerebral blood flow in mechanically ventilated preterm neonates: Comparison of near infrared spectroscopy and ^{133}Xenon clearance. *Paediatr Res* 1990; 27:445–449.
47. Carson KJ, Cunningham P, Wickramasinghe YABD, Rolfe P: Time resolved near infrared measurements for spectroscopy and imaging. *NIRSI Newsletter* 1993; 1:44.
48. Gopinath SP, Robertson CS, Grossman RG, Chance B: Near-infrared spectroscopic localization of intracranial hematomas. *J Neurosurg* 1993; 79:43–47.

CHAPTER 13

ANESTHESIA IN HEAD INJURY

Lewis A. Coveler
Sally R. Raty

SYNOPSIS

The anesthetic management of head-injured patients begins in the emergency room with an aggressive and informed approach to airway management. Special attention is focused on patients with facial trauma or an unstable cervical spine. In the operating room, control of intracranial pressure, careful management of hemodynamics, and an awareness of associated injuries enables the surgical team to care for critically ill patients. Planning for awakening and extubation begins early in the procedure. Attention to details helps the surgical team achieve a successful outcome.

PREOPERATIVE MANAGEMENT

The first and probably the most critical contact between an individual who has sustained neurotrauma and an anesthesiologist takes place in the emergency room. Rapid assessment of hemodynamic stability and respiratory gas exchange, along with the establishment of an artificial airway and manually or mechanically supplemented ventilation, when these interventions are indicated, can maximize the probability of recovery.

Patient Assessment

In contrast to patients undergoing elective neurosurgical procedures, the assessment of a neurotrauma victim is often compromised by the urgency of the situation and the complexity of the injury. As with any trauma patient, a clear understanding of the mechanism of injury is important for the anesthesiologist. Patient assessment is frequently undertaken concurrently with resuscitation and stabilization. These simultaneous activities often limit access to the patient while requiring rapid and timely intervention before a complete evaluation is feasible.

History and physical examination

The backbone of management by the anesthesiologist is a rapidly conducted investigation of the patient's history in conjunction with the performance of a relevant physical examination. Information about the day-to-day performance of the patient's cardiovascular and pulmonary systems may be elicited along with historical data about renal, hepatic, and endocrine dysfunction. Exercise tolerance; work history; drug, alcohol, and tobacco use or abuse; and the allergic and surgical history are also investigated. If the anesthesiologist is unable to obtain this information because of the patient's condition or is too involved in the early resuscitation to interview others, a member of the surgical team can obtain this essential information from family members and/or other sources and report it to the entire trauma team. However, all too often no reliable historical information is available during the early management of a neurotrauma victim.

Physical examination by the anesthesiologist is of necessity focused on the head, neck, and chest. Auscultation of the heart and lungs along with palpation of the neck, face, and chest will reveal injuries that require immediate intervention or injury-specific action by the anesthesiologist. The remainder of the physical examination is performed by other members of the trauma team and is reported to the anesthesiologist.

Certain aspects of the patient's history are of special

importance to the anesthesiologist and are detailed below.

Anesthetic history

If either the patient or the patient's immediate family has been exposed to surgical anesthesia, important information may be available. The interviewer must ask the broadest questions to avoid limiting the response of the historian. For example, instead of asking only whether the patient has experienced difficulties with anesthesia, the interviewer should ask whether the patient has had any problems with anesthesia *or* surgery. This type of question will often uncover problems that the lay public does not associate with anesthesia but may associate with the surgical experience. Specific inquiries about intraoperative and postoperative fevers, drug reactions, transfusion reactions, prolonged awakening, difficult airway management, and postoperative care in an intensive care unit are also helpful in evaluating the importance of what might have been an unrecognized sentinel event in the patient's surgical experience.

NPO status

While special attention is focused on the timing of the patient's last oral intake, it is probably safer to assume that a neurotrauma patient has a full stomach and act accordingly. This is important when the patient has a depressed level of consciousness or requires sedation for diagnostic or therapeutic procedures. It is also very important if the patient must undergo endotracheal intubation, especially awake intubation associated with sedation and topical anesthesia of the airway. Patients who are sufficiently obtunded or sedated and anesthetized to tolerate the placement of an endotracheal tube can usually tolerate the presence of gastric contents or other foreign bodies in the airway.

Substance abuse

The combination of anesthetic agents, adjuvants, and recreational drugs, including alcohol, can contribute to the development of an unstable cardiovascular system. The neurological examination, especially the examination of mental status, and the ability of the patient to give a history are further compromised by these agents. In the authors' institution there is a strong association between alcohol and/or cocaine abuse and head trauma. Errors in formulation by street vendors compound the problems of the surgical team because a mixture of unidentified drugs and other substances, all in unknown concentrations, might have been ingested or injected. Alpha and beta blockers, vasodilators, catecholamines, and vasopressors may all be required at various stages of the patient's care to maintain cardiovascular stability.

A substance-intoxicated head-injured patient may benefit from pulmonary artery catheterization if he or she is hemodynamically unstable, although if emergent surgical intervention is required, surgery should not be delayed to permit placement of the catheter.

Airway Assessment and Management

After the history and physical examination, however abbreviated, the anesthesiologist may be called on to provide an artificial airway to prevent tracheal soilage, guarantee a high concentration of inspired oxygen, and permit controlled ventilation.

Anticipation of difficult intubation

As with any patient requiring endotracheal intubation, examination of the airway before anesthetic intervention is the only way to prevent the potentially lethal consequences of a failed intubation in an anesthetized and apneic patient. Even after careful examination of the airway in an elective surgical patient, failed intubation occurs in up to 1 in 3000 intubation attempts. If a head-injured patient is pregnant and near term, the incidence of failed intubation rises to as high as 1 in 300 attempts. This is due to a combination of effects, including a protuberant abdomen which causes cephalad displacement of pregnancy-enlarged breasts and hormonally induced edema of the airway mucosa.

Mallampati et al.[1] described a scoring system to help predict the degree of difficulty that can be anticipated during oral endotracheal intubation. Others have subsequently modified or added to this technique.[2] During airway assessment, it is important to note the presence of foreign bodies, dentures, food, candy, or chewing gum in the mouth and the soundness of the teeth. An estimate of the ability of the patient to flex and extend the neck must be made. This flexibility may be compromised in a head-injured patient because of an associated or suspected cervical spine injury or by the presence of a neck collar or another stabilizer. Examination of the submandibular space for overall size and volume as well as measurement of the hyoid-mental distance completes the basic airway assessment.

Cervical spine

When possible, the cervical spine (c-spine) should be evaluated by x-ray before endotracheal intubation. Frequently, however, this is not possible because of an urgent need for controlled ventilation and oxygenation. The presence of associated injuries, as discussed later, often dictates a modification of routine techniques for airway management.

INTUBATION TECHNIQUES

The anesthesiologist should have a high level of skill with several techniques for endotracheal intubation. These techniques can be tailored to the management of the individual patient.

Awake versus Asleep

Two major decisions must be made before the patient can be intubated. The first concerns the degree of sedation required, up to and including the formal induction of general anesthesia. Uncooperative patients and/or those requiring oral intubation are candidates for heavy sedation or, in the authors' institution, general anesthesia. Heavy sedation may result in a rise in intracranial pressure caused by hypoventilation-induced hypercarbia, predisposes the patient to silent aspiration, and places the patient at a high risk of developing hypoxemia.

Rapid Sequence Induction of General Anesthesia

Because patients undergoing the induction of general anesthesia are placed at risk of aspiration, a rapid sequence induction is indicated. Preoxygenation before the administration of induction agents is mandatory. This helps maintain the patient's arterial saturation during the inevitable period of apnea associated with intubation. Cricoid pressure is applied before the development of unconsciousness to help prevent gastric reflux before endotracheal intubation. Once applied, cricoid pressure should be released only after confirmation of the intratracheal position of the endotracheal tube.

The second major decision required before intubation involves the selection of the route to be used. Several factors must be considered, including the stability of the cervical spine, associated injuries, facial trauma, state of consciousness, expected degree of elevation of intracranial pressure, presence of spontaneous ventilation, cardiovascular stability, and the experience and skill of the anesthesiologist.

Direct Vision

Intubation under direct vision using a rigid laryngoscope, with in-line cervical traction in case there is a suspected or documented cervical spine injury, permits the rapid establishment of an artificial airway. The endotracheal tube can be placed orally or nasally. Nasal intubation can be facilitated by using intubating forceps to guide the endotracheal tube into the correct position. A lighted stylet placed in the endotracheal tube, with the light source at the distal end of the tube, can provide additional lighting during intubation through a soiled airway.

Blind

"Blind" endotracheal intubation is performed, using the nasal route, in spontaneously breathing patients. The authors use the Endotrol[3] endotracheal tube for this procedure because of the ability to deflect the tip of the tube during intubation attempts. Increasingly loud breath sounds heard through the endotracheal tube are the major guide for this approach. One technique the authors have found helpful is the placement of an acoustic amplifier on the proximal end of a nasally placed endotracheal tube.[4] This increases the likelihood of correct positioning of the endotracheal tube, especially in the noisy emergency room setting.

Lighted Stylet

Another helpful technique for blind intubation involves the use of a light-tipped flexible guidewire. This technique transilluminates the larynx, with the light on the inside, when the tip of the tube is placed in the trachea. Sometimes, however, the lights in the room must be lowered, temporarily interrupting patient care.

Fiber-optic Guided

Use of a fiber-optic bronchoscope to facilitate endotracheal intubation is quite popular and successful in the management of elective surgery patients. The bronchoscope is used during oral and, more commonly, nasal intubation. Drawbacks include the necessity of having a cooperative patient and the problems of visualizing the trachea when the airway has been soiled with blood and/or vomitus. Practice is mandatory to develop speed and attain a high success rate. Most emergency rooms do not have this fragile and expensive equipment immediately available. The authors have a fully equipped cart designed especially for fiber-optic intubations, including television monitoring, which can be brought to the emergency room on a dedicated elevator within 90 to 120 s. In spite of the drawbacks, this technique is especially useful for intubating a patient with an unstable c-spine. When necessary, the bronchoscope can be passed nasally under direct vision even in patients who have sustained midface trauma. The difficulties associated with the soiled airway may be reduced by blowing oxygen through the bronchoscopic suction port instead of using the small lumen for suction.

Management of Failed Intubation

Even during the controlled circumstances of an elective and well-planned anesthetic induction, endotracheal intubation can sometimes be impossible. Therefore, in the emergency room under less controlled circumstances, failed intubation becomes more likely, especially after a limited patient assessment. Options for obtaining control of the airway in this circumstance must be established in anticipation of the event. Several devices are available that may be useful with an apneic patient, perhaps anesthetized and pharmacologically paralyzed, who cannot be quickly intubated or ventilated by conventional bag-valve-mask techniques.

Combitube

The Combitube[5] is a short double-cuffed, double-lumen tube designed for blind placement into the airway. If the short distal portion of the tube enters the trachea, ventilation proceeds as usual. The distal cuff seals the trachea around the tube. If the distal portion of the tube enters the esophagus, ventilation is maintained through the fenestrated proximal portion of the tube. The distal cuff seals the esophagus around the tube. A larger proximal cuff seals the oropharynx, allowing positive-pressure ventilation of the lungs. Limitations include a less than perfect seal in the airway and the esophagus, resulting in compromised ventilation if lung and/or chest compliance is poor.

Laryngeal Mask Airway

Another airway adjunct is the Laryngeal Mask Airway[6] (LMA). The LMA, like the Combitube, is designed for blind transoral placement. It also has a cufflike air seal in the oropharynx. Unlike the one-sized Combitube, this device comes in several different sizes, allowing its use in patients ranging in size from infants to very large adults. Aspiration can occur before, during, and after placement of the LMA, and in the face of poor lung compliance, there is reduced ventilation of the lungs. High airway pressures will result in gastric distension during use of the LMA. After the LMA is in place and the patient is receiving adequate ventilation, a small endotracheal tube can be advanced, either blindly or under fiber-optic control, via the shaft of the LMA into the trachea.

Transtracheal Jet Ventilation

Emergency ventilation can be provided by using an IV catheter or a needle placed percutaneously into the trachea through the cricothyroid membrane. Oxygen pressure proximal to the catheter may be as high as 50 pounds per square inch to provide adequate ventilation. Misplacement of the catheter will result in the injection of a large amount of oxygen into the subcutaneous tissues or the mediastinum. Once ventilation is established by this technique, a more effective and permanent method of airway maintenance must be chosen. Flexible or rigid laryngoscopy or the retrograde technique described below may be performed during transtracheal jet ventilation.

Retrograde Technique

With this technique, a long flexible wire is introduced into the trachea by passing it through a needle or catheter inserted into the trachea through the cricothyroid membrane. The wire is directed retrograde through the larynx and into the pharynx, from where it is retrieved with forceps. An endotracheal tube may then be advanced over the wire into the trachea, or the wire may be passed retrograde through the suction channel of a flexible bronchoscope onto which an endotracheal tube has been loaded. The wire is then used to help guide the flexible bronchoscope into the trachea. An endotracheal tube can thus be introduced into the tracheal lumen, and its position can be confirmed under direct vision through the bronchoscope.

Cricothyrotomy

When other techniques fail or the nature of the patient's injuries dictates a surgical airway, cricothyrotomy must be performed.

Monitoring during Intubation

During the induction of general anesthesia and subsequent endotracheal intubation in the operating room, the patient's vital signs are measured frequently and repetitively. In the emergency room, patients undergoing endotracheal intubation should have the same monitoring.

Electrocardiogram

At least one lead of the ECG should be monitored. Dysrhythmia or other ECG findings, such as ST segment changes, may signal an impending cardiovascular collapse or rising intracranial pressure.

Blood Pressure

Systemic blood pressure should be measured, utilizing an automated noninvasive device or, when immediately available, an arterial catheter. During sedation or general anesthesia administered to facilitate intubation, the noninvasive unit should be operated at the maximum rate or in the "STAT" mode, measuring blood pressure as frequently as once per minute.

Oxygen Saturation

Pulse oximetry is a required monitoring technique. Along with beat-to-beat detection of the pulse rate, it provides almost instantaneous detection of the presence of a dysrhythmia and a prompt warning of developing arterial desaturation.

End-Tidal Carbon Dioxide (ET_{CO_2})

In the operating room, detection of ET_{CO_2} is the accepted standard for confirming the intratracheal placement of an endotracheal tube.[7] In the emergency room or elsewhere within the hospital, ET_{CO_2} detection can be performed with a portable electronic qualitative device or a disposable semiquantitative photochemical detector. Except during cardiac arrest, when ET_{CO_2} may normally be absent or too low to measure with these devices, they are cost-effective and efficient when used to confirm the correct placement of an endotracheal tube.

Associated Injuries

Open Globe

A victim of head trauma can sustain injury to the orbit and its contents, resulting in an "open globe" injury. Any technique that could raise the intraocular pressure and result in the extrusion of intraocular contents is contraindicated. It has been shown that the intravenous administration of a small dose of a nondepolarizing muscle relaxant followed by an induction agent and succinylcholine will result in satisfactory and safe intubating conditions.[8] This avoids the prolonged paralysis associated with large doses of nondepolarizing muscle relaxants. Given to permit intubation without raising intraocular pressure, these long-acting neuromuscular blocking drugs prevent serial neurological examinations. The brief and limited rise in both intraocular pressure and intracranial pressure associated with succinylcholine administration does not appear to be clinically significant. The rapid achievement of intubating conditions and the prompt institution of controlled ventilation and airway protection seem to outweigh the theoretical adverse effects.

Vascular Injury or Exsanguinating Hemorrhage

Associated truncal trauma, long bone fractures, and even a large scalp laceration may leave a neurotrauma victim with a markedly reduced circulating blood volume. Hypovolemia requires a reduction in depressant drugs if these drugs are needed for intubation, since the administration of a full dose of an anesthetic induction agent or the institution of controlled ventilation may result in profound hypotension. The blood pressure may require pharmacological support during volume resuscitation to maintain cerebral perfusion. Limited vascular access may make large-volume fluid infusion unavailable as an option during this stage of resuscitation.

Facial Trauma

Patients who have experienced blunt trauma to the face and head should, when possible, undergo oral endotracheal intubation, avoiding the nasal route with its potential for contamination of the cranial vault, or even intracranial placement of the endotracheal tube. When the oral route and the nasal route are both unavailable, a surgical airway will be necessary.

Pediatric Patients

An in-depth discussion of pediatric patients appears in Chap. 59. However, some specific anesthetic concerns should be mentioned here.

Vascular Access

Although starting an IV in most adults is fairly simple, this may not be the case in hypovolemic or obese youngsters. Atropine and succinylcholine can be given intramuscularly to facilitate intubation, and certain resuscitation drugs can be given intratracheally, such as lidocaine and epinephrine. Fluid administration requires access to the circulation. When IV placement is difficult or time-consuming, a bone marrow aspiration needle can be percutaneously inserted into the marrow canal of the tibia. This intraosseous needle can usually be placed within 1 min, allowing fluid resuscitation and drug administration.[9] Once standard venous access has been obtained, the intraosseous needle is removed, although it may be retained for as long as 24 h if necessary.

Central venous catheterization is a quick way of obtaining reliable vascular access in children with limited peripheral venous access. Femoral, subclavian, or jugular (internal or external) venous catheterization can be performed with a 20-gauge 5-in.-long catheter, using the modified Seldinger technique.[10] In larger children, a 16-gauge 8-in.-long catheter can be placed, using the same technique. The femoral vein is easily located because it has a constant relationship to the femoral arterial pulse. Inadvertent femoral artery puncture can provide needed access to the arterial circulation.

Airway management

The larynx in a young child differs somewhat from that in an adult. The narrowest part of the child's larynx is at the cricoid ring. This permits the use of uncuffed endotracheal tubes. The practitioner will choose the size on the basis of the child's age or height and weight or may use the size of the child's little finger as a guide. Adenoidal hypertrophy can make nasal intubation very difficult or traumatic in young children.

Airway equipment requires special consideration in pediatric patients. Almost all the airway management techniques described above, except for the Combitube, are available for children. The 2.1-mm flexible fiberoptic endoscope does not have a suction port, making its use in a soiled airway frustrating. Pretreatment of the patient with glycopyrrolate (Robinul), if time permits, can help reduce secretions and improve laryngeal visualization.

Endotracheal tubes ranging from 2.0 to 6.0 uncuffed and 4.0 to 6.0 cuffed should suffice for children. Appropriately sized oral airways, stylets, laryngoscopes, and masks must be available as well. Small catheters for transtracheal jet ventilation are mandatory if this technique is to be used.[11]

Pregnant Patients

An in-depth discussion of how the physiology of pregnancy relates to trauma is beyond the scope of this chapter.[12] However, a few basic patient management considerations, as they differ from those for nonpregnant patients, will be presented.

Physiological considerations

The treatment or prevention of supine hypotension utilizing left uterine displacement begins at the gestational age at which pregnancy becomes obvious to the observer in the emergency room. A pregnant patient should be treated as a "full stomach" for purposes of airway management, regardless of the length of her fast, especially after trauma. Fetal monitoring equipment should be used, if time permits and the equipment is available, during anesthetic drug administration, endotracheal intubation, or prolonged radiological studies. If the injury pattern allows it, the fetus can be shielded from x-rays by a lead apron placed on the mother's abdomen. The location of the x-ray source should be noted when the pelvic shield is placed. The physiological anemia of pregnancy may complicate the diagnosis of hemorrhage.

Triage: mother versus fetus

As the patient approaches term, cardiopulmonary resuscitation (CPR) becomes relatively ineffective. The uterus must be emptied by cesarean section, a procedure that the authors have performed in the emergency room while attempting to save the life of an unborn child after the mother died in a motor vehicle accident. The authors have developed a special protocol for triage of a traumatized parturient and her fetus when fetal distress or the nature of the trauma dictates emergent surgery or cesarean section and the patient is not undergoing CPR. If the fetus is viable and the mother is considered unlikely to survive, the infant is delivered in the obstetric unit because of the proximity of the neonatal intensive care unit and neonatal resuscitation equipment. If the fetus is dead and the mother is expected to survive, the fetus is delivered in the main operating room because of the availability of specialized equipment and personnel.

Transportation to the Operating Room

A trip to the operating room (OR) often follows the completion of the initial resuscitative and diagnostic measures which usually include a computed tomographic (CT) scan of the head. When indicated, portions of the spine (especially cervical), chest, and abdomen are imaged as well. A decrease in vigilance during the transportation phase is related to the changing focus of the trauma team as plans for operative intervention are formulated. The transfer of the patient may be the responsibility of less experienced individuals, while the senior members of the trauma team go to the operating room to don OR attire and discuss any special requirements with the OR staff. Attention must be directed toward stabilization of the c-spine during patient transfer as well as to the details of controlled ventilation. Portable monitoring equipment should be available for hemodynamically unstable patients. Minimum capabilities should include ECG, pulse oximetry, and invasive or noninvasive blood pressure measurement. The choice of monitoring devices and monitored parameters is dependent on the status of the patient at the time of the initiation of the transfer to the operating room.

INTRAOPERATIVE MANAGEMENT

Monitoring

The objective for intraoperative monitoring of a head-injured patient is to continuously evaluate the patient's circulatory status, oxygenation, ventilation, and temperature. Intraoperative positioning and surgical draping of a head-injured patient make it difficult to place catheters for invasive monitoring or for vascular access after the start of the surgical procedure. The authors are therefore aggressive with the preoperative placement of invasive monitoring catheters (intraarterial, central venous, and pulmonary artery) because this may be the only opportunity to place such catheters in a controlled and sterile environment.

Electrocardiogram

Cardiac rate, rhythm, and ischemia are best monitored with a continuously displayed two-lead electrocardiogram with strip-recording capabilities. Lead II of the electrocardiogram facilitates the detection of dysrhythmias, while precordial lead IV or V is used to detect ischemia. Strip recording permits comparison of the ECG findings over several hours and documents any changes noted during the operative procedure.

Systemic blood pressure

Changes in blood pressure can lead to cerebral or myocardial ischemia. The placement of an intraarterial catheter preoperatively allows more precise control of blood pressure during anesthetic induction and endotracheal intubation. Large variations in systolic pressure may be related to associated injuries, changing intracranial dynamics, or occult substance abuse. If the patient arrives in the operating suite without an intraarterial catheter, induction, intubation, and surgical preparation may proceed with the use of a noninvasive blood pressure monitor if the patient's condition demands rapid intervention. However, in the authors' experience, the intraarterial catheter can usually be placed in the 1 or 2 min before the induction of anesthesia while other essential monitors are being placed and the patient is undergoing preoxygenation. Intraoperatively, an arterial catheter allows fast and convenient serial sampling of the patient's arterial blood for evaluation of oxygenation and ventilation and measurement of electrolytes and hematocrit.

The zero reference point for the arterial pressure transducer should be established at the level of the circle of Willis (external auditory meatus). Placing the electronic zero at this location assures that arterial blood pressure readings will reflect the pressure to which the brain is exposed. In the supine position, the brain and the heart are in the same vertical plane and there is no hydrostatic pressure gradient between them. However, in the head-up position that is frequently used in neurosurgery, the brain may be 20 to 30 cm above the heart. In this position, the brain and heart are exposed to different blood pressures because of the hydrostatic pressure gradient between them.

Cerebral perfusion pressure

Cerebral perfusion pressure (CPP) is defined as the difference between systemic mean arterial pressure (MAP) and intracranial pressure (ICP). In an uninjured normotensive patient, a CPP of 40 to 50 mmHg is considered adequate. At this perfusion pressure, autoregulation is functional and cerebral blood flow (CBF) is maintained within a narrow range. Below this level of CPP, the compensatory mechanisms of the cerebral circulation are inadequate and reductions in CBF occur. In a severely head injured patient, the lower limit of CPP that provides adequate perfusion in the face of elevated ICP is higher than it is in an uninjured patient. Some investigators estimate that in a head-injured patient a threshold CPP of at least 70 mmHg should be maintained to optimize perfusion.[13] Other investigators have found that continuous monitoring of jugular bulb mixed venous oxygen saturation (Sjv_{O_2}) allows more precise identification of this threshold for CPP.[14] The use of such monitoring intraoperatively may provide valuable information to the anesthesiologist during the first few hours after an injury.

Central venous pressure

The administration of mannitol and/or furosemide to head-injured patients makes urine output an unreliable indicator of intravascular volume. The placement of a central venous catheter permits accurate monitoring of right-sided heart filling pressures. Placement of the catheter in the subclavian vein rarely leads to venous obstruction and is easier than placement of an antecubital catheter. The subclavian catheter should be placed whenever possible without the use of Trendelenburg's position, as this will increase intracranial pressure. If the head-down position is necessary, as it often is in hypovolemic patients, it should be maintained for the shortest time possible. The internal jugular approach is avoided since it is often used in the authors' institution for Sjv_{O_2} monitoring (Chap. 36).

Pulmonary Artery Pressures

A pulmonary artery catheter may better reflect the intravascular volume status in certain patients, such as those who have sustained massive trauma or spinal cord injury or have coexisting heart disease. A pulmonary artery catheter allows repetitive determination of cardiac output. Additional parameters, such as systemic or pulmonary vascular resistance, may be calculated from the data obtained. If vasoactive drugs are necessary for circulatory support or manipulation, the information gained from the pulmonary artery catheter helps determine the effectiveness of the treatment and helps guide changes in therapeutic interventions. An oximetry-capable pulmonary artery catheter provides continuous measurement of mixed venous oxygen saturation, providing information about oxygen extraction in the peripheral tissues.

Urine Output

Sometimes information about the status of a patient's intravascular volume can be obtained from a urine catheter. In a trauma patient who has not received diuretics, a urine output of 0.5 to 1.0 ml/kg/h is primarily an indicator of adequate renal perfusion and secondarily an indicator of adequate volume replacement. However, in a head-injured patient who has received large doses of loop or osmotic diuretics, copious amounts of urine are produced despite a marginal intravascular volume status. Therefore, the clinician should not interpret urine output greater than 0.5 ml/kg/h as a reassuring sign that the patient's volume status is adequate. Conversely, low urine output in the face of diuretic therapy may indicate severe volume depletion and/or the release of antidiuretic hormone.

Pulse Oximetry for Sp_{O_2}

Oxygenation is monitored continuously by a pulse oximeter that uses several wavelengths of light to determine the ratio of oxygenated to deoxygenated hemoglobin. The pulse oximeter accurately reflects changes in Sp_{O_2} when the blood is between 70 and 100 percent saturated with oxygen. Above a Pa_{O_2} of about 70 mmHg, the oxygen hemoglobin dissociation curve flattens. Further increases in oxygen partial pressure cause little change in the percent saturation, making it impossible to track arterial oxygen tension with the pulse oximeter above a Pa_{O_2} of 70 kPa (Table 13-1). An accurate assessment of oxygenation is obtained from serial arterial blood gases. The clinician can also compare the patient's actual Pa_{O_2} with the expected PA_{O_2} (derived from the alveolar gas equation), gaining information about the efficiency of the patient's oxygenation (Table 13-2).

TABLE 13-1 A Comparison of Pa_{O_2} and Sp_{O_2} in Normal Adults

Arterial Oxygen Partial Pressure (Pa_{O_2})	% Peripheral Oxygen Saturation (Sp_{O_2})
26	50
40	75
50	83
60	90
100	97

TABLE 13-2 The Relationship Between Fi_{O_2} and Pa_{O_2}

Fi_{O_2}	Pa_{O_2}
0.2	102
0.4	245
0.6	388
0.8	530
1.0	673

Capnography for ET_{CO_2}

Capnography is used to measure the partial pressure of CO_2 in the patient's inspired and expired gas. The end-tidal CO_2 (ET_{CO_2}) is only an approximation of the arterial CO_2, which is the real indicator of the adequacy of alveolar ventilation. The typical ET_{CO_2}-Pa_{CO_2} gradient is 5 to 10 mmHg with the ET_{CO_2} lower than the Pa_{CO_2}. This gradient can be caused by ventilation-perfusion mismatching, pulmonary emboli (fat, air, thrombus, amniotic fluid), gas sampling errors, chronic obstructive pulmonary disease, bronchoconstriction, and hypoperfusion states.

Mass Spectrometry for ET_{N_2}

Mass spectrometry provides an analysis of nitrogen concentrations in both inspired and expired gases. The detection of nitrogen during an anesthetic administered with oxygen and other non-nitrogen-containing gases provides strong evidence of an intravenous air embolism (see below).

Temperature

Central, or "core," temperature can be monitored by using temperature probes in the rectum, bladder, esophagus, nasopharynx, tympanic membrane, or bloodstream (pulmonary artery catheter). The authors usually employ the esophageal temperature probe/stethoscope. Hypothermia from posttraumatic exposure or hyperthermia from an adverse drug reaction or CNS dysfunction can be detected and managed appropriately.

Blood loss

Monitoring blood loss during craniotomy and most other neurosurgical procedures performed for trauma is extremely difficult because of the noncavitary nature of the surgery. Blood and irrigating fluids are collected in a drainage system which forms part of the surgical drapes. There is no way to measure these losses accurately. The best guide to blood loss in these cases is the determination of serial hematocrits. The patient is transfused as appropriate on the basis of age, underlying disease states, and hemodynamic stability.

Neuromuscular junction

A peripheral nerve stimulator provides a means of evaluating the extent of neuromuscular blockade. Close control of muscle relaxation will allow prompt antagonism of the blockade, permitting immediate neurological assessment of the patient at the end of the surgical procedure.

Laboratory studies

As noted above, serial blood samples from the arterial catheter can provide information about blood gases, electrolytes, and hematocrit. The monitoring of coagulation functions is essential if excessive bleeding develops, since coagulopathies are not uncommon in neurosurgical trauma patients (Chap. 46).

Intracranial pressure monitoring

The monitoring of ICP may be undertaken in comatose head-injured patients who are undergoing surgery for extracranial problems. It is important for the anesthesiologist to avoid the use of a monitoring system which provides a continuous fluid flush, as do the standard monitoring sets used for invasive pressure monitoring. Careful attention is paid to the correct adjustment of the zero reference, as a small change in pressure in this low-pressure system can mandate intervention. ICP monitoring is not usually performed during craniotomy.

Anesthetic Induction and Endotracheal Intubation

Endotracheal intubation

During the induction of anesthesia, after the patient is unconscious but before the trachea is intubated, the patient is at risk of regurgitation and aspiration of gastric contents. All patients presenting to the operating suite for an anesthetic can be classified with regard to their risk for aspiration. Low-risk adults, or "empty" stomachs, have been NPO for 6 to 8 h, are not obese or pregnant, and do not have a history of esophageal reflux, hiatal hernia, diabetes, or autonomic dysfunction. High-risk adults, or "full" stomachs, have ingested solids or liquids within 6 h; are obese or pregnant; have a history of reflux, hiatal hernia, diabetes, or autonomic dysfunction; have intraabdominal pathological conditions (appendicitis or small bowel obstruction); have taken depressant recreational pharmaceuticals or have had similar drugs administered therapeutically; or have sustained trauma. Because head-injured patients are considered to be at high risk for aspiration, their anesthetic induction requires modification.

The most common modification is to perform a "rapid sequence induction" (RSI). During RSI, the patient is required to preoxygenate and denitrogenate by breathing 100% oxygen. The patient is rendered unconscious by the rapid administration of an intravenous induction agent and then is immediately given a rapidly acting neuromuscular blocking agent. The patient is intubated without an attempt at manual ventilation, since mask ventilation can force anesthetic gases into the stomach, leading to gastric dilatation, regurgitation, and aspiration of gastric contents.

During RSI, an assistant applies pressure to the cricoid cartilage in the anteroposterior direction, occluding the esophagus and helping to prevent passive regurgitation while simultaneously moving the glottis into view to facilitate endotracheal intubation. This application of cricoid pressure, known as the Sellick maneuver, is started before induction and is discontinued only after proper placement of the endotracheal tube is confirmed by the presence of CO_2 in the patient's exhaled gases. If the patient cannot be intubated quickly and begins to desaturate, gentle mask ventilation with less than 20 cmH_2O pressure can be instituted while cricoid pressure is maintained. Subsequent attempts to intubate are performed while cricoid pressure is maintained.

All severely head injured patients who arrive in the operating suite should be presumed to have elevated ICP. Endotracheal intubation can further elevate ICP in these patients. Maneuvers that may attenuate this increase include pretreatment with narcotics and/or intravenous lidocaine (1.5 mg/kg) and skillful, gentle, abbreviated instrumentation of the airway during laryngoscopy.

Induction agents

Thiopental (Pentothal)

Thiopental is a lipophilic sulfur-containing, short-acting barbiturate whose primary clinical role is the rapid induction of general anesthesia. It is especially useful in controlling elevated ICP that is resistant to other modes of therapy. The usual induction dose of thiopental, 3 to 5 mg/kg, renders the patient unconscious and apneic in 30 s or less. This dose of thiopental causes a decrease in sympathetic outflow, leading to a decrease in systemic vascular resistance, venous return, cardiac preload, cardiac output, and MAP. The decrease in blood pressure can be offset by the carotid-mediated baroreceptor reflex, resulting in mild tachycardia. Thiopental can be a dangerous induction agent for patients with suspected hypovolemia because these patients are unable to compensate for its vasodilatory effects. These patients often experience a large and rapid decrease in blood pressure. Thiopental decreases CBF, the cerebral metabolic rate, (CMR_{O_2}) and ICP. Its net effect on CPP is limited because of its tendency to lower both mean arterial and intracranial pressures. Used at much higher doses (30 mg/kg), thiopental is the drug of choice for treating increased ICP that is resistant to other forms of treatment, such as ventricular drainage and diuretics.

Etomidate (Amidate)

Etomidate is a carboxylated imidazole-containing compound that is used for the induction of general anesthesia (0.3 mg/kg). Etomidate is a direct cerebral vasoconstrictor, decreases CMR_{O_2}, and lowers previously elevated ICP. Unlike thiopental, etomidate is associated with cardiovascular stability, causing minimal changes in heart rate, stroke volume, and cardiac output, though MAP may decrease slightly secondary to a decrease in peripheral vascular resistance. Up to 80 percent of patients experience pain on injection, and 33 percent have myoclonic movements that are not associated with EEG changes.[15] A single intubating dose of etomidate appears to suppress the 11-beta-hydroxylase enzyme responsible for the conversion of cholesterol to cortisol for 4 to 8 h. There is considerable controversy regarding whether this adrenocortical suppression is clinically significant. However, in patients who are septic or experience hemorrhage, suppression of cortisol production may be detrimental. Finally, etomidate is associated with a higher incidence of postoperative nausea and vomiting than is thiopental.

Propofol (Diprivan)

Propofol is a substituted isopropylphenol that renders patients unconscious within 30 s after an induction dose of 2.0 to 2.5 mg/kg. The 1% aqueous solution of propofol contains 10% soybean oil, 2.25% glycerol, and 1.2% purified egg phosphatide.[16] In patients with a brain injury, an anesthetic induction dose followed by a continuous infusion of propofol (150 μg/kg/min) causes a decrease in MAP, ICP, CBF, and CMR_{O_2}. CPP may be adversely affected. Propofol is associated with pain on injection (10 percent), has a very low incidence of postoperative nausea and vomiting, and does not cause adrenocortical suppression.

Midazolam (Versed)

Midazolam is a water-soluble benzodiazepine that is two to three times more potent than diazepam. In patients with decreased intracranial compliance, induction doses of midazolam (0.1 to 0.3 mg/kg) cause little or no change in ICP. CBF and CMR_{O_2} are decreased in a dose-dependent manner. Hemodynamic changes after midazolam induction are similar to those after thiopental. Hypovolemic patients may have an exaggerated decrease in blood pressure after induction.

Control of Hemodynamics During Endotracheal Intubation

Neither thiopental, etomidate, propofol, nor midazolam has analgesic qualities and thus will not prevent increases in heart rate and blood pressure in response to tracheal intubation. Because autoregulation in a patient with head injury is often defective, the rise in blood pressure that accompanies intubation can lead to an increase in ICP that may further compromise the brain. Several techniques may be used to attenuate increases in blood pressure during intubation. Administration of a narcotic, intravenous or intratracheal lidocaine (1.5 mg/kg), or esmolol, (0.5 to 1.0 mg/kg), a short-acting beta blocker, before intubation can blunt the response to intubation. When a patient comes to the operating room with established hypertension or a history of poorly controlled hypertension, adjuvant drugs such as nitroglycerin and nitroprusside should be readily available. Extreme caution must be exercised in lowering blood pressure in a head-injured patient since hypotension is much more dangerous to these patients than hypertension.

Anesthetic Maintenance

Neuromuscular Blocking Drugs

There are two basic classes of neuromuscular blocking agents: depolarizing and nondepolarizing blockers.

Depolarizing Neuromuscular Blockers

Of the two depolarizing muscle relaxants available for clinical use, succinylcholine is the more widely used. Succinylcholine (1.0 to 1.5 mg/kg) produces optimum

TABLE 13-3 Contraindications to the Administration of Succinylcholine

Absolute	Relative
Cerebrovascular Accident with residual muscle weakness	Open eye injury
Hyperkalemia	Intracranial hypertension
Crush injury	Abnormal plasma cholinesterase
Burn injury	
Denervation injury (such as paraplegia) > 48 h old	
Personal or family history of malignant hyperthermia	
Known allergy to succinylcholine	

intubating conditions in 60 to 90 s. The cardiovascular side effects include bradycardia, junctional rhythms, escape beats, and asystole. Pretreatment with atropine or glycopyrrolate eliminates most of these side effects. Other important side effects include increases in intragastric, intraocular, and intracranial pressures and the potential for hyperkalemia. The rise in intracranial pressure caused by succinylcholine is blunted by pretreatment with a small dose of a nondepolarizing muscle relaxant (e.g., *d*-tubocurarine 3 mg). Serum potassium concentrations increase 0.5 to 1.0 mEq/liter after an intubating dose of succinylcholine. For patients with high serum potassium levels (e.g., renal failure patients) this increase may precipitate a hyperkalemic cardiac dysrhythmia. Patients with antecedent denervation injuries, spinal cord trauma, cerebral vascular accident, closed head injury, burns, upper motor neuron lesions, peritonitis, crush injuries, or protracted immobility are at increased risk for an exaggerated hyperkalemic response. These patients may begin with a potassium concentration within normal limits but may exhibit a large increase in the serum potassium concentration after the administration of succinylcholine. These effects are not usually seen in an acutely injured patient but may occur during reoperation several days after the injury.

Despite the side effects, succinylcholine is the relaxant of choice during an RSI unless a specific contraindication, such as those listed in Table 13-3, is present.

Nondepolarizing Neuromuscular Blockers

After intubation, a long-acting nondepolarizing muscle relaxant is usually administered. Table 13-4 lists the common nondepolarizing muscle relaxants, dose ranges, and significant side effects. Rational choice of an agent requires consideration of the duration of action of the drug and the side effect profiles, which may be either beneficial or detrimental to the patient. For example,

TABLE 13-4 Nondepolarizing Neuromuscular Blockers

Drug	Intubating Dose, mg/kg	Onset, min	Duration, min	Heart Rate Change	Histamine Release	Excretion Renal/Hepatic, %
d-Tubocurarine	0.6	3–5	60–90	Slight decrease	Moderate	45/10–40
Atracurium (Tracrium)	0.4–0.5	3–5	20–35	Increase*	Slight	NS/NS
Mivacurium (Mivacron)	0.16	2–3	12–20	Increase*	Slight	NS/NS
Rocuronium (Zemuron)	0.6–1.2	0.4–6	15–85	None	None	NS/100
Vecuronium (Norcuron)	0.1	3–5	20–35	None	None	15–25/40–75
Doxacurium (Nuromax)	0.05–0.08	4–6	60–100	None	None	70/unknown
Pancuronium (Pavulon)	0.1	3–5	60–90	Increase 10–25%	None	80/5–10
Pipecuronium (Arduan)	0.14	3–5	60–90	None	None	70/20

* Heart rate change is the result of histamine release, not a direct effect at the muscarinic or nicotinic receptor.

TABLE 13-5 Infusion Drugs for the Control of Blood Pressure and Cardiac Output

Drug	Action	Dose	Advantages	Disadvantages	Indications	Miscellaneous
Nitroglycerin (Tridil)	Direct-acting vasodilator	0.1–7.0 µg/kg/min *Preparation:* 50 mg of drug 250 ml of D5W	Decreases myocardial oxygen demand Useful in acute congestive heart failure (CHF) Dilates pulmonary vasculature	Can decrease blood pressure (BP) by decreasing preload Can cause reflex tachycardia Methemoglobinemia can develop with high doses Tachyphylaxis	CHF Hypertension	Venodilation much more than arterial vasodilatation
Sodium nitroprusside (Nipride)	Direct-acting vasodilator	0.1–8.0 mcg/kg/min *Preparation:* 50 mg of drug 250 ml of D5W	Systemic and pulmonary vasodilator Greater decrease in afterload than preload at lower dose Short duration of action (1–2 min)	Cyanide and thiocyanate toxicity Reflex tachycardia Can increase ICP Rebound hypertension Inhibits platelet function	Refractory hypertension	Signs of toxicity include tachyphylaxis, metabolic acidosis, elevated mixed venous O_2 Taper dose to avoid rebound hypertension
Dopamine	Direct alpha 1 and 2 beta 1 and 2 Dopaminergic Indirect Induces release of stored Norepinephrine from nerve terminalis	> 10 µg/kg/min 3–10 µg/kg/min 1–3 µg/kg/min *Preparation:* 200 mg of drug 500 ml of D5W	Increase Renal Blood Flow and Urine Output at lower doses Less vasodilating effect than isoproterenol	Tachycardia and dysrhythmias can occur Less potent inotrope than epi or isoproterenol At higher doses, renal effects are overridden	Hypotension due to low CO or SVR Renal failure or insufficiency	
Dobutamine (Dobutrex)	Synthetic catecholamine Direct Alpha 1 Beta 1 and 2	2–20 µcg/kg/min *Preparation:* 200 mg of drug 500 ml of D5W	Less tachycardia than with isoproterenol, dopamine, or epinephrine May increase RBF via beta effect No MAO metabolism	Hypotension can occur due to beta 2 effect Vasodilatation may cause shunts to develop Coronary steal may lead to ischemia	Low CO states with high SVR or PVR	Administration via central line is preferable

TABLE 13-5 Infusion Drugs for the Control of Blood Pressure and Cardiac Output *(Continued)*

Drug	Action	Dose	Advantages	Disadvantages	Indications	Miscellaneous
Epinephrine	Direct Alpha 1 and 2 Beta 1 and 2	>10 μg/min 1–2 μcg/min (both) 2–10 μcg/min *Preparation:* 1 mg of drug 250 ml of D5W	Very potent inotrope Potent bronchodilator	Tachycardia and dysrhythmias can occur Organ ischemia secondary to vasoconstriction Risk of myocardial ischemia	Cardiogenic shock Cardiac arrest Anaphylaxis	Often used with a vasodilator At high levels may cause Cerebrovascular Accident or Myocardial Infarction May be given IV (central line), per Endotracheal Tube or subcutaneously
Isoproterenol (Isuprel)	Synthetic catecholamine Direct beta	0.5–20 μg/min *Preparation:* 1 mg of drug 250 ml of D5W	No alpha effect Most potent beta agonist per μcg Pulmonary vasodilator Bronchodilator	Beta 2 effect often lowers BP while CO increases Tachycardia Dysrhythmias Can cause systemic shunts Can unmask accessory Atrioventricular conduction pathways May cause coronary steal and ischemia	Pulmonary hypertension Low CO in patients for whom tachycardia is not detrimental Status asthmaticus	

several nondepolarizing muscle relaxants cause histamine release, which may lead to a sudden decrease in peripheral vascular resistance and blood pressure. This decrease in blood pressure may adversely affect the CPP. Furthermore, histamine release should be avoided in patients with a history of reactive airway disease. Because sudden unexpected movement of the patient during neurosurgical procedures can be disastrous, the patient's neuromuscular status must be monitored with a peripheral nerve stimulator.

On occasion, the neurosurgeon must examine a patient immediately after surgery. The anesthesiologist is usually asked to pharmacologically antagonize the patient's muscle relaxation to allow the patient to follow commands. The authors have found that a continuous infusion of a nondepolarizing muscle relaxant with the concomitant use of a peripheral nerve stimulator allows for precise control of neuromuscular blockade, providing adequate intraoperative relaxation yet permitting timely reversal.

Maintenance Agents

The primary objectives during the maintenance phase of anesthesia are to ensure hypnosis, amnesia, and analgesia to limit the morbidity of both the injury and the procedure; and to provide optimum operating conditions. Commonly, a combination of inhalation and intravenous agents is used to maintain anesthesia.

Inhaled Anesthetic Agents

There are four potent inhalation agents available in the United States: enflurane, halothane, isoflurane, and desflurane. Sevoflurane is a potent inhalation agent that is being used in Japan but is unavailable in the United

States. All four of the agents available in the U.S. cause cerebral vasodilatation and decrease the cerebral metabolic rate. Of the three most commonly used agents, the most potent cerebral vasodilator is halothane, followed by enflurane and then isoflurane. The cerebral vasodilatory effects are important in a head-injured patient with abnormal intracranial elastance because any increase in CBF could lead to a large increase in ICP. The decrease in the cerebral metabolic rate seen with these agents tends to decrease CBF. The net effect of these agents on CBF is a balance between these two factors. Isoflurane appears to decrease the metabolic rate to a larger extent than does either halothane or enflurane. Furthermore, enflurane has been shown to induce seizure-like activity on EEG.[17] This activity is exacerbated during hypocarbia. One study with desflurane showed an increase in ICP in patients with a supratentorial mass lesion despite hypocapnia.[18] Currently, isoflurane at concentrations of $\leq$1.15% is the most commonly used inhalation agent for neurotrauma.

Intravenous Agents

The intravenous agents commonly used for the maintenance of anesthesia include narcotics, benzodiazepines, thiopental, and etomidate. After a loading dose of narcotic (fentanyl 5 to 10 μg/kg or sufentanil 0.5 to 1.0 μg/kg), a continuous infusion (fentanyl 3 to 5 μg/kg/h or sufentanil 0.3 to 0.5 μg/kg/h) provides adequate analgesia without hemodynamic perturbation. Since most severely head injured patients remain intubated and mechanically ventilated for at least 12 h postoperatively, this narcotic infusion can be continued until the end of surgery and, if desired, postoperatively.

CONTROL OF HEMODYNAMICS

Of primary importance is the prevention of ischemic brain injury. Hemodynamic instability, regardless of the cause, should be treated aggressively. Table 13-5 provides a list of commonly used vasoactive drugs, dose ranges, indications, and complications. The authors frequently encounter a head-injured patient whose blood pressure remains elevated despite administration of the maximum recommended doses of inhalation agents and an adequate dosage of narcotics. Small intermittent doses of benzodiazepines (midazolam 0.015 to 0.03 mg/kg) often lower the blood pressure to an acceptable level. Thiopental loading is occasionally requested by the surgeon when measures such as diuretics, head-up positioning, and hyperventilation have failed to reduce the volume of the brain. A loading dose of thiopental (5 to 25 mg/kg) is often followed by a continuous maintenance infusion (4 to 10 mg/kg/h). Hypotension and myocardial depression may result from this dosage regimen. Treatment should include both vasopressors (e.g., dopamine 5 μg/kg/min) and judicious volume loading guided by CVP or PA (pulmonary artery) pressure monitoring.

MAINTENANCE OF CARDIAC OUTPUT

Maintenance of cardiac output helps ensure adequate tissue perfusion and oxygenation and therefore is of primary importance to the anesthesiologist. The use of a pulmonary artery catheter allows measurement of the cardiac output and computation of the cardiac index (cardiac output divided by body surface area) and systemic vascular resistance. While a full discussion of the factors affecting cardiac output is beyond the scope of this chapter, a brief discussion of the therapeutic modalities available for the maintenance of cardiac output is appropriate. A cardiac index (CI) of 2.5 to 3.5 liters/m^2/min is normal, and a CI below 2 liters/m^2/min requires evaluation and treatment. A normal Sv_{O2} might justify a period of further observation. Several factors may be associated with a state of low cardiac output.

Preload

Preload may be inadequate. In the trauma setting, the most common cause of an insufficient preload is hypovolemia, as indicated by low right-sided and left-sided heart filling pressures, tachycardia, and a blood pressure that varies with respiration. Clearly, the treatment for a hypovolemic patient involves the administration of fluid, either crystalloid or colloid.

Afterload

Afterload may be excessive. While there are several determinants of afterload, systemic vascular resistance (SVR) provides a useful estimate. Systemic vascular resistance is calculated by using the following formula after determining the cardiac output: $SVR = [(MAP - CVP) \times 79.9])/CO$. CVP is central venous pressure, and CO is the measured cardiac output. Normal SVR is 1200 to 1500 dynes sec/cm. Increased SVR can lead to a low CO. Treatment of an elevated SVR involves the administration of vasodilating drugs such as nitroglycerin and nitroprusside. Nitroglycerin is more potent as a venodilator than as an arterial vasodilator and may not be the best choice for lowering SVR. Nitroprusside has balanced venous and arterial dilating activity. Doses, side effects, and toxicities of both drugs are listed in Table 13-5.

Contractility

Contractility is defined as the inotropic state of the heart independent of preload, afterload, and heart rate. A low CO in the face of normal filling pressures and a normal SVR is probably due to poor cardiac contractility and is best treated with an inotropic drug such as dopamine, dobutamine, epinephrine, or isoproterenol. Doses, side effects, and toxicities are given in Table 13-5.

Management of Combined Operations

Often a head-injured patient requires other surgical procedures or further diagnostic evaluation or examination before undergoing a definitive neurosurgical procedure. This places an extra burden on the anesthesiology team, since many of the principles of management of truncal or extremity trauma are inconsistent with good management for a closed head injury, such as light anesthesia, crystalloid volume resuscitation, avoidance of hyperventilation, and use of the head-down position.

ICP Monitoring

ICP monitoring is mandatory if intracranial hypertension is present or expected and another procedure is planned, such as laparotomy or fracture stabilization. The placement of an intraventricular catheter allows accurate measurement of ICP as well as urgent decompression of the brain if that becomes necessary. The selection and administration of anesthetic drugs, adjustment of mechanical ventilation, volume replacement, and control of hemodynamics may all be influenced by the ICP.

Posture

The head-elevated position may compromise the surgical management of intraabdominal injuries. The optimal head position is somewhat controversial and may vary from patient to patient and even from time to time in an individual patient. In any case, blood pressure should be measured at the level of the head.

Hemorrhage

Blood replacement should be guided by the hematocrit and the presence of cardiovascular instability. Clotting factors may be administered if an intracranial procedure is pending and excessive bleeding is noted. Intraabdominal packing to control hemorrhage may result in a rise in ICP because of elevated intraabdominal pressures and should be avoided in these patients if possible.

Hypothermia

Mild hypothermia may offer protection to the ischemic brain but can create other problems, especially with the clotting cascade. Active heating of the patient should begin as soon as the patient reaches the operating room, if not before, using a fan-forced warm air heater.[19]

Complications

Venous Air Embolism

Whenever the surgical field is 5 cm or more above the heart, there is a risk of venous air embolism. The tendency for neurotrauma patients to be hypovolemic from both blood loss and volume contraction through the use of diuretics makes the likelihood of a venous air embolism even greater. Air can pass from the surgical site to either the right side of the heart and the pulmonary circulation or to the left side of the heart via a patent foramen ovale (paradoxical venous air embolism). The most sensitive device available for detecting a venous air embolism is the transesophageal echocardiogram, which is not yet in routine use during surgery for neurotrauma. A precordial Doppler placed over the right atrium will give early warning of a venous air embolism.

Another sign of air embolism is a sudden decrease in ET_{CO_2} as measured by capnography. The intravenous entrainment of room air (79% N_2 and 21% O_2) also causes an increase in ET_{N_2} that is detectable by mass spectroscopy. This increase in ET_{N_2} is difficult to detect if the patient is receiving air as part of the inspired gas mixture. In the case of a venous air embolism, air can cause "foaming" of the blood within the ventricle with marked hypotension, or can traverse a patent foramen ovale entering the coronary arteries and causing changes in the ST segment, cardiac dysrhythmias, or complete cardiovascular collapse. In any case, the surgeon must be notified immediately and the surgical field should be flooded with sterile solution to stop the entrainment of air. If possible, the surgical field should be lowered at least to the level of the heart. Aspiration from a central venous catheter can often evacuate the air.

Coagulopathy

In patients who have sustained severe brain injury, tissue thromboplastin from the brain enters the circulation and can lead to the consumption of coagulation factors and fibrinolysis. Early diagnosis requires monitoring of the prothrombin time, partial thromboplastin time, platelet count, and fibrin split products or D-dimer. Treatment of this coagulopathy is accomplished with fresh-frozen plasma, cryoprecipitate, platelets, and packed red blood cells (Chap. 46).

POSTOPERATIVE MANAGEMENT

Emergence and Extubation

Many of the authors' head-injured patients have been emergently intubated either on the scene or in the emergency room. In these cases there is usually no attempt to extubate the patient immediately after operation. However, for patients who arrive unintubated in the operating suite, the decision to allow the patient to emerge from anesthesia in the immediate postoperative period should be considered. Because of their "full stomach" status and unpredictable postoperative mental status, these patients are not candidates for extubation asleep but must be following commands before extubation. If extubation is planned, narcotic infusions should be discontinued 60 to 90 min before the completion of surgery. With 20 to 30 min remaining in the procedure, all potent inhalation agents can be discontinued and a propofol infusion of 120 to 180 μg/kg/min can be started. After placement of the surgical dressing, the neuromuscular blockade is antagonized. Extubation should proceed if the patient is hemodynamically stable, follows commands, is able to demonstrate adequate reversal of the neuromuscular blockade, and has maintained adequate oxygenation, as assessed by pulse oximetry, during spontaneous ventilation.

Transportation to the Intensive Care Unit

During transportation of the patient from the operating suite to the neurosurgical intensive care unit, where the authors' patients recover after neurosurgical procedures, ECG and intraarterial blood pressure should be monitored. If the patient has been extubated, an oxygen tank, face mask oxygen, and continuous verbal contact with the patient during transportation are necessary. Transportation of an intubated patient requires the addition of a device for providing controlled ventilation. The authors transport patients in the head-up position. Vasoactive drug infusions are continued during transport. Additional drugs should be available if hemodynamic instability develops during transport.

Airway Management after Difficult Intubation

A patient with a difficult airway preoperatively provides a challenge at the time of extubation. If the endotracheal tube is removed and the patient requires reintubation, it may be impossible to replace the endotracheal tube. These patients should undergo careful assessment to evaluate their readiness for extubation. A hollow jet stylet can be placed into the trachea via the endotracheal tube. A jet ventilator connected to the stylet permits controlled ventilation with 100% oxygen through the stylet. Before the endotracheal tube is slid out of the trachea while the stylet is left in place, a brief trial of jet ventilation should be performed. After the endotracheal tube is removed, a face shield or mask is placed on the patient's face and the patient is allowed to breathe on his or her own during this trial of extubation. The stylet is left in place until arterial blood gas and vital signs confirm that the patient is able to breathe adequately without the endotracheal tube. Upon completion of this trial of spontaneous breathing, the jet stylet can be removed. However, if the patient fails this trial of extubation, the stylet can be used to oxygenate and ventilate the patient and as a guide for the rapid reinsertion of an endotracheal tube.

References

1. Mallampati SR, Gatt SP, Gugino LD: A clinical sign to predict difficult tracheal intubation: A prospective study. *Can Anesth Soc J* 32:429–434, 1985.
2. Oates JD, Macleod AD, Oates PD, et al: Comparison of two methods for predicting difficult intubation. *Br J Anaesth* 66(3):305–309, 1991.
3. Endotrol® Tracheal Tube, manufactured by Mallinkrodt Medical, Inc., Mallinkrodt Anesthesiology Division, St. Louis, MO 63042.
4. Beck Airway Airflow Monitor Mark VI®, manufactured by Great Plains Ballistics, Inc., P.O. Box 16485, Lubbock, TX 79490.
5. Combitube® manufactured by Sheridan Catheter Corporation, Argyle, NY 12809.
6. Laryngeal Mask Airway distributed by Gensia Pharmaceuticals, Inc., 1-800-788-7999.
7. *Standards for Basic Intraoperative Monitoring.* American Society of Anesthesiologists, Park Ridge, IL. Oct. 13, 1993.
8. *Int Anesthesiol Clin* 28(2):83–88, 1990.
9. Jamshidi® Intraosseous Needle manufactured by Baxter Healthcare Corporation, Pharmaseal Division, Valencia, CA 91355.
10. Arrow® Pediatric Jugular Puncture Kit manufactured by Arrow International, Inc., Reading, PA 19605.
11. Lebowitz PW: Muscle relaxants and the open globe, in Calobrisi BL, Lebowitz PW (eds): *Advanced Trauma Life Support Program for Physicians.* Chicago: Committee on Trauma, American College of Surgeons, 1993.
12. Baker BW: Trauma, in Chestnut DH, editor: Obstetric Anesthesia: Principles and Practice, 1st. ed. St. Louis, Mosby, (53):996–1005.
13. Rosner J, Daughton S: Cerebral perfusion pressure management in head injury. *J Trauma* 30(8):933–941, 1990.
14. Chan Kwan-Hon et al: The effect of changes in cerebral perfusion upon middle cerebral artery blood flow velocity

and jugular bulb venous oxygen saturation after severe brain injury. *J Neurosurg* 77:55–61, 1992.

15. Holdcroft A, Morgan M, Whitwam JG, Lumley J: Effect of dose and premedication on induction complications with etomidate. *Br J Anaesth* 48:199–205, 1976.
16. Sebel PS, Lowden JD: Propofol: A new intravenous anesthetic. *Anesthesiology* 71:260–277, 1989.
17. Michenfelder JD, Cucchiara RF: Canine cerebral oxygen consumption during enflurane anesthesia and its modification during induced seizures. *Anesthesiology* 40:575–580, 1974.
18. Muzzi D, Losassa T, Dietz NM, et al: The effect of desflurane and isoflurane on cerebrospinal fluid pressure in humans with supratentorial mass lesions. *Anesthesiology,* 76(5):720–724, 1992.
19. Giesbrecht G, Ducharme M, McGuire J: Comparison of forced-air patient warming systems for perioperative use. *Anesthesiology* 80(3):671–679, 1994.

CHAPTER 14

SURGICAL ASPECTS OF THE HEAD INJURED

Alex B. Valadka
Raj K. Narayan

SYNOPSIS

Cranial trauma can present with a variety of pathological entities that require prompt surgical intervention. This chapter describes the technical aspects of the surgical management of closed and penetrating head injury. Certain medical issues related to surgery are also reviewed.

BACKGROUND

Closed vs. Open

Because of some fundamental differences in surgical techniques and objectives between open and closed head injuries, these two types of injury will be discussed separately. Each section will begin with a brief review of the more common pathological entities, followed by specific discussions of the actual surgical technique. This chapter then concludes with comments applicable to all intracranial operations for trauma.

Frequency of Surgery

Most series report that roughly one-third of patients with severe closed head injuries (excluding those dead on arrival) require immediate craniotomy for mass lesions.[1] The most common of these is an acute subdural hematoma. Although the mortality rate in patients with subdural hematomas may be as high as 50 to 90 percent, one series has reported a mortality rate of 30 percent if surgery is performed within 4 hours of injury.[2]

Some victims of head injury may undergo craniotomy on a somewhat less urgent basis. These include those with depressed skull fractures and patients whose injury is clinically mild or moderate, but whose CT scans reveal sizable hematomas. Other patients whose initial CT scans are relatively unimpressive may proceed to develop delayed hematomas that require surgical interventions.[3–5]

Unless they harbor a mass lesion, victims of gunshot wounds to the head need not be taken to the operating room (OR) immediately. Debridement of entrance and exit wounds may be done semi-electively or, in some cases, in the intensive care unit. It is often wise to stabilize patients and to make certain that they are neurologically salvageable before beginning general anesthesia for a craniotomy.[6] The increasing incidence[7] and brutality of shootings in the United States may well change the patterns of the resultant pathology in that an increase in immediate mortality may result in fewer gunshot victims being taken to the OR. Conversely, increased intracranial ricocheting of bullets may raise the number of intracranial hematomas that require immediate evacuation.

Timing of Surgery

The question of whether to operate on a closed head injury—as with any type of invasive procedure—is based on the risk : benefit ratio, i.e., the likelihood of helping the patient without causing unnecessary risk. The urgency of the procedure is dictated by the patient's condition. With head injuries, the questions of necessity and timing are inextricably linked.

The speed with which diagnosis and treatment must proceed is dictated by the patient's neurological exam and history. For example, those who arrive comatose or who deteriorate rapidly while in the emergency room need an immediate CT scan, and those who are found

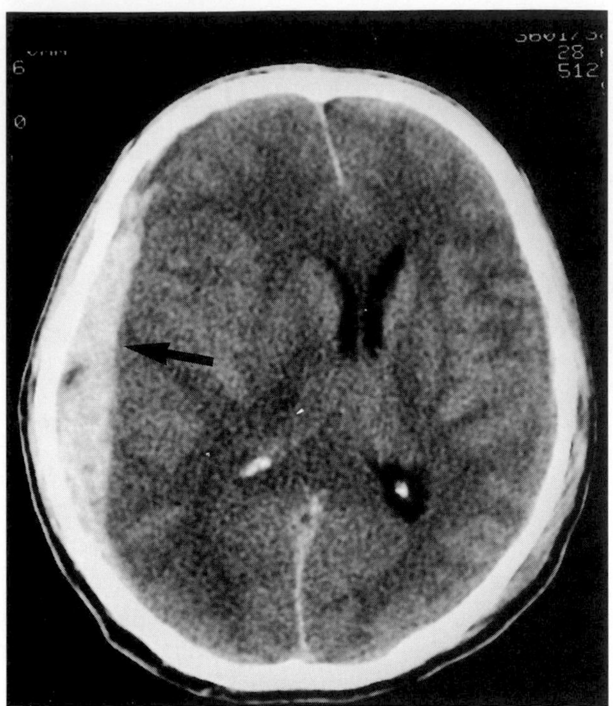

Figure 14-1. Axial CT scan demonstrating large acute subdural hematoma *(arrow)* causing considerable midline shift.

to have a significant hematoma should be taken immediately to surgery[8] (Fig. 14-1). Patients who are still conscious but whose symptoms are found to be due to a subdural hematoma also require prompt craniotomy, but perhaps without the extreme urgency of the preceding case. Finally, those who appear neurologically intact and who may have only a small hematoma may not require evacuation at all (Fig. 14-2, 14-3).

The importance of prompt evacuation of subdural hematomas has been demonstrated in clinical studies.[2] Although other studies have not reproduced the statistical significance of improved outcome following prompt surgery, a trend in this direction was still evident.[9] The fact remains that prompt evacuation of a significant hematoma optimizes the environment in which the brain's reparative processes may begin to work. Removal of the solid clot may also provide precious additional intracranial volume into which the brain can expand without elevating the intracranial pressure (ICP). Studies using multimodality monitoring (ICP, jugular oxygen saturation, near-infrared spectroscopy, etc.) also demonstrate the physiological benefits of early evacuation of significant hematomas (Fig. 14-4).

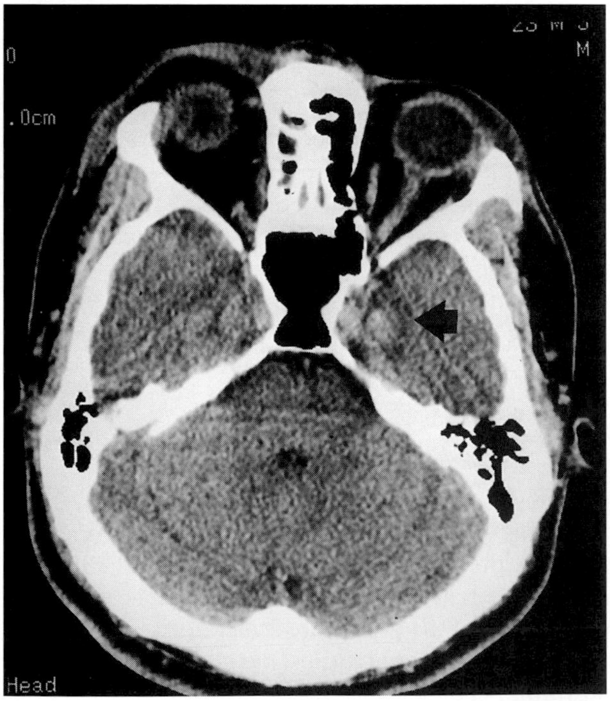

Figure 14-2. Axial CT scan demonstrating medial temporal contusion *(arrow)*. Despite the worrisome location of this lesion, this patient never required surgical evacuation of the contusion. He presented with a Glasgow Coma Score of 15 and never suffered any neurological deterioration.

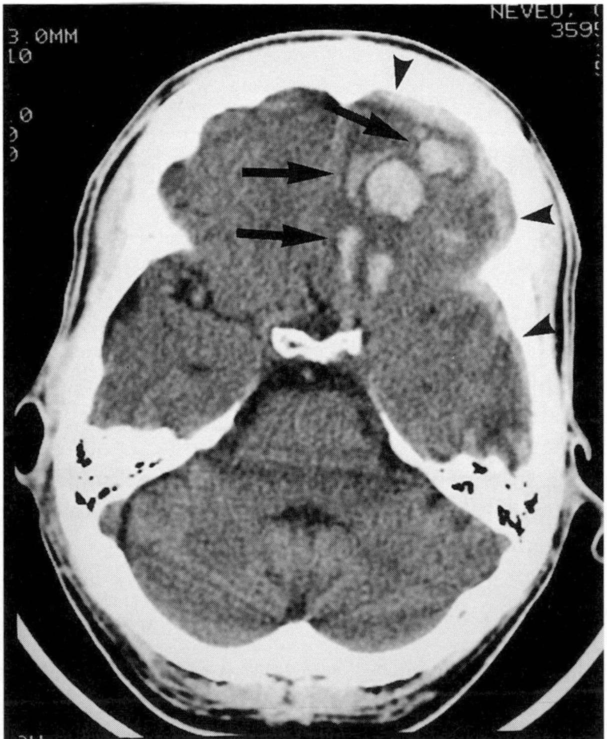

Figure 14-3. Axial CT scan demonstrating sizable subfrontal contusions and hematomas *(arrows)* and moderate subdural hematoma *(arrowheads)*. Because this patient did not arrive at the hospital until several days after his injury and was always obeying commands, he was managed nonsurgically and had an uneventful hospital course.

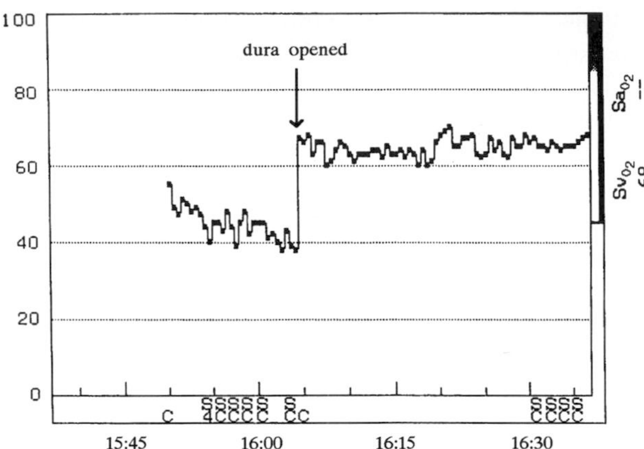

Figure 14-4. Recording of jugular venous oxygen saturation demonstrating dramatic improvement in oxygenation as soon as the dura is opened during an emergency craniotomy for evacuation of a hematoma. (Courtesy of Dr. C. S. Robertson.)

CLOSED HEAD INJURIES

Types of Lesions

Contusions

In the majority of operated head injuries, a craniotomy is undertaken to evacuate a contusion or hematoma. Although hematomas consist of a localized collection of blood from an injured vessel or vessels, contusions are composed of actual brain tissue that has been "bruised," i.e., in which the blood-brain barrier has been focally disrupted.[10] On CT scan, this mixture of blood and parenchyma creates a characteristic, heterogeneous "salt and pepper" appearance (Fig. 14-5). Contusions are most frequently located in the basal frontal lobe and the anterior and basal temporal lobe.

Hematomas

Although classic teaching holds that the various types of intracranial hematomas are each due to a specific pattern of bleeding,[11] this clear-cut relationship is in fact sometimes blurred. Subdural hematomas (SDH) are generally said to arise from tearing of a bridging vein from the cortex to the venous sinuses, but in reality a cortical artery may be the actual source of hemorrhage. Much to the unease of the surgeon, sometimes no actively bleeding vessel can be found. An epidural hematoma (EDH) classically arises in the temporal fossa from laceration of the middle meningeal artery. In our experience, however, EDH is more common in locations other than the temporal fossa (Fig. 14-6). The only apparent cause may be the oozing of blood from the edges of a skull fracture. The classic association between an expanding EDH and a so-called posttraumatic lucid interval is not commonly encountered. Intracerebral hematoma (ICH) may occur posttraumatically in almost any region of the brain. The most dangerous are those in the posterior fossa and near the basal cisterns; as these swell, they can cause hydrocephalus or lethal compression of the brainstem. For the same reason, extra care must be taken with EDHs and SDHs of the posterior fossa.

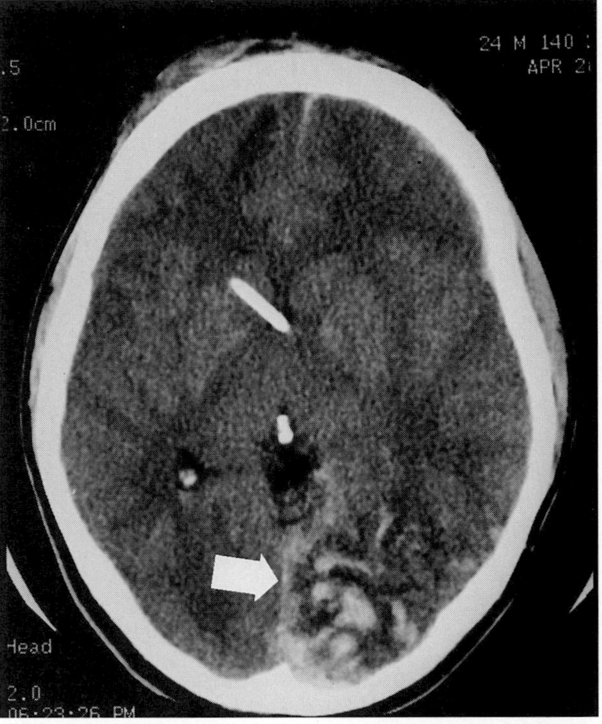

Figure 14-5. Axial CT scan demonstrating large contusion in the occipital pole *(arrow)*. Although the location of this contusion is atypical, its mottled "salt and pepper" appearance is classic.

General Indications for Surgery

In general, hematomas causing significant mass effect should be evacuated promptly (Fig. 14-1). "Significant mass effect" may be arbitrarily defined in radiographic terms as displacement of intracranial structures more than 5 mm across the midline[12] or as compression or effacement of basal cisterns.[13] Surgery is undertaken more readily in the temporal fossa and in the posterior fossa, where a smaller lesion may prove lethal via compression of the brainstem and/or obstruction of CSF flow. Clinically, mass effect is significant when it causes symptoms. However, the association between symptoms and the degree of mass effect is an unpredictable one and cannot be relied upon as the sole indicator of the need for surgery.

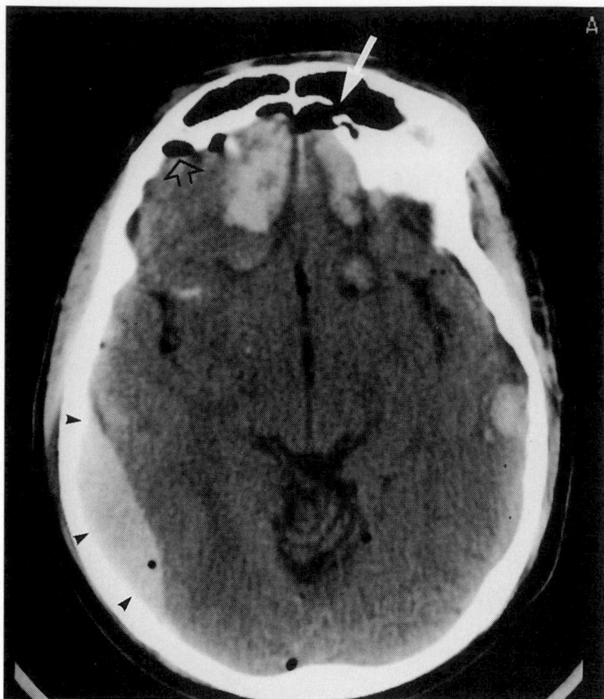

Figure 14-6. Axial CT scan with several interesting findings. An epidural hematoma is visible on the right *(arrowheads)*. This was not evacuated because the patient had remained alert during the many hours between his injury and his arrival in the emergency room. Scattered contusions and hematomas are seen. Pneumocephalus *(open arrow)* is due to a fracture of the posterior wall of the left frontal sinus *(straight arrow)*.

Subdural Hematoma

Indications

As stated above, an acute SDH requires removal when it causes significant mass effect, which is arbitrarily defined as a midline shift of 5 mm or more. Smaller lesions are often removed when the ICP is elevated and the brain appears swollen on CT scanning; in these cases, evacuation of even a small hematoma may provide enough extra room to keep ICP low. Smaller lesions that have shown significant enlargement on serial CT scanning may also be candidates for surgical evacuation.

Technique

A craniotomy for a SDH is performed with the patient supine and the head turned to the appropriate side and placed on a doughnut (Fig. 14-7, 14-8). A roll is placed under the shoulder to facilitate turning of the head. When a cervical spine fracture is known or suspected, a three-point head holder may be used to facilitate fixing the neck in as neutral a position as possible. Hematomas in atypical locations may require different positioning, such as prone (for posterior fossa cases) or supine with the head neutral (for subfrontal approaches). We recommend clipping all the hair to facilitate contralateral craniotomy or placement of a ventriculostomy, should these become necessary.

The anesthesia team faces a difficult task in these cases, for the incompleteness of the preoperative history and screening in most trauma patients stands in direct contrast to the usually meticulous preparation preferred by the anesthesiologist. Provisions must be made to notify the anesthesiologist of all lab results as soon as they become available. The start of the case is also the best time for the neurosurgeon to request that all anesthetic agents be reversed or metabolized by the end of the procedure. If used, prophylactic antibiotics should be administered prior to incising the skin. To reduce the incidence of seizures during the first 8 days post-injury,[14] prophylactic anticonvulsants also may be administered at this time.

Craniotomies for SDHs require a large bone flap. The uncertainty as to the exact type of pathology that might be present, along with the large number and variety of possibilities, requires that the cranial contents be accessible from the skull base to the sagittal sinus. This exposure is best obtained through the reverse question-mark flap. Although some surgeons advocate smaller flaps, we have found that the problems caused by the inadequate exposure more than outweigh the putative advantages of this approach.

The quickest method of opening involves dividing and reflecting the scalp and temporalis muscle as a single unit. Hemostasis may be obtained with Raney clips and/or with dilute epinephrine injected preoperatively along the planned line of incision. Depending on the type of drill used, the appropriate number of burr holes is made and the underlying dura stripped away. The saw is used to create a beveled flap except at the pterion, the contour of which necessitates fracturing the flap off. The bone flap may be stored until closure in a sponge moistened with saline or with antibiotic solution. To save time, dural tack-up sutures are not placed until after the hematoma has been evacuated.

Initial opening of the dura is done with a #15 scalpel blade while the dura is carefully lifted off the underlying cortex with fine-tipped forceps or with a small stitch placed through the outer layer of dura. Often, solid clot is immediately evident. This serves as a protective layer over the cortex while the remainder of the dural opening is completed with shielded Metzenbaum or tenotomy scissors. The dura is continually elevated away from the cortex with Penfield or Cushing forceps. Care is taken to cauterize and divide any small bridging veins. Reflection of the dural flap is maintained by small hemostats hung from sutures placed through the corners of the flap.

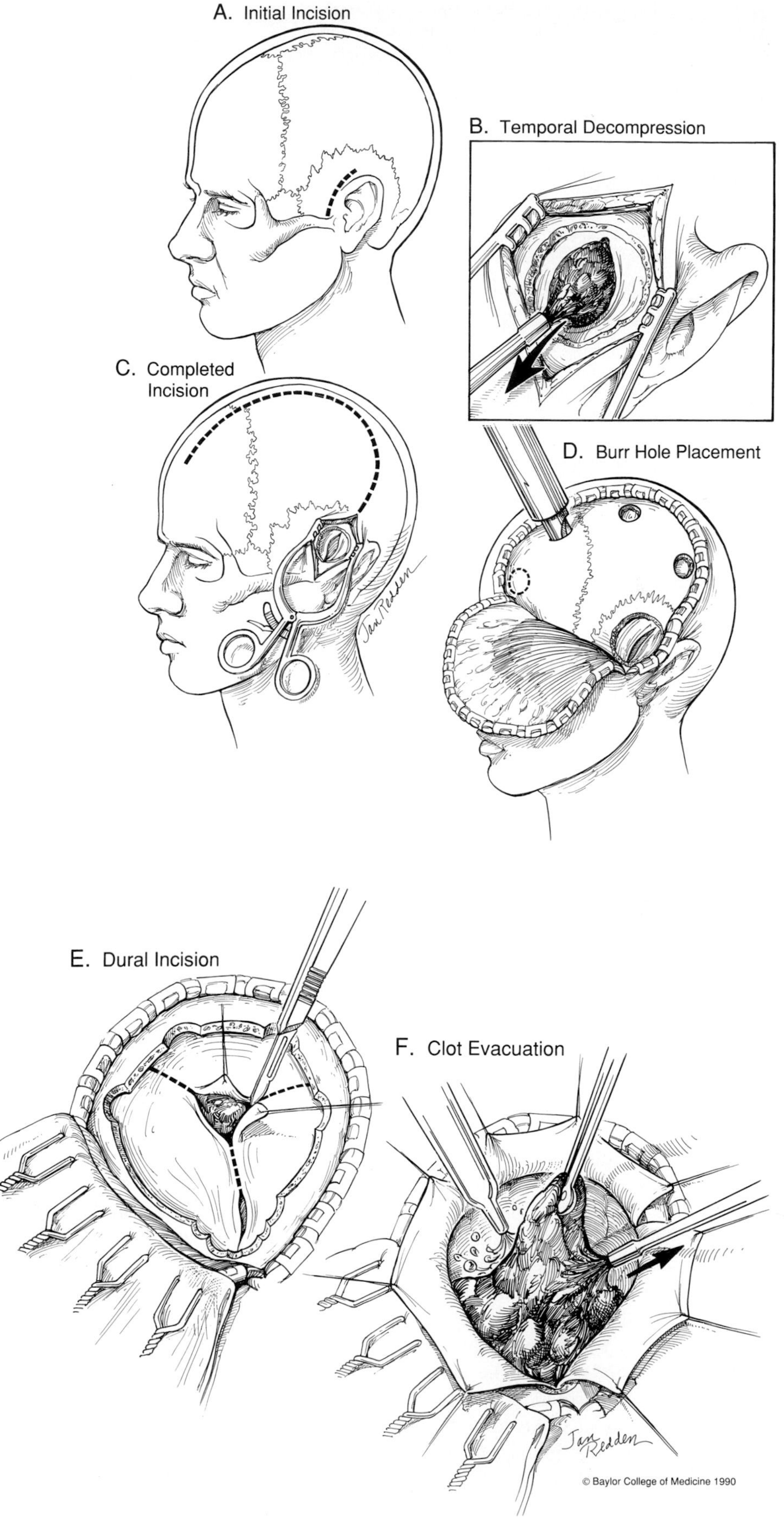

Figure 14-7. Evacuation of an acute subdural hematoma. *A.* In the event of rapid neurological deterioration from a herniation syndrome, temporal decompression is recommended as the first step. An incision just anterior to the ear is taken down to the zygoma, which marks the floor of the temporal fossa. *B.* After a burr hole is made, a quick craniectomy is performed. The dura is incised, and as much clot as possible is aspirated. *C.* The incision is then extended superiorly to form a large question mark, the medial extent of which lies on the midline. *D.* Additional burr holes are made. The medial ones are placed 1.5 cm off the midline to avoid injury to major venous structures and granulations. The anterior burr hole is placed above the frontal sinus, the position of which is estimated from the preoperative CT scan. *E.* The dura is opened with an X-, Y-, or horseshoe-shaped incision, with a flap based on the superior sagittal sinus. *F.* The subdural hematoma is gently evacuated with suction, irrigation, or other mechanical means. Sources of bleeding are identified and cauterized. Contused brain is debrided, and pial edges are carefully cauterized. Ultrasound is used to search for occult intracerebral or contralateral hematomas. (Reproduced, with permission, from Narayan RK: Head injury, in Grossman RG, Hamilton WJ (eds): *Principles of Neurosurgery*. New York: Raven Press, 1991: 259.)

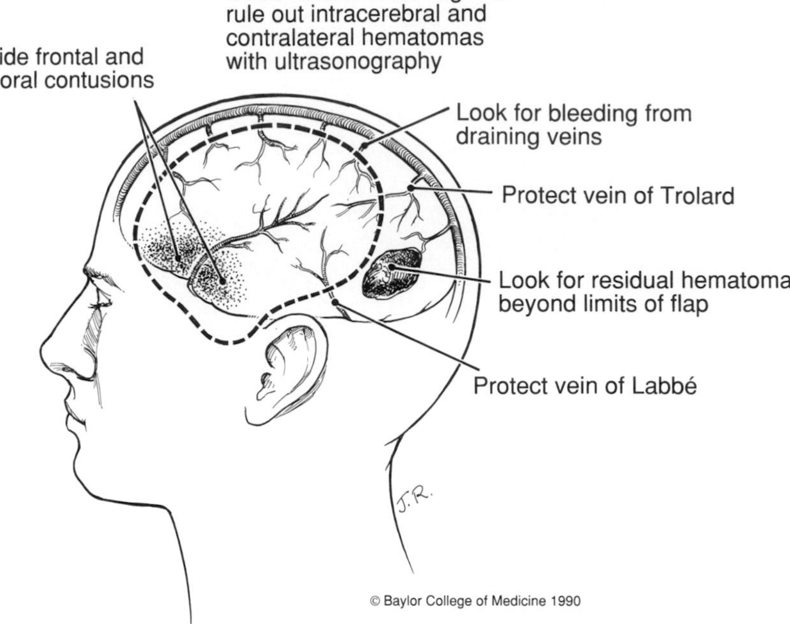
Observe brain swelling and rule out intracerebral and contralateral hematomas with ultrasonography
Debride frontal and temporal contusions
Look for bleeding from draining veins
Protect vein of Trolard
Look for residual hematomas beyond limits of flap
Protect vein of Labbé
J.R.
© Baylor College of Medicine 1990

Figure 14-8. Precautions to be taken during a craniotomy for subdural hematoma. (Reproduced, with permission, from Narayan RK: Head injury, in Grossman RG, Hamilton WJ (eds): *Principles of Neurosurgery*. New York: Raven Press, 1991: 260.)

A SDH may now be removed by careful suctioning on the clot. More complete removal of any clot under the dural edges is accomplished by copious irrigation. If necessary, a wide ribbon retractor can be used to gently depress the underlying cortex while the hematoma is floated off. Careful use of suction and of cup forceps persuades most recalcitrant hematomas to come out. Coaxial headlamp illumination is very useful for carefully searching under the edges of bone and dura.

Occasionally, small portions of hematoma may appear adherent to underlying cortex or may be difficult to remove for other reasons. These are best left alone since their removal does not warrant the risk of cortical damage.

Whenever possible, the origin of the hematoma must be sought and identified. The bleeding most difficult to control is that from the midline. Considerable patience is required to position cottonoids and retractors so as to identify and cauterize the bleeding vessels. When this is not possible, Gelfoam or Surgicel may be used to tamponade the bleeding. Prior to closure, however, the surgeon must make certain that all bleeding has in fact been stopped. A Valsalva maneuver is helpful in verifying the security of the hemostasis.

After dural closure, dural tack-up sutures (Dandy's "sleep stitches") are placed around the periphery of the bony exposure and also in the center of the flap. Epidural drains may be placed if the patient's coagulation status is questionable. The bone flap is replaced tightly with heavy suture or fine wire. After a subgaleal drain is placed, the temporalis fascia is closed, followed by the galea and skin.

Epidural Hematoma

Indications

Because EDHs have a propensity for rapid enlargement, we are aggressive in operating upon relatively small lesions in patients who present shortly after trauma. However, if an EDH has remained small for several hours by the time the patient presents to the emergency room, we are more inclined to watch the patient carefully in the ICU without surgical evacuation of the hematoma.

Technique

These cases begin as described in the preceding section. After the first burr hole is drilled, a sucker can be used to partially evacuate the subjacent portion of the hematoma. Removal of the bone flap affords access to the remainder of the clot. A diligent search must be made for the lacerated vessel that is causing the bleeding. A small (<1 cm) opening may be made in the dura to rule out the presence of a significant subdural hematoma.

In patients with EDHs, a greater than usual number of dural tack-up sutures may be advisable, and epidural drains also may be used. If the brain parenchyma has not been injured, we may not use prophylactic anticonvulsants.

Intracerebral Hematoma

Indications

The indications for surgical evacuation of intracerebral hematomas have not been conclusively defined. Some authors advocate 2 cm as the size limit beyond which surface contusions should be evacuated when encountered at craniotomy. Lesions causing a midline shift of ≥5 mm are also considered candidates for craniotomy and evacuation.[15] These numbers are useful, but only as rough guidelines. For example, little benefit generally accrues from evacuation of a deep hematoma. Likewise, it may be possible to manage hematomas with little mass effect, or those that are more than approximately 24 hours old, without surgical evacuation. However, clots that are expanding are best removed.

Technique

Although some authors describe stereotactic[16] or endoscopic[17] methods of evacuating these lesions, open craniotomy is the most widely used technique.

Depending on coexistent pathology, a smaller craniotomy flap is often adequate for these cases. If the hematoma has not broken through to the surface, the site of corticectomy must be chosen so as to minimize the amount of brain to be traversed. Small malleable retractors are used for brain retraction and for exposure of the hematoma during evacuation. Loupes and headlamps are useful adjuncts. Some authors prefer the operating microscope for greater magnification and illumination.[18] With either technique, complete removal of the hematoma is unlikely, but reduction of mass effect through removal of most of the clot is a readily obtainable goal.

Examination of the walls of these hematoma cavities may occasionally uncover a tangle of abnormal vessels suggestive of an arteriovenous malformation (AVM). These should be resected and sent for pathological examination, for in an occasional trauma patient the accident may have been secondary to a sudden neurological deficit caused by hemorrhage from an AVM.

Surgery for ICP Control

Indications

Surgical procedures for ICP control are heroic measures that should be contemplated only when the full range of conservative measures has failed. The assumption behind these operations is that, if given adequate volume into which to expand, an injured brain may swell without suffering the ill effects of elevated intracranial pressure. The two basic approaches for accomplishing this objective are either resection of brain parenchyma or removal of a portion of the skull. Initial reports that extensive calvarial resection for severe head injuries with diffuse brain swelling improved outcome[19] have not withstood the test of time,[20] and enthusiasm for this practice has remained limited. Lobectomy in head-injured patients has been purported to be of some value as a salvage procedure in certain instances.[21] For cases of focal ischemia, such as that occurring in the distribution of a single carotid artery or in one of its main divisions, there are anecdotal reports that outcome is improved by permitting expansion of the injured region of brain following hemicraniectomy.[22,23] Again, rigorous validation of these anecdotal reports is lacking.

Technique

In undertaking lobectomy as treatment of uncontrollable ICP from diffuse brain swelling, it is generally best to begin with obviously infarcted, contused, or edematous areas, as demonstrated by CT or MRI. If such areas of parenchymal abnormality are not evident or are located in eloquent regions, then noneloquent tissue, typically the right (or nondominant) anterior frontal and anterior temporal lobes, is resected.

The scope of a decompressive craniectomy can range from a simple subtemporal decompression (unilateral or bilateral) to removal of the total calvarium. In a unilateral calvariectomy, access is sought to as much of the calvarium as possible, from the midline to the skull base and from the inion to as close to the glabella as possible. All this exposed bone is then removed. If a prior craniotomy has been done, it may be necessary to remove a second bone flap after the original one is removed. The bone is carefully wrapped and stored in a sterile fashion in a freezer. The dura is incised widely, with relaxing incisions placed at right angles at regular intervals along the dural edge. A large piece of cadaver dura or dural substitute is laid over the exposed cortex and the edges tucked underneath the edges of the bony opening. This is deliberately not closed in the standard watertight fashion, but two or three sutures are often useful to keep this graft from migrating. The galea and skin are closed as usual. If needed, subgaleal drains may be laid on top of the dural graft. If clinically indicated, a ventriculostomy may be placed.

Several weeks may be allowed to pass for the cerebral edema to subside, for the patient's neurological status to improve, and for the surgeon to ensure that no post-operative infection has occurred. At reoperation, the same incision is reopened and the dura closed. The bone flap is replaced and secured in position. Some surgeons choose to autoclave the bone flap prior to replacement.

INTRAOPERATIVE BRAIN SWELLING

One tragic intraoperative event not discussed elsewhere is "malignant" cerebral edema, i.e., the sudden extracranial herniation of brain parenchyma past the edges of the craniotomy. Although the etiology of malignant cerebral edema remains unclear, the speed with which it can appear suggests a defect in vascular autoregulation. If this is anticipated at the start of surgery, it may be minimized by making a smaller initial dural opening in the temporal region so that any brain extrusion occurs in a relatively silent area.[24] Immediate measures must be instituted to attempt to reverse the brain swelling. Systemic causes must be ruled out, including hypoventilation, ventilator malfunction, and occluded cerebral venous drainage.[25] The possibility of another expanding intracranial hematoma also should be considered.[26] Standard therapeutic maneuvers include mannitol and hyperventilation.[26] Barbiturates are often used in this situation because of their ability to effect rapid reductions in ICP,[27] but in our experience results have been mixed, at best. Some authors advocate induced hypotension to a systolic blood pressure of 60 to 90 mmHg for a brief period,[24,26] but others condemn this practice as adding further insult to an already injured brain.[25] Hypotension may occur after the rapid intravenous administration of barbiturates, and in fact preexistent hypotension is a contraindication to the administration of pentobarbital.[26] Perhaps etomidate or another more hemodynamically forgiving drug may be found to play a role in this situation. As a last resort, frontal or temporal lobectomy may be performed, but in many cases there appears to be no end to the fungating parenchyma that must be removed. Although some surgeons will not replace the bone flap in these cases, the swollen brain then strangulates at the bony and dural edges. Moreover, extensive decompressive craniectomy has not been shown to improve outcome in cases of head injury (see above). We simply close as rapidly as possible and immediately transport these patients to the neurosurgical ICU for subsequent management.

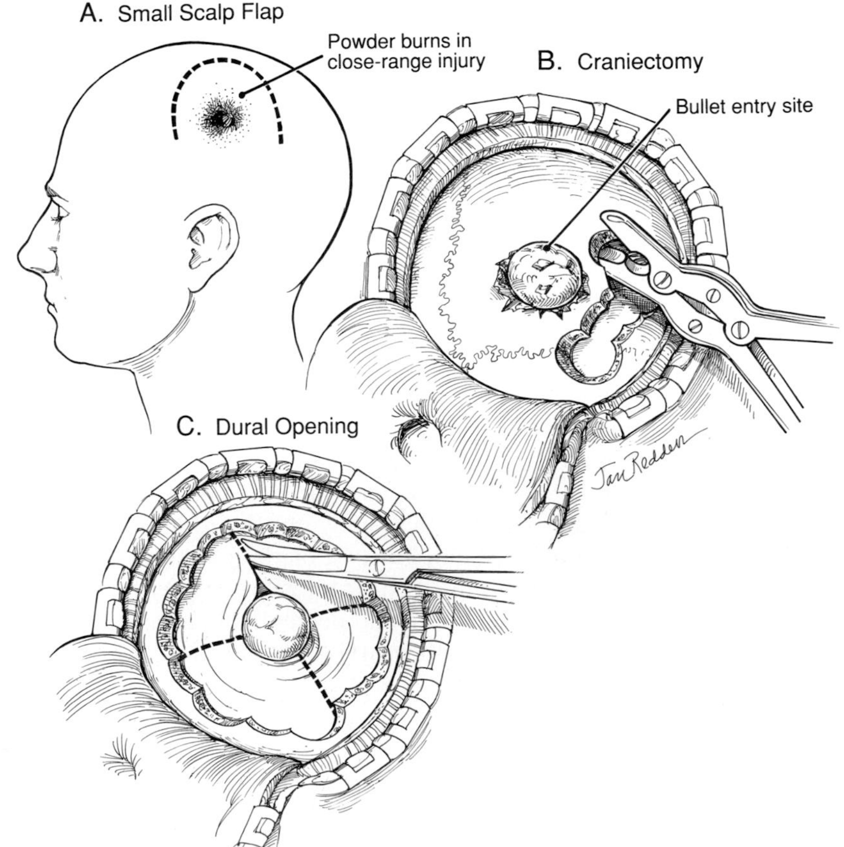

Figure 14-9. Surgery for penetrating head injury (PHI). The approach to PHI is somewhat different than that for closed head injury because the damage tends to be more focal in PHI. The entry and exit wounds are treated similarly. *A.* Either a small linear or S-shaped incision incorporating the entry wound or a small horseshoe-shaped scalp flap around the wound may be used. *B.* A craniectomy is performed at the entry site. *C.* The dura is opened in a cruciate fashion.

PENETRATING HEAD INJURIES

Gunshot Wounds

Civilian gunshot wounds to the head are particularly common in the United States, and the magnitude of the problem is growing. In some areas, head injuries from gunshot wounds have become more common than those from automobile accidents.[7]

Penetrating head injuries (PHI) result in exposure of the cranial contents to the environment. Injury to large cerebral vessels may also result in the formation of intracranial hematomas. These are discussed in another chapter.

Perioperative Care

Because patients with PHI are at high risk for seizures, we immediately administer prophylactic anticonvulsants. For those who receive immediate surgery, antibiotics may be deferred until the wound has been cultured. Otherwise, broad antibiotic coverage against staphylococci, streptococci, common gram-negative bacilli, and anaerobes[28,29] is begun as soon as possible and continued for several days. CT scans are obtained every few days in the immediate postoperative period to monitor the possible formation of an abscess. Early detection and aggressive treatment of infection is important in these cases, since such a complication significantly increases mortality.[28,30]

Surgical Technique

In many cases, it is best to extend one or both ends of the open wound to gain surgical exposure, often through a lazy-S incision. This works quite well for more limited debridements in cases without accompanying mass lesions. Cases that require greater intradural access may require the creation of a craniotomy flap centered on the wound (Fig. 14-9). Generous debridement and copious irrigation are important adjuncts. After necrotic brain

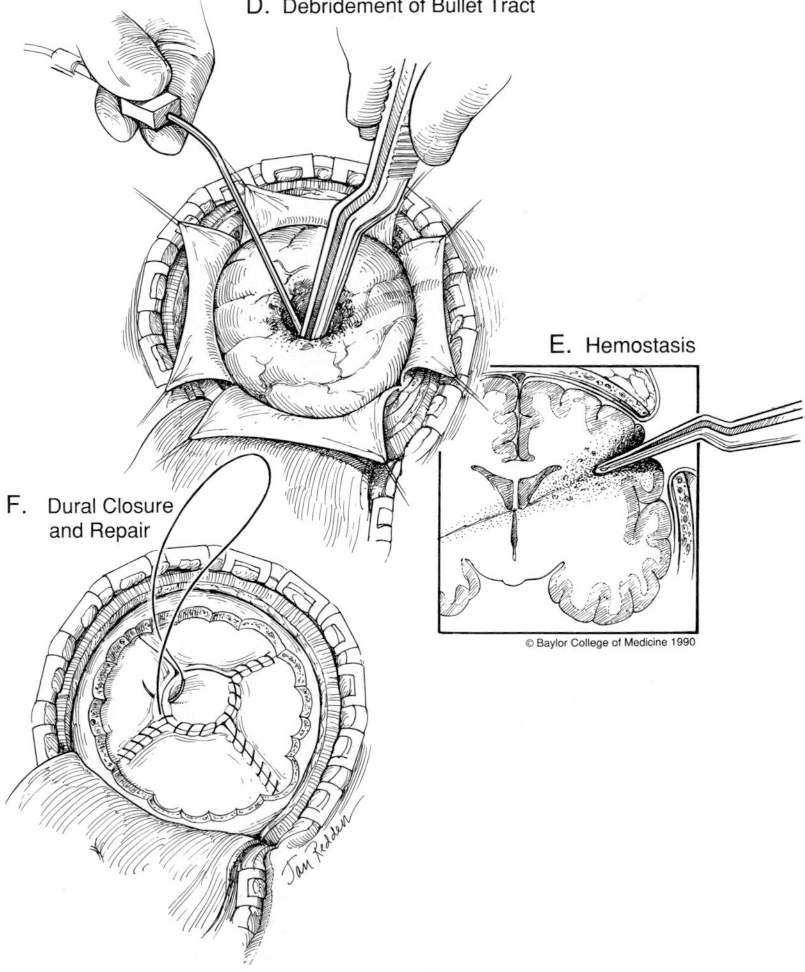

Figure 14-9. (*continued*) *D.* Blood, necrotic brain, and bone and bullet fragments along the path of injury are debrided. *E.* Hemostasis is secured with bipolar cautery and hemostatic agents. *F.* Dural repair is completed using pericranium or other materials as needed. (Reproduced, with permission, from Narayan RK: Head injury, in Grossman RG, Hamilton WJ (eds): *Princples of Neurosurgery*. New York: Raven Press, 1991: 263.)

parenchyma has been resected and hemostasis has been achieved, watertight dural closure is preferred to prevent infection and CSF leak. If excessive dura has been lost through traumatic avulsion or necessary debridement, pericranium is the best choice for duraplasty. Other choices include temporalis fascia, fascia lata, or cadaveric allograft, such as lyophilized dura.

Any small bone fragments are removed. At the surgeon's discretion, larger fragments in relatively uncontaminated wounds may be replaced, using suture, fine wire, or miniplates. Less contaminated wounds may permit the standard two-layer scalp closure, with absorbable material used for the galea. Alternatively, the skin and galea may be closed as a single layer, using 2-0 nylon placed as interrupted vertical mattress sutures. Drains are placed as needed, but these cases often do not require drainage. When fracture of the skull base results in leakage of CSF, postoperative lumbar drainage may be used. A ventriculostomy or other monitoring device will be needed in some cases. The indications for this are similar to those discussed below for closed head injuries.

Surgical Timing and Indications

Different considerations arise in evaluating the necessity and timing of surgical intervention in penetrating head injuries. Even patients with relatively minor injuries may need operative exploration, debridement, and closure in order to minimize the risk of spread of infection to the underlying nervous system. On the other hand, for those unfortunate patients who remain in deep coma with a Glasgow Coma Scale (GCS) of 3 or 4 despite aggressive resuscitation, one may question the value of CT scanning. Even if the scan reveals a hematoma treatable by surgical evacuation, coexistence of such a mass lesion with significant parenchymal destruction from the cavitation effects of the projectile may very well render surgical intervention futile.[31,32]

Often, the surgeon's first instinct is to rush the patient immediately to the operating room. However, in the absence of a significant mass lesion, this is not necessary and may occasionally be unwise. Patients suffer no harm if their surgical debridement and closure are delayed until they have been stabilized and their injuries have been thoroughly evaluated. Because many of these patients are injured at night, it is reasonable to schedule the operation for first thing in the morning, when the surgeon and other OR personnel are fresh. Data from the Lebanese conflict suggest that an interval of a few hours between injury and surgery does not increase the risk of infection in PHI.[28] It must be emphasized that immediate surgery is imperative in the presence of a mass lesion.

VENTRICULOSTOMIES

The details of placement and use of ventriculostomies vary in different institutions. Because the indications and techniques of ICP monitoring are discussed in another chapter, we will make only a few brief comments here (Fig. 14-10). We attempt placement of a ventriculostomy routinely in all patients with a GCS of 8 or less. In patients who do not undergo craniotomy, a ventriculostomy is placed after the prothrombin time (PT), partial thromboplastin time (PTT), platelet count, and sometimes bleeding time are checked. In those patients who undergo emergency craniotomy, the surgeon may decide to forego ventriculostomy if excessive intraoperative bleeding has suggested the presence of a hemorrhagic diathesis. Otherwise, a ventriculostomy is placed after closure of the craniotomy, usually on the contralateral side. We generally choose to avoid the side of the craniotomy for several reasons. It is preferable not to pass a ventricular catheter through a fresh operative site. Also, avoiding the bone flap removes the concern that any subsequent infection will involve the bone flap. Waiting until the end of the case gives the surgeon his greatest chance of successfully cannulating the ventricle, since it is hoped that any mass effect has been eradicated by the surgical procedure. Unless intraoperative brain swelling occurs, placement of a ventriculostomy any sooner provides little useful information, since the open dura precludes proper calibration of zero pressure and since at that point no therapeutic decisions would be based on the results of ventricular pressure readings.

If intraoperative brain swelling has necessitated the placement of a ventricular catheter, the surgeon may have no choice but to bring it out through a burr hole through or adjacent to the bone flap. Tunneling the catheter subcutaneously for some distance may help to prevent infection.

The use of prophylactic antibiotics in patients with ventriculostomies is subject to controversy.[33] Whether prophylactic antibiotics are used or not, regular sampling of the CSF is used to screen for infection. Any rise in CSF white cell count or any other suspicious finding initiates a full set of CSF studies. Empirical treatment with broad-spectrum antibiotics should be initiated if the patient is not already on them. Although in the past we routinely changed ventriculostomies after 5 to 7 days, evidence is accumulating that this may not be necessary.[34] Because the full extent of cerebral edema and elevated ICP may not become manifest for several days after injury, ICP monitoring is usually continued for at least 2 or 3 days in patients who remain comatose and whose ICP remains low.

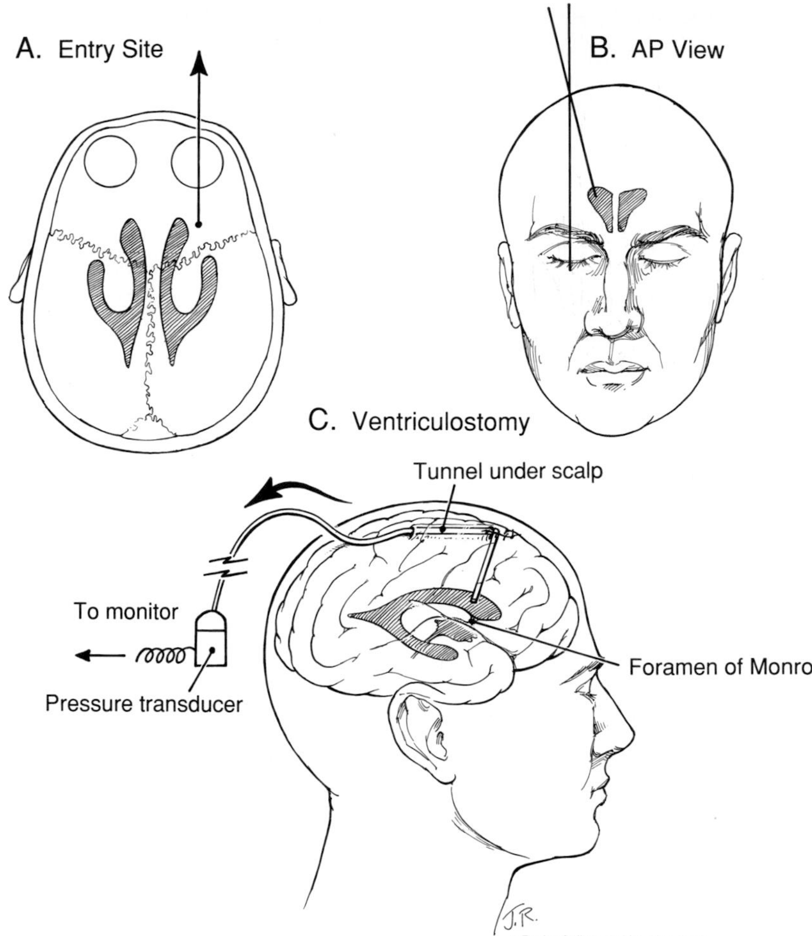

Figure 14-10. Anatomic landmarks for a ventriculostomy. *A.* For the preferred frontal approach, a twist-drill hole is made in the midpupillary line just anterior to the coronal suture. *B.* In the coronal plane, the drill is directed toward the nasion. In the parasagittal plane, the drill is directed toward the tragus of the ipsilateral ear. *C.* The ventricle is entered with a cannula or ventriculostomy catheter passed up to a depth of roughly 7 cm. If the first pass is unsuccessful at cannulating the ventricle, successive passes may be directed more anteriorly and either more laterally or more medially. If the ventricle has not been entered after three passes on each side, the procedure should be abandoned. (Reproduced, with permission, from Narayan RK: Head injury, in Grossman RG, Hamilton WJ (eds): *Principles of Neurosurgery*. New York: Raven Press, 1991: 251.)

SPECIAL SITUATIONS

Neurosurgical vs. General Surgical Priorities

The neurosurgeon's sense of urgency in obtaining an immediate CT scan of the head sometimes conflicts with the general surgeon's need to fully evaluate the trauma patient before he or she leaves the emergency room (ER).[35] Continuous communication between the specialties is the optimal method of solving and minimizing these potential conflicts, along with a mutual desire to keep the patient's best interests tightly in focus. When a comatose patient presents with obvious lateralizing signs, a DPL and other such studies can be done on the CT table or on the operating table. At the other extreme, patients with significant thoracoabdominal trauma but only questionable head injury require full stabilization in the ER or OR before proceeding to CT (Fig. 14-11).

In these latter cases, as well as in situations where CT scanning is not possible, some have advocated bypassing CT by performing immediate exploratory burr holes.[36,37] If a hematoma is found, the patient undergoes immediate craniotomy. If trephination is negative, more pressing diagnostic and therapeutic procedures are carried out. In either case, CT scanning is deferred for quite some time. However, CT scanning is by far the preferable option because of its lower risk and greater diagnostic accuracy. If this is for some reason not possible, then air ventriculography or even cerebral angiography via direct carotid injection can usually be performed.[8]

Suspected or Known Spinal Injury

Approximately 2 to 6 percent of head-injured patients have a fracture of the cervical spine.[38–40] Because a lateral cervical spine x-ray that visualizes the first thoracic vertebra is said to detect at least 85 percent of these fractures (and probably a higher proportion of

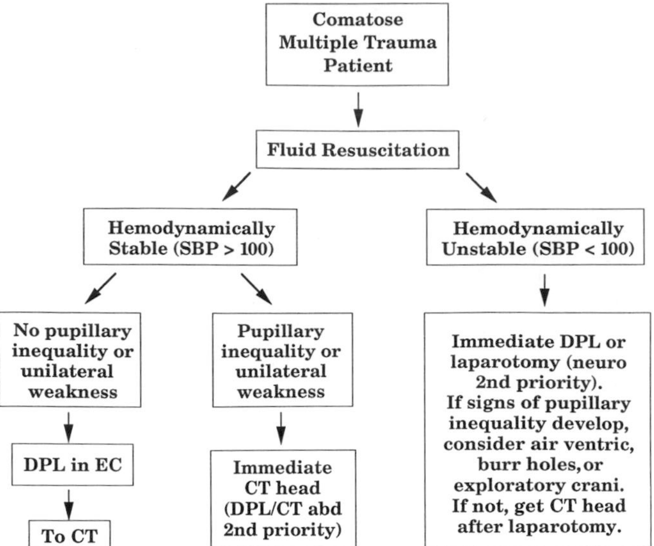

Figure 14-11. Algorithm for use in the emergency room to assist in prioritizing CT scanning of the head versus evaluation of possible abdominal injury. SBP = systolic blood pressure; DPL = diagnostic peritoneal lavage.

unstable injuries),[41] it is imperative that such a radiograph be attempted while the patient is still in the emergency room. If the patient's condition permits, or as soon as possible after stabilization, additional cervical spine films are obtained. Tomography or CT scanning may be required to complete the evaluation or to investigate areas that appear abnormal on roentgenography.

Those operations or procedures that are necessary to stabilize a patient usually cannot be postponed simply because a spinal fracture is present. Because patients with spinal column fractures are at risk of developing neurological deficits even after admission to the hospital,[42] the discovery of a fracture alerts hospital personnel to document carefully the patient's initial neurological function and to transport and position the patient carefully for any surgeries or diagnostic procedures. Neurosurgical consultation should be sought whenever possible to assist with these procedures. With adequate immobilization, definitive surgical treatment of the spinal fracture (if needed) may often be delayed until more pressing problems have been addressed. However, if surgery is not undertaken within the first few days, the window of opportunity for promptly performing a spinal fusion may be lost if the patient subsequently develops pneumonia, urinary tract infection, or other infectious complication. The optimal timing of spinal surgery in these circumstances is unclear and controversial.

Injury of Venous Sinus

These injuries are often quite serious. A recent review of almost 1000 cases of severe closed head injury found that patients with dural sinus injuries had an overall mortality rate of 41 percent and an intraoperative mortality of 20 percent.[43] Sixty-six percent of the dural sinus injuries occurred in the anterior and central superior sagittal sinus, 8 percent in the posterior superior sagittal sinus, and 18 percent in the transverse sinus.

Anticipation of massive hemorrhage is most important in the operative treatment of these injuries. Analysis of the location of fractures or other lesions should alert the surgeon to the possibility of venous sinus injury (Fig. 14-12). These are approached with caution. Advance preparation of numerous long strips of thrombin-soaked Gelfoam is advisable. In conjunction with long cottonoids, these are quite useful for tamponading bleeding from the sinuses. Those planning anesthesia should be alerted to the possibility of sudden, copious blood loss. The anesthesiologist can also adjust the position of the operating table so that the head is uppermost. Although this position minimizes venous bleeding, it also increases the likelihood of venous air embolism, which is discussed below.

Most injuries to the sinus can be managed by tamponading the site of bleeding with hemostatic agents and/or small pieces of crushed muscle. Small tears may be amenable to direct primary suture or to the tacking

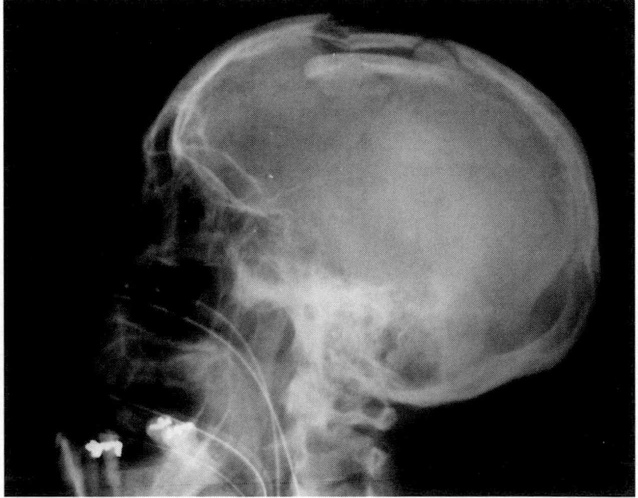

Figure 14-12. Lateral skull film showing depressed skull fracture overlying the superior sagittal sinus. Such an injury should alert the surgeon to the possibility of sudden, massive blood loss. (Reproduced, with permission, from Narayan RK: Head injury, in Grossman RG, Hamilton WJ (eds): *Principles of Neurosurgery*. New York: Raven Press, 1991: 261).

in place of patching or tamponading agents, such as a leaf of dura, pericranium, or temporalis muscle or fascia. Such techniques may be used as long as the sinus retains at least 50 percent of its cross-sectional area.[44,45] Ligation, which may generally be performed relatively quickly and easily, may be the optimal treatment for injuries to noncritical areas, such as the nondominant transverse sinus. A well-known neurosurgical dictum maintains that the anterior third of the sagittal sinus may also be ligated when needed. Experience from a series of patients in Vietnam suggests that as much as the anterior half of the superior sagittal sinus may be taken when necessary.[46]

More complicated injuries may require reconstruction of the sinus. Hemostasis for this procedure is easiest to obtain by simple digital pressure. A Fogarty catheter may be inserted into the lumen either through the rent in the sinus or through a sinotomy just barely large enough to admit a no. 7 Fogarty catheter.[44,45] Shunting may be necessary for those areas in which blood flow is critical. Such a shunt may be fashioned from a pediatric anode endotracheal tube in which the ends have been replaced with two short pediatric tracheostomy tube cuffs.[44,45]

Autogenous vein grafts, typically from the saphenous vein, are the favored material for sinus reconstruction. Ideally, the need to harvest such tissues should be anticipated prior to the operation so that a suitable donor site may be included in the initial preparation and draping. Vein grafts are secured in place in such a fashion that the shunt can be removed at the very end of the repair. Care must be taken to tack up the corners of the graft to make it less vulnerable to thrombosis from compression and subsequent occlusion.[44,45]

Air Sinus Injury

Injuries to the frontal sinus constitute the most common type of sinus injury seen by neurosurgeons (Fig. 14-6). Even so, they are relatively uncommon, comprising 2 to 12 percent of cranial fractures, with severely comminuted fractures of the frontal sinus occurring in roughly 1 to 2 percent of cases of craniocerebral trauma.[47] They may be divided into three general types: fracture of only the anterior wall of the sinus; fracture of the posterior wall (with or without anterior wall fracture); and injury to the nasofrontal duct in conjunction with either of the above two types.[47]

Although nondisplaced anterior wall fractures may be successfully treated nonsurgically,[47,48] the likelihood of residual cosmetic deformity makes surgical reduction the treatment of choice for even moderately displaced fractures of the anterior wall.[48,49] Similarly, nondisplaced fractures of the posterior wall of the frontal sinus may often be amenable to conservative treatment.[47,50] Some surgeons report that CSF leakage associated with a nondisplaced posterior wall fracture spontaneously resolves within a week in roughly one-half of such cases, thus justifying a trial of conservative management.[48] Other surgeons, however, view CSF leakage as an indication for surgical exploration regardless of the type of fracture.[49] Opinion is somewhat more uniform that significantly displaced fractures of the posterior wall require exploration to address the frequently accompanying dural and cerebral injury and to prevent such potential late complications as meningitis, CSF fistula, and mucocele.[47,51] A consensus also exists that damage to the nasofrontal duct (which may be inferred from appropriate findings on a CT scan) probably requires definitive surgical intervention in order to prevent subsequent formation of a mucocele.[47,49,51]

Although the preponderance of opinion seems to favor the necessity of exploration in cases of nasofrontal duct compromise and in the most severe posterior wall fractures, the operative management of these cases still remains a matter of considerable debate. Some authors advocate "cranialization" of the sinus, i.e., removal of the posterior wall, thorough removal of residual mucosa via burring the base and anterior wall of the sinus, and plugging the nasofrontal duct with temporalis muscle or fascia.[49] However, especially when the nasofrontal duct is compromised, other authors favor obliteration of the sinus by mucosal exenteration followed by packing. Suggested materials to use for filling the sinus have included acrylic, cartilage, Proplast, Dacron, plaster of Paris, Gelfoam, Surgicel or, most commonly, cancellous bone, muscle, or fat.[47,51] Packing is often followed by sealing off the sinus with a pericranial graft from the scalp flap.[52] Some surgeons place nothing in the exenterated sinus, relying instead on spontaneous osteoneogenesis to gradually obliterate the sinus in these cases.[53] Because a given case may be amenable only to one or the other of these approaches, it would behoove the neurosurgeon to include in his or her operative armamentarium several different techniques for dealing with frontal sinus injuries. It is also worth emphasizing that either approach requires complete exenteration of the mucosa of the sinus and plugging of the nasofrontal duct. It should be reiterated that obliteration of the sinus applies only to cases of occlusion of the nasofrontal duct and/or severe comminution of the posterior wall of the frontal sinus. Whenever possible, reconstruction of the sinus is preferable to obliteration.

Risk to OR Personnel from HIV

The likelihood of OR personnel acquiring HIV infection through routine job-related duties depends on three main factors: the prevalence of HIV infection in the population served; the likelihood of acquiring HIV infection after percutaneous inoculation; and the frequency of percutaneous injury.[54] The first of these is related to the particular city, neighborhood, and patient population of a given hospital. Studies have shown that victims of trauma have a higher prevalence of HIV infection than does the general population. For example, almost 5 percent of all patients requiring emergency surgery at the Johns Hopkins Hospital were found to have occult HIV infection.[55] A physician or operating room nurse or technician can do little to change this—other than perhaps moving to a city or hospital with a low prevalence of HIV infection.

For OR personnel, the question of the likelihood of acquiring an HIV infection after percutaneous exposure arises most commonly after an accidental needle stick. For most such exposures with surgical instruments or with the solid needles used for suturing, the likelihood of acquiring the infection is probably about 0.4 percent, or 1 in 250.[54]

Thus, the only area in which an OR worker can directly minimize his or her own chances of acquiring job-related HIV infection is by avoiding accidental exposure. The widely implemented universal precautions, which spell out numerous detailed steps to avoid exposing skin and mucous membranes to any patient's body fluids, are a step in this direction.[56] Preventing accidental needle sticks, which may occur as often as once in every 20 to 40 procedures,[54] is more difficult. Many surgeons will allow only themselves and one nurse to scrub on operations on patients known to carry the HIV virus, thus minimizing the chances of accidental sticks from an assistant. Other methods are available to minimize risk, such as modifications in the handling and passing of instruments and use of blunt-tipped needles and impermeable gloves made of wire mesh.[54]

In summary, the best preventive step available to OR personnel is to act carefully and deliberately whenever sharp objects are handled.

Air Embolism

Although neurosurgeons and anesthesiologists traditionally associate venous air embolism with procedures performed in the sitting position, this may occur at any time, even in cases without obvious risk factors.[57] Air embolism has even been attributed to the small puncture wounds in the calvarium caused by placement of a pin for a head-holding device,[58] presumably from aspiration of air through venous diploic channels. One study found an incidence of 10 percent for prone cases and 25 percent for sitting cases.[59] However, the incidence of clinically significant venous air embolism is much lower.

The diagnosis of air embolism may be confirmed by observing the end-tidal CO_2 monitor, which shows a decrease in end-tidal CO_2 because the air embolized to the lungs creates ventilation-perfusion mismatch and an increase in physiological deadspace.[60] A more sensitive indicator, and one that appears sooner than the drop in end-tidal CO_2, is a sudden 1 to 2 percent increase in the expired nitrogen concentration as the nitrogen diffuses from the embolized air bubbles into the alveoli.[61] Precordial Doppler ultrasonography is also quite useful in the detection of air embolus to the right atrium,[62] but for the detection of paradoxical embolism across a patent foramen ovale, only transesophageal echocardiography has proved useful.[63]

Preoperatively, when the neurosurgeon is especially concerned about this complication and when the patient's condition permits, traditional wisdom recommends placing a large-bore right atrial catheter for the possible aspiration of embolized air. However, placement of a central venous catheter for the sole purpose of managing potential venous air embolism remains controversial for several reasons.[57] These include the practical difficulty of placing such a catheter in the precise location required for this purpose, the improvement in techniques of successful prevention and early detection of air embolism, and the uncertainty as to whether prompt aspiration of intraatrial air improves outcome.

Ensuring an adequate central venous blood volume and avoiding unnecessary and/or extreme elevation of the head above the level of the heart are standard methods of minimizing the occurrence of air embolism. When this is diagnosed intraoperatively, the surgeon's first step in treatment is flooding the operative field with saline, followed by packing of the field with wet sponges and occluding raw surfaces of bone with bone wax. The head is lowered below the level of the heart. Animal experiments demonstrate the value of the left lateral decubitus position for trapping air in the apex of the right ventricle (instead of in the pulmonary outflow tract),[64] but this positioning is difficult to achieve in the operative setting. While the surgeon concentrates on these maneuvers, the anesthesiologist immediately discontinues any nitrous oxide that might be in use because this gas rapidly diffuses into all air-containing spaces throughout the body, which may significantly increase the size and thus the danger of embolized gas bubbles.[65,66] The patient is placed on 100 percent oxygen to facilitate diffusion of nitrogen gas from bubbles to alveoli.[67] β-adrenergic agonists may be effective both in lowering the resistance of the pulmonary vasculature and in preventing right-heart failure in cases of sudden, severe pulmonary hypertension.[68] Some authors have advocated positive end-expiratory pressure (PEEP) as both a preventive measure and a treatment for air embolism. Although this may promote venous bleeding, they feel that this effect is outweighed by a presumed concomitant increased resistance to air embolism. However, both clinical and laboratory research have failed to document the efficacy of PEEP in this regard[57] and in fact suggests that higher levels of PEEP may predispose these patients to paradoxical air embolism by causing right atrial pressure to become elevated.[69]

Bone Flap Infections

Fortunately, bone flap infections are relatively uncommon, even after emergency surgery on contaminated wounds. Most series report an incidence of approximately 5 percent or less.[70] In one series, although the infection rate between osteoplastic and free bone flaps was the same, the likelihood of successfully treating the infection without removing the flap was 80 percent for osteoplastic flaps vs. 50 percent for free flaps.[71] Irrigation with copious amounts of saline containing antibiotics may be helpful as prophylaxis in situations of obvious contamination. Generous debridement at the time of surgery is another traditional surgical technique for minimizing wound complications.

Bone flap infections generally appear several weeks after surgery, but both longer and shorter intervals are possible. Superficially, they may cause fever, localized erythema, and painful fluctuance of the scalp overlying the bone flap. Spread of infection to deeper tissues may mimic an epidural abscess, with localized headache a prominent symptom. The CSF may demonstrate increased protein and cellularity, consistent with a parameningeal inflammatory process. Serious infections may produce significant mass effect.

A subgaleal fluid collection in the early stages of infection may be aspirated and cultured in hopes of curing the infection with aggressive antibiotic therapy, initially broad-spectrum and later more organism-specific. Most infections, however, require reoperation for removal of the bone flap, culture of the infected tissues, aggressive debridement and irrigation, and closure of the soft tissues. Most surgeons discard infected bone flaps because of reluctance to reimplant previously infected tissue and because of the denaturation of bone proteins and resultant likely resorption caused by the process of autoclaving. However, if certain precautions are followed, cold-cycle ethylene may represent a more acceptable vehicle with which to sterilize skull.[72] Cranioplasty should not be performed until the infection has been completely eradicated. Conventional wisdom advises waiting 6 to 12 months to verify that no nidus of infection remains.

Cranioplasty

When bony defects are especially large or are situated in cosmetically important areas, it is necessary to repair them with a cranioplasty. Materials that have been used include artificial substances such as methylmethacrylate,[73] hydroxyapatite,[74,75] titanium plus acrylic,[76] and various metals and metallic meshes,[72] as well as bone allografts from such sites as calvarium,[77] ribs,[78] and iliac crest, among others. After calvarial loss from open injury, most neurosurgeons defer cranioplasty with synthetic materials for 6 to 12 months postinjury so that the presence of any possible infection can be definitively excluded. When autologous material is used for calvarial reconstruction, several series report good results with early, single-stage, combined neurosurgical and reconstructive procedures.[79,80] Good results have been reported with this technique, even with injuries involving the frontal sinus[81] or open depressed skull fractures.[82] When ceramic materials are used for repair of defects involving the frontal sinuses, the risk of infection becomes significant.[83] In children under 3 years, the possibility of osseous regeneration from an underlying intact outer leaf of dura has prompted the recommendation that any artificial cranial implants not be placed for at least 1 year.[84]

For large defects, such as those greater than approximately 50 cm^2,[85] proper contour and fit of a ceramic prosthesis may be sought via computer-assisted designs.[85–87] This method is reportedly more effective than the use of molds and casts, a technology adapted from the creation of dental prostheses.[87,88] Some have suggested covering ceramic prostheses with periosteal flaps of cranial bones in an attempt to enhance induction of the bone to hydroxyapatite.[86] However, the use of molds and casts and of computer-based designs has not become widespread, perhaps because most surgeons currently use methylmethacrylate or autologous bone.

The utility of autologous bone versus artificial materials remains controversial. Some authors favor ceramic materials because of the tendency to resorb seen in bone that is orthotopically transplanted to the skull. This is especially prominent in bone autografts that have been autoclaved.[89] Other groups, however, dispute that storage in a freezer and then autoclaving produce clinically significant deleterious effects on the viability of autogenous cranial grafts.[90] Other options, especially suited to countries without sophisticated facilities for storage of bone flaps, include storage in the subcutaneous tissues of the abdomen[91,92] or, in uncontaminated cases in which the bone flap is not replaced because of marked intraoperative brain swelling, under the scalp.[93] These techniques avoid the possibility of bacterial seeding while the flap is in storage and thereby also eliminate concerns about autoclaving prior to reimplantation, but the essential problem of removing the bone from its blood supply remains unsolved.

Reopening the previous incision generally provides adequate access to the bony defect, which must be exposed throughout its perimeter. The bone edge must be exposed at least in its superficial aspect, with care being taken not to violate the underlying scarred dura and thereby cause a CSF leak. A small ledge is created along the bone edge by drilling or rongeuring off the superficial bone.

When methylmethacrylate is used, it may be necessary in large defects to mold several small sponges and lay them over the dura to recreate the normal contour of the skull. A thin sheet of plastic is next laid over these (or directly on the dura of smaller defects). The liquid polymer is poured onto the plastic and rapidly and carefully molded to the appropriate size and shape. Considerable amounts of cool irrigation are needed during the most exothermic part of the hardening process. Any excess plastic may be removed with a high-speed drill, which is also used to create small holes around the perimeter for suture or wire. Some advocate the impregnation of the acrylic flap with antibiotic powder such as tobramycin or gentamicin.[94,95] Clinical and laboratory studies verify the safety of this practice in terms of maintenance of blood levels of the antibiotic well within the therapeutic range and in terms of no resultant neuro-, nephro-, or ototoxicity.[96,97] However, routine implementation of this practice has not been shown to reduce infection rates significantly.[97]

If ribs are to be used for the cranioplasty, they are split longitudinally after harvest. They can then be bent and contoured as necessary to give optimal cosmetic results (Fig. 14-13). Special care must be taken to secure the pieces firmly together and to the calvarium. Any irregularities can be made smooth with a high-speed drill.

When the split calvarial technique is used, calvarium is generally harvested from behind the hairline so as to minimize any subsequent cosmetic defects (Fig. 14-13). Smaller pieces of bone may be harvested with a craniotome or osteotome; larger pieces may be obtained by carefully splitting the outer table from the inner table with a curved osteotome. The more cosmetically suitable half of the split-thickness graft is used to cover the original defect; the other half is replaced over the donor site.

For reconstruction of extensive calvarial defects or those that may have a marginal blood flow, some authors use vascularized tissue grafts in order to obliterate the space between dura and skull with living tissue and/or to graft autologous bone with its blood supply intact.[98] They feel that the extra time and effort necessary to construct the vascular anastomosis pays off in terms of a lower likelihood of complications, such as resorption of the bone graft.

Both autologous bone and methylmethacrylate grafts may be secured in place with miniaturized plates and screws. Besides being quick and easy to use and providing excellent fixation, these devices avoid the need to gain access under the bony edge to pass suture or wire. Epidural scarring often makes such access difficult and carries the risk of dural violation and CSF leak.

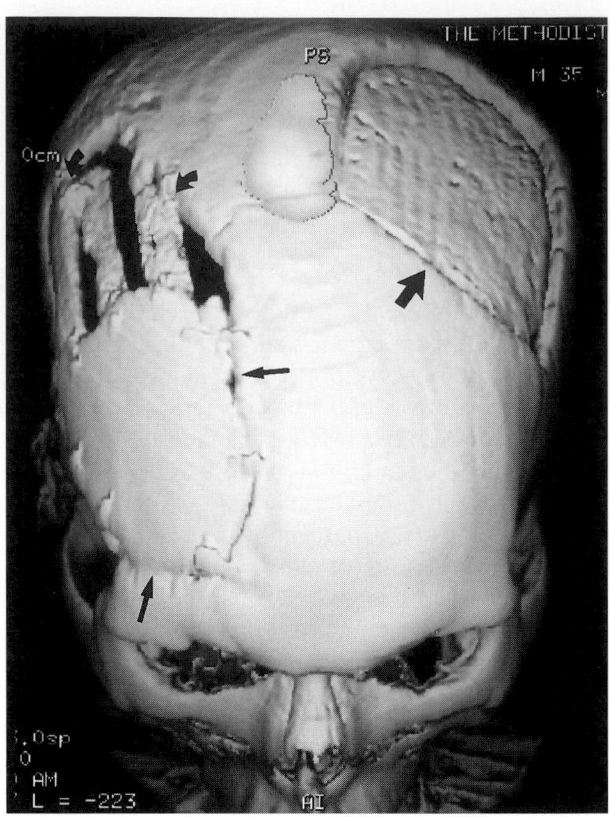

Figure 14-13. Three-dimensional reconstructed CT scan showing large right-sided calvarial defect corrected with several combined techniques. Left parietal bone was harvested for split calvarial graft. Inner table was replaced *(large arrow)*, and outer table was used to reconstruct anterior part of defect *(small arrows)*. Posterior part of defect was reconstructed with autologous rib grafts *(curved arrows)*.

INTRAOPERATIVE MEDICATIONS

Prophylactic Antibiotics

The rate of infection after clean neurosurgical procedures has been shown to be lower when intravenous antibiotics have been administered prior to incision of the skin.[99] There is no reason to exclude emergency craniotomies from this conclusion. Many neurosurgeons empirically place victims of gunshot wounds to the head on broad-spectrum antibiotics for several days. This practice is based on the assumption that the in-driven bone and other tissue cause greater bacterial seeding of the brain parenchyma and therefore merit a greater degree of prophylactic treatment with antibiotics. Although studies documenting this assumption are few,[29] the liberal use of antibiotics to treat suspected bacterial inoculation in these cases seems preferable to the alternative of aggressive surgical debridement of bone fragments, which entails the risk of injury to otherwise viable brain tissue.[100] The exact role of prophylactic antibiotics in penetrating or closed head injury awaits clarification.

Prophylactic Anticonvulsants

Many neurosurgeons routinely place all victims of head injury on prophylactic anticonvulsants. This therapy is often continued for months or even years, even in patients who have never had a seizure. Recent evidence suggests that in many cases such a lengthy duration of treatment may not be effective. Temkin et al. found that prophylactic phenytoin reduced the incidence of seizures only during the first 8 days after injury in head-injured patients who had not undergone craniotomy.[14] However, the numbers in any one subgroup were small, so that it was not possible to compare different types of pathology. Also, only one anticonvulsant medication was investigated. Nevertheless, in patients who have never had a seizure, it seems reasonable to taper their anticonvulsant regimen after the first week. This practice may also apply to those who sustained only immediate seizures (i.e, a seizure within the first 15 minutes of injury) and none subsequently, since immediate seizures are said to indicate no increased risk for subsequent fits.[101]

Mannitol

Mannitol is used to decrease ICP. Classic teaching holds that its mechanism of action is through its osmotic effect, which is said to extract water from the brain parenchyma. However, this has been difficult to prove, and in fact there exists evidence showing no change in brain water content after the administration of mannitol.[102] A more tenable mechanism of action is that the improvement in blood viscosity from mannitol infusion causes compensatory constriction of the cerebral vasculature without compromise of cerebral blood flow.[103] It is this decrease in the volume of intracerebral blood that results in a lowering of ICP.

A dosage as low as 0.25 gm/kg of mannitol has been shown to be effective in lowering ICP in some patients.[104] However, others respond only to doses ≥1.0 gm/kg. There is some evidence that slower infusion rates produce a more sustained decrease in ICP, whereas more rapid rates of infusion at higher doses (1.0 gm/kg) cause a more sizable reduction in ICP.[105] Mannitol may be given as often as needed provided that serum osmolality remains below 320 mOsm/L. Renal failure and systemic acidosis become much more of a concern when serum osmolality exceeds this level.[106]

Hyperventilation

It is well known that the cerebral blood vessels constrict in response to hypocapnia. Because constriction of the vasculature decreases the volume of intracranial blood, ICP can be lowered by this technique.

This physiological response can be quite useful in neurological emergencies. In patients with acutely elevated ICP, short-term hyperventilation may transiently lower ICP long enough to obtain a CT scan and to institute definitive treatment. Normocapnia should be restored as soon as possible, for in some patients the degree of vasoconstriction may be so severe that cerebral ischemia results.[107] Moreover, in the face of continuous hyperventilation, the reflex constriction of the vessels can eventually disappear, with the vessels returning to their normal diameter.[108] Their response to even greater hyperventilation becomes markedly diminished. Because CBF has been shown to be markedly diminished during the first 24 hours after injury,[109] there is concern that aggressive hyperventilation may worsen cerebral perfusion. How to modulate the degree of hyperventilation during this early phase remains uncertain.

Barbiturates

Although the exact mechanism of action of barbiturates and related compounds is unknown,[110] they have been used in severely head-injured patients in hopes of protecting neuronal elements from the effects of uncontrollably elevated intracranial pressure.[111–113] However, a randomized prospective trial of immediate pentobarbital administration to all severely head-injured patients found no improvement in outcome in the group receiving pentobarbital.[114] Hypotension was also significantly more common in this group. In a comparison of mannitol versus pentobarbital as the initial treatment of elevated ICP, the Toronto group found pentobarbital to be less effective than mannitol.[115] However, a five-center study did demonstrate a significant effect of pentobarbital treatment in terms of controlling ICP in certain patients after all conventional therapeutic measures had failed.[116] Intraoperative barbiturates are used by some surgeons to decrease malignant brain swelling.[25,26]

Etomidate seems to be more promising in both the intensive care unit and in the operating room. This steroid analogue produces the same depression of cerebral electrical activity as the barbiturate compounds, but with a much lower incidence of hypotension than pentobarbital and with only a fraction of the duration of action of phenobarbital. Preliminary evidence obtained from heavily monitored patients who had intracranial space-occupying lesions and who were undergoing endotracheal intubation in the operating room has shown that etomidate can significantly lower ICP without affecting mean arterial pressure or heart rate.[117]

SURGICAL ACCESSORIES

Hemostasis

The best technique of ensuring adequate hemostasis is the meticulous identification and cauterization or tamponade of vascular structures. Neurosurgeons have come to favor the bipolar coagulator because of its precision, its compatibility with irrigation, and its restriction of current spread when compared to monopolar irrigation. Another frequently helpful maxim is that bridging vessels from the dura to cortex are best divided closer to the cortex because bleeding following division of a vessel is easier to control when it arises from brain parenchyma than from dura or venous sinuses.

Hemostasis in trauma craniotomies presents its own set of problems. Large surfaces of parenchyma may be raw and oozing from laceration, contusion, and/or ischemia of the underlying tissue. The surgeon may be forced to operate with such speed that the usual meticulous hemostasis is impossible. Finally, as discussed in another chapter, many victims of head injury are coagulopathic.

These considerations may force the surgeon to employ methods of hemostasis which, while not as meticulous nor as satisfying as direct cauterization of the vessel, are still effective. All neurosurgeons are familiar with the technique of placing a small piece of Gelfoam (absorbable gelatin sponge-Upjohn) or Surgicel (oxidized regenerated cellulose-Johnson & Johnson) over a bleeding area and then applying gentle pressure through a cottonoid pledget. More persistent ooze may require Avitene (microfibrillar collagen-Avicon) in place of Gelfoam or Surgicel. A detailed analysis of chemical methods of achieving hemostasis in neurosurgery has been presented elsewhere.[118] Many neurosurgeons tamponade larger areas of injured or oozing brain with cotton balls soaked in half-strength hydrogen peroxide. Others simply irrigate a wet or oozing area with warm saline. Finally, in addition to these direct surgical methods of controlling bleeding, the surgeon must always be aware that any underlying coagulopathy requires treatment with fresh frozen plasma and with other blood products as indicated.

Ultrasound

Because virtually all patients taken to the operating room for a traumatic hematoma have undergone CT scanning to identify and localize the intracranial pathology, and because speed is essential in these cases, ultrasound is not routinely used to pinpoint a hematoma prior to opening the dura. However, once the mass effect has been relieved, ultrasound is useful in detecting residual clot and in guiding further surgical removal. When the brain still seems "tight" despite apparently adequate removal of hematoma, an ultrasound examination may reveal distant hematomas that have formed or enlarged since the CT scan was performed.

Dural Substitutes

Dural substitutes may be needed for a variety of reasons. Often, the cheapest and most readily available material is autologous pericranium or temporalis fascia. If the need for such material is anticipated prior to making the scalp incision, it is often possible to fashion an opening in such a way as to maximize access to pericranial tissue or to temporalis fascia. Fascia lata may also be harvested with good results, but this does require a second incision.[119] Autologous materials carry the advantage of ready availability with no additional cost and no added risk of infection from allogeneic substances.

Various allogeneic materials such as dura or pericardium are commercially prepared in a variety of sizes so as to minimize waste. However, these carry a risk, albeit very small, of possible transmission of infectious agents, such as slow viruses.[120] Among the various xenogeneic materials used are lyophilized calf pericardium[121,122] and porcine peritoneum.[123] These may prove to be valuable when autologous or allogeneic materials are unavailable.

Numerous synthetic materials also have been used, including tantalum foil,[124] fibrin film,[125] amnioplastin,[126] aliphatic polyurethane and polysiloxane-carbonate block copolymer,[127] and Silastic (silicone rubber-coated woven Dacron mesh). Silastic dural substitutes were often used in the past, but numerous reports describing large subjacent hematomas as a long-term complication[128–133] have turned many neurosurgeons away from this type of dural prosthesis.

Although early work with various collagen products was limited by a sometimes severe chronic inflammatory response,[134] newer materials have shown promising early results. These include the use of collagen sponges,[135] resorbable bilayered human placental collagen,[136] bovine collagen-coated vicryl mesh,[137,138] and irradiated bovine collagen-coated polyester.[139] These studies found few, if any, adhesions between the cortex and the dural graft. However, these experimental results await validation in the clinical setting. Moreover, experience with Silastic has demonstrated that lengthy follow-up will be needed for the proper assessment of complications.

When it becomes necessary to use a dural graft, it should be incorporated into the closure in the same watertight fashion as a standard dural closure. An exception is the finding of significant brain swelling at surgery. Especially when this is due to a focal insult, some advocate making many relaxing incisions in the dura and then laying down a large piece of dural substitute over the exposed portions of the swollen cortex. This is placed loosely, with no sutures or perhaps with only a few sutures to prevent migration of the graft. The bone flap is not replaced until the brain swelling decreases, at which point the patient is taken back to surgery, the dural substitute removed, the patient's dura reapproximated, and the bone flap replaced (See "Surgery for ICP Control," above).

References

1. Marshall LF, Gautille T, Klauber MR, et al: The outcome of severe closed head injury. *J Neurosurg* 1991; 75(Suppl):S28–S36.
2. Seelig JM, Becker DP, Miller JD, et al: Traumatic acute subdural hematoma: major mortality reduction in patients treated within four hours. *N Engl J Med* 1981; 304:1511–1518.
3. Bullock R, Golek J, Blake G: Traumatic intracerebral hematoma—which patients should undergo surgical evacuation? *Surg Neurol* 1989; 32:367–372.
4. Elsner H, Rigamonti D, Corradino G, et al: Delayed traumatic intracerebral hematomas: "Spät-Apoplexie." *J Neurosurg* 1990; 72:813–815.
5. Gentleman D, Nath F, Macpherson P: Diagnosis and management of delayed traumatic intracerebral hematomas. *Br J Neurosurg* 1989; 3:367–372.
6. Carey ME, Young HF, Mathis JL: The neurosurgical treatment of craniocerebral missile wounds in Vietnam. *Surg Gynecol Obstet* 1972; 135:386–390.
7. Levy ML, Masri LS, Levy KM, et al: Penetrating craniocerebral injury resulting from gunshot wounds: Gang-related injury in children and adolescents. *Neurosurgery* 1993; 33:1018–1025.
8. Narayan RK: Emergency room management of the head-injured patient, in Becker DP, Gudeman SK (eds): *Textbook of Head Injury.* Philadelphia: WB Saunders, 1989: 23–66.
9. Wilberger JE Jr, Harris M, Diamond DL: Acute subdural hematoma: Morbidity and mortality related to timing of operative intervention. *J Trauma* 1990; 30:733–736.
10. Ribas GC, Jane JA: Traumatic contusions and intracerebral hematomas. *J Neurotrauma* 1992; 9(Suppl 1): S265–S278.
11. Rosenblum WI: Pathology of human head injury, in Becker DP, Gudeman SK (eds): *Textbook of Head Injury.* Philadelphia: WB Saunders, 1989: 525–537.
12. Narayan RK, Kishore PRS, Becker DP, et al: Intracranial pressure: To monitor or not to monitor? A review of our experience with severe head injury. *J Neurosurg* 1982; 56:650–659.
13. van Dongen KJ, Braakman R, Gelpke GJ: The prognostic value of computerized tomography in comatose head-injured patients. *J Neurosurg* 1983; 59:951–957.
14. Temkin NR, Dikmen SS, Wilensky AJ, et al: A randomized, double-blind study of phenytoin for the prevention of post-traumatic seizures. *N Engl J Med* 1990; 323:497–502.
15. Becker DP: Common themes in head injury, in Becker DP, Gudeman SK (eds): *Textbook of Head Injury.* Philadelphia: WB Saunders, 1989: 1–22.
16. Niizuma H, Shimizu Y, Yonemitsu T, et al: Results of stereotactic aspiration in 175 cases of putaminal hemorrhage. *Neurosurgery* 1989; 24:814–819.
17. Auer LM, Deinsberger W, Niederkorn K, et al: Endoscopic surgery versus medical treatment for spontaneous intracerebral hematoma: A randomized study. *J Neurosurg* 1989; 70:530–535.
18. Kaneko M, Tanaka K, Shimada T, et al: Long-term evaluation of ultra-early operation for hypertensive intracerebral hemorrhage in 100 cases. *J Neurosurg* 1983; 58:838–842.
19. Ransohoff J, Benjamin MV, Gage EL Jr, Epstein F: Hemicraniectomy in the management of acute subdural hematoma. *J Neurosurg* 1971; 34:70–76.
20. Cooper PR, Rovit RL, Ransohoff J: Hemicraniectomy in the treatment of acute subdural hematoma: A re-appraisal. *Surg Neurol* 1976; 5:25–28.
21. Litofsky NS, Chin LS, Tang G, et al: The use of lobectomy in the management of severe closed-head trauma. *Neurosurgery* 1994; 34:628–633.
22. Rengachary SS, Batnitzky S, Morantz RA, et al: Hemicraniectomy for acute massive cerebral infarction. *Neurosurgery* 1981; 8:321–328.
23. Kondziolka D, Fazi M: Functional recovery after decompressive craniectomy for cerebral infarction. *Neurosurgery* 1988; 23:143–147.
24. Gade GF, Becker DP: Surgical management of acute head injuries, in Schmidek HH, Sweet WH (eds): *Operative Neurosurgical Techniques: Indications, Methods, and Results,* 2d ed. Philadelphia: WB Saunders, 1988: 19–31.
25. Aldrich EF, Eisenberg HM: Acute subdural hematoma, in Apuzzo MLJ (ed): *Brain Surgery: Complication Avoidance and Management.* New York: Churchill-Livingstone, 1993: 1283–1298.
26. Shapiro HM, Galindo A, Wyte SR, et al: Rapid intraoperative reduction of intracranial pressure with thiopentone. *Br J Anaesth* 1973; 45:1057–1061.
27. Gudeman SK, Young HF, Miller JD, et al: Indications for operative treatment and operative technique in closed head injury, in Becker DP, Gudeman SK (eds): *Textbook of Head Injury.* Philadelphia: WB Saunders, 1989: 138–181.

28. Taha JM, Haddad FS, Brown JA: Intracranial infection after missile injuries to the brain: Report of 30 cases from the Lebanese conflict. *Neurosurgery* 1991; 29:864–868.
29. Carey ME, Young H, Mathis JL: A bacteriological study of craniocerebral missile wounds from Vietnam. *J Neurosurg* 1971; 34:145–154.
30. Rish B, Caveness W, Dillon J, et al: Analysis of brain abscesses after penetrating craniocerebral injuries in Vietnam. *Neurosurgery* 1981; 9:535–541.
31. Grahm TW, Williams FC Jr, Harrington T, Spetzler RF: Civilian gunshot wounds to the head: A prospective study. *Neurosurgery* 1990; 27:696–700.
32. Clark WC, Muhlbauer MS, Watridge CB, Roy MW: Analysis of 76 civilian craniocerebral gunshot wounds. *J Neurosurg* 1986; 65:9–14.
33. Haines SJ: Duration of intracranial pressure monitoring does not predict risk of infectious complications: Comment. *Neurosurgery* 1993; 33:430–431.
34. Winfield JA, Rosenthal P, Kanter RK, Casella G: Duration of intracranial pressure monitoring does not predict daily risk of infectious complications. *Neurosurgery* 1993; 33:424–431.
35. Thomason M, Messick J, Rutledge R, et al: Head CT scanning versus urgent exploration in the hypotensive blunt trauma patient. *J Trauma* 1993; 34:40–45.
36. Andrews BT, Pitts LH, Lovely MP, Bartkowski H: Is computed tomographic scanning necessary in patients with tentorial herniation? *Neurosurgery* 1986; 19:408–414.
37. Mahoney BD, Rockswold GL, Ruiz E, Clinton JE: Emergency twist drill trephination. *Neurosurgery* 1981; 8:551–554.
38. Michael DB, Guyot DR, Darmody WR: Coincidence of head and cervical spine injury. *J Neurotrauma* 1989; 6:177–189.
39. O'Malley KF, Ross SE: The incidence of injury to the cervical spine in patients with craniocerebral injury. *J Trauma* 1988; 28:1476–1478.
40. Soicher E, Demetriades D: Cervical spine injuries in patients with head injuries. *Br J Surg* 1991; 78:1013–1014.
41. Martin RR, Barcia PJ, Johnson EA: Making matters worse: Complications of initial evaluation, treatment, and delayed diagnosis, in Mattox KL (ed): *Complications of Trauma.* New York: Churchill-Livingstone, 1994: 139–154.
42. Marshall LF, Knowlton S, Garfin SR, et al: Deterioration following spinal cord injury: A multicenter study. *J Neurosurg* 1987; 66:400–404.
43. Meier U, Gartner F, Knopf W, et al: The traumatic dural sinus injury—a clinical study. *Acta Neurochir (Wien)* 1992; 119:91–93.
44. Kapp J: Surgical management of dural sinus lacerations, in Schmidek HH, Sweet WH (eds): *Operative Neurosurgical Technique: Indications, Methods, and Results.* Philadelphia: WB Saunders, 1988: 877–879.
45. Kapp JP: Nonseptic venous occlusive disease, in Wilkins RH, Rengachary SS (eds): *Neurosurgery.* New York: McGraw-Hill, 1985: 1300–1307.
46. Kapp JP, Gielchinsky I: Management of combat wounds of the dural venous sinuses. *Surgery* 1972; 71:913–917.
47. Sataloff RT, Sariego J, Myers DL, Richter HJ: Surgical management of the frontal sinus. *Neurosurgery* 1984; 15:593–596.
48. Heckler FR: Frontal sinus fractures: Guidelines to management: Discussion. *Plast Reconstr Surg* 1987; 80:509–510.
49. Luce EA: Frontal sinus fractures: Guidelines to management. *Plast Reconstr Surg* 1987; 80:500–508.
50. Riefkohl R, Georgiade GS, Georgiade NG: Facial fractures, in Wilkins RW, Rengachary SS (eds): *Neurosurgery.* New York: McGraw-Hill, 1985: 1629–1637.
51. Wolfe SA, Johnson P: Frontal sinus injuries: Primary care and management of late complications. *Plast Reconstr Surg* 1988; 82:781–789.
52. Ciric IS, Rosenblatt S: Supratentorial craniotomies, in Apuzzo MLJ (ed): *Brain Surgery: Complication Avoidance and Management.* New York: Churchill-Livingstone, 1993: 51–70.
53. Rohrich RJ, Hollier LH: Management of frontal sinus fractures. Changing concepts. *Clin Plast Surg* 1992; 19:219–232.
54. Schiff SJ: A surgeon's risk of AIDS. *J Neurosurg* 1990; 73:651–660.
55. Kelen GD, Fritz S, Qaqish B, et al: Unrecognized human immunodeficiency virus infection in emergency department patients. *N Engl J Med* 1988; 318:1645–1650.
56. Centers for Disease Control: Recommendations for prevention of HIV transmission in health-care settings. *MMWR* 1987; 36(Suppl 2):1–18.
57. Marco AP, Furman WR: Anesthetic problems: Venous air embolism, airway difficulties, and massive transfusion. *Surg Clin North Am* 1993; 73:213–228.
58. Cabezudo JM, Gilsanz F, Vaquero J, et al: Air embolism from wounds from a pin-type head-holder as a complication of posterior fossa surgery in the sitting position. Case report. *J Neurosurg* 1981; 55:147–148.
59. Albin M, Carroll R, Maroon J: Clinical considerations concerning detection of venous air embolism. *Neurosurgery* 1978; 3:380–384.
60. Bedford RF, Marshall WK, Butler A, et al: Cardiac catheters for diagnosis and treatment of venous air embolism. *J Neurosurg* 1981; 55:610–614.
61. Matjasko J, Petrozza P, Mackenzie CF: Sensitivity of end-tidal nitrogen in venous air embolism detection in dogs. *Anesthesiology* 1985; 63:418–423.
62. English J, Westenskow D, Hodges M, et al: Comparison of venous air embolism monitoring methods in supine dogs. *Anesthesiology* 1978; 48:425–429.
63. Cucchiara RF, Nugent M, Seward JB, et al: Air embolism in upright neurosurgical patients: Detection and localization by two-dimensional transesophageal echocardiography. *Anesthesiology* 1984; 60:353–355.
64. Durant TM, Long J, Oppenheimer MJ: Pulmonary (venous) air embolism. *Am Heart J* 1947; 33:269–281.
65. Munson ES: Effect of nitrous oxide on the pulmonary circulation during venous air embolism. *Anesth Analg* 1971; 50:785–791.

66. Munson E, Merrick H: Effect of nitrous oxide on venous air embolism. *Anesthesiology* 1966; 27:783–787.
67. O'Qiunn RJ, Lakshminarayan S: Venous air embolism. *Arch Intern Med* 1982; 142:2173–2176.
68. Bonsignore M, Jerome E, Culver P, et al: Effects of β-adrenergic agents in lungs of normal and air-embolized awake sheep. *J Appl Physiol* 1988; 64:2647–2652.
69. Perkins N, Bedford R: Hemodynamic consequences of PEEP in seated neurosurgical patients—implications for paradoxical air embolism. *Anesth Analg* 1984; 63:429–432.
70. Blomstedt GC: Craniotomy infections. *Neurosurg Clin North Am* 1992; 3:375–385.
71. Rasmussen S, Ohrstrom JK, Westergaard L, Kosteljanetz M: Post-operative infections of osteoplastic compared with free bone flaps. *Br J Neurosurg* 1990; 4:493–495.
72. Prolo DJ: Cranial defects and cranioplasty, in Wilkins RH, Rengachary SS (eds): *Neurosurgery.* New York: McGraw-Hill, 1985: 1647–1656.
73. Oliver LC, Blaine G: A new one-staged method of cranioplasty with acrylic plastic. *Med Press (London)* 1948; 220:167.
74. Yamashima T: Modern cranioplasty with hydroxylapatite ceramic granules, buttons, and plates. *Neurosurgery* 1993; 33:939–940.
75. Waite PD, Morawetz RB, Zeiger HE, Pincock JL: Reconstruction of cranial defects with porous hydroxylapatite blocks. *Neurosurgery* 1989; 25:214–217.
76. Malis LI: Titanium mesh and acrylic cranioplasty. *Neurosurgery* 1989; 25:351–355.
77. Kulali A, Kayaalp S: Single-table autogenous calvarial grafting for cranioplasty. *J Craniomaxillofac Surg* 1991; 19:208–211.
78. Kawakami M, Takahara N, Yamanouchi Y, et al: Split-rib cranioplasty. *No Shinkei Geka (Neurological Surgery)* 1989; 17:1023–1027.
79. Robotti E, Dagi TF, Ravegnani M, Bocchiotti G: A new prospect on the approach to open, complex, craniofacial trauma. *J Neurosurg Sci* 1992; 36:89–99.
80. Benzil DL, Robotti E, Dagi TF, et al: Early single-stage repair of complex craniofacial trauma. *Neurosurgery* 1992; 30:166–171.
81. Stanley RB Jr: Management of severe frontobasilar skull fractures. *Otolaryngol Clin North Am* 1991; 24:139–150.
82. Blankenship JB, Chadduck WM, Boop FA: Repair of compound-depressed skull fractures in children with replacement of bone fragments. *Pediatr Neurosurg* 1990–91; 16:297–300.
83. Benzel EC, Thammavaram K, Kesterson L: The diagnosis of infections associated with acrylic cranioplasties. *Neuroradiology* 1990; 32:151–153.
84. Olin MS: Repair of defects of the skull, in Schmidek HH, Sweet WH (eds): *Operative Neurosurgical Techniques: Indications, Methods, and Results.* Philadelphia: WB Saunders, 1988: 11–17.
85. van Putten MC Jr, Yamada S: Alloplastic cranial implants made from computed tomographic scan-generated casts. *J Prosthet Dent* 1992; 68:103–108.
86. Ono I, Gunji H, Kaneko F, et al: Treatment of extensive cranial bone defects using computer-designed hydroxyapatite ceramics and periosteal flaps. *Plast Reconstr Surg* 1993; 92:819–830.
87. Joffe JM, McDermott PJ, Linney AD, et al: Computer-generated titanium cranioplasty: Report of a new technique for repairing skull defects. *Br J Neurosurg* 1992; 6:343–350.
88. Joffe JM, Aghabeigi B, Davies EH, Harris M: A retrospective study of 66 titanium cranioplasties. *Br J Oral Maxillofac Surg* 1993; 31:144–148.
89. Prolo DJ, Oklund SA: The use of bone grafts and alloplastic materials in cranioplasty. *Clin Orthop* 1991; 268:270–278.
90. Osawa M, Hara H, Ichinose Y, et al: Cranioplasty with a frozen and autoclaved bone flap. *Acta Neurochir (Wien)* 1990; 102:38–41.
91. Kreider GN: Repair of cranial defects by a new method. *JAMA* 1920; 74:1024.
92. Häuptli J, Segantini P: Neue Aufbewahrungsart von Schädelkalottenstücken nach dekompressiver Kraniotomie. *Helv Chir Acta* 1980; 47:121–124; cited in Prolo DJ: Cranial defects and cranioplasty, in Wilkins RH, Rengachary SS (eds): *Neurosurgery.* New York: McGraw-Hill, 1985; 1647–1656.
93. Korfali E, Aksoy K: Preservation of craniotomy bone flaps under the scalp. *Surg Neurol* 1988; 30:269–272.
94. Aziz TZ, Mathew BG, Kirkpatrick PJ: Bone flap replacement vs acrylic cranioplasty: A clinical audit. *Br J Neurosurg* 1990; 4:417–419.
95. Mann W, el-Khatieb AA: Cranioplasty with Palacos R in reconstruction of frontal sinus defects. *J Laryngol Otol* 1988; 102:824–827.
96. Ronderos JF, Wiles DA, Ragan FA, et al: Cranioplasty using gentamicin-loaded acrylic cement: A test of neurotoxicity. *Surg Neurol* 1992; 37:356–360.
97. Shapiro SA: Cranioplasty, vertebral body replacement, and spinal fusion with tobramycin-impregnated methylmethacrylate. *Clin Orthop* 1991; 268:270–278.
98. Netscher DT, Stal S, Shenaq S: Management of residual cranial vault deformities. *Clin Plast Surg* 1992; 19:301–313.
99. Haines SJ: Efficacy of antibiotic prophylaxis in clean neurosurgical procedures. *Neurosurgery* 1989; 24: 401–405.
100. George ED, Dagi TF: Penetrating missile injuries of the head, in Schmidek HH, Sweet WH (eds): *Operative Neurosurgical Techniques: Indications, Methods, and Results,* 2d ed. Philadelphia: WB Saunders, 1988: 49–55.
101. Jennett B: *Epilepsy After Non-Missile Head Injuries,* 2d ed. Chicago: Year Book, 1975.
102. Tagaki H, Saito T, Kitahara T, et al: The mechanism of the ICP-reducing effect of mannitol. Presented at the 5th International Symposium on Intracranial Pressure, Tokyo, Japan, 1982.
103. Muizelaar JP, Wei EP, Kontos HA, Becker DP: Mannitol causes compensatory vasoconstriction and vasodilation to blood viscosity changes. *J Neurosurg* 1983; 59:822–828.
104. Marshall LF, Smith RW, Rauscher LA, Shapiro HM:

Mannitol dose requirements in head-injured patients. *J Neurosurg* 1978; 48:169–172.

105. Node Y, Nakazawa S: Clinical study of mannitol and glycerol on raised intracranial pressure and on their rebound phenomenon, in Long D, et al (eds): *Advances in Neurology,* Vol. 52. New York: Raven Press, 1990: 359–363.
106. Feig PN, McCurdy DK: The hypertonic state. *N Engl J Med* 1977; 297:1449.
107. Miller JD, Dearden NM, Piper IR, Chan KH: Control of intracranial pressure in patients with severe head injury. *J Neurotrauma* 1992; 9(Suppl 1):S317–S326.
108. Muizelaar JP, van der Poel HG, Li Z, et al: Pial arteriolar vessel diameter and CO_2 reactivity during prolonged hyperventilation in the rabbit. *J Neurosurg* 1988; 69:923–927.
109. Bouma GJ, Muizelaar JP, Stringer WA, et al: Ultra-early evaluation of regional cerebral blood flow in severely head-injured patients using xenon-enhanced computerized tomography. *J Neurosurg* 1992; 77: 360–368.
110. Moskopp D, Ries F, Wassmann H, Nadstawek J: Barbiturates in severe head injuries? *Neurosurg Rev* 1991; 14:195–202.
111. Marshall LF, Smith RW, Shapiro HM: The outcome with aggressive treatment in severe head injuries. Part 2: Acute and chronic barbiturate administration in the management of head injury. *J Neurosurg* 1979; 59:26–30.
112. Rockoff MA, Marshall LF, Shapiro M: High-dose barbiturate therapy in humans: A clinical review of 60 patients. *Ann Neurol* 1979; 6:194–199.
113. Rea GL, Rockswold GL: Barbiturate therapy in uncontrolled intracranial hypertension. *Neurosurgery* 1983; 12:401–404.
114. Ward JD, Becker DP, Miller JD, et al: Failure of prophylactic barbiturate coma in the treatment of severe head injury. *J Neurosurg* 1985; 62:383–388.
115. Schwartz ML, Tator CH, Rowed DW, et al: The University of Toronto head injury treatment study: A prospective, randomized comparison of pentobarbital and mannitol. *Can J Neurol Sci* 1984; 11:434–440.
116. Eisenberg HM, Frankowski RF, Contant CF, Marshall LF, Walker MD, and the Comprehensive Central Nervous System Trauma Centers: High-dose barbiturate control of elevated intracranial pressure in patients with severe head injury. *J Neurosurg* 1988; 69:15–23.
117. Modica PA, Tempelhoff R: Intracranial pressure during induction of anaesthesia and tracheal intubation with etomidate-induced EEG burst suppression. *Can J Anaesth* 1992; 39:236–241.
118. Arand AG, Sawaya R: Intraoperative chemical hemostasis in neurosurgery. *Neurosurgery* 1986; 18:223–233.
119. Thammavaram KV, Benzel EC, Kesterson L: Fascia lata graft as a dural substitute in neurosurgery. *South M J* 1990; 83:634–636.
120. Martinez-Lage JF, Sola J, Poza M, Esteban JA: Pediatric Creutzfeldt-Jakob disease: Transmission by a dural graft. *Childs Nerv Syst* 1993; 9:239–242.
121. Parizek J, Mericka P, Spacek J, et al: Xenogeneic pericardium as a dural substitute in reconstruction of suboccipital dura mater in children. *J Neurosurg* 1989; 70:905–909.
122. Laun A, Tonn JC, Jerusalem C: Comparative study of lyophilized human dura mater and lyophilized bovine pericardium as dural substitutes in neurosurgery. *Acta Neurochir (Wien)* 1990; 107:16–21.
123. Xu BZ, Pan HX, Li KM, et al: Study and clinical application of a porcine biomembrane for the repair of dural defects. *J Neurosurg* 1988; 69:707–711.
124. Robertson RCL, Peacher WG: The use of tantalum foil in the subdural space. *J Neurosurg* 1945; 2:281–284.
125. Ingraham FD, Bailey OT, Cobb CA Jr: The use of fibrin film as a dural substitute and in the prevention of meningocerebral adhesions. Further studies and clinical results. *JAMA* 1945; 128:1088–1091.
126. Chao YC, Humphreys S, Penfield W: A new method of preventing adhesions. The use of amnioplastin after craniotomy. *Br Med J* 1940; 1:517–519.
127. Sakas DE, Charnvises K, Borges LF, Zervas NT: Biologically inert synthetic dural substitutes. Appraisal of a medical-grade aliphatic polyurethane and a polysiloxane-carbonate block copolymer. *J Neurosurg* 1990; 73:936–941.
128. Banerjee T, Meagher JN, Hunt WE: Unusual complications with use of Silastic dural substitute. *Am Surg* 1974; 40:434–437.
129. Adegbite AB, Paine KWE, Rozdilsky B: The role of neomembranes in formation of hematoma around Silastic dural substitute. *J Neurosurg* 1983; 58:295–297.
130. Ng TH, Chan KH, Leung SY, Mann KS: An unusual complication of Silastic dural substitute: Case report. *Neurosurgery* 1990; 27:491–493.
131. Fontana R, Talamonti G, D'Angelo V, et al: Spontaneous hematoma as unusual complication of Silastic dural substitute. Report of 2 cases. *Acta Neurochir (Wien)* 1992; 115:64–66.
132. Ohbayashi N, Inagawa T, Katoh Y, et al: Complication of Silastic dural substitute 20 years after dural plasty. *Surg Neurol* 1994; 41:338–341.
133. Berrington NR: Acute extradural hematoma associated with Silastic dural substitute: Case report. *Surg Neurol* 1992; 38:469–470.
134. Kline DG: Dural replacement with resorbable collagen. *Arch Surg* 1965; 91:924–929.
135. Narotam PK, Van Dellen JR, Bhoola K, Raidoo D: Experimental evaluation of collagen sponge as a dural graft. *Br J Neurosurg* 1993; 7:635–641.
136. Laquerriere A, Yun J, Tiollier J, et al: Experimental evaluation of bilayered human collagen as a dural substitute. *J Neurosurg* 1993; 78:487–491.
137. Meddings N, Scott R, Bullock R, et al: Collagen vicryl—a new dural prosthesis. *Acta Neurochir (Wien)* 1992; 117:53–58.
138. San-Galli F, Darrouzet V, Rivel J, et al: Experimental evaluation of a collagen-coated vicryl mesh as a dural substitute. *Neurosurgery* 1992; 30:396–401.
139. Pietrucha K: New collagen implant as dural substitute. *Biomaterials* 1991; 12:320–323.

CHAPTER 15

MAXILLOFACIAL AND SCALP INJURY IN NEUROTRAUMA

Saleh M. Shenaq
Tue Dinh

SYNOPSIS

Brain injuries are commonly associated with injuries of the face and scalp. Current principles of management emphasize early soft tissue repair, precise anatomic fixation via wide exposure, and, when appropriate, one-stage reconstruction. This chapter summarizes the specific issues relative to the various maxillofacial and scalp injuries seen in the head-injury patient.

INTRODUCTION

The management of complex craniomaxillofacial fracture and facial soft tissue injury has evolved rapidly in the past two decades. Previous beliefs in delayed operative procedure and minimal surgery have been replaced. The new principles include:

1. Early soft tissue repair.
2. Precise anatomic fixation via wide exposure.
3. One-stage reconstruction.

Head trauma patients often have associated maxillofacial injuries (up to 80 percent in one study).[1] In patients with head trauma, the goal of early, one-stage definitive repair should be kept in the context of the patient's overall stability and prognosis. The Glasgow Coma Scale can provide information regarding the ultimate prognosis. However, unless the prognosis is very grave, a low score does not argue against an attempt to restore facial integrity. When intracranial pressure is maintained at 25 mmHg or less, the patient can tolerate anesthesia without increased complications.[2]

EARLY AND EMERGENT CARE

As with any trauma patient, consideration should be given first to the traditional ABCs of trauma care.

Airway

Injuries to the maxillofacial and oral regions can obstruct the airway and compromise life. Debris should be cleaned from the mouth, and the tongue should be pulled forward and occasionally secured with sutures as needed to prevent the tongue from falling backwards.

Early intubation is indicated, and a tracheostomy is preferred in severe facial injuries.

Hemorrhage

This is the next relevant consideration in patients with maxillofacial injuries. Bleeding can be copious and the blood loss very significant. The source of the bleeding can include multiple facial vessels such as the labial artery, facial artery, or external maxillary artery. Initially, bleeding can be controlled by the application of direct pressure. Direct clamping and ligation of the artery is accomplished only when the source is clearly visible. Ligation of the external carotid artery is rarely required. In mandibular fractures, bleeding can occur from the inferior alveolar artery, and this sometimes can be controlled only via reduction of the fracture.

Timing

Repair of maxillofacial injuries should be planned in conjunction with other surgery. Close consultation with other services is essential. In general, the most serious injuries have priority. Maxillofacial injuries (except those compromising life) are managed later during the same operative procedure, after more serious injuries are managed. Operative procedures have the goal of definitive repair.

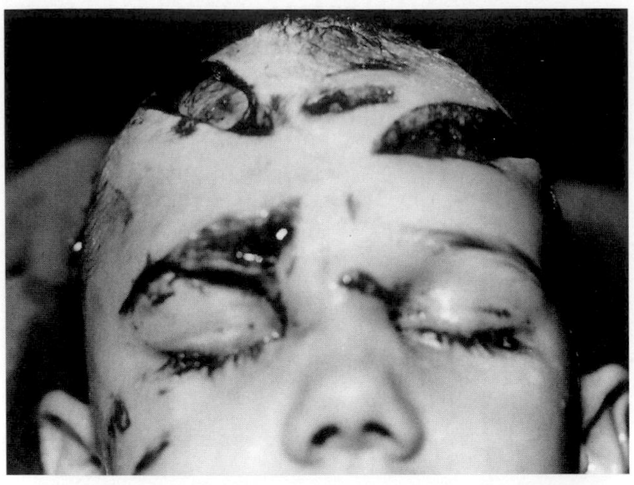

A

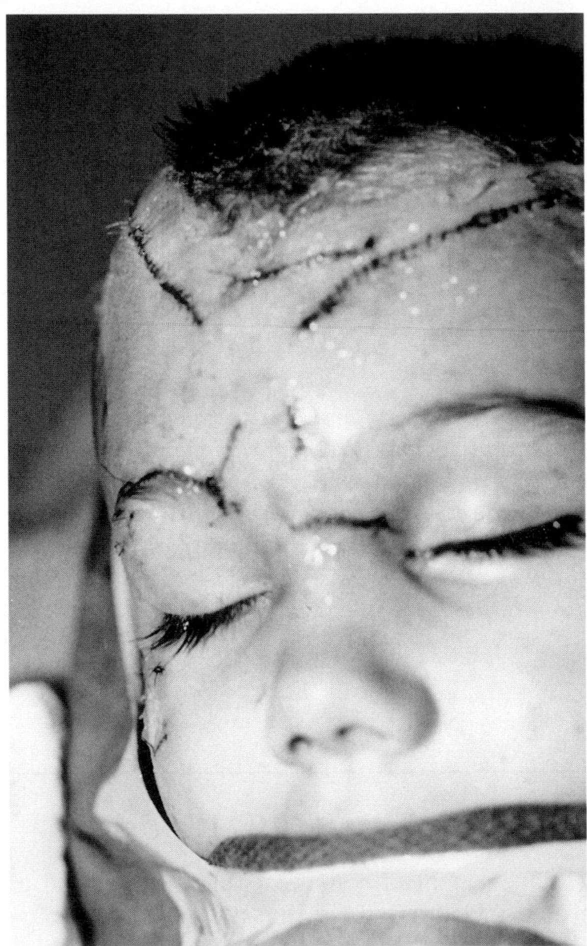

B

Figure 15-1. Eight-year-old boy with multiple facial and scalp lacerations after MVA. *A*. Prior to repair. *B*. Immediately after repair in OR.

SOFT TISSUE INJURIES

The old dictums that soft tissue repair should be delayed so that edema can resolve have not improved results.[3] Instead, soft tissue shrinkage has made late reconstruction more difficult. All soft tissue facial injuries should be closed at the earliest opportunity, either in the emergency center or the operating room. In the emergency center, regional block is preferred over infiltration anesthesia to lessen the amount of tissue distortion (see Fig. 15-1).

Facial Soft Tissue Injuries

Simple Laceration

All simple lacerations should be irrigated vigorously prior to closure. All foreign bodies should be removed, and any nonviable skin edges should be trimmed. Closure should be done in layers under no tension. Before closure, branches of the facial nerve and, if appropriate, the parotid duct should be examined. Injuries to any of these structures should be repaired in the operating room (see Fig. 15-2).

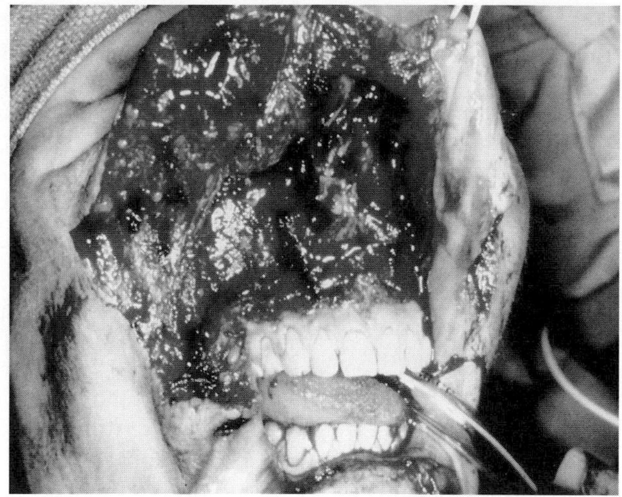
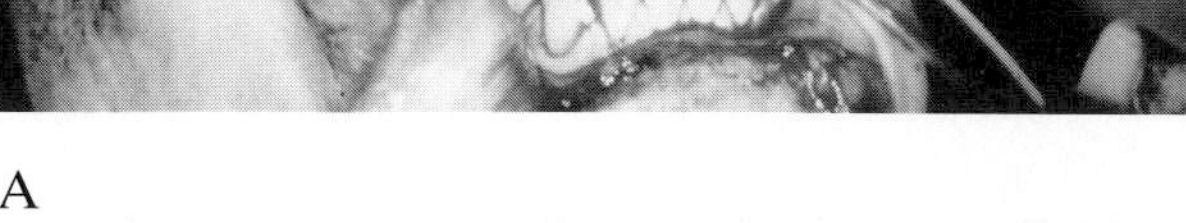

A

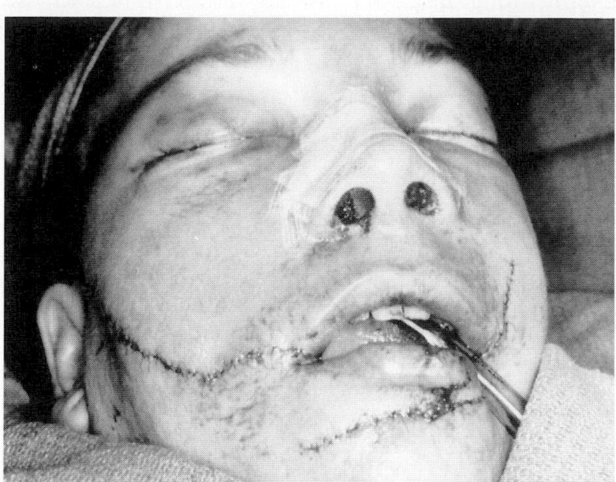

B

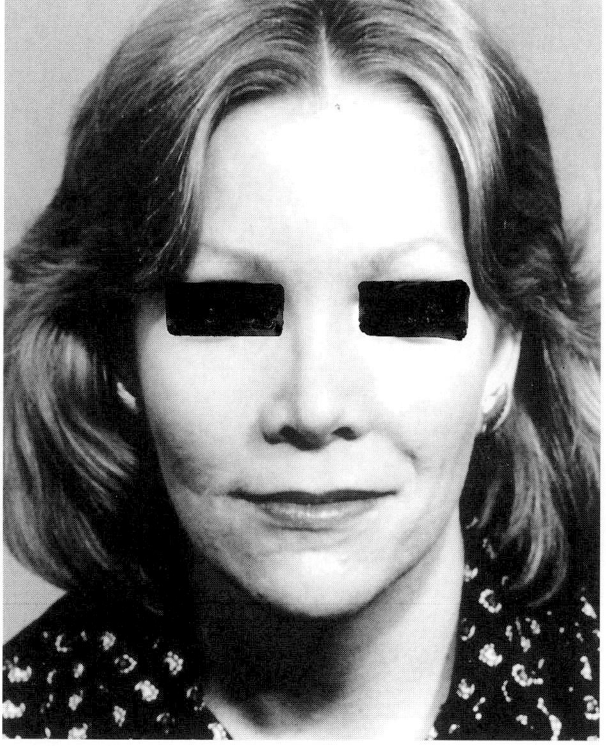

C

Figure 15-2. Thirty-three-year-old woman with midface soft tissue avulsion and maxillary fracture. (Courtesy of Drs. M. Spira and M. Breiner). *A*. Prior to repair. *B*. Immediately after ORIF of maxillary fracture and repair of soft tissue. *C*. Late follow-up.

Abrasion

The main objective for treating abrasions is minimization of scarring and prevention of late deformity. All foreign material, such as dirt or gravel, should be removed during the first treatment. This can be done either with a scrub brush or a dermabrader. Occasionally, removal of each piece of foreign material is indicated. This tedious procedure is worthwhile in preventing traumatic tattoo because late correction is often inadequate. Superficial abrasion can be treated with the application of an antibiotic ointment and protective gauze.

Contusion

A simple contusion or even a small hematoma can be treated with just cold compresses. A large hematoma, however, needs to be evacuated via an incision along the skin crease. The hematoma is then evacuated by pushing along the cavity toward the incision. The resultant cavity should be irrigated and allowed to heal spontaneously.

AVULSION

Avulsion injury is common in windshield accidents. If the avulsed area is small, closure along skin tension line is often possible and desirable. When large avulsed tissue is recovered and is too large to survive as a composite graft, it should be de-fatted and reapplied as a full-thickness skin graft to the injured area.

SCALP AND CRANIAL INJURIES

ANATOMY

The scalp is composed of five layers—skin, dense connective tissue, galea aponeurotica, loose connective tissue, and pericranium. The scalp has an abundant blood supply from the posterior auricular, superficial temporal, and occipital arteries. The first division of the fifth cranial nerve supplies the anterior scalp; the second cervical nerve supplies the posterior portion. The region around the ear including the ear itself is supplied by the great auricular nerve and the zygomatico-temporal branch (from cranial nerve V) that supplies the temporal area. These nerves can be anesthetized to provide regional block.

LACERATION

These should be irrigated and explored. If the galea is torn, it should be closed separately with absorbable sutures. The skin layer can then be closed with through-and-through nylon suture.

AVULSION

Scalp avulsions usually occur through the loose areolar tissue between the galea aponeurotica and the pericranium. These injuries can be accompanied by massive amounts of blood loss and shock, which requires resuscitation. Owing to the extensive vascular supply to the scalp, partial avulsions usually do not require microvascular repair. Unless the base of the avulsed scalp is very small, the avulsed portion of the scalp will survive if it is irrigated, replaced on top of the bone, and secured in place under no tension. Total avulsion of the scalp will require microsurgical reanastomosis of the blood vessels. Usually reconnection of one supplying artery and two draining veins is recommended. If the scalp avulsion cannot be replaced and results in loss of the scalp, skin grafts can be placed over the cranium if the periosteum is intact. If this is not the case, dressing changes can be performed and fenestrations of the outer table of the cranium can be done to allow the diploë to grow outward and cover the exposed bone with granulation tissue. The skin graft will adhere to this tissue. For more protection, transfer of muscle or musculocutaneous free flap with microvascular anastomosis can be performed.

SPECIFIC INJURIES

EAR INJURY

Hematoma of the ear usually results from blunt trauma. The perichondrium is separated from the cartilage, and blood is collected in between. This blood should be aspirated; then a bolus dressing should be applied and secured in place with suture to hold the skin tight to the cartilage and eliminate the dead space. This will prevent the late complication of cauliflower ear. In avulsion of the ear, it is important to maintain any skin connection with the avulsed part if possible, since this can function as a venous drainage channel. For complete avulsion, the avulsed part needs to be assessed for viability prior to reattachment. In general, any segment longer than 2 cm in width will not survive as a composite graft. The avulsed ear or the large portion of the avulsed ear could be dermabraded and implanted under the retroauricular skin to keep the cartilage alive; it is revascularized and used for reconstruction at a later date. Occasionally, a flap is needed to provide blood supply for this cartilage; the temporalis fascia is a useful rotational flap in this area to cover the exposed ear cartilage.

EYELID INJURY

The care of any injuries around the eye should involve an opthalmologist who can perform the ocular examination prior to any repair. Since it protects the cornea, the upper eyelid is more important to function than the lower eyelid. Eyelid lacerations should be examined to see if the levator palpebrae is injured. Laceration to this muscle should be repaired prior to laceration closure to prevent ptosis of the lid. The lacrimal canaliculus can be repaired using a Worst stent. Torn medial canthal ligament needs to be repaired by reattachment with the nasal bone. Dacryocystorhinostomy (DCR) is needed to provide lacrimal drainage if the nasolacrimal ducts are beyond repair.

PAROTID DUCT INJURY

The parotid duct surface marking is found in a line drawn from the tragus to the middle of the upper lip. The parotid duct runs with the buccal branch of the facial nerve, and these two usually are injured simultaneously. In laceration injuries of the parotid duct, a sialocele cyst can develop due to leakage of saliva. This injury should be repaired in the operating room. The duct is repaired over a stent, and the stent is then left in place for 3 weeks.

Facial nerve injury

Injury to the facial nerve should be suspected with any laceration injury to the cheek, and examination should be directed toward this diagnosis. If necessary, exploration under optical magnification of the branches of the facial nerve is indicated. If a nerve is lacerated, it should be repaired in the operating room by coaptation of the two nerve ends. Excellent function can be restored if this repair is done early and there are no other significant injuries to the nerve. In more serious injuries, a nerve graft may be necessary to repair the gap between two nerves. Some patients may have temporary paralysis of the facial muscle due to neurapraxia secondary to contusion of the nerve. The function should return with conservative therapy.

CRANIOMAXILLOFACIAL FRACTURES

Increased survival after severe trauma has increased the need for treatment of combined, complex craniofacial injuries. Currently, we advocate treatment of craniofacial injuries within the first 24 to 48 hours. Patients with combined neurological injuries will have the neurosurgical procedure accomplished first (see Fig. 15-3). Fractures of the skull and facial skeleton are then treated. The goal of treatment in combined injuries of the cranium and facial skeleton is the correct anatomic restoration of the maxillary position in relation to the cranial base above and to the mandible below. This is performed prior to treatment of any other associated craniofacial or zygomatic fracture (see Fig. 15-4). All fractured bones are exposed and assessed by direct visualization; then the surgical plan is decided.[5]

If there is a fracture but no loss of the cranial bone, the cranial bone is first stabilized; then the maxillofacial skeleton is reattached to the cranial vault and fixed.

If the cranial bone has missing portions, we follow a reverse order. The midface and the mandible are repaired first and normal occlusion is re-established. Next the reconstructed facial complex is reattached to the cranium; any missing cranial bone is then assessed and reconstructed with autogenous bone grafts.

Diagnosis

Most facial fractures are suspected during the history and physical examination. Frequently the force that produces neurotrauma also causes injuries to the surrounding bony structure. Examination includes palpation and an examination of the facial skeleton, the teeth, and their occlusion. Routine facial x-ray can diagnose facial fractures quickly; however, CT scan is indicated for complex facial fractures, especially those in the middle third of the face, to provide accurate radiographic location and assessment of severity of injury. Long-term results and healing of the bony union can also be evaluated with CT scan and occasionally by bone scan.

Fracture of the Frontal Sinus

Frontal sinus fractures occur in approximately 10 percent of all maxillofacial injuries. The incidence is increased in high-velocity injuries. The fracture of the frontal sinus usually does not cause any immediate life-threatening problem; however, improper treatment will result in severe complications such as meningitis, pneumocephalus, or brain abscess. Physical findings in a frontal sinus fracture may include depressed forehead, deep laceration to the supraorbital ridge or lower forehead, and bony crepitus upon palpation of the lower forehead. Signs of CSF rhinorrhea should be noted and nasal fluid checked by the "halo" test. If the nasal discharge contains CSF, the fluid will create a halo effect when put on a cloth surface. Radiographs using caudal and lateral views are helpful; thin-cut CT scans will identify the extent and location of the frontal sinus fracture. This fracture can include only the anterior table, both anterior and posterior tables, or the nasofrontal ducts.

Nondisplaced anterior table fractures occurring alone without any obvious deformity can be treated conservatively. Displaced anterior sinus wall fractures are exposed, usually through a bicoronal incision. The sinus is irrigated, the mucosa excised, and the anterior table is then reduced and secured in place with microplates. Nasofrontal duct injuries and obstructions can be identified by instilling fluorescein into the frontal sinus. If the fluorescein does not drain into the nose, the duct is obstructed. We follow the suggestions of Rohrich[6] in the treatment of an obstructed nasofrontal duct. This involves obliteration of the sinus mucosa and removal of the inner cortex of the sinus with a burr and sinus obliteration with spontaneous osteoneogenesis.

If both anterior and posterior tables of the frontal sinus are involved, possible CSF leak should be evaluated carefully. If there is a leak, approximately one week (with patient on antibiotics) should be allowed to see if the leak will resolve spontaneously (approximately 50 percent will do so). If the leak is persistent, it must

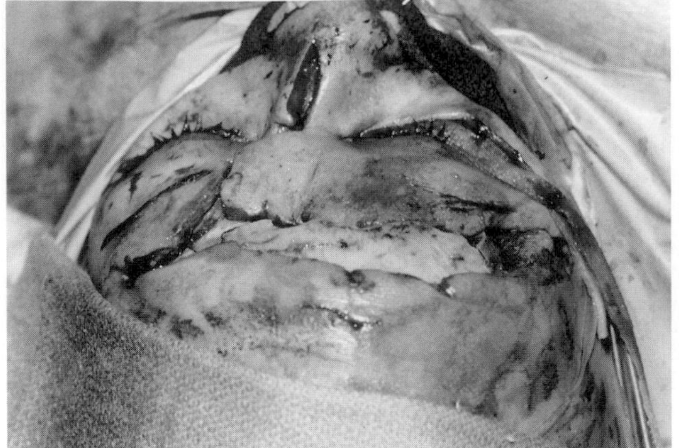

A

B

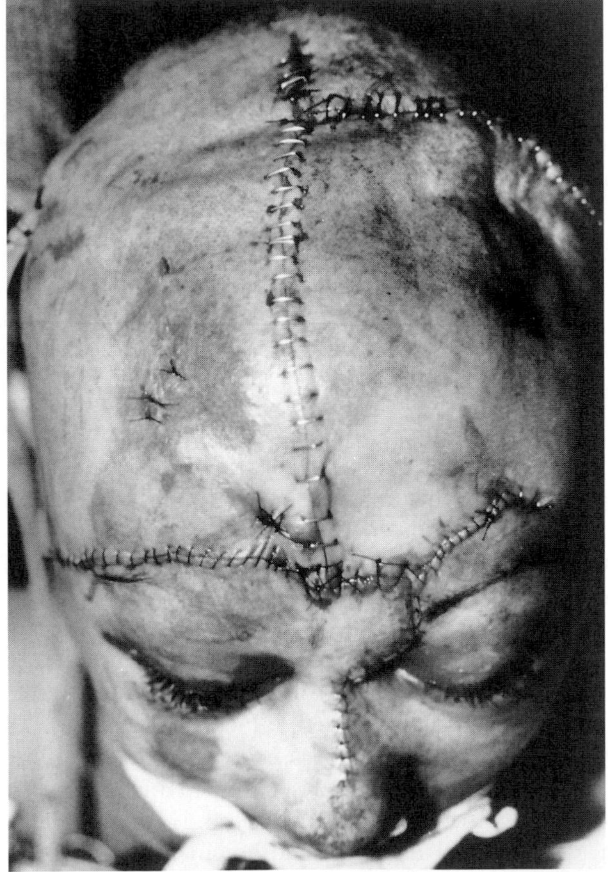

C

Figure 15-3. Forty-year-old woman with blunt trauma to face and head resulting in frontal sinus fracture and depressed skull fracture (Courtesy Dr. M. Anous). *A*. Prior to repair. *B*. Fixation of anterior frontal sinus table with plates after sinus obliteration (exposure via traumatic lacerations). *C*. Immediate postoperative view after both neurosurgical and maxillofacial procedures.

be treated to prevent complications such as meningitis and brain abscess. Treatment usually is by cranialization of the sinus via a frontal craniotomy and the creation of a pericranial flap. The dural repair is done next prior to removal of all the sinus mucosa. The nasofrontal ducts are obliterated and a pericranial flap is then rotated to the floor of the sinus to provide additional division between the nose and the new cranial cavity.

If a combined anterior and posterior wall fracture does not have a CSF leak and no dural injury is found, the posterior wall can be left without surgical intervention if the displacement is less than one width of the posterior wall. Otherwise, the fracture must be reduced and fixed and any injury to the nasofrontal duct treated with sinus obliteration. Complications of sinus repair include sinusitis, meningitis, and brain abscess. Sinusitis

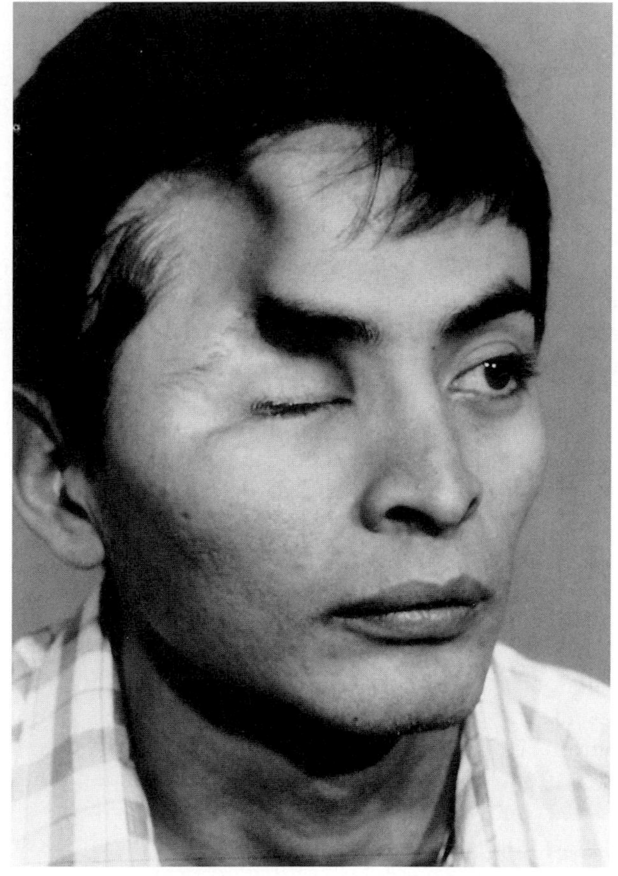

A

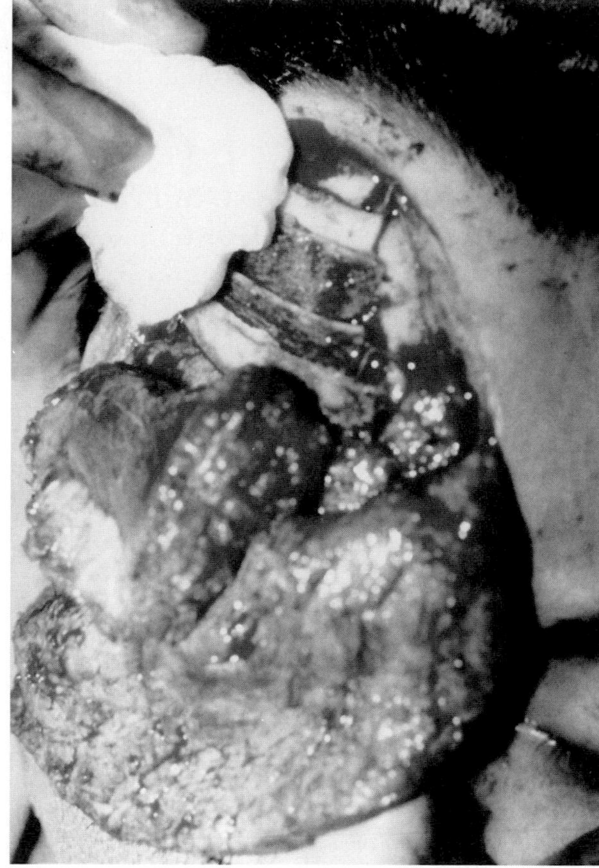

B

C

Figure 15-4. Late orbitozygomatic deformity after gunshot wound with deficient soft tissue and bone in a 28-year-old man. *A*. Before reconstruction. *B*. Reconstruction with split-rib graft and iliac crest osteomusculocutaneous flap. *C*. Late follow-up.

should first be treated with antibiotics and decongestants; however, sinus obliteration may be needed. Other late complications are best treated with cranialization of the frontal sinus.

Fracture of Teeth and Supporting Alveolar Bone

Fracture of teeth and alveolar process are common in facial injuries. Partially fractured teeth can be stabilized using arch bars or wiring. A completely avulsed tooth can be replanted if done after a short period (1 hour). The tooth should be implanted in a clean socket with an intact periodontal membrane.

Alveolar process fractures should be reduced, stabilized, and fixed. Usually the easiest method to stabilize alveolar fractures is with arch bars. Any soft tissue laceration over the alveolar fracture should be reapproximated to protect the bone.

Mandibular Fracture

The mandible is a U-shaped bone with two unique joints to allow both rotational and translational movement. The mandible is usually fractured at its weakest point—mainly the parasymphysis, the angle, and the subcondylar region where the bone is thin or the roots of the teeth weaken it. The stability of any mandibular fracture is determined by the pull of the surrounding muscles. Mandibular fractures are divided into two categories, favorable or unfavorable, depending on whether the muscle pull will reduce the fracture.[7] In general, a horizontal fracture is favorable if, as the fracture extends from the lateral to medial, it goes from posterior to anterior. Any fracture occurring in the opposite direction is unfavorable owing to the pull of the pterygoid muscle. Favorable vertical fracture goes anteriorly as it extends from superior to inferior. Mandibular fractures are also classified into Class I, II, and III. Class I fracture has teeth on both sides of the fracture; Class II fracture has teeth only on one side; and Class III fracture happens in an area without any teeth. All mandibular fractures that traverse dental roots are considered open fractures and need antibiotic therapy. If the tooth is mobile, it should be removed.

The mandible is subject to frequent multiple fractures secondary to the "contrecoup" effect. Over 50 percent of all mandibular fractures are multiple. Mandibular fracture is easy to diagnose because patients often complain that the teeth do not fit together correctly. Physical exam reveals malocclusion, ecchymosis on the floor of the mouth, and occasionally obvious deformity at the region of the fracture. Anesthesia over the area innervated by the mandibular nerve should alert the clinician to mandibular fracture. The fracture can most easily be identified by a Panorex x-ray.

The goals of treatment include adequate union of the fracture, restoration of the normal occlusion, and facial symmetry. The management of a mandibular fracture ranges from very conservative therapy (i.e., soft diet) to intermaxillary fixation (either via arch bar, wire, or elastic bands), to open reduction and internal fixation with plates and screws, to mandibular reconstruction plates to replace the missing bone and provide contour and stability. Dental splints can be used for fixation in an edentulous mandible.

The location and orientation of the fracture determines its management. Generally, nondisplaced and favorable fractures stabilized by the natural pull of the surrounding muscles can be fixed by intermaxillary fixation; nonstable and unfavorable fractures are repaired with internal fixation.

The treatment of condylar fractures is still controversial. If the patient has good occlusion, soft diet is all that is indicated. If there are deformities of the mandible or malocclusion, intermaxillary fixation (IMF) for about 3 weeks is recommended. In general, when a patient continues to have malocclusion oı deviation of the mandible after closed reduction, then open reduction is indicated. Condylar fracture with the condylar head still located in the fossa can usually be treated with closed reduction; if the condylar head is dislocated, which can interfere with the movement of the mandible, open reduction is indicated. Other indications for ORIF include bilateral condylar fracture associated with midfacial fracture and bilateral condylar fracture in an edentulous patient. Therapy should start 3 weeks post-injury to maintain joint motion.

Fracture of the angle of the mandible can be treated with closed reduction and IMF when the fracture is not displaced. Angle fracture posterior to the last tooth (Class II fracture) will require open, rigid fixation.

Fracture of the body of the mandible is very common and usually can be treated with closed reduction if the fracture is favorable. One should keep in mind the use of mandibular reconstruction plates if there is a missing segment of bone. Bone graft can be added later to restore the integrity of the mandible.

Fracture of the coronoid process is rare and often is associated with other fractures. Isolated fracture of the coronoid process usually can be treated with soft diet.

Treatment of fractures of edentulous mandible is difficult because of the lack of teeth for intermaxillary fixation. For favorable and minimally displaced fracture, the use of the denture for IMF is adequate. With unfavorable fracture of bilateral fracture, internal fixation is required in addition to IMF. Extraskeletal fixation works well in these cases. Open reduction to repair comminuted fracture of the edentulous mandible is not recommended.

Maxillary Fracture

Maxillary fractures have been classified by Lefort as I, II, or III, or as horizontal fracture, pyramidal fracture, or craniofacial disjunction. In fact, many maxillary fractures are a combination of these classic types. The development of CT scan with high resolution has helped greatly in the accurate diagnosis of complex midface fractures. The goal of treatment is to restore facial contour and the natural buttresses that provide support and definition of the midface. The supporting buttresses include the nasomaxillary buttress, the zygomaticomaxillary buttress, and the pterygomaxillary buttress. Approaches for open reduction and internal fixation of maxillary fractures are determined by their severity. Small, isolated fractures can be treated via access provided by conjunctival, subciliary orbital rim, or labial sulcus incisions. More complex repairs can be approached by bicoronal flap mobilized over the zygomatic arches, the orbital rims, and the nasoethmoid areas.

In general, management of complex facial fractures starts with fixation of the mandible to obtain occlusion, followed by management of periorbital fracture prior to treatment of midfacial fracture. Next come reduction and fixation of the zygomatic arches and restoration of all the fractured bone segments into their proper place and alignment and stabilization with wire or plates. Plate fixation is preferred to maintain the buttresses laterally. Any bone deficit more than 5 mm can be grafted with autogenous bone obtained from the rib, the iliac, or split calvarial bone.

Nasal Fracture

This is the most common fracture of the face. During the initial evaluation, edema sometimes prevents the immediate detection of nasal fractures. Any step-off, deviation, or instability is indicative of fracture. Facial x-rays and CT scans further delineate the extent of the injury. Nasal fractures can be treated either immediately after trauma, before the edema or obstruction of the airway occurs, or approximately 4 days later, when soft tissue edema decreases. In evaluating any nasal fracture, the clinician should look for septal hematoma. This is a collection of blood under the nasal mucosa and mucoperichondrium. Drainage is required to prevent necrosis of the septal cartilage.

The nose is divided anatomically and physiologically into three vaults.[8] The lower vault contains the inferior buttress; the middle vault includes the midseptum and the lateral nasal cartilages; and the upper vault contains the superior buttress and the adjacent ethmoid bones. Injuries to the nose can affect each of the vaults separately or all three. Nasal necrosis secondary to fracture is rare, since the blood supply to the nose is sufficiently abundant—the major vessels are the sphenopalatine and the posterior lateral nasal arteries, which are protected by the nasal bone.

Diagnosis of nasal injuries should start with observation. Any swelling, ecchymosis, or deviation of the nose is highly suggestive of underlying nasal fractures. Next, palpation can detect any instability or displacement of the nasal bone. X-rays (nasal view and CT scan) can demonstrate the extent of a complex nasal fracture. Finger pressure on the dorsum of the nose can detect the collapse of the three different vaults.

For simple, nondisplaced fracture, digital reduction can be performed with or without instrumentation or anesthesia. By reversing the direction of the force that produces the nasal injury, the minimally displaced bone can be pushed back into place. One should be careful not to convert a greenstick fracture into a full-thickness fracture by too much force. Intranasal packing is not needed if the fracture is stable after reduction. In selected cases, oxidized cellulose can be used for packing.

Septal realignment after severe, acute displacement can be done with forceps or a Dingman septal displacer. The superior displacement is corrected first because it is more easily done; next the caudal septal misalignment is corrected. If this cannot be done, bilateral small incisions through the mucoperichondrium can be made to expose the caudal septum and to realign it. Sutures may be needed to ensure stability.

Open reduction is usually necessary to free any impacted or displaced bone fragments. Exposure can be obtained via intranasal incision, an external laceration, or as in open rhinoplasty. The repair in complex injuries of the nose starts with the upper vault, continues with the middle, and then concludes with the lower vault. The nasofrontal articulation is re-established first and stabilized with either a plate or screw. Distally, the nasal bone fragment can be reduced with direct pressure and then stabilized with microplates or wires. The lower nose can be exposed via intranasal incision through which the caudal septum is brought back into alignment and the nasal cartilage tip is repaired.

In some cases with total nasal collapse and multiple comminution, a bone graft may be needed to reconstruct the nose. Bone grafts can be obtained from either the rib or the calvarium, and cartilage graft can also be obtained from the ear. Cantilever grafts can be used to reconstruct the dorsum of the nose, and the graft can be placed over the nasal bone (overlay cantilever bone graft), or an underlay graft may be used where the bone is placed underneath the nasal bone and nasal cartilages.

Orbitozygomatic Fracture

The zygoma is important in facial aesthetics, and it also provides the support for the anterolateral portion of the orbit. Treatment of the zygoma is aimed both at restoring a natural-appearing facial projection and avoiding complications relating to the orbit.

The two muscles that exert their pull on the zygoma are the masseter and the temporalis. Repair of any zygomatic fracture must overcome the pull of these muscles to optimize healing of the fracture. The zygoma articulates with the frontal bone, the sphenoid bone, the maxilla and the temporal bone. Correction of zygomatic fracture must include correct alignment and stabilization of all these points.

As with other facial fractures, history is important to confirm the extent of the damage. High-velocity facial injuries that affect the zygoma have a high incidence of associated facial injury. Palpation of the zygoma is the most important step in diagnosis. An ophthalmologic exam should also be performed. Any malocclusion of the teeth or malalignment of the maxilla and mandible should be examined to rule out associated arch fracture or coronoid process fracture. Nerve compression due to pressure on the infraorbital nerve is common. Facial x-rays should include the submental vertex, Waters, Caldwell, and lateral views. If a fracture is detected, thin-slice CT scan in both the axial and coronal planes should be ordered.

Isolated zygomatic arch fracture can be detected via x-ray in the submental vertex view and by palpation. Treatment of simple zygomatic arch fracture can be done with reduction only. This includes low-velocity, noncomminuted fractures that are stable after reduction. Close follow-up is mandated to detect any later displacement. Alternatively, reduction is via a Dingman elevator through a small excision in the temporal hairline. If the arch is unstable after reduction, a spinal needle can be passed transcutaneously beneath the arch to provide support for 10 days.[9] Other orbital zygomatic fractures that include high-velocity injuries require open reduction and internal fixation. The method of fixation preferred is via miniplates or microplates fixation.

Displaced fractures are treated via wide exposure. An upper blepharoplasty incision can be used; sometimes a bicoronal approach is required for panfacial fracture with comminution and excessive displacement. The zygomaticomaxillary buttress can be approached via an intraoral incision.

The orbital floor can be approached through a subtarsal incision. The orbital floor should be examined and, if necessary, reconstructed with autologous bone graft placed on the posterior edge of the orbit or with titanium mesh. The goal is reduction of the fracture and rigid fixation in at least two fracture sites. The repair is begun from superior to inferior and from lateral to medial. The initial plate is applied at the zygomaticofrontal fracture. Next, the zygomaticomaxillary fracture is fixed; if necessary, autologous bone is used for defects over 5 mm. It is necessary to check the accuracy of reduction by continuing to assess the reduction at all the articulating points during the fixation. Rarely, in extensive fracture with loss of facial projection, plating of the zygomatic arch is necessary. This can be perfomed through a transcoronal approach.

Nasoethmoid Orbital Fracture (NOE Fracture)

Nasoethmoid orbital fracture (NOE fracture) continues to be one of the most challenging to treat. Successful outcome depends on accurate and early diagnosis. The nasoethmoid orbital region in the central upper midface provides the connection between the nose, both orbits, the maxilla, and the cranium. Its main support is the angular process of the frontal bone plus the frontal process of the maxilla. Around this relatively strong bone, multiple thin delicate bones, including the lacrimal bone, the lamina papyracea, and the ethmoid bone, are connected. Facial fractures are classified as a NOE fracture if there is an isolated central bone fragment attached to the medial canthal tendon. This produces telecanthus, a widening of the distance between the eyes.

NOE fracture should be suspected with any blunt trauma to the midface. Usually localized edema is present. The fracture is diagnosed by both physical exam and CT scan. Several signs are indicative of injuries to the NOE complex. Displacement of the nasopyramid that produces significant loss of nasal projection and height and flattening of the nasodorsum are both suspicious signs. Concomitant neurological injuries are common, resulting in pneumocephalus or cerebrospinal fluid rhinorrhea.

All NOE fractures require CT scan. Examination of the fracture will determine whether it is stable or displaced. This will point toward the need for open reduction and fixation. Bimanual examination using a Kelly clamp placed inside the nose against the medial orbital rim with pressure will produce movement of the fractured central bone segment that can be detected by a finger placed externally over the medial canthal tendon insertion. If there is movement of the canthus-bearing bone segment, the fracture is unstable and operative repair is required. Any displaced fracture detected by the CT scan will also require open repair.

NOE fractures are classified into three patterns.[10] Pattern I consists of a single central fragment connected to the medial canthus. This fracture could be unilateral, bilateral, incomplete, or complete. A Type II pattern fracture can have multiple fragments but also has one single bone segment that is connected to the canthus, and this is used in the reconstruction. In Type III pattern fracture there is comminution of the bone with the canthus, and the fracture extends beneath the canthal tendon insertion. Usually the bone fragment is too small to use for reconstruction and will require a bone graft.

After the fractures are identified and the extent of the injury determined by CT scan, the repair can proceed based on the pattern of the fracture. Three incisions can be used to expose all the fractured bones, which include the coronal incision, the lower eyelid subciliary incision, and the maxillary gingivobuccal sulcus incision. Type I fractures can be repaired easily with plate and screw; any lateral displacement of the bone segment can be reduced using transnasal reduction wire. Type II injuries require exposure via both superior and inferior incisions. Transnasal wires are then placed to repair the telecanthus. All the fragmented bone segments are then linked with interfragment wire.

In Type III fractures, the bone attached to the canthal tendon is too small to be used for reconstruction. The medial canthus is detached to allow better exposure of the fractured bones underneath. After all the bones are reduced and realigned, they are secured in place with wire. Additional transnasal reduction wire must be used in each canthus for reattachment. For each canthus, the attachment will require two reduction wires. Bone grafts using rib or calvarial bone are usually needed in combination with either orbital plates or mesh. It is important to perform the transnasal wiring posterior to the reconstructed medial canthus.

In general, the treatment for NOE fractures depends on early and accurate diagnosis of the type of fracture and exposure of all bone fragments. Reduction and fixation of all bone fragments and reattachment of the canthus—if necessary, via transnasal wiring—will decrease late deformity and telecanthus.

Orbital Fracture

The patient with orbital fracture usually complains of diplopia, uneveness of the two eyes, enophthalmos, difficulty in the upward rotation of the eye (entrapment), and paraesthesia of the ipsilateral cheek. The orbit has been functionally divided into four orbital components, superior, inferior, lateral, and medial. The superior wall of the orbit is composed of the frontal bone, which is relatively thick. Isolated superior wall fractures can be repaired via a superior orbital incision and plate fixation.

The lateral wall of the orbit has the lowest frequency of fracture in all orbital fractures. Such injury usually is associated with fractures of the zygomatic bone. Fractures of this area can be associated with superior orbital fissure syndrome in which the paralysis of the third, fourth, fifth, and sixth nerves occur due to compression inside the orbital fissure. These patients have ptosis of the upper lid, ophthalmoplegia, and dilatation of the pupil. This fracture can be treated via a temporal incision as in the zygomatic fracture. The medial wall of the orbit is relatively thin and composed of fragile bone. This fracture can be treated as a simple NOE fracture.

The inferior orbital wall is the most vulnerable to injury. Owing to the thinness of the maxillary roof and the inferior orbital canal, the floor of the orbit can easily buckle and break. With blow-out fracture, enophthalmos can occur. This condition is due to the increased volume of the orbit and can be repaired after the fracture segment is reduced to obtain the normal orbital volume.

New advances in the treatment of orbital fracture have included the use of both autogenous and biocompatible synthetic graft. Autogenous bone graft includes calvarial graft, iliac crest graft, split rib graft and cartilage graft. Such grafts have a lower infection rate. The disadvantages are the difficulty in constructing an appropriate contour for the fracture segment, the additional donor site morbidity, and late graft resorption. When autogenous graft material is used, rigid fixation with plates is preferred to decrease the amount of late graft resorption.

The use of biocompatible synthetic material has greatly expanded the ability to accurately reconstruct orbits that lack bony support.[11] Biocompatible synthetic alloys include titanium and vitallium. This synthetic mesh can be molded to fit the contour of the orbit accurately. Some advocate the use of absorbable implants such as polyethylene to support the mesh and to provide padding between the extraocular muscle and the synthetic material. In general, accurate repair of the orbital fracture provides excellent results.

SPECIFIC INJURIES

Gunshot Wound Injury

A gunshot wound to the face and head once was managed by serial debridement and treatment of soft tissue initially, without reconstruction. These procedures result in less than optimal repair of the injury. Currently, the preferred treatment is the definitive repair of all bony and soft tissue injuries within the first 48 hours if the patient's condition permits. Most civilian gunshot injuries are low-velocity (i.e., hand-gun) or intermediate velocity (i.e., shotgun). One must carefully evaluate all four components of the gunshot injury: the injury to the soft tissue and bone, and the loss of soft tissue and bone.

Most low-velocity gunshot injuries affect soft tissue and bone without much loss. Such injuries generally are treated as a fracture of the facial skeleton with overlying lacerations. The fractures are reduced and fixed, and the soft tissues are repaired primarily. The track of the bullet is excised, closed, and drained.

The intermediate or high-velocity gunshot injury can result in severe tissue loss. Serial debridements may be needed initially; however, it is optimal that the soft tissue injury be closed within the first 48 hours. "Second look" surgery should be performed within the first 48 hours and definitive reconstruction done at this time, if possible. Between the surgeries, soft tissue on the face should be closed loosely over drains, if necessary. All the fractures should be initially stabilized. Reconstruction of missing bone can be done at the definitive reconstructive procedure, either with autogenous bone or with a fixator device to maintain soft tissue contour. The bone gap can be treated at a later date; however, the bony contour should be rigidly maintained with either a plate or an external fixator.

In conclusion, the goal of treatment of a gunshot wound to the face is early closure of the soft tissue injuries and restoration of the bony contour.

Pediatric Facial Fractures

Treatment of a pediatric facial fracture poses problems different from those in adults owing to the differences in the child's maxillofacial structure, the consideration of a dynamic growing skeleton, and the different types of injuries that occur in this population. A high index of suspicion should be maintained in any pediatric facial injury, and one should not hesitate to order CT scans in such cases. The resiliency of a pediatric facial skeleton decreases significantly after the age of 3 owing to mineralization of the bone. In children under 5 years, facial fractures tend to occur in large blocks without much comminution. The fractures tend to be of the greenstick type and frequently extend to the frontal bone. As the child grows older and sinuses become aerated and the teeth become adult-like, the fracture tends to resemble the adult pattern.

Because of the different types of injuries in the pediatric population, i.e., mostly greenstick fracture without much comminution, one must more carefully consider the role of conservative therapy.[12] Minimally displaced or nondisplaced fractures can be treated conservatively in children. Greenstick fractures may be treated only with reduction without fixation. Severely displaced fractures should be reduced and fixed; however, the exposure should be minimal and the method of fixation should be chosen so that the minimum amount of bone is rigidly immobilized. Many pediatric patients can tolerate a small amount of latitude because of their growing skeleton. Wire fixation has a greater role in these patients. If plate and screw fixation is used, interval removal of the plate and screws should be seriously considered to decrease any growth disturbances and "resorption of the plate" into the growing bone.

Acute bone grafting is indicated for obvious contour deficiencies and lack of support of the facial skeleton; however, for minimal deficiency, consideration should be given to late bone grafting after completion of growth. Autogenous bone is preferred over any alloplastic material.

One should also pay attention to the developing tooth buds. The child's teeth should be preserved if at all possible, and care must be taken in the placement of plate, screws, or wire to avoid any injuries to the developing tooth buds. Any children with facial injuries should be followed long-term for the detection of any growth abnormalities and growth disturbances so that appropriate corrective action can be effected in a timely manner.

CONCLUSION

Opportunities to manage complex craniomaxillofacial injuries have increased recently with the increased survival of multi-trauma patients. With very few exceptions, most of these patients deserve early and definitive repair of their injuries. Optimal results are obtained by early soft tissue repair and one-stage reconstruction of all bony and soft tissue deficiency via restoration of the anatomy.

References

1. Moylan JA, Deteman DE, Rose J, Schultz R: Evaluation of the quality of hospital care for major trauma. *J Trauma* 1976; 16:517.
2. Manson PN: Management of facial fractures. *Perspect Plast Surg* 1988; 2:1.
3. Gruss JS: Complex craniomaxillofacial trauma: Evolving concepts in management: A trauma unit's experience—1989 Fraser B. Gurd lecture. *J Trauma* 1990; 30:377.
4. Steuber K, Salcman M, Spence RJ: The combined use of the latissimus dorsi musculocutaneous free flap and split rib grafts for cranial vault reconstruction. *Ann Plast Surg* 1985; 15:155.
5. Gruss JS, Bubak PJ, Egbert MA: Craniofacial fractures: An algorithm to optimize results. *Clin Plast Surg* 1992; 19:195.

6. Rohrich RJ, Hollier LH: Management of frontal sinus fractures: Changing concepts. *Clin Plast Surg* 1992; 19:219.
7. Olson RA, Fonseca RJ, Zeitler DL, Osborn DB: Fractures of the mandible: A review of 580 Cases. *J Oral Maxillofac Surg* 1982; 40:23.
8. Sheen JH: *Aesthetic Rhinoplasty.* St. Louis: CV Mosby, 1978: 4.
9. Watumull D, Rohrich RJ: Zygoma fracture fixation: A graduated approach to management based on recent clinical and biomechanical studies, in Manson PN (ed): *Problems in Plastic and Reconstructive Surgery.* Philadelphia, JB Lippincott, 1991.
10. Markowitz BL, Manson PN, Sargent LA, et al: Management of the medial canthal tendon in nasoethmoid orbital fractures: The importance of the central fragment in classification and treatment. *Plast Reconstr Surg* 1991; 87:843.
11. Glassman RD, Manson PN, Vanderkolk CA, et al: Rigid fixation of internal orbital fractures. *Plast Reconstr Surg* 1990; 86:1103.
12. Kaban LB, Mulliken JB, Murray JE: Facial fractures in children: An analysis of 122 fractures in 109 patients. *Plast Reconstr Surg* 1977; 59:15.

CHAPTER 16

OPHTHALMOLOGIC INJURIES IN THE HEAD-INJURED PATIENT

M. Bowes Hamill

SYNOPSIS

Damage to the eye and adnexa occurs frequently with head trauma, and a physician caring for these patients should be familiar with the management of common ocular injuries. The ophthalmic history in head trauma patients should be directed toward determining the presence of an eye injury as well as estimating the risk of occult eye trauma. The examination of a traumatized eye differs somewhat from a routine eye exam, and the need for a comprehensive evaluation of the lids, globe, and orbit cannot be overemphasized. Chemical injuries of the eye, orbital hemorrhage, and occlusion of the central retinal artery are the three most emergent ophthalmic conditions likely to be encountered in a head trauma patient, and the physician should be familiar with the initial therapy for these conditions. The management of almost all other traumatic eye conditions can generally be deferred for minutes to hours until an ophthalmic consultant is available. The few exceptions include a lacerated globe, which should be protected with a rigid shield to prevent further damage, and orbital compartment syndromes that compromise retinal blood flow and may require lateral canthotomy or cantholysis to decrease the intraocular pressure and restore retinal perfusion.

It has been estimated that between 1 and 5 percent of patients with head trauma also have an injury to the visual system.[1–3] *Unfortunately, few series have addressed this issue per se. In a study of ocular injuries associated with periorbital fractures, Petro et al found that in 230 cases of periorbital fracture, 23 patients (10 percent) had ocular injuries.*[4] *Three of these cases were bilateral. In a similar study, Holt et al. reviewed 1436 cases of blunt facial trauma at the University of Texas at San Antonio.*[5] *In this series, of the 727 (51 percent) of patients who had a formal ophthalmologic evaluation, 487 (67 percent) had ocular injuries. A breakdown of Holt's cases revealed that in patients who had an ophthalmic evaluation, ophthalmic injuries were most commonly seen with frontal fractures followed by midfacial fractures, with yields of 89 percent and 76 percent positive, respectively. Seventy-nine percent of the ocular injuries were minor, 18 percent were serious (resulting in sustained visual loss or adnexal trauma requiring repair), and 3 percent resulted in blindness. All the patients whose ophthalmic injuries resulted in blindness sustained midfacial, supraorbital, or frontal sinus fractures.*

EXAMINATION OF AN OPHTHALMOLOGICALLY INJURED PATIENT

Because eye injuries may be associated with head injuries, an eye exam is mandatory in all head trauma patients. In general, errors in the management of traumatic ophthalmic injuries are due to omission rather than commission, and the treating physician therefore must maintain a high index of suspicion for unexpected or occult tissue damage. Because of progressive vitreous hemorrhage, traumatic cataract, or bleeding into the anterior chamber, the initial examiner may be the only one who is able to obtain a visual acuity or inspect the ocular fundus. For this reason, the importance of the initial examination in the evaluation and management of an eye trauma patient is self-evident. Additionally, the results of the initial evaluation determine the direction of the subsequent workup and early management. The initial examination therefore should be as comprehensive as possible, given the individual circumstances. To ensure that no finding is missed or overlooked, the examiner should follow a logical, orderly sequence. The goals of the examination are as follows:

A. Recognition of life-threatening injuries
B. Complete evaluation of the eye and adnexa
   1. Recognition of emergent ocular conditions
      a. Chemical injuries
      b. Central retinal artery occlusion
      c. Ruptured globe
   2. Appreciation of the full extent of the injury
C. Identification of factors that could confound the evaluation or management of the injury
   1. Glaucoma
   2. Bleeding disorders
   3. Sickle cell hemoglobinopathy
   4. Atherosclerotic cardiovascular disease
   5. Diabetes
   6. Infectious diseases
      a. AIDS
      b. Hepatitis
D. Identification of the need for further testing
   1. Laboratory
   2. Radiological
   3. Ultrasonographic

The History

After life-threatening injuries have been ruled out or treatment has been initiated, the ocular examination begins with the history. Of all the information the examiner gathers during the initial evaluation, perhaps the most important single item is a detailed description of the traumatic incident. A conscious paient should be asked to describe the exact circumstances of the injury to allow the examiner to develop a complete mental image of the event. Family members and witnesses should also be questioned to ensure that all relevant details have been collected. Several questions should be asked specifically, including questions about the use of spectacles or contact lenses by the patient at the time of injury, the possibility of foreign body trauma, and any exposure to chemicals. This information permits the examiner to make risk assessments for the presence of occult injury (retained ocular or orbital foreign bodies or posterior ruptures) and recognize emergent ocular conditions (chemical injuries or lacerating injuries of the globe).

After the description of the traumatic event, the past ocular history should be elicited. The patient should be questioned about any previous ocular surgery. After ocular surgery, the cornea and sclera never regain their full strength; therefore, previous surgery such as cataract extraction, corneal transplantation, or even radial keratotomy (surgery for nearsightedness) may make the eye significantly more vulnerable to severe damage despite seemingly mild trauma.[6] The patient should be questioned about the presence of periocular or intraocular appliances such as intraocular lenses, scleral buckle materials, and orbital implants, as these materials may become dislodged and complicate patient evaluation or management.

The presence of preexisting ocular disease may also make the management of some patients more complex and should be addressed. For example, unlike a normal patient, a patient with glaucoma is at significant risk for loss of peripheral or central vision from even a modest increase in intraocular pressure, as is commonly seen after ocular trauma. These patients must be recognized to prevent an unfortunate result. The best preinjury visual acuity should be established so that the examiner can judge the visual loss caused by the injury. This is especially important in cases where litigation may be an issue. The patient should be questioned about a history of strabismus or amblyopia, as this may help account for otherwise confusing or contradictory findings, such as unexplained visual loss or oculomotor palsy.

The patient's general medical history should be explored. Several medical conditions have a direct bearing on the ophthalmologic management of an injured patient. Any history of clotting disorders or anticoagulant medications should be noted, especially in patients with hyphema (bleeding into the anterior chamber) or vitreous hemorrhage. Patients with hyphema should be questioned about a family history of sickle cell disease. Women of childbearing age should be asked about the possibility of pregnancy, which may influence the choice of medications used to treat the injury. Additionally, patients with atherosclerotic cardiovascular disease should be identified, as the antifibrinolytic agents commonly used in the treatment of hyphema are contraindicated in those individuals. All the patient's medications and medication allergies should be recorded. Finally, patients with penetrating injuries of the eye or adnexa should be queried about their tetanus immunization status.

In addition to these general inquiries, several types of injuries, such as blunt trauma, injury from a foreign body, and injuries involving chemical exposure, merit specialized questions.

History in Blunt Trauma Patients

The historical inquiry in the setting of blunt trauma should be directed toward determining the amount of energy transferred to the tissues and the physical characteristics of the weapon or injuring object. In determining the energy transfer, consideration should be given not only to the amount of energy transferred but also to the force vectors involved and the area over which the energy was applied. For example, in trauma involving a two-by-four piece of lumbar versus a 1-in.-diameter iron pipe of the same weight and speed, it would be expected that the impact of the pipe would produce a more localized but deeper injury. In addition to area of impact, the anatomic location may provide information concerning the presence of deep tissue injury, such as optic nerve contusion resulting from blunt trauma to the lateral brow (discussed later in this chapter).

History in Patients with Foreign Body Injuries

The potential for foreign bodies must be estimated in all cases of ocular injury. When foreign bodies or projectiles are suspected, four characteristics should be determined: (1) the chemical composition of the foreign body, (2) how the foreign body was produced, (3) the probable trajectory, and (4) the risk of microbial contamination. The determination of the chemical composition of the foreign material has a direct bearing on the management. While glass, lead, plastic, and the like are relatively inert, materials such as iron and copper are toxic to ocular tissues and require early removal. The circumstances surrounding the production of the foreign bodies are also important. An understanding of how the foreign bodies were formed allows a determination of the relative size, speed, and physical characteristics of the fragments so that assessments can be made about the probable trajectory, the relative energy, and the probability of ocular penetration. Finally, the risk of microbial contamination should be estimated. Foreign material arising from farm or agricultural equipment should be considered contaminated, while high-speed hot metal fragments from machining or grinding operations may be sterile.

History in Patients with Chemical Exposure

Chemical injuries are ophthalmic emergencies, and patients suspected of having been exposed to chemicals should have treatment initiated concurrently with the evaluation. The history should attempt to determine the nature and amount of the chemical compound involved and the duration of contact. In general, alkalis are more destructive than acids, although some acids can result in severe injuries. Additionally, the examiner should determine the physical characteristics of the agent, including whether the chemical was in liquid, gel, or particulate form. The evaluation and treatment of chemical trauma are addressed later in this chapter.

The Ocular Examination

For several reasons, the ocular examination in the emergent setting is a modification of the usual office procedure in terms of both order and testing technique. Unfortunately, most trauma occurs at night, and as a result of this and the emergent setting, both the patient and the examiner are often fatigued and anxious. The patient may be under the influence of drugs or alcohol and thus be uncooperative or combative. Some patients may be unconscious or obtunded, limiting the amount of information available. For these reasons, each examiner should develop a logical step-by-step approach to the ophthalmic examination to ensure that a complete evaluation is performed while maintaining a high index of suspicion for the presence of occult injury. A suggested sequence is listed in Table 16-1.

The physical facilities necessary for the examination of patients with ocular injuries are not extensive. While every emergency room should have equipment available for the examination of ophthalmic patients, a fully equipped eye examining room is not necessary. A selection of basic instruments and supplies is sufficient to permit the initial evaluation of an injured patient even if the patient is stretcher-bound. Suggestions for the components of a portable examination kit are listed in Table 16-2.

The External Examination

The ocular examination of a patient with head trauma begins with a general inspection for the presence of life-

TABLE 16-1 The "Eight-Point" Eye Examination in Head Trauma

1. External examination
2. Visual acuity
3. Pupillary reflexes
4. Ocular motility
5. Visual fields (by confrontation)
6. Penlight examination
   - Eyelids
   - Conjunctiva
     - Palpebral
     - Bulbar
   - Cornea
   - Anterior chamber
   - Iris
   - Lens
7. Ocular fundus (direct ophthalmoscopy)
   - Vitreous
   - Retina
   - Optic Nerve
8. Intraocular pressure (optional)

TABLE 16-2 Eye Trauma Examination Kit

Equipment	Supplies
Near reading card	0.5% proparacaine
Pinhole	2.5% Phenylephrine hydrochloride (Neo-Synephe-rine®)
Penlight	1% tropicamide
Desmarres lid retractors (2)	Fluorescein strips
Direct ophthalmoscope	Sterile ocular irrigant
	Tape
	Cotton tip applicators (sterile)
	Eye pads (sterile)
	Rigid eye shield

threatening injuries. Special attention should be given to the airway, sites of hemorrhage, and any other significant injury. Inspection should continue with an examination of the face, orbits, and globe. All periocular wounds and areas of ecchymosis or hemorrhage should be documented in the record by either descriptions or drawings. The position of the globes relative to the orbital rims should be examined, and the presence of exophthalmos or enophthalmos should be noted. Anomalies in canthal anatomy should be sought, as this finding may indicate underlying orbital trauma. In addition to inspection of the face, gentle palpation of the orbital rims may reveal a fracture. Areas of facial numbness corresponding to branches of the trigeminal nerve may also indicate and localize underlying fractures. During palpation, the examiner should note the presence of subcutaneous emphysema or crepitus, which should alert the examiner to the possibility of sinus fractures. The patient's clothing, hair, and skin should be inspected carefully for the presence of foreign bodies or debris, which suggests the possibility of foreign body injury.

After the initial inspection, the patient's face and lids should be cleaned of all blood and debris so that small wounds can be seen more readily. All periocular lacerations and puncture wounds should be probed gently to verify that there is no involvement of the globe or penetration into the intraorbital space.

Vision

After the completion of the external examination, the patient's vision should be tested. The importance of this initial measurement is twofold. First, it may be the most accurate measurement of the patient's acuity, which later may become compromised by intraocular hemorrhage. Second, because of the increasingly litigious nature of the trauma patient population, this initial pretreatment test of visual acuity verifies the presenting vision and serves as a baseline against which postintervention vision can be compared. This simple measurement prevents a trauma patient with a poor outcome caused by trauma from claiming that his or her visual deficit was caused by the treating physician.

The object of vision testing is to obtain the best objective measurement of the patient's visual acuity. While ideally a wall chart should be used, these charts are rarely available in the emergent setting. Any objective measure is acceptable; the patient can be asked to read newsprint, the examiner's watch, or local signage, and the patient's vision compared with the examiner's. Keep in mind that patients over 40 years old often require reading glasses for small print. If the patient is a spectacle lens wearer, his or her glasses should be used during vision testing. If the glasses have been lost or broken during the injury, the use of a pinhole can act as a "universal lens" so that an estimation of corrected vision can be obtained. If no pinhole lens is available, one can be constructed by perforating a stiff paper card with a group of 6 to 10 holes within a 1-in. diameter with a 20-gauge needle. The patient is instructed to hold the card directly in front of his or her eye (1 to 2 cm anterior to the cornea), and distance acuity is then tested. If the patient's vision is sufficiently poor to preclude reading print or signs, the acuity can be measured as the distance at which the patient is able to count fingers or detect hand motion accurately. This should be recorded, for example, as "finger counting at 3 ft" or "hand motion at 5 ft." If the patient is unable to see hand motion, the ability to detect light and identify the light source's direction should be tested. This is recorded as "light perception with projection" or, if the patient can see light but not identify its direction, "bare light perception." If the patient cannot see the brightest available light, his or her vision is recorded as "no light perception" (NLP).

Pupils

The next step is the examination of the pupils. The pupillary diameters should be measured in dim light with the patient fixing at a distant target to avoid the pupillary constriction associated with near synkinesis. Any abnormalities in the pupillary shape, such as an oval or displaced pupil, should be recorded, as this may indicate a rupture in the eye wall. Pupillary responses to light and near, using the brightest available light source, should be tested and recorded. The convention for pupillary reflexes is to grade a normal, brisk response as 4+ and a lack of response as 0. Finally, the presence or absence of an afferent pupillary defect (APD) should be evaluated.

Ocular motility

Because of the risk of prolapse of intraocular contents, the testing of ocular motility should be deferred until the examiner is certain that no rupture of the anterior eye wall is present. Motility testing should begin with an assessment of the alignment of the eyes in primary gaze. The patient should be instructed to look up, right, down, and left, and each eye should be evaluated for a full range of movement. The presence of any limitation of gaze or diplopia should be noted. Abnormalities of the extraocular muscles are covered in more detail in Chap. 43.

Visual fields

The evaluation of peripheral vision should be a part of every injured patient's initial evaluation. In general, visual field testing by finger confrontation is sufficient to uncover significant abnormalities and can pick up some subtle central defects as well. More formal testing should be deferred until the patient is stabilized, as most testing equipment requires that the patient be seated for accurate results. In some situations, such as hysteria and malingering, testing by tangent screen can be very helpful in establishing an etiology for unexplained visual loss.

Penlight/slit lamp evaluation

The lids, conjunctiva, and globe should be carefully examined in a logical, orderly sequence. The examiner should not immediately examine the most visible trauma but instead should develop a step-by-step routine which should be followed for every patient. Initially, the lids should be inspected for the presence of lacerations or foreign material. With gentle eversion of the lids, the palpebral (lid) and bulbar (globe) conjunctiva can be seen. The bulbar conjunctiva should be scrutinized for the presence of subconjunctival hemorrhage or pigment, which could indicate an underlying rupture or perforation. All abnormalities should be sketched in the chart.

As an initial step, the presence of any visible corneal or scleral lacerations should be noted and the examination should be halted at that point. If no violation of the eye wall is noted, the corneal luster and light reflex should be inspected for the presence of abrasions and the corneal clarity should be evaluated. If an abrasion is suspected, fluorescein dye can be instilled into the tear film, allowing the area of epithelial defect to be seen clearly. Foreign material should be noted, and attempts should be made to irrigate the material from the surface of the eye. If there is a corneal abrasion or retained corneal or conjunctival foreign matter, the examination can be greatly facilitated by the instillation of a topical anesthetic (0.5% proparacaine) into the conjunctival cul-de-sac. It should be stressed that although the use of a topical anesthetic provides rapid and significant relief from pain, under *no* circumstances should the patient be prescribed or allowed to take home anesthetics. The self-directed use of topical ocular anesthetics can result in severe ocular complications.

The anterior chamber should be inspected with attention paid to the clarity of the view of anterior segment structures and the presence of blood or foreign material within the chamber. The iris should be assessed with respect to the pupillary shape and the presence of defects in the iris stroma. The crystalline lens lies immediately behind the iris and generally is not visible to penlight examination. After trauma, however, the lens may become opaque or dislocated. The examiner may note a pupillary opacity in the event of a cataract, or the edge of the lens may become visible within the pupillary aperture after subluxation.

Intraocular pressure

While measurement of intraocular pressure (IOP) is important, estimation by a nonophthalmologist in the setting of ocular injury is only rarely useful. One such situation occurs in the case of an acute orbital compartment syndrome when a decision regarding lateral canthotomy must be made. In this setting, the measurement of IOP by palpation in combination with inspection of the optic nerve head for arterial pulsations is sufficient. Before *any* measurement of IOP, the examiner must be sure that there is no defect in the eye wall, as the checking of IOP can itself result in prolapse of intraocular contents if a rupture is present. To estimate pressures by palpation, the index fingers of both hands should be used with gentle alternating pressure to ballotte the globe through the closed lids. The patient's globe should be compared via self-ballottement with the examiner's pressure. A globe with normal IOP should feel like a peeled hard-boiled egg when palpated through the lids. Significantly elevated pressure results in a decidedly firm globe.

Fundus examination

All patients with significant ocular trauma should have an evaluation of the ocular fundus through dilated pupils if this is neurologically permissible. While many agents are available for pupillary dilation, a suggested regimen is 2.5% phenylephrine hydrochloride (Neo-Synephrine) drops in combination with 1.0% tropicamide drops. This choice of medications results in excellent dilation and wears off in 4 to 6 h. The examiner should document in the chart the drugs used and the time when they were instilled. In the setting of a confused, obtunded, or unconscious patient, the drugs and times should be recorded on a piece of 1- or 2-in. adhesive tape and applied to the patient's forehead to ensure that subsequent examiners are aware of pharmacological pupillary dilation.

After dilation, the examiner should inspect the vitreous, retina, and optic nerve by direct ophthalmoscopy. The vitreous should be evaluated for the presence of hemorrhage, which may indicate a posterior rupture or intraocular foreign bodies. The retina should be examined for tears, holes, or detachments in addition to hemorrhages or exudates. A characteristic response of the retina to blunt trauma is retinal edema. This postconcussive swelling appears as focal whitening or pallor of the normally pink color of the fundus. The optic nerve should be examined with respect to the clarity of the disk margins, the character of the entering and exiting vasculature, the cup/disk ratio, the presence of peripapillary splinter hemorrhages, and evidence of elevation of the nerve.

Ancillary Testing

After completion of the history and ocular examination, the physician must determine whether further testing is needed. While plain skull films may be of benefit in recognizing major fractures, computed tomography (CT) scanning has become the initial radiological test of choice in ophthalmic injuries for several reasons. The image quality of CT scans is far superior to that of plain films in both the detection and the delineation of orbital fractures and the visualization of orbital soft tissues. The combination of axial and coronal views with overlapping cuts will detect even small radiopaque foreign bodies with precise localization of foreign material within the globe or orbit. CT also allows visualization of the optic canals along their entire length far better than plain films can do in cases of suspected optic nerve contusion.

Magnetic resonance imaging (MRI) is a relatively new addition to the ophthalmic diagnostic armamentarium. The usefulness of this technique in the setting of acute injuries is somewhat limited, however, by the fact that while some soft tissue changes, such as optic nerve contusion, can be detected, fractures and foreign bodies are not well seen. In an experimental study, foreign bodies of Lucite, Teflon, and wood were implanted within the orbit, and CT and MRI were performed. All foreign bodies were well visualized by CT scanning but not by MRI.[7] The high magnetic fields required for MRI imaging also limit the applicability of this technique in the setting of retained ferrous foreign bodies. Kelly and associates reported a case in which a 3-mm ferromagnetic foreign body was overlooked on initial CT scanning and the performance of a subsequent MRI resulted in vitreous hemorrhage and loss of vision.[8] MRI may be of significant benefit, however, in the evaluation of posttraumatic visual loss, for example, in chiasmal injury.[9]

SPECIFIC OCULAR INJURIES

Ocular Emergencies

If ocular emergencies are defined as situations in which *immediate* intervention by trained personnel can prevent loss of vision, there are only two conditions which qualify as true ocular emergencies: chemical injuries of the eye and occlusion of the central retinal artery. It is imperative that individuals managing ocular trauma be sufficiently familiar with these conditions to immediately render the appropriate therapy.

Chemical injuries of the eye

Of all of the traumatic injuries, chemical injuries are the most emergent. While strong acids can cause significant tissue damage, alkalis are generally considered more destructive. The destructive character of alkali chemicals is due to the ease with which they penetrate ocular tissue and saponify plasma membranes (Fig. 16-1). Al-

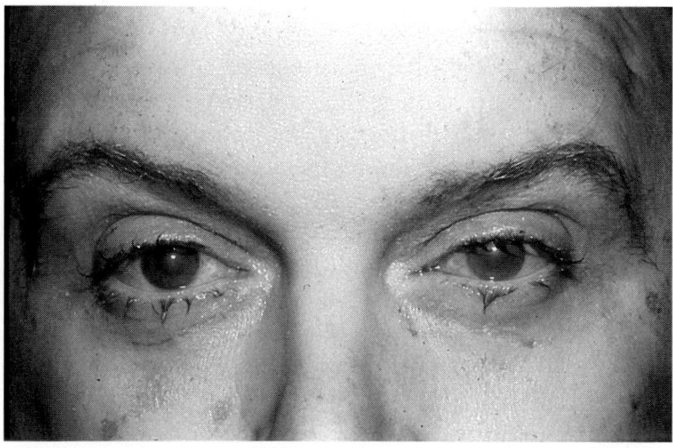

Figure 16-1. This patient had an alkali splash injury involving the face and eyes. Chemical injuries are one of the true ocular emergencies and require immediate irrigation to flush as much of the chemical from the ocular surface as possible. Note the frosted, opalescent appearance of the corneas. This is the characteristic appearance of a moderate to severe ocular alkali burn.

kali applied to the surface of the eye can begin to raise intracameral pH within seconds. This rapidity of penetration results in full-thickness tissue damage as well as destruction of intraocular tissue. In any setting in which chemical injuries are a possibility, the patient should be questioned about the possibility of chemical exposure and the nature of the chemical agent. Chemical injuries are one of the few situations in ophthalmology in which therapy is instituted before the completion of a full history and ocular examination. Once the examiner is satisfied that no rupture of the anterior ocular surface is present, lavage should be instituted immediately with any clean, nontoxic aqueous solution in an attempt to rinse all residual chemicals from the surface of the eye and conjunctiva. This is most easily accomplished in the emergency room setting by positioning the patient supine, applying topical anesthetic to the eye, placing a self-retaining wire lid speculum to hold the lids open, and irrigating the ocular surface, including the conjunctival fornices, with a freely running IV solution. The IV solution used for irrigation is not critical. Special attention should be given to the nature of the chemical, and if the chemical is a gel or particulate, the fornices should be swept with a moistened cotton tip applicator to remove residual chemical and foreign material. Irrigation should be continued until the ophthalmology consultant has evaluated the patient.

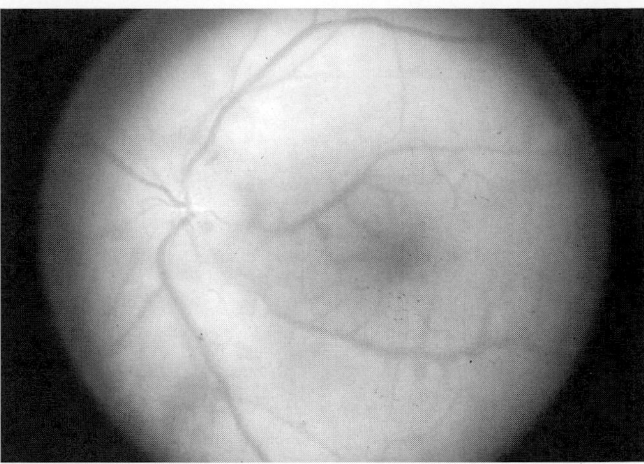

Figure 16-2. Central retinal artery occlusion. Note the pale retinal edema obscuring the choroidal vascular details, enlarged veins, and narrow thready arterioles. Note also the "cherry red spot" in the foveola. This spot is not a red-pigmented area per se but an area of edematous retina which, because of the thinness of neural retina in the foveola, allows the choroidal pigmentation to show through.

Central retinal artery occlusion

Occlusion of the central retinal artery interrupts the blood supply to the inner retina and severely compromises retinal function. Central retinal artery occlusion (CRAO) is a sudden, painless event whose only symptom is an abrupt loss of visual acuity. In general, artery occlusion is associated with embolic phenomena from cardiac sources, atherosclerotic disease of the great vessels, and inflammatory diseases of the smaller arteries such as temporal arteritis. Compromise of arterial flow can also be seen in the traumatic setting when the IOP is raised to nearly arterial pressure levels. This can occur in orbital compartment syndromes in which the intraorbital pressure is abruptly raised and pressure is transmitted to both the globe and the ophthalmic artery. The finding of arterial pulsations at the optic nerve head indicates that IOP elevation is sufficiently high to potentially compromise retinal perfusion. Therefore, the examiner should maintain a high index of suspicion that CRAO may occur in settings of abrupt and significant elevation of intraorbital pressure.

The clinical picture of CRAO is characterized by pale retinal edema obscuring the underlying choroidal vascular details, dilated retinal veins, sluggish flow through thready retinal arteries, and a "cherry red spot" in the foveolar area of the macula (Fig. 16-2). Once artery occlusion has occurred, blood flow must be restored within 60 min to prevent irreversible vision loss. Emergency therapy is directed at causing vasodilation and maximizing the intraocular-intraarterial pressure differential to cause enlargement of the vascular lumen and allow intravascular obstructions to move downstream. Initial treatment should include ocular massage, intravenous mannitol, topical beta blockers, and acetazolamide IV or PO to decrease IOP. Additionally, administration of carbogen gas or rebreathing into a paper bag should be employed to cause vasodilation. Ophthalmology should be consulted on an emergent basis as aspiration of intraocular fluid may be a helpful adjunct therapy to abruptly lower the IOP and move the obstruction.

Nonemergent Injuries

Eyelid lacerations

Trauma to the eyelids is a common occurrence, especially when the impact of trauma has been to the face (Fig. 16-3). It is important to appreciate the fact that eyelid injuries per se, even though quite gruesome, are not emergent and that management can be deferred for hours (or days in some selected cases). The most important aspect of initial management is to ensure that penetrating injury to the globe or orbit has not occurred and that the patient's tetanus immunization is adequate.

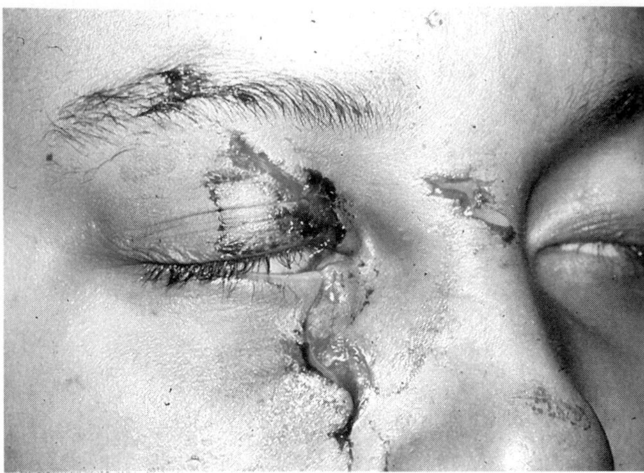

Figure 16-3. This patient was involved in a motor vehicle accident and suffered several lid lacerations. One of the most important aspects in the management of these injuries is ascertaining whether injury to the globe has occurred. If the globe is intact, lid repair can be delayed until definitive reconstruction can be performed.

For management purposes, eyelid lacerations can be divided into three types: nonmarginal, marginal, and canalicular. Nonmarginal injuries involve the tissue of the eyelids without involvement of the eyelid margin. These lacerations can be shallow or deep, depending on the circumstances, and can be quite extensive. When faced with these injuries, it is incumbent on the examiner to determine whether the eye or intraorbital space has been entered. The presence of fat in an eyelid laceration provides evidence that the orbital septum has been violated and that steps to rule out orbital foreign bodies and injuries to deeper structures must be taken. Nonmarginal eyelid wounds can be closed utilizing standard wound management techniques, taking care to direct suture tension parallel to the eyelid margin to prevent distortion of the margin.

When the eyelid margin is involved, the closure must ensure that its contour is preserved. The margin should be approximated first with three interrupted 7/0 silk sutures to appose the anterior and posterior margins. These sutures should be cut long (1 to 2 cm) to allow the free ends to be positioned away from the palpebral fissure to prevent corneal abrasions from the suture ends. The remainder of the laceration can then be closed in one or two layers as necessary.

A special subset of marginal lacerations consists of injuries involving the canalicular system. The canaliculi connect the punctae to the lacrimal sac and run medially from each puncta just below the tissue of the eyelid margin. Unrepaired damage to the drainage system can result in epiphora and require extensive secondary nasolacrimal reconstruction. If these injuries are appreciated in the acute setting, successful primary repair can frequently be performed. It is recommended that an ophthalmologist be consulted for all suspected canalicular injuries and lacerations involving the eyelid margin.

INJURIES TO THE GLOBE

While the globe is relatively well protected within the bony orbit, blunt trauma to the face or foreign body injuries frequently result in damage to the eye. The spectrum of injury ranges from the relatively benign, such as corneal abrasion, to the severe, such as a ruptured globe.

Corneal Abrasion

The cornea is covered by a thin (five to seven cell layers) epithelium overlying a basement membrane (Bowman's membrane). With abrasive trauma, the epithelium is removed, Bowman's membrane is exposed, and a corneal abrasion results. Because of the degree of innervation of the corneal surface, removal of the epithelium results in severe pain out of proportion to the degree of tissue injury. Bowman's membrane is relatively tough, and if it remains intact, the epithelium will heal without corneal scarring. The diagnosis of abrasion is confirmed by the instillation of fluorescein dye into the tear film and examination of the cornea with a blue light. Areas of epithelial defect will fluoresce a bright apple green/yellow (Fig. 16-4). Therapy consists of instillation of a cycloplegic agent to promote patient comfort and application of a tight patch to the eye. The patch

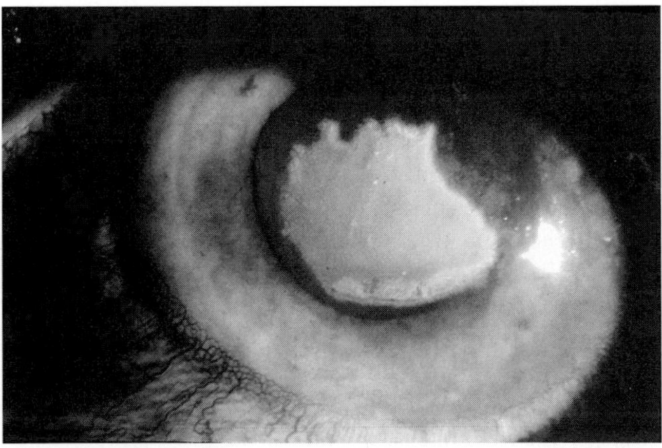

Figure 16-4. Corneal abrasions are one of the most common eye injuries. Areas of epithelial loss can frequently be seen with the penlight as areas of irregular corneal light reflex or areas where the corneal light reflex has lost its usual luster. After application of fluorescein dye, however, the area of epithelial loss shows up as an area of bright apple green fluorescence.

should be tight enough to prevent voluntary opening of the lid. The patient should be seen in follow-up after 24 h of tight patching.

Hyphema

With the application of force to the anterior ocular structures, the lens/iris diaphragm is forced posteriorly, the anteroposterior (AP) axis of the eye is shortened, and the equatorial region expands. This leads to tears in the iris root and filtration angle. If blood vessels are involved, hemorrhage occurs into the anterior chamber, leading to hyphema (Fig. 16-5). Hyphemas can be minimal, with only a trace amount of layered blood, or can completely fill the anterior chamber, a so-called eight ball hyphema. An ophthalmologist should be consulted in all cases of hyphema because although in most cases the blood clears spontaneously over a few days, several complications are possible. The red blood cells in the anterior chamber may occlude the trabecular meshwork, leading to a rise in IOP. If the elevation is significant, or is only moderate but the patient has a history of glaucoma, irreversible damage to the optic nerve can occur. If the IOP is sufficiently elevated and/or there has been endothelial trauma, blood breakdown products (hematoporphyrin) can be driven into the corneal stroma. This appears as an opaque brown-green discoloration of the cornea which can lead to a marked reduction in visual acuity. In most cases, blood staining gradually resolves over 1 to 2 years, although some residual discoloration may remain. In children this complication can result in intractable amblyopia, requiring corneal transplantation for prevention. Finally, as the clot matures, clot retraction can result in rebleeding, leading to increased blood in the anterior chamber and increased risks of the previously discussed complications.

Globe Rupture/Laceration

With the application of sufficient concussive force or with an injury from an edged weapon or projectile, the wall of the eye (sclera or cornea) may be violated. These are always serious injuries and generally require surgical repair. The goal of the initial management of globe rupture is early detection and prevention of complications. The most common situations resulting in a ruptured globe in an urban setting are blunt trauma and gunshot wounds. The examiner should suspect rupture, however, in any setting where the force of impact is sufficient to cause the injury or there is evidence of injury as a result of foreign bodies or sharp objects. Lacerations of the cornea and limbus (cornea-sclera junction) are generally visible to a penlight inspection (Fig. 16-6), although the actual corneal wound may be obscured by prolapsed lens, vitreous, or uveal tissue (Fig. 16-7). Findings in posterior injuries, however, may be quite subtle. Signs indicative of a scleral rupture include hemorrhagic chemosis and subconjunctival pigment from prolapsed uveal tissue. A peaked or dislocated pupil also provides indirect evidence for scleral rupture.

Once a rupture or laceration is noted or suspected, the eye should be protected from external pressure, which could cause further prolapse of intraocular contents. Several types of aluminum or plastic eye shields are manufactured for this purpose. If one is not avail-

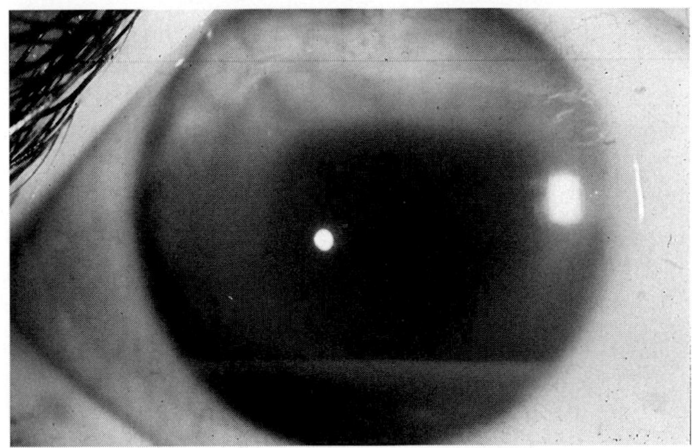

Figure 16-5. Hyphema. Bleeding into the anterior chamber obscures the examiner's view of iris details and can result in a visible blood cell layer. This patient was struck in the eye 2 h before the photo was taken, and both diffuse hemorrhage and the beginnings of a layered hyphema can be seen. The main complications from this injury include increased intraocular pressure, rebleeding, and corneal blood staining.

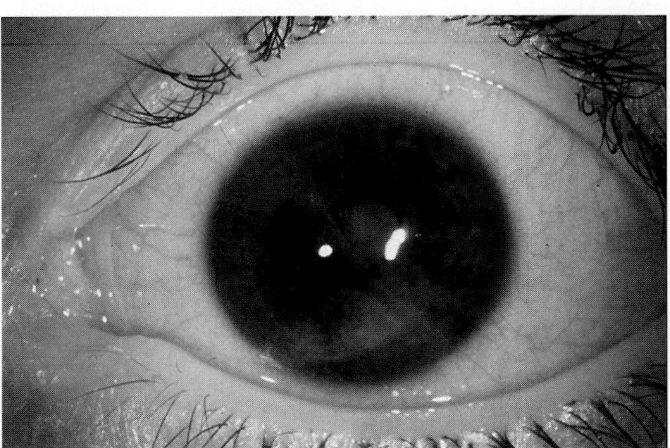

Figure 16-6. With any significant trauma to the eye, the examiner must be alert to the possibility of rupture to the globe. In this photograph, the cornea has been lacerated by a sharp object. While the laceration can be clearly seen in this case, the irregularity of the pupil is an important indication that a rupture may have occurred.

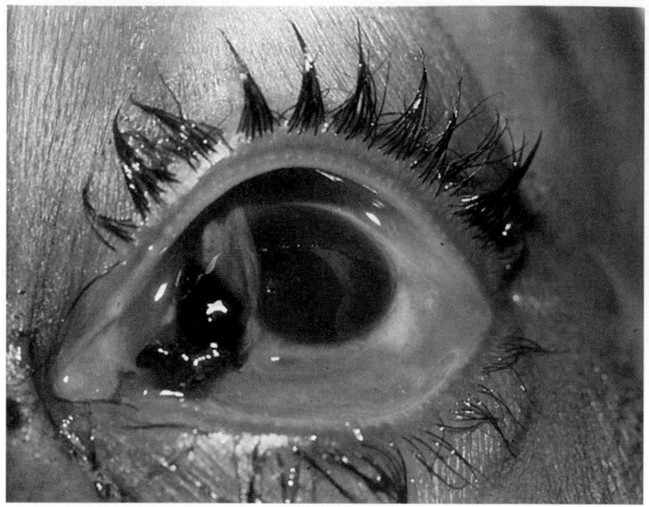

Figure 16-7. This patient also has a ruptured globe. In this case, the cornea is intact while the sclera has ruptured as a result of blunt trauma. Any dark pigment on the ocular surface may indicate an underlying rupture. In this case, both iris and ciliary body have partially prolapsed through the laceration in the sclera and are visible as a dark mass on the bulbar conjunctiva.

able, a satisfactory cover can be made from a Styrofoam or cardboard coffee cup and tape. Ophthalmology should be consulted for any patient suspected of having a corneal or scleral rupture.

Vitreous Hemorrhage/Retinal Detachment

While bleeding in the anterior chamber results in hyphema, bleeding in the posterior segment causes vitreous hemorrhage. Blood in the vitreous may severely limit the patient's vision and completely obscure the examiner's view of the retina and optic nerve. Although the vision may be quite poor because of vitreous hemorrhage, hemorrhage into the vitreous per se does not generally cause an APD. The presence of an APD should alert the examiner that additional damage has occurred, generally to the retina or optic nerve. In most cases, vitreous hemorrhage will resolve over weeks to months, although surgical removal may be necessary in some patients.

The retina can also be involved in both blunt and penetrating trauma. Holes or tears in the retina caused either by penetrating injuries or vitreoretinal traction may lead to detachment of the retina (Fig. 16-8). The detached retina appears as a gray, diaphanous vascular membrane within the vitreous. In the majority of cases, however, traumatic retinal detachments are obscured from direct ophthalmoscopy by overlying vitreous hemorrhage.

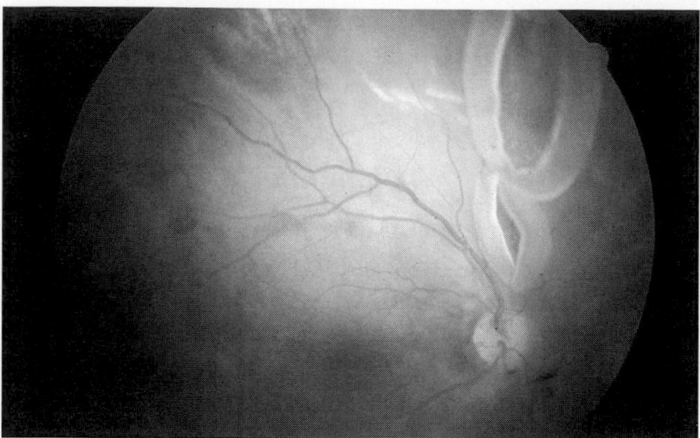

Figure 16-8. This patient was an amateur boxer who noted sudden loss of vision in his right eye after a bout. Examination of the retina reveals two large radial tears with surrounding retinal detachment. This case is unusual in that the tears are radial and are easily seen.

Injury to the Optic Nerve

As a result of its posterior location within the bony orbit and the protection afforded by the optic canal, the optic nerve is rarely injured directly except via penetrating trauma. One exception, however, is optic nerve contusion from blunt head trauma.

Optic Nerve Contusion

The association between blunt trauma to the frontal area and loss of vision has been described since the time of Hippocrates.[10] The etiology of this phenomenon, however, is not completely clear. While damage to the optic nerve has been noted after orbital fractures,[11] there is a subgroup of patients who have the typical blunt injury and optic nerve dysfunction but no evidence of damage to the bony orbital structures. Anderson et al., using holographic interferometry, investigated the orbital effects of force loading to the frontal area of dried human skulls.[12] Their data indicated that with increased loads above the brow region, stresses were concentrated near the optic foramen. Gross et al. postulated that with blunt impact to the lateral brow region, the forces are concentrated adjacent to the optic foramen, causing downward displacement of the orbital roof.[13] With release of the force load, the tissues return to their preload positions. This return is accompanied by tissue oscillations. The elastic time constant of a rigid material such as the bone of the optic canal is much shorter than that of the surrounding soft tissues, the optic nerve. This disparity in tissue oscillation frequency may cause local cavitation and resultant tearing of small vessels and hemorrhage, leading to intracanalicular nerve compression.[13]

Management of these injuries is controversial. Any patient suspected of having an optic nerve contusion should receive a complete eye exam and orbital CT scan with attention to the optic canal. If no fracture or hematoma of the canal is noted, most authorities recommend medical therapy alone. A variety of therapeutic regimens have been suggested, most based on Anderson's "megadose" steroid protocol, in which he recommends dexamethasone phosphate 0.75 mg/kg body weight initially followed by 0.33 mg/kg body weight every 6 h for 24 h. The dose of dexamethasone (Decadron) is then reduced to 1 mg/kg/day for the subsequent 48 h.[12] The author's current protocol for optic nerve contusion is based on doses used in spinal cord injury studies and entails an initial dose of 30 mg/kg methylprednisolone over 15 min. This loading dose is followed 45 min later by 15 mg/kg methylprednisolone IV every 6 h for 48 h.[14] If no improvement in vision is noted within 72 h, the steroid is discontinued.

If an orbital fracture or optic nerve sheath hematoma is present on CT scan (Fig. 16-9) and no improvement is noted with steroid therapy or if there is an initial improvement on steroids followed by loss of vision when the steroids are tapered, consideration should be given to surgical exploration of the optic canal. Results and recommendations for surgical intervention in this condition have been mixed. Some authors, such as Fukado,[15] have had excellent results and recommend routine surgical intervention. Others, such as Hughes,[16] feel that surgery offers no benefit over medical therapy. A series of patients undergoing optic nerve decompression via a transethmoidal approach has been reported.[17] The results in these 14 ptients were quite favorable, and decompression by this route may have some advantages compared with more traditional approaches. A prospective randomized trial of the role of surgical decompression in optic nerve injury is required, but the limited number of cases would make even a multicenter trial difficult to complete with adequate statistical power.

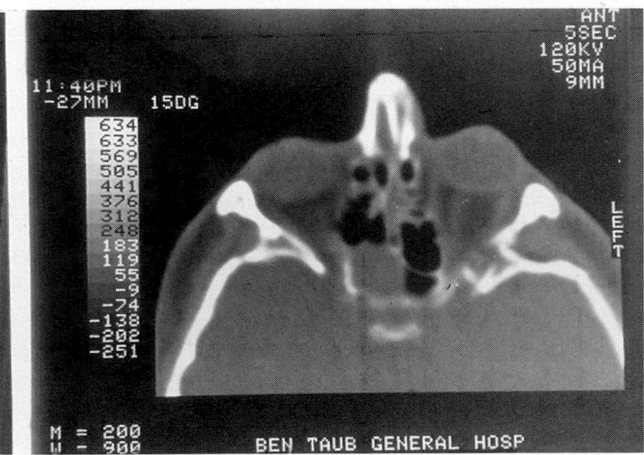

Figure 16-9. Optic nerve contusion can occur after typical blunt trauma to the forehead. This patient was struck in the brow area with a tree branch and noted delayed loss of vision. The CT scan shows a fracture of the optic canal.

Chiasmal Injury

Trauma to the optic nerve may also occur at the level of the chiasm; this type of injury has been estimated as the cause of decreased vision in 0.3 percent of head injury patients.[9] The etiology of chiasmal damage can be compressive, contusive, mechanical, or ischemic.[18] Patients generally have severe frontal head trauma and associated facial and clinoid fractures. The finding of decreased visual acuity combined with bitemporal hemianopia should suggest this diagnosis.

ORBITAL INJURIES

Orbital Fractures

Concussive and penetrating trauma of the face and the periorbital area frequently causes injury to the bony orbit and orbital soft tissues. The most common orbital fractures are those of the floor and medial wall. Two mechanisms have been proposed for these fractures. In the first, a blow to and occlusion of the orbital opening causes a rapid rise in intraorbital pressure, resulting in a "blowout" fracture of the floor and/or medial wall. The second mechanism proposes a similar transmission of bony stresses from force loading of the malar area with resultant fracture, as has been proposed for forehead impact in optic nerve contusion injuries.[12] The clinical findings in patients with floor fractures include enophthalmos (which may be masked by hemorrhage or swelling of the orbital contents), infraorbital hypoesthesia (the most reliable sign of orbital floor fracture), and in some cases limitation of or pain in upward or downward gaze. Surgical treatment should be delayed until the acute swelling subsides. Patients with floor or medial wall fractures should be cautioned against nose blowing in the early postinjury period, as the rapid increase in nasopharyngeal air pressure during nose blowing or sneezing may result in air being driven with force into the orbital space, causing sudden (and frightening) exophthalmos and a potentially very high IOP.[19]

Roof fractures have a greater potential for significant complications than do fractures of the floor or medial wall. The typical injury consists of impact to the supraorbital area, causing a rim fracture extending into the roof of the orbit. These fractures may extend to the ethmoid or frontal sinuses as well as to the inner table of the skull. Patients with orbital roof fractures can exhibit enophthalmos, exophthalmos (which may be pulsatile because of herniation of brain into the orbit if the fracture is large), blepharoptosis, and forehead anesthesia. If the inner table has been involved, CSF rhinorrhea can occur. Occasionally, orbital soft tissue injuries due to penetrating trauma are associated with roof fractures. Common agents for this type of injury include sticks, pencils, umbrella points, and firearm projectiles. As was discussed earlier, it is imperative that in any setting of potential penetrating injury, the skin of the patient be meticulously cleaned and all wounds be located and probed for possible orbital extension. If such an injury is suspected, CT scanning is indicated.

Orbital Compartment Syndromes

Functionally, the orbit is a box closed posteriorly by bone and anteriorly by the orbital septum and globe. As a result of the relative inelasticity of these tissues, any increase in orbital volume is accompanied by an increase in intraorbital pressure and anterior movement of the globe. Any pressure rise in the orbit is transmitted directly to the optic nerve, the ophthalmic artery, and the globe. With moderate increases in intraorbital volume, anterior movement of the globe is sufficient to compensate for the additional volume and keep pressures below dangerous levels. With more marked volume increases, however, the anterior movement of the globe is restricted by the eyelids and orbital septum and the resultant pressure elevation may begin to compromise blood flow through the small nutrient optic nerve vessels and eventually the ophthalmic and central retinal arteries. This situation is indicated by decreased vision, the presence of an APD, a globe that is very firm to palpation, little or no retropulsion of the globe, and arterial pulsations or occlusions visible on inspection of the optic nerve head by ophthalmoscopy. In this situation, the IOP must be abruptly lowered by lateral canthotomy and inferior cantholysis. This procedure involves severing the lateral tendinous attachments of the lids, allowing additional lid opening and anterior movement of the globe and expansion of orbital volume. In this setting, CT scanning should be performed to look for an orbital hematoma, which, if found, should be drained.

Exposure Keratitis

One of the most common ophthalmic complications of head trauma is corneal exposure. Whether as a result of obtundation or neurological deficits, head injury patients frequently have poor lid closure. As the corneal and conjunctival epithelium dry, epithelial defects result in the exposed areas. With loss of the corneal epithelium, the first line of defense against ocular infection is compromised and severe corneal infections may result. These infections are all the more difficult to treat because they frequently result from contamination with hospital-acquired resistant organisms. For this reason, all patients with poor blink reflexes or inadequate lid closure should have artificial ocular lubricants applied routinely. Ointments rather than drops are generally recommended because ointments remain longer in the preocular tear film. These agents should be applied liberally every 2 h around the clock. The ointment should be a nonmedicated lubricating preparation to avoid ocular drug toxicity.

References

1. Russell WR: Injury to cranial nerves including the optic nerves and chiasm, in Brock S (ed): *Injuries of the Skull, Brain, and Spinal Cord: Neuro-psychiatric, Surgical and Medicolegal Aspects.* Baltimore: Williams & Wilkins, 1940: 113–122.
2. Turner JWA: Indirect injuries of the optic nerve. *Brain* 66:140, 1943.
3. Gjerris F: Traumatic lesions of the visual pathways, in Vinken PJ, Bruyn CW (eds): *Handbook of Clinical Neurology,* vol 24. Amsterdam: North Holland, 1976: 27–57.
4. Petro J, Tooze FM, Bales CR, Baker G: Ocular injuries associated with periorbital fractures. *J Trauma* 19(10):730–733, 1979.
5. Holt JE, Holt GR, Bludgett JM: Ocular injuries sustained during blunt facial trauma. *Ophthalmology* 90(1):14–18, 1983.
6. Pearlstein ES, Agapitos PJ, Cantrill HL, et al: Ruptured globe after radial keratotomy. *Am J Ophthalmol* 106:755–756, 1988.
7. Wilson WB, Dreisbach JN, Lattin DE, Stears JC: Magnetic resonance imaging of nonmetallic orbital foreign bodies. *Am J Ophthalmol* 105(6):612–616, 1988.
8. Kelly WM, Paglen PG, Pearson JA, et al: Ferromagnetism of intraocular foreign body causes unilateral blindness after MR study. *AJNR* 7:243, 1986.
9. Tang RA, Kramer LA, Schiffman J, et al: Chiasmal trauma: Clinical and imaging considerations. *Surv Ophthalmol* 38(4):381–383, 1994.
10. Chadwick J, Mann WN: *The Medical Works of Hippocrates.* Oxford, UK: Blackwell, 1950.
11. Lipkin F, Woodson GE, Miller RH: Visual loss due to orbital fracture. *Otolaryngol Head Neck Surg* 113:81–83, 1987.
12. Anderson RA, Panje WR, Gross CE: Optic nerve blindness following blunt forehead trauma. *Ophthalmology* 89(5):445–455, 1982.
13. Gross CE, DeKock JR, Panje WR, et al: Evidence for orbital deformity that may contribute to monocular blindness following minor frontal head trauma. *J Neurosurg* 55:963–966, 1981.

14. Spoor TC, Hartel WC, Lensink DB: Treatment of traumatic optic neuropathy with corticosteroids. *Am J Ophthalmol* 110(6):665–669, 1990.
15. Fukado Y: Results in 400 cases of surgical decompression of the optic nerve. *Mod Probl Ophthalmol* 14:474–481, 1975.
16. Hughs B: Indirect injury of the optic nerves and chiasm. *Bull Johns Hopkins Hosp* 111:98–126, 1962.
17. Joseph MP, Lessel S, Rizzo J, Momose KJ: Extracranial optic nerve decompression for traumatic optic neuropathy. *Arch. Ophthalmol* 108:1091–1093, 1990.
18. Neetens A: Traumatic bitemporal hemianopsia. *Neuroophthalmology* 12:375–383, 1992.
19. Hunts JH, Patrinely JR, Holds JB, Anderson RL: Orbital emphysema: Staging and acute management. *Ophthalmology* 101(5):960–966, 1994.

CHAPTER 17

TEMPORAL BONE INJURIES

Newton J. Coker
Glenn W. Knox

SYNOPSIS

Often subtle and sometimes overlooked in the emergency management of trauma patients, temporal bone injuries can lead to significant morbidity. Early recognition and intervention may minimize the complications. This chapter addresses the evaluation of, clinical findings in, and management of blunt and penetrating injuries of the temporal bone, cochlea, labyrinth, and facial nerve.

EVALUATION OF TEMPORAL BONE TRAUMA

The initial care of a head injury is usually the responsibility of the neurosurgeon, and the management of temporal bone trauma is deferred until the more critical intracranial problems have been addressed. Nevertheless, complete evaluation of the temporal bone and consultation with an otolaryngologist may minimize the morbidity caused by hearing loss, vestibular dysfunction, facial paralysis, CSF otorrhea, and infection which may spread from the temporal bone into the CNS.

Essential elements in the initial evaluation of temporal bone trauma include documentation of symptoms and signs; careful inspection of the external auditory canal, tympanic membrane, and middle ear; cranial nerve assessment, in particular, nerves VII and VIII; and examination for CSF leakage. Subsequent evaluation includes pure-tone and speech audiometry or auditory brainstem evoked response testing, depending on the neurological status of the patient. Neurophysiological testing when complete facial paralysis is present and vestibular assessment of vertigo or dysequilibrium also may be useful.

The symptoms of temporal bone trauma include otalgia, hearing loss, aural fullness, tinnitus, vertigo, and dysequilibrium. Common signs of injury include bleeding from the ear canal, CSF otorrhea or otorhinorrhea, bony deformities of the osseous canal, perforation of the tympanic membrane, hemotympanum, nystagmus, facial weakness, and Battle's sign (ecchymosis over the mastoid region). Battle's sign may not develop immediately after trauma but instead may appear as a late sign.

Examination of temporal bone trauma begins with careful inspection of the external and middle ear. To visualize the osseous canal, tympanic membrane, and middle ear, blood and debris are removed from the external auditory canal. An external auditory canal or middle ear disorder which impedes the transmission of sound to the cochlea results in a conductive hearing loss. A disorder of the cochlea or cranial nerve VIII frequently results in sensorineural hearing loss. In an alert patient, a Weber's test screens for hearing loss. A vibrating 512-CPS tuning fork is placed in the center of the forehead. In a patient with normal hearing, the tone is perceived symmetrically in both ears. If the patient complains of hearing loss in one ear, the sound will lateralize to that ear in the presence of a conductive hearing loss; it will lateralize to the opposite ear if a sensorineural hearing loss exists in the injured ear. The Rinne test compares the loudness of the vibrating fork held 1 in. lateral to the external canal to the loudness with the stem of the fork placed on the mastoid. If the bone conduction is perceived better than the air conduction is, a conductive hearing loss of at least 25 dB is present. Cranial nerve assessment focuses on cranial nerves V through XII, or those nerves within or adjacent to the temporal bone. During the examination of extraocular movements, nystagmus should be documented in the direction of the fast phase. The direction of the nystagmus is toward the dominant labyrinth. Trauma to the temporal bone can produce an irritative or destructive lesion in the vestibular system. In the case of an irritative lesion, the nystagmus is directed toward the involved ear. However, if the nystagmus is directed toward the noninvolved ear, a destructive labyrinthine lesion on the same side as the trauma is suspected.

Facial nerve function should be documented as soon as the patient can cooperate with facial expressions or be made to grimace from painful stimuli. Both sides of the face are compared for symmetry and tone in repose and symmetry of movement in the distribution of the temporal, zygomatic, buccal, mandibular, and cervical branches of the facial nerve. Too often the status of the facial nerve immediately after trauma is unknown. The initial status is often the key to later management. Paresis of the facial nerve generally has a good prognosis for satisfactory recovery, while an immediate and complete facial paralysis carries a higher probability of no return of movement or residual weakness and synkinesis.

Any leakage of clear fluid from the ear canal or nose suggests CSF leakage and provides presumptive evidence of a fracture of the skull base. Drops of fluid allowed to fall onto filter paper can be screened for CSF. Spinal fluid diffuses more rapidly than do blood and mucus, thus producing concentric staining rings on the paper. If the fluid can be collected, the specimen should be analyzed for glucose content or beta transferrin to confirm the presence of CSF.[1]

Temporal bone trauma frequently leads to deficits in auditory and vestibular function. Tests of hearing and balance are the key to the diagnosis and management of cochleovestibular disorders and are crucial to documentation for legal and other purposes. Pure-tone bone conduction and air conduction thresholds and speech discrimination are measured as soon as is practical. For a comatose or uncooperative patient, auditory brainstem evoked response evaluation estimates the hearing level. For patients suffering from dizziness or dysequilibrium, vestibular tests such as electronystagmography (ENG), rotary testing, and posturography document the site of pathology (central versus peripheral) and the extent of dysfunction.

Imaging

The primary imaging modality for temporal bone trauma is high-resolution computed tomography (CT).[2] Both thin-section axial and coronal views are helpful in identifying fracture planes, ossicular discontinuity, infringement of the fallopian canal, and pneumolabyrinth.[2,3] Fractures may be missed without thin-section and biplanar scanning. The incidence of vascular injuries resulting from penetrating wounds of the temporal bone approaches 33 percent.[4] Carotid angiography may therefore be indicated to identify vascular injury, such as vessel laceration, thrombosis, traumatic aneurysm, and arteriovenous fistula.

CT with intrathecal water-soluble contrast usually localizes the site of CSF leakage in high-flow states. In the temporal bone, the site of leakage often correlates with a fracture step deformity along the floor of the middle fossa or across the posterior cortical plate of the temporal bone. When a CSF leak is suspected but its location in the skull base cannot be identified, a radioactive tracer study may be helpful. A radioactive tracer injected intrathecally is recovered on cotton pledgets placed in the ear canals, at the opening of the eustachian tubes, and along the nasal vault. Higher radioactivity counts on specific pledgets may point to the site of leakage.

HISTOPATHOLOGY OF TEMPORAL BONE TRAUMA

Temporal bone fractures can produce a myriad of pathological events in the middle and inner ear, including bleeding into the middle ear and mastoid, ossicular fracture and discontinuity, stapes subluxation into the vestibule, perilymphatic fistulae, tympanic membrane perforation, hemorrhage into the endolymphatic or perilymphatic spaces, endolymphatic hydrops, disruption of the membranous labyrinth, osseofibrogenesis of the perilymphatic spaces, labyrinthitis ossificans, fibrous union of the otic capsule, loss of hair cells and spiral ganglion cells, and contusion or transection of the cochleovestibular and facial nerves[5–7] (Fig. 17-1*A* and 1*B*). Concussive injury without fractures may produce high-frequency hearing loss as a consequence of acoustic energy transmission to the cochlea and damage to the hair cells.[8]

TEMPORAL BONE INJURIES

Temporal Bone Fractures

Temporal bone fractures are classified in accordance with the orientation of the fracture plane to the long

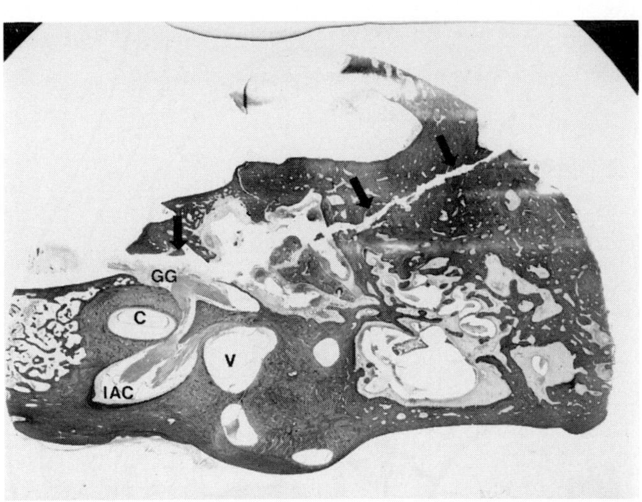

A

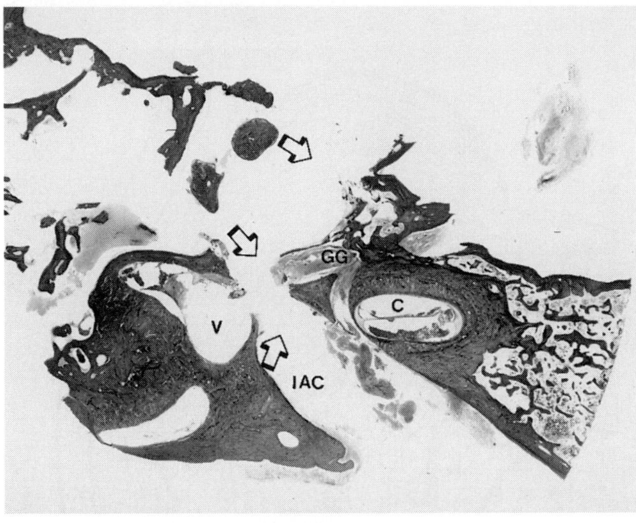

B

Figure 17-1. Temporal bone fractures. *A*. Longitudinal fracture lateral to otic capsule (arrows). *B*. Transverse fracture through internal auditory canal, vestibule, and tympanic segment of facial nerve (arrows). Human specimens: hemoxylin and eosin stain. V = vestibule; C = cochlea; GG = geniculate ganglion; IAC = internal auditory canal. (Used with permission from Morgan et al.[5])

axis of the petrous pyramid. In general, longitudinal fractures extend parallel to the long axis and lateral to the otic capsule; transverse fractures cross the long axis and violate the otic capsule or internal auditory canal.

LONGITUDINAL TEMPORAL BONE FRACTURES

Longitudinal fractures are the most common type of temporal bone fracture resulting from blunt head trauma.[9] Approximately 70 to 90 percent of all presenting temporal bone fractures are longitudinal in nature and usually originate from blows to the temporal region or parietal region.[9–12] Classically, the fracture extends from the squamous portion of the temporal bone through the posterosuperior osseous external auditory canal, across the middle ear to the region of the geniculate ganglion, and then into the middle fossa (Fig. 17-2*A*). The fracture plane runs lateral to the otic capsule. Variations of the classical longitudinal presentation are common, and other structures may be involved in the injury, including the eustachian tube, temporomandibular joint, carotid canal, and jugular fossa. Facial paralysis occurs in approximately 20 percent of patients with longitudinal fractures, and the site of injury is at the geniculate ganglion in over 90 percent of cases.[13,14] A second site of injury may result from fractures extending through the posterior osseous canal into the facial canal in the mastoid. Conductive hearing loss is a characteristic finding in this type of fracture and is due to a torn tympanic membrane, disruption of the ossicles, or blood in the middle ear.[14,15] Sensorineural hearing loss caused by acoustic or concussive injury to the cochlea often coexists with the conductive loss.[8,16–18]

TRANSVERSE FRACTURES

Transverse fractures account for 10 to 30 percent of all presenting temporal bone fractures and represent a more severe form of trauma.[9–11] Transverse fractures are less common because patients often do not survive the severe blows to the head that produce them. Direct blows to the occiput are the most frequent cause; however, frontal blows can also dissipate the force across the axis of the petrous pyramids. The fracture typically extends from the jugular fossa across the posterior aspect of the temporal bone into the otic capsule and vestibule or through the internal auditory canal and into the otic capsule (Fig. 17-2*B*). Blood or CSF behind an intact eardrum is frequently seen in these fractures. Because of the violation of the internal auditory canal or otic capsule, severe sensorineural hearing loss is common and signs of vestibular dysfunction, vertigo, and nystagmus are often present. Not all transverse fractures result in profound hearing loss. Early documentation of hearing is important, as a perilymph fistula represents a possible etiology of sensorineural hearing loss and vertigo and repair may save hearing in an otherwise

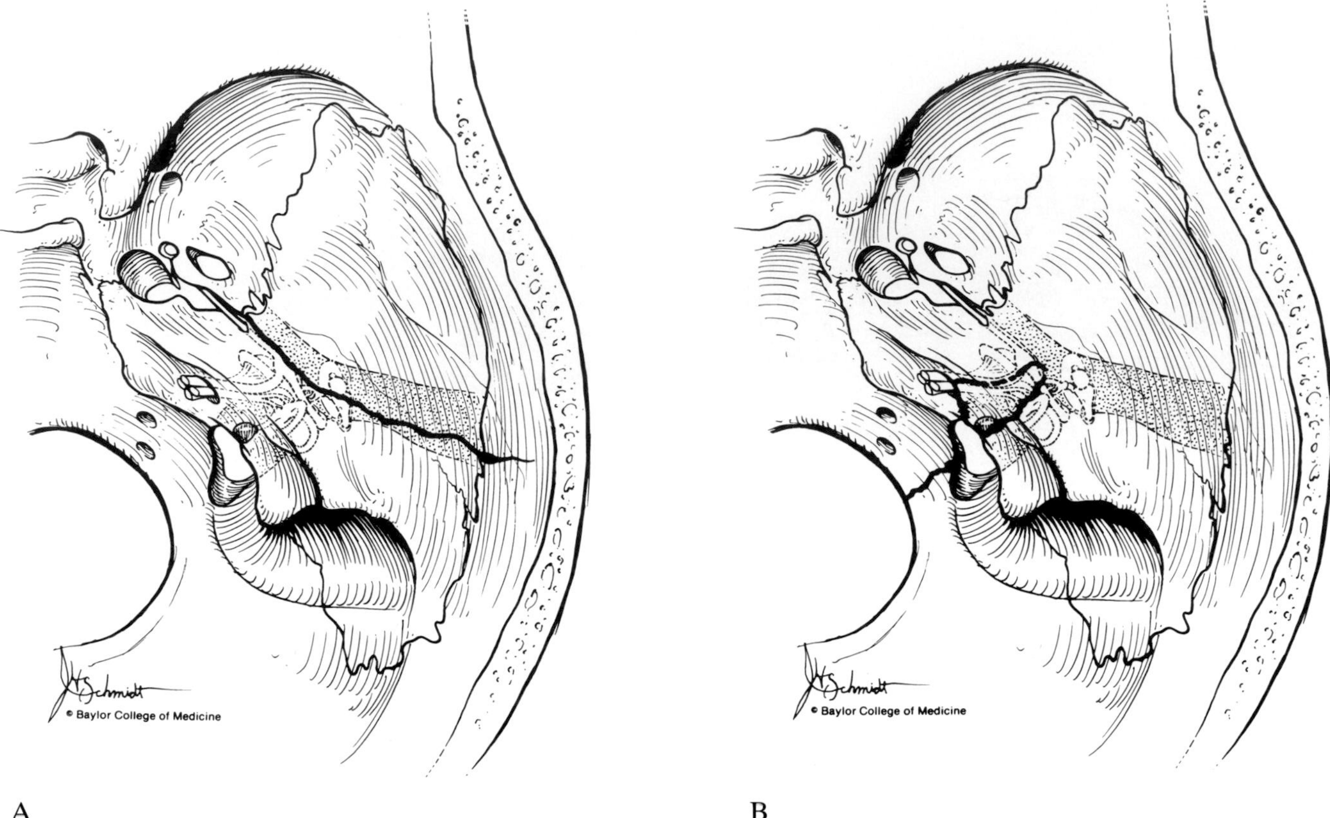

Figure 17-2. Temporal bone fractures. *A*. Longitudinal fractures extend along the roof of the external canal, across the middle ear to the perigeniculate region, and into the carotid canal or eustachian tube. *B*. Transverse fractures extend through the labyrinth or internal auditory canal and tend to involve the facial nerve in the perigeniculate and tympanic segments. (Used with permission from Coker et al.[14])

progressive loss.[3] Facial paralysis occurs in half these cases. Dual sites of injury to the facial nerve are commonly identified in the geniculate region and the tympanic segment above the oval window. CSF leakage is more common in this fracture type and typically presents as otorhinorrhea.

Although most fractures can be classified as longitudinal or transverse, the radiographic features of both may be evident on CT. These hybrid, or mixed, fractures produce clinical findings common to both primary types. The incidence of bilateral temporal bone fractures approaches 29 percent,[19] necessitating close examination of both ears in closed head injuries.

Gunshot Injuries of the Temporal Bone

The incidence of temporal bone involvement in gunshot wounds to the head has been estimated to be 20 percent.[20] Entrance wounds are usually found in the face below the orbit or lateral to the temporal bone. Highly destructive injuries result directly from the missile and its fragmentation and indirectly from the kinetic energy imparted to the temporal bone. Most missiles to the temporal bone produce comminuted or mixed fractures.[4] Loss of hearing is common as a result of damage to the sound conduction mechanism of the middle ear or injury to the cochlea. (Fig. 17-3, *A* to *C*) CT scanning is imperative in the assessment of the middle ear, cochlea, labyrinth, and facial nerve. CT determines missile location, ballistic traverse, and intracranial problems such as hematoma, contusion, edema, pneumocephalus, and metallic or bony fragments.

Carotid arteriography, including analysis of the venous phase, is indicated in gunshot injuries of the temporal bone. Vascular injuries are evident in as many as one-third of these cases, including injury to the internal and external carotid artery or its branches, transverse or sigmoid sinus, and internal jugular vein.[4] Sigmoid sinus injuries can, when necessary, be accessed through a craniotomy or mastoid approach. Methods to control bleeding consist of compression and packing with tem-

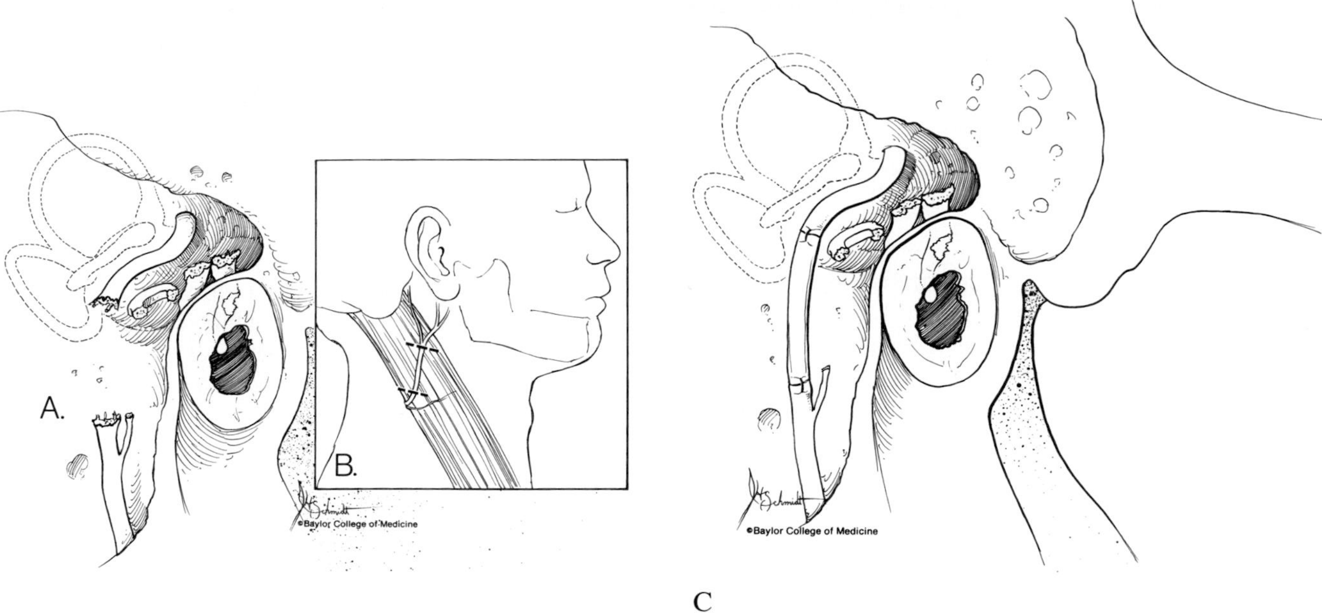

C

Figure 17-3. Gunshot injury to the middle ear and mastoid. *A*. Missile traverses the middle ear and mastoid, disrupting the ossicular chain and transecting the mastoid segment of the facial nerve. *B*. Location of greater auricular nerve coursing from Erb's point toward the external auditory canal.*C*. Interpositional nerve graft repair of injured facial nerve using bony canal as a stent. (Used with permission from Duncan et al.[4])

poralis muscle and ligation of the sinus. Persistent arterial bleeding in the skull base mandates control by compression, vessel ligation, or repair.

Many gunshot wounds require immediate exploration for the purposes of debridement of devitalized tissue, foreign bodies, and impacted skin and management of vascular injuries or CSF leakage. Injuries to the facial nerve occur in approximately 50 percent of these patients.[4] The most commonly injured segments are the tympanic and the mastoid. In patients presenting with facial paralysis, the nerve is almost always transected or severely contused, requiring interpositional grafting for facial reanimation.[21]

In an ear with an intact osseous canal, the eardrum may be reconstructed to protect the middle ear from infection. Ossicular reconstruction corrects conductive hearing loss. Because of the highly destructive nature of gunshot injuries, however, radical mastoidectomy is the most frequently performed procedure.[4]

Management of Facial Paralysis

The controversies regarding the appropriate management of traumatic paralysis, the significance of neurophysiological testing, the timing of surgical intervention, and the most effective techniques for repair remain unresolved with few exceptions.[11,12,22,23] At issue is the quality of the return of facial nerve function.

Documentation of facial nerve function on the initial examination is critical. Immediate paralysis differs from delayed paralysis in prognosis and management. Facial weakness or paresis is indicative of a subtotal lesion, and the prognosis for spontaneous recovery is good. Progression of the weakness to a complete paralysis heralds nerve ischemia, which, if unabated, leads to complete degeneration and a guarded prognosis for satisfactory return of function. An immediate and complete facial paralysis signifies a more complete lesion to the nerve.

The following general statements guide the decision about surgical intervention:

1. Immediate and complete facial paralysis associated with temporal bone fractures which demonstrate progressive degeneration on neurophysiological testing warrants exploration of the injury site.[22] Fractures which show disruption or step deformities of the fallopian canal on CT have a poorer prognosis for spontaneous recovery.
2. Immediate and complete facial paralysis associated with penetrating injuries of the temporal bone is associated with transection or severe contusion.[4,21]
3. Delayed facial paralysis generally is followed by a

successful return of facial function, although exceptions exist.[22,24,25]

4. Facial paralysis associated with transverse fractures has a poorer prognosis than does paralysis associated with longitudinal fractures.
5. Facial nerve injury secondary to gunshot wounds has the poorest prognosis of all temporal bone traumas.[14,21]

The status of hearing dictates the surgical approach toward exploration of a degenerating facial nerve[14] (Fig. 17-4). In ears with a good cochlear reserve, all intratemporal segments of the facial nerve can be explored by means of transmastoid and middle cranial fossa approaches to the fallopian canal. In longitudinal fractures, the facial nerve is usually damaged in the perigeniculate region. This area is best examined via a middle cranial fossa approach with removal of bone over the internal auditory canal, the geniculate ganglion, and the labyrinthine and tympanic segments of the facial nerve. The most common findings are contusion, intraneural hematomas, and bony spicules embedded in the nerve substance. Decompression with removal of hematomas and bone fragments provides a better environment for neural regeneration[10,13,14] (Fig. 17-5). Occasionally, temporal lobe contusion or edema precludes the use of this approach in the first month after an injury.

In a deaf ear the facial nerve can be explored via transmastoid and translabyrinthine routes to the fallopian canal. These approaches are applicable to transverse fractures and penetrating injuries with sensorineural hearing loss and facial paralysis. Entry into the subarachnoid space should be avoided in an infected ear until the infection has been treated. Direct approaches to the intratemporal facial nerve are not advised in only-hearing ears (a situation in which a patient is deaf in one ear but can hear in the other).

Severely contused or transected nerves require grafting to provide a conduit for regenerating motoneurons. The greater auricular and sural nerves provide suitable donor-free grafts for this purpose. Principles of neurorrhaphy include the following: All neuronal tissue should be handled atraumatically with microinstruments designed for neural repair; the approximation of nerve endings is best performed under the illumination and magnification of the operating microscope; exact end-to-end approximation should be accomplished without tension on the anastomosis; and a 9/0 or 10/0 monofilament suture is used for either type of repair.[26] Return of function after grafting in the temporal bone may not be clinically evident for 6 to 9 months. Two years may be necessary to derive the full benefit of regeneration. Interpositional grafting is the preferred method of neural reanimation when the injured ends are accessible for repair. Even under the best conditions, residual forehead weakness and synkinesis or mass movement may be anticipated after grafting.[21]

Cochlear Concussion

The occurrence of injuries to the inner ear in the absence of a fracture may be explained on the basis of concussion. Because of sudden acceleration and deceleration, the membranes of the inner ear may experience violent displacement.[8] Trauma may produce concussive cochlear damage even on the side contralateral to the blow. Vibratory energy of great intensity causes peripheral sensorineural hearing loss by damaging the organ of Corti and hair cells and is most severe in the high frequencies. The histopathology of damage to the co-

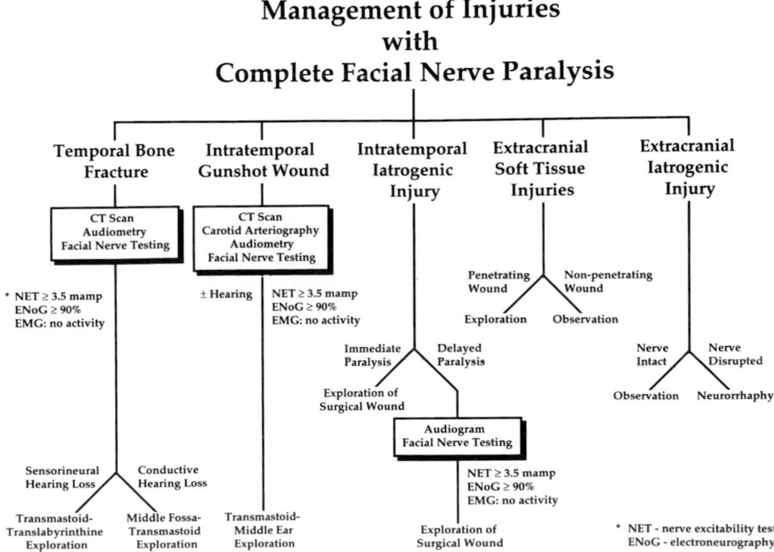

Figure 17-4. Algorithm for the management of complete facial paralysis. Neurophysiological tests are used to determine the level of degeneration. Surgical exploration is recommended for progressive or complete paralysis. NET = nerve excitability test; ENoG = electroneurography; EMG = electromyography.

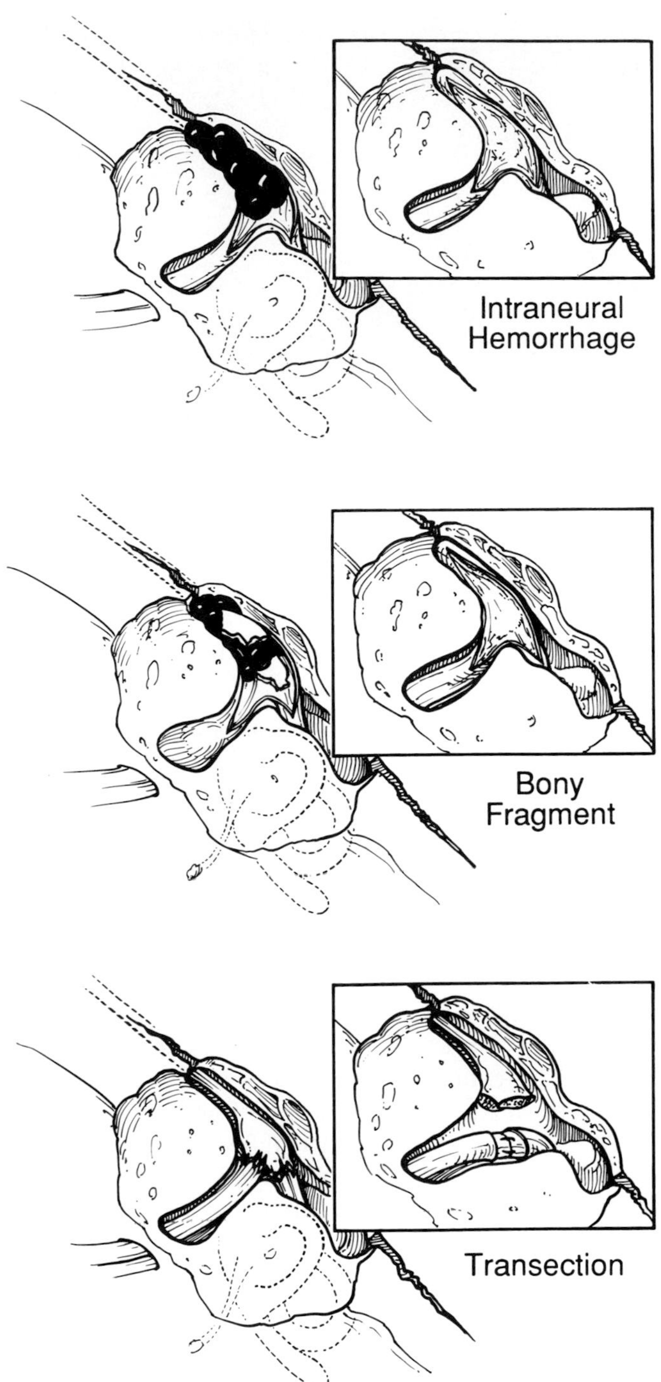

Figure 17-5. Longitudinal temporal bone fracture injuring the facial nerve at the geniculate ganglion. The most common causes of injury are intraneural hemorrhage and compressive bony spicules, which require removal with nerve decompression. An end-to-end anastomosis or graft is used to repair a transectional injury.

chlea both in experimental animals and in human autopsy findings is similar to that caused by prolonged exposure to high-intensity noise.[7] The hearing loss is typically found around the frequency of 4000 Hz (common test range of 250 to 8000 Hz, or cycles per second). As the energy increases, the spectrum widens.

Sensorineural hearing loss occurs very frequently in head injury patients. An audiometric evaluation is of great importance in determining the degree of sensorineural, conductive, or mixed hearing loss. The prognosis for recovery of sensorineural hearing loss in this setting is very poor. It is important to address any correctable sources of conductive hearing loss first and then offer amplification for any residual sensorineural hearing loss. As with noise-induced hearing loss, sensorineural hearing loss from head trauma is often associated with tinnitus. If it persists beyond the acute phase of management, the tinnitus tends to be lifelong and often is exacerbated by multifactorial events such as noise exposure, caffeine, nicotine, alcohol, stress, anxiety, and illnesses of any nature. Often amplification with a hearing aid masks the tinnitus perceived by the patient.

Labyrinthine Dysfunction

The vestibular dysfunction associated with head injury is highly variable in nature. Damage can occur at a number of points along the vestibular pathway: end organ, vestibular nerve, vestibular nuclei, and cerebellum. Symptoms vary with the site of pathology and the extent of damage.

An interesting form of positional dizziness seen in head trauma patients is benign paroxysmal positional vertigo, or cupulolithiasis.[27] The patient typically exhibits spontaneous, abrupt vertigo after rotation of the head. Characteristic features of this vertigo are a 10- to 15-s delayed onset after a change in head position and reproducibility and fatigability on subsequent head maneuvers. When the patient is placed in a supine position, the vertigo and rotary nystagmus are precipitated by placing the involved ear in an undermost position. Schuknecht's theory proposes that calcium carbonate crystals which have broken free of the macula of the utricle or saccule to float in the endolymphatic fluid fall against the cupula of the posterior semicircular canal and stimulate this canal. The condition is remedied by Cawthorne head exercises designed to disperse the crystalline fragments. Recalcitrant cases are treated by singular or vestibular neurectomy to denervate the labyrinth.

Vestibular dysfunction due to longitudinal fractures is usually mild and transient. However, transverse fractures violate the labyrinth and semicircular canals or damage the vestibular nerve, resulting in unilateral denervation and causing vertigo and loss of balance associated with nausea and vomiting. Through the process of compensation, the vestibular nuclei adjust to unilateral input from the one intact system over the course of 2 to 3 months, and in the interim symptomatic treatment suffices. Residual unilateral vestibular end-organ disorders that are unresponsive to vestibular exercises and symptomatic treatment can be managed effectively with vestibular neurectomy. The procedure is contraindicated in vestibular dysfunction of central origin.

Vertigo after head injury can be of both immediate and long-term significance. Postinjury vertigo may have its origin in sources outside the labyrinth. For example, in whiplash injuries the head is free and never strikes another object. Experimentation with whiplash injury in animals has demonstrated marked ecchymosis and edema of the brainstem and cerebral and cerebellar cortical areas. Vertigo occurring with various head positions is a commonly seen physiological finding that may be related to stimuli originating in the soft tissues of the neck and skull.[16] Although temporal bone fractures can cause acute disturbance in equilibrium, long-lasting chronic disturbances may not arise from this source.[17] Many head-injured patients exhibit a mixed central and peripheral disequilibrium.

Perilymphatic Fistula

Leakage of perilymph from the inner ear to the middle ear leads to a deterioration in auditory and vestibular function. This entity is a consideration in the pathogenesis of hearing loss and imbalance in every case of head trauma. Different mechanisms can account for the development of fistulae at the round or oval windows: an increase in CSF pressure transmitted to the perilymphatic space via the cochlear aqueduct or internal auditory canal, an increase in middle ear pressure resulting from Valsalva maneuvers, subluxation of the stapes (Fig. 17-6), and fractures of the otic capsule.[3,28] The hearing loss is sensorineural in type but may be seen in combination with conductive loss due to ossicular or eardrum abnormalities. The hearing loss may be progressive or fluctuating initially, but wth time it tends to stabilize at a severe level. The vertigo is nondescript but may manifest as fleeting moments of vertigo, positional dizziness, or chronic dysequilibrium. The diagnosis requires a high index of suspicion. A fistula test performed by altering the pressure in the external auditory canal with a pneumatic otoscope may elicit nystagmus or the feeling of imbalance. Serial audiograms demonstrate changes in pure-tone thresholds or speech discrimination. ENG may show a weakness to caloric stimulation in the involved ear but may also demonstrate nonspecific findings. The existence of a fistula is determined by surgical exploration of the middle ear and observation of the oval and round windows. Collection of perilymph for beta transferrin analysis is confirmatory.[1] Fistulae represent a treatable cause of cochleovestibular dysfunction, and closure of the defects in the labyrinthine windows often stabilizes or improves hearing and alleviates dysequilibrium.[15,29]

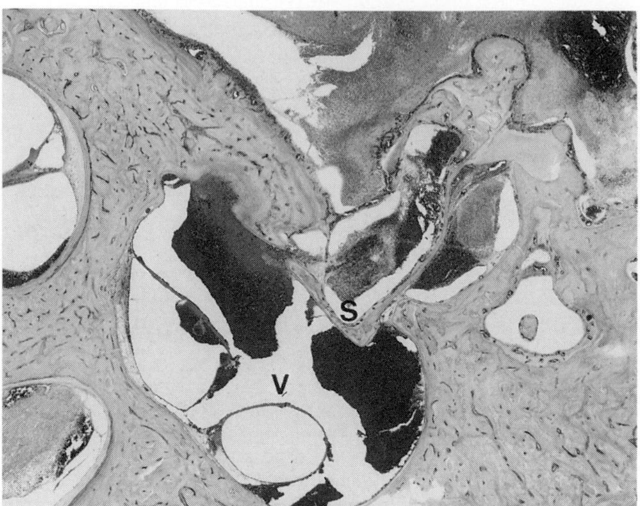

Figure 17-6. Perilymphatic fistula created by subluxation of the stapes (S) into the vestibule (V). Note hemorrhage into middle ear and vestibule. (Used with permission from Morgan et al.[5])

Cerebrospinal Otorrhea

CSF leaks present as otorrhea or otorhinorrhea and result from temporal bone fractures and penetrating causes. This complication is more commonly observed after transverse fractures than after fractures of the longitudinal type. Over 90 percent of leaks respond to conservative measures. Leaks originating from the middle fossa tend to close more quickly than do those from the posterior fossa, as the abundant arachnoid tissue promotes fibrosis in the middle fossa.

Conservative measures include bed rest with elevation of the head of the bed, stool softeners, cough suppressants, and avoidance of any activity which increases intracranial pressure. High-flow or persistent leaks often respond to the use of an indwelling lumbar subarachnoid drain over the course of 1 to 2 weeks. Leaks due to penetrating injuries or bony spicules usually require operative intervention to repair the dural defect. Other indications for repair include large leaks persisting for more than about 10 to 14 days, meningitis, and brain or meningeal herniation through a bony defect. However, the indications for surgical intervention have not been clearly established and are subject to the judgment of the treating surgeon or surgeons.

The efficacy of prophylactic antibiotics is unproven.

For contaminated gunshot wounds to the temporal bone or fractures complicated by middle ear infection, antibiotic coverage of gram-positive organisms is preferred.

CSF leakage unresponsive to observation or subarachnoid drainage requires repair. Options include craniotomy with dural repair; packing with muscle, fat, and fibrin glue; and a radical mastoidectomy with obliteration of the middle ear and mastoid.[30]

Tympanic Membrane Perforations

Rupture of the eardrum results from temporal bone fractures, compression of air in the external canal (e.g., blast injuries or blows to the ear), and penetrating injuries. Bleeding into the ear canal and hearing loss are consequences. Close inspection delineates the defects in the eardrum. Linear tears require protective measures to prevent water contamination in the middle ear. Stellate perforations should be inspected carefully to remove any foreign materials from the edges or the middle ear. Occasionally, large perforations demonstrate infolding of the torn edges which precludes spontaneous healing. Such situations are best managed by unfurling the edges and supporting them in place with Gelfoam in the middle ear or a paper patch applied to the lateral surface of the eardrum. Spontaneous healing occurs in approximately 90 percent of traumatic perforations within 3 months. Exceptions include perforations associated with burns, lightning, welding injuries, or infection. For persistent perforations, formal tympanoplasty is recommended to restore conductive hearing loss and protect the middle ear from infection.

A tympanic membrane perforation discovered in conjunction with vertigo or sensorineural hearing loss is a danger sign of inner ear injury. Audiometric evaluation and middle ear exploration are indicated as soon as possible, as timely closure of a perilymph fistula in the round window or repair of stapes subluxation may save hearing and restore equilibrium.

Ossicular Disruption

Ossicular injury is commonly associated with head injury. The most common of these injuries are separation of the incudostapedial joint and fracture of the stapes arch. Nevertheless, injury can involve fracture of any of the three ossicles or separation of their two joints, incudostapedial and incudomalleal.

Conductive hearing loss results from a tympanic membrane perforation, a hemotympanum, or ossicular discontinuity such that in the initial stages of management, the existence of the ossicular injury may be masked by other pathological conditions in the tympanic membrane and middle ear. High-resolution thin-section CT occasionally demonstrates the ossicular abnormality, but because of the limits of resolution, imaging cannot give all details of the ossicular chain. After closure of the tympanic membrane and resolution of fluid (blood or CSF) from the middle ear, a persistent conductive hearing loss documented on pure-tone bone and air conduction thresholds provides clear evidence of ossicular dysfunction. In such cases, middle ear exploration and ossiculoplasty are warranted to restore hearing.

References

1. Skedros DG, Cass SP, Hirsch BE, Kelly RH: Beta-2 transferrin assay in clinical management of cerebral spinal fluid and perilymphatic fluid leaks. *J Otolaryngol* 22:341–344, 1993.
2. Schubiger O, Valavanis A, Stuckmann G, Antonucci F: Temporal bone fractures and their complications: Examination with high resolution CT. *Neuroradiology* 28:93–99, 1986.
3. Lyos AT, Marsh MA, Jenkins HA, Coker NJ: Progressive hearing loss following transverse temporal bone fracture. *Arch Otolaryngol Head Neck Surg* (in press).
4. Duncan NO, Coker NJ, Jenkins HA, Canalis RF: Gunshot injuries of the temporal bone. *Otolaryngol Head Neck Surg* 94:47–55, 1986.
5. Morgan WE, Coker NJ, Jenkins HA: Histopathology of temporal bone fractures: Implications for cochlear implantation. *Laryngoscope* 104:426–432, 1994.
6. Khan AA, Marion M, Hinojosa R: Temporal bone fractures: A histopathologic study. *Otolaryngol Head Neck Surg* 93:177–186, 1985.
7. Ward PH: The histopathology of auditory and vestibular disorders in head trauma. *Ann Otol Rhinol Laryngol* 78:227–238, 1969.
8. Schuknecht HF, Neff WD, Perlman HB: An experimental study of auditory damage following blows to the head. *Ann Otol Rhino Laryngol* 60:273–289, 1951.
9. Cannon CR, Jahrsdoerfer RA: Temporal bone fractures: Review of 90 cases. *Arch Otolaryngol* 109:285–288, 1983.
10. Fisch U: Management of intratemporal facial nerve injuries. *J Laryngol Otol* 94:129–134, 1980.
11. Maiman DJ, Cusick JF, Anderson AJ, Larson SJ: Nonoperative management of traumatic facial nerve palsy. *J Trauma* 25(7):644–648, 1985.
12. Adour KK, Boyajian JA, Kahn ZM, Schneider GS: Surgical and nonsurgical management of facial paralysis following closed head injury. *Laryngoscope* 87:380–390, 1977.
13. Lambert PR, Brackmann DE: Facial paralysis in longitudinal temporal bone fractures: A review of 26 cases. *Laryngoscope* 94:1022–1026, 1984.
14. Coker NJ, Kendall KA, Jenkins HA, Alford BR: Traumatic intratemporal facial nerve injury: Management rationale for preservation of function. *Otolaryngol Head Neck Surg* 97:262–269, 1987.
15. Bellucci RJ: Traumatic injuries of the middle ear. *Otolaryngol Clin North Am* 16:633–650, 1983.

16. Barber HO: Head injury: Audiological and vestibular findings. *Ann Otol Rhinol Laryngol* 78:239–252, 1969.
17. Nelson JR: Neuro-otologic aspects of head injury, in Thompson RA, Green JR (eds): *Advances in Neurology*, vol 22. New York: Raven Press, 1979: 107–128.
18. Lindsay JR, Zajtchuk J: Concussion of the inner ear. *Ann Otol Rhinol Laryngol* 79:699–709, 1970.
19. Griffin JE, Altenau MM, Schaefer SD: Bilateral longitudinal temporal bone fractures: A retrospective review of seventeen cases. *Laryngoscope* 89:1432–1435, 1979.
20. Byrnes DP, Crockard HA, Gordon DS, Gleadhill CA: Penetrating craniocerebral missile injuries in the civil disturbances in Northern Ireland. *Br J Surg* 61:169–176, 1974.
21. Backous DD, Jenkins HA, Coker NJ: Gunshot injuries to the intratemporal facial nerve. *Proceedings of the VII International Symposium on the Facial Nerve. Eur Arch Otorhinolaryngol* (suppl) 287–289, 1994.
22. Coker NJ, Jenkins HA: On the prognostication of return of function following facial nerve trauma, in Castro D (ed): *The Facial Nerve*. Amsterdam: Kugler and Ghedini, 1990: 273–275.
23. Brodsky L, Eviatar A, Daniller A: Post-traumatic facial nerve paralysis: Three cases of delayed temporal bone exploration with recovery. *Laryngoscope* 93:1560–1565, 1983.
24. Grobman LR, Pollak A, Fisch U: Entrapment injury of the facial nerve resulting from longitudinal fracture of the temporal bone. *Otolaryngol Head Neck Surg* 101:404–408, 1989.
25. Eby TL, Pollak A, Fisch U: Histopathology of the facial nerve after longitudinal temporal bone fracture. *Laryngoscope* 98:717–720, 1988.
26. Coker NJ: Management of traumatic injuries to the facial nerve, in Weisman RA, Stanley RB Jr. (eds.): *Otolaryngol Clinics North Am* 24:215–227, 1991.
27. Schuknecht HF: Cupulolithiasis. *Arch Otolaryngol* 90:765–778, 1969.
28. Goodhill V, Brockman SJ, Harris I, Hantz O: Sudden deafness and labyrinthine window ruptures: audio-vestibular observations. *Ann Otol Rhinol Laryngol* 82:2–12, 1973.
29. Glasscock ME, McKennan KX, Levine SC: Persistent traumatic perilymph fistulas. *Laryngoscope* 97:860–864, 1987.
30. Coker NJ, Jenkins HA, Fisch U: Obliteration of the middle ear and mastoid cleft in subtotal petrosectomy: Indications, technique, and results. *Ann Otol Rhinol Laryngol* 95:5–11, 1986.

CHAPTER 18

MANAGEMENT OF ASSOCIATED SPINE INJURIES IN HEAD-INJURED PATIENTS

Charles H. Tator

SYNOPSIS

The prevalence of concomitant head and spine injuries is quite high: Approximately 5 to 10 percent of head-injured patients have an associated spinal injury, while 25 to 50 percent of spinal injury patients have an associated head injury. The detection of these concomitant injuries requires extreme vigilance in physical examination and careful selection and interpretation of imaging studies. The prognosis for neurological recovery, especially from the cord injury, may be worse in those with concomitant injuries. Treatment priorities must be individualized for optimum management of these patients.

A fundamental tenet of the management of injuries is to be aware of the possibility of an associated spinal injury, especially in an unconscious or inebriated patient who is unable to provide an accurate history or reliably report symptoms.[1,2] *Indeed, one must assume that all unconscious patients have an associated spinal injury until proven otherwise.*[3] *There is less risk of overlooking an associated head injury in a patient with a spinal injury because such a patient can accurately report the history and symptoms.*

INCIDENCE AND NATURE OF CONCOMITANT HEAD AND SPINAL INJURIES

Michael et al.[4] performed a comprehensive analysis of all head injuries and cervical spine injuries in patients admitted to the Detroit Receiving Hospital in 1987 and found that there were 359 head injuries and 92 cervical spine injuries, with 22 patients having both. Thus, 6 percent of head injury patients had associateed cervical spinal injuries and 24 percent of cervical spine injury patients had associated head injuries: 2.4 percent of comatose patients [Glasgow Coma Scale (GCS) < 8] had concomitant cervical spine injuries. Motor vehicle accidents accounted for 13 of the 22 patients with both head and spinal injuries, and there were also eight falls and 1 assault. Concussion with GCS > 8 occurred in 18 of 22 cases, and only 2 patients had a GCS < 8. Five had skull fractures, and one had a cerebral contusion with a small surface clot. The levels of injury paralleled the usual distribution, with 8 of the 22 patients having injuries at C1, C1-C2, or C2 and 8 patients having injuries at C5 or C5-C6. Seventeen had cervical fractures or dislocations. Thirteen patients had no neurological deficit associated with the spinal injury, and there were six patients with incomplete quadriparesis (including three with the central cord syndrome) and three with complete quadriplegia. Three of the 22 patients died. These results are similar to those of other series[1,5] in which the majority of the combined injuries were sustained in motor vehicle accidents rather than in sports-recreational accidents such as diving.

It is likely that the biomechanical forces which produced the head injuries differed from those which produced the spine injuries, although there is some evidence from experimental[6] and clinical studies[7] that the same blow can cause both cerebral and cervical cord injuries.

In the author's series[1] of 144 patients with spinal cord injuries, the associated head injuries included 51 patients (35 percent) with simple concussion and 7 (5 percent) with more severe injuries, including 4 with cerebral contusion, 2 with skull fractures, and 1 with a subdural hematoma. Several of the concomitant head and spine patients had additional injuries, the most common of which were chest injuries (e.g., hemothorax) and abdominal injuries (e.g., ruptured spleen and bowel laceration). Five of the seven patients had cervical injuries, and two patients had thoracic injuries. Three of the seven patients died. This study documented a higher incidence of more severe cord injuries, a higher incidence of hypotension on admission, and a higher mortality rate in those with multiple injuries than in those with cord injuries alone. Also, the multiple trauma groups showed less neurological recovery of the cord injury compared with the group with cord injuries alone, and it was hypothesized that this might have been due to hypotension, hypoxia, or a delay in treating the cord injury caused by the need to treat a life-threatening concomitant injury first.

Several other investigators have reported the incidence of concomitant head and spinal injuries and have generated somewhat differing figures depending on whether they were reporting a series of primarily head or spinal injuries.[8–10] Shrago[10] reported a higher incidence of upper cervical than lower cervical injuries in association with head injuries, but this has not been confirmed in other series.[1,4] Schneider and colleagues[7,11] detailed a number of patients with concomitant injuries to the head and upper cervical cord, many with interesting and complex clinical syndromes, including the onion skin pattern of facial sensory loss and Bell's cruciate paralysis.

Pagni and Massaro[5] provided one of the most complete accounts of concomitant head and spinal injuries in their review of 2304 patients seen during a 7-year period, which included 2027 patients (88 percent) with head injuries alone, 110 (5 percent) with spinal injuries alone, and 167 (7 percent) with combined head and spinal injuries. In the latter group, 121 patients (5 percent) had a vertebral fracture and/or dislocation with or without neurological impairment and 46 (2 percent) had a cervical sprain. Motor vehicle accidents were the most common sources of injury, followed by falls and then sports. Cervical, thoracic, thoracolumbar, and lumbosacral cases accounted for 49 percent, 22 percent, 25 percent, and 4 percent, respectively.

Thus, the incidence of concomitant injuries is quite high, with about 5 to 10 percent of head-injured patients having an associated spinal injury and 25 to 50 percent of spinal injury patients having an associated head injury.

CLINICAL EXAMINATION OF A HEAD-INJURED PATIENT TO DETECT AN ASSOCIATED SPINAL INJURY

As was noted above, it is prudent to assume that a spinal injury is present in every head-injured victim, especially in comatose patients. Clues to the presence of a spinal injury in comatose patients can be obtained from a careful physical examination (Tables 18-1 and 18-2). The vital signs may provide evidence of a spinal cord injury, especially if signs of neurogenic spinal shock are present, such as systemic hypotension and bradycardia (due to unopposed vagotonia) and low body temperature with a high skin temperature (due to sympathectomy effect of a cervical cord injury).[12] In contrast, patients with severe head injuries with space-occupying lesions and high intracranial pressure show systemic hypertension and bradycardia (the Cushing response).

Palpation of the *entire* vertebral column should be performed, including the neck, thoracic region, and lumbosacral spine. The examiner can carefully palpate the entire spine without moving the spine, even in a supine patient, and therefore can proceed without the risk of worsening an injury. In palpating the spine, the examiner is looking for evidence of a spinal injury, including tenderness (in those with lighter coma), crepitus, deformity such as a "step," and bogginess (suggestive of a

TABLE 18-1 Clinical Clues to the Presence of an Associated Spinal Injury in a Head-Injured Patient

1. Neurogenic spinal shock: hypotension and bradycardia instead of hypertension and bradycardia
2. Paradoxical respiration
3. Low body temperature and high skin temperature
4. Priapism
5. Bilateral paralysis of arms and legs, especially flaccid
6. Bilateral paralysis of arms only or of arms more than legs, especially flaccid
7. Bilateral paralysis of legs, especially flaccid
8. Lack of response to painful stimuli
9. Presence of a level of response to painful stimuli
10. Painful stimulation producing only head movement or facial grimacing
11. Sweating level
12. Horner's syndrome
13. Brown-Séquard syndrome

TABLE 18-2 Initial Evaluation of the Spine in Head Injury Patients

1. Inspection and palpation of the entire spine.
2. Radiological examination of entire spine, including AP and lateral views in comatose patients. In awake patients who give a reliable history, only painful parts of the spine need to be radiographed.
3. Do not perform flexion and extension views in comatose patients.
4. Consider evoked potentials, if available, in suspected cord injuries.
5. Search for other injuries which may be "masked," e.g., intraabdominal hemorrhage.

hematoma). Also, the examiner should attempt direct viewing of as much of the spine as possible to look for ecchymosis, which is uncommon except in conditions such as ankylosing spondylitis. Respiratory movements should be observed carefully for the presence of paradoxical respiration, which usually indicates a severe lesion at C5 or below. Priapism is frequently present in patients with major cord injuries but is never a manifestation of cerebral injury. If the paralysis is bilateral, especially if it is flaccid and the deep tendon reflexes are diminished or absent, the lesion is more likely to be in the spinal cord than in the brain. Flaccidity is quite common after major spinal cord injury and is due to spinal shock. In contrast, most severe brain injuries produce hypertonicity, even in the early stages, although major trauma to the brainstem can produce flaccid paralysis. Bilateral paralysis of the arms only or of the arms more than the legs (central cord syndrome) occurs commonly after a spinal cord injury,[13] although lesions at the cervical medullary junction can produce a similar picture (Bell's cruciate paralysis). Although patients with a severe head injury and a GCS of 3 have no response to painful stimulation, patients with less severe injuries usually respond in some way. Accordingly, a complete lack of response to painful stimulation is a clue to a spinal cord injury, especially if the examiner detects a sensory level below which there is no response but above which there is a response to painful stimulation. Similarly, if there is only head movement or facial grimacing in response to a painful stimulus, this is a clue to the possibility of an incomplete spinal cord injury with motor paralysis but preserved sensation. Although testing for a "sweat level" with iodine is seldom done, it is possible to detect a sweat level by feeling the moisture of the skin: Loss of sweating below a definite level denotes the sympathectomy effect of a spinal cord injury. Similarly, Horner's syndrome is frequently present in patients with major cervical cord injuries but is rare in those with head injuries. Unfortunately, ptosis, which is the most obvious feature of Horner's syndrome, is very difficult to detect in supine or comatose patients. Thus, there are numerous clues to the possibility of a spinal cord injury in comatose patients.

WHAT CONSTITUTES APPROPRIATE RADIOLOGICAL EXAMINATION OF THE SPINE IN A HEAD-INJURED PATIENT?

The question of "how to clear the spine" in head-injured patients has always been of major importance in the field of neurotraumatology.[14,15] Several studies have determined the rates of false-negatives or "missed fractures" in this population of patients. There is a significant risk of failure in detection because of the difficulty of obtaining adequate radiological visualization of the spine, especially the cervical spine, in head-injured patients. Urgency in the treatment of other life-threatening conditions, lack of cooperation, and involuntary movements such as decerebrate rigidity and generalized muscle spasm may all impair visualization of the spine. Head-injured victims often are young muscular males, and this compounds the problem of radiological evaluation of the lower cervical and upper thoracic spine on lateral views because of well-developed shoulder musculature.

For the cervical spine, the combination of anteroposterior (AP) and lateral and open-mouth odontoid views,[14] and for the thoracic and lumbosacral areas, AP and lateral views, provide only limited sensitivity. In *all* comatose head-injured patients, *all* areas of the spine should be radiologically examined in both AP and lateral planes (Table 18-2). Areas of poor visualization on the plane views must be subjected to further examination by conventional or computed tomography, preferably with reformatted views.[14] The timing of this further testing is determined by the urgency of treating the head injury or other associated injuries. In the cervical spine, the upper and lower levels have the highest incidences of missed lesions.[14,15] Thus, particular attention must be focused on obtaining excellent radiographic display in two planes of the C1-C2 region including the odontoid and of the C7-T1 region. Flexion-extension views of the spine should *never* be obtained in comatose patients in the acute phase.

Neurophysiological examination of the spine by evoked potentials can provide additional information about the presence of a concomitant spinal cord injury by showing an absence or a marked decrease of amplitude of an increase in the latency of the somatosensory evoked potential.[16] Unfortunately, this technology is seldom available on an acute basis in most centers.

There should be a thorough search for other injuries, especially chest and intraabdominal injuries, which may be "masked" by the absence of typical physical findings such as abdominal rigidity. Liberal use of minilaparotomy is recommended in these circumstances.

TREATMENT

Treatment of these gravely injured patients with concomitant known or suspected head and spinal injuries, particularly in the acute phase, is a great challenge.

TABLE 18-3 Treatment of Known or Suspected Concomitant Head and Spinal Cord Injuries

1. Priorities of trauma management: airway, breathing, and circulation
2. Early use of invasive monitoring
3. Immobilization of spine: collars, fracture boards, halo vests, etc.
4. Log rolling every 2 h
5. Bladder and stomach intubation
6. Operate first on most life-threatening injury
7. Give steroids early
8. Operative cases: immobilization intraoperatively and fiber-optic intubation

There is much to be accomplished and pitfalls to be avoided both in the field by rescue workers and by emergency personnel in the acute care hospital (Table 18-3). The priorities in trauma management of airway, breathing, and circulation (ABC) are especially important not only because of the need to maintain or restore homeostasis for life support but also for specific support of the metabolically compromised brain and spinal cord by maintenance of adequate oxygenation, arterial pressure, and blood flow.[17] Hypotension and hypoxia are particularly damaging to patients with head injury[18] and those with spinal cord injury.[1]

Establishment of an airway in a comatose patient with a known or suspected spinal injury may be extremely difficult and hazardous. However, if the neck is maintained in a neutral position during intubation, the risks can be minimized. If there is time, fiber-optic intubation is always preferable. However, if there is no time, airway establishment and maintenance of adequate breathing take precedence; if limited movement of the neck is required to accomplish this, the risk must be taken. Assisted ventilation to avoid respiratory failure is especially important if the cord injury has weakened or paralyzed the diaphragm and intercostal muscles. Hypotension from spinal shock has to be treated with a combination of fluids, vasopressors, and anticholinergics (to overcome the unopposed vagotonia); this is especially important for maintaining adequate blood flow to the brain and spinal cord.[5,12] The use of invasive monitoring including arterial lines and Swan-Ganz catheters is recommended to guide management of fluid therapy, vasopressors, inotropes, and anticholinergic medications.[12]

Immobilization of the spine can be accomplished with rigid plastic collars, tongs and traction, halo vests, and the like. The author has found that early placement of patients in halo vests is of particular advantage in both operative and nonoperative patients, including intensive care management of patients with concomitant head and cervical spine injuries.[19] The two-hr rule for log rolling must be considered for skin care, even from the start, to prevent pressure sores. Bladder and stomach intubation are also essential early maneuvers. Steroids should be administered early and in large doses to those suspected or known to have a cord injury.

The first operative priority in the treatment of concomitant lesions is the management of intracranial space-occupying lesions. Whenever possible, cervical dislocations should be reduced concomitantly by traction followed by immobilization in tongs or a halo. Cervical traction cannot be applied in patients who require extensive craniotomy. In general, spinal lesions requiring surgical decompression should be given the next priority, perhaps within days of the craniotomy. Spinal lesions requiring operative treatment for stability alone should receive a lower priority, and surgery can usually be delayed for 1 to 2 weeks. The optimal timing of surgical intervention in spinal injury patients remains controversial, as does the issue of surgical versus nonsurgical stabilization (halo vest, etc.). In special circumstances, surgical treatment of the spinal injury may be favored over nonoperative treatment, as in the case of a patient with a depressed skull fracture, which could prevent the use of a halo or tongs.[5]

In the series of Pagni and Massaro,[5] 62 of the 121 patients with combined injuries required surgical treatment: 6 for head and spinal injuries, 27 for the head injury only, and 29 for the spinal injury only. In the 33 patients requiring surgical treatment for head injuries, surgery was required in a lower percentage of the cervical spinal injuries than in the thoracic or thoracolumbar injuries. This reflected the higher incidence in their series of more severe head injuries in association with thoracic and thoracolumbar injuries than in association with cervical injuries. In contrast, Harris[20] found that the more severe head injuries occurred in association with cervical injuries.

References

1. Meguro K, Tator CH: Effect of multiple trauma on mortality and neurological recovery after spinal cord or cauda equina injury. *Neurol Med Chir* (*Tokyo*) 28:34–41, 1988.
2. Tator CH, Rowed DW, Schwartz ML, et al: Management of acute spinal cord injuries. *Can J Surg* 27:289–294, 1984.
3. Tator CH: Acute spinal cord injury: First aid management, diagnosis and treatment. *Medicine* (*Baltimore*) 33:3118–3122, 1983.
4. Michael DB, Guyot DR, Darmody WR: Coincidence of head and cervical spine injury. *J Neurotrauma* 6:177–189, 1989.
5. Pagni CA, Massaro F: Concomitant cranio-cerebral and vertebro-medullary injuries: Analysis of 121 cases. *Acta Neurochir* (*Wien*) 111:1–10, 1991.

6. Gosch HH, Gooding E, Schneider RC: Cervical spinal cord hemorrhages in experimental head injuries. *J Neurosurg* 33:640–645, 1970.
7. Schneider RC, Gosh HH, Norrell H, et al: Vascular insufficiency and differential distortion of brain and spinal cord caused by cervicomedullary football injuries. *J Neurosurg* 33:363–375, 1970.
8. Bohlman HH: Acute fractures and dislocations of the cervical spine. *J Bone Joint Surg* 61A:1119–1142, 1979.
9. Bachulis BL, Long WL, Hynes GD, et al: Clinical indications for cervical spine radiographs in the traumatized patient. *Am J Surg* 153:473–477, 1987.
10. Shrago GG: Cervical spine injuries: Association with head trauma, a review of 50 patients. *AJR* 118:670–673, 1973.
11. Schneider RC: Concomitant craniocerebral and spinal trauma, with special reference to the cervicomedullary regions. *Clin Neurosurg* 17:266–309, 1970.
12. Kiss ZHT, Tator CH: Neurogenic shock, in Geller ER (ed): *Shock and Resuscitation*. Ed E.R. New York: McGraw-Hill, 1993: 421–440.
13. Tator CH: Spinal cord syndromes: Physiologic and anatomic correlations, in Menezes AH, Sonntag VKH (eds.): *Principles of Spinal Surgery*. New York: McGraw-Hill, 1995.
14. Woodring JH, Lee C: Limitations of cervical radiography in the evaluation of acute cervical trauma. *J Trauma* 34:32–39, 1993.
15. Macdonald RL, Schwartz ML, Mirich D, et al: Diagnosis of cervical spine injury in motor vehicle crash victims: How many x-rays are enough? *J Trauma* 30:392–397, 1990.
16. Houlden DA, Schwartz ML, Klettke KA: Neurophysiologic diagnosis in uncooperative trauma patients: Confounding factors. *J Trauma* 33:244–251, 1992.
17. Tator CH, Fehlings MG: Review of the secondary injury theory of acute spinal cord trauma with special emphasis on vascular mechanisms. *J Neurosurg* 75:15–26, 1991.
18. Chestnut RM, Marshall LF, Klauber MR, et al: The role of secondary brain injury in determining outcome from severe head injury. *J Trauma* 34:216–222, 1993.
19. Tator CH, Ekong CEU, Rowed DW, et al: Halo devices for the treatment of acute cervical cord injuries, in Tator CH (ed): *Early Management of Acute Spinal Cord Injury*. New York: Raven Press, 1982: 231–256.
20. Harris P: Associated injuries in traumatic paralysis and tetraplegia. *Paraplegia* 5:215–220, 1968.

CHAPTER 19

ORTHOPEDIC INJURIES

Ronald W. Lindsey
Camille Cash

SYNOPSIS

Orthopedic injuries frequently complicate the management of patients with head injury. Some evidence suggests that the rate of fracture healing is accelerated in patients with a severe head injury, although the mechanism for this phenomenon is conjectural. In general terms, orthopedic injuries should be treated as early as possible. However, in a multiple trauma patient a certain delay is common because of conflicting priorities. Whenever possible, the neurological and hemodynamic condition of the patient should be stabilized before an orthopedic procedure is undertaken. During and after surgery, care should be taken to monitor the patient's blood pressure, hematocrit, and serum sodium. If the possibility of a developing mass lesion is a concern, intracranial pressure monitoring should be considered. Management strategies for different fractures and subluxations are outlined.

INTRODUCTION

Closed head injuries (CHI) is frequently result from high-energy trauma and are associated with multiple injuries.[1] Among the most common concomitant injuries are limb fractures.[2]

The unresponsive nature of severe CHI patients and other therapeutic priorities sometimes make the identification of these fractures extremely challenging, and many injuries may go undiagnosed initially[2] (Fig. 19-1). Once they are detected, displaced or comminuted fractures frequently must await stabilization of the patient's cardiopulmonary and neurological status before definitive treatment, sometimes resulting in the fracture healing in poor functional alignment.

The rate of fracture healing in a head-injured patient may differ dramatically from fracture healing in other patients.[3–13,18,19] Although the reasons for this are poorly understood, evidence suggests that fracture healing may be enhanced in head and spinal cord injury.[4,9,10,13–20] This enhanced bone formation (EBF) may represent functional callus formation or heterotopic ossification.[15]

Heterotopic ossification (HO) is defined as new bone formation in tissues that typically do not ossify.[5] Mature HO closely resembles mature fracture callus both radiographically and histologically. Like fracture callus, HO can be painful during its inflammatory phase and, with maturity, can produce a prominent callus mass. However, HO does not necessarily restore bone continuity, although it can restrict joint or soft tissue mobility.[5,6,21,22]

Therefore, EBF merits special attention in the management of fractures in CHI. Knowledge of the problems specific to these patients is essential, and standard treatment methods may require modification to avoid complications and maximize function.

THE ASSOCIATION OF CHI AND FRACTURES

In a review by Lewin of 821 patients with CHI, associated injuries occurred in 33 percent of the patients.[23] Irving and Irving reported that 47 percent of CHI patients suffered one or more significant injuries aside

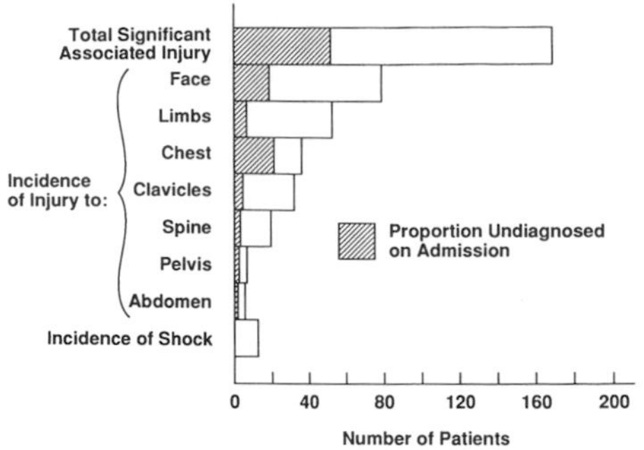

Figure 19-1. In a series of 354 CHIs, the frequency of specific types of associated injuries and the proportion of missed diagnoses at admission were tabulated by Irving and Irving.[2]

from the head injury, and with the exception of facial injuries, fractures of the extremities constituted the most prevalent of these associated injuries.[2] Weissman and Khermosh identified 47 CHIs in 114 polytrauma patients admitted to the orthopedic surgery service.[24]

Modern critical care management of CHI has dramatically improved patient survival as a result of early therapeutic interventions.[22,25] A similarly aggressive approach is necessary in the management of CHI-associated orthopedic fractures, as the ultimate prognosis for neurological recovery cannot always be determined after the initial assessment.[25] Brink and colleagues studied the physical recovery in 344 CHI patients who were initially comatose and were then followed prospectively for at least 12 months. Seventy-three percent of the patients resumed independent ambulation and self-care, while only 19 percent remained dependent or comatose. These authors concluded that recovery from head injury was probable if the coma lasted less than 3 months and suggested that fractures should not be treated with indifference or the expectation of functional compromise.[26]

Unfortunately, the role of the orthopedic surgeon in the early care of a trauma patient is not always well defined. The life-threatening concerns of polytrauma patients may obscure fracture recognition, and once they are detected, care of the fractures may be deferred or may not receive standard treatment. Orthopedic involvement should begin immediately upon the patient's admission to the hospital. This permits musculoskeletal concerns to be included in other diagnostic or therapeutic efforts. The prolonged morbidity or functional compromise of the limb fracture may constitute a more debilitating long-term problem than does the head injury.[22] Early intervention in the fracture care of these patients may prevent some of the complications endemic to this group.

SPECIAL FRACTURE MANAGEMENT CONSIDERATIONS IN CHI

As was previously stated, the basic premise of fracture management in CHI patients is that the final neurological prognosis cannot be accurately determined, and so fractures should be treated with the assumption that full neurological recovery will occur.[25] General anesthesia must not be induced until it is possible to establish a neurological baseline.[22] Spinal anesthesia is generally contraindicated because of potential alterations in CSF dynamics and the risk of herniation.[25] Consequently, orthopedic treatment which may inflict pain or require a sterile environment is delayed until the most life-threatening general and neurological concerns have been addressed.

However, a physician providing fracture care is confronted with conflicting priorities; beyond a couple of days, the longer the delay before fracture reduction and stabilization lasts, the more challenging even the most mundane fracture may become. This is due in part to the reported tendency of CHI fractures to heal with rapid and overabundant callus formation.[4,16–20] Late correction of consolidated but poorly aligned fractures can be extremely difficult.[4,6,22]

Early achievement of acceptable fracture alignment is far more important than rigid fixation or immobilization. Newman and coworkers reported 13 long bone fractures in CHI patients treated by closed methods that healed with unusual rapidity.[10] In a separate review of paraplegic patients, not only did fracture union occur more rapidly than is normally seen, there was considerably more callus despite little or no immobilization.[27] These authors surmised that a greater fracture healing response seemed to be inherent in neurologically impaired patients and that timely orthopedic intervention was essential.

ALTERED FRACTURE HEALING IN CHI

The concept of EBF in patients with fractures and neurological impairment was first reported by Riedel in 1883.[28] Numerous authors have since suggested EBF in patients with a variety of neurological disorders, including spinal cord injury,[19] closed head injury,[5,7,21,29–37] and peripheral nerve injury.[38,39] Even without the presence of bony injury, EBF in the form of ectopic bone formation is exceedingly common in head-injured patients.[5,21,29,30,32–37]

However, somewhat subjective clinical studies have formed the basis for the widespread opinion that CHI fractures heal differently, and scientific confirmation of this phenomenon has been limited.[15] The issues to be resolved include the following: (1) Does altered healing represent callus or heterotopic ossification?[40,41] (2) is callus produced to a greater extent? (3) do CHI-associated fractures heal more reliably?[20,39] (4) do CHI-associated fractures heal at a more rapid rate?[9,10,15,17,22,41]

The fact that rapid callus formation occurs in fractures in patients with significant neurological insult was first reported in 1963 by Benassy and associates in paraplegic and CHI patients.[3] An enhanced rate of healing was reported by Eichenholtz in paraplegic versus nonparaplegic patients.[27] Calandriello reviewed a group of 13 CHI patients with fractures that were thought to heal usually rapidly,[4] and Newman and colleagues identified a similar CHI group with fractures which also appeared to unite exceptionally rapidly despite simple closed treatment methods.[10] Eichenholtz's analysis of the accelerated callus which formed in several patients suggested that the bone differed from normal callus.[27] Histologically, the new bone appeared to be in a permanent intermediate stage between coarse fibrous bone of recent osteoid deposition and adult cortical compact bone.

In addition to rapid callus formation, fracture healing in neurologically impaired patients may be more abundant.[4,11,16–20,27,39,42] Comarr and colleagues documented more exuberant callus in lower extremity fractures sustained at the time of spinal cord injury or after spinal cord injury compared with fractures in neurologically intact patients.[42]

Perkins and Skirving prospectively quantitated excessive callus formation and more rapid union in a radiographic assessment of consecutive femur fractures in patients with and without head injuries.[11] Similarly, Spencer radiographically calculated a significant increase in callus size and time to union in patients with head injury compared with those without such injury.[18] The abundant callus observed in 75 percent of patients appeared to occur in patients with more severe cerebral injuries.

Several animal models have been used to replicate EBF in neurologically impaired patients. Herold and coworkers induced head injury in guinea pigs, created a standard bone defect in the radius with the ulna left intact, and measured the amount of subsequent callus formation with serial x-rays at weekly intervals.[9] Although excessive callus was not demonstrated conclusively, brain injury appeared to accelerate fracture healing (Table 19-1).

A feline model was used in another study in which a stereotactic brain lesion was induced by using a thermocoagulation lesion generator.[19] Unilateral spastic lesions were produced, and bilateral fibular osteotomy healing was analyzed by x-ray, histomorphometry, biochemistry, and hormonal assay. Bone formation appeared to occur faster and be more pronounced in spastic limbs (Table 19-2).

Frymoyer and Pope employed a unilateral denervated rat limb model to assess the nature and quality of healing of bilateral fibula osteotomies.[38] Specimens were sacrificed at varying times after osteotomy (5 to 30 days) and subjected to histological and biomechanical analysis. Histologically, the denervated animals demonstrated better callus and quality of union than did control limbs at 15 to 20 days (Table 19-3). Biomechanically, fracture stress (load per unit area), energy to failure, and stiffness also were significantly increased in the neurologically ipmaired animals during the same period (Fig. 19-2). These authors concluded that flaccid paralysis, as opposed to spasticity, still induced EBF and suggested a systemic rather than a local basis for altered bone healing.

These findings were corroborated by Quilis and Gonzalez in denervated rat limbs, with both histology and radiography demonstrating more advanced healing in the denervated limbs despite flaccidity.[39] Therefore, although it remains to be conclusively shown how or why this phenomenon occurs, the treatment plan in CHI-

TABLE 19-1 Correlation of Brain Damage and Rapidity of Callus Formation

Group of Animals	No. Bone Defects Studied	No. Weeks Till First Appearance of Callus on X-rays, mean ± SD	No. Weeks Till Complete Filling of Bone Defects mean ± SD
Control	38	4.76 ± 2	8.31 ± 2.3
Moderate brain damage (cauterized 2 s)	42	3.9 ± 1 $t = 2.56$ $p < .05$	7.1 ± 2 $t = 2.6$ $p < .05$
Severe brain damage	22	4.7 + 2 $p > .05$	7.8 ± 2.4 $p > .05$

TABLE 19-2 Mean Values of FHR, Union Time, and New Bone Mass (Group 2)

	Right, ±SD	Left, ±SD	Statistical Analysis
Greatest value of FHR (A/B) (mean, n = 11)	2.08 (0.21)	1.85 (0.22)	Wilcoxson signed ranks test (p = .0209)
Union time (weeks; mean, n = 11)	5.27 (0.65)	6.17 (0.60)	Sign test (p = .0020)
New bone mass (g; mean, n = 11)	0.28 (0.12)	0.19 (0.09)	Wilcoxon (nonparametric; p = .0039)

TABLE 19-3 Comparison of Histological Gradings of Experimental and Control Animals 15 Days after Injury

Histological	Control, mean ± SD	Experimental, mean ± SD	Significance, p
Variable			
Clot	2.8 ± .53	3.8 ± .38	.001
Union	1.0 ± .21	2.0 ± .83	.005
Callus	2.6 ± .36	3.2 ± .75	.025
Compact bone	0.6 ± .15	1.5 ± .98	.001
Total score	6.4 ± .89	10.6 ± 2.5	.002

associated fractures must assume that these fractures may heal faster and to a greater extent than do fractures in neurologically intact patients.

HETEROTOPIC OSSIFICATION

HO is a phenomenon characterized by the deposition of calcium and soft tissue outside the skeleton.[43] Neurogenic HO can occur with closed head or spinal cord injury, and its etiology is unknown. The incidence of HO can range from 10 to 75 percent, depending on the frequency of x-ray examinations. CHI-associated HO affects the upper and lower extremities equally; however, spinal cord injury (SCI) HO usually involves the lower extremity, particular the hip joint.

This entity has been reported in a variety of clinical settings, including burns,[44] musculoskeletal fractures and dislocations,[45] meningitis,[46] encephalitis,[47] poliomyelitis,[48] tuberculosis,[48] arthroplasty,[45,49] spinal cord injury,[27,42] and closed head injury.[5,10,21,30,35,50] HO may occur in periarticular sites with trauma, renal failure, pseudogout, and tumoral calcinosis.[29] The joints usually affected include the hip, knee, shoulder, and elbow.

Since the first report of this condition in a paraplegic patient by Riedel in 1883,[28] HO has been called "paraosteoarthropathy,"[51] "myositis ossificans neurotica,"[52,53] "neurogenic ossifying fibromyositis,"[54] "neurogenic osteoma,"[55] and "periarticular new bone formation."[32] The clinical presentation of HO is similar to that of an acute fracture. Localized soft tissue swelling with warmth and redness precedes the onset of radiographic ossification.[43] Because of this pronounced early inflammation, HO can easily be mistaken for septic arthritis,[56] cellulitis,[56] superficial thrombophelebits,[48] or deep

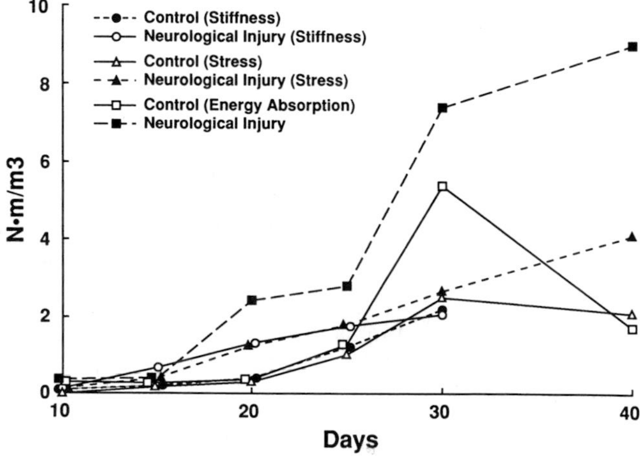

Figure 19-2. Biomechanically, fracture stiffness, stress (load per unit area), and energy to failure were significantly increased in the experimental (denervated) limb at 15 to 20 days.

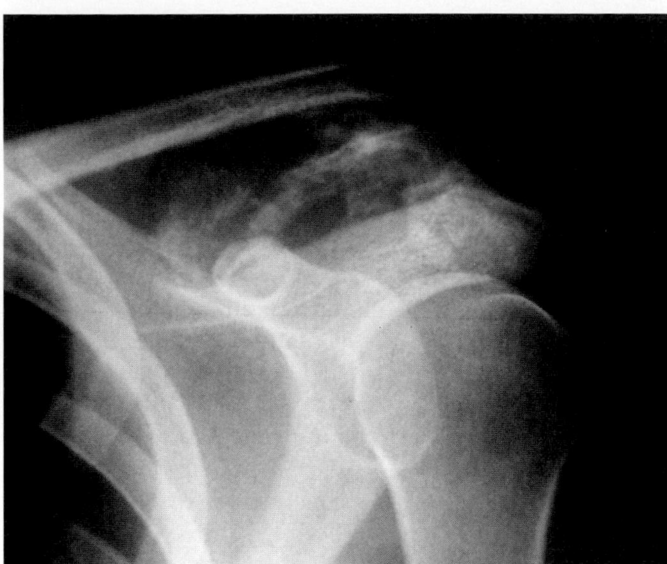

Figure 19-3. Radiograph of a 22-year-old female with CHI status after grade III acromyoclavicular dislocation without fracture with HO along the clavicle diaphysis, demonstrating dense peripheral ossification and a lucent zone between the mass and the cortex.

venous thrombosis.[57] Radiographically, HO can be confused with bone tumors, soft tissue infection, or fracture callus proliferation.[58]

The histological features that distinguish HO from other entities were described by Goldman and coworkers and include (1) an intact diaphyseal cortex, (2) ossification about the diaphysis with or without an obvious fracture, (3) a lucent zone between the diaphyseal cortex and the ossifying mass, (4) peripheral localization of the dense calcification, and (5) shrinking of the zone of ossification with maturity (Fig. 19-3).

Heterotopic bone formation has been most commonly reported in association with SCI.[59] Extensive bone formation, especially about the hips, restricts joint mobility, causes pressure sores, and limits sitting or transfer potential with significant compromise of rehabilitation.

Ossification establishes a cleavage plane at the periphery of muscle groups without direct muscle infiltration. Histologically, this new bone between muscle fascicles appears to be derived from the connective tissue.

It may be advisable to allow the HO to mature before inflicting additional trauma (surgery, aggressive manipulation). However, HO activity can persist for 1 to 5 years, and clinical determination of HO maturity can be challenging. Adequate x-ray visualization of the developing HO lesion does not occur until calcification becomes apparent 2 to 5 weeks after the initiation of the process. The initial inflammatory stage of HO presents radiographically as diffuse swelling within the fat planes.[9] Over time, radiographs progress from ill-defined, hazy regions of calcification with poorly defined trabecular formation to sharply defined trabecular masses with distinct margins. However, visible opacity alone does not accurately reflect HO maturity. Serum alkaline phosphatase levels are elevated because of increased new bone formation. However, normalization of alkaline phosphatase levels is a poor indicator of HO maturity.

Ultrasound is a noninvasive and precise indicator of small soft tissue changes and is useful in the diagnosis of impending or established HO. Three-phase scintigraphy provides the earliest and most accurate identification of HO but is not specific for lesion localization or sizing (Fig. 19-4). Although bone scans can detect a decrease in HO activity, this may not be a reliable predictor of mass maturity. Computed tomography (CT) may assist in planning surgical resection by more precise sizing and localization of the soft tissue mass.[60]

The prevention of HO is both difficult and extremely controversial.[5] Diphosphonates given prophylactically cannot prevent the formation of an osteoid matrix which

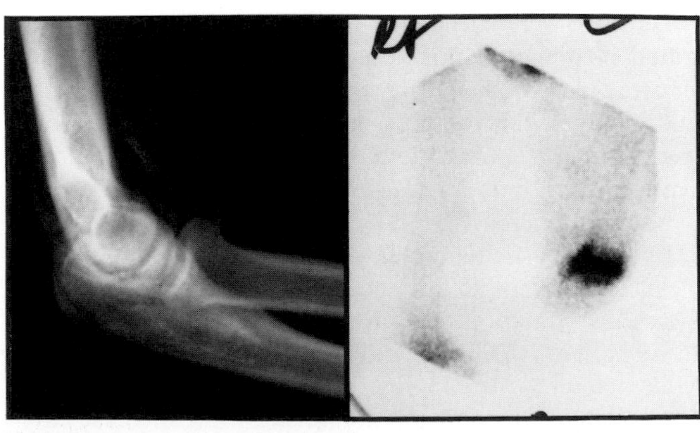

Figure 19-4. *A.* Lateral elbow radiograph of 26-year-old male CHI patient suggests faint HO. *B.* Bone scan clearly demonstrates the active nature of the inflammatory process.

mineralizes upon the completion of treatment.[5] Similar findings were cited by Nollen,[61] who studied the effects of etidronic acid (ethylhydroxydiphosphonate, EHDP) in 25 patients undergoing HO resection. EHDP had a favorable effect on preventing early ossification and maintaining function. However, remineralization of the osteoid occurred after the termination of treatment.[61]

Salicylates are only marginally effective in preventing HO. Indomethacin is more effective; however, it must be given almost immediately after the injury.[5,62] Surgical resection is the sole form of definitive management for a severe symptomatic lesion.[5,49] Prevention of postsurgical recurrence occasionally requires low-dose radiation which begins several days postoperatively and consists of 1000 rad given in 10 sessions.[63] Mild HO recurrence is probable even after adequate radiotherapy if surgical resection is attempted before HO maturity.[64,65]

HO, whether it occurs adjacent to long bones or joints, is not always symptomatic or a functional impediment. Positioning joints in flexion should be avoided, and early passive range-of-motion exercises should be initiated. Patients who demonstrate spasticity require special attention and efforts to maintain functional limb alignment. Regardless of the early severity of the HO, premature surgical excision is contraindicated. Prophylaxis with salicylates or diphosphonates is reasonable during the inflammatory phase to permit vigorous therapy but is a necessity after surgical excision. Frequently, HO management consists more of limiting the process than of preventing or reversing it.

FRACTURE HEALING NOT ALTERED IN CHI?

Several reports by Garland and colleagues suggest that fracture healing in CHI may not differ from healing in other patients.[15,41,66] In a study of tibial diaphyseal fractures with CHI, increased callus formation or accelerated healing was not noted.[66] Similar findings were reported in a review of forearm fractures.[41] In a separate study of femoral fractures, increased callus formation was noted in 52 percent of CHI patients treated operatively, but in nonoperative cases there was no difference in fracture healing.[8]

Even in spastic hemiplegic patients, Garland and associates could not identify accelerated healing or excessive callus formation.[8] In Garland's opinion, CHI predisposed patients to HO but did *not* enhance bone healing. After a review of a 15-year CHI experience, Garland and colleagues could not demonstrate an increase in callus formation or a decrease in time to union in long bone fractures treated nonoperatively.[15] Spencer and coworkers also hypothesized that the increase healing response in CHI was not actually callus but more closely resembled HO.[19] Although the healing response appears to be typical in nature, those authors surmised that the term "callus" is probably inappropriate.

The fracture healing response in patients with SCI is also not universally thought to be enhanced compared with that in patients without neurological injury. One report even suggested that compared to the excessive callus in CHI, SCI may inhibit fracture healing.[5] In this study, SCI patients were actually at greater risk for delayed union, nonunion, and deformity with nonoperative treatment.

After his review of patients with SCI, Garland insisted that the apparent exuberant callus which formed had all the radiographic characteristics of HO, that is, a circumferential bridge of peripheral ossification, usually at a distance from the fracture, in limbs that were treated nonoperatively.[40] Traditional callus was often absent from the fracture site, and Garland concluded that delayed union or nonunion, especially in the femur and tibia, was more prevalent in SCI.

POSSIBLE MECHANISMS OF ALTERED FRACTURED HEALING IN CHI

If fracture healing in CHI is altered, the etiology of this phenomenon is unknown. A number of theories exist in regard to the cause of EBF in CHI, but none have been universally accepted. The more popular theories include spasticity or excess motion at the fracture,[16] hormonal alterations,[67] diminished sympathetic control of local blood flow,[42] metabolic alkalosis,[10] decreased carbon dioxide tension,[68] and resting muscle paralysis.[3] Numerous theories exist,[4,14,30,42,55,67,68] but a single, generally accepted theory has not been identified. Calandriello speculated that loss of neurological function disrupted the regulation of osteogenesis and that a fracture healing moderator or inhibitory factor was altered.[4] Weisz and colleagues also supported the neurogenic theory as they clinically observed enhanced callus formation in patients with cerebral fat embolism.[13] Comarr and associates hypothesized that a diminished sympathetic outflow after SCI enhanced fracture healing with loss of sympathetic tone and increased local blood flow to the fracture site.[42] Excessive fracture site motion, usually from spasticity, has been cited as the cause of enhanced callus formation.[16] Glenn and coworkers noted hyperplastic callus formation as early as 2 weeks after injury in spastic patients.[16] Lindholm and associates manipulated fractured rat tibias daily and found rapid, more abundant callus formation than was the case in nonmanipulated fractures.[69] In a feline fracture model, Spencer and colleagues demonstrated increased bone formation in spastic versus nonspastic limbs.[19] However, these authors could not conclusively attribute the greater callus formation to interfragmentory motion alone and admitted that biomechanical or endocrine factors may have an effect.[18]

The additional trauma of surgical dissection, bleeding, and residual bone debris has been shown to affect local new bone formation.[16,30] Although femur fracture healing seemed to be potentiated by CHI, Glenn and coworkers found that this response was even greater in operatively stabilized injuries.[16] Brumback and colleagues, who cited similar findings, also suggested that an unidentified local and/or systemic factor may be responsible for altered bone response.[30]

Recent evidence has identified a possible humoral factor as the cause of EBF in CHI. Bidner and associates obtained serum samples from patients with CHI alone, CHI and fractures, and fractures only.[14] Growth factor activity was assessed by determining the effect of serum on the incorporation of H thymidine and on osteoblast cell cultures from the calvaria of fetal rats. Samples of serum from the two head injury groups demonstrated a dose-dependent increase in both mitogenic activity and cell number compared with the other two groups. The level of osteoblast activity remained elevated throughout the duration of the neurological insult.

Frymoyer and coworkers used denervated rat limbs as a model to assess subsequent fracture healing.[38] By transecting the sciatic nerve, these authors produced flaccid paralysis, eliminating spasticity or excessive motion as a possible variable. However, these denervated rat limbs still produced more rapid and abundant callus formation. The enhanced fracture healing with only peripheral nerve transection suggests that a neurohumoral mechanism alone is not the probable cause of this phenomenon. Frymoyer and coworkers thought that changes in the local vascular supply secondary to flaccid paralysis promoted fracture healing.

It has been suggested that increased p_{O_2} induced by controlled ventilation stimulates osteogenesis. In a study of manually fractured rat femurs, Yablon and Cruess compared fracture healing in specimens placed in a hyperbaric tank with heating in those subjected to room air only. The specimens exposed to hyperbaric oxygen not only healed faster but healed with more abundant callus than did controls.[70]

However, there is other evidence that diminished oxygenation may stimulate bone formation. Benassy[53] analyzed the O_2, CO_2, and pH of arterial and venous blood in paralytic limbs. He noted that the O_2 level in venous and arterial blood was approximately the same and postulated that a decrease in oxygen at the tissue level may affect fracture repair. These findings were further supported in a study of paralyzed muscle by Armstrong-Ressy and associates that demonstrated reduction in local metabolism, lower CO_2 tension, and a relative alkalosis, all of which favor mineral salt deposition.[68] Changes in local and systemic pH present an interesting explanation for fracture healing regulation.[17] Calcium phosphate is maximally active at pH 7.6 or alkaline where it is less soluble. Using high-resolution phosphorous nuclear magnetic resonance spectroscopy to noninvasively monitor the local pH changes in vivo in rats, these authors documented a 3-week pH shift from acidic to alkaline (7.2 to 7.5), culminating in callus deposition. This change from acidic to alkaline did *not* occur in a hematoma created by direct injection of blood.

Swenson and Claff created fractures in the canine femur and established differences in the pH of the fracture hematoma versus an injected hematoma at varying points in time.[71] At 2½ h the fracture hematoma pH was acidic, but it gradually changed to alkaline over time in a shift that coincided with initial callus formation. In 1987, Neuman and associates also cited alkalosis secondary to traumatic or iatrogenic hyperventilation as the probable etiology of EBF-enhanced fracture healing.[10]

Armstrong-Ressy and associates also identified local and systemic alkalosis as the probable cause of altered healing.[68] They hypothesized that alkalosis occurred locally when inactivity and decreased metabolism of paralyzed muscle lowered carbon dioxide tension and systemically as a result of the hyperventilation employed to decrease intracranial pressure.

GENERAL PRINCIPLES OF FRACTURE MANAGEMENT IN PATIENTS WITH CHI

Although the management of a CHI has usually been granted top priority, it has been recognized that orthopedic problems also warrant early recognition and treatment within a reasonable time frame.[25] Bellamy and Brower appreciated the inaccuracy of attempts to predict final neurological outcome in CHI on the basis of the initial clinical examination.[25]

Because the long-term functional recovery in CHI is uncertain, Wood and Hoffer, in a report of CHI patients with tibia fractures, advised that meticulous care be given to maintaining excellent alignment.[72] Weissman and Khermosh recognized that many injuries to the musculoskeletal system in CHI are entirely missed.[24] Finally, even after more life-threatening injuries have stabilized, continued apprehension often prevents optimal treatment of detected fractures.

Wray and Davies reviewed 75 CHI patients with fractures and recommended only minimal treatment (splints, casts, traction, and elevation) for all noncritical musculoskeletal injuries for the first 48 h.[73] Kernohan and colleagues reported a polytraumatized 44-year-old CHI patient with a neglected anterior shoulder dislocation.[74] Although the patient's head injury resolved, his shoulder required multiple complex reconstructions and his functional prognosis remained guarded at best. To alleviate the confusion over the indications for immediate skeletal surgery, these authors established the following simple criteria: (1) compound fractures, (2) fractures with arterial insufficiency, and (3) major joint dislocations.

The management of limb fractures in CHI can be separated into three distinct phases: acute, recovery, and stable.[22] In the *acute phase,* or the initial hospitalization, fractures must be diagnosed and early treatment must be initiated. In the *recovery phase,* which can last for 12 to 18 months, joint deformities must be prevented or corrected. In the *stable phase,* reconstructive surgery may be needed to correct limb deformities. The success of rehabilitation and the need for reconstructive surgery are substantially affected by the quality of acute-phase interventions.

The diagnosis of skeletal injury in comatose patients requires a strong index of suspicion by the primary treating physician. The initial examination should always include a clinical assessment of all four extremities for gross evidence of fracture. Bone injury may present as obvious limb instability or malalignment or as local warmth, swelling, erythema, or ecchymosis. A negative initial clinical examination does not necessarily indicate an intact skeleton. Fractures in close proximity to joints may not inhibit normal joint motion, multiple fractures in the same limb can be easily overlooked, and centrally located injuries (hip, pelvis, shoulder) can be masked by the surrounding soft tissue.

In a review of 91 CHI patients with a variety of fractures, 66 patients were ultimately capable of independent ambulation.[22] Carey and associates[75] reviewed 6194 general inpatients from 22 rehabilitation facilities and found that the CHI patients were capable of making major functional gains. However, skeletal injuries that are of minimal significance in an otherwise normal patient seem to have profound implications in a neurologically compromised patient.[75]

The agitation and confusion frequently experienced by CHI patients can wreak havoc on efforts to temporarily control limb alignment. These patients often thrash about, pull at external supports, and in essence struggle against all perceived restraints. Splints must be made extremely secure; casts, although more stable, must be restrained to avoid self-inflicted injury; and traction has to be monitored and/or adjusted constantly. The obvious concern is that these patients are at increased risk for nonunion, malunion, secondary neurovascular injury, or needless violation of the soft tissue envelope (a closed fracture becoming an open one). The general patient care concern with traction or splints is restricted mobility that compromises nursing care and transport for necessary diagnostic procedures. Skeletal fixation (internal or external) is preferred when feasible, as it does not limit patient movement or positioning and facilitates overall patient care.

Positioning of joints requires as much attention as does long bone alignment if these patients are to achieve maximum functional recovery. Joints should *never* be maintained in a flexed position, especially in a patient with significant spasticity or rigidity. Acceptable immobilization alignment for major joints includes the following: elbow, 135 degrees (45 degrees of flexion from full extension); wrist, neutral; metacarpophalangeal joints, 45 to 60 degrees; interphalangeal joints, neutral (full extension); thumb, extended/abducted; and hips, knees, and ankles, neutral. Conservatively managed fractures can often displace, shorten, or angulate while maintaining joint extension, making internal fixation even more desirable.

The treatment options for fractures in CHI patients are operative versus nonoperative and closed versus open. Nonoperative treatment, which implies that the fracture can be treated closed or without direct disruption of the soft tissue envelope, is feasible when fractures are stable and adequately aligned or can be easily reduced and both the fracture and the adequately aligned or can be easily reduced and both the fracture and the adjacent joint can be held in alignment by external methods (splint, cast, traction, or bed rest). If more aggressive measures are required to reduce and stabilize a limb injury (surgical incision, excessive traction or manipulation), a general anesthetic is necessary to minimize pain and allow less traumatic realignment. When anesthesia is risked, the orthopedic surgeon must select stabilization methods that guarantee that proper alignment will be maintained.

Nonoperative Treatment

Splints are adequate for initial immobilization, but only in a stable, peripheral fracture will this suffice as definitive treatment. A combative patient has considerable mobility within a splint and will often remove it. More proximally located limb fractures are best treated in a cast which is not so easily discarded. However, if the cast is too tight, CHI patients are not likely to alert the physician to impending pressure sores or other complications.[76] Therefore, casts must be constantly monitored, bivalved prophylactically if excessive swelling is evident, and changed repeatedly to maintain a snug fit.

The authors reserve this treatment for simple, stable fractures in minimally agitated patients.

Traction as the definitive fracture treatment is usually ill advised in CHI patients, as all aspects of patient care are severely compromised. If traction is unavoidable, skin traction is always contraindicted. Skeletal traction, with percutaneous pin placement through bone, is more secure and allows a better transfer of load to the affected limb. This is essential, as traction is primarily indicated for large central fractures (pelvis, hip, femur) which require considerably more weight to maintain alignment. Some authors have combined a cast and traction to control length and rotation while preventing joint contractures.[76]

Operative Treatment

Regardless of the severity of a CHI, the most effective fracture management often consists of internal fixation because of the unreliability of the patient, the unknown functional outcome, and the constant monitoring and readjustments associated with splints, casts, and traction. However, surgical fixation requires general anesthesia, with its attendent risks in this patient group, including difficulties in monitoring and maintaining the patient's neurological and hemodynamic status.

When elective general anesthesia is contemplated in a patient with a CHI, the following guidelines have been recommended[22,76]:

1. Documentation of normal intracranial pressure; magnetic resonance imaging (MRI) or CT negative for intracranial hemorrhage and/or mass
2. A stable neurological status for at least 24 h to avoid masking or potentiating a progressive lesion
3. An anesthesiologist experienced in neuroanesthesia to ensure adequate ventilation, minimize vasodilatation with proper anesthetic selection, maintain proper fluid status and avoid hypotension and hyponatremia.

The optimal time for surgical intervention is unclear and must be individualized according to intracranial pressure, presence of intracranial mass, stability of neurological status, and associated injuries. Most deaths that are a direct consequence of CHI occur in the first week; death thereafter results from associated medical complications.[76] Virtually all CHI patients can undergo orthopedic surgery within 2 weeks. If there is cause to delay surgery beyond 2 weeks in light of possible accelerated fracture healing, the neurosurgeon and orthopedist should discuss the changing risks and/or benefits in terms of the final neurological and functional outcome.

Ideally, the standard care for specific fractures associated with CHI should be similar to that used in the general population.[77] In addition to the previously discussed preoperative considerations, the management of CHI-associated fractures may require special diagnostic, therapeutic, or rehabilitation considerations specific to the particular injury. Upper extremity fractures have been reported to be less common than are lower extremity injuries in CHI.[22] Although upper extremities are non-weight-bearing limbs, they are frequently essential for crutch and/or walker support during rehabilitation and should not be viewed as "less" of a priority. Not only are lower extremity injuries often more severe fractures,[22] requirements for gait demand precision in restoring acceptable limb length, alignment, and joint function.

Open Fractures

A fracture is considered open when the bone or fracture hematoma communicates with the external environment through disrupted skin and soft tissue.[78] Because open fractures are contaminated and predisposed to deep wound infection, *immediate* surgical debridement, intravenous antibiotics, and immobilization are essential. Without urgent debridement, the incidence of nonunion and infection is extremely high.[79] It should be emphasized that antibiotics are only an adjuvant to early surgical debridement.[80] Immobilization must provide reliable stability to permit neovascularization of the wound and endosteal/periosteal blood supply. The initial debridement is most effective when performed within 8 h of injury. Initial irrigation of the wound with antibiotic solution is advisable until definitive sharp debridement and deep wound lavage are performed.

Joint Dislocations

Joint dislocations in conjunction with CHI merit special mention. If it is unrecognized and left unreduced, a dislocated joint can become extremely painful with limited range of motion or stability. Later reduction is difficult because of soft tissue scarring, and early articular joint degeneration is inevitable. Clinical inspection of the four extremities will suggest many dislocations because of awkward limb alignment (ankle, wrist), difficult passive motion (hip, shoulder), or gross instability (knee, elbow). Routine radiographs are mandatory to distinguish a simple dislocation from a fracture dislocation. Neurovascular compromise is common with many dislocations and always should be assessed *before* reduction.[81,82] An early attempt at closed reduction should be made after complete assessment of the injury. This will alleviate pressure and/or tension on local neurovascular structures, permit soft tissue healing to occur with the joint reduced, avoid a more traumatic late reduction, and enhance the chances for a functional joint. After reduction, extremes of motion should be gently applied to the limb to determine the extent and direction of the instability, thus assisting with rehabilitation. Efforts must be made to maintain the joints in as functional a position as the instability pattern allows. This will limit loss of functional motion resulting from contractures or HO while maintaining joint alignment. Finally, all closed dislocated joints that are reduced should be assessed for joint congruity and the presence of an intraarticular body.

TREATMENT OF SPECIFIC FRACTURES

The *shoulder girdle* is the prevalent site of upper extremity injury in CHI patients. Except for the superficial clavicle, the prominent muscular envelope can obscure these injuries. Occasionally, they are detected inadvertently on chest radiographs. Routine x-rays views of this region include an anteroposterior (AP), a lateral (LAT), and the axillary shoulder, or "Y" scapula, views. A stress AP view with downward pull on the arm may be necessary to detect an unstable acromioclavicular dislocation or unstable lateral clavicle fracture. More complex injuries may be best assessed with a CT scan, which can easily be obtained when the patient undergoes a head CT. Major injury to the shoulder girdle should always alert the physician to the possibility of a brachial plexus injury that can be masked by coma.

Clavicle fractures usually respond well to sling immobilization, even when extensive comminution is present. More aggressive treatment is warranted only for select fractures which threaten to perforate the overlying skin and lateral fractures associated with disruption of the coracoclavicular ligament and vertical migration of the medial clavicular fragment.[83] *Scapula fractures* also respond to simple sling immobilization unless a glenoid fracture disrupts shoulder joint stability.[84] These fractures often are associated with chest, rib, lung, or neurovascular injuries, which must be ruled out.

Proximal humerus fractures can be treated with a sling if there is minimal displacement or angulation (<1 cm displacement or 45 degrees of angulation) of the four major components: humeral head, shaft, greater tuberosity, and lesser tuberosity[85] (Fig. 19-5). Significant displacement requires bony reduction and repair of the rotator cuff injury, if present. Either alone or in conjunction with a fracture, a dislocation is easily missed. Fractures in conjunction with dislocation are at greater risk for local neurovascular injury.

Unlike fractures of the shoulder girdle, *humerus shaft fractures* are readily detected clinically because of gross malalignment or instability. Radial nerve injury is prevalent with this type of fracture as a result of its close proximity to bone and must be considered until its function can be established. Routine treatment in the general population usually consists of closed sling, splint, or cast support, which allows excellent healing potential and reasonable functional accommodation of mild shortening or angulation.[86] More aggressive stabilization is reserved for patients presenting with agitation, polytrauma, deteriorating radial nerve function, or the need for immediate shoulder or elbow rehabilitation.

Elbow fractures can have profound functional effects in CHI.[87] Fracture instability is not always readily appreciated clinically, but soft tissue swelling and ecchymosis can be easily detected and fractures can be confirmed by plain radiographs. Closed fracture treatment requires that the joint be both stable and congruous and that adequate alignment be maintained while early motion is permitted. Even in the absence of spasticity, prolonged closed treatment may cause flexion contractures, which can be further complicated by HO. Therefore, immobilization should never exceed 45 degrees of flexion. Operative reduction and fixation of

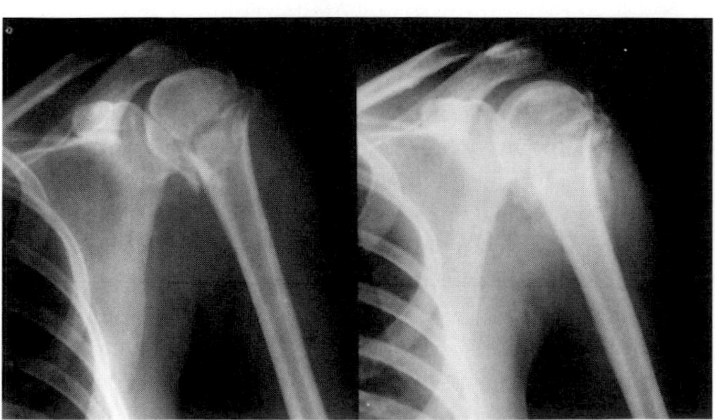

Figure 19-5. *A.* A 30-year-old female CHI patient also sustained a comminuted, minimally displaced proximal humerus fracture. *B.* Within 6 weeks, exuberant callus was evident on x-ray and passive and active motion were possible.

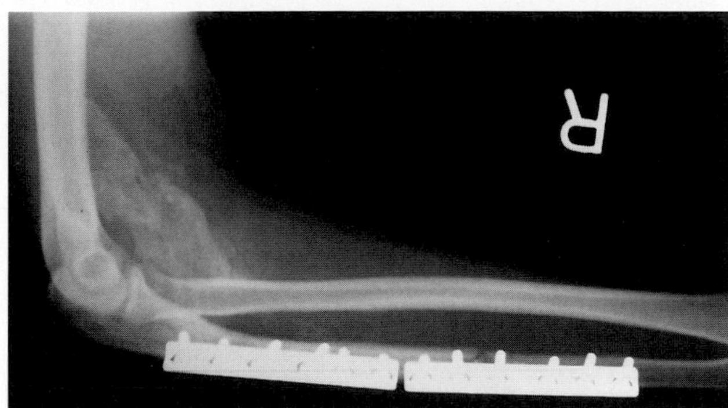

Figure 19-6. A female CHI patient sustained an ulnar fracture with volar dislocation of the radial head (Monteggia fracture dislocation pattern). Despite uneventful open reduction and fixation of the ulna and closed radial head reduction, fulminant elbow HO prevented acceptable elbow function and had to be excised upon mass maturity.

the distal humerus or proximal olecranon or radius are preferred because it allows early active or passive motion to offset the tendency toward contracture. Patients with concomminant elbow dislocation are especially at risk for ectopic bone formation[7] (Fig. 19-6). Ulnar nerve injury, either primary or iatrogenic, is common with these injuries and merits close observation until its function is assured.

In *forearm fractures,* obvious limb instability and malalignment make clinical diagnosis and radiographic confirmation relatively easily. Operative reduction and fixation are absolutely essential if proper limb function is to be restored. The objective in forearm fracture management is to achieve and maintain the anatomic alignment necessary for forearm rotation (pronation/supination) to occur.[50] An isolated simple radius or ulna fracture may be amenable to closed treatment if the patient is not spastic or agitated, but fragment alignment in the presence of concomitant ulna and radius fractures is difficult to ensure even in a compliant patient.[41] Also, adequate closed treatment requires prolonged immobilization of both the elbow and the wrist.

Surgical fixation of both bone forearm fractures can be performed directly with plates and screws or indirectly with intramedullary nails. The authors prefer plates and screws, as anatomic reduction can be ensured. Garland and Waters support intramedullary nail fixation to minimize the risk of synostosis formation, which they feel can be significant in one-third of head injury patients[76] (Fig. 19-7). To minimize the risk of synostosis, early passive motion should be alternated with splint and/or brace immobilization in a neutral rotation alignment.

Distal radius fractures usually present with deformity and swelling, can be confirmed by radiographs, and are amenable to early closed reduction and splinting. When the fracture pattern is extraarticular, without comminution, and the patient is tolerant of splint or cast immobilization, closed treatment should be sufficient if acceptable distal radial length and alignment can be maintained.[88] Unstable fractures and intraarticular fractures are better treated with pin, plate, and/or external fixation devices.[89] The distal radius has two joints which require congruous reduction and alignment: the radiocarpal and the distal radial-ulnar joints. Although neither is subjected to large axial loads, both must tolerate repetitive shear stresses from normal wrist flexion-extension and forearm pronation-supination. Posttraumatic carpal tunnel syndrome or median neuropathy may result from injury or treatment if cast and/or splints are tightly or poorly positioned.

The clinical diagnosis of carpal injury in the wrist and/or hand is less likely, and x-rays are not always conclusive; therefore, carpal fractures may go undetected.[90] In the acute setting, efforts should focus on injury detection and splinting, with definitive treatment to follow initial stabilization of the CHI. A technetium bone scan more than 72 h after injury can be helpful in documenting and localizing injury in this region. Scaphoid fractures can be casted if they are adequately aligned. Surgical stabilization is required if the fracture is displaced or unstable.[91] It is important to identify carpal dislocation (scaphoid, lunate), as simple closed treatment will not suffice.

Functional consideratons are especially important in treating *metacarpal* and *phalangeal fractures.* After initial splinting, radiographs are assessed to determine if the fractures involved the metacarpal base and/or head, metacarpal shaft with comminution, phalangeal base and/or head, or phalangeal shaft comminution. Recognition of these injuries would suggest surgical intervention, even if only for simple percutaneous pinning, in order to avoid metacarpal and/or phalanx shortening or malrotation.[92] Wrist and/or hand injuries are not usually life-threatening and can be addressed semiurgently. If later reconstruction becomes unavoidable, it is usually less complicated than is the case with a more proximal neglected injury.

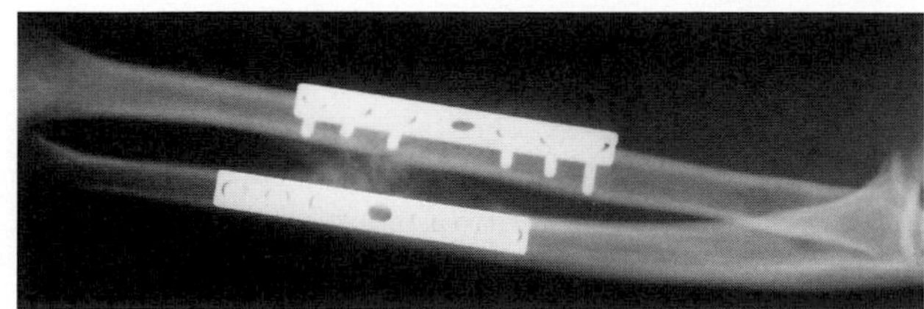

Figure 19-7. A male CHI patient with closed bone fractures of both forearms treated with plate fixation developed ectopic ossification which progressed into synostosis and limited forearm rotation.

Fractures of the *pelvis* can produce significant vascular, neurological, and visceral injury and constitute a significant source of morbidity and mortality which can rival that from an acute head injury. Simple or stable pelvic fractures respond to symptomatic treatment. However, unstable pelvis fractures may result in enormous loss of blood and require emergency volume replacement, pelvis slings, external fixation, and/or angiography with selective embolization.[87] Plain radiographs usually detect pelvic injury; however, CT scans are frequently necessary to establish the extent of injury and determine stability. Acute management often consists of early external fixation and perhaps application of MAST trousers to decrease intrapelvic volume and tamponade bleeding. Longitudinal skeletal traction, although not ideal, is often essential to prevent cephalad migration of the hemipelvis and subsequent discrepancies of leg length.

Pelvic injuries which require surgery warrant well-coordinated efforts between neurosurgery and orthopedic surgery physicians. A CHI patient must be able to withstand a prolonged anesthetic and a surgical dissection which may cause massive blood loss. Despite stabilization, the major subsequent complication of these injuries is the continued risk of thromboembolic disease because of limited mobilization potential. Anticoagulation may be contraindicated as a result of bleeding, and a vena caval filter should be considered. The major late complication is grossly malaligned healing, which can compromise both gait and sitting or subject the patient to the significant morbidity of late reconstructive efforts.

Fractures of the *acetabulum* possess all the problems of pelvic fractures with the additional need to restore the stability, congruity, and motion of a major weight-bearing joint. The central location of this fracture in an unresponsive patient increases the likelihood that it will not be detected. After x-ray diagnosis, ipsilateral limb traction can assist in maintaining temporary alignment and reduction. Sciatic nerve palsy is common and should be suspected until an adequate examination is possible.

After the CHI has stabilized, the displaced or unstable injury requires surgical reduction and fixation.[93] Maintaining joint alignment, even if anatomic congruity is impossible, is of benefit, as it makes later reconstructive efforts less complicated. Posttraumatic arthritis, HO, pain, and loss of motion are the most prevalent complications related to acetabulum injury. Neglected or unrecognized acetabular fractures can both shorten and ankylose, further compromising both the sitting and the ambulatory potential of the patient.

With a fractured hip, the affected limb will clinically present as markedly shortened and malrotated. After x-ray confirmation of injury, the limb should be placed in traction during the acute head injury phase. Definitive treatment consists of either internal fixation or prosthetic replacement, depending on the viability of the femoral head's vascularity. Fractures amenable to fixation must be internally stabilized as soon as possible to ensure fracture union and a normal joint. Prosthetic joint replacements can be delayed for a while, but traction must be maintained to preserve limb length. Regardless of the treatment, patient mobilization is compromised until surgery can be performed. Aside from the usual complications of nonunion or avascular necrosis, CHI patients are at risk for HO, and early passive motion can be of enormous benefit.

Fractures of the *femur* are clinically suggested by thigh swelling, erythema, instability, pain, and/or malalignment. Skeletal traction is employed acutely to maintain length, provide temporary stability, and permit initial management of the head injury. However, traction will not suffice as a definitive treatment because of the restraints placed on overall CHI management, an inability to assure acceptable alignment, and the prolonged immobilization necessary before cast application. CHI patients with unstabilized femurs in traction are at acute risk for fat emboli and respiratory compromise, and later thromboembolism is a concern.

The preferred surgical fixation can await stabilization of the head injury for up to 2 weeks but should not be delayed needlessly, as closed intramedullary nailing, the fixation of choice, becomes more difficult.[94] HO is common even when the fracture can be fixed by closed indirect methods. If open fracture reduction and nailing are necessary, HO can develop more extensively and threaten knee motion through quadriceps scarring (Fig. 19-8). After fixation, passive motion of the limb can begin while one awaits resolution of the coma.

Intraarticular injuries of the *knee* require clinical suspicion, restoration of joint congruity, and early motion if reasonable function is to be achieved. Clinically, the patient presents with a knee effusion, warmth, or instability.[95] Joint aspiration of a hemarthrosis confirms the injury and will provide some symptomatic relief. Radiographs may reveal bony injuries but occasionally do not depict the complexity of injury without tomograms or CT scans. Immobilization in plaster or a cast brace will suffice for ligamentous injuries until a more in-depth evaluation can be performed. If early passive motion is possible, definitive elective ligamentous surgical reconstruction can be delayed and performed electively. Fractures also can await initial CHI management but should be addressed more urgently, before passive motion. The major functional complication is residual joint instability or posttraumatic arthritis.

The superficial location of the *tibia* makes it highly susceptible to fracture, and as in the general population, the initial focus is the extent of soft tissue injury: open versus closed fracture, compartment syndrome, and distal neurovascular status. Clinical diagnosis of a fracture is usually obvious, and the bony aspect of the injury can be assessed adequately with plain x-rays. The initial

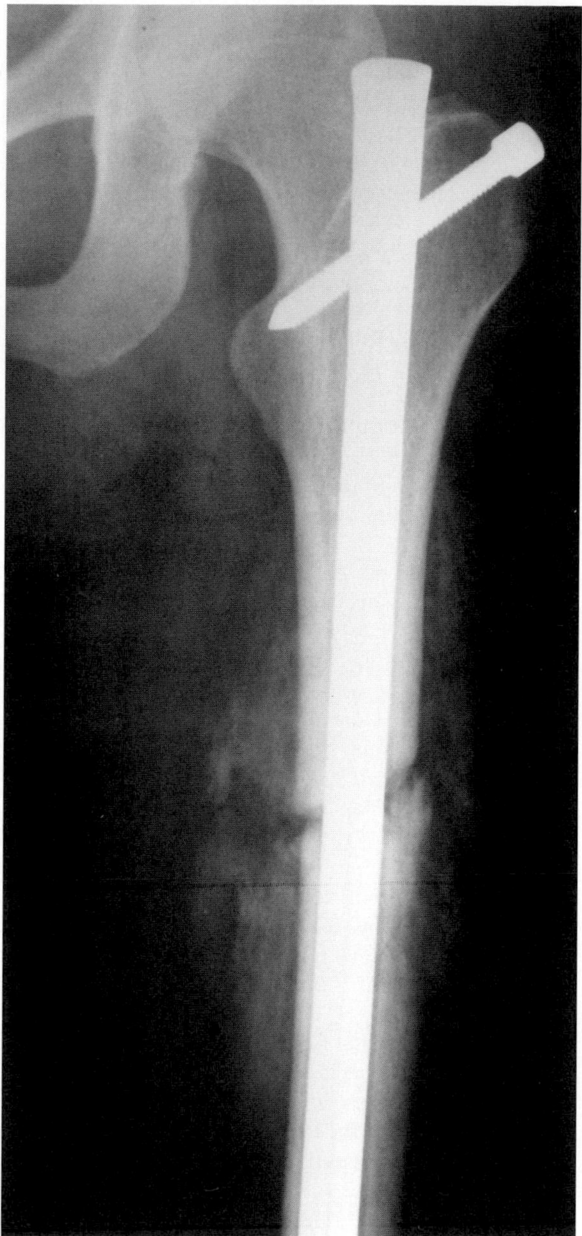

Figure 19-8. The status of a 22-year-old male CHI patient 3 weeks after closed nailing of a left femur fracture demonstrates abundant early ossification which radiographically could be termed either callus or HO. Regardless, early passive or active knee motion is essential to minimize quadriceps muscle scarring.

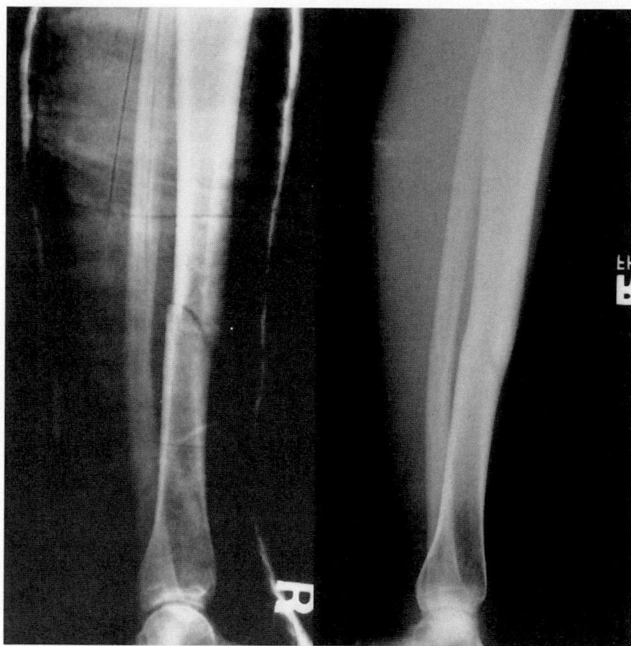

Figure 19-9. *A.* A male CHI patient with a stable short oblique closed midshaft tibial fracture amenable to cast immobilization. *B.* Fracture healing occurred in acceptable alignment without abundant callus formation.

treatment consists of plaster splint immobilization which accommodates further soft tissue swelling and initial management of the head injury. Definitive treatment depends on the fracture's stability. Garland and Toder demonstrated that acceptable union rates in tibial fractures can be achieved with conventional plaster cast methods if alignment can be maintained[66] (Fig. 19-9). A malaligned/unstable injury is best managed with an intramedullary nail (closed fracture) or external fixation (open fractures) (Fig. 19-10). The complications usually encountered include malalignment, delayed or nonunion healing, and infection. Reconstructive procedures of the tibia can be complicated and lengthy and are best avoided by means of proper initial treatment.

Prominent soft tissue swelling and intraarticular disruption with joint instability are the primary problems associated with an acute *ankle fracture.* Clinical examination may suggest injury, and an x-ray should confirm the fracture. Splint immobilization acutely minimizes pain, fracture displacement, and additional swelling. When the CHI has stabilized, surgical fixation is warranted in all but nondisplaced, stable injuries.[96] The treatment can defer to considerations associated with the CHI, as later fixation of these fractures can still be extremely successful if proper immobilization and nonweight bearing are adhered to. Posttraumatic arthritis, if it occurs, responds well to ankle arthrodesis.

Although fractures of the *foot* merit a relatively low priority in the acute management of CHI, they should not be completely ignored, as prominent soft tissue swelling, a compartment syndrome, or wound contamination may culminate in a needless amputation. The initial clinical assessment should determine the status of foot vascularity, skin viability, and compartment swelling. X-rays provide sufficient imaging for most fractures; calcaneus or talus fractures may benefit from CT scan assessment. Aside from closed reduction of obvious major joint dislocations (subtalar, talonavicular, meta-

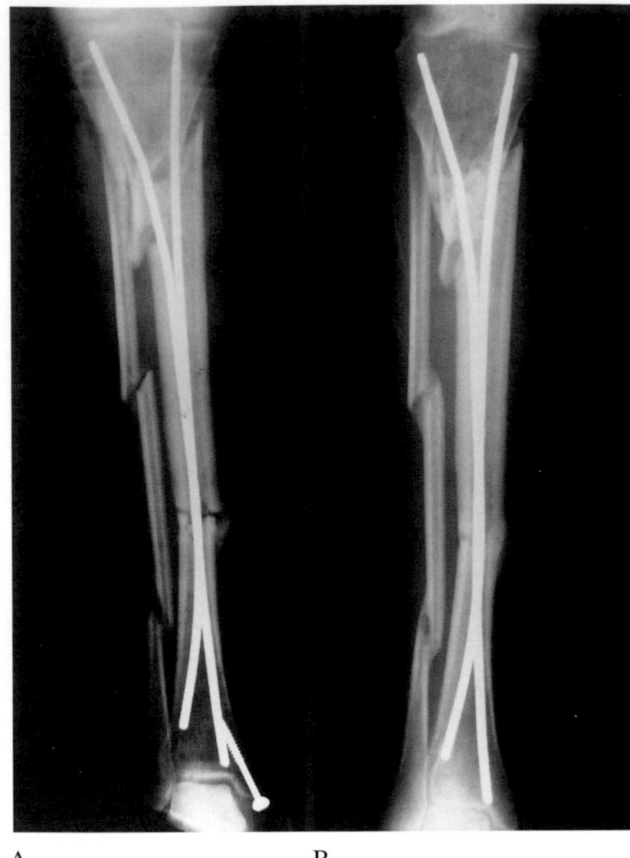

Figure 19-10. *A.* A closed segmental tibia fracture with gross instability in a male CHI patient treated with Ender's nails. *B.* Despite the fractures' gross instability and the usual tendency for delayed or nonunion healing, rapid healing occurred at both fracture sites.

carpal-phalangeal, etc.), simple plaster splinting and elevation constitute adequate initial care until definitive treatment can be entertained. Displaced fractures of the hindfoot (calcaneus or talus) respond better to reduction and internal fixation, especially if the injuries involve a joint, and usually can wait 1 to 2 weeks before surgery.[97,98] Midfoot fractures (navicular, cuneiform, cuboidal) can be treated with percutaneous pinning to maintain bone and joint alignment. Forefoot injuries (tarsometatarsal, phalanges) also are amenable to percutaneous pin fixation once the CHI is stable. Hindfoot and midfoot malunion/nonunion generally can be addressed with fusions; residual forefoot problems are also suitable for fusion or resection.

References

1. Glenn MB, Rosenthal M: Rehabilitation following severe traumatic brain injury. *Semin Neurol* 5:233–246, 1985.
2. Irving MH, Irving PM: Associated injuries in head injuries patients. *J Trauma* 7:500–511, 1967.
3. Benassy J, Mazabraud A, Diverres J: L'osteogenese neurogene. *Rev Chir Orthop* 49, 1963.
4. Calandriello B: Callus formation in severe brain injuries. *Istituto Ortopedico Toscano* "P. Palagi" 170–175, 1964.
5. Cope R: Heterotopic ossification. *South Med J* 83:1058–1064, 1990.
6. Garland DE, Miller G: Fractures and dislocations about the hip in head-injured adults. *Clin Orthop* 186:154–158, 1984.
7. Garland DE, O'Hollaren RM: Fractures and dislocations about the elbow in the head-injured adult. *Clin Orthop* 168:38–41, 1982.
8. Garland DE, Rothi B, Waters RL: Femoral fractures in head-injured adults. *Clin Orthop* 166:219–225, 1982.
9. Herold HZ, Tadmor A, Hurvitz A: Callus formation after acute brain damage. *Isr J Med Sci* 6:163–166, 1970.
10. Newman RJ, Stone MH, Mukherjee SK: Associated fracture union in association with severe head injury. *Br J Accident Surg* 18:241–246, 1987.
11. Perkins R, Skirving AP: Callus formation and the rate of healing of femoral fractures in patients with head injuries. *J Bone Joint Surg* 69B:521–524, 1987.
12. Smith R: Head injury, fracture healing, and callus. *J Bone Joint Surg* 69B:518–520, 1987.
13. Weisz GM, Fishman J, Steiner E: Callus formation in cases of cerebral fat embolism (a contribution to the theory of neurogenic influence on osteogenesis). *Conf Neurol* 31:362–369, 1969.
14. Bidner SM, Rubins IM, Desjardins JV, et al: Evidence for a humoral mechanism for enhanced osteogenesis after head injury. *J Bone Joint Surg* 72A:1144–1149, 1990.
15. Garland DE: Clinical observations on fractures and heterotopic ossification in spinal cord and traumatic brain injured population. *Clin Orthop* 233:86–101, 1988.
16. Glenn JN, Miner ME, Peltier LF: The treatment of fractures of the femur in patients with head injuries. *J Trauma* 13:958–961, 1973.
17. Newman RJ, Phil D, Duthie RB, Francis MJO: Nuclear magnetic resonance studies of fracture repair. *Clin Orthop* 198:297–303, 1985.
18. Spencer RF: The effect of head injury on fracture healing. *J Bone Joint Surg* 69B:525–528, 1987.
19. Spencer RF, Bullock R, Cooper K, et al: The effect of a brain lesion on bone healing. *J Orthop Res* 8:646–650, 1990.
20. Wilkes JA, Hoffer MM: Clavicle fractures in head-injured children. *J Orthop Trauma* 1:55–58, 1987.
21. Garland DE, Blum CE, Waters RL: Periarticular heterotopic ossification in head-injured adults. *J Bone Joint Surg* 62A:1143–1146, 1980.
22. Garland DE, Rhoades ME: Orthopedic management of brain-injured adults. *Clin Orthop* 131:111–122, 1978.
23. Lewin W: Factors in the mortality of closed head injury. *Br Med J* 1:1239–1244, 1953.
24. Weissman SL, Khermosh O: Orthopedic aspects in multiple injuries. *J Trauma* 10:377–385, 1970.

25. Bellamy R, Brower TD: Management of skeletal trauma in the patient with head injury. *J Trauma* 14:1021–1028, 1974.
26. Brink JD, Imbus C, Woo-Sam J: Physical recovery after severe closed head trauma in children and adolescents. *J Pediatr* 97:721–727, 1980.
27. Eichenholtz SN: Management of long-bone fractures in paraplegic patients. *J Bone Joint Surg* 45A:299–310, 1963.
28. Riedel B: Demonstration eines durchachtagiges Umhergenhen total destruirten Kniegelenkes von einem Patienten mit Stichverletzung des Ruckens. *Verh Dtsch Ges Chir* 12:93–96, 1883.
29. Asselmeier J, Light TR: Heterotopic para-articular ossification of the proximal interphalangeal joint. *J Hand Surg* 17A:154–157, 1992.
30. Brumback RJ, Wells JD, Lakatos R, et al: Heterotopic ossification about the hip after intramedullary nailing for fractures of the femur. *J Bone Joint Surg* 72A:1067–1073, 1990.
31. Marks PH, Paley D, Kellam JF: Heterotopic ossification around the hip with intramedullary nailing of the femur. *J Trauma* 28:1207–1214, 1988.
32. Mendelson L, Grosswasser Z, Najenson T, et al: Periarticular new bone formation in patients suffering from severe head injuries. *Scand J Rehabil Med* 7:141–145, 1974.
33. Mital MA, Garber JE, Stinson JT: Ectopic bone formation in children and adolescents with head injuries: Its management. *J Pediatr Orthop* 7:84–90, 1987.
34. Roberts PH: Heterotopic ossification complicating paralysis of intracranial origin. *J Bone Joint Surg* 50B:70–79, 1968.
35. Sazbon L, Najenson T, Tartakovsky M, et al: Widespread periarticular new-bone formation in long-term comatose patients. *J Bone Joint Surg* 63B:120–125, 1981.
36. Wainapel SF, Rao PU, Schepsis AA: Ulnar nerve compression by heterotopic ossification in a head-injured patient. *Arch Phys Med Rehabil* 66:512–514, 1985.
37. Wenner SM: Heterotopic ossification of the shoulder following head injury. *Clin Orthop* 212:231–236, 1986.
38. Frymoyer JW, Pope MH: Fracture healing in the sciatically denervated rat. *J Trauma* 17:355–361, 1977.
39. Quilis AN, Gonzalez AP: Healing in denervated bones. *Acta Orthop Scand* 45:820–835, 1974.
40. Garland DE: Correspondence. *J Bone Joint Surg* 74(1):152–153, 1992.
41. Garland DE, Dowling V: Forearm fractures in the head-injured adult. *Clin Orthop* 176:190–196, 1983.
42. Comarr AE, Hutchinson RH, Bors E: Extremity fractures of patients with spinal cord injuries. *Am J Surg* 103:732–739, 1962.
43. Conner JM: *Soft Tissue Ossification.* New York: Springer-Verlag, 1983.
44. Johnson JTH: A typical myositis ossificans. *Acta Pathol Microbiol Scand* 74:11–25, 1957.
45. Rosendahl S, Christoffersentk NM: Periarticular ossification following hip replacement: *Acta Orthop Scand* 48:400–404, 1977.
46. Lorber J: Ectopic ossification in tuberculous meninigitis. *Arch Dis Child* 28:98–103, 1953.
47. Storey G, Tegner WS: Paraplegic para-articular calcification. *Ann Rheum Dis* 14:176–182, 1955.
48. Stoikovic JP, Bonfiglio M, Paul WD: Myositis ossificans complicating poliomyelitis. *Arch Phys Med Rehabil* 36:236–243, 1955.
49. Hamplen DL: Ectopic ossification, in Ling RSM (ed): *Complications of Total Hip Replacement.* London: Churchill-Livingstone, 1984:108.
50. Anderson L, Sisk T, Tooms R, Park W: Compression-plate fixation in acute diaphyseal fractures of the radius and ulna. *J Bone Joint Surg* 57(A):287–297, 1975.
51. Déjérine J, Ceillier A: Para-osteo-arthropatnies des paraplegiques par lesion medullaire (etude clinique et radiographique). *Ann Med Intern (Paris)* 5:497–535, 1918.
52. Meyer P: Dystrophische Muskelver Kalkung und Vernocherung (Myositis ossificans neurotica) und 'Kal Kmetastasen der Nieren nach Querschnittslasion des Ruckenmarks. *Bruns Beitr Klin Chir* 138:233–254, 1927.
53. Miller LF, O'Neill CJ: Myositis ossificans in paraplegies. *J Bone Joint Surg Am* 31:283–294, 1949.
54. Soule AB Jr: Neurogenic ossifying fibromyopathies: A preliminary report. *J Neurosurg* 2:485–497, 1945.
55. Benassy J: Ossifications and fracture healing in paraplegics and brain injuries. *Proc Annu Clin Spinal Cord Inj Conf* 15:55–70, 1966.
56. Goldberg MA: Heterotopic ossification mimicking acute arthritis after neurologic catastrophes. *Arch Intern Med* 137:619–621, 1977.
57. Distunno JF, Venier LH: Heterotopic ossification presenting as deep vein thrombophlebitis in the paraplegic—a report of 2 cases. *Arch Phys Med Rehabil* 51:719, 1970.
58. Hendrix RW, Calinoff L, Lederman RB, et al: Radiology of pressure sores. *Radiology* 138:351–256, 1981.
59. Bressler EL, Marn CS, Gore RM, Hendrix RW: Evaluation of ectopic bone by C.T. *AJR* 148:931–935, 1987.
60. Kirkpatrick JS, Koman LA, Rovere GD: The role of ultrasound in the early diagnosis of myositis ossificons: A case report. *Am J Sports Med* 15:179–181, 1987.
61. Nollen AJG: Effects of ethylhydroxydiphosphonate (EHDP) on heterotopic ossification. *Acta Orthop Scand* 57:358–381, 1986.
62. Schmide SA, Kjaersgaard-Anderson P, Pedersen NW, et al: The use of indomethacin to prevent the formation of heterotopic bone after total hip replacement. *J Bone Joint Surg [Am]* 70:834–838, 1988.
63. VorenKamp SE, Nelson TL: Ulnar nerve entrapment due to heterotopic bone formation after a severe burn. *J Hand Surg* 12A:378–380, 1987.
64. Ayers DG, Evarts CM, Parkinson JR: The prevention of heterotopic ossification in high-risk patients by low-dose radiation therapy after total hip arthroplasty. *J Bone Joint Surg [Am]* 68:1423–1430, 1986.
65. Brunner R, Morscher E, Huing R: Para-articular ossification in total hip replacement: An indication for radiation therapy. *Arch Orthop Trauma Surg* 106:102–107, 1987.
66. Garland DE, Toder L: Fractures of the tibia diaphysis in adults with head injuries. *Clin Orthop* 150:198–202,1980.

67. Haas HG: Skelet und Mineralsoffwechsel, in Siegenthalar W (ed): *Klinische Pathophysiologie.* Stuttgart: Thieme, 867, 1970.
68. Armstrong-Ressy CT, Weiss AA, Ebel A: Results of surgical treatment of extra-osseous ossification in spinal cord injuries. *Proceedings of the 6th Annual Clinical Paraplegia Conference,* V.A. Hospital, Richmond, Va. October 12–17, 1957.
69. Lindholm RV, Lindholm TS, Toikkanen S, et al: Effect of forces on fragmental movements on the healing of tibial fractures in rats. *Acta Orthop Scand* 40:721–728, 1969.
70. Yablon IG, Cruess RL: The effect of hyperbaric oxygen on fracture healing in rats. *J Trauma* 8:186–202, 1968.
71. Swenson O, Claff CL: Changes in the hydrogen ion concentration of healing fractures. *Proc Soc Exp Biol Med* 61:151–154, 1946.
72. Wood D, Hoffer MM: Tibial fractures in head-injured children. *J Trauma* 27:65–68, 1987.
73. Wray JB, Davies CH: The management of skeletal fractures in the patient with a head injury. *South Med J* 53:748–753, 1960.
74. Kernohan J, Dakin PK, Beacon JP, Bayley JIL: Treatment of major skeletal injuries in patients with a severe head injury. *Br Med J* 288:1822–1823, 1984.
75. Carey RG, Seibert JH, Posavac EJ: Who makes the most progress in inpatient rehabilitation? An analysis of functional gain. *Arch Phys Med Rehabil* 69:337–343, 1988.
76. Garland DE, Waters RL: Extremity fractures in head injured adults, in Meyers, M.H. (ed.): *The Multiply Injured Patient with Complex Fractures.* Philadelphia, Lea & Febiger, 1984:134–155.
77. Rockwood CA, Green DP, Bucholz RW: *Fractures in Adults,* 3d ed. Philadelphia: Lippincott, 1991.
78. Gregory CF: Open fractures, in Rockwood CA, Green DP (Eds): *Fractures.* Philadelphia: Lippincott, 119–155, 1975.
79. Gustilo RB, Anderson JT: Prevention of infection in the treatment of one thousand and twenty-five open fractures of long bones. *J Bone Joint Surg* 58A:453–458, 1976.
80. Patzakis MJ, Harvey JP, Ivler D: The role of antibiotics in the management of open fractures. *J Bone Joint Surg* 56A:532–533, 1974.
81. Gariepy R, Derome A, Lurin CA: Brachial plexus paralysis following shoulder dislocation. *Can J Surg* 5:418–421, 1962.
82. Jardon OM, Hood LT, Lynch RD: Complete avulsion of the axillary artery as a complicaton of shoulder dislocation. *J Bone Joint Surg* 55A:189–192, 1973.
83. Neer CS: Fractures of the distal third of the clavicle. *Clin Orthop* 58:43–50, 1968.
84. Kummel BM: Fractures of the glenoid causing chronic dislocation of the shoulder. *Clin Orthop* 69:189–191, 1970.
85. Neer CS II: Displaced proximal humeral fractures: II. Treatment of the three-part and four-part displacement. *J Bone Joint Surg* 52(A):1090–1103, 1970.
86. Spak I: Humeral shaft fractures—treatment with a simple hand sling. *Acta Orthop Scand* 49:234–239, 1978.
87. Flint L, et al: Definitive control of bleeding from severe pelvic fractures. *Ann Surg* 189:709–716, 1979.
88. Sarmiento A, Pratt G, Berry N, Sinclair W: Colles' fractures—functional bracing in supination. *J Bone Joint Surg* 57A:311–317, 1975.
89. Green D: Pins and plaster treatment of comminuted fractures of the distal end of the radius. *J Bone Joint Surg* 57A:304, 1975.
90. Dobyns JH, Linscheid RL, Chad EYS, et al: Traumatic instability of the wrist. *AAOS Instructional Course Lecture* 24:182–199, 1975.
91. Melone CP: Scaphoid fractures: Concepts of management. *Clin Plast Surg* 8:83–94, 1981.
92. Green DP, Rowland SA: Fractures and dislocations of the hand, in Rockwood, C.A.; and Green, D.P. (eds): *Fractures.* Philadelphia: Lippincott, 1975.
93. Letournel E: Acetabulum fractures—classification and management. *Clin Orthop* 151:81–106, 1980.
94. Hansen S, Winquist R: Closed intramedullary nailing of the femur—Kuntscher technique with reaming of the femur. *Clin Orthop* 138:56–61, 1979.
95. Reckling F, Peltier L: Acute knee dislocations and their complications. *J Trauma* 9:181–191, 1969.
96. Muller M, Allgower M, Schneider R, Willenegger H: *Manual of Internal Fixation.* Berlin: Springer-Verlag, 1979:282–300.
97. Franklin J, Johnson K, Hansen ST Jr: Open ankle fractures treated by immediate internal fixation. Presented at the American Academy of Orthopedic Surgeons Annual Meeting, Anaheim, 1983.
98. McReynolds IS: The case for operative treatment of fractures of the os calcis, in Leach RE, Hoaglund FT, Riseborough EJ (eds): *Controversies in Orthopaedic Surgery.* Philadelphia: Saunders, 1982:232–254.

CHAPTER 20

THORACIC VASCULAR INJURY IN PATIENTS WITH NEUROLOGICAL INJURY

Kenneth L. Mattox
Matthew J. Wall, Jr.

SYNOPSIS

Thoracic vascular injury accounts for a significant proportion of trauma morbidity and mortality. Patients' recovery and treatment decisions may be markedly altered by a concomitant neurological injury. The common presentations consist of bleeding, embolization, and thrombosis of vessels that supply neurological structures. The neurological complications of thoracic vascular injury also include syndromes associated with the close approximation of nervous structures to the great vessels as well as anatomic anomalies related to the arterial supply of neurological structures. The overall outcome of these patients is determined to a great extent by aggressive evaluation and judgment regarding appropriate repair.

Trauma is a leading cause of death and is responsible for more years of life lost than are the next several causes combined, including heart disease, cancer, atherosclerosis, and infections (including AIDS).[1–3] *Thoracic injury accounts for about 25 percent of trauma-associated deaths, and thoracic complications contribute to death in an additional 25 percent of patients.*[4–6] *Neurosurgeons treating patients with head injuries or consulting about trauma patients with neurological complications must understand the etiology of neurological deficits secondary to a thoracic vascular injury.*

MECHANISM OF INJURY AND THORACIC GREAT VESSEL INJURY

Blunt injury to the innominate artery, the left carotid artery at the thoracic outlet, or the descending thoracic aorta is secondary to (1) transfer of energy from forward impact deceleration, falls from great heights, or auto-pedestrian accidents or (2) a pincer movement between the sternum and the thoracic spine incurred during a frontal impact. The significant forces that cause a deceleration injury to the descending thoracic aorta also may cause a contusion to the adjacent spinal cord.[7–11] Contusion of the thoracic spinal cord with associated spinal column compartment syndrome may be a significant contributing factor to the paraplegia that occurs in up to 20 percent of patients who require repair of a descending thoracic aorta injury.[12–19]

Penetrating wounds of the chest account for the majority of thoracic vascular injuries seen in urban centers.[4,5,20–29] Wounds may be from a diverse spectrum of household objects, industrial instruments (such as a screwdriver), icepicks, and knives (Fig. 20-1). With the ready availability of firearms of increasing caliber and

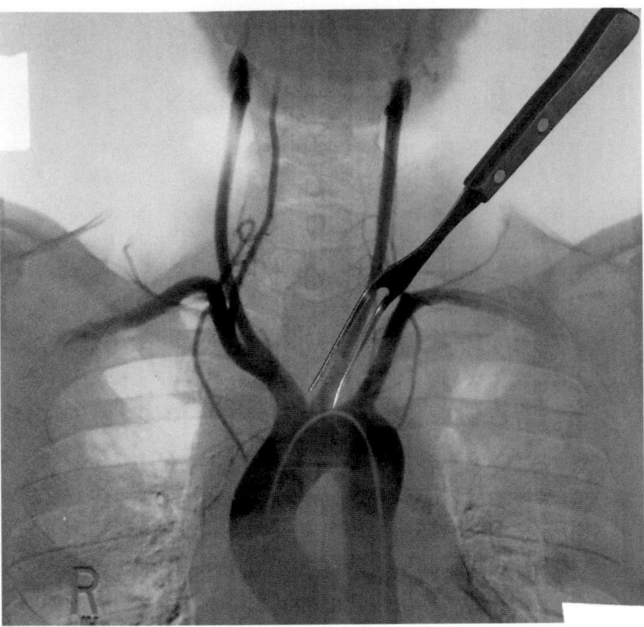

Figure 20-1. Thoracic aortogram with barbecue fork overlay in a patient with an injury to the aortic arch.

velocity, penetrating thoracic injuries secondary to this etiology have become very common in the United States. In one major U.S. city, police estimate that 50 percent of automobile occupants have firearms in their vehicles.[77]

Penetrating wounds of the chest with injury to the thoracic great vessels cause immediate exsanguination and death in a majority of cases. Among patients arriving at a hospital alive, only 15 percent require a thoracotomy.[4,5,25,26] Among those requiring a thoracotomy, cardiac or great vessel injury occurs in a significant number.[4–6,24–26] Concomitant thoracic cervical, thoracic, and/or lumbar spinal cord injury occurs in approximately 2 to 5 percent of patients with a penetrating thoracic great vessel injury. Even with control and repair of the vascular injury, return of full function is extremely rare in patients with such injuries.

Prehospital and Emergency Center Factors

The use of an antishock garment for patients with a penetrating thoracic injury is contraindicated and increases the probability of death rather than aiding in survival.[30–34] Contrary to the rapid fluid resuscitation dogmas that once were adhered to, restriction of preoperative fluids has been shown to be beneficial in patients with a penetrating truncal injury.[29,35–42] A patient with a potential thoracic great vessel injury is frequently brought to the hospital on a backboard with a cervical collar in place.[1,2,21,29–31] Radiologists and neurosurgeons in the emergency center are frequently called on to assist in clearing the cervical and thoracic spine. In some neurologically intact patients with a documented unstable cervical spine fracture, the presence of a thoracic vascular injury requiring urgent lateral thoracotomy presents special problems in regard to cervical stabilization. In such situations, communication between the paramedics, emergency physicians, thoracic surgeons, anesthesiologists, and neurosurgeons is essential to prevent compounding of the cervical injury. If there is suspected thoracic aortic injury, diagnosis is accomplished by arteriography, *not* computed tomography (CT) scan, magnetic resonance imaging (MRI), or transesophageal echocardiography.[7–11]

Indications for aortography after a blunt thoracic injury are broad and liberal, as the consequence of "missing" an acute aortic injury may be death. These indications are based on patient history, physical examination, and/or radiographic clues. If the patient was ejected from or hit by an automobile, fell from a significant height, had a history of transitory paralysis, or presented with a strong suggestion of energy transfer, aortography must be considered. Aortography is also considered in patients with blunt trauma and spinal shock, intrascapular murmurs, upper extremity hypertension, and/or a steering wheel imprint on the sternum. The presence of radiographic suggestions of a mediastinal hematoma—mediastinal wounding, loss of the aortic knob contour, depression of the left main stem bronchus, and loss of the aortopulmonary window—mandates that an aortogram be performed (Fig. 20-2).

Pneumothorax, hemothorax, and hemopneumothorax are commonly diagnosed on physical examination or radiologically in patients with a thoracic vascular injury. Once this is diagnosed, tube thoracostomy is accomplished in the emergency center or operating room. If more than 1500 ml of blood is aspirated on initial tube insertion, the possibility of a great vessel injury should be considered and the patient should undergo an urgent thoracotomy.

Aortic Arch Injury

In patients with a penetrating or blunt injury to the ascending aortic arch or the branch vessels off the aortic arch, hypotension, vascular occlusion, or embolism may create a neurological deficit before arrival at the hospital.[20,23,24,28,43–49] With a blunt innominate or carotid artery injury, intimal dissection may result in a prehospital neurological deficit, even to the point of a fixed deficit with deep coma. These injuries may be precipitated by seat belt compression or other pressure to the carotid or the base of the neck.[50–57] In the majority of cases,

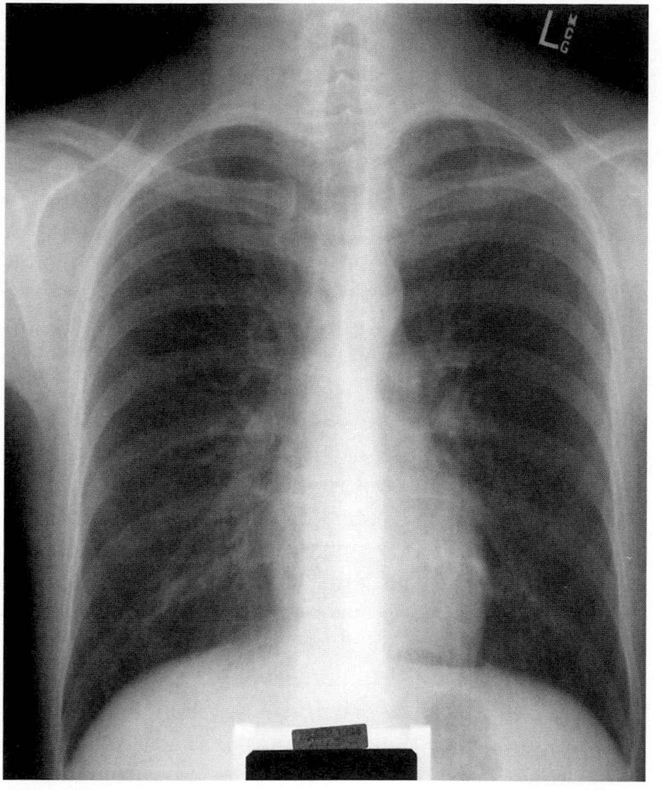

A

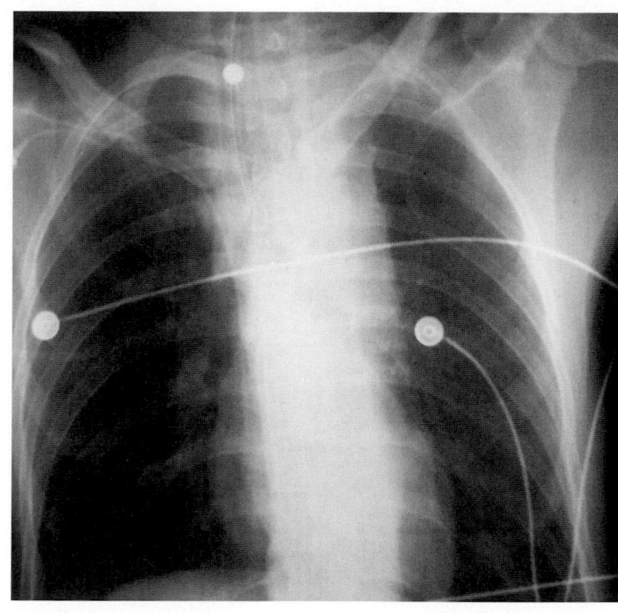

B

Figure 20-2. Two comparative chest roentgenograms. Note (*A*) the normal-appearing mediastinum on the left and (*B*) the abnormally widened mediastinum and loss of aortic knob contour of the x-ray on the right.

reconstruction of the ascending aorta and aortic arch requires cardiopulmonary bypass with its concomitant systemic heparinization. Cerebral contusion and the concomitant cervical spine or closed head injury may result in further bleeding into the head or spinal cord canal during the period of total body anticoagulation. Therefore, in the presence of concomitant injuries, most trauma surgeons recommend against using total body heparinization.

Injuries to the innominate and left common carotid arteries usually are managed with a bypass from the ascending aorta to the distal innominate or carotid artery[26,44,46] (Fig. 20-3). Hypothermia, temporary shunts, heparinization, and cardiopulmonary bypass are not necessary. Embolization and/or postoperative neurological symptoms that were not present preoperatively are extremely rare. In a select group of patients, nonoperative or delayed operative management may be a consideration in a multiply injured patient.

Injury to the Descending Thoracic Aorta

The majority of injuries to the descending thoracic aorta are secondary to deceleration. Eighty-five percent of these patients die before reaching a treatment facility.[6,58,59] Patients surviving when they reach the hospital have a mortality rate of 1 percent per hour over the next 48 h if the lesion is unrecognized and untreated. A small number of patients develop chronic traumatic aneurysms. A few highly selected patients with multisystem and head injury may be treated with temporizing measures because of extensive associated injuries.[15,16,60–63] Among patients reaching the hospital alive with a descending thoracic aortic injury, approximately 15 percent die and up to 20 percent have resultant paraplegia.[8,12,13,15–18,61,63–67] Although extensively debated, the standard perioperative management adjuncts are not major determinants of whether postoperative neu-

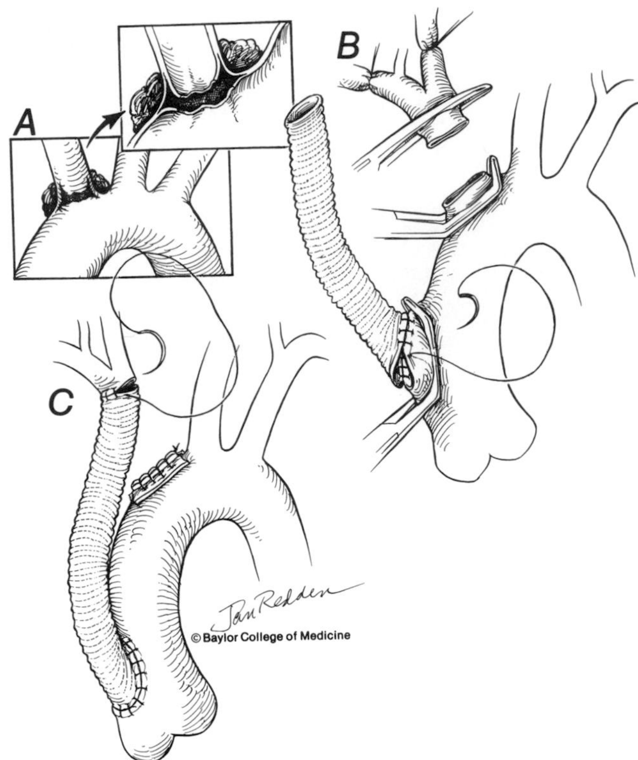

Figure 20-3. Drawing depicting the bypass principle for innominate artery injuries. (*A*) close-up of injury and hematoma. (*B*) clamp and control sequence. (*C*) completion of reconstruction.

rological complications are seen. Clamp repair, temporary shunt bypass, and the use of a pump bypass are accepted operative techniques, and each technique carries with it the possibility of postoperative neurological complications. Approximately 85 percent of these patients require substitute conduits.

The etiologies and factors contributing to paraplegia after surgery on the descending thoracic aorta have been and continue to be the subject of debate.[12–18,61,65,66,68–70] Attempts to settle this debate have focused on the experimental animal laboratory, the operating room, the intensive care unit, surgical conferences, and, unfortunately, the courtroom. This debate has led to strategies for the prediction and prevention of the complication of paraplegia. None of these strategies, including somatosensory evoked potentials, drainage of CSF, use of complex bypass shunts, hypothermia, cardiopulmonary bypass, and attempts at more rapid surgery, have statistically decreased the rate of paraplegia. The often quoted "thirty-minute safe period for descending thoracic aortic cross-clamping" has never been demonstrated to be a direct contributing factor to paraplegia. The length of the cross-clamp time is more a function of the complexity of the injury, with the complexity being a greater contributor to paraplegia. Undoubtedly, a more complex injury has a greater potential for concomitant contusion of the adjacent spinal cord and its variable anatomy.

In the past, one of the contributing factors to paraplegia was thought to be declamping hypotension at the conclusion of a procedure. It is now recognized that declamping hypotension is undoubtedly a manifestation of "spinal shock" syndrome rather than being the etiology of paraplegia. Paraplegia may be manifest preoperatively, may develop within a short period after the aorta is cross-clamped, or may not appear until 2 to 5 days after surgery.

Several factors are strongly associated with the appearance of paraplegia. In an upper thoracic aortic injury, concomitant contusion of the spinal cord from the same decelerative forces that caused the aortic tear undoubtedly could be a significant factor. In the numerous reported series of patients undergoing emergency thoracotomy and cross-clamping of the descending thoracic aorta for penetrating thoracic wounds, the occurrence of paraplegia is virtually never cited. Paraplegia occurring in association with blunt trauma to this aortic location implies that factors other than cross-clamping of the aorta are major contributors to neurological complication. In cases of emergency center thoracotomy with cross-clamping of the aorta, patients are not on cardiopulmonary bypass or centrifugal pumps and do not have temporary shunts. They are not systematically heparinized or treated with any special monitoring techniques.[71] Additionally, cross-clamp times may be lengthy. The data from this group of patients and the obvious conclusions that can be derived have been completely ignored and/or omitted from consideration in reports stating that cross-clamp times over 30 min result in paraplegia.

Perhaps the greatest contributing factor to paraplegia in patients with a blunt injury to the descending thoracic aorta is the variable anatomy of the anterior spinal artery, which allows the development of an unpredictable ischemic injury. This unfavorable anatomy in conjunction with spinal cord contusion and spinal cord compartment syndrome may significantly contribute to a subsequent neurological injury. This simple observation can also explain in part the delayed appearance of paralysis in some patients.

The single anterior spinal artery is more rudimentary than are the paired posterior spinal arteries. The anterior spinal artery may be tenuous or even interrupted in its course and is supplied by approximately nine segmental anterior radicular arteries. The anterior radicular artery or anterior spinal artery may be segmentally absent. Thus, in a patient with a spinal artery anomaly, the area between the clamps is at risk whether or not shunts, pumps, or heparin is used (Fig. 20-4).

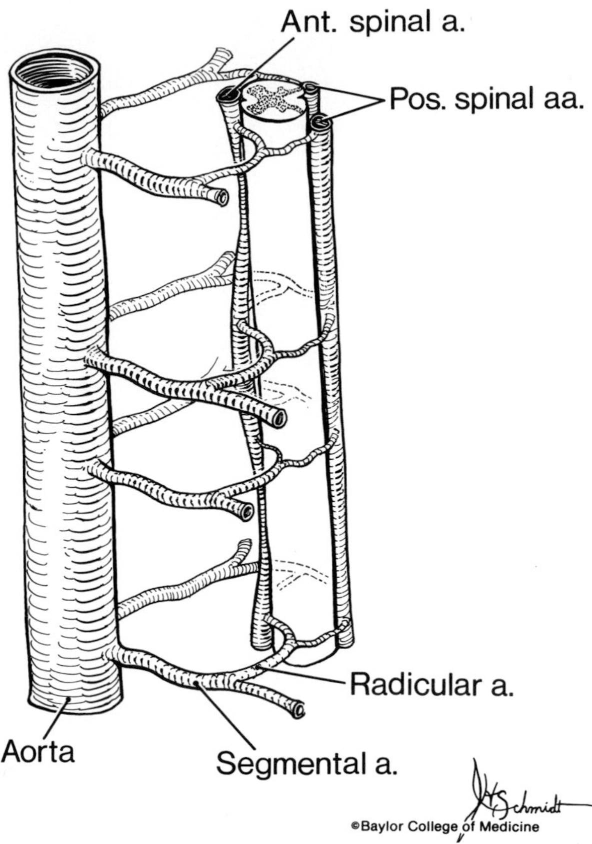

Figure 20-4. Drawing of the anatomy of the radicular and spinal arteries illustrating the primitive and tenuous characteristics of these vessels.

All consultants, especially neurologists and neurosurgeons, should recognize that the mortality rate is considerably higher when patients with an acute blunt injury have total body heparinization. When cardiopulmonary bypass is used for a thoracic great vessel injury, the mortality rate greatly increases as a result of associated injuries in the pelvis, chest, and head. Intracerebral hemorrhage also may occur during total body heparinization.

Systemic Embolization of Foreign Bodies

Embolization of material into the systemic circulation has been described, although it occurs only rarely. Various externally introduced fragments may enter the pulmonary veins, heart, or great vessels and embolize to the distal circulation. Embolization to the spinal cord and to the carotid arteries, sometimes with fatal results, has also been described[72,73] (Fig. 20-5). In evaluating a thoracic great vessel injury, angiography catheters may also embolize atheromatous debris to the peripheral or abdominal circulation or the spinal cord, creating limb ischemia, abdominal catastrophes, and/or neurological deficits.

Systemic Air Embolization

When intrapulmonary pressure exceeds 60 mmHg in a patient with penetrating injuries to the lung, systemic embolization of air from a bronchiolar or alveolar to a pulmonary vein fistula may produce symptoms of confusion, cardiac arrhythmias, asystole, and cardiovascular collapse (Fig. 20-6). In such instances, air may be seen on retinal examination, in the arterial monitoring line, or in the coronary arteries if an emergency thoracotomy is performed for resuscitation. The cerebral manifesta-

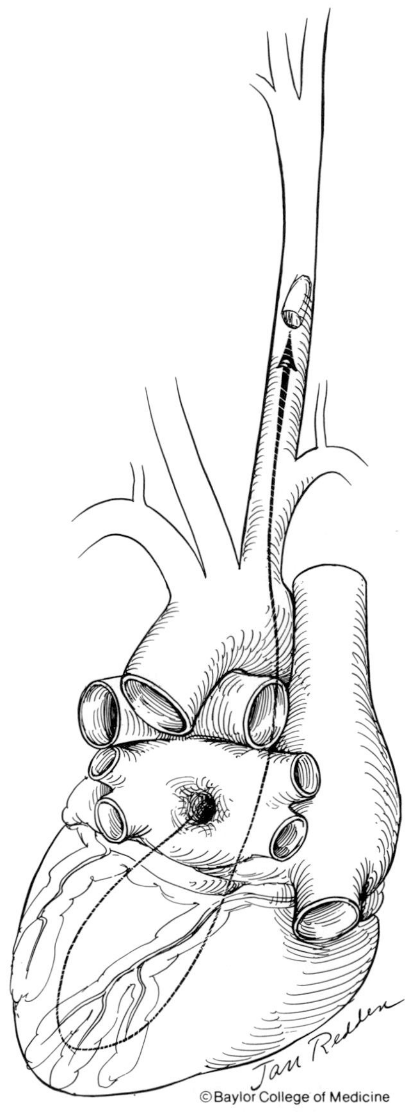

Figure 20-5. Drawing illustrating a bullet embolism from the left atrium to the left carotid artery. This patient died of a cerebral infarction.

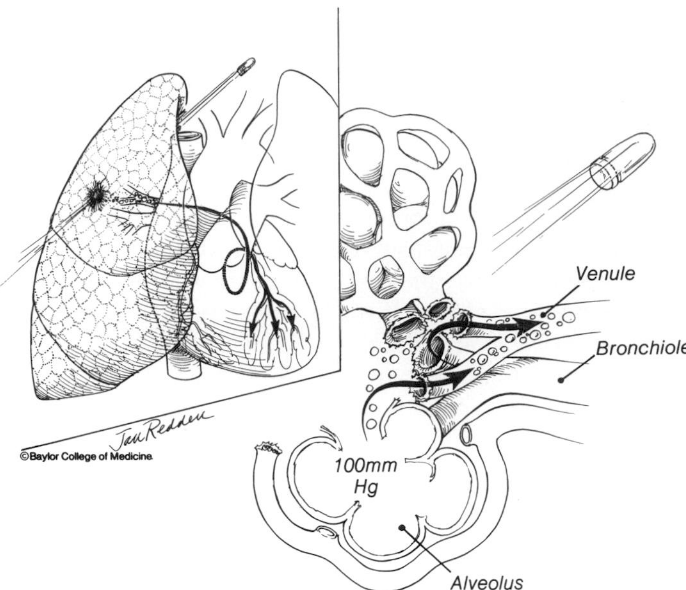

Figure 20-6. Drawing depicting the mechanism of systemic air embolism in a patient with lung penetration and forced positive-pressure ventilation greater than 60 mmHg.

tions of confusion, seizure, or coma may be the first symptoms of systemic air emboli. Although thoracic surgeons may perform an immediate thoracotomy in a patient with systemic air emboli from these etiologies, survival is rare. This deadly complication is best prevented by avoiding ventilatory pressures greater than 60 mmHg during times of resuscitation and in patients who have a closed pulmonary injury.[74,75]

Venous Air Embolization

Venous air embolization occurs in the right-sided circulation when air is introduced into the heart from a central line; this can occur when the central line is disconnected and central venous pressure is low. Venous air embolization produces an air lock from the frothing of the blood in the right atrium and right ventricle, with reduction of pulmonary flow and subsequent cardiac arrest from the failure of blood to get through the lungs.[76] In some instances, with a patent foramen ovale or with the frothy air going through the pulmonary circulation, systemic air embolization also may occur. The diagnosis of venous air embolization may be aided by aspiration of air from the right side of the heart. At times the first manifestation of venous air emboli may be hypotension, cardiac arrest, and/or neurological and cerebral symptoms.

Multidisciplinary Approach to Patients with a Thoracic Great Vessel Injury

Management of patients with a suspected or confirmed thoracic great vessel injury requires close communication, cooperation, and therapeutic interaction among the trauma surgeon, thoracic surgeon, interventional radiologist, neurosurgeon, anesthesiologist, and other members of the trauma team. Most neurological complications of a thoracic great vessel injury are secondary to the complexity of the original injury itself and are not due to therapeutic misadventures. Unfortunately, one of the most litigious areas involves a patient with an acute injury to the thoracic great vessels and concomitant neurological complications or even a neurological manifestation of the thoracic great vessel injury. The older thoracic surgery and trauma literature adds to the confusion, since this is an area that continues to evolve rapidly as new clinical and basic research is performed.

Complications of Thoracic Vascular Injury

Recurrent Laryngeal/Phrenic Nerves

Injury to the phrenic, vagus, or recurrent laryngeal nerves may occur secondary to a direct injury, a stretch injury from an expanding hematoma or an aneurysm, or a surgical injury during control, exposure, or repair. The vagus nerve, its recurrent laryngeal branch, or the phrenic nerve can be injured directly or indirectly. The resultant hoarseness or diaphragmatic paralysis can be a nuisance and may result in significant disability. Treatments for these complications include diaphragm plication and injection of the paralyzed vocal cord.

Causalgia

Patients with a thoracic outlet vascular injury, those with a "trapdoor" or "book" incision, and those with partial injury to the brachial plexus may develop causalgia. This reflex sympathetic dystrophy can be extremely disabling and resistant to physical therapy. Causalgia in the upper extremities may respond to chemical and/or surgical sympathectomy. Transthoracic sympathectomy via a second interspace axillary incision or via thoracoscopy must remove the lower half of the stellate ganglion and all thoracic ganglia down to the third ganglion, as the intercostal brachial nerves to the inner surface of the arm carry cross-linking sympathetic fibers. This procedure relieves symptoms in 35 to 60 percent of cases of upper extremity causalgia. Other surgical therapies include dorsal column stimulation and occasionally intrathecal morphine via a continuous infusion pump.

Radicular incisional pain

Neurosurgeons may see patients who have recovered from surgery for a thoracic vascular injury but have severe radicular intercostal pain. Radiculitis in the distribution of the intercostal nerves may be secondary to pericostal sutures encircling the ribs above and below the incision. The pain is usually in the distribution of the intercostal nerve just below the intercostal incision. The entrapped nerve may require chemical or surgical ablation to achieve pain relief.

Transverse myelopathy and thoracic incisions

Rarely, a transverse myelopathy may develop at the level of a thoracic intercostal incision or intercostal nerve block. Since the dura may have outpouchings through the spinal foramina and may even extend a short distance under the posterior rib margins, incisions and injections into the posterior intercostal region can cause damage. As an intercostal incision is widened using a rib spreader retractor, temporary packing is used. As the ribs are reapproximated at the end of the thoracotomy, such bleeding often ceases. The use of topical hemostatic material to "pack" the angle of the incision and electrocoagulation has contributed to a transverse myelopathy. While neurosurgeons may be asked to evaluate this uncommon finding, transverse myelopathy in this setting is usually nonreversible.

References

1. *Advanced Trauma Life Support Course, Instructor Manual.* Chicago: American College of Surgeons Committee on Trauma, 1989.
2. American College of Surgeons Committee on Trauma Resources for Optimal Care of the Injured Patient: Chicago, 1993.
3. Trunkey D: Trauma. *Sc Am* 249:28–35, 1983.
4. LoCicero J: Epidemiology of thoracic trauma. *Surg Clin North Am* 69:15–20, 1989.
5. Mattox KL: Thoracic great vessel injury. *Surg Clin North Am* 68:693–703, 1988.
6. Kulshrestha P, Iyer KS, Das B, et al: Chest injuries: A clinical and autopsy profile. *J Trauma* 28:844–847, 1988.
7. Agee CK, Metzler MH, Churchill R, Mitchell F: Computed tomographic evaluation to exclude traumatic aortic disruption. *Ann Surg* 172:1002–1006, 1970.
8. Mattox KL: Fact and fiction about management of aortic transection. *Ann Thorac Surg* 48:1–3, 1989.
9. Miller FB, Richardson JD, Thomas HA: Role of CT in the diagnosis of major arterial injury after blunt thoracic trauma. *Surgery* 106:596–603, 1989.
10. Mirvis SE, Bidwell JK, Buddemeyer EU, et al: Imaging diagnosis of traumatic aortic rupture: A review and experience at a major trauma center. *Invest Radiol* 22:187–196, 1987.
11. Moore EH, Webb WR, Verrier ED, et al: MRI of chronic posttraumatic aneurysms of the thoracic aorta. *AJR* 143:1195–1196, 1984.
12. Cowley RA, Turney SZ, Hankins JR, et al: Rupture of thoracic aorta caused by blunt trauma: A 15-year experience. *J Thorac Cardiovasc Surg* 100:652–661, 1990.
13. Duhaylongsod FG, Glower DD, Wolfe WG: Acute traumatic aortic aneurysm: The Duke experience from 1970 to 1990. *J Vasc Surg* 15:331–343, 1992.
14. Mattox KL: Reply to Mayo Clinic letter to editor re clamp/repair of traumatic transection of descending aorta. *Ann Thorac Surg* 43:351–352, 1987.
15. Mattox KL, Holzman M, Pickard LR, et al: Clamp/repair: A safe technique for treatment of blunt injury to the descending thoracic aorta. *Ann Thorac Surg* 40:456–463, 1985.
16. Merrill WH, Lee RB, Hammon JW, et al: Surgical treatment of acute traumatic tear of the thoracic aorta. *Ann Surg* 207:699–706, 1988.
17. Oka Y, Takashi M: Prevention of spinal cord injury after cross-clamping of the thoracic aorta. *Jpn J Surg* 14:159–162, 1984.
18. Shenaq SA, Svensson LG: Paraplegia following aortic surgery. *J Cardiovasc Vasc Anesth* 7:81–94, 1993.
19. Svensson LG, Von Ritater CM, Groeneveld HT, et al: Crossclamping of the thoracic aorta: Influence of aortic shunts, laminectomy, papaverine, calcium channel blockers, allopurinol, etc, on blood flow and paraplegia. *Ann Surg* 204:38–47, 1986.
20. Blass DZ, James EC, Reed RJ, et al: Penetrating wounds of the neck and upper thorax. *J Trauma* 18:2–7, 1979.
21. Durham LA, Richardson RJ, Wall MJ, et al: Emergency center thoracotomy: Impact of prehospital resuscitation. *J Trauma* 32:775–779, 1992.
22. Flint LM, Snyder WH, Perry MO: Management of major vascular injuries in the base of the neck. *Arch Surg* 106:407–413, 1973.
23. George SM Jr, Croce MR, Fabian TC, et al: Cervicothoracic arterial injuries: Recommendations for diagnosis and management. *World J Surg* 15:134–140, 1991.
24. Imamoglu K, Read RC, Huebl HC: Cervicomediastinal vascular injury. *Surgery* 61:274–279, 1967.

25. Mattox KL: Priorities in repairing a penetrated chest. *Emerg Med* 14:282–288, 1982.
26. Mattox KL: Approaches to trauma involving the major vessels of the thorax. *Surg Clin North Am* 69:77–92, 1989.
27. Mattox KL, Feliciano DV, Beall AC, et al: Five thousand seven hundred sixty cardiovascular injuries in 4459 patients: Epidemiologic evolution 1958–1988. *Ann Surg* 209:698–705, 1989.
28. Mavroudis C, Roon AJ, Baker CC, Thomas AN: Management of acute cervicothoracic vascular injuries. *J Thorac Cardiovasc Surg* 80:342–349, 1980.
29. Border JR, Lewis FR, Aprahamian C, et al: Prehospital trauma care—stabilization or scoop and run. *J Trauma* 23:708–711, 1983.
30. Pepe PE, Wyatt CH, Bickell WH, et al: The relationship between total prehospital time and outcome in hypotensive victims of penetrating injuries. *Ann Emerg Med* 16:293–297, 1987.
31. Trunkey DD: Is ALS necessary for prehospital trauma care? *J Trauma* 24:86–87, 1984.
32. Mackersie RC, Christensen JM, Lewis FR: The prehospital use of external counterpressure: Does MAST make a difference? *J Trauma* 24:882–888, 1984.
33. Mattox KL, Bickell W, Pepe P, et al: Prospective MAST study in 911 patients. *J Trauma* 29:1104–1112, 1989.
34. McSwain NE: Pneumatic anti-shock garment: State of the art 1988. *Ann Emerg Med* 17:506–525, 1988.
35. Bickell WH, Shaftan GW, Mattox KL: Intravenous fluid administration and uncontrolled hemorrhage. *J Trauma* 29:409, 1989.
36. Bickell WH, Bruttig SP, Millnamoro GA, et al: The detrimental affects of intravenous crystalloid after aortotomy in swine. *Surgery* 110:529–536, 1991.
37. Crawford ES: Ruptured abdominal aortic aneurysm (editorial). *J Vasc Surg* 13:348–350, 1991.
38. Gross D, Landau EH, Assalia A, et al: Is hypertonic saline resuscitation safe in "uncontrolled" hemorrhagic shock? *J Trauma* 28:751–756, 1988.
39. Kowalenko T, Stern S, Dronen S, Wang X: Improved outcome with hypotensive resuscitation of uncontrolled hemorrhagic shock in a swine model. *J Trauma* 33:349–353, 1992.
40. Lewis FL: Prehospital intravenous fluid therapy: Physiologic computer modeling. *J Trauma* 26:804–811, 1986.
41. Martin RR, Bickell WH, Pepe PE, et al: Prospective evaluation of preoperative fluid resuscitation in hypotensive patients with penetrating truncal injury: A preliminary report. *J Trauma* 33:1–9, 1992.
42. Mattox KL, Maningas PA, Moore EE, et al: Prehospital hypertonic saline/dextran infusion for post-traumatic hypotension. *Ann Surg* 213:482–491, 1991.
43. Bosher LH, Freed TA: The surgical treatment of traumatic rupture or avulsion of the innominate artery. *J Thorac Cardiovasc Surg* 54:732–739, 1967.
44. Graham JM, Feliciano DV, Mattox KL, et al: Innominate vascular injury. *J Trauma* 22:647–655, 1982.
45. Graham JM, Feliciano DV, Mattox KL, et al: Management of subclavian vascular injuries. *J Trauma* 20:537–544, 1980.
46. Johnston RH, Wall MJ, Mattox KL: Innominate artery injury: A thirty year experience. *J Vasc Surg* 17:134–140, 1993.
47. Klein SR, Bongard FS, White RA: Neurovascular injuries of the thoracic outlet and axilla. *Am J Surg* 156:115–118, 1988.
48. Samaan HA: Vascular injuries of the upper thorax and the root of the neck. *Br J Surg* 58:881–886, 1971.
49. Strum JT, Perry JF: Brachial plexus injuries from blunt thoracic trauma—a harbinger of vascular and thoracic injury. *Ann Emerg Med* 16:404–406, 1987.
50. Baik S, Uku JM, Joo KG: Seat belt injuries to the left common carotid artery and left internal carotid artery. *Am J Forensic Med Pathol* 9:38–39, 1988.
51. Beatty RA: Dissecting hematoma of the internal carotid artery following chiropractic cervical manipulation. *J Trauma* 17:248, 1977.
52. Chedid MK, Deeb ZL, Rothfus WE, et al: Major cerebral vessels injury caused by a seatbelt shoulder strap: Case report. *J Trauma* 29:1601–1603, 1989.
53. Dragon R, Saranchak H, Lakin P, et al: Blunt injuries to the carotid and vertebral arteries. *Am J Surg* 141:497–500, 1981.
54. Englund R, Harris JP, May J: Blunt trauma to the internal carotid artery. *Ann Vasc Surg* 2:362–366, 1988.
55. Pozzati E, Giuliani G, Poppi M, Faenza A: Blunt traumatic carotid dissection with delayed symptoms. *Stroke* 20:412–416, 1989.
56. Silvernail WI, Croutcher DL, Byrd BR, Pope DH: Carotid artery injury produced by blunt neck trauma. *South Med J* 68:310–311, 1975.
57. Weimann S, Rumpl E, Flora G: Carotid occlusion caused by seat belt trauma. *Eur J Vasc Surg* 2:193–196, 1988.
58. Parmley LF, Mattingly TW, Marion WC, et al: Nonpenetrating traumatic injury to the aorta. *Circulation* 17:1086–1101, 1958.
59. Parmley LF, Mattingly TW, Marion WC: Penetrating wounds of the heart and aorta. *Circulation* 17:953–973, 1958.
60. Fisher RD, Mattox KL: Conservative management of aortic laceration due to blunt trauma. *J Trauma* 30:1562–1566, 1990.
61. Hilgenberg AD, Logan DL, Akins CW, et al: Blunt injuries of the thoracic aorta. *Ann Thorac Surg* 53:233–239, 1992.
62. McCollum CH, Graham JM, Noon GP, DeBakey ME: Chronic thoracic aneurysm of the thoracic aorta: An analysis of 50 patients. *J Trauma* 19:248, 1979.
63. Williams TE, Vasko JS, Kakos GS, et al: Treatment of acute and chronic traumatic rupture of the descending thoracic aorta. *World J Surg* 4:545, 1980.
64. Olivier HF Jr, Maher TD, Liebler GA, et al: Use of the BioMedicus centrifugal pump in traumatic tears of the thoracic aorta. *Ann Thorac Surg* 38:586–591, 1984.
65. Pate JW: Traumatic rupture of the aorta: Emergency operation. *Ann Thorac Surg* 39:531, 1985.
66. Soyer R, Bessou JP, Bouchart F, et al: Long term results

of surgical treatment of traumatic rupture of the thoracic aorta: 47 cases. *J Cardiovasc Surg* 31(suppl):102, 1990.
67. Walls JT, Curtis JJ, Boley T: Sarns centrifugal pump for repair of thoracic aorta injury: Case report. *J Cardiovasc Surg* 29:1283–1285, 1989.
68. Adamkiewicz A: Die blutgefasse de menschlichen ruckenmarkesoerflache. *Sitz Acad Urss Wien Math* 85:101, 1882.
69. Crawford ES, Svensson LG, Hess KR, et al: A prospective randomized study of cerebrospinal fluid drainage to prevent paraplegia after high-risk surgery on the thoracoabdominal aorta. *J Vasc Surg* 13:36–46, 1991.
70. Donahoo JS, Brawley RK, Gott VL: The heparin-coated vascular shunt for thoracic aortic and great vessel procedures: A ten-year experience. *Ann Thorac Surg* 23:507, 1977.
71. Garcia-Rinaldi R, Defore WW, Mattox KL, Beall AC Jr: Unimpaired renal myocardial and neurologic function after cross-clamping of the thoracic aorta. *Surg Gynecol Obstet* 143:249–252, 1976.
72. Graham JM, Mattox KL: Right ventricular bullet embolectomy without cardiopulmonary bypass. *J Thorac Cardiovasc Surg* 82:310–313, 1981.
73. Mattox KL, Beall AC, Ennix CL, DeBakey ME: Intravascular migratory bullets. *Am J Surg* 137:192–195, 1979.
74. Graham JM, Beall AC Jr, Mattox KL, Vaughn GD: Systemic air embolism following penetrating trauma to the lung. *Chest* 72:449–454, 1977.
75. Graham JM, Mattox KL, Feliciano DV, Beall AC Jr: Air embolism following penetrating thoracic trauma. *Curr Concepts Trauma Care* 2(3):7–9, 1979.
76. Mattox KL, Bricker DS: Air embolism following subclavian catheterization. *Tex Med* 66:74–76, 1970.
77. Brown L: Personal communication, 1985.

CHAPTER 21

ABDOMINAL INJURIES

Darrell C. Boone
Andrew B. Peitzman

SYNOPSIS

The identification of a significant abdominal injury in a trauma patient with a head injury may be difficult, as a patient with an altered sensorium may have an unreliable abdominal examination.[1–4] *Early recognition and prompt treatment of abdominal injury in these patients are vital. The abdominal injury in and of itself contributes to the ultimate morbidity and mortality of a multiply injured patient. Furthermore, it may contribute to hypoxia and hypotension, leading to a secondary brain insult and having a detrimental effect on the outcome.*[5,6] *The decision to investigate for possible abdominal injury must be expeditious, and the means of evaluation must not delay appropriate characterization and treatment of the head injury, especially if craniotomy for an intracranial mass lesion is indicated. Appropriate management of patients with combined head and abdominal injuries requires not only concurrent evaluation and treatment of all life-threatening injuries but prioritization of the evaluation and definitive treatment of multiple injuries: head, abdominal, and others. Each injury must be definitively addressed at the most appropriate time during both the evaluation and the resuscitation of a patient with multiple injuries.*

PREVENTABLE TRAUMA DEATHS

Over the past four decades, there have been numerous reports of deaths after trauma that might have been prevented if more appropriate medical care had been rendered.[7] Reports reviewing deaths from vehicular accidents have identified inadequate resuscitation of patients with abdominal injury, delay in diagnosis of abdominal injury, or delay in surgical treatment of an already diagnosed abdominal injury as being responsible for 22 to 50 percent of preventable trauma deaths.[7] The combination of abdominal and head injuries was found to be particularly lethal. In an early report,[8] the mortality rate in patients with blunt abdominal trauma was four times greater when an associated head injury was present. More than half the deaths caused by a missed abdominal injury in that series occurred in patients with a coexistent head injury that was thought to have masked recognition of the intraabdominal injury.

These reports of preventable deaths prompted the recognition that hypotension in a patient with a head injury should never be initially ascribed to the head injury. In addition, potentially lethal intraabdominal injuries may not have consistent manifestations on abdominal physical examination. In fact, even without head injury, 46 percent of trauma patients with normal abdominal examinations have significant abdominal visceral injury at laparotomy.[9] Conversely, 48 percent of patients with positive abdominal findings on initial physical examination may have negative findings at laparotomy.[9] In response to these observations, more accurate and rapid means of diagnosing intraabdominal injury have evolved; their appropriate and timely application to patients with a head injury are discussed below.

INITIAL ASSESSMENT

Protocols for the resuscitation of trauma victims, such as those provided by the Advanced Trauma Life Support

(ATLS) course,[10] have been established to maximize resuscitative efforts and avoid missing life-threatening injuries. ATLS protocols prescribe a primary survey to identify immediately life-threatening injuries. Resuscitation is initiated simultaneously. This is followed by a secondary survey for a more thorough evaluation of the patient from head to toe. The definitive care of the identified injuries completes the initial assessment (Table 21-1). Evaluation and reevaluation of the patient, particularly if the clinical status deteriorates, are important. A "tertiary survey" during the patient's first 24 to 48 h in the hospital has been advocated to detect injuries which might have been missed during the initial assessment.[11]

The goals of the primary survey are establishment of a patent airway, adequate ventilation, maintenance of circulation, and assessment of global neurological function. Hypotension should be vigorously treated, and intravenous fluids should not be restricted in a hypovolemic patient with an associated head injury. Inadequate resuscitation of patients who are hypovolemic from undetected associated injuries and deliberate fluid restriction in patients assumed to have an isolated head injury may contribute to hypoperfusion and secondary brain injury.

Once the goals of the primary survey have been achieved, the secondary survey and continuing resuscitation can commence. A patient with an intraabdominal injury may occasionally present with a distended abdomen and signs of hemorrhagic shock. Maintenance of circulation may not be possible without rapid transfer to the operating room and immediate laparotomy to control bleeding. In these patients, a complete secondary survey may be delayed until the laparotomy has been completed. Otherwise, a more complete history of the mechanism of injury may be obtained and a more thorough examinaton may be performed.

With respect to the abdominal evaluation, the secondary survey includes inspection, auscultation, and palpation of the exposed abdominal region as well as passage of a nasogastric or orogastric tube, rectal examination, passage of a urinary catheter (if no meatal blood is present and the prostate is not "high-riding"), and examination of the Anterior-Posterior (AP) chest and pelvic x-rays. Blood is obtained for type and crossmatch, complete blood count, platelet count, prothrombin time (PT), partial thromboplastin time (PTT), electrolytes, blood urea nitrogen (BUN), creatinine, arterial blood gas determination, and a toxicology screen if indicated. A urinalysis is also performed. The findings of this secondary survey may prompt further diagnostic procedures to identify possible intraabdominal injury.

TABLE 21-1 Trauma Resuscitation Sequence

Primary survey
Airway patency with c-spine control
Breathing
Circulation
Disability (neurological examination)
Exposure
Resuscitation
Secondary survey
Head and skull
Face
C-spine
Chest
Abdomen
Rectal exam
Extremities
Neurological exam
Stabilization
Definitive care
Continuing reevaluation

SOURCE: Modified from Advanced Trauma Life Support Program, American College of Surgeons.[10]

WHO SHOULD BE INVESTIGATED FOR POSSIBLE ABDOMINAL INJURY?

Head injuries are common among patients treated at trauma centers. Among almost 50,000 patients reported from the Major Trauma Outcome Study (MTOS), 34 percent had a head injury but the incidence of isolated head injury was only 6 percent. Among those with a head injury, 39 percent had a significant extracranial injury manifested by an Abbreviated Injury Scale (AIS) of 3 or more.[12] It is necessary to determine which of these patients deserves investigation for a possible intraabdominal injury and, conversely, which patients with an obvious abdominal injury and a decreased level of consciousness require investigation for a possible head injury.

Clinicians managing head-injured patients who may have associated extracranial injuries are faced with a management dilemma: Should a cranial computed tomography (CT) scan or a diagnostic peritoneal lavage (DPL) be carried out first? Setting priorities in this situation depends in part on the relative likelihood of head or abdominal injury. A recent study from Toronto[13] addressed relative incidences of intracranial and extracranial injury in the trauma patient population.

The authors found that trauma patients younger than 30 years of age were more likely to have an extracranial injury requiring operation than an intracranial mass lesion, while patients over the age of 70 were more likely to have an intracranial mass lesion than an extracranial injury. Patients who were tachycardic or hypotensive were more likely to have an extracranial injury, possibly abdominal, than an intracranial mass lesion. Patients injured in a motor vehicle accident (MVA) were more likely to have a torso injury than an intracranial mass lesion, although in the MTOS group, the incidence of head injury in those sustaining an injury in an MVA, a motorcycle accident, or an automobile-pedestrian accident was higher than the average incidence of head injury for the entire MTOS population.[12] Patients who fall are less likely to have sustained an abdominal injury than an intracranial mass lesion. Patients who present with lateralizing neurological signs have a relatively high probability of an intracranial lesion, with one-third requiring craniotomy.[14] Trauma patients with arterial base deficits <-3 mEq/liter and associated major chest trauma or pelvic fractures have a significantly increased chance of having an intraabdominal injury.[15]

The decision to investigate for possible abdominal injury depends on the mechanism of injury, the findings on physical examination, the laboratory and x-ray findings, and the identification of injuries known to be associated with a high incidence of abdominal injury. Patients with a head injury who fall into any of these categories for a high risk of abdominal injury should be considered candidates for further investigation (Table 21-2).

TABLE 21-2 High-Risk Features for Associated Abdominal Injury in a Head-Injured Patient

Significant mechanism of injury: motor vehicle, motorcycle, or pedestrian-automobile accident
Associated major chest trauma
Associated pelvic fracture
Presence of hypotension or tachycardia
Arterial base deficit <-3 mEq/l

DIAGNOSTIC MODALITIES

Diagnostic laparotomy, peritoneal lavage, CT, ultrasound, and diagnostic laparoscopy as well as other techniques may be utilized in the identification of an abdominal injury. The diagnostic approaches to blunt and penetrating abdominal trauma are different, and the two will be discussed separately.

Blunt Abdominal Trauma

Exploratory Laparotomy

Patients with a head injury undergoing primary resuscitation who are found to be hypotensive and tachycardiac without evidence of external blood loss or hemothorax on chest x-ray and with an obviously distended abdomen require a secure airway, adequate ventilation, and immediate laparotomy for control of hemorrhage and prevention of further secondary injury (Fig. 21-1). Simulta-

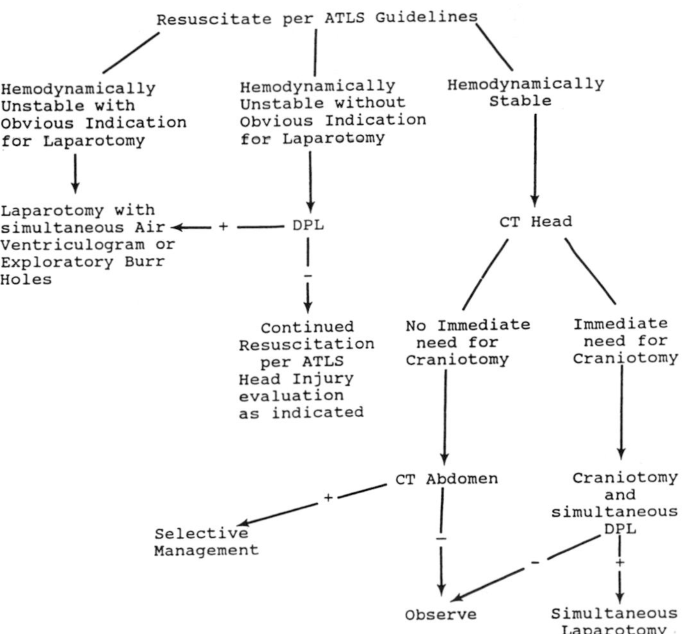

Figure 21-1. Algorithm for the management of a head-injured patient with a suspected blunt abdominal injury.

neous evaluation for a possible intracranial lesion requiring surgical intervention can be done in the operating room. Exploratory burr holes, especially if there are signs of tentorial herniation or upper brainstem dysfunction (ipsilateral pupillary dilatation with loss of the light reflex and contralateral hemiparesis[16]), or an air ventriculogram may be performed rapidly, with the findings dictating further management. If craniotomy is indicated, it is carried out concurrently with the laparotomy.

Although serious head injury is present in 40 percent of hypotensive blunt trauma patients, intracranial mass lesions requiring urgent surgical intervention are uncommon (about 2.5 percent in one report).[17]

Diagnostic Peritoneal Lavage

In the absence of an obvious indication for an immediate laparotomy, a hemodynamically unstable head-injured patient should continue to be resuscitated, and DPL should be performed rapidly (Fig. 21-1). DPL should also be carried out on a hemodynamically stable patient who has an intracranial mass lesion which requires craniotomy and also has an indication for further abdominal diagnostic evaluation. In this scenario, the DPL should be performed in the operating room as the neurosurgical procedure is being carried out in order to avoid delayed treatment of the head injury.

Introduced by Root et al. in 1965,[18] DPL provides a rapid, inexpensive, accurate, and relatively safe, although invasive, modality of diagnosis of intraabdominal injuries in blunt trauma victims. Under local anesthesia, a small infraumbilical incision is made into the abdominal fascia through which a catheter is placed into the peritoneal cavity. The catheter is aspirated, and if less than 10 ml of blood is obtained, 1 liter of saline is instilled and then allowed to drain (more than 750 ml must be recovered for validity). If analysis of the effluent reveals a red blood cell (RBC) count $> 100{,}000/mm^3$, a white blood cell (WBC) count $> 500/mm^3$ (although it may take up to 3 h after a hollow viscus injury for WBCs to migrate into the peritoneal cavity) and amylase $>$ 200 IU/liter or enteric contents or if more than 10 ml of blood is initially aspirated, the test is positive and the patient should proceed directly to laparotomy with simultaneous evaluation of the head injury as previously described.

RBC counts $< 50{,}000/mm^3$ and WBC counts $< 200/mm^3$ are considered negative. RBC counts of 50,000 to $100{,}000/mm^3$ and WBC counts of 200 to $500/mm^3$ are equivocal, and as 10 to 15 percent of patients with DPL values in this indeterminate range have a serious injury,[19] these patients merit reevaluation with a delayed repeat DPL or CT if hemodynamic stability has been ultimately achieved or urgent exploratory laparotomy if it has not. Visceral injury is present in over 95 percent of blunt trauma victims with RBC counts $> 100{,}000/mm^3$ but in less than 5 percent of those with RBC counts $< 20{,}000/mm^3$.[20–24] Significant morbidity rates from DPL itself are consistently below 1 percent but may be higher if a "closed" percutaneous method is utilized.[19]

DPL is contraindicated if there is an obvious need for laparotomy or if there have been multiple previous abdominal operations and should be performed supraumbilically in pregnant patients and in patients with a pelvic fracture. DPL has the disadvantages of oversensitivity and lack of specificity, which may result in a nontherapeutic laparotomy rate of 15 to 20 percent. It is also unreliable in detecting diaphragmatic[25] and retroperitoneal injuries.[26,27]

Computed Tomography

A hemodynamically stable patient with a head injury who has undergone CT of the head and has no immediate indication for neurosurgical intervention but does have an indication for further abdominal evaluation should undergo an abdominal CT scan with oral and intravenous contrast (Fig. 21-1).

CT evaluation for blunt abdominal trauma has been utilized increasingly since the initial reports in the early 1980s. Its advantages include noninvasiveness, the ability to reveal and anatomically characterize solid viscus injury (allowing nonoperative management in selected cases), the ability to quantitate free intraabdominal fluid, and superior assessment of retroperitoneal injuries. However, it is somewhat costly, is time-consuming, requires specialized personnel, and is of questionable ability in detecting hollow viscus injuries and early pancreatic injuries. Reports of accuracy vary, but studies with modern scanners and experienced interpreters have reported an accuracy of 92 to 98 percent.[28–30]

Ultrasound Evaluation

Indications for abdominal ultrasound evaluation are identical to those for CT. Ultrasound has been used extensively in Europe and Japan over the past 20 years and has the advantage of being a noninvasive bedside test. It is not widely utilized in North America, as its reported sensitivity (84 percent) and specificity (88 percent) are well below those of DPL.[31]

Penetrating Abdominal Trauma

Eight to 10 percent of patients who sustain penetrating abdominal wounds have a massive injury or life-threatening hemorrhage requiring immediate laparotomy.[32] The remaining 90 percent require an appropriate means of determining the need for operative intervention. In a patient with a clear sensorium, serial physical examinations are performed with operative intervention indicated for the development of peritoneal signs. A head-injured patient with an altered sensorium obviously requires an alternative approach. Surgical exploration to rule out visceral penetration is much more readily undertaken in such cases.

GUNSHOT WOUNDS

The likelihood of intraabdominal visceral injury is as high as 98 percent in patients who have a bullet traverse the peritoneal cavity.[33] All patients with gunshot wounds to the abdomen should undergo prompt laparotomy. Evaluation of the concurrent head injury may proceed as outlined in Blunt Abdominal Trauma, above (Fig. 21-2).

STAB WOUNDS

Only one-third of patients who sustain stab wounds to the abdomen have a visceral intraabdominal injury. Patients with hypotension, peritoneal signs, or evisceration after an abdominal stab wound require laparotomy. In a patient who has incurred an abdominal stab wound but has a benign examination, serial examination is an accepted method of management. However, a head-injured patient is not a candidate for serial examination to identify the need for laparotomy; in this setting, a more invasive method of management is necessary.

If the patient has a benign abdominal examination, the anterior abdominal stab wound may be explored locally to determine if the abdominal fascia has been penetrated. If it can be determined with confidence that no fascial penetration has occurred, the risk of an intraabdominal injury is negligible and laparotomy is not required. Appropriate evaluation and treatment of the head injury may progress as indicated.

If the fascia has been penetrated, laparotomy may be carried out with concurrent head injury evaluation as was previously described; however, as the likelihood of a nontherapeutic laparotomy is at least 20 to 25 percent,[32] one may elect to proceed with evaluation of the head injury and subsequently carry out a DPL. Various values of RBC counts have been suggested as a threshold for exploration after stab wounds to the abdomen, ranging from > 1000 RBCs/mm^3 to > 100,000 RBCs/mm^3.[28] In general, a higher sensitivity and a higher negative laparotomy rate result from the lower threshold values (Fig. 21-2).

In general, CT is not useful in the evaluation of penetrating abdominal trauma, with a reported sensitivity as low as 14 percent.[34] However, a triple-contrast CT (oral, rectal, and intravenous contrast) may be of value in the evaluation of a hemodynamically stable patient with a posterior wound[35] (Fig. 21-2).

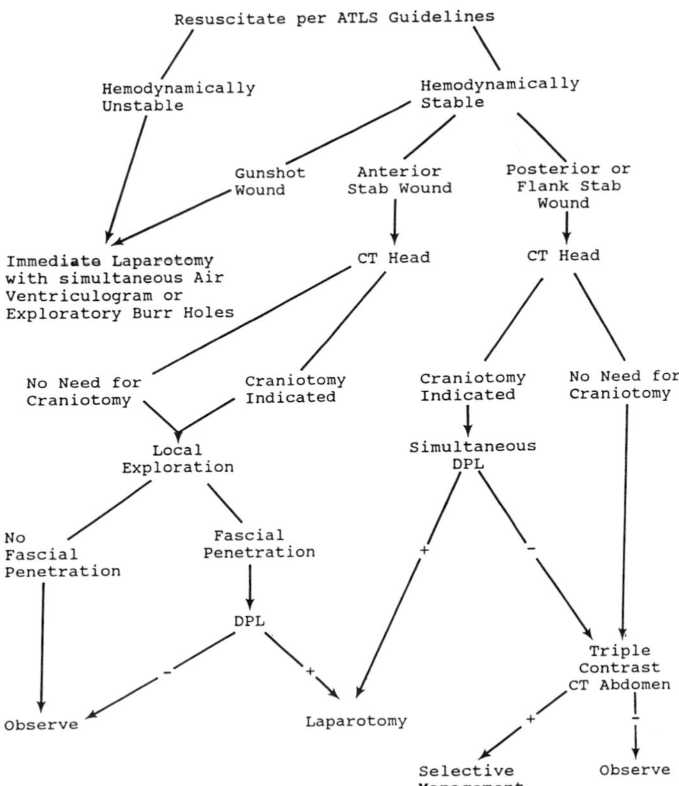

Figure 21-2. Algorithm for the management of a penetrating abdominal injury in a head-injured patient.

SPECIFIC ORGAN INJURIES

Diaphragmatic rupture is associated with high-speed MVAs and may be difficult to diagnose if it is not immediately obvious on chest x-ray after the placement of an orogastric tube. Real-time ultrasound examination may assist in the diagnosis. Laparoscopy may be used in cases of penetrating thoracoabdominal trauma. All these patients should undergo laparotomy for repair. Mortality (40 percent) and morbidity (80 percent) are due primarily to associated injuries.[36]

Gastric injury rarely results from blunt trauma but may be diagnosed by chest x-ray (free intraabdominal air), DPL, or CT findings. Most of these injuries can be primarily repaired with laparotomy, with a good outcome expected. Small bowel injury is a more common injury with blunt trauma (5 to 15 percent incidence)[37] and may be similarly diagnosed and treated by primary repair. Postoperative morbidity is rare, with an anastomotic leak rate of only 1 percent and a bowel obstruction rate of 1 to 2 percent.[38]

Colonic injury may be diagnosed from x-ray, CT, or DPL findings, while rectal injury may be identified on proctoscopy prompted by the finding of blood on rectal examination or the presence of a displaced pelvic fracture. In a hemodynamically stable patient, an isolated colonic injury with minimal fecal spillage may be primarily closed. However, with associated injuries, shock, or contamination, a policy of exteriorization or colostomy should be followed. Rectal injury should be treated with diverting sigmoid colostomy, presacral drainage, and repair. Morbidity is in proportion to the magnitude of the original injury and includes a 5 to 17 percent incidence of intraabdominal abscess and a mortality rate of 20 to 50 percent for combined pelvic and rectal injuries.[38–40]

The diagnosis of duodenal injury is often delayed but may be prompted by the detection of retroperitoneal air on plain x-ray or CT scan, along with periduodenal hemorrhage or contrast extravasation. These findings may be confirmed by contrast duodenography. This injury may be missed intraoperatively unless the duodenum is adequately mobilized and exposed. Simple injuries can be closed primarily or repaired by onlay jejunal patch techniques. More serious injuries can be managed with lateral tube duodenostomy or pyloric exclusion and gastrojejunostomy. The 40 percent mortality associated with a delayed diagnosis can be reduced to 11 percent if surgery is performed within 24 h.[41]

Pancreatic injury is relatively uncommon after blunt trauma and may be very difficult to diagnose on the basis of DPL or CT findings. Suspicion of injury should prompt endoscopic retrograde cholangiopancreatography or exploratory laparotomy with adequate exposure, visualization, and palpation of the gland. Ductal injuries generally require distal resection and drainage.[41]

Splenic injury is readily diagnosed by DPL or CT and is the most common indication for laparotomy after blunt trauma. Grade I or II injuries (Table 21-3) in a hemodynamically stable patient without an indication for laparotomy may be treated nonoperatively. When an operation is indicated, splenic preservation should be the goal.[42] If splenectomy is required, pneumococcal

TABLE 21-3 Splenic Injury Scale

Grade*		Injury Description†
I.	Hematoma	Subcapsular, nonexpanding <10% surface area
	Laceration	Capsular tear, nonbleeding, <1 cm parenchymal depth
II.	Hematoma	Subcapsular, nonexpanding, 10–50% surface area Intraparenchymal, nonexpanding, <2 cm in diameter
	Laceration	Capsular tear, active bleeding; 1–3 cm parenchymal depth which does not involve a trabecular vessel
III.	Hematoma	Subcapsular, >50% surface area or expanding; ruptured subcapsular hematoma with active bleeding; intraparenchymal hematoma >2 cm or expanding
	Laceration	>3 cm parenchymal depth or involving trabecular vessels
IV.	Hematoma	Ruptured intraparenchymal hematoma with active bleeding
	Laceration	Laceration involving segmental or hilar vessels producing major devascularization (>25% of spleen)
V.	Laceration	Completely shattered spleen
	Vascular	Hilar vascular injury which devascularizes spleen

* Advance one grade for multiple injuries to the same organ.

† Based on the most accurate assessment at autopsy, laparotomy, or radiological study.

SOURCE: Moore EE, Shackford SR, Pachter HL, et al: Organ injury scaling: Spleen, liver, and kidney. *J Trauma* 29:1665, 1989, with permission.

TABLE 21-4 Liver Injury Scale

Grade*		Injury Description†
I.	Hematoma	Subcapsular, nonexpanding <10% surface area
	Laceration	Capsular tear, nonbleeding, <1 cm parenchymal depth
II.	Hematoma	Subcapsular, nonexpanding, 10–50% surface area Intraparenchymal, nonexpanding, <2 cm in diameter
	Laceration	Capsular tear, active bleeding; 1–3 cm parenchymal depth, <10 cm in length
III.	Hematoma	Subcapsular, >50% surface area or expanding; ruptured subcapsular hematoma with active bleeding; intraparenchymal hematoma >2 cm or expanding
	Laceration	>3 cm parenchymal depth
IV.	Hematoma	Ruptured intraparenchymal hematoma with active bleeding
	Laceration	Parenchymal disruption involving 25–50% of hepatic lobe
V.	Laceration	Parenchymal disruption involving >50% of hepatic lobe
	Vascular	Juxtahepatic venous injuries, i.e., retrohepatic vena cava/major hepatic veins
VI.	Vascular	Hepatic avulsion

* Advance one grade for multiple injuries to the same organ.

† Based on the most accurate assessment at autopsy, laparotomy, or radiological study.

SOURCE: Moore EE, Shackford SR, Pachter HL, et al: Organ injury scaling: Spleen, liver, and kidney. *J Trauma* 29:1665, 1989, with permission.

vaccine should be administered postoperatively to guard against overwhelming postsplenectomy sepsis.[43,44]

Similarly, liver injuries are readily characterized by CT or diagnosed at laparotomy prompted by DPL findings. Nonoperative treatment with bed rest and serial hematocrit determinations is generally successful in a hemodynamically stable patient regardless of the grade of injury (Table 21-4). If operative management is required, hepatotomy with individual suture ligation of bleeders and nonanatomic debridement of devitalized tissue is preferred. Mortality correlates with the grade of injury (Table 21-4) and can be as high as 80 percent for grade V injuries.[45]

CONCLUSION

The MTOS study reported that 67.8 percent of deaths in patients with head injury treated at trauma centers were due to the head injury alone, 6.6 percent were due to extracranial injury alone, and 25.6 percent were due to the combination of injuries.[12] To optimize the outcome in patients with multiple injuries, a high index of suspicion for intraabdominal injury must be maintained, especially in a comatose patient. These patients should be adequately volume-resuscitated. Diagnostic evaluation of the abdomen in a hemodynamically stable patient should not delay prompt evaluation and care of the head injury. Emergent laparotomy in a hemodynamically unstable patient with head and abdominal injuries should be combined with simultaneous neurosurgical evaluation and operative treatment if indicated. Management that is guided by these principles provides optimal results with this combination of injuries.

References

1. Wilson CB: The management of abdominal injuries in the presence of head injury. *West J Med* 3:343–346, 1969.
2. Belin RP, Richardson JD, Griffen WO: Reducing lethality of simultaneous head injury and blunt abdominal trauma. *South Med J* 65:976–981, 1972.
3. Butterworth JF, Maull KI, Miller JD, et al: Detection of occult abdominal trauma in patients with severe head injuries. *Lancet* 1980:759–762.
4. Nicholson R, Golden G: Blunt abdominal trauma in head injuries. *Lancet* 1966:793–794.
5. Miller JD, Becker DP: Secondary insults to the injured brain. *J R Coll Surg Edinb* 27:292, 1982.
6. Siegal JH, Gens DR, Mamantov T, et al: Effect of associated injuries and blood volume replacement on death, rehabilitation needs and disability in blunt traumatic brain injury. *Crit Care Med* 19:1252, 1991.
7. Cales RH, Trunkey DD: Preventable trauma deaths. *JAMA* 254:1059–1063, 1985.
8. Wilson CB, Vidrine A, Rives JD: Unrecognized abdominal trauma in patients with head injuries. *Ann Surg* 161:608–613, 1965.

9. Olsen WR, Hildreth DH: Abdominal paracentesis and peritoneal lavage in blunt abdominal trauma. *J Trauma* 11:824, 1971.
10. Advanced Trauma Life Support Program. Chicago: American College of Surgeons, 1993.
11. Enderson BL, Reath DB, Meadors J, et al: The tertiary trauma survey: A prospective study of missed injury. *J Trauma* 30:666–669, 1990.
12. Gennarelli TA, Champion HR, Sacco WJ, et al: Mortality of patients with head injury and extracranial injury treated in trauma centers. *J Trauma* 29:1193–1202, 1989.
13. Gutman MB, Moulton RJ, Sullivan I, et al: Relative incidence of intracranial mass lesions and severe torso injury after accidental injury: Implications for triage and management. *J Trauma* 31:974–977, 1991.
14. Wisner DH, Victor NS, Holcroft JW: Priorities in the management of multiple trauma: Intracranial versus intra-abdominal injury. *J Trauma* 35:271–276, 1993.
15. Mackersie RC, Tiwary AD, Shackford SR, et al: Intra-abdominal injury following blunt trauma: Identifying the high-risk patient using objective risk factors. *Arch Surg* 124:809–813, 1989.
16. Andrews BT, Pitts LH, Lovely MP, et al: Is computed tomographic scanning necessary in patients with tentorial herniation? *Neurosurgery* 19:408–413, 1986.
17. Thomason M, Messick J, Rutledge R, et al: Head CT scanning versus urgent exploration in the hypotensive blunt trauma patient. *J Trauma* 34:40–45, 1993.
18. Root HD, Hauser CW, McKinley CR, et al: Diagnostic peritoneal lavage. *Surgery* 57:633, 1965.
19. McAnena OJ, Moore EE, Marx JA: Initial evaluation of the patient with blunt abdominal trauma. *Surg Clin North Am* 70:499–500, 1990.
20. Alyono D, Perry JF: Value of quantitative cell count and amylase activity of peritoneal lavage fluid. *J Trauma* 21:345, 1981.
21. Caffee HH, Benfield JR: Is peritoneal lavage for the diagnosis of hemoperitoneum safe? *Arch Surg* 103:4, 1971.
22. Fischer RP, Bererlin BC, Engrav LH, et al: Diagnostic peritoneal lavage: Fourteen years and 2586 patients later. *Am J Surg* 136:701, 1978.
23. Gomez GA, Alvarez R, Plasencia AR, et al: Diagnostic peritoneal lavage in the management of blunt abdominal trauma: A reassessment. *J Trauma* 27:1, 1987.
24. Thal ER, Shires GT: Peritoneal lavage in blunt abdominal trauma. *Am J Surg* 125:64, 1973.
25. Freeman T, Fischer RP: The inadequacy of peritoneal lavage in diagnosing acute diaphragmatic rupture. *J Trauma* 16:538, 1976.
26. Flint LM, McCoy M, Richardson JD, et al: Duodenal injury: Analysis of common misconceptions in diagnosis and treatment. *Ann Surg* 191:697, 1980.
27. Lucas CE, Ledgerwood AM: Factors influencing outcome after blunt duodenal injury. *J Trauma* 15:839, 1975.
28. Feliciano DV: Diagnostic modalities in abdominal trauma. *Surg Clin North Am* 71:248, 1991.
29. Peitzman AB, Makaroun MS, Slasky S, et al: Prospective study of computed tomography in initial management of blunt abdominal trauma. *J Trauma* 26:590, 1986.
30. Meyer DM, Thal ER, Weigelt JA, et al: Evaluation of computed tomography and diagnostic peritoneal lavage in blunt abdominal trauma. *J Trauma* 29:1168, 1989.
31. Gruessner R, Mentges B, Duber C, et al: Sonography versus peritoneal lavage in blunt abdominal trauma. *J Trauma* 29:242, 1989.
32. Nance FC: Penetrating abdominal trauma, in Cameron JL (ed.): *Current Surgical Therapy* (4th ed). St. Louis: Mosby Year Book, 835–839, 1992.
33. Moore EE, Moore JP, Van Duzer-Moore S, et al: Mandatory laparotomy for gunshot wounds penetrating the abdomen. *Am J Surg* 140:847, 1980.
34. Marx JA, Moore EE, Jorden RC, et al: Limitations of computed tomography in the evaluation of acute abdominal trauma: A prospective comparison with diagnostic peritoneal lavage. *J Trauma* 25:933, 1985.
35. Phillips T, Sclafani SJ, Goldstein A, et al: Use of the contrast-enhanced CT enema in the management of penetrating trauma to the flank and back. *J Trauma* 26:593, 1986.
36. Maull KI: Diaphragmatic rupture, in Cameron JL (ed.): *Current Surgical Therapy* (4th ed). St. Louis: Mosby–Year Book, 840–843, 1992.
37. Thal ER, Meyer DM: Blunt abdominal trauma, in Cameron JL (ed.): *Current Surgical Therapy* (4th ed). St. Louis: Mosby Year Book, 829–834, 1992.
38. Flint LM: Small and large bowel injuries, in Cameron JL (ed.): *Current Surgical Therapy* (4th ed). St. Louis: Mosby Year Book, 853–857, 1992.
39. Mucha P: Pelvic fractures, in Mattox KL, Moore EE, Feliciano DV (eds.): *Trauma*. Norwalk, CT: Appleton and Lange, 505–518, 1988.
40. Richardson JD, Harty J, Amin M, et al: Open pelvic fractures. *J Trauma* 22:533, 1981.
41. Carrico CJ, Jurkovich GJ: Pancreatic and duodenal injuries, in Cameron JL (ed.): *Current Surgical Therapy* (4th ed). St. Louis: Mosby–Year Book, 849–852, 1992.
42. Richardson JD, Miller FB: Spleen injury, in Cameron JL (ed.): *Current Surgical Therapy* (4th ed). St. Louis: Mosby–Year Book, 858–860, 1992.
43. Pearce WH, Moore EE, Moore FA: Injury to the spleen, in Mattox KL, Moore EE, Feliciano DV (eds.): *Trauma*. Norwalk, CT: Appleton and Lange, 443–458, 1988.
44. Caplan ES, Boltansky H, Snyder MJ, et al: Response of traumatized splenectomized patients to immediate vaccination with a polyvalent pneumococcal vaccine. *J Trauma* 23:801, 1983.
45. Trunkey DD: Liver injury, in Cameron JL (ed.): *Current Surgical Therapy* (4th ed). St. Louis: Mosby–Year Book, 844–848, 1992.

CHAPTER 22

GENITO-URINARY INJURIES

Michael Coburn

SYNOPSIS

The diagnosis and staging of genitourinary injuries depend on obtaining an accurate urologic history and physical examination and appropriate imaging studies; this requires a high degree of suspicion and a thorough knowledge of common patterns of injury. Selection of operative versus nonoperative management for many urologic injuries must be individualized on the basis of the anatomy of the injury, the hemodynamic and metabolic stability of the patient, and the presence and significance of other, nonurologic injuries. The diagnosis of genitourinary injuries in a head-injured patient may be challenging if the patient is unable to provide historical information or describe the symptomatology after the trauma; the establishment of standard criteria for the evaluation of hematuria and other objective findings of urinary tract injury is of greater importance in this setting.

INTRODUCTION

The diagnosis and management of genitourinary injury present special challenges in head-injured patients. The history and physical examination may not be obtainable in the usual manner, and the prioritization of injuries is complex, requiring subtle clinical judgments regarding the relative morbidity of the diagnostic and therapeutic maneuvers being considered and the patient's capacity to tolerate nonneurosurgical procedures when the seriousness of the neurological injury is uncertain or evolving.

Genitourinary injury may be dramatic in presentation, as is the case when gross hematuria is present on catheter insertion, or it may be subtle and delayed, as is seen in evolving peritonitis or pelvic infection with a missed bladder injury. Occult injuries represent a special challenge in a patient with head injury, in whom typical symptoms, such as flank or suprapubic pain, may not be accurately reportable. With the exception of occasional cases of exsanguinating hemorrhage of renal origin, urologic injury is an uncommon cause of early mortality. However, delayed diagnosis of urinary tract injuries may result in substantial morbidity from urosepsis, loss of renal function, or long-term disability from lower tract dysfunction. Potential delayed mortality from septic or hemorrhagic complications is generally preventable with appropriate diagnosis and management. Further iatrogenic damage may be prevented through recognition of the urologic injury, for example, by avoiding injudicious attempts at urethral catheterization before excluding a urethral injury.

Current trends in urologic trauma management focus on careful and complete staging of urologic injuries by means of appropriately selected imaging studies, followed by the selection of nonoperative versus open surgical, endoscopic, or radiological management. The use of temporizing measures to delay definitive management of urologic injuries in a polytrauma patient represents a major challenge to the urologist and requires active interaction between the various specialists involved in the patient's care. Particularly in the case of concomitant head injury, the patient's overall clinical status must be assessed to determine the safest timing and method for the management of a urologic injury.

INCIDENCE AND PATTERN OF UROLOGIC INJURY

As in all forms of trauma, urologic injury is manifested in certain patterns, and knowledge of this process can substantially reduce the problem of delayed diagnosis. For example, injuries that result from major forces of deceleration or acceleration classically produce a renal pedicle injury. As a result of the kidney's mobility in the retroperitoneum, sudden deceleration, as occurs in high-speed motor vehicle accidents and falls from a height, may produce traction on the renal pedicle, resulting in renal arterial intimal disruption with thrombosis. Renal pedicle laceration or avulsion also may be seen after such mechanisms of injury. While isolated renal arterial occlusion from blunt trauma may present with subtle signs and without hematuria, vascular avulsion is more likely to result in hemodynamic instability from major retroperitoneal hemorrhage. Specific injuries more commonly observed in the pediatric population include vascular pedicle avulsion, ureteropelvic junction avulsion, and forniceal avulsion in which the entire collecting system may be separated from the renal parenchyma.

Renal parenchymal injury caused by blunt trauma most commonly results from crush forces during abdominal impact, with compression of the kidney between an external object and bony structures such as the lower ribs or the spine. Associated findings may include fracture of the thoracolumbar spinal column, spinal transverse process, or lower rib. Concomitant injury to the liver, spleen, duodenum, or lower thoracic cavity may result from the same forms of impact. Renal parenchymal injuries vary greatly in grade and gravity and are discussed in detail below. A kidney with an underlying abnormality is more prone to significant injury from a seemingly minor trauma. For example, rupture of the renal pelvis with massive urinary extravasation may result from relatively minor abdominal impact to a kidney with marked renal pelvic dilation from a previously unrecognized underlying obstruction of the ureteropelvic junction. Similarly, renal neoplasms may be a source of gross hematuria after minimal trauma. Ureteral injury from blunt trauma is rare but may be seen if prior surgery or retroperitoneal inflammatory disease has resulted in tissue fixation and the loss of the normal mobility of the upper urinary tract.

Urethral or bladder injury is commonly associated with pelvic fracture caused by the fascial attachment of the lower urinary tract organs in the pelvis and the shear forces that accompany such high-energy injuries or, less commonly, with direct penetration by bony spicules. Pelvic fractures are most often seen in association with extraperitoneal bladder rupture, generally involving the lower bladder segment anterolaterally. Intraperitoneal bladder rupture results from direct impact to the lower abdomen with a full bladder and almost invariably involves the bladder dome, which ruptures as a result of the sudden increase in intravesical pressure. Concomitant extraperitoneal and intraperitoneal rupture can be seen when both mechanisms occur during pelvic trauma. Posterior urethral disruption is classically associated with pelvic fracture as well, occurring most commmonly when significant and multiple pubic rami fractures and/or pubic diastasis are involved. These injuries are much more common in males because of the attachment of the prostate retropubically and the vulnerability of the male prostatomembranous and deep bulbous urethra to such trauma. In females, injury to the vaginal vault with concomitant urethral or bladder neck injury may result from a major pelvic fracture. Occasionally, avulsion of the bladder neck may be seen as an isolated injury or in addition to other lower urinary tract injuries, especially when pelvic fracture involves massive pubic diastasis or significant abduction injuries. Visceral injury involving the rectum, vagina, or major pelvic vasculature greatly complicates the management of a urinary tract injury. Crush injury involving the scrotal contents may result from direct genital, perineal, or pelvic trauma and may be missed in the early postinjury period because of the typical degree of scrotal edema, hematoma, and ecchymosis seen after a major pelvic injury, making careful examination of the scrotal contents difficult.

Similar patterns of injury apply to penetrating urologic trauma. Approximately 10 to 15 percent of penetrating abdominal traumas involve the urinary tract; conversely, 80 to 90 percent of penetrating abdominal urologic injuries involve injury to other, nonurologic intraabdominal organs. Penetrating renal and upper ureteral injury may be seen commonly in combination with trauma to great vessels, liver, spleen, stomach, colon, duodenum, and small intestine. Lower ureteral and bladder damage may be commonly seen with iliac vessel, sigmoid colon, rectal, and small intestinal injury. Urethral and external genital injury is often accompanied by injury to the thigh, occasionally involving the femoral vessels.

Appreciation of these typical mechanisms and patterns of genitourinary injury in both the blunt and penetrating trauma settings increases one's awareness of the settings in which specific organ injuries are common. It also can decrease the risk of missing important injuries by appropriately increasing one's suspicion and affecting the diagnostic approach.

CLINICAL PRESENTATION

Genitourinary injuries may be plainly observable on presentation, as in the case of major genital trauma, or may require a high degree of suspicion followed by diagnostic testing, as with renal lacerations. The typical history and physical findings in patients with urologic injuries and the special problems encountered in a head-injured patient must be appreciated to achieve diagnostic accuracy.

Patients with blunt injury to the kidney may complain of flank or abdominal pain, often associated with tenderness in the costovertebral angle posteriorly or below the costal margin anteriorly and laterally. Eliciting tenderness anteriorly by deep palpation during inspiration may be useful diagnostically. Flank ecchymosis may be noted. If there has been significant retroperitoneal hemorrhage from a renal or other urologic injury, hypotension and tachycardia may be present. The delayed emergence of hemodynamic instability after renal injury is an ominous sign and has a major impact on management decisions. Progressive abdominal distention may be indicative of the enlargement of a retroperitoneal hematoma from a renal injury, ileus resulting from abdominal trauma with a urologic or abdominal visceral injury, or urinary extravasation from a renal or bladder injury. Progressive urinary extravasation typically produces an ileus, and patients with delayed extravasation after operative management of urologic injuries or during observation in a nonoperative management approach often develop fever, abdominal distension, nausea, and vomiting from ileus, or frank signs of intraabdominal sepsis.

Patients with head injury may fail to complain of pain, voiding abnormalities, or other typical symptoms of urologic injury because of altered mental status. Thus, the typical symptomatology may be masked.

SIGNS AND SYMPTOMS OF UROLOGIC INJURY

UPPER TRACT INJURY

Hematuria is the cardinal sign of urinary tract trauma, but excessive reliance on this finding to rule in or rule out significant injury can lead to an unreliable and inaccurate diagnosis. It is important to think anatomically in one's view of hematuria in the trauma setting; that is, the presence of blood in bladder urine after an upper tract injury depends on a flow of urine from the injured renal unit down the ureter and into the bladder. As such, a major renal injury with extensive disruption of the renal parenchyma and collecting system resulting from a blunt or penetrating trauma may not consistently result in a magnitude of hematuria that is commensurate with the degree of renal injury, since urine from the injured kidney may be accummulating in the retroperitoneum rather than being conducted down the ureter. The same is true of renal pedicle injuries, in which the kidney may be nonperfused, with arterial occlusion from an intimal arterial injury or even free bleeding into the retroperitoneum from pedicle avulsion or laceration without the consistent presence of hematuria. A completely transected ureter may not result in hematuria for the same reason, while urine freely enters the retroperitoneum or peritoneal cavity. Disappearance of hematuria early after injury is often considered a sign that a minor injury has occurred, while persistence is thought to indicate a more significant injury. While this is generally true, it is not always the case.

Hematuria is generally present after a bladder injury, although the degree does not correlate well with the severity of the bladder injury. For example, with delayed presentation, an intraperitoneal bladder rupture may temporarily seal off with omentum or bowel adherent to the dome rupture, with the transient resolution of hematuria but with the continued potential for substantial morbidity when the minimal fibrinous adhesions lyse and massive intraperitoneal urinary extravasation continues. Similarly, blood at the external urethral meatus or in the vaginal or rectal vault is an important sign of lower tract injury after a pelvic fracture, but its absence does not confirm the absence of a significant urethral injury.

In general, however, hematuria is an important sign of urinary tract injury. Recent data indicate that after blunt trauma, the presence of microscopic hematuria alone, in the absence of hypotension any time after injury, predicts a very low risk of significant renal injury, and renal imaging studies have a very low yield.[1–4] This rule cannot be safely applied to a pediatric patient or a penetrating trauma patient. A more conservative view would amend this simple rule to include deceleration trauma; the presence of long bone, pelvic, or transverse spinal process or lower rib fracture; and loss of consciousness or altered mental status as further indications to evaluate microhematuria after blunt trauma.

As was indicated above, pain and tenderness in the flank or upper abdomen are important indicators of possible upper tract injury but may be obscured in a head-injured patient. A mass effect in the flank or upper abdomen, the presence of ecchymoses, and penetrating injury to the lower chest or abdomen are important potential indicators of urinary tract injury.

Hemodynamic instability after multiple trauma in patients in whom urinary tract injury is suspected is problematic, as it may be difficult to assign it to a specific cause. When combined with a dropping hematocrit and the presence of signs of abdominal injury, renal damage should be suspected and appropriately excluded by means of imaging studies or laparotomy if that is elected by the trauma surgeon.

Lower Tract Injury

The signs and symptoms of lower urinary tract injury may include failure to void, urinary retention after an injury, hematuria, blood at the urethral meatus, abdominal distension, scrotal mass or pain, perineal hematoma or urinoma, and abnormalities on rectal examination. Blood at the urethral meatus is commonly seen with urethral injury and should prompt retrograde urethrography for confirmation before the insertion of a Foley catheter. Abdominal distension may indicate urinary retention from a full bladder after urethral trauma or may reflect intraperitoneal urine or extravasated extraperitoneal urine with an expanding pelvic hematoma after bladder rupture. Scrotal swelling and pain may occur after testicular rupture or may simply reflect blood in the scrotal wall after pelvic trauma, most often after a pelvic fracture. After posterior urethral disruption, the prostate may be difficult to palpate on digital rectal examination because of cephalad migration of the prostate and the surrounding pelvic hematoma. A definitive diagnosis of these common forms of urologic injury often requires specific imaging studies for confirmation and selection of the management approach.

DIAGNOSIS OF GENITOURINARY INJURY

Urologists are fortunate to have an ample armamentarium of diagnostic imaging studies available to fully assess the urinary tract and thus "stage" urologic injuries and allow a fully informed selection of therapeutic options.

Hematuria

As was indicated previously, gross hematuria after injury or microscopic hematuria accompanied by hypotension or the other relative indications for investigation should prompt a thorough urologic evaluation to exclude significant injury. The standard approach, as in the elective evaluation of nontraumatic hematuria, involves both upper and lower urinary tract imaging studies to assess the renal parenchyma and collecting system, ureters, and bladder. The selection of appropriate imaging studies for the specific clinical situation is important for an accurate and cost-effective diagnosis.

Upper Tract Injury

Intravenous pyelography

Intravenous pyelography (IVP) by a bolus infusion technique has long been the standard means of upper tract assessment after injury. After it has been determined that there is no known allergy to iodinated contrast, a scout film of the abdomen is obtained, followed by intravenous administration of 1 to 2 ml/kg of iodinated contrast. Films are then obtained at varying intervals, depending on the information desired; 5, 10, and 20 min after injection is typical. Normally, bilateral nephrograms are observed, followed by contrast excretion and opacification of the upper collecting systems and ureters and then by the cystographic phase with bladder filling. Nonvisualization of either kidney may indicate arterial occlusion from intimal disruption, major parenchymal disruption, severe contusion, congenital absence, or nonfunction resulting from nontraumatic causes. Loss of a portion of the cortical outline may indicate a renal laceration or hematoma or may reflect a suboptimal study with the renal anatomy obscured by bowel gas or soft tissue shadowing. Extravasation from the calyces, pelvis, or ureter may be seen on the delayed films. Limitations of IVP in regard to trauma include poor imaging of the perinephric space, failure to gain information about other solid abdominal viscera, and nonspecific information from the finding of renal nonvisualization or loss of cortical outline. IVP is, however, readily available, can be performed in the emergency room setting with basic radiographic equipment, is relatively inexpensive, and will stage a large proportion of renal injuries adequately, at least for the initiation of therapy. In the setting of a patient for whom laparotomy is planned for a urologic or nonurologic indication, and especially after penetrating trauma, IVP is quite useful preoperatively to assure the surgeon that there are two functioning renal units in case the operative findings raise the possibility of nephrectomy for the injured kidney.

Abdominal computed tomography

Computed tomography (CT) has moved to the forefront as the study of choice for the most precise, accurate staging of blunt renal trauma and in the penetrating trauma setting when nonoperative management of renal injury is contemplated. While IVP provides adequate diagnostic information in many cases of upper urinary tract injury, CT scan has many advantages. Imaging of other upper abdominal viscera, such as the liver and spleen, is excellent. The presence of free intraperitoneal fluid is often appreciable. Detailed examination of the status of the renal parenchyma and perinephric space is possible, allowing detection of a perinephric hematoma

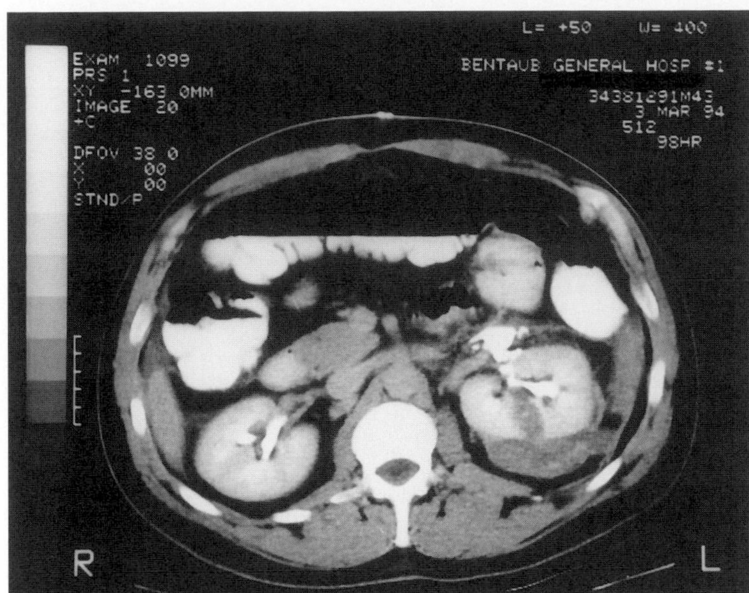

Figure 22-2. CT scan showing deeper laceration through the medulla with contrast extravasation anteriorly and a perinephric hematoma posteriorly.

and devitalized renal parenchyma. Nonperfusion of the renal parenchyma can be documented clearly after intravenous contrast administration as a likely indication of renal arterial occlusion, as opposed to the analogous finding of nonvisualization of IVP, which leaves open the question whether the kidney is absent, contused, crushed, or nonperfused. CT scanning is quite sensitive for visualizing contrast extravasation of parenchymal or collecting system origin. In the penetrating trauma setting, the determination of whether a tangential abdominal injury has penetrated the peritoneal cavity may be achieved by recognizing the tissue tract. In cases of penetrating renal trauma in which the presence or absence of associated intraabdominal injury will determine the selection of operative versus nonoperative management, such information may be critical. As these features that are notable on CT can help one select operative versus nonoperative management for renal trauma, CT is now widely considered the gold standard for renal injury staging (Figs. 22-1 through 22-3), although the cost of CT is significantly greater than that of IVP. However, IVP still plays an important role in urgent imaging in the emergency room setting, in cases in which the need for other solid organ imaging is not critical, and when the precise staging afforded by CT for selection is not relevant to operative versus nonoperative decision making.

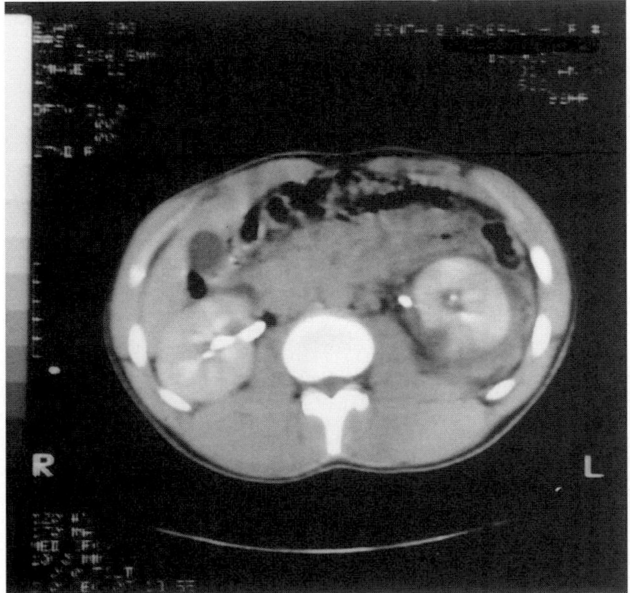

Figure 22-1. CT scan with contrast showing minor parenchymal laceration in the posterior portion of the left kidney. A small perinephric hematoma is present. Such injuries generally are managed nonoperatively with a low complication rate.

When operative intervention for abdominal trauma is planned and if the patient's condition allows it, a preoperative CT scan can obviate the need for a renal exploration at the time of laparotomy if careful staging shows that the injury has a high likelihood of being successfully handled nonoperatively.

Arteriography

In the past, renal arteriography was utilized extensively for assessing major renal injuries and documenting renal pedicle injury from blunt trauma. With the advent of CT scanning, arteriography is used much less often. It is still useful when embolization is contemplated for nonoperative management of early or delayed renal bleeding after trauma or when one is considering the

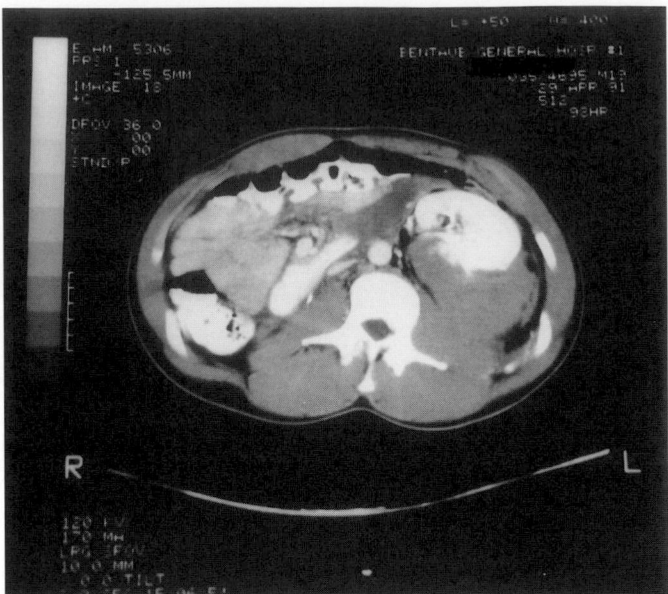

A

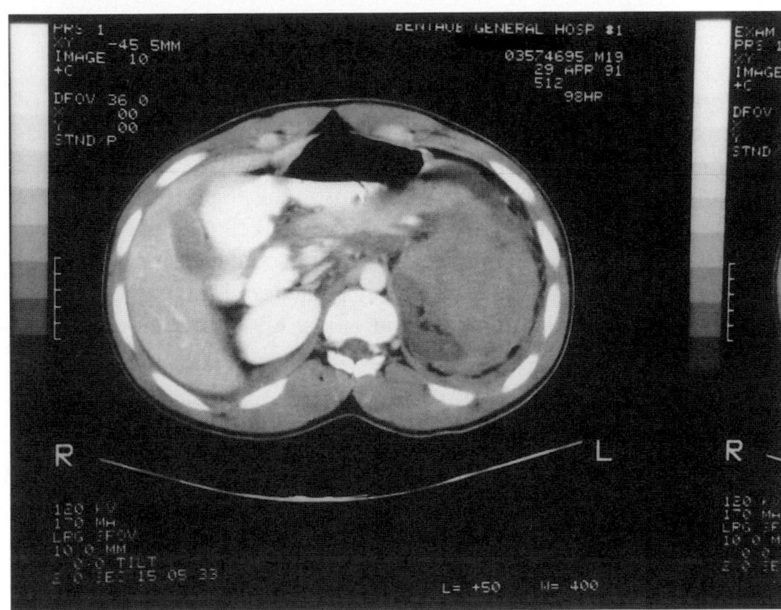

B

Figure 22-3. *A.* CT scan reveals a large left perinephric hematoma but normal perfusion of parenchyma. *B.* More cephalad view of same patient demonstrates a large hematoma with devascularization of a significant parenchymal fragment of the upper pole. The patient underwent evacuation of the hematoma and upper pole nephrectomy; operative findings showed avulsion and infarction of the upper pole with active bleeding from segmental branch renal vessels.

placement of vascular stents in selected cases of renovascular trauma. In some cases of major renal injury, arteriography can provide useful information regarding perfusion and document avulsion or distraction of parenchymal fragments if the CT scan does not provide such information adequately.

Ultrasound

There is increasing interest in ultrasound for imaging a traumatized abdomen both in urology and in general surgery. In many European trauma centers, ultrasound is the mainstay of diagnostic imaging for abdominal trauma. Ultrasound is often readily available and demonstrates the intactness of the renal parenchyma adequately in most cases, though the presence of a significant perinephric hematoma may obscure other anatomic details. However, urinary extravasation cannot be appreciated without a contrast study unless the presence of a large urinoma or free abdominal fluid allows such a diagnostic inference. Doppler flow imaging may allow the determination of renal arterial patency but is operator-dependent and may be technically difficult. In general, ultrasound is a useful initial screening test after trauma but probably does not afford the degree of specificity or sensitivity that would make it a plausible alternative to CT in most centers.

Nuclear scan

In a contrast-allergic patient, nuclear scanning may provide a key to the presence of urinary extravasation and clearly demonstrate nonperfusion of a kidney, but without the diagnostic accuracy of CT scanning. Nuclear scanning is not readily available in most hospitals off hours and at short notice. Its relevance in the acute trauma setting is limited.

Retrograde pyelography

Retrograde pyelography performed cystoscopically or during an open surgical procedure through an open bladder is the gold standard for contrast imaging of the ureter and collecting system. It is relevant when IVP or CT demonstrates a contrast extravasation pattern suggestive of renal pelvic disruption, ureteropelvic avulsion, or forniceal avulsion (all more common in the pediatric population) after blunt trauma and for the definitive staging of blunt or penetrating trauma when the intactness of the upper collecting cannot be definitively established from noninvasive imaging studies.

Lower Tract Injury

Retrograde urethrography

Retrograde urethrography is the study of choice for imaging the urethra and bladder outlet after trauma. The study is performed by instilling radiopaque contrast into the urethral meatus through a catheter inserted into the fossa navicularis and allowing the entire urethra to fill and distend in this manner. Extravasation of contrast and areas of abnormal narrowing may be demonstrative of urethral injury. Voluntary or involuntary constriction of the external sphincter may occur in an awake patient in response to anterior urethral distension, preventing contrast from entering the bladder; this must be distinguished from a true anatomic obstruction. Posterior urethral disruption may be recognized after a pelvic fracture and may be complete or partial. Anterior urethral trauma may result from straddle injuries, with direct blunt impact against the perineum, or from penetrating injury to the perineum or genitalia. The presence of blood in the urethra or at the urethral meatus is a cardinal sign of urethral injury, and when it is noted, a retrograde urethrogram should be performed before any attempt is made to catheterize the urethra; the injudicious attempts to pass a catheter without recognition that the area has suffered a traumatic injury may result in inadvertent urethral damage.

Stress cystography (retrograde, antegrade)

A stress cystogram involves filling the bladder with radiopaque contrast, usually through a urethral catheter, for the purpose of detecting a bladder injury (Figs. 22-4 through 22-7). The study must fully distend the urinary bladder to reliably demonstrate or exclude an injury, since a significant bladder rupture may temporarily seal off with blood, fibrinous debris, omentum, or bowel, and incomplete distension during cystography may produce a false-negative study. The goal is to produce pressures typical of normal voiding to determine that the bladder wall has not been compromised. In an adult, this usually is best performed by filling the bladder by gravity through an indwelling catheter and then instilling 30 to 60 ml of additional contrast after gravity filling ceases. Alternatively, if the patient has normal sensation and can describe a sensation of bladder fullness or an urge to void, filling can be halted and a radiograph can be obtained. An adequate cystogram also can be obtained by CT, but again, full distension is needed. The entire abdomen should be included on the radiographic image obtained after bladder filling so that one can observe contrast that may have flowed into the upper abdomen, outlining the liver or filling the lateral colic gutters if an intraperitoneal rupture is present, or observe contrast that may extravasate into the lower pelvis or perineum as seen in the extraperitoneal bladder ruptures most commonly associated with pelvic fracture. After the film with a full bladder is assessed, a "washout" study is obtained by draining all the contrast from the bladder and irrigating the bladder with normal saline. Extravasation may be seen on the washout film that can be missed on the filling study if the extravasated contrast is anterior or posterior to the bladder and is obscured by the intraluminal contrast. A stress cystogram also may be obtained through a suprapubic cystostomy tube placed percutaneously for the treatment of a urethral disruption. The importance of evaluation of the bladder in this setting must not be overlooked.

Scrotal ultrasound

Scrotal ultrasonography is useful in determining whether testicular rupture is present in settings in which scrotal wall swelling and hematoma obscure anatomic landmarks, making physical examination unreliable.

Cystoscopy

Because of the availability of radiographic imaging studies to evaluate the intactness of the lower urinary tract, cystoscopy is not often utilized in the acute trauma setting. Exceptions include the use of cystoscopy and retro-

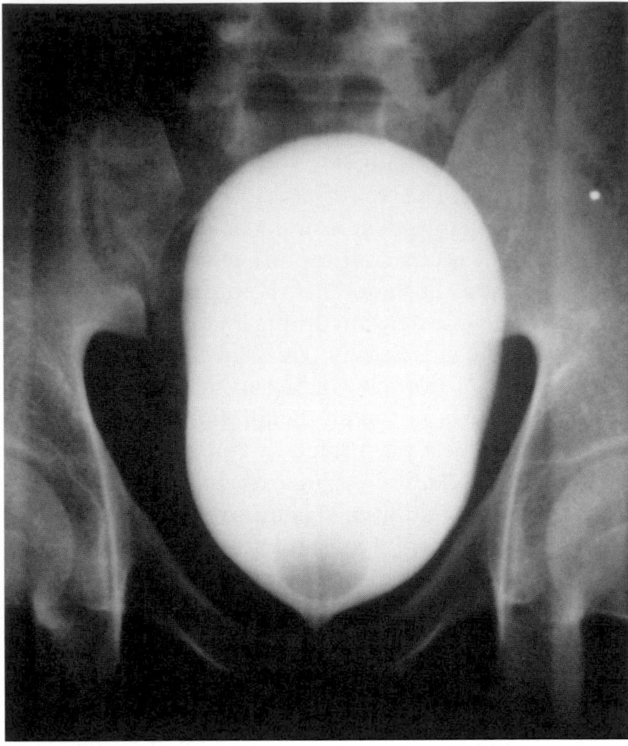

Figure 22-4. Normal stress cystogram. The bladder if fully distended; the Foley catheter balloon is visible near the bladder neck.

grade pyelography to assess the upper collecting system and the occasional use of cystoscopy to assess urethral or bladder injuries for selection of nonoperative management in either the blunt or the penetrating trauma setting.

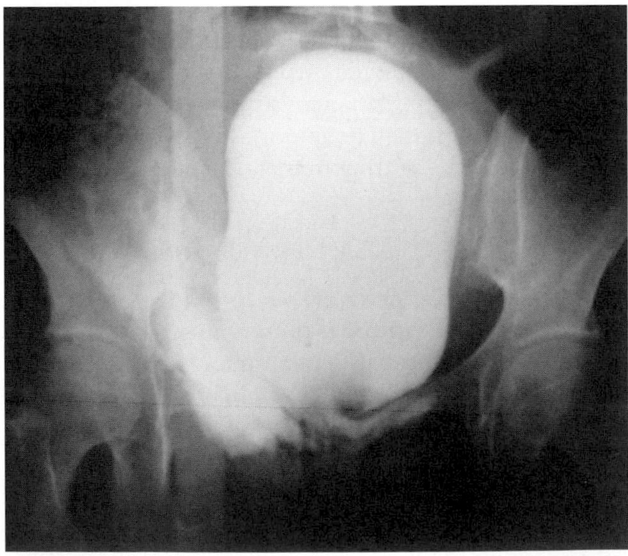

Figure 22-5. Stress cystogram revealing extraperitoneal bladder rupture. Note contrast lateral to the lower bladder segment.

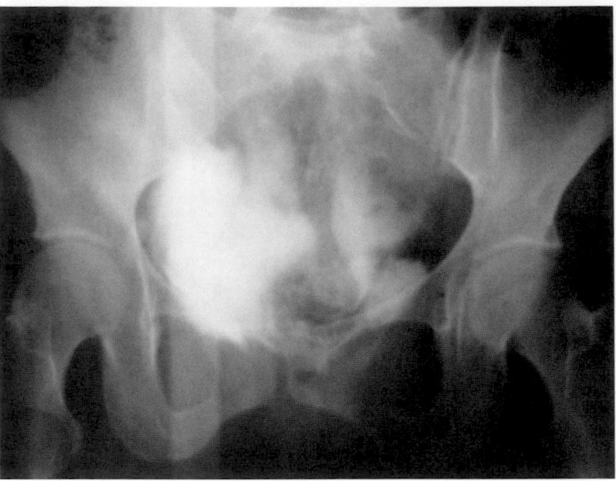

Figure 22-6. Washout film after cystography reveals significant extraperitoneal extravasation.

MANAGEMENT

Management of urogenital injuries must be integrated into the overall management plan of a patient with multiple injuries. In general, an aggressive approach to the diagnosis and staging of urinary tract trauma is appropriate in selecting patients for operative versus nonoperative management. Categorizing urologic injuries into those which present an immediate threat to life and those for which delayed or semielective management is

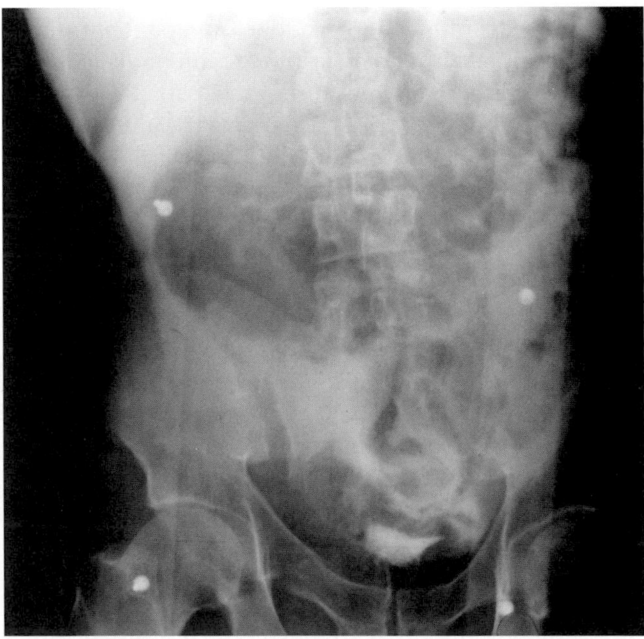

Figure 22-7. Stress cystogram demonstrating the classic findings of intraperitoneal bladder rupture. Contrast can be seen surrounding loops of intestine, in the right colic gutter, and around the liver in the right upper quadrant.

acceptable is critical. Management considerations will be discussed below in regard to organ site and mechanism of injury.

Renal Trauma

Blunt renal injury may result in contusion, minor or major laceration, avulsion of parenchymal fragments, comminuted fractures with complete destruction of the kidney, and pedicle injuries. Appropriate staging of renal injuries, as discussed above, allows the intelligent selection of a management approach for each of these forms of renal trauma. Renal contusions and minor lacerations (involving only the renal cortex) usually are managed nonoperatively with observation and bed rest. More significant lacerations (involving the deep cortex, medulla, and/or collecting system) also are often manageable nonoperatively as long as the patient is hemodynamically stable and is not suffering significant blood loss from the renal injury. Patients with major renal lacerations managed nonoperatively need to be closely observed, preferably initially in an intensive care unit setting, with frequent determination of vital signs and hematocrit. Bed rest for several days usually is instituted. One must always be prepared to alter one's approach and move on to operative management if ongoing blood loss or complications such as urinoma formation become evident. Patients whose renal injuries involve extensive destruction of parenchyma with multiple lacerations, significant avulsed/distracted parenchymal fragments, and massive contrast extravasation are poorer candidates for nonoperative management, as the complication rate is significantly higher when such injuries are managed nonoperatively. While such radiographic findings may constitute relative indications for operative exploration and reconstruction, partial nephrectomy, or nephrectomy, hemodynamic instability indicative of significant blood loss is the primary absolute indication for surgery in renal trauma. In general, approximately 80 percent of renal injuries may be managed nonoperatively, 5 to 10 percent require immediate surgery for significant bleeding, and 10 to 15 percent are in the "gray zone" in which the risk of observation is increased and patients must be monitored very closely and possibly progress to surgery or radiographic intervention if complications arise. The development of a urinoma often can be managed by percutaneous drainage under CT or ultrasound guidance, and renal bleeding sometimes can be managed successfully with selective angiographic embolization. The selection of operative versus radiological intervention for complications of renal trauma must be individualized and depends on the skill and experience of the radiology staff, the patient's clinical condition, and the specific anatomic features of the injury.

Penetrating injuries to the kidney have traditionally been managed operatively, although recent data suggest that a significant proportion may be manageable nonoperatively, as is done for blunt trauma.[5–7] For renal gunshot wounds, the risk of concomitant intraabdominal visceral injury is at least 85 percent; since laparotomy usually is performed for the evaluation and treatment of nonurologic injuries in such cases, the kidney is often explored as well. Stab wounds to the back or flank more often present an opportunity to manage penetrating renal injury nonoperatively; CT scanning is extremely useful in selecting such patients.

Renal pedicle injuries which involve arterial occlusion resulting from intimal disruption with resultant thrombosis may be surgically revascularized if the kidney can be expected to remain viable; this requires that no more than a few hours elapse between the time of arterial thrombosis and the time of repair. The difficulty lies in determining when complete thrombosis and warm ischemia time actually begin, since this process may occur immediately after injury or hours later. In general, revascularization attempts occurring more than 8 to 12 h after injury have a low likelihood of success, while those performed within 4 h of injury are much more likely to result in a viable, functioning kidney. Assessment of the general condition of the patient is critical in choosing to revascularize a kidney after a pedicle injury. One may conclude that general anesthesia and operative intervention represent too high a risk after major head injury if the contralateral kidney is uninjured. Avulsion injuries to the pedicle often result in substantial retroperitoneal bleeding, typically requiring urgent operative intervention.

Ureteral Trauma

As was noted previously, blunt ureteral injury is uncommon except in the pediatric age group, in which ureteropelvic or forniceal avulsion and renal pelvic rupture may be seen. Most of these injuries are managed operatively with surgical repair. Penetrating ureteral injury is usually encountered during laparotomy for a nonurologic injury, and operative repair is routine. Middle and upper ureteral injuries generally are managed by means of primary anastomosis; distal injuries usually require reimplantation into the bladder because of concern about the viability of the distal stump.

Bladder Trauma

Selection of the management approach for bladder injury depends largely on whether the rupture is intraperitoneal or extraperitoneal and on the presence or absence of adjacent organ injury.[8,9] Intraperitoneal bladder rupture is almost always repaired surgically to prevent continued entry of urine into the abdomen. Extraperitoneal bladder ruptures can be managed nonoperatively in more than 90 percent of cases by allowing them to heal with an indwelling urethral or suprapubic catheter.[10] Indications for operative repair include combined intra- and extraperitoneal injury, failure to achieve adequate catheter drainage because of ongoing bleeding and clot occlusion, and concomitant vaginal or rectal injury.

Urethral Trauma

The approach to the management of posterior urethral disruption has evolved over the last three decades[11–16] from an era in which morbid, traumatic attempts at early open surgical realignment were routine to the current approach of suprapubic tube diversion followed by delayed urethroplasty 3 to 6 months after an injury. There has been increasing interest in endoscopically guided approaches to earlier urethral realignment, but data regarding urethral patency after such endoscopic repairs do not clearly demonstrate their appropriateness in the treatment of urethral injury.[17] The standard approach is still delayed elective reconstruction of obliterated strictures after initial suprapubic diversion. Anterior urethral injuries from blunt or penetrating trauma can be managed with primary excision and repair or with suprapubic tube or urethral catheter placement, depending on the patient's condition and the experience of the surgeon.[18]

Genital Trauma

Blunt or penetrating penile or testicular injuries are managed operatively if rupture is suspected or verified by imaging studies. Injuries to the corpus cavernosum of the penis are primarily sutured to avoid future deformity, pain, and erectile dysfunction; testicular ruptures are repaired surgically if adequate parenchyma can be salvaged and the blood supply to the testis is intact.[19,20] Loss of genital skin may present a plastic surgical challenge and usually is managed initially with conservative debridement and wound cleansing followed by delayed coverage with split-thickness or full-thickness skin grafts or local tissue transfer flap techniques.[21,22]

References

1. Nicolaisen GS, McAninch JW, Marshall GA, et al: Renal trauma: Reevaluation of the indications for radiographic assessment. *J Urol* 133:183, 1985.
2. Peterson NE, Schulze KA: Selective diagnostic uroradiography for trauma. *J Urol* 137:449, 1987.
3. Mee SL, McAninch JW: Indications for radiographic assessment in suspected renal trauma. *Urol Clin North Am* 16:187, 1989.
4. Mee SL, McAninch JW, Robinson AL, et al: Radiographic assessment of renal trauma: A 10 year prospective study of patient selection. *J Urol* 141:1095, 1989.
5. Heyns CD, van Vollenhoven P: Increasing role of angiography and segmental embolization in the management of renal stab wounds. *J Urol* 147:1231, 1992.
6. Scott R Jr, Carlton CE Jr, Goldman M: Penetrating injuries of the kidney: An analysis of 181 patients. *J Urol* 101:247, 1969.
7. Baniel J, Schein M: Collective Review: The management of penetrating trauma to the urinary tract. *J Am Coll Surg* 178:417, 1994.
8. Cass AS: Bladder trauma in the multiple injured patient. *J Urol* 115:667, 1976.
9. Carroll PR, McAninch JW: Major bladder trauma: Mechanisms of injury and a unified method of diagnosis and repair. *J Urol* 132:254, 1984.
10. Corriere JN Jr, Sandler CM: Mechanisms of injury, patterns of extravasation and management of extraperitoneal bladder rupture due to blunt trauma. *J Urol* 139:43, 1988.
11. Morehouse DD, MacKinnon KJ: Management of prostatomembranous urethral disruption. *J Urol* 123:173:1980.
12. Turner-Warwick R: Complex traumatic posterior urethral strictures. *J Urol* 118:564, 1977.
13. Waterhouse K, Abrams HG, Hackett RE, et al: The transpubic approach to the lower urinary tract. *J Urol* 109:486, 1973.
14. Webster GD, Sihelnik S: The management of strictures of the membranous urethra. *J Urol* 134:469, 1985.
15. Webster GD, Mathes GL, Selli C: Prostatomembranous urethral injuries: A review of the literature and a rational approach to their management. *J Urol* 130:898, 1985.
16. Johansen B: Reconstruction of the male urethra in strictures. *Acta Chir Scand* Suppl 176:1, 1953.
17. Marshall FF, Chang R, Gearhart JP: Endoscopic reconstruction of traumatic membranous urethral transection. *J Urol* 138:306, 1987.
18. Pontes JE, Pierce JM: Anterior urethral injuries: Four years of experience at the Detroit General Hospital. *J Urol* 120:563, 1978.
19. Gross M: Rupture of the testicle: The importance of early surgical treatment. *J Urol* 101:196, 1969.
20. Albert NE: Testicular ultrasound for trauma. *J Urol* 124:558, 1980.
21. Jordan GH, Gilbert DA: Male genital trauma. *Clin Plast Surg* 14:431,1988.
22. McAninch JW: Management of genital skin loss. *Urol Clin North Am* 16:387, 1989.

ICU Management

CHAPTER 23

CARDIOPULMONARY MANAGEMENT OF THE HEAD-INJURED PATIENT

MariaElaina Sumas
Raj K. Narayan

SYNOPSIS

The improved outcomes from head injury over the past few decades are generally attributed to improved triage and patient transport, rapid surgical evacuations of lesions, and better management of intracranial pressure (ICP). However, there is little doubt that more aggressive application of critical care techniques have played a major role in this regard. In this chapter, the cardiac and pulmonary management of the head-injured patient have been reviewed with an emphasis on the more common problems encountered.

INTRODUCTION

The care of critically ill "neurotraumatized" patients requires a working knowledge of neurosurgery, neurology, critical care, anesthesiology, physiology, cardiology, and pulmonary medicine. The general medical problems which frequently occur in this population, often due to immobilization, include aspiration, sepsis, pulmonary embolism, myocardial ischemia, electrolyte abnormalities, and blood pressure abnormalities. The recognition and prevention of systemic complications, such as hypotension (systolic blood pressure < 90), hypoxia (Pa_{O_2} < 70 mmHg), hypercarbia (Pa_{CO_2} > 45 mmHg), and hyperthermia, which can cause secondary injury to the already traumatized brain cannot be overemphasized. This chapter reviews the common cardiopulmonary problems that afflict the head-injured patient, and the treatments that may be used in their management.

THE CARDIOVASCULAR SYSTEM IN HEAD INJURY

Monitoring Techniques

ECG Monitoring

As with other intracranial pathologies, such as subarachnoid hemorrhage, stroke, and intracerebral hemorrhage, the cardiovascular system can also be affected by head injury. Proper management of the comatose patient should consist of electrical and hemodynamic monitoring combined with the appropriate clinical examination in order to minimize the negative consequences of cardiac dysrhythmias and blood pressure changes on an already "traumatized" brain. A baseline 12-lead electrocardiograph (ECG) should be obtained on admission to the intensive care unit (ICU) followed by continuous ECG monitoring in lead II. An acute myocardial infarction should be ruled out if there is any evidence to suggest that an ischemic event has occurred, especially when the history suggests that a fall, seizure, or syncopal episode preceded the head injury. Furthermore, in the patient with multiple trauma where an associated chest injury with myocardial contusion is suspected, echocardiography may be of value in assessing the cardiac status and guiding subsequent decision making.[1] The patient with an unexplained ECG abnormality will need an echocardiogram to help determine if there is a dyskinetic or hypokinetic heart segment.

While experimental studies have shown several cardiovascular abnormalities following head injury,[2,3] the common abnormalities include peaked T waves, long Q-T intervals, and prominent U waves. Hypothalamic control of cardiac repolarization[4] and stimulation of the sympathetic system[5] are thought to be the cause of these changes. Atrial and ventricular arrythmias, including premature atrial contractions, atrial flutter, atrial fibrillation, supraventricular tachycardia, ventricular tachycardia, ventricular fibrillation, intraventricular conduction defect, and atrioventricular block, can be seen after head injury.[6] In addition sinus bradycardia may indicate a Cushing response due to raised intracranial pressure. While the rapid appearance and disappearance of ECG changes suggest a neural rather than humoral or primary cardiac etiology, these phenomena may result in sudden unexpected death in adults.[7]

Arterial blood pressure monitoring

Hemodynamic monitoring in patients with severe head injury generally requires invasive devices, including an arterial line, central venous pressure catheter, and even a pulmonary artery catheter (PAC). The volume status and blood pressure must be closely regulated to ensure adequate cerebral perfusion pressure (CPP). A catheter inserted into the patient's bladder can be used as an indirect indicator of volume status. The urinary output should be >0.5 ml/kg/h. A Foley catheter should be inserted in all comatose patients, elderly patients with a history of cardiac or renal disease, and in hypotensive patients in shock in order to monitor urinary output and, indirectly, renal perfusion.

The standard practice in comatose head-injured patients is to measure the arterial pressure directly via catheters placed in the radial artery or occasionally the femoral or dorsalis pedis artery. Arterial catheters are particularly indicated in patients with hemodynamic instability or those requiring vasopressor, vasodilator, or inotropic medications. The radial artery is preferred because it is superficial, accessible, compressible, and the skin site is easy to keep clean. Furthermore, the hand receives collateral flow through the ulnar artery and the palmar arch, so that occlusion of the radial artery rarely causes ischemic damage of the hand and digits. Ischemic necrosis is extremely rare.[8–10] Nevertheless, arterial occlusion has been reported in 25 percent of radial artery cannulations[9] with occlusion permanent in 3 percent of cases.[10] The brachial artery should rarely be used since it is the sole blood supply to the forearm and hand. The dorsalis pedis artery is less popular in adults because of the distortion produced in the pulse waveform at this site.[11] In addition to allowing for continuous monitoring of systolic, diastolic, and mean arterial blood pressure, arterial catheters are commonly used to obtain serial arterial blood gases and other blood test samples.

Central venous pressure monitoring

The most common form of central venous pressure (CVP) monitoring is via cannulation of the superior vena cava with a multiple lumen catheter. This is clearly needed in patients with poor peripheral venous access and in those that require rapid fluid resuscitation, vasoactive therapy, or total parenteral nutrition (TPN). The subclavian vein is the most common site for central venous cannulation using the subclavicular or supraclavicular approach with equal success (Fig. 23-1). While the advantages include ease of insertion and patient comfort, at least 1 to 2 percent of atttempted insertions result in pneumothorax and 1 percent in subclavian artery puncture.[12] This is partly related to the expertise of the person inserting the catheter, although complications can and do occur even in very experienced hands.

The internal jugular vein (IJV) can be entered near

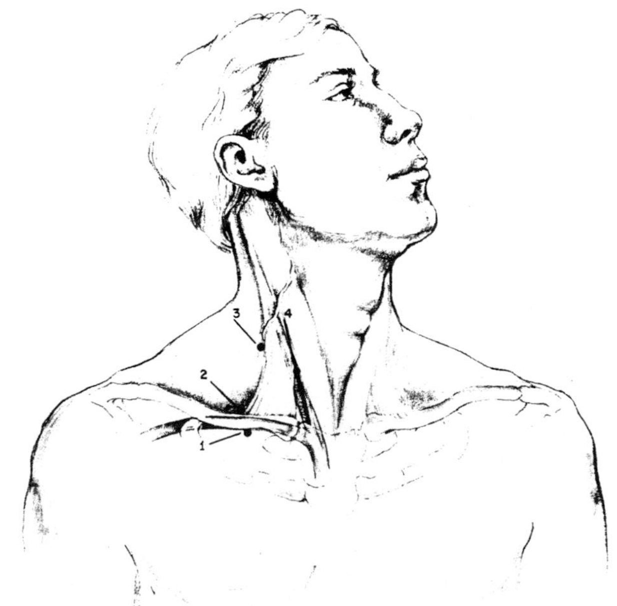

Figure 23-1. Surface anatomy for percutaneous cannulation of the subclavian (points 1 and 2) and the jugular veins (points 3 and 4). (From Marino PL: *The ICU Book*. Philadelphia: Lea & Febiger, 1991: 42, with permission.)

the base of the neck just before it joins the subclavian vein under the sternoclavicular joint (Fig. 23-1). Patients with an IJV line often complain of limited neck mobility. Inappropriate neck flexion can lead to thrombosis of the line and secretions from a tracheostomy can contaminate the catheter insertion site. Apart from the risk of a pneumothorax (less than 0.1 percent),[13] the major risk is carotid artery puncture (2 to 10 percent of insertions), which can occasionally have serious consequences.[14] Rare complications of IJV cannulation include carotid artery cannulation, endotracheal tube cuff puncture, cannulation of the spinal cord, neck hematomas causing severe compression and obliteration of the trachea, and embolism of fragmented cannula components.[15] A post-insertion chest x-ray (CXR) should generally be obtained to assess catheter tip position and to check for any complications, especially a pneumothorax. While the normal central venous pressure is 2 to 8 mmHg, patients with underlying cardiac or pulmonary diseases will often require Swan Ganz catheters since the CVP may not be an accurate assessment of their volume status or left heart function.[16]

Pulmonary Artery Catheters

In 1970 Swan, Ganz, and colleagues introduced a flow-directed, balloon flotation catheter which allowed right heart catheterization to be performed at the bedside.[17] This pulmonary artery catheter (PAC) provides an estimate of left ventricular filling pressures, measures pulmonary pressures, allows assessment of cardiac function, allows for optimization of hemodynamic performance, and may serve as an early detector of impending organ dysfunction. Recent developments include the addition of leads with pacemaker functions and the continuous measurement of mixed venous saturation through a fiberoptic catheter. Using the oximetric pulmonary artery catheter, a continuous trend of the mixed venous saturation is obtained, which may aid in maximizing oxygen delivery and cardiac output (CO).

Normal saturation of mixed venous blood ranges from 65 to 75%. A drop in $S\dot{V}_{O_2}$ to below 60% lasting for 5 min or longer indicates a dramatic compromise in at least one of the determinants of oxygen transport (cardiac output, hemoglobin concentration, or arterial oxygenation) or an uncompensated increase in oxygen consumption. Clinically, this may occur in patients with decreased oxygen delivery due to left ventricular failure, significant bleeding, hypoxemia, or increased oxygen consumption as a result of hyperthermia, violent shivering, seizures, or agitation. Higher values of $S\dot{V}_{O_2}$ indicate an increase in oxygen delivery relative to demand. This may occur in patients in the hyperdynamic phase of sepsis, delirium tremens, neuromuscular paralysis, hypothermia, and hyperoxia. An increase in $S\dot{V}_{O_2}$ may also suggest diminished extraction of oxygen by the tissues as well as a relative maldistribution of CO (peripheral left to right shunting).[16]

The PAC may be inserted percutaneously or via the basilic, brachial, femoral, subclavian, or internal jugular veins. The subclavian and internal jugular veins are the most common routes. Once the catheter tip is in the right atrium (RA), the balloon is inflated with the recommended amount of air or carbon dioxide. The catheter advancement should then be continued until the right ventricular (RV) pressure tracing is seen on the monitor (Fig. 23-2). While catheter passage into and through the RV is associated with a risk of arrythmias, ventricular irritation is minimized by keeping the balloon inflated.[18] However, monitoring of vital signs and the ECG is necessary throughout the entire insertion procedure. The catheter advancement is continued until the diastolic pressure tracing rises above that seen in the RV (see Fig. 23-2), indicating passage into the pulmonary artery (PA). With further advancement, when a fall in systolic pressure is noted, the balloon has wedged into the pulmonary artery branch. This is the pulmonary capillary wedge pressure (PCWP).

Once the PCWP is obtained, the balloon is immediately deflated and the pulmonary artery waveform should reappear. Usually the pulmonary artery diastolic pressure (PADP) and PCWP are reasonably close, within 3 mmHg.[19] With correct positioning of the catheter, no marked fluctuation in the wedge pressure should occur with respiratory variation. A CXR should confirm the catheter tip located at or below the level of the left atrium[20] with the tip not more than 3 to 5 cm from the midline. Daily CXRs are recommended to assess whether peripheral catheter migration has occurred.[18]

The following measurements can be obtained directly from the PAC and do not require any calculations: cen-

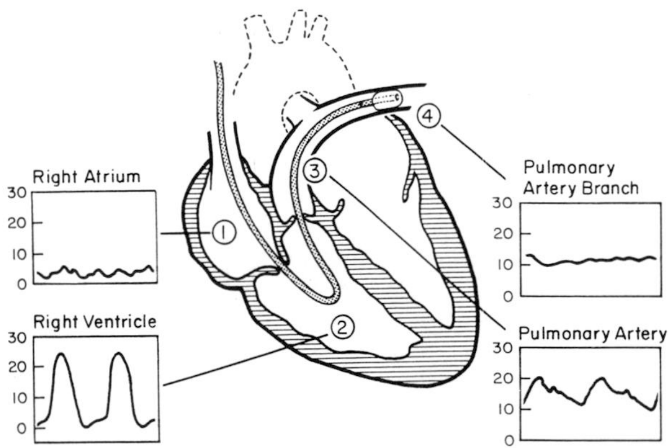

Figure 23-2. Representative pressure waveforms seen with advancement of pulmonary artery catheter. (From Marino PL: *The ICU Book*. Philadelphia: Lea & Febiger, 1991: 103, with permission.)

tral venous pressure (CVP), pulmonary capillary wedge pressure (PCWP), cardiac output (CO), and mixed venous oxygen saturation ($S\dot{V}_{O_2}$). Table 23-1 illustrates the range of normal values obtained with the PAC.

The CVP is recorded from the proximal port of the catheter situated in the right atrium. Provided there is no obstruction between the right atrium and ventricle, the right atrial pressure should equal the right ventricular end-diastolic pressure (RVEDP) (CVP=RVEDP). The PCWP is the pressure at the distal end when the balloon is lodged in a small branch of the pulmonary artery. This pressure should equal the left atrial pressure or the left ventricular end-diastolic pressure (PCWP = LVEDP). The thermistor at the distal end of the catheter can be used to measure cardiac output by monitoring the change in temperature of the blood flowing in the pulmonary arteries after bolus injection of a dextrose or saline solution that is cooler than blood through the proximal port of the PAC. Lastly, the oxygen saturation in the pulmonary artery can be measured either in vivo by using a special PAC or in vitro using a blood sample obtained from the distal port of the catheter. The mixed venous oxygen saturation ($S\dot{V}_{O_2}$) is used as an index of the oxygen extracted by tissues from the peripheral microcirculation.[21]

By performing some simple calculations on the above parameters, a set of hemodynamic parameters such as the ones lisetd in Table 23-2 are derived. All the variables are "indexed" or adjusted to body surface area (BSA).

The cardiac index (CI) is the average cardiac output divided by the BSA.

$$CI = CO/BSA$$

The systemic vascular resistance (SVR) is the measure of the force which opposes ventricular contraction (afterload) for the left ventricle. It is obtained from the following equation:

$$SVR = SAP - RAP/CO$$

where SAP = mean systemic arterial pressure and RAP = right atrial pressure. Systemic vascular resistance index (SVRI) is the vascular resistance across both arterial and venous circuits.

$$SVRI = (MAP - CVP)/CI \times 80$$

The factor of 80 converts pressure and volume to dynes · s/cm^5

Oxygen delivery ratio ($\dot{D}O_2$) is the amount of oxygen delivered to the capillaries per minute, calculated as the cardiac index and the oxygen content of arterial blood (Ca_{O_2}).

$$\dot{D}O_2 = CI \times Ca_{O_2}$$

Oxygen uptake ($\dot{V}O_2$) is the amount of oxygen taken up by the tissues from the capillaries per minute. This is calculated as the product of cardiac index and oxygen content difference across the capillaries ($Ca_{O_2} - C_{VO_2}$).

$$\dot{V}O_2 = CI \times (Ca_{O_2} - C_vO_2)$$

Although the $\dot{V}O_2$ is often called the "oxygen consumption," it is not necessarily a measure of the metabolic consumption of oxygen. Oxygen extraction ratio (O_2ER) is the fractional uptake of oxygen from the capillaries, or the balance between oxygen delivery ($\dot{D}O_2$) and oxygen uptake ($\dot{V}O_2$).

$$O_2ER = \dot{V}O_2/\dot{D}O_2$$

The function of each ventricle can be evaluated using the ventricular filling pressures or preload (which is CVP for the RV and PCWP for the LV), the systemic and pulmonary resistance or afterload (which is PVRI for the RV and SVRI for the LV), and the stroke volume (SVI for both ventricles). The mean arterial blood pressure is a function of flow and resistance where MAP = CI × SVRI. Changes in these variables can help identify and treat different forms of clinical shock. Furthermore, the changes in O_2 delivery ($\dot{D}O_2$) and O_2 uptake ($\dot{V}O_2$) are valuable in the diagnosis and management of clinical shock. In hemorrhagic shock the $\dot{D}O_2$ and $\dot{V}O_2$ are low

TABLE 23-1 Normal Values with a Pulmonary Artery Catheter

Right atrium (RA)	0–6 mmHg
Right ventricle (RV) systolic/diastolic	15–30/0–6 mmHg
Pulmonary artery (PA)	15–30/6–12 mmHg
Pulmonary artery mean	10–18 mmHg
Pulmonary wedge (PCWP)	6–12 mmHg
Cardiac output (CO)	4–6 l/min
Mixed venous oxygen saturation ($S\dot{V}_{O_2}$)	65–75%

TABLE 23-2 Selected Derived Cardiopulmonary Parameters

Parameter	Normal Range
Cardiac index (CI)	2–4 $L/min/m^2$
Systemic vascular resistance index (SVRI)	1200–2500 dyne · $s/cm^5/m^2$
Oxygen delivery rate ($\dot{D}O_2$)	500–600 $ml/min/m^2$
Oxygen uptake ($\dot{V}O_2$)	110–160 $ml/min/m^2$
Oxygen extraction ratio (O_2ER)	22–32%

m^2 is indexed to body surface area

SOURCE: Marino PL: *The ICU Book*. Philadelphia: Lea & Febiger, 1991: 104.

with a resultant high O_2ER. In septic shock the $\dot{D}O_2$ and $\dot{V}O_2$ are high with a low O_2ER.[22]

The catheterization of the pulmonary artery is not without side effects, but few are life threatening.[23–25] While many of these complications are nonspecific and are seen with all types of intravascular catheters, a few complications are specific to the PACs. When catheters are passed through the right side of the heart, ventricular arrythmias can occur in more than 50 percent of insertions.[25] Since these arrythmias are usually benign and disappear when the catheter is withdrawn, prophylactic therapy with antiarrythmic agents is not necessary.[26,27] While right bundle branch block develops in about 3 percent of insertions, it usually disappears within 24 h.[28] The rare complication of pulmonary artery rupture (10 reported cases in the first 10 years of catheter use),[29] whose usual presentation is acute hemoptysis, is often a fatal condition. While cases have been managed without surgery, thoracotomy is usually required. Although therapeutic intervention may be refined by the use of pulmonary artery catheters, a survival advantage is not necessarily conferred, owing to interpretation errors and complications associated with placement.[30]

Severe closed head injury (SCHI) patients, with Glasgow Coma Scale (GCS) $\leq$ 8, should have their CPP maintained at $\geq$ 70 mmHg. A PAC is suggested for patients > 50 years old; with a history of cardiac disease and/or multiple trauma (especially chest or abdominal injuries); or when vasopressors or high-dose barbiturates are used. In those patients who do not meet these criteria, often a CVP line is adequate. Colloids may be given to further maximize volume status, if needed. If the CVP is >10 mmHg, or the PCWP is >14, and the blood pressure and hence the CPP is still inadequate, then induced hypertension with a pressor is indicated.

Cardiovascular Disturbances

Types of Shock

Shock is a state of inadequate tissue oxygenation with the three basic shock syndromes; hypovolemic, cardiogenic, and vasogenic. Their respective hemodynamic findings are shown in Table 23-3.

With hypovolemic shock there is a low PCWP due to hypovolemia and a decrease in ventricular filling. This results in a decrease in the cardiac output (CO), which then produces vasoconstriction and an increase in systemic vascular resistance. In cardiogenic shock there is a decrease in cardiac output which leads to venous congestion with a high PCWP and a high SVR from peripheral vasoconstriction. Vasogenic shock results from a variety of causes, including sepsis, where there is a loss of vascular tone in the arteries. This produces a low SVR and a variable degree of loss of vascular tone in the veins resulting in a low PCWP. The CO is often elevated but can vary. If venous tone is not altered, or if the ventricle is stiff, the PCWP may be normal. In addition to sepsis the vasogenic shock pattern is commonly caused by multiorgan failure, postoperative state, pancreatitis, trauma, adrenal crisis, and anaphylaxis. A patient may have a combination of these shock syndromes.

TABLE 23-3 Differentiating Between the Types of Shock*

Type of Shock	CO	PCWP	SVR
Hypovolemic	Low	<u>Low</u>	High
Cardiogenic	<u>Low</u>	High	High
Vasogenic	High	Low	<u>Low</u>

* The primary problem is underlined
CO = cardiac output; PCWP = pulmonary capillary wedge pressure; SVR = systemic vascular resistance

Treatment of Shock

The treatment of these shock states depends on the condition present. Since fluids are always preferred to drugs, a patient with a low or normal PCWP should be given a volume infusion prior to initiating vasoactive drugs. Recall that an $alpha_1$-adrenergic agonist causes peripheral vasoconstriction and an $alpha_2$ agonist exerts antihypertensive effects by interacting with $alpha_2$ receptors within the brainstem sympathetic centers that regulate blood pressure. A $beta_1$ receptor agonist leads to vasodilation and cardiac stimulation, a $beta_2$ agonist causes vasodilation and bronchodilation. A dopamine-1 receptor agonist mediates vasodilation in the renal, mesenteric, coronary, and cerebral vascular beds. The table below illustrates this further with specific examples of each (Table 23-4).

One should first look at the hemodynamic problem, determine what is needed to correct it, and then decide which treatments will accomplish this. A patient with a low CO and high SVR without hypertension should be started on dobutamine which will increase the CO, decrease the SVR, and not elevate the BP. However, if the patient has severe hypotension, then a beta agonist with some alpha constriction is more likely to increase the BP because the alpha influence prevents the SVR from decreasing in response to the increase in CO. The patient with a low CO and normal SVR should be started on dopamine. The patient with a low SVR and low or normal CO will need an alpha-beta agent, while the patient with a low SVR and high CO will need an alpha agent. In general it is best to avoid pure vasoconstrictors because the small vessel constriction from these

TABLE 23-4 Adrenergic and Dopaminergic Effects

Receptor	Main Effect	Agonists
Adrenergic		
Alpha$_1$	Vasoconstriction	Phenylephrine, dopamine
Alpha$_2$	Centralon brainstem	Clonidine
Beta$_1$	Stimulates HR and contractility	Dobutamine, dopamine
Beta$_2$	Vasodilation, bronchodilation	Albuterol
Dopaminergic	Renal vasodilation	Dopamine

agents will not be reflected in the SVR. Therefore when vasoconstriction is needed, a combined alpha-beta agent is preferred to a pure alpha agent to decrease the tendency for profound vasoconstriction. For this reason dopamine (an alpha-beta agonist) is often preferred because it stimulates special dopamine receptors in the kidneys, which may help to preserve renal blood flow. The cardiac parameters, of which CO (or CI) and SVR are the most important, will dictate which hemodynamic drugs are needed. Dopamine, dobutamine, norepinephrine, and phenylephrine are most commonly used with head injury patients (Table 23-5).

Dopamine (Intropin), one of the most versatile hemodynamic drugs presently available, is part of the metabolic pathway which leads to norepinephrine (NE) synthesis. This endogenous catecholamine has both alpha and beta effects, depending on the dose used. Dopamine stimulates adrenergic receptors both directly and through the release of NE. At 2 μg/kg/min dopaminergic receptors are stimulated to produce selective vasodilatation in the cerebral, renal, and splanchnic circulations with a resultant increase in urinary output. At doses of 2 to 5 μg/kg/min dopamine has both chronotropic and inotropic effects on the heart by beta$_1$ receptor stimulation. At doses of 5 to 20 μg/kg/min significant alpha receptor stimulation occurs with a resultant increase in SVR due to peripheral vasoconstriction. High doses produce vasoconstriction via peripheral alpha receptor stimulation. Tachyarrhythmias are the most common adverse effects, and at very high doses profound vasoconstriction can occur with a loss of the improved renal perfusion seen at low doses. Dopamine is indicated for cardiogenic and septic shock, and in the first few hours of oliguric renal failure an increase in urine output is seen when given in dopaminergic doses ($<$2 μg/kg/min).[31]

Dobutamine (Dobutrex), a synthetic catecholamine introduced in 1978, is a selective beta$_1$ agonist of primarily inotropic action with mild beta$_2$ stimulation (peripheral vasoconstriction) and minimal alpha activity. Dobutamine produces a dose-related increase in CO up to an infusion rate of 40 μg/kg/min with few side effects.[32] While SVR decreases through reflex mechanisms,[33] preload decreases from the improved cardiac performance.

TABLE 23-5 Commonly Used Vasoactive Drugs

Vasoactive Drugs	Dosage	Effect
To Raise BP		
Dopamine	0.5–2 μg/kg/min	dopaminergic
	2–5 μg/kg/min	beta$_1$
	5–20 μg/kg/min	primarily alpha, some beta$_1$
Dobutamine	2.5–40 μg/kg/min	selective beta$_1$ (contractility > HR)
		mild beta$_2$
		minimal alpha$_1$
Norepinephrine	2–12 μg/min	primarily alpha, some beta
Phenylephrine	20–200 μg/min	alpha agonist
To Lower BP		
Nitroprusside	0.5–10 μg/kg/min	direct vasodilation
Nitroglycerin	10–20 μg/min	vasodilator
Hydralazine	20–40 mg IV prn	direct arterial dilation
Labetalol	20 mg IVP (max: 300 mg)	selectively blocks alpha$_1$
		nonselectively blocks beta
Enalaprilat	1.25 mg IVP up to 5 mg q6 prn	ACE inhibitor

The heart rate is usually unchanged, but tachycardia can be prominent when patients are hypovolemic. The change in CO and peripheral resistance are equal and opposite, leaving the BP unchanged. Compared to dopamine, dobutamine produces more of an increase in CO and is less arrhythmogenic.[34] This greater increase in CO is the result of the absence of vasoconstriction. The usual range is 5–15 μg/kg/min. The adverse effects include occasional ventricular arrythmias and tachycardia which can be prominent in hypovolemic patients.

Norepinephrine (Levophed), predominantly an alpha agonist, can produce profound vasoconstriction in all vascular beds, including the renal circulation.[35] Norepinephrine can also stimulate cardiac beta receptors in low doses (less than 2 μg/min). While norepinephrine causes a profound vasoconstriction which should limit its use, the addition of low-dose dopamine (1 μg/kg/h) helps to preserve renal blood flow.[36] Norepinephrine is indicated for septic shock that is refractory to volume and dopamine therapy. One should start at 8 μg/min and increase the dose to the desired effect, with vascular responses often diminished in septic shock. An effective dose in one human study was 0.5–1 μg/kg/h or 35–70 μg/min for an average-sized adult.[36] Adverse effects include renal failure and other manifestations of peripheral vasoconstriction. Norepinephrine is contraindicated in hypotension associated with peripheral vasoconstriction such as hypovolemic shock.

Phenylephrine (Neo-Synephrine) is a pure alpha sympathomimetic that increases BP by increasing SVR via vasoconstriction. A reflex increase in parasympathetic tone results in a slowing of the heart rate (HR). Phenylephrine's lack of beta actions implies there is no inotropic effect, no cardiac acceleration, no relaxation of bronchial smooth muscle and the CO and renal blood flow may decrease. This is useful for hypotension with associated tachycardia such as atrial tachyarrhythmias. The usual dosage range is 1–5 μg/kg/min.

Treatment of Hypertension[37]

While chronic hypertension can be damaging to the brain and other organs and/or tissues, one does not want to treat BP elevations in brain-injured patients too aggressively as this can compromise CPP. However, when better control of BP is warranted and this is not possible with analgesics like morphine sulfate, then antihypertensives like labetalol or hydralazine may be used prior to starting a nitroprusside drip (Table 23-5).

The following table shows some parenteral antihypertensive agents grouped according to their effect on ICP[38,39] (Table 23-6).

Nitroprusside (NTP or Nipride) is the primary agent for most hypertensive emergencies. Nitroprusside raises ICP in patients with intracranial mass lesions[40] due to direct vasodilation, with arterial > venous and small coronaries > large. Nitroprusside may preferentially dilate peripheral vessels before cerebral vessels and therefore produce a "cerebral steal" phenomenon. While nitroprusside acts within seconds, its duration of action is 3 to 5 min. Side effects with prolonged use include thiocyanate and cyanide toxicity which may cause neurologic deterioration[41] or hypotension. Thiocyanate levels should be checked if NTP is more than 24 h, at a rate of greater or equal to 10 μg/kg/min, or in renal failure. If levels are >10 mg/dl it should then be stopped. Other side effects include tachycardia, tachyphylaxis, and hypotension which can extend an myocardial infarction (MI) via "coronary steal." In addition, this should be avoided in pregnancy because of the fear of cyanide toxicity. The IV drip rate is 0.25 to 8 μg/kg/min with an average of 3 μg/kg/min. To reduce the risk of cyanide toxicity, one could start at a very low rate of 0.3 μg/kg/min and not give the maximum rate of 10 μg/kg/min for more than 10 min.

TABLE 23-6 Antihypertensive Drugs and ICP

Agents More Likely to Raise ICP (Vasodilators)	Agents Less Likely to Raise ICP
Nitroprusside (Nipride)	Labetalol (Normodyne)
Hydralazine (Apresoline)	Methyldopa (Aldomet)
Nitroglycerin (NTG)	Trimethaphan (Arfonad)

Hydralazine (Apresoline) is a direct vasodilator with arterial > venous and also increases ICP. This is less predictable than other parenterals and thus, for IV use, nitroprusside is preferred. The IV onset of action is 10 to 30 min with a 2 to 4 h duration. Its main use is in pregnancy. Side effects include a marked reflex tachycardia with possible angina which can be countered with beta blockers. The dosages are 10 to 20 mg intravenous push (IVP) prn, or 10 mg IM, which may be repeated every 2 to 4 h, incrementing each time up to 60 mg, or 10 mg PO every 6 h, increasing gradually to a range of 40 to 200 mg/day.

Nitroglycerin (NTG) is a vasodilator with venous > arterial and large coronaries > small. While it also raises ICP, the increase is less than with nitroprusside due to preferential venous action.[40] As a result there is a decrease in the left ventricle (LV) filling pressure or preload. Furthermore, unlike nitroprusside, NTG does not cause "coronary steal." The usual dose is 10 to 20 μg/min as an IV drip, which can be decreased by 5–10 μg/min every 5 to 10 min.

Methyldopa (Aldomet) inhibits sympathomimetics in the brainstem vasomotor center to decrease SVR. While Aldomet maintains renal perfusion and does not alter CO, it is not for acute hypertension since it has a slow onset of 4 to 6 h and lasts 10 to 16 h after injection. A rebound hypertension may be seen on withdrawal. Side effects include sedation, confusion, and fluid retention. The dose is 250 to 500 mg IVPB every 6 h or 500 to 3000 mg/day PO in divided doses.

Labetalol (Normodyne, Trandate) selectively blocks $alpha_1$ receptors and nonselectively blocks beta receptors with a potency less than propanolol. Labetalol either reduces or causes no change in ICP.[42] There is a decrease or no change in pulse rate and no change in CO. Side effects include fatigue, dizziness, and orthostatic hypotension. Labetalol should not be used in patients with congestive heart failure, asthma, greater than first-degree heart block, cardiogenic shock, or severe bradycardia. With IV administration the onset is 5 min, with a peak in 10 min, and a duration of 3 to 6 h. Each IV dose should be given over 2 min every 10 min until the desired BP is achieved. The patient should be supine with the dosing sequence of 20, 40, 80, 80, and then 80 mg up to a total of 300 mg. Once the BP is controlled the same total dose can be given IVP every 8 h. Alternatively, a 2 mg/min drip can be given, up to 300 mg, with bradycardia limiting the dose.

Enalaprilat (Vasotec) is an angiotensin-converting enzyme inhibitor which is the active metabolite of the orally administered drug enalapril. This acts within 15 min of administration. Hyperkalemia occurs in approximately 1 percent of patients and should not be used in pregnancy. The IV dose should start with 1.25 mg over 5 min and then be increased up to 5 mg every 6 h as needed.

Cardiac Arrythmias

As discussed above, both atrial and ventricular arrythmias may be seen with head injury. However each arrythmia should be worked up as if the head injury itself was not the cause. The more common dysrhythmias and their treatment have been discussed in detail elsewhere[43,44] and will be briefly reviewed below.

Sinus Tachycardia

The heart rate is usually in the rate of 100 to 180 beats per minute and is regular. Critically ill patients may have sinus tachycardia for a number of reasons including fever, pain, hypoxemia, volume depletion, cardiac tamponade, pulmonary embolism, pneumothorax, emotion, thyrotoxicosis, drugs, and shock. In general no treatment is required since it is usually a physiological adjustment to maintain CO. Primary treatment should be directed to the underlying cause.

Sinus Bradycardia

The heart rate is less than 60 beats per minute and is regular. This may be seen normally in young athletic individuals. Sinus bradycardia can result from carotid sinus massage. It also may occur in response to: drugs, including morphine, reserpine, beta-blockers, calcium channel blockers, and digoxin; increased vagal tone; increased intracranial pressure as a Cushing response; sinus node dysfunction; hypothermia; hypothyroidism; and inferior myocardial infarction and other forms of cardiac disease. Treatment is required only when this is hemodynamically significant. Atropine is the drug of choice with 0.5 to 1 mg IV given as a bolus which can be repeated every 5 min for a maximum dose of 2 mg. If pharmacologic therapy is ineffective, then external or transvenous pacing may be needed.

Premature Atrial Contractions (PACs)

The premature abnormal P wave signifies that the impulse for contraction originates in the atria outside of the sinus node. Ventricular conduction may be variable with pauses or an early, widened QRS. PACs may result from digitalis, hypoxia, or sympathetic stimulation. They frequently mark the emergence of an underlying problem. Usually no treatment is required if infrequent.

Supraventricular Tachyarrhythmias (SVT)

These are regular, narrow QRS tachycardias with rates usually less than 200 beats per minute. SVT associated with hypotension, angina, or congestive heart failure is unstable and requires emergency cardioversion. Currently adenosine 6 mg IV push over 2 to 3 s, followed by one or two 12 mg IV boluses every 1 to 2 min, if necessary, is the drug of choice for stable SVT. If this is not successful, verapamil (5 mg IV followed in 15 to 20 min by an additional 10 mg IV) can be tried. If verapamil is unsuccessful, then elective cardioversion, digoxin, beta blockers, and therapeutic pacing should be considered.

Atrial Flutter

The atrial rate is regular and usually 250 to 300 beats per minute with the ventricular rate usually half the atrial rate at 150 beats per minute. The classic P wave morphology is characterized by a zigzag or sawtooth appearance (flutter waves). Atrial flutter can be seen in patients with rheumatic heart disease, coronary artery disease, hypertensive heart disease, cardiomyopathy, pulmonary disease, hyperthyroidism, and pericarditis. Digoxin 0.5 mg IV followed by 0.25 mg every 4 to 6 h for a total of 1.0 to 1.25 mg is most frequently used for treatment of the hemodynamically stable patient. Verapamil in 2.5 to 5.0 mg doses IV, or propanolol IV in 1 mg doses every 5 min can then be used to restore normal sinus rhythm. Alternatively, elective cardioversion or atrial overdrive pacing are additional options. Cardioversion is recommended for the unstable patient.

Atrial Fibrillation

This is completely chaotic atrial activity with a very rapid rate of 400 to 700 beats per minute which usually cannot be counted. While atrial fibrillation may occasionally be seen in normal individuals and is associated with rheumatic heart disease, pericarditis, hyperthyroidism and hypertension, it is usually found in patients with cardiovascular or pulmonary disease. The treatment of this condition is determined by the condition of the patient. Emergent electrical cardioversion is required when atrial fibrillation with rapid ventricular response is associated with angina, congestive heart failure, or hypotension. However, the condition is usually benign and digoxin is the pharmacological treatment of choice. Patients should be loaded with 0.5 mg IV and then be given 0.25 mg IV every 4 to 6 h for a total of 1.0 to 1.25 mg. If digoxin fails to slow the ventricular response adequately, a second drug, such as propanolol 20 to 40 mg PO every 6 h or verapamil 5 to 10 mg IV, may be given. For patients who remain in atrial fibrillation with a controlled ventricular rate, quinidine or procainamide can be given. If the patient does not convert by 36 h, then electrical cardioversion can be attempted.

Premature Ventricular Contractions (PVCs)

These are wide complex premature QRS complexes which have unusual morphologies. The QRS complex is usually greater than 0.12 s in duration. PVCs are not preceded by a PAC. PVCs are caused by hypokalemia, hypomagnesemia, acidemia, alkalemia, hypoxia, hypercapnia, myocardial ischemia or infarction, endocrine disorders, digitalis toxicity, the mechanical stimulation of the pulmonary artery catheter, and a variety of drugs including cocaine, phenothiazines, sympathomimetic agents, and tricyclic antidepressants. Treatment should be directed toward the underlying cause. Isolated PVCs only require treatment if their frequency causes a significant bradycardia. Treatment with lidocaine 1 mg/kg IV is recommended for PVCs which are increasing in frequency, are multifocal, occur in couplets, exhibit R on T phenomenon, or develop a bigeminal pattern. Procainamide and bretylium should be administered if up to 3 mg/kg of lidocaine is not effective.

Ventricular Tachycardia (VT)

This is three or more consecutive PVCs at a rate of 100 or more beats per minute. VT is common in the early phase of acute anterior and inferior MIs and in the setting of significant left ventricular dysfunction. As with PVCs, treatment should begin with looking for the possible causes. Immediate DC cardioversion is recommended for the hemodynamically unstable patient, including those with chest pain, dyspnea, hypotension, congestive heart failure, ischemia, or myocardial infarction. For the stable VT patient lidocaine 1 mg/kg IV followed by 0.5 mg/kg every 8 min until VT resolves or up to 3 mg/kg is recommended. If unsuccessful, then procainamide 20 mg/min is administered until VT resolves or up to 1000 mg is the next step prior to cardioversion as in the unstable patient.

Atrioventricular Blocks (A-V Block)

A-V block is grouped by measurement of the PR interval and the frequency of interference with the normal conduction of electrical impulses from the atria to the ventricle. There are many causes such as coronary artery disease, increased vagal tone, drugs (including beta blockers, digitalis, and calcium channel blockers), hyperkalemia, hypoxia, endocarditis, thyrotoxicosis, and trauma. First-degree A-V block and type I (Wenckebach) second-degree A-V block only require treatment when hemodynamically significant. Type II second-degree A-V block and third-degree A-V block should always be treated with atropine 0.5 to 1.0 mg IV up to a maximum of 2 mg. If ineffective then external pacing or transvenous pacing is recommended.

THE RESPIRATORY SYSTEM IN HEAD INJURY

The cardiopulmonary management of the head injury patient should begin at the accident scene with the emergency medical technicians (EMTs). Adequate airway, breathing, and circulation (ABC) should be established prior to transportation, whenever possible. The upper airways should be cleared of vomitus, foreign bodies, and blood. Pulmonary complications are one of the leading causes of avoidable deaths in hospitalized head injury patients.[45] These complications, including hypoxia, pulmonary edema, insufficient respiration, and aspiration pneumonia leading to respiratory failure, occur in 20 percent of head-injured patients.[46]

Ventilatory Support

Intubation

Tracheal intubation is indicated for maintenance of airway patency, protection of the airway from aspiration, secretion clearance, and provision of mechanical respiratory support. All comatose patients [Glasgow Coma Scale (GCS) score of 8 or less] should be routinely intubated. Orally placed endotracheal (ET) tubes are preferred to nasally placed tubes so as to avoid sinusitis as a complication. Nasotracheal intubation is relatively contraindicated in the presence of severe maxillofacial injuries or basilar skull fractures, since the tube may be inadvertently placed into the cranial vault.[47] The ET tube protects the airway from aspiration and airway obstruction, aids in tracheal suctioning, and is mandatory for controlled ventilation.

Routine pulmonary care

Head injury patients who are intubated should ideally be on continuous pulse oximetry, have frequent CXRs, and have at least a daily arterial blood gas (ABG). An end-tidal CO_2 monitor can be useful in following the degree of hyperventilation and reducing the need for frequent ABGs. The CXR must be of acceptable quality with all portions of the chest visible to check for new infiltrates, follow atelectasis and/or effusions, and confirm the position of all tubes and catheters. The CXR of the multiple trauma patient should especially be inspected for evidence of barotrauma, namely, pneumothorax, pneumomediastinum, tracheal deviation, broken ribs, or subcutaneous emphysema.

Patients with significant cardiac arrythmias or an increase in ICP associated with suctioning[48] may be premedicated with atropine or lidocaine intravenously or endotracheally. Bronchodilators may be needed when wheezing is a problem. Respiratory alkalosis is common in patients receiving mechanical ventilation and can result in hypophosphatemia.[49] Transient episodes of cerebral hypoxia occur in about half of all severe head injury patients. This is best detected with jugular oxygen saturation monitoring. A jugular venous oxygen saturation of less than 50% denotes significant cerebral hypoxia.[50] This is discussed in detail in Chap. 36.

Ventilator settings

Once the airway is secured, mechanical ventilation will aid in the maintenance of good oxygenation and normocapnia, the prevention of atelectasis and subsequent pneumonia, and the treatment of pulmonary edema and adult respiratory distress syndrome (ARDS).[51] While there are three types of ventilators (volume-cycled, flow-cycled, and time-cycled), the volume-cycled ventilators are preferred in head-injured patients since they can deliver a constant volume of gases in the presence of changing lung mechanics.[52–54] When mechanical ventilation is initiated, the respiratory therapist will request the mode of ventilation, inflation volume, respiratory rate, and inspired oxygen level. For the comatose patient the "assist/control" mode of ventilation is usually used first and allows the patient to initiate the mechanical breath by generating a small negative intrathoracic pressure (assist mode), and also provides adequate ventilation if the patient is unable to breath at all (control mode).[55]

Sedation with drugs like morphine sulfate is often needed for patients with a high respiratory rate that are "fighting" the respirator. There is evidence to suggest that sedation is preferable to paralysis in patients with severe head injury.[56] Paralysis is used when sedation is inadequate to control the patient or their ICP. Alternatively intermittent mandatory ventilation (IMV), which intersperses spontaneous breaths with forced breaths, may be used and has become the most popular method of weaning patients off ventilatory support. The inflation volumes delivered during mechanical ventilation are at least twice the volume of normal tidal breathing with ventilator tidal volume (V_T) of 12 to 15 ml/kg versus the normal V_T of 5 to 6 ml/kg. The ventilator rate is usually set at 12 to 14 breaths/min and is adjusted as needed to maintain the P_{CO_2} required for management. When the patient is able to initiate the ventilator breaths, the machine rate serves only as a backup system in the event that the patient is no longer able to breath adequately. The initial fraction of inspired oxygen (FI_{O_2}) should be set at 80 percent or higher and then decreased by 10 to 20 percent until a safe level (below 60 percent) is attained. It is recommended to wait at least 20 min between FI_{O_2} changes to allow the arterial P_{O_2} to reach a new steady state level.

PEEP

The addition of a low level of positive end-expiratory pressure (PEEP) increases arterial P_{O_2}, allows the FI_{O_2} to be lowered to less toxic levels, and increases dead space ventilation (V_D/V_T) by overdistending alveoli in normal lung regions. However, PEEP in excess of approximately 10 cmH_2O increases intrathoracic pressure and may decrease systemic blood pressure and cardiac output, in addition to possibly causing barotrauma (pneumothorax, pneumomediastinum, and subcutaneous emphysema), fluid retention, and intracranial pressure elevation.[57] ICP is usually only increased by higher levels of PEEP in patients with decreased cerebral compliance as determined by the volume-pressure response.[58] When 33 severe head injury patients were studied to determine whether the use of PEEP would cause an increase in ICP, the mean ICP did not increase in the 8 patients with a ICP over 20. In addition there was an increase in the mean ICP of only 1.33 mmHg with a decrease in the mean CPP of 2 mmHg, both of which were clinically insignificant.[59] In general while a PEEP of up to 10 cmH_2O will probably not affect one's ICP, each patient's needs should be individualized with respect to the level of PEEP used and its risk-benefit ratio.

Weaning

As with much of medicine there are often a variety of ways to reach the same goal and weaning a patient off ventilatory support is no exception. A survey of ICU directors conducted in 1987 showed that the IMV is the most popular method of weaning in the United States. From a neurosurgical viewpoint this method is gradual and allows for close monitoring of the patient's respiratory and neurological condition. The Fi_{O_2} should be 40 to 50 percent with satisfactory levels of arterial P_{O_2} before considering a weaning trial. Once the patient's level of consciousness is such that s/he can protect his or her airway (with GCS > 8), then the respiratory rate (RR) can be decreased by 2 as often as every 20 min down to an RR of 4. Initially the pulse oximeter can be followed and kept >94 percent. Once at an IMV of 4 an ABG should be checked in addition to the weaning parameters listed in Table 23-7 below. If both are satisfactory the patient can be extubated or converted to a T piece for an additional 30 min of observation before being extubated. If the patient is given a T piece trial, an ABG can be checked prior to extubation. While being weaned, the patient should be assessed for tachypnea, hypoxia, and hypercapnia.

Tracheostomy

Tracheostomy is a valuable adjunct to continued respiratory support. The decision to perform a tracheostomy is determined by weighing the benefits and risks of the procedure. The benefits of tracheostomy include sparing further laryngeal injury from the translaryngeal tube, facilitating airway suctioning and mouth care, increasing patient mobility by providing a more secure tube, facilitating transfer from the ICU setting, improving comfort, permitting speech, facilitating oral nourishment, and providing psychological benefit. The translaryngeal route is clearly preferable if the anticipated need of the artificial airway is less than 10 days. Since the majority of comatose patients require prolonged intubation, the oral or nasotracheal tube should generally be converted to a tracheostomy if more than 21 days of ventilation is expected.[63] The optimal time for performing a tracheostomy remains somewhat controversial and practice in this regard remains quite variable.

Tracheostomy is associated with serious complications in up to 5 percent of cases[64] and has a reported mortality of up to 2 to 3 percent.[63] Immediate postoperative complications include pneumothorax (five percent), stomal hemorrhage (5 percent), and accidental decannulation.[63,64] Figure 23-3 illustrates the complications of endotracheal intubation and tracheostomy.

TABLE 23-7 Bedside Criteria for Weaning

Parameter	Required to Wean	Reference
$Pa_{O_2} - FI_{O_2}$	>60 mmHg	
Tidal Volume	>5 ml/kg	60
Vital Capacity	>10 ml/kg	60
Minute Ventilation	<10L/min	61
Negative Inspiratory Pressure	>−30 mmHg	62

SOURCE: Marino PL: *The ICU Book*. Philadelphia: Lea & Febiger, 1991; 400

Pulmonary Problems

Aspiration

Patients are usually intubated while comatose to protect against aspiration of oropharyngeal secretions, blood, or vomitus. Aspiration can often occur at the scene of the injury, even prior to intubation. It is also possible to aspirate some upper airway contents around the cuff.[65] Prevention is the most satisfactory approach to the problem and can be accomplished by nasogastric and oropha-

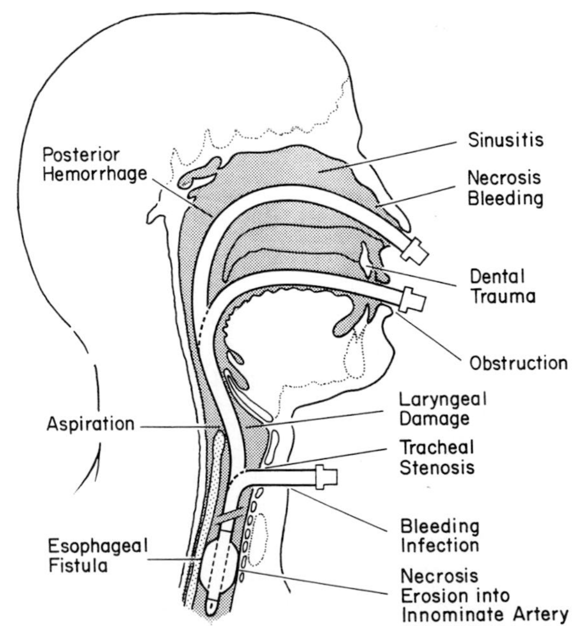

Figure 23-3. Complications of endotracheal intubation and tracheostomy. (From Marino PL: *The ICU Book*. Philadelphia: Lea & Febiger, 1991: 384, with permission.)

ryngeal suctioning.[66] Although elevating the patient's head 30 degrees may help to reduce its incidence, aspiration is still said to occur in approximately 20 percent of head-injured patients.[67] After aspiration of gastric contents the patients may develop acute respiratory distress with tachypnea, tachycardia, wheezing, and cyanosis. This may be followed in 3 to 4 h with radiographic evidence of pulmonary edema due to alveolar damage.

Atelectasis

Patients on mechanical ventilation are generally treated with frequent suctioning, position changes, and chest percussion to prevent atelectasis and superimposed infections. However, the data on the value of chest percussion remains limited. Mucus plug formation is a frequent complication in mechanically ventilated patients, especially when there is a diminished cough reflex due to a decreased level of consciousness, neuromuscular weakness, or paralysis. If a mucus plug is not recognized and treated it can result in lung atelectasis, hypoxia, and pneumonia. The removal of mucus plugs may require bronchoscopy.

Pneumonia

Despite aggressive therapy and newer antibiotics pneumonia remains a lethal hospital-acquired (nosocomial) infection with a mortality rate of up to 50 percent.[68–72] Nosocomial pneumonias are the most common cause of acute respiratory failure and older patients have a poorer prognosis. The prevalence of gram-negative bacillary pneumonia in hospitalized patients has increased dramatically[73] with more than 50 percent of cases due to gram-negative rods, followed in incidence by gram-positive cocci (coagulase positive streptococci). Bacteria can be introduced into the trachea by aspiration of oropharyngeal contents, during endotracheal intubation, and during tracheal suctioning. The depressed cough reflex and mucus retention which are common in head injury patients increases the risk of pneumonia. The radiographic appearance should be combined with the physical examination, sputum production, temperature, white blood cell count, and sputum gram's stain and culture, in order to make a definitive diagnosis.

Adult respiratory distress syndrome (ARDS)

Adult respiratory distress syndrome is estimated to cause 150,000 cases of respiratory failure each year.[74] Since over 50 percent of patients will not survive ARDS, this places ARDS in the same class as lung cancer (100,000 deaths per year) as one of the most lethal pulmonary conditions.[75] The adult respiratory distress syndrome is defined by diffuse bilateral roentgenographic pulmonary infiltrates, hypoxemia poorly responsive to supplemental oxygen, the absence of heart failure, a normal pulmonary artery wedge pressure, and normal cardiac function. The most prominent feature is an increase in pulmonary vascular resistance. These findings suggest that widespread pulmonary microvascular occlusion is the cause. In a recent angiographic study of nine patients with posttraumatic ARDS, 78 percent had multiple pulmonary artery filling defects.[76] Adult respiratory distress syndrome is thought to develop in response to microembolization to the lungs of fibrin-rich material which is thought to increase vascular permeability and cause progressive interstitial and alveolar edema, which ultimately leads to pulmonary insufficiency.[77] Aspiration pneumonia, pulmonary edema, and pulmonary contusion directly damage the lung tissue, while allergic reaction, pancreatitis, blood transfusion reaction, and sepsis cause indirect damage.[78] In the initial phase of ARDS the arterial blood gases (ABGs) may be abnormal with a normal CXR. However, with disease progression, lung compliance decreases, hypoxic respiratory failure develops, and a characteristic "white lung" (diffuse fluffiness of pulmonary edema) pattern is seen on CXR. The destruction of alveoli starts with interstitial fibrosis in the late phase.

While there is no effective therapy for reversing the capillary damage in ARDS, management goals are to reduce edema, maintain tissue oxygenation, prevent oxygen toxicity, and prevent adverse occurrences while specific therapy is directed at the underlying causes. While common underlying causes for ARDs in head-injured patients are sepsis, aspiration, major trauma, and pneumonia; less common causes include neurogenic pulmonary edema, fat embolism, pancreatitis, burns, multiple transfusions, disseminated intravascular coagulopathy, irritant gas or smoke inhalation, and oxygen toxicity.[79]

Pulmonary edema

Pulmonary edema refers to a transudation of fluid into the alveoli at a rate which exceeds normal clearance mechanisms. This results in increased extravascular lung water and often leads to the clinical syndrome of hypoxia, dyspnea, and audible rales in the chest. Iatrogenic pulmonary edema after severe head injury frequently is caused by overaggressive fluid replacement. Pulmonary edema is less likely if fluid replacement is accomplished with blood products and isotonic saline solutions. Whenever possible, CVP or PCWP should be monitored during fluid replacement and kept below 20 cm of H_2O. Cardiogenic pulmonary edema can occur with massive fluid infusions in elderly patients or those with preexisting cardiac disease.

Neurogenic pulmonary edema (NPE)

Neurogenic pulmonary edema is a relatively uncommon condition associated with a variety of intracranial pathologies including intraparenchymal and subarachnoid hemorrhages, seizures, and head injury. It results in respiratory failure which is relatively refractory to oxygen therapy. This can occur almost immediately after intracranial trauma and is usually seen in young, healthy individuals with no underlying cardiac or renal pathology. While its pathophysiology is not completely understood, it is felt that a sudden increase in ICP or a hypothalamic injury may cause a massive alpha-adrenergic discharge mediated from the hypothalamus leading to a generalized release of catecholamines which cause vasoconstriction and hypertension. The pulmonary capillary pressure increases because of pulmonary venous and arterial hypertension, which then damages capillary membranes. This results in transudation of fluid into the pulmonary interstitum and alveoli and leads to pulmonary edema.[80] Treatment is primarily supportive using measures like PEEP in addition to normalizing ICP. A PAC is usually useful to closely monitor CO and PCWP and to aid in avoiding hypervolemia. A recent case report discusses the successful treatment of a case of NPE using a dobutamine infusion supplemented with furosemide as needed.[81] NPE may be more common in victims of penetrating head injuries, having been diagnosed in only 2 of 2100 patients with closed head injuries[82] versus 17 of 20 patients with penetrating head injuries.[83]

Pulmonary embolism (PE)

A common cause of death among immobile hospitalized patients is a massive PE.[84] Furthermore, subclinical PE can cause adult respiratory distress syndrome in addition to other pulmonary problems.[85] Pulmonary thromboembolism should be considered in the patient who suddenly develops hypoxia and in older patients with progressive deterioration in mental function. Pulmonary thromboembolism from deep venous thrombosis in the deep pelvic vessels or lower extremities is common in immobilized neurosurgical patients. Deep vein thrombosis (DVT) is the source of the embolism in most patients who die of PE.[86] Depending on the diagnostic criteria used, the reported incidence of DVT is 20 to 90 percent and that of PE is 4 to 22 percent in trauma patients.[87] The length of time on assisted ventilation has been correlated with the development of DVT[84] as has the duration of immobility[88] with head injury patients at risk for developing DVT because they frequently are immobilized for long periods. Unfortunately the diagnosis of DVT and/or PE is very difficult in this setting.

Venous thrombi which embolize into the pulmonary arteries or their major branches can cause ventilation-perfusion mismatch that manifests as hemoptysis, hypotension, cardiovascular collapse, or sudden death. While the classic triad for a pulmonary embolism includes hemoptysis, pleuritic chest pain, and dyspnea, this is rarely seen in the intubated comatose patient. However pulmonary embolism must be considered whenever sudden dyspnea, tachypnea, tachycardia, third or fourth heart sounds, and rales occur. One must check for thrombophlebitis and deep venous thrombosis as a source and remember that shock and congestive heart failure (which may mimic a myocardial infarction) may indicate a massive life-threatening pulmonary embolus.

Unfortunately no laboratory findings are entirely specific for a PE. The ECG usually illustrates nonspecific ST and T segment changes and rarely the classic $S_1Q_3T_3$ (deep S in limb lead I and prominent Q in lead III with inversion of T in III). The CXR will be normal in 30 percent of cases; abnormal CXRs usually show an infiltrate and elevated hemidiaphragm. A $P_{O_2} > 90$ on room air virtually excludes a significant pulmonary embolus. While the definitive techniques to diagnose a DVT and PE are venography and pulmonary angiography, respectively, these procedures are invasive and often unnecessary in the majority of cases. A technically adequate negative ventilation perfusion (VQ) scan can virtually exclude a significant PE.

Anticoagulation with heparin is normally indicated if the diagnosis of PE is highly suspected. However, this is usually not possible in head injury patients due to the risk of intracranial hemorrhage. When heparin is contraindicated a Greenfield filter may be necessary. The patient with a massive PE may be hemodynamically unstable and require ICU care, a PAC, and pressors. Thrombolytic therapy may be of benefit for those with a massive PE or extensive proximal DVT.[89] Prophylaxis for DVT-PE includes anticoagulants, leg compression devices, or filters placed in the inferior vena cava. Comatose head-injured patients should generally have pneumatic sequential compression devices placed over their lower extremities. Intermittent inflation of these simulates the normal pumping action of the calf muscles. Dennis and coworkers evaluated intermittent pneumatic compression therapy versus minidose heparin versus control in posttrauma patients. Risk was reduced from 16.7 to 1.4 percent in the head injury group, with no additional bleeding complications when instituted on the first postoperative day.[90] Mini- or low-dose heparin (5000 IU) may be given subcutaneously every 8 to 12 h until the patient is ambulatory. Coagulation tests (PT, PTT) do not need to be monitored since this dose will inhibit thrombin formation from prothrombin by activating antithrombin III with little or no risk of bleeding.

Heparin-induced thrombocytopenia, an important

drug-related problem,[91] occurs in 3 to 30 percent of patients receiving therapeutic doses. The drug exposure may be as minimal as flushes of a venous line with dilute heparin. Bovine heparin has been found to cause this more often than porcine heparin. While the mechanism is uncertain, a complement-mediated mechanism may be responsible.[92,93] The platelet count, which occasionally decreases to below 50,000/mm^3, usually occurs 2 days after the initiation of therapy and often quickly reverses within a day of stopping the heparin. Since dangerous hemorrhagic and arterial thrombotic complications may develop, daily platelet counts are recommended. Heparin-dependent immune injury to endothelial cells may play a role in thrombocytopenia and arterial thromboses.[94]

FAT EMBOLISM SYNDROME (FES)

Long bone fractures occur in 32 percent of patients with severe head injury.[95] While fat embolism syndrome (FES) is most often seen after a long bone fracture, such as a femur fracture, it also may occur after a clavicular, tibial, and even an isolated skull fracture. Fat embolism syndrome may occur in as many as 28 percent of trauma victims with skeletal fractures.[96] The syndrome is usually mild or subclinical with only 10 to 20 percent of cases being severe. The fulminant form can lead to multiple organ failure. Respiratory distress is the most important component of FES and the diagnosis of fat embolism should be considered in any trauma patient with long bone or pelvic fractures who develops respiratory insufficiency. The clinical findings usually appear within 12 to 72 h of injury and do not always include the complete classic clinical triad of acute respiratory failure, global neurological dysfunction, and petechial rash. In up to 75 percent of cases the only manifestation of FES may be acute respiratory failure, including hypoxemia, tachypnea, and dyspnea, with diffuse pulmonary infiltrates usually seen as bilateral fluffy infiltrates. The mental status change may include lethargy, seizures, and confusion with a Pa_{O_2} usually not low enough to account for these changes.[97] A petechial rash may be seen over the thorax 24 to 72 h after the fracture. Other possible findings include pyrexia and retinal fat emboli. Posttraumatic release of fat into the bloodstream often is associated with platelet activation and intravascular coagulation which can both compromise the pulmonary microcirculation and lead to respiratory distress.[98] Asymptomatic or subclinical forms of fat embolism are common. Four out of six postmortem studies of multiple trauma victims demonstrated having intravascular fat in their pulmonary arteries.[99]

While there is no specific test for FES, fat globules in the urine (positive in 1 in 3)[100] and serum and serum lipase activity have been proposed with poor sensitivity and specificity. In situations of unexplained neurological or pulmonary abnormalities, FES may be diagnosed, if on bronchoalveolar lavage, >5 percent of cells in the washings stain for neutral fat with red oil O.[101] Nonspecific ABG findings include hypoxemia, hypocarbia from hyperventilation, and respiratory alkalosis.

Treatment consists of pulmonary support with oxygen and mechanical ventilation if needed, including the use of PEEP, as well as early stabilization of fractures. Early operative fixation of long bone fractures may reduce the incidence of FES.[102] But given the relatively low rate of diagnosis of this condition, the value of any intervention is difficult to prove.

The outcome is usually related more to the underlying injuries. While FES is usually compatible with a good recovery, a mortality rate of up to 10 percent is usually quoted. In nonfatal cases, the symptoms usually resolve spontaneously in 3 to 4 days.

ACKNOWLEDGMENT

The authors wish to thank Dr. Samuel Krachman for his helpful comments in the preparation of this chapter.

REFERENCES

1. *Advanced Trauma Life Support (ATLS) Course for Physicians: Instructors' Manual.* American College of Surgeons. Chicago, IL, 1988.
2. Evans DE, Alter WA, Shatsky SA, et al: Cardiac arrythmias resulting from experimental head injury. *J Neurosurg* 1976; 45:609–616.
3. Fernando OU, Mariano GT, Gurdjian ES, et al: Electrocardiographic patterns in experimental cerebral concussion. *J Neurosurg* 1969; 31:34–40.
4. Hugenholtz PG: Electrocardiographic abnormalities in cerebral disorders: Report of six cases and review of the literature. *Am Heart J* 1962; 63:451–461.
5. Hawkins WE, Clower BR: Myocardial damage after head trauma and simulated intracranial hemorrhage in mice: The role of the autonomic nervous system. *Cardiovasc Res* 1971; 5:524–529.
6. VanderArk GD: Cardiovascular changes with acute SDH. *Surg Neurol* 1975; 3:305–308.
7. Narayan RK, Gopinath SP, Robertson CS: Intracranial complications, in Mattox KL (ed): *Complications of Trauma.* New York, Churchill Livingstone, 1994: 351–367.
8. Russell JA, Joel M, Hudson RJ, et al: Prospective evaluation of radial and femoral artery catheterization sites in critically ill adults. *Crit Care Med* 1983; 11:936–939.
9. Slogoff S, Keats AS, Arlund C: On the safety of radial artery cannulation. *Anesthesiology* 1983; 59:42–47.

10. Weiss BM, Gattiker RI: Complications during and following radial artery cannulation: A prospective study. *Intensive Care Med* 1986; 12:424–428.
11. Park MK, Robotham JL, German VF: Systolic pressure amplification in pedal arteries in children. *Crit Care Med* 1983; 11:286–289.
12. Marino PL: *The ICU Book*. Philadelphia: Lea & Febiger, 1991: 41–42.
13. Venus B, Mallory DL: Vascular cannulation, in Civetta JM, Taylor RW, Kirby RR (eds): *Critical Care*. Philadelphia, JB Lippincott Company, 1992: 149–169.
14. Seneff MG: Central venous catheterization: A comprehensive review: II. *Intensive Care Med* 1987; 2:218–232.
15. McGee WT, Mallory DL: Cannulation of the internal and external jugular veins. *Probl Crit Care* 1988; 2:217–221.
16. Ermakov S, Hoyt JW: Pulmonary artery catheterization. *Crit Care Clin* 1992; 8:773–806.
17. Swan HJC, Ganz W, Forrester JS, et al: Catheterization of the heart in man with the use of flow directed balloon-tipped catheters. *N Engl J Med* 1970; 283:447–451.
18. Voyce SJ, Urbach D, Rippe JM: Pulmonary artery catheters, in Rippe JM, Irwin RS, Alpert JS, Finch MP (eds): *Intensive Care Medicine*. Boston: Little, Brown, 1991: 48–72.
19. Forrester JS, Diamond G, McHugh TJ, Swan HJ: Filling pressures in the right and left sides of the heart in acute myocardial infarction: A reappraisal of central venous pressure monitoring. *N Engl J Med* 1971; 285:190–193.
20. Marini JJ: Hemodynamic monitoring with the pulmonary artery catheter. *Crit Care Clin* 1986; 2:551–572.
21. Marino PL: *The ICU Book*. Philadelphia: Lea & Febiger, 1991: 103–104.
22. Marino PL: *The ICU Book*. Philadelphia: Lea & Febiger, 1991: 105–108.
23. Sladen A: Complications of invasive hemodynamic monitoring in the intensive care unit. *Curr Probl Surg* 1988; 25(2):69–145.
24. Putterman C: The Swan-Ganz catheter: A decade of hemodynamic monitoring. *J Crit Care* 1989; 4:127–146.
25. Patel C, Laboy V, Venus B, et al: Acute complications of pulmonary artery catheter insertion in critically ill patients. *Crit Care Med* 1986; 14:195–197.
26. Gill JB, Cairns JA: Prospective study of pulmonary artery balloon flotation catheter insertion. *J Intensive Care Med* 1988; 3:121–128.
27. Iberti TJ, Benjamin E, Gruppi L, et al: Ventricular arrhythmias during pulmonary artery catheterization in the intensive care unit. *Am J Med* 1985; 78:451–454.
28. Marino PL: *The ICU Book*. Philadelphia: Lea & Febiger, 1991: 108.
29. Paulson DM, Scott SM, Sethi GK: Pulmonary hemorrhage associated with balloon flotation catheters. *J Thorac Cardiovasc Surg* 1980; 80:453–458.
30. Swan HJC: The pulmonary artery catheter. *Dis Mon* 1991; 37(8):473–543.
31. Schwartz LB, Gewertz BL: The renal response to low dose dopamine. *J Surg Res* 1988; 45:574–588.
32. Abdul-Rasool IH, Chamberlain JH, Swan PC, et al: Cardiorespiratory and metabolic effects of dopamine and dobutamine infusions in dogs. *Crit Care Med* 1987; 15:1044–1050.
33. Leier CV, Unverferth DV: Dobutamine. *Ann Intern Med* 1983; 99:490–496.
34. Leier CV, Heban PT, Huss P, et al: Comparative systemic and regional hemodynamic effects of dopamine and dobutamine in patients with cardiomyopathic heart failure. *Circulation* 1978; 58:466–475.
35. Higging TL, Chernow B: Pharmacotherapy of circulatory shock. *Disease-a-Month* 1987; 33:314–360.
36. Desjars P, Pinaud M, Potel G, et al: A reappraisal of norepinephrine therapy in human septic shock. *Crit Care Med* 1987; 15:134–137.
37. Greenberg MS: *Handbook of Neurosurgery*. Lakeland: Greenberg Graphics, 1994:6–8.
38. Drugs for hypertensive emergencies. *Med Letter* 1987; 29:18–20.
39. Ferguson RK, Vlasses PH: Hypertensive emergencies and urgencies. *JAMA* 1986; 255:1607–1613.
40. Cottrell JE, Patel K, Turndorf H, Ransohoff J: ICP changes induced by sodium nitroprusside in patients with intracranial mass lesions. *J Neurosurg* 1978; 48:329–331.
41. Ram Z, Spiegelman R, Findler G, et al: Delayed postoperative neurological deterioration from prolonged sodium nitroprusside administration. *J Neurosurg* 1989; 71:605–607.
42. Orlowski JP, Shiesley D, Vidt DG, et al: Labetalol to control blood pressure after cerebrovascular surgery. *Crit Care Med* 1988; 16:765–768.
43. Becker RC, Gore JM: Cardiac rhythm disturbances: Recognition and treatment, in Rippe JM, Irwin RS, Alpert JS, Finch MP (eds): *Intensive Care Medicine*. Boston: Little, Brown, 1991:217–228.
44. Davis WR: Cardiac dysrhythmias, in Civetta JM, Taylor RW, Kirby RR (eds): *Critical Care*. Philadelphia: JB Lippincott Company, 1992: 1185–1189.
45. Jeffreys RV, Jones JJ: Avoidable factors contributing to the death of head injury patients in general hospitals in Mersey region. *Lancet* 1981; 2:459–461.
46. Baigelman W: Pulmonary effect of head trauma. *Neurosurgery* 1981; 9:729–740.
47. Gallagher TJ: Endotracheal intubation. *Crit Care Clin* 1992; 8:665–676.
48. Demers RR: Complications of respiratory therapy: Complications of ET suctioning procedures. *Respir Care* 1982; 27:453–457.
49. Marino PL: *The ICU Book*. Philadelphia: Lea & Febiger, 1991: 508.
50. Gopinath SP, Robertson CS, Contant CF, et al: Jugular venous desaturation and outcome after head injury. *J Neurol Neurosurg Psychiatry* 1994; 57:717–723.
51. Ducker TB, Redding JS: Pulmonary complications in neurosurgery. *Clin Neurosurg* 1976; 23:483–493.
52. Grum CM, Chauncey JB: Conventional mechanical ventilation. *Clin Chest Med* 1988; 9:37–54.
53. Jardin F, Farcot JC, Gueret P, et al: Cyclic changes in arterial pulse during respiratory support. *Circulation* 1983; 68:266–274.
54. Synder JV, Carroll GC, Shuster DP, et al: Mechanical

ventilation: Physiology and application. *Curr Prob Surg* 1984; 21(3):1–87.

55. Marino PL: *The ICU Book.* Philadelphia: Lea & Febiger, 1991: 361.
56. Hsiang JK, Chesnut RM, Crisp CB, et al: Early, routine paralysis for intracranial pressure control in severe head injury: Is it necessary? *Crit Care Med* 1994; 22(9):1471–1476.
57. Pacult A, Gudeman SK: Medical management of head injuries, in Becker DP, Gudeman SK (eds): *Textbook of Head Injury.* Philadelphia, WB Saunders, 1989: 192–220.
58. Apuzzo MLJ, Weiss MH, Petersons V, et al: Effect of positive and expiratory pressure ventilation on intracranial pressure in man. *J Neurosurg* 1977; 46(2):227–232.
59. Cooper KR, Boswell PA, Choi SC: Safe use of PEEP in patients with severe head injury. *J Neurosurg* 1985; 63:552–555.
60. Benedixen HH, et al: *Respiratory Care*. St. Louis: C. V. Mosby Co. 1965: 137–156.
61. Stetson JB: Introductory essay in prolonged tracheal intubation. *Int Anesthesiol Clin* 1970; 8:767–779.
62. Sahn SA, Lakshminarayan S: Bedside criteria for discontinuation of mechanical ventilation. *Chest* 1973; 63:1002–1005.
63. Consensus conference on artificial airways in patients receiving mechanical ventilation. *Chest* 1989; 96:178–180.
64. Heffner JE, Miller KS, Sahn SA: Tracheostomy in the intensive care unit: Parts I and II. *Chest* 1986; 90:269–274, 430–436.
65. Logemann JA: Aspiration in head and neck surgical patients. *Ann Otol Rhinol Laryngol* 1985; 94:373–376.
66. Wynne JW, Modell JH: Respiratory aspiration of stomach contents. *Ann Intern Med* 1977; 87:466–474.
67. Cooper KR, Boswell PA: Reduced functional residual capacity and abnormal oxygenation in patients with severe head injury. *Resp Care* 1984; 29:263–269.
68. Bartlett JG, O'Keefe P, Tally FP: Bacteriology of hospital-acquired pneumonia. *Arch Intern Med* 1986; 146:868–871.
69. Craven DE, Driks MR: Nosocomial pneumonia in the intubated patient. *Semin Respir Med* 1987; 2:20–33.
70. Hessen MT, Kaye D: Nosocomial pneumonia. *Crit Care Clin* 1988; 4:245–257.
71. Ruiz-Santana S, Jiminez AG, Esteban A, et al: ICU pneumonias: A multi-institutional study. *Crit Care Med* 1987; 15:930–932.
72. Verghese A, Berk SL: Bacterial pneumonia in the elderly. *Medicine* 1983; 62:271–285.
73. Pierce AK, Edmonson EB, McGee G, et al: An analysis of factors predisposing to gram-negative bacillary necrotizing pneumonia. *Am Rev Resp Dis* 1966; 94:309–315.
74. Weidemann HP, Matthay MA, Matthay RA (eds): Acute lung injury. *Crit Care Clin* 1986; 2:377–667.
75. Marino PL: *The ICU Book*. Philadelphia: Lea & Febiger, 1991: 293.
76. Vesconi S, Rossi GP, Pesenti A, et al: Pulmonary microthrombosis in severe adult respiratory distress syndrome. *Crit Care Med* 1988; 16:111–113.
77. Modig J: Posttraumatic pulmonary insufficiency caused by microembolism syndrome. *Acta Chir Scand Suppl* 1980; 499:57–65.
78. Shapiro BA, Harrison RA, Trout CA: *Clinical Application of Respiratory Care.* Chicago: Year Book Medical Publisher, 1979.
79. Cooper KR: Respiratory complications in patients with serious head injuries, in Becker DP, Gudeman SK (eds): *Textbook of Head Injury*. Philadelphia: WB Saunders, 1989: 255–264.
80. Epstein FM, Ward JD, Becker DP: Medical complications of head injury, in Cooper PR (ed): *Head Injury*. Baltimore: Williams and Wilkins, 1987:390–421.
81. Knudsen F, Jensen HP, Petersen PL: Neurogenic pulmonary edema: Treatment with dobutamine. *Neurosurgery* 1991; 29:269–270.
82. Graf CJ, Rossi NP: Pulmonary edema and the central nervous system: A clinicopathological study. *Surg Neurol* 1975; 4:319–325.
83. Simmons RL, Martin AM Jr, Heisterkamp CA III, Ducker TB: Respiratory insufficiency in combat casualties: II. Pulmonary edema following head injury. *Ann Surg* 1969; 170:39–44.
84. Kaufman HH, Satterwhite T, McConnell BJ, et al: Deep vein thrombosis and pulmonary embolism in head injured patients. *Angiology* 1983; 34:627–638.
85. Vesconi S, Rossi GP, Pesenti A, et al: Pulmonary microthrombosis in severe adult respiratory distress syndrome. *Crit Care Med* 1988; 16:111–113.
86. Sevitt S, Gallagher N: Venous thrombosis and pulmonary embolism: A clinico-pathologic study in injured and burned patients. *Br J Surg* 1969; 48:475–489.
87. Shackford SR, Moser KM: Deep venous thrombosis and pulmonary embolism in trauma patients. *J Inten Care Med* 1988; 3:87.
88. Coon WW, Willis PW: Recurrence of venous thromboembolism. *Surgery* 1973; 73:823–827.
89. Volgesang GB, Bell WR: Treatment of pulmonary embolism and deep vein thrombosis with thrombolytic therapy. *Clin Chest Med* 1984; 5:487–494.
90. Dennis JW, Menawat S, Von Thron J, et al: Efficacy of deep venous thrombosis prophylaxis in trauma patients and identification of high-risk groups. *J Trauma* 1993; 35:132–139.
91. King DJ, Kelton JG: Heparin-associated thrombocytopenia. *Ann Intern Med* 1984; 100:535–540.
92. Bell WR, Royall RM: Heparin-associated thrombocytopenia: A comparison of three heparin preparations. *N Engl J Med* 1980; 303:902–907.
93. Cines DB, Kaywin P, Bina M, et al: Heparin-associated thrombocytopenia. *N Engl J Med* 1980; 303:788–795.
94. Cimo PL, Moake JL, Winger RS, et al: Heparin-induced thrombocytopenia: Association with a platelet aggregating factor and arterial thromboses. *Am J Hematol* 1979; 6:125–133.
95. Miller JD, Sweet RC, Narayan RK, Becker DP: Early

insults to the injured brain. *JAMA* 1978; 240:439–442.
96. Alho A: Fat embolism syndrome: A variant of posttraumatic pulmonary insufficiency. *Ann Chir Gynaecol Suppl* 1982; 196:31–36.
97. Fabian TC, Hoots AV, Stanford DS, et al: Fat embolism syndrome: Prospective evaluation of 92 fracture patients. *Crit Care Med* 1990; 18:42–46.
98. Shier MR, Wilson RF: Fat embolism syndrome: Traumatic coagulopathy with respiratory distress. *Surg Annu* 1980; 12:139.
99. Lepisto P, Lahti R: Lipids in the pulmonary circulation after fatal trauma: A postmortem study. *Ann Chir Gynaecol* 1978; 67:17–21.
100. Dines DE, Burgher LW, Okazaki H: The clinical and pathologic correlation of fat embolism syndrome. *Mayo Clin Proc* 1975; 50:407–411.
101. Chastre J, Fagon JY, Soler P, et al: Bronchoalveolar lavage for rapid diagnosis of the fat embolism syndrome in trauma patients. *Ann Intern Med* 1990; 113:583–588.
102. Riska EB, Myllynen P: Fat embolism in patients with multiple injuries. *J Trauma* 1982; 22:891–894.

CHAPTER 24

FLUID AND ELECTROLYTE MANAGEMENT IN THE HEAD-INJURED PATIENT

Brian T. Andrews

SYNOPSIS

The management of fluids and electrolytes is an important aspect of the intensive care of patients with intracranial disease and injury because the CNS plays a critical role in fluid, electrolyte, and acid-base homeostasis and in turn is affected by it. Head injury therefore often results directly in perturbations in this homeostasis, as may treatment such as the use of intravenous diuretics, controlled hyperventilation, and fluid restriction. Conversely, the consequences of fluid, electrolyte, and acid-base disturbance on the abnormal brain are profound, influencing the development of cytotoxic or vasogenic brain edema, loss of cerebral autoregulation, increased intracranial pressure or decreased perfusion pressure, and altered level of consciousness. Recognition and effective management of fluid, each of these complications and improving overall recovery from the primary insult. This chapter reviews fluid, electrolyte, and acid-base balance; their common disturbances in neurosurgical disorders; and their practical management.

NORMAL FLUID AND ELECTROLYTE DISTRIBUTION

Normally, total body water (TBW) accounts for about 60 percent of body weight in adults, varying somewhat with leanness and age. Newborns and young children have higher TBW, while women and the obese have lower TBW as a result of a lower amount of water in adipose tissue. Normally, about two-thirds of TBW is intracellular fluid (ICF) and one-third is extracellular fluid (ECF), with 25 percent of the ECF in the intravascular compartment and 75 percent in the interstitial space. So-called third-space fluid includes water in the gastrointestinal and biliary tracts, CSF, and lymphatics.[1] The term "third-space fluid" is also used to describe ECF accumulating as a result of injury or inflammation that is functionally not a part of the normal ECF.

Total body sodium (Na^+) is about 40 mEq/kg with a concentration gradient of 98% extracellular and 2% intracellular. The extracellular [Na^+] normally ranges from 135 to 145 mEq/liter, with an intracellular concentration of 5 to 15 mEq/liter. Total body potassium (K^+) is about 50 mEq/kg, has a concentration gradient opposite to that of sodium, and is 98% intracellular and 2% extracellular, with an intracellular [K^+] of 140 to 150 mEq/liter and an extracellular concentration of 3.5 to 5.0 mEq/liter. The high intracellular to extracellular gradients of sodium and potassium are necessary to maintain normal resting membrane potential, and are regulated by the Na^+,K^+-ATPase pump.

NORMAL FLUID AND ELECTROLYTE REGULATION

Regulation of Body Water and Osmolality

Plasma sodium and osmolality are maintained within narrow ranges of normal by adjustments of TBW that keep it in balance with sodium. TBW is regulated by central monitoring of ECF osmolality (total concentration of all solutes in water), intravascular volume, and intravascular pressure. Normal osmolality is maintained at 285 to 295 mOsm/liter. Because most cell membranes are freely permeable to water, osmolality is a major determinant of water distribution between the ICF and the ECF. Osmotic pressure is the force of water movement generated by differences in osmolality across membranes. Oncotic pressure is osmotic pressure that is due only to differences in protein concentration. ECF hypo-osmolality is an excess of free water relative to the concentration of solutes, and hyperosmolality is a relative deficiency in ECF. The primary extracellular solutes are sodium, its anions chloride and bicarbonate, glucose, and urea [blood urea nitrogen (BUN)]. Their contribution to ECF osmolality can be calculated as follows:

$$\text{Effective osmolality (mOsm/kg)} = [\text{Na}^+] \times 2 + [\text{glucose}]/18 + [\text{BUN}]/2.8$$

The concentration of any other osmotically active solute, such as mannitol or alcohol, can be added to this value to calculate effective osmolality. Osmoreceptors in the organum vasculosum laminae terminalis of the anterior hypothalamus are sensitive to changes in tonicity, which are communicated to the magnicellular neurons in the supraoptic and paraventricular nuclei of the hypothalamus. Axons from these nuclei descend in the hypothalamo-hypophyseal tract to terminate in the neurohypophysis of the pituitary gland. These neurons release arginine vasopressin, or antidiuretic hormone (ADH), into the bloodstream in response to increases in ECF osmolality. ADH acts on the collecting ducts of the renal tubules to increase water absorption, adding free water to the ECF and correcting hyperosmolar states.

Under hypo-osmolar conditions, ADH release usually falls to zero below an osmotic threshold of about 280 mOsm/kg, decreasing water absorption by the renal collecting tubules and permitting excretion of maximally dilute urine. Thus, less water is returned to the ECF, and the hypo-osmolar state is corrected. There are, however, numerous other mechanisms for the release of ADH which may override osmotic stimuli and produce water retention to preserve intravascular volume *despite hypotonic ECF and worsening hypo-osmolality*. The magnicellular neurons also integrate information regarding intravascular volume and pressure that is sensed by cardiac and arterial baroreceptors. Hypotension and hypovolemia are potent stimuli for the massive release of ADH. Pain, stress, nausea, emesis, hypoxia, and drugs such as barbiturates, narcotics, and carbamazepine can also stimulate ADH release.[2] These factors may explain, along with pathological states such as the syndrome of inappropriate ADH (SIADH; see below) and cerebral salt wasting (see below), why hyponatremia and hypo-osmolar states are so common after head injury and other intracranial insults despite a "normal" amount of fluid intake.

Under hyperosmolar conditions, thirst and drinking behavior are also important in the maintenance of water balance. Even in the absence of ADH, plasma osmolality can be maintained if the patient is able to drink to thirst. This may be influenced, however, by the patient's level of consciousness and physical capacity for drinking.

In patients with a head injury, hypo- and hyperosmolar states are common clinical problems caused primarily by disturbances in water balance or by therapeutic measures such as dehydration and the use of mannitol. Although effective osmolality can be estimated easily by using plasma sodium, glucose, and BUN, direct measurement of osmolality is useful in patients receiving mannitol for the treatment of increased intracranial pressure (ICP). This is particularly true when patients are receiving high or repeated doses of mannitol, which may lead to increased brain edema[3] or mannitol-induced renal failure[4] if plasma osmolality remains above about 340 mOsm/kg. As a general rule, a goal of therapy should be to maintain plasma osmolality below this level.[1]

Regulation of intracellular volume

Cellular homeostasis in the brain includes mechanisms that balance changes in plasma (ECF) osmolality with changes in intracellular solute concentration.[1,5,6] These mechanisms may be important in controlling brain volume under hypo- and hyperosmolar conditions. Under hypo-osmolar conditions, the intracellular solute concentration decreases by means of increased binding of Na^+, K^+, and Cl^- and the extrusion of those electrolytes to normalize osmolality with the ECF and prevent cellular swelling.[5] Under hyperosmolar conditions, the intracellular solute concentration increases by means of the influx of electrolytes across the cell membrane, decreased intracellular binding, and increased amino acid concentration, preventing cellular dehydration.[1,6] Cellular injury due, for example, to head trauma may disrupt these mechanisms, leading to exacerbated cellular swelling and brain edema during hypo-osmolar states or excessive cellular dehydration during aggressive osmolar therapy, potentially with negative consequences.

Regulation of sodium

The goal of sodium regulation is the maintenance of adequate blood pressure and volume. Two physiological systems maintain normal blood pressure and volume by allowing for sodium retention and causing vasoconstriction: the renin-aldosterone system and the sympathetic nervous system. It is the net balance of these two systems that determines the final response. A third system, which is less well defined, may be mediated by atrial natriuretic factor (ANF or atriopeptin) and other factors which promote natriuresis and vasodilation and inhibit other mechanisms of sodium retention.[7]

Baroreceptors in the preglomerular arterioles of the kidney respond to a decrease in blood pressure by releasing renin. Increased sympathetic tone (a response to the hypotensive state) and tubular sodium concentration sensed by the nephron also modulate renin release.[8] Renin stimulates the conversion of angiotensinogen to angiotensin I, which is rapidly metabolized to angiotensin II. Angiotensin II has multiple effects in which it (1) acts as a potent direct vasoconstrictor, (2) stimulates increased secretion of aldosterone from the adrenal medulla, and (3) stimulates hypothalamic thirst mechanisms. Aldosterone acts at the distal renal tubule to promote the reabsorption of sodium. The sympathetic nervous system, in addition to stimulating renin release, also directly promotes sodium retention in the renal tubule. The overall effect of hypotension therefore is to promote sodium reabsorption, retention of free water passively with sodium, vasoconstriction, and increased thirst.

ANF may counterbalance these systems by promoting sodium excretion. ANF is released from the atrium of the heart in response to increased atrial pressure[7] and appears to promote natriuresis and diuresis, vasodilation, and decreased thirst and antagonize the release of ADH, renin, and aldosterone. ANF is also present in the CNS in areas such as the hypothalamus, median eminence, midbrain, choroid plexus, and spinal cord and may act as a neuromodulator in the central regulation of sodium and volume homeostasis.[9] ANF locally released in the CNS also appears to play an important role in the control of intracellular volume in the brain[10] and decreases brain capillary permeability, thus reducing brain water after ischemic insults. Other, less well-defined central and peripheral natriuretic factors may also interfere with sodium transport through inhibition of Na^+,K^+-ATPase.[1]

Regulation of Potassium

The regulation of potassium secretion occurs in the kidney and is based on the concentration in the distal tubule. Aldosterone release is also stimulated by elevated serum potassium levels and acts at the distal renal tubule to promote not only reabsorption of sodium but also potassium excretion. Acid-base balance influences the distribution of potassium between the intracellular and extracellular spaces. Alkalosis, as may occur with hyperventilation therapy, leads to the movement of potassium into cells, lowering plasma levels and promoting renal excretion, possibly resulting in hypokalemia.

Regulation of Other Electrolytes

Other electrolytes important in the management of patients with a head injury include calcium, magnesium, and phosphate. Calcium circulates in the blood 50 percent as an ionized fraction, 40 percent bound to protein (mostly albumin), and 10 percent chelated to other ions; the ionized fraction is thought to be the physiologically important and regulated component. Serum Ca^{2+} is regulated by parathyroid hormone (PTH) and vitamin D. PTH promotes calcium release from bone, renal reabsorption, and gastrointestinal (GI) absorption. Release of PTH is suppressed by hypercalcemia, hypo- or hypermagnesemia, and metabolites of vitamin D. Vitamin D is either absorbed by the GI tract or synthesized in the skin; after conversion by the liver and kidney to 1,25-dihydrovitamin D, its action is similar to that of PTH, promoting an increase in serum Ca^{2+}.

Magnesium also circulates as ionized (55 percent), protein-bound (30 percent), and chelated (15 percent) components, and homeostasis is maintained by means of renal excretion. Urinary loss of magnesium occurs with expansion of the ECF, hypermagnesemia, hypercalcemia, phosphate depletion, metabolic acidosis, and the use of diuretics.

Phosphate is controlled by regulated resorption in the proximal renal tubules, and excretion is stimulated by expansion of ECF, PTH, and drugs such as dextrose, digoxin, and corticosteroids.

FLUID AND ELECTROLYTE MANAGEMENT

Changes in fluids and electrolytes are commonly associated with head trauma, particularly severe head injury, and may be compounded by other systemic injuries that cause alterations in blood pressure, volume states, or hematocrit. Among head-injured patients, dehydration, hemorrhage, and the stress of injury often lead to salt and water retention as neurohumeral, renal, and cardiovascular mechanisms act to preserve intravascular volume and maintain organ perfusion. Activation of the renin-angiotensin system and secretion of aldosterone and ADH decrease the excretion of sodium and free water. As a consequence of these changes, such patients may become edematous, gain weight, and develop hyponatremia in response to fluid resuscitation.[11] Patients with head trauma compounded by multisystem injury may have an increase in vascular permeability causing third-space fluid retention and have increased initial fluid requirements. Later, reabsorption of this fluid may be associated with intravascular congestion and pulmonary edema. Treatment with diuretics such as mannitol and furosemide to decrease brain edema may aggravate free water and sodium losses.

Whereas in the past there was a philosophy of keeping neurosurgical patients dehydrated by means of hypovolemic hemoconcentration or an attempt to decrease cerebral edema, more recently the goals have been to maintain intravascular volume at normal levels and maintain cerebral perfusion and normal metabolic function regardless of intracranal pathology.[12] Important to the correct management of fluids and electrolytes is an assessment of ongoing requirements. Among the parameters to consider are body weight assessed on a daily basis, fluid intake and output, measured serum electrolytes, glucose and arterial blood gases, renal function, and cardiopulmonary hemodynamics. The types and volumes of fluid administered should be continually reevaluated and adjusted to restore and maintain normal water and electrolyte balance as well as acid-base balance and tissue oxygenation.

Fluid requirements are divided into three components: maintenance needs, ongoing losses, and deficits. Maintenance water requirements in an uncomplicated patient are about 30 to 35 ml/kg/day. This provides a balance against urinary losses of 800 to 1500 ml/day, GI losses of up to 250 ml/day, and insensible losses from the lungs and skin of 600 to 900 ml/day. In a critically ill patient, each of these requirements may change: Fever may increase insensible water loss by 30 percent, whereas controlled ventilation may decrease insensible loss from the lungs to near zero.[1] Patients with a head injury are extremely catabolic,[12] with increased production of free water through tissue breakdown. Thus, repeated assessment is necessary to monitor these varying conditions.

Initial Maintenance Fluids

Initial maintenance fluids in a neurosurgical patient who is not taking oral nutrition consist of an intravenous infusion of normal (0.9%) saline solution with or without supplemental K^+. Patients with ongoing losses or an initial volume deficit may require additional boluses of fluid. In these patients, it is preferable to have central venous pressure (CVP) monitoring established to allow an accurate assessment of intravascular volume, with a goal of achieving a CVP of 1 to 4 mmHg.[12] In patients with subarachnoid hemorrhage, severe multisystem injury, or spinal cord injury and those requiring barbiturate therapy to control elevated ICP, the placement of a Swan-Ganz catheter allows additional measurement of pulmonary arterial wedge pressures and cardiac output. The rate of maintenance fluids may become difficult to determine in severely head injured patients, as they are predisposed to impaired water excretion and hyponatremia. Repeated assessment of volume status and serum electrolytes every 6 to 12 h and daily weight assessment are useful to guide ongoing fluid administration.

Resuscitation from Shock

Patients with hemorrhagic shock require rapid volume restoration to correct hypotension and increased fluid administration to account for ongoing losses.[13] *The presence of a head injury should not preclude the administration of the volume required to correct shock*, as secondary injury due to hypotension is more deleterious to the injured brain than is increased cerebral edema due to added fluids.[12] While vigorous fluid administration should be used initially, a poor response to fluid administration should prompt a search for ongoing hemorrhage into the chest or abdominal cavity or for alternative causes of hypotension, such as cardiac tamponade and contusion.

Determination of the optimal volume needed for resuscitation from hemorrhagic shock may be difficult. Many trauma protocols involve the use of isotonic crystalloids up to 2000 ml by intravenous infusion with observation of the effect on blood pressure, pulse, and other signs of shock, such as skin color, temperature, and capillary refill. Assessment of blood pressure alone may be misleading, as endogenous catecholamine release can result in nearly normal blood pressure despite profound blood loss. A sudden drop in pressure may then occur as compensatory mechanisms are exhausted. Assessment of pulse only may also be unreliable, as pulse may be elevated as a result of pain or, in some patients, may be misleadingly low despite massive injury and blood loss.[13] Other measures of volume status are usually impractical in the emergency setting, although early institution of CVP monitoring has been used. Repeated assessment of hematocrit is often performed, but it is frequently not truly reflective of ongoing blood loss.

The type of fluid used for volume resuscitation from shock remains controversial.[13–15] Some authors have suggested that the use of colloids rather than crystalloids minimizes secondary injury to the brain and may decrease posttraumatic pulmonary dysfunction.[16] Others, however, consider the available data inconclusive regarding the potential benefits of colloids[13] and warn that such solutions may leak into the pulmonary extravascular space and exacerbate pulmonary edema.[14,17] Colloids may also negatively affect cardiac and renal function and the immune system.[13,18,19] The most common practice currently employed with multitrauma patients with hemorrhagic shock is to give isotonic crystalloid solutions because of their efficacy, ease of administration, low rate of complications, and low cost.[13]

Interest has been generated in the use of low-volume hypertonic crystalloid solutions, such as 7.5% saline, for early resuscitation of multitrauma patients with severe head injury.[20–22] The effect of such solutions on the cardiovascular system in shock is profound. Volumes as little as one-tenth those normally needed for isotonic solutions may have a marked effect on blood pressure and cardiac output as the hypertonic solution rapidly draws free water into the vascular spaces of the ECF.[13] The use of colloids such as Dextran 70 may prolong this effect for several hours.[22] Hypertonic solutions also appear to have a direct effect on cardiac contractility and output.[23] In patients with a severe head injury, these resuscitation fluids may be ideal because blood pressure is restored without excessive free water to exacerbate cerebral edema, while hypertonic saline may have a mannitol-like effect of lowering ICP.[24,25] Indeed, these reports suggest that ICP is lowered, cerebral perfusion pressure is improved, and brain water content is decreased, as measured by nuclear magnetic resonance.[24,25] A randomized study of prehospital fluid resuscitation of hypotensive head-injured patients indicated a trend toward improved outcome with the use of 7.5% saline/dextran solution.[26] Some concerns about the effect of rapid cellular dehydration on cerebral function remain,[13] especially with repeated boluses or prolonged resuscitation, and these issues are being explored.

Other Considerations

Clinical studies of severe head injury have shown that moderately severe hyperglycemia (>200 to 250 mg/dl) is associated with a poor outcome, perhaps because of increased lactate production and lactic acidosis in marginally perfused tissue subject to anaerobic metabolism.[27–29] Therefore, initial maintenance fluids in severely head injured patients at risk for secondary injury due to cerebral ischemia should be dextrose-free.

Patients with spinal cord injury and spinal shock require special consideration as a result of the loss of sympathetic tone, which often results in systemic hypotension combined with bradycardia. Such patients are commonly overresuscitated with a crystalloid infusion in an attempt to obtain a normal blood pressure, resulting in hyponatremia, pulmonary edema, and third-space fluid losses. Such patients often require Swan-Ganz catheterization and monitoring, along with judicious fluid resuscitation combined with the use of vasopressors such as phenylephrine (Neo-Synephrine), which restore adrenergic tone and peripheral vasoconstriction.[12,30]

Ongoing fluid requirements and replacement should be based on repeated assessment of fluid status, as outlined above. Ongoing fluid losses usually occur as a result of gastrointestinal losses, use of osmotic diuretics, and third-space fluid losses and must be replaced.[1] Optimally, such losses can be measured and their electrolyte content can be assessed.

FLUID AND ELECTROLYTE DISORDERS

Hyponatremia

Hyponatremia with a measured serum sodium below 135 mEq/liter is extremely common in neurosurgical patients and should be carefully monitored because the associated decrease in extracellular osmolality may cause cellular swelling, increased cerebral edema, and impaired brain function.[1] Hyponatremia usually is due to increased ADH release combined with the use of replacement fluids which are hypotonic (i.e., 0.45% saline). The result is increased absorption of free water and lowered serum sodium. As was noted earlier, ADH secretion may be increased by a variety of stimuli, such as pain and surgical stress, and may override the usual osmotic regulation of ADH and result in continued release despite a hypo-osmolar and hyponatremic state. This condition may merge with SIADH (see below), which often results from head injury, where the incidence of hyponatremia is 5 to 12 percent.[2,31,32] In children with head trauma, the incidence of SIADH may be as high as 25 percent.[33] Hyponatremia is also very common after aneurysm rupture[34,35] and spinal cord injury.[36–38]

Hyponatremia can also be seen in other states where there is an increase in total body water, such as congestive heart failure and hepatic cirrhosis, or where the ECF volume is contracted as a result of gastrointestinal or renal losses of sodium in excess of losses of water[2,7,9,10] or hypopituitarism.[39] Table 24-1 outlines common clinical conditions that can produce water retention or sodium loss.

The evaluation of hyponatremia has usually been approached by clinical assessment of daily weights, volume status, and measurement of urinary electrolytes and osmolality, as outlined in Table 24-2. Urinary sodium measurement is used to differentiate various salt-retaining states, such as heart failure and cirrhosis, from conditions characterized by excessive urinary salt loss.[2]

TABLE 24-1 Causes of Hyponatremia

Water retention
- Hyperosmolar states (mannitol, alcohol, hyperlipidemia)
- Pain and stress
- Congestive heart failure
- Hepatic cirrhosis
- Pregnancy
- Drugs
- SIADH

Sodium loss
- Diuretics
- Mineralocorticoid insufficiency
- Glucocorticoid insufficiency (hypopituitarism)
- Hypothyroidism
- Salt-wasting nephropathies
- Cerebral salt wasting
- Elevated ANF

Syndrome of Inappropriate ADH

SIADH is a state of expanded or normal intravascular volume, hypo-osmolar hyponatremia, and continued ADH release, resulting in the secretion of excessively concentrated urine, with a urinary sodium greater than 25 mEq/liter. SIADH is common in a variety of neurosurgical disorders, particularly head injury,[31–33] where the incidence is 5 to 12 percent. In children, the incidence of SIADH may be as high as 25 percent.[40] In head-injured patients, increased levels of ADH are detected in the blood, CSF, and urine.[33,40,41]

The definition of SIADH requires that renal disease, hypothyroidism, and adrenal insufficiency be excluded, as increased ADH levels may occur in these disorders and hyponatremia may occur with "normal" levels of free water intake.[2] Hypopituitarism must also be ruled out, where suppressed glucocorticoid release results in excessive urinary losses of sodium.[39]

The diagnosis of SIADH in critically ill patients may be a problem because volume status may be difficult to assess, and extracellular volume may vary as a result of ongoing blood loss, the use of diuretics, and the presence of peripheral edema. SIADH may occur despite the presence of contracted intravascular volume, such as in sepsis, multiple trauma, or hypoalbuminemia, when overall volume is increased. However, the diagnosis can presumptively be confirmed by fluid restriction and repeated assessment of serum and urinary sodium. In the case of SIADH, there will be an increase in serum sodium and a reduction in absolute urinary sodium loss, although the urinary concentration of sodium may remain high.

The occurrence of a high urinary sodium level in SIADH has not been explained fully. Possible contributions may arise from an increased glomerular filtration rate with an increased filtered load of sodium, decreased aldosterone secretion, and decreased sodium reabsorption caused by the effect of ANF.[2] Both plasma and CSF levels of ANF have been shown to be elevated in SIADH associated with aneurysmal subarachnoid hemorrhage.[39,42,43] Thus, elevated ANF levels appear to occur in diseases and injuries of the brain and result in increased urinary excretion of sodium despite plasma hyponatremia and hypo-osmolality. Of interest, ANF appears to also be involved in the development of so-called cerebral salt wasting, a state similar to hyponatremia except that extracellular volume and overall volume status are contracted (see below).

Treatment of SIADH

SIADH typically has been treated with restriction of fluid intake to 800 to 1000 ml per day in adults, using isotonic intravenous fluid such as normal saline. For patients receiving enteral feedings, additional intravenous fluids should be minimized and IV drugs should be made up in normal saline. Patients on nasogastric tube feeding will probably need additional salt intake, as most standard enteric feeding solutions contain only a small amount of sodium.[2] Care should be taken to observe a patient undergoing fluid restriction for signs

TABLE 24-2 Volume Status, Daily Body Weight, and Urinary Sodium in Hyponatremia and Hypo-Osmolality

Diagnosis	Volume Status	Weight	Urinary Sodium, mEq/L
SIADH	Increased	Increased	>25
Congestive heart failure	Increased	Increased	<10
Hepatic cirrhosis	Increased	Increased	<10
Renal disorders (diuretics, cerebral salt wasting, adrenal insufficiency)	Decreased	Decreased	>25
Hyponatremic dehydration	Decreased	Decreased	<10
Pituitary insufficiency	Decreased	Decreased	>25

of hypotension or hypovolemia in case the patient has cerebral salt wasting rather than SIADH and is dehydrated to begin with. If there is any question about volume status, monitoring of the CVP or pulmonary artery wedge pressure should be used to assess the situation.

Severe, symptomatic hyponatremia (<120 mEq/liter) can be corrected by using an infusion of hypertonic 3% saline (1 ml per kilogram of body weight per hour) and intravenous furosemide or mannitol, which will increase free water diuresis relative to sodium retention. Treatment is directed toward reducing the elevation in total body water, and the main goal of using a hypertonic solution is to facilitate diuresis rather than directly raise serum sodium.[2] A point of controversy is the rate at which hyponatremia should be corrected. Rapid correction has been associated with the development of central pontine myelinolysis and the "osmotic demyelination syndrome."[44–46] Numerous factors are involved in this case, such as the rate of development of hyponatremia, its duration and severity before treatment, and the rapidity of correction.[46] This insult probably reflects cellular adaptation to a chronic or severe hypo-osmolar state, with overly rapid correction of serum hyponatremia leading to cellular dehydration and resulting injury.[2] It appears that patients with the acute development of hyponatremia can be corrected quickly, as fast as 1–2 mEq/liter/h, to serum levels of 130 to 134 mEq/liter, followed by a slower and more complete correction using volume restriction. More severe or long-standing hyponatremia should probably be corrected no more than about 12 mEq/24 h (≤0.5 mEq/liter/h).[46] During correction, serum electrolytes should be carefully reassessed at least every 4 to 6 h to prevent overcorrection. Hypertonic saline should be discontinued when signs and symptoms have resolved or mild hyponatremia has been achieved.

An adjunct to the treatment of chronic SIADH is oral demeclocycline hydrochloride (200 to 400 mg tid), a tetracycline analogue which induces nephrogenic diabetes insipidus and chronic diuresis.[47,48] Demeclocycline should be used with caution in patients with renal disease.[2] Another method of treatment is to increase salt intake and use oral fludrocortisone (Florinef) (0.1 to 0.4 mg/day).[54]

Cerebral Salt Wasting

The syndrome of cerebral salt wasting was first described in the 1950s[49,50] but fell into disregard until much more recently. Careful analysis of both patients and laboratory models with various brain insults, including head injury, revealed a syndrome of hyponatremia and hypo-osmolality associated with depleted intravascular volume and contracted ECF.[50–55] Such patients may appear normal clinically but in reality are dehydrated, at times to the point of hypotension. In these patients, persistent urinary loss of sodium occurs even during restricted fluid intake, and treatment appropriate for SIADH results in further hypovolemia without correction of the hyponatremia. Nelson et al.,[51] in an experimental model of subarachnoid hemorrhage in primates, indicated that in cerebral salt wasting the levels of ADH are not elevated and are more likely the result of an increased effect of ANF.

Treatment of Cerebral Salt Wasting

Treatment of cerebral salt wasting requires reexpansion of the depleted intravascular volume and total body sodium, using isotonic (0.9%) intravenous saline for mild hyponatremia or hypertonic (3%) saline solution for more severe cases.[52,53,55] Others have found that head-injured patients with this syndrome benefit from the use of increased salt intake combined with oral fludrocortisone (0.1 to 0.4 mg/day) to increase renal sodium and water retention.[54] Some reports suggest that many patients with hyponatremia presumed to be due to SIADH actually may have cerebral salt wasting with a depleted intravascular volume.[51,53] Therefore, treatment of hyponatremia should be predicated on a careful assessment of volume status before one chooses between fluid restriction and rehydration with salt-rich solutions. Patients for whom fluid restriction causes symptoms or signs of volume depletion or in whom hyponatremia is not corrected should be reassessed for cerebral salt wasting and treated accordingly.

Hypernatremia and Hyperosmolality

The most common hyperosmolar states in patients with neurosurgical disorders are due to hypernatremia as a result of excessive diuresis, often therapeutically induced by the use of mannitol or furosemide. These patients may also have increased loss of free water due to fever or increased insensible losses from the lungs. They may receive excessive salt in intravenous fluids or enteral feedings, particularly when combined with overall fluid restriction. Hypernatremia may also occur as a result of diabetes insipidus caused by an insult or injury to the hypothalamus or pituitary stalk.

Clinical signs of hypernatremia are usually seen only when serum Na^+ is higher than 160 mEq/liter and serum osmolality is higher than 330 mOsm/liter. Symptoms usually include confusion, lethargy, restlessness, and occasionally seizures. Acute hypernatremia with dehydration may result in brain shrinkage and occasionally the development of subdural or intraparenchymal hemorrhages.[56] In the setting of chronic hypernatremia, intracellular sodium is increased, and subsequent rapid correction of serum sodium may result in cerebral edema[2] or seizures.[57]

Treatment of hypernatremia is based on calculation of the free water deficit followed by replacement at an appropriate rate. The free water deficit is calculated by using the following formula:

$$\text{Free water deficit (kg or L)} = \frac{[0.6 \times \text{wt (kg)}] \times \text{serum Na}^+}{140 - \text{serum Na}^+}$$

Once the free water deficit has been calculated, replacement can be achieved safely if half the deficit is replaced initially, using intravenous 5% dexrose in water or 0.2% saline, and the remainder is replaced over the next 24 h.[2] Serum sodium should be carefully followed during such resuscitation because prior use of mannitol or hyperglycemia may have resulted in a total body loss of sodium, and additional sodium may be required along with restitution of total body water to achieve a normotonic state.

Other hyperosmolar states may occur as a result of hyperglycemia, which is usually caused by insulin resistance due to sepsis or the administration of glucocorticoids such as dexamethasone or total parenteral nutrition with an increased glucose load. Severe hyperglycemia also results in urinary osmotic diuresis, with additional loss of free water and sodium, and may result, as was noted above, in a deficit of both total body water and sodium that requires replacement.

Diabetes Insipidus

Diabetes insipidus (DI) results from injury to the anterior hypothalamus or the pituitary stalk and neurohypophysis, resulting in a decrease in or a total loss of circulating ADH. The result is an excessive loss of water from the renal tubules that is unresponsive to changes in serum osmolality or hypotension, the usual stimuli for ADH secretion. The most common causes of DI are pituitary region tumors such as pituitary adenomas and their surgical treatment and cranial trauma.[58–62] The incidence of DI after severe closed head injury is reported as only 2 percent but appears to be more likely to occur if there are fractures in and about the sella turcica.[60,61] Patients with markedly elevated ICP and clinical brain death also commonly develop DI.[63,64] It should be remembered that other causes of DI may be present concurrently in a neurosurgical intensive care patient, including phenytoin use, alcohol intoxication, and bacterial meningitis.[65]

The clinical diagnosis of DI is defined as polyuria (>30 ml/kg/h or, in an adult, >200 ml/h) with a low urinary specific gravity (<1.005) associated with elevated serum sodium (>145 mEq/liter). The onset of clinical DI usually begins no sooner than in 6 to 8 h and may be delayed as long as 24 h after an injury, as endogenous ADH will still be circulating for this long even with an acute transection of the pituitary stalk.[61] Injury to the hypothalamus or tuber cinereum usually results in permanent DI, whereas injury to the neurohypophysis or lower stalk often results in only transient DI, as secretion of ADH from the hypothalamus is reestablished.

Patients with complete untreated DI usually have 10 to 15 liters/day of dilute urine, which can rapidly lead to hemodynamic instability due to dehydration. Thus, DI must be recognized and corrected rapidly, especially in poorly responsive or uncommunicative patients. Patients who are awake and communicative usually complain of intense thirst and, if able, drink adequate volume to compensate for urinary losses because the thirst mechanism, which is responsive to both serum osmolality and hypotension, is usually preserved.

Patients with partial DI may have the onset of polyuria later and at a lower volume compared with those with complete DI. However, their urine remains dilute with a low specific gravity (<1.005), and if this is not treated, serum sodium will rise above normal. In this case, other causes of polyuria must also be considered, including the use of osmotic diuretics such as mannitol or iodinated contrast agents, hyperglycemia, mobilization of third-space fluids (usually several days after injury or surgery), and fluid overload.[2] In these situations, the urinary specific gravity is usually higher (>1.009) and the urine is less dilute. The distinction between these conditions and DI can be made by measurement of serum and urinary glucose and repeated assessment of serum electrolytes and clinical volume status. In this circumstance, monitoring the CVP or pulmonary capillary wedge pressures with a Swan-Ganz catheter is particularly helpful in both diagnosis and subsequent fluid management.[12] Patients who are fluid overloaded respond to simple fluid restriction with normalization of serum sodium and reconcentration of their urine as the volume status is corrected.

The diagnosis of either complete or partial DI can be confirmed by the administration of vasopressin (aqueous pitressin) or the synthetic analogue of ADH, desmopressin acetate (DDAVP). In DI there is usually a rapid response to administered vasopressin, with decreased output of more concentrated urine. Once the diagnosis of DI is established, subsequent management (Table 24-3) includes careful hourly monitoring of overall fluid intake and output, with replacement of the existing free water deficit and ongoing urinary losses using D5-0.2% saline, monitoring of serum electrolytes every 4 to 6 h, and administration of vasopressin. The initial use of aqueous pitressin (4 to 10 units SC or IM,

TABLE 24-3 Management of Diabetes Insipidus

Initial calculation and replacement of free water deficit
Hourly monitoring and replacement of ongoing urinary volume loss
Monitoring of serum electrolytes every 4 to 6 h
Administration of vasopressin or DDAVP as needed to control polyuria

q 6 h, prn) is recommended because of the shorter half-life of this medication, thus allowing for titration of the dosage every 6 h. In cases of complete DI, where significant injury to the hypothalamus or upper pituitary stalk is thought likely, or after several days of initial management using aqueous pitressin, one may consider the use of DDAVP.[66] With a duration of effect of 8 to 12 h, DDAVP can be used either intravenously (0.5 to 2 μg, IV, q 8 to 12 h, prn) or by nasal inhalation. It is important to avoid overzealous treatment, which can result in fluid retention and hyponatremia, aggravating cerebral edema after a head injury.

HYPOKALEMIA

Hypokalemia is one of the most common electrolyte disorders in patients with a head injury, commonly resulting from decreased dietary intake or absorption or increased losses from either the GI tract or the kidney. Renal excretion is increased by the administration of loop diuretics such as furosemide, osmotic diuretics such as mannitol, glucocorticoids, some antibiotics, catabolic losses in systemic trauma, and fluid overload. Excessive renal losses also occur with hypovolemia, alkalemia, and hypomagnesemia.[2] Hypokalemia has been reported to occur in a large percentage of patients with severe head injury and is also a common occurrence in patients with other brain insults caused by increased adrenergic stimulation that results in an intracellular shift of potassium.[67]

Clinical findings with hypokalemia include cardiac manifestations reflected in the ECG, including conduction blocks, and arrhythmias. Chronic hypokalemia may result in generalized weakness, hyporeflexia, decreased GI motility, and impaired renal water retention.

Treatment of hypokalemia is usually recommended when K^+ is less than 3.5 mEq/liter, using carefully monitored boluses of K^+ (10 to 30 mEq/h for 3 or 4 h) through a large-bore peripheral vein or central venous access with interval reassessment of serum potassium levels. Additional K^+ can also be added to the maintenance intravenous solution (10 to 40 mEq/liter). Severe, symptomatic hypokalemia (K^+ <2.0 mEq/liter) may be treated with doses of KCl as high as 80 to 100 mEq/h, usually through multiple sites of IV access.[2] In less acute settings, K^+ can be added to enteral feedings to correct serum potassium and replace ongoing losses. A serum magnesium level should also be measured with persistent hypokalemia, as both electrolytes may be depleted and require simultaneous replacement.

HYPERKALEMIA

Hyperkalemia usually results from impaired renal function, hypoadrenalism, or systemic acidosis, with release of intracellular K^+ into the ECF. Serum K^+ can be reduced rapidly by the administration of glucose, insulin, and bicarbonate to increase absorption into cells. Urinary potassium excretion can be promoted by the use of either loop or osmotic diuretics or ion-exchange resins. If these measures are inadequate, renal dialysis may be needed. Loss of pituitary function usually results in chronic hyperkalemia and may require the use of a mineralocorticoid such as fludrocortisone to promote renal excretion of potassium.

HYPOCALCEMIA

Hypocalcemia (<8.5 mEq/liter) is extremely common during any critical illness and results from a wide variety of causes, including the administration of chelating agents such as albumin, bicarbonate, and citrate (such as with blood transfusions); alkalosis; pancreatitis; vitamin D deficiency; sepsis; hypomagnesemia; and hypoparathyroidism.[68] Hypocalcemia is clinically important only when the physiologically active ionized component is reduced. The remainder is bound to albumin (50 percent) or chelated (10 percent). Ionized hypocalcemia cannot be easily predicted by measurement of total calcium or calculations of ionized calcium corrected for the serum albumin level.[69] Hypoalbuminemia lowers measured serum calcium levels, whereas ionized calcium remains normal and the patient remains asymptomatic.[70]

The symptoms and signs of hypocalcemia include hypotension and heart failure, bradycardia and other arrhythmias, bronchospasm, laryngospasm, and neurological manifestations such as muscle weakness and spasms, tetany, hyperreflexia, parasthesias, agitation, confusion, and seizures.[68,70,71]

Before treatment for hypocalcemia begins, hypomagnesemia should be excluded, as patients with low magnesium respond poorly to calcium replacement.[2,69] Severe hypocalcemia should be treated with intravenous calcium chloride or calcium gluconate (1 g IV over 10 min followed by an infusion of 1 to 2 mg/kg/h) until the serum calcium is normalized. Excessively rapid infusion of calcium may cause hypertension, bradycardia, or cardiac conduction block or may precipitate digitalis toxicity. Less severe hypocalcemia may be safely treated with oral calcium supplements such as calcium carbonate (up to 1200 mg PO tid).

Hypercalcemia occurs rarely but can result from prolonged immobilization, hyperparathyroidism, renal failure, or excessive administration of exogenous calcium. Management includes treatment of the underlying cause and increasing renal excretion of calcium with loop or osmotic diuretics and intravenous hydration.

Hypomagnesemia

Hypomagnesemia (<1.5 mg/dl) results most often from increased urinary excretion induced by diabetes insipidus or the use of diuretics, mannitol, volume expansion, and some antibiotics, such as the aminoglycosides. This electrolyte disorder may also result from sepsis, alkalosis, or inadequate magnesium replacement or enteral supplementation and is more common in malnourished or alcoholic populations.

Symptoms of hypomagnesemia include muscle weakness, spasms or tetany, hypotension, heart failure, and increased digitalis toxicity. The neurological manifestations include tremor, hyperreflexia, parasthesias, agitation, confusion, coma, and seizures.[72]

Like calcium, magnesium is partially bound to proteins and chelated, with a physiologically active ionized form (55 percent of the total). Therefore, measurement of total plasma magnesium is physiologically inaccurate, although levels <1.0 mg/dl are associated with increased mortality and should lead to replacement therapy.[88] Hypocalcemia and refractory hypokalemia are often associated with hypomangesemia and should be addressed concurrently.

Treatment of severe hypomagnesemia is usually done with intravenous infusion of 25% magnesium sulfate (2 g/h) over several hours. Milder cases may be treated with oral replacement using magnesium oxide (20 to 80 mEq/day).

Hypophosphatemia

Hypophosphatemia (<2.7 mg/dl) can result from increased renal loss, insufficient dietary intake or administration, or intracellular shifts of phosphate due to prolonged hyperventilation (respiratory alkylosis)[73] or carbohydrate loading. Renal excretion is increased, as in the case of other electrolytes, by the use of diuretics, diabetic ketoacidosis, hypomagnesemia, hyperparathyroidism, and renal tubular defects. Poor intake alone rarely results in hypophosphatemia but may aggravate the effects of increased excretion. Malnourished or alcoholic patients are at much greater risk for developing clinical hypophosphatemia. Drugs such as phosphate-binding antacids and corticosteroids are commonly associated with hypophosphatemia.

Clinical signs and symptoms are usually not noted until phosphate levels are <1.0 mg/dl and can include muscle weakness, ventricular dysfunction, tremor, altered mental status, seizures, coma, respiratory insufficiency, rhabdomyolysis, and hemolysis. As with magnesium and calcium, serum phosphate measurement does not accurately reflect total body stores. Therefore, the initial treatment is empirical, and levels should be monitored. Treatment in acutely ill patients remains controversial, especially when a low phosphate level is associated with an intracellular shift such as with hyperventilation.[74] Treatment of severe hypophosphatemia should begin with intravenous replacement (20 mmol over 4 to 6 h). Potential complications of phosphate administration include hypocalcemia and hypotension. Patients with less severe deficits can be treated with various enteric or oral preparations or by adding phosphate to standard total parenteral nutrition (TPN) formulas as needed.

Hyperphosphatemia is usually seen with renal failure or massive cell lysis and results in hypocalcemia, with symptoms resulting from calcium depletion. Treatment includes limiting phosphate intake, using oral phosphate-binding agents, and increasing excretion through the use of intravenous saline hydration and diuretics.

ACID-BASE DISORDERS

Acid-base disorders are common after many neurosurgical disorders, including severe head injury, and are often induced by complications such as sepsis and tissue ischemia or by a treatment such as hyperventilation. In this setting, acid-base disorders are usually acute and may exacerbate electrolyte imbalance, organ failure, and altered function of the nervous system. The reader is referred to other, more detailed reviews of this topic.[75,76] Acid-base disorders are commonly divided into those due to respiratory disturbances and those due to metabolic disturbances.

Respiratory Disturbances

Acute respiratory changes that affect arterial Pa_{CO_2} result in a rapid alteration in extracellular acid-base balance. With rising Pa_{CO_2}, acidosis develops, and with decreasing Pa_{CO_2}, alkalosis develops. Because of rapid diffusion of CO_2 across the blood-brain barrier, extracellular and intracellular pH follow arterial Pa_{CO_2}, and this has an important effect on cerebral blood flow (CBF).

As Pa_{CO_2} decreases, causing alkalosis, vasoconstriction occurs, with a consequent decrease in CBF and cerebral blood volume. As Pa_{CO_2} increases, causing acidosis, vasodilation occurs with an increase in CBF and cerebral blood volume.[75–77] Compensatory mechanisms exist that return tissue pH toward normal over the course of hours by means of increased lactate production and changes in tissue bicarbonate. These mechanisms explain why cerebral arterial caliber, blood flow, and blood volume return to nearly normal within 24 h after the initiation of continuous hyperventilation.[78]

The most frequently utilized example of this physiological principle is the therapeutic use of hyperventilation (Pa_{CO_2} <30 mmHg). This causes respiratory alkalosis, resulting in vasoconstriction and a decrease in CBF and cerebral blood volume. As a result, elevated ICP may be reduced.[12] The therapeutic use of hyperventilation for the control of ICP is outlined in other chapters of this book and has been reviewed elsewhere.[12] Many patients with a head injury spontaneously hyperventilate as a result of their CNS injury or associated pulmonary complications, fever, or pulmonary embolism.[79] The respiratory alkalosis induced by hyperventilation also may be exacerbated by concurrent use of diuretics, nasogastric suction, or glucocorticoids. Extreme hypocapnia may result in parasthesias, altered mental status, seizures, and a regional or global decrease in cerebral blood flow with resulting ischemic brain injury.[12,80,81] For these reasons, hyperventilation to a Pa_{CO_2} lower than 20 mmHg is generally avoided, and hyperventilation is utilized only until other methods of intracranial pressure control can be established.[66] Among patients with central hyperventilation, altering the parameters of controlled ventilation often does little to normalize Pa_{CO_2}, and the use of narcotics to calm an agitated patient or suppress an elevated respiratory drive has been recommended by some.[2]

Respiratory acidosis results from hypercarbia (Pa_{CO_2} >45 mmHg) and hypoventilation. This may result from a variety of insults, such as airway obstruction, chest wall injury, excessive use of sedatives, central hypoventilation due to the CNS insult, or a spinal cord injury causing paralysis of the muscles of respiration. Hypercarbia is a serious problem in neurosurgical patients because the resulting acidosis ($pH < 7.36$) causes cerebral vasodilation, increased blood volume, and potentially an increase in ICP. This is often compounded by hypoxia, which increases ischemic-hypoxic tissue injury and aggravates metabolic lactic acidosis.[12,82] In addition to its adverse effect on the CNS, respiratory acidosis may impair cardiac function and cause hypotension.[2] Thus, monitoring for hypercarbia and its correction are critical to the management of neurosurgical patients; in the intensive care unit, serial arterial blood gases analysis and capnography are essential. Treatment includes the establishment of a protected airway. In mildly head injured patients, this may require only the reversal of sedation and oral airway management. In more critically ill patients, the use of endotracheal intubation and mechanical ventilation may be necessary, adjusted to normalize the arterial Pa_{CO_2} and systemic pH. Correction of arterial hypoxia and metabolic acidosis is also necessary to protect the brain fully from secondary injury.[12]

Metabolic Disturbances

Unlike plasma CO_2, which rapidly crosses the blood-brain barrier and affects the acid-base balance of the brain and its blood vessels, hydrogen and bicarbonate ions by themselves cross the blood-brain barrier poorly. Thus, the brain and its vasculature are relatively unaffected by acute metabolic acidosis or alkalosis. In addition, respiratory compensation for acute metabolic disorders, such as hyperventilation in the case of metabolic acidosis, results in a paradoxical shift of brain pH in the direction opposite that of the metabolic insult.[2]

Metabolic Alkalosis

Metabolic alkalosis (plasma HCO_3^- >30 mEq/liter) is the most common acid-base disturbance and is divided into chloride-responsive and chloride-resistant types.[83,84] Chloride-responsive alkalosis results from the loss of chloride ion from the kidney or the GI tract, with a compensatory increase in absorption of bicarbonate from the kidney. Common causes in neurosurgical patients include nasogastric suctioning or emesis with loss of HCl and repeated use of diuretics with renal loss of chloride. Volume contraction may compound the problem by increasing renal reabsorption of bicarbonate with sodium and free water as potassium and hydrogen ions are excreted.[2] Chloride-resistant alkaloses are less common and result from the use of glucocorticoids with mineralcorticoid activity, such as methylprednisolone in spinal cord injury, which promotes renal sodium and bicarbonate reabsorption.

Complications of metabolic alkalosis include compensatory hypoventilation, which may aggravate increased ICP in patients with head injury;[66] hypokalemia; and impaired O_2 delivery due to increased binding of oxygen to hemoglobin.[2] Severe metabolic alkalosis may be associated with an altered mental status and seizures.[85]

Treatment of metabolic alkalosis includes correction of the underlying cause, such as treatment of emesis or decreasing the use of nasogastric suctioning; replacement of lost volume; administration of H2 blockers such as famotidine; and decreased use of diuretics.[2] For chloride-responsive alkalosis, especially when aggravated by volume contraction, the administration of normal saline and potassium is beneficial. Severe metabolic alkalosis has also been treated with intravenous HCl.[84]

METABOLIC ACIDOSIS

Metabolic acidoses (plasma HCO_3^- <25 mEq/liter) are divided into those with an anion gap and those without an anion gap. The anion gap ($Na^+ - [Cl^- + HCO_3^-]$) is the sum of all unmeasured ions in plasma, including negatively charged albumin, sulfate, phosphate, and organic ions,[2] and is usually 10 to 14 mEq/liter. The most common cause of metabolic acidosis in patients with a head injury is lactic acidosis due to decreased tissue perfusion or prolonged hyperventilation (respiratory alkalosis) with metabolic compensation. Lactic acidosis causes metabolic acidosis with an increased anion gap. Lactic acidosis is aggravated by hyperglycemia, which is extremely common after a head injury and in patients treated with corticosteroids and has been associated with a worsened prognosis in both stroke and head injury.[12,86,87] Other causes of acidosis with an increased anion gap include diabetic ketoacidosis and acute renal failure.[2] Non-anion-gap acidoses are those with increased chloride in plasma and may be seen with prolonged hyperventilation, large-volume or hypertonic saline administration, diarrhea, or the administration of TPN. Mixed anion gap and non-anion-gap acidoses may also occur.

Symptoms, signs, and effects of metabolic acidosis may include reflex hyperventilation, hypotension due to myocardial depression,[2] altered mental status, seizures, and, as noted above, a worsened prognosis for CNS recovery from injury or ischemia.[12,86,87] Treatment of metabolic acidosis is first directed at correction of the underlying cause, such as correction of tissue ischemia, ketoacidosis, or azotemia. Patients with severe acidosis ($pH < 7.2$) due primarily to lactic acidosis should be treated with sodium bicarbonate, with the immediate goal of raising the pH to at least 7.3. One should avoid overcorrection, which may result in paradoxical CSF acidosis due to hypoventilation, and alkalosis-related complications such as hypokalemia, hypocalcemia, and hypernatremia.[2] A simple formula for the amount of bicarbonate needed to raise pH to acceptable levels[88] is as follows:

$$\text{Dose in mEq} = (1/2\, Pa_{CO_2} - [HCO_3^-]) \times 0.5 \text{ body wt (kg)}$$

Treatment should be monitored with repeated assessment of arterial blood gases and should be modified as needed. Hyperchloremic acidosis due to hyperventilation is corrected with simple normalization of ventilation and arterial Pa_{CO_2}. TPN-related acidosis is corrected with alteration in the TPN formula to minimize the use of chloride salts.[2]

REFERENCES

1. Darby JM, Nelson PB: Fluid, electrolyte, and acid-base balance in neurosurgical intensive care, in Andrews BT (ed): *Neurosurgical Intensive Care.* New York: McGraw-Hill, 1993:133–162.
2. Robertson GL: The regulation of vasopressin function in health and disease. *Recent Prog Horm Res* 33:333, 1977.
3. Stuart FP, Torres E, Fletcher R, et al: Effects of single, repeated and massive mannitol infusion in the dog: Structural and functional changes in the kidney and brain. *Ann Surg* 172:190, 1970.
4. Dorman HR, Sondheimer JH, Cadnapaphornchai P: Mannitol-induced acute renal failure. *Medicine (Baltimore)* 69:153, 1990.
5. Cserr HF, dePasquale M, Patlak CS: Volume regulatory influx of electrolytes from plasma to brain during acute hyperosmolality. *Am J Physiol* 253:F530, 1987.
6. Thurston JH, Hauhart RE: Brain amino acids decrease in chronic hyponatremia and rapid correction causes brain dehydration: Possible clinical significance. *Life Sci* 40:2539, 1987.
7. Needleman P, Grenwald JE: Atriopeptin: A cardiac hormone intimately involved in fluid, electrolyte and blood-pressure homeostasis. *N Engl J Med* 314:828, 1986.
8. DiBona GF: Neural regulation of renal tubular sodium reabsorption and renin release. *Fed Proc* 44:2816, 1985.
9. Samson WK: Atrial natriuretic factor and the central nervous system. *Endocrinol Metab Clin North Am* 16:145, 1987.
10. Doczi T, Joo F, Szerdahelyi P, Bodosi M: Regulation of brain water and electrolyte content: The possible involvement of central atrial natriuretic factor. *Neurosurgery* 21:454, 1987.
11. Hamlyn JM, Harris DW, Ludens JH: Purification and characterization of a digitalis-like factor from human plasma. *Hypertension* 12:336, 1988.
12. Andrews BT: The intensive care management of patients with head injury, in Andrews BT (ed): *Neurosurgical Intensive Care.* New York: McGraw-Hill, 1993:227–242.
13. Wisner DH: The intensive care management of multisystem injury, in Andrews BT (ed): *Neurosurgical Intensive Care.* New York: McGraw-Hill, 1993:252–290.
14. Sturm JA, Wisner DH: Fluid resuscitation of hypovolemia. *Intensive Care Med* 11:227, 1985.
15. Wisner DH, Busche F, Sturm JA, et al: Traumatic shock and head injury: Effects of fluids resuscitation on the brain. *J Surg Res* 46:49, 1989.
16. Albright AL, Latchaw RE, Robinson AG: Intracranial and systemic effects of osmotic and oncotic therapy in experimental cerebral edema. *J Neurosurg* 60:481, 1984.
17. Holcroft JW, Trunkey DD: Extravascular lung water following hemorrhagic shock in the baboon: Comparison between resuscitation with Ringer's Lactate and plasmanate. *Ann Surg* 180:408, 1974.
18. Dahn MS, Lucas CE, Legerwood AM, et al: Negative ionotropic effects of albumin resuscitation for shock. *Surgery* 86:235, 1979.

19. Lucas CE, Weaver D, Higgins RF, et al: Effects of albumin versus non-albumin resuscitation on plasma volume and renal excretory function. *J Trauma* 18:564, 1978.
20. Wisner DH, Shuster L, Quinn C: Hypertonic saline resuscitation of head injury: Effects on cerebral water content. *J Trauma* 30:75, 1990.
21. DeFelippe J, Timoner J, Velasco IT, et al: Treatment of refractory hypovolemic shock by 7.5% sodium chloride injections. *Lancet* 2:1002, 1980.
22. Maningas PA, Mattox KL, Pepe PE, et al: Hypertonic saline-dextran solutions for the prehospital management of traumatic hypotension. *Am J Surg* 157:528, 1989.
23. Templeton GH, Mitchell JH, Wildenthal K: Influence of hyperosmolarity on left ventricular stiffness. *Am J Physiol* 222:1406, 1972.
24. Battistella FD, Wisner DH: Combined hemorrhagic shock and head injury: Effects of hypertonic saline (7.5%) resuscitation. *J Trauma* 31:182, 1991.
25. Wisner DH, Battistella FD, Freshman SP, et al: Nuclear magnetic resonance as a measure of cerebral metabolism: Effects of hypertonic saline resuscitation. *J Trauma* 32:351, 1992.
26. Vassar MJ, Perry CA, Gannaway WL, Holcroft JW: 7.5% sodium chloride/dextran for resuscitation of trauma patients undergoing helicopter transport. *Arch Surg* 126:1065, 1991.
27. Young B, Ott L, Dempsey R, et al: Relationship between admission hyperglycemia and neurologic outcome of severely brain-injured patients. *Ann Surg* 210:466, 1989.
28. Lam AM, Winn HR, Cullen BF, Sundling N: Hyperglycemia and neurological outcome in patients with head injury. *J Neurosurg* 75:545, 1991.
29. Robertson CS, Goodman JC, Narayan RK, et al: The effect of glucose administration on carbohydrate metabolism after head injury. *J Neurosurg* 74:43, 1991.
30. Mackenzie CF, Shin B, Krishnaprasad D, et al: Assessment of cardiac and respiratory function during surgery on patients with acute quadriplegia. *J Neurosurg* 62:843, 1985.
31. Doszi T, Tarjanyi J, Huszka E, Kiss J: Syndrome of inappropriate secretion of antidiuretic hormone (SIADH) after head injury. *Neurosurgery* 10:685, 1982.
32. Steinbok P, Thompson GB: Metabolic disturbances after head injury: Abnormalities of sodium and water balance with special reference to the effects of alcohol intoxication. *Neurosurgery* 3:9, 1978.
33. Padilla G, Leake JA, Castro R, et al: Vasopressin levels and pediatric head trauma. *Pediatrics* 83:700, 1989.
34. Wijdicks EFM, Van Dongen KJ, Vangijn J, et al: Enlargement of the third ventricle and hyponatremia in aneurysmal subarachnoid hemorrhage. *J Neurol Neurosurg Psychiatry* 51:516, 1988.
35. Takaku A, Shindo K, Tanaka S, et al: Fluid and electrolyte disturbances in patients with intracranial aneurysms. *Surg Neurol* 11:349, 1979.
36. Sica D, Zawada E, Midha M, et al: Hyponatremia in the cord injured patient—a neglected phenomenon. *Kidney Int* 24:137, 1984.
37. Leehey DJ, Picache AA, Robertson GL: Hyponatremia in quadriplegic patients. *Clin Sci* 75:441, 1988.
38. Williams HH, Wall BM, Horan JM, et al: Nonosmotic stimuli after osmoregulation in patients with spinal cord injury. *J Clin Endocrinol Metab* 71:1536, 1990.
39. Oelkers W: Hyponatremia and inappropriate secretion of vasopressin (antidiuretic hormone) in patients with hypopituitarism. *N Engl J Med* 321:492, 1989.
40. Shimoda M, Yamada S, Yamamoto I, et al: Atrial natriuretic polypeptide in patients with subarachnoid hemorrhage due to aneurysm rupture: Correlations to hyponatremia. *Acta Neurochir* (*Wien*) 97:53, 1989.
41. Mather H, Ang V, Jenkins JS: Vasopressin in plasma and CSF of patients with subarachnoid hemorrhage. *J Neurol Neurosurg Psychiatry* 44:216, 1981.
42. Diringer MN, Kirsch JR, Ladenson PW, et al: Cerebrospinal fluid atrial natriuretic factor in intracranial disease. *Stroke* 21:1550, 1990.
43. Diringer MN, Ladenson PW, Stern B, et al: Plasma atrial natriuretic factor and subarachnoid hemorrhage. *Stroke* 19:1119, 1988.
44. Messert B, Orrison WW, Hawkins MJ, Cuaglieri CE: Central pontine myelinolysis: Considerations of etiology, diagnosis and treatment. *Neurology* 29:147, 1979.
45. Norenberg MD, Leslie KO, Robertson AS: Association between rise in serum sodium and central pontine lyelinolysis. *Ann Neurol* 11:128, 1982.
46. Sterns RH, Riggs JE, Schochet SS: Osmotic demyelination syndrome following correction of hyponatremia. *N Engl J Med* 314:1535, 1986.
47. De Troyer A: Demeclocycline. *JAMA* 237:2723, 1977.
48. Forrest JN, Cox M, Hong C, et al: Superiority of demeclocycline over lithium in the treatment of chronic syndrome of inappropriate secretion of antidiuretic hormone. *N Engl J Med* 298:173, 1978.
49. Cort JH: Cerebral salt wasting. *Lancet* 1:752, 1954.
50. Peters JP, Welt LG: A salt wasting syndrome associated with cerebral disease. *Trans Assoc Am Physicians* 63:57, 1950.
51. Nelson PB, Seif S, Gutai J, Robinson AG: Hyponatremia and natriuresis following subarachnoid hemorrhage in a monkey model. *J Neurosurg* 60:23, 1984.
52. Wijdicks EFM, Ropper AH, Hunnicut EJ, et al: Atrial natriuretic factor and salt wasting after aneurysmal subarachnoid hemorrhage. *Stroke* 22:1519, 1991.
53. Vingerhoets F, De Tribolet N: Hyponatremia hypoosmolarity in neurosurgical patients: "Appropriate secretion of ADH" and "cerebral salt-wasting syndrome" *Acta Neurochir* (*Wien*) 91:50, 1988.
54. Ishikawa SE, Saito T, Aneko K, et al: Hyponatremia responsive to fludrocortisone acetate in elderly patients after head injury. *Ann Intern Med* 106:187, 1987.
55. Nelson PB, Seif SM, Maroon JC, Robinson AG: Hyponatremia in intracranial disease: Perhaps not the syndrome of inappropriate secretion of antidiuretic hormone (SIADH). *J Neurosurg* 55:938, 1981.
56. Bingham WF: The limits of cerebral dehydration in the treatment of head injury. *Surg Neurol* 25:340, 1986.
57. Kahn A, Brachet E, Blum D: Controlled fall in natremia and risk of seizures of hypertonic dehydration. *Intensive Care Med* 5:27, 1979.
58. Balestrieri FJ, Chernow B, Rainey T: Postcraniotomy

diabetes insipidus: Who's at risk? *Crit Care Med* 10:108, 1982.
59. Coculescu M, Dumitrescu C: Etiology of cranial diabetes insipidus in 164 patients. *Endocrinologie* 22:135, 1984.
60. Edwards OM, Clark JA: Post-traumatic hypopituitarism. *Medicine (Baltimore)* 65:281, 1986.
61. Notman DD, Mortek MA, Moses AM: Permanent diabetes insipidus following head trauma: Observations on ten patients and an approach to the diagnosis. *J Trauma* 20:599, 1980.
62. Levitt MA, Fleischer AS, Meislin HW: Acute post-traumatic diabetes insipidus: Treatment with continuous intravenous vasopressin. *J Trauma* 24:532, 1984.
63. Fiser DH, Jiminez JF, Wrape V, Woddy R: Diabetes insipidus in children with brain death. *Crit Care Med* 15:551, 1987.
64. Outwater KM, Rockoff MA: Diabetes insipidus accompanying brain death in children. *Neurology* 34:1243, 1984.
65. Tindall GT, Barrow DL: *Disorders of the Pituitary*. St. Louis: Mosby, 1986:461–467.
66. Shucart WA, Jackson I: Management of diabetes insipidus in neurosurgical patients. *J Neurosurg* 44:65, 1976.
67. Pomeranz S, Constantini S, Rappaport ZH: Hypokalemia in severe head injury. *Acta Neurochir (Wien)* 97:62, 1989.
68. Zaloga GP, Chernow B: Hypocalcemia in critical illness. *JAMA* 256(14):1924, 1986.
69. Zaloga GP, Wilkens R, Tourville J, et al: A simple method for determining physiologically active calcium and magnesium concentrations in critically ill patients. *Crit Care Med* 15:813, 1987.
70. Zaloga GP, Chernow B, Cook D, et al: Assessment of calcium homeostasis in the critically ill surgical patient. *Crit Care Med* 12:236, 1984.
71. Sugar O: Central neurological manifestations of hypoparathyroidism. *Arch Neurol Psychiatry* 70:86, 1953.
72. Chernow B, Smith J, Rainey TG, Finto C: Hypomagnesemia: Implications for the critical care specialist. *Crit Care Med* 10:193, 1982.
73. Gadisseux P, Sica DA, Ward JD, Becker DP: Severe hypophosphatemia after head injury. *Neurosurgery* 17:35, 1985.
74. Knochel JP: The clinical status of hypophosphatemia. *N Engl J Med* 313:447, 1985.
75. Fencl V, Rossing TH: Acid-base disorders in critical care medicine. *Annu Rev Med* 40:17, 1989.
76. Narins RG, Emmett M: Simple and mixed acid-base disorders: A practical approach. *Medicine (Baltimore)* 59:161, 1980.
77. Arieff AI, Kerian A, Massry SG, DeLima J: Intracellular pH of brain: Alterations in acute respiratory acidosis and alkylosis. *Am J Physiol* 230:804, 1976.
78. Muizelaar JP, van der Poel HG, Li Z, et al: Pial arteriolar vessel diameter and CO_2 reactivity during prolonged hyperventilation in the rabbit. *J Neurosurg* 69:923, 1988.
79. Frost EAM: The physiopathology of respiration in neurosurgical patients. *J Neurosurg* 50:699, 1979.
80. Marion D, Darby J, Yonas H: Acute regional cerebral blood flow changes caused by severe head injury. *J Neurosurg* 74:407, 1991.
81. Kennealy JA, McLennan JE, Loudon RG, McLaurin RL: Hyperventilation-induced cerebral hypoxia. *Am Rev Respir Dis* 122:407, 1980.
82. North JB, Jennett S: Abnormal breathing patterns associated with acute brain damage. *Arch Neurol* 31:338, 1974.
83. Rimmer JM, Gennari GJ: Metabolic alkylosis. *Intensive Care Med* 2:137, 1987.
84. Friedman BS, Lumb PD: Prevention and management of metabolic alkylosis. *Intensive Care Med* 5(suppl):S22, 1990.
85. Lubash GD, Coehn BD, Young CW: Severe metabolic alkylosis with neurologic abnormalities. *N Engl J Med* 258:1050, 1958.
86. Marie C, Bralet J: Blood glucose level and morphological brain damage following cerebral ischemia. *Cerebrovasc Brain Metab Rev* 3:29, 1991.
87. Merguerian P, Perel A, Wald U, et al: Persistent nonketotic hyperglycemia as a grave prognostic sign in head-injured patients. *Crit Care Med* 9:939, 1981.
88. Hazard RB, Griffin JP: Calculation of sodium bicarbonate requirement in metabolic acidosis. *Am J Med Sci* 283(1):18, 1982.

CHAPTER 25

NUTRITIONAL AND METABOLIC MANAGEMENT OF THE HEAD-INJURED PATIENT

Byron Young
Linda Ott

SYNOPSIS

Patients with a head injury must overcome central and systemic insults. Systemic insults include hypermetabolism, hypercatabolism, the acute-phase response, a decreased immune state, altered glucose metabolism, and increased cytokine and hormone levels. The organ functions of the lung, liver, and gut are altered so that normal physiological processes are affected. The study of the metabolic response to head injury has improved our knowledge of optimal nutrient administration, which is associated with a better outcome in these patients.

The goals of nutritional support are to provide an optimal environment for repair and regeneration of the brain, prevent secondary brain injury, and decrease negative systemic effects. Enteral support is the preferred method of feeding patients with a head injury and is tolerated better when administered into the small intestine. Parenteral nutrition is safe and can be used when enteral support is not possible. Future work will combine nutrient support with the administration of growth factors and pharmacological and/or physiological agents to provide an optimal environment for the brain and improve overall organ function.

INTRODUCTION

During the past decade, the metabolic and nutritional management of patients with a head injury has been studied in detail. Despite advances in our knowledge base, many unanswered questions pertaining to head injury, metabolism, and nutrition persist. After a head injury, a systemic response to the injury occurs and is mediated neurally and chemically. The systemic effects, which can affect mortality and morbidity rates, include increased energy expenditure, increased protein turnover, altered vascular permeability, increased cytokine and hormone release, altered gastric emptying, altered mineral metabolism, altered immune status, altered glucose metabolism, a hyperdynamic cardiovascular state, and gastric ulceration. These systemic effects, such as hyperglycemia, may also cause secondary injury to the brain (Fig. 25-1).

Improved neurological function occurs after injury as a result of axon sprouting and system reorganization.[1] Therefore, providing an optimal environment for neural repair after head injury is essential. Nutritional intervention may play an important role in the provision of adequate nutrients and minerals for optimal neural regeneration. Nutrient and metabolic modification may prevent secondary damage such as that caused by hyperglycemia, cytokine elevation, or hormone elevation.

The systemic responses observed after head injury may be more intense and/or prolonged than those observed after other types of injuries. This is speculated to occur because the brain is the control center for many physiological processes. Stimuli that act centrally may elicit a more profound response than do those that act peripherally and indirectly trigger a central response. For example, the response to interleukin-1 (IL-1) administered intraventricularly is severalfold higher than the response to IL-1 administered through the peripheral venous system.[2] Damage to the pituitary area of the brain has been linked to depressed growth hormone levels.[3,4] Administering growth hormone releasing factor cannot stimulate growth hormone levels in head-injured patients with poor outcomes.[5] The production of insulin-like growth factor-1 (IGF-1) is not stimulated

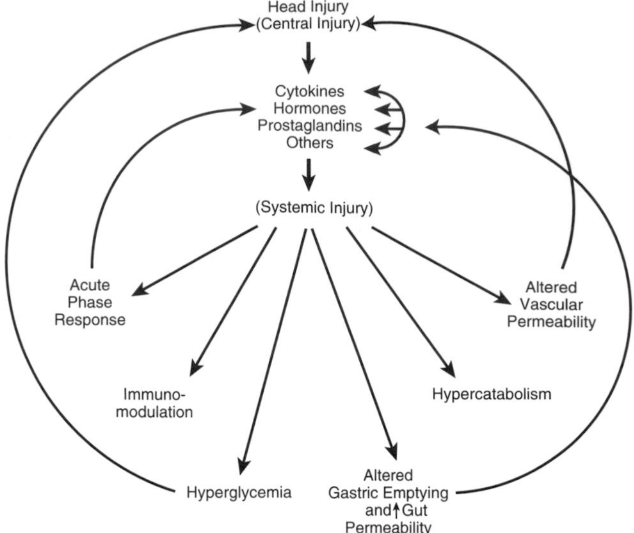

Figure 25-1. Metabolic consequences of head injury.

by the infusion of growth hormones in most head injury patients. Haider and coworkers suggested that brain injury (apallic) patients have increased metabolic rates for as long as 1 year after the injury.[6]

Head injury affects systemic organs such as the gut, liver, and lung. The gut is affected by altered gastric emptying, decreased pH, and increased gut permeability.[7] The results of liver function tests are elevated after head injury,[8,9] evidencing mild liver injury that most likely is caused by inflammatory cytokine effects such as tumor necrosis factor (TNF). After a head injury, the liver stimulates hepatic acute-phase responses (synthesis of acute-phase proteins, decreased synthesis of negative acute-phase proteins).[10] Altered gene expression occurs with the synthesis of acute-phase reactants and a decrease in the production of albumin and hepatic drug metabolites such as cytochrome p450.[11] An altered reprioritization of hepatic protein synthesis and gene expression is mediated through cytokines such as TNF, IL-1, and IL-6. The lung is affected in several ways, including alveolar edema, hemorrhage, and congestion.[12] Ventilatory support is required by most severely head-injured patients to manage the secondary pulmonary sequelae of the primary brain injury.

The goals of nutritional and metabolic support are to achieve caloric balance; establish positive or neutral nitrogen balance; prevent weight loss; decrease the acute-phase response; maintain gut function, immune status, and glucose homeostasis; decrease harmful cytokine and hormone release; decrease negative secondary effects; and lower morbidity and mortality rates. The following sections describe our current knowledge about the prevention of these negative secondary effects of head injury.

Achieving Caloric Balance

Energy expenditure has been studied in patients with head injury more than it has in any other patient population.[6,13–34] Despite the publication of more than 20 articles on measured energy expenditure (MEE) and head injury, unanswered questions pertaining to this issue persist. Energy expenditure is increased after head injury, with an average increase of 40 percent over that calculated for an uninjured person of similar age, sex, and height. Although the energy requirements of most patients with severe head injuries are elevated, some patients have energy requirements closer to normal values. Conflicting conclusions have been reached on the basis of the available data about the length of time energy expenditure is increased after a head injury, the effect of this increased energy expenditure on morbidity and mortality, and the best nutritional substrate and route of administration to provide for this increased energy expenditure.

Haider and associates suggested that the energy expenditure levels of patients with brain lesions that cause an apallic syndrome remain elevated for as long as 1 year after a brain injury.[6] Deutschman and colleagues suggested that energy expenditure is elevated for only 5 to 7 days after a head injury and that extraneous factors such as infection, steroid therapy, and the thermic effect of nutrients cause prolonged increases in the metabolic rate.[19,20] Research from the authors' group on over 200 patients with a severe head injury suggests that metabolic rate normalizes an average of 3 months after a head injury. Certain individuals had a short-term increase in metabolic rate, others had prolonged increases (for example, patients who had decerebrate posturing), and certain patients did not have any elevations (these patients were almost always on medications such as barbiturates or sedatives).[16,17] Most studies indicate that the variables suggested by Deutschman and coworkers and noted previously play at most a minor role in the increase in metabolic rate.

Diet can markedly affect metabolic rate. Fruin and colleagues[21] and Robertson and associates,[15] however, found no relationship between nutrient intake and an increase in metabolic rate in patients with a severe head injury. Steroid administration is known to affect protein metabolism, but its impact on energy requirements has not been studied in detail. Robertson and associates found no significant difference in metabolic rate between steroid-treated and non-steroid-treated patients.[32] Greenblatt and coworkers found higher MEE levels in head injury patients receiving steroids; however, the large variation in measured levels rendered any statistical comparisons insignificant.[33] The effect of infection on metabolic rate in stressed patients is unclear. Popp and Brennan found that in all types of patients (except those with burns) infection causes a more extensive increase in metabolic rate.[35] The authors studied MEE in 108 patients with severe head injury and found no significant difference in the measured to predicted energy expenditure ratio before (1.58 ± 0.07), during (1.45 ± 0.07), or after (1.42 ± 0.06) infection. In general, patients who are sedated or are in a pharmacologically induced coma have the lowest energy expenditure levels (mean of 90 percent of predicted), whereas those who decerebrate and decorticate have very high energy expenditure levels (mean of two to three times the predicted level).

Clifton and associates developed a nomogram for estimating caloric expenditure during the first 2 weeeks after a head injury, with the most potent predicting factors the Glasgow Coma Scale score and the number of days since the injury.[31] Sunderland and Heilbrun used several methods in an effort to determine the best way of calculating metabolic rate after head injury[34] (Table 25-1). The best predictive measure was that derived from Clifton and associates; however, Sunderland and Heilbrun suggested that clinically significant discrepancies exist between MEE and predictive formulas. They further suggested that the ability to decipher the meaning of specific metabolic indicators and make reasonable clinical decisions regarding specific caloric supplementation is tenuous when one is estimating energy expenditure with predictive formulas (Table 25-1). We suggest that the increase in MEE is unique for each patient and that indirect calorimetry is a useful way of determining MEE in a patient with a head injury. Although the cost of indirect calorimetry is nominal, an experienced person is required to perform the test and evaluate the results.

Several factors may be involved in the observed increase in metabolic rate after a severe head injury. Bucci et al. found a strong correlation between increased intracranial pressure and increased MEE in these patients.[30] Whether this is a direct or an indirect effect is unknown. Hormonal surge, cytokine increase, or brain inflammation could mediate the increase in metabolic rate. Robertson et al. correlated the severity of head injury, temperature, catecholamine level, resting muscle tone, spontaneous muscle activity, and drugs such as barbiturates and musculoskeletal blocking agents to metabolic rate.[15]

Pharmacologically induced paralysis and sedation affect metabolic rate. In 10 patients with severe head

TABLE 25-1 Ways to Determine Energy Requirements

Author	Method
Sunderland and Heilbrun[34]	Best → indirect Calorimetry
Moore et al.[28]	$y = 950 + 10.5x$*
Clifton et al.[14,31]	GCS ≤ 7
	%RME = 152 − 14(GCS) + 0.4(HR) + 7(DSI)
	GCS > 7
	%RME = 90 − 3(GCS) + 0.9(HR)
Robertson et al.[15]	Paralyzed head injury = 128% (of predicted)*
	Head injury nonparalyzed = 152% (of predicted)
	Barbiturate coma = 96% (of predicted)
Touho et al.[25]	Overall 131% (of predicted)
Clifton et al.[14]	Nonsedated = 138% (of predicted)
	Sedated = 89% (of predicted)
Bruder et al.[22]	Sedated = 1.04% (of predicted)
	No sedation = 1.34% (of predicted)
Dempsey et al.[26]	Barbiturate coma = 86 ± 28% (of predicted)
	No barbiturate coma = 126 ± 36% (of predicted)
Chiolero et al.[29]	Overall 126% (of predicted)
Young et al.[16]	Overall 140% (of predicted)
Fruin et al.[21]	Barbiturate coma = 108% (of predicted)
	Abnormal motor activity = 191% (of predicted)

y = estimated energy expenditure; x = patient weight in pounds; RME = resting metabolic expenditure; HR = heart rate; DSI = days since injury.

* Predicted = Harris-Benedict equation.

injury, Dempsey et al. found that MEE was significantly lower in patients who received barbiturates than in those who did not.[26] Bucci et al. also showed a significant difference in metabolic rate in head injury patients who were in a pharmacologically induced coma versus those who were not.[30] Bruder et al. found a 22 percent average increase in metabolic rate in 8 patients with severe head injury who were no longer sedated.[22] Barbiturate therapy could lower metabolic rate through its effects on either systemic cellular metabolism or cerebral metabolism. Since cerebral metabolism accounts for 20 percent of total energy expenditure, a depression in it alone could decrease overall energy expenditure. Barbiturates could also suppress neuronal substrates that control systemic circulation or decrease effects such as prolonged posturing, which is known to increase metabolic rate. However, Clifton et al. found that certain patients with head injury continued to have increased MEE despite pharmacologically induced paralysis, suggesting that muscle tone alone cannot fully explain hypermetabolism.[31]

Hormonal surge, including increased levels of serum insulin, cortisol, glucagon, and catecholamines, is observed after head injury.[13,36–39] These hormones have been speculated to cause an increase in metabolic rate. Bessey et al. found that infusion of triple hormone in normal healthy humans caused an increase in metabolic rate.[40] Interestingly, Hadfield et al. found that continuous administration of vecuronium bromide (a nondepolarizing muscle relaxant) caused mean metabolic rate to be nearly normal in 13 head injury patients.[13] Variations in the metabolic rate were seen, and some patients had a significantly elevated metabolic rate despite pharmacologically induced paralysis. Hormonal surge was measured in these patients at the same time metabolic rate was evaluated. Plasma concentrations of cortisol, glucagon, insulin, and catecholamines were significantly above normal 1 to 2 weeks after the injury. These results demonstrate that induced paralysis cannot consistently decrease metabolic rate in head injury patients and that hormonal surge may not be the primary causative factor for increased metabolic rate.

Cytokines are known to be elevated after head injury and may play a role in causing an increased metabolic rate.[41–45] The role these peptides play in the metabolic rate of patients with a head injury is unclear at present. Growth factor administration may decrease metabolic rate in these patients. Strock et al. found that IGF-1 administration decreased metabolic weight and weight loss in burned rats.[46] In the authors' study of patients with head injury, we found no difference in metabolic rate between patients who were given IGF-1 and those who were not, but weight seemed to be better preserved in patients who received IGF-1 than in those who did not.

Chiolero et al. showed that propranolol administration produces a decrease in both heart rate and resting metabolic rate, thus reducing hypermetabolism by approximately 25 percent.[29] Since a hyperdynamic state is present along with hypermetabolism, these findings may indicate the degree to which the hyperdynamic response affects metabolic rate. This may also partially implicate catecholamines in the increase in metabolic rate.

In summary, the increase in metabolic rate after head injury is most probably caused by many factors, including but not limited to hormones, cytokines, and movement. How to decrease metabolic rate and what effect this reduction might have on patient outcome are unclear. Standard nutritional therapy includes measurement of metabolic rate and the administration of calories to meet this metabolic requirement. Future therapy may include antihormonal or cytokine agents, administration of growth factors, and other methods to decrease metabolism.

Achieving Positive or Neutral Nitrogen Balance

Nitrogen balance is a global assessment of the body's protein equilibrium.[47] By comparing the measured urinary output of nitrogen and estimated bodily nitrogen loss with nitrogen input, one can make an estimate of protein balance. A normal, healthy individual is in neutral or zero nitrogen balance. A growing child, a pregnant woman, or a body builder is in positive nitrogen balance. Individuals with large urinary losses of nitrogen or inadequate nitrogen intake are in negative nitrogen balance.

Patients with a severe head injury lose weight, with a decrease in muscle mass and biochemical evidence of decreased visceral protein levels, which are signs of increased protein turnover. Increased urinary nitrogen loss occurs in patients with a severe head injury.[14,16–20,22,25,31–33,48–57] The cause of this increased nitrogen loss has been debated. Protein turnover at the cellular level has not been measured in these patients. Urinary nitrogen loss, total body and compartment measurements of plasma amino acid levels, and forearm muscle flux indicate increased protein turnover.[19,20,50,58–62]

The following questions are often raised: (1) Does steroid therapy cause nitrogen loss in this patient population? (2) Is the loss of weight and muscle caused by immobility? and (3) Can positive nitrogen balance be achieved in a patient with a severe head injury?

Many investigators have observed increased urinary nitrogen loss in patients with a severe head injury. Nitrogen excretion peaks approximately 10 days to 2 weeks after an injury. Kaufman et al. suggested that nitrogen

TABLE 25-2 Comparison Studies of Metabolic Effects of Steroid Administration

Author	Type of Study and Dosing of Steroids	Steroid Effects
Greenblatt et al.[33]	Retrospective review, 16–24 mg/day Dexamethasone (n = 16)	Significant nitrogen balance difference No difference in blood glucose, insulin, creatinine, 3-MH, albumin
Deutschman et al.[20]	Retrospective review, 50–120 mg/day Prednisolone (n = 16)	Significant difference in UUN, 3-MH, L/P ratio, blood glucose level, amino acid change
Zagara et al.[63]	Prospective, randomized control trial, 0.36 mg/kg/day Dexamethasone (n = 24)	No difference in weight, blood glucose, albumin, creatinine, UUN
Robertson et al.[32]	Prospective, randomized trial, 100 mg/m^2/day Methylprednisolone (n = 20)	No difference in weight, albumin, anthropometrics Significant difference in fasting UUN, TLC; no difference in fed UUN
Hausmann et al.[50]	Prospective, randomized trial, 24 mg/day Dexamethasone	Significant difference in nitrogen, lactate level, amino acid profiles

3-MH = 3-methylhistidine; UUN = urinary urea nitrogen; L/P = lactate pyruvate; TLC = total lymphocyte count.

loss in patients with a head injury is associated with poor neurological status, but no statistical significance was detected.[51] Hadfield et al. found that urinary nitrogen excretion was positively correlated with metabolic rate when moribund patients were excluded.[13] Chiolero et al. found that nitrogen balance correlated negatively with urinary adrenaline, noradrenaline, and plasma glucagon levels in 14 patients with a severe head injury.[37]

Urinary nitrogen loss increases whether or not steroids are administered to a patient with a severe head injury. At least five studies have compared nitrogen dynamics in patients who were given steroids with those in patients who did not receive steroids[20,32,33,50,63] (Table 25-2). In a retrospective review, Greenblatt et al. found that patients who received steroids had a significantly greater negative nitrogen balance compared with patients who did not.[33] In another retrospective review, Deutschman et al. found significantly higher urinary nitrogen loss in head injury patients who were given steroids than in those who were not.[20] In a prospective, randomized trial, Hausmann and associates found a significant difference in nitrogen loss between patients who received steroid therapy and those who did not.[50] In another retrospective review, Robertson found that fasting urinary nitrogen loss was 30 percent higher in patients who received steroids than in those who did not.[32] The difference disappeared when feedings were initiated. Zagara and coworkers could find no difference in urinary nitrogen loss when 12 head injury patients who were prospectively randomized to receive steroids were compared with 12 head injury patients who were not.[63] Robertson, Hausmann, and Deutschman also found that other alterations were more abnormal in the steroid group, including lactate levels, amino acid profiles, and blood glucose.[20,32,50] Although the results were not consistent in these studies, steroids seem to potentiate nitrogen loss in patients with a head injury.[16]

Urinary nitrogen excretion has long been used as an indicator of increased protein turnover in critically ill patients. Popp and Brennan suggested that the effects of immobilization on urinary nitrogen loss have not been taken into account in all types of trauma.[35] A head injury patient who is flaccid or in a state of pharmacologically induced paralysis could have some nitrogen loss that is attributed to immobility.[64,65] The immediate increase in nitrogen excretion after a head injury suggests that immobilization does not play an important role immediately after the injury. A patient with movement or decerebrate posturing would not fit the immobilization theory. Bessey compared known MEE rates and nitrogen losses in patients with various forms of injury.[66] Interestingly, head injury patients had the highest cumulative nitrogen loss in a 10-day period but fell in the middle range of MEE increase. What this means is unclear, but it may be an indication of the effects of immobilization. If this is the case, approximately 25 percent of the nitrogen loss can be attributed to the atrophy of immobility.

In normal, healthy humans, nitrogen loss can be decreased by nutrient intake.[47] This does not seem to be the case in head injury patients. As early as 1959, McLaurin et al. suggested that patients with a head injury have decreased nitrogen efficiency, as evidenced by increased output despite adequate nitrogen intake.[52] Clifton et al. found that the level of intake of nitrogen and calories influenced nitrogen excretion more strongly than did any other variable.[31] In separate studies, Twyman et al. and Clifton et al. tested whether high protein intake can cause positive nitrogen balance.[67,68] Although nitrogen balance was improved by high protein intake, positive nitrogen balance could not be achieved. Bivins et al. found that nitrogen excretion was significantly correlated with nitrogen intake.[69] Urinary nitrogen excretion was not decreased by increasing caloric intake up to and beyond two times the basal energy expenditure.

Despite adequate caloric intake and high protein intakes (2 g/kg/day), positive nitrogen balance cannot be achieved in a patient with a severe head injury for as long as 2 or 3 weeks after the injury. Nutrient intake improves nitrogen balance but does not cause positive nitrogen balance in the early periods of head injury; this is also true for other trauma patients.[66] Further modulation is required to achieve positive nitrogen balance. This may include nutrient, pharmacological, or physiological manipulation. Investigators have suggested that these patients should be put in a decreased metabolic state with drugs such as barbiturates and propranolol to decrease metabolic rate and nutrient need during the first 2 weeks after a head injury. Fried et al. found that barbiturate therapy decreased nitrogen loss in patients with a head injury.[70] This is an unexpected finding, because one would expect nitrogen excretion to increase as a result of the immobility and atrophy caused by barbiturate coma. The authors' group has reported that IGF-1 infusion in patients with head injury can cause positive nitrogen balance in the early periods of a head injury.[71] Positive nitrogen balance correlates significantly with increased levels of serum IGF-1. Other future therapies may include cyclooxygenase inhibitors, growth factor administration, anticytokine agents, and other agents that may override the catabolic response to stress and facilitate nitrogen balance.[45,72] Current therapy includes the administration of adequate nutrients, both calories and protein, in an effort to improve nitrogen balance.

Preventing Weight Loss

Weight change is a common phenomenon after severe trauma.[16] The loss of less than 10 percent of preinjury weight leads to little disability, but severe weight loss of 40 percent of preinjury weight is associated with death. Patients with head trauma experience an average weight loss of 15.6 ± 5.9 lb during the hospitalization period. Despite the provision of adequate caloric intake, weight loss persists in this patient population. Future work will further define how weight loss may be decreased in this patient population. Preliminary data from the authors' group showed that the infusion of IGF-1 was associated with a trend toward decreased weight loss in these patients.

Weight Gain from Head Injury

After a 3-month period, weight loss reaches a plateau, and then weight gain is often observed.[73] Hyperphagia is a common finding in patients with head injury during the rehabilitation period. Some of these patients are insatiable, and weight gain above preinjury weight is often observed. Patients with poor recovery often undergo long-term tube feedings. These patients either maintain or gain weight, depending on the amount of feeding.

Decreasing the Acute-Phase Response

The acute-phase response occurs after severe head injury and is identified by fever without evidence of infection, increased levels of positive acute-phase proteins, decreased levels of negative acute-phase proteins, hypozincemia, hyperzincuria, and hypercupria.[10] The effects of these metabolic alterations after head injury vary: Some effects are beneficial, and others are detrimental to recovery. This response has been attributed to increased levels of interleukins, specifically IL-1, IL-6, and TNF.[74] IL-6 causes a dose- and time-dependent increase in the synthesis of serum alpha$_2$-macroglobulin, fibrinogen, cysteine proteinase inhibitor, C-reactive protein, and alpha$_1$-acid glycoprotein and a decrease in serum albumin.[75] IL-1 and IL-6 have been found to be elevated in the serum and ventricular fluid of patients with a severe head injury.[41–43] The increase in the plasma level of IL-6 is inversely related to the Glasgow Coma Scale score. Thus, the more severe the head injury, the higher the increase in IL-6 activity and the greater the acute-phase response. The Glasgow Coma Scale score of head injury patients has also been significantly inversely related to temperature level, indicating that the severity of the head injury and the intensity of the systemic response are correlated.[10]

The authors found no significant correlation between serum zinc level and level of head injury, but the patients we studied were all moderately to severely injured. We have not studied the acute-phase response in patients with a minor injury.[75] Lin and colleagues found that serum zinc levels were significantly more depressed in head injury patients with Glasgow Coma Scale scores of 4 to 8 than in patients with scores of 9 to 13.[76] This difference was apparent until day 15 after the injury. Hypozincemia and hyperzincuria occur in patients with a head injury and are associated with the acute-phase response. There may be several reasons for this response. Wannemacher originally suggested that the immediate depression of the serum zinc and iron levels, the subsequent increase in copper and ceruloplasmin levels, and the increased uptake of plasma amino acids in individuals with typhoid fever are protective mechanisms designed to preserve host function yet deter the proliferation and growth of bacterial organisms through the absence of essential nutrients such as zinc and iron.[77] Zinc is very important in a number of processes, including wound healing, protein synthesis, membrane stabilization, and the maintenance of vascular endothelium and immune status.[78,79] Zinc is also vitally important for normal brain function. Zinc modulates N-methyl-D-aspartate (NMDA) receptors, interacts with calcium-binding proteins, is a component of nerve growth factors, stimulates axonal transport, induces assembly of microtubules, is a component of presynaptic vesicle-associated zinc pools in the hippocampus and other brain regions, modulates the binding of several neurotransmitters to their receptors, activates metalloenzymes, and regulates gene transcription.[80–82] Administering supplemental zinc after a head injury to provide adequate zinc for priority functions such as healing, immune status, and other functions necessary for survival may enhance recovery. Sixty-eight patients entered a randomized, prospective, double-blind controlled trial of supplemental zinc (12 mg/day intravenously) or standard zinc (2.5 mg/day) for 3 months after injury.[83] Serum zinc levels were not significantly different between the two groups. Although urinary zinc excretion was higher in the zinc-supplemented group, zinc balance was more positive in that group. One month after injury, the mortality rate was 23 percent in the standard zinc group and 12 percent in the zinc-supplemented group. Glasgow Coma Scale scores improved more quickly in the zinc-supplemented group. Serum retinol-binding protein and thyroxine-binding prealbumin levels were significantly higher in the zinc-supplemented group 3 weeks after injury. These results indicate that zinc supplementation during the immediate postinjury period improves the rate of neurological recovery and improves visceral protein levels in patients with a severe closed head injury.

Serum albumin depression is a negative effect of the acute-phase response.[84] Albumin is important in a number of processes, including maintenance of oncotic pressure, drug transport, and tolerance of enteral feeding. Albumin supplementation in trauma and critically ill patients improves the serum albumin level. Brown and associates found that albumin supplementation in critically ill patients causes a twofold reduction in complication rates.[85] Ford et al. found that albumin supplementation improves enteral feeding tolerance in pediatric patients.[86] Foley et al., however, found no difference in the complication rate, duration of hospital and intensive care unit stay, ventilator dependence, and tolerance of enteral feeding between patients given albumin and those in the control group.[87] Albumin supplementation has not been studied in patients with head injury in a prospective randomized trial.

Hypoalbuminemia is probably mediated by cytokine elevation. Intravenous injection of recombinant TNF into normal rabbits causes a dose-dependent depression of serum albumin levels. In vitro exposure to murine IL-1 and TNF increases endothelial permeability to albumin and causes a time- and dose-dependent albumin leakage.[88] IL-1 and IL-6 decrease the synthesis of mRNA for albumin.[74,89] Thus, albumin depression probably occurs because of increased vascular permeability and decreased synthesis. The current therapy for decreased serum albumin levels includes adequate nutrient supplementation. Early after a head injury, plasma levels of albumin are influenced more by the cytokine-mediated acute-phase response than by nutritional intake. Future therapy may include specific anticytokine agents.

The reason for some of the other changes in plasma protein concentrations may be the production of a protective or demarcating zone around areas of tissue destruction.[10] Both proteinases released from leukocytes and lysosomes released from destroyed cells are inhibited by proteinase inhibitors such as alpha$_1$-antitrypsin and alpha$_2$-macroglobulin. An increase in fibrinogen provides adequate substrate for the formation of fibrin and blood coagulation at the wound site. Moreover, some of these proteins may play a regulatory role in the acute-phase response. Alpha$_1$-acid glycoprotein has been shown to decrease IL-1 activity in vivo.[90] The increase in serum C-reactive protein level may be important in the immune stimulation required after an injury. Thus, a variety of biological functions have been postulated for the evolutionary development of the acute-phase response after infection and injury. It is unclear how the acute-phase response could be altered and what effect, if any, altering one aspect would have on the other components of the system.

MAINTAINING GUT FUNCTION

During critical illness, increased gut permeability occurs.[91–94] Increased gut permeability, atrophy of the gastrointestinal tract, antibiotic therapy, and other factors lead to bacterial translocation. Bacterial translocation can increase morbidity and assist in the development of infection or the multiple organ failure syndrome.[92–94] Gut permeability seems to be altered in patients with head injury. The authors' studied gut permeability using the noninvasive marker ^{99m}technetium–diethylenetriamine pentacetate. Normally, when this marker is administered orally or through a gastric tube, less than 3 percent of the marker is absorbed in the small intestine. Patients with head injury demonstrated markedly increased gut permeability on admission, with over 25 percent absorption of the marker. Gut permeability improved during the hospital course and was in the normal range by day 15.

A patient with a head injury has alterations in gastric emptying.[7] Studies in these patients show a high predominance of delayed gastric emptying with an altered biphasic response similar to that in patients who have undergone a vagotomy or pyloroplasty. This response may hinder the delivery of enteral feedings. Possible mediators of decreased gastric emptying include cytokines, opioids, hormones, and neural control mechanisms.

After trauma, glutamine, an important source of fuel for the gut, may become a conditionally essential nutrient[91] because the utilization of this amino acid exceeds its synthesis. Head injury patients were found to have depressed plasma glutamine levels for approximately 1 week after injury. Decreased plasma glutamine levels were also observed in burn patients, and this was suggested to be an indicator of glutamine deficiency. Several studies indicate that glutamine supplementation supports the gut mucosal barrier and enhances gut immune function.[95–97] Supplementation of glutamine has not been studied in patients with a head injury.

Growth factors have been found to have positive effects on the gut. Epidermal growth factor has been found to be effective in reversing gut hyperplasia and inducing intestinal hypertrophy.[98] Neurotensin administration increased small intestine weight, DNA content, and protein content.[99] Increases were also observed in brush border enzymes (maltase, sucrase, and leucine amino peptidase). Additionally, neurotensin has been shown to prevent small intestine atrophy and improve biliary secretion of IgA and IgM in parenterally fed animals. IGF-1 has potent trophic effects on the gut. Lemmey and colleagues found that IGF-1 increases the weight of the stomach and residual duodenum, cecum, and colon in animals with 80 percent bowel resection.[100] Seidel and colleagues doubled ileal mucosal mass, cellularity, and protein content in rats via intraluminal administration of IGF-1.[101] Preliminary work from the authors' group suggests that IGF-1 administration in patients with head injury decreases the incidence of diarrhea.

Thus, gut function is altered after head injury. Future work should determine how this response can be attenuated by nutrient or pharmacological manipulation.

Maintaining Immune Status

Depression of immune function is a secondary effect of injury, occurring during a period when the body requires improved immune status to defend itself from infections that increase morbidity or mortality. Approximately 60 percent of severely head-injured patients become infected, with 35 percent of late deaths in this population attributed to infection.[102,103] Improving the immunostatus is important in preventing infections.

Skin anergy to antigens occurs in almost all patients with a severe head injury for as long as 3 weeks after the injury.[104] Imhoff et al. found that the anergy rate is related to the severity of the injury.[105] Miller et al. found that lymphocyte activation and production of IL-2 receptor are suppressed after head injury.[106] Quattrocchi et al. found that interferon-γ production, which is necessary for cell-mediated immunity, is also depressed in the serum of these patients.[107] They also found that lymphocyte blastogenesis, T-cell expression, helper T-cell expression, IL-2 production, and interferon-γ production are significantly depressed in head-injured patients.[108] They found no significant depression in immunoglobulin and complement levels. Hoyt et al. found a reduction in the proliferative response of T cells to mitogen stimulation in 27 patients with severe head injury. The B-cell response was unaffected.[109] These researchers also found a diminished expression of early activation antigens (IL-2 receptor and transferrin receptor) and late antigen (HLA-DR). In 20 patients with severe head injury, Maerker et al. found no decrease in IgG, IgA, IgM, and the complement factors.[110] The depression in immune function is speculated to result from a nutrient, mineral, or cytokine deficit. Miller et al. found that lymphokine-activated killer T-cell cytotoxicity is diminished after incubation with IL-2.[106] Cellular dysfunction of suppressor cells may also be involved in immune depression.

Nutrient modification may affect immune status. Zinc is known to be necessary for proper functioning of the immune system. Zinc deficiency has been correlated with T-lymphocyte dysfunction. The amino acid arginine has also been shown to have an immunomodulatory function in animals.[111] Daly and colleagues showed enhanced T-lymphocyte responsiveness in patients receiving enteral feedings supplemented with arginine.[112] The type of lipid administered may also affect immune status. Fish oil, which is rich in omega-3 fatty acids, is immunostimulatory. Early data obtained from animal models demonstrated that enteral diets containing fish oils can reduce the incidence of septic complications after experimental burn injury.[113]

Growth factors may also play a regulatory role. Timsit and associates found that IGF-1 administration and adequate nutrition improved the ratio of helper to suppressor cells in patients with severe head injury (personal communication).[114]

Maintaining Glucose Homeostasis

After injury, endogenous glucose production by the liver is increased, glucose oxidation is more than doubled, and there is an overall increase in glucose flow through the extracellular compartment.[66] This increase in glucose flow is termed "the diabetes of injury" and is related to the severity of injury. A patient with moderate or severe head injury has hyperglycemia. The degree of hyperglycemia is related to the severity of injury and correlates with a poorer outcome in patients with head injury.[115–118]

Ischemic cells metabolize glucose anaerobically. Lactate is the end product of the anaerobic metabolism of glucose. In patients with neurological injury, lactate and acidosis may play a role in causing secondary damage to ischemic nerve cells or in eliciting a cellular cascade that promotes secondary injury.[119,120] Preventing hyperglycemia in patients with head injury may improve outcome.

Several factors may be responsible for the occurrence of hyperglycemia. Triple hormone infusion in normal, healthy humans causes hyperglycemia.[40] Infusion with cytokines such as TNF has been shown to cause the glucose flow of injury in rats.[121] Both cytokines and hormones have been shown to increase in patients with a severe head injury.

Insulin administration, nutrient modification, pharmacological agents, and growth factors have been used to decrease hyperglycemia in head injury patients.[122] These attempts have met with only limited success. Initially, patients should be resuscitated with a fluid that does not contain glucose. Insulin decreases blood glucose levels in most patients. Persistent hyperglycemia during insulin administration ("insulin resistance") is a poor prognostic sign.[115,116]

Robertson and coworkers randomized 21 patients with severe head injury to alimentation with or without glucose.[123] There were no differences in blood or CSF glucose concentrations between the two groups, but ketone bodies were used more extensively by the brain in the saline group. The CSF lactate concentration was lower in the patients treated with saline. Since hyperglycemia occurs as part of the stress response, withholding a small amount of glucose (5 percent) does not significantly affect the serum glucose level. Glucose administration, however, may affect the cerebral metabolism of glucose, ketones, and lactate. In a study of trauma patients, Singer and associates noted that the infusion of glycerol compared to glucose as a protein-sparing agent significantly decreased blood glucose levels without affecting nitrogen retention.[124] This decrease was associated with an increased level of blood glycerol. This technique has not been tried in patients with head injury.

Rosner and Becker found that the infusion of tromethamine in rats with a head injury improved outcome.[125] This agent, which counteracts acidosis, may be useful in future studies. In head injury patients, tromethamine decreased the incidence of increased intracranial pressure and the requirements for barbiturate administration.[126]

Hyperglycemia is a stress-induced response to head injury that may cause secondary neuronal injury. Prospective randomized trials should be performed to determine whether treating hyperglycemia improves outcome.

Decreasing Cytokine and Hormone Levels

After head injury, cytokines and hormones are found in significantly higher concentrations in blood, urine, and cerebroventricular spinal fluid.[13,36–39,41–43] These peptides mediate some of the systemic effects of head injury and may be involved in secondary neuronal injury (Table 25-3). Clifton et al. found that patients with head injury alone have norepinephrine levels as high as seven times normal.[38] Chiolero et al. found that isolated head injury induces a full response in the secretion of the counterregulatory hormones, including serum glucagon, insulin, cortisol, and urinary adrenaline and noradrenaline, that was similar to that observed in patients with head injury plus multiple injury.[37] Hadfield and colleagues found significantly elevated concentrations of plasma glucose, lactate, nonesterified fatty acids, cortisol, glucagon, and insulin in patients with head injury.[13] Goodman et al. found significantly elevated TNF levels in the serum of head-injured patients during the first week after injury.[42] The authors observed increases in the levels of plasma and ventricular IL-1, IL-6, and IL-8 in head-injured patients.[41,43] Damage to the brain alters the hypothalamic-pituitary axis, with alterations in feedback mechanisms, excesses in catabolic hormones, and deficiencies in follicle-stimulating hormone, luteinizing hormone, and growth hormone.[3,4]

In trauma and burn patients, hypercortisolemia and hyperglucagonemia are related to injury severity.[127,128] Hypermetabolism correlates with urinary catecholamine excretion.[129] One hormone alone cannot explain the complex metabolic response to injury, but a triple hormone infusion of cortisol, glucagon, and epinephrine in normal, healthy humans induced metabolic changes similar to those observed after injury.[40] These individuals had increased resting heart rate, widened pulse pressure, increased minute ventilation, hypermetabolism, negative potassium balance, increased endogenous glu-

TABLE 25-3 Cytokine and Hormonal Profile in Patients with Head Injury

Cytokine or Hormone	Level in Patients with Head Injury	Effects
Cytokines		
Interleukin-1	↑	Coagulation Inflammation Tissue injury Tissue repair Induction of other cytokines Acute-phase response Hypermetabolism Hypercatabolism Induces liver for acute-phase response
Interleukin-6	↑	Acts on B cells to augment immunoglobulin production May be involved in tissue injury
Tumor necrosis factor	↑	Cytotoxicity Modulation of endothelial cells and granulocyte function Differentiation of myeloid cell lines Metabolic activation of macrophages and osteoclasts Growth of B lymphocytes Tissue repair Angiogenesis Induction of collagenase release Induces other cytokines Acute-phase response Glucose, fat, and protein metabolism
Interleukin-8	↑	Stimulation of respiratory burst leading to superoxide and hydrogen peroxide formation Exocytosis leading to release of storage proteins from neutrophils Shape changes enabling neutrophils to adhere to endothelium and migrate
Interferon-γ	Unknown	Enhances oxidation activities of blood monocytes Enhances cytotoxicity of circulating monocytes toward tumor cells Hypertriglyceridemia, hepatic impairment, fever, headache
Hormones		
Catecholamines	↑	Hypermetabolism Hyperdynamic state ↑ glucose production ↑ glycolysis ↑ lipolysis ↑ ketogenesis
Glucagon	↑	↑ gluconeogenesis ↑ glycogenesis ↑ lipolysis
Cortisol	↑	↑ protein turnover Body and muscle wasting
Insulin	↑	Maintains protein homeostasis Maintains glucose and fatty acid metabolism Major anabolic hormone Insulin insensitivity after injury
Growth hormone	↓	↑ protein synthesis, ↓ protein breakdown DNA and RNA synthesis Enhancement of nitrogen and mineral retention Stimulation of lipolysis Protein synthesis Immune function Neural growth

TABLE 25-3 Cytokine and Hormonal Profile in Patients with Head Injury *(Continued)*

Cytokine or Hormone	Level in Patients with Head Injury	Effects
Insulin-like growth hormone	↓	Stimulates glucose uptake, glycogen synthesis, amino acid transport ↑ net protein synthesis DNA synthesis and cellular proliferation Immune function Neural growth

cose production, insulin resistance, sodium retention, leukocytosis, and negative nitrogen balance. Herndon and associates demonstrated reduced cardiac work in a group of burned children receiving pharmacological alpha- and beta-adrenergic blockade.[130] In septic rats, glucocorticoid blockade decreased protein catabolism without affecting protein synthesis.[131] Future work will determine the positive or negative effects that can be attained by modulation and blocking of the hormonal response to injury.

Cytokines are extracellular signaling proteins secreted by numerous cells.[44,74,132–134] Their primary function is to modify the behavior of other cells in both pathological and normal states. Cytokines signal cells through various intermediates, which include but are not limited to the endocrine hormones, arachidonic acid metabolites, and neuropeptides. Cytokines have overlapping biological activities, and the actions of combinations of cytokines are complex. They include cell proliferation, immune system modulation, and the acute-phase response.

The cytokines that have been studied in patients with head injury are IL-1, IL-6, and TNF. The levels of these cytokines are known to be elevated both in the brain and in the systemic circulation of animals and humans with a head injury.[41–43,135,136] IL-1 and IL-6 are known to stimulate the acute-phase response of injury. IL-6 infusion is known to have a dose- and time-dependent relationship with many of the alterations in the acute-phase response.[89] IL-1 is involved in the acute-phase response and was originally named endogenous pyrogen because its administration causes fever. The IL-1 receptor antagonist in an animal model completely blocked the induction of C-reactive protein (CRP) and serum amyloid, moderately decreased the induction of complement C3 and alpha$_1$-acid glycoprotein, and enhanced the induction of fibrinogen in vitro. Partial blocks in the down-regulatory effects of negative acute-phase proteins albumin and transferrin also occurred.[135] A small amount of IL-1 injected directly into the brain is much more potent than the systemic intravenous administration of this agent.[133] IL-1 works centrally and may be a neuromodulator in the CNS pathways that cause the metabolic response to stress.[137] Studies to determine the exact role of IL-1 in protein metabolism and hypermetabolism have yielded conflicting results. Baracos et al. suggested that IL-1 may cause increased muscle proteolysis, but Moldawer et al. could find no effect of IL-1 on protein breakdown.[138,139] Watters and colleagues administered etiocholanolone, which is known to stimulate IL-1 production, to humans.[140] The subjects manifested the acute-phase response, but no effects on protein turnover or metabolic rate were observed. The combination of catabolic hormones and etiocholanolone infusion stimulated the acute-phase response, increased protein breakdown, and increased metabolic rate. The last finding underscores the complex mediator pattern in the metabolic response to stress.[141]

TNF is a peptide that is also involved in the metabolic response to stress. Administration of TNF in normal, healthy humans causes headache, fever, tachycardia, and stimulation of the adrenal-pituitary axis.[142] Warren et al. infused TNF into normal, healthy humans and found increased serum CRP levels, decreased serum zinc levels, doubled forearm efflux of amino acids (primarily the gluconeogenic amino acids alanine and glutamine), and depressed arterial levels of amino acids.[143] TNF infusion enhances glucose flux in animals.[121] TNF, IL-1, and IL-6 are involved in the stimulation of lipolysis and cause increased levels of serum triglyceride and very low density lipoproteins.[144] This metabolic effect may be a positive homeostatic mechanism, since lipids are known to bind endotoxin and various bacteria.

The cytokines IL-1, TNF, and IL-6 also may be involved in causing secondary organ injury.[145] Tumor necrosis infusion in animals causes metabolic and multisystem dysfunction comparable to the effects of clinical sepsis. In the endotoxemic baboon model, serum TNF and IL-6 levels were increased.[146] Observed effects included decreased vascular resistance and blood pressure, increased blood lactate levels, decreased circulating neutrophils, organ dysfunction, thrombocytopenia, and decreased hematocrit levels. Pretreatment with TNF Mab, an anti-TNF monoclonal antibody, prevented increases in detectable serum TNF levels; disturbances in cardiovascular function; dysfunction of kidney, liver, and coagulation systems; increases in IL-6 levels; and death.[147] IL-1 and TNF infusion are associated with the development of brain edema and increased blood-brain barrier vasculature.[148,149] IL-1 administration also causes organ damage to the lungs and brain.[150–152] TNF administration causes lung and liver dysfunction and may be involved in the multisystem organ dysfunction observed after head injury.[153,154]

Cytokines may also be involved in the repair and regeneration process.[44,45,74] After head injury, cytokine infusion can elevate the levels of growth factors such as nerve growth factor. IL-1 stimulates astrocyte proliferation. TNF infusion stimulates wound healing. Cytokines cause organ dysfunction and are involved in the repair process, underscoring their complex role after an injury.

Work in this field is expanding at a rapid pace. New cytokines are being discovered, and their role in the metabolic response to brain injury will be elucidated. Cytokines are involved in a complex cascade that is precipitated by injury. In a head injury patient, cytokines are involved in the system metabolic response, organ dysfunction, and the repair process.

Decreasing Negative Secondary Effects

The primary injury to the CNS initiates a cascade of events both in the brain and in the periphery, which may later cause a secondary injury (Table 25-4). The release of cytokines may further damage the brain by enhancing the permeability of the blood-brain barrier. Increased systemic protein breakdown may deprive the brain of necessary protein substrate in a period of enhanced repair. Hyperglycemia may cause secondary neural injury. The consequences of hyperglycemia may include increased lactate production and cellular acidosis, both of which are known to negatively affect neural tissue. Hypozincemia may deprive the brain of a nutrient required for protein turnover and immune status. Hypoalbuminemia may be involved in poor drug transport, intolerance to enteral feedings, and enhanced fluid retention. Altered plasma amino acid levels may allow an inappropriate amount of certain amino acids to enter the brain. Excitatory amino acids such as glutamate and aspartate may cross the blood-brain barrier in excessive amounts and cause secondary injury.[155] Immunodepression may make the host susceptible to infection.

Thus, the systemic metabolic and local sequelae of injury can affect the process of brain repair, reorganization, and regeneration (Fig. 25-1). Future studies will elucidate exactly how these responses can be modulated through nutrient, physiological, pharmacological, or growth factor intervention to further improve the outcome of patients with a head injury.

TABLE 25-4 Mediators of Neural Secondary Injury

Lipid peroxidation
Cell calcium influx
Cell potassium release
Lactate accumulation/acidosis
Hyperglycemia
Cellular swelling
Excitatory amino acid excess
Neurotransmitter release
Increase in catabolic hormones
Increase in cytokine levels
Ionic destabilization
Prostaglandin synthesis
Decreased immune status
Increased systemic metabolic requirements
Opioid excess
Deficiency of trophic factors
Anabolic hormone deficiencies
Deficiency of intracellular magnesium
Zinc deficiency
Glutamine and alanine alterations

INFLUENCE OF NUTRITIONAL SUPPORT ON OUTCOME

To date, six studies of humans with head injury have examined the effect of nutritional support on outcome after head injury. In 1983, Rapp et al. prospectively randomized patients with severe head injury to receive enteral or parenteral nutrition.[104] The group that received enteral nutrition did not tolerate feedings because of abnormal gastric emptying; thus, significantly fewer calories and less protein were administered to these patients than to parenterally fed patients. The mortality rate in the patients receiving enteral nutrition was significantly higher than that in the patients fed parenterally. The data indicated that inadequate feedings in the enteral group increased the mortality rate. In a later prospective, randomized, controlled trial, the same authors attempted to reproduce these study results.[156] Although nutrient delivery systems were improved in the enteral group, patients fed by the parenteral method had significantly better calorie and protein intake and an improved nutritional status. Because of this better nutritional support, the parenteral group experienced a more rapid improvement in outcome. Hadley et al. also randomized patients with head injury to receive parenteral or enteral nutrition.[157] An improved nitrogen balance was observed in the parenteral group. No difference was observed in caloric intake, morbidity, or mortality between groups. In a retrospective analysis, Kaufman et al. found no relationship between nutrient intake and neurological outcome.[51] In separate retrospective reviews, Waters et al. and Balzola et al. found better neurological outcomes in head-injured patients who were provided with a higher nutrient intake.[158,159] The potential mechanisms by which nutrient intake affects outcome after a head injury are multifactorial. Nutrient substrates may be essential for immune system function, cellular membrane integrity, cellular repair, neural reorganization, and other restorative functions necessary for host survival.

Route of Nutrient Supplementation

The optimal route of nutrient supplementation in a patient with a head injury is a topic of debate. Early gastric enteral feedings were inadequate in patients with head injury because the abnormal gastric emptying that follows head injury may delay nutritional support for 1 to 2 weeks.[67,68,104,160–162] Parenteral nutrition, however, was speculated to be involved in initiating the cascade of secondary injury, including fluid retention, hyperglycemia, cerebral edema, and electrolyte disorders.[163,164] Until the outcome study published by Rapp et al. in 1983, patients with head injury were poorly fed, and nutrition was not a primary concern in the medical treatment of these patients.[104] Since 1983, neurosurgeons have begun to realize the importance of nutrient delivery in these patients. Studies by Combs et al. in animals and by Young et al. in humans found that parenteral nutrition does not cause hyperglycemia, increase cerebral edema, or increase intracranial pressure.[165,166] Combs et al. found that parenteral nutrition did not increase specific gravity measurements of the brain in a rat model of cold injury. Young et al. randomized 96 patients to receive parenteral or enteral nutrition and found no difference in glucose levels, calculated serum osmolality, or intracranial pressure between the groups. The cause of enteral feeding intolerance was further assessed. Patients who do not tolerate feedings have abnormal gastric emptying that may preclude feeding directly into the stomach.[7] Feeding intolerance was also related to the severity of injury and to increased intracranial pres-

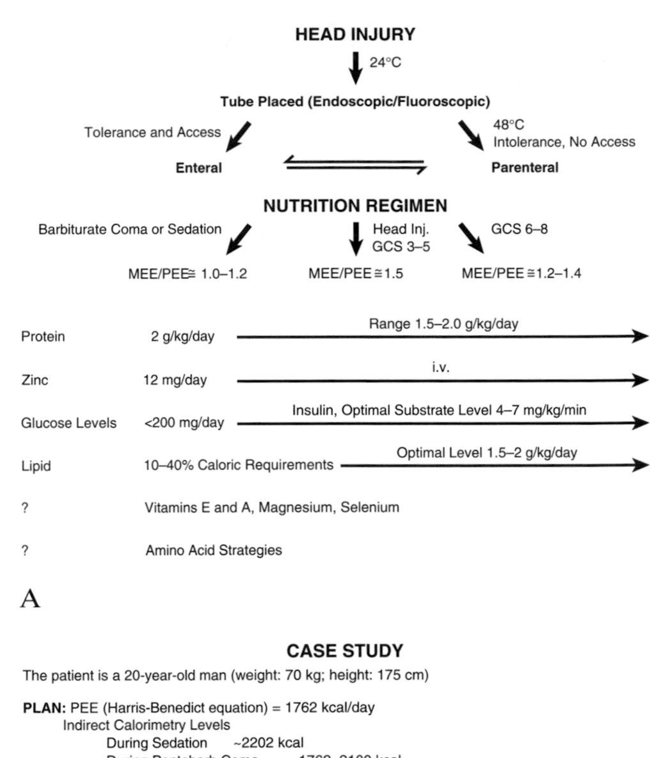

A

CASE STUDY

The patient is a 20-year-old man (weight: 70 kg; height: 175 cm)

PLAN: PEE (Harris-Benedict equation) = 1762 kcal/day
Indirect Calorimetry Levels
During Sedation ~2202 kcal
During Pentobarb Coma 1762–2100 kcal
During Posturing ~3524–6000 kcal
Overall 40% increase, 2400 kcal
Or use formula of Clifton et al.[102] for patients with head injury
GCS ≤ 7: % RME (MEE) = 152 - 14 (GCS) + 0.4(HR) + 7(DSI)
GCS > 7: % RME (MEE) = 90 - 3(GCS) + 0.9(HR)

NUTRITIONAL REGIMEN
Enteral = high-calorie, high-protein per fluid volume (into small intestine)
Ex: TraumaCal, Ensure Plus, 2 cal, Osmolite HN
CCs required:
TraumaCal = 1800 ml - 2100 ml; protein: 2g/kg/day; 2700–3150 total kcal
Sustacal HC = 1800 ml - 2100 ml; protein: 1.6 g/kg/day; 2700–3150 total kcal
2 Cal = 1440 ml; protein: 1.7 g/kg/day; 2880 total kcal
Osmolite HN = 2400 ml -2600 ml; protein: 1.5 g/kg/day; 2544–2756 total kcal
TPN: 6.1% amino acids; D25/500 ml; 20% lipid/day
RATE: 75 ml/h with lipid 1 day; 1000 kcal lipid (1.4 g/kg/day); protein 1.62 g/kg/day; 1530 kcal dextrose (~3 mg/mg/min)

B

Figure 25-2. *A.* Recommended nutritional regimen during the acute period for patients with severe head injury. PEE = Harris-Benedict equation: male = 66 + (13.7 × weight in kg) + (5 × height in cm) − (6.8 × age); female = 655 + (9.6 × weight in kg) + (1.7 × height in cm) − (4.7 × age). i.v. = intravenous. *B.* Case study of a patient with a severe head injury based on recommendations in *A*. GCS = Glascow Coma Scale score; HR = heart rate; DSI = days since injury.

sure.[160] Turner suggested that feeding into the small bowel is feasible for head-injured patients.[167] Kirby et al. and Grahm et al. fed all patients enterally by bypassing the stomach and feeding into the small intestine.[168,169] Grahm and associates achieved early enteral feeding into the small intestine through nasoendoscopic means, and Kirby et al. did this by means of the insertion of percutaneous endoscopically placed gastrostomies.

Indeed, most of these patients tolerated feedings through the placement of an endoscopic or fluoroscopic small intestine feeding tube by day 3 after injury. This, however, was not early enough for enteral nutrition to attenuate the metabolic response to stress observed in burn patients who were administered oral feedings by 24 h after an injury.[170]

If early enteral feedings are to occur, an efficient system for placing tubes, replacing tubes, and monitoring these patients is necessary. Whether feeding into the small bowel decreases the incidence of aspiration pneumonitis is unclear.[171,172] No studies have compared the costs of enteral nutrition with those of parenteral nutrition, including the cost of this labor-intensive process and endoscopy. Because of nutrient-dense formulas, enteral nutrition may also be a way to provide more calories per fluid volume in patients who often have fluid limitations. Enteral feedings are more physiological and should be used whenever possible. Evidence suggests that feeding trauma and burn patients within 24 h after injury can attenuate the metabolic response to stress and improve immune function. Enteral feedings may decrease gut atrophy.

CONCLUSION

The past decade has improved our knowledge of the metabolic and nutritional treatment of patients with head injury (Fig. 25-2). Patients with a head injury must overcome a central neurological insult and a systemic metabolic response. The systemic response includes hypermetabolism, hypercatabolism, altered vascular permeability, increased hormone and cytokine release, altered gastric emptying, altered mineral metabolism, altered glucose metabolism, and altered immune status. This response may initiate mechanisms that lead to secondary brain injury and may adversely affect the function of the lung, gut, liver, and brain. The goals of nutritional support are to provide an optimal environment for repair and regeneration of the brain and to prevent secondary brain injury. Nutritional support improves the outcome of patients with head injury. Parenteral and enteral support are both safe therapies in patients with head injury. Enteral support can be tolerated within 3 days after injury in most of these patients if it is administered through the small intestine. Future work will be directed toward modulation of the metabolic response to injury through the administration of nutrients and physiological, pharmacological, and growth factors.

References

1. Davis JN: Neuronal rearrangements after brain injury: A proposed classification, in Beckers DP, Povlishock JT (eds): *Central Nervous System Trauma Status Report*. Bethesda, MD: National Institutes of Neurological and Communicative Disorders and Stroke, 1985: 491–502.
2. Turchik JB, Bornstein OL: Role of the central nervous system in acute-phase responses to leukocyte progress. *Infect Immun* 30:439, 1980.
3. Clark JDA, Raggatt PR, Edwards OM: Hypothalamic hypogonadism following major head injury. *Clin Endocrinol (Oxf)* 29:153, 1988.
4. Edwards OM, Clark JDA: Post-traumatic hypopituitarism: Six cases and a review of the literature. *Medicine (Baltimore)* 65:281, 1986.
5. Gottardis M, Nigitsch C, Schmutzhard E, et al: The secretion of human growth hormone stimulated by human growth hormone releasing factor following severe cranio-cerebral trauma. *Intensive Care Med* 16:163, 1990.
6. Haider W, Lackner F, Schlick W, et al: Metabolic changes in the course of severe acute brain damage. *Eur J Intensive Care Med* 1:91, 1975.
7. Ott L, Young B, Phillips R, et al: Altered gastric emptying in the head injured patient: Relationship to feeding intolerance. *J Neurosurg* 74:738, 1991.
8. Zagara G, Vignazia M, Crespi G, et al: Hepatic insufficiency in patients with cranial injuries. *Minerva Anestesiol* 53(10):559, 1987.
9. Hill DB, Stokes BD, Ott L, et al: Liver dysfunction and plasma cytokine activity following head injury (abstr). *Gastroenterology* 102:A821, 1992.
10. Young B, Ott L, Beard D, et al: The acute phase response of the brain-injured patient. *J Neurosurg* 69:375, 1988.
11. Toler SM, Young B, McClain CJ, et al: Head injury and cytochrome p450 enzymes. Differential effect on mRNA and protein expression in the Fischer-344 rat. *Drug Metab Dispos* 21:1064, 1993.
12. Demling R, Riessen R: Pulmonary dysfunction after cerebral injury. *Crit Care Med* 18:768, 1990.
13. Hadfield JM, Little RA, Jones RAC: Measured energy expenditure and plasma substrate and hormonal changes after severe head injury. *Injury* 23(3):177, 1992.
14. Clifton GL, Robertson CS, Grossman RG, et al: The metabolic response to severe head injury. *J Neurosurg* 60:687, 1984.
15. Robertson CS, Clifton GL, Grossman RG, et al: Oxygen utilization and cardiovascular function in head-injured patients. *J Neurosurg* 15:307, 1984.
16. Young B, Ott L, Norton J, et al: Metabolic and nutritional sequelae in the non-steroid treated head injury patient. *Neurosurgery* 17:784, 1985.
17. Gadisseux P, Ward J, Young H, et al: Nutrition and the neurosurgical patient. *J Neurosurg* 60:219, 1984.
18. Long CL, Schaffel N, Geiger JW, et al: Metabolic response to injury and illness: Estimation of energy and

protein needs from indirect calorimetry and nitrogen balance. *JPEN* 3:452, 1979.
19. Deutschman CS, Konstrantinides FN, Raup S, et al: Physiological and metabolic response to isolated closed-head injury: I. Basal metabolic state: Correlations of metabolic and physiological parameters with fasting and stressed controls. *J Neurosurg* 64:89, 1986.
20. Deutschman CS, Konstantinides FN, Raup S, et al: Physiological and metabolic response to isolated closed-head injury: II. Effects of steroids on metabolism: Potentiation of protein wasting and abnormalities of substrate utilization. *J Neurosurg* 66:388, 1987.
21. Fruin AH, Taylor C, Pettis S: Caloric requirements in patients with severe head injuries. *Surg Neurol* 25:25, 1986.
22. Bruder N, Damon JC, Francois G: Evolution of energy expenditure and nitrogen excretion in severe head-injured patients. *Crit Care Med* 19:43, 1991.
23. Kahn RC, Koslow M, Butcher S: Metabolic studies in head injured patients (abstr.). *JPEN* 11(suppl):9, 1987.
24. Durr D, Hunt D, Rowlands B, et al: Energy supply and demand following head injury: Balancing the metabolic budget (abstr.). *JPEN* 11(suppl):5, 1987.
25. Touho H, Karasawa J, Nakagawara J, et al: Measurement of energy expenditure in the acute stage of head injury (Part 1). *No To Shinkei* 39:739, 1987.
26. Dempsey DT, Guenter P, Mullen JL, et al: Energy expenditure in acute trauma to the head with and without barbiturate therapy. *Surg Gynecol Obstet* 160:128, 1985.
27. Gerold K, Grankenfield D, Turney S, et al: Energy expenditure in acute severe head injury (abstr.). *JPEN* 13(suppl):20, 1989.
28. Moore R, Najarian P, Konvolinka C: Measured energy expenditure in severe head trauma. *J Trauma* 29:1633, 1989.
29. Chiolero RL, Breitenstein E, Thorin D, et al: Effects of propranolol on resting metabolic rate after severe head injury. *Crit Care Med* 17:328, 1989.
30. Bucci MN, Dechert RE, Arnoldi DK, et al: Elevated intracranial pressure associated with hypermetabolism in isolated head trauma. *Acta Neurochir (Wien)* 93:133, 1988.
31. Clifton GL, Robertson CS, Choi SC: Assessment of nutritional requirements of head-injured patients. *J Neurosurg* 64:895, 1986.
32. Robertson CS, Clifton GL, Goodman JC: Steroid administration and nitrogen excretion in the head injured patient. *J Neurosurg* 63:714, 1985.
33. Greenblatt SH, Long CL, Blakemore RS, et al: Catabolic effect of dexamethasone in patients with major head injuries. *JPEN* 13:372, 1989.
34. Sunderland PM, Heilbrun P: Estimating energy expenditure in traumatic brain injury: Comparison of indirect calorimetry with predictive formulas. *Neurosurgery* 31:246, 1992.
35. Popp MB, Brennan MF: Metabolic response to trauma and infection, in Fischer JE (ed): *Surgical Nutrition*. Boston: Little, Brown, 1983: 479–514.
36. Hortnagl H, Hammerle AF, Hackl JM, et al: The activity of the sympathetic nervous system following severe head injury. *Intensive Care Med* 6:169, 1980.
37. Chiolero R, Schutz Y, Lemerchand T, et al: Hormonal and metabolic changes following severe head injury and noncranial injury. *JPEN* 13:5, 1989.
38. Clifton GL, Ziegler MG, Grossman RG: Circulating catecholamines and sympathetic activity after head injury. *Neurosurgery* 8:10, 1981.
39. Haider MN, Benzer H, Krystof G, et al: Urinary catecholamine excretion and thyroid hormone blood level in the course of severe acute brain damage. *Eur J Intensive Care Med* 1:115, 1975.
40. Bessey PQ, Watters JM, Aoki TT, et al: Combined hormonal infusion stimulates the metabolic response to injury. *Ann Surg* 200:264, 1984.
41. McClain CJ, Cohen D, Ott L, et al: Ventricular fluid interleukin-1 activity in patients with head injury. *J Lab Clin Med* 110:48, 1987.
42. Goodman JC, Robertson CS, Grossman RG, et al: Elevation of tumor necrosis factor in head injury. *J Neuroimmunol* 30:213, 1990.
43. McClain CJ, Cohen D, Phillips R, et al: Increased plasma and ventricular fluid interleukin-6 levels in patients with head injury. *J Lab Clin Med* 118:225, 1991.
44. Klasing KC: Nutritional aspects of leukocytic cytokines. *J Nutr* 118:1436, 1988.
45. Dinarello CA, Neta R: An overview of interleukin-1 as a therapeutic agent. *Biotherapy* 1:245, 1989.
46. Strock LL, Singh H, Abdullah A, et al: The effect of insulin-like growth factor I on postburn hypermetabolism. *Surgery* 108:161, 1990.
47. Elwyn DH: Protein metabolism and requirements in the critically ill patient. *Crit Care Clin* 3:57, 1987.
48. Boop FA, Andrassy RJ, Brown WE, et al: Excessive nitrogen losses in severe brain injury (abstr.). *Neurosurgery* 16:725, 1985.
49. Fell D, Benner B, Billings A, et al: Metabolic profiles in patients with acute neurosurgical injuries. *Crit Care Med* 12:649, 1984.
50. Hausmann D, Mosebach O, Caspari R, et al: Effects of steroid on nitrogen loss and plasma amino acid profiles after head injury (abstr.). *JPEN* 11:10S, 1987.
51. Kaufman HH, Bretaudiere JP, Rowlands BJ, et al: General metabolism in head injury. *Neurosurgery* 20:254, 1987.
52. McLaurin RL, King L, Tutor FT, et al: Metabolic response to intracranial surgery. *Surg Forum* 10:770, 1959.
53. Miller SL: The metabolic response to head injury. *S Afr Med J* 65:90, 1984.
54. Schiller WR, Long CL, Blakemore WS: Creatinine and nitrogen excretion in seriously ill and injured patients. *Surg Gynecol Obstet* 149:561, 1979.
55. Hadfield JM, Little RA: Substrate oxidation and the contribution of protein oxidation to energy expenditure after severe head injury. *Injury* 23:183, 1992.
56. Kolpek JH, Ott L, Record KE: Comparison of urinary urea nitrogen excretion and measured energy expendi-

ture in spinal cord injury and nonsteroid-treated severe head trauma patients. *JPEN* 13:277, 1989.

57. Dickerson RN, Fried RC, Guenter PA, et al: Increased caloric contribution of protein to resting energy expenditure following head injury (abstr). *JPEN* 10:10S, 1986.
58. Ott M, Schmidt J, Young B, et al: Nutritional and metabolic variables correlate to amino acid forearm flux in patients with severe head injury. *Crit Care Med* 22:393, 1994.
59. Ott L, Schmidt J, Young B, et al: Comparison of administration of two standard intravenous amino acid formulas to severely brain-injured patients. *Drug Intell Clin Pharm* 22:763, 1988.
60. Piek J, Lumenta CH, Bock WJ: Amino acid metabolism in patients with severe head injury (abstr). *Acta Neurochir (Wien)* 68:165, 1983.
61. Rowlands B, Hunt D, Roughneen P, et al: Intravenous and enteral nutrition with branched chain amino acid enriched products following multiple trauma with closed head injury. *JPEN* 10:4S, 1986.
62. Twyman D, Young B, Ott L, et al: Plasma amino acid profiles in non-steroid treated head injury patients (abstr.). *J Parenter Ent Nutr* 9:121, 1985.
63. Zagara G, Scaravilli P, Bellucci CM, et al: Effects of dexamethasone on nitrogen metabolism in brain-injured patients. *J Neurosurg Sci* 31:207, 1987.
64. Deitrick JE, Whedon GD, Shorr E: Effects of immobilization upon various metabolic and physiologic functions of normal men. *Am J Med* 4:3, 1948.
65. Schonheyder F, Heilskov NSC, Olesen K: Isotopic studies on the mechanism of negative nitrogen balance produced by immobilization. *Scand J Clin Lab Invest* 6:178, 1954.
66. Bessey PQ: Parenteral nutrition and trauma, in Rombeau JL, Caldwell MD (eds): *Parenteral Nutrition* (2d ed). Philadelphia: Saunders, 1993: 538–565.
67. Twyman D, Young B, Ott L, et al: High protein enteral feedings: A means of achieving positive nitrogen balance in head-injured patients. *JPEN* 9:679, 1985.
68. Clifton GL, Robertson CS, Constant CF: Enteral hyperalimentation in head injury. *J Neurosurg* 62:186, 1985.
69. Bivins B, Twyman D, Young B: Failure of non-protein calories to mediate protein conservation in brain-injured patients. *J Trauma* 26:980, 1986.
70. Fried R, Dempsey D, Guenter P, et al: Barbiturates improve nitrogen balance in patients with severe head trauma (abstr.). *JPEN* 8:86, 1984.
71. Luer MS, Hatton J, Rapp RP, et al: Positive nitrogen balance in moderate to severe closed head injury following administration of insulin-like growth factor-1 (abstr. 114). *Pharmacotherapy* 13:285, 1993.
72. Goldberg AL: Factors affecting protein balance in skeletal muscle in normal and pathological states, in Blackburn GL, Grant JP, Young VR (eds): *Amino Acids: Metabolism and Medical Applications.* Boston: John Wright PSG, 1983: 201–211.
73. Holt K, Yingling B, McClain CJ, et al: Hyperphagia and excess weight gain (abstr). *JPEN* 15:34S, 1991.
74. Fong Y, Moldawer LL, Shires T, et al: The biologic characteristics of cytokines and their implication in surgical injury. *Surg Gynecol Obstet* 170:363, 1990.
75. McClain CJ, Twyman D, Ott L, et al: Serum and urine zinc response in head injured patients. *J Neurosurg* 64:224, 1986.
76. Lin C-N, Howng S-L, Hu S-H, et al: Assessments of nutritional status and immunological responses in head trauma: Alterations in zinc and C-reactive protein. *Kao Hsiung J Med Sci* 8:195, 1992.
77. Wannemacher RW: Key role of various individual amino acids in host response to infection. *Am J Clin Nutr* 30:1269, 1977.
78. Lindeman RD, Mills BJ: Zinc homeostasis in health and disease. *Miner Electrolyte Metab* 3:223, 1980.
79. Wolman SL, Anderson GH, Marliss EB, et al: Zinc in total parenteral nutrition: Requirements and metabolic effects. *Gastroenterology* 76:458, 1979.
80. Frederickson CJ, Klitenick MA, Manton WI, et al: Cytoarchitectonic distribution of zinc in the hippocampus of man and the rat. *Brain Res* 273:335, 1983.
81. Slevin JT, Kasarskis EJ: Effects of zinc on markers of glutamate and aspartate neurotransmission in rat hippocampus. *Brain Res* 334:281, 1985.
82. Kasarskis EJ: Regulation of zinc homeostasis in rat brain, in Frederickson CJ, Howell GA, Kasarskis EJ (eds): *The Neurobiology of Zinc. Part A: Physiochemistry Anatomy and Techniques.* New York: Liss, 1984: 27–37.
83. Ranseen JD, Schmitt FA, Holt K, et al: Zinc supplementation and early outcome following severe brain injury (abstr.). *J Clin Exp Neuropsychol* 12:34, 1990.
84. McClain CJ, Hennig B, Ott L, et al: Mechanisms and implications of hypoalbuminemia in head-injured patients. *J Neurosurg* 69:386, 1988.
85. Brown RO, Bradley JE, Bekemeyer WB, et al: Effect of albumin supplementation during parenteral nutrition on hospital morbidity. *Crit Care Med* 16:1177, 1988.
86. Ford EG, Jennings LM, Andrassey RJ: Serum albumin (oncotic pressure) correlates with enteral feeding tolerance in the pediatric surgical patient. *J Pediatr Surg* 22:597, 1987.
87. Foley EF, Borlase BC, Dzik WH: Albumin supplementation in the critically ill. *Arch Surg* 125:739, 1990.
88. Hennig B, Honchel R, Goldblum SE, et al: Tumor necrosis factor-mediated hypoalbuminemia in rabbits. *J Nutr* 118:1586, 1988.
89. Castell JV, Gomez-Lechon MJ, David M, et al: Recombinant human interleukin-6 (IL-6/BSF-2/HSF) regulates the synthesis of acute phase proteins in human hepatocytes. *FEBS Lett* 232:347, 1988.
90. Bories PN, Guenounou M, Feger J, et al: Human alpha 1-acid glycoprotein-exposed macrophages release interleukin-1 inhibitory activity. *Biochem Biophys Res Commun* 147:710, 1987.
91. Dudrick PS, Souba WW: Special fuels in parenteral nutrition, in Rombeau JL, Caldwell MD (eds): *Parenteral Nutrition* (2d ed). Philadelphia: Saunders, 1993: 209–222.

92. Border JR, Hassett J, LaDuca J, et al: The gut origin septic states in blunt multiple trauma (ISS=40) in the ICU. *Ann Surg* 206:427, 1987.
93. Deitch EA: The role of intestinal barrier failure and bacterial translocation in the development of systemic infection and multiple organ failure. *Arch Surg* 125:403, 1990.
94. Meyer J, Yurt RW, Duhaney R, et al: Differential neutrophil activation before and after endotoxin infusion in enterally versus parenterally fed volunteers. *Surg Gynecol Obstet* 167:501, 1988.
95. O'Dwyer ST, Smith RJ, Hwang TL, Wilmore DW: Maintenance of small bowel mucosa with glutamine-enriched parenteral nutrition. *JPEN* 13:579, 1989.
96. Grant JP, Snyder PJ: Use of L-glutamine in total parenteral nutrition. *J Surg Res* 44:506, 1988.
97. Ziegler TR, Young LS, Benfell K, et al: Clinical and metabolic efficacy of glutamine-supplemented parenteral nutrition after bone marrow transplantation: A randomized, double-blind, controlled study. *Ann Intern Med* 116:821, 1992.
98. Goodlad RA, Wilson TJG, Lenton W, et al: Proliferative effects of urogastrone-EGF on the intestinal epithelium. *Gut* 28:37, 1987.
99. Wood JG, Hoang HD, Bussjaeger LJ, et al: Neurotensin stimulates growth of small intestine in rats. *Am J Physiol* 255:G813, 1988.
100. Lemmey AB, Martin AA, Read LC, et al: IGF-1 and the truncated analogue des-(1-3) IGF-1 enhance growth in rats after gut resection. *Am J Physiol* 260:E213, 1991.
101. Seidel ER, Chaurasia O, Groblewski GE: Intraluminal IGF-1 and stimulation of gastrointestinal mucosal growth (abstr.). *2nd International Symposium on the Insulin-like Growth Factors/Somatomedins* 2:54, 1991.
102. Clifton GL, McCormick WF, Grossman RG: Neuropathology of early and late deaths after head injury. *Neurosurgery* 8:309, 1981.
103. Helling RS, Evans LL, Fowler DL, et al: Infectious complications in patients with severe head injury. *J Trauma* 28:1575, 1988.
104. Rapp RP, Young B, Twyman D, et al: The favorable effect of early parenteral feedings on survival in head-injured patients. *J Neurosurg* 58:906, 1983.
105. Imhoff M, Gahr RH, Hoffmann P: Delayed cutaneous hypersensitivity after multiple injury and severe burn. *Ann Ital Chir* 61:525, 1990.
106. Miller CH, Quattrocchi KB, Frank EH, et al: Humoral and cellular immunity following severe head injury: Review and current investigations. *Neurol Res* 13:117, 1991.
107. Quattrocchi KB, Frank EH, Miller CH, et al: Suppression of cellular immune activity following severe head injury. *J Neurotrauma* 7:77, 1990.
108. Quattrocchi KB, Frank EH, Miller CH, et al: Impairment of helper T-cell function and lymphokine-activated killer cytotoxicity following severe head injury. *J Neurosurg* 75:766, 1991.
109. Hoyt DB, Ozkan AN, Hansbrough JF, et al: Head injury: An immunologic deficit in T-cell activation. *J Trauma* 30:759, 1990.
110. Maerker AG, Beckmann H, Richard KE, et al: Humoral immunodeficiency syndrome in patients with severe head injury. *Neurosurg Rev* 12:420, 1989.
111. Barbul A: Arginine and immune function. *Nutrition* 6:53, 1990.
112. Daly JM, Reynolds J, Thom A, et al: Immune and metabolic effects of arginine in the surgical patient. *Ann Surg* 208:512, 1988.
113. Gorlin R: The biological actions and potential clinical significance of dietary omega-3 fatty acids. *Arch Intern Med* 148:2043, 1988.
114. Timsit J, Savino W, Safieh B, et al: Growth hormone and insulin-like growth factor-1 stimulate hormonal function and proliferation of thymic epithelial cells. *J Clin Endocrinol Metab* 75:183, 1992.
115. Merguerian P, Perel A, Wald U, et al: Persistent nonketotic hyperglycemia as a grave prognostic sign in head-injured patients. *Crit Care Med* 9:838, 1981.
116. Pentel'enyi T, Kammerer L, Stutzel M, et al: Alterations of the basal serum insulin and blood glucose in brain-injured patients. *Injury* 10:201, 1979.
117. Young B, Ott L, Dempsey R, et al: Relationship between admission hyperglycemia and neurological outcome of severe brain-injured patients. *Ann Surg* 210:466, 1989.
118. Lam AM, Winn HR, Cullen BF, et al: Hyperglycemia and neurological outcome in patients with head injury. *J Neurosurg* 75:545, 1991.
119. DeSalles AA, Kontos HA, Becker DP, et al: Prognostic significance of ventricular CSF lactic acidosis in severe head injury. *J Neurosurg* 65:615, 1986.
120. Sieber FE, Traystman RJ: Special issues: Glucose and the brain. *Crit Care Med* 20:104, 1992.
121. Lang CH, Dobrescu C, Bagby GJ: TNF impairs insulin action on peripheral glucose disposal and hepatic glucose output. *Endocrinology* 130:43, 1992.
122. LeRoith D, Clemmons D, Nissley P, et al: Insulin-like growth factors in health and disease. *Ann Intern Med* 116:854, 1992.
123. Robertson CS, Goodman JC, Narayan RK, et al: The effect of glucose administration on carbohydrate metabolism after head injury. *J Neurosurg* 74:43, 1991.
124. Singer P, Bursztein S, Kirvela O, et al: Hypercaloric glycerol in injured patients. *Surgery* 112:509, 1992.
125. Rosner MJ, Becker DP: Experimental brain injury: Successful therapy with the weak base, tromethamine. *J Neurosurg* 60:961, 1984.
126. Wolf AL, Levi L, Marmarou A, et al: Effect of THAM upon outcome in severe head injury randomized prospective clinical trial. *J Neurosurg* 78:54, 1993.
127. Vaughan GM, Becker RA, Allen JP, et al: Cortisol and corticotrophin in burned patients. *J Trauma* 22:263, 1982.
128. Wilmore DW, Lindsey CA, Moylan JA, et al: Hyperglucagonaemia after burns. *Lancet* 1:73, 1974.
129. Harrison TS, Seaton JF, Feller I: Relationship of in-

creased oxygen consumption to catecholamine excretion in thermal burns. *Ann Surg* 165:169, 1967.
130. Herndon DN, Barrow RE, Rutan TC, et al: Effect of propranolol administration on hemodynamic and metabolic responses of burned pediatric patients. *Ann Surg* 208:484, 1988.
131. Hall-Angeras M, Hasselgren PO, Angeras U, et al: Glucocorticoid receptor blocker RU-38486 decreased muscle protein breakdown in sepsis. *Surg Forum* 41:26, 1990.
132. Dinarello CA: Biology of Interleukin I. *FASEB J* 2:108, 1988.
133. Le J, Vilcek J: Tumor necrosis factor and interleukin 1: Cytokines with multiple overlapping biological activities. *Lab Invest* 56:234, 1987.
134. Bendtzen K: Interleukin I, interleukin 6 and tumor necrosis factor in infection, inflammation and immunity. *Immunol Lett* 19:183, 1988.
135. Gershenwald JE, Fong Y, Fahey TJ, et al: Interleukin-1 receptor blockade attenuates the host inflammatory response. *Proc Natl Acad Sci USA* 87:4966, 1990.
136. Ramadori G, Damme J, Rieder H, et al: Interleukin 6, the third mediator of acute-phase reaction, modulates hepatic protein synthesis in human and mouse: Comparison with interleukin 1 beta and tumor necrosis factor alpha. *Eur J Immunol* 18:1259, 1988.
137. Breder CD, Dinarello CA, Saper CB: Interleukin-I immunoreactive innervation of the human hypothalamus. *Science* 240:321, 1988.
138. Baracos V, Rodeman HP, Dinarello CA, et al: Stimulation of muscle protein degradation and prostaglandin E2 release by leukocytic pyrogen (interleukin-1): A mechanism for the increased degradation of muscle proteins during fever. *N Engl J Med* 308:553, 1983.
139. Moldawer LL, Svaninger G, Gelin J, et al: Interleukin-I and tumor necrosis factor do not regulate protein balance in skeletal muscle. *Am J Physiol* 253:766, 1987.
140. Watters JM, Bessey PQ, Dinarello CA, et al: The induction of interleukin-1 in humans and its metabolic effects. *Surgery* 98:298, 1985.
141. Watters JM, Bessey PQ, Dinarello CA, et al: Both inflammatory and endocrine mediators stimulate host responses to sepsis. *Arch Surg* 121:179, 1985.
142. Michie HR, Manogue KR, Spriggs DR, et al: Detection of circulating tumor necrosis factor after endotoxin administration. *N Engl J Med* 318:1481, 1988.
143. Warren RS, Starnes F, Gavrilove JL, et al: The acute metabolic effects of tumor necrosis factor administration in humans. *Arch Surg* 122:1396, 1987.
144. Feingold KR, Grunfeld C: Role of cytokines in inducing hyperlipidemia. *Diabetes* 41:97, 1992.
145. Rodriguez JL, Miller CG, Miller BS, et al: Correlation of the local and systemic cytokine response with clinical outcome following thermal injury. *J Trauma* 34:684, 1993.
146. Lindsey DC, Emerson TE, Thompson TE, et al: Characterization of an endotoxemic baboon model of metabolic and organ dysfunction. *Circ Shock* 34:298, 1991.
147. Emerson TE Jr, Lindsey DC, Jesmok GJ, et al: Efficacy of monoclonal antibody against tumor necrosis factor alpha in an endotoxemic baboon model. *Circ Shock* 38:75, 1992.
148. Shibata M, Leffler CW, Busija DW: Recombinant human interleukin I alpha dilates pial arterioles and increases cerebrospinal fluid prostanoids in piglets. *Am J Physiol* 259:H1486, 1990.
149. Megyeri P, Abraham CS, Temesvari P, et al: Recombinant human tumor necrosis factor alpha constricts pial arterioles and increases blood-brain barrier permeability in newborn piglets. *Neurosci Lett* 148:137, 1992.
150. Goldblum SE, Jay M, Yoneda K, et al: Monokine-induced acute lung injury in rabbits. *J Appl Physiol* 63:2093, 1988.
151. Khoruts A, Stahnke L, McClain CJ, et al: Circulating tumor necrosis factor, interleukin-1 and interleukin-6 concentrations in chronic alcoholic patients. *Hepatology* 13:267, 1991.
152. Ott MT, Vore M, Barker DE, et al: Monokine depression of the bile flow in the isolated perfused rat liver. *J Surg Res* 47:248, 1989.
153. Remick DG, Kunkel RG, Larrick JW, et al: Acute in vivo effects of human recombinant tumor necrosis factor. *Lab Invest* 56:583, 1987.
154. Tracey J, Beutler B, Lowry SF, et al: Shock and tissue injury induced by recombinant human cachectin. *Science* 234:470, 1986.
155. Robertson CS, Clifton GL, Grossman RG, et al: Alterations in cerebral availability of metabolic substrates after severe head injury. *J Trauma* 28:1523, 1988.
156. Young B, Ott L, Twyman D, et al: The effect of nutritional support on outcome from severe head injury. *J Neurosurg* 67:668, 1987.
157. Hadley MN, Grahm TW, Harrington T, et al: Nutritional support and neurotrauma: A critical review of early nutrition in forty-five acute head injury patients. *Neurosurgery* 19:367, 1986.
158. Waters DC, Dechert R, Bartlett R: Metabolic studies in head injury patients: A preliminary report. *Surgery* 100:531, 1986.
159. Balzola F, Boggio BD, Solerio A, et al: Dietetic treatment with hypercaloric and hyperproteic intake in patients following severe brain injury. *J Neurosurg Sci* 24:131, 1980.
160. Norton J, Ott L, McClain CJ, et al: Intolerance to enteral feeding in the brain injured patient. *J Neurosurg* 69:375, 1988.
161. Hunt D, Rowlands B, Allen S: The inadequacy of enteral nutritional support in head injury patients during the early post-injured period (abstr.). *JPEN* 9:121, 1985.
162. Olivares L, Segovia A, Revuelta R: Tube feeding and lethal aspiration in neurological patients: A review of 720 autopsy cases. *Stroke* 5:654, 1974.
163. Lutz H, Peter K, Van Ackern K: Total parenteral alimentation in neurosurgical and neurological patients, in Manni C, Magalina SI, Scrascio E (eds): *Total Parenteral Alimentation.* Amsterdam: Excerpta Medica, 1976: 214–217.
164. Waters DC, Hoff JT, Black KL: Effects of parenteral

nutrition on cold-induced vasogenic edema in cats. *J Neurosurg* 64:460, 1986.

165. Young B, Ott L, Haack D, et al: Effect of total parenteral nutrition upon intracranial pressure in severe head injury. *J Neurosurg* 67:76, 1987.
166. Combs DJ, Ott L, McAninch PS, et al: The effect of total parenteral nutrition on vasogenic edema development following cold injury in rats. *J Neurosurg* 70:623, 1989.
167. Turner WW: Nutritional considerations in the patient with disabling brain disease. *Neurosurgery* 16:707, 1985.
168. Kirby D, Turner J, Barrett J, et al: Early enteral feeding with PEG/J's in severe head injury. *JPEN* 15:298, 1991.
169. Grahm TW, Zadrozny DB, Harrington T: The benefits of early jejunal hyperalimentation in the head-injured patient. *Neurosurgery* 25:729, 1989.
170. Alexander JW, MacMillan BG, Stinnett JD, et al: Beneficial effects of aggressive protein feeding in severely burned children. *Ann Surg* 192:505–517, 1980.
171. Strong RM, Namihas N, Matsuyama R, et al: Random, prospective assessment of aspiration risk for percutaneous endoscopic gastrojejunostomy (abstr.). *JPEN* 14:18, 1990.
172. Lazarus BA, Murphy JB, Culpepper L: Aspiration associated with long-term gastric versus jejunal feeding: A critical analysis of the literature. *Arch Phys Med Rehabil* 71:46, 1990.

Therapeutic Interventions

CHAPTER 26

CONVENTIONAL DRUG THERAPIES FOR HEAD INJURY

Ann-Christine Duhaime

SYNOPSIS

This chapter reviews some of the pharmacological agents used in conventional head injury management. The history of the introduction of these agents and subsequent studies attempting to document their mechanism of action, efficacy, and toxicity are discussed. Controversies regarding optimal use and appropriate settings for each agent are reviewed. Specific classes of drugs covered in this chapter include steroids, sedatives and analgesics, paralytic agents, diuretics, and barbiturates. Management schemes including perfusion pressure therapy are mentioned. The difficulties inherent in the evaluation of efficacy of drugs used for head injury management are discussed.

INTRODUCTION

"Put him to bed
And cover his head
With vinegar and brown paper."
—*English nursery rhyme*

Prior to the modern medical era, a variety of nostrums were used to treat patients who had suffered from traumatic injury to the head. These included boiling oil, cold compresses, calomel, and brandy.[1,2] As understanding of the pathophysiology of the injured brain evolved, treatment shifted from empiric therapies to those designed to maximize "support" of the patient, in order to prevent further physiological insults to the brain and to allow optimum spontaneous recovery to occur. More recent discoveries have held out hope for therapies that are specific to the injured brain that may limit ongoing damage after the initial traumatic event.

A variety of common pharmacological agents have been included in the armamentarium available to the clinician caring for the head-injured patient. However, choice and optimal use of these agents has not always met with uniform agreement. The goal of this chapter is to provide an overview of the various "standard" drug therapies for head injury, particularly in the more severely injured patients. Rationale and experimental evidence for the efficacy of these agents will be reviewed, and controversies relating to the pharmacological management of traumatic brain injury in the emergency and intensive care settings will be discussed. Newer experimental treatments have been covered in the next chapter.

CAUSES OF DAMAGE AFTER TRAUMATIC BRAIN INJURY

Neuronal loss related to trauma has traditionally been divided into "primary" and "secondary." The former term is applied to the immediate, irreversible tissue loss that occurs at the time of trauma. Brain laceration is the most obvious and indisputable example of this kind of injury. Secondary injury is damage that does not occur immediately, but rather takes place in otherwise viable tissue due to additional systemic or local insults, such as shock, hypoxia, or increased intracranial pressure. The essential goal of supportive care is to limit the extent of secondary damage.

More recent insights into the pathophysiology of a

variety of brain insults, including ischemia, hypoxia, hpoglycemia, status epilepticus, and mechanical trauma, suggest that the characterization of injury as primary and secondary is oversimplified. Rather than occurring in a strictly biphasic sequence, cell death after trauma likely occurs in more of a continuum. This is because it has been shown that the actual death of injured neurons is often not immediate, but rather occurs some time after the insult has occurred, when processes initiated by the disturbance come to completion and result in death of the cell. Newer neuroprotective therapies seek to take advantage of a possible therapeutic window provided by this "delayed primary" injury by blocking steps in the biochemical cascades initiated but not completed at the time of the insult.[3,4] Likewise, adjacent or even distant tissue sites may succumb over time to an accumulation of deleterious factors, some of which have been regarded as "secondary" insults, including shock and other causes of focal and global ischemia, hypoxia, and increased intracranial pressure. Apart from these newer cascade-oriented strategies, current "conventional" medical management of trauma patients attempts to optimize conditions in both sublethally injured and uninjured regions of the brain, thus reducing the amount of tissue eventually lost after head injury. The role of specific pharmacological agents in this scheme is detailed below.

GOALS OF TREATMENT WITH CONVENTIONAL DRUG THERAPY

Standard pharmacological agents have been used in head-injured patients in an attempt to achieve the following goals: (1) to gain physiological control of the patient in order to optimize substrate delivery to the brain and prevent paroxysmal increases in intracranial pressure (paralytics, analgesics, pressors); (2) to prevent or treat brain swelling (diuretics, barbiturates); (3) to decrease secondary (or delayed primary) damage (steroids); (4) to treat symptoms associated with brain injury (sedatives, stimulants); and (5) to prevent or treat complications of brain injury (anticonvulsants, antibiotics).

The rationale for the treatment of increased intracranial pressure and the efficacy of measures designed for this purpose have been much debated, and will be discussed in more detail elsewhere in this volume.[5] Suffice it to say that to date both conventional and experimental strategies in head injury management have emphasized the control of intracranial pressure as a central theme. However, drug therapy is but one treatment modality, and these agents are used in an individualized treatment plan in which other parameters are varied, including ventilation, fluids, and nutrition. Conventional treatments generally have been applied in escalating intensity, beginning with a variable combination of sedation, paralysis, ventricular drainage, hyperventilation, osmotherapy, and barbiturates.[6,7] This chapter will deal with all conventional medications except anticonvulsants and antibiotics, which have been described elsewhere in this text.

STEROIDS

The use of glucocorticoids in head injury dates to the 1960s, when their efficacy in reducing brain swelling associated with tumors had become established.[8,9] For the following two decades a variety of animal and human studies provided evidence for and against the use of steroids in head injury. The prolonged controversy surrounding steroids highlights the problems inherent in head injury research in general and drug treatment in particular. These include: (1) the limitations of animal models in reproducing the pathophysiology of clinically occurring trauma; (2) the heterogeneity of head injury; (3) the frequent lack of suitable control populations in clinical trials; (4) the difficulties in comparing studies that used different doses, administration times, and types of agents; (5) the variability of outcome measures; and (6) an incomplete understanding of both beneficial and detrimental drug actions.

With respect to animal models, those involving substantial focal edema, such as cold lesions, have shown the greatest degree of success in demonstrating reduction of edema using corticosteroids. However, most of the studies in which efficacy could be demonstrated involved experiments in which the drug was given before the lesion occurred, thus limiting the drug's potential clinical usefulness.[10–12] In addition, the difficulties in extrapolating from edema around cold lesions in rodents and cats to the pathophysiology of brain swelling in human head injury are apparent.[13]

In attempting to more closely model conditions relevant to trauma, steroids have been tested in other animal paradigms of impact and acceleration/deceleration injury. While edema from impact in cats has been influenced minimally by dexamethasone, motor abilities at 1 h after impact injury in mice was improved by methylprednisolone.[13,14] Increased duration of survival and decreased edema also were reported in impacted monkeys treated with dexamethasone after injury.[15]

Clinical trials have been particularly difficult to interpret because of differing doses, inclusion criteria, and outcome measures. Several early studies which concluded that steroids improved outcome were comprised of small numbers of patients who were compared to historical controls.[8,9] At the time of these studies, steroids were generally considered relatively benign, with complications limited largely to a mildly increased risk of medical problems often seen in the setting of severe injury anyway, such as pneumonias and gastrointestinal hemorrhage.

Because of the poor outcome of severe head injuries, the potential risk/benefit ratio was widely felt to favor use of the agents, and steroid administration became widespread in the 1970s.[16] However, more carefully contolled and prospective studies in adults and children with severe head injuries failed to show substantial benefit from steroid use with respect to intracranial pressure effects or clinical outcome at 6 months, even when large doses were used.[17–20] Other studies have noted trends in improved outcome for certain subpopulations of head-injured patients given high-dose steroids, but the exact characterization of which patients might benefit is incomplete, especially with respect to selecting patients prospectively for steroid therapy.[21–23] In other studies, steroid use was found to be not only ineffective, but also to correlate with worse neurological outcome in some groups of patients.[20,22]

Metabolic changes associated with high-dose short-term steroids adversely affect nitrogen balance in both adults and children with head injury, although the influence of this effect on outcome is less clearly demonstrated.[24–26] Corticosteroids also have been shown to potentiate ischemic insults in animals, probably related to hyperglycemia.[27] Because of these theoretical risks and lack of clear benefit in well-controlled clinical trials, most centers have abandoned the routine use of standard corticosteroids in head-injured patients.[5,20] An exception is made for head-injured patients with known or suspected spinal cord injury, in whom methylprednisolone is usually administered because of its apparent beneficial effect on the latter injury. It is of interest that a variety of newer synthetic steroid compounds designed to capitalize on the theoretical beneficial actions of older corticosteroids in the setting of traumatic brain injury are now being tested, and will be discussed in the chapter on experimental agents.

SEDATIVES AND ANALGESICS

In the trauma setting, head-injured patients may manifest responses to ongoing painful or noxious stimuli which can interfere with optimal management. In all but the most severely impaired, pain is associated with elevations in both intracranial pressure and blood pressure. Excessive hypertension may increase the risk of intracranial hemorrhage and brain swelling. Posturing or agitation with excessive motor activity and straining often is associated with elevations in intracranial pressure. Abnormal motor activity may elevate the temperature, and shivering can hinder the implementation of therapeutic hypothermia. Resistance to controlled ventilation interferes with the effectiveness and predictability of this intervention. For these reasons, drugs which act as sedatives and analgesics are often used in the setting of acute head injury, and sometimes in the more chronic recovery stage as well.

The primary disadvantage of these agents is that their desired action also obscures the neurological exam, and their use sometimes precipitates the need for increased invasive monitoring. Even when invasive monitoring is performed, deterioration due to tissue shifts or mass lesions can be masked. Of nearly equal concern is the depressant effect of many of these drugs on cardiovascular parameters, particularly blood pressure. Some authors believe these drugs to be underutilized in the acute setting, where they might be protective against episodic increases in intracranial pressure. Others have cautioned that use of sedatives without careful attention to their hemodynamic effects may contribute to episodes of decreased cerebral perfusion pressure resulting in cerebral ischemia.[28–30] To date, a beneficial effect on outcome from sedatives and analgesics independent of other factors has not been clearly demonstrated, although studies of this issue are scarce, and often are hindered by the administration of multiple drugs simultaneously.[30,31]

The most frequently used narcotic in the acute setting is intravenous morphine. Its advantages include rapid efficacy in analgesic effect when pain is present, a long history of safety when titrated correctly, and rapid reversibility. It has been also shown to be effective in curtailing episodes of sympathetic discharge associated with extensor posturing.[32] In sedative doses, particularly when ventilation is controlled, it does not appear to cause significant increases in intracranial pressure, which have been noted in some synthetic narcotics used for neuroanesthesia. However, when pharmacological reversal is necessary, intracranial pressure and cerebral blood flow may increase acutely.[30]

Fentanyl, sufentanil, and several similar agents are rapidly metabolized synthetic narcotics that have as a theoretical advantage a brief duration of action, making them suitable for use in transient painful events such as bedside procedures or the induction of anesthesia. These agents are associated with a mild but reproducible elevation in intracranial pressure, and it has been suggested that they should be used with caution in situations in which intracranial pressure is dangerously elevated.[29,33]

Two newer agents deserve mention in the context of the acute management of head-injured patients. While the use of benzodiazepines previously was avoided in most instances of head injury management because of their depressant action and irreversibility, the advent of new antagonists has brought this class into use in trauma patients. For example, midazolam is a potent benzodiazepine that has gained increasing use in intensive care, particularly for patients requiring ventilatory support. It can be titrated by continuous intravenous infusion, produces minimal ventilatory depression or hypotension, and is also an effective anticonvulsant. Midazolam can be reversed by the benzodiazepine antagonist flumazenil, but as with narcotic antagonists, the effects of reversal on intracranial pressure dynamics must be monitored closely.[34] In addition, these agents may have a prolonged duration of action in critically ill head-injured patients.[35]

Propofol is an intravenous anesthetic agent whose effects are nearly entirely limited to its duration of infusion, and therefore has been used for anesthesia during painful procedures in head-injured patients. Unlike narcotics, it does not appear to produce increases in intracranial pressure, although, like many other agents, it has been associated with decrease in cerebral perfusion pressure.[36]

Lidocaine's action is probably central when administered intravenously, but it appears to blunt the intracranial pressure response elicited by endotracheal suctioning.[37,38] Bolus doses of lidocaine intravenously (1 mg/kg) or endotracheally prior to pulmonary care have become routine in the intensive care management of patients with severe head injury. Response to tracheal suctioning can also be blunted by prior intravenous administration of thiopental, 1 to 3 mg/kg.[38,39]

Small doses of barbiturates are very effective as sedatives and have a salutary effect on intracranial pressure, but like other sedatives decrease blood pressure as well. These will be discussed in more detail below.

PARALYZING AGENTS

Much has been written about various paralyzing agents and their use in resuscitation, intubation, and administration of surgical anesthesia for head-injured or multiply injured patients.[40–42] Muscle relaxants including succinylcholine, vecuronium, curare, pancuronium, and atracurium have been shown to differ in their tendency to cause histamine release, hypotension, and increased intracranial pressure.[40,43,44] Decisions regarding choice of agents in the field or emergency department depend on the patient's overall status, including vital signs and volume status, neurological condition, and predicted duration of required paralysis, with the shorter-acting agents usually preferred.[39]

The use of muscle relaxants in the post-resuscitation stage of head injury, though widely practiced, has been less well characterized. The rationale for the use of these agents in the intensive care unit is that excessive motor activity related to agitation or to posturing is associated with increases in intracranial pressure. Pharmacological paralysis aids in control of this contribution to intracranial hypertension, and also facilitates ventilatory control.[5,45] For this purpose, longer-acting agents such as pancuronium are often utilized. It must be remembered that paralysis alone will block neither the patient's perception of nor response to noxious stimuli, and adequate sedation also must be provided, even in patients with depressed consciousness.

The use of muscle relaxants severely limits clinical examination and, depending on the dose and schedule of administration, may not always prove immediately reversible. Their use is limited, therefore, to severely injured patients whose intracranial pressure is being monitored continuously. As with sedatives, controlled trials proving the efficacy of this intervention in controlling intracranial pressure and affecting outcome have not been performed. For these reasons, while some centers routinely paralyze all severely head injured patients, others prefer to use relaxants only in situations in which motor activity appears correlated with unacceptably sustained increases in intracranial pressure.

DIURETICS

Osmotic Diuretics

The link between intravenously administered hypertonic solutions and intracranial pressure has been studied since the early part of the twentieth century.[46] Agents such as urea, albumin, and glycerol given orally or intravenously have been used to treat cerebral edema during the 1940s through the 1970s, but a variety of systemic effects such as renal and hemodynamic disturbances have limited their usefulness.[47–49] Urea was one of the earliest osmotic agents tried for brain swelling, and was found to be quite effective.[48,50] However, its side effects including hematuria, skin sloughing with infiltration, and elevated prothrombin times were more troublesome than those found with mannitol, and so the latter agent has largely supplanted its use.[51]

Glycerol has the advantage of oral or intravenous

administration, and was used originally for brain swelling in the setting of intracranial tumors or pseudotumor. Unlike mannitol, it is liquid at room temperature and thus does not crystallize in and directly damage the renal tubules. For this reason, serum osmolarity is not strictly limited to a maximum of 320 mOsm when glycerol is used, although hemolysis and other adverse effects of intravascular hypertonicity will still occur at higher levels. In comparative studies, intravenous glycerol has been shown to effectively lower intracranial pressure, although the immediate reduction is less pronounced than with mannitol infusion. Rebound phenomenon, which will be discussed further below, has been inconsistently reported.[52,53] The efficacy of glycerol relative to mannitol with respect to intracranial pressure control in severe head injury, or its effect on outcome, has not been studied. In addition, intravenous glycerol is not currently approved for use in the United States except as an "experimental" drug.

The use of mannitol for the treatment of brain swelling in head-injured patients has been reported since the early 1960s.[54] Unlike urea, mannitol is a hyperosmotic agent which is not metabolized and therefore remains in the extracellular space. It has been shown to be effective in rapidly reducing intracranial pressure in the setting of head injury.[55,56] By the mid-1970s it was used routinely to treat elevated intracranial pressure, usually administered as bolus doses of 1 gm/kg of 20% mannitol intravenously every 3 to 4 h as needed to keep the intracranial pressure below 20 mmHg and serum osmolarity between 310 and 320 mOsm per liter.[57] However, the use of mannitol has also generated controversy, and many studies have been carried out to answer questions regarding its physiological effects, mechanism of action, optimal dosing schedule, interactions with other therapies, and deleterious effects.

One of the early questions regarding mannitol's use in head injury related to its mechanism of action. While the ability of the agent to lower intracranial pressure was not disputed, it remained unclear whether this effect had to do with water being "drawn out" of the interstitial fluid into the vascular bed by an osmotic gradient or was due to some other mechanism. Further, if water were being drawn out, was it from the injured area or the preserved, "good brain" distant from the lesion? The answers have not been entirely clear, with some authors finding dehydration of injured tissue after mannitol, and others finding modest water loss only in uninjured white matter.[58,59] These discrepancies, like those found in studies of the effectiveness of steroids, may be partly explained by differences in experimental variables such as lesion types, endpoints, and species differences.

Because of the arguments that dehydration occurs in a time course and magnitude which is too slow to explain mannitol's almost immediate effect on intracranial pressure, other authors have investigated the drug's effect on other physiological parameters, such as cerebrospinal fluid production, cerebral blood volume, and cerebral blood flow. Both cerebral blood volume and cerebral blood flow increase transiently after mannitol administration.[60-62] Some authors have suggested that these changes, along with reductions in blood viscosity, lead to a reduction in intracranial pressure after mannitol administration which is mediated by vasoconstrictive, rather than osmotic factors.[59,63,64]

Because of these discrepancies, attempts have been made to understand the relationship between mannitol's various physiological effects and its ability to provide a desired therapeutic effect in a particular clinical setting. This relates in part to the complex relationship between brain swelling in a given patient and the relative contributions of increased blood flow, increased blood volume, and increased water content (edema).[65] It has been suggested that mannitol may be most beneficial in patients with high intracranial pressure and focal injuries, often associated with edema, in whom cerebral blood flow is low.[65,66] Similarly, measurement of arteriovenous oxygen content difference (AVD_{O_2}) or jugular bulb oxygen saturation has led some authors to propose mannitol as the treatment of choice for those patients without global cerebral hyperemia in whom intracranial pressure is elevated. Likewise, because of the resultant increase in cerebral blood flow, mannitol may help protect the brain against ischemia when hyperventilation is utilized to decrease intracranial pressure.[28,67] In contrast, hypnotic agents such as barbiturates, along with hyperventilation, may be the treatment of choice when blood volume or blood flow is already elevated, as often is the case in younger patients with more diffuse injuries.[65]

Another question regarding the use of mannitol has been the possibility of a so-called "rebound effect" after its administration.[68] This refers to the tendency for intracranial pressure to exceed its baseline value after the effects of the diuretic wear off. A variety of studies have been performed in an attempt to verify and quantitate this effect, but with mixed results. As with other drug studies, the variability in conclusions regarding the rebound phenomenon likely arises in part because of differences in experimental models, doses, and schedules of administration of the drug. However, several recent studies suggest that this effect, if present, is modest, and treatment with mannitol need not be avoided in patients in whom the drug is otherwise likely to be useful.[52,53]

The optimal dose and dosing schedule of mannitol also have generated controversy. Some authors have advocated use of smaller doses, since these may be adequate to control intracranial pressure; others have shown that maximal acute reduction in intracranial pressure occurs with larger bolus doses of 1 g/kg.[66,69,70] Continuous infusion schedules have also been advocated.[71] In one study, which was limited by patient numbers, mannitol administered intermittently in response to intracranial pressure greater than 25 mmHg was not found to favorably influence outcome compared to that administered empirically on a regular schedule. However, using a lower intracranial pressure threshold for treatment may favorably influence outcome.[72,73] Regardless of the exact dose and schedule, common experience suggests that "keeping ahead" of the intracranial pressure by frequent use of mannitol appears to make management of intracranial pressure easier, and may improve outcome, although studies specifically addressing this effect are incomplete.[72,73]

On the negative side, rapid infusion of mannitol has been associated with an acute elevation in intracranial pressure, cerebral blood volume, and cerebral blood flow, coupled with a decline in systemic arterial blood pressure, especially in the setting of hypovolemia.[60,64] This combination of effects has been shown in some studies to lower cerebral perfusion pressure, and it has been demonstrated that periods of cerebral ischemia may result.[28] As increasing evidence accumulates that such episodes may adversely affect outcome, weighing various factors such as the patient's intravascular volume status, oxygenation, ventilation parameters, and cerebral compliance becomes important.[74] In addition, contrary to the suggestion that mannitol may be most useful in more focal injuries, concern has been generated that the resultant increase in cerebral blood flow may convert areas of contusion into frank hemorrhages as the increased flow through fragile tissue breaks through the tenuous vascular barrier.

As yet the specific conditions under which mannitol is effective and safe are not completely elucidated. It appears likely that continuous monitoring of jugular venous oxygen saturation or other parameters of cerebral oxygenation will enable more careful monitoring of potentially deleterious consequences of therapy, although these techniques fail to fully characterize the heterogeneous nature of a given patient's injury.[28,74,75] In addition, a trend toward more widespread use of ventricular fluid drainage or the use of newer neuroprotective strategies may modify the need for this conventional pharmacological intervention for raised intracranial pressure.

Furosemide

Another approach to the problems inherent in mannitol therapy has been to use nonosmotic diuretics, either alone or in combination with osmotic agents. There is some evidence that furosemide potentiates the effect of mannitol.[70] Another theoretical advantage is that furosemide, unlike mannitol, is not associated with increased cerebral blood flow, and for this reason is perhaps less likely to potentiate hemorrhage into contused parenchyma. However, furosemide acts less rapidly and reduces intracranial pressure to a lesser extent than do mannitol and other osmotic agents, and so is generally used in cases of more mild elevations in intracranial pressure, or as an adjunct to other therapies.

Hypertonic Saline

This agent has been studied most thoroughly as a resuscitation fluid in patients with shock in the setting of multiple organ system injuries. In this setting it has been found in both clinical and experimental studies to restore hemodynamic stability with much lower intravenous volumes than that required using more dilute solutions, and to be associated with less elevation of intracranial pressure.[43,76] As with any hypertonic solution, renal or hematological consequences can occur and must be monitored carefully.

Hypertonic saline also has been used to treat elevated intracranial pressure in experimental head injury and in the intensive care setting as treatment of refractory intracranial pressure in humans. While early reports show some promise, more evaluation is needed before this agent becomes more widely used.[77,78]

BARBITURATES

The protective effect of barbiturates in experimental models of cerebral ischemia began to be reported in the 1970s.[79–82] The ability of these agents to reduce cerebral blood flow, cerebral metabolism, and intracranial pressure have been well studied in a variety of experimental and clinical settings.[83–85] By the late 1970s, reports of the successful use of barbiturates to control elevations in intracranial pressure refractory to hyperventilation, cerebrospinal fluid drainage, steroids, and osmotherapy in severely head injured patients began to appear.[85,86] According to these series, refractory intracranial pressure could be controlled with high-dose continuous pentobarbital coma in 75 percent of patients, with a greater than 50 percent good outcome in this group. Compared with historical controls in the treating institutions, these results were felt to represent a significant improvement in outcome related to the introduction of aggressive management of intracranial pressure with barbiturate therapy.

However, these studies were criticized on several grounds. First, outcome in these series was not very different from overall outcome in other large series of similarly injured patients at other centers who were not treated with barbiturates. Second, the studies were neither prospective nor blinded. Third, it remained unclear whether control of intracranial pressure was really the critical parameter in determining patient outcome. Finally, the complications and complexity of barbiturate coma, during which patients require continuous intracranial pressure monitoring, Swan-Ganz catheters, pressors, and other invasive maneuvers were inadequately documented.[87]

Several subsequent studies performed during the 1980s sought to address some of these questions. Several principles emerged or were reinforced by these studies. First, more aggressive control of intracranial pressure at lower levels (e.g., 15 mmHg) with standard maneuvers (cerebrospinal fluid drainage, osmotic diuretics, etc.) appears to meliorate overall control of intracranial pressure.[73,88] Second, barbiturates administered prophylactically are of no benefit and have side effects, most notably hypotension, which can adversely affect outcome.[88] However, a large, multicentered, controlled study showed benefit of high-dose barbiturates, with reduction in mortality, in the small percentage of patients truly refractory to other conventional management of intracranial pressure. Thus, while barbiturate coma may in fact reduce mortality in some instances, the number of patients for whom this aggressive therapy is indicated is distinctly smaller than the original enthusiasm suggested, and is estimated at 12 percent of severely head injured patients.[7]

Criticisms of high-dose barbiturate therapy continue as side effects become apparent, including decreased perfusion pressure and possible ischemia; hepatic, renal, and pulmonary dysfunction; hypokalemia; and infectious complications.[28,65,89] Questions also remain regarding the quality of life of patients salvaged by barbiturate coma, although the small numbers reported along with common experience suggest that at least some patients enjoy good outcomes. In some severely injured patients, a secondary delayed rise in intracranial pressure occurs which may represent more severe underlying damage and a poorer prognosis regardless of intervention; this phenomenon revives the argument of intracranial pressure as an "epiphenomenon" which merely indicates the degree to which the brain has been compromised.[90] The use of low-dose, intermittent bolus barbiturates has been incompletely studied, but is widely practiced; this may be associated with fewer adverse systemic consequences. Whether newer neuroprotective agents will further reduce the need for barbiturate therapy remains to be seen.

PERFUSION PRESSURE MANAGEMENT

While ischemia has long been recognized as a complicating factor in a high proportion of serious head injuries, several recent efforts have focused on the iatrogenic exacerbation of ischemia during the acute phase of patient management.[74,75,91] This may be related to inadequate volume resuscitation and to the use of agents such as diuretics, sedatives, analgesics, and hypnotics which can all have the effect of decreasing systemic arterial pressure. The result of this therapy may be counterproductive, as decreased perfusion pressure leads to cerebral ischemia which then causes reflex vasodilation and a worsening of the intracranial hypertension.

To combat this problem, some authors have suggested that a primary management focus on perfusion pressure, with attention to the blood pressure side of the equation, may decrease the frequent occurrence of in-hospital ischemia and thus improve outcome.[28,63,92] In this scheme, patients are nursed with the head flat, the intravascular volume is expanded, and catecholamine pressors are added to the equation in order to elevate the arterial pressure. While elevated intracranial pressure is treated with cerebrospinal fluid drainage and osmotic diuretics, pressures higher than those previously stressed as dangerous are tolerated if the perfusion pressure can be maintained. While improved outcome has been reported in small noncontrolled series using this strategy, controlled trials are needed to validate the superiority of this approach over conventional management. In addition, other studies contradict aspects of this treatment strategy, such as keeping the head of the bed flat.[93] Nonetheless, improved recognition of preventable ischemic insults appears to hold promise of benefit in head injury care.

SUMMARY

The variability in clinical head injury makes evaluation of a particular intervention difficult, and complex management schemes involving multiple simultaneous therapies provide even greater analytic complexity. Nonetheless, it appears that conventional medical management, when individualized and applied with the pathophysiology of the individual patient's injury in mind, is effective in preventing some of the morbidity and mortality that would otherwise occur in severely head injured patients. Recognition of the limitations and complications of aggressive pharmacotherapy and the availability of increasingly sophisticated monitoring techniques may further improve our ability to tailor therapy to an individual patient's needs. The effect of these agents on outcome will continue to be difficult to evaluate, especially as new agents are added to the treatment plan. The efficacy of interventions may ultimately have to be assessed by their ability to produce measurable improvements in cerebral physiological parameters.

References

1. Spector B: One hour of medical history: Selected excerpts. *Surg Neurol* 1990; 33:64–73.
2. Zellem RT: Wounded by bayonet, ball, and bacteria: Medicine and neurosurgery in the American Civil War. *Neurosurgery* 1985; 17:850–860.
3. Siesjo BK: Pathophysiology and treatment of focal cerebral ischemia: Part II. Mechanisms of damage and treatment. *J Neurosurg* 1992; 77:337–354.
4. Bullock R, Fujisawa H: The role of glutamate antagonists for the treatment of CNS injury. *J Neurotrauma* 1992; 9(suppl 2):S443–S473.
5. Chestnut RM, Marshall LF: Treatment of abnormal intracranial pressure. *Neurosurg Clin North Am* 1991; 2(2):267–284.
6. Marmarou A, Anderson RL, Ward JD, et al: NINDS Traumatic Coma Data Bank: Intracranial pressure monitoring methodology. *J Neurosurg* 1991; 75:S21–S27.
7. Eisenberg HM, Frankowski RF, Contant CF, et al: High-dose barbiturate control of elevated intracranial pressure in patients with severe head injury. *J Neurosurg* 1988; 69:15–23.
8. Sparacio RR, Lin TH, Cook AW: Methylprednisolone sodium succinate in acute craniocerebral trauma. *Surg Gynecol Obstet* 1965; 121:513–516.
9. French LA: Steroids in the treatment of cerebral edema. *Bull N Y Acad Med* 1966; 42(4):301–311.
10. Nelson SR: Effects of drugs on experimental brain edema in mice. *J Neurosurg* 1974; 41(2):193–199.
11. Dick AR, McCallum ME, Maxwell JA, Nelson SA: Effect of dexamethasone on experimental brain edema in cats. *J Neurosurg* 1976; 45(2):141–147.
12. Maxwell RE, Long DM, French LA: The effects of glucosteroids on experimental cold-induced brain edema: Gross morphological alterations and vascular permeability changes. *J Neurosurg* 1971; 34:477–487.
13. Tornheim PA, McLaurin RL: Effect of dexamethasone on cerebral edema from cranial impact in the cat. *J Neurosurg* 1978; 48(2):220–227.
14. Hall ED: High-dose glucocorticoid treatment improves neurological recovery in head-injured mice. *J Neurosurg* 1985; 62(6):882–887.
15. Kobrine AI, Kempe LG: Studies in head injury: Part II. Effect of dexamethasone on traumatic brain swelling. *Surg Neurol* 1973; 1:38–42.
16. Marshall LF, King J, Langfitt TW: The complications of high-dose corticosteroid therapy in neurological patients: A prospective study. *Ann Neurol* 1977; 1:201–203.
17. Gudeman SK, Miller JD, Becker DP: Failure of high-dose steroid therapy to influence intracranial pressure in patients with severe head injury. *J Neurosurg* 1979; 51:301–306.
18. Cooper PR, Moody S, Clark WK, et al: Dexamethasone and severe head injury: A prospective double-blind study. *J Neurosurg* 1979; 51:307–316.
19. Braakman R, Schouten HJA, Dishoeck MB, Minderhoud JM: Megadose steroids in severe head injury: Results of a prospective double-blind clinical trial. *J Neurosurg* 1983; 58:326–330.
20. Dearden NM, Gibson JS, McDowall DG, et al: Effect of high-dose dexamethasone on outcome from severe head injury. *J Neurosurg* 1986; 64:81–88.
21. Giannotta SL, Weiss MH, Apuzzo ML, Martin E: High-dose glucocorticoids in the management of severe head injury. *Neurosurgery* 1984; 15(4):497–501.
22. Saul TG, Ducker TB, Salcman M, Carro E: Steroids in severe head injury: A prospective randomized clinical trial. *J Neurosurg* 1981; 54:596–600.
23. Du Plessis JJ: High-dose dexamethasone therapy in head injury: A patient group that may benefit from therapy. *Br J Neurosurg* 1992; 6:145–147.
24. Robertson CS, Clifton GL, Goodman JC: Steroid administration and nitrogen excretion in the head-injured patient. *J Neurosurg* 1985; 63:714–718.
25. Deutschman CS, Konstantinides FN, Raup S, Cerra FB: Physiologic and metabolic response to isolated closed head injury: Part 2. Effects of steroids on metabolism. Potentiation of protein wasting and abnormalities of substrate utilization. *J Neurosurg* 1987; 66:388–395.
26. Ford EG, Jennings LM, Andrassy RJ: Steroid administration potentiates urinary nitrogen losses in head-injured children. *J Trauma* 1987; 27(9):1074–1077.
27. Sapolsky RM, Pulsinelli WA: Glucocorticoids potentiate ischemic injury to neurons: Therapeutic implications. *Science* 1985; 229:1397–1400.
28. Chan K, Dearden NM, Miller JD, et al: Multimodality monitoring as a guide to treatment of intracranial hypertension after severe brain injury. *Neurosurgery* 1993; 32(4):547–553.
29. Sperry RJ, Bailey PL, Reichman MV, et al: Fentanyl and sufentanil increase intracranial pressure in head trauma patients. *Anesthesiology* 1992; 77(3):416–420.
30. Chiolero RL, de Tribolet N: Sedatives and antagonists in the management of severely head injured patients. *Acta Neurochir (Wien)* 1992; 55:43–46.
31. Nakayama DK, Waggoner T, Venkataraman ST, et al: The use of drugs in emergency airway management in pediatric trauma. *Ann Surg* 1992; 216(2):205–211.
32. Rossitch EJ, Bullard DE: The autonomic dysfunction syndrome: Aetiology and treatment. *Br J Neurosurg* 1988; 2(4):471–478.
33. Weinstabl C, Mayer N, Richling B, et al: Effect of sufentanil on intracranial pressure in neurosurgical patients. *Anaesthesia* 1991; 46(10):837–840.
34. Schulte am Esch J, Kochs E: Midazolam and flumazenil in neuroanesthesia. *Acta Anaesthesiol Scand* 1990; 92(suppl):96–102.
35. Malacrida R, Fritz ME, Suter PM, Crevoisier C: Pharmacokinetics of midazolam administered by continuous intravenous infusion to intensive care patients. *Crit Care Med* 1992; 20(8):1123–1126.
36. Pinaud M, Lelausque JN, Chetanneau A, et al: Effects of propofol on cerebral hemodynamics and metabolism in patients with brain trauma. *Anesthesiology* 1990; 73(3):404–409.
37. Yano M, Nishiyama H, Yokota H, et al: Effect of lido-

caine on ICP response to endotracheal suctioning. *Anesthesiology* 1986; 64(5):651–653.

38. White PF, Schlobohm RM, Pitts LH: A randomized study of drugs for preventing increases in intracranial pressure during endotracheal suctioning. *Anesthesiology* 1982; 57:242.
39. Pilmer SL, Duhaime AC, Raphaely RC: Intracranial pressure control, in Eichelberger MR (ed): *Pediatric Trauma: Prevention, Acute Care, Rehabilitation.* St. Louis: Mosby-Year Book, 1993: 200–216.
40. McGill WA: Anesthesia, in Eichelberger MR (ed): *Pediatric Trauma: Prevention, Acute Care, Rehabilitation.* St. Louis: Mosby-Year Book, 1993: 217–225.
41. Redan JA, Livingston DH, Tortella BJ, Rush BFJ: The value of intubating and paralyzing patients with suspected head injury in the emergency department. *J Trauma* 1991; 31(3):371–375.
42. Syverud SA, Borron SW, Storer DL, et al: Prehospital use of neuromuscular blocking agents in a helicopter ambulance program. *Ann Emerg Med* 1988; 17(3):236–242.
43. Ducey JP, Mozingo DW, Lamiell JM, et al: A comparison of the cerebral and cardiovascular effects of complete resuscitation with isotonic and hypertonic saline, hetastarch, and whole blood following hemorrhage. *J Trauma* 1989; 29(11):1510–1518.
44. Stirt JA, Maggio W, Haworth C, et al: Vecuronium: Effect on intracranial pressure and hemodynamics in neurosurgical patients. *Anesthesiology* 1987; 67(4):570–573.
45. Werba A, Klezl M, Schramm W, et al: The level of neuromuscular block needed to suppress diaphragmatic movement during tracheal suction in patients with raised intracranial pressure: A study with vecuronium and atracurium. *Anaesthesia* 1993; 48(4):301–303.
46. Weed LH, McKibben PS: Pressure changes in the cerebrospinal fluid following intravenous injection of solutions of various concentrations. *Am J Physiol* 1919; 48:512–530.
47. Gates EM, Craig WM: The use of serum albumin in cases of cerebral edema: Preliminary report. *Proc Staff Meet Mayo Clin* 1948; 23:89–93.
48. Javid M, Settlage P: Effect of urea on cerebrospinal fluid pressure in human subjects: Preliminary report. *JAMA* 1956; 160:943–949.
49. Cantore GP, Guidetta B, Verno M: Oral glycerol for the reduction of intracranial pressure. *J Neurosurg* 1964; 21:278–283.
50. Javid M: Urea in intracranial surgery: A new method. *J Neurosurg* 1961; 18:51–57.
51. Mason MS, Raaf J: Physiological alterations and clinical effects of urea-induced diuresis. *J Neurosurg* 1961; 18:645–653.
52. Node Y, Nakazawa S: Clinical study of mannitol and glycerol on raised intracranial pressure and on their rebound phenomenon. *Adv Neurol* 1990; 52:359–363.
53. Garcia-Sola R, Pulido P, Capilla P: The immediate and long-term effects of mannitol and glycerol. *Acta Neurochir* (*Wien*) 1991; 109:114–121.
54. Shenkin HA, Goluboff B, Haft H: The use of mannitol for the reduction of intracranial pressure in intracranial injury. *J Neurosurg* 1962; 19:897–901.
55. James HE, Langfitt TW, Kumar VS: Treatment of intracranial hypertension: Analysis of 105 consecutive, continuous recordings of intracranial pressure. *Acta Neurochir* 1977; 36:189–200.
56. McGraw CP, Howard G: Effect of mannitol on increased intracranial pressure. *Neurosurgery* 1983; 13:269–271.
57. Becker CP, Miller JD, Young HF, et al: Diagnosis and treatment of head injury in adults, in Youmans JR (ed): *Neurological Surgery.* Philadelphia: WB Saunders, 1981: 1938–2083.
58. Nath F, Galbraith S: The effect of mannitol on cerebral white matter water content. *J Neurosurg* 1986; 65:41–43.
59. Hartwell RC, Sutton LN: Mannitol, intracranial pressure, and vasogenic edema. *Neurosurgery* 1993; 32(3):444–450.
60. Ravussin P, Archer DP, Tyler JL, et al: Effects of rapid mannitol infusion on cerebral blood volume. *J Neurosurg* 1986; 64:104–113.
61. Bruce DA, Langfitt TW, Miller JD, et al: Regional cerebral blood flow, intracranial pressure, and brain metabolism in comatose patients. *J Neurosurg* 1973; 38:131–144.
62. Johnston IH, Harper AM: The effect of mannitol on cerebral blood flow: An experimental study. *J Neurosurg* 1973; 38:461–471.
63. Rosner MJ, Coley I: Cerebral perfusion pressure: A hemodynamic mechanism of mannitol and the postmannitol hemogram. *Neurosurgery* 1987; 21:147–156.
64. Muizelaar JP, Lutz HAI, Becker DP: Effect of mannitol on ICP and CBF and correlation with pressure autoregulation in severely head-injured patients. *J Neurosurg* 1984; 61:700–706.
65. Miller JD, Piper IR, Dearden NM: Management of intracranial hypertension in head injury: Matching treatment with cause. *Acta Neurochir* 1993; 57(suppl):152–159.
66. Mendelow AD, Teasdale GM, Russell T, et al: Effect of mannitol on cerebral blood flow and cerebral perfusion pressure in human head injury. *J Neurosurg* 1985; 63:43–48.
67. Cruz J, Miner ME, Allen SJ, et al: Continuous monitoring of cerebral oxygenation in acute brain injury: Injection of mannitol during hyperventilation. *J Neurosurg* 1990; 73:725–730.
68. Troupp H, Valtonen S, Vapalahti M: Intraventricular pressure after administration of dehydrating agents to severely brain-injured patients: Is there a rebound phenomenon? *Acta Neurochir* (*Wien*) 1971; 24:89–95.
69. Marshall LF, Smith RW, Shapiro HM: Mannitol dose requirement in brain-injured patients. *J Neurosurg* 1978; 48:169–172.
70. Roberts PA, Pollay M, Engles C, et al: Effect on intracranial pressure of furosemide combined with varying doses and administration rates of mannitol. *J Neurosurg* 1987; 66:440–446.
71. Becker DP, Gade GF, Young HF, Feuerman TF: Diagnosis and treatment of head injury in adults, in Youmans JR (ed): *Neurological Surgery.* Philadelphia: WB Saunders, 1990: 2017–2148.
72. Smith HP, Kelly DLJ, McWhorter JM, et al: Comparison of mannitol regimens in patients with severe head injury undergoing intracranial monitoring. *J Neurosurg* 1986; 65:820–824.

73. Saul TG, Ducker TB: Effect of intracranial pressure monitoring and aggressive treatment on mortality in severe head injury. *J Neurosurg* 1982; 56:498–503.
74. Robertson CS, Contant CF, Narayan RK, Grossman RG: Cerebral blood flow, AVDO2, and neurologic outcome in head-injured patients. *J Neurotrauma* 1992; 9 (suppl) 1:S349–358.
75. Chan K, Miller JD, Dearden NM, et al: The effect of changes in cerebral perfusion pressure upon middle cerebral artery blood flow velocity and jugular bulb venous oxygen saturation after severe brain injury. *J Neurosurg* 1992; 77:55–61.
76. Prough DS, Johnson JC, Stump DA, et al: Effects of hypertonic saline versus lactated Ringer's solution on cerebral oxygen transport during resuscitation from hemorrhagic shock. *J Neurosurg* 1986; 64:626–632.
77. Freshman SP, Battistella FD, Matteucci M, Wisner DH: Hypertonic saline (7.5%) versus mannitol: A comparison for treatment of acute head injuries. *J Trauma* 1993; 35(3):344–348.
78. Worthley LIG, Cooper DJ, Jones N: Treatment of resistant intracranial hypertension with hypertonic saline: Report of two cases. *J Neurosurg* 1988; 68:478–481.
79. Yatsu FM, Diamond I, Graziano C, Lindquist P: Experimental brain ischemia: Protection from irreversible damage with a rapid-acting barbiturate (Methohexital). *Stroke* 1972; 3:726–732.
80. Hoff JT, Smith AL, Hankinson HL, Nielsen SL: Barbiturate protection from cerebral infarction in primates. *Stroke* 1975; 6:28–33.
81. Moseley JI, Laurent JP, Molinari GF: Barbiturate attenuation of the clinical course and pathologic lesions in a primate stroke model. *Neurology* 1975; 25:870–874.
82. Smith AL, Nielson SL, Larson CP: Barbiturate protection in acute focal cerebral ischemia. *Stroke* 1974; 5:1–7.
83. Weschler RL, Dripps RD, Kety SS: Blood flow and oxygen consumption of the human brain during anesthesia produced by thiopental. *Anesthesiology* 1951; 12:308–314.
84. Kassell NF, Hitchon PW, Gerk MK, et al: Alterations in cerebral blood flow, oxygen metabolism, and electrical activity produced by high-dose sodium thiopental. *Neurosurgery* 1980; 7:598–603.
85. Marshall LF, Smith RW, Shapiro HM: The outcome with aggressive treatment of severe head injury: Part II. Acute and chronic barbiturate administration in the management of head injury. *J Neurosurg* 1979; 50:26–30.
86. Rockoff MA, Marshall LF, Shapiro HM: High-dose barbiturate therapy in humans: A clinical review of 60 patients. *Ann Neurol* 1979; 6:194–199.
87. Miller JD: Barbiturates and raised intracranial pressure. *Ann Neurol* 1979; 6(3):189–193.
88. Ward JD, Becker DP, Miller JD, et al: Failure of prophylactic barbiturate coma in the treatment of severe head injury. *J Neurosurg* 1985; 62:383–388.
89. Schalen W, Messeter K, Nordstrom CH: Complications and side effects during thiopentone therapy in patients with severe head injuries. *Acta Anaesthesiol Scand* 1992; 36:369–377.
90. Unterberg A, Kiening K, Schmiedek P, Lanksch W: Long-term observations of intracranial pressure after severe head injury: The phenomenon of secondary rise of intracranial pressure. *Neurosurgery* 1993; 32(1):17–24.
91. Graham DI, Adams JH, Doyle D: Ischaemic brain damage in fatal non-missile head injuries. *J Neurol Sci* 1978; 39:213–234.
92. Rosner MJ, Daughton S: Cerebral perfusion pressure management in head injury. *J Trauma* 1990; 30(8):933–941.
93. Feldman Z, Kanter MJ, Robertson CS, et al: Effect of head elevation on intracranial pressure, cerebral perfusion pressure, and cerebral blood flow in head-injured patients. *J Neurosurg* 1992; 76:207–211.

CHAPTER 27

EXPERIMENTAL DRUG THERAPIES FOR HEAD INJURY

Ross Bullock

SYNOPSIS

Major advances have recently been made in understanding the pathophysiology of central nervous system (CNS) trauma, and a rapidly expanding range of diverse pharmacological agents have been shown to ameliorate these pathophysiological processes in the laboratory. At least 24 clinical trials with different agents have been performed or are in progress. Trial design has now progressed from an initial "blanket neurophylaxis" approach to an attempt to target therapy at mechanisms of pathophysiology and drug action. In this chapter, the strengths and weaknesses of 17 animal models relevant to CNS trauma are reviewed. The pathomechanisms that have become the focus of clinical trials, e.g., calcium flux, free radical activation, excitatory amino acids, and ion-channel modulation, are discussed with the relevant clinical trials. Future prospects for therapy, such as microcirculatory modulation, cytokines, first- and second-generation glutamate antagonists, and synergistic therapy, are reviewed. Clinicians who care for CNS trauma patients face the challenge of translating the enormous potential of the newer neuroprotective agents, now in the laboratory, into clinical benefit.

INTRODUCTION

There have been many attempts to reduce brain damage after severe head trauma using pharmacological therapy. In 1954, Ward et al. reported the use of atropine in over 1000 severely head-injured patients, based on prior evidence demonstrating increased acetylcholine levels in cerebrospinal fluid after severe head trauma.[1,2] Unfortunately this trial failed to show benefit because of inadequate design. Presently, at least 24 trials of pharmacological therapy in severe head injury have been reported or are ongoing (Tables 27-1 and 27-2). Most of these trials have been based on sound evidence of prior efficacy in in vitro studies (for example, tissue binding, receptor affinity, and tissue culture neuroprotection studies). Most trials have also been based on evidence of efficacy in a number of animal models, which replicate different aspects of human head injury.[3] However, this has not always been the case, and some clinical trials have in fact been performed, even in recent years, with minimal evidence of efficacy in animal models.

Targeted Pharmacotherapy Versus Blanket Chemoprophylaxis

For the majority of trials performed to date in severe head trauma, the pathophysiological mechanism against which the drug is being directed has not been ascertained. The trials have been based on evidence of improved outcome in animal models of neurotrauma. Under these circumstances, the strategy of "blanket" chemoprophylaxis has been used. The drug is given to large numbers of all types of head-injured patients in a pragmatic trial format, and an improvement in outcome is sought. Before embarking on this type of trial, a lack of harmful effect by the trial medication must first be demonstrated. However, this approach is expensive and time-consuming because very large numbers of patients are necessary to demonstrate drug efficacy. In this type of trial, a dominant consideration should be the avoidance of a Type-II statistical error—that is, falsely concluding that no significant difference exists between two

TABLE 27-1 Completed "Neuroprotection" trials in Human Severe Head Injury

Investigator, and Year	Agent	No. of Patients	Outcome/Comments
1. Ward, et al, 1954	Scopolamine	940	Uncontrolled, no benefit
2. Six authors	Corticosteroids	365 (summary of 6 trials)	Controlled, no benefit
3. Schwartz, et al, 1984	Mannitol versus Pentobarbital	59	Randomized crossover permitted, Mannitol group had better outcome.
4. Ward, et al, 1985	Barbituates (Prophylaxis)	53	Controlled, Prophylactic No benefit
5. Eisenberg, et al, 1988	Barbituates (Therapeutic)	73	Controlled (high ICP patients only) ICP lowered
6. Wolf, et al, 1993	THAM (Tromethamine Buffer)	149	Controlled, ameliorates danger of hyperventilation ICP control better
7. Teasdale, et al, 1992	Nimodipine (Hit I) Calcium antagonist	255	Double blind Controlled, No benefit
8. Braakman, 1993	Nimodipine (Hit II)	840	Double blind Controlled, No benefit
9. Muizelaar, et al, 1993	PEG-SOD-Free Radical Scavenger (Phase II)	94	Double blind Controlled, ICP lower, Outcome better
10. Muizelaar, et al, 1994	PEG-SOD-Free Radical Scavenger (Phase III)—3 Dose Levels	463	Double blind Controlled Outcome was 90% better in drug than placebo ($P = 0.15$)
11. Bullock, et al, 1995	CGS 19755 (Glutamate NMDA Antagonist)	113	Double blind Controlled ICP lower, CPP better (Outcome awaited)
12. Alves, W, Jane, JA, 1995	Tirilazad (Amino-steroid Antioxidant)	1170	Double blind Controlled Enrollment complete, Outcome awaited (USA, Canada)
13. Marshall, L, 1995	Tirilazad	1128	As above (Europe, Australia)

TABLE 27-2 Ongoing Clinical Neuroprotection Trials (in Head Injury ⟨1995⟩)

Investigators	Agent/Category	Projected No. Of Patients		Comments
Muizelaar, P.	PEG-SOD-conjugat-anti-oxidant enzyme	450	Trial 006	Severe head injury (GCS 3-8) (single dose)
Cohadon, F.	Eliprodil Synthelabo-	100	Initial Europe	Severe head injury
Miller, J. D.	Polyamine-site glutamate antagonist	400	Phase III	CGS 4-8
Mendelow, A. Pickard, J. D.	D-CPP-ene-Sandoz (NMDA glutamate antagonist)	>50 Swiss/UK	Phase II	Severe head injury
Bullock, R., et al	CGS19755 (Selfotel) (NMDA glutamate antagonist)	900 USA, Israel	Phase III	Severe head injury, GCS 4-8, with focal lesions on CT.
Marshall, L., Marshall, S.	CGS 19755 (Selfotel)	900 Europe, Australia, Canada	Phase III	As above
Teasdale, G. M., Clifton, G.	CNS 1102 (Noncompetetive NMDA Glutamate antagonist)	16	Phase II	Severe head injury
Takakura, K.	Tirilazad	40 Japan	Phase II	Severe and moderate head injury CGS 4-12
Takakura, K.	OPC-14117 antioxidant	40 Japan	Phase II	Moderate head injury GCS 9-14
Nichols, J., et al	"Brady Cor"-Cortech (Bradykinin antagonist)	60 USA	Phase II	Focal Contusion Patients-ICP and point
Kelly, D., et al	Propofol (IV Short-acting anesthesia induction agent) vs. Morphine	100 USA	Phase II	Severe and moderate head injury (ICP end point)

groups, because the group sizes were too small for the magnitude of difference sought (see Chap. 64). Some of the trials listed in Table 27-1 suffer from this problem.

More recently, efforts have been focused on designing *mechanism-driven trials*, where evidence of a certain pathophysiological process has been shown in either animal models or in human head injury, and drug therapy has then been targeted at those patients in whom the pathophysiological mechanism has been shown to be operative (Fig. 27-1).[3,4] With this approach, smaller numbers of patients may be sufficient to show significant beneficial effects, and large numbers of patients who are not expected to benefit from the drug are not exposed to their unwanted side effects. This targeted approach will be discussed further for glutamate antagonists, in particular (see below).

In recent years, there has been an exponential increase in the number of laboratory studies conducted in models relevant to human head trauma. Many of these studies have shown beneficial effects from drug therapy. These studies have yielded important insights into the scope and range of neuroprotection, such as the limitations of pharmacokinetics and brain penetration, the temporal windows of opportunity, and the vulnerability for different pathophysiological processes. Laboratory studies have shown that combinations of drugs may even create difficulties due to *antagonistic* rather than synergistic interactions.[5,6]

There has also been a more gradual increase in our knowledge of the pathophysiological events that cause brain damage following human head trauma. This has come about because of neuropathological studies with careful clinicopathological correlation, as well as through monitoring and imaging studies in head-injured patients. This information, coupled with an increasing awareness of the nuances of head injury trial design, now presents clinicians who care for patients with head injury with the challenge of converting the enormous laboratory benefits demonstrated from drug therapy into tangible benefits for the head-injured patient.

Surrogate End-Points

Owing to the difficulties inherent in obtaining reliable long-term follow-up in head-injured patients and the multiple extraneous factors that may affect outcome, investigators have sought indices that may be measurable "on-line," and that may detect immediate evidence of drug effect. For example, calcium antagonists were thought to have an effect on arterial vasospasm after both subarachnoid hemorrhage and trauma, so that transcranial Doppler was used to seek evidence of a drug effect in trauma patients in various trials.[7,8] Currently, a popular surrogate end-point is intracranial pressure, and both the free radical scavenger PEG-SOD and the glutamate NMDA antagonist CGS19755 have been shown to reduce intracranial pressure in severely head-injured patients[9,10] (Fig. 27-2). The aim of testing drug effects upon surrogate end-points is twofold: (1) to detect mechanisms on which the drug may be acting, and thus choose more accurately the population in whom the drug may be effective; (2) to shorten the duration and reduce the cost of clinical trials. For example, an agent that lowers intracranial pressure may be ineffective, or

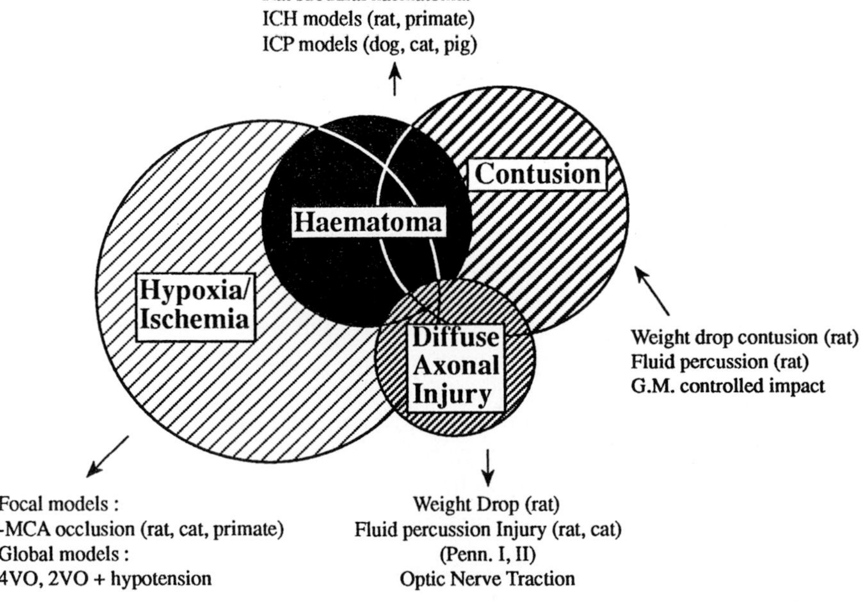

Figure 27-1. Composite venn diagram to show the multiple overlapping causes of brain damage in fatal human head injury and some of the major animal models that depict each type of brain damage.

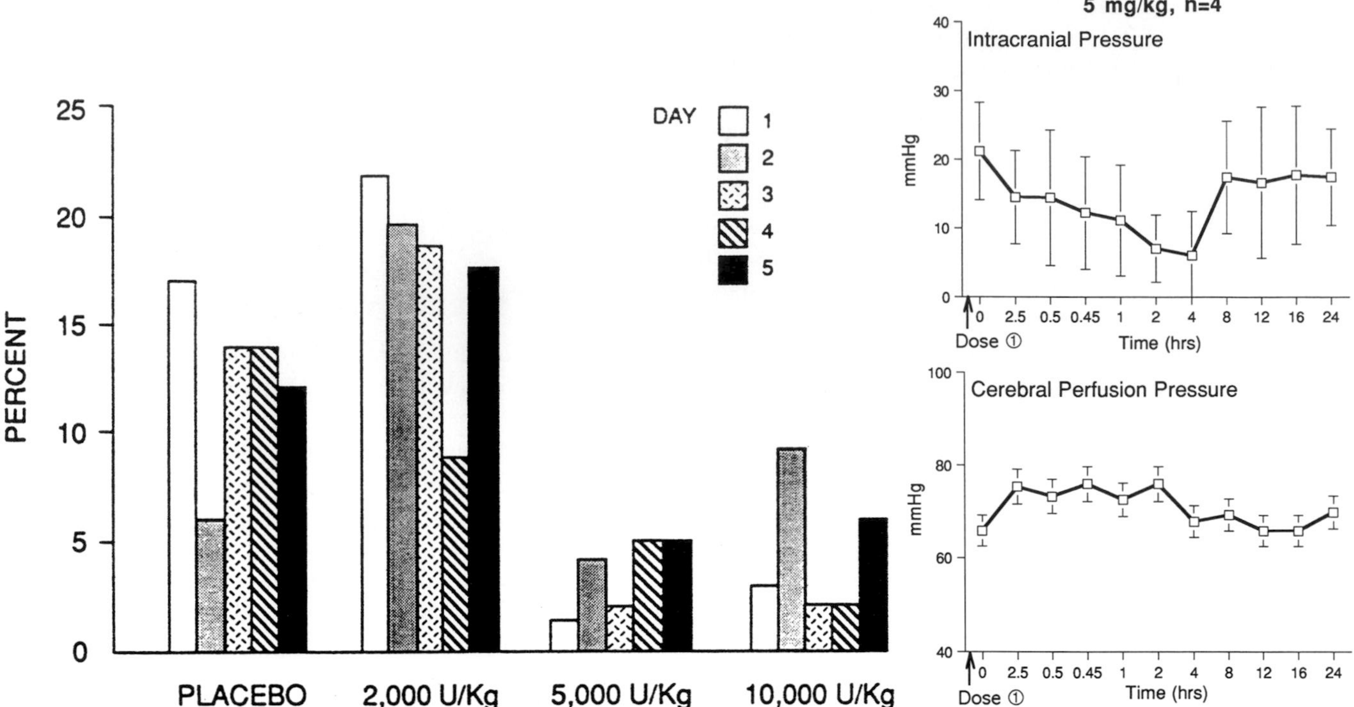

Figure 27-2. Effect of two putatively neuroprotective drugs on intracranial pressure (ICP) after severe head trauma: *Left.* Effect of the free radical scavenger PEG-SOD on ICP. *Right.* Effect of the NMDA glutamate antagonist CGS19755 (Selfotel) 5 mg/kg on mean ICP (n = 5).

not indicated, in patients without raised intracranial pressure.

Selecting Drugs from Model Data

In order to select potentially neuroprotective drugs from the ever-increasing range of compounds developed by the pharmaceutical industry, it is necessary to have a clear idea of the pathophysiological processes that cause brain damage. It is also necessary to administer the drugs such that they will achieve adequate brain concentrations when the damaging process is thought to be occurring. Figures 27-1 and 27-3 provide a pathological and a biochemical overview of the processes probably responsible for most of the damage in patients with severe injury. In those who die, ischemic brain damage is overwhelmingly the most important factor seen, and 60 to 70 percent of patients have sustained high intracranial pressure during their clinical course.[11] Clearly, pathophysiological processes that operate in *moderate* head trauma will *also* be operative in most patients with severe head injury, but they may be exacerbated or overshadowed by the severe ischemia induced by a hematoma, high intracranial pressure, or hypoxic ischemic episodes.

Because few patients with moderate head injury die, the pathophysiological processes that lead to the long-term cognitive and behavioral sequelae in this group must largely be inferred from animal model studies. In the few patients subjected to detailed postmortem neuropathological studies (patients who have died of unrelated, extracranial causes, such as pulmonary embolism), the only structural abnormalities consistently reported are small basal contusions, and scattered retraction balls and microglial stars, suggestive of mild diffuse axonal injury.[12,13]

The Choice of Animal Models

Once a candidate compound has been cleared through appropriate short-term and/or long-term toxicology and mutagenicity testing by the pharmaceutical industry, the next goal usually is the demonstration of neuroprotective efficacy in the model most appropriate for the indication being considered. For compounds being evaluated for anti-ischemic efficacy, middle cerebral artery occlusion in the mouse, rat, and cat, used in a stepwise fashion, has proved effective in discriminating neuroprotective effects.[14] Because of the importance of focal ischemia in severe head trauma patients, this approach is also very valid for neurotrauma. Anti-ischemic efficacy alone, however, is not sufficient for newer compounds currently under development; some compounds already in trials have shown powerful effects not only in ischemia models, but also in fluid percussion injury[3] and impact/contusion[15] models, which would indicate likely effects in human neurotrauma.

For the free radical scavenging compound, Tirilazad, currently in clinical trials, the most significant early evidence of efficacy was obtained in impact injury models (Fig. 27-5); more recently, ischemia models also showed excellent benefits from this compound.[16,17] Fluid percussion injury (FPI) models have been discussed extensively elsewhere in this book. Although the FPI model may be used in different configurations to produce "pure" shearing trauma with almost no contusional brain damage, it may also be administered to cause significant focal contusions.[18,19] The difficulty with using FPI for neuroprotection studies revolves around endpoints. Because structural changes are largely absent,

TABLE 27-3 Animal Models Relevant to Human Traumatic Brain Injury

Animal Model and Species	Author (References)	Human Head Injury Component Tested	End Points	Pathomechanisms Shown	Response to Drug Therapy
Subdural Hematoma: Rat	Miller (23) Bullock	Subdural Hematoma Focal Ischemia	Histology Neurochemical CBF ICP Glucose Use	Focal Ischemia Hippocampal Necrosis Delayed High ICP	+++
Intracerebral Hematoma: Rat	Bullock (70) Mendelow Ropper (71)	Intracerebral Hematoma Focal Ischemia	Histology ICP CBF	Focal Ischemia High ICP	+++
Middle Cerebral Artery Occlusion: Rat	Tamura (72)	Focal Ischemia	Histology	Focal Ischemia	++++
Cat	(73)	Focal Ischemia	CBF		++++
Primate	Symon (74) Sundt. (75)	Focal Ischemia	Glucose Use Neurochemical		
Global Forebrain Ischemia: Rat Cat Dog Primate	Smith/Siesjo (76) Pulsinelli (77) Michenfelder (78)	Global Ischemia	Histology-cell counts Glucose Use Neurochemical	Global Ischemia -hippocampal, cortical necrosis	+++ + +
Fluid Percussion: Rat	Dixon (18) McIntosh (19)	"Contusion" Mild DAI Cognitive Effects	Behavioral Neurochemical	Mild DAI Ion Flux	++++
Cat	Sullivan (67) Povlishock	Cognitive Effects	CBF Glucose Use	DAI metabolism	?
Pig	Povlishock Gennarelli	Moderate DAI	Histology	DAI	?
"Penn I, II" Primate	Gennarelli (68) Thibault	Severe DAI Subdural Hematoma Brain Swelling	Histology, EM, Macroscopic, Morphology	Severe DAI Hippocampal Necrosis	---
GM Controlled Impact: Rat	Dixon (25) Lighthall	Contusion	Histology, EM	Delayed Contusion Focal Atrophy	?
Focal Impact: Rat	Nilsson (69) Hillered	Contusion	Histology	Ion Flux	?
Weight Drop: Rat	Marmarou (20) Foda (21) (22)	DAI Hippocampal Necrosis Global Ischemia/Secondary Insult	Behavior, Histology, ICP, CBF	DAI Ischemic Necrosis Wallerian Change Brain Atrophy	++
Mouse	Hall (15)	Neurologic Function	Neurologic Function		+++

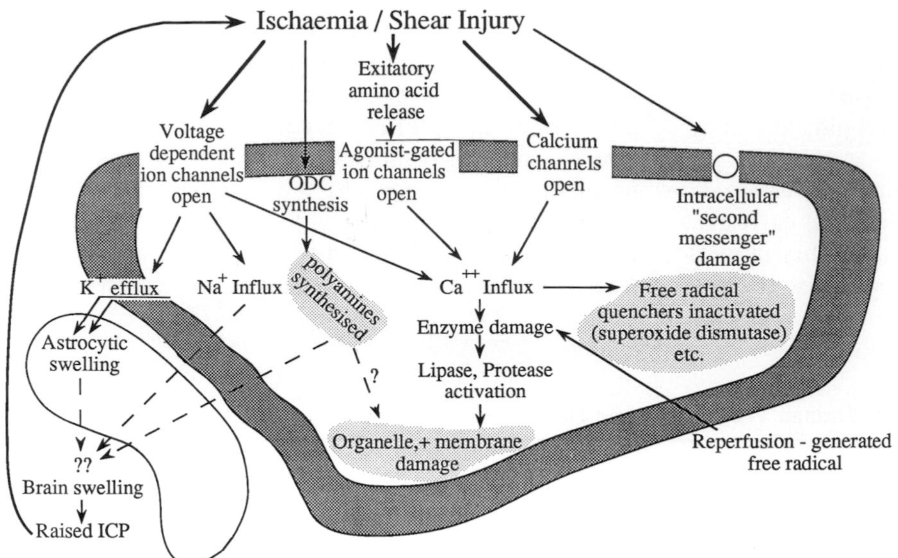

Figure 27-3. Some of the major cerebral biochemical mechanisms against which clinical trials are currently directed.

behavioral end-points have conventionally been used, and these are subject to training effects, inter-observer and inter-test variability, and the subtle effects of strain, species, and testing conditions.

Recently, the Marmarou rat weight-drop model has been devised to mimic severe human head injury.[20,21] This model produces extensive structural changes in the form of retraction balls, neuronal necrosis, cerebral atrophy, and ventricular enlargement, as well as long-lasting behavioral deficits. Although the ability of this model to discriminate drug effects has not yet been well explored, its potential for assessing putatively neuroprotective compounds is considerable.[22]

The rat subdural hematoma model has proved effective for detecting neuroprotective properties in NMDA antagonists, but the variability of the infarction induced by subdural hematoma means that relatively larger numbers of animals must be used to avoid Type-II statistical error.[23] This model may have its greatest value in evaluating compounds that may reduce platelet aggregation and intravascular clotting in the microcirculation, because the ultrastructural microcirculation changes induced by the model are identical to those seen in humans.[24]

The General Motors controlled impact model, described by Dixon et al., has been shown to produce large focal contusions and late tissue deficit at the site of impact.[25] This model may thus reproduce severe human focal injury, and it also may prove useful in testing drugs that affect the microcirculation after trauma.

New compounds being considered for clinical trials in head trauma should demonstrate efficacy across a *wide variety* of models. In Table 27-3, the comparative strengths and weaknesses of current trauma models are shown.

Biochemical Mechanisms for Neuroprotection Trials

Considerable advances have been made in understanding the mechanisms responsible for the patterns of brain damage seen after human head injury (Fig. 27-1). These are considered in detail in other chapters of this text.

In Fig. 27-3, some of the major mechanisms and their interrelationships with pathological events are shown. Currently, drugs targeted at the effects of free radicals, calcium antagonists, and glutamate antagonists have entered clinical trials. Ion channel blockers, adenosine agonists, and drugs active at the microcirculation, such as leucotriene antagonists are being developed for future studies. These six categories of drugs are reviewed in this chapter. Agents that nonspecifically depress brain metabolism (and thus ionic flux), such as barbiturates, etomidate, propofol, and other anesthetic agents, do not necessarily improve outcome after neurotrauma (Chap. 26). Hypothermia has become a focus of interest in this "metabolic" area (Chap. 29).

GLUTAMATE ANTAGONISTS

The amino acid, glutamate, is the most important and widely distributed neurotransmitter in the mammalian brain. It is primarily excitatory, acting via three ionophore-linked receptors [the N-methyl-D-aspartate channel, the kainate channel, and the AMPA channel], and also via a second messenger-linked-"metabotropic" receptor. There are now considerable experimental

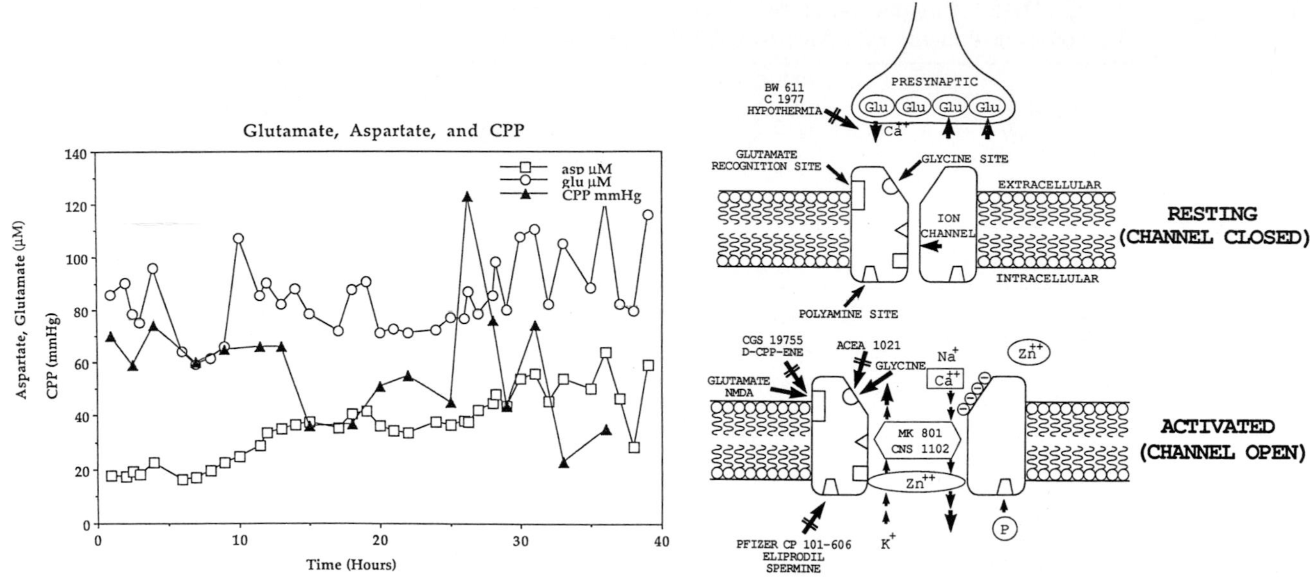

Figure 27-4. *Left.* Pattern of extracellular glutamate release measured by microdialysis, and cerebral perfusion pressure changes, over time, in severe brain injury after a motor vehicle accident (normal glutamate in ECF = 2 ± 1 μl). *Right.* The NMDA channel and associated receptor sites.

data, and limited human data, to support the excitotoxic hypothesis postulated by Olney et al.[26,27] Excessive glutamatergic activation of ionophore-linked receptors may be rapidly toxic to postsynaptic neurons because of excessive calcium influx, as well as excessive metabolic demands placed on neurons and astrocytes by the need to restore ionic homeostasis after glutamate release. Electrophysiological evidence also suggests that excessive glutamatergic neuronal firing may contribute to this process.[28] After trauma, disturbed cerebrovascular control and possibly microcirculatory compression may mean that blood flow is temporarily inadequate to meet these increased metabolic demands, thus leading to cell death.[29,30]

Homeostatic glutamate reuptake mechanisms in the presynaptic dendritic and axonal terminals, and in adjacent astrocytes, act to remove glutamate rapidly from the extracellular space, thus keeping glutamate levels at around 2 μmol in the ECF.[31] Recently, we and others have shown 10- to 50-fold increases in extracellular glutamate levels after human head injury, which persist for up to 4 days after injury[32] (Fig. 27-4).

Several animal models depicting different aspects of the pathophysiological events that follow human brain injury have also demonstrated excessive ECF glutamate and aspartate release and transient increases in glucose utilization in traumatized tissue.[33,34] These models include global cerebral ischemia, focal cerebral ischemia, subdural hematoma, fluid percussion injury, and cortical impact contusion (Tables 27-4 and 27-5). Of greatest interest, however, has been the demonstration in over 300 laboratory studies, using a variety of different models, that these detrimental "excitotoxic" consequences of excitatory amino acid release may be ameliorated or abolished by pre- and post-injury treatment with a variety of glutamate antagonist drugs[3,4] (Fig. 27-4). Such

TABLE 27-4 Comparison of the Effects of Tirilazad Mesylate on the 3-Month Mortality in Patients with Aneursymal Subarachnoid Hemorrhage

Vehicle N = 61		*TIR 0.6 mg/kg/day N = 51*		*TIR 2.0 mg/kg/day N = 42*		*TIR 6.0 mg/kg/day N = 91*	
n	%	n	%	n	%	n	%
			Mortality				
8	14%	4	8%	2	5%	18	20%

Note: The lowest mortality was observed in the 2.0 mg/kg/day dosing group.

TABLE 27-5 Comparison of the Effects of Tirilazad Mesylate on Symptomatic Vasopasm in Patients with Aneursymal Subarachnoid Hemorrhage

Vehicle N = 59		*TIR 0.6 mg/kg/day N = 51*		*TIR 2.0 mg/kg/day N = 42*		*TIR 6.0 mg/kg/day N = 90*	
n	%	n	%	n	%	n	%
Symptomatic Vasospasm							
24	41%	16	31%	8	19%	34	38%

Note: There was a statistically significant difference (P = 0.02) between the placebo and the 2.0 mg/kg/day dosing group.

magnitude and consistency of efficacy (in the laboratory) had not been achieved previously for any other class of neuroprotective compound. The first and best known of the glutamate antagonists is the Merck, Sharp and Dohme compound, MK801, which is now widely used in laboratory studies as the "positive control" or "gold standard" against which other neuroprotective compounds are evaluated. However, this compound has been withdrawn from clinical evaluation because of its side effect profile, although similar compounds have entered Phase II human testing.

Competitive NMDA Antagonists

These have been extensively evaluated in neurotrauma models, and two agents, CGS19755 or "Selfotel" (Ciba-Geigy) and D-CPP-ene (Sandoz), have been evaluated in Phase II clinical studies of severe human head trauma (Fig. 27-2).[3] Both of these agents are high-affinity, potent NMDA-receptor antagonists, with a long brain half-life, probably 12 to 24 hours. However, because of their hydrophilic characteristics, both have relatively poor brain penetration, although this may be greater in areas where blood-to-brain transport has been enhanced due to trauma or ischemia.

All NMDA antagonists are likely to affect behavior because of their high receptor affinity and the widespread distribution of the receptors in behavioral areas of cortex, such as the hippocampus and limbic system. This is in marked contrast to most antiepileptic agents, some of which are glutamate antagonists, but which have uniformly weak receptor binding affinities. Deoxyglucose studies and receptor binding autoradiography have shown that these agents cause activation of limbic structures and suppression of activity in the rest of the cortex, particularly the frontal lobes.[35] In high doses, the drugs also influence the extrapyramidal motor system; in animals, these agents cause psychomotor agitation combined with a catatonic-like immobile state. In both normal human volunteers and patients with CNS pathology, these agents generally cause lethargy and sedation, and occasional visual hallucinations, although most individuals regard these as benign "vivid dreams." These effects may be controlled by concomitant therapy with major tranquilizers, e.g., haloperidol. The activation of the limbic system seems to be readily blocked by most forms of anesthesia, such as volatile agents and barbiturates.[35] These effects are most prominent with MK801, but they were also seen with Selfotel in stroke patients in whom psychomotor effects were the limiting factor in dose escalation.[36]

In 1987, Olney reported that large, single, intravenous bolus doses of high-affinity NMDA antagonists, such as MK801, phencyclidine, CPP, and ketamine, when given to rats, produced a reversible cytoplasmic neuronal vacuolation visible only with careful plastic embedding histology techniques, disappearing within 12 hours.[37] It was shown subsequently that very high doses of MK801 could produce permanent necrosis in a few neurons (1 to 2 percent) in the cingulate cortex. These phenomena have now been extensively investigated, and it has been shown that vacuolation does not occur in higher gyrencephalic animals, such as dogs or primates, whatever dosing paradigm is used. It is probable that vacuolation represents an epiphenomenon associated with the massive (up to 200 percent) increase in metabolism in these neurons.[35] Thus, the rapidity of onset of receptor blockade appears to be a factor in determining the side effects for this group of compounds.

Potential Therapeutic Advantages of Glutamate Antagonists for Head Trauma

Neuroprotective doses of these compounds are sedative. This may be a particular advantage for the treatment of agitated, restless head trauma patients, and preliminary experience in Phase II studies suggests that these agents reduce the amount of conventional sedation required for such patients. The compounds are also anticonvulsants and may increase cerebral blood flow, both effects having therapeutic advantages. Animal studies have shown that these agents do not increase intracranial pressure when Pa_{CO_2} is controlled.[38,39]

Clinical studies

Preliminary Phase II dose-escalation safety studies have been completed with both CGS19755 and D-CPP-ene. CGS19755 exerts an ICP-lowering effect at 5 mg/kg (Fig. 27-2), and because the compound did not affect blood pressure, cerebral perfusion pressure was improved. Phase III studies have begun for CGS19755 (Selfotel).

Noncompetitive NMDA Antagonists

In contrast to competitive NMDA antagonists, which have slow brain penetration and a long brain half-life, the noncompetitive agents, e.g., MK801 and CNS1102, penetrate the brain extremely rapidly, depending on cerebral blood flow. They have high receptor affinity (Ki 3 nm for MK801, 28 nm for CNS1102), and CNS1102 appears to be active in the brain for only 3 to 4 hours after an IV bolus. These agents may thus be theoretically "ideal" neuroprotectives. They would need to be given concomitantly with anesthesia in patients at risk, or during the period at risk, and should then rapidly clear the brain, so that the patient's neurological status could be evaluated within a few hours of the dose.

Because these agents bind *within* the ion channel, their receptor blockade is use-dependent, such that their binding is greatly enhanced in the presence of high glutamate concentrations, as occurs in such situations as head injury and stroke (Fig. 27-4). The potency of these agents may, however, mean that they are most suited to concomitantly sedated patients or those under anesthesia.[35]

CNS1102 (Cambridge Neuroscience) is currently under Phase II evaluation for severe head injury and stroke, and Phase III efficacy studies are planned.

Glycine Site NMDA Antagonists

The ubiquitous structural amino acid, glycine, is a necessary coagonist for activation of the NMDA receptor, and blockade of the so-called glycine modulatory site (Fig. 27-4*B*) has been shown to be neuroprotective in tissue culture experiments and in animal studies with middle cerebral artery occlusion. Recently, glycine antagonists with good brain penetration and high receptor affinity have been developed, and these agents may be less likely to cause psychomotor agitation and hallucinations than competitive and noncompetitive glutamate NMDA blockers. If a similar degree of neuroprotective efficacy can be shown for these compounds, they may possess advantages for therapy of conscious patients with stroke and head injury, particularly the moderately head-injured. New high-affinity glycine NMDA antagonists have demonstrated excellent neuroprotective efficacy in animal models (e.g., ACEA1021), and these agents are about to enter Phase I clinical testing.[40]

Polyamine Site NMDA Antagonists

Polyamines such as spermine, spermidine, and putrescine, have been shown to modify the NMDA receptor allosterically such that sensitivity to glutamate binding is enhanced and opening of the ionophore is facilitated.[41] This receptor has been localized to the F-3 subunit of the NMDA complex, and high-affinity antagonists have been synthesized that have demonstrated excellent neuroprotective effects. What remains unclear, however, is the degree to which supraphysiological concentrations of polyamines may influence events at this receptor. Increased polyamine synthesis has been shown intracellularly, but no increase in polyamines has been shown extracellularly in models of both global and focal ischemia.[42] These compounds have not been fully studied in other trauma models. However, no evidence of use-dependency has been demonstrated at this receptor.

As with glycine-site antagonists, these polyamine-site glutamate antagonists may cause fewer behavioral side effects in conscious patients.

Clinical studies

The Synthelabo compound, Eliprodil, is currently in Phase II testing for severe human head injury in France and the U.K. (Table 27-1). A newly synthesized compound (Pfizer CP101-606-27) with improved brain penetration and receptor affinity has demonstrated the ability to reduce ICP and brain swelling in a model of focal cerebral contusion, and is currently undergoing Phase I human testing and evaluation in trauma models.

Non-NMDA Glutamate Antagonists

Recently, high-affinity antagonists for the AMPA and kainate glutamate receptors have been developed and have demonstrated neuroprotective efficacy in *global and* focal cerebral ischemia, in contrast to the NMDA receptor blockers, which have not consistently demonstrated protection against global ischemia.[43] These compounds are of interest for neurotrauma, because a substantial component of the ischemic damage seen in severe head trauma is global in nature, owing to raised intracranial pressure. The pro-drug in this series, NBQX, is unlikely to be developed clinically because of nephrotoxicity and relatively poor brain penetration. Similar compounds, such as GYKI52466 and LY293558

(Eli Lilly), are potent neuroprotective agents and may prove suitable for clinical use.[44]

Presynaptic Glutamate Release Blockers

Blockade of presynaptic release of glutamate secondary to trauma, ischemia, or increased neuronal activity (e.g., seizures) offers a theoretically attractive strategy for neuroprotection (Fig. 27-4). The success of this approach, however, depends on the premise that most of the pathologically released glutamate during trauma, ischemia, and seizures is of vesicular origin. Studies in animal models have shown that presynaptic glutamate release antagonists, such as BW1003, BW619 (Burroughs-Wellcome) and Enadoline-CI977 (Parke-Davis), are neuroprotective in models of fluid percussion injury, middle cerebral artery occlusion, and global ischemia. These compounds also demonstrate suppression of glutamate release, as detected by microdialysis in the same models, thus elegantly demonstrating a putative mechanism for the neuroprotection.[45] Such mechanistic studies are required in humans. BW619 is now poised to enter Phase II efficacy studies in human stroke and head trauma, and Enadoline, a kappa-opioid agonist with substantial analgesic effect and ability to suppress presynaptic glutamate release, has completed Phase I studies. Because of their different mechanisms of action, both these agents may be free of the behavioral side effects shown by the direct NMDA antagonists.

CALCIUM ANTAGONISTS AND NEUROTRAUMA

Many of the compounds currently being evaluated as neuroprotective agents act by blocking the entry of calcium into cells via different ion channels. By convention, calcium antagonists are those compounds that block calcium entry via the specific L-, N-, and M-type calcium channels, which constitute three of the 14 or more different types of ion channels identified thus far in neuronal membranes.[46]

Dihydropyridine Calcium Antagonists

The dihydropyridine calcium antagonist, Nimodipine (Bayer), was the first compound that conclusively demonstrated neuroprotective efficacy in humans. Five trials to date have demonstrated that Nimodipine improves outcome and reduces the incidence of infarction following subarachnoid hemorrhage when given prophylactically.[47] Subsequent studies from Japan with other calcium antagonists have confirmed these findings for subarachnoid hemorrhage.

Subsequently, two major trials were performed with Nimodipine for severe head injury (Table 27-1). The first of these, in which 351 patients were enrolled, was conducted in the United Kingdom and Finland.[48] Nimodipine was commenced within 24 hours of injury. Although this trial demonstrated a trend toward better outcome in the Nimodipine-treated patients, this was not statistically significant, and therefore, a larger trial in which 850 patients were enrolled, was conducted in more than 20 neurosurgical centers throughout Europe. Nimodipine was given within 12 hours of the injury, and outcome was tested at 6 months, but in this study no conclusive benefit was found.[49] It is, however, interesting that in the subgroup of patients with post-traumatic subarachnoid hemorrhage demonstrable by CT scan, there was significant evidence of benefit in the Nimodipine-treated group. Therefore, a small exploratory study is being performed in Germany to see whether administration of Nimodipine specifically to patients who have CT-demonstrated post-traumatic subarachnoid hemorrhage will demonstrate a beneficial effect.

Dihydropyridine calcium antagonists are limited by brain penetration. Mild hypotension has also been seen in clinical use, although this was not problematical in the head injury trials. Consequently, more recent laboratory efforts have been directed at evaluating different calcium channel blockers, including agents that block multiple calcium channels. These agents are being evaluated particularly for stroke. The potential for this group of compounds in neurotrauma needs further evaluation.

Conotoxins

Omega conotoxin is a 27-amino acid peptide derived from the venom of the fish hunting cone snail; the agent blocks neuronal N-type high-voltage-dependent calcium channels, but not low-voltage T channels.[41] These agents have been used to characterize calcium channels and they are able to block neurotransmitter release and calcium entry into cultured neurons, using the FURA2 method. They have recently been evaluated in CNS trauma models, and have shown efficacy in reducing calcium accumulation and cell death.[50] These compounds are currently under development (Neurex Corp.) and may offer a promising avenue for future therapy in neurotrauma, although their toxicity, pharmacokinetics, brain penetration, and mutagenicity need to be determined.

ADENOSINE ANTAGONISTS

The last few years have seen a tremendous increase in numbers of publications addressing the role of adenosine in both neurological and cardiac function. Adenosine has long been known to act as a local metabolic mediator (autacoid), but its effects are most marked in nervous tissue and the heart. Adenosine is a pyridine nucleotide with a central role in high energy phosphate metabolism (ATP). It freely diffuses through neurons and the extracellular space, but not from the intravascular compartment across endothelial cells, so that its penetration into the brain is limited. Within the CNS, it acts as an inhibitory neuromodulator with the following actions:

1. Reduces neuronal activity (and hence glucose utilization).
2. Reduces levels of excitatory amino acid and other neurotransmitters in the extracellular space.
3. Increases regional cerebral blood flow by vasodilatation (smooth muscle effect).
4. Reduces platelet stickiness within the microvasculature.
5. Reduces leukocyte adherence and activation within the microvasculature.
6. Regulates many intracellular processes by activating second-messenger systems such as adenylate cyclase and G-proteins.[51]

Adenosine acts via specific receptors, the A_1 and A_2 receptors (and possibly the A_3 receptor), which are distributed heterogeneously in the brain. The maximum density of A_1 receptors is in tissues that are maximally vulnerable to focal cerebral ischemia, e.g., hippocampus.

In view of its diverse functional effects, both on neuronal activity and the microvasculature, a potentially neuroprotective role for adenosine is easy to envisage. Unfortunately, adenosine itself is evanescent in the peripheral circulation (t1/2 less than 5 seconds) and it penetrates the brain poorly. Current interest has, therefore, been focused on manipulating adenosine activity via drugs that augment its levels within the tissue by blocking the enzymes that degrade it (e.g., adenosine deaminase) or enzymes that convert it to ATP (e.g., adenylate cyclase).

In addition, specific receptor site agonists have been developed. Compounds that enhance the action of adenosine (adenosine agonists) have been shown to be neuroprotective in a variety of in vitro and in vivo systems such as middle cerebral artery occlusion, global brain ischemia, etc. Unfortunately, most of these agents have poor brain penetration and need to be administered directly via microdialysis or intraventricular injection.

Adenosine antagonists, such as caffeine and theophylline, activate CNS neurons, promote seizures, and in some studies worsen the effects of middle cerebral artery occlusion and in vitro ischemia. Candidate adenosine agonists are being evaluated for future clinical testing as neuroprotective agents.

Adenosine and the Heart

Adenosine is a powerful cardioprotective, increasing myocardial tolerance for ischemia and reducing the effects of reperfusion damage. These agents are also hypotensive, and they dilate the pulmonary vasculature—an effect that can be beneficial in chronic left heart failure. In Phase II studies with patients undergoing coronary artery bypass grafting, the cardioprotectant adenosine release promotor arasine (Acadesine, Gensia Pharmaceuticals) has been shown to produce a significantly lower incidence of myocardial infarction. These agents are also in trials for cardiac arrest therapy. The potential benefits of a neuro- and cardioprotective agent are easily seen, but brain penetration appears to be the major limiting factor with the agents currently available.

ION CHANNEL BLOCKERS

Magnesium

Magnesium is a ubiquitous cation in biological systems, with a large hydration shell, and it occupies a central role in the functioning of the NMDA ionophore (Fig. 27-4*B*). Magnesium is loosely bound by hydrostatic forces within the ion channel, acting as a partial block to prevent the passage of other ions, such as sodium, potassium, calcium, and chloride. For the NMDA receptor to become permeable, the magnesium ion must be displaced from the ionophore, and this is achieved by two main mechanisms: (1) the ionophore undergoes conformational changes when glutamate binds to its receptor, such that the magnesium ion is displaced; (2) partial depolarization of the cell membrane weakens the hydrostatic forces that bind magnesium in the ion channel so that the block is weakened. This creates the possibility that partial depolarization of the cell membrane, due to mechanical forces or energy failure, may reduce the magnesium block and thus potentiate the effects of glutamate on the NMDA receptor, thus allowing ion flux, particularly calcium.[52] It is thus attractive to speculate that neurotrauma may potentiate glutamate neurotoxicity via magnesium displacement.

The therapeutic potential of magnesium revolves around increasing its concentration in extracellular fluid so that its blockade effect on the ion channel can thus be increased. Administration of magnesium sulfate, intravenously, increases the concentration of ECF magnesium, but the problem with this strategy is that magnesium has an extremely narrow therapeutic window. Magnesium rapidly becomes toxic because of neuromuscular blockade, the heart and skeletal musculature being particularly vulnerable. Overdose of magnesium can thus cause cardiac arrest and can weaken respiratory and neuromuscular effort. Despite these limitations, Pinard et al. have shown that magnesium administration can reduce the severity of infarction after middle cerebral artery occlusion, in comparison with a control group; its magnitude of effect was similar to that of MK801.[53] Magnesium has long been used clinically as an anticonvulsant, particularly for seizures due to eclampsia of pregnancy. Gennarelli et al. are currently engaged in a trial of magnesium augmentation in neurotrauma patients. The magnesium was administered orally in this study, thus eliminating the dangers of overdosage with intravenous administration.[68]

ZINC

Zinc is also a ubiquitous cation in biological systems. In addition to its role as a metallo-protein cofactor in many enzymic reactions within cells, zinc also has a weaker modulatory effect on the NMDA receptor and other ion channels. Zinc augmentation may thus stabilize ion channels. Young et al.[5] are engaged in studies to test the hypothesis that zinc augmentation improves outcome after severe head injury.

DRUGS DIRECTED AT NEUTRALIZING FREE RADICAL ACTIVITY

Several hundred in vitro and in vivo animal studies have documented different aspects of free radical activity in the brain, and in cultured neurons, in such pathological conditions as trauma and ischemia.[15–17] Unfortunately, because of the evanescent nature of these highly-charged reactive molecular species, indirect methods must be used to demonstrate their existence and effects (Fig. 27-3). It has thus far been impossible to show concrete evidence of their role in human trauma. The pathobiology of free radicals in trauma is discussed elsewhere in this text. Blockade of free radical activity in the brain has now become possible with the development of effective *antioxidant* molecules, e.g., the amino-steroid series, such as Terelazad (U74006F, Upjohn). Natural antioxidants, such as Vitamins A and C, have also been shown to blunt the effects of free radical generation (Fig. 27-5). These large lipophilic molecules become incorporated into cell walls, where they are preferentially broken down by free radicals, thus preserving the integrity of the intra- and extracellular structures.[15]

An alternative approach has been to employ specific free radical *scavengers.* These are molecules with higher affinity for free radical species than the surrounding tissue components. Thus, the scavengers are themselves either broken down by radical activity or enzymically catalyze the conversion of free radical species to metabolites such as water and oxygen, thus protecting such vulnerable cellular structures as membranes and enzymes.[15] The naturally occurring enzymes, superoxide dismutase and catalase, for example, convert the hydroxyl radical in the following reaction:

$$O_2^{\cdot} + O_2^{\cdot} + 2H^+ \xrightarrow{\text{SOD}} H_2O_2 +$$
$$O_2^{\cdot} \text{ and } H_2O_2 \xrightarrow{\text{catalase}} H_2O + O_2$$

The thiol, dimethyl-thiourea acts in a similar way, such that the thiol groupings are broken down by free radical activity. These substances have been extensively studied in vivo and in vitro[46,54] and have shown potent neuropro-

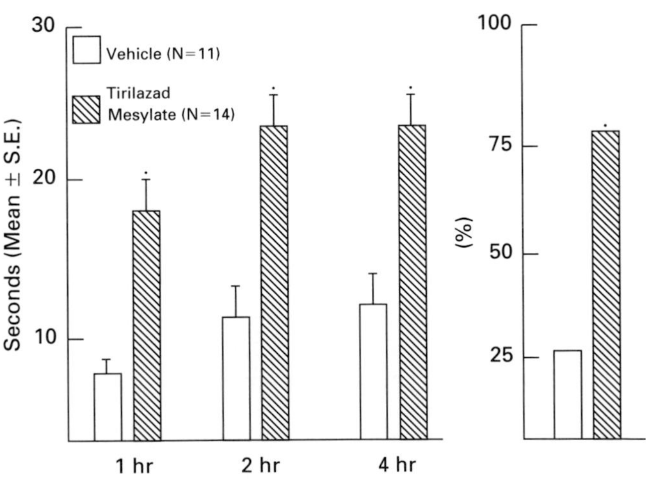

Figure 27-5. The effect of Tirilazad mesylate (U74006F) on early neurological recovery (*left*) grip score, and one-week survival (*right*) in mice subjected to severe concussive head injury. Vehicle or drug was given by IV injection, 5 minutes and 1.5 hours post-injury.[16]

tective effect in studies using middle cerebral artery occlusion in the cat.[55]

Polyethylene Glycol-Conjugated Superoxide Dismutase (PEG-SOD)

Native superoxide dismutase enzyme with a molecular weight of 64,000D has been purified, and it may be extracted in high concentrations from bovine tissues. When this enzyme is administered systemically, it has a short half-life—around 30 minutes—but when conjugated to polyethylene glycol, its half-life is extended to around 48 hours, and its penetration into brain is enhanced.[9] Evidence suggests that this compound, PEG-SOD, exerts its maximal beneficial effect on the microvasculature and on perivascular astrocytes.

Clinical studies

PEG-SOD (Sterling-Winthrop Pharmaceuticals) has now been evaluated for a number of indications in humans, including rheumatoid arthritis, organ preservation in transplantation surgery, and severe head trauma.[9] Allergic side effects are very rare.

In an important recent Phase II safety study performed at the Medical College of Virginia and in Maryland, this agent showed a trend toward improved outcome and easier control of intracranial pressure in a placebo-controlled multiple-dose study in 104 severely head-injured patients.[9] This is the first study in which a significant improvement in outcome has been shown in severe human head injury (Fig. 27-2*B*). Based on this evidence, two Phase III studies, involving 30 different U.S. centers, have recently been completed. In the first of these, (*Protocol 005*) outcome was 9 percent better in the 10,000μ PE SOD group, than placebo ($p = 0.15$) at 3 months. Outcome was improved across all categories of the Glasgow outcome scale. This is an extremely important finding, because PEG-SOD is a single-dose, safe drug, suitable for use by emergency personnel, even at the roadside. The results of the larger 480 patient per group protocol 006, are therefore awaited with great interest.

Antioxidants—Amino Steroids

These large molecular weight synthetic derivatives of Vitamin E have demonstrated in vitro and in vivo efficacy in animal models of neurotrauma (fluid percussion and impact contusion types) and cerebral ischemia, using both structural and behavioral end-points.[15–17,54] There is clear evidence that these compounds reduce damage to the microvasculature and reduce vasospasm in models of subarachnoid hemorrhage, and the incidence of neurological deficit in primates after SAH was reduced by Tirilazad in one study.[53]

Clinical studies

A large European multicenter placebo-controlled three-arm trial with Tirilazad, after human subarachnoid hemorrhage, has shown a convincing 50 percent reduction in the incidence of neurological deficits due to vasospasm (Table 27-3). Outcome was also significantly improved in this study.

Three large multicenter trials in head injury have recently been completed (Table 27-1). For these studies, both severe and moderately injured patients were enrolled, and analysis will be stratified accordingly. Analysis and follow up is currently ongoing, and no data is currently available (July, 1995).

FUTURE DEVELOPMENTS

Current preclinical research is directed toward the development of new drugs that may act at different sites within the brain. Some of those that appear promising are listed below:

Agents that Hyperpolarize the Cellular Membrane

Evidence from several studies has begun to suggest that depolarization of neuronal and glial membranes occurs due to mechanical deformation of tissue, such as that following neurotrauma.[56] Although this initial depolarization phase may be brief and short-lived, cellular membranes may be rendered more vulnerable to subsequent depolarization by agonists, owing to *structural conformational changes* in ion channels.

Several studies have also shown that depolarization of cell membranes occurs when energy metabolism fails due to ischemia or hypoxia.[55] Our group has recently confirmed that very low levels of regional cerebral perfusion occur in the periphery of focal contusions, suggesting that ischemia may be an important mechanism in perpetuating ion flux, and leading to consequent cell swelling, and mass effect.[57] Several pharmacological strategies can be proposed to influence transmembrane depolarization and ion flux. For example, increasing the extracellular magnesium levels may augment the "magnesium block" which renders the NMDA receptor more resistant to depolarization.

Agents that block the passage of ions through voltage-operated channels may also stabilize cell membranes. The neurotoxins, tetrodotoxin and ouabain, are examples, but these toxins could never be considered for development as drugs because of their nonselective action and the extremely narrow margin between the ED50 and LD50. Many anticonvulsants, such as phenytoin, phosphenytoin, and sodium valproate, also act by this mechanism. Recently, specific 5HT1A agonists that act by stabilizing cell membrane have been evaluated in this context.

Kimelberg et al. have shown that the formation of cytotoxic edema can be reduced in trauma models by the administration of compounds with diuretic properties similar to furosemide, which block the chloride and sodium channels in neural membranes and have good brain penetration.[58] These compounds may be particularly suitable for combination therapy together with specific ion channel blockers such as NMDA antagonists.

New Drugs Active at the Microcirculation and Endothelium

Recently, pathophysiological studies have shown that a profound early reduction of global cerebral blood flow occurs in the majority of severely head-injured patients.[59] In patients with focal lesions such as acute subdural hematoma, hemispheric brain swelling, and focal cerebral contusion, this early reduction in regional CBF persists for long periods, sufficient to cause subsequent ischemic damage.[57] Human ultrastructural studies have shown that the microvasculature is grossly abnormal in patients with focal lesions, and this accords with the regional CBF changes.[60] The principal microcirculatory abnormalities are: (1) leukocyte plugging and increased leukocyte adherence to the endothelium; (2) perivascular astrocyte swelling; and (3) compression or collapse of the lumen of the microvasculature. These ultrastructural changes have been seen as early as 6 hours after injury.[60] Similar microvascular abnormalities have been reported in animal models of focal and global brain ischemia, and trauma.[61] In vivo confocal microscopy studies have shown that leukocytes and platelets become increasingly adherent to the endothelium, with increased endothelial pseudopodial activity and leukocyte activation.[62]

Shear damage to endothelial cells may result in the release of mediators such as cytokines, for example, platelet aggregating factor, leukotrienes, and the interleukins.[63] Recently, there has been a surge of interest in the gaseous neurotransmitter, nitric oxide, which has been demonstrated in large concentrations within endothelial cells (although nitric oxide is primarily a vasodilator in the microcirculation).[64]

Neuroprotection studies using interleukin antagonists and platelet aggregating factor antagonists have shown that the volume of ischemic damage is reduced after middle cerebral artery occlusion.[63] Prostaglandin antagonists that decrease platelet aggregation (such as indomethacin) have long been recognized as agents that may reduce the extent of brain edema formation in trauma models and ischemia—both focal and global.[63]

Recently, studies with a model of intracerebral hematoma have demonstrated that the extent of perilesional edema and neuronal damage are reduced by whole-body irradiation in the rat, which reduces the leukocyte count and platelet numbers.[64,65] This accumulation of evidence incriminating the microcirculation suggests that early therapy with agents directed at stabilizing the endothelium, preventing free radical or cytokine activation within the endothelium, and leukocyte activation, will play an important role in reducing the degree of ischemic damage after human head injury. Candidate compounds in this category include: PAF antagonists, PEG-SOD, leukotriene LT_4 antagonists, and antibodies directed at cytokines.[63] Recently, human Phase I trials have been completed with an LT_4 antagonist, and Phase II mechanistic studies in trauma, are planned.

SYNERGISTIC THERAPY—THERAPEUTIC "COCKTAILS"

Neurosurgeons often indicate that the concept of a polyfunctional therapeutic "cocktail" is attractive for neurotrauma patients. Such a cocktail may include therapies directed at blocking free radicals, excitatory amino acids, and even a calcium channel blocking component. A putatively neuroprotective mixture was previously advocated—"the Sendai cocktail" for high-risk cerebrovascular surgery—but its efficacy was never demonstrated by a controlled trial.[65]

There are two reasons why such an approach is unlikely to be demonstrably effective, at least for the next 5 years:

Very few animal studies have been designed to seek synergistic effects between different forms of neuroprotective therapy. Recently, Buchan et al. tested the combination of MK801 and NBQX in a rat global ischemia model, and the combination of the two agents proved less effective than either drug alone.[6] Similarly, Young et al. have demonstrated in their spinal cord injury model that the addition of the ganglioside GM-1 to therapy with methylprednisolone counteracted the benefits of methylprednisolone, worsening outcome.[5] The design of such experiments to seek synergistic effects is extremely difficult. Considerations of power analysis require much larger numbers of animals because the magnitude of effect in each group may be small, and multiple comparisons necessitate that significance can be drawn only at higher p values.

The second reason that synergistic studies will be difficult to conduct is that the pharmaceutical industry remains resistant to the idea of trials with combinations of therapy across different companies, for obvious commercial reasons.

Despite these problems however, there is clearly an urgent scientific need for such studies because of the theoretical advantage that simultaneous blockade of calcium channels and glutamate operated channels, for example, may confer, or that the simultaneous blockade of free radical generation and ion flux could be beneficial. Such experiments, therefore, need to become an important focus for the next 5 years, in anticipation of single neuroprotective agents being shown to confer at least some benefit in neurotrauma.

PEDIATRIC CONSIDERATIONS

Although neurotrauma is a major cause of death and disability in children, at present no "neuroprotection" trials are currently being performed in the pediatric age group. This is primarily because of the legal and ethical restraints on clinical experiments in children. NMDA antagonists, furthermore, theoretically may inhibit synaptogenesis in the developing nervous system. Nevertheless, new therapies must be tried in this age group, and the weak noncompetitive NMDA antagonist, dextrorphan, or the safe free radical agents PEG-SOD and Tirilazad, are obvious choices.

CONCLUSIONS

Pharmacological agents can never provide a "magic bullet" for an injury process, which is the consequence of excessive shearing forces upon a poorly supported, vulnerable brain. However, there is now a real prospect, for the first time in clinical neuroscience, that improved pathophysiological knowledge will lead to successful targeted "neuroprotective therapies." The situation may prove to be analogous to the introduction of antibiotics into clinical practice over 50 years ago. However, the potential benefit of such agents on outcome can be realized only in patients who receive optimal prehospital care, resuscitation, speedy diagnosis, and optimized ICU management. Rigorously designed clinical trials are mandatory to evaluate the increasing number of candidate neuroprotective compounds. There is little doubt that during the next decade, the enormous advances in neuroprotective pharmacology of the last 10 years will fundamentally alter care of patients who suffer CNS trauma and stroke.

REFERENCES

1. Ward A Jr: Atropine in the treatment of closed head injury. *J Neurosurg* 1950; 7:398–402.
2. Sachs E Jr: Acetylcholine and serotonin in the spinal fluid. *J Neurosurg* 1957; 14:22–27.
3. Bullock R, Fujisawa H: The role of glutamate antagonist for the treatment of CNS injury. *J Neurotrauma* 1992; 9(suppl 2):S443–S461.
4. Bullock R: Opportunities for neuroprotective drugs in clinical management of head injury. *J Emerg Med* 1993; 11:23–30.
5. Constantini S, Young W: The effects of methylprednisolone and the ganglioside GN1 on acute spinal cord injury in rats. *J Neurosurg* 1994; 80:97–112.
6. Xue D, Hung Z, Barnes K, et al: Delayed treatment with AMPA but not NMDA antagonists reduces neocortical infarction. *J Cereb Blood Flow Metab* 1994; 14:251–261.
7. Braakman R et al: A multicenter trial of the efficacy of nimodipine on outcome after severe head injury. *J Neurosurg* 1994; 80.
8. Grossett DG, O'Shaughnessy D, Picard JG, Bullock MR: Effect of intravenous calcitonin gene-related peptide upon cerebral vasospasm following severe head injury, in, Avezaat CJ, Van Eijndhoven JHM, Maas AIR, Jans JJ. (eds). *Intracranial Pressure VIII.* Berlin: Springer Verlag, 1993; 322–326.
9. Muizelaar JP, Marmarou A, Young HF, et al: Improving the outcome of severe head injury with the oxygen radical scavenger polyethylene glycol conjugated superoxide dismutase: A phase II trial. *J Neurosurg* 1993; 78:375–382.
10. Bullock R, Katake A, Stewart L, et al: The glutamate antagonist CGS 19755 lowers ICP and improves CPP in severely head injured humans, in Nagai H, Kamiya K, Ishiis (eds): *Intracranial Pressure IX.* Tokyo: Springer Verlag, 1994; 238–241.
11. Miller JD, Becker DP, Ward JD, et al: Significance of intracranial hypertension in severe head injuries. *J Neurosurg* 1977; 47:503–516.
12. Povlishock JT, Becker DP, Cheng CLY, Vaughan GW: Axonal change in minor head injuries. *J Neuropathol Exp Neurol* 1983; 42:225–242.
13. Adams JH, Graham DI, Murray LS, Scott G: Diffuse axonal injury due to nonmissile head injury in humans. *Ann Neurol* 1982; 12:557–563.
14. McCulloch J, Bullock R, Teasdale GM: Excitate amino acid antagonists: Opportunities for the treatment of is-

chemic brain damage in man, in Meldrum BS (ed): *Excitatory Amino Acid Antagonists.* London: Blackwell Scientific, 1991:287–327.

15. Hall ED, McCall JM, Means ED: Therapeutic potential of the lazaroids [21-amino steroids] in acute CNS trauma, ischemia and subarachnoid hemorrhage. *Adv Pharmacol* 1994; 28:221–268.
16. Hall ED, Yonkers PA, McCall JM, Braughler JM: Effects of the 21-amino steroid U-74006 Terezezad on experimental head injury in mice. *J Neurosurg* 1988; 68:456–461.
17. Park CK, Hall ED: Dose response analysis of the effect of 21-amino steroid Terelazad mesylate [U-74006F] upon neurological outcome and ischemic brain damage in permanent focal cerebral ischemia. *Brain Res* 1994.
18. Dixon LE, Lyeth BG, Povlishock JT: A fluid percussion model of experimental brain injury in the rat. *J Neurosurg* 1987; 67:110–119.
19. McIntosh TK, Vink R, Noble L: Traumatic brain injury in the rat: Characterization of a lateral fluid percussion model. *Neuroscience* 1989; 28[1]:233–244.
20. Marmarou A, Foda AM, VandenBrink W, et al: A new model of diffuse brain injury in rats. Part I: Pathophysiology and Biomechanics. *J Neurosurg* 1994; 80:291–301.
21. Foda AM, Marmarou A: A new model of diffuse brain injury in rats. Part II: Morphological Classification. *J Neurosurg* 1994; 80:302–314.
22. Shirotani T, Foda AM, Marmarou A: Effect of VA-045 on behavioral outcome following rodent impact acceleration injuries. In, Nagai H, Kamiyak K, Ishii S, (eds). *Intracranial Pressure IX.* Tokyo: Springer Verlag, 1994; 409–412.
23. Miller JD, Bullock R, Graham DI, et al: Ischemic brain damage in a model of acute subdural hematoma. *Neurosurgery* 1990; 27:433–439.
24. Fujisawa H, Maxwell WG, Graham DI, et al: Focal microvascular occlusion after acute subdural hematoma in the rat: A mechanism for ischemic damage and brain swelling? *Acta Neurochir* 1994; S60:193–197.
25. Dixon CE, Clifton GL, Lighthall JW, Yaghmai AA: A controlled cortical impact model of traumatic brain injury in the rat. *J Neurosci Methods* 1991; 39:253–262.
26. Olney JW, Ho OL, Rhee Z: Cytotoxic effects of acidic and sulphur-containing amino acids on the infant mouse central nervous system. *Exp Brain Res* 1991; 14:61–76.
27. Rothman SM, Onley JW: Glutamate and pathophysiology of hypoxic-ischemic brain damage. *Ann Neurol* 1986; 19:105–111.
28. Rothman S: Synaptic release of excitatory amino acid neurotransmitter mediates ischemic neuronal death. *J Neurosci* 1984; 4:1884–1891.
29. Kuroda Y, Bullock R: Failure of cerebral blood flow-metabolism coupling after acute subdural hematoma in the rat. *Neurosurgery* 1992; 31:1062–1071.
30. Ginsberg MD: Local metabolic responses to cerebral ischemia. *Cereb Brain Metab Rev* 1990; 2:58–93.
31. Nicholls D, Atwell D: The release and uptake of excitate amino acids. *Trends Pharmacol Sci* 1990; 11:462–468.
32. Bullock R, Zauner A, Woodward JJ, et al: Excitate amino acid release in severe human head trauma: The role of intracranial pressure and cerebral perfusion pressure changes. In, Nagai H, Kamiya K, Ishii S (eds): *Intracranial Pressure IX.* Tokyo: Springer-Verlag, 1994; 264–267.
33. Yoshino A, Hovda DA, Kawamata T, et al: Dynamic changes in local cerebral glucose utilization following cerebral concussion in rats: Evidence of a hyper and subsequent hypo metabolic state. *Brain Res* 1991; 561:106–119.
34. Katayama Y, Becker DP, Tamura T, Hovda DA: Massive increase in extracellular potassium and the indiscriminate release of glutamate following concussive brain injury. *J Neurosurg* 1990; 73:889–900.
35. McCulloch J, Iversen LL: Autoradiographic assessment of the effects of N-methyl-D-aspartate [NMDA] receptor antagonist *in vivo. Neurochem Res* 1991; 16:951–963.
36. Grotta J and the CGS19755 study group: Safety and tolerability of the glutamate antagonist CGS19755 in acute stroke patients. *Stroke* 1994; 25[Abstract 52]:12.
37. Onley JW, Labruyere J, Price MT: Pathological changes induced in cerebral cortical neurons by phencyclidine and related drugs. *Science* 1989; 244:1360–1362.
38. Stewart L, Bullock R, Jones M, et al: The cerebral hemodynamic and metabolic effects of the competitive NMDA antagonist CGS 19755 in humans with severe head injury. *J Neurotrauma* 1993; 10[suppl 1]:S104.
39. Kuroda Y, Fujisawa H, Strebel S, et al: Effect of neuroprotective N-methyl-D-aspartate antagonist on increased intracranial pressure: Studies in the rat acute subdural hematoma model. *Neurosurgery* 1994; 35:1–7.
40. Johnson JW, Ascher P: Glycine potentiates the N-methyl-D-aspartate response in cultured mouse brain neurons. *Nature* 1987; 325:529–531.
41. Carter C, Benavidies J, Dana C, et al: Noncompetitive NMDA receptor antagonists acting on the polyamine site, in excitate amino acid antagonists. Meldrum BS (ed): Oxford: Blackwell Scientific, 1991:130–163.
42. Paschen W: Polyamine metabolism in reversible cerebral ischemia. *Cerebrovasc Brain Metab Rev* 1992; 4[1]:59–88.
43. Buchan AM, Lee IH, Cho S, Pulsinelli WA: Blockade of the AMPA receptor prevents CA1 hippocampal injury following severe but transient forebrain ischemia in adult rats. *Neurosci Lett* 1991; 132:255–258.
44. Bullock R, Graham DI, Swanson S, McCullough J: Neuroprotective effect of the AMPA receptor antagonist LY-293558 in focal cerebral ischemia in the cat. *J Cereb Blood Flow Metab* 1994; 14:466–471.
45. Leach MJ, Swan JH, Eisenthal D, Dapson M, Nobbs M: BW619 C89, a glutamate release inhibitor protects against focal cerebral ischemic damage. *Stroke* 1993; 24:1063–1067.
46. Siesjo BK: Pathophysiology and treatment of focal cerebral ischemia: Part I. *J Neurosurg* 1992; 77:169–184.
47. Pickard JG, Mae GD, Illingworth R: Effect of a calcium antagonist on cerebral infarction and outcome after subarachnoid hemorrhage: British aneurysm nimodipine trials. *Br Med J* 1989; 298:636–642.
48. Teasdale G, Bailey I, Bell A, et al: The effect of nimodipine on outcome after head injury: A prospective randomized controlled trial. The British/Finnish Coopera-

tive Head Injury Trial Group. *Acta Neurochir (Wien)* 1990; 51:315–316.
49. Takeda K, Nordmann JJ: Omega conotoxin: Calcium currents and neurosecretion, in Cann PM (ed): *Methods in Neurosciences, Vol. 8, Neurotoxins.* San Diego: Academic Press, 1992:202–223.
50. Badie H, Fu K, Samii A, Hovda DA: A selective internal calcium blocker attenuates the injury induced accumulation of calcium following experimental brain injury. *J Neurosurg* 1993; 10:S161.
51. Miller LP, Shu C: Therapeutic potential for adenosine receptor activation in ischemic brain injury. *J Neurotrauma* 1992; 9(suppl 2):S563–S577.
52. Foster AC: Channel blocking drugs for the NMDA receptor, in Meldrum BS (ed): *Excitate Amino Acid Antagonists.* Oxford: Blackwell Scientific, 1991:164–179.
53. Pinard E, Izumi Y, Roussel S, Seylaz J: Comparative effects of magnesium chloride and MK-801 on infarct volume after MCA occlusion in Fisher-344 rats, in Globus MY, Dietrich WD (eds): *The Role of Neurotransmitters in Brain Injury.* New York: Plenum Press, 1992:93–98.
54. Siesjo BK: Pathophysiology and treatment of focal cerebral ischemia. Part II: Mechanisms of damage and treatment. *J Neurosurg* 1992; 77:334–344.
55. Braughler JM, Pregenzer JF, Chase RL, et al: Novel 21-amino steroids as potent inhibitors of iron-dependent peroxidation. *J Biol Chem* 1987; 262:10438–10440.
56. Sachs F: Mechanical transduction by membrane ion channels: A mini review. *Mol Cell Biochem* 1991; 104:57–60.
57. Bullock R, Schroeder ML, Muizelaar JP, et al: Pericontusional brain edema: Evidence for microvascular hypoperfusion in humans. In, Nagai H, Kamiya K, Ishii S (eds.): *Intracranial Pressure IX.* Tokyo: Springer-Verlag, 1994; 276–279.
58. Kimelberg HK, Rose JW, Barron KD, et al: Astrocytic swelling in traumatic-hypoxic brain injury-beneficial effects of an inhibitor of anion exchange transport and glutamate uptake in glial cells. *Mol Chem Neuropathol* 1989; 11:1–31.
59. Bouma GJ, Muizelaar JP, Stringer WA, et al: Ultra-early evaluation of regional cerebral blood flow in severely head injured patients using stable Xenon-enhanced computerized tomography. *J Neurosurg* 1992; 77:360–368.
60. Bullock R, Maxwell WL, Graham DI, et al: Glial swelling following human cerebral contusion: An ultrastructural study. *J Neurol Neurosurg Psychiatry* 1991; 54:427–434.
61. Giulian D, Chen J, Ingeman JE, et al: The role of mononuclear phagocytes in wound healing after traumatic injury to adult rodent brain. *J Neurosci* 1989; 9:4416–4429.
62. Lorenzl S, Koedel U, Dirnagl U, et al: Imaging of leukocyte endothelium interaction using *in vivo* confocal laser scanning microscopy during the early phase of experimental meningitis. *J Infect Dis* 1993; 168(4):927–933.
63. Rothwell NJ, Relton JK: Involvement of Interleukin-1 and lipocortin-1 in ischemic brain damage. *Cerebrovasc Brain Metabol Rev* 1993; 5:178–198.
64. Snyder SH: Nitric oxide: First in a new class of neurotransmitters. *Science* 1992; 24:257(5069)494–496.
65. Kochanek PM, Dutka AJ, Hallenbeck JM: Indomethacin, prostacyclin, and heparin improved post-ischemic cerebral blood flow without effecting early post-ischemic granulocyte accumulation. *Stroke* 1987; 18:634–637.
66. Kane PJ, Modah P, Strachan RD, et al: The effect of immunosuppression with whole body and regional irradiation on the development of cerebral edema in the rat model of intracerebral hemorrhage. *Acta Neurochir (Wien)* 1990; (suppl)51:52–54.
67. Sullivan HG, Martinez J, Becker DP: Fluid percussion injury model of mechanical brain injury in the cat. *J Neurosurg* 1976; 45:520–534.
68. Gennarelli TA, Thibault LE, Adams JH, et al: Diffuse axonal injury and traumatic coma in the primate. *Ann Neurol* 1982; 12:564–574.
69. Nilsson P, Hillered L, Olsson Y, et al: Regional changes in interstitial and calcium levels following cortical compression contusion trauma in rats. *J Cereb Blood Flow Metab* 1993; 13:183–192.
70. Bullock R, Mendelow AD, Teasdale GM, Graham DI: Intracranial hemorrhage induced arterial pressure in the rat. Part I. Description of technique, ICP changes and neuropathological findings. *Neurol Res* 1984; 6:184–188.
71. Ropper AH, Zervas NT: Cerebral blood flow after experimental basal ganglia hemorrhage. *Ann Neurol* 1982; 11:266–271.
72. Tamura A, Graham DI, McCullough J: Focal cerebral ischemia in the rat: II. Regional cerebral blood flow determined by 14C-iodoantipyrine autoradiography following middle cerebral artery occlusion. *J Cereb Blood Flow Metab* 1981; 1:61–69.
73. Weinstein PR, Anderson GG, Telles DA: Neurological deficit and cerebral infarction of temporary middle cerebral artery occlusion in unanesthetized cats. *Stroke* 1986; 17:318–324.
74. Symon L, Pasztor E, Branston NM: The distribution and density of reduced cerebral blood flow following acute middle cerebral artery occlusion: An experimental study by the technique of hydrogen clearance in baboons. *Stroke* 1974; 5:355–364.
75. Sundt TM Jr, Michenfelder JD: Focal transient cerebral ischemia in the squirrel monkey. Effect on brain adenosine triphosphate and lactate levels with electrocorticography and pathologic correlation. *Circ Res* 1972; 30:703–712.
76. Smith ML, Auer RN, Siesjo BK: The density and distribution of ischemic brain injury in the rat following two to ten minutes of forebrain ischemia. *Acta Neurol Pathol* 1984; 64:319–332.
77. Pulsinelli WA, Brierley JB, Plum F: Temporal profile of neuronal damage in a model of transient forebrain ischemia. *Ann Neurol* 1982; 11:491–498.
78. Steen PA, Newberg LA, Milde JH, Michenfelder JD: Nimodipine improves cerebral blood flow and neurologic recovery after complete cerebral ischemia in the dog. *J Cereb Blood Flow Metab* 1983; 3:38–43.

CHAPTER 28

HYPERBARIC OXYGEN THERAPY IN HEAD INJURY

Gaylan L. Rockswold

SYNOPSIS

A review of the medical literature suggests that hyperbaric oxygen (HBO) therapy may have some benefit in the treatment of brain injury. Possible mechanisms of action include reduction in intracranial pressure due to cerebral vasoconstriction, improvement in glucose metabolism, and reduction of cerebral edema. However, HBO also has a potentially harmful effect on the injured brain by supplying oxygen for free radical reactions that result in iron-catalyzed lipid peroxidation. Further basic and clinical research is required to define the ideal HBO treatment paradigm, study potential toxicity, and evaluate combination treatments that may ameliorate its toxic effects.

INTRODUCTION

The history of hyperbaric oxygen (HBO) for the treatment of brain injury is long and somewhat checkered. However, a survey of this published material suggests that this modality may indeed have some potential use in brain injury therapy. This chapter reviews the clinical studies that relate to HBO in brain injury, discusses its potential mechanisms of action, and finally, defines the studies required to determine what role hyperbaric oxygen has in the treatment of brain injury in the future.

REVIEW OF CLINICAL STUDIES

Mogami et al. described the use of HBO in 66 patients, 51 of whom had severe head injuries.[1] The HBO treatment was usually given at a pressure of 2 atmospheres absolute (ata) for 1 hour once or twice daily; six of the treatments, however, were given at 3 ata for 30 minutes. In total, 143 treatments were given to the 66 patients. The treatment schedule or number of treatments given to each patient was not stated. During HBO, 33 patients (50 percent) showed clinical improvement, 21 of them to "a remarkable degree." The most impressive responses were increased awareness and responsiveness. Patients who were comatose rapidly became responsive to painful stimuli and simple commands. However, most of the favorable responses were temporary, and regression occurred immediately after decompression. There were three cases in which HBO appeared to be of permanent benefit. In one case described, a severely head-injured patient received HBO treatments seven times during five days, which was well above the average number of treatments per patient.

A clinical trial performed by Holbach in Germany suggests that HBO applied systematically may improve outcome in severe head injuries.[2] Of 99 patients with a traumatic mid-brain syndrome, every second patient was treated with HBO. Patients received from one to seven HBO treatments at 1.5 atmospheres (atm) for 20 to 30 minutes. In most cases the treatments were given between the second and tenth day of hospitalization. The overall mortality for the 49 HBO-treated patients was 33 percent; for the 50 control patients it was 74 percent ($p \leq 0.01$ by Chi-squared analysis). Patients under 30 years old with cerebral contusions particularly benefited from HBO. Functional outcome was also improved and 33 percent of the HBO patients made a good recovery, as compared with 6 percent of the control ($p \leq 0.01$ by 1-tailed Fisher's exact test). Injury severity was not well assessed and the randomization process was not adequate. Nonetheless, the study suggested a definite beneficial effect.

Artu et al. also attempted a prospective controlled study of the effect of HBO in 60 severely head-injured patients.[3] They were unable to demonstrate any statistically significant difference in the treated versus control group except in patients under 30 years old who had a "brain stem contusion" without supratentorial mass lesions. There were several problems with this study. Treatment was administered at 2.5 ata for 60 minutes. This high pressure resulted in the interruption of treatment of 11 patients because of pulmonary toxicity. In addition, there was an average time delay of 4.5 days before HBO treatment was instituted. This would appear to be the critical time for the development of cerebral edema and increased intracranial pressure. Other studies have shown that 2.5 ata does not provide for optimal cerebral glucose metabolism or reduction in intracranial pressure.

Sukoff and Ragatz reported 50 patients with traumatic cerebral edema who were treated with HBO.[4] Intracranial pressure monitoring was carried out in 10 patients. In these 10 patients, clinical improvement during and following treatment was observed in most. In the 40 patients who did not undergo ICP monitoring in the HBO chamber, 22 patients reportedly improved clinically while undergoing their treatments. However, specific categorization such as Glasgow recovery scales or control groups were not given.

In 1983 we undertook a prospective, randomized clinical trial to evaluate the treatment of severely head-injured patients with HBO.[5] During the next 6 years, 168 patients were randomized into the study. Patients were included if they had a total Glasgow coma scale (GCS) score of 9 or less for at least 6 hours. Patients were not randomized into the study during the first 6 hours following hospital admission because rapid neurological improvement or deterioration can occur at this time. After the GCS score was established and consent obtained, the patient was randomized, stratified by GCS score and age, into the treatment or control group. All patients received intensive neurosurgical care, according to protocol, covering stabilization in the emergency department, surgical management, medical treatment, and the management of intracranial pressure (ICP). Medical management was consistent with standardized management practices in institutions that routinely treat severely head-injured patients.[6] HBO treatments were given in a Sechrist monoplace hyperbaric chamber. Compression with 100 percent oxygen to 1.5 ata occurred at a rate of 1 pound per square inch (psi) per minute. The patient was kept at depth for 60 minutes and was decompressed at the same rate. Treatments were given every 8 hours for 2 weeks or until the patient was brain-dead or could consistently follow simple commands. When it became apparent that ICP was not decreasing during the HBO treatments as anticipated, we postulated that ear pain might be a contributing factor. Therefore, bilateral myringotomies were performed in the last 46 of the 84 patients in the HBO group.

The subjects were divided into broad age categories: 0–29 years, 30–59 years, and 60 years and older. The GCS strata included individual entry scores of 3 through 9. This preassigned stratification gave some protection against the chance development of significant imbalance between the HBO and the control groups in terms of age and initial severity of injury. Although the subjects were examined several times during their recovery, comparisons were based on the 12-month follow-up. We conducted separate statistical analyses for the treatment effects on subjects with entry GCS scores of 3, 4, 5, and 6 and the group of values 7 to 9.

One hundred sixty-eight patients were entered into the study: 84 into the HBO treatment group and 84 into the control group (Table 28-1). Indicators of injury severity and prognosis were very similar for the two groups.

The average amount of time from injury to the first HBO treatment was 26 hours. Eighty patients received a total of 1688 HBO treatments, for a per-patient average of 21 treatments.[5] Twenty-two patients experienced 24 protocol deviations; the most frequent deviation was in the administration of the HBO (Table 28-2).

Considering the number of treatments delivered, relatively few complications occurred. The most frequent complication was pulmonary, manifested by an increasing FiO_2 requirement and chest x-ray infiltrates. In ten patients, HBO had to be stopped permanently. Only two patients had an isolated generalized seizure. All study patients were treated with phenytoin sodium. Two

TABLE 28-1 Characteristics of 168 Head-Injured Patients in this Series

Factor*	*Treatment Group* Hyperbaric O_2	Control
No. of patients	84	84
Average age (yrs)	32	33
Sex (males)	77%	71%
Average entry GCS score	6.2	6.2
Operative mass lesion(s)	39%	49%
Multiple trauma	37%	41%
15- to 24-years-old	33%	33%
ICP persistently >20 mmHg	52%	46%
Unreactive pupils	29%	29%
Unilateral	8%	5%
Bilateral	22%	24%
Poor-outcome BAEP	6%	10%
Poor-outcome SSEP	44%	37%

* Abbreviations: GCS = Glasgow Coma Scale[31]; ICP = intracranial pressure; BAEP = brain-stem auditory evoked potentials; SSEP = somatosensory evoked potentials.

Reprinted with permission.[5]

TABLE 28-2 Deviations from the Protocol

Deviation	No. of Cases
Moribund at time of randomization	2*
Medical condition not compatible with study and/or hyperbaric O_2 therapy	5
Delayed randomization	1*†
Wrong age group	1*†
No head injury, removed from study	1
Hyperbaric O_2 treatment depth, duration, and/or frequency	14
Total cases	24

* Assigned to hyperbaric O_2 therapy group but did not receive therapy.

† Also deviated from protocol in "hyperbaric O_2 treatment depth, duration, and/or frequency" category.

Reprinted with permission.[5]

patients had hemotympanum. One patient's family requested that HBO therapy be discontinued.

Table 28-3 presents the mean observed peak ICPs by treatment group. A simple t-test comparing peak ICP values between HBO and control subjects found no statistically significant difference ($t = 0.92$ with 154 degrees of freedom). However, when the group of subjects with HBO plus myringotomy are separated, some significant differences can be detected. It can be seen that the group with the lowest peak ICP value is the HBO plus myringotomy group, which was significantly smaller than either the HBO only group ($t = 2.84$, $p < 0.05$) or the control group ($t = 2.48$, $p < 0.05$). The HBO plus myringotomy group also showed the least variability in these peak values (SD = 11.7).

The entire study population of 168 patients was tracked through the 12-month post-injury follow-up interval. Two control patients were lost to follow-up; therefore, 12-month outcome analyses were based on data from 84 HBO patients and 82 controls, for a total of 166 patients. The difference in overall mortality between the HBO and control groups was statistically significant, with comparisons between certain subgroups revealing significant differences (Table 28-4). The mortality rate for the 84 HBO-treated patients was 17 percent and for the 82 control patients was 32 percent (Chi-squared 1 df, $p = 0.037$). The log-rank (Mantel-Haenszel) test for comparing the differences between two survival curves indicated a difference with a p value of 0.017. Of the 40 patients who died (both groups), 90 percent died of cerebral causes. If the patient was vegetative, death was attributed to a neurological cause even if the patient died of intercurrent illnesses (e.g., pulmonary embolus). HBO treatment was related to a significant difference in mortality for two specific subgroups: patients with entry GCS scores of 4 to 6 and patients with ICPs consistently greater than 20 mmHg. The difference in mortality between the HBO and control patients with GCS scores 4 to 6 was significant (Chi-square, 1 df, $p = 0.04$) and by the log-rank (Mantel-Haenszel) test for equality of survival curves ($p = 0.02$). HBO patients with ICPs persistently higher than 20 mmHg (above 20 mmHg at several observations throughout the day and unrelated to such interventions as suction or turning the patient) had a mortality rate of 21 percent compared with 48 percent for the control group (Chi-square, 1 df, $p = 0.02$).

Although the difference in mortality between the HBO and control patients with surgical mass lesions was not statistically significant by two-tailed chi-squared analysis ($p = 0.09$), it was found significant when probability of survival was compared using the log-rank (Mantel-Haenszel) test ($p = 0.03$). One control patient with a surgical mass lesion died after his 12-month follow-up; his death is not reflected in Table 28-3 but was included in the Mantel-Haenszel analysis.

No statistically significant differences resulted between HBO treated and control patients when favorable outcome was analyzed at 12 months (Table 28-5).

In this study, HBO dramatically reduced the mortality rate among the severely head-injured patients so treated. The mortality rate for the 84 HBO patients was

TABLE 28-3 Mean Peak ICP in Each Treatment Group*

Treatment Group	No. of Cases	Mean Peak ICP (mmHg)	t-Test Value	p Value
Hyperbaric O_2 & myringotomy	42	22.1 ± 11.7		
Only hyperbaric O_2	37	33.0 ± 20.6	2.84	<0.05
Control	77	30.3 ± 24.3	2.48	<0.05
All subjects	156	28.7 ± 21.0		

* Intracranial pressure (ICP) expressed as mean ± standard deviation. All statistical comparisons are to the hyperbaric O_2 plus myringotomy group.

Reprinted with permission.[5]

TABLE 28-4 Patient Mortality Data at 12 Months*

Category	Treatment Group: Hyperbaric O_2	Treatment Group: Control†	p Value‡
All patients	14/84 (17%)	26/82 (32%)	0.04
GCS score 3	3/4 (75%)	4/4 (100%)	1.00
GCS score 4 to 6	7/42 (17%)	16/38 (42%)	0.04
GCS score 7 to 9	4/38 (11%)	7/39 (18%)	0.55
Mass lesions	8/33 (24%)	19/41 (46%)	0.09
Contusions	6/51 (12%)	7/41 (17%)	0.67
ICP ≤20 mmHg	3/32 (9%)	5/35 (14%)	0.81
ICP >20 mmHg	10/47 (21%)	19/40 (48%)	0.02
Fixed pupil(s)	9/23 (39%)	13/23 (57%)	0.38

* Abbreviations: GCS = Glasgow Coma Scale[31]; ICP = intracranial pressure.

† Two patients lost to follow-up study.

‡ Chi-squared analysis.

Reprinted with permission.[5]

17 percent, compared with 32 percent for the 82 control patients. In particular, HBO resulted in an approximately 50 percent reduction in mortality for patients with GCS scores of 4 to 6, those with mass lesions, and those with increased ICP. These three factors are interrelated; mortality rate would be highest in these groups of patients, since all three are indicative of severe brain injury. Thus, HBO, through reducing ICP and probably allowing more aerobic glucose metabolism to occur, allows these very severely brain-injured patients to survive.

However, the functional recovery of the salvaged patients was not satisfactory, i.e., the increased survivors did not make it into the good recovery or moderately disabled categories. We cannot say whether this was because the severely damaged brain lacked the potential for further recovery or because there was a secondary harmful effect by the HBO, such as increased free radical production and peroxidation.

MECHANISM OF ACTION

Inadequate oxygen supply to the traumatized brain results in the conversion of aerobic glucose metabolism to anaerobic metabolism.[7] Anaerobic metabolism results in acidosis and depletion of cellular energy. As the demands for energy production are no longer met, the brain cells lose their ability to maintain normal ionic

TABLE 28-5 Favorable Outcome at 12 Months*

Category	Treatment Group: Hyperbaric O_2	Treatment Group: Control†	p Value‡
All patients	44/84 (52%)	44/82 (54%)	0.99
GCS score 3	1/4 (25%)	0/4 (0%)	1.00
GCS score 4 to 6	17/42 (40%)	16/38 (42%)	0.94
GCS score 7 to 9	26/38 (68%)	28/39 (72%)	0.94
Mass lesions	15/33 (45%)	14/41 (34%)	0.45
Contusions	29/51 (57%)	30/41 (73%)	0.16
ICP ≤20 mmHg	17/32 (53%)	25/35 (71%)	0.20
ICP >20 mmHg	23/47 (49%)	16/40 (40%)	0.54
Fixed pupil(s)	4/23 (17%)	4/23 (17%)	0.70

* Favorable outcome defined as a Glasgow Outcome Scale[15] score of 1 (good recovery) or 2 (moderately disabled). Abbreviations: GCS = Glasgow Coma Scale[31]; ICP = intracranial pressure.

† Two patients lost to follow-up study.

‡ Chi-squared analysis.

Reprinted with permission.[5]

homeostasis. Abnormally high intracellular concentrations of calcium result. This abnormal cellular environment causes the formation of highly reactive free radicals that are extremely damaging to cell membranes.[8,9] When ischemia is immediate and profound, as from cerebral vascular occlusion, the above events occur rapidly; however, there is evidence that ischemia can occur days after the initial head injury.[10] HBO may improve the availability of oxygen to the injured brain and so maintain the aerobic metabolism of cerebral glucose. Still viable but nonfunctioning tissue could possibly be preserved by supporting the aerobic processes of the threatened cells.

The potential benefits of HBO in the treatment of severe head injury are several. Hyperbaric oxygen increases the amount of oxygen dissolved in the plasma, depending on the absolute pressure used. At 2 atmospheres absolute (ata), it increases arterial oxygen tension to 1000–1250 mmHg[11] and decreases cerebral blood flow (CBF) in the normal individual by approximately 22 percent.[12–16] The reduction in the CBF is due to cerebral vasoconstriction; several investigators have demonstrated that it is not dependent on hypocarbia.[17–19] When cerebral autoregulation is lost, CBF no longer decreases with the administration of HBO.[20,21]

Corresponding with the reduction in CBF secondary to cerebral vasoconstriction, there is experimental and clinical evidence that reduction in the intracranial pressure (ICP) occurs. Miller et al. demonstrated in several laboratory studies that ICP decreases by about one-third of the control value with the application of HBO.[11,18] Both cold lesions of the cerebral cortex and extradural balloons were used in these experiments. Sukoff and Ragatz reported on a series of 50 patients with traumatic cerebral edema who were treated with HBO.[4] In 10 of these, ICP was systematically monitored. The ICPs during HBO were consistently lower than those before HBO ($p \leq 0.001$), and the reductions were sustained for 2 to 4 hours after HBO in most cases. Other investigators have not reported such a consistent response. Hayakawa et al. measured cerebrospinal fluid pressure via a needle inserted in the cisterna magna in 26 dogs.[22] They found a consistent decrease in pressure during the first 20 to 30 minutes of HBO, but then a tendency for the pressures to return toward baseline. However, these animals were treated at 3 ata, and Miller found ICP reduction relatively resistant at pressures greater than 2 ata.[11] Hayakawa et al. also studied the changes in cerebrospinal fluid pressure with HBO in 13 patients suffering acute cerebral damage.[22] In nine of these patients who had sustained closed-head injury, pressure decreased at the beginning of HBO but reverted rapidly with decompression. There was a tendency to some rebound after cessation of treatment.

Holbach et al. studied glucose metabolism in 23 patients who had acute cerebral injuries.[23] While the patients breathed air and oxygen at normobaric pressure and then again at 1.5 and 2.0 ata, the cerebral arteriovenous differences for oxygen, glucose, lactate, pyruvate, blood gas pressures, and pH values were measured. There was a distinctly increased cerebral glycolysis while patients breathed air, indicating insufficient oxygen delivery to the brain. The change from breathing air to oxygen resulted in a distinct inhibition of cerebral glycolysis, indicating improved cerebral oxygenation and energy production. At an inspiratory oxygen pressure of 1.5 ata, cerebral glucose metabolism was nearly balanced, indicating optimal cerebral oxygenation and energy formation. A further increase in inspiratory oxygen pressure to 2.0 ata increased cerebral glycolysis considerably. This was assumed to be due to cerebral oxygen poisoning resulting in disturbed oxidative energy formation. Artu et al. studied similar parameters in brain-injured patients treated with HBO at 2.5 ata.[24] His results are less consistent and less suggestive that HBO is beneficial in cerebral glucose metabolism. However, the study of Holbach et al. suggests that 2.5 ata is an excessive pressure for ideal glucose metabolism.[23]

Contreras et al. documented that exposure to HBO increased the overall glucose utilization in a freeze traumatized rat brain.[25] Local cerebral glucose utilization was measured with the autoradiographic 2-deoxy-glucose technique. Treatment of lesioned animals with HBO was at 2 ata for 90 minutes on each of four consecutive days. A potentially important and novel finding of the study was the fact that the increase in glucose utilization persisted for at least 24 hours after termination of HBO exposure.

CURRENT RESEARCH AND FUTURE DIRECTIONS

In spite of the considerable amount of literature quoted above suggesting the potential benefit of HBO in the treatment of traumatic brain injury, many questions regarding its application and efficacy persist. The ideal HBO treatment paradigm, in terms of the depth of the dive, the duration of the treatment, or frequency of treatments has never been systematically determined. In addition, whether there is a "window of opportunity" following head injury, in which HBO has to be administered to be effective, has likewise not been determined. The number of days that treatment should be continued may vary with the severity of the injury and is likewise unknown. Further investigation is required to elucidate the effect of HBO on cerebral glucose metabolism, cerebral blood flow, and intracranial pressure.

As noted earlier, HBO is potentially harmful to the injured brain by supplying oxygen for free radical reactions that result in iron-catalyzed lipid peroxidation.[8,26–28] The brain is particularly vulnerable to this process because its membrane lipids are rich in polyunsaturated fatty acids which are susceptible to free-radical attack. The brain is rich in iron, and the iron-catalyzed Haber-Weiss reaction is the probable mechanism of the initiation of lipid peroxidation. The timing of HBO treatment in relation to the injury occurrence, as well as the amount of oxygen given, is most likely important in the amount of harmful peroxidation that could occur. The evaluation of HBO in conjunction with a brain protectant agent that could reduce its potential toxic effects on the injured brain would seem logical. HBO in combination with an agent such as tirilazad, which is a potent antiperoxidation agent, may act synergistically to improve outcome by reducing oxygen toxicity and exerting their own therapeutic effects.

At the present time, we have ongoing experimental and clinical protocols attempting to answer these remaining questions. Our preliminary results would suggest that it is important to give HBO early after injury. HBO delivered at 1.5 ata for periods as short as 30 minutes seem to be more effective than HBO at 2 atmospheres for 90 minutes.

Since HBO has been shown clinically to significantly improve survival rate after severe head injury but does not lead to favorable outcomes in the survivors, an effective treatment paradigm and/or a combination treatment must be found before HBO therapy can be accepted as a treatment for traumatic brain injury.

References

1. Mogami H, Hayakawa T, Kanoi N, et al: Clinical application of hyperbaric oxygenation in the treatment of acute cerebral damage. *J Neurosurg* 1969; 31:636–643.
2. Holbach KH, Wassman H, Kolberg T: Improved reversibility of the traumatic mid-brain syndrome with application of hyperbaric oxygen pressure. *Acta Neurochir* 1974; 30:247–256.
3. Artu F, Charcornac R, Deleuze R: Hyperbaric oxygenation for severe head injuries. Preliminary results of a controlled study. *Eur Neurol* 1976; 14:310–318.
4. Sukoff MH, Ragatz RE: Hyperbaric oxygenation for the treatment of acute cerebral edema. *Neurosurg* 1982; 10:29–38.
5. Rockswold GL, Ford SE, Anderson DC, et al: Results of a prospective randomized trial for treatment of severely brain-injured patients with hyperbaric oxygen. *J Neurosurg* 1992; 76:929–934.
6. Bergman TA, Rockswold GL, Haines SJ, et al: Outcome of severe closed head injury in the Midwest. A review and comparison with other major head trauma studies. *Minn Med* 1987; 70:397–401.
7. Muizelaar JP: Cerebral blood flow, cerebral blood volume, and cerebral metabolism after severe head injury, in Becker DP, Gudeman SK (eds): *Textbook of Head Injury*. Philadelphia: WB Saunders, 1989:221–240.
8. Ikeda Y, Long DM: The molecular basis of brain injury and brain edema: The role of oxygen free radicals. *Neurosurgery* 1990; 27:1–11.
9. Seisjo BK, Agardh CD, Bengtsson F: Free radicals and brain damage. *Cerebrovasc Brain Metab Rev* 1989; 1:165–211.
10. Robertson CS, Narayan RK, Gokaslan ZL, et al: Cerebral arteriovenous oxygen difference as an estimate of cerebral blood flow in comatose patients. *J Neurosurg* 1989; 70:222–230.
11. Miller JD: The effects of hyperbaric oxygen at 2 and 3 atmospheres absolute and intravenous mannitol on experimentally increased intracranial pressure. *Eur Neurol* 1973; 10:1–11.
12. Kety SS, Schmidt CF: The effects of altered arterial tensions of carbon dioxide and oxygen on cerebral blood flow and cerebral oxygen consumption of normal young men. *J Clin Invest* 1948; 27:484–492.
13. Lambertson CJ, Kough RH, Cooper DY, et al: Oxygen toxicity: Effects in man of oxygen inhalation at 1 and 3.5 atmospheres upon blood gas transport, cerebral metabolism. *J Appl Physiol* 1953; 5:471–486.
14. Jacobson K, Harper AM, McDowall DG: The effects of oxygen under pressure on cerebral blood-flow and cerebral venous oxygen tension. *Lancet* 1963; 2:549.
15. Jacobson K, Harper AM, McDowall DG: The effects of O^2 at 1 and 2 atmospheres on the blood flow and oxygen uptake of the cerebral cortex. *Surg Gynecol Obstet* 1964; 119:737–742.
16. Reivich M, Holling HE, Roberts B, et al: Reversal of blood flow through tex vertebral artery and its effect on cerebral circulation. *N Engl J Med* 1961; 265:878–885.
17. Harper AM, Glass HI: Effect of alterations in arterial carbon dioxide tension on the blood flow through the cerebral cortex at normal and low arterial blood pressures. *J Neurol Neurosurg Psychiatry* 1965; 28:449–452.
18. Miller JD, Fitch W, Ledingham IM, et al: The effect of hyperbaric oxygen on experimentally increased intracranial pressure. *Neurosurgery* 1970; 33:287–296.
19. Miller JD, Ledingham IM: Reduction of increased intracranial pressure. Comparison between hyperbaric oxygen and hyperventilation. *Arch Neurol* 1971; 24:210–216.
20. Kanai N, Hayakawa T, Mogami H: Blood flow changes in carotid and vertebral arteries by hyperbaric oxygenation. *Neurology* 1973; 23:159–163.
21. Nagao S, Okumura S, Nishimoto A: Effects of hyperbaric oxygenation on cerebral vasomotor tone in acute intracranial hypertension: An experimental study. *Resuscitation* 1975; 4:51–59.
22. Hayakawa T, Kanai N, Kuroda R, et al: Response of cerebrospinal fluid pressure to hyperbaric oxygenation. *J Neurol Neurosurg Psychiatry* 1971; 34:580–586.
23. Holbach KH, Caroli A, Wassman H: Cerebral energy

metabolism in patients with brain lesions at normo- and hyperbaric oxygen pressures. *J Neurol* 1977; 217:17–30.
24. Artu F, Philippon B, Gau F, et al: Cerebral blood flow, cerebral metabolism and cerebrospinal fluid biochemistry in brain-injured patients after exposure to hyperbaric oxygen. *Eur Neurol* 1976; 14:351–364.
25. Contreras FL, Kakekaro M, Eisenberg HM: The effect of hyperbaric oxygen on glucose utilization in a freeze-traumatized rat brain. *J Neurosurg* 1988; 65:615–624.
26. Noda Y, McGeer PL, McGeer GE: Lipid peroxide distribution in brain and the effect of hyperbaric oxygen. *J Neurochem* 1983; 40:1329–1332.
27. Becker N, Glavin SF: Effect of oxygen rich atmospheres on cerebral lipid peroxides. *Aerospace Med* 1962; 33:985–987.
28. Zalaska MM, Floyd RA: Regional lipid peroxidation in rat brain in vitro: Possible role of endrogenous iron. *Neurochem Res* 1984; 10:397–410.

CHAPTER 29

HYPOTHERMIA FOR THE TREATMENT OF HEAD INJURY

Guy L. Clifton
Ronald L. Hayes

SYNOPSIS

The historical background and recent clinical experience with the use of hypothermia has been reviewed. The Phase II trials of this modality in the treatment of severe head injury have been detailed. A Phase III prospective, randomized, multicenter trial has been initiated, based on encouraging early results.

HISTORICAL BACKGROUND

Profound hypothermia (10–20°C) is a well-established and highly effective means of cerebral protection from global ischemia. Bigelow et al., in 1950, first described protection from global cerebral ischemia by producing total cardiac arrest in dogs for 15 minutes at 20°C.[1] This experiment was done before the pump oxygenator became available and was investigated as a strategy to permit surgical entry of the heart. By 1959, Drew and Anderson had reported clinical trials in which circulation was completely stopped for up to 45 minutes at 13 to 15°C using a pump but no oxygenator.[2] Hypothermic perfusion without an oxygenator was then abandoned owing to operative mortalities.[3] Following a proposal by Shumway and Lower, moderate hypothermia (30°C) came into wide clinical use in conjunction with the membrane oxygenator (with selective cardiac cooling).[4] Surface cooling to profound levels was never used clinically because ventricular fibrillation occurred at temperatures below 27°C.[3,5] From 1974 to 1980, large series reported successful total circulatory arrest at 10 to 20°C for up to 50 minutes in repair of cardiac anomalies in children less than 1 year of age.[6,7] Since then, total circulatory arrest at temperatures of 8 to 10°C has been used in repair of adult ascending aortic arch aneurysms.[8] These techniques, based on the cerebral protective effects of profound hypothermia against global ischemia, are in current use.

In 1969 and 1973, White and colleagues demonstrated in primates that profound hypothermia (15°C) with circulatory arrest for periods of 30 minutes was tolerated with no neurological sequelae. This increased neurosurgical interest in hypothermia.[9] However, the neurosurgical experience with profound hypothermia did not result in clinical utility. Between 1964 and 1976, the neurosurgical literature reported 111 patients who were operated on under profound hypothermia with circulatory arrest using cardiopulmonary bypass to cool and rewarm.[10–20] Most of these patients had surgically difficult intracranial aneurysms. The problem of intracranial hemorrhage during rewarming, coupled with the necessity of large vessel cannulation, led to the virtual abandonment of profound hypothermia.

Moderate hypothermia with surface cooling to 30°C was investigated in the treatment of human and experimental brain injury from 1955 to 1974. Rosomoff et al. showed that surface-induced systemic hypothermia to 30°C in dogs reduced the mortality rate induced by a cortical cold injury if administered within 6 hours of injury.[21] Clasen et al. and Laskowski et al. demonstrated that systemic hypothermia substantially reduced cerebral edema associated with cortical cold injury in primates and dogs.[22,23] Rosomoff showed that hypothermia decreased brain volume.[24] From 1958 to 1974, five publications reported 121 patients treated with sustained surface cooling after severe brain injury.[25–30] Temperatures ranged from 28 to 34°C and durations of hypothermia from 2 to 10 days. Mortality rates of these series were from 43 to 72 percent. Cooling was usually begun 12 to 24 hours after injury. In most cases, patients who were believed to have sustained mortal injuries were treated. Twenty-three of 66 deaths occurred during rewarming and 13 during hypothermia itself. In no case was death attributed to hypothermia. No occurrence of ventricular fibrillation was reported. Since control groups were not used, it was not possible to reach any conclusion as to effectiveness, though each author felt benefit was derived. Thus, because of bleeding complications with profound hypothermia and because of lack of clinical trials designed to detect efficacy of moderate hypothermia, these techniques of cerebral protection remained virtually unused in neurosurgery.

POTENTIAL CLINICAL TOXICITY

Brief periods of moderate hypothermia in humans are associated with little cardiovascular, hematological, metabolic, or neurological toxicity. Potential causes of toxicity from systemic hypothermia may be deduced from an extensive literature. The limiting factor in depth of hypothermia is ventricular ectopy and fibrillation. At 30°C, ventricular conduction and refractory period increase by 50 percent, but at 25°C by 300 percent.[31] Disparities in conduction velocity and refractory period may lead to ventricular fibrillation.[32] Myocardial contractility actually increases as temperature decreases until a temperature of 28°C, after which it falls.[33,34] At 30°C, cardiac output falls to 55 percent due to bradycardia, although stroke volume increases.[35] Blood pressure remains constant as a result of an increase in systemic vascular resistance.[35] When surface cooling without cardiopulmonary bypass was used in cardiac surgery, as many as 25 percent of patients fibrillated at temperatures of 27°C; therefore, 30 to 33°C was accepted as the safe lower limit of surface cooling.[5,36] In a literature of over 150 cases of patients with neurological diseases who were surface-cooled to levels of 28 to 32°C, a single case of ventricular fibrillation was reported.[25–30,37–39]

Rheologic changes during hypothermia have led some investigators to use hemodilution in experimental studies of focal cerebral ischemia.[40,41] In dogs, blood viscosity is increased by 50 percent at 25°C, but at 30°C it is increased by only 25 percent.[42] Platelet counts decrease during cardiopulmonary bypass and with surface cooling.[42] Viscosity changes are due to increased vascular resistance and to increased hematocrit.[43] In dogs, prothrombin time and partial thromboplastin time are normal at 30°C for 24 hours.[44] With continued cooling for 72 hours, however, a severe coagulopathy develops, and animals die of multi-organ hemorrhage and congestion.[44] The problem with postoperative intracranial hemorrhage in neurosurgery was related to the combination of profound hypothermia and the use of heparin necessitated by cardiopulmonary bypass. At moderate levels of hypothermia (30°C) for brief periods, the literature has suggested little toxicity.

LABORATORY BASIS FOR CLINICAL TESTING

The recent resurgence of interest in moderate hypothermia has resulted from the consistent finding of very high levels of cerebral protection in well-established models of global ischemia. The finding by Busto et al. in 1987 of marked neuronal protection by 3 to 4°C hypothermia in the rat model of four-vessel occlusion was rapidly confirmed by at least three other laboratories that had ongoing experience in the study of global ischemia.[45–49] In our laboratory, 2 to 3°C hypothermia provided more protection from Ca_1 hippocampal loss in the gerbil model of forebrain ischemia than we had been able to achieve pharmacologically.[46] The finding of marked protection by even mild hypothermia may explain many of the contradictory conclusions among laboratories regarding pharmacological protection in these models. Not only is intraischemic mild hypothermia protective in these models, but postischemic hypothermia also is protective.[50–52] Hypothermia of 30°C for 3 hours induced immediately after 10 minutes of four-vessel occlusion eliminates severe neuronal loss.[51] In the rat model of carotid occlusion with hypotension, postischemic hypothermia of 27°C greatly reduces neuronal loss.[52] In Safar's laboratory, Leonov found that postischemic mild hypothermia provided behavioral and neuronal protection superior to that of moderate hypothermia.[48]

Cerebral ischemia is a common occurrence in human brain injury. Pathological studies have shown arterial boundary zone and diffuse ischemic changes in 40 to 90 percent of autopsied brains.[53] Adams et al. concluded that ischemia occurred soon after injury since these changes occurred more commonly in those with hypotension and hypoxia soon after injury.[53] Miller et al. have shown that early hypoxic and hypotensive events are associated with a markedly worse outcome.[54] Robertson et al. found 22 percent of patients with severe brain injury to have ischemia based on a characteristic pattern of cerebral blood flow, cerebral oxygen utilization, and cerebral lactate excretion.[55] Overgaard et al. identified regions of ischemic blood flow (<20 ml/100 qr/min) in 61 percent of 23 patients with poor outcome from brain injury. In these studies, ischemic flow values were rarely found in those who subsequently had a good outcome.[56] Muizelaar et al. reported that 18 percent of 55 patients undergoing hyperventilation to Pa_{CO_2} 23 mmHg showed widened arteriovenous oxygen difference, concluding that these patients were on the brink of ischemia.[57] Therefore, it is likely that global cerebral ischemia occurs early after brain injury with great frequency and occurs transiently thereafter in many patients. The effectiveness of moderate hypothermia in treatment of experimental global ischemia is, therefore, relevant to therapy of human brain injury.

Post-injury hypothermia also exerts strong behavioral protection in models of brain injury without ischemia. In the fluid percussion model of mild to moderate brain injury in the rat, we have shown a marked reduction in performance deficits for 5 days after injury by systemic hypothermia induced after injury.[58]

The mechanisms of hypothermic protection observed following brain injury are probably multifactorial. Investigators of hypothermic protection following ischemia have proposed a number of possible processes. For example, hyperthermia has been shown to increase and hypothermia to decrease intracellular acidosis during ischemia and reperfusion.[59–61] However, significant acidosis has not been reported in the fluid percussion model of brain injury.[62,63] Hypothermia is known to reduce brain metabolic requirements which may diminish the impact of substrate-limiting neural insults such as edema, hypoxia, and hypoglycemia. However, substrate limitation in moderate brain injury has not been demonstrated.[62,63] In models of global ischemia, blood-brain barrier alterations are very prominent and are diminished markedly by intraischemic and postischemic hypothermia.[64,65] Blood-brain barrier opening also is prominently found in both cat and rat models of fluid percussion injury, and hypothermia diminishes blood-brain barrier opening in experimental models of brain injury.[66]

A substantial body of evidence indicates that excitotoxic processes initiated by excessive release of excitatory neurotransmitters may mediate neural injury following ischemia and traumatic brain injury. Inhibition of pathological neurotransmitter release may be a particularly important mechanism of moderate hypothermia. Cerebral hypothermia of 30°C and 33°C has been shown to completely inhibit the sevenfold increase in brain glutamate and produce a 60 percent attenuation of 500-fold increase in dopamine after global ischemia.[67] Neurotransmitter surges (glutamate, acetylcholine) have also been reported following brain injury in the rat.[68–70] Additionally, pharmacological blockade of NMDA glutamate receptors or muscarinic cholinergic receptors has reduced behavioral deficits following brain injury in the rat.[68,71,72] Thus, reduction of receptor-mediated pathology by inhibition of excessive neurotransmitter release is one plausible mechanism mediating hypothermic protection, while the closing of the blood-brain barrier is another.

CLINICAL TRIALS

Operative Cases[73]

Based on the clinical data and current laboratory data outlined, we conducted three series of clinical trials to evaluate potential toxicity and potential treatment effect of moderate hypothermia in patients with severe brain injury.[73–75]

Twenty-one patients underwent elective craniotomy (large tumors, large aneurysms, or arteriovenous malformations) performed by the authors in an 18-month period (January 1990–July 1991). Of the patients undergoing surgery, three had arteriovenous malformations, 14 had tumors, three had large aneurysms (>2 cm), and one had symptomatic carotid stenosis with contralateral carotid occlusion. Those patients likely to require carotid arterial occlusion, those requiring prolonged dissection, those with large tumors (>4 cm diameter) causing brain compression, and those with large arteriovenous malformations were selected for hypothermia. Hypothermia was not used on routine craniotomies. Anesthesia was with fentanyl and isoflurane plus muscle relaxants with vecuronium. Cooling blankets were placed above and below the patient and turned to 5°C after anesthesia induction and positioning. Temperature was measured by esophageal probe or Swan-Ganz catheter, and blood pressure was measured by intra-arterial monitoring. Pulse oximetry was routine. The target esophageal temperature was 32 to 33°C, and cooling blankets were turned off when the temperature was 34°C. The patients would continue to cool 1 to 2°C after the cooling blankets were turned off. Blankets were turned to 37°C 30 minutes before closing the craniotomy or 1.5 hours before completion of the procedure. At conclusion of surgery, muscle relaxants were not reversed, and patients were left in the operating room intubated until core temperature reached 35°C or greater. At this time, muscle relaxants were reversed or discontinued, and patients were extubated. Warming units were used in the recovery room to accelerate rewarming. In this series, cooling rates varied from

0.5°C/h to 2°C/h, with a mean of 1.6°C/h. Rewarming rates varied from 1°C/h to 3.5°C/h, with a mean of 1.6°C/h. The duration of hypothermia (a core temperature of 33°C or less) varied from 1 to 8 hours (mean 4 hours). There were no complications attributable to hypothermia, specifically cardiac arrhythmias or intracerebral hemorrhage. We concluded that moderate hypothermia could be induced rapidly and safely with surface cooling.

Severe Brain Injury (Phase I)[75]

Based on the lack of toxicity found in operative patients, ten patients with a GCS of 4 to 8 who had traumatic brain injury without major systemic injuries were randomized into two groups, normothermia and hypothermia (30–32°C). Informed consent was obtained from family members. Cooling was begun within 6 hours of injury by cooling blankets set at 5°C on the patient's dorsal and ventral surfaces. Iced saline lavage of the stomach was used to accelerate cooling in most cases. Temperatures were maintained at 30 to 32°C for 24 hours, with gradual warming over 12 to 18 hours. Glasgow Outcome Scale (GOS) was assessed at 3 months.[76] Patients had Swan-Ganz catheters, jugular bulb catheters, and either ventriculostomies or fiberoptic catheters for intracranial pressure measurement. Patients undergoing hypothermia were treated with metocurine (10–20 mg) and morphine (5–10 mg IV) every hour. General management principles included early intubation, early surgery for mass lesions, jejunal or IV alimentation within 72 hours of injury, maintenance of pulmonary capillary wedge pressure ≥12 mmHg, maintenance of Pa_{CO_2} at 35 mmHg, and maintenance of $Pa_{O_2} > 100$ mmHg. Blood gases were corrected to patient temperature. Hyperventilation to 30 mmHg was used for intracranial pressure greater than 20 mmHg. Increased intracranial pressure was managed with mannitol and CSF drainage, while adjusting hyperventilation to avoid jugular bulb venous saturation <50 percent. All patients had therapeutic phenytoin levels. Intravascular temperatures from the Swan-Ganz catheters were used to guide the depth of hypothermia.

There were no differences in types or rates of complications between the two groups except for the occurrence of ventricular tachycardia at 31.5°C in one patient. This patient underwent cardioversion and recovered without sequelae. One patient developed atrioventricular block at 31.7°C and was warmed to 33°C, with resolution of this finding. No delayed bleeding occurred in any patient. Other complications were the same in both groups. Based on GOS at 3 months, the hypothermia group did at least as well as the control group neurologically. Based on the occurrence of ventricular arrhythmias at temperatures below 32°C, we concluded that to avoid cardiac arrhythmias temperature must be kept no lower than 32°C.

Severe Brain Injury (Phase II)[74]

To determine potential toxicity and to estimate the level of neurological protection that may be achieved with systemic cooling, we performed a randomized study of moderate hypothermia in 46 patients with GCS 4–7. Twenty-two control patients with standardized management were maintained at 37 to 38°C. The treatment protocol was modified from our first Phase I study. Twenty-four patients with standardized management were cooled by cooling blankets to an intravascular temperature of 32 to 33°C for 48 hours and rewarmed over 12 to 16 hours.

Inclusion criteria were patients aged 16 to 60 with post-resuscitation GCS 4–7 after nonpenetrating brain injury. Exclusion criteria were hypoxia (O_2 saturation < 94 percent for >30 minutes), major systemic injuries requiring laparotomy, pulmonary failure, or sustained hypotension (systolic blood pressure ≤90 mmHg for ≥2 hours). Patients were excluded if cooling could not be initiated within 6 hours of injury. Randomization was stratified into two groups, GCS 4–5 and GCS 6–7, to obtain balance in injury severity in the two groups. Initial patient management consisted of rapid intubation and ventilatory support (usually done prior to admission), early computerized tomographic (CT) scanning, and surgical procedures for hematomas. Either fiberoptic or ventricular catheters were placed for intracranial pressure (ICP) monitoring. Ninety-five percent of the patients were transported by helicopter from the roadside or from another hospital's emergency department within 2 hours of injury. CT scans were performed in the emergency department and craniotomies for hematomas were performed immediately. Placements of arterial catheters, internal jugular catheters, and Foley catheters were routine. Patients undergoing hypothermia or requiring treatment with mannitol also had placement of Swan-Ganz catheters. In the absence of increased ICP, Pa_{CO_2} was maintained at 30 to 35 mmHg. Increased ICP was managed first by hyperventilation to a Pa_{CO_2} of 25 to 30 mmHg using jugular venous saturation of 50 percent to determine the lowest level of hyperventilation. Morphine-sulfate (10–20 mg) and metocurine (10–20 mg) intravenously were used hourly to control ventilation. Mannitol was given for ICP >20 mmHg after hyperventilation until a serum osmolality of ≥315 mosm was reached. Fluids were replaced so that pulmonary capillary wedge pressure was ≥8 mmHg. All patients were given phenytoin (18 mg/kg body weight) and maintained at therapeutic phenytoin blood levels thereafter. Feeding was begun within 72 hours of injury by nasojejunal tube placed endoscopically, or by parenteral nutrition. Serum glucose was maintained <200 mg/dl in all patients.

Patients who were treated with standard management at normothermia were kept at 37°C by use of cooling blankets (Baxter Pharmaceuticals, Valencia, CA) and acetaminophen for 80 hours after injury. In the hypothermia group, cooling was induced by wrapping the patients securely in cooling blankets set at 5°C. Metocurine (10 mg/h) and morphine-sulfate (10 mg/h) were given continuously. These medications were discontinued when the patient was warmed to a temperature of 35°C unless ICP was >20 mmHg. Intravascular temperatures from the Swan-Ganz catheter were used for temperature measurement in the hypothermia group. Bladder or rectal temperatures were used in the normothermia group. Warming was begun 48 hours after a temperature of 33°C was first reached, and patients were warmed at 1°C every 4 hours thereafter. Serum potassium was measured every 6 hours during the first 72 hours and maintained at 3.5 to 5.0 mEq/L by intravenous potassium administration. Blood gases were not corrected for temperature but were measured and interpreted at 37°C. Complete blood count, prothrombin time, and partial thromboplastin time were measured daily for 4 days for all patients and again at 37°C. Records of all complications during hospitalization were kept. Therapy intensity level is a numerical score quantifying Pa_{CO_2}, mannitol dosage, muscle relaxant use, and sedation as treatments for elevated ICP.[77] This was computed hourly for all patients during ICP monitoring. Glasgow Outcome Scale (GOS) was assessed at 3 months after injury.[73] GOS was assessed by a neuropsychologist who was blinded to the treatment arm.

Glasgow Outcome Scale score distribution between groups was compared by chi-square test. Physiological and laboratory data were analyzed in four blocks of time: the first 12 hours (cooling), the next 48 hours (steady state at 32–33°C), the next 12 hours (rewarming), and the subsequent 12 hours (steady state after rewarming) for a total of 84 hours after injury. Bonferroni's t-test was used to compare the mean values for each patient in each time block for both laboratory and physiological data. Repeated measured analyses of variance showed interaction effects between treatment and time period for all variables except ICP, for which $.05 < p < .10$. Therefore, we tested the differences between treatments at each of the four time periods using Bonferroni's t-test.

The characteristics of the two groups that most affect outcome are shown in Table 29-1. Age (Wilcoxon's rank-sum, $p > 0.95$) and GCS distribution (chi-square analysis, $p = 0.54$) were not significantly different in the two groups. Distribution by pupillary reactivity and primary diagnosis was similar. The mean temperature on admission for all patients was 36.2 ± 1.3°C (SE) at 2.7 ± 1.6 hours after admission. Figure 29-1 shows the mean temperature in the two groups as compared to heart rate at four different time intervals. Error bars show standard error. In the hypothermia group, temperatures were measured intravascularly. In the normothermia group, temperatures were measured by bladder or

TABLE 29-1 Phase II Trial of Hypothermia in Severe Head Injury—Clinical Features

	Normothermia (N = 22)	Hypothermia (N = 24)
Age		
15–25	11	12
26–35	4	7
36–45	3	4
46–55	3	1
>55	1	0
Glasgow Coma Scale Score		
4–5	9	12
6–7	13	12
Primary Diagnosis		
Epidural hematoma	1	0
Subdural hematoma	5	8
Intracerebral hematoma	1	0
Diffuse brain injury	15	16
Pupillary Reactivity		
Reactive	17	16
Unilaterally nonreactive	2	(4 orbital injuries)
Bilaterally nonreactive	3	4

HEART RATE (bpm)

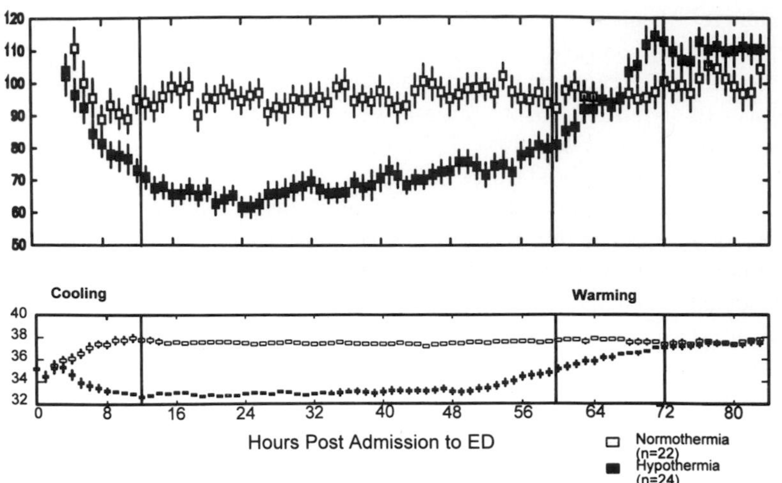

Figure 29-1. Mean temperatures with standard error are shown for the first 84 hours after injury and compared to heart rate at four different time periods. The first time period is the 12 hours from admission, during which time patients were cooled to 33°C. Eight hours were required for most patients. The second time period is a 48-hour steady state condition. The third time period is the 12 hours of rewarming and the fourth time period is a 12-hour steady state period after re-warming. In the hypothermia group, temperatures are intravascular. In the normothermia group, temperatures are bladder or rectal. Heart rate (beats/min) ± SE is shown in the first panel. There was significant bradycardia in the hypothermia group in the second time period ($p < .001$) (Table 29-2).

rectal probe. Time zero is the time of emergency department admission. To bring patients to 33°C required 7.88 ± 0.61 (SE) hours from admission. Rewarming was started 48 hours after the patient's temperature reached 33°C, and 12 to 14 hours were used to bring patients from 33°C to 37°C. Heart rate was significantly lower in the hypothermia group only in the second time period when hypothermia resulted in bradycardia (Fig. 29-1, Table 29-2). Mean arterial pressure (MAP) was significantly different in the two groups only in the third time

TABLE 29-2 Phase II Trial of Hypothermia in Severe Head Injury—Physiological Parameters

	Normothermia		*Hypothermia*		
H After ER Admission	**mean**	**SE**	**mean**	**SE**	**Bonferroni p-value**
Temperature					
0–11	36.98	.021	34.69	0.26	$p < .001$
12–59	37.51	0.12	33.05	0.14	$p < .001$
60–71	37.70	0.16	35.35	0.25	$p < .001$
72–83	37.52	0.16	37.05	0.19	NS
Heart Rate					
0–11	95.71	3.67	88.47	3.18	NS
12–59	97.20	3.35	71.49	3.16	$p < .001$
60–71	97.45	4.25	97.92	3.80	NS
72–83	101.45	4.84	110.61	3.88	NS
Mean Arterial Pressure					
0–11	96.95	3.16	97.00	2.10	NS
12–59	92.00	3.07	87.10	2.20	NS
60–71	96.01	2.50	83.37	1.83	$p < .001$
72–83	96.06	3.04	87.99	2.28	NS
Intracranial Pressure					
0–11	11.02	1.91	10.80	0.97	NS
12–59	18.32	3.61	12.96	0.99	NS
60–71	17.04	2.06	18.09	1.49	NS
72–83	19.19	2.34	16.11	0.82	NS
Cerebral Perfusion Pressure					
0–11	87.13	3.61	87.32	2.34	NS
12–59	80.44	2.21	74.23	2.13	NS
60–71	80.90	3.42	64.96	2.13	$p < .001$
72–83	77.07	4.56	73.52	2.27	NS

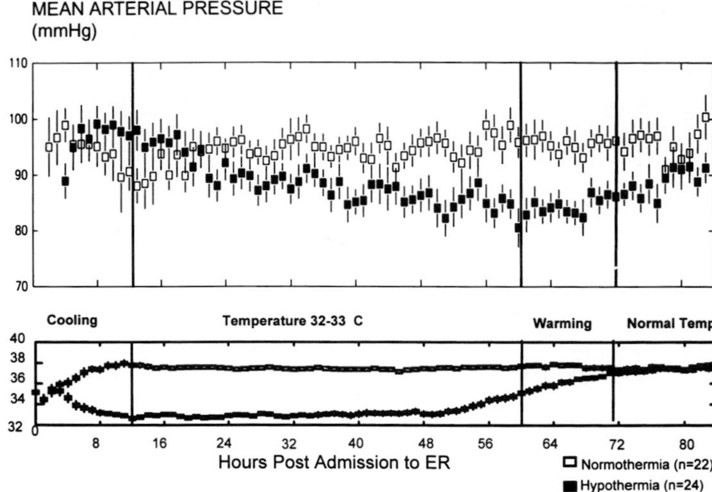

Figure 29-2. Temperature is compared to mean arterial pressure. Mean arterial pressure was lower in the hypothermia group in the third time period ($p < .001$) (Table 29-2).

period with a 13 mmHg lower MAP in the hypothermia group (Fig. 29-2). Figure 29-3 shows temperature and ICP in both groups. There were no differences in ICP at any time period (Fig. 29-3, Table 29-2). Therapy intensity level was 3.81 ± .4 for normothermia and 6.10 ± .23 for hypothermia in the second time period, reflecting the routine administration of morphine and metocurine in the hypothermia group.[75] Cerebral perfusion pressure was 16 mmHg lower in the hypothermia group in the third time period, with a mean value in normothermia of 80.9 ± 3.42 mmHg, and in the hypothermia group of 64.96 ± 2.13 mmHg (Fig. 29-4). Morphine and metocurine doses were higher in the hypothermia group in the first three time periods. Mean Pa_{CO_2} was 31.0 ± .89 mmHg in the normothermia group and 30.8 ± .83 mmHg in the hypothermia group in the second time period.

Hypothermia is known to induce an intracellular shift of potassium, and cooling of blood prolongs prothrombin time and partial thromboplastin time.[37] Table 29-3 details the mean and standard error of prothrombin time, partial thromboplastin time (PTT), serum potassium, and serum glucose in the two groups of patients. Prothrombin time (PT) was measured daily for 4 days and was slightly, but significantly, prolonged in the third and fourth time periods (normal 11.1 to 13.1 seconds). PTT was normal and not different in the two groups in the first time block and the second time period (normal 25.0 to 35.0 seconds). PTT in the normothermia group in the third time period was 32.62 ± 1.14 seconds and slightly prolonged at 34.62 ± 1.01 seconds in the hypothermia group ($p < 0.025$). PTT was also slightly prolonged in the fourth time period in hypothermia patients with a PTT in normothermia patients of 31.66 ± 0.61 seconds and in the hypothermia group of 37.05 ± 3.11 seconds ($p < 0.001$). Serum potassium was within a normal range in both groups in the first three time periods. Serum potassium was slightly increased after re-

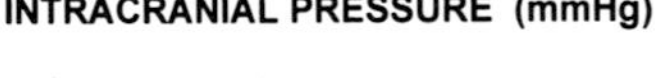

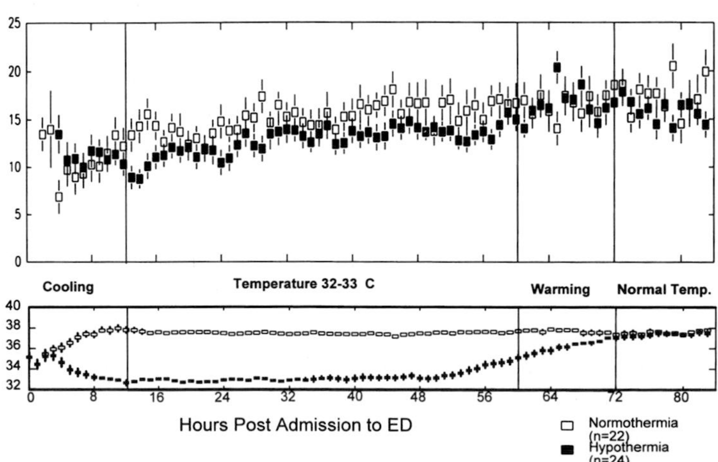

Figure 29-3. Temperature is compared to intracranial pressure. There were no significant differences (Table 29-2).

CEREBRAL PERFUSION PRESSURE (mmHg)

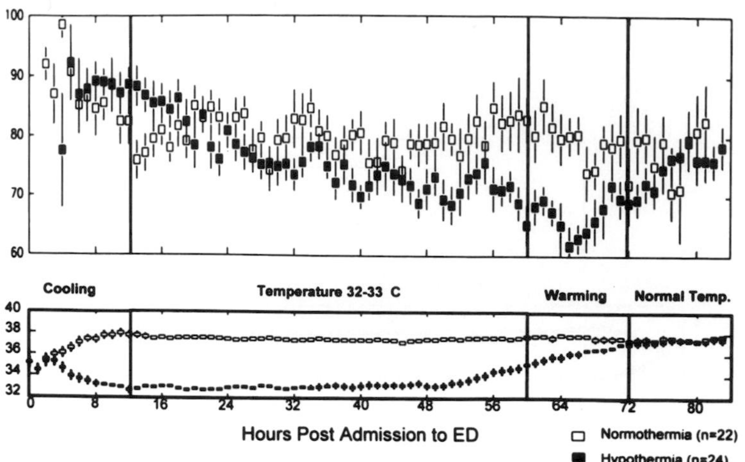

Figure 29-4. Temperature is compared to cerebral perfusion pressure (CPP). CPP was significantly lower in the third time period (Table 29-2).

warming in the fourth time period in the hypothermia group (Table 29-3). This was due to potassium replacement in the hypothermia group during cooling with potassium mobilization during rewarming. The hypothermia group received 65 percent more potassium than the normothermia group during the 84 hours of measurement. Serum glucose was increased in the hypothermia group in the second time period (normothermia, 158.31 ± 5.79 mg/dl and hypothermia, 195.38 ± 9.30 mg/dl, $p < 0.01$).

Complications are shown in Table 29-4. The incidence of sepsis was higher in the hypothermia group, although the difference was not statistically different. The incidence of seizures was lower in the hypothermia group (Fisher's exact test, $p = 0.019$). The mortality rate was 8/22 or 36 percent in the normothermia group and 8/23 or 35 percent in the hypothermia group. There were no cardiac complications or coagulopathy-related complications in either group.

There was an indication of improved neurological

TABLE 29-3 Phase II Trial of Hypothermia in Severe Head Injury—Laboratory Parameters

	Normothermia		*Hypothermia*		
H After ER Admission	**mean**	**SE**	**mean**	**SE**	**Bonferroni p-value**
Prothrombin Time					
0–11	13.80	.23	13.31	.19	NS
12–59	13.02	.17	13.04	.12	NS
60–71	12.47	.29	12.86	.21	$p < .05$
72–83	12.13	.30	12.93	.23	$p < .001$
Partial Thromboplastin Time					
0–11	30.93	1.03	28.65	.92	NS
12–59	30.88	.57	33.13	1.13	NS
60–71	32.62	1.14	34.62	1.01	$p < .025$
72–83	31.66	.61	37.05	3.11	$p < .001$
Potassium					
0–11	3.79	.07	3.65	.10	NS
12–59	3.80	.05	3.75	.05	NS
60–71	3.76	.08	4.03	.13	NS
72–83	3.80	.09	4.24	.14	$p < .005$
Glucose					
0–11	186.82	12.31	177.52	13.34	NS
12–59	158.31	5.79	195.38	9.30	$p < .01$
60–71	154.72	8.03	194.05	20.62	NS
72–83	174.74	12.17	206.91	20.23	NS

TABLE 29-4 Phase II Trial—Complications

Complications	Normothermia	Hypothermia
Acute respiratory distress syndrome	2	2
Pneumonia	7	9
Sepsis	4	9
Seizures	5	0
Pancreatitis	1	0
Cardiac arrhythmias	1	0
Renal failure	1	2
Uncontrollable ICP	6	7

TABLE 29-5 Phase II Trial—Outcome

		GOS Distribution	
		GR/MD	**S/V/D**
Normothermia	N	8	14
	%	36.4	63.6
Hypothermia	N	12	11
	%	52.2	47.8

outcome in the hypothermia group. GOS scores were combined into two categories: Good Recovery/Moderate Disability (GR/MD), and Severe Disability/Vegetative/Dead (SD/V/D). In the normothermia group, 36.4 percent of patients were in the GR/MD group and 63.6 percent were in the SD/V/D group. In the hypothermia group, 52.2 percent were in the GR/MD group and 47.8 percent were in the SD/V/D group. These differences were not significant by chi-square analysis ($p = 0.287$) but do show a trend. GOS distributions are illustrated in Table 29-5.

CONCLUSION

These studies show that induction of systemic hypothermia to 32 to 33°C when beginning cooling within 6 hours of injury increased the absolute percentage of patients in the good outcome category by 16 percent at 3 months after injury. This is a 30 percent increase in the percentage of patients in the good outcome group. Statistically there was a significant decrease in early seizure incidence in the hypothermia group. There were no cardiac arrhythmias at 32 to 33°C. While a statistically significant increase in the partial thromboplastin time and prothrombin time, just out of the normal range, was found during and after rewarming, there were no clinically significant problems with bleeding. The incidence of sepsis was increased in the hypothermia group, but the difference was not statistically significant.

Use of systemic hypothermia may affect management decisions regarding potassium and acid-base balances. Hypothermia drives potassium intracellularly, thereby producing hypokalemia.[37] We chose to replace potassium until serum potassium was normalized. The possibility of rebound hyperkalemia during rewarming concerned us, and this did occur, but because of very slow rewarming (1°C/4 h), the potassium levels were not out of the normal range. Acid-base management was guided by blood gas analysis, which was not corrected for temperature, but was instead measured at 37°C. In order to maintain Pa_{CO_2} 30–35 mmHg, ventilatory rates were decreased during hypothermia because of systemic hypometabolism.

While using a depth of hypothermia of 32 to 33°C is well established by our experience and that of others, the optimal duration of hypothermia is not as certain nor is the optimal time after injury for treatment. We took the approach that therapy should be started as soon after injury as possible; therefore, a designated entry criterion in this study was that cooling begin within 6 hours of injury. Mild hypothermia was usually present upon admission.

Forty-eight hours was selected as the longest time period for treatment that still might have minimal morbidity in patients. In animals, toxicity from moderate hypothermia occurs both as the temperature is decreased and as the duration of hypothermia is increased.[40,41] In this clinical study, 48 hours of hypothermia proved to produce minimal complications with evidence of benefit in functional outcome.

Finally, in a similarly designed study of hypothermia to 32°C for 24 hours in 46 patients with severe brain injury, Marion et al. found a similar level of functional improvement with minimal toxicity.[78] A Phase III randomized, multicenter trial of the use of hypothermia in patients with severe head injury has been initiated.

REFERENCES

1. Bigelow WG, Callaghan JC, Hopps VA: General hypothermia for experimental intracardiac surgery: Use of artificial pacemaker for cardiac standstill and cardiac rewarming in general hypothermia. *Ann Surg* 1950; 132:531–543.
2. Drew CE, Anderson IM: Profound hypothermia in cardiac surgery: Report of three cases. *Lancet* 1959; 1:748–750.
3. Mohri H, Merendino KA: Hypothermia with or without

a pump oxygenator, in Gibbon JH, Sabiston DC, Spencer FC (eds): *Surgery of the Chest.* Philadelphia: WB Saunders, 1969:643–673.
4. Shumway WE, Lower RR: Topical cardiac hypothermia for extended periods of anoxic arrest. *Surg Forum* 1959; 10:563.
5. Bailey CP, Cookson BA, Downing DF, Neptune WB: Cardiac surgery under hypothermia. *J Thorac Surg* 1954; 27:73–95.
6. Castaneda AR, Lamberti J, Sade RM, et al: Open-heart surgery during the first three months of life. *J Thorac Cardiovasc Surg* 1974; Part 2, 68:719–731.
7. Smith DL, Wilson JM, Ebert PA: Cardiac surgery in infants up to one year old. *Cardiovasc Med* 1978; Part 2, 3:925–940.
8. Crawford ES, Saleh SA: Transverse aortic arch aneurysm. Improved results of treatment employing new modifications of aortic reconstruction and hypothermic cerebral circulatory arrest. *Ann Surg* 1981; 194:180–188.
9. White RJ, Massopust LA, Wolin LR, et al: Profound selective cooling and ischemia of primate brain without pump or oxygenator. *Surgery* 1969; 66:224–232.
10. Adams JE, Wylie EJ: Value of hypothermia and arterial occlusion in the treatment of intracranial aneurysms. *Surg Gynecol Obstet* 1959; 108:631–635.
11. Connolly JE, Boyd RJ, Calvin JW: The protective effect of hypothermia in cerebral ischemia: Experimental and clinical application by selective brain cooling in the human. *Surgery* 1962; 51(1):15–23.
12. Drake CG, Barr WK, Coles JC, Gergely NF: The use of extracorporeal circulation and profound hypothermia in the treatment of ruptured intracranial aneurysm. *J Neurosurg* 1964; 21:575–581.
13. McMurtry JG, Housepian EM, Bowman FO Jr, Matteo RS: Surgical treatment of basilar artery aneurysms: Elective circulatory arrest with thoracotomy in 12 cases. *J Neurosurg* 1974; 40:486–494.
14. Patterson RH, Ray BS: Profound hypothermia for intracranial surgery: Laboratory and clinical experiences with extracorporeal circulation by peripheral cannulation. *Ann Surg* 1962; 156:377–393.
15. Selker RG, Wolfson SK, Maroon JC, Steichen FM: Preferential cerebral hypothermia with elective cardiac arrest: Resection of "Giant" aneurysm. *Surg Neurol* 1976; 6:173–179.
16. Silverberg GD, Reitz BA, Ream AK, et al: Operative treatment of a giant cerebral artery aneurysm with hypothermia and circulatory arrest: Report of a case. *J Neurosurg* 1980; 6(3):301–305.
17. Sundt TM Jr, Pluth JR, Gronert GA: Excision of giant basilar aneurysm under profound hypothermia. *Mayo Clin Proc* 1972; 47:631–634.
18. Uihlein A, MacCarty CS, Michenfelder VD, et al: Deep hypothermia and surgical treatment of intracranial aneurysms. *JAMA* 1966; 195:127–129.
19. Uihlein A, MacCarty CS, Michenfelder JD, et al: Deep hypothermia and surgical treatment of intracranial aneurysms. *JAMA* 1966; 195(8):127–129.
20. Williams BN, Turner EA: Report of 10 operations under local cerebral hypothermia. *J Neurol Neurosurg Psychiatry* 1970; 33:647–655.
21. Rosomoff HL, Shulman K, Raynor R, Grainger W: Experimental brain injury and delayed hypothermia. *Surg Gynecol Obstet* 1960; 110:27–32.
22. Clasen RA, Pandolfi S, Russell J, et al: Hypothermia and hypotension in experimental cerebral edema. *Arch Neurol* 1968; 19:472–486.
23. Laskowski EJ, Klatzo I, Baldwin M: Experimental study of the effects of hypothermia on local brain injury. *Neurology* 1960; 10:499–505.
24. Rosomoff HL, Gilbert R: Brain volume and cerebrospinal fluid pressure during hypothermia. *Am J Physiol* 1955; 183:19–22.
25. Drake CG, Jory TA: Hypothermia in the treatment of critical head injury. *Can Med Assoc J* 1962; 87(17):887–891.
26. Hendrick EB: The use of hypothermia in severe head injuries in childhood. *Arch Surg* 1959; 79:362–364.
27. Lazorthes G, Campan L: Hypothermia in the treatment of craniocerebral traumatism. *J Neurosurg* 1958; 15:162–167.
28. Sedzimir CB: Therapeutic hypothermia in cases of head injury. *J Neurosurg* 1959; 16:407–414.
29. Shapiro HM, Syte SR, Loesser J: Barbiturate-augmented hypothermia for reduction of persistent intracranial hypertension. *J Neurosurg* 1974; 40:90–100.
30. Strachan RD, Whittle IR, Miller JD: Hypothermia and severe head injury. *Brain Inj* 1989; 3(1):51–55.
31. Mouritzen CV, Andersen MN: Mechanisms of ventricular fibrillation during hypothermia: Relative changes in myocardial refractory period and conduction velocity. *J Thoracic Cardiovasc Surg* 1966; 51:585–589.
32. Covino BG, D'Amato HE: Mechanism of ventricular fibrillation in hypothermia. *Circ Res* 1962; 148–155.
33. Badeer HS: Effect of hypothermia on the contractile "capacity" of the myocardium. *J Thorac Cardiovasc Surg* 1967; 53:651–656.
34. Remensnyder JP, Austen WG: Diastolic pressure-volume relationships of the left ventricle during hypothermia. *J Thorac Cardiovasc Surg* 1965; 49(2):339–351.
35. Blair E: *Clinical Hypothermia.* New York: McGraw-Hill, 1964:206–213.
36. Lewis JF, Varco RL, Taufic M: Repair of atrial septal defects in man under direct vision with the aid of hypothermia. *Surgery* 1954; 36:538–552.
37. Benson DW, Williams GR, Spencer FC, Yates AJ: The use of hypothermia after cardiac arrest. *Anesth Analg* 1959; 38(6):423–428.
38. Lundberg N, Nielsen KC, Nilsson E: Deep hypothermia in intracranial surgery. *J Neurosurg* 1956; 13:235–247.
39. Williams GR Jr, Spencer FC: The clinical use of hypothermia following cardiac arrest. *Ann Surg* 1958; 148(3):462–466.
40. Steen PA, Mide JH, Michenfelder JD: The detrimental effects of prolonged hypothermia and rewarming in the dog. *Anesthesiology* 1980; 52:224–230.
41. Steen PA, Soule EH, Michenfelder JD: Detrimental effect of prolonged hypothermia in cats and monkeys with

and without regional cerebral ischemia. *Stroke* 1979; 10:522–529.

42. Sands MP, Mohri H, Sato S, et al: Hematorheology during deep hypothermia. *Cryobiology* 1979; 16:229–239.
43. Chen RYZ, Chien S: Hemodynamic functions and blood viscosity in surface hypothermia. *Am J Physiol* 1978; Part 1, 235:H136–H143.
44. Gray TC: Reflections on circulatory control. *Lancet* 1957; 383–389.
45. Busto R, Dietrich WD, Globus MY, et al: Small differences in intraischemic brain temperature critically determine the extent of ischemic neuronal injury. *J Cereb Blood Flow Metab* 1987; 7:729–738.
46. Clifton GL, Taft WC, Blair RE, et al: Conditions for pharmacologic evaluation in the gerbil model of forebrain ischemia. *Stroke* 1987; 20(11):1545–1552.
47. Dempsey RJ, Combs DJ, Maley ME, et al: Moderate hypothermia reduces postischemic edema development and leukotriene production. *Neurosurgery* 1987; 21(2):177–181.
48. Leonov Y, Sterz F, Safar P, et al: Mild cerebral hypothermia during and after cardiac arrest improves neurologic outcome in dogs. *J Cereb Blood Flow Metab* 1990; 10:57–70.
49. Minamisawa H, Smith ML, Siesjo BK: The effect of moderate hypothermia (39°C) and hypothermia (35°C) on brain damage following 10–15 minutes of forebrain ischemia. *J Cereb Blood Flow Metab* 1989; 9(suppl 1):S265.
50. Busto R, Dietrich WD, Globus MY, Ginsberg MD: The importance of brain temperature in cerebral ischemic injury. *Stroke* 1989; 20(8):1113–1114.
51. Busto R, Dietrich WD, Globus MY, et al: Postischemic moderate hypothermia inhibits CA1 hippocampal ischemic neuronal injury. *J Cereb Blood Flow Metab* 1989; 9(suppl 1):S266.
52. Moller BF, Smith ML, Siesjo BK: Effects of hypothermia on brain ischemia: A comparison of intraischemic and postischemic hypothermia. *J Cereb Blood Flow Metab* 1989; 9(suppl 1): S276.
53. Adams JH, Graham DI, Gennarelli TA: Contemporary neuropathological considerations regarding brain damage in head injury, in Becker DP, Povlishock JT (eds): *Central Nervous System Trauma Status Report.* 1985:65–77. NIH/NINCD
54. Miller JD, Butterworth JF, Gudeman SK, et al: Further experience in the management of severe head injury. *J Neurosurg* 1981; 54:289–299.
55. Robertson CJ, Grossman RJ, Goodman JC, Narayan RK: The predictive value of cerebral anaerobic metabolism with cerebral infarction after head injury. *J Neurosurg* 1987; 67:361–368.
56. Overgaard J, Mosdal C, Tween WA: Cerebral circulation after head injury. Part 3. Does reduced regional cerebral blood flow determine recovery of brain function after blunt head injury? *J Neurosurg* 1981; 55:63–74.
57. Muizelaar JP, Obrist WD: Cerebral blood flow and metabolism with brain injury, in Becker DP, Povlishock JT (eds): *Central Nervous System Trauma Status Report.* 1985:123–137. NIH/NINCD
58. Clifton GL, Jiang JY, Lyeth BG, et al: Marked protection by moderate hypothermia after experimental traumatic brain injury. *J Cereb Blood Flow Metab* 1991; 11:114–121.
59. Chopp M, Knight R, Tidwell CD, et al: The metabolic effects of mild hypothermia on global cerebral ischemia and recirculation in the cat: Comparison to normothermia and hyperthermia. *J Cereb Blood Flow Metab* 1989; 9:141–148.
60. Chopp M, Welch KMA, Tidwell CD, et al: Effect of mild hypothermia on recovery of metabolic function after global cerebral ischemia in cats. *Stroke* 1988; 19:1521–1525.
61. Norwood WI, Norwood CR: Influence of hypothermia on intracellular pH during anoxia. *Am J Physiol* 1982; 243:C62–C65.
62. Ishige N, Pitts LH, Pogliani L, et al: Effects of hypoxia in traumatic brain injury in rats: Part 2. Changes in high energy phosphate metabolism. *Neurosurgery* 1987; 20:854–858.
63. Vink R, McIntosh TK, Weiner MW, Faden AI: Effects of traumatic brain injury on cerebral high-energy phosphates and pH: A ^{31}p magnetic resonance spectroscopy study. *J Cereb Blood Flow Metab* 1987; 7:563–571.
64. Dietrich WD, Busto R, Halley M, Valdez I: The importance of brain temperature in alterations of the blood–brain barrier following cerebral ischemia. *J Neuropathol Exp Neurol* 1993; 49:486–497.
65. Dietrich WD, Busto R, Valdes I, Loor Y: Neuropathological consequences of normothermic versus mild hyperthermic transient forebrain ischemia in rats. *Stroke* 1990; 21(9):1318–1325.
66. Povlishock JT: The morphopathologic responses to head injuries of varying severity, in Becker DP, Povlishock JT (eds): *Central Nervous System Status Report.* 1985:443–452. NIH/NINCD
67. Busto R, Globus MY, Dietrich WD, et al: Effect of mild hypothermia on ischemia-induced release of neurotransmitters and free fatty acids in rat brain. *Stroke* 1989; 20(7):904–910.
68. Faden AL, Demediuk P, Panter SS, Vink R: The role of excitatory amino acids and NMDA receptors in traumatic brain injury. *Science* 1989; 244:798–800.
69. Gorman LK, Fu K, Hovda DA, et al: Analysis of acetylcholine release following concussive brain injury in the rat. *J Neurotrauma* 1989; 6:203.
70. Katayama Y, Cheung MK, Gorman L, et al: Increase in extracellular glutamate and associated massive ionic fluxes following concussive brain injury. *Soc Neurosci Abstr* 1988; 14:1154.
71. Hayes RL, Jenkins LW, Lyeth BG, et al: Pretreatment with phencyclidine, an N-methyl-D-aspartate receptor antagonist, attenuates long-term behavioral deficits in the rat produced by traumatic brain injury. *J Neurotrauma* 1988; 5(4):287–302.
72. Lyeth BG, Dixon CE, Jenkins LW, et al: Effects of scopolamine treatment on long-term behavioral deficits following concussive brain injury to the rat. *Brain Res* 1988; 452:39–48.

73. Clifton GL, Christensen ML: Use of moderate hypothermia during elective craniotomy. Texas Med 1993; 88(12):66–69.
74. Clifton GL, Allen S, Barrodale P, et al: A phase II trial of systemic hypothermia in severe brain injury. *J Neurotrauma* 1993; 10(3):263–271.
75. Clifton GL, Allen S, Berry J, Koch SM: Systemic hypothermia in treatment of brain injury. *J Neurotrauma* 1992; 9(2):S487–S495.
76. Jennett B, Bond M: Assessment of outcome after severe brain damage. *Lancet* 1985; 1:480–487.
77. Marmarou A, Anderson RL, Ward JD, et al: NINDS Traumatic Coma Data Bank: Intracranial pressure monitoring methodology. *J Neurosurg* 1991; 75:S21.
78. Marion DW, Obrist WD, Carlier PM, et al: The use of moderate therapeutic hypothermia for patients with severe head injuries: A preliminary report. *J Neurosurg* 1993; 79:354–362.

Monitoring and Treatment

CHAPTER 30

PATHOPHYSIOLOGY OF INTRACRANIAL PRESSURE

Anthony Marmarou

SYNOPSIS

This chapter reviews the mathematical basis of ICP dynamics to help clarify the sequence of events leading to raised intracranial pressure and subsequent cerebral ischemia. It must be emphasized that although much has been learned over the past 25 years of research in this field, the basic question of which factors are the most important in causing brain swelling has not been fully answered. As a result, brain edema and vascular engorgement have been used interchangeably to explain increased brain volume and subsequent rise in ICP. As we now have strong evidence that CSF parameters play a relatively minor role in ICP elevation, it is necessary to shift the focus to the cerebral vasculature, to better understand its role in the genesis of elevated intracranial pressure. Finally, the relative contribution of both ICP elevation and systemic hypotension in accounting for cerebral perfusion pressure reduction is beginning to emerge.

INTRODUCTION

Uncontrollable intracranial pressure (ICP) remains a frequent cause of death in the severely head-injured patient, and in survivors the poor prognosis associated with sustained elevations of ICP has been well documented.[1,59,65,66,71,92] Intracranial hypertension (ICH) is a problem in at least half of patients with mass lesions and in one-third of patients with diffuse injury. Half of patients who develop high ICP die despite surgical decompression and other therapies. Recent data provide compelling evidence that outcome and morbidity from severe head injury is directly related to time above the critical threshold of 20 mmHg.[53] As ICP increases, the gradient of pressure available for perfusion of the brain decreases, and it is this reduction of cerebral perfusion pressure (CPP), ie., the difference between arterial pressure and the ICP, which is considered the critical event. Sustained elevation of ICP may have direct effects on neural tissue despite adequate perfusion. However, the major emphasis in ICP management has focused on maintaining cerebral perfusion pressure above a certain minimum threshold.

The objective of this chapter is to describe the pathophysiology of intracranial pressure in traumatic brain injury and to provide a mathematical basis for estimating parameters essential to understanding the mechanisms responsible for ICH.

INTRACRANIAL PRESSURE—DEFINITION AND MEASUREMENT

By classic definition the intracranial pressure is the cerebrospinal fluid pressure, which in turn is defined as the pressure that must be exerted against a needle introduced into the cerebrospinal fluid space to just prevent escape of fluid.[6] Lundberg[38] introduced the practice of ICP monitoring, and ICP measured by direct cannulation of the ventricular system is the standard of reference to which all other pressures within the cranial cavity are compared. Other so-called intracranial pressures may include fluid pressures measured in the cisterna magna or subdural space, or directly in tissue. Alternative measures of ICP are necessary in those cases where ventricular catheterization is not possible or perhaps not desirable. These include subarachnoid bolts[45] or epidural devices[46,48] as well as fully implantable devices. The subarachnoid bolt has been widely used in many head injury centers; however, bolt pressures may underestimate the ICP when fluid coupling is lost through tissue impaction of the screw device. Epidural pressure underestimates ICP at high levels of pressure and thus is used less frequently in trauma, but is sometimes chosen for patients with liver failure and concomitant coagulopathy.[7]

At equilibrium, it is considered that the fluid within the brain parenchyma is in continuity with the cerebrospinal fluid and, as such, the ventricular and parenchymal pressures are identical, or at least very similar. The advent of fiberoptic devices and other new miniaturized ICP devices now allow measurement of brain tissue pressure.[32,76,110] The main disadvantages of tissue pressure measurement alone is that it obviates drainage of CSF for pressure control and cannot be verified in vivo without simultaneous ventricular pressure monitoring. The primary advantage of such devices is their ease of insertion and maintenance.

Pulsatile and Baseline Components

The physiological basis of ICP is best explained by a doctrine describing the interaction between CSF, blood, and brain tissue. This doctrine, expressed by Kellie and Monroe,[41,70] states that the intracranial tissue compartments are normally in a state of volume equilibrium. A disruption of this volume equilibrium by an increase in the volume of blood, interstitial space, CSF, or a mass must be compensated for by one or more of the other fluids such that the total intracranial volume remains constant. Simply stated,

(1)
$$\text{Total intracranial volume } (V_T) = V_{\text{blood}} + V_{\text{CSF}} + V_{\text{tissue}}$$

(2) $$V_T = \Delta V_{\text{blood}} + \Delta V_{\text{CSF}} + \Delta V_{\text{tissue}} + \Delta V_{\text{mass}}$$

Disturbance of compartmental volume equilibrium disrupts pressure equilibrium, and the magnitude of pressure change will depend on the magnitude and rate of volume interchange as well as the compliance of each compartment. Under normal physiological conditions, volume compartments remain relatively constant; thus, the ICP remains constant in the range of 8 to 10 mmHg above atmospheric level.[22]

Pulsatile Components of ICP

The exceptions to complete volume equilibrium are the constant volume fluctuations synchronous with cardiac and respiratory rates that produce the pulsatile components of ICP. Thus, the intracranial pressure consists of a baseline level, above atmospheric pressure, on which is superimposed a cardiac and respiratory pulse. The pulsatile component of ICP is clearly discerned with high fidelity pressure monitors and is in the range of 3 to 5 mmHg, peak to trough. Pulsatile components of the CSF pressure were recognized in the late 1800s; however, attempts to measure amplitude accurately were blunted by the older recording systems that required large volume change. As electronic gauges were developed, the pulsations were more accurately identified, and the amplitudes were noted to range from 20 to 40 mm saline.[2,31]

Early workers focused on the choroid plexus as the driving force necessary for pulsation; however, more recent studies have discounted the choroid plexus as the source of pulsation. It still remains undecided as to whether the pulse is primarily arterial[20] or venous[35] or both arterial and venous.[13,15]

Regardless of source, the pulsatile component of ICP is hydraulically transmitted throughout the brain tissue and is clearly visualized in both CSF and parenchymal pressure measurements. Most important, it is seen to rise in amplitude as the ICP increases, a phenomenon that will be described in detail in the section dealing with pressure-volume relationships.

THE CEREBROSPINAL FLUID SYSTEM

The physiological mechanisms governing volume homeostasis of the cerebrospinal fluid system are fundamental to the understanding of intracranial pressure. Comprehensive in-depth reviews of CSF physiology are covered in other texts.[14,24,30,63] Briefly, the CSF spaces consist of two continuous compartments: the interstitial space, which surrounds cellular elements; and the larger compartmental volumes of CSF, which include the ventricles, major cisterns, and subarachnoid space. The cerebrospinal fluid flows through the ventricles, exiting to the cisterna magna and basal cisterns to the subarachnoid spaces of the cerebral convexity and finally toward the arachnoid villi, where it is reabsorbed.

Choroidal and Extrachoroidal CSF Production

While the origin of cerebrospinal fluid remains unclear, two sites of formation are known to exist. These are the choroid plexus and the ventricular ependyma. Estimates of percentage of fluid formed by these two sources vary widely. Earlier studies attributed most if not all of formation to the choroid plexus.[108] The transient reduction of CSF formation by as much as 50 percent by acetazolamide[75,81] suggested that CSF formation by the choroid plexus and extrachoroidal sources may be equal. However, other workers have concluded that extrachoroidal formation accounts for about one-third of newly formed CSF.[62] Thus, the issue of percentage contribution of extrachoroidal sources remains unresolved.

Under normal conditions, rates of CSF formation in man have been estimated to equal 0.35 ml/min or approximately 500 ml per day.[9,64,90] The total volume of CSF in the adult is estimated at 150 ml. Thus, the CSF volume is turned over approximately every 8 hours.

CSF Absorption

The sites of cerebrospinal fluid egress have been studied extensively, and the classic textbook description is that CSF absorption takes place at the arachnoid villi, where the CSF is returned to the blood via the dural sinus. However, more recent studies utilizing magnetic resonance technology have challenged these earlier concepts, as will be discussed later. Studies into the mechanism of absorption indicated that compounds of different molecular weight were absorbed into the blood at the same rate, implicating a bulk flow process.[85] It has been established that drainage into the dural sinuses occurs only in the presence of a positive gradient between CSF and dural sinus pressure.[97] This is the basis for the Masserman method for estimating rates of CSF formation.[61] Because no absorption takes place when ICP is below dural sinus pressure, a known amount of fluid is removed and the time necessary to return to baseline pressure provides a linear estimate of the rate of formation.

Circulation of the Cerebrospinal Fluid

The driving force propelling fluid along the CSF pathways generally has been attributed to arterial pulsations, and this early notion was derived mainly by observation during surgical procedures.[72] The results of isotope cisternography gave further credence to an active circulation, but with limited interpretation.[16] Although workers generally accept an arterial component, a more precise explanation of how the arterial pulsation acts to expel CSF from the ventricular system and eventually over the convexities remains elusive.

A concept that held for several decades was put forth by Bering,[2] who proposed that expansion of the choroid plexus serves to pump fluid out of the ventricles. Others postulated the existence of a third ventricular pump[72] as well as a fourth pump in the basal cistern due to brain expansion.[17,19] The third ventricular pump was considered to provide a mixing action between fluid in the third ventricle and basal cisterns. Subsequent observations with air and cisternography by du Boulay demonstrated pulse-synchronous pulsations in the upper cervical region with small or absent pulsations in the ventricles. Antegrade flow during systole and retrograde flow during diastole were observed in the aqueduct. The amplitude of the pulsations in the cervical region were graded ten times larger than those observed in the aqueduct.[18,19]

The advent of magnetic resonance imaging (MRI) techniques fostered new phase imaging investigations into the flow of cerebrospinal fluid. Utilizing these methods, flow in the foramen magnum, aqueduct, and pontine cistern was studied in normal volunteers.[34] According to these studies, the large pulsations observed in the foramen magnum, which start before pulsations in the aqueduct and pontine cistern, were not consistent with the assumption by earlier workers that ventricular pulsations were the driving force behind CSF circulation. These studies demonstrated that systolic expansion of the brain combined with a downward movement during the systolic pulse propels the extraventricular CSF, with the entire brain acting as a piston. It was also concluded that bulk flow in the anterior and posterior part of the spinal canal was small.

The mechanism of spinal circulation, which has been considered bi-directional, also remains controversial. Tracers injected into the lumbar area are transported cephalad, and those in the ventricle are transported caudad at speeds significantly greater than could occur by simple diffusion. In one study, a bi-directional flow could not be demonstrated and no consistent bulk flow component could be measured, although these levels of flow were bordering on the accuracy of the technique.[72] Undoubtedly, further research will be required before an accurate description of CSF circulation is achieved. Clearly, MRI will contribute greatly to this field of study. An excellent review of CSF circulation and new concepts utilizing phase imaging is provided by Greitz.[33]

BRAIN INTERSTITIAL FLUID MOVEMENT

It was stated earlier that the CSF spaces may be considered as two compartments, the fluid surrounding cellular elements or interstitium and the larger CSF volumes. As these compartments are in continuity, an increase in interstitial fluid volume (or edema fluid) adds an additional burden toward maintaining volume homeostasis. Thus, it is important to consider the mechanisms by which both the fluid and solute constituents that lead to brain edema enter the brain tissue.

Three possible mechanisms have been identified for the clearance of fluid and extravasated protein from the extracellular space—pressure-driven bulk flow into the CSF,[4,87,88] glial and neuronal uptake of the protein compounds,[23,37,43,47,63] and reverse vesicular transport from the extracellular space to the blood via transendothelial passage.[106,107] Among these pathways, the role of bulk flow propelling fluid from the interstitium across the ependyma to the ventricular CSF has been demonstrated by many workers and is believed to be the most important.[4,54,74,87] The concept of bulk flow was further emphasized by investigators demonstrating clearance of different size molecules from brain at a similar rate.[8] Furthermore, other immunocytochemical studies have confirmed movement of particulate matter not only toward the ventricle, but also toward the glial limitans as well as the extracellular space of the cortical neuropil.[73] Thus, fluid migration extends not only toward the ventricle but also toward the subarachnoid space.

This movement was observed to occur in the absence of pressure gradients. Because the movements of high and low molecular tracers were observed, it was concluded that this movement occurred by a process of diffusion. These results point further to the CSF pathway as the primary route responsible for the egress of extracellular edema fluid. Thus, the volume challenge to the CSF absorptive systems is not only the newly formed cerebrospinal fluid, but the added edema fluid that engorges the extracellular space following traumatic brain injury. Routes of egress include diffusion through the extracellular space of the cortical neuropil; bulk flow through the extracellular space into ventricular CSF, and bulk flow through the perivascular spaces into the subarachnoid CSF.[73] Few data are available to describe how the efficiency of these pathways is altered with trauma. In one study of head-injured patients, cerebrospinal fluid production, estimated by the techniques to be described in this chapter, was within normal limits except for two patients whose CSF production was estimated to be twice normal. However, in general, the rate of new CSF formation in most brain-injury patients, including the edema component of interstitial flow, is very small.[8] Considering the degree of brain swelling that is prevalent with trauma, it would appear that the resolution of edema may be seriously compromised.

DEVELOPMENT OF MATHEMATICAL MODELS TO DESCRIBE ICP DYNAMICS

Although the Monroe-Kellie equations describing a constant intracranial volume appear simple, the implications in terms of pressure equilibrium are far-reaching and mathematically complex. Efforts to model the dynamic behavior of various compartments, specifically the CSF system, under various conditions has developed into a special field of research, and each investigation has provided incremental understanding of the relationship of ICP in trauma and disease.[2,13,15,20,22,24,31,32,35,41,63,70,76,86,104,105,110] In the following sections, a physiological model of the cerebrospinal fluid system will be presented that has stood the test of time and contains several parameters used routinely in the clinical setting.[56] In an earlier section, the ICP was defined as a base level above atmospheric, on which are superimposed respiratory and cardiac components. The model to be presented deals only with the steady-state level of ICP and not the pulsatile component. The changes in amplitude of the pulsatile component will be dealt with separately in the pressure-volume section.

Factors Governing the Steady-State Level of ICP

Pressure equilibrium is directly related to volume equilibrium, and efforts to describe the steady state or basal level of ICP in essence describe the delicate balance between all fluids entering and leaving the intracranial cavity. Since ICP is defined as the pressure of the cerebrospinal fluid, the dynamic flow characteristics of CSF will be discussed first. For mathematical purposes, the mechanisms of formation, storage, and absorption of CSF can be understood by electrical analogy (Fig. 30-1). The electrical analogy subdivides the physical mechanisms into three major categories: formation, storage, and absorption. As the newly formed cerebrospinal fluid (I_f) is developed, a component (I_s) can either be stored, which acts to increase ventricular volume and compress brain, or a component (I_a) can be absorbed. Mathematically this balance between formation, storage, and absorption can be expressed as shown in Equa-

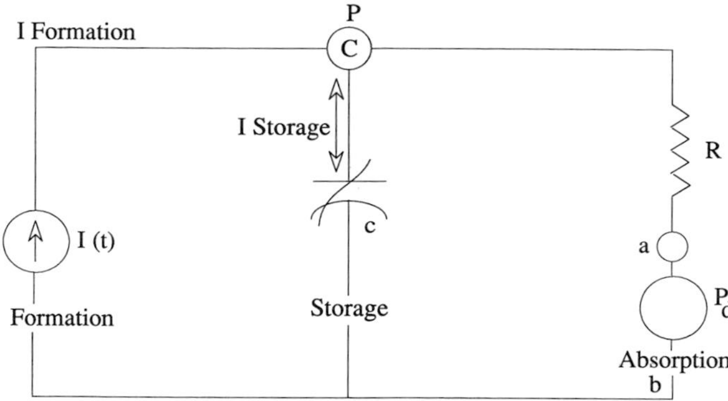

Figure 30-1. The major parameters of the CSF system are depicted as an electrical analog. CSF formation is represented as a constant current source and is independent of pressure. The newly formed fluid (I formation) is either stored (I storage) into a compliant chamber or absorbed (I absorbed) through a resistance element representing the hydraulic resistance offered to the absorption of fluid. The fluid that is absorbed eventually sinks into the dural sinus, which is depicted at a constant pressure (Pd).

tion 3, where the amounts stored or absorbed must equal the amount formed:

(3) $$I_f = I_s + I_a$$

Referring to the electrical analog, both choroidal and extrachoroidal sources of fluid are "lumped" into a single pump which continuously provides fluid into the CSF space. As no feedback paths are included, it is considered that the rate of fluid formation remains constant and independent of the pressure head seen by the pump mechanism. Note that the pressure at the juncture of this space represented by the node (*c*) is equal to the intracranial pressure denoted as (*P*).

Under normal conditions the rate of formation is equally balanced by an equal rate of absorption. This condition of equilibrium results in the storage component to equal zero, and thus both the resting pressure and the resting CSF volume remain unchanged.

Critical to the model is the physiological principle governing the absorption of CSF. This was defined by Davson,[14] who stated that the rate of absorption (I_a) is dependent on the gradient of pressure between CSF space (P) and the dural sinus (Pd) and the resistance (R) offered to the egress of fluid. Expressed mathematically,

(4) $$I_a = (P - Pd)/R.$$

From this physiological relationship, the equation was solved for P and it was concluded[56] that at equilibrium, the level of the intracranial pressure (P) is governed by the pressure of the dural sinus and the production of formation rate and resistance to outflow. Thus, Equation 5 represents the steady state equation for the level of intracranial pressure at equilibrium:

(5) $$P = (I_f \times R) + Pd$$

The assumption implicit in this relationship is that CSF formation, dural sinus pressure, and the resistance to outflow remain constant and time invariant. Many investigators have shown that bulk absorption of fluid is linearly related to the pressure gradient, further substantiating the formula and thus yielding the steady state equation utilized for ICP analysis.[58] Although there is general agreement concerning the dependence of CSF outflow on the available pressure gradient, the pressure independence of CSF formation—and for that matter outflow resistance—remained a topic of controversy for many years. A review of this issue and the approach used by other investigators has been published.[55] At present, the relationship is generally accepted and, in fact, is the basis for the Katzman and Hussey test for measurement of CSF absorption.[40] Interestingly, these investigators focused on the rate of pressure rise and plateau for a specific rate of infusion as a qualitative measure of CSF block. Other investigators quantified the outflow resistance by accepting the notion that the difference between initial and final steady-state pressures divided by the infusion rate is a quantitative measure of outflow. As the rate of CSF formation, or in this case an infusion pump, rate is increased in stepwise fashion to a new constant rate, the ICP will transiently increase and will stabilize at a new steady-state level. The linear slope of the formation vs ICP relationship represents the resistance to outflow of CSF expressed in mmHg/ml/min and can be simply computed by noting the change in steady-state pressure and dividing by the change in infusion rate. This method of outflow resistance measure has been applied for diagnosis of hydrocephalus but is less useful in assessment of Ro changes in traumatic injury because of the required infused volume and the necessity for raising pressure to a higher steady-state level for a prolonged period.

What Parameters Are Likely to Contribute to Raised ICP?

It is interesting at this point to speculate how this dynamic equilibrium is altered in the case of raised intracranial pressure. According to the model equation, a sustained increase in pressure must be accompanied by an increase in at least one of three parameters: rate of formation, resistance to outflow of fluid, and an elevation in dural sinus pressure. In a previous section, the contribution of interstitial flow caused by edema adding to the newly formed fluid was not considered to affect overall fluid formation dramatically. Thus, it appears unlikely that ICP elevation results from sharp increases in rate of fluid formation. On the other hand, it is clear from clinical observations in the patient with subarachnoid hemorrhage that ICP is elevated as a result of increased outflow resistance, and studies have clearly shown this to be the case.[29,36,43] Perhaps the most difficult to comprehend is the increased pressure that accompanies diffuse brain injury where outflow resistance may not be elevated. This leaves the final parameter, dural sinus pressure, suspect for alteration under these conditions, and this is discussed more fully in the section of vascular contribution to raised ICP.

Pressure-Volume Theory: Intracranial Compliance

Thus far, the relationship of intracranial pressure at equilibrium has dealt only with three parameters: rate of formation, resistance to absorption, and dural sinus pressure. With formation and absorption in balance, there is no alteration in the amount stored, and compartmental volumes remain unchanged. As long as volumes remain constant, pressure remains constant. When the CSF volume is altered, the CSF pressure will change, and the amount of pressure change will depend on three factors: the rate of volume change, the amount of volume change, and the intracranial compliance. The change in CSF volume per unit change in CSF pressure defines the intracranial compliance. Expressed mathematically,

(6)
Compliance C = change in volume/change in pressure
$= \Delta V/\Delta P.$

The term "elastance" is simply the reciprocal of compliance or

(7) Elastance = change in pressure/change in volume
$= \Delta P/\Delta V$

An ideal container in biophysical terms is one in which pressure changes linearly with volume; however, it has been shown by several investigators that intracranial pressure and volume are not linearly related, but that intracranial pressure changes exponentially with volume[45,68,69,94,98,99] (Fig. 30-2). The exponential variation of pressure with volume shown in Fig. 30-2 offers an explanation why pulse pressure increases as ICP increases. The same volume change on the horizontal axis due to a net intracranial volume perturbation will be reflected as a pulsatile change in pressure which increases as ICP increases. The intracranial compliance can be quantified by first plotting the exponential curve on a logarithmic axis and computing the slope as shown in Fig. 30-3. The slope of this straight line given by the

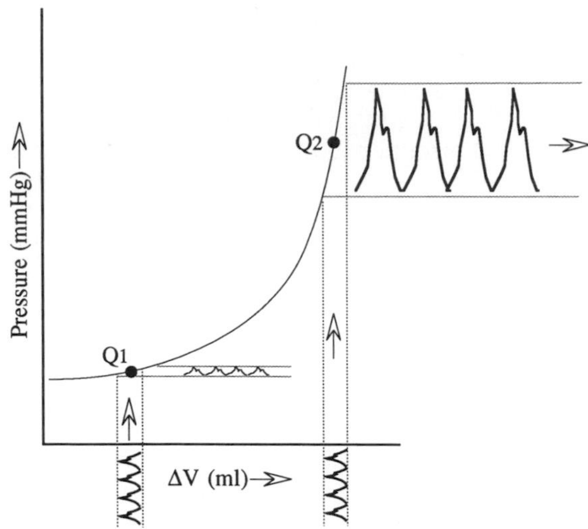

Figure 30-2. Intracranial pressure and CSF volume are exponentially related. Pressure and volume equilibrium can be depicted as a point *(Q1)* on the curve. Volume changes introduced by cardiac and respiratory pulsation are reflected in pressure according to the slope at the *Q1* region of the curve. An increase in pressure shifts the operating point to a new region of the curve *(Q2)*. Note, the same level of volume changes reflect in higher pulsations due to the increase in the slope of the curve. This is why pulsatile pressure increases with increasing pressure.

change in volume (ΔV) to the change in pressure from an initial level Po to a new peak level Pp was defined as the pressure volume index or (PVI).[56,94]

Expressed mathematically,

(8) $$\text{PVI} = \Delta V/\{\log \text{Pp}/\text{Po}\}\ \text{ml}$$

The volume pressure ratio (VPR) is another compliance index which describes the slope of the pressure volume

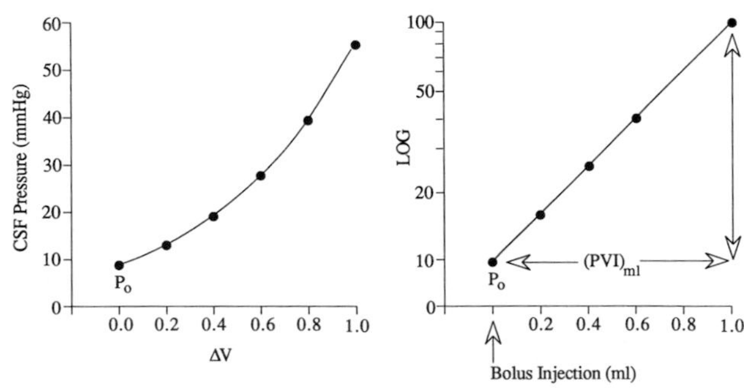

Figure 30-3. The exponential pressure volume curve *(A)* plotted on a logarithmic axis *(B)* yields a straight line where the slope of the line is defined as the pressure volume index. The normal value of PVI is approximately 25 ml in man. The PVI is determined by noting the peak pressure reached in response to bolus injection or by measuring the pressure response to rapid infusion.

curve at a given level of ICP and is defined as the change in pressure achieved by a 1-ml bolus addition of CSF volume.[67,68] If the shape of the pressure-volume curve remains fixed, the VPR will vary linearly with pressure as a natural consequence of the exponential curve. As it defines the slope at a specific level, the change in elasticity or the VPR must be related to the pressure at which the elastance is evaluated. The VPR and the PVI at a steady-state pressure level Po are related by the following equation,

$$\text{VPR} = \text{Po}/(0.434\ \text{PVI}) \quad (9)$$

MEASUREMENT OF BRAIN COMPLIANCE

Since brain compliance refers to the relationship of volume change to pressure change, it can be measured by injecting small quantities of fluid into the CSF space and recording the instantaneous rise in ICP. Two conditions are necessary for obtaining the pressure volume curve. First, the rate of volume addition must be considerably higher than the rate of formation; second, the magnitude of volume addition must not exceed that level which causes vasodilation or alteration of the original resting pressure. In the clinical setting, PVI measures are obtained by first removing 2.0 ml and noting the reduction in pressure. By this technique, the PVI can be estimated. After deciding on a peak pressure that should not be exceeded, a maximum volume injection can be calculated from Equation 8. Ordinarily, the PVI measures are obtained by repeated injections of 2 or 3 ml and the average PVI is calculated from multiple injections. Injection of fluid into the CSF space is not performed when ICP exceeds 25 mmHg. In those cases, PVI is obtained from withdrawal of known quantities of fluid. As expected, PVI measures from withdrawal of CSF are close to PVI measures obtained from injection.[60]

Recently, other methods that provide a continuous estimation of compliance have been developed.[80] This is accomplished by utilizing multiple time-averaged small-volume pulses introduced by a computer-controlled pressure generator. The small volumes are of advantage because less perturbation in pressure is produced. However, time averages of compliance tend to underestimate levels of compliance obtained by more conventional methods and most incorporate a compensating factor, which fortunately is a constant value.

MEASUREMENT OF CSF PARAMETERS BY VOLUME CHANGE

The mathematical determination of compliance allows the prediction of how pressure will change in response to any CSF volume disturbance. For example, if fluid is added to the system, pressure will increase and the magnitude of increase depends on the PVI. Following the increase of pressure, the rate of return to original baseline will depend on a complex function which includes terms of compliance and the resistance to absorption. These mathematical relationships can now be used to advantage by introducing small volume changes, observing the pressure responses, and from specific measures of pressure the major parameters of resistance to CSF outflow and dural sinus pressure can be obtained. As an example, the resistance to outflow can be measured from the pressure response to bolus injection by injecting a known volume (ΔV), measuring the initial (Po) and peak pressure (Pp) and a pressure (P2) on the response curve at a selected time (T2) (Fig. 30-4). Inserting these elements into the equation shown in the figure will provide the resistance to CSF outflow. The methods by which other parameters can be measured using these pressure responses to known volume additions are summarized in Fig. 30-4. Although the bolus method is preferred for studies of head-injured patients, new methods based on these basic equations been developed which utilize infusion and instant computer computation of both compliance and resistance parameters.[12] In addition to these new techniques, sophisticated waveform analysis has been applied to on-line analysis of brain compliance measures.[77] These methods hold promise for less invasive assessment, which is most desirable for detecting pending herniation and further characterizing parameters leading to raised intracranial pressure.

AN EXPANDED PRESSURE-VOLUME MODEL

The pressure-volume theory that has been described in this chapter is based fundamentally on the exponential portion of the pressure-volume curve which embodies the normal physiological range of pressure. If, however, a considerable amount of CSF volume is withdrawn, the pressure volume curve tends to flatten, and at very low pressures, the slope increases. Conversely, as pressure increases to very high levels, where cerebral perfusion pressure is compromised, the normally exponential rise tends to flatten. Friden has developed a mathematical relationship that accurately describes the pressure volume curve at the lower extreme and that includes the middle exponential rise of the curve[27] (Fig. 30-5). His equation describing the parameters of the curve is

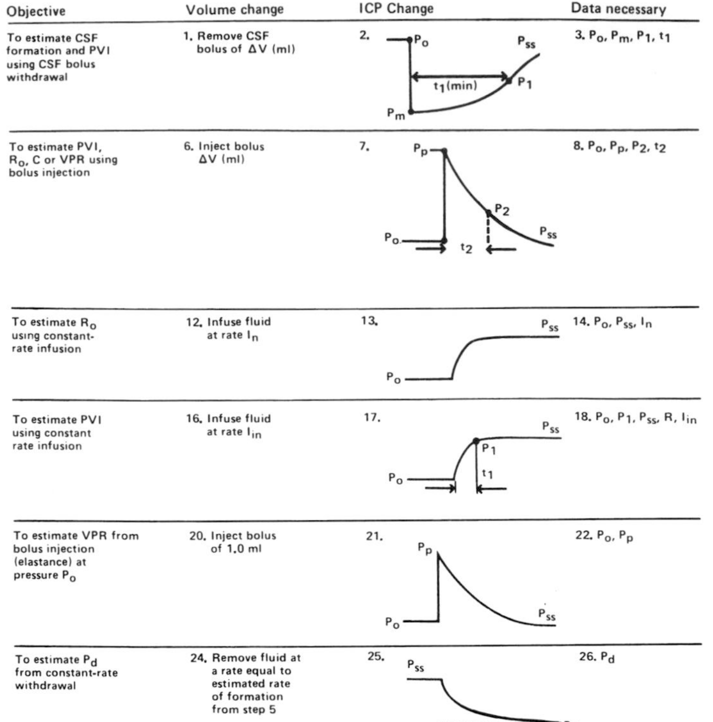

Summary of ICP dynamics

Objective	Volume change	ICP Change	Data necessary	Equations	Normal values of adults
To estimate CSF formation and PVI using CSF bolus withdrawal	1. Remove CSF bolus of ΔV (ml)	2. P_o, P_{ss}, t_1(min), P_1, P_m	3. P_o, P_m, P_1, t_1	4. $PVI = \frac{\Delta V}{\log_{10} P_o/P_m}$ 5. $I_{form} = \frac{PVI}{t_1}(\log P_1/P_m)$	25-30 ml 0.3-0.4 ml/min
To estimate PVI, R_o, C or VPR using bolus injection	6. Inject bolus ΔV (ml)	7. P_p, P_2, P_{ss}, P_o, t_2	8. P_o, P_p, P_2, t_2	9. $PVI = \frac{\Delta V}{\log_{10} P_p/P_o}$ 10. $R_o = \frac{t_2 P_o}{(PVI) \log \left[\frac{P_2}{P_p} \cdot \frac{P_p - P_o}{P_2 - P_o}\right]}$ 11. $C = \frac{.4343\ PVI}{P_o}$ and $VPR = \frac{1}{C}$	25-30 ml 2-12 mm Hg/ml/min 0.25-1.5 ml/mm Hg
To estimate R_o using constant-rate infusion	12. Infuse fluid at rate I_n	13. P_{ss}, P_o	14. P_o, P_{ss}, I_n	15. $R_o = \frac{P_{ss} - P_o}{I_n}$	2-12 mm Hg/ml/min
To estimate PVI using constant rate infusion	16. Infuse fluid at rate I_{in}	17. P_{ss}, P_1, P_o, t_1	18. P_o, P_1, P_{ss}, R, I_{in}	19. $PVI = \frac{\Delta I\ P_{sst}}{(P_o - P_{ss}) \log \left[\frac{P_o(P_{ss} - P_1)}{P_1(P_{ss} - P_o)}\right]}$	25-30 ml
To estimate VPR from bolus injection (elastance) at pressure P_o	20. Inject bolus of 1.0 ml	21. P_p, P_o, P_{ss}	22. P_o, P_p	23. $VPR = \frac{\Delta P}{\Delta V} = P_p - P_o$ $VPR = \frac{1}{C}$	0-3 mm Hg/ml up to 30 mm Hg
To estimate P_d from constant-rate withdrawal	24. Remove fluid at a rate equal to estimated rate of formation from step 5	25. P_{ss}, P_d	26. P_d	27. Estimate of dural sinus pressure P_d equals ICP level after reaching equilibrium following withdrawal of fluid at rate estimated CSF formation (I_{form}).	

Figure 30-4. A summary of the ICP dynamical relationships and the procedures necessary to calculate parameters describing the cerebrospinal fluid system. For example, the top of the table illustrates the means by which CSF formation can be estimated by removing a known volume of CSF (Step 1), recording the response of pressure (Step 2), extracting the data from the curve (Step 3), and using the equations to calculate PVI and formation rate (Step 4).

given by

$$\text{(10)} \quad \begin{aligned} Pc(t) &= Poffset + Amin/[Vmin - Vc(t)] \\ &\quad + Amax/[Vmax - Vc(t)] \\ &\quad [Vmin < Vc(t) < Vmax]. \end{aligned}$$

The first term is an offset term related to cerebral venous pressure. The second and third terms describe the relationship as CSF volume approaches its minimum and maximum levels. The terms Amin and Amax define the bending function at its extremes and is related to the work to fully drain or fill the CSF system.

ICP Pulse Waveform Analysis

The ICP pulsation can be described using spectral analysis techniques consisting of a complex sum of sinusoidal waves, each with a specific amplitude and phase. This form of analysis has led to a new field of study. It has been shown that spectral properties of the ICP pulse vary as a function of compliance, vascular delay between inflow and outflow, autoregulation, cerebral perfusion pressure, and site of measurement.[10,11,78,79,82,83,84] As the complexity of the wave increases, so does the number of harmonic components. The major components of the ICP waveform can be identified by one fundamental and five harmonics. The fundamental, as expected, occurs at the heart rate frequency and the higher harmonics at multiples of this frequency. Other investigators have focused on simply the pulse amplitude in relation to the mean ICP. As described earlier, the pulse amplitude at any ICP level is determined by the tangent slope of the pressure volume curve. As ICP increases, the pulse amplitude will increase in direct proportion for a true exponential. Investigators have used this relationship to detect reduced cerebral perfusion pressure as the pressure volume curve plateaus. In the study by Czosnyka et al., a simple transmission coefficient described the ratio of compartmental compliances and is given by the following equation,

$$\text{(11)} \quad \text{transmission} = Ca/(Ca + Ci).$$

In this relationship, Ca represents a lumped arterial compliance and Ci the compliance of the CSF compartment. Combining this principle with the correlation co-

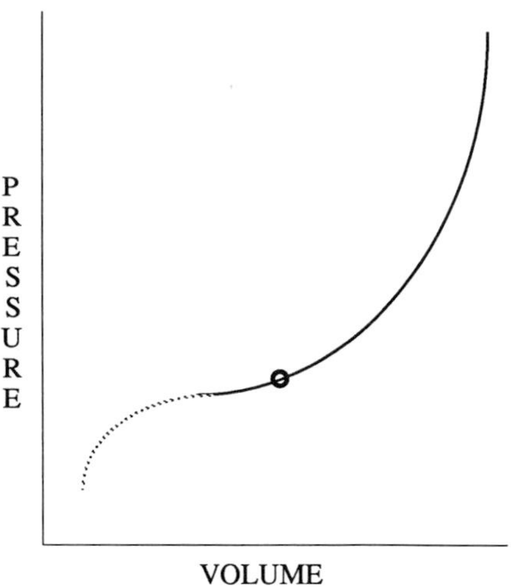

Figure 30-5. A new expression developed by Fridén describes both the exponential portion and the lower segment *(broken line)* of the pressure volume curve (see text).

efficient (RAP) between pulse amplitude and mean ICP, studies of head-injured patients revealed marked changes of RAP as cerebral perfusion pressure was compromised. More important, there were distinct patterns of RAP associated with Glasgow outcome score.[10]

Measurement of Brain Compliance by the Volume Accounting Method

An alternative technique that has had limited use for validation of the compliance and resistance parameters is the method of volume accounting.[28] The technique requires an accounting of the net CSF volume change caused by endo- and exogenous flows of CSF into and out of the CSF system. The assumptions essential to the technique are: the mean CSF volume does not change when the mean CSF pressure is constant; if the CSF pressure has been changed by CSF volume changes, the return of the CSF pressure to the former value has been caused by a return of the CSF volume to its former value. The mathematical basis of the method is structured on the equation

$$(12)\quad \mathrm{Vnet}(t) = \mathrm{Vinput}(t) + \mathrm{Vform}(t) - \mathrm{Vabs}(t)$$

where all volume parameters are a function of time. In this relationship Vnet is the net volume change, Vinput is the volume added or drained from the system, Vform is the volume of the newly formed fluid, and Vabs is the volume absorbed according to the Davson equation. As an example, if Vinput and Vform are a constant value, then the right-hand side of the equation represents the volume that is not absorbed and results in an elevation of pressure. The compliance curve can be obtained by plotting the intracranial pressure corresponding to the net volume as a function of time. This method is more appropriate when combined with either the longer duration constant pressure or constant infusion studies.[26]

INFUSION TECHNOLOGY FOR MEASUREMENT OF CSF PARAMETERS

As described earlier, the relationship between the intracranial pressure, rate of formation, resistance to CSF absorption and dural sinus pressure is given by Equation 5.

The three parameters of interest, If, Ro, and Pd, can be derived by a variety of methods, among them the techniques described in Fig. 30-4. Other methods include constant pressure infusion and lumbar-ventricular perfusion. The constant pressure infusion method[21] can also provide measures of CSF formation rate, resistance to outflow, and indirect measure of dural sinus pressure. In the constant pressure method, two needles are inserted in the L3–L4 interspace, and free passage of fluid by aspiration of 2 ml and replacement by artificial CSF is determined. The patient is allowed to lie supine with the zero reference level at the cranial sagittal center. Drainage of CSF and infusion of artificial CSF is made from a continuously-weighed bottle. The pressure in the bottle is regulated by an electronic control system acting on the fluid within it by means of air pressure from a pump. The CSF pressure is determined following a 10-minute stable period, usually following a 30- to 60-minute recording. Subsequently, the pressure in the bottle is altered to different levels and the resulting inflow of CSF measured. Within a few minutes a stable inflow at a stable pressure is obtained, and the pressure is altered to a new level. From these data, the slope of the pressure/flow values is equal to the CSF conductance or the reciprocal of the resistance to outflow. The CSF formation rate is determined by lowering the bottle below the pressure of the sinus (0 mmHg) for a period of time to measure a stable pressure and outflow to the bottle. By extrapolating the curve to zero flow, one can estimate the dural sinus pressure. This constant pressure technology has the advantage of obtaining multiple points to assess the CSF parameters. The major disadvantages are the complexity of the instrumentation and study duration.

LUMBAR-VENTRICULAR PERFUSION

The lumbar-ventricular perfusion method is also a constant pressure infusion technique[3] and is carried out by introducing a constant rate infusion with an overflow cannulae through a ventricular catheter raised to the desired height. Artificial CSF is infused through the lumbar catheter. In this method, the CSF absorption is calculated as the difference between the infusion rate and outflow rate. The amount of absorption is given by the equation

$$\text{Vabs} = \text{Vin} + \text{qf} - \text{Vout} \tag{13}$$

where Vin is the infused CSF volume, qf the CSF formation rate, and Vout the CSF collected via the ventricular catheter.

To some degree, the application of the specific method depends on the application. In cases of traumatic injury, the time required by the constant pressure or constant infusion method is too long in duration and the bolus technique is more applicable. However, these other methods find their place in applications requiring vigorous assessment of CSF parameters when time and complexity is not a consideration.

CLINICAL APPLICATION OF CSF PARAMETERS

With traumatic brain swelling, the compensatory reserves of the cranial cavity approach exhaustion, and brain compliance is gradually reduced. One of the most important applications of these mathematical tools is to isolate the cause of ICP rise. In head injury, several studies have applied these measures for determining the need for surgical decompression,[67] documenting elevation of outflow resistance in subarachnoid hemorrhage,[29,36,43,57] establishing the prognostic value of PVI in head-injured patients,[93,101] and isolating the contribution of CSF and vascular parameters to ICP rise.[8] These investigations are only a few examples to illustrate the clinical use of CSF parameter measurement. At present, the PVI is measured routinely in certain head-injury centers to follow the course of brain swelling and its response to treatment.

Contribution of CSF and Vascular Components to ICP Rise in Traumatic Brain Injury

The steady state equation describing intracranial pressure can be subdivided into two major components: CSF and vascular. The CSF component consists of the formation resistance product and the vascular component the dural sinus level. Studies of head-injured patients utilizing the methods described in this chapter were conducted to study which factor, CSF or vascular, was most responsible for ICP rise.[8] *It was found that, with exception of those patients with subarachnoid hemorrhage, CSF parameters accounted for approximately one-third of the ICP rise after severe head injury and that a vascular mechanism was the predominant factor in elevation of the ICP.* Interestingly, CSF formation rate remained within normal limits over the 4 days following injury, with only a mild reduction seen at elevated pressure. Although outflow resistance was elevated above normal levels, it did not account for appreciable ICP rise. Evaluating the vascular component by controlled withdrawal technique (see Fig. 30-4), it was determined that the major contributor was not the CSF component given by CSF formation resistance product but the vascular component of ICP identified in the steady state equation as dural sinus pressure. As it was determined that CSF parameters played a relatively minor role in elevations of ICP, it was recommended that future research focus on vascular mechanisms.

Bolus Injection Overshoot in Traumatic Brain Injury

As described earlier, the recovery of pressure to the initial injection can be used to estimate outflow resistance to cerebrospinal fluid. Recent studies have shown that in some cases of TBI, the ICP recovery behaves differently, with a secondary increase starting 8 to 10 seconds after bolus injection and lasting for minutes.[100] This paradoxical response was studied in a group of 34 severely head-injured patients, and the association of this pattern to other clinical variables was assessed. The mean ICP for the group studied averaged 21.95 mmHg ± 7.94 (s.d.) and the average maximal overshoot equaled 37.04 mmHg ± 14.66 (s.d.). It was concluded that the paradoxical response (PR) was a frequent finding in TBI and was associated with patients in whom PVI was low and with a greater incidence of absent or compressed cisterns. The brief overshoot and eventual return suggests a vascular phenomenon and a persistent paradoxical response is associated with poor prognosis. Investigators have utilized mathematical modeling to study the paradoxical response and have attributed the complex change to a combination hemodynamic instability at the arteriolar level and autoregulatory phenomenon. Simply explained, the injection maneuver in patients with preserved autoregulation elicits arterial vasodilation and an increase in blood volume which accounts for the secondary rise in pressure. An opposite paradoxical response (vasoconstriction with a delayed reduction in cerebral blood volume and ICP) is evident in the same patients following withdrawal of fluid.[102,103]

Cerebrovenous Pressure in Traumatic Brain Injury

The contribution of the cerebrovenous system, particularly the outflow pathways, to the ICP and cerebral blood flow is unclear. Early workers were focused on the behavior of the superior sagittal sinus at raised pressure conditions on the premise that collapse of the sinus would lead to diminution of cerebral blood flow. Langfitt et al. showed that the level of cerebral blood flow reduction depends on the ICP and how rapidly it developed.[44] However the precise anatomic site of vascular obstruction in the presence of adequate perfusion pressure had not been identified. Cerebral perfusion pressure (CPP) has long been considered the difference between mean arterial and intracranial pressure, and justification for this estimate was given by the work of Johnston and co-workers,[39] who measured the cortical vein pressure of monkeys and found that the pressure was close to that of the ICP. Thus, the substitution of ICP for cortical vein pressure was introduced for cerebral perfusion. These studies were supported by similar findings by other workers.[95,96] Earlier, we described the fundamental equation relating ICP to the product of formation rate and outflow resistance added to a vascular component long considered the pressure of the dural sinus. Studies were described in which the "CSF component" of ICP accounted for only one-third of ICP elevation, while the remaining two-thirds were attributed to a "vascular" component. In theory, the Pv term in this equation should indeed be the pressure of the sagittal sinus, and thus these studies implied that sagittal sinus pressure was elevated. Attempts to confirm elevated sinus pressure were made by measuring the pressure of the jugular bulb and studies showed that hourly averages of ICP and jugular bulb pressures were equal.[51] A subsequent investigation measured sagittal sinus pressure by direct cannulation of the sagittal sinus utilizing radiological techniques, and it was observed that sinus pressure was elevated with elevated ICP. Moreover, it was concluded that the jugular bulb pressure is a close estimate of sinus pressure level.[49] The observation that sagittal sinus pressure is elevated has important implications to our current understanding of ICP pathophysiology and is fertile area for continued study.

Summary of Factors Leading to Raised ICP

Clearly, a precise description of the sequence of events leading to ICP elevation remains elusive. However an attempt to unify many of the concepts described in the literature is presented in Fig. 30-6. In the schema of Fig. 30-6, traumatic brain injury initiates several types of insults. First, the rise in ICP due to CSF factors, including CSF resistance and absorption of fluid, is one pathway. In general, this pathway contributes up to one-third of ICP rise, as stated earlier; however, the contribution can increase markedly with subarachnoid hemorrhage. The remaining two-thirds of ICP rise is attributed to a vascular component that can either be manifested directly by an increase in vascular stability leading to an increase in blood volume (second pathway) or indirectly by increased tissue water (pathways 3, 4, and 5),

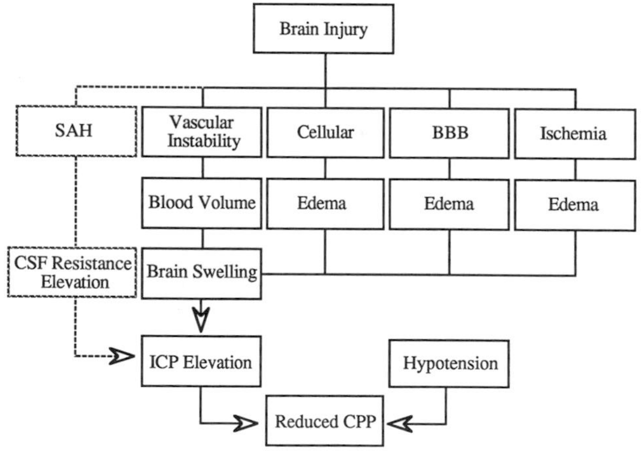

Figure 30-6. A current concept of those factors responsible for ICP rise and subsequent reductions of cerebral perfusion pressure. The effect of increased CSF resistance leading to ICP rise has been well documented *(dashed line)* and clearly understood. The remaining factors are less understood, particularly those compartments responsible for brain swelling. Blood volume and three types of edema contribute to brain swelling and subsequent ICP rise, although their relative contribution remains unknown. Recent studies (see text) indicates that hypotension, occurring during the course of management is a major factor leading to CPP reduction and must be avoided.

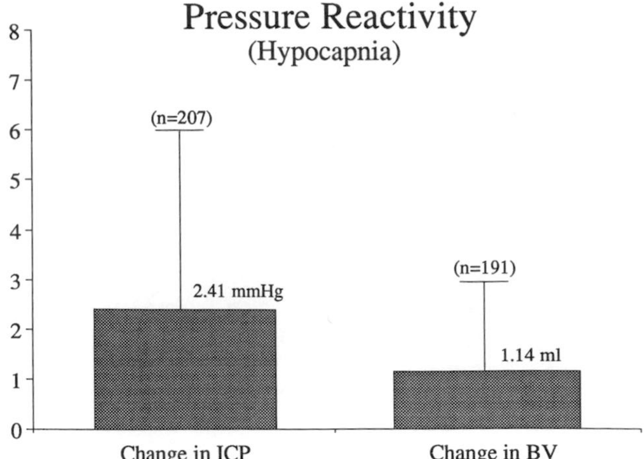

Figure 30-7. Intracranial pressure is remarkably sensitive to small changes in blood volume as indicated by studies of pressure reactivity in head-injured patients. In these studies, the average PVI of the patient group equaled 21 ml. Thus, a 1.14-ml change in blood volume results in a 2.41 mmHg change. Based on this average reactivity, it would only require 5.0-ml change of blood volume to raise ICP from a normal level of 10 mmHg to the treatment threshold of 20 mmHg.

acting to compress the cerebrovasculature. The increase in blood volume or engorgement contributes directly to brain swelling and the exquisite sensitivity of ICP to changes in blood volume is illustrated in Fig. 30-7. According to these studies, an increase in blood volume of 1 ml would result in an increase in ICP of 1.56 mmHg. Thus, it would only require an uncompensated blood volume increase in 6.4 ml to raise ICP from a normal value of 10 mmHg to the treatment threshold of 20 mmHg.[52,109]

The increase in tissue water can be subdivided into three types of edema—neurotoxic, BBB, and ischemic. Neurotoxic and ischemic forms of edema are considered to be of cellular origin. Traumatic edema as produced by compromise of the blood brain barrier is considered to be extracellular. All three types contribute to the swelling process and can be mutually interactive, eventually leading to ICP rise.

Finally, the contribution of hypotension (pathway 6), which may be present upon admission or occur spontaneously,[53] detracts further from cerebral perfusion pressure. Its importance should not be underestimated, as emphasized by the next section.

Effect of ICP and Hypotension in Head Injury on Outcome

In the head-injury literature, considerable evidence has accumulated that high levels of ICP are associated with poor outcome and that aggressive treatment is essential to reduce risk of mortality and improve neurological outcome. However, in studies of relatively small numbers of patients, it is difficult to directly measure the putative influence of raised ICP on outcome because of the multiplicity of other factors involved. A large-scale study of ICP involving 1030 patients was conducted as part of the Traumatic Coma Data Bank (TCDB).[16] Of this group, ICP data were studied from 428 patients that met monitoring criteria.[53] As expected, age at admission, motor score, and abnormal pupils were highly significant in explaining outcome. Beyond these factors, the percentage time that ICP was above 20 mmHg was highly significant ($p < 0.0001$). The next factor that was most significant was the percentage time that arterial blood pressure was below a mean level of 80 mmHg. The individual effect of these parameters on prognosis is illustrated in Fig. 30-8. As cerebral perfusion pressure combines both ICP and arterial pressure, it was not mathematically possible to separate ICP and CPP. However, taking these findings in concert and subtracting the critical ICP threshold of 20 mmHg from the critical threshold of 80 mmHg arterial pressure, the cortical cerebral perfusion pressure approximates 60 mmHg.

Contribution of ICP and Blood Pressure to Reduction of Cerebral Perfusion Pressure

The studies described in the previous section provided substantive data identifying the treatment thresholds for ICP and blood pressure. However, the observation that head-injured patients experienced brief periods of hypotension after resuscitation and during management was unexpected. As a result of these and other studies,[89] vigilance for hypotensive episodes in the intensive care setting has been heightened and the importance of CPP management emphasized.[5] This focused effort by investigators to study the relative contribution of raised ICP and reduced arterial pressure to reductions of CPP during the acute management period.[50] From these studies, which included the TCDB cohort, it was found that the percentage of time that CPP was compromised below a threshold of 60 mmHg was related to the severity of injury as identified by the GCS. For the entire cohort, the percentage time that CPP was reduced below the critical threshold during the first 72 hours approached 14.2 percent. Most important, the incidence of hypotension during these episodic reductions of CPP ranged from 76.6 to 89.5 percent and was related to the severity of injury. The incidence of raised ICP during periods of reduced CPP ranged from 33 to 41 percent, and outcome was worse in these patients. It was concluded from these results that reduced blood pressure was the

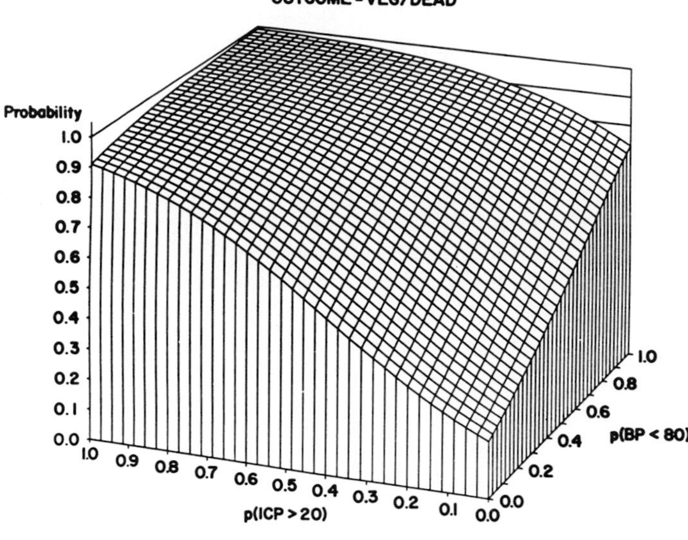

Figure 30-8. Using stepwise logistic regression techniques, the computer selected the percentage time above 20 mmHg as the critical threshold affecting outcome when factors of motor score, age, and pupil reactivity are held constant. In addition, the next critical factor was the percentage time spent below a mean blood pressure level of 80 mmHg. The three-dimensional graph depicts the interrelationship of these two parameters vs. probability of a poor outcome (GOS veg/dead). As time above 20 mmHg increases (0 to 100 percent), probability of poor outcome increases. At any percentage time above 20 mmHg value, percent time below 80 mmHg also increases probability of poor outcome.

predominant cause of reduced cerebral perfusion pressure and that the incidence of combined hypotension and raised ICP occurs approximately one-third of the time. The mechanisms responsible for these periodic hypotensive episodes remain unclear.

References

1. Becker DP, Miller JD, Ward JD, et al: The outcome from severe head injury with early diagnosis and intensive management. *J Neurosurg* 1977; 47:491–502.
2. Bering EA: Choroid plexus and arterial pulsation of cerebrospinal fluid. *Arch Neurol Psychiat* 1955; 73:165–172.
3. Borgesen SE, Gjerris F, Sorensen SC: The resistance to cerebrospinal fluid absorption in humans. A method of evaluation by lumboventricular perfusion, with particular reference to normal pressure hydrocephalus. *Acta Neurol Scand* 1978; 57:88–96.
4. Bruce DA, Ter Weeme C, Kaiser G, et al: The dynamics of small and large molecules in the extracellular space and cerebrospinal fluid following local cold injury of the cortex, in Pappius HM, Feindel W (eds): *Dynamics of Brain Edema.* Berlin: Springer-Verlag, 1976:122–128.
5. Chesnut RM, Marshall LF, Klauber M, et al: The role of secondary brain injury in determining outcome from severe head injury. *J Trauma* 1993; 34:216–222.
6. Cohadon F, Castel JP, Nouillant A, et al: Volume pressure relationship in clinical and experimental condition of raised ICP, in Lundberg N, Pontén U, Brock M (eds): *Intracranial Pressure II.* Berlin: Springer-Verlag, 1975:107–110.
7. Cormio M, Marmarou A, Fisher R: Intracranial monitoring in hepatic encephalopathy and liver transplant patients. *Crit Rev Neurosurg* 1994.
8. Cserr HF: Convection of brain interstitial fluid, in Ishii S (ed): *Hydrocephalus.* Tokyo: Excerpta Medica, 1983:24–30.
9. Cutler RWP, Page LK, Galicich J, Waters GV: Formation and absorption of cerebrospinal fluid in man. *Brain* 1968; 91:707–720.
10. Czosnyka M, Guazzo E, Kirkpatrick P, et al: Prognostic significance of the ICP pulse waveform analysis after severe head injury, in Nagai H, Kamiya K, Ishii S (eds): *Intracranial Pressure IX.* Tokyo: Springer-Verlag, 1994:200–203.
11. Czosnyka M, Price JD, Williamson M: Monitoring of cerebrospinal dynamics using continuous analysis of intracranial pressure and cerebral perfusion pressure in head injury. *Acta Neurochir (Wien)* 1994; 126:113–116.
12. Czosnyka M, Batorski L, Laniewski P, et al: A computer system for the identification of cerebrospinal compensatory model. *Acta Neurochir (Wien)* 1990; 105:112–116.
13. Dardenne G, Dereymaeker A, Lacheron JM: Cerebrospinal fluid pressure and pulsatility. *Europ Neurol* 1969; 2:193–216.
14. Davson H: *Physiology of the Cerebrospinal Fluid.* Edinburgh: Churchill, 1967:337.
15. Dereymaeker A, Stevens A, Rombouts JJ, et al: Study on the influence of the arterial pressure upon the morphology of cisternal CSF pulsations. *Europ Neurol* 1971; 5:107–114.
16. Di Chiro G: Observations on the circulation of the cerebrospinal fluid. *Acta Radiol* 1966; 5:988–1002.
17. du Boulay G, O'Connell J, Currie J, et al: Further investigations on pulsatile movements in the cerebrospinal fluid pathways. *Acta Radiol* 1972; 13:496–523.

18. du Boulay GH: Pulsatile movements in the CSF pathways. *Br J Radiol* 1966; 39:255–262.
19. du Boulay GH: Specialisation broadens the view. The significance of a CSF pulse. 2nd Glyn Evans Memorial Lecture. *Clin Radiol* 1972; 23:401–409.
20. Dunbar HS, Guthrie TC, Karpel B: A study of the cerebrospinal fluid pulse wave. *Arch Neurol* 1966; 14:624–630.
21. Ekstedt J: CSF hydrodynamic studies in man. 1. Method of constant pressure CSF infusion. *J Neurol Neurosurg Psychiatry* 1977; 40:105–119.
22. Ekstedt J: CSF Hydrodynamic studies in man. 2. Normal hydrodynamic variables related to CSF pressure and flow. *J Neurol Neurosurg Psychiatry* 1978; 41:345–353.
23. Fenstermacher JD, Patlak CS: The exchange of material between cerebrospinal fluid and brain, in Cserr HF, Fenstermacher JD, Fencl V (eds): *Fluid Environment of the Brain.* New York: Academic Press, 1975:215–224.
24. Fishman RA: Physiology of the cerebrospinal fluid, in *Cerebrospinal Fluid in Diseases of the Nervous System,* 2d ed. Philadelphia: WB Saunders, 1992:23–42.
25. Foulkes MA, Eisenberg HM, Jane JA, et al: The traumatic coma data bank: Design, methods, and baseline characteristics. *J Neurosurg* 1991; 75:S8–S13.
26. Fridén H: The Hydrodynamics of the Cerebrospinal Fluid in Man. Umeå University Medical Dissertations. New series No. 416-ISSN 0346-6612, 1994.
27. Fridén H, Ekstedt J: CSF dynamics modeling in man, in Nagai H, Kamiya K, Ishii S (eds): *Intracranial Pressure IX.* Tokyo: Springer-Verlag, 1994:502–503.
28. Fridén H, Eksted J: Volume accounting: A method for the study of CSF-hydrodynamics. An aid for parameter estimation and validation of pressure/flow models, in: Miller JD, Teasdale GM, Rowan JO et al (eds): *Intracranial Pressure VI.* Berlin: Springer-Verlag, 1986:54–61.
29. Fuhrmeister J, Ruether P, Dommasch D, et al: Alterations of CSF hydrodynamics following meningitis and subarachnoid hemorrhage, in Shulman K, Marmarou A, Miller JD (eds): *Intracranial Pressure IV.* Berlin: Springer-Verlag, 1980:241–244.
30. Go KG: *Cerebral Pathophysiology.* Amsterdam: Elsevier, 1991.
31. Goldensohn ES, Whitehead RW, Parry TM, et al: Studies on diffusion respiration. IX. Effect of diffusion respiration and high concentrations of CO_2 on cerebrospinal fluid pressure of anesthetized dogs. *Am J Physiol* 1951; 165:334–340.
32. Gopinath SP, Cherian L, Robertson CS, et al: Evaluation of a microsensor intracranial pressure transducer. *J Neurosci Methods* 1993; 49:11–15.
33. Greitz D: *Cerebral Spinal Fluid Circulation and Associated Intracranial Dynamics.* Doctoral Thesis, Stockholm, 1993.
34. Greitz D, Nordell B, Ericsson A, et al: Notes on the driving forces of the CSF circulation with special emphasis on the piston action of the brain. *Neuroradiology* 1991; 33:178–181.
35. Hamer J, Alberti E, Hoyer S, Wiedemann K: Influence of systemic and cerebral vascular factors in the cerebrospinal fluid pulse waves. *J Neurosurg* 1977; 46:36–45.
36. Hase U, Reulen JH, Fenske A, et al: Intracranial pressure and pressure volume relation in patients with subarachnoid hemorrhage (SAH). *Acta Neurochir* 1978; 44:69–80.
37. Johansson B, Li C-L, Olsson Y, et al: The effect of acute arterial hypertension on the blood-brain barrier to protein tracers. *Acta Neuropathol (Berl)* 1970; 16:117–124.
38. Johnston I, Gilday DL, Paterson A, et al: The definition of a reduced CSF absorption syndrome: clinical and experimental studies, in Lundberg N, Pontén U, Brock M (eds): *Intracranial Pressure II.* Berlin: Springer-Verlag, 1975:50–53.
39. Johnston HI, Rowan JO: Raised intracranial pressure and cerebral blood flow. 3. Venous outflow tract pressures and vascular resistances in experimental intracranial hypertension. *J Neurol Neurosurg Psychiatry* 1974; 37:392–402.
40. Katzman R, Hussey F: A simple constant-infusion manometric test for measurement of CSF absorption. I. Rationale and method. *Neurology* 1970; 20:534–544.
41. Kellie G: An account of the appearances observed in the dissection of two of three individuals presumed to have perished in the storm of the 3D, and whose bodies were discovered in the vicinity of Leith on the morning of the 4th of November 1821 with some reflections on the pathology of the brain. *Trans Med Chir Sci Edinb* 1824; 1:84–169.
42. Klatzo I, Chui E, Fujiwara K, et al: Resolution of vasogenic brain edema, in Cervos-Navaro, Ferszt R (eds): *Advances in Neurology, 28, Brain Edema.* New York: Raven Press, 1980:359–373.
43. Kosteljanetz M: CSF dynamics in patients with subarachnoid and/or intraventricular hemorrhage. *J Neurosurg* 1984; 60:940–946.
44. Langfitt TW, Weinstein JD, Kassell NF, et al: I. Dural sinus pressures, in Langfitt TW: *Compression of Cerebral Vessels,* Acta Neurochirurgica, Vol XV, Fasc. 3-4, 213-222, 1966.
45. Langfitt TW, Weinstein JD, Kassell NP, et al: Cerebral vasomotor paralysis produced by intracranial hypertension. *Neurology* 1965; 15:622–641.
46. Lim ST, Potts DG, Deonarine V, et al: Ventricular compliance in dogs with and without aqueductal obstruction. *J Neurosurg* 1973; 39:463–473.
47. Liu HM: Neovasculature and blood-brain barrier in ischemic brain infarct. *Acta Neuropathol (Berl)* 1988; 75:422–426.
48. Lofgren J, von Essen C, Zwetnow NN: The pressure-volume curve of the cerebrospinal fluid space in dogs. *Acta Neurol Scand* 1973; 49:557–574.
49. Marmarou A and Allen C: The Measurement of Raised Cerebrovenous Pressure and Intracranial Pressure in Brain Injured Patients. Surgery of the Intracranial Venous System 145–151, 1995.
50. Marmarou A, Bullock R, Young HF, et al: The contribution of raised ICP and hypotension to reduced cerebral perfusion pressure in severe brain injury, in Nagai H, Kamiya K, Ishii S (eds): *Intracranial Pressure IX.* Tokyo: Springer-Verlag, 1994:302–304.
51. Marmarou A, Foda A, Bandoh K, et al: Elevated venous

outflow pressure in head injured patients, in Avezaat CJJ, van Eijndhoven JHM, Maas AIR, Tans JTJ (eds): New York: Springer Verlag, 1993.

52. Marmarou A: Increased intracranial pressure in head injury and influence of blood volume. *J Neurotrauma* 1992; 9:S327–S332.

53. Marmarou A, Eisenberg HM, Foulkes MA, et al: Impact of ICP instability and hypotension on outcome in patients with severe head trauma. *J Neurosurg* 1991; 75:S59–S66.

54. Marmarou A, Nakamura T, Tanaka K: Kinetics of fluid movement through brain tissue. *Semin Neurol* 4; No. 4, 1984.

55. Marmarou A: Progress in the analysis of intracranial pressure dynamics and application to head injury. *Central Nervous System Trauma Status Report:* 79–87, 1985. Becker DP and Povlishock JT, eds. Washington, D.C. National Institute of Neurological Coma Disorders and Stroke

56. Marmarou A, Shulman K, Rosende RM: A nonlinear analysis of the cerebrospinal fluid system and intracranial pressure dynamics. *J Neurosurg* 1978; 48:332–344.

57. Marmarou A, Shapiro K, Shulman K: Isolation of factors leading to sustained elevations of the ICP, in Beks JWF, Bosch DA, Brock M (eds): *Intracranial Pressure III.* Berlin: Springer-Verlag, 1976:33–36.

58. Marmarou A: A theoretical and experimental evaluation of the cerebrospinal fluid system. Ph.D. Thesis, Drexel University, 1973.

59. Marshall LF, Smith RW, Shapiro HM: The outcome with aggressive treatment in severe head injuries. Part I. The significance of intracranial pressure monitoring. *J Neurosurg* 1979; 50:20–25.

60. Maset AL, Marmarou A, Ward JD, et al: Pressure-volume index in head injury. *J Neurosurg* 1987; 67:832–840.

61. Masserman JH: Cerebrospinal hydrodynamics. IV. Clinical experimental studies. *Arch Neurol Psychiatr* 1934; 32:226–234.

62. Milhorat TH: Cerebrospinal fluid and the brain edemas. New York: *Neuroscience Society of New York,* 1987.

63. Milhorat TH, Hammock MK: Cerebrospinal fluid as reflection of internal milieu of brain, in Wood JH: *Neurobiology of Cerebrospinal Fluid 2.* New York: Plenum Press, 1983:1–23.

64. Milhorat TH: *Hydrocephalus and the Cerebrospinal Fluid.* Baltimore: Williams & Wilkins, 1972.

65. Miller JD, Butterworth JF, Gudeman SK, et al: Further experience in the management of severe head injury. *J Neurosurg* 1981; 54:289–299.

66. Miller JD, Becker DP, Ward JD, et al: Significance of intracranial hypertension in severe head injury. *J Neurosurg* 1977; 47:503–516.

67. Miller JD, Pickard JD: Intracranial volume-pressure studies in patients with head injury. *Injury* 1974; 5:265–269.

68. Miller JD, Garibi J, Pickard JD: Induced changes of cerebrospinal fluid volume. *Arch Neurol* 1973; 28:265–269.

69. Miller JD, Garibi J: Intracranial volume-pressure relationship during continuous monitoring of ventricular fluid pressure, in: Brock M, Dietz H (eds): *Intracranial Pressure.* Berlin: Springer-Verlag, 1972:270–274.

70. Monro A: *Observations on the Structure and Function of the Nervous System.* Edinburgh: Creech & Johnson, 1783.

71. Narayan RK, Greenberg RP, Miller JD, et al: Improved confidence of outcome prediction in severe head injury. A comparative analysis of the clinical examination, multimodality evoked potentials, CT scanning, and intracranial pressure. *J Neurosurg* 1981; 54:751–762.

72. O'Connell JEA: The vascular factor in intracranial pressure and the maintenance of the cerebrospinal fluid circulation. *Brain* 1943; 73:165–172.

73. Ohata K, Marmarou A: Clearance of brain edema and macromolecules through the cortical extracellular space. *J Neurosurg* 1992; 77:387–396.

74. Ohata K, Marmarou A, Povlishock JT: An immunocytochemical study of protein clearance in brain infusion edema. *Acta Neuropathol* 1990; 81:162–177.

75. Oppelt WW, Patlak CS, Rall DP: Effect of certain drugs on cerebrospinal fluid production in the dog. *Am J Physiol* 1964; 206:247–250.

76. Ostrup RC, Luerssen TG, Marshall LF, Zornow MH: Continuous monitoring of intracranial pressure with a miniaturized fibre optic device. *J Neurosurg* 1987; 67:206–209.

77. Piper IR, Chan KH, Whittle IR, Miller JD: Differential effect of hypercarbia and hypertension on cerebrovascular pressure transmission and craniospinal compliance, in Avezaat CJJ, van Eijndhoven JHM, Maas AIR, Tans JTJ (eds): *Intracranial Pressure VIII.* Berlin: Springer-Verlag, 1993:382–389.

78. Piper IR, Chan KH, Whittle IR, Miller JD: An experimental study of cerebrovascular resistance, pressure transmission, and craniospinal compliance. *Neurosurgery* 1993; 32:805–816.

79. Piper IR, Miller JD, Dearden NM, et al: Systems analysis of cerebrovascular pressure transmission: An observational study in head injured patients. *J Neurosurg* 1990; 73:871–880.

80. Piper IR, Miller JD, Whittle IR, Lawson A: Automated time-averaged analysis of craniospinal compliance. *Acta Neurochir (Wien)* 1990; 51:387–390.

81. Pollay M, Davson H: The passage of certain substances out of the cerbrospinal fluid. *Brain* 1963; 86:137–150.

82. Portnoy HD, Chopp M, Branch C: Hydraulic model of myogenic autoregulation and the cerebrovascular bed: The effects of altering systemic arterial pressure. *Neurosurgery* 1983; 13:482–498.

83. Portnoy HD, Chopp M, Branch C, Shannon MB: Cerebrospinal fluid pulse waveform as an indicator of cerebral autoregulation. *J Neurosurg* 1982; 56:668–678.

84. Portnoy HD, Chopp M: Cerebrospinal fluid pulse wave form analysis during hypercapnia and hypoxia. *Neurosurgery* 1981; 9:14–27.

85. Prockop LD, Schanker LS, Brodie BB: Passage of lipid-insoluble substances from cerebrospinal fluid to blood. *J Pharmacol Exp Ther* 1962; 135:266–270.

86. Rekate HL, Brodkey JA, Chizeck HJ, et al: Ventricular volume regulation: A mathematical model and computer simulation. *Pediatr Neurosci* 1988; 14(2):77–84.

87. Reulen HJ, Tsuyumu M, Tack A, et al: Clearance of edema fluid into cerebrospinal fluid: A mechanism for resolution of vasogenic brain edema. *J Neurosurg* 1978; 48:754–764.
88. Rosenberg GA, Kyner WT, Estrada E: Bulk flow of brain interstitial fluid under normal and hyperosmolar conditions. *Am J Physiol* 1980; 238:F42–F49.
89. Rosner MN, Daughton S: Cerebral perfusion pressure management in head injury. *J Trauma* 1990; 30:933–941.
90. Rubin RC, Henderson ES, Walker MD, Rall DP: The production of cerebrospinal fluid in man and its modification by acetazolamide. *J Neurosurg* 1966; 25:430–436.
91. Ryder HW, Epsey FP, Kimbell ED, et al: The mechanism of the change in cerebrospinal fluid pressure following an induced change in the volume of the fluid space. *J Lab Clin Med* 1953; 41:428–435.
92. Saul TG, Ducker TB: Effects of intracranial pressure monitoring and aggressive treatment on mortality in severe head injury. *J Neurosurg* 1982; 56:498–503.
93. Shapiro K, Marmarou A, Shulman K: Characterization of clinical CSF dynamics and neural axis compliance using the pressure-volume index. 1. The normal pressure-volume index. *Ann Neurol* 1977; 7:508–514.
94. Shulman K, Marmarou A: Pressure-volume considerations in infantile hydrocephalus. *Dev Med Child Neurol* 1971; 13(Suppl 25):90–95.
95. Shulman K, Verdier GR: Cerebral vascular resistance changes in response to cerebrospinal fluid pressure. *Am J Physiol* 1967; 213:1084–1088.
96. Shulman K: Small artery and vein pressures in the subarachnoid space of the dog. *J Surg Res* 1965; 5:56–61.
97. Shulman K, Yarnell P, Ransohoff J: Dural sinus pressure in normal and hydrocephalic dogs. *Arch Neurol* 1964; 10:575–580.
98. Sklar FH: Non-steady state measurements of cerebrospinal fluid dynamics, in Wood JH (ed): *Neurobiology of Cerebrospinal Fluid.* New York: Plenum Press, 1980:365–379.
99. Sklar FH, Beyer Jr. CW, Clark WK: Physiological features of the pressure-volume function of brain elasticity in man. *J Neurosurg* 1980; 53:166–172.
100. Stocchetti N, Rossi S, Ceccarelli P, et al: Time pattern of ICP after bolus injection as an indicator of intracranial disturbances, in Nagai H, Kamiya K, Ishii S (eds): *Intracranial Pressure IX.* Tokyo: Springer-Verlag, 1994:172–174.
101. Tans JJ, Poortvl DCJ: Intracranial volume-pressure relationship in man. Part 2: Clinical significance of the pressure-volume index. *J Neurosurg* 1983; 59:810–816.
102. Ursino M, DiGiammarco P: A mathematical model of the relationship between cerebral blood volume and intracranial pressure changes: the generation of plateau waves. *Ann Biomed Eng* 19:15–42.
103. Ursino M, Rossi S, Stocchetti N: Paradoxical responses to pressure volume tests: Analysis with a mathematical model, in Nagai H, Kamiya K, Ishii S (eds): *Intracranial Pressure IX.* Tokyo: Springer-Verlag, 1994:510–511.
104. Ursino M: Computer analysis of the main parameters extrapolated from the human intracranial basal artery blood flow. *Comput Biomed Res* 1990; 23(6):542–559.
105. Ursino M: A mathematical study of human intracranial hydrodynamics. Part II—Simulation of clinical tests. *Ann Biomed Eng* 1988; 16(4):403–416.
106. Van Deurs B: Vesicular transport of horseradish peroxidase from brain to blood in segments of the cerebral microvasculature in adult mice. *Brain Res* 1977; 124:1–8.
107. Vorbrodt AW, Lossinsky AS, Wisniewski HM, et al: Ultrastructural observations on the transvascular route of protein removal in vasogenic brain edema. *Acta Neuropathol (Berl)* 1985; 66:265–273.
108. Welch K: Secretion of cerebrospinal fluid by choroid plexus of the rabbit. *Am J Physiol* 1963; 205:617–624.
109. Yoshihara M, Bandoh K, Marmarou A: Cerebrovascular CO_2 reactivity assessed by ICP dynamics in severely head injured patients. *J Neurosurg.* In Press. 1995.
110. Yoshihara M, Marmarou A, Dunbar J, et al: A fiberoptic device suitable for subdural pressure measurement, in Avezaat CJJ, van Eijndhoven JHM, Maas AIR, Tans JTJ (eds): *Intracranial Pressure VIII.* Berlin: Springer-Verlag, 1993:20–24.

CHAPTER 31

ICP MONITORING: INDICATIONS AND TECHNIQUES

J. Douglas Miller
Ian R. Piper
Patrick F. X. Statham

SYNOPSIS

This chapter reviews the historical background and development of intracranial pressure (ICP) monitoring, describing methods that have been and are being used. The authors present the current indications for ICP monitoring and discuss the interpretation of findings and the role they play in patient management. Other physiological measurements that are required for the interpretation of ICP data and other monitoring systems that amplify the information from ICP monitoring are also described. Finally, the chapter assesses the techniques and forms of analysis that have developed from straightforward continuous recording of ICP, stress and infusion tests, and forms of data analysis that will shed more light on the genesis and prediction of intracranial hypertension.

The development of intermittent positive-pressure ventilation and a strain gauge transducer that could produce a continuous record of intraarterial pressure with appropriate amplification and recording led to the development of general intensive care units for the monitoring and management of critically ill patients in the 1960s. The introduction of continuous monitoring of intracranial pressure (ICP) in the 1970s into clinical neurosurgical practice led to the recognition of neurological critical care as a specific branch of critical care medicine. While opinions still vary about the contribution of continuous monitoring of ICP to a reduction in mortality and morbidity after head injury, few would deny that this technique allows more informed decisions about patient management to be made.

HISTORICAL BACKGROUND

Although the technique of continuous monitoring of ICP is relatively new, interest in the pathophysiology of raised ICP extends back over 200 years. More than a hundred years ago, direct measurements of ICP were made with manometric systems. The concept of a compensatory phase of normal ICP during the initial slow expansion of an intracranial lesion followed by progressive decompensation and a steepening rise in pressure as spatial buffering mechanisms were exhausted was an established belief by the end of the last century.[1] Landmark studies in the twentieth century included those of Weed and associates[2] and the Evans and Ryder group in Cincinnati and Chicago, who carried out specific studies of the effects of induced changes in CSF volume and in arterial P_{CO_2} and of the effect of therapies aimed at reducing ICP.[3]

However, credit must be given to Guillaume and Janny in Clermont Ferrand, France, for introducing into clinical neurosurgical practice the technique of continuous monitoring of intracranial CSF pressure using an indwelling intraventricular catheter attached to an external strain gauge transducer, amplifying system, and chart recorder.[4] The work of these authors was published in French and initially received little notice outside Europe. In 1960 Nils Lundberg from Lund, Sweden, published a landmark thesis entitled "Continuous Recording and Control of Ventricular Fluid Pressure in Neurosurgical Practice."[5] In this 193-page monograph,

Lundberg reviewed previous investigations of ICP over the previous 100 years, acknowledged the major contribution of Pierre Janny, and described in detail his technique for ventricular puncture and continuous recording of intraventricular pressure. He went on to present clinical observations of 143 patients. A majority of those patients suffered from brain tumors, but his material also included patients with intracranial infection, cerebral trauma, abnormalities of CSF circulation, and benign intracranial hypertension.

Lundberg clearly showed that ICP can rise to extremely high levels in patients with a variety of intracranial disorders and that even severe intracranial hypertension cannot be predicted reliably by clinical examination of the patient, although there were some subtle correlative changes. Perhaps Lundberg's most notable contribution was his clear demonstration of the variability of ICP over time (which emphasized the importance of obtaining a continuous record of pressure) and description of three discernible patterns of ICP variation. The most important of these were the plateau waves, or A waves, as they were defined by Lundberg. They consisted of a rapid rise in ICP from normal or nearly normal levels to peak levels which remained at 50 mmHg or more for 5 to 20 min or occasionally longer, followed by an equally abrupt spontaneous reduction in ICP back to normal or nearly normal levels (Fig. 31-1). Lundberg also described B waves, which consist of sharply peaked waves in which the ICP rises again from normal or nearly normal levels to 30 mmHg or more and then falls again equally rapidly, with the process being repeated every 1 or 2 mins. This waveform pattern was associated with periodic respiration in some but not all cases. The third waveform pattern described by Lundberg consisted of C waves in which there were rhythmic waves of ICP occurring five to six times per minute which corresponded with the Traube-Hering-Mayer waves of changing blood pressure. This pattern would appear and disappear spontaneously in patients with a variety of brain disorders.

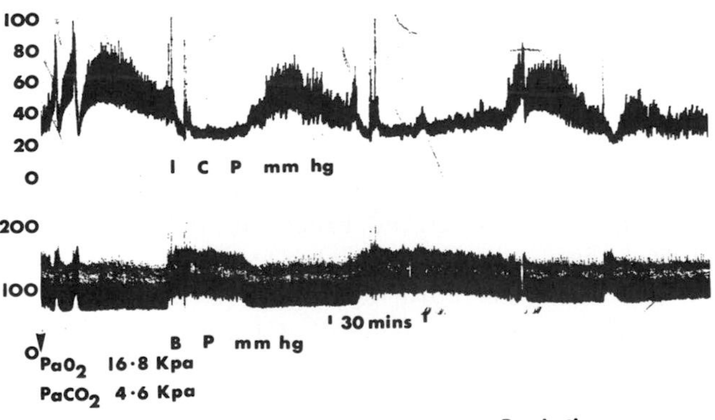

Figure 31-1. Recording of blood pressure and intracranial pressure from a head-injured patient during spontaneous respiration, exhibiting "A" waves, as first described by Lundberg.

Through meticulous attention to detail, Lundberg obtained reliable recordings in a large number of patients with a very low incidence of infection. However, despite his monograph and other papers, the technique of ICP monitoring was not immediately adopted in Sweden or elsewhere.

During the period 1964–1969, Langfitt and Kassell and their associates at the University of Pennsylvania published an important series of papers on intracranial dynamics in experimental animals that were subjected to experimental brain compression using inflatable balloons or infusion of fluids under pressure.[6] This group provided clear graphic evidence of the progression of brain compression which illustrated the theories that had been held about this process since the end of the previous century. Langfitt introduced the term "vasomotor paralysis" to define the end stage of severe intracranial hypertension when cerebral blood vessels were dilated and ICP was highly pulsatile yet cerebral blood flow was reduced considerably.[7] At that stage the vessels were held to be unreactive to normally vasoactive stimuli such as lowered arterial P_{CO_2} and induced changes in arterial pressure and ICP reacted passively to changes in arterial pressure. The other major contribution of the Philadelphia group was the clear demonstration of the development of gradients of ICP during the expansion of supratentorial mass lesions, in which supratentorial pressure rose progressively while infratentorial pressure, measured from the cisterna magna or the lumbar subarachnoid space, rose at first, plateaued, and then began to fall.[8] This occurred because the infratentorial compartments were anatomically separated from the supratentorial compartment by the blockage of the cisterna ambiens induced by tentorial herniation. The process of tentorial herniation, with its effects on midbrain and pupillary function, had already been well described by Jefferson and investigated in humans by Johnson and Yates[9] and in experimental animals by Jennett and Stern.[10] It was the Langfitt group, however, that clearly showed the way in which this process is accompanied by the development of a pressure gradient. This in turn implied that for patients with any form of mass lesion in the cerebral hemispheres, the only accurate way of obtaining a measure of ICP was to measure the pressure above the tentorium either in the lateral ventricle or over the surface of the brain.

In the course of his studies, Langfitt came across Lundberg's monograph, realized its importance for neurosurgical practice, and publicized it widely in the United States and internationally. It is fair to say that the widespread adoption of continuous monitoring ICP stems from the combined efforts of Janny, Lundberg, and Langfitt.

By 1970 Jennett and colleagues in Glasgow had published a paper describing ICP changes after head injury and the value of this form of monitoring.[11] Their findings paralleled experience with head injury patients already reported by Lundberg, Vapalahti, and Troupp.[12,13] Jennett's study pointed to the value of ICP monitoring in the diagnosis either of the nature of the process or of changes in that state. Particular value was ascribed to the discovery that ICP could be normal in cases in which it had been clinically suspected to be high and, conversely, high when that had not been suspected clinically. ICP monitoring was also seen to be of value in treatment to demonstrate the efficacy or nonefficacy of therapeutic measures and in prognosis by identifying patients in whom a poor outcome might be anticipated because of persistent intracranial hypertension.

METHODS OF ICP MONITORING

Methods for Comparing Intracranial Pressure Sensors

There are two areas to consider in comparing pressure sensors: static and dynamic characteristics. Static characteristics include zero drift, linearity, sensitivity, and accuracy; dynamic characteristics include frequency response and damping. Considering the static characteristics first, all pressure sensors have some measurable drift caused by temperature- and humidity-dependent fluctuations in strain gauge resistance or shape. Most manufacturers quote sensor drifts in the region of 1 to 2 mmHg per day, which can be insignificant if the drift is random; however, a systematic drift in any single direction can produce serious errors, particularly when one is measuring small pressure levels such as ICP. If allowed to continue unchecked, a large enough error can accrue and fail to reflect the occurrence of ICP raised above a treatment threshold. Systems that do not provide routine in vivo zero checking must have zero drift confirmed in both bench test and clinical studies where, as a minimum, the sensor drift is recorded just after removal of the sensor from the patient (while held at the zero reference point) and followed by a bench test zero drift study.

Linearity is rarely a problem with strain gauge sensors; however, it creates difficulties with some fiberoptic systems, which often use correction algorithms over the calibrated pressure range to ensure linearity. Most systems, both analogue and digital, are sufficiently sensitive to resolve pressures less than 1 mmHg, which is accurate enough for most clinical monitoring. However, depending on the application, resolution better than 1 mmHg is sometimes required. For example, if measurement of craniospinal compliance is carried out with small CSF volume injections and if patients have high compliance, small ICP rises of only a few mmHg will be produced. In such cases, pressure measurement errors of 1 mmHg can produce significant variation in measured compliance.

When determining how accurate a given sensor is, it is customary to compare it against a "gold standard" system. For ICP measurement, the measurement site of choice is usually intraventricular pressure. A single site comparison is intrinsically limited, as it assumes no significant pressure gradient within the cranium. Although this may be true for the supratentorial compartment in head-injured patients with diffuse brain injury, it is unclear whether pressure gradients exist around focal lesions. Nonetheless, in making comparisons, it is important to consider more than just the absolute pressure of the test system against the gold standard system, as two systems can be highly correlated but mask a systematic bias against the test system. This occurs because such correlative associations are usually constant under deviations of scale or bias. A better measure involves calculating the difference between the two systems for each reading and then calculating the 95 percent confidence interval (agreement) for the difference between the systems.[14]

Dynamic characteristics of pressure sensors must also be considered. The general criteria for the accuracy of pressure recording have been well reviewed by Fry,[15] Geddes,[16] and Gabe.[17] The weakest link in the pressure recording system is often the catheter-transducer system used for monitoring pressure. This system consists of a pressure transducer and any fluid-filled linkages (needles, tubing, three-way taps) that may separate the pressure source from the pressure sensor. A catheter-transducer system can be described as a second-order mechanical system consisting of a mass of fluid which acts against the viscous (damping) and elastic properties of the walls of both the catheter and the pressure transducer dome.

Hanson and Warburg[18] demonstrated that a fluid-filled catheter-transducer system, if underdamped, oscillates at its own natural frequency and can produce significant pressure waveform amplitude and phase distortion. The degree of distortion depends on the damping factor (β) of the system. The natural frequency and damping properties of a system can be tested by applying a step or transient pressure to the input of the system and recording the output pressure response. This transient response, or "pop" test, technique can show that for most purposes a damping factor of 0.64 (optimal damping) is desirable, as the amplitude error will be less than 2 percent for up to two-thirds of the natural frequency of the system and the phase lag will be approximately linear over this range.

Catheter-tip pressure sensors—that is, catheters with the sensing element at the tip of the catheter and in close proximity to the pressure source—do not have significant fluid linkages and thus generally have high resonant frequencies. These frequencies are sufficiently high to avoid significant amplitude and phase distortion at the frequencies of physiological interest (<30 Hz). However, fluid-filled catheter-transducer systems do have resonant frequencies within reach of physiological frequencies of interest, and if pressure pulse harmonics higher in frequency than the fundamental or heart rate frequency are to be studied, the damping characteristics of these systems should be measured and then corrected if they are found to be suboptimal. One simple device capable of adjusting the damping characteristics of catheter-transducer systems is the Acudynamic adjustable damping device.[19] This three-way taplike device acts as an adjustable air bubble which, when placed in series with the catheter-transducer system, can be used to adjust the damping characteristics of the system.

Finally, one aspect of pressure sensor systems that is sometimes overlooked is system reliability. ICP sensors often receive a considerable amount of "rough handling" in the operating room, in intensive care, and during patient transport. Any weakness in the strain relief design will soon lead to system failure. Often, such problems are not detected until sensors are tested in the "real world" during clinical studies.

Fluid-Coupled Systems

The system described by Lundberg[5] involved making a burr hole in the frontal bone anterior to the coronal suture, behind the hairline, 2 to 3 cm in front of the bregma, and 1.5 to 2 cm lateral to the midline, usually in line with the pupil of the eye. In patients with a head injury in whom a degree of compression of the lateral ventricles is anticipated, the burr hole should be made somewhat more medially, in line with the inner edge of the iris. Lundberg advocated making a small opening in the dura and other meninges, just sufficient to permit passage of the canula. He used a ventricular needle which was passed through a rubber plug that anchored the system in the burr hole. Currently, a more flexible plastic tubing is passed from the surface of the brain to the lateral ventricle with the aid of a stylet. The ventricular catheter is first connected to a stopcock, then to fluid-filled tubing, and finally to an externally located transducer which is placed for its zero reference at the level of the foramen of Monro. The transducer is connected in turn to an amplification and recording system. This method of continuously recording intraventricular CSF pressure remains the gold standard for measurements of ICP, against which any new method must be assessed. Over the years, a number of alternative methods have been introduced, and some are reviewed here.

In head-injured patients, the lateral ventricles may be small and difficult to locate. No more than three attempts should be made to locate the lateral ventricle. In the first attempt, the tip of the catheter is directed toward the inner canthus of the ipsilateral eye; in the second pass, toward the bridge of the nose; and in the third, toward the inner canthus of the opposite eye. If the ventricle has not been located at this point, a common practice has been to pass the fluid-filled catheter over the surface of the brain to record from the subdural or subarachnoid space. Satisfactory pulsatile recordings of pressure can be obtained in this way; however, a careful study by Barlow and associates in Glasgow showed that when true ICP rose above 30 mmHg, the subdural recording gave a progressively greater underreading of ICP.[20] Such underreading of ICP is not necessarily associated with the appearance of a damped record showing a low pulse pressure; therefore, it is difficult to know when the subdural catheter is underreading (Figs. 31-2 and 31-3). For this reason, the method is being used less and less.

An alternative system of recording ICP that was used in Leeds and Richmond involves the insertion of a threaded screw into the burr hole, with lateral openings in the case of the Leeds bolt and an end opening in the case of the Richmond bolt.[21,22] Both devices are fluid-filled and record subdural pressure. The dura is opened

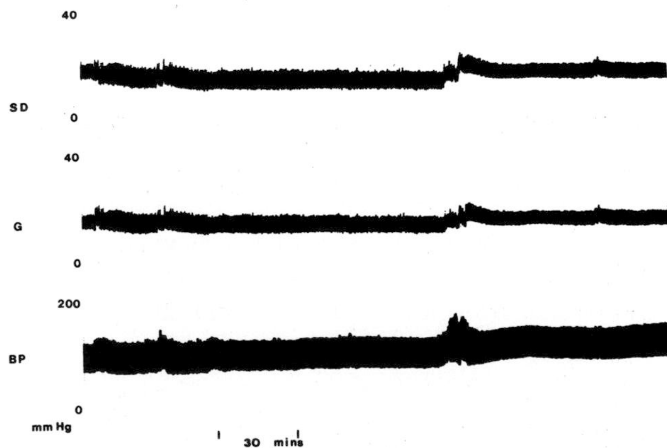

Figure 31-2. Recording of intracranial pressure through a subdural fluid-filled catheter (SD), showing a similar pressure and pulse waveform shape compared with a Gaeltec catheter-tip subdural sensor.

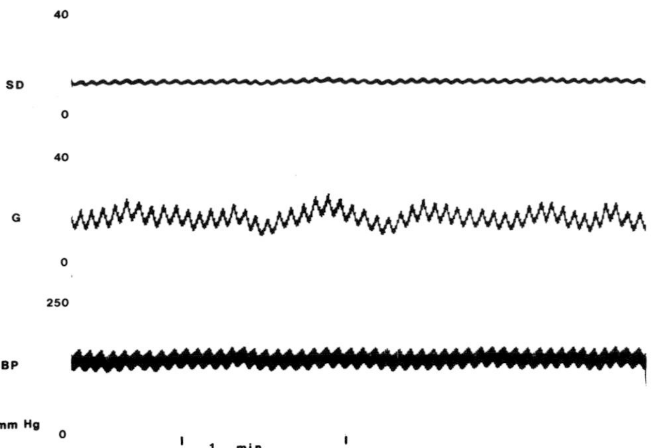

Figure 31-3. Recording of intracranial pressure through a subdural fluid-filled catheter (SD), exhibiting underreading of pressure and an overdamped pulse waveform compared with a Gaeltec catheter-tip subdural sensor.

in a cruciate manner. Comparative recordings of intraventricular and subdural bolt pressure have shown the same tendency to underread elevated ICP when levels rise above 30 mmHg. At levels below this, the bolt system usually works satisfactorily.

Non-Fluid-Coupled Systems

A large number of devices have been developed over the last 20 years in which a miniature transducer is placed directly within the cranial cavity or some form of solid-state sensing system involving the use of fiber optics is connected to an external system that transduces changes in reflected light into a pressure recording. Some of these devices have been designed for recording ICP from the epidural space, assuming that pressure from the subdural and subarachnoid compartments is transmitted accurately across the dura. Schettini and Walsh emphasized the importance of surrounding the transducer with a ring that was coplanar with the inside of the skull and would absorb dural tension so that the transducer was recording only transmitted ICP and was not reflecting dural tension.[23] A number of workable epidural systems have been tried, but most are very sensitive to any collection of blood or bone dust on the dural surface. Furthermore, the principal drawback of most systems is that they cannot be recalibrated in situ.

Gaeltec developed an implantable transducer surrounded by a latex envelope that allows rezeroing in situ. Although unique in its design and one of the few systems offering a means of correcting for transducer drift in situ, the early Gaeltec systems suffered problems with mechanical failure.[24] Recently, a new epidural pressure sensor has been produced by Spiegelberg which also offers correction for zero drift.[25] This system measures pressure by means of a small air pouch partially filled with approximately 0.1 ml of air. Pressure equilibrates across the thin bag membrane and is sensed via flexible tubing connected to an external pressure transducer. Every hour, the transducer automatically rezeroes to atmosphere and volume is added or removed to maintain a constant air bag volume. This maintains the partially collapsed state of the bag and assures approximate coplanar alignment with the dura. Early reports showed improved performance over other epidural sensors, although little is known about how well this system correlates with ventricular pressure. Clinical studies validating this system against fiber-optic sensors are needed. A ventricular version of the system is planned.

Over the years, a number of workers have attempted to obtain accurate measurements of ICP from within the parenchyma of the brain. When fluid-filled systems are used, the catheter has to be filled with fine fibers that allow transmission of pressure within the fluid between the fibers but prevent the ingress of brain tissue to block the catheter. Comparisons with pressure recordings of ventricular fluid show that measurements of brain tissue pressure using wick catheters tend to underread the true pressure unless the fluid within the catheter is held at 20 mOsm above plasma.[26] This suggests that the tissue catheter has caused a small amount of damage in the system with passage of oncotically active molecules into the extracellular space. With the introduction of fiber-optic recording systems, accurate measurements of intraparenchymal brain pressure have become possible and have been shown to give values that correspond with intraventricular pressure.[27,28]

In current ICP monitoring, fiber-optic systems can accurately record pressure from within the lateral ventricle, from the subdural space over the surface of the cerebral hemisphere, and from within the brain tissue itself.[27,28] Typically, these systems can be electronically rezeroed but have to be calibrated before insertion and after removal. Comparative studies show close correspondence among recordings taken from these three sites. In a recent study by Midgley and Statham,[28a] fiber-optic catheter systems were placed both parenchymally and in the ventricle and then were compared simultaneously with a fluid-filled intraventricular catheter as the gold standard measurement. Comparison of both mean pressure and the first 10 harmonic components of the ICP pressure waveform demonstrated good correlation between all three sites of measurement, with a maximum bias of 2 mmHg between the sites of measurement. Further work needs to be done in groups of patients with unilateral mass lesions to ascertain whether under certain clinical conditions significant pressure gradients exist between the intraparenchymal and intraventricular compartments.[26]

INDICATIONS FOR ICP MONITORING AFTER HEAD INJURY

Attempts to define the indications for ICP monitoring in head-injured patients have essentially been based on data concerning the prevalence of raised ICP in various categories of head injury and the observed links between raised ICP and increased mortality and morbidity. Measurement of the prevalence of intracranial hypertension after injury is not sufficient, as continuous ICP data may not be available; even if ICP is measured continuously, the hard copy record available for analysis may consist only of digital values of ICP recorded periodically by the nursing staff onto the intensive care data sheet, thus missing transient ICP surges. In their 1977 paper describing the management and outcome of 160 patients with severe head injury, Miller et al. detected raised ICP in 44 percent of these patients.[29] In 1981, Miller et al. described management and outcome in 225 patients scoring Glasgow Coma Scale (GCS) 8 or less after resuscitation, and the prevalence of ICP levels in excess of 20 mmHg for 5 min or longer was 54 percent.[30] In both series of patients, however, there were subgroups in whom raised ICP was found in the majority of cases. These included patients with intracranial mass lesions and coma who had required surgical evacuation of the hematoma (postoperatively, between 52 and 70 percent of such patients had intracranial hypertension) and patients without intracranial hematomas who showed abnormal motor responses consisting of abnormal flexion or extension.[29,30] These data were obtained only because ICP monitoring was carried out in all comatose head-injured patients in the two Richmond series. The study performed by Teasdale et al.[31] found that intracranial hypertension was also evident in a majority of comatose patients whose CT scans showed obliteration of the basal cisterns and loss of the image of the third ventricle.[31]

After these studies, Miller and Narayan et al. attempted to make a more selective definition of the head-injured patients in whom ICP monitoring was most likely to be useful.[32,33] Miller suggested that all patients who are artificially ventilated should have ICP monitoring.[32] This would include comatose patients with a hematoma and/or a GCS < 6 and patients in whom the CT scan showed loss of the perimesenphalic cisterns, a midline shift of more than 5 mm, and/or dilatation of the contralateral ventricle. In the study of Narayan et al.,[33] the incidence of raised ICP in patients with severe head injury was 53 to 63 percent if the initial CT scan showed a high- or low-density abnormality. If the scan was normal, the incidence of raised ICP was only 13 percent. However, in the normal CT group, the incidence of ICP elevation was 60 percent if the patients demonstrated two or more of the following features: age over 40 years, unilateral or bilateral motor posturing, and blood pressure less than 90 mmHg. If only one or none of these features was present, the incidence of intracranial hypertension was only 4 percent. It was suggested that comatose patients without such features may not require ICP monitoring because their risk of intracranial hypertension is so low.

In the prospective Traumatic Coma Data Bank study, further information was obtained on the incidence of intracranial hypertension in patients with a severe head injury.[34] An incidence figure of 72 percent for raised ICP was obtained when ICP monitoring was conducted in all patients scoring 8 or less on the GCS after early resuscitation. In another prospective study in Edinburgh designed to detect and record the severity and duration of a wide variety of secondary insults, including arterial hypotension, intracranial hypertension, hypoxemia, and pyrexia, Jones and colleagues found an incidence of intracranial hypertension of over 80 percent.[35] O'Sullivan et al. identified a small number of comatose head-injured patients in whom the initial CT was essentially normal, showing a preserved CSF space around the midbrain, and yet intracranial hypertension occurred.[36]

It can be concluded from these reports that the more assiduously evidence for intracranial hypertension is sought, the more likely it is that it will be found, and that there is no subgroup of comatose head-injured patients who can be considered to be entirely free from the risk of raised ICP. Therefore, it is the authors' current recommendation that all comatose head-injured patients receive continuous monitoring of ICP.

COMPLICATIONS OF ICP MONITORING

Although most ICP monitoring devices can be inserted in the intensive care unit (ICU), this procedure may involve moving the patient to the operating room, giving a local or general anesthetic, and placing it in the appropriate intracranial location. ICP may be raised for up to 2 weeks, and so the device must be durable and may need replacement. Complications can develop at any of these stages. Therefore, it is important that the indications for monitoring be clear-cut and that an appropriate system be used. For instance, a fluid-coupled system inserted into the lateral ventricle would be particularly appropriate in a head-injured patient in whom previously undetected aqueduct stenosis was seen on initial imaging but less appropriate in a patient with a large mass lesion with evidence of distortion of the anterior horns of the lateral ventricles. Secondary insults occur if the patient is not resuscitated adequately before the insertion of a monitoring device; therefore, resuscitation takes priority. Some devices, such as the intraparenchymal fiber-optic monitor, can be inserted by the bedside, avoiding the risks of transfer to an operation room.

Complications of catheter insertion include failure of correct placement, brain swelling caused by repeated attempts to cannulate the ventricle, and intracerebral or subdural hematoma, particularly in patients with disorders of hemostasis. These complications can be minimized by means of a suitable choice of device when ventricles are distorted, limitation to three attempts at ventricular placement, and checking the coagulation screen before insertion. In one large study, the incidence of intracerebral hemorrhage secondary to ventriculostomy placement was 1.4 percent.[33]

Infection is an important complication of ventriculostomy and relates most clearly to the duration of monitoring. Mayhall et al. found that 85 percent of ventriculostomy-related infections in patients with a severe head injury occurred in patients who had been monitored for over 5 days but that no infections occurred in patients monitored for 3 days or less.[37] This has led to the practice of removing a ventriculostomy after about 5 days and placing a new catheter through a separate burr hole. Another factor associated with infection may be the frequency of sampling of ventricular fluid; the more frequent the sampling of CSF, the higher the risk of infection.[37,38] Placement of a subdural fluid-coupled system under the craniotomy bone flap may increase the risk of subsequent bone flap infection. Infection in non-fluid-coupled systems is rare, except for local contamination of the wound edges. Intraparenchymal fiber-optic catheters have been used for up to 2 weeks without reports of infectious complications.

Non-fluid-coupled systems are prone to mechanical failure, which may occur at the sensor or at its connection. The glass fibers of fiber-optic systems can be damaged by severe kinking of the tubing or overtightening at the bolt. It is particularly important when using these systems to interpret the data with care and not to rely on the data in isolation. Calibration before insertion is a sensible precaution, if only to reassure the clinician that the device is accurate. If there is a significant discrepancy between ICP measurement and other evidence, it is safest to remove the system and insert a newly zeroed, calibrated system. However, the amount of drift and calibration error has been a maximum of 6 mmHg in both clinical and laboratory tests in catheters used for up to 5 days. All systems, except for fully implantable devices, must be firmly secured to avoid accidental dislodgment of the catheter, which usually occurs while the patient is being turned. The risk of epilepsy associated with an intraventricular or intraparenchymal catheter is about 2 to 3 percent.[39] In head-injured patients, the additional risk posed by the ICP monitoring device is difficult to quantify because of concomitant factors such as intracranial hemorrhage, dural penetration, and prolonged posttraumatic amnesia, which are themselves associated with an increased risk of epilepsy.

INTERPRETATION OF ICP DATA

In the early days of continuous ICP monitoring in patients with a head injury, two aspects were emphasized: (1) defining the threshold level of ICP above which corrective measures should be undertaken and (2) detecting intermittent waves of increased ICP that might indicate a state of reduced craniospinal compliance or another pathophysiological disturbance requiring treatment. To establish thresholds, it is first necessary to define the upper limit of normal ICP. Lundberg defined this at 15 mmHg, equivalent to 200 mmH_2O or 2 kPa. However, this definition applied only to adults. Welch has pointed out that in children, the upper limit of normal ICP is much lower (5 mmHg in children age 1 to 5 years and 3 mmHg in neonates).[40]

With the normal range defined, at which threshold level can ICP be considered unequivocally elevated? While some would hold that any level above 15 mmHg is abnormally high, the majority would probably regard ICP values of 20 mmHg as the threshold above which ICP is definitely elevated. Above this level, steps should be undertaken to verify that the ICP is indeed elevated and easily correctable factors should be attended to. If ICP exceeds 25 mmHg despite this initial intervention, most clinicians will begin treatment to reduce ICP.

However, the situation is not always as simple as this, and other factors must be taken into account in determining threshold levels for abnormal ICP and its therapy. These factors include the level of cerebral perfusion pressure (CPP) and the relationship between ICP and the processes of brain shift and herniation, particularly tentorial herniation.

The pressure in the thin-walled cerebral veins coursing through the subarachnoid space before their entry into the dural venous sinuses must remain slightly in excess of cranial pressure during intracranial hypertension or the veins will collapse and the cerebral circulation will cease. For that reason, the true CPP is represented by the difference between the pressure within the internal carotid and vertebral arteries after they have entered the cranial cavity and the pressure in the cerebral venous system before it reaches the dural venous sinuses.[41] The perfusion pressure is not the difference between carotid artery and jugular venous pressure, since jugular venous pressure is invariably close to atmospheric pressure regardless of conditions within the craniospinal axis. Therefore, the CPP can be well approximated by the difference between mean arterial pressure recorded from a radial artery or another peripheral artery and the mean ICP, since ICP and cerebral venous pressure change in parallel, with cerebral venous pressure remaining 2 or 3 mmHg higher.[42] This has been verified over a range of ICP levels between 0 and 100 mmHg. The absolute height of ICP, then, if it is evenly distributed within the craniospinal axis, is less important than the difference between ICP and arterial pressure, since this is the effective driving force of the cerebral circulation, which in head-injured patients may need to be held at a higher than normal level because of an increase in peripheral resistance. The causes of the increase in vascular resistance have not been fully established. Contributing factors include spasm or partial occlusion in the microcirculation and edema with microvascular compression or distortion. Experimental and clinical studies have suggested that in normal subjects CPP values of 40 or 50 mmHg suffice to maintain an adequate level of cerebral blood flow, whereas in head-injured patients recent studies using Doppler ultrasonography of the middle cerebral arteries indicate that reactive changes in flow pattern begin when CPP falls below 70 mmHg and are well established when CPP is less than 60 mmHg.[43] Therefore, the ICP level must be interpreted in the context of the current arterial blood pressure.[44]

In patients with localized brain swelling or compression, particularly when it affects the temporal lobes, there is an important interaction between ICP and tentorial herniation. As the brain swells around the tentorial hiatus and the CSF space in the cisterna magna is progressively obliterated, pressure gradients can develop in which the supratentorial pressure is higher than the infratentorial, and this pressure difference helps propel the temporal lobe structures downward through the tentorial hiatus and also facilitates downward axial movement of the brainstem.[8] The absolute level of supratentorial ICP at which these processes occur seems to be widely variable. In the case of temporal lobe contusions, ipsilateral pupillary dilatation, which signals the development of lateral tentorial herniation, has been observed to develop with ICP below 20 mmHg.[45] However, in clinical practice, infratentorial CSF pressure is not generally measured, and thus the magnitude of the pressure gradient in tentorial herniation is unknown.

For these reasons, one must be reluctant to rely on definitions of threshold levels of ICP alone to determine when therapeutic action should be taken.

ADDITIONAL MEASUREMENTS IN PATIENTS UNDERGOING ICP MONITORING

It is clear from the above discussion that ICP should not be considered in isolation. The intensive management of a severely head injured patient should, if possible, be based on pathophysiological information rather than being determined empirically. To elucidate the pathophysiology, a number of measurements can be made in addition to ICP. These can be separated into two groups: those which are essential and those which may be helpful or are still considered to be under development. A continuous measurement of intraarterial pressure from an indwelling cannula is essential for the management of a severely head injured patient, as ICP data must be regarded as relatively incomplete without simultaneous information on the level of arterial pressure. The arterial line also provides the necessary access for frequent withdrawals of blood samples to measure the levels of arterial P_{CO_2}, P_{O_2}, and pH. These intermittent measurements are important in checking on the validity of continuous recordings of end-tidal CO_2 and arterial oxygen saturation obtained noninvasively by pulse oximetry.

Body temperature must be monitored continuously, with recordings of both core and peripheral temperature. Elevation of body temperature increases the risk of intracranial hypertension and is one of the correctable factors in its management. Pyrexia is also a factor of considerable adverse prognostic significance in traumatic brain injury.[35]

In the literature on experimental brain ischemia, there are indications of the additional importance of obtaining a measurement of brain tissue temperature, which may differ from systemic core temperature.[46] However, such measurements in head-injured patients are considered developmental at present.

The ECG should be monitored continuously not only to obtain a measure of the heart rate but also because of the known association between traumatic intracranial hemorrhage and ECG abnormalities that can include prolongation of the QT interval, ST segment elevation, and frank arrhythmias.[47]

Concomitant measurements that would be regarded as desirable include the continuous monitoring of oxygen saturation in the jugular bulb (Sjv_{O_2}), which can now be carried out using a fiber-optic catheter system.[48] A recording of high levels of oxygen saturation (more than 75%) in jugular venous blood is suggestive of cerebral hyperemia and, in the presence of intracranial hypertension, would support the use of hyperventilation or barbiturate therapy as a means of lowering ICP. Levels of oxygen saturation between 45 and 50% indicate increased oxygen extraction, usually a response to reduced cerebral blood flow, while oxygen saturation levels below 40% are indicative of global brain ischemia.[49] Gopinath et al. have defined jugular venous desaturation as an Sjv_{O_2} less than 50% for more than 10 min.[50] In these circumstances, hyperventilation should not be employed and arterial hypotension should not be allowed to occur. Continuous monitoring of Sjv_{O_2} is not a simple exercise, however. The location of the catheter tip in the jugular bulb must be verified radiographically, and the continuous readout of oxygen saturation values must be accompanied by readings of adequate light intensity. Every 8 to 12 h the system should be recalibrated against direct measurements of oxygen saturation made by co-oximetry on samples of blood withdrawn from the jugular bulb through the same catheter system.[48]

Transcranial Doppler sonography of middle cerebral artery flow velocity (systolic, diastolic, and mean) and calculation of the pulsatility index (S-D/M) can be obtained continuously by using an appropriate headband to hold the probe securely in position over the temporal scalp. Measurements may be made continuously over several hours. Such a system may be useful in the detection of low-flow states, hyperemia, and possibly the development of vasospasm in the middle cerebral arteries.[51] This is signaled by the development of very high levels of mean blood flow velocity in excess of 130 cm/s compared with the normal value of around 65 cm/s.[52,53]

One of the major problems in managing comatose, artificially ventilated head-injured patients in the ICU is a lack of information about the level of brain function, particularly if the patients are receiving multiple relaxant drugs. In such cases, only the pupillary light responses are available for assessment. Under these circumstances, a continuous record of brain electrical activity can be valuable despite the known difficulties in its assessment. These difficulties arise because changes in body temperature and brain metabolism caused by drug therapy can interfere with the interpretation of a particular EEG frequency or amplitude. The same problems arise in the interpretation of event-related evoked potential responses. Nevertheless, even crude measures of EEG wave amplitude can be valuable in providing a rapid warning of impaired brain function that corresponds to reductions in CPP.

DEVELOPMENTS IN ICP MONITORING

Observation of high ICP or of a sudden rise in ICP is clearly valuable in the management of a head-injured patient, but very often by the time treatment has been delivered, harm to the brain may already have occurred. It would clearly be more beneficial to be able to predict the likelihood of raised ICP in a patient whose ICP is still normal or only mildly elevated. It would also be helpful if the monitoring of ICP, with or without additional measurements, could indicate the mechanism of any rise in ICP and in particular could differentiate between vascular and nonvascular causes. Knowledge of the cause of increased ICP could then be translated into selection of the most appropriate therapy, since ideal therapy for raised ICP should be correct the first time.[54] The rapidity with which brain ischemia causes loss of function and evident damage in the brain may not permit the empirical approach of sequentially trying different therapies until one is found that successfully reduces ICP.

Two main approaches have been used to derive more information from ICP monitoring. The first has been to challenge the craniospinal axis with small volumes of fluid delivered or aspirated in known periods of time, observe the results, and use the data to predict what the effect of larger volumetric changes on ICP might be. The second approach has been a systems analysis approach in which the craniospinal axis is regarded as a closed box of which the input is the arterial blood pressure waveform and the output is the ICP waveform. Both the arterial and intracranial pressure waveforms are then subjected to spectral analysis to resolve them into their fundamental and higher harmonic waves so that the changes in amplitude and phase shift that occur as the waves pass through the cerebrovascular bed in the cranial cavity can be analyzed.

Miller et al. conducted a series of studies which investigated the effect on ICP of the introduction of 1 ml of saline into the ventricular CSF over a period of 1 s in patients in whom ICP was being recorded continuously by the Lundberg technique. In 16 patients with head injury, it was found that this volume-pressure response (VPR) ranged from 1.0 to 13.7 mmHg/ml.[55] There was a weak correlation between the height of the baseline ICP and the VPR in that all VPR values above 2 mmHg/ml were obtained in patients with raised ICP. However, it was also noted that the highest values of VPR were observed in patients with intracranial mass lesions and midline brain shift due either to swollen brain contusions or to formed intracranial hematomas. A stronger correlation was observed between the height of the VPR and the extent of midline brain shift.

This approach was taken further by Shulman and Marmarou, who observed that there was an exponential relationship between the CSF pressure and the addition of volume to the CSF space; this was determined first in experimental animals and confirmed later in humans[56] (Fig. 31-4). Marmarou used this relationship to develop a pressure-volume index (PVI) measured in milliliters. The PVI represented the notional volume of fluid which, when added to the craniospinal contents, would produce a 10-fold rise in ICP (Fig. 31-5). The great advantage of the PVI was that unlike the VPR, its value was independent of the baseline level of ICP at which the test measurement took place (Fig. 31-6). Marmarou and colleagues have shown that reduced levels of PVI are not uncommon after head injury, and when they fall to levels below 15 ml, they are highly predictive of intracranial hypertension and indicate a state of seriously reduced craniospinal compliance.[57]

Marmarou et al. went on to demonstrate that after the bolus addition of a small volume of CSF and the resultant rapid increase in ICP from baseline to peak values, there was an exponential decay in pressure back to baseline, the rate of which was largely determined by CSF outflow resistance.[58] In this way, Marmarou et al. provided an opportunity to rapidly measure CSF outflow resistance, using a method well suited to investigations in patients. Up to this point, such measurements of CSF resistance had required steady-state infusion techniques that demanded stable conditions over many minutes. While Sullivan et al. and Takisawa and colleagues showed that the bolus technique of measuring CSF outflow resistance tended to underestimate the outflow resistance calculated by steady-state techniques under normal conditions in the craniospinal axis, there was close correlation between the bolus and infusion techniques under conditions of raised ICP and reduced CSF buffering capacity such as frequently occur after a traumatic brain injury.[59,60] Marmarou's dynamic technique of estimating CSF outflow resistance can there-

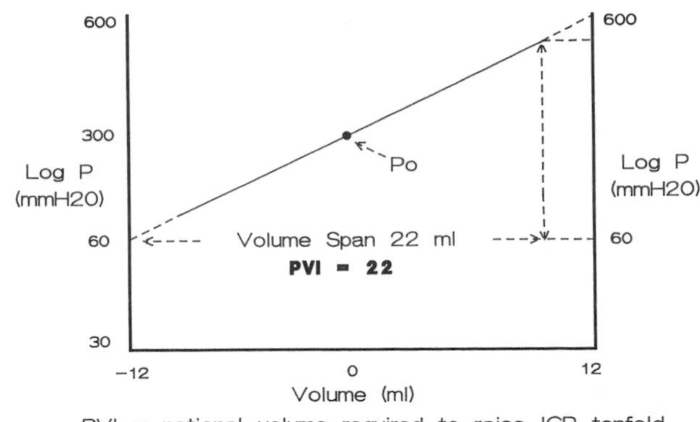

Figure 31-5. Log ICP versus volume relationship described by Marmarou. The PVI is the volume in millimeters of fluid which, when added to the CSF space, results in a 10-fold rise in pressure.

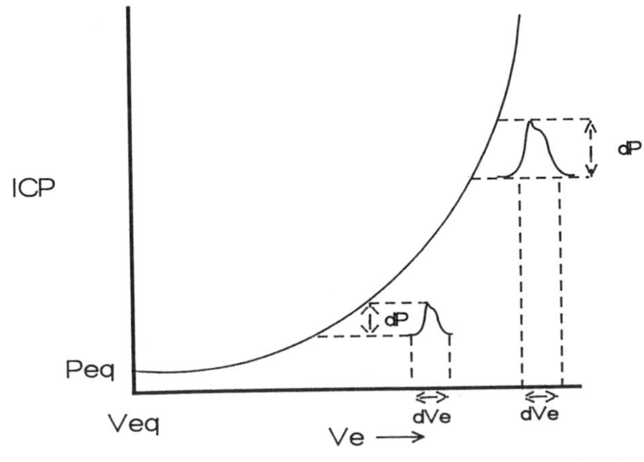

The exponential volume–pressure relationship is described mathematically:

$$\text{equation 1)} \quad P = Peq\ e^{E1\ dVe} + Po$$

where: P = ICP
Peq = equilibrium ICP
E1 = Elastic coefficient
Ve = elastic volume (addition to total volume)
Po = constant term

Figure 31-4. Exponential craniospinal volume-pressure relationship demonstrating that for the same increment in intracranial volume (dVe), a larger intracranial pulse pressure (dP) results when Ve is injected farther up the volume-pressure relationship. Equation 1 describes this volume-pressure relationship mathematically.

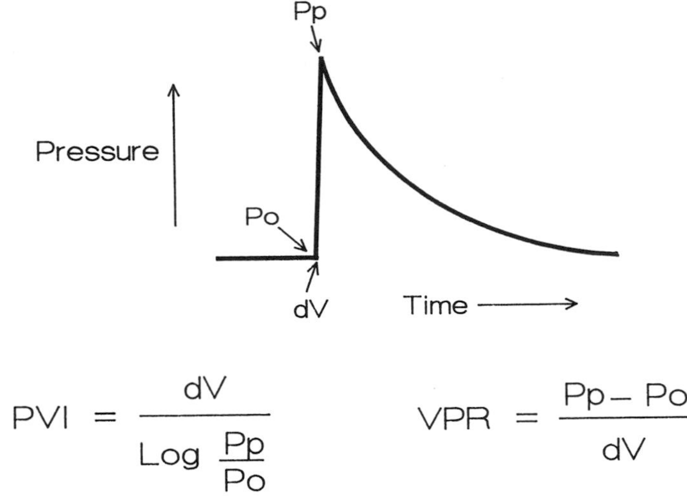

Figure 31-6. The PVI and VPR techniques are based on the manual injection of known volumes (dV) of fluid into the CSF space, resulting in an increase in pressure (Pp) relative to a baseline pressure (Po).

fore be applied in human subjects after a traumatic brain injury to estimate the contribution of CSF flow obstruction to raised ICP.

Marmarou et al. added a third measurement to their armamentarium by aspirating CSF from the craniospinal axis and measuring the time needed for CSF pressure to return to baseline levels. From this, they calculated the CSF formation rate. Then, by continuously aspirating CSF from the patient at the calculated CSF formation rate, they arrived at a new, lower steady-state level of pressure that was thought to represent sagittal sinus venous pressure. From these calculations, this group obtained an estimate of the proportions of the patient's CSF pressure that are due to vascular and nonvascular factors. Marmarou et al. have calculated that in patients with raised ICP after head injury, vascular factors account for 70 percent of the observed ICP.[61]

CURRENT RESEARCH INTO ICP AND CRANIOSPINAL COMPLIANCE

From this landmark work of Marmarou and colleagues, it was suggested that knowledge of a patient's craniospinal VPR could be an important adjunct to ICP measurement for predicting states of raised ICP. However, with these volume injection techniques, the variability between measurements is high, as it is difficult to manually inject and withdraw consistent volumes of fluid rapidly at a constant rate. Therefore, an average of repeated measures is usually required, which, with the time required for ICP to return to baseline between tests, makes these methods time-consuming and erratic.

In an effort to find an improved and less invasive means of obtaining similar data, Avezaat, Van Eijndhoven, and coworkers[62,63] systematically studied the ICP waveform pulse amplitude (ICP_{plse}) as a measure of craniospinal elastance, the inverse of compliance. The rationale behind this concept is as follows: With each heartbeat there is a pulsatile increase in cerebral blood volume, which is the equivalent of a small intracranial volume injection; the ICP_{plse} is the ICP response to that volume increment and therefore should be directly related to the craniospinal elastance (dP/dV). That is, as craniospinal elastance increases (compliance decreases), the ICP_{plse} should increase. Avezaat and Van Eijndhoven described the mathematical relationship between ICP_{plse} and ICP by substituting ICP_{plse} for elastance (dP/dV) and substituting pulsatile blood volume for the volume injection. This relationship was verified in both clinical and experimental studies in which they found that the ICP_{plse} increased linearly with ICP up to a pressure of 60 mmHg, after which a breakpoint occurred (Fig. 31-7). Above 60 mmHg, the ICP_{plse} increased more rapidly with increasing ICP. Avezaat and Van Eijndhoven argue that the breakpoint is a marker for loss of cerebral blood flow (CBF) autoregulation, postulating that the onset of vasomotor paralysis causes a decreased arteriolar inflow resistance which results in an increased

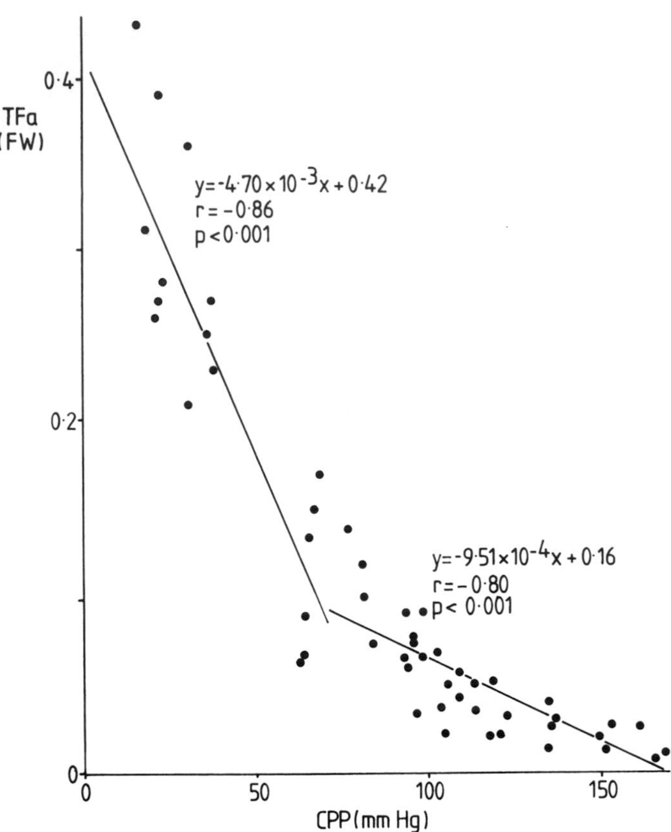

Figure 31-7. Relationship between cerebral perfusion pressure (CPP) and the amplitude transfer function for the fundamental harmonic (TFa), which is approximately equivalent to the ratio of ICP pulse to BP pulse, exhibited in a feline model of diffusely raised ICP. Note the increase in the slope of the TFa versus CPP relationship above 70 mmHg.

phase shift between inflow and outflow pulsatile blood volume. This translates to an overall increased intracranial pulsatile blood volume and tends to increase the slope of the relationship of ICP_{plse} to ICP. Largely as a consequence of the dependence of this relationship on the pulsatile blood volume, the clinical utility of this technique as a measure of lumped craniospinal elastance is limited unless a clinically practical measure of pulsatile blood volume can be monitored simultaneously and controlled in patients. Such a measure of blood volume is not currently available.

Chopp and Portnoy[64] recognized the importance of measurement of the input function in an analysis of the ICP_{plse} and were the first to apply a systems analysis approach to the ICP waveform. Their method assumes that the blood pressure (BP) waveform is the chief input signal to the cerebrovascular system and that the ICP waveform is the output response to that stimulus. Both BP and ICP waveforms are converted into the frequency domain by Fourier analysis, and the resulting frequency spectra are used in the calculation of the amplitude transfer function, which is a measure of how much pressure is transmitted through the cerebrovascular bed over a range of frequencies. Using these methods, Portnoy and Chopp[65] found in an experimental model of raised ICP in cats that arterial hypercarbia and hypoxia produced an increase in ICP_{plse} and an increase mainly in the amplitude transfer function of the fundamental harmonic. Through a series of experimental studies,[65,66] they attributed this alteration in pressure transmission chiefly to functional autoregulatory tone of the precapillary cerebral resistance vessels.

Bray et al. and Robertson et al., also using Fourier analysis of the ICP waveform in patients, identified a high-frequency band (4 to 15 Hz) in the ICP waveform power spectrum.[67,68] The centroid (power-weighted average frequency) of this high-frequency band correlated inversely with the PVI as a measure of craniospinal compliance. As compliance decreased, the high-frequency centroid increased, with the percentage of time the centroid spent at greater than 9 Hz correlating exponentially to increased mortality.[68] However, the utility of this technique as a measure of compliance is regarded as uncertain because recent studies by this group and others have indicated that the high-frequency centroid is also highly dependent on the heart rate, a change in which could account for at least some of the measured centroid response.

Adapting the systems analysis method of Portnoy and Chopp to a clinical study of cerebrovascular pressure transmission, Piper et al.,[69] in an observational study of 1500 pressure records in 30 severely head injured patients, identified four patterns of amplitude transfer function. Both forms showing an elevated fundamental pressure transmission from BP to ICP were associated with raised ICP, whereas the remaining forms with a normal fundamental amplitude transfer function were associated with ICP below 15 mmHg. After this work, a further explanatory experimental study was performed in cats, demonstrating that the fundamental amplitude transfer function can be increased by active arteriolar vasodilation, by loss of autoregulatory vascular tone, or through reduced cerebrovascular transmural pressure.[70] It may be possible to distinguish these mechanisms on the basis of the observed phase shift between the fundamental of the BP and ICP waveforms. In this experimental model, active arteriolar vasodilation was followed by an increasingly negative phase shift, decreased transmural pressure resulted in no overall phase shift, and impaired autoregulation showed that an increased fundamental amplitude was accompanied by a positive phase shift. Further studies are needed to correlate these ICP waveform measures with CBF and pressure autoregulation in head-injured patients.

Another area of research showing promise concerns the continuous measure of transcranial middle cerebral artery (MCA) flow velocity and its correlation with CPP. Chan et al.[49] demonstrated that in continuously monitored head-injured patients, the MCA Doppler pulsatility index (PI), when plotted against CPP, showed a breakpoint at 70 mmHg, below which the PI increases. Simultaneous measurement of jugular venous oxygen saturation in the same patients demonstrated a fall in jugular venous saturation toward ischemic levels below

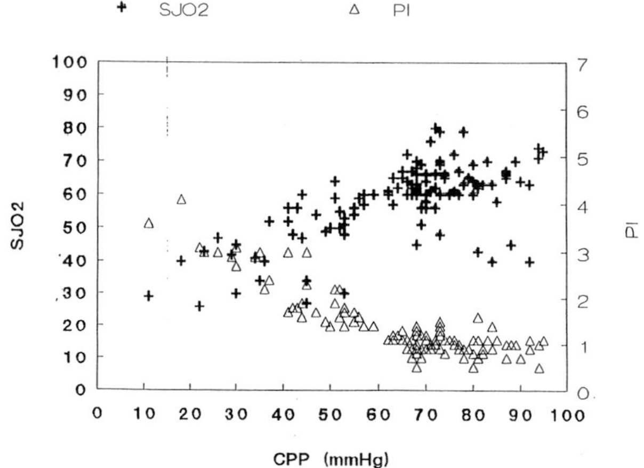

Figure 31-8. MCA Doppler pulsatility index (PI), when plotted against CPP, showed a breakpoint at 70 mmHg, below which the PI increases. Simultaneous measurement of jugular venous oxygen saturation in the same head-injured patients demonstrated a fall in jugular venous saturation toward ischemic levels from the same CPP breakpoint.

the same CPP breakpoint (Fig. 31-8). These data indicate that below a CPP threshold of 70 mmHg, autoregulation in these patients became exhausted. This information is useful, as it provides a means for determining the optimal CPP threshold for treating raised ICP at any time during the management of head-injured patients. A similar relationship between CPP and the exhaustion of autoregulation may also be identified through analysis of the ICP waveform. Although this relationship is currently under study in head-injured patients, it confirms the earlier experimental study in cats by Takizawa et al.[71] which demonstrated that the fundamental amplitude transfer function showed a positive correlation to raised ICP and an inverse correlation to CPP, with the latter demonstrating a breakpoint phenomenon as CPP exceeded 60 mmHg.

Much of the work just described shows promise for elucidating the status of cerebral autoregulation in head-injured patients; nonetheless, we are no closer to improving on the methods developed by Marmarou and Miller for assessment of the craniospinal volume-pressure status. However, some of the limitations of these manual volume-pressure techniques are being overcome as a result of innovative applications of computer technology. For example, Smielewski et al.[72] reported a new method of measuring craniospinal compliance and CSF outflow resistance in hydrocephalus patients that is based on controlled CSF drainage. This system uses an electromagnetically driven clamp which opens or closes the outlet of the lumbar drain under computer control, permitting on-line controlled drainage of CSF and measurement of CSF pressure and volume. This automated drainage method does not raise ICP and thus overcomes the risk of provoking the uncontrolled rises in ICP associated with the continuous infusion or bolus techniques. Similarly, Piper et al.[73] reported an automated method for measuring craniospinal compliance that is based on an electronic square-wave pressure generator triggered under computer control and able to produce small (0.05 ml) volume injection/withdrawal sequences into the CSF space. In this method, the compliance is calculated from the amplitude of the ICP response to this small volume increment. The resulting pressure response itself is small (1 to 2 mmHg) and is isolated from background noise through the use of computer-controlled signal averaging. Using this technique, work is under way to develop a practical clinical device for measuring craniospinal compliance in patients at risk of raised ICP. Thus, current research on multimodality monitoring and applied computer technology is a promising approach to the study of raised ICP and may prove to be a powerful aid in the investigation of cerebrovascular pathophysiology and craniospinal volume-pressure relationships.

References

1. Von Bergmann E: Uber den Hirndruck. *Arch Klin Chir* 32:705–732, 1885.
2. Weed LH: Some limitations of the Monro-Kellie Hypothesis. *Arch Surg* 18:1049–1068, 1929.
3. Ryder HW, Espey FF, Kimball FD, et al: Mechanism of the change in cerebrospinal fluid pressure following an induced change in the volume of fluid space. *J Fab Clin Med* 41:428–435, 1953.
4. Guillaume J, Janny P: Manometrie intracranienne continue: Interet de la methode et premiers resultats. *Rev Neurol (Paris)* 84:131–142, 1951.
5. Lundberg N: Continuous recording and control of ventricular fluid pressure in neurosurgical practice. *Acta Psychiatr Scand [Suppl]* 36(suppl 149):1–193, 1960.
6. Langfitt TW: Increased intracranial pressure. *Clin Neurosurg* 16:436–471, 1969.
7. Langfitt TW, Weinstein JD, Kassell NF: Cerebral vasomotor paralysis produced by intracranial hypertension. *Neurology* 15:622–641, 1965.
8. Langfitt TW, Weinstein JD, Kassell NF, Simeone FA: Transmission of increased intracranial pressure: I. Within the craniospinal axis. *J Neurosurg* 21:989–997, 1964.
9. Johnson RT, Yates PO: Brain stem hemorrhages in expanding supratentorial conditions. *Acta Radiol* 46:250–256, 1956.
10. Jennett WB, Stern WE: Tentorial herniation, the mid brain and the pupil: Experimental studies in brain compression. *J Neurosurg* 17:598–608, 1960.
11. Johnston IH, Johnston JA, Jennett WB: Intracranial pressure following head injury. *Lancet* 2:433–436, 1970.
12. Lundberg N, Troupp H, Lorin H: Continuous recording of the ventricular fluid pressure in patients with severe acute traumatic brain injury. *J Neurosurg* 22:581–590, 1965.
13. Troupp H: Intraventricular pressure in patients with severe brain injuries. *J Trauma* 5:373–378, 1965.
14. Altman DG, Bland JM. Measurements in Medicine: the analysis of method comparison studies. *Statistician* 32:307–317, 1983.
15. Fry DL: Physiological recording by modern instruments with particular reference to pressure recording. *Physiol Rev* 40:753–788, 1960.
16. Geddes LA: *The Direct and Indirect Measurement of Blood Pressure.* Chicago: Year Book, 1970.
17. Gabe IT: Pressure measurement in experimental physiology, in *Cardiovascular Fluid Dynamics.* PA Bergel ed. pp 11–50 London: Academic Press, 1972.
18. Hanson AT, Warburg E: The theory for elastic liquid membrane manometers: General part. *Acta Physiol Scand* vol. 19: 306–332, 1950.
19. Allan MWB, Gray WM, Ashbury AJ: Measurement of arterial pressure using catheter-transducer systems: Improvement using the acudynamic adjustable damping device. *Br J Anaesth* 60:413–418, 1988.
20. Barlow P, Mendelow AD, Lawrence AE, et al: Clinical evaluation of two methods of subdural pressure monitoring. *J Neurosurg* 63:578–582, 1985.
21. Vries JK, Becker DP, Young HF: A subarachnoid screw for monitoring intracranial pressure. *J Neurosurg* 39:416–419, 1973.
22. North B, Reilly P: Comparison among three methods of intracranial pressure recording. *Neurosurgery* 18:730–732, 1986.
23. Schettini A, Walsh EK: Pressure relaxation of the intracranial system in vivo. *Am J Physiol* 225:513–517, 1973.
24. Barlow P, Mendelow AD, Rowan JO, et al: Clinical evaluation of the Gaeltec ICT/b Pressure transducer placed subdurally, in Miller JD, Teasdale GM, Rowan JO, et al (eds): *Intracranial Pressure.* Berlin: Springer-Verlag, 1986:181–183.
25. Hermann HD, Spiegelberg A: Brain pressure monitor. *Neurosurgery* 33:1111–1112, 1993.
26. Reulen HJ, Graham R, Klatzo I: Development of pressure gradients within brain tissue during the formation of vasogenic brain edem, in Lundberg N, Ponten U, Brock M (eds): *Intracranial Pressure II.* Berlin: Springer-Verlag, 1975:233–238.
27. Sundberg G, Nordstrom CH, Messeter K, Soderstrom S: A comparison of intraparenchymatous and intraventricular pressure recording in clinical practice. *J Neurosurg* 67:841–845, 1987.
28. Crutchfield JS, Narayan RK, Robertson CS, Michael LH: Evaluation of a fiberoptic intracranial pressure monitor. *J Neurosurg* 72:482–487, 1990.

28a. Statham PFX, Midgley S, Dearden NN, et al. A clinical evaluation of an intraparenchymal intracranial pressure transducer, in Avezaat CJJ, van Eijndhoven JHM, (eds): *AIR Maas and JTJ Taus.* Berlin: Springer-Verlag, 1993: 7–10.

29. Miller JD, Becker DP, Ward JD, et al: Significance of intracranial hypertension in severe head injury. *J Neurosurg* 47:503–516, 1977.
30. Miller JD, Butterworth JF, Gudeman SK, et al: Further experience in the management of severe head injury. *J Neurosurg* 54:289–299, 1981.
31. Teasdale E, Cardoso E, Galbraith S, Teasdale G: CT scan in severe diffuse head injury: Physiological and clinical correlations. *J Neurol Neurosurg Psychiatry* 47:600–603, 1984.
32. Miller JD: ICP monitoring—current status and future directions. *Acta Neurochir (Wien)* 85:80–86, 1987.
33. Narayan RK, Kishore PRS, Becker DP, et al: Intracranial pressure: To monitor or not to monitor: A review of our experience with severe head injury. *J Neurosurg* 56:650–659, 1982.
34. Marmarou A, Anderson RL, Ward JD, et al: NINDS Traumatic Coma Data Bank: Intracranial pressure monitoring methodology. *J Neurosurg* 75:S21–27, 1991.
35. Jones PA, Andrews PJD, Midgley S, et al: Measuring the burden of secondary insults in head injured patients during intensive care. *J Neurosurg Anesth* 6:4–14, 1994.
36. O'Sullivan MG, Statham PF, Jones PA, et al: Role of intracranial pressure monitoring in severely head injured patients without signs of intracranial hypertension on initial computerized tomography. *J Neurosurg* 80:46–50, 1994.
37. Mayhall CG, Archer NH, Lamb VA, et al: Ventriculostomy related infections. *N Engl J Med* 310:553–559, 1984.

38. Sundbärg G, Kjällquist A, Lundgerg N, Ponten U: Complications due to prolonged ventricular fluid pressure recording in clinical practice, in Brock M, Dietz H (eds): *Intracranial Pressure.* Berlin: Springer-Verlag, 1972:348–352.
39. Leggate JRS, Baxter P, Minns RA, et al: The role of a separate subcutaneous cerebrospinal fluid reservoir in the management of hydrocephalus. *Br J Neurosurg* 2:327–337, 1988.
40. Welch K: The intracranial pressure in infants. *J Neurosurg* 52:693–699, 1980.
41. Miller JD, Stanek AE, Langfitt TW: Concepts of cerebral perfusion pressure and vascular compression during intracranial hypertension, in Meyer JS, Schade JP (eds): *Progress in Brain Research,* vol 35: *Cerebral Blood Flow.* Amsterdam: Elsevier, 1972:411–432.
42. Johnston IH, Rowan JO: Raised intracranial pressure and cerebral blood flow: III. Venous outflow tract pressures and vascular resistances in experimental intracranial hypertension. *J Neurol Neurosurg Psychiatry* 37:392–402, 1974.
43. Chan KH, Miller JD, Dearden NM, et al: The effect of changes in cerebral perfusion pressure upon middle cerebral artery blood flow velocity and jugular venous oxygen saturation after severe brain injury. *J Neurosurg* 77:55–61, 1992.
44. Contant CF, Robertson CS, Gopinath SP, et al: Determination of clinical important thresholds in continuously monitored patients in head injury. *J Neurotrauma* 10(suppl 1):S57, 1993.
45. Marshall LF, Cotten JM, Bowers-Marshall S, Seelig JM: Pupillary abnormalities; Elevated intracranial pressure and mass location, in Miller JD, Teasdale GM, Rowan JO, et al (eds): *Intracranial Pressure VI.* Berlin: Springer-Verlag, 1986:656–660.
46. Dietrich WD, Busto R, Alonso O, et al: Intra-ischemia but not post-ischemia brain hypothermia protects chronically following global forebrain ischemia in rats. J. *CBF Metab* 13:541–549, 1993.
47. Connor RCR: Heart damage associated with intracranial lesions. *Br Med J* 3:29–31, 1968.
48. Andrews PJD, Dearden NM, Miller JD: Jugular bulb cannulation: Description of a cannulation technique and validation of a new continuous monitor. *Br J Anaesth* 67:553–558, 1991.
49. Chan KH, Dearden NM, Miller JD, et al: Multimodality monitoring as a guide to treatment of intracranial hypertension after severe head injury. *Neurosurgery* 32:547–553, 1993.
50. Gopinath SP, Robertson CS, Contant CF, et al: Jugular venous desaturation and outcome after head injury. *J Neurol Neurosurg Psychiatry* 57:717–723, 1994.
51. Chan KH, Dearden NM, Miller JD: The significance of post-traumatic increase in cerebral blood flow velocity: A transcranial doppler ultrasound study. *Neurosurgery* 30:697–700, 1992.
52. Chan KH, Miller JD, Dearden NM: Intracranial blood flow velocity after head injury: Relationship to severity of injury, time, neurological status and outcome. *J Neurol Neurosurg Psychiatry* 55:787–791, 1992.
53. Martin NA, Doberstein C, Zane C, et al: Posttraumatic cerebral arterial spasm: Transcranial Doppler ultrasound, cerebral blood flow, and angiographic findings. *J Neurosurg* 77:575–583, 1992.
54. Miller JD, Dearden NM, Piper IR, Chan KH: Control of intracranial pressure in patients with severe head injury. *J Neurotrauma* 9:(suppl 1):S317–326, 1992.
55. Miller JD, Garibi J, Pickard JD: Induced changes of cerebrospinal fluid volume: Effects during continuous monitoring of ventricular fluid pressure. *Arch Neurol* 28:265–269, 1973.
56. Shulman K, Marmarou A: Pressure-volume considerations in infantile hydrocephalus. *Dev Med Child Neurol* 13(suppl 25):90–95, 1971.
57. Maset AL, Marmarou A, Ward JD, et al: Pressure volume index in head injury. *J Neurosurg* 67:832–840, 1987.
58. Marmarou A, Shulman K, Lamorgese J: Compartmental analysis of compliance and outflow resistance of the cerebrospinal fluid outflow system. *J Neurosurg* 43:523–534, 1975.
59. Sullivan HF, Miller JD, Griffith RL, et al: Bolus vs steady state infusion for determination of CSF outflow resistance. *Ann Neurol* 5:228–238, 1979.
60. Takizawa H, Gabra-Sanders T, Miller JD: Validity of measurements of CSF outflow resistance estimated by the bolus injection method. *Neurosurgery* 17:63–66, 1995.
61. Marmarou A, Maset AL, Ward JD, et al: Contribution of CSF and vascular factors to elevation of ICP in severely head-injured patients. *J Neurosurg* 66:883–890, 1987.
62. Avezaat CJJ, Van Eijndhoven JHM, Wyper DJ: Cerebrospinal fluid pulse pressure and intracranial volume-pressure relationships. *J Neurol Neurosurg Psychiatry* 42:687–700, 1979.
63. Avezaat CJJ, Van Eijndhoven JHM: Cerebrospinal fluid pulse pressure and craniospinal dynamics: A theoretical, clinical and experimental study. Thesis: Erasmus University, Rotterdam, 1984.
64. Chopp M, Portnoy H: Systems analysis of intracranial pressure: Comparison with volume-pressure test and CSF-pulse amplitude analysis. *J Neurosurg* 53:516–527, 1980.
65. Portnoy HD, Chopp M: Cerebrospinal fluid pulse wave form analysis during hypercapnia and hypoxia. *Neurosurgery* 9:14–27, 1981.
66. Portnoy HD, Chopp M, Branch C, Shannon MB: Cerebrospinal fluid pulse waveform as an indicator of cerebral autoregulation. *J Neurosurg* 56:668–678, 1982.
67. Bray RS, Sherwood AM, Halter JA, et al: Development of a clinical monitoring system by means of ICP waveform analysis, in Miller JD, Teasdale GM, Rowan JO, et al (eds): *Intracranial Pressure VI.* Berlin: Springer-Verlag, 1986:260–264.
68. Robertson CS, Narayan RK, Contant CF, et al: Clinical experience with a continuous monitor of intracranial compliance. *J Neurosurg* 71:673–680, 1989.
69. Piper IR, Miller JD, Dearden NM, et al: Systems analysis of cerebrovascular pressure transmission: An observational study in head injured patients. *J Neurosurg* 73:871–880, 1990.

70. Piper IR, Chan KH, Whittle IR, Miller JD: An experimental study of cerebrovascular resistance, pressure transmission and craniospinal compliance. *Neurosurgery* 32:805–816, 1993.
71. Takizawa H, Gabra-Sanders T, Miller JD: Changes in the cerebrospinal fluid pulse wave spectrum associated with raised intracranial pressure. *Neurosurgery* 20:355–361, 1987.
72. Smielewski P, Czosnyka M, Maksymowicz W., et al: Identification of the cerebrospinal compensatory mechanisms via computer controlled drawings of cerebrospinal fluid, in Avezaat CJJ, van Eijndhoven JHM, (eds): *AIR Maas and JTJ Tans.* Berlin: Springer-Verlag, 1993:766–770.
73. Piper IR, Miller JD, Whittle IR, Lawson A: Automated time-averaged analysis of craniospinal compliance. *Acta Neurochir* [*Suppl*] (*Wien*) 51:387–390, 1990.

CHAPTER 32

TREATING RAISED INTRACRANIAL PRESSURE IN HEAD INJURY

Randall M. Chesnut

SYNOPSIS

Monitoring intracranial pressure (ICP) and controlling intracranial hypertension are fundamental in preventing herniation and avoiding ischemic secondary brain insults in severely head injured patients. Particular attention should be paid to maintaining adequate cerebral perfusion pressure (CPP). As a first approximation, ICP generally should be maintained below 20 to 25 mmHg and CPP above 70 mmHg, although these values appear to vary between patients and over time. A significant goal of neurotrauma critical care is to develop methods to identify and quantify the various underlying pathological conditions and the appropriate treatment approaches for individual patients (targeted therapy). A fairly effective approach to controlling ICP has evolved over the past two decades. Most of these techniques, however, have potentially detrimental side effects, and balancing the risk-benefit ratio of such therapeutic maneuvers is critical to optimizing outcome beyond simply lowering ICP. The physiological ramifications of the various "traditional" techniques and several newer approaches are discussed to guide the clinician in developing and tailoring ICP/CPP management strategies.

INTRODUCTION

The measurement of intracranial pressure (ICP) and the treatment of intracranial hypertension are fundamental in the modern management of severe head injury. Few physicians would deny that profound or refractory intracranial hypertension is commonly associated with serious brain injury and is a strong predictor of a poor outcome.[1–5] However, some argue that the absence of a prospective double-blind study demonstrating that the treatment of intracranial hypertension improves outcome after traumatic coma indicates that monitoring ICP is not necessary. Nevertheless, a large body of clinical experience indirectly supports the correlation between ICP control and improvement in outcome. From a pragmatic standpoint, therefore, the argument against ICP monitoring in severely head injured patients appears to be founded more on nihilism than on parsimony. Indeed, the majority of neurotraumatologists feel so strongly about the necessity of treating ICP in severe head injury patients that ethical considerations make it difficult if not impossible to perform a randomized clinical trial of ICP monitoring.

There is significant indirect evidence supporting the treatment of intracranial hypertension in severely head injured patients. Narayan et al. suggested that the treatment of small rises in ICP can allay the subsequent development of profound intracranial hypertension.[3] In a communitywide study addressing various methods of managing head injury in a noncontrolled fashion, Marshall et al. reported a significant improvement in outcome in patients whose ICP was maintained below 15 mmHg compared with those whose ICP exceeded 40 mmHg for 15 min or more.[6,7] Saul and Ducker, in a sequential study of ICP control at two different levels, strongly suggested an improvement in outcome for patients who were treated at an ICP of 15 mmHg compared with 25 mmHg.[8] Marmarou's analysis of data from the Traumatic Coma Data Bank (TCDB)* showed that the proportion of ICP measurements greater than 20 mmHg was the fourth most powerful predictor of outcome, after age, admission Glagow Coma Scale motor score, and admission pupillary examination.[2] Furthermore, when he analyzed which ICP value was most strongly related to outcome based on the Glasgow Outcome Score, 20 mmHg showed the strongest association. Since all centers in the TCDB aggressively treated intracranial hypertension, this at least indirectly suggests that patients whose ICP remained within control values had improved outcomes. This is supported by a recent report by Contant et al., who found an ICP threshold for outcome prediction at 25 mmHg.[9]

Data recently collected in neurotrauma patients over a 2-year period at Cornell by Ghajar et al., while measurement of ICP and treatment of intracranial hypertension in neurotrauma patients over a 2-year period was or was not performed depending on the admitting physician, found a significant improvement in outcome in patients who were monitored and treated for intracranial hypertension and whose other modalities of treatment were fairly comparable between groups (J. Ghajar, unpublished observations, 1993).

Reports such as this strongly, although indirectly, support monitoring of ICP and treatment of intracranial hypertension in head injury patient's and are the raison d'être of this chapter. The approach to the measurement of intracranial hypertension is based on protocols practiced at the UCSD Medical Center in San Diego, California. Although such protocols remain in a constant state of evolution and are not suggested as the only or even the optimal approaches in all situations, a body of evidence arising from the TCDB indicates that these paradigms are effective.[10] This approach is presented as an operational framework in an attempt to outline the clinical treatment of intracranial hypertension in light of its scientific and pragmatic underpinnings in order to facilitate the adaptation of the individual procedural steps in this chapter.

* Throughout this chapter references are made to the TCDB. The TCDB is an NINDS collaborative project involving four clinical centers—the Medical College of Virginia at Richmond, the University of California at San Diego, the University of Virginia at Charlottesville, and the University of Texas Medical Branch at Galveston—with a coordinating center within the Biometry and Field Studies Branch, NINDS. These centers prospectively studied all severely head injured patients admitted between April 1983 and April 1988. The operational definition of severe head injury was a Glasgow Coma Scale (GCS) score of 8 or less occurring on admission (postresuscitation) or during the ensuing 48 h. In addition to data for the acute care course, prehospital information and rehabilitation follow-up results were collected. Outcome was rated using the GCS. One thousand thirty patients were admitted to the TCDB. Of these, 284 were brain-dead on admission, did not survive resuscitation, or suffered a gunshot wound to the brain, leaving 746 patients in the overall cohort. Data collection ended in 1988, and the data became available to the principal investigator for analysis shortly thereafter. A number of monographs that have been appearing arise from this large database and address a number of important statistical questions involving the head-injured population.

INTRACRANIAL HYPERTENSION IN SEVERE HEAD INJURY

Intracranial hypertension can have two effects on an injured brain. Elevation of ICP, if untreated, often results in herniation of brain tissue through the incisura, the foramen magnum, or subfalcine, resulting in distortion of brain material and injury to vital brain structures. Thus, treatment of intracranial hypertension represents an attempt to establish an early warning system for herniation syndromes.

In contrast to herniation, which may be viewed as essentially an end result, the production of secondary insults lies on a continuum of intracranial hypertension. As ischemia becomes increasingly recognized as a major factor in producing the pathological conditions associated with severe head injury, a number of mechanisms are being recognized. Systemic insults such as hypoxia and hypotension are surprisingly common and are seriously detrimental to outcome.[11,12] In addition, derangements of internal blood flow during the early postinjury phases appear to be intrinsic consequences of trauma, the exact mechanisms of which are poorly understood.[13,14] As a compounding factor, intracranial hypertension is an antagonist of intracranial perfusion and can produce secondary ischemia, both global and focal.

Although we are limited in our understanding of the mechanisms controlling cerebral blood flow and cannot easily obtain real-time data on regional perfusion, the fundamental goal of ICP treatment is to minimize or eliminate the secondary insults resulting from ischemia. Hence, the focus has shifted somewhat from ICP per se to cerebral perfusion pressure (CPP). As this concept becomes recognized, unfortunately, many of the treatment modalities that have classically been employed and are known to be effective in lowering ICP appear to have the potential of potentiating or exacerbating cerebral ischemia. As a result, although we have become increasingly effective in controlling intracranial hypertension, our understanding of the proper methods for doing so in an individual patient lags behind.

In this light, the focus of this chapter will be twofold. The first goal is to outline a safe and effective method for dealing with intracranial hypertension that is applicable to the majority of patients in a reasonably straightforward fashion. The second is to outline the physiological mechanisms supporting these methods in order to foster an understanding of the doubled-edged nature of many of these therapies.

SELECTION OF PATIENTS FOR INTRACRANIAL PRESSURE MONITORING

In general, any patient with a severe head injury, defined as a GCS score of 8 or less, should be considered for monitoring of ICP.[3] Patients presenting with this degree of posttraumatic neurological impairment who are younger than 40 years, have no evidence of abnormal motor activity, have normal pupillary examinations, have no significant history of secondary hypoxic/ischemic brain insults, and receive a head computed tomography (CT) scan that demonstrates no pathology and open basilar cisterns, however, represent a select group of patients who may be managed without ICP monitoring if their neurological examinations can be continuously monitored in an intensive care unit (ICU).[3,15,16]

In addition, a subset of patients with moderate head injuries (GCS scores 9 to 12) should also have ICP monitoring. Patients with absent or compressed basilar cisterns or 5 mm or more of midline shift are at significant risk of intracranial hypertension and should be monitored.[17] Patients with nonsurgical mass lesions (e.g., intracerebral contusions/hematomas of less than 25 ml with minimal mass effect) in the deep frontal or temporal regions should also be monitored because of the propensity of such lesions to compress brainstem structures early in their evolution and at lower ICP values (see below).[18] Finally, any patient with a moderate head injury and an abnormal CT scan who cannot be clinically monitored for a significant period as a result of emergency diagnostic or therapeutic procedures that require paralysis and/or anesthesia should also be considered for ICP monitoring.

The decision to monitor ICP in patients who have only a moderate risk of developing intracranial hypertension obviously involves a trade-off between risk and benefit, and therefore it is desirable to minimize the complications associated with the monitoring system. In such cases, the Camino intraparenchymal pressure monitor and other accurate, minimally invasive ICP measuring devices have considerable advantages over ventriculostomy, with its attendant risks of parenchymal hemorrhage and infection, in situations where the indications for ICP monitoring are less than absolute.

DEFINITION OF INTRACRANIAL HYPERTENSION

The definition of intracranial hypertension has never been conclusively established, and the critical threshold in a given patient most likely is patient-specific and will vary over the patient's course. As was noted previously, values from 15 to 25 mmHg are the most widely reported.[2,3,8–10,18] Generally, 20 mmHg is felt to be the threshold of intracranial hypertension and was the value most highly correlated with GCS scores in the TCDB.[2] The authors characteristically initiate treatment at this value, with the exception of situations involving contusions or hematomas in the deep frontal or temporal regions. Because of the propensity of such lesions to cause brainstem compression at lower ICP levels,[18] the authors set our threshold at 15 mmHg in such situations, moving to surgical evacuation of the lesion if the pressure cannot be controlled at this value.

"EXPECTANT" MANAGEMENT OF SUSPECTED INTRACRANIAL HYPERTENSION

The management of ICP in a patient at risk of intracranial hypertension (ICH) should not be delayed until ICP can be proved. This is particularly true during initial contact, triage, and the early stages of resuscitation. It is in this light that many of the modalities that are applicable to established ICH in a targeted fashion may be applied prophylactically during these early times when the patient is at risk (Fig. 32-1*A*). Although not risk-free, moderate early hyperventilation and the administration of mannitol, as well as sedation with or without pharmacological paralysis, are useful measures to buy time in patients with a reasonable probability of developing ICH. Although obviously indicated in patients with evidence of herniation, such modalities should be applied to any patient who meets the previously discussed indications for ICP monitoring as a means of temporizing until the risk of ICH can be established definitively.

Particular care should be taken during the intubation of head-injured patients. The insertion of an endotracheal tube is an extremely noxious stimulus and can precipitate marked ICH and transtentorial herniation in patients with diminished intracranial compliance. It is easy to be misled into thinking that a patient who

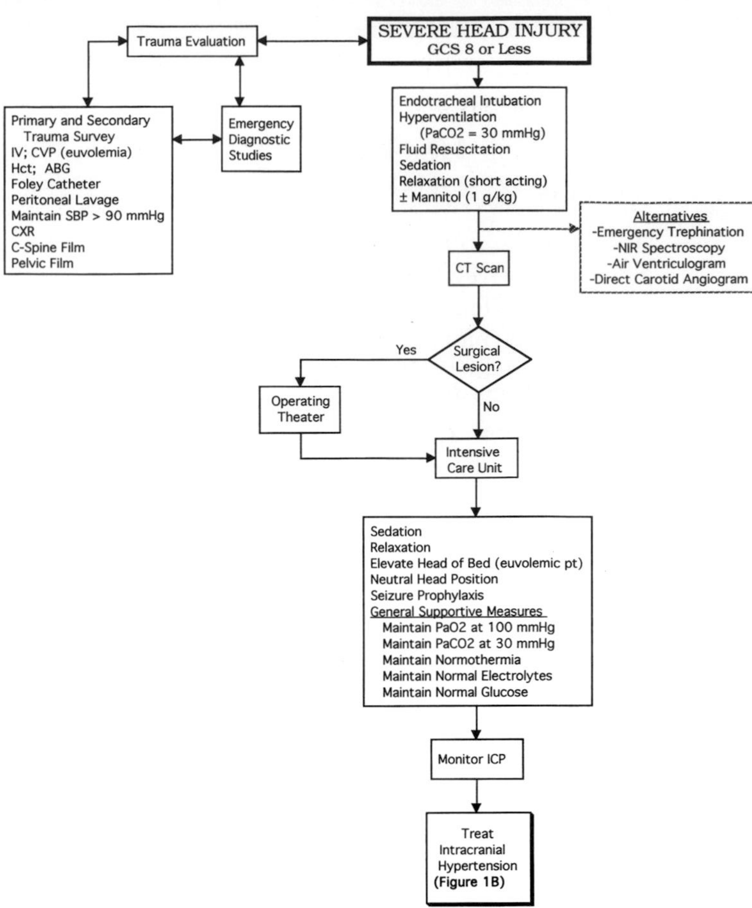

A

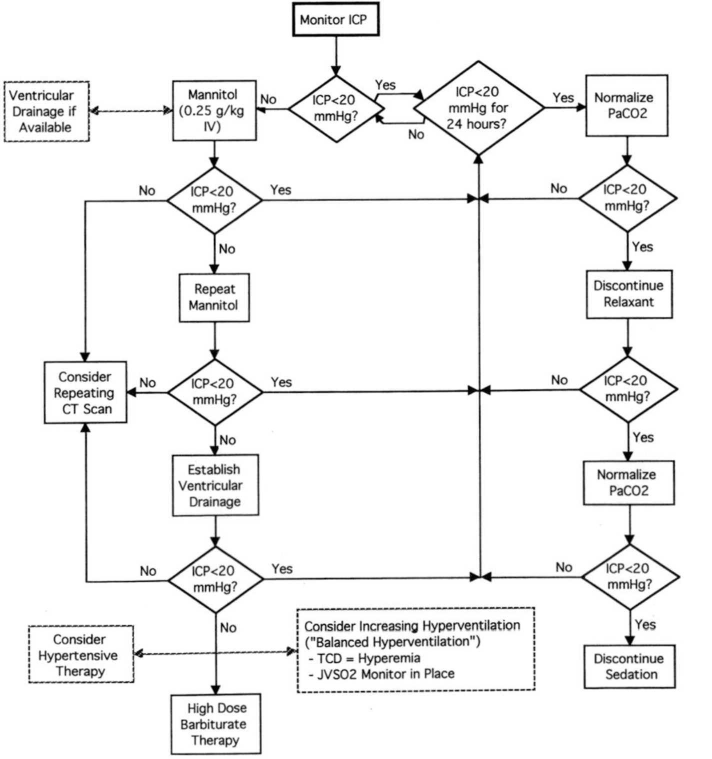

B

Figure 32-1. An algorithm for the evaluation and treatment of a patient with a severe head injury. *A* encompasses the period from admission and resuscitation through the establishment of ICP monitoring. *B* covers the treatment of ICH. The rationales behind individual steps and their sequencing are discussed in the text. (Adapted from Chesnut RM et al., in Eisenberg HM, Aldrich F (eds): *Head Injury, Neurosurg Clin North Am,* Saunders, 2:267–284, 1991, with permission.)

does not respond externally to intubation is not affected by it. Therefore, whenever possible, intubation should be performed with sedation and depression of airway reflexes in a rapid sequence fashion, and the patient should be closely observed for signs of neurological compromise.

TARGETED THERAPY

As will be discussed below, the "classic" approach to the treatment of elevated ICP has been the sequential application of various modalities as ICP control becomes increasingly difficult (Fig. 32-1*A* and *B*). After such a serial approach, a patient might be initially treated with sedation and mild hyperventilation. If ICP control is not satisfactory, CSF drainage might be initiated and, subsequently, further hyperventilation, mannitol, and the like, could be added.

Fundamental to such a treatment scheme is the assumption that all brain injuries are essentially similar. However, it has become evident that this is not true, and this has given rise to the concept of targeted therapy. Targeted therapy accepts the fact that several subcategories of head injury differ significantly in their underlying pathophysiologies and are optimally treated using different treatment schemes (Fig. 32-2). Targeted therapy allows a parallel approach to the pathological processes thought to be responsible for an individual case of ICH. In particular, patients with head injuries best treated with modalities that are traditionally used at the end of a sequential treatment pattern are subjected to a considerable period in which secondary insults occur or continue as their ICH proves refractory to the earlier, less applicable treatments.

The existence of subclasses of head injury patients is strongly supported by the recent report of Marshall et al. demonstrating a correlation between intracranial diagnosis by CT imaging and remarkably different constellations of predictors of outcome.[17] These CT diagnostic categories are outlined in Table 32-1 and Fig. 32-3. While age and admission GCS motor score were the most powerful predictors of outcome for TCDB patients admitted with a surgical mass lesion, patients whose primary intracranial pathological condition con-

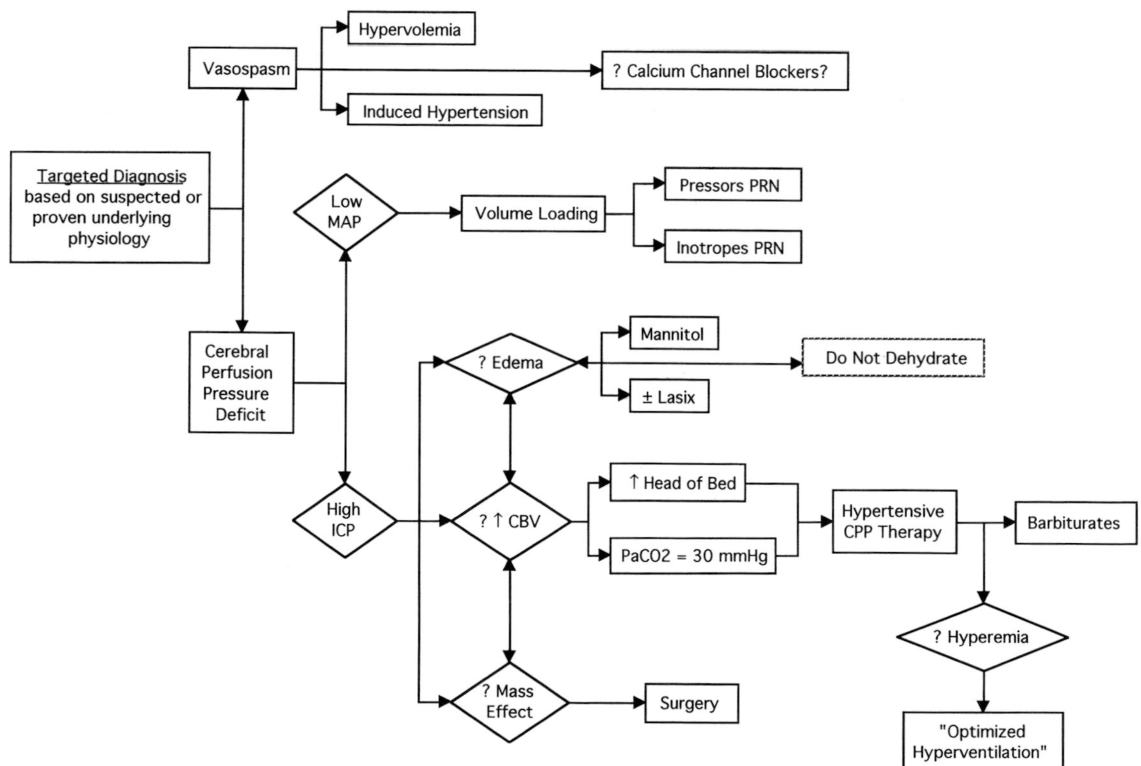

Figure 32-2. An algorithm demonstrating targeted ICP therapy. The parallel nature of this approach should be compared with the serial nature of the algorithm in Fig. 32-1*A* and 1*B*. Targeted therapy attempts to apply treatments specific to pathological processes thought to be responsible for ICH with the caveat that these processes are poorly understood and difficult to differentiate (see text for details).

TABLE 32-1 Head Injury Diagnostic Categories Based on Abnormalities Visualized on CT

Diffuse Injury I	No visible pathology seen on CT
Diffuse Injury II	Cisterns are present with shift 0–5 mm; no high- or mixed-density lesion >25 ml; may include bone fragments and foreign bodies
Diffuse Injury III (swelling)	Cisterns compressed or absent; shift 0–5 mm; no high- or mixed-density lesion > 25 ml
Diffuse Injury IV (shift)	Shift >5 mm; no high- or mixed-density lesion >25 ml
Evacuated mass lesion	Any lesion surgically evacuated
Nonevacuated mass lesion	High- or mixed-density lesion >25 ml not surgically evacuated
Brain-dead	No brainstem reflexes; flaccid; fixed, nonreactive pupils: no spontaneous respirations with normal Pa_{CO_2}; spinal reflexes permitted

SOURCE: Adapted from Marshall LF, et al: *J Neurosurg,* 75:S14–S20, 1992, with permission.

sists of compression of the basilar cisterns with or without midline shift have their prognosis most strongly determined by the degree of ICH.[10,17] Feeling that such patients are better treated with a combination of hyperventilation and hypnotics than with osmotic diuretics, the authors have managed a number of young patients presenting with severe ICH and absent or compressed cisterns by means of the early initiation of barbiturate coma and have found this to be effective in selected instances.[19] Along a very similar path of reasoning, Miller's group in Edinburgh has suggested that young patients with an active EEG, a diffuse injury pattern on CT, jugular venous saturation > 75%, and ICH should be considered for early hyperventilation/hypnotic therapy, whereas patients not meeting these criteria should be treated differently.[20,21]

There are, of course, a number of pathophysiological assumptions underlying such decisions. Modalities such

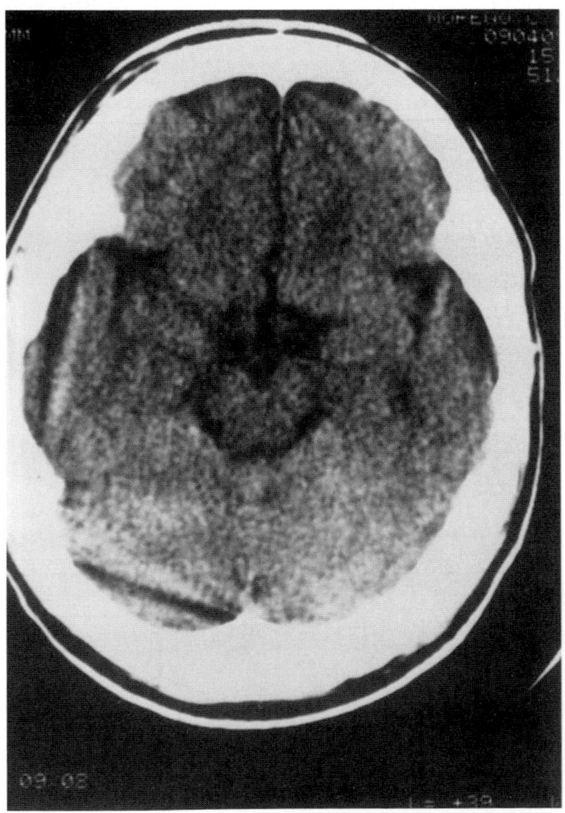

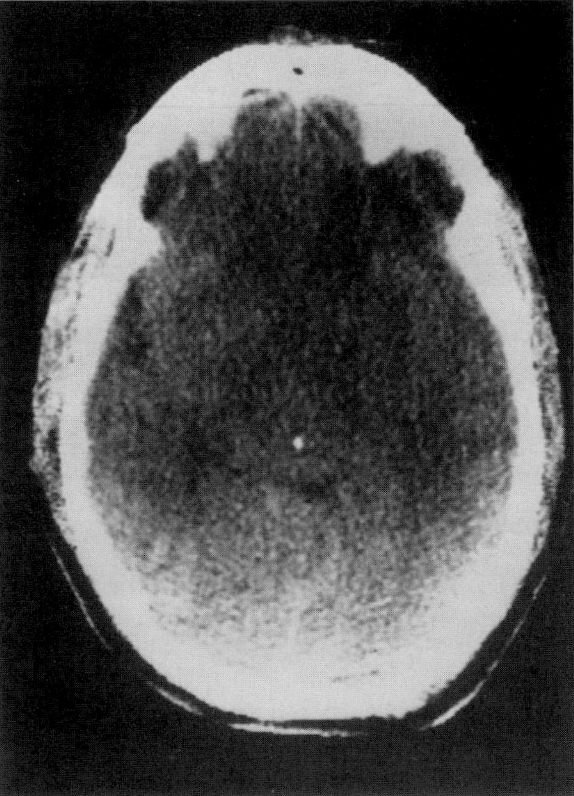

Figure 32-3. CT images contrasting basal cisterns of normal shape and symmetry (*left*) and cisterns compressed to the extent that they are not visualized (*right*). According to the classification scheme in Table 32-1, the left scan would be either a Diffuse Injury I or II and the right scan would be a Diffuse Injury III or IV, depending on the findings in other images in each sequence.

as hyperventilation and hypnotics, which work primarily by modifying cerebral blood flow and cerebral blood volume, and flow-metabolism coupling would be the treatment of choice in patients whose underlying pathophysiology centers on loss of autoregulation with resultant increased cerebral blood volume. Alternatively, patients whose ICH results from alterations of tissue compliance, such as cerebral edema, would be better treated with agents such as mannitol.

Unfortunately, we remain significantly hampered by our rudimentary understanding of the pathology of human head injury. It is naive to assume that there are only two types of head-injured patients. Not only will the majority of patients manifest more than one pathophysiological mechanism, the relative importance of these mechanisms undoubtedly changes over time and as a result of treatment. Certainly, patients best treated with hyperventilation and hypnotics may subsequently become "mannitol patients" at a later stage. An additional impediment to targeted therapy is the rudimentary status of our ability to identify underlying pathophysiological mechanisms in a clinically useful fashion. Nevertheless, although the sequential method of managing ICH as presented in this chapter and commonly applied today remains an effective and proven approach for head injury patients in toto, it is anticipated that we will move toward more targeted therapy as our understanding of head injury improves and as better agents become available for treating each pathophysiological abnormality.

ICP AND CPP

Cerebral perfusion pressure (CPP) represents the perfusion pressure gradient across the intracranial compartment and is defined as mean arterial pressure (MAP) minus ICP (MAP − ICP = CPP). Although it ignores a number of intracranial mechanisms and inhomogeneities, it is a very useful concept for following and managing cerebral perfusion. It is becoming increasingly well recognized that the determination of CPP is the major use for ICP. Although transtentorial herniation is a direct result of abnormal ICP, not CPP, the exquisite sensitivity of the injured nervous system to ischemic insults makes maintenance of CPP critical.[11,12,22,23] Therefore, the use of treatment modalities that lower ICP at the expense of blood pressure (and thus CPP) will probably not result in an optimal outcome despite preventing acute herniation.

Since support of CPP often depends on maintenance of an optimal MAP, this topic will be discussed briefly here. It appears that since even episodes that are notably brief and seemingly mild can be associated with a significantly poorer outcome,[11,12] every attempt must be made to avoid any fluctuations in CPP and immediate attention must be paid to rapidly correcting abnormally low values. A level of vigilance and a rapidity of response that are acceptable for patients without a head injury appear to be inadequate in the neurotrauma setting.

The primary mechanism for maintenance of adequate CPP is strict avoidance of hypovolemia. The poorly founded but widely held notion that head-injured patients should be mildly to moderately dehydrated should be discarded. Indeed, it is generally desirable to maintain such patients in a mild state of isotonic hypervolemia. Adequate volumes of crystalloid, colloid, or blood products (if appropriate) should be administered to maintain adequate cardiac preload. To this end, head-injured patients with ICH should have central venous pressure monitoring supplemented with pulmonary artery pressures, systemic vascular resistance, and cardiac output monitoring with a Swan-Ganz catheter if there is any question that central venous pressure monitoring may not adequately reflect the cardiovascular or central volume status. In general, central venous pressures should be kept at 8 or above and pulmonary capillary wedge pressures (PCWP) should be kept at 12 or more. For many patients, this will be all the treatment necessary to maintain a satisfactory CPP.

In some instances, however, further treatment modalities may be required to optimize CPP. In instances where euvolemia or mild hypervolemia is not sufficient to maintain an adequate MAP, it is advisable to monitor cardiac output and systemic vascular resistance. In patients with decreased systemic vascular resistance, very commonly patients with spinal cord injury or sepsis, pressors such as dopamine or phenylephrine may be required. Dopamine is a useful first-line agent, as it preserves splanchnic blood flow but becomes increasingly contaminated with varying degrees of alpha and beta effects as the dose is increased (Table 32-2). If levels over 10 to 15 μg/kg/min are required to maintain MAP, the dopamine may be reduced to 4 μg/kg/min or less and a second agent can be added.

The most commonly employed second agent is phenylephrine. Unfortunately, various degrees of resistance to this drug exist, and tachyphylaxis tends to develop over time. If necessary, norepinephrine (levarterenol) can be substituted for phenylephrine. Norepinephrine is a very effective agent but has a significant risk of producing end-organ ischemia (e.g., splanchnic or renal), particularly if intravascular volume is not maintained. Although it is generally well tolerated in younger

TABLE 32-2 Pharmacological Mechanisms and Physiological Actions of Pressors and Inotropes Used in Cerebral Perfusion Pressure Management

			Physiological Actions†									
			Cardiac		*Vascular*		*Effect on Clinical Parameters†*					
Agent	**Dose**	**Receptors***	**Int**	**Cht**	**Vcon**	**Vdil**	**HR**	**MAP**	**CO**	**SVR**	**UO**	**RBF**
Dobutamine	2–10 μg/kg/min	1α; 3β_1; 2β_2	3+	1+	1+	2+	↑	↑	↑	↔↓	↑	↑
Dopamine	1–4 μg/kg/min	3D; 1β_1	2+	1+	0	1+	↔	↔	↔	↔	↑↑	↑↑
	5–20 μg/kg/min	3D; 3β_1; 2β_2	4+	2+	0	1+	↑	↑	↑	↔	↑↑	↑↑
	>10–20 μg/kg/min	3$\alpha_{1,2}$; 3β_1; 1β_2	3+	3+	3+	0	↑	↑	↑	↑	↑↓	↑↓
Norepinephrine	2–20 μg/min	4α; 2β_1	1+	2+	4+	0	↔↑↓	↑↑↑	↔↑↓	↑↑↑	↓	↓
Phenylephrine (Neo-Synephrine)	20–200 μg/min	4α	0	0	4+	0	↓	↑↑	↔↑↓	↑↑	↓	↓

* Action on α, β, or D (dopaminergic) receptors. Strength of action is rated from 1 (weak) to 4 (very strong).

† Cardiac = inotropic (Int) and chronotropic (Cht); vascular = vasoconstriction (Vcon) or vasodilation (Vdil). Strength of action is rated from 1 (weak) to 4 (very strong).

‡ Heart rate (HR), mean arterial pressure (MAP), cardiac output (CO), systemic vascular resistance (SVR), urinary output (UO), and renal blood flow (RBF). Actions include no change (↔), increase (↑), or decrease (↓). Strength of action is rated as weak (↑ or ↓), moderate (↑↑ or ↓↓), or strong (↑↑↑ or ↓↓↓).

patients, it should be used sparingly and with caution in elderly patients and patients with compromised circulation.

In instances of deficient cardiac output due to antecedent disease, cardiac trauma, and the like, dobutamine can be used to increase cardiac output. Agents directed primarily at afterload reduction should be avoided because of the potential for hypotension.

Although the importance of CPP is becoming increasingly well recognized, the optimal CPP in head injury remains unclear. In normal, nonneurotrauma patients, a minimum pressure of 50 mmHg appears to be the lower limit of normal.[24,25] Based largely on anecdotal evidence from a number of centers, including ours, however, it is generally accepted that 50 mmHg is too low in neurotrauma, and levels of 70 mmHg or more are generally postulated. Such suggestions are based largely on noncontrolled studies of the effect of elevating CPP above 50 mmHg on ICP, jugular venous saturation, and intracranial compliance. Recently, however, Chan et al. have demonstrated systematically collected transcranial Doppler and jugular venous saturation evidence suggesting that a reasonably consistent breakpoint exists in head trauma patients that has a mean value of approximately 70 mmHg.[26] It is notable, however, that significant inter- and intrapatient variability exists, and values as high as 90 mmHg may be encountered (K. H. Chan and M. Dearden, personal communication, 1992). These data suggest that there is a point at which autoregulation appears to be maintained in a significant percentage of neurotrauma patients and that this point seems to be significantly higher than the lower breakpoint in normals. These authors did not determine the particular utility of this lower breakpoint in the treatment of head injury, although their research suggests that such a value would be useful as a minimum CPP. Unfortunately, there is no highly practical method for easily determining such a breakpoint for individual patients in a general clinical setting, although when it occurs, desaturation of jugular venous blood suggests that such a threshold has been passed.

Since the alteration of MAP in an attempt to optimize CPP involves the use of agents that have inherent risks and complications, it is important to maintain a pragmatic viewpoint. Although it appears to be critical to maintain a minimum CPP of at least 50 mmHg and optimally 70 mmHg, the attendant risks of using pressors and inotropes to elevate CPP beyond these values must be balanced against the unproven benefits of maintaining an above-normal CPP.

TREATMENT OF ELEVATED ICP

GENERAL MEASURES

An algorithm presenting a simple and effective approach to treating severely head-injured patients is presented in Fig. 32-1*A* and *B*. This algorithm is applicable to the majority of severely head injured patients, but the order in which the parts are used may differ in individual patients.

Patients undergo early intubation with mild hyperventilation, sedation, and often pharmacological paralysis either at the accident scene or on arrival in the emergency room. In patients whose CT scan does not reveal surgical intracranial pathology but who are felt to be at risk of ICH, an ICP monitor is inserted. If a monitor is not felt to be indicated or if the patient has a normal ICP after being stabilized in the ICU, pharmacological paralysis is discontinued and the patient is observed under sedation during the return of motor function. If the exam and ICP remain acceptable, particularly if the patient is localizing or following commands, the remainder of the ICP control protocol (see below) is aborted and the patient is allowed to emerge from sedation under continuous observation.

As early as possible during the course of treatment of a head-injured patient, physiological parameters consistent with normal homeostasis should be attained and maintained. Euvolemia should be established, and attention should be applied to avoiding secondary ischemic or hypoxic insults. Continuous peripheral oxygen saturation should be monitored. End-tidal CO_2 monitoring is also useful, but its accuracy must be regularly confirmed with arterial blood gas values. The development of continuous Pa_{O_2} and Pa_{CO_2} monitoring via indwelling arterial systems is proving useful in such patients, particularly hyperventilated patients with unstable pulmonary pictures.

Elevations of body temperature should be corrected, and euthermia should be maintained. The ICP will increase by several mmHg for every 1°C of fever. Additionally, it has been suggested that hyperthermia per se is detrimental to neurological recovery independent of the underlying etiology (C. F. Contant, personal communication, 1993).

The etiology of the hyperdynamic state in patients presenting with hypertension and/or tachycardia must be ascertained before treatment. Young patients in particular may present with profoundly hyperdynamic indexes in compensation for hypovolemia, and their cardiovascular picture will normalize on adequate volume resuscitation. In other instances, pain or anxiety may be contributory and may respond to analgesics or mild sedation. The authors generally do not correct hypertension unless it is exceptionally severe. If the patient was hypertensive as a preexisting state, restoration of "normal" blood pressures may result in ischemia. In addition, some patients appear to exhibit hypertension as a reflex attempt to "perfuse their brains" in the face of ICH. In such cases, the hypertension will resolve with successful ICP treatment. In all instances, treatment of systemic hypertension must be performed very cautiously to avoid hypotension.

In cases of hypertension without an obvious explanation, the hyperdynamic state may reflect the elevated levels of circulating catecholamines that often result from head trauma.[27–31] The idea that the cardiac consequences of this adrenergic storm can be detrimental is suggested by the finding of elevated myocardial enzymes, ECG changes, and histological evidence of myocardial cellular damage in head injury patients without direct cardiac trauma.[29,32,33] In light of such evidence, severely hyperdynamic patients without evidence of any of the underlying etiologies mentioned above may be cautiously treated with selective short-acting beta blockers such as labetalol, which may be administered in 10-mg doses. Hypotension must be avoided during such treatment.

Seizure Prophylaxis

Although they are commonly administered, the efficacy of prophylactic anticonvulsants in reducing the incidence of delayed development of posttraumatic epilepsy is unproven.[34–36] During the early postinjury period, however, particularly in the face of ICH, the occurrence of epileptiform activity and the associated profound intracerebral hyperemic response can compromise ICP control significantly. Transtentorial herniation can also be precipitated. If the patient is under pharmacological paralysis, the occurrence of epileptiform activity is manifested only by tachycardia, transient hypertension, and fluctuations in ICP and may easily be missed. Therefore, one should consider treating all acute head injury patients with anticonvulsants during the course of ICP control. In patients who are pharmacologically paralyzed, monitoring EEG or compressed spectral array data can be useful when occult seizure behavior is suspected. The issue of anticonvulsant therapy in head injury is discussed in greater detail in Chap. 42.

Head Position

Elevation of the head of the bed to between 15 and 30 degrees from horizontal is an effective means of lowering ICP.[37–41] Euvolemia must be established before elevating the head of the bed, however, as the beneficial effects of decreasing the cerebral venous outflow resistance can be negated if the MAP and CPP drop when the head of the bed is elevated in a hypovolemic patient.[42]

The neck must be maintained in a neutral position, and compression of the jugular venous system, such as by an overly tight cervical orthosis or tracheostomy tape, must be avoided.[39,41] In patients with possible thoracic or lumbar spine fractures, the head of the bed may be raised, using a reverse Trendelenburg's position.

Sedation and Pharmacological Paralysis

Sedation and pharmacological paralysis are very useful tools in treating a severely head-injured patient. Since they alter or eliminate the neurological examination, however, they must be used with discretion. Agitation or uncontrolled movement can result from the brain injury, intoxication, or pain and not only interferes with ICP control but can hamper or prevent diagnostic or therapeutic maneuvers and may put the patient at risk. Morphine is an excellent analgesic and a strong depressant of airway reflexes when endotracheal intubation and nasotracheal suction are needed. However, it is only a fair sedative. A steady-state level of sedation is best achieved by means of constant intravenous infusion, which should be initiated at 4 mg/min and may be increased as needed. Unfortunately, tachyphylaxis per se requires dose escalation, and the development of tolerance necessitates slow withdrawal of the drug when it is no longer needed.

Physiological dependence develops rapidly and so withdrawal must be performed slowly when a patient has been under morphine for several days. The dose should be decreased by no more than 20 percent per day. Signs of overly rapid withdrawal of narcotics include tachycardia, agitation, hypertension, tremulousness, and diarrhea.

When sedation is the primary requirement, a continuous intravenous infusion of midazolam can be used, either alone or in addition to a morphine infusion. An intravenous test dose of 2 mg is useful to determine the efficacy and the systemic response, with the goal of initiating a continuous intravenous infusion at between 2 and 4 mg/h. Care must be taken to avoid hypotension when one is adding midazolam, particularly in combination with morphine. Midazolam can be reversed with flumazenil if necessary, although this must be done very cautiously, as uncontrolled ICH could result from an overly rapid reversal.

Pharmacological paralysis is a useful addition to sedation in patients with refractory ICH. It is also valuable in situations where complete absence of motor activity is required (such as diagnostic imaging) and in patients who are "bucking" the ventilator. The downside of pharmacological paralysis is the complete elimination of the neurological examination, a tendency to prolong the ICU stay, and an elevated incidence of ICU-associated complications such as pneumonia and sepsis.[43]

Many patients arrive at the hospital or ICU having already been treated with sedation and pharmacological paralysis in a "prophylactic" fashion. In such patients, the necessity of continuing paralysis should be assessed. Patients who are not felt to be at risk of ICH or whose monitor demonstrates normal ICP should have their pharmacological paralysis reversed under observation, as was noted previously. Continuation of pharmacological paralysis in such patients is unnecessary and potentially hazardous.

In patients who have ICH or do not tolerate weaning from pharmacological paralysis, paralysis should be maintained by using a constant infusion of neuromuscular blocking agents. If discontinuation of paralysis in the near future is anticipated, the use of a short-acting agent such as vecuronium bromide or atracurium besylate is useful. Pancuronium bromide may be used in patients whose paralysis will be more protracted and has the advantage of being significantly less expensive than the newer, shorter-acting agents. If tachycardia remains with the use of pancuronium, vecuronium may be substituted; alternatively, metocurine iodide may be mixed with the pancuronium in a 4:1 ratio, and this inexpensive solution can be used as the paralyzing infusion. Significant savings can be achieved by carefully selecting the paralyzing agent in cases where substitution is acceptable (Table 32-3). At UCSD, the authors have saved over $30,000 in 6 months by substituting neuromuscular blocking agents.

Overdosage of pharmacological paralysis agents should be avoided. There is a growing body of evidence indicating that overadministration of neuromuscular blockers can profoundly prolong weaning[44,45] and produce detrimental effects on the immune system.[46,47] Overdosage can be avoided by monitoring the depth of paralysis. Bedside monitoring with a peripheral nerve stimulator on a scheduled basis affords an objective method for evaluating the efficacy of pharmacological paralysis. ICP control is generally accomplished when paralysis is titrated to one to two twitches out of a train-of-four.

It is critical that pharmacologically paralyzed patients be adequately sedated. Agitation or pain, as well as an improving level of consciousness in an unsedated but paralyzed patient, is very difficult to recognize objectively, will interfere with ICP control, and can be the sole cause of ICH. This reinforces the disadvantage of

TABLE 32-3 Daily Expenses Associated with Routine Dosing of Various Neuromuscular Blocking Agents*

Neuromuscular Blocking Agent	Dose, μg/kg/min	Cost per mg, $	Cost per 24 h, $
Pancuronium bromide (Pavulon)	1	0.124	12.50
Vecuronium bromide	1.5	1.73	261.58
Atracurium besylate	7	0.378	266.72
Metocurine iodide (Metubine Iodide)	4	0.50	201.60
Pancuronium : metocurine mixture @ 4:1	0.05 + 2	0.124 + $0.50	107.05

* Pharmacy costs, not including hospital markup, administrative costs, etc., for UCSD Medical Center, 1994.

losing the neurological examination and the need for continuously reassessing the requirement for continued pharmacological paralysis and discontinuing it as soon as possible.

Hyperventilation

Hyperventilation is an established and effective mechanism for decreasing ICP. Unfortunately, a growing body of evidence suggests that inappropriate or excessive hyperventilation can produce or exacerbate cerebral ischemia and negatively influence outcome.[48–50] The mechanism of action of hyperventilation involves metabolic autoregulation, which is characteristically preserved in most instances of severe head injury even when pressure autoregulation has been disrupted.[49,51–55] The decrease in cerebral blood volume that results from hyperventilation-induced cerebral vasoconstriction lowers the ICP, consistent with the Monro-Kellie doctrine. The alterations in cerebral blood flow caused by this vasoconstriction, however, have effects on regional and global cerebral blood flow that are unquantified and have the potential of producing ischemic secondary insults. In addition, regional inhomogeneities in the preservation of metabolic autoregulation within an injured brain may result in "steal" and "inverse steal" phenomena, depending on the direction of change in Pa_{CO_2}.[48] On a global basis, when flow-metabolic coupling is measured by jugular venous oxygen sampling, whole-brain indexes do not commonly suggest ischemia.[56,57] Unfortunately, the averaging implicit in this technique can miss significant areas of focal ischemia, and so it should be used very cautiously in the presence of obvious focal brain injuries and must not be overinterpreted in general.

An additional caveat with respect to the use of hyperventilation is the general occurrence of tachyphylaxis over a time period of 72 to 96 h after the induction of hyperventilation as the CSF compensates for the systemic alkalosis.[58,59] This compensation has the dual effect of diminishing the tonic effect of the established level of hypocapnia on the cerebral vasculature and making weaning from hyperventilation more difficult, since rebound CSF acidosis and associated vasodilatation will occur during the restoration of eucapnia. In some instances, the compensation will allow the safe establishment of further degrees of hyperventilation in treating refractory ICH, but since the effect of compensation on hyperventilation-induced vasoconstriction cannot be quantified, further hyperventilation should not be performed without some index of flow-metabolic coupling such as jugular venous oxygen saturation monitoring (see below).

Finally, hyperventilation also has systemic consequences. A rapid induction of hypocapnia can induce hypotension and profound hypocapnea can significantly interfere with oxygen delivery via the Bohr effect, although this does not appear to be a problem at the levels of hyperventilation commonly used in severe head injury.[57] This is of particular concern during the initial stages of resuscitation, when there is a tendency to overventilate.

In an attempt to utilize hyperventilation to control ICP without inducing ischemia, the authors initiate hyperventilation to a Pa_{CO_2} of approximately 30 mmHg. The degree of hyperventilation is continuously monitored using end-tidal CO_2 monitoring or, more recently, an intraarterial CO_2-sensitive monitor (PB3300® Continuous Intra-Arterial Blood Gas Monitor) with frequent confirmation using blood gas values. Overhyperventilation during maneuvers such as preoxygenation for bronchoscopy is carefully avoided, and "bagging" in response to acute episodes of acute ICH is not performed unless signs of herniation are present. Jugular venous saturation is also monitored (see below) to optimize hyperventilation.[56,60,61] Both the risk of hyperventilation-induced global cerebral ischemia and the potential of gaining therapeutic benefit from further hyperventilation in diffuse injury situations can be estimated with this technique.

Diuretics

The administration of diuretics is an effective means of decreasing ICP. The most commonly used diuretic is mannitol. As an intravascular agent that does not easily cross the blood-brain barrier, it osmotically draws fluid from both normal and abnormal brains.[62,63] The rapidity of its effect on ICP, however, suggests that it may work through mechanisms other than its osmotic load. One possibility is that mannitol also increases erythrocyte membrane flexibility, which decreases blood viscosity, resulting in reflex vasoconstriction and decreased cerebrovascular volume.[64] These effects are potentiated when mannitol is administered in bolus form.

Several potential problems are associated with the administration of mannitol. The significant osmotic diuresis can result in volume contraction and hypotension. Mannitol should therefore not be administered to hypovolemic patients. The fluids lost after mannitol-induced diuresis should be fully replaced with solutions slightly hypertonic to the urine so that the patient's overall volume status is not compromised.

Repeated dosage of mannitol will increase serum osmolarity. Not only does this decrease the effectiveness of mannitol, it may precipitate acute renal failure.[65] Additionally, protracted use of osmotic diuretics can wash out the renal medullary gradient and cause nephrogenic diabetes insipidus. Finally, the blood-brain barrier is not absolute with respect to mannitol, particularly after trauma, and prolonged or repeated administration will result in tissue sequestration, which may cause rebound ICH as a result of osmotically driven fluid influx into the extracellular compartment.[66,67]

These considerations mandate restraint in mannitol dosing. In terms of lowering ICP, doses of 0.25 g/kg appear to be as efficacious as doses of 1.0 g/kg, although the duration of action is shorter.[68] Serum osmolarity should be monitored and maintained below 320 mOsm/kg, and serum sodium should be maintained within the normal range.

Furosemide is a loop diuretic that is also effective in lowering ICP, although to a lesser extent than mannitol.[69] It does not appear to have the other beneficial actions of mannitol with respect to inducing reflex vasoconstriction. It too can result in significant dehydration and also induces potassium wasting, which must be monitored and controlled. Additionally, furosemide is potentially ototoxic, particularly when used in high doses with rapid and repeated administration. In general, mannitol appears to be the preferable agent when a single diuretic is desired for ICP control. There is, however, evidence that furosemide works synergistically with mannitol in a superadditive manner to lower ICP.[70,71] This synergism may be useful when the response to mannitol alone is unsatisfactory.

Since the more protracted actions of diuretics on ICP are mediated primarily by dehydration of the brain, it is to be expected that they are more efficacious in situations where ICH is a manifestation of increased extracellular and/or intracellular tissue fluid than in cases where ICP is elevated as a result of dysautoregulatory states that result in increased cerebral blood volume (Fig. 32-2). The development of an accurate and reliable method for identifying such situations is an unrealized prerequisite for targeted ICP therapy. Although there is some evidence that ICP waveform analysis might be usable in detecting this distinction, these data remain preliminary.[72,73]

Steroids

Steroids continue to be administered to a significant percentage of head-injured patients despite the lack of literature to support their efficacy (J. B. G. Ghajar and R. J. Hariri, personal communication, 1992). Numerous reports have demonstrated no beneficial effects of steroids administered in the setting of head injury, and trends toward increased risks of infection and gastrointestinal (GI) hemorrhage have been noted.[74–80] The systemic metabolic effects and the depression of the immune response resulting from steroid administration are also undesirable in the setting of acute trauma. At present, there is no indication for the routine administration of steroids in severe head trauma patients.

However, in keeping with the increasing recognition of the role of lipid peroxidation in producing neuronal damage after ischemic or mechanical insults in experimental animals and bolstered by the results of the NASCIS-II study reporting some degree of efficacy of methylprednisolone sodium succinate in promoting neurological recovery after spinal cord injury, there is continued interest in the possibility that certain newer forms and administration patterns of steroids might be efficacious in strictly defined trials on human head injury victims. A multicenter study in the United States and a multinational study on the efficacy of nonglucocorticoid 21-aminosteroids (tirilazad) in human head injury are nearing completion. These agents are powerful inhibitors of free radical formation and lipid peroxidation.[81,82] These studies are phase 3 randomized prospective trials using early administration in a controlled dose-escalation fashion, and their results are awaited with interest.

It should be pointed out that tirilazad is not comparable with conventional steroids with respect to either tissue bioavailability or mechanism of action, and the ongoing tirilazad trials should not be viewed as supporting the general use of steroids in head injury.

CSF Drainage

Drainage of CSF is an effective method of lowering ICP, particularly when ventricular size has not been compromised. Since it requires penetration of the brain parenchyma in patients who often have abnormal clotting indexes early in the posttraumatic course, there is a risk of developing a procedure-related hematoma that requires surgical evacuation when a ventricular catheter is placed during the acute postinjury period.[3,83] In addition, there is a 2 to 10 percent risk of infection with ventricular catheters in general, which goes up to 40 percent when ventricular drainage is employed in patients who require surgery for open depressed skull fractures.[84,85] Finally, as brain swelling progresses, the ventricular system is often compressed and the ability to drain CSF is compromised. This may be exacerbated by overdrainage, in which the ventricular walls or the choroid plexus may actually occlude the orifices of the catheter. Catheter patency may be better preserved by not draining at a zero or negative gradient and limiting drainage to a short, set interval (e.g., 2 min).

The precise role of CSF drainage in treating ICH depends to some extent on the method used for the initial determination of ICP. At centers using ventriculostomies, CSF drainage is an early and integral part of ICP management and in some instances may be the only therapeutic modality required during a patient's course. It has been the authors' experience, however, that the efficacy of CSF drainage in controlling ICP diminishes over the first several postinjury days in patients with severe ICH and that the ability to drain CSF becomes compromised as the ventricles are compressed. Nevertheless, if ventriculostomy is the initial ICP monitor, CSF drainage should be pursued vigorously in the initial treatment of ICH.

If ICP monitoring techniques are chosen that do not provide the ability to drain CSF, the role of CSF drainage as a treatment option (and the need for ventricular access) becomes a separate issue (Fig. 32-1*B*). At the authors' institution, where we insert Camino intraparenchymal devices as our first-line ICP monitors, CSF drainage is not established if the patient responds well to mild hyperventilation and mannitol administration. CSF diversion is established in patients who do not respond to these modalities and whose CT scans demonstrate targetable ventricles. In actual clinical experience, the authors have found that a majority of patients are now treated without CSF drainage, which does not appear to have increased the complexity of their management and has essentially eliminated iatrogenic intracranial hemorrhage and meningitis/ventriculitis as complications (R. M. Chesnut, unpublished observations, 1992). Nevertheless, given the risks associated with hyperventilation and mannitol, CSF drainage as an early or first-line treatment for ICH remains a very useful approach.

Barbiturates

A significant controversy surrounds the use of barbiturates in the treatment of ICH. A plethora of clinical evidence suggests that barbiturates are effective in decreasing ICP.[86–90] The best evidence comes from a prospective double-blind trial of barbiturates in the control of ICH. This study showed that barbiturates, as administered, clearly lowered ICP.[86] Barbiturates do not appear to be effective in improving outcome when they are randomly substituted for mannitol as the first-line agent for treatment of ICH[91] or administered in a prophylactic fashion to severe head injury patients without proven ICH.[92]

Mechanism of Action

Barbiturates have a number of physiological mechanisms of action in head-injured patients. In addition to their action as a sedative, barbiturates reduce CMR_{O_2}, have important vasoconstrictive properties, and appear to inhibit free radical–induced lipid peroxidation.[92–98] The sedative activity is accompanied by a decrease in cerebral metabolism, as evidenced by depression of CMR_{O_2}. This metabolic depression is accomplished by suppressing the activation component of cerebral metabolism.[95–97] The activation component constitutes approximately 40 percent of the total neuronal metabolism, and therefore, even total elimination of the activation component will still leave 60 percent of neuronal metabolism unaltered. Nevertheless, the barbiturate-induced CMR_{O_2} depression results in a lowering of cerebral blood flow through flow-metabolic coupling with a resultant decrease in cerebral blood volume and therefore ICP. Additionally, the lowered metabolic demands of the brain under these conditions allow the brain to tolerate a lower CPP (e.g. 50 mmHg) without flow-metabolic mismatching.

Complications

Unfortunately, high-dose barbiturate therapy has a significant potential for serious complications (Table 32-4). The most common side effect is hypotension, which results from lowering of the systemic vascular resistance and depression of the myocardium.[86,91,92] Despite the

TABLE 32-4 Complications of Barbiturates

Sepsis in an anergic patient
- Patient may not mount fever or develop elevated WBC
- Signs of sepsis
  - Falling platelet count
  - Rising serum glucose
  - Elevated PT or PTT
  - Hypotension–falling SVR
  - Rising CO
  - Falling AVD_{O_2}
- Suspect
  - Pneumonia
  - Urosepsis
  - Sinusitis
  - Occult GI pathology
  - CNS infection
  - Line septis

Hypotension (SBP $<$ 90 mmHg; CPP $<$ 50–70* mmHg)
- Barbiturates
- Sepsis
- Blood loss
- Third spacing
- Myocardial infarction
- Pulmonary embolism
- If due to barbiturates, may be multifactorial
  - Falling CO
    - Treat with dobutamine
  - Falling SVR
    - Treat initially with dopamine
    - Phenylephrine/levarterenol if dopamine not effective

* See text.

CVP = central venous pressure; PAS = pulmonary artery systolic pressure; PAD = pulmonary artery diastolic pressure; PCWP = pulmonary capillary wedge pressure; SVR = systemic vascular resistance; AVD_{O_2} arteriovenous oxygen difference; CO = cardiac output.

SOURCE: Adpated from Chesnut RM, Marshall LF, Bowers, Marshall S, Medical Management of claustal intracranial pressure, in Cooper PR (ed): *Head Injury* (3d ed.) pp. 225–276. Baltimore: Williams & Wilkins, 1992, with permission.

cerebral protective effects of barbiturates, hypotension has the potential to rapidly eliminate any beneficial effects. Indeed, the one proven contraindication to the initiation of barbiturate coma is the occurrence of cardiovascular compromise, including episodes of hypotension, before the administration of barbiturates.[86]

As a result of the significant tendency of barbiturates to lower the blood pressure and the recognizably deleterious effects of hypotension on injured neurons, an adequate CPP must be assiduously maintained throughout the course of barbitrate therapy. Barbiturates must not be administered to patients who are hypovolemic. Because of the profound systemic and myocardial effects of these agents, insertion of a pulmonary artery catheter should be accomplished before the administration of barbiturates. Particular care must be taken if there is a history of systemic cardiovascular disease or previous hypotension. The authors characteristically have dopamine attached to a venous infusion line and a solution of phenylephrine mixed and in the patient's room before the initiation of barbiturate therapy so that the response time can be minimized if blood pressure starts to fall. With such precautions, barbiturate coma may be managed entirely without hypotension, although not without significant effort.

The other major complication associated with barbiturate coma is systemic infection. The necessity of a protracted and intense ICU course, coupled with the induced immunologic anergy characteristic of high-dose barbiturate administration, places these patients at risk of infections ranging from pneumonia and line infections to sepsis. Since these patients tend to become hypothermic and often require pressors and/or inotropic agents to maintain an adequate CPP, the most common and easily recognized early manifestations of sepsis, such as fever, leukocytosis, and a hyperdynamic state, are masked. Secondary indicators such as hyperglycemia, coagulopathy, thrombocytopenia, and an unexplained fall in systemic vascular resistance or a decrease in systemic oxygen extraction may therefore represent the first clinical signs of sepsis. A high level of suspicion coupled with close clinical, laboratory, and radiological surveillance is needed to allow early diagnosis of infections in barbiturate coma patients. When evidence of infection arises, all systems (e.g., blood, sputum, urine, drains, CSF) should be thoroughly cultured and broad-spectrum antibiotic coverage should be initiated, with subsequent targeting of the antibiotic coverage after accurate identification of the causative organisms.

TECHNIQUE

Adequate preparation for the initiation of barbiturate coma includes stable mechanical oxygenation and ventilatory status, euvolemia with an indwelling pulmonary artery catheter, sufficient vascular access to allow vigorous fluid administration concomitantly with medication administration, and the standard accouterments appropriate to an ICU patient (Table 32-5). Some form of EEG monitoring capabilities, such as a compressed spectral array display or a four- or eight-channel EEG machine, is very useful as a guide in titrating the patient to burst suppression. In addition, the authors generally include jugular venous saturation monitoring, some capability for continuously monitoring ventilation (end-tidal CO_2 or intraarterial CO_2-sensitive monitor), and monitoring of cerebral saturation (INVOS 3100 cerebral oximeter, Somanetics Corporation, Troy, Michigan). Finally, the patient must be situated in an intensive care setting with the capability of continuous close neurological and systemic observation, preferably on a one-to-one nursing basis. In general, if the above conditions cannot be met, the risks of barbiturate coma may outweigh the potential benefits.

Monitoring of electrical brain activity is useful prognostically and therapeutically in barbiturate coma. Barbiturate coma is generally not effective in patients who do not have significant high-frequency activity.[21] In addition, as burst suppression is a useful therapeutic goal in guiding barbiturate dosing (see below), a bedside EEG machine or compressed spectral array display is recommended. The recognition of burst suppression in

TABLE 32-5 Patient Preparation for Barbiturates

Endotracheal intubation: oral intubation preferable (versus sinusitis)
Mechanical ventilation
Arterial line: blood pressure monitoring and frequent blood gases
Pulse oximeter
Pulmonary artery catheter: monitoring of CVP, PAS, PAD, PCWP
  Frequent measurement of CO, SVR, AVD_{O_2}
Bedside EEG monitor: monitor burst suppression
  Standard EEG or compressed spectral array
Adequate IV access
  Include large-bore line for bolus fluids
Pressors and inotropes
  Dopamine mixed and connected for infusion
  Phenylephrine, levarterenol, dobutamine available
Temperature probe: avoid hypothermia
Vigorous pulmonary care
DVT and decubitus prophylaxis
One-to-one nursing: preferable

WBC = white blood cell; PT = prothrombin time; PTT = partial thromboplastin time; SVR = systemic vascular resistance; AVD_{O_2} = arteriovenous oxygen difference; GI = gastrointestinal; CNS = central nervous system; SBP = systolic blood pressure; CPP = cerebral perfusion pressure; CO = cardiac output.

SOURCE: Adapted from Chesnut RM et al., in Cooper PR (ed): *Head Injury* (3d ed). Williams & Wilkins, 1992, with permission.

a compressed spectral array format is not always straightforward, and viewing the two-lead raw EEG display is often helpful.

The initiation of barbiturate therapy is accomplished through the administration of a loading dose of 10 mg/kg of pentobarbital sodium over 30 min. This is followed by an infusion of 5 mg/kg/h for the next 3 h. The patient is then started on a continuous IV infusion of 1 mg/kg/h. This can be increased as indicated for ICP control or EEG burst suppression to 2 to 3 mg/kg/h or higher in selected instances.

If the physician is at the bedside and fluid and pharmacological mechanisms for responding to downward trends in blood pressure are readily available, the initiation of barbiturate coma can be hastened by performing the loading dose by means of the administration of 100- to 200-mg bolus aliquots of pentobarbital sodium by hand. This allows the most rapid induction of barbiturate coma, but significant caution must be taken to guard against hypotension.

The goal of barbiturate coma is ICP control. The progress of coma can be tracked by monitoring EEG suppression. Serum pentobarbital levels can also be followed on a 12- or 24-h basis. Satisfactory levels are generally between 3 and 4 mg/dl, but the authors have seen levels as high as 9 mg/dl in some patients requiring higher infusion rates for ICP control.

In patients who have been titrated to burst suppression without achievement of adequate ICP control, further barbiturate administration, to the point of EEG flatline, may be associated with improvement in ICP. A possible explanation for this has been reported by Walker et al., who noted increases in middle cerebral artery transcranial Doppler flow velocity phase linked to the bursts in patients with burst suppression patterns on EEG.[99] This suggests that flow-metabolic coupling may be occurring during these bursts with a concomitant transient increase in cerebral blood volume. Suppressing even these bursts may result in a net decrease in cerebral blood volume, producing better ICP control.

The serum levels of pentobarbital sodium generally obtained during barbiturate coma characteristically produce miosis. At higher levels, however, mydriasis may raise the specter of bilateral third nerve palsies caused by transtentorial herniation, which must be ruled out as well as possible on the basis of other factors.

When ICP has come into satisfactory control for 24 to 48 h, withdrawal of barbiturate therapy may be initiated. Despite the long half-life and significant adipose depot of pentobarbital sodium, profound refractory rebound ICH can occur if withdrawal proceeds too rapidly. A suggested regimen is to decrease the hourly infusion by 50 percent per day. As serum barbiturate levels drop, reinitiation of sedation with or without pharmacological paralysis may become necessary. Withdrawal of barbiturates has also been associated with seizures, and the administration of anticonvulsant medications may be required if the patient is not already receiving them prophylactically. During withdrawal of barbiturate sedation, the pupillary light response recovers first, with corticospinal voluntary motor control recovering later.

A number of nursing issues are critical in caring for a patient in a barbiturate coma. These patients become poikilothermic, and while moderate hypothermia is associated with neuronal protection from a variety of insults, a decreased body temperature depresses the immune response, interferes with the coagulation system, alters systemic metabolism, and prolongs the half-life of drugs. Therefore, an effort should be made to keep the patient's body temperature above 35°C unless hypothermic therapy is specifically desired. Skin care issues are also critical, as these patients not only are immobile but often are also receiving pressor agents that may decrease skin perfusion and increase the likelihood of pressure ulceration. Finally, prolonged immobilization also increases the risk of deep venous thrombosis and pulmonary embolism.

Early Initiation of Barbiturate Coma as Targeted Therapy

The CT classification studies from the TCDB have revealed that patients with compressed or absent cisterns, plus or minus midline shift of 5 mm or more (Diffuse Injury III and IV), have a unique profile of outcome predictors, with ICP being the most powerful.[17] The authors have noted that patients presenting with such CT images tend to be young, manifest ICH very early in their course, are not well controlled with mannitol, and characteristically have intact pressure and metabolic autoregulation. In our experience, these patients respond very well to barbiturate therapy, but when they are treated according to the sequential approach, a significant delay obtains before the administration of pentobarbital. As a result, we have initiated early barbiturate therapy in a number of these patients in the manner of targeted therapy (Fig. 32-2). Barbiturate loading has been initiated within 6 h of admission, and although our results remain anecdotal, a significant proportion of very satisfactory outcomes has been obtained.

The early administration of barbiturates, however, destines the patient to a very intensive ICU course. In the study of Eisenberg et al., the patient's course was significantly more complex because of complications if barbiturate therapy was initiated within 52 h of patient contact.[86] These patients characteristically are in a barbiturate coma course for up to 7 days, and the majority develop pneumonia and require the administration of pressors for some part of their course to maintain adequate CPP. Indeed, CPP management is critical in these patients, who tend to demonstrate improvement in ICP and jugular venous saturation when CPP is maintained at 80 mmHg or above.

Early administration of barbiturates in this type of patient represents an attempt to target therapy at patients with severe, potentially intractable ICH who have some degree of intact autoregulation and therefore should respond to mild hyperventilation, elevated CPP, and barbiturates. Given the absence of significant intraparenchymal lesions on their presenting CT scans, the authors believe that the actual parenchymal injury either is not devastating or is reversible and that these patients succumb primarily to secondary insults. Nevertheless, because of the high complication rate and very difficult course of these patients, the early initiation of barbiturate therapy in this patient group, while very encouraging, cannot be recommended as a primary treatment protocol.

WITHDRAWAL OF ICP THERAPY

The withdrawal of ICP therapy in a patient who has required significant treatment for ICH must be predicated on the attainment of stable intracranial dynamics for 24 to 48 h. The response of ICP during withdrawal of the various treatment modalities not only can reflect unacceptable intracerebral events but also can be due to the patient's "waking up." Therefore, initiating the withdrawal of ICP therapy requires a patient whose ICP course is acceptable and stable, whose ICP waveform or other compliance information has normalized, and who has been weaned from the more extreme therapies, such as barbiturate coma and profound ("balanced") hyperventilation. This generally is a patient who is sedated, has a Pa_{CO_2} of approximately 30 mmHg, and may or may not be pharmacologically paralyzed. In patients with neuromuscular blockers on board, the blockers are discontinued while sedation is maintained to prevent agitation or bucking on the endotracheal tube during the return of neuromuscular control.

The return of the neurological examination is invaluable in assessing the continued progress of withdrawal of ICP treatment. Patients who are following commands can be weaned in a straightforward fashion without significant concern if ICP rises to some extent during this process. Patients who are not following commands, however, are more difficult and must be observed very carefully while Pa_{CO_2} is normalized. As a result of the previously discussed CSF compensation for hyperventilation, ICP characteristically increases during normalization of Pa_{CO_2}, and other indicators, such as status of the cisterns on the patient's CT scan, the ICP waveform, and the neurological examination, must be used to determine whether the associated ICP elevations are expected and acceptable.

If the patient tolerates normalization of Pa_{CO_2}, sedation is withdrawn and ICP monitoring is discontinued. If at any point during withdrawal of ICP therapy there is evidence of decompensation, the withdrawal pattern can be reversed.

ALTERNATIVE AGENTS AND METHODS FOR TREATING ICH

Lidocaine

Lidocaine decreases synaptic transmission either directly or through blockade of sodium channels, decreases CMR_{O_2} and glucose consumption, and has been reported to have direct action as a vasoconstrictor.[100–102] Lidocaine had reduced ICH resulting from acute ischemia in experimental animals[101] and has been reported to decrease ICP elevations resulting from head injury and other intracranial disturbances in humans, although many of these patients had little or no initial ICH.[103] Lidocaine acts to lower ICP in the authors' clinical experience, but its efficacy over time and in comparison to other agents has not been established in humans. In addition, its depressant action on the myocardium and its lowering of the seizure threshold are serious considerations in this patient population. At present, although it may be useful in selected situations, it cannot be generally recommended for ICP control. When used, it is administered at 1 to 2 mg/min as a continuous intravenous infusion.

In contrast to continuous infusion for ICP control, intravenous lidocaine is very effective in blunting ICP responses to transient noxious stimuli such as invasive procedures and endotracheal suctioning when it is administered shortly before such occurrences.[104–106] When used prophylactically for the performance of pulmonary toilet, it may also be administered intratracheally and may be somewhat more effective.[105,106]

Propofol

Propofol is a sedative-hypnotic with a very rapid onset and a short duration of action. It depresses CMR_{O_2}, although not as effectively as do the barbiturates and etomidate. Studies in head injury patients have revealed that the administration of propofol decreases ICP in patients with normal or elevated pressures, but unfortunately, there is characteristically an accompanying fall in systemic blood pressure that generally results in a net decrease of CPP, often of significant magnitude.[107–112] Since propofol does decrease the CMR_{O_2}, the overall effect of its intracranial and systemic response on flow-metabolism matching is unclear and has not been determined in the head-injured population.

Although its rapid onset and short duration of action are desirable in neuroanesthesia, the tendency of propofol to lower CPP, coupled with its less powerful CMR_{O_2} depressant activities compared with barbiturates and etomidate, limits this agent's utility in treating ICH. If it is to be used, hypovolemia must be corrected before its administration.[110]

Etomidate

Etomidate is a sedative-hypnotic with rapid onset and a short duration of action. It compares very favorably with barbiturates and is without many of the complicating CNS side effects. It is effective in reducing ICP in patients with ICH caused by mass lesions or head injury.[113–116] As with barbiturates, the reduction in ICP parallels depression of the EEG, and etomidate is not effective in reducing ICP in patients with initial suppression of cerebral electrical activity.[117–119] The mechanism of ICP reduction appears to be a reduction in cerebral blood volume mediated by means of flow-metabolic coupling in response to etomidate-induced depression of the CMR_{O_2}.[120]

The mild tendency of etomidate to lower systemic blood pressure appears to be powerfully countered by its profound ability to lower ICP so that significant drops in CPP do not occur when etomidate is administered in adequately hydrated patients without preexisting EEG depression.[113–117,121] Its powerful ability to lower ICP without concomitant depression of arterial blood pressure constitutes an advantage over barbiturates and propofol, which have a much greater tendency to lower CPP.

Etomidate was used widely for sedation and ICP control in head-injured patients outside the United States until 1984, at which time circumstantial evidence associating long-term use with increased mortality due to infectious complications in ventilated patients was reported.[122] Subsequent investigations demonstrated a severe, reversible direct suppression of the adrenal cortex by etomidate that results in decreased circulating plasma cortisol and a blunting of the cortisol release to pharmacological stimulation or surgical stress.[123–127] Addisonian-type hypotensive episodes that responded to steroid administration occurring in patients receiving long-term etomidate infusion have been reported.[123,125] Given the concern that long-term infusion of etomidate can produce an iatrogenic addisonian syndrome and immunologic suppression, the use of etomidate has been curtailed despite suggestions that corticosteroid replacement therapy could be used to cover the adrenal suppression.[127,128] With its highly desirable CNS effects, however, etomidate remains the most exciting candidate for a replacement for barbiturates in treating ICH, and single-center trials supplementing etomidate infusion with corticosteroid replacement are under way, with promising early results.

Hyperbaric Oxygen

Studies on the use of hyperbaric oxygen in treating closed head injuries have produced mixed results.[129–135] Prospective double-blind studies have shown very limited beneficial effects in head-injured patients.[129,131] Although ICP can be lowered by hyperbaric oxygen therapy, these effects are neither profound nor lasting, and no well-controlled study on patients with elevated ICP has been done.[130,131] Although mortality is reported to be decreased by this form of therapy, the additional survivors are reported to remain severely disabled or vegetative rather than making good recoveries.[134]

Performance of hyperbaric treatments is expensive and logistically difficult; a hyperbaric chamber is a less than optimal location for taking care of a seriously ill head-injured patient. Additionally, the beneficial effects of modulating cerebral blood volume and decreasing cerebral edema appear to be offset by the neurotoxicity of hyperoxygenation. Finally, the frequency, duration, pressure, and number of treatments necessary are not clear. Although further investigation into this method of treatment is indicated, hyperbaric therapy for head-injured patients cannot be recommended at this time.

Decompressive Craniectomy

Decompressive craniectomy as a method of "giving room to the swelling brain" has been reported to be beneficial in a number of neurological disorders, including head injury,[136,137] cerebral infarction,[138–140] spontaneous intracerebral hemorrhage,[141] Reye's syndrome,[142] and subarachnoid hemorrhage.[143] In a severe head injury patient, there is no doubt that decompressive craniectomy results in a significant decrease in ICH.[136,137,144] Although the mortality associated with the intractable ICH for which decompressive craniectomy was performed is generally significantly decreased,[136,144] this is not universally the case,[145] and the high morbidity among the survivors raises serious questions about the utility of this procedure in general.[144,145] Certainly, the literature suggests that early decompressive craniectomy in response to massive brain swelling may merely convert mortalities into vegetative survivors.[136,144,145]

One report, however, suggests that decompressive craniectomy in patients with intractable hypertension who have survived several days into their treatment may be beneficial in terms of mortality and morbidity.[146] This is in accordance with the authors' experience, which suggests that selected patients with refractory ICH who have CT scans showing diffuse injury patterns without significant areas of infarction or contusion have characteristically responded well to decompressive craniectomy. In terms of a sequential treatment paradigm, decompressive craniectomy may be considered in selected cases in patients with ICH and "potentially salvageable brains" as an alternative to barbiturate coma therapy in those who are not good candidates for this treatment or as a subsequent choice in patients who do not tolerate or respond well to barbiturates.

After decompressive craniectomy with durotomy or dural augmentation, the brain tends to mushroom into the operative site. Although this looks unpleasing on CT, the anticipated infarction of the bulging brain does not characteristically occur. The question of whether decompressive craniectomy actually increases edema in the underlying brain is unresolved.[147,148]

It is desirable to retain the removed bone for subsequent replacement. Although bone banking can be used, if available, the authors have found burying the removed bone in the subcutaneous adipose tissue of the abdomen or thigh to be a safe and convenient alternative that has the benefit of potentially maintaining the osteoinductive properties of the bone flap. For infectious reasons, bone flap replacement should probably be delayed approximately 12 weeks.[149] Interestingly, varying degrees of neurological improvement have been reported after cranioplasty in patients with reasonable neurological function after decompressive craniectomy.[149–151]

ALTERNATIVE CONCEPTS AND TECHNIQUES FOR TREATING ELEVATED ICP

VASOSPASM AND TRANSCRANIAL DOPPLER

The technique of transcranial Doppler velocity measurement in the major arteries of the circle of Willis has become widely used in neurosurgery. Increased flow velocity in an artery can result either from an actual increase in blood flow or from narrowing of the vessel lumen. Since increased flow with a normal diameter (hyperemia) results in increased distal delivery whereas increased flow velocity due to vessel narrowing (vasospasm) may result in decreased distal delivery, distinguishing between these two situations is important. In an attempt to differentiate hyperemia from vasospasm, the Lindegaard ratio has been developed.[152] This is the ratio between the middle cerebral artery (MCA) and ipsilateral extracranial internal carotid artery (ICA) velocities (MCA/ICA) and has a normal value of 1.7 ± 0.4.[153] Transcranial Doppler MCA velocities that are significantly higher than the ipsilateral ICA will result in a high Lindegaard ratio (>3) and are suggestive of vasospasm, whereas comparable elevations in flow velocities in both arteries are more consistent with hyperemia.

Unfortunately, the absolute values of both the MCA velocities and the Lindegaard ratio in terms of proper diagnosis are unclear. The incidence of vasospasm will vary directly with the thresholds set. MCA velocities from 100 to 200 have been suggested in various disease entities.[154–158] If the value of 120 is used, estimates of cerebral vasospasm in head trauma have been as high as 26.7 percent.[156] Ratios of 200 or greater will significantly lower the incidence rate and appear much more likely to be associated with severe angiographic changes and signs of infarction although not necessarily with clinical deterioration.[159,160] Alternatively, it has been suggested that the rate of increase in MCA velocity (i.e., over 50 cm/s per 24 h) is a stronger indicator of the development of vasospasm.[161]

Vasospasm does appear to be a significant entity in head trauma.[20,162–164] There may be two forms of vasospasm after brain trauma. An early mechanical form has been reported in the proximal arteries of the circle of Willis, particularly the basilar circulation.[162] This "early vasospasm" may present in a protean fashion with signs of brainstem dysfunction suggesting herniation. More recently, attention has been focused on the delayed form of vasospasm, which is very similar to that occurring in subarachnoid hemorrhage.[156]

With head injury, the authors characteristically become suspicious of vasospasm when we see day-to-day progression in MCA velocities of 20 percent or more with a rising Lindegaard ratio. If the flow velocity goes over 160 and the Lindegaard ratio is above 3:1, we generally perform confirmatory angiography. If the velocity is above 200 and the Lindegaard ratio is above 5:1, we always proceed to angiography. In the absence of the ability to perform regional cerebral blood flow studies, angiography is the usual confirmatory test.

If vasospasm is detected, hypertensive-hypervolemic therapy, similar to that used in subarachnoid hemorrhage is the general treatment protocol. This is generally accompanied by the addition of calcium channel blockers. Of note, a forme fruste of hypertensive-hypervolemic therapy is integrally included in our standard head injury protocol.

Although the potential for vasospasm to produce ischemia is straightforward, the involvement of vasospasm-induced ischemia as a causative agent in posttraumatic ICH has not been conclusively proved. Nevertheless, vasospasm can result in ICP elevation through ischemia-related cellular swelling or if cerebral blood volume increases when autoregulatory mechanisms attempt to compensate for the decreased cerebral blood flow distal to regional areas of vasospasm. It is therefore reasonable to suspect vasospasm when ICH cannot be explained by more conventional mechanisms.

Hyperemia and "Optimized Hyperventilation"

The role of hyperemia in head injury is also unclear. Hyperemic transcranial Doppler indexes (high flow velocities in both the MCA and the ipsilateral ICA with a low Lindegaard ratio) are not uncommon in severe head injury, particularly after surgical removal of an ipsilateral extraaxial hematoma. Hyperemia is, however, generally an incidental finding that is not associated with ICH. If it is asymptomatic, no treatment is indicated. However, if hyperemia is felt to be responsible for elevated ICP on the basis of increased cerebral blood volume, it has been suggested that "optimized hyperventilation" can be used as the treatment.[56,165,166] If jugular venous oxygen saturation is measured in the situation of true hyperemia, saturation values above 70% [arteriovenous oxygen content (AVD_{O_2}) values below 5.9 g/dl] will be noted. In "optimized hyperventilation" the ventilatory rate is increased such that the Pa_{CO_2} falls below 30 mmHg and even below 25 mmHg until the ICP comes under control or the jugular venous oxygen saturation reaches the lower limit of its normal range of 50 to 70% (AVD_{O_2} reaches the upper limit of its normal range of 5 to 8.5 vol%).[56,167]

"Optimized hyperventilation" is based on the mismatch between perfusion and metabolism that results in abnormally high oxygen saturation in the jugular outflow from the brain. The accompanying excess cerebral blood volume can be diminished by increasing vasoconstriction through further lowering of the Pa_{CO_2}. Although the potential for ischemia resulting from indiscriminate use of hyperventilation is well recognized (see above), the use of optimized hyperventilation represents an attempt to prevent iatrogenic hypoperfusion by avoiding jugular venous desaturation during progressive increases in hyperventilation. It is notable that this assumes reasonable homogeneity of flow-perfusion coupling throughout the brain, limiting the use of optimized hyperventilation to patients with diffuse injury patterns with or without small associated nonsurgical intracerebral irregularities. Unfortunately, there is evidence that significant flow inhomogeneities can exist in patients with such CT findings, although their association with actual ischemia is less clear.[13,48–50,168] In addition, the assumption of homogeneity does not address the possibility of significant focal uncoupling that is not related to lesions definable on early CT images such as might occur during excitotoxic glutamate release in the hippocampus. Nevertheless, in diffuse injury cases where ICH is associated with hyperemia, optimized hyperventilation can be a useful method of controlling ICP if used in moderation.

Hypertensive CPP Therapy

The extent to which pressure autoregulation is maintained after severe head injury is unclear. There is mounting evidence that pressure autoregulation remains intact in many instances.[26,50,169–171] Figure 32-4 illustrates this concept. The normal autoregulatory curve is represented by the solid line, which has breakpoints at 50 mmHg and 150 mmHg. The disrupted state of autoregulation resulting from brain trauma is represented by the dashed line. In the situation of complete disruption of autoregulation, where the system becomes pressure-passive, the curve will appear linear without a breakpoint (line A). If the trauma has not completely disrupted autoregulation, the situation will be as represented by the dashed curve, with a breakpoint at 80 mmHg* and an autoregulatory plateau from 80 to 150 mmHg (line B). As can be seen in the figure, CPP values between 50 and 80 mmHg result in ischemia in the injured brain although they would be well tolerated by the normal brain. The response to CPP values above 80 mmHg depends on the curve. If the system is pressure-passive (line A), raising the CPP will increase cerebral blood flow (CBF) and the cerebral blood volume (CBV) and ICP will rise. If the system autoregulates (line B), raising the CPP will maintain a steady CBF through autoregulatory vasoconstriction. Since vasoconstriction actually decreases CBV, the ICP will often fall as CPP rises.

A number of confounding factors have clouded this issue. Not only is this a difficult problem to study in humans, but the apparent strong dependency of autoregulatory phenomena on Pa_{CO_2} and commonly used pharmacological agents, coupled with the uncertain and variable breakpoints of the flow-pressure curve in head-

* It should be noted that 80 mmHg is used for illustration and does not represent the breakpoint in any given patient. This value varies between patients and perhaps within patients as a function of time, evolution of the intracranial situation, and the administration of vasoactive agents or hyperventilation.

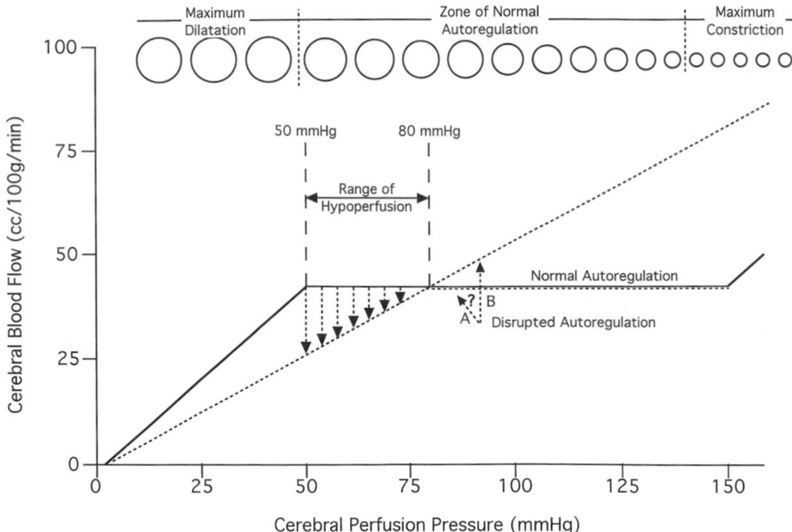

Figure 32-4. An illustrative diagram demonstrating two possible effects of brain injury on pressure autoregulation. Normal-pressure autoregulation is represented by the solid curve with breakpoints at 50 mmHg and 150 mmHg. Complete disruption of pressure autoregulation (pressure-passive system) is represented by the straight dashed curve where CBF varies linearly with CPP (line A). A "reset" pressure autoregulatory curve is represented by line B in which a plateau is maintained between 80 and 150 mmHg but the range between 50 and 80 mmHg is abnormally pressure-passive. In this range, ischemia will result despite a CPP that would be adequate in a normal brain. The circles represent the mean vessel diameter in the normal situation. Below the lower breakpoint of 50 mmHg, the vessels are maximally vasodilated. In the range of pressure autoregulation (50 to 150 mmHg), the vessels constrict as CPP rises to increase cerebrovascular resistance and keep CBF constant. In the situation of brain insult with some preservation of pressure autoregulation (line B), vasoconstriction will occur only over the range of 80 to 150 mmHg. The decrease in mean vessel diameter results in decreased cerebral blood volume (see text).

injured patients, has made the published data very difficult to understand or apply in individual instances. In the situation of a patient with an intact autoregulatory system, it is the authors' experience that the ICP will generally rise in response to spontaneous or induced elevations of CPP if CPP remains below the breakpoint where autoregulation becomes active (pressures below 80 mmHg in Fig. 32-4). However, as CPP becomes elevated above this point, the ICP response will flatten or often become negative. If vasodilatation is maximum below the breakpoint, the ICP response can be understood as a pressure-passive relationship over this range. As the breakpoint is passed, however, active autoregulatory vasoconstriction occurring in response to CPP elevation will decrease cerebral blood volume, resulting in a fall in ICP in patients with intact autoregulation (R. M. Chesnut and E. Lang, unpublished observations, 1993).

The importance of such relationships is twofold. First, the determination of the breakpoint can be used to set the minimum CPP for a given patient at the time of testing. Second, manipulation of CPP within the autoregulatory plateau above the breakpoint can be useful in lowering ICP through CPP manipulation alone.

There are several ways to attempt to determine the breakpoint if it exists in a patient. Chan et al. have demonstrated two methods of estimating this breakpoint.[26] They found that the pulsatility index of the transcranial Doppler velocity from the MCA decreases steadily until a certain CPP point, after which it plateaus. They showed that the rise in jugular venous saturation that occurs with increasing CPP tends to plateau at a similar CPP in a given patient. They also suggested that this CPP value represents the breakpoint for the autoregulation curve. Recent work at UCSD has revealed that if CPP is pharmacologically elevated in steps of 10 mmHg, a point is often reached above which ICP drops as CPP is elevated (R. M. Chesnut and E. Lang, unpublished observations, 1993). This point appears to correspond with the TCD-PI breakpoint of Chan et al., and pushing the CPP above this level has been found to be useful in lowering ICP ("hypertensive CPP therapy," R. M. Chesnut and E. Lang, unpublished observations, 1993).

The concept of treating ICH by artificially elevating CPP beyond the autoregulatory breakpoint involves a number of unsettled issues. The possibility of worsening cerebral edema or precipitating intracranial hemorrhage has not been quantified. In addition, once adequate cerebral perfusion has been attained, the absolute ICP value to be targeted is unclear. Nevertheless, hypertensive CPP therapy for ICH appears practical and may become useful in a wider sense as more data are acquired on its utility.

References

1. Miller JD: Significance and management of intracranial hypertension in head injury, in Ishii S, Nagai H, Brock M (eds): *Intracranial Pressure V.* Berlin: Springer-Verlag, 1983:44–53.
2. Marmarou A, Anderson RL, Ward JD, et al: Impact of ICP instability and hypotension on outcome in patients with severe head trauma. *J Neurosurg* 75:S159–S66, 1991.
3. Narayan R, Kishore P, Becker D, et al: Intracranial pressure: To monitor or not to monitor? A review of our experience with head injury. *J Neurosurg* 56:650–659, 1982.
4. Eisenberg HM, Cayard C, Papanicolaou A, et al: The effects of three potentially preventable complications on outcome after severe closed head injury, in Ishii S, Nagai H, Brock M (eds): *Intracranial pressure V.* Berlin: Springer-Verlag, 1983, 549–553.
5. Becker DP, Miller JD, Ward JD, et al: The outcome from severe head injury with early diagnosis and intensive management. *J Neurosurg* 47:491–502, 1977.
6. Marshall LF, Smith RW, Shapiro HM: The outcome with aggressive treatment in severe head injuries: I. the significance of intracranial pressure monitoring. *J Neurosurg* 50:20–25, 1979.
7. Marshall LF: Treatment of brain swelling and brain edema in man. *Adv Neurol* 28:459–469, 1980.
8. Saul TG, Ducker TB: Effects of intracranial pressure monitoring and aggressive treatment on mortality in severe head injury. *J Neurosurg* 56:498–503, 1982.
9. Contant CF, Robertson CS, Gopinath SP, et al: Determination of clinically important thresholds in continuously monitored patients in the neurosurgical intensive care unit, in *Proceedings of the Second International Neurotrauma Symposium,* Glasgow, Scotland, 1993:O4.
10. Marshall LF, Gautille T, Klauber MR, et al: The outcome of severe head injury. *J Neurosurg* 75:S28–S36, 1991.
11. Chesnut RM, Marshall LF, Klauber MR, et al: The role of secondary brain injury in determining outcome from severe head injury. *J Trauma* 34:216–222, 1993.
12. Piek J, Chesnut RM, Marshall LF, et al: Extracranial complications of severe head injury. *J Neurosurg* 77:901–907, 1992.
13. Bouma GJ, Muizelaar JP, Stringer WA, et al: Ultra-early evaluation of regional cerebral blood flow in severely head-injured patients using xenon-enhanced computerized tomography. *J Neurosurg* 77:360–368, 1992.
14. Yoshino A, Hovda DA, Kawamata T, et al: Dynamic changes in local cerebral glucose utilization following cerebral conclusion in rats: Evidence of a hyper- and subsequent hypometabolic state. *Brain Res* 561:106–119, 1991.
15. Haar FL, Sadhu VK, Sampson J, Gildenberg PL: Can CT scan findings predict ICP in closed head injury patients? in *Proceedings of the Thirtieth Annual Meeting of the Congress of Neurological Surgeons,* Houston, Texas, 1980:122–124.
16. Marshall LF, Marshall SB: Medical management of intracranial pressure, in Cooper PR (ed): *Head Injury.* Baltimore: Williams & Wilkins, 1986:177–196.
17. Marshall LF, Bowers-Marshall S, Klauber MR, et al: A new classification of head injury based on computerized tomography. *J Neurosurg* 75:S14–S20, 1991.
18. Marshall LF, Barba D, Toole BM, Bowers SA: The oval pupil: Clinical significance and relationship to intracranial hypertension. *J Neurosurg* 58:566–568, 1983.
19. Chesnut RM, Marshall LF: Management of head injury: Treatment of abnormal intracranial pressure. *Neurosurg Clin North Am* 2:267–284, 1991.
20. Miller JD, Dearden NM, Piper IR, Chan KH: Control of intracranial pressure in patients with severe head injury. *J Neurotrauma* 1:S317–326, 1992.
21. Dearden NM, Miller JD: Paired comparison of hypnotic and osmotic therapy in the reduction of intracranial hypertension after severe head injury, in Hoff JT, Betz AL (eds): *Intracranial Pressure VII.* Berlin: Springer-Verlag, 1989:474–481.
22. Miller JD, Sweet RC, Narayan R, Becker DP: Early insults to the injured brain. *JAMA* 240:439–442, 1978.
23. Miller JD, Becker DP: Secondary insults to the injured brain. *J R Coll Surg Edinb* 27:292–298, 1982.
24. Mchenry LCJ, West JW, Cooper ES, et al: Cerebral autoregulation in man. *Stroke* 5:695–706, 1974.
25. Lassen N: Cerebral blood flow and oxygen consumption in man. *Physiol Rev* 39:183–238, 1959.
26. Chan KH, Miller JD, Dearden NM, et al: The effect of changes in cerebral perfusion pressure upon middle cerebral artery blood flow velocity and jugular bulb venous oxygen saturation after severe brain injury. *J Neurosurg* 77:55–61, 1992.
27. Beckman DL, Iams SG: Circulating catecholamines in cats before and after lethal head injury. *Proc Soc Exp Biol Med* 160:200–202, 1979.
28. Graf CJ, Rossi NP: Catecholamine response to intracranial hypertension. *J Neurosurg* 49:862–8, 1978.
29. Hortnagl H, Hammerle AF, Hackl JM, et al: The activity of the sympathetic nervous system following severe head injury. *Intensive Care Med* 6:169–167, 1980.
30. Neil DG, Cruickshank J, Stott A, Brice J: The urinary catecholamine and plasma cortisol levels in patients with subarachnoid haemorrhage. *J Neurol Sci* 22:375–382, 1974.
31. Rosner MJ, Newsome HH, Becker DP: Mechanical brain injury: The sympathoadrenal response. *J Neurosurg* 61:76–86, 1984.
32. Schulte am Esch J, Murday H, Pfeifer G: Haemody-

namic changes in patients with severe head injury. *Acta Neurochir (Wien)* 54:243–250, 1980.
33. Cruickshank JM, Neil DG, Hayes Y, et al: Stress/catecholamine-induced cardiac necrosis: Reduction by beta 1-selective blockade. *Postgrad Med* 83:140–147, 1988.
34. North JB, Penhall RK, Hanieh A, et al: Phenytoin and postoperative epilepsy: A double-blind study. *J Neurosurg* 58:672–677, 1983.
35. Temkin NR, Dikmen SS, Wilensky AJ, et al: A randomized, double-blind study of phenytoin for the prevention of post-traumatic seizures. *N Engl J Med* 323:497–502, 1990.
36. Young B, Rapp RP, Norton JA, et al: Failure of prophylactically administered phenytoin to prevent late post-traumatic seizures. *J Neurosurg* 58:236–241, 1983.
37. Durward QJ, Amacher AL, DelMaestro RF, Sibbald WJ: Cerebral and cardiovascular responses to changes in head elevation with intracranial hypertension. *J Neurosurg* 59:938–944, 1983.
38. Feldman Z, Kanter MJ, Robertson CS, et al: Effect of head elevation on intracranial pressure, cerebral perfusion pressure, and cerebral blood flow in head-injured patients. *J Neurosurg* 76:207–211, 1992.
39. Hulme A, Cooper R: The effects of head position and jugular vein compression on intracranial pressure, in Beks J, Bosch DA, Brock M (eds): *Intracranial Pressure III.* Berlin: Springer-Verlag, 1976:259–263.
40. Ropper AH, O'Rourke D, Kennedy SK: Head position, intracranial pressure and compliance. *J Neurol* 32:881–886, 1982.
41. Shapiro HM: Intracranial hypertension: Therapeutic and anesthetic considerations. *Anesthesiology* 43:445–471, 1975.
42. Rosner MJ, Coley IB: Cerebral perfusion pressure, intracranial pressure, and head elevation. *J Neurosurg* 60:636–641, 1986.
43. Hsiang J, Chesnut RM, Crisp CB, et al: Early, routine paralysis for ICP control in severe head injury: Is it necessary? in (eds): *J Crit Care Med* vol 22:471–76; *Proceedings of the Second International Neurotrauma Symposium,* Glasgow, 1993:O75.
44. Segredo V, Caldwell JE, Matthay MA, et al: Persistent paralysis in critically ill patients after long-term administration of vecuronium. *N Engl J Med* 327:524–528, 1992.
45. Partridge BL, Abrams JH, Bazemore C, Rubin R: Prolonged neuromuscular blockade after long-term infusion of vecuronium bromide in the intensive care unit. *Crit Care Med* 18:1177–1179, 1990.
46. Krumholz W, Kabisch S, Biscoping J: The effect of pancuronium bromide on polymorphonuclear neutrophil adherence in vitro. *Anaesthesist* 37:246–248, 1988.
47. Bardosi L, Bardosi A, Gabius AJ: Changes of expression of endogenous sugar receptors by polymorphonuclear leukocytes after prolonged anaesthesia and surgery. *Can J Anaesth* 39:143–150, 1992.
48. Marion DW, Bouma GJ: The use of stable xenon-enhanced computed tomographic studies of cerebral blood flow to define changes in cerebral carbon dioxide vasoresponsivity caused by a severe head injury. *Neurosurgery* 29:869–873, 1991.
49. Muizelaar JP, Marmarou A, Ward JD, et al: Adverse effects of prolonged hyperventilation in patients with severe head injury: A randomized clinical trial. *J Neurosurg* 75:731–739, 1991.
50. Bouma GJ, Muizelaar JP: Cerebral blood flow, cerebral blood volume, and cerebrovascular reactivity after severe head injury. *J Neurotrauma* 1:S333–348, 1992.
51. Obrist WD, Langfitt TW, Jaggi JL, et al: Cerebral blood flow and metabolism in comatose patients with acute head injury: Relationship to intracranial hypertension. *J Neurosurg* 61:241–253, 1984.
52. Overgaard J, Tweed WA: Cerebral circulation after head injury: I. Cerebral blood flow and its regulation after closed head injury with emphasis on clinical correlations. *J Neurosurg* 41:531–541, 1974.
53. Nordstrom CH, Messeter K, Sundbarg G, et al: Cerebral blood flow, vasoreactivity, and oxygen consumption during barbiturate therapy in severe traumatic brain lesions. *J Neurosurg* 68:424–431, 1988.
54. Messeter K, Nordstrom CH, Sundbarg G, et al: Cerebral hemodynamics in patients with acute severe head trauma. *J Neurosurg* 64:231–237, 1986.
55. Enevoldsen EM, Jensen FT: Autoregulation and CO_2-responses of cerebral blood flow in patients with acute severe head injury. *J Neurosurg* 48:689–703, 1978.
56. Cruz J, Raps EC, Hoffstad OJ, et al: Cerebral oxygenation monitoring. *Crit Care Med* 21:1242–1246, 1993.
57. Cruz J, Gennarelli TA, Hoffstad OJ: Lack of relevance of the Bohr effect in optimally ventilated patients with acute brain trauma. *J Trauma* 33:304–310, 1992.
58. Havill JH: Prolonged hyperventilation and intracranial pressure. *Crit Care Med* 12:72–74, 1984.
59. Van der Poel H: Cerebral vasoconstriction is not maintained with prolonged hyperventilation, in Hoff JT, Betz AL (eds): *Intracranial Pressure VII.* Berlin: Springer-Verlag, 1989:899–903.
60. Cruz J: Continuous versus serial global cerebral hemometabolic monitoring: Applications in acute brain trauma. *Acta Neurochir [Suppl] (Wien)* 42:35–39, 1988.
61. Sheinberg M, Kanter MJ, Robertson CS, et al: Continuous monitoring of jugular venous oxygen saturation in head-injured patients. *J Neurosurg* 76:212–217, 1992.
62. Nath F, Galbraith S: The effect of mannitol on cerebral white matter water content. *J Neurosurg* 65:41–43, 1986.
63. Bell BA, Smith MA, Kean CM, et al: Brain water measured by magnetic resonance imaging. *Lancet* 1:66, 1987.
64. Muizelaar JP, Wei EP, Kontos HA, et al: Mannitol causes compensatory cerebral vasoconstriction and vasodilatation in response to blood viscosity changes. *J Neurosurg* 59:822–828, 1983.
65. Stuart F, Torres E, Fletcher R, et al: Effects of single, repeated, and massive mannitol infusion in the dog: Structural and functional changes in kidney and brain. *Ann Surg* 172:190–204, 1970.
66. Kaufmann AM, Cardoso ER: Aggravation of vasogenic cerebral edema by multiple-dose mannitol. *J Neurosurg* 77:584–589, 1992.
67. Wise B, Perkins R, Stevenson E, Scott K: Penetration of 14C-labelled mannitol from serum into cerebrospinal fluid and brain. *Exp Neurol* 10:264–270, 1964.
68. Marshall LF, Smith RW, Raucher LA, Shapiro HM:

Mannitol dose requirements in brain-injured patients. *J Neurosurg* 48:169–172, 1978.

69. Levin A: Treatment of increased intracranial pressure: A comparison of different hyperosmotic agents and the use of thiopental, in *Proceedings of the American Association of Neurological Surgeons Annual Meeting,* p 174 New Orleans, 1978.
70. Wilkinson HA, Rosenfeld SR: Furosemide and mannitol in the treatment of acute experimental intracranial hypertension. *Neurosurgery* 12:405–410, 1983.
71. Pollay M, Fullenwider C, Roberts PA, Stevens FA: Effect of mannitol and furosemide on blood-brain osmotic gradient and intracranial pressure. *J Neurosurg* 59:945–950, 1983.
72. Piper IR, Dearden NM, Miller JD: Can waveform analysis of ICP separate vascular from non-vascular causes of intracranial hypertension, in Hoff JT, Betz AL (eds): *Intracranial Pressure VII.* Berlin: Springer-Verlag, 1989:157–163.
73. Piper IR, Dearden NM, Leggate JRS, Miller JD: Methodology of spectral analysis of the intracranial pressure waveform in a head injury intensive care unit, in Hoff JT, Betz AL (eds): *Intracranial Pressure VII.* Berlin: Springer-Verlag, 1989:668–671.
74. Cooper P, Moody S, Clark W, et al: Dexamethasone and severe head injury: A prospective double blind study. *J Neurosurg* 51:307–316, 1979.
75. Dearden NM, Gibson JS, McDowal DG, et al: Effect of high-dose dexamethasone on outcome from severe head injury. *J Neurosurg* 64:81–88, 1986.
76. Gudeman S, Miller J, Becker D: Failure of high-dose steroid therapy to influence intracranial pressure in patients with severe head injury. *J Neurosurg* 51:301–306, 1979.
77. Marshall L, King J, Langfitt T: The complications of high-dose corticosteroid therapy in neurosurgical patients: A prospective study. *Ann Neurol* 1:201–203, 1977.
78. Miller J, Leech P: Effects of mannitol and steroid therapy on intracranial volume pressure relationships in patients. *J Neurosurg* 42:275–281, 1975.
79. Pitts E, Katkis J: Effects of megadose steroids on ICP in traumatic coma, in Shulman K, Marmarou A, Miller A (eds): *Intracranial Pressure IV.* New York: Springer-Verlag, 1972:638–642.
80. Saul T, Ducker T, Saleman M, Carro E: Steroids in severe head injury: A prospective, randomized clinical trial. *J Neurosurg* 54:596–600, 1981.
81. Hall ED, Yonkers PA, Andrus PK, et al: Biochemistry and pharmacology of lipid antioxidants in acute brain and spinal cord injury. *J Neurotrauma* 2:S425–442, 1992.
82. Hall ED, Braughler JM, McCall JM: Antioxidant effects in brain and spinal cord injury. *J Neurotrauma* 1:S165–172, 1992.
83. Kaufman HH, Moake JL, Olson JD, et al: Delayed and recurrent intracranial hematomas related to disseminated intravascular clotting and fibrinolysis in head injury. *Neurosurgery* 7:445–449, 1980.
84. Luerssen TG, Chesnut RM, Van Berkum-Clark M, et al: Post traumatic cerebrospinal fluid infections in the Traumatic Coma Data Bank: The influence of type and management of ICP monitors, in Avezaat CJJ, van Eijndhoven JHM, Maas AIR, et al (eds): *Intracranial Pressure VIII.* New York: Springer-Verlag, 1993:42–45.
85. Mayhall CG, Archer NH, Lamb VA, et al: Ventriculostomy-related infections: A prospective epidemiologic study. *N Engl J Med* 310:553–559, 1984.
86. Eisenberg H, Frankowski R, Contant C, et al: The Comprehensive Central Nervous System Trauma Centers: High-dose barbiturate control of elevated intracranial pressure in patients with severe head injury. *J Neurosurg* 69:15–23, 1988.
87. Marshall L, Smith R, Shapiro H: The outcome with aggressive treatment in severe head injuries: Acute and chronic barbiturate administration in the management of head injury. *J Neurosurg* 50:26–30, 1979.
88. Rea G, Rockswold G: Barbiturate therapy in uncontrolled intracranial hypertension. *Neurosurgery* 12:401–404, 1983.
89. Rockoff M, Marshall L, Shapiro M: High-dose barbiturate therapy in humans: A clinical review of 60 patients. *Ann Neurol* 6:194–199, 1979.
90. Shapiro HM, Galindo A, Wyte SR, Harris AB: Rapid intraoperative reduction of intracranial pressure with thiopentone. *Br J Anaesth* 45:1057–1062, 1973.
91. Schwartz M, Tator C, Towed D, et al: The University of Toronto Head Injury Treatment Study: A prospective, randomized comparison of pentobarbital and mannitol. *Can J Neurol Sci* 11:434–440, 1984.
92. Ward J, Becker D, Miller J, Choi S, et al: Failure of prophylactic barbiturate coma in the treatment of severe head injury. *J Neurosurg* 62:383–388, 1985.
93. Smith DS, Rehncrona S, Siesjo BK: Barbiturates as protective agents in brain ischemia and as free radical scavengers in vitro. *Acta Physiol Scand [Suppl]* 492:129–134, 1980.
94. Majewska MD, Strosznajder J, Lazarewicz J: Effect of ischemic anoxia and barbiturate anesthesia on free radical oxidation of mitochondrial phospholipids. *Brain Res* 158:423–434, 1978.
95. Lafferty JJ, Keykhah MM, Shapiro HM, et al: Cerebral hypometabolism obtained with deep pentobarbital anesthesia and hypothermia (30 C). *Anesthesiology* 49:159–164, 1978.
96. Michenfelder JD: The interdependency of cerebral functional and metabolic effects following massive doses of thiopental in the dog. *Anesthesiology* 41:231–236, 1974.
97. Pierce E, Lambertsen C, Deutsch S: Cerebral circulation and metabolism during thiopental anesthesia and hyperventilation in man. *J Clin Invest* 41:1664–1671, 1962.
98. Flamm ES, Demopoulos HB, Seligman ML, Ransohoff J: Possible molecular mechanisms of barbiturate-mediated protection in regional cerebral ischemia. *Acta Neurol Scand [Suppl]* 64:150–151, 1977.
99. Walker DAJ, Isley MR, Lucas WJ, Kafer ER: Cerebral blood flow velocity is coupled to EEG activity during hypothermic cardiopulmonary bypass. *Anesthesiology* 75:A177, 1991.
100. Astrup J, Sørensen PM, Sørensen HR: Inhibition of cerebral oxygen and glucose consumption in the dog

by hypothermia, pentobarbital, and lidocaine. *Anesthesiology* 55:263–268, 1981.
101. Evans DE, Kobrine AI: Reduction of experimental intracranial hypertension by lidocaine. *Neurosurgery* 20:542–547, 1987.
102. Rasool N, Faroqui M, Rubinstein EH: Lidocaine accelerates neuroelectrical recovery after incomplete global ischemia in rabbits. *Stroke* 21:929–935, 1990.
103. Donegan MF, Bedford RF: Intravenously administered lidocaine prevents intracranial hypertension during endotracheal suctioning. *Anesthesiology* 52:516–518, 1980.
104. Bedford RF, Persing JA, Pobereskin L, Butler A: Lidocaine or thiopental for rapid control of intracranial hypertension? *Anesth Analg* 59:435–437, 1980.
105. White PF, Schlobohm RM, Pitts LH, Lindauer JM: A randomized study of drugs for preventing increases in intracranial pressure during endotracheal suctioning. *Anesthesiology* 57:242–244, 1982.
106. Yano M, Nishiyama H, Yokota H, et al: Effect of lidocaine on ICP response to endotracheal suctioning. *Anesthesiology* 64:651–653, 1986.
107. Van Hemelrijck J, Van AH, Plets C, et al: The effects of propofol on intracranial pressure and cerebral perfusion pressure in patients with brain tumors. *Acta Anaesthesiol Belg* 40:95–100, 1989.
108. Weinstabl C, Mayer N, Hammerle AF, Spiss CK: Effekte von Propofolbolusgaben auf das intrakranielle Druckverhalten beim Schadel-Hirn-Trauma. *Anaesthesist* 39:521–524, 1990.
109. Pinaud M, Lelausque JN, Chetanneau A, et al: Effects of propofol on cerebral hemodynamics and metabolism in patients with brain trauma. *Anesthesiology* 73:404–409, 1990.
110. Merlo F, Demo P, Lacquaniti L, et al: Il propofol in singolo bolo nel trattamento della ipertensione endocranica. *Minerva Anestesiol* 57:359–363, 1991.
111. Herregods L, Verbeke J, Rolly G, Colardyn F: Effect of propofol on elevated intracranial pressure: Preliminary results. *Anaesthesia* 43:107–109, 1988.
112. Hartung HJ: Intrakranielles Druckverhalten bei Patienten mit Schadel-Hirn-Trauma nach Propofol-bzw. Thiopental-Applikation. *Anaesthesist* 36:285–287, 1987.
113. Dearden NM, McDowall DG: Comparison of etomidate and althesin in the reduction of increased intracranial pressure after head injury. *Br J Anaesth* 57:361–368, 1985.
114. Moss E, Powell D, Gibson RM, McDowall DG: The effect of etomidate on intracranial pressure and cerebral perfusion pressure. *Br J Anaesth* 51:347–352, 1979.
115. Moss E, Gibson JS, McDowal DG, Gibson RM: Intensive management of severe head injuries. *Anaesthesia* 38:214–225, 1983.
116. Prior JG, Hinds CJ, Williams J, Prior PF: The use of etomidate in the management of severe head injury. *Intensive Care Med* 9:313–320, 1983.
117. Bingham RM, Procaccio F, Prior PF, Hinds CJ: Cerebral electrical activity influences the effects of etomidate on cerebral perfusion pressure in traumatic coma. *Br J Anaesth* 57:843–848, 1985.
118. Krugler J, Doenicke A, Laub M: The EEG after etomidate, in Doenicke A (ed): *Etomidate.* Berlin: Springer-Verlag, 1977:31–48.
119. Modica PA, Tempelhoff R: Intracranial pressure during induction of anaesthesia and tracheal intubation with etomidate-induced EEG burst suppression. *Can J Anaesth* 39:236–241, 1992.
120. Renou AM, Vernheit J, Macrez P, et al: Cerebral blood flow and metabolism during etomidate anaesthesia in man. *Br J Anaesth* 50:1047–1051, 1978.
121. Schulte am Esch J, Pfeifer G, Thiemig I, Entzian W: The influence of intravenous anaesthetic agents on primarily increased intracranial pressure. *Acta Neurochir (Wien)* 45:15–25, 1978.
122. Ledingham IM, Watt I: Influence of sedation on mortality in critically ill multiple trauma patients (letter). *Lancet 1*:1270, 1983.
123. Allolio B, Stuttmann R, Fischer H, et al: Long-term etomidate and adrenocortical suppression (letter). *Lancet* 2:626, 1983.
124. Fellows IW, Byrne AJ, Allison SP: Adrenocortical suppression with etomidate (letter). *Lancet* 2:54–55, 1983.
125. Fellows IW, Bastow MD, Byrne AJ, Allison SP: Adrenocortical suppression in multiply injured patients: A complication of etomidate treatment. *Br Med J [Clin Res]* 287:1835–1837, 1983.
126. Fellows IW, Yeoman PM, Selby C, Byrne AJ: The effect of anaesthetic induction with etomidate on the endocrine response to surgical trauma. *Eur J Anaesthesiol* 2:285–290, 1985.
127. Wagner RL, White PF, Kan PB, et al: Inhibition of adrenal steroidogenesis by the anesthetic etomidate. *N Engl J Med* 310:1415–1421, 1984.
128. Miranda DR, Stoutenbeek CP: Etomidate in the intensive care unit (letter). *Lancet* 2:684–685, 1983.
129. Artru F, Chacornac R, Deleuze R: Hyperbaric oxygenation for severe head injuries: Preliminary results of a controlled study. *Eur Neurol* 14:310–318, 1976.
130. Sukoff MH, Ragatz RE: Hyperbaric oxygenation for the treatment of acute cerebral edema. *Neurosurgery* 10:29–38, 1982.
131. Brown JA, Preul MC, Taha A: Hyperbaric oxygen in the treatment of elevated intracranial pressure after head injury. *Pediatr Neurosci* 14:286–290, 1988.
132. Holbach KH, Schroder FK, Datene G, Dohr H: Hyperbaric oxygenation: A treatment in neurosurgery. *J Neurol Neurosurg Psychiatry* 33:717, 1970.
133. Moody RA, Mead CO, Ruamsuke S, Mullan S: Therapeutic value of oxygen at normal and hyperbaric pressure in experimental head injury. *J Neurosurg* 32:51–54, 1970.
134. Rockswold GL, Ford SE, Anderson DC, et al: Results of a prospective randomized trial for treatment of severely brain-injured patients with hyperbaric oxygen. *J Neurosurg* 76:929–934, 1992.
135. Mogami H, Hayakawa T, Kanai N, et al: Clinical application of hyperbaric oxygenation in the treatment of acute cerebral damage. *J Neurosurg* 31:636–643, 1969.
136. Gower DJ, Lee KS, McWhorter JM: Role of subtemporal decompression in severe closed head injury. *Neurosurgery* 23:417–422, 1988.

137. Ransohoff J, Benjamin MV, Gage ELJ, Epstein F: Hemicraniectomy in the management of acute subdural hematoma. *J Neurosurg* 34:70–76, 1971.
138. Kondziolka D, Fazl M: Functional recovery after decompressive craniectomy for cerebral infarction. *Neurosurgery* 23:143–147, 1988.
139. Delashaw JB, Broaddus WC, Kassell NF, et al: Treatment of right hemispheric cerebral infarction by hemicraniectomy. *Stroke* 21:874–881, 1990.
140. Rengachary SS, Batnitzky S, Morantz RA, et al: Hemicraniectomy for acute massive cerebral infarction. *Neurosurgery* 8:321–328, 1981.
141. Dierssen G, Carda R, Coca JM: The influence of large decompressive craniectomy on the outcome of surgical treatment in spontaneous intracerebral haematomas. *Acta Neurochir (Wien)* 69:53–60, 1983.
142. Ausman JI, Rogers C, Sharp HL: Decompressive craniectomy for the encephalopathy of Reye's syndrome. *Surg Neurol* 6:97–99, 1976.
143. Miyata I, Tsuno K, Masaoka T, et al: Effect of external decompression on the development of delayed ischemic neurological deficits after subarachnoid hemorrhage. *Neurol Med Chir (Tokyo)* 29:735–739, 1989.
144. Venes JL, Collins WF: Bifrontal decompressive craniectomy in the management of head trauma. *J Neurosurg* 42:429–433, 1975.
145. Cooper PR, Rovit RL, Ransohoff J: Hemicraniectomy in the treatment of acute subdural hematoma: A reappraisal. *Surg Neurol* 5:25–28, 1976.
146. Gaab MR, Rittierodt M, Lorenz M, Heissler HE: Traumatic brain swelling and operative decompression: A prospective investigation. *Acta Neurochir [Suppl] (Wien)* 51:326–328, 1990.
147. Cooper PR, Hagler H, Clark WK, Barnett P: Enhancement of experimental cerebral edema after decompressive craniectomy: Implications for the management of severe head injuries. *Neurosurgery* 4:296–300, 1979.
148. Rinaldi A, Mangiola A, Anile C, et al: Hemodynamic effects of decompressive craniectomy in cold induced brain oedema. *Acta Neurochir [Suppl] (Wien)* 51:394–396, 1990.
149. Yamaura A, Sato M, Meguro K, et al: Cranioplasty following decompressive craniectomy—analysis of 300 cases (author's transl). *No Shinkei Geka* 5:345–353, 1977.
150. Simonetti G, Fiume D, Di BA, et al: Complicanze di ampie craniectomie decompressive: Caso clinico. *Riv Neurol* 56:14–18, 1986.
151. Tabaddor K, LaMorgese J: Complication of a large cranial defect: Case report. *J Neurosurg* 44:506–508, 1976.
152. Lindegaard KF, Nornes H, Bakke SJ, et al: Cerebral vasospasm after subarachnoid haemorrhage investigated by means of transcranial Doppler ultrasound. *Acta Neurochir [Suppl] (Wien)* 42:81–84, 1988.
153. Aaslid R, Markwalder TM, Nornes H: Noninvasive transcranial Doppler ultrasound recording of flow velocity in basal cerebral arteries. *J Neurosurg* 57:769–774, 1982.
154. Weber M, Grolimund P, Seiler RW: Evaluation of posttraumatic cerebral blood flow velocities by transcranial Doppler ultrasonography. *Neurosurgery* 27:106–112, 1990.
155. Rozsa L, Gombi R, Szabo S, Sztermen M: Vasospasm after head injury studied by transcranial Doppler sonography. *Radiol Diagn (Berl)* 30:151–157, 1989.
156. Martin NA, Doberstein C, Zane C, et al: Posttraumatic cerebral arterial spasm: Transcranial Doppler ultrasound, cerebral blood flow, and angiographic findings. *J Neurosurg* 77:575–583, 1992.
157. Gomez CR, Backer RJ, Bucholz RD: Transcranial Doppler ultrasound following closed head injury: Vasospasm or vasoparalysis? *Surg Neurol* 35:30–35, 1991.
158. Compton JS, Teddy PJ: Cerebral arterial vasospasm following severe head injury: A transcranial Doppler study. *Br J Neurosurg* 1:435–439, 1987.
159. Seiler RW, Grolimund P, Aaslid R, et al: Cerebral vasospasm evaluated by transcranial ultrasound correlated with clinical grade and CT-visualized subarachnoid hemorrhage. *J Neurosurg* 64:594–600, 1986.
160. Aaslid R, Huber P, Nornes H: A transcranial Doppler method in the evaluation of cerebrovascular spasm. *Neuroradiology* 28:11–16, 1986.
161. Grosset DG, Straiton J, du TM, Bullock R: Prediction of symptomatic vasospasm after subarachnoid hemorrhage by rapidly increasing transcranial Doppler velocity and cerebral blood flow changes. *Stroke* 23:674–679, 1992.
162. Marshall LF, Bruce DA, Bruno L, Langfitt TW: Vertebrobasilar spasm: A significant cause of neurological deficit in head injury. *J Neurosurg* 48:560–564, 1978.
163. Muizelaar JP, Marmarou A, DeSalles AA, et al: Cerebral blood flow and metabolism in severely head-injured children: I. Relationship with GCS score, outcome, ICP, and PVI. *J Neurosurg* 71:63–71, 1989.
164. Obrist WD, Gennarelli TA, Segawa H, et al: Relation of cerebral blood flow to neurological status and outcome in head-injured patients. *J Neurosurg* 51:292–300, 1979.
165. Cruz J, Miner ME, Allen SJ, et al: Continuous monitoring of cerebral oxygenation in acute brain injury: Assessment of cerebral hemodynamic reserve. *Neurosurgery* 29:743–749, 1991.
166. Cruz J, Gennarelli TA, Alves WM: Continuous monitoring of cerebral oxygenation in acute brain injury: Multivariate assessment of severe intracranial "plateau" wave—case report. *J Trauma* 32:401–403, 1992.
167. Gibbs EL, Lennox WG, Nims LF, et al: Arterial and cerebral venous blood: Arterial-venous differences in man. *J Biol Chem* 144:325–332, 1942.
168. Cruz J: Brain ischemia in head injury (letter). *J Neurosurg* 78:522–523, 1993.
169. Bouma GJ, Muizelaar JP, Bandoh K, Marmarou A: Blood pressure and intracranial pressure-volume dynamics in severe head injury: Relationship with cerebral blood flow. *J Neurosurg* 77:15–19, 1992.
170. Rosner MJ, Becker DP: Origin and evolution of plateau waves: Experimental observations and a theoretical model. *J Neurosurg* 60:312–319, 1984.
171. Rosner MJ, Daughton S: Cerebral perfusion pressure management in head injury. *J Trauma* 30:933–940, 1990.

CHAPTER 33

XENON TECHNIQUES FOR CBF MEASUREMENT IN CLINICAL HEAD INJURY

Walter D. Obrist
Donald W. Marion

SYNOPSIS

The theoretical and practical aspects of cerebral blood flow (CBF) measurement by three Xenon-based methods have been described. These are the intracarotid ^{133}Xe method, the noninvasive (inhalation or intravenous) ^{133}Xe method, and the stable (nonradioactive) xenon-CT method. The advantages and limitations of each are discussed and the clinical experience with each is reviewed, with particular emphasis on the study of head injury.

INTRODUCTION

Cerebral blood flow (CBF) is generally considered an important pathophysiological factor in acute brain trauma, alterations of which may contribute to secondary brain damage. Impetus has been given to CBF measurement in head-injured patients because of its potential prognostic and therapeutic relevance. Among the several techniques available for clinical research, the most widely used involve the administration of xenon gas, either in its radioactive or stable forms. The present chapter concerns three of these CBF methods: (1) the intracarotid ^{133}Xe injection technique; (2) the "noninvasive" ^{133}Xe technique (inhalation or IV injection); and (3) the stable xenon-computed tomography method (Xe/CT).

CBF measurement with either radioactive or stable xenon is based on the same principle as the pioneer nitrous oxide method of Kety and Schmidt[1]; namely, that the rate of uptake and clearance of an inert diffusible gas is proportional to blood flow in the tissue. Whereas the nitrous oxide technique yields global estimates of cerebral flood flow, based on the concentration of gas in arterial and jugular venous blood, the use of a radioactive tracer or transmission tomography permits external monitoring of tissue concentration, thus providing estimates for particular brain regions.

The first systematic studies of cerebral blood flow in human head injury were performed in the early 1970s by the intracarotid (IC) technique,[2] using multiple extracranial detectors. Carried out in conjunction with carotid angiography—widely practiced at the time—this method provided a wealth of new pathophysiological information that served to stimulate and guide subsequent research.

Because of its invasiveness and the declining use of carotid angiography, the IC method was soon replaced by less invasive routes of ^{133}Xe administration, i.e., inhalation or intravenous injection.[3] The majority of CBF head injury studies published to date have utilized this noninvasive approach which, because of its portability and repeatability, is especially suited to use in the intensive care unit.

The desire for higher spatial resolution, particularly in deep brain structures, has prompted employment of the Xe/CT method[4] in recent head injury studies. This technique has the distinct advantage of permitting direct morphological/blood flow correlations in the same tomographic image.

The following sections describe and compare the methodology of the several xenon techniques, and briefly discuss the clinical research findings of each.

INTRACAROTID ^{133}Xe METHOD

Methodology

This technique, introduced by Lassen and Ingvar,[2] involves a bolus injection of ^{133}Xe/saline into one internal carotid artery. Extracranial monitoring of gamma radiation is performed by multiple collimated detectors placed over the injected hemisphere.[2,5–7] As shown in Fig. 33-1 (upper graph), a rapid rise in count rate is seen as the bolus enters the brain, followed by a slower decline over the next 10 min as the isotope clears. Little recirculation of ^{133}Xe occurs because the cerebral venous blood is diluted by isotope-free blood from the rest of the body, and because of efficient elimination of the gas by the lungs. Quantitative analysis of the resulting clearance curves assumes that CBF does not change during the 10 to 15 min measurement interval, i.e., a steady state prevails.

Calculation of cerebral blood flow is based on equations derived from the mass balance relationship, as presented in detail elsewhere.[8] Estimates of mean blood flow in the tissue "seen" by a detector are obtained from the height-over-area formula, where the initial height of the clearance curve is divided by the area under it, i.e., the integral from time zero (injection) to infinity.[2,5] Extrapolation to infinity can be avoided by integrating the curve to the end of recording (10–15 min), with a corresponding adjustment of its height. Fig. 33-1 illustrates this computational procedure.

Because the brain contains two tissues, gray and white matter, that have distinctly different clearance rates, it is possible to perform a biexponential analysis in which separate estimates of flow are obtained for the fast (gray) and slow (white) clearing compartments.[5] An alternative approach for estimating gray matter flow is to determine the initial slope of the curve, which over the first minute is dominated by the fast clearing compartment and approximates a single exponential.[2] This procedure is also illustrated in Fig. 33-1.

Owing to the difficulty of separating fast and slow tissue compartments, especially in pathological conditions, the more reliable height-over-area method has generally been used in preference to biexponential analysis.[9] Height-over-area estimates of CBF are in excellent agreement with those obtained by the Kety-Schmidt technique, yielding comparable normal values of 50 ml/100 g/min.[5,6]

Clinical Research Findings

The intracarotid ^{133}Xe method was the primary CBF technique in head injury research during the 1970s. Performed only during angiography, the studies were necessarily limited in their sample size, and in the timing and frequency of examinations. Anatomic correlations were difficult to make in the absence of morphological brain imaging which was not available at the time, and because CBF measurements were usually confined to one hemisphere. In spite of these limitations, considerable data were collected that established the importance of cere-

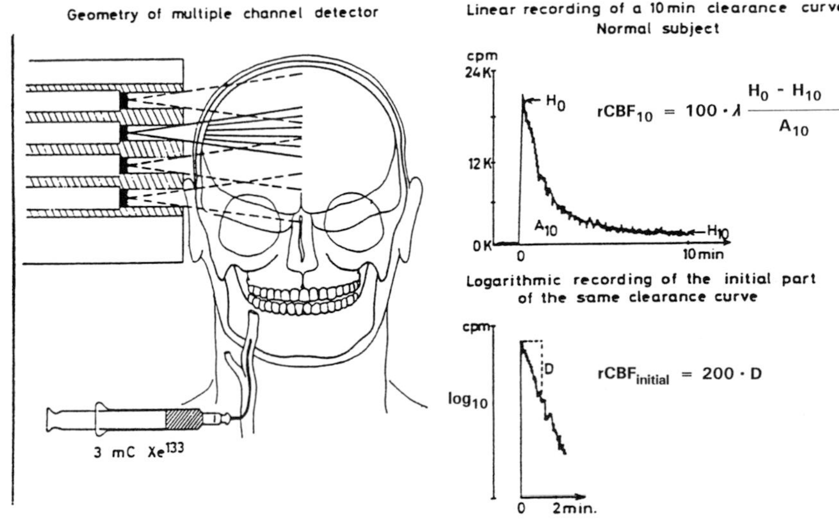

Figure 33-1. *Left:* Collimated scintillation detectors placed over the hemisphere ipsilateral to a ^{133}Xe carotid injection. *Right upper:* Clearance curve showing the height-over-area calculation. λ = brain-blood partition coefficient for ^{133}Xe, H_0 = initial height, H_{10} = ordinate value at 10 min, A_{10} = area under the curve from time 0 to 10 min. *Right lower:* Logarithmic recording showing the initial slope calculation. The linear decrease over the first minute is multiplied by 200, a constant representing 100 times the product of λ, the assumed gray matter partition coefficient (0.87), and the factor for converting base 10 to natural logarithms. (From McHenry,[7] modified with permission.)

bral circulatory disturbances in acute brain trauma. Of particular interest was the ability to obtain regional as well as global CBF information, and to correlate the findings with cerebral metabolic rate for oxygen (CMR_{O_2}), calculated as the product of mean hemispheric CBF and the arteriojugular venous O_2 difference (AVD_{O_2}).

Variations in CBF level

A frequent observation was the wide variation in blood flow, ranging from subnormal to supernormal levels, during the acute phase of severe head injury.[10–13] This variability contrasted with the consistently low CMR_{O_2} found in such patients,[10,14–16] suggesting that the lower flows were coupled with depressed metabolism, while the higher flows were uncoupled.[15] Indeed, Lassen[17] introduced the concept of "luxury perfusion" (high flow relative to metabolic need), based in part on observations in acute head injury.

Attention was given to the occurrence of a very low CBF (<20 ml/100 g/min) that might indicate cerebral ischemia and contribute to secondary neurological deterioration. Some authors argued[10,13] that globally reduced blood flow simply reflects a low cerebral metabolism, as found in patients with diffuse hypoxic/ischemic insult[18] and/or chronic coma.[19] On the other hand, an association of poor outcome with marked CBF reductions in the early hours posttrauma suggested the possibility of ischemia.[12]

Unlike previous inconclusive studies involving only a few detectors,[10,11] those of Overgaard and coworkers[20] obtained significant regional information, based on 35 detectors over the injected hemisphere. Fourteen of 23 patients who died or remained in persistent coma had focal decreases in the early hours postinjury (the majority <17 ml/100 g/min), compared with only 4 of 40 cases who recovered consciousness. These foci were primarily in arterial boundary-zone regions.[21] As the authors noted, in the absence of regional metabolic data, the occurrence of focal CBF reductions cannot prove the existence of ongoing ischemia. Such foci may simply reflect the reduced flow of already severely damaged tissue. Even with the later development of more sophisticated technology, this important issue remains largely unresolved.

Normal or supernormal CBF in the presence of coma, designated as hyperemia, was first observed with the IC method.[17] Hyperemia usually appeared on the second or third days postinjury,[11] in contrast to the reduced flow found in the first 24 hours.[12] It was associated with early filling veins on angiography,[13] elevated jugular P_{O_2},[16] and increased intracranial pressure (ICP).[11] Moderate global hyperemia was not incompatible with recovery, but marked CBF elevations were considered a poor prognostic sign.[11,12]

Based on compartmental analysis of the initial portion of the clearance curve,[22,23] Enevoldsen et al.[13] identified a very fast clearing component in areas adjacent to contusions and previously evacuated hematomas. This "tissue-peak hyperemia" suggested compensatory vasodilation in the vicinity of ongoing or just-preceding local ischemia. The occurrence of these high-flow regions paralleled the patient's clinical course, such that they increased in extent with deterioration and decreased with improvement.

The first CBF measurements in brain death were made by the intracarotid technique.[24] Although not practical for the diagnosis of this condition,[18] they can provide useful prognostic information in head-injured patients with "impending brain death." In the presence of normal perfusion pressure, extremely low blood flows of 5 to 10 ml/100 g/min have been recorded that are incompatible with cerebral survival.[25]

Autoregulation and CO_2 reactivity

At the time of these early studies, there was considerable interest in mechanisms regulating the cerebral circulation, impairment of which was considered an important factor in the pathophysiology of acute head injury. Both systemic arterial pressure and arterial P_{CO_2} were manipulated as a means of testing, respectively, CBF autoregulation and CO_2 reactivity.

Autoregulation was regarded as defective when a significant CBF change could be induced by >20 percent alteration of cerebral perfusion pressure (mean arterial pressure minus ICP). Over half of severely head injured patients showed defective autoregulation during the acute phase,[10–12] a finding that was not related to prognosis. Beyond 5 days postinjury, however, autoregulation returned to normal. Impairment during the acute phase argued for maintenance of normal perfusion pressure as a means of avoiding cerebral ischemia or severe hyperemia.[11,12,26]

Regional impairment of autoregulation was found in a high proportion of cases.[26] Induced hypertension evoked or augmented focal hyperemia in the vicinity of contusions.[13] Figure 33-2 illustrates such a regional response, observed by Bruce and coworkers.[10] Following a 33 mmHg increase in perfusion pressure, the detector adjacent to a temporal lobe contusion revealed a 40 percent CBF increase, indicating defective autoregulation. Other regions showed normal autoregulatory responses, i.e., no significant CBF change. Figure 33-2 also illustrates the effect of intravenous mannitol, found to produce a general augmentation of flow in 11 of 14 cases. The greater CBF response shown in the temporal

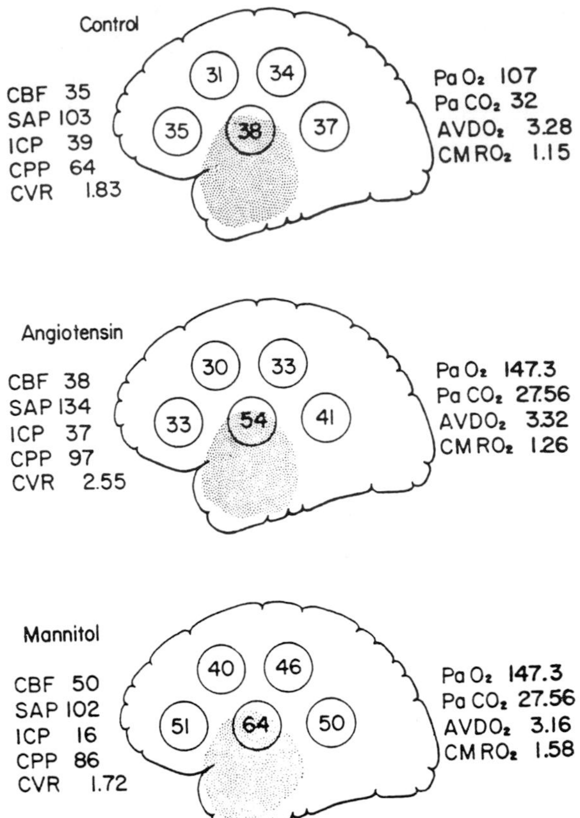

Figure 33-2. Regional cerebral blood flow (ml/100 g/min) from the left hemisphere of a patient one day after head injury resulting in a temporal lobe contusion. *Shaded area* indicates location of the lesion. *Top,* baseline values; *middle,* during angiotensin-induced blood pressure increase; *bottom,* after intravenous mannitol. CBF = cerebral blood flow, SAP = systemic arterial pressure, ICP = intracranial pressure, CPP = cerebral perfusion pressure, CVR = cerebral vascular resistance, Pa_{O_2} and Pa_{CO_2} = arterial oxygen and carbon dioxide tensions, AVD_{O_2} = cerebral arteriovenous oxygen difference, CMR_{O_2} = cerebral metabolic rate for oxygen. (From Bruce et al,[10] with permission.)

lobe is consistent with the increased perfusion pressure and loss of autoregulation in that region. This is one of the early human CBF studies on mannitol.

Normal CO_2 reactivity is approximately 3 percent CBF change per mmHg change in arterial P_{CO_2}. Most studies agreed that CBF responsiveness is preserved following severe brain injury.[11–13,27] Although reactivity may be lower in the first days posttrauma, especially in deeply comatose patients,[27,28] it usually returns to normal within a week.[11,12,27] The magnitude of response has little prognostic value, except that near or total loss of reactivity is associated with a very poor outcome.[12] A dissociation was sometimes found between autoregulation and CO_2 reactivity, in that impairment of one could occur with preservation of the other.[11,28]

Observations were made on hyperventilation, used therapeutically to control intracranial hypertension. The expected decline in CBF was accompanied by increased AVD_{O_2}, there being no consistent change in CMR_{O_2}.[14] Although cerebrospinal fluid (CSF) lactate increased with sustained 24-h hyperventilation, CSF acid-base parameters did not show adaptation.[27] Hyperemic foci were particularly sensitive to hypocapnia, decreasing in extent or disappearing completely,[13] which resulted in more homogeneous regional patterns.[29] An inverse steal was occasionally seen in low-flow areas; i.e., a shunting of blood from more reactive regions.[29] Although hyperventilation was effective in reducing ICP among patients with very low CBF, it increased the number of regions with values <20 ml/100 g/min, suggesting a deleterious effect in such cases.[30]

Advantages and Limitations

Advantages of the intracarotid method are: low radiation dose, repeatability within minutes, excellent counting statistics, well-developed quantitative methods, and the ability to separate fast and slow clearing tissue components. Owing to the weak gamma radiation of ^{133}Xe, the underlying cortex is seen better than tissues at that depth. This makes the technique quite sensitive to cortical blood flow, which can be extracted by compartmental or initial slope analysis. Multiple small detectors permit high resolution cortical topography.

The obvious disadvantage is its invasiveness, which limits the method to special situations where puncture of the carotid artery or transfemoral catheterization can be justified. This has resulted in small sample sizes, infrequent serial observations, and few normal controls. CBF measurements are usually confined to one hemisphere, and information about deeper brain structures is not obtainable. An additional limitation discussed below is the "look-through" phenomenon,[31] such that blood flow in tissues surrounding a lesion become averaged. Thus, small ischemic or hyperemic foci could be missed, although larger regional variations are easily detected.

NONINVASIVE ^{133}Xe METHOD

Methodology

This technique is an extension and modification of the intracarotid (IC) method, employing multiple detectors over each hemisphere. Rather than a selective injection of ^{133}Xe into one internal carotid artery, the isotope is introduced into the systemic circulation, either by a brief (1–2 min) inhalation[32] or by intravenous injection.[33] These two noninvasive routes are theoretically the same and give equivalent results.[34] They differ, however, from the IC method in a very important respect—the duration of isotope input. Instead of a rapid bolus that directly enters the brain and clears with minimal recirculation, the input from either inhalation or IV injection is distributed over time and includes considerable recirculation. Clearance curve analysis must therefore take account of the arterial input, which can be estimated noninvasively by continuous monitoring of the expired (end-tidal) air.[3,34]

Based on the Fick principle, Kety[35] derived a generalized equation for the uptake and clearance of an inert diffusible gas, in which the arterial input is convoluted with an exponential function. This convolution was first applied to noninvasive CBF studies by Obrist and coworkers,[3] who proposed a two-compartment model that contains both fast and slow clearing tissue components. Thus:

$$C(t) = \sum_{i=1}^{2} P_i \int_0^t C_A(u)e^{-K_i(t-u)}du \qquad (1)$$

where $C(t)$ and $C_A(t)$ are the measured cerebral and end-tidal ^{133}Xe concentrations, respectively, P_1 and P_2 are weighting coefficients, and K_1 and K_2 are the clearance rates for the two compartments. Computer solutions for the linear coefficients and nonlinear clearance rates are easily obtained by a least-squares curve-fitting procedure.

Multiplying the rate constant of the fast clearing compartment, K_1, by the assumed ^{133}Xe partition coefficient for gray matter, λ_1, yields an estimate of gray matter blood flow: $f_1 = \lambda_1 K_1$.[3] Such estimates, which approximate 80 ml/100 g/min in normals, are highly correlated with those obtained by the IC method.[8] In contrast, values for white matter flow derived from the slow clearing compartment ($f_2 = \lambda_2 K_2$) tend to be underestimated, owing to the presence of extracerebral (scalp) components.

In severe pathological conditions, f_1 and f_2 become unstable owing to shifts in compartment size. More reliable estimates can be obtained from noncompartmental indices based on slope or height-over-area determinations. The most commonly used indices are Risberg's ISI,[36] the slope between 2 and 3 min on the curve, and CBF_{15},[8] a height-over-area formulation similar to that of the intracarotid technique. CBF_{15} provides an estimate of mean tissue flow that is relatively immune to pathological variations in compartment size, while minimizing the influence of extracerebral contamination.

Figure 33-3 illustrates ^{133}Xe clearance curves obtained by IV injection in a head-injured patient before and following clinical brain death.[37] The upper curves,

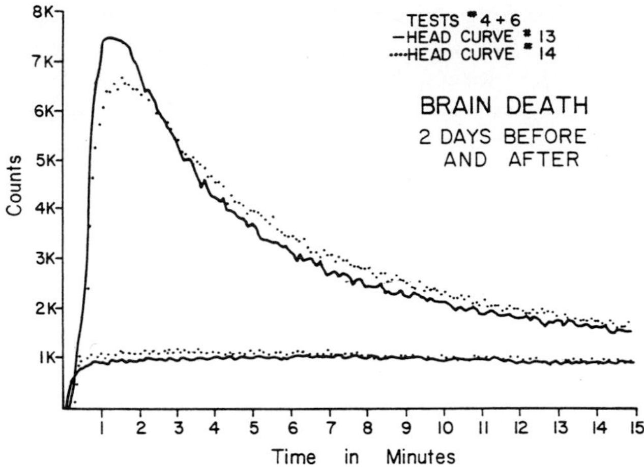

Figure 33-3. Clearance curves recorded from the left (#13) and right (#14) temporal regions of a head-injured patient 2 days before (*upper curves*) and following brain death (*lower curves*). Each point represents ^{133}Xe counts accumulated over a 6-s sampling interval. The same intravenous dose was injected on each occasion. A significant left > right asymmetry is seen in the upper curves, which gave CBF_{15} values of 40 and 32 ml/100 g/min, respectively. Values for the lower curves averaged 6 ml/100 g/min, consistent with scalp circulation only. (From Obrist et al,[37] with permission.)

taken from homologous detectors over the left and right temporal regions, reveal a distinct asymmetry, both in their clearance rates and computed blood flows. The lower curves, recorded after brain death, show minimal uptake and clearance, which is compatible with purely scalp circulation.

Clinical Research Findings

The ability to make repeated bedside measurements during intensive care allowed the noninvasive method to confirm and considerably extend the head injury findings of the IC technique. More readily observed was the time course of CBF changes and their relationship to neurological status, to treatment modalities, and to other physiological parameters. Larger sample sizes and the availability of control data facilitated statistical evaluation. As with the IC method, CMR_{O_2} was estimated as the product of AVD_{O_2} and mean regional CBF, except that the latter involved the average of both hemispheres.

Variations in CBF Level

Attention was directed to extreme levels of blood flow that might play a role in the acute pathophysiology of head injury. Based on measurements of arteriojugular venous O_2 difference, Obrist and coworkers[37,38] examined the adequacy of CBF relative to the brain's metabolic need. Since AVD_{O_2} represents the ratio of metabolism to flow ($AVD_{O_2} = CMR_{O_2}/CBF$), values above or below the normal range can indicate, respectively, global ischemia or hyperemia. These authors found few instances of global ischemia (increased AVD_{O_2}) in physiologically stable ICU patients. Rather, more than half of comatose patients in the first days postinjury had AVD_{O_2} values below the normal range, indicating blood flow in excess of metabolic need. Patients with subnormal flow showed the expected coupling (correlation) of CBF and metabolism, while those with normal or elevated flows revealed uncoupling.[38] Unfortunately, the erratic schedule of studies did not permit insight into the time course of CBF changes during the acute phase, as there were relatively few observations in the early hours postinjury.

Based on a large series that included early studies, Bouma et al.[39,40] reported initially reduced flows (<12 h), which progressed into the normal range on subsequent days. Because a number of patients had CBF values ≤18 ml/100 g/min, the assumed threshold for cerebral infarction, these authors suggested the occurrence of early posttraumatic ischemia. The use of an ischemic threshold of 18, however, is problematical, since AVD_{O_2} values in that study were for the most part normal, indicating that CBF was coupled to a low metabolism. Thus, the poor outcome of patients with early blood flow reductions[39,40] might be attributed to the correlation between outcome and acute CMR_{O_2},[41] rather than to ischemia per se.

Based on longitudinal observations, the present authors[42] confirmed the above findings, as there was a remarkable consistency of low CBF in the first 12 h, followed by a period of elevated flow (hyperemia) that peaked on the second or third day. The early reduced flows were accompanied by normal AVD_{O_2}'s appropriate for the arterial P_{CO_2}. The occurrence of a normal AVD_{O_2} does not, however, rule out ischemia as a factor in secondary brain injury, since ischemia might well occur on a regional basis (not detected by global measurements), or before stabilization in the ICU. Delayed ischemia secondary to cerebral vasospasm may occur in some cases.[43]

A relationship between acute CMR_{O_2} and scores on the Glasgow Coma Scale (GCS) has been observed in both adults[38] and children,[44] the lowest scores being found when metabolism is severely depressed. CBF, in contrast, was related to GCS motor score only during the first day postinjury,[45] especially the first 12 h,[39] a correlation that disappeared with time. A strong association was obtained between low CMR_{O_2} and poor outcome,[41,44] the prognostic value of metabolism approaching that of age.[41] Acute CBF measurements, however, were related to outcome only when hyperemic flows were excluded.[41] It appears that blood flow is related to both GCS and outcome by virtue of its coupling to metabolism, there being little correlation during periods of hyperemia when uncoupling occurs. Early reductions in CMR_{O_2}, and hence CBF, are probably a function of injury severity.[46]

The rise in CBF on the second and third days postinjury was accompanied by a decrease in AVD_{O_2} below the normal range (hyperemia),[39,44] a trend that reversed by the fifth day.[42] It is difficult to attribute the blood flow elevation to lactic acidosis, as suggested earlier,[17] since CSF lactate significantly declines during the period of rising CBF.[47] An inflammatory process has been implicated in the blood flow increase.[48] Head-injured patients with anemia (hemoglobin <10 g/dl) have decreased AVD_{O_2} in association with reduced CMR_{O_2},[49] suggesting a limitation in oxygen availability rather than hyperemia. Since CBF in children is appreciably higher than adults (30 percent greater at 10–15 y),[50] the limits of hyperemic flow require upward adjustment.[44]

An association has been reported between the occurrence of hyperemia and intracranial hypertension, defined as persistent elevations of ICP >20 mmHg.[38,51] A number of exceptions were noted, however, in that one-third of patients with consistently low ICP developed hyperemia. Longitudinally, there is a clear trend for higher ICP and increased treatment intensity during the period of elevated flow (second and third days),[42] but a cause and effect relationship has not been established. In children of heterogeneous ages, no correlation could be found between CBF level and simultaneous ICP recordings.[44] Brain compliance (pressure-volume index) was only weakly related to CBF level; cases with the lowest compliance, however, had extremely high flows.[44] There is some evidence that CBF elevations after the first day are greater in patients with low GCS scores,[44] and that patients with relatively low AVD_{O_2} have unfavorable outcomes.[41] A negative relationship has been reported between acute hyperemia and cognitive function at 3 months postinjury.[52]

CT scan evidence of cerebral swelling has also been related to the occurrence of hyperemia,[51] but again, exceptions were noted; almost half of severe injuries with minimal swelling developed hyperemia. Diffuse brain swelling in late adolescence is accompanied by significantly higher blood flow, relative to the absence of such swelling.[53] The association of hyperemia with both intracranial hypertension and CT brain swelling has been attributed to increased cerebral blood volume (CBV).[38,53] Although there is a trend for blood flow and blood volume to follow the same time course,[54] the relationship between CBF and CBV is complex, the two being correlated only under certain conditions.[44,45] Depending on the status of autoregulation, alterations in perfusion pressure or blood viscosity can affect CBF and CBV quite differently, as does cerebral vasospasm.

These factors, along with variations in other intracranial compartments (tissue water, CSF), may explain the inconsistent relationship of CBF to ICP and brain swelling.

Although the noninvasive method has provided regional data in a number of applications,[8] only a few head injury studies have systematically examined regional CBF changes. This is perhaps due to the few detectors utilized in ICU studies, which permit only gross localization. Hemispheric asymmetries are the most frequent finding. During periods of reduced flow, CBF is lower on the side of major CT scan lesions (hematomas, contusions).[55,56] During the hyperemic phase, however, there is a reversal of this asymmetry, i.e., CBF is higher in the hemisphere with the primary lesion.[56,57] Figure 33-4 illustrates such a case. Test #1 at 9 h postinjury shows significantly lower blood flow in the right hemisphere, the site of a previously evacuated subdural hematoma (SDH). In accordance with earlier SDH findings,[46] a normal AVD_{O_2} was obtained (7.2 vol-percent), indicating that CBF was adequate for the low $CMRO_2$ (1.3 ml/100 g/min). At 68 h (Test #6), there is global hyperemia, at which time the previously depressed right hemisphere had significantly higher flows.

A reversal of the normal anterior-posterior gradient (lower frontal lobe CBF) has been observed during deep coma, which normalizes with recovery of consciousness.[56,58] Several acute studies have been performed on minor head injury, where consciousness is only minimally impaired (responsive to commands).[37,59,60] A mild global reduction of blood flow was found, with some patients having superimposed focal or asymmetrical abnormalities. Follow-up studies 3 to 8 weeks later revealed significant increases in flow, which were accompanied by improvements in coma score,[37] neuropsychological function,[59] and regional CBF pattern.[60]

Autoregulation and CO_2 Reactivity

In agreement with earlier findings by the IC technique, defective autoregulation was observed in approximately 50 percent of both adults[40] and children[61] during the acute phase of head injury, the occurrence of which was unrelated to outcome. Defective autoregulation was also unrelated to GCS and time postinjury.[40,61] In children, however, there was a trend for greater impairment at very high and low CBF levels.[61]

Although of little prognostic significance, the status of autoregulation is important for the maintenance of adequate blood flow and control of intracranial hypertension. When defective, CBF rises or falls in concert with the blood pressure change, there being a corresponding change in ICP.[62] With intact autoregulation (CBF relatively constant), decreases in blood pressure precipitate a rise in ICP, presumably because of compensating vasodilation, i.e., increased CBV.[62] The opposite effect (ICP reduction with BP increase) is less likely to occur with intact autoregulation, possibly because the induced vasoconstriction produces smaller CBV changes.[62] These findings are of considerable rele-

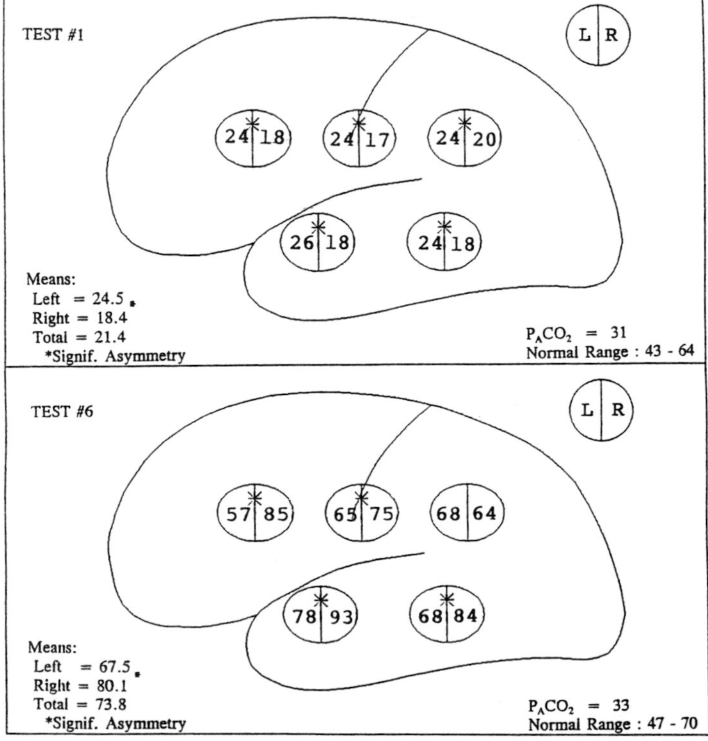

Figure 33-4. Regional cerebral blood flow (IV technique) in a 42-year-old male examined at bedside with five homologous detectors over each hemisphere; L = left, R = right. *Test #1:* 9 h postinjury following evacuation of a large right subdural hematoma (GCS = 3). *Test #6:* 68 h postinjury (GCS = 4). Values represent the initial slope (100 × min^{-1}) of the impulse equivalent curve, an index of fast compartment flow.[8] The early study reveals globally reduced CBF with significantly lower values in the right hemisphere. By the third day there is global hyperemia with a reversal of the previous asymmetry, i.e., the right side now has higher flows. Data from the present authors.

vance to the management of acutely injured patients, and give emphasis to the need for maintaining adequate perfusion pressure.

Based on experimental evidence that mannitol evokes cerebral vasoconstriction in response to blood viscosity changes, Muizelaar and coworkers[63] postulated that the effect of mannitol on CBF and ICP in head-injured patients would depend on the status of autoregulation. In patients with intact autoregulation, blood flow did not change following mannitol, but ICP decreased as expected. When autoregulation was defective, however, CBF increased and ICP underwent a much smaller decline.[63] These results could not be attributed to changes in cardiac output.[64] The above findings appear at variance with another study[65] that found increased CBF after mannitol in a majority of patients, especially in those with elevated ICP and/or low perfusion pressure. As suggested by the authors, impaired autoregulation could have influenced their results.

Essentially normal CO_2 reactivity was found in the acute phase of severe head injury, the response being greater in patients with higher flows.[38] Marked impairment of reactivity occurred only in preterminal stages accompanying neurological deterioration. During aggressive hyperventilation (mean Pa_{CO_2} = 23 mmHg), patients with an already reduced CBF showed wide AVD_{O_2}'s (9–12 vol-percent) and very low jugular P_{O_2}'s (mean = 22 mmHg), consistent with global cerebral ischemia.[38] Such abnormal values were not obtained at higher CBF levels. These findings suggested that patients with reduced flow may be at risk of ischemia when hyperventilated vigorously.

In a randomized trial,[66] 5 days of prophylactic hyperventilation (mean Pa_{CO_2} = 26 mmHg) resulted in significantly fewer cases with favorable outcomes at 3 and 6 months postinjury, relative to normally ventilated controls. AVD_{O_2} measurements, however, showed no evidence of global ischemia, being consistently <9 vol-percent. Of interest are the results of a comparison group where the weak base tromethamine (THAM) was administered, which prevented CBF adaptation to prolonged hypocapnia. In this group the blood flow reductions were sustained over 5 days. This comparison group also showed little evidence of ischemia (wide AVD_{O_2}), but in addition, did not differ in outcome from the controls.[66] The fact that patients with more sustained CBF reductions (hyperventilation plus THAM) did not experience poorer outcomes argues against the detrimental effect of reduced blood flow, per se. Other possibilities considered were CSF acid-base changes and greater ICP lability in the hyperventilated group.[66]

A comparison was made between cerebral hemodynamic and metabolic responses to hyperventilation and those produced by barbiturate therapy (intravenous thiopental).[67,68] Patients with normal CO_2 reactivity showed matched reductions in CBF and CMR_{O_2} following barbiturate administration.[68] In contrast, patients with impaired CO_2 reactivity responded to barbiturate therapy with significantly less CBF decline and no change in CMR_{O_2}. Neurological outcome was better in the CO_2 responsive group, attributed in part to better control of intracranial hypertension.[68] An unexpected finding was that hyperventilation increased CMR_{O_2} in patients with impaired CO_2 reactivity. The authors had no explanation except for possible methodological error.

Another study also found increased CMR_{O_2} during hyperventilation,[69] but independent of CO_2 responsiveness. Methodological error specific to the ^{133}Xe technique seemed unlikely, since similar results were obtained by the nitrous oxide method. CMR_{O_2} increased because the CBF reductions induced by hyperventilation were offset by relatively greater increases in AVD_{O_2}.[69] Hyperventilation improves interregional homogeneity, primarily because of the enhanced responsivity of regions with higher flow.[69,70] Greater CO_2 reactivity has been observed in the hemisphere with unilateral CT scan lesions, especially when associated with cerebral swelling.[71]

Advantages and Limitations

The noninvasive ^{133}Xe method enjoys most of the technical advantages of the intracarotid technique, but in addition, has the further capability of making repeated bedside measurements, as described in the section above. The CBF information obtained has proved of particular value when combined with measurements of other physiological parameters, thus providing a more comprehensive picture of cerebral hemodynamic and metabolic alterations.

Not exploited to its full extent is the ability to record bilateral data from multiple brain regions. In addition to requiring an array of small detectors (now available with improved design), a normative database is necessary for the statistical evaluation of focal and asymmetrical patterns. Such data, although relatively easy to obtain, have not always been acquired by investigators.

A specific limitation of the noninvasive method is the small amount of extracerebral contamination originating from overlying tissues (scalp, bone) and from scattered radiation in the airways (nasopharynx, throat). Their effects can be minimized by appropriate analysis of the clearance curve, as described in detail elsewhere.[3,8]

A major limitation, also applicable to the IC technique, is an insensitivity to local alterations in flow due to the averaging of multiple tissues in view of the detector, i.e., the look-through phenomenon.[8,31] Thus, the computed values may not represent the magnitude of blood flow changes in and around a lesion, and areas of zero flow may go undetected. Even so, significant regional increases or decreases in flow can be appreciated that bear a meaningful relation to neurological and anatomic findings.

STABLE Xe/CT METHOD

METHODOLOGY

This technique involves the inhalation of 30 to 35 percent concentrations of stable (nonradioactive) xenon during sequential brain scanning by x-ray computed tomography. Xenon has a high radiodensity, being comparable to that of iodine. By measuring changes in x-ray attenuation over time, the rate of uptake and clearance of the gas can be determined, from which estimates of cerebral blood flow are derived. The underlying principles are the same as those employed by other inert diffusible gas techniques.

The first quantitative measurements of stable xenon uptake and clearance were attempted by Drayer and coworkers.[72] This was soon followed by the systematic development of the method in a number of laboratories, notably by Gur and associates,[4] who introduced techniques for the rapid computation and display of CBF images.

Data acquisition usually consists of one or two baseline scans, followed by four to six scans at 1-min intervals during xenon inhalation, or alternatively, during inhalation and subsequent clearance.[73] Enhancement values in Hounsfield units (HU) are obtained by subtracting the baseline image, pixel by pixel, from each of the later images. This yields uptake and/or clearance curves that are proportional to xenon concentration in the tissue. Since three or more sections can be scanned during each 1-min interval, data are obtainable at different brain levels. Arterial xenon concentration is estimated from the expired end-tidal air, measured by a thermoconductivity analyzer. These measurements are then converted into CT enhancement units, based on knowledge of the blood hematocrit.[74]

Calculation of blood flow employs the same convolution integral as the ^{133}Xe method, except that only one tissue compartment is assumed:[4]

$$C(t) = \lambda K \int_0^t C_A(u)e^{-K(t-u)}du \qquad (2)$$

where $C(t)$ and $C_A(t)$ are the measured cerebral and end-tidal concentrations of stable xenon, respectively, λ is the xenon partition coefficient, and K is the clearance rate. Computer solutions for λ and K are obtained by a least-squares curve-fitting procedure. The blood flow, f, in each CT voxel is then determined by $f = \lambda K$. Computational speed is gained by fitting the end-tidal xenon curve with an exponential function, which permits an analytic solution of the convolution integral.[75]

A major difficulty in estimating CBF by the Xe/CT method is the presence of random noise, attributable to x-ray counting statistics and tomographic reconstruction.[76] Additional noise is introduced by the image subtraction procedure. Typically, the maximum enhancement after 5 min of 33% xenon inhalation is 8 HU, with smaller values on the rising slope of the curve. Since the standard deviation of CT noise is approximately 1 HU, blood flow estimates for a single pixel may vary by as much as 100 percent. A reduction in variability can be achieved by smoothing filters, applied to both the raw enhancement values and computed blood flows.[4] Since this involves a weighted average of values in the vicinity of a pixel, spatial resolution is thereby reduced.

Figure 33-5 shows the effect of random noise on CBF measurements.[4] Six uniform phantoms loaded with different iodine concentrations were sequentially scanned to simulate data points on a xenon uptake curve, representing a given CBF level.[77] Measurement variability attributable to CT noise was assessed by calculating blood flow in multiple regions of interest (ROI) of equal and specified size. As shown in Fig. 33-5, the relative error (coefficient of variation) of computed blood flows approaches 100 percent for a single 1-mm^2 pixel. Larger ROIs have progressively less error, so that regions exceeding 100 mm^2 approach 10 percent, which is an ac-

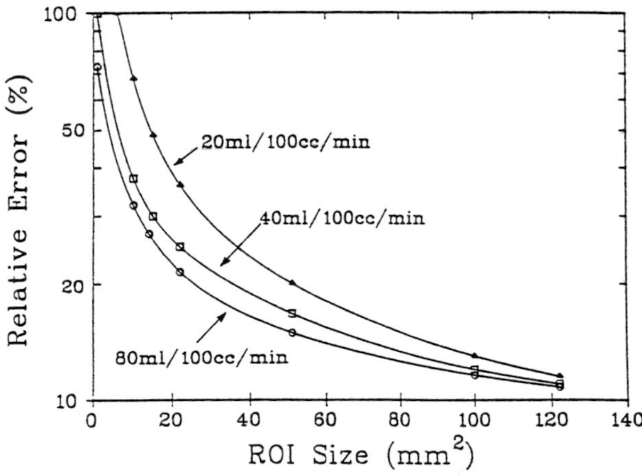

Figure 33-5. Relative error (coefficient of variation) of blood flow measurements plotted as a function of region of interest (ROI) size. The data were generated by sequential scanning of phantoms which simulated xenon uptake curves.[77] Variations in computed flow are entirely attributable to random CT noise. Three CBF levels are compared. (From Gur et al.[4] with permission.)

ceptable amount. The error is less for higher levels of flow owing to a better signal-to-noise ratio. These findings have clear implications for human Xe/CT studies—reliable CBF measurements cannot be obtained from regions smaller than 100 mm^2, especially when the blood flow is low.

Tissue heterogeneity is another factor influencing the variability of CBF measurements.[76] The mathematical model assumes one compartment, yet a given voxel may include tissues with different levels of flow. Smoothing the raw enhancement values effectively increases tissue heterogeneity. Computer simulations reveal that a 50/50 mixture of gray and white matter (worst case) results in a 10 percent attenuation of the computed values.[73,76] Tissue heterogeneity also affects the mean CBF for a region of interest, and depending on the tissue mix, adjacent ROIs can differ by two- or threefold.

Because blood flow for each pixel is calculated from sequential scans, misalignment of the pixels due to head motion may create artifact in the curves.[4] This is less of a problem in comatose head-injured patients than in conscious subjects, where the subanesthetic effects of 30 to 35% xenon (paresthesias, euphoria, light-headedness)[78,79] may induce head movement.

As with other inert gases, stable xenon is vasoactive, producing CBF increases of 15 to 30 percent at standard concentrations in normal volunteers.[79,80] Increases in blood flow velocity (transcranial Doppler) are of similar magnitude, but the onset of the velocity changes is delayed for 2 min after starting xenon inhalation.[81] Computer simulations of such delayed activation reveal only small increases (<5 percent) in calculated CBF,[82] presumably because data points in the first 2 min are minimally affected.

In normal volunteers, blood flow estimates by Xe/CT are comparable to those obtained by other CBF methods, including age-related declines.[83,84] High correlations have been reported between measurements made by Xe/CT and the intravenous ^{133}Xe method in both normal controls[85] and head-injured patients.[86]

Clinical Research Findings

The stable Xe/CT method has only recently been employed in head injury research. As already demonstrated in cerebrovascular disease, this technique has the potential for providing new insight into cerebral pathophysiology by virtue of its ability to observe local blood flow alterations in direct relation to morphological CT findings.

Variations in CBF Level

The first systematic observations in severe brain trauma were reported by Marion and coworkers.[87] They clearly documented early reductions in blood flow (1 to 4 h postinjury) that were followed by significant increases over the next 24 h. Patients with multiple bihemispheric contusions had the lowest flows. CBF was asymmetrically higher on the side of previously evacuated subdural hematomas.

These findings were confirmed by another series of early (admission) Xe/CT studies,[88] where an attempt was made to detect cerebral ischemia, defined as CBF ≤ 18 ml/100 g/min. Thirty-one percent of severely injured patients had such reductions either globally or regionally, which were significantly related to an unfavorable short-term outcome. The inference that these patients suffered from ischemia, however, is not convincing in the absence of global or regional metabolic measurements. Although a blood flow of 18 is an appropriate threshold for infarction in vasospasm patients, referred to by the authors,[88] a much lower value may apply to severely injured, deeply comatose patients with an already depressed CMR_{O_2}.

Regional ischemia may nevertheless occur in patients with subdural hematomas, where CBF is asymmetrically reduced in the hemisphere with the mass,[88,89] and in cases with large hemorrhagic contusions, where a low blood flow is found adjacent to the lesion.[88,89] Figure 33-6 presents the CT scan and corresponding CBF image of a patient with a large edematous contusion in the right frontal lobe. Of special interest is the extended area of reduced flow adjacent to the lesion, where the CT scan shows normal density. Whether this is a primary CBF reduction (oligemia), or a decrease secondary to incomplete neuronal loss and/or dysfunction can only be speculated.

CO_2 Reactivity and Xenon Effects

As previously observed with ^{133}Xe methods, CO_2 reactivity is generally preserved following severe head injury.[87,90] Responsiveness is greater in patients with elevated flow, particularly after evacuation of a subdural hematoma, where it is higher on the ipsilateral side. Bihemispheric contusions are associated with lower CO_2 reactivity. An inverse steal has been reported during hyperventilation,[91] such that a presumed ischemic area developed hyperemia as CBF declined in normally reactive regions. Of particular interest is the large interregional variation in CO_2 responsiveness,[90] the significance of which deserves further investigation.

Since xenon is vasoactive, the question arises whether this might have an adverse effect on intracranial pressure. An early study noted ICP increases of 50 to 81 percent in head-injured patients during 7 min of stable xenon inhalation.[92] Unfortunately, ICP levels and arterial P_{CO_2} were not reported. Subsequent studies employing only 4.5 min of inhalation failed to find a signifi-

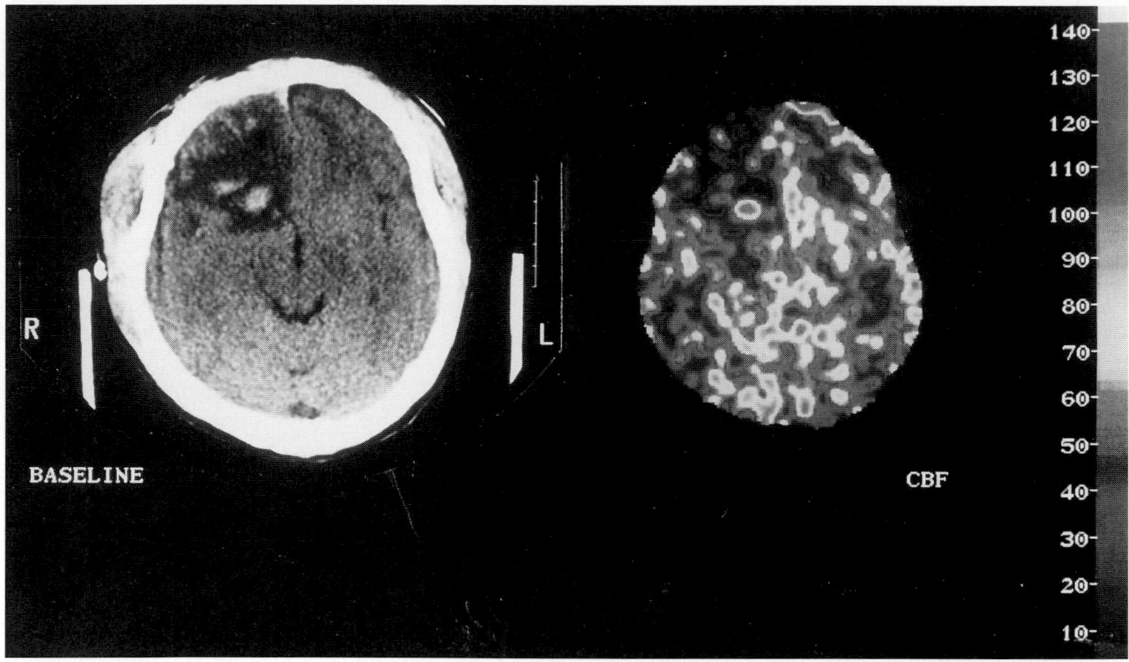

Figure 33-6. CT scan (*left*) and Xe/CT CBF image (*right*) in a 24-year-old male (GCS = 7) following elevation of a depressed comminuted fracture of the right frontal bone. CBF is color-coded in ml/100 g/min. A large edematous contusion is seen in the right frontal lobe, where blood flow averages 19 ml/100 g/min. Adjacent areas within 1 cm of the contusion (normal CT density) have CBF values averaging 28 ml/100 g/min. This contrasts with a mean of 43 obtained elsewhere in the hemisphere and 44 in the contralateral hemisphere. Data from the present authors.

cant increase in ICP during either moderate[93] or mild[94] hypocapnia, even in patients with initially high pressures. Because CBF activation is delayed,[81] brief xenon inhalations should have less effect on ICP and, as the results indicate, can be considered safe.

Combined Techniques

Cerebral blood volume (CBV) is an important factor in intracranial pressure dynamics, but its measurement in critically ill trauma patients has been difficult to achieve. Recently a method has been proposed[95] that combines Xe/CT blood flow determinations with estimates of mean cerebral transit time, obtained by rapid scanning of an intravascular iodinated bolus. Blood volume is determined by the relationship: $CBV = CBF \times \bar{t}$, where $\bar{t}$ is the mean transit time of the bolus, estimated by fitting a gamma variate function to the time-density curve. Although not yet validated, preliminary studies suggest that this technique has considerable potential.

Using this technique, observations have been made on the relationship of blood volume to CBF, ICP, and brain compliance,[96] the latter being measured by the pressure-volume index (PVI). Whereas blood flow is poorly related to ICP and PVI, cerebral blood volume reveals higher correlations, particularly with PVI. Patients with subdural hematomas have reduced CBV in association with a low CBF,[97] suggesting compression of the microcirculation. Following evacuation of the hematoma, both CBV and CBF increase.

Although Xe/CT measurements are conveniently made during routine CT scanning, requiring only an additional 20 min, frequent repeated studies are not practical. This has prompted some investigators to recommend a combination of the Xe/CT and noninvasive ^{133}Xe methods,[86,98] thus taking advantage of their complementary characteristics. Local Xe/CT measurements have recently been used to evaluate continuous CBF monitoring by the thermal diffusion technique.[99]

Advantages and Limitations

The principal advantage of the Xe/CT method is its ability to estimate blood flow within and around a lesion, and to correlate such measurements with morphological CT findings. Not possible with two-dimensional ^{133}Xe techniques is the delineation of subcortical structures, including basal ganglia, brainstem, and white matter. Clearly, such anatomic specificity is needed in studies on traumatic brain injury.

The primary limitation of the method is the poor signal-to-noise ratio and the few data points (scans) available on xenon uptake and clearance curves. This necessitates computational smoothing, which reduces spatial resolution. It also requires averaging relatively large regions of interest in order to achieve statistically reliable estimates. In spite of these limitations, spatial resolution and measurement stability are adequate for most investigational purposes. The challenge is to take full advantage of the regional information available by detailed quantitative analysis of the CBF images.

References

1. Kety SS, Schmidt CF: The nitrous oxide method for the quantitative determination of cerebral blood flow in man: Theory, procedure and normal values. *J Clin Invest* 1948; 27:476–483.
2. Lassen NA, Ingvar DH: Radioisotopic assessment of regional cerebral blood flow. *Prog Nucl Med* 1972;1: 376–409.
3. Obrist WD, Thompson HK Jr, Wang HS, et al: Regional cerebral blood flow estimated by ^{133}xenon inhalation. *Stroke* 1975; 6:245–256.
4. Gur D, Yonas H, Good WF: Local cerebral blood flow by xenon-enhanced CT: Current status, potential improvements, and future directions. *Cerebrovasc Brain Metab Rev* 1989; 1:68–86.
5. Hoedt-Rasmussen K: Regional cerebral blood flow: The intra-arterial injection method. *Acta Neurol Scand* 1967; 43(suppl 27):1–81.
6. McHenry LC, Jaffee ME, Goldberg HI: Regional cerebral blood flow measurements with small probes: I. Evaluation of the method. *Neurology* 1969; 19:1198–1206.
7. McHenry LC: *Cerebral Circulation and Stroke.* St. Louis: Warren H Green, 1978.
8. Obrist WD, Wilkinson WE: Regional cerebral blood flow measurement in humans by xenon-133 clearance. *Cerebrovasc Brain Metab Rev* 1990; 2:283–327.
9. Bruce DA, Schutz H, Vapalahti M, et al: Pitfalls in the interpretation of xenon CBF studies in head-injured patients, in Langfitt TW, McHenry LC, Reivich M, et al (eds): *Cerebral Circulation and Metabolism.* New York: Springer-Verlag, 1975: 406–408.
10. Bruce DA, Langfitt TW, Miller JD, et al: Regional cerebral blood flow, intracranial pressure, and brain metabolism in comatose patients. *J Neurosurg* 1973; 38:131–144.
11. Fieschi C, Battistini N, Beduschi A, et al: Regional cerebral blood flow and intraventricular pressure in acute head injuries. *J Neurol Neurosurg Psychiatry* 1974; 37:1378–1388.
12. Overgaard J, Tweed WA: Cerebral circulation after head injury: Part 1. Cerebral blood flow and its regulation after closed head injury with emphasis on clinical correlations. *J Neurosurg* 1974; 41:531–541.
13. Enevoldsen EM, Cold G, Jensen FT, et al: Dynamic changes in regional CBF, intraventricular pressure, CSF pH and lactate levels during the acute phase of head injury. *J Neurosurg* 1976; 44:191–214.
14. Gordon E, Bergvall U: The effect of controlled hyperventilation on cerebral blood flow and oxygen uptake in patients with brain lesions. *Acta Anaesth Scand* 1973; 17:63–69.
15. Overgaard J, Tweed WA: Cerebral circulation after head injury: Part 2. The effects of traumatic brain edema. *J Neurosurg* 1976; 45:292–300.
16. Cold GE: Cerebral metabolic rate of oyxgen ($CMRO_2$) in the acute phase of brain injury. *Acta Anaesth Scand* 1978; 22:249–256.
17. Lassen NA: The luxury-perfusion syndrome and its possible relation to acute metabolic acidosis localised within the brain. *Lancet* 1966; 2:1113–1115.
18. Brodersen P, Jorgensen EO: Cerebral blood flow and oxygen uptake, and cerebrospinal fluid biochemistry in severe coma. *J Neurol Neurosurg Psychiatry* 1974; 37:384–391.
19. Ingvar DH, Ciria MG: Assessment of severe damage to the brain by multiregional measurements of cerebral blood flow. *Ciba Found Symp* 1975; 34:97–120.
20. Overgaard J, Mosdal C, Tweed WA: Cerebral circulation after head injury: Part 3. Does reduced regional cerebral blood flow determine recovery of brain function after blunt head injury? *J Neurosurg* 1981; 55:63–74.
21. Overgaard J, Tweed WA: Cerebral circulation after head injury: Part 4. Functional anatomy and boundary-zone flow deprivation in the first week of traumatic coma. *J Neurosurg* 1983; 59:439–446.
22. Kasoff SS, Zingesser LH, Shulman K: Compartmental abnormalities of regional cerebral blood flow in children with head trauma. *J Neurosurg* 1972; 36:463–470.
23. Enevoldsen EM, Jensen FT: Compartmental analysis of regional cerebral blood flow in patients with acute severe head injuries. *J Neurosurg* 1977; 47:699–712.
24. Brock M, Schurmann K, Hadjidimos A: Cerebral blood flow and cerebral death: Preliminary report. *Acta Neurochir* 1969; 20:195–209.
25. Overgaard J, Tweed WA: rCBF in impending brain death. *Acta Neurochir* 1975; 31:167–175.
26. Cold GE, Jensen FT: Cerebral autoregulation in unconscious patients with brain injury. *Acta Anaesth Scand* 1978; 22:270–280.
27. Cold GE, Jensen FT, Malmros R: The cerebrovascular CO_2 reactivity during the acute phase of brain injury. *Acta Anaesth Scand* 1977; 21:222–231.
28. Enevoldsen EM, Jensen FT: Autoregulation and CO_2 responses of cerebral blood flow in patients with acute severe head injury. *J Neurosurg* 1978; 48:689–703.
29. Cold GE, Jensen FT, Malmros R: The effects of $PaCO_2$ reduction on regional cerebral blood flow in the acute phase of brain injury. *Acta Anaesth Scand* 1977; 21:359–367.
30. Cold GE: Does acute hyperventilation provoke cerebral oligaemia in comatose patients after acute head injury? *Acta Neurochir* 1989; 96:100–106.
31. Skyhoj Olsen T, Larsen B, Skriver EB, et al: Focal cere-

bral ischemia measured by the intra-arterial ^{133}xenon method: Limitations of 2-dimensional blood flow measurements. *Stroke* 1981; 12:736–744.
32. Mallett BL, Veall N: The measurement of regional cerebral clearance rates in man using xenon-133 inhalation and extracranial recording. *Clin Sci* 1965; 29:179–191.
33. Austin G, Horn N, Rouhe S, et al: Description and early results of an intravenous radioisotope technique for measuring regional cerebral blood flow in man. *Eur Neurol* 1972; 8:43–51.
34. Obrist WD, Wang HS: Comparison of 133-xenon inhalation and IV-injection in regional CBF studies, in Meyer JS, Lechner H, Reivich M, et al (eds): *Cerebral Vascular Disease 3.* Amsterdam: Excerpta Medica, 1981: 140–144.
35. Kety SS: The theory and applications of the exchange of inert gas at the lungs and tissues. *Pharmacol Rev* 1951; 3:1–41.
36. Risberg J, Ali Z, Wilson EM, et al: Regional cerebral blood flow by ^{133}xenon inhalation: Preliminary evaluation of an initial slope index in patients with unstable flow compartments. *Stroke* 1975; 6:142–148.
37. Obrist WD, Gennarelli TA, Segawa H, et al: Relation of cerebral blood flow to neurological status and outcome in head-injured patients. *J Neurosurg* 1979; 51:292–300.
38. Obrist WD, Langfitt TW, Jaggi JL, et al: Cerebral blood flow and metabolism in comatose patients with acute head injury: Relation to intracranial hypertension. *J Neurosurg* 1984; 61:241–253.
39. Bouma GJ, Muizelaar JP, Choi SC, et al: Cerebral circulation and metabolism after severe traumatic brain injury: The elusive role of ischemia. *J Neurosurg* 1991; 75:685–693.
40. Bouma GJ, Muizelaar JP: Cerebral blood flow, cerebral blood volume, and cerebrovascular reactivity after severe head injury. *J Neurotrauma* 1992; 9(suppl 1):S333–S348.
41. Jaggi JL, Obrist WD, Gennarelli TA, et al: Relationship of early cerebral blood flow and metabolism to outcome in acute head injury. *J Neurosurg* 1990; 72:176–182.
42. Obrist WD, Marion DW, Aggarwal S, et al: Time course of cerebral blood flow and metabolism in comatose patients with acute head injury. *J Cereb Blood Flow Metab* 1993; 13(suppl 1):S571.
43. Martin NA, Doberstein C, Zane C, et al: Posttraumatic cerebral arterial spasm: Transcranial Doppler ultrasound, cerebral blood flow, and angiographic findings. *J Neurosurg* 1992; 77:575–583.
44. Muizelaar JP, Marmarou A, DeSalles AA, et al: Cerebral blood flow and metabolism in severely head-injured children: Part 1. Relationship with GCS score, outcome, ICP, and PVI. *J Neurosurg* 1989; 71:63–71.
45. Muizelaar JP, Obrist WD: Cerebral blood flow and metabolism with brain injury, in Becker DP, Povlishock JT (eds): *Central Nervous System Trauma Status Report.* Bethesda, MD: National Institutes of Health, 1985: 123–137.
46. Salvant JB, Muizelaar JP: Changes in cerebral blood flow and metabolism related to the presence of subdural hematoma. *Neurosurgery* 1993; 33:387–393.
47. DeSalles AA, Muizelaar JP, Young HF: Hyperglycemia, cerebrospinal fluid lactic acidosis, and cerebral blood flow in severely head-injured patients. *Neurosurgery* 1987; 21:45–50.
48. Uhl MW, Biagas KV, Grundl PD, et al: Effects of neutropenia on edema, histology, and cerebral blood flow after traumatic brain injury in rats. *J Neurotrauma* 1994; 11:303–315.
49. Cruz J, Jaggi JL, Hoffstad OJ: Cerebral blood flow and oxygen consumption in acute brain injury with acute anemia: An alternative for the cerebral metabolic rate of oxygen consumption? *Crit Care Med* 1993; 21:1218–1224.
50. Ogawa A, Sakurai Y, Kayama T, et al: Regional cerebral blood flow with age: Changes in rCBF in childhood. *Neurol Res* 1989; 11:173–176.
51. Uzzell BP, Obrist WD, Dolinskas CA, et al: Correlation of acute ICP and CBF with CT scan and neuropsychological recovery in severe head injury, in Miller JD, Teasdale GM, Rowan JO, et al (eds): *Intracranial Pressure VI.* Berlin/Heidelberg: Springer-Verlag, 1986: 687–690.
52. Uzzell BP, Obrist WD, Dolinskas CA, et al: Relationship of acute CBF and ICP findings to neuropsychological outcome in severe head injury. *J Neurosurg* 1986; 65:630–635.
53. Bruce DA, Alavi A, Bilaniuk L, et al: Diffuse cerebral swelling following head injuries in children: The syndrome of "malignant brain edema." *J Neurosurg* 1981; 54:170–178.
54. Kuhl DE, Alavi A, Hoffman EJ, et al: Local cerebral blood volume in head-injured patients: Determination by emission computed tomography of ^{99m}Tc-labeled red cells. *J Neurosurg* 1980; 52:309–320.
55. Obrist WD, Dolinskas CA, Gennarelli TA, et al: Relation of cerebral blood flow to CT scan in acute head injury, in Popp AJ, Bourke RS, Nelson LR, et al (eds): *Neural Trauma.* New York: Raven Press, 1979: 41–50.
56. Obrist WD, Dolinskas CA, Jaggi JL, et al: Serial cerebral blood flow studies in acute head injury: Application of the intravenous ^{133}Xe method. *Functional Radionuclide Imaging of the Brain.* New York: Raven Press, 1983: 145–150.
57. Beyda SH: Regional cerebral blood flow in pediatric patients with acute severe head injuries. *J Cereb Blood Flow Metab* 1987; 7(suppl 1):S645.
58. Deutsch G, Eisenberg HM: Frontal blood flow changes in recovery from coma. *J Cereb Blood Flow Metab* 1987; 7:29–34.
59. Arvigo F, Cossu M, Fazio B, et al: Cerebral blood flow in minor cerebral contusion. *Surg Neurol* 1985; 24:211–217.
60. Korner E, Marguc K, Ott E, et al: Alterations of cerebral blood flow in slight head injury, in Hartmann A, Hoyer S (eds): *Cerebral Blood Flow and Metabolism Measurement.* Berlin/Heidelberg: Springer-Verlag, 1985: 92–97.
61. Muizelaar JP, Ward JD, Marmarou A, et al: Cerebral blood flow and metabolism in severely head-injured children: Part 2. Autoregulation. *J Neurosurg* 1989; 71:72–76.
62. Bouma GJ, Muizelaar JP, Bandoh K, et al: Blood pressure and intracranial pressure-volume dynamics in severe head injury: Relationship with cerebral blood flow. *J Neurosurg* 1992; 77:15–19.

63. Muizelaar JP, Lutz HA, Becker DP: Effect of mannitol on ICP and CBF and correlation with pressure autoregulation in severely head-injured patients. *J Neurosurg* 1984; 61:700–706.
64. Bouma GJ, Muizelaar JP: Relationship between cardiac output and cerebral blood flow in patients with intact and with impaired autoregulation. *J Neurosurg* 1990; 73:368–374.
65. Mendelow AD, Teasdale GM, Russell T, et al: Effect of mannitol on cerebral blood flow and cerebral perfusion pressure in human head injury. *J Neurosurg* 1985; 63:43–48.
66. Muizelaar JP, Marmarou A, Ward JD, et al: Adverse effects of prolonged hyperventilation in patients with severe head injury: A randomized clinical trial. *J Neurosurg* 1991; 75:731–739.
67. Messeter K, Nordstrom C-H, Sundbarg G, et al: Cerebral hemodynamics in patients with acute severe head trauma. *J Neurosurg* 1986; 64:231–237.
68. Nordstrom C-H, Messeter K, Sundbarg G, et al: Cerebral blood flow, vasoreactivity, and oxygen consumption during barbiturate therapy in severe traumatic brain lesions. *J Neurosurg* 1988; 68:424–431.
69. Obrist WD, Clifton GL, Robertson CS, et al: Cerebral metabolic changes induced by hyperventilation in acute head injury, in Meyer JS, Lechner H, Reivich M, et al (eds): *Cerebral Vascular Disease 6.* Amsterdam: Elsevier, 1987: 251–255.
70. Cold GE: Measurements of CO_2 reactivity and barbiturate reactivity in patients with severe head injury. *Acta Neurochir* 1989; 98:153–163.
71. Jaggi JL, Obrist WD, Gennarelli TA, et al: CBF-CO_2 reactivity in relation to CT findings in acute head injury. *J Cereb Blood Flow Metab* 1991; 11(suppl 2):S833.
72. Drayer BP, Wolfson SK, Reinmuth OM, et al: Xenon enhanced CT for analysis of cerebral integrity, perfusion, and blood flow. *Stroke* 1978; 9:123–130.
73. Polacin A, Kalender WA, Eidloth H: Simulation study of cerebral blood flow measurements in xenon-CT: Evaluation of washin/washout procedures. *Med Phys* 1991; 18:1025–1031.
74. Kelcz F, Hilal SK, Hartwell P, et al: Computed tomographic measurement of the xenon brain-blood partition coefficient and implications for regional cerebral blood flow: A preliminary report. *Radiology* 1978; 127:385–392.
75. Good WF, Gur D: Errors in cerebral blood flow determinations by xenon-enhanced computed tomography due to estimation of arterial xenon concentrations. *Med Phys* 1987; 14:377–381.
76. Good WF, Gur D: The effect of computed tomography noise and tissue heterogeneity on cerebral blood flow determination by xenon-enhanced computed tomography. *Med Phys* 1987; 14:557–561.
77. Good WF, Gur D, Herron JM, et al: The development of a xenon/computed tomography cerebral blood flow quality assurance phantom. *Med Phys* 1987; 14:867–869.
78. Yonas H, Grundy B, Gur D, et al: Side effects of xenon inhalation. *J Comput Assist Tomogr* 1981; 5:591–592.
79. Hartmann A, Dettmers C, Schuier FJ, et al: Effect of stable xenon on regional cerebral blood flow and the electroencephalogram in normal volunteers. *Stroke* 1990; 22:182–189.
80. Obrist WD, Jaggi JL, Harel D, et al: Effect of stable xenon inhalation on human CBF. *J Cereb Blood Flow Metab* 1985; 5(suppl 1):S557–S558.
81. Giller CA, Purdy P, Lindstrom WW: Effects of inhaled stable xenon on cerebral blood flow velocity. *AJNR* 1990; 11:177–182.
82. Good WF, Gur D: Xenon-enhanced CT of the brain: Effect of flow activation on derived cerebral blood flow measurements. *AJNR* 1991; 12:83–85.
83. Yonas H, Darby JM, Marks EC, et al: CBF measured by Xe-CT: Approach to analysis and normal values. *J Cereb Blood Flow Metab* 1991; 11:716–725.
84. Meyer JS, Imai A, Ichijo M, et al: Local cerebral blood flow and local lambda values change with normal advancing age, in Yonas H (ed): *Cerebral Blood Flow Measurement with Stable Xenon-Enhanced Computed Tomography.* New York: Raven Press, 1992: 89–92.
85. Yonas H, Obrist W, Gur D, et al: Cross-correlation of CBF derived by 133-Xe and Xe/CT in normal volunteers. *J Cereb Blood Flow Metab* 1989; 9(suppl 1):S409.
86. Stringer WA, Marion DW, Bouma GJ, et al: Correlation of xenon-133 and stable xenon-enhanced computed tomographic cerebral blood flow measurements in patients with severe head injury, in Yonas H (ed): *Cerebral Blood Flow Measurement with Stable Xenon-Enhanced Computed Tomography.* New York: Raven Press, 1992: 233–237.
87. Marion DW, Darby J, Yonas H: Acute regional cerebral blood flow changes caused by severe head injuries. *J Neurosurg* 1991; 74:407–414.
88. Bouma GJ, Muizelaar JP, Stringer WA, et al: Ultra-early evaluation of regional cerebral blood flow in severely head-injured patients using xenon-enhanced computerized tomography. *J Neurosurg* 1992; 77:360–368.
89. DuTrevou MD, Bullock MRR, VanDellen JR, et al: Regional cerebral blood flow determination by computed tomography and xenon gas inhalation after severe head injury: Report of 2 cases. *S Afr J Surg* 1987; 25:95–98.
90. Marion DW, Bouma GJ: The use of stable xenon-enhanced computed tomographic studies of cerebral blood flow to define changes in cerebral carbon dioxide vasoresponsivity caused by a severe head injury. *Neurosurgery* 1991; 29:869–873.
91. Darby JM, Yonas H, Marion DW, et al: Local "inverse steal" induced by hyperventilation in head injury. *Neurosurgery* 1988; 23:84–88.
92. Harrington TR, Manwaring K, Hodak J: Local basal ganglia and brain stem blood flow in the head injured patients using stable xenon enhanced CT scanning, in Miller JD, Teasdale GM, Rowan JO (eds): *Intracranial Pressure VI.* Berlin/Heidelberg: Springer-Verlag, 1986: 680–686.
93. Darby JM, Yonas H, Pentheny S, et al: Intracranial pressure response to stable xenon inhalation in patients with head injury. *Surg Neurol* 1989; 32:1–3.
94. Marion DW, Crosby K: The effect of stable xenon on ICP. *J Cereb Blood Flow Metab* 1991; 11:347–350.
95. Bouma GJ, Fatouros PP, Muizelaar JP, et al: Determina-

tion of cerebral blood volume by simultaneous xenon-enhanced computed tomographic cerebral blood flow measurement and dynamic computed tomography enhanced by intravenous contrast, in Yonas H (ed): *Cerebral Blood Flow Measurement with Stable Xenon-Enhanced Computed Tomography*. New York: Raven Press, 1992: 100–104.

96. Bouma GJ, Muizelaar JP, Schuurman R, et al: Cerebral blood volume in acute head injury: Relationship to CBF and ICP, in Avezaath CJJ (ed): *Intracranial Pressure VIII*. Berlin/Heidelberg: Springer-Verlag, 1992: 529–534.

97. Schroder ML, Muizelaar JP, Kuta AJ: Documented reversal of global ischemia immediately after removal of an acute subdural hematoma: Report of two cases. *J Neurosurg* 1994; 80:324–327.

98. Marion DW, Obrist WD, Carlier PM, et al: The use of therapeutic moderate hypothermia for patients with severe head injuries: A preliminary report. *J Neurosurg* 1993; 79:354–362.

99. Schroder ML, Muizelaar JP: Monitoring of regional cerebral blood flow (CBF) in acute head injury by thermal diffusion. *Acta Neurochir* 1993; 59(suppl)47–49.

CHAPTER 34

NITROUS OXIDE SATURATION TECHNIQUE FOR CBF MEASUREMENT

Claudia S. Robertson

SYNOPSIS

Measurements of global cerebral blood flow (CBF) using the nitrous oxide saturation method can be performed in the intensive care unit. In patients with a severe head injury, these measurements have provided a better understanding of the pathophysiology and the physiological effects of various drug treatments. The average value for CBF in 282 patients with severe head injury was normal at 51 ± 23 ml/100 g/min, while cerebral oxygen consumption (CMR_{O_2}) was significantly reduced, averaging 2.1 ± 1.2 ml/100 g/min. Serial measurements of global CBF during the first 5 days after an injury have shown several patterns of behavior. Most important, the development of a low CBF during the first 5 days after an injury has been correlated with a poor neurological outcome.

Cerebral blood flow (CBF) measurements have contributed significantly to the understanding of the pathophysiology of head trauma. The Kety-Schmidt technique, which was described in 1945, was the first method for accurately measuring CBF in humans.[1] Despite the development of newer techniques, that permit regional measurement of CBF or continuous measurement of local CBF, the Kety-Schmidt technique remains a useful method for measuring global CBF in the intensive care unit (ICU).

THEORY

The Kety-Schmidt method of CBF measurement is based on the Fick principle, which states that the amount of tracer taken up by the brain in a given period must equal the amount delivered by arterial blood minus the amount removed by cerebral venous blood in the same period. Since the amount delivered (milligrams per minute) equals flow (milliliters per minute) multiplied by concentration (milligrams per milliliter), it is possible to make an estimate of CBF if the brain content can be determined. The brain content is determined by assuming that brain concentration (milligrams of tracer/100 g of brain) is proportional to tracer concentration in cerebral venous blood if sufficient time is given to allow tissue-blood equilibration. The proportionality constant, the blood-brain partition coefficient λ, was determined in vitro. Flow is then expressed per unit mass of brain tissue (ml/100 g/min). The equation for this relationship is

$$(C_b)_T = (C_v)_T\,\lambda = \text{CBF}\int_0^T (C_a - C_v)\,dt \qquad (1)$$

where $(C_b)_T$ is the brain concentration at time T, the time needed to achieve tissue saturation; $(C_v)_T$ is the cerebral venous concentration at time T; CBF is the cerebral blood flow per unit of brain mass (ml/100 g/min); and C_a and C_v are arterial and cerebral venous concentrations, respectively, drawn at various times t between t = 0 and T.

Kety and Schmidt used 15% nitrous oxide (N_2O) as a tracer, given by continuous inhalation for 10 min, a time assumed to be adequate for brain–cerebral venous equilibration (as evidenced by Cv = Ca). During inhalation, samples were taken intermittently from a peripheral artery and from the jugular bulb, and curves, such as the one shown in Fig. 34-1, were constructed. The quantity $\int_0^{10} (Ca - Cv)\,dt$ is obtained by measuring the area between the arterial and venous saturation curves,

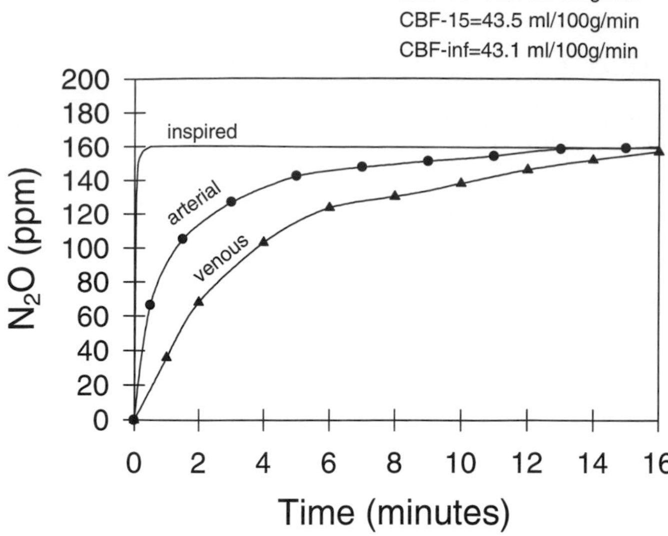

Figure 34-1. Example of arterial and jugular venous saturation curves for N_2O.

TABLE 34-1 Formulas for Calculating Cerebral Metabolic Parameters

Parameter (units)*	Formula	Conversion Factor	Normal Values: Reference[2] (n = 14)	Normal Values: Reference[57] (n = 50)	Normal Values: Reference[58] (n = 8)	Head Injury Values (n = 282)
CBF (ml/100 g/min)			54 ± 12		52 ± 12	51 ± 23
Ca_{O_2} (ml/dl)	$1.34*Hgb*Sa_{O_2} + .0031*Pa_{O_2}$	$\frac{Ca_{O_2}\text{ (ml/dl)}}{2.24} = Ca_{O_2}\ (\mu\text{mol/ml})$		19.6 ± 1.2	16.9 ± 1.5	14.1 ± 2.4
Cjv_{O_2} (ml/dl)	$1.34*Hgb*Sjv_{O_2} + .0031*Pjv_{O_2}$	$\frac{Cjv_{O_2}\text{ (ml/dl)}}{2.24} = Cjv_{O_2}\ (\mu\text{mol/ml})$		12.9 ± 1.3		9.7 ± 2.3
AVD_{O_2} (ml/dl)	Ca_{O_2} (ml/dl)-Cjv_{O_2} (ml/dl)	$\frac{AVD_{O_2}\text{(ml/dl)}}{2.24} = AVD_{O_2}\ (\mu\text{mol/ml})$	6.3 ± 1.2	6.7 ± 0.8	6.5 ± 1.8	4.4 ± 1.6
CMR_{O_2} (ml/100 g/min)	$\frac{AVD_{O_2}\text{ (ml/dl)*CBF (ml/100 g/min)}}{100}$	$\frac{CMR_{O_2}\text{ (ml/100 g/min)}}{2.24} = CMR_{O_2}\ (\mu\text{mol/g/min})$	3.3 ± 0.4		3.3 ± 0.6	2.1 ± 1.2
O_2ER (%)	$\frac{AVD_{O_2}\text{ (ml/dl)*100\%}}{Ca_{O_2}\text{ (ml/dl)}}$			34 ± 4		31 ± 10
AVDG (ml/dl)	ArtGluc (ml/dl)-JVGluc (ml/dl)	$\frac{\text{AVDG (ml/dl)}}{18} = \text{AVDG}\ (\mu\text{mol/ml})$		9.6 ± 1.7	11.0 ± 2.3	7.2 ± 3.6
CMRG (ml/100 g/min)	$\frac{\text{AVDG (ml/dl)*CBF (ml/100 g/min)}}{100}$	$\frac{\text{CMRG (ml/100 g/min)}}{18} = \text{CMRG}\ (\mu\text{mol/g/min})$			5.5 ± 1.1	3.5 ± 2.4
AVDL (ml/dl)	ArtLact (ml/dl)-JVLact (ml/dl)	$\frac{\text{AVDL (ml/dl)}}{9} = \text{AVDL}\ (\mu\text{mol/ml})$		−1.7 ± 0.9	−0.5 ± 0.9	−0.5 ± 1.2
CMRL (ml/100 g/min)	$\frac{\text{AVDL (ml/dl)*CBF (ml/100 g/min)}}{100}$	$\frac{\text{CMRL (ml/100 g/min)}}{9} = \text{CMRL}\ (\mu\text{mol/g/min})$			−0.23 ± 0.37	−0.25 ± 0.73
LOI	$\frac{-\text{AVDL}\ (\mu\text{mol/ml})}{AVD_{O_2}\ (\mu\text{mol/ml})}$			.06 ± .03		.02 ± .05

* All average values are given in the units used in the first column.

Abbreviations: CBF = cerebral blood flow; Ca_{O_2} = arterial oxygen content; Cjv_{O_2} = jugular venous oxygen content; Sa_{O_2} = arterial oxygen saturation; Sjv_{O_2} = jugular venous oxygen saturation; Hgb = hemoglobin concentration; Pa_{O_2} = arterial P_{O_2}; Pjv_{O_2} = jugular venous P_{O_2}; AVD_{O_2} = arterial venous oxygen difference; CMR_{O_2} = cerebral metabolic rate of oxygen; O_2ER = oxygen extraction ratio; ArtGluc = arterial glucose concentration; JVGluc = jugular venous glucose concentration; AVDG = arterial venous glucose difference; CMRG = cerebral metabolic rate of glucose; ArtLact = arterial lactate concentration; JVLact = jugular venous lactate concentration; AVDL = arterial venous lactate difference; CMRL = cerebral metabolic rate of lactate; LOI = lactate : oxygen index.

and $(C_b)_T$ is taken as $(C_v)_{10}\,\lambda$. CBF is then calculated by the formula

$$CBF = \frac{(C_v)_{10}\,\lambda}{\int_0^{10} (C_a - C_v)\,dt} \tag{2}$$

Once CBF is known, the cerebral metabolic rates of glucose, lactate, and oxygen (CMR_G, CMR_L, and CMR_{O_2}, respectively) can be calculated by multiplying the arteriovenous difference by the CBF (Table 34-1).

MAJOR ASSUMPTIONS

Jugular Bulb Blood Is Mixed Cerebral Venous Blood

The Kety-Schmidt method gives values for mean CBF if the venous blood samples obtained from one internal jugular vein are representative of mixed cerebral venous blood. Although the dural sinuses join at the torcular in most people, there may not always be sufficient mixing so that the blood in the two lateral sinuses is similar. Kety and Schmidt[2] measured CBF simultaneously from both the right and left jugular bulbs in 10 patients. There was not a significant difference in the two measurements. Others, however, have found consistent differences in CBF measured in the right and left jugular bulbs.[3]

There Is Minimal Extracerebral Contamination of Jugular Bulb Blood

Shenkin and associates[4] found that the amount of extracerebral contamination of jugular venous blood averaged only 2.7 percent (range, 0 to 6.6 percent) in normal adults. In a few anecdotal cases, however, extracerebral contamination has been found to be considerable.[5] Proper catheter position is important. Jakobsen and Enevoldsen[6] showed that when a catheter that had been placed in the jugular bulb was pulled back more than 2 cm from the base of the skull, oxygen saturation in blood drawn from the catheter increased over 10% in 4 of 13 patients, indicating major extracerebral contamination.

Equilibration of Brain and Cerebral Venous Blood Occurs by 10 Min

Kety and Schmidt[2] observed equilibration of arterial and venous N_2O concentrations by 10 min in subjects with normal CBF. Later investigators, using more sensitive assays for N_2O, found that arterial and venous N_2O concentrations do not equilibrate completely even by 60 min.[7] Lassen and Klee[8] observed that the CBF calculated from 10-min saturation curves overestimated CBF by 10 to 15 percent but that this potential error could be minimized by prolonging the saturation period to 14 to 16 min and extrapolating the saturation curves to infinity.

Blood-Brain Partition Coefficient of N_2O Is 1.0

The blood-brain partition coefficient for nitrous oxide has been studied in a variety of circumstances and has been found to be close to 1.0 in all circumstances studied, 0.98 in in vivo studies, 1.03 in the dog in vitro, and 1.06 in the human in vitro.[9]

ADVANTAGES AND DISADVANTAGES OF THE KETY-SCHMIDT TECHNIQUE

The Kety-Schmidt method for measuring CBF is easily applied in the ICU with a minimum of equipment and uses an indicator that is widely available, inexpensive, and nontoxic. For these reasons, CBF measurements can be repeated frequently and therefore can be used to examine serial changes in CBF and the effect of various treatments on global CBF and metabolism. This method has been applied to both adult and pediatric patients.[10,11] Theoretically, it is more valid for obtaining cerebral metabolic parameters, since the blood obtained for the arteriovenous differences of the metabolites is drawn from the same distribution in the brain from which the CBF measurement is obtained.

However, the Kety-Schmidt CBF is a global CBF measurement and cannot be used to detect regional differences in CBF. Areas with no flow are ignored. In addition, the measurement is invasive, requiring a jugular bulb and arterial catheter for sampling blood. The measurement is time-consuming, and the patient must be in a steady state during the measurement; thus, rapidly changing states cannot be studied.

METHODS

The patient must be in a steady state during the entire 15 to 16 min of the CBF measurement. Intracranial pressure (ICP), blood pressure (BP), and end-tidal CO_2 (ET_{CO_2}) should be recorded continuously during the CBF measurement, and arterial and jugular venous blood gases should be obtained at the beginning and end of the CBF measurement to assure that a steady state was maintained.

Introduction of N_2O

Ten to fifteen percent N_2O is introduced into the inspired gases in a stepwise fashion. The precise concentration of N_2O is not crucial; between 10 and 15 percent is sufficient to obtain blood levels that can be assayed accurately. However, the addition of the N_2O must be stepwise over a period of less than 15 s, and thereafter the inspired N_2O concentration must be kept constant for 16 min.

One practical method for introducing N_2O in ventilated patients is via the oxygen inlet of the ventilator, using an external blender to mix oxygen and N_2O. The advantage of this setup is that a drop in the inspired fraction of oxygen (Fi_{O_2}) caused by the amount of N_2O added to the inspired gases can be used as a signal to start the timing of the blood sampling.

Blood Sampling

At known time intervals after the introduction of N_2O in the inspired gases, 0.5 ml of arterial and jugular venous blood is drawn anaerobically into heparinized 1 ml sy-

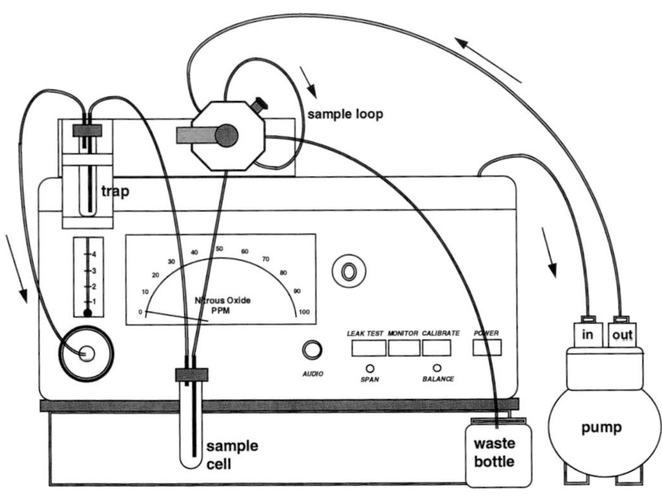

A

EQUIPMENT:
1. Trace Nitrous Analyzer (Traverse Medical Monitors)
2. Pump (Air Cadet)
3. Valve (8-port injection Hamilton valve)
4. Sample cell and trap (12x75mm culture tubes)

Figure 34-2. Measurement of N_2O concentration in blood samples. *A.* Diagram of extraction device for separating N_2O from the blood sample. *B.* Details of the air flow through the Hamilton valve as the blood sample is being injected (left) and as the N_2O concentration is being measured (right).

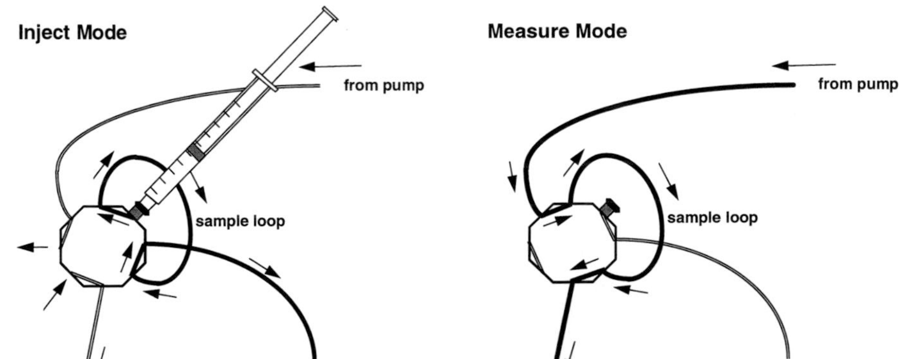

INSTRUCTIONS:
1. Let the N_2O analyzer warm-up for 5 minutes before using.
2. With the valve handle in ***Inject*** position (left diagram), allow the tubing to be flushed with air, or oxygen if the room air is contaminated with significant amounts of N_2O. Place a new culture tube as sample cell.
3. With the valve handle in ***Measure*** position (right diagram), zero the N_2O analyzer.
4. With the valve handle in ***Inject*** position, inject the blood sample until some of the sample enters the waste tubing. Make certain that there are no air bubbles in the sample loop.
5. Turn the valve handle to ***Measure*** position.
6. Vortex the blood sample which has fallen into the culture tube for 2-3 seconds.
7. After the N_2O readings have stabilized (15-20 seconds), record the N_2O value.

B

ringes. Since the arterial concentration of N_2O changes most rapidly just after N_2O is added to the inspired gases, better saturation curves are obtained if the blood is sampled more frequently during the first 2 min. A practical schedule is 0, 0.5, 1.5, 3, 5, 7, 9, 11, 13, and 15 min for the arterial samples and 0, 1, 2, 4, 6, 8, 10, 12, 14, and 16 min for the venous samples. A total of 10 ml of blood is drawn for the CBF measurement, and one operator can collect both the arterial and the venous samples since the times are staggered.

Measurement of N_2O in Blood Samples

Kety and Schmidt measured N_2O in blood samples by using the Van Slyke–Neil manometric technique.[1] N_2O can also be analyzed using gas chromatography, mass spectroscopy, or infrared spectrophotometry. The third method may be more convenient in the ICU setting. For this type of analysis, N_2O must be extracted from the blood samples into air circulating through the analyzer (Trace Nitrous Monitor, Traverse Medical Monitors). A diagram of a typical extraction setup appears in Fig. 34-2.

NORMAL VALUES

Normal values for CBF and CMR_{O_2} using the Kety-Schmidt technique were initially reported in 1945[1] and similar values have been reproduced by numerous investigators since then. Representative values are shown in Table 34-1.

HEAD INJURY VALUES

After a severe head injury, CMR_{O_2} is consistently reduced by one-third to one-half, while CBF can be reduced, normal, or elevated relative to normal. The relative reduction in CMR_{O_2} is proportional to the decrease in the Glasgow Coma Scale (GCS).[12] Table 34-1 lists the average values for global CBF and the cerebral metabolic parameters in a group of 282 severely head injured patients (n = 2242 CBF values).

In addition, CBF and CMR_{O_2} are not necessarily constant after a head injury. CMR_{O_2} tends to be the highest very early after the injury and decreases over the first 1 to 5 days. This tendency for CMR_{O_2} to decrease is not artifactual, resulting from decreasing hemoglobin concentration, as suggested by Cruz and colleagues,[13] since it has been observed even when hemoglobin concentration has remained constant (Table 34-2). CMR_{O_2} increases later in patients who improve neurologically.

CBF also evolves over time. Very early after an injury (less than 6 h), marked global hypoperfusion can occur.[14] After 6 h after the injury, global ischemia is uncommon except when it is associated with secondary insults.

One of the advantages of the Kety-Schmidt technique is the ability to perform serial measurements of CBF over time. Several patterns of CBF behavior were observed using serial measurements of global CBF during days 1 through 10 in 102 severely head injured patients at Ben Taub General Hospital (BTGH).[15] Twenty-five (25 percent) had a reduced CBF, 47 (47 percent) had a normal CBF, and 30 (30 percent) had an elevated CBF. The mean CBF of the normal CBF group was 0.41 ± 0.10 ml/g/min, compared with 0.62 ± 0.14 ml/g/min in the elevated CBF group and 0.29 ± 0.05 ml/g/min in the reduced CBF group. The intergroup differences in CBF were inversely related to differences in the arterial venous oxygen difference (AVD_{O_2}), which averaged 2.1 ± 0.7 μmol/ml in the reduced CBF group, 1.9 ± 0.5 μmol/ml in the normal CBF group, and 1.6 ± 0.4 μmol/ml in the elevated CBF group.

Figure 34-3 shows frequency histograms of the individual CBF and AVD_{O_2} measurements among the three groups of patients. The distributions of CBF and AVD_{O_2} indicate separation of the patients into distinct groups with differences not only in CBF level but also in the ratio between CBF and cerebral metabolism, as reflected by the AVD_{O_2}.

TABLE 34-2 Changes in CBF and Cerebral Metabolism during First 5 Days after Injury in 22 Patients

Parameter	Day 1	Day 2	Day 3	Day 4	Day 5
CBF (ml/100 g/min)	42.6 ± 20.4	60.1 ± 30.7	47.5 ± 28.0	45.7 ± 21.5	44.5 ± 18.1
CMR_{O_2} (μmol/g/min)	0.88 ± 0.41	0.85 ± 0.36	0.81 ± 0.37	0.75 ± 0.26	0.78 ± 0.27
Hemoglobin (ml/dl)	10.1 ± 1.5	10.1 ± 1.2	10.5 ± 1.4	10.4 ± 0.9	10.3 ± 1.1
CMRG (μmol/g/min)	0.162 ± 0.083	0.159 ± 0.082	0.159 ± 0.062	0.155 ± 0.056	0.146 ± 0.069
CMRL (μmol/g/min)	−0.016 ± 0.023	−0.012 ± 0.021	−0.222 ± 0.097	−0.023 ± 0.022	−0.016 ± 0.020

SOURCE: Robertson et al.[59]

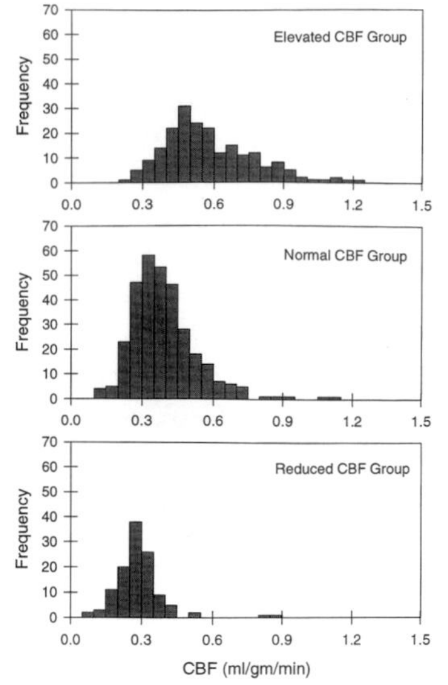

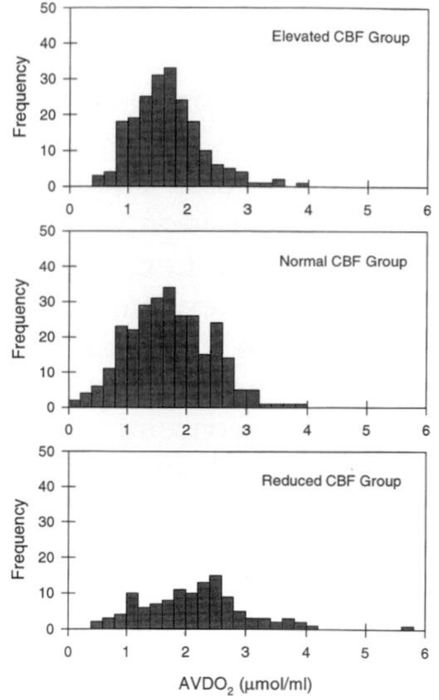

Figure 34-3. Frequency histograms of CBF (*left*) and AVD_{O_2} (*right*) measurements in 100 patients with severe head injury. (Used with permission from Robertson et al.[15])

Figure 34-4 shows box-plot graphs of the distribution of the CBF values obtained during successive 8-h periods for the reduced, normal, and elevated CBF groups. The horizontal line across the box depicts the median CBF for the 8-h period; the top and bottom of the box represent the 75th and 25th percentiles, respectively; and the error bars mark the 90th and 10th percentiles. Outlying points are shown as filled circles. A normal CBF was present throughout the period of monitoring in 47 patients (Fig. 34-4, *middle*).

A reduced CBF was typically present on the initial measurement of CBF (16 patients; see Fig. 34-4, *top*) or developed within the first 48 h after injury (7 patients). In the latter group, the initial CBF was elevated in two patients and was normal in the remaining five. Two additional patients who were not comatose and therefore were not monitored on admission to the hospital later deteriorated to coma. Initial CBF values were found to be reduced on the fifth and sixth postinjury days when they neurologically deteriorated. CBF tended to remain reduced throughout the acute recovery phase in these patients. In the patients who died of intracranial hypertension, CBF fell to very low values as the ICP became uncontrollable. In only three patients did the CBF recover to normal values during the period of monitoring.

An elevated CBF was present on the initial measurements of CBF (15 patients) or developed within the first 24 to 48 h (15 patients; see Fig. 34-4, *bottom*). Four patients with elevated CBF who developed intracranial hypertension refractory to treatment with hyperventilation, mannitol, and CSF drainage and who were treated with barbiturates all had early elevations of CBF that persisted for many days. Other patients, however, had CBF elevations without significant intracranial hypertension. The hyperemia tended to be more transient in the patients with normal ICP.

COUPLING OF CBF AND METABOLISM

NORMAL REGULATION OF CBF

In normal individuals, CBF is closely coupled to and regulated by CMR_{O_2}. Local CBF is increased or decreased, depending on the tissue metabolic requirements.[16] In certain altered physiological states, such as seizures, changes in brain temperature, and some types of anesthesia, CBF remains coupled to CMR_{O_2}.[17] If the cerebral metabolic rate is decreased by barbiturate anesthesia, for example, CBF also will decrease, since requirements for metabolic substrates are less. If the cerebral metabolic rate is increased, for example, by fever, CBF also will increase. Because the ratio between CMR_{O_2} and CBF does not change if these parameters are normally coupled, the cerebral arteriovenous difference of oxygen remains constant. Figure 34-5 (*left*) shows data from laboratory studies where CMR_{O_2} was varied by different experimental paradigms. CBF increased and decreased with CMR_{O_2}, and AVD_{O_2} remained relatively unchanged. Similar findings have been observed in humans with hypothermia and barbiturate anesthesia.

MECHANISMS OF NORMAL COUPLING OF CBF AND CMR_{O_2}

The concept that regulation of the cerebral circulation is at least in part mediated by the products of cerebral metabolism and CBF is adjusted to local cerebral metabolism is more than a century old. In 1890, Roy and Sherrington[18] stated, "The chemical products of cerebral metabolism contained in the lymph which bathes

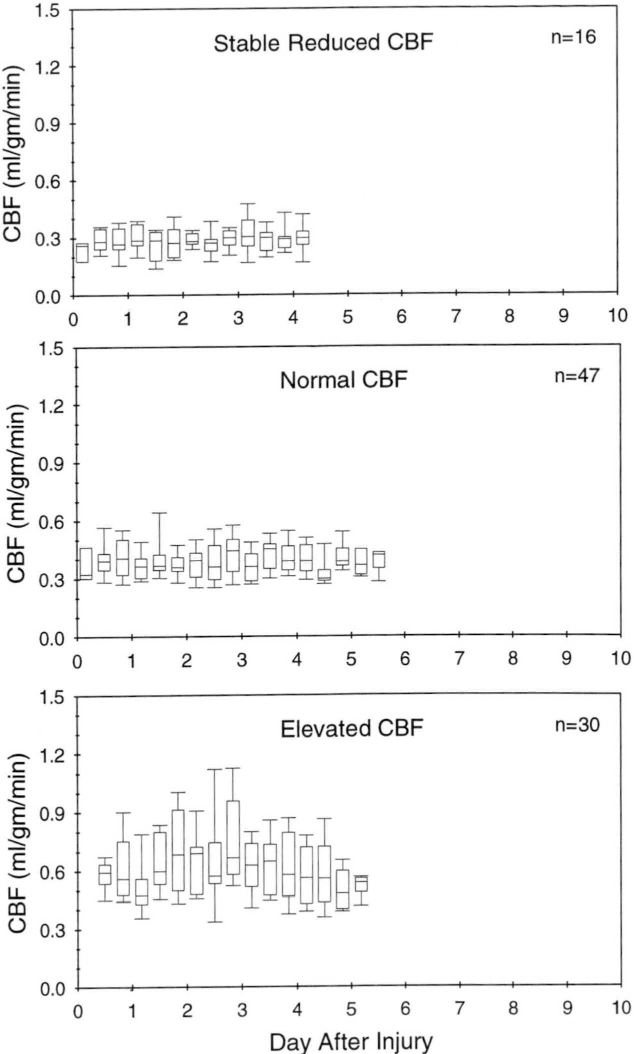

Figure 34-4. Box-plot graphs of the distribution of the CBF values obtained during successive 8-h periods for patients with reduced (*top*), normal (*middle*), or elevated (*bottom*) CBF. The horizontal line across the box depicts the median CBF for the 8-h period; the top and bottom of the box represent the 75th and 25th percentiles, respectively; and the error bars mark the 90th and 10th percentiles. (Used with permission from Robertson et al.[15])

the walls of the arterioles of the brain can cause variations in the calibre of the cerebral vessels. In the reaction the brain possesses an intrinsic mechanism by which its vascular supply can be varied locally in correspondence with local variations of functional activity."

The principal metabolic products that may be responsible for the coupling of cerebral metabolism and blood flow are P_{O_2}, P_{CO_2}, extracellular pH, and adenosine. The levels of these agents are directly influenced by local energy metabolism. In addition, K^+ has been proposed as a possible coupler, although extracellular K^+ is involved only indirectly in energy metabolism through its role in membrane function in neurons and smooth muscle cells.

Nitric oxide (NO), which is synthesized from L-arginine by the enzyme NO synthase, activates guanylate cyclase to dilate many vascular beds and also has been investigated as a mediator of the coupling of CBF and metabolism during neuronal activation. Recent studies have shown that activation of the *N*-methyl-D-aspartate (NMDA) receptor can cause local release of NO.[19] Cerebral vasodilation in response to NMDA was inhibited by dizocilpine maleate (MK-801), an NMDA receptor antagonist, and by L-NNA, an inhibitor of NO synthase, suggesting that the vasodilation was dependent on neuronal activity and was mediated by NO. In other studies in cats, administration of L-NAME, an NO synthase inhibitor, produced complete blockade of the hyperemia associated with spreading depression but no change in the increase in the neuronal firing rate.[20]

Uncoupling of CBF and CMR_{O_2} after Head Injury

In a patient with a severe head injury, CMR_{O_2} is typically reduced from a normal value of 1.5 μmol/g/min to between 0.6 and 1.2 μmol/g/min.[5,12,21] If CBF remains coupled to CMR_{O_2}, CBF will be equally reduced. However, normal coupling of CBF is retained in only 45 percent of comatose head-injured patients.[12] In the majority of patients, CBF regulatory mechanisms are abnormal, and rather than being coupled to CMR_{O_2}, CBF is increased or decreased independent of the reduced cerebral metabolic rate. In this situation, the ratio between CMR_{O_2} and CBF varies.

The mechanism of the uncoupling of CBF and metabolism in an injured brain is not completely understood. Acidosis may play a role in causing vasodilation. It has been reported that hyperventilation, which would ameliorate cerebral acidosis, restores normal autoregulation.[22] Neuronal innervation, particularly from the trigeminal ganglion, may play a role in the development of hyperemia.[23] Cerebral vasoconstriction has many potential mediators.[24]

Because CBF changes occur independent of cerebral metabolism, measurements of the reciprocal changes in AVD_{O_2} have been used as an indicator of CBF adequacy.[12] The brain extracts oxygen more completely than do most tissues, and the normal cerebral AVD_{O_2} ranges from 1.8 to 3.9 μmol/ml.[2] A normal AVD_{O_2} suggests that CBF is normally coupled to CMR_{O_2}, a decreased AVD_{O_2} indicates that CBF is excessive for cerebral metabolic requirements, and an elevated AVD_{O_2} indicates a decreased CBF. Figures 34-5 (*right*) and 34-6 (*right*) illustrate the nonlinear relationship between CBF and AVD_{O_2} that would be expected in normal and pathophysiological conditions by displaying a

Normal Coupling of CBF and $CMRO_2$

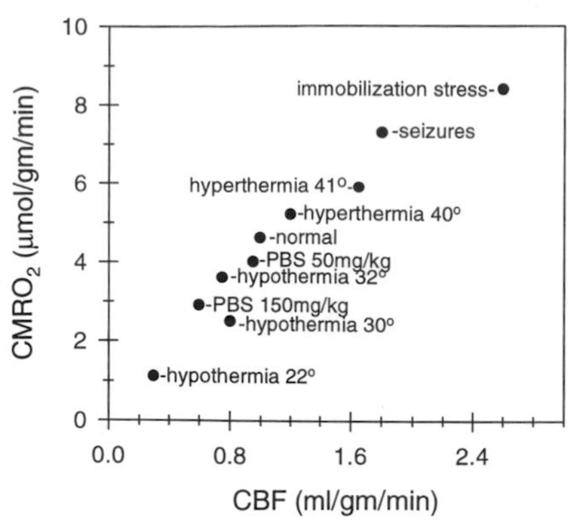

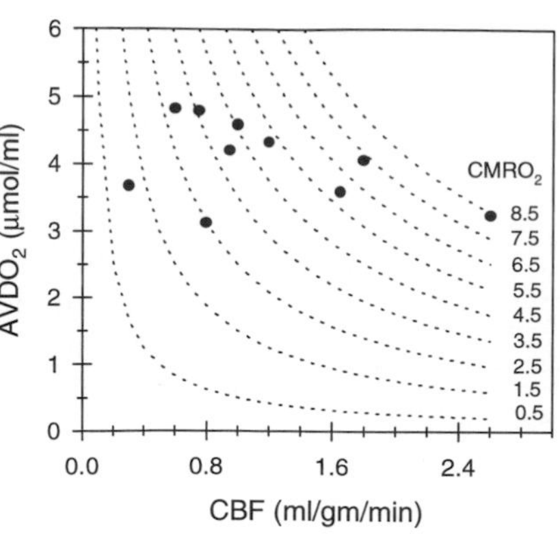

Figure 34-5. Normally, CBF is tightly coupled to CMR_{O_2}. The graphs show data from laboratory studies in rats where CMR_{O_2} was varied by different experimental paradigms (data from Nilsson et al.[60]). CBF increased and decreased with CMR_{O_2}, and AVD_{O_2} remained relatively unchanged.

series of curves, each described by the formula $AVD_{O_2} = CMR_{O_2}/CBF$. Each individual curve defines the relation between AVD_{O_2} and CBF that would occur if CMR_{O_2} were held constant at a particular value and CBF were varied. If a coupled change in CMR_{O_2} and CBF occurs (Fig. 34-5, *right*), AVD_{O_2} remains unchanged and the relationship between CBF and AVD_{O_2} simply shifts to a new CMR_{O_2} curve. If an uncoupled change in CBF occurs, changes in AVD_{O_2} reflect the variations in CBF (Fig. 34-6, *right*).

The relationship between CBF and AVD_{O_2} was studied in a group of 100 comatose patients,[21] and there was the expected nonlinear correlation between the Kety-Schmidt CBF and AVD_{O_2} ($n = 313$, $r = -0.74$, $p < .01$). These patients had a mean CMR_{O_2} of 0.82 ± 0.21 μmol/g/min regardless of the level of the CBF and could be divided into three CBF categories by the level of AVD_{O_2}. Patients with an $AVD_{O_2} < 1.3$ μmol/ml had an elevated or hyperemic CBF, averaging 0.529 ± 0.181 ml/g/min. Patients with an AVD_{O_2} between 1.3 and 3.0 μmol/ml had a normal CBF, averaging 0.416 ± 0.124 ml/g/min. Patients with an $AVD_{O_2} > 3.0$ μmol/ml had a low CBF, averaging 0.234 ± 0.069 ml/g/min.

Changes in cerebral metabolism parameters during episodes of ischemia are illustrated in Fig. 34-7 by a patient who developed refractory intracranial hypertension. As CBF decreases, AVD_{O_2} proportionally increases as the brain compensates for the decreased flow by extracting a greater amount of oxygen. As long as increased extraction of oxygen completely compensates for the decreased blood flow, CMR_{O_2} remains unchanged (*hypoperfusion pattern*). However, a point will be reached at which further decreases in CBF cannot be compensated for by increased oxygen extraction. Ischemia, manifested by a fall in CMR_{O_2} and an increase in cerebral lactate production, results (*ischemia pattern*). Initially, these metabolic changes of ischemia may be reversible. However, as time passes, irreversible ischemic injury or infarction develops (*infarction pattern*). The time required for the changes to become irrevers-

CBF and $AVDO_2$ After Head Injury

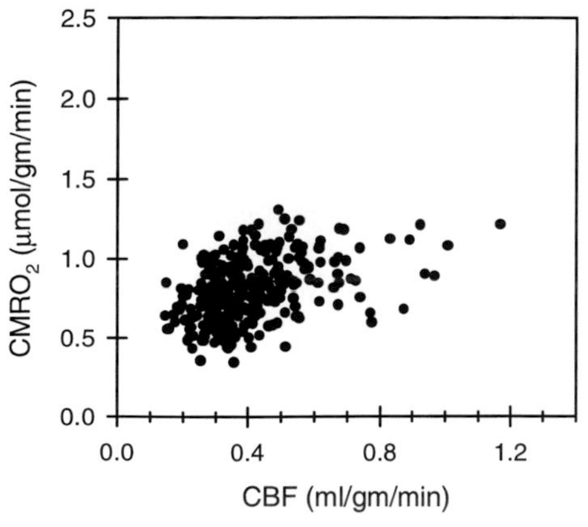

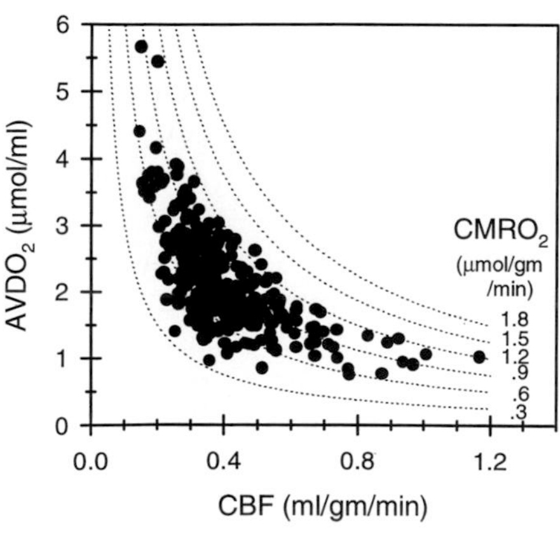

Figure 34-6. After a severe head injury, CBF may vary independently of CMR_{O_2}, and AVD_{O_2} reflects the changes in CBF. Patients with an elevated CBF can be identified by a low AVD_{O_2}, while patients with a reduced CBF can be identified by a widened AVD_{O_2}.

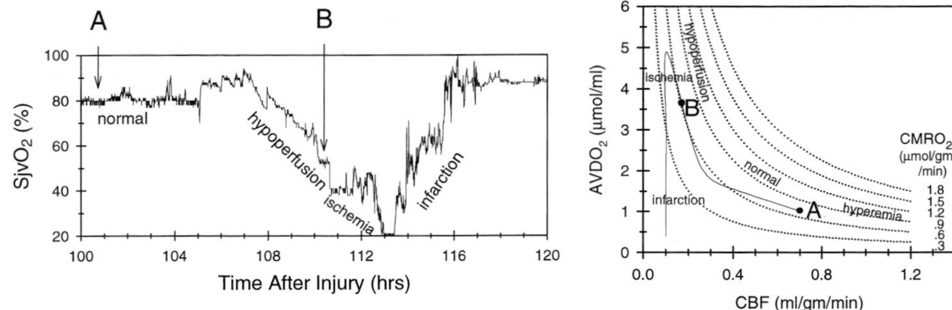

Figure 34-7. Example of the changes in cerebral metabolism that were observed in a patient who developed global ischemia as a result of refractory intracranial hypertension. On the left is the tracing of Sjv_{O_2} and the values for CBF, CMR_{O_2}, and CMRL before and during the episode of ischemia. On the right the same data are plotted on the CBF/AVD_{O_2} graph, showing that the patient went through all four stages of metabolism (normal → hypoperfusion → ischemia → infarction).

ible depends on the severity of the reduction in CBF. As the tissue dies, CMR_{O_2} falls, while cerebral lactate production may remain elevated. Increases in CBF after the tissue has infarcted do not result in a significant increase in CMR_{O_2} but instead are expressed as a decrease in AVD_{O_2}.

The *hypoperfusion pattern* may be the most important to recognize clinically. The increased AVD_{O_2} suggests that the brain is compensating for the decreased blood flow by extracting oxygen more completely, but because anaerobic metabolism is not increased and because CMR_{O_2} does not change as CBF is increased, the low blood flow does not appear to alter overall cerebral energy metabolism. Although these patients are not truly ischemic at the moment of the CBF measurement, they have exhausted the brain's compensatory mechanism for maintaining cerebral metabolism in the presence of decreased oxygen availability. In such cases, small decreases in either CBF or arterial oxygen content can produce significant cerebral ischemia.

The *ischemia/infarction pattern* is also important to identify because this pattern is sometimes reversible. Because AVD_{O_2} is low, this pattern is often thought to indicate that brain tissue is irreversibly injured and that CBF is adequate for the markedly reduced metabolic requirements. Although this is often the case, the presence of reversible ischemic changes is best determined by a trial of increasing CBF. The reason for the low AVD_{O_2} in patients with reversible ischemia is not entirely clear. It may be that the blood flow is not homogeneous and that areas of very low flow and markedly increased oxygen extraction are mixed with areas of normal oxygen extraction. Alternatively, with very low CBF, venous blood in the jugular bulb may be contaminated with more extracerebral blood than occurs when blood flow is normal.

ISCHEMIC THRESHOLDS

Ischemic Thresholds in Normal Subjects

The functional and metabolic effects of ischemia depend on the severity and duration of the reduction in CBF. When CBF decreases below 58 percent of normal, or below 23 to 30 ml/100 g/min, alterations in the EEG and consciousness develop.[25] The EEG becomes isoelectric at a CBF less than 33 percent of normal, or below 18 ml/100 g/min.[26] Evoked potentials disappear at a CBF less than 10 percent of normal. Below this critical threshold, cellular ionic homeostasis is altered, resulting in an increase in extracellular K^+ and an increase in intracellular Na^+ and Ca^{2+}.

The duration of the CBF reduction is also crucial in determining whether irreversible injury will occur. For example, flow distal to a middle cerebral artery occlusion must remain less than 12 ml/100 g/min for at least 2 h before infarction develops.[27] In general, the lower the CBF, the shorter the time required for irreversible injury to develop.

Ischemic Thresholds after Head Injury

Ischemic thresholds have not been definitively established in head-injured patients. Because cerebral metabolic requirements are reduced after a head injury, some researchers have speculated that ischemic thresholds may occur at a lower value of CBF. However, since hemoglobin concentration may be lower than normal in head-injured patients, actual oxygen delivery may be lower for any given CBF value than it is in normal persons. This might be expected to result in ischemic thresholds at a higher value of CBF.

RELATIONSHIP OF CBF AND OUTCOME

An extremely low CBF, less than the ischemic threshold of 0.18 ml/g/min, has almost always been associated with a poor neurological outcome. Bouma and coworkers[14] found a CBF < 0.18 ml/g/min of 11 of 31 patients studied within 6 h of an injury. Early mortality was significantly related to the presence of a CBF < 0.18 ml/g/min. Overgaard and associates,[28] using intracarotid xenon CBF measurements, showed that rCBF values < 0.20 ml/g/min occurred in 61 percent of patients who died or were severely disabled or vegetative but in only 10 percent of patients with a good outcome. Overgaard and Tweed[29] reported that patients who died or remained vegetative often had very low rCBF in arterial boundary zones and as a group had lower global CBF values than did patients who recovered.

Extremely elevated CBF levels have also been related to a poor neurological outcome. Fieschi and coworkers[30] reported that an initially low CBF returned to normal in patients who recovered and increased to elevated levels in patients who died of a cerebral injury. Overgaard and Tweed[29] reported a good outcome in only 1 of 12 patients with elevated CBF in their series. Uzzell and colleagues[31] observed that hyperemic patients suffered greater neuropsychological impairment than did patients with a reduced CBF.

Exclusive of these two extremes, the optimal level for the CBF after a head injury is controversial. Some studies suggest that reduced CBF is associated with a favorable outcome. Langfitt and associates[32] and Obrist and coworkers[33] found that the early reduced CBF returned to normal in patients who recovered from injury and decreased in patients who died. Obrist and colleagues[12] suggested that a lower CBF was appropriate for the lower cerebral metabolic rate of a comatose patient and offered the normal AVD_{O_2} as evidence. A reduced CBF was associated with a lower incidence of intracranial hypertension. However, other studies have suggested that reduced CBF is associated with an unfavorable outcome. Tabaddor and colleagues[34] found that CBF and CMR_{O_2} were lower in patients who died of a head injury. Muizelaar[35] found that in the first 24 h after an injury, patients with a good neurological outcome had a higher CBF than did those with a poor neurological outcome. After 24 h there was no relationship between CBF and outcome.

In the BTGH series of 102 patients with severe head injury, the Kety-Schmidt CBF level has been correlated with outcome.[15] In patients with a reduced CBF, the mortality rate was 32 percent 3 months after the injury, compared with 21 percent in patients with a normal CBF and 20 percent in patients with an elevated CBF. The patients with a reduced CBF also were more likely to have an outcome of severe disability or persistent vegetative state: 48 percent compared with 39 percent in patients with a normal CBF and 27 percent in patients with an elevated CBF. Twenty percent of patients with a reduced CBF had a good recovery or moderate disability 3 months after the injury, compared with 53 percent of patients with an elevated CBF and 41 percent of patients with a normal CBF. In a subsequent series of 116 patients at BTGH, those with a reduced CBF were twice as likely to have transient periods of ischemia identified by continuous monitoring of Sjv_{O_2}.[36]

CBF CHANGES AFTER THERAPY

Because Kety-Schmidt CBF measurements can be repeated, the technique has been used to evaluate the cerebrovascular effects of the therapies used in head-injured patients.

Treatment of Ischemia

Forty-nine of the patients in the BTGH series had serial measurements of CBF every 8 h during the first 5 to 10 days after injury, prospectively looking for global ischemia.[2] When changes of ischemia were identified, therapy was instituted to increase CBF, and then repeat measurements of CBF and metabolism were obtained to evaluate the effects of treatment.

Eleven (22 percent) of the 49 patients were identified as having the characteristic changes of compensated hypoperfusion: decreased CBF, $AVD_{O_2} > 3.0$ μmol/ml, but a normal lactate : oxygen index (LOI). CBF averaged 0.221 ± 0.038 ml/g/min. One patient with intracranial hypertension who was being treated with mechanical hyperventilation was treated by permitting the P_{CO_2} to increase to 35 mmHg. The remainder of the patients were treated with hypervolemic hemodilution, and one also was treated with dopamine-induced hypertension. All the patients had an increase in CBF with treatment, to a mean value of 0.336 ± 0.050 ml/g/min. In all the patients, AVD_{O_2} decreased into the normal range as CBF was increased by the therapy from 3.92

± 0.84 to 2.61 ± 0.39 μmol/ml. CMR_{O_2} was unchanged by the CBF treatment, confirming the conclusion obtained from the normal cerebral lactate production that these patients were not truly ischemic but were able to compensate for the low CBF by means of increased extraction of oxygen.

Four (7 percent) of the 49 patients studied developed an ischemia/infarction CBF pattern after having an initially normal CBF. In one of these patients, the ischemia was due to severe intracranial hypertension that developed 24 h after the evacuation of a traumatic intracerebral hematoma. A second patient developed ischemia caused by vasospasm 72 h after a subarachnoid hemorrhage. The other two patients developed cerebral ischemia 2 to 3 days after a closed head injury. Regardless of the etiology, all four patients changed from a pattern of normal CBF, with a normal AVD_{O_2} and a normal cerebral lactate production to a pattern of infarction between the routine CBF measurements (approximately 8 h). CBF dropped from 0.342 ± 0.035 to 0.214 ± 0.042 ml/g/min, CMR_{O_2} decreased from 0.76 ± 0.09 to 0.18 ± 0.13 μmol/g/min, and cerebral lactate production increased from −0.020 ± 0.017 to −0.042 ± 0.007 μmol/g/min. AVD_{O_2} decreased from 2.23 ± 0.36 to 0.81 ± 0.54 μmol/ml, which, interpreted alone, might suggest that CBF had increased. However, the LOI increased dramatically from 0.03 ± 0.02 to 0.36 ± 0.29, indicating the presence of ischemia/infarction and demonstrating that AVD_{O_2} would not accurately reflect CBF. In each case, a lateral skull x-ray documented that the venous catheter remained in the jugular bulb; however, it cannot be ruled out that with the drop in CBF, increased extracerebral contamination of the jugular venous blood might have accounted for the increase in venous oxygen saturation.

Ten (20 percent) of the 49 patients prospectively evaluated for ischemia had an ischemia CBF pattern on the initial CBF measurement or developed cerebral ischemia during the subsequent hospital course. In two patients who had cerebral ischemia caused by intractable intracranial hypertension, it was not possible to follow treatment of the ischemia with CBF measurements because these patients died despite aggressive treatment. In the remaining eight patients, nine separate episodes of treatment of cerebral ischemia were documented with CBF measurements before and after treatment. The treatments that were examined included increasing P_{CO_2} to 35 mmHg (three patients), hypervolemic hemodilution (five patients), and dopamine-induced hypertension (one patient). CBF increased with treatment in all nine cases, from 0.163 ± 0.038 to 0.303 ± 0.107 ml/g/min. With five of the episodes of ischemia, an increase in CMR_{O_2} accompanied the increase in CBF from a mean value of 0.26 ± 0.17 to 0.68 ± 0.14 μmol/g/min. In four of the patients, CMR_{O_2} remained unchanged, although CBF was increased by the therapy. The change in AVD_{O_2} was quite variable, and it was not possible to determine whether CMR_{O_2} was improved from the changes in AVD_{O_2}. However, the LOI decreased in the five episodes of cerebral ischemia where treatment resulted in an increase in CMR_{O_2} and, in contrast, increased in the four patients in whom CMR_{O_2} remained unchanged. Both patients whose CMR_{O_2} did not change with treatment eventually died of neurological injury. In the four patients whose improvement in CMR_{O_2} was sustained for the remainder of the CBF monitoring, LOI decreased to less than 0.08, clearly into the nonischemic range, while in the patient whose improvements in cerebral metabolism were transient despite continued treatment, LOI decreased only from 0.45 to 0.13.

Hyperventilation

Induced hyperventilation constricts cerebral blood vessels, reducing global CBF and cerebral blood volume. The effect of changes in P_{CO_2} on cerebral vessels is mediated by the change in pH induced in the extracellular fluid.[37] CO_2 reactivity is preserved in most patients with a severe head injury, and therefore hyperventilation can rapidly lower ICP by reducing cerebral blood volume.

Hyperventilation reduces ICP at the expense of cerebral perfusion. Whether hyperventilation can actually result in cerebral ischemia in head-injured patients is controversial. Hyperventilation (to P_{CO_2} of 20 mmHg) was shown to have a detrimental effect on outcome in one randomized trial.[38] The authors of this study recommended using hyperventilation only in patients with intracranial hypertension rather than in all head-injured patients. In a study of 27 comatose patients, Cold reported that hyperventilation increased the frequency of finding rCBF values less than 0.2 ml/g/min from 5 percent to 16 percent.[39] A low rCBF before hyperventilation predisposed to this increased frequency.

The relationship of hyperventilation and global cerebral blood flow using the Kety-Schmidt technique has been examined in a series of a 171 head-injured patients during the first 10 days after injury.[40] Of 1212 CBF measurements in these patients, 132 (10 percent) were less than 0.25 ml/g/min. Among the 132 low CBF values, 71 (54 percent) were appropriately reduced relative to the lower CMR_{O_2}, while 61 (46 percent) were associated with increased oxygen extraction and/or increased cerebral lactate production, suggesting a relative inadequacy of perfusion. The incidence of an inadequate CBF steadily increased as the P_{CO_2} decreased and was 2, 4, 8, and 23 percent when the P_{CO_2} was greater than 30 mmHg, 25 to 30 mmHg, 20 to 25 mmHg, and less than 20 mmHg, respectively. The incidence of an inadequate CBF was twice as high during the first 24 h than on any other day (8 percent compared with 4 percent). The incidence was highest in patients with a reduced CBF: 11 percent compared with 2 percent in patients with normal or elevated CBF. These studies suggested that hyperventilation should be reserved for patients who actually develop intracranial hypertension and that P_{CO_2} should not be reduced to less than 25 mmHg unless Sjv_{O_2} is monitored to make certain that it does not produce ischemia.

Head Elevation

Elevation of the head of the bed and keeping the head in a neutral position to minimize compression of venous return from the brain have been standard neurosurgery practice for the management of ICP. However, the ideal head position for patients with a head injury has been disputed in recent years. Rosner and associates have advocated keeping patients' heads flat as part of an overall treatment program intended to maximize cerebral perfusion pressure (CPP).[41,42] Other studies have shown a reduction in ICP without a reduction in either CPP or CBF in most patients with elevation of the head to 30 degrees.[43,44] The effects of head position on ICP and cerebral hemodynamics using the Kety-Schmidt technique have been studied in 22 patients with severe head injury.[43] Elevation of the head to 30 degrees reduced ICP and BP without changing CPP or CBF in most patients.

Antihypertensive Agents

Systemic hypertension associated with a head injury is common. It is characterized by a systolic blood pressure increase greater than the diastolic increase and is associated with a hyperdynamic state that includes tachycardia and increased cardiac output. It is unwise to reduce systemic blood pressure in patients with hypertension associated with untreated intracranial mass lesions, because cerebral perfusion is maintained by the higher blood pressure. However, treatment of systemic hypertension (systolic blood pressure $>$ 160 mmHg) during the postoperative course after a head injury is recommended by many neurosurgeons. Since autoregulation is frequently impaired after a severe head injury, systemic hypertension may increase CBF and ICP[45] and may exacerbate cerebral edema.[46] However, others have emphasized the importance of maintaining CPP even at the expense of a higher ICP.[47,48]

Systemic hypertension often resolves with sedation. If antihypertensives are required, it is important to remember that vasodilating antihypertensives, including hydralazine and sodium nitroprusside, consistently increase ICP.[49,50] Sympathetic blocking antihypertensives such as beta blocking agents (propranolol and labetalol) and centrally acting alpha agonists (clonidine and α-methyldopa) are preferred because they reduce blood pressure without affecting ICP.[51] The effects of labetalol and hydralazine have been compared in nine hypertensive head-injured patients.[52] While both antihypertensives reduced blood pressure by approximately 20 mmHg, ICP increased from 16 $\pm$ 1 to 24 $\pm$ 1 mmHg with hydralazine but did not change significantly with labetalol. As shown in Table 34-3, the increase in ICP with hydralazine was accompanied by an increase in CBF and a decrease in cerebrovascular resistance (CVR) and AVD_{O_2}. In addition, the systemic cardiovascular abnormalities resolved with labetalol but were exaggerated with hydralazine.

Barbiturate Coma

Barbiturate coma is another treatment modality that has been used to lower ICP in head-injured patients. Barbiturates are protective during periods of cerebral hypoxia. While routine use of barbiturates in unselected patients has not been consistently effective in reducing morbidity or mortality after a severe head injury, a randomized multicenter trial demonstrated that instituting barbiturate coma in patients with refractory intracranial

TABLE 34-3 Comparison of Hydralazine and Labetalol as Antihypertensives in Head-Injured Patients

	Hydralazine		*Labetalol*	
	Before	**After**	**Before**	**After**
ICP (mmHg)	16 $\pm$ 1	24 $\pm$ 3	16 $\pm$ 2	18 $\pm$ 3
CBF (ml/g/min)	0.51 $\pm$ 0.11	0.68 $\pm$ 0.12	0.54 $\pm$ 0.07	0.45 $\pm$ 0.05
CVR (mmHg/ml/g/min)	2.9 $\pm$ 0.6	1.8 $\pm$ 0.5	2.6 $\pm$ 0.4	2.6 $\pm$ 0.4
AVD_{O_2} (μmol/ml)	0.8 $\pm$ 0.3	1.4 $\pm$ 0.1	1.9 $\pm$ 0.4	2.3 $\pm$ 0.3
CMR_{O_2} (μmol/g/min)	0.88 $\pm$ 0.12	0.92 $\pm$ 0.12	0.90 $\pm$ 0.12	0.94 $\pm$ 0.14

hypertension resulted in a twofold greater chance of controlling ICP.[53]

Because of the hypotensive complications associated with barbiturates and because the neurological examination is unavailable during treatment, barbiturate coma is usually reserved for patients with intracranial hypertension that is resistant to other modalities. Pentobarbital sodium is given in both loading and maintenance doses. The loading dose is 10 mg/kg given over 30 min, followed by 5 mg/kg every hour for three doses. This typically provides a therapeutic level after the fourth dose. The maintenance dose is 1 to 2 mg/kg/h or is adjusted so that the serum level is in the therapeutic range of 30 to 50 μg/ml or so that the EEG demonstrates a burst suppression pattern. Pulmonary wedge pressure and cardiac output are monitored in all patients. Hypotension caused by pentobarbital is treated first with volume replacement and then with dopamine if necessary.

The mechanism of ICP reduction by barbiturates is not entirely clear but is usually considered to be hemodynamic because of the immediate effect on ICP. Studies by Messeter and colleagues have suggested that the reduction in ICP with barbiturates is closely tied to the retention of CO_2 reactivity by the brain.[54,55]

The effects of pentobarbital on cerebral hemodynamics using the Kety-Schmidt technique have been examined in 29 patients with refractory intracranial hypertension.[56] The loading dose of pentobarbital decreased ICP and BP by 11 and 15 mmHg, respectively. Dopamine was required to treat systemic hypotension in 20 (69 percent) of the 29 patients. CPP was improved in only 11 (38 percent) of the patients and was decreased or unchanged in 18 (62 percent) patients. For the whole group, CPP averaged 65 $\pm$ 15 mmHg before treatment and 62 $\pm$ 13 mmHg after the loading dose of pentobarbital. CBF and CMR_{O_2} were also significantly decreased after the loading dose of pentobarbital: by 25 percent and 34 percent, respectively. The reduction in CMR_{O_2} and CBF was directly related to the pretreatment values, suggesting that if CMR_{O_2} was already very low because of a severe injury, the barbiturates had very little effect.

References

1. Kety SS, Schmidt CF: The determination of cerebral blood flow in man by the use of nitrous oxide in low concentrations. *Am J Pysiol* 143:53–66, 1945.
2. Kety SS, Schmidt CF: The nitrous oxide method for the quantitative determination of cerebral blood flow in man: Theory, procedure, and normal values. *J Clin Invest* 27:476–483, 1948.
3. Himwich WA, Hamburger E, Maresca R, et al: Brain metabolism in man: Unanesthetized and in pentothal narcosis. *Am J Psychiatry* 103:689–696, 1946.
4. Shenkin GA, Harmel MH, Kety SS: Dynamic anatomy of the cerebral circulation. *Arch Neurol Psych* 60:240–252, 1948.
5. Lassen N: Cerebral blood flow and oxygen consumption in man. *Physiol Rev* 39:183–238, 1959.
6. Jakobsen M, Enevoldsen E: Retrograde catheterization of the right internal jugular vein for serial measurements of cerebral venous oxygen content. *J Cereb Blood Flow Metab* 9:717–720, 1989.
7. Hoyer S: Metabolism of the human brain: The principles and limitations of global measurements, in Hartmann A, Hoyer S (eds): *Cerebral Blood Flow and Metabolism Measurement.* Berlin: Springer-Verlag, 1985: 382–390.
8. Lassen NA, Klee A: Cerebral blood flow determined by saturation and desaturation with krypton^{85}. *Circ Res* 16:26–32, 1965.
9. Kety SS, Harmel MH, Broomell HT, et al: The solubility of nitrous oxide in brain and blood. *J Biol Chem* 173:487, 1948.
10. Sharples PM, Stuart AG, Aynsley Green A, et al: A practical method of serial bedside measurement of cerebral blood flow and metabolism during neurointensive care. *Arch Dis Child* 66:1326–1332, 1991.
11. Robertson CS, Grossman RG, Goodman JC, et al: The predictive value of cerebral anaerobic metabolism with cerebral infarction after head injury. *J Neurosurg* 67:361–368, 1987.
12. Obrist WD, Langfitt T, Jaggi J, et al: Cerebral blood flow and metabolism in comatose patients with acute head injury: Relationship to intracranial hypertension. *J Neurosurg* 61:241–253, 1984.
13. Cruz J, Jaggi JL, Hoffstad OJ: Cerebral blood flow and oxygen consumption in acute brain injury with acute anemia: An alternative for the cerebral metabolic rate of oxygen consumption. *Crit Care Med* 21:1218–1224, 1993.
14. Bouma GJ, Muizelaar JP, Stringer WA, et al: Ultra-early evaluation of regional cerebral blood flow in severely head-injured patients using xenon-enhanced computerized tomography. *J Neurosurg* 77:360–368, 1992.
15. Robertson CS, Contant CF, Gokaslan ZL, et al: Cerebral blood flow, arteriovenous oxygen difference, and outcome in head injured patients. *J Neurol Neurosurg Psychiatry* 55:594–603, 1992.
16. Raichle ME, Grubb RLJ, Gado MH, et al: Correlation between regional cerebral blood flow and oxidative metabolism: In vivo studies in man. *Arch Neurol* 33:523–526, 1976.
17. Nilsson B, Rehncrona S, Siesjo BK: Coupling of cerebral metabolism and blood flow in epileptic seizures, hypoxia, and hypoglycaemia, in Purves M (ed): *Cerebral Vascular Smooth Muscle and Its Control.* CIBA Foundation Symposium 56 (New Series). Amsterdam: Elsevier, 1978: 199–214.
18. Roy CW, Sherrington CS: On the regulation of the blood supply of the brain. *J Physiol* 11:85–108, 1890.
19. Garthwaite J, Charles SL, Chess-Williams R: Endothelium-derived relaxing factor release on activation of NMDA receptors suggests a role as intercellular messenger in the brain. *Nature* 336:385–388, 1988.
20. Goadsby PJ, Kaube H, Hoskin KL: Nitric oxide synthesis

couples cerebral blood flow and metabolism. *Brain Res* 595:167–170, 1992.

21. Robertson CS, Narayan RK, Gokaslan Z, et al: Cerebral arteriovenous oxygen difference as an estimate of cerebral blood flow in comatose patients. *J Neurosurg* 70:222–230, 1989.
22. Paulson OB, Olesen J, Christensen MS: Restoration of autoregulation of cerebral blood flow by hypocapnia. *Neurology* 22:286–293, 1972.
23. Macfarlane R, Tasemiroglu E, Moskowitz MA, et al: Chronic trigeminal ganglionectomy or topical capsaicin application to pial vessels attenuates postocclusive cortical hyperemia but does not influence postischemic hypoperfusion. *J Cereb Blood Flow Metab* 11:261–271, 1991.
24. Findlay JM, MacDonald RL, Weir BK: Current concepts of pathophysiology and management of cerebral vasospasm following aneurysmal subarachnoid hemorrhage. *Cerebrovasc Brain Metab Rev* 3:336–361, 1991.
25. Morawetz RB, Krowell RH, DeGirolami U, et al: Regional cerebral blood flow thresholds during cerebral ischemia. *Fed Proc* 38:2493–2494, 1979.
26. Astrup J, Symon L, Branston NM, et al: Cortical evoked potential and extracellular K^+ and H^+ at critical levels of brain ischemia. *Stroke* 8:51–57, 1977.
27. Morawetz RB, DeGirolami U, Ojemann RG, et al: Cerebral blood flow determined by hydrogen clearance during middle cerebral artery occlusion in unanesthetized monkeys. *Stroke* 9:143–149, 1978.
28. Overgaard J, Molsdal C, Tweed TA: Cerebral circulation after head injury: 3. Does reduced regional cerebral blood flow determine recovery of brain function after blunt head injury? *J Neurosurg* 55:63–74, 1981.
29. Overgaard J, Tweed WA: Cerebral circulation after head injury: 4. Functional anatomy and boundary-zone flow deprivation in the first week of traumatic coma. *J Neurosurg* 59:439–446, 1983.
30. Fieschi C, Battistini N, Bedushi A, et al: Regional cerebral blood flow and intraventricular pressure in acute head injuries. *J Neurol Neurosurg Psychiatry* 37:1378–1388, 1974.
31. Uzzell BP, Obrist WD, Dolinskas CA, et al: Relationship of acute CBF and ICP findings to neuropsychological outcome in severe head injury. *J Neurosurg* 65:630–635, 1986.
32. Langfitt TW, Obrist WD, Gennarelli TA, et al: Correlation of cerebral blood flow with outcome in head-injured patients. *Ann Surg* 186:411–414, 1977.
33. Obrist WD, Gennarelli TA, Segawa H, et al: Relation of cerebral blood flow to neurological status on outcome in head-injured patients. *J Neurosurg* 51:292–300, 1979.
34. Tabaddor K, Bhushan C, Pevsher PH, et al: Prognostic value of cerebral blood flow (CBF) and cerebral metabolic rate of oxygen (CMR_{O_2}) in acute head trauma. *J Trauma* 12:1053–1055, 1972.
35. Muizelaar JP: Cerebral blood flow, cerebral blood volume, and cerebral metabolism after severe head injury, in Becker DP, Gudeman SK (eds): *Textbook of Head Injury.* Philadelphia: Saunders, 1989: 221–240.
36. Gopinath SP, Robertson CS, Contant CF, et al: Jugular venous desaturation and outcome after head injury. *J Neurol Neurosurg Psychiatry* 57:717–723, 1994.
37. Kontos HA, Raper AJ, Patterson JL Jr: Analysis of vasoactivity of local pH, P_{CO_2}, and bicarbonate on pial vessels. *Stroke* 8:358–360, 1977.
38. Muizelaar JP, Marmarou A, Ward JD, et al: Adverse effects of prolonged hyperventilation in patients with severe head injury: A randomized clinical trial. *J Neurosurg* 75:731–739, 1991.
39. Cold GE: Does acute hyperventilation provoke cerebral oligemia in comatose patients after acute injury? *Acta Neurochir (Wien)* 96:100–106, 1989.
40. Hayes C, Robertson CS, Narayan RK, et al: The effect of hyperventilation on cerebral blood flow in head injured patients. *Am Assoc Neurol Surg Abstr* 1992.
41. Rosner M: Cerebral perfusion pressure: Link between intracranial pressure and systemic circulation, in Wood JH (ed): *Cerebral Blood Flow.* New York: McGraw-Hill, 1987: 425–448.
42. Rosner MJ, Coley IB: Cerebral perfusion pressure, intracranial pressure, and head elevation. *J Neurosurg* 65:636–641, 1986.
43. Feldman Z, Kanter MJ, Robertson CS, et al: Effect of head elevation on intracranial pressure, cerebral perfusion pressure, and cerebral blood flow in head-injured patients. *J Neurosurg* 76:207–211, 1992.
44. Durward QJ, Amacher AL, Del Maestro RF, et al: Cerebral and cardiovascular responses to changes in head elevation in patients with intracranial hypertension. *J Neurosurg* 59:938–944, 1983.
45. Enevoldsen EM, Jensen JT: Autoregulation and CO_2 responses of cerebral blood flow in patients with severe head injury. *J Neurosurg* 48:689–703, 1978.
46. Durward QJ, Del Maestro RF, Amacher AL, et al: The influence of systemic arterial pressure and intracranial pressure on the development of cerebral vasogenic edema. *J Neurosurg* 59:803–809, 1983.
47. Changaris DG, McGraw CP, Richardson JD, et al: Correlation of cerebral perfusion pressure and Glasgow Coma Scale to outcome. *J Trauma* 27:1007–1013, 1987.
48. Rosner MJ, Daughton S: Cerebral perfusion pressure management in head injury. *J Trauma* 30:933–941, 1993.
49. Cottrell JE, Patel K, Turndorf H, et al: Intracranial pressure changes induced by sodium nitroprusside in patients with intracranial mass lesions. *J Neurosurg* 48:329–331, 1978.
50. Overgaard J, Skinhoj E: A paradoxical cerebral hemodynamic effect of hydralazine. *Stroke* 6:402–404, 1975.
51. Robertson CS, Clifton GL, Taylor AA, et al: Treatment of hypertension associated with head injury. *J Neurosurg* 59:445–460, 1983.
52. Gokaslan ZL, Villareal C, Robertson CS, et al: Treating hypertension in neurosurgical patients. *Congr Neurol Surg Abstr* 1991.
53. Eisenberg HM, Frankowski RF, Contant CF, et al: High-dose barbiturate control of elevated intracranial pressure in patients with severe head injury. *J Neurosurg* 69:15–23, 1988.

54. Messeter K, Nordstrom CH, Sundbarg G, et al: Cerebral hemodynamics in patients with acute severe head trauma. *J Neurosurg* 64:231–237, 1986.
55. Nordstrom CH, Messeter K, Sundbarg G, et al: Cerebral blood flow, vasoreactivity, and oxygen consumption during barbiturate therapy in severe traumatic brain lesions. *J Neurosurg* 68:424–431, 1988.
56. Gokaslan ZL, Robertson CS, Narayan RK, et al: Barbiturates, cerebral blood flow, and intracranial hypertension, in Hoff JT, Betz AL (eds): *Intracranial Pressure VII.* Berlin: Springer-Verlag, 1989: 894–897.
57. Rowe GG, Maxwell GM, Castillo CA, et al: A study in man of cerebral blood flow and cerebral glucose, lactate, and pyruvate metabolism before and after eating. *J Clin Invest* 38:2154–2158, 1959.
58. Gibbs EL, Lennox WG, Nims LF, et al: Arterial and cerebral venous blood: Arterial-venous differences in man. *J Biol Chem* 144:325–332, 1942.
59. Robertson CS, Goodman JC, Narayan RK, et al: The effect of glucose administration on carbohydrate metabolism after head injury. *J Neurosurg* 74:43–50, 1991.
60. Nilsson B, Rehncrona S, Siesjo BK: Coupling of cerebral metabolism and blood flow in epileptic seizures, hypoxia and hypoglycemia, in Purves M (ed): *Cerebral Vascular Smooth Muscle and its Control.* Ciba Foundation Symposium. Amsterdam: Elsevier, 1978: 119–218.

CHAPTER 35

REGIONAL CEREBRAL BLOOD FLOW TECHNIQUES

Panayiotis J. Sioutos
Jose A. Orozco
L. Philip Carter

SYNOPSIS

Cerebral blood flow (CBF) is an objective measurement of cerebral perfusion. Many intermittent techniques have been used to measure CBF clinically in patients with traumatic brain injury (TBI), including nitrous oxide, radioactive Xe clearance, stable Xe computed tomography, single-photon emission computed tomography (SPECT), and positron emission tomography (PET). Through these studies, it has been demonstrated that patients with TBI may have ischemia or hyperemia. Patients with prolonged symptoms have more persistent abnormalities in CBF than do those who completely recover from TBI. Normalization of CBF has been shown to have favorable prognostic significance. Continuous monitoring of CBF can be accomplished with either laser-Doppler flowmetry (LDF) or thermal-diffusion flowmetry (TDF). TDF has been used in head-injured patients to help guide therapeutic decisions and has demonstrated that normalization of CBF is statistically related to a better prognosis as defined by the Glascow Outcome Score (GOS).

INTRODUCTION

Cerebral blood flow (CBF) measurement and monitoring is one way to assess brain function in an objective fashion. Under most conditions, CBF and brain metabolism (CMR_{O_2}) are functionally coupled. In normal humans and experimental animals, increased CMR_{O_2} increases CBF and decreased CMR_{O_2} has the opposite effect. In many pathological situations, though, CBF and CMR_{O_2} are not directly linked. Head injury results in consistently depressed brain metabolism. Normal coupling of CBF and CMR_{O_2} in head-injured comatose patients is retained in only 45 percent of cases. Thus, in the majority of these patients, changes in CBF occur independently of reduced CMR_{O_2}.

Many methods of determining CBF have been developed over the last decades. These methods either report CBF directly in units of milliliters per 100 g of tissue per minute (quantitative methods) or provide three-dimensional images of CBF with or without mapping flow and metabolism (qualitative methods). CBF recordings can be either intermittent or dynamic. Dynamic recordings should recognize "real-time" changes of CBF (continuous measurement). CBF measurement techniques can provide an average of whole-brain flow values (global CBF) or local flow values (regional CBF). Normal flow values of the whole brain are on the order of 50 ml/100 g/min. The flow values of the gray matter are significantly higher (60 to 90 ml/100 g/min) than those of the white matter (20 to 30 ml/100 g/min).

In 1945 Kety and Schmidt made the first quantitative measurements of brain blood flow in humans, using the nitrous oxide technique.[1] Subsequently, the krypton-85 clearance technique was developed by Lassen and Munck in 1955 and was applied for the measurement of cerebral, myocardial, and renal blood flow.[2–4] With the development of methods of external recording of the clearance of radioactive tracers, measurements of regional CBF became possible.

INTERMITTENT MEASUREMENT OF REGIONAL CBF

History

Early intermittent studies of regional CBF (rCBF) consisted of external recording of the clearance of radioactive krypton (^{85}Kr) and xenon (^{133}Xe), which were injected into the carotid arteries. Blood flow through a hemisphere of brain was observed.[5–8] The use of ^{85}Kr was abandoned early, since it is such a weak beta emitter that a small craniotomy was necessary for the completion of the study. ^{133}Xe became the most widely used tracer for regional CBF measurements. One to two mCi of ^{133}Xe dissolved in isotonic saline was injected directly into the internal carotid artery through a thin, heparinized polyethylene catheter or a Teflon catheter and in some cases through a fine needle.[8–10] The tissue clearance of the isotope was recorded for 15 min by scintillation detectors placed extracranially over the areas of interest. The counts were simultaneously stored on a magnetic tape so that they could be used for electronic data processing. The invasiveness of the technique was, however, a major drawback and led to the development of atraumatic methods for the measurement of regional CBF, utilizing ^{133}Xe.

Xe Inhalation and Intravenous Techniques

Atraumatic ^{133}Xe methods for the measurement of rCBF include the ^{133}Xe inhalation and intravenous injection techniques. Both have the added advantage of measuring gray and white matter flow of different regions of the whole brain, including brainstem and cerebellar regions, rather than only the part of hemisphere perfused by the injected carotid artery.

The ^{133}Xe inhalation method was first introduced by Mallett and Veall.[11,12] The major advantage of this method is that it is noninvasive and repeatable. The gas passes through the brain, and the clearance curve is analyzed by sensors placed over the calvarium. The major drawback of the technique as it was described originally is the contamination of the clearance curves by radioactivity from the scalp and other extracerebral sources, which may result in significant measurement error. Obrist and coworkers, in an effort to overcome this problem, introduced three-compartmental analysis of the curves.[13] The first two compartments represented the faster-clearing gray and white matter, and the third compartment represented the slower extracerebral sources. The authors reported a flow of 74.5 ml/100 g/min in the gray matter and 24.8 ml/100 g/min in the white matter. This modification of the technique, though, required extended periods of recording (up to 40 min or more) and was unsuitable in clinical situations. To overcome this difficulty, Obrist and coworkers proposed a shorter and simpler method in which ^{133}Xe clearance was monitored extracranially for 10 min after a 1-min inhalation.[14,19] This technique is limited to CBF measurements of the gray matter only but is suitable to clinical conditions. It has been used to evaluate rCBF in the intensive care unit and operating room. Sharbrough and coworkers used this technique to demonstrate the level of CBF when EEG changes occurred during carotid endarterectomy.[15]

^{133}Xe inhalation allows measurement of CBF as a one-time event. To identify changes, multiple evaluations must be performed. The differences identified between the two hemispheres have been particularly useful in detecting areas of ischemia.[16] In addition, activation of CBF with either acetazolamide (Diamox) or CO_2 may demonstrate the "reserve" of CBF.[17]

The intravenous administration of ^{133}Xe described by Agnoli and coworkers allows serial determinations of CBF at the bedside with minimal discomfort to the patient.[18] The hemispheric CBF is determined after intravenous administration of ^{133}Xe, followed by a rapid injection of 20 ml of isotonic saline. Clearance of the radioactive agent is monitored from both parietotemporal regions and expired air. The CBF data are automatically calculated from the clearance curves by conventional bicompartmental analysis and a delayed-start fit time according to the method of Obrist and coworkers.[14,19]

Although both the ^{133}Xe inhalation and intravenous techniques proved to be very useful for the intermittent measurement of rCBF, there are some technical problems common to the use of radioactive tracers in which emission from the brain is detected by means of the use of external probes. The primary disadvantages of these techniques include "see-through" in areas with markedly reduced blood flow which results from contamination by radioactivity from structures adjacent to the focus and "cross-talk" which results from the contamination by radioactivity from the opposite hemisphere. Furthermore, flow evaluation involves only the cortical flow, and deep structures are not seen. There are additional problems that lessen the accuracy of rCBF measurements in abnormal brain because tissue–blood partition coefficients (solubility) are not measured and frequently are altered in an abnormal brain.[20] These ^{133}Xe studies also are relatively insensitive to low-flow areas.[21]

Xe/CT Technique

These limitations led a number of investigators to develop methods that take advantage of the excellent resolving powers of conventional x-ray transmission computed tomography (CT) scanners by combining them with the contrast properties of stable xenon gas, which diffuses readily across the blood-brain barrier after inhalation. Since stable xenon has a high atomic number of 54, this allows image enhancement. The Xe/CT method of measurement of rCBF has been studied by several groups.[20,22–26] The technique combines direct anatomic information with blood flow information in a single examination. A conventional series of 10-mm-thick scans is first obtained, from which three levels may be selected for blood flow imaging. At each level, two baseline images are obtained. Then a mixture of 33% xenon and 67% oxygen is administered. Four to six enhanced scans are obtained at each level at approximately 30-s intervals, beginning 40 s after the initial detection of xenon in the expired air. The rate of enhancement within the brain is defined on a pixel-by-pixel basis. An iterative algorithm simultaneously generates both xenon tissue solubility and flow. The flow values are finally displayed on a quantitative, continuous gray scale.[27]

This technique has many advantages for the measurement of rCBF: (1) It is noninvasive, (2) it can derive fairly high resolution flow maps (6 to 9 mm Full Width–Half Maximum) from anatomic sections that can be displayed adjacent to the routine CT image for comparison, (3) it can estimate the local partition coefficients (λ), which have been demonstrated to vary considerably in pathological tissues, (4) it can be performed in a relatively simple manner over a short period since the additional time needed to obtain functional blood flow information may be as little as 10 min, and (5) it is relatively inexpensive because of the modest cost of xenon. The Xe/CT technique has been used to locate regions of low CBF near epileptic foci interictally and increased CBF during seizure, thus guiding epilepsy surgery; has been helpful in evaluating CBF around intracranial tumors so that new therapeutic modalities such as hyperthermia can be varied, depending on the CBF; and has been applied to the diagnosis of brain death. Limitations of the technique include (1) radiation which averages 10 to 20 rad per study and accumulates with repeated studies, (2) artifacts created by motion and breathing that may significantly affect the results, (3) side effects of xenon gas inhalation, which include sedation and "funny feelings," and (4) the fact that xenon inhalation itself may affect blood flow.

SPECT Technique

Single-photon emission computed tomography (SPECT) is a noninvasive, qualitative three-dimensional study of rCBF. Lipophilic radiopharmaceuticals that emit single photons are injected intravenously and are trapped in the brain in proportion to regional perfusion. Rotating cameras are then used to detect the single photons with spatial resolution.[28] The radioisotopes used are *N*-isopropyl-*p*-iodo-amphetamine (IMP), hydroxy-iodo-benzylpropanediamine (HIPDM), and hexamethylpropyleneamine oxime (HMPAO). IMP and HIPDM are labeled with iodine-123, which makes them expensive and inconvenient to obtain, whereas HMPAO is labeled with ^{99m}technetium by a kit procedure which makes it convenient to use. A cold object (no uptake) in a hot area (increased uptake) can be recognized if it is larger than 2 cm. A hot object in a cold area can be recognized regardless of its size. SPECT studies have the advantage of being able to freeze CBF at one point in time with the isotope injection. Scanning may be done later, and comparisons between the two hemispheres are readily apparent. This is of great importance in the evaluation of epilepsy patients, since the isotope can be injected at the time of seizure discharge and the scanning is carried out in the nuclear medicine facility at a later time, after the seizure (Fig. 35-1). SPECT is also helpful in considering patients for cerebral revascularization, predicting the outcome from cerebral trauma, and allowing assessment of brain death.[29–32] In a study of severe head injury patients between 3 and 36 months after the injury, it was found that SPECT showed many more lesions than did CT or magnetic resonance imaging (MRI). The most severely disabled patients showed the highest number of SPECT lesions, which were either contusional or ischemic. The authors of this study concluded that SPECT has a greater value than MRI in the assessment of patients seen late after a head injury.[33] This is an important finding because of the lower overall cost of SPECT compared with MRI. The main disadvantage of SPECT is that it is a nonquantitative study for CBF measurement and cannot be repeated at short intervals. The time limit for repeating the study depends on the type of the radioisotope used. With HMPAO, the study can be repeated after 24 h.

PET Technique

Positron emission tomography (PET) employs positron-emitting radionuclides and positron imaging devices to obtain three-dimensional representations of rCBF.[34] Since positron-emitting radionuclides such as ^{11}C, ^{13}N, and ^{15}O can be tagged to a number of metabolically active compounds, this study allows the assessment of local metabolism at the same time rCBF is evaluated (functional brain mapping). Because of the short half-life of these radioisotopes, ready access to a cyclotron is necessary. This makes PET an expensive study which is not readily available. Functional brain maps based on PET suffer from limited spatial and temporal resolution.[35]

One clinical area where PET has been useful is the preoperative evaluation of patients with medically intractable epilepsy. In 75 percent of patients with com-

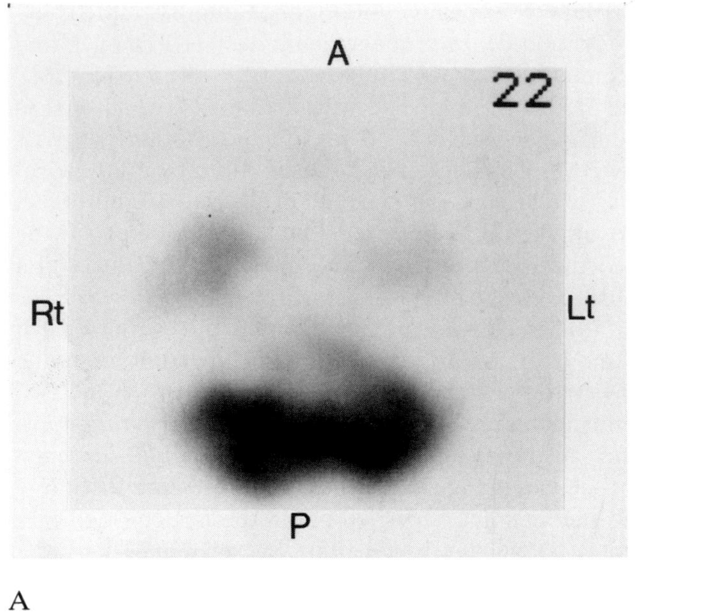

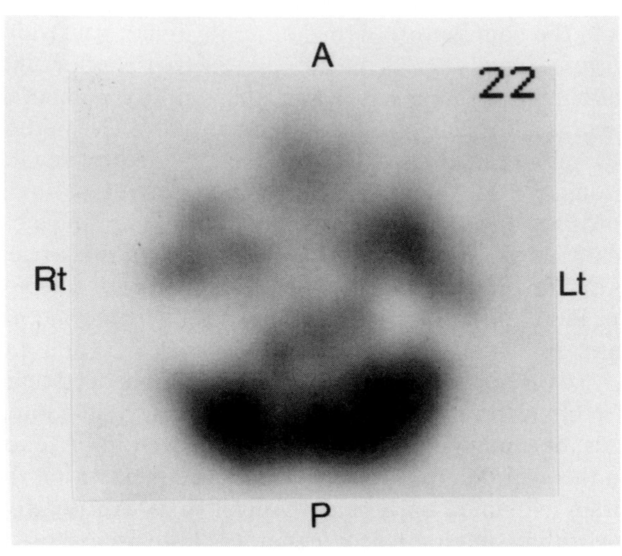

A B

Figure 35-1. SPECT scan, axial view, of patient G.C., showing decreased left temporal lobe CBF interictally (*A*) and increased CBF in the left temporal lobe with seizure (*B*). A = anterior; P = posterior; Rt = right; Lt = left.

plex partial seizures, unilateral temporal hypometabolism ipsilateral to the EEG focus has been found.[36] Interictal focal hypometabolism also has been found in a small percentage of patients with complex partial seizures originating away from the temporal lobe. Patients with intractable complex partial seizures who demonstrate focal hypometabolism on PET scan and EEG findings that indicate a definite site of origin of the seizures can be operated on without invasive preoperative monitoring. This reduces the total cost and potential risk of the workup. In patients with nonlocalized surface EEG seizure origin, the PET findings may help plan and modify the strategy for invasive preoperative monitoring.

Another clinical area in which PET has been helpful is the differentiation of high-grade glioma recurrence as a result of radiation necrosis. The recurrence of a high-grade glioma and radiation-induced necrosis have similar appearances and cannot be distinguished on conventional brain imaging studies. On PET, however, the recurrent tumor is hypermetabolic whereas radiation necrosis is hypometabolic. This information may be helpful in planning future treatment.

EPI Technique

Rapid sequence MRI in the form of gradient-echo echoplanar imaging (EPI) is a rapidly developing technique which provides information on rCBF similar to that derived from the Xe/CT method without requiring contrast injection. This technique uses the effects of changes in blood oxygenation. Deoxygenated blood, which is more paramagnetic than is oxygenated blood, acts as an endogenous contrast agent. An increase of signal implies a decrease of deoxyhemoglobin within the voxel, and this correlates with the change in rCBF.[37,38] In experiments with cats undergoing anoxia, a change from 100% arterial hemoglobin oxygen saturation to 40% saturation was associated with a 15 percent decrease in image intensity in brain gray matter for an echo time of 40 ms.[39] The effects of photic stimulation on the visual cortex in humans have been studied by means of gradient-echo EPI. These studies showed an increase in signal intensity in the visual cortex during stimulation that corresponded to an increase of blood oxygenation in regions of increased neural activity.[38,40,41] High-resolution functional brain mapping based on EPI is expected to have widespread clinical application for studies of rCBF in ischemia and epilepsy. Early detection of infarcted areas could certainly be useful in evaluating patients who are thought to have suffered a stroke.

Transcranial Doppler Monitoring

Transcranial Doppler (TCD) allows assessment of flow velocities in large intracranial vessels. This technique uses a 2-mHz transducer which is held over small, thin bone "windows" in the temporal bone and the foramen magnum. Flow velocities of the anterior, middle, and posterior cerebral and the vertebral arteries can be assessed with the TCD technique. In a neurosurgical practice, the greatest value of this technique is the evaluation of the degree of vasospasm, particularly in patients with subarachnoid hemorrhage. As vasospasm develops, flow velocities increase. TCD studies in patients with aneurysmal subarachnoid hemorrhage have found that a middle cerebral artery (MCA) velocity greater than 200 cm/s is associated with ischemic neurological defects.[42] The regional nature of the study is not as well defined as that of studies which actually assess capillary flow.

CONTINUOUS MEASUREMENT OF REGIONAL CBF

The previously described methods of rCBF measurement are by nature intermittent, generally requiring a period of time to develop a saturation and desaturation curve. This clearance is then analyzed and yields one value of CBF. The whole process must then be repeated to recognize changes in CBF. However, techniques exist that monitor surface blood flow in the brain and allow observation of dynamic "real-time" changes in cortical blood flow (CoBF). No clearance curve is necessary, and so changes in flow are seen immediately. The two techniques available for continuous surface monitoring are laser-Doppler flowmetry (LDF) and thermal-diffusion flowmetry (TDF). These techniques depend on the assessment of cortical capillary flow in one region of the cortex and consequently are limited by the assumption that this area is representative of the brain tissue of interest.

Laser-Doppler Flowmetry

LDF works on the principle of directing a laser beam at the tissue to be assessed. The light is reflected from static sources differently from the way it is reflected from moving red blood cells. Photons are scattered and undergo a frequency shift. The photons are then collected and delivered to a photo detector. The electrical output of the photo detector yields a continuous recording proportional to CBF. This technique was first described by Riva and coworkers in retinal vessels.[43] Subsequently, Stern studied LDF and concluded that it could be used in the evaluation of the microcirculation.[44] LDF has been used to measure blood flow in skin[45,46] and has been compared to hydrogen clearance with good correlation in measuring intestinal mucosal blood flow.[47] Dirnagl and coworkers studied LDF in the cortical capillary bed and concluded that absolute regional flow did not correlate well with autoradiography but that changes and the percentage of changes seemed to correlate very well.[48] The LDF probe was placed by Haberl and coworkers through a cranial window port in the cat.[49] They demonstrated the appropriate changes with hyperventilation and hypotension and found good correlation with the hydrogen clearance technique. Dirnagl and Pulsinelli studied autoregulation of CBF with focal ischemia with LDF,[50] demonstrating loss of autoregulation in ischemic areas and good autoregulation in normal areas. Skarphedinsson and coworkers studied CoBF in hypertensive rats with LDF[51] and found that movement and external light interfered with the optimal use of LDF. When these factors were controlled, LDF correlated quite well with a slow component of hydrogen clearance. Saeki and coworkers found that LDF is easily applied in small animals, since the probe is very small and can be easily placed on the cortex.[52] They demonstrated the effect of sympathetic stimulation on CoBF.

Rosenblum and coworkers were the first to report the intraoperative use of LDF in a patient with an arteriovenous malformation (AVM) of the brain.[53] Blood flow was measured in six cortical regions around the AVM before and after the excision of the malformation. Before the excision, blood flow in those six sites was estimated to be from 18.6 to 48.0 ml/100 g/min. After the excision of the AVM, blood flow ranged from 60.0 to 168.0 ml/100 g/min. These authors pointed out the need to avoid large surface vessels, since the Doppler broadening from the large-volume, high-velocity vessels dominated the Doppler signals from the microcirculation, resulting in inaccurate measurements of the blood flow of the microcirculation. Rosenblum et al. also discussed the need for gentle contact of the probe with the cortical surface and the cautious way the probe should be moved since excessive motion can lead to artifacts.

Arbit and coworkers were the first to study CBF in tumors during craniotomy using the LDF technique.[54] These authors measured CBF intraoperatively across two tissue regions, normal and tumorous, in 12 patients who had high-grade gliomas (4 patients), meningioma (1 patient), and metastatic disease (7 patients). These authors stated that the LDF technique was very motion sensitive and was affected by the operating room lights. They found reduced tumor CBF values compared with adjacent normal brain flow values in all cases except two (a meningioma and a melanoma). They also found inconsistent responses among tumors to blood pressure alterations (autoregulation) and a normal response among tumors to Pa_{CO_2} changes. They concluded that the LDF technique is simple to employ and can be easily used intraoperatively for CBF studies. No LDF study has been reported in head injury patients.

LDF offers real-time continuous monitoring of blood

flow to a depth of a few millimeters. It does appear to be qualitative, and most authors do not consider it quantitative; however, in addition to the concerns noted above, since the flow is based on moving particles, a correction for hematocrit may be necessary.

Thermal-Diffusion Flowmetry

TDF dates back to 1933, when Gibbs first described the use of a thermal probe constructed of thermocouples to measure cerebral perfusion.[55] Subsequently, Grayson demonstrated that the thermal conductivity of tissue was constant without blood flow but that with increased blood flow, the thermal conductivity increment was a linear function of the rate of flow in the tissue.[56] In 1955, Carlyle and Grayson demonstrated autoregulation of the brain with thermal probes.[57] In 1962, Perl studied the theory of tissue blood flow determined by heat clearance and provided further mathematical confirmation of the method.[58] In 1966, Betz and coworkers compared TDF with krypton-85 clearance.[59] They did not find a good correlation, and this was attributed to local vascular geometry caused by the small size of the thermal sensor they employed. Brawley subsequently described a thermal probe constructed of a Peltier stack which created a thermal gradient between heated and cooled plates.[60] The temperature difference between the plates was correlated with blood flow in a qualitative fashion. Wullenweber, using a thermal-diffusion probe, was the first to report CBF measurements of the white mater intraoperatively.[61]

Carter and Atkinson constructed a flow probe similar to the one described by Brawley and compared it to ^{133}Xe fast flow in cats.[62] They found a correlation and concluded that the thermal sensor was quantitative. Their Peltier probe was the first surface probe that gave a quantitative measure of CoBF. Using TDF, these authors found that deep inhalational anesthesia with halothane produced less reduction in CoBF than did two other techniques of controlled hypotension. Subsequently, Carter and Atkinson studied autoregulation and hyperemia of CBF with TDF and demonstrated the effectiveness of the technique in measuring rCoBF.[63] Further studies comparing TDF and radioactive clearance techniques yielded the mathematical model $\mathrm{CoBF} = K(1/\Delta v - 1/\Delta v_o)$, where K = constant, Δv = voltage difference, and Δv_o = voltage difference with no flow.[64] The voltage difference, Δv, was the thermocouple output in microvolts.

Gaines and coworkers compared the TDF and hydrogen clearance techniques for the measurement of rCBF in cats.[65] They found a close correlation between rCBF values obtained by the two methods and concluded that since the hydrogen clearance technique was accepted as quantitative, TDF was also a reliably quantitative method for rCBF measurement. Cusick and Myklebust also reported a linear relationship between thermal-determined and hydrogen clearance–determined rCBF with a miniaturized probe that incorporated both methods.[66] When TDF is compared with the isotope or hydrogen clearance techniques in regard to measuring CoBF, TDF has many advantages: It is more accurate at lower flows, it can demonstrate abrupt changes in flow, there is no need to perforate the pial membrane, and it is easy to use. TDF can be applied in the operating theater and gives continuous real-time dynamic changes in regional surface flow.

Gopinath and coworkers reported their experience with CBF measurement in 10 adult patients with severe head injury using both TDF and the nitrous oxide saturation method.[67] They found that although the thermal-diffusion CBF values tended to be slightly higher than the nitrous oxide saturation values, there was a significant correlation between the two CBF measurements. They further stated that although cortical CBF measurements are not identical to global measurements, TDF has the advantage of being continuous and easy to perform.

In 1978, Carter and coworkers reported the first series of 32 patients undergoing craniotomy for various brain lesions who had intraoperative rCoBF measurement with the TDF technique.[68] In 1984, Carter et al. reported a comparison of somatosensory evoked potentials (SSEPs) and CoBF measured with TDF during craniotomy for vascular disease.[69] A relationship between the central conduction time (CCT) and reduction in cortical potentials was found, with changes noted in surface-monitored CoBF. Three of the four patients with a long CCT had a low CoBF. Takemae and coworkers were the first to report the postoperative monitoring of rCoBF with TDF.[70] They monitored postoperative aneurysm patients to evaluate the effects of vasospasm. Ohmoto et al. reported 12 patients operated on for intracranial aneurysms in whom temporary arterial occlusion was applied.[71] When CoBF fell below 30 ml/100 g/min, they recommended keeping the occlusion time below 15 min and concluded that TDF was of value in estimating temporary occlusion tolerance. Barnett and coworkers reported the intraoperative use of TDF in surgery for AVMs.[72] They studied 18 patients, using a Peltier stack type of thermal diffusion flow probe. The mean preexcision CoBF was 62.9 ± 6.7 ml/100 g/min near the AVM and 43.0 ± 4.2 ml/100 g/min away (>2 cm) from the AVM. The mean postexcision CoBF near the AVM remained stable (55.8 ± 5.1 ml/100 g/min), but the CoBF away from the AVM increased significantly after excision (57.2 ± 6.8 ml/100 g/min). Two patients who developed normal perfusion pressure breakthrough syndrome (NPPBS) had low CoBF and disturbed CO_2 reactivity before the excision of the AVM and a significant increase of CoBF after the excision. These authors concluded that intraoperative measurement of CoBF and CO_2 reactivity may be useful in predicting which patients may develop NPPBS.

Tamaki and coworkers measured CoBF in 16 patients with an AVM intraoperatively.[73] TDF was used in 14 patients, and LDF in 2 patients. Blood flow measurements were done in several regions around the lesion, about 2 cm away from the AVM, in each patient. These authors determined the ratio of postexcision/preexcision cortical blood flow in each patient. Two patients with large AVMs who developed postoperative hematoma had flow ratios higher than 1.9. In four patients with large AVMs and initial flow ratios higher than 2, Silverstone clamps or special clamps were applied in the extracranial carotid or the main feeding arteries of the lesion, respectively. In this way, these authors were able to reduce the flow ratio in those patients to less than 1.5, thus avoiding postoperative hemorrhagic complications. Nine patients with small AVMs had low (below 1.5) flow ratios and did not develop postoperative hemorrhagic complications. These authors concluded that intraoperative continuous measurement of CoBF coupled with this flow modulation technique allowed safe, one-stage excision of high-flow AVMs without postoperative development of NPPBS.

TDF has been used in the operative theater in the evaluation of patients with epilepsy. It has been demonstrated that in the interictal period a seizure focus has reduced blood flow. However, when seizure discharge occurs, the blood flow reaches marked supranormal values, presumably as a result of the cerebral metabolic demand. Weinand and coworkers reported their experience with TDF measurement of CoBF in patients undergoing burr hole placement of strip subdural monitoring leads.[74] They found that a significant reduction of blood flow occurred in the areas of epileptogenic focus interictally. In monitoring epilepsy patients with subdural strip electrodes and TDF probes, the authors of this chapter have found a significant increase of rCoBF during the epileptogenic activity.

The most recent models of TDF monitoring equipment use a small probe since the Peltier stack has been eliminated. The surface area beneath the probe must remain relatively large (3 to 5 mm in diameter) to average the rCoBF and eliminate the effects of local vascular architecture. In isocaloric probes, there is a constant power input and the temperature difference between a neutral plate and a heated plate is monitored. The temperature difference is correlated with blood flow. In isothermal probes, there is a constant temperature between a neutral plate and a heated plate. The current required to maintain this temperature gradient is correlated with blood flow. In the authors' studies, we use the isocaloric probe without the Peltier stack. We rely on a confidence check to ensure that the two contact plates are in apposition to the cortex. When the heating element is turned off, the heated plate and the neutral plate become equivalent. If both plates are in touch with the same tissue, that is, cortex, the temperature will be the same. If one contact surface is partially in touch with CSF or air, the temperature between the two plates will vary (poor confidence factor). This confidence check is present in the commercially available equipment produced by Flowtronics, Inc., of Phoenix, Arizona. The confidence factor is particularly helpful if the probes for postoperative monitoring have been implanted in an area where the probe position in relation to the cortex cannot be readily assessed.

In 1991 Kuwayama and coworkers reported the development of a modified thermal-diffusion flow probe for the continuous measurement of rCBF.[75] Their modification included a constantan wire as a heat source to make a miniature probe. The pair of thermocouples used to detect the heat gradient between two gold plates was elongated to avoid heat conduction between them. These authors compared their thermal-diffusion flow probe in rabbits with the hydrogen clearance technique of monitoring rCBF and demonstrated a very good correlation. They also applied their technique to the clinical situation and demonstrated the development of vasospasm and brain death in aneurysm patients, confirming previous reports.[76] They also showed that changes in cortical temperature do not affect the measurement of CoBF.

TDF sensors are larger than LDF probes and produce more of an averaging effect over the surface of the brain. TDF experiences artifact with irrigation, with loss of contact with the brain, and when large surface vessels are in contact with the probe. It is not clear whether different brain pathological conditions have the thermal properties as normal brain. However, movement, light, and contact with large cortical vessels create significant artifact with LDF. The smaller size of the LDF probe is an advantage but can cause difficulty in practice because of the pulsatile nature of the cortical surface. Since LDF is based on moving particles, changes in hematocrit can produce artifacts. Both techniques have demonstrated reduced blood flow around brain tumors in a normal brain and increased blood flow after the excision of AVMs. TDF has been used both intra- and postoperatively in patients with cerebral aneurysms. Postoperative monitoring in the intensive care unit is more easily performed at present with TDF; however, the loss of contact of the probe with the brain surface remains a significant problem.

Continuous monitoring of rCBF aids in the recognition of immediate changes in cortical perfusion. This could be a significant addition to the diagnostic armamentarium of the neurosurgeon and intensivist for the treatment of diseases and injuries of the brain.

CBF IN HEAD INJURIES

Efforts to improve the outcome in patients with severe head injuries have focused on the prevention and treatment of secondary insults such as anoxia/hypoxia, hypotension, intracranial hypertension, and brain ischemia. Ischemic brain damage has been found on neuropathologic examination in 88 percent of patients with a head injury.[77,78] The development of different CBF monitoring methods has led many investigators to evaluate cerebral perfusion in head injury patients and has raised questions about the benefits of standard treatment modalities such as hyperventilation.

N_2O Saturation Technique

The N_2O saturation technique has been employed for the measurement of global CBF in head injury patients by a number of investigators. Gokaslan and coworkers at Baylor used this technique in 91 head-injured comatose patients.[79] They found that 51 percent of the patients had a normal global CBF, while low and high CBFs were observed in 28 percent and 21 percent of their patients, respectively. These authors questioned the safety of hyperventilation in the treatment of increased intracranial pressure (ICP) in patients with a reduced CBF pattern. Sheinberg and coworkers, also at Baylor, subsequently updated their experience with CBF in 45 head-injured comatose patients.[80] Thirty-six percent of their patients had reduced CBF, 20 percent had normal CBF, and 44 percent had elevated CBF. There was no significant difference in age, initial Glasgow Coma Scale (GCS) score, or type of injury among the three CBF categories. Fifty-six percent of patients with reduced CBF died, compared with 33 percent of those with normal CBF and 20 percent of those with elevated CBF.

^{133}Xe Injection and Inhalation Techniques

The intraarterial ^{133}Xe injection method was used by Fieschi and coworkers to study rCBF in 12 head-injured comatose patients.[81] Ten patients were studied from 7 to 35 h after the injury, and two patients were examined for the first time on the third and tenth postinjury days. These authors divided their patients into three prognostic groups and correlated the rCBF patterns with each group. In cases of cerebral death, rCBF increased to reach high values (hyperemia) between 36 and 96 h, indicating that late hyperemia is a bad prognostic factor. In cases of extracerebral death, rCBF slowly increased toward normal after the second day, without instances of hyperemia. In the recovery group, a similar course of rCBF was observed except for a milder CBF impairment in the early stages. These authors concluded that in patients with neurological recovery, the course of CBF is roughly parallel with clinical status.

Enevoldsen and coworkers used the intracarotid ^{133}Xe injection method to measure rCBF in 23 patients with severe head injury.[82] Most patients in this study had reduced rCBF. The ^{133}Xe clearance curves from areas of severe cortical lesions had very fast initial components called tissue peaks. The tissue-peak areas correlated with areas of early veins in the angiograms, an indication of relative hyperemia which was called "tissue-peak" hyperemia. The peaks increased in number during clinical deterioration and disappeared during improvement.

The inhalation ^{133}Xe technique was used by Barclay and coworkers to measure CBF in 12 alert, responsive patients both 2 to 13 months after head injury and 1 to 12 months after they regained consciousness.[83] Global CBF was significantly decreased in patients with head injury relative to age-matched normal controls. Barclay et al. concluded that the chronic sequelae of head trauma include decreased CBF which correlates with the neuropsychological impairment.

Obrist and coworkers measured rCBF in 36 head-injured comatose patients, using the intravenous ^{133}Xe method.[84] Without exception, CBF declined to very low levels in the nine patients who died. One patient who remained in a persistent vegetative state continued to demonstrate depressed CBF 4 months after the injury. Almost all the patients (25 of 26) who recovered consciousness showed increases in CBF. Obrist et al. found that early hyperemia was associated with either diffuse cerebral swelling or recovery from profound systemic shock. Late hyperemia was associated with mass lesions on CT scan, focal seizures, or deterioration of neurological status.

In another study of 75 head-injured, comatose patients, Obrist and coworkers measured rCBF with the intravenous ^{133}Xe method.[85] They also measured the arteriojugular venous oxygen differences (AVD_{O_2}), which provided estimates of the cerebral metabolic rate for oxygen (CMR_{O_2}). The simultaneous measurement of rCBF and AVD_{O_2} permitted the assessment of the balance between metabolism and CBF. All patients were studied acutely within 96 h after injury. Fifty-five percent of the patients developed acute hyperemia, and 45 percent had subnormal values. Obrist et al. defined hyperemia as a normal or supernormal CBF in the presence of coma, a definition that was independently confirmed by narrow AVD_{O_2} values. All comatose patients had significant depression in CMR_{O_2}. A significant association was found between hyperemia and high ICP (>20 mmHg). In the group of patients with reduced CBF values, a coupling of CBF and CMR_{O_2} was found. In 10 of these patients, hyperventilation resulted in an increase of AVD_{O_2}, suggesting true ischemia.

Bouma and coworkers measured rCBF in 186 head-injured comatose patients by using the intravenous ^{133}Xe technique and AVD_{O_2} within the first 6 h after injury.[86] The earliest measurement was performed 4 h after injury. CBF values found between 4 and 6 h after injury were significantly lower than those obtained at any later time. The CBF values increased significantly during the first 24 h. By contrast, AVD_{O_2} values were initially above normal and decreased rapidly in the first 24 h. Patients with low motor scores in their neurological examination had the highest AVD_{O_2} values early after injury and the steepest decline in AVD_{O_2} during the first 24 h. In 13 percent of these patients, ischemia, defined as a global CBF less than 18 m/100 g/min in the absence of low cerebral perfusion pressure, was found at some point after injury. Ischemia was found in one-third of the studies obtained between 4 and 6 h after injury. Bouma et al. reported a significant correlation between low CBF values and poor outcome of their patients. They concluded that early hyperventilation or lowering of blood pressure to prevent brain edema may be harmful in the management of severely head injured patients.

In another study, Bouma and coworkers measured CBF in 35 comatose patients as early as 4 hours after injury, using the Xe/CT method.[87] Global or regional ischemia (CBF <18 ml/100 g/min) was found in 31.4 percent of their patients. Ischemia was significantly associated with early mortality, whereas normal or high CBF values were not predictive of a favorable short-term outcome. Bouma et al. concluded that ischemia is an important secondary insult in head injury and argued against the use of hyperventilation and antihypertensive drugs in the initial management of these patients. Their conclusions supported the findings of an earlier study by Muizelaar and coworkers, also from the Medical College of Virginia, who found poorer outcomes in patients with severe head injury who were prophylactically hyperventilated.[88]

PET Technique

PET has been used in the evaluation of brain function in head-injured patients. Langfitt and coworkers described the results of CT, MRI, PET, intravenous ^{133}Xe measurement of CBF, and neuropsychological assessments in three head trauma patients.[89] These authors found that MRI was superior to CT in identifying the precise location and extent of the brain hemorrhage and the associated swelling. The extent of encephalomalacia in the chronic stages of brain injury was also defined better with MRI. PET identified regions of brain injury, as manifested by decreased glucose metabolism, that were not apparent on CT or MRI. Every structural lesion identified by CT and MRI, except for the small brain hemorrhages seen on MRI, was associated with a reduction of metabolism. Of particular importance was the finding of hypometabolism in both anterior temporal lobes with sparing of the posterior temporal lobes in all three patients during the acute stage of injury. The rCBF studies failed to show a number of abnormalities seen on MRI and CT and did not detect the hypometabolic disturbance shown by PET.

SPECT Technique

SPECT also has been employed for the assessment of cerebral perfusion in patients with head trauma. Reid and coworkers studied 13 patients with ^{99m}technetium HMPAO scanning.[30] CT scanning was also done in nine patients. In all cases, SPECT showed defects with a quality equivalent to or greater than that shown on CT. Reid et al. concluded that HMPAO-SPECT may predict the degree of permanent injury and predict which patients may develop postinjury headaches. These authors also described the use of SPECT for the diagnosis of brain death. Newton and coworkers studied 19 patients with ^{99m}technetium HMPAO-SPECT and compared it with CT and MRI.[33] SPECT identified more focal brain lesions than did CT or MRI alone or in combination. Most defects shown by SPECT were not apparent on CT or MRI. Newton et al. found that the number of rCBF defects and the global CBF correlated with the functional status of their patients: The most disabled patients had the highest number of lesions on SPECT.

Transcranial Doppler Monitoring

Transcranial Doppler ultrasound monitoring was used in the evaluation of head-injured patients by Martin and coworkers,[90] who studied 30 patients with GCS scores ranging from 3 to 15. Cerebral blood flow measurements were also done using the intravenous ^{133}Xe technique in 16 of these patients. Vasospasm (defined as MCA velocity over 120 cm/s) was found in 26.7 percent of these patients. Severe vasospasm (defined as MCA velocity above 200 cm/s) was found in 10 percent of the patients and was confirmed by angiography. Most of the patients with vasospasm and all the patients with severe vasospasm also had traumatic subarachnoid hemorrhage. Martin et al. found a significant correlation between the lowest CBF and the highest MCA velocity in patients with vasospasm and concluded that vasospasm is an important secondary postinjury insult. They further stated that traumatic severe vasospasm in a patient with neurological deterioration could be treated with hypervolemic-hemodilutional/hypertensive therapy coupled with nimodipine or balloon dilatation angioplasty. The findings of this study, along with the findings of earlier angiographic studies which showed vasospasm of the large conducting arteries in 30 to 40 percent of head-injured patients, may establish new frontiers in the treatment of the comatose brain injury patients.[91,92] Early hyperventilation and arbitrary lowering of the mean arterial blood pressure may prove dangerous in head-injured patients whose cerebral perfusion is already compromised.

Thermal-Diffusion Flowmetry

A few studies have been conducted on the continuous measurement of rCBF in head-injured patients, and all have employed the TDF method. Gopinath and coworkers studied 10 adult patients with severe head injury for 2 to 4 days.[67] All patients were operated on for evacuation of a hematoma. A TDF probe was placed on the area of interest during craniotomy. These authors also measured the global CBF with the N_2O saturation technique and jugular venous oxygen saturation (Sjv_{O_2}). A significant correlation between the two CBF measurements was found. The TDF measurements were also significantly correlated with the Sjv_{O_2} trends during most of the monitoring periods.

Dickman and coworkers monitored rCBF and ICP continuously with a combined TDF probe/ICP monitor in 12 patients with a mean GCS score of 6 on admission.[93] The TDF/ICP probes were placed during craniotomy in 11 patients and were placed in the intensive care unit (ICU) in 1 patient. The brain injuries included seven subdural hematomas, four contusions, and one epidural hematoma. No probe-related complications were reported. Reduced rCBF values occurred in 33 percent of these patients. One patient had transient, nonsustained fluctuations of rCBF (20 to 140 ml/100 g/min), and 50 percent of the patients had elevated rCBF values. These CBF patterns were observed in patients with a GCS score equal to or below 9. One patient with a GCS score of 12 had a normal rCBF pattern. In half the patients with reduced CBF values, there were increased ICP patterns. Posttraumatic cerebral arterial vasospasm in one patient was detected by CBF monitoring and confirmed by angiography. In six patients who progressed to brain death, rCBF patterns disappeared. Five of six patients with hyperemia had high ICP values. In two of these patients, increases in rCBF preceded rises in ICP, leading these authors to assume that loss of autoregulation is the underlying mechanism in the development of malignant brain edema. They found an association between hyperemia and a poor outcome but stated that no firm conclusion regarding prognosis could be established on the basis of their preliminary data.

In the authors' series of continuous CBF measurement in head injury patients with TDF, patients who require a craniotomy undergo a stab incision in the scalp, and the probe is tunneled subgaleally toward the craniotomy site (Fig. 35-2). The probe is placed under the dura so that the plates are in contact with a gyral surface of the cortex of interest and away from large surface vessels. When the TDF probe is not combined with the ICP monitor, a ventriculostomy or a subdural ICP monitor probe is placed through a separate skin incision. The dura is closed routinely, and the bone flap is replaced. Notching the bone flap with either a rongeur or a high-speed drill at the exit sites of the TDF and the subdural ICP probes facilitates seating the flap. A purse-string silk suture at the skin entry of the probe(s) prevents CSF leakage.

For continuous monitoring of ICP and CBF in trauma patients who do not require a craniotomy, the authors place a right frontal ventriculostomy and insert the CBF sensor at the same time (Fig. 35-3). The procedure is performed in the operating room because of the need

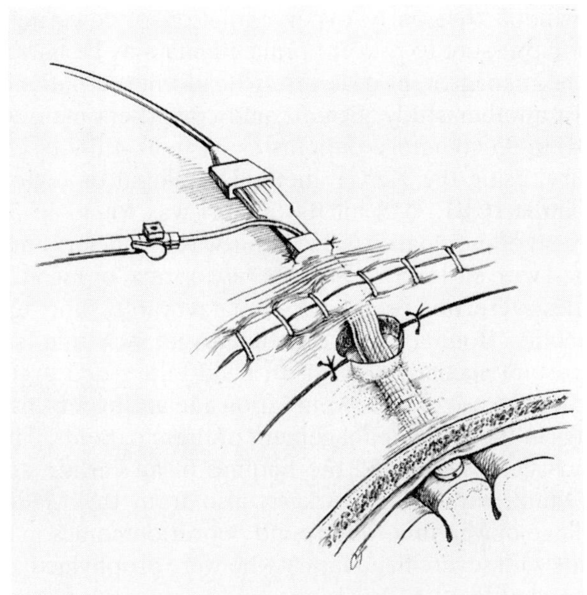

Figure 35-2. A TDF probe with a pressure port left in the craniotomy site. The probe rests on the cortex under the dura and exits through a burr hole and a stab wound in the scalp. Pressure monitoring for the subdural space can be performed with this technique.

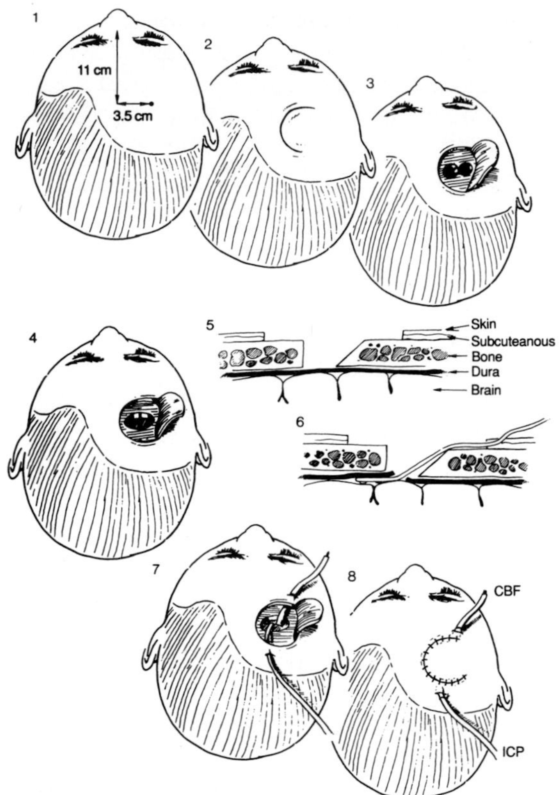

Figure 35-3. The TDF probe and ventriculostomy catheter placement in patients who do not require a craniotomy. (1) The right frontal region is shaved. The center of the skin flap is 11 cm above the nasion and 3.5 cm from the midline. (2) Skin flap. (3) Two burr holes are placed next to each other. (4) The two burr holes are connected. (5) The anterior margin of the lateral burr hole is beveled. (6) The TDF probe is passed through a stab wound anterior to the flap and threaded beneath the dura posteriorly. (7) The TDF sensor and the ventriculostomy catheter in place. (8) Skin flap turned back and closed.

for adequate lighting, suction, and cautery. The patient's right frontal region is shaved and sterilely prepped. We turn a small skin flap centered 11 cm above the nasion and 3.5 cm from the midline. Two burr holes are placed next to each other. The bony bridge between the burr holes is rongeured away, and the lateral burr hole is beveled so that the anterior margin allows a straight track to the cortex. The dura is opened, and the edges are coagulated. The thermal sensor is passed through a stab wound anterior to the flap and threaded beneath the dura posteriorly. The ventriculostomy is then passed in the usual fashion and tunneled. The small flap is closed and dressed. The patient is then transferred to the ICU for monitoring.

In our series of 37 head-injured patients (31 men and 6 women), continuous rCBF monitoring was started as early as 1 h and as late as 7 days (in one case) after injury.[94] In 15 patients monitoring was started within 8 h after injury, and in 28 patients it was started within 24 h after injury. The age range of our patients was 5 to 75 years (mean, 37.5; median, 35). The admission GCS score ranged from 3 to 15 (mean, 8.7; median, 8). Four patients had epidural hematomas, 21 had subdural hematomas, 10 had cerebral contusions, and 2 had intracerebral hematomas. The number of patients, according to the GOS, the admission GCS score, and the diagnosis, is shown in Table 35-1.[94] There was no significant difference in the mean initial rCBF values between the comatose (admission GCS score 3 to 7) and the noncomatose (admission GCS score 8 to 15) patients ($p > 0.05$) (Table 35-2).[94] Initial mean rCBF in the good outcome (GOS 4 to 5) and poor outcome (GOS 1 to 2) patients was similar ($p > 0.05$) (Table 35-2). Comparison of final rCBF between the poor-outcome and good-outcome groups revealed a trend toward normal rCBF in those with a good outcome. The change in mean rCBF (final minus initial) in good-outcome patients (19.8 ml/100 g/min) was significantly greater than that in poor-outcome

TABLE 35-1 Patients According to Outcome, Admission GCS score, and Diagnosis

No. Patients	Outcome	Admission GCS (range)	Admission GCS (mean)	*Diagnosis* EDH	SDH	C	ICH
9	1	3–9	5		6	2	1
2	2	7	7		1	1	
6	3	4–15	8	1	3	2	
8	4	8–14	11	2	5	1	
12	5	3–15	9	1	6	4	1

EDH = epidural hematoma; SDH = subdural hematoma; C = contusions; ICH = intracerebral hematoma.

Outcome: 1 = death; 2 = persistent vegetative state; 3 = severe disability; 4 = moderate disability; 5 = good outcome.

TABLE 35-2 Initial and Final rCBF in Comatose and Noncomatose Admissions, Good and Poor Outcomes

	Admission GCS 3–7	Admission GCS 8–15	p
Initial rCBF (mean ± standard error)	37.9 ± 6.10	39.8 ± 5.42	.815
	Outcome 1–2	**Outcome 4–5**	
Initial rCBF (mean ± standard error)	37.8 ± 7.42	38.6 ± 5.30	.934
Final rCBF (mean ± standard error)	30.6 ± 9.42	58.4 ± 9.52	.065
Final − initial rCBF (mean ± standard error)	−7.18 ± 6.51	19.8 ± 5.14	.004

CBF in ml/100 g/min.

patients (−7.18 ml/100 g/min) ($p < 0.05$). Thirty-three percent of the comatose patients in this study whose monitoring started within 8 h after injury had initial rCBF values ≤ 18 ml/100 g/min, the threshold for infarction. The patients with acute subdural hematomas showed improved rCBF during the course of their hospitalization, a finding consistent with that of Salvant and Muizelaar, who measured rCBF in patients with acute subdural hematomas by using either the inhalation or the intravenous ^{133}Xe technique.[95] Thirty-three percent of our patients with acute subdural hematomas had initial rCBF values ≤ 18 ml/100 g/min, compared with 9 percent of the patients of Salvant and Muizelaar.[95] An example of continuous monitoring in a postoperative acute subdural hematoma is shown in Fig. 35-4.

Possible complications related to TDF include infection, retained sensors, and CSF leakage. Among 56 head-injured patients who underwent TDF probe placement in our service, there were only 3 cases of infection of the scalp entry sites (5 percent). These patients were treated with antibiotics and were cured.

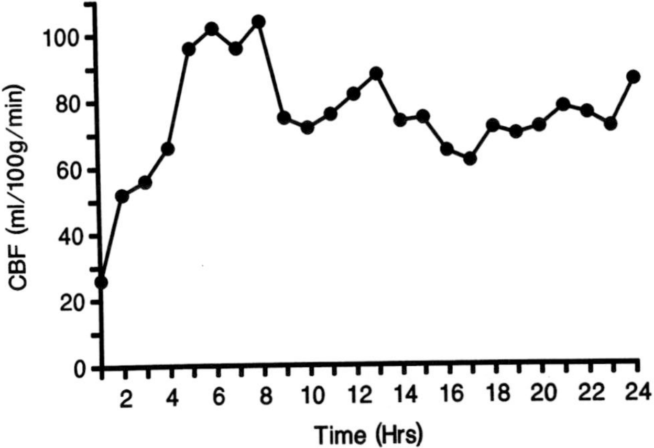

Figure 35-4. Postoperative continuous CBF monitoring in a patient with acute subdural hematoma. Admission GCS score was 11, and outcome was 4. CBF in the beginning of the recording was in the low 20s. At 5 to 8 h, a hyperemic phase developed, and then the flow normalized into range of 60 to 80. Flow monitoring was done for only 24 h since the patient responded well. The P_{CO_2} value was similar at the beginning and during the monitoring (23 to 26 mmHg).

Our data confirm that significant ischemia is a secondary insult in the early hours after a severe head injury. They also support the findings of other trials regarding the normalization trend of the final rCBF in patients with a good outcome. Continuous rCBF monitoring with TDF is a new parameter for following head-injured patients. It is fairly easy to perform and safe, since there is no significant morbidity. TDF may help the neurosurgeon and intensivist decide which forms of therapy (such as hyperventilation, osmotherapy, and early barbiturate coma) may be of value in the treatment of intracranial hypertension in comatose head-injured patients.

References

1. Kety SS, Schmidt CF: Determination of cerebral blood flow in man by use of nitrous oxide in low concentrations. *Am J Physiol* 143:53–66, 1945.
2. Lassen NA, Munck O: The cerebral blood flow in man determined by the use of radioactive krypton. *Acta Physiol Scand* 33:30, 1955.
3. Tybjaerg-Hansen A, Haxholdt BF, Husfeldt E, et al: Measurement of coronary blood flow and cardiac efficiency in hypothermia by use of radioactive krypton[85]. *Scand J Clin Lab Invest* 8:182, 1956.
4. Brun C, Crone C, Davidsen HG, et al: Renal blood flow in anuric human subject determined by use of radioactive krypton[85]. *Proc Soc Exp Biol Med* 89:687, 1955.
5. Hoedt-Rasmussen K, Skinhoj E: Transneural depression of the cerebral hemispheric metabolism in man. *Acta Neurol Scand* 40:41–46, 1964.
6. Ingvar D, Obrist W, Chivian E, et al: General and regional abnormalities of cerebral blood flow in senile and presenile dementia. *Scand J Clin Lab Invest* 22(suppl 102):12B, 1968.
7. Lewis BM, Sokoloff L, Wechsler RL, et al: A method for the continuous measurement of cerebral blood flow in man by means of radioactive krypton. *J Clin Invest,* 39:707–716, 1960.
8. Hoedt-Rasmussen K, Sueinsdotter E, Lassen NA: Regional cerebral blood flow in man determined by intra-

arterial injection of radioactive inert gas. *Circ Res* 18:237–247, 1966.
9. Hoedt-Rasmussen K: Regional cerebral blood flow: The intra-arterial injection method. *Acta Neurol Scand* 27(suppl):1–81, 1967.
10. Olesen J, Paulson OB, Lassen NA: Regional cerebral blood flow in man determined by the initial slope of the clearance of intra-arterially injected ^{133}Xe. *Stroke* 2:519–540, 1971.
11. Mallett BL, Veall N: Measurement of regional cerebral clearance rates in man using xenon-133 inhalation and extracranial recording. *Clin Sci* 29:179–191, 1965.
12. Veall N, Mallett BL: Regional cerebral blood flow determination by ^{133}Xe inhalation and external recording: The effect of arterial recirculation. *Clin Sci* 30:353–369, 1966.
13. Obrist WD, Thompson HK Jr, King CH, et al: Determination of regional cerebral blood flow by inhalation of 133-xenon. *Circ Res* 20:124–135, 1967.
14. Obrist WD, Thompson HK Jr, Wang HS, et al: A simplified procedure for determining fast compartment rCBFs by ^{133}Xe inhalation, in Russell RWR (ed): *Brain and Blood Flow: Proceedings of the Fourth International Symposium.* London: Pitman, 1971:11–15.
15. Sharbrough FW, Messicle JM, Sundt TM: Correlation of continuous electroencephalograms with cerebral blood flow measurements during carotid endarterectomy. *Stroke* 4:674–683, 1973.
16. Ewing JR, Robertson WM, Brown GG, et al: 133-xenon inhalation: Accuracy in detection of ischemic cerebral regions and angiographic lesions, in Wood JH (ed): *Cerebral Blood Flow: Physiologic and Clinical Aspects.* New York: McGraw-Hill, 1987:202–219.
17. Barnett GH, Little JR, Ebraham ZY, et al: Cerebral circulation during arteriovenous malformation operation. *Neurosurgery* 20:836–842, 1987.
18. Agnoli A, Precipe M, Priori AM, et al: Measurements of rCBF by intravenous injection of ^{133}Xe: A comparative study with the intra-arterial injection method, in Brock M, Fieschi C, Ingvar DH, et al (eds): *Cerebral Blood Flow: Clinical and Experimental Results.* Berlin/Heidelberg/New York: Springer-Verlag, 1969:31–34.
19. Obrist WD, Thompson HK Jr, Wang HS, et al: Regional cerebral blood flow estimated by ^{133}xenon inhalation. *Stroke* 6:245–256, 1975.
20. Meyer JS, Hayman LA, Amano T, et al: Mapping local blood flow of human brain by CT scanning during stable xenon inhalation. *Stroke* 12:426–435, 1981.
21. Ackerman RH: Of cerebral blood flow, stroke and SPECT. *Stroke* 15:1–4, 1984.
22. Drayer BP, Wolfson SK, Reinmuth OM, et al: Xenon enhanced CT for analysis of cerebral integrity, perfusion, and blood flow. *Stroke* 9:123–130, 1978.
23. Drayer BP, Gur D, Wolfson SK, et al: Experimental xenon enhancement with CT imaging: Cerebral applications. *AJR* 134:39–44, 1980.
24. Gur D, Wolfson SK Jr, Yonas H, et al: Progress in cerebrovascular disease: Local cerebral blood flow by xenon enhanced CT. *Stroke* 13:750–758, 1982.
25. Segawa H, Susumu W, Tamura A, et al: Computed tomographic measurement of local cerebral blood flow by xenon enhancement. *Stroke* 14:356–362, 1983.
26. Yonas H, Good WF, Gur D, et al: Mapping cerebral blood flow by xenon-enhanced computed tomography: Clinical experience. *Radiology* 152:435–442, 1984.
27. Wozney P, Yonas H, Latchaw RE, et al: Central herniation revealed by focal decrease in blood flow without elevation of intracranial pressure: A case report. *Neurosurgery* 17:641–644, 1985.
28. Holman BL, Hill TC: Profusion imaging with single-photon emission computed tomography, in Wood JH (ed): *Cerebral Blood Flow: Physiologic and Clinical Aspects.* New York: McGraw Hill, 1987:243–256.
29. Peterman SB, Taylor A Jr, Hoffman HC Jr: Improved detection of cerebral hypoperfusion with internal carotid balloon test occlusion and 99m Tc-HMPAO cerebral perfusion SPECT imaging. *AJNR* 12:1035–1041, 1991.
30. Reid RH, Guleychyn KY, Ballinger JR, et al: Cerebral perfusion imaging with technetium-99 m HMPAO following cerebral trauma: Initial experience. *Clin Nucl Med* 15:383–388, 1990.
31. Abdel-Dayem HM, Sadek SA, Kouris K, et al: Changes in cerebral perfusion after acute head injury: Comparison of CT with Tc-99 m HM-PAO SPECT. *Radiology* 165:221, 1987.
32. Reid RH, Gulenchyn KY, Ballinger JR: Clinical use of technetium-99 M HM-PAO for determination of brain death. *J Nucl Med* 30:1621, 1989.
33. Newton MR, Greenwood RJ, Britton KE, et al: A study comparing SPECT with CT and MRI after closed head injury. *J Neurol Neurosurg Psychiatry* 55:92–94, 1992.
34. Herscovish P, Powers WJ: Measurement of regional cerebral blood flow by positron emission tomography, in Wood JH (ed): *Cerebral Blood Flow: Physiologic and Clinical Aspects.* New York: McGraw-Hill, 1987:257–271.
35. Belliveau JW, Kennedy DN, McKinstry RC, et al: Functional mapping of the human visual cortex by magnetic resonance imaging. *Science* 254:716–719, 1991.
36. Engel J Jr, Brown WJ, Kuhl DE, et al: Pathological findings underlying focal temporal lobe hypometabolism in partial epilepsy. *Ann Neurol* 12:518–529, 1982.
37. Bandettini PA, Wong EC, Hinks RS, et al: Time course EPI of human brain function during task activation. *Magn Reson Med* 25:390–397, 1992.
38. Turner R, Jezzard P, Wen H, et al: Functional mapping of the human visual cortex at 4 and 1.5 tesla using deoxygenation contrast EPI. *Magn Reson Med* 29:277–279, 1993.
39. Turner R, Le Bihan D, Moonen CTW, et al: Echo-planar time course MRI of cat brain oxygenation changes. *Magn Reson Med* 22:159, 1991.
40. Kwong KK, Belliveau JW, Chesler DA, et al: Dynamic magnetic resonance imaging of human brain activity during primary sensory stimulation. *Proc Natl Acad Sci USA* 89:5675–5679, 1992.
41. Frahm J, Merboldt KD, Hänicke W: Functional MRI of human brain activation at high spatial resolution. *Magn Reson Med* 29:139–144, 1993.

42. Seiler RW, Grolimund P, Aaslid R, et al: Cerebral vasospasm evaluated by transcranial ultrasound correlated with clinical grade and CT-visualized subarachnoid hemorrhage. *J Neurosurg* 64:594–600, 1986.
43. Riva C, Ross B, Benedek GB: Laser-doppler measurements of blood flow in capillary tubes and retinal arteries. *Invest Ophthalmol* 11:936–944, 1972.
44. Stern MD: In vivo evaluation of microcirculation by coherent light scattering. *Nature* 254:56–58, 1975.
45. Englehart M, Kristensen JK: Evaluation of cutaneous blood flow responses by ^{133}Xe washout and a laser-doppler flowmeter. *J Invest Dermatol* 80:12–15, 1983.
46. Johnson JM, Taylor WF, Shepherd AP, et al: Laser-doppler measurement of skin blood flow: Comparison with plethysmography. *J Appl Physiol Respir Environ Exerc Physiol* 56:798–803, 1984.
47. Kvietys PR, Shepherd AP, Granger DN: Laser-doppler H_2 clearance and microsphere estimates of mucosal blood flow. *Am J Physiol* 249:G221–227, 1985.
48. Dirnagl U, Kaplan B, Jacewicz M, et al: Continuous measurement of cerebral cortical blood flow by laser-doppler flowmetry in a rat stroke model. *J Cereb Blood Flow Metab* 9:589–596, 1989.
49. Haberl RC, Heizer MC, Marmarou A, et al: Laser-doppler assessment of brain microcirculation: Effect of systemic alternatives. *Am J Physiol* 256:H1247–1254, 1989.
50. Dirnagl U, Pulsinelli W: Autoregulation of cerebral blood flow in experimental focal brain ischemia. *J Cereb Blood Flow Metab* 10:327–336, 1990.
51. Skarphedinsson JO, Hardins HJ, Thoren P: Repeated measurements of cerebral blood flow in rats: Comparison between the hydrogen clearance method and laser-doppler flowmetry. *Acta Physiol Scand* 143:133–142, 1988.
52. Saeki Y, Sato A, Sato Y, et al: Effects of stimulation of cervical sympathetic trunks and various frequencies on the local cortical cerebral blood flow measured by laser-doppler flowmetry in the rat. *Jpn J Physiol* 40:15–32, 1990.
53. Rosenblum RB, Bonner RF, Oldfield EH: Intraoperative measurement of cortical blood flow adjacent to cerebral AVM using laser-doppler velocimetry. *J Neurosurg* 66:396–399, 1987.
54. Arbit E, DiResta GR, Bedford RF, et al: Intraoperative measurement of cerebral and tumor blood flow with laser-doppler flowmetry. *Neurosurgery* 24:166–170, 1989.
55. Gibbs FH: A thermoelectric blood flow recorder in the form of a needle. *Proc Soc Exp Biol Med* 31:141–146, 1933.
56. Grayson J: Internal calorimetry in the determination of thermal conductivity and blood flow. *J Physiol* 118:54–72, 1952.
57. Carlyle A, Grayson J: Blood pressure and the regulation of brain blood flow. *J Physiol* 127:15P-6, 1955.
58. Perl W: Heat and matter distribution in body tissues and the determination of tissue blood flow by local clearance methods. *J Theor Biol* 2:201–235, 1962.
59. Betz E, Ingvar EH, Lassen NA, et al: Regional blood flow in the cerebral cortex, measured simultaneously by heat and insert gas clearance. *Acta Physiol Scand* 67:1–9, 1966.
60. Brawley BW: The pathophysiology of intracerebral steal following carbon dioxide inhalation, an experimental study. *Scand J Lab Clin Invest* 22(suppl 102):13B, 1968.
61. Wullenweber R: Observations concerning autoregulation of central blood flow in man. *Acta Neurol Scand* 41(suppl 14):111–115, 1965.
62. Carter LP, Atkinson JR: Cortical blood flow in controlled hypotension as measured by thermal diffusion. *J Neurol Neurosurg Psychiatry* 36:906–913, 1973.
63. Carter LP, Atkinson JR: Autoregulation and hyperemia of cerebral blood flow as evaluated by thermal diffusion. *Stroke* 4:917–922, 1973.
64. Carter LP, Erspamer RJ, Bro WJ: Cortical blood flow thermal diffusion vs isotope clearance. *Stroke* 12:513–551, 1981.
65. Gaines C, Carter LP, Crowell RM: Comparison of local cerebral blood flow determined by thermal and hydrogen clearance. *Stroke* 14:66–69, 1983.
66. Cusick J, MyklebURST J: Continuous quantitative local cerebral blood flow measurement: Calibration of chemical conductivity measurements by the hydrogen clearance method. *Stroke* 11:661–664, 1980.
67. Gopinath SP, Robertson CS, Narayan RK, et al: Continuous monitoring of cerebral cortical blood flow in head-injured patients. Poster 1262, AANS 1993 Annual Meeting, April 24–29, 1993, Boston.
68. Carter LP, White WL, Atkinson JR: Regional cortical blood flow at craniotomy. *Neurosurgery* 2:223–229, 1978.
69. Carter LP, Raudzeus PA, Gaines C, et al: Somatosensory evoked potentials and cortical blood flow during craniotomy for vascular disease. *Neurosurgery* 15:22–28, 1984.
70. Takemae T, Kobayashi S, Otsabo H, et al: Intra- and postoperative cortical blood flow monitoring in the cerebrovascular surgery. *J Cereb Blood Flow Metab* 7(suppl 1):S550, 1987.
71. Ohmoto T, Nagao S, Mino S, et al: Monitoring of cortical blood flow during temporary arterial occlusion in aneurysm during surgery by the thermal diffusion method. *Neurosurgery* 28:49–55, 1991.
72. Barnett GH, Little JR, Ebraham ZY, et al: Cerebral circulation during arteriovenous malformation operation. *Neurosurgery* 20:836–842, 1987.
73. Tamaki N, Ehara K, Fujita K, et al: Cerebral hyperperfusion during surgical resection of high-flow arteriovenous malformations. *Surg Neurol* 40:10–15, 1993.
74. Weinand ME, Carter LP, Oommen KJ, et al: Surface monitoring of cerebral cortical blood flow in epilepsy. *Neurology* 42(suppl 3):81, 1992.
75. Kuwayama N, Takaku A, Harada J, et al: Modified thermal diffusion flow probe for the continuous monitoring of cortical blood flow: Technical report. *Neurosurgery* 29:583–589, 1991.
76. Carter LP, Graham T, Zabramski JM, et al: Postoperative monitoring of cerebral blood flow in patients harboring intracranial aneurysms. *Neurol Res* 12:214–218, 1990.
77. Graham DI, Adams JH: Ischaemic brain damage in fatal head injuries. *Lancet* 1:265–266, 1971.
78. Graham DI, Ford I, Adams JH, et al: Ischaemic brain damage is still common in fatal non-missile head injury. *J Neurol Neurosurg Psychiatry* 52:346–350, 1989.

79. Gokaslan ZL, Robertson CS, Narayan RK, et al: Prognostic, pathophysiological, and therapeutic implications of CBF patterns in head injury. *J Neurosurg* 70:323A, 1989.
80. Sheinberg M, Kanter MJ, Robertson CS, et al: Continuous monitoring of jugular venous oxygen saturation in head-injured patients. *J Neurosurg* 76:212–217, 1992.
81. Fieschi C, Battistini N, Beduschi A, et al: Regional cerebral blood flow and intraventricular pressure in acute head injuries. *J Neurol Neurosurg Psychiatry* 37:1378–1388, 1974.
82. Enevoldsen EM, Cold G, Jensen FT, et al: Dynamic changes in regional CBF, intraventricular pressure, CSF pH and lactate levels during the acute phase of head injury. *J Neurosurg* 44:191–213, 1976.
83. Barclay L, Zemcov A, Reichert W, et al: Cerebral blood flow decrements in chronic head injury syndrome. *Biol Psychiatry* 20:146–157, 1985.
84. Obrist WD, Gennarelli TA, Segawa H, et al: Relation of cerebral blood flow to neurological status and outcome in head-injured patients. *J Neurosurg* 51:292–300, 1979.
85. Obrist WD, Langfitt TW, Jaggi JL, et al: Cerebral blood flow and metabolism in comatose patients with acute head injury: Relationship to intracranial hypertension. *J Neurosurg* 61:241–253, 1984.
86. Bouma GJ, Muizelaar PJ, Choi SC, et al: Cerebral circulation and metabolism after severe traumatic brain injury: The elusive role of ischemia. *J Neurosurg* 75:685–693, 1991.
87. Bouma GJ, Muizelaar PJ, Stringer WA, et al: Ultra-early evaluation of regional cerebral blood flow in severely head-injured patients using xenon-enhanced computerized tomography. *J Neurosurg* 77:360–368, 1992.
88. Muizelaar JP, Marmarou A, Ward JD, et al: Adverse effects of prolonged hyperventilation in patients with severe head injury: A randomized clinical trial. *J Neurosurg* 75:731–739, 1991.
89. Langfitt TW, Obrist WD, Alavi A, et al: Computerized tomography, magnetic resonance imaging, and positron emission tomography in the study of brain trauma. *J Neurosurg* 64:760–767, 1986.
90. Martin NA, Doberstein C, Zane C, et al: Posttraumatic cerebral arterial spasm: Transcranial doppler ultrasound, cerebral blood flow, and angiographic findings. *J Neurosurg* 77:575–583, 1992.
91. MacPerson P, Graham DI: Correlation between angiographic findings and the ischaemia of head injury. *J Neurol Neurosurg Psychiatry* 41:122–127, 1977.
92. Suwanwela C, Suwanwela N: Intracranial arterial narrowing and spasm in acute head injury. *J Neurosurg* 36:314–323, 1972.
93. Dickman CA, Carter LP, Baldwin HZ, et al: Continuous regional cerebral blood flow monitoring in acute craniocerebral trauma. *Neurosurgery* 28:467–472, 1991.
94. Sioutos P, Orozco J, Carter LP, et al: Continuous regional cerebral cortical blood flow monitoring in head-injured patients. *Neurosurgery* vol 36: 943–950, 1995.
95. Salvant JB Jr, Muizelaar JP: Changes in cerebral blood flow and metabolism related to the presence of subdural hematoma. *Neurosurgery* 33:387–393, 1993.

CHAPTER 36

JUGULAR VENOUS OXYGEN SATURATION MONITORING

Troy Woodman
Claudia S. Robertson

SYNOPSIS

Global cerebral oxygenation can be measured by means of a catheter placed in the internal jugular vein with the tip positioned in the jugular bulb. Jugular venous oxygen saturation (Sjv_{O_2}) can be measured intermittently by drawing a blood sample through the catheter or continuously by using a fiber-optic oxygen saturation catheter. Sjv_{O_2} monitoring is useful for detecting episodes of cerebral hypoxia/ischemia, allowing early treatment. Sjv_{O_2} monitoring can also help direct the treatment of intracranial hypertension toward the underlying pathophysiology and identify the optimal level of cerebral perfusion pressure and P_{CO_2} for the individual patient. Sjv_{O_2} monitoring is a relatively low-risk high-yield technique, and the cost is modest.

Many factors contribute to the long-term neurological disability incurred by a patient who has sustained a severe head injury. The primary pathological condition produced by the injury, secondary insults, and the age of the patient have all been identified as determinants of outcome after head injury.

Recent studies have suggested that secondary insults resulting in hypoxia/ischemia of the brain may also contribute significantly to a poor outcome.[1–4] At least some of these secondary insults may be prevented or the resulting injury may be minimized by recognizing and treating the underlying causes at the earliest possible time. Because the technology for monitoring venous oxygen saturation continuously by means of a fiber-optic catheter has become available, jugular venous oxygen saturation (Sjv_{O_2}) is used increasingly to detect ischemic episodes in patients with a head injury.

PHYSIOLOGY OF JUGULAR VENOUS OXYGEN SATURATION

Oxygen Extraction Ratio

Sjv_{O_2} is theoretically a useful monitor for cerebral hypoxia/ischemia because it reflects the balance between oxygen delivery to the brain and oxygen consumption by the brain. Because both delivery and consumption parameters can be abnormal after a head injury, the relative balance between these two parameters often provides more valuable information than does the absolute level of either parameter alone.

The oxygen extraction ratio (O_2ER) is the parameter that describes the relative balance between oxygen consumption and delivery and is calculated by the formula

$$O_2ER = \frac{O_2\ \text{consumption}}{O_2\ \text{delivery}}$$

This formula can be simplified to

$$O_2ER = \frac{AVD_{O_2} \times CBF}{Ca_{O_2} \times CBF} = \frac{AVD_{O_2}}{Ca_{O_2}}$$

where AVD_{O_2} is the arteriovenous difference of oxygen, Ca_{O_2} is the arterial oxygen content, and CBF is cerebral blood flow. AVD_{O_2} is generally determined by radial arterial oxygen saturation and P_{O_2} (Sa_{O_2} and Pa_{O_2}), jugular venous oxygen saturation and P_{O_2} (Sjv_{O_2} and Pjv_{O_2}), and hemoglobin concentration (Hgb) by the following formula:

$$AVD_{O_2} = (Sa_{O_2} - Sjv_{O_2}) \times 1.34 \times Hgb + (Pa_{O_2} - Pjv_{O_2}) \times .0031$$

If the small contribution of dissolved oxygen to arterial and venous oxygen content (*in italics*) is ignored, O_2ER can be simplified as follows:

$$O_2ER = \frac{AVD_{O_2}}{Ca_{O_2}} = \frac{(Sa_{O_2} - Sjv_{O_2}) \times 1.34 \times Hgb}{Sa_{O_2} \times 1.34 \times Hgb} \frac{+\, \mathit{(Pa_{O_2} - Pjv_{O_2}) \times 0.0031}}{+\, \mathit{Pa_{O_2} \times .0031}} = \frac{Sa_{O_2} - Sjv_{O_2}}{Sa_{O_2}}$$

These relationships are depicted in Fig. 36-1, which shows a balance beam with oxygen delivery on one end and oxygen consumption or cerebral metabolic rate of oxygen (CMR_{O_2}) on the opposite end. Any disturbance that increases cerebral oxygen consumption or decreases oxygen delivery may decrease Sjv_{O_2}. A disturbance that decreases cerebral oxygen consumption or increases oxygen delivery may increase Sjv_{O_2}.

Cerebral Oxygen Consumption

CMR_{O_2} is typically reduced from the normal value of 1.5 μmol/g/min to an average of 0.9 μmol/g/min in patients with a severe head injury. The reduction in CMR_{O_2} is directly related to the severity of the injury.[5] Two complications, however, can significantly increase CMR_{O_2} after a head injury: fever and seizures. In addition, two treatment modalities sometimes used to manage intracranial hypertension—barbiturate coma and hypothermia—can significantly reduce CMR_{O_2}.

Fever increases the body's metabolic rate by approximately 10 to 13 percent per degree Centigrade. The effect of fever on CMR_{O_2} has been studied in neonatal

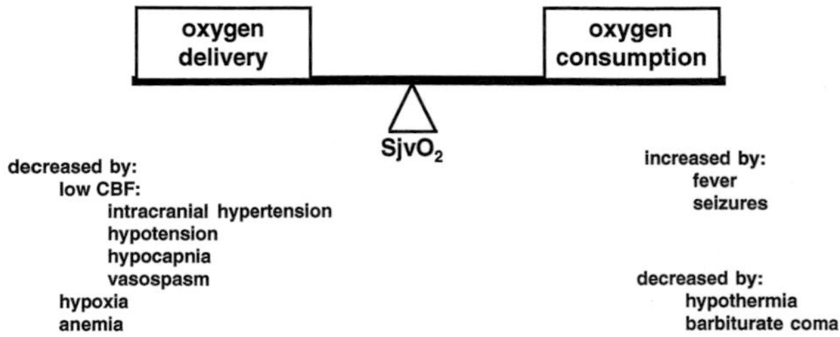

Figure 36-1. Sjv_{O_2} reflects the balance between cerebral oxygen delivery and oxygen consumption (CMR_{O_2}). An increase in CMR_{O_2} or a decrease in oxygen delivery can decrease Sjv_{O_2}.

pigs.[6] Increasing temperature from 38 to 42°C increased CBF by 97 percent and CMR_{O_2} by 65 percent.

Seizures can also dramatically increase CMR_{O_2}. When seizures were induced in rats by administering bicuculline, CMR_{O_2} increased by 150 to 250 percent.[7]

The administration of thiopental sodium to normal adults in a dose of 35 mg/kg reduced cerebral oxygen consumption approximately 50 percent from a normal value of 3.3 to 1.5 ml/100 g/min.[8] Barbiturate coma in patients with refractory intracranial hypertension after head injury reduced CMR_{O_2} an average of 34 percent from 0.93 ± 0.45 to 0.61 ± 0.25 μmol/g/min.[9]

As a general rule, hypothermia decreases CMR_{O_2} by approximately 5 percent per degree Centigrade reduction in body temperature. More precisely, the effect of hypothermia on CMR_{O_2} is expressed as Q10, the factor by which metabolism is altered after a 10°C change in temperature. Between 37 and 27°C, Q10 is 2.2 in experimental studies.[10] In a study of patients under midazolam and fentanyl anesthesia who were cooled to 27°C using cardiopulmonary bypass, CMR_{O_2} was decreased 64 percent from 1.4 ± 0.3 to 0.5 ± 0.2 ml/100 g/min.[11] In patients with a severe head injury, moderate hypothermia to 32 to 33°C reduced CMR_{O_2} approximately 11 percent.[12]

Cerebral Oxygen Delivery

Cerebral oxygen delivery is a product of CBF and arterial oxygen content. The latter is calculated from arterial oxygen saturation and hemoglobin concentration and is normally around 22 ml/dl. In head-injured patients, arterial oxygen saturation is usually maintained at normal values by controlled ventilation with supplemental oxygen. However, pulmonary complications such as atelectasis, pulmonary edema, pneumonia, and adult respiratory distress syndrome can result in hypoxia. It is desirable to maintain hemoglobin concentration at least in the lower than normal range of 9 to 10 g/dl by using blood transfusions, if necessary. However, complications such as gastrointestinal bleeding and bleeding into the retroperitoneal space or from long bone fractures can result in significant and sudden anemia.

CBF has been studied extensively in head-injured patients and is described in detail in other chapters in this book. Briefly, CBF can be reduced, normal, or elevated relative to normal values.[5,13] Furthermore, CBF can be normally coupled to the cerebral metabolic rate or can be completely unrelated.[5]

Because so many of these factors affecting oxygen delivery and consumption can be abnormal in patients with a head injury (Table 36-1), O_2ER or Sjv_{O_2} is more useful than any other single parameter as a measure of cerebral oxygenation.

TABLE 36-1 Changes in Cerebral Oxygen Delivery and Oxygen Consumption Parameters after Head Injury

Determinants of Cerebral Oxygenation	Normal Values	Changes in Head Injury
Oxygen consumption (CMR_{O_2})	1.5 μmol/g/min	50% decrease but can be increased by fever, seizures
Oxygen delivery		
CBF	0.54 ml/g/min	Can be increased, decreased, or normal
Sa_{O_2}	98%	Usually maintained at normal with supplemental oxygen
Hemoglobin	14–15 g/dl	Usually maintained at slightly less than normal, 10 g/dl
Sjv_{O_2} and Derived Parameters Used to Monitor Cerebral Oxygenation	**Normal values (n = 50 male adults)**	**Average Head Injury Values (n = 149 patients)**
Sjv_{O_2}	62 ± 4% (range, 55–71%)	68 ± 10% (range, 32–96%)
AVD_{O_2}	6.7 ± 0.8 ml/dl (range, 4.5–8.5 ml/dl)	4.5 ± 1.6 ml/dl (range, 0.5–12.1 ml/dl)
O_2ER	35%	31 ± 10% (range, 3–69%)

Changes in Cerebrovascular Hemodynamics with Decreases in Arterial Oxygen Content

In normal subjects

Arterial oxygen content (Ca_{O_2}) can be reduced by two conditions: anemia and hypoxia. The cerebrovascular effects of both conditions have been studied extensively in normal experimental animals and normal humans. In both conditions, until the decrease in Ca_{O_2} is extreme, the primary mechanism for compensation for the decrease in Ca_{O_2} is an increase in CBF (Fig. 36-2).

Progressive normovolemic anemia has been studied in the laboratory. In the rat, a reduction in Ca_{O_2} from 22 to 5 ml/dl was produced by removing blood and replacing the loss with an equal volume of plasma.[14] The primary compensation for the decrease in Ca_{O_2} was an increase in CBF from 114 ± 6 ml/100 g/min at a normal Ca_{O_2} of 22 ml/dl to 510 ± 40 ml/100 g/min at a markedly reduced Ca_{O_2} of 5 ml/dl. O_2ER remained unchanged until the Ca_{O_2} decreased below 8 ml/dl, at which time O_2ER increased from 40 to 51 percent.

In normal humans, normovolemic hemodilution sufficient to decrease the hematocrit by 26 percent had cerebrovascular effects similar to those in animal studies.[15] The primary compensatory mechanism was CBF. CBF was increased by 19 percent, while CMR_{O_2}, Sjv_{O_2}, and Pjv_{O_2} remained unchanged.

Severe hypoxia has also been studied in the laboratory. In the rat, a decrease in arterial P_{O_2} from a normal value of 140 to 24 mmHg was accomplished by reducing the Fi_{O_2}.[16] The primary compensation for the decrease in Ca_{O_2} was an increase in CBF from 114 ± 6 ml/100 g/min at a normal Ca_{O_2} of 22 ml/dl to 516 ± 41 ml/100 g/min at a markedly reduced Ca_{O_2} of 4 ml/dl. Because the Sa_{O_2} was markedly decreased with the low P_{O_2} values, the Sjv_{O_2} decreased from a normal value of 60 percent to 10 percent. However, the O_2ER remained unchanged until Ca_{O_2} decreased below 5 ml/dl, at which time O_2ER increased slightly from 44 to 50 percent.

In normal adults, the cerebrovascular effects of hypoxia have been studied by reducing Fi_{O_2}.[17,18] At an Fi_{O_2} of 0.10 (corresponding to a P_{O_2} of 40 mmHg), CBF is increased by 35 percent,[17] and at an Fi_{O_2} of 0.09 (P_{O_2} of 35 mmHg), CBF is increased by 70 percent.[18]

In head-injured subjects

Because the primary compensation for decreases in arterial oxygen content is normally an increase in CBF, head injury might be expected to impair the ability of the brain to compensate for both hypoxia and anemia. Levels of hypoxia, which in a normal animal have no adverse consequences, are neurologically devastating to an animal that has suffered a mild head injury.[19,20] Epidemiological studies suggest that hypoxia on admission to the hospital emergency room or during hospitalization increases the risk of a poor outcome after a head injury.[1,21,22]

Studies in the laboratory have shown that at least part of the mechanism of this increased susceptibility to decreases in arterial oxygen content is the inability of an injured brain to respond by increasing CBF. Therefore, for any given level of hypoxia or anemia, oxygen delivery to the brain is lower in an injured animal than in a normal animal.

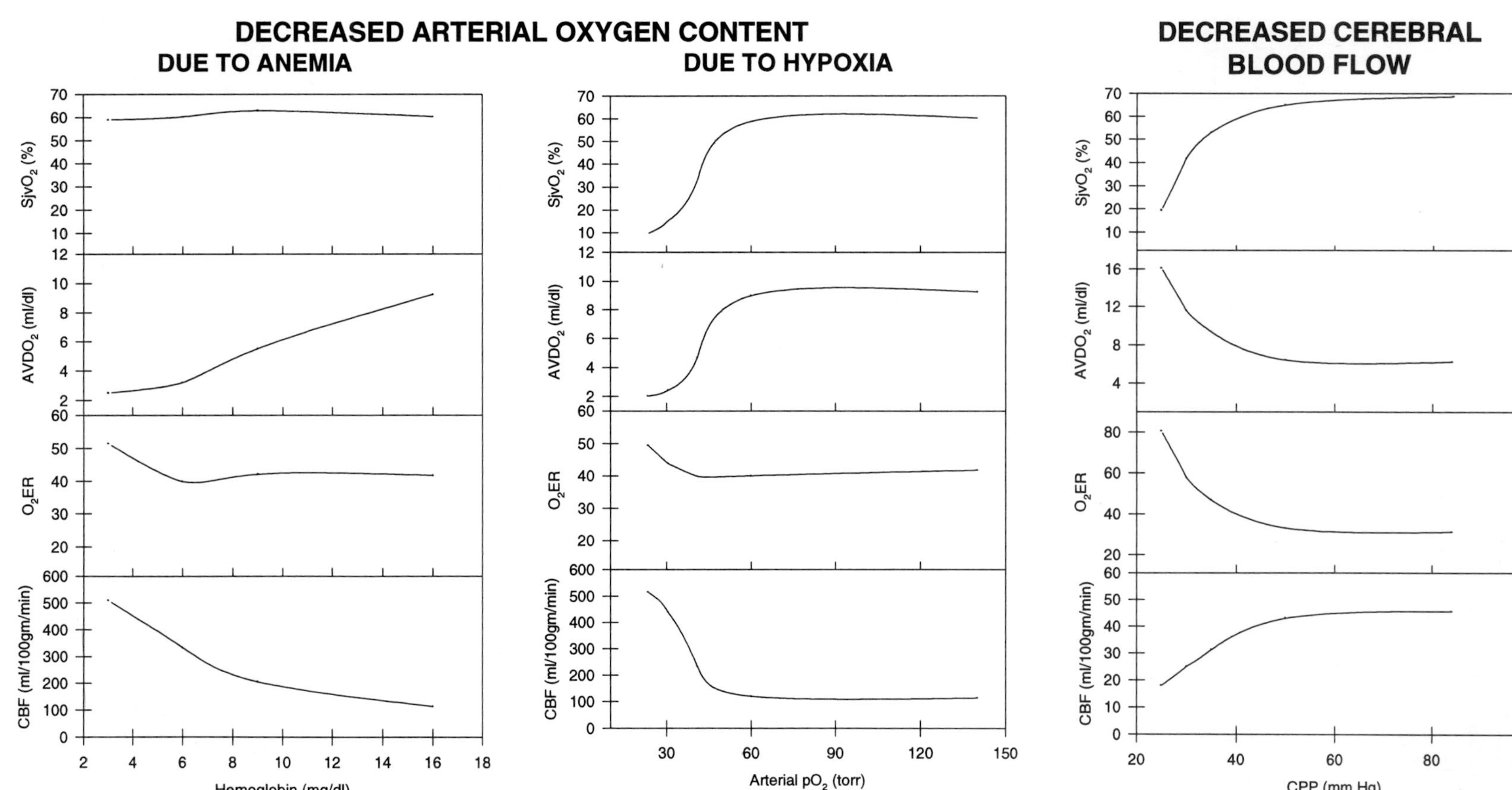

Figure 36-2. In the normal brain, decreases in arterial oxygen content are well compensated by an increasing CBF and O_2ER does not change until the decrease in arterial oxygen content is extreme. (Data from Refs. 16 and 48.) In head-injured patients, however, in whom CBF may not be able to increase in response to decreased oxygen availability, Sjv_{O_2} may decrease and O_2ER may increase at a lower reduction in arterial oxygen content.

Lewelt et al.[23] examined the effects of mild and severe fluid percussion injury on the CBF response to hypoxia. The mild fluid percussion injury resulted in an increase in CBF, while the severe injury caused CBF to decrease. However, both levels of injury severely impaired the ability of the brain to increase CBF during hypoxia.

DeWitt et al.[24] compared the effects on CBF of an acute hemorrhage of 30 percent of the total blood volume followed by resuscitation with an equal volume of hetastarch (hydroxyethyl starch) in normal cats and in cats with a moderate fluid percussion injury. The animals with a head injury had significantly lower blood pressures, CBF, and cerebral oxygen delivery than did the noninjured animals.

Changes in Cerebral Hemodynamics with Ischemia

In Normal Subjects

As CBF decreases as a result of intracranial hypertension or systemic hypotension, the primary compensatory mechanism is increasing oxygen extraction (Fig. 36-2). In normal adults in whom blood pressure was reduced from a mean of 84 to 35 mmHg by infusion of hexamethonium, CBF decreased from 45.6 to 31.3 ml/100 g/min.[25] CMR_{O_2} remained constant, and AVD_{O_2} increased from 6.24 to 9.35 ml/dl. If CBF continues to decrease, a point is eventually reached at which the brain is no longer able to completely compensate for decreased CBF by further increases in oxygen extraction. At this point, CMR_{O_2} decreases and cerebral lactate production increases.

In Head-Injured Subjects

The sequence of cerebrovascular changes is similar to that described in normal subjects.[26] Initially, increasing oxygen extraction compensates for the reduced CBF, and there is no effect on cerebral metabolism. At this stage, AVD_{O_2} and O_2ER are increased, Sjv_{O_2} is decreased, and CMR_{O_2} is unchanged. As CBF decreases further, the brain can no longer compensate fully by increasing oxygen extraction, and CMR_{O_2} falls and cerebral lactate production increases. The major difference from normal subjects is that after a head injury CBF decreases at less severe reductions in cerebral perfusion pressure (CPP).

Lewelt et al.[27] showed in a fluid percussion injury model that autoregulation was severely impaired after both low-level and high-level injuries. Normally, CBF is constant until CPP falls below 60 mmHg. After the fluid percussion injury, CBF decreased proportional to the CPP below 80 mmHg.

Chan et al.[28] described similar findings in patients with head injury, with middle cerebral artery (MCA) flow velocity measured by transcranial Doppler and Sjv_{O_2} decreasing as CPP was reduced below 70 mmHg.

Indications and Contraindications for Sjv_{O_2} Monitoring after Head Injury

Indications

Because the monitoring of Sjv_{O_2} is invasive, it should be reserved for patients at significant risk of ischemic insults that might be identified with such monitoring. In a prospectively monitored series of 149 patients at Ben Taub General Hospital (BTGH) with a Glasgow Coma Scale (GCS) ≤ 8 on admission or within 48 h after a severe head injury, 58 (39 percent) had at least one documented episode of jugular venous desaturation ($Sjv_{O_2} < 50$ percent for at least 10 min). Table 36-2 shows that the risk of jugular desaturation was the same in patients with an admission GCS 3 to 5 and those with a GCS of 6 to 8. The risk of jugular desaturation was somewhat lower in patients who were admitted with a GCS > 8 but who deteriorated to coma after admission and were then monitored. The risk of jugular desaturation was greatest in patients with a focal injury, intermediate in patients with a diffuse injury, and lowest in patients with a gunshot wound, but these differences were not statistically significant. The presence of intracranial hypertension increased the risk of desaturation from 26 to 55 percent. Therefore, Sjv_{O_2} monitoring seems to be most appropriate for patients admitted with a GCS ≤ 8, especially patients with intracranial hypertension.

Contraindications

Sjv_{O_2} catheters should be placed with great care in patients with cervical spine injuries, since the head usually has to be turned to insert the catheter, and in patients with significant coagulopathies. The presence of a tracheostomy is a relative contraindication because of the increased potential for infection.

TABLE 36-2 Incidence of Jugular Desaturation in 149 Patients with Severe Head Injury

Category	Number of Episodes of Desaturation		
	None	One	Multiple
Number	91(61%)	36(24%)	22(15%)
Admission GCS			
3–5	32(59%)	15(28%)	7(13%)
6–8	35(58%)	16(27%)	9(15%)
9–15	24(68%)	5(14%)	6(17%)
Type of injury			
Closed head injury			
Diffuse	29(63%)	12(26%)	5(11%)
Focal	46(58%)	20(25%)	14(18%)
Gunshot wound	16(70%)	4(17%)	3(13%)
Intracranial pressure			
Normal	35(74%)	6(13%)	6(13%)
Increased but controllable	47(67%)	18(26%)	5(7%)
Increased and refractory to treatment	9(28%)	12(48%)	11(34%)

IN VIVO OXIMETRY TECHNOLOGY

When Sjv_{O_2} was first sampled in the 1930s and 1940s, the jugular bulb was directly punctured by a needle that was inserted 1 cm below and anterior to the mastoid process.[29] More recently, placement of an internal jugular vein catheter similar to the type used for central venous pressure monitoring but directed cephalad into the jugular bulb has allowed repetitive sampling of Sjv_{O_2} without repeated needle punctures.[5,26,30–32] Most recently, the development of in vivo reflectance oximetry using fiber-optic catheters has allowed continuous monitoring of Sjv_{O_2} without sampling blood, except for calibration purposes.[33–35] A new technology called near-infrared spectroscopy is being investigated as an additional way to monitor brain tissue oxygen saturation noninvasively.[36]

Oxygen saturation in blood is measured in a co-oximeter by means of a technology called transmission spectroscopy. Light with 2–4 wavelengths is directed through a cuvette containing the blood sample. A sensor on the opposite side of the cuvette measures the absorbance of light by the blood sample at those wavelengths. Then, using Beer's law, the oxygen saturation is calculated from the absorbance of the light by the hemoglobin.

The in vivo measurement of oxygen saturation is similar except that it uses reflectance rather than transmission spectroscopy. A catheter containing two fiber-optic cables is placed in the blood vessel of interest. Light with 2–3 wavelengths is directed into the flowing stream of blood in the vessel by one of the fiber-optic cables. The light reflected by the hemoglobin is directed to an external sensor by another fiber-optic cable. The oxygen saturation is calculated from the absorbance of the light by the hemoglobin.

Three groups of investigators have reported their experience with the accuracy of fiber-optic catheters placed in the jugular bulb.[33,34,37] In general, the correlation is not as good as it is when the catheters are placed in the pulmonary artery ($r = \sim 0.90$ in jugular bulb, compared with 0.99 in the pulmonary artery), but trends in Sjv_{O_2} can be monitored and the precise Sjv_{O_2} can be obtained by drawing a blood sample through the catheter.

TECHNIQUE OF Sjv_{O_2} MONITORING

Anatomy of the Cerebral Venous Circulation

Ideally, the venous blood sampled for global cerebral oxygen saturation monitoring should be representative of the entire brain and should be free of extracerebral contamination. It is important to know the anatomy of the venous drainage of the brain in order to understand these potential limitations of Sjv_{O_2} monitoring. A diagram of the venous drainage of the brain appears in Fig. 36-3.

On the convex and medial surfaces of the brain there are 8 to 12 pairs of veins passing into the superior sagittal sinus. The inferior half of the brain has many large veins,

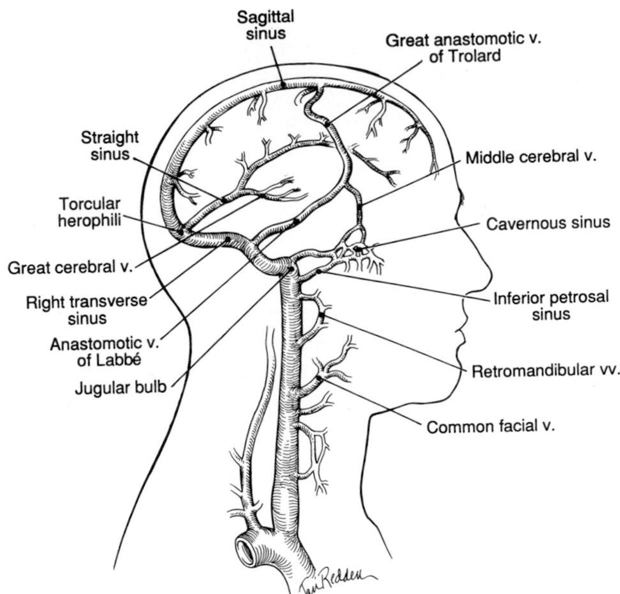

Figure 36-3. Venous drainage of the head and neck.

the principal one being the middle cerebral vein, which runs in the sylvian fissure and ends in the cavernous sinus. This large vessel also communicates with the superior sagittal sinus through the great anastomotic vein of Trolard and with the transverse sinus through the large vein of Labbé. The deep, or central, veins are drained principally through the great cerebral vein into the straight sinus. The principal dural sinuses, which collect blood from these sources (the superior sagittal sinus and the straight sinus) join to form the torcular Herophili. The two lateral sinuses take origin from the torcular and course laterally to reach the jugular bulbs. Of the two lateral sinuses, the right is usually the larger (62 percent larger on the right, 26 percent larger on the left, and 12 percent same size).[38] The cavernous and circular sinuses at the base of the brain have equally free communication from side to side and drain through the petrosal sinuses to the jugular bulbs.

The internal jugular vein exits the base of the skull through the jugular foramen and enters the carotid sheath dorsally with the internal carotid artery. It then courses posterolaterally to the artery, running beneath the sternocleidomastoid muscle. The vein lies medial to the anterior portion of the sternocleidomastoid muscle in its upper part and then runs beneath the triangle formed by the two heads of the muscle in its medial portion before entering the subclavian vein near the medial border of the anterior scalene muscle beneath the medial border of the clavicle.

Anatomic structures close to the internal jugular vein that may be injured during catheterization include the internal carotid artery, which runs just medial to the vein; the stellate ganglion and cervical sympathetic trunk, which lie behind the internal carotid artery just outside the sheath; and the phrenic nerve and pleural dome, which lie caudal to the junction of the internal jugular vein and subclavian vein.

Is Blood Obtained from the Jugular Bulb Representative of the Whole Brain?

Although the dural sinuses join at the torcular in most people, there has been controversy about whether there is sufficient mixing to ensure that the blood in the two lateral sinuses is similar. Gibbs and Gibbs[39] examined the torcular and associated veins from 25 human autopsy specimens and observed that blood from the straight sinus (draining subcortical areas) tended to flow into the left lateral sinus and that blood from the superior sagittal sinus (draining cortical areas) tended to flow into the right lateral sinus. These anatomic studies suggested that there may be differences in the oxygen saturation in the two jugular veins because the metabolic rates of cortical and subcortical tissues are different. However, in later studies,[40] the same authors compared oxygen saturation in blood obtained simultaneously from the right and left jugular bulbs in 25 patients with a variety of diagnoses. They found similar oxygen saturations in all except four patients with psychoses and four patients with organic pathological conditions associated with epilepsy.

Shenkin et al.[41] performed dynamic studies of the cerebral venous circulation by injecting Evan's blue dye into the internal carotid artery in five patients and comparing the appearance of the dye in the different cerebral venous structures. These studies suggested that on average, two-thirds of the blood from a single internal carotid artery was drained by the ipsilateral internal jugular vein and one-third was drained by the contralateral jugular vein.

These early studies suggested that either jugular bulb would provide similar Sjv_{O_2} information in most normal people. However, in patients who may have focal lesions, such as those in the study of Gibbs et al.[40] who had psychoses or epilepsy, there may be a significant difference in the oxygen saturation obtained in the right and left jugular bulbs. Stocchetti et al.[42] recently compared simultaneous measurements of Sjv_{O_2} in the right and left jugular bulbs of 32 patients with severe head injury. The average difference in Sjv_{O_2} between the right and left jugular bulbs was 5 percent. Fifteen patients had a maximal right-to-left difference in Sjv_{O_2} greater than 15 percent. Three additional patients had differences greater than 10 percent. It was not possible to predict on the basis of computed tomography (CT) information which patients would have significant differences in Sjv_{O_2} or which jugular bulb would have the most abnormal values.

Extracerebral Contamination of Jugular Venous Blood

Extracerebral contamination of blood in the jugular bulb can come from two sources. Blood drained into the jugular vein from the sigmoid sinus is mixed to a slight degree with extracerebral blood. The superior sagittal sinus receives blood from emissary and frontal veins. The sigmoid sinus and the superior bulb of the internal jugular vein are connected to the cavernous sinus through the petrosal sinuses. The cavernous sinus communicates with the ophthalmic veins and the pterygoid plexus. Below the superior bulb, the internal jugular vein receives influx from the facial and retromandibular veins; this can be a source of substantial extracerebral contamination if blood sampling is done below the jugular bulb. Shenkin et al.[41] quantified the amount of extracerebral contamination of jugular venous blood. In eight patients, Evan's blue dye was injected into the external carotid artery to estimate the amount of extracerebral contamination in blood obtained in the jugular bulb. An average of only 2.7 percent (range, 0 to 6.6 percent) of the blood in the internal jugular veins was derived from extracerebral sources. However, in a few anecdotal cases the extracerebral contamination has been found to be considerable.[43] Since the technique for obtaining blood was a blind needle stick in these early studies, it is not clear that these exceptional cases always involved true jugular venous blood. Jakobsen and Enevoldsen[44] showed that when a catheter which had been placed in the jugular bulb was pulled back more than 2 cm from the base of the skull, oxygen saturation in blood drawn from the catheter increased more than 10 percent in 4 of 13 patients, indicating major extracerebral contamination.

Insertion of the Jugular Bulb Catheter

On the basis of these anatomic considerations, several conventions have been used to determine which internal jugular vein should be catheterized. If the injury is diffuse, there is general agreement that the catheter should be placed on the side of the dominant venous drainage, which in most cases is the right side. Two methods are commonly used to verify which internal jugular vein accommodates the highest flow. In the first method, the problem is approached from a functional standpoint by employing sequential manual compression of each internal jugular vein.[45] The vein that upon compression elicits the greater elevation in intracranial pressure is identified as the dominant side carrying the larger portion of cerebral venous outflow. The second method utilizes the admission head CT scan to visualize which of the two jugular foramina is the largest, assuming that the larger foramen houses the larger jugular bulb.[42]

If the injury is focal, some investigators place the catheter on the side of the most severe injury, arguing that this provides the best chance of obtaining the most abnormal values; others continue to place the catheter on the dominant side, arguing that this monitors the greatest portion of the brain and gives the highest blood flow, which may improve the performance of the continuous oximetry catheters. Recent bilateral catheterization studies by Stocchetti et al.[42] suggest that there is not a reliable way to determine which internal jugular vein will have the most abnormal values; therefore, the latter convention may be the most logical.

Three approaches to catheterization of the internal jugular vein have been described: the anterior, central, and posterior approaches.[46] The most direct method for retrograde cannulation of the jugular bulb is the central approach to the internal jugular vein. The patient is placed in a supine or slight Trendelenburg's position with the head gently rotated to the contralateral side. The surface anatomy is identified (Fig. 36-4), including the triangle formed by the two heads of the sternocleidomastoid muscle and the clavicle. The internal jugular vein usually runs directly beneath the triangle just lateral to the carotid pulsation and can be entered quickly and easily at that point. Some investigators have advocated using two-dimensional ultrasound to localize the internal jugular vein, since as many as 8 percent of patients may not have the expected anatomic relationships.[47] This is not usually necessary for an experienced operator but may be considered in a difficult patient. The area from the chin to the nipple is prepped and draped in a sterile fashion. The puncture site is identified at the apex of the triangle or 1 to 2 cm cephalad of the apex. With the 4.5F introducer kit, the introducer needle is 20-gauge; therefore, a "finder" needle is not necessary. With the operator's left hand retracting the carotid artery medially, the introducer needle is inserted at a 45-degree angle to the frontal plane. The vein is typically entered within a depth of 1 to 1.5 cm; the needle should not be passed deeper than 4 cm. If venipuncture does not occur on the initial penetration, the angle of entry should be adjusted 5 to 10 degrees laterally for the next attempt. If this approach also fails, a cautious attempt slightly medial to the initial attempt is appropriate as long as the plane of the needle remains parallel and lateral to the carotid artery pulsation.

Once the vein has been punctured, the fiber-optic oxygen saturation catheter is inserted into the internal jugular vein via a 4.5F peel-away introducer, using the Seldinger technique, as shown in Fig. 36-5. An alternative method is to use an introducer that remains in the

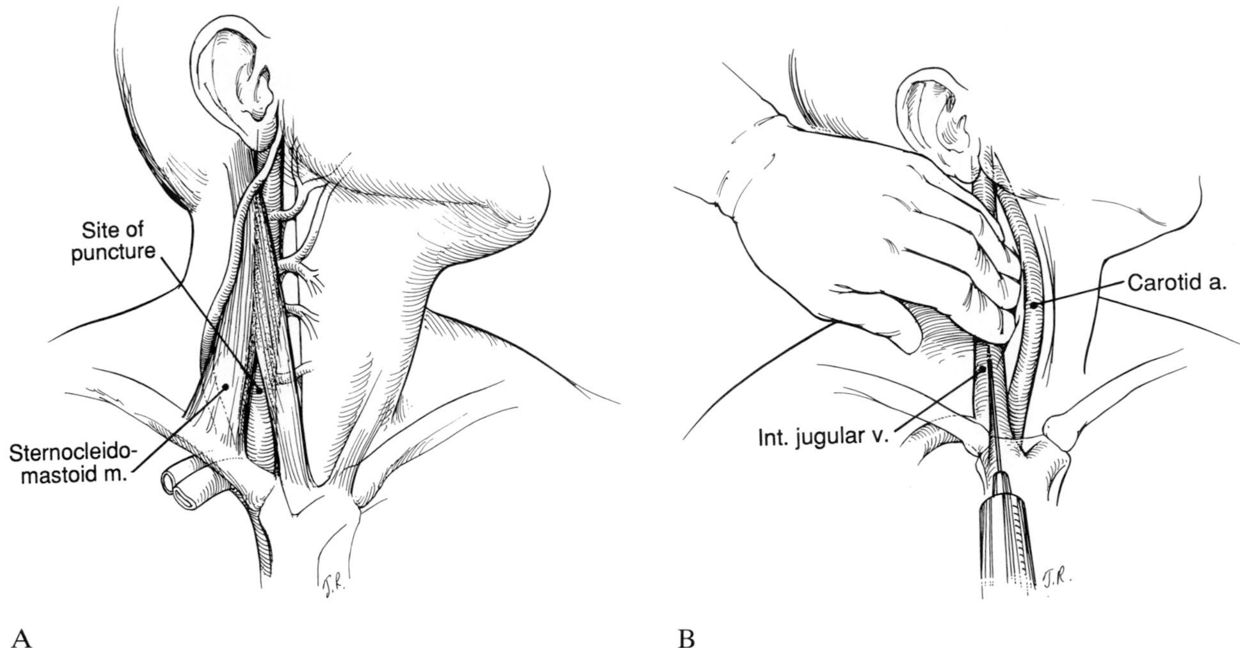

Figure 36-4. *A*. The external landmark for the central approach to the internal jugular vein is the triangle formed by the two heads of the sternocleidomastoid muscle and the clavicle. *B*. Diagram of puncture of the internal jugular vein by the central approach.

jugular vein. This permits easier repositioning of the catheter if necessary, but the introducer is of larger diameter than the catheter alone and requires an additional saline flush for the introducer. The catheter is advanced until the tip is properly positioned in the jugular bulb. A slight resistance usually can be felt when the catheter tip meets the roof of the jugular bulb (typically 13 to 15 cm from the skin). It is best not to advance the catheter more than 15 cm, as the catheter may loop in the internal jugular vein. The best catheter position is obtained if the catheter is pulled back 0.5 to 1 cm from the point at which the roof of the jugular bulb is felt. A lateral skull x-ray should be obtained to confirm the position of the catheter tip within the jugular bulb. Radiographically, this landmark is slightly medial to the mastoid bone and is curved in the medial direction at the level of the mastoid base.[44]

Maintenance of the Jugular Bulb Catheter

Once it has been inserted, the catheter is connected to a continuous flush device to keep the lumen patent. To minimize the risk of thrombosis of the vein, no medications or potassium supplements are given through the catheter. The catheter is used only for Sjv_{O_2} monitoring and blood sampling.

Sjv_{O_2} monitoring has been used for up to 14 days, although the average length of monitoring is 4 to 5 days. As with all intravascular catheters, the risk of infection increases with the duration of monitoring. Changing catheters every 5 to 7 days in patients who require prolonged monitoring may be considered. In addition, catheters should be removed if there is suspicion of catheter sepsis or thrombosis of the internal jugular vein.

POTENTIAL COMPLICATIONS OF Sjv_{O_2} MONITORING

Potential complications can be divided into those associated with insertion of the catheter, including carotid artery puncture, injury to nerves in the neck, and pneumothorax, and those associated with the catheter remaining in the jugular vein, including infection, an increase in intracranial pressure (ICP), and thrombosis.

Carotid puncture is the most common complication associated with the internal jugular vein catheterization. However, it rarely has serious consequences, and the risk can be minimized by making certain that the puncture is lateral to the carotid pulsation. In a study of 123 pediatric patients, Goetting and Preston[48] documented only four (3 percent) accidental carotid punctures while attempting to cannulate the internal jugular vein. Stocchetti et al.[49] recorded puncture of the carotid artery in

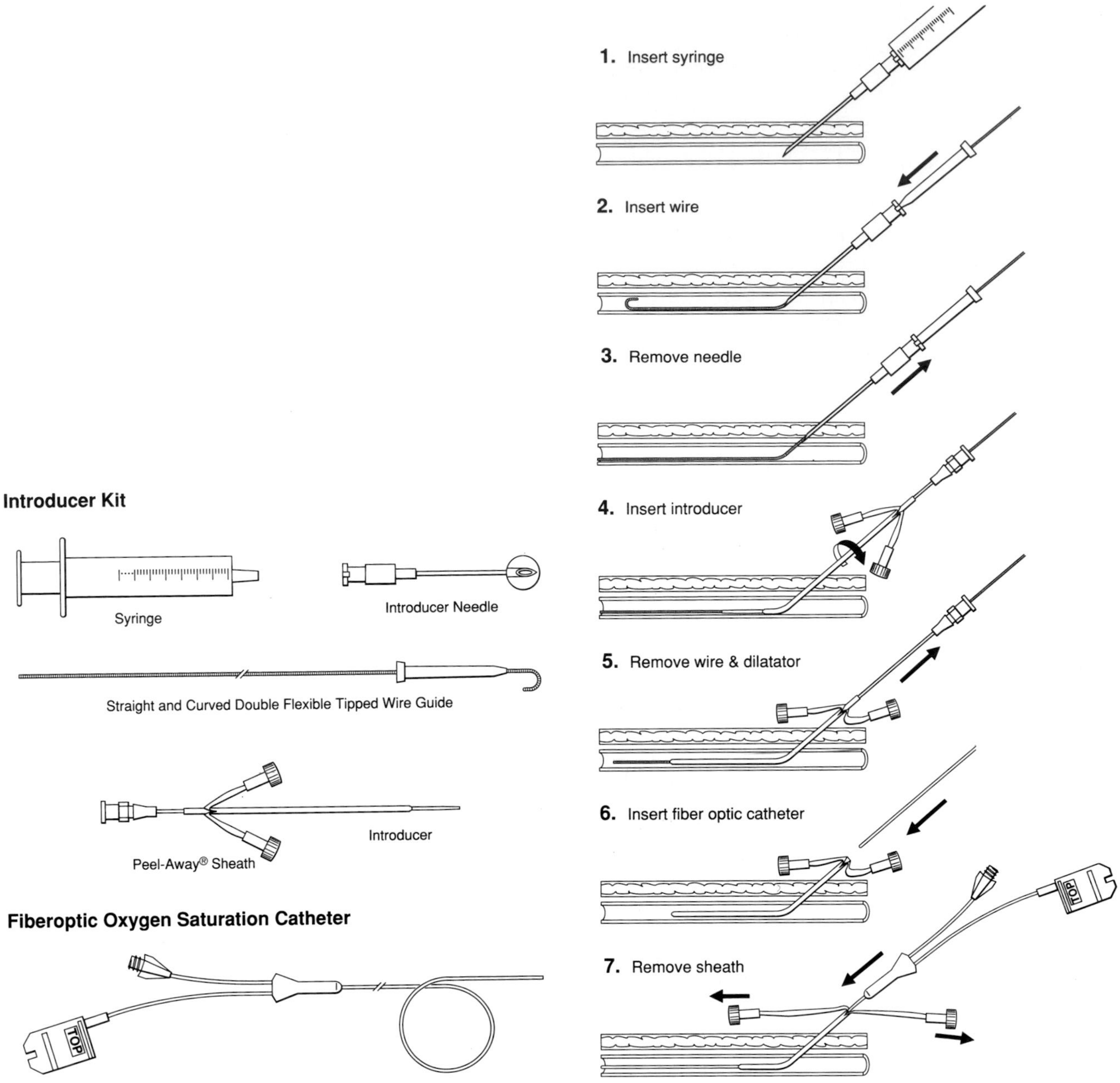

Figure 36-5. *A*. Peel-away introducer kit and fiber-optic oxygen saturation catheter. *B*. Steps in the insertion of the catheter through a peel-away introducer, using the Seldinger technique. (1) Puncture the internal jugular vein with the introducer needle. (2) Slide the wire guide through the introducer needle into the vein. (3) Leaving the wire guide in place, remove the introducer needle. (4) Slide the sheath introducer over the wire and advance the introducer into the vein. (5) Leaving the sheath in place, remove the introducer and wire guide. (6) Introduce the fiber-optic catheter into the sheath and advance the catheter until the tip meets the roof of the jugular bulb. (7) Peel the sheath away from the catheter.

2 (4 percent) of 45 attempts. There were no sequelae in either series. The vast majority of arterial punctures can be managed conservatively without sequelae by applying local pressure for 10 min.

No cases of Horner's syndrome, phrenic or recurrent laryngeal nerve damage, or pneumothorax have been reported with jugular bulb cannulation, but these complications are possible and have occurred in large series of internal jugular vein catheterizations for central venous pressure monitoring.[46]

Line sepsis is a complication that is commonly associated with all types of indwelling catheters. Most studies have reported an overall rate of 0 to 5 episodes of infection per 100 catheters.[46] In the study of Goetting and Preston,[48] no cases of line sepsis were observed over a mean catheter duration of 2.5 ± 1.6 days. In the study of Stocchetti et al.,[49] catheter-induced infection occurred in 1.8 percent of 45 patients. Proper sterile technique in the placement and maintenance of the jugular bulb catheter should minimize this risk.

ICP can be increased by maneuvers that obstruct venous return from the brain, and it is reasonable to be concerned that a catheter in the jugular vein might raise ICP. However, the 4F catheter used for Sjv_{O_2} monitoring is quite small relative to the lumen of the internal jugular vein. Stocchetti et al.[49] reported that there was a slight increase in ICP "of no clinical significance" during catheter insertion. Goetting and Preston[50] found no evidence that jugular bulb catheterization caused jugular venous obstruction sufficient to exacerbate elevated ICP.

Thrombosis of the internal jugular vein has not been reported with jugular bulb catheters but could have serious consequences. Depending on the normal flow to the thrombosed internal jugular vein, the obstruction could impair venous return from the head and elevate ICP. Based on experience with other intravascular catheters, the larger the catheter relative to the size of the vessel and the lower the flow through the vessel, the greater the risk of thrombosis.

NORMAL Sjv_{O_2} AND ISCHEMIC THRESHOLDS

Normal Sjv_{O_2} Values

Gibbs et al.[29] studied 50 normal young males and observed that their Sjv_{O_2} ranged from 55 to 71 percent (mean of 61.8 percent). This is lower than normal mixed venous oxygen saturation, suggesting that the brain normally extracts oxygen more completely from arterial blood than do many other organs.

Relationship between Sjv_{O_2} and Derived Parameters and CBF in Head-Injured Patients

When arterial oxygen saturation and hemoglobin concentration are relatively constant, changes in Sjv_{O_2} are generally reflective of changes in CBF. In a study of 100 patients with severe brain injury,[26] the relationship between CBF and AVD_{O_2} was examined. There was a curvilinear relationship between CBF and Sjv_{O_2}, AVD_{O_2}, and O_2ER (Fig. 36-6).

In patients with a head injury, other factors may potentially affect the relationship between Sjv_{O_2} and CBF. The effects of pH and hemoglobin concentration have been studied.

Effect of pH

Alkalosis, such as that induced by hyperventilation, can shift the oxyhemoglobin dissociation curve to the left so that tissues are less able to extract oxygen completely. Very low jugular venous P_{O_2} (Pjv_{O_2}) values indicating cerebral ischemia could theoretically occur at an Sjv_{O_2} that might not be considered low. Cruz et al.[51] examined the relationship between Pjv_{O_2} and Sjv_{O_2} in their series of patients and reported that unless pH is >7.6, Sjv_{O_2} adequately reflects Pjv_{O_2}.

In the BTGH series, similar results were found by examining the relationship between Pjv_{O_2} and Sjv_{O_2} at different PjvH levels (Fig. 36-7). The oxyhemoglobin dissociation curve was similar at PjvH values of 7.2 to 7.5, with the P50 ranging from 22 to 25. Below a PjvH of 7.2, the oxyhemoglobin curve was shifted to the right, with a P50 of 28. There were not enough PjvH values above 7.5 for an evaluation.

These two studies suggest that unless alkalosis is severe, Pjv_{O_2} and Sjv_{O_2} reflect changes in CBF in a similar manner.

Effect of hemoglobin concentration

Cruz et al.[52] observed that anemia can result in AVD_{O_2} values that may underestimate the reduction in CBF. Although AVD_{O_2} increases as CBF decreases in an anemic patient, abnormally high values may not be reached even with very low Sjv_{O_2} values. Examples of this phenomenon are shown in Fig. 36-8, where at equivalent reductions in Sjv_{O_2}, AVD_{O_2} is significantly lower in anemic patients.

Therefore, while under all conditions that affect cerebral oxygenation (Fig. 36-2) AVD_{O_2} reflects changes in CBF better than the other parameters do, the absolute values of AVD_{O_2} may underestimate the severity of the reduction in CBF, and O_2ER or Sjv_{O_2} may be better reflections of the effects of CBF reduction on brain oxygenation.

Ischemic Thresholds for Sjv_{O_2} in Normal Subjects

Experimental studies have extensively examined the ischemic thresholds for CBF. This topic is discussed in other chapters in this book. A few studies have examined the Sjv_{O_2} threshold associated with the depletion of energy stores in animals and with loss of consciousness or EEG changes during anoxia in normal humans (Fig. 36-9).

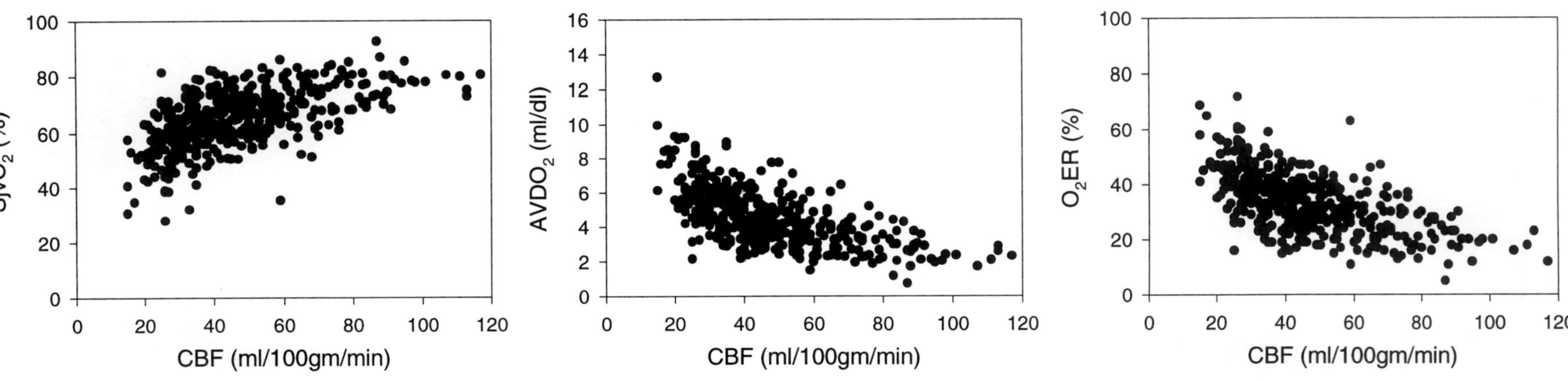

Figure 36-6. Relationships between CBF and Sjv_{O_2} (*left*), AVD_{O_2} (*center*), and O_2ER (*right*).

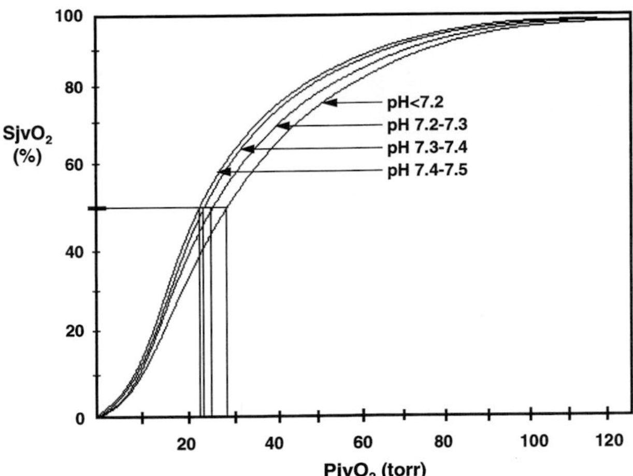

Figure 36-7. The effect of PjvH on the oxyhemoglobin dissociation curve.

Experimental studies in cats in which CPP was decreased by cisternal infusion of saline suggested that energy stores become depleted at a jugular venous oxygen content level below 2 ml/dl.[53] At a hemoglobin concentration of 10 g/dl, this value would be equivalent to an Sjv_{O_2} of approximately 15 percent. Values of Sjv_{O_2} this low are rarely seen in patients.

Meyer et al.[54] found that during breathing of 100% nitrogen EEG changes occurred with a Pjv_{O_2} below 19 mmHg. This Pjv_{O_2} would be approximately equivalent to an Sjv_{O_2} of 40 percent. Lennox et al.[55] found that confusion developed during anoxia or with orthostatic hypotension when Sjv_{O_2} decreased below 45 percent and that unconsciousness developed when Sjv_{O_2} decreased below 24 percent.

Optimal Values for Sjv_{O_2} after Head Injury

In head-injured patients, the range for Sjv_{O_2} is considerably wider than it is in normal subjects, and it is not clear what the optimal value for Sjv_{O_2} is or what value of Sjv_{O_2} is clearly dangerous. In the BTGH series of patients with continuous measurement of Sjv_{O_2} for the first 5 to 10 days after a severe head injury, Sjv_{O_2} averaged 68.1 ± 9.7 percent (range, 32 to 96 percent) in 1329 measurements. Pjv_{O_2} averaged 37 ± 7 mmHg (range, 22 to 85 mmHg). These mean values are slightly higher average values than those reported in normal adults, and the range is much wider (Table 36-1).

Since head-injured patients already have significant neurological deficits, it has been difficult to determine the levels of Sjv_{O_2} that are associated with neurological changes. Cruz[37] observed clear-cut neurological deterioration in patients with Sjv_{O_2} that was decreased below 30 percent.

To begin to answer this question, the BTGH series has examined the relationship between the occurrence of jugular desaturation ($Sjv_{O_2} < 50$ percent for at least 10 min) and neurological outcome as well as the relationship between the length of time Sjv_{O_2} is below the thresholds of 50 percent, 40 percent, and 30 percent and neurological outcome.

The relationship between the occurrence of episodes of jugular venous desaturation and outcome was examined and is shown in Table 36-3. Even a single episode of desaturation was associated with a doubling of the mortality rate, and with multiple episodes the mortality rate increased four times. One episode of desaturation increased the risk of a poor outcome from 55 to 70 percent. With multiple episodes of desaturation, a good outcome was rare (9 percent).

The relationship between the length of time Sjv_{O_2} is below a threshold of 50 percent, 40 percent, and 30 percent and neurological outcome is shown in Fig. 36-10. The length of time Sjv_{O_2} was below the thresholds of 50 percent and 40 percent was significantly greater in patients who were vegetative or dead as a result of their injuries.[3] There were very few times when Sjv_{O_2} was below 30 percent.

These data suggesting that a decrease in Sjv_{O_2} below 50 percent is associated with a worse outcome are similar to the results of a study done in patients undergoing a carotid endarterectomy with monitoring of oxygen saturation in the lateral sinus. Lyons et al.[56] monitored oxygen saturation in 50 patients undergoing carotid endarterectomy and found that neurological dysfunc-

TABLE 36-3 Relationship between Occurrence of Episodes of Jugular Venous Desaturation and Neurological Outcome

	No. Episodes of Desaturation		
3-Month Glasgow Outcome Scale	**None**	**One**	**Multiple**
Good recovery/moderate disability	41(45.1%)	12(33.3%)	2(9.1%)
Severe disability/vegetative	33(36.3%)	11(30.6%)	4(18.2%)
Dead	17(18.7%)	13(36.1%)	16(72.7%)
Total	91(100%)	36(100%)	22(100%)

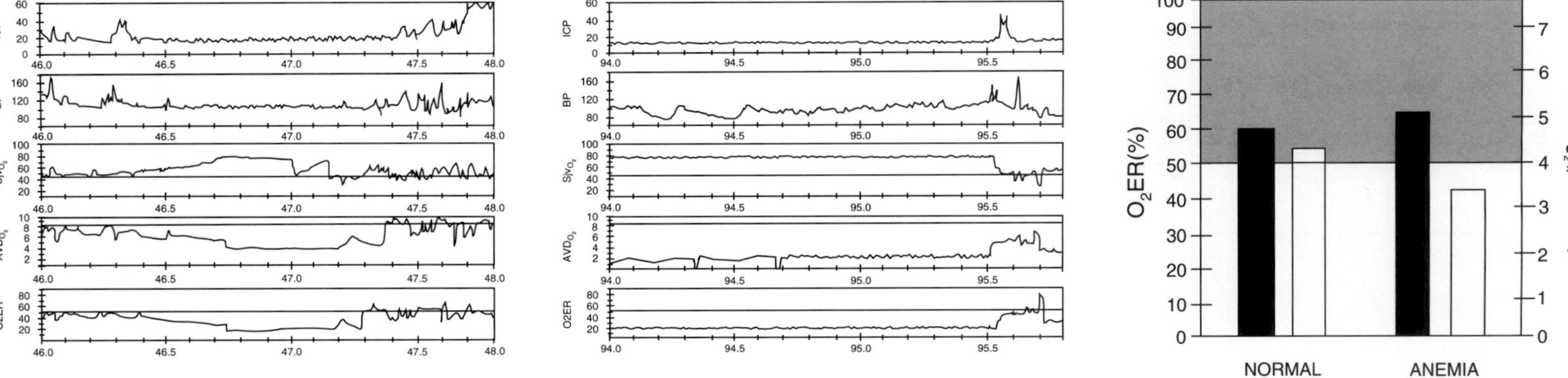

Figure 36-8. The effect of anemia on oxygen saturation parameters. On the left is an example of changes in Sjv_{O_2}, AVD_{O_2}, and O_2ER during jugular venous desaturation in a patient with a normal hemoglobin; in the center is a similar example in a patient with low hemoglobin. While the changes in Sjv_{O_2} and O_2ER are similar, AVD_{O_2} changes less in anemic patients. On the right, mean values for AVD_{O_2} (white bars) and O_2ER (black bars) during 47 episodes of jugular desaturation are shown.

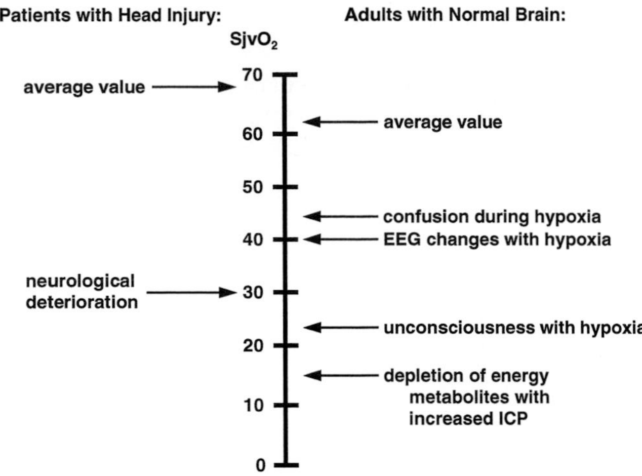

Figure 36-9. Thresholds for neurological changes associated with decreased Sjv_{O_2}. The left column describes associations that have been reported in head-injured patients. The right column describes changes that have been reported in studies of normal humans and animals. (Data from Refs. 37 and 53–55.)

tion was associated with lateral sinus oxygen saturation below 50 percent. No neurological dysfunction was observed when saturation was equal to or above 60 percent.

Although an exact threshold for Sjv_{O_2} cannot be pinpointed with the present information, the data currently available suggest that Sjv_{O_2} should be maintained above 50 percent.

DIAGNOSIS AND MANAGEMENT OF JUGULAR DESATURATION

Figure 36-11 shows an algorithm for diagnosing and treating jugular desaturation. Whenever Sjv_{O_2} falls below 50 percent, the catheter light intensity value is checked to exclude poor catheter position as the cause. If the light intensity is unsatisfactory, the patient's head and/or the catheter may be repositioned. If the catheter position is determined to be correct, a sample of blood

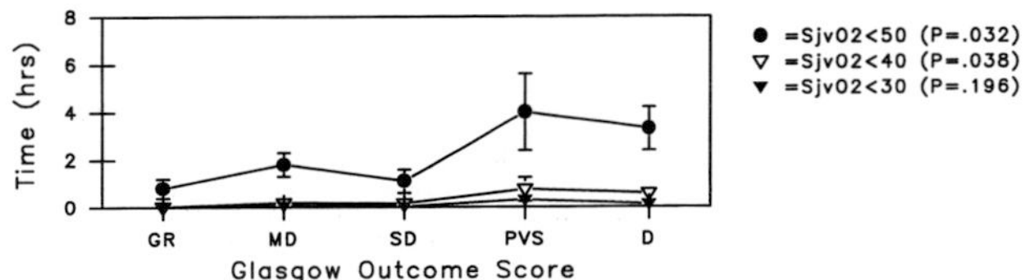

Figure 36-10. The durations of times Sjv_{O_2} was <50 percent and times Sjv_{O_2} was <40 percent were associated with an outcome of vegetative or dead.

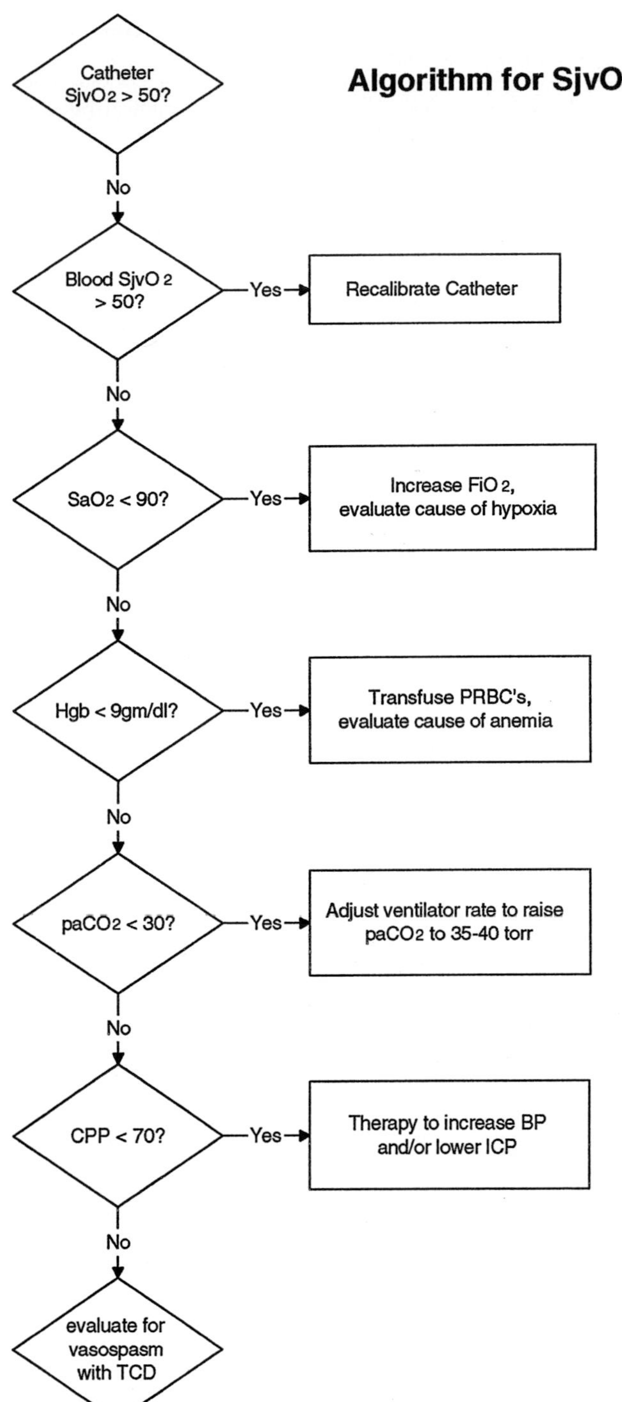

Figure 36-11. Algorithm for diagnosing the cause of jugular venous desaturation.

is withdrawn through the jugular venous catheter to verify the appropriate calibration of the catheter. If the Sjv_{O_2} value measured by the co-oximeter is more than 4 percent different from the catheter value, the catheter is recalibrated. If the Sjv_{O_2} is confirmed to be <50 percent, the cause of desaturation is systematically sought.

TABLE 36-4 Causes of Episodes of Jugular Desaturation in 149 Patients with Severe Head Injury

No. Episodes	Cause of Episodes
Systemic causes, 43(45%)	
12	Hypotension
6	Hypoxia
24	Hypocarbia
1	Anemia
Cerebral causes, 46(48%)	
45	Intracranial hypertension
1	Vasospasm
Systemic and cerebral causes, 7(7%)	
7	Combinations of decreased CPP, hypocarbia, and anemia
Total 96	

Causes for a reduced arterial oxygen content are examined first. Arterial hypoxia is ruled out by measuring arterial oxygen saturation. If Sa_{O_2} is below 90 percent, the condition is corrected by increasing Fi_{O_2} or adding positive end-expiratory pressure (PEEP). Hemoglobin concentration is measured to make sure values are at least 9 mg/dl. If arterial oxygen content is not sufficiently reduced to explain the desaturation, treatable causes of reduced CBF are sought. Hypocapnia, hypotension, and intracranial hypertension are looked for and appropriately treated. Cerebral vasospasm might be considered in cases where no other systemic cause can be found and ICP is not increased sufficiently to impair CPP.

In the BTGH series of 149 patients, 96 episodes of desaturation were identified, diagnosed, and treated. The causes of these episodes, which were both systemic and cerebral, are listed in Table 36-4. Artifactual readings due to catheter malpositioning continue to be a technical problem in certain patients. Efforts are under way to improve catheter design to reduce the impaction of the catheter tip against the vessel wall.

OTHER TREATMENT APPLICATIONS

Matching Treatment of Intracranial Hypertension to the Underlying Pathophysiology

Miller et al.[57] proposed that since there are two major causes of ICP—vascular engorgement and cerebral edema—the optimal treatment should be directed at the cause. In a study of 17 patients, several factors predicted whether hypnotic agents (treatment of vascular engorgement) or mannitol (treatment of cerebral edema) was more successful in lowering ICP. Sjv_{O_2} was helpful in this regard. An elevated Sjv_{O_2} suggested that the underlying pathophysiology was vascular engorgement and that hypnotic agents would be more effective. A normal or low Sjv_{O_2} suggested that cerebral edema was the underlying cause of the increased ICP and that mannitol would be more effective.

Individualizing Hyperventilation

Hyperventilation has been used for many years as a treatment of intracranial hypertension. It has been reported that routine hyperventilation may have detrimental effects on outcome,[58] and it has become clear that in some patients hyperventilation can cause ischemia.[2,26] In the BTGH series, hyperventilation (average P_{CO_2} = 24 mmHg) was the most common systemic cause of jugular desaturation. Cruz[35] suggested that hyperventilation should be optimized in all patients by lowering P_{CO_2} until the O_2ER is normal. While most neurotrauma physicians currently do not use hyperventilation unless the ICP requires treatment, Sjv_{O_2} can identify patients with a marginal CBF who should not be hyperventilated.

Optimizing Cerebral Perfusion Pressure

While normal adults can maintain a normal CBF at a CPP as low as 50 mmHg, patients with a severe head injury can have autoregulation curves that are shifted to a higher pressure range or can have impaired autoregulation at all pressures. Most patients require a CPP of 60 to 70 mmHg, but some require a higher CPP to perfuse the brain normally.[59,60] Sjv_{O_2} can be useful in identifying the optimal CPP for the individual patient.[59]

Diagnosing Cerebral Vasospasm in Head-Injured Patients

Transcranial Doppler has been used to identify cerebral vasospasm by the characteristic increase in flow velocity caused by vasoconstriction of cerebral vessels. However, increases in CBF are very common after head injury, with the incidence peaking on days 2 and 3 after the injury,[13] and can also increase flow velocity.

The distinction between hyperemia and vasospasm is critical, since the treatments may be vastly different. Several methods have been used to distinguish these conditions. First, the flow velocity pattern is different.[61] The flow velocity waveform has a distinct diastolic notch in patients with increased flow velocity due to vasospasm, while a diastolic notch is absent in patients with increased flow velocity due to hyperemia. Second, with vasospasm the increased flow velocity can be localized to individual vessels, while hyperemia is usually diffuse.[62] Third, with cerebral vasospasm the increased flow velocity is found in the intracranial vessels more often than it is in the internal carotid artery, while hyperemia increases flow velocity in all vessels. The ratio between the MCA and internal carotid artery flow velocity has been used to distinguish this characteristic.[63] Sjv_{O_2} can be another factor in distinguishing hyperemia from cerebral vasospasm. With an increase in CBF, Sjv_{O_2} will be elevated. With cerebral vasospasm, Sjv_{O_2} will be normal or low.[59]

LIMITATIONS

The major limitations of Sjv_{O_2} in detecting cerebral hypoxia/ischemia are the anatomic restrictions. Sjv_{O_2} monitors global cerebral oxygenation. Regional ischemia can be present and may not be detected by changes in Sjv_{O_2}. Also, because jugular venous blood may not be truly mixed cerebral blood, ischemia could occur in a part of the brain being drained by the opposite jugular vein. In addition, as CBF decreases, the amount of extracerebral contamination may become proportionally greater, artificially increasing Sjv_{O_2}.

Despite these limitations, Sjv_{O_2} monitoring allows physicians to detect episodes of cerebral hypoxia which were not identifiable previously. There appears to be a very strong association between these episodes of desaturation and a poor outcome. It is hoped that the early detection of ischemia will permit prompt therapy before cerebral function is permanently compromised.

References

1. Piek J, Chesnut RM, Marshall LF, et al: Extracranial complications of severe head injury. *J Neurosurg* 77:901–907, 1992.
2. Gopinath SP, Robertson CS, Contant CF, et al: Jugular venous desaturation and outcome after head injury. *J Neurol Neurosurg Psychiatry* 57:717–723, 1994.
3. Contant CF, Robertson CS, Gopinath SP, et al: Determination of clinically important thresholds in continuously monitored patients with head injury. *J Neurotrauma* 10(suppl 1):S57, 1993.
4. Jones PA, Piper IR, Corrie J, et al: Microcomputer based detection of secondary insults and 12 month outcome after head injury. *J Neurotrauma* 10(suppl 1):S102, 1993.
5. Obrist WD, Langfitt T, Jaggi J, et al: Cerebral blood flow and metabolism in comatose patients with acute head injury: Relationship to intracranial hypertension. *J Neurosurg* 61:241–253, 1984.
6. Busija DW, Leffler CW, Pourcyrous M: Hyperthermia increases cerebral metabolic rate and blood flow in neonatal pigs. *Am J Physiol* 255:H343–H346, 1988.
7. Meldrum BS, Nilsson B: Cerebral blood flow and metabolic rate early and late in prolonged seizures induced in rats by bicuculline. *Brain* 99:523–542, 1976.
8. Pierce EC, Lambertsen CJ, Deutsch S, et al: Cerebral circulation and metabolism during thiopental anesthesia and hyperventilation in man. *J Clin Invest* 41:1664–1671, 1962.
9. Gokaslan ZL, Robertson CS, Narayan RK, et al: Barbiturates, cerebral blood flow, and intracranial hypertension, in Hoff JT, Betz AL (eds): *Intracranial Pressure VII.* Berlin: Springer-Verlag, 1989: 894–897.
10. Michenfelder JD, Milde JH: The relationship among canine brain temperature, metabolism, and function during hypothermia. *Anesthesiology* 75:130–136, 1991.
11. Croughwell N, Smith LR, Quill T, et al: The effect of temperature on cerebral metabolism and blood flow in adults during cardiopulmonary bypass. *J Thorac Cardiovasc Surg* 103:549–554, 1992.
12. Marion DW, Obrist WD, Carlier PM, et al: The use of moderate therapeutic hypothermia for patients with severe head injuries: A preliminary report. *J Neurosurg* 79:354–362, 1993.
13. Robertson CS, Contant CF, Gokaslan ZL, et al: Cerebral blood flow, arteriovenous oxygen difference, and outcome in head injured patients. *J Neurol Neurosurg Psychiatry* 55:594–603, 1992.
14. Borgstrom L, Johannsson H, Siesjo BK: The influence of acute normovolemic anemia on cerebral blood flow and oxygen consumption of anesthetized rats. *Acta Physiol Scand* 93:505–514, 1975.
15. Paulson OB, Parving HE, Olesen J, et al: Influence of carbon monoxide and of hemodilution on cerebral blood flow and blood gases in man. *J Appl Physiol* 35:111–116, 1973.
16. Johannsson H, Siesjo BK: Cerebral blood flow and oxygen consumption in the rat in hypoxic hypoxia. *Acta Physiol Scand* 93:269–276, 1975.
17. Kety S, Schmidt CF: The effects of altered arterial tensions of carbon dioxide and oxygen on cerebral oxygen consumption of normal young man. *J Clin Invest* 27:484–492, 1948.
18. Cohen PJ, Alexander SC, Smith TC, et al: Effects of hypoxia and hypocarbia on cerebral blood flow and metabolism in conscious man. *J Appl Physiol* 23:183–189, 1967.
19. Ishige N, Pitts L, Pogliani L, et al: Effect of hypoxia on traumatic brain injury in rats: II. Changes in high energy phosphate metabolism. *Neurosurgery* 20:854–858, 1987.
20. Ishige N, Pitts L, Hashimoto T, et al: Effect of hypoxia on traumatic brain injury in rats: I. Changes in neurological function, electroencephalograms, and histopathology. *Neurosurgery* 20:848–853, 1987.
21. Kohi YM, Mendelow AD, Teasdale GM, et al: Extracra-

nial insults and outcome in patients with acute head injury—relationship to the Glasgow Coma Scale. *Injury* 16:25–29, 1984.
22. Miller JD, Sweet RC, Narayan RK, et al: Early insults to the injured brain. *JAMA* 240:439–442, 1978.
23. Lewelt W, Jenkins LW, Miller JD: Effects of experimental fluid-percussion injury of the brain on cerebrovascular reactivity to hypoxia and to hypercapnia. *J Neurosurg* 56:332–338, 1982.
24. DeWitt DS, Prough DS, Taylor CL, et al: Reduced cerebral blood flow, oxygen delivery, and electroencephalographic activity after traumatic brain injury and mild hemorrhage in cats. *J Neurosurg* 76:812–821, 1992.
25. Finnerty FA, Witkin L, Fazekas JF: Cerebral hemodynamics during cerebral ischemia induced by acute hypotension. *J Clin Invest* 33:1227–1232, 1954.
26. Robertson CS, Narayan RK, Gokaslan Z, et al: Cerebral arteriovenous oxygen difference as an estimate of cerebral blood flow in comatose patients. *J Neurosurg* 70:222–230, 1989.
27. Lewelt W, Jenkins LW, Miller JD: Autoregulation of cerebral blood flow after experimental fluid percussion injury of the brain. *J Neurosurg* 53:500–506, 1980.
28. Chan KH, Miller JD, Dearden NM, et al: The effect of changes in cerebral perfusion pressure upon middle cerebral artery blood flow velocity and jugular bulb venous oxygen saturation after severe brain injury. *J Neurosurg* 77:55–61, 1992.
29. Gibbs EL, Lennox WG, Nims LF, et al: Arterial and cerebral venous blood: Arterial-venous differences in man. *J Biol Chem* 144:325–332, 1942.
30. Robertson CS, Grossman RG, Goodman JC, et al: The predictive value of cerebral anaerobic metabolism with cerebral infarction after head injury. *J Neurosurg* 67:361–368, 1987.
31. Cruz J: Continuous versus serial global cerebral hemometabolic monitoring: Applications in acute brain trauma. *Acta Neurochir [Suppl] (Wien)* 42:35–39, 1988.
32. Garlick R, Bihari D: The use of intermittent and continuous recordings of jugular venous bulb oxygen saturation in the unconscious patient. *Scand J Clin Lab Invest [Suppl]* 188:47–52, 1987.
33. Sheinberg M, Kanter MJ, Robertson CS, et al: Continuous monitoring of jugular venous oxygen saturation in head-injured patients. *J Neurosurg* 76:212–217, 1992.
34. Andrews PJD, Dearden NM, Miller JD: Jugular bulb cannulation: Description of a cannulation technique and validation of a new continuous monitor. *Br J Anaesth* 67:553–558, 1991.
35. Cruz J: Combined continuous monitoring of systemic and cerebral oxygenation in acute brain injury: Preliminary observations. *Crit Care Med* 21:1225–1232, 1993.
36. McCormick P, Stewart M, Goetting M, et al: Noninvasive cerebral optical spectroscopy for monitoring cerebral oxygen delivery and hemodynamics. *Crit Care Med* 19:89–97, 1991.
37. Cruz J: On-line monitoring of global cerebral hypoxia in acute brain injury: Relationship to intracranial hypertension. *J Neurosurg* 79:228–233, 1993.
38. Hatiboglu MT, Anil A: Structural variations in the jugular foramen of the human skull. *J Anat* 180:191–196, 1992.
39. Gibbs EL, Gibbs FA: The cross section areas of the vessels that form the torcular and the manner in which blood is distributed to the right and to the left lateral sinus. *Anat Rec* 54:419, 1934.
40. Gibbs EL, Lennox WG, Gibbs FA: Bilateral internal jugular blood: Comparison of A-V differences, oxygen-dextrose ratios and respiratory quotients. *Am J Psychol* 102:184–190, 1945.
41. Shenkin GA, Harmel MH, Kety SS: Dynamic anatomy of the cerebral circulation. *Arch Neurol Psych* 60:240–252, 1948.
42. Stocchetti N, Paparella A, Bridelli F, et al: Cerebral venous oxygen saturation studied using bilateral samples in the jugular veins. *Neurosurgery* 34:38–44, 1994.
43. Lassen N: Cerebral blood flow and oxygen consumption in man. *Physiol Rev* 39:183–238, 1959.
44. Jakobsen M, Enevoldsen E: Retrograde catheterization of the right internal jugular vein for serial measurements of cerebral venous oxygen content. *J Cereb Blood Flow Metab* 9:717–720, 1989.
45. Dearden NM: Jugular bulb venous oxygen saturation in the management of severe head injury. *Curr Opin Anaesth* 4:279–286, 1991.
46. Seneff MG, Rippe JM: Central venous catheters, in Rippe JM, Irwin RS, Alpert JS, et al. (eds): *Intensive Care Medicine.* Boston: Little, Brown, 1985: 16–33.
47. Denys BG, Uretsky B: Anatomical variations of internal jugular vein location: Impact on central venous access. *Crit Care Med* 19:1516–1519, 1991.
48. Goetting MG, Preston G: Jugular bulb catheterization: Experience with 123 patients. *Crit Care Med* 18:1220–1223, 1990.
49. Stocchetti N, Barbagallo M, Gordon CR, et al: Arterio-jugular difference of oxygen and intracranial pressure in comatose, head injured patients: I. Technical aspects and complications. *Minerva Anestesiol* 57:319–326, 1991.
50. Goetting MG, Preston G: Jugular bulb catheterization does not increase intracranial pressure. *Intensive Care Med* 17:195–198, 1991.
51. Cruz J, Gennarelli TA, Hoffstad OJ: Lack of relevance of the Bohr effect in optimally ventilated patients with acute brain trauma. *J Trauma* 33:304–310, 1992.
52. Cruz J, Jaggi JL, Hoffstad OJ: Cerebral blood flow and oxygen consumption in acute brain injury with acute anemia: An alternative for the cerebral metabolic rate of oxygen consumption. *Crit Care Med* 21:1218–1224, 1993.
53. Sutton LN, McLaughlin AC, Dante S, et al: Cerebral venous oxygen content as a measure of brain energy metabolism with increased intracranial pressure and hyperventilation. *J Neurosurg* 73:927–932, 1990.
54. Meyer JS, Gotoh F, Ebihara S, et al: Effects of anoxia on cerebral metabolism and electrolytes in man. *Neurology* 15:892–901, 1965.
55. Lennox WG, Gibbs FA, Gibbs EL: Relationship of unconsciousness to cerebral blood flow and to anoxemia. *Arch Neurol Psych* 34:1001–1013, 1935.
56. Lyons C, Clark LC Jr, McDowell H, et al: Cerebral ve-

nous oxygen content during carotid thrombintimectomy. *Ann Surg* 160:561–567, 1964.

57. Miller JD, Piper IR, Dearden NM: Management of intracranial hypertension in head injury: Matching treatment with cause. *Acta Neurochir [Suppl] (Wien)* 57:152–159, 1993.
58. Muizelaar JP, Marmarou A, Ward JD, et al: Adverse effects of prolonged hyperventilation in patients with severe head injury: A randomized clinical trial. *J Neurosurg* 75:731–739, 1991.
59. Chan KH, Dearden NM, Miller JD, et al: Multimodality monitoring as a guide to treatment of intracranial hypertension after severe brain injury. *Neurosurgery* 32:547–552, 1993.
60. Rosner M: Cerebral perfusion pressure: Link between intracranial pressure and systemic circulation, in Wood JH (ed): *Cerebral Blood Flow*. New York: McGraw-Hill, 1987: 425–448.
61. Chan KH, Dearden NM, Miller JD, et al: Transcranial Doppler waveform differences in hyperemic and nonhyperemic patients after severe head injury. *Surg Neurol* 38:433–436, 1992.
62. Chan KH, Dearden NM, Miller JD: The significance of posttraumatic increase in cerebral blood flow velocity: A transcranial Doppler ultrasound study. *Neurosurgery* 30:697–700, 1992.
63. Lindegaard KF, Nornes H, Bakke SJ, et al: Cerebral vasospasm diagnosis by means of angiography and blood velocity measurements. *Acta Neurochir (Wien)* 100:12–24, 1989.

CHAPTER 37

TRANSCRANIAL DOPPLER ULTRASONOGRAPHY IN HEAD INJURY

Curtis Doberstein
Neil A. Martin

SYNOPSIS

Transcranial Doppler ultrasonography (TCD) is a noninvasive monitoring technique that can determine the direction and velocity of blood flow in the large conducting arteries at the base of the brain. This technique can be used to study the incidence, severity, and time course of posttraumatic cerebral vasospasm, a common finding after head injury. In addition, TCD can be used as a continuous monitoring device to determine autoregulatory function and CO_2 reactivity and to provide an index of relative changes in cerebral blood flow. Furthermore, features of the Doppler waveform can be used to estimate intracranial pressure, and TCD has become a reliable method for confirming the diagnosis of brain death. These features make TCD particularly useful for the study of the complex cerebral hemodynamic changes that frequently occur after a head injury.

INTRODUCTION

In 1843, Christian Doppler postulated the wave theory of light and described the effects moving objects have on the frequency of reflected light and sound.[1] This principle has become known as the Doppler effect. In clinical use, a Doppler probe or transducer emits ultrasonic waves that are reflected by moving blood cells and are detected again by the probe. The Doppler shift, which describes the frequency increase when the reflecting element comes closer to the probe and the frequency decrease when it moves away from the probe, is the basic principle behind present-day transcranial Doppler ultrasonography (TCD). The magnitude of the frequency change correlates with blood flow velocity. Blood flow velocity, which must be distinguished from flow volume, can be calculated automatically and displayed by most modern TCD machines.

The blood flow velocity can be calculated from the Doppler shift by using equation 1:

$$F = \frac{2 \times V \times F_o \times \cos \Theta}{C} \qquad (1)$$

where F = the Doppler shift (Hz), F_o = mean frequency of transmitted ultrasound, V = actual blood flow velocity (cm/s), Θ = angle between the transmitted ultrasound and the direction of blood flow, and C = velocity of ultrasound in brain tissue (1550 m/s). It can be seen that the determinants of the Doppler frequency shift in clinical practice are blood flow velocity and the angle of insonation of the Doppler probe. When the emitting frequency and angle of insonation remain constant, the Doppler shift is directly proportional to blood flow velocity. In some of the older literature, Doppler values are given in Hertz units. When equation 1 is used, the correction factor needed to calculate velocity (cm/s) from F (Hz) can be determined. For example, if a 2-MHz Doppler probe is used and the angle of insonation is 0, the correction factor for converting Hz to velocity is 3.88. Equation 1 shows that the angle of insonation can have an effect on Doppler velocity measurements. However, the large arteries at the base of the brain generally can be examined with an angle of insonation less than 30 degrees by using a probe placed over typical TCD testing sites (cranial windows). This results in an acceptable measurement error (less than 15 percent).

BACKGROUND

For many years Doppler ultrasound was used to assess flow in the heart and peripheral blood vessels, but it was assumed that the skull was impenetrable to sound waves. In 1982, however, Aaslid and coworkers discovered that low-frequency ultrasound (in the 2-MHz range) could be transmitted through thin areas of the calvarium, such as the temporal region. They introduced TCD as a noninvasive method to measure blood flow velocity in the basal cerebral arteries.[2] Since its inception, TCD has been employed to identify feeding arteries of arteriovenous malformations, detect vasospasm after an aneurysmal subarachnoid hemorrhage, measure the hemodynamic alterations associated with stroke, and monitor the cerebral circulation during surgical procedures.[3–9]

Transcranial Doppler has unique capabilities that are particularly useful in the study of head trauma patients. First, TCD allows continuous monitoring of flow velocity in brain arteries and can be used to record second-to-second changes in flow velocity. This feature has been used to measure autoregulatory function, CO_2 responsivity, and treatment-induced changes. Second, flow velocity alterations can be used to detect arterial narrowing. Thus, TCD has been used to study the incidence, severity, and time course of posttraumatic cerebral arterial vasospasm. Transcranial Doppler also can be used to diagnose stenosis caused by traumatic arterial dissection. Third, features of the systolic/diastolic flow velocity waveform (e.g., the pulsatility index) can be used to make inferences about cerebral vascular resistance; this may be useful for ICP estimation. Fourth, TCD can detect cerebral circulatory arrest and thus confirm the clinical diagnosis of brain death.

TECHNIQUE OF TCD EXAMINATION AND ANALYSIS OF RECORDINGS

Transcranial Doppler has several distinct advantages compared with other cerebral blood flow (CBF) monitoring methods. It provides quantitative information about the velocity and direction of blood flow, does not require administration of intravenous contrast agents or exposure to radiation, can be performed at the bedside so that patient transport is not required, and is relatively inexpensive. There have been no reports of complications resulting from its use to date. Because it is safe and noninvasive, TCD can be repeated frequently or used as a continuous monitoring technique.

As with all monitoring techniques, TCD has limitations. The quality of the examination and the analysis of recordings are dependent on the experience and knowledge of the examiner. It takes time and practice to master the techniques required for assessment of the intracranial arteries, particularly in subjects with a pathological condition or altered vessel anatomy. Patients must be relatively still during the examination, which can be a problem in a head-injured victim with altered mental status. Doppler velocities may be altered by several factors, including the angle of insonation of the artery, the diameter of the vessel, and the variables that influence CBF (P_{CO_2}, hematocrit, cerebral metabolic rate, age, etc.).

TCD utilizes a pulsed ultrasonic signal of low frequency (1 to 2 MHz) to allow penetration through thin areas of the skull. Therefore, to assess the cerebral vasculature, natural cranial windows (thin skull areas) and foramina must be utilized. Three conventional areas have been described: the transtemporal window,[1] the transorbital window,[10] and the suboccipital or transforaminal window.[11] In addition, the extracranial internal carotid artery can be assessed at the base of the skull in the submandibular region. These windows are shown in Fig. 37-1.

The transtemporal window is located above the zygoma in front of the ear. This window has been subdi-

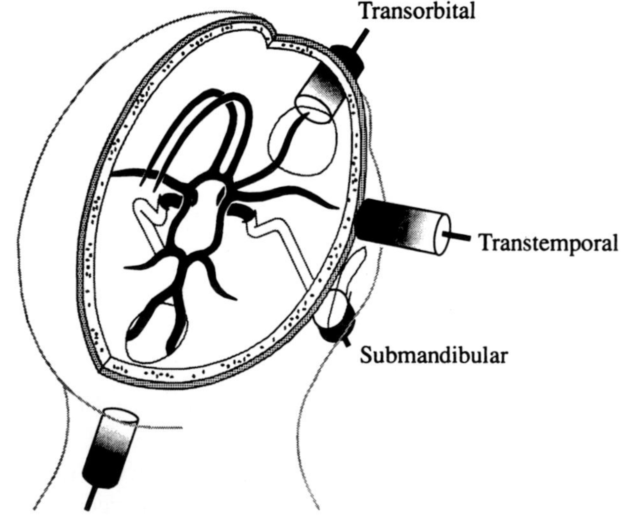

Figure 37-1. The natural intracranial windows through which an ultrasonic beam can pass to allow detection of the direction of blood flow and blood flow velocity in the large arteries at the base of the brain. (With permission from Fujioka KA, Douville CM: Anatomy and freehand examination techniques in Newell DW, Aaslid R (eds): *Transcranial Doppler.* New York: Raven Press, 1992: pp 9–31.)

vided into three regions: anterior, middle, and posterior. The region with the best penetration and the best reflected signal (highest acoustical intensity) should be used, and this varies from patient to patient. It should be noted that in approximately 10 percent of subjects, particularly older women, the ultrasonic beam cannot penetrate the temporal bone as a result of increased bone thickness and density. In cases where it is difficult to obtain an adequate temporal signal, it is important to perform a thorough examination encompassing all portions of the temporal bone. Of practical importance in postsurgical patients is obstruction of the temporal window caused by a head dressing. In these cases the dressing may have to be cut to allow proper placement of the Doppler probe. If this is necessary, it is recommended that the dressing be opened 3 to 4 cm anterior to the root of the zygoma so that the incision site, which usually is just in front of the ear in typical trauma scalp incisions, remains covered. In addition, postoperative patients often have significant temporal soft tissue swelling that adds 1 to 2 cm to the usual depth required for vessel identification.

Most portions of the anterior circle of Willis can be assessed through the temporal window, including the distal segment of the supraclinoid internal carotid artery (ICA), proximal middle cerebral artery (MCA), posterior communicating artery (PCoA), posterior cerebral artery (PCA), the A1 segment of the anterior cerebral artery (ACA), and occasionally the anterior communicating artery (ACoA). A working knowledge of the anatomic location and direction of flow in all major branches from the supraclinoid ICA is required to correctly identify and interpret signals from these vessels. It is easiest to initially identify the proximal portion of the MCA (M1 segment), which travels in a lateral and slightly anterior horizontal plane, with the direction of flow toward the Doppler probe. The M1 segment is typically identified at a depth of 45 to 55 mm and can be followed proximally to allow identification of the other basal arteries. The ICA bifurcation is found at a depth of 55 to 65 mm, and the ACA at a depth of 60 to 80 mm.

The transorbital window, which is assessed by gently placing the Doppler transducer over the closed eyelid and directing it toward the optic canal, can determine flow velocity in the ophthalmic artery and the siphon region of the intracranial ICA. The power intensity should be reduced to limit ultrasonic eye exposure. The ophthalmic artery has a characteristic extracranial waveform (high resistance, low diastolic flow) and is usually located at a depth of 40 to 50 mm. This artery can then be followed posteriorly to allow identification of the carotid siphon.

The vertebral and basilar arteries can be studied through the foramen magnum via the transforaminal window. This window is greatly affected by patient posture and can be increased by flexing the subject's head. An initial search for the vertebral artery is made at a depth of 60 to 70 mm, and the basilar artery can be identified at a depth of 80 to 120 mm or more.

Although the main focus of TCD is the intracranial circulation, the authors recommend evaluation of the extracranial ICA in all cases. The extracranial ICA is easy to insonate at a depth of 40 to 70 mm with the probe aimed at the skull base near the angle of the jaw (submandibular window). Assessment of this portion of the ICA is important in trauma patients because it can identify traumatic dissections involving this segment and provide an index of hemispheric blood flow. The use of extracranial ICA velocities is reviewed in more detail in the discussion of the detection of cerebral vasospasm, below.

ESSENTIAL CEREBRAL HEMODYNAMICS AND INTERPRETATION OF TCD RECORDINGS

Before analyzing and interpreting Doppler recordings, it is necessary to understand the basic hemodynamic principles that pertain to TCD. These fundamental principles not only provide a background for understanding TCD technology but also illustrate some of the limitations of TCD as an investigative tool for assessing CBF.

TCD detects the velocity (in centimeters per second) and direction of blood flow in cerebral arteries but not actual flow volume (in milliliters per second). The relationship between flow volume (Q) and flow velocity (V) is described in equation 2:

$$Q = V \times \pi r^2 \tag{2}$$

This demonstrates that flow volume Q (ml/s) is equal to the product of velocity V (cm/s) and the cross-sectional area of the arterial lumen (cm^2). If this equation is rearranged to solve for velocity, we obtain equation 3:

$$V = \frac{Q}{\pi r^2} \tag{3}$$

Thus, the major determinants of blood flow velocity are flow volume and arterial radius. It should be noted from equation 3 that the velocity of blood flow is inversely proportional to the square of the vessel radius. In practical terms, this means that TCD velocities increase markedly in an area where the cross-sectional luminal diameter is reduced, such as an area of focal narrowing caused by cerebral vasospasm. According to the law of the maintenance of mass and because of the incompressibility of fluids, flow velocity increases across a stenosis by an amount that is inversely proportional to the square of the vessel radius (provided that a constant flow is maintained through the stenotic area). This is depicted in equation 4 and Fig. 37-2, where r(1) and v(1) are equal to the radius and velocity before the area of narrowing and r(2) and v(2) are the radius and velocity in the area of vessel narrowing:

$$r(1)^2 \times v(1) = r(2)^2 \times v(2) \qquad (4)$$

It must be stressed that this applies only if flow volume remains constant. Investigations of arterial stenosis have shown that there is no decrease in blood flow volume until the cross-sectional area is narrowed by more than 80 percent.[12–14] Before reaching this degree of critical stenosis, progressive compensatory increases in flow velocity are able to maintain a fairly constant flow volume. When resistance from stenosis reaches a hemodynamically critical level, flow volume is progressively reduced. This negates the effect of vessel narrowing on velocity and acts to reduce flow velocity (Fig. 37-3).

The interpretation of high flow velocity also may be influenced by flow volume. It is important to remember, particularly in head trauma patients, that a TCD recording of high velocity may be caused by arterial narrowing (as in posttraumatic vasospasm), by high volume flow (as in posttraumatic hyperemia), or by a combination of the two. Proper interpretation of flow velocity therefore requires knowledge (or an accurate estimation) of one of these factors. In clinical practice, flow volume is usually estimated by measuring cerebral blood flow or by recording flow velocity in extracranial arteries (because extracranial arteries are not prone to spasm and have a relatively constant diameter, flow velocity changes in these vessels are proportional to flow volume

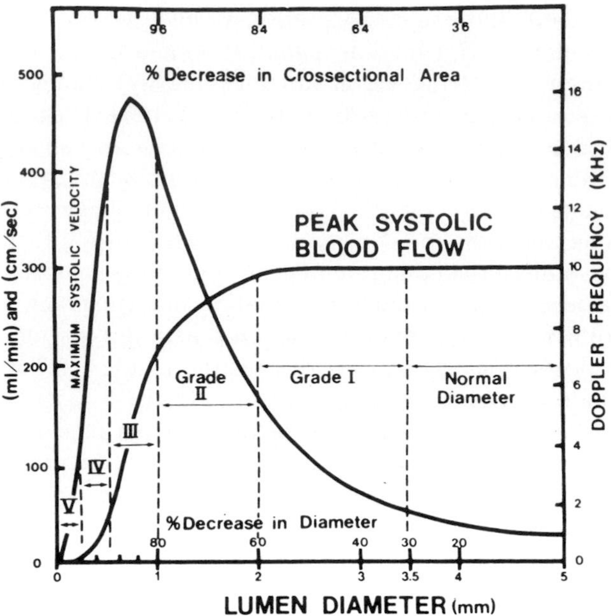

Figure 37-3. Relationship between blood velocity and flow in human carotid artery stenosis. Note that before reaching a critical degree of stenosis (greater than 80 percent reduction in cross-sectional area), compensatory velocity increases are able to maintain flow volume. (With permission from Spencer MP, Reid JM: Quantification of carotid stenosis with continuous-wave (C-W) Doppler ultrasound. *Stroke* 10:326–330, 1979.)

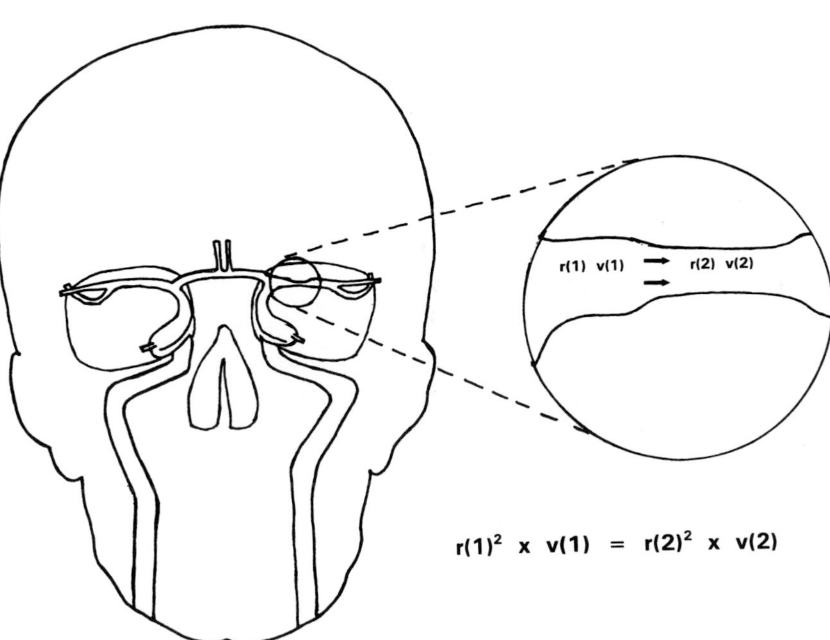

Figure 37-2. In areas of vessel stenosis where a constant volume of blood flow is maintained, the velocity of blood flow increases in an amount that is inversely proportional to the square of the vessel radius.

changes). The relationship between flow velocity, flow volume, and CBF is considered further in the next section.

Because flow volume affects flow velocity, several physiological parameters must be taken into account in studying TCD recordings. Factors that alter CBF and therefore volume flow include cerebral metabolic activity, arterial P_{CO_2}, age, and hematocrit. CBF (except in states of ischemia and hyperemia) is generally coupled to cerebral metabolism. Many physiological alterations can influence CBF, but P_{CO_2} is the most influential and clinically significant variable. Several investigators have demonstrated the great effect P_{CO_2} alterations may have on TCD velocities, with velocities increasing as P_{CO_2} rises between 20 and 60 mmHg.[15,16] CBF does not increase until P_{O_2} falls below 50 mmHg and does not significantly change with elevated P_{O_2} levels, making correction based on this variable unnecessary. Velocity varies according to age, with the highest values occurring between the ages of 4 to 6 and declining with age thereafter.[17,18] This is similar to CBF data that demonstrate that blood flow is highest in the first decade and progressively declines during adulthood.[19,20] Hematocrit can affect TCD velocity measurements, with anemia resulting in increased velocity.[21] The effect of a low hematocrit on TCD velocities should be taken into account in head-injured patients with dilutional anemia after fluid resuscitation for hemorrhagic shock. Although the precise flow velocity correction factors for P_{CO_2} and hematocrit in head injury patients are unknown, the effects of these factors must be kept in mind in comparing groups of patients and recording serial velocity changes in individuals.

Most modern TCD machines display flow velocities in a spectral fashion, and it is necessary to know the fundamental features of this waveform. A typical MCA recording with a schematic summarizing the major features is shown in Fig. 37-4. Peak systolic flow velocity

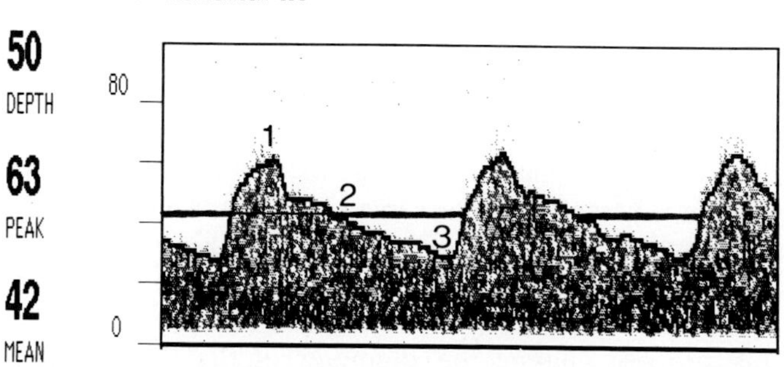

Figure 37-4. A characteristic TCD recording from the middle cerebral artery. The labeled numbers indicate features of the waveform. 1 = peak systolic velocity (V_{sys}); 2 = mean velocity of blood flow (V_{mean}); and 3 = end-diastolic velocity (V_{dias}).

(V_{sys}) is the maximal velocity obtained during left ventricular contraction. End-diastolic velocity (V_{dias}) is the maximal velocity recorded at the end of diastole, just before the acceleration phase of systole. The velocity of diastolic blood flow is dependent on the peripheral resistance and is greatest in vascular systems with low distal resistance (such as the intracranial circulation). Peripheral vascular systems have higher resistance and demonstrate little flow during diastole. Mean flow velocity (V_{mean}) is the time-averaged maximum velocity over the entire cardiac cycle. *Pulsatility* is a term that describes the variability in the maximal flow velocities (V_{sys} and V_{dias}) throughout the cardiac cycle and is an index of the resistance in the distal vasculature. The closer V_{sys} and V_{dias} are to each other, the lower the pulsatility, and conversely, the farther they are from each other, the greater the pulsatility. In an attempt to quantify pulsatility, Gosling and King[22] defined a *pulsatility index* (PI) that is calculated by equation 5:

$$PI = \frac{(V_{sys} - V_{dias})}{V_{mean}} \tag{5}$$

Although the PI can be influenced by many factors, including cardiac contractility and extracranial arterial stenosis, it generally reflects resistance in the distal cerebral vessels. It is elevated in states of increased distal resistance such as intracranial hypertension and is decreased in states of reduced distal vascular resistance such as hyperemia.

DOPPLER VELOCITIES AS AN INDEX OF CEREBRAL BLOOD FLOW

Disturbances of CBF play an important role in the pathophysiology of craniocerebral trauma. After an injury, the CNS is vulnerable to a variety of secondary insults that adversely affect outcome. Trauma-induced blood flow changes such as ischemia and hyperemia may compound damage in an injured brain. Furthermore, the normal adaptive mechanisms of the cerebral vasculature may be impaired after traumatic brain injury so that events such as elevated ICP, systemic hypotension, and increased blood viscosity may lead to ischemic complications. It is clinically important to distinguish states of low blood flow and high blood flow in patients with a head injury, as the management principles can differ vastly. Many investigators have demonstrated that low CBF can occur after head trauma,[23–25] and Bouma and Muizelaar have recently shown that severe reductions in CBF can be seen very early after an injury.[26] In patients with low CBF, caution must be exercised before deliberately inducing therapies such as fluid restriction and hyperventilation for the control of elevated ICP because these maneuvers may worsen cerebral perfusion. Hyperemia, which is defined as CBF exceeding the brain's metabolic demands, has been observed in many head injury patients and may be associated with raised ICP.[24,27,28] It is thought to occur secondary to impaired cerebral autoregulation resulting in increased brain blood volume.

Most previous blood flow studies have utilized quantitative CBF techniques such as ^{133}Xe and stable xenon computed tomography to characterize alterations in CBF after a head injury. These techniques have the advantage of providing quantitative measurement of tissue perfusion, but they necessitate radiation exposure, may require patient transport, and cannot be used for continuous monitoring of CBF. Because TCD is noninvasive, is portable, and can be repeated frequently or used continuously, it is ideal for the assessment of cerebral hemodynamics in critically ill head injury patients.

Blood flow volume (Q) and blood flow velocity (V) are related as shown in equation 2. The radius of the insonated vessel must be accurately known to permit calculation of absolute blood flow volume in milliliters per minute. This, of course, is not generally known. In addition, the perfusion territory of the vessel being examined and the contribution from vessels providing collateral blood flow, both of which may vary in pathological states, must be known. Therefore, in most clinical situations, TCD cannot provide an accurate quantitative measure of regional tissue perfusion. Despite these issues, several investigators have attempted to correlate TCD velocity and CBF measurements. Sorteberg and associates[29] studied normal subjects and compared absolute maximum TCD velocities from the MCA, ACA, PCA, and extracranial ICA to CBF measurements obtained using ^{133}Xe inhalation single photon emission tomography (SPECT). They analyzed TCD and CBF data by regression analysis and found a statistical correlation between absolute Doppler velocities and quantitative regional CBF in the vascular distribution of each artery when the studies were corrected for normal P_{CO_2} values. Bishop and coworkers[30] and Halsey and colleagues[31] have examined the correlation between absolute Doppler velocities and CBF studies in patients with cerebrovascular disease. While there was a fair statistical correlation in the study by Bishop and coworkers[30] ($r = 0.424$, $p < .01$), Halsey and colleagues[31] found that there was a significant correlation between the two studies only when CBF was lower than 20 ml/100 g/min. The authors have correlated absolute Doppler velocities and CBF, as determined by intravenous ^{133}Xe measurements, in 44 head-injured patients and have found a variable correlation between the two techniques.[32] The authors found that extracranial carotid TCD measurements showed a better correlation with hemispheric CBF than did MCA velocities. The strongest correlation identified was between extracranial ICA end-diastolic velocity (V_{dias}) and ipsilateral hemispheric CBF. This coincides with the studies of Risberg and Smith,[33] who identified a strong correlation between extracranial ICA V_{dias} and CBF in patients free of cerebrovascular disease. The relatively poor correlation between CBF measurements and MCA velocities can be explained partially by the confounding effects of MCA vasospasm, which is a common posttraumatic finding. Although statistically significant correlations can be found, the relationship between CBF measurements and TCD is too variable to permit accurate determination of absolute CBF from Doppler velocities in individual cases.[34]

Although the correlation between TCD velocities and absolute CBF measurements is not accurate enough to be of practical clinical use, serial changes in Doppler velocities in individual patients appear to be promising for assessing short-term, relative changes in CBF. Bishop and coworkers[30] examined the relationship of TCD velocities and ^{133}Xe measurements made at rest and during induced hypercapnia. They observed only a fair correlation between the absolute baseline measurements using the two techniques but found that the relative blood flow changes to hypercapnia measured by TCD and ^{133}Xe correlated well. Kirkham and colleagues[16] studied the relationship of P_{CO_2} and time-averaged Doppler frequencies in 38 normal subjects. They found that velocity changes that occurred in response to changes in P_{CO_2} over the range of 20 to 60 mmHg were very similar to those which have been reported for CBF studies, providing further evidence that changes in MCA velocities may reliably monitor relative changes in flow.

To determine relative CBF changes, it is not necessary to know the arterial diameter. However, it is assumed that significant changes in the diameter of the insonated artery do not occur during the measurement of velocity change. It has been shown that most acute CBF changes are related to changes in vasomotor activity in the distal arterial system (e.g., arterioles and capillaries), not to changes in the diameter of the large conductance vessels being assessed by TCD. This has been confirmed angiographically in a study by Huber and Haneda[35] that demonstrated that changes in P_{CO_2} produced drastic changes in the distal cerebral vasculature but did not change the diameter of the larger basal vessels to a significant degree. Giller[8] reported that MCA diameter measured visually during craniotomy did not change significantly in response to varying CO_2 concentrations. Therefore, it appears that short-term alterations (over minutes or hours) in relative CBF estimated by TCD and related to changes of P_{CO_2} are reliable.

However, in the case of trauma patients, velocity measurements made over longer time intervals may not accurately estimate relative CBF changes because of the confounding effects on flow velocity of intracranial arterial spasm and because of changes in the perfusion territory of the artery being assessed. For long-term monitoring (days or weeks) of relative CBF changes, Doppler evaluation of the extracranial ICA is more suitable. The extracranial carotid artery has a constant diameter because it generally is not affected by posttraumatic spasm (although it may rarely be damaged by traumatic dissection) and probably has a more constant perfusion territory. The authors routinely record the flow velocity of the extracranial ICA in trauma patients and use this measurement as an index of CBF.

ASSESSMENT OF CEREBRAL AUTOREGULATION

The ability of resistance-regulating arterioles of the cerebral circulation to maintain a constant level of CBF in the face of blood pressure fluctuation is referred to as autoregulation. It has previously been shown, using classic CBF methods, that severely head injured patients may have impaired cerebral autoregulation.[36] When autoregulation is impaired, CBF changes in response to alterations in mean arterial pressure. Under this circumstance, blood pressure changes may result in ischemia or hyperemia, which may cause deleterious secondary brain injury.[25,37]

Aaslid and colleagues described a noninvasive method for evaluating the autoregulatory response with transcranial Doppler.[38] Bilateral thigh blood pressure cuffs are inflated for several minutes and then abruptly released, causing a rapid fall in arterial blood pressure (BP). This drop in BP, which is due to muscular vasodilation and reactive hyperemia, persists for approximately 10 s. During this maneuver, the cerebral hemodynamic response is assessed by continuous measurement of MCA flow velocity using TCD. This provides a dynamic assessment of relative CBF changes in response to the transient BP drop. When autoregulation is intact, V_{MCA} briefly drops and then returns toward its baseline value, usually within 5 s and well before BP returns to normal (Fig. 37-5). This confirms that autoregulation is a fast and effective mechanism.[39] In cases where autoregulation is completely impaired, V_{MCA} does not return to baseline and fluctuates passively and in parallel with changes in systemic BP (Fig. 37-5).

The cerebrovascular resistance (CVR) and the rate of the autoregulatory response can be calculated. *Cerebrovascular resistance*, which is calculated by dividing V_{MCA} by the arterial BP, changes in a linear fashion 1 to 5 s after the induced BP drop. If the CVR can decrease and fully compensate for the fall in BP, CBF rapidly returns to baseline (intact autoregulation). Conversely, if CVR does not correct for the fall in BP, CBF does not return to baseline (impaired autoregulation). Using the calculated CVR, an index of the *rate of regulation* (*RoR*) can be determined from the change in CVR (per unit time) divided by the change in BP (per unit time) and has a normal value of 20.0 percent (± 3.0 percent) per second.[38] An RoR of 0 indicates completely

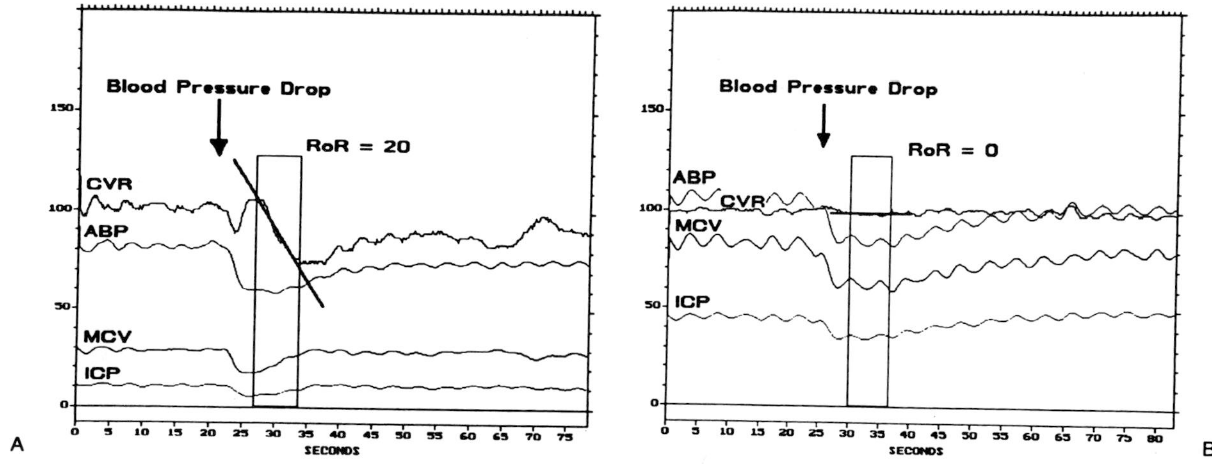

Figure 37-5. *A.* Middle cerebral artery velocity response to an induced blood pressure drop in a patient with intact autoregulation. *B.* Middle cerebral artery velocity response to an induced blood pressure drop in a patient with absent autoregulation. (With permission from Newell DW, Seiler RW, Aaslid R.[40])

impaired autoregulation, whereas values ranging from 1 to 15 percent per second imply decreasing degrees of impairment. Newell and coworkers applied this technique to head injury patients and found that autoregulation could be normal, absent, or impaired to various degrees.[40] Lundar and associates measured MCA flow velocity continuously in head injury patients during changes in cerebral perfusion pressure (CPP).[41] Five of their 12 patients demonstrated pressure-passive blood velocity changes at all levels of CPP, indicating dysfunctional autoregulation. The other patients, however, maintained stable blood velocity levels until CPP dropped below 40 to 45 mmHg.

The relationship between impaired autoregulation and outcome in head injury patients remains unclear. Overgaard and Tweed[42] noted that if cerebral autoregulation remains intact during the first week after an injury, the clinical prognosis is good, but they could not identify a clear relationship between defective autoregulation and outcome. However, Fieschi and associates[43] found that 50 percent of their head injury patients had defective autoregulation between 2 and 4 days after injury and that this was adversely associated with outcome.

Although the relationship between defective autoregulation and outcome remains unclear, knowledge of the status of autoregulation is important in determining treatment strategies for elevated ICP in head-injured patients. For example, the effect of mannitol in reducing ICP elevations is more pronounced when autoregulation is intact because the mannitol-induced decrease in blood viscosity leads to vasoconstriction and decreased cerebral blood volume.[44] This vascular effect adds to the osmotic effect of mannitol. Furthermore, the presence or absence of autoregulatory impairment may help determine the optimal BP for management of ICP after a severe head injury. If autoregulation is defective in the face of elevated mean arterial blood pressure, lowering of the systemic BP may help decrease ICP by reducing cerebral blood volume. (This, of course, must be done cautiously, because lowering of BP in this setting can cause ischemic damage.) However, if autoregulation is shown to be intact, lowering of BP leads to vasodilation and increased cerebral blood volume, which may cause further elevations in ICP. Although more research needs to be done, TCD appears to be a promising technique for the assessment of autoregulation.

CO_2 RESPONSE

Hyperventilation is frequently employed in head-injured patients in an effort to reduce raised ICP. However, cerebrovascular CO_2 reactivity can be impaired early after a traumatic brain injury.[45] Newell and colleagues found that the MCA velocity response to CO_2 changes in head-injured patients was variable: absent in some, moderately impaired in others, and normal in many.[40] Absent CO_2 reactivity was generally found in patients with severe brain injury or extensive lesions in an MCA distribution. Lundar and associates, using TCD, found normal blood velocity responses to CO_2 change (approximately 3 percent change in velocity for each 1 mmHg change in arterial P_{CO_2}) in two-thirds of their head trauma patients.[41] Four severely injured patients showed markedly reduced blood velocity responsivity (less than 1 percent for each mmHg of P_{CO_2}). All these patients also had abolished autoregulation, and all had a poor outcome. Klingelhofer and Sander studied CO_2 reactivity in 40 patients with severe intracranial hemorrhage, 27 of whom were head injury patients.[46] They found that CO_2 reactivity was lower in the intracranial hemorrhage patients (2.0 percent change in V_{MCA}/mmHg P_{CO_2}) than in controls (3.7 percent change

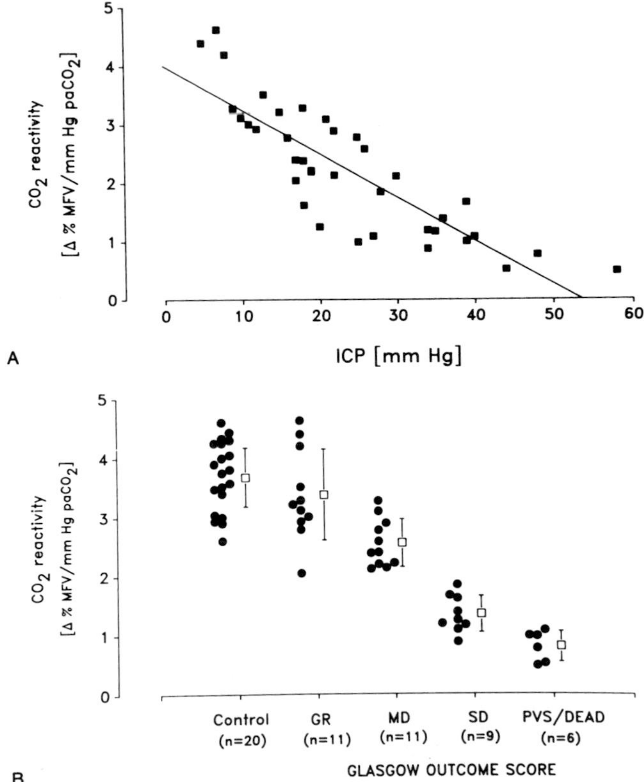

Figure 37-6. *A*. Scatterplot showing relation between relative CO_2 reactivity and ICP ($r = -0.89$, $p < .001$). Each point represents one patient with a severe intracranial hemorrhage. *B*. Plot showing the relation between relative CO_2 reactivity and outcome according to the Glasgow Outcome Scale at 3 months after an injury. Filled circles represent individual patients, and open squares represent the mean values for each group. (With permission from Klingelhofer J, Sander D.[46])

in V_{MCA}/mmHg P_{CO_2}).There was a good correlation between ICP and CO_2 reactivity and between outcome and CO_2 reactivity (Fig. 37-6). While patients with a good outcome showed nearly normal reactivity, patients in the bad outcome group (persistent vegetative state or dead) had significantly reduced reactivity (0.8 percent change in V_{MCA}/mmHg P_{CO_2}).

DETECTION OF POSTTRAUMATIC ARTERIAL SPASM

Before the advent of computed tomography (CT), angiography was a routine diagnostic study for the initial evaluation of head injury patients. Previous angiographic studies revealed that spasm of the intracranial arteries occurred in approximately 5 to 10 percent of severe head injury patients.[47,48] However, angiography was performed only as a preliminary diagnostic test and was not usually repeated, and so it might be expected that the incidence of posttraumatic vasospasm was actually higher than reported. In fact, several reports utilizing TCD to study patients suffering from craniocerebral trauma have indicated that arterial narrowing can be identified in approximately 30 percent of cases in the days to weeks after the injury.[23,49]

During arterial spasm, TCD velocities increase through the narrowed segment proportionally to the reduction in the vessel's cross-sectional area (equation 4). MCA velocities exceeding 120 cm/s generally are associated with vasospasm. Values greater than 200 cm/s, which are associated with a greater than 50 percent reduction in vessel diameter,[50] indicate severe vessel narrowing. However, reliance solely on intracranial velocity measurements to detect vasospasm may be misleading because MCA velocities also can be elevated by increased volume flow (as in hyperemia). Elevation of flow velocity resulting from arterial narrowing can be differentiated reliably from high flow velocity resulting from hyperemia by measuring the CBF concurrently. The measurement of low CBF associated with high flow velocity eliminates hyperemia as a consideration and establishes the presence of vasospasm. In the absence of direct CBF measurement, the difficulty in differentiating hyperemia from vasospasm may be partially overcome by assessing Doppler velocities in the extracranial ICA at the base of the skull with a submandibular approach. A "hemispheric index" or *Lindegaard ratio* can be calculated by dividing the MCA velocity by the velocity obtained in the extracranial ICA (V_{MCA}/V_{ICA}).[51] This ratio has a normal value of around 1.7 but may range from 1.1 to 3.0.[6,51,52] Lindegaard and colleagues[6] found angiographic evidence of MCA narrowing after an aneurysmal subarachnoid hemorrhage to be associated with a V_{MCA}/V_{ICA} ratio greater than 3. Posttraumatic vasospasm results in increased TCD velocities through the narrowed vessel but is associated with normal or reduced extracranial ICA measurements. In cases of intracranial cerebral hyperperfusion or hyperemia without vasospasm, both the intracranial and extracranial velocities are affected in a similar fashion, and the hemispheric index is stable (<3).

Similar to the vasospasm that follows aneurysmal rupture, arterial spasm after a head injury is commonly associated with subarachnoid hemorrhage (SAH) and typically involves the large arteries at the base of the brain. Although the authors have identified mild vasospasm in some patients without evidence of traumatic SAH, all patients with *severe* arterial narrowing have had evidence of SAH. Weber and associates found a statistically significant relationship to MCA spasm and the presence of CT-visualized SAH or intracerebral blood,[49] and the authors' experience has shown that posttraumatic vasospasm is strongly associated with blood in an intradural location (including the subarachnoid, subdural, intraparenchymal, and intraventricular compartments). In a study of severe head injuries reported from the National Institute of Health Traumatic Coma Data Bank, CT evidence of SAH was found in 39 percent of the patients.[53] The presence of SAH in that series was found to be a strong independent predictor of death, which may have been related to ischemia caused by vasospasm.

The arterial segments affected by posttraumatic vasospasm in the authors' experience are all areas typically affected by aneurysmal SAH, such as the supraclinoid ICA, MCA, ACA, and basilar artery (Fig. 37-7). The time course of spasm after a head injury is also similar to that after an aneurysmal SAH. Elevated velocities first appear several days after injury, peak around 2 weeks after the injury, and resolve after approximately 3 weeks (Fig. 37-8). Taken as a whole, these findings provide strong evidence that cerebral arterial spasm after a head injury is closely related to the spasm seen after an aneurysmal SAH and reinforce a common pathophysiological connection with periarterial blood of any cause.

In a study of angiograms in patients who died after a head injury, Macpherson and Graham[54] found a significant correlation between angiographic arterial narrowing and postmortem ipsilateral ischemic hemispheric damage. This provides further evidence that vasospasm can be an important secondary brain insult and can lead to brain infarction. The authors previously reported their initial experience with TCD and ^{133}Xe CBF studies in head-injured patients and found that there was a significant correlation between high TCD velocities during vasospasm and low CBF measurements, confirming that posttraumatic arterial spasm is

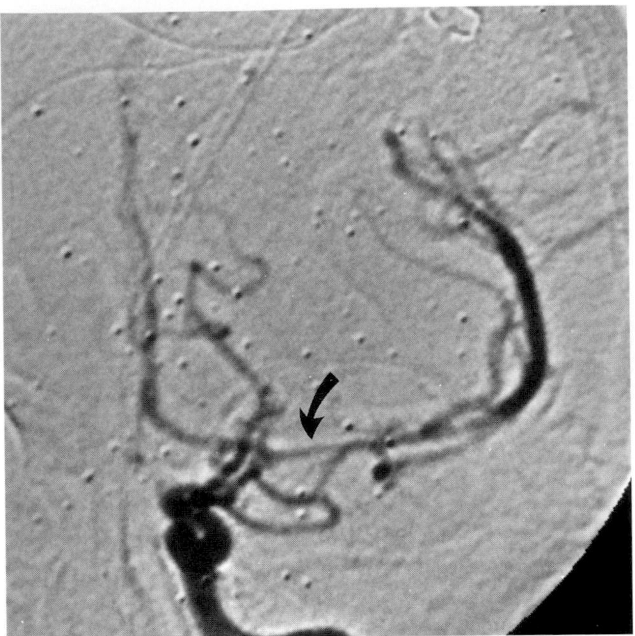

Figure 37-7. Posttraumatic vasospasm has an appearance similar to that of the arterial narrowing seen after an aneurysmal subarachnoid hemorrhage. In this case, vasospasm involved the anterior circulation and was most severe in the middle cerebral artery (arrow).

associated with impaired cerebral perfusion.[23] In fact, the authors observed one patient with severe TCD-detected spasm who went on to develop postmortem evidence of infarction in territories supplied by the arteries affected by spasm. In summary, vasospasm is a relatively common complication of craniocerebral trauma; may be associated with decreased CBF, ischemic damage, and an adverse outcome; and can be detected effectively by transcranial Doppler. Undoubtedly, future investigations will evaluate the effectiveness of therapies aimed at improving CBF in TCD-detected posttraumatic vasospasm, such as hypervolemia, induced arterial hypertension, calcium channel blockers, and balloon angioplasty, all of which have been shown at least anecdotally to be effective in reducing ischemic complications after an aneurysm rupture.

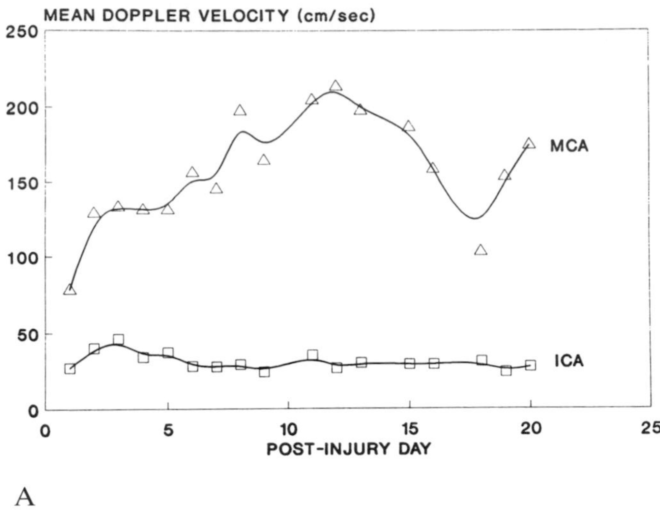

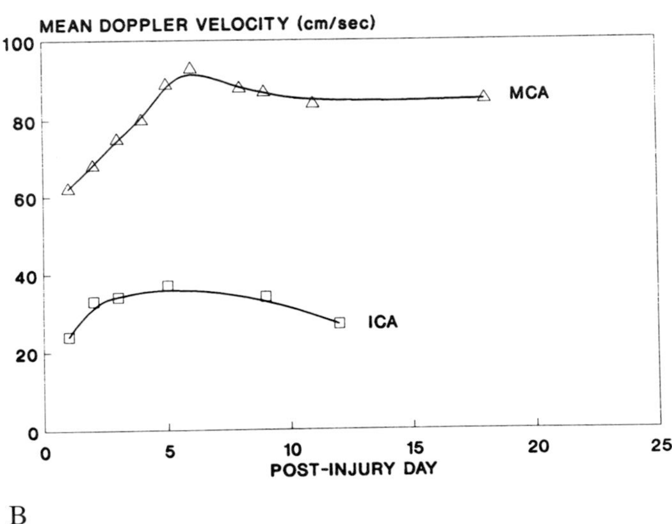

Figure 37-8. *A.* Time course of middle cerebral artery transcranial Doppler velocities in head-injured patients with vasospasm. Note that the time course is similar to that seen after an aneurysmal subarachnoid hemorrhage and that the MCA velocities increase whereas the extracranial ICA velocities decrease during arterial narrowing. *B.* Transcranial Doppler velocities in head-injured patients without vasospasm. Note that the MCA and extracranial ICA velocities change only slightly and are in parallel.

DETECTION OF RAISED INTRACRANIAL PRESSURE AND CONFIRMATION OF BRAIN DEATH

The most frequent cause of death in head injury patients is intractable intracranial hypertension,[55,56] and the reduction of high ICP is one of the major intensive care unit (ICU) treatment strategies employed for severe head injuries. Prolonged elevation of ICP can lead to ischemia resulting from reduced cerebral perfusion and is associated with a poor outcome.[57,58] In the extreme case, high ICP may result in cessation of brain perfusion. Current ICP monitoring devices, such as ventricular catheters and subdural and intraparenchymal fiber-optic monitors, are invasive and are associated with a small

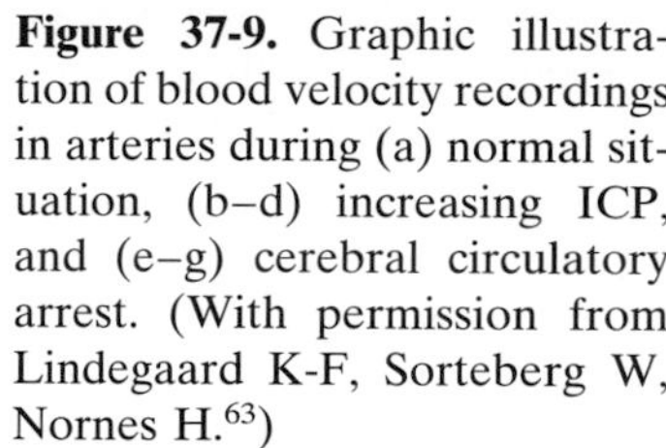

Figure 37-9. Graphic illustration of blood velocity recordings in arteries during (a) normal situation, (b–d) increasing ICP, and (e–g) cerebral circulatory arrest. (With permission from Lindegaard K-F, Sorteberg W, Nornes H.[63])

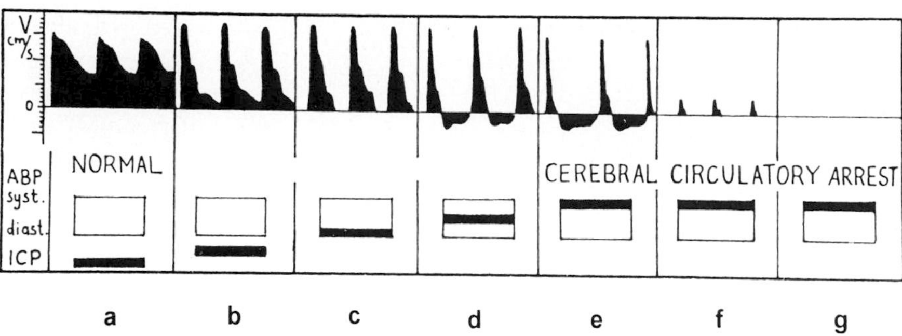

but definite risk to the patient. The development of TCD has made it possible to assess intracranial physiology noninvasively. The assessment of ICP and cerebral circulatory arrest employing TCD has been examined by several authors and appears to be promising.[59–62]

An elevation in ICP causes an increase in cerebrovascular resistance, probably as a result of microcirculatory or venous compression. Increasing ICP causes a stereotyped sequence of changes in the intracranial arterial blood velocity waveform[59,63] (Fig. 37-9). As the ICP approaches diastolic blood pressure, the systolic velocity increases slightly and the diastolic velocity decreases. This change results in an increase in the PI. When ICP reaches the level of diastolic blood pressure, diastolic flow in the intracranial arteries ceases (Fig. 37-10). With a further increase in ICP, a to-and-fro flow pattern may appear. In this situation, the cerebral arteries become distended by forward flow driven by systolic pressure. Because critically high ICP and CVR prevent normal outflow, the distended intracranial arteries eject blood in a retrograde direction during diastole. When net forward flow is seriously reduced, this situation leads to severe ischemic brain damage or brain death. With persistence of this level of intracranial hypertension, the intracranial waveform degrades to become a small systolic spike and then disappears altogether.

Because the CBF velocity waveform changes in a predictable fashion as ICP increases, TCD-recorded parameters have been evaluated quantitatively for their correlation with ICP or CPP.[61,62] The correlation of PI with ICP has been studied by several investigators. Homburg and associates examined the relationship between ICP and PI in 10 head injury patients.[61] They found a positive, statistically significant association with a correlation coefficient of 0.82 (Fig. 37-11). They also studied the change in PI and ICP over time during mannitol infusion in one patient and found a remarkably tight relationship between the two parameters (Fig. 37-

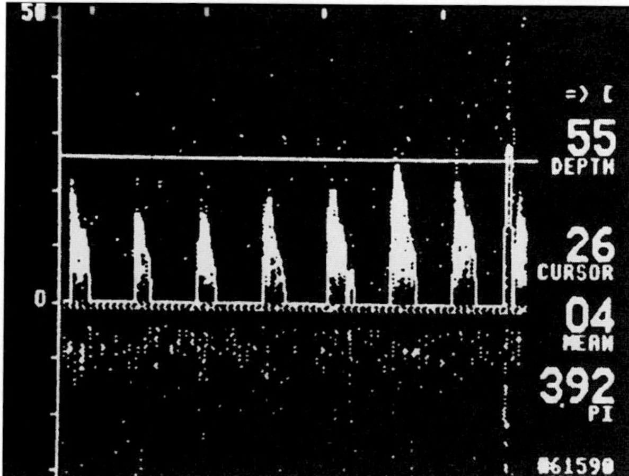

Figure 37-10. Characteristic transcranial Doppler waveform of cerebral circulatory arrest. Note the loss of diastolic blood flow on the waveform.

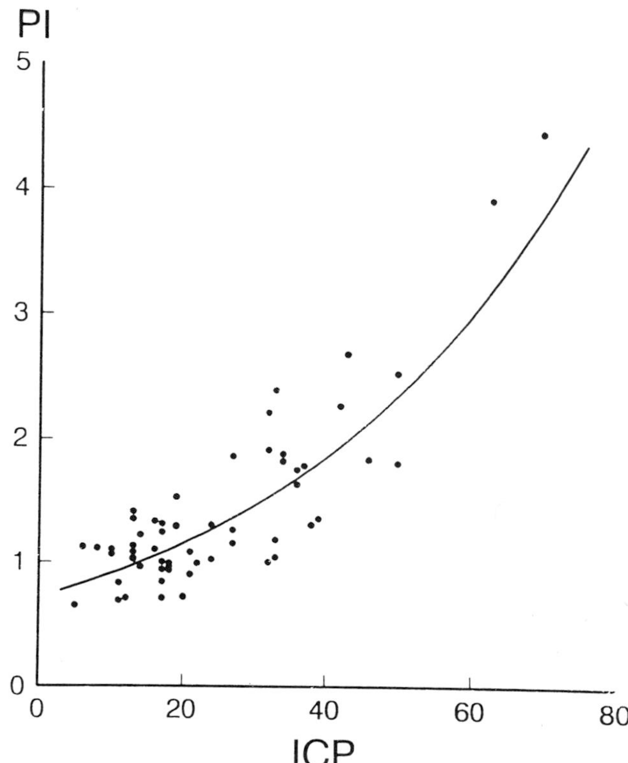

Figure 37-11. The relation between PI and ICP in 10 head-injured patients. (r = 0.82, $p < .001$). (With permission from Homburg AM, Jakobsen M, Enevoldsen E.[61])

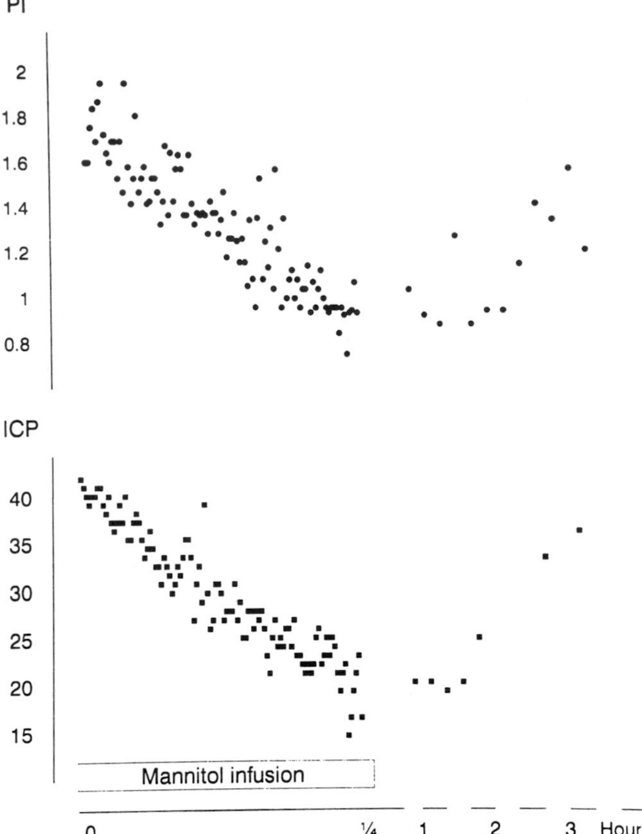

Figure 37-12. Changes in PI and ICP during mannitol infusion related to time in a head-injured patient. (With permission from Homburg AM, Jakobsen M, Enevoldsen E.[61])

12). Kwan-Hon and associates found an analogous relationship between CPP and PI.[62] While the overall correlation between ICP (or CPP) and PI is good, the variability of the relationship is such that it is possible in clinical practice to use only the PI to separate patients with normal ICP (≤20 mmHg) from those with critically high ICP (≥40 mmHg). It is not possible to estimate the ICP accurately in the range of 10 to 35 mmHg. The authors' experience with ICP and PI substantiates this concept.[64] There are simply too many other factors, such as cardiac output, proximal arterial resistance, cerebral vasospasm, and arterial P_{CO_2}, that influence the PI in addition to ICP.

The guidelines set forth for the determination of brain death by the President's Commission state that the diagnosis of brain death must be made on the basis of clinical findings and that blood flow studies should be used only as confirmatory tests.[65] Nevertheless, several investigators have shown that TCD is useful in confirming the diagnosis of brain death.[59,66,67] Newell and coworkers[66] found that in 12 clinically brain dead subjects, a TCD pattern of reverberating flow was always associated with absent CBF measured by radioactive technetium scanning. Powers and coworkers[68] and Kirkham and colleagues[69] both found that no patients survived if mean MCA flow velocity was less than 10 cm/s. However, it should be noted that cerebral circulatory arrest may occur for brief periods as a result of transient elevations in ICP and may be associated with clinical recovery. Grote and Hassler[70] described a patient with rebleeding from a ruptured cerebral aneurysm who had TCD evidence of to-and-fro flow for 2 min that gradually returned to normal. This patient eventually went on to make a clinical recovery. Arrest of the supratentorial circulation has been noted to occur before the loss of brainstem reflexes and in some cases has progressed to brain death.[67,71] Conversely, devastating brainstem lesions occasionally can lead to the diagnosis of brain death even though blood flow in the supratentorial compartment is present. Ropper and associates[72] found to-and-fro flow patterns in 19 of 24 brain-dead patients. Three patients had absent brainstem function but persistent EEG activity. In these patients TCD waveforms appeared normal, and they probably had some remaining cortical activity that persisted for a period of time.

It is evident, then, that clinically determined brain death is not synonymous with intracranial circulatory arrest, although certainly when the arrest of the cerebral circulation is prolonged, brain death will ensue. Nevertheless, TCD studies are useful in studying the intracranial circulation and provide objective confirmation of clinically diagnosed brain death. Transcranial Doppler evaluation can be extremely helpful in establishing cerebral circulatory arrest in cases where the clinical examination is obscured or unreliable because of the presence of certain drugs or medications. The demand for organ transplant donors continues to grow, but many potential donor candidates are refused because a delay in the diagnosis of brain death can lead to multiple organ failure. Early recognition of irreversible cerebral death may well be possible using TCD, but further investigations are needed.

References

1. Doppler CA: Uber das fabrige licht der Doppelsterne and einiger anderer Gestirne des Himmels. *Abhandl Konigl Bohm Ges Wiss,* 1842.
2. Aaslid R, Markwalder TM, Nornes H: Noninvasive transcranial Doppler ultrasound recording of flow velocity in basal cerebral arteries. *J Neurosurg* 57:769–774, 1982.
3. Lindegaard KF, Grolimund P, Aaslid R, Nornes H: Evaluation of cerebral AVM's using transcranial Doppler ultrasound. *J Neurosurg* 65:335–344, 1986.

4. Petty GW, Massaro AR, Tatemichi TK, et al: Transcranial Doppler ultrasonographic changes after treatment for arteriovenous malformations. *Stroke* 21:260–266, 1990.
5. Harders AG, Gilsbach JM: Time course of blood velocity changes related to vasospasm in the circle of Willis measured by transcranial Doppler ultrasound. *J Neurosurg* 66:718–728, 1987.
6. Lindegaard KF, Nornes H, Bakke SJ, et al: Cerebral vasospasm diagnosis by means of angiography and blood velocity measurements. *Acta Neurochir (Wien)* 100:12–24, 1989.
7. Kushner MJ, Zanette EM, Bastianello S, et al: Transcranial Doppler in acute hemispheric brain infarctions. *Neurology* 41:109–113, 1991.
8. Giller CA: Transcranial Doppler monitoring of cerebral blood flow velocity during craniotomy. *Neurosurgery* 25:769–776, 1989.
9. Steiger HJ, Schaffler L, Boll J, Liechti S: Results of microsurgical endarterectomy: A prospective study with transcranial Doppler and EEG monitoring, and elective shunting. *Acta Neurochir (Wien)* 100:31–38, 1989.
10. Spencer MP, Whisler D: Transorbital Doppler diagnosis of intracranial arterial stenosis. *Stroke* 17:916–921, 1986.
11. Arnold BJ, von Reutern GM: Transcranial Doppler sonography: Examination techniques and normal reference values. *Ultrasound Med Biol* 12:115–123, 1986.
12. Berguer R, Hwang NHC: Critical arterial stenosis: A theoretical and experimental solution. *Ann Surg* 180:39–50, 1974.
13. May AG, de Weese JA, Robb CG: Hemodynamic effects of arterial stenosis. *Surgery* 53:513–524, 1963.
14. May AG, van de Berg L, de Weese JA, et al: Critical arterial stenosis. *Surgery* 54:250–258, 1963.
15. Markwalder TM, Grolimund P, Seiler RW, et al: Dependency of blood flow velocity in the middle cerebral artery on end-tidal carbon dioxide partial pressure—a transcranial Doppler ultrasound study. *J Cereb Blood Flow Metab* 4:368–372, 1984.
16. Kirkham FJ, Padayachee TS, Parsons S, et al: Transcranial measurement of blood velocities in the basal cerebral arteries using pulsed Doppler ultrasound: Velocity as an index of flow. *Ultrasound Med Biol* 12:15–21, 1986.
17. Bode H, Wais U: Age dependence of flow velocities in basal cerebral arteries. *Arch Dis Child* 63:606–611, 1988.
18. Grolimund P, Seiler RW: Age dependence of the flow velocity in the basal cerebral arteries—a transcranial Doppler ultrasound study. *Ultrasound Med Biol* 14:191–198, 1988.
19. Leenders KL, Perani D, Lammertsma AA, et al: Cerebral blood flow, blood volume and oxygen ultilization: Normal values and effect of age. *Brain* 113:27–47, 1990.
20. Matsuda H, Maeda T, Yamada M, et al: Age matched normal values and topographic maps for regional cerebral blood flow measurements by Xe-133 inhalation. *Stroke* 15:336–342, 1984.
21. Brass L, Pavlakis S, DeVivo D, et al: Transcranial Doppler measurements of the middle cerebral artery: Effect of hematocrit. *Stroke* 19:1466–1469, 1988.
22. Gosling RG, King DH: Continuous wave ultrasound as an alternative and complement to x-rays in vascular examinations, in Reman RE (ed): *Cardiovascular Applications of Ultrasound.* Amsterdam: North-Holland, 1974.
23. Martin NA, Doberstein C, Zane C: Posttraumatic cerebral arterial spasm: Transcranial Doppler ultrasound, cerebral blood flow, and angiographic findings. *J Neurosurg* 77:575–583, 1992.
24. Obrist WD, Langfitt TW, Jaggi JL, et al: Cerebral blood flow and metabolism in comatose patients with acute head injury: Relationship to intracranial hypertension. *J Neurosurg* 61:241–253, 1984.
25. Muizelaar JP: Cerebral blood flow, cerebral blood volume, and cerebral metabolism after severe head injury, in Becker DP, Gudeman SK (eds): *Textbook of Head Injury.* Philadelphia: Saunders, 1989: 221–240.
26. Bouma GJ, Muizelaar JP: Ultra-early evaluation of regional cerebral blood flow in severely-injured patients using xenon-enhanced computerized tomography. *J Neurosurg* 77:360–368, 1992.
27. Bruce DA, Alavi A, Bilaniuk L, et al: Diffuse cerebral swelling following head injury in children: The syndrome of "malignant brain edema." *J Neurosurg* 54:170–178, 1981.
28. Muizelaar JP, Ward JD, Marmarou A, et al: Cerebral blood flow and metabolism in severely head-injured children: 2. Autoregulation. *J Neurosurg* 71:72–76, 1989.
29. Sorteberg W, Lindegaard KF, Rootwelt K, et al: Blood velocity and regional blood flow in defined cerebral artery systems. *Acta Neurochir (Wien)* 97:47–52, 1989.
30. Bishop CCR, Powell S, Rutt D, Browse NL: Transcranial Doppler measurement of middle cerebral artery blood flow velocity: A validation study. *Stroke* 17:913–915, 1986.
31. Halsey JH, McDowell HA, Gelmon S, Morawetz RB: Blood velocity in the middle cerebral artery and regional cerebral blood flow during carotid endarterectomy. *Stroke* 20:53–58, 1989.
32. Zane CJ, Doberstein CE, Martin NA, et al: Prediction of cerebral blood flow using Doppler velocity measurements. *J Cereb Blood Flow Metab* 11:2, 1991.
33. Risberg J, Smith P: Prediction of hemispheric blood flow from carotid velocity measurements: A study with the Doppler and inhalational ^{133}Xe techniques. *Stroke* 11(4):399–402, 1980.
34. Aaslid R: Cerebral hemodynamics, in Newell DW, Aaslid R (eds): *Transcranial Doppler.* New York: Raven Press, 1992: 49–56.
35. Huber P, Haneda J: Effect of contrast material, hypercapnia, hyperventilation, hypertonic glucose and papaverine on the diameter of cerebral arteries—angiographic determination in man. *Invest Radiol* 2:17–32, 1967.
36. Enevoldsen EM, Jensen FT: Autoregulation and CO_2 responses of cerebral blood flow in patients with acute severe head injury. *J Neurosurg* 48:689–703, 1978.
37. Doberstein CE, Hovda DA, Becker DP: Clinical considerations in the reduction of secondary brain injury. *Ann Emerg Med* 22:993–997, 1993.
38. Aaslid R, Lindegaard KF, Sorteberg W, Nornes H: Cere-

bral autoregulation dynamics in humans. *Stroke* 20:45–52, 1989.
39. Aaslid R: Developments and principles of transcranial Doppler, in Newell DW, Aaslid R (eds): *Transcranial Doppler.* New York: Raven Press, 1992: 1–8.
40. Newell DW, Seiler RW, Aaslid R: Head injury and circulatory arrest, in Newell DW, Aaslid R (eds): *Transcranial Doppler.* New York: Raven Press, 1992: 109–122.
41. Lundar T, Lindegaard K-F, Nornes H: Continuous monitoring of middle cerebral artery blood velocity in clinical neurosurgery. *Acta Neurochir (Wien)* 102:85–90, 1990.
42. Overgaard J, Tweed TA: Cerebral circulation after head injury: I. Cerebral blood flow and its regulation after closed head injury with emphasis on clinical correlations. *J Neurosurg* 41:531–541, 1974.
43. Fieschi C, Battistini N, Beduschi A, et al: Regional cerebral blood flow and intraventricular pressure in acute head injuries. *J Neurol Neurosurg Psychiatry* 37:1378–1388, 1974.
44. Muizelaar JP, Wei EP, Kontos HA, et al: Mannitol causes compensatory vasoconstriction and vasodilation in response to blood viscosity changes. *J Neurosurg* 59:822–828, 1983.
45. Marion DW, Bouma GJ: The use of stable xenon-enhanced computed tomographic studies of cerebral blood flow to define changes in cerebral carbon dioxide vasoresponsivity caused by severe head injury. *Neurosurgery* 29:869–873, 1991.
46. Klingelhofer J, Sander D: Doppler CO_2 test as an indicator of cerebral vasoreactivity and prognosis in severe intracranial hemorrhages. *Stroke* 23:962–966, 1992.
47. Wilkins RH: Cerebral vasospasm in conditions other than subarachnoid hemorrhage. *Neurosurg Clin North Am* 1:329–334, 1990.
48. Wilkins RH, Odom GL: Intracranial arterial spasm associated with craniocerebral trauma. *J Neurosurg* 32:626–633, 1970.
49. Weber M, Grolimund P, Seiler RW: Evaluation of posttraumatic cerebral blood flow velocities by transcranial Doppler ultrasonography. *Neurosurgery* 27:106–112, 1990.
50. Newell DW, Winn HR: Transcranial Doppler in cerebral vasospasm. *Neurosurg Clin North Am* 1:319–328, 1990.
51. Lindegaard KF, Bakke SJ, Grolimund P, et al: Assessment of intracranial hemodynamics in carotid artery disease by transcranial Doppler ultrasound. *J Neurosurg* 63:890–898, 1985.
52. Sorteberg W, Langmoen IA, Lindegaard KF, Nornes H: Side-to-side differences and day-to-day variations of transcranial Doppler parameters in normal subjects. *J Ultrasound Med* 9:403–409, 1990.
53. Eisenberg HM, Gary HE, Aldrich EF, et al: Initial CT findings in 753 patients with severe head injury: A report from the NIH Traumatic Coma Data Bank. *J Neurosurg* 73:688–698, 1990.
54. Macpherson P, Graham DI: Correlation between angiographic findings and the ischemia of head injury. *J Neurol Neurosurg Psychiatry* 41:122–127, 1978.
55. Becker DP, Miller JD, Ward JD, et al: The outcome from severe head injury with early diagnosis and intensive management. *J Neurosurg* 47:491–502, 1977.
56. Marshall LF, Smith RW, Shapiro HM: The outcome with aggressive treatment in severe head injuries: I. The significance of intracranial pressure monitoring. *J Neurosurg* 50:20–25, 1979.
57. Miller JD, Becker DP, Ward JD, et al: Significance of intracranial hypertension in severe head injury. *J Neurosurg* 47:503–516, 1977.
58. Miller JD, Butterworth JF, Gudeman SK, et al: Further experience in the management of severe head injury. *J Neurosurg* 54:289–299, 1981.
59. Hassler W, Steinmetz H, Gawlowski J: Transcranial Doppler in raised intracranial pressure and in intracranial circulatory arrest. *J Neurosurg* 68:745–751, 1988.
60. Saunders FW, Cledgett P: Intracranial blood velocity in head injury: A transcranial ultrasound Doppler study. *Surg Neurol* 29:401–409, 1988.
61. Homburg AM, Jakobsen M, Enevoldsen E: Transcranial Doppler recordings in raised intracranial pressure. *Acta Neurol Scand* 87:488–493, 1993.
62. Kwan-Hon C, Miller JD, Dearden NM, et al: The effect of changes in cerebral perfusion pressure upon middle cerebral artery blood flow velocity and jugular bulb venous oxygen saturation after severe head injury. *J Neurosurg* 77:55–61, 1992.
63. Lindegaard K-F, Sorteberg W, Nornes H: Transcranial Doppler in neurosurgery. *Adv Tech Stand Neurosurg* 20:39–73, 1993.
64. Doberstein C, Martin NA, Zane C, et al: Prediction of intracranial pressure from Doppler ultrasonography. Presented at the 1991 annual meeting of the American Association of Neurological Surgeons, New Orleans, LA, 1990.
65. President's Commission: Guidelines for the determination of brain death. *JAMA* 246:2184–2187, 1981.
66. Newell DW, Grady S, Sirotta P, Winn HR: Evaluation of brain death using transcranial Doppler. *Neurosurgery* 24:509–513, 1989.
67. Petty GW, Mohr JP, Pedley TA, et al: The role of transcranial Doppler in confirming brain death: Sensitivity, specificity, and suggestions for performance and interpretation. *Neurology* 40:300–303, 1990.
68. Powers AD, Graeber MC, Smith RR: Transcranial Doppler ultrasonography in the determination of brain death. *Neurosurgery* 24:884–889, 1989.
69. Kirkham FJ, Levin SC, Padayachee TS, et al: Transcranial pulsed Doppler ultrasound findings in brainstem death. *J Neurol Neurosurg Psychiatry* 50:1504–1513, 1987.
70. Grote E, Hassler W: The critical first minutes after subarachnoid hemorrhage. *Neurosurgery* 22:654–661, 1988.
71. Pillay PK, Wilberger J: Transcranial Doppler evaluation of brain death (letter). *Neurosurgery* 25:482–483, 1989.
72. Ropper AH, Kehne SM, Weschler L: Transcranial Doppler in brain death. *Neurology* 37:1733–1735, 1987.

CHAPTER 38

CBF AND MANAGEMENT OF THE HEAD-INJURED PATIENT

J. Paul Muizelaar

SYNOPSIS

This chapter explains the relationships between cerebral blood flow, cerebral metabolism, and arterio-venous oxygen differences, and summarizes current understanding of how these parameters can be helpful in the management of patients with severe head injury. The frequency of cerebral ischemia in the first few hours after the injury is emphasized. The reasons for the current disenchantment with severe prophylactic hyperventilation are detailed. However, it is suggested that hyperventilation may be the treatment of choice in children with raised intracranial pressure.

INTRODUCTION

In the past decade a large body of data has become available that has deepened out insight into the pathophysiology of severe head injury and impacted on the management of its acute stage. Part of this new knowledge stems from randomized clinical trials and part from the careful analysis of data generated by new monitoring techniques, especially of cerebral blood flow (CBF) and metabolism. Although the conclusions drawn from these analyses regarding optimal management are logical, their effect on clinical outcome has not been tested in a rigorous fashion and thus the analyses should be regarded with caution.

RELATIONSHIPS BETWEEN CBF, CEREBRAL METABOLISM, AND CEREBRAL OXYGEN EXTRACTION

With regard to the following data, a few principles should be kept in mind. The first is that cerebral metabolism is almost entirely dependent on the oxidation of glucose and requires a constant supply of oxygen by cerebral blood flow. Thus,

$$CMRO_2 = CBF \times AVDO_2 \qquad (38\text{-}1)$$

where $CMRO_2$ is the cerebral metabolic rate of oxygen and $AVDO_2$ is the arteriovenous difference of oxygen. Under most circumstances $CMRO_2$ is constant at approximately 3.2 ml (of O_2)/100g (of brain tissue)/min[1]. $CMRO_2$ is much lower, but still constant, during coma and much higher during seizures. $AVDO_2$ is approximately 6.5 vol% (ml of O_2/100 ml of blood)[1] and the brain has a very strong tendency to keep this constant, independent of $CMRO_2$ or CBF. Thus, if we consider $AVDO_2$ as a constant in Equation (1), CBF will have to follow changes in $CMRO_2$ (metabolic autoregulation or metabolic coupling). However, owing to compensatory mechanisms under circumstances of constant $CMRO_2$, the CBF remains constant despite changes in perfusion pressure (pressure autoregulation)[2] or in blood viscosity (viscosity autoregulation).[3] This leads us to the second principle to be kept in mind, namely the factors that govern CBF:

$$CBF = K \frac{CPP \times d^4}{8 \times l \times v} \qquad (38\text{-}2)$$

where k is a constant, CPP is cerebral perfusion pressure (defined as mean arterial blood pressure [MABP] minus intracranial pressure (ICP)), d is diameter of blood vessels, 1 is the length of the blood vessels (which, of course, is practically constant), and v is blood viscosity. By far the most powerful factor in this equation is vessel diameter. For instance, the maximum constriction that can be obtained by hyperventilation is approximately 20 percent from normal baseline,[4] but this leads to a decrease in CBF of almost 60 percent from a normal value of 50 ml/100g/min to 20 ml/100g/min. It should be noted that practically all of this diameter regulation takes place in the microcirculation, especially in the arterioles that have a diameter of 300-μ down to 15 μ.[4,5] The interaction between diameter changes in the larger conducting arteries and changes in the microcirculation (which sometimes occur in opposite directions) and their relationship with $CMRO_2$, $AVDO_2$, and ICP are discussed elsewhere,[6] and are summarized in Table 38-1.

The third important factor to be kept in mind is that whereas in both metabolic and pressure autoregulation the vessel diameter changes are compensatory responses which maintain a constant $AVDO_2$, in CO_2 responsivity the diameter changes are primary and CBF and $AVDO_2$ will follow passively. Thus, CO_2 reactivity differs from any type of autoregulation in that the $AVDO_2$ changes, and that it is not some sort of adaptation response of the brain to changing circumstances. Whereas the "purpose" of autoregulation can be quite obvious, e.g., protect the brain against the occurrence of ischemia during shock, the physiological "purpose" of CO_2 reactivity is unclear.

TABLE 38-1 Changes in Cerebral Blood Flow (CBF), Cerebral Blood Volume (CBV), and Arteriovenous Difference of Oxygen ($AVDO_2$) with Primary Reduction in the Cerebral Metabolic Rate of Oxygen ($CMRO_2$), Cerebral Perfusion Pressure (CPP), blood viscosity, $PaCO_2$, and with Vasospasm

Primary Reduction	CBF	CBV	$AVDO_2$
$CMRO_2$	↓	↓	=
CPP (autoregulation intact)	=	↑	=
CPP (autoregulation defective)	↓	↓	↑
Blood viscosity (autoregulation intact)	=	↓	=
Blood viscosity (autoregulation defective)	↑	=	↓
Pa_{CO_2}	↓	↓	↑
Conductance vessel diameter ("vasospasm")	↓	↑	↑

TABLE 38-2 Time Course of Regional Ischemia*

Time of Study	Total	Regional Ischemia	No Ischemia
0.7–4 Hours	58	16 (28%)	42 (72%)
4–8 Hours	15	3 (20%)	12 (80%)
8–24 Hours	29	0 (0%)	29 (100%)

* Regional ischemia = cerebral blood flow of ≤ 18 ml/100g/min in one entire lobe or basal ganglia or brain stem.

EARLY POSTINJURY ISCHEMIA

It had been suspected for a long time that cerebral ischemia, defined as CBF not being able to meet the metabolic demands of the brain tissue, played an important role after severe head injury. This suspicion was based, for the most part, on autopsy findings of histological damage indicative of cerebral ischemia in 80 percent of patients who died following severe head injury, even though most of those patients had an adequate CPP during the period in which this was monitored.[7] However, in a large number of studies in which CBF was measured intermittently, flow values below the threshold of ischemia (usually taken as 18 ml/100g/min)[8] were hardly ever found.[9–17]

Moreover, in the first study to report on a sizeable number of $AVDO_2$ measurements, critically high values of $AVDO_2$ indicative of ischemia were also extremely rare.[17] We speculated, however, that most of these measurements were not obtained early enough after injury, and the preliminary data supporting this view were published in 1984.[18] Later, we presented results of measurements of CBF in 186 adult patients, using the ^{133}Xe technique in the intensive care unit (ICU).[19] These data are summarized in Table 38-2. Although the average $AVDO_2$ in the first few hours was 7.1 vol%, it should be noted that in those head-injured patients in poor clinical condition (Glasgow Coma Score 3 and 4),[20] it

TABLE 38-3 Initial CT Findings and Incidence of Regional Ischemia*

CT Findings	No. of Cases	Ischemia (%)
Epidural hematoma	5	0
Subdural hematoma	22	41
Focal contusions	36	6
Diffuse swelling	16	50
Normal	13	0

* Regional ischemia = cerebral blood flow of ≤ 18 ml/100g/min in one entire lobe or basal ganglia or brain stem.

TABLE 38-4 Outcome Modalities of Patients with and without Regional Ischemia*

	Regional Ischemia		*No Ischemia*	
Outcome	**48 Hours**	**6 Months**	**48 Hours**	**6 Months**
Dead	14	14	4	17
Comatose	5	2	57	5
Awake	0	3	11	45

* Regional ischemia = cerebral blood flow of less or equal than 18 ml/100g/min in one entire lobe or basal ganglia or brain stem.

was 8 vol%, thus indicating cerebral ischemia.[19] Obviously, the incidence of ischemia very rapidly diminishes over time; since the earliest measurements with ^{133}Xe were done at 4 hours post-injury, the question as to what the situation would be even earlier after injury remained unanswered from that study. Moreover, no patients with intracranial mass lesions, in whom the highest incidence of ischemia could be expected, were included in the study.

Using the stable Xenon-CT technique, CBF can now be calculated during the initial diagnostic CT scan. Patients with mass lesions still *in situ* can also be studied with this technique, but the additional 10 to 30 minutes needed for the CBF study leads to an under-representation of those with very large lesions causing major brain shift or those with ominous clinical signs such as pupillary abnormalities, because these patients are taken to the operating room without the slightest delay. Results from stable Xenon-CT scanning in 32 patients were presented and extensively discussed earlier,[21] but this initial series has now been expanded to 92 patients, whose data are shown in Tables 38-3, 38-4, and 38-5. It should be noted that all 92 patients, including the 32 discussed earlier,[21] are represented in these tables, except for the 6-months outcome data in Table 38-5, which were not yet available for all subjects. It can be assumed, however, that the number of comatose and awake patients will increase but that proportion between the two will remain about the same, while the proportion of dead patients will drop because most deaths occur within 2 to 3 months after injury. The following conclusions can be drawn:

1. Cerebral ischemia is a very early event after severe head injury and becomes less common after operative evacuation of mass lesions.[22]
2. Acute subdural hematoma and diffuse cerebral swelling (absence of basal cisterns) are the CT diagnoses most often associated with cerebral ischemia. The low incidence of ischemia with epidural hematoma is most likely due to the fact that in patients with urgent indication for operation CBF was not measured.
3. The prognosis for patients with ischemia is extremely poor.

Although it has been argued that our definition of ischemia (CBF < 18 ml/100g/min) would not necessarily indicate insufficient cerebral perfusion, but might be a normal adjustment of CBF to extremely low $CMRO_2$ (coupling of CBF and $CMRO_2$)[23], we feel that our early high $AVDO_2$ values argue against such a position[24] and that measures should be taken at least not to aggravate ischemia and rather to possibly prevent or treat it altogether.

TABLE 38-5 Cerebral Blood Flow and Arteriovenous Blood Oxygen Differences in Head-Injured Patients Measured at 6-Hour Intervals Postinjury*

Hours Post-injury	CBF (ml/100gm/min)	$AVDO_2$ (ml/100 ml)	No. of Cases	No. (%) with Ischemia
4–6	22.5 ± 5.2†	7.1 ± 1.5™	12	4 (33%)
6–12	29.0 ± 10.0	6.3 ± 2.5™	74	8 (11%)
12–18	33.3 ± 11.0	4.7 ± 1.6	50	0 (0%)
18–24	34.8 ± 11.4	4.7 ± 1.6	37	2 (5%)
24–30	33.9 ± 10.4	4.4 ± 2.4	29	1 (3%)
30–36	33.2 ± 12.0	4.6 ± 1.4	23	1 (4%)
36–42	36.9 ± 12.7	4.2 ± 1.7	19	1 (5%)
42–48	34.8 ± 14.7	3.9 ± 1.1	11	0 (0%)
>48	33.6 ± 12.2	4.4 ± 1.6	129	7 (5%)

* CBF = Cerebral blood flow; $AVDO_2$ = arteriovenous difference of oxygen content. Ischemia is defined as CBF ≤ 18 ml/100gm/min.
† Significantly lower than values at all later time intervals (Newman-Keuls' test, $p < 0.05$).
™ $AVDO_2$ values in the first 12 hours postinjury were significantly higher than values of later intervals (Newman-Keuls' test, $p < 0.05$).
Adapted from Bouma et al.[19] with permission.

MANAGEMENT OF EARLY ISCHEMIA

It is not practical under most circumstances to measure CBF during the first diagnostic CT scan, and this should be considered research, albeit with very practical applications. Moreover, the other method to detect cerebral ischemia, i.e., determination of $AVDO_2$ or $SjvO_2$ (saturation of jugular venous oxygen, see below), is also not easily accomplished during the first few hours postinjury, exactly at the time that ischemia most frequently occurs. Thus, we should simply assume that cerebral ischemia is present, until proved otherwise. The principles to treat this by improving CBF can easily be grasped by considering Equation (2), and some of these treatments are clearly in contrast with earlier teachings, when most emphasis was placed on diminishing ICP and prevention of brain edema. The first factor in Equation (2) that can be manipulated to raise CBF is CPP, determined by MABP and ICP. Of course, rapid evacuation of intracranial mass lesions to decrease ICP and thus improve CPP is still the cornerstone of early efforts to improve CBF and prognosis, and is widely accepted to be effective.[22,25,26] Another means of decreasing ICP is by diminishing cerebral blood volume (CBV), which can be accomplished with hyperventilation. CO_2 reactivity is usually intact after severe head injuries, albeit diminished in the first few hours.[27] However, despite the increase in CPP, CBF practically always goes down with hyperventilation,[17,27] owing to the fact that vessel diameter in Equation (2) is to the fourth power. Moreover, we have shown that *preventive hyperventilation retards clinical improvement* after severe head injury,[28] although we do not want to imply here that that occurs because of induction or aggravation of early ischemia. Finally, Obrist has published data showing that in a severely head injured patient with a low CBF and a low $AVDO_2$ (and thus a low $CMRO_2$) (further) hyperventilation leads to further decrease in CBF with concomitant rise in $AVDO_2$.[29] However, in a number of patients, the relative rise in $AVDO_2$ was larger than the relative decrease in CBF, resulting in a paradoxical and unexplained increase in $CMRO_2$. Whether this increased $CMRO_2$ with hyperventilation is an improvement is debatable and, in fact, we feel it is detrimental. Suppression of $CMRO_2$ early after injury by inducing mild hypothermia may lead to improved outcome, as has been shown by Marion and co-workers.[30] Taken together, unless there is a unilateral pupillary abnormality, we advocate normocapnia early after severe head injury, although impaired pulmonary function often forces us to use mild hyperventilation ($Pa_{CO_2} \simeq 35$ mmHg) in order to maintain optimal arterial oxygenation.

Another way of increasing CPP would be by raising MABP. In the past, and also recently, it has been advocated to treat the arterial hypertension that often accompanies severe head injuries, mostly in the hope of diminishing cerebral edema caused by blood-brain barrier breakdown.[31–33] However, there are no data to indicate that the blood-brain barrier is indeed defective after severe head injury, and we actually have data indicating the contrary, except in cases of contusions (unpublished data, Marmarou A and Muizelaar JP). Moreover, treating arterial hypertension under these circumstances has not been put to the test in any clinical trial, and it is almost certain to aggravate (borderline) cerebral ischemia if present—which is 30 to 50 percent of the time. Therefore, we consider arterial hypertension early postinjury as a physiological response to cerebral ischemia (Cushing response) until otherwise proved and should best be left alone. It should be emphasized here, however, that such a management policy is based solely on interpretation of early CBF, $AVDO_2$, and $CMRO_2$ data and has also not been put to the test in any rigorous fashion.

The treatment of hypotension is a completely different matter. If autoregulation is defective, CBF is directly and linearly related to blood pressure; if autoregulation is intact, arterial hypotension can lead to considerable increase in ICP.[34,35] Thus, depending on the status of autoregulation, maintaining a normal blood pressure or inducing some arterial hypertension can lead to improved CBF or diminished ICP or both.[18,19,34–39] A final way to influence CBF is by manipulating blood viscosity, which is also linearly related to CBF. Thus, when ischemia and viscosity autoregulation are absent,[3] we can double the prevailing CBF by slashing blood viscosity in half. The latter occurs when hematocrit (Hct) is reduced from 45 to 50 percent to 30 to 33 percent, although this reduction also leads to a decrease in arterial oxygen content by 30 percent. However, doubling the flow of blood with only 70 percent of the oxygen still leads to an increase of 40 percent in total oxygen delivery, and therefore we always aim to maintain Hct between 30 and 35 percent. Reductions of Hct below 30 percent do not result in much further viscosity change while oxygen content falls precipitously. Through its effect on Hct and also on erythrocyte volume and deformability, mannitol has a considerable beneficial influence on blood viscosity.[40] Combined with its cerebral dehydrating effect, mannitol therefore either diminishes ICP or increases CBF or both, with the balance between the two effects partly dependent on the status of autoregulation. When we consider that mannitol is also a scavenger of the hydroxyl anion oxygen radical species and consider the role of oxgyen radicals after severe head injury,[41] the generous use of mannitol can be easily justified, especially early after injury when raised blood osmolality is of no concern as yet.

SUBACUTE POSTINJURY CEREBRAL ISCHEMIA OR HYPOXIA: MONITORING

With most established techniques for CBF measurements, such as nitrous oxide clearance, ^{133}Xe clearance or stable Xe-CT scanning, it is impossible to monitor CBF continuously and impractical to even do this frequently. Thermodilution CBF monitoring is a technique yielding continuous data,[42,43] but it demands that an epicortical probe be left behind at surgery or implanted in a separate procedure, while it also only gives very local CBF values and its usefulness after severe head injury has not been established.[44] Blood velocity measurement with transcranial Doppler (TCD) ultrasound is a noninvasive, easily applied technique that can give some indication of CBF, especially when the Lindegaard index[45] is used; and Martin et al. have shown that TCD is useful for the detection of ischemia caused by cerebral arterial vasospasm.[46] However, vasospasm as the primary cause for ischemia appears to be uncommon, and when it occurs, can be detected with $SjvO_2$ monitoring (see below).

The search for a continuous monitor for the adequacy of cerebral oxygenation has led to the introduction of measuring the oxygen saturation of venous blood in the jugular bulb.[47–49] When one considers Equation (1) and assumes that $CMRO_2$ remains unchanged with sufficient oxygen supply, $AVDO_2$ can be used as an estimate of CBF.[50] Venous oxygen content, in turn, can be estimated from oxygen saturation, which can be measured continuously with a fiberoptic catheter similar to that used for umbilical vein monitoring in the newborn (Oximetrics, Abbott Labs), but now introduced in the jugular vein and placed retrograde in the jugular bulb. A good correlation between *changes* in $SjvO_2$ and CBF has also been described.[51] When saturation is low (generally considered low when $SjvO_2 < 50–55$ percent), this means that $AVDO_2$ is abnormally high, indicative of ischemia, unless arterial saturation is also very low, or (arterial) hemoglobin level is very low. Whatever the case may be, $SjvO_2$ monitoring can tell whether oxygen supply to the brain is matched with metabolism; if it is low, the cause for this mismatch must be found (after checking and calibration of the catheter) and corrected.

TABLE 38-6 Jugular Desaturation <50% in 116 Patients

Systemic Causes	
Hypocarbia	21
Hypotension	8
Aterial Hypoxia	6
Anemia	1
Cerebral Causes	
Intracranial Hypertension	34
Cerebral Vasospasm	1
Combination of Systemic and Cerebral Causes	6
Total Number	77

* Adapted from Gopinath et al.[51] with permission.

Others have defined jugular bulb desaturation as $SjvO_2 < 50$ percent for 5 minutes or longer, and we have adopted these guidelines as well. When this occurs, one should first check the light intensity of the fiberoptic device. In a very large number of cases, light intensity is too low because the catheter is lodged against the wall of the blood vessel. Simply by rotating the patient's head slightly or wiggling the catheter a little, this can be corrected. If the light intensity is sufficient or if the above-mentioned measures are insufficient, one should draw a blood sample through the catheter, together with an arterial sample, to calibrate the device. In general, the correlation between the apparatus' reading and the actual blood gases is very good, but for an in-depth discussion of the validity and representativeness of the jugular bulb oxygen tension, the reader is referred to the article by Stocchetti et al.[52] An important point, not discussed in that article, is that the number of "false alarms" with this monitoring technique is high (>50 percent, CS Robertson, personal communication), but the number of missed periods of ischemia appears to be extremely low or nonexistent. Thus, no false sense of security is induced, but at the cost of frequent "unnecessary" checks.

Recently, the Baylor College of Medicine group has

TABLE 38-7 Jugular Desaturation <50% in 116 Patients*

No. of Desaturation	Good Recovery/ Moderate Disability	Severe Disability Vegetative	Dead
0	45%	39%	16%
1	26%	32%	42%
Multiple	10%	20%	70%

* Relationship between confirmed episodes of jugular desaturation and outcome at 3 months in 116 patients. (*Adapted from Gopinath et al.[51] with permission).

provided an update on their experience with $SjvO_2$ monitoring.[51] As noted above, desaturations were defined as $SjvO_2 < 50$ percent for at least 5 minutes and confirmed with a jugular blood sample measurement. Most of these desaturations took place during the first 48 hours of monitoring and did not last much longer than 15 minutes because corrective measures were successful. An exception was the desaturation due to high ICP, which generally occurred later (up to 7 days) and would last much longer as high ICP was sometimes intractable.

Table 38-6 indicates the reasons for jugular bulb desaturations, and in Table 38-7, generated by the same group, the strong correlation between the number of desaturations per patient and poor outcome is clearly depicted.

MANAGEMENT OF SUBACUTE POST-INJURY CEREBRAL ISCHEMIA OR HYPOXIA

Depending on the cause for the desaturation, appropriate therapeutic action can be taken. When too vigorous hyperventilation is present, the CO_2 can be allowed to rise, or, if hypocapnia is still necessary for ICP control, it can be combined with mannitol so as to both decrease ICP and stimulate CBF.[53] Gopinath et al.[51] also described how the use of a diuretic (furosemide) leads to hypotension secondary to hypovolemia with low central venous pressure (CVP), resulting in desaturation. This could be corrected by rapid administration of fluids such as albumin solution, rather than by using an alpha-adrenergic drug to raise the blood pressure. For some other causes of desaturation, the treatment is quite obvious: give blood for anemia, adjust ventilator settings for arterial hypoxia, and raise the blood pressure for vasospasm (similar to treatment of vasospasm with subarachnoid hemorrhage[36]). Maintaining CPP over 70 mmHg, even if ICP cannot be kept below 20 mmHg, by raising the MABP ("CPP management") as proposed by Rosner and Daughton,[54] probably is also beneficial through its prevention of jugular bulb desaturations. Again, in practice, this is accomplished in the same way as vasospasm after SAH is treated: maintain good volume status with ample fluids including albumin solution to keep CVP at 10 to 15 cm H_2O, and use an alpha-adrenergic drug to induce hypertension. There are data supporting the use of albumin 25–50 ml/hr over other colloid solutions,[55] while we prefer phenylephrine (Neo-Synephrine) 80 mg/250 or 500 ml normal saline for reasons explained elsewhere.[36] However, CPP management has not been subjected to a randomized trial to prove its beneficial effect. Nevertheless, along with other changes in treatment based on measurements of CBF, $AVDO_2$, $CMRO_2$ and $SjvO_2$, CPP management has taken its place in our armamentarium to improve outcome.[55a]

CONSIDERATION OF CBF IN THE HEAD-INJURED CHILD

It has been proposed that the relationship between ICP and CBF is even more important in children than in adults.[56,57] In children, elevated ICP is caused mainly by increased cerebral blood volume (CBV). Increased CBV, in turn, is believed to be secondary to hyperemia. Diminished Pa_{CO_2} will lead to diminished CBF by vasoconstriction, so that high ICP can be treated almost exclusively with vigorous hyperventilation. This treatment was held responsible for the exceptionally good results reported by Bruce et al.[56,57] On the other hand, these authors dismissed the use of mannitol to treat high ICP in children, as this agent had been found by the same group of investigators to increase CBF in a number of patients with brain injury.[10] However, several objections to their interpretation can be made. First, from Table 38-1 it can be seen that mannitol, in the absence of autoregulation, indeed raises CBF, but this is *not* accompanied by a rise in CBV; thus, mannitol will still decrease ICP by its dehydrating effect. Secondly, Bruce et al. had performed CBF measurements in only six children.[56,57] We later published data on a series of 32 children;[6,58] within 24 hours post-injury, only a single child had CBF in the range of "absolute hyperemia" according to the criteria of Obrist et al. (CBF above mean + 2 SD of normal adults),[17] and actually the average flow in all the children was below the "normal" value in this time period. After 24 hours there were indeed three children with high flows (80 to 116 ml/100g/min), but the majority were still in the range of relative hyperemia (average ± 2 SD from normal young adults). Moreover, no correlation could be established[6] between CBF and ICP or a measure of intracranial compliance, the pressure volume index (PVI).[59,60] Third, the normative data for CBF were derived from young adults. However, in a series of 125 normal children ranging in age from 4 days to 15 years, Susuki found that CBF starts around 40 ml/100g/min, rises to 65 ml/100g/min at 6 months, 80 ml/100g/min at 1 year, reaches a peak of 108 ml/100g/min between 2 and 4 years, and then slowly declines again to 85 ml/100g/min at age 8 years and 70 ml/100g/min at 14 years.[61] Thus, relative hyperemia is extremely uncommon in children. This was recently confirmed in another larger series of severely head-injured children in whom measurements of CBF, $AVDO_2$, and $CMRO_2$ were perfomed.[62,63] Fourth, as pointed out earlier, the relationship between CBF and CBV is not at all linear under most circumstances.[6]

In spite of all the above, it must be stated that indeed $AVDO_2$ is usually very low in the brain-injured child and that hyperventilation actually is a good and safe means of controlling ICP in this population. Nevertheless, we feel that the same safeguards should be used as in adults, of which monitoring of jugular oxygen saturation is the most important. Only with a thorough knowledge and understanding of the normal physiology and of the pathophysiology of the brain can the best results be obtained.[35]

ACKNOWLEDGMENTS

Many of the studies mentioned in this manuscript were supported by NIH Grants #NS-12587, 154600-1758-A1 and NS29412-02 and the Lind Lawrence Fund. Large parts of this manuscript were published earlier in the *Journal of Neurosurgery* and the *Canadian Journal of Neurological Sciences*.

REFERENCES

1. Kety SS, Schmidt CF: Effects of altered arterial tensions of carbon dioxide and oxygen on cerebral blood flow and cerebral oxygen consumption of normal young men. *J Clin Invest* 1948; 27:484–492.
2. McHenry LC, West JW, Cooper ES, et al: Cerebral autoregulation in man. *Stroke* 1974; 5:695–706.
3. Muizelaar JP, Wei EP, Kontos HA, Becker DP: Cerebral blood flow is regulated by changes in blood pressure and in blood viscosity alike. *Stroke* 1986; 17:44–48.
4. Kontos HA, Raper AJ, Patterson JL: Analysis of local pH, pCO_2, and bicarbonate in pial vessels. *Stroke* 1977; 8:358–360.
5. Kontos HA, Wei EP, Navari RM, et al: Responses of cerebral arteries and arterioles to acute hypotension and hypertension. *Ann J Physiol* 1978; 234:H371–H383.
6. Muizelaar JP, Marmarou A, DeSalles AAF, et al: Cerebral blood flow and metabolism in severely head-injured children. Part I: Relation with GCS, outcome, ICP and PVI. *J Neurosurg* 1989; 71:63–71.
7. Adams JH, Graham DI. The pathology of blunt head injury, in Critchley M, O'Leary JL, Jennett B (eds): *Scientific Foundations of Neurology*. London: Heinemann, 1972:488–491.
8. Jones TH, Morawetz RB, Crowell RM, et al: Thresholds of focal cerebral ischemia in awake monkeys. *J Neurosurg* 1981; 54:773–782.
9. Kasoff SS, Zingesser LH, Shulman K: Compartmental abnormalities of regional cerebral blood flow in children with head trauma. *J Neurosurg* 1972; 36:463–470.
10. Bruce DA, Langfitt TW, Miller JD, et al: Regional cerebral blood flow, intracranial pressure and brain metabolism in comatose patients. *J Neurosurg* 1973; 38:131–144.
11. Fieschi C, Battistini N, Beduschi A, et al: Regional cerebral blood flow and intraventricular pressure in acute head injuries. *J Neurol Neurosurg Psychiatry* 1974; 37:1378–1388.
12. Overgaard J, Tweed WA: Cerebral circulation after head injury. Part I: CBF and its regulation after closed head injury with emphasis on clinical correlations. *J Neurosurg* 1974; 41:531–541.
13. Enevoldsen EM, Cold GE, Jensen FT, Malmros R: Dynamic changes in regional cerebral blood flow, intraventricular pressure, cerebrospinal fluid pH and lactate levels during the acute phase of head injury. *J Neurosurg* 1976;44:191–214.
14. Enevoldsen EM, Jensen FT: Compartmental analysis of regional cerebral blood flow in patients with severe head injuries. *J Neurosurg* 1977; 47:699–712.
15. Obrist WD, Gennarelli TA, Segawa H, et al: Relation of cerebral blood flow to neurological status and outcome in head-injured patients. *J Neurosurg* 1979; 51:292–300.
16. Overgaard J, Mosdal C, Tweed WA: Cerebral circulation after head injury. Part 3: Does reduced regional CBF determine recovery of brain function after blunt head injury? *J Neurosurg* 1981; 55:63–74.
17. Obrist WD, Langfitt TW, Jaggi JL, et al: Cerebral blood flow metabolism in comatose patients with acute head injury. *J Neurosurg* 1984; 61:241–253.
18. Muizelaar JP, Becker DP, Lutz HA, Newlon PG: Cerebral ischemia after severe head injury: Its role in determining clinical status and its possible treatment, in Villani R (ed): *Advances in Neurotraumatology*. Amsterdam: Excerpta Medica, 1984:92–98.
19. Bouma GJ, Muizelaar JP, Choi SC, et al: Cerebral blood flow and metabolism after severe traumatic brain injury: The elusive role of ischemia. *J Neurosurg* 1991; 75(5):685–693.
20. Teasdale GM, Jennett B: Assessment of coma and impaired consciousness. A practical scale. *Lancet* 1974; 2:81–84.
21. Bouma GJ, Muizelaar JP, Stringer WA, et al: Ultra-early evaluation of regional cerebral blood flow in severely head-injured patients using stable xenon-enhanced computerized tomography. *J Neurosurg* 1992; 77:360–368.
22. Schröder ML, Muizelaar JP, Kuta AJ: Reversal of global ischemia after removal of an acute subdural hematoma documented with cerebral blood flow and cerebral blood volume measurement. *J Neurosurg* 1994; 80:324–327.
23. Cruz J: Brain ischemia in head injury. *J Neurosurg* 1993; 78:522–523 (letter).
24. Muizelaar JP: Brain ischemia in head injury. *J Neurosurg* 1993; 78:521 (letter).
25. Becker DP, Miller JD, Ward JD, et al: The outcome from

severe head injury with early diagnosis and intensive management. *J Neurosurg* 1977; 47:491–502.
26. Seelig JM, Greenberg RP, Becker DP: Traumatic acute subdural hematoma; major mortality reduction in comatose patients treated under four hours. *N Engl J Med* 1981; 304:1511–1518.
27. Marion DW, Bouma GJ: The use of stable xenon-enhanced computed tomography studies of cerebral blood flow to define changes in cerebral carbon dioxide vasoresponsitivity caused by severe head injury. *Neurosurgery* 1991; 29(6):869–873.
28. Muizelaar JP, Marmarou A, Ward JD, et al: Adverse effects of prolonged hyperventilation in patients with severe head injury: A randomized clinical trial. *J Neurosurg* 1991; 75:731–739.
29. Obrist WD, Clifton GL, Robertson CS, Langfitt TW: Cerebral metabolic changes induced by hyperventilation in acute head injury, in Meyer JS (ed): *Cerebral Vascular Disease 6.* Amsterdam: Elsevier, 1987:251–255.
30. Marion W, Obrist WD, Carlier PM, et al: The use of moderate therapeutic hypothermia for patients with severe head injuries: a preliminary report. *J Neurosurg* 1993;79:354–362.
31. Marshall WJS, Jackson JLF, Langfitt TW: Brain swelling caused by trauma and arterial hypertension. *Arch Neurol* 1969; 21:545–553.
32. Simard JM, Bellefleur M: Systemic arterial hypertension in head trauma. *Am J Cardiol* 1989; 63:32C–35C.
33. Robertson CS, Clifton GL, Taylor AP, Grossman RG: Treatment of hypertension associated with head injury. *J Neurosurg* 1983; 59:455–461.
34. Muizelaar JP, Lutz HA, Becker DP: Effect of mannitol on ICP and CBF and correlation with pressure autoregulation in severely head injured patients. *J Neurosurg* 1984; 61:700–706.
35. Bouma GJ, Muizelaar JP, Bandoh K, Marmarou A: Blood pressure and intracranial pressure-volume dynamics in severe head injury: Relationship with cerebral blood flow. *J Neurosurg* 1992; 77:15–19.
36. Muizelaar JP, Becker DP: Induced hypertension for the treatment of cerebral ischemia after subarachnoid hemorrhage. Direct effect on CBF. *Surg Neurol* 1986; 25:317–325.
37. Muizelaar JP: Induced arterial hypertension in the treatment of high ICP, in Hoff JT, Betz AL (eds): *Intracranial Pressure VII.* Heidelberg: Springer-Verlag, 1989; 508–509.
38. Bruce DA, Schutz H, Vapalahti M, Langfitt TW: Pitfalls in the interpretation of xenon CBF studies in head-injured patients, in Langfitt TW, McHenry LC, Reivich M, Wollman H (eds): *Cerebral Circulation and Metabolism.* Berlin: Springer-Verlag, 1975:406–408.
39. Muizelaar JP, Wei EP, Kontos HA, Becker DP: Mannitol causes compensatory vasoconstriction and vasodilation in response to blood viscosity changes. *J Neurosurg* 1983; 59:822–828.
40. Burke AM, Quest DO, Chien S, et al: The effects of mannitol on blood viscosity. *J Neurosurg* 1981; 55:550–553.
41. Muizelaar JP, Marmarou A, Young HF, et al: Improving the outcome of severe head injury with the oxygen free radical scavenger PEG-SOD. A phase II trial. *J Neurosurg* 1992; 78:375–382.
42. Carter LP, Erspamer R, Bro WJ: Cortical blood flow: Thermal diffusion vs. isotope clearance. *Stroke* 1981; 12:513–518.
43. Dickman CA, Carter LP, Baldwin MZ, et al: Continuous blood flow monitoring and intracranial pressure monitoring in acute craniocerebral trauma. *Neurosurgery* 1991; 28:467–472.
44. Schröder ML, Muizelaar JP: Monitoring of regional cerebral blood flow (CBF) in acute head injury by thermal diffusion. *Acta Neurochir (Wien)* 1993(Suppl); 59:47–49.
45. Lindegaard KF, Nornes H, Bakke SJ, et al: Cerebral vasospasm diagnosis by means of angiography and blood velocity measurements. *Acta Neurochir* 1989; 100:12–24.
46. Martin NA, Doberstein C, Zane C, et al: Posttraumatic cerebral arterial spasm: Transcranial Doppler ultrasound, cerebral blood flow, and angiographic findings. *J Neurosurg* 1992; 77:575–583.
47. Cruz J: Continuous versus serial global cerebral hemometabolic monitoring: Applications in acute brain trauma. *Acta Neurochir* 42:35–39, 1988.
48. Cruz J, Miner ME, Allen SJ, et al: Continuous monitoring of cerebral oxygenation in acute brain injury: Assessment of cerebral hemodynamic reserve. *Neurosurgery* 1991; 29:743–749.
49. Sheinberg M, Kanter MJ, Robertson CS, et al: Continuous monitoring of jugular venous oxygen saturation in head-injured patients. *J Neurosurg* 1992; 76:212–217.
50. Robertson CS, Narayan RK, Gokaslan ZL, et al: Cerebral arterial oxygen difference as an estimate of cerebral blood flow in comatose patients. *J Neurosurg* 1989; 70:222–230.
51. Gopinath SP, Robertson CS, Contant CF, et la. Transient jugular venous desaturation and outcome after head injury. *J Neurol Neurosurg Psychiatry.* 1994; 57:717–723.
52. Stocchetti N, Paparella A, Bridelli F: Cerebral venous oxygen saturation studied with bilateral samples in the internal jugular veins. *Neurosurgery* 1994; 34:38–44.
53. Cruz J, Miner ME, Allen SJ, et al: Continuous monitoring of cerebral oxygenation in acute brain injury: Injection of mannitol during hyperventilation. *J Neurosurg* 1990; 73:725–730.
54. Rosner MJ, Daughton S: Cerebral perfusion pressure management in head injury. *J Trauma* 1990; 30:933–941.
55. Trumble ER, Muizelaar JP, Myseros JS, et al: Coagulopathy and morbidity with the use of hetastarch in the treatment of aneurysmal vasospasm. *J Neurosurg* 1995;82:44–47.
55a. Rosner MJ, Rosner SD, Johnson AH: Cerebral perfusion pressure: management protocol and clinical results. *J Neurosurgery* 1995; 83:949–962.
56. Bruce DA, Alavi A, Bilaniuk L, et al: Diffuse cerebral swelling following head injuries in children: The syndrome of "malignant brain edema." *J Neurosurg* 1981; 54:170–178.
57. Bruce DA, Raphaely RC, Goldberg AI, et al: Pathophys-

iology, treatment and outcome following severe head injury in children. *Childs Brain* 1979; 5:174–191.
58. Muizelaar JP, Ward JD, Marmarou A, et al: Cerebral blood flow and metabolism in severely head injured children. Part 2: Autoregulation. *J Neurosurg* 1989; 71:72–76.
59. Marmarou A, Shulman K, Rosende RM: A nonlinear analysis of the cerebrospinal fluid system and intracranial pressure dynamics. *J Neurosurg* 1978; 48:332–344.
60. Maset AL, Marmarou A, Ward JD, et al: Pressure-volume index in head injury. *J Neurosurg* 1987; 67:832–840.
61. Susuki K: The changes of regional cerebral blood flow with advancing age in normal children. *Nagoya Med J* 1990; 34:159–170.
62. Sharples PM, Stuart AG, Matthews DSF, et al: Cerebral blood flow and metabolism in severely head injured children. Part 1: Relationship to age, Glasgow coma score, outcome, intracranial pressure and time after injury. *J Neurol Neurosurg Psychiatry* 1995; 58:145–152.
63. Sharples PM, Stuart AG, Matthews DSF, et al: Cerebral blood flow and metabolism in severely head injured children. Part 2: Cerebrovascular resistance and determinants. *J Neurol Neurosurg Psychiatry* 1995; 58:153–159.

CHAPTER 39

ELECTROPHYSIOLOGICAL MONITORING IN HEAD INJURY

Pauline G. Newlon

SYNOPSIS

In traumatic brain injury, standard EEG studies are the most useful method for determining brain death. Although quantitative methods of EEG analysis hold future promise, at present the most useful electrophysiological tests for severely head-injured patients are sensory evoked potentials. These tests provide important diagnostic and prognostic information early after injury in unconscious patients. Severe abnormalities in early-latency auditory and somatosensory potentials can pinpoint significant subcortical damage. However, middle- and long-latency hemispheric potentials must be included in any evoked potential test battery in which a complete evaluation of the severity and extent of brain dysfunction is desired. Early-latency potentials are the most reliably recorded, but it is likely that hemispheric evoked potentials are the most sensitive monitors of brain function for the prevention of secondary insults in the intensive care setting.

INTRODUCTION

The application of electrophysiological techniques to the diagnosis, prognosis, and monitoring of patients suffering traumatic brain injury (TBI) has intuitive appeal, since these techniques yield a direct measure of brain function in patients whose neurological status might otherwise be difficult to evaluate. Indeed, reports of EEG findings in head-injured patients date back to the 1940s.[1] During the 1970s, the performance of evoked potential (EP) studies in these patients became feasible when the difficulties of electrical recording in an intensive care environment were surmounted. Reports then emerged suggesting that EP results could improve the diagnosis of the location, severity, and extent of brain damage and aid in prognostic decisions.[2–11] Most of these investigations were performed in comatose TBI patients in the early posttraumatic period.

Since that time many studies have demonstrated the diagnostic and prognostic accuracy of EPs.[12–29] Discussions in the literature revolve around which tests should be performed, how the studies should be interpreted or quantified, the timing of tests with respect to injury, and the appropriate patient groups in which to use them. The last two decades of research have reliably demonstrated a practical utility of electrophysiological testing in severely head injured patients, although the clinical advantage in milder forms of injury has not been determined. Recent research on severe TBI patients has centered on the use of EEG or EPs as dynamic monitors of brain function.[30] Therefore, efforts are being made to develop hardware and software that will permit computer-assisted monitoring and analysis of brain electrical activity with minimal human intervention and interpretation. Progress in this area awaits technological development, and there are questions regarding the validity and reliability of some EPs in this context.

Clinical neuroscientists must be able to make informed decisions regarding the appropriate use of EEG and EPs in head-injured patients. Below, guidelines for their use are provided, based on findings that have gained some validation.

ELECTROENCEPHALOGRAPHY

STANDARD EEG

The standard scalp-recorded EEG, a measure of spontaneous brain electrical activity, has had its greatest utility in the head injury population for determining brain death. A description of the literature on this topic can be found elsewhere.[31–33] Although a positive correlation between the degree of EEG abnormality and the severity of head injury is well documented, these recordings have had limited diagnostic and prognostic value in head-injured patients in the moderate and severe injury categories, particularly in the early period after an injury. Altered consciousness and the drugs that are routinely used in the clinical management of these patients cause profound alterations in the spontaneous EEG that preclude a clear view of injury-specific dysfunction. Thus, the EEG is vulnerable to many of the same factors that compromise the utility of the neurological examination in these patients.

CHARACTERISTIC EEG PATTERNS

The goal of EEG research has been to correlate characteristic EEG patterns with injury severity and resolution of coma and to predict outcome and/or the development of posttraumatic epilepsy. There are clearly some EEG patterns with prognostic value, although skilled interpretation of waveforms is required. Most patients in acute traumatic coma show a classic pathophysiological pattern of diffuse EEG slowing known as delta waves.[31] This pattern is not in itself a particularly useful discriminator of the outcome of a TBI patient, since its mere presence does not imply a poor outcome. The higher the proportion of EEG that is attributable to delta, the more likely is a poor prognosis, but quantifying that proportion from the standard EEG paper output may be difficult.

Across the continuum of TBI severity, EEG slowing may be focal or generalized. Focal findings are more common in mild or moderate injury cases or in the presence of contusion or local ischemia rather than in diffuse injury with prolonged unconsciousness. EEG abnormalities found in mild, concussive injury may indicate subtle functional deficits that are not readily apparent clinically. However, in most of these patients (and certainly in animal research paradigms of concussion), EEG patterns normalize quickly.[33] Therefore, since extensive neuropsychological testing is available to assess cognitive deficits, the practical diagnostic advantage of EEG in mild head injury may be limited.

UNFAVORABLE EEG PATTERNS

One EEG pattern that may be seen after TBI is alpha coma, which is characterized by a predominance of alphalike activity in an unconscious patient. This abnormal pattern can be differentiated from the normal alpha activity that predominates over the posterior scalp because it is unreactive to sensory stimulation. Another classic pattern, burst suppression, also may be seen in severely head injured patients and is recognizable by periods of electrical silence interspersed with brief bursts of activity. These abnormal patterns are indicative of severe anoxic insult and carry a poor prognosis. It is important to note that burst suppression can be pharmacologically induced by barbiturates, in which case it clearly is not prognostic. However, the EEG is very useful in assessing the level of barbiturate coma when it is used as a therapeutic modality.

FAVORABLE PATTERNS OF ACTIVITY

Spindle activity, a pattern seen in normal subjects during transition states between waking and sleep, is another EEG finding occasionally observed in head-injured patients. Unlike alpha coma and burst suppression patterns, it is a favorable prognostic sign. The reappearance of sleep cycles in the EEG of these patients early after injury is also generally indicative of a favorable outcome, as is EEG reactivity, or the ability to induce change in EEG patterns with auditory, visual, or somatosensory stimuli.

Some investigators recommend performing multiple EEGs since *changes* in the EEG, especially toward normal patterns, are the most useful prognostic indicators. A theme put forth by most investigators who have evaluated electrophysiological testing is that the validity of the tests increases with repeated measures within the same patient in which a course of improvement or deterioration can be defined. Conditions change rapidly and dramatically during the acute management of a head-injured patient, and any measure of brain function is limited to the window during which it is recorded.

One of the most common uses of standard EEG in head-injured patients is in the diagnosis of posttraumatic epilepsy. In this case, EEG is usually performed weeks or months after the injury. An early appearance of epileptiform activity in these patients is not commonly reported except in very severe injuries with high mortality, although the widespread prophylactic administration of anticonvulsant drugs in the routine care of these patients may mask the incidence.

There is no firm evidence that a standard EEG study can reliably pinpoint specific functional deficits such as hemiparesis or visual dysfunction or predict their resolution when they are apparent early in a head-injured patient. Sensory evoked potential studies that test the integrity of specific sensory pathways are somewhat more useful in this regard.

Quantitative EEG

Reports from evaluations of computer-assisted mathematical transformation and quantification of scalp-recorded EEG[34] suggest a potential use in a subset of head-injured patients. Such quantification of the EEG signal, as is shown in Fig. 39-1, enables reduction of a complex waveform into numeric values and often provides additional comparative topographic analysis of activity across brain regions that is not readily available from an analog EEG waveform.[35] Examples of quantitative indexes include amplitude measures of absolute and relative *power* (μv^2) over the four EEG frequency bands (delta, theta, alpha and beta), hemispheric *symmetry* of EEG amplitude (or the lack thereof), and *phase* or *coherence* of the EEG either within a hemisphere or between the two hemispheres. The latter two measures reflect the temporal relationship between EEG frequencies from homologous brain areas, information that cannot be appreciated by a visual inspection of the analog EEG. Theoretically, these temporal characteristics of the EEG are indicative of synchronous activation of spatially separate brain regions linked by common neural pathways. Therefore, abnormalities indicate relatively subtle deficits in conduction or synchronous activation that may have implications for the recovery of function. Since many of these measures examine differences between one hemisphere and the other or one electrode site and another within the same hemisphere, they are less vulnerable to the generalized drug effects or altered consciousness that may otherwise significantly compromise the interpretation of EEG.

Thatcher and colleagues[36] compared a number of routine clinical and radiographic indexes of head injury severity with quantitative EEG results in a sample of 162 patients with closed head injury (Glasgow Coma Scale 4 to 15). They found that EEG *phase* was one of the most accurate predictors of 1-year outcome as assessed by the Rappaport Disability Rating Scale.[37] The amplitude measures, the absolute and relative power, and the brainstem auditory evoked potential (BAEP, discussed below) were less accurate in predicting outcome.

If phasic abnormalities or other derived measures of the EEG are validated as prognosticators, the EEG may regain a role in the early evaluation of head-injured patients in a quantitative form that can be more easily communicated between clinicians and the critical care staff. Equipment that provides quantitative output is available, although it is more expensive than a basic polygraph. No additional procedures are required for recording EEG for use in subsequent quantitative analysis. The computer analysis itself does not need to be performed at the patient's bedside, and so no additional "on-line" time is required. These studies require about 20 to 30 min of quality EEG recording from which a number of samples are used for analysis. It is not known whether repeated or continuous monitoring of EEG under these circumstances would provide a clinical advantage.

Practical aspects must be considered in the use of quantitative EEG as a monitor. The calculation of derived values such as symmetry and coherence, as well as any topographic analyses, may require a full montage of 19 to 21 electrode placements (and channels of EEG) for statistically valid computation. However, it may be difficult to maintain the recording integrity of so many electrodes over time in an intensive care unit (ICU) environment. Therefore, an abbreviated electrode array with only a few channels of EEG may be more desirable. In such a circumstance, one must ascertain whether the equipment is designed or configured so that a reduction in the number of recorded channels will not compromise the validity of the waveform analysis. Since the application of quantitative EEG for monitoring has not been thoroughly studied, the minimum number of electrodes or channels required to obtain a sample of activity sufficient to assess whole-brain functional integrity is not known. This is an area of application that will undoubtedly benefit from future research.

SENSORY EVOKED POTENTIALS

Comparison with the Spontaneous EEG

A second electrophysiological means of evaluating neural integrity after head injury involves sensory evoked potentials (SEPs). While the EEG represents random, spontaneous brain activity, an EP reflects electrical activity in a specific sensory pathway that is activated by controlled stimulation of a peripheral or cranial nerve. With the assistance of computer averaging techniques, an electrical signal emerges from the background EEG that reflects not only neocortical excitatory and inhibitory postsynaptic potentials such as those exhibited in scalp-recorded EEG but also compound action potentials generated all along the sensory pathway being stimulated. Therefore, the EP has an advantage over the

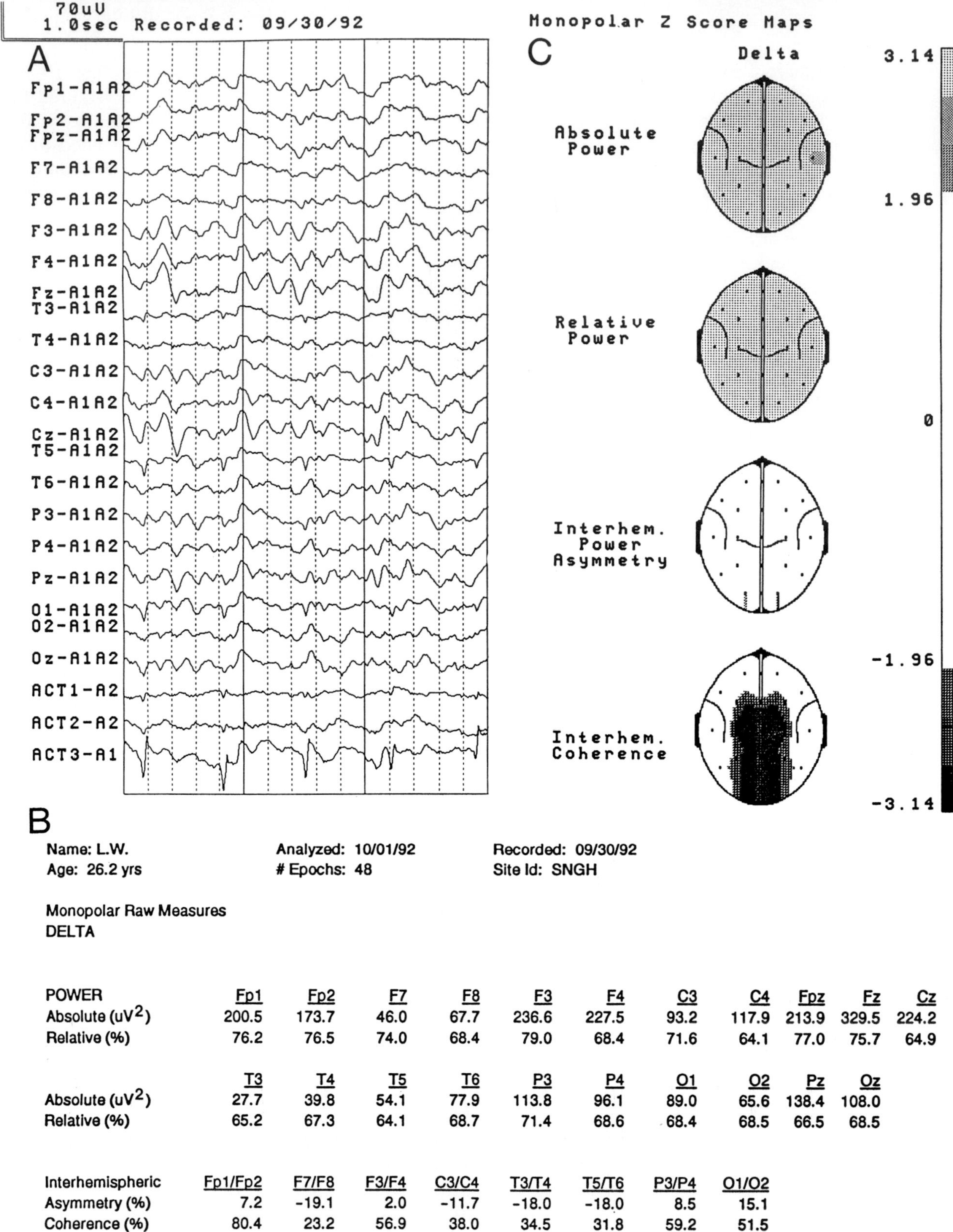

B

Name: L.W.	Analyzed: 10/01/92	Recorded: 09/30/92
Age: 26.2 yrs	# Epochs: 48	Site Id: SNGH

Monopolar Raw Measures
DELTA

POWER	Fp1	Fp2	F7	F8	F3	F4	C3	C4	Fpz	Fz	Cz
Absolute (uV^2)	200.5	173.7	46.0	67.7	236.6	227.5	93.2	117.9	213.9	329.5	224.2
Relative (%)	76.2	76.5	74.0	68.4	79.0	68.4	71.6	64.1	77.0	75.7	64.9

	T3	T4	T5	T6	P3	P4	O1	O2	Pz	Oz
Absolute (uV^2)	27.7	39.8	54.1	77.9	113.8	96.1	89.0	65.6	138.4	108.0
Relative (%)	65.2	67.3	64.1	68.7	71.4	68.6	68.4	68.5	66.5	68.5

Interhemispheric	Fp1/Fp2	F7/F8	F3/F4	C3/C4	T3/T4	T5/T6	P3/P4	O1/O2
Asymmetry (%)	7.2	-19.1	2.0	-11.7	-18.0	-18.0	8.5	15.1
Coherence (%)	80.4	23.2	56.9	38.0	34.5	31.8	59.2	51.5

Figure 39-1. Quantitative EEG in a TBI patient. *A*. Twenty-one channels of EEG are recorded from standard electrode placements, along with three channels of eye muscle and ECG (bottom three traces). Forty-eight, 2-s samples (3 s is shown here) of the analog waveforms are subjected to Fourier transformation to yield values describing power, symmetry, and coherence for each of the EEG frequency bands. *B*. Delta values generated from analysis of the analog waveform in *A*. Values are generated for each electrode or, in the

EEG since more of the CNS can be accessed. For example, SEPs obtained by electrical stimulation of the dorsal column system via the median nerve allow assessment of the integrity of the peripheral nerve, spinal cord, brainstem, thalamus, and the primary as well as secondary sensory areas of cortex. Similarly, the visual evoked potential (VEP) can track conduction and elaboration of neural activity from the retina to the calcarine region and beyond. Since the origins of some EP peaks are known and the latencies at which they occur after stimulation can be measured with great accuracy, one can directly examine conduction within the CNS. This provides a means with which to evaluate damage to axons in long track pathways as well as polysynaptic systems such as the auditory pathway through the brainstem. The routine EEG does not allow this evaluation.

Additional practical advantages of the EP include an immunity of many EP components to altered consciousness and drugs. Although the effects of CNS depressants on EP latency and amplitude can be expected and drug regimens such as high-dose barbiturates can substantially compromise the cortical peaks of EPs,[38,39] many components remain well elaborated. EPs also show less contamination from muscle activity, which tends to average out during EP acquisition but may cause difficulty in EEG interpretation.

There are also disadvantages of EPs compared with the EEG. The equipment is more expensive, requiring stimulating, recording, and computer averaging components. Some EP protocols take much longer to perform, and since stimulation of the patient is required, patient cooperation plays a greater role in the ability to obtain high-quality data. A TBI patient who is unconscious, intubated, and sedated or is receiving paralytic agents may be an excellent candidate for study. However, in patients who are obtunded and/or disoriented and in whom sedation is not indicated, the task of obtaining high-quality recordings is challenging and sometimes impossible. A technician must often devise novel strategies for obtaining data and work between bouts of restlessness; this adds time. The cost-benefit ratio of EP application in an uncooperative patient must always be kept in mind, since it is possible to spend a great deal of time gathering uninterpretable data.

Another technical drawback of EPs is the inability to use routine EEG filtering for noise reduction, leading to a requirement for other methods of artifact control. The cell populations contributing to an EP are much smaller than those generating an EEG, making greater amplification of the signal a requirement. Also, the cellular generators of EPs are often located far from the recording site, in the thalamus or brainstem, lying in anatomic configurations that are unfavorable to the generation of large field potentials. Hence, large numbers of stimulus repetitions may be required to resolve these potentials, adding time to the testing protocol.

Decisions about which tests to use, whether one is choosing between EEG and EPs or between sensory modalities within an EP test battery, must be tempered by these practical factors and by a clear understanding of the goal of testing. A particular testing protocol may be advantageous or useless, depending on that goal. General diagnosis and prognosis may be best achieved by performing multimodality EPs. However, if one wishes to do repeated testing and use the EPs as a dynamic monitor, a single test in a modality that taps function in the areas of concern is preferable. Undoubtedly, some investigators fail to find utility in EP testing in a head-injured patient because of misapplication of the tests or expectations beyond the limitations of the technique.

EEG and Evoked Potentials in Mild and Moderate Head Injury

Most clinical neuroscientists would probably agree that in mild and moderate head injury, a complete clinical neurological examination coupled with neuropsychological assessment of cognitive function is adequate for the diagnosis of functional deficits. EEG is sometimes useful in mildly injured patients, although the findings are normal in many cases. Additional research in this area is required.

In moderately head injured obtunded patients, another issue arises. Some moderate TBI patients show evidence of a mass lesion or contusion without an initial indication for surgery. These conditions can progress rapidly and cause significant neurological deterioration, requiring immediate intervention. Regular or continuous EEG monitoring may be useful in those patients.

---

case of symmetry and coherence, for two homologous electrode pairs. This example shows delta values only. *C.* With the equipment shown here (Cadwell Laboratories, Inc.), one can generate topographical "*z* score" maps with schematized heads (nose toward the top) showing areas containing abnormal values. The shaded scale to the right is calibrated to shade 2 standard deviations above or below a normative mean. In this case, absolute and relative delta power are abnormally high at all leads, and delta coherence is abnormally low over the central, parietal, and occipital regions. The coherence abnormality is not apparent in the analog waveform but becomes so with a look at the *z* score maps.

EEG changes such as increased slow activity and loss of coherence may forewarn of troublesome events, although such an application of the EEG in this sample of patients has not been systematically evaluated. A more practical advantage of the EEG may also apply. Moderately injured TBI patients are difficult subjects for EP testing early after injury. These patients are generally unable to cooperate and are easily aggravated by stimulation of any kind. Sedation may not be clinically desirable, particularly if they are not intubated. The EEG does not require sustained stimulation of the patient once electrodes have been placed and may be a more realistic choice as a monitor in this instance.

There is some evidence that in moderate TBI, long-latency electrical activity from specific EP tests may be useful in tracking deficits such as amnesia.[40] However, there is not enough literature in this area to recommend these studies for routine use. In clinical practice, one must question whether EPs provide information beyond that available from existing means of neurological assessment. Scientifically, however, objective and quantifiable measures of brain function are always needed.

SEVERE HEAD INJURY

EPs are most useful in a severely head-injured patient, early after injury, in whom other measures of neurological function are limited.[41,42] This limitation may be due to coma, brain damage to speech areas, or the use of any of the therapeutic agents required for adequate clinical and/or ventilatory management. There is a substantial literature on the use of EPs in these patients, and the prognostic accuracy of EPs in this subset of patients has been reported to be equal to[16,28] and in some reports more accurate[14,18,20] than that of the clinical examination. When a clinical examination cannot be obtained, EPs become a powerful clinical tool. A specific strength of EPs in this regard is that while a certain number of falsely pessimistic prognostic errors will be made by clinical indicators (the patient is doing poorly but then makes an unexpected recovery), EPs do not demonstrate this type of error. Some falsely optimistic errors of prediction are unavoidable with any indicator because of the occurrence of unforeseen secondary insults. EPs gain their prognostic power from their ability to discriminate viable from inviable neural populations early after TBI and to assess functional changes that affect outcome.

The EP tests that are currently available to the clinical neuroscientist can be categorized by pathways, or modalities of stimulation (auditory, visual, or somatosensory), or by the anatomic origins of activity, either subcortical or hemispheric. Since outcome from TBI depends so heavily on which regions of brain are compromised, it is useful to discuss them here with respect to their anatomic origins.

SUBCORTICAL POTENTIALS

Potentials that appear early in recordings, between 0 and 40 ms after the presentation of a stimulus in any modality, usually represent activity in the precortical portions of that pathway. In the auditory and somatosensory systems, early-latency potentials are relatively easy to obtain and yield reliable measures in normal individuals. From these pathways one can record activity that represents compound action potentials traveling along the ascending lemniscal tracts through brainstem and diencephalic structures. Early activity in the visual geniculostriate pathway is not readily recordable as it is obscured by the large, slow electroretinogram. Therefore, the most commonly used early latency EPs are the brainstem auditory evoked potential (or response) (BAEP or BAER) obtained by click or tone stimulation and the somatosensory early latency (SEL) response to electrical stimulation of the median nerve. Early-latency activity in response to stimulation of nerves in the lower extremities can also be recorded over the back, but these EPs are not commonly used in head injury. They are technically more difficult to record reliably and provide information that is redundant with the upper extremity SEL above the spinal cord. Lower extremity EPs from posterior tibial or peroneal nerves are more apt to be applied in the diagnosis of spinal cord injury or during operative procedures on the spine.

The peaks that make up the BAEP occur within 10 ms of stimulation, and those of the SEL occur within 20 ms. Methods for recording the potentials vary, and several different electrode pairings can be used for this purpose, especially the SEL. These technical differences affect the latencies and even the polarity of the peaks recorded. A discussion of the technical aspects of EP recording is beyond the scope of this chapter and is not included here. However, in practice, most investigators transform peak latency values into interpeak latencies or conduction times, and those indexes partially circumvent idiosyncratic differences in recording techniques.

A number of papers describe an assessment of these tests in samples of head-injured patients.[9–13,15,20,21,23–28,43] Abnormalities in the early-latency potentials may be manifested as latency delays, amplitude reductions, or actual loss of peaks. Most studies have focused on the presence or absence of peaks and the latency of peaks as indicators of subcortical conduction. These are the most reliable aspects of the waveform. Peak amplitudes vary more readily with nonneurological factors. In the clinical situation of TBI, variability in the amplitude of

EPs may be particularly difficult to interpret. Peripheral nerve integrity and the extent to which maximal activation of the nerve has been achieved are often questionable, and this precludes an emphasis on amplitude. Attempts to circumvent peripheral problems and analyze central conduction have led most investigators to use interpeak latencies (IPLs). The time difference between peaks of known origin reflects conduction through prescribed regions of brain. For the BAEP, this is usually the wave I through V IPL, which reflects conduction from eighth nerve insertion at the pons to the inferior colliculus in the midbrain (IPL approximately 4 ms) and includes several synaptic delays. In the SEL, the "central conduction time"[15] (CCT) can be measured in a variety of electrode configurations and includes an interpeak latency that is indicative of conduction from the cervical spinal cord to the first cortical volley. The normal values for the SEL are 3 to 5 ms (depending on how it is measured), and this test essentially includes only the thalamic synaptic delay. Hence, the SEL more purely reflects white matter conduction over a substantial extent of subcortical tissue.

Despite dependence on CCTs to avoid peripheral delays, peripheral activation problems are unavoidable in some TBI patients. The existing literature on the BAEP in TBI suggests that as many as 10 to 20 percent of ears will not be assessable because of an absence of sufficient eighth nerve activation.[10,13,23,29] Luckily, this is a crossed pathway, and one intact ear can often provide sufficient information about brainstem integrity. This is not the case with the somatosensory system, which is largely unilateral, and although the incidence is less well documented, some percentage of somatosensory pathways will be inaccessible as a result of peripheral nerve, brachial plexus, or spinal neuropathy.

BAEP

Most published reports of application of EPs to head injury have utilized the auditory brainstem potential, and abnormality is usually defined by a delay in the interpeak latency of I through V or by a grading system of abnormality that ranges from a normal waveform and interpeak latency to an absent response.[5,9,10,12,20–23,25,26] Considering the small amount of brain tissue represented by this test (a few centimeters rostrocaudal extent), it is surprising that so much interest has been shown in its application. One reason for the BAEP's popularity may be that it is very reliable. This response is readily obtained with little variability in latency in a normal population and is immune to drugs and nonpathological factors such as attention and consciousness. Of course, the potential disadvantage of any highly reliable measure is that it may not be sufficiently sensitive to be useful, and this is a drawback of the BAEP. Only a small proportion of severely head injured patients demonstrate significant BAEP abnormalities early after injury, and anywhere from 50 to 80 percent, despite clear clinical evidence of CNS dysfunction, have normal responses.[12,19,28,29,43] BAEPs have been shown to persist for a number of hours in patients who have reached clinical and standard EEG criteria of brain death.[44] Thus, while a severely abnormal BAEP is an accurate indicator of discrete damage to the brainstem or global problem, such as herniation, the presence of a normal potential does not rule out dysfunction, especially in brain areas other than those traversed by this pathway. Primary brainstem injury is not the predominant etiology of patients surviving TBI, and any test that does not tap hemispheric function thus is limited in applicability in this population of patients.

Perhaps one of the most appealing aspects of the BAEP has been the potential to link electrophysiology with existing clinical indicators of subcortical dysfunction: oculocephalic and pupillary reflexes and decerebrate posturing. The existing literature suggests that the best correlation of BAEP abnormality is with pupillary abnormalities, while correlations with oculocephalic reflex integrity are less consistently reported, except at the extremes of normal and absent.[9,23,28,29] BAEP abnormalities are not correlated with abnormal motor responses, nor is there a precise correlation between BAEP abnormality and the Glasgow Coma Scale, although a very low GCS (3 to 4) is usually associated with abnormal BAEPs.

As a prognostic indicator, the BAEP is most useful when it is severely abnormal. Mild delays in conduction seen on BAEP early after injury can later normalize and are not associated with a poor outcome.[10,12,19,20] The use of BAEPs to monitor patients with serial studies has not received much attention in the literature, although a few reports are available.[10,19,21,26,29] Repeated evaluations in the first few weeks after injury can indicate important clinical changes, but there is some evidence that a BAEP recorded several months after injury has no real prognostic value.[43] The reliability of BAEP makes it appealing as a potential monitor of function, but as will be seen below, the use of the BAEP by itself is always of limited utility in a severely head-injured patient.

SEL

Attempts to assess the diagnostic and prognostic utility of early-latency somatosensory potentials and related conduction values show similar findings to those involving the BAEP. That is, most patients show normal conduction times, but loss of waves or extreme delays in conduction indicate significant subcortical dysfunction and carry a poor prognosis.[15,24,27,28] In many such cases, this information only confirms an existing dismal clinical picture, since the SEL shows a better correlation with the GCS than does the BAEP.[28] As with the BAEP, mild delays in conduction on SEL may be seen that are transient and not prognostic,[15,27,28] and the SEL also has limitations in sensitivity. Normal SELs may still be associated with a poor outcome, particularly when hemispheric injury and dysfunction are guiding the patient's course.

Although there is some overlap in the areas of the brainstem and midbrain through which the SEL and BAEP pathways course, they are not entirely redundant and the combined use of SEP and BAEP enhances the rostrocaudal view of subcortical function. The BAEP checks conduction only up to the diencephalon, while the IPL generated from the somatosensory test reflects conduction beyond the thalamus through the internal capsule to the cortex. Fig. 39-2 provides a clinical example of how these two tests demonstrate differential sensitivity on the basis of the anatomic source of dysfunction. The data presented were obtained during 5 days of continuous monitoring of a 21-year-old male who was comatose after a severe brain injury. He demonstrated no mass lesions but had bifrontal contusions. Routine monitoring included intracranial pressure (ICP), median nerve SEP, and BAEP. Dynamic ICP studies had shown that this patient had abnormal outflow resistance of CSF, and he was being treated with sustained periods of continuous CSF drainage as part of ICP management. During the early part of monitoring, the somatosensory IPL showed significant delays whenever ICP rose above 10 mmHg. The BAEP I through V IPL showed a trend toward delays but never exceeded normal limits, defined as 2 standard deviations above the normative mean. It is quite possible that contused, edematous frontal areas were focally vulnerable and had less functional tolerance of pressure increases. This was better indicated by axonal conduction through the internal capsule than by that through the pontine/midbrain region. When continuous CSF drainage was applied in this patient, the SEP IPL would reliably normalize. Another interesting aspect of this effect was that the exquisite vulnerability of the SEP to pressure resolved by day 5, and conduction through this area was thereafter unaffected by such subtle changes in ICP. This suggests a possible role of EPs in helping to define critical windows of vulnerability within an individual patient. But for this individual, the BAEP was not the most sensitive monitor. To the extent that the SEL and BAEP represent only subcortical activity, exclusive reliance on these tests will never attain the diagnostic and prognostic accuracy that is afforded when they are combined with additional hemispheric testing.

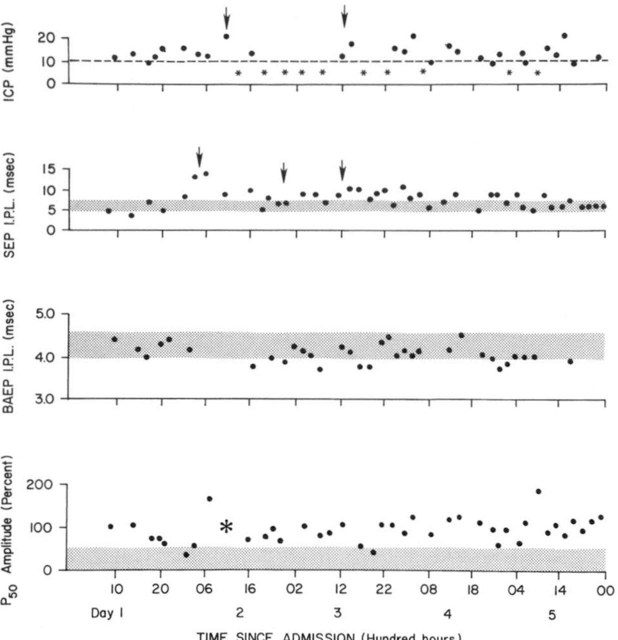

Figure 39-2. Differential sensitivity of EP indexes in a TBI patient during 5 days of ICU monitoring. Graphs, from top to bottom, are ICP, somatosensory interpeak latency, auditory interpeak latency, and amplitude of a positive cortical peak in the somatosensory evoked potential, expressed as a percentage of that obtained on an admission study. Shaded areas for the IPL graphs indicate the range of normal (±2 SD). The shaded area for the amplitude graph marks a ≧50 percent reduction in amplitude, considered to be a significant drop. In this patient, the ICP was relatively low and reached 20 mmHg only on two occasions, but the SEP abnormality preceded it when ICP was still 10 to 15 mmHg (arrow). Periods of CSF drainage (asterisks in the ICP graph) were associated with normalization of the IPL (arrow 2), but each time drainage was interrupted, conduction slowed (arrow 3). This sensitivity of the SEP resolved by day 5, when the IPL became more stable despite ICP fluctuations. During monitoring, the BAEP IPL did not exceed normal limits. The SEP cortical P_{50} disappeared when ICP reached 20 mmHg (asterisk, bottom graph) but showed variable amplitudes otherwise and rarely dropped below 50 percent of baseline amplitude. Since the cortical peak is dependent on the integrity of conduction in the ascending lemniscal pathways, P_{50} variability might have been secondary to the conduction disturbances observed in the IPL. (Reprinted with permission from Newlon et al.[41])

Hemispheric potentials

Evoked potentials generated by cortical cell populations can be obtained in any modality and are manifested in waves occurring later than 20 to 30 ms after stimulation. Small differences in stimulation and recording parameters distinguish these tests from early-latency protocols.

Depending on which modalities and peaks are evaluated, one can use these tests to assess the functional integrity of primary sensory receiving areas and secondary association areas of cortex. The fact that a number of cortical regions can be assessed with multimodality testing allows a thorough evaluation of the extent of dysfunction, providing important information on the etiology.[2–4,6–8,13,16,18,20] For example, global anoxic insults present in multimodality EPs as a loss of hemispheric activity in all modalities, while the impact of a subdural hematoma over the parietal lobe may be limited to the SEP response on one side. In addition, morphologically "silent" contrecoup injury in the hemisphere opposite a mass lesion often can be detected. The extent of injury affects the prognosis, and the accuracy of outcome determination is enhanced by the use of several modalities of stimulation. There is, however, a practical trade-off, since each new test adds time to the testing procedure. Again, the specific goal of testing must be clearly defined in order to determine which battery might best answer the questions at hand. An initial early diagnostic and prognostic study should include all modalities to determine the severity and extent of cortical dysfunction. These results can be extremely useful for communicating with the family and in planning rehabilitation. Subsequent evaluations may include a limited protocol designed to track the recovery of a dysfunctional area or assure the stability of normal function during the early course of ICU care. If one is limited to a single modality for testing, the somatosensory potential is the best choice, since the course traveled by the dorsal column system covers all levels of the neuroaxis.

A general rule for the diagnostic and prognostic significance of hemispheric abnormalities in a head-injured patient is not whether latencies are delayed or amplitudes are reduced but whether waves are present or absent.[6,8,13,16–18] This is partly due to the fact that hemispheric potentials are inherently more variable, even between normal subjects, and more vulnerable to attentional and pharmacological factors. Because of this, many investigators simply count the numbers of peaks present in various cortical modalities when using these tests for diagnostic and prognostic purposes.

The inability to activate and obtain EPs from a portion of a primary sensory cortical region is significant and highly predictive of persistent deficits in that sensory system. Somatosensory potentials are also predictive of motor deficits, undoubtedly as a result of the proximity of sensory and motor areas of the cortex and the diffuse nature of brain injury. Hence, these tests provide important information about recovery early after injury, when these systems cannot otherwise be tested. Hemiparesis resolution can be predicted by the SEP,[6] while visual dysfunction is linked to VEP abnormalities.[4] When one is combining the results of many EP tests to determine the overall outcome, the worst response often dictates the ultimate result 1 year after injury. If severe abnormalities are focal, the worst case may involve a focal dysfunction in, for example, one extremity. However, severe diffuse abnormalities are usually associated with devastating disability or a vegetative state.

It is difficult to assess the integrity of frontal and temporal cortical association areas early after injury. To the extent that cells in these areas contribute to late activity of the cortical potentials (>100 ms), one can comment about whether this activity is present or absent during diagnostic testing. Some investigators have built this into their grading systems, and the absence of late activity defines a mild or moderate abnormality.[5,7,8,13,16,17] Unfortunately, these peaks are subject to pharmacological effects. When late activity is asymmetrical, that is, present with SEP from one side and not the other, this is not likely to be pharmacological but instead may indicate a lack of functional integrity in the association areas of the affected pathway. General examination of the presence or absence of late activity in several modalities can provide a hint as to whether this is a significant finding.

There is good evidence that serial evoked potential studies provide useful information about the recovery of function in areas that are originally intact but dysfunctional.[17–19,30] This is particularly true in the early period after injury, and EPs are sensitive measures of secondary insult.[3,16,19,22,29,30,45] Persistent moderate abnormalities in hemispheric potentials that are basically intact may predict a slower recovery or moderate disability.[18,19] An important aspect of the appopriate use of EP testing in severe head injury is that the EP indexes usually precede the clinical manifestation of functional integrity. This attribute imparts prognostic power to these tests but also means that discrepancies between the clinical and electrophysiological portraits of a patient will be encountered. In practice, it is tempting for clinicians who are confronted with such a discrepancy to believe their eyes (the apparent clinical condition) rather than the EP results, particularly when the EPs offer a more favorable prognosis than do the clinical signs. In such instances, it must be emphasized that the EP reflects the *potential* for recovery. Hence, the discrepancy represents an opportunity for aggressive clinical management to change the clinical picture.

In comparing the utility of early- versus long-latency cortical EPs, it appears that the subcortical potentials are more reliable and less sensitive, while hemispheric potentials are somewhat less reliable between individuals but may be the most sensitive monitors of functional brain integrity within an individual over time.

THE FUTURE OF EPs IN HEAD INJURY: DYNAMIC MONITORS OF BRAIN FUNCTION

At an informal gathering of a TBI research group some years ago, Dr. J. Douglas Miller described the evolution of critical care of head injury patients in head injury centers as a natural progression through three stages (unpublished communication). During stage I, about twenty years ago, patient care was highly variable, with each patient being treated differently, largely as a result of benign ignorance. Anything that seemed to have a beneficial effect without hurting the patient was tried, but in the absence of specific guidelines based on scientific evidence. Stage II, which began in the late 1970s, was characterized by the application of state-of-the-art standardized care with an emphasis on clinical research, so that scientific evidence supporting procedures and modalities of treatment could be obtained and scrutinized. The standardization of care was an absolute prerequisite for valid scientific determination of useful therapies. In stage III, individualized care would stage a comeback, but now based on knowledge of the important variables to measure, the methods at hand for measuring them, and appropriate therapies with which to treat them. TBI patient care is now perched somewhere between stages II and III. It is now known that mass lesions must be removed quickly and that ICP, blood flow, blood pressure, and CO_2 must be managed carefully. However, the *relative* importance of each of these factors for a particular patient and the immediate impact on recovery of the brain is not fully known.

Most patients who reach the ICU survive with disability ranging anywhere from subtle cognitive deficits to a persistent vegetative state. At present, it is difficult to state what proportion of neurons that are alive and dysfunctional on arrival at the ICU go on to survive or die. The goal of early ICU management is to provide the environment necessary to maximize those which survive. Defining that ideal environment for an individual is a likely future role of electrophysiological monitoring in TBI patients. While this is perhaps the most exciting and clinically useful role EPs may play in neurological patient care, it is also the least studied area of their application. There are technological limitations on automated monitoring, and there is not an adequate database available to dictate standards for the most reliable and valid monitors. It seems likely that EP monitoring will have to be individualized to the nature, severity, and extent of injury.

In monitoring, the emphasis is on changes that occur in specific EP parameters in an individual over time. To serve as monitors of neurological function, EPs must be reliable in appearance in the absence of untoward clinical events and be sensitive to events that are known to compromise neuronal integrity, such as compression (by hematoma, edema, or elevated ICP) and ischemic processes. The sensitivity of EPs to elevated ICP and compression is well documented.[45,46] As was discussed earlier and as is shown in Fig. 39-2, studies of continuous monitoring in head-injured patients suggest that EPs may help define the tolerable range of ICP for an individual. Figure 39-3 gives another example of this sensitivity, but in the VEP.

In this case, the latency of an early cortical response, the N_{70} peak, was monitored over several days during continuous monitoring of a head-injured patient. During this time, the patient's ICP varied between 3 and 35 mmHg, and the relationship between the VEP component and ICP or cerebral perfusion pressure (CPP = mean arterial blood pressure − ICP) was assessed. In the figure, the boxed-in areas show the normal range of latency for this peak: between 60 and 80 ms. This patient required an ICP of 10 or below to normalize the N_{70} latency. This translated into a CPP requirement of 100 mmHg or above, well beyond the minimal 60 mmHg that is commonly considered a critical cutoff for preventing frank ischemia. In this case, the relationship with CPP was quite linear ($r = 0.805$). It is not known whether this linearity could be expected in all patients, although there is some evidence of this in the literature.[45]

Similar effects can be seen with regard to blood flow. Some degree of hyperventilation is viewed as beneficial

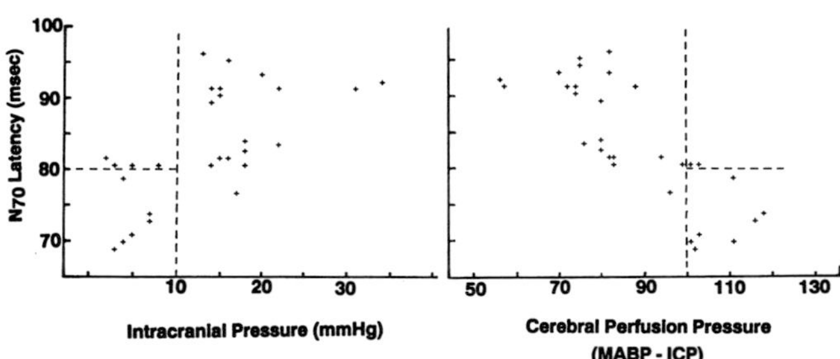

Figure 39-3. Intracranial pressure and VEP latency in a TBI patient over 3 days of monitoring. Ordinate: latency of the N_{70} peak of the VEP in response to flash stimuli. Abscissa: left, ICP; right, cerebral perfusion pressure (CPP). Vertical dotted lines at 10 mmHg ICP and 100 mmHg CPP are for reference. The horizontal dotted lines indicate 2 SD above a normative mean latency of 70 ms. This patient had a mildly abnormal VEP on admission and showed delays in N_{70} on the majority of tests. However, when the ICP was particularly low (or CPP was high), the latency normalized. The relationship is more clear when the data are plotted against CPP, a more meaningful physiological endpoint. Since these data represent recordings obtained over several days, undoubtedly other variables affected the latency as well. The centroparietal SEP in this patient was normal and unresponsive to ICP changes, suggesting that optic pathways were most vulnerable to secondary compromise.

in a severely head injured patient to reduce ICP and combat acidosis. However, extreme reductions in CO_2 with hyperventilation can ultimately lead to significant cerebral vasoconstriction and ischemia. Determining the optimum degree of hyperventilation for an individual is difficult since bedside cerebral blood flow (CBF) studies are uncommon. Furthermore, areas of brain already compromised by injury may be highly susceptible to reductions in flow that would not be critical for normal tissue. EPs can help define the impact of such manipulations on brain function. Figure 39-4 shows data obtained from an individual patient who received continuous monitoring of SEP over 5 days that yielded 50 repeated tests. This patient showed cerebral ischemia early in his course and was managed to keep CBF within the normal range. In the figure, the amplitudes of two middle-latency components of the SEP are plotted against end-tidal CO_2 as an indicator of serum CO_2 levels (ET_{CO_2} usually ran slightly lower than blood levels). SEP amplitudes were dramatically reduced when CO_2 dropped below 25 mmHg, particularly the N_{80} peak. Increases in ET_{CO_2} above 35 mmHg also resulted in reduced amplitude. Hence, for this individual, ET_{CO_2} between 33 and 35 mmHg was maximal for functional brain integrity. It is conceivable that a protocol could be devised to obtain sufficient numbers of EPs to define the curve for an individual so that optimal parameters could be assured.

The data provided here in regard to EP sensitivity come from cortical potentials, which were described earlier as being more variable between and within normal individuals. A paradox seems to occur in a head-injured patient who is unconscious. There is less variability in values from repeated studies in the same patient under stable conditions than is customarily reported in normals. A lack of consciousness may afford an advantage in this case, removing the influences of attentional factors. Because they are reliable in this context, it is likely that the hemispheric potentials will be more useful than subcortical brainstem potentials in the early detection of subtle, subclinical changes in brain function. The choice of tests for monitoring ultimately depends on the nature and extent of injury. Hence, it is worthwhile to have a variety of EP tests available to choose from.

NOVEL APPLICATIONS

The guidelines described here are limited to those which are clearly documented with regard to the clinical utility of EP testing in a head-injured patient. There are several other topics of potential interest to clinical neuroscientists. These include novel experimental techniques, the use of EPs as surrogate endpoints in clinical trials, and the use of EPs in rehabilitation. Experimental applications include motor evoked potentials that involve either electrical or magnetic stimulation of motor cortex coupled with recording of either electromyography (EMG) or peripheral motor nerve action potentials. Such an application in head injury has not been sufficiently investigated to show utility in this context. There are technical concerns, and it is important to ask whether these tests would provide information to the clinician that is not obtainable by other means. Clearly, in the case of spinal cord injury, there is a great deal of information to be gained by evaluating ventral pathways in addition to testing the dorsal columns of the spinal cord. But in diffuse head injury, it is not clear whether unique

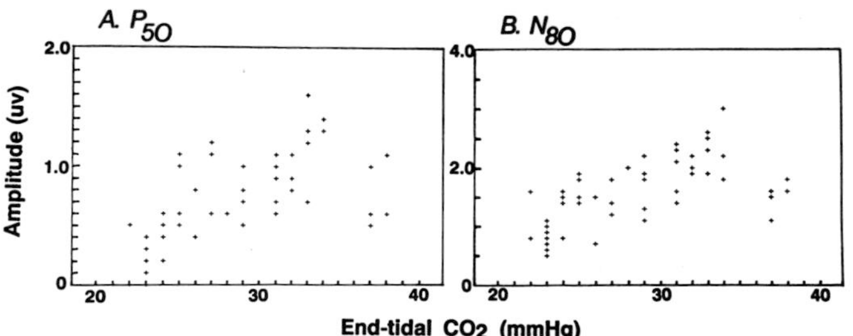

Figure 39-4. Relationship of SEP amplitude and end-tidal CO_2 (ET_{CO_2}) in a TBI patient. Ordinates: peak amplitude in microvolts. Abscissa: ET_{CO_2} associated with various degrees of hyperventilation. The P_{50} and N_{80} are part of a primary cortical complex recorded over centroparietal regions of the scalp with somatosensory stimulation. Each point represents a separate SEP obtained from this patient over 5 days of ICU monitoring. These scatter plots show a general curvilinear relationship of SEP amplitude and ET_{CO_2}. The best SEP response (highest amplitude) is seen at ET_{CO_2} between 33 and 35 mmHg, and amplitude drops above and below these levels. With vigorous hyperventilation (23 to 24 mmHg), the peaks almost disappear completely.

information about motor systems is required to the exclusion of that provided by a general sampling of brain by sensory EPs. Furthermore, there may be some risk in directly stimulating the cortex of a head-injured patient in whom the seizure threshold may be reduced. More work is required in this area before routine application of these tests can be done.

The use of EPs as functional endpoints in clinical trials of therapy in TBI patients is an idea that is becoming more popular as a means to acquire rapid feedback about safety and therapeutic efficacy. This application is limited to institutions involved in such research. The present trend in head injury research toward multicenter clinical trials will further increase a need for early, objective endpoints of brain function, and it is possible that EPs will be used more in those circumstances.

Another area of ongoing research is the use of EPs in the rehabilitative setting. It is not clear whether specific EP tests might provide unique information about cognitive processes[7,18,40] that cannot be obtained by behavioral analysis. To the extent that EPs can confirm the physiological basis and location of dysfunction, they are advantageous in any setting. It will be interesting to see whether specialized EP protocols can quantify cognitive function and become useful in the late phases of patient care.

References

1. Williams D: The electro-encephalogram in acute head injuries. *J Neurosurg Psychiatry* 4:107, 1941.
2. Walter S, Arfel G: Responses aux stimulations visuelles dans les etats de coma aigu et de coma chronique. *Electroencephalogr Clin Neurophysiol* 32:27, 1972.
3. Larson SJ, Sances A, Ackmann JJ, Reigel DH: Noninvasive evaluation of head trauma patients. *Surgery* 74:34, 1973.
4. Feinsod M, Auerbach E: Electrophysiological examinations of the visual system in the acute phase after head injury. *Eur Neurol* 9:56, 1973.
5. Greenberg RP, Mayer DJ, Becker DP, Miller JD: Evaluation of brain function in severe human head trauma with multimodality evoked potentials: Evoked brain injury potentials, methods and analysis. *J Neurosurg* 47:150, 1977.
6. Greenberg RP, Becker DP, Miller JD, Mayer DJ: Evaluation of brain function in severe human head trauma with multimodality evoked potentials: II. Localization of brain dysfunction and correlation with post-traumatic neurological conditions. *J Neurosurg* 47:163, 1977.
7. Rappaport M, Hall K, Hopkins HK, et al: Evoked brain potentials and disability in brain damaged patients. *Arch Phys Med Rehabil* 58:333, 1977.
8. De la Torre JC, Trimble JL, Beard RT, et al: Somatosensory evoked potentials for the prognosis of coma in humans. *Exp Neurol* 60:304, 1978.
9. Uziel A, Benezech J: Auditory brain-stem responses in comatose patients: Relationship with brain-stem reflexes and levels of coma. *Electroencephalogr Clin Neurophysiol* 45:515, 1978.
10. Seales DM, Rossiter VS, Weinstein ME: Brainstem auditory evoked response in patients comatose as a result of blunt head trauma. *J Trauma* 19:347, 1979.
11. Hume AL, Cant BR, Shaw NA: Central somatosensory conduction time in comatose patients. *Ann Neurol* 5:379, 1979.
12. Tsubokawa T, Nishimoto H, Yamamoto T, et al: Assessment of brain-stem damage by the auditory brain stem response in acute severe head injury. *J Neurol Neurosurg Psychiatry* 43:1005, 1980.
13. Greenberg RP, Newlon PG, Hyatt MS, et al: Prognostic implications of early multimodality evoked potentials in severe head injury patients: A prospective study. *J Neurosurg* 55:227, 1981.
14. Narayan RK, Greenberg RP, Miller JD, et al: Improved confidence of outcome prediction in severe head injury: A comparative analysis of the clinical examination, multimodality evoked potentials, CT and ICP. *J Neurosurg* 54:751, 1981.
15. Hume AL, Cant BR: Central somatosensory conduction after head injury. *Ann Neurol* 10:411, 1981.
16. Lindsay KW, Carlin J, Kennedy I, et al: Evoked potentials in severe head injury: Analysis and relation to outcome. *J Neurol Neurosurg Psychiatry* 44:796, 1981.
17. Rappaport M, Hall K, Hopkins HK, Belleza T: Evoked potentials and head injury: I. Rating of evoked potential abnormality. *Clin Electroencephalogr* 12:154, 1981.
18. Rappaport M, Hopkins HK, Hall K, Belleza T: Evoked potentials and head injury: II. Clinical applications. *Clin Electroencephalogr* 12:167, 1981.
19. Newlon PG, Greenberg RP, Hyatt MS, et al: The dynamics of neuronal dysfunction and recovery following severe head injury assessed with multimodality evoked potentials. *J Neurosurg* 57:168, 1982.
20. Anderson DC, Bundlie S, Rockswold GL: Multimodality evoked potentials in closed head trauma. *Arch Neurol* 41:369, 1984.
21. Hall JW, Mackey-Hargadine J: Auditory evoked responses in severe head injury. *Semin Hearing* 5:313, 1984.
22. Mackey-Hargadine J, Hall JW: Sensory evoked responses in head injury. *J Am Paralysis Assoc* 2:187, 1985.
23. Papanicolaou AC, Loring DW, Eisenberg HM, et al: Auditory brain stem evoked responses in comatose head-injured patients. *Neurosurgery* 18:173, 1986.
24. Whittle IR, Johnston IH, Besser M: Short latency somatosensory-evoked potentials in children: III. Findings following head injury. *Surg Neurol* 27:29, 1987.
25. Rumpl E, Prugger M, Gerstenbrand F, et al: Central somatosensory conduction time and acoustic brainstem tranmission time in post-traumatic coma. *J Clin Neurophysiol* 5:237, 1988.
26. Facco E, Munari M, Liviero MC, et al: Serial recordings of auditory brainstem responses in severe head injury: Relationship between test timing and prognostic power. *Intensive Care Med* 14:422, 1988.

27. Judson JA, Cant BR, Shaw NA: Early prediction of outcome from cerebral trauma by somatosensory evoked potentials. *Crit Care Med* 18:363, 1990.
28. Lindsay K, Pasaoglu A, Hirst D, et al: Somatosensory and auditory brain stem conduction after head injury: A comparison with clinical features in prediction of outcome. *Neurosurgery* 26:278, 1990.
29. Barelli A, Valente MR, Clemente A, et al: Serial multimodality-evoked potentials in severely head-injured patients: Diagnostic and prognostic implications. *Crit Care Med* 19:1374, 1991.
30. Moulton R, Kresta P, Ramirez M, Tucker W: Continuous automated monitoring of somatosensory evoked potentials in posttraumatic coma. *J Trauma* 31:676, 1991.
31. Tyner FS, Knott JR, Mayer WB: Head trauma, in *Fundamentals of EEG Technology*, vol. 2: *Clinical Correlates*. New York: Raven Press, 1989:227–244.
32. Bauer G: Coma and brain death, in Niedermeyer E, Lopes da Silva F (eds): *Electroencephalography* (3d ed). Baltimore: Williams & WIlkins, 1993:445–459.
33. Rumpl E: Craniocerebral trauma, in Niedermeyer E, Lopes da Silva F (eds): *Electroencephalography* (3d ed). Baltimore: Williams & Wilkins, 1993:383–403.
34. John ER, Karmel B, Corning W, et al: Neurometrics. *Science* 196:1393, 1977.
35. Duffy FH (ed): *Topographic Mapping of Brain Electrical Activity*. Boston: Butterworth, 1986.
36. Thatcher RW, Cantor DS, McAlaster R, et al: Comprehensive predictions of outcome in closed head-injured patients: The development of prognostic equations. *Ann NY Acad Sci* 620:82, 1991.
37. Rappaport M, Hall KM, Hopkins K, et al: Disability rating scale for severe head trauma: Coma to community. *Arch Phys Med Rehabil* 63:118, 1982.
38. Sutton LN, Frewen T, Marsh R, et al: The effects of deep barbiturate coma on multimodality evoked potentials. *J Neurosurg* 57:178, 1982.
39. Newlon PG, Greenberg RP, Enas GP, Becker DP: Effects of therapeutic pentobarbital coma on multimodality evoked potentials recorded from severely head injured patients. *Neurosurgery* 12:613, 1983.
40. Papanicolaou AC, Levin HS, Eisenberg HM, et al: Evoked potential correlates of posttraumatic amnesia after closed head injury. *Neurosurgery* 14:676, 1984.
41. Newlon PG, Greenberg RP, Gudeman SK: Evoked potentials in the management of severely head-injured patients, in Becker DP, Gudeman SK (eds): *The Textbook of Head Injury*. Philadelphia, Saunders, 1989:278–308.
42. Stone JL, Ghaly RF, Hughes JR: Evoked potentials in head injury and states of increased intracranial pressure. *J Clin Neurophysiol* 5:135, 1988.
43. Shin DY, Ehrenberg B, Whyte J, et al: Evoked potential assessment: Utility in prognosis of chronic head injury. *Arch Phys Med Rehabil* 70:189, 1989.
44. Goldie WD, Chiappa KH, Young RR, Brooks EB: Brainstem auditory and short-latency somatosensory response in brain death. *Neurology* 31:248, 1981.
45. York D, Legan M, Benner S, Watts C: Further studies with a noninvasive method of intracranial pressure estimation. *Neurosurgery* 14:456, 1984.
46. Nagao S, Kuyama H, Honma Y, et al: Prediction and evaluation of brainstem function by auditory brainstem responses in patients with uncal herniation. *Surg Neurol* 27:81, 1987.

CHAPTER 40

BIOCHEMICAL MONITORING IN HEAD INJURY

J. Clay Goodman
Richard K. Simpson, Jr.

SYNOPSIS

Monitoring of neurochemical markers of primary and secondary brain injury may provide basic insights into the pathophysiological mechanisms operative in neurotrauma. In the clinical setting, neurochemical monitoring provides information about the magnitude and nature of tissue injury, permitting prognostication and the design of rational therapy. This chapter will discuss progressively more proximate loci of neurochemical monitoring in head injury, starting with systemic biochemical derangements, moving to alterations of blood and CSF caused by the release of analytes from the injured brain, and ending with a discussion of biochemical alterations within the brain monitored using microdialysis. The primary focus of this chapter is neurochemical monitoring using microdialysis.

INTRODUCTION

Monitoring and management of the harmful biochemical derangements of systemic and cerebral metabolism set into motion by a head injury constitute a major new aspect of neurotraumatology. Head injury is a process driven by biochemical and cellular alterations evolving over days to weeks rather than an event spanning milliseconds at the time of the initial injury. For example, diffuse axonal injury matures over hours to days, implying an ongoing cellular pathophysiological process rather than an abrupt axonal shearing event at the instant of impact. Similarly, complex systemic hypercatabolic derangements evolve over days to weeks after a head injury, compelling vigorous nutritional support. Finally, injured brain exhibits many neurochemical features seen in ischemic injury, including anaerobic metabolism, elevated extracellular excitotoxic amino acids, and increased extracellular potassium. Secondary brain injury due to ischemia is a common and serious accompaniment of traumatic head injury, and traumatically injured tissue may be more susceptible to ischemic injury. The relatively indolent tempo of these injurious cellular processes may provide a physician with an opportunity to forestall or reverse damage. Meaningful intervention is contingent on detection of neurochemical abnormalities through clinically relevant, reasonably simple, cost-effective biochemical monitoring. Biochemical monitoring of head injury ranges in complexity from the analysis of changes in blood and CSF that reflect neural tissue destruction and altered metabolism to direct measurement of neurochemical alterations in the brain. Biochemical monitoring of the brain using microdialysis in the intensive care unit is a field in its infancy that has made a promising start and is the primary focus of this chapter.

BIOCHEMICAL MECHANISMS IN NEURAL INJURY

Ischemia and trauma have many neurochemical similarities, suggesting that common biochemical mechanisms are at work in both processes. Increasingly, investigators of stroke and trauma find themselves at the same meetings, presenting work about the same neurochemical mechanisms, and grappling with the same difficult therapeutic issues.[1] Evidence is accumulating that ischemia and trauma act *synergistically* through a common set of neurochemical pathways.[2,3] A fundamental assumption in contemporary neurotraumatology is that damage set into motion by trauma (primary injury) is exacerbated by ischemia (secondary injury) acting through these common pathways. Ischemia and trauma both lead to increased anaerobic energy generation, excitatory amino acid neurotransmitter release, and increased polyamine production, which act synergistically to produce tissue damage.[4–8] There is substantial evidence that focal brain trauma acutely results in decreased cerebral blood flow sufficient to produce ischemic injury. Hence, trauma may initiate ischemic injury, which in turn augments the damaging neurochemical cascades. An overview of these destructive metabolic processes produced by traumatic or ischemic injury is shown in Fig. 40-1.

Anaerobic metabolism generates a feeble trickle of energy while producing tissue lactic acidosis.[9,10] Outcome after ischemic injury correlates with lactate elevation, and injury can be limited by restricting glucose availability or inhibiting lactate dehydrogenase, the enzyme that produces lactic acid. Hyperglycemia augments focal and global ischemic injury by supplying substrate for the production of lactic acid, and partial ischemia results in greater production of lactate compared with complete ischemia by continuing the delivery of glucose.[4] Tissue and microdialysate levels of lactate increase 10-fold to 20-fold in ischemia and are also elevated after trauma.[11,12] Lactate accumulation exerts potent cytotoxic effects, and the precise mechanism of this toxicity remains under intense study.[7–9,12–16] Lactic acidosis leads to increased cellular swelling, potentially compromising cerebral perfusion, and impaired recovery of mitochondrial energy metabolism, excacerbating energy failure. Tissue lactic acidosis decreases cerebral utilization of glucose, while systemic lactic acidosis leads to increased cerebral blood flow.[17] Elevation of parenchymal extracellular lactate has been demonstrated with microdialysis in experimentally produced ischemia and cortical impact, using high-performance liquid chromatography.[5,14]

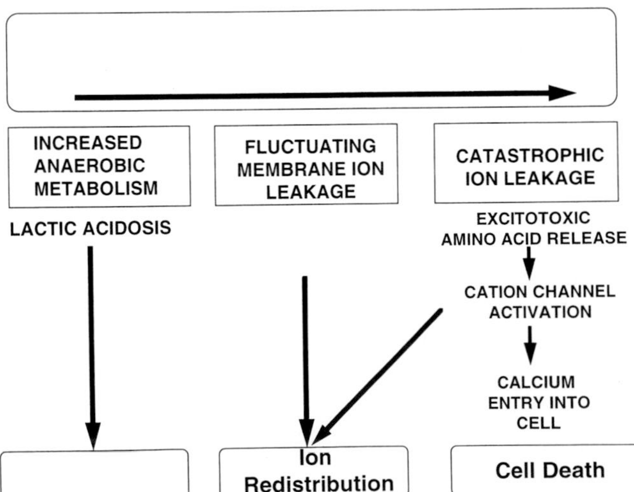

Figure 40-1. Traumatic and ischemic brain injury set into motion a destructive cascade of neurochemical processes, including acidosis, ion leakage, and excitotoxicity.

Adenosine is elevated 10-fold to 40-fold in ischemia and trauma as a result of impaired adenosine triphosphate regeneration during energy failure.[5,18] Adenosine elevation is a sensitive indicator of energy insufficiency and has been measured with microdialysis. Unlike lactic acid, adenosine may exert cytoprotective effects by dilating cerebral vessels and decreasing neuronal excitability. Activation of the high-affinity A_1 adenosine receptor may inhibit the release of excitatory amino acids during ischemia, but activation of the low-affinity A_2 adenosine receptor may enhance the release of amino acids under these circumstances. A much more pronounced elevation in adenosine has been reported after cortical impact compared with middle cerebral artery occlusion, causing some authors to hypothesize that trauma leads to mechanical disruption of cells with release of purines into the extracellular space, where adenosine cannot be converted to inosine and hypoxanthine. In ischemia, in contrast, the purines remain inside cells, where interconversion can take place, leading to elevations of adenosine, inosine, and hypoxanthine.[19–21]

Energy failure results in membrane instability, permitting the release of potassium into the extracellular space and elevation of the extracellular potassium concentration up to 80-fold.[19–23] Potassium leakage is accompanied by electrical hyperexcitability, which increases energy demand, worsening the mismatch between energy production and demand. This potassium elevation occurs before the catastrophic collapse of membrane ion gradients and therefore may provide a warning that tissue is at risk. Large increases in extracellular potassium have been measured using microdialysis after fluid percussion injury in rats. The elevation in extracellular potassium correlated with percussion intensity but was transient unless protracted apnea supervened. The elevation in potassium was paralleled by an elevation in glutamate, suggesting that the increase in extracellular potassium leads to excitatory amino acid release.[24] Other investigators demonstrated that application of potassium to the cerebral cortex via cortical cup superfusate induces an efflux of neurotransmitter amino acids and purines, suggesting that elevated extracellular potassium may be one of the primary early events in tissue injury.[25]

The membrane resting potential is maintained by energy-dependent redistribution of ions by membrane-bound transporters. If energy sources are inadequate, membranes depolarize, with dissipation of the normal asymmetrical ion distributions and release of the excitatory amino acid neurotransmitters—glutamate and aspartate—into the extracellular space. Tenfold elevations of the normal concentrations may be seen. Repeated episodes of ischemia lead to increasing larger elevations of extracellular amino acids and are potentially very harmful.[1,6,26] These neurotransmitters activate ligand-gated cation channels, which augment membrane depolarization, resulting in more neurotransmitter release and thus establishing a pathological self-perpetuating cycle.[27–29] Extracellular ions, including sodium, chloride, and calcium, enter the cell through these activated channels. Increased intracellular calcium activates proteases, quenches mitochondria, and disrupts intracellular signaling. While calcium is widely regarded as an intracellular assassin which must be tightly regulated, there is recent intriguing evidence that calcium entry is essential for vesicle-mediated membrane repair.[30] When a hole is poked in the cell membrane, allowing calcium to enter, intracellular vesicles move from cytoskeletal attachments to the cell membrane, where they fuse with the membrane and restore its integrity. This may be an evolutionarily ancient cellular response to membrane injury, and modification of this response may have led to neurotransmission via calcium-mediated neurotransmitter vesicle fusion with the cell membrane. Cellular protein synthesis is inhibited, and cytoplasmic proteins are degraded. Cells attempting to restore membrane ion gradients consume energy, worsening lactate production. The operation of membrane-bound amino acid transporters that normally reabsorb glutamate and aspartate from the extracellular space is dependent on the transmembrane sodium gradient. With membrane depolarization and abolition of the sodium gradient, excitotoxic amino acids cannot be reabsorbed and their pathological effects are prolonged. Extrusion of calcium from the cell is also an energy-dependent process. Blockade of excitatory amino acid receptors reduces lactate production in ischemic tissue by reducing the amount of calcium which must be pumped out of the cell. Administration of excitatory amino acid antagonists via microdialysis reduces the increase in glucose utilization normally seen after a concussive head injury.[31] Elevations in extracellular excitatory amino acids have been demonstrated using microdialysis by numerous investigators in both trauma and ischemia.[5,24,32–36] Defective electron transport in mitochondria and activation of xanthine oxidase during ischemia lead to free radical generation, which may in turn damage membrane integrity through lipid peroxidation.[6,37]

Other neurotransmitters are altered after head injury. Acetylcholine levels increase in brain tissue, extracellular space, and CSF in experimental and clinical head injury. The elevated acetylcholine levels may impair consciousness, and in experimental studies, administration of muscarinic acetylcholinergic blockers reduces posttraumatic seizures and behavior deficits. Monoaminergic neurotransmitters are increased and may modulate excitotoxicity, vascular reactivity, and thrombogenesis.[1,6,33]

The polyamines putrescine, spermidine, and spermine are produced sequentially by a set of enzymatic reactions activated in response to stress. The synthesis of all three polyamines is known as the "complete" polyamine synthesis response, which promotes neuronal survival after injury. Polyamine synthesis is disrupted in ischemia and trauma, where the major polyamine produced by this "incomplete" polyamine synthesis response is putrescine.[38–47] Putrescine increases calcium influx, triggers synaptosomal excitotoxic neurotransmitter release, increases electrical hyperexcitability, and disrupts the blood-brain barrier.[48] Putrescine positively modulates excitatory amino acid receptors, augmenting excitotoxicity. Putrescine elevation occurs 24 to 48 h after injury and appears to participate in delayed neuronal death. Inhibition of putrescine synthesis by the ornithine decarboxylase inhibitor difluoromethyl-ornithine (DFMO) reduces infarct size in middle cerebral artery occlusion, thus confirming the active participation of putrescine in tissue damage. An "incomplete" putrescine response is also seen after contusive injury in which the severity of neurological injury correlates with putrescine elevation, and improved outcome is seen in animals treated with the ornithine decarboxylase inhibitor DFMO.[47,49]

BIOMECHANICAL CHANGES IN BLOOD AND CSF IN HEAD INJURY

Injury leads to a systemic hypermetabolic response which may influence recovery and must be considered in the metabolic and nutritional management of a head-injured patient. The primary and secondary mechanisms of neural injury may lead to tissue death with the resultant release of cellular structural proteins and enzymes into the blood and CSF. Indeed, with severe injury, gross fragments of brain tissue can sometimes be seen in blood or CSF. Measurement of released proteins in the blood and CSF may provide information about the volume of necrotic brain tissue and may help in prognostication and the detection of ongoing secondary injury. Injury that is insufficient to cause tissue death but results in metabolic dysfunction may be detected by measuring substances such as lactate, amino acids, and ions, which serve as neurochemical signatures of tissue injury.

Alterations Reflecting the Systemic Response to Injury

Injury evokes a systemic metabolic response characterized by a hypermetabolic state with increased energy expenditure, nitrogen mobilization, elevated catabolic hormones, and elevated serum cytokines. Skeletal muscle and visceral proteins are mobilized, urinary nitrogen losses increase, and hepatic synthesis of plasma proteins is shifted to acute-phase reactants. The elevated acute-phase proteins include alpha$_2$-macroglobulin, fibrinogen, cysteine proteinase inhibitor, C-reactive protein, and alpha$_1$-glycoprotein. The redirection of hepatic protein synthesis to the acute-phase reactants occurs at the expense of albumin synthesis, leading to hypoalbuminemia. Serum and urinary zinc are depressed during the acute-phase reaction. The acute-phase response is driven by elevated serum interleukin-1 and interleukin-6.

The systemic stress response leads to nitrogen mobilization and increased urinary nitrogen loss, which may impair wound healing, muscle strength recovery (including respiratory muscle strength), and immune function.

Hyperglycemia is a part of the systemic stress response and is driven by hypercatecholaminemia and insulin resistance. Hyperglycemia imperils injured brain by exacerbating ischemic injury. The systemic hypercatabolic response to head injury is discussed in Chap. 25.[50]

Alterations Indicative of Damage to Brain Tissue

Tissue necrosis and an altered metabolic state may be reflected in the biochemical composition of the blood and CSF. When cells die, they release structural proteins and enzymes in proportion to the amount of tissue necrosis and the rapidity of tissue death. Measurements of liver and cardiac enzymes have long been part of medical practice, but measurement of nervous system proteins in the blood and CSF is a much less developed field. Ideally, proteins indicative of injury should be relatively specific for the organ of interest and should be elevated in proportion to the extent of tissue injury. In the case of the brain, creatine kinase, lactate dehydrogenase, glial fibrillary acidic protein (GFAP), S100, neuron-specific enolase, and myelin basic protein have been measured in blood and CSF in a variety of diseases. A limited number of studies have reported alterations in these substances after traumatic injury. The elevation of these proteins is roughly proportional to the amount of tissue damage but is not specific to the mechanism of injury.

Creatine Kinase

The brain isoenzyme of creatine kinase (CK-BB) has been studied extensively as a potential enzymatic marker of cerebral injury. Creatine kinase (CK) is a mitochondrial and cytoplasmic enzyme that catalyzes phosphate transfer from creatine phosphate to adenosine diphosphate (ADP) to generate adenosine triphosphate (ATP). CK is a dimer composed of monomeric subunits designated M and B. These subunits dimerize to form three isoenzymes: CK1 (CK-BB), CK2 (CK-MB), and CK3 (CK-MM). CK-BB is the predominant isoenzyme in brain tissue, CK-MM is the major isoenzyme found in skeletal muscle, and CK-MB is contained predominantly in myocardial muscle. In head injury, CK-BB is elevated in proportion to the quantity of cerebral tissue injured. Elevation is measurable within 24 h of injury, and early elevation reflects primary injury. Later elevations may indicate secondary injury. The prognosis correlates with the degree of elevation of this isoenzyme. CK-BB elevation is seen in subarachnoid hemorrhage or even with neurosurgical manipulation as subtle as ventricular shunt catheter placement. It is important to recognize that CK determination without isoenzyme differentiation can be misleading because head trauma patients often have skeletal muscle injury that leads to massive elevations of CK-MM. Also, in head injury and subarachnoid hemorrhage, subendocardial necrosis may occur, leading to elevations of CK-MB. The brain is not the sole potential source of CK-BB; viscera, including the gastrointestinal tract, uterus, kidney, prostate, and lung, are rich in CK-BB. In a multitrauma patient, these viscera may be damaged, leading to elevated serum CK-BB. Elevations may also be seen with childbirth, hypothermia, and cardiopulmonary resuscitation. Because of the importance of CK isoenzyme measurements in cardiac disease, this assay is widely available and usually has a rapid turnaround time.[51–53]

CK can also be measured in CSF, and elevations have been described in brain tumors, infarcts, meningitis, and head trauma. CSF CK-BB levels correlate with the Glasgow Coma Scale score and tend to be maximal in the first 24 h after injury. The degree of elevation correlates with survival in that patients with values greater than 200 U/liter always die, those with levels between 100 and 200 U/liter are moderately to severely disabled, and those with levels below 100 U/liter may have a good recovery.

Lactate dehydrogenase

Lactate dehydrogenase (LDH) catalyzes the interconversion of pyruvate and lactate and therefore plays a central role in energy metabolism. This ubiquitous enzyme has five isoenzymes, but studies of LDH elevations after head injury have concentrated on total LDH activity. Elevations of total serum LDH in a trauma patient are much less specific than are elevations of CK isoenzymes and play no role in monitoring head injury. CSF LDH levels are elevated in head injury, but correlations with the Glasgow Coma Scale score and outcome are considerably weaker than with CK isoenzyme measurements. CSF LDH elevations can also be seen in primary and metastatic brain tumors, seizures, stroke, hemorrhage, hydrocephalus, and meningitis. LDH measurement is widely and rapidly available but has no advantages over CK isoenzyme determination.[51,53]

Neuron-specific enolase

Despite the fact that the name suggests neuronal specificity of this enzyme, neuron-specific enolase (NSE) is widely distributed throughout the body. Indeed, some disparagingly refer to NSE as *n*on*s*pecific *e*nolase. This glycolytic enzyme, also known as phosphopyruvate hydratase, has been used as an immunohistochemical and serum tumor marker for tumors of neuroendocrine origin, including neuroblastoma, pheochromocytoma, small cell carcinoma of the lung, carcinoid, medullary thyroid carcinoma, malignant melanoma, and neuroendocrine tumors of the pancreas. After brain injury from trauma, stroke, subarachnoid hemorrhage, or meningitis, serum NSE is elevated. The assay is a radioimmunoassay, with the upper limit of normal being 12.5 μg/ml. This assay has limited availability and a slow turnaround time.

Myelin basic protein

Myelin basic protein (MBP) is one of the major protein components of myelin. Myelin is synthesized by oligodendroglia and invests axons, permitting saltatory conduction. White matter injury leads to release of MBP into the CSF and blood. Most investigations of MBP elevations have concentrated on demyelinating disorders, but a limited number of studies in head injury have disclosed a correlation between the degree of MBP elevation and the volume of brain tissue damaged. Poor prognosis is associated with marked elevated MBP. This assay is widely available, but the turnaround time is relatively slow.[51,54]

Other proteins

GFAP is the major cytoskeletal intermediate filament constituent in astrocytes. Like other structural and enzymatic protein indicators of tissue injury, GFAP increases with tissue necrosis. GFAP is found almost exclusively in astrocytes and is therefore specific for CNS tissue damage. This assay is not available except in a research setting. Elevated neural cell adhesion molecule (NCAM) and S100 have been reported in head trauma, but measurement of these proteins is confined to the research setting.[55]

Alterations Indicative of Abnormal Cerebral Metabolism

The composition of the CSF represents the pooled metabolic activity of the brain, and as a result of the rather indolent fluid dynamics of the CSF circulation, changes in composition are slow to develop. Elevations of lactate in the CSF have been reported after head injury, and marked elevations are consistently associated with a poor outcome. Elevations of lactate in the first 24 h after injury probably reflect primary damage, whereas later elevations may indicate ischemic injury. The CSF lactate-pyruvate ratio is normally 20 or less, but during increased glycolysis associated with injury, the ratio is higher. Lactate elevation in the CSF is not specific for traumatic or ischemic brain injury; marked elevations can be seen in meningitis and subarachnoid hemorrhage. Red blood cells are devoid of mitochondria and are exclusively dependent on glycolysis for energy production; therefore, erythrocytes in the CSF elevate CSF lactate. Cerebral metabolism is reflected in arteriovenous differences of metabolites and in oxygen saturation of the venous efflux; these are discussed in Chaps. 34 and 37.[11,13,49,56,57] One of the very damaging mechanisms of ischemic injury is free radical generation with subsequent membrane lipid peroxidation. Measurement of lipid peroxidation using the thiobarbituric acid assay in jugular venous blood indicates that free radical injury does take place in severe head injury, and the degree of free radical generation correlates with decreased jugular venous oxygen saturation.[58]

DIRECT MONITORING OF THE BIOCHEMICAL MILIEU OF THE BRAIN

While the neurochemistry of ischemic and traumatic injury has been studied extensively in animals, work in humans is more limited. Studies of human tissues obtained at surgery or postmortem are confined to single time points in the patient's course, and there are recognized confounding changes in metabolites and neurotransmitters in such tissues.[59] Positron emission tomography (PET) and nuclear magnetic resonance spectroscopy studies can be performed in neurosurgical patients and are providing valuable insights into brain injury and stroke. However, these methods are cumbersome and expensive, and only a few time points can be evaluated during the patient's course. Measurements of metabolites and neurotransmitters in venous efflux from the brain or in CSF yield valuable information but are limited because these sources reflect neurochemical activity of large volumes of brain. CSF dynamics are sufficiently indolent that measurements of metabolites poorly reflect the time course of neurochemical events in the brain.[56]

The neurochemistry of injury can be pursued with measurements directly in the brain parenchyma. Electrodes can be used to measure pH, oxygen tension, ion composition, and some electroactive neurotransmitters, such as the catecholamines. Immobilized enzyme electrodes can be used to measure metabolites, amino acids, and neurotransmitters. None of these methods have been used to any significant extent in clinical head injury monitoring, as there are major difficulties with electrode calibration and stability. An alternative to having the sensor directly in the brain is to use a technique which allows frequent or continuous sampling of the extracellular space with subsequent off-line analysis. A variety of cortical cups, push-pull cannulas, diatrodes, and microdialysis probes have been used in experimental animals, but only microdialysis probes have been used in humans. Microdialysis is a sampling method which allows *continuous* acquisition of samples with good temporal resolution from a *limited area* of brain. This technique has been used extensively in animals, and has recently been used in humans.[60–69] Microdialysis represents a compromise between the highly desirable omnipotence of the ideal and currently unachievable neurochemical monitoring situation in which detailed information would be available continuously about all volume elements of the brain and the study of brain biochemistry by examination of the effluvium of the CSF or blood (Fig. 40-2).

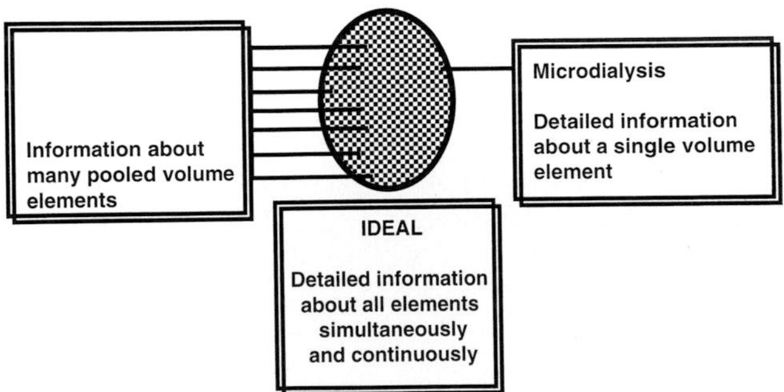

Figure 40-2. Neurochemical monitoring would ideally provide detailed continuous information about all the volume elements of the brain. Examination of blood and CSF provides pooled information from a large number of elements and obscures heterogeneity. Microdialysis provides detailed information about a single small-volume element of the brain.

MICRODIALYSIS: PRINCIPLES, TECHNIQUES, AND LIMITATIONS

Over the past decade, microdialysis has been used extensively in experimental neuroscience to acquire information regarding neurochemical alterations in the extracellular space of neural tissue.[60] This technique permits the acquisition of samples for days to weeks with minimal disruption of the structural or biochemical mileau of the tissue under investigation. The analytes are generally low-molecular-weight compounds including neurotransmitters, intermediary metabolites, small peptides, and pharmaceuticals. The biochemical analytic methods employed are wide-ranging, but the methods used must have high sensitivity and must be compatible with small sample sizes. Given these constraints, high-pressure liquid chromatography (HPLC) has been the most widely used analytic technique.

The principles of microdialysis are straightforward, but important nuances must be borne in mind. A microdialysis probe consists of a tube through which dialysate fluid is pumped at a low rate (2 to 10 μl/min). A portion of the tubing residing in the tissue has a small segment of dialysis membrane which is permeable to low-molecular-weight compounds. The dialysate has an ionic composition similar to that in the extracellular fluid so that no net exchange of ions or water occurs across the probe membrane, but compounds present in the extracellular space but not in the dialysate flow down their concentration gradients and enter the dialysate. The steepness of the concentration gradient is contingent on the flow rate of the dialysate so that analyte recovery varies as a function of flow rate. Microdialysate is collected over specified epochs (usually 5 to 30 min) and stored over subsequent analysis (Fig. 40-3).

Several microdialysis probe geometries are available.

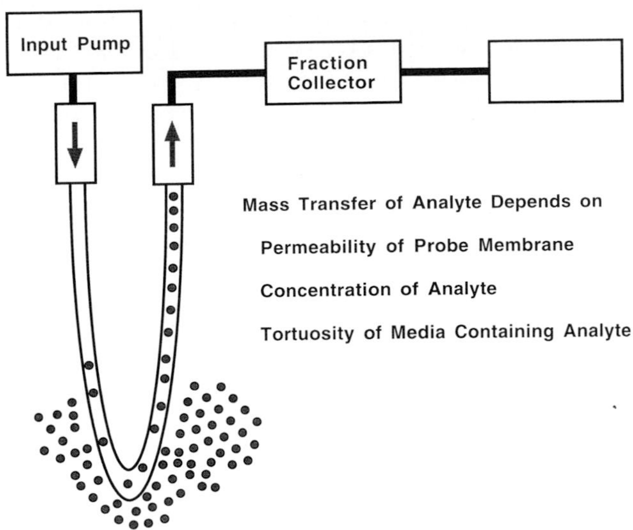

Figure 40-3. Microdialysis probes collect compounds from the extracellular space of the brain. Substances move from the brain into the microdialysate according to the flow rate of the microdialysate, the permeability of the probe membrane, the molecular weight of the compound, and the geometry of the tissue adjacent to the probe (tortuosity).

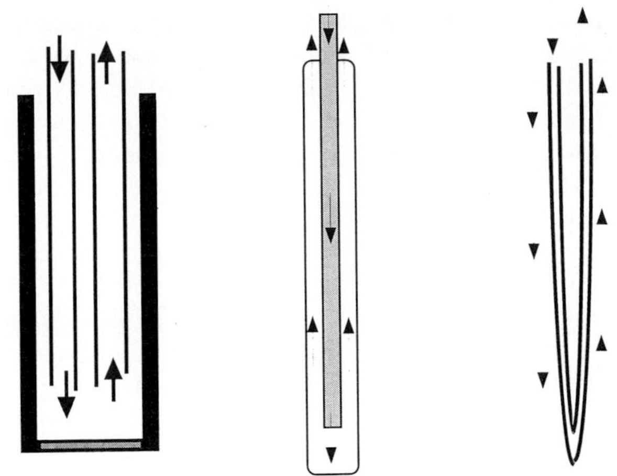

Figure 40-4. Microdialysis probes may be constructed in the side-by-side, concentric, or loop arrangement. Most commercially available probes are side-by-side or concentric, whereas "homemade" probes are usually loops.

Straight microdialysis tubing with active sampling restricted to one zone by coating the surface of the tubing with impermeants has been used extensively in experimental systems in which the tubing is simply threaded through the tissue of interest. Investigations using this technique have involved through-and-through placement in the brain and spinal cord. Alternatively, straight tubing has been placed on the surface of the brain in experimental and clinical studies, but exclusion of CSF contamination of results has been troublesome in this setting. Most investigators use loop, concentric, or side-by-side microdialysis probes, which permit a single perforation of the tissue under study (Fig. 40-4). Probes of this design can be chronically implanted and have been used extensively in experimental studies and increasingly in clinical studies.

Microdialysis probes have been used for continuous sampling of adipose tissue, muscle, blood, and, most extensively, brain and spinal cord. Minimal tissue damage is incurred by probe placement, and after a brief period of increased anaerobic metabolism, the cells adjacent to the probe resume normal metabolic operations. In neural tissues, microdialysis probes can be used to monitor extracellular concentrations of neurotransmitters, including amino acids, biogenic amines, substance P, and acetylcholine, in response to pharmacological manipulation or electrophysiological stimulation, as well as to monitor pathological conditions. The relative contribution of glycolysis to energy production can be monitored by measuring extracellular lactate and pyruvate. Adenosine, uric acid, free radicals, and polyamines also have been successfully measured in brain using this technique.

As a result of the small size of the probe and the low flow rates normally used, the net mass exchange of analyte at the site of sampling is small and the volume interrogated is limited to a very small domain immediately around the active site of the probe. In addition to the restricted size of the volume element sampled by the probe, the complex geometry of the extracellular space in tissue (especially neural tissue) has importance in the interpretation of data from microdialysis experiments. As was mentioned earlier, the recovery of analyte depends on the flow rate of dialysate through the probe. Probe recovery can be measured in vitro by placing the probe in a solution of known analyte concentration and then measuring the concentration of the compound in the microdialysate. As molecules of the compound of interest are taken away by the microdialysis system, a local concentration gradient in the immediate vicinity of the probe active site is established such that fewer molecules are present in the volume immediately around the probe. Molecules from the surrounding fluid, however, can move unimpeded down this concentration gradient, immediately reestablishing the original concentration of the analyte. In contrast, in tissue where the extracellular space may constitute only 10 to 15 percent of the volume surrounding the probe and this volume is disposed in a complex geometry, molecules of analyte are impeded in their journey to the probe. This restraint on molecular movement imposed by the complex geometry of the media is known as tortuosity.[60,61] The impact of tortuosity on microdialysis measurements is substantial, so that failure to account for tortuosity will result in a fivefold to 10-fold underestimation of the absolute concentration of the analyte in the extracellular space. Tortuosity is difficult to measure, although some data are available in experimental systems. If the tortuosity of the tissue under study is unknown, the microdialysis data can still be used to study relative changes of the analyte over time or with manipulation, and most investigators take this approach rather than attempt to extrapolate to the absolute concentration of the analyte in the extracellular space. Tortuosity also may vary as a pathological process evolves so that changes in the concentrations in the microdialysate could reflect tortuosity changes rather than alterations in the absolute extracellular analyte concentrations. Thus, microdialysis sampling has major limitations.

1. The volume of tissue sampled is very small and may not reflect neurochemical events occurring elsewhere in the brain. Clinical information and data from other clinical monitoring methods are used to identify focal pathological processes adjacent to the probe. The fact that the microdialysis probe samples only a very small volume of brain may not be as significant a limitation as it first might appear because there is strong evidence that blood flow, glucose consumption, and electrophysiological activity are widely disrupted after head injury. PET and magnetic resonance imaging (MRI) abnormalities are usually substantially larger and more widespread than would be anticipated from the computed tomography (CT) scan alone, and EEG abnormalities are frequently widespread.
2. Microdialysis does not provide a direct measurement of the absolute concentrations of analytes in the extracellular space because of tortuosity and probe recovery characteristics. Tortuosity may vary as pathological processes evolve so that changes in the concentrations in the microdialysate may reflect tortuosity changes rather than alterations in the absolute extracellular analyte concentrations. Changes in an individual analyte's concentration are more likely to reflect actual changes occurring in the tissue, whereas if all the analytes' concentrations change at the same time, tortuosity fluctuations may account for the changes. Pathological processes leading to concentration changes are expected to lead to elevations in some analytes and to reductions in others. For example, increased anaerobic metabolism raises lactate and adenosine while lowering pyruvate. In the authors' preliminary studies, elevations of lactate were accompanied by declines in pyruvate, suggesting that the lactate elevations were in fact reflecting anaerobic metabolism rather than changes in tortuosity, since increased tortuosity would decrease the microdialysate levels of all the compounds. Similarly, among the amino acids, the neurotransmitter amino acids—glutamate, aspartate, glycine, and gamma-aminobutyric acid (GABA)—are all released by ischemia-induced membrane depolarization, but neutral amino acids such as valine and isoleucine are not increased. Tortuosity changes would be expected to change all amino acid concentrations in the same direction. In the authors' preliminary studies, glutamate and aspartate, taurine, and glycine changed together during pathophysiological events but GABA did not, suggesting that altered tortuosity was not the cause of the amino acid elevations.

Differences in probe recovery of analytes may hinder comparison of results from different centers. Since recovery is determined by dialysate flow rate and probe membrane characteristics, investigators should report flow rates and probe recoveries in order to facilitate comparison of results. Calculation of absolute extracellular analyte concentrations based on probe recovery may also allow comparison of results, although the analyte concentrations reported should not be taken too literally, as the effects of tortuosity are not accounted for by this approach.

CLINICAL MICRODIALYSIS

Hundreds of papers using microdialysis in experimental systems have been published in the last decade. In the past 5 years, several investigators have reported microdialysis investigations in humans with Parkinson's disease, epilepsy, brain tumors, subarachnoid hemorrhage, and head injury. Microdialysis probes have been kept in place in these patients for up to 21 days without adverse effects. Four Parkinson's disease patients had placement of a microdialysis probe during thalamotomy for tremor, and thalamic extracellular levels of dopamine, 3,4-dihydroxyphenylacetic acid DOPAC, homovanillic acid (HVA), 5-hydroxyindoleacetic acid (5-HIAA), hypoxanthine, inosine, guanosine, adenosine, GABA, taurine, aspartate, and glutamate were successfully measured.[63] Seven patients with intractable epilepsy were monitored concurrently with electrodes and microdialysis; during seizures, dramatic elevations in extracellular aspartate, glutamate, glycine, and serine were seen.[35] Lactate and pyruvate were also measured in two of these patients during seizures, and small changes relative to those seen in trauma or ischemia were observed, suggesting that energy metabolism is not deranged in focal seizures of limited duration. Similar studies using a combination depth electrode–microdialysis probe on 15 patients with intractable complex partial seizures disclosed ictal increases in excitatory amino acids and the purine adenosine and ictal decreases in the inhibitory amino acid GABA.[70] As many as 50 epilepsy patients have also been monitored intraoperatively using pial and depth microdialysis probes.[71] Microdialysis probes have been used in three patients with malignant gliomas to deliver chemotherapy, with the probes remaining in place without complications for up to 21 days.[72]

Of greater relevance to neurotraumatologists is the microdialysis study of Persson and Hillered on three head trauma patients and one subarachnoid hemorrhage patient.[73] Microdialysis was performed from 2.3 to 8.3 days after the ictus, and the energy-related metabolites lactate, pyruvate, and hypoxanthine were measured. Amino acids were also measured in the subarachnoid hemorrhage patient. Elevations of lactate and the lactate-pyruvate ratio correlated with clinical events such as increased intracranial pressure, seizures, hemodynamic instability, pneumothorax, and withdrawal of barbiturate coma. The excitatory amino acids glutamate and aspartate were elevated up to 25-fold during energy metabolism derangement, corresponding to periods of elevated intracranial pressure and increased lactate-pyruvate ratios. Taurine also increased during these pathophysiological derangements. This alteration is of interest because taurine has been implicated as an osmole important in astrocyte volume regulation. Studies by these authors on microdialysis of human frontal lobe before and after resection for tumor demonstrated elevation of excitatory amino acids and lactate after resection with interruption of perfusion.[73–75] Energy-related metabolite levels changed rapidly in microdialysates but lagged and were of smaller magnitude in CSF in middle cerebral artery occlusion in rats; therefore, microdialysis should be superior to CSF measurements in the clinical setting.[56]

The authors have studied 20 patients with severe head injury, using microdialysis. The injuries included subdural and epidural hematomas, cerebral contusions, and gunshot wounds with brain laceration. Microdialysate lactate levels increased, pyruvate levels decreased, and the lactate-pyruvate ratio increased during periods of increased intracranial pressure, jugular venous oxygen desaturation, and herniation. Barbiturate coma decreased the lactate levels. A poor outcome (severely impaired or dead) at 3 months was linked to peak microdialysate lactate levels greater than 1.0 μmol/liter. Patients with lactate levels below 1.0 μmol/liter had good outcomes (good recovery or moderate disability)

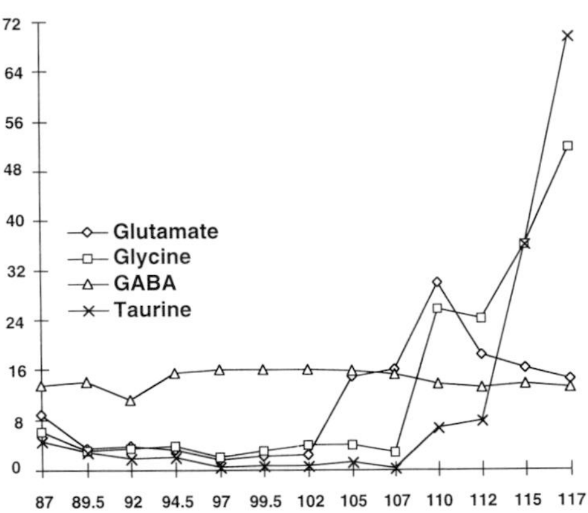

Figure 40-5. The microdialysate concentrations of the amino acids glutamate, glycine, and taurine increased dramatically during cerebral ischemia, as indicated by jugular venous oxygen desaturation.

at 3 months. In parallel with the elevations of lactate, the excitatory amino acids glutamate and aspartate increased during periods of physiological deterioration. These elevations were accompanied by elevations of glycine and taurine but were not accompanied by increased GABA or neutral amino acids (Fig. 40-5). The authors have measured polyamines in five patients thus far, and elevations were seen only in one patient who died of a gunshot wound. Only putrescine was increased, indicating the presence of the potentially damaging "incomplete" polyamine response. The remaining four patients did not have elevations of any of the polyamines, and all had a good to moderate recovery. These clinical studies indicate that microdialysis permits the measurement of pathological neurochemical events in critically injured patients.

Practical Aspects of Clinical Microdialysis

Clinical microdialysis is a rapidly developing field which will undoubtedly undergo substantial technical and conceptual evolution. This method of biochemical monitoring is technically demanding, and seemingly trivial "tricks of the trade" may make the difference between success and failure. The authors have been performing microdialysis monitoring in the neurosurgical intensive care unit at the Ben Taub General Hospital since April 1993 and as of this writing have investigated 20 patients. The following points represent our experience with this technique.

The microdialysis probe is placed at the time of craniotomy or placement of an intracranial pressure transducer. The right frontal cortex is usually selected for placement of pressure transducers and is therefore the most common probe insertion site. The active surface of the probe is 5 mm long, and since the average human cerebral cortex is 3 to 4 mm thick, the probe resides predominantly in the cerebral cortex. No subcortical structures are sampled. The dialysis probe consists of a 0.2-mm-diameter flexible tubing with a molecular weight cutoff of 6000 daltons. This delicate tubing runs through clear 2-mm polyethylene tubing which serves as an umbilical cord connecting the insertion site with the microdialysis pump and fraction collector. The probe penetrates 5 mm below the cortical surface, and the microdialysis tubing is lightly anchored to the dura. The tubing is tunneled in a subgaleal plane, externalized at a skin site separate from the burr hole or craniotomy site, and dressed under sterile technique. The delicate microdialysis tubing is shielded by the polyethylene tubing where it emerges from the dressing. The umbilical tubing is essential, since the microdialysis probe inflow and outflow tubes are very fragile and are easily disrupted during patient manipulations such as turning, physical therapy, and x-rays. The components of the clinical microdialysis system are shown in Fig. 40-6.

Microdialysis probes can be purchased from any of several vendors or can be handmade locally. The authors manufacture and gas sterilize our probes, but other centers use manufactured probes. The manufactured probes have concentric or side-by-side geometry and are slightly smaller in diameter than our homemade loop probes, but they are somewhat more rigid and are quite expensive. Investigators considering entry into the field should try both approaches in experimental animals and should honestly assess their ability and aptitude for manufacturing these delicate little devices.

The dialysis tubing is perfused with a 0.9% sodium chloride solution. The solution is commercially available medical intravenous fluid. In preliminary investigations,

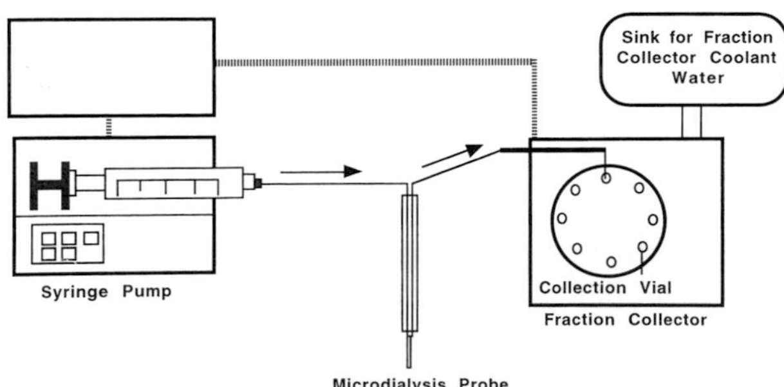

Figure 40-6. In the NICU, the microdialysate pump and fraction collector are adjacent to one another at the head of the patient's bed. The pump delivers microdialysate to the probe, and the fraction collector stores 30-min samples. The pump and collector are computer-controlled, and the fraction collector is thermoelectrically cooled, necessitating cooling water from a nearby sink.

the authors found that this perfusate results in stable microdialysis studies in animals and is virtually free of contaminating polyamines and amino acids. Since this fluid is manufactured for medical use, it is pyrogen-free, sterile, and rigorously controlled in composition, reducing the safety concerns associated with the manufacture of perfusate in the pharmacy or research laboratory.

The microdialysis infusion pump (CMA100, CMA/Microdialysis, Stockholm, Sweden; sold in the United States by Bioanalytical Systems, Inc., West Lafayette, IN) is a syringe pump providing perfusate at a rate of 2.0 μl/min, and fraction collection is performed using a cooled microfraction collector especially designed for the minute fluid-handling requirements of microdialysis (CMA170, CMA/Microdialysis, Stockholm, Sweden). The perfusion, probe, and collection array constitute a closed system during operation. Periodic maintenance of perfusate requires placement of fresh syringes filled with 0.9% saline in the pump, temporarily opening the system. This procedure is performed under sterile precautions.

Microdialysis fractions are collected in 30-min epochs (60-μl samples) into sealed, labeled collection vials. Samples are stored at −70°C until biochemical analysis is performed. The vials must be labeled with waterproof ink since they often become moist with condensate as they thaw before analysis. An enormous number of samples can be generated during a relatively brief period of microdialysis monitoring. For example, if microdialysis probes are left in place for 5 days, up to 240 samples will be generated.

Microdialysis monitoring is terminated when intracranial pressure monitoring is no longer required. The microdialysis probe is carefully pulled out under aseptic conditions in the same way pressure transducers and ventricular catheters are removed. Removal is done in the neurosurgical intensive care unit (NICU) and does not require anesthesia.

Safety Issues

No immediate benefit can be anticipated for individual patients enrolling in current microdialysis protocols, since the neurochemical analyses are performed off-line. The risks of the monitoring are very small and consist of the possibility of producing a hematoma or infection. The microdialysis probe is considerably smaller than the intraventricular catheters and intraparenchymal pressure transducers used in the NICU, and these devices rarely produce significant injury. Patients in the NICU are monitored clinically by intracranial pressure (ICP) measurement, inspection of CSF drainage for blood, and neuroimaging procedures so that the formation of a hematoma can be detected. Infection has not been seen in the series reported from other centers or in the authors' experience. The microdialysis system is continuously flushed during operation, reducing the possibility of microbial adhesion to the tubing or probe. The probe dialysis membrane is not permeable to bacterial and fungi and serves as a barrier to brain invasion in the unlikely event of contamination of the perfusate. NICU patients are monitored closely for the development of infections by clinical examination, temperature monitoring, ICP measurement, and daily leukocyte counts. Patients exhibiting clinical deterioration suggestive of infection or elevation of white blood cell count are examined for infection, and appropriate cultures are taken. If hemorrhagic or infectious complications ensue in conjunction with microdialysis monitoring, the probe should be removed and not replaced.

The removed probe is cultured. Potential long-term complications of microdialysis probe placement are local gliosis and epileptogenesis. The authors anticipate that this complication will be less common than it is with pressure transducer placement in view of the size disparity between these devices. In experimental animals, no such long-term adverse effects have been described. A potential complication which has not been described in experimental or clinical systems is biochemical derangement of the extracellular space caused by excessive transport of substances into the probe or entry of water from the perfusate. The perfusate is osmotically balanced with CSF so that net fluid transport is unlikely. Furthermore, the volume of effect of the probe is very limited so that any such complications should be confined to the immediate volume surrounding the probe.

ANALYTIC METHODS

Biochemical measurement techniques used in conjunction with microdialysis must have high analytic sensitivity and low sample volume requirements. HPLC using a variety of separation protocols and detectors (spectrophotometric, fluorescence, electrochemical) has been the primary analytic technique used. HPLC has enormous flexibility in terms of the types of compounds that can be analyzed, the sample requirements are very low (10 to 30 μl), and the sensitivity of the technique is high. Since the microdialysis samples have already passed through a microdialysis membrane, they are of high-molecular-weight compounds which normally have to be removed before HPLC annalysis of metabolites and neurotransmitters. In the case of lactate and pyruvate, the microdialysate samples can be injected directly into the HPLC system. Many compounds, including amino acids and polyamines, require chemical derivatization in order to be detected; therefore, some sample manipulation is necessary. Some investigators have reported systems in which microdialysate is collected directly into an HPLC system's injection loop, permitting on-line analysis. HPLC systems exist which allow for on-line sample derivatization as well, and so we can envision the possibility of continuous on-line analysis of a variety of analytes. Such systems are formidable in their complexity, cost, and propensity to malfunction and are therefore unlikely to be used for "routine" neurochemical monitoring in the NICU setting. It is more likely that if a limited number of compounds are proved to be informative by the microdialysis systems in research NICUs, in-line arrays of analyte-specific electrodes will be developed for insertion into the microdialysis stream to permit continous monitoring.

Other analytic techniques, including radioimmunoassay and enzyme-linked immunoassays, have been used to detect compounds in microdialysate samples from experimental animals. Only a limited number of samples can be analyzed using these techniques, and the analyses are by necessity off-line. There are promising developments in antibody-linked electrode technology which may make on-line analysis possible.[76]

Finally, while HPLC has low sample volume requirements, this technique is being challenged by capillary electrophoresis (CE), which has similar sensitivity but requires samples in the nanoliter volume range. CE offers the prospect of measuring a larger number of analytes from smaller microdialysate samples representing shorter collection intervals. Improved temporal resolution as a result of shortened collection intervals may permit detection of transient biochemical processes which would be overlooked by techniques requiring longer collection times. The greatest challenge in CE lies in the difficulty of physically manipulating the incredibly small sample volumes involved.

Analytic methods for several of the compounds that have been studied thus far are reviewed below.

Lactate and pyruvate measurements are performed by HPLC using a 25-μl injection of unprocessed microdialysate onto a BioRad HPX87 anion exchange organic acid column perfused isocratically with dilute sulfuric acid (BioRad Laboratories, Hercules, CA). Detection is performed by absorbance at 210 nm, using peak area measurement with a three-point standard curve. The method requires no sample preparation when applied to microdialysis specimens and has a run time of 17 min, permitting substantial analytic throughput. The mobile phase is inexpensive and is continuously recirculated, simplifying system maintainence. The authors and others have used this method extensively in the analysis of microdialysate samples.[14,74,76–78]

Purine measurements encompassing adenosine, inosine, xanthine, and hypoxanthine are performed by isocratic reverse-phase HPLC with ultraviolet detection at 254 nm. No sample preparation is required, and adenosine elutes 8 min after injection. This method permits simultaneous measurement of all the purines of interest in assessing energy metabolism.[70]

Ions, including sodium, potassium, and calcium, can be measured directly in microdialysate by using a small ion-specific electrode system (World Precision Instruments, Sarasota, FL).[24]

Amino acid analysis is performed using precolumn phenyl isothiocyanate (PITC), dansyl chloride, or orthophthalaldehyde (OPA) derivatization with subsequent gradient programmed reverse-phase HPLC with absorbance or fluorescence detection. Electrochemical detection of OPA or tert-butylthiol amino acid derivatives also has been used. The techniques using fluorescence and electrochemical detection are more sensitive than are those employing absorbance detection, but the PITC derivatization technique is satisfactory for clinical microdialysis. Derivatization is labor-intensive, and the reagents and standards are moderately expensive. The mobile phases are expensive, require helium sparging, and are consumed in substantial quantities. The cost, long analytic run time, and labor intensity limit the number of amino acid analyses that can be performed. These techniques have, however, been used extensively for amino acid quantification in microdialysis samples.[26,29,32,34,64,79,80]

Polyamine analysis is performed by precolumn extraction and derivatization with dansyl chloride with subsequent gradient programmed reverse-phase chromatography and fluorescence detection. Quantitation is done by peak area analysis, using a two-point standard and an internal standard (diaminohexane). Putrescine, cadaverine, spermine, and spermidine are measured using this method. Experience with this analytic technique in microdialysis samples is very limited. Grimaldi and associates measured cerebral microdialysate putrescine, spermidine, and spermine in a rat model of transient forebrain ischemia using this derivatization method.[81,82] The authors have successfully measured polyamines in both tissue extracts and microdialysis samples using this technique. The analytic technique is very labor-intensive and requires great attention to technique to avoid contamination by ubiquitous polyamines. For microdialysis perfusate preparation, the authors have found that sterile microfiltered water prepared for human physiological infusions is relatively free of endogenous polyamines, whereas commercially available analytic or HPLC-grade water is seriously contaminated. The reagents are moderately expensive, and the analytic run time is about 30 min.

Fluctuations in analyte concentrations in microdialysis may reflect actual pathophysiological events or may simply indicate changes in tissue tortuosity. Tortuosity alterations can be compensated for by measuring ratios of analytes of similar molecular migration characteristics, as changes in tortuosity should not alter the ratios of these compounds. For example, lactate and pyruvate are measured in pairs, and their ratio is computed. A decrease in tissue tortuosity reflecting increased extracellular space volume would lead to an increase in the concentrations of both compounds in the microdialysate. Inspection of the elevated lactate concentration alone would lead to the erroneous conclusion that increased anaerobic metabolism was occurring, but evaluation of the lactate-pyruvate ratio would reveal that the concentrations of both compounds had increased but that the ratio was preserved. If the lactate went up in response to increased anaerobic metabolism, the pyruvate would be expected to decrease and the ratio of these metabolites would increase. Similar ratio methods can be used to compare amino acids, using neutral amino acids such as valine and isoleucine in relationship to the excitotoxic amino acids. No such internal ratio evaluation is available with the polyamines; however, the tortuosity can be evaluated using the lactate-pyruvate ratio's since the polyamines and the organic acids have similar molecular migration properties.

CONCLUSIONS

The brain is an oxygen-hungry, glucose-consuming, biochemically complex organ. When injured, it emits neurochemical signatures of damage which are coming under increased scrutiny using the techniques described here and elsewhere in this book. At present, clinical microdialysis is a formidably complicated undertaking, and it is unlikely that this technique will soon find application outside the research NICU setting. The broad range of analytes which can be studied by this method may allow identification of a few critical biochemical markers of tissue injury which are strongly predictive of outcome or indicative of ongoing damage that is amenable to intervention. Once these sentinel analytes are identified, more "user-friendly" monitoring equipment can be developed. Sample acquisition may continue to rely on microdialysis, but analysis could potentially be simplified to make bedside on-line analysis possible. Alternatively, once the important compounds are identified, analyte-specific electrodes or electrode arrays could be placed directly in or on the brain. Other promising technologies include reflectance spectroscopy and miniaturized optrodes that permit in situ optical spectroscopy. The field of biochemical monitoring of head-injured patients will require the combined efforts of neurosurgeons, neurochemists, intensivists, physicists, and biomedical engineers spanning the gamut of basic and applied science.

ACKNOWLEDGMENTS

The excellent and dedicated support of the nursing staff, house officers, and research fellows of the neurosurgical intensive care unit, Ben Taub General Hospital, is gratefully acknowledged, for without their hard work, our clinical microdialysis work would not be possible. Thanks also to Ms. Mary V. Williams for carrying out the biochemical analyses and to Drs. Robert Grossman, Claudia Robertson, and Raj Narayan for their support and encouragement.

REFERENCES

1. Globus MYT, Dietrich WD: *The Role of Neurotransmitters in Brain Injury* (1st ed). New York: Plenum, 1992.
2. Jenkins LW, Moszynski K, Lyeth BG, et al: Increased vulnerability of the mildly traumatized rat brain to cerebral ischemia—the use of controlled secondary ischemia as a research tool to identify common or different mechanisms contributing to mechanical and ischemic brain injury. *Brain Res* 477:211–224, 1989.
3. Hovda DA, Becker DP, Katayama Y: Secondary injury and acidosis. *J Neurotrauma* 9:47–60, 1992.
4. Gardiner M, Smith ML, Kagstrom E: Influence of blood glucose concentration on brain lactate accumulation during severe hypoxia and subsequent recovery of brain energy metabolism. *J Cereb Blood Flow Metab* 2:429–438, 1982.
5. Nilsson P, Hillered L, Ponten U, Ungerstedt U: Changes in cortical extracellular levels of energy-related metabolites and amino acids following concussive brain injury in rats. *J Cereb Blood Flow Metab* 19:631–637, 1990.
6. Pitts LH, McIntosh TK: Dynamic changes after brain trauma, in Braakman R (ed): *Head Injury*. New York: Elsevier, 1990:65–100.
7. Siesjo BK: Pathophysiology and treatment of focal cerebral ischemia: I. Pathophysiology. *J Neurosurg* 77:169–184, 1992.
8. Siesjo B: Pathophysiology and treatment of focal cerebral ischemia: II. Mechanisms of damage and treatment. *J Neurosurg* 77:337–354, 1992.
9. Kraig RP, Chesler M: Astrocytic acidosis in hyperglycemia and complete ischemia. *J Cereb Blood Flow Metab* 10:1–11, 1988.
10. Ginsberg MD: Glycolytic metabolism in brain ischemia, in Weinstein PR, Faden AI (eds): *Protection of the Brain from Ischemia*. Baltimore: Williams & Wilkins, 1990:37–48.
11. Inao S, Marmarou A, Clarke GD, et al: Production and clearance of lactate from brain tissue, cerebrospinal fluid, and serum following experimental brain injury. *J Neurosurg* 69:736–744, 1988.
12. Smith M-L, von Hawehr R, Siesjö BK: Changes in extra- and intracellular pH in the brain during and following ischemia in hyperglycemic and in moderately hypoglycemic rats. *J Cereb Blood Flow Metab* 6:574–583, 1986.
13. Siesjö BK, Ekholm A, Katsura K, Theander S: Acid-base changes during complete brain ischemia. *Stroke* 21:194–199, 1990.
14. Robertson CS, Goodman JC, Grossman RG, Priessman A: Reduction in spinal cord post-ischemic lactic acidosis and functional improvement with dichloroacetate. *J Neurotrauma* 7:1–12, 1990.
15. Norenberg MD, Mozes LW, Gregorios JB, Norenberg LB: Effects of lactic acid on astrocytes in primary culture. *J Neuropathol Exp Neurol* 46:154–165, 1987.
16. Marmarou A: Intracellular acidosis in human and experimental brain injury. *J Neurotrauma* 9:551–562, 1992.
17. Van Nimmen D, Weyne J, Demeester G, Leusen I: Local cerebral glucose utilization during intracerebral pH changes. *J Cereb Blood Flow Metab* 6:584–589, 1986.
18. Phillis JW: Adenosine, inosine, and the oxypurines in cerebral ischemia, in Schurr A, Rigor BM (eds): *Cerebral Ischemia and Resuscitation*. Boca Raton: CRC, 1990:189–204.
19. Goldberg MP, Monyer H, Weiss JH, Choi DW: Adenosine reduces cortical neuronal injury induced by oxygen or glucose deprivation in vitro. *Neurosci Lett* 89:323–327, 1988.
20. Miller LP, Hsu C: Therapeutic potential for adenosine receptor activation in ischemic brain injury. *J Neurotrauma* 9:563–578, 1992.
21. Rudolphi KA, Schubert P, Parkinson FE, Fredholm BB: Adenosine and brain ischemia. *Cerebrovasc Brain Metab Rev* 4:346–369, 1992.
22. Astrup J, Symon L, Branston NM: Cortical evoked potential and extracellular K and H at critical levels of brain ischemia. *Stroke* 8:51–57, 1977.
23. Branston NM, Strong AJ, Symon L: Extracellular potassium activity, evoked potential and tissue blood flow. *J Neurol Sci* 32:305–321, 1977.
24. Katayama Y, Becker DP, Tamura T, Hovda DA: Massive increases in extracellular potassium and the indiscriminate release of glutamate following concussive brain injury. *J Neurosurg* 73:889–900, 1990.
25. Phillis JW, Perkins LM, O'Regan MH: Potassium evoked efflux of transmitter amino acids and purines from rat cerebral cortex. *Brain Res Bull* 31:547–552, 1993.
26. Nakata N, Kato H, Kogure K: Effects of repeated cerebral ischemia on extracellular amino acid concentrations measured with intracerebral microdialysis in the gerbil hippocampus. *Stroke* 24:458–464, 1993.
27. Rothman SM, Olney JW: Glutamate and the pathophysiology of hypoxic-ischemic brain damage. *Ann Neurol* 19:105–111, 1986.
28. Goldberg MP, Monyer H, Choi DW: Hypoxic neuronal injury in vitro depends on extracellular glutamine. *Neurosci Lett* 94:52–57, 1988.

29. Benveniste H: The excitotoxin hypothesis in relation to cerebral ischemia. *Cerebrovasc Brain Metab Rev* 3:213–245, 1991.
30. Steinhardt RA, Bi G, Alderton JM: Cell membrane resealing by a vesicular mechanism similar to neurotransmitter release. *Science* 263:390–393, 1994.
31. Kawamata T, Katayama Y, Hovda DA, et al: Administration of excitatory amino acid antagonists via microdialysis attenuates the increase in glucose utilization seen following concussive brain injury. *J Cereb Blood Flow Metab* 12:12–24, 1992.
32. Faden A, Panter S: Elevations in extracellular amino acids following spinal contusion. *Science* 244:798–800, 1989.
33. Hayes RL, Jenkins LW, Lyeth BG: Neurotransmitter-mediated mechanisms of traumatic brain injury: Acetylcholine and excitatory amino acids. *J Neurotrauma* 9:173–188, 1992.
34. Palmer AM, Marion DW, Botscheller ML, et al: Traumatic brain injury-induced excitotoxicity assessed in a controlled cortical impact model. *J Neurochem* 61:2015–2024, 1993.
35. Ronne EE, Hillered L, Flink R, et al: Intracerebral microdialysis of extracellular amino acids in the human epileptic focus. *J Cereb Blood Flow Metab* 12:873–876, 1992.
36. Shimada N, Graf R, Rosner G, Heiss WD: Ischemia-induced accumulation of extracellular amino acids in cerebral cortex, white matter, and cerebrospinal fluid. *J Neurochem* 60:66–71, 1993.
37. Zini I, Tomasi A, Grimaldi R, et al: Detection of free radicals during brain ischemia and reperfusion by spin trapping and microdialysis. *Neurosci Lett* 138:279–282, 1992.
38. Gilad GM, Gilad VH: Polyamines can protect against ischemia-induced nerve cell death in gerbil forebrain. *Exp Neurol* 111:349–355, 1991.
39. Gilad GM, Gilad VH: Polyamines in neurotrauma—ubiquitous molecules in search of a function. *Biochem Pharmacol* 44:401–407, 1992.
40. Gilad GM, Casero RA, Busto R, Globus MYT: Polyamines in rat brain extracellular space after ischemia. *Mol Chem Neuropathol* 18:27–33, 1993.
41. Gilad GM, Gilad VH, Wyatt RJ: Accumulation of exogenous polyamines in gerbil brain after ischemia. *Mol Chem Neuropathol* 18:197–210, 1993.
42. Paschen W, Schmidt KR, Hallmayer J, Djuricic B: Polyamines in cerebral ischemia. *Neurochem Pathol* 9:1–20, 1988.
43. Paschen W, Rohn G, Meese CO, et al: Polyamine metabolism in reversible cerebral ischemia: Effect of alpha-difluoromethylornithine. *Brain Res* 453:9–16, 1988.
44. Paschen W, Csiba L, Rohn G, Bereczki D: Polyamine metabolism in transient focal ischemia of rat brain. *Brain Res* 566:354–357, 1991.
45. Paschen W, Bengtsson F, Rohn G, et al: Cerebral polyamine metabolism in reversible hypoglycemia of rat—relationship to energy metabolites and calcium. *J Neurochem* 57:204–215, 1991.
46. Paschen W, Widmann R, Weber C: Changes in regional polyamine profiles in rat brains after transient cerebral ischemia (single versus repetitive ischemia): Evidence for release of polyamines from injured neurons. *Neurosci Lett* 135:121–124, 1992.
47. Shohami E, Nates JL, Glantz L, et al: Changes in brain polyamine levels following head injury. *Exp Neurol* 117:189–195, 1992.
48. Hossmann KA, Paschen W: Disturbances of protein and polyamine metabolism after reversible cerebral ischemia, in Bazan NG, Braquet P, Ginsberg MD (eds): *Neurochemical Correlates of Cerebral Ischemia.* New York: Plenum, 1992:59–80.
49. Bakay RAE, Sweeney KM, Wood JH: Pathophysiology of cerebrospinal fluid in head injury: II. Biochemical markers for central nervous system trauma. *Neurosurgery* 18:376–382, 1986.
50. Ott L, Young B: Neurosurgery, in Zaloga GP (ed): *Nutrition in Critical Care.* St. Louis: Mosby, 1994:691–706.
51. Bakay RAE, Sweeney KM, Wood JH: Pathophysiology of cerebrospinal fluid in head injury: I. Pathological changes in cerebrospinal fluid solute composition after traumatic head injury. *Neurosurgery* 18:234–243, 1986.
52. Cooper PR, Chalif DJ, Ramsey JF, Moore RJ: Radioimmunoassay of the brain type isoenzyme of creatine phosphokinase (CK-BB): A new diagnostic tool in the evaluation of patients with head injury. *Neurosurgery* 12:536–541, 1983.
53. Moss DW, Henderson AR: Enzymes, in Burtis CA, Ashwood ER (eds): *Tietz Textbook for Clinical Chemistry.* Philadelphia: Saunders, 1994:735–896.
54. Thomas DG, Rabow L, Teasdale G: Serum myelin basic protein, clinical responsiveness, and outcome of severe head injury. *Acta Neurochir [Suppl] (Wien)* 28:93–95, 1979.
55. Aurell A, Rosengren LE, Wikkelso C: The S100 protein in cerebrospinal fluid: A simple ELISA method. *J Neurol* 89:157–164, 1989.
56. Hillered L, Kotwica Z, Ungerstedt U: Interstitial and cerebrospinal fluid levels of energy-related metabolites after middle cerebral artery occlusion in rats. *Exp Med* 191:219–225, 1991.
57. Robertson CS, Contant CF, Narayan RK, Grossman RG: Cerebral blood flow, AVDO2, and neurological outcome in head-injured patients. *J Neurotrauma* 9:349–358, 1992.
58. Bochicchio M, Latronico N, Zani DG, et al: Free radical induced lipoperoxidation and severe head injury. *Intensive Care Med* 16:444–447, 1990.
59. Bird ED, Iversen LL: *Human Brain Postmortem Studies of Neurotransmitters and Related Markers* (2d ed). New York: Plenum, 1982.
60. Benveniste H, Huttemeier PC: Microdialysis—theory and application. *Prog Neurobiol* 35:195–215, 1990.
61. Hamberger A, Jacobson I, Nystrom B, Sandberg M: Microdialysis sampling of the neuronal environment in basic and clinical research. *J Intern Med* 230:375–380, 1991.
62. Lonnroth P: Microdialysis—a new and promising method in clinical medicine. *J Intern Med* 230:363–364, 1991.

63. Meyerson BA, Linderoth B, Karlsson H, Ungerstedt U: Microdialysis in the human brain: Extracellular measurements in the thalamus of parkinsonian patients. *Life Sci* 46:301–308, 1990.
64. Robinson TE, Justice JB Jr: *Microdialysis in the Neurosciences* (1st ed). New York: Elsevier, 1991.
65. Ungerstedt U, Hallstrom A: In vivo microdialysis—a new approach to the analysis of neurotransmitters in the brain. *Life Sci* 41:861–864, 1987.
66. Ungerstedt U: Introduction to intracerebral microdialysis, in Robinson TE, Justice JB Jr (eds): *Microdialysis in the Neurosciences*. New York: Elsevier, 1991:450.
67. Ungerstedt U: Microdialysis—principles and applications for studies in animals and man. *J Intern Med* 230:365–373, 1991.
68. Whittle IR: Intracerebral microdialysis: A new method in applied clinical neuroscience research (editorial). *Br J Neurosurg* 4:459–462, 1990.
69. Pickar D: A clinical perspective on microdialysis. *Prog Neuropsychopharmacol Biol Psychiatry* 14 Suppl:S59–62, 1990.
70. During MJ: In vivo neurochemistry of the conscious human brain: Intrahippocampal microdialysis in epilepsy, in Robinson TE, Justice JB Jr (eds): *Microdialysis in the Neurosciences*. New York: Elsevier, 1991:450.
71. Hamberger A, Jacobson I, Larsson S, et al: Microdialysis techniques for studying brain amino acids in the extracellular fluid: Basic and clinical studies, in Robinson TE, Justice JB Jr (eds): *Microdialysis in the Neurosciences*. New York: Elsevier, 1991:450.
72. Ronquist G, Hugosson R, Sjolander U, Ungerstedt U: Treatment of malignant glioma by a new therapeutic principle. *Acta Neurochir (Wien)* 114:8–11, 1992.
73. Persson L, Hillered L: Chemical monitoring of neurosurgical intensive care patients using intracerebral microdialysis. *J Neurosurg* 76:72–80, 1992.
74. Hillered L, Persson L: Microdialysis for metabolic monitoring in cerebral ischemia and trauma: Experimental and clinical studies, in Robinson TE, Justice JB Jr (eds): *Microdialysis in the Neurosciences*. New York: Elsevier, 1991:450.
75. Hillered L, Persson L, Ponten U, Ungerstedt U: Neurometabolic monitoring of the ischaemic human brain using microdialysis. *Acta Neurochir (Wien)* 102:91–97, 1990.
76. Wise DL: *Bioinstrumentation—Research, Developments, and Applications* (1st ed). Stoneham, MA: Butterworth, 1990.
77. Korf J, de Boer J: Lactography as an approach to monitor glucose metabolism on-line in brain and muscle. *Int J Biochem* 22:127–138, 1990.
78. Hallstrom A, Carlsson A, Hillered L, Ungerstedt U: Simultaneous determination of lactate, pyruvate, and ascorbate in microdialysis samples from rat brain, blood, fat, and muscle using high-performance liquid chromatography. *J Pharmacol Methods* 22:113–124, 1989.
79. Fabricius M, Jensen LH, Lauritzen M: Microdialysis of interstitial amino acids during spreading depression and anoxic depolarization in rat neocortex. *Brain Res* 612:61–69, 1993.
80. Simpson RK, Robertson CS, Goodman JC: Spinal cord ischemia-induced elevation of amino acids: Extracellular measurement with microdialysis. *Neurochem Res* 15:635–639, 1990.
81. Zini I, Zoli M, Grimaldi R, et al: Evidence for a role of neosynthetized putrescine in the increase of glial fibrillary acidic protein immunoreactivity induced by a mechanical lesion in the rat brain. *Neurosci Lett* 120:13–16, 1990.
82. Grimaldi R, Zini I, Zoli M, et al: Neuron-astroglia interactions in physiopathological conditions: Possible role of volume transmission, in Fuxe K, Agnati LF (eds): *Volume Transmission in the Brain: Possible Novel Mechanisms for Neural Transmission*. New York: Raven Press, 1991:247–256.

Complications and Sequelae

CHAPTER 41

POSTCONCUSSION SYNDROME AND WHIPLASH INJURIES

Randolph W. Evans

SYNOPSIS

Two of the most controversial clinical topics discussed in this book are the postconcussion syndrome and whiplash injuries. According to a recent nationwide survey in the United States,[1] the average number of patients with postconcussion syndrome seen per month is 5.1 by neurologists and 4.0 by neurosurgeons. The corresponding numbers of patients with whiplash injuries are 10.3 and 7.0, respectively. Although physicians readily recognize acute symptoms after mild head injuries and whiplash-type neck injuries, the cause of persistent symptoms has long been a subject of debate. The evaluation, management, and medicolegal aspects of these conditions have also been controversial. This chapter considers the historical aspects of both topics and reviews their causation, symptoms and signs, testing, prognosis, medicolegal aspects, and treatment.

HISTORICAL ASPECTS

Railway Spine

Although the sequelae of mild head and neck injuries have been recognized for centuries,[2] the origins of the present-day controversy can be traced back 130 years.[3] In 1866 John Erichsen, a London surgeon, published a series of six lectures entitled "Certain obscure injuries of the nervous system commonly met with as the results of shocks of the body received in collisions on railways" that subsequently were expanded into a book published in 1882.[4] He believed that minor injuries to the head and spine could result in severe disability as a result of "molecular disarrangement" or anemia of the spinal cord. Although only 17 of the 52 patients Erichsen described in his book sustained injuries in railway accidents, these types of injuries became known as railway spine or railway brain.

Rigler observed an increased incidence of posttraumatic invalidism after a system of financial compensation was established for accidental injuries on the Prussian railways in 1871. In 1879, Rigler countered Erichsen's view, arguing that the symptoms were due to a compensation neurosis.[5] In the United States in 1881, Hodges also challenged the organicity of railway spine and separated the alleged injuries into different categories: "so-called 'spine cases,' familiar to lawyers and courts of law as well as to physicians. . . . The fourth class includes those of functional disorder, presenting symptoms, the knowledge of which is obtained not from observation, but from the statements of patients. . . ."[6] In 1883 Putnam distinguished hysteria from malingering in medicolegal cases.[7]

In 1889, Oppenheim popularized the notion of traumatic neurosis, in which a strong afferent stimulus results in impairment of function in the CNS. Charcot disagreed, arguing that the impairment described was actually due to hysteria and neurasthenia.

Postconcussion Syndrome

In 1892, Friedmann proposed that posttraumatic cases with features of headache, dizziness, vasomotor instability, and intolerance to alcohol be labeled a "vasomotor symptom complex" caused by disordered intracranial circulation.[8] The first use of the term "postconcussion syndrome" found by this author was in the landmark 1934 paper by Strauss and Savitsky.[9] Those authors argued that concussion can occur without loss of consciousness and also discussed the interrelationships of head injury, premorbid personality, and the stress resulting from dealing with the aftermath of an injury.

Two opposing viewpoints from the 1960s are still widely cited. In a well-known 1961 paper, Miller described the postconcussion syndrome as an accident neurosis: "The most consistent clinical feature is the subject's unshakable conviction of unfitness for work. . . ."[10] In 1962, Symonds took a strong opposing position: "It is questionable whether the effects of concussion, however slight, are ever completely reversible."[11] Symonds is also well known for a 1937 statement emphasizing the importance of variables within the individual: "The symptom picture depends not only upon the kind of injury, but upon the kind of brain."[12]

Whiplash

Nineteenth-century controversies about railway spine have evolved into similar twentieth-century arguments about whiplash injuries. The whiplash mechanism of hyperextension-flexion injury may have been recognized first in U.S. Navy pilots after World War I.[13] When their planes were launched from the decks of ships by catapults, these pilots developed hyperextension-flexion injuries. The Navy was quickly able to prevent problems by providing the pilots with a shoulder harness and headrest. Civilian automakers took 50 more years to routinely provide the same protective devices.

An orthopedist, Harold Crowe, reported in 1964 that he first used the term "whiplash" in a 1928 paper before the Western Orthopedic Association.[14] However, the first use of the term in the medical literature to this author's knowledge was in a 1945 article by another orthopedist, Davis.[15] In a pioneering series of staged rear-end collisions using humans and dummies in 1955, Severy and coworkers made a number of important observations about the nature of whiplash injuries.[16] They correctly identified the sequence of hyperextension followed by flexion of the neck, which prior investigators had reversed.[17] Unfortunately, treatment has not changed much in the last 40 years. A 1955 article recommended heat, cervical traction, cervical collars, muscle relaxants, aspirin and codeine, and trigger point injections with procaine.[18] (It should be added that the terms "trigger point" and "myofascial pain" were first used by an American orthopedist, Steindler, in 1939.[19])

THE POSTCONCUSSION SYNDROME

Perhaps 50 percent of patients with a mild head injury develop the postconcussion syndrome.[20] Loss of consciousness does not have to occur for the syndrome to develop. One or more of the following symptoms and signs constitute this syndrome: headaches, dizziness, vertigo, tinnitus, hearing loss, blurred vision, diplopia, convergence insufficiency, light and noise sensitivity, diminished taste and smell, irritability, anxiety, depression, personality change, fatigue, sleep disturbance, decreased libido, decreased appetite, memory dysfunction, impaired concentration and attention, slowing of reaction time, and slowing of information-processing speed (Table 41-1).[21] Rare sequelae of mild head injury include subdural and epidural hematomas,[22] seizures,[23]

TABLE 41-1 Sequelae of Mild Head Injury

Headaches
Muscle contraction type
Migraine
Cluster
Occipital neuralgia
Supraorbital and infraorbital neuralgia
Secondary to neck injury
Secondary to temporomandibular joint syndrome
Owing to scalp laceration or local trauma
Mixed
Cranial nerve symptoms and signs
Dizziness
Vertigo
Tinnitus
Hearing loss
Blurred vision
Diplopia
Convergence insufficiency
Light and noise sensitivity
Diminished taste and smell
Psychological and somatic complaints
Irritability
Anxiety
Depression
Personality change
Fatigue
Sleep disturbance
Decreased libido
Decreased appetite
Cognitive impairment
Memory dysfunction
Impaired concentration and attention
Slowing of reaction time
Slowing of information-processing speed
Rare sequelae
Subdural and epidural hematomas
Seizures
Transient global amnesia
Tremor
Dystonia

SOURCE: Evans RW: Post-concussion syndrome, in Evans RW, Baskin DS, Yatsu FM (eds): *Prognosis of Neurological Disorders*. New York: Oxford University Press, 1992, p 98; with permission.

movement disorders (tremor and dystonia),[24–26] and transient global amnesia.[27]

Many physicians are appropriately concerned about the use of the term "postconcussion syndrome" for a syndrome consisting of many vague subjective symptoms because the term can easily be overused and used inappropriately. In response to the statement that the postconcussion syndrome is a clearly defined syndrome with a solid basis for determining the prognosis, only 23.6 percent of neurologists and 29.1 percent of neurosurgeons agreed.[1] The postconcussion syndrome refers to a heterogeneous patient population with varying degrees of injury to the brain and head. A variety of individual patient characteristics, including age, gender, personality profile, educational level, intelligence quotient, occupation, socioeconomic class, prior head injury, psychiatric history, and drug and alcohol abuse, may alter the expression of the injury.[28]

Causation

During the last 40 years, the organicity of the postconcussion syndrome has been increasingly well documented by abnormalities in neuropathologic, neurophysiological, neuroimaging, and neuropsychological studies discussed in other chapters in this book. However, many physicians still have doubts about the organicity of the syndrome and the cases of individual patients.

Some of the responses from the survey of physicians in the United States illustrate these differences of opinion.[1] In response to the statement "I personally tend to question the authenticity of patients' reports of symptoms with postconcussion syndrome," 16.5 percent of neurologists and 20.5 percent of neurosurgeons agreed. Neurologists and neurosurgeons believe that other physicians are skeptical, judging by their 63.5 percent and 48.1 percent agreement, respectively, with the statement "Most physicians tend to question the authenticity of patients' reports of symptoms with postconcussion syndrome."

Symptoms and Signs

Headaches

Different studies have variably reported the incidence of headaches after mild head injury as ranging from 30 to 90 percent of patients (see Table 41-2). Headaches may occur more often and have a longer duration after a mild head injury compared with more severe degrees of trauma.[29] Some patients have more than one distinct form of headache.[30] Headaches with both migraine and muscle contraction features can occur.

Muscle Contraction Type

Perhaps 85 percent of posttraumatic headaches are of the muscle contraction type,[20] often associated with greater occipital neuralgia. Because head injuries are commonly associated with neck and occasionally temporomandibular joint trauma, the headache may arise from myofascial injury, intervertebral disks, and facet joints. Headaches can also be referred from trigger points in other neck muscles, including the semispinalis cervicis, the digastric, and the sternocleidomastoid.

Migraine

Recurring attacks of migraine with and without an aura can develop hours to weeks after a mild head injury with or without loss of consciousness in patients who often have a positive family history of migraine.[31] Acute episodes of migraine can be triggered by mild head injuries occurring in a variety of sports, including soccer,[32] American football,[33] rugby,[34] and boxing.[28] After a mild head injury, children, adolescents, and young adults can develop four clinical types of transient neurological sequelae that are not always associated with headache: hemiparesis; somnolence, irritability, and vomiting; transient blindness often precipitated by occipital impacts; and brainstem signs.[35]

Other Types of Headaches

Dysesthesias over scalp lacerations frequently occur and can last for weeks or months. Rarely, cluster headaches can develop after a mild head injury.[36] Other rare headaches described include dysautonomic cephalgia[37] and orgasmic cephalgia.[21]

Cranial nerve symptoms and signs

Dizziness and Hearing Loss

Dizziness frequently occurs after a mild head injury and is reported by 53 percent of patients within 1 week[38] of the injury and by 18 percent after 2 years.[39] A peripheral injury such as benign positional vertigo[40] or labyrinthine concussion can be responsible.[41] Rarely, perilymph fistulas can occur. Hearing loss of both the conductive and sensorineural types can also occur occasionally.

Visual Symptoms

After a mild head injury, blurred vision is reported by 14 percent of patients.[42] Convergence insufficiency is the most common cause.[43] Mild head injury can infrequently cause diplopia as a result of third, fourth, and sixth cranial nerve palsies.[44] Findings of diminished visual acuity and hue discrimination can be due to optic nerve contusions.

Other Symptoms

The most common cause of anosmia is head trauma.[45] More than 5 percent of patients report decreased smell and taste after a mild head injury.[39] Fourteen days after a mild head injury, light and noise sensitivity were reported, respectively, by 7.2 percent and 15 percent of patients.[46]

Psychological and Somatic Complaints and Cognitive Impairment

Irritability, personality change, anxiety, and depression are commonly reported within 3 months of injury[47] and can be quite persistent, with an incidence of 15 percent after 3 years.[48] Posttraumatic stress disorder, which has some symptoms similar to those of postconcussion syndrome, may also occur.[49,50] Fatigue is reported by 29 percent of patients 4 weeks after the injury and by 23 percent at 6 months.[39] Frequently, disruption of sleep patterns occurs after a mild head injury, especially with difficulty in falling asleep and arousals.[51]

Four weeks after a mild head injury, 19 percent of patients complain of loss of memory and 21 percent complain of difficulty with concentration.[39] Deficits in cognitive functioning have been documented, including a reduction in information-processing speed,[43] attention,[52] reaction time,[53] and memory for new information.[35] Cognitive impairment is discussed in detail in Chap. 50.

Testing

The indications for radiological and other forms of testing after a mild head injury, both acutely and with persistent symptoms, continue to be controversial.[54,55] In the acute setting, the incidence of abnormal studies is very low. The incidence of neurosurgical complications among patients presenting to the emergency room is between 0.3 percent and 3 percent.[56,57]

Skull X-Rays

In a health care system such as that of Great Britain, where computed tomography (CT) scanners are not readily available, a skull x-ray has been considered a reasonable screening study.[58] A fracture has been reported to increase the risk of intracranial hematoma in patients who are fully conscious when first evaluated by 176 times for adults and by 80 times for children.[59] Conversely, Rosenorn and colleagues in Denmark found no significant difference in intracranial complications in patients with or without a fracture detected by skull x-ray.[60]

CT Scanning

In a setting where a CT scan is available, early CT scanning without obtaining skull x-rays can significantly increase the diagnosis of intracranial complications.[61] Using early CT scanning routinely without skull x-rays as a triage strategy has been shown to significantly and safely reduce the number of hospital admissions for observation while being almost as cost-effective as strategies employing routine skull x-rays with liberal hospital observation guidelines.[62]

MRI

Although magnetic resonance imaging (MRI) is more sensitive in detecting intracranial abnormalities than is CT at all stages of evaluation, MRI is rarely more sensitive than CT in detecting surgical candidates. However, the parenchymal and extraparenchymal lesions detected by MRI may have prognostic significance for neurobehavioral recovery[63] and may be helpful in documenting injury in medicolegal cases. These advantages entail an additional 20 to 30 percent increase in cost.

EEG

Although often obtained, EEG studies after mild head injuries without a suspicion of a seizure disorder have very limited sensitivity and specificity and rarely alter patient management. The abnormalities demonstrated are nonspecific, may resolve with time, and have no prognostic value for predicting time lost at work.[64] In addition, because of the significant percentage of abnormalities seen on EEG studies performed before a mild head injury, abnormalities seen afterward may be incorrectly attributed to the injury.[65]

ABR

Auditory brainstem responses (ABR) have been reported as being abnormal after mild head injuries. Montgomery and coworkers reported an abnormal I-V interval in about half of a group of patients; it persisted in most for at least 6 weeks.[53] However, Schoenhuber and colleagues found abnormal results in only about 10 percent of patients.[66] No specific pattern of abnormality was detected, although interpeak latency I-III was most often affected. Although abnormal ABR confirm a disturbance of brainstem function in some patients, routine use outside a research setting cannot be recommended since there is no correlation between abnormal results and postconcussion symptoms.[67]

EEG Brain Mapping

Abnormalities in EEG power spectral analyses have been reported in two studies of patients after mild head injury.[49,68] These studies are intriguing and certainly warrant additional evaluation in a research setting. However, the Therapeutics and Technology Assessment Subcommittee of the American Academy of Neurology does not recommend the routine use of brain mapping for evaluation of a mild head injury, concluding: "On the basis of the present medical literature, the sensitivity and specificity fail to substantiate a role for these tests in the clinical diagnostic evaluation of individual patients. . . ."[69] Erroneous diagnosis using EEG discriminant analysis can occur for a variety of reasons[70] and can lead to abuse in the courtroom.[71]

Neuropsychological Testing

When performed by a knowledgeable and experienced psychologist, neuropsychological testing can be helpful. However, in some cases, psychologists who are not knowledgeable and experienced come to inappropriate conclusions, especially in medicolegal cases.[72,73] Malingering continues to represent a major challenge to assessment.[74] Neurologists and neurosurgeons should become more familiar with the uses and abuses of neuropsychological testing[75] and assess the qualifications of the psychologists to whom they refer patients.

Prognosis

During the last 50 years, multiple prognostic studies have been performed. However, comparison among them is difficult because of differences, including the definition of mild head injury, the testing used, the study design, and subject characteristics.[76]

Persistent symptoms and neuropsychological deficits are not predicted by whether the patient is only dazed or alternatively has loss of consciousness of varying duration up to 1 hour.[45,77] The duration of posttraumatic amnesia has been reported as being predictive[39] and not predictive[78] of sequelae.

Many subject characteristics may influence the prognosis, including age, gender, occupation, socioeconomic status, personality, intelligence, history of prior head injuries, prior use of alcohol or illicit drugs, social adversity,[79] and multiple trauma. Age over 40 years is a risk factor for slower recovery from cognitive deficits[80] and for increased number and duration of postconcussion symptoms.[69] Women have late symptoms more often than men do.[81] A number of variables are significant predictors for return to work by 1 to 24 months in patients with a mild head injury, including older age; higher level of education, employment, and socioeconomic status; and greater income.[82,83]

Table 41-2 presents data on the persistence of headache, dizziness, memory problems, and irritability.[84,85] Although most patients recover within 3 to 6 months, a significant minority have persistent deficits of cognitive functioning that may persist for well over a year.[68] Chapter 50 provides additional information about the prognosis for cognitive functioning.

The Effect of Litigation and Compensation Claims

Neurologists and neurosurgeons often are reluctant to become involved in litigation as treating physicians and less often as expert witnesses. Many specialists have strong opinions about the effect of litigation on postconcussion complaints. In the survey, 12 percent of neurologists and 23.3 percent of neurosurgeons agreed that litigation is the most important factor responsible for symptoms in the postconcussion syndrome.[1] In response to the statement "Once litigation is settled, symptoms quickly resolve in patients with postconcussion syndrome," 23.6 percent of neurologists and 31.2 percent of neurosurgeons agreed.

As noted in the historical section, in 1961, Henry Miller reported his conclusions based on seeing 200 consecutive cases of mild head injury for medicolegal examination in Newcastle upon Tyne, England. Of the 200, 47 patients were reported to have gross and unequivocally psychoneurotic complaints. Miller believed that these patients had an accident neurosis: "The most consistent clinical feature is the subject's unshakable conviction of unfitness for work, a conviction quite unrelated to overt disability even if his symptomatology is accepted at its face value. At a later stage the patient will declare his fitness for light work, which is often not available. . . . Another cardinal feature is an absolute refusal to admit any degree of symptomatic improvement."[10]

Miller's observations are still widely quoted by defense attorneys. Unfortunately, although Miller's subjective and judgmental conclusions apply to a small minority of patients, such broad generalizations were improperly drawn from a flawed study of a biased sample of patients.[67] In a later study of 398 consecutive head injury patients examined in connection with a claim for compensation, Guthkelch identified accident neurosis in only 6.8 percent.[86]

Patients with litigation and compensation claims are quite similar to those without. Both groups have similar symptoms that improve with time[68,87,88] and similar cognitive test results.[68,79] In a study from Harare, Africa,

TABLE 41-2 Percentage of Patients with Persistence of Symptoms after a Mild Head Injury

	1 Week	1 Month	6 Weeks	2 Months	3 Months	6 Months	1 Year	2 Years	3 Years	4 Years	5 Years
Headache	71[38]* 36[39]	90[48] 31.3[42] 56[38]	24.8[81]	31.5[84]	78[82] 47[38]	21.6[42] 27[39]	35[48] 8.4[81] 18[39]	22[48] 24[39]	20[48]	24[78]	12[85] (headaches and/or dizziness)
Dizziness	53[38] 19[39]	12[48] 21.9[42] 35[38]	14.5[81]	23[84]	22[38]	13.1[42] 22[39]	26[48] 4.6[81] 14[39]	18[48] 18[39]	16[48]	18[78]	
Memory problems		18.8[42]	8.3[81]		59[82]	15.3[42]	3.8[81]			19[78]	
Irritability		24.7[42]	9[81]			19.6[42]	5.3[81]				

* Superscript numbers refer to references.

SOURCE: Evans RW: The post-concussion syndrome, in Evans RW, Baskin DS, Yatsu FM (eds): *Prognosis of Neurological Disorders.* New York: Oxford University Press, 1992, p 102; with permission.

claimants for compensation did not have increased symptoms compared with nonclaimants.[89] In another study, patients with posttraumatic migraine both with and without pending litigation responded similarly to appropriate treatment.[28]

However, pending litigation is stressful for many claimants and may result in an increased frequency of symptoms after the settlement.[90,91] The end of litigation does not mean the end of symptoms or a return to work for many claimants; they are not cured by a verdict.[81,82] In a study of 50 patients with chronic posttraumatic headaches, 100 percent reported persistent headache symptoms 1 year or more after a legal settlement.[92] Older patients and/or those employed in more dangerous occupations often do not return to work after the settlement.[93]

Although "pure" compensation neurosis or malingering is uncommon, secondary gain should always be considered in patients with persistent complaints after a mild head injury. Patients with premorbid neuroticism, inadequate or histrionic personalities, and psychosocial problems can certainly exaggerate or fabricate complaints.[94,95] Since some patients with underlying organic disease may have seemingly hysterical signs and symptoms, the diagnosis of accident or conversion neurosis should be made with trepidation.[96]

Physicians involved in medicolegal cases should strive to be fair and independent of plaintiff and defense attorneys and insurance companies. If a patient's disability is based only on symptoms, it should be clearly explained to the jury and/or judge that the physician's opinion is based on information that cannot be objectively verified. At the other extreme, to dismiss a patient's complaints solely because of pending litigation or a compensation claim is unfair to an individual who can also become a victim of an adversarial judiciary process.

TABLE 41-3 Treatments for Postconcussion Syndrome

Muscle contraction–type headaches
Simple analgesics
NSAID*
Antidepressants
Muscle relaxant
TENS unit*
Barbiturates-narcotics (with caution)
Biofeedback
Migraine-type headaches
Prophylactic drugs
Beta blockers
Antidepressants
NSAID*
Calcium channel blockers
Valproic acid
Abortive drugs
Ergotamine
Dihydroergotamine
Sumatriptan
Isometheptene
Barbiturates-narcotics (with caution)
Occipital neuralgia
Greater occipital nerve block
NSAID*
Muscle relaxants
Carbamazepine
TENS unit*
Rarely surgical
Psychological support
Cognitive rehabilitation
Education for all involved

* NSAID = nonsteroidal anti-inflammatory drug; TENS = transcutaneous electrical nerve stimulator.

SOURCE: Evans RW: Some observations on whiplash injuries. *Neurol Clin North Am* 10:839, 1992; with permission.

TREATMENT

After the patient's specific problems are diagnosed, treatment is individualized for each problem (Table 41-3). Since most patients improve within a few months, reassurance can be the most important treatment. Many physicians have doubts about the efficacy of treatment, especially for chronic cases. In response to the statement "Effective treatment is available for postconcussion syndrome," only 35.3 percent of neurologists and 17.2 percent of neurosurgeons agreed.[1]

Headaches

Posttraumatic muscle contraction and migraine-type headaches may respond to the usual prophylactic medications, such as amitriptyline, nortriptyline, maprotiline, and propranolol.[28,97,98] Tricyclic antidepressants may also be helpful for symptoms that often are associated with headaches, such as depression, insomnia, anxiety, fatigue, and irritability. Muscle contraction–type headaches may respond to nonsteroidal anti-inflammatory drugs and muscle relaxants. Intravenous dihydroergotamine and metoclopramide may constitute an effective treatment for posttraumatic headaches.[99] Other drugs that may be helpful for prophylactic and abortive treatment of migraines are listed in Table 41-3.

Greater occipital neuralgia frequently responds to a nerve block with a local anesthetic.[100] Transcutaneous electrical nerve stimulators,[101] physical therapy, and manipulation[102] may also help. Carbamazepine or baclofen may reduce painful paroxysms of shooting pain. Greater occipital nerve section or decompression is rarely indicated.[103]

A short course of biofeedback may be worthwhile for patients with persistent headaches that do not respond to the usual medications. In single reports, acupuncture[104] and naltrexone[105] have been reported to be helpful.

Psychological Approaches

When psychological symptoms are particularly prominent or persistent, supportive psychotherapy and psychotropic medications may be useful. The use of cognitive retraining for cognitive difficulties after a mild head injury is controversial.[106] In view of the expense, until prospective studies demonstrating the efficacy of cognitive rehabilitation are reported, widespread use cannot be recommended.

The Hollywood Head Injury Myth and Education

The public is often misinformed about the effects of mild head injury in movies and on television because of what Evans has termed "the Hollywood head injury myth."[76] Head injuries are presented in two contexts in the movies and on television. In the first, the trauma appears to be serious but does not result in significant sequelae, as in detective, action, martial arts, Western, and boxing films. The public is led to overestimate the dose of head trauma that results in brain injury. In the second context, in cartoons and slapstick sequences in films, head trauma not only is not serious but can be extremely funny. When the public has been so misinformed, education can be difficult. Perhaps the use of counterexamples such as technical knockouts and the punch-drunk state in boxers and concussions in football players would be helpful.

Education of the patient and family members should be routine. A treatment program of education, short-term bed rest, and timely follow-up may help in the recovery process in some patients.[39] Physicians, employers, attorneys, and representatives of insurance companies also may benefit from education and a review of the literature on mild head injury over the last 20 years.

WHIPLASH INJURIES

Terminology

Whiplash refers to the hyperextension followed by flexion of the neck that occurs when an occupant of a motor vehicle is hit from behind by another vehicle. The term is also used to describe other types of collisions in which the neck is subjected to different sequences and combinations of flexion, extension, and lateral motion. Some physicians prefer other terms, such as cervical sprain, acceleration/deceleration injury, hyperextension injury, and myofascial pain syndrome. There are terms for this type of injury in other languages: in French, *le coup du lapin* ("rabbit blow"); in German, *Schleudertrauma* ("sling or catapult trauma"); in Italian, *colpo di frusta* ("whiplash"); and in Spanish, *latigazo* ("whiplash").[107]

Many physicians are skeptical about the existence of a chronic whiplash syndrome.[108] In response to the statement that whiplash is a "clearly defined syndrome with a solid basis for determining prognosis," only 18.9 percent of neurologists and 17.2 percent of neurosurgeons agreed.[1]

Epidemiology

Whiplash injuries occur commonly worldwide. In the United States in 1993, there were 11.9 million motor vehicle accidents including 2.75 million rear-end collisions.[109] Rear-end collisions are responsible for about 85 percent of all whiplash injuries.[110] Side and front impact collisions are responsible for the other 15 percent. Although only rough estimates exist, perhaps 1 million people sustain whiplash-type injuries per year in the United States.[111] Women have persistent neck pain more often than do men, especially in the 20- to 40-year age group, by a ratio of 70 percent to 30 percent.[112] Women may be more susceptible to injury because they have a narrower neck with less muscle mass supporting a head of roughly the same volume as that of men.[113]

Seventy-three percent of occupants wearing a seat belt develop neck pain compared with 53 percent not wearing a seat belt.[114] However, front seat occupants without a seat belt may be propelled into the dashboard or windshield and sustain a more severe head injury while avoiding a whiplash injury. Proper use of headrests can reduce the incidence of neck pain in rear-end collisions by 24 percent.[115] Unfortunately, many people use the headrest to rest their heads at traffic lights and do not properly set the head restraint at the proper level. If an adjustable headrest is too low, it can act as a fulcrum, resulting in a more severe hyperextension injury.

Pathology

Both animal and human studies have revealed structural damage from whiplash-type injuries.[116] In different species of monkeys, experimentally caused acceleration/extension injuries have produced a variety of lesions, including muscle tears, avulsion, and hemorrhages; rupture of the anterior longitudinal and other ligaments, especially between C4 and C7; avulsions of disks from vertebral bodies and disk herniations; retropharyngeal hematoma; intralaryngeal and esophageal hemorrhage; cervical sympathetic nerve damage associated with injury to the longus colli; nerve root injury; cervical spinal cord contusions and hemorrhages; cerebral concussion; and gross hemorrhages and contusions over the surface of the cerebral hemispheres, brainstem, and cerebellum.[117,118]

Human studies have revealed similar injuries.[119] An MRI study of selected patients done within 4 months of a whiplash-type injury revealed ruptures of the anterior longitudinal ligament; horizontal avulsions, separation of the disk, and occult fractures of the horizontal endplate; acute posterolateral cervical disk herniations; focal muscular injury of the longus colli muscle; posterior interspinous ligament injury; and prevertebral fluid collections.[120] Autopsy series have demonstrated clefts in the cartilage plates of the intervertebral disks, posterior disk herniation through a damaged annulus fibrosis, and hemarthrosis in facet joints.[121,122]

Symptoms and Signs

Table 41-4 lists the sequelae of whiplash trauma, which include neck and back injuries; headaches; dizziness; paresthesias; cognitive, somatic, and psychological sequelae; and rare sequelae.[123]

Neck Pain

After a motor vehicle accident, 62 percent of patients presenting to the emergency room complain of neck pain.[98] The onset of neck pain occurs within 6 h in 65 percent of these patients, within 24 h in an additional 28 percent, and within 72 h in the remaining 7 percent.[102]

Most neck pain is due to myofascial injury. Cervical spine fractures and dislocations and cervical disk herniations are uncommon.[124] Upper cervical trauma to the atlas, axis, and associated ligaments is much less common than is lower cervical injury.[125]

Cervical facet joint injury may also be an important source of pain[126] in an undetermined percentage of patients and may be assessed by comparative local anesthetic blocks.[127] Like trigger points,[128] facet joints at different levels can produce characteristic patterns of referred pain over various parts of the occipital, posterior cervical, shoulder girdle, and scapular regions.[129]

Headaches

In a prospective study of 180 patients seen within 4 weeks of a whiplash injury, 82 percent complained of

TABLE 41-4 Sequelae of Whiplash Injuries

Neck and back injuries
Myofascial
Fractures and dislocations
Disk herniations
Spinal cord compression
Spondylosis
Radiculopathy
Facet joint injury
Increased development of spondylosis
Headaches
Muscle contraction type
Greater occipital neuralgia
Temporomandibular joint injury
Migraine
Dizziness
Vestibular dysfunction
Brainstem dysfunction
Cervical origin
Hyperventilation syndrome
Paresthesias
Trigger points
Thoracic outlet syndrome
Brachial plexus injury
Cervical radiculopathy
Facet joint
Carpal tunnel syndrome
Ulnar neuropathy at the elbow
Weakness
Radiculopathy
Brachial plexopathy
Entrapment neuropathy
Reflex inhibition
Cognitive, somatic, and psychological sequelae
Memory, attention, and concentration impairment
Nervousness and irritability
Sleep disturbances
Fatigability
Depression
Personality change
Compensation neurosis
Visual symptoms
Convergence insufficiency
Oculomotor palsies
Abnormalities of smooth pursuit and saccades
Horner's syndrome
Vitreous detachment
Other rare sequelae
Torticollis
Transient global amnesia
Esophageal perforation and descending mediastinitis
Hypoglossal nerve palsy

SOURCE: Modified from Evans RW: Some observations on whiplash injuries. *Neurol Clin North Am* 10:981, 1992; with permission.

headaches that were occipitally located in 46 percent, were generalized in 34 percent, and were in other locations in 20 percent.[130] Fifty percent of these patients reported that pain was present more than half the time.

These headaches are usually of the muscle contraction type. Greater occipital neuralgia or referred pain from trigger points from suboccipital muscles can produce a pattern of pain radiating variably over the occipital, temporal, frontal, and retroorbital distribution. Third occipital nerve headache can produce a similar headache.[131] Whiplash injuries can also injure the temporomandibular joint, and this can become a source of headaches.[132] Occasionally, whiplash injuries can precipitate recurring common, classic, and basilar migraines *de novo*.[28,133,134] The headaches can begin immediately or within a few days after the injury. The longer the onset of migraine after the injury, the more tenuous the causal link.

Dizziness

In a study of 262 patients with persistent neck pain and headaches for 4 months or longer after an injury, symptoms were reported as follows: vertigo, 50 percent; floating sensations, 35 percent; tinnitus, 14 percent; and hearing impairment, 5 percent.[135] Posttraumatic dysfunction of the vestibular apparatus, brainstem, cervical sympathetics, vertebral insufficiency, and cervical proprioceptive system have all been postulated as causing dizziness.[136] In patients who are in pain and anxious, hyperventilation syndrome is a common cause of dizziness, which at times is associated with paresthesias that can be symmetrical and bilateral as well as unilateral.

Paresthesias

Paresthesias of the upper extremities are commonly reported after whiplash injuries. In one study, 33 percent of patients with symptoms but no objective findings complained of paresthesias acutely and 37 percent reported paresthesias after a mean follow-up of 19.7 months.[137] Trigger points, brachial plexopathy, facet joint disease, entrapment neuropathies, cervical radiculopathy, and spinal cord compression can all cause paresthesias.

Whiplash injuries can precipitate a thoracic outlet syndrome[138,139] that occurs more often in women than in men.[140] Thoracic outlet syndrome has been controversial,[141] since at least 85 percent of cases are of the nonspecific neurogenic or so-called disputed type. The disputed type is a diagnosis of exclusion based on reproduction of symptoms by provocative tests on physical examination. Similar symptoms can be due to a myofascial pain syndrome with referred pain from the anterior neck muscles, such as the anterior scalene, or from the shoulder girdle muscles, such as the pectoralis minor.[142] Neural or vascular compression occurs in only a small minority of cases.

Entrapment neuropathies can also cause paresthesias. Carpal tunnel syndrome may develop immediately or within 2 weeks of the accident[143] as a result of hyperextension of the wrists caused by holding the steering wheel in a collision.[144] If the patient has a cervical radiculopathy or neurogenic thoracic outlet syndrome from the injury, a double crush syndrome resulting in carpal tunnel syndrome or cubital tunnel syndrome can ensue.[145] A cervical radiculopathy can certainly occur after a whiplash injury as a result of a cervical disk herniation.

Weakness

After whiplash injuries, patients frequently complain of weakness, heaviness, or fatigue when there is no evidence of radiculopathy, plexopathy, or entrapment neuropathy. The nonspecific neurogenic type of thoracic outlet syndrome may be the basis of these complaints. In addition, patients may have a sensation of weakness because of reflex inhibition of muscles caused by pain[146] that can be overcome by more central effort.[106] It should be emphasized that a whiplash injury can be associated with quadriparesis or quadriplegia in patients with a narrow cervical canal[147] or a large central disk herniation.

Cognitive and Psychological Symptoms

In a study of patients with chronic symptoms after a whiplash injury, the following proportions of patients complained of the following symptoms: 67 percent, nervousness and irritability; 50 percent, cognitive disturbances; 44 percent, sleep disturbances; 40 percent, fatigability; and 37 percent, symptoms of depression.[148] Obviously, these symptoms are also common in chronic pain syndromes, depression, and neurosis. Cognitive impairment after whiplash injuries has been variably attributed to damage to basal frontal and upper brainstem structures[149] and the medication effect.[150] Although many physicians believe that chronic symptoms are psychogenic in origin rather than being due to a real injury,[1] a prospective study of 78 consecutive patients with whiplash injuries demonstrated that psychosocial factors, negative affectivity, and personality traits were not significant in predicting the duration of symptoms.[151]

Back Pain

Interscapular pain and low back pain are frequent complaints after whiplash injuries and are reported in 20 percent and 35 percent of patients, respectively, after the injury.[152] After a mean follow-up of 2 years, one study reported a 25 percent incidence of persistent back pain.[153]

Other Sequelae

Visual symptoms, especially blurred vision, are common and usually are due to convergence insufficiency, although oculomotor palsies occasionally occur.[154] Rarely, torticollis has been precipitated by whiplash injuries, with the onset occurring within 6 days of the trauma.[155,156] Other rare sequelae include esophageal perforation,[157] descending mediastinitis,[158] transient global amnesia,[159] and hypoglossal nerve palsy.[160]

Radiographic Studies

Although cervical spine x-rays are routinely obtained after whiplash injuries, the yield of abnormalities is quite low in patients who are alert and have no focal findings on exam. Algorithms have been suggested to safely decrease the number of cervical spine series obtained.[161–163]

Frequently it is difficult to determine which findings are new and which findings are preexisting in radiographic studies. Cervical spondylosis and degenerative disk disease occur with increasing frequency with older age and are often asymptomatic.[164,165] Cervical disk protrusions are common in the general population and are often asymptomatic. Protrusions occur in 20 percent of patients 45 to 54 years of age and in 57 percent of patients older than 64 years.[166] Most studies have reported that whiplash injuries can accelerate the development of cervical spondylosis with degenerative disk disease,[135,167,168] although one retrospective study did not show such a relationship.[169]

Prognosis

Studies on the prognosis of whiplash injuries are difficult to compare because of multiple methodological differences, including selection criteria for patients, prospective and retrospective designs, patient attrition rates, duration of follow-up, and treatments used.[106,170] Although most patients may have only soft tissue injuries,[107] imaging studies other than plain spine films have not been performed routinely.

Symptoms

Neck pain and headaches persist in significant numbers of patients (Table 41-5). Patients with neck pain after 1 year probably will not show significant improvement with longer follow-up.[171] Neck pain present 2 years after the injury is still present after 10 years.[148]

Risk Factors

Three characteristics of the accident have been associated with more severe symptoms: an unprepared occupant, a rear-end collision, and a rotated or inclined head position at the moment of impact.[172] The following risk factors have been reported for persistent symptoms: older age of patient,[148,173] interscapular or upper back pain,[154,174] occipital headache,[154] multiple symptoms or

TABLE 41-5 Percentage of Patients with Persistence of Neck Pain and Headaches after a Whiplash Injury

	1 Week	1 Month	2 Months	3 Months	6 Months	1 Year	2 Years	10 Years
Neck pain (%)	92[114]* 88[153]	64[114]	63[174]	51[114]	43[114]	26[114]	29[153,173] 44[124]† 81[124]‡ 90[124]§	74[167]
Headaches (%)	54[153]	82[130]		73[130]			9[173] 37[124] 37[124]† 70[124]§	33[167]

* Superscript numbers refer to references.

† Subgroup of patients with subjective symptoms only after a mean follow-up of 19.7 months.

‡ Subgroup with subjective symptoms and a reduced cervical spine range of movement after a mean follow-up of 23.9 months.

§ Subgroup with subjective symptoms, reduced cervical range of movement, and objective neurological loss after a mean follow-up of 24.7 months.

SOURCE: Evans RW: Whiplash syndrome, in Evans RW, Baskin DS, Yatsu FM (eds): *Prognosis of Neurological Disorders.* New York: Oxford University Press, 1992, p 624; with permission.

paresthesias at presentation,[154] reduced range of movement of the cervical spine,[111] objective neurological deficit,[111,154] preexisting degenerative osteoarthritic changes,[111,175] and upper-middle compared with lower and higher occupational categories.[176] The duration of symptoms was similar in patients involved in rear-end collisions compared with other types of collisions.[177] There is only a minimal association of a poor prognosis with the speed or severity of the collision and the extent of vehicle damage.[178]

Litigation and symptoms

Many clinicians and certainly the insurance industry and defense attorneys believe that pending litigation is a major cause of persistent symptoms that promptly resolve once the litigation is completed. In response to the statement "Once litigation is settled, symptoms quickly resolve," 31.7 percent of neurologists and 33 percent of neurosurgeons agreed.[1] However, the literature does not support this position. Litigants and nonlitigants have similar recovery rates.[158] The majority of plaintiffs who have persistent symptoms at the time of settlement of their litigation are not cured by a verdict.[111,135,154,169]

Certainly there are patients who exaggerate or lie about persisting complaints to help or make a legal case. The clinician should evaluate the merits of each case. However, the available evidence does not support bias against patients just because they have pending litigation.[179]

Treatment

Practice Patterns

Most physicians are skeptical about the effectiveness of treatment for whiplash injuries. According to the survey, only 44.7 percent of neurologists and 15 percent of neurosurgeons agreed that effective treatment is available.[1] A variety of treatments and referrals were endorsed as being sometimes recommended by the neurology and neurosurgery respondents (Table 41-6).

Cervical collars are recommended for the following maximum duration by neurologists and neurosurgeons, respectively: less than 2 weeks, 38.3 percent and 25.7 percent; 2 to 4 weeks, 32.7 percent and 43.4 percent; and 4 weeks or more, 29 percent and 30.9 percent. Neurologists and neurosurgeons, respectively, endorse the following lengths of time to gain the maximum benefit from physical therapy: 3 months or less, 67.1 percent and 76.6 percent; 4 to 6 months, 25 percent and 17.5 percent; and more than 6 months, 8.4 percent and 7.4 percent.

Studies

Unfortunately, limited treatment recommendations can be made from the very few prospective controlled studies available.[180] Early mobilization of the neck using the Maitland technique, followed by local heat and neck exercises, has been reported to produce more rapid improvement after acute injuries than does the use of a

TABLE 41-6 Percentage of Neurologists and Neurosurgeons Reporting Treatments or Referrals Sometimes Recommended for Whiplash Injuries

Treatment	Neurologists, %	Neurosurgeons, %
Nonsteroidal anti-inflammatory drugs	96.5	95.7
Muscle relaxants	78.8	85.9
Narcotics	22.4	22.8
Tricyclics	89.4	54.3
Massage	81.2	78.3
Stretch and spray	42.4	25.0
Range-of-motion exercises	80.0	68.5
Hot shower, heating pad	80.0	70.7
Cervical traction	48.2	55.4
Cervical collars	54.1	58.7
Trigger point injections	47.1	38.0
Occipital nerve blocks	17.6	20.7
TENS units	47.1	43.5
Acupuncture	9.4	6.5
Biofeedback	35.3	31.5
Chiropractors	16.5	13.0
Psychologists	47.1	21.7
Psychiatrists	29.4	12.0
Pain clinic	64.7	51.1

cervical collar and rest[181] and to be as effective as physical therapy performed during the first 8 weeks after the injury.[182] Cervical traction may be no more effective than exercises alone.[158] Intraarticular injection of corticosteroids is not an effective therapy for chronic pain from the facet joints after a whiplash injury.[183]

In uncontrolled studies, trigger point injections with local anesthetics[184] and dry needling can be beneficial for acute and chronic myofascial pain.[185] Trigger point injections with sterile water may also be helpful in chronic whiplash patients.[186] Transcutaneous electrical nerve stimulators (TENS) may be worthwhile.[187]

According to one estimate, 94 percent of patients with chronic whiplash symptoms see more than one specialist.[117] Patients desperate for pain relief or a sympathetic approach may seek treatment from both physicians and other healers.[188] Controlled prospective studies of current conventional[189] and unconventional treatments and more effective treatments for chronic pain are greatly needed.

References

1. Evans RW, Evans RI, Sharp MJ: The physician survey on the post-concussion and whiplash syndromes. *Headache* 34:268–274, 1994.
2. Trimble MR: *Post-Traumatic Neurosis: From Railway Spine to the Whiplash.* Chichester, UK: Wiley, 1981.
3. Evans RW: The postconcussion syndrome: 130 years of controversy. *Semin Neurol* 14:32–39, 1994.
4. Erichsen JE: *On Concussion of the Spine: Nervous Shock and Other Obscure Injuries of the Nervous System in Their Clinical and Medico-Legal Aspects.* London: Longmans Green, 1882.
5. Rigler J: *Ueber die Verletzungen auf Eisenbahnen Insbesondere der Verletzungen des Rueckenmarks.* Berlin: Reimer, 1879.
6. Hodges RM: So-called concussion of the spinal cord. *Boston Med Surg J* 104:361–365, 1881.
7. Putnam JJ: Recent investigations into the pathology of so-called concussion of the spine, with cases illustrating the importance of seeking for evidences of typical hysteria in the chronic as well as in the acute stages of the disease. *Boston Med Surg J* 109:217–220, 1883.
8. Friedmann M: Ueber eine besondere schwere Form von Folgezustanden nach Gehirnerschutterung und uber den vasomotorischen Symptomencomplex bei derselben im Allgemeinen. *Arch Psychiatr* 23:230–267, 1892.
9. Strauss I, Savitsky N: Head injury: Neurologic and psychiatric aspects. *Arch Neurol Psych* 31:893–955, 1934.
10. Miller H: Accident neurosis. *Br Med J* 1:919, 1961.
11. Symonds C: Concussion and its sequelae. *Lancet* 1:1–5, 1962.
12. Symonds C: The assessment of symptoms following head injury. *Guys Hosp Gazette* 51:464, 1937.
13. McIntire RT: Opening remarks of the Symposium on Whiplash Injuries. *Int Rec Med* 169:2, 1956.
14. Crowe H: A new diagnostic sign in neck injuries. *Calif Med* 100:12–13, 1964.
15. Davis AG: Injuries of the cervical spine. *JAMA* 127:149–156, 1945.
16. Severy DM, Mathewson JH, Bechtol CO: Controlled automobile rear-end collisions, an investigation of related engineering and medical phenomena. *Can Serv Med J* 11:727–759, 1955.
17. Gay JR, Abbott KH: Common whiplash injuries of the neck. *JAMA* 152:1698–1704, 1953.
18. Lipow EG: Whiplash injuries. *South Med J* 48:1304–1311, 1955.
19. Steindler A: The interpretation of sciatic radiation and the syndrome of low-back pain. *J Bone Joint Surg* 22:28–34, 1940.
20. Mandel S: Minor head injury may not be "minor." *Postgrad Med* 85:213–225, 1989.
21. Evans RW: The postconcussion syndrome and the sequelae of mild head injury. *Neurol Clin North Am* 10:815–847, 1992.
22. Jennett B, Teasdale G, Murray G, et al: Head injury, in Evans RW, Baskin DS, Yatsu FM (eds): *Prognosis of Neurological Disorders.* New York: Oxford University Press, 1992: 86.
23. Annegers JF, Grabow JD, Groover RV, et al: Seizures after head trauma: A population study. *Neurology* 30:683–689, 1980.
24. Goetz CG, Pappert EJ: Trauma and movement disorders. *Neurol Clin North Am* 10:907–919, 1992.
25. Lee MS, Rinne JO, Ceballos-Baumann A, et al: Dystonia after head trauma. *Neurology* 44:1374–1378, 1994.
26. Jankovic J: Post-traumatic movement disorders: Central and peripheral mechanisms. *Neurology* 44:2006–2014, 1994.
27. Haas DC, Ross GS: Transient global amnesia triggered by mild head trauma. *Brain* 109:251–257, 1986.
28. Dikmen SS, Levin HS: Methodological issues in the study of mild head injury. *J Head Trauma Rehabil* 8(3):30–37, 1993.
29. Yamaguchi M: Incidence of headache and severity of head injury. *Headache* 32:427–431, 1992.
30. Packard RC: Posttraumatic headache. *Semin Neurol* 14:40–45, 1994.
31. Weiss HD, Stern BJ, Goldberg J: Post-traumatic migraine: Chronic migraine precipitated by minor head or neck trauma. *Headache* 31:451–456, 1991.
32. Matthews WB: Footballer's migraine. *Br Med J* 2:326–327, 1972.
33. Bennett DR, Fuenning SI, Sullivan G, et al: Migraine precipitated by head trauma in athletes. *Am J Sports Med* 8(3):202–205, 1980.
34. Ashworth B: Migraine, head trauma and sport. *Scott Med J* 30:240–242, 1985.
35. Haas DC, Lourie H: Trauma-triggered migraine: An explanation for common neurological attacks after mild head injury. *J Neurosurg* 68:181–188, 1988.
36. Turkewitz LJ, Wirth O, Dawson GA, Casaly JS: Cluster headache following head injury: A case report and review of the literature. *Headache* 32:504–508, 1992.
37. Vijayan N: A new post-traumatic headache syndrome:

Clinical and therapeutic observations. *Headache* 17(1):19–22, 1977.
38. Levin HS, Mattis S, Ruff RM, et al: Neurobehavioral outcome following minor head injury: A three-center study. *J Neurosurg* 66:234–243, 1987.
39. Cartlidge NEF: Post-concussional syndrome. *Scot Med J* 23:103, 1978.
40. Baloh RW, Honrubia V, Jacobson K: Benign positional vertigo: Clinical and oculographic features in 240 cases. *Neurology* 37:371–378, 1987.
41. Tuohimaa P: Vestibular disturbances after acute mild head injury. *Acta Otolaryngol [Suppl] (Stockh)* 359:1–59, 1978.
42. Minderhoud JM, Boelens MEM, Huizenga J, et al: Treatment of mild head injuries. *Clin Neurol Neurosurg* 82:127–140, 1980.
43. Krohel GB, Kristan RW, Simon JW, et al: Posttraumatic convergence insufficiency. *Ann Ophthalmol* 18:101–104, 1986.
44. Keane JR, Baloh RW: Posttraumatic cranial neuropathies. *Neurol Clin North Am* 10:849–867, 1992.
45. Hendriks APJ: Olfactory dysfunction. *Rhinology* 26:229–251, 1988.
46. Gronwall D, Wrightson P: Delayed recovery of intellectual function after minor head injury. *Lancet* 2:605–609, 1974.
47. Slagle DA: Psychiatric disorders following closed head injury: An overview of biopsychological factors in their etiology and management. *Int J Psychiatry Med* 20:1–35, 1990.
48. Denker PG: The postconcussion syndrome: Prognosis and evaluation of the organic factors. *NY State J Med* 44:379–384, 1944.
49. Merskey H: Psychiatric aspects of the neurology of trauma. *Neurol Clin North Am* 10:895–905, 1992.
50. Chibnall JT, Duckro PN: Post-traumatic stress disorder in chronic post-traumatic headache patients. *Headache* 34:357–361, 1994.
51. Rutherford WH, Merrett JD, McDonald JR: Sequelae of concussion caused by minor head injuries. *Lancet* 1:1–4, 1977.
52. Gentilini M, Nichelli P, Schoenhuber R: Assessment of attention in mild head injury, in Levin HS, Eisenberg HM, Benton AL (eds): *Mild Head Injury.* New York: Oxford University Press, 1989: 163–175.
53. Montgomery EA, Fenton GW, McClelland RJ, et al: The psychobiology of minor head injury. *Psychol Med* 21:375–384, 1990.
54. Young WB, Silberstein SD: Imaging and electrophysiologic testing in mild head injury. *Semin Neurol* 14:46–52, 1994.
55. Duus BR, Lind B, Christensen H, Nielsen OA: The role of neuroimaging in the initial management of patients with minor head injury. *Ann Emerg Med* 23:1279–1283, 1994.
56. Dacey RG, Alves WM, Rimel RW, et al: Neurosurgical complications after apparently minor head injury. *J Neurosurg* 65:203–210, 1986.
57. Jeret JS, Mandell M, Anziska B, et al: Clinical predictors of abnormality disclosed by computed tomography after mild head trauma. *Neurosurgery* 32:9–16, 1993.
58. Jennett B: Skull x-rays after mild head injuries. *Arch Emerg Med* 4:133–135, 1987.
59. Teasdale GM, Murray G, Anderson E, et al: Risks of acute traumatic intracranial hematoma in children and adults: Implications for managing head injuries. *Br Med J* 300:363–367, 1990.
60. Rosenorn J, Duus B, Nielsen K, et al: Is a skull x-ray necessary after milder head trauma? *Br J Neurosurg* 5:135–139, 1991.
61. Stein SC, Ross SE: Mild head injury: A plea for routine early CT scanning. *J Trauma* 33:11–13, 1992.
62. Stein SC, O'Malley KF, Ross SE: Is routine computed tomography scanning too expensive for mild head injury? *Ann Emerg Med* 20:1286–1289, 1991.
63. Levin HS, Williams DH, Eisenberg HM, et al: Serial MRI and neurobehavioral findings after mild to moderate closed head injury. *J Neurol Neurosurg Psychiatry* 55:255–262, 1992.
64. Dow RS, Ulett G, Raaf J: Electroencephalographic studies immediately following head injury. *Am J psychiatry* 101:174–183, 1944.
65. Lorenzoni E: Electroencephalographic studies before and after head injuries. *Electroencephalogr Clin Neurophysiol* 28:216, 1970.
66. Schoenhuber R, Gentilini M, Scarano M, et al: Longitudinal study of auditory brainstem response in patients with minor head injuries. *Arch Neurol* 44:1181–1182, 1987.
67. Schoenhuber R, Gentilini M, Orlando A: Prognostic value of auditory brainstem responses for late postconcussion symptoms following minor head injury. *J Neurosurg* 68:742–744, 1988.
68. Thatcher RW, Walker RA, Gerson I, et al: EEG discriminant analyses of mild head injury. *Electroencephalogr Clin Neurophysiol* 73:94–106, 1989.
69. American Academy of Neurology: EEG brain mapping. *Neurology* 39:1100–1101, 1989.
70. Nuwer MR, Hauser HM: Erroneous diagnosis using EEG discriminant analysis. *Neurology* 44:1998–2000, 1994.
71. Epstein C: Computerized EEG in the courtroom. *Neurology* 44:1566–1569, 1994.
72. McCaffrey RJ, Williams AD, Fisher JM, Laing LC: Forensic issues in mild head injury. *J Head Trauma Rehabil* 8(3):38–47, 1993.
73. Fisher JM, Williams AD: Neuropsychologic investigation of mild head injury: Ensuring diagnostic accuracy in the assessment process. *Semin Neurol* 14:53–59, 1994.
74. Ruff RM, Wylie T, Tennant W: Malingering and malingering-like aspects of mild closed head injury. *J Head Trauma Rehabil* 8(3):60–73, 1993.
75. Prigatano GP, Redner JE: Uses and abuses of neuropsychological testing in behavioral neurology. *Neurol Clin North Am* 11:219–231, 1993.
76. Evans RW: The post-concussion syndrome, in Evans RW, Baskin DS, Yatsu FM (eds): *Prognosis of Neurological Disorders.* New York: Oxford University Press, 1992: 97–107.
77. Leininger BE, Gramling SE, Farrel AD, et al: Neuropsychological deficits in symptomatic minor head injury

patients after concussion and mild concussion. *J Neurol Neurosurg Psychiatry* 53:293–296, 1990.

78. Edna T-H, Ceppelen J: Late postconcussional symptoms in traumatic head injury: An analysis of frequency and risk factors. *Acta Neurochir (Wien)* 86:12–17, 1987.
79. Fenton G, McClelland R, Montgomery A, et al: The postconcussional syndrome: Social antecedents and psychological sequelae. *Br J Psychiatry* 162:493–497, 1993.
80. Gronwall D: Cumulative and persisting effects of concussion on attention and cognition, in Levin HS, Eisenberg HM, Benton AL (eds): *Mild Head Injury.* New York: Oxford University Press, 1989: 153–162.
81. Rutherford WH, Merrett JD, McDonald JR: Symptoms at one year following concussion from minor head injuries. *Injury* 10:225–230, 1978.
82. Rimel RW, Giordani B, Barth JT, et al: Disability caused by minor head injury. *Neurosurgery* 9:221–228, 1981.
83. Dikmen SS, Temkin NR, Machamer JE, et al: Employment following traumatic head injuries. *Arch Neurol* 51:177–186, 1994.
84. Denny-Brown D: Disability arising from closed head injury. *JAMA* 127:429–436, 1945.
85. Steadman JH, Graham JG: Rehabilitation of the brain-injured. *Proc Soc Med* 63:23–28, 1969.
86. Guthkelch AN: Post-traumatic amnesia, post-concussional symptoms and accident neurosis. *Eur Neurol* 19:92–102, 1980.
87. Merskey H, Woodforde JM: Psychiatric sequelae of minor head injury. *Brain* 95:521–528, 1972.
88. McKinlay WW, Brooks DN, Bond MR: Post-concussional symptoms, financial compensation and outcome of severe blunt head injury. *J Neurol Neurosurg Psychiatry* 46:1084–1091, 1983.
89. Mureriwa J: Head injury and compensation: A preliminary investigation of the postconcussional syndrome in Harare. *Cent Afr J Med* 36:315–318, 1990.
90. Fee CRA, Rutherford WH: A study on the effect of legal settlement on post-concussion symptoms. *Arch Emerg Med* 5:12–17, 1988.
91. Mendelson G: Not "cured by a verdict": Effect of legal settlement on compensation claimants. *Med J Aust* 2:132–134, 1982.
92. Packard RC: Posttraumatic headache: Permanency and relationship to legal settlement. *Headache* 32:496–500, 1992.
93. Kelly R, Smith BN: Post-traumatic syndrome: Another myth discredited. *J R Soc Med* 74:275–277, 1981.
94. Binder LM: Persisting symptoms after mild head injury: A review of the postconcussive syndrome. *J Clin Exp Neuropsychol* 8:323–346, 1986.
95. Lishman WA: Physiogenesis and psychogenesis in the "post-concussional syndrome." *Br J Psychiatry* 153:460–469, 1988.
96. Gould R, Miller BL, Goldberg MA, et al: The validity of hysterical signs and symptoms. *J Nerv Ment Dis* 174:593–597, 1986.
97. Tyler GS, McNeely HE, Dick ML: Treatment of post-traumatic headache with amitriptyline. *Headache* 20:213–216, 1980.
98. Label LS: Treatment of post-traumatic headaches: Maprotiline or amitriptyline? *Neurology* 41(suppl 1):247, 1991.
99. McBeath JG, Nanda A: Use of dihydroergotamine in patients with postconcussion syndrome. *Headache* 34:148–151, 1994.
100. Sjaastad O: The headache of challenge in our time: Cervicogenic headache. *Funct Neurol* 5:155–158, 1990.
101. Solomon S, Guglielmo KM: Treatment of headache by transcutaneous electrical stimulation. *Headache* 25:12–15, 1985.
102. Jensen OK, Nielsen FF, Vosmar L: An open study comparing manual therapy with the use of cold packs in the treatment of post-traumatic headache. *Cephalgia* 10:241–250, 1990.
103. Graff-Radford SB, Jaeger BJ, Reeves JL: Myofascial pain may present clinically as occipital neuralgia. *Neurosurgery* 19:610–613, 1986.
104. Chilvers CD: Acupuncture in the post-concussional syndrome. *NZ Med J* 98:658, 1985.
105. Tennant FS, Wild J: Naltrexone treatment for post concussional syndrome. *Am J Psychiatry* 144:813–814, 1987.
106. Levin HS: Cognitive rehabilitation: Unproved but promising. *Arch Neurol* 47:223–224, 1990.
107. Evans RW: Whiplash around the world. *Headache* 35:262–263, 1995.
108. Pearce JMS: Polemics of chronic whiplash injury. *Neurology* 44:1993–1997, 1994.
109. National Safety Council. *Accident Facts.* National Safety Council. Itasca, IL, 1992.
110. Deans GT, McGalliard JN, Rutherford WH: Incidence and duration of neck pain among patients injured in car accidents. *Br Med J* 292:94–95, 1986.
111. O'Neill B, Haddon W, Kelley AB, et al: Automobile head restraints—frequency of neck claims in relation to the presence of head restraints. *Am J Public Health* 62:403, 1972.
112. Pearce JMS: Whiplash injury: A reappraisal. *J Neurol Neurosurg Psychiatry* 52:1329–1331, 1989.
113. Kahane CJ: *An Evaluation of Head Restraints.* U.S. Department of Transportation. National Highway Traffic Safety Administration Techical Report DOT HS-806-108. Springfield, VA: National Technical Information Service, 1982.
114. Deans GT, McGalliard JN, Kerr M, Rutherford WH: Neck sprain—a major cause of disability following car accidents. *Injury* 18:10–12, 1987.
115. Nygren A: Injuries to car occupants: Some aspects of the interior safety of cars. *Acta Otolaryngol (Stockh)* 395(suppl):1–164, 1984.
116. Barnsley L, Lord S, Bogduk N: The pathophysiology of whiplash. *Spine* 7:329–353, 1993.
117. MacNab I: Acceleration injuries of the cervical spine. *J Bone Joint Surg* 46A:1797–1799, 1964.
118. Ommaya AK, Faas F, Yarnell P: Whiplash injury and brain damage—an experimental study. *JAMA* 204:285–289, 1968.
119. Barnsley L, Lord S, Bogduk N: The pathophysiology of whiplash. *Spine* 7:329–353, 1993.
120. Davis SJ, Teresi LM, Bradley WG, et al: Cervical spine hyperextension injuries: MR findings. *Radiology* 180:245–251, 1991.

121. Taylor JR, Kakulas BA: Neck injuries. *Lancet* 338:1343, 1991.
122. Taylor JR, Twomey LT: Acute injuries to cervical joints: An autopsy study of neck sprain. *Spine* 18:115–122, 1993.
123. Evans RW: Some observations on whiplash injuries. *Neurol Clin North Am* 10:975–997, 1992.
124. Norris SH, Watt I: The prognosis of neck injuries resulting from rear-end vehicle collision. *J Bone Joint Surg* 65B:608–611, 1983.
125. Shkrum MJ, Green RN, Nowak ES: Upper cervical trauma in motor vehicle collisions. *J Forensic Sci* 34:381–390, 1989.
126. Lord S, Barnsley L, Bogduk N: Cervical zygapophysial joint pain in whiplash. *Spine* 7:355–372, 1993.
127. Barnsley L, Lord S, Bogduk N: Comparative local anaesthetic blocks in the diagnosis of cervical zygapophysial joint pain. *Pain* 55:99–106, 1993.
128. Bogduk N, Simons DG: Neck pain: Joint pain or trigger points? in Voeroy H, Merskey H (eds): *Progress in Fibromyalgia and Myofascial Pain.* Amsterdam: Elsevier, 1993: 267–273.
129. Dwyer A, Aprill C, Bogduk N: Cervical zygapophysial joint pain patterns: I. A study in normal volunteers. *Spine* 15:453–457, 1990.
130. Balla J, Karnaghan J: Whiplash headache. *Clin Exp Neurol* 23:179–182, 1987.
131. Lord SM, Barnsley L, Wallis BJ, Bogduk N: Third occipital headache: A prevalence study. *J Neurol Neurosurg Psychiatry* 57:1187–1190, 1994.
132. Brooke RI, LaPointe HJ: Temporomandibular joint disorders following whiplash. *Spine* 7:443–454, 1993.
133. Jacome DE: Basilar artery migraine after uncomplicated whiplash injuries. *Headache* 26:515–516, 1986.
134. Winston K: Whiplash and its relationship to migraine. *Headache* 27:452–457, 1987.
135. Oosterveld WJ, Kortschot HW, Kingma GG, et al: Electronystagmographic findings following cervical whiplash injuries. *Acta Otolaryngol* (*Stockh*) 111:201–205, 1991.
136. Toglia JU: Acute flexion-extension injury of the neck: Electronystagmographic study of 309 patients. *Neurology* 26:808–814, 1976.
137. Norris SH, Watt I: The prognosis of neck injuries resulting from rear-end vehicle collision. *J Bone Joint Surg* 65B:608–611, 1983.
138. Capistrant TD: Thoracic outlet syndrome in whiplash injury. *Ann Surg* 185:175–178, 1977.
139. Capistrant TD: Thoracic outlet syndrome in cervical strain injury. *Minn Med* 69:13–17, 1986.
140. Pollack EW: Surgical anatomy of the thoracic outlet syndrome. *Surg Gynecol Obstet* 150:97–103, 1980.
141. Wilbourn AJ: The thoracic outlet syndrome is overdiagnosed. *Arch Neurol* 47:328–330, 1990.
142. Hong CZ, Simons DG: Response to treatment for pectoralis minor myofascial pain syndrome after whiplash. *J Musculoskeletal Pain* 1:89–129, 1993.
143. Haas DC, Nord SG, Bome MP: Carpal tunnel syndrome following automobile collisions. *Arch Phys Med Rehabil* 62:204–206, 1981
144. Label LS: Carpal tunnel syndrome resulting from steering wheel impact. *Muscle Nerve* 14:904, 1991.
145. Osterman AL: The double crush syndrome. *Orthop Clin North Am* 19:147–155, 1988.
146. Aniss AM, Gandevia SC, Milne RJ: Changes in perceived heaviness and motor commands produced by cutaneous reflexes in man. *J Physiol* 397:113–126, 1988.
147. Eismont FJ, Clifford S, Goldberg M, Green B: Cervical sagittal spinal canal size and spine injury. *Spine* 9:663–666, 1984.
148. Kischka U, Ettlin TH, Heim S: Cerebral symptoms following whiplash injury. *Eur Neurol* 31:136–140, 1991.
149. Ettlin TM, Kischka U, Reichmann S, et al: Cerebral symptoms after whiplash injury of the neck: A prospective clinical and neuropsychological study of whiplash injury. *J Neurol Neurosurg Psychiatry* 55:943–948, 1992.
150. Radanov BP, Di Stefano G, Schnidrig A, et al: Cognitive functioning after common whiplash: A controlled follow-up study. *Arch Neurol* 50:87–91, 1993.
151. Radanov BP, Di Stefano G, Schnidrig A, et al: Role of psychosocial stress in recovery from common whiplash. *Lancet* 338:712–715, 1991.
152. Hohl M: Soft tissue injuries of the neck in automobile accidents: Factors influencing prognosis. *J Bone Joint Surg* 56A:1675–1682, 1974.
153. Hildingsson C, Toolanen G: Outcome after soft-tissue injury of the cervical spine. *Acta Orthop Scand* 61:357–359, 1990.
154. Burke JP, Orton HP, West J, et al: Whiplash and its effect on the visual system. *Graefes Arch Clin Exp Ophthalmol* 230:335–339, 1992.
155. Truong DD, Dubinsky R, Hermanowicz N, et al: Posttraumatic torticollis. *Arch Neurol* 48:221–223, 1991.
156. Goldman S, Ahlskog JE: Posttraumatic cervical dystonia. *Mayo Clin Proc* 68:443–448, 1993.
157. Stringer WL, Kelly DL, Johnston FR, et al: Hyperextension injury of the cervical spine with esophageal perforation. *J Neurosurg* 53:541–543, 1980.
158. Totstein OD, Rhame FS, Molina E, et al: Mediastinitis after whiplash injury. *Can J Surg* 29:54–56, 1986.
159. Fisher CM: Whiplash amnesia. *Neurology* 32:667–668, 1982.
160. Dukes IK, Bannerjee SK: Hypoglossal nerve palsy following hyperextension neck injury. *Injury* 24:133–134, 1993.
161. Ringenberg BJ, Fischer AK, Urdaneta LF, Midthun MA: Rational ordering of cervical spine radiographs following trauma. *Ann Emerg Med* 17:792–796, 1988.
162. Mirvis SE, Diaconis JN, Chirico PA, et al: Protocol-driven radiologic evaluation of suspected cervical spine injury: Efficacy study. *Radiology* 170:831–834, 1989.
163. Diliberti T, Lindsey RW: Evaluation of the cervical spine in the emergency setting: Who does not need an x-ray? *Orthopedics* 15:179–183, 1992.
164. Irvine DH, Fisher JB, Newell DJ, et al: Prevalence of cervical spondylosis in a general practice. *Lancet* 1:1089–1092, 1965.
165. Friedenberg ZB, Miller WT: Degenerative disc disease

of the cervical spine: A comparative study of asymptomatic and symptomatic patients. *J Bone Joint Surg* 45A:1171–1178, 1963.

166. Teresi LM, Lufkin RB, Reicher MA, et al: Asymptomatic degenerative disk disease and spondylosis of the cervical spine: MR imaging. *Radiology* 164:83–88, 1987.
167. Gargan MF, Bannister GC: Long term prognosis of soft tissue injuries of the neck. *J Bone Joint Surg* 72B:901–903, 1990.
168. Hamer AJ, Gargan MF, Bannister GC, Nelson RJ: Whiplash injury and surgically treated cervical disc disease. *Injury* 24:549–550, 1993.
169. Parmar HV, Raymakers, R: Neck injuries from rear impact road traffic accidents: Prognosis in persons seeking compensation. *Injury* 2:75–78, 1993.
170. Evans RW: Whiplash syndrome, in Evans RW, Baskin DS, Yatsu FM (eds): *Prognosis of Neurological Disorders.* New York: Oxford University Press, 1992: 621–631.
171. Bannister G, Gargan M: Prognosis of whiplash injuries: A review of the literature. *Spine* 7:557–569, 1993.
172. Sturzenegger M, DiStefano G, Radanov BP, Schnidrig A: Presenting symptoms and signs after whiplash injury: The influence of accident mechanisms. *Neurology* 44:688–693, 1994.
173. Maimaris C, Barnes MR, Allen MJ: Whiplash injuries of the neck: A retrospective study. *Injury* 19:393–396, 1988.
174. Greenfield J, Ilfeld FW: Acute cervical strain: Evaluation and short term prognostic factors. *Clin Orthop* 122:196–200, 1977.
175. Miles KA, Maimaris C, Finlay D, et al: The incidence and prognostic significance of radiological abnormalities in soft tissue injuries to the cervical spine. *Skeletal Radiol* 17:493–496, 1988.
176. Balla JI: The late whiplash syndrome. *Aust N Z J Surg* 50:610–614, 1980.
177. Pennie BH, Agambar LJ: Whiplash injuries: A trial of early management. *J Bone Joint Surg* 72B:277–279, 1990.
178. Kenna C, Murtagh J: Whiplash *Aust Fam Physician* 16:727, 1987.
179. Shapiro AP, Roth RS: The effect of litigation on recovery from whiplash. *Spine* 7:531–556, 1993.
180. Teasell RW, Shapiro AP, Mailis A: Medical management of whiplash injuries: An overview. *Spine* 7:481–499, 1993.
181. Mealy K, Brennan H, Fenelon GCC: Early mobilization of acute whiplash injuries. *Br Med J* 292:656–657, 1986.
182. McKinney LA, Dornan JO, Ryan M: The role of physiotherapy in the management of acute neck sprain following road-traffic accidents. *Arch Emerg Med* 6:27–33, 1989.
183. Barnsley L, Lord SM, Wallis BJ, Bogduk N: Lack of effect of intraarticular corticosteroids for chronic pain in the cervical zygapophyseal joints. *N Engl J Med* 330:1047–1050, 1994.
184. Garvey TA, Marks MR, Wiesel SW: A prospective, randomized double-blind evaluation of trigger-point injection therapy for low-back pain. *Spine* 14:962–964, 1989.
185. Lewitt K: The needle effect in the relief of myofascial pain. *Pain* 6:83–90, 1979.
186. Byrn C, Olsson I, Falkheden L, et al: Subcutaneous sterile water injections for chronic neck and shoulder pain following whiplash injuries. *Lancet* 341:449–452, 1993.
187. Graff-Redford SB, Reeves JL, Baker RL, et al: Effects of transcutaneous electrical nerve stimulation on myofascial pain and trigger point sensitivity. *Pain* 37:1–5, 1989.
188. Murray RH, Rubel AJ: Physicians and healers—unwitting partners in health care. *N Engl J Med* 326:61–64, 1992.
189. Newman PK: Whiplash injury: Long term prospective studies are needed and meanwhile, pragmatic treatment. *Br Med J* 301:2–3, 1990.

CHAPTER 42

POST-TRAUMATIC SEIZURES

Nancy R. Temkin
Michael Haglund
H. Richard Winn

SYNOPSIS

Post-traumatic seizures are a relatively frequent complication of severe head injury. They can complicate the management of patients in the acute phase by increasing ICP and may significantly impair the quality of life of the survivors. Penetrating brain injury, intracerebral hematomas, subdural hematomas, depressed skull fractures, and seizures during the first week are strong risk factors for the development of late post-traumatic seizures, with over one-third of patients with one or more of these factors having at least one subsequent seizure.

Treatment with phenytoin, begun with intravenous loading soon after the injury, has been shown to be effective in preventing post-traumatic seizures in the first week after injury. Unfortunately, no regimen has yet been proved effective for preventing post-traumatic seizures in the long term. Both newer antiepileptic drugs and therapies aimed at preventing the brain damage that underlies the development of seizures need to be studied to find an effective way of preventing this common and troublesome complication.

HISTORY

Early post-traumatic seizures have been known as a complication of head injury since at least the time of Hippocrates, and possibly since Egyptian times.[1] They were considered an indicator of very poor prognosis, usually death. The connection between head injury and delayed seizures, beginning months or years after the injury was described by the fourteenth century. Currently, head injury is known to be a major cause of epilepsy, accounting for about 5.5 percent of cases.[2]

DEFINITIONS

Seizures that occur soon after a head injury have been recognized as having a character different from those occurring later. Although not entirely consistent, the most common nomenclature is that *early post-traumatic seizures* occur within the first 7 days after injury and *late post-traumatic seizures* occur later. *Immediate seizures* occurring within hours of injury are sometimes considered separately from other early seizures.[3,4] The term "post-traumatic epilepsy" is frequently used interchangeably with "post-traumatic seizures" although, more technically, the term "epilepsy" is reserved for two or more unprovoked—in this case, late—seizures.

COMPLICATIONS CAUSED BY POST-TRAUMATIC SEIZURES

Up to 40 percent of patients with severe closed head injuries will have increases in intracranial pressure.[5] Since many of these patients have low intracranial compliance, the prevention of seizures in the early period may be particularly important. Seizures are not only known to increase cerebral metabolic rate, but also dramatically increase cerebral blood flow.[6] These changes in a critically ill patient may lead to secondary insults, including ischemia and plateau waves of increased intracranial pressure.[7,8] In patients who are sedated and paralyzed for treatment of increased intracranial pressure, a rare cause of sustained intracranial pressure can be epilepsia partialis continua. After other causes of increased ICP are ruled out, an EEG evaluation is sometimes warranted to determine if these sustained seizures are occurring.[8]

In addition to the medical consequences, late post-traumatic seizures can have negative effects on the cognitive, psychosocial, and emotional well-being of the patients.

Many cognitive deficits caused by the head injury can be worsened by epilepsy, causing a partial setback in recovery.[9] Memory is most likely to be affected, but distractibility, word-finding difficulty, psychomotor slowing, and decreased reasoning and problem-solving ability also have been associated with complex partial seizures. Additionally, all seizures that impair consciousness interrupt the patient's ability to receive and process information. Postictal depression can extend the period of decreased cognitive ability.

The loss of driving privileges that usually results from late post-traumatic seizures causes major changes in the life-style of most adults, limiting mobility and increasing their dependence on others. The loss of a driver's license—or the seizures themselves—can lead to job loss. Additional changes, such as avoiding alcohol or increasing sleep to avoid exacerbating the seizures, can disrupt relationships with friends. In a 15-year followup of World War II veterans, those with epilepsy were more likely to be nondrivers, nonparticipants in the community, unmarried and teetotalers as compared to those with similar head injuries but without epilepsy.[10]

Emotionally, seizures lead to a loss of the sense of control over one's life. This is especially true when there is no warning before a seizure. Emotional problems associated with epilepsy can compound those already present due to the head injury. Dealing with both can be an overwhelming handicap.

POST-TRAUMATIC SEIZURES AS INDICATOR OF INTRACRANIAL LESIONS IN MILD HEAD INJURY

Although post-traumatic seizures occur more frequently with increasing injury severity, in mild injury, the occurrence of an early post-traumatic seizure can alert the neurosurgeon to a possible intracranial lesion. In a series of 4232 adults with GCS of 13–15 in the emergency room and no compound depressed skull fracture or penetrating injury, 100 experienced early post-traumatic seizures.[11] These 100 cases had a CT scan, yielding 41 cases with intracerebral hemorrhage (including 17 with subdural hematomas), three with epidural hematomas, and three with subarachnoid hemorrhage. In seven cases (three epidural, four subdural), craniotomy was performed because of a mass effect that caused a significant midline shift. Although the possibility of a surgically-correctable lesion is relatively low, an untreated lesion can be devastating. This suggests that a CT scan should be performed in patients with mild head injury if they experience early post-traumatic seizures.

PATHOPHYSIOLOGICAL MECHANISMS

The structural and physiological changes that lead to post-traumatic epilepsy are not well understood; however, many of the initiating factors and resulting changes are known.[12,13] At the most basic level, the extent of the injury is determined by the magnitude of the kinetic energy imposed on the brain. The kinetic energy leads to cavitation and propagation of a pressure wave through the brain tissue elements.[14–16] The forces are not applied at right angles, but involve strong lateral and rotational forces. These strong forces result in shearing injury to fiber tracts and blood vessels, and contusional hemorrhages.[17] The histopathological examination of brain tissue after trauma reveals reactive gliosis, axon retraction balls, Wallerian degeneration, neurological scar formation, and cystic white matter lesions.[18,19] Two pathophysiological mechanisms that may underlie the development of post-traumatic seizures are iron deposition and activation of the arachidonic acid cascade.

The direct contact of blood with cortical tissue has been strongly associated with epileptogenesis. The presence of intracerebral hemorrhage appears in many studies as a key factor in the development of post-traumatic epilepsy. These hemorrhages and the resulting deposition of iron liberated from hemoglobin may be one of the key features in the development of post-traumatic epilepsy.[20–22] This supposition is supported by animal models where injection of iron salts into the rodent cortex or application to the cortical surface leads to acute epileptiform discharges.[23,24]

Iron and other compounds have been found to affect intracellular calcium concentration. For example, cultured glial cells from human epiletogenic brain tissue demonstrate rapid calcium oscillations and calcium waves when exposed to glutamate.[25] The same oscillation and waves are present at a much lower frequency in glial cell cultures exposed to iron in either its ferric or ferrous form.[26]

Pretreatment of animals with the antioxidants α-tocopherol and selenium prevents seizures, suggesting that the initiation and propagation of lipid peroxidation, especially activation of the arachidonic acid cascade, may play an important role in epileptogenesis.[27–29] The protective effects of antioxidants were observed following ferrous chloride injection into the rat hippocampus[30] and after compression and cold-induced edema in the rat brain.[28,31] Activation of the arachidonic acid cascade leads to formation of diacylglycerol (DAG) and inositoltidyl phosphytate (IP3). Increases in IP3 cause the release of intracellular calcium stores and modification of calcium channels which further elevates the intracellular calcium concentration. Rising intracellular calcium concentrations appear to be involved in excitotoxic damage to neurons. Neuronal death and reactive gliosis clearly can lead to a glial scar formation, which forms the epicenter of the hyperexcitable focus[32] (Fig. 42-1).

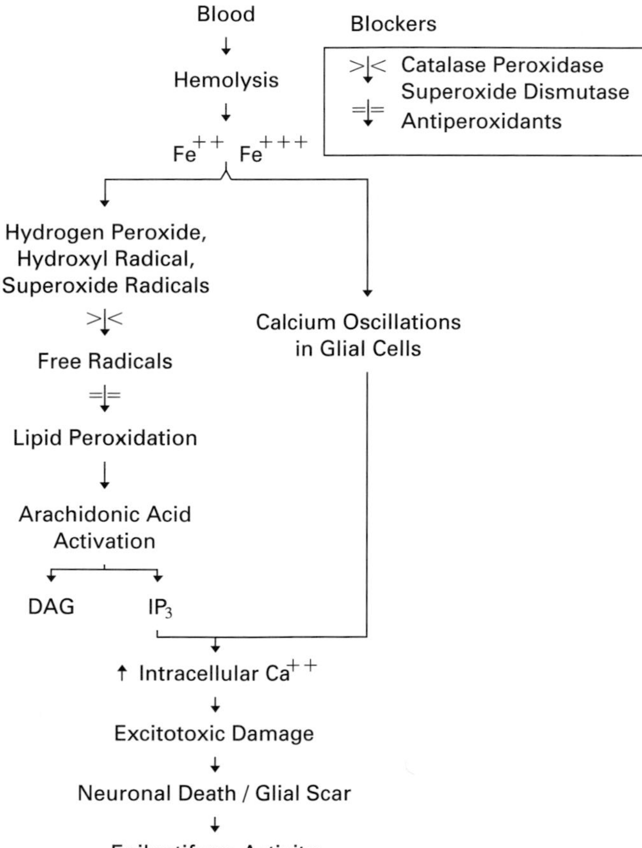

Figure 42-1. Schematic of possible changes leading to epilepsy and interventions to inhibit them. (From Temkin, Haglund, Winn.[39])

EPIDEMIOLOGY OF POST-TRAUMATIC SEIZURES

Early Seizures

Timing of early seizures

Although early seizures can occur any time during the first week after injury, their occurrence is not uniform in that period. About one-third occur in the first hour post-injury, one-third between 1 and 24 hours, and one-third between 1 and 7 days. Adults tend to have early seizures somewhat later than children do.[4,33] Patients with intracerebral hematomas or hemorrhagic contusions are more likely to have early seizures after 24 hours than are those without intracranial hematomas.[34]

Incidence

Early seizures occur in about 2 percent of unselected cases of head injury receiving medical attention.[35] Among those admitted to hospital, the rate is 3 to 6 percent, with the higher incidence in series limited to children.[4,34,36,37] The highest rates—7 to 9 percent—are found in children under the age of 5.[4,33] Many incidence studies have been performed on different populations. (See Yablon[38] for a more comprehensive review.)

Risk factors

Patient Characteristics

Age is the major patient characteristic affecting the risk of early post-traumatic seizures. Children, especially young children, have a higher incidence than adults with the same severity of injury.[4,33,37]

Injury Characteristics

Severity is the most potent risk factor for early as well as late post-traumatic seizures. Early post-traumatic seizures are rare after mild injuries with only brief disruption of consciousness, except in young children.[4] The risk of early post-traumatic seizures is increased with prolonged unconsciousness, skull fractures, hematomas, hemorrhagic contusions, and focal neurological signs.[4,39]

Seizure types

Focal seizures with or without secondary generalization are seen in 60 to 80 percent of people with early post-traumatic seizures, with generalized tonic-clonic seizures occurring in most of the rest. Focal seizures are most common in children and in patients with missile wounds.[40] Status epilepticus occurs in about 10 percent of adults and 4 percent of children under 5 with early post-traumatic seizures.[40,41]

Late Seizures

Timing of Late Seizures

The risk of new-onset seizures decreases with time following injury. In the Viet Nam series, 18 percent developed their seizures within the first month and 57 percent began within the first year.[21] A similar distribution was reported by Jennett.[4] The risk remains elevated for quite some time. Annegers et al.[35] demonstrated an increased risk through 4 years and a trend beyond that in mostly mild civilian cases. Salazar et al.[21] reported a seizure risk 25 times that expected even 10 to 15 years after combat injuries. They have not yet published data from later periods.

Incidence

At least one late post-traumatic seizure occurs in about 2 percent of cases receiving any medical attention for head injury[35] and in about 5 percent of hospitalized civilian cases.[4] The rate is much higher—34 to 53 percent—among those with combat missile wounds.[21,42,43]

Risk Factors

Patient Characteristics

Adults are at higher risk for late post-traumatic seizures than are children.[35] Family history of seizures has been reported to be associated with modestly increased risk for post-traumatic seizures in some studies,[4,43] but the finding is not supported by others,[21] suggesting that it is, at most, a weak effect.

Injury Characteristics

Missile wounds, especially those obtained in combat, yield the highest risk of late post-traumatic seizures. Brain volume loss is highly predictive, with late post-traumatic seizures occurring in 79 percent of patients losing over 75 ml, but only 40 percent of patients losing under 25 ml of brain tissue. After controlling for brain volume lost, additional risk factors are focal neurological signs, hematoma, retained metal fragments, and location of the lesion.[21,44]

The main risk factors in civilian (usually blunt) head injury are hematomas, depressed fracture, focal signs, and early seizures. Table 42-1 shows the rate of late post-traumatic seizures for patients with different characteristics of their injury. Except as noted, these figures are derived from the authors' series of 323 adults followed to 2 years.[45] All patients with a feature are included, regardless of other risk factors present. For degree of coma, especially, the association with late post-traumatic seizures may be attributable to association with other factors. In patients with no other risk factors, prolonged or deep coma was associated with about 2 percent risk.[4,39,46] Several authors provide methods for estimation of seizure risk based on several factors simultaneously and also offer estimates of future risk, given the interval seizure-free since injury.[4,47,48]

TABLE 42-1 Factors Associated with Late Post-Traumatic Seizures

Data from the authors' series of 233 cases followed post 8 days unless indicated otherwise.

	Incidence of Late Post-traumatic Seizures (%)
Penetrating missile wound[21]	53
Early seizure	47
Intracerebral hematoma	40
Subdural hematoma	33
Glasgow Coma Scale ≤10	32
Depressed skull fracture	31
Cortical contusion	28
Epidural hematoma	26
Linear fracture[49]	5
Mild concussion[4]	<1

SOURCE: Temkin, Haglund, Winn.[39]

Seizure Types

Unlike early post-traumatic seizures, 60 to 70 percent of late seizures are generalized convulsive seizures with or without focal onset.[40] The rest are simple or complex partial seizures, with other generalized seizures occurring very rarely.

Recurrence and Persistence

About 23 percent of patients having an initial remote symptomatic seizure, such as a late post-traumatic seizure, never have another seizure.[50] One-third to one-half of patients experience three or fewer seizures.[4,43] The fewer seizures early on, the less likely they will persist. For example, only about one-third of patients with one or two seizures in the first year are still having seizures by 8 years after injury as compared to two-thirds of those with three or more seizures in the first year.[4,51] Epilepsy that develops shortly after the injury, i.e., in the first year, is more likely to remit than will later-developing seizures.[4]

TREATMENT

Early Seizures

Early post-traumatic seizures need not be treated unless they are prolonged or are causing difficulties in the patient's management. Early seizures requiring treatment should be treated as status epilepticus.[52] At the authors' institution, the initial treatment of choice is intravenous lorazepam, 1–2 mg per minute up to 10 mg. Long-term treatment is not generally started for early post-traumatic seizures.

Late Seizures

Before treatment for late post-traumatic seizures is considered, a definitive diagnosis needs to be reached. In many cases, clinical observations are sufficient, but the varied manifestations of post-traumatic seizures sometimes makes diagnosis difficult. Diagnosis of partial seizures may be especially difficult in patients with significant cognitive or behavioral impairments. Nonepileptic seizures, nonepileptic myoclonus, or syncopal episodes can all be mistaken for seizures. In difficult cases, long-term video-EEG recording may be required to obtain a definite diagnosis.[38]

Once a diagnosis of unprovoked seizure is made, late post-traumatic seizures are treated like any other unprovoked seizure of the same type.[53] Some choose not to treat the first late seizure, since this is the only seizure in over 20 percent of the cases.[50,54] At the authors' institution, the usual policy is to begin long-term treatment, most often with carbamazepine or phenytoin, following the first late seizure. An initial low dose is increased gradually to minimize side effects.[53]

PREVENTION

Almost since effective drugs were found to treat seizures, neurosurgeons have tried to prevent the onset of post-traumatic seizures by administering antiepileptic drugs to patients with severe head injury. Early reports from nonrandomized studies suggested an over 80 percent reduction in seizure rates.[55–59] The most commonly used drugs are phenytoin and phenobarbital, alone or in combination.

Ten well-controlled studies of seizure prophylaxis following head trauma have been found.[45,60–67] All the studies have used patients at high risk for seizures and have employed a parallel-group design comparing one or two active drugs to placebo or no drug. Treatment began within 24 hours in all but two studies.[61,67] While not entirely consistent, the results have been fairly discouraging, at least as far as late seizures are concerned (Table 42-2).

Effectiveness

Early seizures

Of the four studies that report results on early seizures separately, the carbamazepine study[64] and two phenytoin studies[45,66] show significant reductions in early post-traumatic seizures with the active drug, while the remaining phenytoin study shows low but identical rates.[62] A meta-analysis of the phenytoin studies[65] indicates that their results are compatible and give a combined estimated 57 percent reduction in early seizures with phenytoin (95 percent confidence interval: 39 to 82 percent reduction).

Late seizures

Less consistent results are found in results concerning late seizures. Some of the studies are small, and combined with a low seizure rate in the placebo group, have little power to detect a modest effect of the drug. Thus it is important to look at the totality of evidence and especially at confidence intervals indicating the changes in seizure rate that are consistent with the results of the studies. A substantial positive effect was found in the Pechadre et al. study,[66] while three others had nonsignificant positive findings and six actually reported a higher seizures rate with the active drug. The disparate results are especially confusing because the Pechadre and four other studies tested phenytoin in populations that appear similar. The designs were also similar, except that the Pechadre study was less well controlled, using no treatment rather than placebo, and no blinding. A meta-analysis[65] indicates that the Pechadre et al. study, with an estimated 86 percent reduction in seizures (95 percent confidence interval: 40 to 97 percent reduction), is not compatible with the other four phenytoin studies, which demonstrated a combined estimated 10 percent increase in late post-traumatic seizures (95 percent confidence interval: 25 percent reduction to 61 percent increase). Close examination of the studies is needed to determine whether details of the treatments

TABLE 42-2 Summary of Well-Controlled Studies of Prophylaxis of Post-traumatic Seizures

				Seizure Rates					
			Length of Treatment/	Early			Late		
Investigator (City)	Active Treatment	Patients (N)	Followup Mos.	Active %	Placebo %	P	Active %	Placebo %	P
Brackett et al (Kansas City, KS)	Low dose pb/pht	125	18/36				23*	13	ns
Brackett et al (Kansas City, KS)	Ther pb/pht	49	6/18				14*	39	0.09
McQueen et al (Edinburgh, New Castle, UK)	Ther pht	164	12/24				10	9	ns
Marshall et al (San Diego, CA)	Ther ph/pht	154	6/18				24*	16	τ
Locke et al (Los Angeles, CA)	Ther pb, pht, pb/pht	303	6/18				4*	12	τ
Young et al (Lexington, KY)	Ther pht	244	18/18	4	4	ns	12	11	ns
Temkin et al (Seattle, WA)	Ther pht	404	12/24	4	14	0.001	27	21	ns
Glötzner et al (Wurzburg, Germany)	Ther cbz	139	24/24	10	25	0.016	27	33	ns
Manaka (Tokyo, Japan)	Ther pb	126	24/60				16	11	ns
Pechadre et al (Clermont-Ferrand, France)	Ther pht	86	3-12/24	6	24	.05	6	42	.001

Abbreviations: * = rate for early and late seizures combined, τ = significance test accounting for loss to follow-up not available, pht = phenytoin, pb = phenobarbital, Ther = therapeutic levels, ns = not significant, cbz = carbamazepine.

SOURCE: Temkin, Haglund, Winn,[39] adapted from Temkin, Dikmen, Winn.[65]

or populations suggest a more beneficial policy for prophylaxis. Differences are not readily apparent, although the alternate-day treatment assignment and lack of blinding could allow biases in the Pechadre et al. study. At present, our best estimate of the effectiveness of phenytoin for preventing late post-traumatic seizures in patients at high risk following head trauma comes from combining all five controlled studies. This yields a small, nonsignificant reduction of 15 percent with phenytoin (95 percent confidence interval: 40 percent reduction to 22 percent increase).

Adverse Effects

Prophylactic use of antiepileptic drugs is not without cost in terms of adverse effects. The sedative effects of phenobarbital can depress the patient's level of consciousness, confusing the management of head-injured patients, and can decrease the effectiveness of rehabilitation efforts. Phenytoin causes rashes in almost 10 percent of cases.[45] It also causes adverse effects on cognitive and psychomotor functioning, especially relatively soon after a severe head injury.[68] Other drugs have not been evaluated similarly in head-injured patients, so one does not know whether their neurobehavioral effects would be similar.

Conclusions

As summarized above and reinforced by two studies[69,70] of prophylaxis following craniotomy for a variety of reasons, empirical evidence indicates phenytoin (and, likely, carbamazepine) prevent early post-traumatic seizures. Therapeutic levels of phenytoin usually can be obtained initially with an intravenous loading dose of 18 mg/kg administered at a rate not exceeding 40 mg/min. They usually can be maintained by a dose of 5 mg/kg/day, but patients with severe multisystem injuries may hypermetabolize the drug and require significantly higher maintenance doses. Administration of other drugs, such as steroids, can also alter metabolism. Total phenytoin blood levels should be checked periodically and doses altered to maintain levels in the therapeutic range of 40–80 mmol/L (10–20 mg/L). Prophylactic administration of phenytoin can be stopped after 1 to 2 weeks. Currently, there is no regimen that has been shown to prevent late post-traumatic seizures.

FUTURE DIRECTIONS

Post-traumatic seizures are a frequent and disruptive complication of head injury. Although prior efforts have been unsuccessful in demonstrating effective prophylaxis of late post-traumatic seizures, many other avenues remain to be explored. Other antiepileptic drugs may prove effective. Valproate prevents development of a kindled focus in rodents[71] and is under investigation by the authors for prophylaxis of post-traumatic seizures in humans. Additional new drugs have recently been approved or are under development. They warrant evaluation in animal models to see if they show antieleptogenesis effects. Our increasing knowledge of the brain and its response to injury may yield other strategies that interrupt the formation of a seizure focus. Some interesting possibilities include chelation, antioxidants and antiperoxidants such as α-tocopherol, selenium, and superoxide dismutase.[29,32,72] Perhaps one of these strategies will greatly decrease the risk of post-traumatic seizures, thereby increasing the quality of life of head-injured patients.

REFERENCES

1. Temkin O: *The Falling Sickness: A History of Epilepsy from the Greeks to the Beginnings of Modern Neurology*, 2d ed. Baltimore: Johns Hopkins Press, 1971.
2. Hauser WA, Annegers JF, Kurland LT: Incidence of epilepsy and unprovoked seizures in Rochester, Minnesota: 1935–1984. *Epilepsia* 1993; 34:453–468.
3. Elvidge AR: Remarks on post-traumatic convulsive state. *Trans Am Neurol Assoc* 1939; 65:125–129.
4. Jennett B: *Epilepsy After Nonmissile Injuries*, 2d ed. Chicago: Year Book, 1975.
5. Miller JD, Becker DP, Ward JD, et al: Significance of intracranial hypertension in severe head injury. *J Neurosurg* 1977; 47:503–516.
6. Lassen NA: Control of cerebral circulation in health and disease. *Circ Res* 1974; 34:749–760.
7. Graham DI, Ford I, Adams JH, et al: Ischemic brain damage is still common in fatal non-missile head injury. *J Neurol Neurosurg Psychiatry* 1989; 52:346–350.
8. Chesnut RM, Marshall LF, Marshall SB: Medical management of intracranial pressure, in Cooper PR: *Head Injury*. Baltimore: Williams & Wilkins, 1993:225–246.
9. Bennett TL: Post-traumatic epilepsy: Its nature and implications for head injury recovery. *Cognitive Rehab* 1987; September/October:12–18.
10. Walker AE, Erculei F: *Head Injured Men: Fifteen Years Later*. Springfield IL: Charles C Thomas, 1969.
11. Lee S-T, Lui T-N: Early seizures after mild closed head injury. *J Neurosurg* 1992; 76:435–439.
12. Dichter MA, Ayala GF: Cellular mechanisms of epilepsy: A status report. *Science* 1987; 237:157–164.
13. Willmore LJ: Post traumatic epilepsy. *Neurol Clin* 1992; 10:869–878.
14. Pudenz RH, Shelden CH: The lucite calvarium—a direct observation of the brain. *J Neurosurg* 1946; 3:487–505.
15. Lindgren SO: Experimental studies of mechanical effects in head injury. *Acta Chir Scand* 1966; (Suppl) 360:1–100.
16. Willmore LJ: Post traumatic epilepsy: Cellular mechanisms and implications for treatment. *Epilepsia* 1990; 31 (Suppl 3):S67–S73.
17. Gennarelli TA, Thibaulat LE, Adams JH, et al: Diffuse axonal injury and traumatic coma in the primate. *Ann Neurol* 1982; 12:564–574.
18. Langfitt TW, Weinstein JD, Kassell NF: Vascular factors in head injury: Contribution to brain swelling and intracranial hypertension, in Caveness WF, Walker AE (eds): *Head Injury*. Philadelphia: JB Lippincott, 1966:172–194.
19. Tornheim PA, Liwnicz BH, Hirsch SC, et al: Acute responses to blunt head trauma. *J Neurosurg* 1983; 59: 431–438.
20. Jennett B: Epilepsy and acute traumatic intracranial hematoma. *J Neurol Neurosurg Psychiatry* 1975; 38: 378–381.
21. Salazar AM, Jabbari B, Vance SC, et al: Epilepsy after penetrating head injury. I Clinical correlates: A report of the Vietnam Head Injury Study. *Neurology* 1985; 35:1406–1414.
22. Faught E, Peters D, Bartolucci A, et al: Seizures after primary intracerebral hemorrhage. *Neurology* 1989; 39:1089–1093.
23. Willmore LJ, Sypert GW, Munson JB: Recurrent seizures induced by cortical iron injection: A model of posttraumatic epilepsy. *Ann Neurol* 1978; 4:329–336.
24. Reid SA, Sypert GW: Acute FeC13-induced epileptogenic foci in cats: electrophysiological analyses. *Brain Res* 1980; 188:531–542.
25. Lee S, Magge S, Spencer DD, et al: Laser photobleach-recovery shows increased gap junction coupling on astrocytes from human epileptic foci which exhibit hyperexcitable calcium responses. *Soc Neurosci Abstr* 1992; 18:164.
26. Kraemer DL, Kim WT, Spencer DD, et al: Iron model of epilepsy revisited: Role of astrocytes. *Epilepsia* 1993; 34(Suppl 6):127.
27. Fishman RA, Chan PH, Lee J, et al: Effects of superoxide free radicals on the induction of brain edema. *Neurology* 1979; 29:546.
28. Chan PH, Fishman RA: Transient formation of superoxide radicals in polyunsaturated fatty acid-induced brain swelling. *J Neurochem* 1980; 35:1004–1007.
29. Willmore LJ, Rubin JJ: Antiperoxidant pretreatment and iron-induced epileptiform discharges in the rat: EEG and histopathologic studies. *Neurology* 1981; 31:63–69.

30. Willmore LJ, Sypert GW: Epileptiform activity initiated by peel iontophoresis of ferrous and ferric chloride into rat cerebral cortex. *Brain Res* 1978; 152:406–410.
31. Yoshida S, Busto R, Ginsberg MD, et al: Compression-induced brain edema: Modification by prior depletion and supplementation of Vitamin E. *Neurology* 1983; 33:166–172.
32. Willmore LJ, Triggs WJ, Gray JD: The role of iron-induced hippocampal peroxidation in acute epileptogenesis. *Brain Res* 1986; 382:422–426.
33. De Santis A, Pagni CA: Osservazioni su 134 casi di traumatizzati cranici in eta infantile con crisi convulsive precoci. Atti del VII Congresso Naz. della Soc. Ital Neuropsich Infantile Ediz Centro Min Medica, Torino, 1976:269–273.
34. De Santis A, Pagni CA: Valore prognostico delle crisi convulsive precoci nel coma traumatico. *Riv Neurol* 1976; 46:400.
35. Annegers JF, Grabow JD, Groover RV, et al: Seizures after head trauma: A population study. *Neurology* 1980; 30:683–689.
36. Hendrick EB, Harris L: Post-traumatic epilepsy in children. *J Trauma* 1968; 8:547–556.
37. De Santis A, Cappricci E, Granata G: Early posttraumatic seizures in adults. Study of 84 cases. *J Neurosurg Sci* 1979; 23:207–210.
38. Yablon SA: Posttraumatic seizures. *Arch Phys Med Rehabil* 1993; 74:983–1001.
39. Temkin NR, Haglund M, Winn HR: Post-traumatic epilepsy, in Youmans JR (ed): *A Textbook of Neurosurgery*, 3d ed. Philadelphia: WB Saunders, 1994: Chap. 77.
40. Pagni CA: Posttraumatic epilepsy. Incidence and prophylaxis. *Acta Neurochir* 1990; Suppl 50:38–47.
41. Jennett B, Teasdale G: *Management of Head Injuries.* Philadelphia: FA Davis, 1981:284–285.
42. Walker AE, Jablon S: *A Follow-up Study of Head Wounds in World War II.* Washington: Veterans Administration, 1961.
43. Caveness WF: Onset and cessation of fits following craniocerebral trauma. *J Neurosurg* 1963; 20:570–583.
44. Salazar AM, Amin D, Vance SC, et al: Epilepsy after penetrating head injury: Anatomic correlates. *Neurology* 1985; 35 (Suppl 1):230.
45. Temkin NR, Dikmen SS, Wilensky AJ, et al: A randomized double-blind study of phenytoin for prevention of post-traumatic seizures. *N Engl J Med* 1990; 323:497–502.
46. De Santis A, Sganzerla E, Spagnoli D, et al: Risk factors for late posttraumatic epilepsy. *Acta Neurochir* 1992; Suppl 55:64–67.
47. Feeney DM, Walker AE: The prediction of post-traumatic epilepsy: A mathematical approach. *Arch Neurol* 1979; 36:8–12.
48. Weiss GH, Feeney DM, Caveness WF, et al: Prognostic factors for the occurrence of post-traumatic epilepsy. *Arch Neurol* 1983; 40:7–10.
49. Jennett WB: *Epilepsy After Blunt Head Injuries.* London: Heinemann, 1962.
50. Annegers JF, Shirts SB, Hauser WA, Kurland LT: Risk of recurrence after an initial unprovoked seizure. *Epilepsia* 1986; 27:43–50.
51. Weiss GH, Caveness WF: Prognostic factors in the persistence of post-traumatic epilepsy. *J Neurosurg* 1972; 37:164–169.
52. Working Group on Status Epilepticus: Treatment of convulsive status epilepticus: Recommendations of the Epilepsy Foundation of America's working group on status epilepticus. *JAMA* 1993; 270:854–859.
53. Laidlaw J, Richens A, Oxley J: *A Textbook of Epilepsy*, 3d ed. Edinburgh: Churchill-Livingstone, 1988:452–456.
54. Hauser WA, Hesdorffer DC: *Epilepsy: Frequency, Causes and Consequences.* Epilepsy Foundation of America. New York: Demos, 1990.
55. Rapport RL, Penry JK: Pharmacologic prophylaxis of posttraumatic epilepsy: A review. *Epilepsia* 1972; 13:295–304.
56. Wohns RNW, Wyler AR: Prophylactic phenytoin in severe head injuries. *J Neurosurg* 1979; 51:507–509.
57. Servit Z, Musil F: Prophylactic treatment of post-traumatic epilepsy: Results of a long term followup in Czechoslovakia. *Epilepsia* 1981; 22:315–320.
58. Murri L, Arrigo A, Bonuccelli U, et al: Phenobarbital in the prophylaxis of late posttraumatic seizures. *Ital J Neurol Sci* 1992; 13:755–760.
59. Price DJ: The efficiency of sodium valproate as the only anticonvulsant administered to neurosurgical patients, in Parsonage MJ, Caldwell ADS (eds): *The Place of Sodium Valproate in the Treatment of Epilepsy.* London: The Royal Society of Medicine International Congress and Symposium Series, Number 30, 1980:23–34.
60. Penry JK, White BG, Brackett CE: A controlled prospective study of the pharmacological prophylaxis of posttraumatic epilepsy. *Neurology* 1979; 29:600–601.
61. McQueen JK, Blackwood DHR, Harris, P, et al: Low risk of late post-traumatic seizures following severe head injury: Implication for clinical trials of prophylaxis. *J Neurol Neurosurg Psychiatry* 1983; 46:899–904.
62. Young B, Rapp RP, Norton JA, et al: Failure of prophylactically administered phenytoin to prevent early posttraumatic seizures. *J Neurosurg* 1983; 58:231–235.
63. Young B, Rapp RP, Norton JA, et al: Failure of prophylactically administered phenytoin to prevent late posttraumatic seizures. *J Neurosurg* 1983; 58:236–241.
64. Glötzner FL, Haubitz I, Miltner F, et al: Anfallsprophylaxe mit carbamazepin nach schweren schädelhirnverletzungen. *Neurochirurgia* 1983; 26:66–79.
65. Temkin NR, Dikmen SS, Winn HR: Posttraumatic seizures. *Neurosurg Clin North Am* 1991; 2:425–435.
66. Pechadre JC, Lauxerois M, Colnet G, et al: Prevention de l'epilepsie post-traumatique tardive par phenytoine dans les traumatismes craniens graves: Suivi durant 2 ans. *Presse Med* 1991; 20:841–845.
67. Manaka S: Cooperative prospective study on posttraumatic epilepsy: Risk factors and the effect of prophylactic anticonvulsant. *Jpn J Psychiatry Neurol* 1992; 46:311–315.
68. Dikmen SS, Temkin NR, Miller B, et al: Neurobehavioral effects of phenytoin prophylaxis of posttraumatic seizures. *JAMA* 1991; 265:1271–1277.
69. North JB, Penhall RK, Hanieh A, et al: Phenytoin and

postoperative epilepsy: A double-blind study. *J Neurosurg* 1983; 58:672–677.

70. Foy PM, Chadwick DW, Rajgopalan N, et al: Do prophylactic anticonvulsant drugs alter the pattern of seizures after craniotomy? *J Neurol Neurosurg Psychiatry* 1992; 55:753–757.

71. Silver JM, Shin C, McNamara JO: Antiepileptogenic effects of conventional anticonvulsants in the kindling model of epilepsy. *Ann Neurol* 1991; 29:356–363.

72. Chan PH, Longar S, Fishman RA: Protective effects of liposome-entrapped superoxide dismutase on post traumatic brain edema. *Ann Neurol* 1987; 21:540–547.

CHAPTER 43

TRAUMA TO THE CRANIAL NERVES AND BRAINSTEM

Sophia M. Chung
Glen A. Fenton
John G. Schmidt
John B. Selhorst

SYNOPSIS

Studies have reported that the incidence of cranial nerve injury among head trauma patients ranges between 5 and 23 percent.[1] *The same studies suggest that the first, seventh, and eighth cranial nerves are the ones most often injured and that the lower cranial nerves are the least frequently affected. Cranial nerve injuries occur when the forces of impact are absorbed by the skull and transmitted along its base. Neuroimaging studies are often unable to demonstrate the mode of injury to the cranial nerve or the adjacent bone. Therefore, the treating physician should be thoroughly familiar with the clinical manifestations of cranial neuropathies and the possible mechanisms of the injury. This requires a thorough understanding of the anatomic course of each cranial nerve along the base of the skull. This chapter describes and illustrates the pathway of each cranial nerve from its origin in the brainstem to its course through the skull (Fig. 43-1). It also outlines the common presentation and management of each cranial nerve deficit. Although they occur less frequently, injuries involving the posterior skull and primarily affecting the brainstem or cerebellum are also discussed in this chapter.*

CRANIAL NERVE INJURIES

Olfactory Nerve (Cranial Nerve I)

Injury to the olfactory nerve occurs in 5 to 10 percent of all head injuries, making this the most commonly injured cranial nerve.[2–6] In general, the presence of anosmia correlates with the severity of the injury. Sumner[4] found a loss of olfaction in nearly 20 percent of patients whose posttraumatic amnesia lasted more than 7 days. However, a loss of smell after minor trauma also occurs. Many of these patients are unaware of their hyposmia, and so detection is dependent on olfactometry.[7] Quantitative methods of assessment have been defined and are commercially available.[8] Although this usually is present immediately after the injury, a delayed onset of the loss of smell by several months or more has been observed by several authors.[9,10]

Frontal and, more often, occipital blows are the most common type of injury producing anosmia.[2,4,5] With or without fracture of the cribriform plate, these direct and contrecoup injuries produce such severe acceleration/deceleration forces that stretching or shearing of the olfactory nerve roots occurs as depicted in Fig. 43-2.[2,5,9,11] Fractures of the cribriform plate may also compress or lacerate olfactory rootlets. Alternatively, anosmia results from edema, hematoma, ischemia, or direct injury to the olfactory bulb and tract.[12–14] Many patients with anosmia experience CSF rhinorrhea from paranasal sinus fractures,[5] and this establishes anosmia as a potential risk factor for posttraumatic meningitis.[15] Parosmia, a distorted sense of smell, sometimes accompanies hyposmia and is occasionally a permanent symptom.[16] Nearly 40 percent of these patients recover from the loss of smell, and although most do so within 3 months, several years may pass for some patients. This recovery reflects dysfunction from the direct effects of trauma, such as concussion, edema, or hemorrhage, and in later stages it indicates regeneration of olfactory axons. In patients who do not recover the sense of smell, the migrating axons of the olfactory neurons in the nasal mucosa are often unable to reconnect with the olfactory bulb because of severe disruption of the lamina cribosa

Cranial Nerves & Skull Base

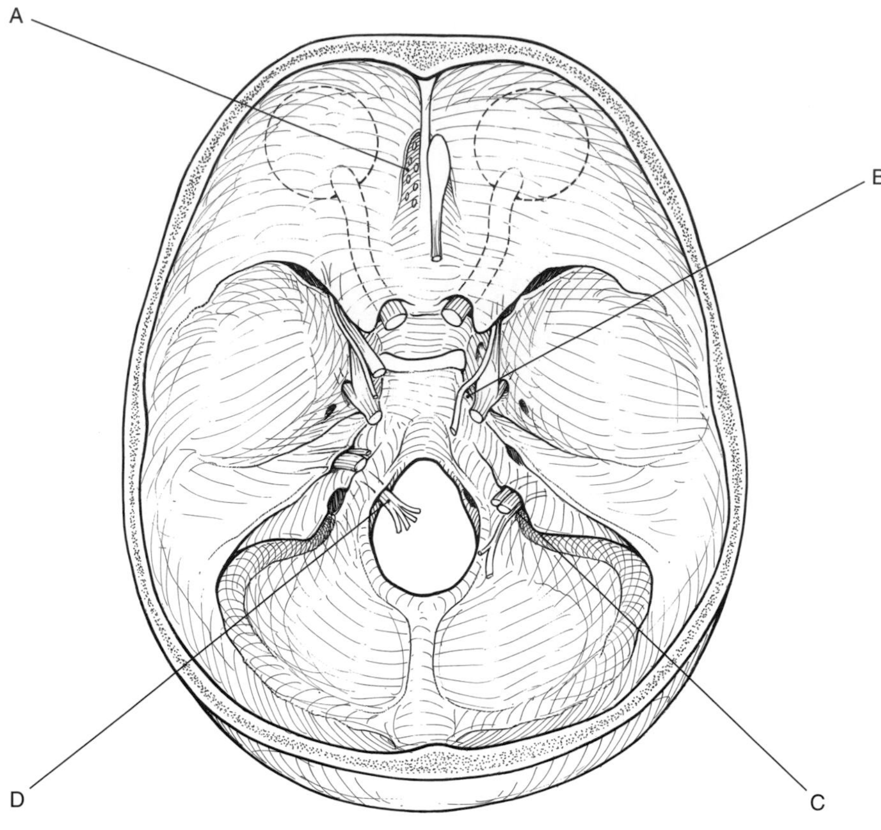

Figure 43-1. The courses of cranial nerves I through XII are shown in their subarachnoid and dural pathways and along the base of the skull. Through fenestrations of the cribriform plate (*A*), olfactory rootlets enter the intracranial cavity. The optic nerve makes a subtle S shape between the globe and the optic canal at the apex of the orbit. Omission of the third and fourth cranial nerves indicates their superior position above the sixth cranial nerve (*B*), which passes medial to the trigeminal ganglion and across the petrous apex. Below the auditory foramen, which normally contains cranial nerves VII and VIII (unlabelled), cranial nerves IX, X, and XI (*C*) enter the jugular foramen. Cranial nerve XII (*D*) is shown in the lower portion of the occipital bone as it approaches the hypoglossal canal.

Olfactory Nerve (I)

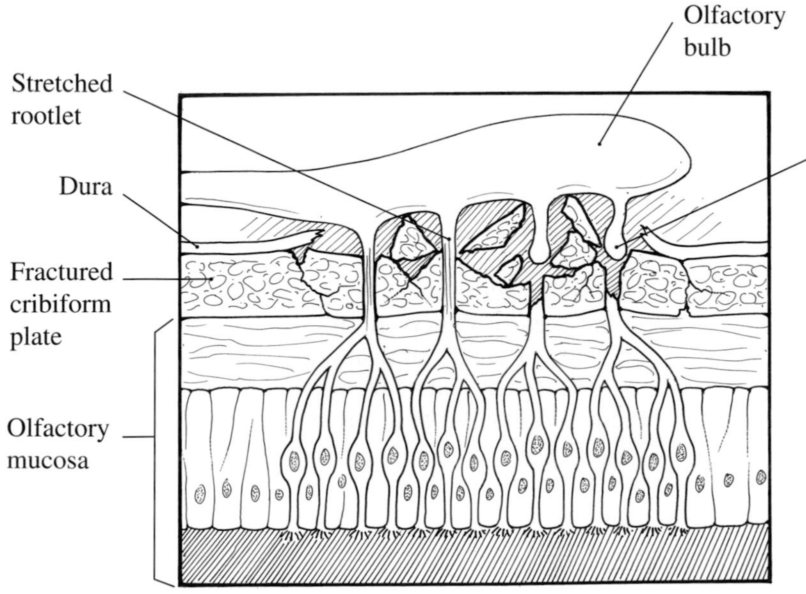

Figure 43-2. Damage to the olfactory nerve includes injury to the first-order neurons in the nasal mucosa but also occurs through stretching or shearing of the delicate unmyelinated rootlets that pass through the cribriform plate of the frontal bone.

or excessive fibrotic tissue around the fractured cribriform plate.[13] Less often, both olfactory bulbs are too damaged to allow for recovery.

Optic Nerve (Cranial Nerve II)

The optic nerve measures approximately 4.5 to 5.0 cm in length and may be divided into intraocular, intraorbital, intracanalicular, and intracranial segments. The intraocular portion is only 1 mm in length and is readily visualized with the ophthalmoscope as the optic disk. The longest segment is the 25- to 30-mm intraorbital portion, which has a slender S-shaped configuration (Fig. 43-1). This allows for mobility of the globe and prevents undue stretching by posterior orbital edema or hemorrhage. Orbital fat and ocular muscles provide additional protection for the nerve. As the nerve enters the optic canal, its dural covering becomes contiguous with the periosteum of the optic canal and orbit. The intracanalicular portion of the optic nerve measures approximately 5 to 9 mm. Here, the immobile nerve can be stretched, sheared, or contused by displacement of the brain and optic chiasm or fracture across the optic canal, making the intracanalicular segment the most susceptible to injury in closed head trauma. The optic nerve exits the canal as the 9- to 10-mm intracranial segment and unites with the contralateral optic nerve in the chiasm.

The optic nerve, the largest and perhaps the most important cranial nerve, is injured in approximately 1.6 percent of all head injuries.[3] Direct injury causes about 25 percent of traumatic optic neuropathies and results from penetrating objects, usually missiles from firearms.[1] Indirect optic nerve injury usually refers to monocular visual loss from the transmitted effects of trauma on contiguous structures. Kline and associates divided indirect optic nerve injuries into anterior and posterior categories.[17] Anterior indirect injuries are recognized by involvement of the anterior optic nerve or retina, especially when the central retinal artery is involved. Optic nerve avulsion sometimes occurs with seemingly trivial trauma to high-velocity injuries. Funduscopy reveals a deep round hole where the nerve once exited the globe. Coexisting central retinal artery involvement may result in ischemic infarction of the macula; the resulting edema highlights the normal fovea, causing it to stand out as a cherry-red spot. The mechanism of the avulsion is uncertain but probably includes anterior displacement, torque of the globe, and a sudden rise in intraocular pressure with perforation of the lamina cribrosa.[18,19] Traumatic ischemic optic neuropathy is diagnosed in patients with sudden loss of vision and a swollen papilla.[20,21] Traumatic injury to the posterior ciliary arteries, which supply the optic disk, is assumed.

In posterior indirect optic nerve injury, patients have poor visual acuity but have a normal funduscopic examination. Posterior optic nerve injuries typically occur in the setting of severe head trauma with loss of consciousness. The blow to the head is usually frontal, especially around the outer brow, but occasionally involves the ipsilateral temporal bone.[3,22,23]

The diagnosis of optic nerve injury is often difficult in patients with multisystem injuries and altered levels of consciousness. Visual acuity is frequently unobtainable or inaccurate. Pupillary examination is sometimes compromised by miosis or mydriasis. However, if the pupillomotor pathways along the oculomotor nerve are intact, examination of the pupil is essential for the early recognition of optic nerve injury. Depending on the degree of injury, the pupil on the affected side normally reacts sluggishly or is fixed, but a relative afferent pupillary defect is often demonstrable with the swinging flashlight test. That is, if a light is swung from the normal eye to the impaired eye, the pupil initially dilates rather than constricts. In alert patients, confrontation visual fields are useful, and according to Hughes,[22] inferior altitudinal defects are present in 75 percent of traumatic optic neuropathies. Although the initial funduscopic examination is normal, traces of optic nerve pallor appear within 1 to 2 weeks; however, optic atrophy is not readily apparent for 1 to 2 months. Patients with severe head trauma and any suggestion of an orbital injury require a complete ophthalmologic examination to evaluate for injuries such as a ruptured globe, vitreous hemorrhage or retinal edema, hemorrhage, and detachment.

After bedside evaluation, high-resolution computed tomography (CT) of the head and orbits in both axial and coronal planes is obtained to identify fractures of the optic canal or adjacent bones (Fig. 43-3), intraorbital foreign bodies, and compressive hematomas within the orbit, apex, or dural sheath. The incidence of optic canal fractures in posterior traumatic optic neuropathies varies from 6 to 92 percent.[22,24,25] However, a fracture is not necesary for injury to the optic nerve to occur; histological studies have shown hemorrhages within the nerve, dura, and sheath; tears of optic nerve axons; and contusion necrosis.[24,26,27] These injuries often carry a poor prognosis. Conversely, loss of vision is potentially due to conduction block from less severe structural injuries, allowing for spontaneous recovery.[22,28] In some patients, visual loss is delayed for several hours and rarely may occur weeks to months after the initial injury as a result of the development of a traumatic aneurysm or mucocele.

The treatment of indirect posterior optic nerve injuries remains controversial because of its uncertain natural history. Up to one-third of these injuries may improve spontaneously. Thus, treatment options range

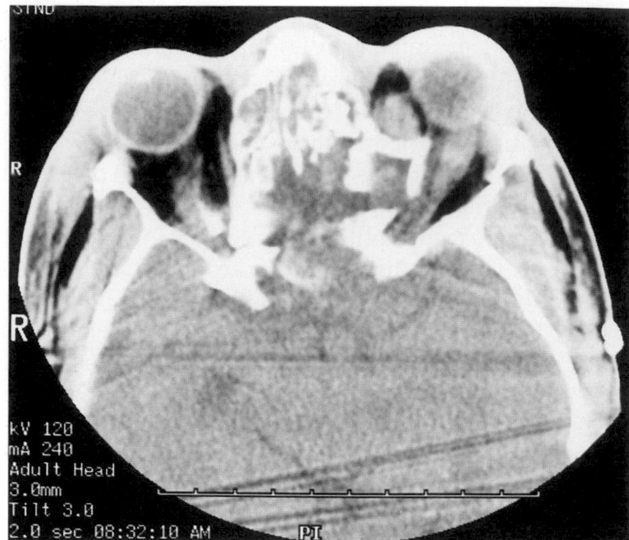

Figure 43-3. CT scanning shows multiple fractures and bone fragments in a patient who was blind in each eye. After removal of intraorbital fragments on the left, vision improved to 20/40, but it remained at no light perception after optic canal decompression on the right.

from conservative observation to megadose intravenous corticosteroids or surgical decompression. In 1982, Anderson and colleagues[29] advocated an initial dose of 0.75 mg of dexamethasone sodium phosphate per kilogram of body weight, followed by 0.33 mg/kg every 6 h for the next 24 h. Continued treatment was dependent on the patient's response. Subsequent, uncontrolled studies have claimed a benefit with similar doses of corticosteroids.[28,30–32] The proposed protective mechanisms of corticosteroids are reduction of edema, cell membrane stabilization, and decreased circulatory spasm.[33]

Surgical decompression of the optic canal is indicated when identifiable bony fragments and hematomas are present.[34] In their absence, the rationale for decompressing the canalicular segment of the optic nerve is loss of vision caused by swelling and secondary ischemia, especially indicated by progressive loss of vision. Hence, a vigorous interventional approach to anterior head and orbital injuries necessitates measuring visual acuity as early as possible and sequentially until vision is established as stable over several intervals in the first 24 to 48 h after injury. Optic nerve exploration and decompression vary, with transcranial, transorbital, transethmoidal, transsphenoidal, and endonasal-transethmoidal approaches.[25,35–37] Reports of benefits from surgical decompression are numerous[28,30,35,36,38]; the Japanese literature provides the most enthusiastic results.[25,32] Fukado[25] reported that all 400 patients undergoing decompression of the optic canal experienced visual improvement. His method of patient selection, however, is unclear. Fujitani et al.[32] described improvement after decompression in 25 percent of patients who initially had no light perception. The same authors also advocated surgery for patients who fail 3 weeks of corticosteroid therapy. A controlled, randomized clinical trial studying the natural history and the choice of proper treatment for traumatic optic neuropathy is clearly needed[17,39] to compare placebo, systemic corticosteroids, and surgical decompression by a uniform and standard approach.

Although chiasmal injuries are rare after closed head trauma, a number have been reported.[23,40–46] Often there is a history of severe head trauma to the frontal or temporal bone with loss of consciousness and multiple facial fractures. Signs of hypothalamic dysfunction, such as diabetes insipidus, are sometimes present. Hemiparesis and other cranial neuropathies are also common. As the patient's sensorium clears, visual complaints, often asymmetrical, are voiced. Then bitemporal visual field defects are found along with diminished vision in one or both eyes because of concurrent optic nerve injury. Several weeks after the injury, optic nerve pallor is apparent, especially along the nasal margin, because this portion of the optic disk head selectively serves the crossing fibers in the chiasm. The mechanism of chiasmal trauma is attributed to either separation of the chiasm by lateral opposing traction on the optic nerves or ischemic infarction. Chiasmal tears have been reproduced by forcibly separating the optic foramina[47] or mechanically stretching the chiasm.[48] Traquair and coauthors,[40] however, have proposed that interruption of the vascular supply to the chiasm best accounts for the visual impairment and concurrent hypothalamic dysfunction.

Oculomotor Nerve (Cranial Nerve III)

Injury to the oculomotor nerve presents with a spectrum of findings as a result of the complexity of its anatomy. The oculomotor nerve arises from the nuclei in the midbrain ventral to the cerebral aqueduct. Subnuclei selectively innervate individual ocular muscles. Important points for localization are that the superior recti are supplied by the contralateral subnucleus and that both levator palpebrae superioris muscles receive axons from a conjoined midline structure known as the central caudal nucleus. The fascicles of the oculomotor nerve travel ventrally through the red nucleus and cerebral peduncle into the interpeduncular fossa. The nerve then passes between the posterior cerebral and superior cerebellar arteries into the cavernous sinus. There, the nerve separates into the superior and inferior divisions and enters the orbit. The superior division innervates the superior rectus and levator palpebrae superioris, while the inferior division supplies the inferior and medial recti and the inferior oblique muscle. The inferior division also carries presynaptic parasympathetic axons to the ciliary ganglion, which, with the short ciliary nerves, supplies the sphincter pupillae and the ciliary muscle.

Caution must be exercised in overdiagnosing a third nerve palsy in a patient with orbital swelling from direct trauma and a traumatic mydriasis. In this setting, the pattern of the eye movement must conform to the third nerve, which means that orbital edema must not be so severe that it prevents full adduction. Otherwise, time must be allowed to lapse for the orbital swelling to resolve before a definitive diagnosis is made. Specific ocular signs can be of great localizing value. A nuclear lesion is identified by bilateral ptosis, a contralateral superior rectus weakness, and ipsilateral paresis of the remaining muscles supplied by the third nerve. A contralateral tremor in the presence of a third nerve paresis indicates an injury to the red nucleus, while a contralateral hemiplegia localizes the point of trauma to the cerebral peduncle.

Head trauma accounts for 8 to 16 percent of all oculomotor palsies.[49–52] Among children, acquired third nerve palsies are due to trauma in 12 to 20 percent of cases.[53,54] Oculomotor palsies often result from compression of the nerve by a temporal lobe which is swollen by contusion or hemorrhage and is herniating through the tentorial notch. Concurrent alteration in consciousness is invariably present. In such circumstances, an examiner encounters a mydriatic pupil with varying degrees of ptosis and extraocular muscle weakness. An avulsion or stretch injury of the nerve is suggested by the rapid recovery of consciousness in an otherwise complete oculomotor nerve palsy.[55]

A few weeks to months after a third nerve injury, a new pattern of eye movements sometimes appears because, with regeneration, axons may terminate in inappropriate structures. This phenomenon of aberrant regeneration includes elevation of the ptotic lid with adduction or downgaze, adduction with attempted elevation or depression, and a pupil that is poorly reactive to light but constricts during adduction.[56] The management of an incompletely resolved third nerve paresis is often difficult because of variability of presentations, the number of muscles involved, and incomitance of strabismus. Extraocular muscle surgery may be offered to achieve binocular single vision in the primary position and/or the reading position.

Trochlear Nerve (Cranial Nerve IV)

Trochlear nerve palsies are not well recognized but account for one-third of all traumatic ocular motor palsies.[57–60] The trochlear nerve's susceptibility to trauma is determined by its anatomic course. The trochlear nerve is the smallest and longest of the ocular motor nerves and is the only cranial nerve that exits the brainstem on its dorsal surface. It decussates in the anterior medullary velum, exits dorsally, and sweeps laterally around the midbrain in the free edge of the tentorium. After a sudden deceleration injury or blow to the head, the brain may move backward and impact against the bony cranium, resulting in an injury of the fourth nerve in the dorsal midbrain or in the free edge of the tentorium. In blows to the head along the midline, bilateral trochlear palsies are common and nearly always result from trauma.[57,61,62] The degree of head injury varies. Most patients have moderate to severe head trauma with loss of consciousness. However, minor head trauma without alteration of consciousness may also occasionally result in fourth nerve palsies. Fourth nerve palsies are rarely identified during the initial comatose phase following a severe head injury and are almost always diagnosed after the patient recovers consciousness.

Patients with unilateral trochlear palsies report seeing double images that are vertically or obliquely oriented to each other. Rarely, they complain that the environment slants, and others unconsciously adopt a head tilt contralateral to the paretic muscle. The symptoms may be exacerbated when reading or walking downstairs. Examination reveals a hypertropia (affected eye is higher) on the affected side that worsens in opposite gaze. Bilateral fourth nerve palsies often show smaller vertical deviations. They are identified by the presence of alternating hyperdeviations (upward deviation of one eye) in various positions of gaze, a V-pattern esotropia (visual axes converge), and excyclotorsion (external rotation of globes) of 10 or more degrees on ophthalmologic examination.

The prognosis associated with fourth nerve palsies is variable. Sydnor et al.[63] reported that 65 percent of unilateral palsies recover spontaneously, while only 25 percent of bilaterally affected persons have a satisfactory improvement. Eye patches or prisms that paste onto spectacles may be used to eliminate or lessen the symptoms. After 12 months, if there is incomplete resolution, permanent prisms or surgery to restore binocular single vision is required.

Trigeminal Nerve (Cranial Nerve V)

The trigeminal nerve is not commonly damaged in head injury. The distal branches, especially the inferior alveolar, supraorbital, and infraorbital nerves (Fig. 43-4) are much more frequently injured than is the gasserian ganglion or nerve root.[3,64] Direct facial trauma causes most distal branch injuries, whereas penetrating objects, espe-

Trigeminal Nerve (V)

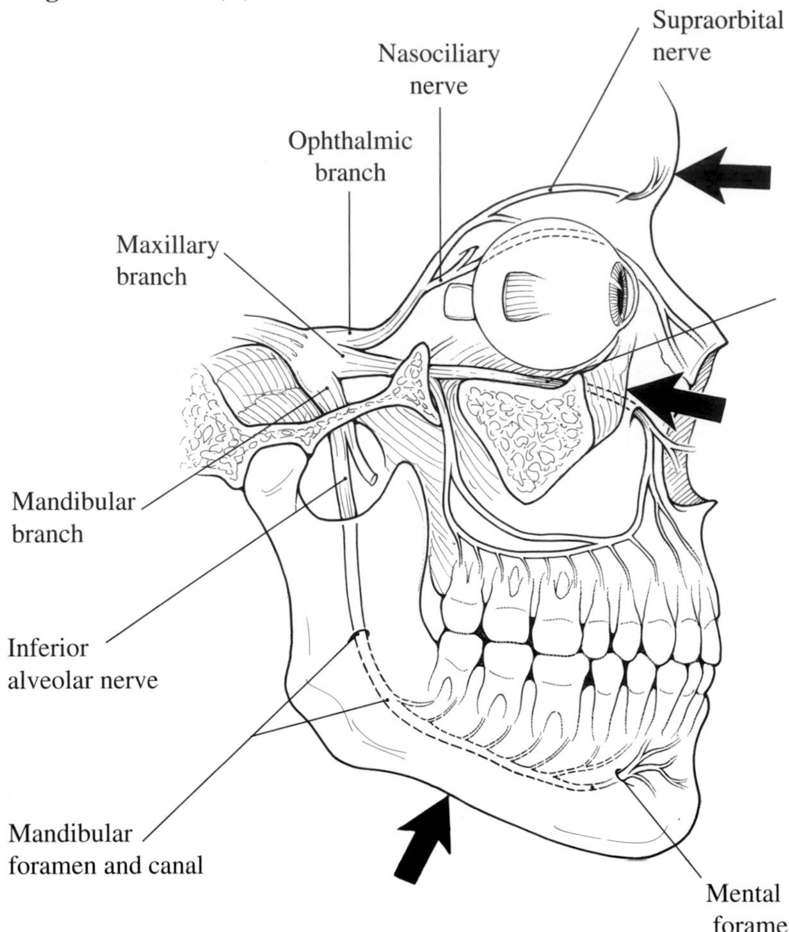

Figure 43-4. The peripheral branches, their three divisions, and the ganglion of the trigeminal nerve are depicted in their course from the skin through the anterior bony structures of the face along the base of the skull. Arrows indicate bony abutments near the course of sensory nerves around which trauma is common.

cially gunshot wounds, can damage any portion of the trigeminal system.[65] Impairment of the trigeminal nerve or one of its branches also has been reported in 29 percent of traumatic carotid-cavernous sinus fistulae.[66]

The trigeminal nerve root bends over the petrous ridge as it courses toward its ganglion. Lying in close approximation to the petrous apex, the ganglion sits in a reflection of the dura known as Meckel's cave. Fractures which extend from the temporal bone to the clivus therefore sometimes injure the ganglion or root.[67] Forceful blows to the posterior third of the skull, especially the mastoid, may crush the petrous apex against the lateral edge of the dorsum sellae and in so doing damage the ganglion.[65,68] Sixteen of Jefferson and Schorstein's[65] patients suffered ganglionic injury from either penetrating or blunt injuries. The injury, which often was incomplete, involved one or more of the three sensory divisions of the trigeminal nerve. Most of these patients suffered damage to other cranial nerves as well, particularly the abducens. In addition to lasting facial anesthesia, a serious potential complication of trigeminal nerve injury is neuroparalytic keratitis, which results from the loss of corneal sensation. In patients with an impaired corneal reflex, appropriate protective steps must be taken, including lubricating drops, protective lenses, moisture chambers, and, if necessary, tarsorrhaphy, to prevent undue exposure and infection of the cornea.

Supraorbital nerve injuries were present in 45 of 1000 head-injured patients in Russell's series.[64] Most of these patients had soft tissue damage to the eyebrow, which directly injured the nerve where it enters the supraorbital notch, resulting in unilateral anesthesia of the brow and the anterior scalp. The nasociliary nerve may be injured as a result of a severe compound fracture of the frontal bone, usually with extensive comminution of the frontal and ethmoidal sinuses.[65] The resultant anesthesia involves the tip of the nose. The infraorbital nerve is damaged before it enters the foramen or within its bony canal, producing anesthesia of the cheek and upper lip. It is commonly injured in fractures of the zygomatic tripod but also may be affected by impacts around its foramen despite the overlying lower orbital ridge, which rises to protect the eye.[65,69] Trauma to the orbit is known to result in a "blowout" of the inferior orbital floor, in which case loss of sensation over the cheek occurs along with diplopia caused by contusion or entrapment of the inferior rectus muscle. Surgical intervention is indicated if ocular restriction persists, but only after orbital edema resolves. Conversely, barotrauma of the maxillary sinus is another cause of infraorbital nerve injury.[70] Clinically, injury to the infraorbital nerve is distinguished from more posterior maxillary nerve trauma by retention of sensation on the roof of the mouth.

Posterior fractures of the horizontal ramus of the mandible may injure the inferior alveolar nerve in its canal and produce anesthesia of the lower lip, chin, distal gum, and teeth. Fortunately, many jaw fractures occur anteriorly to the mandibular canal so that injury to the trunk of this nerve is infrequent. Any of these peripheral branch injuries can potentially be treated by interposing a nerve graft. However, the surgical approach is often difficult compared with the limited disability of a nerve branch injury.

Abducens Nerve (Cranial Nerve VI)

Head trauma accounts for 3 to 17 percent of sixth nerve palsies.[50,52,71,72] Moreover, the abducens nerve is the most frequently involved ocular motor nerve, being damaged in 2.7 percent of head injuries.[22] Its long intracranial route up the clivus and over the petrous ridge, along with its strong dural attachments in the cavernous sinus, explains its vulnerability to stretching and displacement by trauma. The nucleus is just lateral to the midline of the pons. Two cell populations reside in the nucleus; a group of small cells that provide axons for the medial longitudinal fasciculus innervate a subpopulation of medial rectus neurons in the contralateral third nerve nucleus, and a larger group of neurons innervate the ipsilateral lateral rectus. The axons of the latter neurons course ventrally to exit at the pontomedullary junction, ascend in the prepontine cistern to the petrous bone, and enter Dorello's canal by piercing the dura. Traveling through the inferior cavernous sinus, the sixth nerve is lateral to the internal carotid artery and medial to the trigeminal ganglion (Fig. 43-1). The nerve then enters the orbit via the superior orbital fissure.

Schneider and Johnson[73] suggested that a "severe upward thrust from the base of the skull impact(s) [sic] the sixth nerve against the rather thin and rigid petrosphenoidal ligament, accounting [sic] for injury to the sixth nerve." However, Arias[74] proposed that the rigid dural hole and petrous ridge are the sites of nerve contusion or avulsion. Thus, either mode of injury may account for stretch or tear injuries to the nerve and lead to its dysfunction (Fig. 43-5).

A patient with a sixth nerve injury presents with variable degrees of consciousness and typically complains of binocular horizontal diplopia greater at distance and lesser for fixation on near objects. Testing of extraocular movements demonstrates a primary position esotropia (the visual axes converge) and limitation of abduction (Fig. 43-6). Resolution may be complete or incomplete. Occlusion therapy to eliminate diplopia, prisms to achieve binocular single vision in primary position, and botulinum therapy for the antagonist medial rectus to restore the primary position in persisting esotropia are used to alleviate troublesome symptoms of double images. Surgery is offered only after an observation period of 6 to 12 months to allow sufficient time for

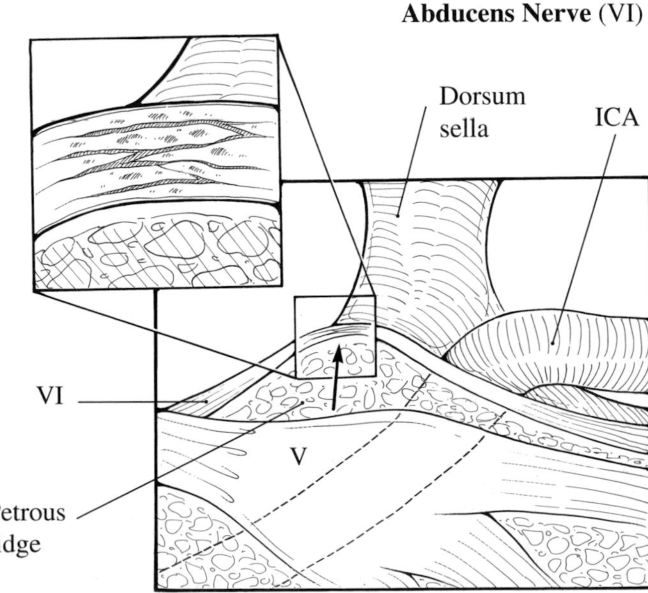

Figure 43-5. An attenuated sixth nerve is shown as it ascends over the clivus, turns anteriorly at the apex of the petrous ridge, and runs laterally to the internal carotid artery (ICA). In the inset, an enlargement of the thinned nerve reveals stretched and separated axons in which pectechial hemorrhages have occurred.

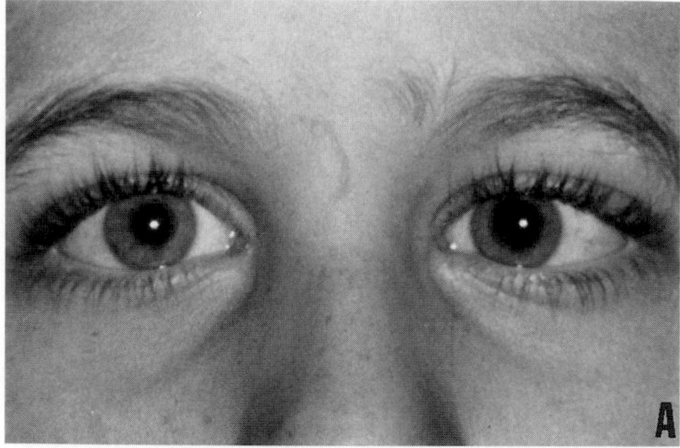

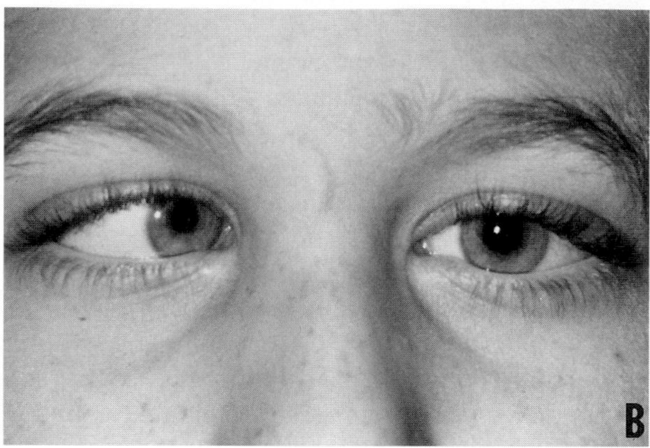

Figure 43-6. A 10-year-old child sustained a left orbital apex injury, resulting in a traumatic optic neuropathy, a third nerve paresis (*A*: shows the mydriatic pupil, primary position), and a sixth nerve palsy (*B*: left gaze reveals the left lateral rectus palsy). Without medical or surgical therapy, the vision in the left eye improved from light perception to 20/25 and the ocular muscle dysfunction resolved completely.

maximal spontaneous recovery. For mild to moderate degrees of paralysis, a resection of the affected lateral rectus combined with a recession of the antagonist medial rectus may be offered. Severe degrees of paralysis require transposition of the superior and inferior recti to the lateral rectus.

Combined Traumatic Ocular Palsies: Carotid-Cavernous Fistulae

Combined traumatic ocular motor injuries are found particularly in carotid-cavernous (C-C) sinus fistulae. These are abnormal communications between the intracavernous portion of the internal carotid artery or its branches and the cavernous sinus. The fistulae result in arterialized blood under high pressure flowing directly into a low-pressure venous system, producing exophthalmos, ophthalmoplegia, conjunctival hyperemia, chemosis, pain, and a cephalic bruit (Fig. 43-7). Although C-C fistulae can occur spontaneously, especially among the elderly, trauma accounts for a large majority of them. Most of these patients are young men who are in good health but have sustained blunt trauma to the head. Often, there is a coexisting basilar skull fracture. Penetrating injury occasionally causes a C-C fistula.

C-C fistulae are rarely life-threatening, but they frequently compromise visual function. The signs and symptoms can develop dramatically over several hours but, somewhat surprisingly, typically appear weeks to months after the initial head injury. The heightened retrograde pressure in the superior ophthalmic vein causes hyperemia and swelling (chemosis) of the conjunctiva, which are often the initial manifestations of a C-C fistula. Proptosis ranges typically from 3 to 10 mm, but as much as 16 mm has been reported.[75] Seventy-five percent of these patients complain of hearing a "swishing" noise. Typically, a thrill is palpable over the

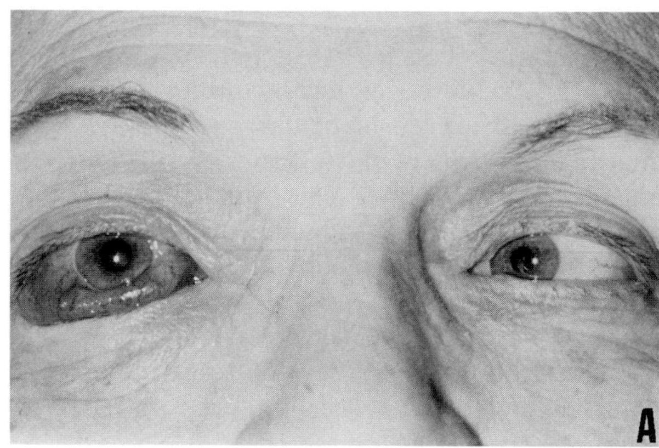

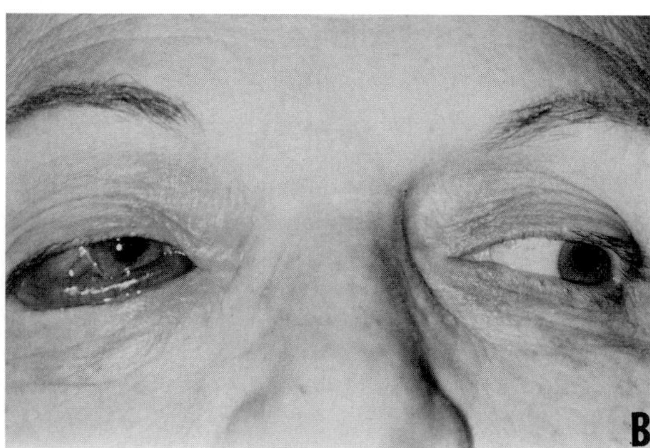

Figure 43-7. A 67-year-old woman sustained a head injury several months before developing diplopia, proptosis, chemosis, and conjunctival hyperemia. An audible bruit indicated a cavernous sinus fistula. Right (*A*) and left (*B*) gaze show lateral and medial rectus palsy caused by compression of the sixth and third cranial nerves.

orbit, and a bruit is audible by auscultation. Retroorbital pain or ipsilateral headache is common and often necessitates medicinal relief. Diplopia results from intraorbital edema that restricts ocular movements and from compression of the ocular nerves by the high pressure of the arterialized cavernous sinus. The sixth nerve is more vulnerable because it runs within the sinus itself, while the third and fourth cranial nerves course in its lateral dural reflection.

Visual loss results from corneal exposure, ocular hypoxia, and changes in the retinal circulation. The fundus may develop signs of venous stasis retinopathy: dilated retinal veins, widespread hemorrhages, disk edema, and retinal edema. Severe orbital congestion and highly elevated intraocular pressure contribute to occlusion of the central retinal artery or vein, with a devastating loss of vision.

Diagnosis is readily made by the clinical findings. Ancillary studies such as orbital ultrasonography demonstrate a dilated superior ophthalmic vein (SOV) and symmetrically engorged extraocular muscles.[76] Both are evident by contrast-enhanced CT and magnetic resonance imaging (MRI).[77,78] Bulging of the lateral wall of the cavernous sinus is also sometimes identified. However, the definitive study in such patients is selective carotid angiography with magnification and subtraction techniques.[79] Most fistulae arise from the horizontal intracavernous portion of the internal carotid artery or from the junction of the horizontal and ascending segments of the internal carotid artery.[80]

Spontaneous closures are sometimes induced by temporarily raising venous pressure with manual compression of the jugular vein.[75,81] More often, however, traumatic fistulae require therapeutic intervention. Carotid ligation and trapping procedures have generally been replaced by catheter-directed embolization of the fistula.[80–82] A detachable balloon is typically passed transarterially via the femoral artery and threaded into the internal carotid artery, where it is inflated and disengaged from the catheter. The internal carotid artery is preserved, and successful closure is attained in over 80 percent of these patients. Complications, however, may arise from balloon deflation or incomplete deflation with pseudoaneurysmal formation and migration of the catheter tip with inadvertent occlusion of the internal carotid artery. In one reported series, 20 percent of patients suffered a transient oculomotor nerve palsy in the hours after treatment and 3 percent suffered permanent neurological complications such as cerebral infarction and intracranial hemorrhage.[80] Alternative means of inducing thrombosis of the cavernous sinus in high-flow fistulae include the use of cotton, Gelfoam, oxidized cellulose, and thrombogenic wire.[83,84] These materials are placed in the cavernous sinus transdurally, require craniotomy, and are not currently used in most centers.

Facial Nerve (Cranial Nerve VII)

The facial nerve is the second most commonly damaged cranial nerve in head-injured patients and the most commonly damaged motor cranial nerve. It is affected in 1 to 3 percent of patients who sustain a head trauma.[3,85,86] A rising incidence is associated with increasing motorized transportation (i.e., automobile, motorcycle, airplane). Facial nerve injury results from either blunt or penetrating trauma to the petrous part of the temporal bone. The majority of intracranial facial nerve injuries result from blunt trauma received in automobile and motorcycle accidents. Facial palsy appears immediately or can be delayed in onset. Weakness of the facial muscles is partial or complete, unilateral or bilateral. Penetrating injuries such as gunshot wounds are less common, although, unfortunately, their incidence in the United States is increasing.[87] Cases of traumatic facial palsy are nearly always accompanied by fracture of the temporal bone. Conversely, among temporal bone fractures, 25 to 50 percent have associated facial paralysis.[85,88] Petrous bone fractures are divided into three types: longitudinal, transverse, and mixed (oblique). Longitudinal fractures are produced by a blow to the temporoparietal area. The fracture line is along the long or horizontal axis of the petrous bone and tends to involve the nerve in its perigeniculate region (Fig. 43-8). These fractures are the most common type, accounting for about 70 to 80 percent of all petrous temporal fractures.[89] The incidence of facial paresis in these fractures is only 15 percent.[90] Facial nerve dysfunction can be caused by intraneural hematoma (40 to 50 percent), nerve disruption (9 to 26 percent), contusion (36 percent), or an impinging bony fragment (17 to 45 percent).[91–93] When facial weakness is delayed with this type of fracture, as is often the case, the prognosis is more favorable.[94,95] Because the auditory nerve also courses with the facial nerve in the petrous portion of the bone, conductive hearing loss frequently occurs.

Transverse fractures are less common, accounting for 20 percent of all temporal bone fractures. However, the facial nerve is affected in about half these fractures.[89] Blows to the frontal or occipital area are usually reported,[96,97] with a greater injury being necessary to affect the temporal bone. Consequently, these patients have more severe brain damage and remain unconscious for longer periods.[98] The fracture line is perpendicular to the longitudinal axis of the petrous bone so that the horizontal section of the facial nerve is affected. Facial paralysis is most often immediate and complete,[97] reflecting the greater tendency for this type of injury to cause nerve transection or laceration by bony fragments.[96,99] Rarely, the facial nerve root is avulsed from its exit from the brainstem. Loss of hearing and labyrinthine function is very common and frequently perma-

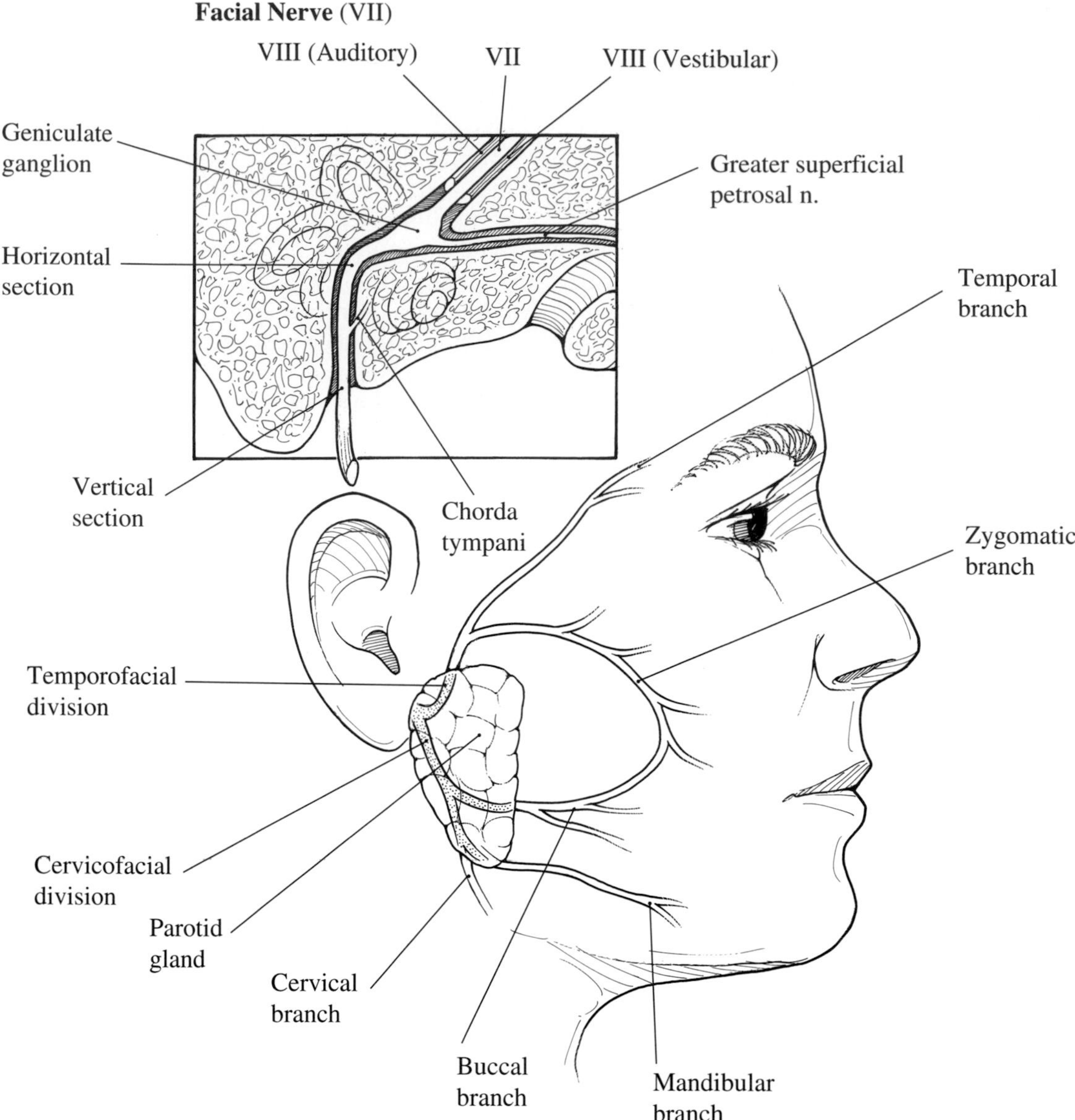

Figure 43-8. The facial nerve exits from the stylomastoid foramen and divides into two trunks which anastomose in the parotid plexus. The inset shows the relationship of the geniculate ganglion to the horizontal and vertical segments of the facial nerve and its branches. It also depicts the close relationship to the auditory and the vestibular portion of the eighth cranial nerve in the internal auditory canal.

nent. The prognosis for spontaneous recovery is much worse than in longitudinal fractures.

Many, if not most, patients with temporal bone fractures actually have mixed rather than distinct longitudinal or transverse fractures.[100] An experimental study which simulated automobile-related impact injuries using cadavers frequently uncovered mixed fractures.[101] High-resolution CT scanning is identifying more of these mixed complex fractures.[102]

Penetrating injuries, such as gunshot wounds, to the temporal bone are an uncommon but sadly increasing cause of traumatic facial paralysis. They account for 6 percent of temporal bone fractures[94] and 2 percent of facial nerve injuries.[87] In civilian life, most gunshot injuries are caused by handguns which propel relatively low-velocity missiles. The most common missile trajectory involves facial entrance below the orbit, but postauricular entry sites also occur.[103] As a result of the low missile velocity, the bullet often lodges in the petrous bone and affects the facial nerve anywhere along its course. Treatment is individualized, depending on the mechanism and site of injury, and consists of decompression or anastomosis with or without graft interposition.

Facial weakness on initial presentation usually indicates a direct nerve injury which is less likely to resolve spontaneously. Facial trauma and edema, however, sometimes obscure identification of facial weakness. Nonetheless, recognition of the delayed onset of a facial nerve palsy is important because its recovery is complete in up to 94 percent of patients.[104] Topographic assessment is used to determine the site of nerve injury along its bony pathway through the internal auditory canal, inner ear, and facial canal. Weakness of the upper and lower half of the face indicates injury of the facial nerve between its nucleus in the pons and its division into multiple branches behind the parotid gland. At the geniculate ganglion, the greater superficial petrosal nerve departs to supply the lacrimal gland. Lesions at or proximal to the ganglion impair lacrimation, which is determined by applying litmus paper to the conjunctiva to quantitate the amount of tearing (Schirmer's test). The nerve to the stapedius muscle departs from the facial nerve in the facial canal. Its injury results in a sensitivity to sounds (hyperacusis) or a failure in the stapedial reflex by impedance testing. The latter is not possible if hearing is impaired. The chorda tympani also exits the facial canal and allows the perception of taste on the anterior two-thirds of the tongue. Taste is determined by applying various chemicals to the tongue or by using an electrical gustometer.

High-resolution CT scanning provides an excellent means for identifying small fractures. Hence, it is indicated in all patients with a traumatic facial palsy to delineate the site and extent of petrous bone damage.[100,102,105] MRI with gadolinium enhancement is also useful for evaluating soft tissue injury,[106] but its advantages over CT scanning in this setting have not been demonstrated.

Methods of assessing facial nerve function and recovery assist in selecting patients for surgical intervention. Salivary flow studies are accurate but labor-intensive, limiting their regular use.[98] Various neurophysiological methods have been described, including the nerve excitability test and electroneuronography. Electrical stimulation of the proximal, injured facial nerve is compared with that of the unaffected nerve. The strength of the stimulus needed to elicit contraction of the denervated muscles is normal for the first 3 to 4 days after injury, as excitability is maintained in nerves distal to a severed nerve for a short time.[107] Subsequently, wallerian degeneration is indicated by a difference in current stimulation thresholds of at least 3.5 mA between the normal and affected nerves.[96] Alternatively, as an indication of recovery, electroneuronography utilizes maximal stimulation to achieve at least 10 percent of the amplitude of compound muscle action potentials compared with normals. Electromyography of facial muscles, showing signs of reinnervation, is useful 2 to 3 weeks after injury to identify ongoing recovery and a favorable outcome.

A great deal of controversy exists regarding the selection and timing of patients who require surgical intervention for recovery.[86–88,91–93,95,97,98,107–112] Pertinent is Turner's report[104] of a nonsurgical approach in which 85 percent of facial nerve injuries completely recovered; in patients with a delayed onset, recovery was complete in 94 percent. Thus, the majority of patients do not require surgical treatment. Patients with incomplete paralysis routinely recover full facial motility without intervention.[108] In patients with complete paralysis, most authors base treatment decisions on early versus delayed onset, blunt versus penetrating injury, and the results of electrical tests. Since recovery continues up to 18 months after injury, the benefit of surgical intervention is difficult to show.

The following are guidelines for surgical exploration and decompression of the facial nerves. In patients with penetrating injury and immediate complete paralysis, intervention is justifiable. The timing of operation varies. McKennan and Chole[109] debride the wound immediately, but other authors advocate observation with antibiotic treatment and surgical intervention 21 days after an injury if severe nerve degeneration is supported by electrical studies.[103,113] The latter approach is also advocated in patients with nonpenetrating injuries.[95,114] Injuries that show adequate nerve functioning on repeated electrical testing are not explored unless there is absolutely no evidence of recovery by 2 to 3 months after the injury.[97] McCabe[115] has proposed that the timing of surgery should be at the height of axonal regeneration, which occurs 21 days after injury. Experimental studies have shown better results when grafting is performed early but also have confirmed previously held notions that benefit follows from surgery delayed as long as several months.[116,117] The procedures used are discussed in Chap. 17.

For all patients with facial paralysis, frequent application of artificial tears during the day and an ointment at night is advocated to reduce the discomfort of corneal drying from inadequate tear secretion or exposure from a weakened orbicularis oculi. If symptoms of a keratitis persist, a temporary tarsorrhaphy is indicated and is effective in providing relief.

Extracranial Facial Nerve Injury

The facial nerve also can be injured at any point after its exit from the temporal bone at the stylomastoid foramen. Causes include lacerations, stab wounds, gunshots, soft tissue avulsion, and contusion.[114,118,119] Because of the rich anastomotic crossover as the nerve traverses the parotid gland, many incomplete injuries do not require treatment. Furthermore, nerve contusion resulting from blunt injury usually recovers spontaneously. However, disruption of the main trunk or either of its divisions (temporofacial and cervicofacial) results in significant impairment and should be repaired. The temporal division especially requires repair because of the need to protect the cornea from eyelid weakness. Likewise, marginal mandibular branch injuries are usually repaired to prevent troublesome drooling resulting from lower lip weakness.

Repair should be undertaken as soon as possible, optimally at the time of closure of the soft tissue defect.[114] If primary repair is not possible in the first 3 days, the optimal time for repair may be at 21 days after injury because of the dynamics of axonal regeneration.[96] When repair must be delayed, the nerve stumps should be tagged with metal clips or colored nonabsorbable sutures at the time of presentation so that they can be easily identified later.

Direct end-to-end anastomotic repair affords the greatest likelihood of full recovery as long as it is accomplished without tension on the nerve. Mobilization of the intratemporal portion of the facial nerve affords 2 to 3 extra mm of length, if necessary. Injuries which result in the loss of longer nerve segments require interpositional nerve grafting.[96,114] The quality of recovery is best if the lesion is singular and distal and is repaired within 21 days.

Acoustic Nerve (Cranial Nerve VIII)

Trauma to the eighth cranial nerve varies from concussion of the cochlea and semicircular ducts to fractures of the petrous bone. Labyrinthine concussion with vertigo occurs frequently even with mild head injury and in the absence of a skull fracture.[120,121] Recovery is usually complete within a few months, although vertigo or disequilibrium from gait instability is occasionally persistent. Transmission of pressure waves alone can disrupt the housing of the inner ear, also producing loss of hearing and balance. Transverse fractures extending across the internal auditory canal may result in severe hearing loss and vertigo from contusion, compression, or avulsion of the auditory and vestibular components of the eighth cranial nerve. The facial nerve is also frequently involved. Commonly, the fracture also disrupts the ossicles in the middle ear, and a hematotympanum is apparent on examination. A clue to a longitudinal fracture of the petrous segment of the temporal bone is ecchymosis over the mastoid process (Battle's sign). The tympanic membrane is sometimes lacerated, and the external auditory canal becomes misaligned because of an interdicting fracture. In lesser injuries, statoconia are dislodged from the utricle and settle on the cupola of the posterior semicircular canal, causing brief but intense vertigo with sudden changes in position of the head. Positional exercises are recommended to hasten suppression by the CNS. In distinction to positional vertigo, some patients describe the onset of an intense spinning sensation that is heralded by tinnitus and a popping sound or periaural discomfort. These symptoms vary from time to time and are typically provoked by straining because of the association of a perilymphatic fistula between the subarachnoid space and the endolymphatic duct. This vertiginous condition is remediable by surgical repair, as is conductive hearing loss from dislocation of the ossicles.

Glossopharyngeal Nerve, Vagus Nerves, and Spinal Accessory Nerves (Cranial Nerves IX, X, and XI)

Traumatic injury to cranial nerves IX, X, and XI, is infrequent and usually follows from damage during their passage through the jugular foramen (Fig. 43-9). Trauma to this trio of cranial nerves is probably underes-

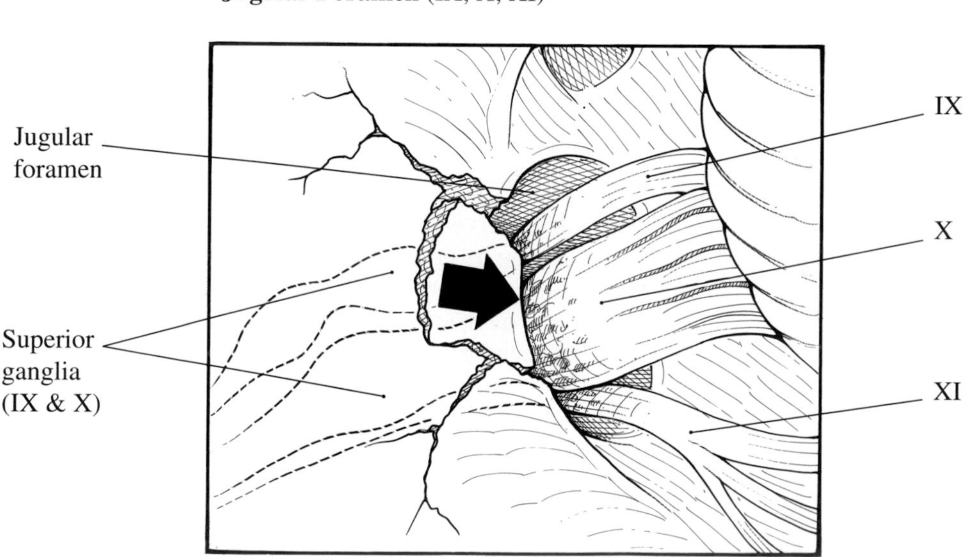

Figure 43-9. Contusion and compression by a fragment of the occipital bone at the edge of the jugular foramen impairs cranial nerves IX, X, and XI and accounts for Vernet's syndrome.

timated.[122] The resulting clinical picture is known as Vernet's syndrome of dysarthria, dysphagia, and paralysis of the trapezius and sternocleidomastoid muscles. If fractures are not detected by CT, the prognosis is favorable. In patients with this syndrome, videofluoroscopy is useful to guard against aspiration and to guide rehabilitation and diet modification.[123] Injuries of the ninth, tenth, and eleventh nerves may also occur with stab wounds, blunt trauma, and stretch injuries to the extracranial portions of these nerves.[124]

Hypoglossal Nerve (Cranial Nerve XII)

Isolated injury to the hypoglossal nerve with dysarthria and wasting of one-half of the tongue is rare.[125] A gunshot wound or trauma from neck surgery is frequently responsible. CT often reveals fractures of the occipital condyle. The prognosis is generally favorable.

Collet-Sicard syndrome

Hashimoto and associates have reported patients with unilateral lower cranial nerve injuries involving cranial nerves IX through XII.[126] Fractures of the occipital condyle or bullet wounds are usually responsible for this syndrome in trauma patients. Axial and coronal CT scanning with bone windows shows the injury to the occipital condyle. Because of the position of these lower nerves at the posterior base of the skull, management is limited to dealing with the symptoms. Unfortunately, the prognosis is poor and aspiration is common.

BRAINSTEM INJURIES

Traumatic injury to the brainstem is "primary," being direct on impact, or "secondary," resulting from complications that usually involve the cerebral hemispheres.[127] Rotational forces are a major factor in producing primary injuries such as axonal shearing, ischemic necrosis, and microhemorrhage in tegmental areas of the brainstem. Conversely, secondary injuries resulting from compression and distortions of the brainstem are more often found in paramedian areas. Axonal disconnections are principally evident in the junctions of the midbrain to the pons, the pons to the medulla, and the medulla to the cervical spinal cord.[128,129] Primary brainstem injury is clinically recognized in patients with persistent coma, decerebrate rigidity, alterations in pupillary size and reactivity, and impaired oculovestibular reflexes, especially in the absence of neuroimaging studies that reveal a compromising pathological condition in the cerebral hemispheres. The following discussion is directed toward primary and focal rather than diffuse injuries of the brainstem.

Diencephalon

The hypothalamus and pituitary are the most frequently injured portions of the diencephalon. Pathological studies show evidence of localized ischemia or hemorrhage in 42 percent of patients with fatal closed head injuries.[130] The syndrome of inappropriate antidiuretic hormone (SIADH), is a well-recognized but poorly understood complication of head injury.[131,132] The hormone is secreted in the supraoptic and paraventricular nuclei of the hypothalamus. Its hypersecretion results in expanded intravascular volume with low serum sodium, low serum osmolality, high urine sodium, and high urine osmolality. The mainstay of treatment is moderate to severe fluid restriction of 500 to 1000 ml/day. Severe anterior hypothalamic injury results in inadequate ADH secretion and diabetes insipidus (DI), a condition in which excretion of large volumes of dilute urine results in hypernatremia and high serum osmolality. The onset after trauma is immediate or delayed over several months.[133] Among patients with DI, head injury is the cause in 17 percent, and concurrent anterior pituitary dysfunction is found in 80 percent of these patients.[134,135] Replacement with vasopressin corrects the DI, which is fortunately often transient.

Midbrain, Pons, and Medulla

Trauma affecting the lower brainstem is usually mixed with trauma to the cerebral hemispheres.[136,137] Isolated substantial lower brainstem injuries are rare. One example was reported in a patient with total deafness from bilateral contusion of the inferior colliculi.[138] The deafness was permanent. Another example was a patient with midbrain tremor in whom a cavity extended from the low pons to the upper midbrain.[139] In a recent study, midbrain tremors were observed in children with lesions shown by CT in the tectum of the midbrain and the pons.[140] This homolateral movement disorder is sometimes quite dramatic and is remediable with propanolol or dopamine agonists, although it often subsides spontaneously. Most important, it is aggravated by dopamine antagonists, including metoclopramide. Pontine lesions usually result from secondary hemorrhages caused by herniation or downward displacement that tears pontine vessels upon impact.[141] Hyperextension injuries are known to stretch the long tracts between the medulla and the pons. Although trauma to the medulla is recognized by neuropathologic study, solitary medullary injuries are rarely identified clinically.

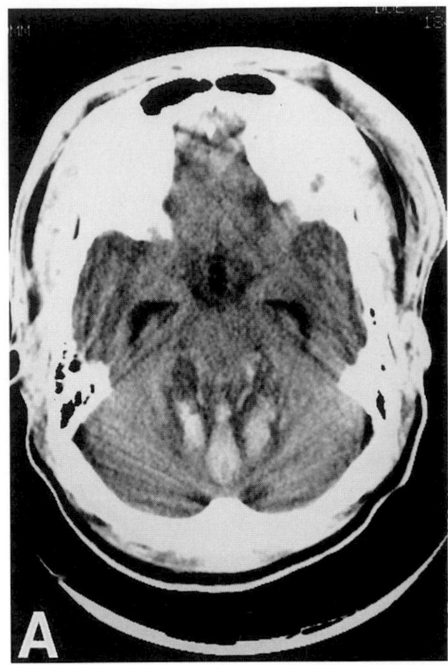

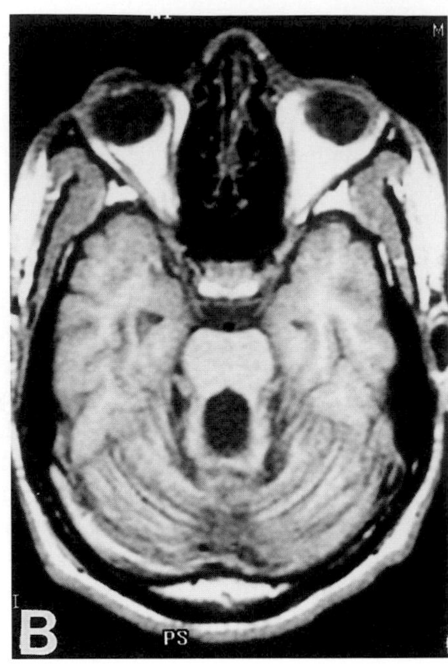

Figure 43-10. *A*. Midline hemorrhage and edema are evident in the cerebellar vermis immediately after injury. *B*. Six months later, marked dilation of the fourth ventricle is accompanied by diffuse atrophy of the cerebellar folia.

Cerebellar Injury

The cerebellum is not part of the brainstem proper, but it is on rare occasion subject to posterior fossa injury. For example, unilateral ataxia has been reported with a lesion of the superior cerebellar peduncle.[142] Cerebellar contusion, lacerations, and hematomas are usually due to occipital blows. These conditions are often fatal because of concurrent compression or direct injury to the brainstem. An example of a relatively isolated cerebellar injury is shown in Fig. 43-10. The patient was struck with a crowbar in the occiput. He retains good mentation but has severe dysarthria and rigidity and when upright, has severe projectile vomiting.

References

1. Keane JR, Baloh RW: Post-traumatic cranial neuropathies, in Evans RW (ed): *The Neurology of Trauma*. Philadelphia: Saunders, 1992:849–868.
2. Leigh AD: Defects of smell after head injury. *Lancet* 244:38–40, 1943.
3. Turner JWA: Indirect injuries of the optic nerve. *Brain* 66:140–151, 1943.
4. Sumner D: Post-traumatic anosmia. *Brain* 87:107–120, 1964.
5. Lewin W: Cerebrospinal fluid rhinorrhoea in closed head injuries. *Br J Surg* 42:1–18, 1954.
6. Hughes B: The results of injury to special parts of the brain and skull: The cranial nerves, in Rowbotham GF (ed): *Acute Injuries of the Head*. Baltimore: Williams & Wilkins, 1964:408–410.
7. Levin HS, High WM, Eisenberg HM: Impairment of olfactory recognition after closed head injury. *Brain* 108:579–591, 1985.
8. Doty RL, Shaman P, Kimmelman CP, Dann MS: University of Pennsylvania smell identification test: A rapid quantitative olfactory function test for the clinic. *Laryngoscope* 94:176–178, 1984.
9. Hagan PJ: Posttraumatic anosmia. *Arch Otolaryngol* 85:107–111, 1967.
10. Schechter PJ, Henkin R: Abnormalties of taste and smell after head trauma. *J Neurol Neurosurg Psychiatry* 37:802–810, 1974.
11. Griffith IP: Abnormalities of smell and taste. *Practitioner* 217:907–913, 1976.
12. Goland PP: Olfactometry in cases of acute head injury. *Arch Surg* 35:1173–1182, 1937.
13. Jafek BW, Eller PM, Esses BA, Moran DT: Post-traumatic anosmia. *Arch Neurol* 46:300–304, 1989.
14. Nakashima T, Kimmelman C, Snow J: Histopathology of the olfactory pathway due to ischemia. *Laryngoscope* 94:171–175, 1984.
15. Mendelow AD: Clinical examination in traumatic brain damage, in Braakman R (ed): *Handbook of Clinical Neurology*, vol. 57: *Head Injury*. Amsterdam: Elsevier, 1990:123–142.
16. Sumner D: Disturbance of the senses of smell and taste after head injuries, in Vinken PJ, Bruyn BW (eds): *Handbook of Clinical Neurology*, vol. 24: *Injuries of the Brain and Skull*, part 2. Amsterdam: Elsevier, 1976:1–25.
17. Kline LB, Morawetz RB, Swaid SN: Indirect injury of the optic nerve. *Neurosurgery* 14:756–764, 1984.
18. DeVries-Knoppert WAEJ: Evulsion of the optic nerve. *Doc Ophthalmol* 72:241–245, 1989.
19. Duke-Elder S: *System of Ophthalmology*. St. Louis: Mosby, 1972: 187–194.

20. Hedges TR, Gragouda ES: Traumatic anterior ischemic optic neuropathy. *Ann Ophthalmol* 13:625–628, 1975.
21. Wyllie AM, McLeod D, Cullen JF: Traumatic ischemic optic neuropathy. *Br J Ophthalmol* 56:851–853, 1972.
22. Hughes B: Indirect injury of the optic nerves and chiasm. *Bull Johns Hopkins Hosp* 111:98–126, 1962.
23. Noble MJ, McFadzean R: Indirect injury to the optic nerves and optic chiasm. *Neuroophthalmology* 7:341–348, 1987.
24. Edmund J, Godtfredsen E: Unilateral optic atrophy following head injury. *Acta Ophthalmol (Copenh)* 41:693–697, 1963.
25. Fukado Y: Results in 400 cases of surgical decompression of the optic nerve. *Mod Problems Ophthalmol* 14:474–481, 1975.
26. Crompton MR: Visual lesions in closed head injury. *Brain* 93:785–792, 1970.
27. Pringle JH: Monocular blindness following diffused violence to the skull: Its causation and treatment. *Br J Surg* 4:373–385, 1916.
28. Lessell S: Indirect optic nerve trauma. *Arch Ophthalmol* 107:382–386, 1989.
29. Anderson RL, Panje WR, Gross CE: Optic nerve blindness following blunt forehead trauma. *Ophthalmology* 89:445–455, 1982.
30. Spoor TC, Hartel WC, Lensink DB, Wilkinson MJ: Treatment of traumatic optic neuropathy with corticosteroids. *Am J Ophthalmol* 110:665–669, 1990.
31. Lam BL, Weingeist TA: Corticosteroid-responsive traumatic optic neuropathy. *Am J Ophthalmol* 109:99–101, 1990.
32. Fujitani T, Inoue K, Takahashi T, et al: Indirect traumatic optic neuropathy: Visual outcome of operative and nonoperative cases. *Jpn J Ophthalmol* 30:125–134, 1986.
33. Braughler JM, Hall ED: Current application of "high-dose" steroid therapy for CNS injury. *J Neurosurg* 62:806–810, 1985.
34. Guy J, Sherwood M, Day AL: Surgical treatment of progressive visual loss in traumatic optic neuropathy. *J Neurosurg* 70:799–801, 1989.
35. Joseph MP, Lessell S, Rizzo J, Momose KJ: Extracranial optic nerve decompression for traumatic optic neuropathy. *Arch Ophthalmol* 108:1091–1093, 1990.
36. Kennerdell JS, Amsbaugh GA, Myers EN: Transantral-ethmoidal decompression of optic canal fracture. *Arch Ophthalmol* 94:1040–1043, 1976.
37. Niho S, Yasuda K, Sata T, et al: Decompression of the optic canal by the transethmoidal route. *Acta Soc Ophthalmol Jpn* 64:2607–2627, 1966.
38. Spoor TC, Hartog RH: Restoration of vision after optic canal decompression. *Arch Ophthalmol* 104:804–806, 1986.
39. Miller NR: The management of traumatic optic neuropathy. *Arch Ophthalmol* 108:1086–1087, 1990.
40. Traquair HM, Dott NM, Russell WR: Traumatic lesions of the optic chiasma. *Brain* 58:398–411, 1935.
41. Savino PJ, Glaser JS, Schatz NJ: Traumatic chiasmal syndrome. *Neurology* 30:963–970, 1980.
42. Louw GJ: Traumatic bisection of the optic chiasma. *S Afr Med J* 28:971–975, 1954.
43. Anderson DL, Lloyd LA: Traumatic lesions of the optic chiasma: A report of four cases. *Can Med Assoc J* 90:110–115, 1964.
44. Wuest FC: Bitemporal hemianopsia following a traumatic lesion of the optic chiasm. *Arch Ophthalmol* 63:173–175, 1960.
45. Logan WC, Gordon DS: Traumatic lesions of the optic chiasma. *Br J Ophthalmol* 51:258–260, 1967.
46. Fisher NF, Jampolsky A, Scott AB: Traumatic bitemporal hemianopsia. *Am J Ophthalmol* 65:237–242, 1968.
47. Coppez H: Le mechanisme des lesions du chiasma dans les fractures du crane. *Arch Ophthalmol* 46:705–716, 1929.
48. Osterberg G: Traumatic bitemporal hemianopia (sagittal tearing of the optic chiasma). *Acta Ophthalmol (Copenh)* 16:466–474, 1938.
49. Rucker CW: Paralysis of the third, fourth and sixth cranial nerves. *Am J Ophthalmol* 46:787–794, 1958.
50. Rucker CW: The causes of paralysis of the third, fourth and sixth cranial nerves. *Am J Ophthalmol* 61:1293–1298, 1966.
51. Green WR, Hackett ER, Schlezinger NS: Neuro-ophthalmologic evaluation of oculomotor nerve paralysis. *Arch Ophthalmol* 72:154–167, 1964.
52. Rush JA, Younge BR: Paralysis of cranial nerve III, IV and VI: Cause and prognosis in 1000 cases. *Arch Ophthalmol* 99:76–80, 1981.
53. Miller NR: Solitary oculomotor nerve palsy in childhood. *Am J Ophthalmol* 83:106–111, 1977.
54. Harley RD: Paralytic strabismus in children: Etiologic incidence and management of the third, fourth and sixth nerve palsies. *Ophthalmology* 87:34–43, 1980.
55. Memon MY, Paine KWE: Direct injury of the oculomotor nerve in craniocerebral trauma. *J Neurosurg* 35:461–464, 1971.
56. Walsh FB: Third nerve regeneration: A clinical evaluation. *Br J Ophthalmol* 41:577–598, 1957.
57. Younge BR, Sutula F: Analysis of trochlear nerve palsies: Diagnosis, etiology and treatment. *Mayo Clin Proc* 52:11–18, 1977.
58. Khawan E, Scott AB, Jampolsky A: Acquired superior oblique palsy. *Arch Ophthalmol* 77:761–768, 1967.
59. Burger LJ, Kalvin NH, Smith JL: Acquired lesions of the fourth cranial nerve. *Brain* 93:567–574, 1970.
60. Mansour AM, Reinecke RD: Central trochlear palsy. *Surv Ophthalmol* 30:279–297, 1986.
61. Chapman LI, Urist MJ, Folk ER, Miller MT: Acquired bilateral superior oblique muscle palsy. *Arch Ophthalmol* 84:137–142, 1970.
62. Lee J, Flynn JT: Bilateral superior oblique palsies. *Br J Ophthalmol* 69:508–513, 1985.
63. Sydnor CF, Seaber JH, Buckley EG: Traumatic superior oblique palsies. *Ophthalmology* 89:134–138, 1982.
64. Russell WR: Injury to the cranial nerves and optic chiasm, in Brock S (ed): *Injuries of the Brain and Spinal Cord and Their Coverings* (4th ed). Baltimore: Williams & Wilkins, 1960:118–126.

65. Jefferson G, Schorstein J: Injuries of the trigeminal nerve, its ganglion and its divisions. *Br J Surg* 42:561–581, 1955.
66. Parker L: Neuro-ophthalmological aspects of carotid-cavernous fistula, in Smith RR, Haerer AF, Russell WF (eds): *Vascular Malformations and Fistulas of the Brain.* New York: Raven Press, 1982:181–195.
67. Ghorayeb BY, Yeakley JW, Hall JW, Jones BE: Unusual complications of temporal bone fractures. *Arch Otolaryngol Head Neck Surg* 113:749–753, 1987.
68. Summers CG, Wirtschafter JD: Bilateral trigeminal and abducens neuropathies following low velocity, crushing head injury. *J Neurosurg* 50:508–511, 1979.
69. Ungley HG, Suggit SC: Fractures of the zygomatic tripod. *Br J Surg* 32:287–299, 1944.
70. Murrison AW, Smith DJ, Francis TJR, Counter RT: Maxillary sinus barotrauma with fifth cranial nerve involvement. *J Laryngol Otol* 105:217–219, 1991.
71. Shrader EC, Schlezinger NS: Neuro-ophthalmologic evaluation of abducens nerve paralysis. *Arch Ophthalmol* 63:108–115, 1960.
72. Keane JR: Bilateral sixth nerve palsy: Analysis of 125 cases. *Arch Neurol* 33:681–683, 1976.
73. Schneider RC, Johnson FD: Bilateral traumatic abducens palsy: A mechanism of injury suggested by the study of associated cervical spine fractures. *J Neurosurg* 34:33–37, 1971.
74. Arias MJ: Bilateral traumatic abducens nerve palsy without skull fracture and with cervical spine fracture: Case report and review of the literature. *Neurosurgery* 16:232–234, 1985.
75. Kupersmith MJ, Berenstein A, Flamm E, Ransohoff J: Neuroophthalmologic abnormalities and intravascular therapy of traumatic carotid cavernous fistulas. *Ophthalmology* 93:906–912, 1986.
76. Phelps CD, Thompson HS, Ossoinig KC: The diagnosis and prognosis of atypical carotid-cavernous fistula. *Am J Ophthalmol* 93:423–436, 1982.
77. Grove AS: The dural shunt syndrome: Pathophysiology and clinical course. *Ophthalmology* 90:31–44, 1983.
78. Sergott RC, Grossman RI, Savino PJ, et al: The syndrome of paradoxical worsening of dural-cavernous sinus arteriovenous malformation. *Ophthalmology* 94:205–212, 1987.
79. Takahashi M, Nakana Y: Magnification angiography of dural carotid-cavernous sinus fistulae: With emphasis on clinical and angiographic evolution. *Neuroradiology* 19:249–256, 1980.
80. Debrun GM, Vinuela F, Fox AJ, et al: Indications for treatment and classification of 132 carotid cavernous fistulas. *Neurosurgery* 22:285–289, 1988.
81. Kwan E, Hieshima GB, Higashida RT, et al: Interventional neuroradiology in neuro-ophthalmology. *J Clin Neurol* 9:83–97, 1989.
82. Uflacker R, Lima S, Ribas G, Piske R: Carotid-cavernous fistulas: Embolization through the superior ophthalmic vein approach. *Radiology* 159:175–179, 1986.
83. Albert P, Polaina M, Trujillo F, Romero J: Direct carotid sinus approach to treatment of bilateral carotid-cavernous fistulas. *J Neurosurg* 69:942–944, 1988.
84. Mullan S: Treatment of carotid cavernous fistulas by cavernous sinus occlusion. *J Neurosurg* 50:131–144, 1979.
85. Potter JM: Facial palsy following head injury. *J Laryngol Otol* 78:654–657, 1964.
86. Adegbite AB, Khan MI, Tan L: Predicting recovery of facial nerve function following injury from a basilar skull fracture. *J Neurosurg* 75:759–762, 1991.
87. Kamerer DB: Intratemporal facial nerve injuries. *Otolaryngol Head Neck Surg* 90:612–615, 1982.
88. May M: Trauma to the facial nerve. *Otolaryngol Clin North Am* 16:661–670, 1983.
89. Goodwin WJ: Temporal bone fractures. *Otolaryngol Clin North Am* 16:651–659, 1983.
90. McCabe BF: Injuries to the facial nerve. *Laryngoscope* 82:1891–1896, 1972.
91. Fisch U: Facial paralysis in fractures of the petrous bone. *Laryngoscope* 84:2141–2154, 1974.
92. Lambert PR, Brackmann DE: Facial paralysis in longitudinal temporal bone fractures: A review of 26 cases. *Laryngoscope* 94:1022–1026, 1984.
93. Coker NJ, Kendall KA, Jenkins HA, Alford BR: Traumatic intratemporal facial nerve injury: Management rationale for preservation of function. *Otolaryngol Head Neck Surg* 97:262–269, 1987.
94. Cannon CR, Jahrsdoerfer RA: Temporal bone fractures: Review of 90 cases. *Arch Otolaryngol* 109:285–288, 1983.
95. Lindeman RC: Temporal bone trauma and facial paralysis. *Otolaryngol Clin North Am* 12:403–413, 1979.
96. Adkins WY, Osguthorpe JD: Management of trauma of the facial nerve. *Otolaryngol Clin North Am* 24:587–611, 1991.
97. Harker LA, McCabe BF: Temporal bone fractures and facial nerve injury. *Otolaryngol Clin North Am* 7:425–431, 1974.
98. Glasscock ME, Wiet RJ, Jackson CG, Dickins JRE: Rehabilitation of the face following traumatic injury to the facial nerve. *Laryngoscope* 89:1389–1404, 1979.
99. Miehlke A: Typical sites of facial-nerve lesions. *Arch Otolaryngol* 89:122–126, 1969.
100. Aguilar EA, Yeakley JW, Ghorayeb BY, et al: High resolution CT scan of temporal bone fractures: Association of facial nerve paralysis with temporal bone fractures. *Head Neck Surg* 9:162–166, 1987.
101. Travis LW, Stalnaker RL, Melvin JW: Impact trauma of the human temporal bone. *J Trauma* 17:761–766, 1977.
102. Schubiger O, Valavanis A, Stuckmann G, Antonucci F: Temporal bone fractures and their complications, examination with high resolution CT. *Neuroradiology* 28:93–99, 1986.
103. Duncan NO, Coker NJ, Jenkins HA, Canalis RF: Gunshot injuries of the temporal bone. *Otolaryngol Head Neck Surg* 94:47–55, 1986.
104. Turner JWA: Facial palsy in closed head injuries. *Lancet* 246:756–757, 1944.
105. Leslie PA, Zinreich SJ: Facial nerve imaging. *Otolaryngol Clin North Am* 24:571–585, 1991.
106. Haberkamp TJ, Harvey SA, Daniels DL: The use of gadolinium-enhanced magnetic resonance imaging to

determine lesion site in traumatic facial paralysis. *Laryngoscope* 100:1294–1300, 1990.
107. McGovern FH: Facial nerve injuries in skull fractures. *Arch Otolaryngol* 88:536–542, 1968.
108. Adour KK, Boyajian JA, Khan ZM, Schneider GS: Surgical and nonsurgical management of facial paralysis following closed head injury. *Laryngoscope* 87:380–390, 1977.
109. McKennan KX, Chole RA: Facial paralysis in temporal bone trauma. *Am J Otol* 13:167–172, 1992.
110. Rosenwasser RH, Liebman E, Jimenez DF, et al: Facial reanimation after facial nerve injury. *Neurosurgery* 29:568–574, 1991.
111. Yanagihara N: Transmastoid decompression of the facial nerve in temporal bone fracture. *Otolaryngol Head Neck Surg* 90:616–621, 1982.
112. Jongkees LBW: On peripheral facial nerve paralysis. *Arch Otolaryngol* 95:317–323, 1972.
113. Hagan WE, Tabb HG, Cox RH, Travis LW: Gunshot injury to the temporal bone: An analysis of thirty-five cases. *Laryngoscope* 89:1258–1272, 1979.
114. Coker NJ: Management of traumatic injuries to the facial nerve. *Otolaryngol Clin North Am* 24:215–227, 1991.
115. McCabe BF: Facial nerve grafting. *Plast Reconstr Surg* 45:70–75, 1970.
116. Barrs DM: Facial nerve trauma: Optimal timing for repair. *Laryngoscope* 101:835–848, 1991.
117. Brodsky L, Eviatar A, Daniller A: Post-traumatic facial nerve paralysis: Three cases of delayed temporal bone exploration with recovery. *Laryngoscope* 93:1560–1565, 1983.
118. Milford ML, Loizeaux AD: Facial paralysis secondary to mandibular fracture: Report of case. *J Oral Surg* 30:605–607, 1972.
119. Goin DW: Facial nerve paralysis secondary to mandibular fracture. *Laryngoscope* 90:1777–1785, 1980.
120. Griffiths MV: The incidence of auditory and vestibular concussion following minor head injury. *J Laryngol Otol* 93:253–265, 1979.
121. Browning GG, Swan RC, Gatehouse S: Hearing loss in minor head injury. *Arch Otolaryngol* 198:474–477, 1982.
122. Simoncelli C, Altissimi G, Frenguelli A, et al: Post-traumatic paralytic syndromes of the jugular and condylar foramina. *Rev Laryngol* 110:115–118, 1989.
123. Smoot EC, Konrad HR: Dysphagia associated with head and neck trauma: Report of a case. *J Oral Maxillofac Surg* 47:190–194, 1989.
124. Berry H, MacDonald EA, Mrazek AC: Accessory nerve palsy: A review of 23 cases. *Can J Neurol Sci* 18:337–341, 1991.
125. Delamont RS, Boyle RS: Traumatic hypoglossal nerve palsy. *Clin Exp Neurol* 26:239–241, 1989.
126. Hashimoto T, Watanabe O, Takase M, et al: Collet-Sicard syndrome after minor head injury. *Neurosurgery* 23(3):367–370, 1988.
127. Adams JH, Mitchell D, Graham DI, Doyle D: Diffuse brain damage of the immediate impact type: Its relationship to "primary brain stem" damage in head injury. *Brain* 100:484–502, 1977.
128. Crompton MR: Brain stem lesions due to closed head injury. *Lancet* 1:669–673, 1971.
129. Adams JH: Brain damage in fatal non-missile head injury in man, in (eds) PJ Vinken and GW Bruyn *Handbook of Clinical Neurology*. Amsterdam, Elsevier Science Publications, vol.13, 1990:43–63.
130. Crompton MR: Hypothalamic lesions following closed head injury. *Brain* 94:165–172, 1971.
131. Carter NW, Rector FC, Seldin DW: Hyponatremia in cerebral disease resulting from the inappropriate secretion of antidiuretic hormone. *N Engl J Med* 264:67–72, 1961.
132. Fox JL, Falik JL, Shalhoub RJ: Neurosurgical hyponatremia: The role of inappropriate antidiuresis. *J Neurosurg* 34:506–514, 1971.
133. Griffin JM, Hartley JH, Crow RW, Schatten WE: Diabetes insipidus caused by craniofacial trauma. *J Trauma* 16:979–984, 1976.
134. Moses AM, Miller M, Streeten DHP: Pathophysiologic and pharmacologic alterations in the release and action of ADH. *Metabolism* 25:697–721, 1976.
135. Barreca T, Perria C, Sannia A, et al: Evaluation of anterior pituitary function in patients with post-traumatic diabetes insipidus. *J Clin Endocrinol Metab* 51:1279–1282, 1980.
136. Ropper AH, Miller DC: Acute traumatic midbrain hemorrhage. *Ann Neurol* 18:80–86, 1985.
137. Caplan LR, Zervas NT: Survival with permanent midbrain dysfunction after surgical treatment of traumatic subdural hematoma: The clinical picture of a Duret hemorrhage? *Ann Neurol* 1:587–589, 1977.
138. Jani NN, Launeno R, Mark AS, et al: Deafness after bilateral midbrain contusion: A correlation of magnetic resonance imaging with auditory brain stem evoked responses. *Neurosurgery* 29:106–109, 1979.
139. Samie MR, Selhorst JB, Koller WC: Post-traumatic midbrain tremors. *Neurology* 40:62–66, 1990.
140. Johnson SJL, Hall DMB: Post-traumatic tremor in head-injured children. *Arch Dis Child* 67:227–228, 1992.
141. Turazzi S, Bricolo A: Acute pontine syndromes following head injury. *Lancet* 2:62–64, 1977.
142. Chester CS, Reznik BR: Ataxia after severe head injury: The pathological substrate. *Ann Neurol* 22:77–79, 1987.

CHAPTER 44

TRAUMATIC CEREBROSPINAL FLUID FISTULAS

Bruce McCormack
Paul R. Cooper

SYNOPSIS

CSF fistulas are an infrequent complication of head injury. They result most commonly from a tear of the dura and arachnoid at the base of the skull along with an associated fracture of the adjacent bony structures of the frontal or middle fossa. CSF fistulas must be diagnosed promptly because the same break in the protective covering overlying the brain that permits the escape of CSF may allow the entry of pathogenic bacteria into the CNS. While most fistulas cease with nonoperative management, those which persist must be localized accurately with appropriate imaging studies and treated aggressively with an operation. Although intracranial repair was once the preferred method of operative treatment, the extracranial approach is now favored by many authors because it avoids the morbidity of a craniotomy and is at least as effective as a craniotomy in closing a fistula.

INTRODUCTION

CSF fistulas are most commonly caused by trauma, either accidental or iatrogenic. Eighty percent are caused by accidents, and the remainder occur after surgery.[1] Traumatic CSF fistulas can be managed with either nonoperative or operative means. The most appropriate treatment depends on the size and location of the fistula and the likelihood that it will cease spontaneously without resulting in meningitis. The majority resolve without intracranial infection and may be managed with nonoperative therapy.

Surgical dural repair is a proven method of preventing intracranial infection, and if a fistula fails to stop spontaneously or with temporary CSF diversion, the site must be localized and operative repair must be performed.[2] Surgery may be indicated even if the leak resolves, because spontaneous closure by adhesions or herniations of brain may remain a source of intracranial infection weeks or years later. However, such latent leaks are difficult to identify or prove.

Traditionally, surgical repair has been performed by neurosurgeons utilizing an intracranial approach.[2–5] Recently, however, extracranial procedures performed by otolaryngologists have become more popular because of their improved success rate and reduced morbidity and mortality compared with craniotomy.[1,6–13] The development of nasal endoscopes and the accompanying endoscopic instruments has further enabled otolaryngologists to repair these defects precisely with minimal morbidity.[14–17]

This chapter will review the epidemiology, pathophysiology, diagnosis, and treatment of accidental traumatic CSF fistulas.

PATHOPHYSIOLOGY

CSF fistulas result from a break in meningeal continuity. The great majority of leaks occur at the base of the skull, where the dura adheres firmly to the bone and is likely to be lacerated with a fracture. The sinuses, which are contiguous with the base of the skull, communicate with the nasopharynx and thus permit egress of CSF. The lower incidence of CSF fistulas in children may occur because the base of the growing skull is more flexible and the paranasal sinuses are incompletely developed compared with adults.[18]

Otorrhea

Temporal bone fractures are most often parallel to the long axis of the petrous bone and pass through the external canal, middle ear, and mastoid. The ossicular chain is usually dislocated and results in moderate to severe conductive hearing loss and occasionally vertigo. A facial paralysis may result from injury to the seventh cranial nerve. This fracture usually causes tympanic membrane rupture, and if there is a dural tear, CSF enters the mastoid air cells and exits through the external ear canal. This is termed otorrhea. If the tympanic membrane remains intact, CSF escapes through the eustachian tube into the nose, a condition known as otorhinorrhea.

Transverse temporal bone fractures pass at right angles to the petrous ridge and break through the internal auditory canal or laterally through the cochlea and the medial wall of the inner ear. The cochlea and vestibular components are usually injured with complete loss of eighth nerve function. The tympanic membrane remains intact, and hemtotympanum may be observed from bleeding into the middle ear space. If the dura is torn, a pathway between the CNS and the middle ear exists. Otorhinorrhea may result, or the communication may be an occult source of meningitis because it involves the otic capsule, which contains endochondral bone and heals poorly with fibrous proliferation rather than by osteogenesis. An episode of otitis media any time after such a fracture can cause meningitis.[19]

Rhinorrhea

Frontal fractures that extend to the floor of the anterior fossa tend to involve the thin ethmoid roof, specifically the cribriform plate and crista galli, which are just medial to the ethmoid complex. The high incidence of cribriform plate "fractures" associated with rhinorrhea reported in the literature actually represents fractures of the cribriform-ethmoid junction or fractures through the ethmoid itself[20,21] (Fig. 44-1).

The posterior wall of the frontal sinus is another common fracture site through which CSF can escape via the nasofrontal duct into the nose. Middle cranial fossa fractures can cause rhinorrhea through the sphenoid sinus, particularly the lateral extensions of this sinus.[22] Fistulas from this area are difficult to localize, and many patients have been subjected to multiple surgical procedures without closure of the fistula. CSF fistulas into the sphenoid sinus are unusual after accidental trauma but are seen commonly after pituitary surgery.

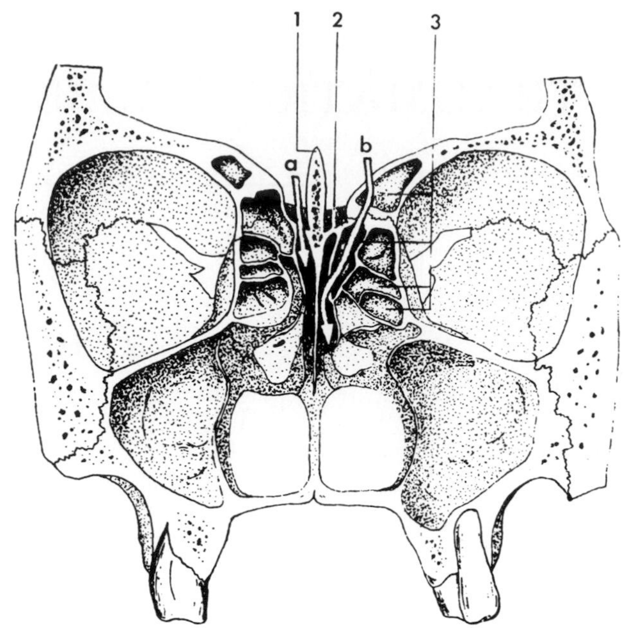

Figure 44-1. Fracture of the cribriform plate (a). Fracture through the ethmoid air cells (b), the more common fracture type. 1 = Crista galli; 2 = cribriform plate; 3 = ethmoid roof. (Reproduced with permission from Markham JW.[24]) Pneumocephalus, in Vinken PJ, Bruyn GW (eds): *Handbook of Clinical Neurology,* vol. 24: *Injuries of the Brain and Skull.* New York: American Elsevier, 1976:201–213.

If posttraumatic osseous and dural defects are small, normal healing is possible with cessation of the leak. CSF leakage may fail to resolve as a result of the presence of (1) large dural or bony defects, (2) inadequate bony support of incompetent dura, (3) impaired tissue healing (usually due to chronic disease, metabolic disorders, or nutritional deficits), and (4) raised intracranial pressure.[1]

The phenomenon of delayed traumatic CSF fistulas is less well understood. One theory of delayed fistula formation holds that a temporary seal is provided by a blood clot, inflammatory or granulation tissue, cerebral adhesions, cerebral herniations, or mucocele formation. With time, several possible mechanisms may lead to reopening of the fistula, including (1) progressive maturation and contraction of the wound, (2) devascularization with necrosis of the soft tissue or bony wound edges, and (3) resolution of the edema, inflammation, and hematoma associated with the initial injury.[1]

A fracture also may occur without a complete tear of the dura, and in time, the pulse waves of the intracranial contents allow herniation of the dura into the unhealed fracture site, eventually causing separation of the dural fibers and the CSF fistula. Additional trauma or any activity that elevates intracranial pressure, such as coughing, sneezing, and straining, as well as sinus infections may precipitate a fistula.[1]

Pneumocephalus

Two pathophysiological mechanisms have been used to explain the etiology of pneumocephalus after a head injury.[23,24] Straining, coughing, or sneezing can force air up from the nasopharynx into the cranium through a fistulous tract with a "ball-valve" mechanism that allows air to enter but not exit. Another theory holds that egress of CSF through a fistula can cause pneumocephalus in the same manner that occurs when a bottle is inverted: Air enters as a liquid escapes, rapidly filling the empty space and compensating for negative pressure. This has been termed the "inverted bottle" mechanism. Both mechanisms may be present in the same individual. Any factor that predisposes to CSF loss (e.g., CSF lumbar drainage) or to large fluctuations of CSF pressure (e.g., postural changes) across a fistula or minimizes internal tamponade may facilitate pneumocephalus.[25]

CLINICAL PRESENTATION

CSF fistulas occur in approximately 2 percent of patients with head injuries and 11 percent of patients with skull base fractures.[26–30] Motor vehicle accidents account for the majority of cases (61 percent), followed by falls (19 percent), assaults (5 percent), and, less frequently, gunshot injuries.[31] The majority of these patients are young males. The severity of the head injury has little correlation with the appearance of a fistula. CSF fistulas may occur in patients who suffer no loss of consciousness or acute neurological dysfunction.[1]

A CSF fistula occurs in 70 percent of patients within 48 h of the trauma, and 98 percent of fistulas occur within 3 months of an accident.[1,27,29,32,33] Rhinorrhea may be delayed many months or even years after injury. Early posttraumatic fistulas resolve spontaneously within a week in 70 percent of patients, and in the vast majority of patients they heal by 6 months. However, there is a 10 percent recurrence of rhinorrhea after initial spontaneous cessation.[29,47] Otorrhea almost always resolves spontaneously, and delayed otorrhea is rare.

Meningitis

Meningitis develops in 9 to 46 percent of traumatic fistulas,[28,35–39] and repeated episodes, especially pneumococcal meningitis, may be the sole presenting symptom.

Pneumocephalus

Pneumocephalus is present in approximately 30 percent of patients with a CSF fistula.[1,2,32] Other symptoms include headaches, decreased hearing, and a salty taste in the mouth.[11]

HISTORY AND PHYSICAL EXAMINATION

The initial diagnosis of a CSF fistula is established by the history. Patients who complain of a nasal discharge after a head injury should be assumed to have a CSF fistula, particularly if there is clinical evidence of a basal skull fracture. A history of gushing of fluid from the nose when a patient changes head position suggests a collection of fluid in one of the larger sinuses, particularly the frontal or sphenoid sinus. A sensation of ear fullness or hearing loss may be due to a collection of CSF in the middle ear.

The site of an anterior fossa CSF fistula sometimes can be directly visualized in the office, utilizing nasal endoscopy, which provides enhanced illumination and an angled, magnified view of the sinuses.[3,14,40]

Neurological signs may be helpful in localizing the fistula site. Anosmia indicates an injury in the anterior fossa near the olfactory area. Normal olfaction, however, does not exclude a fracture in the cribriform plate region.[8] Impaired cochlear or vestibular function or facial paralysis suggests a fracture of the temporal bone. Optic nerve injury localizes the defect in the region of the tuberculum sellae, sphenoid sinus, or posterior ethmoid sinus. Sensory loss in the first or second division of the trigeminal nerve suggests a defect in the anterior fossa or middle fossa, respectively.

Bilateral periorbital ecchymosis (raccoon sign) indicates a fracture of the anterior fossa. Ecchymosis over the mastoid process (Battle's sign) indicates a petrous bone fracture. A contour defect over the forehead suggests a frontal sinus defect. The ears should be examined carefully for blood, fluid, or air bubbles behind the tympanic membrane or laceration of the tympanic membrane with otorrhea.

When leakage is profuse and clear, the diagnosis is unmistakable. However, the nostril from which CSF drips does not necessarily indicate the site of the fistula. In one review, the site of leakage was contralateral to the nasal drip in 5 of 21 patients.[8] This can occur if there is disruption of the cribriform-ethmoid roof with respect to the midline or dislocation of the vomer from the crista galli that allows fluid that leaks from one cribriform plate to cross to the opposite nostril. Similarly, CSF from one eustachian tube may drain to the opposite nostril.

Small and intermittent fistulas may be overlooked or misinterpreted, especially if they are mixed with blood or nasal secretions. Allergic rhinitis may cause copious nasal secretions, which may be confused with CSF. If the secretions produce a clear "halo" that surrounds a central blood stain on an absorbant surface such as a handkerchief or cotton gauze, the fluid may be assumed to be CSF. Fistula drainage may be initiated or augmented by a Valsalva maneuver or by compressing both jugular veins. Rhinorrhea often can be demonstrated by flexing the neck of a patient who has moved from a supine to a sitting position. Succussion splash with head movement is pathognomonic for pneumocephalus.

Traditionally, the glucose content in a suspected nasal discharge has been used to determine whether it consists of CSF. If enough fluid that is uncontaminated by blood can be obtained, the discharge may be assumed to be CSF if it contains over 30 mg/100 ml of glucose.[41] Glucose oxidase papers are unreliable because a positive reaction occurs in 45 to 75 percent of normal nasal secretions. A negative paper strip test for glucose, however, effectively eliminates the possibility of CSF rhinorrhea.[42]

A more specific test to identify a fluid sample as CSF is by immunofixation of β_2 transferrin.[43] A high proportion of transferrin in CSF exists as a carbohydrate-free isoform, or β_2 transferrin, which is not present in tears and ear and nose exudates. β_2 transferrin detection in such fluids is indicative of CSF leakage. Only a small sample is needed (<1 ml), and no special handling or refrigeration is required.

RADIOGRAPHIC STUDIES AND FISTULA LOCALIZATION

Routine skull series may disclose an osseous defect, a fracture fragment, air-fluid levels in a sinus, or pneumocephalus. These findings help direct further diagnostic studies.

For the purpose of localizing the fracture site (and the fistula), computed tomography (CT) is better than magnetic resonance imaging (MRI) because bone is best visualized with CT. High-resolution CT scanning at 3-mm intervals can localize the site of the fistula in 50 percent of patients.[11] The plane of the scan is determined by the suspected location of the fistula. The frontal sinus is best visualized with axial CT scanning. The ethmoid-cribriform complex, sphenoid sinuses, and tegmen of the middle ear are evaluated with coronal CT scanning.

To firmly establish the presence of a fistula and better define the location for operative planning, three tracers can be injected into the subarachnoid space: (1) fluorescein, (2) indium, and (3) iopamidol. All studies are dependent on active leaking through the fistula site. Because many fistulas leak intermittently, false-negative studies are common. Maneuvers which increase intracranial pressure increase the probability of CSF leakage at the time of the study. This may be achieved by having the patient cough or strain or by placing the patient's head in a dependent position. Lumbar intrathecal infusion of artificial CSF also has been used to increase intracranial pressure and enhance the likelihood of abnormal findings on these studies.[41,44,45]

CT scanning with iopamidol cisternography is the best technique to localize active CSF fistulas and can identify the site of the fistula in 46 to 81 percent of patients[1,34,46,48] (Fig. 44-2). A baseline CT scan is performed before the infusion of subarachnoid contrast to better differentiate between small bones and thin tracks of contrast medium on the subsequent contrast study.[46]

Radionuclide cisternography is the preferred diagnostic study for evaluating questionable or intermittent fistulas.[49] Indium (In-111 DTPA) is the most frequently used radioisotope. The fistula site is identified by recovering the radionuclide on pledgets that have been strategically placed in the nose after approximately 24 h. Thus, if the patient leaks at any point during this period, activity will be detected on one of the pledgets. If the pledget in the anterior nasal roof is saturated, a fistula exists at the cribriform plate or the anterior ethmoid roof. When the pledgets placed in the posterior nasal roof and sphe-

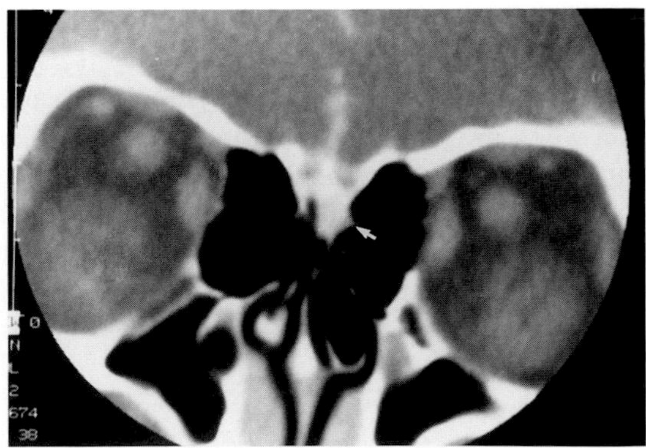

Figure 44-2. Coronal CT scanning with iopamidol cisternography identifies the fistula site (arrow) at the cribriform-ethmoid complex.

noethmoid recess are stained, the posterior ethmoid region or sphenoid sinus is involved. Radionuclide staining of a cottonoid placed on the middle meatus indicates a fistula through the frontal sinus. If the cottonoid below the posterior end of the inferior turbinate is saturated, a leak in the eustachian tube is probable.

Radionuclide cisternography has been reported to localize the fistula in approximately 50 percent of patients.[11,45] Other researchers have reported localization in less than one-third of patients and have found the study useful only if the diagnosis of CSF fistula is in doubt.[8] False localization results from oversaturation of the anatomically placed pledgets and gross nuclide staining of the tissues surrounding the actual fistulous tract.

Various intrathecal vital dyes (indigo carmine, methylene blue, and fluorescein) have been used to identify the site of a fistula. Intrathecal fluorescein is still widely used, either with cotton pledgets placed in the nose[11,13,49] or with nasal endoscopy.[50] A lumbar puncture is performed, and spinal fluid is withdrawn and mixed with 0.5 ml of 5% fluorescein, which is then slowly reinjected into the intrathecal space. After patients have been recumbent for about 30 min, the nose is examined and the cottonoid pledgets are removed. The area of cottonoid staining identifies the site of the fistula. Alternatively, nasal endoscopy is performed after intrathecal injection, and the site of the fistula is identified by the egress CSF, which appears bright yellowish-green. In one reported series, intrathecal fluorescein and cottonoid pledgets were successful in preoperatively localizing the site of the fistula in five of eight patients.[11] Complications are infrequent when fluorescein is used in appropriate doses.[14]

NONOPERATIVE MANAGEMENT

It is the authors' belief that a trial of nonoperative management is warranted in the vast majority of patients because many CSF fistulas stop spontaneously and because most patients do not develop complications. Moreover, surgery does not guarantee closure; if repair is performed via an intracranial approach, it carries the risk of a craniotomy and frequently results in the loss of olfaction.[1,8,38,45,51,60]

The authors begin treatment with a 2-week trial of bed rest in a semisitting position. Patients are cautioned against nose blowing, straining, and sneezing, which may elevate intracranial pressure. Laxatives are prescribed. A trial of CSF diversion with an indwelling lumbar catheter may be attempted if the fistula does not cease after 72 h.

Other researchers advocate immediate surgical repair for all patients with CSF fistulas because of the delayed risk of meningitis in untreated patients.[3,28,35,37] Further studies are needed on the long-term risk of intracranial infection in patients with a traumatic CSF fistula to justify operative repair for all patients. In the future, more frequent surgical intervention may be justified because early experience with nasal endoscopic surgery indicates that precise repair can be performed with minimal morbidity.[14,15,17,40]

Prophylactic Antibiotics

The use of prophylactic antibiotics for patients with a CSF fistula is controversial.[52] Early publications emphasized the importance of antibiotics to reduce the risk of meningitis on the basis of the perceived or theoretical risk of infection.[16,28]

However, there are several strong arguments against the use of prophylactic antibiotics. Antibiotics have been prescribed most often in doses that are too low to be effective, and some of the most commonly used drugs, the penicillins and cephalosporins, penetrate poorly into the subarachnoid space in the absence of meningeal inflammation. Inadequate CSF antibiotic levels may explain why patients have developed meningitis caused by pathogens that were sensitive to the prophylactic antimicrobials they were receiving.[26,30] Even when patients have received large doses of intravenous penicillin or chloramphenicol, meningitis due to sensitive pneumococci has been reported.[30] Furthermore, the optimal duration of antibiotic treatment is unclear because the theoretical risk of meningitis extends beyond the duration of the CSF leak. Finally, antibiotics eradicate the bacteria that colonize the nasopharynx, the sites from which the organisms that cause meningitis presumably originate, and cause a risk of colonization by bacteria resistant to the prophylactic antibiotic.[53,54] Infection with unusual pathogens has been reported after the routine use of prophylactic antibiotics.[47]

MacGee and coworkers[55] reported a 14 percent incidence (46 of 325 patients) of meningitis in patients with either CSF rhinorrhea or otorrhea who had received prophylactic antibiotics compared with a 5 percent incidence (4 of 77) in untreated patients; this difference was not statistically significant.[55] Based on the results of their own experience as well as a review of the literature published before 1970, these authors did not recommend antibiotic prophylaxis. Among seven more recent publications,[31,33,38,52,53,56,57,58] only two demonstrated a benefit from prophylaxis.[31,38] The reduced infection rate in one study may have been due to the benefits of early surgery, not the use of antibiotics.[38] The other study documented an increased incidence of gram-negative meningitis.[31] To date, only one prospective, randomized, double-blind placebo-controlled trial has been published.[52] Meningitis developed in none of 26 patients who received antibiotics and in 1 of 26 who received placebos. These results obviously do not support or refute the efficacy of antibiotic prophylaxis, although these authors argued against prophylaxis. All studies to date are flawed by limited numbers.

At this time, the weight of evidence does not appear to favor the routine administration of prophylactic antibiotics. Most authors agree that if antibiotics are to be used, penicillin is preferred to avoid the development of meningitis with drug-resistant organisms.[47] The controversy surrounding the role of prophylaxis will be resolved only by a prospective, double-blind randomized trial comparing placebo with an appropriate antibiotic prescribed in adequate doses in a large cohort of patients. This will probably require a multicenter trial, because no single institution is likely to see enough patients to achieve adequate statistical power.

Facial Fractures and CSF Fistulas

In the past, repair of facial fractures in patients with CSF fistulas was delayed until the fistula resolved for fear that an early operation would disrupt the fracture site and prevent spontaneous resolution of the fistula.[32] Collins has shown that early reduction of facial fractures does not adversely affect spontaneous resolution of the fistula.[58] CSF leakage may increase temporarily but more often resolves sooner or is decreased after reduction. Delayed surgery increased the risk of infection with hospital organisms, reduced the chance of primary healing of fractures, and made reconstruction more difficult because of partial healing. In addition, later reduction may cause a closed dural fistula to reopen.[59]

OPERATIVE MANAGEMENT

Indications for Operation

Patients with open wounds that communicate with the dura should have immediate surgery because of the risk of infection. Similarly, the presence of an intracranial abscess associated with a dural fistula requires prompt operative management. Patients with intracranial hemorrhages who require craniotomy should have simultaneous repair of any associated CSF fistula if it is accessible.

Extensive fractures that involve the frontal skull base are unlikely to heal on their own and should be treated with operation. CSF fistulas which are delayed in onset several days to years after the trauma are unlikely to heal spontaneously and also should be explored immediately.[1] Some authors believe that patients with pneumocephalus warrant surgery because the presence of intracranial air implies a more extensive dural tear which is less likely to close spontaneously and is more likely to result in meningitis.[1]

Indications for surgical repair in patients who are initially treated conservatively are (1) persistent or increased CSF leakage over 1 or 2 weeks, (2) persistent or enlarging pneumocephalus, and (3) meningitis. Although meningitis is an indication for repair, an operation should not be undertaken until the meningitis is adequately treated with antibiotics.

Extracranial versus Intracranial Repair

Dandy reported the first successful intracranial repair of a CSF fistula in 1926.[4] The first series of cases treated by the Grant-Dandy technique of transcranial extradural repair using fascia lata was published by Hugh Cairns in 1937.[3] In 1941, Eden reported the technique of intradural repair, which is currently the means of treatment of CSF fistula preferred by neurosurgeons.[5] In 1990, Eljamel and Foy[2] reported the largest series of traumatic CSF fistulas treated with intracranial exploration (149 patients). Initial repair was successful in 90 percent of patients; the remaining patients required an additional procedure. The operative morbidity and mortality were 24.9 percent and 1.3 percent, respectively.[2]

The intracranial approach employs uni- or bilateral frontal bone flaps. This technique has the advantage of permitting direct visualization of the dural tear and inspection and treatment of the adjacent brain injury. An intracranial approach is particularly appropriate in the presence of an open wound that communicates with the brain or in the presence of an intracranial hemorrhage that necessitates craniotomy.

However, intracranial operations have a number of disadvantages. Sphenoid sinus fistulas are approached with great difficulty and may be inaccessible to intracranial approaches because of the presence of adjacent neural and vascular structures. Exposure of the skull base and the necessity for brain retraction during intracranial procedures carry a significant risk of anosmia, postoperative intracerebral hemorrhage, and brain edema. Leech and Paterson reported 23 percent morbidity and 3 percent mortality from craniotomy.[38] A failure rate of 27 percent after initial repair and an overall failure rate of 10 percent after multiple procedures have been reported in one series.[60] Another study documented a persistent fistula in one-third of patients treated with craniotomy.[45] The main causes of surgical failure are inability to find the defect, multiple defects, and inadequate repair.[29,51]

The first extracranial approach to the repair of CSF rhinorrhea was reported in 1948 by Dohlman, who repaired a defect in the cribriform plate through a nasoorbital incision used for external ethmoid surgery.[61] Before 1948, only nasal cauterization had been used to treat this entity, with limited success.[62] In 1952, Hirsch described two patients with sphenoid sinus CSF leaks who had successful endonasal repair, using a mucosal flap from the nasal septum that was folded into the sphenoid sinus.[63] In the years that followed, Montgomery,[12,13] Calcaterra et al.,[64,65] and others[6,9,66] established the efficacy of the extracranial approach for the repair of a CSF fistula in the otolaryngology literature.

There was scant mention of the extracranial approach in the neurosurgical literature until 1985, when Hubbard et al. reported success in treating spontaneous rhinorrhea with transethmoidal and transsphenoidal repair in 15 of 17 patients (76 percent).[8] McCormack et al. subsequently reported successful repair in 36 of 37 patients (97 percent), of whom 32 (86 percent) were repaired with one procedure.[11]

Extracranial repair produces less morbidity than does the intracranial approach and does not generally result in anosmia. The extracranial approach provides the best exposure of the sphenoid, parasellar, and posterior ethmoid areas and excellent visualization of fistulas of the posterior wall of the frontal sinus, the cribriform plate, and the fovea ethmoidalis.

The major disadvantage of the extracranial approach is that one is unable to visualize adjacent posttraumatic cerebral damage. The presence of intracranial lesions can, however, be objectively documented with MRI and CT. Therefore, one can determine preoperatively those patients in whom an intracranial exploration or a combined intracranial and extracranial approach might be more appropriate. However, these patients represent a minority of the total number of patients with CSF fistulas. There are few complications specifically related to extracranial repair. These include postoperative sinusitis and cranial nerve injury; neurological morbidity is virtually nil.

Endoscopic Repair

In 1989, Papay and coworkers described closure of anterior fossa CSF fistulas in four patients with fat, muscle, and fascia lata, using a rigid fiber-optic nasal endoscope.[15] In 1990, Mattox and Kennedy successfully treated four patients with anterior fossa CSF fistulas and two patients with encephaloceles through an endoscope, using free or pedicled mucosal grafts. One patient required an additional procedure before the fistula was stopped.[14] Others have reported endoscopic closure of CSF fistulas after ethmoidectomy.[17,40]

Endoscopic repair of an anterior fossa CSF fistula has several advantages over conventional external ethmoid or transseptosphenoid procedures. An external incision is avoided, there is reduced blood loss, operating time is shorter, and morbidity is minimal. The endoscope provides improved visualization compared with the standard binocular surgical telescope and ensures accurate localization and debridement of the defect, along with precise repair. Endoscopy also can be used as an adjunct in open procedures for improved visualization. A contraindication to endoscopic repair is the inability to visualize the defect with the scope. On the basis of the success of endoscopic surgery in these small series, many surgeons believe that this will become the initial procedure of choice for closure of anterior fossa CSF fistulas in appropriate patients.[14,15]

Intracranial Hypertension

All operative procedures to repair CSF fistulas are likely to fail in the presence of untreated intracranial hypertension. In one study, 7 of 10 patients who leaked despite multiple surgical procedures were ultimately treated successfully when their abnormal CSF dynamics were corrected.[45] Therefore, all patients with a CSF fistula should be evaluated for impaired CSF absorption. This occurs commonly with a spontaneous CSF fistula but also can be seen after trauma, particularly if it is complicated by a subarachnoid hemorrhage or meningitis.

Unfortunately, evaluation for hydrocephalus is difficult, as the drainage of CSF through the fistula prevents the development of enlarged ventricles or intracranial hypertension. Ventricular reflux on cisternography is an indication of impaired CSF absorption. A shunt may also be indicated if previous repairs have failed.[45] A shunt provides a low-resistance diversion of CSF and thus facilitates spontaneous closure of a dural tear and eliminates the stress of increased intracranial pressure. The only relative contraindication to shunting is the presence of a profuse fistula because of the potential risk of tension pneumocephalus. Although this is a theoretical risk, no evidence suggests that shunting increases the risk of meningitis by suctioning bacteria through the fistula into the intracranial cavity.[45]

OPERATIVE TECHNIQUE

INTRACRANIAL TECHNIQUES OF OPERATIVE REPAIR

Intracranial repair may be used when a CSF fistula has been localized to the base of the frontal fossa, the frontal sinus, or the petrous portion of the temporal bone.

FRONTAL FOSSA

If the site of the fistula has been localized by preoperative studies to the floor of the frontal fossa and the fistula is unilateral, a unilateral frontal bone flap is fashioned on the side of the fistula. The bone flap must be as low as possible to facilitate exposure of the base of the frontal fossa and should not be compromised to avoid the frontal sinus. Mannitol is administered shortly before the scalp incision is made to maximize relaxation of the brain. If a spinal drain was previously placed to reduce the volume of the fistula, it is opened to produce further relaxation of the brain and minimize brain retraction when the frontal fossa is explored.

The dura is opened, and intradural exploration of the floor of the frontal fossa is performed. Although an extradural exploration may be done, the authors believe that an initial intradural exploration is preferred; extradural dissection of dura off the bone of the floor of the frontal fossa may produce factitious tears that cannot be distinguished from those responsible for the CSF fistula.

A systematic search for the tear is made, using the operating microscope if necessary. Particular attention is paid to areas of adherence of the undersurface of the frontal lobe to the base and to sites of fracture identified on preoperative imaging studies. When the tear is located, intradural repair may be difficult or impossible. This is frequently the case when the tear is located medially and posteriorly in the frontal fossa. In this situation, repair from an extradural approach may be more easily achieved.

If primary repair using nonabsorbable suture material is not possible, a graft of pericranium or fascia lata is placed over the site of the dural tear. This may be done from an intradural or extradural approach or both. If there is a bony defect, it should be repaired with wire mesh before dural repair is carried out. Methyl methacrylate should never be used because of the potential for bacterial contamination.

When there are bilateral fractures of the frontal base or when the site of the CSF fistula cannot be localized with imaging studies, a bicoronal scalp incision is made and a bilateral frontal bone flap is fashioned. The dura is opened as anteriorly as possible, and the most anterior portion of the sagittal sinus is doubly ligated and cut. The falx is cut, and systematic bilateral exploration of the frontal fossa is carried out as described in the preceding paragraphs. If the source of the fistula cannot be identified after intradural exploration, the floor of the frontal fossa is covered with a piece of fascia lata or pericranium. A lumbar subarachnoid catheter is inserted if the patient does not already have one, and spinal drainage is continued for 3 to 5 days to minimize the chances of a recurrent fistula.

FRONTAL SINUS

CSF rhinorrhea may result from a tear of the dura adjacent to a fracture of the posterior wall of the frontal sinus. Exploration and repair are carried out utilizing a bicoronal scalp flap and a low bilateral frontal bone flap. The site of the fracture and fistula is approached extradurally. The fractured posterior wall of the frontal sinus is resected; dural lacerations usually can be repaired primarily. If the dura has been extensively torn, a graft of pericranium or fascia lata may be necessary to achieve a watertight closure. The mucosa of the frontal sinus is exenterated, the sinus is plugged with muscle or fat, and closure is performed in routine fashion. A spinal drain is placed for 3 to 5 days.

PETROUS BONE

In patients with CSF otorrhea which has not stopped spontaneously within 7 to 10 days after injury, a bone flap is fashioned to expose the dura mater at the site of the fistula at or adjacent to the petrous bone in the middle or posterior fossa. Exploration is begun extradurally according to the principles discussed above for anterior cranial fossa fistulas.

EXTRACRANIAL TECHNIQUES OF OPERATIVE REPAIR

In the authors' opinion, extracranial surgical techniques are the preferred operative treatment for CSF fistulas in patients who do not require treatment of intracranial injuries.[11] The procedures are performed to repair fistulas from four anatomic sites: (1) frontal sinus, (2) cribriform plate and ethmoid roof, (3) sphenoid sinus, and (4) petrous bone.

After the induction of general endotracheal anesthesia, a lumbar subarachnoid catheter is placed. About 30 min before the anticipated exposure of the dural leakage site, 0.5 ml of 5% fluorescein mixed with spinal fluid is slowly injected. By the time the fistula is exposed, a discrete flow of fluorescein-stained spinal fluid will be seen exiting from the dural defect. The anesthesiologist can augment this flow by applying prolonged positive-pressure ventilation to the patient. The indwelling catheter serves a second purpose by permitting CSF drainage for 3 to 4 days after the operation, maintaining a low CSF pressure and enhancing dural healing.[11]

Regardless of the site of the fistula, a number of principles should be followed in the repair of CSF fistulas. Once a dural fistula is exposed, nonviable tissue should be debrided. Although an attempt should be made to suture the dura directly, this is not possible in the majority of patients. In these patients, the site of the dural fistula is covered with fascia, which is tucked under the bony margin. Fat, muscle, pedicled mucosal flaps, or free mucosal grafts are then placed over the area. The tissue selected depends on the site of the fistula and the method of exposure. Combinations of various tissues often are used. Whenever possible, a flap is used instead of a free graft. Fat is preferred to muscle for the obliteration of sinus cavities. Tissue adhesives are used to provide better graft adhesion and improve the initial seal during healing.

Frontal sinus

Fractures through the posterior table of the frontal sinus are repaired by the frontal osteoplastic sinusotomy technique.[7] The frontal sinus is approached through a coronal scalp or eyebrow incision. Once the bony anterior table of the frontal sinus is exposed, the superior margin of the frontal sinus is outlined, and the bony anterior table is fractured anteriorly and inferiorly, pedicled on a pericranial flap. The sinus mucosa is then exenterated. A high-speed drill is used to ensure complete removal of the mucosa and remove the entire cortical lining of the frontal sinus to obtain an adequate blood supply for an adipose implant (Fig. 44-3). The sinus is then explored, and the site of the CSF fistula is identified. The bony margins of a fracture or dehiscent posterior table may be widened, and comminuted free bone fragments that surround a large fistula are removed. Hairline fractures are left undisturbed. The dural tear is exposed by resecting bone around the fracture site. The fistula site is then repaired as outlined previously. The sinus is obliterated with abdominal fat, which has the advan-

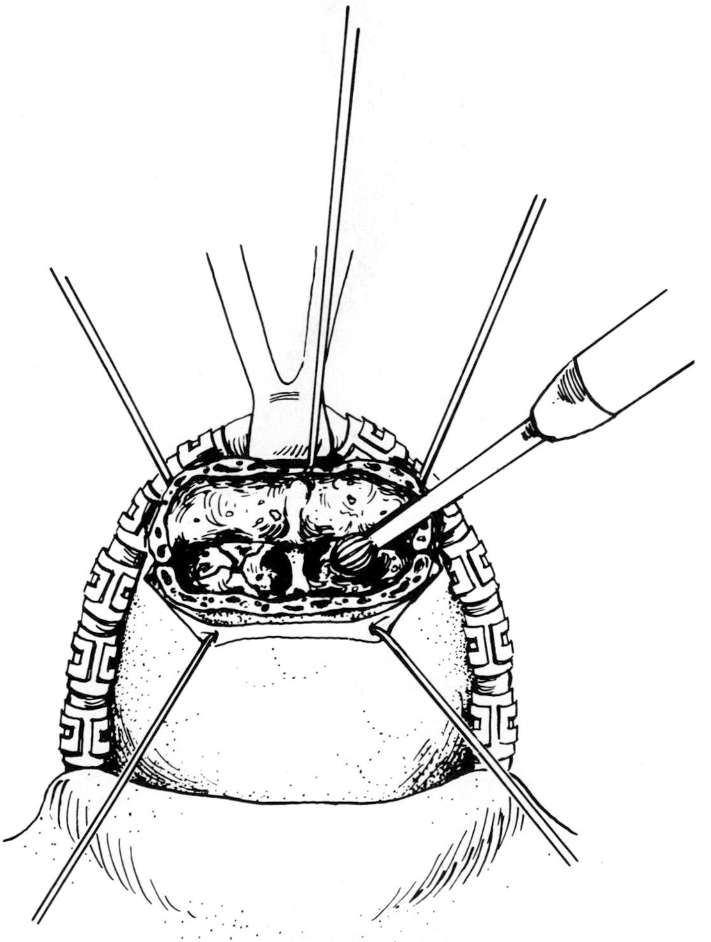

Figure 44-3. The frontal bone flap is pedicled on the lower part of the periosteum. The sinus mucosa is exenterated with a high-speed drill, and the fracture site is identified.

tage of buttressing the anterior table. The anterior wall of the sinus is then secured into its anatomic position.

Cribriform plate and ethmoid roof

Fistulas of the ethmoid and the cribriform plate are approached through a medial orbital incision (Fig. 44-4). The orbital contents are dissected posteriorly in a subperiorbital plane to the level of the optic foramen. The anterior and posterior ethmoid neurovascular bundles are sacrificed to provide additional exposure and allow mobilization of the orbital contents. During this dissection, the frontoethmoid suture line is easily identified and delineates the level of the cribriform plate (Fig. 44-5). The ethmoid labyrinth is entered by perforating the thin lacrimal bone and lamina papyracea with a sharp curette, and the bones of the anterior and posterior ethmoid sinus are exenterated (Fig. 44-6).

The roof of the ethmoid sinus, which also forms the floor of the anterior cranial fossa, is exposed. The superior nasal septum is identified, as is the cribriform plate, which is immediately lateral (Fig. 44-7). The defect is identified with the operating microscope. If the defect is large enough, a free graft of fascia lata is inserted and tucked beneath the margins of bone within the anterior cranial fossa. The site is then covered with a pedicled flap of nasoseptal mucoperiosteum (Fig. 44-8). A flap fashioned from the middle turbinate also may be used to cover the ethmoid defect. Alternatively, the middle turbinate can be removed and the cribriform plate and ethmoid roof can be covered with a posteriorly based mucoperiosteal flap from the nasal septum, as described

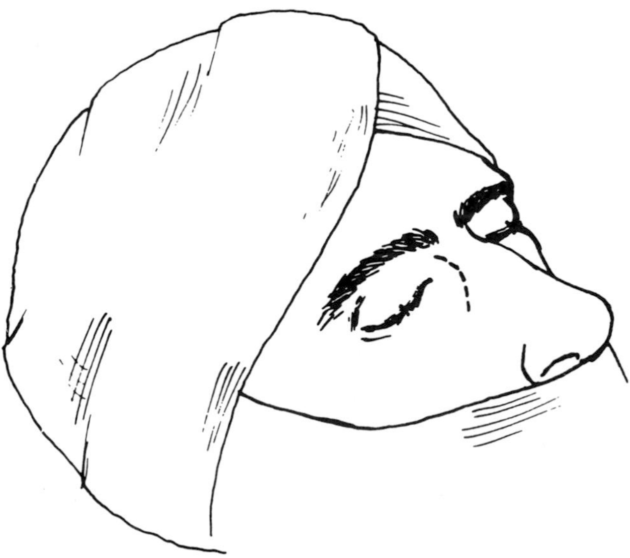

Figure 44-4. Medial orbital incision used for the exposure of fistulas in the cribriform plate, ethmoid roof, and sphenoid sinus.

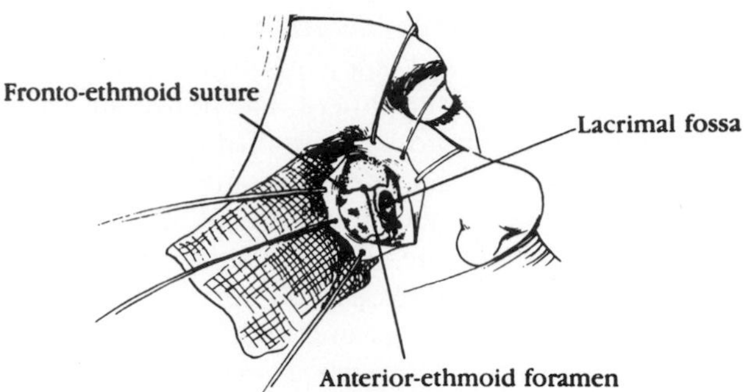

Figure 44-5. The external ethmoidectomy approach, showing bony landmarks. The frontoethmoid suture line delineates the level of the cribriform plate and the floor of the anterior fossa.

by Montgomery.[13] McCabe described a flap from the middle turbinate containing attached turbinated bone which was rotated laterally against the ethmoid roof and secured with packing.[10]

If these techniques are not feasible, an additional piece of fascia lata may be placed over the site of the fistula and covered with a free graft of middle turbinate mucosa or nasal septal mucosa. Once the graft is secured into place, it is covered with Gelfoam and buttressed with nasal packing, which is left in place for 10 days. Administration of antibiotics is continued during this period, and the patient is given stool softeners and cautioned to refrain from strenuous activity.

Sphenoid sinus

A transseptosphenoid approach to the sphenoid sinus is used. The surgical approach is through either a sublabial or a transnasal route and has been well described

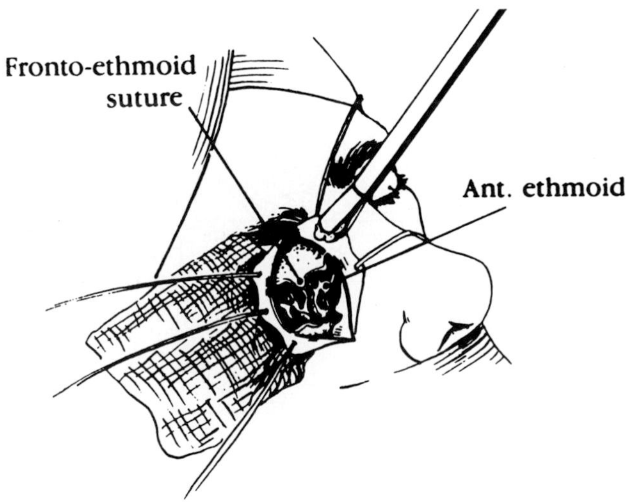

Figure 44-6. Exenteration of ethmoid air cells.

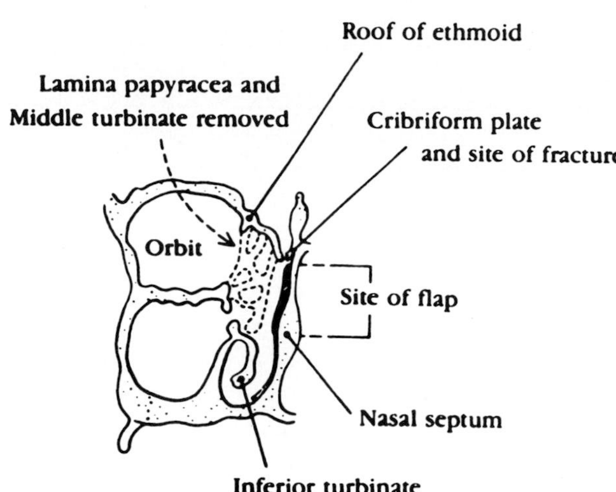

Figure 44-7. Coronal view of the operative approach to a cribriform plate fistula. The lamina papyracea, middle turbinate (dotted lines), and ethmoid air cells are exenterated to expose the fistula site.

in the literature.[67] This avoids a facial incision and allows sphenoid sinus packing without an open communication with the nasal cavity. If the fistula cannot be localized to the sphenoid sinus by preoperative studies, it is preferable to approach the region through an external ethmoidectomy. In either case, the intersinus septum is removed and the sphenoid sinus is denuded of its mucosa, utilizing the operating microscope or endoscope. Typically, a fascia graft is placed against the dural tear and then buttressed with fat. Occasionally, lateral pneumatization of the sphenoid sinus extends to the pterygoid recesses, which must be carefully packed with fat.

Petrous Bone

Otorrhea and otorhinorrhea are repaired extracranially through a mastoidectomy approach. The surgeon can easily identify the fistula site by the egress of fluorescein dye, a far easier task from an extracranial than from an intracranial exposure. Seventh and eighth cranial nerve function is preserved in patients with normal nerve function preoperatively.

The extent of mastoid surgery depends on the location of the dural defect and whether the patient has functional hearing. If the patient has functional hearing, the cochlea should be preserved at all costs. The mastoid air cells are removed with a high-speed drill, and the dura surrounding the fistula is widely exposed so that a graft of temporalis fascia can be placed tightly against the fistula and secured with tissue adhesive. The mastoid cavity and epitympanum are then packed with fat.

When a CSF fistula exists with total permanent hearing loss, as in a transverse petrous bone fracture, a CSF fistula can be stopped by obliterating the middle ear and eustachian tube.[65] Because the mastoid air cell system is sterile, the presence of CSF in the mastoid cells is not likely to cause meningitis as long as there is no communication with the upper respiratory tract.

Fistulas of Uncertain Location

When a fistula cannot be localized to the sphenoid sinus by preoperative studies, the base of the skull is best approached through the ethmoid sinuses.[11] The operative approach described for ethmoid and cribriform sinus fistulas is used. After ethmoidectomy, the anterior wall of the sphenoid sinus is also removed and the sphenoid sinus mucosa is exenterated. This exposes the undersurface of the floor of the anterior fossa from the most anterior portion of the ethmoid sinus to the anterior clinoid processes in an anteroposterior direction. The medial-lateral exposure is from the midline to the lateral border of the supraorbital ethmoid sinuses. The dural dehiscence is repaired as described previously, and the sphenoid sinus is packed with fat.

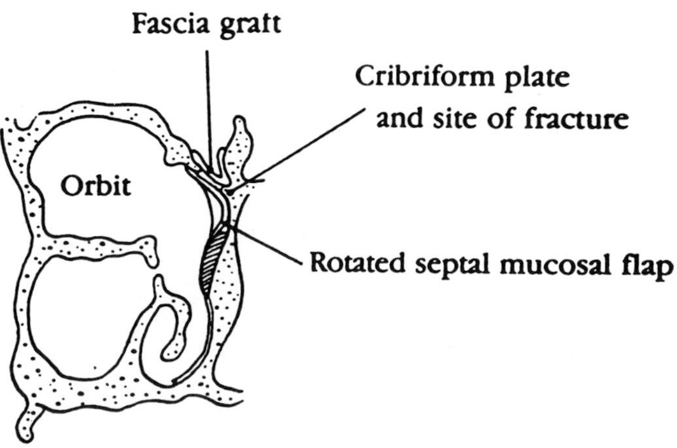

Figure 44-8. Coronal view demonstrating repair of a cribriform plate fistula. Fascia lata is tucked into the anterior fossa overlying the fistula. A rotated septal mucosa flap is used to cover the site, and the repair is held in place with nasal packing (not illustrated).

COMPLICATIONS

Meningitis

Bacterial meningitis is the major complication of traumatic CSF fistulas and occurs in 9 to 46 percent of cases[28,31,35,37,38] (Table 44-1). In one study, the overall incidence of meningitis before surgical dural repair was 31 percent and the cumulative risk exceeded 85 percent at 10 years follow-up (Fig. 44-9). In this same report, meningitis was recurrent in 31 percent.[31]

The most common pathogen is pneumococcus, which is the causative organism in 40 to 54 percent of cases.[1,31,70] Gram-negative organisms and negative cultures are more common in patients treated with antibiotic prophylaxis.[31]

Despite the use of modern antibiotics, meningitis still carries a mortality rate approaching 20 percent[37,70,71] and a morbidity as high as 29 percent.[71] In one study, 10 percent of patients with bacterial meningitis developed intracranial abscess and 10 percent developed hydrocephalus.[2] Stroke, epilepsy, and deafness are other sequelae.

Risk factors for developing meningitis have not been clearly defined. Eljamel and Foy reported that patients with CSF fistulas that persisted beyond 1 week were no more likely to develop meningitis than were those whose fistulas resolved within 1 week.[31] There is some evidence to suggest that patients with the delayed onset of a CSF fistula are more likely to develop meningitis. Park and coworkers reported a 20 percent incidence of meningitis in patients with immediate onset of CSF rhinorrhea but an incidence of 57 percent in those with delayed fistulas.[1]

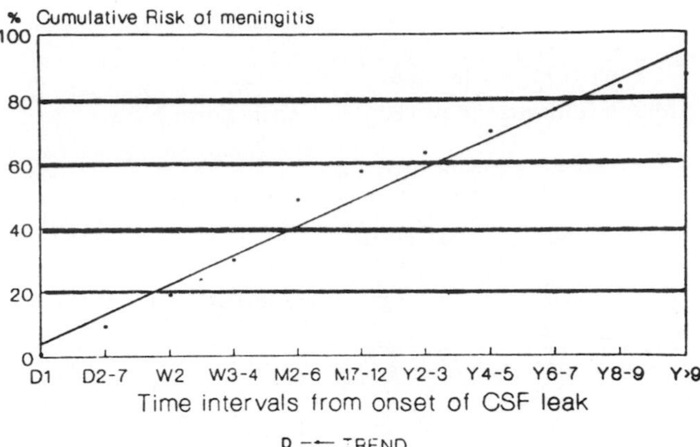

Figure 44-9. The cumulative risk of meningitis as the period of follow-up increases: D1 = day one; W = week; M = month; Y = year of follow-up before surgical dural repair (Reproduced with permission from Eljamel MS, Foy PM.[31]) Acute traumatic CSF fistulae: The risk of intracranial infection. *Br J Neursurg* 4:381–385, 1990.

This may be due to the increased duration of exposure. Patients with pneumocephalus have been reported to have a higher incidence of meningitis,[1] although other studies have not confirmed this finding.[31]

Pneumocephalus

The incidence of pneumocephalus has been reported to range from 0.5 to 0.88 percent in a series of unselected head-injured patients examined with skull x-rays.[24] The incidence was 7.8 percent, or 10 times higher, in Lewin's series of 308 patients with fractures of the base of the skull.[28]

TABLE 44-1 Risk of Meningitis after Traumatic CSF Rhinorrhea

Author	Total No. Patients	*Patients with Meningitis, %*		
		No.	Fatal	Recurrence
Calvert and Cairns[35]	11	4 (36)	2 (50)	
Lewin[32]	84	16 (25)	4 (25)	2 (12.5)
Ray and Bergland[60]	11	(24)		
Brisman et al.[27]	9	3 (33)		
Grahane[36]	13	(46)		
MacGee et al.[55]	23	2 (9)	1 (50)	
Robinson[68]	59	13 (22)		2 (15)
Leech and Paterson[38]	118	11 (9)		
Westmore and Whittam[39]	81	28 (35)	(1.2)	
Manelfe et al.[69]	19	6 (32)		3 (50)
Park et al.[1]	29	8 (30)		
Eljamel and Foy[2]	160	49 (31)	2 (4)	15 (31)

SOURCE: Reproduced with permission from Eljamel MS, Foy PM[2]. Post-traumatic CSF fistulas, the case for surgical repair. *Br J Neurosurg* 4:479–483, 1990.

In 1977, Steudel and Hacker reported pneumocephalus in 49 of 508 patients (9.7 percent) with an acute head injury examined with CT scan.[72] The high incidence of pneumocephalus in this study probably reflects the sensitivity of CT in detecting as little as 0.5 ml of intracranial air.[73] Patients were also examined within a few hours of injury, the period in which the likelihood of detecting pneumocephalus is greatest. This is consistent with the finding that small amounts of intracranial air can resolve over several hours.

Acute traumatic pneumocephalus or intracranial air that occurs within several hours of injury provides prima facie evidence of a basal skull fracture. In most cases, the air resolves over several hours or days without sequelae. Its presence does not affect patient outcome, and patients with pneumocephalus fare as well as do those with head injuries of similar severity who do not have pneumocephalus.

The presence of multiple air bubbles in different intracranial locations is a sign of severe trauma and is generally associated with a worse prognosis compared with injuries with a well-delineated gas collection or pneumatoceles.[72] Late pneumocephalus, or intracranial air appearing several days after a head injury, suggests the presence of a persistent CSF fistula.

Tension pneumocephalus develops in patients in whom air collects continuously in the cranium and produces a mass effect and a neurological deficit. The symptoms are nausea, vomiting, headache, and impaired consciousness. Plain skull x-rays, MRI, and CT will confirm the presence of increasing volumes of air. For patients with profound deficits, treatment consists of craniotomy or burr hole drainage. The dural defect is repaired simultaneously.

In patients who are less critically ill, nonoperative maneuvers include bed rest and 100% oxygen therapy. High inspiratory oxygen washes nitrogen out of the bloodstream and results in a prompt reduction in the volume of intracranial gas as the nitrogen in the intracranial air pocket diffuses into the bloodstream.[41] Localizing studies and elective surgery are performed after the resolution of intracranial hypertension.

References

1. Park J, Strelzow VV, Friedman WH: Current management of cerebrospinal fluid rhinorrhea. *Laryngoscope* 93:1294–1300, 1983.
2. Eljamel MS, Foy PM: Post-traumatic CSF fistulae, the case for surgical repair. *Br J Neurosurg* 4:479–483, 1990.
3. Cairns H: Injuries of the frontal and ethmoidal sinuses with special references to cerebrospinal rhinorrhea and aerocele. *J Laryngol* 52:589–623, 1937.
4. Dandy WE: Pneumocephalus (intracranial pneumatocele or aerocele). *Arch Surg* 12:949–982, 1926.
5. Eden K: Traumatic cerebrospinal rhinorrhea: Repair of the fistula by a transfrontal intradural operation. *Br J Surg* 290:299–303, 1941.
6. Briant TDR, Snell E: Diagnosis of cerebrospinal rhinorrhea and the rhinologic approach to its repair. *Laryngoscope* 77:1390–1409, 1976.
7. Calcaterra TC: Extracranial surgical repair of cerebrospinal rhinorrhea. *Ann Otol* 89:108–116, 1980.
8. Hubbard JL, McDonald TJ, Pearson BW, Laws ER: Spontaneous cerebrospinal fluid rhinorrhea: Evolving concepts in diagnosis and surgical management based on the Mayo Clinic experience from 1970 through 1981. *Neurosurgery* 16:314–321, 1985.
9. Hudson WR, Hughes LA: Cerebrospinal rhinorrhea: Diagnosis and management. *South Med J* 68:1520–1523, 1975.
10. McCabe BF: The osteo-mucoperiosteal flap in repair of cerebrospinal fluid rhinorrhea. *Laryngoscope* 86:537–539, 1980.
11. McCormack BM, Cooper PR, Persky M, Rothstein S: Extracranial repair of cerebrospinal fluid fistulas: Technique and results in 37 patients. *Neurosurgery* 27:412–417, 1990.
12. Montgomery WW: Cerebrospinal fluid rhinorrhea. *Otolaryngol Clin North Am* 6:757–771, 1973.
13. Montgomery WW: Surgery for cerebrospinal fluid rhinorrhea and otorrhea. *Arch Otolaryngol* 84:538–550, 1966.
14. Mattox DE, Kennedy DW: Endoscopic management of cerebrospinal fluid leaks and cephaloceles. *Laryngoscope* 100:857–862, 1990.
15. Papay FA, Benninger M, Levine H, et al: Transnasal transseptal endoscopic repair of sphenoidal cerebral spinal fluid fistula. *Orolaryngol Head Neck Surg* 101:595–597, 1989.
16. Rowbothom GF: *Acute Injuries of the Head.* Edinburgh: E & S Livingstone, 1964.
17. Stankiewicz JA: Cerebrospinal fluid fistula and endoscopic sinus surgery. *Laryngoscope* 101:250–256, 1991.
18. Caldicott WJH, North JB, Simpson DA: Traumatic cerebrospinal fluid fistulas in children. *J Neurosurg* 38:1–9, 1983.
19. Hough JVD: Otologic trauma, in Pavalla M, Shumarch DA (eds): *Otolaryngology.* Philadelphia: Saunders, 1973:241–262.
20. Johnson RT, Dutt P: On dural laceration over paranasal and petrous air sinuses. *Br J Surg* (*War Suppl*) 1:141–167, 1947.
21. Morley TP, Hetherington RF: Traumatic cerebrospinal fluid rhinorrhea and otorrhea, pneumocephalus, and meningitis. *Surg Gynecol Obstet* 104:88–98, 1957.
22. Morley TP, Wortzman G: The importance of the lateral extensions of the sphenoid sinus in post-traumatic cerebrospinal rhinorrhea and meningitis: Clinical and radiological aspects. *J Neurosurg* 22:326–332, 1965.
23. Lunsford LD, Maroon JD, Sheptok PE, Albin MS: Sub-

dural tension pneumocephalus. *J Neurosurg* 50:525–527, 1979.

24. Markham JW: Pneumocephalus, in Vinken PJ, Bruyn GW (eds): *Handbook of Clinical Neurology: Injuries of the Brain and Skull,* vol. 24. New York: American Elsevier, 201–213, 1976.
25. Walker FO, Vern BA: The mechanism of pneumocephalus formation in patients with CSF fistula. *J Neurol Neurosurg Psychiatry* 49:203–205, 1986.
26. Brawley BW, Kelly WA: Treatment of basal skull fractures with and without CSF fistula. *J Neurosurg* 26:57–61, 1967.
27. Brisman R, Hughes JE, Mount LA: Cerebrospinal fluid rhinorrhea. *Arch Neurol* 22:245–252, 1966.
28. Lewin W: Cerebrospinal fluid rhinorrhea in closed head injuries. *Br J Surg* 42:1–18, 1954.
29. Lowe F, Pertuiset B, Chaumier EE, Jacksche H: Traumatic, spontaneous and postoperative CSF rhinorrhea, in Symon L (ed): *Advances and Technical Standards in Neurosurgery.* Vienna, New York: Springer-Verlag, 169–207, 1984.
30. Mincy JE: Post-traumatic CSF fistula of the frontal fossa. *J Trauma* 6:618–621, 1966.
31. Eljamel MS, Foy PM: Acute traumatic CSF fistulae: The risk of intracranial infection. *Br J Neurosurg* 4:381–385, 1990.
32. Lewin W: Cerebrospinal fluid rhinorrhea in nonmissile head injuries. *Clin Neurosurg* 12:237–252, 1964.
33. Zrebeet HAK, Huang PS: Prophylactic antibiotics in the treatment of fractures at the base of the skull. *Del Med J* 58:741–748, 1986.
34. Prere J, Puech JL, Deroover N, et al: Rhinorrhea and meningitis due to post-traumatic osteo-meningeal defects in the anterior cranial fossa: Diagnosis with water-soluble CT cisternography. *J Neuroradiol* 13:278–285, 1986.
35. Calvert CA, Cairns H: Discussion on injuries of the frontal and ethmoidal sinuses. *Proc R Soc Med* 35:805–810, 1942.
36. Grahane B: Traumatic cranionasal fistulas, persistent cerebrospinal fluid rhinorrhea and their repair with frontal sinus osteoplasty. *Acta Otolaryngol* (*Stockh*) 70:392–400, 1970.
37. Prere J, Peuch JL, Deroover N, et al: Death from bacterial meningitis. *Br Med J* 1:453, 1974.
38. Leech PJ, Paterson A: Conservative and operative management for cerebrospinal fluid leakage after closed head injury. *Lancet* 1:1013–1016, 1973.
39. Westmore GA, Whittam DE: Cerebrospinal fluid rhinorrhea and its management. *Br J Surg* 69:489–492, 1982.
40. Wigand ME: Transnasal ethmoidectomy under endoscopic control. *Rhinology* 19:7–15, 1981.
41. Spetzler RF, Wilson CB: Dural fistula and their repair, in Youmans JR (ed): *Neurological Surgery,* vol. 4 (2d ed). Philadelphia: Saunders, 2209–2227, 1982.
42. Gadenholt H: The reaction of glucose-oxidase test paper in normal nasal secretions. *Acta Otolaryngol* (*Stockh*) 58:271–272, 1964.
43. Ryall RG, Peacock MK, Simpson DA: Usefulness of B2-transferrin assay in the detection of cerebrospinal fluid leaks following head injury. *J Neurosurg* 77:737–739, 1992.
44. Magnaes B, Solheim D: Controlled overpressure cisternography to localise cerebrospinal fluid rhinorrhea. *J Nucl Med* 18:109–111, 1977.
45. Spetzler RF, Wilson CB: Management of recurrent CSF rhinorrhea of the middle and posterior fossa. *J Neurosurg* 49:393–397, 1978.
46. Colquhoun IR: CT cisternography in the investigation of cerebrospinal fluid rhinorrhea. *Clin Radiol* 47:403–408, 1993.
47. Price DJ, Sleigh JD: Control of infection due to Klebsiella aerogenes in a neurosurgical unit by withdrawal of all antibiotics. *Lancet* 2:1213–1215, 1970.
48. Schaefer SD, Diehl JT, Briggs WH: The diagnosis of CSF rhinorrhea by metrizamide CT scanning. *Laryngoscope.* 90:871–875, 1980.
49. Kirchner FR, Proud GO: Method of identification and localization of cerebrospinal fluid, rhinorrhea, and otorrhea. *Laryngoscope* 70:921–930, 1960.
50. Messerklinger W: Nasenendoscpie: Nachweis, lokalisation und defferentialdiagnose der nasalen liquorrhoe. *HNO* 20:268–270, 1972.
51. Naidich TP, Moran CJ: Precise anatomic localization of atraumatic sphenoethmoidal cerebrospinal fluid rhinorrhea by metrizamide CT cisternography. *J Neurosurg* 53:222–228, 1980.
52. Klastersky J, Sadeghi M, Brihaye J: Antimicrobial prophylaxis in patients with rhinorrhea or otorrhea: A double-blind study. *Surg Neurol* 6:111–114, 1976.
53. Ignelzi RJ, VanderArk GD: Analysis of the treatment of basilar skull fractures with and without antibiotics. *J Neurosurg* 43:721–726, 1975.
54. Ronwig DA, Voth DW, Liu C, et al: Bacterial flora and infection in patients with brain injury. *J Neurosurg* 38:710–716, 1973.
55. MacGee EE, Cauthen JC, Brackett CE: Meningitis following acute traumatic cerebrospinal fluid fistula. *J Neurosurg* 33:312–316, 1970.
56. Dagi TF, Meyer FB, Poletti CA: The incidence and prevention of meningitis after basilar skull fracture. *Am J Emerg Med* 3:295–298, 1983.
57. Einhorn A, Mizrahi EM: Basilar skull fractures in children: The incidence of CNS infection and the use of antibiotics. *Am J Dis Child* 132:1121–1124, 1978.
58. Collins WF: Dural fistulae and their repair, in Youmans, JR (ed): *Neurological Surgery.* Philadelphia: Saunders, 981–992, 1973.
59. Dingman RO: Maxillofacial injuries, in Youmans JR (ed): *Neurological Surgery.* Philadelphia: Saunders, 931, 1973.
60. Ray BS, Bergland RM: Cerebrospinal fluid fistula: Clinical aspects, techniques of localization and methods of closure. *J Neurosurg* 30:399–405, 1969.
61. Dohlman G: Spontaneous cerebrospinal rhinorrhea. *Acta Otolaryngol* [*suppl*] (*Stockh*) 67:20–23, 1948.
62. Fox N: Cure in case of cerebrospinal rhinorrhea. *Arch Otolaryngol* 17:85–86, 1933.
63. Hirsch O: Successful closure of cerebrospinal fluid rhi-

norrhea by endonasal surgery. *Arch Otolaryngol* 56:1–13, 1952.

64. Calcaterra TC, Moseley JI, Rand RW: Cerebrospinal rhinorrhea: Extracranial surgical repair. *West J Med* 127:279–283, 1977.
65. Calcaterra TC, Rand RW: Tympanic cavity obliteration for cerebrospinal otorhinorrhea. *Arch Otolaryngol* 97:388–390, 1973.
66. Aboulker P, Lebeau J, Sterkers JM, Elbaz P: Treatment of ethmoidofrontal meningeal fistulas: Fifteen cases with successful operation by the exocranial route. *Ann Otolaryngol Chir Cervicofac* 83:27–32, 1966.
67. Hardy J: Transsphenoidal hypophysectomy. *J Neurosurg* 34:582–594, 1971.
68. Robinson RG: Cerebrospinal fluid rhinorrhea and pneumocephalus due to nonmissile injuries. Aust NZ *J Surg* 37:328–334, 1970.
69. Manelfe C, Cellerier P, Sobel D, et al: Cerebrospinal fluid rhinorrhea: Evaluation with metrizimide cisternography. *AJR* 138:471–476, 1982.
70. McKenzie P, Love WC, Jemieson WM, et al: Cephaloridine in pneumococcal and other forms of pyogenic meningitis. *Postgrad Med J* 43(suppl):142–145, 1967.
71. Levin S, Nelson KE, Spies HW, Lepper MH: Pneumococcal meningitis, the problem of unseen cerebrospinal fluid leakage after closed head injury. *Am J Med Sci* 264:319–327, 1972.
72. Steudel WI, Hacker H: Prognosis, incidence and management of acute traumatic intracranial pneumocephalus: A retrospective analysis of 49 cases. *Acta Neurochir* (*Wien*) 80:93–99, 1986.
73. Osborne A, Daines J, Wing S, et al: Intracranial air on computed tomography. *J Neurosurg* 48:355–359, 1978.

CHAPTER 45

CEREBROVASCULAR COMPLICATIONS IN THE HEAD-INJURED PATIENT

Joshua L. Dowling
Adam P. Brown
Ralph G. Dacey, Jr.

SYNOPSIS

The head-injured patient often presents with a variety of neurological findings. While most are due to direct cerebral trauma, the possibility of vascular injury should always be considered. For most of these lesions, accurate diagnosis requires a high index of suspicion coupled with a thorough awareness of the clinical settings and presentations of vascular injuries. Neurological deficits not explained by CT scan, or occurring days to weeks following trauma, should prompt consideration of vessel trauma. In most instances cerebral angiography is needed. Other diagnostic modalities can often reveal the diagnosis of vascular injury; however, angiography offers the necessary detail for treatment planning. In many cases, particularly in vertebral artery injuries and traumatic arteriovenous fistulae, angiography makes possible definitive treatment using endovascular techniques.

INTRODUCTION

Although the advent of computed tomography (CT) has generally improved the diagnosis and management of head injury, the resultant decrease in routine angiography has made the detection of associated vascular injury more difficult. The presence of injury to cerebrovascular structures, usually considered with penetrating trauma, is often overlooked in nonpenetrating head injury. The potential for life-threatening ischemic or hemorrhagic complications, sometimes even in the setting of mild or trivial head trauma, demands a high index of suspicion from the neurosurgeon. A delay in the onset of symptoms often results in delayed diagnosis, and the opportunity to treat these injuries before the patient has sustained any permanent deficit may be missed. Even with prompt diagnosis, management of these lesions can be problematic, with options frequently limited by accompanying trauma or by the location of the lesion. Nevertheless, the development of newer surgical and endovascular techniques has produced an expanded choice of treatments and the possibility of improved outcome from these injuries. For these reasons, a thorough knowledge of potential vascular complications is essential for the proper management of the head-injured patient.

CERVICAL VASCULAR INJURIES

Extracranial Carotid Artery Injuries

Extracranial carotid artery injuries are the most common neurovascular injury. In one series of carotid artery injuries, penetrating trauma involved the common carotid artery 75 percent of the time, whereas nonpenetrating trauma involved the carotid bifurcation or the internal carotid artery in 93 percent of cases.[1,2]

Nonpenetrating trauma

Nonpenetrating injury to the carotid arteries has an incidence of about 0.08 percent within the general blunt trauma population.[3] About 3 to 5 percent of all carotid injury is caused by blunt trauma.[1,4,5] The mean age of affected individuals is 36 years.[5] Men outnumber women, as in most trauma populations; however, in one series the number of women was out of proportion to the percentage of women in the general trauma population, leading the authors to speculate that women may be more susceptible to carotid artery dissection.[6]

Blunt carotid trauma has been reported in many settings, but almost all studies identify motor vehicle accidents as the most common mechanism of injury.[2,6,7] Other settings include falls, fist-fights, strangulation, blunt intraoral trauma, chiropractic manipulation, and local surgery.[2,6–12] These mechanisms can produce injury to the carotid artery either by direct trauma or by stretch. Although direct trauma is clearly implicated in some settings, such as strangulation, local surgery, or intraoral trauma, in many instances the exact manner in which the artery is injured is not entirely clear. Stringer and Kelly proposed that injury was most commonly caused by hyperextension with contralateral flexion causing stretching over the transverse processes of the upper cervical vertebrae.[9] This theory is consistent with the biomechanics of motor vehicle accidents. Batzdorf et al., however, questioned the role of hyperextension, noting the lack of associated central cord syndrome in earlier reports.[13] Moreover, in cadaver experiments, they were unable to reproduce the results of a previous study demonstrating distortion or stretching of the internal carotid artery with neck extension.[13,14]

The internal carotid artery may also be injured as a result of compression between the lateral processes of the upper cervical vertebrae and the angle of the mandible.[5] The reported association between internal carotid artery dissection and mandibular fractures supports this putative mechanism, although these injuries may be independently related to a common mechanism of trauma.[15]

Several studies from the Mayo Clinic have examined internal carotid artery injuries due to blunt trauma and have noted the proximity of these injuries to a prominent styloid process.[7,16] Stundt et al. noted that traumatic aneurysms or pseudoaneurysms, found in 30 percent of dissections of the internal carotid artery, frequently occurred in this region (Fig. 45-1) and in some cases were adherent to the styloid process.[16] Thus, arterial damage could result when sudden rotation of the head forces the styloid process against the internal carotid artery.[7,16]

Regardless of the precise mechanism of injury, the initial pathology usually involves intimal disruption.[2,9,12,15] Intimal injury can act as a nidus for thrombosis, which can progress to occlusion or become a source for emboli.[9] Dissections can also occur, if, upon disruption of the intima, blood tracks subintimally. The expanding false lumen can result in stenosis or occlusion of the artery. Depending on the degree of involvement of the arterial media or adventitia, a traumatic aneurysm, pseudoaneurysm, or fistula can result. Traumatic aneurysms more commonly result from dissections of the distal internal carotid, and only rarely occur with more proximal dissections.[16] Thus, dissection, stenosis, occlusion, and aneurysm can all result from similar mechanisms of injury, with intimal damage as the common initial pathology.

Cerebral ischemic complications are clearly the most serious sequelae of blunt carotid artery injuries. Ischemia can result from inadequate perfusion due to stenosis or occlusion in patients with insufficient collateral circulation. Additionally, thromboembolism can occur. The typical delay from the time of injury to the onset of ischemic symptoms is thought to represent the time during which thrombus formation progresses to occlusion, severe stenosis, or embolism.[12] Of these, embolization is probably the most frequent cause of delayed symptoms.[7]

Given the infrequent occurrence of blunt carotid artery injury relative to blunt trauma in general, some factors may predispose certain individuals to this type of injury. As mentioned above, a prominent styloid process may play a role in some patients.[16] Prominent lateral processes may be necessary for internal carotid artery injury by hyperextension.[9,13] Sullivan et al. reported one case in which the internal carotid artery was noted at surgery to be adherent to the lateral process of the atlas, which may have contributed to that patient's injury.[15] Although the relative youth of patients suffering from internal carotid artery dissections may be a reflection of the average age of the trauma population, some have speculated that the greater mobility of the cervical spine, as well as the greater elasticity of the arteries, may be relevant factors.[17,18] Atheromas have been noted at the site of many dissections.[13,19] Other underlying diseases that might predispose to traumatic injury include fibromuscular dysplasia, Marfan's syndrome, cystic medial degeneration, homocystinuria, and syphilis.[10]

Symptoms of focal cerebral ischemia, either transient ischemic attacks or stroke, are the most common presentation for patients with nonpenetrating carotid artery injury. These occurred 71 percent of the time in one series.[20] A delay in the onset of ischemia is typical of these patients, ranging from hours to years after the injury, thus throwing the causality into question.[9,10,19,21] Headache is another common presenting complaint. It is usually focal, involving frontal, orbital, and periorbital areas, and often unilateral, occurring ipsilateral to the

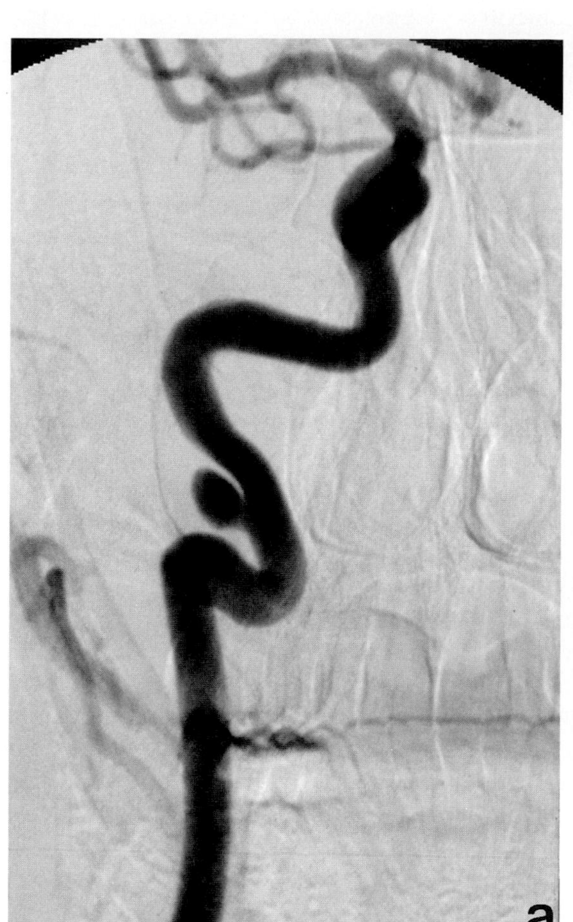

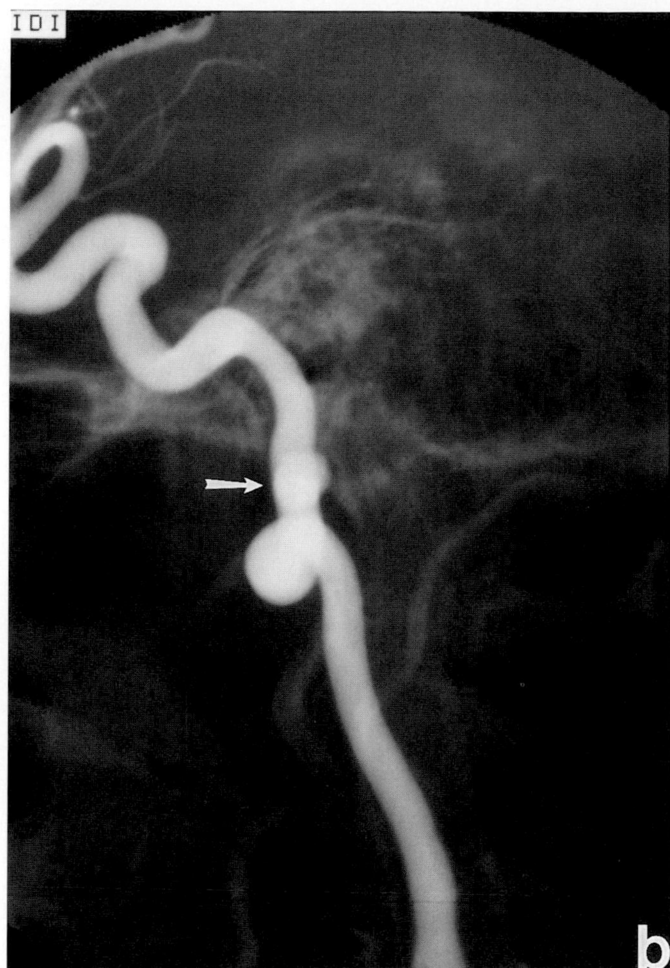

Figure 45-1. Post-traumatic extracranial aneurysm formation. This 19-year-old female was involved in a motor vehicle accident and sustained a loss of consciousness. A right cervical bruit was present. CT scan of the head demonstrated subarachnoid hemorrhage. A cerebral angiogram was obtained. *A*. Digital subtraction angiography (DSA), AP projection, of the right internal carotid artery demonstrates a post-traumatic pseudoaneurysm at the skull base. The pseudoaneurysm projects laterally as the artery enters the carotid canal of the petrous bone. The remaining portions of the artery appear normal, with no luminal abnormalities. *B*. Lateral digital angiogram of the right internal carotid artery shows the same aneurysm (*arrow*) at the skull base. The lesion was treated with internal carotid artery occlusion by endovascular techniques using balloons and coils. A previously performed test occlusion of the internal carotid artery demonstrated no neurological deficit after 30 minutes. (Courtesy of DeWitte T. Cross III, M.D., St. Louis, MO.)

injury.[7,20] Other presenting symptoms include Horner's syndrome, cervical bruit, neck pain, and amaurosis fugax.[6–8,10,12]

External evidence of cervical injury is present in only about 50 percent of patients, and in many of these only a skin abrasion is noted.[2,19] In one study, only 7 percent of 96 patients could recall any neck trauma.[2] This is not surprising given that the mechanism of carotid injury in many cases is indirect stretch of the artery. Nevertheless, a neck hematoma when present should raise suspicion for a vascular injury.[8,12]

Head injury frequently accompanies blunt carotid artery injuries. One series found a history of head injury in 75 percent of patients; 23 percent of these injuries were severe.[19] As a result, neurological deficits due to vascular injury often are erroneously attributed to intracranial pathology.[2] Patients with focal deficits due to blunt carotid artery trauma, however, usually remain alert, whereas intracranial trauma causing focal deficits usually produces obtundation.[8,12] Needless to say, the patient with both severe intracranial and severe cervical vascular injury can be problematic.

Blunt carotid artery injury is frequently misdiagnosed. One series found accurate admission diagnoses in only 6 percent of patients.[2] The low overall incidence of carotid artery injury in blunt trauma is undoubtedly partly responsible for this initial error. However, several other features make accurate diagnosis difficult. As noted above, the onset of symptoms is frequently delayed.[13] Also, signs of cervical trauma may be trivial or lacking.[19] The presence of associated head injury may further complicate the clinical picture. For these reasons, a high index of suspicion is essential for the proper diagnosis of blunt trauma to the extracranial carotid artery. Possible vascular injury should be considered in any patient presenting with a neurological deficit following trauma, especially if the injury involves any of the mechanisms or presentations discussed above. Thus, Horner's syndrome, unilateral headache, cervical bruit, or the complaint of head noise synchronous with pulse (subjective bruit) occurring in the setting of head or neck injury should prompt consideration of carotid artery injury.[7,11,13] Basilar skull fracture, mandibular fracture or dislocation, or facial injuries are also suggestive.[7] Following head injury, a CT scan usually is performed. The presence of focal neurological deficit with a normal CT scan should prompt further work-up for vascular injury, especially if the patient is alert and oriented.[2,6,11]

In cases of suspected blunt injury to the extracranial carotid artery, angiography remains the diagnostic study of choice.[5,6,11] Angiography clearly defines the injury and identifies any coexisting cerebrovascular abnormalities, including the presence of distal emboli.[5] It also offers an opportunity to assess collateral circulation through balloon occlusion testing. In some cases, angiography provides the setting for definitive treatment using endovascular techniques.

Improvements in magnetic resonance imaging (MRI) and MR angiography (MRA) have prompted some to advocate the use of this noninvasive technique to diagnose blunt carotid artery trauma. Axial MRI has been shown to be sensitive to dissections of the internal carotid artery.[22,23] Arterial dissections on MRI demonstrate hyperintensity within the false lumen on T1- and T2-weighted images, thought to be due to methemoglobin.[23] Typically, the semilunar hyperintense false lumen is seen to displace the signal void of the residual true lumen. MRA may in fact be more sensitive than angiography in demonstrating the full extent of dissection and in detecting residual low flow through a highly stenotic vessel.[22] Also, with MRI the vascular lesion and the cerebral ischemic changes can be demonstrated in a single study.[23] In spite of these potential advantages, MRI and MRA cannot provide the same clarity of information regarding collateral circulation and are inadequate for planning treatment. However, there may be a role for MRA in following lesions already defined by angiography.

Duplex ultrasound scanning has been advocated by some as a noninvasive screening test for extracranial carotid artery injury.[8] Although this technique can accurately diagnose many abnormalities, difficulties with visualization of the distal internal carotid artery render this approach inadequate.[24,25] Transcranial Doppler ultrasound (TCD) can be used to monitor blood flow, even in distal internal carotid and intracranial arteries.[25] Although TCD cannot provide as much information as angiography regarding the adequacy of collateral flow and the presence of other abnormalities, it is a valuable tool in monitoring pathology already visualized angiographically.[25]

There is no universally accepted treatment approach to lesions caused by blunt trauma to the extracranial carotid artery. Although some advocate conservative treatment in virtually all cases,[6] others have advocated a more aggressive surgical approach. Treatment options include expectant management, anticoagulation, surgery, or, in some cases, endovascular treatment. Several factors must be evaluated prior to treatment, including the precise nature of the lesion or lesions as identified by angiography, the adequacy of collateral circulation, the neurological status of the patient, and the presence of other injuries. Treatment must be tailored to individual situations. Regardless of the treatment approach, outcome correlates primarily with pre-treatment neurological status.

The patient's neurological status is often the major determinant of treatment. As stated above, most patients with blunt carotid artery lesions present with symptoms of focal cerebral ischemia. Patients with severe, fixed neurological deficits have a poor prognosis regardless of treatment.[6,26] Surgery for revascularization in these instances may worsen the outlook because of the risk of reperfusion hemorrhage.[2,27,28] Reperfusion hemorrhage probably results from endothelial damage and loss of cerebral autoregulation secondary to ischemia.[26] These factors may take several hours to become relevant.[26] Thus, even in cases of severe neurological deficit, some would consider revascularization if the symptoms are of very recent onset.[2,12,26] Unfortunately, this treatment window is often lost through delays in diagnosis. In patients who are asymptomatic, conservative treatment can be considered. Some advocate the use of antiplatelet drugs in these cases, although their benefit has not been proved in controlled studies.[7] In patients with minor deficits or transient ischemic attacks (TIAs), anticoagulation and observation are reasonable options[5,7]; however, the presence of other injuries often precludes anticoagulation.[7] In cases of continued ischemic episodes or progressive deficits, surgical treatment should be given serious consideration.

The precise findings on angiography will strongly influence treatment. In patients with neurological deficits, angiography may be able to determine whether the ischemia is due to hemodynamic factors, as in the case of occlusion or severe stenosis, or whether thromboembolism from intimal damage, the more common etiology, has occurred. Anticoagulation may be appropriate in the latter circumstance, but would be ineffective in the former, in which case surgery might be indicated. The location of the lesion is also important. Surgery might be considered even with minor or no neurological symptoms in patients with easily accessible lesions. Frequently, however, dissections extend to the distal internal carotid artery or are associated with pseudoaneurysm at the skull base (Fig. 45-1). In these instances, surgical access can be very difficult, and in thromboembolism unresponsive to anticoagulation, some have advocated carotid ligation, with or without vascular bypass.[16,29,30] Assessment of adequate collateral perfusion by balloon occlusion testing during angiography is essential, since unselected carotid ligation has been associated with stroke rates as high as 30 percent.[16] Even in patients who tolerate balloon occlusion testing, 5 to 20 percent may develop ischemic complications.[30] The presence of bilateral injuries increases this risk even further.[30] Thus, some have advocated augmentation of perfusion with superficial temporal artery to middle cerebral artery (STA-MCA) bypass.[29] However, this procedure may not provide enough blood flow or may create abnormal watershed perfusion areas, which could result in intracranial vessel thrombosis.[30] For these reasons, other surgical approaches including direct repair of distal lesion with or without interposition grafting,[16] or ligation with saphenous vein bypass grafting[30] have been proposed. In cases of distal internal carotid artery pseudoaneurysms, once the patient has developed symptoms of thromboembolism, the risk of stroke is high, and surgery should be seriously considered.[16,31] Endovascular treatment of surgically inaccessible lesions is also an option. Unfortunately, placement of coils or balloons into pseudoaneurysms in an attempt to spare the arterial lumen is often ineffective because the aneurysm wall consists of hematoma instead of the firm tissue found in true aneurysms.[32] In these cases, endovascular trapping can be performed, but still carries the same risks for ischemia as ligation without bypass.[30,32]

In summary, considerable variability exists in treatment options. Conservative treatment usually consists of supportive therapy in patients with severe, fixed neurological deficits.[2,28] Asymptomatic patients may receive no treatment or may be placed on antiplatelet drugs.[7] Anticoagulation is used in patients with evidence of distal thromboembolization.[7] Surgical repair can be performed in patients who fail anticoagulation, in patients with severe deficits of very short duration, or even in patients with mild or no symptoms when the lesion is easily accessible.[2,7,8] In difficult to access lesions of the distal carotid artery, options include direct repair[16] or ligation, which may or may not be accompanied by bypass.[29,30] Trapping of these lesions by endovascular techniques is also an option.[32] Follow-up can include TCD to monitor the progression of stenosis or the patency of vascular grafts. For more proximal lesions, duplex ultrasound provides a noninvasive means for assessing dissection, occlusion, or stenosis. Angiography probably should be repeated in most patients after 1 or 2 months, and, in patients with aneurysms treated conservatively, repeat angiography after 1 or 2 years also should be considered.[7]

Reported outcome from blunt trauma to the extracranial carotid arteries varies considerably among studies, owing largely to selection criteria as well as the small numbers of patients in most series. In a review of the 96 patients reported in the British literature up to 1980, Krajewski and Hertzer reported that blunt carotid trauma carried a 30 percent mortality, while 42 percent of the patients were left with severe neurological deficits.[2] This grim picture was not echoed in the series by Mokri et al., in which 78 percent of patients at follow-up were either asymptomatic or had only mild problems.[7] The mode of treatment may affect outcome, as some have shown more favorable outcomes in surgically treated patients.[2,19] However, this may not be a fair comparison, since patients with severe, fixed deficits have the worst outcomes and are unlikely to be considered for surgical treatment. As stated earlier, the best predictor of outcome is pre-treatment neurological status; those with mild or no deficits usually do well, while those with more serious deficits tend to do poorly.[6,26]

PENETRATING TRAUMA

Penetrating cervical trauma, usually by stabbing or gunshot wound, is the most common cause of injury to the extracranial carotid artery. Injury usually involves the common carotid artery.[1,26] Young males predominate.[26]

In contrast to the subtleties of nonpenetrating carotid injuries, the signs of penetrating injuries of the carotid artery are often immediately evident on presentation. A rapidly expanding hematoma, often with airway compression, is typical. Pulsatile bleeding and shock frequently are present. Even in the absence of these signs, any penetrating neck wound should prompt consideration of carotid artery injury. Associated injuries to aerodigestive structures, brachial plexus, cranial nerves, veins, and spinal cord can occur in up to 30 percent of cases.[10]

In many instances, the diagnosis of carotid artery injury is made clinically. Hypotension, airway compression, active bleeding, or an expanding hematoma require immediate surgical exploration, precluding any further diagnostic work-up. Other times, the site of injury determines management. Penetrating injuries to the neck are often managed in relation to three anatomic zones: zone I extends from the base of the neck to the cricoid cartilage; zone II lies between the cricoid cartilage and the angle of the mandible; zone III extends from the angle of the mandible to the base of the skull. In patients in whom arterial injury is not readily apparent, angiography should be performed in all cases of injury to zones I and III of the neck, since physical exam alone cannot reliably detect vascular trauma in these areas.[26] For injuries of zone II, angiography should be performed when the injury is in proximity to vascular structures.[26,33] Because of the reliability of physical examination in detecting vascular injuries of zone II, some authors have discouraged use of angiography for penetrating trauma in this region.[34] As with blunt injuries, angiography not only defines the pathology, it also provides the setting for balloon occlusion evaluation of collateral circulation, and in some cases for endovascular treatment of injuries. Findings on angiography may include laceration, occlusion, arteriovenous fistula, pseudoaneurysm, and distal embolization of thrombus or bullet fragments[10,26] (Fig. 45-2).

Many studies have demonstrated the superiority of repair over ligation with respect to outcome.[28,35] Even patients with severe deficits and total occlusion should probably be repaired since rapid transport, resuscitation, and diagnosis usually allow for surgical intervention when symptoms are still of short duration and the risk of reperfusion hemorrhage is minimal.[33] In patients with no deficit and total occlusion, repair may be contraindicated because of the risk of distal embolization.[26] Also, because injuries to the spinal cord, brachial plexus, or cranial nerves occur in 20% of patients with carotid artery lesion, neurological deficit may not be of vascular origin.[26] Nevertheless, treatment of penetrating carotid injuries should include arterial repair whenever possible. In cases of distal internal carotid artery injury where direct repair is not feasible, ligation can be performed,[33] with or without bypass.[28] In patients undergoing angiography, treatment of arteriovenous fistulae often can be performed endovascularly with coils or detachable balloons (Fig. 45-3).

Penetrating carotid injury carries an overall mortality rate of 10 to 30 percent.[26] As with blunt injuries, preoperative neurological status has the greatest predictive value. In a summary of earlier studies, Pierce and Whitehill found that in addition to neurological status, whether or not the patient was treated with ligation also had a strong influence on outcome. They found that of patients with mild or no deficits, repair of the injured vessel was associated with successful outcome 91 percent of the time, compared with 60 percent for ligation. In patients with severe deficits or coma, the difference was not significant as repair and ligation were associated with 34 percent and 33 percent successful outcome, respectively.[26]

Vertebral Artery Injuries

Nonpenetrating Trauma

Vertebral artery injuries due to blunt trauma occur predominantly in women,[36,37] and most patients are between 30 and 50 years old—features that distinguish it from blunt carotid injury.[36] The incidence of vertebral artery injuries due to blunt trauma is difficult to estimate, since most cases probably are asymptomatic and go undiagnosed.

Nonpenetrating injury to the vertebral artery commonly involves rotation of the head. Thus, injuries have been reported to occur with chiropractic manipulation, calisthenics, archery, and head turning while driving.[36,38] Dissections have also been reported following cervical spine injuries.[39] The vertebral artery is commonly divided into four segments: the V1 segment extends from the origin of the artery to its entrance into the foramen transversarium of C6; V2 lies within the foramina transversaria from C6 to C2; V3 runs from C2 to the dura; V4 includes the entire intradural vertebral artery.[37] The V3 segment of the vertebral artery is most commonly involved in nonpenetrating injuries,[36,40] probably relating to the stretching and compression that normally occur at the atlanto-occipital and atlantoaxial joints during head rotation.[41] In some cases, intimal injury results, and, as with blunt carotid artery injuries, this can progress to thrombosis, with subsequent occlusion or embolization, or to dissection with resulting stenosis, occlusion, or pseudoaneurysm. Because of the redundancy of vertebral artery flow to the basilar artery, unilateral occlusion is often asymptomatic. Lesions can become symptomatic by thromboembolism, or by involvement of the posterior inferior cerebellar artery (PICA). Also, patients with congenital anomalies of the vertebral arteries or PICA are susceptible to vertebrobasilar insufficiency, even with unilateral injury. Congenital atresia or hypoplasia occurs 3.1 percent of the time on the left and 1.8 percent on the right.[42] Underlying vascular diseases such as fibromuscular dysplasia, cystic medial necrosis, Marfan's syndrome, homocystinuria, and syphilis may predispose patients to this injury.[41]

Pain is a frequent symptom of traumatic vertebral artery dissections, occurring in 66 percent of cases in one series,[40] and can be either immediate or delayed by hours to days.[36,37,40] The pain is severe and nonthrobbing, typically involving the upper neck and occipital region ipsilateral to the dissection. In the absence of ischemia, symptoms are often attributed to musculoskeletal injury. Ischemic symptoms, if they develop, are frequently delayed hours to weeks beyond the onset of pain. Any pattern of vertebrobasilar ischemia can be seen; however, lateral medullary syndrome occurs in up to 50 percent of cases.[36,42]

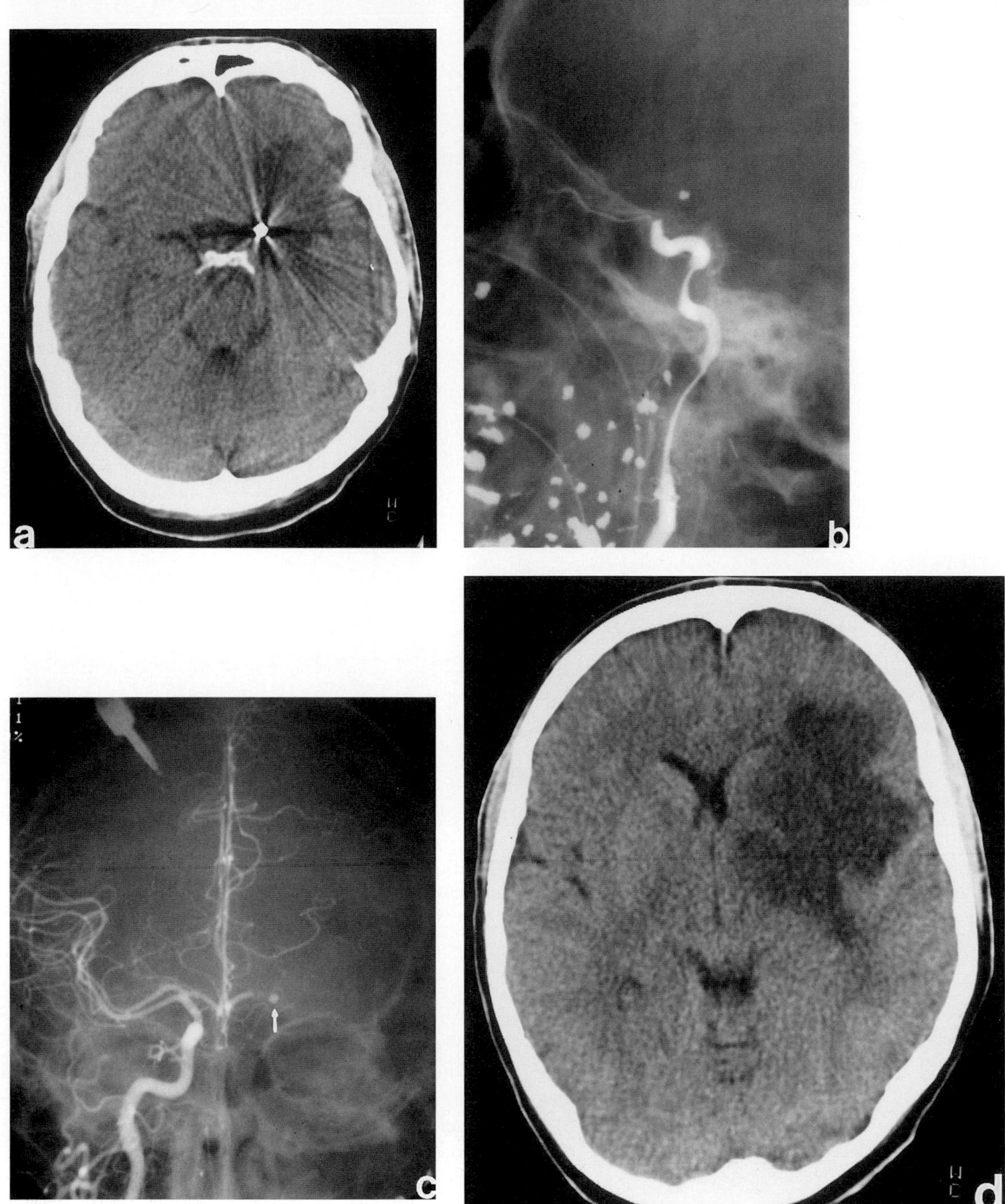

Figure 45-2. Gunshot wound to the neck. This 32-year-old male sustained a shotgun blast to the neck in a drive-by shooting. *A*. CT scan demonstrates an intracranial shotgun pellet with surrounding edema. During the CT examination the patient became hypotensive and was taken emergently to the operating room for repair of the carotid artery. *B*. A postoperative lateral angiogram of the left common carotid artery demonstrates focal spasm in the extracranial internal carotid artery (ICA) as well as in the cavernous carotid. There is no intracranial filling of the supraclinoid ICA. The pellet seen on the CT projects above the sella turcica. Multiple bullet fragments are also seen in the upper cervical and facial regions. *C*. A right injection of the common carotid artery (AP view) demonstrates filling of the right intracranial vessels, as well as the left anterior cerebral artery via the anterior communicating artery. No opacification of the left middle cerebral artery is seen secondary to occlusion of the proximal middle cerebral artery (MCA) by the embolized shotgun pellet (*arrow*). *D*. A postoperative CT scan of the head demonstrates a hypodense region in the distribution of the anterior division of the left MCA. This is consistent with a cerebral infarction secondary to vascular occlusion.

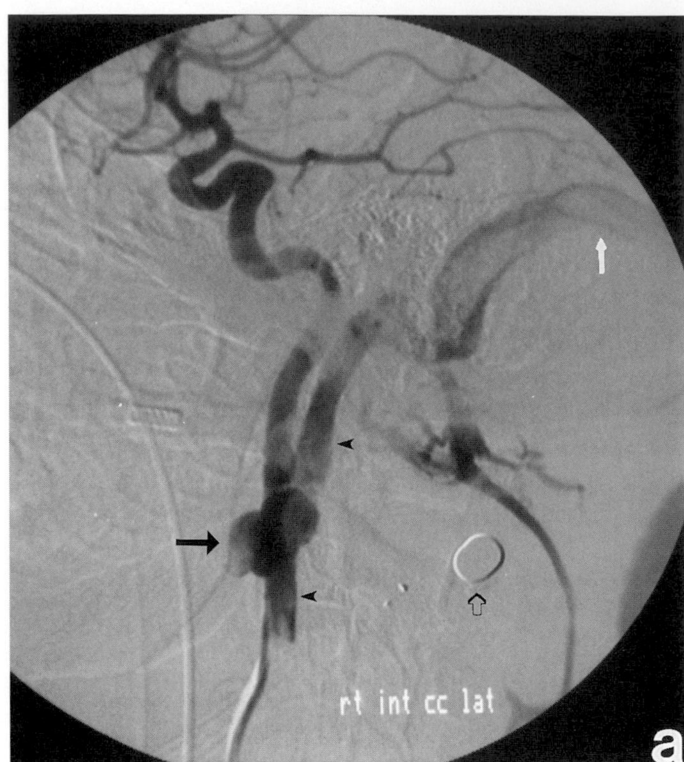

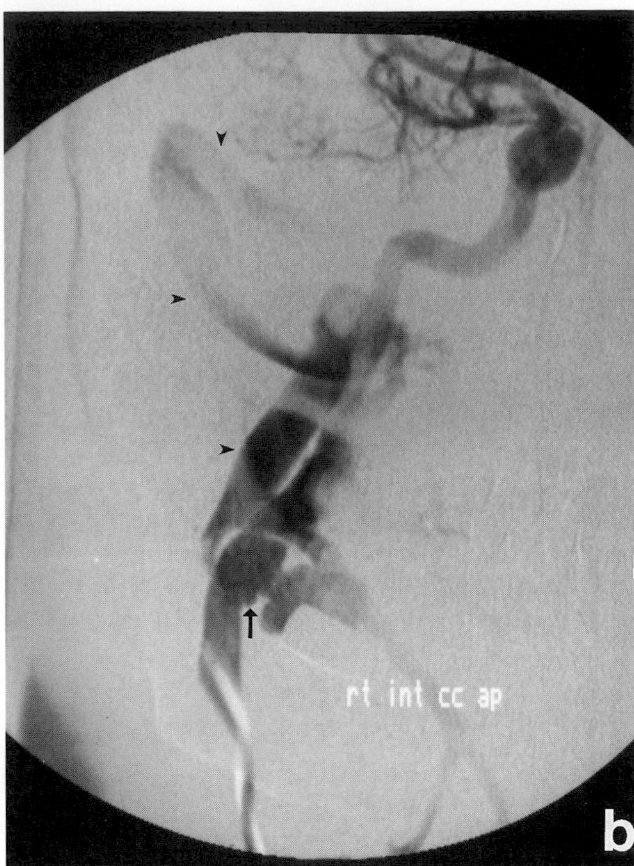

Figure 45-3. Carotid artery to jugular vein fistula following penetrating injury to the neck. This 25-year-old male sustained a gunshot wound to the neck. The bullet entered the right lateral neck at the level of the hyoid bone and fractured the lateral mass of C2. *A*. DSA, lateral projection, of the right internal carotid injection demonstrates the carotid-jugular fistula. There is an aneurysmal dilatation, or fistula, between the two vessels (*arrow*). There is antegrade and retrograde filling of the ipsilateral jugular vein (*arrowheads*). The retrograde filling continues rostrally to the level of the transverse sinus (*white arrow*). The bullet fragment is at the level of the spinous process of C2 (*clear arrow*). *B*. An AP view of the carotid artery to jugular vein fistula. Note the aneurysmal dilatation of the fistula (*arrow*). There is retrograde filling of the jugular vein, sigmoid sinus, and transverse sinus (*arrowheads*). (Courtesy of Christopher J. Moran, M.D., St. Louis, MO.)

Unfortunately, the diagnosis of vertebral artery dissection is usually considered only after vertebrobasilar ischemia has occurred. Once the diagnosis is suspected, angiography is suggested. Typical findings on angiography include stenosis, occlusion, pseudoaneurysm, and "double lumen,"[36,40] most commonly occurring at the V3 segment.[36]

Most patients with blunt vertebral artery injuries can be treated conservatively.[36,37,40] Anticoagulation is the preferred treatment, but subarachnoid hemorrhage from vertebral dissection must be excluded.[36] One study found no difference in outcome when either anticoagulation or antiplatelet drugs were used; however, the number of patients in that study was small.[40] In cases of failed conservative treatment, either surgical or endovascular occlusion of the affected artery can be attempted.[42] Some have stressed the need for both proximal and distal occlusion. In instances of bilateral involvement or inadequate collateral flow due to anomalous vessels, bypass can be considered.[30]

Mortality for blunt traumatic vertebral artery injury in one series was 21 percent[36]; however, other series have found much lower rates of unfavorable outcome.[37]

Penetrating Trauma

The majority of penetrating injuries to the vertebral arteries are caused by gunshot wounds. The patients are predominantly young males.

Vertebral artery injuries often are not apparent on presentation. Hemorrhage, if present, is often attributed to carotid artery injury. Because of the redundancies of the vertebrobasilar system, the injuries are usually neurologically asymptomatic.[44] In one series, 74 percent of patients presented with no signs of vertebral artery injury other than the presence of a penetrating neck wound and, in some, a stable hematoma. The remaining 26 percent, however, had an expanding hematoma or overt hemorrhage.[44] Seventy-two percent of these patients had injuries to other cervical structures. When the diagnosis is initially missed, the injury may later present as an enlarging neck mass or with symptoms of vertebrobasilar ischemia.[38]

When not precluded by hemorrhage or shock, angiography should be performed. A four-vessel study is needed to demonstrate any anomalies of the vertebral arteries and PICAs, and also to examine the distal segment of an occluded vertebral artery for evidence of arteriovenous fistula or pseudoaneurysm.[38] The vertebral venous plexus predisposes these injuries to the formation of arteriovenous fistulae. If missed initially, these lesions tend to enlarge by recruitment and become more difficult to treat.[38] The most common finding on angiography is occlusion of the injured vessel, although the angiographic lesions in one study did not always correlate with the findings at surgery.[44]

Conservative treatment consisting of anticoagulation or antiplatelet drugs can be employed in patients with minimal vessel wall abnormalities, normal flow, and no evidence of pseudoaneurysm.[44] Patients with total occlusion who are asymptomatic can also be treated conservatively, as long as the contralateral vertebral artery is normal and there is no evidence of arteriovenous fistula or pseudoaneurysm distal to the occlusion.[38] When angiography demonstrates pseudoaneurysm, arteriovenous fistula or other evidence of vessel wall disruption, treatment usually involves trapping the affected segment.[38,44,45] Proximal occlusion of the injured vessel alone is inadequate, since the distal segment can later develop an arteriovenous fistula or pseudoaneurysm.[38,44] Proximal and distal occlusion can often be performed endovascularly at the time of initial angiogram.[38,41,45] In cases where distal occlusion cannot be achieved endovascularly, surgery is indicated. Patients with symptoms of vertebrobasilar ischemia who have an anomalous contralateral vertebral artery or bilateral injuries may require arterial repair or bypass.[30,38]

Mortality associated with penetrating vertebral artery injury has been reported to be about 18 percent[26]; however, many deaths were attributable to concomitant injuries. One study reporting an overall mortality of 12 percent found that only 4.7 percent was attributable to the vertebral artery injury.[44]

INTRACRANIAL VASCULAR INJURIES

INTRACRANIAL INTERNAL CAROTID ARTERY LESIONS

NONPENETRATING TRAUMA

Injury to the intracranial carotid artery due to blunt trauma is rare. Patients are predominantly young males.[46] The exact incidence is unknown. Given that computed tomography (CT) has supplanted angiography for the acute evaluation of head trauma, it is likely that many instances of internal carotid artery injury are missed.

Intracranial internal carotid artery injuries can have a variety of causes, including fist-fights, motor vehicle accidents, sporting activities, and falls.[46–48] Arterial injury characteristically occurs in two anatomic settings. The first is in proximity to skull fractures. Fractures of the petrous temporal bone can injure the intracavernous or petrous carotid artery. The supraclinoid carotid can be injured in fractures of the cribriform plate and anterior clinoid process.[46] The second anatomic site involves transition points between mobile and immobile, or less mobile, carotid artery. These include the carotid canal entrance point, the point of dural penetration, and the point of attachment to the circle of Willis.[46] As with extracranial carotid artery injuries, pathology generally involves the intima. Intimal damage can produce thromboembolism, or dissection can develop, resulting in stenosis, occlusion, or progression of dissection to terminal branches.[46] Aneurysms can also develop following trauma, but will be discussed separately below.

In many patients the onset of symptoms following trauma is delayed.[46] About one-third experience ischemic symptoms immediately, another third have a delay of less than 24 hours, while the remainder experience a delay of days to weeks. Patients may experience headache prior to or at the onset of symptoms.[21] Signs of cerebral ischemia may be transient, or the patient may present with a completed stroke.[46]

Diagnosis requires a degree of clinical suspicion. Clues to vascular injury that should prompt angiography include a focal neurological deficit in an otherwise alert patient, deficit after minor head injury, focal deficit with basilar skull fracture, and neurological deficit not explained by findings on CT.[46]

Most authors advocate conservative treatment including anticoagulation unless contraindicated.[46–48] There may be a role for EC-IC bypass, particularly in cases of bilateral disease.[30,46]

The reported mortality of 60 percent may be high

owing to the number of postmortem diagnoses compared with the number of missed diagnoses.[46] Nevertheless, these lesions have the potential for catastrophic sequelae, including severe permanent neurological deficits and death.

Carotid-Cavernous Fistulae

Direct carotid-cavernous (C-C) fistula is the most common injury to the intracranial internal carotid artery.

C-C fistulae can occur following both penetrating and nonpenetrating trauma, but are more often a result of blunt trauma.[43] Traumatic C-C fistulae are of the direct type (Barrow type A—see Table 45-1), with flow from the internal carotid artery directly into the cavernous sinus.[10,50] Venous drainage is usually through the superior ophthalmic vein, the petrosal sinuses, and the pterygoid venous plexus, but may involve cortical veins, causing venous hypertension and risk of hemorrhage[10] (Fig. 45-4). Venous hypertension involving the cavernous sinus and the superior ophthalmic vein can lead to impairment of cranial nerves II, III, IV, or VI. Serious complications of C-C fistulae include cerebral ischemia from vascular steal, subarachnoid hemorrhage, loss of vision, and parenchymal hemorrhage secondary to venous hypertension and severe epistaxis.[10,43]

Patients usually present with symptoms of raised intraorbital pressure. These include chemosis, proptosis, diplopia, headache, and decreased visual acuity.[10,43] Multiple cranial nerve deficits may be present on examination. Ocular bruits are frequently present.

Diagnosis can be made on the basis of the characteristic clinical findings described above. Angiography should be performed to define the fistulous communication, as well as to identify abnormal drainage through cortical veins. These lesions are often well visualized on MRI; however, angiography is superior for planning treatment as most traumatic fistulae will be treated endovascularly.

TABLE 45-1 Barrow Classification of Carotid-Cavernous Fistulas*

Category	Definition
Type A	Direct high flow fistulas resulting from a tear between the internal carotid artery and the cavernous sinus. Usually traumatic.
Type B	Dural shunts between meningeal branches of the internal carotid artery and the cavernous sinus. Spontaneous.
Type C	Dural shunts between meningeal branches of the external carotid artery and the cavernous sinus. Spontaneous.
Type D	Dural shunts between meningeal branches of both the internal and external carotid arteries and the cavernous sinus. Spontaneous.

SOURCE: Barrow et al.[49]

Traumatic C-C fistulae are less likely to spontaneously resolve than indirect fistulae.[51,52] Surgical treatment involves trapping the fistula by occlusion of the internal carotid artery in the neck and intracranially. Because the ophthalmic artery is often unavoidably included in the trapped segment, this procedure may be associated with blindness in the ipsilateral eye.[10,43] Newer endovascular techniques, which permit selective occlusion of the fistula with preservation of the internal carotid and ophthalmic arteries[10,50,51] have now become the treatment methods of choice. The lesion can be approached through the internal carotid artery, the inferior petrosal sinus, or the superior ophthalmic vein. Surgery need only be used for lesions in which endovascular treatment has failed.[50]

Outcome following treatment of C-C fistulae is generally favorable, with one series of more than 200 cases treated endovascularly reporting complete closure of the fistula in 99 percent of cases, with a 5 percent rate of complications consisting primarily of strokes and symptomatic pseudoaneurysms.[32,43]

Other Intracranial Vascular Injuries

Traumatic Intracranial Aneurysms

Traumatic intracranial aneurysms are uncommon lesions. Benoit and Wortzman reported that only 4 of 850 aneurysms in their series were traumatic in origin.[53] One series found an incidence of 3.2 percent among civilian victims of penetrating head trauma.[54] These lesions are found predominantly in young males,[55] perhaps reflecting their relative number in the head injury population.

These lesions have been reported in blunt trauma as a result of assault, motor vehicle accidents, falls, iatrogenic injury, and in association with penetrating trauma, primarily gunshot wounds.[54,56] Blunt mechanisms predominate in adults, accounting for 60 to 70 percent of the cases.[54,55] Aneurysms are classified as true, false (pseudo-), or mixed, depending on the degree of medial or adventitial disruption. True aneurysms have an intact adventitia, whereas the wall of a pseudoaneurysm is formed by hematoma.[56] A mixed aneurysm occurs when a true aneurysm ruptures and forms a pseudoaneurysm. Most traumatic aneurysms are pseudoaneurysms.[55] Unlike nontraumatic aneurysms, these lesions usually do not involve branching points,[56] instead occurring more peripherally along the course of the artery. They also have a greater tendency to rupture.[54] Ninety-four per-

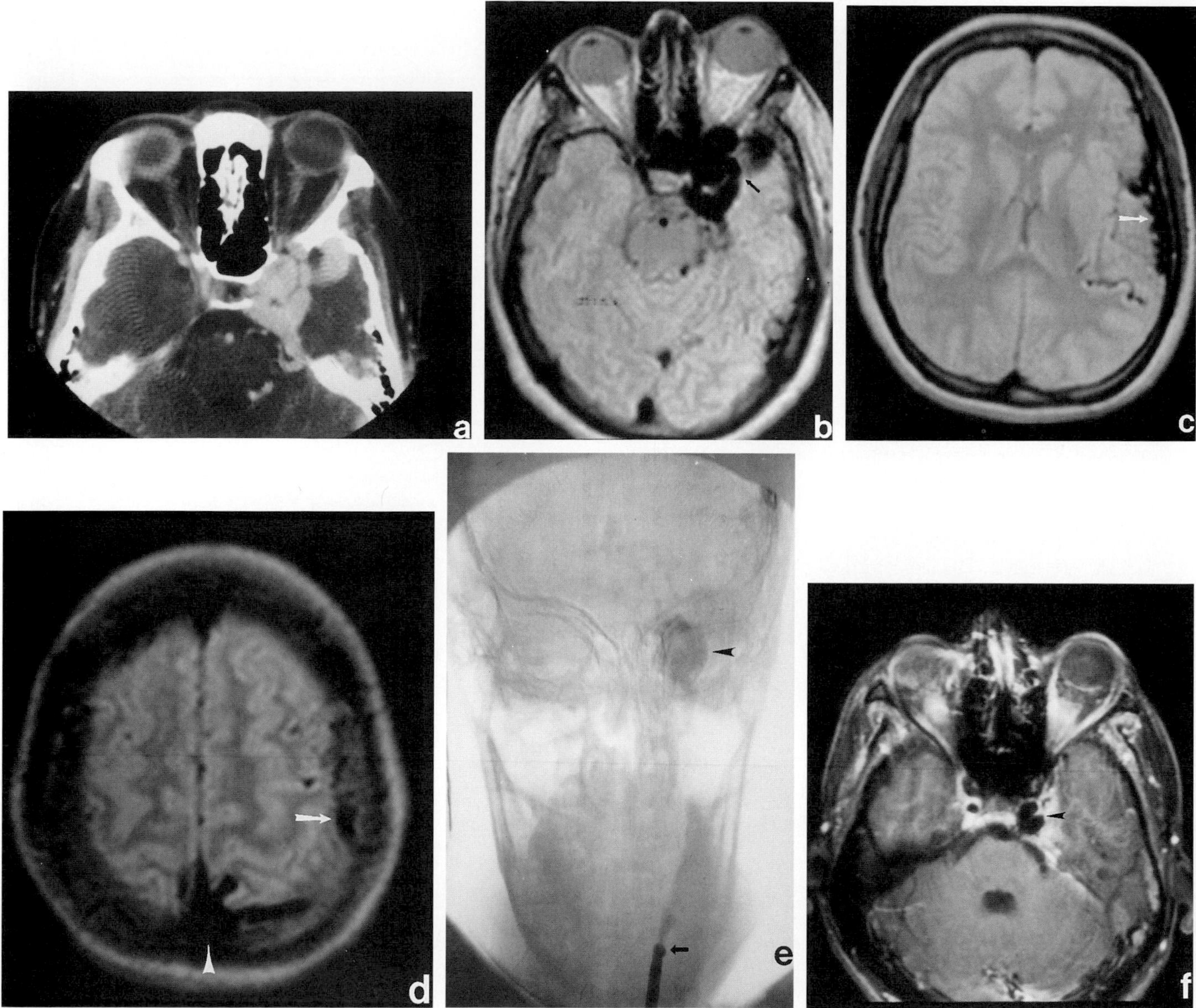

Figure 45-4. Delayed carotid-cavernous (C-C) fistula following a motor vehicle accident. This 32-year-old female was involved in a motor vehicle accident approximately 2 years prior to the onset of a headache associated with an intracranial bruit. A work-up was performed. *A*. An enhanced axial CT scan of the brain demonstrates large, tortuous vessels in the left anterior temporal region. *B*. Proton density weighted MRI of the brain shows the extensive flow voids of the fistula (*arrow*). *C*., *D*. Rostral images of the same MR scan show serpiginous flow voids over the left cerebral cortex (*arrows*). These vessels represent the cortical venous drainage of the fistula. The veins drain into the superior sagittal sinus (*arrowhead in D*). *E*. A subtracted AP carotid angiogram of the fistula demonstrates the high flow lesion projecting over the left orbit. Note the injection of dye in the internal carotid artery just above the bifurcation (*arrow*). The difficulty opacifying the fistula (*arrowhead*) is secondary to the high flow through the lesion. The fistula was treated with balloon occlusion. The patient's symptoms resolved. *F*. A second C-C fistula is demonstrated in this MRI scan of the brain.

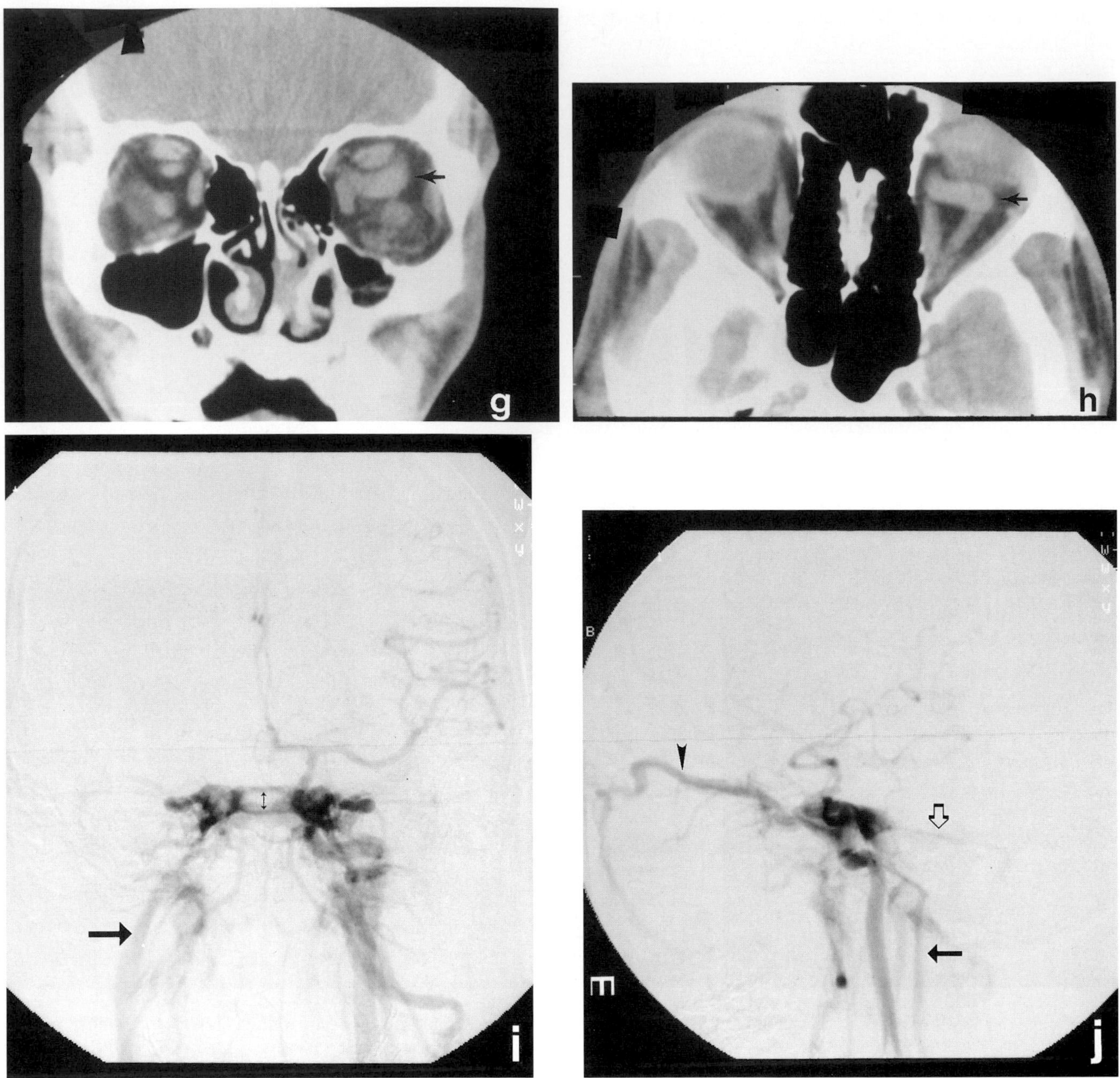

A smaller flow void is seen in the region of the cavernous sinus on the left (*arrowhead*). *G., H.* CT scans from this second case in the coronal (*G*) and axial (*H*) views demonstrate a dilated superior ophthalmic vein (arrows) commonly seen in C-C fistulas. *I., J.* AP (*I*) and lateral (*J*) angiographic images of a third C-C fistula. The left internal carotid artery injection fills the ipsilateral and contralateral cavernous sinuses, via the circular sinuses (*double-headed arrow*). The jugular vein (*arrows*) fills via drainage of the inferior petrosal sinus (*clear arrow*). There is drainage anteriorly (see *J*) into the superior ophthalmic vein (*arrowhead*) and subsequently into the facial vein. (Courtesy of Miles B. Koby, M.D., St. Louis, MO.)

cent of these lesions are associated with other serious intracranial pathology,[55] which in many instances is the most important factor determining outcome. In penetrating injury, direct trauma is the usual cause of these aneurysms, which then occur adjacent to the injured brain.[55] In blunt trauma, damage can be caused by movement of the brain, resulting in compression of arteries against relatively fixed structures.[55] Thus, the pericallosal artery can be injured by the edge of the falx, the middle cerebral artery by the sphenoidal edge, and the supraclinoid carotid by the anterior clinoid process[55] (Fig. 45-5).

Traumatic intracranial aneurysms usually occur with severe head injury. Onset of symptoms, most commonly due to aneurysmal rupture, frequently follows a delay ranging from 5 days to 10 years, with a mean interval of 21 days.[55]

Clinical suspicion for a traumatic aneurysm should be raised in instances of delayed deterioration following head injury, delayed intracranial hemorrhage, or vigorous arterial bleeding during hematoma removal. Angiography is usually required to make the diagnosis. Angiographic features of traumatic aneurysms differ from those of congenital aneurysms. As stated previously, they tend to be more peripheral and do not usually involve arterial bifurcation. Also, there is often no neck. Delayed filling and emptying are also characteristic.[56]

When diagnosed, traumatic aneurysms should be treated surgically, as conservative management carries a 50 percent mortality rate.[56] Because of the lack of a neck and their peripheral location, these lesions are usually treated with trapping or excision rather than clipping.

The surgical mortality for these lesions is 24 percent versus 50 percent for conservative treatment.[56] Poor outcome is often a result of associated cerebral injury or infarction in the distribution of the involved vessel.

Vasospasm

The incidence of vasospasm in nonpenetrating head injury has ranged in reports from 5 to 41 percent.[57] This wide variation can be attributed to differences in injury severity, in timing of angiography, and in the definition of vasospasm used.[57] The incidence of vasospasm in one series of penetrating injuries with subarachnoid hemorrhage evident on CT scan was 16 percent.[54]

Post-traumatic vasospasm, like that seen following aneurysmal hemorrhage, correlates with the amount of subarachnoid blood,[58] and similarly is felt to be related to the direct effects of blood and its decomposition products on the artery.[59,60] Post-traumatic vasospasm, however, may follow a different time course for development and resolution. Weber et al., following patients with transcranial Doppler, found that post-traumatic vasospasm tended to develop earlier, after about 48 hours.[57] Another series, also employing TCD, distinguished two different patterns of vasospasm.[61] The first was associated with SAH and was similar in time course and severity to that seen with aneurysmal rupture. The second pattern was not associated with SAH and tended to be short-lived, with a mean duration of 1.25 days (see Fig. 45-2*B*).[61] Although post-traumatic vasospasm has been described primarily in association with the anterior cerebral circulation, Marshall et al. reported six cases of vertebrobasilar vasospasm that significantly contributed to neurological deficit. Surprisingly, all but one of these patients had clear ventricular cerebrospinal fluid.[62]

The diagnosis of post-traumatic vasospasm should be considered in head injury patients with significant SAH. Diagnosis can be confirmed with serial TCD measurements or with angiography.

The treatment of post-traumatic vasospasm can be problematic. The accepted treatment for vasospasm due to aneurysmal subarachnoid hemorrhage, consisting of hypervolemia, hypertension, and hemodilution,[60] has not been proved to be clearly effective in post-traumatic vasospasm and is complicated in trauma patients who frequently have intracranial hypertension. The use of nimodipine may have a beneficial effect in post-traumatic vasospasm,[63] but further study is needed to prove its efficacy.

The presence of ischemic lesions corresponding to the territories of vessels demonstrating vasospasm has led some to conclude that post-traumatic vasospasm has a definite adverse effect on outcome.[57,61,64] Statistically, this correlation has been more difficult to demonstrate. Vasospasm has been shown to correlate with the amount of subarachnoid blood, and subarachnoid blood is associated with poor outcome, but post-traumatic vasospasm has not been shown to be independently predictive of outcome.[57,61] Thus, the exact role of post-traumatic vasospasm requires further elucidation.

Dural sinus injuries

The exact incidence of dural sinus injury is highly dependent on the population examined. In wartime situations incidence has been reported to be 4 to 12 percent of penetrating craniocerebral trauma.[65,66] whereas the incidence in civilian populations is lower, around 1 percent.[65] One study with a preponderance of blunt trauma found a 4 percent incidence of dural sinus injury.[65] The mean age in this group was 35 years, and the patients were predominantly male.[65]

The dural sinuses can be injured in both penetrating trauma, primarily gunshot wounds, and blunt trauma, including motor vehicle accidents, falls, and assaults (Fig. 45-6). Trauma can result in thrombosis, laceration, or transection of the sinus, or it can lead to the develop-

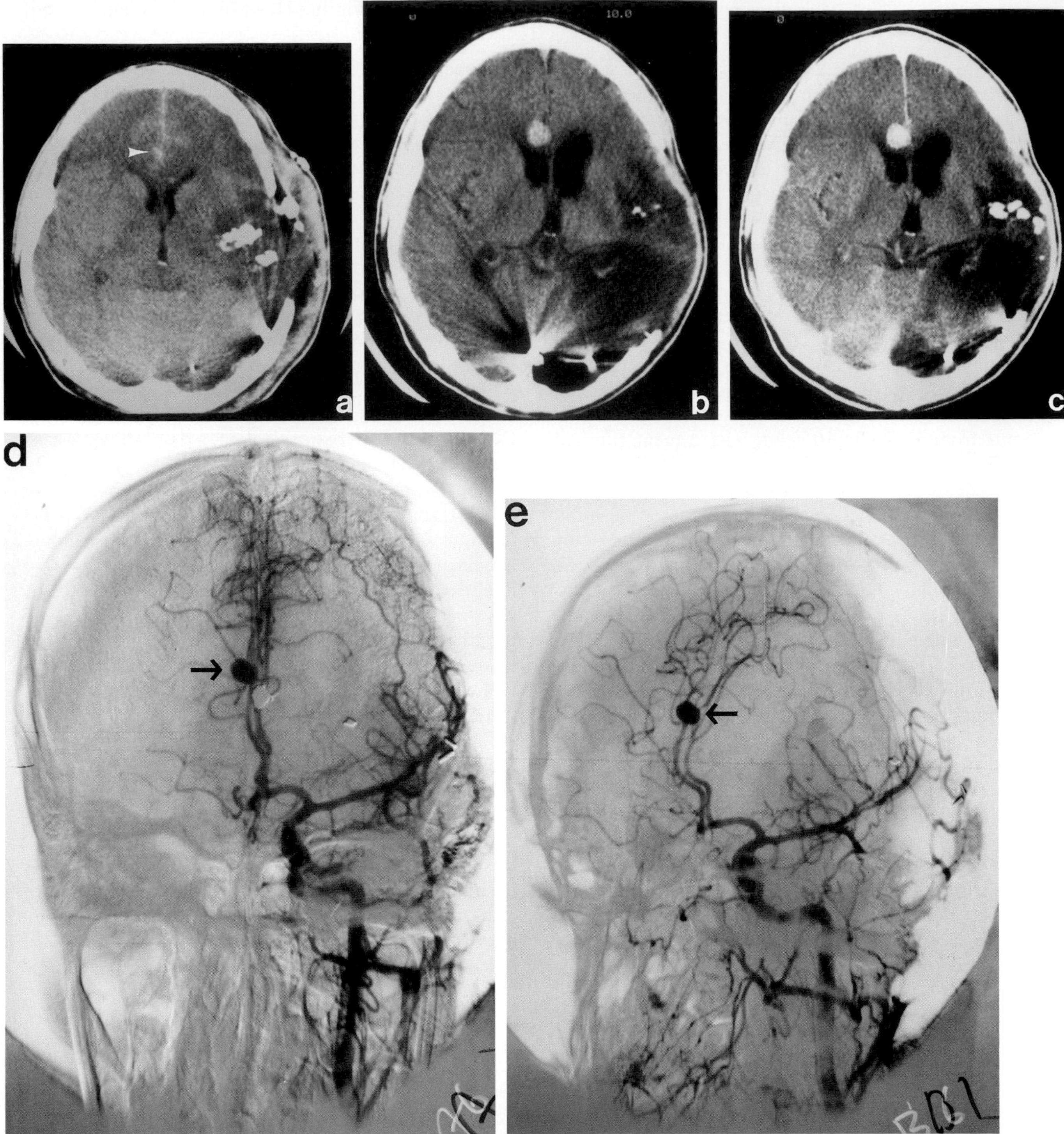

Figure 45-5. Post-traumatic intracranial aneurysm formation, secondary to penetrating injury to the cranium. This 17-year-old male sustained a gunshot wound to the left temporal region. He underwent craniotomy and partial debridement of the necrotic tissue. *A*. An axial CT scan of the head demonstrates postoperative changes along with some retained bone fragments. There is marked edema in the left temporal region. A focal area of high density in the interhemispheric fissure anterior to the right frontal horn of the ventricle is noted (*arrowhead*). *B*., *C*. A follow-up CT scan was performed eight months later. Unenhanced (*B*) and enhanced CT scans (*C*) show the enlarging interhemispheric lesion, which takes up intravenous contrast. *D*., *E*. An AP (*D*) and oblique (*E*) subtracted cerebral angiogram demonstrate a post-traumatic aneurysm of the pericallosal artery on the right (*arrow*). Bullet fragments are present. The patient underwent surgical clipping without sequelae. (Courtesy of Miles B. Koby, M.D., St. Louis, MO.)

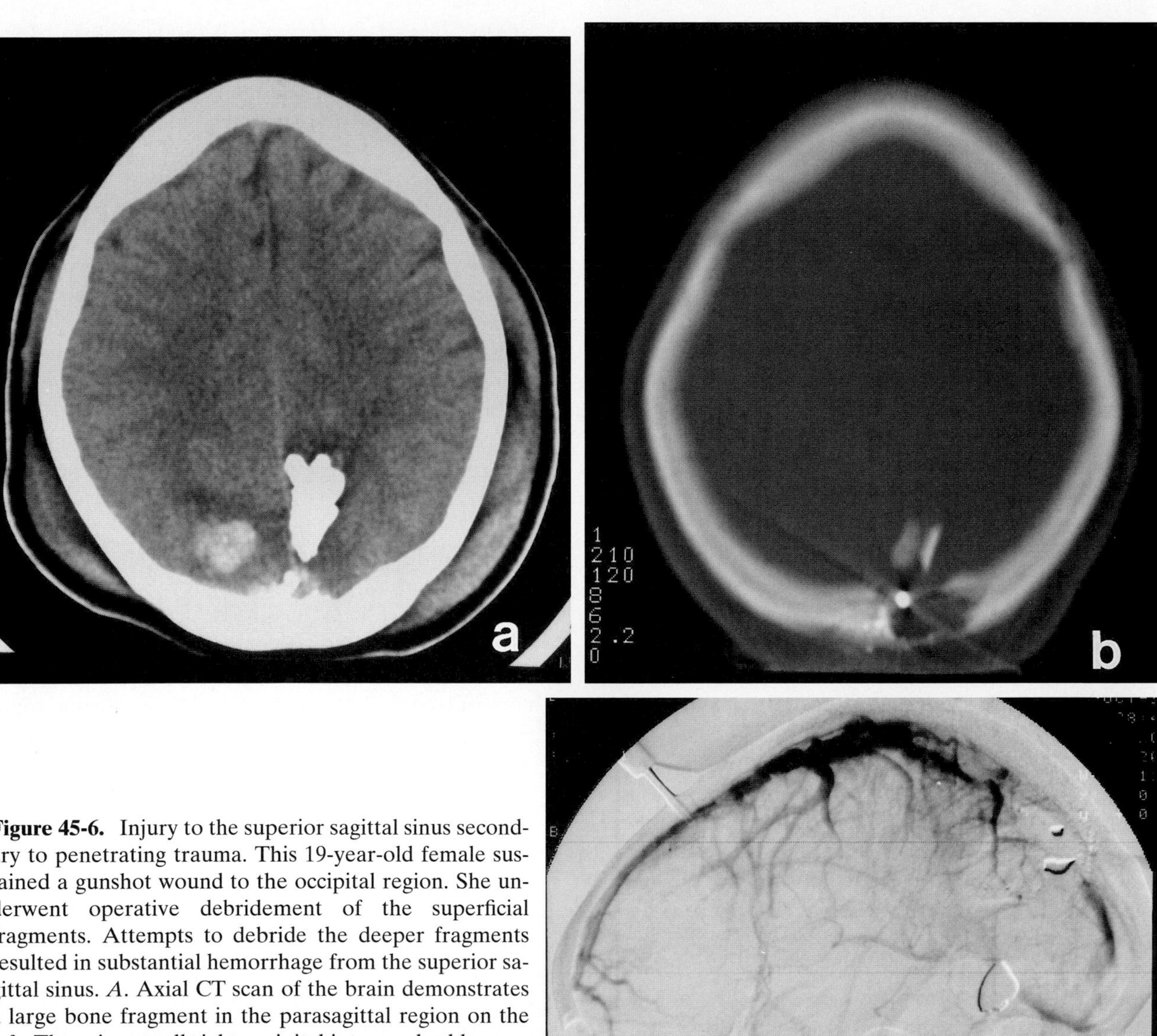

Figure 45-6. Injury to the superior sagittal sinus secondary to penetrating trauma. This 19-year-old female sustained a gunshot wound to the occipital region. She underwent operative debridement of the superficial fragments. Attempts to debride the deeper fragments resulted in substantial hemorrhage from the superior sagittal sinus. *A*. Axial CT scan of the brain demonstrates a large bone fragment in the parasagittal region on the left. There is a small right occipital intracerebral hemorrhage. *B*. A bone window of the CT scan shows a superficial bullet fragment with a deeper bone fragment in the parasagittal region. *C*. A lateral cerebral angiogram in the venous phase illustrates a 5-cm defect of the superior sagittal sinus. There is retrograde filling of cortical veins draining the sinus. Multiple bullet fragments are present in the occipital region.

ment of a dural arteriovenous fistula. In penetrating trauma, laceration or transection of the sinus can result in life-threatening hemorrhage, subdural hematoma, or progressive thrombosis.[66] In blunt trauma, thrombosis can occur by a number of mechanisms. First, there is a high incidence of associated skull fracture, which often is depressed.[67] This can produce traumatic rifts that occlude the sinus or can damage the endothelium, leading to thrombosis.[67] Occlusion also can result from sinus compression due to edema or bleeding or from extension of thrombus from damaged emissary veins.[67] Even in the absence of skull fracture, thrombosis can result from coagulopathy or secondary to intramural hemorrhages caused by rupture of small sinusoids.[67,68]

Once obstruction of a dural sinus has occurred, symptoms depend largely on the exact location of the occlusion. If occlusion occurs in the anterior superior sagittal sinus or in a nondominant transverse sinus, the patient may have no symptoms referable to the sinus injury. If, however, significant venous outflow obstruction occurs, venous engorgement can result in increased intracranial pressure, cerebral edema, and hydrocephalus.[68,69] Propagation of thrombus from the sinus into cortical veins can produce venous infarction.[68]

Dural arteriovenous fistula is thought to result from damage to adjacent meningeal vessels, usually in close proximity to a skull fracture.[70] Recruitment can involve meningeal, cortical, or scalp vessels.[70] Although these lesions are often asymptomatic and can regress spontaneously, neurological deficit can result from ischemia due to vascular steal, from hydrocephalus due to increased superior sagittal sinus pressure, or from increased intracranial pressure due to venous hypertension.[70]

Dural sinus injuries often present in severe head injury, whether penetrating or nonpenetrating. In instances of penetrating trauma, hemorrhage from the wound may be apparent. Otherwise, symptoms may be difficult to attribute to the sinus injury alone. Penetrating injuries to the middle one-third of the sagittal sinus are sometimes associated with spastic paresis of the legs, while cortical blindness can be seen with trauma to the posterior one-third.[66] In both blunt and penetrating trauma, sinus injury can present as subdural hematoma.[65] In nonpenetrating trauma, sinus thrombosis may be missed initially or may occur in a delayed fashion. In those cases the injury may be asymptomatic or the patient may present secondarily with delayed or persistent headache, vomiting, papilledema, ataxia, or confusion.[67,68] Traumatic dural arteriovenous fistulae frequently are asymptomatic initially, presenting after an interval as long as months to years.[70] Many of these close spontaneously, but otherwise can present with headache, dementia, bruit, or neurological deficit produced by the mechanisms discussed above.[70]

In penetrating trauma, the site of injury, including entrance and exit wounds and missile tracts of gunshot wounds, usually prompts consideration of a dural sinus injury. In cases of blunt trauma, skull films will frequently demonstrate fracture, often depressed, crossing the injured sinus. CT may demonstrate hyperdensity in thrombosed sinuses,[67] but because of the plane of imaging, injuries to the superior sagittal and transverse sinuses may be missed. MRI may demonstrate dural sinus injury more reliably, but is not generally employed in the evaluation of head trauma. Sinus injury should be considered in instances of unexplained intracranial hypertension or severe edema, as well as in cases of delayed or persistent headache, vomiting, papilledema, or ataxia. When the patient's condition permits, angiography should be considered. Even in cases of penetrating trauma, angiography can be helpful in determining the extent of injury. In blunt trauma, the exact site of thrombosis may not be known without angiography. Caution is necessary in interpreting the angiogram, however, since several anatomic variants can occur, including an absent or hypoplastic transverse sinus, usually on the left.[71] If arteriovenous fistula is suspected, angiography is essential for defining involved vessels.[70]

Treatment of dural sinus injuries depends largely on the location of the injury and the condition of the patient. Treatment can include conservative management, ligation, or repair. Although some suggest that the anterior one-half of the superior sagittal sinus can be occluded safely, others feel that only the anterior one-third is safe, whereas the middle one-third carries risk, and the posterior one-third should never be ligated.[69] Also, a nondominant transverse sinus can often be occluded without problem; however, determining dominance angiographically in the presence of unilateral occlusion can be difficult.[69]

Regardless of location, many authors recommend repair whenever possible.[65,69] Repair of sinuses can be complicated owing to active bleeding from the sinus, the risk of air embolism, and the presence of numerous bridging veins along the course of the sinuses. In addition, occlusion on the sinus during surgery can result in excessive brain swelling. In cases of simple laceration, direct suture repair of the sinus is often possible. Avulsion of a wall of the sinus may require patching, which can be accomplished using autologous saphenous vein graft.[66,69,72] Control of bleeding often can be achieved with simple digital pressure on the sinus.[66] Some authors have advocated the use of a shunt during repair to prevent venous stasis and to decrease intraoperative blood loss.[66,69,72] Removal of thrombus can be achieved by digital expulsion, gentle suction, or by use of a Fogarty catheter.[66,69]

Treatment of traumatic dural arteriovenous fistulae can be complicated. Many of these lesions close spontaneously, so an initial conservative approach may be warranted. However, because these lesions can grow by recruitment and can eventually produce neurological deficits, treatment is necessary for those that do not regress. Ligation of proximal feeders alone is generally inadequate since collateral flow will usually develop.[70] Radical isolation of the sinus is advocated by some, and may require resection of a portion of the sinus.[70] Because of the alteration in venous drainage secondary to high sinus pressures in longstanding fistulae, sacrifice of the sinus in these instances may not carry the usual risks.[70] This also argues for an initially conservative approach.[73]

Outcome from dural sinus injuries varies considerably depending on the population studied. Factors affecting outcome include the location of the sinus injury and the extent of coexisting cerebral injury. As expected, most studies demonstrate significantly higher mortality for injuries involving the posterior superior sagittal sinus compared with those to the anterior superior sagittal sinus.[65,68,74] Exact mortality rates vary significantly among studies, reflecting differences in populations as well as improvements in operative techniques. For example, Meirowski reported mortality associated with dural sinus injuries during the Korean conflict to be 11.6 percent.[74] Kapp et al., reporting on dural sinus injuries during the Vietnam war, found a mortality of 27 percent from 1968 to 1970 as compared to 6 percent from 1971 to 1972 following introduction of vein grafting and sinus shunting.[69] In many cases, mortality is due to concomitant cerebral injury. Patients without severe cerebral injury tend to have good outcomes.[66] In patients with delayed thrombosis of a sinus following mild head injury, complete resolution of symptoms often occurs as a result of recanalization of the sinus.[67] Thus, although dural sinus injuries are associated with significant morbidity and mortality, the overall outlook for many patients is favorable.

ACKNOWLEDGMENTS

We would like to thank Miles B. Koby, M.D., for his assistance in reviewing the radiographs in this manuscript.

References

1. Rubio PA, Ruel JG Jr, Beall AC Jr, et al: Acute carotid artery injury: 25 years experience. *J Trauma* 1974; 14:967.
2. Krajewski LP, Hertzer NR: Blunt carotid artery trauma: Report of two cases and review of the literature. *Ann Surg* 1980; 191:341–346.
3. Davis JW, Holbrook TL, Hoyt DB, et al: Blunt carotid artery dissection: Incidence, associated injuries, screening, and treatment. *J Trauma* 1990; 30:1514–1517.
4. Fry WJ, Fry RE: Extracranial carotid artery injuries. *Surgery* 1980; 88:581–586.
5. Zelenock GB, Kazmers A, Whitehouse WM, et al: Extracranial internal carotid artery dissections. *Arch Surg* 1982; 117:425–432.
6. Watridge CB, Muhlbauer MS, Lowery RD: Traumatic carotid artery dissection: Diagnosis and treatment. *J Neurosurg* 1989; 71:854–857.
7. Mokri B, Piepgras DG, Houser OW: Traumatic dissections of the extracranial internal carotid artery. *J Neurosurg* 1988; 68:189–197.
8. Martin RF, Eldrup-Jorgensen J, Clark DE, Bredenberg CE: Blunt trauma to the carotid arteries. *J Vasc Surg* 1991; 14:789–795.
9. Stringer WL, Kelly DL: Traumatic dissection of the extracranial internal carotid artery. *Neurosurgery* 1980; 6:123–130.
10. O'Sullivan RM, Graeb DA, Nugent RA, et al: Carotid and vertebral artery trauma: Clinical and angiographic features. *Australas Radiol* 1991; 35:47–55.
11. Fakhry SM, Jacques PF, Proctor HJ: Cervical vessel injury after blunt trauma. *J Vasc Surg* 1988; 8:501–508.
12. Jernigan WR, Gardner WC: Carotid artery injuries due to closed cervical trauma. *J Trauma* 1971; 11:429–435.
13. Batzdorf U, Bentson JR, Machleder HI: Blunt trauma to the high cervical carotid artery. *Neurosurgery* 1979; 5:195–201.
14. Hughes JT, Brownell B: Traumatic thrombosis of the internal carotid artery in the neck. *J Neurol Neurosurg Psychiatry* 1968; 31:307–314.
15. Sullivan HG, Vines FS, Becker DP: Sequelae of indirect carotid injury. *Radiology* 1973; 109:91–98.
16. Sundt TM Jr., Pearson BW, Piepgras DG, et al: Surgical management of aneurysms of the distal extracranial internal carotid artery. *J Neurosurg* 1986; 64:169–182.
17. Batnitzky S, Price HI, Holden RW, et al: Cervical internal carotid artery injuries due to blunt trauma. *AJNR* 1983; 4:292–295.
18. Batjer HH, Giller CA, Kopitnik TA, et al: Intracranial and cervical vascular injuries, in Cooper PR (ed): *Head Injury,* 3d ed. Baltimore: Williams & Wilkins, 1993: 373–404.
19. Yamada S, Kindt GW, Youmans JR: Carotid artery occlusion due to nonpenetrating injury. *J Trauma* 1967; 7:333–342.
20. Mokri B: Traumatic and spontaneous extracranial internal carotid artery dissections. *J Neurol* 1990; 237:356–361.
21. Hart RG, Easton JD: Dissections of cervical and cerebral arteries. *Neurol Clin* 1983; 1(1):155–182.
22. Gelbert F, Assouline E, Hodes JE, et al: MRI in spontaneous dissection of vertbral and carotid arteries. *Neuroradiology* 1991; 33:111–113.
23. Nelson JR, Boundy KL: Magnetic resonance imaging in carotid dissection. *Australas Radiol* 1992; 36:40–43.
24. Padberg F: Comment following Martin RF, Eldrup-Jorgensien J, Clark DE, Bredenberg CE: Blunt trauma to the carotid arteries. *J Vasc Surg* 1991; 14:789–795.
25. Müllges W, Ringelstein EB, Leibold M: Non-invasive diagnosis of internal carotid artery dissections. *J Neurol Neurosurg Psychiatry* 1992; 55:98–103.
26. Pierce WH, Whitehill TA: Carotid and vertebral arterial injuries. *Surg Clin North Am* 1988; 68:705–723.
27. Wylie EJ, Hein MF, Adams JE: Intracranial hemorrhage following surgical revascularization for treatment of acute strokes. *J Neurosurg* 21:212–215.
28. Richardson JD, Simpson C, Miller FB: Management of carotid artery trauma. *Surgery* 1988; 104:673–680.
29. Fein JM, Flamm E: Planned intracranial revascularization before proximal ligation for traumatic aneurysm. *Neurosurgery* 1979; 5:254–258.
30. Morgan MK, Sekhon LH: Extracranial-intracranial saphenous vein bypass for carotid or vertebral artery dissections: A report of six cases. *J Neurosurg* 1994; 80:337–346.
31. Mokri B, Piepgras DG, Sundt TM, et al: Extracranial internal carotid artery aneurysms. *Mayo Clin Proc* 1982; 57:310–321.
32. Higashida RT, Halbach VV, Tsai FY, et al: Interventional neurovascular treatment of traumatic carotid and vertebral artery lesions: Results in 234 cases. *AJR* 1989; 153:577–582.
33. Rao PM, Ivatury RR, Sharma P, et al: Cervical vascular injuries: A trauma center experience. *Surgery* 1993; 114:527–531.
34. Menawat SS, Dennis JW, Laneve LM, Frykberg ER: Are arteriograms necessary in penetration zone II neck injuries? *J Vasc Surg* 1992; 16:397–401.

35. Liekweg WG, Greenfield LJ: Management of penetrating carotid arterial injuries. *Ann Surg* 1978; 188:587–592.
36. Hinse P, Thie A, Lachenmayer L: Dissection of the extracranial vertebral artery: Report of four cases and review of the literature. *J Neurol Neurosurg Psychiatry* 1991; 54:863–869.
37. Mas JL, Bousser MG, Hasboun D, Laplane D: Extracranial vertebral artery dissections: A review of 13 cases. *Stroke* 1987; 18:1037–1047.
38. Golueke P, Sclafani S, Phillips T, et al: Vertebral artery injury: Diagnosis and management. *J Trauma* 1987; 27:856–865.
39. Schwarz M, Buchinger W, Gaudernak T, et al: Injuries to the cervical spine causing vertebral artery trauma: Case reports. *J Trauma* 1991; 31:127–133.
40. Josien E: Extracranial vertebral artery dissection: Nine cases. *J Neurol* 1992; 239:327–330.
41. Davis JM, Zimmerman RA: Injury of the carotid and vertebral arteries. *Neuroradiology* 1983; 25:55–69.
42. Halbach VV, Higashida RT, Dowd CF, et al: Endovascular treatment of vertebral artery dissections and pseudoaneurysms. *J Neurosurg* 1993; 79:183–191.
43. Halbach VV, Higashida RT, Hieshima GB: Interventional neuroradiology. *AJR* 1989; 153:467–476.
44. Reid JD, Weigelt JA: Forty-three cases of vertebral artery trauma. *J Trauma* 1988; 28:1007–1012.
45. Blickenstaff KL, Weaver FA, Yellin AE, et al: Trends in the management of traumatic vertebral artery injuries. *Am J Surg* 1989; 158:101–106.
46. Morgan MK, Besser M, Johnston I, Chaseling R: Intracranial carotid artery injury in closed head trauma. *J Neurosurg* 1987; 66:192–197.
47. Pozzati E, Gaist G, Servadei F: Traumatic aneurysms of the supraclinoid internal carotid artery. *J Neurosurg* 1982; 57:418–422.
48. Ajir F, Tibbetts JC: Post-traumatic occlusion of the supraclinoid internal carotid artery. *Neurosurgery* 1981; 9:173–176.
49. Barrow DL, Spector RH, Braun IF, et al: Classification and treatment of spontaneous carotid-cavernous sinus fistulas. *J Neurosurg* 1985; 62:248–256.
50. Debrun GM, Viñuela F, Fox AJ, et al: Indications for treatment and classification of 132 carotid-cavernous fistulas. *Neurosurgery* 1988; 22:285–289.
51. Rambo WM, Simpson RK: Carotid-cavernous sinus fistula complicating shotgun injuries to the head. *Neurochir* 1993; 36:96–100.
52. Mullan S: Carotid-cavernous fistulas and intracavernous aneurysms, in Wilkins RH, Rengachary SS (eds): *Neurosurgery.* New York: McGraw-Hill, 1985: 1483–1494.
53. Benoit BG, Wortzman G: Traumatic cerebral aneurysms: Clinical features and natural history. *J Neurol Neurosurg Psychiatry* 1973; 36:127–138.
54. Levy ML, Rezai A, Masri LS, et al: The significance of subarachnoid hemorrhage after penetrating craniocerebral injury: Correlations with angiography and outcome in a civilian population. *Neurosurgery* 1993; 32:532–540.
55. Asari S, Nakamura S, Yamada O, et al: Traumatic aneurysm of peripheral cerebral arteries: Report of two cases. *J Neurosurg* 1977; 46:795–803.
56. Parkinson D, West M: Traumatic intracranial aneurysms. *J Neurosurg* 1980; 52:11–20.
57. Weber M, Grolimund P, Seiler RW: Evaluation of posttraumatic cerebral blood flow velocities by transcranial Doppler ultrasonography. *Neurosurgery* 1990; 27: 106–112.
58. Steiger HJ, Aaslid R, Stooss R, Seiler RW: Transcranial Doppler monitoring in head injury: Relations between type of injury, flow velocities, vasoreactivity, and outcome. *Neurosurgery* 1994; 34:79–86.
59. Muttaqin Z, Kazunori A, Uozumi T, et al: Vasospasm after traumatic subarachnoid haemorrhage: Transcranial Doppler evaluation: Case report. *Neurosurg Rev* 1991; 14:321–325.
60. Kassell NF, Peerless SJ, Durward QJ, et al: Treatment of ischemic deficits from vasospasm with intravascular volume expansion and induced arterial hypertension. *Neurosurgery* 1982; 11:337–343.
61. Martin NA, Doberstein C, Zane C, et al: Posttraumatic cerebral arterial spasm: Transcranial Doppler ultrasound, cerebral blood flow, and angiographic findings. *J Neurosurg* 1992; 77:575–583.
62. Marshall LF, Bruce DA, Bruno L, Langfitt TW: Vertebrobasilar spasm: A significant cause of neurological deficit in head injury. *J Neurosurg* 1978; 48:560–564.
63. Kostron H, Rumpl E, Stampfl G, et al: Treatment of cerebral vasospasm following severe head injury with the calcium influx blocker nimodipine. *Neurochir* 1985; 28:103–109.
64. MacPherson P, Graham DI: Arterial spasm and slowing of the cerebral circulation in the ischaemia of head injury. *J Neurol Neurosurg Psychiatry* 1973; 36:1069–1072.
65. Meier U, Gärtner F, Knopf W, et al: The traumatic dural sinus injury: A clinical study. *Acta Neurochir* 1992; 119:91–93.
66. Rish BL: The repair of dural venous sinus wounds by autogenous venorrhaphy. *J Neurosurg* 1971; 35:392–395.
67. Taha JM, Crone KR, Berger TS, et al: Sigmoid sinus thrombosis after closed head injury in children. *Neurosurgery* 1993; 32:541–546.
68. Kinal ME: Traumatic thrombosis of dural venous sinuses in closed head injuries. *J Neurosurg* 1967; 27:142–145.
69. Kapp JP, Gielchinsky I, Deardourff SL: Operative techniques for management of lesions involving the dural venous sinuses. *Surg Neurol* 1977; 7:339–342.
70. Feldman RA, Hieshima G, Giannotta SL, Gade GF: Traumatic dural arteriovenous fistula supplied by scalp, meningeal, and cortical arteries: Case report. *Neurosurgery* 1980; 6:670–674.
71. Björnebrink J, Liliequist B: Traumatic lateral sinus thrombosis. *Angiology* 1976; 27:688–697.
72. Kapp JP, Gielchinsky I, Petty C, McClure C: An internal shunt for use in the reconstruction of dural venous sinuses. *J Neurosurg* 1971; 35:351–354.
73. Brawley BW: Comment following Feldman RA, Hieshima G, Giannotta SL, Gade GF: Traumatic dural arteriovenous fistula supplied by scalp, meningeal, and cortical arteries: Case report. *Neurosurgery* 1980; 6:670–674.
74. Meirowski AM: Wounds of dural sinuses. *J Neurosurg* 1953; 10:496–514.

CHAPTER 46

COAGULATION DISORDERS IN THE HEAD-INJURED PATIENT

W. Keith Hoots

SYNOPSIS

Coagulation disorders are encountered frequently in patients with severe head injury. Also, the outcome in patients with such abnormalities is clearly worse than is the case when a normal coagulation status is maintained. The cause-or-effect question has been answered only in part. The coagulation pathways are immensely complex. This chapter summarizes current knowledge relating to the physiology and pathophysiology of coagulation in patients with a head injury.

INTRODUCTION

It has been recognized for more than two decades that significant traumatic insults to brain tissue may result in substantive systemic coagulation abnormalities.[1–9] This systemic coagulopathy is most commonly referred to as disseminated intravascular coagulation (DIC). Goodnight and coworkers further classified this so-called consumption coagulopathy as DIC with defibrination, and their report demonstrated that the amount of fibrin clot breakdown as measured by standardized laboratory techniques correlates with the severity of brain tissue destruction.[10] This and other clinical studies indicated that primary damage to brain cells and surrounding tissue engenders a chain of events culminating in a combination of the following: (1) reduction in the measured amount of clotting proteins in the circulation, (2) generation of localized brain clots and in many instances clots in non-CNS or systemic organs as well, and (3) evidence of defibrination that includes consumed fibrinogen (hypofibrinogenemia) with elevated circulating fibrin degradation products. From a laboratory and clinical perspective, this promulgation of the clotting process with or without actual thrombogenesis is virtually indistinguishable from the DIC syndrome induced by other disparate etiologies, such as sepsis-induced release of bacterial endotoxin.[11,12]

Early attempts to explain this phenomenon of abnormal clotting after brain injury focused on the likely release of thromboplastic materials (presumed to be tissue thromboplastin) into the bloodstream. It had been known for decades that brain homogenate is capable of inducing whole blood or plasma to clot.[13] Quick utilized this observation in 1935 to develop the one-stage prothrombin time.[14] For the first time a correlation could be made between in vivo bleeding and abnormality of an in vitro laboratory test. A major constituent of this test is *brain* extract of porcine or bovine origin which induces the patient's plasma in the test tube to clot. Hence, it may be true that an injury that introduces tissue thromboplastin into the circulation will produce extensive intravascular clotting. No compelling evidence to exclude this as an explanation for DIC after head injury has been forthcoming despite the fact that much more is known now about the triggering of DIC by multiple stimuli. This straightforward explanation does not, however, exclude a myriad of contributing factors that ultimately may determine the extent of this morbidity. Some of these possible confounding factors will be explored in the following discussion, as will the interplay between the clotting system and other inflammatory responses associated with brain injury.

Diseases other than head injury may induce the release of endogenous tissue factor (the source of tissue thromboplastic activity) into the circulation, producing a DIC with defibrination.[15] In obstetric medicine, retained dead fetus syndrome is a well-characterized example. In this syndrome, necrotic fetal tissue and enzymes associated with its breakdown are released into the uterine and maternal systemic circulation, activating the procoagulant system. Although not wholly analogous to the brain injury model for the induction of DIC, the rapid and rampant cellular and enzymatic activation that either insult induces has a similar capacity to induce DIC. Florid activation by such insults probably overwhelms the normal homeostatic mechanisms of the host. In addition to the intravascular entry of exogenous cells and proteins, both types of injury may produce significant damage to the vascular system and endothelial cells. This vascular injury may then trigger an overwhelming DIC. A more complete understanding of this process requires knowledge not only of the triggering event but also of the type and extent of the vascular injury. Vascular cells may indeed hold the key to mitigating or blunting any systemic or inflammatory response, as will be discussed in the following section.

THE PHYSIOLOGY OF HEMOSTASIS

Before analyzing in greater detail the evidence for the association between head injury and abnormalities in hemostasis and thrombosis, it is necessary to explore in greater detail the relationship between coagulation biology and the more generalized inflammatory response that animals (including humans) exhibit in response to injury and disease. Efforts to differentiate the clotting response from the overall inflammatory response may be not only simplistic but also naive regardless of whether the initiating event is brain trauma or endoxin-induced shock. The extraordinary complexity of the processes involved necessitates a selective focus on the response to vascular injury and the regulatory mechanisms that attempt to localize the insult.

Blood clotting exists to preserve vascular integrity after an injury.[16] This obvious conclusion may be stated in another way: Hemostatic mechanisms exist to maintain blood components in the vascular space and to ensure that any impedance to optimal blood flow or perfusion is minimal and of short duration. An integrated system of cellular and protein responses exists to achieve and maintain this homeostasis. However, though they are completely integrated and interdependent, these individual biological responses often must be analyzed to understand this complex phenomenon. An understanding of the extreme hemostatic challenge produced by DIC probably requires such a step-by-step examination. Since the focus in this chapter is head injury, a summary of the predominant mechanisms will be provided.

In response to injury, three parallel yet integrated components must be activated for effective hemostasis to occur. These responses—vascular, platelet, and procoagulant—work in concert to staunch hemorrhage and, with the concomitant activation of the fibrinolytic system, restore normal downstream perfusion. In addition, the degree of each component's activation is closely regulated by biological inhibitory or feedback systems that ensure that the clotting is proportionate to the injured area and is localized exclusively to that site. Each component will be discussed succinctly. Emphasis will be placed on the pathways responsible for both up and down regulation of clotting, since both forms of regulation are critical for preventing the overwhelming systemic activation of clotting, a DIC.

VASCULAR PHASE

When a vessel is damaged, a number of nearly simultaneous events occur at the injury site.[17] Proximal smooth vessel contractions occur when arterial and arteriolar vessels are injured to stem blood flow.[18,19] Undamaged endothelial cells proximal to the injury in any type of vessel (artery, vein, or capillary) begin to express tissue factor (TF), and TF also is released from the subendothelium.[20,21] This TF expression can be substantially increased when the associated injury induces monocytes to secrete tissue necrosis factor (TNF) and interleukin-1 (IL-1).[16,22] In addition, catecholamine release from the adrenal glands and the release of vasoactive peptides from the posterior pituitary (e.g., vasopressin) can induce the release of adhesive proteins (called integrins) that are necessary for cell attachment to the site of injured endothelium.[23]

The prototype integrin for the initial phases of hemostasis is von Willebrand's factor (VWF), which allows circulating platelets to stick to each other and adhere to injured endothelium. The endothelial cells secrete VWF continuously and release more of it in response to hormonal stimuli. VWF is the "bridge" that localizes platelets to the injury site. Other classes of integrins (e.g., laminins) released from the subendothelium help anchor other essential elements of tissue repair (e.g., fibroblasts) to sites where the endothelium has been damaged.

Important homeostatic mechanisms exist to ensure that unwanted thrombosis does not occur physiologically. These vasoactive and antiplatelet adherent processes may be compromised by endothelial injury, temporarily making the site susceptible to platelet adherence and altering critical downstream blood flow. Examples of such important regulatory chemicals include prostacyclin (PGI_2) and nitrous oxide (endothelial relaxing factor).[24,25]

PLATELET PHASE

The role that platelets play as the "thumb in the dike" in injured vascular tissue is implied by these strategic adhesive events. Clearly, the sticking of platelets to the exposed subendothelium provides the initial "plug" that prevents extravasation of blood. Also important, however, are the roles platelets play in the injury response: (1) provision of the essential phospholipid surface for the localization of circulating procoagulants to the injury site and (2) release of cytokines to induce other biochemical events necessary for localization of the biological response to injury and the induction of tissue repair.[26] In addition, a break in the endothelial surface exposes collagen molecules in the subendothelium that facilitate further platelet binding through specific collagen receptors on the platelets.[27]

Without the binding of the circulating clotting proteins to the platelet surface, the acceleration in the production of activated clotting enzymes needed for clot formation does not occur efficiently. Other white blood cells may play a role in providing alternative surfaces for clotting activation and fibrin clot generation; however, the bleeding that invariably occurs with extreme thrombocytopenia implies that this is an essential role for platelets.[22] The cytokines released from platelets have a myriad of real or potential roles in inflammation. These include (1) proteins that work to slow platelet aggregation and procoagulant activation (e.g., platelet factor 4, α_1-antitrypsin),[28] (2) proteins that enhance platelet adhesion and aggregation (e.g., thrombospondin, platelets, VWF),[26,29] (3) procoagulant proteins (e.g., fibrinogen, factor V, factor XI),[30–33] (4) enhancers and inhibitors of fibrinolysis (e.g., plasminogen, α_2-antiplasmin), and (5) growth factors capable of inducing DNA synthesis (e.g., platelet-derived growth factors).[34–36] Indeed, platelets and leukocytes share some of these secretory roles.[22,37,38] These manifold functions indicate the complexity of the roles shared by the cellular and protein components of inflammation. From a holistic perspective, however, it appears that when the normal regulatory balance between each of these actions is threatened, there is a significant potential for inordinate tissue and organ damage. Presumably, in DIC such a remarkable imbalance is perpetuated because the vascular injury is diffuse and extensive and because the inflammatory mediators lead to further vascular injury and damage to the associated tissue.

Procoagulant Phase

The procoagulant/anticoagulant phase of ciotting induced by tissue injury (particularly vascular) generates a fibrin clot around and between the platelets aggregated at the site of a vascular injury. Like the platelet phase, however, this phase cannot be separated completely from other components of the inflammatory response. The subtleties of the biochemistry (particularly the stoichiometry of the enzyme-substrate interactions in vivo) are not completely understood. However, a better understanding of the sequence of events that leads to the generation of thrombin (IIa), the key enzyme for converting fibrinogen to a cross-linked fibrin clot, now exists because of several key observations. The sequence of these enzyme cleavages is very important.[29] Vascular injury induces the release of membrane-localized TF from both subendothelium and direct endothelial secretion.[21,26,39] This membrane-bound TF then binds circulatory factor VII as well as trace amounts of factor VIIa. The new formed TF:VII:VIIa complex can efficiently cleave factors X and IX to their active forms [tenase (Xa) and IXa, respectively]. The Xa generated in this process then cleaves activation peptides from prothrombin (which has been localized through weak binding to the platelet surface from its soluble, circulating state) to produce active thrombin. This rapid and early generation of thrombin on or near the surface of the adherent and aggregated platelets induces profound amplification of further IIa generation through direct action on several key substrates. This initial generation of IIa results in the direct activation of the serine protease factor XI, thus inducing intrinsic pathway activation of factor IX.[31] Simultaneously, other IIa molecules activate factors V and VIII, neither of which is a serine protease. By contrast to the active serine enzymes, factors VIIIa and Va dramatically increase the reaction rates of their respective reaction steps. The biochemical acceleration of Xa and IIa generation relies on the capacity of these large glycoproteins to assemble the target proteases in close proximity to each other on the platelet surface.[29] This accelerated production of IIa rapidly results in the cleavage of platelet-localized fibrinogen (concentrated from the large circulating pool) to fibrin monomer.[32] These fibrin monomers cross-link side to side and end to end to form a fibrin clot matrix in and around the adherent platelets. Thrombin also cleaves a circulating factor XIII to its active form, XIIIa, which converts the soluble fibrin meshwork into an insoluble, permanent clot by converting the cross-linked fibrin attachments into irreversible covalent bonds. The clot that is formed remains until the fibrinolytic enzyme plasmin lyses it as part of the repair and restoration phase of vascular injury. Thrombin also has other functions that enhance the inflammatory matrix that will be discussed in the context of the excessive IIa generation that occurs during clinical DIC.[17–19,40–45]

Protease Inhibitors of Inflammation and Coagulation

The most important circulating natural inhibitor of thrombin (and probably Xa and other serine proteases as well) is antithrombin III (ATIII).[46] This inhibitor protein with a molecular weight of approximately 58,000 is one of a special class of serine protease inhibitors, or *serpines,* that are essential for ensuring that hemostasis does not extend beyond the minimum needed to preserve vascular perfusion. The serpines serve as the protein vanguard against systemic thrombosis, just as the endothelial cell and its secretion products (e.g., PGI_2) provide the cellular barriers against systemic thrombosis. (Naturally, either system or both may be taxed excessively when the flow rate becomes inordinately low or when chronic vascular injury precludes complete restoration of an intact endothelium.) Antithrombin III binds both IIa and Xa very avidly and quickly when these proteins are present in a soluble form in the circulation. More important from a physiological point of view are the localizing of ATIII molecules on the endothelium at or near the site of injury. This is accomplished when endothelial cells express heparinlike molecules (glycosaminoglycans) that bind ATIII and markedly enhance the binding capacity of this serpine for IIa and Xa (and to a lesser degree other serine proteases, such as IXa, as well).[47] Hence, the excess of these activated protease molecules that are generated by the acceleration of the cascade by VIIIa and Va are quickly and irreversibly neutralized by the ATIII-heparinoid complex. This confers protection against downstream clot propagation.

A second mechanism for rapidly quelling the generation of IIa is provided by the presence of intact endothelium proximal to the site of injury. Endothelial cells express a IIa-specific receptor, thrombomodulin (TM), that complexes the protease rapidly and totally.[48] The IIa-TM complex formed in this manner plays a secondary but critically important role in slowing IIa generation as well. The IIa-TM complex initiates its own pathway for decreasing the rate of thrombin formation. Protein C, when complexed to its cofactor protein S (a second vitamin K–dependent zymogen), is activated in the fluid phase by the IIa-TM complex on the endothelial surface. Activated protein C (APC) is a very potent inactivator of factors V and VIII. Hence, the acceleration that permits rapid generation of IIa and markedly enhances the cleavage of fibrinogen to form fibrin is dramatically decelerated by APC, ensuring that inordinate thrombogenesis does not occur.

A third critical natural inhibitor of thrombin generation and thrombogenesis is tissue factor pathway inhibitor. Work by Broze and others has demonstrated that this circulating molecule functions to inactivate the VIIa-tissue factor-X complex, the pathway that is essential in producing Xa (tenase) activation of prothrombin.[28]

In addition to the thrombomodulin receptor on the cell surface of systemic endothelial cells, there appears to be a second thrombin-specific receptor on endothelial cells in the brain and CNS. Work by Cunningham and associates has demonstrated that this receptor, known as protease nexin-1 (PN-1), is primarily a brain protein

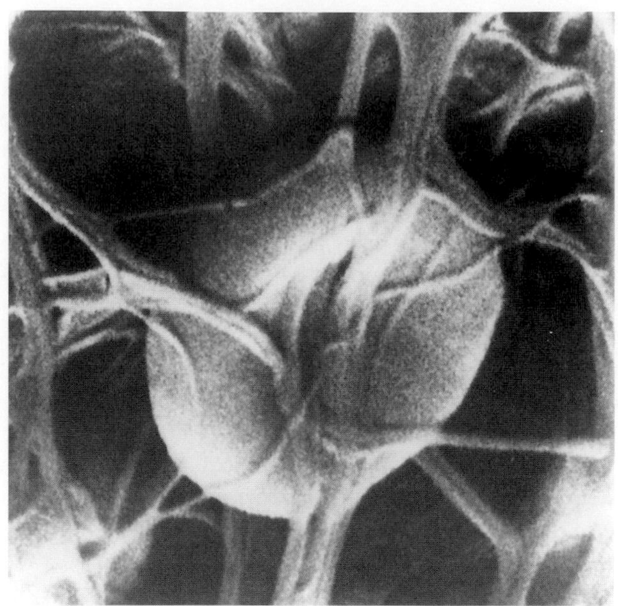

Figure 46-1. Fibrin strands enlarged about 20,000 diameters enmesh a red blood cell in an electron micrograph. (Emil O. Bernstein and Eila Kairinen of the Gillette Research Institute.)

and is abundant around cerebral blood vessels.[49] It appears to play a role in localizing and inactivating IIa to the endothelial surface (perhaps in an analogous sense to the IIa-TM complex) (Fig. 46-1); however, the PN-1-IIa complex also appears to have physiological importance in initiating the response to injury. Experiments conducted in the author's laboratory indicate the following: (1) PN-1 and thrombin can regulate neurite outgrowth from neurons and neuroblastoma cells, (2) PN-1 and IIa also regulate astroglial proliferation and control the stellate processes in these cells, (3) the primary effect is due to IIa, (4) thrombin retracts processes on neurons and astroglial cells and is mitogenic for those cells, and (5) PN-1 causes process outgrowth and modulates the mitogenic response as a result of its ability to inhibit or inactivate IIa. This and other evidence indicate that this protease nexin-1-thrombin complex is important in the local physiology that regulates the response of brain cells to injury.

FIBRINOLYSIS

Just as stopping hemorrhage is critical to the survival of an injured animal or human, restoration of blood flow as quickly as possible to organ or tissue sites distal to the site of injury is essential for the preservation of structure and function. When the zymogen plasminogen is converted to the enzyme plasmin by the action of released tissue plasminogen activator (t-PA), the bonds of the fibrin clot are cleaved.[50] Monocytes and macrophages then remove the residual fibrinolytic debris. The release of the initiator t-PA is stimulated by inflammatory hormones such as epinephrine. There are two important regulators of the generation of enzymatically active plasmin: (1) Plasminogen activator inhibitor-1 (PA-1) inactivates t-PA, and (2) α_2-antiplasmin is the most potent of several natural inhibitors of plasmin. Localization of t-PA onto the fibrin meshwork helps localize plasmin activation to the site of a newly formed or older clot rather than accentuating such activation of the enzyme in the plasma itself.

Contact Pathway Activation

To conclude this summary of hemostasis and its close incorporation into the overall inflammatory response to injury, a brief discussion of the contact phase of coagulation (the traditional entry into the intrinsic pathway of the clotting cascade) is in order. Not only does this pathway play a specific role in inducing fibrinolysis (as was noted above), but factor XII, prekallikrein, high-molecular-weight kininogen (HMWK), factor XI, and the inhibitor of the first component of complement (C1-INH) play a major role in the activation and mediation of surface-dependent pathways.[51] These surface-sensitive reactions are important since they often play a critical role in the amplification of the events that follow extreme vascular or organ damage. Hence, there is special relevance to DIC pathogenesis.

DISSEMINATED INTRAVASCULAR COAGULATION

DIC as a clinical finding in overwhelming disease was first described by Walter H. Seegers in 1950[13] in the context of a release of placental thromboplastin into the circulation of a delivering mother. The syndrome has been extended to include many life-threatening insults that result in direct activation of the clotting system (e.g., snake bite), massive tissue or organ injury (e.g., burns), or a combination of the two. The purpose here is not to provide a discussion of the multifaceted etiologies of DIC but to examine common pathogenetic characteristics of the syndrome (regardless of etiology) in an effort to elucidate the induction of DIC after head injury.

The DIC syndrome is present when a significant injury to an individual or animal gives rise to a majority of the following:

1. Induction of a massive localized or generalized inflammatory response which gradually or dramatically becomes a systemic inflammatory response.
2. Large-scale vascular injury with extensive damage of endothelial cells of many blood vessels (probably including an extensive arterial, venous, and capillary insult).[15]
3. Activation of coagulation pathways with the excessive generation of thrombin.[29]
4. Because of extreme clotting activation that is beyond the capacity of the natural inhibitors to quell, localization of thrombus formation exclusively to injury sites is gradually lost. Microthrombi form distal to the initial injury site in many disparate vascular sites.
5. The microthrombi occlude small vessels, thus compromising downstream perfusion. This induces tissue ischemia, which may evolve to infarction; infarction may lead to dramatic progression to multiple organ failure (MOF).[52] Ironically, MOF itself may provide the initiating event of DIC in certain disease processes.
6. Release of an extraordinary amount of cytokines, secretagogues, and hormones from multiple inflammatory and vascular cell types (including but not limited to endothelium, monocytes/macrophages/glial cells, T lymphocytes, polymorphonuclear leukocytes, and mast cells).[15,53–57]
7. Massive vasodilatation with concomitant loss of tight junctions between the endothelial cells, extravasation of plasma proteins and cells, and microangiopathic hemolytic anemia[24,44,58] (Fig. 46-1).
8. Massive fibrinolysis and defibrination with the production of a large quantity of circulating fibrin degradation products that impede further fibrin clot formation.[10]
9. Hemorrhage into tissues, organs, and damaged integument secondary to the depletion ("consumption") of platelets and procoagulants and the presence of fibrin degradation products (FDPs). By this stage, failure to remove the initiating insult makes organism death imminent.

This sequence of events is not invariable, and the initiating stimulus probably determines which pathogenetic events predominate. Nonetheless, an examination of some of the biochemical and cellular events that give rise to each event provides some insight into the extraordinary complexity of the DIC syndrome and may offer clues to the difficulties which face a clinician who attempts to curtail this escalating phenomenon in a patient.

In the preceding discussion about hemostatic mechanisms, extensive evidence was provided about the integration of the coagulation system with other components of inflammation. Much of the information about the enzymatic and other chemical links between these responses that once were considered disparate has only recently been gleaned from exhaustive work in in vitro systems. New pathways linking these systems coupled with new data about noncoagulant cell (e.g., leukocyte) secretion of procoagulants are one example of how highly integrated all the facets (including hemostasis) of inflammation are.[22] Presumably, only such a tightly regulated system can preserve the capacity of the host organism to respond to an infinite number of injuries or assaultive insults with a finite but carefully proportionate response system designed to keep the insult or injury localized. Any insult massive enough or specifically directed enough to exhaust the regulatory chemicals that ensure such localization through a specific, tailored response has the potential to create a spiraling and consumptive induction of an even greater inflammatory response. The more inflammation there is, the more likely it becomes that localization of the biochemical response is lost. This becomes particularly likely when the regulatory or inhibitory proteins are being depleted by the excessive inflammation. For example, massive vessel injury ensures extensive loss of the endothelial protective barrier and resultant marked contact activation.[50] This in turn induces generation of intrinsic pathway clotting, extraordinary polymorphonuclear neutrophil (PMN) activation, and generation of massive quantities of vasoactive peptides such as bradykinin that can induce a dramatic fall in systemic blood pressure. This fall in blood pressure compromises perfusion and extends the stimulus for inflammatory activation because of the resultant organ infarction. This represents one of many simultaneous responses to the initial stimulus that has the potential to further engender inflammation. Thus, DIC progresses.

The importance of vascular injury to the induction of the DIC syndrome cannot be overstated. The endothelial cell lining of blood vessels is critical to maintaining physiological function. As was stated previously, the many regulatory tasks for this cell type (e.g., thrombomodulin receptor, PGI_2) and the barrier it provides against the contact of blood with enzymatic activators

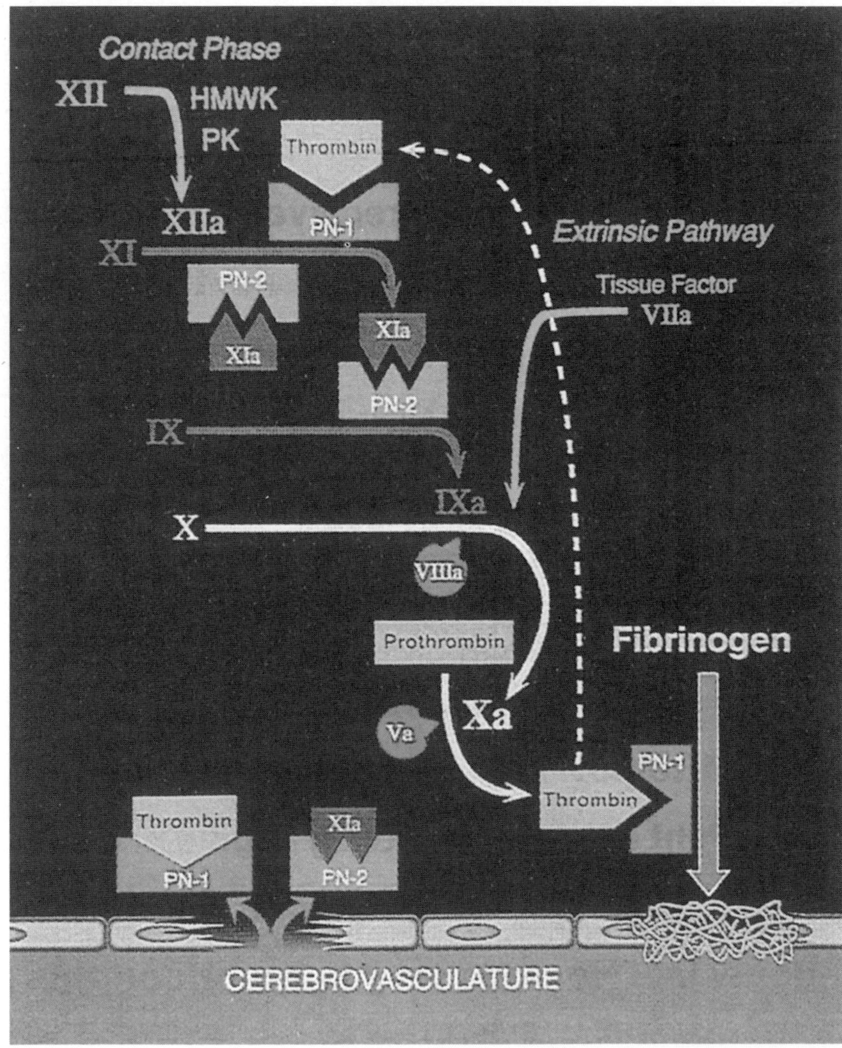

Figure 46-2. Schema for protease nexin inactivation of thrombin in the cerebral vasculature. (Used with permission of Dennis Cunningham, MD of Science.)

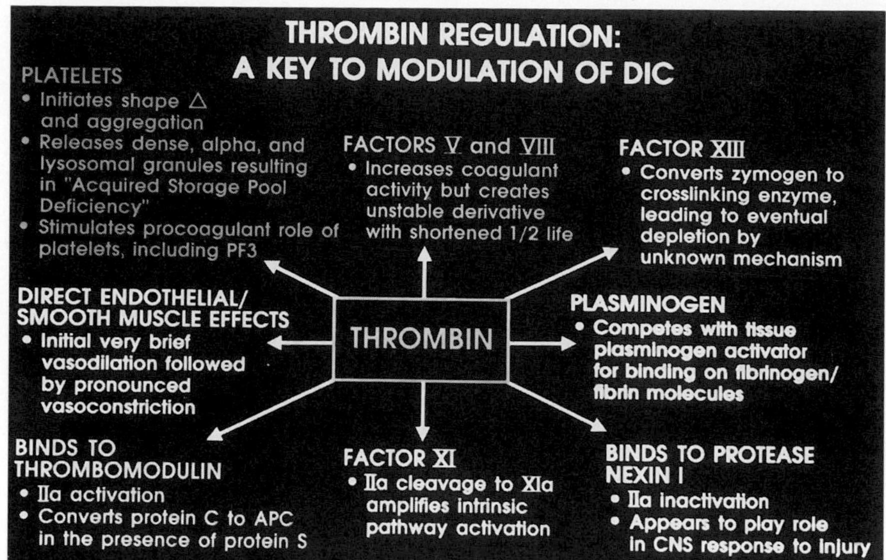

Figure 46-3. Thrombin activities that enhance coagulopathy and increase the inflammatory response.

in the underlying tissue matrix imply that propagation of injury to an even larger number of endothelial cells will ensure escalating thrombogenesis, the sine qua non for DIC.[18] It has been suggested from both clinical and animal experience (particularly the endotoxin/bacterial lipopolysaccharide DIC experimental model) that preservation of intact endothelium is an essential element in preventing propagation of clotting and the other components of the inflammatory response.[17,26,41,43]

If small vessel thrombogenesis is the sine qua non for DIC, the generation of thrombin is similarly essential. Figure 46-2 summarizes the myriad actions of this pluripotent serine protease. Naturally, foremost among these actions is the generation of fibrin clots from circulating fibrinogen. Additional actions that require binding of IIa or its enzymatic cleavage of multiple substrates guarantee that excessive thrombin will induce remarkable cellular and vascular responses as well[18,40,42,49] (Fig. 46-3). The presence of excessive thrombin in the circulation can induce injury to vascular tissues that is similar to that caused by bacterial lipopolysaccharide.[59] Each can initiate the rampant release of vasoactive peptides [e.g., tumor necrosis factor (TNF) and anaphylotoxins C3a and C5a][60] (Fig. 46-4). This implies that no effort to abort the DIC syndrome therapeutically will be successful unless it ensures that adequate inhibitors are present to inactivate circulating thrombin molecules that are no longer localized at or near the site of the initial injury.

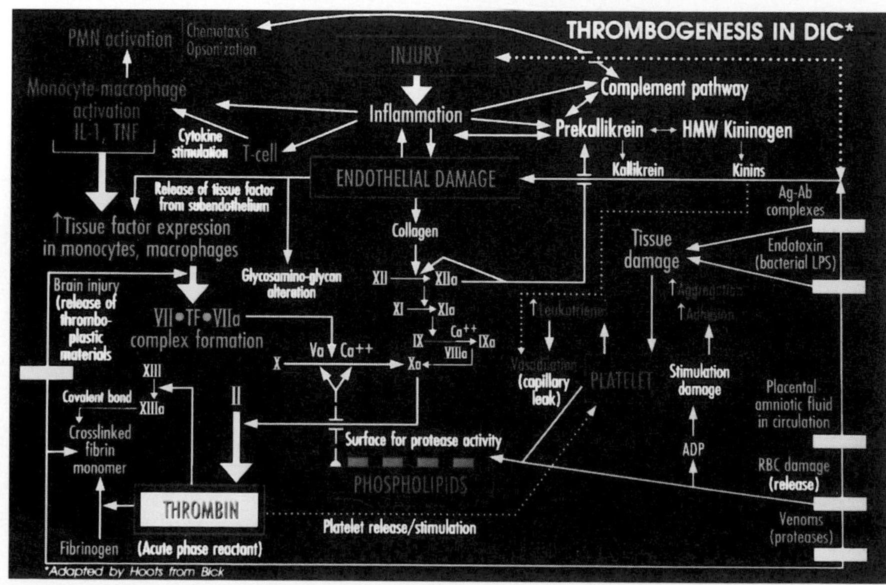

Figure 46-4. Physiologic pathways in injury and inflammation that enhance thrombin generation.

Multiple organ failure is a common consequence of severe DIC. In addition, Risberg and colleagues cite evidence that extensive local thrombogenesis in certain organs can predispose to dissemination of the clotting response.[52] An example is adult respiratory distress syndrome (ARDS), in which microemboli in the lung parenchyma create alveolar membrane leaks and localized fibrin deposition.[37] The secondary inflammatory response that ARDS induces may then give rise to DIC and MOF.

Our understanding of the role of cytokines in inducing and modifying inflammation has increased dramatically in recent years. With the onset of DIC, there is a sudden secretion of both IL-1 and TNF in response to thrombin stimulation of monocytes.[25,61] These secretagogues enhance the susceptibility of endothelium to thrombosis by inducing tissue factor expression from the endothelium and by initiating monocyte adherence to and egress between endothelium.[22] Each of these processes will "stoke the furnace" of a consumptive coagulopathy. For example, the vasoactive peptides induced in response to these cytokines enhance the tendency for the development of shock.[50] The resultant decreased hydrostatic pressure in small blood vessels that already are partially occluded with clots further impairs perfusion and predisposes to organ failure.

In fulminant DIC, small vessel thrombosis quickly becomes irreversible. This can be explained in part by the depletion of plasmin available to lyse occlusive clots.[9] The drastically increased demand for plasmin to lyse these clots inevitably exhausts the hepatic capacity to replete the circulating plasminogen. The life span of the clots lengthens, and the perfusion emergency grows for the organ. Paradoxically, the already strained capacity of the liver to provide even greater quantities of plasminogen, procoagulants, and procoagulant inhibitors becomes further compromised because this synthetic organ is susceptible to damage from DIC.[13] Equally critical (and perhaps even more significant as a physiological focus for therapeutic intervention) is the inevitable depletion of the key inhibitory proteins for all the components of the exploding inflammation.[62] Studies have demonstrated the almost invariable depletion of each of the following as DIC progresses: ATIII, protein C, protein S, α_2-antiplasmin, PAI-1, C1-INH, decreased glycosamino-glycans (perhaps secondary to endothelial injury), α_1-antitrypsin, and α_2-macroglobulin.[47,59,63] Other inhibitory proteins for cytokine production also are likely to be in short supply if the cells that produce them cluster as aggregates in damaged organs. Hence, in the simplest sense, DIC represents profound consumption of protease and cytokine inhibitors. Further, prospects for interrupting the process are dependent on repleting these regulatory or inhibitory proteins. For this reason, fresh frozen plasma, which is a reservoir for all serpines and related proteins, remains the mainstay of therapy for DIC.

Finally, no discussion of the pathogenesis of DIC is complete without an examination of the impact of even greater hemorrhage. The model presented here has been built on thrombosis and escalating inflammation. Bleeding in DIC occurs as a late phenomenon. Its presence usually indicates that consumption of procoagulants (particularly fibrinogen) and platelets has continued unabated and that preexistent organ damage is likely to be very substantial. Exceptions exist when the liver or bone marrow (critical sites of the production of these components) are the primary sites of injury so that these components are already in deficit when the DIC begins.[39] Otherwise, the appearance of severe bleeding signals extremely morbid DIC and often implies that if substantial progress is not being made toward removing the initiating cause, prospects for patient survival are poor.[64] At this stage, therapeutic intervention for the "consumptive coagulopathy" involves simultaneous replenishment of procoagulants, platelets, and the natural inhibitors of thrombin generation and inflammation acceleration. Naturally this must accompany progress in removing or alleviating the initiating injurious event or events and treating the associated complications of the primary insult.

DIC IN HEAD-INJURED PATIENTS

The DIC that may follow a severe head injury has been produced experimentally in animal models.[65] After minor experimental head injury, fibrin microthrombi were demonstrable in the brain and lungs of rats. As was discussed above, the prevailing hypothesis is that blunt or penetrating injury of the brain produces an inoculation of a thromboplastic material into the circulation. Supporting this inference are data demonstrating that the injection of homologous tissue thromboplastin produces a reversible acute DIC in dogs.[66] In this study, the authors were able to demonstrate the generation of a few nanomoles of thrombin in vivo, with its subsequent inactivation by the major thrombin inhibitors (e.g., ATIII). Further, pretreatment with the ATIII cofactor heparin effectively inhibited the development of the tissue thromboplastin-induced DIC.

In addition to the release of thromboplastin into the circulation with associated activation of factor VII (see above), extensive endothelial injury occurs in brain trauma with activation of the contact factor pathway and stimulation of platelet release.[67] This establishes a pathway for amplification of the clotting mechanisms

TABLE 46-1 Association Between Status on Admission and Delayed Brain Injury

	Delayed Brain Injury		
	Present	**Absent**	**Difference (p value)**
Admission computed tomography scan*			
Normal (%)	10.7	16.0	NS
Skull fracture (%)	34.2	28.7	NS
Contusion, swelling (%)	61.1	55.9	NS
Subdural hematomas (%)	14.1	2.1	<0.001
Intracerebral hematomas (%)	8.1	3.2	NS
Epidural hematomas (%)	6.0	4.3	NS
Subarachnoid or intraventricular hemorrhage (%)	5.4	7.4	NS
Other lesion (%)	16.8	16.0	NS
Admission coagulation studies			
Mean prothrombin time(s)	14.3	12.7	<0.001
Mean partial thromboplastin time(s)	34.8	28.2	<0.001
Mean platelet count ($\times 10^3$)	284.0	315.6	<0.05
With coagulopathy (%)	57.4	8.7	<0.001

* Totals > 100%; some patients had multiple lesions.

SOURCE: Stein SC, et al: Delayed and progressive brain injury in closed-head trauma: Radiological demonstration. *Neurosurgery* 32(1):25–31, 1993.

(as previously described) with thrombotic occlusions and perhaps DIC-induced hemorrhage. In addition, there are signs of neurohumoral alterations after brain injury that may further confound the rapidly evolving coagulopathy.[9] A catecholamine surge may play a role in vascular damage and stimulation of platelet release, further fueling the incipient DIC.[67]

Extensive clinical studies over the last two decades support the prevalence of coagulopathic abnormalities in patients after a head injury.[2,3,5,6,10,64,68–71] Further, the degree of such coagulopathy appears to be proportionate to the extent of brain injury as indicated by surrogate markers for severity such as the Glasgow Coma Scale.[72,73] In addition, the work of Stein and coworkers and Kaufman and colleagues indicates that the presence of coagulopathy predicts the prevalence of delayed brain injury[74,75] (Table 46-1). This conclusion is supported by the presence of new or progressive lesions on follow-up computed tomography (CT) scans of injuries which had not been present on the initial CT scan that was performed in the immediate postinjury period.[76] Most important, there were highly statistically significant correlations not only with the appearance of delayed cerebral insults but also with the severity of the initial injury and the presence of coagulopathy at admission. Each event correlated with higher mortality, slowed recovery, and poorer outcome at 6 months.

This association between coagulopathy after injury and poor outcome is consistent with data from a large, prospectively followed head injury cohort assembled by colleagues at the author's institution between 1979 and 1982.[67,69,75,77,78] Approximately 2900 injured individuals of all ages were assessed on arrival in our emergency center after an isolated head injury or a head injury associated with multiple trauma. Approximately 2100 of these individuals survived long enough for entry in the trauma registry, and all these individuals underwent hemostatic evaluation within 24 h of injury. Ninety percent of these individuals were admitted to the hospital within 4 h of injury, and 50 percent had blood taken for coagulation testing within 3 h of the injury. In each case, the coagulation testing consisted minimally of the following clotting tests: prothrombin time, activated partial thromboplastin time, thrombin clotting time, platelet count, plasma fibrinogen level, and fibrin degradation products. The battery was performed on arrival and sequentially every 8 to 12 h thereafter until the patient was clinically stable or expired. In addition, a subset of randomly selected individuals were assessed serially with an extensive battery of tests designed to assess ongoing procoagulant activation and/or consumption (e.g., fibrinopeptide A and multiple factor assay), inhibitor status (e.g., ATIII), fibrinolysis (e.g., plasminogen), and platelet activation (beta-thromboglobulin). Some newer tests, such as measurement of thrombin-antithrombin complexes (TAT) and soluble fibrin monomers, had not been developed at the time of the study.

During the 3 years of the study, patients with different injury types (Table 46-2) and multiple ages (Table 46-

TABLE 46-2 Etiology of Head Injury

Etiology	Number (%)
Traffic accident	111 (42)
Gunshot wounds	66 (25)
Fall	58 (22)
Assault	13 (5)
Other	15 (6)
Total	263

SOURCE: Olson et al (1989).

TABLE 46-3 Patients Studied

Age	No.	Male, %
0–10	55	75
11–20	55	75
21–30	78	85
31–40	33	85
41–50	23	74
51–60	10	90
61–70	8	63
71–80	4	75
81–100	2	100
	268*	79%

* One male did not have his age recorded.

SOURCE: Olson et al (1989).

3) were evaluated. The clinical severity of the injuries was distributed over the entire range as measured by the Glasgow Coma Scale (GCS).[69] A DIC score was calculated for each injured person. The score for each patient was obtained by categorizing the laboratory results of the following six clotting tests as normal (0), mildly abnormal (1), moderately abnormal (2), or severely abnormal (3). Hence, the possible aggregate DIC score for a head-injured patient ranged from 0 to 18. A striking association was demonstrated between a high DIC score at enrollment and the ultimate outcome (survival versus mortality) (Fig. 46-6). A similar yet expected predictive correlation was also seen with GCS (Fig. 46-7). In addition, both scores correlated with subjective assessments of injury severity. By contrast, there were individuals in whom there was discordance between GCS and DIC scores for whom the DIC score accurately predicted a fatal outcome. Some who had strikingly abnormal coagulation tests but were ambulatory and fully cognizant on arrival in the emergency center died within several days after the injury.[79] These "talk and die" individuals appeared to indicate that the coagulopathy we were measuring not only was reflective of the degree of brain injury but perhaps also was contributing significantly to subsequent morbidity and mortality. This inference was further supported by a statistical analysis using a logistic regression model to predict survival based on enrollment GCS and the extent of coagulopathy (DIC score or variations on it) (Table 46-4). Figure 46-5 demonstrates the accuracy of the model in predicting survival. Among young head-injured patients less than 16 years of age, the model had a sensitivity of 93 percent and a specificity of 87 percent in predicting who would or would not survive his or her injury at the time of arrival in the emergency center (regardless of whether it was an isolated head injury or a head injury plus multiple trauma). The remarkable accuracy of this model in predicting outcome raised the question of whether early, aggressive intervention to improve the coagulopathy might affect survival.

Autopsy studies performed on 16 individuals from the UT-Houston/Hermann Hospital cohort initially failed to indicate small vessel thrombogenesis despite the presence of abnormal DIC screening tests.[80] However, when the tissue slides from brain, lung, liver, kidney, and pancreas were stained with an immunoperoxidase technique using rabbit-antihuman fibrinogen antiserum, microthrombi were demonstrated almost universally (88 percent of individuals) and almost invariably in sections from each respective organ. Small vessels in the brain had the highest incidence of microthrombi, whereas distal organs exhibited the highest density of small clots. Newer endothelial histopathologic techniques (perhaps including examination of endothelial glycosoaminoglycan expression at these various organ sites) must be applied to confirm the conclusions of these studies. Remarkable technological advances in this area may provide an opportunity to examine more fully the sequence of events and pathogenetic progression of this injury-associated phenomenon.

Further data supportive of the conclusion about the impact of DIC on the survival of the subjects enrolled in the University of Texas Houston/Hermann Hospital study were gleaned from the few randomly chosen individuals on whom more extensive coagulation testing was performed. Abnormalities of plasma at the level of ATIII, like DIC, proved to be a fairly effective surrogate marker or prediction for mortality (Table 46-5). This phenomenon of ATIII depletion (a presumed consumption) occurred despite the early laboratory assessment done in the emergency center and the fact that ATIII behaves initially as an acute-phase reactant such as fibrinogen, rising acutely with the catecholamine surge that follows an injury (unpublished data). Hence, a rapid depletion from this acute physiologically high level of ATIII implies that ATIII is a strong indicator of a rapidly progressing thrombogenesis that has the potential to become full-blown clinical DIC. Plasma plasminogen levels appear to behave similarly to ATIII (rapidly rising and then acutely falling in the most severely injured),

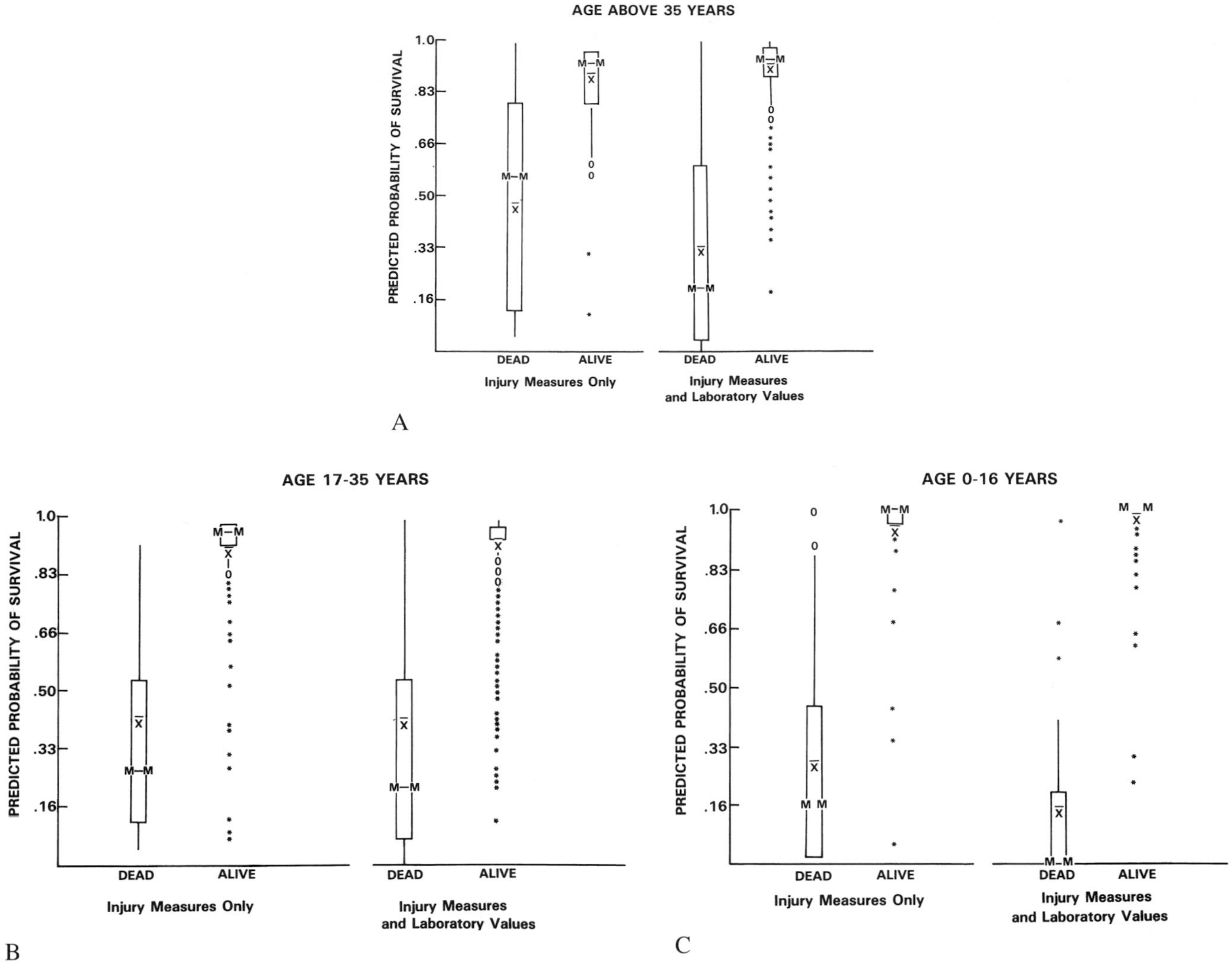

Figure 46-5. The relative predicted probability of survival at the first assessment after an injury of coma/motor score versus coma/motor scores plus stepwise logistic regression models that also include coagulation laboratory parameters, by age. *A*. Age above 35 years. *B*. Age 17 to 35 years of age. *C*. Age 0 to 16 years.

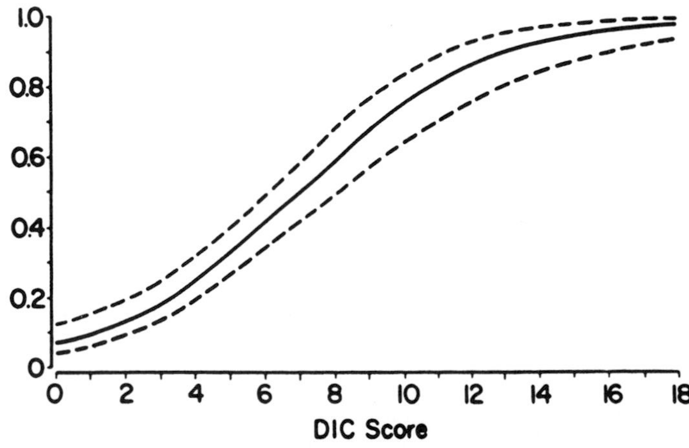

Figure 46-6. The probability of death as predicted by the initial DIC score assessed in the immediate hours after injury (mean, 4 h after injury). The initial coma score and DIC scores were assessed simultaneously. (From Olson et al., 1989.)

TABLE 46-4 Variables Examined by Stepwise Logistic Regression

Glascow Coma Scale
Fibrinogen
Platelet count
Fibrin degradation products
Thrombin clotting time
Prothrombin time
Activated partial thromboplastin time
DIC score

SOURCE: Olson et al (1989).

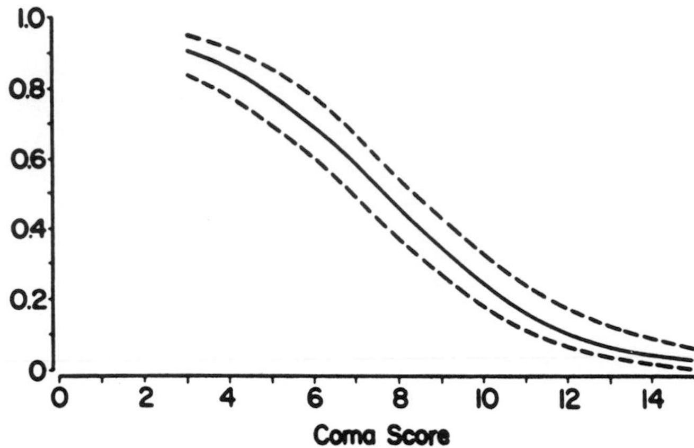

Figure 46-7. The probability of death as predicted by the initial coma score assessed in the immediate hours after injury (mean, 4 h after injury). The initial coma score and DIC scores were assessed simultaneously. (From Olson et al., 1989.)

supporting the hypothesis that rapidly engendered fibrinolysis is another indicator of an incipient DIC. Other clinical studies have shown similar kinetic behavior of ATIII, plasminogen, and other natural inhibitors of coagulation and fibrinolysis in incipient DIC syndromes, whether from sepsis, trauma, or abruption.[62,81–88] In addition, Wada and associates demonstrated that in severely ill intensive care unit (ICU) patients, the presence of subtle markers of excess thrombin generation preceded and predicted subsequent DIC development as much as 3 to 5 days later.[89] Therefore, even though the inducing insult for DIC among head-injured subjects may be unique, it appears that the usually accepted laboratory markers for its development in this syndrome are not pathognomonic of the injury. This conclusion is important for two reasons. First, it provides a further indication that the coagulopathy is not exclusively a reflective phenomenon of the degree of brain damage. Instead, it appears to have the capacity to markedly enhance local injury through the mechanisms described above and to extend the injury processes to distal organ sites. Second, it implies that an aggressive effort to abort this thrombogenic/inflammatory process as soon as possible after injury is an essential component of therapy for head injury.

Recent work by Bredbacka and colleagues at the Karolinska Institute in Stockholm has corroborated earlier work on the high prevalence of DIC in association with head trauma as measured by several established and a few more laboratory coagulation markers (e.g., plasma fibrin monomer and thrombin-antithrombin levels).[90–93] Figure 46-8 shows data from this study relating this specific coagulation marker of thrombin activation to the clinical outcome. As was noted, a low GCS predicts for abnormal coagulation markers and a poorer Glasgow Outcome Score. This is highly consistent with the studies from the 1980s and adds credence to the conclusion that coagulopathy often is both a result of head injury and an insult added to the ultimate clinical outcome of the injured individual.

TABLE 46-5 Antithrombin Levels in Head-Injured Patients at the University of Texas-Houston/Hermann Hospital, 1979–1982

Antithrombin III Level*	*N*	Mortality, %
≤75 IU/ml	15	87
>75 IU/ml	45	36
Total	60	

* On arrival at emergency center.

Plasma ATIII Levels, Mean ± SD**
Survivors 98.6 IU/ml ± 16.6
Decedents 80.5 IU/ml ± 21.4

* *N* = number of head injured patients.
** On the 60 individuals cited above.

Therapy for Head Trauma–Associated Coagulopathy

Traditional therapy for the coagulation dysfunction that follows a head injury has consisted of replacement of the consumed plasma and cellular constituents. In most instances in U.S. trauma centers, this has consisted of the judicious but aggressive administration of blood components. Fresh frozen plasma (FFP), platelets, and packed red blood cells are administered to treat both the blood loss from trauma and the ongoing microangiopathic hemolytic anemia. In many instances, rapid treatment of thrombocytopenia with platelets and replacement of natural inhibitors of thrombin generation (e.g., ATIII) and plasminogen activation (e.g., α_2-antiplasmin, PAI-1) with infusion of large volumes of FFP will permit early and extensive neurosurgery to be per-

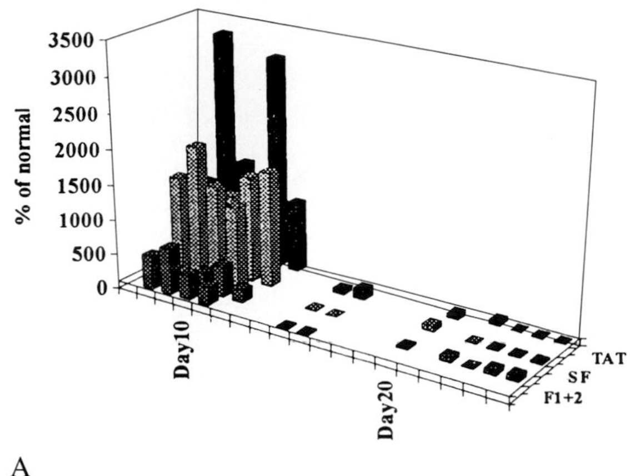

A

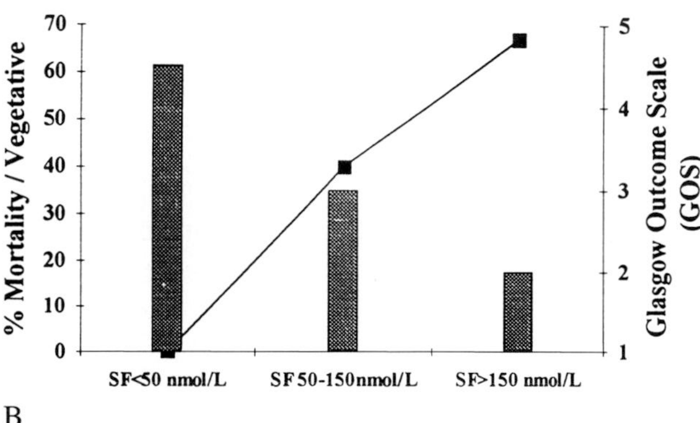

B

Figure 46-8. *A.* Elevations of selected biochemical products of coagulation activation in patients with head trauma. (TAT = thrombin-antithrombin complex; SF = soluble fibrin; F1 + 2 = prothrombin fragment 1 + 2) in the 25 days following injury. (Bredbacka, Hypercoagulation in anaesthesia and intensive care. Karolinska, Stockholm, 1993.) *B.* Correlations between circulating soluble fibrin levels and initial mortality/vegetative state (■—■) and Glascow Outcome Scale (bar graph) in individuals after a head injury. (Bredbacka, Hypercoagulation in anaesthesia and intensive care. Karolinska, Stockholm, 1993.)[91]

formed without life-threatening hemorrhage. However, the potential that FFP may be providing insufficient mitigation of ongoing microthrombogenesis in the brain and elsewhere has not been studied extensively. Hence, some neurosurgeons and trauma experts have undertaken to enhance the clotting inhibition with specific component therapies.

Aggressive use of component therapy designed to decrease the risk of an accelerating coagulopathy has been employed in European and Japanese trauma centers. In many instances, this has consisted of the administration of ATIII concentrates with or without the addition of heparin.[71,94] Several clinical case reports and small series have indicated (through not scientifically proved) the efficacy of such administration of ATIII concentrates in shortening the period of clinical DIC.[95] The rationale is, of course, that by blunting the generation of thrombin with associated clotting and inflammatory actions, one may be able to reduce the secondary injury complications (see above). Despite the fact that laboratory models have demonstrated the therapeutic benefit of ATIII concentrate infusion in aborting impending DIC, randomized, prospective, controlled studies that demonstrate once and for all the clinical efficacy of ATIII administration have not been performed. This lack of proven efficacy includes not only DIC associated with head trauma but also DIC from any acquired injury or disease.[84] The conclusion that the therapeutic efficacy of ATIII concentrate administration is lessening short-term and long-term morbidity and ultimately providing a possible benefit in reducing mortality after head injury awaits further study. Such a randomized, placebo-controlled, double-blind study of ATIII in moderately to severely injured head injured subjects is needed. New information about the benefit or lack of benefit of aggressive replenishment of ATIII in patients with post-traumatic DIC awaits the results of such a large multicenter clinical trial.

References

1. Keimowitz RM, Annis BL: Disseminated intravascular coagulation associated with massive brain injury. *J Neurosurg* 39:178–180, 1973.
2. Strinchini A, Baudo F, Nosari AM, et al: Defibrination and head injury. *Lancet* ii:957, 1974.
3. Preston FE, Malia RG, Sworn MJ, et al: Disseminated intravascular coagulation as a consequence of cerebral damage. *J Neurol Neurosurg Psychiatry* 37:241–248, 1974.
4. Vecht CJ, Smit Sibinga CT, Minderhoud JM: Disseminated intravascular coagulation head injury. *J Neurol Neurosurg Psychiatry* 38:567–571, 1975.
5. Watts C: Disseminated intravascular coagulation. *Surg Neurol* 8:258, 1977.
6. Clark JA, Finelli RE, Netsky MG: Disseminated intravascular coagulation following cranial trauma. *J Neurosurg* 52:266–269, 1980.
7. McGauley JL, Miller CA, Penner JA: Diagnosis and treatment of diffuse intravascular coagulation following cerebral trauma: Case report. *J Neurosurg* 43:374–376, 1975.
8. Tikk A, Noormaa U: The significance of cerebral and systemic disseminated intravascular coagulation in early prognosis of brain injury. *Acta Neurochir (Wien)* 28:96–97, 1978.
9. Nachmann RL, Hajjar KA, Silverstein RL, et al: Interleukin 1 induces endothelial synthesis of plasminogen activator inhibitor. *J Exp Med* 163:1595–1600, 1986.
10. Goodnight SH, Kenoyer G, Rapaport SI, et al: Defibrin-

ation after brain-tissue destruction. *N Engl J Med* 290(19):1043–1047, May 1974.
11. Rickles FR, Levin J, Hardin JA, et al: Tissue factor generation by human mononuclear cells: Effects of endotoxin and dissociation of tissue factor generation from the mitogenic response. *J Lab Clin Med* 89:792–803, 1977.
12. Marbet GA, Griffith MJ: Tissue thromboplastin induced reversible DIC and heparin-enhanced inhibitors in dogs. *Thromb Haemost* 55(1):78–85, 1986.
13. Bick RL: Disseminated intravascular coagulation and related syndromes: A clinical review. *Semin Thromb Hemost* 14(4):299–338, 1988.
14. Quick AJ: Determination of prothrombin. *Proc Soc Exp Biol Med* 42:788–789, 1939.
15. Bick RL: Disseminated intravascular coagulation. *Hematol Oncol Clin North Am* 6(6):1259–1285, 1992.
16. Conkling PR, Greenberg CS, Weinberg JB: Tumor necrosis factor induces tissue factor-like activity in human leukemia cell line U937 and peripheral blood monocytes. *Blood* 72:128–133, 1988.
17. Glusa E: Vascular effects of thrombin. *Semin Thromb Hemost* 18(3):296–304.
18. Glusa E, Markwardt F: Studies on thrombin-induced endothelium-dependent vascular effects. *Biomed Biochim Acta* 47:623–630, 1988.
19. Nakamura K, Hatano Y, Mori K: Thrombin-induced vasoconstriction in isolated cerebral arteries and the influence of a synthetic thrombin inhibitor. *Thromb Res* 40:715–720, 1985.
20. Drake TA, Morissey JH, Edgington TS: Selective expression of tissue factor in human tissues. *Am J Pathol* 134:1087–1097, 1989.
21. Edgington TS, Mackman N, Brand K, et al: The structural biology of expression and function of tissue factor. *Thromb Haemost* 66:67–79, 1991.
22. Edwards RL, Rickles FR: The role of leukocytes in the activation of blood coagulation. *Semin Hematol* 29(3):202–212, 1992.
23. Hawiger J: Adhesive interactions of blood cells and the vascular wall, in Colman RW, Hirsch J, Marder VJ, Salzman EW (eds): *Hemostasis and Thrombosis*, 3d ed. Philadelphia: JB Lippincott, 1994: 781–787.
24. Clauss M, Gerlach M, Gerlach H, et al: Vascular permeability factor: A tumor-derived polypeptide that induces endothelial cell and monocyte procoagulant activity, and promotes monocyte migration. *J Exp Med* 172:1535–1545, 1990.
25. Nawroth P, Stern D: Modulation of endothelial cell hemostatic properties by tumor necrosis factor. *J Exp Med* 164:740–745, 1986.
26. Jaffe EA, Grulich J, Weksler BB, et al: Correlation between thrombin-induced prostacyclin production and inositol triphosphate and cytosolic free calcium levels in cultured human endothelial cells. *J Biol Chem* 262:8557–8565, 1987.
27. Harmon JT, Jamieson GA: Activation of plates by α-thrombin is a receptor mediated event. *J Biol Chem* 261:15928–15933, 1986.
28. Broze G Jr, Girard TJ, Novotny WF: The lipoprotein-associated coagulation inhibitor. *Prog Hemost Thromb* 10:243–268, 1991.
29. Mann KG, Krishnaswamy S, Lawson JH: Surface-dependent hemostasis. *Semin Hematol* 29(3):213–226, 1992.
30. Nemerson Y: The tissue factor pathway of blood coagulation. *Semin Hematol* 29(3):170–176, 1992.
31. Walsh PN: Factor XI: A renaissance. *Semin Hematol* 29(3):189–201, 1992.
32. Mosesson MW: The roles of fibrinogen and fibrin in hemostasis and thrombosis. *Semin Hematol* 29(3):177–188, 1992.
33. Broze G Jr: Binding of human factor VII and VIIa to monocytes. *J Clin Invest* 70:526–535, 1982.
34. Edgington TS, Helin H, Gregory SA, et al: Cellular pathways and signals for the induction of biosynthesis by cells of the monocyte lineage of initiators of the coagulation protease cascade, in van Furth R (ed): *Mononuclear Phagocytes.* Boston: Martinis Nijhoff, 1985:687–696.
35. DeMoerloose PA, Reber GM, Rickles FR: Interferongamma induces procoagulant activity in macrophage cell lines (abstr). *Thromb Haemost* 54(suppl):1173, 1985.
36. Kornberg A, Catane R, Peller S, et al: Tuftsin induces tissue factor-like activity in human mononuclear cells and monocytic cell lines. *Blood* 76:814–819, 1990.
37. Chapman HA, Allen CL, Stone OL, et al: Human alveolar macrophages synthesize factor VII in vitro: Possible role in interstitial lung disease. *J Clin Invest* 75:2030–2037, 1985.
38. Edwards RL, Rickles FR: The role of human T cells (and T cell products) for monocyte tissue factor generation. *J Immunol* 125:606–616, 1980.
39. Deykin D: The role of the liver in serum induced hypercoagulability. *J Clin Invest* 45:256–263, 1966.
40. Shuman MA: Thrombin-cellular interactions. *Ann NY Acad Sci* 485:228–239, 1986.
41. Carney DH, Steirnberg J, Fenton JW II: Initiation of proliferative events by human thrombin requires both receptor binding and enzymic activity. *J Cell Biochem* 26:181–195, 1984.
42. Kohno M, Yasunari K, Yokokawa K, et al: Thrombin stimulates the production of immunoreactive endothelin-1 in cultured human umbilical vein endothelial cells. *Metabolism* 39:1003–1005, 1990.
43. Glusa E: Thrombin induces endothelium-dependent relaxation of pig coronary arteries. *Folia Haematol (Leipz)* 115:101–105, 1988.
44. Gebremedhin D, Ballagi-Pordany G, Hadhazy P, et al: Species specificity of thrombin-induced changes in vascular tone. *Eur J Pharmacol* 132:71–74, 1986.
45. Haver VM, Namm DH: Characterization of the thrombin-induced contraction of vascular smooth muscle. *Blood Vessels* 21:53–63, 1984.
46. Buller HR, Ten Cate JW: Acquired antithrombin III deficiency: Laboratory diagnosis, incidence, clinical implications, and treatment with antithrombin III concentrate. *Am J Med* 87(suppl 3B):44S–60S, 1989.
47. Faulk WP, Labarre CA: Antithrombin III in normal and transplanted human hearts: Indications of vascular disease. *Semin Hematol* 31(suppl):26–34, 1994.
48. Broze G, Miletich J: Biochemistry and physiology of

protein C, protein S, and thrombomodulin, in Colman RW, Hirsch J, Marder V, Salzman E (eds): *Hemostasis and Thrombosis: Basic Principles and Clinical Practice*, 3d ed. Philadelphia: Lippincott, 1994:259–276.

49. Cunningham DD, Pulliam L, Vaughan PJ: Protease nexin-1 and thrombin: Injury-related processes in the brain. *Thromb Haemost* 70(1):168–171, 1993.
50. Sundsmo JS, Fair DS: Relationships among the complement, kinin, coagulation and fibrinolytic systems in the inflammatory reaction. *Clin Physiol Biochem* 1:225–284, 1983.
51. Schmaier AH, Silverberg M, Kaplan AP, Colman RW: Contact activator and its abnormalities, in Colman RW, Hirsh J, Marder VJ, Salzman EW (eds): *Hemostasis and Thrombosis,* 2d ed. Philadelphia: Lippincott 1987: 18–38.
52. Risberg B, Andreasson S, Eriksson E: Disseminated intravascular coagulation. *Acta Anaesthesiol Scand* 35(suppl 95):60–71, 1991.
53. Van Ginkel CJW, Zeijlemaker WP, Stricker LAM, et al: Enhancement of monocyte thromboplastin activity by antigenically stimulated lymphocytes—A link between immune reactivity and blood coagulation. *Eur J Immunol* 11:579–583, 1981.
54. Karpati J, Varadi K, Elodi S: Effect of granulocyte proteases on human coagulation factors IX and X: The protective effect of calcium. *Hoppe Seylers Z Physiol Chem* 363:521–525, 1982.
55. Geczy CL, Jones A: Procoagulant induction by human lymphokine and interferon g/PMA on a myelomonocytic cell line, RC2a. *Br J Haematol* 70:211–218, 1988.
56. Cozzolino F, Torcia M, Miliani A, et al: Potential role of interleukin-1 as the trigger for diffuse intravascular coagulation in acute nonlymphoblastic leukemia. *Am J Med* 84:240–250, 1988.
57. Geczy CL: Induction of macrophage procoagulant by products of activated lymphocytes. *Haemostasis* 14:400–411, 1985.
58. Colvin RB, Dvorak HF: Role of the clotting system in cell-mediated hypersensitivity: II. Kinetics of fibrinogen/fibrin accumulation and vascular permeability changes in tuberculin and cutaneous basophil hypersensitivity reactions. *J Immunol* 114:377–387, 1975.
59. Moore KL, Andreoli SP, Esmon NL, et al: Endotoxin enhances tissue factor and suppresses thrombomodulin expression on human vascular endothelium in vitro. *J Clin Invest* 79:124–130, 1987.
60. Brett J, Gerlach H, Nawroth P, et al: Tumor necrosis factor/cachectin increases permeability of endothelial cell monolayers by a mechanism involving regulatory G proteins. *J Exp Med* 169:1977–1991, 1989.
61. Nawroth P, Handley D, Esmon C, et al: Interleukin 1 induces endothelial cell procoagulant while suppressing cell surface anticoagulant activity. *Proc Nat Acad Sci USA* 83:3460–3464, 1986.
62. Albert J, Blomqvist H, Gardlund B, et al: The effect of haemostatic variables of antithrombin concentrate in critically ill patients with low antithrombin levels. *Acta Anaesthesiol Scand* 36(8):745–752, 1992.
63. Semeraro N, Colucci M: Changes in the coagulation-fibrinolysis balance of endothelial cells and mononuclear phagocytes: Role in disseminated intravascular coagulation associated with infectious diseases. *Int J Clin Lab Res* 21(3):214–220, 1992.
64. Touho H, Hirakawa K, Hino A, et al: Relationship between abnormalities of coagulation and fibrinolysis and postoperative intracranial hemorrhage in head injury. *Neurosurgery* 19(4):523–531, 1986.
65. Van der Sander JJ, Emeis JJ, Lindemar J: Intravascular coagulation: A common phenomenon in minor experimental head injury. *J Neurosurg* 54(1):21–25, 1981.
66. Marbet GA, Griffith MJ: Tissue thromboplastin induced reversible DIC and heparin-enhanced inhibitors in dogs. *Thromb Haemost* 55(1):78–85, 1986.
67. Kaufman HH, Mattson JC: Coagulopathy in head injury, in Becker DP (ed): *Central Nervous System Trauma Status Report.* Besthesda, MD.: National Institute of Neurological and Communicative Disorders and Stroke. 1985:187–206.
68. Drayer BP, Poser CM: Disseminated intravascular coagulation and head trauma: Two case studies. *JAMA* 231:174–175, 1975.
69. Olson JD, Kaufman HH, Moake J, et al: The incidence and significance of hemostatic abnormalities in patients with head injuries. *Neurosurgery* 24:825–832, 1989.
70. Pitts LH: Medical complications of head injury, in Cooper PR (ed): *Head Injury.* Baltimore: Waverly Press, 1982:333–334.
71. Kumura E, Sato M, Fukuda A, et al: Coagulation disorders following acute head injury. *Acta Neurochir (Wien)* 85:23–28, 1987.
72. Greenwald B, Brooks DM, Barnes T, et al: The effect of age on the development of coagulopathy in severely head-injured patients. American Association of Neurosurgeons, Poster 1262, p. 371. San Francisco.
73. Keimowitz RM, Annis BL: Disseminated intravascular coagulation associated with massive brain injury. *J Neurosurg* 39:178–180, 1973.
74. Stein SC, Young GS, Talucci RC, et al: Delayed brain injury after head trauma: Significance of coagulopathy. *Neurosurgery* 30(2):160–165, 1992.
75. Kaufman HH, Moake JL, Olson JD, et al: Delayed and recurrent intracranial hematomas related to disseminated intravascular clotting and fibrinolysis in head injury. *Neurosurgery* 7(5):445–449, 1980.
76. Stein SC, Spettell C, Young G, Ross SE: Delayed and progressive brain injury in closed-head trauma: Radiological demonstration. *Neurosurgery* 32(1):25–31, 1993.
77. Miner ME, Kaufman HH, Graham SH, et al: Disseminated intravascular coagulation fibrinolytic syndrome following head injury in children: Frequency and prognostic implications. *J Pediatr* 100:687–691, 1982.
78. Kaufman HH, Makela ME, Lee KF, et al: Gunshot wounds to the head: A perspective. *Neurosurgery* 18(6):689–695, 1986.
79. Hoots WK, Contant C, Mattson J, et al: The "talk and die" phenomenon: Disseminated intravascular coagulation as a possible explanation for dramatic deterioration among head trauma patients. *Blood* 62(suppl 1)1003:275a, 1983.

80. Kaufman HH, Kin-Sang H, Mattson JC, et al: Clinicopathological correlations of disseminated intravascular coagulation in patients with head injury. *Neurosurgery* 15(1):34–42, 1984.
81. Bredbacka S: *Hypercoagulation in Anesthesia and Intensive Care: Risk Estimation and Prediction of Outcome.* Thesis from Congle. Karolinska Medico Chirugiska Institute, Stockholm, 1993.
82. Schipper HG, Jenkins CSP, Kahle LH, et al: Antithrombin-III transfusion in disseminated intravascular coagulation. *Lancet* 2:854–856, 1978.
83. Brandt P, Jespersen J, Gregersen G: Postpartum haemolytic-uraemic syndrome successfully treated with antithrombin III. *Br Med J* 280:44, 1980.
84. Buller HR, Weenink AH, Treffers PE, et al: Severe antithrombin III deficiency in a patient with pre-eclampsia. *Scand J Haematol* 25:81–86, 1980.
85. Laursen B, Mortensen JZ, Frost L, et al: Disseminated intravascular coagulation in hepatic failure treated with antithrombin III. *Thromb Res* 22:701–704, 1981.
86. Miller RS, Weatherford DA, Stein M: Antithrombin III and trauma patients: Factors that determine low levels. *Journal of Trauma* 37(3):442–445, 1994.
87. Dickneite G, Pâques E-P: Reduction of mortality with antithrombin III in septicemic rates: A study of klebsiella pneumoniae induced sepsis. *Thromb Haemost* 69(2):98–102, 1993.
88. Fourrier F, Chopin C, Goudemand J, et al: Septic shock, multiple organ failure, and disseminated intravascular coagulation: Compared patterns of antithrombin III, protein c, and protein s deficiencies. *Chest* 101:816–823, 1992.
89. Wada H, Minamikawa K, Wakita Y, Nakase T, et al: Hemostatic study before onset of disseminated intravascular coagulation. *Am J Hematol* 43:190–194, 1993.
90. Bredbacka S, Blombäck M, Wiman B, Pelzer H: Laboratory methods for detecting disseminated intravascular coagulation (DIC): New aspects. *Acta Anaesthesiol Scand* 37:125–130, 1993.
91. Bredbacka S, Blombäck M, Wiman B: Soluble fibrin: A predictor for the development and outcome of multiple organ failure. *American Journal of Hematology* 46(4):289–294, 1994.
92. Bredbacka S, Blombäck M, Wiman B, Pelzer H: Disseminated intravascular coagulation in neurosurgical patients: Diagnosis by new laboratory methods. *J Neurosurg Anesthesiol* 4:128–133, 1992.
93. Bredbacka S, Edner G: Soluble fibrin and D-dimer as detectors of hypercoagulability in patients with isolated brain trauma, (submitted for publication).
94. Hanada T, Abe T, Takita H: Antithrombin III concentrates for treatment of disseminated intravascular coagulation in children. *Am J Pediatr Hematol Oncol* 7(1):3–8, 1985.
95. Blauhut B, Necek S, Vinazzer H, Bergmann H: Substitution therapy with an antithrombin III concentrate in shock and DIC. *Thromb Res* 27:271–278, 1982.

CHAPTER 47

DELAYED TRAUMATIC INTRACRANIAL HEMATOMA

Timothy I. Cohen
Steven K. Gudeman

SYNOPSIS

Delayed traumatic intracranial hematomas, including delayed traumatic intracerebral, epidural, and subdural hematomas, have been increasingly recognized since the advent of CT scanning and can be a significant source of morbidity and mortality in head-injured patients. They are treated using principles similar to those employed for most intracranial mass lesions and require meticulous care to minimize damage from secondary injury. In this chapter, the pathogenesis, diagnosis, management, and outcome of these lesions are reviewed. Delayed hematomas are associated with a worse prognosis. Potential diagnostic and therapeutic strategies are outlined.

DELAYED TRAUMATIC INTRACEREBRAL HEMATOMA

Delayed traumatic intracerebral hematomas (DTICHs) were originally described by Bollinger in 1891 as "*traumatische spat apoplexie*." The entity of late traumatic apoplexy was defined by Bollinger in his original work as an apoplectic event preceded by a history of trauma and a relatively asymptomatic period without preexisting vascular pathology. His original work described three patients at autopsy with delayed hemorrhage and fourth ventricular blood, and a fourth patient with a parieto-occipital hemorrhage with ventricular extension.[1] Bollinger hypothesized that necrotic softening occurred near a vessel, causing delayed rupture and hemorrhage. Traumatic late apoplexy was later applied throughout the literature to a number of conditions, including rupture of congenital or traumatic aneurysms, late-onset cranial nerve palsies, and even episodes of somnolence and confusion, to which it did not apply.[2]

The early development of the concept of DTICH has occurred in a number of stages that have been outlined by Duret.[3] The original work of Bollinger was refuted by Langerhans, who thought these hemorrhages occurred secondary to an undiagnosed vascular anomaly.[2]

In 1904 a significant contribution was presented by Lafforgue,[4] who thought that delayed hemorrhage occurred as a result of an earlier hemorrhage. Pathological confirmation of this was provided by von Holder, who showed that vascular integrity was compromised in areas of the brain with resultant microhematoma after a head injury.[5]

The focus from the earlier years of mainly operative or autopsy findings has changed recently to radiographic features. This change, which has been caused by dramatically improved imaging, explains the increased recognition of DTICH. The definition, pathogenesis, and treatment also have undergone significant changes with advancing technology and imaging.

DEFINITION

The definition of DTICH has evolved from a clinical diagnosis with autopsy verification to a primarily radiographic one. In Bollinger's original definition, an apoplectiform event with prior head trauma and an asymptomatic period in the absence of vascular pathology with findings of intraparenchymal and intraventricular blood at autopsy satisfied the criteria of "*traumatisch spat apoplexy*." The term was later applied to patients with delayed neurological deterioration with ventriculographic, angiographic, operative, or autopsy diagnosis of intracerebral hematoma.[3–15] Computed tomography (CT) scanning, with its ability to identify areas of hemorrhage as well as preexisting small focal abnormalities, has revolutionized the concept of DTICH. However, there is still no uniform definition of DTICH, and this makes a concise evaluation of its incidence and pathophysiology difficult. Neurotraumatologists tend to use many different subjective criteria for inclusion in this category. The spectrum of cases can range from patients without a clearly explainable course to the exclusion of patients with any abnormality on initial CT.[14,17,18] An appropriate definition of DTICH based on head CT, although arbitrary, is that of Lipper and coworkers. Their series included patients with no lesion, or a lesion less than 1 cm on initial CT, who developed high-density intraparenchymal lesions on follow-up CT.[13] Magnetic resonance imaging (MRI), with its improved resolution and earlier detection of lesions, may help further define and predict DTICH in the future.[19]

Incidence

The detection of DTICH has increased steadily with improved imaging. Before the advent of CT scanning, DTICH was thought to be rare. In the series by Baratham and Dennyson in 1972, only 21 of 7866 head injuries were complicated by the development of DTICH.[10] The primary reasons for the low detection rates were numerous and included (1) poor imaging capabilities, (2) poor survival from the initial insult, and (3) strict criteria for patients who were asymptomatic or had a minimal deficit after a closed head injury with subsequent decline and a radiographically and pathologically proven hematoma.

Improved imaging, the use of prehospital and hospital care, and wider recognition of this entity by clinicians have enhanced the identification of DTICH. The incidence, though increased, is still variable and is based on a number of factors, including patient selection, CT resolution, the timing and frequency of CT scanning, and the inclusion criteria.[11,13]

Understandably, studies with more severely injured patients, such as the series of Cooper and colleagues[11] and Gudeman and associates,[20] show a greater incidence of DTICH than do studies with less severely injured patients. The series of Cooper and Gudeman, which define an identical group of patients with a Glasgow Coma Scale (GCS) ≤ 8, when combined show an incidence of approximately 10 percent. As illustrated by Young et al.[21] the resolution of a CT scanner can alter incidence through the identification of small areas of cerebral contusion on initial head CT. Furthermore, the timing and frequency of CT scanning can have a considerable effect on incidence figures, as DTICH usually occurs within the first 72 h after a head injury.[20] A head CT obtained no later than 1 to 2 h after an injury may show a hematoma that was not initially present. It has been noted in several studies that regularly established intervals for CT scanning reveal larger numbers of DTICHs.[10,12,20] The increase in numbers of DTICHs is a result of the identification of lesions that caused no deterioration or were thought to be traumatic brain edema with increased intracranial pressure (ICP).[22] Finally, as was noted earlier, the range of definitions of DTICH can make the assessment of incidence difficult.[13]

The population most commonly stricken with DTICH seems to show a bimodal distribution in a number of series.[8–10,20,23] Baratham and Dennyson in the pre-CT era, with 21 of 7866 head-injured patients, showed that DTICH occurred predominantly in the 70- to 80-year age range.[10] More recent studies by Gudeman and associates show an average age in the thirties to forties.[20]

Imaging

DTICH originally was described on a clinical and autopsy basis. Early investigators noted an association between fracture as noted on plain skull x-rays and DTICH. The concurrence in one series was as high as 72 percent.[23] Fractures occurring anywhere in the skull increase the risk of DTICH, especially frontal, temporal, and occipital fractures. (Fig. 47-1, *A* to *D*).[23,24] Ventriculography represented the next improvement in imaging. Somewhat greater accuracy in localizing the hematoma and the possibility of draining the DTICH after burr hole placement were the major benefits of this method.[9] Angiography was also a useful means of diagnosis for Baratham and Dennyson because of the usual frontal or temporal location of the clot.[10]

CT scanning, which is currently the method of choice, replaced all imaging modalities because of its speed and definition. A noncontrasted head CT usually is adequate after a trauma. Severe injury and developing neurological deficits generally call for sequential scans. These follow-up scans usually increase the detection of DTICH. Evaluation of the ability of contrast-enhanced CT to predict future sites of DTICH has shown that only 50% of abnormally enhanced areas become intracerebral hemorrhages. High-density lesions on noncontrasted head CT usually occur in the frontal and temporal lobes secondary to a coup-countrecoup type of injury.

The next technical advance in the imaging of DTICH appears to be MRI. Improved resolution and the ability to detect small lesions early have shown some promise, as illustrated by Tanaka and associates.[19] In this study,

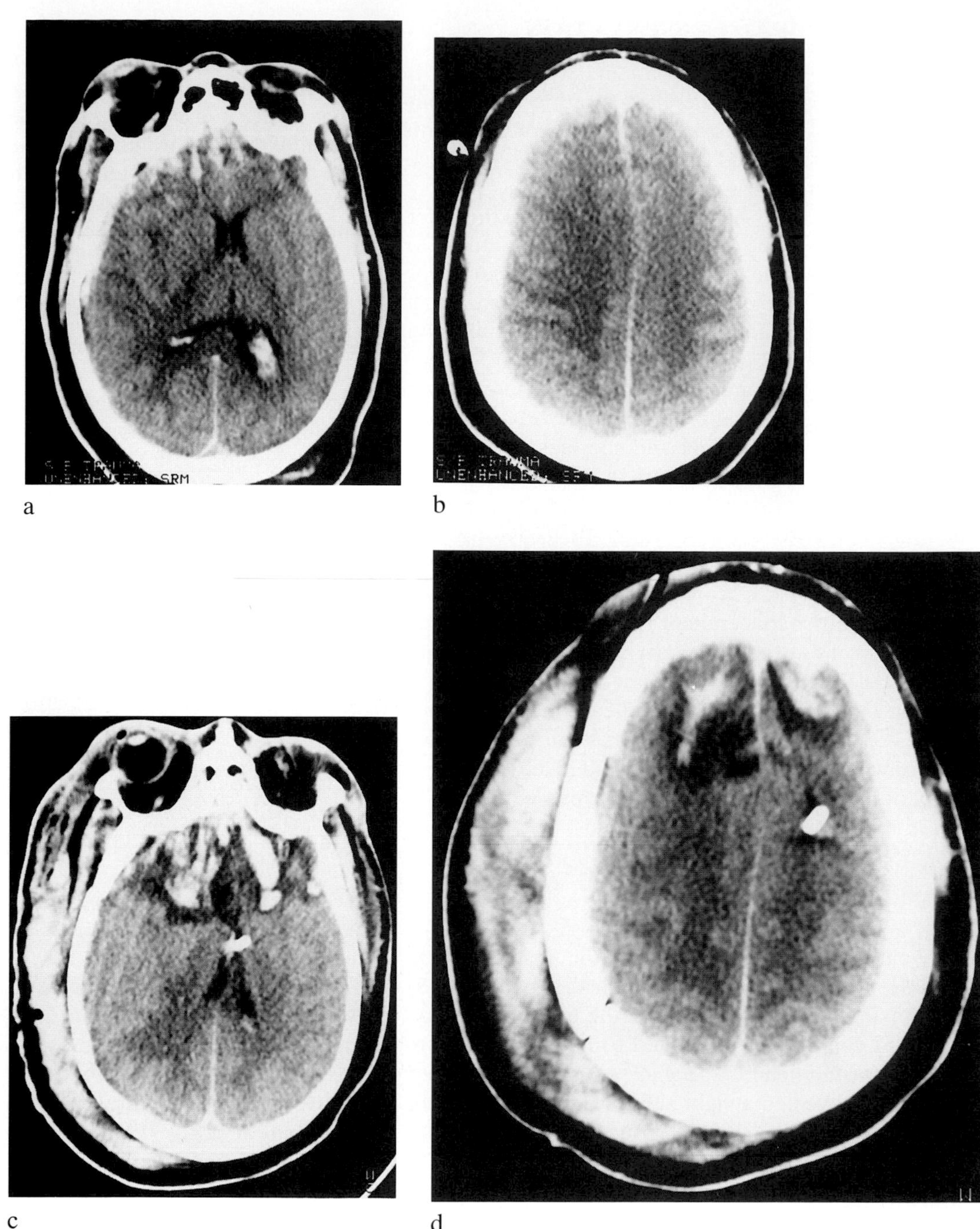

Figure 47-1. *A* and *B*. Case 1. Admission CT scan showing a right subdural hematoma with a right-to-left midline shift of 8 mm with small bifrontal, subdural, and bifrontal interhemispheric subarachnoid blood and left trigonal intraventricular hemorrhage. *C* and *D*. Axial CT scan of the head 72 h after admission showing the development of bifrontal DTICH, a left frontal ventriculostomy, and changes consistent with a right trauma craniotomy.

six patients whose exams did not fit with CT findings underwent MRI. In four of these patients, MRI showed high-intensity lesions on T_2 scans, which all subsequently developed into DTICH. In the other two patients there were no abnormalities on the T_2-weighted images, with follow-up CT correlating this finding. As MRI develops with improved speed of acquisition and patient monitoring, it will undoubtedly augment and/or replace CT in the assessment of head injury neurotrauma. It also may facilitate the diagnosis of impending DTICH and possibly allow the development of prophylactic strategies.

Clinical Presentation

The clinical presentation of patients with DTICH is variable but appears to be best stratified into four groups. Group I patients are those who present with minor or moderate head injury (GCS > 8) and have DTICH discovered on routine head CT.

Group II patients, who are well described in the older literature,[1,2,5] are relatively asymptomatic for hours to weeks. They subsequently suffer an apoplectic event or a progressive neurological deficit requiring intervention or autopsy. In an analysis of patients who "talk and deteriorate," only 12 percent suffered from DTICH.[25] Groups I and II predominate in the early literature on DTICH. The high mortality rate from severe brain injury associated with DTICH and the lack of sophisticated imaging were major factors in this poor survival.

Group III patients are best defined in the study by Gudeman and associates, in which 10 to 12 severely head-injured patients who were unable to obey simple commands and speak words (GCS ≤ 8) developed DTICH without a concomitant rise in ICP or a decline in neurological status.[16] Patients with medically manageable increased ICP also are included in this group.

Group IV patients are severely head-injured persons with a GCS ≤ 8 who develop a decline in neurological status, have medically uncontrollable ICP, or show signs of impending herniation.[9,21,23,26] An example of DTICH is presented in Case 1.

Case 1

A 42-year-old male was found on the road. He was transported by the emergency medical service (EMS) to an outside hospital and then to the authors' facility. On arrival, the patient was noted to have a GCS of 6. A noncontrasted head CT (Fig. 47-1*A* and *B*) obtained at that time revealed a right subdural hematoma with a right-to-left midline shift of about 8 mm with a small bifrontal subdural hematoma, bifrontal interhemispheric subarachnoid blood, fourth ventricular blood, and a linear nondepressed left suboccipital skull fracture. The patient was emergently taken to the operating room for evacuation of the right acute subdural hematoma via a right frontotemporoparietal craniotomy. At surgery, he was noted to have a superficial right temporal contusion with approximately 1-cm right acute subdural and right hemispheric edema. A left frontal ventriculostomy was placed on completion of the case, and the patient was transferred to the intensive care unit (ICU), where he was treated with CSF drainage and intermittent mannitol. His neurological exam improved somewhat with intermittent localization, ICP running in the midteens to the high twenties, and cerebral perfusion pressures in the range of 70 to 100 mmHg. On the third postoperative day, the patient developed seizures and right pupillary dilation with increased ICP into the mid-sixties. The patient underwent a repeat CT scan (Fig. 47-1*C* and *D*), which showed the development of bifrontal delayed traumatic intracerebral hemorrhages. The patient was treated with increased intermittent mannitol and continued CSF drainage and subsequently improved to the point of following commands.

Treatment

The guidelines for the treatment of DTICH are not significantly different from those for the treatment of other traumatic intracranial hematomas. These strategies can be broken down along the lines of the four clinical groups, with patients crossing over into groups in accordance with the progression of their neurological status. Group 1 patients without or with a minimal deficit, that presents incidentally or secondary to seizures, should have a period of observation and treatment of seizures with close clinical follow-up. Group II patients who present with a relatively good GCS but abruptly decompensate, require immediate operative intervention with peri- and intraoperative management to prevent secondary insults. Postoperatively, these patients should receive maximal medical therapy with ICP monitoring and follow-up head CT for any significant neurological or ICP changes. Group III patients who present with GCS less than or equal to 8 and show no discernible neurological change or medically uncontrollable increase in ICP, require close monitoring of neurological status and ICP. This group should be treated with maximal medical management to prevent increasing ICP and a worsening neurological status. Group III patients who do not respond to maximal medical therapy with an improvement in neurological status or a decrease in ICP are treated as Group IV patients.

Group IV patients are those who present with a poor neurological status (GCS less than or equal to 8) and have progressive neurological deterioration or medically uncontrollable ICP. These patients require hematoma evacuation with maximal peri- and intraoperative medical therapy. However, these general guidelines for treatment must be tailored to the specific situation. Perioperatively, a patient's clinical status must be optimized (i.e., attempts must be made to correct hypoxia, coagulopathies, hypovolemia, and associated injuries) to ensure the best outcome and prevent secondary injury.[20,21,23]

Etiology and Pathogenesis

As was noted earlier, the pathogenesis of DTICH has not been clearly elucidated. It has been suggested that several pathological processes contribute to the formation of DTICH. Bollinger, in his first description of late traumatic apoplexy, felt that the underlying event occurred as a result of necrotic brain softening. This necrotic softening occurred adjacent to a vessel wall, with subsequent rupture and the formation of an intercerebral hematoma.[1] Von Holder proposed that at primary injury there are small areas of vascular and parenchymal compromise, leading to extravasation of blood and focal hemorrhages, which ultimately coalesce to form an enlarging hematoma.[5] This theory of coalescence of extravasated microhematomas was augmented by the concept of dysautoregulation put forth by Gudeman and associates[20] and Evans and Scheinker.[27] The model proposed by Gudeman and associates describes a previously injured brain with failed mechanisms for the regulation of cerebral blood flow that when exposed to hypotension and hypoxia causes vasodilation with increased intravascular pressure and rupture with hemorrhage. This breakdown in the blood-brain barrier can cause an enlargement of the hematoma through the self-perpetuating cycle of increasing hemorrhaging causing increased hypoxia and decreased perfusion.

The presence of a local or systemic coagulopathy also causes enlargement of a hematoma secondary to poor hemostasis.[28] Bullock and colleagues showed hematoma enlargement in their report of 12 out of 13 patients who had a coagulopathy that was verified or was presumed to be secondary to alcohol intoxication with associated platelet dysfunction.[29]

The local method of hematoma enlargement involves exposure to the thromboplastic substances of the brain that produce intravascular coagulation. The vascular occlusion, with the resultant infarct formation, results in an enlarging area of regionally injured brain, which ultimately continues on to hematoma formation by the mechanisms mentioned above.

The theory of vascular occlusion with subsequent hematoma formation was hypothesized secondary to the large number of intracerebral hematomas, which were demonstrated to occur after decompression of an extracerebral hematoma.[23] It was felt that in cases in which patients presented with epidural or subdural hematomas, venous thrombi with infarction occurred; upon removal of the extracerebral hematoma. This was substantiated by the work of Czernicki and Koznieska, which reproduced the effect of epidural compression with an inflatable balloon. Intracerebral hemorrhages occurred after balloon deflation in the cat model. Their explanation for intracranial hemorrhage (ICH) was the disruption of the blood-brain barrier secondary to cerebral ischemia and an intravascular clot.[30]

Outcome

A review of the literature shows that patients with DTICH have a universally poor outcome.[17,19,23,26] Mortality associated with DTICH ranges from 50 to 75 percent, with a high number of the surviving patients having poor outcomes. Mortality and vegetative rates seem to have remained fairly constant despite the advent of CT scanning. Thus, as suggested by Diaz and coworkers[26] and Gudeman and associates,[20] DTICH may be an epiphenomenon associated with secondary insults that compound the injury to an already damaged brain. However, these hypotheses remain conjectural.

DELAYED EPIDURAL HEMATOMA

Definition

Delayed epidural hematomas are now more frequently seen, probably as a result of improved transport times and the liberal use of head CT in head-injured patients.[31–33] The current definition of a delayed epidural hematoma is made primarily on the basis of the CT scan and includes lesions that are not apparent on the initial CT scan after a head injury, but are evident on follow-up CT. The absence of a radiologically identifiable skull fracture does not exclude the possibility of the formation of a delayed epidural hematoma.

Incidence and Epidemiology

Epidural hematomas are uncommon in children.[34] In adults, Teasdale and Galbraith[35] noted an overall incidence of intracranial hematomas in head injury patients that ranged from approximately 1 to 30 percent in patients with head trauma, depending on the institution's referral base. At least 20 to 30 percent of the hematomas were epidural.[35] Chan and coworkers[36] evaluated 1178 adolescents with head injury and noted that 13 developed ICH, with only 1 developing a delayed epidural hematoma (DEDH) in conjunction with subdural and intracerebral hemorrhages. This prospective study showed a 1.1 percent incidence of epidural hematomas in adolescents, with the overall incidence of DEDH being 0.08 percent of the total number of adolescents with head injuries and 10 percent of the patients with epidural hematomas.[36] The single patient with DEDH died, while all nine patients with acute epidural hematomas survived with good recovery.

The occurrence of DEDHs in adults in a number of series appears to be between 5 and 10 percent of that of acute epidural hematomas.[31,33] There is a male-to-female preponderance, as would be expected from most incidences of head injury. The average age across a number of large series is 27 years, with a range from 9 to 70 years.[1–3] This is significant, because it is thought that the dura of the elderly population is more adherent to the inner table of the skull than is the case in the younger age group. This appears to be a protective feature among the elderly in regard to acute epidural hematomas (AEDHs). The inciting events in order of frequency are typically motor vehicle or pedestrian accidents, falls, and focal head traumas. A fracture overlying a DEDH is typical, although there are several cases in the literature with no overlying fracture.

AEDHs have classically occurred in the temporal region secondary to fracture of the thin overlying temporal squama with a subsequent tear of the middle meningeal artery in its bony groove. These patients deteriorate rapidly because of the high pressure associated with arterial bleeding and rapidly increasing ICP.

It is also known that the vein running with the artery in the bony groove contributes to a large number of epidural hematomas, as do venous sinuses and diploic veins. The remainder of AEDHs occur in the frontal and occipital regions with approximately equal frequency. DEDHs occur most commonly and with equal frequency in the temporal, frontal, and parietal regions.

Imaging

The more liberal use of CT scanning will undoubtedly increase recognition of DEDHs and improve patient outcome.

The association between a skull fracture and both acute and delayed epidural hematomas has been well described in the literature.[31,36,37] However, the absence of a skull fracture does not necessarily rule out the development of an epidural hematoma. The use of CT scanning therefore cannot be overrated in patients with a closed head injury as an aid to the diagnosis of increased ICP or declining neurological status.

Clinical Presentation

There appears to be no distinct clinical presentation of patients with a DEDH. Patients range from those, as illustrated by Ashkenazi and associates,[37] who suffered from severe headache but were without a neurological deficit to those, as described by Meguro and colleagues[38] and Feuerman and coworkers,[39] whose GCS scores ranged from 4 to 9 and who underwent operative intervention for other intracranial pathology and subsequently developed delayed contralateral epidural hematomas with brain herniation. The delayed hematoma may appear anywhere from minutes to 16 days after an injury, as identified by Sparacio and coworkers.[40] The three patients described by Ashkenazi and associates were admitted to the hospital after a head injury and recovered with a GCS of 15 without a neurological deficit; however, they all complained of continued severe headaches and for that reason underwent CT scanning. All three patients were found to have DEDHs that were evacuated via a craniotomy. These patients were subsequently discharged in excellent condition.[37]

Patients with DEDH also may present with neurological deterioration and, after the discovery of an epidural hematoma on CT, undergo operative removal. This group of patients tend to display a good recovery in the absence of associated extra- and intracranial pathology.

Case 2

A 7-year-old white male was struck by a truck while riding his bicycle. On presentation to an outside emergency room (ER), he had a GCS of 14, losing a point for verbal score with some disorientation. He was otherwise neurologically intact and underwent a head CT (Fig. 47-2*A* and *B*) which was thought to be normal. The patient deteriorated over the next hour and was intubated and transferred to the authors' facility. On arrival, the patient was noted to have a GCS of 7, and underwent an immediate head CT, which showed a large left frontal epidural hematoma (Fig. 47-2*C* and *D*). The patient was then taken to the operating room (OR) for evacuation of the delayed epidural hematoma. The patient improved over the next 24 h and was extubated. He left the hospital 4 days later without a neurological deficit. At 3 months after injury, the patient remained neurologically intact and was doing well.

Etiology and Pathogenesis

DEDHs form as a result of several contributing factors. They occur more commonly in a younger population, as would be expected because of the looser adherence of the dura mater to the skull. Typically, AEDHs as well as DEDHs are associated with an overlying fracture; however, while this is the usual case, a fracture may not be identified, as illustrated by Case 2. The initial trauma is the inciting event, at which time a source of bleeding is created that eventually manifests itself when the system is no longer able to compensate for the insult. Evaluation of the causes of DEDH include the source of the bleeding, a tamponade effect and its release, and the systematic pathology that contributes to the formation of delayed clots.

The bleeding was classically thought to originate from a tear of the middle meningeal artery secondary to a fracture of the inner table of the temporal squama. Venous bleeding from the vein running with the middle meningeal from the dural sinuses, from small venules, or from diploic veins also provides a low-pressure source for a slowly growing hematoma. The resultant accommodation by the brain and CSF to slowly increasing

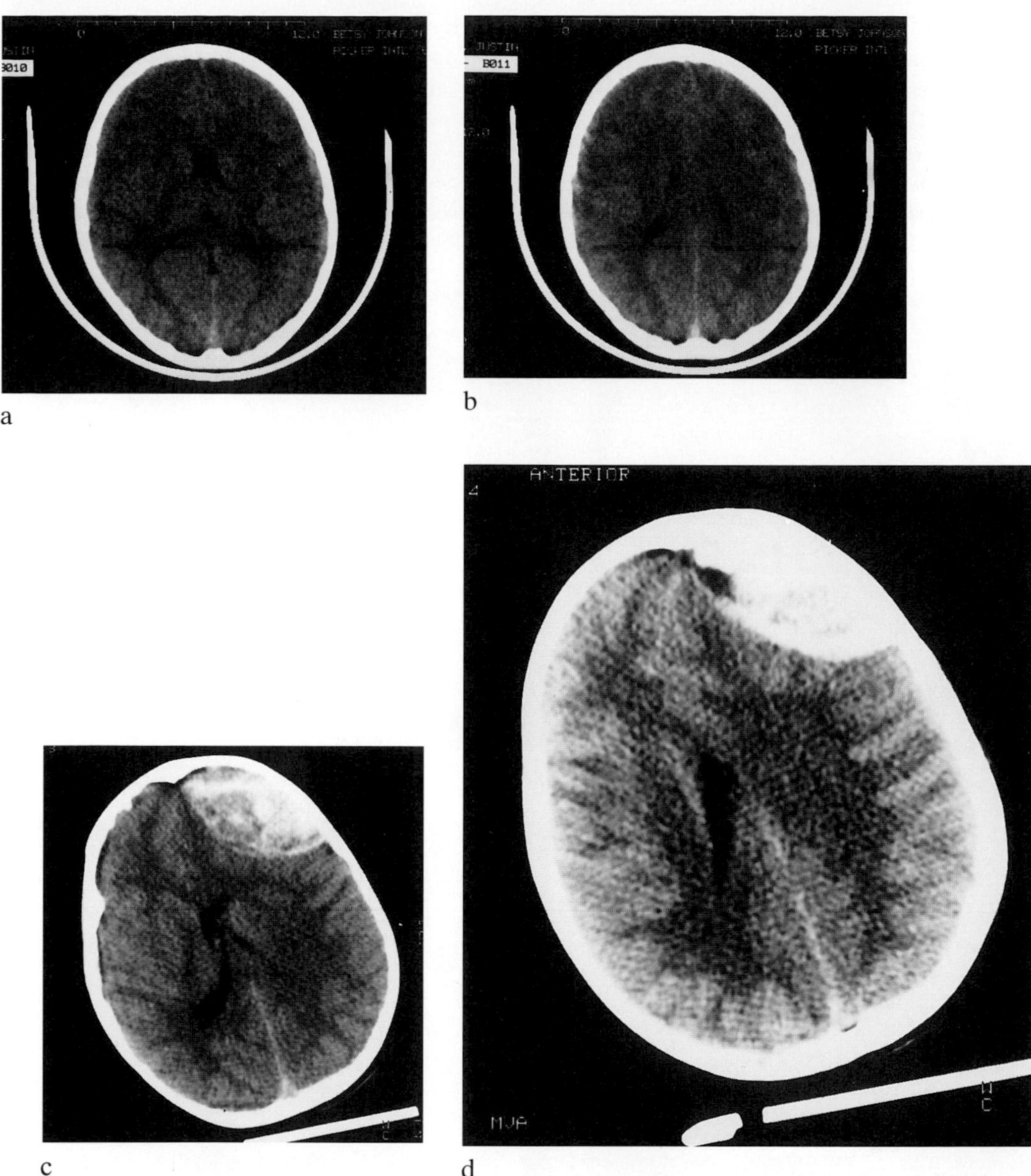

Figure 47-2. *A* and *B*. Case 2. Admission axial head CT showing a normal exam. *C* and *D*. Axial head CT 4 h after trauma showing a large left frontal delayed epidural hematoma with 1 cm of midline shift.

ICP may explain the many patients who present with worsening headache, with or without slowly progressive neurological deficits. Delayed bleeding rarely occurs from other sources as well, including traumatically induced pseudoaneurysms and traumatic arteriovenous fistulae, which rupture at a later time.[41,42]

The association of both AEDH and DEDH is well noted. The fracture overlying the source of bleeding may actually be beneficial after an injury, allowing decompression of the epidural blood into the subgaleal space and temporalis muscle. This decompression through a fracture works in an opposite direction to the tamponade effect, which basically implies that secondary to a number of reasons (including brain edema and a contralateral hematoma), ICP is increased, providing a tamponade effect to the source of bleeding with a subsequent delay in hematoma formation. The brain edema in patients with significant head injury serves to increase the force on the dura, with a resultant decrease in the rate of bleeding into the epidural space, which is not evident on acute CT scanning after the injury. This protective mechanism can be counteracted, as shown by Mendelow et al.[43], with the administration of mannitol.

Another novel method of decreasing tamponade was

described by Borovich et al.[33] in two of their patients with traumatically induced CSF leaks. The CSF leaks contributed to DEDH formation by lowering ICP and releasing the tamponade on the previously injured vessel or vessels.

The removal of a contralateral hematoma has been well described in the literature by Meguro and colleagues,[38] and Feuerman and coworkers,[39] and is thought by some researchers to be a completely separate entity. This subgroup of DEDHs fits the criteria for inclusion in this group and portrays the pathophysiology behind the tamponade effect. A heightened awareness of this entity allows rapid diagnosis and always should be included in the differential diagnosis when brain be-

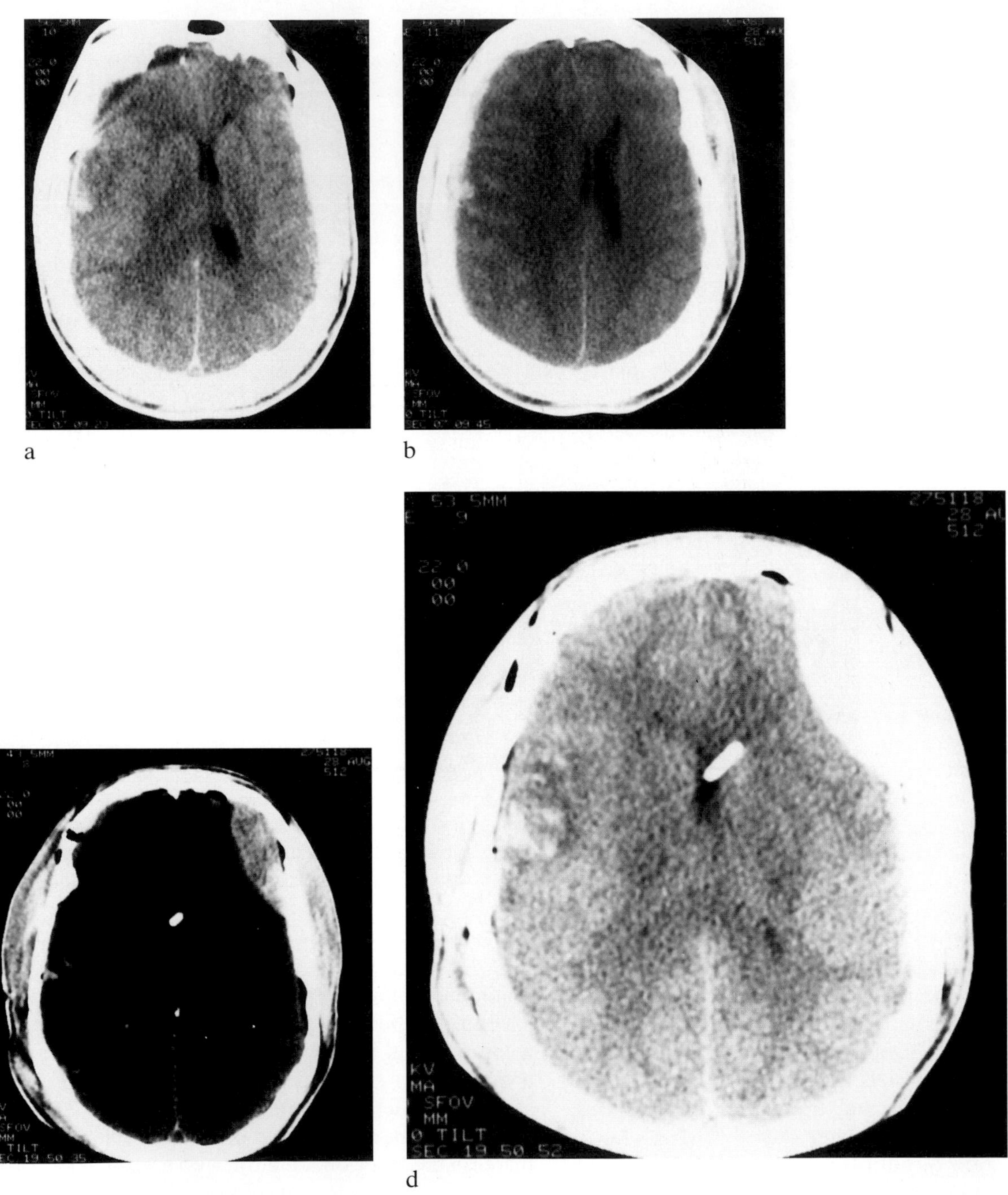

Figure 47-3. *A* and *B*. Case 3. Axial head CT on admission showing right acute subdural hematoma with 1 cm of midline shift, and small ventricles in a right temporoparietal contusion with edema. *C* and *D*. Axial head CT postoperatively shows left frontal epidural hematoma and a left frontal ventriculostomy in place.

gins to herniate through a craniotomy performed for a previously diagnosed traumatic lesion, with cerebral edema and hyperemia occurring secondary to a number of local and systematic causes. A variant of this description is illustrated by Case 3.

Case 3

A 26-year-old white male who was involved in a single-car motor vehicle accident (MVA) presented to the emergency room intubated and hemodynamically stable with a GCS of E1, VT, M5 for 7T, with 4-mm bilaterally reactive pupils, and other cranial nerves intact. Associated injuries included an open left femur fracture, a right pneumothorax, and an acute abdomen with a positive diagnostic peritoneal lavage. The patient's head CT (Fig. 47-3*A* and *B*) showed a right acute subdural hematoma with approximately 1 cm of midline shift, small ventricles, and a right temporoparietal contusion with edema. The patient was taken to the OR immediately, where a right frontotemporoparietal craniotomy was performed with evacuation of the right subdural hematoma. A left frontal ventriculostomy was placed for ICP monitoring. Concurrently, an exploratory laparotomy was performed, which revealed a small laceration of the spleen that was repaired primarily. Immediate postoperative CT (Fig. 47-3*C* and *D*) showed that the patient had a small left frontal epidural hematoma, which secondary to his low ICP and generally poor condition was managed conservatively in the ICU. The patient's ICP began to rise while he was receiving medical therapy over the next day, and he was taken to the OR, where a left frontal craniotomy for evacuation of the epidural hematoma was performed. Postoperatively, the patient's ICP remained low, he improved neurologically to following commands, and he was extubated after being weaned from the ventilator over a 5-day period. He subsequently recovered with a good outcome.

Systemic pathology is thought to contribute significantly to the formation of a DEDH. It has been noted in several studies that patients who initially presented hypotensive with negative head CTs later developed epidural hematoma on resuscitation. Hypotension may serve as a protective mechanism in patients with a torn middle meningeal artery, as the pressure head may not be forceful enough to strip the dura from the inner table; upon correction of patients to normotensive and hypertensive levels in the effort to raise cerebral perfusion pressure (CPP), the hemorrhagic force overpowers the adherent force of the dura to the inner table, with the subsequent formation of a DEDH. Venous sources of bleeding would be affected similarly, as standard treatment for a hypotensive trauma patient includes intubation with positive end-expiratory pressure (PEEP) and increased intrathoracic and subsequently venous pressures. Fluid resuscitation also increases venous pressure, allowing DEDH formation by the sequence mentioned above.

A second identifiable systematic contributor to DEDH formation is disseminated intravascular coagulopathy (DIC). The formation of DEDH in patients with DIC has been described by Frankhauser and Kiener.[32] Patients with multisystem trauma and head injuries are especially susceptible to DIC, and a heightened awareness in all practitioners caring for these patients allows for rapid diagnosis and treatment with an improved outcome.

Outcome

The mortality from DEDH ranges from 20 percent in the series of patients discussed by Askhenazi and associates,[37] to 45 percent in the review by Milo and coworkers.[31] The differences between these two series are undoubtedly due to a number of factors. The levels of consciousness on admission and just before surgical intervention are important predictors of outcome. Other important determinants are associated intra- and extracranial lesions and delay in the diagnosis of the DEDH.

DELAYED ACUTE SUBDURAL HEMATOMA

Definition

Delayed acute subdural hematomas (DASDHs) have not received the critical examination in the literature that both DTICH and DEDH have received. The lack of focus on DASDHs as a separate entity probably stems from a number of factors, including the inclusion of DASDH in the broad category of acute subdural hematomas,[44] the inability to demonstrate DASDHs in the pre-CT era in the acute phase of trauma care, and the occurrence of relatively asymptomatic DASDHs which remain unidentified until progression into the subacute or chronic subdural stage.

A DASDH probably is best defined as an acute subdural hematoma that is not apparent on the initial CT scan, but appears on a follow-up CT scan during the patient's postinjury course. This definition is based primarily on the use of CT for the evaluation of patients with head trauma. In the pre-CT era, the difficulties in diagnosing an acute subdural hemorrhage as a delayed event were obvious, given the limited resolution of ventriculography and arteriography. This limited resolution allowed small ASDHs to go unnoticed. Our ability to diagnose DASDHs has improved greatly with the advent of CT scanning. The incidence of this entity will undoubtedly change as availability and the speed of acquisition make MRI the modality of choice in evaluating trauma patients.

The incidence of operatively treated DASDH is approximately 0.5 percent of operatively treated acute subdural hematomas at the authors' institution. These hematomas are typically associated with other intracranial lesions, including intracerebral hemorrhage, accompanying mass lesions, and brain edema.

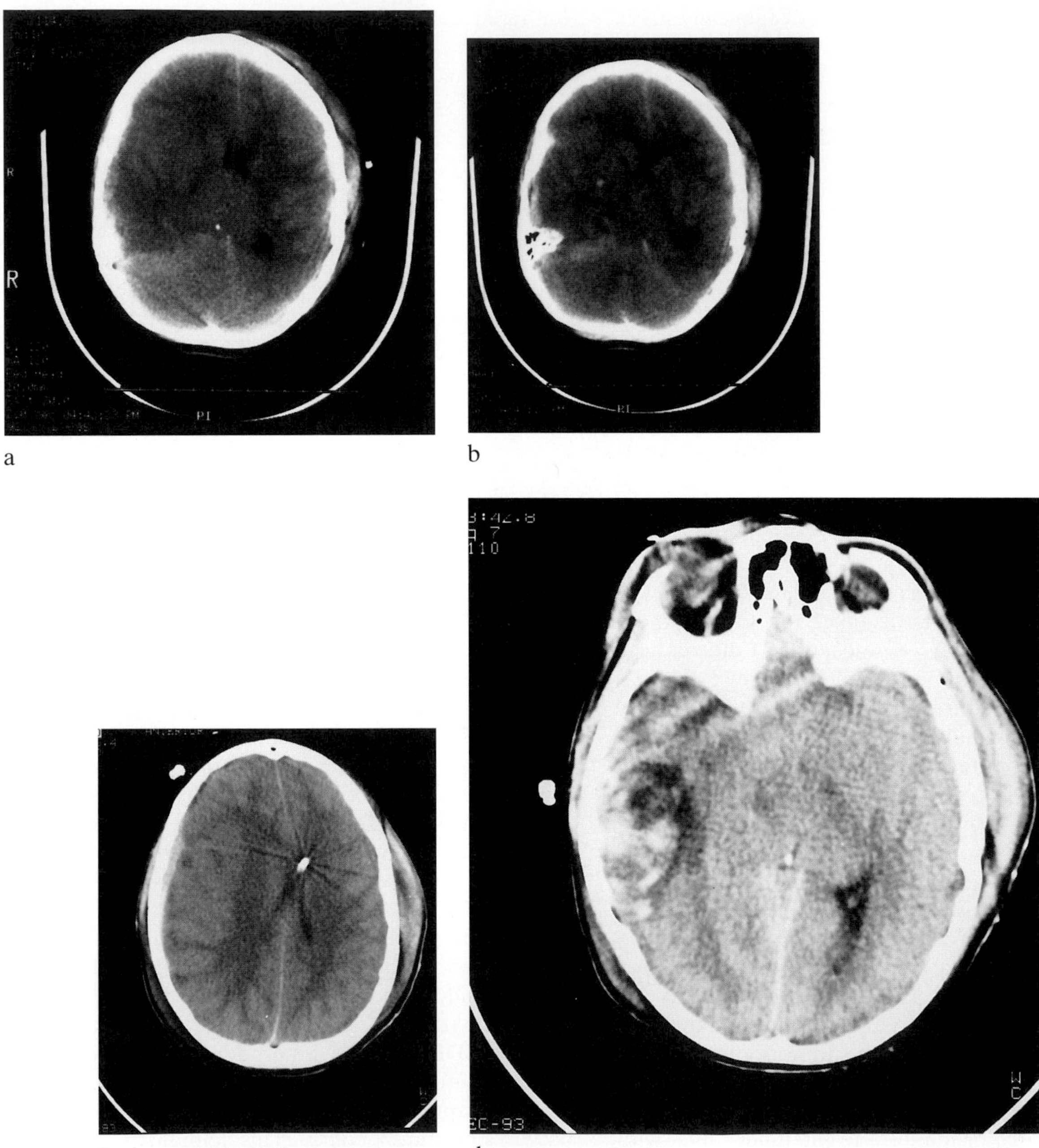

Figure 47-4. *A* and *B*. Case 4. Axial head CT showing right hemispheric edema with 7 mm of midline shift. *C* and *D*. Axial head CT showing a right posterior DTICH with rupture into the subdural space and a delayed subdural hematoma with a left frontal ventriculostomy with 1 cm of midline shift.

Etiology and Pathogenesis

DASDHs occur secondary to a number of occurrences that are similar to those of their counterpart, delayed epidural hematomas. A torn bridging vein in the presence of systemic hypotension and low central venous pressure secondary to trauma-induced hemorrhage delay the appearance of an acute subdural hematoma on CT. The appearance of an acute subdural hematoma (ASDH) also progresses slowly in the face of tamponade by brain edema. The removal of the tamponade effect by the administration of mannitol, the evacuation of the accompanying mass lesion or lesions, and CSF decompression via a CSF leak or through the placement of a ventriculostomy all serve to promote the formation of a DASDH. The presence or development of a coagulopathy in a multisystem trauma patient enhances hematoma formation.

Traumatically induced vascular malformations, including arteriovenous fistula and traumatic aneurysms,[45] have been identified as the underlying cause of a DASDH after a trauma. The appearance of a DASDH is undoubtedly influenced by a number of these factors in the individual patient. The patient in Case 4 demonstrates the contribution of edema to a tamponade effect while decompression using mannitol and a ventriculostomy with CSF drainage led to the development of a DASDH and a DTICH.

Case 4

A 12-year-old white male was an unbelted passenger involved in an MVA in which he was ejected from the car. On admission to an outside ER, he displayed a GCS of 5. The patient was hemodynamically stable but displayed an arterial blood gas (ABG) of pH 7.21, P_{CO_2} 44, P_{O_2} 48, hemoglobin and hematocrit 10.8 and 32 with 200,000 platelets, and prothrombin time/partial thromboplastin time 15.3 and 38 (slightly elevated).

The patient was transferred to the authors' facility, where on arrival he was noted to have a GCS of 3, was hemodynamically stable, and had improved ABG with pH 7.27, P_{CO_2} 36, and P_{O_2} 149. The patient was transported to CT scan; Fig. 47-4*A* and *B* shows right hemispheric edema with approximately 7 mm of midline shift. There was a right basal ganglia contusion and a traumatic subarachnoid hemorrhage. The patient was admitted to the pediatric ICU, where a ventriculostomy was placed with medical management of ICP. The patient's ICP became uncontrollable with standard management over the next 6 h, and an emergent repeat CT (Fig. 47-4*C* and *D*) displayed a right posterior temporal delayed traumatic intracerebral hematoma with apparent rupture into the subdural space that caused a delayed subdural hematoma. The venticulostomy is seen in place in the left frontal horn of the lateral ventricle with continued midline shift. The patient was taken to the OR emergently, where a right frontotemporal parietal craniotomy was performed with evacuation of the ASDH and intracerebral hematoma with a partial temporal lobectomy. The patient eventually was diagnosed with posttraumatic hydrocephalus, underwent a ventriculoperitoneal shunt, and remains in a coma with a GCS of 5.

Treatment and Outcome

The treatment of DASDHs follows the same guidelines used for other intracranial mass lesions. Patients who develop small delayed subdural hematomas, have stable neurological exams, and have medically controllable ICP probably are best managed conservatively. Patients who display a significant deficit and develop progressive neurological deficits and/or medically uncontrollable ICP require operative treatment. Preoperative therapy should include treatment of coexisting problems, including hypotension, hypoxia, and coagulopathies, to prevent secondary brain injury. The outcome of patients who develop a DASDH apppears to be quite variable, although it is difficult to clearly define because of the paucity of outcome data.

CONCLUSIONS

The detection of delayed intracranial hematomas has greatly improved with the advent of CT scans for head injury. Delayed traumatic intracranial hematomas may occur in any patient with head trauma, but especially in more severely injured patients. Coexisting or associated pathologies include hypoxia, hypotension, coagulopathies, and other intracranial lesions. Patients with these associated pathologies require particular vigilance, since they seem to be at heightened risk for developing a DTICH.

The diagnosis of delayed hematomas is usually made after clinical deterioration or through routine sequential head CT scans. The management of these patients is dictated by their neurological status, the location of the hemorrhage, associated injuries, metabolic abnormalities, the presence of coagulopathies, and the response to conservative therapy.

Surgical treatment consists of craniotomy for hematoma evacuation with ICP monitoring, in most cases postoperatively. The general care of these patients must be meticulous to limit the risk of secondary injury and a subsequently poor outcome.

Diagnostic advances such as the use of MRI for head trauma and better physiological monitors may improve the speed of diagnosis. Earlier diagnosis of these lesions combined with improved treatment may lead to an improved outcome. Rapid transportation of a patient with a head injury to the hospital, with the first CT performed within an hour of the injury, is likely to increase the possibility of hematomas that were not apparent on the first scan showing up on subsequent studies.

References

1. Bollinger O, Lebenjahres, Berlin A: *Ueber Traumatische Spatapoplexie*: Ein Beitrag zur Lehre von der Hirnerschutterung, in Internationale Beitrage zur Wissenschaftlichen Medizin, Festschrift, Rudolf Virchow Gewidmet zur Vollendung Seines. Berlin: Hirschwald, 70:457–470, 1891.
2. Langerhans R, Berlin A: *Die Traumatische Spatapoplexie*. Berlin: Hirschwald, 1903.
3. Duret H: Traumatismes cranio-cerebraux: Accidents primitifs, leurs grandes syndromes. Paris: Felix Alcan 833–851, 1922.
4. Lafforgue E: Hemorragies intra-craniennes traumatiques evoluant en deux temps. *Bull Med Paris* 18:875–878, 1904.
5. Von Holder H: *Pathologische Anatomie der Gehirnerschutterung Beim Menschen.* Stuttgart: J. Weise, 1904.
6. Bailey P: Traumatic apoplexy. *Medical Record* Oct. 1, 1904, pp 528–529.
7. Symonds CP: Delayed traumatic intracerebral haemorrhage. *Br Med J* 1:1048–1051, 1940.
8. Courville CB, Blomquist OA: Traumatic intracerebral hemorrhage with particular reference to its pathogenesis and its relation to "delayed traumatic apoplexy." *Arch Surg* 41:1–28, 1940.
9. McLaurin RL, McBride BH: Traumatic intracerebral hematoma–review of 16 surgically treated cases. *Ann Surg* 143:294–305, 1956.
10. Baratham G, Dennyson WG: Delayed traumatic intracerebral haemorrhage. *J Neurol Neurosurg Psychiatry* 35:698–706, 1972.
11. Cooper PR, Maravilla K, Moody S, Clark WK: Serial computerized tomographic scanning and the prognosis of severe head injury. *Neurosurgery* 5:566–569, 1979.
12. Hirsh LF: Delayed traumatic intracerebral hematomas after surgical decompression. *Neurosurgery* 5:653–655, 1979.
13. Lipper MH, Kishore PRS, Girevendulis AK, et al: Delayed intracranial hematoma in patients with severe head injury. *Neuroradiology* 133:645–649, 1979.
14. Morin MA, Pitts FW: Delayed apoplexy following head injury ("Traumatische Spat-Apoplexie"). *J Neurosurg* 33:542–547, 1970.
15. Cooper PR: Delayed traumatic intracerebral hemorrhage. *Neurosurg Clin North Am* 3:659–665, 1992.
16. Yamaki T, Hirakawa K, Ueguchi T, Tenjin H, Kuboyama T, and Nakagawa Y: Chronological evaluation of acute traumatic intracerebral haematoma. *Acta Neurochir (Wien)* 103:112–115, 1990.
17. Fukamachi A, Kohno K, Wakao T: Traumatic intracerebral hematomas: A classification according to the dynamic changes on sequential CTs. *Neurol Med Chir (Tokyo)* 19:1039–1051, 1979.
18. Gentleman D, Nath F, MacPherson P: Diagnosis and management of delayed traumatic intracerebral haematomas. *Br J Neuosurg* 3:367–372, 1989.
19. Tanaka T, Hakai T, Vemura A, Fujishima I, Yamamoto T: MR Imaging as predictor of delayed posttraumatic cerebral hemorrhage. *J Neurosurg* 69:203–209, 1988.
20. Gudeman SK, Kishore PR, Miller JD, and Girevendulis AK: The genesis and significance of delayed traumatic intracerebral hematoma. *Neurosurgery* 5:309–313, 1979.
21. Young HA, Gleave JRW, Chir B, et al: Delayed traumatic intracerebral hematoma: Report of 15 cases operatively treated. *Neurosurgery* 14:22–25, 1984.
22. Unterberg A, Kiening K, Schmiedek P, Lanksch W: Long-term observations of intracranial pressure after severe head injury: The phenomenon of secondary rise of intracranial pressure. *Neurosurgery* 32:17–24, 1993.
23. Ninchoji T, Uemura K, Shimoyama I, Hinokuma K, Bun T, and Nakajima S: Traumatic intracerebral haematomas of delayed onset. *Acta Neurochir (Wien)* 71:69–90, 1984.
24. Young HA, Schmidek HH: Complications accompanying occipital skull fracture. *J Trauma* 22:914–920, 1982.
25. Rockswold GL, Leonard PR, Nagib M: Analysis of management in thirty-three closed head injury patients who "talked and deteriorated." *Neurosurgery* 21:51–55, 1987.
26. Diaz FG, Yock DH Jr, Larson D, Rockswold GL: Early diagnosis of delayed posttraumatic intracerebral hematomas. *J Neurosurg* 50:217–223, 1979.
27. Evans JP, Scheinker IM: Histologic studies of the brain following head trauma: II. Posttraumatic petechial and massive intracerebral hemorrhage. *J Neurosurg* 3:101–113, 1946.
28. Kaufman HH, Moake JL, Olsen JD, Miner ME, duCret RP, Pruessner JL, and Gildenberg PL: Delayed and recurrent intracranial hematomas related to disseminated intravascular clotting and fibrinolysis in head injury. *Neurosurgery* 7:445–449, 1980.
29. Bullock R, Hannemann OC, Murray L, et al: Recurrent hematomas following craniotomy for traumatic intracranial mass. *J Neurosurg* 72:9–14, 1990.
30. Czernicki Z, Koznieska E: Disturbances in the blood-brain-barrier and cerebral blood flow after rapid brain decompression in the cat. *Acta Neurochir (Wien)* 36:181–187, 1977.
31. Milo R, Razon N, Schiffer J: Delayed epidural hematoma: A review. *Acta Neurochir (Wien)* 84:13–23, 1987.
32. Frankhauser H, Kiener M: Delayed development of extradural hematomas. *Acta Neurochir (Wien)* 60:29–35, 1982.
33. Borovich B, Braun J, Guilburd JN, Zaaroor M, Michich M, Levy L., Lemberger A, Grushkiewicz, and Feinsod M: Delayed onset of traumatic extradural hematoma. *J Neurosurg* 63:30–34, 1985.

34. Choux M: Extracerebral hematomas in children, in Vigoroux RP, McLaurin RL (eds): *Advances in Neurotraumatology*, vol. 1. New York: Springer-Verlag, 173–208, 1986.
35. Teasdale G, Galbraith S: Acute traumatic intracranial hematomas, in Krayenbuhl H, Zurich Maspes PE, Milan, Sweet WH, Boston (eds): *Progress in Neurological Surgery,* vol 10. Basel: Karger, 1980.
36. Chan K, Mann K, Yeu C, et al: The significance of skull fracture in acute traumatic intracranial hematomas in adolescents: A prospective study. *J Neurosurg* 72:189–194, 1990.
37. Ashkenazi E, Constantini S, Pomeranz S, et al: Delayed epidural hematoma without neurologic deficit. *J Trauma* 30:613–615, 1990.
38. Meguro K, Kobayashi E, Maki Y: Acute brain swelling during evacuation of subdural hematoma caused by delayed contralateral extradural hematoma: Report of two cases. *Neurosurgery* 20:326–328, 1987.
39. Feuerman T, Wackym PA, Gade GF, et al: Intraoperative development of contralateral epidural hematoma during evacuation of traumatic extraaxial hematoma. *Neurosurgery* 23:480–484, 1988.
40. Sparacio R, Khatib R, Chiu J, et al: Chronic epidural hematoma. *J Trauma* 12:435–439, 1972.
41. Handa J, Shimizu Y, Sato K, Handa H: Traumatic aneursym and arteriovenous fistula of the middle meningeal artery. *Clin Radiol* 21:39–41, 1970.
42. Higazi I, El-Banhawy A, El-Nady F: Importance of angiography in identifying false aneurysm of the middle meningeal artery as a cause of extradural hematoma: Case report. *J Neurosurg* 30:172–175, 1966.
43. Mendelow AD, Teasdale GD, Russell T, et al: Effect of mannitol on cerebral blood flow and cerebral perfusion pressure in human head injury. *J Neurosurg* 63:43–48, 1985.
44. Shenkin MD: Acute subdural hematoma: Review of 39 consecutive cases with high incidence of cortical artery rupture. *J Neurosurg* 57:224–257, 1982.
45. Aoki N, Sakai T, Kaneko M: Traumatic aneurysm of the middle meningeal artery presenting as delayed onset of acute subdural hematoma. *Surg Neurol* 37:59–62, 1992.

CHAPTER 48

INFECTIOUS COMPLICATIONS AFTER HEAD INJURY

Stephen B. Greenberg
Robert L. Atmar

SYNOPSIS

Infections after head trauma, whether extracranial, cranial, or intracranial, are associated with increased morbidity and mortality. Extracranial and cranial infections include wound infections, subgaleal abscesses, and osteomyelitis of the skull. Although relatively uncommon in this setting, infections require early diagnosis and aggressive local surgical management as well as antibiotic therapy. The predominant source of these infections is skin flora, such as staphylococcus. Meningitis may occur posttraumatically, postoperatively, or after the placement of catheters and other intracranial devices. The most common cause of meningitis after a closed head injury is pneumococcal infection. Gram-negative bacilli and staphylococci are more commonly associated with postoperative or shunt-related infections.

Other intracranial infections, such as brain abscess, epidural abscess, and subdural abscess, following neurotrauma are uncommon but constitute potentially life-threatening complications. Mixed infections with both aerobes and anaerobes are common in these localized intracranial infections. Nosocomial infections occur frequently, with the most common sources occurring in the urinary tract, the respiratory tract, and intravenous catheters. Empirical antibiotic therapy should be based on the prevalent local flora and bacterial resistance patterns.

Antibiotic selection for CNS infections should be based on CNS penetration, spectrum of activity, side effects, and cost. Beta-lactam antibiotics such as penicillins and cephalosporins are commonly used in high doses for these CNS infections. Early diagnosis and appropriate intervention may aid in a more rapid and complete recovery from these potentially devastating infections.

INTRODUCTION

The significant morbidity and mortality after major head trauma are primarily related to the trauma itself. However, infectious complications that follow trauma, including cranial, extracranial, and intracranial infections, and discrete or systemic hospital-acquired infections can certainly compound the problem.[1–4] Infections may follow either minor or major trauma, may be acute or chronic, and may involve any part of the head from the outer skin to the parenchyma of the brain. Effective treatment of these infections requires an understanding of the principles of antimicrobial therapy. To provide a basis for management, this chapter reviews the pathophysiology, epidemiology, microbiology, clinical features, diagnosis, and treatment of several common extracranial, cranial, intracranial, and nosocomial infections.

EXTRACRANIAL AND CRANIAL INFECTIONS

WOUND INFECTIONS

Wound infections after neurosurgical procedures have been reported in approximately 1 percent of cases. In one of the only published case-control series, reported risk factors associated with wound infections in over 9000 operations were (1) CSF leaks, (2) concomitant non-CNS infections, and (3) perioperative infections.[5] Over 60 percent of the reported postoperative wound infections were due to staphylococcal species, and about 5 percent were due to gram-negative bacilli. Other factors thought to be important in the development of wound infections included the placement of foreign objects, a surgical procedure with paranasal sinus entry, and the use of postoperative drains.

Early scalp wound infections after neurotrauma usually result from insufficient wound debridement. Late scalp wound infections may be associated with systemic signs and symptoms of infection. Deeper infection involving subcutaneous tissue or bone should be considered if a scalp wound infection appears weeks after a traumatic event.

The choice of therapy for wound infections should relate to the culture and sensitivity of the bacteria isolated. Empirical coverage with antibiotics before the microbiology is known should employ antibiotics that treat staphylococcal infections. Although there have been few controlled studies on the effects of perioperative antibiotics on wound infections, most reviews suggest that these antibiotics do in fact reduce the incidence of wound infection after intracranial neurosurgical procedures.[6]

Subgaleal Abscess

Bacteria inoculated into a scalp laceration or puncture wound can grow in the subgaleal spaces. Occasionally, subgaleal abscesses have been reported after hematogenous spread from skull osteomyelitis or with fetal monitoring. Few reported series have defined the microbiology of subgaleal abscesses, but staphylococci, streptococci, and anaerobes are the species most frequently recovered.[7–9] The treatment of choice is incision and drainage, with irrigation of the abscess cavity. Parenteral antibiotics should provide coverage for gram-positive cocci and anaerobes. If there is no associated osteomyelitis, antibiotic treatment should be given for 10 to 14 days.

Osteomyelitis of the Skull

Osteomyelitis of the skull is relatively uncommon after cranial trauma. In one large series reported by Bullitt and Lehman,[10] only 3 of 18 patients with osteomyelitis of the skull had a history of cranial trauma. Most presentations were subacute, with sinus or incisional drainage, local swelling, and tenderness being the most common signs and symptoms. Headache also was present. Unlike the acute presentation of osteomyelitis at other sites, fever and malaise were uncommon. Meningitis occurred in one patient. The osteomyelitis developed 2 months to 32 years after an inciting event in 16 patients, but it presented acutely in 2 patients. No leukocytosis or elevated erythrocyte sedimentation rate (ESR) was observed. The organisms cultured from the bones of the skull were predominantly *Staphylococcus aureus* and *S. epidermidis*, with a few mixed infections and an occasional diphtheroid isolate. Skull x-rays showed changes consistent with osteomyelitis. This series was published before computed tomography (CT) and magnetic resonance imaging (MRI) were available. The authors suggested that the preferred treatment was complete surgical debridement with the removal of the entire bone flap and treatment with antibiotics. Antibiotic therapy is generally given for a total of 6 weeks; at least 10 to 14 days of therapy is given postoperatively and should be based on the bacteriology of the wound culture.

INTRACRANIAL INFECTIONS

Meningitis

Meningitis has been described following neurotrauma as a postoperative complication or in association with catheters or other intracranial devices. Neurosurgeons need to be aware of the epidemiology, pathogenesis, and microbiology of these different presentations of meningitis so that appropriate antibiotics and surgical treatment may be employed. The following sections will examine the importance of each of these underlying risk factors for meningitis in the neurosurgical patient.

Posttraumatic meningitis

The reported incidence of meningitis after head trauma varies from 0.2 to 17.8 percent.[11] CSF leak is a significant risk factor for the development of posttraumatic meningitis, with meningitis occurring in 2 to 9 percent of these patients.[12,13] The longer the duration of the CSF leak, the greater seems to be the cumulative risk of bacterial meningitis. Rhinorrhea is a more common sign of CSF leak than is otorrhea. In one series of patients seeking medical attention for head injury, approximately 25 percent had a basilar skull fracture, 10 percent of whom had a CSF leak.[14] Rhinorrhea occurred three times more frequently than did otorrhea.

The pathogenesis of posttraumatic meningitis relates to the anatomy of the dura on the floor of the cranium.[14,15] The dura is adherent to bone in this area, and thus when fractures of the cranial base occur, the dura is also lacerated, causing a fistula. The bacterial flora of the nasopharynx or inner ear can thus gain access to the meninges. The thinness of the bony roof of the paranasal sinuses also predisposes to CSF leak when fractures occur in this area. The petrous bone is contiguous with the auditory canal, and a fracture in this area can cause otorrhea. CSF leakage in either of these areas may less commonly occur weeks to years after the initial trauma.

The symptoms of posttraumatic meningitis are the same as those of nontraumatic meningitis. CSF is needed to identify the causative organism. Because there is often an interruption of normal CSF flow in trauma patients, lumbar CSF may not reflect activity in the basal cisterns or the ventricles. In addition, the finding of normal CSF from ventriculostomies does not completely rule out meningitis. An increased number of white blood cells and/or neutrophils in the CSF suggests infection but may be a nonspecific finding. Special tests (latex agglutination and counterimmunoelectrophoresis) for the diagnosis of commonly found bacterial organisms, such as *Hemophilus influenzae, Neisseria meningitidis,* and *Streptococcus pneumoniae,* are available. A limulus lysate test may detect the presence of gram-negative bacilli because of the presence of endotoxin on the outer cell wall of these organisms. If rhinorrhea or otorrhea is present, a CSF leak is the usual cause. Intracranial air with a history of trauma also suggests a CSF leak. The best test for finding the site of leakage is high-resolution CT scan with water-soluble contrast injection into the CSF. The glucose content in rhinorrhea does not reliably distinguish CSF from nasal mucus.

Organisms isolated from posttraumatic meningitis are predominantly from the nasopharynx (Table 48-1). In one study *S. pneumoniae* (pneumococcus) accounted for over 80 percent of all posttraumatic meningitis occurring after a closed head injury.[16] *H. influenzae, S. pyogenes,* and *N. meningitidis* have been found with increased frequency, especially when CSF rhinorrhea is present.[17,18] *S. pneumoniae*–associated meningitis often is associated with bacteremia. Staphylococci, gram-negative bacilli, and nonhemolytic streptococci also have been reported, but staphylococci and gram-negative bacilli rarely cause meningitis after a basilar skull fracture.[19] If the meningitis occurs within 3 days of injury, the cause is almost always *S. pneumoniae*. The meningitis that occurs with otorrhea commonly begins within 48 h of an injury. Cases of posttraumatic meningitis associated with rhinorrhea may occur within a few days or months to years after the traumatic episode.[20]

Only a small percentage of persistent CSF leaks require surgical repair. If the meningitis is caused by *S. pneumoniae,* penicillin (20 to 24 MU/day) is the drug of choice. In areas where there is a significant incidence of penicillin-resistant pneumococci, a third-generation cephalosporin should be used. When *H. influenzae* is suspected, a third-generation cephalosporin usually is indicated. Before the result of cultures, empirical coverage with nafcillin or vancomycin with ceftazidime covers the most likely organisms. Although there has not been a prospective controlled trial of prophylactic antibiotics in patients with a basilar skull fracture, several studies suggest a decline in the incidence of posttraumatic meningitis when antibiotics are given.[21] Leech reported a 0 percent incidence of posttraumatic meningitis in antibiotic-treated patients with rhinorrhea versus 16.6 percent in untreated patients.[22] Similarly, in patients with otorrhea who were given prophylactic antibiotics, there was a 5.2 percent incidence of posttraumatic meningitis compared with 41.7 percent in untreated patients. However, other uncontrolled studies have failed to show a benefit of prophylactic antibiotics in this clinical situation and the Infection in Neurosurgery Working Party of the British Society for Antimicrobial Chemotherapy recommends that antibiotics be withheld and patients be monitored closely for signs and symptoms of early meningitis.[11,23,23a] The mortality rate of posttraumatic meningitis, despite treatment, appears to be approximately 10 percent. Patients with CSF leak–associated meningitis need reevaluation after the meningitis has cleared to determine whether surgery is necessary to correct a persistent leak. Ten percent of CSF leaks persist for longer than 1 month, but 90 percent close within 7 to 10 days.[24,25] However, in patients with recurrent meningitis after head trauma, reevaluation for a CSF leak is mandatory.

TABLE 48-1 Meningitis in Neurosurgery Patients

Mechanism	Common Infecting Organisms	%
Posttraumatic	*Streptococcus pneumoniae*	70–85
	Hemophilus influenzae	0–15
	Neisseria meningitidis	0–6
	Staphylococci	0–5
	Gram-negative bacilli	0–5
Postoperative	Gram-negative bacilli	80
	Staphylococci	10–15
Shunt infections	Staphylococci	65–85
	Gram-negative bacilli	5–20
	Diphtheroids	1–14
	Streptococcus sp.	10
	Streptococcus pneumoniae, *Hemophilus influenzae*, *Neisseria meningitidis*	2–8

Postoperative Meningitis

The incidence of postoperative meningitis after "clean" neurosurgery has been reported to be approximately 0.5 to 0.7 percent.[5,26–29] In clean-contaminated cases, the incidence has been 0.4 to 2.0 percent. One study reported an overall incidence of 0.3 percent after craniotomy. The pathogenesis of postoperative meningitis usually involves direct contamination from the sinuses, nasal mucosa, or contaminated scalp. Because gram-negative bacilli commonly colonize some of these sites in hospitalized patients, they are frequent etiologic agents in postoperative meningitis. Hematogenous spread as a cause of postoperative meningitis is probably rare. Half of the cases of postoperative meningitis occur within 2 days of surgery, and the onset may be subtle. Fever is present in most cases. Bloodstream and CSF leukocytosis are common laboratory findings.

Diagnosis requires culture of the CSF, but an MRI or CT scan must be obtained to exclude the possibility of brain abscess. Common abnormalities in CSF include elevated protein (100 to 500 mg/dl), white blood cell counts greater than 1000/mm^3 (75 percent neutrophils), decreased glucose (less than 40 mg/dl) in 85 percent, and a positive Gram's stain in 50 to 80 percent. The most common gram-negative organisms isolated have been *Klebsiella pneumoniae, Enterobacter* species, and *Pseudomonas aeuriginosa* (Table 48-1).

Third-generation cephalosporins are the standard treatment, with a cure rate greater than 70 percent. Development of resistance on therapy has occurred. Some investigators suggest that an aminoglycoside be added in appropriate intrathecal doses to treat gram-negative meningitis.

A few studies of the use of prophylactic antibiotics in neurosurgery have suggested a reduction in postoperative infections when antibiotics have been given.[30] The use of vancomycin plus gentamicin or cefazolin has resulted in a reduction in postoperative infection rates from 3.5 percent to less than 1 percent.[31] Therefore, when neurosurgery is performed for cranial trauma, perioperative antibiotics probably should be employed, although a prospective randomized trial of this practice is lacking.

External devices and shunt infections

The incidence of infections following the use of external CNS devices or shunts is 4.5 to 14 percent.[32–37] The rate of infection with lumboperitoneal shunts is lower than that recorded with ventriculoperitoneal or ventriculovenous shunts.[38] A 5 to 7 percent incidence of infection has been reported for external devices. Risk factors for infection related to the use of external devices include increased intracranial pressure, intraventricular hemorrhage, and monitoring for more than 5 days.[35,39] With implanted CSF reservoirs, the incidence of infection appears to be 3 to 15 percent, and most infections occur within 30 days of placement. Most studies support the use of antibiotics to reduce the incidence of shunt infections although the greatest effect appears to have been seen in studies with high infection rates in the placebo group.[23a,40–43]

Several factors are associated with the pathogenesis of these infections. First, retrograde infection probably accounts for most of the infections associated with external devices.[33,34] Repeated flushing of these devices can lead to a breakdown of sterile technique. The breakdown of wounds or overlying skin may allow direct access of bacteria into shunts. Rarely, hematogenous spread occurs. While shunts may become infected following bacteremia, colonization with skin organisms at the time of surgery probably accounts for the majority of these infections. The length of the operation and the experience of the surgeon appear to be additional factors affecting the incidence of these infections.

In shunt infections, fever is almost always present. Other features include headache, nausea, lethargy, and changes in mental status. Meningeal symptoms are rare with infected ventricular shunts but seem to be more common with lumboperitoneal shunts.

Infected vascular shunts almost always have associated bacteremia. Patients with ventriculoperitoneal shunts frequently have associated abdominal symptoms that may mimic an acute abdomen. Fungal shunt infections may present with more subtle signs and symptoms; obstruction of the shunt may be the only sign of infection. Culture of the shunt, the shunt fluid, or the tissue contiguous to the shunt is necessary to make a correct diagnosis. Negative Gram's stains are common.

The organisms isolated from shunts include predominantly *Staphylococcus* species, with *S. epidermidis* being twice as common as *S. aureus* (Table 48-1). Gram-negative bacilli occur in 5 to 20 percent of shunt infections. The organisms most commonly reported in posttraumatic meningitis—*S. pneumoniae, N. meningitidis,* and *H. influenzae*—account for only 2 to 8 percent of shunt infections. Diphtheroids have been reported in as many as 14 percent of cases, and anaerobes have been reported in 6 percent. Ten to 15 percent of cases have involved mixed infections, with both gram-positive and gram-negative organisms. Predisposing factors for fungal infections of shunts include prior antibiotic use, hyperalimentation, leukemia, diabetes mellitus, and the use of steroids.[33]

Treatment of shunt infections should include parenteral antibiotics and shunt replacement. This approach gives a 75 percent or greater cure rate.[44] Antibiotics alone have resulted in a cure rate greater than 90 percent for infections associated with external drainage devices, although a second infection can occur if the device remains in place.[45] If intracranial pressure monitoring is still needed, a new device should be inserted at a different site. The initial antibiotic treatment for a presumed shunt infection is determined by examination of the CSF. CSF may be obtained directly or by tapping the shunt, and a Gram's stain of this fluid should be performed. If gram-positive cocci are observed, antistaphylococcal antibiotics should be given. If gram-negative organisms are found, therapy with a third-generation cephalosporin should be initiated. If the Gram's stain is negative and the cell count shows pleocytosis with abnormal chemistries and the patient is ill, empirical coverage for both staphylococci and gram-negative bacilli is required. If the patient is not ill, treatment can be directed only against staphylococci. If the Gram's stain is negative and there are abnormal chemistries or pleocytosis but wound infection or cellulitis is present, antistaphylococcal therapy should be given. If the CSF appears normal but distal symptoms exist, one should look for proximal symptoms. The presence of proximal symptoms suggests dysfunction of the shunt. If the shunt dysfunctions, revision should be made and operative cultures should be obtained to direct therapy. Some investigators add rifampin (600 to 1200 mg/day) for additional coverage in the treatment of staphylococcal infections. Intraventricular antibiotics for shunt infection have not been well studied; nevertheless, some investigators recommend intrathecal vancomycin (5 to 10 mg) or gentamicin (1 to 10 mg). With fungal infections, intrathecal administration of amphotericin B (0.25 to 0.50 mg) has been recommended as well. The duration of intrathecal therapy is based on the duration of signs and symptoms and the results of repeated cultures. The duration of systemic therapy should probably be 7 to 10 days. The patient should be recultured 3 days after the completion of antibiotic therapy.

Epidural and Subdural Abscesses

The epidural space is located between the dura and the overlying bone; the subdural space is between the dura mater and the arachnoid surrounding the brain. Either space can be infected after neurotrauma. Infections in these spaces are most often complications of paranasal sinusitis but can occur after head trauma, after neurosurgery, with osteomyelitis of the skull, or after bacteremia from another focus.[46–54]

Subdural and intracranial epidural abscesses are less common than are brain abscesses. Intracranial epidural abscesses, unlike subdural empyemas, are rare in young children. Both infections affect males more commonly than they affect females. Trauma is probably a predisposing factor in 10 to 15 percent of all subdural empyemas.[55]

The clinical presentation may be confused with other infectious and noninfectious processes. Fever and headache are reported in 90 percent of these patients. Nausea, vomiting, and lethargy also are reported. Papilledema is found in approximately one-third of these patients. Diagnosis is made by CT scan or MRI. However, MRI is more sensitive and better than CT in differentiating a subdural abscess from an epidural abscess.

Although the microbiology of these infections is not well defined, streptococci and staphylococci are the predominant organisms recovered.[56] Gram-negative bacilli have been isolated in 8 to 10 percent of patients. Sterile cultures have been reported in up to 30 percent of cases, but this may reflect a failure to obtain anaerobic cultures.

Lumbar puncture is neither sensitive nor specific in diagnosing subdural or epidural abscesses. Gram's stain is rarely positive, and the causative organism is rarely recovered from CSF cultures. A polymorphonuclear pleocytosis is common, but mononuclear cells predominate in one-third of cases. An elevated protein and normal glucose are common findings.

Antibiotic treatment should begin immediately upon diagnosis and should be chosen to treat staphylococci, streptococci, and anaerobes. Operative treatment for the drainage of pus should be performed as quickly as possible. The relative benefits of burr holes, craniotomy, and craniectomy as optimal therapy are debated.[57,58] Antibiotics should be continued for 2 to 4 weeks after drainage.[59] Mortality rates with a combined antibiotic and early surgical approach range from 10 to 40 percent; morbidity can be severe, with long-term seizure disorders being reported in up to one-third of patients.[49]

Brain Abscesses

Although morbidity and mortality have declined with the availability of more sensitive diagnostic techniques and refined neurosurgical procedures, brain abscess continues to be a serious infection. Brain abscesses usually complicate a suppurative focus distinct from the brain itself.[60,61] The most common sources of infection are ear, nose, and throat infections.[62] Neurosurgery and trauma account for 20 percent of brain abscesses. However, brain abscess as an intracranial complication is the least common infection after head trauma or neurosurgery. In 10 percent of cases, no source is found. After a penetrating cranial injury, the risk of brain abscess increases. In Vietnam, 3 percent of the cranial injuries in military personnel resulted in brain abscesses.[63,64] Other combat series have reported the incidence of brain abscess to be 3 to 17 percent.[31,65–71] Risk factors for brain abscess after cranial injury include (1) gunshot wounds, (2) multiple injuries, and (3) wound complications such as hematoma or fluid collections. Retained bone fragments are an additional risk factor. Multiple types of cranial trauma are associated with the development of brain abscesses and include depressed skull fractures and trauma from animal bites and sharp objects such as pencil points and lawn darts.[72–82]

In the antibiotic era, the incidence of brain abscess has been stable. Two age peaks have been noted in several series: the first two decades of life and from age 50 to age 70. Many series have documented a male predominance in all age groups. While early studies failed to demonstrate the importance of anaerobic bacteria in the microbiology of most brain abscesses,[83,84] more recent studies have reported the recovery of anaerobes in more than 60 percent of appropriately cultured brain abscesses.[16,85–89] When the abscess is secondary to otitis media or mastoiditis, streptococci, *Bacteroides fragilis,* and aerobic gram-negative bacilli predominate. With sinusitis, similar organisms are recovered, along with staphylococci and *Hemophilus* species. After cranial trauma or neurosurgery, *S. aureus,* streptococci, gram-negative bacilli, and clostridia are the organisms most commonly recovered.

Clinical manifestations may be subtle or acute and alarming. Symptoms have been reported for only a few hours or several weeks before the diagnosis was made. Less than half of all patients have the triad of fever, headache, and focal neurological deficits. Other signs and symptoms, such as nausea, vomiting, seizures, and/or papilledema, are reported in less than half of these patients. The most common focal neurological deficits are hemiplegia and cranial nerve palsies. Few patients are comatose at the time of diagnosis. The differential diagnosis usually includes other CNS infections and cerebrovascular diseases. Brain abscess should be considered when these typical clinical manifestations follow cranial trauma.

Early diagnosis of brain abscesses has been enhanced by the introduction of CT scans.[90] Other noninvasive tests, such as skull x-rays, EEGs, and brain scans, are less sensitive.[90] However, in the detection of early cerebritis, MRI is much more sensitive than CT scan.[60] On CT, brain abscesses have characteristic hypodense centers outlined by ring enhancement and hypodense zones of brain edema. MRI is useful in both the diagnosis and the follow-up of brain abscesses.[91] It is also better than CT for defining posterior fossa lesions and following the resolution of abscesses and is associated with less toxicity because of the contrast agents employed.

CSF analysis and other laboratory tests are not diagnostic for brain abscesses. In fact, lumbar puncture is contraindicated when a brain abscess is strongly suspected. Clinical deterioration has been reported to occur in 20 percent of patients undergoing lumbar puncture who have an underlying brain abscess.[92] An MRI or CT scan should be performed promptly when a brain abscess is suspected. If pyogenic meningitis is also suspected, blood cultures and empirical parenteral antibiotics should be given before a CT scan is obtained.

There are no published controlled trials of antimicrobial therapy for brain abscesses.[93,94] Empirical therapy is based on a knowledge of the most likely bacteriology and the pharmacology of the antimicrobial agents.[95–98] The antibiotics with the longest history of use are penicillin and chloramphenicol. High-dose penicillin (24 MU/day) achieves sufficient CNS concentrations in pus to treat susceptible bacteria. Chloramphenicol also achieves significant concentrations in CNS pus at doses of 50 to 100 mg/kg/day.

Metronidazole is active against anaerobes recovered from brain abscesses and achieves high CNS levels at a dose of 750 mg every 8 h. Other antibiotics, such as trimethoprim-sulfamethoxazole and vancomycin, also reach CNS concentrations sufficient to treat susceptible gram-negative bacilli and aerobic staphylococci and streptococci, respectively. The newer third-generation cephalosporins provide good CNS concentrations that should treat susceptible aerobic gram-negative bacilli, but there is little in vivo experience with brain abscess–treated patients. Imipenem-cilastatin has not been used to treat many brain abscesses and therefore cannot be recommended as first-line therapy.

Parenteral therapy with high-dose penicillin and metronidazole or chloramphenicol is an appropriate initial regimen for treating brain abscesses. Adding coverage for gram-negative bacilli depends on the location of the brain abscess and the underlying condition of the patient. If staphylococci are suspected, nafcillin or vancomycin should be used. Although the duration of therapy is dependent on etiology, location, and concomitant surgical intervention and drainage, 6 to 8 weeks of antibiotics is usually recommended.

Surgical drainage of brain abscesses is recommended, but the timing and the procedure to be used remain controversial.[99–101] Stereotactic-guided CT aspiration has been reported to be successful and provides a specific bacteriological diagnosis in most cases.[60]

The use of corticosteroids in the management of brain abscess is also controversial. In patients with neurological deterioration, steroids may be of value in reducing intracranial edema. However, they also may decrease CNS entry of antibiotics and may confuse the interpretation of the sequential CT scans used to assess the therapeutic response.[102]

Mortality from brain abscesses has been reduced to 5 percent since the introduction of the CT scan.[92] Nevertheless, significant morbidity has been reported in 30 to 50 percent of treated patients.[103] Seizures occur in more than one-third of successfully treated patients, and behavioral abnormalities are commonly reported in treated children. Fortunately, early diagnosis with CT and the institution of appropriate parenteral antibiotics and surgical drainage have improved the overall prognosis for this previously highly fatal infection.

NOSOCOMIAL INFECTIONS

Nosocomial infections are common complications after head trauma. One study found that 10 percent of patients admitted with acute head trauma developed a nosocomial infection, and infection rates have been even higher in those receiving mechanical ventilation, steroids, and certain other therapies.[104–107] The most common sites affected are the urinary tract, lung, and bloodstream.[108] An awareness of the risk factors associated with the acquisition of common nosocomial infections and the manifestations and management of such infections is important in the care of patients with head trauma.

URINARY TRACT INFECTIONS

Forty to sixty percent of all nosocomial infections occur in the urinary tract.[109,110] The most common risk factor for the development of a urinary tract infection (UTI) is the use of a urinary catheter.[111] The placement of bladder catheters facilitates the entry of bacteria into the bladder. Bacteria may be introduced into the bladder at the time of catheter insertion, through reflux of contaminated urine through the catheter, or by retrograde migration outside the catheter in the mucus of the periurethral sheath.[111] This latter method of bacterial entry predominates.[112,113] Conditions such as increased age, female gender, severe illness, and lack of systemic antibiotic use are associated with an increased colonization of the periurethral area with potentially pathogenic bacteria and also are risk factors for UTIs. Other risk factors include duration of catheterization, reason for catheterization, hospital service caring for the patient, and baseline renal function.[114–116]

Ten percent or more of patients who have an indwelling catheter for more than 1 day become bacteriuric, but only 30 percent of these patients become symptomatic.[111] By 30 days of catheterization, most patients will have had an episode of bacteriuria.[117] *Escherichia coli, P. aeruginosa, Enterococcus* sp., yeasts, and other gram-negative organisms are the most common organisms isolated after short-term colonization, while *Providencia stuartii, Proteus* sp., *E. coli,* and *P. aeruginosa* are found most commonly with long-term (>30 days) catheterization.[117] Bacteriuria also is more frequently polymicrobic with long-term catheterization.

The diagnosis of a UTI can be difficult in a neurosurgical patient. Symptoms such as dysuria, urinary frequency, and flank pain often cannot be elicited or are absent. Fever and peripheral leukocytosis may be present because of other conditions. Thus, the urine culture is the single most helpful diagnostic test, but the physician also must use clinical judgment to exclude other possible sources of infection in a febrile patient.[111]

Treatment of symptomatic nosocomial UTIs consists of systemic antibiotic therapy with a drug to which the infecting organism is sensitive and removal of the urinary catheter, if possible. When fever, leukocytosis, or other systemic signs of infection are present, intravenous broad-spectrum antibiotic therapy should be given and other potential sites of infection should be excluded. The antibiotics may be changed after the antibiotic susceptibility of the infecting organism or organisms is known.

The most effective way to prevent nosocomial UTIs is by avoiding prolonged or unnecessary use of urinary catheters. The introduction of closed catheter systems in the 1960s significantly reduced the incidence of catheter-associated UTIs, but other modifications to the catheter or collection system (including the use of sealed closed systems, silver-impregnated catheters, and antiseptics in the collection bag) have not consistently decreased infection rates.[111,113,118,119] Antibiotic prophylaxis to prevent bacteriuria has shown only transient beneficial effects with short-term catheterization and has not changed the incidence of bacteriuria or fever with long-term catheterization.[111,112,117] Bladder irrigants and antiseptics also have been ineffective with long-term catheterization. Antibiotic prophylaxis should not be used, because its continued use has resulted in colonization of the bladder with resistant organisms.[111,117]

PNEUMONIA

Pneumonia is the second most common cause of nosocomial infection and is the most frequent nosocomial infection causing death.[120] Aspiration of oropharyngeal or gastric contents is the predominant manner by which the lung becomes infected, but hematogenous, aerosolized, and contiguous spread of infection to the lung also may occur. Pneumonia in patients with head trauma usually follows aspiration and causes one of two clinical syndromes: aspiration pneumonia or ventilator-associated pneumonia.

ASPIRATION PNEUMONIA

Aspiration of small amounts of oropharyngeal or gastric contents occurs frequently during sleep or during surgery without demonstrable sequelae.[121] Studies in which dye was placed in the stomachs of patients undergoing surgery or radiocontrast was placed in the mouths of sleeping patients have shown that these materials reach the tracheobronchial tree.[122,123] Pneumonia occurs when larger volumes of material are aspirated, if the aspirate is toxic to the respiratory epithelium, and/or if mechanisms for clearance of the aspirate are impaired. Aspiration pneumonia has been a leading cause of death after head injury.[124] Risk factors for aspiration pneumonia include impaired level of consciousness (seen in association with trauma, anesthesia, seizures, etc.), nasotracheal or nasogastric intubation, impaired swallowing (seen after a cerebrovascular accident), and tracheostomy.[125]

Three distinct clinical syndromes that follow aspiration have been identified and are related to the type of material aspirated: toxic pneumonitis, pneumonitis after aspiration of an inert material, and bacterial pneumonitis. Toxic pneumonitis occurs most commonly after the aspiration of gastric acid.[121] Mendelson first described this syndrome in obstetric patients who aspirated gastric contents while anesthetized, and it has since been shown that the pH of the fluids must be less than 2.5 to trigger a toxic reaction.[70,121,125,126] The clinical picture of gastric acid aspiration is characterized by the sudden onset of dyspnea, bronchospasm, and frothy, nonpurulent sputum production.[121] Chest x-rays reveal densities in dependent areas of the lung, typically the lower lobes. Patients are usually hypoxic, with an arterial P_{O_2} ranging from 35 to 50 mmHg. Occasionally, adult respiratory distress syndrome results. Treatment is primarily supportive, with supplemental oxygen, assisted ventilation, and frequent suctioning to maintain a clear airway.[121] Steroids have been used to reduce inflammation after acid aspiration, but controlled clinical studies in animals and humans have not shown consistent benefits of this therapy.[125]

Clinical symptoms after the aspiration of nontoxic, inert materials usually are caused by blockage of the airways. Aspiration of small quantities of neutral-pH fluids causes only transient respiratory distress in anesthetized animals, while aspiration of larger amounts can produce suffocation.[121] Similarly, aspiration of particulate matter may cause obstruction of large or small airways, depending on the size of the aspirate. The initial symptom of cough may be followed by the development of pneumonia in the area of the lung behind the obstruction. Treatment consists of removal of the aspirated material, using suctioning for liquids and removing particulate matter by extraction (usually with a bronchoscope).[121]

Bacterial pneumonitis may occur after aspiration of oropharyngeal or gastric materials. Pneumonia results because the bacteria present in these secretions are not cleared by local defense mechanisms. The principal symptoms are purulent sputum production and fever. The onset of symptoms is more gradual than that seen after acid aspiration. The causative organisms are those found in the oropharyngeal and gastric secretions. Anaerobes are often the cause of pneumonia after aspiration, though aerobic gram-positive and gram-negative pneumonias also occur, especially in hospitalized patients. Treatment of the pneumonia is directed at the infecting organism; clindamycin probably is superior to penicillin for the treatment of anaerobic pneumonias.[27]

VENTILATOR-ASSOCIATED PNEUMONIA

Endotracheal intubation presents the greatest risk for the development of nosocomial pneumonia, increasing the incidence sevenfold to 21-fold compared with nonintubated patients.[127] Intubation predisposes a patient to infection in a number of ways: It circumvents the normal defense mechanisms that filter the air and clear material from the airways, causes mechanical irritation of the respiratory mucosa that may allow increased colonization with potential bacterial pathogens, and may serve as a source of bacterial contaminants.[128]

The incidence of nosocomial pneumonia in patients receiving mechanical ventilation ranges from 3 to 54 percent.[128–133] Differences in the infection rates are due to the different patient populations studied and different definitions used for the diagnosis of pneumonia. In most patients, including those with head injury, pneumonia occurs within the first 7 to 10 days after intubation.[130,134] Risk factors associated with the development of ventilator-associated pneumonia include prolonged mechanical ventilation (>3 days), more than one intubation during mechanical ventilation, a prior episode of gastric acid aspiration, the use of an H_2 antagonist, the presence of an intracranial pressure monitor, underlying chronic obstructive pulmonary disease, hospitalization during the fall or winter, the use of positive end-expiratory pressure, and mechanical ventilator circuit changes every 24 h.[127,131] The mortality rate is 20 to 50 percent and has been as high as 80 percent.[120] Individuals with an ultimately fatal underlying disease, respiratory failure worsened by the pneumonia, septic shock, inappropriate antibiotic treatment, and noncardiac surgery have increased mortality rates.[131]

Nosocomial pneumonia is frequently a mixed bacterial infection. Aerobic gram-negative bacilli, including *P. aeruginosa, K. pneumoniae, Enterobacter* sp., and *E. coli,* are isolated in more than 50 percent of cases; *S. aureus* is also a common pathogen. *Acinetobacter* sp. and *Legionella* sp. are important pathogens in some centers.[120,127] Respiratory viruses (e.g., influenza virus, respiratory syncytial virus, and parainfluenza viruses) may cause up to 20 percent of nosocomial pneumonias, especially in pediatric patients, but their role in ventilated patients has not been well studied.[120,135]

The most common sources for bacterial contamination of the lung are the oropharynx, the stomach, and respiratory equipment. Colonization of the oropharynx with gram-negative bacilli occurs early during hospitalization and is more common in individuals who are critically ill, have received antibiotics, are elderly, have had major surgery, or have one of a variety of underlying diseases (including diabetes mellitus, alcoholism, and chronic obstructive pulmonary disease).[127,136] Colonization of the stomach with gram-negative bacilli occurs more frequently in individuals receiving H_2 antagonists or antacids and is associated with an increased rate of nosocomial pneumonia.[104,120,127,129] However, in at least one study of neurosurgical trauma patients, the stomach did not appear to be an important source of pulmonary pathogens.[137] In-line nebulizers, ventilation tubing, resuscitation bags, spirometers, and oxygen analyzers are all potential sources for pathogenic bacteria.[127]

The diagnosis of pneumonia should be suspected in a patient with new or progressive pulmonary infiltrates and purulent sputum, fever, and leukocytosis. However, critically ill patients frequently are at increased risk for pulmonary infiltrates from other causes, including acute respiratory distress syndrome and congestive heart failure; purulent sputum may be a result of tracheobronchitis. Autopsy studies have shown that pneumonia has been overdiagnosed in some series and underdiagnosed in others.[120] Identification of the responsible pathogen may be even more difficult. The use of a protected specimen brush with a quantitative bacterial culture has been useful both in the identification of patients with pneumonia ($>10^3$ pfu/ml) and in the identification of the pathogen.[120,138–141] Bronchoalveolar lavage with quantitative bacteriology has not been consistently effective in diagnosing nosocomial pneumonia.[120,142]

Treatment of nosocomial pneumonia is directed at the likely causative organisms. Since aerobic gram-negative bacilli cause the majority of pneumonias, an extended-spectrum penicillin or third-generation cephalosporin with or without an aminoglycoside should be used until bacteriological data become available. Treatment for *S. aureus* with nafcillin (or, if methicillin-resistant *S. aureus* is prevalent, with vancomycin) also should be considered. Knowledge of the prevalent nosocomial pathogens also should direct therapy, so that antibiotic choices are modified on the basis of antibiotic resistance patterns and the presence of organisms such as *Legionella* species.

Several approaches to the prevention of nosocomial pneumonia have been advocated, including maintenance of an effective infection control program, prevention of colonization with pathogenic bacteria, prevention of aspiration, and improvement of host defense mechanisms.[143] Several infection control measures, many of which are now standard, may decrease the incidence of nosocomial pneumonia and include the following: sterilization or disinfection of respiratory therapy equipment, cleansing and drying of in-line medication nebulizers after each use, use of sterile gloves and catheters for suctioning, and hand washing after each patient contact.[143] Topical antibiotics have been used to prevent colonization with gram-negative bacilli in the hope that the incidence of pneumonia would decrease.[144–147] Recent studies used a combination of polymyxin B, gentamicin, and amphotericin B or nystatin or systemic antibiotics with or without topical antibiotics and showed a decrease in the incidence of colonization with gram-negative bacilli and pneumonia.[127,144,148] Further studies are needed to determine whether the emergence of resistant organisms continues to be a problem with these newer regimens. The maintenance of gastric acidity through the use of sucralfate, in place of H_2 antagonists or antacids, for stress ulcer prophylaxis also may decrease the incidence of colonization with gram-negative bacilli and pneumonia.[104] However, critically ill patients may have problems with gastric acidification even when sucralfate is used.[148] The role of methods to decrease aspiration and self-extubation, including 30-degree elevation of the head of the bed, sedation, and the use of restraints, must be defined. Immunoprophylaxis by active or passive immunization has had only limited success in preventing gram-negative infections but still holds promise.[109,127,149] Other approaches to the prevention of nosocomial pneumonia need to be developed to decrease the morbidity and mortality associated with this infection.

Decubitus Ulcers

Decubitus ulcers, or pressure sores, are a common preventable complication after head trauma. Although not an infectious complication, a decubitus ulcer is a break in the body's barrier defense system and is associated with a number of infectious complications, including soft tissue infections, osteomyelitis, and bacteremia.[150,151] The ulcers occur most frequently over bony prominences in dependent areas, including the sacrum and coccyx, the greater trochanters of the femurs, and the ischial tuberosities.[151] Decubitus ulcers usually can be prevented by good nursing care practices, such as relief of pressure by frequent rotation of the patient, reduction of shearing forces by lifting (not dragging) patients, and care to prevent the skin from becoming too moist or too dry.[151]

Bacteremia/Sepsis

Bacteremia is the fourth most common nosocomial infection after UTIs, pneumonia, and surgical wound infections.[108,110] The most common identifiable sources for bacteremia are the urinary tract and intravascular catheters,[152] but the lung, skin, gastrointestinal tract, and CNS also may be sources of secondary bacteremia. Sepsis is the clinical response to a bacterial infection; symptoms include fever or hypothermia, tachypnea, and tachycardia. Septic shock is defined as the symptoms of sepsis accompanied by hypotension. Sepsis and septic shock frequently occur in the absence of demonstrable bacteremia or fungemia, with the clinical syndromes resulting from the effects of the release of various cytokines in response to infection.[153]

Catheters

Central venous catheters are more common sources of bacteremia than are peripheral venous or arterial catheters.[154] Local catheter infections and exit-site infections are also common. To identify a catheter as the primary source of a bacteremia, one of several criteria must be met: (1) presence of an exit site or tunnel infection caused by the organism isolated from the bloodstream, (2) cessation of clinical symptoms within 48 h after removal of the catheter when no antibiotics are being administered or after the patient has failed more than 72 h of appropriate antibiotic therapy, (3) implication of the catheter as the source of the infection by quantitative cultures.[154] Quantitative cultures may be done with the roll-plate method, showing more than 15 bacterial colonies per catheter tip, or by drawing blood cultures from a peripheral site and through the catheter and demonstrating a tenfold or greater increase in the number of organisms in the culture drawn through the catheter.[155,156]

Catheter-related infection may occur as a result of bacterial colonization of any of four potential sites: the skin insertion site, the catheter hub, hematogenous seeding of the catheter, or contaminated infusate. The skin insertion site and the catheter hub are the two most important sources of infection.[154] Risk factors associated with catheter infection include prolonged catheterization, type of catheter material, use of multilumen catheters, site of catheterization, use of transparent plastic dressings, frequent catheter manipulation, employment of improper aseptic techniques for catheter insertion or maintenance, and use of contaminated skin solutions.[154] Catheter infection rates may be decreased by using topical disinfectants or antibiotics at the insertion site and insertion and maintenance of catheters by an infusion therapy team. Protective modifications to the catheter (such as silver impregnation of the cuff, coating of the catheter with antiseptics or antibiotics, and changing the material from which the catheter is made) also may be protective.[154,157] Routine exchange of a central venous catheter over a guide wire does not decrease the risk of catheter infection and may even increase that risk.[158]

Catheter infections are treated with antibiotics directed against the causative organism and in most cases by removal of the catheter. Gram-positive organisms (*Staphylococcus* sp.) are the most common infecting organisms, but gram-negative bacilli and yeast infections also occur frequently. Infections caused by *S. epidermidis* often can be treated successfully without removal of the catheter, though the risk of recurrence of infection is greater than is the case when the catheter is removed.[154] Resolution of infections with other organisms usually requires catheter removal in addition to antibiotic therapy.[154,159] If a patient is febrile and has a central venous catheter and other potential sources of infection, the catheter may be exchanged over a guide wire and the exchanged catheter tip may be cultured quantitatively. If more than 15 colony forming units (CFU) of bacteria are cultured, the new catheter should be removed and a replacement should be inserted at a different site.[158,160]

The principal treatment for sepsis and septic shock consists of the prompt administration of appropriate antimicrobial therapy and is associated with improved survival.[161] The etiologic agent can be suspected on the basis of the results of a physical cxamination and radiological studies. Initial therapy should include antibiotics active against both gram-positive and gram-negative organisms if no focus of infection is apparent. The administration of fluids, pressors, supplemental oxygen, and other supportive care is frequently required for a septic patient.[162] Several controlled studies have demonstrated that the use of steroids in sepsis is not associated with long-term benefits.[163,164] Treatment directed against endotoxin or cytokines is still investigational.

PRINCIPLES OF ANTIMICROBIAL THERAPY

Blood-Brain Barrier

Passage of certain antibiotics into the CSF and the extracellular fluid of the brain parenchyma is inhibited by the specialized anatomy of the CNS.[165,166] Because the capillary beds of the brain are nonfenestrated, a barrier exists for the transport of many compounds into the CNS. The capillary endothelium is highly fenestrated at the choroid plexus. However, the continuous tight junctions at the apical side of the epithelium prohibit the passage of certain compounds.[167–169] Thus, the blood-brain and blood-CSF barriers have similar physiological effects in spite of anatomic differences. Since there is usually concordance between substances that penetrate poorly into the extracellular fluid of the brain and those which penetrate poorly into the CSF, the terms "blood-brain barrier" and "blood-CSF barrier" are considered equivalent.

Four major characteristics of antimicrobial agents affect passage into the CSF: (1) lipid solubility, (2) degree of ionization, (3) degree of serum protein binding, and (4) molecular weight.[89] Lipid-soluble antimicrobial agents are able to penetrate the membranes of the capillary endothelium or the epithelium of the choroid plexus. Water-soluble agents such as ionized molecules penetrate the CNS less easily. Antimicrobial agents with higher molecular weights penetrate the CSF poorly in the absence of inflammation. Agents with increased binding to serum proteins have a lesser ability to leave the bloodstream. An active transport system at the level of the choroid plexus eliminates beta-lactam antibiotics. Since reduced inflammation leads to a corresponding decrease in CSF penetration of many antibiotics, the dose of the chosen antimicrobial agent should not be reduced with clinical improvement.[170]

The concentration of antibiotic that kills an organism is called the minimum bactericidal concentration (MBC). The lowest concentration of an antibiotic that inhibits the growth of an organism is the minimum inhibitory concentration (MIC). When the MBC and MIC are low and equal, the antibiotic is considered to be bactericidal. When the MBC is considerably higher than the MIC, the antibiotic is considered bacteriostatic. Beta-lactam antibiotics such as penicillins and cephalosporins usually are bactericidal. Chloramphenicol is bactericidal against gram-negative rods such as *K. pneumoniae* and *E. coli.*

Besides antibiotic concentration and organism sensitivity, other local factors usually are important in the recovery from bacterial infections. Two of these factors—complement and immunoglobulin—are lower in CSF than in serum.[171] This makes the use of bactericidal antimicrobial agents a necessity in most CNS infections.

Specific Antimicrobial Agents

The choice of antibiotics is based on the source of infection, the likely organisms, and whether the infection was acquired nosocomially or was present on admission to the hospital. For CNS infections resulting from neurotrauma, the antibiotics of choice should be based on the attainable CSF concentrations, the physiological status of the patient, and the bacteria involved. The spectrum of antibacterial activity and the major adverse effects should be taken into consideration in selecting antibiotic therapy (Table 48-2).

Penicillins

The presence of the 6-aminopenicillanic nucleus in all penicillins is the criterion for calling pencillins "beta-lactam" antibiotics. Penicillins work by inhibiting the synthesis of the bacterial cell wall in actively dividing bacteria. Penicillin G is highly active against *S. pneumoniae, N. meningitidis,* and other streptococci, except *Enterococcus* sp. Penetration of penicillin G into the CSF is poor, with peak CSF levels being approximately 1 to 2 μg/ml with high-dose antibiotic given intravenously (24 MU/day in adults or 300 to 400 thousand U/kg/day in children).[172] Although this level is well above the MBC for susceptible organisms, it is obtained only with relatively frequent administration of high-dose penicillins. With the cessation of inflammation in the CNS, the penicillin concentration reaching the CSF is diminished. Thus, it is important to maintain a schedule of high-dose, frequently administered penicillin throughout the treatment course. Less is known about the penetration of penicillins into pus, but penicillin appears to achieve therapeutic concentrations when high doses are given.[97,98] Common toxicities associated with penicillins include allergic phenomena related to skin rashes and anaphylaxis. Seizures have been reported, but only in patients receiving high-dose penicillin who have concurrent diminished renal function. With renal insufficiency, the dose of penicillin should be decreased.

Ampicillin is active not only against *S. pneumoniae* and *N. meningitidis* but also against *Enterococcus* sp. and non-beta-lactamase-producing strains of *Hemophilus* sp. It appears to be less active against gram-negative bacilli than are the extended-spectrum penicillins. The toxicity of ampicillin appears to be the same as that of penicillin. The dose of ampicillin given intravenously for CNS infections is usually 150 mg/kg/day in divided doses.[173,174]

Semisynthetic antistaphylococcal penicillins such as nafcillin, oxacillin, and methicillin have increased activity against most strains of *S. aureus.* These semisynthetic penicillins are not degraded by staphylococcal penicillinase and therefore retain good activity, in contrast to penicillin G, which has markedly decreased activity against *S. aureus.* Although these newer drugs are also active against *S. pneumoniae* and group A streptococci, penicillin G still has greater activity against these particular bacteria. When nafcillin is given at 150 to 200 mg/kg/day in divided doses, CSF levels are reached that will kill most *S. aureus.*[175–178] The significant risk of interstitial nephritis and hemorrhagic cystitis precludes the use of high-dose methicillin. Little is known about the penetration of semisynthetic penicillins into pus. Because excretion of nafcillin occurs mainly through the biliary tract, only a minimal reduction in dose is needed for patients with renal insufficiency. Toxicities associated with the semisynthetic penicillins are similar to those of penicillin but also include an increased incidence of neutropenia in patients receiving these drugs over an extended period.

TABLE 48-2 Antimicrobial Therapy for CNS Infections

Antimicrobial Agents	Therapeutic CSF Level	Spectrum of Activity	Major Adverse Reactions
Penicillins			
Penicillin	Yes	Pneumococcus, meningococcus	Anaphylaxis, skin rash
Ampicillin	Yes	Pneumococcus, meningococcus, hemophilus	Anaphylaxis, skin rash
Nafcillin	Yes†	Staphylococcus	Anaphylaxis, skin rash
Ticarcillin	Yes†	Gram-negative rods	Anaphylaxis, skin rash
Mezlocillin	Yes†	Gram-negative rods	Anaphylaxis, skin rash
Piperacillin	Yes	Gram-negative rods	Anaphylaxis, skin rash
Cephalosporins			
Cefuroxime	Yes	Hemophilus, pneumococcus	Skin rash
Ceftriaxone	Yes	Gram-negative rods, pneumococcus	Skin rash
Cefotaxime	Yes	Gram-negative rods	Skin rash
Ceftazidime	Yes	Gram-negative rods	Skin rash
Imipenem-cilastatin	Yes†	Gram-negative rods, gram-positive cocci	Seizures
Vancomycin	No▲	Staphylococcus, pneumococcus	Nephrotoxicity, leukopenia
Aminoglycosides	No▲	Gram-negative rods	Nephrotoxicity, ototoxicity
Chloramphenicol	Yes	Pneumococcus, meningococcus	Anemia
Quinolones	Yes	Gram-negative rods	Encephalopathy, skin rash
Metronidazole	Yes	Anaerobes	Encephalopathy
Sulfonamides	Yes	Gram-negative rods, nocardia	Anemia
Rifampin	Yes	Staphylococci	Hepatitis
Amphotericin B	Yes	Candida, cryptococcus, histoplasmosis	Renal insufficiency, hypothalemia
Imidazoles			
Fluconazole	Yes	Candida, cryptococcus	
Itraconazole	No▲	Histoplasmosis, coccidioidomycosis	

† Inadequate pseudomonas coverage
▲ Efficacy demonstrated in specific CNS infections

The broad-spectrum penicillins include ticarcillin, piperacillin, azlocillin, and mezlocillin. Their pharmacokinetics are similar to that of penicillin G, but these antibiotics are active against gram-negative bacilli. Again, they are unable to easily penetrate the blood-brain barrier, and so larger doses are necessary.[179,180] When there is renal insufficiency, the dose must be reduced because of toxicities similar to those seen with penicillin G. Platelet dysfunction also has been described with each of these antibiotics, resulting in a potential for increased bleeding disorders. These extended-spectrum penicillins generally should not be used alone to treat CNS infections. However, in some instances they can be used in combination with an aminoglycoside to treat gram-negative CNS infections.

Cephalosporins

Cephalosporins are also bactericidal beta-lactam antibiotics. Over the past 20 years, new cephalosporins have been developed that have different pharmacokinetics and antibacterial spectra. Cefazolin is a typical first-generation cephalosporin. The first-generation cephalosporins demonstrate good activity against gram-positive cocci but limited activity against gram-negative bacilli. They are not active against *P. aeruginosa* and are not useful for CNS infections because they do not attain therapeutic levels in CSF. Second-generation cephalosporins include cefoxitin, cefotetan, and cefuroxime. Although cefoxitin and cefotetan penetrate into CSF, their MBCs for gram-negative organisms are so high that therapeutic concentrations are not reached.[176,180a–180d] Cefuroxime has better penetration and is effective for *H. influenzae* meningitis. However, it has been replaced by ceftriaxone because of the broader spectrum of activity of ceftriaxone.

Third-generation cephalosporins are very active against gram-negative bacilli, and CSF concentrations are reached that are inhibitory for many gram-negative bacilli. Third-generation cephalosporins used for the treatment of gram-negative CNS infection include cefotaxime, ceftriaxone, and ceftazidime, and ceftazidime is active against *P. aeruginosa.* The toxicities of the cephalosporins are similar to those of the penicillins, with allergy and neutropenia being the most commonly reported. Thus, the third-generation cephalosporins have become the drugs of choice for gram-negative meningitis.[181–187]

VANCOMYCIN

Vancomycin is a bactericidal glycopeptide that is active only against gram-positive cocci, including *S. aureus* and *S. epidermidis.* It inhibits cell wall synthesis and probably impairs RNA synthesis. It is the drug of choice for infections caused by *S. epidermidis.* Peak serum levels of 25 to 35 μg/ml and 12-h levels of 5 to 10 μg/ml are reached after infusion. Toxicities include renal impairment, rash, leukopenia, and hearing loss. With rapid infusion of the drug, a "red neck" syndrome and hypotension have been reported. Levels are not found in the CSF in the presence of uninflamed meninges, and variable bactericidal levels are obtained in the CSF of patients with meningitis.[188,189] Some investigators have given vancomycin intrathecally (3 to 5 mg) for significant ventriculitis or meningitis resulting from susceptible organisms.

AMINOGLYCOSIDES

Aminoglycosides are bactericidal antibiotics that are active mainly against gram-negative bacilli. The aminoglycosides are used as adjunctive therapy for CNS infections because even with meningeal inflammation, their penetration into the CSF is limited.[190–192] If used, they must be given intrathecally to achieve therapeutic levels (4 to 8 mg for gentamicin or tobramycin or 10 to 15 mg for amikacin).[193–195] Toxicities associated with systemic administration of aminoglycosides include acute tubular necrosis and vestibular and cochlear toxicities.

IMIPENEM-CILASTATIN

Imipenem-cilastatin is a carbepenem antibiotic that has broad-spectrum antibacterial activity and is bactericidal. Penetration into the CSF with inflamed meninges is good but variable.[196,197] Mean CNS concentrations of 1.75 μg/ml have been found. This concentration is sufficient for the treatment of meningitis caused by susceptible strains but is below the MBC of many of the *P. aeruginosa* strains seen in CSF infections. Drug-induced seizures have been reported in patients receiving imipenem but usually occur in individuals who are older, have an underlying disease, or have a history of a seizure disorder. One study demonstrated that children receiving imipenem for acute bacterial meningitis developed seizures at a significantly higher percentage than did those receiving other antibiotics.[196]

AZTREONAM

Aztreonam is a monobactam that contains only the beta-lactam ring and is active only against gram-negative bacilli; it is inactive against anaerobes and gram-positive cocci. Aztreonam penetrates the CSF of patients with meningitis, but the concentrations usually are only 5 percent of the concomitant serum concentration, making its use in gram-negative meningitis questionable.[198]

CHLORAMPHENICOL

Chloramphenicol has a long history of use in both systemic and CNS infections. It appears to be bactericidal against pneumococci but is bacteriostatic for several organisms that can infect the CNS. Because it is a lipid-soluble antibiotic, it penetrates the CSF when there is no inflammation. Its use as an agent against gram-negative meningitis has been superseded by the use of third-generation cephalosporins. Nevertheless, it may be useful as an adjunct antibiotic in nontraumatic brain abscess or subdural empyema secondary to sinusitis. No dose adjustment is necessary for patients with renal insufficiency because of its hepatic metabolism; the serum levels are equivalent whether the drug is given orally or intravenously. The usual dose is 50 to 100 mg/kg/day in divided doses. The toxicities are well known and may include severe hematological problems. Idiosyncratic aplastic anemia is the most feared toxic effect of chloramphenicol; it occurs in about 1 in 40,000 people and is nonreversible.[199]

SULFONAMIDES

Among the sulfonamides in use today, trimethoprim-sulfamethoxazole has the greatest potential for use against certain gram-negative organisms that can infect the CNS. Trimethoprim-sulfamethoxazole appears to be bactericidal against *E. coli* and many *Proteus* and *Enterobacter* species. It is given in a dose of 20 mg/kg/day intravenously in four divided doses (based on the trimethoprim concentration). Toxicities include nausea, vomiting, diarrhea, and hypersensitivity reactions, specifically rash. The sulfamethoxazole component of the drug reaches concentrations in the CSF and brain tissue that have activity against many organisms, including *Nocardia.*[200,201]

QUINOLONES

The newer fluoroquinolones have been reported to achieve significant CSF levels in patients with meningitis. The quinolones are bactericidal and have broad-spectrum activity, especially against gram-negative bacilli.[23,202] They show little activity against anaerobes. The fluoroquinolones that penetrate the CSF and brain tissue include ciprofloxacin, ofloxacin, and pefloxacin. Concentrations of pefloxacin in the CSF in patients with normal meninges are similar to those of patients with meningitis, suggesting that this antibiotic is highly lipid-soluble.[203,204] Although the pharmacokinetics suggest that the quinolones might play a role in the treatment of gram-negative meningitis and CNS infections, only anecdotal experiences have been reported.[205–207]

Tetracyclines

Because tetracyclines are only moderately lipid-soluble, they do not penetrate into the CSF or brain very well. Animal data suggest that the more lipid-soluble drugs, such as doxycycline and minocycline, could penetrate the CNS better than do the older tetracycline compounds. There is insufficient information in humans to warrant their use in specific CNS infections.[208,209]

Metronidazole

Metronidazole is a highly lipid-soluble antibiotic that penetrates the CSF even in the absence of inflammation. CSF concentrations were reported as 6 to 9 μg/ml in patients with meningitis receiving 500 mg intravenously.[172,210] Penetration into brain tissue is as efficient as penetration into the CSF. Metronidazole is active primarily against anaerobes. Adverse reactions are rarely encountered but may include seizures, encephalopathy, a disulfiram reaction with alcohol, and pancreatitis. Oral administration provides similar serum and CSF levels compared with intravenous administration.

Rifampin

Although rifampin is highly lipid-soluble, there is poor penetration of inflamed meninges. Most of our understanding of CSF rifampin levels has been obtained from the treatment of tuberculous meningitis.[211,212] This antimicrobial may be used in conjunction with other agents for the treatment of staphylococcal meningitis.

Antifungal agents

Until recently, treatment of CNS fungal infections required the administration of amphotericin B intravenously and/or intrathecally. Amphotericin B probably works by altering membrane permeability of the fungus. Amphotericin B is active in candidiasis, cryptococcosis, histoplasmosis, coccidioidomycosis, and other invasive fungal infections. Most of the amphotericin B is degraded in the body; only a small percentage is excreted in the urine or bile. Hemodialysis does not alter blood concentrations. There is poor penetration of normal and inflamed meninges.[213,214] Therefore, the need for intrathecal administration must be considered in selected cases. The principal toxicities are azotemia, hypokalemia, fever, and chills. The newer imidazole antifungal agents can be given orally and have good CNS penetration.[215,216] Future studies will determine whether they can replace amphotericin B for all CNS fungal infections.

References

1. Miller JD: Infection after head injury, in Vinken PJ, Bruyn GW (eds): *Handbook of Clinical Neurology.* Vol 24: *Injuries of the Brain and Skull, Part II.* Amsterdam: North-Holland, 1976: 215–230.
2. Tunkel AR, Scheld WM: Acute infectious complications of head trauma, in Braakman R (ed): *Handbook of Clinical Neurology: Head Injury.* New York: Elsevier, 1990: 317–326.
3. Katz PM, Cooper PR: Infectious complication of neurosurgical trauma. *Infect Surg* 4:22–27, 1985.
4. Gallagher M, Colohan ART: Infectious complications of head injury, in Barrow DL (ed): *Complications and Sequelae of Head Injury.* Park Ridge, IL: American Association of Neurological Surgeons, 1992: 61–89.
5. Mollman HD, Haines SJ: Risk factors for postoperative neurosurgical wound infection: A case-control study. *J Neurosurg* 64:902–906, 1986.
6. Savitz MH, Katz SS: Prevention of primary wound infection in neurosurgical patients: A 10-year study. *Neurosurgery* 18:685–688, 1986.
7. Goodman SJ, Cahan L, Chow AW: Subgaleal abscess: A preventable complication of scalp trauma. *West J Med* 127:169–172, 1977.
8. Wiley JF II, Sugarman JM, Bell LM: Subgaleal abscess: An unusual presentation. *Ann Emerg Med* 18:785–787, 1989.
9. Razzouk A, Collins N, Zirkle T: Chronic extensive necrotizing abscess of the scalp. *Ann Plast Surg* 20:124–127, 1988.
10. Bullitt E, Lehman RA: Osteomyelitis of the skull. *Surg Neurol* 11:163–166, 1979.
11. Kaufman BA, Tunkel AR, Pryor JC, et al: Meningitis in the neurosurgical patient. *Infect Dis Clin North Am* 4:677–701, 1990.
12. Appelbaum E: Meningitis following trauma to the head and face. *JAMA* 173:1818–1822, 1960.
13. Dagi TF, Meyer FB, Poletti CA: The incidence and prevention of meningitis after basilar skull fracture. *Am J Emerg Med* 1:295–298, 1983.
14. Raaf J: Posttraumatic cerebrospinal fluid leaks. *Arch Surg* 95:648–651, 1967.
15. Saito H: Late posttraumatic rhinogenic meningitis: Temporal bone findings of meningogenic labyrinthitis. *Adv Otorhinolaryngol* 31:175–183, 1983.
16. Hand WL, Sanford JP: Posttraumatic bacterial meningitis. *Ann Intern Med* 72:869–874, 1970.
17. Leblanc W, Heagarty MC: Posttraumatic meningitis due to *Haemophilus influenzae* type A. *J Natl Med Assoc* 75:995–1000, 1983.
18. Bryan CS, Jernigan FE: Posttraumatic meningitis due to ampicillin-resistant *Haemophilus influenzae. J Neurosurg* 51:240–241, 1979.

19. Jones SR, Luby JP, Sanford JP: Bacterial meningitis complicating cranial-spinal trauma. *J Trauma* 13:895–900, 1973.
20. Sengupta RP, Garvan N: Recurrent fulminating meningitis 20 years after head injury: Case report. *J Neurosurg* 41:758–761, 1974.
21. Langley JM, LeBlanc JC, Drake J, et al: Efficacy of antimicrobial prophylaxis in placement of cerebrospinal fluid shunts: Meta-analysis. *Clin Infect Dis* 17:98–103, 1993.
22. Leech P: Cerebrospinal fluid leakage, dural fistulae and meningitis after basal skull fractures. *Injury* 6:141–149, 1974.
23. Helling TS, Evans LL, Fowler DL, et al: Infectious complications in patients with severe head injury. *J Trauma* 28:1575–1577, 1988.
23a. Infection in Neurosurgery Working Party of the British Society for Antimicrobial Chemotherapy. Antimicrobial prophylaxis in neurosurgery and after head injury. *Lancet* 344:1547–1551, 1994.
24. Hyslop NE, Montgomery WW: Diagnosis and management of meningitis associated with cerebrospinal fluid leaks, in Remington JS, Whitley RJ (eds): *Current Clinical Topics in Infectious Diseases.* New York: McGraw-Hill, 1982: 185–254.
25. McGee EE, Cauthen JC, Brackett CE: Meningitis following acute traumatic cerebrospinal fluid fistula. *J Neurosurg* 33:312–316, 1970.
26. Gorse GJ: Management of posttraumatic and postoperative meningitis. *Infect Surg* 4:740–746, 1985.
27. Levison ME, Mangura CT, Lorber B, et al: Clindamycin compared with penicillin for the treatment of anaerobic lung abscess. *Ann Intern Med* 98:466–471, 1983.
28. Swartz MN, Dodge PR: Bacterial meningitis—a review of selected aspects. *N Engl J Med* 272:725–731, 779–787, 842–848, 898–902, 1965.
29. Durand ML, Calderwood SB, Weber DJ, et al: Acute bacterial meningitis in adults: A review of 493 episodes. *N Engl J Med* 328:21–28, 1993.
30. Young RF, Lawner PM: Perioperative antibiotic prophylaxis for the prevention of postoperative neurosurgical infections: A randomized clinical trial. *J Neurosurg* 66:701–705, 1987.
31. Geraghty J, Feely M: Antibiotic prophylaxis in neurosurgery. *J Neurosurg* 60:724–726, 1984.
32. Aoki N: Lumboperitoneal shunt: Clinical applications, complications, and comparison with ventriculoperitoneal shunt. *Neurosurgery* 26:998–1004, 1990.
33. Kaufman BA, McLone DG: Infections of cerebrospinal fluid shunts, in Scheld WM, Whitley RJ, Durack DT (eds): *Infections of the Central Nervous System.* New York: Raven Press, 1991: 561–585.
34. Mayhall CG, Archer NH, Lamb VA, et al: Ventriculostomy-related infections: A prospective epidemiologic study. *N Engl J Med* 310:553–559, 1984.
35. Noetzel MJ, Baker RP: Shunt fluid examination: Risks and benefits in the evaluation of shunt malfunction and infection. *J Neurosurg* 61:328–332, 1984.
36. Forward KR, Fewer D, Stiver HG: Cerebrospinal fluid shunt infections: A review of 35 infections in 32 patients. *J Neurosurg* 59:389–394, 1983.
37. Venes JL: Infections of CSF shunt and intracranial pressure monitoring devices. *Infect Dis Clin North Am* 3:289–299, 1989.
38. Schoenbaum SC, Gardner P, Shillito J: Infections of cerebrospinal fluid shunts: Epidemiology, clinical manifestations, and therapy. *J Infect Dis* 131:543–552, 1975.
39. Chan KH, Mann KS: Prolonged therapeutic external ventricular drainage: A prospective study. *Neurosurgery* 23:436–438, 1988.
40. Wyler AR, Kelly WA: Use of antibiotics with external ventriculostomies. *J Neurosurg* 37:185–187, 1972.
41. Smith RW, Alksne JF: Infections complicating the use of external ventriculostomy. *J Neurosurg* 44:567–570, 1976.
42. Shapiro M: Prophylaxis in otolaryngologic surgery and neurosurgery: A critical review. *Rev Infect Dis* 13(suppl 10):S858–S868, 1991.
43. Clark WC, Muhlbauer MS, Lowrey R, et al: Complications of intracranial pressure monitoring in trauma patients. *Neurosurgery* 25:20–24, 1989.
44. Walters BC, Hoffman HJ, Hendrick EB, et al: Cerebrospinal fluid shunt infection: Influences on initial management and subsequent outcome. *J Neurosurg* 60:1014–1021, 1984.
45. James HE, Walsh JW, Wilson JD, et al: Prospective randomized study of therapy in cerebrospinal fluid shunt infection. *Neurosurgery* 7:459–463, 1980.
46. Anagnostopoulos DI, Gortvai P: Intracranial subdural abscess. *Br J Surg* 60:50–52, 1973.
47. Greenlee JE: Subdural empyema, in Mandell GL, Douglas RG Jr, Bennett JE (eds): *Principles and Practice of Infectious Diseases,* 3d ed. New York: Churchill Livingstone, 1990: 788–791.
48. Harris LF, Haws FP, Triplett JN Jr, et al: Subdural empyema and epidural abscess: Recent experience in a community hospital. *South Med J* 80:1254–1258, 1987.
49. Helfgott DC, Weingarten K, Hartman BJ: Subdural empyema, in Scheld WM, Whitley RJ, Durack DT (eds): *Infections of the Central Nervous System.* New York: Raven Press, 1991: 487–488.
50. Khan M, Griebel R: Subdural empyema: A retrospective study of 15 patients. *Can J Surg* 27:283–288, 1984.
51. Mauser HW, Van Houwelingen HC, Tulleken CA: Factors affecting the outcome in subdural empyema. *J Neurol Neurosurg Psychiatry* 50:1136–1141, 1987.
52. Miller ES, Dias PS, Uttley D: Management of subdural empyema: A series of 24 cases. *J Neurol Neurosurg Psychiatry* 50:1415–1418, 1987.
53. Renaudin JW, Frazee J: Subdural empyema—importance of early diagnosis. *Neurosurgery* 7:477–479, 1980.
54. Weisberg L: Subdural empyema: Clinical and computed tomographic correlations. *Arch Neurol* 43:497–500, 1986.
55. Gellin BG, Weingarten K, Gamache FW Jr, et al: Epidural abscess, in Scheld WM, Whitley RJ, Durack DT (eds): *Infections of the Central Nervous System.* New York: Raven Press, 1991: 499–514.
56. Coonrod JD, Dans PE: Subdural empyema. *Am J Med* 53:85–91, 1972.

57. Bok APL, Peter JC: Subdural empyema: Burrholes or craniotomy? A retrospective computerized tomography-era analysis of treatment in 90 cases. *J Neurosurg* 78:574–578, 1993.
58. Feuerman T, Wackym PA, Gade GF, et al: Craniotomy improves outcome in subdural empyema. *Surg Neurol* 32:105–110, 1989.
59. Bannister G, Williams B, Smith S: Treatment of subdural empyema. *J Neurosurg* 55:82–88, 1981.
60. Wispelwey B, Dacey RG Jr, Scheld WM: Brain abscess, in Scheld WM, Whitley RJ, Durack DT (eds): *Infections of the Central Nervous System.* New York: Raven Press, 1991: 457–486.
61. Wispelwey B, Scheld WM: Brain abscess. *Clin Neuropharmacol* 10:483–510, 1987.
62. Ariza J, Casanova A, Fernandez-Viladrich P, et al: Etiological agent and primary source of infection in 42 cases of focal intracranial suppuration. *J Clin Microbiol* 24:899–902, 1986.
63. Carey ME, Young H, Mathis JL, et al: A bacteriological study of craniocerebral missile wounds from Vietnam. *J Neurosurg* 34:145–154, 1971.
64. Rish BL, Caveness WF, Dillon JD, et al: Analysis of brain abscess after penetrating craniocerebral injuries in Vietnam. *Neurosurgery* 9:535–541, 1981.
65. Cairns H, Calvert CA, Daniel P, et al: Complications of head wounds with special reference to infection. *Br J Surg (War Surg)* Suppl 1:198–243, 1947.
66. Grahm TW, Williams FC Jr, Harrington T, et al: Civilian gunshot wounds to the head: A prospective study. *Neurosurgery* 27:696–700, 1990.
67. Hagan RE: Early complications following penetrating wounds of the brain. *J Neurosurg* 34:132–141, 1971.
68. Harsh GR III: Infection complicating penetrating craniocerebral trauma, in Coates JB, Meirowsky AM (eds): *Neurological Surgery of Trauma.* Washington, D.C.: U.S. Government Printing Office, 1965: 135–142.
69. Kaufman HH, Makela ME, Lee F, et al: Gunshot wounds to the head: A perspective. *Neurosurgery* 18:689–695, 1952.
70. Teabeaut JR II: Aspiration of gastric contents: An experimental study. *Am J Pathol* 28:51–67, 1952.
71. Wannamaker GT, Pulaski EJ: Pyogenic neurosurgical infections in Korean battle casualties. *J Neurosurg* 15:512–518, 1958.
72. Alpert G, Sutton LN: Brain abscess following cranial dog bite. *Clin Pediatr (Phila)* 23:580, 1984.
73. Berkowitz FE, Jacobs DWC: Fatal case of brain abscess caused by rooster pecking. *Pediatr Infect Dis J* 6:941–942, 1987.
74. Duffy GP, Bhandari YS: Intracranial complications following transorbital penetrating injuries. *Br J Surg* 56:685–688, 1969.
75. Fanning WL, Willett LR, Phillips CF, et al: Puncture wound of the eyelid causing brain abscess. *J Trauma* 16:919–920, 1976.
76. Foy P, Scharr M: Cerebral abscesses in children after pencil-tip injuries. *Lancet* 2:662–663, 1980.
77. Jennett B, Miller JD: Infection after depressed fracture of the skull: Implications for management of nonmissile injuries. *J Neurosurg* 36:333–339, 1972.
78. Lew JR, Wiedermann BL, Sneed J, et al: Aerotolerant *Clostridium tertium* brain abscess following a lawn dart injury. *J Clin Microbiol* 28:2127–2129, 1990.
79. Miller JD, Jennett WB: Complications of depressed skull fracture. *Lancet* 2:991–995, 1968.
80. Pencek TL, Burchiel KJ: Delayed brain abscess related to a retained foreign body with culture of *Clostridium bifermentans. J Neurosurg* 64:813–815, 1986.
81. Tay JS, Garland JS: Serious head injuries from lawn darts. *Pediatrics* 79:261–263, 1987.
82. Tiffany KK, Kline MW: Mixed flora brain abscess with *Pseudomonas paucimobilis* after a penetrating lawn dart injury. *Pediatr Infect Dis J* 7:667–669, 1988.
83. Nielsen H, Gyldensted C, Harmsen A: Cerebral abscess: Aetiology and pathogenesis, symptoms, diagnosis and treatment–a review of 200 cases from 1935–1976. *Acta Neurol Scand* 65:609–622, 1982.
84. Webster JE, Schneider RC, Lofstrom JE: Observations on early type of brain abscess following penetrating wounds of the brain. *J Neurosurg* 3:7–14, 1946.
85. Anderson D, Strong AJ, Ingham HR, et al: Fifteen year review of the mortality of brain abscess. *Neurosurgery* 8:1–6, 1981.
86. Brand B, Caparosa RJ, Lubic LG: Otorhinological brain abscess therapy—past and present. *Laryngoscope* 94:483–487, 1984.
87. DeLouvois J: The bacteriology and chemotherapy of brain abscess. *J Antimicrob Chemother* 4:395–413, 1978.
88. DeLouvois J, Gortvai P, Hurley R: Bacteriology of abscesses of the central nervous system: Multicentre prospective study. *Br Med J* 2:981–984, 1977.
89. Ingham JR, Selkon JB, Roxby CM: Bacteriological study of otogenic cerebral abscesses: Chemotherapeutic role of metronidazole. *Br Med J* 2:991–993, 1977.
90. Miller ES, Dias PS, Uttley D: CT scanning in the management of intracranial abscess: A review of 100 cases. *Br J Neurosurg* 2:439–446, 1988.
91. Britt RH, Enzmann DR: Clinical stages of human brain abscesses on serial CT scans after contrast infusion: Computerized tomographic, neuropathological, and clinical correlations. *J Neurosurg* 59:972–989, 1983.
92. Samson DS, Clark K: A current review of brain abscess. *Am J Med* 54:201–210, 1973.
93. Brewer NS, MacCarty CS, Wellman WE: Brain abscess: A review of recent experience. *Ann Intern Med* 82:571–576, 1975.
94. Mampalam TJ, Rosenblum ML: Trends in the management of bacterial brain abscesses: A review of 102 cases over 17 years. *Neurology* 23:451–458, 1988.
95. Black P, Graybill JR, Charache P: Penetration of brain abscess by systemically administered antibiotics. *J Neurosurg* 38:705–709, 1973.
96. DeLouvois J, Gortvai P, Hurley R: Antibiotic treatment of abscesses of the central nervous system. *Br Med J* 2:985–987, 1977.
97. DeLouvois J, Hurley R: Antibiotic concentration in intracranial pus: A collaborative project, in Williams JD, Geddes AM (eds): *Chemotherapy: Pharmacology of Antibiotics.* New York: Plenum Press, 1975: 66–71.

98. Holm SE, Kourtopoulos H: Penetration of antibiotics into brain tissue and brain abscesses: An experimental study in steroid treated rats. *Scand J Infect Dis Suppl* 44:68–70, 1985.
99. Garfield J: Management of supratentorial intracranial abscess: A review of 200 cases. *Br Med J* 2:7–11, 1969.
100. Rosenblum ML, Mampalam TJ, Pons VG: Controversies in the management of brain abscesses. *Clin Neurosurg* 33:603–632, 1986.
101. Yildizhan A, Pasaoglu A, Ozkul MH, et al: Clinical analysis and results of operative treatment of 41 brain abscesses. *Neurosurg Rev* 14:279–282, 1991.
102. Yoshikawa TT, Quinn W: The aching head: Intracranial suppuration due to head and neck infections. *Infect Dis Clin North Am* 2:265–277, 1988.
103. Jefferson AA, Keogh AJ: Intracranial abscesses: A review of treated patients over 20 years. *Q J Med* 46:389–400, 1977.
104. Driks MR, Craven DE, Celli BR, et al: Nosocomial pneumonia in intubated patients given sucralfate as compared with antacids or histamine type 2 blockers: The role of gastric colonization. *N Engl J Med* 317:1376–1382, 1987.
105. Braakman R, Schouten HJA, Blaauw-van Dishoeck M, et al: Megadose steroids in severe head injury: Results of a prospective double-blind clinical trial. *J Neurosurg* 58:326–330, 1983.
106. DeMaria EJ, Reichman W, Kenney PR, et al: Septic complications of corticosteroid administration after central nervous system trauma. *Ann Surg* 202:248–252, 1985.
107. Braun SR, Levin AB, Clark KL: Role of corticosteroids in the development of pneumonia in mechanically ventilated head-trauma victims. *Crit Care Med* 14:198–201, 1986.
108. Pories SE, Gamelli RL, Mead PB, et al: The epidemiologic features of nosocomial infections in patients with trauma. *Arch Surg* 126:97–99, 1991.
109. Stamm WE, Martin SM, Bennett JV: Epidemiology of nosocomial infections due to gram-negative bacilli: Aspects relevant to the development and use of vaccines. *J Infect Dis* 136(suppl):S151–S160, 1977.
110. Haley RW, Hooton TM, Culver DH, et al: Nosocomial infections in U.S. hospitals, 1975–1976: Estimated frequency by selected characteristics of patients. *Am J Med* 70:947–959, 1981.
111. Garibaldi RA: Hospital-acquired urinary tract infections: Epidemiology and prevention, in Wenzel RP (ed): *Prevention and Control of Nosocomial Infections.* Baltimore: Williams & Wilkins, 1987:335–343.
112. Garibaldi RA, Burke JP, Dickman ML, et al: Factors predisposing to bacteriuria during indwelling urethral catheterization. *N Engl J Med* 291:215–219, 1974.
113. Thompson RL, Haley CE, Searcy MA, et al: Catheter-associated bacteriuria: Failure to reduce attack rates using periodic instillation of a disinfectant into urinary drainage systems. *JAMA* 251:747–751, 1984.
114. Platt R, Polk BF, Murdock B, et al: Mortality associated with nosocomial urinary-tract infection. *N Engl J Med* 307:637–642, 1982.
115. Shapiro M, Simchen E, Sacks TG: A multivariate analysis of risk factors for acquiring bacteriuria in patients with indwelling urinary catheters for longer than 24 hours. *Infect Control* 5:525–532, 1984.
116. Platt R, Polk BF, Murdock B, et al: Risk factors for nosocomial urinary tract infection. *Am J Epidemiol* 124:977–985, 1986.
117. Warren JW: Nosocomial urinary tract infections, in Mandell GL, Douglas RG Jr, Bennett JE (eds): *Principles and Practice in Infectious Diseases,* 3d ed. New York: Churchill Livingstone, 1990: 2205–2215.
118. Classen DC, Stevens LE, Bass SA, et al: Lack of efficacy of a silver oxide-coated catheter in the prevention of catheter-associated bacteriuria: A large randomized clinical trial (abstr). *Programs and Abstracts of the 30th ICAAC.* Atlanta, Abstract 710:204, 1990.
119. Classen DC, Larsen RA, Burke JP, et al: Prevention of catheter-associated bacteriuria: Clinical trial of methods to block three known pathways of infection. *Am J Infect Control* 19:136–142, 1991.
120. Scheld WM, Mandell GL: Nosocomial pneumonia: Pathogenesis and recent advances in diagnosis and therapy. *Rev Infect Dis* 13(suppl 9):S743–S751, 1991.
121. Bartlett JG, Gorbach SL: The triple threat of aspiration pneumonia. *Chest* 68:560–566, 1975.
122. Culver GA, Makel HP, Beecher HK: Frequency of aspiration of gastric contents by the lungs during anesthesia. *Ann Surg* 133:289–292, 1951.
123. Amberson JB: Aspiration bronchopneumonia. *Int Clin* (47) 3:126–138, 1937.
124. Maciver IN, Frew IJC, Matheson JG: The role of respiratory insufficiency in the mortality of severe head injuries. *Lancet* 1:390–393, 1958.
125. Wynne JW, Modell JH: Respiratory aspiration of stomach contents. *Ann Intern Med* 87:466–474, 1977.
126. Mendelson CL: The aspiration of stomach contents into the lungs during obstetric anesthesia. *Am J Obstet Gynecol* 52:191–205, 1946.
127. Craven DE, Steger KA: Nosocomial pneumonia in the intubated patient. *Infect Dis Clin North Am* 3:843–866, 1989.
128. Pennington JE: Hospital-acquired pneumonia, in Wenzel RP (ed): *Prevention and Control of Nosocomial Infections.* Baltimore: Williams & Wilkins, 1987: 321–334.
129. Craven DE, Kunches LM, Kilinsky V, et al: Risk factors for pneumonia and fatality in patients receiving continuous mechanical ventilation. *Am Rev Respir Dis* 133:792–796, 1986.
130. Hsieh A-H, Bishop MJ, Kubilis PS, et al: Pneumonia following closed head injury. *Am Rev Respir Dis* 146:290–294, 1992.
131. Torres A, Aznar R, Gatell JM, et al: Incidence, risk, and prognosis factors of nosocomial pneumonia in mechanically ventilated patients. *Am Rev Respir Dis* 142:523–528, 1990.
132. George DL: Epidemiology of nosocomial ventilator-associated pneumonia. *Infect Control Hosp Epidemiol* 14:163–169, 1993.
133. Deppe SA, Kelly JW, Thoi LL, et al: Incidence of colonization, nosocomial pneumonia, and mortality in criti-

cally ill patients using a Trach Care closed-suction versus an open-suction system: Prospective, randomized study. *Crit Care Med* 18:1389–1393, 1990.

134. Langer M, Mosconi P, Cigada M, et al: Long-term respiratory support and risk of pneumonia in critically ill patients. *Am Rev Respir Dis* 140:302–305, 1989.
135. Valenti WM, Hall CB, Douglas RG Jr, et al: Nosocomial viral infections: I. Epidemiology and significance. *Infect Control* 1:33–37, 1979.
136. Johanson WG, Pierce AK, Sanford JP: Changing laryngeal bacterial flora of hospitalized patients: Emergence of Gram-negative bacilli. *N Engl J Med* 281:1137–1140, 1969.
137. Reusser P, Zimmerli W, Scheidegger D, et al: Role of gastric colonization in nosocomial infections and endotoxemia: A prospective study in neurosurgical patients on mechanical ventilation. *J Infect Dis* 160:414–421, 1989.
138. Montravers P, Fagon J-Y, Chastre J, et al: Follow-up protected specimen brushes to assess treatment in nosocomial pneumonia. *Am Rev Respir Dis* 147:38–44, 1993.
139. Fagon J-Y, Chastre J, Hance AJ, et al: Detection of nosocomial lung infection in ventilated patients: Use of a protected specimen brush and quantitative culture techniques in 147 patients. *Am Rev Respir Dis* 138:110–116, 1988.
140. Wimberley N, Faling LJ, Bartlett JG: A fiberoptic bronchoscopy technique to obtain uncontaminated lower airway secretions for bacterial culture. *Am Rev Respir Dis* 119:337–343, 1979.
141. Teague RB, Wallace RJ Jr, Awe RJ: The use of quantitative sterile brush culture and Gram stain analysis in the diagnosis of lower respiratory tract infection. *Chest* 79:157–161, 1981.
142. Chastre J, Fagon J-Y, Soler P, et al: Diagnosis of nosocomial bacterial pneumonia in intubated patients undergoing ventilation: Comparison of the usefulness of bronchoalveolar lavage and the protected specimen brush. *Am J Med* 85:499–506, 1988.
143. Septimus EJ: Nosocomial bacterial pneumonias. *Semin Respir Infect* 4:245–252, 1989.
144. Klastersky J, Carpentier-Meunier F, Kahan-Coppens L, et al: Endotracheally administered antibiotics for gram-negative bronchopneumonia. *Chest* 75:586–591, 1979.
145. Feely TW, Du Moulin GC, Hedley-Whyte J, et al: Aerosol polymyxin and pneumonia in seriously ill patients. *N Engl J Med* 293:471–475, 1975.
146. Greenfield S, Teres D, Bushness LS, et al: Prevention of gram-negative bacillary pneumonia using aerosol polymyxin as prophylaxis. *J Clin Invest* 52:2934–2940, 1973.
147. Klastersky J, Huysmans E, Weerts D, et al: Endotracheally administered gentamicin for the prevention of infections of the respiratory tract in patients with tracheostomy: A double-blind study. *Chest* 65:650–654, 1974.
148. Flaherty J, Nathan C, Kabins SA, et al: Pilot trial of selective decontamination for prevention of bacterial infection in an intensive care unit. *J Infect Dis.* 162:1393–1397, 1990.
149. Pennington JE: Nosocomial respiratory infection, in Mandell GL, Douglas RG Jr, Bennett JE (eds): *Principles and Practice of Infectious Diseases,* 3d ed. New York: Churchill Livingstone, 1990: 2199–2205.
150. Galpin JE, Chow AW, Bayer AS, et al: Sepsis associated with decubitus ulcers. *Am J Med* 61:346–350, 1976.
151. Reuler JB, Cooney TG: The pressure sore: Pathophysiology and principles of management. *Ann Intern Med* 94:661–666, 1981.
152. Eykyn SJ, Gransden WR, Phillips I: The causative organisms of septicaemia and the epidemiology. *J Antimicrob Chemother* 25(suppl C):41–58, 1990.
153. Bone RC: The pathogenesis of sepsis. *Ann Intern Med* 115:457–469, 1991.
154. Raad II, Bodey GP: Infectious complications of indwelling vascular catheters. *Clin Infect Dis* 15:197–210, 1992.
155. Maki DG, Weise CE, Sarafin HW: A semiquantitative culture method for identifying intravenous catheter-related infections. *N Engl J Med* 296:1305–1309, 1977.
156. Wing EJ, Norden CW, Shadduck RK, et al: Use of quantitative bacteriologic techniques to diagnose catheter-related sepsis. *Arch Intern Med* 139:482–483, 1979.
157. Goldmann DA, Pier GB: Pathogenesis of infections related to intravascular catheterization. *Clin Microbiol Rev* 6:176–192, 1993.
158. Cobb DK, High KP, Sawyer RG, et al: A controlled trial of scheduled replacement of central venous and pulmonary-artery catheters. *N Engl J Med* 327:1062–1068, 1992.
159. Benezra D, Kiehn TE, Gold JWM, et al: Prospective study of infections in indwelling central venous catheters using quantitative blood cultures. *Am J Med* 85:495–498, 1988.
160. Armstrong CW, Mahall CG, Miller KB, et al: Prospective study of catheter replacement and other risk factors for infection of hyperalimentation catheters. *J Infect Dis* 154:808–816, 1986.
161. Parrillo JE, Parker MM, Natanson C, et al: Septic shock in humans: Advances in the understanding of pathogenesis, cardiovascular dysfunction, and therapy. *Ann Intern Med* 113:227–242, 1990.
162. Harris RL, Musher DM, Bloom K, et al: Manifestation of sepsis. *Arch Intern Med* 147:1895–1906, 1987.
163. Bone TC, Fisher CJ, Clemmer TP, et al: A controlled clinical trial of high-dose methylprednisolone in the treatment of severe sepsis and septic shock. *N Engl J Med* 317:653–658, 1987.
164. Veterans Administration Systemic Sepsis Cooperative Study Group: Effect of high-dose glucocorticoid therapy on mortality in patients with clinical signs of systemic sepsis. *N Engl J Med* 317:659–665, 1987.
165. Haines DE, Harkey HL, Al-Mefty O: The "subdural" space: A new look at an outdated concept. *Neurosurgery* 32:111–120, 1993.
166. Selkow JB, Barling RWA: The cerebrospinal fluid penetration of antibiotics. *J Antimicrob Chemother* 4:204–227, 1978.
167. Oldendorf WH: Blood-brain barrier permeability to drugs. *Annu Rev Pharmacol* 4:239–248, 1974.

168. Oldendorf WH: Permeability of the blood-brain barrier, in Tower DB (ed): *The Nervous System,* vol. 1. New York: Raven Press, 1975: 279–289.
169. Rall DP, Stabenau JR, Zubrud CG: Distribution of drugs between blood and CSF: General methodology and effects of pH gradients. *J Pharmacol Exp Ther* 125:185–195, 1959.
170. Heiber JP, Nelson JD: A pharmacologic evaluation of penicillin in children with purulent meningitis. *N Engl J Med* 297:410–413, 1977.
171. Simberkoff MS, Moldover NH, Rahal JJ Jr: Absence of detectable bactericidal and opsonic activities in normal and infected human cerebrospinal fluids. *J Lab Clin Med* 96:362–372, 1980.
172. Everett ED, Strasbaugh LJ: Antimicrobial agents and the central nervous system. *Neurosurgery* 6:691–714, 1980.
173. Bakken JS, Bruun JN, Gaustad P, et al: Penetration of amoxicillin and potassium clavulanate into the CSF of patients with inflamed meninges. *Antimicrob Agents Chemother* 21:551–553, 1982.
174. Strasbaugh LJ, Girgil NI, Mikhail IA, et al: Penetration of amoxicillin into CSF. *Antimicrob Agents Chemother* 14:899–902, 1978.
175. Fossieck BE Jr, Kane JG, Diza CR, et al: Nafcillin entry into human cerebrospinal fluid. *Antimicrob Agents Chemother* 11:965–967, 1977.
176. Frame PT, Watanakunakorn C, McLaurin RL, et al: Penetration of nafcillin, methicillin and cefazolin into human brain tissue. *Neurosurgery* 12:142–147, 1983.
177. Kane JG, Parker RH, Jordan GW, et al: Nafcillin concentration in cerebrospinal fluid during treatment of staphylococcal infections. *Ann Intern Med* 87:307–311, 1977.
178. Ruiz DE, Warner JF: Nafcillin treatment of *Staphylococcus aureus* meningitis. *Antimicrob Agents Chemother* 9:554–555, 1976.
179. Decazes JM, Meulemans A, Burea F, et al: Penetration of piperacillin into CSF of patients with purulent meningitis. *Presse Med* 13:261–264, 1984.
180. Modai J, Pierre J, Bergogne-Berezin E, et al: CSF penetration of mezlocillin. *Arzheim-Forsch/Drug Res* 29:1967–1969, 1979.
180a. Liu C, Hinthorn DR, Hodges GR, et al: Penetration of cefoxitin into human CSF: Comparison with cefamandole, ampicillin and penicillin. *Rev Infect Dis* 1:127–131, 1979.
180b. Galvao PA, Lomar AV, Francisco W, et al: Cefoxitin penetration in CSF in patients with purulent meningitis. *Antimicrob Agents Chemother* 17:526–529, 1980.
180c. Netland A, Muller C, Andrew E: Concentration of cefuroxime in CSF in patients with bacterial meningitis. *Scand J Infect Dis* 13:273–275, 1981.
180d. Beam TR Jr: Cephalosporins in adult meningitis. *Bull NY Acad Med* 60:380–393, 1984.
181. Overturf GD, Cable DC, Forthal DN, et al: Treatment of bacterial meningitis with ceftizoxime. *Antimicrob Agents Chemother* 25:258–262, 1984.
182. Chandrasekar PH, Rolston KVI, Smith BR, et al: Diffusion of ceftriaxone into the CSF of adults. *J Antimicrob Chemother* 14:427–430, 1984.
183. Danker EM, Conner JD, Sawyer M, et al: Treatment of bacterial meningitis with once daily ceftriaxone therapy. *J Antimicrob Chemother* 21:637–645, 1988.
184. Fong IW, Tomkins KB: Penetration of ceftazidime into the CSF of patients with and without meningeal inflammation. *Antimicrob Agents Chemother* 26:115–116, 1984.
185. McCracken GH, Sande MA, Lentnek A, et al: Evaluation of new anti-infective drugs for the treatment of acute bacterial meningitis. *Clin Infect Dis* 15(suppl 1):S182–S188, 1992.
186. Modai J, Meulemans A, Vittecoq D: Treatment of *Pseudomonas aeruginosa* meningitis with ceftazidime. *J Antimicrob Chemother* 11:198–199, 1983.
187. Yogev R, Shulman ST, Chadwick EG, et al: Once daily ceftriaxone for CNS infections and other serious infections. *Pediatr Infect Dis J* 5:416–420, 1986.
188. Hawley B, Gump DW: Vancomycin therapy of bacterial meningitis. *Am J Dis Child* 126:261–264, 1973.
189. Levy RM, Gutin PH, Baskin DS, et al: Vancomycin penetration of a brain abscess: Case report and review of the literature. *Neurosurgery* 18:632–636, 1986.
190. Briedis DJ, Robson HG: Cerebrospinal fluid penetration of amikacin. *Antimicrob Agents Chemother* 13:1042–1043, 1978.
191. Kaiser AB, McGee ZA: Aminoglycoside therapy of gram-negative bacillary meningitis. *N Engl J Med* 293:1215–1220, 1975.
192. Neuwelt EA, Horaczek A, Pagel MA: The effect of steroids on gentamicin delivery to brain after blood-brain disruption. *J Neurosurg* 72:123–126, 1990.
193. Gilbert BE, Beals JD, Natelson SE, et al: Treatment of cerebrospinal fluid leaks and gram-negative bacillary meningitis with large doses of intrathecal amikacin and systemic antibiotics. *Neurosurgery* 18:402–406, 1986.
194. McCracken GH Jr, Mize SG, Threlkeld N: Intraventricular gentamicin therapy in gram-negative bacillary meningitis of infancy: Report of the second neonatal meningitis cooperative study group. *Lancet* 1:787–791, 1990.
195. Rahal JJ, Hyams PJ, Simberkoff MS, et al: Combined intrathecal and intramuscular gentamicin for gram-negative meningitis. *N Engl J Med* 290:1394–1398, 1974.
196. Wong VK, Wright HT Jr, Ross LA, et al: Imipenem/cilastatin treatment of bacterial meningitis in children. *Pediatr Infect Dis J* 10:122–125, 1991.
197. Modai J, Vittecoq D, Decazes JM, et al: Penetration of imipenem and cilastatin into CSF of patients with bacterial meningitis. *J Antimicrob Chemother* 16:751–755, 1985.
198. Duma RJ, Berry AJ, Smith SM, et al: Penetration of aztreonam into CSF of patients with and without inflamed meninges. *Antimicrob Agents Chemother* 26:730–733, 1984.
199. Rahal JJ, Simberkoff MS: Bactericidal and bacteriostatic action of chloramphenicol against meningeal pathogens. *Antimicrob Agents Chemother* 16:13–18, 1979.

200. Levitz RE, Quintiliani R: Trimethoprim-sulfamethoxazole for bacterial meningitis. *Ann Intern Med* 100:881–890, 1984.
201. Svedhem A, Iwarson S: Cerebrospinal fluid concentrations of trimethoprim during oral and parenteral treatment. *J Antimicrob Chemother* 5:717–720, 1979.
202. Scheld WM: Quinolone therapy for infections of the central nervous system. *Rev Infect Dis* 11(suppl 5):S1194–S1202, 1989.
203. Segev S, Barzilai N, Rosen N, et al: Pefloxacin treatment of meningitis caused by gram-negative bacteria. *Arch Intern Med* 149:1314–1316, 1989.
204. Wolff M, Regnier B, Daldoss C, et al: Penetration of pefloxacin into cerebrospinal fluid of patients with meningitis. *Antimicrob Agents Chemother* 26:289–291, 1984.
205. Norrby SR: 4-Quinolones in the treatment of infections of the central nervous system. *Rev Infect Dis* 10(suppl):S253–S255, 1988.
206. Schonwald S, Beus I, Lisic M, et al: Ciprofloxacin in the treatment of gram-negative bacillary meningitis. *Am J Med* 87(suppl):248S–249S, 1989.
207. Wolff M, Boutron L, Singlas E, et al: Penetration of ciprofloxacin into CSF of patients with bacterial meningitis. *Antimicrob Agents Chemother* 31:899–902, 1987.
208. Wood WS, Kipnis GP: The concentration of tetracycline, chlortetracycline and oxytetracycline in the CSF after intravenous administration, in Welch H, Martí-Ibañez F (eds): *Antibiotics Annual 1953–1954. Proceedings of the Symposium on Antibiotics.* New York: Medical Encyclopedia, Inc., 1953: 98–101.
209. Yim CW, Flynn NM, Fitzgerald FT: Penetration of oral doxycycline into the CSF of patients with latent or neurosyphilis. *Antimicrob Agents Chemother* 28:347–348, 1985.
210. Hoffman HF, Forster D, Muirhead B: Metronidazole concentration of the CSF from slightly inflamed meninges. *Arsimittel-Forsch* 34:830–831, 1984.
211. D'Oliveira JS: CSF concentrations of rifampin in meningeal tuberculosis. *Am Rev Respir Dis* 106:432–437, 1972.
212. Sippel JE, Mikhail IA, Girgis NI, et al: Rifampin concentrations in cerebrospinal fluid of patients with tuberculous meningitis. *Am Rev Respir Dis* 109:579–580, 1974.
213. Atkinson AJ Jr., Bennett JE: Amphotericin B pharmacokinetics in humans. *Antimicrob Agents Chemother* 13:271–276, 1978.
214. Diamond RD, Bennett JE: A subcutaneous reservoir for intrathecal therapy of fungal meningitis. *N Engl J Med* 288:186–188, 1973.
215. Dismukes WE: Azole antifungal drugs: Old and new. *Ann Intern Med* 109:177–179, 1988.
216. Tucker RM, Williams PI, Arathoon EG, et al: Pharmacokinetics of fluconazole in cerebrospinal fluid and serum in human coccidioidal meningitis. *Antimicrob Agents Chemother* 32:369–373, 1988.

CHAPTER 49

ASSESSMENT OF OUTCOME FROM HEAD INJURY

H. Julia Hannay
Mark Sherer

INTRODUCTION

The importance of measuring the outcome after head injury cannot be denied.[1,2] Outcome is measured in order to determine the extent to which head injury constitutes a public health problem. Outcome must be evaluated to improve our basic knowledge of head injury and to provide professionals and family members with prognostic information that will aid them in decision-making at various stages in the recovery process. Outcome is measured in order to assess the efficacy of various interventions. With the advent of health care reform in the United States, it is likely that professionals treating the patient during the acute stages of head injury and the rehabilitative phase will be required to demonstrate the efficacy of their treatments not only in terms of a reduction of impairments but also in terms of a reduction of disabilities or handicaps and improved quality of life if the use of such treatments is to be approved and reimbursed. This chapter critically evaluates the measurement of outcome with emphasis on: defining outcome, measurement of impairment including neuropsychological, emotional, social, and behavioral impairment, measures of disability, measures of handicap, measures of global outcome, and other issues such as defining severity of injury, control groups for outcome research, and endpoints for outcome studies. The section on neuropsychological impairment not only critiques commonly used measures but addresses many issues including approaches to neuropsychological assessment, research vs. clinical batteries, criteria for impairment, threats to the validity of neuropsychological assessment, assessment in the intensive care unit, testing quadriplegic patients, and testing children. The assessment tools reviewed were selected on the basis of their frequent use in research and/or clinical assessment with head trauma survivors, adequacy of existing reliability and validity data, and/or promise as new measures pending demonstration of adequate reliability and validity. More extensive reviews of these and similar measures are available.[3–7]

DEFINING OUTCOME

A key issue in measurement of outcome following head injury is first to define outcome so that it can then be assessed objectively. If outcome refers to mortality rate, or the presence of neurological, physical, cognitive, or behavioral impairments, it is relatively easy to measure. In contrast, changes in performance at school, at work, in productivity, etc.—that is, in disabilities or handicaps or quality of life—are more difficult to define and thus to measure.

The International Classification of Impairments, Disabilities, and Handicaps (ICIDH)[8] offers an attractive model for conceptualizing measurement of outcome following head injury. An important contribution of the ICIDH is the notion that any illness may have an impact at four levels: pathology, impairment, disability, and handicap.[7] Pathology refers to damage or abnormal processes occurring in an organ or organ system within the body, such as bilateral temporal lobe contusions following a closed head injury. Impairment is a loss or abnormality of psychological, physiological, or anatomic structure or function and is thus a consequence of pathology—i.e., the pathology of bilateral temporal contusions might, among other memory deficits, result in a list-learning deficit. Impairments are determined by comparing performance of the patient against some normative standard. Impairments can have a negative effect on the patient's life, which represents a disability. Disability refers to any restriction or lack of ability to perform an activity within the range considered normal for a human being.[8] Disability is the effect of pathology or impairment on actions that have meaning to the person.[7] An impairment in list-learning from temporal lobe contusions might manifest itself as a disability in which the patient failed to recall and thus carry out a number of instructions in an everyday setting. Handicap is a disadvantage for an individual resulting from an impairment or disability that limits or prevents fulfillment of a role that is normal for that individual in his/her social context (depending on age, sex, social and cultural factors).[8] Handicap reflects the cultural, socioeconomic, and environmental consequences of impairment and disability.[7] Inability to recall and carry out verbally presented instructions is a disability that might result in a vocational handicap such as inability to hold a job.

Pathology, impairment, disability, and handicap are not directly linked. Poorly understood factors intervene between pathology and impairment so that apparently identical neuropathology may be manifested in different cognitive or behavioral impairments in different patients. Similarly, factors such as motivation and emotional state intervene between impairment and disability so that persons with similar degrees of cognitive impairment may have quite different degrees of disability. The relationship between disability and handicap is the most complicated, because factors outside the individual such as social support, environmental demands, and cultural expectations influence this relationship. Thus, acute findings of bilateral temporal lobe contusions will not always result in memory impairment, particularly in the postacute phase. Memory impairment as detected by a neuropsychological test requiring word list-learning may or may not be manifested in a disability for recall of verbal instructions. In turn, a disability to recall verbal instructions will not invariably result in vocational handicap, particularly if the employer is willing to provide written instructions.

An important implication of the ICIDH schema is that the focus of assessment should change with the passage of time.[7] Immediately following a closed head injury, pathology and impairment are of crucial importance. Appropriate assessments include neurological examinations and CT or MRI scans to detect intracranial pathology, and the Glasgow Coma Scale (GCS) to rate the degree of impaired consciousness. Once the patient is medically stable and responsive, the focus of assessment will shift to cognitive and behavioral impairments. These impairments are generally assessed with neuropsychological tests. Both early[9] and late[10] neuropsychological assessment can be useful in predicting later outcome and in guiding patient management. As the patient enters rehabilitation, disability and handicap become the key issues. With few exceptions, measures of disability and handicap are less well developed than measures of impairment. The Functional Independence Measure (FIM)[11] is a commonly used measure of disability, while the Craig Handicap Assessment and Reporting Technique (CHART)[12] is a recently developed measure of handicap that shows promise. Existing global outcome rating scales such as the Disability Rating Scale (DRS)[13] combine measures of impairment, disability, and handicap in an overall score, although not providing a detailed assessment of any of them.

Another issue is whether measurement of outcome should focus on a delineation of specific cognitive deficits or on the functional implications of these deficits in real world environments. An argument can be made for determining both deficits and functional implications. Certainly, it might be possible to show a significant reduction in an impairment, in say, memory, as the result of a pharmacological or physiological intervention or cognitive rehabilitation, but the intervention might or might not have a significant effect on the patient's everyday life and might or might not result in the patient being less disabled or handicapped. Yet researchers or clinicians could be asked to demonstrate a change in the level of disability or handicap to receive funding for a particular treatment because the effects of the impairments on the individual's life understandably could be considered to be more important than the impairments themselves. So why measure impairments at all? As mentioned earlier, impairment measures provide indices of outcome at early stages of recovery that are predictive of later outcome. Also, impairment measures will still need to be included to understand the reasons for various disabilities or handicaps since impairments resulting from damage to different areas and systems of the nervous system (which could have different pharmacological implications) can be the basis for the same disability or handicap in patients and may be amenable to different forms of rehabilitation.

MEASURES OF IMPAIRMENTS

Impairments or deficits following head injury can be classified as neurological, physical but non-neurological, neuropsychological, and emotional, psychosocial, and behavioral. Measurement of neurological and physical but non-neurological impairments is covered in detail in other chapters in this text. The discussion of impairment that follows here will thus focus on issues involved in neuropsychological assessment and the measurement of neuropsychological, emotional, psychosocial, and behavioral impairments.

Approaches to Neuropsychological Assessment

Neuropsychologists generally use a fixed or flexible battery approach to assessment.[14] The fixed battery approach refers to the administration of the same group of tests to all individuals. The most commonly used batteries are the Halstead-Reitan Neuropsychological Battery (HRNB)[15] and the Luria Nebraska Neuropsychological Battery (LNNB).[16] Data are collected on a normative group and on patients and these data are then used to develop guidelines for making diagnostic decisions. The obvious advantages to these batteries are the development of a common data base and their amenability to administration by a technician. Such fixed batteries, however, may provide insufficient coverage of some areas; for instance, the aphasia screening test of the HRNB does not provide a description of the nuances of aphasic disturbances. Additionally, these batteries preclude the replacement of individual tests based on patient requirements or new advances. Instead, these batteries are often supplemented with recently developed tests.[17,18]

The flexible battery approach involves a common core of tests given to all patients and additional groups of tests based on the type of disorder and the patient's particular set of symptoms. Less time is required for administration since there does not have to be extensive testing in areas of intact functioning. However, it does have the disadvantage in a clinical setting of involving the psychologist more in the testing, since a technician will not be able to make the decision about what tests over and above the core should be given to each patient to explore areas of impairment. Today, flexible rather than fixed batteries are used by most neuropsychologists[19,20] in clinical practice. Such an approach is also useful in research settings, including multicenter studies in which researchers can agree on a core battery but not on the entire battery because they study populations with different demographic characteristics, have different theoretical and test biases, or have different experimental questions to answer. In such cases, a core battery can be used across centers and supplemented to meet individual research questions.

Criteria for Impairment

Neuropsychologists differ in the criterion or operational definition for deciding if performance on a test or group of tests is impaired. For instance, Heaton, Grant, and Mathews[18] define an impairment (or deficit) as a score one standard deviation below the mean for one's age, gender, and educational level. This criterion reportedly results in a 15 percent false-positive rate, but, in their opinion, provides good sensitivity and specificity plus a balance between false-positives and false-negatives. Lezak[3] prefers to describe an impairment on individual tests as a statistically significant change in the performance of an individual from his/her premorbid level, whether based on actual previous performance or on an estimate, given the individual's age, gender, and education. A change of one to two standard deviations is described as suggestive of a deficit, while a two or more standard deviation change is considered significant. Both would agree, however, that differential diagnosis depends on the pattern of deficits and that impaired performance on one or two tests is not likely to be meaningful. If rates of impairment are reported for various groups in a study, those rates will vary with the criterion for impairment. If the outcome measure is rate of impairment, the impairment criterion employed should be clearly stated to facilitate both an understanding and comparison of test results. The alternative is to present the means and standard deviations for the performance of individuals in various groups, to include age, gender, and education and other demographic characteristics as covariates in the analysis of group differences, and to examine group differences in performance. This does not require the researcher to specify a criterion for impairment. But, while it tells us about group differences, it does not tell us whether these group differences are clinically significant.

Research vs. Clinical Batteries

Research batteries are usually designed to test specific hypotheses concerning head injury and not to provide broad information about intellectual, cognitive, psychosocial, and academic deficits and strengths that are required in order to answer clinical questions about an individual and to plan rehabilitation. While research batteries are sometimes not as extensive as clinical batteries, a common core data base is developed for all patients.

Examples of clinical batteries used in some well-known centers for neurobehavioral and neuropsychological research can be found in Jones' and Butters' work.[14] Most of the batteries include a large array of tests that can be used to assess intelligence; academic performance; auditory, visual and somatosensory perception; language, visuospatial and visuoconstructional ability; motor functions; attentional processes; concept formation; and personality.

Test batteries that have come out of meetings sponsored by the National Institutes of Health–National Institute of Neurological Disorders and Stroke (NIH-

TABLE 49-1 Outcome Measures Recommended for Clinical Trials with Moderately and Severely Head-Injured Patients

Impairment Measures	
Attention	Digit Symbol Substitution
	*Paced Auditory Serial Addition Test
Memory	Selective Reminding Test
	Rey-Osterreith Complex Figure Test
Language	Controlled Oral Word Association
Mental Processing	Trail Making B
	*Wisconsin Card Sorting
Motor	Grooved Pegboard
Behavior	Neurobehavioral Rating Scale
Disability Measures	Glasgow Coma Scale
	Disability Rating Scale

* Given to patients with moderate injuries only.

NINDS) are perhaps typical of smaller fixed batteries specifically designed for assessing head-injured populations. In this context, researchers developing various pharmacological and physiological interventions for head-injured patients have attempted to identify outcome measures that could be used in multicenter clinical trials or that would, in general, permit easier comparison of findings across centers. Clifton et al.[21] reported the results of a two-day conference held in Houston, TX, in 1991. A relatively short neuropsychological test battery was recommended to assess cognitive, motor, and behavioral impairments commonly associated with moderate and severe head injury. The battery was designed to take only 1.5 hours to administer so as to be portable and to maximize patient compliance and ease of follow-up while minimizing cost of administration (Table 49-1). In addition, traditional measures of global outcome, the Glasgow Outcome Scale (GOS)[22] and the Disability Rating Scale (DRS)[13] were recommended, since they have established validity for use with head-injured patients and adequate test-retest and inter-rater reliability. The battery is first given when the patient obtains a score ≥76 on the Galveston Orientation and Amnesia Test (GOAT)[23] on two consecutive days. At this point posttraumatic amnesia is considered to have ended and the patient is generally capable of participating in a neuropsychological examination. It was suggested that the battery be given to severely head-injured patients at baseline, 3, 6, and 12 months as well, and to moderately injured patients at baseline, 3, and 6 months.

Such a protocol, however, provides a barebones assessment which, while useful for clinical trials, may not provide an adequate description of the strengths and weaknesses of individual patients for clinical as well as research purposes. The protocol also does not deal with the fact that some patients are discharged from the hospital while still quite disoriented. To obtain outcome data on a reasonable number of severely head-injured patients while they are still in the hospital. Hannay et al.[24] developed a short battery for acute stage testing. Pilot work had demonstrated that patients with a GOAT of 30 to 40 could not be expected to complete any psychological tests. Patients who had reached a GOAT of 40 or greater could understand the instructions of at least some tests, so an acute battery was put together that included measures of language comprehension,[25] attention,[26] short-term memory, visual acuity, and tracking (Table 49-2). These researchers found that it was possible to give their acute battery to about twice as many severely head-injured patients as were able to complete a full neuropsychological test battery before discharge. This finding suggests that the development of a short battery for testing patients in an acute care setting has some potential. However, the usefulness of neuropsychological test data collected at this stage of recovery has yet to be demonstrated. Hannay et al.[24] also found that the number of days until a patient achieved a GOAT score ≥ 40 was significantly related to GOS score at discharge, 1, and 3 months postinjury as well as to the DRS score at discharge and at 1 month postinjury. The number of days to a GOAT score ≥ 76, the

TABLE 49-2 Percentage of Severely Head-Injured Patients Completing, Attempting, and Having Missing Data on an Acute Battery

Test	% Completing	% Attempting	% Missing Data
Complex Ideational Material	100	0	0
Auditory Number Search	87.5	8.3	4.2
Digit Span	87.5	0	12.5
Visual Screening	83.3	0	16.7
Visual Number Search	70.8	4.2	25
Trail Making A	50	20.8	29.2
Trail Making B	29.2	29.2	41.7

score commonly used to decide when patients are ready for extensive testing, was related only to discharge GOS and 1 month DRS scores, although this may be due to the fact that the sample size was much smaller for these correlations since fewer patients reached a GOAT score of 76. It is interesting to note that when patients achieve a GOAT score ≥ 40 a high percentage of them have recovered remote memory for personal information (name, date of birth, street address and city) and the year, but not knowledge for events surrounding their accident or other items of temporal orientation.[24] This suggests that reaching a GOAT score ≥ 40 may be clinically important.

A subcommittee appointed by the NIH-NINDS National Head Injury Centers recently considered these and other issues in the measurement of outcome.[27] The committee recommended that patients first be assessed with the GOAT on a daily basis once they reached a best motor score of 6 on the GCS. Levin[28] has criticized the GOAT for relying too heavily on verbal processing and verbal responding in determining the end of posttraumatic amnesia (PTA) and has suggested the inclusion of nonverbal items. Thus, it was also recommended that the GOAT be supplemented with the visual memory items from the Oxford/Westmead Scale[29,30] to help determine the end of PTA. If centers have difficulty keeping patients until a standard battery can be given and the patients are likely to be lost to follow-up, some testing during the acute stage of recovery at 1 month postinjury was recommended. The formal neuropsychological battery recommended by the committee was designed to be somewhat more extensive than the clinical trial batteries described by Clifton et al.[21] It provides a broader measurement of various types of impairments experienced by head-injured patients (Table 49-3) so as to provide information that might be useful to the clinician managing the patient as well as to the researcher. The DRS and GOS were again recommended as measures of global outcome. However, as discussed later in this chapter, it was recognized that the DRS and GOS provide only gross measures of disability, and primarily assess changes in motor functioning, not changes in life circumstances.[31] To remedy this, structured interviews with the patient and the family were included. These interviews provide information about preinjury factors such as psychosocial functioning, which can be used as covariates in any analysis of outcome data much as demographic factors, medical, and drug history are now. Also, the interviews provide information about changes in living arrangements, work, school, and psychosocial functioning. Additionally, a measure of handicap was included, the CHART.[12] Completing the test battery, the interview, and the handicap measure with the patient takes about 3.5 hours. Completing the interview and handicap measure with a family member takes about .75 hour. The interview with a family member concerning the patient's preinjury behavior and status is conducted shortly after the injury. The follow-up interviews and evaluation of disability and handicap would occur each time the patient was fully assessed neuropsychologically, that is, at 3, 6, 12, and 24 months, if possible. Longer follow-up would, of course, provide us with more information about the eventual consequences of head injury.[32,33]

Retention of patients in long-term studies of outcome is of major concern to researchers. The committee[27] also considered this, and recommended that a full-time neuropsychology technician be hired who has experi-

TABLE 49-3 Assessment Procedures Recommended by the Outcome Measures Subcommittee of the NIH-NINDS Head Injury Centers

A. Neuropsychological
  Orientation
  1. Galveston Orientation and Amnesia Test
  2. Oxford/Westmead Memory Items
  Attention
  1. 2 and 7 Test (with large numbers)
  2. Digit Symbol Modalities Test
  3. Paced Auditory Serial Addition Test
  4. Simple and Complex Reaction Time
  Memory
  1. Selective Reminding Test
  2. Rey-Osterreith Complex Figure Test (immediate and delayed memory)
  Language
  1. Token Test
  2. Visual Naming Test
  3. Controlled Oral Word Association
  Visual Perception, Visuospatial, and Visuoconstructive Ability
  1. Visual Form Discrimination Test
  2. Rey-Osterreith Complex Figure Test (copy)
  Mental Processing
  1. Trail Making Test B
  2. Wisconsin Card Sorting Test
  Motor
  1. Finger Tapping Test
  2. Grooved Pegboard
B. Behavioral/Psychosocial
  1. Neurobehavioral Rating Scale
  2. N.Y.U. Head Injury Family Interviews (HI-FI)—Follow-up Interviews with the Patient and Significant Other
C. Pre-Injury Status
  1. N.Y.U. Head Injury Family Interview (HI-FI)—Preinjury Patient Version
D. Disability and Handicap
  1. Disability Rating Scale
  2. Glasgow Outcome Scale
  3. Craig Handicap Assessment and Reporting Device

ence in working with families and who can be trained to do assessment as well. If necessary, the technician should also be bilingual. The role of such a technician and the procedures to be followed in dealing with the family and the patient are clearly defined in the report.

THREATS TO THE VALIDITY OF NEUROPSYCHOLOGICAL ASSESSMENT

Results of neuropsychological assessment must be valid if they are to be useful in characterizing a patient's current function and predicting extra test behaviors such as capacity for return to work. Several factors other than severity of acquired brain injury may affect performance on neuropsychological tests. Such factors include preexisting cognitive impairments, such as learning disability or mental retardation, premorbid or postmorbid substance use, effects of prescribed medications, psychiatric disturbance such as schizophrenia or depression, poor cooperation with testing procedures, and intentional exaggeration of impairments. This information can then be used either to aid the interpretation of clinical test results, to exclude subjects in research, or to form covariates for subsequent data analyses in research. The first three factors can generally be detected if a thorough history is obtained. The latter three factors may be more vexing.

While severe premorbid psychiatric disturbance may be revealed by a careful review of the patient's history, more subtle premorbid disturbance or psychiatric symptomatology that is reactive to the traumatic event that caused the head injury may be more difficult to assess. Some patients see themselves as dramatically changed by a traumatic event and, as a result, report numerous symptoms that they believe are due to the trauma. A common example is the reporting of normal forgetfulness as a significant memory impairment attributable to head trauma. This phenomenon of "symptom magnification" or "unintentional malingering" may be most common following mild head trauma. It may be contributed to by a mild premorbid psychiatric disturbance. Tests such as the Minnesota Multiphasic Personality Inventory-2 (MMPI-2)[34] may be useful in addressing this issue.

Poor cooperation with testing procedures may be manipulative or nonmanipulative. The former phenomenon is malingering. The latter may be seen in patients who have suffered true traumatic brain injury. Occasionally such patients fail to see the need for neuropsychological testing or find it threatening. In either case, patient awareness of the effects of the head trauma is the culprit. Patients who have anosognosia or unawareness of their deficits following head trauma may see no reason to submit to neuropsychological evaluation and thus are uncooperative. Other patients who have at least limited awareness of their deficits may actively resist neuropsychological evaluation as their poor performances confront them with deficits they would prefer to deny. These problems may be avoided if the neuropsychologist takes some time to develop rapport with the patient and to explain supportively the reasons for the evaluation. In some cases, it may be helpful to involve family members in securing the patient's cooperation.

The malingering patient intentionally performs poorly on neuropsychological assessment. Such dissimulation is motivated by desire for gain, such as a financial settlement in personal injury litigation. Detection of possible malingering is most difficult in mild closed head injury cases where objective findings may be absent. In a typical case, the neurological examination, CT, and MRI studies are normal and there is no reliable informant regarding possible loss of consciousness or post-traumatic amnesia. A number of recent studies[35–38] investigated special techniques for detecting malingering. Typically, in these techniques, the subject is confronted with a task that appears more difficult than it actually is and where random responding would result in 50 percent correct responses. Performance on these tests that is poorer than would be expected by chance or worse than those produced by patients with severe traumatic brain injury are suggestive of malingering. Malingering can also be detected by considering the performance of patients on the tests usually found in a neuropsychological examination. Clinicians look for atypical performance on individual tests or a pattern of performance overall that is not consistent with the injury,[17,39–44] although this effort does not appear to be entirely successful.[45–48] Some tests such as the MMPI-2[34] have validity scales built into them that can aid in detecting malingering.[49–52]

ASSESSMENT IN THE NEURO-INTENSIVE CARE UNIT (NICU)

Severely head-injured patients who achieve a best motor score of 6 on the GCS in the NICU may not be initially testable with the GOAT or any other measures of PTA for a variety of reasons. They may be too confused, agitated, aphasic, tracheostomized, or intubated. In these cases, PTA tasks given in a multiple choice format may be useful. For instance, there is a multiple choice GOAT that involves all the items but the ones assessing PTA and retrograde amnesia (RA); thus the total possible GOAT score is 80. There are no standardized rules for creating the multiple choice items for the GOAT, but they do have to be tailored to the particular patient. While formal neuropsychological testing can be carried out in the NICU, it is not without difficulty. Patients are easily distracted by the activities of personnel and the sounds of their own and others' monitors, and the data thus obtained are sometimes of questionable validity. The most valid test results are best achieved in a quiet room set aside for testing.

Testing Quadriplegic Patients

Patients who are quadriplegic cannot be given all the tests in a standard neuropsychological battery. They obviously cannot carry out tests that assess reaction time, motor speed, and coordination; they also have difficulty with cognitive tests requiring a manual motor response. These include but are not limited to such tests as the Rey-Osterreith Complex Figure Test of memory,[3] the Token Test[53] of auditory comprehension, the Trail Making Tests[15] of speed of visual search, the Symbol Digit Modalities Test[54] of visuomotor speed, and the Wisconsin Card Sorting Test[55,56] of concept formation. Some of these tests can be or have been modified for administration to such patients. For instance, the Symbol Digit Modalities Test has both written and oral versions. The Rey-Osterreith Complex Figure test cannot be so modified, and another test of immediate and long-term memory would have to be substituted that involves a yes-no or multiple choice response. The scores from substitute tests, while useful clinically, should not be used to replace the results of the original tests in a research data base, even if scores from the original and substitute tests are converted to a common unit such as standard deviations, since different cognitive processes are likely to be involved.

Testing Children

Injury to a child occurs in the context of the child's normal developmental process. The development of various motor and cognitive functions progresses at dissimilar rates in the normal child. Thus, outcome measures used to test an infant, young child, older child, and adolescent are likely to be different or to involve a modification of a basic procedure. For instance, to assess motor skills, the Bayley Scales of Infant Development Motor Scale[57] might be used with infants,[58] the McCarthy Scales of Children's Abilities Motor Scale[59] with young children,[58] and tests such as Finger Tapping[15] and the Grooved Pegboard[60] with older children and adolescents.

A head-injured child might not show deficits in performance on a test until that child reaches a stage at which other children normally exhibit a particular behavior and the head-injured child does not[61]. As a result, it is possible that the full range of deficits resulting from a head injury will not be known until the child reaches adolescence or later. This suggests that follow-up studies with children need to span many years. Finally, since different tests or modified tests are given at various ages, it is not possible to compare test scores directly. Some have transformed test scores to z-scores, using normative data and then have completed the analyses on the transformed scores. As mentioned earlier, this may not be an entirely satisfactory solution to the problem, since tests given to different age groups may involve different cognitive and/or motor processes and be normed on quite different populations. The reader is referred to several sources for a discussion of assessment of head-injured children[58,62,63] and to the NIH-NINDS sponsored workshop on Consequences of Traumatic Head Injury in Children: Variability in Short-Term and Long-Term Outcome.[64]

COMMONLY USED NEUROPSYCHOLOGICAL MEASURES FOR THE ASSESSMENT OF HEAD INJURY

The neuropsychological tests mentioned here have, for the most part, been the subject of extensive research. Thus, information concerning test administration, interpretation, reliability, and normative data can be found in general sources[3,4] and will not be reviewed here.

Measures of Posttraumatic Amnesia

Posttraumatic Amnesia (PTA) refers to the interval from the time of injury until an individual has continuous memory for ongoing events.[65,66] The duration of PTA provides a measure of severity of injury and is related to outcome.[67,68] Initially, the duration of PTA was estimated from retrospective accounts of recovered head-injured patients; perhaps not surprisingly, such estimates were not in agreement with the results of prospective testing of memory for ongoing events.[69] As a result, researchers[23,29,30,70] have developed measures of orientation and memory that define the resolution of PTA as improvement of the patient's score into the normal range (23).

The Galveston Orientation and Amnesia Test (GOAT)

The GOAT is widely used and consists of a series of questions about orientation for person, place, and time as well as questions that attempt to provide a rough estimate of retrograde amnesia (RA) and anterograde amnesia (AA).[23] Several criticisms of the GOAT have been made. Unfortunately, there is no way of verifying the answers to questions concerning the last event the patient recalls before the injury and the first event the patient can remember after the injury. This makes these questions difficult to score, correct answers being ones that seem plausible to the clinician. Also, a patient can score in the normal range without being able to answer these amnesia questions. Some patients still have anterograde amnesia for ongoing events even though they have a normal GOAT score.[69,70] The GOAT thus primarily assesses disorientation, not memory. It also consists only of verbal items, and even a transient impairment of receptive language could affect the score.[28] It could be supplemented with memory and verbal items. A multiple choice alternative format is used when there are expressive problems. GOAT scores with the regular format can range from −8 to 100, since 108 error points are possible. Normal orientation corresponds to a GOAT score ≥76, since this score was exceeded by 92 percent of the normative sample. The duration of PTA is related to the best motor and best verbal responses on the Glasgow Coma Scale (GCS)[71] on admission and to Glasgow Outcome Scale (GOS)[67] measures of long-term global outcome, thus validating its usefulness as a measure of injury severity and a predictor of outcome. Interobserver reliability is satisfactory.

The Children's Orientation and Amnesia Test (COAT)

The COAT has somewhat different questions of general orientation than the GOAT, but includes questions of orientation to person, place, and time as well as immediate and remote memory.[72] COAT scores proved to be related to verbal and nonverbal memory at baseline, 6, and 12 months postinjury, and were a better predictor of memory than GCS score at 6 and 12 months. Duration of PTA was related to GOS score. Interobserver reliability was .98. The COAT was normed on children in a school setting, but a recent study[73] renormed it on hospitalized children with non-neurological injuries.

The Oxford/Westmead Scale

Unlike the GOAT, the Oxford scale[29] and the Westmead variant of it[30] include a procedure for testing the patient's recall and recognition memory for pictures of objects and the examiner's name and face to determine when anterograde amnesia has actually ended, in addition to questions of orientation. PTA is judged to have ended on the first of three successive days of correct recall. While Shores[74] has published a short report on the ability of this measure of PTA to predict outcome, more research on the validity and reliability of these techniques is needed. Recently it has been found that the scale can be administered to children over the age of 7 and its use with head-injured children is being pursued.[75]

Test Batteries

The two most frequently used standardized test batteries are the Halstead-Reitan Neuropsychological Battery[15] and the Luria-Nebraska Neuropsychological Battery.[16]

The Halstead-Reitan Neuropsychological Battery (HRNB)

The HRNB, as it is used nowadays, consists of the Category Test, the Tactual Performance Test, the Seashore Rhythm Test, the Speech Sounds Perception Test, the Finger Tapping Test from the original Halstead battery along with the Aphasia Screening Test, the Sensory-Perceptual Examination, Grip Strength, Trail Making Test (A & B), the Wechsler Adult Intelligence Scale (WAIS), and the Minnesota Multiphasic Personality Inventory (MMPI) added by Reitan.[15] Excluding the WAIS and the MMPI, which together involve about 3 hours of the patient's time, this battery takes about 4 to 6 hours to administer. As discussed earlier, clinicians also supplement the HRNB with other tests,[5,17] such as memory tests, since the battery does not adequately cover all functional areas.[17] This is an extremely important addition since head-injured patients frequently have memory deficits. Not all the tests, such as the Rhythm Test and Speech Sounds Perception Test, may be useful in assessing head-injured patients or other patients.[76] Some of the tests are so useful that they are recommended for general clinical practice[3,4] or short research batteries.[21,74] More detailed information about the battery and the performance of the head-injured patient is provided by a variety of sources.[5,15,17,77,78,81]

Luria-Nebraska Neuropsychological Battery (LNNB)

The LNNB[16] represents an attempt to standardize psychometrically the procedures of Alexandr Luria's clinical examination. It is based on Luria's procedures as written down by Anne Lise-Christensen,[82] but should not be confused with her work in making Luria's theory of brain organization availabile to the clinician. The battery consists of 248 individual items (269 items if other scorings of 26 items are included) rather than subtests. The patient's response to each item is classified as normal (0), weak evidence of brain disorder (1), or strong evidence of brain disorder (2). From these responses, clinical scales, summary scales, localization scales, and factor scales are created. The clinical scales include motor function, rhythm, tactile functions, visual functions, receptive speech, expressive speech, writing, reading, arithmetic, intellectual processes, intermediate memory (only Form II), spelling (optional), and motor writing (optional). The summary scales include the pathognomonic, left-hemisphere, right-hemisphere, profile elevation, and impairment scales. There are eight localization scales. The 28 factor scales represent an attempt to divide the rather heterogeneous items in the clinical scales into more homogeneous sets of items. Administration time is usually 2.5 hours, but can take from 1.5 to 6 hours. The battery has been the subject of much criticism, including concerns that items in particular scales measure functions other than the one named by the scale, and therefore a patient's disorder might not be adequately or appropriately described.[83–87] Relatively few studies have used this battery to determine the deficits of head-injured patients.[88,89]

Language

Aphasia batteries are not usually administered to head-injured patients since aphasia is not a common sequela.[90–92] Rather, neuropsychologists test visual naming, word fluency, and auditory comprehension, which tend to be impaired with head injury[93–95] and possibly represent a subclinical aphasic disorder that may be evident during testing but not during conversational speech. Clinicians add an aphasia battery such as the Boston Diagnostic Aphasia Examination (BDAE),[25] the Multilingual Aphasia Examination (MAE),[96] or the Neurosensory Center Comprehensive Examination for Aphasia (NCCEA)[97] if a frank aphasic disorder is present. Representative subtests for auditory comprehension and verbal fluency from the MAE will be discussed here along with the Boston Naming Test of visual naming.

Token Test

This test measures auditory comprehension, which can be impaired with head injury.[93–95] It consists of a set of large and small circles and squares colored black, green, yellow, red, and white. The tokens are laid out in front of the patient in rows with the large circles at the top, then the large squares, followed by the small circles and then the small squares, all in a particular order by color. The patient is asked to manipulate the tokens with 22 oral commands.

Controlled Oral Word Association (COWA)

This test measures verbal fluency.[96] Over 60 seconds the patient must give as many words as possible that begin with a particular letter without giving proper nouns or just changing the suffix so that the word is essentially the same word. The letters C, F, and L are used. Reduced word fluency can be another consequence of head injury.[93–95,98,99]

Boston Naming Test

This test consists of 85 black-and-white drawings of items which are for the most part familiar.[100] The patient is shown a drawing (e.g., whistle). If unable to give the name, a stimulus cue is given (e.g., used for blowing). If still unable to give the name, a phonemic cue is given (e.g., wh). Shortened versions of the test have been developed.[101,102] Visual naming difficulties have been demonstrated on the Boston Naming Test.[98,103]

Attention

Attention is known to be a multidimensional concept.[104–108] Several types of attention have been distinguished by theorists, and perhaps the types most often mentioned are focused attention, sustained attention (vigilance), and divided attention and alertness (arousal). The tests used by most clinicians to assess attention have not been derived from theories of attention,[106] and researchers do not always agree as to which type of attention is measured by a particular test. Clinicians assessing the head-injured generally give tests measuring focused and divided attention, giving tests of sustained attention[109,110] or alertness[105] less often.

Digit span

This test is thought of as a measure of attention-concentration as well as immediate memory span.[111] In digits-forward a series of digits is read aloud and the patient simply repeats the series. In digits-backward a series of digits is read aloud and the patient must repeat them backwards. For both tasks, the length of the series is increased over trials. Reduced forward and backward digit span have been reported in many studies of the head-injured,[112] and some patients pass digits-forward while failing digits-backward.[113]

Digit cancellation 2s and 7s

A variety of cancellation tasks have been developed[3] to assess focused attention.[105] The 2s and 7s test requires subjects to cross out numerical targets (2 and 7) embedded in blocks of digits or letters, and poor performance is seen in severe head injuries.[9,108]

Symbol digit modalities test (SDMT)

This test is said to measure divided attention. The patient has to fill in a number below each of the geometric figures in a page of rows of geometric figures as quickly as possible, stopping at 90 sec. There are nine geometric figures, and the key linking the numbers 1–9 to the figures is given at the top of the page. The SDMT is given in a written and oral version. For the oral administration, the examiner fills in the answers given by the patient. Poor performance on the written version requires readministration with the oral version. This test has proved to be useful in assessing the effects of head injury and subsequent recovery.[104,115,116]

Paced auditory serial addition test (PASAT)

The PASAT[69,117,118] provides a measure of information processing speed and divided attention. One version[119] consists of a tape with four different sets of 50 numbers from 1 to 9 in random order. The subject is required to add the number heard now to the number immediately preceding it. This is a much more difficult task than just simply adding up the numbers when one hears them and keeping a running total. In fact, some subjects have difficulty understanding the task, even with practice trials, or revert to keeping a running total part way through. This task is thus not recommended for severely head-injured patients in the early stages of recovery. The rate at which the stimuli are presented increases over the four sets producing progressively shorter inter-digit intervals of 2.4s, 2.0s, 1.6s, and 1.2s, and thus increasing processing demands. A children's version has been developed.[120,121] PASAT tasks have proved to be sensitive to the effects of mild head injury[69,118,122] as well as to more severe head injuries.[104,109]

Learning and Memory

In earlier years the standard clinical device for memory assessment was the Wechsler Memory Scale (WMS),[123] which measured personal and current information, orientation for place and time, ability to repeat automatized sequences and to count by threes, digit span, immediate memory for short prose passages and geometric designs, and verbal paired associate learning. It did not provide measures of delayed memory, although Russell[124] added this feature. The Wechsler Memory Scale-Revised (WMS-R)[125] updated the stimuli in some of these subtests and added immediate memory for figural stimuli, visual paired associate learning, and visual digit span as well as providing more extensive norms. Despite this update, many clinicians do not give the whole battery but select tests from it to add to their memory battery, which often includes a list-learning test and a test of visual memory with a more complex stimulus. For this reason, only Logical Memory and Visual Reproduction from the WMS-R will be discussed along with list-learning tests, the Rey-Osterreith Complex Figure Test,[3,126,127] and the Continuous Recognition Memory Test.[128] It is important to assess recognition memory as well as recall, not only to help determine whether a deficit in recall is a consequence of storage or retrieval deficits but to obtain a measure of visual memory when patients have a motor impairment that interferes with the reproduction of figures required for the recall of visual stimuli.

The Selective Reminding Test (SRT),[131,132] the California Verbal Learning Test (CVLT),[133] and the Auditory Verbal Learning Test (AVLT)[3,134] have proved to be useful in assessing verbal learning and memory, and most neuropsychologists choose to include one of them in their battery. There are quite a few differences between the tasks, and these have been outlined by Lezak,[3] who uses the AVLT. The reader is referred to the test manual of the CVLT for information on reliability, validity, and norms[133] as well as to Lezak[3] and to research articles for its use with head-injured patients.[135,136] For similar information on the AVLT, the reader is referred to Lezak[3] and to several head-injury studies.[122,137,138] Children's versions of the AVLT,[139] the CVLT,[140] and the SRT[141,142] have been developed. Only the SRT will be discussed here.

Logical memory

This subtest of the WMS and WMS-R can measure immediate and delayed memory for two short prose passages. The patient attempts to recall each story as closely as possible after each has been read aloud. The patient is told to try to remember the stories and, after a 30-minute delay, is asked to recall them again. Impaired performance is often noted with head injury.[9,108,125,130]

Selective reminding test (SRT)

A list of words is read aloud to the subject who attempts to recall them in any order. Then the subject is reminded only of the words not recalled, and is then asked again to recall the entire list. This selective reminding procedure[131,132] is followed until the entire list is learned to some criterion or until a specified number of trials is reached. There are several versions of the test.[3,4] One commonly used with adolescents and adults[143,144] consists of 12 unrelated words presented for 12 trials or until the subject correctly recalls the list on two or three consecutive trials. This is followed by cued recall and multiple choice recognition trials and a 30-minute delayed recall trial. SRT procedures have been used widely with head-injured patients,[145–149] and performance is related to severity of injury[148] and to outcome.[149]

Visual reproduction I and II

These subtests of the WMS-R measure immediate and delayed recall of four visual designs of varying complexity. Each design is displayed for 10 seconds; immediately after its removal, the patient draws it from memory. The patient is asked to try to remember the designs and, after a 30-minute delay is asked to draw them again. Head injury can cause reduced immediate and delayed memory.[81,149]

Rey-Osterreith complex figure test

This test[126,127] was developed to assess visuoconstructive ability and visual memory. A complex black-and-white drawing of a geometric figure is placed in front of the patient, who is asked to copy it. Then the figure and the copy are removed. The patient is not told to remember the figure but later is required to reproduce it without warning. Many clinicians give both immediate and delayed recall trials; some give only a delayed recall trial.[3,4] Head injury can cause deficits in performance.[122,137,150,151]

Continuous recognition memory test (CRM)

Several visual recognition memory tests[3] that have quite different stimulus characteristics have been used to assess head-injured patients. The Continuous Recognition Memory Test[128,152] consists of 120 line drawings of familiar things (e.g., fish, flowers, birds). Eight of the drawings in the first block of trials appear once again in each succeeding block of trials along with drawings that are similar to them. Each drawing is presented for a brief time, and the patient calls each drawing either "new" (appearing for the first time) or "old" (reappearing in the deck). This test was specifically designed to assess memory deficits in head-injured patients, to not require a motor response, and to be sensitive to the severity of diffuse damage rather than to the presence of a lateralized mass lesion. In these respects, the test has been rather successful.[128,152–154]

Motor Skills

Neuropsychologists often measure several types of motor function—for instance, fine motor speed, fine motor coordination, and grip strength.

Finger tapping

This test is also known as the Finger Oscillation Test and measures fine motor speed.[15] It requires the patient to tap a key as rapidly as possible for 10 seconds for five consecutive trials, first with the index finger of the preferred hand and then with the nonpreferred hand—although more trials may have to be administered to get five consecutive trials within five taps of each other with each hand. This test is sensitive to the effects of head injury.[81,155,156]

Grooved pegboard

This test of fine motor coordination consists of a board of five rows of five slotted holes with the slots angled in different directions.[157] The patient picks up one peg at a time and puts it in the holes by row as quickly as possible, rotating it in his/her fingers so that its ridge will match up with and fit into the slot in the hole. The task is completed first with the preferred hand and then with the nonpreferred hand, and the time taken to complete the task is recorded. Performance can be affected by head injury.[151]

Grip strength

Grip strength is measured on two trials with the preferred and nonpreferred hands, using a hand dynamometer.[15] The device is adjusted to fit the size of the patient's hand, held at the patient's side, and squeezed as hard as possible. Reduced grip strength has been noted with head injury.[155]

Mental Flexibility and Concept Formation

The Wisconsin Card Sorting Test[55,56] and the Category Test[15] are frequently used to assess abstraction ability, but they cannot be substituted for each other. While both involve response-contingent feedback, the principles to be derived are more difficult in the Category Test. Also, on the WCST the patient is required to shift principles without warning, and the WCST provides measures of mental flexibility or ability to shift set (in the form of perseverations).[4] The tests share little common variance.[3] The Trail Making Tests also provide measures of mental flexibility.

Wisconsin card sorting test (WCST)

This test measures concept formation, but also the ability to switch set (as measured by perseverations) and to maintain set.[58,59,158] Four key cards are placed in front of the patient. The key cards consist of one red triangle, two green stars, three yellow crosses, and four blue circles. Patients are given two decks of 64 different cards, which contain one, two, three, or four triangles, stars, crosses, or circles printed in red, green, yellow, or blue. The patient must take a card off the top of the deck, one at a time, and place it under one of the key cards so that it matches. The examiner does not give any information about how to match the cards but tells the patient whether the match is right or wrong; the patient uses that information to decide what to do next. The patient must sort according to color, form, and then number—and then repeat this. This test has been used to assess head-injured patients.[156,159]

Category test

This test, taken from the HRNB,[15] is generally thought of as a test of concept formation, and is more difficult than the Wisconsin Card Sorting Test. Patients can take a very long time to complete it, even an hour or two. The original adult version consists of 208 items presented as slides and divided into seven subtests that involve various principles. The patient looks at the figure(s) on the page and decides what number (1–4) is suggested. The patient must figure out what principle is involved, using feedback provided after making a response on each trial. There are shortened forms,[3] intermediate, and children's forms of the test as well as a booklet form.[160,161] Head-injured patients can have difficulty figuring out the concepts involved.[81,122,163]

Trails making A & B

For Part A of this test, the patient draws lines sequentially, joining the 25 numbered circles placed all over a sheet. This test measures speed of visual search. For Part B of this test, the patient draws lines on a piece of paper so as to join numbered and lettered circles in order while alternating between the numbers from 1 to 13 and the letters from A to L. This test[15] measures speed of visual search but also ability to switch set. Difficulties on both tasks have been noted with head injury.[81,151,163,164]

Personality

A variety of personality tests are available, but the Minnesota Multiphasic Personality Inventory-2 (MMPI-2)[34] continues to be used widely by clinicians, in part because of the need for a test with built-in validity scales for forensic work.

Minnesota multiphasic personality inventory-2 (MMPI-2)

This test is a revision of the most highly used personality test, the MMPI.[165] It is a self-report personality inventory. It consists of 567 true-false items. It takes about 1 to 1.5 hours to complete if the patient has no cognitive difficulties. While it has proved very useful clinically, it is probably not an appropriate assessment device for many head-injured patients. It requires reading comprehension possibly as high as a 9th grade level[49,66] and is only appropriate for individuals 18 years of age and older, although there is an adolescent version. There are four validity scales, ?, L, F, and K, which have been useful in detecting malingering as well as in assessing defensiveness.[167,168] There are 10 clinical scales—Hypochondriasis (Hs), Depression (D), Hysteria (Hy), Psychopathic-Deviate (Pd), Masculinity-Femininity (Mf), Paranoia (Pa), Psychasthenia (Pt), Schizophrenia (Sc), Hypomania (Ma), and Social Introversion (Si), and many supplementary scales. The pattern of scores on the 10 clinical scales is interpreted by comparing it to the patterns of normals and various diagnostic groups of psychiatric patients. Among brain-injured patients, relatively high mean scores can be expected on scales Hs, D, Hy, Pt, and Sc,[3,169,170] but the usual interpretation of elevations of such scales has been questioned[169–172] because some of the items are descriptive of neurological dysfunction. MMPI short forms have not been recommended for use with head-injured patients.[173]

Emotional, Social and Behavioral Impairment

Measures of emotional, social, and behavioral impairment are the General Health Questionnaire, the Katz Adjustment Scale–Relative form, the Neurobehavioral Rating Scale, and the Portland Adaptability Index. These measures address the behavioral effects of traumatic brain injury that play a critical role in determining the degrees of social and occupational handicap.

General health questionnaire

The General Health Questionnaire (GHQ)[174] has been used in a number of studies to assess psychological distress in the relatives of head injury survivors. Such studies have generally found that head injury frequently results in significant psychological distress for the family members of the head-injured person.[175] This finding is important because the degree of family support after head injury is a significant mediating factor between disability and handicap. For example, an individual who is unable to drive and has no mass transit available may not suffer a vocational handicap if family members provide transportation to and from work. Psychological distress may be a determinant of family members' ability to provide ongoing support. While a number of measures have been used to assess family response to head injury,[175] the GHQ is the best validated.

The GHQ was developed by Goldberg[174] to assess inability to carry out one's normal healthy functions and the appearance of new phenomena of a distressing nature.[176] The scale consists of 60 items that fall into four categories of psychological distress: depression, anxiety, social impairment, and hypochondriasis. The respondent rates his difficulty over the past few weeks with each item on a four-point scale, generally ranging from "no difficulty" to "much more than usual." Sample items include "lost much sleep over worry" and "felt constantly under strain." The scale is of British origin, but several items have been reworded for American use.

The GHQ appears to be a reliable[177,178] and valid scale[179] which also may be appropriate for use with mild traumatic brain survivors who have persistent symptoms. For such patients, subjective psychological distress is frequently a major component of their complaints. As a self-report measure, the GHQ will frequently be inappropriate for severe head injury survivors owing to the cognitive demands of completing the scale[7] and possible problems with impaired self-awareness.

Katz Adjustment Scale–Relatives Form

The Katz Adjustment Scale–Relatives Form (KAS-R)[180] is part of a set of inventories developed for assessing adjustment and social behavior in psychiatric patients. Some of these inventories (Patient form) are completed by the patient; others (Relatives form) are completed by a relative of the patient. Only the latter scales have been used with head trauma survivors. In a study of closed head injury patients, Klonoff, Costa, and Snow[183] found that various KAS-R scores are predicted by initial severity of brain injury, presence of frontal lobe lesions, seizure disorder, and motor performance on neuropsychological tests. Other studies with head trauma survivors have shown that KAS-R scores are predictive of return to work,[9,184] social isolation,[185] and marital adjustment.[186]

While originally developed for use with another patient population, the KAS-R has been shown to be useful in research and clinical assessment with head-injured patients. Additional study of the scale's reliability,[180] validity,[180,182] and factor structure[180] is needed. An advantage of the KAS-R is that it is completed by a relative rather than by the patient and thus may be used with more severely impaired survivors.

Neurobehavioral Rating Scale

The Neurobehavioral Rating Scale (NRS)[187] was developed to assess the behavioral manifestations of traumatic brain injury. The scale includes items from the Brief Psychiatric Rating Scale[188] and additional items to assess neurobehavioral disturbances commonly seen with head-injured patients. The NRS consists of 27 items that are clinician-rated on a seven-point scale ranging from "not present" to "extremely severe." Sample items include "memory deficit," "inaccurate insight and self-appraisal," and "depressed mood." Items are to be rated based on the subject's responses in a structured interview.

Reliability and validity studies[187,189] of the NRS have generally produced positive findings. Levin et al.[187] found interrater correlations ranging from .88 to .90 with 89.9 to 96.1 percent agreement on degree of behavioral disturbance. In their factor analysis of the NRS with 101 mild, moderate, and severe closed head injury patients, Levin et al.[187] found four factors: cognition/energy, metacognition, somatic concern/anxiety, and language. Levine, Van Horn, and Curtis[190] factor-analyzed the NRS with a sample of 40 moderate closed head injury patients and obtained a three-factor solution that differs significantly from Levin et al.'s results. Perhaps this apparent discrepancy is the result of inadequate sample size for factor analysis of 27 items in both studies. Levin et al.[187] had fewer than four subjects per item, while Levine et al.[190] had fewer than two subjects per item. Validity of the NRS is supported by Levin et al.'s findings that NRS scores are modestly correlated with initial severity of brain injury and that the NRS is sensitive to behavioral recovery in head trauma patients. Levin et al.[187] also found tentative evidence that the NRS is sensitive to differential behavioral impairments in patients with predominantly frontal as opposed to predominantly nonfrontal lesions. It is also useful with patients having dementia[141] and HIV infection.[192]

Portland Adaptability Index

The Portland Adaptability Index (PAI)[193] was developed to assess social, personality, and emotional dysfunction following traumatic brain injury. Rehabilitation professionals generally agree that social, emotional, and behavior impairments are more predictive of level of handicap than are cognitive and physical impairments. The PAI consists of 24 items divided into three categories: temperament and emotionality, activities and social behavior, and physical capabilities. Each item is rated by the clinician on a four-point scale ranging from "no impairment" to "severe impairment." Lower scores indicate less impairment. Ratings are based on interviews with the patient, clinician observations, and reports from third parties such as family members or medical personnel. Temperament and emotionality items assess such issues as irritability, anxiety, and depression. Activities and social behavior items assess significant relationships, type of residence, work or school activities, leisure activities, and other issues. Physical capacity items assess such issues as ambulation, vision, and aphasia.

Several studies of the PAI have been conducted in recent years. Lezak[193] reported PAI results for 42 head trauma survivors over a five-year period, but failed to report interrater reliability or test-retest reliability data. Her findings do provide preliminary evidence of validity of the PAI as a measure of social and behavioral problems. The PAI does appear to have high internal consistency[194] and Malec and Thompson[195] provide data on the concurrent validity of the PAI whose scores are significantly related to DRS[13] ratings. Malec, Smigielski, and DePompolo[196] found that PAI scores rated at entry to a postacute brain injury program were predictive of vocational outcome at graduation. However, PAI scores were not predictive of likelihood that patients would drop out of the program. The relationship of PAI scale scores to vocational/academic scores has been reported elsewhere.[197]

MEASURES OF DISABILITY

Measures of disability are the Functional Independence Measure, the Functional Assessment Measure, and the Sickness Impact Profile. These scales assess the degree of disability to perform routine daily tasks.

Functional Independence Measure

The Functional Independence Measure (FIM)[198] was developed as a measure of personal disability. It is intended for use in clinical assessment, outcome research, and program evaluation. The FIM was developed for use with all disability groups and it is part of the Uniform Data System for Medical Rehabilitation. It has been used in studies of head trauma and is included in the data set for the Traumatic Brain Injury Model System projects. The FIM consists of 18 items, 13 measuring motor functions and 5 measuring cognitive functions. Areas of motor functioning assessed are feeding, grooming, bathing, dressing (2 items), toileting, bladder management, bowel management, transfers (3 items), and locomotion (2 items). Areas of cognitive functioning assessed are communication (2 items), social interaction, problem solving, and memory. Scores are clinician ratings for each item on a seven-point scale ranging from complete dependence to complete independence (Table 49-4).

Studies of the FIM have found excellent interrater reliability with an interrater correlation of .97 for total FIM score[199] and interrater agreement on level of dis-

TABLE 49-4 Functional Independence Measure (FIM)

	Levels	
	No Helper	
LEVELS	7 Complete Independence (Timely, Safely) 6 Modified Independence (Device)	NO HELPER
	Helper	
	Modified Dependence 5 Supervision 4 Minimal Assist (Subject = 75%+) 3 Moderate Assist (Subject = 50%+) Complete Dependence 2 Maximal Assist (Subject = 25%+) 1 Total Assist (Subject = 0%+)	HELPER

Self Care	
A. Eating	☐
B. Grooming	☐
C. Bathing	☐
D. Dressing-Upper Body	☐
E. Dressing-Lower Body	☐
F. Toileting	☐
Sphincter Control	
G. Bladder Management	☐
H. Bowel Management	☐
Mobility	
Transfer:	
I. Bed, Chair, Wheelchair	☐
J. Toilet	☐
K. Tub, Shower	☐
Locomotion	
L. Walk/wheel Chair	w☐ c☐ ☐
M. Stairs	☐
Communication	
N. Comprehension	a☐ v☐ ☐
O. Expression	v☐ n☐ ☐
Social Cognition	
P. Social Interaction	☐
Q. Problem Solving	☐
R. Memory	☐
Total FIM	☐

NOTE: Leave no blanks; enter 1 if patient not testable due to risk.

ability of 88 percent.[200] Internal consistency is also excellent, with a Cronbach alpha of .95.[201] Validity studies of the FIM have also produced positive findings. Whitlock[202] found total FIM score at discharge to be correlated .51 with admission GCS score, although Hall et al.[200] found weaker relationships between FIM scores and measures of initial severity of injury. The FIM also correlated .50 with Levels of Cognitive Functioning Scale score and .84 with GOS category. Hall et al.[200] found that FIM motor total correlated .653 with the DRS while FIM cognitive total correlated .704 with the DRS. FIM scores have been found to be predictive of need for care in MS patients[203] and stroke patients.[204] The FIM has been found to be sensitive to functional gains made during rehabilitation.[201]

The FIM is a reliable and valid measure of disability that is easily obtained by clinician ratings. It is most useful for assessment of progress during inpatient rehabilitation because it may be insensitive to significant functional gains in the later stages of recovery. The DRS appears to be a better choice when following patients long-term,[200] and the Sickness Impact Profile is more predictive of general life satisfaction.[204] Additional investigation of the relationship of FIM ratings to eventual community functioning is needed.

Functional Assessment Measure

The Functional Assessment Measure (FAM)[200] is a set of items to be added to the FIM to improve assessment of deficits in cognition, psychosocial adjustment, and communication following brain injury.[205] While both FIM and FAM items assess disability, as opposed to handicap, some FAM items appear more closely related to community functioning (e.g., car transfers, employability, community mobility). The FAM consists of 12 items (3 motor and 9 cognitive) to be added to the 18 FIM items (13 motor and 5 cognitive). FAM items are clinician-rated on a seven-point scale, ranging from completely dependent to just like the FIM items.

Preliminary investigation of the FAM has found interrater agreement to be only 67 percent as compared to 88 percent for the FIM.[200] However, the authors note that raters did not receive specific training in rating of FAM items. The only published validity study of the FAM[200] did not evaluate FAM validity separately from the combined FIM + FAM. FIM + FAM scores were correlated with measures of severity of brain injury and outcome such as initial GCS, length of coma, length of PTA, DRS, and LCFS rating. However, these correlations do not appear to differ from those for FIM scores alone. Indeed, FIM motor total correlated .992 with FIM + FAM motor total while FIM cognitive total correlated .952 with FIM + FAM cognitive total.

Sickness Impact Profile

The Sickness Impact Profile (SIP)[206] was developed as a measure of the behavioral impact of sickness. The SIP is a well-researched scale that has been used with a variety of clinical populations, including traumatic brain injury survivors. The SIP consists of 136 statements in 12 categories. The 12 categories are sleep and rest, eating, work, home management, recreation and pastimes, ambulation, mobility, body care and movement, social interaction, alertness behavior, emotional behavior, and communication. The SIP can be administered by an interviewer or self-administered. Respondents simply indicate whether each item pertains to them. Each item has been assigned a weight based on judges' ratings. Scores for each category are obtained by summing the weights of all items and multiplying by 100. A SIP total score may also be calculated.

Studies of the SIP have found excellent reliability. Test-retest reliability correlations have been reported as .97 for the interview administered SIP and .87 for the self-administered version.[206] Internal consistency (as measured by Cronbach's coefficient alpha) has been reported to be .93 to .96.[207] Validity studies have also been very positive. Granger et al.[203] found the SIP to be predictive of patients' need for care and self-report of life satisfaction in stroke survivors. Stambrook et al.[184] found the SIP to be predictive of employment status in head injury survivors. Temkin et al.[207] found relationships between the SIP and measures of severity of traumatic brain injury (GCS score and time to follow commands). Furthermore, the SIP discriminated brain injury survivors from a control group with 91 percent accuracy at 1 month postinjury and 78 percent accuracy at 1 year postinjury.

MEASURES OF HANDICAP

Two new measures of handicap, the Craig Handicap Assessment and Reporting Technique and the Community Integration Questionnaire, are available. These scales represent the best attempts to quantify the WHO concept of handicap. Measures of handicap, along with assessment of emotional functioning, address the ill-defined notion of "quality of life."

Craig Handicap Assessment and Reporting Technique

The Craig Handicap Assessment and Reporting Technique (CHART)[12] was designed to quantify extent of handicap. The CHART assesses five of the six dimensions of handicap described by WHO.[8] These six dimensions are: (1) orientation—the individual's ability to orient himself in relation to his surroundings; (2) physical independence—the individuals' ability to sustain a customarily effective independent existence; (3) mobility—the individual's ability to move about effectively in surroundings; (4) occupation—the individual's ability to occupy time in the manner customary to his age, sex, and culture; (5) social integration—the individual's ability to participate in and maintain customary social relationships; and (6) economic self-efficiency—the individual's ability to sustain customary socioeconomic activity and independence. The CHART does not assess orientation because the authors believed that orientation is difficult to measure objectively and is integral to other dimensions such as mobility and occupation.[12]

The CHART assesses each dimension based on reports of how the individual actually functions from day to day. For example, employment is assessed by asking how many hours the respondent works per week rather than by a clinician's rating of *capacity* to work, as with the Glasgow Outcome Scale (GOS).[208] The CHART consists of 27 questions. Each of the CHART dimensions is scored from "0" to "100," with 100 representing no handicap as compared to a normative sample of the able-bodied individuals. A total CHART score may also be calculated by summing scores on the five dimensions.

The CHART was originally developed for use with spinal cord-injured individuals, but it has also been used with head trauma survivors. In a study of spinal cord-injured persons, Whiteneck et al.[12] found test-retest reliability to be excellent with a correlation of .93 for total CHART score at a 1-week interval. CHART scores based on patient responses were highly correlated with scores based on responses from a family member or significant other with the exception of the social integration dimension. In a study of moderate and severe head injury survivors, Boake and High[209] found that average score on the five CHART dimensions correlated .71 with GOS ratings and −.69 with DRS ratings. CHART dimensions were appropriately predictive of behavioral indicators of walking, transportation, productivity, and relationships. Furthermore, the CHART was more predictive of levels of disability than the GOS.

Community Integration Questionnaire

The Community Integration Questionnaire (CIQ)[210] is a measure of community integration that was specifically developed for use with traumatic brain injury survivors. The authors consider community integration to be the converse of the WHO concept of handicap. Thus, the CIQ may be considered to be a measure of handicap similar to the CHART. The CIQ consists of 15 questions that assess home integration, social integration, and productive activities. Questions for each dimension were developed by panels of rehabilitation professionals, researchers, and consumers. The three-dimensional structure of the CIQ was confirmed by factor analysis.[210] CIQ items are similar to CHART items in that the respondent reports actual behaviors rather than presumed capacities. The CIQ produces a score for each of the three dimensions and a total score.

In their study of the CIQ with brain injury survivors, Willer et al.[210] found somewhat marginal internal consistency for the CIQ, with a coefficient alpha of .76. The test-retest correlations for a 10-day interval was .91 for survivor responses and .97 for family member responses for a sample of 16. In the same sample, total CIQ scores based on survivor responses or on family member report were significantly correlated with total CHART score with correlations of .62 and .70, respectively. In a larger sample of 94 survivors, the correlation between total CIQ based on survivor responses and total CIQ based on family member responses was .89. Scores on all three CIQ dimensions differed between a nondisabled sample and groups of brain injury survivors.

As with the CHART, studies of reliability and validity of the CIQ are at an early stage. The authors of the CIQ suggest that the CHART is better suited for use with spinal cord injury survivors while the CIQ is more appropriate for brain injury survivors.

MEASUREMENT OF GLOBAL OUTCOME

Available measures of global outcome are the Glasgow Outcome Scale, the Disability Rating Scale, and the Levels of Cognitive Functioning Scale. With these measures, patients are placed in a functional category based on a mixture of impairment, disability, and handicap issues.

Glasgow Outcome Scale

The Glasgow Outcome Scale (GOS)[22] is the most widely used global outcome measure in studies of traumatic brain injury. The GOS classifies patients in five categories: death, persistent vegetative state, severe disability (conscious but disabled), moderate disability (disabled but independent), or good recovery. A detailed description of the basis for categorizing patients is provided by Jennett.[211] This description indicates that categories are based on a mixture of impairment, disability, and handicap. Ratings typically are obtained on patients at 3, 6, and 12 months postinjury.

Studies of the GOS have found better than 95 percent interrater agreement.[208] Studies have not addressed test-retest reliability, but this can be inferred to be excellent from the finding that less than 10 percent of patients change category between 6-month and 12-month ratings.[208] Validity of the GOS as a measure of brain injury outcome is supported by its strong correlations with length of coma, initial severity of injury (as measured by the Glasgow Coma Scale), and type of intracranial lesion.[212] GOS category is also correlated with length of posttraumatic amnesia.[208] Evidence of concurrent validity of the GOS is provided by its significant correlations with other outcome measures such as the Disability Rating Scale[213] and the Functional Independence Measure.[202]

The primary criticism of the GOS is its relative insensitivity to clinically significant improvements in patient condition, particularly after 6 months postinjury.[213] Furthermore, the GOS is inconsistent with current concepts of handicap in that the patient is rated on what she/he *could* do rather than on what she/he is actually doing. For example, patients are rated as having "good recovery" if they are judged to have the "capacity" to work, even if they are not working.[208] The strengths of the GOS are that it can be quickly and reliably rated and has been demonstrated to be related to various measures of initial severity of brain injury. The scale is well suited to large studies of general factors contributing to brain injury outcome, but it is inappropriate for ongoing clinical assessment of progress for the individual patient.

Disability Rating Scale

The Disability Rating Scale (DRS)[13] was developed for the purpose of assessing disability in severe head trauma patients from coma through return to the community. The authors sought to create a global outcome measure that would be more sensitive to changes in function than the Glasgow Outcome Scale (GOS). The DRS has been used in many studies of head trauma outcome.

The DRS assesses level of arousal and responsivity, cognitive ability to perform self-care activities, dependence on others, and psychosocial adaptability. Scores range from "0" to "30," with lower scores representing less disability. Based on the numerical score, patients are assigned to one of ten disability categories ranging from no disability to death. No explanation is given for the establishment of numerical cut-offs for the disability categories. Level of arousal and responsivity are measured by the Glasgow Coma Scale (GCS)[71] with scoring reversed so that lower scores indicate less impairment. Cognitive ability for self-care activities is rated by a clinician for each of feeding, toileting, and grooming on a four-point scale ranging from "complete ability" to "no ability." Dependence on others is rated on a six-point scale ranging from completely "independent" to "totally dependent." Psychosocial adaptability is rated on a four-point scale ranging from "not restricted" to "not employable." While descriptors for this scale relate to employability, the authors indicate that ability to carry out home responsibilities or responsibilities as a student should be rated on the same scale.

Studies of the DRS have found interrater correlations of .97 to .98[13,214]; however, the issue of interrater agreement on disability category assigned has not been addressed. Test-retest reliability is reported to be excellent with a correlation of .92.[214] Validity of the DRS is supported by significant correlations with electrophysiological measures of brain function,[13] the GOS,[214] and employment status at follow-up.[215]

As with other global outcome measures, the DRS may fail to detect differential improvement in different functional areas. The DRS has been criticized for mixing assessment of impairment and disability[7] and for being insensitive to change as patients approach normal levels of function.[205] Strengths of the DRS are that it is quickly and reliably rated and it has been shown to be more sensitive to patient change, particularly past 6 months postinjury, than the GOS.[213]

Levels of Cognitive Functioning Scale

The Levels of Cognitive Functioning Scale (LCFS) or Rancho Scale[216] was developed to categorize general cognitive or language sequelae of traumatic brain injury. With this scale, clinicians rate patients as being at one of eight cognitive levels: no response; generalized response; localized response; confused-agitated; confused, inappropriate, nonagitated; confused-appropriate; automatic-appropriate; or purposeful and appropriate based on their predominant behaviors[217] (Table 49-5). Ratings are based primarily on impairments and to some extent on disability. The LCFS has been used in outcome studies of head trauma, but it probably is most commonly used for treatment planning and tracking patient recovery.[214] Hagen[217] recommended that the LCFS be used to determine when more lengthy assessments should be administered.

Gouvier et al.[214] found interrater correlations of .87 to .94 for the LCFS, but failed to report the percentage of patients classified at the same cognitive level by different raters. Findings regarding validity of the LCFS are mixed. LCFS scores at admission to rehabilitation were not significantly correlated with measures of severity of brain injury such as length of coma or initial GCS.[218] The LCFS is significantly correlated with other measures of outcome such as the Functional Independence Measure

TABLE 49-5 Ranchos Los Amigos Scale

Level I	No response to stimuli. Appears in deep sleep.
Level II	Generalized response. First reaction may be to deep pain. Has delayed, inconsistent responses.
Level III	Localized response. Inconsistent responses but reacts in more specific manner to stimulus. Might follow simple command "squeeze my hand."
Level IV	Confused, agitated. Reacts to own inner confusion, fear, disorientation. Excitable behavior, may be abusive.
Level V	Non-agitated, confused, inappropriate. Usually disoriented. Follows tasks for 2 to 3 minutes, but easily distracted by environment, frustrated.
Level VI	Confused, appropriate. Follows simple directions consistently. Memory and attention increasing. Self-care tasks performed without help.
Level VII	Automatic, appropriate. If physically able, can carry out routine activities. Appears normal. Needs supervision for safety.
Level VIII	Purposeful, alert, oriented. May have decreased abilities relative to premorbid state.

(FIM)[202] and eventual return to work.[219] Gouvier et al.[214] found that LCFS ratings at admission for rehabilitation correlated .57 with GOS ratings at discharge.

The LCFS has been criticized for being insensitive to subtle changes in patient condition and for the fact that patients may exhibit many behaviors associated with different cognitive levels at the same time.[220] Nonetheless, Timmons et al.[221] found the LCFS to be more sensitive to functional improvements than the GOS. While the LCFS may have adequate reliability and validity, other scales, such as the DRS, are better choices for use in outcome studies. The LCFS has some limited usefulness in clinical assessment of patients' progress; however, it may be most useful as a teaching aid to instruct family members and significant others about general phases of recovery following traumatic brain injury.

RESEARCH ISSUES

Defining Severity of Head Injury

If we are to continue to study how outcome is related to severity of head injury, it will be necessary to agree on the definition of severity of head injury. The Glasgow Coma Scale (GCS)[71] is currently the most widely used measure of head injury severity. Traditionally, a score of 3 to 8 represents a severe head injury, 9 to 12 represents a moderate head injury, and 13 to 15 represents a mild head injury. But various researchers differ, for instance, as to which patients are included in the mild and moderate groups. Does a patient with a GCS score of 13 to 15 but abnormalities on a CT scan, MRI, or a neurological examination have a mild head injury or a moderate head injury? Should we classify such a patient as a complicated mild head injury? Williams et al.[222] found complicated mild head injury patients to be similar to mild but not moderate head injury patients in terms of duration of coma and PTA. In contrast, complicated mild head injury patients had significantly lower word fluency, visual recognition memory, and information processing speed scores than mild head injury patients but were similar to moderate head injury patients in this regard. While mild head injury patients had significantly lower verbal memory scores than did moderate head injury patients, patients with complicated mild head injury performed in between these groups. Mild head injury patients also had significantly better Glasgow Outcome Scale scores than did complicated mild or moderate head injury patients who had similar outcome scores. These findings suggest a need to separate complicated mild head-injured patients from mild head-injured patients for clinical and research purposes in order to predict their outcomes more precisely.

Control Groups for Outcome Studies

Outcome studies should include a nontrauma control group for several reasons. Trauma patients could show changes on measures of outcome that are related to nonspecific effects of head trauma, for instance, being confined to a hospital or having other injuries such as broken bones. Secondly, trauma patients could evidence significant improvements on outcome measures such as cognitive tests that are not due to recovery of cognitive function but to practice effects from repeated testing with multiple follow-up points. When a nontrauma control group is also tested at the same follow-up points, it is possible to partial out the effects of these variables. Thirdly, nonstandardized tests, ones for which there are few normative data, or tests that have been standardized on populations with different demographic characteristics than the patients in the current study, are sometimes included in the test batteries to answer specific questions about the effects of the head injury. By testing control patients with similar risk factors and demographic characteristics, it is possible to determine with greater certainty whether scores on these outcome measures are abnormal.[223]

The selection of an appropriate control group for outcome studies is not without problems. Most neuropsychological tests have been normed on subjects who are considered "normal" because they do not have a history of a major psychiatric disorder, neurological disorders, learning disability, or drug and alcohol abuse. At first glance such subjects might seem to constitute an appropriate control group. However, individuals who suffer a head injury may have different risk factors than such a group, and having such physical injuries as a broken arm or other injuries other than the brain injury may themselves predispose the patient to develop various neurobehavioral and psychiatric disorders, and additionally to produce family stressors that in turn affect the patient. It thus seems reasonable to include control groups that might have similar demographics and risk factors as the head-injured patients as well as injuries to other systems. Patients with orthopaedic injuries or injuries other than a head injury might be appropriate controls.[223–225] In fact, in the study of mild head injury, including such a control group has proved to be a very important research strategy and has resulted in neuropsychologists being more skeptical about long-term effects of a truly mild head injury.[223]

Endpoints for Outcome Studies

When should follow-up assessments occur? For adult patients with mild or moderate head injuries, outcome is most frequently assessed at baseline when the patient has achieved a GOAT $\geq$ 76[23] and at 3, 6, and 12 months postinjury. For severely head-injured patients, baseline measurement might not be possible until 3 months postinjury, and further measurements are typically made at 6 and 12 months postinjury.[21] Should we follow patients further—perhaps for 5, 10, or even more years? While different patterns of recovery have been noted neuropsychologically early on,[9] concern has now been raised[32] that the course of head injury is one of some improvement of function in the early years, followed by relatively stable functioning, and then an "exacerbated decline" many years later that depends on the site of the brain injury, age at injury, and the injury-test interval. However, long-term follow-up is not without problems. Clearly, the longer a patient is followed, the more likely he/she is to be lost to follow-up because of a move to a new address, city, or country, because of death, further head injuries, or serious illness, or because of unwillingness to continue to cooperate in a research venture. While some researchers have gone to extraordinary means to follow patients for as long as 23 years,[33] tracking 76 percent of the patients, this is not likely to be the case for many researchers, and the resulting group may represent a biased picture of recovery. Even Klonoff et al.[33] were unable to do more than a telephone interview with these patients, and thus obtained only subjective estimates of the frequencies of chronic difficulties rather than objective psychometric results. The fall-out rate can perhaps be reduced by giving patients remuneration, by providing transportation to facilities, or by going to the homes of patients to complete follow-up interviews and assessments.

References

1. Langfitt TW: Measuring the outcome from head injury. *J Neurosurg* 1978; 48:673.
2. Levin HS, Hamilton W, Grossman RG: Outcome after head injury, in Braakman R (ed): *Handbook of Clinical Neurology.* Amsterdam: Elsevier, 1990: 367–394.
3. Lezak MD: *Neuropsychological Assessment,* 3d ed. New York: Oxford University Press, 1995.
4. Spreen O, Strauss E: *A Compendium of Neuropsychological Tests.* New York: Oxford University Press, 1991.
5. Franzen MD: *Reliability and Validity in Neuropsychological Assessment.* New York: Plenum, 1989.
6. McDowell I, Newell C: *Measuring Health: A Guide to Rating Scales and Questionnaires.* Oxford: Oxford University Press, 1987.
7. Wade DT: *Measurement in Neurological Rehabilitation.* Oxford: Oxford University Press, 1992.
8. World Health Organization: *International Classification of Impairments, Disabilities, and Handicaps: A Manual of Classification Relating to the Consequences of Disease.* Geneva: World Health Organization, 1980.
9. Ruff RM, Marshall LF, Crouch J, et al: Predictors of outcome following severe head trauma: Follow-up data from the Traumatic Coma Data Bank. *Brain Inj* 1993; 7:101.
10. Brooks NR, McKinlay W, Symington C, et al: Return to work within the first seven years of severe head injury. *Brain Inj* 1987; 1:5.
11. Granger CV, Hamilton BB, Sherwin FS: *Guide for the Use of the Uniform Data Set for Medical Rehabilitation.* Buffalo, NY: Uniform Data System for Medical Rehabilitation Project Office, 1986.
12. Whiteneck GC, Charlifue SW, Gerhart KA, et al: Quantifying handicap: A new measure of long-term rehabilitation outcomes. *Arch Phys Med Rehabil* 1992; 73:519.
13. Rappaport M, Hall KM, Hopkins K, et al: Disability rating scale for severe head trauma: Coma to community. *Arch Phys Med Rehabil* 1982; 63:118.
14. Jones BP, Butters N: Neuropsychological assessment, in Hersen M, Kadzin AE, Bellack AS (eds): *The Clinical Psychology Handbook.* New York: Pergamon, 1983; 377–396.
15. Reitan RM, Davison LA: *Clinical Neuropsychology: Current Status and Applications.* New York: Hemisphere, 1974.
16. Golden CJ, Purisch AD, Hammeke TA: *Luria-Nebraska Neuropsychological Battery: Forms I and II.* Los Angeles: Western Psychological Services, 1985.
17. Jarvis PE, Barth JT: *Halsted-Reitan Test Battery: An*

Interpretative Guide, 2d ed. Odessa: Psychological Assessment Resources, 1994.

18. Heaton RK, Grant I, Mathews CG: *Comprehensive Norms for an Expanded Halstead-Reitan Battery.* Odessa: Psychological Assessment Resources, 1991.
19. Sweet JJ, Moberg PJ: A survey of practices and beliefs among ABPP and non-ABPP clinical neuropsychologists. *Clin Neuropsychol* 1990; 4:101.
20. Guilmette TJ, Faust D, Hart K, Arkes HR: A national survey of pscyhologists who offer neuropsychological services. *Clin Neuropsychol* 1990; 5:373.
21. Clifton GL, Hayes RL, Levin HS, et al: Outcome measures for clinical trials involving traumatically brain-injured patients: Report of a conference. *Neurosurgery* 1992; 31:975.
22. Jennett B, Bond M: Assessment of outcome after severe brain damage. A practical scale. *Lancet* 1975; 2:480.
23. Levin HS, O'Donnell VM, Grossman RG: The Galveston Orientation and Amnesia Test: A Practical scale to assess cognition after head injury. *J Nerv Ment Dis* 1979; 167:675.
24. Hannay HJ, Struchen MA, Contant CF, et al: Assessment of severely head injured patients and the prediction of outcome. Paper presented at the 22nd Annual INS meeting, Cincinnati, OH, February 1994.
25. Goodglass H, Kaplan E: *Assessment of Aphasia and Related Disorders*. Philadelphia: Lea & Febiger, 1972.
26. Levin HS, Hannay HJ, Martin A, Kreutzer J: Acute battery tests for the Army Penetrating Head Injury Project. Unpublished manuscript, 1988.
27. Hannay HJ, Ezrachi O, Contant CD, Levin HS: Outcome measures for clinical trials involving traumatically brain-injured patients revisited. Report of a Subcommittee of the NIH-NINDS National Head Injury Centers, Los Angeles, October 1994.
28. Levin HS: Posttraumatic amnesia: Conceptualization and measurement. Paper presented at the NIH-NINDS Conference on Outcome Measures in Head Injury Clinical Trials, Houston TX, October 8, 1991.
29. Artiola I, Fortuny L, Briggs M, et al: Measuring the duration of post-traumatic amnesia. *J Neurol Neurosurg Psychiatry* 1980; 43:377.
30. Shores EA, Marosszeky JE, Sandanam J, Batchelor J: Preliminary validation of a clinical scale for measuring the duration of post-traumatic amnesia. *Med J Aust* 1986; 144:569.
31. Gouvier WD: Comments on the Glasgow Outcome Scale and Outcome Measures. Discussion presented at the NIH Conference on Outcome Measures in Head Injury Clinical Trials, Houston, TX, October 8, 1991.
32. Corkin S, Rosen JT, Sullivan EV, Clegg RA: Penetrating head injury in young adulthood exacerbates cognitive decline in later years. *J Neurosci* 1989; 9:3876.
33. Klonoff H, Clark C, Klonoff PS: Long-term outcome of head injury: A 23 year followup study of children with head injuries. *J Neurol Neurosurg Psychiatry* 1993; 56:410.
34. Hathaway Sr, McKinley JC: *Minnesota Multiphasic Personality Inventory-2. Manual for Administration and Scoring.* Minneapolis: University of Minnesota, 1989.
35. Binder LM, Willis SC: Assessment of motivation following financially compensable minor head trauma. *Psychol Assessment* 1991; 3:175.
36. Binder LM: Assessment of malingering after mild head trauma with the Portland Digit Recognition Test. *J Clin Exp Neuropsychol* 1993; 15:170.
37. Hiscock M, Hiscock CK: Refining the forced-choice method for the detection of malingering. *J Clin Exp Neuropsychol* 1989; 11:967.
38. Prigatano GP, Amin K: Digit memory test. Unequivocal cerebral dysfunction and suspected malingering. *J Clin Exp Neuropsychol* 1993; 15:537.
39. Bernard LC: Prospects for faking believable memory deficits on neuropsychological tests and the use of incentives in simulation research. *J Clin Exp Neuropsychol* 1990; 12:715.
40. Hannay HJ, James CM: Simulation of a memory deficit on the continuous recognition memory test. *Percept Mot Skills* 1981; 53:51.
41. Benton AL, Spreen O: Visual memory test. *Arch Gen Psychiatry* 1961; 4:79.
42. Mensch AJ, Woods DJ: Patterns of feigning brain damage on the LNNB. *Int J Clin Neuropsychol* 1986; 8:59.
43. Goebel RA: Detection of faking on the Halstead-Reitan Neuropsychological Test Battery. *J Clin Psychol* 1983; 39:731.
44. Heaton RK, Smith HH Jr, Lehman RAW, Vogt AT: Prospects for faking believable deficits on neuropsychological testing. *J Consult Clin Psychol* 1978; 46:892.
45. Guilmette TJ, Guiliano AJ: Taking the stand: Issues and strategies in forensic neuropsychology. *Clin Neuropsychol* 1991; 5:197.
46. Faust D, Hart K, Guilmette TJ: Pediatric malingering: The capacity of children to fake believable deficits on neuropsychological testing. *J Consult Clin Psychol* 1988; 56:578.
47. Bigler ED: Neuropsychology and malingering: Comment on Faust, Hart, and Guilmette. *J Consult Clin Psychol* 1994; 58:244.
48. Perry GG, Kinder BN: The susceptibility of the Rorschach to malingering: A critical review. *J Personality Assess* 1990; 54:47.
49. Greene RL: The MMPI-2/MMPI. An Interpretative Manual. Needham Heights, MS: Allyn & Bacon, 1991.
50. Graham JR: *MMPI-2. Assessing Personality and Psychology.* New York: Oxford University Press, 1990.
51. Berry D, Baer R, Harris M: Detection of malingering on the MMPI: A meta-analysis. *Clin Psychol Rev* 1991; 11:585.
52. Wetter MW, Baer RA, Berry DTR, et al: Sensitivity of MMPI-2 validity scales to random responding and malingering. *Psychol Assess* 1992; 4:369.
53. Benton AL, Hamsher K deS: *Multilingual Aphasia Examination. Manual of Instructions.* Iowa City: AIA Associates, 1983.
54. Smith A: *Symbol Digit Modalities Test. A Manual.* Los Angeles: Western Psychological Services, 1973.
55. Berg EA: A simple objective technique for measuring flexibility in thinking. *J Gen Psychol* 1948; 39:15.
56. Grant DA, Berg EA: A behavioral analysis of degree

of reinforcement and ease of shifting to new responses in a Weigl-type card sorting problem. *J Exp Psychol* 1948; 38:404.
57. Bayley N: *Manual for the Bayley Scales of Infant Development.* New York: Psychological Corporation, 1969.
58. Ewing-Cobbs L, Miner ME, Fletcher JM, Levin HS: Intellectual, motor, and language sequelae following closed head injury in infants and preschoolers. *J Pediatr Psychol* 1989; 14:531.
59. McCarthy D: *McCarthy Scales of Children's Abilities.* New York: Psychological Corporation, 1977.
60. Mathew CG, Klove H: Instruction Manual for the Adult Neuropsychological Test Battery. Madison: University of Wisconsin Medical School, 1964.
61. Fletcher JM: Variations in outcome: A development perspective. Paper presented at the NIH-NINDS Workshop on Consequences of Traumatic Head Injury in Children: Variability in Short- and Long-Term Outcomes. Bethesda, November 1993.
62. Rourke BP, Fisk J, Strong JD: *Neuropsychological Assessment of Children: A Treatment-Oriented Approach.* New York: Guilford, 1986.
63. Ewing-Cobbs L, Fletcher JM: Neuropsychological assessment of head injury in children. *J Learn Disabil* 1987; 20:526.
64. Fletcher JM: Variations in outcome: A developmental perspective. Paper presented at the NIH-NINDS Conference on Consequences of Traumatic Head Injury in Children: Variability in Short- and Long-Term Outcomes, Bethesda, MD, November 18–19, 1993.
65. Russell WR: *The Traumatic Amnesias.* New York: Oxford University Press, 1971.
66. Russell WR, Smith A: Post-traumatic amnesia in closed head injury. *Arch Neurol* 1961; 5:4.
67. Jennett B: Assessment of severity of head injury. *J Neurol Neurosurg Psychiatry* 1976; 39:647.
68. Bishara SN, Partridge FM, Godfrey HPD, Knight RG: Post-traumatic amnesia and Glasgow Coma Scale related to outcome in survivors in a consecutive series of patients with severe closed head injury. *Brain Inj* 1992; 6:373.
69. Gronwall D, Wrightson P: Duration of post-traumatic amnesia after mild head injury. *Clin Neuropsychol* 1980; 2:51.
70. Corrigan JD, James A, Annett JA, Forrester G: Reality orientation for brain injured patients: Group treatment and monitoring recovery. *Arch Phys Med Rehabil* 1985; 66:626.
71. Teasdale G, Jennett B: Assessment of coma and impaired consciousness: A practical scale. *Lancet* 1974; 2:81.
72. Ewing-Cobbs L, Levin HS, Fletcher J, et al: The Children's Orientation and Amnesia Test: Relationship to severity of acute head injury and to recovery of memory. *Neurosurgery* 1990; 27:683.
73. Baryza MJ, Haley SM: Use of the Children's Orientation and Amnesia Test at hospital discharge for children with neurological and non-neurological traumatic injuries. *Brain Inj* 1994; 8:167.
74. Shores EA: Comparison of the Westmead PTA Scale and Glasgow Coma Scale as predictors of neuropsychological outcome following extremely severe blunt head injury. *J Neurol Neurosurg Psychiatry* 1989; 52:126.
75. Marosszeky NEV, Batchelor J, Shores JE, et al: The performance of hospitalized non head-injured children on the Westmead PTA Scale. *Clin Neuropsychol* 1993; 7:85.
76. Sherer M, Parsons OA, Nixon SJ, Adams RL: Clinical validity of the Speech-Sounds Perception Test and the Seashore Rhythm Test. *J Clin Exp Neuropsychol* 1991; 13:741.
77. Russell EW, Neuringer C, Goldstein G: *Assessment of Brain Damage.* New York: Wiley-Interscience, 1970.
78. Reitan RM, Wolfson D: *The Halstead-Reitan Neuropsychological Test Battery: Theory and Clinical Interpretation.* Tucson: Neuropsychology Press, 1993.
79. Dikmen S, Machamer J, Temkin N, McLean A: Neuropsychological recovery in patients with moderate to severe head injury: 2 year follow-up. *J Clin Exp Neuropsychol* 1990; 12:507.
80. Dikmen S, McLean A, Temkin N: Neuropsychological and psychosocial consequences of minor head injury. *J Neurol Neurosurg Psychiatry* 1986; 49:1227.
81. Dikmen S, Machamer JE, Winn RH, Temkin NR: Neuropsychological outcome at 1-year post head injury. *Neuropsychology* 1995; 9:80.
82. Christensen AL: *Luria's Neuropsychological Investigation*, 2d ed. Copenhagen-Munksgaard, 1979.
83. Adams KM: In search of Luria's battery: A false start. *J Consult Clin Psychol* 1980; 48:511.
84. Golden CJ: In reply to Adams' "In search of Luria's battery: A false start." *J Consult Clin Psychol* 1980; 48:517.
85. Spiers PA: Have they come to praise Luria or to bury him? The Luria-Nebraska controversy. *J Consult Clin Psychol* 1981; 49:331.
86. Crosson B, Warren RL: Use of the Luria-Nebraska neuropsychological battery in aphasica. A conceptual critique. *J Consult Clin Psychol* 1982; 50:22.
87. Delis DC, Kaplan E: The assessment of aphasia with the Luria-Nebraska neuropsychological battery: A case critique. *J Consult Clin Psychol* 1982; 50:40.
88. Harrington DE, Levandowski DH: Efficacy of an educationally-based cognitive retraining programme for traumatically head-injured as measured by LNNB pre- and post-test scores. *Brain Inj* 1987; 1:65.
89. Franzen MD, Harris CV: Neuropsychological rehabilitation: Application of a modified multiple baseline design. *Brain Inj* 1993; 7:525.
90. Heilman KM, Safran A, Geschwind N: Closed head trauma and aphasia. *J Neurol Neurosurg Psychiatry* 1971; 34:256.
91. Arsini C, Constantinovici A, Iliescu D, et al: Considerations on posttraumatic aphasia in peace time. *Psychiatria Neurologia Neurochirurgia* 1970; 73:105.
92. Sarno MT, Levin HS: Speech and language disorders after closed head injury, in Darby JK (ed): *Speech and Language Evaluation in Neurology: Adult Disorders.* Orlando: Grune & Stratton, 1985; 323–339.
93. Levin HS, Grossman RG, Kelly PJ: Aphasic disorder

with closed head injury. *J Neurol Neurosurg Psychiatry* 1976; 39:1062.

94. Sarno MT: The nature of verbal impairment after closed head injury. *J Nerv Ment Dis* 1980; 168:685.
95. Sarno MT: Verbal impairment after closed head injury. *J Nerv Ment Dis* 1984; 172:475.
96. Benton AL, Hamsher K deS: *Multilingual Aphasia Examination. Manual of Instructions.* Iowa City: AIA Associates, 1983.
97. Spreen O, Benton AL: *Neurosurgery Center Comprehensive Examination for Aphasia.* Victoria, Neuropsychological Laboratory, Department of Psychology, University of Victoria, 1969.
98. Jordan FM, Murdoch BE: Linguistic status following closed head injury in children: A follow-up study. *Brain Inj* 1990; 4:147.
99. Ewing-Cobbs L, Levin HS, Eisenberg HM, Fletcher JM: Language functions following closed head injury in children and adolescents. *J Clin Exp Neuropsychol* 1987; 9:575.
100. Kaplan EF, Goodglass H, Weintraub S: *The Boston Naming Test.* Malvern: Lea & Febiger, 1993.
101. Huff FJ, Collins C, Corkin S, Rosen TJ: Equivalent forms of the Boston Naming Test. *J Clin Exp Neuropsychol* 1986; 8:556.
102. Thompson LL, Heaton RK: Comparison of different versions of the Boston Naming Test. *Clin Neuropsychol* 1989; 3:184.
103. Jordan FM, Ozanne AE, Murdoch BE: Performance of closed head-injured children on a naming task. *Brain Inj* 1990; 4:27.
104. Ponsford J, Kinsella G: Attentional deficits following closed head injury. *J Clin Exp Neuropsychol* 1992; 14:822.
105. Cooley EL, Morris RD: Attention in children: A neuropsychologically based model for assessment. *Devel Neuropsychol* 1990; 6:239.
106. van Zoomeren AH, Brouwer WH: *Clinical Neuropsychology of Attention.* New York: Oxford University Press, 1994.
107. Mirsky AF, Anthony BJ, Duncan CC, et al: Analysis of the elements of attention: A neuropsychological approach. *Neuropsychol Rev* 1991; 2:109.
108. Davies DR, Jones DM, Taylor A: Selective and sustained-attention tasks: Individual and group differences, in Parasuraman R, Davies DR (eds): *Varieties of Attention.* Orlando FL: Academic, 1984.
109. Levin HS, High WM, Goldstein FC, Williams DH: Sustained attention and information processing speed in chronic survivors of severe closed head injury. *Scand J Rehab Med* 1988; 17(suppl):33.
110. Ewing R, McCarthy D, Gronwall D, Wrightson P: Persisting effects of minor head injury observable during hypoxic stress. *J Clin Neuropsychol* 1980; 2:147.
111. Wechsler D: *Wechsler Adult Intelligence—Revised Manual.* San Antonio: Psychological Corporation, 1981.
112. Levin HS, Benton AL, Grossman RG: *Neurobehavioral Consequences of Closed Head Injury.* New York: Oxford University Press, 1982.
113. Mandleberg IA, Brooks DN: Cognitive recovery after severe head injury. I. Serial testing on the Wechsler Adult Intelligence Scale. *J Neurol Neurosurg Psychiatry* 1975; 38:1121.
114. Ruff RM, Evans RW, Light RH: Automatic detection vs controlled search. *Percept Mot Skills* 1986; 62:407.
115. Gouvier WD, Maxfield MW, Schweitzer JR, et al: Psychometric prediction of driving performacne among the disabled. *Arch Phys Med Rehabil* 1989; 70:745.
116. Siviak M, Hill CS, Henson DL, et al: Improved driving performance following perceptual training in persons with brain damage. *Arch Phys Med Rehabil* 1984; 65:163.
117. Gronwall D: Paced auditory serial addition task: A measure of recovery from concussion. *Percept Mot Skills* 1977; 44:367.
118. Gronwall D, Sampson H: *The Psychological Effects of Concussion.* Auckland: Auckland Unviersity Press, 1974.
119. Levin, Mattis, Ruff, Eisenberg, Marshall, Tsbaddor, High, Frankowski, 1982. Pasat tape
120. Dyche GM, Johnson DA: Development and evaluation of CHIPASAT, an attention test for children: II. Test-retest reliability and practice effect for a normal sample. *Percept Mot Skills* 1991; 72:563.
121. Johnson DA, Rofthig O, Johnston K, Middleton J: Development and evaluation of an attention test for head-injured children: 1. Information processing capacity in a normal sample. *J Child Psychol Psychiatry* 1988; 29:199.
122. Leininger BE, Grambling SE, Farrell AD, et al: Neuropsychological deficits in symptomatic mild head injury patients after concussion and mild concussion. *J Neurol Neurosurg Psychiatry* 1990; 53:293.
123. Wechsler D, Stone CP: *Wechsler Memory Scale.* New York: Psychological Corporation, 1945.
124. Russell EW: A multiple scoring method for the assessment of complex memory functions. *J Consult Clin Psychol* 1973; 43:800.
125. Wechsler D: *Wechsler Memory Scale—Revised Manual.* San Antonio: Psychological Corporation, 1987.
126. Rey A: L'examen psychologique dans les cas d'encephalopathie traumatique. *Arch de Psychologie* 1941; 28:286.
127. Osterreith PA: Le test de copie d'une figure complexe. *Arch Psychologie* 1944; 30:206.
128. Hannay HJ, Levin HS, Grossman RG: Impaired recognition memory after head injury. *Cortex* 1979; 15:269.
129. Brooks DN: Wechsler Memory Scale performance and its relationship to brain damage after severe closed head injury. *J Neurol Neurosurg Psychiatry* 1976; 39:593.
130. Wilson B, Vizor A, Bryant T: Predicting severity of cognitive impairment after severe head injury. *Brain Inj* 1991; 15:189.
131. Buschke H: Selective reminding for analysis of memory and learning. *J Verbal Learn Verbal Behav* 1973; 12:543.
132. Buschke H, Fuld PA: Evaluating storage, retention, and retrieval in disordered memory and learning. *Neurology* 1974; 24:1019.
133. Delis DC, Kramer JH, Kaplan E, Ober BA: *California Verbal Learning Test.* San Antonio: *Psychological Corp.*, 1987.

134. Rey A: L'examen psychologique dans les cas d'encephalopathie traumatique. *Arch Psychologie* 1941; 28:286.
135. Crosson B, Novack TA, Trenerry MR, Craig PL: California Verbal Learning Test (CVLT) performance in severely head-injured and neurologically normal adult males. *J Clin Exp Neuropsychol* 1988; 10:754.
136. Crosson B, Novack TA, Trennery MR, Craig PL: Differentiation of verbal memory deficits in blunt head injury using the recognition trial of the California Verbal Learning Test: An exploratory study. *Clin Neuropsychologist* 1989; 3:29.
137. Bigler ED, Rosa L, Schultz R, et al: Rey-Auditory learning and Rey-Osterreith complex figure design performance in Alzheimer's disease and closed head injury. *J Clin Psychol* 1989; 45:277.
138. Lezak MD: Recovery of memory and learning functions following traumatic brain injury. *Cortex* 1979; 15:63.
139. Talley JL: *Children's Auditory Verbal Learning Test—2 (CAVLT-2).* Odessa, FL: Neuropsychological Assessment Resources, 1993.
140. Delis DC, Kramer J, Kaplan E, Ober BA: *California Verbal Learning Test—Children's Version.* San Antonio: Psychological Corporation, 1994.
141. Clodfelter CJ, Dickson AL, Wilkes C, Johnson RB: Alternate forms of selective reminding for children. *Clinical Neuropsychologist* 1987; 1:243.
142. Morgan SF: Measuring long-term memory storage and retrieval in children. *J Clin Neuropsychol* 1982; 4:77.
143. Hannay HJ, Levin HS: Selective Reminding Test: An examination of the equivalence of four forms. *J Clin Exp Neuropsychol* 1985; 7:251.
144. Levin HS: Learning and memory, in Hannay HJ (ed): *Experimental Techniques in Human Neuropsychology.* New York: Oxford University Press, 1986.
145. Levin HS, Grossman RG: Effects of closed head injury on storage and retrieval in memory and learning of adolescents. *J Pediatr Psychol* 1976; 1:38.
146. Paniak CE, Shore DL, Rourke BP: Recovery of memory after severe closed head injury: Dissociations in recovery of memory parameters and predictors of outcome. *J Clin Exper Neuropsychol* 1989; 11:631.
147. Brooks N, McKinley W, Symington C, et al: Return to work within the first seven years of severe head injury. *Brain Inj* 1987; 1:5.
148. Dikmen S, Temkin N, McLean A, et al: Memory and head injury severity. *J Neurol Neurosurg Psychiatry* 1987; 50:1613.
149. Levin HS, Grossman RG, Rose JE, Teasdale G: Long-term neuropsychological outcome of closed head injury. *J Neurosurg* 1979; 50:412.
150. Brooks DN: Memory and head injury. *J Nerv Ment Dis* 1972; 155:350.
151. Clifton GL, Kreutzer JS, Choi SC, et al: Relationship between Glasgow Outcome Scale and neuropsychological measures after brain injury. *Neurosurgery* 1993; 33:34.
152. Hannay HJ, Levin HS: *The Continuous Recognition Memory Test. A Manual.* Houston: Neuropsychology Resources, 1988.
153. Levin HS, Eisenberg HM, Wigg NR, Kobayashi K: Memory and intellectual ability after head injury in children and adolescents. *Neurosurgery* 1982; 11:668.
154. Levin HS, High WM Jr, Ewing-Cobbs L, et al: Memory functioning during the first year after closed head injury in children and adolescents. *Neurosurgery* 1988; 22:1043.
155. Haaland KY, Temkin N, Randahl G, Dikmen S: Recovery of simple motor skills after head injury. *J Clin Exper Neuropsychol* 1994; 16:448.
156. Grafman J, Jonas B, Salazar A: Wisconsin Card Sorting Test performance based on location and size of neuroanatomical lesion in Vietnam veterans with penetrating head injury. *Percept Mot Skills* 1990; 71:1120.
157. Mathews CG, Klove H. *Instruction Manual for the adult neuropsychology* test battery. Madison: University of Wisconsin Medical School, 1964.
158. Heaton RK: *Wisconsin Card Sorting Test. Manual.* Odessa, FL: Psychological Assessment Resources, 1981.
159. Goldstein FC, Levin HS, Boake C: Conceptual encoding following severe closed head injury. *Cortex* 1989; 25:541.
160. DeFilippis NA, McCampbell E: *Manual for the Booklet Category Test.* Odessa, FL: Psychological Assessment Resources, 1979.
161. DeFilippis NA, McCampbell E, Rogers P: Development of a booklet form of the Category Test. *J Clin Neuropsychol* 1979; 1:339.
162. MacNiven E, Finlayson MAJ: The interplay between emotional and cognitive recovery after closed head injury. *Brain Inj* 1993; 3:241.
163. Brouwer WH, Ponds RWHM, Van Wolffelaar PC, Van Zoomeren AH: Divided attention 5 to 10 years after closed head injury. *Cortex* 1989; 25:219.
164. des Rosiers G, Kavanaugh D: Cognitive assessment in closed head injury: Stability, validity and parallel forms for two neuropsychological measures of recovery. *Int J Clin Neuropsychol* 1987; 9:162.
165. Hathaway SR, McKinley JC: *MMPI Manual (Rev Ed).* New York: Psychological Corporation, 1967.
166. Blanchard JS: Readability of the MMPI. *Percept Mot Skills* 1981; 52:985.
167. Greene RL: *The MMPI-2: An Interpretative Manual.* Boston: Allyn & Bacon, 1991.
168. Graham JR: *MMPI-2 Assessing Personality and Psychopathology.* New York: Oxford University Press, 1990.
169. Lezak MD, Glaudin V: Differential effects of physical illness on MMPI profiles. *Newsletter Res Psychol* 1969; 11:27.
170. Mack JL: The MMPI and neurological dysfunction, in Newmark CS (ed): *MMPI: Current Clinical and Research Trends.* New York: Praeger, 1979.
171. Gass CS: MMPI-2 interpretation and closed head injury: A correction factor. *Psychol Assess* 1991; 3:27.
172. Alfano DP, Paniak CE, Finlayson MAJ: A neurocorrected MMPI for closed head injury. Poster presented at the 20th Annual Meeting of the International Neuropsychological Society, San Diego, February 7, 1992.
173. Alfano DP, Finlayson MAJ: Comparison of standard and abbreviated MMPIs in patients with head injury. *Rehab Psychol* 1987; 32:67.
174. Goldberg D: *The Detection of Psychiatric Illness by*

Questionnaire. London: Oxford University Press, 1972.
175. Livingston MG, Brooks DN: The burden on families of the brain injured: A review. *J Head Trauma Rehabil* 1988; 3:6.
176. Goldberg D, Hillier VF: A scaled version of the General Health Questionnaire. *Psychol Med* 1979; 9:139.
177. Goldberg D: *Manual of the General Health Questionnaire.* Windsor, England: NFER Publishing, 1978.
178. Chan DW, Chan TSC: Reliability, validity and the structure of the General Health Questionnaire in a Chinese context. *Psychol Med* 1983; 13:363.
179. McDowell I, Newell C: *Measuring Health: A Guide to Rating Scales and Questionnaires.* Oxford: Oxford University Press, 1987.
180. Katz MM, Lyerly SB: Methods for measuring adjustment and social behavior in the community: 1. Rationale, description, discriminative validity and scale development. *Psychol Rep* 1963; 13:503.
181. Fabiano RJ, Goran DA: A principal component analysis of the Katz Adjustment Scale in a traumatic brain injury rehabilitation sample. *Rehab Psychol* 1992; 37:75.
182. Hogarty GE, Katz MM: Norms of adjustment and social behavior. *Arch Gen Psychiatry* 1971; 25:470.
183. Klonoff PS, Costa LD, Snow WG: Predictors and indicators of quality of life in patients with closed-head injury. *J Clin Exp Neuropsychol* 1986; 8:469.
184. Stambrook M, Moore AD, Peters LC, et al: Effects of mild, moderate and severe closed head injury on long-term vocational status. *Brain Inj* 1990; 4:183.
185. Oddy M: Head injury and social adjustment, in Brooks N (ed): *Closed Head Injury: Psychological, Social, and Family Consequences.* New York: Oxford, 1984.
186. Peters LC, Stambrook M, Moore AD, Esses L: Psychosocial sequelae of closed head injury: Effects on the marital relationship. *Brain Inj* 1990; 4:39.
187. Levin HS, High WM, Goethe KE, et al: The Neurobehavioral Rating Scale: Assessment of the behavioral sequelae of head injury by the clinician. *J Neurol Neurosurg Psychiatry* 1987; 50:183.
188. Overall JE, Gorham DR: The brief psychiatric rating scale. *Psychol Rep* 1992; 10:799.
189. Corrigan JD, Dickerson J, Fisher E, Meyer P: The Neurobehavioral Rating Scale: Replication in an acute, inpatient rehabilitation setting. *Brain Inj* 1990; 4:215.
190. Levine MJ, Van Horn KR, Curtis AB: Developmental models of social cognition in assessing psychological adjustments in head injury. *Brain Inj* 1993; 7:153.
191. Stultzer DL, Levin HS, Mahler ME, et al: Assessment of cognitive, psychiatric, and behavioral disturbances in patients with dementia: The Neurobehavioral Rating Scale. *J Am Geriatr Soc* 1992; 40:549.
192. Hilton G, Sisson R, Freeman E: The Neurobehavioral Rating Scale: An interrater reliability study in the HIV seropositive population. *J Neurosci Nurs* 1990; 22:36.
193. Lezak MD: Relationships between personality disorders, social disturbances, and physical diability following traumatic brain injury. *J Head Trauma Rehabil* 1987; 2:57.
194. Kaplan SP: Adaptation following serious brain injury. An assessment after one year. *J Applied Rehabil Counsel* 1988; 19:3.
195. Malec JF, Thompson JM: Relationship of the Mayo-Portland Adaptability Inventory to functional outcome and cognitive performance measures. *J Head Trauma Rehabil* 1994; 9:1.
196. Malec JF, Smigielski JS, DePompolo RW: Goal attainment scaling and outcome measurement in post-acute brain injury rehabilitation. *Arch Phys Med Rehabil* 1991; 72:138.
197. Walker MI, Hannay HJ, Davidson K: PAI and the prediction of level of vocational/academic outcome post CHI. Paper presented at the 20th Annual Meeting, San Diego, February 8, 1992.
198. Hamilton BB, Granger CV, Sherwin FS, et al: A uniform national data system for medical rehabilitation, in Fuhrer MJ (ed): *Rehabilitation Outcomes: Analysis and Measurement.* Baltimore, Brookes, 1987.
199. Hamilton BB, Laughlin JA, Granger CV, Kayton RM: Interrater agreement of the seven level Functional Independence Measurement (FIM). *Arch Phys Med Rehabil* 1991; 72:572.
200. Hall KM, Hamilton BB, Gordon WA, Zasler ND: Characteristics and comparisons of functional assessment indices: Disability Rating Scale, Functional Independence Measure, and Functional Assessment Measure. *J Head Trauma Rehabil* 1993; 8:60.
201. Dodds TA, Martin DP, Stolov WC, Deyo RA: A validation of the Functional Independence Measure and its performance among rehabilitation inpatients. *Arch Phys Med Rehabil* 1993; 74:531.
202. Whitlock JA: Functional outcome of low-level traumatically brain-injured admitted to an acute rehabilitation programme. *Brain Inj* 1992; 6:447.
203. Granger CV, Cotter AC, Hamilton BB, et al: Functional assessment scales: A study of persons with multiple sclerosis. *Arch Phys Med Rehabil* 1990; 71:870.
204. Granger CV, Cotter AC, Hamilton BB, Fiedler RC: Functional assessment scales. A study of persons after stroke. *Arch Phys Med Rehabil* 1993; 74:133.
205. Hall K: Overview of functional assessment scales in brain injury rehabilitation. *Neuro Rehabil* 1992; 2:98.
206. Bergner M, Bobbitt RA, Carter WB, Gilson BS: The Sickness Impact Profile: Development and final revision of a health status measure. *Med Care* 1981; 19:787.
207. Temkin N, McLean A, Dikmen S, et al: Development and evaluation of modifications to the Sickness Impact Profile for head injury. *J Clin Epidemiol* 1988; 41:47.
208. Jennett B, Snoek J, Bond MR, Brooks N: Disability after severe head injury: Observations on the use of the Glasgow Outcome Scale. *J Neurol Neurosurg Psychiatry* 1981; 44:285.
209. Boake C, High WM: Measuring outcome following traumatic brain injury rehabilitation. Denver, Meeting of American Congress of Rehabilitation Medicine, 1993.
210. Willer B, Rosenthal M, Kreutzer JS, et al: Assessment of community integration following rehabilitation for traumatic brain injury. *J Head Trauma Rehabil* 1993; 8:75.

211. Jennett B: The measurement of outcome, in Brooks N (ed): *Closed Head Injury: Psychological, Social, and Family Consequences*. New York: Oxford University Press, 1984.
212. Gennarelli TA, Spielman GM, Langfitt TW, et al: Influence of the type of intracranial lesion on outcome from severe head injury: A multicenter study using a new classification system. *J Neurosurg* 1982; 56:26.
213. Hall K, Cope DN, Rappaport M: Glasgow Outcome Scale and Disability Rating Scale: Comparative usefulness in following recovery in traumatic head injury. *Arch Phys Med Rehabil* 1985; 66:35.
214. Gouvier WD, Blanton PD, LaPorte KL, Nepomuceno C: Reliability and validity of the Disability Rating Scale and the Levels of Cognitive Functioning Scale in monitoring recovery from severe head injury. *Arch Phys Med Rehabil* 1987; 68:94.
215. Cope DN, Cole JR, Hall KM, Barkans H: Brain injury: Analysis of outcome in a post-acute rehabilitation system. Part 1: General analysis. *Brain Inj* 1991; 5:111.
216. Hagen C, Malkmus D: Intervention strategies for language disorders secondary to head trauma. Atlanta, American Speech-Language-Hearing Association Convention Short Course, 1979.
217. Hagen C: Language-cognitive disorganization following closed head injury: A conceptualization, in Trexler LE (ed): *Cognitive Rehabilitation: Conceptualization and Intervention.* New York: Plenum, 1982.
218. Spivack G, Spettell CM, Ellis DW, Ross SE: Effects of intensity of treatment and length of stay on rehabilitation outcomes. *Brain Inj* 1992; 6:419.
219. Rao N, Kilgore KM: Predicting return to work in traumatic brain injury using assessment scales. *Arch Phys Med Rehabil* 1992; 73:911.
220. Horn S, Shiel A, McLellan L, Campbell M, et al: A review of behavioral assessment scales for monitoring recovery in and after coma with pilot data on a new scale of visual awareness. *Neurol Rehabil* 1993; 3:121.
221. Timmons M, Gasquoine L, Scibak JW: Functional changes with rehabilitation of very severe traumatic brain injury survivors. *J Head Trauma Rehabil* 1987; 2:64.
222. Williams DH, Levin HS, Eisenberg HM: Mild head injury classification. *Neurosurgery* 1990; 27:422.
223. Bijur PE, Haslum M, Golding J: Cognitive and behavioral sequelae of mild head injury in children. *Pediatrics* 1990; 86:337.
224. Rutter M, Chadwick O, Shaffer D, Brown G: A prospective study of children with head injuries: I. Design and methods. *Psychol Med* 1980; 10:633.
225. Dikmen SS, Temkin NR, Machamer JE, et al: Employment following traumatic head injuries. *Arch Neurol* 1994; 51:177.

CHAPTER 50

OUTCOME FROM MILD HEAD INJURY

Harvey S. Levin

SYNOPSIS

This chapter discusses the outcome of mild head injury from a neurobehavioral perspective and considers the definition of a mild head injury, particularly in regard to the integration of the Glasgow Coma Scale with the results of neuroimaging. The epidemiology of mild head injury as elucidated in population-based studies is reviewed, and methodological issues in neurobehavioral outcome studies of mild head injury are discussed; this is followed by a synthesis of the empirical findings. In addition to the cognitive outcome of mild head injury, the frequency and persistence of specific postconcussional symptoms are considered and base rates of postconcussional symptoms are reviewed, including their relationship to psychiatric sequelae. Finally, guidelines for the postacute management of patients who sustain a mild head injury are extrapolated from the literature on neurobehavioral outcome.

DEFINITION OF MILD HEAD INJURY

Consistent with previous research[1] and Stein's classification of head injury, Chapter 3 in this volume, a mild head injury can be defined as an injury caused by blunt trauma and/or sudden acceleration/deceleration which produces a period of unconsciousness for 20 min or less, a Glasgow Coma Scale[2] score of 13 to 15, no focal neurological deficit, no intracranial complications, and computed tomography (CT) findings limited to a skull fracture without evidence of a contusion or hematoma. Since Rimel and coworkers[3] at the University of Virginia defined a mild closed head injury (CHI) in terms of the Glasgow Coma Scale (GCS) score, investigators have adopted a similar definition. As reflected in the neuropsychological literature, this definition has evolved since the publication of the study by Rimel et al.[3] Several outcome studies have also specified a maximum duration of hospitalization of 48 h to exclude major extracranial injuries. Variation across studies in the definition of mild head injury primarily reflects differences in the screening of CT findings and the use of exclusionary criteria to mitigate preexisting conditions, including a previous head injury (Table 50-1). Despite the dissemination of research diagnostic criteria, ambiguities are inherent in defining mild head injury and accruing patients. First, estimating the duration of unconsciousness is difficult when witnesses are not available. Second, intoxication at the time of hospital admission can obscure the contribution of a head injury to the impairment of consciousness. Third, there is a difficulty in studies limited to patients hospitalized for mild head injury. Although outcome studies have focused on hospitalized patients, Strang et al.[4] estimated that five patients were treated in emergency rooms for every patient who was hospitalized for a mild head injury. In view of neurosurgical studies indicating that delayed complications are extremely rare in patients with normal CT scans, it is likely that fewer patients will be hospitalized for mild head injury.

EPIDEMIOLOGY

Kraus and Nourjah[5] reported that uncomplicated mild head injury constituted 80 percent of all hospital admis-

TABLE 50-1 Summary of Major Studies Concerning Neuropsychological Outcome of Mild Head Injury

Authors	Samples	Postinjury Interval	Procedure	Major Findings	Critique
Rimel et al.[3] (Charottesville)	n = 424, GCS = 13–15	3 months	GOS, neuropsychology, interview	Mild to severe neurobehavioral deficits were present in ⅔ of the series, and ⅓ were unemployed. Disability was less severe in older patients.	No control group. No screening for antecedent conditions. 31% had previous head injury.
Levin et al.[1] (three centers)	n = 57, GCS = 13–15, normal CT; 56 controls	<1 week, 3 months	Memory, attention, interview	Cognitive deficits at 1 week resolved by 1–3 months; memory was the most common deficit. Somatic and affective symptoms improved over 3 months, but 47% still complained of headaches, 22% of dizziness, and 22% of reduced energy.	Only 32 patients returned at 3 months; controls were tested only once.
Hugenholtz et al.[6] (Ottawa)	n = 36 (14 dropouts) with PTA but not hospitalized; 22 controls	<72 h, 7–10 days, 14–17 days, 28–31 days, 88–90 days	Simple and choice visual reaction time (RT); interview	Patients had slower complex RTs than controls for the first three exams, but the difference was not significant on any RT measure by visit 5 (3 months). Mean duration of postconcussion symptoms was 13 days (range 2–89 days).	Of the series, 7 had a previous concussion. Controls tended to slow their RTs across sessions. Questionable reliability of PTA measurement.
Gentilini et al.[7]	n = 50, GCS = 13–15, 50 controls	1 month (3 months)	Attention, memory	Differences between patients and controls were limited to selective attention, but the overall comparison was not significant. Execution time was slower in 22 patients who returned at 3 months. On a distributed attention test, patients responded more quickly than controls at 5 months after injury.	Selective attrition could have influenced results. Marked inconsistency between data at 3 months and 5 months.
Dikmen et al.[8]	n = 20, GCS = 12–15, 19 controls	1 month, 1 year	Memory, attention, other neuropsychology measures, psychosocial assessment, interview	Controls performed above the level of patients on 2 of 21 measures at 1 month after injury. There were no differences in cognitive performance at 1 year. Daily activities (e.g., return to work) were reduced at 1 month, but no difference was present by 1 year. Patients reported more postconcussional symptoms than controls at 1 month but not at 1 year. Multiple trauma contributed to the disability at 1 month.	Subgroups with versus without multiple trauma had small sample size.
Gronwall and Wrightson[9,10]	PTA < 1 h, no complications, n = 237	Serial testing until 3 months	Paced auditory serial addition task (PASAT)	About 75% of patients recovered to a normal rate of information processing by 4–6 weeks; the remainder, by 3 months. Recovery on PASAT concussional symptoms. Consecutively treated patients recover more rapidly than cases referred due to persistent postconcussional symptoms.	Limited to a single cognitive measure; no CT scan.

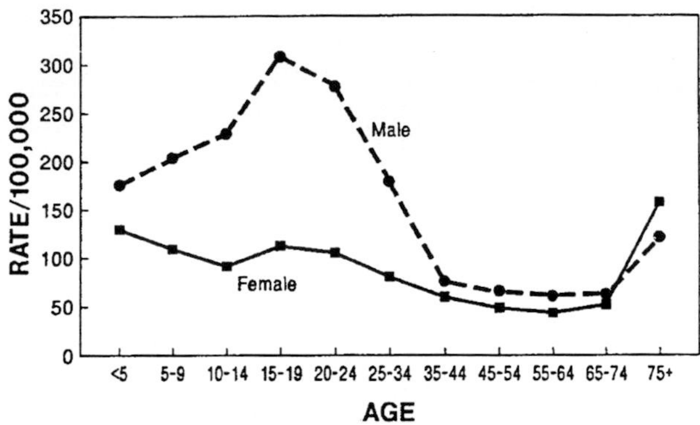

Figure 50-1. Age-specific mild head injury rates per 100,000 by gender in San Diego County, California, in 1981. (From Kraus and Nourjah[5] with permission.)

sions for head injury in San Diego County. The incidence rate for mild head injury was 130.8 in 100,000 per year. As reflected in Fig. 50-1, the age- and gender-specific incidence was highest for young men, followed by a secondary peak for both men and women older than age 65 years. Kraus and Nourjah[5] also found that 64 percent of their patients were intoxicated according to the legal definition based on the blood alcohol level.

OUTCOME OF MILD HEAD INJURY

Reports by Rimel and colleagues[3] at the University of Virginia alerted the neurosurgical and rehabilitation communities to sequelae of mild head injury which had not been widely appreciated. Analysis of the 3-month outcome of mild head injury disclosed that mild to severe residual neurobehavioral deficits existed in two-thirds of the patients and that one-third of the patients were unemployed (Table 50-1). The assets of the research by Rimel et al.[3] included basing the diagnostic criteria primarily on the GCS score and the collection of outcome data from 424 patients who were consecutively hospitalized for mild head injury. Although the Virginia work was a milestone in research on mild head injury, interpretation of the findings was complicated by (1) the lack of an appropriate comparison group selected from the same community and tested on the same neurobehavioral measures, (2) the inclusion of patients who had been hospitalized previously for head injury, and (3) the lack of screening or separate analysis of patients who had a preexisting neuropsychiatric disorder, such as alcohol abuse, which could have contributed to their cognitive deficits.

The studies summarized in Table 50-1 can be differentiated according to (1) whether they included a comparison group of uninjured persons, (2) the length of the follow-up interval, (3) the definition of a mild head injury, (4) screening for preexisting neuropsychiatric disorders, and (5) outcome measures. All the studies included a comparison group except the Charlottesville study, which relied on published normative data to evaluate the presence of cognitive deficits. However, the high rate of cognitive impairment reported by Rimel et al.[3] might have been due in part to their use of normative data collected from samples which were demographically different from their head-injured patients. Among the studies summarized in Table 50-1 which employed demographically matched comparison groups and screened for preexisting neuropsychiatric disorders, it can be seen that consistent evidence exists for recovery of the cognitive deficit within 1 to 3 months after a mild CHI.

To illustrate the time course for the resolution of a cognitive deficit after a mild head injury, the results of the three-center study[1] for verbal memory and the information-processing rate are summarized in Fig. 50-2. The verbal memory test involved recalling a list of 12 words over 12 trials. After the examiner presented the entire list on the first trial, subsequent presentations were limited to the words the patient failed to recall on the preceding trial. The total number of words recalled across the 12 trials was entered for each patient and control. The box plot for verbal memory (left) shows that the mild head injury patients were initially impaired at baseline but recovered by 1 to 3 months. The variation in the level of verbal recall across the three centers is evident for the normal control data. It can be seen that the controls in the Bronx tended to recall words at a level similar to that of the mild CHI patients in the other centers.

The information-processing rate was evaluated by the Paced Auditory Serial Addition Task (PASAT), in which the patient was asked to add single-digit numbers which were presented at progressively faster rates. The number of correct additions per second of presentation provided a measure of the information-processing rate. The initial slowing of the information-processing rate in the mildly injured patients improved at 1 and 3 months after injury to within the range of normal controls. The patients at the Galveston and Bronx centers recovered to levels of the processing rate which did not differ from these of controls by 1 month after injury. Consistent with the impression that the information-processing rate remained slow among the San Diego patients, their performance remained impaired relative to that of their local control group. The investigators found evidence for selective attrition in the San Diego

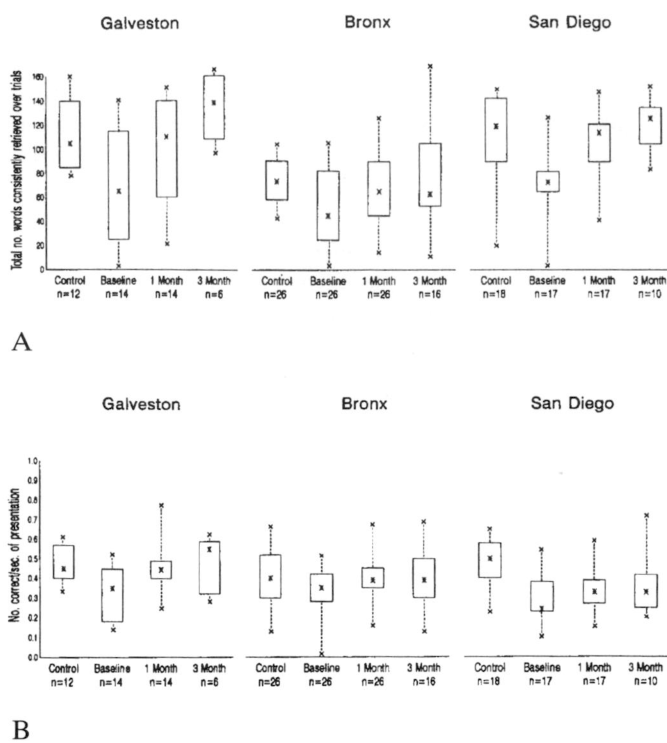

Figure 50-2. *A.* Distribution of verbal memory retrieval scores for control and head-injured groups studied in Galveston, the Bronx, and San Diego at 1 week (baseline), 1 month, and 3 months after injury. Asterisks (*) signify the median, whereas the upper and lower horizontal lines of each bar indicate the 75th and 25th percentile scores, respectively. Maximum/minimum scores are depicted by X's, and n = number of patients. *B.* Distribution of information-processing rate scores for control and head-injured groups studied in Galveston, the Bronx, and San Diego at 1 week (baseline), 1 month, and 3 months after injury. Symbols are as represented in *A.* (From Levin et al.[1] with permission.)

sample, as reflected by the lower level of education of patients who returned for follow-up.

POSTCONCUSSIONAL SYMPTOMS

Likelihood of Postconcussional Symptoms after Mild Head Injury

The most commonly reported postconcussional symptoms (PCSs) are fairly consistent across studies of consecutive patients treated for mild head injury. Using a structured interview, Levin et al.[1] found that the percentage of patients reporting PCSs within 1 week of injury ranged from 82 to 93 percent across three centers. In all these patients, the three most frequent symptoms at all three centers were headache (71 percent), decreased energy (60 percent), and dizziness (53 percent). Although the severity of PCSs diminished over 3 months, mild residual complaints persisted in the cognitive, somatic, and affective domains. The high rate of PCSs reported by all three centers during the first week after mild head injury supports a neurogenic etiology. However, it is important to take into account the prevailing level of headaches and other symptoms associated with mild head injury in the general population. For example, Dikmen et al.[8] found that more than a third of uninjured controls reported symptoms such as headaches, fatigability, and irritability.

Persistence of PCS

Few studies have serially examined consecutive patients after a mild head injury to assess the resolution of PCSs. Rutherford and coworkers in Northern Ireland[11,12] reported 1-year outcome data for 131 patients whom they examined at 24 h and at 6 weeks after injury. These investigators found that 51 percent of the series reported at least one PCS at 6 weeks after injury. Nineteen patients (14.5 percent of the series) complained of at least one PCS at 1 year, including six patients who had one symptom, seven who had two symptoms, and six who reported between four and nine symptoms. Headache (8.4 percent), irritability (5.3 percent), and dizziness (4.6 percent) were the most common symptoms. In regard to the issue of the delayed onset of symptoms, Rutherford et al.[11,12] found that no patient who was symptom-free at 6 weeks reported symptoms at 1 year. The patients who reported PCSs at 1 year consisted of two subgroups, including 10 patients with new symptoms and 9 patients whose symptoms had been present at 6 weeks. Interestingly, 6 of the 10 patients reporting new symptoms at 1 year were involved in litigation. Apart from the patients with new symptoms, the findings by Rutherford et al. indicate PCSs in about 7 percent of patients 1 year after a mild head injury. In view of the prevailing level of similar symptoms in the general population,[8] the etiology of the symptoms reported by patients 1 year after a mild head injury is potentially compromised by intervening events. However, the clinical implications of persistent PCSs were supported by the recent findings by Bohnen et al.,[13] who showed that patients with PCSs persisting for about 6 months performed on attention tests at a level below that of a matched group of mild CHI patients whose PCSs had resolved. Pending replication of this provocative study based on small samples of patients, the interaction between PCSs and cognition may be a major factor in recovery.

PSYCHIATRIC SEQUELAE OF MILD HEAD INJURY

An elucidation of the risk factors for posttraumatic psychiatric disorders and the persistence of these sequelae require a longitudinal investigation of consecutively treated patients. Recent studies, which have used standard methods of psychosocial assessment, have shown that emotional disturbance is common after a mild head injury. Evidence for predisposing factors was provided by Fenton et al.,[14] who found that patients reported a mean of 3 stressful, adverse life events (i.e., illness in the family, moving, divorce) in the year preceding a mild head injury (which they defined according to a PTA duration of <24 h) compared with 1.5 adverse events in a control group taken from the waiting list of a general practitioner. However, the patients and controls did not differ in regard to preinjury psychopathology or social interactions as measured by standard instruments. According to the results of an objective examination for psychopathology administered at 6 weeks after injury, 16 (39 percent) of the head injury patients were identified as psychiatric cases (depression or anxiety states) compared with only 2 (4 percent) controls. Patients who developed depression or anxiety were on the average 10 years older and were more likely to be women than were control patients.

Postconcussional Symptoms in Relation to Psychiatric Sequelae

Fenton and coworkers[14] studied postconcussional symptoms in relation to psychiatric status at 6 weeks after injury as described above. Postconcussional symptoms, which were assessed by means of a symptom checklist at 6 weeks and 6 months, were associated with chronic social difficulties compared with patients whose PCSs had remitted. Fenton et al.[14] also found that persistence of PCSs at 6 months after injury was more common among patients who had been considered depressed or anxious at 6 weeks after injury.

The relationship between PCS and emotional disturbance was further investigated by Bohnen et al.,[15] who studied 71 patients who were consecutively admitted for mild head injury (i.e., unconscious for no longer than 15 min, PTA duration less than 60 min, and GCS score of 15). Of this series, 46 patients were considered to have sustained uncomplicated injuries, whereas 25 patients had a complication (multiple trauma, preexisting emotional problem, previous head injury, or intoxication at the time of injury). A checklist of PCSs was administered 6 to 14 days after injury and was repeated 5 weeks after injury. A principal components analysis (a statistical technique which identifies key dimensions or factors common to several outcome measures) disclosed that the PCS questionnaire items could be divided into postconcussive symptoms (e.g., headaches, dizziness, decreased cognitive status, and decreased work performance) and emotional-vegetative symptoms (e.g., depression, physical manifestations of anxiety). Bohnen et al.[15] found that the scores on both factors improved between the initial examination to the follow-up assessment. Among the complicated cases, patients with a previous head injury had higher scores on both the postconcussive and emotional-vegetative scales than did uncomplicated patients. Patients with preexisting emotional problems also had higher scores on the postconcussive and emotional-vegetative scales than did uncomplicated patients.

POSTACUTE MANAGEMENT

A review of the literature concerning the outcome of mild head injury has implications for the clinical management of postacute patients. Before discharge from the hospital or emergency room, educating the patient and family about the sequelae of and time course for recovery can mitigate secondary problems such as depression. Encouragement to gradually resume activities while refraining from taking on excessive workloads can diminish the frustration, anxiety, and depression surrounding a premature return to activities which involve difficult cognitive tasks and impose time pressure. Stress reduction techniques such as relaxation training are potentially useful, but no controlled studies support the efficacy of this type of intervention in head-injured patients. Informing patients that the first few weeks of convalescence are typically characterized by PCSs and reduced cognitive efficiency which subsequently resolve can be reassuring, particularly when the clinician also points out individual differences in the recovery curves and the contribution of extracerebral injury.

In view of the typical clinical course of improvement over 1 to 3 months, the delayed onset of PCSs can be a sign of depression when neurological complications and the effects of extracerebral injury are ruled out. While a premature return to work or school places the patient at risk for affective changes and persistent PCSs,[16] excessive absence and a focus on somatic complaints also can prolong the period of disability. Although referral for cognitive rehabilitation has been advocated for patients with persistent sequelae after a mild head injury, the efficacy of this treatment remains controversial. Unfortunately, terms such as "traumatic brain injury" and the practice of citing evidence for diffuse axonal injury[17] without placing it in perspective carry connotations which can intensify the somatic concerns of mildly head injured patients unless they are given accurate and complete prognostic information. Extended litigation also may prolong the patient's period of inactivity, increase the level of stress, and diminish the motivation for recovery.

References

1. Levin HS, Mattis S, Ruff R, et al: Neurobehavioral outcome following minor head injury: A three-center study. *J Neurosurg* 66:234–243, 1987.
2. Teasdale G, Jennett B: Assessment of coma and impaired consciousness: A practical scale. *Lancet* 2:81–84, 1974.
3. Rimel RW, Giordani B, Barth JT, et al: Disability caused by minor head injury. *Neurosurgery* 9:221–228, 1981.
4. Strang I, MacMillan R, Jennett B: Head injuries in accident and emergency departments at Scottish hospitals. *Injury* 10:154–159, 1978.
5. Kraus JF, Nourjah P: The epidemiology of mild, uncomplicated brain injury. *J Trauma* 28:1637–1643, 1988.
6. Hugenholtz H, Stuss DT, Stethem LL, et al: How long does it take to recover from a mild concussion? *Neurosurgery* 22:853–858, 1988.
7. Gentilini M, Nichelli P, Schoenhuber R, et al: Neuropsychological evaluation of mild head injury. *J Neurol Neurosurg Psychiatry* 48:137–140, 1985.
8. Dikmen S, McLean A, Temkin N: Neuropsychological and psychosocial consequences of minor head injury. *J Neurol* 49:1227–1232, 1986.
9. Gronwall D, Wrightson P: Delayed recovery of intellectual function after minor head injury. *Lancet* 2:605–609, 1974.
10. Gronwall D, Wrightson P: Memory and information processing capacity after closed head injury. *J Neurol Neurosurg Psychiatry* 44:889–895, 1981.
11. Rutherford WH, Merrett JD, McDonald JR: Sequelae of concussion caused by minor head injuries. *Lancet* 1:1–4, 1977.
12. Rutherford WH, Merrett JD, McDonald JR: Symptoms at one year following concussion from minor head injuries. *Injury* 10:225–230, 1979.
13. Bohnen N, Jolles J, Twijnstra A: Neuropsychological deficits in patients with persistent symptoms six months after mild head injury. *Neurosurgery* 30:692–695, 1992.
14. Fenton G, McClelland R, Montgomery A, et al: The postconcussional syndrome: Social antecedents and psychological sequelae. *Br J Psychiatry* 162:493–497, 1993.
15. Bohnen N, Twijnstra A, Jolles J: Post-traumatic and emotional symptoms in different subgroups of patients with mild head injury. *Brain Injury* 6:481–487, 1992.
16. Wrightson P, Gronwall D: Time off work and symptoms after minor head injury. *Injury* 12:445–454, 1981.
17. Oppenheimer DR: Microscopic lesions in the brain following head injury. *J Neurol Neurosurg Psychiatry* 31:299–306, 1968.

CHAPTER 51

OUTCOME FROM MODERATE HEAD INJURY

Sherman C. Stein

SYNOPSIS

Moderate head injury (MHI) has not been studied as extensively as either the severe or the mild ends of the severity spectrum. Although MHI has arbritarily been defined as a Glasgow Coma Scale (GCS) score of 9 to 12, a case is made in this chapter to include GCS 13 patients into the moderate rather than into the mild head injury group. Approximately 30 percent of MHI patients have intracranial lesions on CT scans, 3.8 to 10.6 percent require a craniotomy, and 10 to 20 percent deteriorate into coma. Only 60 percent of patients make a good recovery, 26 percent are moderately disabled and 7 percent are dead by 6 months. MHI patients may represent the group most likely to benefit from careful observation, invasive monitoring in selected cases, and newer medical therapies.

INTRODUCTION

Positioned as it is between milder and more severe forms of head trauma, moderate head injury (MHI) had seemingly elicited relatively little scientific interest.[1] A recent review of MHI[2] questions its continued existence, as commonly defined, as a separate category at all! Nevertheless, the clinical aspects of MHI from presentation to outcome comprise a distinct entity.

This chapter will review our experience with MHI[3] and offer a defense for the continued use of the moderate category, offer a practical definition and suggest a plan for management of these patients.

DEFINITIONS

Although a few would question MHI as having a severity or risk intermediate between minor and severe, the boundaries of this category have rarely been precisely defined. Some authorities have relied on the duration of unconsciousness or post-traumatic amnesia,[4] but most systems are based on an interval of Glasgow Coma Scale (GCS) scores.[5] However, there is little agreement as to what time after admission the category is assigned[1,6] or whether other clinical events are necessary for a given head injury to be considered moderate.[7–9] Some authors have even recommended changes in the commonly accepted GCS interval of 9 to 12.[2,3] Table 51-1 summarizes these definitions of MHI. Although many of these definitions are significant for research purposes, most require 6 to 48 hours of observation before a category can be assigned. Hence, they are of little value in directing patient management.

In previous publications,[3,10] it has been advocated that, in terms of the incidence of intracranial complications and the need for neurosurgical attention, patients admitted after head injury with a GCS of 13 have more in common with the moderate than the minor head injury category. This chapter thus defines MHI as a GCS of 9 to 13 at the time of hospital admission.

TABLE 51-1 Definitions of Moderate Head Injury (MHI)

	Glasgow Coma Scale (GCS) Score			
Authors	**Lowest**	**Highest**	**Time Determined**	**Other Requirements**
Annegers et al, 1980[4]	—	—	—	Loss of consciousness or post-traumatic amnesia 0.5 to 24 hours
Rimel et al, 1982[1]	9	12	6 hours after admission	—
Tabbador et al, 1984[6]	9	11	if lowest score first 48 hours	—
Kraus et al, 1984[7]	9	12	admission	Hospital stay ≥ 48 hours, or abnormal CT scan or intracranial surgery
Levin et al, 1988[8]	9	12*	admission	*Focal deficit, or intracranial lesion on CT, depressed fracture with dural tear or intracranial surgery
Miller and Jones, 1989[14]	9	12	admission	—
Eisenberg, 1989[51]	9	12*	admission	GCS never below 9 *intracranial complications
Williams et al, 1990[9]	9	12	admission	GCS never below 9
Colohan and Oyesiku, 1992[2]	6	10	—	—
Stein and Ross, 1992[3]	9	13	admission	—

* If GCS > 12, must have at least 1 other requirement.

EPIDEMIOLOGY

Incidence

The incidence of MHI varies from 7 to 28 percent of all head injuries,[3,4,7,11,12] largely depending on whether the source of the data is a population- or hospital-based study.

Demographics

According to Rimel and associates,[1] the patient population is 77 percent male, has a mean of age 33, and a mean blood alcohol level of 0.14 g/dl, 79 percent of the patients having detectable blood alcohol levels. In 42 percent there is a history of prior head injury, 34 percent have a history of alcohol abuse, and 21 percent are chronically unemployed. The demographics from a recent series of 477 MHI patients from our institution are provided in Tables 51.2 and 51.3. There are many more children in our series in that of Rimel,[1] perhaps reflecting the greater proportion of children riding in cars and running on the streets in our predominantly urban and suburban geographical area. Most other epidemiological details agree closely with the exhaustive population review of San Diego County by Kraus and Arzenanian[13] and a survey of hospitalized patients in Edinburgh, Scotland, performed by Miller and Jones.[14]

TABLE 51-2 Mechanism of Trauma in Moderate Head Injury

Mechanism	% Incidence
Motor vehicle accident	42
Motor vehicle vs. pedestrian or bike	22
Fall	20
Sports accident, other	5
Assault	11

Unique Features of MHI

One might speculate about what makes MHI unique. The high incidence of alcohol intoxication could contribute to the relatively low GCS in patients whose head injury might otherwise be minor. The relatively high incidence of intracranial hematoma may also be a factor

TABLE 51-3 Age Distribution of Moderate Head Injuries

Age (yrs)	Number	%
0–9	107	23.9
10–19	68	15.2
20–29	103	23.0
30–39	76	17.0
40–49	32	7.2
50–59	29	6.5
60–69	15	3.4
70+	17	3.8
Total	447	100.0

TABLE 51-4 Incidence of Abnormal Computerized Tomography Scans in Moderate Head Injury

Glasgow Coma Scale Score	No. of Cases	*Cases with Abnormal Scans* No.	Percent
13	106	47	44.3
12	80	28	35.0
11	113	38	33.6
10	83	32	38.6
9	65	35	53.8
totals	447	180	40.3

Reprinted with permission from: Stein SC, Ross SE: Moderate head injury: A guide to initial management. *J Neurosurg* 1992; 77:562–564.

(Table 51-4). One theory to explain the high incidence of intracranial hematoma is that patients, whose initial trauma might appear mild, develop swelling or evolving hematomas associated with their intracranial lesions, and arrive at the hospital later than those in whom the initial impact was great enough to cause impaired consciousness. However, the mean time between injury and arrival was 85.2 minutes for the 33 intracranial hematoma patients in our series versus 89.9 minutes for the other MHI patients.

There are several ways to derive a given total score from the three components of the GCS. Pitts has already pointed out that the mathematical possibilities are greatest toward the center of the scale.[15] This is exactly where the MHI category lies. Therefore, this patient group is most likely to be heterogeneous, and this heterogeneity is likely to complicate categorization.

PATHOLOGY

Pathophysiology

The biochemical and pathophysiological mediators of MHI have been studied intensively in the laboratory setting. In addition to contusions and hematomas, vascular permeability changes; axonal dysfunction; alterations of high-energy metabolites, acid-base balance, and magnesium; abnormal neurotransmitter-receptor interactions; heightened vulnerability to ischemia; and other possible mechanisms may all play a role in the cerebral dysfunction associated with MHI.[2,16,17]

Clinical

A variety of cerebral lesions are reported in MHI patients who come to autopsy.[18] The sorts of lesions encountered are roughly in the same proportions as those seen on a CT scan.

CT scans

Rimel reported intracranial abnormalities in 70 percent of their MHI patients in whom a CT scan was obtained.[1] However, CT scans were performed in only 38 percent of the MHI group, presumably those patients with the most abnormal clinical pictures. As the GCS score decreased, Rimel found an increasing incidence of CT scan abnormalities.

In a series of MHI patients, all of whom had admis-

TABLE 51-5 Lesions Seen on Computerized Tomography Scans in Moderate Head Injury

Lesion	*Glasgow Coma Scale Score* 9	10	11	12	13	Total Cases (N)	%
Fracture							
linear	3	7	9	4	6	29	13.2
basilar	5	2	3	5	5	20	9.1
depressed	2	2	3	1	7	15	6.8
Subarachnoid or intraventricular hemorrhage	6	4	5	2	6	23	10.5
Brain swelling	7	4	9	4	4	28	12.7
Cerebral contusion	14	12	12	11	23	72	32.7
Hematoma							
intracerebral	3	6	0	2	2	13	5.9
subdural	3	2	0	3	4	12	5.5
epidural	2	0	0	1	5	8	3.6
						220	

Reprinted with permission from: Stein SC, Ross SE: Moderate head injury: A guide to initial management. *J Neurosurg* 77:562–564, 1992

TABLE 51-6 Acute Sequelae of Moderate Head Injury

	Glasgow Coma Scale Score					Entire Series
	9	**10**	**11**	**12**	**13**	
Number	65	83	113	80	106	447
% Needing Craniotomy, fracture elevation	4.6	2.4	2.6	1.2	7.5	3.8
% Needing ICP monitor	6.1	1.2	3.5	2.5	7.5	4.3
% Hospital deaths	1.5	1.2	0	1.2	0.9	0.9

sion CT scans, Stein and Ross[3] found intracranial abnormalities in almost 31 percent and skull fractures in an additional 10 percent (Tables 51-4, 51-5). The high abnormality rate associated with a GCS of 13 justifies its inclusion in MHI.

Skull Fracture

Skull fracture has been suggested as a harbinger of intracranial pathology.[19] Indeed, some recent reviews of minor head injury have promoted skull radiography as a screening test prior to CT scanning.[20,21] Among our patients, 42 percent of the 64 with skull fractures had associated intracranial lesions. However, only 20 percent of the 137 patients harboring intracranial abnormalities on CT had a skull fracture, a fact that clearly limits the predictive value of skull radiographs.

SEQUELAE

Acute

Twenty-one percent of patients presenting with MHI on admission will improve to a mild level within 6 hours.[1] The incidences of surgical intervention, deterioration to coma, intracranial pressure monitoring, and mortality among our patients are summarized in Table 51-6. These numbers differ from those of Rimel and associates[1] (Table 51-7). Their higher incidence of CT scan abnormality is probably the result of restricting scans to the most seriously ill patients as opposed to our approach in which all patients were scanned. A similar explanation can be invoked for why more of Rimel's patients required surgical intervention and intracranial pressure monitoring and had a higher mortality. Rimel required that the patient's GCS be 9 to 12 at 6 hours following hospital admission, whereas our MHI population was identified on admission. Hence, they were dealing with a more seriously ill group of patients.

Delayed and Progressive Brain Injuries

Evidence from experimental studies,[22] autopsies,[23] and serial CT scans[24,25] of head-injured humans has supported the presence of progressive pathological changes that begin minutes to hours after the primary impact. Several biochemical and vascular insults have been hypothesized to play important roles in the process. Potential toxins in head trauma include excitatory neurotransmitters,[26] histamine,[27] bradykinin,[28] arachidonic acid,[29] free radicals,[30] leukotrienes,[31] serotonin,[32] cerebral acidosis,[33] intracellular calcium, and other factors.[34]

TABLE 51-7 Acute Sequelae for Moderate Head Injury: Comparison of Two Series

	Rimel et al, 1982[1]	Stein and Ross, 1992[3]
Number	199	447
% Cranial CT scan	37.2	100.0
% Abnormal CT scan	68.9	40.3
% Cranial surgery	10.6	3.8
% ICP monitor	17.6	4.3
% With second CT scan	—	49.6
% Worsening second CT scan	—	32.5
% Hospital deaths	2.5	0.9

TABLE 51-8 Delayed and Progressive Brain Lesions in Moderate Head Injury: CT Scan Evidence

	Glasgow Coma Scale Score					
	9	**10**	**11**	**12**	**13**	**Entire Series**
Number	65	83	113	80	106	447
% Needing second CT scan	73.8	49.4	33.6	40.0	59.4	49.6
% Worsening on second scan	37.5	22.0	18.9	21.9	49.2	32.4

The blood brain barrier can be disrupted by direct injury or secondary to many of the above toxins.[35] The release of platelet activating factor,[36] traumatic vasospasm,[37] or the effects of disseminated intravascular coagulation[24] can cause secondary brain insults. There is increased vulnerability to secondary ischemia after moderate head injury.[38] Some of these mechansims are discussed in relation to moderate head injury by Colohan and Oyesiku[2] and by McIntosh and Vink.[17]

There is clinical evidence to support the concept of delayed brain damage in moderate head injury. We studied serial CT scans in a number of patients with moderate and severe head injury[25] and found progressive clinical and radiological changes in many (Table 51-8).

Case reports

Two examples of patients with delayed and progressive cerebral lesions following MHI are shown in Figs. 51-1 and 51-2.

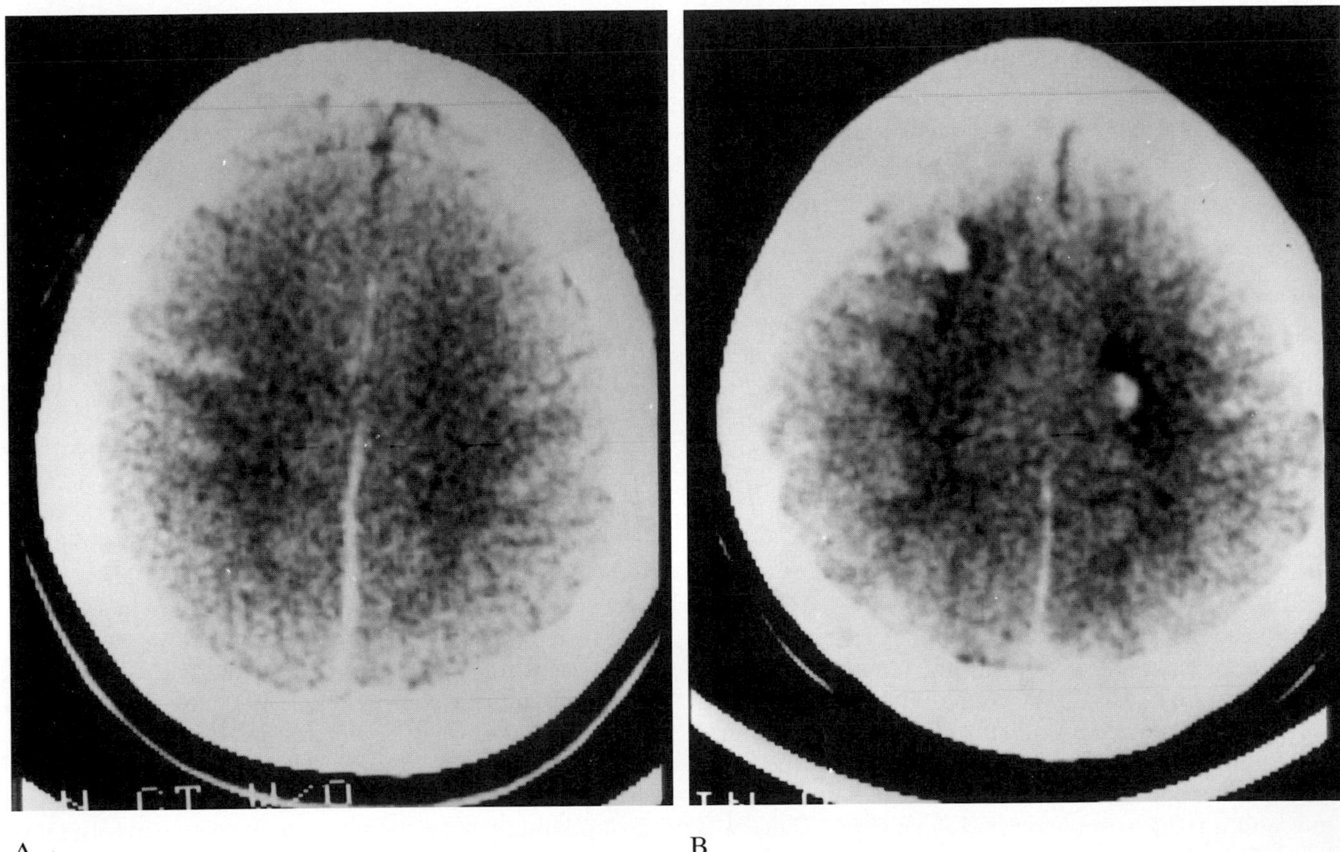

A B

Figure 51-1. *Case 1:* Delayed brain injury. *A.* CT scan on admission shows subarachnoid hemorrhage. *B.* Twelve hours later there are multiple intracerebral hematomas.

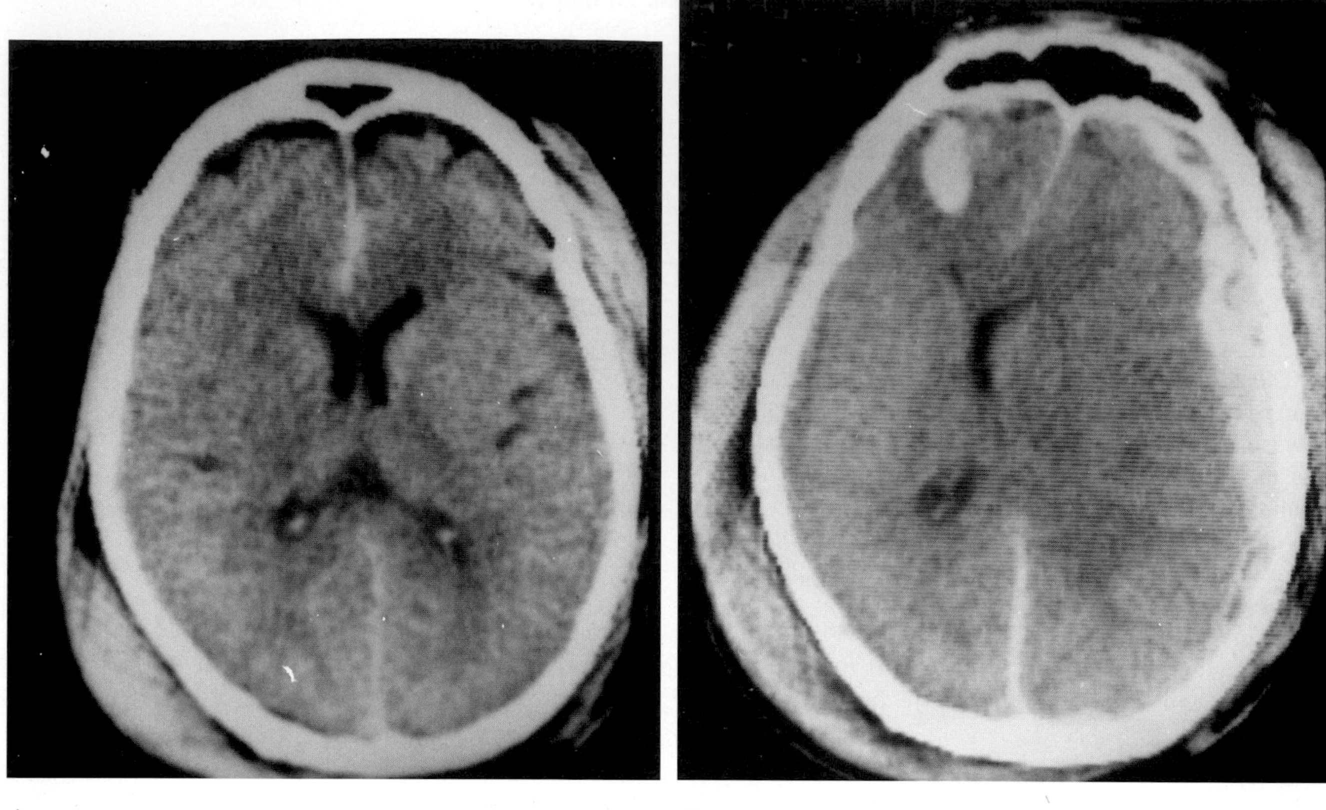

Figure 51-2. *Case 2:* Delayed and progressive brain injuries. *A.* CT scan on admission shows a small interhemispheric subdural hematoma and cerebral atrophy. *B.* Six hours after admission, a large left subdural hematoma and right frontal intracerebral hematoma are evident.

Case 1

This 18-year-old driver, who was not wearing restraints, was involved in a motor vehicle accident. Consciousness was briefly lost, but the GCS score on admission was 13. On initial CT scan, subarachnoid hemorrhage was noted. Twelve hours later, the patient's GCS dropped to 7. Two intracerebral hematomas with surrounding edema were evident, and several more were seen on adjacent slices of the CT scan (Fig. 51-1).

Case 2

A 58-year-old man fell down a flight of stairs. He did not lose consciousness, but did not remember the fall. Admission GCS was 13. A cranial CT scan performed on admission showed a small interhemispheric subdural hematoma and cerebral atrophy. There was no skull fracture. Six hours later, the patient's GCS had dropped to 6 and a right hemiplegia had developed. There was now a large left subdural hematoma and a right frontal intracerebral hematoma (Fig. 51-2).

Chronic

General outcome

Relatively early outcome factors, such as hospital mortality, average length of hospital, stay, and need for a chronic care facility are shown in Table 51-9. Six-month Glasgow Outcome Scale (GOS)[39] determinations were obtained in over 87 percent of the 447 cases (Table 51-10). Sixty percent of the patients made a good recovery, and another 26 percent had moderate disability at 6 months. Approximately 7 percent of the patients had severe disability. There was only one patient in a vegetative state at 6 months, and the combined vegetative and dead cases were just above 7 percent of the total.

Our results are comparable to the outcomes reported by Rimel.[1] Although 38 percent of their patients made a good recovery by 3 months after injury, only 4 percent were symptom-free. Williams and associates[9] reported 55 moderately head-injured patients with 6 month GOS determinations. Seventy-three percent of the patients had made a good recovery, and the rest experienced

TABLE 51-9 Early Outcome in Moderate Head Injury

	Glasgow Coma Scale Score					Entire Series
	9	10	11	12	13	
Mean length of stay (days)	10.5	10.5	7.3	15.4	11.2	10.7
% Hospital mortality	1.5	1.2	0	1.2	0.9	0.9
% Needing inpatient rehab or nursing home	18.5	15.7	12.4	13.7	17.0	15.5

moderate disability. A small group of moderate head injuries reported from the Medical College of Virginia[40] showed a similar incidence of moderate and severe disability.

Neurobehavioral Outcome

Every investigation of performance on neuropsychological test batteries following MHI has shown frequent and profound impairments. Where comparisons are made to mild head injury, patients with MHI recover less rapidly and less completely. One month after trauma, at which time neuropsychological functions of most mild head injury patients have returned to normal, test performances in MHI have been shown to be still quite impaired.[41,42] Scores remain abnormal on most neuropsychological batteries at 3 months[1,40] and many abnormalities persist at 6 months and beyond.[6,9,40] Memory function is particularly slow to recover,[6,8] as is rapidity with which tests can be performed.[43] Return to work has been reported at 31 percent at 3 months after injury.[1] Fifty percent of MHI patients have some emotional or behavioral sequelae at 1 year after injury;[44] subtle problems can persist even longer.[45,46] Levin provides an excellent review of neurobehavioral outcome in MHI.[47]

Recovery from Abnormal Neurodiagnostic Studies

Lesions on CT scan often clear rather quickly, leaving atrophy or a normal appearing brain in their place. This may occur before clinical recovery has even begun. No comprehensive data are available concerning the frequency of parenchymal lesions on MRI scans of patients with MHI, but they are seen with much greater frequency than on CT scan.[48] Recovery from these lesions appears to parallel functional improvement. Cortical evoked responses may remain abnormal for months following MHI.[49–51]

DETERMINANTS OF OUTCOME

Admission Glasgow Coma Scale

Rimel[1] reported a strong association between the GCS at 6 hours after trauma and a variety of outcome parameters. An analysis of these data by Colohan and Oye-

TABLE 51-10 Late Outcome in Moderate Head Injury

	Glasgow Coma Scale Score					Entire Series
	9	10	11	12	13	
Number	65	83	113	80	106	447
Number with 6-month follow-up	57	74	94	64	101	390
	Glasgow Outcome Scale at 6 months					
% Good recovery	68.4	62.2	60.6	64.1	50.5	60.0
% Moderate disability	7.0	23.0	26.6	29.7	35.6	25.9
% Severe disability	17.5	2.7	4.3	4.7	7.9	6.9
% Vegetative/Dead	7.0	12.2	8.5	1.6	5.9	7.2

TABLE 51-11 Effect of Intracranial Complications on Acute Sequelae of Moderate Head Injury

	Initial CT Scan		
	Normal	Abnormal	* Difference (P Value)
Number	310	137	—
% Craniotomy	0	12.4	$p < .001$
% ICP monitor	0	13.9	$p < .001$
% Needing second CT scan	28.1	98.5	$p < .001$
% Worsening on second CT scan	4.5	42.3	$p < .001$
% Hospital deaths	0	2.9	$p < .025$

* Calculated using Chi square (df = 1) with Yates correction coefficient

siku[2] led them to conclude that there is "an apparent dichotomy within the MHI category." They recommended a reclassification of head injury, incorporating patients with a GCS of 9 or 10 with more severe injuries and those whose GCS is 11 or 12 with mild head injury."

However, if admission GCS is used and patients whose GCS is 13 are included as MHI, no such dichotomy is evident. Whether the incidence of intracranial complications is examined (Table 51-5), the need for neurosurgical intervention (Table 51-6), the risk of delayed brain injury (Table 51-8), early outcome parameters (Table 51-9) or late outcome (Table 51-10), admission GCS scores of 9 and 13 are consistently more ominous than are the intervening scores of 10 to 12. The reason for this is not readily apparent; perhaps patients with GCS scores of 9 and 13 represent two distinct populations. The relatively high incidence of intracranial lesions in both groups would contribute to the poor outcome. Patients admitted with a GCS score of 9 may have suffered more cerebral dysfunction at impact, while those with a score of 13 may be beginning to deteriorate from intracranial masses and delayed cerebral insults. Patients with GCS scores of 10 to 12 may be suffering more from the effects of alcohol, a common condition accompanying MHI.[1,52,53]

Intracranial Complications

Table 51-11 compares acute sequelae in 137 patients with intracranial complications (intracranial abnormalities on admission CT scan) against the 310 in whom the CT scan was normal or showed only skull fractures. Patients with intracranial complications had significantly greater risks of requiring surgical intervention, of developing delayed cerebral insults, and of dying before hospital discharge. Similarly, long-term outcome, as determined by the GOS at 6 months, is significantly worse in the group with intracranial complications (Table 51-12).

Rimel et al.[1] reported dismal outcomes in their MHI patients who harbored intracranial hematomas. Levin and his associates found a strong association between several lesions on MRI scan and neurobehavioral impairments in MHI.[48] The presence or absence of intracranial complications may represent the true dichotomy within the MHI category.

Delayed and Progressive Cerebral Injury

Previous work at our institution supports a strong correlation between the presence of delayed and progressive brain lesions as seen on CT scan and poor outcome.[25] This relationship held across the spectrum of head-injury severity and included a moderate head injury group.

Table 51-13 confirms this relationship for MHI. Of the 447 MHI patients, 222 required follow-up CT scan. This was usually to follow lesions noted on the initial CT scan, for clinical deterioration, or for failure to improve at the expected rate. There were 193 patients in whom follow-up information was available 6 months after injury. Almost all the poor outcomes were in the group exhibiting delayed injury, and almost all the good

TABLE 51-12 Effect of Intracranial Complications on Longterm Outcome in Moderate Head Injury

	Initial CT Scan	
	Normal	Abnormal
Number	310	137
Glasgow Outcome Scale at six months:		
% Good recovery	63.5	27.0
% Moderate disability	22.2	23.3
% Severe disability	1.9	19.7
% Vegetative/dead	1.0	18.2
% Unknown	11.3	16.0

Difference calculated using Chi square test (df = 3) $p < .001$

TABLE 51-13 Delayed Brain Lesions and Outcome in Moderate Head Injury

	Progressive Changes on Serial CT Scans	
	Absent	**Present**
Number	150	72
Glasgow Outcome Scale at 6 months		
% Good recovery	65.3	2.8
% Moderate disability	19.3	27.8
% Severe disability	0.7	22.2
% Vegetative/dead	0	37.5
% Unknown	14.7	9.7

Difference calculated using Chi square test (df = 3), $p < .001$

recoveries were in the group without delayed injury. These differences are highly significant ($p < .001$).

Patient Age and Other Factors

Advancing age is associated with a worse prognosis after MHI (Table 51-14). The number of patients is too small to demonstrate statistical significance as plotted. However, if good recovery versus moderate disability or worse is compared in patients above and below the age of 40 years, a significant association emerges between age and outcome ($p < .01$). Other investigators have commented on the influence of age on outcome in MHI[52,53] and have also noted an association between outcome and alcohol abuse, prior head injury, and severe non-neurological injury.

PATIENT MANAGEMENT

The emergency room or trauma physician first encountering the patient with MHI should be aware of the high risk of intracranial complications and the frequency with which neurosurgical intervention is required in this group. Many authorities recommend skull radiography on admission to determine the need for urgent CT scanning in MHI.[14] This author believes that the frequency with which cerebral lesions can occur in MHI without skull fracture is high enough to justify urgent CT scanning as the initial diagnostic test. Therefore, every patient with MHI must be treated at a center that has immediate access to CT and to neurosurgical consultation. If the CT scan is normal or shows only skull fracture, the patient may be admitted for a brief period of observation. Intracranial abnormalities on CT scan require immediate neurosurgical consultation and treatment in a critical care unit. Over 25 percent of such patients require neurosurgical intervention, and 40 percent will develop delayed brain injury (Table 51-11). Any patient who deteriorates clinically or fails to improve to a GCS of 14 or 15 within 12 hours of injury should have a follow-up CT scan.

An additional advantage of identifying MHI patients with intracranial lesions on CT scans is the high incidence of persistent neurobehavioral problems in this group (Table 51-12).[47] It has been recommended that counseling and psychological interventions be focused on these high-risk patients to attempt to lessen persisting disability.[54,55] Several promising, pharmacological agents have been introduced to minimize or prevent delayed brain injury,[17,56–58] and trials have begun for some of these agents in patients who have sustained MHI (Chap. 27). It is hoped that appropriate and early pharmacological intervention will improve outcome in MHI, particularly in those patients with intracranial complications and delayed brain injury.

CONCLUSIONS

MHI is a distinct category of head injury in terms of degree of brain dysfunction, risk of intracranial compli-

TABLE 51-14 Age and Outcome in Moderate Head Injury

	Age Interval (Yrs)			
	0–19	**20–39**	**40–59**	**60+**
Number with 6 months GOS	158	154	49	29
GOS at 6 months				
% Good recovery	67.7	60.4	55.1	24.1
% Moderate disability	26.6	27.9	26.5	10.3
% Severe disability	3.8	9.7	6.1	10.3
% Vegetative/dead	1.9	1.9	12.2	55.2

cations, and short- and long-term outcome. Since all these indices are similar over the range of GCS Scores from 9 to 13, this interval is most appropriate. Furthermore, because of the need to make patient management decisions at or soon after admission, the category should be assigned at that time.

Complications of MHI are common and frequently major. Thirty percent of the patients have intracranial lesions on CT scan. Almost half of the patients require a second CT scan on clinical grounds, and one-third of these show delayed or progressive cerebral lesions. In two series, the proportion of MHI patients that required a craniotomy was 3.8 percent and 10.6 percent. The proportion that underwent ICP monitoring in the same two series was 4.3 percent and 17.6 percent. Mortality during the initial hospitalization ranges between 0.9 to 2.5 percent, but 15 percent of the patients require an extended care facility, and only 60 percent have made a good recovery by 6 months. Almost 70 percent are unable to return to work within 3 months after their head injury. Intracranial complications on CT scan, whether immediate or delayed, are associated with a much worse outcome. The overall 6 month mortality figure in our series was approximately 7 percent.

All patients with MHI should be treated in a hospital where immediate CT scanning and neurosurgical consultation are available, and all such patients deserve urgent CT scans on admission. Those with intracranial lesions should have urgent neurosurgical consultation and admission to critical care units. Some promising pharmacological interventions are being tested in an effort to improve eventual function in this group of patients.

ACKNOWLEDGMENTS

The author wishes to thank the Institute of Brain Injury Research and Training at Mediplex Rehab-Camden for its support. Valuable help in data collection was provided by Jeff Comito, B.A., and Mary Lou Thelmo, B.S., M.P.H.

REFERENCES

1. Rimel RW, Giordani B, Barth JT, et al: Moderate head injury: Completing the clinical spectrum of brain trauma. *Neurosurgery* 1982; 11:344–351.
2. Colohan ART, Oyesiku NM: Moderate head injury: An overview. *J Neurotrauma* 1992; 9(suppl.) S259–S264.
3. Stein SC, Ross SE: Moderate head injury: A guide to initial management. *J Neurosurg* 1992; 77:562–564.
4. Annegers JF, Grabow JD, Kurland LT, et al: The incidence, causes and secular trends of head trauma in Olmstead County, Minnesota, 1935–1974. *Neurology* 1980; 30:912–919.
5. Teasdale G, Jennett B: Assessment of coma and impaired consciousness. A practical scale. *Lancet* 1974; 2:81–83.
6. Tabaddor K, Mattis S, Zazula T: Cognitive sequelae and recovery course after moderate and severe head injury. *Neurosurgery* 1984; 14:701–708.
7. Kraus JF, Black MA, Hessol N, et al: The incidence of acute brain injury and serious impairment in a defined population. *Am J Epidemiol* 1984; 119:186–201.
8. Levin HS, Goldstein FC, High WM Jr, et al: Disproportionately severe memory deficit in relation to normal intellectual functioning after closed head injury. *J Neurol Neurosurg Psychiatry* 1988; 51:1294–1301.
9. Williams DH, Levin HS, Eisenberg HM: Mild head injury classification. *Neurosurgery* 1990; 27:422–428.
10. Stein SC, Ross SE: The value of computed tomographic scans in patients with low-risk head injuries. *Neurosurgery* 1990; 26:638–640.
11. Frankowski RF: Descriptive epidemiological studies of head injury in the United States, 1974–84. *Adv Psychosom Med* 1986; 16:163.
12. Whitman S, Coonley-Hoganson R, Desai BT: Comparative head trauma experiences in two socioeconomically different Chicago-area communities—a population study. *Am J Epidemiol* 1984; 119:570–580.
13. Kraus JF, Kraus JF, Arzemanian S: Epidemiologic features of mild and moderate head injury, in Hoff JT, Anderson TE, Cole TM (eds): *Mild to Moderate Head Injury*. Boston: Blackwell Scientific, 1989:9–28.
14. Miller JD, Jones PA: Management aspects of mild and moderate head injury. *Ibid*:117–124.
15. Pitts LH: Clinical diagnosis of mild to moderate head injury. *Ibid*:107–113.
16. Jenkins LW, Lyeth BG, Hayes RL: The role of agonist-receptor interactions in the pathophysiology of mild and moderate head injury. *Ibid*:47–61.
17. McIntosh TK, Vink R: Biochemical and pathophysiological medianism in mild to moderate traumatic brain injury. *Ibid*:35–46.
18. Graham DI, Lawrence AE, Adams JH, et al: Pathology of mild head injury. *Ibid*:63–75.
19. Miller JD, Murray LS, Teasdale GM: Development of a traumatic intracranial hematoma after a "minor" head injury. *Neurosurgery* 1990; 27:669–673.
20. Servadei F, Vergoni G, Nasi MT, et al.: Management of low-risk head injuries in an entire area: Results of an 18-month survey. *Surg Neurol* 1993; 39:269–275.
21. Reinus WR, Wippold FJ II, Erickson KK: Practical selection criteria for noncontrast cranial computed tomography in patients with head trauma. *Ann Emerg Med* 1993; 22:1148–1155.
22. Baethmann A, Kempski O, Schurer L (eds): *Mechanisms of Secondary Brain Damage. Current State.* Vienna: Springer-Verlag, 1993.
23. Graham DI, Adams JH, Doyle D, et al: Quantification of primary and secondary lesions in severe head injury. *Acta Neurochir* 1993; (Suppl.) 57:41–48.

24. Stein SC, Young GS, Talucci RC, et al: Delayed brain injury following head trauma: Significance of coagulopathy. *Neurosurgery* 1992; 30:160–165.
25. Stein SC, Spettell C, Young GS, et al: Delayed and progressive brain injury in closed-head trauma: Radiological demonstration. *Neurosurgery* 1993; 32:25–31.
26. Hayes RL, Jenkins LW, Lyeth BG: Neurotransmitter-mediated mechanisms of traumatic brain injury: Acetylcholine and excitatory amino acids. *J Neurotrauma* 1992; 9(Suppl 1):S173–S187.
27. Orr EL: Cryogenic lesions induce a mast cell-dependent increase in cerebral histamine levels in the mouse. *Neurochem Pathol* 1988; 8:43–51.
28. Unterberg A, Dautermann C, Baethmann A, et al: The kallikrein-kinin system as a mediator in vasogenic brain edema. *J Neurosurg* 1986; 64:269–276.
29. Baethmann A, Maier-Hauff K, Schurer L, et al: Release of glutamate and of free fatty acids in vasogenic brain edema. *J Neurosurg* 1989; 70:578–591.
30. Chan PH, Longar S, Fishman RA: Protective effects of liposome-entrapped superoxide dismutase on posttraumatic brain edema. *Ann Neurol* 1987; 21:540–547.
31. Moskowitz MA, Kiwak KJ, Hekimian K, et al: Synthesis of compounds with properties of leukotrienes C_4 and D_4 in gerbil brains after ischemia and reperfusion. *Science* 1984; 224:886–889.
32. Pappius HM, Dadoun R: Effects of injury on the indoleamines in cerebral cortex. *J Neurochem* 1987; 49:321–335.
33. Marmarou A, Holdaway R, Ward JD, et al: Traumatic brain tissue acidosis: Experimental and clinical studies. *Acta Neurochir* 1993; (Suppl) 57:160–164.
34. Hallenbeck JM, Dutka AJ: Background review and current concepts of reperfusion injury. *Arch Neurol* 1990; 47:1245–1254.
35. Wahl M, Schilling L, Unterberg A, et al: Mediators of vascular and parenchymal mechanisms in secondary brain damage. *Acta Neurochir* 1993; (Suppl) 57:64–72.
36. Frerichs KU, Lindsberg PJ, Hallenbeck JM, et al: Platelet-activating factor and progressive brain damage following focal brain injury. *J Neurosurg* 1990; 73:223–233.
37. Compton JS, Teddy PJ: Cerebral arterial vasospasm following severe head injury: A transcranial Doppler study. *Br J Neurosurg* 1987; 1:435–439.
38. Jenkins LW, Marmarou A, Lewelt W, et al: Increased vunerability of the traumatized brain to early ischemia, in Baethmann A, Go KG, Unterberg A (eds): *Mechanisms of Secondary Brain Damage.* New York: Plenum Press, 1986:273–281.
39. Jennett B, Bond M: Assessment of outcome after severe brain damage. *Lancet* 1975; 1:480–484.
40. Clifton GL, Kreutzer JS, Choi SC, et al: Relationship between Glasgow Outcome Scale and neuropsychological measures after brain injury. *Neurosurgery* 1993; 33:34–39.
41. Gronwall D, Wrightson P: Delayed recovery of intellectual function after minor head injury. *Lancet* 1974; 2:605–609.
42. Dickman S, McLean A, Temkin NR: Neuropsychological outcome at one month post head injury. *Arch Phys Med Rehab* 1966; 67:507–513.
43. Van Zomeren AH, Deelman BG: Long term recovery of visual reaction time after closed head injury. *J Neurol Neurosurg Psychiatry* 1978; 41:452–457.
44. Middelboe T, Andersen HS, Birket-Smith M, et al: Minor head injury: Impact on general health after 1 year. A prospective follow-up study. *Acta Neurol Scand* 1992; 85:5–9.
45. Rappaport M, Herrero-Backe C, Rappaport ML, et al: Head injury outcome up to ten years later. *Arch Phys Med Rehabil* 1989; 70:885–892.
46. Stuss DT, Ely P, Hugenholtz H, et al: Subtle neuropsychological deficits in patients with good recovery after closed head injury. *Neurosurgery* 1985; 17:41–47.
47. Levin HS: Neurobehavioral outcome of mild to moderate head injury, in Hoff JT, Anderson TE, Cole TM (eds): *Mild to Moderate Head Injury.* Boston: Blackwell Scientific, 1989:153–185.
48. Levin HS, Williams DH, Eisenberg HM, et al: Serial MRI and neurobehavioral findings after mild to moderate closed head injury. *J Neurol Neurosurg Psychiatry* 1992; 55:255–262.
49. Noseworthy JH, Miller I, Murray TJ, et al: Auditory brainstem responses in postconcussion syndrome. *Arch Neurol* 1981; 38:275–278.
50. Papanicolaou AC, Levin HS, Eisenberg HM, et al: Evoked potential correlates of posttraumatic amnesia after closed head injury. *Neurosurgery* 1984; 14:676–678.
51. Montgomery EA, Fenton GW, McClelland RJ, et al: The psychobiology of minor head injury. *Psychol Med* 1991; 21:375–384.
52. Miller JD, Pentland B: The factors of age, alcohol and multiple injury in patients with mild and moderate head injury, in Hoff JT, Anderson TE, Cole TM (eds): *Mild to Moderate Head Injury.* Boston: Blackwell Scientific, 1989:125–133.
53. Berrol S: Other factors: age, alcohol and multiple injuries. *Ibid*:135–142.
54. Teasdale G: Workshop Consensus: Clinical management of mild to moderate head injury. *Ibid:*227–229.
55. Sahgal V, Heinemann A: Recovery of function during impatient rehabilitation for moderate traumatic brain injury. *Scand J Rehabil Med* 1989; 21:71–79.
56. Povlishock J: Workshop consensus: Neurochemistry and neuropathology of mild to moderate head injury. Op. cit., chap 17, pp. 219–225.
57. Muizelaar JP, Marmarou A, Young HF, et al: Improving the outcome of severe head injury with oxygen radical scavenger polyethylene glycol-conjugated superoxide dismutase: A Phase II trial. *J Neurosurg* 1993; 78:375–382.
58. Garcia JH: Prehospital management of head injuries: International perspectives. *Acta Neurochir* 1993; (Suppl) 57:145–151.

CHAPTER 52

OUTCOME FROM SEVERE HEAD INJURY

Donald W. Marion

SYNOPSIS

During the last two decades, elucidation of the pathophysiology of severe traumatic brain injury (TBI) has led to a substantial improvement in the quality of acute care provided to these patients and has resulted in improved outcomes. Several recent clinical trials suggest that effective treatment of secondary brain injury will result in further improvement in outcomes. The severity of TBI has been correlated with acute changes in cerebral blood flow, cerebral oxygen extraction, conduction of evoked potentials, release of neurochemicals into the cerebrospinal fluid, as well as numerous clinical variables. These findings have been used to support early prognostication following TBI. However, early predictions of outcome are often inaccurate except in the most severely injured. Future studies must focus on improving the cognitive and neuropsychological deficits that are common following injury.

INTRODUCTION

The evolution of modern acute care for severe traumatic brain injury (TBI) can be traced through the outcomes of several major series reported during the last 25 to 30 years (Fig. 52-1). Interpretation of outcomes in the earliest series suffered from a lack of standardization in outcome measures or even entry criteria. It was not until Jennett and Teasdale developed the Glasgow Coma Scale (GCS) in 1974 that a common system for the initial evaluation of TBI patients was recognized.[111] Several years later these investigators devised the Glasgow Outcome Scale score (GOS), which has become the most frequently used objective determination of outcome.[46]

In the last two decades, many of the pathophysiological changes caused by TBI have been defined, and standardized high-quality systems of triage and acute care for these patients have been developed. Nonetheless, most victims of severe TBI still cannot function normally months or years after the injury. Many patients described as having made a "good recovery" based on the GOS undergo substantial personality changes that disrupt family relationships and careers.[9,38,39]

The authors of the GOS cautioned that outcome analysis should assess physical and mental disabilities separately, and that the overall social consequence of the injury also should be determined.[49] Indeed, it is the more subtle cognitive and neuropsychological deficits suffered 1 year or more after a TBI that determines the victim's true ability to function normally at work and enjoy life.[59] Neuropsychological recovery from severe TBI usually lags behind physical recovery,[62] but the cognitive and emotional sequelae that emerge after the return of normal speech or extremity function are often the most disabling.

Tate et al. monitored the GOS scores and level of psychosocial reintegration of 87 patients with severe TBI for 6 years after injury.[110] In the group as a whole, 76 percent were classified as having either poor or substantially limited reintegration. Even in those with the best GOS scores (good recovery or moderate disability) only 50 percent were classified as having good reintegration with regard to employment, interpersonal relationships, functional independence, social contacts, and leisure interests. Kaiser and Pfenninger studied outcome in 24 children with severe TBI who received state-of-the-art acute care in a neurointensive care unit.[50] After

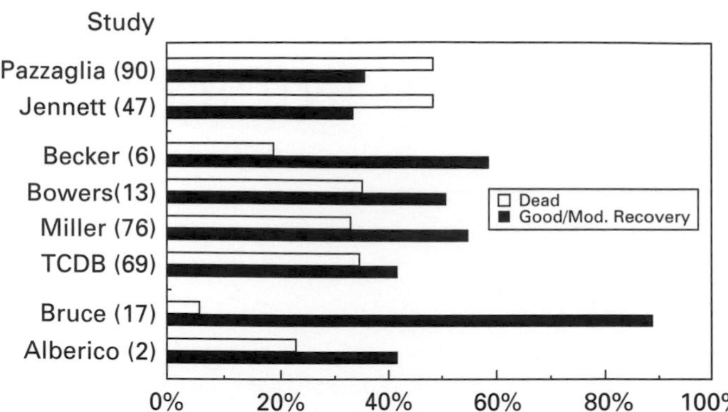

Figure 52-1. A comparison of outcomes in select series of patients with severe traumatic brain injury in which there was inconsistent use of early intubation, ICP monitoring, and other principles of comtemporary acute care,[47,90] series that consistently applied these principles,[6,13,69,76] and series that included only children.[2,17]

2.5 years, 42 percent had residual focal neurological deficits, and 58 percent had measurable neuropsychiatric deficits primarily characterized as altered personality. Despite these deficits, however, few required special education.

The most common cognitive disabilities caused by severe TBI are memory and behavior disturbances, the magnitude of which are related to both the severity of the initial injury (GCS score) and the time from injury.[31,88] The type of brain lesion as defined on computed tomography (CT) images also influences neuropsychological outcome and may predict the likelihood of improvement in deficits such as recall and learning.[116] In many patients, this effect seems to be related to orbital frontal lobe injury.[75,117] The duration of coma and posttraumatic amnesia also affect the incidence of long-term neuropsychological sequelae: coma lasting longer than 1 month significantly worsens social behavior, school performance, and vocational functioning.[36] Verbal and performance intelligence quotient (IQ) scores at 3 and 6 months have been correlated with the duration of posttraumatic amnesia.[65]

In the early 1980s, Langfitt and Gennarelli concluded that there were two principal causes for the neurological damage caused by TBI: mechanical damage of neurons and their processes, and ischemia.[57] Some have suggested that ischemia is the most important cause of secondary brain injury and that in 40 percent of cases, ischemia may be delayed, providing the opportunity for therapeutic intervention.[18] Ischemia initiates several biochemical cascades that lead to the production of oxygen-free radicals. Other mechanisms of secondary brain injury include the release of cytokines such as interleukin 1-β, which initiate the inflammatory response to brain injury, and the increase in tissue lactic acid, which results from anaerobic glycolysis. These mechanisms eventually lead to brain swelling, and high or uncontrolled levels of brain swelling are cited as the most common cause of death and neurological disability following severe TBI.[6,70]

Acute care strategies that emphasize treatment to avoid cerebral ischemia can improve outcome. In a 1982 review, Jane and Rimel pointed out that the outcome of severe TBI was closely related to three preventable or treatable factors: hypoxia, shock, and increased intracranial pressure (ICP), all of which can cause ischemia.[45] Recent reports have found that prolonged hypotension (shock) is associated with a doubling of the mortality rate seen in TBI.[22,56] Investigators at several major trauma centers found that the aggressive, consistent treatment of these problems could reduce the mortality rate to 34 percent and increase the rate of good recovery/moderate disability to 56 percent.[13,76] Thus, although the initial trauma is certainly a factor in determining outcome following severe TBI, the secondary injury that occurs in the first few hours and days also clearly contributes to outcome.

HEMODYNAMIC, NEUROCHEMICAL, AND ELECTROPHYSIOLOGICAL CORRELATES

CEREBRAL BLOOD FLOW AND TBI

Cerebral blood flow (CBF) changes associated with TBI have been described in many reports over the last 25 years.[16,24,34,44,58,78,81,97,109] Several of these studies found that CBF was typically low during the first day after injury and then increased.[16,34] The typical time course of CBF changes during the first 5 days after injury was defined, and a profound reduction of global CBF was correlated with aggressive hyperventilation.[82]

Current studies support the conclusion that CBF, both regionally and globally, typically is very low during the first 24 hours and then increases, peaking at 3 to 4 days after injury.[11,86] The lowest CBF values consistently are observed in those with the most severe injuries and therefore the worst prognosis.[12,67,78,86,87] In one series, local or global CBF values in the ischemic range (<18 ml/100 g/min) were found in 31 percent of patients during the first several hours after severe TBI. These low flow values were not due to a low P_{CO_2} or hypotension, although hypotension has been shown to be associated with low flows.[12] Robertson and colleagues obtained multiple CBF studies for each of 102 patients with severe TBI and found a significant correlation between low CBF and mortality: at 3 months, mortality rates were 32 and 20 percent, respectively, for groups with CBF values of 29 and 62 ml/100 g/min.[98] In this series outcome was more closely correlated with the CBF value than with the type of injury, initial GCS score, or ICP. Jaggi et al. also found a significant positive correlation between acute CBF and functional recovery at 6 months.[44] In addition, low values for the cerebral metabolic rate for oxygen (CMR_{O_2}) correlated significantly with death or persistent vegetative state at 6 months, and these investigators concluded that CMR_{O_2} is a more powerful predictor of outcome than is CBF.

Blood flow in the brain underlying contusions or hematomas typically is lower than in the rest of the brain. Some reports suggest that it may remain low for several days, even if the lesion is evacuated.[19,100] Years before the development of local CBF monitoring techniques, it was theorized that ischemia was the main cause of the brain swelling and high mortality rate associated with acute subdural hematomas, and Langfitt proposed that the sooner the hematoma was evacuated, the less ischemic damage would occur.[57] Schroder et al. recently described the dramatic reversal of low CBF in two patients after the evacuation of subdural hematomas, and Seelig and colleagues found that evacuation of acute subdural hematomas within 2 hours after injury led to 40 percent fewer deaths than among patients whose clots were not removed for 4 or more hours.[101,102]

The significance of low CBF following severe TBI is not entirely clear, however. Obrist et al. determined that low CBF may, in fact, be appropriate for the metabolic demands of the severely injured brain, indicating coupling of CBF with metabolism.[82] In addition, no study has shown that low CBF at any time during the first 5 days after injury accurately predicts outcome. Although low CBF is associated with poor outcome, any large group of TBI patients with low CBF includes a substantial number who ultimately make a good recovery. Also, medications or hypercarbia can be used to elevate low CBF, and the effect of such intervention on outcome is unknown.

The most important contribution of CBF information has been the elucidation of the effects of TBI on acute cerebral physiology. Consequently, the acute care of these patients, and possibly also their outcome, has improved. Prognostication, however, should not rely on CBF measurements. The possible exception to this admonition is in the determination of brain death, although Cruz recently reported a good recovery in a patient whose early CBF values were consistent with no flow.[28] Schroder also described a patient who had a good recovery after evacuation of a subdural hematoma despite extremely low CBF values prior to surgery.[101]

Transcranial Doppler

The measurement of cerebral blood flow velocities using transcranial Doppler ultrasonography (TCD) has helped to define trauma-related hemodynamic changes. In 40 percent of 35 patients with severe TBI, Weber et al. found TCD evidence of middle cerebral artery vasospasm (increased blood flow velocities) which significantly correlated with the presence of subarachnoid hemorrhage.[120] They and others have found that the onset of posttraumatic vasospasm temporally mimics the vasospasm that occurs following aneurysmal subarachnoid hemorrhage 5 to 7 days after injury.[72,120] However, they did not find an association between the occurrence of posttraumatic vasospasm and 6-month outcome. Another recent study of 86 TBI patients also found no correlation between flow velocities and outcome.[106] In addition, none of the patients in this series had vasospasm-related cerebral infarction. However, the association between TCD-defined blood flow velocity changes and outcome remains controversial. Chan et al. noted a significant correlation between middle cerebral artery flow velocities and outcome in 121 patients with TBI.[21] Patients with severe injuries (GCS scores < 8) had significantly lower flow velocities than did those with mild or moderate injuries, and all of the 10 patients in this series who later died had very low flow velocities.

Posttraumatic CBF abnormalities complicate the interpretation of TCD measurements. As previously described, CBF typically is depressed during the first 24 hours after injury and then rises to a maximum value by days 3 to 4. Because both vasospasm and increased CBF can cause an increase in cerebral blood flow velocities, definitive statements about vasospasm based solely on TCD ultrasonography usually are not possible.

Measurement of Jugular Venous Oxygen Content or Saturation

Measurements of cerebral oxygen extraction after TBI frequently are used to determine the adequacy of global cerebral perfusion. Arterial jugular venous oxygen content differences (AVd_{O_2}) can be determined by sampling the O_2 content from the jugular bulb and subtracting it from the O_2 content of arterial blood. Measurements of AVd_{O_2} values have shown that the level of O_2 extraction typically is increased during the first day after a severe TBI, and returns to normal thereafter.[11,24,78,98] Normal values for AVd_{O_2} have been determined, and most agree that values above and below these indicate cerebral ischemia and hyperemia, respectively.[82]

Alternatively, the adequacy of global cerebral perfusion can be gauged by the level of jugular venous oxygen saturation (SjV_{O_2}). This measurement is amenable to continuous monitoring and does not routinely require the withdrawal of blood samples. Normal SjV_{O_2} is > 50 percent, and saturations below 50 percent have been correlated with poor outcome.[27,104] Sheinberg et al. identified the probable causes for such desaturations in 20 patients with TBI[104] as intracranial hypertension and hypocarbia, both of which were potentially treatable. They also have found that the incidence and severity of jugular desaturations correlate significantly with poor outcome.

The primary limitation of both these techniques is their inability to detect regional changes in tissue perfusion. Although many hypotheses about cerebral ischemia or hyperemia are based on measurements of AVd_{O_2} or SjV_{O_2}, at best they reflect only the global average of regional posttraumatic events. For example, the brain underlying a subdural hematoma may be poorly perfused, as xenon/CT CBF studies suggest, but if other areas of the brain are hyperemic, the average values obtained by monitoring AVd_{O_2} or SjV_{O_2} will appear normal. Another problem with these measurements is the assumption that the values obtained from one internal jugular vein accurately represent mixed cerebral venous blood. Stocchetti and co-workers concluded that this assumption was invalid after simultaneously measuring the SjV_{O_2} from both internal jugular veins in 32 patients with TBI.[107] They found bilateral differences of greater than 15 percent in as many as 64 percent of the patients.

As with CBF monitoring after severe TBI, measurements of AVd_{O_2} and SjV_{O_2} have been most useful in helping to guide optimal acute care. They are not useful for prognosis, and many patients with abnormal values will have a good outcome.

Cerebrospinal Fluid Analysis

Several neurochemicals and metabolites are released into the cerebrospinal fluid (CSF) following severe TBI, and the type and level of these neurochemicals have been correlated with the severity of the injury. The CSF of patients who die of a severe TBI typically has three to four times the serum level of CSF creatine kinase BB isoenzyme and 20 to 100 times the CSF level of this isoenzyme found in those who die of asphyxia or cardiac failure.[26,85]

Others have identified high CSF levels of lactate in patients with severe TBI.[30,54,93] Although CSF levels of creatine kinase usually decline within 10 hours after the injury, CSF lactate levels continue to rise for several days in those with a poor outcome.[93] In a study of 19 patients, CSF lactate levels correlated with both ICP and neurological outcome, the highest levels occurring in those who died.[30] Among patients with a good recovery, CSF lactate levels decreased significantly within 48 hours of injury, but no significant decrease occurred in the poor outcome group. Presuming that high CSF lactate levels may contribute to poor neurological outcome, some investigators have attempted to improve outcome by administering systemic alkalinizing agents.[10,89] However, a controlled, randomized study of one such agent, tromethamine (THAM), found no significant improvement in outcome in the group receiving this drug.[123]

Electroencephalography

The effects of trauma on the electrical activity of the brain have been investigated for more than 20 years. The earliest studies found that injury severe enough to cause death was associated with absence of brain waves on the electroencephalogram (EEG), even at high gain. This relationship proved so reliable that EEG was incorporated as part of the original criteria for confirming brain death (Harvard Criteria).[1] Conventional EEG has not been as useful for those with less severe head injuries.[66] Many investigators have attempted to define a role for this technology in the acute care of patients with TBI, possibly as an early warning of elevated ICP or impending herniation. Others have tried to demonstrate a correlation between EEG findings and outcome. However, conventional EEG has never been shown to consistently predict acute events or outcome.

A transformation of continuous EEG recordings known as compressed spectral array (CSA) recently has been found to have a high degree of prognostic accuracy. CSA uses Fourier or similar transforms to convert EEG tracings to a graphic representation of the relative signal amplitude inherent within each frequency band. These data are compressed into an array of tracings that illustrate a spectrum of frequencies and relative power. Thatcher and colleagues compared the prognostic strength of CSA with brainstem auditory evoked potentials (BSAEP), CT, and the GCS scores in a series of 162 patients with TBI.[113] Outcome at 1 year was determined using the Disability Rating Scale score, a somewhat more detailed determination of functional outcome than the GOS.[95] They found that the best single predictor of outcome was CSA, and that it was significantly better than the CT scan, the BSAEP, or the GCS score obtained at 7.5 days after injury. CSA had a 95.8 percent discriminant accuracy between good outcome and death, though it was somewhat less accurate for predicting intermediate outcomes.

Evoked Potentials

Visual, somatosensory, and brainstem-auditory evoked potentials all have been used to investigate the electrophysiological abnormalities caused by TBI. As an early warning of brain swelling and potential herniation and as an outcome predictor during acute care, these techniques are most useful for those with severe TBI. Studies have found them insensitive for predicting the memory deficits, lethargy, or emotional lability that frequently occur after mild TBI.[121]

Visual evoked potentials (VEP) are the least complicated type of evoked potentials to obtain and interpret and were the first type to be studied in patients with TBI. The anatomic location of the potential generators are not well understood, and the waves most commonly monitored are a negative potential at 70 msec (N2) and positive potential at 100 msec (P2). York and colleagues demonstrated that prolongation of the VEP latencies (P2 or N2 waves) bears a linear relationship to increases or decreases in ICP.[125] VEP changes after TBI also correlate with delayed cognitive deficits and psychosocial disturbances.[91,96]

Somatosensory evoked potentials (SSEP) usually are obtained by stimulation of either the posterior tibial, common peroneal, or median nerves. Potential generators with characteristic latencies and positivity or negativity are located in the frontal lobes (P20/22 and N30), parietal lobes (N20), and brainstem (N16). The posttraumatic loss of the parietal or frontal waves has been correlated with poor outcome. Gutling and colleagues examined 50 patients within 72 hours after TBI; by considering frontal and parietal waves together, they correctly predicted the outcomes (mild or no disability vs death or severe disability) in 94 percent of the patients.[37] Facco et al. also found a strong correlation between outcome and dissociation of the parietal and frontal waves.[32]

An advantage of BSAEPs is that they are least likely to be affected by barbiturates, which may be required to treat intracranial hypertension. A disadvantage of this type of evoked potential, however, is that it depends on intact hearing, and studies note a 17 to 56 percent incidence of sensorineural hearing loss following TBI.[25] Continual or serial recordings of BSAEPs during the acute care of patients with TBI may provide an early warning of uncal herniation: alterations in amplitude and latency have been documented minutes or hours before there are changes in the pupils.[5] There is histological (postmortem) evidence that abnormalities of latency and amplitude of waves III, IV, and V are related to lesions in the lower, middle, and upper brainstem, respectively.[108] Nonetheless, the prognostic use of BSAEPs has not been widely accepted. Although abnormal findings do correlate with a poor outcome, normal studies also are common in those who do poorly.[3] When compared with SSEPs, BSAEPs have a much lower predictive power.[105]

The use of evoked potential and EEG monitoring in patients with TBI is often limited by the resources they demand. Their ability to accurately detect signs of acute neurological deterioration or to predict long-term outcome require continual recordings for several days. Technicians skilled in interpreting the recordings must be present around the clock. Since there are no studies that have demonstrated improved outcome with the use of these monitoring techniques, it is not clear that the expense is warranted.

THE EFFECT OF AGE ON OUTCOME

Reports of outcome after severe TBI have consistently demonstrated better outcomes for children (0–19 years) than for adults (Fig. 52-1). In a large prospective study, Alberico et al. found that the 1-year rate of good outcome was 55 percent for patients aged 0 to 19 years but only 21 percent for older patients, despite similar postresuscitation GCS scores for both groups.[2] Even among children, increasing age correlates with poor outcome; those between the ages of 11 and 15 years have the highest mortality rates.[51,64,71]

Outcomes in children and adults are not significantly different in subgroups of patients with subdural hematomas or profound hypotension; however, adults have nearly twice the incidence of subdural hematomas.[2,64] The most common brain injury in children, diffuse swelling,[89] is not associated with the high incidence of poor outcome found among adults with this injury.[51,63] Subdural hematomas in children are most common before the age of 1 year.[94]

Elderly victims of severe TBI have particularly poor outcomes. Among patients entered into the Traumatic Coma Data Bank (TCDB), the mortality rate for those older than 56 years was 80 percent, compared with 36 percent for the entire group.[118] None of the elderly patients had a good outcome. Among 195 elderly victims of TBI, Ross et al. found that all who remained comatose for at least 72 hours died within 6 months.[99] The length of hospital stay, likelihood of dying in the acute-care hospital, and likelihood of discharge to a chronic care facility after TBI are all significantly increased in older persons.[35]

EARLY PROGNOSTICATION

A substantial proportion of comatose TBI patients will die or remain severely disabled years after the injury, and there are obvious humanitarian and economic reasons for providing the patient's family with prognostic information that is farily accurate. When the prognosis is very poor, the physician and family may decide to withhold or withdraw treatment that would preserve vegetative survival, thereby diverting health care resources to those who might improve. Based on data from several large prospective epidemiological studies, the likelihood of death or severe disability usually can be predicted within hours or days after severe TBI.

Choi et al. reviewed the data from the Traumatic Coma Data Bank and found that the presence of a fixed and dilated pupil together with a low motor score on the GCS and age older than 60 years strongly predicted death or severe disability.[23] None of these patients had a good recovery. In a large European database, Braakman et al. also found age, GCS score, pupil reactivity to light, and spontaneous and reflex eye movements to be powerful predictors of outcome.[15] When considered independently, however, the predictive accuracy of these clinical findings was substantially reduced. Jennett et al. assessed the prognostic value of early clinical findings based on outcome at 6 months after injury in a series of 1000 patients.[47] They found that the reliability of predictions on this basis increased along with the time interval between early assessment and injury. Predictions made during the first 24 hours after injury were correct (greater than 97 percent probability) for only 44 percent of the patients.[48] Even predictions based on later assessments were most likely to be correct when limited to only two outcomes: death or survival.

Kaufmann et al. studied 100 patients with severe TBI to determine the prognostic reliability of combined findings from the neurological examination and CT studies obtained during the first 24 hours after injury.[53] Outcome was estimated correctly in only 59 percent of the cases. Thus, they concluded that even with sophisticated clinical and radiological techniques, outcome predictions during the first day were not sufficiently accurate to guide early treatment or treatment-withholding decisions. Based on a related study, they suggested that victims of severe TBI have a protracted period of improvement and that outcome cannot be accurately determined for at least 1 year after the injury.[52] Another group reviewed the medical records of 306 patients with severe TBI and also found a poor correlation between the initial GCS scores and outcome.[119] In this series a substantial number of patients with an initial GCS score of 3 eventually had a good neurological recovery.

The duration of posttraumatic amnesia also has been correlated with recovery. Bishara et al. found this variable to be more reliable than the initial GCS score for describing outcome variance on the GOS at 6 and 12 months after injury.[8]

Marshall et al. proposed that the severity of brain injury as defined by the initial CT images of the head can be used to help predict outcome.[69] The finding of diffuse injuries, diffuse swelling, acute subdural hematomas, or large contusions all correlate with a poor outcome.[61] The appearance of new hyper- or hypodense lesions not detected on the initial head CT also has been correlated with a poor outcome.[55] Additional negative prognostic indicators include the absence of basal cisterns and shift of the midline structures.[126] However, some believe that these findings simply reflect the severity of intracranial mass lesions or hemispheric swelling, and do not independently correlate with outcome.[103]

In children with very severe TBI, the initial CT scan may reveal hypodense diffuse swelling, obliteration of the ambient cisterns and third ventricle, and loss of definition of the basal ganglia as well as the gray-white differentiation. This CT finding is particularly ominous and consistently associated with death or persistent vegetative state.[122]

Others have suggested the use of magnetic resonance imaging (MRI) during the first several days after injury to predict outcome. Although MRI is more sensitive than CT for detecting posttraumatic lesions,[29] MRI scans obtained within 30 days after the injury show many small and temporary lesions that do not correlate with functional outcome.[84] However, MRI may be useful for defining the extent of permanent anatomic damage when obtained several months after the injury.[7]

Ventricular or lumbar CSF sampled within hours or days after severe TBI contains high levels of several compounds not formally found in this fluid. Both the concentration and rate of decline of CSF creatine kinase BB,[26] lactate,[93] catecholamine,[68] and cytokines,[73,74] have been correlated with outcome. In one study, CSF creatinine kinase BB isoenzyme activity was more closely associated with 6-month outcome than were four other risk factors, including the GCS score and age.[43]

The magnitude of increase in CSF catecholamine also has been suggested as an early predictor of outcome.[68] The autonomic response to trauma is well defined, and elevated levels of norepinephrine and epinephrine in the plasma of those with severe injuries may exceed 10 times normal levels. Moreover, posttraumatic levels of norepinephrine and, to a lesser extent, epinephrine, are much higher if the trauma includes TBI.[33,42,129] Markianos and colleagues examined the correlation between outcome and acute CSF levels of norepinephrine, dopamine, serotonin, methoxyhydroxyphenylglycol, homovanillic acid, and 5-hydroxyindoleacetic acid (5HIAA) in 24 patients within 1 to 12 days after severe TBI.[68] They found significantly lower levels of 5HIAA in the 14 patients who had a good recovery compared with the 10 patients who did not. In addition, analysis of variance showed a negative correlation between the GCS score and CSF concentrations of 5HIAA, but not with the other neurotransmitters.

During the last several years, the prognostic utility of several other clinical findings and monitoring techniques has been investigated, but the value of many of these remains inconclusive. Most of these studies are much more accurate for predicting who will die or be left severely disabled than for determining who will recover with minimal or no disabilities. Serial observations of neurological recovery over several months remain the best means to predict complete or near-complete recovery.

The proliferation of reports describing ways to predict outcome based on early assessments has led some to develop outcome prediction models that can be used by acute care physicians. Murray et al. prospectively studied more than 1000 TBI patients admitted to four neurosurgical units in Great Britain from 1986 to 1989.[80] The study was divided into three phases: a baseline period of at least 1 year before the introduction of a computer-based outcome prediction model; 1 year during which outcome predictions were provided to the attending physicians; and the final 6 months, after prediction models were withdrawn. During the period when outcome predictions were provided, the use of osmotic diuretics, ICP monitors, and intubation and/or controlled ventilation increased for patients predicted to have a good outcome and decreased by 39 percent for patients predicted to have a poor outcome.

Thus, exposure to outcome prediction models can affect the care provided to TBI patients. This is cause for some concern because current clinical therapeutic trials have been initiated based on the premise that outcome following TBI can be improved. If outcome prediction models are to become widely used, they must be designed to account for new findings regarding outcome-improving therapy.[14] Clinicians must remember that predictive models are based on the statistical analysis of a large number of patients and may not apply to a specific patient.[20] In addition, the literature concerning outcome prediction can easily be misinterpreted, particularly with regard to the distinction between associations and cause-and-effect. For example, in a study of 102 patients with severe TBI, Robertson et al. found that mortality at 3 months was 32 percent for the subgroup of patients with a mean CBF of 29 ml/100 g/min and 20 percent in the subgroup with a mean CBF of 62 ml/100 g/min.[98] Despite the association between low CBF and poor outcome, their study was not designed to test the hypothesis that a low CBF caused a poor outcome or that all patients with a low CBF had a poor outcome, and it did not show this. In addition, the study did not determine whether outcome could be improved by artificially elevating the CBF when it was low.

CONCLUSIONS

Outcome after severe TBI has improved during the last several decades, undoubtedly because much of the pathophysiology of this disease has been elucidated and acute care principles have been adopted that account for specific pathophysiological derangements. Further improvement is expected as we learn more about the role of ischemia and other biochemical and cellular mediators of secondary brain injury and with the development of therapy that effectively attenuates those mediators. Successful clinical trials must include high-quality, consistent acute care in addition to assessment of experimental treatments. Outcome determinations also must focus on cognitive and neuropsychological issues, since it is becoming increasingly clear that these more subtle deficits remain as severe disabilities even in those who recover from their physical deficits.

ACKNOWLEDGMENT

The author gratefully acknowledges Helene Marion for editing the manuscript.

REFERENCES

1. Ad Hoc Committee of the Harvard Medical School to examine the definition of brain death. A definition of irreversible coma. *JAMA* 1965; 205:337–340.
2. Alberico AM, Ward JD, Choi SC, et al: Outcome after severe head injury. Relationship to mass lesions, diffuse injury, and ICP course in pediatric and adult patients. *J Neurosurg* 1987; 67:648–656.
3. Anderson DC, Bundie S, Rockswold GL: Multimodality evoked potentials in closed head trauma. *Arch Neurol* 1984; 41:369–374.

4. Athiappan S, Muthukumar N, Srinivasan US: Influence of basal cisterns, midline shift and pathology on outcome in head injury. *Ann Acad Med Singapore* 1993; 22:452–455.
5. Barelli A,Valente MR, Clemente A, et al: Serial multimodality-evoked potentials in severely head-injured patients: diagnostic and prognostic implications [see comments]. *Crit Care Med* 1991; 19:1374–1381.
6. Becker DP, Miller JD, Ward JD, et al: The outcome from severe head injury with early diagnosis and intensive management. *J Neurosurg* 1977 47:491–502.
7. Bigler ED, Kurth SM, Blatter D, Abildskov TJ: Degenerative changes in traumatic brain injury: Post-injury magnetic resonance identified ventricular expansion compared to pre-injury levels. *Brain Res Bull* 1992; 28:651–653.
8. Bishara SN, Partridge FM, Godfrey HP, Knight RG: Post-traumatic amnesia and Glasgow Coma Scale related to outcome in survivors in a consecutive series of patients with severe closed-head injury. *Brain Inj* 1992; 6:373–380.
9. Blyth B: The outcome of severe head injuries. *N Z Med J* 1981; 93:267–269.
10. Bondoli A, De Cosmo G, Pietrini D, Magalini SI: An attempt to control cerebrospinal fluid acidosis in coma due to head injury. *Resuscitation* 1980; 8:217–222.
11. Bouma GJ, Muizelaar JP, Choi SC, et al: Cerebral circulation and metabolism after severe traumatic brain injury: The elusive role of ischemia. *J Neurosurg* 1991; 75:685–693.
12. Bouma GJ, Muizelaar JP, Stringer WA, et al: Ultra early evaluation of regional cerebral blood flow in severely head injured patients using xenon enhanced computed tomography. *J Neurosurg* 1992; 77:360–368.
13. Bowers SA, Marshall LF: Outcome in 200 consecutive cases of severe head injury treated in San Diego County: A prospective analysis. *Neurosurgery* 1980; 6:237–242.
14. Braakman R: Early prediction of outcome in severe head injury. *Acta Neurochir (Wien)* 1992; 116:161–163.
15. Braakman R, Gelpke GJ, Habbema JD, et al: Systematic selection of prognostic features in patients with severe head injury. *Neurosurgery* 1980; 6:362–370.
16. Bruce DA, Langfitt TW, Miller JD, et al: Regional cerebral blood flow, intracranial pressure, and brain metabolism in comatose patients. *J Neurosurg* 1973; 38:131–144.
17. Bruce DA, Schut L, Bruno LA, et al: Outcome following severe head injuries in children. *J Neurosurg* 1978; 48: 679–688.
18. Bullock R: Introducing NMDA antagonists into clinical practice: Why head injury trials? *Br J Clin Pharmacol* 1992; 34:396–401.
19. Bullock R, Sakas D, Patterson J, et al: Early post-traumatic cerebral blood flow mapping: Correlation with structural damage after focal injury. *Acta Neurochir (Wien)* 1992; 55:14–17.
20. Butterworth JF, Selhorst JB, Greenberg RP et al: Flaccidity after head injury: Diagnosis, management, and outcome. *Neurosurgery* 1981; 9:242–248.
21. Chan KH, Miller JD, Dearden NM: Intracranial blood flow velocity after head injury: Relationship to severity of injury, time, neurological status and outcome. *J Neurol Neurosurg Psychiatry* 1992; 55:787–791.
22. Chesnut RM, Marshall LF, Klauber MR, et al: The role of secondary brain injury in determining outcome from severe head injury. *J Trauma* 1993; 34:216–222.
23. Choi SC, Narayan RK, Anderson RL, Ward JD: Enhanced specificity of prognosis in severe head injury. *J Neurosurg* 1988; 69:381–385.
24. Cold GE: The relationship between cerebral metabolic rate of oxygen and cerebral blood flow in the acute phase of head injury. *Acta Anaesthesiol Scand* 1986; 30:453–457.
25. Coligado EJ, Wiet RJ, O'Connor CA, et al: Multichannel cochlear implantation in the rehabilitation of post-traumatic sensorineural hearing loss. *Arch Phys Med Rehabil* 1993; 74:653–657.
26. Cooper PR, Chalif DJ, Ramsey JF, Moore RJ: Radioimmunoassay of the brain type isoenzyme of creatine phosphokinase (CK-BB): A new diagnostic tool in the evaluation of patients with head injury. *Neurosurgery* 1983; 12:536–541.
27. Cruz J: On-line monitoring of global cerebral hypoxia in acute brain injury. Relationship to intracranial hypertension. *J Neurosurg* 1993; 79:228–233.
28. Cruz J: Low clinical ischemic threshold for cerebral blood flow in severe acute brain trauma. Case report. *J Neurosurg* 1994; 80:143–147.
29. Derosier C, Brinquin L, Bonsignour JP, Cosnard G: MRI and cranial traumas in the acute phase. *J Neuroradiol* 1991; 18:309–319.
30. DeSalles AA, Kontos HA, Becker DP, et al: Prognostic significance of ventricular CSF lactic acidosis in severe head injury. *J Neurosurg* 1986; 65:615–624.
31. Dikmen S, Temkin N, McLean A, et al: Memory and head injury severity. *J Neurol Neurosurg Psychiatry* 1987; 50:1613–1618.
32. Facco E, Munari M, Dona B, et al: Spatial mapping of SEP in comatose patients: Improved outcome prediction by combined parietal N20 and frontal N30 analysis. *Brain Topogr* 1991; 3:447–455.
33. Feldman Z, Contant CF, Pahwa R, et al: The relationship between hormonal mediators and systemic hypermetabolism after severe head injury. *J Trauma* 1993; 34:806–816.
34. Fieschi C, Battistini N, Beduschi A, et al: Regional cerebral blood flow and intraventricular pressure in acute head injuries. *N Neurol Neurosurg Psychiatry* 1974; 37:1378–1388.
35. Fife D, Faich G, Hollinshead W, Boynton W: Incidence and outcome of hospital-treated head injury in Rhode Island. *Am J Public Health* 1986; 76:773–778.
36. Filley CM, Cranberg LD, Alexander MP, Hart EJ: Neurobehavioral outcome after closed head injury in childhood and adolescence. *Arch Neurol* 1987; 44:194–198.
37. Gutling E, Gonser A, Regard M, et al: Dissociation of frontal and parietal components of somatosensory evoked potentials in severe head injury. *Electroencephalogr Clin Neurophysiol* 1993; 88:369–376.
38. Gensemer IB, McMurry FG, Walker JC, et al: Behav-

ioral consequences of trauma. *J Trauma* 1988; 28:44–49.

39. Gensemer IB, Smith JL, Walker JC, et al: Psychological consequences of blunt head trauma and relation to other indices of severity of injury. *Ann Emerg Med* 1989; 18:9–12.
40. Greenberg RP, Becker DP, Miller JD, et al: Evaluation of brain function in severe human head trauma with multimodality evoked potentials. Part 2: Localization of brain dysfunction and correlation with posttraumatic neurological conditions. *J Neurosurg* 1977; 47:163–177.
41. Greenberg RP, Mayer DJ, Becker DP: Evaluation of brain function in severe human head trauma with multimodality evoked potentials. Part I: Evoked brain injury potentials, methods, and analysis. *J Neurosurg* 1977; 47:150–162.
42. Hadfield JM, Little RA, Jones RA: Measured energy expenditure and plasma substrate and hormonal changes after severe head injury. *Injury* 1992; 23:177–182.
43. Hans P, Albert A, Franssen C, Born J: Improved outcome prediction based on CSF extrapolated creatine kinase BB isoenzyme activity and other risk factors in severe head injury. *J Neurosurg* 1989; 71:54–58.
44. Jaggi JL, Obrist WD, Gennarelli TA, Langfitt TW: Relationship of early cerebral blood flow and metabolism to outcome in acute head injury. *J Neurosurg* 1990; 72:176–182.
45. Jane JA, Rimel RW: Prognosis in head injury. *Clin Neurosurg* 1982; 29:346–352.
46. Jennett B, Snoek J, Bond MR, Brooks N: Disability after severe head injury: Observations on the use of the Glasgow Outcome Scale. *J Neurol Neurosurg Psychiatry* 1981; 44:285–293.
47. Jennett B, Teasdale G, Braakman R, et al: Prognosis of patients with severe head injury. *Neurosurgery* 1979; 4:283–289.
48. Jennett B, Teasdale G, Braakman R, et al: Predicting outcome in individual patients after severe head injury. *Lancet* 1976; 1:1031–1034.
49. Jennett B, Teasdale G, Knill-Jones R: Prognosis after severe head injury. *Ciba Found Symp* 1975; 309–324.
50. Kaiser G, Pfenninger J: Effect of neurointensive care upon outcome following severe head injuries in childhood—a preliminary report. *Neuropediatrics* 1984; 15: 68–75.
51. Kalff R, Kocks W, Pospiech J, Grote W: Clinical outcome after head injury in children. *Childs Nerv Syst* 1989; 5:156–159.
52. Kaufman HH, Bretaudierre JP, Rowlands BJ, et al: Head injury. Variability of course and presence of confounding factors. *Int J Technol Assess Health Care* 1989; 5:631–638.
53. Kaufmann MA, Buchmann B, Scheidegger D, et al: Severe head injury: Should expected outcome influence resuscitation and first-day decisions? *Resuscitation* 1992; 23:199–206.
54. King LR, McLaurin RL, Knowles HC, Jr: Acid-base balance and arterial and CSF lactate following human head injury. *J Neurosurg* 1974; 40:617–625.
55. Kobayashi S, Nakazawa S, Otsuka T: Clinical value of serial computed tomography with severe head injury. *Surg Neurol* 1983; 20:25–29.
56. Kohi YM, Mendelow AD, Teasdale GM, Allardice GM: Extracranial insults and outcome in patients with acute head injury—relationship to the Glasgow Coma Scale. *Injury* 1984; 16:25–29.
57. Langfitt TW, Gennarelli TA: Can the outcome from head injury be improved? *J Neurosurg* 1982; 56:19–25.
58. Langfitt TW, Obrist WD, Gennarelli TA, et al: Correlation of cerebral blood flow with outcome in head injured patients. *Ann Surg* 1977; 186:411–414.
59. Levin HS, Grossman RG, Rose JE, Teasdale G: Long-term neuropsychological outcome of closed head injury. *J Neurosurg* 1979; 50:412–422.
60. Lindsay K, Pasaoglu A, Hirst D, et al: Somatosensory and auditory brain stem conduction after head injury: A comparison with clinical features in prediction of outcome. *Neurosurgery* 1990; 26:278–285.
61. Lipper MH, Kishore PR, Enas GG, et al: Computed tomography in the prediction of outcome in head injury. *Am J Roentgenol* 1985; 144:483–486.
62. Livingston MG, McCabe RJ: Psychosocial consequences of head injury in children and adolescents: Implications for rehabilitation. *Pediatrician* 1990; 17:255–261.
63. Lobato RD, Sarabia R, Cordobes F, et al: Posttraumatic cerebral hemispheric swelling. Analysis of 55 cases studied with computerized tomography. *J Neurosurg* 1988; 68:417–423.
64. Luerssen TG, Klauber MR, Marshall LF: Outcome from head injury related to patient's age. A longitudinal prospective study of adult and pediatric head injury. *J Neurosurg* 1988; 68:409–416.
65. Mandleberg IA: Cognitive recovery after severe head injury. 3. WAIS verbal and performance IQs as a function of post-traumatic amnesia duration and time from injury. *J Neurol Neurosurg Psychiatry* 1976; 39:1001–1007.
66. Marion DW, Bouma GJ: The use of stable xenon-enhanced computed tomographic studies of cerebral blood flow to define changes in cerebral carbon dioxide vasoresponsivity caused by a severe head injury. *Neurosurgery* 1991; 29:869–873.
67. Marion DW, Darby J, Yonas H: Acute regional cerebral blood flow changes caused by severe head injuries. *J Neurosurg* 1991; 74:407–414.
68. Markianos M, Seretis A, Kotsou et al: CSF neurotransmitter metabolites and short-term outcome of patients in coma after head injury. *Acta Neurol Scand* 1992; 86:190–193.
69. Marshall LF, Gautille T, Klauber MR, et al: The outcome of severe closed head injury. *J Neurosurg* 1991; 75:S28–S36.
70. Marshall LF, Smith RW, Shapiro HM: The outcome with aggressive treatment in severe head injuries. I. The significance of intracranial pressure monitoring. *J Neurosurg* 1979; 50:20–25.
71. Martin KM: Predicting short-term outcome in comatose head-injured children. *J Neurosci Nurs* 1987; 19:9–13.

72. Martin NA, Doberstein C, Zane C, et al: Posttraumatic cerebral arterial spasm: Transcranial Doppler ultrasound, cerebral blood flow, and angiographic findings. *J Neurosurg* 1992; 77:575–583.
73. McClain C, Cohen D, Phillips R, et al: Increased plasma and ventricular fluid interleukin-6 levels in patients with head injury. *J Lab Clin Med* 1991; 118:225–231.
74. McClain CJ, Cohen D, Ott L, et al: Ventricular fluid interleukin-1 activity in patients with head injury. *J Lab Clin Med* 1987; 110:48–54.
75. Mendelsohn D, Levin HS, Bruce D, et al: Late MRI after head injury in children: Relationship to clinical features and outcome. *Childs Nerv Syst* 1992; 8:445–452.
76. Miller JD, Butterworth JF, Gudeman SK, et al: Further experience in the management of severe head injury. *J Neurosurg* 1981; 54:289–299.
77. Moulton RJ, Marmarou A, Ronen J, et al: Spectral analysis of the EEG in craniocerebral trauma. *Can J Neurol Sci* 1988; 15:82–86.
78. Muizelaar JP, Marmarou A, DeSalles AA, et al: Cerebral blood flow and metabolism in severely head-injured children. Part 1: Relationship with GCS score, outcome, ICP, and PVI. *J Neurosurg* 1989; 71:63–71.
79. Muizelaar JP, Marmarou A, Young HF, et al: Improving the outcome of severe head injury with the oxygen radical scavenger polyethylene glycol-conjugated superoxide dismutase: A Phase II trial. *J Neurosurg* 1993; 78: 375–382.
80. Murray LS, Teasdale GM, Murray GD, et al: Does prediction of outcome alter patient management? *Lancet* 1993; 341:1487–1491.
81. Obrist WD, Gennarelli TA, Segawa H, et al: Relation of cerebral blood flow to neurological status and outcome in head-injured patients. *J Neurosurg* 1979; 51: 292–300.
82. Obrist WD, Langfitt TW, Jaggi JL, et al: Cerebral blood flow and metabolism in comatose patients with acute head injury. *J Neurosurg* 1984; 61:241–253.
83. Obrist WD, Marion DW, Aggarwal S: Time course of cerebral blood flow and metabolism in comatose patients with acute head injury. *J Cereb Blood Flow Metab* 1993 (Abstract).
84. Ogawa T, Sekino H, Uzura M, et al: Comparative study of magnetic resonance and CT scan imaging in cases of severe head injury. *Acta Neurochir (Wien)* 1992; 55:8–10.
85. Osuna E, Perez-Carceles MD, Luna A, Pounder DJ: Efficacy of cerebro-spinal fluid biochemistry in the diagnosis of brain insult. *Forensic Sci Int* 1992; 52:193–198.
86. Overgaard J, Molsdal C, Tweed WA: Cerebral circulation after head injury. Part 3: Does reduced regional cerebral blood flow determine recovery of brain function after blunt head injury? *J Neurosurg* 1981; 55:63–74.
87. Overgaard J, Tweed WA: Cerebral circulation after head injury. Part 4: Functional anatomy and boundary-zone flow deprivation in the first week of traumatic coma. *J Neurosurg* 1983; 59:439–446.
88. Paniak CE, Shore DL, Rourke BP: Recovery of memory after severe closed head injury: Dissociations in recovery of memory parameters and predictors of outcome. *J Clin Exp Neuropsychol* 1989; 11:631–644.
89. Pascucci RC: Head trauma in the child. *Intensive Care Med* 1988; 14:185–195.
90. Pazzaglia P, Frank G, Frank F, Gaist G: Clinical course and prognosis of acute post-traumatic coma. *J Neurol Neurosurg Psychiatry* 1975; 38:149–154.
91. Pfurtscheller G, Schwartz G, Gravenstein N: Clinical relevance of long-latency SSEPs and VEPs during coma and emergence from coma. *Electroencephalogr Clin Neurophysiol* 1985; 62:88–98.
92. Pietropaoli JA, Rogers FB, Shackford SR, et al: The deleterious effects of intraoperative hypotension on outcome in patients with severe head injuries. *J Trauma* 1992; 33:403–407.
93. Rabow L, DeSalles AF, Becker DP, et al: CSF brain creatine kinase levels and lactic acidosis in severe head injury. *J Neurosurg* 1986; 65:625–629.
94. Raimondi AJ, Hirschauer J: Head injury in the infant and toddler. Coma scoring and outcome scale. *Childs Brain* 1984; 11:12–35.
95. Rappaport M, Hall KM, Hopkins K, et al: Disability rating scale for severe head trauma: Coma to community. *Arch Phys Med Rehabil* 1982; 63:118–123.
96. Rappaport M, Hopkins R, Hall K, et al: Evoked brain potentials and disability in brain damaged patients. *Arch Phys Med Rehabil* 1977; 58:333–338.
97. Robertson CS, Clifton GL, Grossman RG, et al: Alterations in cerebral availability of metabolic substrates after severe head injury. *J Trauma* 1988; 28:1523–1532.
98. Robertson CS, Contant CF, Gokaslan ZL, et al: Cerebral blood flow, arteriovenous oxygen difference, and outcome in head injured patients. *J Neurol Neurosurg Psychiatry* 1992; 55:594–603.
99. Ross AM, Pitts LH, Kobayashi S: Prognosticators of outcome after major head injury in the elderly. *J Neurosci Nurs* 1992; 24:88–93.
100. Salvant JB, Muizelaar JP: Changes in cerebral blood flow and metabolism related to the presence of subdural hematoma. *Neurosurgery* 1993; 33:387–393.
101. Schroder ML, Muizelaar JP, Kuta AJ: Documented reversal of global ischemia immediately after removal of an acute subdural hematoma. *Neurosurgery* 1994; 80:324–327.
102. Seelig JM, Becker DP, Miller JD, et al: Traumatic acute subdural hematoma. Major mortality reduction in comatose patients treated within four hours. *N Engl J Med* 1981; 304:1511–1512.
103. Selladurai BM, Jayakumar R, Tan YY, Low HC: Outcome prediction in early management of severe head injury: An experience in Malaysia. *Br J Neurosurg* 1992; 6:549–557.
104. Sheinberg M, Kanter MJ, Robertson CS, et al: Continuous monitoring of jugular venous oxygen saturation in head-injured patients. *J Neurosurg* 1992; 76:212–217.
105. Shin DY, Ehrenberg B, Whyte J, et al: Evoked potential assessment: Utility in prognosis of chronic head injury. *Arch Phys Med Rehabil* 1989; 70:189–193.
106. Steiger HJ, Aaslid R, Stooss R, Seiler RW: Transcranial

doppler monitoring in head injury: Relations between type of injury, flow velocities, vasoreactivity, and outcome. *Neurosurgery* 1994; 34:79–86.

107. Stocchetti N, Paparella A, Bridelli F, et al: Cerebral venous oxygen saturation studied with bilateral samples in the internal jugular veins. *Neurosurgery* 1994; 34:38–44.
108. Stockard JJ, Rossiter VS: Clinical and pathologic correlates of brainstem auditory response abnormalities. *Neurology* 1977; 27:316–325.
109. Tabaddor K, Bhushan C, Pevsner PH, Walker AE: Prognostic value of cerebral blood flow (CBF) and cerebral metabolic rate of oxygen (CMRO2) in acute head trauma. *J Trauma* 1972; 12:1053–1055.
110. Tate RL, Lulham JM, Broe GA, et al: Psychosocial outcome for the survivors of severe blunt head injury: The results from a consecutive series of 100 patients. *J Neurol Neurosurg Psychiatry* 1989; 52:1128–1134.
111. Teasdale G, Jennett B: Assessment of coma and impaired consciousness. A practical scale. *Lancet* 1974; 2:81–84.
112. Tebano MT, Cameroni M, Gallozzi G, et al: EEG spectral analysis after minor head injury in man. *Electroencephalogr Clin Neurophysiol* 1988; 70:185–189.
113. Thatcher RW, Cantor DS, McAlaster R, et al: Comprehensive predictions of outcome in closed head-injured patients. The development of prognostic equations. *Ann NY Acad Sci* 1991; 620:82–101.
114. Thatcher RW, Walker RA, Gerson I, et al: EEG discriminant analyses of mild head trauma. *Electroencephalogr Clin Neurophysiol* 1989; 73:94–106.
115. Tomei G, Sganzerla E, Spagnoli D, et al: Posttraumatic diffuse cerebral lesions. Relationship between clinical course, CT findings and ICP. *J Neurosurg Sci* 1991; 35: 61–75.
116. Uzzell BP, Dolinskas CA, Wiser RF, Langfitt TW: Influence of lesions detected by computed tomography on outcome and neuropsychological recovery after severe head injury. *Neurosurgery* 1987; 20:396–402.
117. Varney NR: Prognostic significance of anosmia in patients with closed-head trauma. *J Clin Exp Neuropsychol* 1988; 10:250–254.
118. Vollmer DG, Torner JC, Jane JA, et al: Age and outcome following traumatic coma: Why do older patients fare worse? *J Neurosurg* 1991; 75:S37–S49.
119. Waxman K, Sundine MJ, Young RF: Is early prediction of outcome in severe head injury possible? *Arch Surg* 1991; 126:1237–1241.
120. Weber M, Grolimund P, Seiler RW: Evaluation of posttraumatic cerebral blood flow velocities by transcranial doppler ultrasonography. *Neurosurgery* 1990; 27:106–112.
121. Werner RA, Vanderzant CW: Multimodality evoked potential testing in acute mild closed head injury. *Arch Phys Med Rehabil* 1991; 72:31–34.
122. Whyte KM, Pascoe M: Does black brain mean doom? Computed tomography in the prediction of outcome in children with severe head injuries: Benign vs malignant brain swelling. *Australas Radiol* 1989; 33:344–347.
123. Wolf AL, Levi L, Marmarou A, et al: Effect of THAM upon outcome in severe head injury: A randomized prospective clinical trial. *J Neurosurg* 1993; 78:54–59.
124. Woolf PD, McDonald JV, Feliciano DV, et al: The catecholamine response to multisystem trauma. *Arch Surg* 1992; 127:899–903.
125. York DH, Pulliam MW, Rosenfeld JG, et al: Relationship between visual evoked potentials and intracranial pressure. *J Neurosurg* 1981; 55:909–916.
126. Young B, Rapp RP, Norton JA, et al: Early prediction of outcome in head-injured patients. *J Neurosurg* 1981; 54:300–303.

CHAPTER 53

PREDICTING OUTCOME IN THE HEAD-INJURED PATIENT

Sung C. Choi
Thomas Y. Barnes

SYNOPSIS

This chapter discusses the prediction of outcome in head-injured patients. Most prognostic indicators are measured or recorded the first few days after admission and then are utilized in prediction models. This chapter reviews four basic prediction models: the discriminant function method, the logistic regression method, the nearest neighbor method, and the prediction tree method. Selected studies from the literature and some new data have been applied individually to those prediction methods to illustrate their use. The accuracy rates of these four models are also studied, using the Traumatic Coma Data Bank (TCDB) as a common database. The accuracy rate is a measure of the performance and usefulness of a model. TCDB data have also been analyzed to examine the additional predictive power of data collected after admission. It is postulated that the outcome of a head-injured patient may be determined by three variables: the effect of the prognostic factors, the treatment effect, and the random effect. Extremely good or poor outcomes can be predicted with confidence; however, intermediate outcomes are more difficult to predict, and a large number of intermediate outcomes may adversely affect the overall predictive accuracy of a chosen method. Future areas of research that must be explored in the prediction of outcome after head injury include improving the prediction of intermediate outcomes, predicting the patterns and rates of improvement in patients undergoing rehabilitation therapy, and utilizing technological resources to establish computer-intensive prediction systems that can be set up in neurosurgical intensive care units.

INTRODUCTION

Predicting the outcome in head-injured patients and determining the best prognostic indicators are issues of great interest to both clinicians and statisticians and have been dealt with by many investigators.[1–13] Outcome prediction can provide an understanding of the different pathophysiological aspects of head trauma. It can also serve as an objective and continuous measure of the severity of a patient's injury. In addition, prediction of outcome may provide a better basis for therapeutic strategies, as a clinician may select a different therapeutic approach for a patient with a good prognosis compared with a patient with a poor prognosis. Prediction also provides an objective basis for reviewing a patient's progress; if a patient does much better or worse than predicted, a clinician can attempt to determine the possible reasons. Prognostication is important in family counseling as well. Finally, prediction can aid in the assessment of the therapies used in nonrandomized studies by comparing the observed outcomes with the predicted outcomes.

The outcome measures commonly used in head-injured patients include the Glasgow Outcome Score (GOS), the Disability Rating Scale (DRS), the extended GOS, and certain neuropsychological and neurobehavioral scales. The GOS has been widely accepted as a standard means of describing outcome in head injury, having established validity and interobserver variability.[14] However, it is not a very sensitive scale, especially in assessing outcome in a moderate head injury, since a large proportion of moderately injured patients attain good recovery or moderate disability. Nevertheless, it remains the primary endpoint in most clinical studies. It has been customary to measure the GOS at 3 months, 6 months, and 12 months after an injury. The outcomes of head-injured patients are time-dependent dynamic processes. Many investigators prefer measurement of outcome at 6 months after injury because most patients' outcomes are relatively stable by that time. In fact, the 6-months-postinjury GOS was recommended as the primary endpoint for outcome assessment at a recent NIH conference on outcome measures for clinical trials.[15] While the longer the follow-up period, the more convincing the data, this has to be balanced against the reality of patient loss to follow-up.

OUTCOME FROM SEVERE HEAD INJURY

A review of the distribution of GOS at 3, 6, and 12 months after injury is provided in Fig. 53-1, which is based on 786 patients with severe head injury treated between 1976 and 1991 at the Medical College of Virginia (MCV). At 3 months the distribution has a sort of J shape, but the distribution shifts to a U shape at 12 months. The shift of the distribution results from continued improvement of some patients in the first four categories of the GOS, while the proportion of deaths is basically stationary since most deaths occur earlier in the course. Table 53-1 details shifts in GOS distribution from 3 months to 12 months in 448 patients with severe head injury. For example, of the patients who were severely disabled (SD) at 3 months after injury, 23 percent improved to a good recovery (G), 43 percent became moderately disabled (MD), and only 31 percent remained SD at 12 months. Among vegetative (V) patients, 6 percent improved to MD, 47 percent became SD, and the remaining patients either remained vegetative or died (D). The remarkable improvement in severely injured patients between 3 months and 12 months came as a pleasant surprise.

TABLE 53-1 GOS Distribution by Percent at 12 Months after Injury versus Outcome at 3 Months

3-Month Outcome	*n*	*12 Months Postinjury Outcome* G*	MD	SD	V	D
G	100	100.0	0	0	0	0
MD	136	74.3	25.7	0	0	0
SD	141	23.4	43.3	30.5	1.4	1.4
V	71	0	5.6	46.7	23.9	23.9

* G = good recovery; MD = moderately disabled; SD = severely disabled; V = vegetative; D = dead.

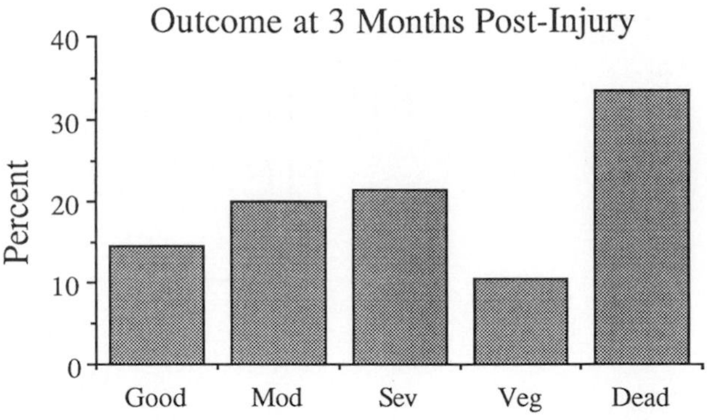

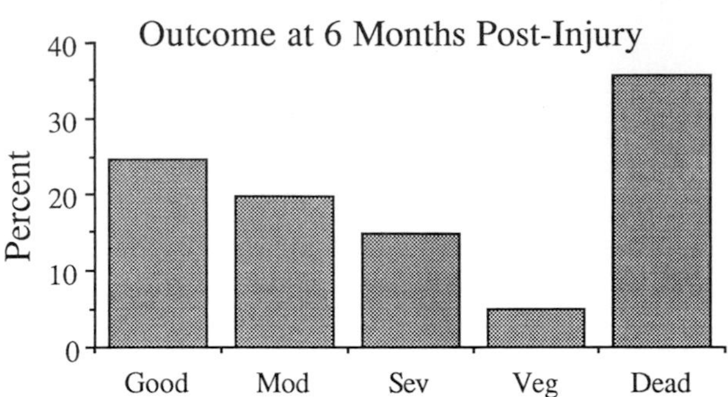

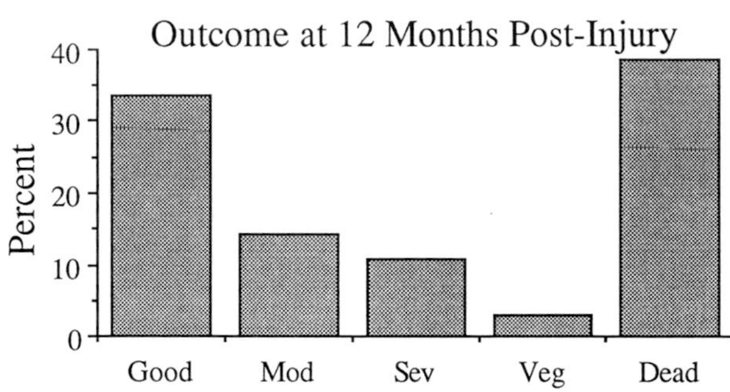

Figure 53-1. Distribution of GOS outcomes at 3, 6, and 12 months after injury, based on 786 severely head injured patients seen at the Medical College of Virginia from 1976 through 1991.

PROGNOSTIC INDICATORS

Many prognostic factors can potentially be used to predict outcome in head injury patients. The emphasis is generally on factors which are measured or recorded within the first few days after a patient's admission, since the value of such predictions depends on how early one can make them. Some well-known prognostic indicators and some other potential factors are summarized in Table 53-2, along with the significance level of the correlation between each factor and the 3-month postinjury GOS. The *p* value is based on the rank correlation when the factor is ordinal or continuous and on a chi-square test when the factor is categorical. Theoretically, each of two or three factors may not be individually significant, but they could be jointly significant. However, this occurs extremely rarely in the authors' experience. Similarly, one does not have to use all individually significant factors because of interfactor correlations. For example, both pupillary response and oculocephalics have a highly significant correlation with the GOS, but only one or the other is required in a prediction model because of the high correlation between them.

Deciding on the ideal number of indicators in the prediction model is not straightforward. There are good reasons for using a relatively low number of predictors. First, the reliability of the data is easier to maintain if one is dealing with a small number. Second, the chance of incompleteness as a result of missing values is less. Third, beyond a point, adding more indicators to the model does not necessarily increase the accuracy in most practical situations. This point is demonstrated in the following sections.

TABLE 53-2 Prognostic Factors in Patients with Severe Head Injury

Factor	Grades and Definitions	*p**
Age	Age in years	0.001
Race	White, black, or Asian-American	NS
Sex	Male or female	NS
Motor response†	6: obeys commands; 5: localizes; 4: normal flexor; 3: abnormal flexor; 2: extensor; 1: none	0.001
Pupillary response	2: bilaterally absent; 1: unilaterally absent; 0: bilaterally normal	0.001
Pupillary size‡	1: mydriatic; 0: normal	0.001
Oculocephalics‡	2: normal; 1: impaired; 0: absent	0.001
Eye opening	4: spontaneous; 3: to sound; 2: to pain; 1 none	0.001
Verbal response	5: oriented; 4: confused; 3: inappropriate words; 2: unintelligible sounds; 1: none	0.001
Midline shift	1: shifted; 0: not shifted	0.001
Intracerebral lesion	1: present; 0: absent	0.001
Extracerebral lesion	1: present; 0: absent	0.001
Intracranial pressure	mmHg	0.001
Systolic blood pressure	mmHg	NS
Diastolic blood pressure	mmHg	NS
Pulse	Beats per minute	0.001
Respiration	Breaths per minute	0.096
Temperature	°C	0.005
Hematocrit	Percent	0.022
P_{CO_2}	Arterial P_{CO_2} in mmHg	NS
P_{O_2}	Arterial P_{O_2} in mmHg	0.017
pH	Arterial blood pH	NS
Blood alcohol	mg/dl	NS
Injury to admission	Time in hours	NS
Multiple injury	1: yes; 0: no	0.072
Intracranial diagnosis	1: Diffuse Injury I (no visible pathology); 2: Diffuse Injury II; 3: Diffuse Injury III (swelling); 4: Diffuse Injury IV (shift); 5: mass lesion	0.001

* NS = not statistically significant.

† Best response from either right or left arm.

‡ Response of the best side.

SOURCE: Modified from Choi et al.[20]

BASIC PREDICTION METHODS

The prediction of outcome in a head-injured patient requires a model or formula that is based on a sample of well-documented patients with known outcomes. The formula essentially uses one or more predictor variables, such as age and the Glasgow Coma Scale (GCS). The primary aim of such an exercise would be to use the model to predict the outcome for a new patient. Four commonly used methods for prediction are described briefly below.

Discriminant Function Method

The discriminant function method consists of forming the outcome prediction groups on the basis of selected predictor variables in such a way that the differences between groups are maximized while each group itself is relatively homogeneous. Once the outcome groups are determined, the data on a patient can be checked to see into which group he or she should be placed for prediction. For example, in Fig. 53-2, age and the GCS are used to form two predictor groups. Theoretically, the underlying assumption is that the distribution of predictor variables is normal. However, the method is often satisfactory for nonnormal data.[16] In addition to the normal distribution assumption, the variances and covariances must be approximately equal between groups to apply a simple form of the method, known as the linear discriminant function, in which boundaries between groups are given by straight lines. If the groups have unequal variances and covariances, the so-called quadratic discriminant function with curvilinear boundaries should be used.

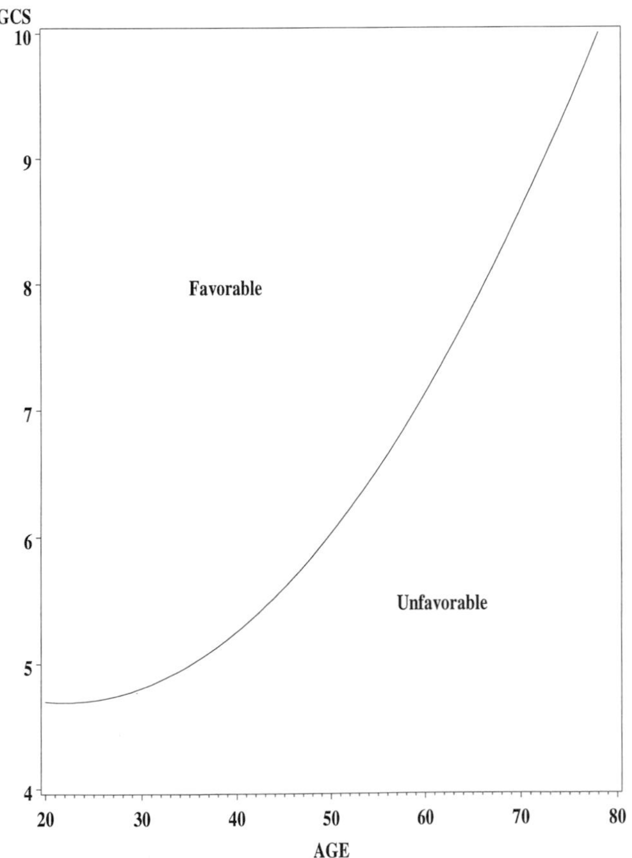

Figure 53-2. Discriminant regions based on a quadratic discriminant analysis, using age and GCS as prognostic factors and a binary outcome at 6 months after injury as the response.

Logistic Regression Method

Logistic regression involves deriving a regression equation which can be used to determine the probability of a patient belonging to each of the outcome groups. This method is particularly convenient when one is dealing with just two groups, as in the case of favorable (G/MD) and unfavorable outcomes (SD/V/D). A logistic regression model can provide the probability of a favorable outcome for a patient with a certain set of prognostic indicators. For example, if the calculated probability of a favorable outcome is 20 percent, the patient is clearly predicted to have an unfavorable outcome, as 50 percent is commonly taken as the cutoff point between the two outcome groups.[16,17] If the probability is 49 percent, the patient is again predicted to have an unfavorable outcome, although the confidence level is much lower since the patient has almost an equal chance for a favorable or an unfavorable outcome.

Nearest Neighbor Method

If a database is available for a relatively high number of patients with known outcomes, the outcome of a new patient can be predicted by using the nearest neighbor method. This consists of identifying a certain fixed number of patients (k) with the closest similarity to the patient in question. Then the outcome of the patient can be predicted by referring to a majority rule on the "neighbors." Clinicians probably apply some form of the nearest neighbor approach in predicting the outcomes of patients. This approach is attractive because it is conceptually simple, the idea makes good sense, and no assumption about the distribution is required. One problem with this approach is in measuring the similarity, which is by no means uniquely defined. The other problem involves choosing an optimal value for k.[16,18]

Prediction Tree Method

In this approach, all patients are initially considered as a single group. The set of prognostic indicators is used to split the group into two subgroups that are based on the most important indicator cut at the most critical value. The two subgroups are then each split, using the most important factor for that subgroup and again determining the most critical value for that factor. This process can be continued to a certain point when the subgroups are reasonably homogeneous. Thus, the process branches out in the manner of tree branches. In using the prediction tree, unlike the other methods described above, different prognostic factors may be used for different patients.[19,20]

ACCURACY RATE

The single most important measure of the performance and usefulness of a prediction rule is its correct prediction rate, or accuracy rate (AR). Any prediction rule whose AR has not been determined is suspect. The AR indicates how well the rule would work in future patients.

A simple approximation of the AR of a method is given by the proportion of patients who were correctly predicted using the same data set from which the rule was developed. The accuracy determined in this manner is called the apparent accuracy rate (AAR). As an illustration, consider the following table, which summarizes the results of predicting the 6-month postinjury outcomes of 730 severely head injured patients admitted to MCV from 1976 to 1991. Again, a favorable outcome is defined as G or MD on the GOS scale. The prediction is based on a logistic regression equation that uses age, GCS, and pupillary response as the prognostic factors.

	Predicted	Actual	Inaccurate Predictions
Favorable	309	226	83
Unfavorable	421	321	100

The AAR is the number of accurate predictions divided by the total number of patients:

$$\frac{226 + 321}{730} = 74.9\%$$

Unfortunately, the AAR tends to overestimate the true accuracy rate, since the data used to calculate the rule are also used in evaluating the rule. That is, the rule tends to work better when it is used to predict patients who were used in its development. In general, the overestimation tends to be more pronounced in a small sample than in a large one. The AAR can nevertheless be used as an optimistic upper limit of the true AR.

There are two common approaches for determining an unbiased AR. One simple procedure is to randomly split the total number of patients into two groups: a design set to develop a rule and a validation set to cross-validate and determine the AR. Although this method makes sense, it is not practical for small databases.

A more complicated approach is the "leave-one-out" procedure, which consists of the following steps:

1. Among all patients in the database, leave out the first patient and develop a rule using the rest of the patients.
2. Determine whether the outcome of the patient who was left out is correctly predicted.
3. Replace the first patient with the second patient and repeat steps 1 and 2.
4. Repeat steps 1 and 2 for each of the remaining patients.
5. An almost unbiased true AR is given by the proportion of patients correctly predicted.

Clearly, the leave-one-out procedure is computer-intensive and is recommended only when the sample is small. In other cases, the authors recommend the first approach.

RESULTS OF PREDICTION BASED ON ADMISSION DATA

The methods described in Basic Prediction Methods, above, are illustrated and discussed here, using selected studies from the literature as well as some new results. The methods described earlier have been applied to data recorded at the time of admission. The data analyzed in these examples were collected over a number of years, using standardized recording forms. The examples described below are by no means exhaustive.

DISCRIMINANT FUNCTION METHOD

Discriminant analysis was used to predict outcomes in a set of 523 patients with severe head injuries.[21,22] The patients were treated at MCV between May 1976 and December 1986. The primary criterion for inclusion was the inability of a patient to obey simple commands even after cardiopulmonary stabilization.

The prognostic factors considered were essentially those listed in Table 53-2, except for intracranial pressure and extracerebral and intracerebral lesions on computed tomography (CT). Model fitting was carried out in a stepwise fashion, with prognostic factors being added to or deleted from the model one at a time until the final model was determined. In an effort to make more specific predictions, four outcome categories were used instead of two. The V and D categories were combined because the V category included relatively few patients. An accurate prediction was said to be specific if it correctly placed a patient into the appropriate outcome category. A prediction was termed grossly accurate if it placed a patient either into the correct outcome group or into a group adjacent to the correct group.

The final model was based on three prognostic factors: age, motor score, and pupillary response. It was recognized that reclassification of the entire sample, using a model derived from that sample, would result in an overly optimistic estimate of predictive accuracy.[16] To correct this, the entire sample was divided randomly into two groups: two-thirds into a design set for model building and one-third into a validation set for cross-validation of the ARs. The specific AR and the gross AR were estimated to be 78.4 percent and 90.4 percent, respectively. Substituting the entire GCS score for the motor score failed to increase the accuracy rates for these data. A figure was presented to facilitate the prediction of outcomes in new patients.[21,22]

Several methods are available for performing a discriminant analysis. Linear and quadratic discriminant functions are among the most powerful and can be used if the set of prognostic factors has a normal distribution. When the model is based on only a few prognostic factors, a graph can be constructed and used to predict the outcomes of patients. For instance, Fig. 53-2 shows a prediction graph for severe head injury patients that uses only age and the GCS as prognostic factors. The predicted 6-month outcome for a given combination of age and GCS can be found by locating the point corresponding to those values on the graph. For example, a 30-year-old patient with an admission GCS of 7 is predicted to have a favorable outcome, while a 50-year-old patient with an admission GCS of 5 is predicted to have an unfavorable outcome. Figure 53-2 shows that elderly patients are expected to fare poorly no matter what their GCS is. Adolescents and young adults stand the best chance of having a favorable outcome as long as their GCS is above 4.

Logistic Regression Method

In using the logistic regression method, the estimated probability of an unfavorable (or favorable) outcome can be determined for each subject. Step-by-step instructions for calculating probabilities by using a logistic regression equation have been reported by Narayan et al.[22] Several studies have used this method to predict outcome in severely head injured individuals. One early study compared logistic regression to sequential Bayes methods for estimating the probability of an unfavorable outcome.[23] Data from 115 patients were analyzed, and 12 prognostic factors were considered, including age, motor score, pupillary light response, pupillary size, and presence or absence of a mass lesion. A logistic regression model based on these data had a 91 percent AAR. These authors[23] listed several advantages of the logistic regression approach over the sequential Bayes method as a predictive model.

A subsequent investigation[24] used a larger data set and supplemented clinical data with other information obtained after admission. In this study, logistic regression was employed in a comparative analysis of the clinical examination, multimodality evoked potentials (MEPs), CT scanning, and intracranial pressure (ICP). A combination of age, GCS score, pupillary response, eye movements, and presence or absence of a surgical mass lesion predicted outcome with an AAR of 82 percent. Models based solely on CT scan data or ICP levels proved to be weak predictors of outcome. However, when used in combination with the clinical parameters, CT and ICP data provided more reliable predictions. MEPs were effective predictors both on their own and in combination with the clinical prognostic factors. These authors[24] concluded that the clinical examination provided the best basis for predicting outcome in severe head injury but that additional information could enhance the reliability of such predictions somewhat.

A third study analyzed clinical and demographic data from 264 patients and used stepwise logistic regression to construct charts for binary outcome prediction.[25] The final model was based on age, GCS score, and oculocephalic response. A somewhat better prediction was achieved when the GCS scores on postinjury days 1 and 4 were used. Therefore, two sets of charts were created, Fig. 53-3*A* for day 1 data alone and Fig. 53-3*B* for day 1 and day 4 data. The probability of a favorable outcome for a patient with a given age, GCS score(s), and oculocephalic response may be read from the appropriate chart. For example, from Fig. 53-3*A*, a 35-year-old patient with a normal oculocephalic response and a GCS of 8 on day 1 would have approximately an 80 percent chance of a favorable outcome. Naturally, this patient would be predicted to have a favorable outcome. The use of Fig. 53-3*B* is more complex, since the abscissa is a function of the day 1 and day 4 GCS scores. Consider a 30-year-old patient with a bilaterally impaired oculocephalic response, a day 1 GCS of 6, and a day 4 GCS of 3. Then $0.35(6) + 0.46(3) = 3.48$, which is the appropriate reference value on the abscissa. This patient has only a 20 percent probability of a favorable outcome.

The expected accuracy of prediction was evaluated by means of computer simulations. Taking 50 percent as the threshold probability for predicting a favorable response, AARs were 79 percent for the day 1 data and 81 percent for the day 1 and day 4 data. The charts provide a visually useful way to examine the effects of age, oculocephalic response, and GCS score on outcome.

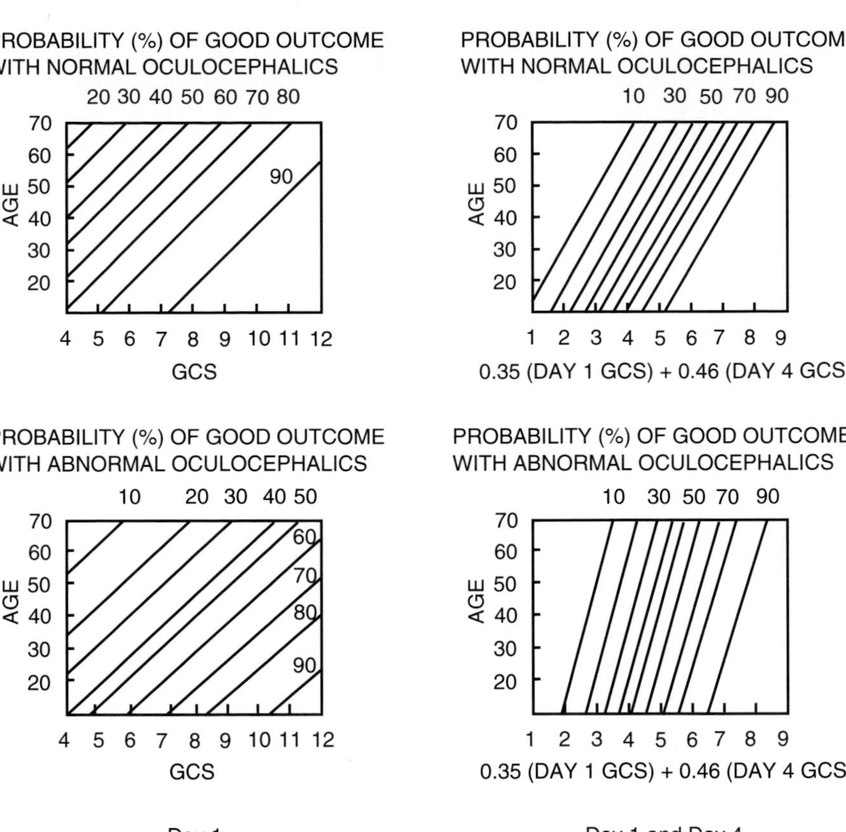

Figure 53-3. *A.* Probability of a good outcome based on oculocephalic response, age, and GCS score on day 1. Upper: outcome probability for a patient with an absent or bilaterally impaired oculocephalic response. Lower: outcome probability for a patient with a normal or unilaterally impaired response. *B.* Probability of a good outcome based on oculocephalic response, age, and GCS score on day 1 and day 4. Upper: outcome probability for a patient with an absent or bilaterally impaired oculocephalic response. Lower: outcome probability for a patient with a normal or unilaterally impaired response. (From Choi et al.[25] with permission.)

Logistic regression provides a flexible framework for investigating the simultaneous impact of several factors on outcome in head injury. A mixture of numerical and categorical factors can be analyzed and ranked in order of prognostic importance.

Nearest Neighbor Method

Enas[18] analyzed data from 133 patients with severe head injuries admitted to MCV between May 1976, and September 1979. He used nearest neighbor discriminant analysis to build a set of classification rules based on these patients and then predicted outcomes in a set of 100 new patients. Although data from CT scans, MEPs, and ICP monitoring were evaluated, his best discriminant models used only age, GCS score, pupillary response, presence or absence of a mass lesion, and normal eye movements. Predictive accuracies were generally 75 percent or higher. Enas[18] also examined procedures to specify the optimal number of "nearest neighbors" for a particular analysis.

Prediction Tree Method

More recently, data from 555 severely head injured patients were used to develop a prediction tree for outcome prediction in severe head injury.[20] These patients were admitted to the MCV neurosurgical service between May 1976, and December 1989, and each had a known GOS outcome at 12 months after injury. The patients were managed aggressively, with emphasis on ventilatory support and control of ICP below 25 mmHg.

A prediction tree relating the prognostic factors obtained at admission to the 12-month GOS outcome is presented in Fig. 53-4, which has been modified from Choi et al.[20] The ovals in this diagram denote intermediate subgroups subject to further splitting, while the prognostic subgroups appear as squares. The numbers below the squares represent the prognostic rank of each subgroup based on the proportion of favorable (G/MD) outcomes. The predicted outcome for a single patient is easily determined by running that patient down the tree. For example, a patient with a bilaterally absent pupillary response and a motor score of 2 or less would go right at the initial split, would go to the left at the next split, and would be placed into prognostic subgroup 9. The predicted outcome for that patient would be V or D. If the motor score had been above 2, the patient would have proceeded down the tree for further splitting based on age and would have wound up in either subgroup 5 or subgroup 7. The predicted outcome would be that corresponding to the appropriate prognostic subgroup.

In the prediction tree, the patients first are split on

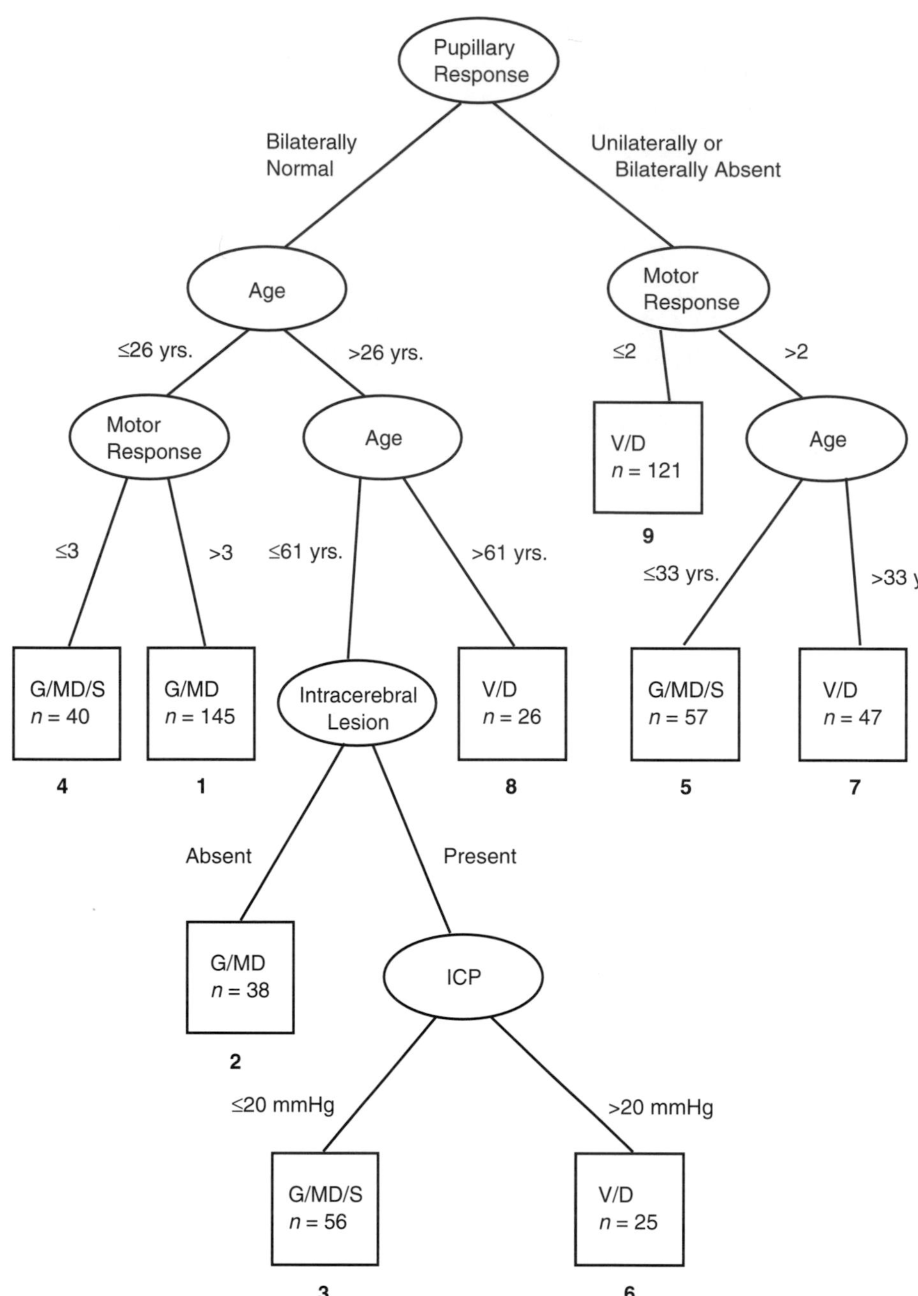

Figure 53-4. Prediction tree based on 555 severely head-injured patients. The predicted 12-month outcomes (defined by the Glasgow Outcome Scale) are G = good recovery; MD = moderately disabled; S = severely disabled; V = vegetative; D = dead. Ovals denote intermediate subgroups subject to further splitting; squares denote final prognostic subgroups. The numbers below the squares represent the prognostic rank of each subgroup based on the proportion of favorable (G/MD) outcomes. (Modified from Choi et al.[20] with permission.)

the basis of their pupillary response, but subsequent splits show different patterns. Patients with bilaterally normal pupillary responses tend to have favorable outcomes unless they are elderly or have an intracerebral lesion and a high ICP. Patients with abnormal pupils tend to have unfavorable outcomes, with motor score and then age as subsequent split variables. Although only five factors were used to construct this tree, other factors, such as pupillary size and oculocephalic response, could be included as "alternative" splits.

The authors calculated the proportion of cases correctly classified in each prognostic subgroup, combining SD and V patients because of the small number of patients in the V state. Overall predictive accuracy was 77.7 percent. The subgroup accuracy rates ranged from 57 percent to 90 percent, with the highest accuracy of prediction occurring in subgroups with very good (subgroup 1) or very poor (subgroup 9) outcomes. The predictive accuracy rate was 82.3 percent for G and 81.5 percent for D but only 60.5 percent for MD. It is generally recognized that intermediate outcomes are harder to predict accurately.[22] The primary benefit of the prediction tree technique remains the characterization of important prognostic factors and their relationship to outcome. Another benefit is that it shows some common prognostic patterns ranked in terms of likely outcomes.

It is interesting to observe that all the existing models of prediction include age and GCS (or motor score). Clearly, these two factors are the two most critical indicators at the time of admission.

COMPARING SEVERAL PREDICTION METHODS

One may wish to compare the accuracy rates of several different prediction techniques using the same database. It is clear that the unbiased comparison of two different prediction methods based on different sets of data would be difficult. Therefore, data from the Traumatic Coma Data Bank (TCDB)[26,27] were analyzed by several different classification methods. This multicenter database contained clinical, intensive care unit (ICU), and outcome data on over 1000 severely head injured patients. Information from CT scans and data describing the incidence of complications such as hypoxia and hypotension were included in these analyses. Logistic regression, linear and quadratic discriminant analyses, nearest neighbor discriminant analyses (with $k = 3$ and $k = 5$), and nonparametric prediction tree analyses were performed. Outcome at 6 months after injury, dichotomized as favorable (G/MD) or unfavorable (SD/V/D), was used.

Exclusions for various reasons (brain-dead on arrival, etc.) left a sample of 742 subjects for analysis. Four hundred sixty-two of these subjects were randomly allocated to a design set for model building, while the remaining 280 made up a validation set for cross-validation. The predictive models were fitted in three stages (Table 53-3). Model A used prognostic data available at the time of admission: the patient's age, motor score, and pupillary response. Model B added hypoxia and hypotension to the set of prognostic factors from model A. Hypoxia was defined as $Pa_{O_2} \leq 60$ mmHg, and hypotension was defined as systolic blood pressure ≤ 90 mmHg. Both were recorded as 0 if absent and 1 if present. Finally, model C added the intracranial diagnosis. A CT-based classification scheme for intracranial diagnosis[28] was used. Briefly, the diagnostic classes were diffuse injury with no visible pathology (D1 I), diffuse injury (D1 II), diffuse injury with swelling (D1 III) diffuse injury with midline shift (D1 IV), and evacuated (MI) or nonevacuated (MII) mass lesion.

The accuracy rates for these analyses are summarized in Table 53-3. These rates ranged from 67 to 75 percent for model A, 68 to 76 percent for model B, and 67 to 76 percent for model C. The logistic, linear, and quadratic discriminant functions had slightly better accuracy rates than did the other approaches. The highest predictive accuracy (75.6 percent) was achieved using a quadratic discriminant function based on model B. The nearest neighbor method with $k = 3$ had the lowest predictive accuracy, below 70 percent for all three models. The differences among various prediction methods in terms of accuracy were rather small. Also, it appears that the addition of hypoxia, hypotension, and CT scan data did little to improve the predictive accuracy. The results suggested that the highest accuracy one can achieve in the early period after a head injury is no more than 80 percent.

Clearly, one cannot expect to achieve a 100 percent accuracy rate in predicting patients' outcomes. It is well recognized that some patients with very good prognostic indicators at the time of admission have unfavorable outcomes. For example, a patient in the teens or early twenties with a GCS of 8 can have an unfavorable outcome. Conversely, a patient who is 60 years old and has a GCS of 4 or 5 cannot be predicted to have a favorable outcome. Although it is unlikely, such a patient can make a remarkable recovery despite the odds against it. This unpredictability is due to the random effect, which will be described in Discussion and Conclusions, below. In most prediction methods, "falsely pessimistic" predictions occurred somewhat more frequently than did "falsely optimistic" ones.

There was some evidence that increasing k, the number of nearest neighbors, could increase the accuracy of that technique. When k was increased from 3 to 5,

TABLE 53-3 Accuracy Rates for Several Methods of Prediction

Method	Model A, %	Model B, %	Model C, %
Logistic	71.8	73.7	72.5
Liner discriminant	73.3	73.3	72.5
Quadratic discriminant	74.8	75.6	75.5
Nearest neighbor ($k = 3$)	67.3	68.1	67.2
Nearest neighbor ($k = 5$)	71.4	68.1	70.2
Prediction tree			68.8

See Table 53-4 for the definitions of the three different models.

the predictive accuracy of model A improved from 67.3 to 71.4 percent and that of model C increased from 67.2 to 70.2 percent. However, no corresponding increase was observed for model B. The reader is referred to Enas[18] for a discussion of optimality considerations in nearest neighbor discriminant analysis. Also, the performance of the prediction tree approach on these data was somewhat disappointing, as it achieved only 69 percent predictive accuracy. Only one split was performed, and it was based on the best motor score. Therefore, there was no new information on possible interactions among the prognostic factors.

EFFECT OF LATER DATA ON PREDICTION

One could speculate that data collected after admission could be used to improve the accuracy of prediction. Variables of interest include ICP, CT scan data, and incidence of complications. The TCDB data were analyzed to examine the additional predictive power provided by considering CT scan data, hypotension, and hypoxia. Outcomes at 3, 6, and 12 months after injury were dichotomized as favorable or unfavorable, as described in Comparing Several Prediction Methods, above. Models A, B, and C (described above) were analyzed, and the same design and validation sets were employed.

Table 53-4 summarizes the predictive accuracy of logistic regression analyses on the TCDB data. Age, motor score, pupillary response, and intracranial diagnosis were found to be significantly related to outcome at 6 and 12 months after injury ($p < .001$), while hypotension was marginally significant ($.05 < p < .15$). The associations between the prognostic factors and outcome at 3 months after injury were almost as strong as ($p < .001$ for motor score, $p < .01$ for age and intracranial diagnosis, $p < .05$ for pupillary response, $p > .40$ for hypotension). Hypoxia was not significantly related to outcome in any of the regression models ($p > .40$). The three models were then used to predict outcomes at 3, 6, and 12 months after injury in the validation set. There was little difference among these rates, all of which fell into the range of 70 to 75 percent. The highest accuracy, 75.4 percent, was achieved by model B at 12 months after injury.

It was observed that the accuracy rates for model C were lower than the corresponding rates for model B. This was actually due to random error, since the ARs for model C, based on an additional prognostic indicator, theoretically cannot be lower than those for a model based on a subset of the indicators. In any event, it was evident that the accuracy rate did not improve when the intracranial diagnosis was added to the model B prognostic factors. However, there are some indications that the "confidence level" of prediction can be improved by adding the additional prognostic data to the three primary factors of model A. These findings are described below.

Subjects were predicted to have an unfavorable outcome if their estimated probability of an unfavorable outcome was greater than or equal to 50 percent. Naturally, one could predict with more confidence when the estimated probability was close to 0 or 100 percent (called "polar" predictions by previous authors[22]) than when it was close to 50 percent ("neutral" predictions). To illustrate this, model A and model C prediction results for several probability levels are presented in Tables 53-5 and 53-6 and in Fig. 53-5. As might be expected, both models attained their highest predictive accuracies at the extremes of the distribution of estimated probabilities. Predictive accuracy rates were much lower in the neutral probability levels. Thus, if the estimated probability was either very low or very high, one would have a high degree of confidence in the corresponding prediction. Conversely, if the estimated probability was near

TABLE 53-4 Accuracy of Prediction by Logistic Regression at Three Time Points

	Model A Admission Data	Model B Further ER Data	Model C ICU Data
	Age Best motor score Pupillary response	Age Best motor score Pupillary response Hypoxia Hypotension	Age Best motor score Pupillary response Hypoxia Hypotension Intracranial DX
3-month accuracy, %	73.6	73.6	70.5
6-month accuracy, %	71.8	73.7	72.5
12-month accuracy, %	73.1	75.4	73.4

TABLE 53-5 Accuracy of Model A Prediction of Probability of an Unfavorable Outcome

Estimated Probability of an Unfavorable Outcome, %	*n*	Correct Predictions No.	Correct Predictions %
0–9	0	—	—
10–29	47	34	72
30–49	60	35	58
50–69	38	19	50
70–89	55	40	73
90–99	66	63	95
Total	266	191	72

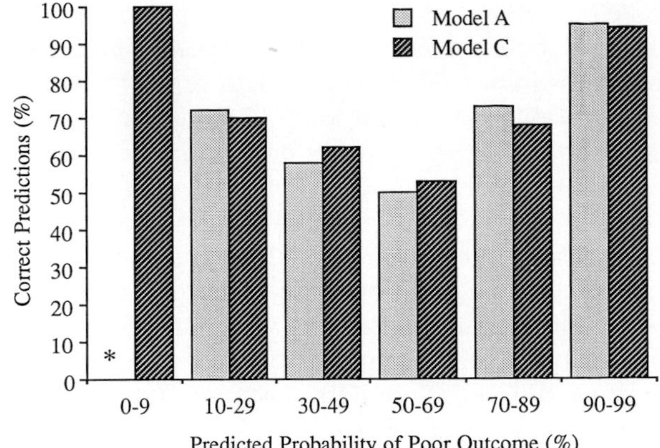

Figure 53-5. Percentage of correct predictions by predicted probability of a poor outcome for model A (using age, best motor score, and pupillary response) and model C (add hypoxia, hypotension, and intracranial diagnosis to prognostic factors from model A). *No patients with predicted probability of a poor outcome 0–9% under model A.

50 percent, one would not be as confident in the prediction. After pooling the results from the intervals of 30 to 49 percent and 50 to 69 percent, it can be seen that model C's "neutral" predictions were slightly more accurate than those of model A (58 percent versus 55 percent). No subject had an estimated probability of an unfavorable outcome less than 10 percent under model A, and only four subjects had such a prediction under model C.

Tables 53-5 and 53-6 and Fig. 53-5 provide information about how accurate a single prediction is likely to be. For example, if a patient has a 92 percent estimated probability of an unfavorable outcome under model C, the chance that this prediction will be correct is approximately 94 percent (Fig. 53-5). If a patient has a 24 percent estimated probability of an unfavorable outcome under model A, the chance that this prediction will be correct is approximately 72 percent. Knowledge of the projected accuracy of a given prediction may then influence the choice of therapeutic strategies. It also could be helpful in reviewing a patient's progress and in family counseling.

The above prediction results, like those of all previous studies, are confined to prognostic factors recorded before a patient's discharge. When follow-up data such as the discharge or the 3-month GOS are available, it is of interest to see if outcome at a future time can be predicted accurately by the outcome at an earlier time point. For the 1976–1991 MCV database, a logistic regression model incorporating age, motor score, pupillary response at the time of admission, and the GOS outcome at discharge as prognostic factors was used to predict favorable or unfavorable outcome at 3, 6, and 12 months after injury. The results are presented in Table 53-7. The predictive accuracy rates for these analyses were 87.2 percent, 83.0 percent, and 88.5 percent, respectively. These rates were substantially higher than those from prediction models using only admitting and CT scan prognostic data. In general, the discharge GOS, age, and pupillary response were significantly associated with subsequent outcomes ($p < .001$ for discharge GOS, $.006 < p < .180$ for age, $.01 < p < .05$ for pupillary response), while motor score was not. Therefore, if one wishes at discharge to predict the outcome at a later time point, it is important to add the discharge data to

TABLE 53-6 Accuracy of Model C Prediction of Probability of an Unfavorable Outcome

Estimated Probability of an Unfavorable Outcome, %	*n*	Correct Predictions No.	Correct Predictions %
0–9	4	4	100
10–29	46	32	70
30–49	45	28	62
50–69	43	23	53
70–89	57	39	68
90–99	70	66	94
Total	265	192	72

TABLE 53-7 Effect of Follow-up Data on Predictive Accuracy at Three Time Points

	Logistic Regression Model	
	Admission Data Plus GOS at Discharge	**Admission Data Plus GOS at 3 Months Postinjury**
3-month accuracy, %	87.2	—
6-month accuracy, %	83.0	93.5
12-month accuracy, %	88.5	93.4

the key baseline prognostic factors. Similarly, a model with age, motor score, pupillary response, and the 3-month postinjury GOS was used to predict favorable or unfavorable outcome at 6 and 12 months after injury. From Table 53-7, the corresponding predictive accuracies were 93.5 percent and 93.4 percent. These accuracy rates also represented a substantial improvement over models using only the admitting prognostic data and models including additional data recorded before discharge. The 3-month postinjury GOS and the pupillary response were significantly associated with later outcomes ($p < .001$ for 3-month postinjury GOS, $.05 < p < .10$ for pupillary response), but age and motor score were not. It should be noted that given the 3-month postinjury GOS, age and motor score are no longer critical for prediction.

The formulas which can be used to determine the probability of an unfavorable outcome at 3, 6, and 12 months after injury, using the admission data and GOS at discharge, are presented below:

Age = age in years
Pupil = pupillary response coded as
  0 = bilaterally normal
  1 = unilaterally absent
  2 = bilaterally absent
GOSDC = GOS at discharge coded as
  0 = good recovery (G)
  1 = moderately disabled (MD)
  2 = severely disabled (SD)
  3 = vegetative state (V)
  4 = dead (D)

For 3-month outcome:

$$P = \frac{1}{[1 + \exp(5.607 - 0.037\text{Age} - 0.542\text{Pupil} - 2.345\text{GOSDC})]}$$

For 6-month outcome:

$$P = \frac{1}{[1 + \exp(7.262 - 0.045\text{Age} - 0.440\text{Pupil} - 2.472\text{GOSDC})]}$$

For 12-month outcome:

$$P = \frac{1}{[1 + \exp(7.453 - 0.026\text{Age} - 0.448\text{Pupil} - 2.528\text{GOSDC})]}$$

Any of the above probabilities can be easily calculated using a pocket calculator.

It should be remarked that the improved predictive accuracy attained by the model that included the discharge GOS and the even greater accuracy attained by the model that included the 3-month GOS were not entirely unexpected. Among other reasons, patients dead at 6 months after injury were likely to be dead at discharge and at 3 months after injury. For example, in a sample of 406 patients from the MCV database, 126 were dead at discharge and at 3 months after injury and only 5 more were dead at 6 months after injury.

DISCUSSION AND CONCLUSIONS

The authors' experience with severe head injury suggests that one can expect to predict the outcomes with about 80 percent accuracy by using the data available at admission. The AR can be increased to about 90 percent if the GOS at discharge is incorporated in the prediction models.

It has been postulated that patient outcome is determined by three major components: effect of prognostic factors, treatment effect, and random effect. The effect of various prognostic factors has been described in this chapter. The treatment effect refers to the effect resulting from different centers, different clinicians, and different treatments. For example, one would expect differences in patient profiles, delay from injury to surgery, management techniques, and other support systems among different centers. Furthermore, almost all the MCV patients were randomized in trials involving a barbiturate, hyperventilation, and Tromethamine. The possible effect of the different therapies used in the trials is not incorporated in the prognostic factors. Incorporation of such therapies would make a prediction model less meaningful because the study therapies were not effective or not universally accepted. The random effect refers to the inherent variability among similar patients. Even if two patients have exactly the same degree of injury and identical prognostic indicators and are treated identically by the same clinician, their outcomes can be different. The random effect also includes the effect of unexpected complications or certain unknown factors. In any event, the random effect is a fact of life.

On the basis of extensive work involving various methods and models for prediction, it would appear that the upper limit of predictive accuracy in severely head injured patients, based on the data recorded at admission and in the ICU, is about 80 percent. The inaccurate predictions of the remaining 20 percent are due to the possible treatment effect (positive or negative) and the random effect. It should be emphasized that even an 80 percent accuracy rate is remarkable and is higher than that for other diseases or injuries. The high accuracy rate in predicting outcomes for severely head injured patients indicates the power of the prognostic factors, including age, GCS (or motor score), and pupillary response. The advent of new diagnostic tools such as magnetic resonance imaging (MRI) may provide new prognostic information which will improve the accuracy of outcome prediction.

It should be mentioned that an 80 percent accuracy rate does not imply that the outcomes of severely head injured patients can be predicted with a high degree of accuracy regardless of patient care. Care that is less than state-of-the-art would decrease the AR because the therapy effect would increase. It also should be remarked that all patients in the database are managed more or less uniformly according to a carefully developed treatment protocol. Thus, the 80 percent accuracy rate applies to patients treated with a state-of-the-art protocol.

In reviewing the prediction results of numerous studies, one finds a definite pattern. Extremely good or extremely poor outcomes can be predicted accurately, but intermediate outcomes such as MD and SD are more difficult to predict. When a large proportion of outcomes lies in this intermediate range, the overall predictive accuracy suffers. For example, if logistic regression is performed, many of these patients will be predicted to have about an equal chance for a favorable outcome or an unfavorable outcome. This leads to an excess of cases in the neutral probability levels, which are known to have relatively poor predictive accuracy, as shown in Fig. 53-5. To illustrate this, a subset of patients from Table 53-6 whose estimated probability of an unfavorable outcome fell between 40 and 59 percent was identified and their actual GOS outcomes were observed. Almost 50 percent of these patients were moderately or severely disabled at 6 months after injury, in contrast to only 33 percent in the entire TCDB validation set. Hence, the overall predictive accuracy for Table 53-6 is only 72 percent. The problem is less serious at 12 months after injury, when the GOS distribution contains a smaller proportion of intermediate outcomes and becomes more U-shaped, as illustrated in Fig. 53-1. Still, improving the prediction of intermediate outcomes would increase the overall predictive accuracy at all time points. This should be a goal of future research.

Many studies of severely head injured patients have attempted to predict outcome at a certain time after injury. In future analyses, investigators may focus on predicting patterns and rates of improvement over time in patients who are undergoing rehabilitation therapy. There is little emphasis on this topic in the current literature.[29] Such research would target moderately and severely disabled subjects, whose outcomes are often difficult to predict. The methods described in Basic Prediction Methods, above, could still be applied but may require modification because of the fact that the levels of the prognostic factors themselves could change over time.

Traditionally, statistical methods for outcome prediction could be implemented on mainframe computers. Today, as a result of significant improvements in computer technology, these techniques are becoming "portable" to personal computers. Computer-intensive approaches such as the prediction tree method are now feasible. The increased availability of these procedures should stimulate interest and lead to further improvements. Also, it would not be difficult to set up a computerized prediction system in the neurosurgical ICU once an effective prediction rule was developed. Current clinical data would be collected and used to continually update the prognoses of all the patients.

References

1. Becker DP, Miller JD, Ward JD, et al: The outcome from severe head injury with early diagnosis and intensive management. *J Neurosurg* 47:491–502, 1977.
2. Bowers SA, Marshall LF: Outcome in 200 consecutive cases of severe head injury treated in San Diego County: A prospective analysis. *Neurosurgery* 6:237–242, 1980.
3. Braakman R, Gelpke GJ, Habbema JDF, et al: Systematic selection of prognostic features in patients with severe head injury. *Neurosurgery* 6:362–370, 1980.
4. Habbema JDF, Braakman R, Avezaat CJJ: Prognosis of the individual patient with severe head injury. *Acta Neurochir [Suppl] (Wien)* 28:158–160, 1979.
5. Jennett B: Prognosis after head injury, in Vinken PJ, Bruyn GW (eds): *Handbook of Clinical Neurology: Injuries of the Brain and Skull, Part II.* Amsterdam: North-Holland, 1976:669–681.
6. Jennett B, Bond M: Assessment of outcome after severe brain damage: A practical scale. *Lancet* 1:480–484, 1975.
7. Jennett B, Teasdale G, Braakman R, et al: Predicting outcome in individual patients after severe head injury. *Lancet* 1:1031–1034, 1976.
8. Klauber MR, Barrett-Conner E, Marshall LF, et al: The epidemiology of head injury: A prospective study of an entire community—San Diego County, California, 1978. *Am J Epidemiol* 113:500–509, 1981.
9. Levati A, Farina ML, Vecchi G, et al: Prognosis of severe head injuries. *J Neurosurg* 57:779–783, 1982.
10. Miller JD, Butterworth JF, Gudeman SK, et al: Further experience in the management of severe head injury. *J Neurosurg* 54:289–299, 1981.
11. Overgaard J, Christensen S, Hvid-Hansen O, et al: Prognosis after head injury based on early clinical examination. *Lancet* 2:631–635, 1973.
12. Teasdale G, Jennett B: Assessment and prognosis of coma after head injury. *Acta Neurochir (Wien)* 34:45–55, 1976.

13. Teasdale G, Jennett B: Assessment of coma and impaired consciousness: A practical scale. *Lancet* 2:81–84, 1974.
14. Maas AIR, Braakman R, Schouten HJA, et al: Agreement between physicians on assessment of outcome following severe head injury. *J Neurosurg* 58:321–325, 1983.
15. Clifton GL, Hayes RL, Levin HS, et al: Outcome measures for clinical trials involving traumatically brain-injured patients: Report of a conference. *Neurosurgery* 31:975–978, 1992.
16. Choi SC (ed): *Statistical Methods of Discrimination and Classification: Advances in Theory and Applications.* Oxford: Pergamon Press, 1986.
17. Hosmer DW, Lemeshow S: *Applied Logistic Regression.* New York: Wiley, 1989.
18. Enas GG: Optimality considerations in nearest neighbor classification. Unpublished Ph.D. dissertation, Richmond, VA: Department of Biostatistics, Virginia Commonwealth University, 1982, pp 95–98.
19. Breiman L, Freidman JH, Olshen RA, et al: *Classification and Regression Trees.* Belmont, CA: Wadsworth, 1984.
20. Choi SC, Muizelaar JP, Barnes TY, et al: Prediction tree for severely head-injured patients. *J Neurosurg* 75:251–255, 1991.
21. Choi SC, Narayan RK, Anderson RL, et al: Enhanced specificity of prognosis in severe head injury. *J Neurosurg* 69:381–385, 1988.
22. Narayan RK, Enas GG, Choi SC, et al: Practical techniques for predicting outcome in severe head injury, in Becker DP, Gudeman SK (eds): *Textbook of Head Injury.* Philadelphia: Saunders, 1989:420–425.
23. Stablein DM, Miller JD, Choi SC, et al: Statistical methods for determining prognosis in severe head injury. *Neurosurgery* 6:243–248, 1980.
24. Narayan RK, Greenberg RP, Miller JD, et al: Improved confidence of outcome prediction in severe head injury: A comparative analysis of the clinical examination, multimodality evoked potentials, CT scanning and intracranial pressure. *J Neurosurg* 54:751–762, 1981.
25. Choi SC, Ward JD, Becker DP: Chart for outcome prediction in severe head injury. *J Neurosurg* 59:294–297, 1983.
26. Marshall LF, Becker DP, Bowers SA, et al: The National Traumatic Coma Data Bank. Part 1: Design, purpose, goals and results. *J Neurosurg* 59:276–284, 1983.
27. Eisenberg HM, Gary HE Jr, Aldrich EF, et al: Initial CT findings in 753 patients with severe head injury: A report from the NIH Traumatic Coma Data Bank. *J Neurosurg* 73:688–698, 1990.
28. Marshall LF, Marshall SB, Klauber MR, et al: A new classification of head injury based on computerized tomography. *J Neurosurg* 75:S14–S20, 1991.
29. Choi SC, Barnes TY, Bullock R, et al: Temporal profile of outcomes in severe head injury. *J Neurosurg,* 81:169–173, 1994.

CHAPTER 54

AGE AND OUTCOME OF HEAD INJURY

John A. Jane
Paul C. Francel

SYNOPSIS

This chapter evaluates and explores the relationship between age and neurological outcome following traumatic brain injury. In some studies age has been noted to be either the most *important variable, or* one *of the most important variables, in determining outcome. Clinical variables known to affect functional outcome for traumatic head injury have been examined and related to outcome. Some of these prognostic indicators included prior medical systemic illness, history of multiple injury at the time of trauma, severity of the injury, mechanism of injury, and the presence of clinical signs such as those evaluated by the GCS score or motor score, pupillary response, presence of hypoxia or hypertension, and skull fractures. Though each of these variables strongly affected neurological outcome and each was affected by age, none singly or in combination could exclude age as an independent variable affecting neurological outcome.*

Evaluation of radiological data shows that hemorrhagic complications that increase with age do not entirely explain the age-dependent effect. It is probable that there are intrinsic characteristics of the aging brain that worsen outcome following head injury. The biological basis for this phenomenon remains unclear. It has been suggested that perhaps the aging brain shows a greater excitotoxic sensitivity per nerve cell than the younger brain, and that the aging brain functions ineffectively after severe head injury because of its reduced neuronal reserve.

INTRODUCTION

Age is one of the most reliable prognostic indicators of mortality and morbidity following traumatic brain injury. There is a progressive age-associated increase in mortality rate following an equivalent head injury: patients older than 65 years will have nearly twice the mortality of patients under 65.[1–16] It has been found that this increased rate does not relate to the neurological examination on admission nor to the presence of extraaxial hematomas on a computerized tomography (CT) scan. When patients of different ages were matched according to admission Glasgow Coma Scale (GCS) score and evidence of extraaxial fluid collections, the older patients always fared worse than the younger ones.[17–20] The vegetative survival rate for all ages appeared to be approximately the same,[9,19] suggesting that the effect of age on outcome is not the result of younger patients surviving in a severely disabled or vegetative state instead of dying, but rather that the aged population suffers greater brain injury from the same trauma.

A large prospectively collected database showed that age made no difference in the injury severity as assessed by motor or GCS score.[17] In the older age group minor head injury produced a significantly higher percentage and severity of postconcussion syndrome at 6 weeks and 1 year.[21] Thus, it can be concluded that age is directly associated with an increase in mortality and morbidity rates following brain injury.

Studies are needed to eliminate other variables that correlate with age.[22,23] For example, is the increased mortality rate seen in the elderly due to injuries of greater severity than those in younger patients, or is it secondary to an increase in frequency of preexisting illness? Possibly the increased mortality rate is a result of more frequent systemic medical complications rather than the effects of brain damage. Does the greater mortality rate seen in older patients correspond to an increased rate of severely disabled or vegetative younger patients, or is age itself an independent variable in determining outcome? We think that age is a key independent variable because of an intrinsic biological difference between the brain of an elderly patient and that of a younger one. In the latter portion of this chapter mechanisms that make central nervous system (CNS) neurons more susceptible to an equivalent injury as they age are evaluated as possibly explaining the effect of age on outcome of head injury.

CLINICAL VARIABLES AND OUTCOME FROM TRAUMATIC HEAD INJURY

A study of 661 patients undertaken by our group,[19] in collaboration with other centers involved in the Traumatic Coma Data Bank,[17,24–33] evaluated the relationship of age and outcome following traumatic coma. The outcome of patients at 6 months postinjury was clearly age-dependent and independent of the cause of injury.[19] Figure 54-1 compares outcome with age using the Glasgow Outcome Scale. In this study, good recovery was seen in 33 percent of 16- to 35-year-old patients and in 0 percent of the greater-than-55-year-olds. Vegetative survival was approximately 3 percent in both these groups, and slightly higher in the middle-age groups. Figure 54-2 illustrates these same points differently by evaluating the age distribution of different Glasgow Outcome Scales. Eighty percent of patients more than 55 years old died within 6 months postinjury, and none showed a good recovery. In marked constant, in the 16-

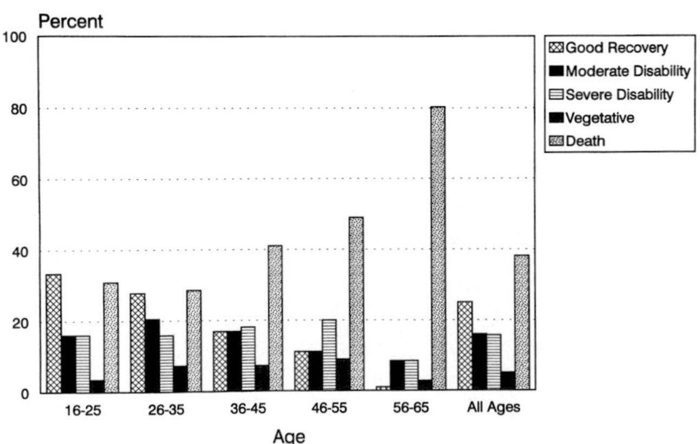

Figure 54-1. Glasgow Outcome Scale vs. Age. This figure subcategorizes age and outcome by evaluating outcomes based on the Glasgow Outcome Scale (GOS), looking at each age group as one unit. The relative proportion of outcomes for each age group is illustrated.

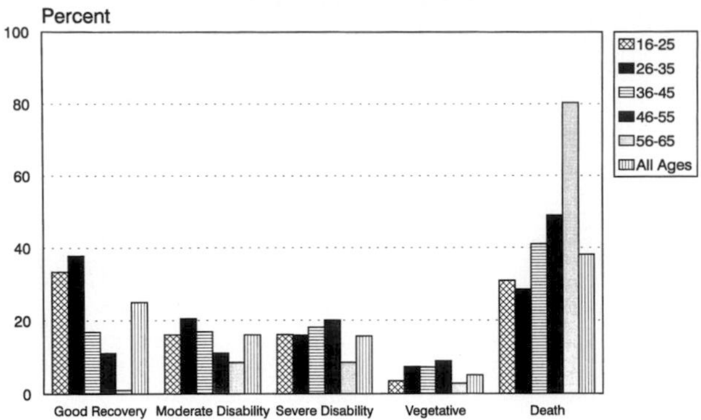

Figure 54-2. Age distribution of different Glasgow outcomes. This figure subcategorizes the data in Fig. 54-1 into groups based on the GOS. These data enable an evaluation of which age groups perform better per each outcome category. For example, vegetative outcome is approximately the same in all the age groups, whereas in the category of good recovery there is a higher percentage of good recovery among the younger age groups and a precipitous fall as the patients age.

to 25-year group, 33 percent showed a good recovery and approximately 31 percent died. Figure 54-2 demonstrates that in the 26- to 35-year group approximately 30 percent of patients died from their severe head injury within 6 months. This death rate increased progressively with age to 80 percent of the over-55 age group.

The over-55 age group showed a markedly different trend in percentage of survival versus days after injury (Fig. 54-3). Death within 48 h of admission was the same in all groups. However, in the ensuing days, the over-55 group showed a progressive decrease in survival until the rate leveled off at approximately 35 percent. In patients under 55 the final survival rate was approximately 80 percent for the 15- to 35-year age group, and slightly worse for patients between 35 and 55. Older patients tended to die over an extended period; younger patients reached a plateau sooner.

There are other possibly age-dependent variables that may affect clinical outcome: significant premorbid diseases (markedly more common in older patients); the presence of multiple injuries; and the mechanism(s) of injury. If any of these shows an age-dependent effect, the effect of age may then be indirect. For example, older people are more often injured in falls that result in acute subdural hematomas, which have the poorest outcome.

Previous medical illness is frequently used to explain why older patients fare worse from head injury, and certainly this age group shows a higher percentage of systemic diseases. In the Traumatic Coma Data Bank

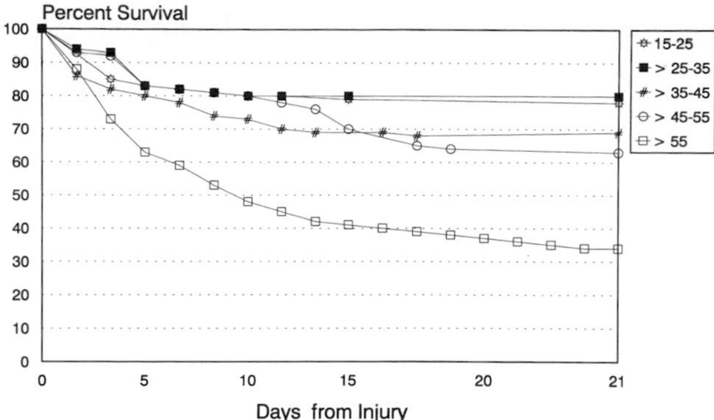

Figure 54-3. Survival curves by age. This figure illustrates the percentage of patient survival by days after severe traumatic head injury. The over-55 age group shows a continual decline over the 21 days of evaluation, whereas the other age groups tend to level off at approximately 60 to 80 percent survival. Note that in the first 24 to 48 h after injury the survival for all groups is nearly the same.

study, 75 percent of the patients over 55 had systemic medical illnesses, whereas this was true for only 5 percent of the 16- to 25-year age group. Analyses show that those who have preexisting systemic disease suffer more fatalities after head injury. If each age group is evaluated separately (Fig. 54-4), there is little difference in the proportion of patients with and without a systemic medical problem, except for the older-than-55 age group, where the proportion with systemic illnesses is much higher. Thus, medical illnesses could be part of the explanation for the poorer outcomes in the over-55 group; however, this has been subjected to a logistic regression analysis, and its inclusion still does not remove age as an independent variable (see below).

Multiple injury is clearly not the explanation (Fig. 54-5), since this is significantly less frequent in older patients. Analysis of the data in the multiple injury categories and each age group reveals that there was no significant difference between the vegetative survival or death outcome of each age group at 6 months, regardless of whether there was multiple injury.[4,6,19,34,35]

Possibly older patients fare less well after traumatic head injury because the mechanism of injury is more severe. This seems unlikely because older patients have multiple injuries less often. In the over-55 category, nearly half of all injuries were from falls, whereas in the younger groups, the vast majority of injuries occurred in motor vehicle accidents[19,35–41] (Fig. 54-6).

Pedestrian accidents were significantly more common in the oldest group, perhaps because of decreased concentration and reaction time. Falls and pedestrian accidents caused slightly worse outcomes than did other mechanisms of injury (data not shown). Still: was the worse outcome from falls and pedestrian accidents intrinsic to the particular injury mechanism, or was the outcome worse because there was a greater proportion of older patients in the fall and pedestrian-accident cate-

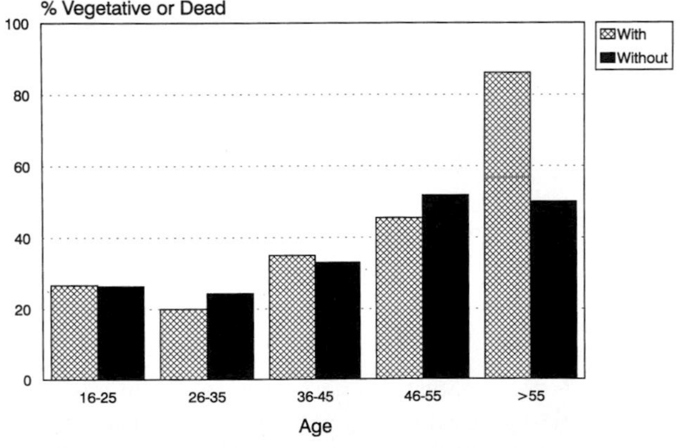

Figure 54-4. Medical systemic illness. This graph shows the vegetative or dead percentages at 6 months. In all the age groups, except older than 55, there is no difference in vegetative or dead percentages, regardless of previous medical systemic illness. Only in the older-than-55 group does previous medical systemic illness appear to increase the vegetative or dead percentage, relative to those without previous medical systemic illness. Also, the vegetative or dead percentage gradually increases with age.

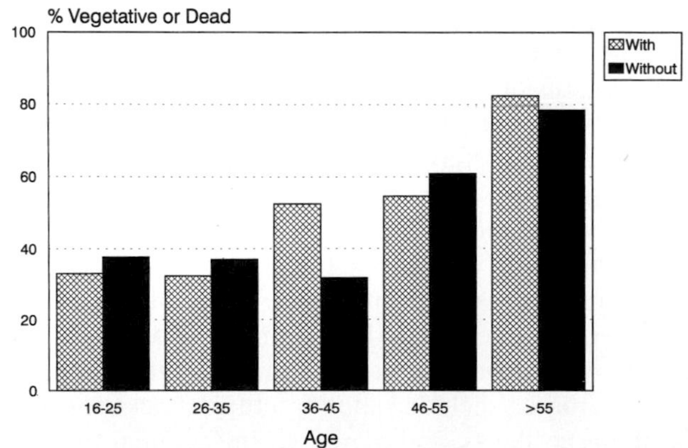

Figure 54-5. Multiple injury. This figure evaluates the relationship between vegetative or dead percentages and the presence or absence of multiple injury. Only in the 36- to 45-year-old group did multiple injury appear to play a role in increasing the vegetative or dead percentage rate. Again, there is an age-dependent increase in this rate, independent of the presence or absence of multiple injury.

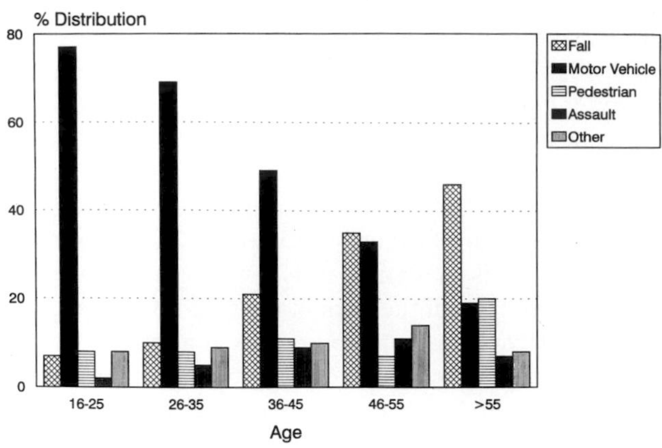

Figure 54-6. Injury mechanism. The figure reveals the distribution of injury mechanisms for each age group. There is a high incidence of motor vehicle accidents in the younger age groups; the percentage of the total injury secondary to motor vehicle accidents decreases dramatically with age. Falls and pedestrian accidents increase with age, and, in the older groups, play a more important role than other mechanisms of injury.

gories than in the other subgroups of mechanism of injury? The latter is more probable. Seventy-eight percent of patients over 55 who had a fall resulting in traumatic coma were either dead or showed vegetative survival 6 months postinjury, whereas 83 percent of this same age group whose traumatic coma had another mechanism were vegetative or dead at 6 months. Therefore, mechanism of injury does not explain the age-dependent effect on outcome.

If injury severity is evaluated based on the GCS, the motor score, or pupillary response, there is essentially no difference between the GCS score and the motor score in the different age groups. However, the frequency of pupillary abnormalities is greater in the older age group. This may be secondary to the higher frequency of mass lesions seen in these patients (see below). Some studies have found the initial GCS to be less reliable, and instead use the postresuscitation GCS, but again there is little difference between age groups.

Other variables related to injury have also been examined, but do not appear to explain the age effect. These variables included skull fracture, shock, postmorbid medical illness, and increased intracranial pressure (ICP).[42–44] Hypoxia, shock, or the presence of a skull fracture, all of which are associated with a higher mortality rate, were not significantly more common in elderly patients. Serious cardiac complications appeared to have a very strong influence on outcome, particularly in younger patients.[19] Although older patients more frequently had serious complications involving other organ systems of the body, these complications did not explain the age-dependent effect on outcome, for again an age-independent effect appeared throughout all these categories. Even increased ICP did not explain the age-dependent effect on outcome, for no significant differences were observed between various age groups and the frequency of elevated ICP.

Overall, this large analysis showed that a significantly increased risk of poor outcome began at the age of 45 years and increased after the age of 55 years. Since none of the above clinical parameters appeared to explain the age-dependent effect, it seems probable that age acts as an independent predictor of outcome—i.e., something intrinsic to the aging process is making the brain more susceptible to severe or lethal injury in head trauma.

MORPHOLOGY AND OUTCOME FROM TRAUMATIC HEAD INJURY

Because it has been difficult to explain the age-dependent effect on outcome, some attention has been directed toward the anatomy and physiology of the aging brain and its ability to cope with traumatic head injury.

Figure 54-7 shows the major subtypes of injuries seen on head CT scans and their effect on outcome. As the

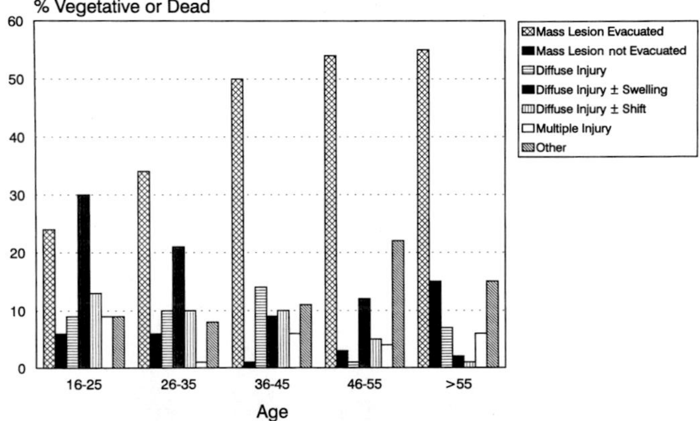

Figure 54-7. Percent distribution of various CT findings based on age. This figure summarizes broad, major categories of head CT abnormalities. As the age of the patient increases, the percentage distribution of mass lesions among severe head injury patients increases. The mass lesions evacuated category in the older age groups shows that increasing age is not a strong deterrent to mass lesion evacuation. For the older age groups, the percentage of incidence of diffuse injury is significantly lower than seen in younger groups. Likewise, in the younger age groups, the percentage of diffuse injury, plus or minus swelling and shift, is relatively higher than in older groups and mass lesions are less common than in the older groups.

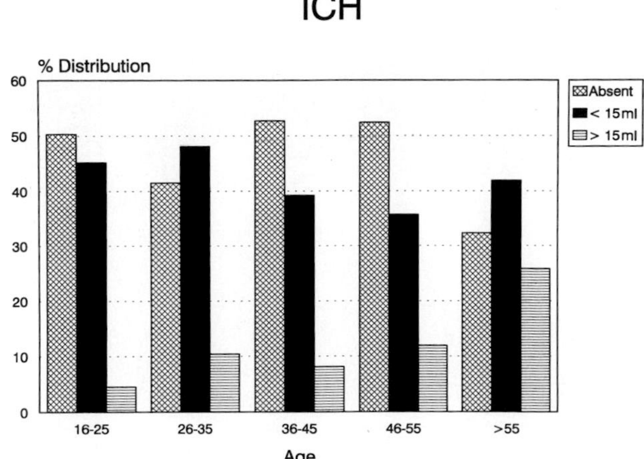

Figure 54-8. Percentage of distribution of intracerebral hematoma. This curve shows that the percentage of intracerebral hematoma increases with age, particularly intracerebral hemorrhage greater than 15 ml. The curves are otherwise similar, with only the oldest age group showing the marked change of much more common large-volume intracerebral hematoma and more frequent intracerebral hematoma.

patient's age increased, so did the mortality associated with surgical mass lesions. Diffuse injury was more common in the younger age groups, especially in children (Fig. 54-8).

The subtypes of mass lesions and the evidence of midline shift, perimesencephalic cistern compression, and ventricular system asymmetry also can be analyzed to evaluate their predictive value on outcome. These subgroups of mass lesions include intracerebral hematomas and contusions, epidural and subdural hematomas, and subarachnoid hemorrhage (SAH). Intracranial and epidural/subdural lesions can be further subdivided into those with less or more than 15 ml of blood. There was a clear age-dependent increase in the number of hematomas greater than 15 ml (Fig. 54-9); SAH (Fig. 54-10); compressed basal cisterns (Fig. 54-11); midline shift of more than 5 mm (Fig. 54-12); and an asymmetrical ventricular system (Fig. 54-13).

Are these morphological diagnoses associated with patient outcome? When Figs. 54-14 through 54-19 are

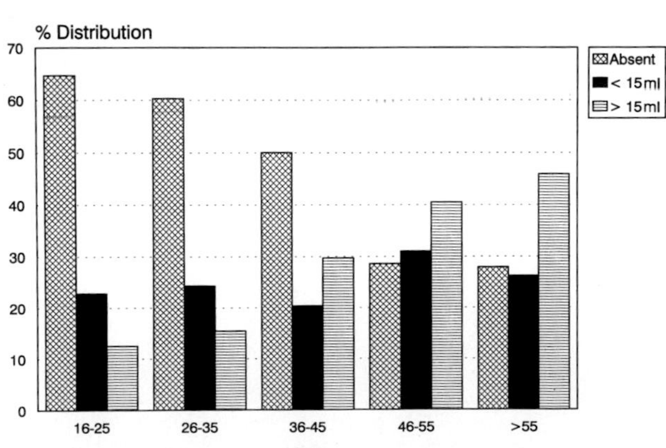

Figure 54-9. Percentage distribution of epidural/subdural hematoma. This figure evaluates epidural/subdural hematoma. The possibility of an extraaxial hemorrhage greater than 15 ml volume increases with age. In addition, there is a trend of increased incidence of mass lesions in older patients with severe head injury.

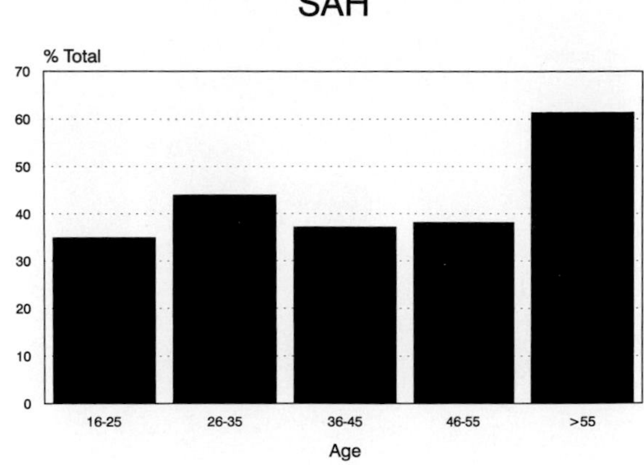

Figure 54-10. Incidence of subarachnoid hemorrhage. This figure shows the percentage of incidence of subarachnoid hemorrhage in patients with severe head injury. The percentage of incidence is approximately the same in all groups until the patient's age is greater than 55, when the incidence increases significantly.

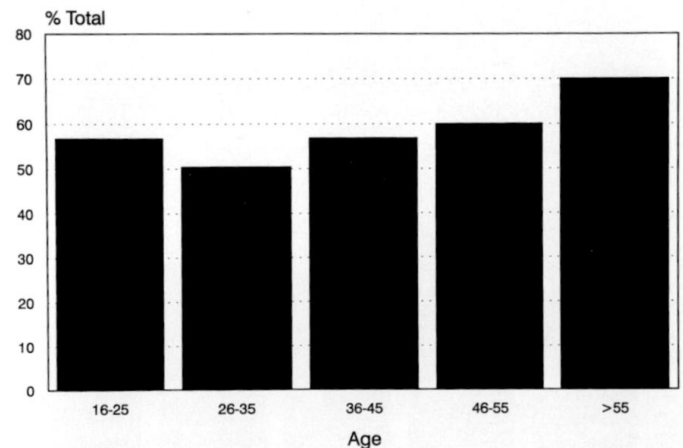

Figure 54-11. Compressed basal cisterns. The percentage of compressed basal cisterns is approximately the same for all age groups, with a mild-to-moderate increase as age increases. This figure may represent a combination of the increased tendency for diffuse swelling observed in younger groups, i.e., the 16- to 25-year group superimposed on a general age trend of increased incidence of compressed basal cisterns as age increases.

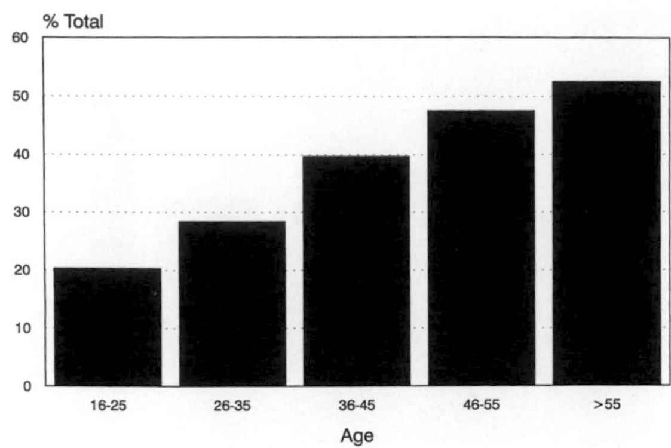

Figure 54-12. Incidence of midline shift greater than 5 mm. There is a marked age-dependent effect on the incidence of midline shift greater than 5 mm, with a 20 percent rate noted in the 16- to 25-year group and greater than 50 percent in the over-55 group.

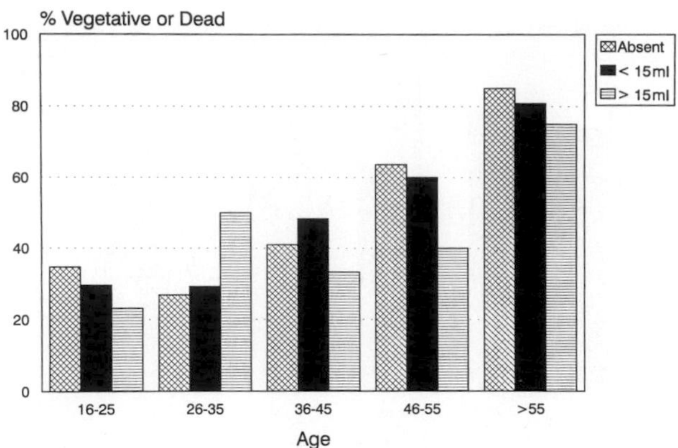

Figure 54-14. Outcome of intracerebral hematoma. The same radiological categories evaluated in several previous figures are now evaluated in terms of the percentages of vegetative or dead at 6 months. A marked age-dependent effect is seen in all these categories, with an increase in percentages of vegetative or dead at 6 months independent of whether an intracerebral hematoma is absent, less than 15 ml, or greater than 15 ml.

examined, such an association is clearly seen. Patients with large extracerebral lesions had a particularly poor outcome, with 50 percent of the 16- to 25-year group and 89 percent of the over-55 group vegetative or dead (Fig. 54-15). However, an age-dependent effect has always been evident in these data; therefore if Figs. 54-14 through 54-19 are evaluated, a worse outcome is seen with increasing age, given the same radiological abnormality. Older patients show more predisposition to intracranial and extraaxial lesions than do younger patients, and subdural hematoma is more common.

Older patients have a greater propensity for hematomas, but the cause for this is not entirely clear. Some of this tendency may be secondary to cerebral atrophy, which is accompanied by alterations in the mechanical properties of bridging veins, changes in the viscoelastic properties of the brain, and stress placed on venous and arterial structures.

The aging brain also has other characteristics that may increase the risk of hematoma formation, including higher mean arterial blood pressure, increased vascular rigidity, and alterations in hemostatic mechanisms. Even the increased volume of the subdural space that occurs

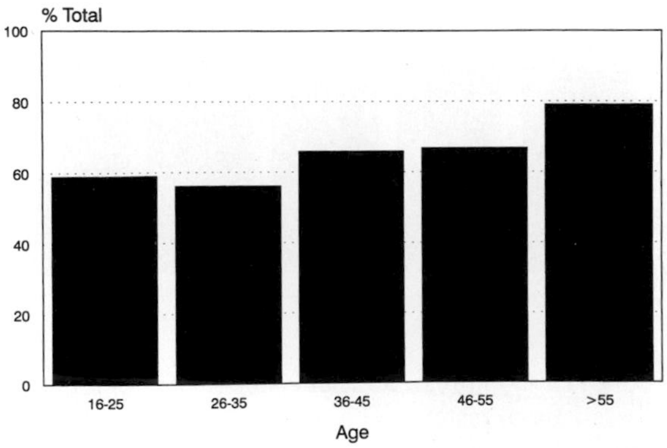

Figure 54-13. Presence of compressed ventricles. The incidence of compressed ventricles increases gradually with age, with the most marked increase occurring in the oldest category.

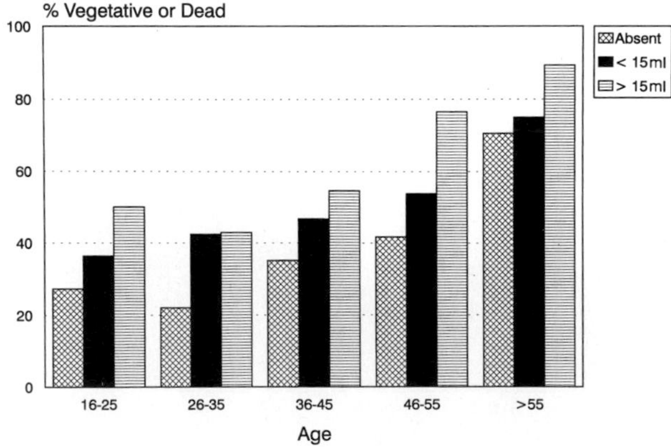

Figure 54-15. Outcome of epidural/subdural hematoma. The vegetative or dead percentages increase dramatically as age increases for all three categories of absent, less than 15 ml, and greater than 15 ml volume of hemorrhage. Again, this suggests an age-dependent effect on survival.

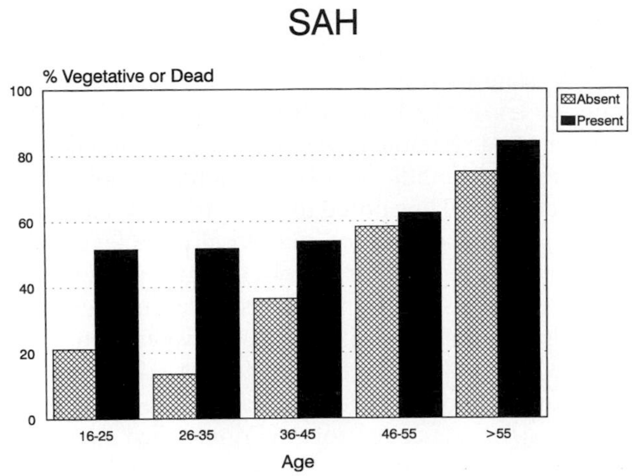

SAH
% Vegetative or Dead
100
80
60
40
20
0
Absent
Present
16-25
26-35
36-45
46-55
>55
Age

Figure 54-16. Outcome of subarachnoid hemorrhage. A clear progression of vegetative or dead percentages occurs as age increases, regardless of whether subarachnoid hemorrhage is present. In the younger age groups, subarachnoid hemorrhage significantly increases the vegetative or dead percentages at 6 months relative to those patients with no subarachnoid hemorrhage. Again, an age-dependent effect is seen.

Midline Shift
% Vegetative or Dead
100
80
60
40
20
0
< 5 mm
> 5 mm
16-25
26-35
36-45
46-55
>55
Age

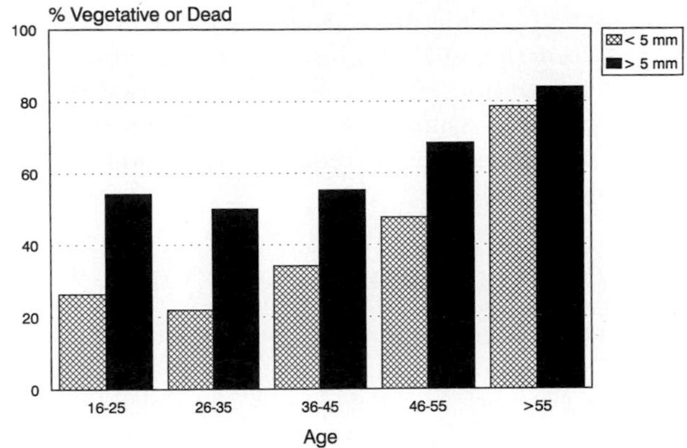

Figure 54-18. Outcome of midline shift. This graph also shows a similar distribution with an age-dependent effect, producing increased percentages of vegetative or dead at 6 months post-injury as age increases. In all patients, a midline shift greater than 5 mm results in a worse outcome, and the differential between greater or lesser shift is more pronounced in the younger groups.

secondary to brain atrophy may contribute to the formation of larger hematomas. Subdural hematomas are more lethal than most other brain lesions and are more commonly seen in older patients. Some increased frequency is probably due to the higher incidence of falls, which effectively induce subdural hematoma formation.[45–49] However, the greater incidence of falls and the propensity to develop more and larger subdural hematomas do not explain the age-dependent poor outcome seen, because if older and younger patients who have these same hematomas are compared, the older patients always fare worse. It can be concluded from these data that the anatomy discernible by CT scan, such as the presence of various types of hematomas in different locations, the compression of the basal cisterns or ventricular system, and the shift of midline structures,

Basal Cisterns
% Vegetative or Dead
100
80
60
40
20
0
Open
Compressed
16-25
26-35
36-45
46-55
>55
Age

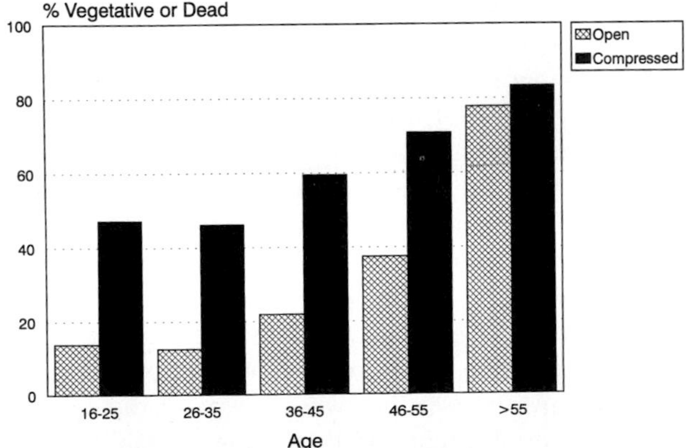

Figure 54-17. Compression of the basal cisterns. As in subarachnoid hemorrhage, a marked age-dependent effect on percentages of vegetative or dead at 6 months is clearly seen. This is independent of the radiological findings. However, younger patients with compressed basal cisterns certainly fare worse than do similar younger patients without compressed basal cisterns.

Ventricles
% Vegetative or Dead
100
80
60
40
20
0
Symmetric
Compressed
16-25
26-35
36-45
46-55
>55
Age

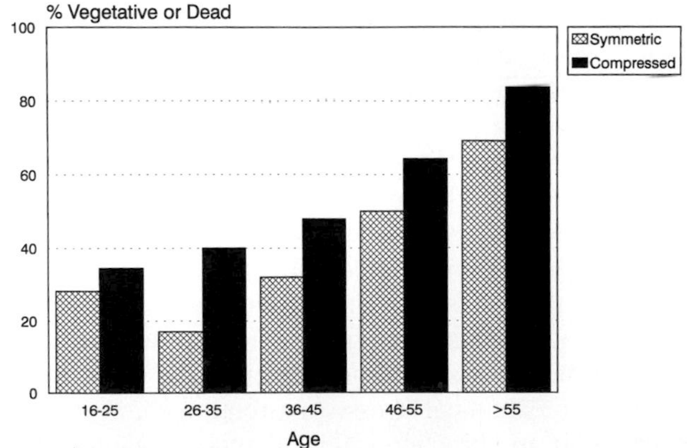

Figure 54-19. Mass effect on the ventricles. There is a marked age-dependent increased percentage of vegetative or dead at 6 months as age increases. Patients who show compressed ventricles have a worse outcome than those with symmetrical ventricles, and the differential between these two categories is more marked in the younger age groups.

all correlate with worse outcome and are more common in the older age groups. However, despite all these variables, aging presents itself as an independent variable.

There is no significant difference in the frequency of surgical evacuation of large hematomas based on age. Therefore, the possibility that older patients are doing less well because of less frequent evacuation of their hematomas is not borne out.

Multivariate Analysis

Vollmer et al. used Traumatic Coma Bank information[19] and performed a multivariate analysis of all the aforementioned factors to determine if any or all of these factors in combination would predict outcome across all age groups. Using age first as a continuous variable and then by categories, they showed that the overall predictive ability and significance of age was equivalent in both models. Their analysis revealed that a significantly increased risk of poor outcome began at 45 years and that this rate of worse outcome increased rapidly after 55 years. Since none of the clinical or radiological parameters studied appeared to adequately explain the age-dependent effect, it seems probable that age acts as an independent predictor of outcome and that something intrinsic to the aging process is making the brain more susceptible to severe or lethal injury from head trauma.

PATHOPHYSIOLOGY OF THE AGING BRAIN

Much of the clinical and radiological information mentioned above suggests that although there are numerous variables that show an age-dependent change, these variables, either alone or in combination, do not completely account for the age-dependent effect on outcome seen in traumatic brain injury. Attention must be focused on the biology of the aging brain to understand the poorer prognosis associated with increasing age. Some possible areas of study should include the effects of aging on intracranial compliance, the generation of cerebral edema, the viscoelastic properties, and on the response to mechanical stress. Age-related changes occur at a cellular and biochemical level, including alterations in the neural populations, neurotransmitter metabolism, microvasculature, dendritic spines and arborization, and in the blood-brain barrier.

To evaluate these parameters, animal models were used to examine how an aging brain responds to head injury. One recent study by Hamm et al. utilized the fluid percussion model to investigate the effect of age on outcome.[50] In this model, young and aging rats were injured, using fluid percussion to induce either low or moderate levels of traumatic brain injury. The investigators then used systemic physiological, neurological, and histopathological indices of brain injury to look at age-related changes. They noted that, in brains given equivalent acute traumatic injury, plasma glucose levels were approximately equivalent in both age groups. Examination at low levels of brain injury showed no significant gross histopathological difference between young and old rats. The older rats showed increased duration of suppression of nonpostural and postural reflexes and of more complex somatomotor functions, such as righting and escape. Old and young rats were similar only in terms of head support. The authors found that the worse outcome seen in older rats was neither secondary to systemic response nor explainable at the gross histopathological level. The only difference in physiological response noted between aging and young rats was in heart rate, but even here there was only a modest age-related change that did not explain the age-associated increase in mortality rate and neurological deficits that occurred following head injury. Therefore, all evidence pointed to change at a cellular level.

The aging brain's particular vulnerability to excitotoxic damage after brain injury appears to explain nearly all the available data. It is known that a mechanical impact to the brain will lead to widespread depolarization of neurons and the release of excitatory neurotransmitters such as glutamate and aspartate.[51] Theoretically, the surge of excitatory neurotransmitters produced during head injury (and brain injury from other causes as well) produces more serious functional damage to the aging brain because of its age-related neuronal loss. The older brain attempts to compensate for this loss and maintain normal function by making the remaining nerve cells increasingly sensitive to stimulation, i.e., by increasing the receptor density on the neurons that remain, altering the allosteric regulation of the receptors, or decreasing the reuptake of the excitatory neurotransmitters. This is an adaptive response under normal conditions, but during the massive release of excitatory neurotransmitters that occurs in brain injury, the excitotoxic effect may be greatly exacerbated. Full proof of this theory awaits experimental validation. Certainly such an adaptive response would explain the effect of brain injury on the aging brain, for it is probable that age is also an independent variable determining outcome in other acute neurological disorders such as stroke and SAH.

This possibility of age effect in excitotoxicity-mediated neuronal death was studied by Olney,[52] who noted that *N*-methyl-D-aspartate (NMDA) receptors are more sensitive in early life and that non-NMDA receptors are more sensitive in adulthood. This suggests that the non-NMDA receptors increase the excitotoxicity seen in the elderly. He theorized that the NMDA receptor may be more involved in processes relating to children with developmental brain abnormalities, whereas the non-NMDA receptors may play a role in the neurodegenerative diseases seen in the elderly.

One other area of investigation focuses on the supporting cells of the brain, i.e., the various types of glia, rather than the neurons, as a partial explanation for the aging brain's greater susceptibility to injury. Topp et al.[53] evaluated the time course and magnitude of astrocytic proliferation following neural trauma in young-adult and middle-aged rats. In this model a needle groove was made in the cortex and hippocampus, and tritiated thymidine was injected at various intervals. Immunohistochemical staining for glial fibrillary acidic proteins (GFAP) was also performed to evaluate the age-related differences in astrocytic proliferation. These investigators showed that, in both young and old rats, astrocytic proliferation occurring during the first 4 postlesion days consisted of an early glial response to neural trauma. Older rats demonstrated greater labeling in the cortex than did younger rats, suggesting that the older animals developed a greater degree of scarring in response to a given injury. If one compares the glial response in these young and old animals to that of very young animals, including embryonic animals, the scarring in embryos is minimal and there is significant regeneration of nerve cells. The older brain is much less plastic than the young brain and, for a given injury, is much less able to induce a regenerative neuronal response; instead, it shows a greater regenerative response in the scar-forming cells of the nervous system (gliosis).

Rudge et al., in their evaluation of wound healing in the CNS,[54–56] isolated, cultured, and characterized cells that responded to trauma by implanting nitrocellulose filters into the brains of neonatal and adult rats under varying conditions. After observation of their response to trauma, cells were harvested from neonatal rats (critical period), adult rats, and rats in which the filters had remained in vivo past the neonatal critical period. It was found that the majority of cells in the cell culture taken from neonatal rats and rats in which the filters remained in vivo past the critical period were astrocytes, whereas the majority of cells in the adult glial and fibroblastic scar were fibroblasts and macrophages. Even the morphology of the astrocytes was different; astrocytes taken from neonatal rats exhibited a more ordered distribution than did the haphazard arrangement of astrocytic processes on the surface of the filters taken from adults rats and from those in which the nitrocellulose filters were left in vivo past the critical period. The cell behavior was also different, with the astrocytes from the neonatal animals showing an epithelioid morphology and clustering together with definite boundaries between astrocytes and endothelial cells. The postcritical period filters had astrocytes that were more elongated and randomly dispersed among the endothelial cells, rather than separated from endothelial cells as in the neonatal critical period filters. In the adult animals, the scar astrocytes exhibited a wide range of morphologies with some tendency to cluster, but with none of the ordered association seen in the neonatal animals. The results of this study strongly indicate that the immature CNS is capable of greater plasticity, partly because of the rapid and ordered cellular response of its astrocytes. The older brain lacks this plasticity because of gliofibroblastic scarring in which fibroblasts and macrophages predominate over astrocytes.

These investigators then used the same implant system to show that glial scar taken from adult rats stimulated only minimal neuritic outgrowth from cultured hippocampal neurons, whereas filters from neonatal rats showed significant neuritic outgrowth. They postulated that the gliofibroblastic scar either directly inhibited growth cones or occluded neurite-promoting factors in the extracellular matrix or on the astrocyte surface. The researchers found that all filters contained the growth-promoting molecules laminin, collagen type IV, and fibronectin. However, only the adult animals contained chondroitin-6 sulfate proteoglycan and cytotactin/tenascin, extracellular matrix molecules that block neurite outgrowth, in the region of the scar colocalized with intensely GFAP-positive astrocytes. This suggests a molecular basis for the lack of neuronal regenerative potential in the adult CNS. Whether these and/or other molecules can further explain the progressive worsening of neurological outcome from a variety of causes of CNS injury remains to be determined.

HEAD INJURY AND NEURODEGENERATIVE DISORDERS

The previous portions of this chapter focused on the grave outcome seen in elderly patients with traumatic brain injury, in particular those patients in traumatic coma. Is it possible that in minor head injury there is no age-dependent change in function? Do minor injuries that occurred in the past have an effect on the functional outcome of patients as they age? Many studies now show that any previous head injury—severe head injury in particular—is a risk factor for the development of Alzheimer's and possibly also Parkinson's disease, although the latter is more speculative.[57–77] This relationship is shown in *dementia pugilistica* (*punch drunk syndrome*), frequently seen in boxers who, after repeated head injury, develop early onset of Alzheimer's disease.[72]

Cerebral amyloid deposition likely plays a key role in the pathogenesis of Alzheimer's disease, but the etiology is not entirely clear. There is an increased risk of Alzheimer's in first-degree relatives of patients with this disease. It has been observed that amyloid precursor protein gene mutations on chromosome 21 seen in some families with Alzheimer's play an important role in producing the heritable form of the disease. However, many cases do not show this genetic predisposition, but rather seem correlated with previous head injury, which causes the release of beta-A4 amyloid protein in the brain within days of the injury.[60,71] It remains to be determined whether this release also triggers the formation of beta-A4 amyloid immunoreactive plaques and other pathological features of Alzheimer's disease already fairly well demonstrated in cases secondary to the amyloid precursor protein mutation. Researchers have suggested that severe head injury hastens the age of onset of Alzheimer's disease, stating that Alzheimer's patients with severe head injury before the age of 65 showed onset of symptoms earlier than did Alzheimer's patients without head trauma. Patients with presenile dementia following head injury and professional boxers in whom dementia develops have antibodies to the beta-A4 amyloid protein. The relationship between head injury and Alzheimer's disease is consistent with the hypothesis that cerebral amyloid deposition leads to the formation of neuritic plaques and neuronal destruction. Amyloid that is deposited freely is thought to competitively inhibit its own proteolysis, which results in an accumulation in neurons that destroys the cell membrane and cytoskeleton and leads to neuronal degeneration.

Frequently, patients with Alzheimer's disease and associated head injury have this head injury within 5 years of the onset of their symptoms. One study showed that the risk of Alzheimer's disease is increased in first-degree relatives of patients whose disease begins before the age of 70, but not for relatives of patients with a later age of onset.[66] Patients over the age of 70 who have head injuries more frequently develop Alzheimer's disease and the odds of having a head injury are significantly higher among elderly patients, particularly those over the age of 70. Possibly head injuries in older individuals lead to different pathological processes than do similar injuries in younger patients. Studies on the effect of advancing age have shown that the metabolism of beta-A4 amyloid can be altered, and there may be reduced capacity for proteolysis of the expressed amyloid.

The relationship between prior history of head trauma and Parkinson's disease is much more tenuous. One study reported a trend toward statistical significance when examining head trauma with alteration of consciousness as a risk factor in the etiology of Parkinson's disease.[62] Other investigators have also suggested this, but the results of these studies are still questionable. At best, the relationship remains unclear.

CONCLUSION

The aging brain is itself an important factor in determining the poor outcome from head injury noted in older patients. To improve this dismal prognosis, experimental and clinical work exploring the molecular, subcellular, and cellular basis of the aging effect is needed so that more effective interventions can be devised. It is suggested that the aging brain shows greater scarring and less regenerative capacity than the younger brain, and also is more susceptible to accelerated neurodegeneration culminating in diseases such as Alzheimer's and possibly Parkinson's disease. Improvement in outcome will require a better understanding of the neurobiology of the aging brain; development of newer pharmacological, medical, and surgical interventions; and a program aimed at the prevention of these injuries through community education and the implementation of effective safety measures.

References

1. Alberico AM, Ward JD, Choi SC, et al: Outcome after severe head injury: Relationship to mass lesions, diffuse injury, and ICP course in pediatric and adult patients. *J Neurosurg* 1987; 67:648–656.
2. Braakman R, Gelpke GJ, Habbema JDF, et al: Systematic selection of prognostic features in patients with severe head injury. *Neurosurgery* 1980; 6:362–370.
3. Bricolo A, Turazzi S, Alexandre A, et al: Decerebrate rigidity in acute head injury. *J Neurosurg* 1977; 47: 680–698.
4. Carlsson CA, von Essen C, Lofgren J: Factors affecting the clinical course of patients with severe head injuries. Part 1: Influence of biological factors. Part 2: Significance of posttraumatic coma. *J Neurosurg* 1968; 29:242–251.
5. Conroy C, Kraus JF: Survival after brain injury: Cause of death, length of survival, and prognostic variables in a cohort of brain-injured people. *Neuroepidemiology* 1988; 7:13–22.
6. Edna TH: Risk factors in traumatic head injury. *Acta Neurochir* 1983; 69:15–21.
7. Heiskanen O, Sipponen P: Prognosis of severe brain injury. *Acta Neurol Scand* 1970; 46:343–348.
8. Hernesniemi J: Outcome following head injuries in the aged. *Acta Neurochir* 1979; 49:67–79.
9. Jennett B, Teasdale G, Braakman R, et al: Prognosis of

patients with severe head injury. *Neurosurgery* 1979; 4:283–289.
10. Levati A, Farina ML, Vecchi G, et al: Prognosis of severe head injuries. *J Neurosurg* 1982; 57:779–783.
11. Luerssen TG, Klauber MR, Marshall LF: Outcome from head injury related to patient's age: A longitudinal prospective study of adult and pediatric head injury. *J Neurosurg* 1988; 68:409–416.
12. Overgaard J, Hvid-Hansen O, Land AM, et al: Prognosis after head injury based on early clinical examination. *Lancet* 1973; 2:631–635.
13. Pazzaglia P, Frank G, Frank F, et al: Clinical course and prognosis of acute post-traumatic coma. *J Neurol Neurosurg Psychiatry* 1975; 38:149–154.
14. Pentland B, Jones PA, Roy CW, et al: Head injury in the elderly. *Age Aging* 1986; 15:193–202.
15. Teasdale G, Skene A, Parker L, et al: Age and outcome of severe head injury. *Acta Neurochir* 1979; (suppl) 28:140–143.
16. Teasdale G, Skene A, Spiegelhalter D, et al: Age, severity, and outcome of head injury, in Grossman RG, Gildenberg PL (eds): *Head Injury: Basis and Clinical Aspects.* New York: Raven Press, 1982: 213–220.
17. Eisenberg HM, Gray HE Jr, Aldrich EF, et al: Initial CT scan findings in 753 patients with severe head injury: A report from the NIH Traumatic Coma Data Bank. *J Neurosurg* 1990; 73:688–698.
18. Espersen JO, Peterson OF: Computerized tomography (CT) in patients with head injuries: Assessment of outcome based upon initial clinical findings and initial CT scans. *Acta Neurochir* 1982; 65:81–91.
19. Vollmer DJ, Torner JC, Jane JA, et al: Age and outcome following traumatic coma: Why do older patients fare worse? *J Neurosurg* 1991; 75:537–549.
20. Narayan RK, Greenberg RP, Miller JD, et al: Improved confidence of outcome prediction in severe head injury: A comparative analysis of the clinic examination, multimodality evoked potentials, CT scanning, and intracranial pressure. *J Neurosurg* 1981; 54:751–762.
21. Rutherford WH, Merrett JD, McDonald JR: Symptoms at one year following concussion from minor head injuries. *Injury* 1979; 10:225–230.
22. Choi SC, Ward JD, Becker DP: Chart for outcome prediction in severe head injury. *J Neurosurg* 1983; 59:294–297.
23. Vollmer DG: Prognosis and outcome of severe head injury, in Cooper PR (ed): *Head Injury.* Baltimore: Williams & Wilkins, 1993: 553–581.
24. Gross CR, Wolf C, Kunitz SC, et al: Pilot Traumatic Coma Data Bank: A profile of head injuries in children, in Dacey RG Jr, Winn HR, Rimel RW, et al (eds): *Trauma of the Central Nervous System.* New York: Raven Press, 1985: 19–26.
25. Foulkes MA, Eisenberg HM, Jane JA, et al: The Traumatic Coma Data Bank: Design, methods, and baseline characteristics. *J Neurosurg* 1991; 75(suppl):S8–S13.
26. Marshall LF, Toole BM, Bowers SA: The National Traumatic Coma Data Bank: Part 2. Patients who talk and deteriorate: Implications for treatment. *J Neurosurg* 1983; 59:285–288.
27. Marshall LF, Becker DP, Bowers SA, et al: The National Traumatic Coma Data Bank: Part 1. Design, purpose, goals, and results. *J Neurosurg* 1983; 59:276–284.
28. Berger MS, Pitts LH, Lovely M, et al: Outcome from severe head injury in children and adolescents. *J Neurosurg* 1985; 62:194–199.
29. Bruce DA, Schut L, Bruno LA, et al: Outcome following severe head injuries in children. *J Neurosurg* 1978; 48:679–688.
30. Jennett B, Bond M: Assessment of outcome after severe brain damage: A practical scale. *Lancet* 1975; 1:480–484.
31. Armitage P: *Statistical Methods in Medical Research.* New York: John Wiley, 1971: 363–365.
32. Freeman DH: *Applied Categorical Data Analysis.* New York: Marcel Dekker, 1987: 72–76.
33. Teasdale G, Jennett B: Assessment of coma and impaired consciousness: A practical scale. *Lancet* 1974; 2:81–84.
34. Baxt WG, Moody P: The differential survival of trauma patients. *J Trauma* 1987; 27:602–606.
35. Becker DP, Miller JD, Ward JD, et al: The outcome from severe head injury with early diagnosis and intensive management. *J Neurosurg* 1977; 47:491–502.
36. Baker SP, Harvey AH: Fall injuries in the elderly. *Clin Geriatr Med* 1985; 1:501–512.
37. Hadley E, Radebaugh TS, Suzman R: Falls and gait disorders among the elderly: A challenge for research. *Clin Geriatr Med* 1985; 1:497–500.
38. Sattin RW, Lambert-Huber DA, DeVito CA, et al: The incidence of fall injury events among the elderly in a defined population. *Am J Epidemiol* 1991; 131:1028–1037.
39. Tinetti ME, Speechley M, Ginter SF: Risk factors for falls among elderly persons living in the community. *N Engl J Med* 1988; 319:1701–1707.
40. Mazzucchi A, Cattelani R, Missale G, et al: Head-injured subjects aged over 50 years: Correlations between variables. *J Neurol* 1992; 239:256–260.
41. Nelson DE, Sattin RW, Langois JA, et al: Alcohol as a risk factor for fall injury events among elderly persons living in a community. *J Am Geriatr Soc* 1992; 40:658–661.
42. Eisenberg H, Cayard C, Papanicolaou A, et al: The effects of three potentially preventable complications on outcome after severe closed head injury, in Ishii S, Nagai H, Brock M (eds): *Intracranial Pressure V.* New York: Springer-Verlag, 1983: 549–553.
43. Hartung HJ, Olenik D: Early prognosis of severe craniocerebral injuries. *J Anaesthetist* 1992; 41:468–473.
44. Miller JD, Sweet RC, Narayan R, et al: Early insults to the injured brain. *JAMA* 1978; 240:439–442.
45. Fell DA, Fitzgerald S, Moiel RH, et al: Acute subdural hematomas: Review of 144 cases. *J Neurosurg* 1975; 42:37–42.
46. Gennarelli TA, Thibault LE: Biomechanics of acute subdural hematoma. *J Trauma* 1982; 22:680–686.
47. Gennarelli TA, Spielman GM, Langfitt TW, et al: Influence of the type of intracranial lesion on outcome from severe head injury. *J Neurosurg* 1982; 56:26–32.
48. McKissock W, Richardson A, Bloom WH: Subdural hematoma: A review of 389 cases. *Lancet* 1960; 1:1365–1369.

49. Seelig JM, Becker DP, Miller JD, et al: Traumatic acute subdural hematoma: Major mortality reduction in comatose patients treated within four hours. *N Engl J Med* 1981; 304:1511–1518.
50. Hamm RJ, Jenkins LW, Lyeth BG, et al: The effect of age on outcome following traumatic brain injury in rats. *J Neurosurg* 1991; 75:916–921.
51. Katayama Y, Becker DP, Tamura T, et al: Massive increases in extracellular potassium and the indiscriminate release of glutamate following concussive brain injury. *J Neurosurg* 1990; 73:889–900.
52. Olney JW: Excitotoxin-mediated neuronal death in youth and old age. *Prog Brain Res* 1990; 86:37–51.
53. Topp KS, Faddis BT, Vijayan VK: Trauma-induced proliferation of astrocytes in the brain of young and aged rats. *J Glia* 1989; 2:201–211.
54. Rudge JS, Silver J: Inhibition of neurite outgrowth on astroglial scars in vitro. *J Neurosci* 1990; 10(11):3594–3603.
55. Rudge JS, Smith GM, Silver J: An in vitro model of wound healing in the CNS: Analysis of cell reaction and interaction at different ages. Center for Neuroscience. *J Exper Neurol* 1989; 103:1–16.
56. McKeon RJ, Schreiber RC, Rudge JS, Silver J: Reduction of neurite outgrowth in a model of glial scarring following CNS injury is correlated with the expression of inhibitory molecules on reactive astrocytes. Department of Neuroscience. *J Neurosci* 1991; 11:3398–3411.
57. Amaducci LA, Fratiglioni L, Rocca WA, et al: Risk factors for clinically diagnosed Alzheimer's disease: A case-control study of an Italian population. *Neurology* 1986; 36:922–931.
58. Buchner DM, Larson EB: Falls and fractures in patients with Alzheimer-type dementia. *JAMA* 1987; 42:412–417.
59. Chandra V, Kokmen E, Schoenberg BS, Beard CM: Head trauma with loss of consciousness as a risk factor of Alzheimer's disease. *Neurology* 1989; 39:1576–1578.
60. Clinton J, Ambler MW, Roberts GW: Post-traumatic Alzheimer's disease: Preponderance of a single plaque type. *Neuropathol Appl Neurobiol* 1991; 17:69–74.
61. Cotman CW, Monaghan DT, Geddes JW: N-methyl-D-aspartate receptors, synaptic plasticity, and Alzheimer's disease. *Drug Dev Res* 1989; 17:331–338.
62. Factor SA, Weiner WJ: Prior history of head trauma in Parkinson's disease. *J Movement Disorders* 1991; 6:225–229.
63. Gedye A, Beattie BL, Tuokko H, et al: Severe head injury hastens age of onset of Alzheimer's disease. *J Am Geriatr Soc* 1989; 37:970–973.
64. Graves AB, White E, Koepssell TD, et al: The association between head trauma and Alzheimer's disease. *Am J Epidemiol* 1990; 131:491–501.
65. Lyeth BG, Jenkins LW, Hamm RJ, et al: Prolonged memory impairment in the absence of hippocampal cell death following traumatic brain injury in the rat. *Brain Res* 1990; 526:249–258.
66. Mayeux R, Ottman R, Tang MX, et al: Genetic susceptibility and head injury as risk factors for Alzheimer's Disease among community-dwelling elderly persons and their first-degree relatives. *J Am Neurol Assoc* 1993; 1:494–500.
67. Molgaard CA, Stanford EP, Morton DJ, et al: Epidemiology of head trauma and neurocognitive impairment in a multi-ethnic population. *J Neuroepidemiol* 1990; 9:233–242.
68. Mortimer JA, French LR, Hutton JT, Schuman LM: Head trauma as a risk factor for Alzheimer's disease. *Neurology* 1985; 35:264–267.
69. Mortimer JA, van Duijn CM, Chandra V, et al: Head trauma as a risk factor for Alzheimer's disease: A collaborative re-analysis of case-control studies. *Int J Epidemiol* 1991; 20:S28–S35.
70. Reider-Groswassere I, Cohen M, Costeff H, Groswasser Z: Late CT findings in brain trauma: Relationship to cognitive and behavioral sequelae and to vocational outcome. *AJR* 1993; 160:147–152.
71. Roberts GW, Gentleman SM, Lynch A, et al: Beta A4 amyloid protein deposition in brain after head trauma. *Lancet* 1991; 338:1422–1433.
72. Roberts GW, Allsop D, Bruton CJ: The occult aftermath of boxing. *J Neurol Neurosurg Psychiatry* 1990; 53:3783–3788.
73. Rutherford WH, Merrett JD, McDonald JR: Symptoms at one year following concussion from minor head injuries. *Injury* 1979; 10:225–230.
74. Rutherford WH, Merrett JD, McDonald JR: Sequelae of concussion caused by minor head injuries. *Lancet* 1977; 1:1–4.
75. van Duijn CM, Tanja TA, Haaxma R, et al: Head trauma and the risk of Alzheimer's disease. *Am J Epidemiol* 1992; 135:775–782.
76. Williams DB, Annegers JF, Kokmen E, et al: Brain injury and neurologic sequelae: A cohort study of dementia, parkinsonism and amyotrophic lateral sclerosis. *Neurology* 1991; 41:1554–1557.
77. Wilson JA, Pentland B, Currie CT, et al: The functional effects of head injury in the elderly. *Brain Inj* 1987; 1:183–188.

ACKNOWLEDGMENTS

The authors would like to acknowledge the expert technical assistance of Melonie Carter and Kim Mann for typing the manuscript, Sherry Richardson for illustration assistance, and Elizabeth Fisher for editorial evaluation.

CHAPTER 55

THE LIMITS OF SALVAGEABILITY IN HEAD INJURY

Zeev Feldman

"... *For it is impossible to make all the sick well ... since men die, some even before calling the physician, from the violence of the disease, and some die immediately after calling him ... and before the physician could bring his art to counteract the disease; it therefore becomes necessary to know the nature of such affections, how far they are above the powers of the constitution* .."

Hippocrates[1]

"... *Whenever therefore a man suffers an illness which is too strong for the means at the disposal of medicine he surely must not expect that it can be overcome by medicine.*"

Hippocrates[2]

SYNOPSIS

This chapter discusses the limits of salvageability in a head-injured patient and the relationship of outcome prediction to these limits. Physicians must rely on the effectiveness of prognostic indicators to predict a poor or good outcome. Certain combinations of prognostic indicators generally provide a fairly accurate means of predicting outcome. The time at which outcome is predicted may play an important role in determining the accuracy of the prediction. Early predictions of outcome generally are less accurate for various reasons, including alcohol and/or drug intoxication, and can be overly pessimistic. Predictions made later in the hospital course are increasingly more accurate. However, no system of outcome prediction is perfect because of the inherent unpredictability of biological events. Furthermore, the experience at one center should not be blindly applied to another patient population. Newer surgical, critical care, and pharmacological therapies can make prediction schemas obsolete. Finally, one must always err toward over-optimistic predictions rather than over-pessimistic ones, especially when declaring a patient to be unsalvageable.

INTRODUCTION

In ancient times the limits of medicine were easier to define and accept. However, modern medicine and evolving technology have expanded our abilities to cure, to control, or at least to treat previously "incurable" diseases. This has resulted in increasing financial burdens and ethical dilemmas on society at a time when resources for medical care are becoming more limited. Difficult decisions, therefore, need to be made regarding who to treat and for how long. Such decisions can raise complex moral, ethical, and legal issues. Patients sustaining severe head injury are, by definition, incompetent to participate in the decision-making process concerning their treatment. Consequently, these vital decisions must be made through a surrogate mechanism. Whoever makes the decisions must base them on a thorough understanding of both the diagnosis and the prognosis of the condition. If death or the vegetative state could be predicted accurately, such patients could be triaged to less aggressive treatment, thus allowing for the optimal use of available resources. However, one needs to beware of the self-fulfilling prophecy of death and its attendant nihilism. Society will be forced to deal with the cost-benefit ratio of treatment and will make judgments regarding where to draw the line.

This chapter reviews some of the factors affecting outcome after severe head injury; it examines several prediction models, their accuracy, and the timing of their application; and it discusses whether guidelines can be drawn as to how and when it can be determined whether a head-injured patient is salvageable. There is no doubt that these guidelines will vary from country to country, and perhaps from one region to another. Nevertheless, certain broad generalizations can be made, and this chapter reviews some current thinking in this field.

PREDICTORS OF OUTCOME AFTER SEVERE HEAD INJURY

Clinical Examination

Glasgow Coma Scale (GCS)

The most commonly used scale for assessing the severity of head injury is the Glasgow Coma Scale (GCS). The GCS was designed to remain fairly consistent when used by different observers. The GCS uses three parameters, i.e., eye opening, verbal responses, and motor responses. Sum scores from 3 to 8 generally indicate a severe head injury, 9 to 12 a moderate injury, and 13 to 15 a mild head injury. There is a strong association between a poor outcome and a low GCS score. About 80 to 87 percent of patients with a closed head injury and an initial GCS score of 3 will die.[3,4] Several modifications of the GCS have been proposed, such as incorporating brainstem reflex evaluation (the Glasgow-Liege Scale) or motor lateralization (the Maryland Coma Scale), but the GCS remains the gold standard for clinical grading of injury severity.[5,6] However, like all other scales, the GCS has some shortcomings. Initially, the Glasgow group determined the GCS score six hours after injury in the belief that earlier assessments might overestimate the severity of injury. But, with most patients now arriving at trauma centers within a couple of hours after injury, and with aggressive treatment being initiated as soon as possible after admission, the National Coma Data Bank chose to use the GCS score soon after cardiopulmonary resuscitation rather than at six hours post-injury.[7] However, this early scoring can reduce the predictive strength of the GCS, since all prognostic systems in head injury work better the further one is into the hospital course. A recent study found considerable variability in the quality of early GCS assessment, thus bringing into question the validity of this measure in making vital management decisions.[8]

Another problem with the use of GCS arises in patients with swollen eyes and endotracheal intubation, as the eye and verbal scores cannot be evaluated. Jane and Rimel found the GCS motor score by itself to be strongly predictive value of mortality in 90 percent of patients with a GCS motor score of 1.[9] Thus, especially in comatose patients, the motor score alone may be preferable to the GCS sum score.

Age

A patient's age greatly influences both the mortality rate and the degree of disability. Teasdale and co-workers found a consistent relationship between increasing age and poor outcome.[10] Other series reported mortality rates of 70 to 90 percent in patients over 56 to 60 years of age.[3,11–16] A tendency for worse outcome was observed in patients under 5 years of age when compared to those in the 6- to 19-year age range.[3] Thus, a patient's age has important prognostic value; however, no decisions concerning the aggressiveness of treatment should be based on age alone.

Pupils reactivity and eye movements

Alteration in consciousness, anisocoria or pupillary unresponsiveness, and abnormal motor response traditionally have been associated with injury or mechanical compression of the upper brainstem (usually from transtentorial herniation) and are associated with a poorer prognosis.[17–21] Andrews and co-workers reviewed functional recovery after traumatic transtentorial herniation[17,22] and reported that 18 percent of 153 patients had a favorable outcome (either good recovery or moderate disability).[22] Two of these moderately disabled patients had bilaterally dilated and fixed pupils on admission. Patients with a favorable outcome are often younger, have anisocoria, and maintain some preservation of upper brainstem function. A favorable outcome may be expected in one of three patients if anisocoria is present at admission, but is uncommon among patients with bilaterally fixed pupils.[22] Impaired eye movements are also an ominous prognostic sign and are associated with a 70 to 90 percent mortality rate.[3,57,12]

At first glance, bilaterally dilated and nonreactive pupils seem to be good indicators of an unsalvageable patient. However, the two patients in Andrews' study who made a favorable recovery, although they comprised only 3.5 percent of the patients with fixed dilated pupils, make it difficult to eliminate these patients from further treatment. Unfortunately, in this study severely disabled, vegetative, and dead patients were grouped together, making it difficult to determine the number of patients with bilaterally fixed pupils who survived with severe disability.

Type of Injury

Diffuse axonal injury

Severe diffuse axonal injury (DAI) is associated with prolonged coma that is not primarily due to mass lesions or ischemic insults. These patients become comatose immediately after a high-velocity injury and often present with motor posturing and autonomic dysfunction.[23] Gennarelli and co-workers reported a 51 percent mortality rate in severely head-injured patients (GCS 3–5), with 14 percent of patients left severely disabled and 8 percent vegetative. Thus, 26 percent had either a good recovery or mild disability.[24]

Cerebral contusions and hematomas

Cerebral contusions are the most frequent lesions following head injury.[25] Temporal lobe contusions and hematomas should be aggressively treated as they can produce brainstem compression with little warning.[3] The most important factor that determines mortality and outcome in different series was the clinical status prior to the operation; unconscious patients clearly have higher mortality rates.[4,26,27]

Acute subdural hematoma

The incidence of acute subdural hematomas in severely head-injured patients varies widely in different series.[26,28,29] In the Traumatic Coma Data Bank (TCDB), 37 percent of the 746 patients with severe closed head injuries had surgically removed hematomas.[30,31] Fifty-eight percent of these hematomas were subdural, 26 percent were intracerebral, and 16 percent were epidural.[31] Recent experience from Baylor College of Medicine demonstrates a much higher incidence of surgically evacuated hematomas (56 percent of 214 patients). Nevertheless, the proportion of hematoma type is similar, i.e., 61 percent subdural, 20 percent intracerebral, and 20 percent epidural (personal communication; Narayan, RK et al., 1994). Patients incurring acute subdural hematomas usually are older than the average head-injured patient, with a mean age of 41 years.[29] The mortality and disability rates of these patients are high and range from 42 to 90 percent.[29,32,33] Factors affecting outcome in patients with acute subdural hematomas are:[34]

1. Age. Older patients have higher mortality and disability rates than younger patients (20 percent mortality for patients under 40; 65 percent for patients over 40).[35] Older patients also demonstrate a volume of hematoma up to five times larger than younger patients and a greater midline shift.[36]

2. Neurological status. As with intracerebral hematomas, conscious patients with acute subdural hematomas did better than patients who were unconscious prior to operation (9 percent vs. 40–65 percent mortality rates, respectively).[53,35] Gennarelli and co-workers observed a mortality rate of 74 percent in patients with acute subdural hematomas whose GCS scores were 4–5 as compared with a mortality rate of 36 percent in patients whose GCS scores were 6–8.[24] Impaired pupillary reactivity also was associated with poorer outcome, although Seelig and colleagues found a 10 percent functional recovery even in patients with bilaterally fixed and dilated pupils.[26,35]

3. Timing of operation. Seelig and associates found a 60 percent lower mortality in their patient population (90 percent vs. 30 percent) when the acute subdural hematoma had been evacuated within four hours after injury.[26,29,35] Haselberger and co-workers found operative mortality to be 47 percent in patients with acute subdural hematoma who were unconscious less than two hours, as compared with 80 percent when the unconscious state lasted for more than two hours.[37] Other authors failed to find such a strong association between timing of operation and outcome, although the same trend was evident.[38]

Epidural hematomas

Epidural hematomas constitute approximately 16 percent of surgically evacuated mass lesions in severe head injury.[31] The reported mortality from epidural hematomas ranges between 5 and 43 percent. Higher mortality rates tend to be associated with older age, presence of intradural lesions, temporal location, large volume of hematoma, mixed density of the hematoma on CT scan, rapid progression of signs, pupillary abnormalities, elevated intracranial pressure (ICP), and unconsciousness.[34]

Gunshot wounds

The incidence of civilian gunshot wounds (GSW) to the head has risen in recent years. The overall mortality rate from civilian GSW head injuries ranges from 30 to 97 percent in different series.[39–43] It has been reported that about 70 percent of patients die at the scene of accident.[41] Factors such as a GCS of 3–5, injury by high-velocity large caliber missiles, injuries to multiple lobes, and coagulation abnormalities have been shown to be associated with a dismal outcome.[44] Overall, between 50 and 66 percent of patients admitted to the hospital will die, and only about 25 percent will have a favorable outcome.[45] Narayan and co-workers found that, at the two ends of the GCS spectrum, the neurological examination was a strong predictor of outcome. Patients with a GCS score of 3–4 almost always died, and only one of the seven survivors had a favorable outcome. Ninety-seven percent of patients with a GCS score of 15 had a good outcome.[43] Helling and associates reported a better outcome in patients who underwent early surgical intervention (36 percent survival), as compared with patients who were not operated on (3 percent survival). However, these results may simply reflect patient selection bias.[46] Aldrich and co-workers reported that 88 percent of 151 patients with penetrating GSW to the head from the NIH Traumatic Coma Data Bank died. Ninety-four percent of these patients had an initial GCS score of 3–5; 70 percent had a GCS score of 6–8. Elevated ICP, midline shift, subarachnoid or intraventricular hemorrhages, and intracerebral hyperdense or mixed density lesions greater than 15 ml were all associated with poor outcome.[47] In conclusion, GSW patients with a GCS of 3, and even perhaps of 4, may indeed constitute a group that is generally unsalvageable with current therapies. Nevertheless, a few patients do survive, even in this group.

Systemic Insults

Associated systemic injuries worsen outcome from severe head injury. Miller and colleagues reported associated systemic injuries in 49 percent of their series. The most frequent were skeletal (30 percent), chest (25 percent), abdominal (17 percent) and spinal injuries (6 percent).[27] Eisenberg and co-workers reported hypotension (systemic blood pressure <90 mmHg) accompanying head injury in 33 percent of patients. Mortality rate from severe head injury associated with hypotension was 83 percent, as compared to only 45 percent in isolated head injury. Hypoxemia (Pa_{O_2} < 60 mmHg) was found in 20 percent of patients and increased the mortality rate by approximately 20 percent.[48] Piek and associates reported that the most common extracranial complications in 746 head-injured patients from the Traumatic Coma Data Bank were electrolyte abnormalities (59.3 percent), pneumonia (40.6 percent), hypotension of at least 30 minutes' duration (29.3 percent), coagulopathies (18.4 percent), and septicemia (10 percent).[49] Chesnut and colleagues recently demonstrated the clearly deleterious effect of hypotension in patients with severe head injury.[50] Furthermore, Gopinath and co-workers, using jugular oxygen saturation monitoring, have shown that episodes of desaturation (Sjv_{O_2} < 50 percent for more than 10 minutes) are common in patients with severe head injury and are strongly associated with poorer outcomes.[51] However, none of these associations predict certain death.

CT Scan and Physiological Measurements

CT scan

Several features appearing on the initial CT scan have been correlated with outcome after severe head injury, including the presence of hematomas, midline shift, and compression or absence of the basal cisterns.[52,53] Mortality rate has been reported as 77 percent in patients with absent cisterns, 39 percent in patients with compressed cisterns, and 22 percent in patients with normal basal cisterns.[52,53] The degree of horizontal shift of the septum pellucidum has been correlated with outcome.[54] Marshall and co-workers recently generated a new classification for head injury based on the initial CT scan.[55] This classification subdivides diffuse injury into four grades based on midline shift and the status of basal cisterns (DI I to DI IV) and employs separate categories for evacuated mass lesions (MI) and nonevacuated mass lesions larger than 25 ml (MII). Using the five categories of the Glasgow Outcome Scale (G/MD/SD/V/D), the authors found that they could correctly predict death in 59 percent of patients by combining this CT classification system with age and motor score.

Intracranial pressure

Elevated ICP can cause death in patients with severe head injury.[32,56] Aggressive treatment of elevated ICP has been associated with improved outcomes.[50,57,58] Furthermore, ICP data has been shown to have a strong predictive value in determining outcome. Marmarou and colleagues after analyzing the Traumatic Coma Data Bank data, found that ICP measurements greater than 20 mmHg were a strong predictor of outcome, independent of other factors such as age, admission motor score, and admission pupillary reactivity.[50,59] Miller and associates found that head-injured patients with ICP > 20 mmHg had a mortality rate of 55 percent as compared to 14 percent in patients with normal ICP.[60] Narayan and co-workers reported that ICP > 20 mmHg was associated with a 44 percent mortality rate, while head injured patients with normal ICP had only a 16 percent mortality rate.[13,84] Patients with persistently elevated ICP refractory to therapy generally do not survive.

However, we have all seen a few patients with ICP over 40 mmHg who eventually survive and even do well. Hence, ICP alone is not a foolproof indicator of unsalvageability unless it reaches the same value as the mean blood pressure, indicating brain death.

EVOKED POTENTIALS

Monitoring evoked potentials (EP) in head-injured patients may be helpful in three ways. It can help to localize the neurological dysfunction, assess the ability of neural tissue to recover, and monitor changes in neural tissue function [Newlon, 1989, 64). Greenberg and colleagues generated a four-point clinical grading system of EP abnormalities, with grade I representing EP values closest to normal and grade IV representing absent EP.[61] In a prospective study of 100 comatose head injured patients, these authors could accurately predict death from cerebral causes early after injury (mean 3.8 days). Patients with normal EP usually do well unless secondary systemic or neurological insult occurs.[62–64] Brainstem auditory evoked potentials (BAEP) were also used to predict outcome from head injury.[65–68] Abnormal BAEP were closely associated with poor outcome with the best prognostic value achieved after three days post-injury.[67] In a study comparing the clinical examination, EP, ICP, and CT scan data in predicting outcome after severe head injury, Narayan and colleagues found the clinical exam to be the most reliable indicator of outcome; but the other data, notably EP, could strengthen the confidence of the prediction.[13] However, EP data are not widely available and may not be uniformly effective as a predictor.[69] This is particularly true when the patient dies of unexpected complications.

CEREBRAL BLOOD FLOW AND JUGULAR BULB OXYGEN SATURATION

Robertson and co-workers measured cerebral blood flow (CBF) during the first 10 days after injury in 102 patients.[70] Twenty-five patients had a reduced CBF averaging 29 ± 5 ml/100g/min; 47 had a normal CBF, averaging 41 ± 1 ml/100g/min; and 30 had an elevated CBF, averaging 62 ± 14 ml/100g/min. Patients with reduced CBF had a mortality rate of 32 percent, as compared to 21 percent and 20 percent in the normal and elevated CBF groups, respectively. Gopinath and associates measured the jugular bulb oxygen saturation (Sjv_{O_2}) in 116 patients.[51] Strong association was found between outcome and transient jugular desaturation reflecting cerebral ischemia. Mortality rates were 17.4 percent for patients with no desaturation episode, 40.7 percent for patients with one episode, and 68.4 percent for patients with multiple episodes of jugular desaturation.

PROGNOSTIC SCALES

It is evident from the above section that no single prognostic indicator will predict outcome with 100 percent accuracy. Over the years, numerous attempts have been made using various statistical methods to strengthen the confidence of prediction by combining different prognostic indicators into the "perfect prognostic scale."

Jennett, Teasdale, and Braakman formed a model based on Bayesian statistics to predict outcome.[71–73] They selected 400 patients from the International Data Bank, assessed over 100 data items for each patient, and used this information to generate their model. This was then employed to predict outcome of another 200 patients from the Data Bank, and the predicted outcome was compared to the actual outcome. When the system was used to predict one of two outcomes (functional vs. dead/vegetative), the model correctly predicted outcome in about 94 percent of patients in the first week after injury. When the 100 data items/patient was reduced to eight, the performance of the model was almost as good.

Braakman and co-workers generated a model that employed a varying number of outcome categories (from two to five) and prognostic indicators that depended on the time point after injury.[74,75] On admission, these authors found that they could predict outcome correctly in 86 percent of 305 patients by using two outcome categories (dead/alive) and three indicators (age, pupillary reactivity, and eye and motor scores of the GCS). By day 28 post-injury, all five categories of the GOS were employed along with five prognostic indicators (pupillary reactivity, GCS eye and motor scores, sex, and age). This model accurately predicted outcome in 96 percent of 177 patients.[75]

Stablein and associates described a logistic regression model for differentiating between good (G/MD/SD) and poor (V/D) outcome.[76] The authors used the presence of a mass lesion on CT scan, necessary surgical decompression, physiological status on admission, age, sex, motor and eye opening response, and pupillary response to predict outcome correctly in 91 percent of 115 cases. Narayan and associates used GCS scores, age, EP data, and ICP to determine outcome accurately in 89 percent of 133 patients.[13]

Choi and colleagues used a stepwise discriminant analysis to predict one of four categories of outcome (good recovery, moderate disability, severe disability and vegetative/dead).[77–79] The analysis included 523 patients, and the final model was based on age, motor score, and pupillary reactivity. For each pupillary reactivity category (bilateral reactive, unilateral absent, bilateral absent), a graph of age vs. motor score was plotted, and each outcome category occupied a different portion of the rectangle formed between the x-axis (the motor score) and the y-axis (the age). For example, in the graph for bilaterally absent pupillary response, most of the area was occupied by the vegetative/dead category. If a prediction fell into the correct outcome category, it was termed specifically accurate. If it fell into an adjacent category, it was termed grossly accurate. The overall specific prediction rate with four outcome categories was 78 percent, and the grossly accurate prediction rate was 90.4 percent.

Baldwin and co-workers analyzed data from 828 patients registered in the Traumatic Coma Data Bank (TCDB) to select a combination of variables that could be used to predict the probability of survival or death.[80] Advanced age, low admission GCS score, presence of pupillary dysfunction, hypotension, and hypoxia were found to be associated with mortality. The authors used the model to calculate the probability of death for each patient. If the probability was calculated to be more than 0.5, death was predicted. The model correctly predicted survival or death in 91.2 percent of the TCDB patients.

A bedside model of outcome prediction was developed by Gibson and Stephenson from Leeds, England (Leeds Prognostic Scale), using seven variables—age, unreactive pupils, ICP, systolic blood pressure, GCS score, presence of extracranial injuries, and the presence of high-density lesions on CT scan(s).[81] Each variable was weighted to reflect its influence on mortality (Table

TABLE 55-1 Variables and Weighting of Leeds Prognostic Scale

Factor	Weighting
Age	
0–40	0
41–60	1
>60	2
UNREACTIVE PUPILS	
Unilateral	1
Bilateral	4
INTRACRANIAL PRESSURE	
<20	0
20–40	2
>40	4
SYSTOLIC BLOOD PRESSURE	
≤80 mmHg	4
GLASGOW COMA SCORE	
≥9	0
6–8	1
3–5	2
OTHER EXTRACRANIAL INJURIES	3
HIGH DENSITY LESIONS ON CT	
Intracerebral	2
Intracerebral and extracerebral	4

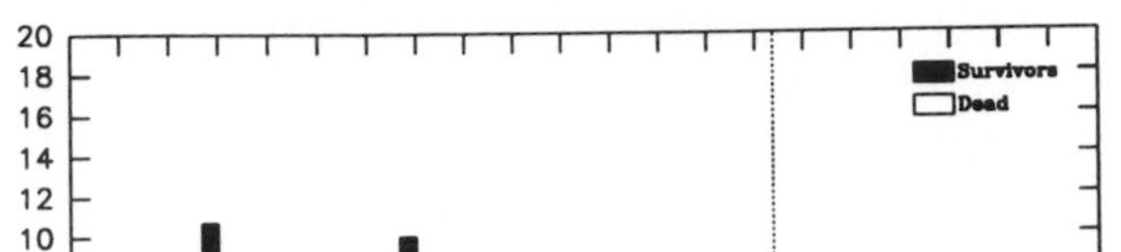
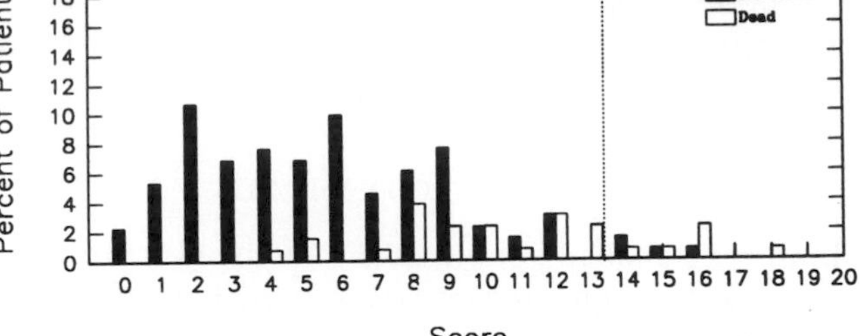

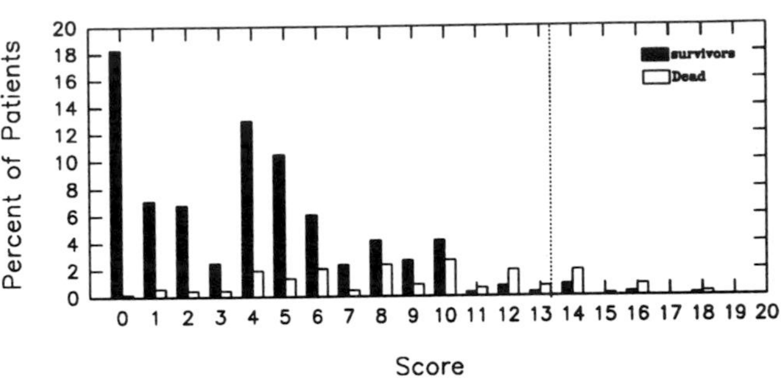

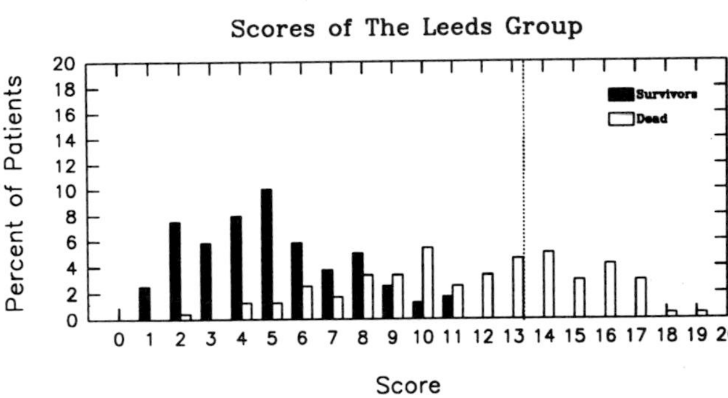

Figure 55-1. Comparison between scores of the Ben Taub group, the Houston-Galveston registry group and the Leeds series.

55-1). Using scores that ranged from 0 (best) to 24 (worst), they reported that none of the patients with a score higher than 11 survived. Allowing for a margin of safety, they concluded that death could be predicted with 100 percent accuracy in patients with scores higher than 13 and proposed withdrawal of active treatment from these patients because in a series of 187 retrospective and 52 prospective patients not one patient with a score of 12 or higher had survived.

To determine the universal applicability of the Leeds Prognostic Scale, we applied it to two patient populations (Fig. 55-1).[82] The first group was composed of 479 patients from the Houston-Galveston head injury registry, the second group included 131 patients studied prospectively at the Ben Taub General Hospital. Only

16 of the 23 patients (69.6 percent) from the Houston-Galveston group who were predicted certainly to die according to the Leeds scale (scores > 13) actually died; 380 (83.3 percent) of 456 patients with scores of 13 or less survived (sensitivity of 18.5 percent and specificity of 98.2 percent). Fourteen survivors had scores greater than 11 (up to a score of 18). Three of these survivors with a score higher than 11 had a good outcome, two were moderately disabled, five severely disabled, and four were in a vegetative state three months post-injury. In the Ben Taub group, only six of the 10 patients predicted to die by the Leeds scale actually died. Ninety-eight of 121 patients (81 percent) with scores of 13 or less survived (sensitivity of 20.68 percent and specificity of 96.07 percent). Eight of the surviving patients had scores greater than 11. Of these patients, two were moderately disabled, two were severely disabled, and four were in a vegetative state three months post-injury.

By reviewing retrospectively 100 patients with penetrating GSW to the head, Levy and co-workers generated a predictive model with eight parameters, including: admission GCS score; age; bihemispheric injury; presence of subarachnoid blood; intracranial hemorrhage; intraventricular hemorrhage; contusion(s); and presence of bone or bullet fragmentation. This logistically derived prognostic model had a positive predictive value of 86 percent and a negative predictive value of 74.2 percent.[83]

DIFFICULTIES IN DECLARING UNSALVAGEABILITY

Timing of Predictions

When should prediction of survival be made, and should this influence management? The question of prognosis prediction and its relationship to patient management was raised in a survey among 59 neurosurgeons. Eighty-nine percent of the participants stated that they attempted to estimate prognosis, and 74 percent did so at 24 hours post-injury. Sixty percent claimed that their estimate "greatly" or "moderately" influenced their decision to operate, and 42 percent used their 24-hour estimate of prognosis to influence management decisions. Fifty-six percent ranked the estimated prognosis first among factors that influence clinical decisions.[84]

Any prognosis estimation has two conflicting goals: accuracy and rapidity. It is obvious that the longer the time elapsed since injury, the more information will be available. However, the longer one waits before prognosis estimation, need for such estimation decreases; resources and effort already have been allocated for treating the patient.

Early predictions may be inaccurate, however, owing to the effects of alcohol and drugs, substances commonly associated with trauma, and head injury in particular. Forty to 60 percent of patients sustaining trauma were found to test positive for alcohol or drugs.[85–87] Both alcohol and drugs often alter the neurological assessment of head-injured patients, and thus any prognosis estimation based on such examination will be erroneous.

Even when facing the most devastating head-injured patients, decisions concerning management are not always clear. Braakman considered prediction of outcome on admission difficult, partly because "admission" is not a sharply defined term; it can mean arrival at a primary facility, or arrival at a neurosurgical service after transfer from a primary facility. Because the magnitude of brain damage soon after injury may be overestimated owing to associated factors such as shock and other extracranial injuries, these authors concluded that the first prognostic statement should be deferred until at least six hours post-injury, when resuscitation has been completed.[88]

Waxman and co-workers examined whether an accurate prediction of outcome could be made from data taken at three time points within six hours after patient arrival, i.e., at the emergency department, after CT scanning, and after a second neurological assessment six hours after arrival at the hospital.[89] Using a stepwise linear logistic regression, these authors concluded that aggressive therapy should be continued for at least six hours after arrival because not all patients with potential for favorable recovery can be identified within this period.

Kaufman and associates used the 24 hours post-injury time point to evaluate prospectively the quality of first-day outcome prediction of 100 consecutive head injured patients.[90] Prognosis estimates were made independently by a neuroradiologist and a neurosurgeon. The neuroradiologist predicted outcome correctly in 59 percent of patients, often overpredicting favorable outcome; the neurosurgeon correctly predicted outcome in 56 percent of patients, often overpredicting unfavorable outcome. In combining the predictions of both the radiologist and clinician, the outcome predictions were found to be correct for 73 percent of patients. They concluded that it was not possible to predict outcome on the first day after injury with sufficient accuracy to guide early management.

As time elapses after the injury, the probability of accurately predicting mortality increases; most deaths will occur in the first few days after injury, and the survivors will begin to "declare" themselves.[14,89,91,92] Carlsson and co-workers and Clifton and associates estimated that between 70 and 75 percent of deaths occurred within the initial 48 hours;[91,92] and Pazzaglia and colleagues reported 50 percent of deaths within 72 hours.[14] In the Waxman series, patients who died did so within an average of 1.7 days post-injury.[89]

Bricolo and co-workers found that 31 percent of 135 patients in coma for two weeks after head trauma had either moderate disability or a good outcome at one-year follow-up; 31 percent were severely disabled, 8 percent were vegetative, and 30 percent had died.[93]

Braakman and associates studied the outcome of 140 patients in a vegetative state one month after the onset of coma.[94] Fifty-nine patients had regained consciousness within one year post-injury, but only 10 percent had become independent; none had made a complete recovery. No patient over 40 years of age had become independent during the first year. In addition, none of the patients in a vegetative state three months after injury became independent.

Bond and Brooks studied the rate of recovery of head-injured patients.[95] They found that most patients with an outcome of severe disability reached a steady state after three months, while only two-thirds of patients with an eventual outcome of good or moderate disability reached this status by three months. Overall, 90 percent of patients had reached a steady state at six months. However, others have reported that significant recovery may occur up to a year and even longer after injury[96,97] (Choi personal communication).

Falsely Optimistic Vs. Falsely Pessimistic Predictions

Narayan and co-workers reported on the probability of falsely optimistic vs. falsely pessimistic predictions of outcome.[79] The authors employed a logistic regression model to calculate prospectively the probability of poor outcome in 100 patients from the Medical College of Virginia from May 1976 to September 1979. The system proved accurate in 82 percent of cases, with 18 percent of the predictions wrong. The probability of a poor outcome in a series of patients with serious head injury can range from 0 percent to 100 percent. The prediction of outcome in a patient whose prognostic signs indicate a very good or a very poor outcome ("polar predictions") is more likely to be accurate than prediction in a patient with a probability estimate closer to 50 percent ("central predictions") (Figure 55-2). This figure clearly illustrates that "polar" predictions (p^{poor} = 0–10 percent or 90–100 percent) are the most accurate (96–100 percent), while "central" predictions (p^{poor} = 31–50 percent) are the least accurate (56 percent). Figure 55-2 also illustrates that it is easier to predict a poor outcome ($p^{poor} > 50$ percent) accurately than to predict a good outcome ($p^{poor} < 50$ percent). Hence, falsely optimistic errors are more likely to occur than are falsely pessimis-

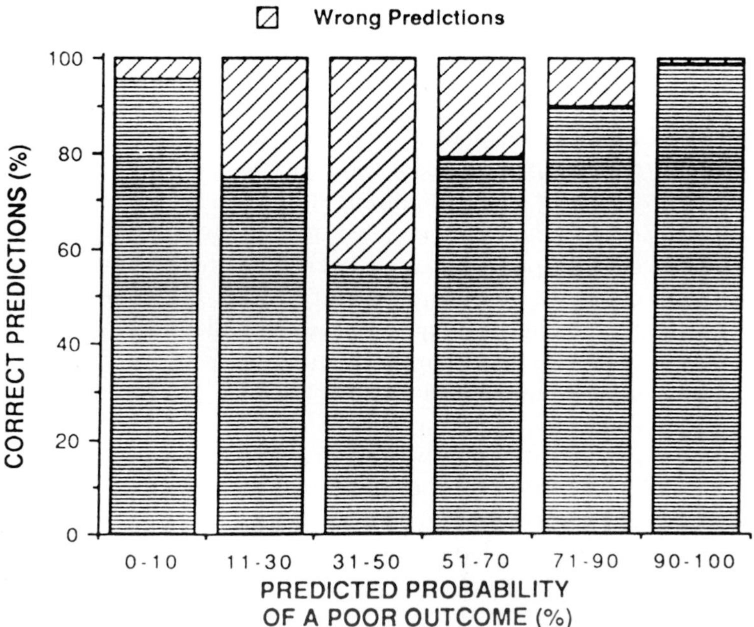

Figure 55-2. Accuracy of outcome predictions in 100 patients with severe head injury.

tic errors. This is because unexpected complications may worsen the outcome in patients who originally had seemed to be doing quite well neurologically.

Effect of Newer Therapies

Extensive research during the last three decades has led to a better understanding of the epidemiology, pathophysiology, and therapy of head-injured patients. The mortality from severe head injury reported in the 1970s to be around 50 percent[71,75] appears to have come down to around 30 to 36 percent in recent series.[58,98,99] Understanding the causes of early death after head injury has led to policy changes that affect where patients with severe head injury are hospitalized and how quickly a CT scan is performed.[100] These policy changes have reduced the mortality of patients with intracranial hematomas from 38 percent to 29 percent and of patients who "talk and die" from 31 percent to 16 percent.

Aggressive medical treatment of intracranial hypertension has been shown to improve outcome from severe head injury.[58,101] Barbiturates have been found to provide brain protection by reducing metabolic rate and to improve outcome in patients without hypotension.[102] Surgical treatment of intracranial hypertension has had mixed results. Hemicraniectomies, bifrontal craniectomies, and circumferential de-roofing have all been tried and generally abandoned. Recently, several authors have reported a beneficial effect of subtemporal bony decompression for patients with medically uncontrollable intracranial hypertension. Alexander and associates performed subtemporal decompression on 15 head injured patients with an ICP of such degree that it could not be managed medically.[103] Seven of the patients had a favorable recovery. Gower and co-workers performed subtemporal decompression on 10 patients who failed to respond to medical treatment of elevated ICP.[104] Four of the patients died (40 percent) as compared to an 82.4 percent mortality rate in patients who were placed in pentobarbital coma. Five of the six survivors made a favorable recovery. Gaab and colleagues prospectively studied 37 selected patients with brain swelling who subsequently underwent extensive craniotomies and a wide opening of the dura. Four of the patients died, and 41 percent achieved an independent recovery.[105] The authors recommended surgical treatment of elevated ICP unresponsive to adequate conservative treatment for younger patients (<40 years) with a GCS score >3, no mass lesion or infarction, preserved fifth wave of the BAER, and no evidence of oscillating flow on transcranial Doppler.

New drugs are being tested for the treatment of head injured patients. THAM (tromethamine tris (hydroxymethyl) aminomethane), by entering the cerebrospinal fluid compartment and reducing cerebral acidosis, has been shown to ameliorate the deleterious effect of prolonged hyperventilation, and helps in ICP control of head injured patients.[106,107] However, no significant difference in outcome between THAM-treated and control groups has been reported. PEG-SOD (Polyethylene glycol conjugated superoxide dismutase), a free radical scavenger, appears promising in improving outcome after severe head injury. Patients receiving 10,000U/kg of PEG-SOD needed less mannitol for ICP control and had shorter periods of time of ICP higher than 20 mmHg compared with the placebo group. At three months post-injury, only 20 percent of patients receiving treatment were either vegetative or dead as compared with 44 percent of the placebo group. At six months, 36 percent of the placebo group were either in a vegetative state or dead, as compared with 21 percent in the treatment group.[108]

Variability In Outcome At Different Hospitals Settings

Colohan and co-workers compared head injury mortality in two centers in the United States and India.[109] The mortality rate, adjusted for initial severity of injury, was 11 percent in New Delhi, India, versus 7.2 percent in Charlottesville, VA. Patients with the most severe or least severe injuries had similar mortality rates. However, in those with a GCS motor score of 5 (localizing), the mortality rate was 12.5 percent in New Delhi versus 4.8 percent in Charlottesville. The relative lack of prehospital emergency care and the delay in admission after head injury in New Delhi are cited as two possible causes for the differences in mortality in this group of patients.

Several authors emphasize the importance of neurosurgical intensive care units in mortality reduction. Superior intensive care was cited by Bowers and Marshall as a vital contribution to the low overall mortality rate reported in the San Diego neurosurgical community.[98] Warme and associates found an increase of 15 to 52 percent in the good outcome category of the GOS in a subgroup of patients with a GCS motor score of 4 or higher after the establishment of a neurosurgical intensive care unit.[110] Similar results showed that patients at moderate risk (with GCS score of 7 or higher), and who were likely to make a useful recovery, had the highest risk of dying if the level of surveillance in the hospital was inadequate.[111]

These data again emphasize that differences in emergency medical services and intensive care can influence outcome, thus making the task of forming universal guidelines for unsalvageability difficult. Furthermore, a patient who may be unsalvageable in one country or center may indeed be salvageable in another setting because of superior facilities and more aggressive management.

Differing Expectations

When addressing the issue of unsalvageability, one has to bear in mind the attitudes of the family toward the injury. Families may have varying perceptions of the outcome after severe head injury. Often, the situation is emotionally charged, and physicians need to be sensitive to the fragile state of the family, which may preclude them from fully and clearly understanding or accepting of the prognosis of the patient. Families are likely to judge the situation emotionally as a result of the distressing condition they are facing, and will not consider rationally the information presented to them. This scenario can be especially delicate. Some families may be thankful that the patient is alive despite the severity of his/her eventual disability; other families may view the severely disabled state as a fate worse than death. In such cases the physician must keep in mind the gap that lies between the objective condition of the patient and the subjective way families perceive it, trying to individualize care.

CONCLUSION

The outcome of severe head injury can be predicted fairly accurately. This prediction is most appropriately used when counseling patients' families, for comparison of the effect of new therapies on outcome, and for the detection and control of variables that might affect and/or improve outcome. The prediction of outcome should be used with extreme caution in determining the individual management of patients. Caution also should be exercised when the experience of one center is applied directly to another. All prediction scales are generated based on a specific population; as population differs with respect to demographic factors, so do mechanism and severity of injury, delay between injury and treatment, management techniques, and other support systems. Providing initial aggressive treatment to all patients on arrival at the hospital may be costly, but this must be compared with the risk of withholding treatment from patients who might be salvageable. Furthermore, by deciding to provide initial aggressive treatment, the physician does not make a personal commitment to treat the patient indefinitely. If sufficient data are collected by frequent neurological assessments and supportive tests to prove that the patient's condition is irreversible, termination of active therapy and life support should be discussed with the patient's family. The guidelines suggested by Edmund D. Pellegrino seem to summarize the best current thinking in this area:[112]

1. The moral onus is on those who move to discontinue treatment. When in serious doubt about prognosis, competence, or the wishes of the patient or surrogate, the patient should be treated.
2. Withhold emergency treatment rarely unless prognosis and other criteria are indisputable.
3. Starting treatment does not entail a commitment to continue to the "bitter end."
4. Allow time for the clinical picture to emerge. Frequent assessments of prognosis, competence, and patient or surrogate wishes are essential. "Vector in" on the decision; don't "jump in."
5. Moral decisions based on diagnosis of brain dysfunction and destruction must be carefully scrutinized, especially in infants and old people. Consultation and confirmation must be sought.
6. Beware of categorizing patients too early or changing their categorization too late.
7. Consult frequently with all parties to a decision.
8. Ask not "Is this what I would want done to me?" but "Is this what I think the patient would want?"
9. Withholding or withdrawing treatment must always be associated with continued care for the patient.
10. Perform ethical postmortems, rethinking your decisions, especially those that had to be made in haste.
11. Examine all formulae and algorithms (including this one) with a critical eye.

References

1. Hippocrates: The book of prognostics, in *The Genuine Works of Hippocrates.* Baltimore: Williams & Wilkins, 1939:42–43.
2. Hippocrates: The art, in *Hippocrates,* vol 2. Cambridge: Harvard University Press, 1967:203–205.
3. Jennett B, Teasdale G, Braakman R, et al: Prognosis of patients with severe head injury. *Neurosurgery* 1979; 4:282–289.
4. Kanter MJ, Scheinberg MA, Kritzer RO, et al: Management of cerebral contusions. Congress of Neurological Surgeons' Annual Meeting, Los Angeles, October 1990.
5. Born MR, Albert A, Hans P, et al: Relative prognostic value of best motor response and brain stem reflexes in patients with severe head injury. *Neurosurgery* 1985; 16:595–601.
6. Salcman M, Schepp RS, Ducker TB: Calculated recovery rates in severe head trauma. *Neurosurgery* 1981; 8:301–308.

7. Marshall LF, Becker DP, Bowers SA, et al: The national traumatic coma data bank. Part 1: Design, purpose, goals, and results. *J Neurosurg* 1983; 59:276–284.
8. Marion DW, Carlier PM: Problems with initial Glasgow Coma Scale assessment caused by prehospital treatment of patients with head injuries: Results of a national survey. *J Trauma* 1994; 36(1):89–95.
9. Jane JA, Rimel RW: Prognosis in head injury, in Weiss MH (ed): *Clin Neurosurg.* vol 29. Baltimore: Williams & Wilkins, 1982; 346–352.
10. Teasdale G, Skene A, Parker L, et al: Age and outcome of severe head injury. *Acta Neurochir* 1979; 28(suppl):140–143.
11. Heiskanen O, Sipponen P: Prognosis of severe brain injury. *Neurol Scand* 1970; 46:343–348.
12. Levati A, Farina ML, Vecchi G, et al: Prognosis of severe head injury. *J Neurosurg* 1982; 57:779–783.
13. Narayan RK, Greenberg RP, Miller JD, Enas GG: Improved confidence of outcome in severe head injury. *J Neurosurg* 1981; 54:751–762.
14. Pazzaglia P, Frank G, Frank F, Gaist G: Clinical course and prognosis of acute post-traumatic coma. *J Neurol Neurosurg Psychiatr* 1975; 38:149–154.
15. Ross AM, Pitts LH, Kobayashi S: Prognosticators of outcome after major head injury in the elderly. *J Neurosci Nurs* 1992; 24:88–93.
16. Vollmer DG, Torner JC, Jane JA, et al: Age and outcome following traumatic coma: Why do older patients fare worse? *J Neurosurg* 1991; 75:s37–s49.
17. Andrews BT, Pitts LH, Lovely MP, Bartowski H: Is computed tomographic scanning necessary in patients with tentorial herniation? Results of immediate surgical exploration without computed tomography in 100 patients. *Neurosurgery* 1986; 19:408–414.
18. Brender SJ, Selverstone B: Recovery frome decerebration. *Brain* 1970; 93:381–392.
19. Gutterman P, Shenkin HA. Prognostic features in recovery from traumatic decerebration. *J Neurosurg* 1970; 32:330–335.
20. Hoff JT, Spetzler R, Winestock D: Head injury and early signs of tentorial herniation—a management dilemma. *West J Med* 1978; 128:112–116.
21. Marshall LF, Barba D, Toole BM, Bowers SA: The oval pupil: Clinical significance and relationship to intracranial hypertension. *J Neurosurg* 1983; 58:566–568.
22. Andrews BT, Pitts LH: Functional recovery after traumatic transtentorial herniation. *Neurosurgery* 1991; 29:227–231.
23. Gennarelli TA: Mechanisms of brain injury. *J Emerg Med* 1993; 11:S5–S11.
24. Gennarelli TA, Spielman GM, Langfitt TW, et al: Influence of the type of intracranial lesion on outcome from severe head injury: A multicenter study using a new classification system. *J Neurosurg* 1982; 56:26–32.
25. Freytag E: Autopsy findings in head injuries from blunt forces. Statistical evaluation of 1367 cases. *Arch Path* 1963; 75:402–413.
26. Jamieson KG, Yelland JDN: Traumatic intracerebral hematoma. Report of 63 surgically treated cases. *J Neurosurg* 1972; 37:528–532.
27. Miller JD, Butterworth JF, Gudeman SK, et al: Further experience in the management of severe head injury. *J Neurosurg* 1981; 54:289–299.
28. Grossman RG: Treatment of patients with intracranial hematomas. *N Engl J Med* 1981; 304:1540–1541.
29. Seelig JM, Becker DP, Miller JD, et al: Traumatic acute subdural hematoma. Major mortality reduction in comatose patients treated within four hours. *N Engl J Med* 1981; 304:1511–1518.
30. Foulkes MA, Eisenberg HM, Jane JA, et al: The traumatic coma data bank: Design, methods and baseline characteristics. *J Neurosurg* 1991; 75:s8–s13.
31. Marshall LF, Gautille T, Klauber MR: The outcome of severe closed head injury. *J Neurosurg* 1991; 75:S28–S29.
32. Becker DP, Miller JD, Ward JD, et al: The outcome from severe head injury with early diagnosis and intensive management. *J Neurosurg* 1977; 47:491–502.
33. Cooper PR, Rovit RL, Ransohoff J: Hemicraniectomy in the treatment of acute subdural hematoma: a reappraisal. *Surg Neurol* 1976; 5:25–28.
34. Cooper PR: Post-traumatic intracranial mass lesions, in: Cooper PR (ed): *Head Injury* (3d ed). Baltimore: Williams & Wilkins, 1993:275–329.
35. McKissock W, Richardson A, Bloom WH: Subdural hematoma. A review of 389 cases. *Lancet* 1960; 1:1365–1369.
36. Howard MAI, Gross AS, Dacey RGJ, et al: Acute subdural hematomas: An age dependent clinical entity. *J Neurosurg* 1989; 71:858–863.
37. Haselberger K, Pucher R, Auer LM: Prognosis after acute subdural or epidural hemorrhage. *Acta Neurochir* 1988; 90:111–116.
38. Wilberger JE, Harris M, Diamond DL: Acute subdural hematoma: Morbidity and mortality related to timing of operative intervention. *J Trauma* 1990; 30:733–736.
39. Crockard HA: Bullet injuries of the brain. *Ann R Coll Surg Engl* 1974; 55:111–123.
40. Goodman JM, Kalsbeck J: Outcome of self inflicted gunshot wounds to the head. *J Trauma* 1965; 5:636–642.
41. Kaufman HH, Makela ME, Lee KF, et al: Gunshot wounds to the head: A perspective. *Neurosurgery* 1986; 18:689–695.
42. Lillard PL: Five years experience with penetrating craniocerebral gunshot wounds. *Surg Neurol* 1978; 9:79–83.
43. Narayan RK, Contant CF, Russell DK, et al: Gunshot wounds to the head: Lessons from a 9-year civilian experience. AANS 60th Annual Meeting, San Francisco, 1992:369.
44. Shaffrey ME, Polin RS, Phillips CD, et al: Classification of civilian craniocerebral gunshot wounds: A multivariate analysis predictive of mortality. *J Neurotrauma* 1992; 9:s279–s285.
45. Cooper PR: Gunshot wounds of the brain, in Cooper PR (ed): *Head injury* (3d ed). Baltimore: Williams & Wilkins, 1993:355–371.
46. Helling TS, Mcnabney WK, Whittaker CK, et al: The role of early intervention in civilian gunshot wound to the head. *J Trauma* 1992; 32:398–400.

47. Aldrich EF, Eisenberg HM, Saydjari C, et al: Predictors of mortality in severely head injured patients with civilian gunshot wounds: A report from the NIH Traumatic Coma data bank. *Surg Neurol* 1992; 38:418–423.
48. Eisenberg HA, Cayard C, Papaniculaou AC: The effect of three potentially preventable complications on severe head injuries, in Ishii S, Nagai H, Brock M (eds). *Intracranial pressure* V. Berlin: Springer-Verlag, 1983:549–553.
49. Piek J, Chesnut R, Marshall LF, et al: Extracranial complications of severe head injury. *J Neurosurg* 1992; 77:901–907.
50. Chesnut RM, Marshall LF, Bowers-Marshall S: Medical management of intracranial pressure, in: Cooper PR (ed). *Head injury,* (3d ed). Baltimore: Williams & Wilkins, 1993:225–246.
51. Gopinath SP, Robertson CS, Contant CF, et al: Jugular venous desaturation and outcome after head injury. *J Neurol Neurosurg Psychiatr* 57:717–723, 1994.
52. Teasdale E, Cardoso E, Galbraith S, et al: CT scan in severe diffuse head injury: Physiological and clinical correlations. *J Neurol Neurosurg Psychiatr* 1984; 47:600–603.
53. Teasdale G, Jennett B: Assessment of coma in impaired consciousness: A practical scale. *Lancet* 1974; 2:81–84.
54. Ross DA, Olsen WL, Ross AM, et al: Brain shift, level of consciousness, and restoration of consciousness in patients with acute intracranial hematoma. *J Neurosurg* 1989; 71:498–502.
55. Marshall LF, Bowers-Marshall S, Klauber MR, et al: A new classification of head injury based on computerized tomography. *J Neurosurg* 1991; 75:s14–s20.
56. Marshall LF, Smith RW, Shapiro HM: The outcome with aggressive treatment in severe head injuries. Part I: The significance of intracranial pressure monitoring. *J Neurosurg* 1979; 50:20–25.
57. Narayan RK, Kishore PRS, Becker DP, et al: Intracranial pressure. To monitor or not to monitor? *J Neurosurg* 1982; 56:650–659.
58. Saul TG, Ducker T: Effect of intracranial pressure monitoring and aggressive treatment on mortality in severe head injury. *J Neurosurg* 1982; 56:498–503.
59. Marmarou A, Anderson RL, Ward JD, et al: Impact of ICP instability and hypotension on outcome in patients with severe head trauma. *J Neurosurg* 1991; 75:s59–s66.
60. Miller JD, Becker DP, Ward JD, et al: Significance of intracranial hypertension in severe head injury. *J Neurosurg* 1977; 47:503–516.
61. Greenberg RP, Mayer DJ, Becker DP, Miller JD: Evaluation of brain function in severe human head trauma with multimodality evoked potentials. Part I: Evoked brain injury potentials, methods, analysis. *J Neurosurg* 1977; 47:150–162.
62. Greenberg RP, Becker DP, Miller JD, Mayer DJ: Evaluation of brain function in severe human head trauma with multimodality evoked potentials. Part 2: Localization of brain dysfunction and correlation with post-traumatic neurological conditions. *J Neurosurg* 1977; 47:163–177.
63. Moulton R, Kresta P, Ramirez M, Tucker W: Continuous automated monitoring of somatosensory evoked potentials in post-traumatic coma. *J Trauma* 1991; 31:676–683.
64. Newlon PG: Utility of multimodality evoked potentials in cerebral injury. Neurol Clin 1985; 3:675–686.
65. Hall JWI, Huangfu M, Gennarelli TA: Auditory function in acute severe head injury. *Laryngoscope* 1982; 92:883–890.
66. Karnaze DS, Weiner JM, Marshall LF: Auditory evoked potentials in coma after close head injury: A clinical-neurophysiologic coma scale for predicting outcome. *Neurology* 1985; 35:1122–1126.
67. Seals DM, Rossiter VM, Weinstein ME: Brain stem evoked response in patients comatose as a result of blunt head trauma. *J Trauma* 1979; 19:347–353.
68. Tsubokawa T, Nishimoto H, Yamamoto T, et al: Assessment of brain stem damage by the auditory brain stem response in acute severe head injury. *J Neurol Neurosurg Psychiatr* 1980; 43:1005–1011.
69. Lindsay KW, Carlin J, Kennedy I, et al: Evoked potentials in severe head injury: Analysis and relation to outcome. *J Neurol Neurosurg Psychiatr* 1981; 44:796–802.
70. Robertson CS, Contant CF, Gokaslan ZL, et al: Cerebral blood flow, arteriovenous oxygen difference, and outcome after head injury. *J Neurol Neurosurg Psychiatr* 1992; 55:594–603.
71. Jennett B, Teasdale G: Prognosis after severe head injury, in Jennett B, Teasdale G (eds). *Management of head injury.* Philadelphia: FA Davis, 1981:317–332.
72. Jennett B, Teasdale G, Braakman R, et al: Predicting outcome in individual patients after severe head injury. *Lancet* 1976; 1:1031–1035.
73. Teasdale G, Jennett B: Assessment and prognosis of coma after head injury. *Acta Neurochir* 1976; 34:45–55.
74. Braakman R, Avezaat CJJ, Maas AIR, et al: Interobserver agreement in the assessment of the motor response of the GCS. *Clin Neurol Neurosurg* 1977; 80:100–106.
75. Braakman R, Gelpke GJ, Habbema JDF, et al: Systematic selection of prognostic features in patients with severe head injury. *Neurosurgery* 1980; 6:362–370.
76. Stablein DM, Miller JD, Choi SC, et al: Statistical methods for determining prognosis in severe head injury. *Neurosurgery* 1980; 6:243–248.
77. Choi SC, Narayan RK, Anderson RL, Ward JD: Enhanced specificity of prognosis in severe head injury. *J Neurosurg* 1988; 69:381–385.
78. Narayan RK: Head injury, in Grossman RG (ed). *Principles of neurosurgery.* New York: Raven Press, 1991:235–291.
79. Narayan RK, Enas GG, Choi SC, Becker DP: Practical techniques for predicting outcome in severe head injury, in Becker DP, Gudeman DK (eds). *Textbook of head injury.* Philadelphia: WB Saunders, 1989:420–425.
80. Baldwin NG, Marmarou A, Marshall LF, Barnes T, Young HF: A mathematical model for early prediction of mortality in severe head injury. AANS 59th Annual Meeting, New Orleans, 1991:456–457.

81. Gibson RM, Stephenson GC: Aggressive management of severe closed head trauma: Time for reappraisal. *Lancet* 1989; 2:369–371.
82. Feldman Z, Contant CF, Robertson CS, et al: Evaluation of the Leeds prognostic score for severe head injury. *Lancet* 1991; 337:1451–1453.
83. Levy M, Rezai A, Tang G, Appuzzo MLJ: A logistically derived model of outcome following penetrating cranicerebral injury. AANS 59th Annual Meeting, New Orleans, 1991:445.
84. Barlow P, Teasdale G: Prediction of outcome and the management of severe head injuries: The attitude of neurosurgeon. *Neurosurgery* 1986; 19:989–991.
85. Rivara FP, Mueller BA, Fligner CL, et al: Drug use in trauma victims. *J Trauma* 1989; 29:462–470.
86. Tardiff K, Gross EM, Wu J, et al: An analysis of cocaine positive fatalities. *J Forensic Sci* 1989; 34:53.
87. Zobeck TS, Williams GD, Bertolucci D: Trends in alcohol-related fatal traffic accidents. *Alcohol Health Res World* 1986; 11:60–62.
88. Braakman R: Early prediction of outcome in severe head injury. *Acta Neurochir* 1992; 116:161–163.
89. Waxman K, Sundine MJ, Young RF: Is early prediction of outcome in severe head injury possible? *Arch Surg* 1991; 126:1237–1242.
90. Kaufman MA, Buchmann B, Scheidegger D, et al: Severe head injury: Should expected outcome influence resuscitation and first day decisions? *Resuscitation* 1992; 23:199–206.
91. Carlsson CA, von Essen C, Lofgren J: Factors affecting the clinical course of patients with severe head injury. *J Neurosurg* 1968; 29:242–251.
92. Clifton GL, Grossman RG, Makela M, et al: Neurological course and correlated computed tomography findings after severe closed head injury. *J Neurosurg* 1980; 52:611–624.
93. Bricolo A, Turazzi S, Feriotti G: Prolonged posttraumatic unconsciousness. *J Neurosurg* 1980; 52:625–634.
94. Braakman R, Jennett B, Minderhound JM: Prognosis of the posttraumatic vegetative state. *Acta Neurochir* 1988; 95:49–52.
95. Bond MR, Brooks DN: Understanding the process of recovery as a basis for investigation of rehabilitation for the brain injured. *Scand J Rehab Med* 1976; 8:127–133.
96. Dikmen S, Reitan RM, Temkin NR: Neuropsychological recovery in head injury. *Arch Neurol* 1983; 40:333–338.
97. Groswasser Z, Sazbon L: Outcome in 134 patients with prolonged posttraumatic unawareness. Part 2: Functional outcome of 72 patients recovering consciousness. *J Neurosurg* 1990; 72:81–84.
98. Bowers SA, Marshall LF: Outcome in 200 consecutive cases of severe head injury treated in San Diego county: A prospective analysis. *Neurosurgery* 1980; 6:237–242.
99. Miller JD, Sweet RC, Narayan RK, Becker DP: Early insults to the injured brain. *JAMA* 1978; 240:439–442.
100. Teasdale G, Galbraith S, Murray L, et al: Management of traumatic intracranial hematoma. *BMJ* 1982; 285: 1695–1697.
101. Marshall LF, Smith RW, Shapiro HM: The outcome with aggressive treatment in severe head injuries. Part 2: Acute and chronic barbiturate administration in the management of head injury. *J Neurosurg* 1979; 50:26–30.
102. Eisenberg HM, Frankowski RF, Contant CF, et al.: High dose barbiturate control of elevated intracranial pressure in patients with severe head injury. *J Neurosurg* 1988; 69:15–23.
103. Alexander E, Ball MR, Laster DW: Subtemporal decompression: Radiological observation and current surgical experience. *Br J Neurosurg* 1987; 1:427–433.
104. Gower DJ, Lee KS, McWhorter JM: Role of subtemporal decompression in severe closed head injury. *Neurosurgery* 1988; 23:417–422.
105. Gaab MR, Rittierodt M, Lorenz M, et al: Traumatic brain swelling and operative decompression: A prospective investigation. *Acta Neurochir* 1990; 51:s326–s329.
106. Muizelaar JP, Marmarou A, Ward JD, Adverse effects of prolonged hyperventilation in patients with severe head injury: A randomized clinical trial. *J Neurosurg* 1991; 75:731–739.
107. Wolf AL, Levi L, Marmarou A, et al: Effect of THAM upon outcome in severe head injury: A randomized prospective clinical trial. *J Neurosurg* 1993; 78:54–59.
108. Muizelaar JP, Marmarou A, Young HF, et al: Improving the outcome of severe head injury with the oxygen radical scavenger polyethylene glycol-conjugated superoxide dismutase: A phase II trial. *J Neurosurg* 1993; 78:375–382.
109. Colohan AR, Alves WM, Gross CR, et al: Head injury mortality in two centers with different emergency medical services and intensive care. *J Neurosurg* 1989; 71:202–207.
110. Warme PE, Bergstrom R, Persson L: Neurosurgical intensive care improves outcome after severe head injury. *Acta Neurochir* 1991; 110:57–64.
111. Marshall LF: The role of aggressive therapy for head injury: Does it matter? In *Clinical Neurosurgery,* vol 34. Baltimore: Williams & Wilkins, 1986:549–559.
112. Pellegrino ED: Withholding and withdrawing treatments: Ethics at the bedside. *Clin Neurosurg* 1987; 35:164–184.

CHAPTER 56

BRAIN DEATH FOLLOWING HEAD INJURY

Howard H. Kaufman

INTRODUCTION

> ... the death of persons—of human persons—is of profound moral importance and ... therefore people generally are very concerned that the criteria of death reflect this importance and provide reliably accurate methods for determining the death of persons.[1]

The question of what is life and when it is lost must be considered first in philosophic and then in physiological terms. In philosophic terms, there is something unique about a human being that is separate from organic or somatic function. This is embodied in the dualist concept of body and soul, which dates from the teachings of Plato and Aristotle. Therefore, it follows that it is necessary to define what is essential to humanity or "personhood" and to determine what must be lost in order to define death. Dagi has updated this concept: "Death is defined as the loss of a metaphysical quality that is preferred to the corporal entity that it endows with humanhood."[2]

In addition, from ancient times it was felt that the locus of this unique quality resided in the brain.[2,3] "The functions ... of the mind ... are thought to be located, on the basis of compelling scientific data, in the brain."[2] Dagi discusses two special functions of the brain, internal integration and external integration, and notes that the first can be replaced by medical support, but not the second.[2] In the current definition of whole brain death, both functions are lost.

There is an imperative to define death when it occurs. Humanism, the dominant secular philosophy of our time, emphasizes the value of the life of each individual.[2] Thus, it follows that the determination of the ending of a life has tremendous importance. On the one hand, a living person should not be treated as dead. On the other hand, a dead person also should not be treated as being alive. Modern developments in supportive techniques for cardiovascular and respiratory function permit the preservation of somatic function long after the brain has been destroyed. This is inappropriate and wasteful of resources now conceded to be limited.

Since no patient has been reported to have survived when the diagnosis of brain death was made using the criteria described below, these criteria can be employed with confidence. The concept that brain death is equivalent to death as diagnosed by the criteria of loss of respiratory and cardiac function is generally accepted by medicine and the law in the United States. Current Judeo-Christian thinking generally supports the concept of brain death.[4–6]

In addition, the concept of a higher brain or neocortical standard of personhood based on consciousness is already being utilized implicitly, if not always explicitly. Descartes stated the concept of higher brain function with elegant simplicity, "Cogito ergo sum." Consciousness has been defined as "our immediate sense of the present and what amounts to memory (the source of the revisions of reality ...)."[7] As to the exact location of consciousness in the brain, "on the basis of modern evidence for the massive parallel processing of information within the brain, ... consciousness is not a unitary phenomenon but rather a continually changing, updated, and edited version of the world that derives from many neurological sources."[7] The problem is that there is no consensus about exactly what constitutes consciousness, how to determine whether it is lost, or how to know that loss is irreversible.[8]

In recent years it has become widely accepted that there are no ethical requirements to give any support to breathing patients, not even water, if the patient is not sentient or will not suffer discomfort.[9] Although this approach alters the way we deal with the living, we have not treated such patients as dead, which would mean they could be buried or have their organs harvested.[2,3] However, a protocol has been developed in which patients in whom life-sustaining treatments are to be stopped are taken to the operating room where cardiopulmonary care is terminated, the patient is allowed to die, and organs are then harvested.[10] There is a task force that includes representatives from the American Academy of Neurology, the American Academy of Pediatrics, the American Neurological Association, the Association of Neurological Surgeons, and the Child Neurology Society, which has formulated a definition of the permanent vegetative state, which could permit such patients to be treated as dead. This has been approved by several of the parent organizations; if the rest approve it, it should set the standard for a higher brain definition of death that will likely be accepted.

A related issue is the status of anencephalics and whether they can be organ donors, which has been much discussed in the past few years.[11–16]

Neurosurgeons are often involved in determining when whole brain death occurs. This chapter will discuss how the concept of brain death evolved, particularly over the last four decades, the reasons to declare brain death, and a definition of and criteria for diagnosing brain death, including those for pediatric patients.

THE DIAGNOSIS OF DEATH

Through time immemorial there has been a fear of the premature declaration of death, which could be imitated by the depressant effects of various medical conditions and drugs.[2,3] In previous times, putrefaction and possibly *rigor mortis* were considered the only reliable indicators of death. Strategies were developed to guarantee the person would not be alive when buried (e.g., embalming, delayed burial, and visiting the newly dead), and devices were placed in the coffin to alert a passerby if the person was still alive.[3]

In early ages, physicians did not follow a patient after he became moribund. In more recent centuries, as physicians' abilities to diagnose and treat improved, and, as the public gained greater confidence in their abilities, they were required to declare death.[3] Tests requiring knowledge and skill were developed to rule out sleeplike states; these included stimulation and evaluation of vegetative functions.[2] Also, from the 18th century on, techniques of resuscitation were developed, including electric shock, artificial respiration, and stimulation of the heart.[3] The diagnosis of death then required failure of resuscitation or the *irreversible* loss of signs of life.[2,3]

Cardiovascular and respiratory support were further developed in this century (and, since the 1950s, localized in intensive care units[17]) so that the vegetative activities of the body could be supported for many weeks. This resulted in a need "to define death by criteria that did not depend primarily on the cardiorespiratory function that life support systems artificially preserved."[2] This could be done by "clarifying the definition of death, or by revising the criteria for terminating treatment of the living."[3]

At the same time, organ transplantation became a reality. Many thousands of patients a year in the United States could benefit from new organs. This created additional pressure to develop, improve, and shorten the criteria for brain death.

HISTORY OF THE DIAGNOSIS OF WHOLE BRAIN DEATH

The modern scientific concept of brain death was first developed from research into the neuropathology of respirator brain at the Massachusetts General Hospital (C. Miller Fischer, personal communication) and by EEG studies of similar patients in France, where the term "coma depassé"—beyond coma—was used to describe irreversible brain damage.[18–20] The first widely recognized criteria on how to define brain death were evolved by the Harvard ad hoc Committee on Brain Death in 1968.[18,21] Various groups in the United States and throughout the world have formulated other criteria.[20] The NIH-funded Collaborative Study developed additional recommendations.[22,23] A group of consultants to the President's Commission for the Study of Ethical Problems in Medicine and Biomedical Research and Behavioral Research further refined the criteria.[24–26] Important exchanges of information occurred during symposia sponsored by the New York Academy of Sciences (1978)[27] and by the Massachusetts Neurological Association (1981). As Lynn points out, the current standard is the guidelines of the President's Commission: "This societal resolution has relied upon the perceived clarity of medical criteria for neurological death (as opposed to the obvious uncertainties and delays with most forms of higher brain death), the pressure to achieve permission to save other lives with transplantation, and the political acceptability of incremental change."[25] These criteria have proved to be reliable, although, theoretically, they may not be proved mathematically.[9,25,28] But their reliability is further supported since they fulfill the requirement stated by Shewman; that is, they are "self-evident on a priori grounds."[28]

The evolution of criteria for the declaration of brain death in children less than 5 years old has been considered problematic. But in the last few years, work has begun in this area and will be described below.

A model brain death law, the Uniform Determination of Death Act (UDDA), was approved in 1980 by the President's Commission, the American Medical Association, the American Bar Association, and the National Conference of Commissioners on Uniform State Laws. This states that brain death is equivalent to death recognized by cardiopulmonary standards. However, it reserves actual criteria and determination to the medical profession. At least 39 states now have brain death laws, and a few others have formally accepted brain death as death in rulings of that state's Supreme Court. Precedents are now so overwhelming that brain death standards probably can be applied anywhere in the United States, although practitioners should know the status of their local laws.

However, it has been pointed out that: (1) there may be viable cells (and, by necessity, blood flow) in patients who meet the current definition of brain death; (2) this is accepted under "a gentleman's agreement that cellular functions did not count"; and (3) this qualification opens the argument that the issue remains the loss of "key functions" versus "higher brain function" which must be defined and agreed upon and then subjected to measurement.[29]

REASONS TO DECLARE BRAIN DEATH

There are compelling ethical and practical reasons for physicians to know the criteria of brain death and to apply them. The determination of brain death has assumed importance for two reasons: the ability to support vegetative functions for prolonged periods after brain death,[30,31] and the need for organs for transplantation.

Cardiac activity can be supported for many days in patients whose brains have irreversibly ceased all function.[32,33] Physiological derangements, namely cardiovascular instability, thermovariability, anterior and posterior pituitary insufficiency, and altered nutritional needs, can be corrected. It is possible to maintain a brain-dead patient for prolonged periods, the record now being 107 days.[30] In general, such treatment is inappropriate because it ignores the reality of the situation, keeps the family and friends in the limbo of uncertainty and false hope, violates the trust of the family and society that the physician can recognize death, requires health care workers to treat a dead body, expends resources without benefit, and might be perceived as an indignity to and abuse of the body. Exceptions have been made in rare circumstances, as in an attempt to salvage a viable fetus.

Recent advances in transplantation provide the opportunity of using the organs of a brain-dead person to improve or even to save the lives of others, as well as to save considerable sums of money because of diminished medical costs and increased productivity.[34–37] The advances currently being made are reflected in the numbers of transplants (now about 20,000/year)[38] and the rates of organ and donor survival (Table 56-1). (See Organ Transplantation, Chap. 57.)

Slowing this effort is the lack of beating-heart donors, who might benefit 60,000 people/year.[38] Cadaver donors remain at about 4000/year, even though more potential donors exist.[41] The causes for this problem are numerous. Currently, donation is based on voluntarism and altruism.[42] But, although surveys have suggested that the public largely understands brain death and generally looks favorably on donation, this is not a universal attitude, particularly among a number of minorities.[34,35,39,43–45] In addition, many people who would wish to donate do not tell their families, while families who have not been told are more reluctant to donate organs.[45] An intensive effort at public education has been proposed to correct this problem.

Many physicians lack full understanding of brain death and/or do not facilitate retrieval because of a failure to realize the desperate need for organs and do not appreciate the consolation the family can gain from donation.[43,44,46] To increase donations, most states have passed "required request" laws, but these have not had much effect.[42,43] In addition, organs are lost when patients were not vigorously resuscitated or supported.

The result is that there are longer and longer lists of potential recipients, many of whom will die waiting for organs.[36] Because of shortages of organs, current criteria for recipients are very strict. However, if more organs were available, many other people might be considered potential recipients.

National laws to promote transplantation include the National Organ Transplantation Act of 1984 (PL 98-507) and Amendments in 1988 (PL 100-607) and 1990 (PL 101-616). They established a national organ procurement network and a scientific registry, as well as a Task Force, which has led to ongoing activities.[34,35,38] The Surgeon General sponsored a workshop in July 1991 whose recommendations included strategies to increase donations.[36,47] There have been many proposals, including improvement in donor identification and care, more effective contact with donor families, universal checking for donor cards, and public education. Other suggested solutions include presumed consent, mandated decision-making, and rewarded gifting.[34,35,42,43,48,49] In several countries, organs are harvested based on "presumed consent," i.e., if the deceased had not previously objected. But it has been suggested that "mandated choice" is a better solution.[50] A recent Gallup poll suggested financial rewards would not be helpful.[45]

Professional obligations, as well as the ethical and religious imperatives of beneficence, charity, and honesty, compel physicians to be proactive and to facilitate transplantation by informing the family about this possibility when it exists. The AMA Code of Medical Ethics (1992) declares, "The voluntary donation of organs in appropriate circumstances is to be encouraged," and organized neurosurgery has supported this approach.

CLINICAL EVALUATION

> ... brain death criteria, used in cases where a human being is maintained on artificial ventilation, are far less detectable or even understandable by the ordinary non-medical person, and therefore subject to far greater suspicion.[1]

There are several excellent recent reviews about the clinical determination of brain death.[20,51,52] The most recent widely accepted criteria for adult brain death are those of the consultants to the President's Commission for the Study of Ethical Problems in Medicine and Biomedical and Behavioral Research (1981), which advocated that laws should define brain death as "irreversible cessation of all functions of the entire brain."[24,26,53] The clinical difference between the 1981 criteria and older sets lies mainly in the rapidity with which brain death can be declared with the former. Since cardiovascular collapse is increasingly likely during observation of a brain-dead body, many transplantable organs may be lost if older standards are used.

The diagnosis of brain death involves clinical evidence of loss of brain function and a period of observation, which can be shortened by confirmatory tests, particularly cerebral blood flow studies. The following procedure for assessment is consistent with the criteria agreed upon by the advisors to the President's Commission (Table 56-1). In cases that fall outside these guidelines, consultation with physicians with particular expertise in this field may be helpful (Table 56-2). Other criteria and tests are also used.

To be declared brain-dead, a patient must first meet accepted clinical criteria for brain death based on cerebral unresponsivity. The patient should be on a respirator and show no signs of respiratory effort. There should be no brain stem reflexes (Table 56-3). There should be no sign of eye-opening, no spontaneous movement, and no movement elicited by noise or painful stimuli to the face or trunk other than spinal cord reflex movements. The pupils should be midposition, not dilated.[54] There should be absence of brain stem reflexes (pupillary, oculocephalic [Doll's eyes], oculovestibular [iced water irrigation], corneal, gag, and cough reflexes). These reflexes may be difficult to test when there are massive facial injuries.

The spinal cord reflexes seen after brain death may be quite disconcerting, and caregivers, as well as friends and family, need to be warned about them. Initially after brain death, a state of spinal shock develops, after which there is a stepwise restoration of spinal reflexes.[55,56] Both visceral and somatic reflexes have been observed. Changes in cardiac and peripheral vascular function from mechanical (neck flexion) and visceral stimulation may include tachycardia, increased blood pressure, increased peripheral resistance, flushing, and sweating.[57–59] Respiration-like movements, thought to be caused by reflex activity in the respiratory muscles and the diaphragm, have been observed during apnea testing,[60] as have changes in pulse and blood pressure.[61,62] A variety of somatic movements have been observed, including neck turning (cervical muscles of Cr N XI), flexion or extension of the back, and movements of upper and lower extremities. These have been unilateral and bilateral, and they have been symmetrical and asymmetrical. They have occurred spontaneously, during apnea testing, during mechanical stimulation, and during noxious stimulation.[56,63–65] They do not preclude the diagnosis of brain death.

If the patient is *under 5 years* of age, the attending physician must be cautious and may well seek consultation with an experienced pediatric neurologist or neurosurgeon. The advisors to the President's Commission suggested that there might be differences in the ability of young brains to recover from clinical states that would be indicative of complete and irreversible loss of brain function in adults.[26] This might be because neurons of the young have more resistance to ischemia or because the brain can swell without generating high intracranial pressure because the unfused skull can stretch. A variety of criteria for the young have been utilized.[66] Criteria for children are discussed later in this chapter.

Determining the cause of apparent brain death can be helpful in establishing that loss of function is not reversible. The most common causes of brain death are trauma, stroke, or ischemia/hypoxia. In most instances the cause is obvious, i.e., a gunshot wound to the head or a cardiac arrest. If the cause is not apparent, such studies as CT or MRI scans or angiography often will clarify the diagnosis.

Significant levels of a variety of exogenous substances such as alcohol, barbiturates and other depressant drugs, neuromuscular blocking agents (which may be given for

TABLE 56-1 A Model Algorithm for Determining Death by Neurological Criteria

Is the patient in deep coma (no eye opening, no spontaneous movement, and no response other than spinal cord reflexes to noxious stimuli) and on a respirator not showing respiratory effort? Does neurological exam confirm absence of brain stem reflexes including pupillary, corneal, oculocephalic (doll's eyes), oculovestibular (50 ml iced water irrigation into external auditory canals), corneal, gag, and cough reflexes?

No—If not possible to evaluate all reflexes, continue protocol, but at some point do cerebral blood flow study or EEG (helpful mostly if it shows activity) or consider consultation with someone with experience in the determination of death by neurological criteria.

Yes

Is patient over 5 years old?

No—If not experienced in the determination of death by neurological criteria in children, consider consultation with a specialist who is.

Yes

Is etiology of coma known (e.g., trauma, stroke, or hypoxia/ischemia)?

No—Elucidate cause (which may require CT or MR scan and/or intracranial arteriography or consultation.

Yes

Is patient free of alcohol, barbiturates, other depressant drugs, neuromuscular blockade, uremia, or other severe metabolic abnormalities that may impair neurological function?

No—Wait until documented elimination of drug or correction of metabolic abnormalities, or consider cerebral blood flow study or EEG (helpful mostly if it shows activity), or consider consultation.

Yes

Does patient have temperature above 90°F (32°C) and systolic blood pressure above 90 mmHg?

No—Correct hypothermia and raise blood pressure or consider cerebral blood flow study or consultation.

Yes

Is patient free of conditions that might impair ventilatory threshold to hypercarbia and hypoxia (e.g., COPD, CHF)?

No—Do cerebral blood flow study or EEG or consider consultation.

Yes

Test for apnea (no spontaneous respirations with $P_{CO_2} \geq 60$ mmHg).

No—If any respiratory effort, patient is not dead.

No—Inadequate test if arrhythmia or hypotension or other untoward effects before $P_{CO_2} \geq 60$. Do cerebral blood flow study or EEG or consider.

Yes

This documents that brain function is absent. Confirm that this is irreversible by any one of the following:

1. At any time, four-vessel intracranial angiography. If no flow, patient is dead.
2. During initial 6 hours after loss of brain function, radionuclide cerebral angiography. If no flow, confirm death by clinical examination, including apnea test, at 6 hours. (Radionuclide angiography can be used as a confirmatory test after this period as well).
3. At end of initial 6 hours after loss of brain stem function, EEG. If electrocerebral silence at least 6 hours after loss of neurological activity, confirm death by clinical examination, including apnea test.
4. At the end of initial 12 hours after loss of brain function, if the cause of coma is clearly established and is other than hypoxia and if clinical examination including apnea test again shows no brain function, the patient is dead. Additional tests are not required.
5. At the end of the initial 24 hours after loss of brain function, if the cause of coma is hypoxia/ischemia to the brain and if clinical examination including apnea test again shows no brain activity, and if the rest of the protocol has been satisfied, the patient is dead. Additional tests are not required.

Documentation: Complete documentation in the hospital record is essential and should include the date and time of the initial clinical evaluation, including apnea test, the results of pertinent laboratory tests and confirmatory tests done, and the date and time of the final clinical evaluation including apnea test. This can be accomplished either by a written note or by using a form.

TABLE 56-2 When to Seek Consultation by Experienced Expert and/or Perform Tests of Intracranial Circulation

Age <5
Etiology unclear
Confounding hypothermia, hypotension, drugs, metabolic abnormalities, inability to complete full neurological evaluation
Need for accelerated observation
Apnea testing not possible/reliable due to cardiac or pulmonary disease

intubation), and metabolic abnormalities, such as those seen in hepatic or renal failure, can reversibly impair neurological functions and might mimic the clinical picture of brain death. One should always maintain a suspicion of the complicating presence of alcohol or drug use, especially in trauma, where such use is common. Common blood and urine toxicology screening tests do not evaluate all possible drugs, and acceptable drug levels are not well established. It is not clear which drugs and metabolic derangements may suppress brain functions, particularly in the already damaged brain.

TABLE 56-3 Brain Stem Reflexes

Pupillary reflex: In a semidark room, a strong source of light should be shone into each eye sequentially while carefully observing for change in pupil size in both eyes.

Extraocular movements: These may be tested initially by turning the patient's head from side to side with the head elevated 30° (oculocephalic or doll's eyes reflex). Since this movement does not provide a maximum stimulus, if this examination shows no doll's eyes response, the ear canals should be irrigated with ice water (oculovestibular reflex, calorics). For this test, the ears must be free of significant wax and the drums should not be perforated. The head is elevated 30° and each ear drum in turn is irrigated with 50 ml of ice water using a syringe and small cannula. Any movement of the eyes demonstrates that some brain stem pathways are functioning.

Corneal reflex: A sterile piece of cotton or other tissue is lightly touched to the cornea (not the conjunctiva). Any eyelid movement during this maneuver suggests some brain stem function.

Gag reflex: A tongue depressor or other object is touched against the back of the pharynx or the endotracheal tube is moved. Movement of the uvula or retching constitutes a positive response and excludes the diagnosis of brain death.

Cough reflex: A cannula is passed through the endotracheal tube into the tracheobronchial tree or the endotracheal tube is irrigated. Any movement or coughing excludes the diagnosis of brain death.

Therefore, if there is any question as to the etiology of apparent brain death, cerebral blood flow studies can be used to confirm the diagnosis of brain death, even in the presence of intoxication or metabolic abnormalities. Without such studies, prolonged observation and consultation may be indicated. Patients in barbiturate coma for the treatment of increased intracranial pressure are especially problematic.

Both hypothermia (≤90°F, 32°C) and hypotension (≤90 mmHg systolic BP) might reversibly suppress neurological activity. However, there are no data about the magnitude of these effects or for how long they persist after correction of temperature and blood pressure. Certainly, the diagnosis of brain death should be delayed until the temperature and blood pressure can be brought up to these thresholds, if possible. It is important to prevent the decrease of temperature and blood pressure because it is often more difficult to restore them than to maintain them.

Part of the clinical examination of brain stem functions involves evaluation for apnea, at least at the end of the period of observation (Table 56-4). There must be a formal apnea test to prove that brain stem function has been lost. A few patients have been reported who met all other criteria of brain death but did show respiratory efforts.[67] On the other hand, in one series 20 percent of patients had nonspecific reflex movements during apnea testing that were of no significance.[68] However, since testing will lead to increased p_{CO_2} and, therefore, possible elevation of intracranial pressure, it should be reserved until the rest of the initial evaluation makes the diagnosis of brain death reasonably certain. Determining apnea requires a specific protocol that ensures

TABLE 56-4 Apnea Test

1. Preoxygenate for at least 10 minutes with 100 percent O_2 and at the same time adjust the respirator so that P_{CO_2} is about 40 mmHg.
2. Disconnect the respirator and give O_2 at 8 to 12 L/min by tracheal cannula.
3. If hypotension and/or arrhythmias develop at any time, stop the test and place the patient immediately back on the respirator. If this happens, EEG or cerebral blood flow tests or consultation should be obtained.
4. During disconnection from a respirator, the patient should be observed continuously for spontaneous respirations. If there are none in 10 minutes, draw blood gases and place the patient back on the respirator. The P_{CO_2} must be greater than 60 mmHg to be sure of stimulating the medullary respiratory centers maximally. If the P_{CO_2} is greater than 60 mmHg and there is no respiratory effort, the patient is apneic.
5. Obviously, if there is any respiratory effort, the patient is not apneic and not brain dead.

that the p_{CO_2} reaches a level that provides maximal respiratory stimulus, i.e., at least approximately 60 mmHg.[69–71] Apnea testing may not be valid if the patient has chronic pulmonary or cardiac disease in which the sensitivity to hypercarbia may be diminished. If there is a history or evidence of these conditions, tests of intracerebral circulation should be considered.

Efforts have been made to understand and refine the apnea test.[61] In patients with obstructive pulmonary disease and abnormal ventilation/perfusion ratios, long preoxygenation may be required. Preoxygenation of 30 minutes has been suggested.[61] Oxygenation must be continued during the test and can be accomplished by using PEEP, a T-piece, or a tracheal catheter.[61] One group has suggested placing the catheter to the level of the carina.[72] Monitoring should be employed to detect desaturation. Changes in O_2 have been plotted, and hypoxia has occasionally been observed.[72,73]

An acute change in pH (due to accumulation of CO_2) from 7.32–7.36 to <7.18 may be required to stimulate the respiratory centers.[74] But the rise in p_{CO_2} in the nonrespired patient, which is most rapid in the first minute, is nonlinear.[72,73] However, by adjusting the pretest p_{CO_2} to well above 40 mmHg, it may be possible to shorten the test to 5 minutes.[72]

A variety of cardiovascular changes have been noted, including rises and falls in heart rate and blood pressure, occasionally requiring reconnecting the ventilator.[61,72,73] Insignificant arrhythmias have been observed. The apparent sympathetic responses have been correlated with a rise in plasma catecholamines (from below normal baseline levels) and have been attributed to a spinal-mediated sympathoadrenal response.[62] But with monitoring, the patient can be prevented from decompensating.

One aspect of brain death that is being better appreciated involves the hormonal changes that occur. An initial stress reaction may occur due to the original insult, followed by diminished function caused by damage to the hypothalamic-pituitary axis. The stress reaction has been reviewed in detail.[75,76] Appreciating and treating this response is part of routine intensive care.

Postmortem examinations of brain dead patients have revealed progressive changes in the hypothalamus with better preservation of both the anterior and posterior pituitary.[77] This may be explained by the extracranial blood supply to the pituitary and by the fact that it can be protected from increased intracranial pressure by the diaphragma sella. Some hypothalamic hormones may also be produced in extracranial sites.[77] This explains why after brain death there is initial preservation of endocrine function, at least in part, followed by progressive decline.[77] It is advisable to recognize hormonal alterations early so that replacement can be utilized in order to keep the patient stable long enough to fulfill the criteria of brain death and to increase the chance of retrieving organs in optimal condition for transplantation. Desmopressin is recommended to treat the diabetes insipidus caused by lack of antidiuretic hormone because it has a long duration of action and a low pressor/antidiuretic ratio.[41,78] It has been suggested that T3, cortisol, and insulin may be helpful for maintaining somatic function and optimizing activity of organs to be transplanted.[79–81]

There are several excellent guidelines available relating to supportive care for brain-dead patients.[34,35,41,82,83]

CONFIRMATORY TESTS

A *period of observation* may sometimes be needed to confirm the irreversibility of loss of neurological functions. Time periods recommended here follow the criteria of the advisors to the President's Commission. They are not supported by careful study but were designed to be very cautious. Without confirmatory tests, and if the diagnosis is uncertain or confusing secondary problems are present (i.e., hypoxia after head injury), it is advisable to wait 12 to 24 hours after the patient first meets the clinical criteria of brain death to make the final declaration. The consultants to the President's Commission contended that if the cause of coma is hypoxia, the period of observation from the time of loss of brain functions should be 24 hours before the declaration of death. On the other hand, in some situations it is not appropriate to carry out prolonged observations. Patients who have suffered severe gunshot injuries to the head or who have large intracerebral hematomas often become unstable, and it is reasonable to consider them for organ donation early.

Use of certain *confirmatory tests* makes it possible to shorten periods of observation.

One family of tests evaluates cerebral blood flow. Inadequate blood flow to the brain results in irreversible brain damage within minutes. Demonstration of absent cerebral blood flow confirms the diagnosis of brain death, even in cases with drug intoxication, altered metabolic status, shock, or hypothermia. Furthermore, the test is easy for families to understand.

For over two decades, *conventional contrast angiography* was used to diagnose brain death and has been accepted as the standard of intracranial blood flow evaluation against which other tests are measured. This test can be used to confirm brain death at any time after loss of clinical neurological functions. However, it is somewhat more complex, costly, and is potentially risky to a patient who is in fact alive, and it sometimes injures the kidneys of a brain-dead donor. Flow may be inaccurately suggested owing to a high-pressure injection of dye or to having the head in a dependent position during the study. Hence, four-vessel angiography is no longer regularly used for this purpose in the United States. It should preferably be performed by an experienced radiologist who is knowledgeable about its application in brain death.

Radionuclide cerebral angiography is noninvasive, safe, and can be rapidly performed in a nuclear medicine suite or at the bedside with equipment that is likely to be available in many hospitals (Table 56-5).[84] Many now view the radionuclide angiogram with radio tracers utilizing technetium as the confirmatory test of choice. The test may not detect minimal flow within the brain, particularly in the brain stem, because of a combination of low counts and attenuation due to interposed tissue. It also requires an experienced interpreter. While (theoretically) it is not quite as accurate as angiography, absence of flow on isotope studies, as interpreted by an experienced specialist, has never been demonstrably in error in diagnosing brain death. This test is recommended as a confirmatory study, linked with 6 hours of observed absence of clinical neurological functions. Most experts now use this technique immediately after neurological examination shows no response and declare brain death without a further period of observation, if there is no intracranial blood flow, particularly in situations where the etiology is clear, the brain damage is overwhelming (i.e., large spontaneous intracerebral hematoma), and there are no complicating features.

TABLE 56-5 Brain Death Study Using Radionuclide Imaging

1. A scintillation camera equipped with a low energy all-purpose collimator is positioned for anterior views of the patient's head and neck.
2. A dose of 20 to 30 mCi of ^{99m}Tc-labeled serum albumin or pertechnetate in a volume of 0.5 to 1.5 ml is injected through a three-way stopcock into a proximal intravenous or central line. The isotope is then flushed into the circulation with 30 ml of normal saline to deliver a bolus.
3. Serial dynamic images are performed at 2-second intervals for approximately 60 seconds.
4. Then "static" images may be obtained with 400,000 counts in both the anterior and lateral positions.
5. A single technically satisfactory IV isotope angiogram that shows termination of the carotid circulation at the base of the skull and unequivocal absence of uptake in the anterior and middle cerebral arteries is sufficient radiographic evidence to confirm clinical brain death. Faint or delayed appearance of contrast in the dural sinuses does not preclude the diagnosis of brain death.

TABLE 56-6 EEG Criteria for the Determination of Brain Death

1. A minimum of 8 scalp electrodes, with interelectrode distances of at least 10 cm, and ear reference electrodes.
2. Interelectrode resistance of 100 to 10,000 ohms.
3. Tested integrity of the recording system by deliberate creation of electrode artifact by manipulation.
4. Gains increased during most of the recording from 7 to 2 μV/mm and inclusion of appropriate calibrations.
5. The use of 0.3 or 0.4 time constants during part of the recording.
6. Recording with an electrocardiograph and other monitoring devices such as a pair of electrodes on the dorsum of the right hand to exclude extracerebral potentials.
7. Test for reactivity to pain, loud noises, or light.
8. Recording by a specially qualified technician for 30 minutes.
9. Repeat record if doubt about electrocerebral silence.
10. EEGs transmitted by telephone are not appropriate for the determination of brain death.

It has also been used to confirm brain death in young children.[85]

Isotope flow studies in a brain-dead patient may nevertheless show uptake in the superior sagittal sinus, and may demonstrate low flow in the posterior fossa.[86]

An *electroencephalogram (EEG)* can be done at the bedside, is without risk, and may be helpful when performed by an experienced electroencephalographer. EEG for brain death should be carried out according to the guidelines of the American Electroencephalographic Society (Tables 56-6, 56-7).[87] One limitation of the EEG is that it does not directly measure brainstem function. On the other hand, the EEG may still show

TABLE 56-7 EEG—Source of Artifacts and Problems

1. **EEG Machine.** With high gain and frequency, the machine should not produce transient deflections >2 μV per second.
2. **Electrodes.** Drying of electrode jelly causes increased impedance 60-Hz artifacts may be introduced if electrode resistance is dissimilar.
3. **Monitors and ventilator**
4. **Patient.** Artifacts from scalp and neck muscles or heartbeat.
5. **Short circuiting of current.** Test by touching each electrode with a pencil point to create an artifact potential at the beginning of the trace. This also tests the integrity of the system and confirms placement of the electrodes and that the patient is connected to the machine.

activity when patients meet the clinical criteria of brain death.[88] Although electrocerebral activity precludes the diagnosis of brain death, electrocerebral silence does not exclude reversible coma (e.g., from intoxication, hypothermia). If the EEG is used as the only confirmatory test, the patient with electrocerebral inactivity should have at least 6 hours of observation showing complete loss of brain function.

Several *newer tests* have been investigated to help confirm the diagnosis of brain death. None has yet been considered in a consensus conference or by a task force, so none yet carries the imprimatur of widespread acceptance.

One such test is a new type of brain scan that employs radiopharmaceuticals that cross the blood brain barrier proportionally to blood flow with high first-pass extraction and maintenance for hours (since they are actually taken up into the cells), and thus reflect the presence of metabolizing cells.[86,89–91] Early experience in adults and children has been encouraging.[86,89,91–93]

Doppler studies may be helpful. Doppler was initially used in 1983 to study brain-dead neonates by insonating the anterior cerebral and common carotid arteries through the anterior fontanelle.[94] Transcranial Doppler, developed in 1982, was first used to evaluate the basal cerebral vessels in brain death in 1987.[95–97] It appears that the intracranial pressure elevation usually seen with brain death shuts down arterial flow from distal to proximal on the basis of venous occlusion and engorgement.[97] As pressure increases, diastolic flow velocity increases. When intracranial pressure equals diastolic pressure, diastolic flow velocity goes to zero. With further rises in pressure, there is backflow during diastole (oscillating flow), and eventually net flow is zero, which is the critical level. Then, systolic spikes diminish and eventually disappear, the surest indicator of brain death. A variety of numerical standards have been developed and used to measure critical flow characteristics.[98–101] So as not to be confused by a local problem, both supratentorial vascular trees, as well as the basilar artery, should be insonated.[95,99,102] Mass lesions that shift the positions of the vessels can confound the study.[96] The most significant finding is loss of flow in a vessel previously insonated.[97] In a small percentage of patients, the middle cerebral arteries cannot be detected because of temporal bone interference. Therefore, if a vessel is not insonated initially, the test cannot be relied on to indicate no flow. Also, flow may be seen with brain death after the patient is decompressed and has a craniotomy defect or after pressure decreases. Because the test is fairly rapid, is becoming readily available, appears to have good reliability, can be repeated, and is relatively inexpensive, it is becoming more widely used.[96,98,99,101–103] It has been compared with isotope flow studies[104] and even angiograms.[102] It has also been used in children.[100]

Other neuroimaging tests, including CT with stable xenon administration, MR spectroscopy using gadolinium enhancement, and even PET scanning using fluorodeoxyglucose (^{18}FDG) have been used to study patients with brain death. However, although helpful in research applications, these tests are too cumbersome and expensive to be widely used.

Evoked potential studies have been studied in the evaluation of brain death. Brain stem auditory evoked potentials (BAEPs), generated primarily by structures below the upper midbrain, are relatively resistant to toxic or metabolic influences.[105] BAEPs may be useful in the intensive care unit to detect brain stem function in patients who have been heavily sedated or placed in barbiturate coma. Because of a variety of technical and physiological issues,[106–108] only if there is preservation of wave I and no other waves is the BAEP useful in the confirmation of brain death. Somatosensory evoked potentials (SEPs) can be recorded at the cervical medullary junction, but it cannot be determined whether this is from a spinal or medullary generator; therefore, the test is not useful.

Apparent contradictions between tests[109] are explainable. For example, EEG activity after clinical brain death may indicate survival of a few cells, and the presence of evoked potentials may indicate survival of a few axons. Blood flow may restart after it has ceased if intracranial pressure drops. Conversely, there may be some clinical activity when the EEG is flat or the radionuclide flow study is negative because of minimal residual brain stem activity—but such patients are not yet brain-dead because they do not meet the clinical criteria. Thus, confirmatory tests should be performed only after the clinical criteria of brain death have been met.

Findings supporting a determination of brain death should be carefully documented in the hospital record. Date and time of observations should be recorded, as well as details of all clinical evaluation (including apnea testing), pertinent laboratory tests, and results of confirmatory tests. It may be useful for hospitals to have written criteria and policies for the declaration of brain death. Some centers suggest or require a checklist form. A computerized algorithm has been developed in Germany to guide the declaration and clarify problems.[110]

BRAIN DEATH IN CHILDREN

The distress of brain death is compounded by the emotions generated by the death of a child—one whose vulnerability and unfulfilled promise magnify the tragedy of any death. Also, the advisors to the President's

Commission suggested that there might be significant, although not well-defined, differences in the brains of those under 5 years of age which allow some functions of the brain to recover from clinical states that would be accepted as indicative of complete and irreversible loss of brain function in adults (see above).[24] The determination remains problematic.[111]

The need for organ retrieval has added to the imperative to develop criteria for brain death in children. The use of cyclosporin for immunosuppression, beginning in 1983, eliminated the devastating side effects of impairment of mental and physical development by the high-dose steroids used previously, and thus made transplantation more attractive for children. But some organs for transplantation for children must be size-matched. Therefore, when the potential recipients are small children, young donors must be identified and utilized. The need for pediatric organs is great. In 1990, almost 1000 children 1–15 years old were awaiting organs,[112] and perhaps 1000 children are born each year with congenital heart or liver problems who could benefit from a transplant. However, 30 to 50 percent of children registered for transplants will die while awaiting them.

On the other hand, children's organs are more likely to be donated than are the organs of adults.[112] At one center, 18 of 18 families of brain-dead children who were asked agreed to donate organs. This was attributed to the commitment and experience of the patients' physicians, open visiting hours which facilitated rapport and trust between medical staff and families, and a focus on the parents as the sole decision-makers to lessen confusion. These parents were of an age to be comfortable with the concept of brain death, as well as transplantation, and they were likely to empathize with the needs of other families.[112]

Current information about neurodevelopment, unique aspects of the newborn brain, and criteria being used to define brain death in children has been reviewed.[66,113] Recognizing that there were no widely accepted criteria for brain death in children under 5 years of age, several organizations that had begun to consider such criteria formed a Task Force on Brain Death in Childhood (1985–1986) which developed guidelines for term newborns more than 7 days old (Table 56-8).[114] These guidelines have been endorsed by the American Academy of Neurology, the Section on Neurology of

TABLE 56-8 Guidelines after Task Force on Brain Death in Children

I. **History**
   A. Proximate cause.
   B. Rule out remediable or reversible conditions (toxic and metabolic disorders, sedative-hypyotic drugs, paralytic agents, hypothermia, hypotension, surgically remediable conditions).

II. **Physical examination**
   A. Coma and apnea must coexist. The patient must exhibit complete loss of consciousness, vocalization, and volitional activity.
   B. Absence of brain stem function as defined by:
      1. Midposition or fully dilated pupils that do not respond to light. Drugs may influence and invalidate pupillary assessment.
      2. Absence of spontaneous eye movements, those induced by oculocephalic and caloric (oculovestibular) testing.
      3. Absence of movement of bulbar musculature including facial and oropharyngeal muscles. The corneal, gag, cough, sucking, and rooting reflexes are absent.
      4. Respiratory movements are absent with the patient on the respirator. Apnea testing using standardized methods can be performed, but is done after other criteria are met.
   C. The patient must not be significantly hypothermic or hypotensive for age.
   D. Flaccid tone and absence of spontaneous or induced movements, excluding spinal cord events such as reflex withdrawal or spinal myoclonus, should exist.
   E. The examination should remain consistent with brain death throughout the observation and testing period.

III. **Observation Periods According to Age.** The recommended observation period depends on the age of the patient and the laboratory tests utilized.

   7 days to 2 months. Two examinations and electroencephalograms (EEGs) separated by at least 48 hours.

   2 months to 1 year. Two examinations and EEGs separated by at least 24 hr. A repeat examination and EEG are not necessary if a concomitant radionuclide flow study demonstrates no visualization of cerebral arteries.

   Over 1 year. When an irreversible cause exists, laboratory testing is not required but an observation period of at least 12 hours is recommended. There are conditions, particularly hypoxic-ischemic encephalopathy, in which it is difficult to assess the extent and reversibility of brain damage. This is particularly true if the first examination is performed soon after the acute event. Therefore, in this situation, a more prolonged period of at least 24 hours of observation is recommended. The observation period may be reduced if the EEG demonstrates electrocerebral silence or if the isotope flow study does not visualize cerebral arteries.

the American Academy of Pediatrics, the American Neurological Association, and the Child Neurology Society.[113] A number of other guidelines have been developed at various centers.[66] It may be reasonable to declare brain death in children over the age of 3 months who fulfill the clinical criteria, once a single EEG has demonstrated electrocerebral silence.[115,116]

A recent study evaluated 30 children in coma (failure to respond to pain, light, or sound) who were less than 1 month old and 10 more reported in the literature (including preterm infants).[117,118] The authors concluded that brain death can be diagnosed on a clinical basis with repeated observations over at least 3 days in a preterm infant (>32 weeks gestation) and 2 days in a term infant, even though EEG activity and cerebral blood flow by radioisotope infusion are present. Electrocerebral silence (once) together with absence of flow or radionuclide infusion testing could shorten the period of observation to 24 hours. EEG and blood flow were seen to return, but with only brief survival.

EEG has been studied extensively.[119] The EEG may give false-positive or false-negative results.[120] Phenobarbital levels above 25 mg/ml may suppress electrocerebral activity. It appears that a phenobarbital level <25 mg/dl may not confound the diagnosis.[113] The radioactive cerebral blood flow examination has been studied extensively in children. It can be employed to confirm brain death and to shorten the examination period.[85,121]

Nevertheless, there is not yet broad professional consensus on the criteria for the diagnosis of brain death in the pediatric population. A knowledgeable specialist using any of the currently employed criteria can probably be accurate, but use of the criteria requires experience and judgment. Thus, consultation with such an individual should be obtained for the diagnosis of brain death in children 5 years of age or less. If research and discussion within the scientific community continue, it may well be possible to evolve a consensus, as was achieved by the President's Commission.

OTHER ISSUES

Who should declare brain death? Not only neurologists and neurosurgeons, but also intensivists, anesthesiologists, and other specialists staffing ICUs and ERs are capable of making this assessment. General medical curricula and testing of physician qualifications should encompass brain death.

Some criteria (and state laws) suggest that two physicians must agree on the diagnosis of brain death, particularly when organ retrieval is being considered. If an EEG is done, the electroencephalographer may be the second physician. However, if the diagnosis is straightforward and clear, and if the physician involved is well-trained and experienced, it would seem reasonable for a single physician to certify brain death.

Once a patient is declared brain dead, life-support can legally be terminated. Some believe that the physician has the authority and responsibility to stop the respirator and other life-sustaining treatment when a patient is dead and that the option to continue care should not be given to the family. Others feel they should ask families for permission to stop care and turn off the respirator. In any case, when managing distraught or otherwise difficult families, it is prudent to listen for and consider objections. The question may arise in these circumstances as to whether one must continue to employ all possible life-sustaining treatment for the patient. Many families may benefit from a short period to adjust to the sudden tragedy and hopelessness of the situation. They may need this opportunity to develop trust in their physician and accept the diagnosis. If the family objects to discontinuation of the respirator, particularly because of stress or religious reasons, it may be wise to delay the withdrawal of support until the family dynamics are clarified and feelings can be addressed. However, the physician should not mislead the family by implying any insecurity regarding the diagnosis and the fact that the patient is dead. Problems arise when a family becomes distrustful or irrational. A consultant may be called. Chaplains and ministers, as well as ethics committees, may be helpful in aiding such families.

REFERENCES

1. Gillon R: Death. *J Med Ethics.* 1990; 16:3–4.
2. Dagi TF: Death-defining acts: Historical and cultural observations on the end of life, in Kaufman HH (ed): *Pediatric Brain Death and Organ/Tissue Retrieval.* New York: Plenum Press, 1989:1–30.
3. Pernick MS: Back from the grave: Recurring controversies over defining and diagnosing death in history, in Zaner RM (ed): *Death: Beyond Whole-Brain Criteria.* Boston: Kluwer Academic, 1988:17–74.
4. Childress JF: Protestant perspectives on organ donation, in Kaufman HH (ed): *Pediatric Brain Death and Organ/Tissue Retrieval.* New York: Plenum Press, 1989:45–53.
5. Paris JJ: Catholic considerations of brain death and organ retrieval, in Kaufman HH (ed): *Pediatric Brain Death and Organ/Tissue Retrieval.* New York: Plenum Press, 1989:35–43.
6. Tendler RM: A Jewish approach to ethical issues in brain death and organ transplantation, in Kaufman HH

(ed): *Pediatric Brain Death and Organ/Tissue Retrieval.* New York: Plenum Press, 1989:31–34.
7. Purves D: Book review of Dennett DC, *Consciousness Explained, 1991. Science* 1992; 257:1291–1292.
8. Zaner RM: Introduction, in Zaner RM (ed): *Death: Beyond Whole-Brain Criteria.* Boston: Kluwer Academic, 1988:1–14.
9. Council on Scientific Affairs and Council on Ethical and Judicial Affairs. Persistent vegetative state and the decision to withdraw or withhold life support. *JAMA* 1990; 263:426–430.
10. Youngner SJ, Arnold RM: Ethical, psychosocial, and public policy implications of procuring organs from non-heart-beating cadaver donors. *JAMA* 1993; 269:2769–2774.
11. Churchill LR, Pinkus RLB: The use of anencephalic organs: Historical and ethical dimensions. *Milbank Q* 1990; 68:147–169.
12. Fost N: Removing organs from anencephalic infants: Ethical and legal considerations. *Clin Perinatol* 1989; 16:331–337.
13. *Hastings Center Report 18* (Oct/Nov) 1988:5–33.
14. Rothenberg LS: The anencephalic neonate and brain death: An international review of medical, ethical, and legal issues. *Transplant Proc* 1990; 22:1037–1039.
15. Shewmon DA, Capron AM, Peacock WJ, et al: The use of anencephalic infants as organ sources; a critique. *JAMA* 1989; 261:1773–1781.
16. The Medical Task Force on Anencephaly: The infant with anencephaly. *N Engl J Med* 1990; 322:669–674.
17. Reiser SJ: The intensive care unit: The unfolding and ambiguities of survival therapy. *Int J Tech Asses Health Care* 1992; 8:382–394.
18. Fisher CM: Brain death—a review of the concept. *J Neurosci Nurs* 1991; 23:330–333.
19. Mollaret P, Goulon M: Le coma depassé. *Rev Neurol* 1959; 101:3–15.
20. Pallis C: Brainstem death: The evolution of a concept. *Semin Thorac Cardiovasc Surg* 1990; 2:135–152.
21. Anonymous: A definition of irreversible coma: Report of the ad hoc Committee of the Harvard Medical School to examine the definition of brain death. *JAMA* 1968; 205:337–340.
22. Anonymous: An appraisal of the criteria of cerebral death: A summary statement. A collaborative study. *JAMA* 1977; 237:982–986.
23. Walker AE: *Cerebral Death,* 3d ed. Baltimore: Urban & Schwarzenberg, 1985.
24. Anonymous: Guidelines for the determination of death. Report of the medical consultants on the diagnosis of death to the President's Commission for the Study of Ethical Problems in Medicine and Biomedical and Behavioral Research. *JAMA* 1981; 246:2184–2186.
25. Lynn J: Brain death: Historical perspectives and current concerns, in Kaufman HH (ed): *Pediatric Brain Death and Organ/Tissue Retrieval.* New York: Plenum Press, 1989:65–72.
26. President's Commission for the Study of Ethical Problems in Medicine and Biomedical and Behavioral Research: Defining death: Medical, legal, and ethical issues in the determination of death. Washington: U.S. Government Printing Office, 1981.
27. Korein J: The diagnosis of brain death. *Semin Neurol* 1984; 4:52–72.
28. Shewman DA: The probability of inevitability: The inherent impossibility of validating criteria for brain death or 'irreversibility' through clinical studies. *Stat Med* 1987; 6:535–553.
29. Veatch RM: The impending collapse of the whole-brain definition of death. *Hastings Cent Rep* 1993; 23:18–24.
30. Bernstein IM, Watson M, Simmons GM, et al: Maternal brain death and prolonged fetal survival. *Obstet Gynecol* 1989; 74:434–437.
31. Nuutinen LS, Alahuhta SM, Heikkinen JE: Nutrition during ten-week life support with successful fetal outcome in a case with fatal maternal brain damage. *JPEN J Parenteral Enteral Nutr* 1989; 13:432–435.
32. Field DR, Gates EA, Creasy RK, et al: Maternal brain death during pregnancy. Medical and ethical issues. *JAMA* 1988; 260:816–822.
33. Parisi JE, Kim RC, Collins GH, et al: Brain death with prolonged somatic survival. *N Engl J Med* 1982; 306:14–16.
34. Rivers EP, Buse SM, Bivins BA, et al: Organ and tissue procurement in the acute care setting: Principles and practice—part 1. *Ann Emerg Med* 1990; 19:78–85.
35. Rivers EP, Buse SM, Bivins BA, et al: Organ and tissue procurement in the acute care setting: Principles and practice—part 2. *Ann Emerg Med* 1990; 19:193–200.
36. The Surgeon General's Workshop on Increasing Organ Donation: Proceedings, U.S. Department of Health and Human Services, 1991.
37. Olson CM: Diagnostic and therapeutic technology assessment (DATTA). Lung transplantation. *JAMA* 1993; 269:931–936.
38. Evans RW, Orians CE, Ascher NL: The potential supply of organ donors. An assessment of the efficiency of organ procurement efforts in the United States. *JAMA* 1992; 267:239–246.
39. Randall T: Too few human organs for transplantation, too many in need ... and the gap widens. *JAMA* 1991; 265:1223, 1227.
40. Handelsman H: Single and double lung transplantation. Health Technology Assessment Report, 5, 1991, Agency for Health Care Policy and Research, US Department of Health and Human Services.
41. Darby JM, Stein K, Grenvik A, et al: Approach to management of the heartbeating 'brain dead' organ donor. *JAMA* 1989; 261:2222–2228.
42. Caplan AL, Virnig B: Is altruism enough? Required request and the donation of cadaver organs and tissues in the United States. *Crit Care Clin* 1990; 6:1007–1018.
43. Caplan A, Siminoff L, Arnold R, et al: Increasing organ and tissue donation: What are the obstacles, what are our options? in, The Surgeon General's workshop on increasing organ donation. Background papers. U.S. Department of Health and Human Services, 1991:199–232.

44. Lange SS: Psychosocial, legal, ethical, and cultural aspects of organ donation and transplantation. *Crit Care Nurs Clin North Am* 1992; 4;(1):25–42.
45. The Gallup Organization, Inc., "The American Public's Attitudes Toward Organ Donation and Transplantation," conducted for The Partnership for Organ Donation, Boston, MA, February 1993.
46. Youngner SJ, Landefeld S, Coulton CJ, et al: Brain death and organ retrieval. A cross-sectional survey of knowledge and concepts among health professionals. *JAMA* 1989; 261:2205–2210.
47. Novello AC: From the surgeon general, U.S. public health service. *JAMA* 1992; 267:213.
48. Spital A: The shortage of organs for transplantation: Where do we go from here? *N Engl J Med* 1991; 325:1243–1246.
49. Veatch RM: Routine inquiry about organ donation—an alternative to presumed consent. *N Engl J Med* 1991; 325:1246–1249.
50. Spital A: Mandated choice: The preferred solution to the organ shortage? *Arch Intern Med* 1992; 152:2421–2424.
51. Black PM: Conceptual and practical issues in the declaration of death by brain criteria. *Neurosurg Clin North Am* 1991; 2:493–501.
52. de Villiers JC: Pitfalls and problems in the diagnosis of cerebral death, in de Villiers JC (ed): *Some Pitfalls and Problems in Neurosurgery. Progress in Neurological Surgery, Vol 13.* New York: Karger, 1990:180–202.
53. Kaufman HH, Lynn J: Brain death. *Neurosurgery* 1986; 19:850–856.
54. Bleck TP: Dilated pupils and brain death. *Ann Intern Med* 1990; 112:632.
55. Crenna P, Conci F, Boselli L: Changes in spinal reflex excitability in brain-dead humans. *Electroencephalogr Clin Neurophysiol* 1989; 73:206–214.
56. Turmel A, Roux A, Bojanowski MW: Spinal man after declaration of brain death. *Neurosurgery* 1991; 28:298–302.
57. Conci F, Procaccio F, Arosio M, et al: Viscera-somatic and viscera-visceral reflexes in brain death. *J Neurol Neurosurg Psychiatry* 1986; 49:695–698.
58. Kuwagata Y, Sugimoto H, Yoshioka T, et al: Hemodynamic response with passive neck flexion in brain death. *Neurosurgery* 1991; 29:239–241.
59. Wetzel RC, Setzer N, Stiff J, et al: Hemodynamic responses in brain dead organ donor patients. *Anesth Analg* 1985; 64:125–128.
60. Urasaki E, Tokimura T, Kumai J, et al: Preserved spinal dorsal horn potentials in a brain-dead patient with Lazarus' sign; case report. *J Neurosurg* 1992; 76:710–713.
61. Belsh JM, Blatt R, Schiffman PL: Apnea testing in brain death. *Arch Intern Med* 1986; 146:2385–2388.
62. Ebata T, Watanabe Y, Amaha K, et al: Haemodynamic changes during the apnea test for diagnosis of brain death. *Can J Anaesth* 1991; 38:436–440.
63. Heytens L, Verlooy J, Gheuens J, et al: Lazarus sign and extensor posturing in a brain-dead patient. Case report. *J Neurosurg* 1989; 71:449–451.
64. Jastremski MS, Powner D, Snyder J, et al: Spontaneous decerebrate movement after declaration of brain death. Letter to editor. *Neurosurgery* 1991; 29:479–480.
65. Patterson KW, McShane A: Reflex spinal cord activity as a cause of a delay in the diagnosis of brain death. *Ir Med J* 1991; 84:27–28.
66. Kaufman HH (ed): *Pediatric Brain Death and Organ/Tissue Retrieval.* New York: Plenum Press, 1989.
67. Earnest MP, Beresford HR, McIntyre HB: Testing for apnea in suspected brain death: Methods used by 129 clinicians. *Neurology* 1986; 36:542–544.
68. Ropper AH: Unusual spontaneous movements in brain-dead patients. *Neurology* 1984; 34:1089–1092.
69. Posner JB: Coma and other states of consciousness: The differential diagnosis of brain death. *Ann NY Acad Sci* 1978; 315:215–227.
70. Ropper AH, Kennedy SK, Russell L: Apnea testing in the diagnosis of brain death. Clinical and physiological observations. *J Neurosurg* 1981; 55:942–946.
71. Schafer JA, Caronna JJ: Duration of apnea needed to confirm brain death. *Neurology* 1978; 28:661–666.
72. Benzel EC, Mashburn JP, Conrad S, et al: Apnea testing for the determination of brain death: A modified protocol. Technical note. *J Neurosurg* 1992; 76:1029–1031.
73. Benzel EC, Gross CD, Hadden TA, et al: The apnea test for the determination of brain death. *J Neurosurg* 1989; 71:191–194.
74. Shapiro BA: The apnea-$PaCO_2$ relationship: Some clinical and medico-legal considerations. *J Clin Anesth* 1989; 1:323–327.
75. Kaufman HH, Timberlake G, Pait TG, et al: Medical complications of head injury. *Med Clin North Am* 1993; 77:43–60.
76. Rowlands BJ, Kaufman HH: Metabolic physiology, pathophysiology, and management, in Wirth FP, Ratcheson RA (eds): *Neurosurgical Critical Care.* Baltimore: Williams & Wilkins, 1987:81–107.
77. Sugimoto T, Sakano T, Kinoshita Y, et al: Morphological and functional alterations of the hypothalamic pituitary system in brain death with long term bodily living. *Acta Neurochir* 1992; 15:31–36.
78. Debelak L, Pollak R, Reckard C: Arginine vasopressin versus desmopressin for the treatment of diabetes insipidus in the brain dead organ donor. *Transplant Proc* 1990; 22:351–352.
79. Koller J, Wieser C, Gottardis M, et al: Thyroid hormones and their impact on the hemodynamic and metabolic stability of organ donors and on kidney graft function after transplantation. *Transplant Proc* 1990; 22:355–357.
80. Novitsky D: Triiodothyronine replacement, the euthyroid sick syndrome, and organ transplantation. *Transplant Proc* 1991; 23:2460–2462.
81. Zaloga GP: Endocrine function after brain death. *Crit Care Med* 1990; 18:785–786.
82. Prager MC: Care of organ donors. *Int Anesthesiol Clin* 1991; 29:1–16.
83. Powner DJ, Darby JM, Stein KL: Organ donor management in the intensive care unit, in Grande CM (ed):

Textbook of Trauma, Anesthesia and Critical Care. St Louis: CV Mosby, 1993:1007–1012.
84. Goodman JM, Heck LL, Moore BD: Confirmation of brain death with portable isotope angiography: A review of 204 consecutive cases. *Neurosurgery* 1985; 16:492–497.
85. Schwartz JA, Brill D, Baxter J: Detection of blood flow to the brain by radionuclide cerebral imaging, in Kaufman HH (ed): *Pediatric Brain Death and Organ/Tissue Retrieval.* New York: Plenum Press, 1989:149–156.
86. Laurin NR, Driedger AA, Hurwitz GA, et al: Cerebral perfusion imaging with technetium-99m HM-PAO in brain death and severe central nervous system injury. *J Nucl Med* 1989; 30:1627–1635.
87. Anonymous: Minimum technical standards for EEG recording in suspected cerebral death. American Electroencephalographic Society. Guidelines in EEG, 1-7 (Revised 1985). *J Clin Neurophysiol* 1986; 3:144–149.
88. Grigg MM, Kelly MA, Celesia GG, et al: Electroencephalographic activity after brain death. *Arch Neurol* 1987; 44:948–954.
89. de la Riva A, Gonzalez FM, Llamas-Elvira JM, et al: Diagnosis of brain death: Superiority of perfusion studies with $^{99}Tc^{m}$–HMPAO over conventional radionuclide cerebral angiography. *Br J Radiol* 1992; 65:289–294.
90. George MS: Establishing brain death: The potential role of nuclear medicine in the search for a reliable confirmatory test. *Eur J Nucl Med* 1991; 18:75–77.
91. Schlake HP, Bottger IG, Grotemeyer KH, et al: Determination of cerebral perfusion by means of planar brain scintigraphy and ^{99m}Tc-HMPAO in brain death, persistent vegetative state and severe coma. *Intensive Care Med* 1992; 18:76–81.
92. Galaske RG, Schober O, Heyer R: Determination of brain death in children with ^{123}I-IMP and Tc-99m HMPAO. *Psychiatry Res* 1989; 29:343–345.
93. Yatim A, Mercatello A, Coronel B, et al: ^{99m}Tc-HMPAO cerebral scintigraphy in the diagnosis of brain death. *Transplant Proc* 1991; 23:2491.
94. McMenamin JB, Volpe JJ: Doppler ultrasonography in the determination of neonatal brain death. *Ann Neurol* 1983; 14:302–307.
95. Ropper AH, Kehne SM, Wechsler L: Transcranial doppler in brain death. *Neurology* 1987; 37:1733–1735.
96. Gawlowski J, Hassler W: Is TC-Doppler a useful method for the determination of brain death? *Neurosurg Rev* 1989; 12(suppl 1):307–310.
97. Hassler W, Steinmetz H, Pirschel J: Transcranial Doppler study of intracranial circulatory arrest. *J Neurosurg* 1989; 71:195–201.
98. Rozsa L, Hassler W: Investigations on oscillating flow spectra as a doppler ultrasonographic sign of intracranial circulatory arrest. *Acta Neurochir* 1991; 112:113–117.
99. Kirkham FJ, Levin SD, Padayachee TS, et al: Transcranial pulsed Doppler ultrasound findings in brain stem death. *J Neurol Neurosurg Psychiatry* 1987; 50:1504–1513.
100. Kirkham FJ, Neville BGR, Gosling RG: Diagnosis of brain death by transcranial Doppler sonography. *Arch Dis Child* 1989; 64:889–890.
101. Powers AD, Graeber MC, Smith RR: Transcranial Doppler ultrasonography in the determination of brain death. *Neurosurgery* 1989; 24:884–889.
102. Zurynski Y, Dorsch N, Pearson I, et al: Transcranial Doppler ultrasound in brain death: Experience in 140 patients. *Neurol Res* 1991; 13:248–252.
103. Petty GW, Mohr JP, Pedley TA, et al: The role of transcranial Doppler in confirming brain death: Sensitivity, specificity, and suggestions for performance and interpretation. *Neurology* 1990; 40:300–303.
104. Newell DW, Grady MS, Sirotta P, et al: Evaluation of brain death using transcranial Doppler. *Neurosurgery* 1989; 24:509–513.
105. Starr A, Achor LJ: Auditory brainstem responses in neurological disease. *Arch Neurol* 1975; 32:761–768.
106. Goldie WD, Chiappa KH, Young RR, et al: Brain stem auditory and short latency somatosensory evoked responses in brain death. *Neurology* 1981; 31:248–256.
107. Klug N, Csecsei G: Brain stem acoustic evoked potentials in the acute midbrain syndrome and in central death, in Morocutti C, Rizzo PA (eds): *Evoked Potentials. Neurophysiological and Clinical Aspects.* Amsterdam: Elsevier, 1985; 203–210.
108. Starr A: Auditory brain-stem responses in brain death. *Brain* 1976; 99:543–554.
109. Nau R, Prange HW, Klingelholfer J., et al: Results of four technical investigations in fifty clinically brain dead patients. *Intensive Care Med* 1992; 18:82–88.
110. Ron G, Schwarz G, Grims R, et al: Braindex: An interactive, knowledge-based system supporting brain death diagnosis. *Methods Inf Med* 1990; 29:193–199.
111. Kohrman MH, Spivak BS: Brain death in infants: Sensitivity and specificity of current criteria. *Pediatr Neurol* 1990; 6:47–50.
112. Morris JA Jr, Wilcox TR, Frist WH: Pediatric organ donation: The paradox of organ shortage despite the remarkable willingness of families to donate. *Pediatrics* 1992; 89:411–415.
113. Ashwal S, Schneider S: Pediatric brain death: Current perspectives. *Adv Pediatr* 1991; 38:181–202.
114. Task Force for the Determination of Brain Death in Children: Guidelines for the determination of brain death in children. *Arch Neurol* 1987; 44:587–588, *Ann Neurol* 1987; 21:616–617, *Pediatr Neurol* 1987; 3:242–243, *Pediatrics* 1987; 80:298–300.
115. Moshe SL: Usefulness of EEG in the evaluation of brain death in children: The pros. *Electrocephalogr Clin Neurophysiol* 1989; 73:272–275.
116. Moshe SL, Alvarez LA, Davidoff BA: Role of EEG in brain death determination in children: The Bronx experience, in Kaufman HH (ed): *Pediatric Brain Death and Organ/Tissue Retrieval.* New York: Plenum Press, 1989:165–175.
117. Ashwal S: Brain death in the newborn. *Clin Perinatol* 1989; 16:501–518.

118. Ashwal S, Schneider S: Brain death in the newborn. *Pediatrics* 1989; 84:429–437.
119. Bennett DR: The EEG in the determination of brain death in pediatric patients: The NIH study, in Kaufman HH (ed): *Pediatric Brain Death and Organ/Tissue Retrieval.* New York: Plenum Press, 1989:157–163.
120. Schneider S: Usefulness of EEG in the evaluation of brain death in children: The cons. *Electroencephalogr Clin Neurophysiol* 1989; 73:276–278.
121. Goodman JM, Heck LL, Nugent SK, et al: Validity of radionuclide cerebral angiography for diagnosing brain death in infants, in Kaufman HH (ed): *Pediatric Brain Death and Organ/Tissue Retrieval.* New York: Plenum Press, 1989:135–148.

CHAPTER 57

ORGAN TRANSPLANTATION

William Graham Guerriero

SYNOPSIS

In the last 25 years, organ transplantation has become accepted as an effective therapeutic option for the treatment of renal, heart, liver and pulmonary failure, and has been shown to improve the quality of life of those with diabetes. Renal transplantation is more cost-effective than dialysis over a 5-year period, and transplantation greatly improves the quality of life in patients with renal failure. Other solid organs are more expensive to transplant, and their transplantations are just beginning to rival conventional treatment in terms of cost.

Transplantation is not the answer for every patient with organ failure. The patient may be too sick or too old, or may have multisystem failure. However the primary reason that solid organ transplantation is not growing more rapidly is a lack of adequate donors. In 1991, 9953 kidneys, 2123 hearts, and 2951 livers were transplanted in the United States. A total of 4500 donors provided these transplants. Sixty-two percent of the donors provided more than one organ type. The median recovery for all organ procurement organizations in 1991 was 19.4 donors per million population. As of December 31, 1993, 24,973 patients were awaiting transplantation.[1]

Another as yet unsolved problem is organ rejection. Powerful drugs are required to prevent acute rejection of the transplanted organ, and immunologic therapy is associated with high risk. Six percent of patients who receive immunosuppression develop tumors, usually lymphomas or other hematologic malignancies. Cyclosporine, the most commonly used immunosuppressive agent, is toxic to the kidney; steroids impair growth and cause GI and orthopedic complications.

Short-term success with organ transplantation is excellent with currently available immunosuppressive agents. However, the problem of chronic rejection has not been solved. New approaches such as simultaneous transplantation and bone marrow infusion, and new immunosuppressive agents, are being developed in an attempt to produce tolerance to the transplant and avoid prolonged immunosuppression. It has long been known that chimerism develops in the recipient as cells are exchanged between the graft and the patient. The patient becomes a combination of himself and the donor. Significant chimerism frequently is seen in patients who are tolerant to solid organ transplants. These are the patients who have long-term success, sometimes surviving for decades without an appreciable change in graft function.

HISTORY OF TRANSPLANTATION

The history of transplantation parallels the history of surgical progress in the 20th century. Transplantation of solid organs became feasible with the development of such surgical techniques as vascular anastomoses and effective implantation of the ureter into the bladder. Transplantation also benefited from the development of immunology and the discovery of immunosuppressive agents, infectious disease therapy, and the development of organ preservation techniques.

The story of transplantation began at the turn of this century. Alexis Carrel, a French surgeon who won the Nobel prize in 1912, reported a technique in 1902 for the successful anastomosis of small blood vessels with suture.[2] At about this same time, other surgeons, particularly in France, worked to develop transplantation techniques. One of the best known French surgeons, Mathieu Jaboulay of Lyon, performed many transplants in animals, and even implanted a pig kidney into the arm of a patient.[3]

The first attempt at human allotransplantation was by a Russian surgeon, U.U. Voronoy. In the middle 1930s, Voronoy transplanted a kidney across blood group barriers. The kidney had a long warm ischemia time. Failure was inevitable, but not due to lack of surgical skill. One might wonder why the kidney was the first organ to be transplanted. The kidney usually has a single artery and vein, is easily excised, and is small enough to be implanted into the arm or leg.

Interest in renal transplantation was stimulated by the development of dialysis for renal failure. In the late 1930s the discovery of cellophane led Wilhelm Kolff of the Netherlands to use its semipermeable characteristics to remove waste products from the blood of patients with acute renal failure. The development of a dialysis machine that was effective for the treatment of acute renal failure led to the birth of the Kidney Research Unit at the Brigham Hospital in Boston under the direction of Peter Thorn and John Merrill. During World War II, Kolff worked on blood transfusion research in the Netherlands. After the war, Merrill and Walter invited Kolff to come to the Brigham Hospital and they jointly developed the Brigham kidney dialysis machine, which was effective for the treatment of patients with acute renal failure. Attachment of the machine to the patient was a problem, as vascular shunts had not been developed and even the Scribner shunt was not available. Long-term dialysis did not appear to be possible. Needle access was rapidly lost, and thus most research in dialysis was directed toward its short-term use.

Coincident with the development of effective hemodialysis, in 1946 an event of some importance took place at the Brigham Hospital. David Hume, Richard Hufnagel, and a urology resident, Landsteiner, transplanted a cadaver kidney into the antecubital fossa of a woman with acute renal failure and coma due to toxemia of pregnancy. The woman survived the treatment and her toxemia. This successful operation led Hume and Merrill in the late 1940s and early 1950s to try a number of cadaver transplants, both in animals and humans. Only one of these transplants could be called successful. That transplant, a kidney graft, lasted 173 days in a pediatrician with chronic renal failure. No immunosuppression was used in any of these transplants.

By the early 1940s, Peter Medawar, a famous British zoologist, had discovered that chimerism existed in cows. Chimerism occurs as a result of the fetal calf sharing a single placenta in utero with its twin, thus exchanging cells during an immunologically permissive period of development. Chimerism leads to complete acceptance of skin grafts, which was clearly demonstrated by Medawar and others.[4]

By 1954, the technique of transplantation of the kidney into the pelvis had become standardized. Joseph Murray, a plastic surgeon took Hume's place as the Director of the Surgical Research Unit at the Brigham Hospital where Hume left the Brigham to serve in the Korean War. John Merrill, a nephrologist, and Hartwell Harrison, a urologist, joined with Murray to perform the first successful kidney transplant between twins, using the principle of chimerism so eloquently described by Medawar.

After a skin graft was performed to test acceptability, the kidney was removed from one twin brother and placed in the groin of the other. This operation took place in December 1954. Other twin transplants followed, but rejection remained inevitable for those patients who did not have access to a twin.

Damecek and Swartz in the late 1950s reported in the journal *Nature* the immunologic suppressive properties of 6-mercaptopurine, a purine analogue. In the early 1960s this discovery rapidly led to the development of a similar drug, azathioprine (Imuran), by Calne. Steroids were also shown to modify the rejection process, and by 1964 attempts at living-related transplantation were taking place in numerous cities in the United States and Europe, particularly in France.

Credit for the first successful transplant program probably should be given to Thomas Starzl, who, using azathioprine, steroids, and a polyclonal antibody (acute lymphocyte globulin), reported better than a 60 percent survival of cadaveric grafts after one year. An explosion of transplant activity and programs followed.

Recognition of transplantation antigens, which reside on the leukocyte, was a result of the work of Medawar, Dosay, Rappaport, and others. The second cornerstone of transplantation immunology was recognition that histocompatibility antigens are under strict genetic control, and that histocompatibility is different for different genetic relationships between donor and recipient. The probability of genetic histocompatibility is highest between siblings, intermediate between parents and children, and lowest between unrelated individuals. The majority of serological specificities carried by the lymphocyte membrane have been proved to belong to one genetic system, now known as HLA. Other histocompatibility antigens have been identified, but the ability to type specific patients and recipients for the HLA system has become the basis for the selection of recipients in most renal transplant programs. It is clearly recognized that the more similar the recipient is to the donor, the better the long-term result will be with transplantation.

HLA typing is quite expensive and today it is less and less utilized as the primary determinant for matching donors and recipients. But most transplant programs still require some antigenic relationship between donor and recipient before selecting that organ for transplantation into a given patient. Similar relationships have been shown for hearts, livers, and lungs, but these organs have traditionally been transplanted on the basis of ABO compatibility and organ size, rather than the presence or absence of similar histocompatibility antigens, because long-term survival is not as important as initial and short-term survival in these patients.

In order to maximally utilize organs, kidneys, hearts, lungs, and livers must be transported between institutions, cities, and even countries. It had long been recognized that cooling of the kidney led to increased survival and protected against acute renal failure. Some permanent damage will occur to a kidney after 30 minutes of warm ischemia secondary to complete occlusion of the renal artery, and kidneys are unusable after 180 minutes of warm ischemia time. Belzer, in 1968, reported a method of pulsatile perfusion of the kidney using cryoprecipitated plasma at 4–7° C. This method was extremely successful in maintaining kidney grafts for up to 72 hours. A static preservation solution based on intracellular electrolyte composition with a slightly increased oncotic pressure was developed by Collins in Europe and modified by others. With his solution, 24 to 36 hours of successful preservation was possible. In recent years, slightly modified solutions have been used to preserve livers for transplantation, and today static preservation with cold electrolyte solutions is the norm for transplantation of all organs.

The explosion of activity in the early 1960s was premature. During this early developmental period, renal transplantation in the United States more frequently resulted in 30 to 50 percent of patients free of dialysis at one year, rather than the results initially reported by Starzl. In the early 1980s, Calne made another tremendous discovery, cyclosporine A. This dramatically successful immunologic agent soon became widely available. By 1984, transplantation of organs other than the kidney, such as heart, liver, lungs, and pancreas, increased in frequency, as the use of cyclosporine resulted in significantly improved survival. Although cyclosporine is not a perfect agent, this drug and the development of monoclonal antibody agents, such as OKT-3, have led to successes in transplantation that were only dreamed of in the 1950s and 1960s. In a short 30 years, 1-year graft survival with cadaveric kidneys has risen to 85 percent and 50 to 75 percent of hearts, lungs, and livers survive at least 1 year.[2]

To facilitate and coordinate the procurement of solid organs, the federal government in 1987 established a franchised private corporation, the United Network of Organ Sharing. It was hoped that this organization would increase the number of organs available for transplantation and decrease competition for donors between transplant programs. However, successful transplantation of solid organs also led to a rapid increase in the number of patients desiring and awaiting transplantation, and soon the demand overwhelmed the static and even declining number of cadaver donors. With a decrease in the number of motor vehicle and motor cycle related deaths and the use of semiautomatic or high-caliber weapons, which decreased the number of gunshot wound victims living long enough to provide organs for transplantation, organ availability has actually declined. Over the last 4 to 5 years the number of donors available for organ procurement has remained at 4000 to 5000 per year. The number of patients listed awaiting transplantation continues to climb, and is now approaching 30,000. Lack of an adequate donor supply has led to increasing numbers of liver and heart patients dying while awaiting transplantation and a rapid politicalization of the transplant donor procurement process, with patient advocate groups lobbying their Congressmen to modify perceived unfairness in the organ donation process. Transplant surgeons have even been labeled as racially biased because of disparities in the percentage of blacks versus whites transplanted, despite clear-cut evidence that this has occurred only because of the infrequency of black donation and an increased frequency of black patients on dialysis. The use of HLA tissue-typing preselects white recipients for white donors, and the combination of these factors has led to a perceived disparity in the number of blacks transplanted versus the number of black patients on transplant lists. Consequently there is more pressure to abandon the HLA system as a criteria for patient selection. Faulting physicians for their attempts to improve graft survival by the use of tissue matching techniques is counterproductive. It is clearly evident that without tissue matching many more grafts would be lost in the long run as chronic rejection takes its toll. But be that as it may, heavy lobbying has taken place over the last 4 to 5 years, directed at correcting perceived unfairness in organ distribution.

Not everyone who dies is a suitable organ donor. On cessation of respiration and heart beat, irreversible changes occur in heart, lung, liver, and kidney, which may make these organs unsuitable for transplantation. Delays in organ procurement, increased age of the donor, or donors less than 3 years of age, systemic infections, cancer, advanced arteriosclerosis, cirrhosis, and hypertensive nephropathy may preclude donation of one or more organs.

The traditional donor for multi-organ transplantation is the heart-beating, brain-dead patient, who has died as a result of trauma, subarachnoid hemorrhage, or neurological cancer (Table 57-1). In Table 57-2 are listed contraindications to cadaveric organ donation. Of the relative criteria seen in Table 57-2, some contraindications are more important than others for individual organs. For example, a patient with alcoholic cirrhosis,

TABLE 57-1 Potential Solid Organ Donors

Stable cardiovascular function in patients who are brain dead following:
1. Head trauma
2. Subarachnoid hemorrhage
3. Neurological malignancy
4. Brain infarction ± herniation

even with decreased renal function secondary to hepatorenal syndrome, can still be a kidney donor in most cases. The patient with hypertension could still be a liver donor and even donate kidneys if renal biopsy shows little change secondary to the hypertension, and if arteriosclerosis is not too far advanced. The organs most sensitive appear to be the lung and liver, but kidneys can be obtained from most brain-death donors, and hearts from most young victims. Each case must be individualized, and transplant surgeons and transplant coordinators on the scene decide which organs may be removed from each individual heart-beating cadaver. The concept of brain death is covered elsewhere in this text, but certain aspects of the terminal events as they relate to transplant donation need to be emphasized.

A limited time is available to obtain organs after brain death. No matter how good the medical management or intensive the support, the heart usually fails within 24 to 72 hours after brain death, and in many instances within a matter of a few hours. Every effort should be made to contact the family, frequently a laborious process, and permission should be sought for organ donation. In addition, legal issues regarding the nature of the patient's death may take precedence over organ donation, producing further delay as the Medical Examiner or Coroner is consulted. After declaration of death, the donor must be stabilized and serologies obtained to be sure hepatitis or AIDS is not present, a process that frequently takes 4 to 6 hours. Organ procurement teams must be assembled, sometimes from distant transplant centers, to remove and preserve organs to be used for transplantation. A schematic time line for transplantation is seen in Fig. 57-1.

As can be seen from this Figure, even in the most favorable scenario, 24 to 48 hours may elapse after the initial injury before any organs can be transplanted. There is more than enough time for the donor to deteriorate or even to suffer a sudden cardiac arrest. A steadily increasing requirement for vasopressors, an imbalance in electrolytes due to diabetes insipidus, or a less than perfect medical management of the patient may make stabilization of the donor difficult and sometimes impossible. It is unfortunate that once the prognosis is found to be hopeless, those caring for the patient may back away, giving less than appropriate fluids, not following blood gases and electrolytes closely, and, in general, minimizing support. When brain death is declared and

TABLE 57-2 Contraindications to Donation

Absolute:
1. Systemic infection (chronic or active), sepsis, tuberculosis, etc.
2. AIDS
3. Systemic malignancy
4. Profound shock, unresponsive to fluids or low doses of vasopressor
5. Renal failure

Relative:
1. Hepatitis, abnormal liver function test
2. CMV positive status
3. Chronic hypertension
4. Arteriosclerotic heart and peripheral vascular disease
5. Localized infection, treated abscess
6. Congestive heart failure

Of the relative criteria on Table 57-2, some contraindications are more important than others for individual organs. For example, a patient with alcoholic cirrhosis, even with decreased renal function secondary to hepatorenal syndrome, can still be a kidney donor in most cases. A patient with hypertension could still be a liver donor and, if biopsy of the kidney shows little damage and arteriosclerosis is not too bad, a donor for kidneys.

The most sensitive organs are lung and liver. Kidneys can be obtained from most brain-dead donors, and the heart from most young trauma victims. However, each case must be individualized.

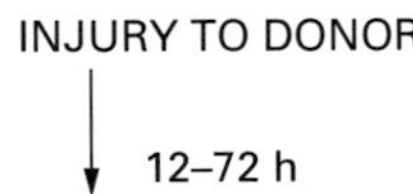

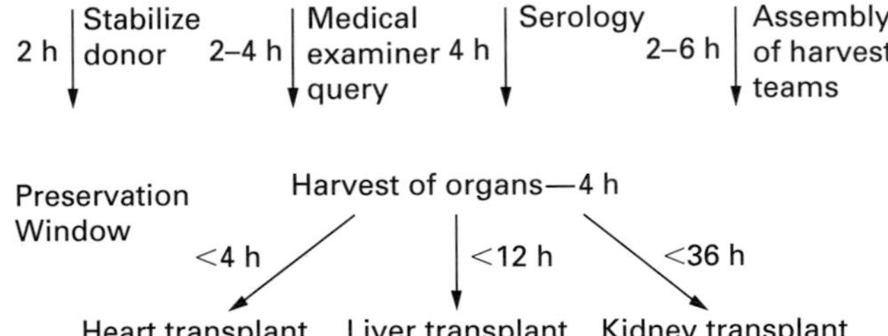

Figure 57-1. Schematic time line for transplantation.

the donor management team assesses the now dead patient, it is not uncommon to find the serum sodium at 170 mg/dl or higher and the blood pressure at barely sustainable levels with the patient receiving large amounts of vasopressors. Many donors are lost because the cardiovascular system cannot be stabilized, and the donor continues to deteriorate while coordinators attempt to assemble harvest teams and prepare for procurement.

It is hard to criticize the primary caregivers in this situation. Their attention is often diverted by numerous other concerns in a busy emergency setting. But many recipients are denied life or freedom from dialysis because of these lost donors.

What should be the role of the neurosurgeon or neurologist in the scenario just described? First, the potential donor's doctor must do everything he can for his patient, with no consideration of the possibility of organ donation. It is assumed that his interest is only in his patient, not in how many organs can be obtained for those awaiting transplantation.

If at the time of declaration of brain death, the patient is properly hydrated, the diabetes insipidus is controlled, and minimal vasopressor support is required, the organ procurement team usually has time to place heart, lungs, two kidneys, liver, pancreas, bones, and eyes. This may save three lives and improve the quality of life of many others. If, on the other hand, the patient is unstable, all of this may be lost.

The role of the neurosurgeon in an organ donation process may seem to present a conflict of interest. However, it is obvious that he must treat the patient's life as his only concern, until death is declared, but every effort should be made to keep the patient in hemodynamically stable condition. Extraordinary measures are rarely necessary. The patient just has to be kept well hydrated with normal electrolyte balance and vasopressors used minimally to give the patient a chance at being an organ donor. If a cardiovascular death precedes a declaration of brain death, no extraordinary methods should be used for resuscitation. An emergency trip to the OR to harvest organs is generally not appropriate.

No assessment of donor suitability is appropriate prior to the declaration of brain death. The Organ Procurement Organization may be alerted that a potential donor exists, but they should not talk to the family or be involved in the patient's care prior to declaration of death.

It is probably best that the patient's physician not be the person who requests organs for transplantation, although there certainly is room for debate about this point. If the physician should desire to show support by being present when the procurement personnel make the request for organs, this may aid the procurement process. But in all studies reported to date, requests for donation are more likely to be successful if they are made by the organ procurement personnel familiar with the questions asked by family members and experienced in answering them. To relinquish control of the family at this emotionally charged moment is difficult for the doctor, but having the organ procurement personnel make the request will lead to the best chance for success and, in addition, maintain a separation of the patient's doctor from the activities following declaration of death. The interest of the physician, not making the request, is seen to be only for the patient and the patient's family.

IMPACT OF DONOR MANAGEMENT ON GRAFT FUNCTION AND SURVIVAL

If powerful vasopressors or large doses of less potent vasopressors are used to support the donor's blood pressure, acute tubular necrosis or even renal shutdown may occur. Acute tubular necrosis is frequently thought to be a problem which will disappear without treatment, but in numerous studies it has been shown clearly that graft survival is reduced and that function at one year is impaired when vasopressors have been used.

No treatment has been found to reverse chronic rejection. Graft function is lost by all patients over time. Fifty percent of cadaver kidneys are lost 8 to 11 years after transplantation. In well-matched living related grafts, 22 years is required for 50 percent of the kidneys to stop functioning sufficiently to support the patient without dialysis. Twenty to 30 percent of patients develop tolerance for the graft, with extended survival and good function. The length of survival of renal grafts depends on the immunologic match of donor and recipient, but even more on the initial condition of the graft. Kidneys with acute tubular necrosis have reduced function. All the gains that we have made with better immunologic agents are lost when acute tubular necrosis occurs. In addition, the cost of transplantation is greatly increased when hospitalization is prolonged and surgical and medical complications multiply.

A similar scenario occurs with heart and liver transplantation, but, of course, the consequence of primary nonfunction is death of the patient—there is no way to support a patient without a heart or a liver.

In summary, great advances have taken place in transplantation, which is now an accepted clinical procedure, not an experiment. However, it is still an expensive treatment option, made more so by reliance on cadaver donors that have suffered agonal brain death. The process of donation of organs is complicated and expensive, with great emotional cost to patients' families and the donor's physician or surgeon. The results of cadaver organ donation can be greatly improved by careful attention to details when caring for patients who are themselves unsalvageable, but who may be able to provide many years of good quality survival to other human beings.[3]

References

1. Suthanthiran, Strom: Medical progress: Renal transplantation. *N Engl J Med* 1989; 3:312–365.
2. Terasaki PI: *History of Transplantation: Thirty-five Recollections.* Los Angeles: UCLA Tissue Typing Laboratory, 1991.
3. Phillips MG: *Organ Procurement, Preservation, and Distribution in Transplantation.* Richmond VA: William Byrd Press, 1991.

Rehabilitation

CHAPTER 58

REHABILITATION OF THE HEAD-INJURED PATIENT

Catherine F. Bontke
Nathan D. Zasler
Corwin Boake

SYNOPSIS

The theoretical basis of rehabilitation for traumatic brain injury (TBI) is briefly reviewed, and several practical issues are then discussed. While much progress has been made in this field, many major issues have not been critically tested. This chapter summarizes the current thinking about TBI rehabilitation and identifies areas for future study.

INTRODUCTION

Advances in neurosurgical care have improved survival from traumatic brain injury (TBI) in the past 20 years. With the increased number of survivors and changes in reimbursement, there has been a proliferation of TBI rehabilitation facilities. Every TBI patient deserves a chance to enhance his or her recovery through high-quality rehabilitation services. This chapter provides an overview of the rehabilitative management of patients with TBI.

NEUROLOGICAL BASIS FOR REHABILITATION AND IMPLICATIONS FOR TREATMENT

Multiple mechanisms have been proposed to explain recovery of function after TBI. However, there is little hard evidence for a causal relationship between the proposed mechanisms and the effects of neurorehabilitative interventions. Resolution of adverse neurophysiological phenomena, including elevated intracranial pressure, edema, and hypoxia, clearly is responsible for some of the improvements noted in the acute postinjury stage of recovery. At a cellular level, modification of synaptic function has been proposed as an explanation for the phenomenon of *diaschsis* (reversible dysfunction in adjacent areas of brain tissue). Alterations in neural connections via axonal regeneration and collateral sprouting also have been proposed as mechanisms that mediate recovery of function. Other theories that have been proposed include functional substitution, vicarious functioning, and redundancy. The overt or covert use of alternative strategies to achieve the desired functional outcome is termed *functional substitution*. In other words, after a CNS insult, patients learn compensatory strategies in order to cope with their functional limitations. *Vicarious functioning* implies that neural structures alter their function in a manner that allows for subserving the direction of new functional tasks. *Redundancy,* by contrast, implies that there are "dormant" neural circuits that have the capability of performing particular functions but do so only when "called on" after a neural insult. *Denervation supersensitivity* and *reactive synaptogenesis* (also called axon collateral sprouting) have both been theorized to play a potential role in neural reorganization; however, it is unclear whether such reorganization is adaptive as opposed to maladaptive.[1,2]

The role of catecholamines, particularly noradrenaline in recovery from TBI-related behavioral deficits is being actively investigated.[3] The exact location where nonadrenergic fibers emanating from the locus coeruleus need to be "stimulated" to mediate accelerated motor recovery is a much debated area of current research. Boyeson and colleagues believe that the critical area is not related to diaschisislike effects in the sensorimotor cortex itself but rather to alterations in noradrenergic function in the cerebellum contralateral to the site of sensorimotor cortex injury.[1,2] Noradrenergic compounds may play a beneficial role if TBI is given after appropriate times and under specific conditions. Conversely, noradrenergic antagonists may actually be detrimental in certain circumstances.[1–4] However, the clinical implications of these findings remain unclear.

Functional recovery may be a consequence of an inherent but poorly defined ability of the CNS to adapt to injury. It is critical to understand the realities of the age-related, genetically driven central processes that underlie functional recovery. Specifically, neuronal sparing mechanisms in early development are quite distinct from those in more mature organisms. In the best of all worlds, with therapies based on a sound scientific rationale, rehabilitationists could intervene in the recovery process to favorably affect outcome. Research suggests that the *rate* of neurological recovery may be more amenable to interventional manipulation than is the *ultimate level* of neurological function. However, faster may not necessarily be better in that there are inherent risks associated with "rushing recovery." Specifically, maladaptive behaviors may be triggered and/or reinforced. Development of a more comprehensive understanding of the pathophysiology of neurological recovery after brain injury is important if rehabilitationists are to intervene most effectively.[2,4]

CONTINUUM OF CARE

The need for a comprehensive continuum of medical and rehabilitative care for persons with varying degrees of TBI must be emphasized.[5] Coordination of services across medical disciplines serves to increase the quality of patient care.

Acute Neurosurgical Care

Ideally, all TBI patients admitted to the hospital for treatment and/or observation, regardless of the severity of injury, should be screened by the rehabilitation medicine consultation service. Proper communication across disciplines has proved to be a critical factor in enhancing the quality of care. Additionally, problems that can lead to potential morbidity may be appropriately evaluated and treated in the acute care setting, allowing for a smoother transition when the patient is transferred to a rehabilitation facility. The major issues of neuromedical management appropriately addressed by the physiatrist include skin care, bowel and bladder management, behavioral management, tone control, maximization of nutritional status, maintenance of joint range of motion, and optimization of the patient's potential for neurological and functional recovery through both pharmacological and nonpharmacological modalities. This type of coordinated approach requires a multidisciplinary neuromedical staff whose members are familiar with and have a heightened awareness of the complications associated with TBI, including but not limited to heterotopic ossification, posttraumatic seizures, spasticity management, neuroendocrine disorders, neuro-ophthalmologic problems, olfactory dysfunction, audiovestibular deficits, orthopedic injuries, dysphagia, tracheostomy management, and posttraumatic psychological as well as psychiatric disturbances.[6,7]

Specifically, aggressive efforts should be made to counteract the adverse effects of immobility. Passive and passive-assisted range-of-motion exercises to decrease muscle atrophy, mobilization efforts, contracture prevention through positioning, range and splinting, positioning protocols to prevent skin breakdown, and deep vein thrombosis prophylaxis are facets of early care directed at avoiding the complications associated with protracted immobilization. Spasticity treatment, including the potential use of neurolytic agents for motor point and/or nerve blocks, also should be a focus of early rehabilitative care.

Acute Brain Injury Rehabilitation

At the discretion of the consulting physiatrist, certain medically stable patients with brain injury may be transferred to an acute inpatient brain injury rehabilitation program.[7,8] Ideally, these units should be dedicated to the patient population in question with regard to the space allocated and the treatment team. Training the staff to be sensitive to medical and psychosocial issues commonly encountered after TBI maximizes treatment efficacy.

Some programs designate a small number of beds or separate units to an "early recovery management program" or "coma management/stimulation program" for patients who are slow to recover neurological function. Ideally, candidates for these types of programs should be admitted within the first 3 months after an injury, as their potential for recovery from the vegetative state and other "low-level" states is much greater than that of patients whose injuries occurred over 3 months earlier.[9,10] Patients who are slow to recover generally should be given a 2- to 3-month trial of inpatient care with a goal of maximizing their recovery potential and minimizing neurological and functional morbidity. If there is no significant improvement, long-term placement must be discussed. Long-term care facilities are typically based in skilled nursing homes and should optimally be staffed by health care professionals familiar with the functional and neuromedical issues relevant to survivors of TBI. Some opportunity for rehabilitative follow-up is critical to assess improvement or decline in neurological or functional status, and to modify existing treatment plans as needed.[7,11,12]

Ideally, a transdisciplinary team approach should be implemented in working with survivors of TBI. With this approach, the team works with the patient and his or her family to maximize recovery from both a neurological and a functional standpoint. The team consists of a variety of medical and nonmedical disciplines. These disciplines include rehabilitation nursing, respiratory therapy, physical therapy, occupational therapy, speech-language pathology, cognitive rehabilitation, neuropsychology, therapeutic recreation, rehabilitation social work, diet, pharmacy, and religious counseling. Team rounds and/or conferences should be held regularly with all treating team members in attendance, if possible. This process increases the team's ability to assess and treat the variety of issues that may arise during an individual's recovery and rehabilitation. Preferentially, team-building activities such as didactic lectures, a journal club, and weekly administrative meetings should be held to promote team cohesiveness.[13]

All patients admitted to an inpatient brain injury rehabilitation unit should receive a full neuromedical workup to fully assess any factors that may be compromising the recovery process. The standard neuromedical workup should consist of a thorough history and physical, including full neurological and functional assessment with electroencephalogram, static brain imaging, and neuroendocrine assessment as indicated. Full nutritional and metabolic evaluation and a comprehensive evaluation to rule out concurrent infection are often valuable. A thorough assessment of medications should be conducted, preferably in conjunction with a pharmacist, to eliminate inappropriate or excessive medications. A psychiatric consultant may be needed for evaluation and treatment of postinjury neurobehavioral sequelae. Preinjury substance abuse issues, which may affect short- and long-term potential, should be addressed as early as possible with the assistance of substance abuse consultants.[14,15]

A critical part of any brain injury rehabilitation program involves family training, regardless of the neurological or functional level of the patient. Families should be encouraged to become active members of the rehabilitation process as early as possible, even before the patient's transfer to the rehabilitation service. Early and ongoing family involvement improves patient outcome and should be encouraged. Institutional as well as community resources should be developed to allow families and patients to cope with the changes that have occurred in their lives. Such resources include in-house support groups and community support groups through organizations such as the Brain Injury Association (formerly the National Head Injury Foundation).

Subacute Rehabilitation

Subacute rehabilitation programs are generally nursing home–based rehabilitation programs that are of lower cost but provide less intensive therapy. They are designed for minimally responsive or slow to recover patients. They incorporate components of a coma treatment program and "slow and steady" rehabilitation protocols. Generally, less than 3 h of therapy per day is provided, with the overall goal of progressing the patient to acute rehabilitation or maintaining the highest level of functioning possible. Patients who eventually plateau over a prolonged period can be transferred to home or a long-term nursing facility. Guidelines for subacute facilities have not been standardized but are being developed by the Commission on Accreditation of Rehabilitation Facilities (CARF) in cooperation with the Head Injury Interdisciplinary Special Interest Group of the American Congress of Rehabilitation Medicine (ACRM) and should be finalized soon.

Postacute Rehabilitation

Most severely head injured adults who do not receive rehabilitation after the acute stage remain unemployed and dependent on their families. However, this outcome should not be accepted as inevitable. It has been shown that with the provision of appropriate rehabilitation through the postacute stage, many severely injured patients improve their level of independence and return to work in some capacity.[16–19] The terms "postacute rehabilitation" and "community reentry" are used for programs or facilities that work with patients after hospital and/or rehabilitation discharge to help improve their vocational and independent living outcomes.

In postacute rehabilitation patients learn to be more independent despite the functional limitations from their permanent impairments. One major postacute rehabilitation technique involves retraining patients to perform lost skills, compensating for their impairments by using new strategies that are based on nonimpaired abilities (e.g., compensating for impaired memory by keeping a memory notebook, using spared reading and writing skills). The second major technique in postacute rehabilitation, termed the "prosthetic environment," entails modifying the patient's environment to place fewer demands on impaired skills (e.g., changing job duties to repetitive tasks). In practice, postacute rehabilitation programs combine both techniques with family counseling, psychotherapy, and other interventions to create an integrated treatment plan. Participants in these programs are often addressed as "clients" (instead of "patients") to encourage them to take an active role in rehabilitation.

The major distinction among postacute rehabilitation programs is whether they are intended to help the clients return to work. Return-to-work programs based on the day treatment model provide prevocational training to help clients obtain employment after leaving the rehabilitation program. Programs based on the supported employment model place clients directly into jobs supervised by a job coach who is gradually faded out over time.[20] Many of these programs are reimbursed by state vocational rehabilitation agencies and can accept appropriate clients regardless of their insurance. For clients who have a poor prognosis for a return to work, postacute rehabilitation programs can provide retraining in independent living skills or modify difficult behaviors that would prevent clients from living at home without constant supervision. Clients with severe behavior or self-care deficits can live in residential (or transitional) rehabilitation facilities in order to receive more intensive training.[21]

Referral of individual patients to appropriate postacute programs requires an assessment of rehabilitation potential, particularly for returning to work. Neuropsychological testing by clinicians familiar with the available postacute programs is often helpful in making this prediction. Clients with reemployment potential should be referred to a return-to-work program, with referral to the state vocational rehabilitation agency for possible funding of these services. For the most impaired patients, who may have poor reemployment potential, insurance coverage will be necessary for enrollment in a postacute facility. A general rule for more impaired patients is that the gains obtained from postacute rehabilitation will be maintained to the extent that the patient has a strong support system and is free of chronic behavior problems (e.g., substance abuse, impaired interpersonal skills).

Chronic Care Options

Acute rehabilitation facilities should operate a follow-up clinic for former inpatients to manage medical complications, make referrals to specialists, and provide consultations for rehabilitation planning. Regular follow-up clinic visits also are a useful way to manage the problems that may arise with patients who are placed in nursing homes (e.g., contractures, overmedication). Although most severely injured patients will live at home and be cared for by family members, there are increasing numbers of spaces available for head-injured patients in group homes and other long-term residential facilities.

EFFICACY AND COST-EFFECTIVENESS OF REHABILITATION

In the current reimbursement environment, the cost-effectiveness of TBI rehabilitation is an increasing concern and may influence patient selection for rehabilitation. Acute rehabilitation programs should be cost-effective to the extent that patients will avoid long-term institutional placement and/or require less supervision, thus costing less per lifetime.[22–25] Compared with nursing home placement, acute rehabilitation can result in considerable cost savings.[22] Ambulatory brain-injured patients usually have a normal life expectancy. Most acute programs are cost-effective if patients can return to gainful employment, although the cost of savings may aptly apply mostly to disability income support.[22] For many patients who live at home, who constitute the vast majority, the benefits of rehabilitation are primarily to improve the quality of life and reduce the overall family burden.

In the past several years, the quality of rehabilitation services has been a significant issue in patient referral and funding, in part because of the rapid proliferation of brain injury rehabilitation programs. The existence of many newer facilities means that fewer staff members are experienced in the care of patients with TBI. Although CARF sets minimum standards for brain injury rehabilitation programs, not all programs choose to undergo CARF accreditation. The National Institute for Disability and Rehabilitation Research (NIDRR) Model System program has designated four federally supported centers that research cost-effective treatment and minimization of disability after TBI. From the recently published summaries of their initial 5 years of data collection,[26] it appears that the average patient requires over $115,000 for both acute and rehabilitation care.[25]

NEUROMEDICAL PROBLEMS IN TBI REHABILITATION

Spasticity

Until the early 1980s, spasticity after brain injury was generally treated in the same way as spasticity after spinal cord injury, that is, with medications causing sedation, such as baclofen and diazepam. Spasticity that results from brain injury is more heavily influenced by factors such as postural changes, body positioning, and labyrinthine and tonic neck reflexes than is the case with spinal cord injuries. Spasticity can be a source of extreme discomfort in patients with a brain injury who have intact sensation. Spasticity can have some beneficial effects, such as maintaining muscle bulk, preventing deep vein thrombosis or osteoporosis, and allowing patients with marginal motor strength to stand and be transferred. It is only when spasticity interferes with function, causes pain, interferes with nursing care, or contributes to the formation of contractures that it needs to be treated. The current trend is away from pharmacological intervention; instead, physical modalities are being used. These modalities include the application of cold or heat; stretching, splinting, and casting (including inhibitory casting); proper positioning; functional electrical stimulation; vibration; relaxation techniques; motor reeducation[27]; and biofeedback.[28,29] In addition, modalities such as chemical neurolysis utilizing nerve blocks and motor point blocks can be tried before drug therapy is begun.[30–35] A newer modality utilizing botulinum toxin has been used successfully in some centers for the control of spasticity as well.[36] When drug therapy is indicated, dantrolene sodium (Dantrium) a peripherally acting agent, is usually the preferred drug, as it appears to have the fewest cognitive or sedating side effects.

Swallowing Disorders (Swallowing, Feeding, Reflux)

The incidence of dysphagia in patients with TBI on transfer to rehabilitation facilities is about 27 percent. In a recent study in which patients were evaluated via video fluoroscopy, 81 percent of patients had a delay or absence of swallowing responses, approximately 50 percent showed reduced tongue control, about one-third had reduced pharyngeal transit times, and 14 percent showed reduced laryngeal closure, elevation, or spasms. Most patients showed two dysfunctional aspects of swallowing, such as impaired tongue control and delayed triggering mechanisms.[37]

Video fluoroscopy has become the gold standard for evaluating patients for dysphagia. This technique allows the clinician to observe the anatomy and physiology of the swallowing mechanism as a bolus consisting of a barium-impregnated liquid or cookie travels from the mouth through the pharynx and into the esophagus. Various dysfunctions, including aspiration, can be documented on the video examination. Compensatory strategies can be tested during the evaluation.[38]

Patients with swallowing difficulties often have concomitant cognitive impairment. They often need to be monitored and reminded to employ compensatory strategies. Their diets need to be changed in a sequential fashion (i.e., from puréed, ground, chopped, soft, to regular) as use of compensatory mechanisms increases and/or the swallowing improves. Treatment efforts focus on compensatory mechanisms. The vast majority of patients improve spontaneously, although this can take several weeks, during which time a patient is at high risk for developing aspiration pneumonia.

Thin liquids are to be avoided in the acute neurosurgical setting, since they are typically the most difficult to handle from a swallowing perspective and can lead to the early complication of aspiration pneumonia.

Patients who fail to progress cognitively, are unable to follow commands, have significant swallowing difficulties, are at high risk for aspiration, or are known aspirators have to be fed via an enteral tube. If enteral feeding is necessary for more than 3 to 4 weeks, a gastrostomy tube is preferable to a nasogastric tube. Prolonged use of a nasogastric tube may lead to nasal ulceration, nasal pharyngeal irritation, and infection. The tube can be placed with an open surgical procedure (gastrostomy) or using an endoscopic technique. The use of a small jejunostomy tube will prevent continued reflux by utilizing the patient's cardiac sphincter (between the esophagus and the stomach) and pyloric sphincter (between the stomach and the duodenum).

Clinically, the use of blue food coloring or methylene blue to dye tube feedings helps identify tracheal aspirations of feedings as opposed to mouth secretions. Continuous feedings can interfere with therapy activities, and therefore a jejunostomy tube is not ideal in this population unless the patient is suffering from severe reflux and aspiration.[29,39] If reflux is a concern, the head of the bed must be elevated and the patient should be tried on various formulas or smaller feedings. The use of metoclopramide (Reglan) should be avoided.[40] This drug is like the phenothiazines, and while it can help initially with reflux by increasing gastric emptying in a small percentage of patients, it is not particularly useful in the long term and is known to cause significant cognitive difficulties for patients, especially those regaining consciousness. It also has potential side effects of extrapyramidal movements and even permanent tardive dyskinesia. In addition to impeded cognitive recovery, patients can develop swallowing difficulties as a result of the use of metoclopramide. If a patient has to be on metoclopramide, its use should be limited to 2 weeks or less.[29,41] Alternatively, erythromycin may be uesful in decreasing gastric transit time by stimulating motility receptors in the stomach. As with most polytrauma patients, a patient with a brain injury has an increased risk of gastrointestinal bleeding secondary to stress ulceration during the acute care phase.[42] It is not unusual for patients to be placed on H_2 antagonist prophylaxis with medications such as cimetidine and ranitidine.[43] Since cognitive and behavioral disturbances have been noted in patients on H_2 antagonists, these medications should be withdrawn once the risk of gastrointestinal bleeding has passed.

Nutritional Status

The high caloric needs of an acutely brain injured patient are well documented in the literature.[42,44] Most trauma centers now take into account the nutritional needs of acutely injured patients when those patients are fed primarily via enteral tube feedings. Patients who have suffered severe visceral trauma can require supplementation by hyperalimentation.[45] They subsequently usually come to the rehabilitation setting in positive nitrogen balance. The physician should consider not only calories and protein but also fiber, vitamins, minerals, and the isotonicity of enteral feedings. Weekly weights are appropriate during the rehabilitation phase, with monthly measurements of serum albumin and protein to monitor nutritional status.[29,41,42,46]

Bowel Management

Fecal incontinence after TBI is fairly common, especially in patients with significant cognitive impairment. After a brain injury, patients can have an uninhibited neurogenic bowel and be unaware of the need to defecate in a timely and appropriate manner. Constipation or diarrhea may also manifest as a significant problem. The development of a daily bowel training program is appropriate regardless of the patient's cognitive status and can be accomplished through the use of high-fiber enteral feedings or oral supplementation of fiber and the use of a glycerin rectal suppository daily or every other day.[47] The use of digital stimulation should be avoided as it can be misinterpreted by patients who have cognitive difficulties.

Diarrhea may result from impaction or osmolar overload from tube feeding or may be due to *Clostridium difficile* colitis. Both osmolar overload and impaction can be prevented through the use of high-protein isotonic feedings that provide essential vitamins and minerals, such as Jevity and Enrich. Patients with brain injury are at an increased risk for the development of *C. difficile* colitis because of the frequent need for antibiotic treatment during the acute care phase. Screening for *C. difficile* toxin is indicated in a patient with a prior history of antibiotic administration and hospital-acquired diarrhea.[48] Treatment is usually successful with metronidazole (Flagyl) or oral vancomycin.

Bladder Management

Neurogenic bladder is uncommon after TBI, and if it does exist, it is usually due to uninhibited detrusor hyperreflexia that causes the patient to void small amounts frequently with complete bladder emptying. Patients can usually be managed adequately with an external collection device such as a condom catheter in males or a diaper in females until they are aware of their surroundings and have sufficient memory to use a commode or bedpan.[49,50] Patients can also have detrusor hyperreflexia as a result of the bladder overdistension that occurs with iatrogenic or traumatic outlet obstruction. These patients usually require prolonged intermittent catheterization (ICP) or an indwelling Foley catheter until this problem has been resolved, which may take weeks to months. It is the rare, primarily brainstem-injured patient with detrusor sphincter dyssynergia who needs intermittent catheterization or prolonged Foley drainage and complete urologic studies.[51]

Respiratory Management

One of the most common complications seen in patients with severe TBI is respiratory failure requiring artificial ventilation for more than 1 week.[52] Pneumonitis, defined radiologically, was the second most common extracerebral complication identified and was associated with a longer length of stay in both acute care and rehabilitation.[52] It is not unusual for brain-injured patients to have a history of pneumonitis, including recurrent pneumonitis, and present to rehabilitation with a tracheostomy in place. Decannulation of patients with a tracheostomy is a frequent consideration. Some recommend maintaining tracheostomies in patients below Rancho III. Nowak and coworkers found increased morbidity and mortality in these patients when they were decannulated.[53] A prospective study by direct endoscopy before decannulation was conducted by these authors and showed that 32 percent of patients had significant laryngeal and tracheal findings, including vocal cord paralysis, tracheal stenosis, subglottic stenosis, glottic stenosis, and tracheal malacia. It is unclear whether these complications resulted from previous intubation, polytrauma, or both.

Most clinicians do not remove the tracheostomy in TBI patients until the patients can safely swallow a regular diet. Decannulation is commonly accomplished by weaning down the tube size, followed by an intermittent tracheostomy tube plugging trial until continuous 24-h plugging can be tolerated, at which point the tracheostomy is removed. Some authors advocate an endoscopic examination of the larynx and trachea to detect granulation tissue that can impair breathing when the tracheostomy tube is removed.[38,54,55] If tracheostomy plugging is to be accomplished safely, it is imperative that a tracheostomy tube of a smaller size be cuffless to prevent accidental suffocation.

Heterotopic Ossification

Neurogenic heterotopic ossification (NHO), the formation of ectopic bone around major joints after CNS injury, is a poorly understood clinical entity that can potentially produce significant morbidity and resultant functional impairment. The incidence of NHO after TBI ranges from 11 to 76 percent depending on the sample studied and the methods used for detection.[56,57] It appears that fewer patients have functionally significant NHO than the numbers suggest.[58] Patients with TBI are at the greatest risk of developing NHO if they have significant spasticity, prolonged coma (more than 2 weeks), long bone fractures, and decreased range of motion. Ectopic bone after TBI usually forms around major joints, including the elbows, shoulders, hips, and knees. As opposed to traumatic myositis ossificans (TMO), which forms within soft tissues, NHO occurs between fascial planes. A genetic predisposition to NHO has been theorized but never proved. Various authors have examined biochemical and neuroendocrine parameters of NHO, but no consistent correlations have emerged.

The diagnosis of NHO after TBI is typically made by following the clinical exam, assessing for elevations in alkaline phosphatase (which may be elevated secondary to concurrent fractures), and confirming calcific changes with radiography. The early clinical presentation may be hallmarked by periarticular warmth and swelling followed by actual changes in "endpoint" range of motion and "feel" (soft versus hard endpoint).[58] Many clinicians rely on early detection of NHO by utilizing triple-phase bone scan technology; specifically, areas demonstrating increased blood flow and soft tissue concentration of the tracer on early imaging (blood flow phase) seem to correlate with sites of subsequent NHO development.[59] Plain radiographs may not show evidence of NHO until 4 to 5 weeks after the injury.[38] However, the exact timing of imaging and accurate assessment of ectopic bone maturity have not been established.

Present treatment options rely on both pharmacological and nonpharmacological interventions. The scientific basis for the treatment efficacy of any intervention in NHO is quite poor; therefore, no absolute treatment recommendations can be made. The mainstay of drug treatment is etidronate disodium (EHDP, Didronel), which has been shown to reduce the incidence and severity of ectopic bone formation with minimal side effects in spinal cord–injured patients and those who have undergone total hip arthroplasty.[60,61] Although optimal drug dose and length of treatment have not been adequately established in TBI, Spielman and Gennarelli suggest using 20 mg/kg/day for 3 months, followed by 10 mg/kg/day for 3 to 6 months, for a total of 6 to 9 months of treatment.[62,63] Prophylaxis with EHDP after TBI is not a routine practice in the United States.[64] In the acute stage of the condition, nonsteroidal anti-inflammatory drugs such as indomethacin can be utilized to alleviate pain and may theoretically decrease the inflammation associated with the pathogenesis of NHO. Several studies have demonstrated the efficacy of indomethacin and salicylates in decreasing ectopic bone formation after hip replacement and pediatric TBI, respectively.[65,66]

Ectopic ossification, when inadequately treated, can delay or prolong rehabilitation efforts through limiting range of motion, joint ankylosis, pain, spasticity, vascular/nerve compression, and lymphedema. It can also cause nerve shortening. Some investigators have theorized that the course and severity of NHO, as well as the response to pharmacological intervention, will vary according to the magnitude of the neurological sequelae. Although this is not yet established through scientific studies, patients who develop NHO that causes significant functional impairment typically end up with less disability if they make a good neurological recovery. Physiatric interventions aimed at decreasing potential functional morbidity include (1) early detection and maintenance of progressive range of motion with adequate analgesia and (2) control of spasticity to help maintain range of motion and function positioning (so that if ankylosis does occur, the joint can fuse in the most functional position). Surgical excision of matured NHO with and without the associated use of EHDP has become the standard treatment in this country for functionally debilitating NHO. However, establishing the diagnosis of mature NHO remains controversial and poorly studied. Other treatment modalities that have been advocated include forceful manipulation under anesthesia and low-dose radiation (postexcision).[67,68]

Central Dysautonomia

The terms "central fever," "neurogenic fever," and "hypothalamic fever" have all been used to describe elevated temperatures caused by abnormal hypothalamic function. In most mammalian species studied, the preoptic area and anterior hypothalamus (PO/AH) were established as the primary loci for thermoregulation. The normal set point for most humans ranges between 96.8 and 100 °F and exhibits a circadian rhythm with a peak body temperature at about 6 p.m. each day. Central fever is a poorly understood cause of hyperthermia in which the hypothalamic set point becomes elevated secondary to local trauma, hemorrhage, tumor, or intrinsic hypothalamic malfunction through a mechanism unrelated to sepsis.[69] Hypothermia is the more common result of hypothalamic damage; however, a few patients with hypothalamic disturbances also have persistent or intermittently elevated body temperatures.[70] Both hypothermic and hyperthermic patients have other abnormal mechanisms of thermoregulation and may exhibit poikilothermia. Clinically, patients with central fever also may demonstrate other signs of abnormal hypothalamic function, such as absent circadian temperature and hormonal rhythm, absence of perspiration, and resistance to antipyretic drugs.

In patients with TBI, it is vital to ensure that the hyperthermia is not a clinical manifestation of infection by obtaining appropriate cultures and doing other laboratory testing. Regardless of the cause, it is vital to decrease the patient's core body temperature. Fever is associated with metabolic dysfunction and potential neurological damage. Different therapeutic options have been developed for the treatment of central fever, including indomethacin, morphine, neuroleptic-type medications, and dopamine agonists such as bromocriptine.[41,46,71]

Posttraumatic Epilepsy

Approximately 5 percent of all hospitalized TBI patients develop posttraumatic epilepsy (PTE). Patients who have depressed skull fractures, acute intracranial hematomas, or seizures during the first week have an increased risk of developing late PTE.[72] Dural tearing, the presence of foreign bodies, focal signs such as aphasia and hemiplegia, and posttraumatic amnesia present for longer than 24 h are also risk factors. Determining the seizure risk of an individual patient is more difficult. In 1979, Feeney and Walker devised a mathematical model for estimating seizure risk that was based on a combination of risk factors.[73] However, this has not proved helpful in most clinical situations. Instead, patients are frequently placed on seizure prophylaxis in an acute neurosurgical setting. Neurosurgeons have traditionally prescribed phenytoin or phenobarbital because these drugs can be administered parenterally and have been in use the longest. Recent studies have shown that phenytoin beyond the first week after a brain injury does not prevent the development of late posttraumatic epilepsy.[74] In addition, the neurobehavioral side effects of phenytoin and other sedating anticonvulsants, such as phenobarbital, can be detrimental to a patient with cognitive and memory deficits and thus hamper the patient's overall progress.[75–78]

Most episodes of posttraumatic epilepsy are either simple partial or complex partial, which is secondarily generalized. Carbamazepine has been shown to be as effective as phenytoin and phenobarbital for generalized tonic-clonic seizures and more effective in controlling partial seizures.[72,77] Carbamazepine is also well tolerated and has fewer side effects (e.g., gastrointestinal distress, headaches, dizziness, diplopia); these effects are usually minimized by starting with a low dose and gradually building up to the therapeutic range. The most limiting side effect of carbamazepine is bone marrow suppression. However, transient leukopenia, primarily a relative neutropenia, can be tolerated and accepted as long as the white blood cell count is above 4000 cells/mm^3 with 50 percent of the white cells being neutrophils for this treatment phenomenon alone.[79] Another disadvantage of carbamazepine is its relatively short half-life, which makes three-times-daily dosing mandatory.[80] This can cause a significant decrease in compliance in patients with a memory impairment. However, memory aids such as beeping pill boxes and alarm watches seem to help with this problem.

Most physiatrists subspecializing in TBI rehabilitation no longer use seizure prophylaxis in patients who have not had seizures beyond the first week. Most now treat the patient only if he or she has a documented seizure and choose the most appropriate antiseizure medication for the patient.[81] Carbamazepine appears to be a good drug to use in this setting.[82–84] Valproic acid, although initially sedating, can be useful as well, since it can have fewer cognitive and behavioral side effects than does carbamazepine. Felbamate (Felbatol) has not been used extensively in the brain-injured population and was recalled after several reports of aplastic anemia. Gabapentin (Neurontin), another new antiepileptic medication, may prove to be helpful, but experience with it is limited.

Neuroendocrine Disorders

Although an array of potential neuroendocrine problems may occur after TBI, most of the commonly encountered problems are transient in nature. Panhypopituitarism is in actuality a rare posttraumatic phenomenon but may be responsible for significant alterations in the patient's level of arousal and awareness. Direct pituitary trauma as an etiology of hypopituitarism is probably less common than is hypothalamic injury. Both anterior and posterior pituitary dysfunction may occur after trauma. Anterior pituitary insufficiency after TBI should be suspected in the presence of anorexia, malaise, hypothermia, hypotension, and bradycardia associated with low serum sodium and glucose.[85,86] Hypothalamic dysfunction also may lead to aberrations in other homeostatic functions, including temperature regulation, appetite and satiety mechanisms, and thermoregulatory processes.

The most commonly encountered endocrine disorder associated with TBI is the syndrome of inappropriate antidiuretic hormone secretion (SIADH).[42,87] This clinical condition, which is related to posterior pituitary dysfunction, is commonly seen in the early phases after an injury and is manifested clinically by hyponatremia.[88] Significant hyponatremia may cause additional neurological problems, such as seizures. Hyponatremia also may be due to "cerebral salt-wasting syndrome." Treatment with mineralocorticoids can be effective in this group of patients. Posttraumatic patients may less commonly experience hypernatremia secondary to problems with central diabetes insipidus (DI), which may manifest clinically with polyuria and elevated serum sodium levels. DI is traditionally treated with desmopressin (DDAVP).[89]

Thyroid dysfunction, commonly in the form of euthyroid disease, may occasionally be seen after a trauma.[90] Sexual dysfunction may be seen in several forms after TBI.[90,91] The most common manifestations include problems with delayed resumption of menstruation and libidinal alterations,[92] although the exact neuroendocrine correlates of these clinical manifestations have not been identified. Studies also suggest that transient hypotestosteronemia is a relatively common occurrence, although the exact clinical significance of this finding on recovery and sexual function has not been delineated.

Communicating Hydrocephalus

Current clinical use of the term "communicating hydrocephalus" implies an abnormality in the absorption of CSF. CSF flows through the ventricular system and cisterns and over the convexities for subsequent absorption into the superior sagittal sinus via the arachnoid villi. If the absorption of CSF is impaired, as can occur with blood clogging up the arachnoid villi, hydrocephalus results. The degree of pressure elevation is quite variable, and the pathogenesis of "normal-pressure" hydrocephalus is incompletely understood.

The incidence of posttraumatic ventriculomegaly (PTV) varies according to the method used in documenting ventricular enlargement, the severity of the neural insult, and the definition used. If one takes into consideration all previous studies without controlling for the severity of injury or method of analysis in those groups, the incidence of posttraumatic ventriculomegaly in severe TBI averages 62 percent.[93] In comparison, the incidence of communicating hydrocephalus requiring shunting is probably about 3 to 8 percent.[94]

Posttraumatic communicating hydrocephalus (PTH) has historically been a difficult clinical entity to diagnose because of the lack of sensitive and definitive clinical diagnostic tests for this condition. Additionally, its presentation tends to be inconsistent, making its identification even more of a challenge, particularly in low-level TBI patients. The main clinical markers for suspecting communicating hydrocephalus are prolonged coma and an arrest in clinical progress.

Posttraumatic hydrocephalus may present in a variety of different ways aside from the classic presentation of normal-pressure hydrocephalus (NPH). The degree of neurological deficit in patients with PTH is variable and extends from deep coma to the dementia, incontinence, and gait disturbance typically associated with NPH.[93,95–97]

Few studies have documented the relationship of PTH and outcome. The available literature suggests that the greater the ventriculomegaly, the worse the performance of patients. Shunting is the mainstay of treatment in posttraumatic hydrocephalus. However, shunts should be inserted only when there is a reversible deficit or a progressive condition. Shunting is not without associated morbidity, including shunt infection and mechanical failure.

If suspicion of the development of PTH is high, serial monthly computed tomography (CT) scans can help clarify the diagnosis.[98,99] The determination of which patients might benefit from shunting is usually based on a constellation of findings and remains an imperfect art. If the patient meets clinical and radiographic criteria for posttraumatic hydrocephalus, a lumbar puncture for craniospinal axis pressure should be obtained. Generally, shunting is successful when the pressure is elevated above 180 mmH_2O or if the ventricles are progressively increasing in size. The patient is also likely to benefit if there is a clinical picture of normal-pressure hydrocephalus.[100] However, in many cases it is difficult to predict whether a patient will benefit from shunt diversion. CT cisternography and radionuclide cisternography may be helpful; however, the reliability of these tests is not universally acknowledged. Bolus infusion studies have not become widely used, although some reports seem to be encouraging.[101]

The use of an adapted version of the CSF tap test[102] has been helpful in some cases. This test involves the utilization of psychometric measures and gait pattern observation before and after a lumbar puncture in which a large quantity of CSF (30 to 60 ml) is removed. Improvement in test results after the removal of fluid implies that successful results will occur if the patient is shunted.

Ocular Care

Patients may sustain direct injuries to the orbital area that can result in cranial nerve and ocular damage. In addition, patients with a decreased ability to communicate are particularly susceptible to corneal injuries. The most deleterious effect of facial nerve injuries is inadequate lid closure. A patient with such an injury is susceptible to exposure keratitis, and if cranial nerve V also has been injured, resulting in corneal sensation being lost, the problem is compounded. It is imperative that the eye be protected by using lubricants and taping the lid closed with eye pads. Unfortunately, this technique is not foolproof and, if not done properly, may cause further damage. Alternatively, the use of an occlusive transparent film that covers the ocular area and creates a "wet chamber" has been utilized successfully in some patients to keep the cornea lubricated. Lid tarsorrhaphy may be necessary to prevent further damage, especially in a low-level patient.

Injury to the motor system of the eye, which is controlled by cranial nerves III, IV, and VI, can occur at several levels, both centrally and peripherally. Secondary insults may occur after impact, as with temporal herniation caused by edema leading to cranial nerve III injury. Strabismus after trauma may be due to cranial nerve injuries, but there are also certain gaze deviations seen in the early stages after brain injury that are not due to cranial nerve injury. Objective testing to determine ocular alignment can be simply determined by noting symmetrical placement of the corneal reflection of a penlight in each of the cardinal eye positions (Herschberg reflex). If the images on both corneas are centered, the visual axes are usually well aligned. A cover/uncover test generally will determine the presence of misalignment of the visual axes when both eyes are viewing, but the need to ensure fixation may limit its utility and agitate a noncooperative patient. Convergence and accommodation testing should be performed when possible. Drug effects, most commonly from phenytoin and phenobarbital, also may impair these reflexes. Diplopia occurring at near vision only may be the result of an impaired vergence system.[103]

It is unclear whether oculomotor exercises utilized by neuro-optometry specialists are of any value in this population since there have been no comprehensive studies to establish their efficacy. However, anecdotal evidence by the authors indicates that such procedures may be helpful. Certainly the use of corrective prisms when a patient's alignment is several diopters off is helpful for patients who can utilize them.

Musculoskeletal Complications

As early as 1970, a study noted that 82 percent of patients with TBI admitted to the hospital sustained one or more extracranial injuries.[104] The Traumatic Brain Injury Model System National Database noted that 71 percent of TBI patients had one or more associated injuries, among which cranial nerve injuries and fractures were the most common. A total of 406 fractures and 100 cranial nerve injuries were recorded in 323 patients.[52] Patients injured in pedestrian/auto and motor vehicle crashes tend to have higher incidences of fractures and cranial nerve injuries than do those injured by other causes.

The physiatrist is often faced with the challenge of diagnosing musculoskeletal injuries in comatose and confused or agitated patients who are unable to cooperate in a complete motor/sensory evaluation or even to complain of pain. Most authors suggest repeating a set of radiographs that include cervical spine, pelvis, hips, and knees to screen for fractures.[46] Routine anterior-posterior radiographs of the extremities in a comatose patient minimize the risk of undiagnosed injuries. Questionable fractures or dislocations require further evaluation. Some authors advocate the use of a bone scan 7 to 10 days after the injury to detect occult fractures.[105] An added advantage of bone scans is that they allow early detection of heterotopic ossification.[41,46] Treatment of musculoskeletal complications should always be based on the presumption that the patient will make a good recovery regardless of prognostic indicators to the contrary.

Management techniques that require prolonged traction are often contraindicated except in unusual circumstances, because they impede the rehabilitation program. Since spasticity usually causes joints to become flexed, immobilization by a cast in a flexed position should be avoided, even if it adequately treats the fracture.[105]

SPECIAL CLINICAL ISSUES IN TBI REHABILITATION

LOW-LEVEL PATIENT

Ninety percent of severely head injured patients who survive the initial phase[106] regain consciousness within 3 to 4 weeks of the injury. The other 10 percent remain unconscious but regain eye-opening and sleep-awake cycles. They also regain reflexes and behaviors that reflect intact brainstem function, including pupillary activity, oculocephalic responses, roving gaze movements, and chewing. Autonomic or vegetative function, such as breathing and control of circulation, is regained, along with bowel and bladder automatic function. These patients, who are no longer comatose, are often classified as being in the *vegetative state.* Vegetative state patients demonstrate arousal without concurrent awareness. Patients who are severely impaired and functionally disabled but show some, albeit intermittent, awareness have been termed minimally responsive. *Permanent* vegetative state is established at 12 months posttrauma and at 3 months after hypoxic insult.

ASSESSING THE LOW-LEVEL PATIENT

Whereas the Glasgow Coma Scale (GCS)[107] is useful in neurotrauma care, it has limited sensitivity as a measure of progress in vegetative and minimally responsive patients. The GCS scores of such patients range only between 7 and 10, depending on the level of motor response to painful stimulation. The Disability Rating Scale[108] has the same limitations because in an unconscious patient, the only scoreable scale components are the eye, motor, and verbal ratings of the GCS. The Rancho Los Amigos Levels of Cognitive Functioning[109] is also insensitive because low-level patients are all categorized as level II or level III. The Coma Near-Coma scale (CNC) developed by Rappaport and colleagues[110] rates the patient's reaction to pain, ability to follow commands, and response to various stimulations in auditory, visual, tactile, and olfactory modalities. Using the CNC, patients are categorized into levels of *extreme* coma, *marked* coma, *moderate* coma, or *near* coma, which are defined as follows:

- Extreme coma—no response to stimulation in any modality and no vocalization
- Marked coma—inconsistent responses to stimulation in one modality without any vocalization or ability to follow commands
- Moderate coma—inconsistent response in two or three modalities, with nonverbal vocalizations possible
- Near coma—consistent responses in two modalities and/or follows commands inconsistently

Alternative rating methods for assessing unconscious patients include the Western Neurosensory Stimulation Profile,[111] the Sensory Stimulation Assessment Measure,[112] and the Coma Recovery Scale.[113]

Neuroimaging and electrophysiological studies contribute to the evaluation of unconscious patients but do not replace the clinical neurological evaluation as the basic method for diagnosis and prognostication. Neuroimaging can reveal correctable causes of unconsciousness and help predict recovery. Standard EEG and evoked potentials can be normal during unconsciousness and therefore may have limited value in diagnosis and prognosis.[7]

It is imperative that unconsciousness be differentiated from conditions that are commonly associated with severe TBI and can interfere with responsiveness. These common conditions include systemic illness, drug-induced sedation, malnourishment, and understimulation. Aphasia, apraxia, or poor comprehension of the examiner's language can also interfere with the ability to follow commands.

OUTCOME STUDIES

In studies of outcome from traumatic coma, recovery of consciousness occurred in 40 to 50 percent of patients, usually within 3 months after the injury. Among the remainder who failed to recover consciousness, 20 to 30 percent did not survive the first year. Recovery of consciousness is probably the most important milestone in neurological recovery, because most patients who regain consciousness continue to recover function and eventually reach the point where they can be discharged from institutional care and live at home. Prolonged traumatic unconsciousness for more than 6 months (i.e., persistent vegetative state) is usually incompatible with a normal life expectancy because such patients are prone to develop significant medical complications, including respiratory tract and urinary tract infections.

COMA MANAGEMENT

The hallmark of good coma management is the reduction of medications that may hinder the recovery of arousal and consciousness. Many medications used to treat seizure disorders, spasticity, and gastrointestinal disturbances in TBI patients have sedating side effects that can decrease a patient's arousal and hinder the recovery of consciousness. A patient's ability to follow commands may be hampered by the use of anticonvulsant prophylaxis and the use of sedating antispasticity medications such as dantrolene sodium, diazepam, and baclofen. Additional examples of drugs with potential sedating side effects are metoclopramide and H_2 antagonists used in low-level patients with reflux and beta blockers such as propranolol used in low-level patients with dysautonomia or primary hypertension. Clonidine, verapamil, and diuretics are better choices for the treatment of hypertension in low-level patients.

Drugs that have anticholinergic side effects, such as amitriptyline, imipramine, and sinequan, usually have some sedating side effects. Although antidepressants could increase the action of some neurotransmitters, such as norepinephrine, these drugs seem to have enough anticholinergic effects to decrease arousal. The same holds true for neuroleptics such as haloperidol (Haldol), chlorpromazine (Thorazine), and thioridazine (Stelazine); therefore, there are limited indications for the use of such drugs in low-level patients.

Several anecdotal reports have described the use of medications to increase arousal and facilitate the recovery of consciousness in some patients.[3,4,39,41,46,119–121] In addition, there have been some limited studies in animal models using dextroamphetamine to improve recovery.[3,4] Arousal-increasing drugs, such as dopaminergic agonists (levodopa, bromocriptine, and amantadine) can certainly be considered once the patient is out of danger from increased intracranial pressure. Drugs such as dextroamphetamine methylphenidate and pemoline may be useful in this regard. In addition, serotonergically acting drugs, in particular fluoxitene (Prozac) and sertraline (Zoloft), may play a role in increasing arousal. An advantage of the dopaminergic drugs is that they may help with central fever, as was noted previously.

The concept of sensory stimulation is no longer accepted as part of coma management. The original rationale for this approach was that stimulation in multiple sensory modalities would increase arousal and responsiveness, thus facilitating emergence from coma. Studies in the United States and abroad have not borne this out.[12,122] However, one component of sensory stimulation that may play a useful role is the system for monitoring patients' responsiveness by multiple team members. The rating scales discussed previously are useful for this purpose. The current view is that the value of sensory stimulation lies only in coordinating the team's assessment of the patient's level of arousal, ability to perceive stimuli, and ability to attend. To ensure consistent monitoring of responses during stimulation sessions, a standard stimulation kit is used and a standard record is completed by team members after each stimulation session.

Agitated Patients

It is not unusual for patients to experience a phase of acute agitation after they regain consciousness. Typically, agitated patients are in posttraumatic amnesia, with confusion and severely impaired recent memory. Agitated patients may thrash about; remove restraints, tubes, or catheters; fall out of bed; or wander away from the rehabilitation unit. They can present a danger to themselves and to others. The underlying causes for this behavior are believed to be severe confusion and absence of continuous memory. Nevertheless, the physician must be alert to the possibility of contributing factors such as sleep disturbances, seizure activity, hydrocephalus, malnutrition, vitamin deficiency, and electrolyte imbalance, which are potentially complicating factors that should be ruled out or treated if found. Conditions that cause discomfort, such as spasticity, unrecognized musculoskeletal injury, and subacute infection, must be ruled out as well. Medications commonly used to control agitation, such as minor tranquilizers, neuroleptics, antihypertensives and medications for the gastrointestinal tract, may actually create unintended problems by increasing confusion, which may in turn worsen the agitation.

The first line of management for an agitated patient is to use one or more of the following behavioral and environmental approaches to create a minimum-stimulation environment: use of a quiet and safe structured area such as a floor bed; removal of noxious stimuli such as tubes, catheters, and restraints; and use of trained attendants to provide physical and verbal reassurance. When behavioral and environmental techniques do not succeed and the patient still presents a danger to himself or herself or to others, pharmacological intervention may be necessary. In recent years, there has been a tendency to move away from the use of sedating medications that may increase confusion. Sutton and colleagues have noted that neuroleptics may contribute to the underlying confused state and have long-term side effects, thus theoretically impeding recovery.[123] Minor tranquilizers may decrease a patient's muscle tone, increase memory deficits, and have paradoxical as well as enhanced side effects. For example, midazolam (Versed) may cause increased respiratory depression in patients with brainstem injuries. Physiatrists experienced in TBI are often more apt to try lorazepam (Ativan), less sedating antidepressants, or serotonergics such as trazadone (Deseryl). Mood stabilizers (e.g., lithium) and psychostimulants could theoretically cause agitation. The physician should consider that since confusion may partly cause agitation, increasing patients' attention to the environment may actually decrease their agitation. If a patient's agitation is not controllable in an acute rehabilitation unit, transfer to a neurobehavioral unit may be indicated. Severe acute agitation, in which the patient becomes so violent and uncontrollable that he or she needs to be restrained by many team members, may be treated with IM or IV administration of haloperidol 5 mg and lorazepam (Ativan) to 2 mg IV every 20 min until the patient is quieted. This should be used only in emergency situations and should be reserved for patients who present an immediate danger to themselves or others.

Cognitive Rehabilitation

Cognitive rehabilitation refers to therapies that are used to treat cognitive impairments resulting from acquired brain injury. Of the two basic approaches used in practice, the accepted approach is based on the concept of learning compensatory strategies, as was mentioned in the discussion of postacute rehabilitation. The second and more controversial approach, termed *cognitive retraining* (or the *process* approach), is based on the concept that the brain's cognitive capacity can be partly restored by the repetitive practice of special exercises. The most controversial form of cognitive retraining involves patients practicing computerized tasks that are designed to remediate their deficits in memory or other specific cognitive functions (e.g., by memorizing lists of words). There already exists a market of cognitive rehabilitation software packages, with minimal efficacy data or user training to justify either their therapeutic claims or their cost. Critics of cognitive retraining state that its efficacy has not been empirically supported, although several evaluation studies have been conducted,[124,125] and that it is not based on known neurobiological mechanisms. Thus, cognitive process training is an investigational form of treatment that requires more empirical and theoretical support.

Unfortunately, many critics of cognitive retraining tend to blur the distinction between cognitive retraining and the compensatory approach, which is based on the relatively noncontroversial concept that patients can learn to be more functional despite their impairments. This approach is similar to the use of compensatory strategies (e.g., transfer training) and environmental modifications (e.g., wheelchair ramps) in rehabilitating physically disabled persons. The compensatory approach is supported by studies showing that chronic brain-injured patients who participate in return-to-work programs have better vocational outcomes.[16,18] The major criticism of the compensatory approach is that while it is possible for brain-injured patients to learn compensatory strategies during therapy, it is likely that some patients will fail to carry over these strategies into the "real world." In particular, patients with a limited ability to generalize strategies may be functional only within highly modified living and working environments. Overall, the available evidence supports the use of compensatory training and environmental modifications, as long as the treatment is directed at realistic goals and is used with patients who have adequate learning potential.

Families of Brain-Injured Patients

Increasing experience with the long-term consequences of brain injury has led clinicians to recognize that adverse effects occur not only in patients but also in the lives of their family members.[126] Particularly high levels of emotional distress, sometimes leading to clinical depression, have been noted in the family members of patients who remain in a vegetative state, have marked personality changes, or require constant supervision at home. While recognizing that many of the consequences of brain injury for the family are inevitable, clinicians can still play an important role in helping family members cope with their predicament, mainly by providing accurate information and being emotionally supportive. The need for information is underlined by family members' complaints in retrospective surveys[127] that they were not kept adequately informed by the acute care team. In the acute stage, prognostic information can be given by stating the range of probable outcomes and acknowledging the uncertainty of long-range predictions. Educating family members about neurobehavioral impairments can help them understand and cope with personality and emotional changes. After the acute stage, the team should take family members' options into account when planning rehabilitation, since the lives of all family members can be affected (e.g., location of acute rehabilitation facility).

Resources for Long-Term Management

Long-term rehabilitation management of severely head injured patients is largely dictated by their reemployment potential and funding resources. As was mentioned above, patients with good reemployment potential should be referred to the state vocational rehabilitation agency for help in returning to work. For patients who have poor reemployment potential, the rehabilitation goals should be to improve the quality of life and minimize dependence on family members. Unfortunately, long-term services for this large category of patients is the weakest link in the continuum of care for head injury survivors in the United States because of the absence of a public rehabilitation system for persons with head injuries and other acquired disabilities. Two new resources that are not yet available in all states are catastrophic rehabilitation funds and long-term residential facilities. Catastrophic funds are government-administered programs, funded through taxes or traffic fines, that pay for rehabilitation services. For example, the Comprehensive Rehabilitation Services program administered by the Texas Rehabilitation Commission funds rehabilitation on the basis of patients' financial need, regardless of their reemployment potential. There is a major need for long-term residential facilities, such as group homes and low-cost apartment programs, for patients who can live in the community with some support services.

Mild Head Injury Rehabilitation

Rehabilitation of a patient with a mild head injury is a controversial topic and has been reviewed in several publications.[128–130] Major factors in rehabilitation planning are objective evidence of brain injury, age, and chronicity. Mild head injury patients (i.e., GCS score of 13 to 15) who have traumatic brain lesions on CT scan may have worse cognitive and functional recoveries, similar to patients with moderate head injury.[131] Elderly persons may recover more slowly and less completely from mild head injury compared with younger adults. Thus, clinicians treating elderly mild head injury patients should have a higher index of suspicion for complications and should extend the periods of close observation and follow-up, as in treating younger patients with moderate head injury.

Most nonelderly patients with an acute mild head injury can be managed with education and temporary activity restriction. Patients and family members should be educated about expected postconcussional symptoms (e.g., irritability, difficulty concentrating). A follow-up clinic visit or phone call is recommended even for patients with apparently uncomplicated injuries to monitor recovery and reinforce earlier education. Patients who have significant cognitive deficits should be given a brief leave from work, school, or even home responsibilities. Prolonged time away from work can be avoided by returning to work part-time or by selective restriction from the most demanding activities (e.g., stressful job duties, school examinations).

Patients who initially present months or years after a mild head injury should not be assumed to have "compensation neurosis." Some chronic patients have occult nonbrain injuries that were undetected in the acute stage and result in persistent unpleasant or even disabling symptoms (e.g., headaches, vertigo). However, the postconcussional complaints of some patients are complicated or caused by malingering or by psychiatric syndromes (e.g., depression, chronic pain syndrome), although the frequency of these problems has been debated.[132]

Ethics

The industry of brain injury rehabilitation has recently had a major shake-up in which ethical violations were exposed in some centers. A common ethical problem is the unjustifiably prolonged treatment of certain patients, often associated with unscrupulous marketing practices aimed at families or payers. The utilization of brain injury rehabilitation is undergoing close scrutiny by third-party payers, and rehabilitation professionals are becoming more accountable in terms of showing functional change as a result of their services. This has led to the development of more stringent documentation of improvement, for example, through the Functional Independence Measure (FIM).[133]

Obviously, there are instances in which patients receive rehabilitation far beyond what is needed, for several years in some cases, with no discernible gain in function. In addition, new guidelines for the removal of feeding tubes in vegetative state patients have been published by the American Academy of Neurology[9,10] that indicate that ethical considerations are now catching up with technical advances. Removal of feeding tubes is usually left to neurosurgeons in the acute care facility, but occasionally physiatrists are called on to make these determinations and support the family through this overwhelming decision. Finally, as patients become more cognizant, they need to play an active role in their rehabilitation and should be actively included in setting their own long-term rehabilitation goals.

SUMMARY

Traumatic brain injury rehabilitation has undergone changes and expansion over the past several years. It is the rare patient who will not benefit from the intervention of a rehabilitation team, if only for family education. Patients who are unconscious should not be transferred to a nursing home "until they wake up." Patients who are treated in this fashion are more prone to complications and have more disability than do those who are aggressively treated in the rehabilitation setting or at least managed in a rehabilitation setting and then sent to a nursing home if they fail to wake up. Their care is easier, their families are calmer, and certainly the care is more humane. Every patient with a traumatic brain injury needs to be given the benefit of the doubt that his or her outcome will be good so that all complications—intracranial or extracranial—will be treated aggressively during the acute phase to prevent and minimize subsequent disability.

References

1. Boyeson MG, Bach-y-Rita P: Determinants of brain plasticity. *J Neurol Rehabil* 3:35–37, 1989.
2. Boyeson MG: Neurochemical alterations after brain in-

jury: Clinical implications for pharmacologic rehabilitation. *Neurorehabilitation* 1:33–43, 1991.
3. Feeney DM, Sutton RL: Pharmacotherapy for recovery of function after brain injury. *CRC Crit Rev Neurobiol* 3:135, 1987.
4. Feeney DM: Pharmacologic modulation of recovery after brain injury: A reconsideration of diaschisis. *J Neurol Rehab* 5:113, 1991.
5. Uomoto J, McLean A: Care continuum in traumatic brain injury. *Rehab Psychol* 34:71–80, 1989.
6. Kreutzer JS, Zasler ND, Devany CW: Neuromedical and psychosocial aspects of rehabilitation after traumatic brain injury, in Fletcher G, Jann B, Wolf S, Banja J (eds): *Rehabilitation Medicine: State of the Art Reviews.* New York: Lea & Febiger, 1992: 63–103.
7. Bontke CF, Boake C: Principles of brain injury rehabilitation, in Braddom R (ed): *Textbook of Physical Medicine and Rehabilitation.* Philadelphia: Saunders, 1995: 1027–1051.
8. Dixon T: Systems of care for the head-injured. *Phys Med Rehabil* 3:169–181, 1995.
9. Multi-Society Task Force on PVS: Medical aspects of the persistent vegetative state (1). *N Engl J Med* 330:1499, 1994.
10. Multi-Society Task Force on PVS: Medical aspects of the persistent vegetative state (2). *N Engl J Med* 330:1572, 1994.
11. Bontke CF, Horn LJ, Sandel B: Sensory stimulation: Accepted practice or expected practice? *J Head Trauma Rehabil* 7:115, 1992.
12. Zasler ND, Kreutzer JS, Taylor D: Coma stimulation and coma recovery: A critical review. *Neurorehabilitation* 1:33, 1991.
13. Zasler ND: A medical perspective on physician training and brain injury rehabilitation, in Durgin CJ, Schmidt ND, Fryer LJ (eds): *Staff Development and Clinical Intervention in Brain Injury Rehabilitation.* Baltimore: Aspen, 1993: 257–269.
14. Sandel ME: Rehabilitation management in the acute care setting. *Phys Med Rehabil* 3:27–42, 1989.
15. Zasler ND, Devany CW: Traumatic brain injury rehabilitation in the military, in Dillingham TW (ed): *Physical Medicine and the Rehabilitative Management of War Casualties.* Borden Institute, 1994.
16. High WM Jr, Boake C, Lehmkuhl LD: Critical analysis of studies measuring the effectiveness of rehabilitation following traumatic brain injury. *J Head Trauma Rehabil* 10:14–26, 1995.
17. Evans RW, Ruff RM: Outcome and value: A perspective on rehabilitation outcomes achieved in acquired brain injury. *J Head Trauma Rehabil* 7:24–36, 1992.
18. Bleiberg J, Cope DN, Spector J: Cognitive assessment and therapy in traumatic brain injury. *Phys Med Rehabil* 3:95–121, 1989.
19. Hall KM, Cope DN: The benefit of rehabilitation in traumatic brain injury: A literature review. *J Head Trauma Rehabil* 10:1–13, 1995.
20. Wehman PH, West MD, Kregel J, et al: Return to work for persons with severe traumatic brain injury: A data-based approach to program development. *J Head Trauma Rehabil* 10:27–39, 1995.
21. Boake C: Transitional living centers in head injury rehabilitation, in Kreutzer JS, Wehman PH (eds): *Community Integration Following Traumatic Brain Injury.* Baltimore: Paul H. Brooks, 1990: 115–124.
22. Aronow HU: Rehabilitation effectiveness with severe brain injury: Translating research into policy. *J Head Trauma Rehabil* 2:24, 1987.
23. Johnston MV: The economics of brain injury: A preface, in Miner ME, Wagner KA (eds): *Treatment and Rehabilitation and Related Issues.* Boston: Butterworths, 1989: 163–185.
24. Ashley MJ, Krych DK, Lehr RP Jr: Cost/benefit analysis for post-acute rehabilitation of the traumatically brain-injured patient. *J Insur Med* 22:156–161, 1990.
25. Lehmkuhl LD, Hall KM, Mann N, Gordon WA: Factors that influence costs and length of stay of persons with traumatic brain injury in acute care and inpatient rehabilitation. *J Head Trauma Rehabil* 8:88–100, 1993.
26. Rosenthal M: The traumatic brain injury model systems of care. *J Head Trauma Rehabil* 8:1–116, 1993.
27. Conine TA, Sullivan T, Mackie T, Goodman M: Effect of serial casting for the prevention of equinus in patients with acute head injury. *Arch Phys Med Rehabil* 71:310, 1990.
28. Gouvier WD, Uddo-Crane M, Brown LM: Base rates of post-concussional symptoms. *Arch Clin Neuropsychol* 3:273, 1988.
29. Glenn MB, Rosenthal M: Rehabilitation following severe traumatic brain injury. *Semin Neurol* 5:233, 1985.
30. Weintraub AH, Opat CA: Motor and sensory dysfunction in the brain injured adult. *Phys Med Rehabil* 3:59, 1989.
31. Lehmkuhl LD, Thoi L, Baize C, et al: Multimodality treatment of joint contractures in patients with severe brain injury. *J Head Trauma Rehabil* 5(2):23–42, 1990.
32. Khalili AA, Betts HB: Peripheral nerve block with phenol in the management of spasticity: Indications and complications. *JAMA* 200:1155, 1967.
33. Loubser PG, Bontke CF, Baize CM: Quadruple motor neurolysis for shoulder and elbow flexor hypertonicity (abstract). *Arch Phys Med Rehabil* 72:826, 1991.
34. Loubser PG, Bontke CF, Baize CM: Intramuscular neurolytic blocks for upper extremity spasticity in head injury (abstract). *Anesthesiology* 71:A763, 1989.
35. Loubser PG, Bontke CF, Vandeventer J: Selective epidural phenol rhizolysis for hip flexor spasticity (abstract). *Arch Phys Med Rehabil* 70:A38, 1989.
36. Yablon SA, Agana BT, Ivanhoe CB, Boake C: Botulinum toxin in severe upper extremity spasticity among patients with traumatic brain injury: An open-labeled trial. *Neurology* (in press).
37. Lazarus C, Logemann JA: Swallowing disorders in closed head trauma patients. *Arch Phys Med Rehabil* 68:79, 1987.
38. Adamovich BB: Treatment of communication and swallowing disorders, in Rosenthal M, Griffith ER, Bond MR, Miller JC (eds): *Rehabilitation of the Adult and*

Child with Traumatic Brain Injury. Philadelphia: Davis, 1990: 374–392.

39. Bontke CF, Baize CM, Boake C: Coma management and sensory stimulation. *Phys Med Rehabil Clin North Am* 3:259, 1992.
40. Anonymous: Metoclopramide (Reglan) for gastrointestinal reflux. *Med Lett Drugs Ther* 27:21, 1985.
41. Bontke CF: Medical advances in the treatment of brain injury, in Kreutzer JS, Wehman PA (eds): *Community Reintegration Following Traumatic Brain Injury.* Baltimore: Paul H. Brookes, 1990: 3–14.
42. Chestnut RM: Medical complications of the head injured patient, in Cooper PR (ed): *Head Injury.* Philadelphia: William & Wilkins, 1993: 225–246.
43. Halloran LG, Zass AM, Gayle WE, et al: Prevention of acute gastrointestinal complications after severe head injury: A controlled trial of cimetidine prophylaxis. *Am J Surg* 139:44, 1980.
44. Clifton GL, Robertson CS, Choi SC: Assessment of nutritional requirements of head-injured patients. *J Neurosurg* 64:895–901, 1985.
45. Graham TW, Zadrozny DB, Harrington T: The benefits of early jejunal hyperalimentation in the head-injured patient. *Neurosurgery* 25:729, 1989.
46. Bontke CF: Medical complications related to traumatic brain injury. *Phys Med Rehabil* 3:1, 1989.
47. Whyte J, Glenn MB: The care and rehabilitation of the patient in a persistent vegetative state. *J Head Trauma Rehabil* 1:39, 1986.
48. Lerman RM, Bontke CF: Clostridium difficile colitis: Nosocomial acquisition and cross infection among head injured patients. *Crit Rev Phys Med Rehabil* 1:247, 1990.
49. Johnson JH: Rehabilitative aspects of neurologic bladder dysfunction. *Nurs Clin North Am* 15:293, 1980.
50. Grinspun D: Bladder management for adults following head injury. *Rehabil Nurs* 18:300, 1993.
51. Anderson JT: Neuro-urological investigation in urinary bladder dysfunction. *Int Urol Nephrol* 9:133, 1977.
52. Bontke CF, Lehmkuhl DL, Englander JS, et al: Medical complications and associated injuries of persons treated in traumatic brain injury model systems programs. *J Head Trauma Rehabil* 8:34, 1993.
53. Nowak P, Cohn AM, Guidice MA: Airway complications in patients with closed-head injuries. *Am J Otolaryngol* 8:91, 1987.
54. Klingbeil GEG: Airway problems in patients with head injury. *Arch Phys Med Rehabil* 69:493, 1988.
55. Garland DE, Bailey S: Undetected injuries in head-injured adults. *Clin Orthop Rel Res* 155:162, 1981.
56. Garland DE, Blum CE, Waters RL: Periarticular heterotopic ossification in head-injured adults. *J Bone Joint Surg* 62A:1143, 1981.
57. Sazbon L, Najenson T, Tartakovsky M, et al: Widespread periarticular new-bone formation in long-term comatose patients. *J Bone Joint Surg* 63B:120, 1981.
58. Buschbacher R: Heterotopic ossification: A review. *Crit Rev Phys Med Rehabil* 4:199, 1992.
59. Freed JH, Hahn H, Menter R, et al: The use of the three-phase bone scan in the early diagnosis of heterotopic ossification (HO) and in the evaluation of Didronel therapy. *Paraplegia* 20:208, 1982.
60. Fingerman G, Krengel W, Lowell JD, et al: Role of diphosphonate EHDP in the prevention of heterotopic ossification after total hip arthroplasty: Preliminary report, in *Proceedings of the Fifth Open Scientific Meeting of the Hip Society.* St. Louis: Mosby, 1977: 222–234.
61. Stover SL, Hahn HR, Miller JM: Disodium etidronate in the prevention of heterotopic ossification following spinal cord injury. *Paraplegia* 14:146, 1976.
62. Gennarelli TA: Subject review: Heterotopic ossification. *Brain Inj* 2:175, 1988.
63. Spielman G, Gennarelli TA, Rogers CR: Disodium etidronate: Its role in preventing heterotopic ossification in severe head injury. *Arch Phys Med Rehabil* 64:539, 1983.
64. Rogers RC: Program idea: Heterotopic calcification in severe head injury: A prevention program. *Brain Inj* 2:169, 1988.
65. Ritter MA, Gioe T: The effect of indomethacin on para-articular ectopic ossification following total hip arthroplasty. *Clin Orthop* 167:113, 1982.
66. Mital MA, Garbar JE, Stinson JT: Ectopic bone formation in children and adolescents with head injury: Its management. *J Pediatr Orthop* 7:83, 1987.
67. Garland DE, Razza BE, Waters RL: Forceful joint manipulation in head-injured adults with heterotopic ossification. *Clin Orthop Rel Res* 169:133, 1982.
68. Coventry MB, Scanlon PW: The use of radiation to discourage ectopic bone. *J Bone Joint Surg* 63:201, 1981.
69. Van Hilten JJ, Roos RAC: Posttraumatic hyperthermia: A possible result of frontodiencephalic dysfunction. *Clin Neurol Neurosurg* 93:223, 1991.
70. Rossitch E, Bullard DE: The autonomic dysfunction syndrome: Etiology and treatment. *Br J Neurosurg* 2:471, 1988.
71. Benedek G, Toth-Daru P, Janaky J, et al: Indomethacin is effective against neurogenic hyperthermia following cranial trauma or brain surgery. *Can J Neurol Sci* 14:145, 1987.
72. Jennett B: Posttraumatic epilepsy, in Rosenthal M, Griffith ER, Bond MR, Miller JD (eds): *Rehabilitation of the Head Injured Adult.* Philadelphia: Davis Company, 1983: 89–93.
73. Feeney DM, Walker AE: The prediction of posttraumatic epilepsy. *Arch Neurol* 36:8, 1979.
74. Temkin NR, Dikmen SS, Wilensky AJ, et al: A randomized, double-blind study of phenytoin for the prevention of posttraumatic seizures. *N Engl J Med* 323:497, 1990.
75. Farwell JR, Lee YJ, Hirtz DG, et al: Phenobarbital for febrile seizures-effects on intelligence and on seizure recurrence. *N Engl J Med* 322:364, 1990.
76. Dikmen SS, Temkin NR, Miller B, et al: Neurobehavioral effects of phenytoin prophylaxis of posttraumatic seizures. *JAMA* 265:1271, 1991.
77. Massagli TL: Neurobehavioral effects of phenytoin, carbamazepine and valproic acid: Implications for use in traumatic brain injury. *Arch Phys Med Rehabil* 72:219, 1991.
78. Andrews DG, Tomlinson L, Elwes RDC, et al: The

influence of carbamazepine and phenytoin on memory and other aspects of cognitive function in new referrals with epilepsy. *Acta Neurol Scand* 69:23, 1984.
79. Pisciotta AV: Hematological toxicity, in Woodbury DM, Penry JK, Pippenger CE (eds): *Antiepileptic Drugs.* New York, Raven Press, 1982: 533–541.
80. Drugs for Epilepsy. *Med Lett Drugs Ther* 28:91–94, 1986.
81. Bontke CF, Reinhard DL, Yablon SA: Anticonvulsant prophylaxis for the prevention of late posttraumatic epilepsy. *J Head Trauma Rehabil* 8:101, 1993.
82. Glenn MB, Wroblewski B: Anticonvulsants for prophylaxis of posttraumatic seizures. *J Head Trauma Rehabil* 1:73, 1986.
83. Ramsey RE: Advances in the pharmacotherapy of epilepsy. *Epilepsia* 34:S9–S16, 1993.
84. Yablon S: Posttraumatic seizures. *Arch Phys Med Rehabil* 74:83, 1993.
85. Barreca T, Perrea C, Sannia A, et al: Evaluation of anterior pituitary function in patients with posttraumatic diabetes insipidus. *J Clin Endocrinol Metab* 51:1279, 1980.
86. Klingbeil GEG, Kleine P: Anterior hypopituitarism: A consequence of head injury. *Arch Phys Med Rehabil* 66:44, 1985.
87. Hansen JR, Cook JS: Posttraumatic neuroendocrine disorders. *Phys Med Rehabil* 7:569, 1993.
88. Doczi T, Tarjanyi J, Huszka E, Kiss J: Syndrome of inappropriate secretion of antidiuretic hormone (SIADH) after head injury. *Neurosurgery* 10:685, 1980.
89. Notman DD, Mortek MA, Moses AM: Permanent diabetes insipidus following head trauma: Observations on ten patients and an approach to diagnosis. *J Trauma* 20:599, 1980.
90. Horn LJ, Glenn MB: Update in pharmacology: Pharmacological intervention in neuroendocrine disorders following traumatic brain injury, Part (B). *J Head Trauma Rehabil* 3:86, 1988.
91. Griffith ER, Cole S, Cole TM: Sexuality and sexual dysfunction, in Rosenthal M, Griffith ER, Bond MR, Miller JD (eds): *Rehabilitation of the Adult and Child with Traumatic Brain Injury.* Philadelphia: Davis, 1990: 206–224.
92. Garden F, Bontke CF: Sexual functioning and marital adjustment after traumatic brain injury. *J Head Trauma Rehabil* 5(2):52–59, 1990.
93. Levin HS, Meyers CA, Grossman RG, et al: Ventricular enlargement after closed head injury. *Arch Neurol* 38:623, 1981.
94. Gudeman SK, Kishore PRS, Backer DP: Computed tomography in the evaluation of incidence and significance of post-traumatic hydrocephalus. *Neuroradiology* 141:397, 1981.
95. Cardoso ER, Galbraith S: Posttraumatic hydrocephalus: A retrospective review. *Surg Neurol* 23:261, 1985.
96. Beyerl B, Black PM: Posttraumatic hydrocephalus. *Neurosurgery* 15:257, 1984.
97. Katz RT, Brander V, Sahgal V: Update on the diagnosis and management of posttraumatic hydrocephalus. *Am J Phys Med Rehabil* 68:91, 1989.
98. Cope DN, Date ES, Mar EY: Serial computerized tomographic evaluations in traumatic head injury. *Arch Phys Med Rehabil* 69:483, 1988.
99. Kishore PRS, Lipper MH, Miller JD, et al: Posttraumatic hydrocephalus in patients with severe head injury. *Neuroradiology* 16:261, 1978.
100. Narayan R, Goskaslan Z, Bontke CF, et al: Delayed neurosurgical sequelae of head injury, in Rosenthal M, Griffith ER, Bond MR, Miller JD (eds): *Rehabilitation of the Adult and Child with Traumatic Brain Injury.* Philadelphia: Davis, 1990: 94–106.
101. Zasler ND, Marmarou A: *Posttraumatic Hydrocephalus: Special Topic Report.* Rehabilitation Research and Training Center, Medical College of Virginia. Richmond, VA, 1992.
102. Wikkelso C, Andersson H, Bloomstrand C, et al: Normal pressure hydrocephalus. *Acta Neurol Scand* 73:566, 1986.
103. Baker RS, Epstein AD: Ocular motor abnormalities from head trauma: Major review. *Surv Ophthalmol* 35:245, 1991.
104. Rimel RW, Jane JA: Characteristics of the head injured patient, in Rosenthal M, Griffith ER, Bond MR, Miller JD (eds): *Rehabilitation of the Head Injured Adult.* Philadelphia: Davis, 1983: 9–21.
105. Hanscom DA: Acute management of the multiply injured head trauma patient. *J Head Trauma Rehabil* 2:1, 1987.
106. Levin HS, Saydjari C, Eisenberg HM, et al: Vegetative state after closed-head injury: A Traumatic Coma Data Bank report. *Arch Neurol* 48:580, 1991.
107. Jennett B, Teasdale G: *Management of Head Injuries.* Philadelphia: Davis, 1981: 77–93.
108. Rappaport M, Hall KM, Hopkins K, et al: Disability Rating Scale for severe head trauma: Coma to community. *Arch Phys Med Rehabil* 63:118–123, 1982.
109. Malkmus D, Booth BJ, Kodimer C: *Rehabilitation of Head Injured Adults: Comprehensive Cognitive Management.* Downey, CA: Professional Staff Association of Rancho Los Amigos Hospital, 1980.
110. Rappaport M, Dougherty AM, Kelting DL: Evaluation of coma and vegetative state. *Arch Phys Med Rehabil* 73:628, 1992.
111. Ansell B, Keenan J: The Western Neuro Sensory Stimulation Profile: A tool for assessing slow-to-recover head injured patients. *Arch Phys Med Rehabil* 70:104, 1989.
112. Rader MA, Ellis DW: *Sensory Stimulation Assessment Measure.* Camden, NJ: Mediplex Rehab-Camden, 1989.
113. Giacino JT, Kezmarsky MA, DeLuca J, Cicerone KD: Monitoring rate of recovery to predict outcome in minimally responsive patients. *Arch Phys Med Rehabil* 72:897, 1991.
114. Braakman R, Jennett WB, Minderhoud JB: Prognosis of the posttraumatic vegetative state. *Acta Neurochir (Wien)* 95:49, 1988.
115. Bricolo A, Turazzi S, Feriotti G: Prolonged posttraumatic unconsciousness: Therapeutic assets and liabilities. *J Neurosurg* 52:625, 1980.

116. Choi SC, Barnes TY, Bullock R, et al: Temporal profile of outcomes in severe head injury. *J Neurosurg* 81:169–173, 1994.
117. Pitts LH: San Francisco General Hospital Medical Center Head Injury Data Bank. Cited in Bartowski M, Lovely MP: Prognosis in coma and the persistent vegetative state. *J Head Trauma Rehabil* 1:1, 1986.
118. Sazbon L, Groswasser Z: Outcome in 134 patients with prolonged posttraumatic unawareness: I. Parameters determining late recovery of consciousness. *J Neurosurg* 72:75, 1990.
119. Lal S, Merbitz CP, Grip JC: Modification of function in head-injured patients with Sinemet. *Brain Inj* 2:225, 1988.
120. Wroblewski BA, Glenn MB: Pharmacological treatment of arousal and cognitive deficits. *J Head Trauma Rehabil* 9:19, 1994.
121. Zasler ND: Update on pharmacology: Acute neurochemical alterations following traumatic brain injury: Research implications for clinical treatment. *J Head Trauma Rehabil* 7:102, 1992.
122. Wilson SL, McMillan TM: A review of the evidence for the effectiveness of sensory stimulation treatment for coma and vegetative states. *Neuropsychol Rehabil* 3:149, 1993.
123. Sutton RL, Weaver MS, Feeney DM: Drug-induced modifications of behavioral recovery following cortical trauma. *J Head Trauma Rehabil* 2:50, 1987.

* The national office of the Brain Injury Association is in Washington, D.C. and can be reached at (202) 296-6443 or at 1-800-444-6443.

124. Butler RW, Namerow N: Cognitive retraining in brain injury rehabilitation: A critical review. *J Neurol Rehabil* 2:97, 1988.
125. Volpe BT, McDowell FH: The efficacy of cognitive rehabilitation in patients with traumatic brain injury. *Arch Neurol* 47(2):220–222, 1990.
126. Williams JM, Kay T: *Head Injury: A Family Matter,* Baltimore: Paul H. Brooks, 1991.
127. Brooks DN: The head-injured family. *J Clin Exp Neuropsychol* 13:155, 1991.
128. Barth JT, Macciocchi SN: Mild traumatic brain injury. *J Head Trauma Rehabil* 8(3):1–87, 1993.
129. Boake C, Bobitec K, Bontke CF: Rehabilitation of the mild traumatic brain injury patient. *Neurorehabilitation* 1:70, 1991.
130. Horn LJ, Zasler ND (Eds.): Rehabilitation of Post-Concussive Disorders. Hanley & Belfus Inc. State of the Art Reviews in PM&R. Philadelphia: 1992: 6(1).
131. Williams DH, Levin HS, Eisenberg HM: Mild head injury classification. *Neurosurgery* 27:422, 1990.
132. Alexander MP: Neuropsychiatric correlates of persistent postconcussive syndrome. *J Head Trauma Rehabil* 7:60, 1992.
133. Hall KM, Hamilton BB, Gordon WA, Zasler ND: Characteristics and comparisons of functional assessment indices: Disability Rating Scale, Functional Independence Measure, and Functional Assessment Measure. *J Head Trauma Rehabil* 8:60–74, 1993.

Special Groups

CHAPTER 59

PEDIATRIC HEAD INJURY

John D. Ward

SYNOPSIS

Pediatric head injury is a common occurrence and a major health problem. Head injuries are a leading cause of death in this age group; thus, it is imperative that persons dealing with head-injured children be knowledgeable in their care and treatment. It is estimated that 200–300 per 100,000 children per year suffer traumatic brain injury, as a result of incidents ranging from auto accidents to child abuse. Reaction of children to injury can be quite different depending on their age. The very young clearly have a different cerebrovascular circulation and respond differently to head injuries than do older children. When evaluating a child with a head injury of any type, five aspects of care need to be addressed: adequate resuscitation and stabilization, prompt diagnosis and evaluation of neurological and associated injuries, appropriate emergency treatment of injuries, intensive care, and rehabilitation.

Child abuse is also a problem that all physicians caring for children need to be aware of. It is increasing in frequency in the United States and is not limited to any particular socioeconomic strata.

Outcome in children is a complex topic. Recovery is usually superimposed on development, and therefore may not be straightforward. Great caution has to be exerted in the evaluation of the mildly injured child in that there may be some preexisting factors that cloud the effect of the injury. In order for a child with a severe head injury to be appropriately treated, differences from the adult need to be recognized and incorporated into their treatment.

INTRODUCTION

Pediatric head injury is a major health problem. Injuries are the leading cause of death in the pediatric age group and those who die of trauma usually do so as a result of brain injury.[1] Thus, it is imperative that persons dealing with the head-injured child be knowledgeable and current in caring for and treating these children.

In many respects the care of the child with a head injury is similar to that of an adult. Therefore, many of the ideas and treatments presented in other chapters of this book are useful and applicable. However, certain aspects of head injury of children are unique and require special emphasis. It is the purpose of this chapter to discuss these unique features.

It is important that persons caring for children with head injuries avoid the two extremes of attitude, ie., children are merely little adults, or that they are totally unique. The truth lies somewhere in between. Much has been learned from the study of adult brain injury that can be useful in caring for injured children. However, head injury in the child occurs in the setting of an immature, developing central nervous system. This will affect the child's response to the injury, as well as the ultimate outcome.

EPIDEMIOLOGY

It has been estimated that unintentional childhood injuries in the United States cost the nation $7.5 billion.[2] Although most pediatric head injuries are mild and involve brief hospital stays,[3] central nervous system (CNS) injury is the most common cause of pediatric traumatic death.[4] It was estimated by Jagger et al. that there are 200–300/100,000 children per year who suffer traumatic brain injuries.[5]

Age is definitely a factor in the distribution of injury severity. The pediatric age group often has milder injuries than the adults (86 vs. 79 percent).[3] Within the pediatric age group there are certain fairly distinct populations. The very young seem to differ from the older children and adolescents in regards to the mechanism, threshold, and location of injury.[6–8]

Automobile accidents account for most fatal injuries, and this prevalence increases significantly from the infant (23 percent) to the adolescent (82 percent).[9] There are many reports of injuries peculiar to the pediatric age group. These include all-terrain vehicles,[10,11] falls,[12,13] walker injuries,[14] in-line skating and skateboarding,[15] and lawn darts.[16] Unfortunately, children and adults share with increasing frequency the problem of penetrating injuries and have a similar high mortality.[17,18]

Child abuse is also a cause of head injury in the pediatric population and unfortunately is one of the most difficult injuries to prevent and treat. Abuse occurs predominantly in the younger pediatric age group. While the exact cause of the injury may be difficult to determine, these children seem to constitute a separate group. One characteristic that all of the above injuries share (almost without exception) is they could potentially have been prevented.

PATHOPHYSIOLOGY

Are there aspects of a child's response to injury that are different from that of an adult? The answer is a qualified "yes." Certainly the older adolescent's response to injury is quite similar to that of an adult. However, in considering younger and younger children, we begin to see increasing differences.

One area of difference is in the child's cerebrovascular response to injury. In 1984 Bruce et al. were among the first groups to put forth the hypothesis that some children developed cerebral swelling of acute onset after a head injury, probably due to hyperemia.[19] This has since been described by others.[20,21] Muizelaar and associates published two papers concerning cerebral blood flow (CBF) in normal and head-injured children.[22,23] They suggested that: (1) the baseline CBF was somewhat higher in the pediatric population and, therefore, a child's brain is less likely to become ischemic; (2) the incidence of hyperemia (defined as two standard deviations above normal) was not as common as first thought; and (3) if autoregulation was intact, the response to raising or lowering blood pressure was similar to that described by Rosner in the adult.[24] Lou et al. reported that even the very young (less than 1 year of age) seemed to have an altered susceptibility to ischemia in that their tolerance is higher than that of older children.[25] The incidence of brain swelling in patients of the Traumatic Coma Data Bank was twice as high in the pediatric population as in the adult.[26] However, the mortality in the adult and the child with brain swelling was similar (46 vs. 53 percent).

EVALUATION

When treating a child with a head injury of any type, five considerations need to be addressed:

1. Immediate and aggressive resuscitation and stabilization.
2. Prompt diagnosis of neurological and associated major injuries.
3. Emergency treatment of such injuries.
4. Intensive care.
5. Rehabilitation.

The first consideration, immediate and aggressive resuscitation and stabilization, differs little from that of the adult. Two points should be remembered when dealing with children, especially of a young age. The first is that their blood volume is small relative to that of an adult. Therefore, what would be a minor blood loss in an adult can have major hemodynamic consequences in a young child. Second, young children can have a difficult time maintaining their body temperature. Often, in the excitement of resuscitation and diagnosis, the child may be left uncovered and may develop clinically significant hypothermia.

If the child is comatose, then a secured airway should be established, generally with endotracheal intubation. Intubating a child is different from intubating an adult. Ideally, only those skilled and experienced in this procedure should attempt intubating a child. If an inexperienced person intubates a child with a tube that is too large or in a way that is too rough, severe permanent tracheal damage can occur. Once a good airway has been established and oxygenation has been initiated, the insertion of reliable venous access lines is imperative. This usually means some type of a central line. Again, the insertion of a large-bore central line in children should be undertaken by experienced personnel whenever possible.

Fluid resuscitation should be sufficient to establish a normal circulation blood volume and blood pressure. One should be familiar with what is considered normal blood pressure in children of varying ages. A newborn has a lower blood pressure than an adolescent. Fluid should not be restricted in a patient with a head injury.[27] To do so merely invites a more serious problem of secondary ischemic insult. Conversely, overloading a child with fluids is easy to do. Hypotonic fluids should be avoided, as in adults.

Once resuscitation has been completed, the task of diagnosing the severity and extent of the neurological injury remains. An initial history should be obtained from those present at the time of the injury. This becomes crucial in trying to determine the exact cause of injury, the degree of force that injured the child, and the circumstances surrounding the injury. If it is a straightforward event, such as an automobile accident, this may take very little time. However, if the child was found unconscious, apparently choked on some food, or found in a tub, and yet there are signs of external trauma, then obviously a more detailed history must be obtained. If there is any suspicion of child abuse, it is crucial to obtain all the facts from as many personnel as appropriate. Detailed documentation of all conversations with the parents and observations of the child should be made because these may form the basis of legal testimony.

The neurological examination aims at answering three questions:

1. What is the extent of injury to this child?
2. Are there any localizing signs?
3. Is the child's neurological examination stabilizing, improving, or getting worse?

This information is usually obtained by use of the Glasgow Coma Score, as well as by some assessment of brainstem function and motor power. For children over the age of 2 to 3 years, this is satisfactory. However, for those under the age of 3, the use of the routine Glasgow Coma Score presents problems. First, it is difficult to interpret the verbalization of a very young child; in an infant under the age of 2, it may be impossible. Second, most of these children are too young to follow commands. Therefore, several scales have been proposed as substitutes for the Glasgow Coma Score in children, including one from the Children's Memorial Hospital in Chicago[28] and another from Australia.[29] Regardless of which scale is used, it should be used repetitively and consistently by all personnel caring for the child. If at this time the child is thought to harbor a mass lesion or is deteriorating, then treatment for elevated ICP is initiated.

After the neurological examination has been performed, appropriate laboratory tests should be obtained, including type and cross-match for possible blood transfusion, electrolytes, and CBC. If appropriate in the adolescent age group, a toxic screen and drug and alcohol levels should also be obtained.

The definitive radiological test in a patient with a severe head injury is the CT scan.[30] This test can almost always identify: (1) a life-threatening mass lesion that has to be evacuated; (2) evidence suggesting elevated ICP; and (3) to some extent, the degree of intracranial injury. Occasionally, time can be taken to obtain plain radiographs of the skull if there is a specific need for them, such as the possibility of a penetrating injury or the presence of a foreign body. However, almost all questions can be answered by the CT scan. In many respects, as in adults, CT has rendered plain radiographs of the skull obsolete. In children who have a very mild injury and a CT scan is not contemplated, there may possibly be a role for plain radiographs of the skull. In such cases the skull film may be used to rule out the presence of a skull fracture in an attempt to assess the risk of deterioration and the need for admission.[31,32] However, if there is any concern regarding an intracranial mass, a CT scan is advisable.

Prior to any manipulation of the child, a set of cervical spine films should be obtained, including a lateral C-spine film and obliques. AP films can be obtained in most cases through the treatment table. The incidence of an adult having a primary head injury with an associated cervical spine injury is about 6 percent.[33] Although this study was done primarily in adults, it is expected that children would have a somewhat similar incidence. If the cervical spine film is normal, the appropriate plain films of the chest, abdomen, and/or extremities are obtained. Minimal time should be used in obtaining these films before obtaining a CT scan. If the patient is unconscious, it is crucial to assume that the child is harboring a mass lesion until proved otherwise. It has been shown that the incidence of mass lesions in children with traumatic coma has remained at about 25 percent. In other words, in children who have a coma score of 8 or less, there is a 1 in 4 chance of a surgical lesion.[34] This is in contrast with adults, in whom there is about a 45 percent chance of harboring a surgical mass lesion.[33]

The immediate care of a pediatric patient with a GCS of 3 or signs of brainstem compression is somewhat controversial. Some investigators have advocated the use of burr holes and ultrasound in place of taking time for a CT scan.[35] Others have pointed out the low incidence of finding a mass lesion and the potential harm that may result from other injuries.[36] However, it would seem that in children with a GCS of 3 and no focal signs of a mass lesion or regression from a higher GCS score, a CT scan before surgery is warranted.

MRI usually is not utilized in the emergency room in the diagnosis of patients with severe head injury. There has been one study of patients with severe head injury who had minimal or no CT abnormalities and Glasgow Coma Scores of 7 or less. In all patients, MRI displayed lesions not evident on the CT scan. While none of the findings resulted in surgical intervention, the MRI was clearly more sensitive in delineating the extent of the patient's injury.[37] Others have examined the MRI and compared it to the neuropsychological outcome in children.[38] In addition, studies have been performed to look at the MRI and relate it to outcome.[39] Nevertheless, to date, the CT scan is the initial imaging study of choice.[30]

Once a complete evaluation has been performed, a decision is made about admission. Table 59-1 lists criteria which suggest a need for admission in a pediatric patient with a head injury.

SPECIAL ISSUES AND TREATMENT

Mild and Moderate Injuries

Mild and moderate head injuries are common in the pediatric age group.[3] Although the overall process of evaluation and treatment, in principle, is the same as for adults, there are some points that need to be clarified in the less severely injured pediatric patient. The first point concerns which children are to be admitted and which should be allowed to go home. There are several studies that suggest that if a child has had a brief interval of unconsciousness and does not have a skull fracture, he/she can be safely discharged with appropriate follow-up.[40,41] A reasonable approach is to establish a list of criteria for admission of the mild/moderately head-injured child. If the child does not meet these, he or she can be discharged[42] (Table 59-1).

Another issue involves the child who has sustained a mild head injury and still wants to participate in contact sports in which head injuries do occur.[43] These sports include football,[44] boxing, or martial arts; or sports with frequent high velocity collisions or falls, as in basketball, soccer, and ice hockey.[43] The decision to allow a child to be exposed to repetitive injury is difficult. The physician often not only has to reason with the patient but also with the parents or coach, who, on occasion, can be more difficult than the child. The underlying principle is that the decision should be made on behalf of the well-being of the child and not on the unrealistic expectations of the parents or coach. Guidelines have been proposed for those children that have suffered a loss of consciousness, and it seems reasonable to adhere to these unless there are extenuating circumstances.[43] (Refer to Sports-Related Head Injury; Chap. 63.)

TABLE 59-1 Criteria for Admission to the Hospital

Coma	Fever associated with a basilar skull fracture
Significant loss of consciousness	Skull fracture
Alteration of consciousness	Severe and persistent headache
Prolonged memory deficit	Possibility of child abuse
Seizures	Focal neurological deficits
Persistent vomiting	

Intracranial Pressure (ICP) Monitoring

The incidence of intracranial hypertension was initially felt to be fairly low in children with severe head injury. However, a more recent series places the incidence at 60 percent.[46] As in the adult, ICP monitoring is generally useful in pediatric patients who have a GCS of 8 or less or whose initial CT scan has findings which suggest that ICP problems are likely to develop. These would include contusions, cerebral swelling, or small extraaxial lesions in patients who are able to follow commands but are lethargic. The risk of ICP monitoring, while real, is quite small, especially when compared to the significant damage that could occur if a patient deteriorates from elevated ICP. If treatment of elevated ICP is expected, an ICP monitor should be inserted.[45]

The treatment of elevated ICP is covered elsewhere in this text. However, in children who do not respond to other maneuvers and have a high refractory ICP with no mass lesions, one technique is the insertion of a lumbar drain.[47] This technique has helped a certain proportion of patients whose raised ICP was resistant to other measures. This technique is quite controversial and is of unproven safety and efficacy; however, it does represent a therapy that may be useful in children but not in adults.

Hyperventilation may be more effective and safe in children than in adults, as discussed in Chap. 38 (CBF and Management of the Head-Injured Patient).

Skull Fracture

Fractures as a rule are diagnosed either by plain radiographs or by CT. The choice of the appropriate test usually is governed by the condition of the child. As was mentioned earlier, if the child has a neurological deficit or if the GCS is less than 13, a CT scan should be done. With the use of bone window techniques, most skull fractures can be diagnosed.

There has been conflicting literature concerning the usefulness of plain radiographs. It has been shown that their yield is quite low in patients who are not badly injured.[48] However, it has also been demonstrated that there is a higher incidence of subsequent problems in those patients who harbor a skull fracture, thus making the films a worthwhile effort because the results may influence the treatment of the child.[49,50] As a basic principle, it is appropriate to err on the side of being overcautious and obtaining a CT scan when there is any suspicion of intracranial pathology.

The linear or minimally depressed skull is important in that, if the fracture is new, the child should have a CT scan of the head. It has been shown that if a linear skull fracture is present, the occurrence of other lesions such as contusions and epidural hematomas is greatly increased.[49,50] In terms of the fracture itself, nothing further needs to be done.

A depressed fracture assumes importance depending on the location, degree of depression, and the integrity of the scalp. If the fracture is depressed at least the full thickness of the skull, consideration should be given to surgical elevation. If there is obvious compression of the brain, a cosmetic deformity such as in the forehead, or if there is CSF or brain tissue coming through a laceration over the fracture, the fracture should be elevated and any dural tear repaired. However, if none of the above conditions exist, then it has been suggested that there is no need for elevation, especially in the young infant whose fracture is over the temporal area. It is thought that, over time, the skull will remodel itself.[51] Further, it has also been suggested that it may not be necessary to be surgically aggressive in pediatric patients with compound depressed skull fractures.[52] This is obviously a judgment call and should be handled on an individual basis.

Basilar skull fractures in the child are treated much as they are in the adult. The child is admitted and serial neurological examinations and examination of the cranial nerves, especially VII and VIII, are performed. If no evidence of meningitis or neurological sequelae occur and any CSF leak abates, the child is discharged, usually after 48 to 72 h. The use of prophylactic antibiotics is controversial. Some prefer to place patients with a CSF leak on antibiotics; others feel that it does nothing to prevent the occurrence of meningitis.[53] However, if the patient develops a fever or any sign of meningitis, the child should have a lumbar puncture and be placed immediately on empiric broad-spectrum antibiotic coverage pending results of the cultures.

Leptomeningeal Cysts

Leptomeningeal cysts, or growing skull fractures as they are commonly called, usually occur in children under the age of 2 years and may be associated with a long diastatic fracture. They are very uncommon.[54] The hallmark of this problem is a palpable nontender swelling in the area of a previous linear or diastatic skull fracture.

A leptomeningeal cyst is believed to represent a tear in the dura with subsequent enlargement and erosion of the bone caused by pulsations of the brain. These are generally repaired surgically[55] by patching the dural tear over the brain hernia. Children under the age of 3 years with a linear or diastatic skull fracture need a follow-up skull film at 2 months postinjury or, at the very least, a return appointment and a close inspection of the area of the skull that was fractured.

Birth Injuries

Neurosurgical lesions more likely to be encountered in neonates are skull fractures, subarachnoid hemorrhage, and epidural and subdural hematomas. Linear fractures are of little importance except as mentioned above. Depressed skull fractures are also treated as indicated above if they are large or causing compression of the brain. In birth trauma, blood can collect underneath the galea (subgaleal hematoma), or under the periosteum (subperiosteal hematoma). If these collections are large, they can cause anemia and hyperbilirubinemia in the newborn. These patients only require observation in the vast majority of cases. There is rarely any indication for intervening surgically in these hematomas. Brachial plexus injuries secondary to traction during childbirth are much less common in developed countries. There are several good summaries of the diagnosis and treatment of this entity.[56,57]

Subdural Hematomas

In the toddler and adolescent, acute subdural hematomas (SDH) resemble those in the adult. However, in the very young infant, the presentation is generally more diffuse. They appear pale with a full fontanelle and may or may not have a focal neurological deficit. In this age group, the diagnosis of acute SDH is made by CT and not by diagnostic taps.[58] Chronic SDH occurs more frequently in children than the acute variety. Injury is still an important factor in terms of etiology, and often it is difficult to determine the exact time and type of injury. The signs and symptoms are typically nonlocalizing and subacute: vomiting; irritability; failure to thrive; seizures; and a growing head in a child whose sutures are not yet closed. The fontanelle in the very young child will also bulge.

In the diagnosis of SDH in the pediatric population, the CT scan is still the procedure of choice. In the pre-CT era, diagnostic subdural taps were used. However, a CT scan outlines the exact pathology and the size of the collection, and provides a baseline for subsequent studies. Once a diagnosis has been made, then therapeutic taps may be employed in certain cases to relieve intracranial pressure and treat the problem.

A variety of opinions exist as to the appropriate treatment of subdural collections. It has been shown that in the appropriate patient, if the subdural collections are tapped only when intracranial pressure is elevated, eventually a good proportion of these subdural hematomas will resolve and the brain will assume its normal configuration.[59] However, if repeated tapping is required over a prolonged period, generally a subdural-peritoneal shunt is performed.

Extradural Hematomas

Approximately 60 percent of patients with extradural hematomas are below the age of 20.[60] The clinical presentation is similar to that in adults. The diagnosis should be made by CT scan if there is time. However, if there is rapid deterioration, the patient should be taken directly to surgery. The bone flap should be large enough to entirely expose and evacuate the clot. As a rule, burr holes alone are not satisfactory. Patients with mass lesions should be given mannitol, intubated, and promptly taken to surgery. There are some patients with epidural hematomas who are asymptomatic or minimally symptomatic with only a headache and perhaps vomiting. If the hematoma is relatively small, there is little or no midline shift, and the patient presents to the hospital a few hours after the injury, a nonsurgical approach is probably justified.[61] However, such patients must be carefully observed, and if any progression occurs, the clot should be evacuated.

Child Abuse

In the care of children with head injury it is important to try to identify those who have suffered abuse. This problem seems to be increasing in frequency in the United States and is not limited to any socioeconomic strata. Child abuse is not always obvious, and often the history is either not available or fabricated. There is often a delay in seeking medical care associated with a history of previous injury upon which the more acute episode is superimposed. One study showed evidence of prior physical abuse or neglect in 71 percent of abused children.[62]

Certain characteristics when seen in an injured child should raise suspicion of child abuse and prompt investigation:

History

- A child seems to have a severe injury and yet the history indicates only minimal or negligible trauma
- History of repeated injury or falls
- The history indicates choking, hypoxia, or anoxia and there is evidence of trauma

Physical exam

- Injuries in areas that are not normally injured in the day-to-day activities of a child, i.e., bruising or injuries between the shoulder blades, circumferentially around the arms, behind the legs, or over the buttocks

Neurological exam

- If a child has minimal signs of trauma accompanied by neurological damage, acute subdural hematoma, and/or retinal hemorrhages[63]

Whereas these findings in the neurological exam may not be pathognomonic in child abuse, they are certainly sufficient to raise grave doubts about how the child suffered the injury. The shaken baby syndrome, initially done by Caffey, described children who arrive with significant neurological injury and not much evidence of external damage.[64] There is a high incidence of acute subdural hematomas and retinal hemorrhages without much external injury. Several articles have described attempts to determine the exact pathophysiology of this syndrome. Some authors have felt that first an impact is required which is then followed by a shaking incident.[65] Others have felt that there is a component of cervicomedullary injury as well as the supratentorial injury[66] from shaking alone. Regardless of the exact pathophysiology, any child who has minimal external signs of trauma with neurological damage, acute subdural hematoma, and retinal hemorrhages should be assumed to have been abused until proved otherwise.

The medical care of the child with suspected abuse does not deviate substantially from that of any other head-injured child. Difficulty may arise from the delay in seeking treatment, the extensiveness of the injury, and from the child's young age. Diagnostic studies can aid in the investigation of a possible child abuse case. Ancillary radiographs of long bones and the chest should be done to look for the presence of old extremity fractures as well as old rib fractures. MRI can play a pivotal role in the diagnosis of child abuse[67] by detecting intracranial lesions of varying vintage. Although a detailed physical examination and history is required in the care of any child with a head injury, it is especially important in child abuse cases. Often months after the occurrence of the injury, there will be legal inquiries into the history that the parents have given, the exact condition of the child, the age of the clots, the need for surgery, and a wide variety of other medical issues. Therefore, it is crucial that the medical personnel involved in these cases be meticulous in their record-keeping and observations.

The severity of injury and the extremely poor outcome in many of these children necessitates that all personnel involved in the care of an abused child be knowledgeable about the situation. It is not appropriate for the neurosurgeon to relinquish all responsibility to the primary care physicians for the resolution of these problems. As an expert in the care of children with neurological injuries, the neurosurgeon should be willing to provide whatever support and medical expertise is required to ensure that these children are protected from further injury and that the persons responsible for the injury receive appropriate counseling and help. Prevention could play a major role in decreasing the number of children with significant intracranial injuries from child abuse.

Seizures

Posttraumatic seizures differ in the child as compared to the adult. The majority seem to occur within the first 24 h.[68] Some predisposing risk factors indicate an increased likelihood of developing early posttraumatic seizures. These include a GCS of less than 8, acute subdural hematoma, cerebral edema, and open depressed skull fracture with parenchymal damage. Prophylactic anticonvulsants may be used if these risk factors are present.

OUTCOME

Clearly, when taken as a group, children do better than adults.[3,69] However, within the pediatric population, there is a difference in outcome. After a severe head injury, the very young seem to do worse than the school-age child,[70] while older adolescents seems to approach the outcome seen in the young adults.

Several principles need to be kept in mind when discussing outcome in children: (1) recovery from injury will be superimposed on normal development. (2) Great caution has to be exerted in the mildly injured child in assigning all subsequent clinical problems in the short and long term exclusively to the head injury. Many of these children have measurable abnormalities prior to the injury.[71] To blame the injury for the entire neuropsychological profile in a child several years after injury may be beneficial for litigation but may not be accurate. It has been shown in age-matched controls that children who get injured may not fall in the normal range prior to the injury.[73] However, this concept is controversial.[72] Not surprisingly, there seems to be a relationship between the severity of the injury and the outcome. It has been shown that very mildly head injured patients may not show any sequelae, while the moderately and severely injured patients may have demonstrable neurobehavioral abnormalities.[74] (3) Children seem to make larger gains in their Glasgow Outcome Score (GOS) from 3 months to 1 year than adults.[33] Therefore, adult recovery profiles should be used with caution in the pediatric population. (4) Finally, it should be remembered that the published outcome figures usually describe patients who have had aggressive, state-of-the-art care. Care should therefore be taken when using outcome data from one center to predict outcomes in another patient population.

References

1. Conroy C, Kraus JF: Survival after brain injury: Cause of death, length of survival, and prognostic variables in a cohort of brain injured people. *Neuroepidemiology* 1988; 7:13–22.
2. Guyer B, Ellers B: Childhood injuries in the United States: Mortality, morbidity, and cost. *Am J Dis Child* 1990; 144:649–652.
3. Luerssen TG, Klauber MR, Marshall LF: Outcome from head injury related to patients's age: A longitudinal prospective study of adult and pediatric head injury. *J Neurosurg* 1988; 68:409–416.
4. Tepas JJ, DiScala C, Ramenofsky ML, Barlow B: Mortality and head injury. *J Pediatr Surg* 1990; 25:92–95.
5. Jagger J, Levine J, Jane J, et al: Epidemiologic features of head injury in a predominantly rural population. *J Trauma* 1984; 24:40–44.
6. Duhaime AC, Alario AJ, Lewander WJ, et al: Head injury in very young children: Mechanism, injury types, and ophthalmologic findings in 100 hospitalized patients younger than 2 years of age. *Pediatrics* 90:179–185.
7. Hahn YS, Chyung C, Barthel MJ, et al: Head injuries in children under 36 months of age: Demography and outcome. *Childs Nerv Syst* 1988; 4:34–40.
8. Rivera FP: Childhood injuries III: Epidemiology of non-motor vehicle head trauma. *Dev Med Child Neurol* 1984; 26:81–87.
9. Lundar T, Nestvold K: Pediatric head injuries caused by traffic accidents: A prospective study with 5 year follow-up. *Childs Nerv Syst* 1985; 1:24–28.
10. Ruddy RM, Selbst SM: Three-wheeled vehicle injuries in children. *Am J Dis Child* 1990; 144:73–71.
11. Kriel RL, Sheehan M, Krach LE, et al: Pediatric head injury resulting from all-terrain vehicle accidents. *Pediatrics* 1986; 78:933–935.
12. Jaffe M, Ludwig S: Stairway injuries in children. *Pediatrics* 1988; 82:457–461.
13. Musemeche CA, Barthel M, Cosentino C, Reynolds M: Pediatric falls from heights. *J Trauma* 1991; 31:1347–1349.
14. Rieder MJ, Schwartz C, Newman J: Patterns of walker use and walker injury. *Pediatrics* 1986; 78:488–493.

15. Retsky J, Jaffe D, Christoffel K: Skateboarding injuries in children: A second wave. *Am J Dis Child* 1991; 145:188–192.
16. Sotiropoulos SV, Jackson MA, Tremblay GF, et al: Childhood lawn dart injuries: Summary of 75 patients and patient report. *Am J Dis Child* 1990; 144:980–982.
17. Beaver BL, Moore VL, Peclet M, et al: Characteristics of pediatric firearm fatalities. *J Pediatr Surg* 1990; 25:97–99.
18. Miner ME, Ewing-Cobbs L, Kopaniky DR, et al: The results of treatment of gunshot wounds to the brain in children. *Neurosurgery* 1990; 26:20–24.
19. Bruce CA, Alavi A, Bilaniuk L, et al: Diffuse cerebral swelling following head injuries in children: The syndrome of "malignant brain edema." *J Neurosurg* 1981; 54:170–178.
20. Humphreys RP, Hendrick EB, Hoffman HJ: The head injured child who "talks and dies." *Childs Nerv Syst* 1990; 6:139–142.
21. Snoek JW, Minderhoud JM, Wilmink JT: Delayed deterioration following mild head injury in children. *Brain* 1984; 107:15–36.
22. Muizelaar JP, Marmarou AM, DeSalles AA, et al: Cerebral blood flow in severely head-injured children: Part I. Relationship with GCS score, outcome, ICP, and PVI. *J Neurosurg* 1989; 71:63–71.
23. Muizelaar PJ, Ward JD, Marmarou AM, et al: Cerebral blood flow in severely head-injured children: Part II. Autoregulation. *J Neurosurg* 1989; 71:72–76.
24. Rosner MJ, Coley IB: Cerebral perfusion pressure, intracranial pressure and head elevation. *J Neurosurg* 1986; 65:636–641.
25. Lou HC, Lassen NA, Fris-Hansen B: Impaired autoregulation of cerebral blood flow in the distressed newborn infant. *J Pediatr* 1979; 94:118–121.
26. Aldrich EF, Eisenberg HM, Saydjart C, et al: Diffuse brain swelling in severely head-injured children: A report from the NIH traumatic coma data bank. *J Neurosurg* 1992; 76:450–454.
27. Ward JD, Moulton RJ, Muizelaar PJ, Marmarou AM: Cerebral homeostasis, in Wirth FP, Ratcheson RA (eds): *Neurosurgical Critical Care: Vol I. Concepts in Neurosurgery.* Baltimore: Williams & Wilkins, 1987: 187–213.
28. Hahn YS, Chyung C, Barthel MJ, et al: Head injuries in children under 36 months of age: Demography and outcome. *Childs Nerv Syst* 1988; 4:34–40.
29. Simpson DA, Cockington RA, Hanieh A, et al: Head injuries in infants and young children: The value of the pediatric coma scale. Review of literature and report on a study. *Childs Nerv Syst* 1991; 7:183–190.
30. Johnson MH, Lee SH: Computed tomography of acute cerebral trauma. *Radiol Clin North Am* 1992; 30:325–352.
31. Chan KH, Yue CP, Mann KS: The risk of intracranial complications in pediatric head injury: Results of multivariate analysis. *Childs Nerv Syst* 1990; 6:27–27.
32. Ros SP, Cetta F: Are skull radiographs useful in the evaluation of asymptomatic infants following minor head injury? *Pediatr Emerg Care* 1992; 8:328–30.
33. Michael DB, Guyot DR, Darmody WR: Coincidence of head and cervical spine injury. *J Neurotrauma* 1989; 6:177–189.
34. Alberico AM, Ward JD, Choi SC, et al: Outcome after severe head injury: Relationship to mass lesions, diffuse injury, and ICP course in pediatric and adult patients. *J Neurosurg* 1987; 67:648–656.
35. Andrews BT, Ross AM, Pitts LH: Surgical exploration before computed tomography scanning in children with traumatic tentorial herniation. *Surg Neurol* 1989; 32:434–438.
36. Johnson DL, Duma C, Sivit C: The role of immediate operative intervention in severely head-injured children with a Glasgow Coma Score of 3. *Neurosurgery* 30:320–324.
37. Wilberger JE Jr, Deeb Z, Rothfus W: Magnetic resonance imaging in cases of severe head injury. *Neurosurgery* 1987; 20:571–576.
38. Levin HS, Amparo EG, Eisenberg HM, et al: Magnetic resonance imaging after closed head injury in children. *Neurosurgery* 1989; 24:223–227.
39. Mendelsohn D, Levin HS, Bruce D, et al: Late MRI after head injury in children: Relationship to clinical features and outcome. *Childs Nerv Syst* 1992; 8:445–452.
40. Rosenthal BW, Bergman I: Intracranial injury after moderate head trauma in children. *J Pediatr* 1989; 115:346–350.
41. Godano U, Serracchioli A, Servadei F, et al: Intracranial lesions of surgical interest in minor head injuries in pediatric patients. *Childs Nerv Syst* 1992; 8:136–138.
42. Dershewitz RA, Kaye BA, Swisher CN: Treatment of children with posttraumatic transient loss of consciousness. *Pediatrics* 1983; 72:602–607.
43. Kelly JP, Nicholas JS, Filley CM, et al: Concussion in sports: Guidelines for the prevention of catastrophic outcome. *JAMA* 1991; 266:2867–2869.
44. Goldberg B, Rosenthal PP, Robertson LS, Nicholas JA: Injuries in youth football. *Pediatrics* 1988; 81:255–261.
45. Kasoff SS, Lansen TA, Holder D, Filippo JS: Aggressive physiologic monitoring of pediatric head trauma patients with elevated intracranial pressure. *Pediatr Neurosci* 1988; 14:241–249.
46. Ward JD: Pediatric head injury: A further experience. *Pediatr Neurosurg* 1993; 458.
47. Baldwin HZ, Rekate HL: Preliminary experience with controlled external lumbar drainage in diffuse pediatric head injury. *Pediatr Neurosurg* 1991–92; 17:115–120.
48. Masters SJ, McClean PM, Arcarese JS, et al: Skull x-ray examinations after head trauma: Recommendations by a multidisciplinary panel and validation study. *N Engl J Med* 1987; 316:84–91.
49. Bonadio WA, Smith DS, Hillman S: Clinical indicators of intracranial lesion on computed tomographic scan in children with parietal skull fracture. *Am J Dis Child* 1989; 143:194–196.
50. Levi L, Guilburd JN, Linn S, Feinsod M: The association between skull fracture, intracranial pathology and outcome in pediatric head injury. *Br J Neurosurg* 1991; 5:617–625.
51. Loeser JD, Kilburn HL, Jolley T: Management of depressed skull fracture in the newborn. *J Neurosurg* 1976; 44:62–64.
52. Van den Heever CM, Van Der Merwe DJ: Management

of depressed skull fractures. *J Neurosurg* 1989; 71:186–190.
53. Hoff JT, Berwin A: Antibiotics for basilar skull fractures. *J Neurosurg* 1976; 44:649.
54. Lende RA, Erickson TC: Growing skull fractures of childhood. *J Neurosurg* 1961; 18:479–489.
55. Locstelli D, Messian AL, Bonfanti N, et al: Growing fractures: An unusual complication of head injury in pediatric patients. *Neurochirurgia* 1989; 32:101–104.
56. Piatt JH Jr, Hudson AR, Hoffman HJ: Preliminary experience with brachial plexus exploration in children: Birth injury and vehicular trauma. *Neurosurgery* 1988; 22:715–723.
57. Piatt JH Jr: Neurosurgical management of birth injuries of the brachial plexus. *Neurosurg Clin North Am* 1991; 2:175–185.
58. Guitierrez FA, Raimondi AJ: Acute subdural hematoma in infancy and childhood. *Child's Brain* 1975; 1:269–290.
59. Aoki N: Chronic subdural hematoma in infancy: Clinical analysis of 30 cases in the CT era. *J Neurosurg* 1990; 73:201–205.
60. Guitierrez FA, McClone DG, Raimondi AJ: Epidural hematomas in infancy and childhood. *Concepts Pediatr Neurosurg* 1981; I:181–188.
61. Pang D, Horton JA, Herron JM, et al: Nonsurgical management of extradural hematomas in children. *J Neurosurg* 1983; 59:958–971.
62. Alexander R, Crabbe L, Sato Y, et al: Serial abuse in children who are shaken. *Am J Dis Child* 1990; 144:58–60.
63. Spaide RF: Shaken baby syndrome: Ocular and computed tomographic findings. *J Clin Neuroophthalmol* 1987; 7:108–111.
64. Caffey J: On the theory and practice of shaking infants. *Am J Dis Child* 1972; 124:161–169.
65. Duhaime AC, Gennarelli TA, Thibault LE, et al: The shaken baby syndrome. *J Neurosurg* 1987; 66:409–415.
66. Hadley MN, Sonntag VKH, Rekate HL, Murphy A: The infant whiplash-shake injury syndrome: A clinical and pathological study. *Neurosurgery* 1989; 24:536–540.
67. Alexander RC, Schor DP, Smith WL Jr: Magnetic resonance imaging of intracranial injuries from child abuse. *J Pediatr* 1986; 109:975–979.
68. Hahn YS, Fuch S, Flannery AM, et al: Factors influencing post traumatic seizures in children. *Neurosurgery* 1988; 22:864–867.
69. Berger MS, Pitts LH, Lovely M, et al: Outcome from severe injury in children and adolescents. *J Neurosurg* 1985; 62:194–199.
70. Kriel RL, Krach LE, Panser LA: Closed head injury: Comparison of children younger and older than 6 years of age. *Pediatr Neurol* 1989; 5:296–300.
71. Dikmen S, McLean A, Temkin N: Neuropsychological and psychosocial consequences of minor head injury. *J Neurol Neurosurg Psychiatry* 1986; 49:1227–1232.
72. Pelco L, Sawyer M, Duffield G, et al: Premorbid emotional and behavioral adjustment in children with mild head injuries. *Brain Inj* 1992; 6:29–37.
73. Bijur PE, Haslum M, Golding J: Cognitive and behavioral sequelae of mild head injury in children. *Pediatrics* 1990; 86:337–344.
74. Jaffe KM, Fay GC, Polissar NL, et al: Severity of traumatic brain injury and early neurobehavioral outcome: A cohort study. *Arch Phys Med Rehabil* 1992; 73:540–547.

CHAPTER 60

CIVILIAN PENETRATING HEAD INJURY

Todd W. Trask
Raj K. Narayan

SYNOPSIS

Penetrating head injuries are becoming increasingly common in the United States as a result of the widespread availability of firearms and the endemic violence in certain segments of society. While military injuries generally are caused by shrapnel and high-velocity missiles, civilian injuries are most commonly associated with handguns. The severity of the injury is related to several factors, including muzzle velocity of the bullet, distance of flight, caliber, trajectory of passage through the cranium, eloquence of the damaged brain, vascular injury, and subsequent complications. Patients with gunshot wounds of the head tend to present at the two ends of the Glasgow Coma Scale spectrum: 3 to 5 and 13 to 15. Consequently, they tend to do very well or very poorly. While it is no longer considered necessary to sacrifice normal brain tissue while searching for embedded bone fragments, a thorough debridement of necrotic tissue and good dural closure still form the cornerstone of surgical therapy. Intracranial pressure monitoring and control are advisable in comatose patients. Prophylactic antibiotics and anticonvulsants are widely used, although the scientific basis for this practice has not been established.

INTRODUCTION

Civilian penetrating head injury is a leading cause of morbidity and mortality and represents a significant public health problem. The devastating nature of these injuries is accentuated by their predilection to affect young and otherwise healthy individuals. The lethal nature of these injuries makes preventive measures the best hope for ameliorating the problem.[1–4] This chapter discusses the epidemiology, pathophysiology, clinical management, and outcomes of civilian penetrating head injuries. The emphasis is on cranial gunshot wounds as the most important category of these injuries. Data from military series of penetrating head injury are included as they pertain to the management of civilian injuries.

EPIDEMIOLOGY

Firearm-related violence is a major public health concern and represents the most important cause of civilian penetrating head injury. Firearms are responsible for approximately 35,000 deaths per year and an even greater number of nonlethal injuries.[2,3,5] The great majority of injuries are either homicides or suicides, although accidental firearm injuries contribute significantly, especially in rural areas where hunting is a popular pastime and in the pediatric population.[6–10] The magnitude of this problem has stirred a national debate over possible solutions, a debate the neurosurgical community has entered.[3,5] The costs incurred by society from these injuries is clearly enormous.

Gunshot wounds to the head are responsible for a large percentage of firearm-related deaths and are second only to motor vehicle accidents as a cause of head injury–associated deaths (14 percent of head injury deaths from 1979 to 1986).[11] The annual incidence of gunshot wound–related head injury deaths has been estimated at 2.4 per 100,000, accounting for approximately 6000 deaths per year in the United States.[10,12]

The incidence is higher in selected population groups and areas, such as among young black males and in urban areas.[7,10] Alcohol and drug use also affect the problem, especially among the young.[1]

PATHOPHYSIOLOGY

Craniocerebral Wound Ballistics

Injury from cranial gunshot wounds occurs as a function of energy transfer from the missile to impacted tissue. This energy transfer can be expressed by the formula

$$KE = \frac{1}{2}M\,(Ventry - Vexit)^2$$

where KE = kinetic energy, M = mass, Ventry = velocity at entry, and Vexit = velocity at exit.[13] This relationship highlights the importance of missile velocity relative to mass (or bullet caliber). Missile velocity at the point of entry is determined by a number of factors, including muzzle velocity of the weapon, distance of flight, and any deflecting barriers to the missile.[14] Military-type rifles and some hunting rifles have muzzle velocities which exceed 2500 ft/s, while civilian-type handguns have muzzle velocities between 800 and 1400 ft/s.[14] Because most civilian gunshot wounds are caused by handguns, civilian injuries have sometimes been termed "low-velocity" and military injuries "high-velocity."[11,15,16] This classification may be misleading in comparisons of military and civilian injuries, as the majority of penetrating wounds incurred during military conflicts are shrapnel injuries from explosive devices.[17,18] Shrapnel fragments are often numerous and can be expected to have variable velocities and complex ballistic characteristics. These characteristics lead to a wide spectrum of injury types and severity and make the data obtained from military series difficult to interpret.

Other important considerations in comparing "low-velocity" and "high-velocity" gunshot wounds include the distance of the shot and any barriers or deflections in the missile's path. Civilian wounds often occur at short range (point-blank in many suicide attempts and execution-type assaults), while the distances involved in firearm-related military wounds may be quite variable (for example, "spent bullets").[14,19,20] Protective helmets utilized by soldiers may alter wound severity.[21] These factors should be considered in comparing military experience with civilian practice.

Cranial gunshot wounds encountered in civilian practice most often result from low-muzzle-velocity weapons, although the increased availability of assault rifles may result in more "high-velocity" injuries. Unfortunately, because of the considerably greater kinetic energy transferred with high-velocity weapons, it is doubtful that many of these patients will be salvageable.[22–24]

Bullet design is also an important aspect of craniocerebral ballistics. Many bullets are designed to deform or fragment after impact, and this increases resistance to their transit through tissue and minimizes or eliminates exit velocity.[25,26] This design capitalizes on the importance of velocity in energy transfer and tissue destruction. Missile "yaw," defined as the deviation of the long axis of the projectile from its line of flight, also may increase tissue destruction by enlarging the cross-sectional area of the missile presented to the tissue.[13]

The energy of the traversing missile is transferred to the surrounding tissue via several mechanisms, resulting in a number of pathophysiological and pathological changes. Injury is initiated by the direct crushing and laceration of tissues as the missile penetrates the skull and brain. In a similar fashion, any indriven bone or tissue fragments cause direct tissue disruption and may be thought of as secondary missiles.[13,25] High-speed shock waves are generated when a missile enters a tissue medium but do not appear to be important in the pathophysiology of cranial gunshot wounds.[25] However, missile energy deposition does result in the formation of a pulsating temporary cavity with subatmospheric intracavitary pressures. The size of this cavity may be many times larger than the diameter of the bullet. In addition to directly injuring tissues adjacent to the cavity by stretching and tearing, the pulsations of the cavity generate pressure waves which may radiate to locations distant from the bullet's path.[13,25,27,28] The magnitude of this temporary cavity is highly dependent on a bullet's impact velocity.

The bullet's path is typically marked by a permanent cavity of highly variable size and configuration, reflecting any internal ricochet, bullet fragmentation, or indriven bone fragments. This cavity is filled with blood, necrotic brain, and indriven debris and may be surrounded by hemorrhagic brain parenchyma.[13,25,29]

Associated Pathology

The brain injury sustained after a cranial gunshot wound is often compounded by concomitant injuries, including scalp lacerations, skull fractures, cerebral contusions, and intracranial hematomas. Operative intervention is frequently indicated for the treatment of these injuries.

Extensive scalp wounds are fortunately uncommon in civilian practice but may be encountered with shotgun injuries.[19,30] Blood loss from scalp wounds can be considerable and may be a cause of hypovolemia and hypotension.

In a significant number of cases in addition to those seen at entry/exit points, skull fractures are seen at

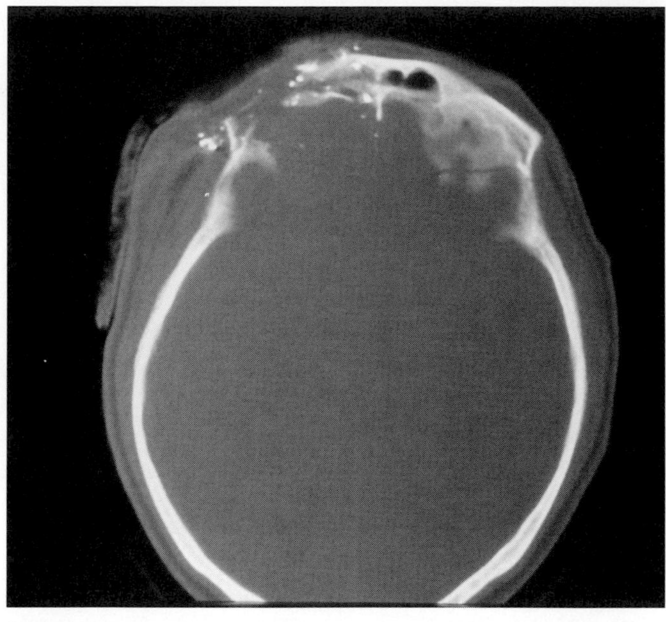

A

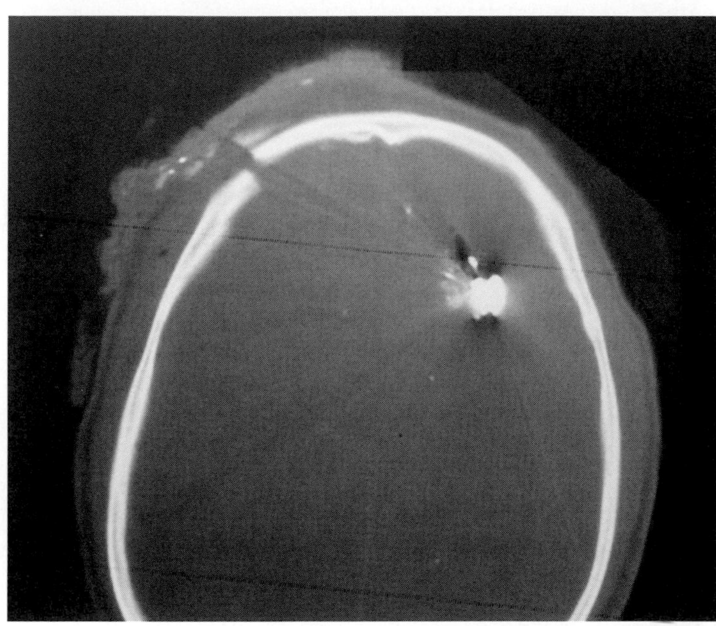

B

Figure 60-1. Bony injuries. Gunshot injuries may result in both local and remote bony fractures. *A*. In this example, the CT with bone windows demonstrates a right frontal entrance with the bullet lodged in the left frontal lobe. *B*. Lower cuts demonstrate a comminuted fracture of the right supraorbital rim and frontal sinus as well as a fracture of the left orbital roof. Such patients are at high risk for the development of CSF leaks and infectious complications.

remote sites, usually in the skull base (Fig. 60-1). Indriven bone fragments and dural lacerations are typical. Dural lacerations may be remote from entry/exit sites. Skull base fractures, presumably resulting from transient increases in intracranial pressure, are also common and may lead to CSF leaks. High-velocity injuries may lead to massive skull fragmentation, which are more commonly reported in military series.[14,25]

Cerebral contusions play an important role in the pathophysiology of cranial gunshot wounds and may be widespread and extensive.[31,32] The common locations for such contusions are at the entry site and contrecoup to the entry site.[14,25] Subfrontal contusions occur in approximately 25 percent of cases and, like skull base fractures, presumably result from a transient craniocaudal displacement at the time of wounding. In addition to contusions apparent at operation or on imaging studies, there may be nonvisualized areas of brain injury which contribute to late neuropsychological dysfunction or posttraumatic epilepsy.[31] Cerebral contusions should be

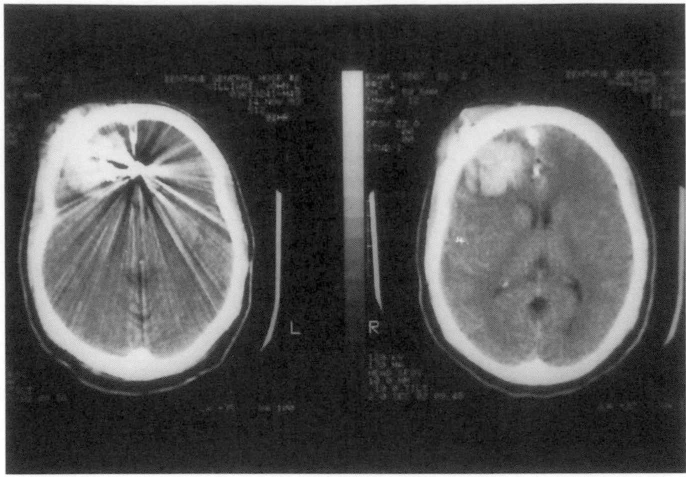

Figure 60-2. Associated hematoma. A large right frontal hematoma is seen secondary to a gunshot wound in this 40-year-old man. The patient's neurological condition (GCS 15) deteriorated after admission but improved after prompt evacuation of the hematoma.

treated as mass lesions when they are reasonably discrete and exert mass effect.

The incidence of intracranial hematomas reported after penetrating head injury has been quite variable and seems to depend partially on the time interval between wounding and assessment. The highest incidence appears to occur between 3 and 8 h after an injury.[33] The advent of computed tomography (CT) has greatly facilitated the diagnosis and treatment of intracranial hematomas.[34] Civilian series of gunshot wounds have reported incidences of intracranial hematomas that range from 10 to 44 percent.[15,33,35] Intracerebral hematomas are the most common, followed by subdural hematomas and the rare epidural hematoma.[19] Data from the NIH Traumatic Coma Data Bank demonstrated a 34 percent incidence of hyperdense lesions greater than 15 ml on CT and found these lesions to be a poor prognostic indicator.[36] Enlarging intracranial hematomas are an important cause of postinjury deterioration and suggest the possibility of associated vascular injury[7,15,33] (Figs. 60-2 through 60-4).

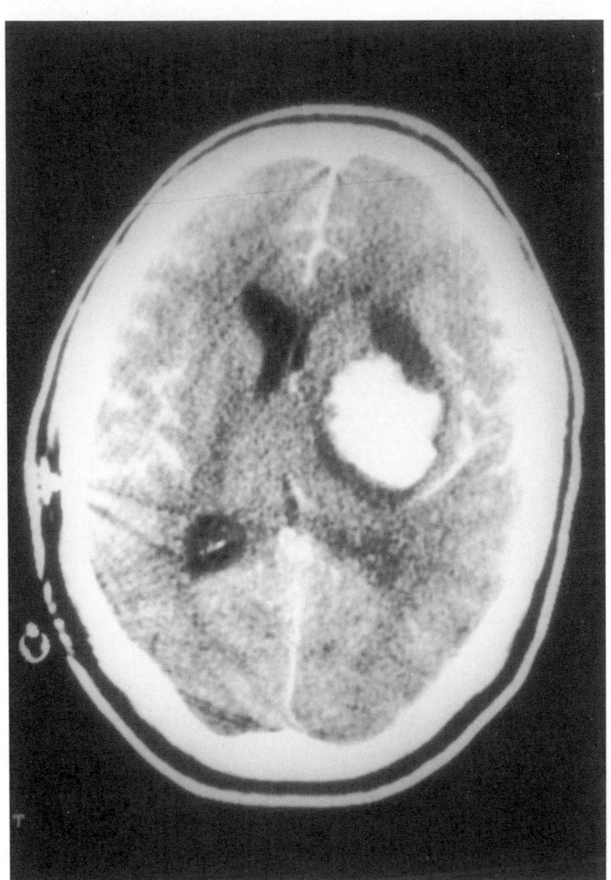

Figure 60-3. Shotgun-related hematoma. Note the large deep-seated hematoma in the region of the left basal ganglia in this 57-year-old man. Note also the midline shift, widespread subarachnoid hemorrhage, and artifact from the pellet over the right parietal skull.

Pathophysiology

Experimental models and autopsy studies have been utilized to study the pathophysiology of missile wounds to the brain. These studies have highlighted postinjury changes in intracranial pressure, systemic responses to injury, and the associated pathological correlates. There are two main areas of interest: the degree of "instantaneous," sometimes irreversible brain injury and the development of postinjury pathophysiological changes which exacerbate the primary injury (secondary insults). This distinction should allow identification of processes that are amenable to therapeutic intervention.

Intracranial pressure (ICP) monitoring studies in experimental animals reveal a high ICP "spike" at the time of wounding, followed by a second, broader peak occurring 2 to 5 min after injury (mean, 47 mmHg).[37] This peak subsides, but ICP does not return to normal values. Concomitantly, a number of systemic changes have been observed in experimental models. A brief period of bradycardia and hypotension is typically followed by a variable period of hypertension. Hypoten-

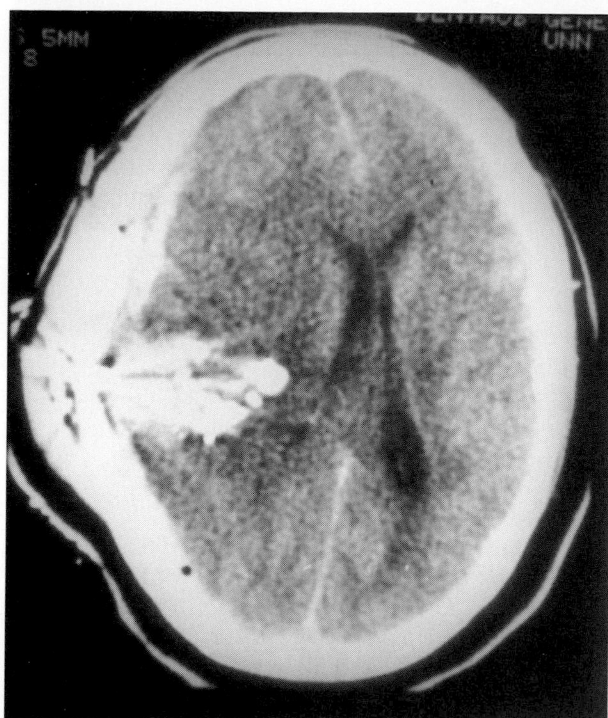

Figure 60-4. Subdural hematoma. A gunshot-related injury can cause a subdural hematoma in addition to the parenchymal injury. When the hematoma is large enough to cause a significant mass effect, as in this case, a large craniotomy is required for evacuation of the subdural hematoma in addition to debridement of the bullet tract.

sion recurs during the terminal phases.[27,38] Cardiac output and contractility are impaired in spite of normal filling pressures and systemic vascular resistance.[38] Impairments of cerebral autoregulation also have been observed.[37,38] As a result of the systemic and intracranial abnormalities, cerebral perfusion pressure and blood flow are reduced. At times, a "vicious cycle" may be established, with cerebral ischemia exacerbating the injury, leading to brain swelling, and contributing to further increases in ICP and thus to further reduction in cerebral blood flow. As expected, the cerebral metabolism of oxygen is reduced after injury, and the metabolism of lactate is increased.[37]

Postwound apnea has also been observed frequently in experimental studies and, when correlated with the bradycardia, has been interpreted as evidence of immediate and sometimes irreversible brainstem injury.[21,27,37] This phenomenon has important clinical implications. "Instantaneous" brainstem injury may explain the neurological devastation that sometimes is observed in the absence of a significant intracranial mass or direct bullet injury to vital structures.[25] The occurrence of postinjury apnea and hypotension establishes the importance of early resuscitation efforts in order to prevent secondary insults from hypoxia and ischemia.[22,35]

Further evidence of immediate brainstem injury at the time of wounding comes from autopsy studies on victims of civilian gunshot wounds (GSWs). These studies frequently reveal the presence of pressure marks on the uncal gyri and cerebellar tonsils, often in the absence of significant cerebral edema or mass lesion.[25,29] These findings are also consistent with a forced craniocaudal displacement of the brain at the time of wounding.

Examination of tissues after experimental missile injury has revealed evidence of widespread and distant damage. The basal ganglia, hypothalamus, midbrain, pons, and cerebellum are the most commonly involved structures.[21] Histologically, these areas show perivascular hemorrhages and staining abnormalities[21]; ultrastructurally, widespread swelling of perivascular astrocytes has been noted.[39]

The etiology of persistent intracranial hypertension observed both experimentally and clinically is most likely multifactorial.[27,37,40] Impaired cerebral autoregulation with increased blood volume, edema, alterations in CSF production or absorption, and intracranial hemorrhage have all been implicated as causes.[27] The importance of postinjury edema has been debated. Autopsy studies have demonstrated the occasionally rapid development of edema after GSWs.[25] However, other experimental studies have downplayed the importance of postinjury edema in the pathophysiology of lower-velocity injuries.[27]

EMERGENCY ROOM MANAGEMENT

Initial Evaluation

The initial evaluation of patients who have suffered penetrating head injuries must accomplish a number of goals in a short period. These goals include a systemic survey, resuscitation, neurological examination, appropriate radiological evaluation, determination of salvageability, and definitive treatment (Table 60-1).

Systemic Survey

A general systemic survey which assesses vital signs and identifies associated injuries must be accomplished quickly. Mechanism of injury, baseline neurological status, past medical history, and allergies should be sought from paramedical personnel and family members when they are available. The patient should be completely undressed and carefully inspected for additional entry/exit wounds, especially when the mechanism of injury has not been clearly established. Radiographic studies

TABLE 60-1 Management Outline

I. Initial assessment
   A. Resuscitation
      1. Stabilize vital signs
      2. Intubate if GCS < 8 or if inadequate airway/ventilation/oxygenation
      3. Pulse oximetry monitor
   B. Examinations
      1. Systemic survey—contact consultants
      2. Neurological examination
         a. GCS score
         b. Pupillary responses, brainstem reflexes
         c. Shave scalp, document entry/exit sites
         d. Check oral cavity
   C. Laboratory studies: CBC, electrolytes, PT/PTT, platelets, type and screen (or cross-match), urinalysis and toxicology screen; consider fibrinogen, fibrin split
   D. Radiological examination
      1. Skull films
      2. CXR, lateral C-spine ± other x-rays
      3. CT head
      4. Consider cerebral angiography
   E. Determine salvageability
      If GCS 3–5, nonreactive pupils, no hematoma—consider no treatment

II. Postoperative care
   A. ICP monitor in patients not following commands
      1. Keep ICP < 20 with ventricular drainage, mannitol, sedation, and neuromuscular blockade
      2. Consider jugular venous saturation monitor
      3. Consider barbiturate coma or lobectomy if refractory intracranial hypertension
      4. Avoid excessive hyperventilation
   B. Follow-up imaging: CT/angiography, especially with increased ICP or neurological deterioration
   C. Antibiotics
   D. Anticonvulsants
   E. Monitor for complications
      1. Delayed hematoma—suspect coagulopathy, TICA
      2. CSF leak, especially craniofacial injuries
      3. Meningitis/abscess
      4. Hydrocephalus
      5. Seizures
      6. Systemic complications

GCS = Glasgow Coma Scale; CBC = complete blood count; PT = prothrombin time; PTT = partial thromboplastin time; CXR = chest x-ray; CT = computed tomography; ICP = intracranial pressure; TICA = traumatic intracranial aneurysm; CSF = cerebrospinal fluid.

such as chest x-ray and lateral C-spine are typically indicated. Appropriate specialists should be involved immediately when there are multiple injuries. Occasionally, a systemic injury takes precedence over the evaluation and management of the cranial wound. For instance, patients with a concomitant thoracic or abdominal GSW may be too unstable to undergo head CT before an operation. Fortunately, patients with multiple penetrating wounds are somewhat less common in civilian practice than in military series.[22,23,41]

RESUSCITATION

Resuscitation proceeds simultaneously with examination and focuses on the restoration of adequate blood pressure and oxygenation. This includes the establishment of adequate intravenous access (central line, if necessary), intubation, and placement of chest tubes as indicated. Intravascular volume is restored with crystalloid, colloid, or blood products as necessary. Some patients require pressor support; however, in the absence of a systemic injury, this is an ominous prognostic indicator.[42] A Foley catheter is placed during this phase. Pulse oximetry is a useful monitoring tool during the resuscitation and evaluation process, ensuring adequate oxygenation at all times.

Routine laboratory studies should be obtained during this phase. These studies generally include complete blood count, electrolytes, coagulation parameters, type and screen (or cross-match), urinalysis, and toxicology screen.

Organized trauma systems represent a significant advance in the management of penetrating head injuries. Many areas have paramedical personnel who initiate resuscitation in the field. In such areas, some of the more severely injured patients arrive at the hospital intubated with intravenous access established.[19,22,24] As was previously noted, many patients who suffer a GSW to the brain can be expected to have a period of apnea and hypotension. Early intubation and resuscitation may reduce the incidence of secondary insults from these changes.[22,35] A study by Kennedy and colleagues examined the incidence of cervical spine injuries in patients with gunshot wounds to the head and found no such injuries in 105 patients with wounds limited to the calvarium. They suggested that cervical spine immobilization during intubation may be unnecessary in patients with isolated cranial gunshot wounds, thus facilitating earlier intubation in the field or emergency room.[43] A proportion of penetrating head injury patients can be expected to develop an expanding intracranial mass lesion. Hence, the rapid transport of these patients to a neurosurgical center, followed by early intervention, may prevent subsequent irreversible neurological deterioration.[33] The use of helicopters in the transport of severely injured patients may aid in reducing the transit time in certain situations.[22,35] While the institution of such measures clearly raises the level of care for these patients, it has been frequently noted that reported in-hospital mortality rates may actually be higher in areas where such systems are in place. This phenomenon undoubtedly occurs because a higher percentage of patients survive to reach the medical facility.[33,35]

Neurological Examination

In conjunction with the systemic survey, a rapid neurological evaluation is performed, including Glasgow Coma Scale (GCS) determination, pupillary responses, and brainstem reflexes. It is important to document when the examination is obscured by hypotension, hypoxia, or pharmacological agents. The scalp should be shaved, and all entry/exit wounds should be carefully documented. Palpation of wounds can help define the presence of fractures, but care must be taken not to disturb loose bone fragments over dural venous sinuses. The oral cavity should always be checked for a hidden entry/exit site. Patients who do not follow simple commands and have GCS scores less than 8 should be intubated if this has not been done in the field. Mannitol should be administered to patients with asymmetrical pupillary or motor examinations and patients who have deteriorated since the time of injury (1 g/kg; patient must be hemodynamically stable). In addition, patients should be loaded with an anticonvulsant and started on intravenous antibiotics in a timely fashion. However, the exact duration, selection, and efficacy of prophylactic anticonvulsants and antibiotics continue to be debated. Seizures that occur during the resuscitation phase may be stopped with intravenous lorazepam. After an adequate neurological examination, it is practical in many cases to sedate and paralyze patients for CT scanning.

Radiological Evaluation

The appropriate initial radiological evaluation depends on the available facilities. Plain films of the skull should be obtained whenever these studies can be performed rapidly in the emergency center. Although of questionable value in closed head injury, skull films are a quick method for the examiner to confirm initial impressions of the nature and trajectory of a penetrating head injury.

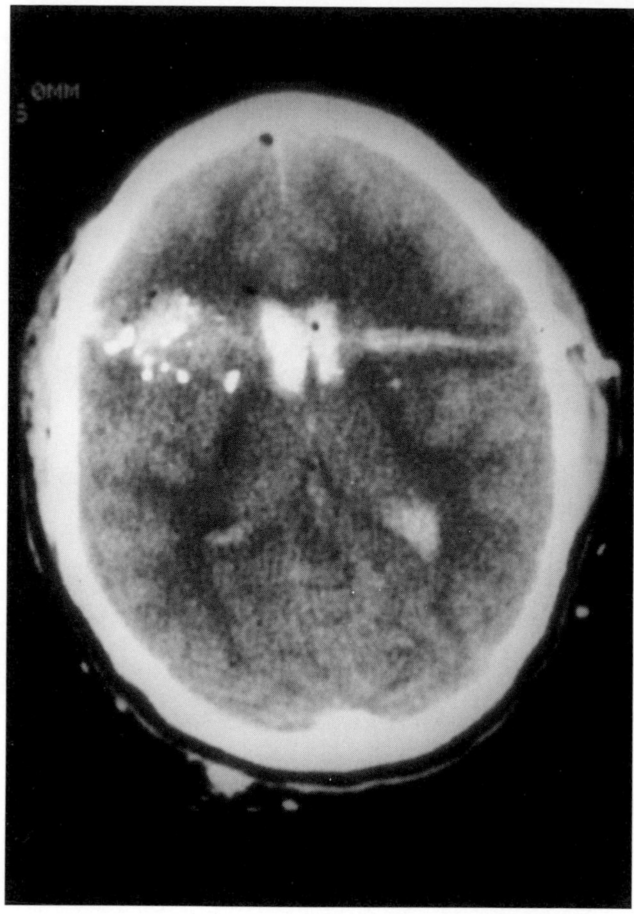

Figure 60-5. Transventricular injury. Note the clear delineation of the bullet tract and the intraventricular blood in this 23-year-old woman. Although the prognosis associated with such injuries is generally poor, this is not always the case.

Ideally, all patients with penetrating head injuries should undergo an immediate CT scan, although this may not be reasonable in patients with impending or completed brain death and unstable vital signs. In patients who present with clearly fatal injuries and do not undergo CT scanning, plain films are useful for confirming the nature and severity of the injury. CT has clearly become the diagnostic imaging modality of choice in the evaluation of penetrating head injuries. It provides excellent resolution of intracranial anatomy and can be utilized to accurately localize the missile tract as well as bone and missile fragments (Fig. 60-5). CT scanning allows the rapid identification of mass lesions such as hematomas and contusions, thus greatly facilitating effective operative management.[16,19,34] CT findings also carry important prognostic information which may affect difficult triage decisions.

Cerebral angiography has been largely supplanted by CT for the initial evaluation of penetrating craniocerebral trauma. However, CT is less effective for the detection of vascular lesions such as traumatic intracra-

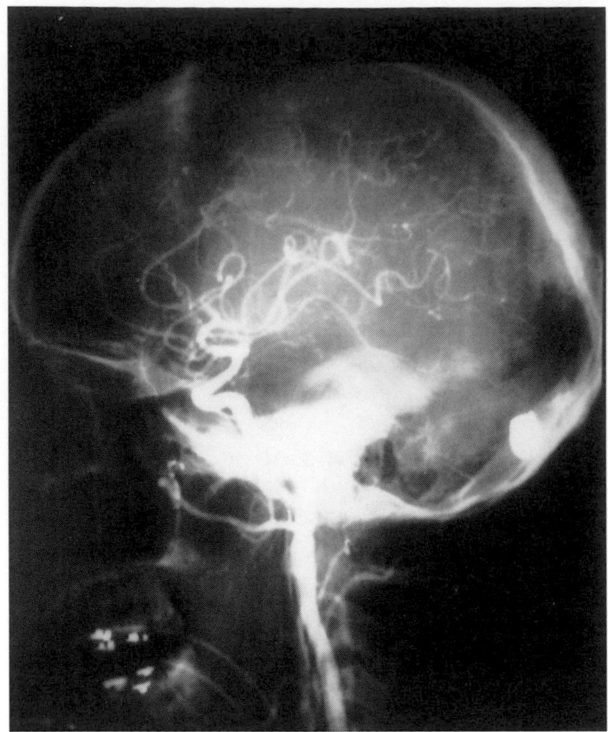

A

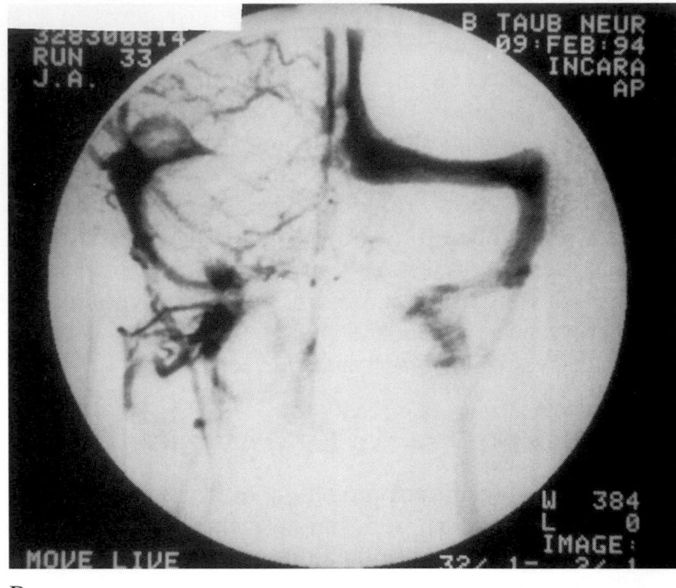

B

Figure 60-6. Vascular injuries. Any missile that traverses the normal location of an arterial or venous structure can potentially cause a vascular injury. In such instances an arteriogram is advisable. In this 20-year-old man with a bullet tracking from the left malar region to the right occiput, the arterial phase did not demonstrate any abnormality (*A*), but the bullet had obviously caused a traumatic occlusion of the right transverse sinus (*B*).

nial aneurysms, arteriovenous fistulas, dural sinus injuries, and other major vascular injuries. Therefore, a high index of suspicion must be maintained for the presence of these lesions, and angiography should be utilized when there are clinical or radiographic reasons to suspect a vascular lesion (Figs. 60-3 and 60-6).

Salvageability

Upon completion of the initial survey, the examiner must be prepared to determine salvageability and select patients appropriate for surgical intervention. The limit of salvageability in civilian penetrating head injury has been a subject of some controversy and is clearly an important issue in an era of increasingly limited resources and overwhelmed trauma centers. Many studies have attempted to identify the critical prognostic factors for penetrating injuries.[4,11,15,24,35,36,44] The level of consciousness after cardiopulmonary resuscitation has consistently been found to be the most important prognostic variable. Circumstances such as suicide attempts, posterior fossa wounds, and through-and-through perforating wounds also have been correlated with poor patient outcome, as has elevated ICP and hypotension on presentation. In addition, the following CT findings have been found to be associated with a poor outcome: bihemispheric injury, transventricular injury, subarachnoid and intraventricular hemorrhage, midline shift, compression of mesencephalic cisterns, and hematomas (hyperdense or mixed-density lesions greater than 15 ml on CT).

In civilian GSW series, patients presenting in coma have repeatedly been observed to have an extremely grim prognosis.[4,15,19,24] This finding has led some authors to advocate a nonaggressive approach to the management of these patients, especially when no mass lesion is present on CT.[19,24,33] However, occasional reports of dramatic recoveries in severely injured patients have prompted some speculation that a "self-fulfilling prophecy" may contribute to the high mortality observed in civilian GSW victims[35]; that is, these patients do not receive aggressive management because it is assumed that their outcome will be poor, and therefore their outcome *is* poor. This speculation has been based on the observation that retrospective reviews of civilian gunshot wounds have revealed that only a minority of comatose GSW patients received aggressive surgical management.[19,24,35]

Grahm and colleagues[22] attempted to answer this dilemma by conducting a prospective trial in which all patients who presented with civilian GSW to the head and maintained at least two neurological signs after resuscitation underwent CT and subsequent operative debridement if brain death did not supervene. In their series of 100 consecutive patients, no patient with a *postresuscitation* GCS of 3 to 5 had a satisfactory (good/moderately disabled) outcome. Likewise, among patients with a GCS of 6 to 8 and bihemispheric or multilobar dominant hemisphere injuries, there were no satisfactory outcomes. On the basis of these results, the authors did not recommend surgical intervention for patients with a GCS of 3 to 5 unless a large hematoma was present and questioned the role of aggressive surgical treatment in patients with a GCS of 6 to 8.

Levy and coworkers[42] also attempted to address this issue with a review of 190 GCS 3 to 5 patients. Sixty of their patients received aggressive surgical and medical management, including pentobarbital coma and lobectomy when needed to control ICP. Patients with intractable hypotension were excluded from surgical intervention. The survival rate of this cohort was significantly improved compared with that of the nonoperative group (38 percent versus <1 percent; however, only two patients achieved a moderately disabled outcome). Both patients had reactive pupils at admission and did not have bihemispheric injury or subarachnoid hemorrhage. The authors felt that operative intervention was unlikely to benefit most GCS 3 to 5 patients but recommended caution in withholding treatment to patients with reactive pupils and favorable CT findings.

The selection of patients appropriate for surgical intervention remains a difficult challenge, and formulistic approaches are unlikely to account for the multitude of variables implicated. While it is clear that the majority of patients with a low GCS cannot currently be helped with surgery, continued efforts must be directed toward the development of methods for the identification of potentially salvageable patients. Care must always be taken to ensure that a surgically treatable mass lesion is not responsible for a patient's poor neurological status. Postinjury deterioration and/or the presence of relatively normal brainstem responses (especially intact pupillary responses) in spite of a low GCS score should alert the examiner to the possibility of an intracranial mass and potential salvage. When any doubt exists, a CT scan must be obtained.

Kaufman and associates performed a mail survey of American neurosurgeons regarding their practice in the management of penetrating head injury.[45] Most neurosurgeons agreed on the use of anticonvulsants and prophylactic antibiotics, and almost all utilized CT scanning in the evaluation of these patients. There was considerably less agreement on the indications for surgical intervention and the limits of salvageability. This was especially true in the management of patients whose GCS was in the middle range of 6 to 8, in which case neurosurgeons were essentially split on the issue of salvageability. A majority of neurosurgeons felt that patients with a GCS of 3 to 5, bilaterally dilated pupils, and deep brain or bihemispheric injuries were not operative candidates. The strongest consideration for surgery in any patient was felt to be the presence of a hematoma.

OPERATIVE MANAGEMENT

Historical Considerations

The basic principles for the operative management of penetrating craniocerebral trauma have been developed and refined largely through the vast experience with these injuries accrued during the major military conflicts of this century. Military techniques have focused on the prevention of devastating postinjury infectious sequelae, and with refinements, these techniques have resulted in progressively lower operative mortality rates through successive conflicts.[23,44,46]

Past military operative techniques focused on thorough debridement of all necrotic tissue, bone fragments, and foreign bodies, followed by meticulous dural and scalp closure, utilizing grafts or rotational flaps as necessary. Debridement of the missile path was continued until it no longer tended to collapse, and mass lesions were always sought and removed. Retained bone fragments on postoperative skull films were felt to be an indication of inadequate debridement and were thought to be associated with an increased incidence of infection; hence, reoperation for further debridement was routinely performed, even at some risk of additional neurological injury. Strict application of these principles led to an operative mortality of approximately 10 percent during the Vietnam war, and the incidence of postoperative infections was low.[23,32,47,48]

A number of technological advances, as well as new data from civilian GSW series, long-term follow-up of Vietnam patients, and follow-up of more recent military conflicts, have resulted in some modifications to these time-honored principles. Technologically, the advent and widespread availability of CT have had a profound effect on many areas of neurosurgery and have also clearly had an impact on the management of penetrating wounds.[34] In addition, there have been a number of advances in the intensive care management of all head-injured patients, most notably the introduction and routine use of ICP monitoring and control. Broad-spectrum and relatively nontoxic antibiotics which exhibit good CSF penetration are now available and may play a role in the prevention of postinjury infections, although this has not been well studied.

A large amount of data has accumulated over recent years on civilian penetrating injuries. Many of these series utilized less aggressive debridement and often removed only bone fragments which were readily available.[15,19,24] A number of authors felt that the low-velocity nature of many of these injuries resulted in less cerebral destruction and a lower propensity toward infection compared with military injuries.[15,19,35] Irrespective of the validity of this argument, while the mortality from civilian GSWs has been high, the morbidity and mortality specifically from infectious complications have not.[7,19,20]

Long-term follow-up data from the Vietnam Head Injury Study have helped clarify the issue. In an analysis of 1221 patients, only 37 cases of brain abscess were found. Eleven of the patients with abscess were noted to have retained bone fragments, but additional risk factors were found in all patients, including CSF fistula, wound complications, facio-orbitocranial/air sinus injuries, multiple surgical procedures, and coma.[48] CSF leak was found to be associated with infectious complications in another large military series.[49] A review of CT scans from long-term Vietnam head injury survivors found retained bone fragments in 23 percent of patients, none of whom had developed an intracranial abscess.[50] Correlation of late postinjury CT scans with neuropsychological and psychiatric outcomes also emphasized the importance of cerebral tissue loss to long-term functioning. Furthermore, reoperation for removal of retained bone fragments has been associated with a significant risk of increased neurological deficit or other complications.[31,32,51]

These observations have led to the application of less aggressive debridement strategies. In the Israeli-Lebanese conflict, Brandvold and colleagues[17] debrided brain, bone, and missile fragments with gentle irrigation and hemostatic maneuvers. Emphasis was placed on the preservation of viable cerebral tissue at the expense of thorough debridement. In 113 patients treated in this fashion, there was only one postoperative intracranial abscess, and this was associated with a CSF fistula. Follow-up CT in 43 patients found a 51 percent incidence of retained bone fragments with no episodes of late abscess formation. Likewise, no association between postinjury seizure disorders and retained bone fragments was identified.[17]

During the same conflict, a series of 32 patients with penetrating missile injuries of the brain were treated with superficial entry wound debridement and closure. This treatment was selected only for patients with a stable neurological exam and a GCS greater than 10. Additionally, the patients had to be evaluated within 6 h of wounding, have entry wounds less than 2 cm, and have no exit wounds or missile tracts which traversed the proximal sylvian fissure. Patients with significant intracranial hematomas were excluded. All patients in this group survived with improved or no neurological deficits. One patient developed a delayed abscess but recovered well after surgical drainage and antibiotic therapy. All patients in this series received 2 weeks of antibiotic therapy.[52]

As a result of such studies and with the now widespread availability of postoperative CT scanning and ICP monitoring, it appears that debridement may be confined to clearly nonviable brain and mass lesions and that bone and missile fragments should be removed only when they are readily accessible. Repeat operation for retained bone fragments is not advocated. However, it must be emphasized that debridement of all clearly necrotic tissue is still advisable. Inadequate debridement may lead to uncontrollable ICP elevation and further brain infarction. In the authors' opinion, the pendulum may be swinging too far in the direction of halfhearted and "sloppy" debridements. The data support not chasing after every hidden bone fragment. Unfortunately, this is often interpreted as justifying a minimalistic surgical approach which is probably unwise.

Goals of Surgery

The current goals for the operative management of penetrating craniocerebral trauma in the civilian population should include the following:

1. Debridement of necrotic scalp, muscle, dura, and brain
2. Removal of accessible indriven bone and bullet fragments (however, not at the expense of an increased neurological deficit or loss of significant amounts of potentially viable cerebral tissue)
3. Evacuation of all significant mass lesions
4. Hemostasis and repair of injured vascular structures
5. Meticulous dural and scalp closure

All operative procedures for penetrating head wounds should begin with wide prepping and draping of the scalp so that additional incisions may be made if more exposure is required. Curvilinear or S-shaped incisions incorporating the entry/exit site are frequently sufficient, but standard scalp flaps may also be utilized when increased exposure is desired. Local craniectomy of entrance and exit sites has been a commonly employed method of bony removal; however, others have favored larger craniotomy flaps centered over the entrance wound.[53] The craniectomy method is best applied to more discrete injuries without large mass lesions or suggestion of vascular or dural sinus injury. Craniotomy is favored for patients with more extensive injuries, as it yields better exposure for debridement, control of injured vascular structures, and evacuation of intracranial hematomas. When craniotomy is performed, the entrance size can be debrided with a small craniectomy and the bone flap can be replaced. Whichever technique is utilized, it is important that the normal dura be exposed circumferentially for later repair.

After an adequate bony opening is obtained, the dura is opened, often in a cruciate manner radiating from the entry hole. Large dural openings are not recommended unless they are designed for a specific purpose such as lobectomy, as they may result in troublesome outward herniation of the brain. Necrotic brain, bone fragments, debris, and foreign materials are then debrided from the bullet tract, using irrigation and gentle suctioning. Debridement is tempered by attempting to preserve all viable brain, especially in eloquent areas. Hemostasis should of course be meticulous, and precise coagulation is preferred to leaving behind hemostatic materials. Unfortunately, intraoperative brain swelling is not an uncommon problem. Attempts to control malignant brain swelling with major cerebral resections are not likely to result in improved outcomes, especially in patients who present with coma and brainstem damage. Intraoperative maneuvers such as raising the head, hyperventilation, and administration of mannitol, furosemide, and barbiturates sometimes can be helpful. Occasionally, frontal or temporal lobectomy may be useful.[42] Intraoperative ultrasound can be utilized to identify hematomas which have arisen since the time of CT scanning.

Upon completion of debridement and evacuation of mass lesions, attention is turned to dural closure. This must be done in a meticulous manner and frequently requires a patch graft. The graft may be obtained from local tissues (pericranium, temporalis fascia), or in the case of more extensive repairs, lyophilized human dura may be utilized. If this is not available, allograft or autologous fascia lata may be employed.

With the exception of shotgun injuries, scalp closure is rarely a problem with civilian injuries. However, when there are large scalp injuries, plastic surgery techniques should be utilized to effect adequate wound coverage.

Exit wounds should be dealt with in a similar manner. Unless there is an underlying hematoma, a small craniectomy with local debridement will suffice. Patients who do not follow commands preoperatively should routinely have a ventriculostomy or the placement of another ICP monitoring device.

Certain patients may be effectively managed with only simple scalp closure. This is most appropriate for patients who have relatively minor injuries, who are in good neurological condition, and in whom operative debridement might incur major risks. For example, small children with bone fragments involving a major dural sinus may easily exsanguinate after debridement, and such fragments may be better left undisturbed. Serial CT scanning can be used to monitor the development of brain abscesses in such patients. The optimal frequency of such scanning has not been established.

POSTOPERATIVE CARE

The postoperative management of patients who have suffered a penetrating head injury is based largely on the principles derived from the management of closed head injuries. In particular, ICP should be monitored routinely in comatose patients and sustained ICP elevations greater than 20 mmHg should be treated aggressively. Continuous monitoring of jugular venous oxygen saturation also may be useful in the prevention of secondary ischemic insults.[54] Ventriculostomy is the preferred method of ICP monitoring, as it allows for the drainage of CSF as an adjunct to ICP control. Intraparenchymal ICP devices may be utilized if the ventricles cannot be cannulated. Bolus infusion of osmotic diuretics such as mannitol as well as the administration of sedatives, narcotics, and neuromuscular blocking agents should be utilized as necessary. The patient's head should remain elevated and straight to avoid impairment of venous outflow.[55] Induced hypocapnia via hyperventilation is most helpful in acute ICP elevations before the evacuation of mass lesions. However, prolonged hypocapnia with P_{CO_2} <25 mmHg can lead to ischemic complications,[56,57] and routine postoperative hyperventilation is not recommended. Periods of hypoventilation and hypercarbia must be avoided to prevent the occurrence of a marked ICP rise. Pentobarbital may be useful in selected cases where these measures fail.[58]

Recognition of delayed intracranial mass lesions is critical in a penetrating head injury patient. Unexpected neurological deterioration or increases in ICP should prompt rapid evaluation by CT scanning. The development of a delayed intracranial hematoma should always arouse suspicion of an unrecognized vascular injury or underlying coagulopathy. All delayed mass lesions should be evacuated promptly.

Antibiotics are now widely used in the postoperative management of penetrating head injuries.[20,22,24,33] However, studies specifically addressing the efficacy, choice, and duration of antibiotic therapy are lacking. Currently, the authors empirically employ a broad-spectrum combination of vancomycin, ceftazidime (Fortaz), and metronidazole (Flagyl) for a 10-day course. This combination adequately accesses the CNS and has been utilized successfully for the prophylaxis of postoperative infections in patients undergoing clean-contaminated craniofacial resections. For thoroughly debrided wounds, this regimen is sometimes simplified to a single agent, such as a first- or second-generation cephalosporin. With the paucity of available data, local preferences will probably prevail.[59–61]

Prophylactic anticonvulsant therapy, usually involving phenobarbital or phenytoin, is widely used in the perioperative period after penetrating craniocerebral trauma. However, even this tenet is sometimes disputed, and the recommended duration of postinjury therapy remains controversial, as does the effectiveness of prophylaxis in preventing posttraumatic epilepsy.[62]

Steroids are still prescribed frequently; however, most studies have not shown benefits from their use. Therefore, because of possible systemic complications, conventional steroid administration is not currently recommended for patients with penetrating head injuries.[45,63]

SPECIFIC MANAGEMENT PROBLEMS

CRANIOFACIAL INJURIES

Penetrating head injury which involves the facial bones, air sinuses, and/or orbits has been recognized as a separate category of injury, as specialized procedures must be utilized to avoid complications. Bullets may enter the cranium after passing through the maxillary, ethmoid, sphenoid, and frontal (most common) sinuses, carrying contaminated mucosal tissue intracranially. Dural laceration may easily give rise to a CSF fistula, a key risk factor for the development of infectious complications.[64,65] Visual loss is also common.[64,66] Operative technique should focus on thorough intracranial debridement and evacuation of hematomas, dural repair, and definitive management of associated sinus and orbit injuries.[65,66] In many instances, a multidisciplinary approach is indicated for the management of these complex cases.

Unilateral frontal, frontotemporal, or bifrontal craniotomy is usually selected, depending on the anatomy of the injury. A bicoronal-type incision with careful preservation of the pericranial layer is helpful when repair of the anterior skull base is anticipated.[59,65] Debridement of the intracranial injury follows previously outlined guidelines. Dural closure or repair is a critical step, and defects in the dura overlying the basal frontal lobes must be sought all the way back to the posterior aspect of the anterior cranial fossa. Large defects are best repaired intradurally, utilizing graft materials.[64,65]

The dogma states that when involved, the frontal sinus should be cranialized by removal of its posterior wall, followed by thorough removal of the mucosa and blockage of the frontonasal ducts with muscle. Pericranial flaps are most useful for isolating the repaired dura and intracranial contents from the opened air sinuses, preventing CSF leaks and encephaloceles.[59] Drainage of CSF via ventriculostomy or lumbar drain also may facilitate healing when the repair is felt to be tenuous.

The potential complications that follow penetrating craniofacial injuries are numerous and include infection (meningitis, abscess, osteomyelitis), CSF leak, subdural and epidural hematoma, encephalocele, mucocele, and carotid-cavernous fistula. Tension pneumocephalus is a potentially life-threatening pre- or postoperative complication which should be considered when there is neurological deterioration.[66] Outcomes from craniofacial penetrating injury are dictated primarily by the severity of the brain injury and by avoidance of postinjury complications.[64–66]

VASCULAR INJURIES

Vascular injuries associated with penetrating craniocerebral trauma can add significantly to morbidity and mortality. Early recognition and treatment of these lesions are essential if preventable deaths are to be avoided. However, the replacement of cerebral arteriography with CT scanning as the primary preoperative imaging modality has in some instances led to a somewhat delayed diagnosis of these lesions.[67] Arterial occlusion, transection and dissection, arteriovenous fistula, traumatic intracranial aneurysms, and dural venous sinus injuries represent the major vascular injuries encountered in penetrating head trauma[67] (Fig. 60-6).

Many minor vascular injuries undoubtedly occur with every penetrating injury as the injured vessels thrombose spontaneously after the initial hemorrhage. Other minor injuries are frequently encountered at surgery and are simply coagulated. However, a small percentage of patients harbor lesions with the potential for massive intraoperative hemorrhage or catastrophic delayed intracranial hemorrhage (ICH), such as traumatic intracranial aneurysms (TICAs). TICAs represent only a very small percentage of intracranial aneurysms, with approximately 25 percent of TICAs being due to penetrating injuries.[68] They are false aneurysms which develop after disruption of the arterial wall followed by periarterial hematoma formation and cavitation. Unlike congenital aneurysms, these aneurysms tend to occur along the course of more peripheral arteries, most commonly around the sylvian candelabra and median hemispheric vessels. Angiography is the diagnostic study of choice, and the aneurysms typically have a well-defined border. A characteristic finding that further distinguishes TICAs from congenital aneurysms is the tendency of TICAs to fill late and have delayed emptying.[69,70]

Aarabi reviewed 223 patients with missile injury undergoing angiography and found 8 TICAs (3.6 percent).[69] A pterional entry site was felt to be an important risk factor. Levy and colleagues performed angiograms on 31 patients with civilian GSWs and subarachnoid hemorrhage on CT and found one TICA (3.2 percent).[68] They concluded that the presence of subarachnoid hemorrhage was not associated with a significant incidence of TICA. In another study, Jinkins and colleagues found five TICAs in a series of just 12 civilian GSWs and concluded that early postinjury angiography may detect vascular injuries in a higher percentage of patients.[67]

Haddad and associates reviewed their experience with TICAs seen during the Lebanese conflict as well as other reported cases.[70] They found TICAs to be associated with an increased incidence of ICH and subdural hematomas (SDHs), with hematomas most frequently occurring in the distal portions of the missile tract. The aneurysms appeared on angiography as early as 2 h after injury or later after an initially negative arteriogram. Approximately 20 percent of TICAs were multiple. These authors and others also have found that the overwhelming majority of TICAs seen in military conflicts are secondary to shrapnel wounds, possibly because low-velocity shrapnel with sharp edges is more likely to scathe an arterial wall and result in an aneurysm.[69–71] Bullet wounds causing TICAs were typically "spent."[71] However, civilian GSWs appear to result in an incidence of TICA similar to that seen in shrapnel wounds.[68]

TICAs appear to have a more malignant natural history than do congenital aneurysms. In addition to the frequently encountered ICH (80 percent) at the time of presentation, these lesions have a high rate of repeat hemorrhage and associated mortality.[69,70] Therefore, surgical or endovascular trapping should be considered when these lesions are encountered. The surgical mortality likewise is higher than that for congenital aneurysms (approximately 20 percent), possibly because of an increased tendency toward intraoperative rupture, since the aneurysmal wall is really a pseudocapsule.[68,69] Overall, outcome is most dependent on the original injury, the preoperative condition of the patient, and the location of the TICA.[70]

A high index of suspicion must be maintained for the occurrence of TICAs. Patients who experience delayed ICH or subarachnoid hemorrhage, have major arterial bleeding at the time of initial debridement, or have an otherwise unexplained deterioration in neurological status should undergo arteriography.[68] The development of significant epistaxis or a delayed cranial nerve palsy should also raise concern about TICA.[72]

Thrombosis, dissection, and transection of major arterial vessels also may result in massive stroke or intraoperative hemorrhage. Bullet trajectories clearly intersecting the proximal sylvian fissure warrant preoperative angiograms if possible, and attention to proximal control of major vessels is obviously critical.[7] An occasional patient may be a candidate for a bypass procedure.

Coagulopathy

Severe head injury is well recognized to cause coagulopathy. The release of tissue thromboplastin is thought to result in the activation of the extrinsic coagulation cascade. Disseminated intravascular coagulation (DIC) may follow with depletion of fibrinogen and platelets, and a catecholamine surge at the time of injury may contribute to the pathophysiology.[73,74] This consumptive coagulopathy may result in increased intraoperative hemorrhage or the development of a delayed intracranial hematoma.[75] Because the degree of coagulopathy is related to the amount of brain tissue injured, the occurrence of DIC is a poor prognostic indicator.[35,74] Routine coagulation parameters which should be checked include prothrombin time, activated partial thromboplastin time, fibrinogen level, fibrin split products, and platelet count. The efficacy of treating abnormal values with blood products remains speculative, but this procedure seems to be reasonable in patients planned for operative procedures and those who develop intra- or postoperative bleeding complications. More recently, experimental efforts have been directed at assaying for and correcting antithrombin III (ATIII) levels in patients with a penetrating head injury.[74]

Tangential Injuries

Tangential craniocerebral gunshot wounds are defined as wounds caused by a missile which passes through tissues adjacent to the cranial cavity and not through the brain itself yet which produces a cerebral injury.[76] Skull fractures and indriven bone fragments may or may not be present. This type of injury has been seen predominantly in the military setting in association with high-velocity missiles but also may be seen in the civilian population with lower-velocity weapons.[61] The brain injury typically consists of an underlying contusion with variable degrees of edema. However, distant contusions and intracerebral and subdural hematomas also may occur.

The occurrence of these occasionally life-threatening injuries highlights the importance of obtaining CT images of the brain in every instance of cranial missile injury, regardless of the presumed trajectory, presence or absence of skull fractures, and neurological status. Even gunshot wounds localized to the face may cause serious intracranial injury.[77] It is not rare for a bullet to be deflected off the skull, travel under the scalp for a variable distance, and then exit the scalp without ever entering the cranium.

Cranial Stab Wound

A variety of nonmissile penetrating brain injuries may occur with weapons ranging from knives to pencils to scissors. A cranial stab wound has been defined as a wound caused by a weapon with a small impact area that has been wielded at low velocity.[78] These injuries have become distinctly less common in most developed countries, presumably because of the availability of more lethal firearms. They remain more common in third world countries and countries with strictly enforced gun control, such as South Africa.[79]

The pathophysiology of these injuries differs significantly from that of bullet wounds. The weapons utilized possess considerably less kinetic energy compared with missiles; therefore, the potential for widespread and distant injury is much lower. Instead, the injury is largely confined to the local area of penetration and any associated hemorrhage. The seriousness of stab injury is critically dependent on the site and depth of penetration, associated vascular injuries, and the occurrence of hematomas. As with other types of penetrating injuries, infectious complications may occur and sometimes dominate the clinical picture, especially when patients present late after injury.[79,80]

On examination, an obvious weapon may be seen protruding from the head (Fig. 60-7), or the entrance site may be barely detectable and misleading. Approximately three-fourths of these patients present with the responsible weapon removed. The removal of the weapon sometimes can increase both the severity of injury and the risk of mortality, possibly because of additional damage resulting from forceful attempts to remove the instrument.[78,80,81]

The radiological examination of these patients in-

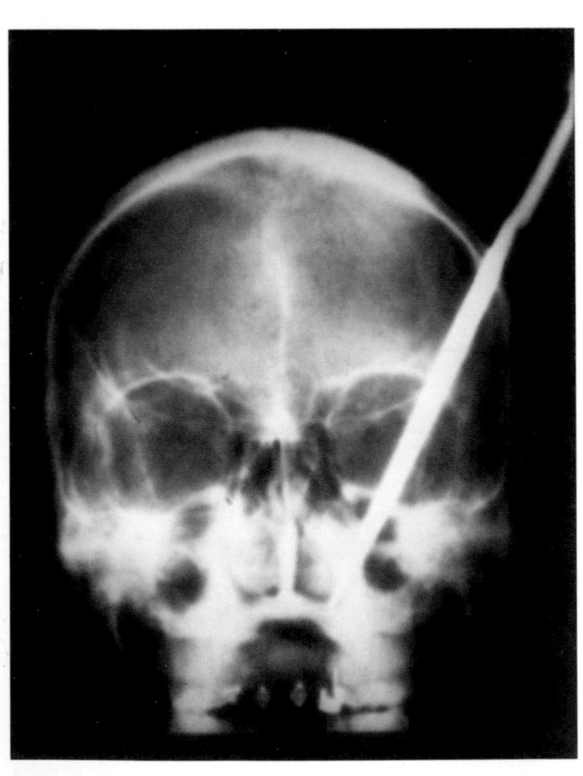

A

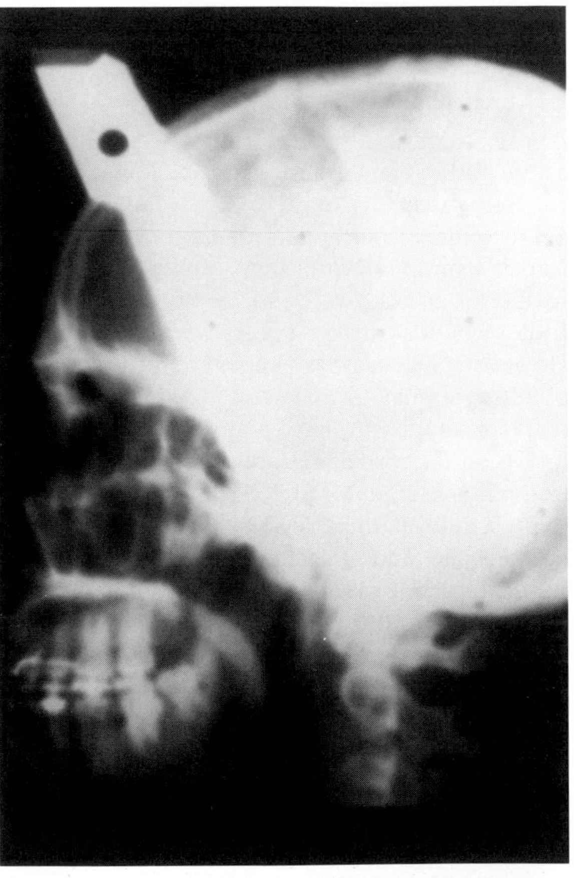

B

Figure 60-7. Stab injury. While he lay asleep in prison, this prisoner's cell mate introduced a scissors blade into his left frontal skull. The patient had a minimal fifth cranial nerve deficit preoperatively. He made a nearly complete recovery after removal of the blade via craniotomy (Reprinted from Becker et al,[94] with permission.) *A.* AP view. *B.* Lateral view.

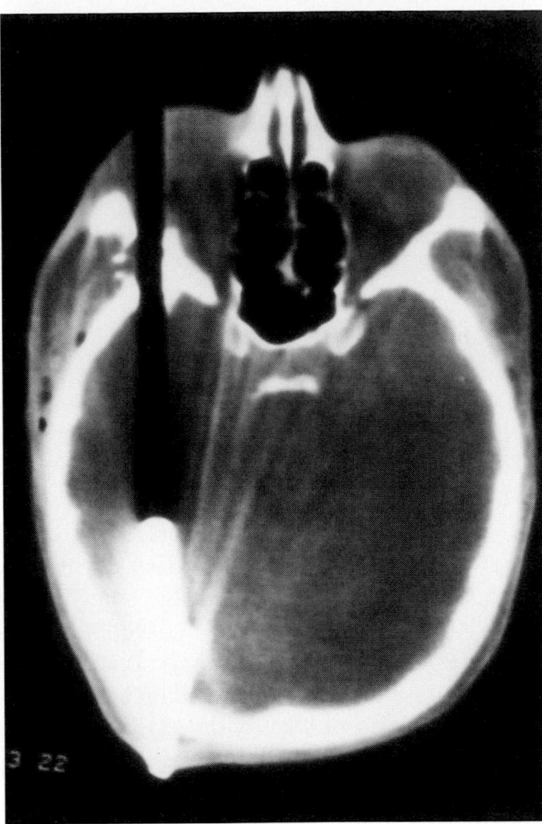

Figure 60-8. Arrow injury. An inebriated 25-year-old man from Oregon who was participating in an initiation rite for an outdoor club attempted to prove his bravery by placing a fuel canister atop his head and allowing his equally inebriated friend to shoot it off with a bow and arrow in a classic "William Tell" maneuver. The arrow missed the can but penetrated the right eye. There was no loss of consciousness. CT of the head is shown above. The cerebral angiogram was unremarkable. A pteriorial flap was performed anteriorly, and a small horseshoe flap was performed posteriorly over the palpable subcutaneous arrow tip. After the arrow was disengaged from the skull, it was cut short and pulled through the skull. A ventriculostomy tube was pulled through the tract with the arrow and was used to irrigate the tract. Dural patch grafts were applied. Apart from a blind right eye and a mild left pronator drift, the patient did well (Reprinted from O'Neill et al,[95] with permission.)

cludes skull films, CT, and arteriography (Fig. 60-8). Plain skull films reveal the characteristic "slot" fractures associated with transcranial stab wounds. CT provides critical information concerning the exact location and extent of injured structures and identifies any associated hematomas.[78]

Depending on the location and trajectory of the offending instrument, cerebral arteriography may be an essential part of the evaluation in these patients and should preferably be performed before operative intervention, except in cases of rapid neurological deterioration. Approximately 30 percent of such patients harbor a detectable vascular abnormality, including pseudoaneurysms (TICA), arteriovenous fistulas, arterial transections and occlusions, and vascular spasm.[78] Traumatic intracranial aneurysms in these patients are more likely to occur at the skull base and, like other TICAs, have a high rate of rehemorrhage and mortality if left untreated. Early angiograms may miss some TICAs because of vasospasm and inadequate visualization of the vasculature, and repeat angiography at a later date is indicated in these instances.[78,80]

The surgical management of stab wounds is similar to that of gunshot injuries. Weapons still in place at the time of presentation should generally be removed under operating room conditions. In cases where the weapon has been removed, tract debridement and hematoma removal are followed by dural repair, and vascular injuries discovered on angiography often can be dealt with in the same operation. Selected patients may require only observation and/or antibiotic therapy.[78,79,81]

The outcome for stab wounds of the head is more favorable than that for gunshot wounds, with approximately two-thirds of patients making a satisfactory recovery [Glasgow Outcome Score (GOS) 1 to 2]. However, mortality rates as high as 26 percent have been observed in patients with the weapon removed and 11 percent in those with the weapon in place. As with gunshot wounds, patients who present in coma frequently have a poor outcome.[78,80]

Dural Sinus Injuries

Dural venous sinus injuries are frequently encountered in penetrating head injuries and often represent challenging surgical problems. Life-threatening hemorrhage from an injured sinus may easily occur in the field or emergency department or during the debridement of depressed bone fragments. Ligation or occlusion of the posterior two-thirds of the superior sagittal sinus or a dominant transverse sinus may result in fatal increases of ICP or massive venous infarcts.[82,83]

The most important step in the management of dural venous sinus injuries is preoperative recognition and appropriate planning. Wide exposure with proximal and distal control of the involved sinus must be secured before debridement in the area. Many smaller rents are easily controlled by packing with Gelfoam or muscle.[83,84] Elevation of the head can temporarily reduce massive hemorrhaging while other maneuvers are pursued (close observation for the occurrence of air embolism is required). The anterior one-third of the sagittal sinus can be ligated when necessary.[83] Extensive injuries to a dominant transverse sinus or posterior sagittal sinus may require microsurgical repair and reconstruction with venous grafts and internal shunting devices.[84] However, such repairs generally are not very practical and should not be lightly attempted. As a general rule, depressed bone fragments involving critical segments of dural sinuses are better left undisturbed unless there is marked compromise of blood flow.[7]

COMPLICATIONS

Penetrating craniocerebral trauma may be associated with a number of medical and surgical complications, including wound infections, osteomyelitis, CSF fistula, meningitis, ventriculitis, cerebritis, intracranial abscess, hydrocephalus, delayed or recurrent hematoma formation, seizures, and the many possible complications associated with critical illness.[7,22,24,47] As was discussed earlier, the infectious complications have traditionally been the most feared. In the literature from Vietnam, retained bone fragments were listed as a complication, and reoperations were routinely performed to remove such fragments.[23] Retained bone fragments do not appear to be major risk factor for infectious complications in civilian injuries, but increased surveillance for the development of abscess may be warranted when retained fragments have been documented.

CSF leaks are a significant risk factor for the development of meningitis and intracranial abscess.[42,48,49] CSF fistulas may be seen most frequently after transbasal or transfacial gunshot wounds causing CSF otorrhea or rhinorrhea. CSF also may leak from inadequately closed wounds or in the presence of hydrocephalus. Many CSF fistulas resolve spontaneously or close with the temporary diversion of CSF via a lumbar or ventricular drain.[22,24] Occasionally, repeat craniotomy with dural repair is required, especially with skull base wounds and otorrhea or rhinorrhea.[64,65]

Intracranial abscess has been a rare complication of civilian penetrating head injuries, occurring in approximately 3 percent of cases.[19,20,33,42] The diagnosis and treatment of intracranial abscess have been greatly facilitated by the advent of CT and modern antimicrobial therapy. Surgical drainage followed by culture-specific antibiotics is the treatment of choice.[20,52]

Hydrocephalus may complicate the acute or chronic phase after penetrating head wounds.[7] GSWs causing hemorrhage into the ventricular system may result in acute hydrocephalus, as may GSWs to the posterior fossa. Subarachnoid hemorrhage after a penetrating injury also may give rise to hydrocephalus and cause cerebral vasospasm in some cases.[68]

Retained intracranial bullets or bullet fragments occasionally migrate within the ventricular system or through the white matter to more dependent locations. Obstructive hydrocephalus or increased neurological deficits may result (Fig. 60-9). Bullet migration is most likely to occur with larger, nondeformed fragments, and removal of such bullets may be indicated in selected circumstances. Fragment migration also has been observed in the setting of brain abscess.[85,86]

OUTCOME

The morbidity and mortality rates associated with civilian penetrating head injury, although improved with the advent of modern therapies, are still unacceptably high in spite of advances in prehospital care, diagnostic studies, and improved postoperative care. In many instances, direct GSWs to the brain are not compatible with life, and victims die at the scene or soon after arrival at an emergency center.[3,11,22] It is unlikely that current medical and surgical therapies can salvage many of these patients.[22,87] Future improvements in outcome probably will derive from improved salvage of more moderately injured patients and from the avoidance of complications in patients who present with better GCS scores.[7] More accurate identification of salvageable patients in the low GCS category should also help in this regard.

In the past, comparison of outcome data between different centers and settings was difficult because the presenting neurological condition of patients was not recorded in a standardized fashion. Similarly, patient outcomes were described with vague terminology. With the introduction of the GCS and GOS, more thorough analysis of results has become possible.

In recent series of civilian gunshot wounds, overall mortality has consistently been near 60 percent in patients presenting to hospitals alive, presumably with significant numbers of victims not surviving to inclusion.[19,22,24,35] An earlier large series found a mortality rate of only 30 percent; again, this presumably was lower because fewer of the more severely injured patients survived to be included.[15] In patients presenting with GCS scores from 3 to 5, mortality is in excess of 90 percent,[22,35,36] although a recent series demonstrated a 40 percent survival rate in a group of these patients who received aggressive surgical and medical treatment (although mortality for the entire cohort remained near 90 percent).[42] Only rare patients in this group have had better than severely disabled outcomes.[22,35,36]

Mortality rates reported for patients presenting with GCS 6 to 8 have been more variable, ranging from 20 to 70 percent.[22,24,36] This variability probably is related to the smaller numbers of patients who present in this category. The majority of patients with cranial GSWs present at one end of the GCS or the other, with relatively fewer patients presenting with intermediate scores. Different management also may account for some of the outcome variability in this group, suggesting

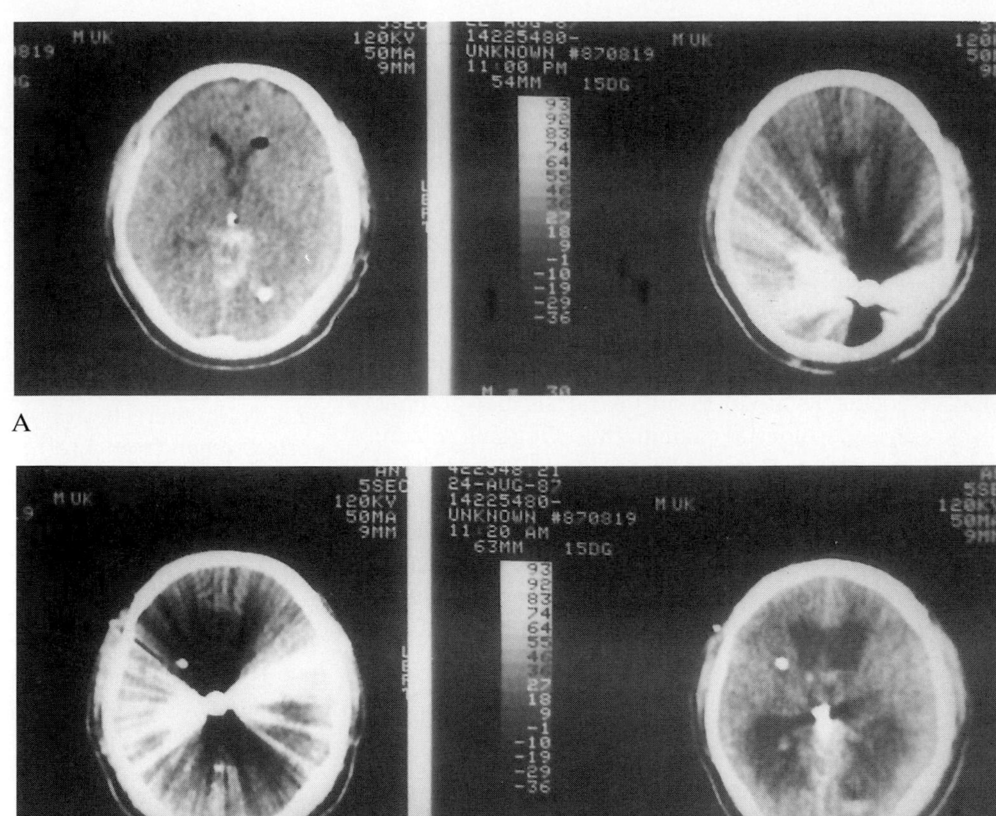

Figure 60-9. Migrating bullet. Intracranial bullets can and often do migrate if they are not embedded in the skull. They are most likely to migrate if they are in the ventricular system or outside the brain. This 50-year-old patient was critically injured and comatose with a bullet in the left parieto-occipital region (*A*). He appeared to be stable until 2 days after admission, when his ventriculostomy began to malfunction and a follow-up CT scan showed that the bullet had migrated into the third ventricle, blocking the aqueduct and causing massive hydrocephalus (*B*). The patient subsequently expired. While it is not always necessary or even advisable to remove intracranial bullets, this case illustrates the unpredictable behavior of such bodies and the difficulty in ascertaining their exact plane because of the metal artifact on the scan.

that more aggressive therapy might salvage additional patients. Overall mortality in patients who present with GCS scores less than 9 exceeds 80 percent in most series.[15,19,20,22,24,35,36] Mortality rates reported for gunshot wounds to the head in the pediatric population have been similar to adult values.[88]

In contrast to the dismal numbers presented above, patients who present in good neurological condition have low mortality rates, approaching zero in those with GCS scores 13 to 15.[22,35] However, in patients who present with GCS scores greater than 9 but then deteriorate, the mortality rate reaches 40 percent.[36] This finding highlights the importance of careful monitoring of these patients and a high index of suspicion for the delayed development of mass lesions.[19,36]

Functional outcome, most commonly reported utilizing the GOS, depends on the presenting level of consciousness, much as mortality rates do. Overall, approximately 30 to 40 percent of patients achieve "satisfactory" outcomes (defined as good or moderately disabled).[19,22,24,35] Among patients with a presenting GCS 9 to 15, approximately half make good recoveries and nearly 90 percent have satisfactory outcomes.[22,24] As with mortality, reported functional outcomes in the middle GCS ranges (6 to 8) are quite variable; however, good recoveries are not common.[22,24,36] As is apparent from these figures, relatively few patients survive vegetative or with severe disability, suggesting an "all or nothing" phenomenon in which most patients either die or make useful recoveries.[7]

INJURY-ASSOCIATED MORBIDITY

Posttraumatic Epilepsy

The occurrence of posttraumatic epilepsy has long been recognized as an important complication of penetrating brain injury, and postinjury seizures may have an impact on a patient's clinical course in a variety of ways. Seizures in the acute postinjury period may result in dangerous increases in ICP and exacerbate ongoing ischemia. A postictal state or Todd's paralysis may at times obscure the neurological examination. Ongoing seizure activity must be detected and abolished in any head injury patient, and most authors recommend the routine loading of patients with a penetrating brain injury with intravenous phenobarbital or phenytoin.[19,22,24,42] Delayed posttraumatic epilepsy impairs patients psychosocially and may increase their level of disability. Furthermore, the life expectancy of patients with posttraumatic epilepsy may be diminished relative to that of the general population and patients without epilepsy.[51,89,90]

The Vietnam Head Injury Study has collected extensive data on many patients who suffered penetrating brain injuries during the Vietnam war.[89] A study of 421 veterans with penetrating injuries followed for an average of 15 years found that 53 percent had posttraumatic epilepsy and 28 percent had "persistent" epilepsy (more than one seizure in the 2-year period before the study). Ninety-two percent of affected patients had more than one seizure, and the duration of the seizure disorders (time interval from the first to the last seizure) averaged 93 months. Fifty-seven percent of patients experienced the first seizure during the first year after injury, but 18 percent had the first seizure more than 5 years later.

The study also identified a number of clinical characteristics which correlated with the occurrence of posttraumatic epilepsy. These characteristics were divided into initial wound characteristics and long-term neurological deficits. Among the wound characteristics associated with postinjury seizure disorders were high brain volume loss evident on CT, early evidence of hematoma, and retained metal fragments. Tangential gunshot wounds, retained bone fragments, presence of a dural graft or cranioplasty, and brain abscess were not associated with an increased incidence of seizures when the data were corrected for volume of brain tissue lost. Brandvold and associates also found no relationship between retained bone fragments and postinjury seizures.[17]

Postinjury neurological deficits associated with an increased incidence of posttraumatic epilepsy in this population included organic mental disorder, visual field loss, aphasia, and hemiparesis. The duration of postinjury unconsciousness was not found to be significantly related. Interestingly, some of the patient groups with the highest likelihood of posttraumatic epilepsy also had the lowest risk for "persistent" seizures. These groups included patients with the highest volume of brain tissue loss, residual aphasia, or organic mental disorders. The most important prognostic indicator for "persistent" seizures appeared to be the number of seizures during the first year after injury.

Information regarding the incidence of posttraumatic epilepsy in the civilian population, especially long-term data, is limited. The reported incidence of seizures reported ranges from 4 to 15 percent, but follow-up times are short.[4,7,19] Further study is required to elucidate any important differences between the military and civilian populations.

The role of prophylactic anticonvulsants in the prevention of posttraumatic epilepsy has been controversial. However, there is no convincing evidence that long-term anticonvulsant therapy can prevent the development of posttraumatic epilepsy or even the occurrence of seizures during therapy. While anticonvulsant administration during the acute phase is widely accepted, the appropriate duration of this therapy in the absence of a seizure disorder remains uncertain. Routine long-term administration of anticonvulsants does not appear to be warranted.[62,89]

Neurological Morbidity

Patients who survive penetrating brain injuries are frequently left with a wide variety of neurological, neuropsychological, and neurobehavioral deficits which subsequently affect their long-term quality of life and level of functioning. Destruction of eloquent areas of the brain will obviously produce predictable neurological deficits. Many survivors of gunshot wounds also show cognitive and behavioral deficits characteristic of more diffuse injuries.[51,91]

In a study of civilian GSW victims, defects in long-term memory for new information were the most common neuropsychological sequelae, while visuospatial and linguistic deficits were related to the side of injury.[91] The side of injury may indeed predict the type of deficit encountered; however, overall functioning and psychosocial adjustment may not differ.[92]

The Vietnam Head Injury Study has assessed a large number of long-term survivors of penetrating brain injury with regard to their postinjury employment record, a measure of overall function.[51] Approximately 56 percent of patients were working 15 years after injury, compared with 82 percent of controls. Six impairments were found to correlate with work status: posttraumatic epilepsy, paresis, visual field loss, verbal memory loss, psychological problems, and violent behavor. Postinjury intelligence and total brain volume loss were also predictive of the degree of disability. While one or two of these impairments usually did not prevent employment, the effects appeared to be cumulative. It has been noted that the neurobehavioral changes following these injuries may at times be more disabling than are specific neurological deficits.[51,92]

Ewing-Cobbs and coworkers[93] studied neurobehavioral outcomes in children after craniocerebral gunshot wounds. Their study group followed 13 patients from 1.5 years to 14 years of age at the time of injury for 3 years and compared younger and older age groups. At 3-year follow-up, 85 percent had moderate disability and 8 percent had severe disability. Outcome was felt to correlate most strongly with the lowest postresuscitation GCS. Intellectual functioning was most impaired in children less than age 5 at the time of injury. The deficits encountered were felt to be commensurate in degree with those found in a population of similar severe closed head injury patients. The authors concluded that young age may not correlate with a better prognosis and that the types of deficits found are affected by the patient's neurological development.

References

1. Brent D, Perper J, Allman C: Alcohol, firearms, and suicide among youth: Temporal trends in Allegheny County, Pennsylvania. *JAMA* 257:3369–3372, 1987.
2. Jagger J, Dietz P: Death and injury by firearms: Who cares? *JAMA* 255:3143–3144, 1986.
3. Kaufman H: Civilian gunshot wounds to the head. *Neurosurgery* 32:962–964, 1993.
4. Lillard P: Five years experience with penetrating craniocerebral gunshot wounds. *Surg Neurol* 9:79–83, 1978.
5. Cotton P: Gun-associated violence increasingly viewed as public health challenge. *JAMA* 267:1171–1174, 1992.
6. Beaver B, Moore V, Peclet M, et al: Characteristics of pediatric firearm fatalities. *J Pediatr Surg* 25:97–100, 1990.
7. Benzel E, Day W, Kesterson L, et al: Civilian craniocerebral gunshot wounds. *Neurosurgery* 29:67–70, 1991.
8. Carter G: Accidental firearm fatalities and injuries among recreational hunters. *Ann Emerg Med* 18:406–409, 1989.
9. Patterson D, Holguin A: Firearm-related deaths among children in Texas: 1984–1988. *J Tex Med* 86:92–97, 1990.
10. Sosin D, Sacks J, Smith S: Head injury-associated deaths in the United States from 1979–1986. *JAMA* 262:2251–2255, 1989.
11. Siccardi D, Cavaliere R, Pav A, et al: Penetrating craniocerebral missile injuries in civilians: A retrospective analysis of 314 cases. *Surg Neurol* 35:455–460, 1991.
12. Cooper P: Gunshot wounds of the brain, in Cooper P (ed): *Head Injury,* 2d ed. Baltimore: Williams & Wilkins, 1987:313–326.
13. Hopkinson D, Marshall T: Firearm injuries. *Br J Surg* 54:344–353, 1967.
14. Dagi T: Emergency management of missile injuries to the brain: Resuscitation, triage, and preoperative stabilization. *Am J Emerg Med* 5:140–148, 1987.
15. Raimondi A, Samuelson G: Craniocerebral gunshot wounds in civilian practice. *J Neurosurg* 32:647–653, 1970.
16. Shoung H, Sichez J, Pertuiset B: The early prognosis of craniocerebral gunshot wounds in civilian practice as an aid to the choice of treatment. *Acta Neurochir (Wien)* 74:27–30, 1985.
17. Brandvold B, Levi L, Feinsod M, George E: Penetrating craniocerebral injuries in the Israeli involvement in the Lebanese conflict, 1982–1985: Analysis of a less aggressive surgical approach. *J Neurosurg* 72:15–21, 1990.
18. Carey M, Young H, Mathis J, Forsythe J: A bacteriologic study of craniocerebral missile wounds from Vietnam. *J Neurosurg* 34:145–154, 1971.
19. Clark W, Muhlbauer M, Watridge C, Ray M: Analysis of 76 civilian craniocerebral gunshot wounds. *J Neurosurg* 65:9–14, 1986.
20. Helling T, McNabney W, Whittakev C, et al: The role of early surgical intervention in civilian gunshot wounds to the head. *J Trauma* 32:398–400, 1992.
21. Allen I, Scott R, Tannel J: Experimental high velocity head injury. *Injury* 14:183–193, 1982.
22. Grahm T, Williams F Jr, Harrington T, Spetzler R: Civilian gunshot wounds to the head: A prospective study. *Neurosurgery* 27:696–700, 1990.
23. Hammon W: Analysis of 2187 consecutive penetrating wounds of the brain from Vietnam. *J Neurosurg* 34:127–131, 1971.
24. Nagib M, Rockswold G, Sherman R, Lagaard M: Civilian gunshot wounds to the brain: Prognosis and management. *Neurosurgery* 18:533–536, 1986.
25. Kirkpatrick J, DiMaio V: Civilian gunshot wounds of the brain. *J Neurosurg* 49:185–198, 1978.
26. Selden B: Craniocerebral wound ballistics. *Indiana Med* 80:150–152, 1987.
27. Carey M, Gurcharan S, Farrell J: Brain edema following an experimental missile wound to the brain. *J Neurotrauma* 7:13–20, 1990.
28. Harvey E: Studies on wound ballistics, in Andrus E, Bronk D, Carden G Jr (eds): *Advances in Military Medicine.* Boston: Atlantic Little Brown, 1948:191–205.
29. Freytag E: Autopsy findings in head injuries from firearms. *Arch Pathol* 76:215–225, 1963.
30. Sights W Jr: Ballistic analysis of shotgun injuries to the central nervous system. *J Neurosurg* 31:25–33, 1969.
31. Carey M, Tutton R, Strub R, et al: The correlation between surgical and CT estimates of brain damage following missile wounds. *J Neurosurg* 60:947–954, 1984.
32. Meirowsky A: Secondary removal of retained bone fragments in missile wounds of the brain. *J Neurosurg* 57:617–621, 1982.
33. Hubschmann O, Shapiro K, Baden M, Schulman K: Craniocerebral gunshot injuries in civilian practice—prognostic criteria and surgical management: Experience with 82 cases. *J Trauma* 19:6–12, 1979.

34. Cooper P, Maravilla K, Cone J: Computerized tomographic scan and gunshot wounds of the head: Indications and radiographic findings. *Neurosurgery* 22:373–380, 1979.
35. Kaufman H, Makela M, Lee K, et al: Gunshot wounds to the head: A perspective. *Neurosurgery* 18:689–695, 1986.
36. Aldrich E, Eisenberg H, Saydjari C, et al: Predictors of mortality in severely head-injured patients with civilian gunshot wounds: A report from the NIH Traumatic Coma Data Bank. *Surg Neurol* 38:418–423, 1992.
37. Crockard H, Brown F, Calica A, et al: Physiological consequences of experimental cerebral missile injury and use of data analysis to predict survival. *J Neurosurg* 46:784–794, 1977.
38. Levett J, Johns L, Repogle R, Mullan S: Cardiovascular effects of experimental cerebral missile injury in primates. *Surg Neurol* 13:59–64, 1980.
39. Allen I, Kirk J, Maynard R, et al: An ultrastructural study of experimental high velocity penetrating head injury. *Acta Neuropathol (Berl)* 59:277–282, 1983.
40. Crockard H: Early intracranial pressure studies in gunshot wounds of the brain. *J Trauma* 15:339–347, 1975.
41. Levi L, Borovich B, Guilbard J, et al: Wartime neurosurgical experience in Lebanon, 1982–1985: I. Penetrating craniocerebral injuries. *Isr J Med Sci* 26:548–554, 1990.
42. Levy M, Masri L, Lavine S, Apuzzo M: Outcome prediction after penetrating craniocerebral injury in a civilian population: Aggressive surgical management in patients with admission Glasgow Coma Scale of 3, 4, or 5. *Neurosurgery* 35:77–85, 1994.
43. Kennedy F, Gonzales P, Beitler A, et al: Incidence of cervical spine injury in patients with gunshot wounds to the head. *South Med J* 87:621–623, 1994.
44. Aarabi B: Surgical outcome in 435 patients who sustained missile wounds during the Iran-Iraq War. *Neurosurgery* 27:692–695, 1990.
45. Kaufman H, Schwab K, Salazar A: A national survey of neurosurgical care for penetrating head injury. *Surg Neurol* 36:370–377, 1991.
46. Cushing H: Notes on penetrating wounds of the brain. *Br Med J* 5:558–684, 1918.
47. Hagan R: Early complications following penetrating wounds of the brain. *J Neurosurg* 34:132–141, 1971.
48. Rish B, Caveness W, Dillon J, et al: Analysis of brain abscess after penetrating craniocerebral injuries in Vietnam. *Neurosurgery* 9:535–541, 1981.
49. Aarabi B: Causes of infections in penetrating head wounds in the Iran-Iraq War. *Neurosurgery* 25:923–926, 1989.
50. Myers P, Brophy J, Salazar A, Jonas B: Retained bone fragments after penetrating brain wounds: Long-term follow up in Vietnam veterans (abstract). *J Neurosurg* 70:319A, 1989.
51. Schwab K, Grafman J, Salazar A, Kraft J: Residual impairments and work status 15 years after penetrating head injury: Report from the Vietnam Head Injury Study. *Neurology* 43:95–103, 1993.
52. Taha J, Saba M, Brown J: Missile injuries to the brain treated by simple wound closure: Results of a protocol during the Lebanese conflict. *Neurosurgery* 29:380–384, 1991.
53. Rish B, Dillon J, Caveness W, et al: Evolution of craniotomy as a debridement technique for penetrating craniocerebral injuries. *J Neurosurg* 53:772–775, 1980.
54. Sheinburg M, Kantor M, Robertson C, et al: Continuous monitoring of jugular venous oxygen saturation in head-injured patients. *J Neurosurg* 76:212–217, 1992.
55. Feldman Z, Kantor M, Robertson C, et al: Effect of head elevation on intracranial pressure, cerebral perfusion pressure, and cerebral blood flow in head-injured patients. *J Neurosurg* 76:207–211, 1992.
56. Turner E, Hilfiker O, Braun V, et al: Metabolic and hemodynamic response to hyperventilation in patients with head injury. *Intensive Care Med* 10:127–132, 1984.
57. Yoshida K, Marmarou A: Effects of tromethamine and hyperventilation on brain injury in the cat. *J Neurosurg* 74:87–96, 1991.
58. Eisenberg H, Frankowski R, Contant C, et al: Comprehensive central nervous system trauma centers: High-dose barbituate control of elevated intracranial pressure in patients with severe head injury. *J Neurosurg* 69:15–23, 1988.
59. Blacklock J, Weber R, Lee Y, Goepfert H: Transcranial resection of tumors of the paranasal sinuses and nasal cavity. *J Neurosurg* 71:10–15, 1989.
60. Carrau R, Snyderman C, Janecka I, et al: Antibiotic prophylaxis in cranial base surgery. *Head Neck Surg* 13:311–317, 1991.
61. Green H, O'Donoghue M, Shaw M, Dowling C: Penetration of ceftazidime into intracranial abscess. *J Antimicrob Chemother* 24:431–436, 1989.
62. Temkin N, Dikmen S, Wilensky A, et al: A randomized, double-blind study of phenytoin for the prevention of post-traumatic seizures. *N Engl J Med* 323:497–502, 1990.
63. Molofsky W: Steroids and head trauma. *Neurosurgery* 15:424–426, 1984.
64. Arendall R, Meirowsky A: Air sinus wounds: An analysis of 163 consecutive cases incurred in the Korean War. *Neurosurgery* 13:377–380, 1983.
65. Dillon J Jr, Meirowsky A: Facio-orbito-cranial missile wounds. *Surg Neurol* 4:515–518, 1975.
66. Sollman W, Seifert V, Haubitz B, Dietz H: Combined orbito-frontal injuries. *Neurosurgery* 12:115–121, 1989.
67. Jinkins J, Dadsefan M, Sener R, et al: Value of acute-phase angiography in the detection of vascular injuries caused by gunshot wounds to the head: Analysis of 12 cases. *AJR* 159:365–368, 1992.
68. Levy M, Rezui A, Masri L, et al: The significance of subarachnoid hemorrhage after penetrating craniocerebral injury: Correlations with angiography and outcome in a civilian population. *Neurosurgery* 32:532–540, 1993.
69. Aarabi B: Traumatic aneurysms of the brain due to high velocity missile head wounds. *Neurosurgery* 22:1056–1063, 1988.
70. Haddad F, Haddad G, Taha J: Traumatic intracranial aneurysms caused by missiles: Their presentation and management. *Neurosurgery* 28:1–7, 1991.
71. Rahimizadeh A, Abtahi H, Daylami M, et al: Traumatic cerebral aneurysms caused by shell fragments: Report

of four cases and review of the literature. *Acta Neurochir (Wien)* 84:93–98, 1987.
72. Buckingham M, Crone K, Ball W, et al: Traumatic intracranial aneurysms in childhood: Two cases and a review of the literature. *Neurosurgery* 22:398–408, 1988.
73. Awasthi D, Rock W, Carey M, Farrell J: Coagulation changes after an experimental missile wound to the brain in the cat. *Surg Neurol* 36:441–446, 1991.
74. Kearney T, Bentt L, Grode M, et al: Coagulopathy and catecholamines in severe head injury. *J Trauma* 32:608–612, 1992.
75. Kaufman H, Maake J, Olsen J, et al: Delayed and recurrent intracranial hematomas related to disseminated intravascular clotting and fibrinolysis in head injury. *Neurosurgery* 7:445–449, 1980.
76. Copley I: Cranial tangential gunshot wounds. *Br J Neurosurg* 5:43–53, 1991.
77. Hadas N, Schiffer J, Roger M, Shperber Y: Tangential low-velocity missile wound of the head with acute subdural hematoma: Case report. *J Trauma* 30:358–359, 1990.
78. Du Trevou M, van Dellen J: Penetrating stab wounds to the brain: The timing of angiography in patients with the weapon already removed. *Neurosurgery* 31:905–912, 1992.
79. Khalil N, Elwany M, Miller J: Transcranial stab wounds: Morbidity and medicolegal awareness. *Surg Neurol* 35:294–299, 1991.
80. Kieck C, Devilliers J: Vascular lesions due to transcranial stab wounds. *J Neurosurg* 60:42–46, 1984.
81. Van Dellen J, Lipshitz R: Stab wounds of the skull. *Surg Neurol* 10:110–114, 1978.
82. Meier V, Gartner F, Klotzer R, Wolf O: The traumatic dural sinus injury—a clinical study. *Acta Neurochir (Wien)* 119:91–93, 1992.
83. Meirowky A: Wounds of dural sinuses. *J Neurosurg* 10:496–514, 1953.
84. Kapp J, Gielchinsky I, Deardourft S: Operative techniques for management of lesions involving the dural venous sinuses. *Surg Neurol* 7:339–342, 1977.
85. Deschamps G, Morano J: Intracranial bullet migration—a sign of brain abscess: Case report. *J Trauma* 31:293–295, 1991.
86. Rengachary S, Carey M, Templer J: The sinking bullet. *Neurosurgery* 30:291–295, 1992.
87. Suddaby L, Weir B, Forsyth C: The management of .22 caliber gunshot wounds of the brain: A review of 49 cases. *Can J Neurol Sci* 14:268–272, 1987.
88. Miner M, Ewing-Cobbs L, Kopaniky D, et al: The results of treatment of gunshot wounds to the brain in children. *Neurosurgery* 26:20–25, 1990.
89. Salazar A, Jabbar B, Vance S, et al: Epilepsy after penetrating head injury: I. Clinical correlates: A report of the Vietnam Head Injury Study. *Neurology* 35:1406–1414, 1985.
90. Walker A: Posttraumatic epilepsy in World War II veterans. *Surg Neurol* 10:110–114, 1978.
91. Kaufman H, Levin H, High W Jr, et al: Neurobehavioral outcome after gunshot wounds to the head in adult civilians and children. *Neurosurgery* 16:754–758, 1985.
92. Tellier A, Adams K, Walker E, Rourke B: Longterm effects of severe penetrating head injury on psychosocial adjustment. *J Consult Clin Psychol* 58:531–537, 1990.
93. Ewing-Cobbs L, Thompson N, Miner M, Fletcher J: Gunshot wounds to the brain in children and adolescents: Age and neurobehavioral development. *Neurosurgery* 35:225–233, 1994.
94. Becker DP, Miller JD, Young HF, et al: Head injury in adults, in Youmans JR (ed): *Neurological Surgery,* 2d ed. Philadelphia: Saunders, 1982, vol 4: 2034.
95. O'Neill OR, Gilliland G, Delashaw JB, Purtzer TJ: Transorbital penetrating head injury with a hunting arrow: Case report. *Surg Neurol* 42:494–497, 1994.

Portions of the text and figures in this chapter have been reproduced or modified from Trask T, Narayan R: Management of penetrating head injuries, in Barrow D, Cooper P, Tindall G (eds): *The Practice of Neurosurgery,* 1st ed. Baltimore: Williams & Wilkins, by permission.

CHAPTER 61

MILITARY HEAD INJURIES

John J. Knightly
Morris W. Pulliam

SYNOPSIS

A large proportion of battlefield mortality and morbidity is related to penetrating craniocerebral injuries. The introduction of antibiotics has significantly reduced the infection rate. Earlier enthusiasm for extensive debridement along the bullet tract has been tempered somewhat. Wide exploration of normal brain in search of bone or bullet fragments is not currently recommended, especially in eloquent brain. However, evacuation of hemotomas, debridement of extensive necrotic brain, careful dural closure, and removal of easily accessible foreign bodies still constitute the accepted surgical approach to these injuries. In this chapter, the current thinking regarding the management of penetrating head injury in the military setting has been reviewed.

INTRODUCTION

Penetrating craniocerebral wounds suffered in combat continue to be a common and lethal military injury. Like many advances made in the surgical treatment of trauma, management techniques in caring for penetrating head injuries have been developed and improved by physicians in the military trying to treat battlefield injuries. However, management of these patients remains as much or more of a challenge for physicians in the civilian setting today, as for those in the military.

For centuries, penetrating head injuries were considered fatal and were essentially not treated, especially if the dura was compromised.[1] Gurdjian found little difference between the reported mortality rate of 71.7 percent for penetrating head wounds in the American Civil War and a deduced 76 percent mortality rate from Homeric times, circa 900 B.C.[2] Although trephining the skull to elevate skull fractures and evacuate hemorrhage has been practiced since antiquity, infection rates were so high that few operations were performed. West reported that one American Civil War series with 4350 head injuries showed only 674 operative interventions.[1] There was some evidence to suggest that patients did better if treated expectantly than with surgery owing to the increased risk of infection in surgical patients.[1–4]

Several developments during the late 1800s and early 1900s led to more aggressive surgical intervention and improved survival rates. By far the most important of these was the development of antiseptic techniques by Lister in 1867 and the development of antibiotics during World War I and II (WWI, WWII).[1] This greatly decreased infection rates and allowed more aggressive surgical intervention. In addition, the development of an ambulance system, first by Larrey serving with Napolean, and advanced by Letterman during the Civil War, allowed injured combatants to be evacuated in an orderly fashion to centralized medical facilities with more competent physicians—the same principles that guide civilian trauma systems today.[1,3] Preventive health measures also led to improved health of combatants and support personnel. As an example, the Union Army lost 225,000 casualties to disease in the American Civil War compared to 110,000 in combat.[3] For WWII, Korea, and Vietnam, 90 percent of U.S. Army deaths were classified as killed in action.[5]

Finally, increased knowledge of the pathophysiology of head injuries allowed more rational medical and surgical management techniques to be developed. Cushing is widely credited with developing the first systematic approach to the management of penetrating head injuries.[1,6] His techniques, refined in later conflicts and by

The views expressed in this article are those of the authors and do not reflect the official policy or position of the Department of the Navy, Department of Defense, or the United States Government.

advances in medical and surgical technology, paved the way for the current treatment regimens used in managing these injuries.

MILITARY ENVIRONMENT VS CIVILIAN

One of the major issues facing neurosurgeons in managing military craniocerebral injuries is the battlefield environment in which they must practice. Facilities available for patient care are widely variable and dependent on the tactical military situation. In some instances, medical treatment facilities (MTF) are as modern and well-equipped as any civilian trauma center, with almost unlimited resources and far from any ongoing hostilities. At the other end of the spectrum, the neurosurgeon may be managing patients in a canvas tent or hastily converted room with minimal, if any, radiographic support, basic instruments, and a real threat of bodily harm from surrounding combat. Whatever the environment, considerable flexibility is needed to adjust to adverse circumstances not usually present in the civilian sector.

In most military units, wounded combatants are evacuated through organized echelons of care. An example of such an organizational plan is found in Table 61-1. At each level, patients are triaged for type and severity of injury. The triage format commonly used is found in Table 61-2. Patients are evacuated to the next appropriate level of care depending on triage status, type of injury, and the medical resources of the treatment facilities.

Treatment of craniocerebral injuries begins at the time of injury with basic first aid given by other soldiers or medics/corpsmen attached to the unit. The patient is transported to an Echelon I MTF where they may be evaluated for the first time by a physician. After appropriate stabilization and treatment, severely injured patients are evacuated to Echelon II or III facilities for definitive care. The decision regarding which level of care the patient is transferred to depends on the capabilities of the different echelons, the time and distance for evacuation, and which MTFs are able to handle additional patients. In many systems, medical regulating teams provide an orderly flow of patients through the different echelons of care and ensure that patients are sent to facilities with appropriate specialty support. When patients are stabilized, they are evacuated to an Echelon IV facility for more specialized care, follow-up treatment, and rehabilitation prior to discharge.

TABLE 61-1 Echelons of Care in the Wartime Environment

Echelon	Description
I.	Aid station or clearing station where initial medical treatment and stabilization beyond basic first aid can begin
II.	Resuscitation and treatment facility with general surgical support and inpatient capabilities
III.	Medical facility with more advanced surgical and inpatient capabilities
IV.	Rear-echelon facility with rehabilitation and definitive surgical capabilities

TABLE 61-2 Triage Requirements for Combat Injuries

Group	Description
Group I (Minimal)	Patients whose injuries are treated easily and can return to duty with minimal delay
Group II (Delayed)	Patient's condition requires modest emergency intervention with little possibility of morbidity/mortality from delayed definitive treatment
Group III (Immediate)	Patient's injuries require immediate intervention and should receive the highest medical priority
Group IV (Expectant)	Patients with massive injuries whose likelihood of survival is negligible even if intense intervention is attempted

The medical sophistication of each echelon is dependent on the resources of the military units they care for. In the case of the United States military, field hospitals are often located near hostilities and have advanced support services such as computerized tomography (CT) and angiography. Such services are also available on hospital ships, such as the USNS COMFORT and MERCY. Other nations' military resources may not support such units, with sophisticated medical support being far removed from the combat units they serve. In the era of "small" regional conflicts, even nations with advanced resources may not have all medical units deployed to regions of military activity, which leads to lengthy evacuations of seriously injured combatants.

Where neurosurgeons are stationed within the system is determined by the resources of the military unit. Like a tank, jet fighter, or CT scanner, a neurosurgeon is viewed as an asset and deployed where most beneficial. If sufficient numbers exist and the tactical situation merits, neurosurgeons can be assigned to Echelon II MTFs. In most instances, neurosurgical care is found in Echelon III or IV facilities.

The evacuation process is important in caring for head-injured patients. Since the advent of evacuation by air, patients can be quickly taken to the appropriate MTF. When craniocerebral injuries are found, lower echelons of care are bypassed, allowing the patient to receive neurosurgical care with minimal delay. However, this assumes that helicopters are available for evacuation missions and that air superiority exists to insure safety of flight crews and their patients. This is not always the case, and patients may have to be cleared through the different echelons of care and moved by any means available.

This "traditional" method of patient evacuation was standard practice during many recent conflicts. Vranković and co-workers, describing their war-injury experience in Croatia during 1991, reported a mean transportation time of 3 hours and 50 minutes (some patients requiring from 10 to 24 hours) to reach their facility.[7] Aarabi reported a mean injury to arrival time of 49 hours (range 7 to 450) during the Iraq-Iran War, 1981–1988.[8,9] Patients in this conflict were transferred to the general hospital, 400 miles from the front, by ground or air after first being evaluated at dressing stations or field hospitals near the front.[9] The Israeli experience during the Lebanon war (1982–1985) showed transit times of 2 to 2.3 hours.[10,11] During the Vietnam war, the United States was able to operate a large helicopter medical evacuation system with transit times of under 2 hours, compared with 2 to 4 hours during the Korean War, when limited helicopter support was available, and 6 to 12 hours during World War II, when no such aircraft were available.[12,13]

Neurosurgical support, and medical and physical support for the neurosurgeon, depend primarily on the capabilities of the military units they support. For efficient care of craniocerebral injuries, an infrastructure is needed to provide prompt evaluation and evacuation of casualties. Material support of the MTFs is similarly crucial. Under wartime conditions, the number of systems that can possibly fail are limitless. Flexibility in the use of limited available resources is needed much more often under these conditions, forcing changes in how craniocerebral injuries are managed compared with the civilian environment.

TYPES OF INJURIES/ CLASSIFICATION

As in civilian trauma, head injuries suffered in combat are classified as open or closed. Closed head injuries can result from the concussive effects of munitions and explosions, falls, and deceleration injuries from motor vehicle accidents. Management of this type of injury is covered elsewhere in this text and will not be discussed here.

With open craniocerebral wounds, injury classification is determined on the basis of both the characteristics of the missile and the anatomic features of injury. For penetrating head wounds, missile projectiles are divided between those coming directly from firearms (gunshot wounds) and shrapnel. Shrapnel projectiles can be further divided into primary fragments from munitions (bomb, grenade, mine, missile, etc.), or secondary fragments projected by the blast force of exploding munitions (stones, pieces of wood or metal, etc.). A third category of penetrating head wound consists of impaling injuries from weapons such as knives, bayonets, spears, or similar objects. While these injuries are relatively uncommon in most modern armed conflicts, they are the major mode of injury in many areas of the world, such as Africa where machetes are common weapons.

The degree of damage a projectile inflicts is related to the kinetic energy (KE) it imparts to the skull and brain. The KE of a projectile is determined by the equation $KE = \frac{1}{2} mV^2$, where m is the mass of the projectile (caliber of bullet in gunshot wounds) and V is velocity at time of impact. As this equation indicates, increasing the velocity of the projectile produces proportionally much more energy than increasing its mass. The amount of energy deposited to the cranial contents (KE_d) is the difference between KE of the projectile at impact and its residual KE when leaving tissue.[14] With most military firearms, muzzle velocity is in the range of 2400 to 3200 ft/sec, whereas the muzzle velocity of most handguns is less than 1000 ft/sec.[15]

Wounding ballistics of a projectile depend on several factors, many of these originally described by Harvey.[16] As the projectile enters tissue, a shock wave is produced ahead and to the side of it. Cavitation (production of a cavity greater than the volume displaced by the missile) occurs from this outward shock wave. Increasing KE_d increases the degree of cavitation accordingly. Cavity formation will also deform surrounding structures.

The flight path of the projectile influences the KE_d and the amount of cavitation. Transfer of energy depends on resistance of the tissue being traversed.[15] The longer the path through tissue, the larger the resistance and the increase in KE_d. If the projectile does not deviate from its course and remains appropriately aligned, less resistance is encountered; accordingly, less energy is deposited. This is rarely the case, especially in the head, where penetration of the skull induces the projectile to roll or tumble. This yaw phenomenon projects a greater surface area for the projectile along its path, increasing resistance from brain and resulting in a higher KE_d to involved brain tissue.[14,15]

Because the brain is contained within a rigid vault, shock wave and cavitation forces generated by projectiles are transferred throughout the confines of the skull. A low velocity (<1500 ft/sec) projectile deposits most of its KE on local structures adjacent to the path of the missile. The degree of neurological injury is influenced mainly by the function of the nervous and soft tissue traversed by the projectile. However, with high-velocity missile wounds, neurological injury can result from damage to tissues distant to the path of the projectile owing to pressure forces transmitted within the skull.[14,15,17] Death from high-velocity craniocerebral injuries usually results from acute pressure waves exerted on the brain stem.[15,18] Pressure waves probably also account for the diffuse cerebral edema seen in areas remote to the injury site, which often develops within minutes of injury.[15]

Until recently, most classifications of combat craniocerebral injuries were anatomically based on physical descriptions of the wound. Cushing (Table 61-3) analyzing his experience in WWI, and later Matson (Table 61-4), reviewing WWII injuries, divided most craniocerebral injuries as tangential (grazing or gutter), penetrating, or perforating missile wounds with associated factors contributing to the severity of the wound.[19,20] Most recent series of combat head injuries use a modification of Matson's classification for grouping patients. Although easy to use, this classification system is often simplistic and does not adequately describe the full extent of the patient's injury. There are several contributing anatomic, radiographic, and clinical findings, listed in Table 61-5, which have been shown to be effective in classifying craniocerebral head injuries in terms of survival outcome.

TABLE 61-3 Cushing's Classification of Craniocerebral Injuries

Grade	Description
I.	Scalp lacerations with or without cerebral contusion, skull intact
II.	Wounds with skull fractures but with intact dura, with or without depression
III.	Wounds with depressed skull fracture and dural laceration
IV.	Wounds with detached and in-driven bone fragments, brain usually extruding
V.	Penetrating wounds with projectile lodged, brain usually extruding
VI.	Wounds penetrating ventricles with:
	(A) bone fragments
	(B) projectile
VII.	Wounds involving:
	(A) orbitonasal region
	(B) auropetrosal region
VIII.	Perforating wounds, cerebral injury severe
IX.	Bursting skull fractures, extensive cerebral contusion

TABLE 61-4 Matson's Classification of Craniocerebral Injuries

Grade	Description
I.	Scalp wound
II.	Skull fracture without dural penetration
III.	Skull fracture with penetration of dura/brain:
	(A) Gutter-type (grazing) wounds—bone fragments in-driven with no retained missile fragments
	(B) Penetrating wounds—missile fragments retained within brain
	(C) Perforating wounds—through-and-through injuries to the brain
IV.	Complicating factors:
	(A) Ventricular penetration
	(B) Fractures of orbit or sinus
	(C) Injury of dural sinus
	(D) Intracerebral hematoma

Grazing, or gutter-type, injuries are caused when the projectile strikes the skull tangentially and exits. Only a portion of the projectile's kinetic energy is deposited on the skull. With low velocity projectiles, a limited scalp wound or skull fracture without dural penetration may result. If the projectile has a high-velocity, a significant amount of energy may be imparted to the skull and underlying soft tissue, leading to significant skull fracturing, dural penetration, and local and distant (contra coup) brain injuries.[21] In addition, KE is transferred to bone fragments and induces them to act as secondary projectiles, leading to injuries deep to the path of the original projectile. Bone fragments acting as secondary projectiles can occur with any type of missile wound to the calvarium.

TABLE 61-5 Factors Complicating Combat Craniocerebral Injuries

Ventricular penetration[10,11,19,20]
Facial/orbital entrance or fracture[19,20,41]
Dural sinus injury[20,28]
Intracerebral mass lesion[22,37]
Low Glasgow Coma Scale on admission[8,10,11,18,22,35]
Abnormal coagulation status[22,37]
Crossing mid-sagittal/mid-horizontal plane[22,37]
Contusion of brain > 10 percent[22]
Pupillary changes[22,37]
Subarachnoid hemorrhage[32,37]
Infection[1,2,8–10,35]
High-velocity projectiles[10,11,13,36]
Diffuse fragmentation[37]
Systemic shock[10,11]
CSF leak[29,35]

Penetrating injuries usually result in retention of the projectile within the confines of the skull. Some low-velocity projectiles lack enough KE to penetrate the skull. Significant penetrating injuries result from missiles fracturing the skull and entering the brain. Significant energy must be deposited by the projectile to penetrate the skull. The projectile may reach the contralateral side and not have enough KE to exit the skull and overlying soft tissue. In these cases, the bullet will lodge in the contralateral skull/soft tissue, and is readily apparent on plain radiographs. In other cases, the projectile will ricochet back into brain, causing further damage.[15] This injury pattern may not be apparent on plain films leading to confusion regarding the projectile's exact path.

Perforating wounds are through-and-through craniocerebral injuries with the projectile exiting the head. In most cases, patients presenting clinically with these types of injuries have wounds resulting from low-velocity projectiles. Perforating wounds from high-velocity projectiles result in massive brain injuries and are usually immediately fatal. As with tangential and penetrating injuries, secondary projectiles from bone fracturing and projectile fragmentation are common with these lesions.

The ability to evacuate combat patients to facilities where CT is available allows classification schemes used in civilian trauma centers to be used in the military environment, thus more effectively triaging patients with craniocerebral injuries. A recent scheme devised by Shaffrey and co-workers combines clinical, radiographic, and laboratory data, including GCS, pupillary response, number and type of anatomic plains traversed by the projectile based on CT images, and coagulation status.[22] By relying on these types of data rather than on an anatomic description alone, a better understanding of a patient's overall clinical status can be achieved.

Classification strategies are important in combat situations where resources are limited and where many patients may need attention. Categorizing patients effectively and understanding prognostic significance of different types of injuries expedites triage of injured patients and directs life-saving resources to those patients with the best chance for useful survival.

INITIAL MANAGEMENT

Stabilization

Successful treatment of craniocerebral injuries sustained in combat begins with prompt recognition of the nature and extent of the wounds and rapid evacuation. Initial care is provided by members of the patient's unit or a medic after first removing the patient and caregiver from threat of danger, which is not a small feat in many instances. A sterile dressing is applied and the patient is taken to an Echelon I MTF, usually a clearing station. Standard protocols for transporting patients in the civilian environment require cervical spine immobilization prior to moving the patient. In combat situations, this is not possible. Arishita et al. in their review of Vietnam combat casualty data found that only 3.7 percent of casualties presenting for care had spinal column injuries and only 1.4 percent possibly benefiting from immobilization.[23] It should be noted that 10 percent of casualties resulted from rendering first-aid to other casualties. Cervical immobilization should be initiated as soon as feasible after removing the patient from risk of further injury.

For serious craniocerebral injuries, establishment and maintenance of a patent airway and providing adequate ventilation is critical. If needed, endotracheal intubation is performed as soon as possible. Intravenous access is obtained for hemodynamic support and administering medications. The remainder of the body is surveyed for other injuries and treated appropriately. A baseline neurological exam should be performed, preferably before any muscle relaxants or other medications are administered. These findings, and any pertinent information concerning circumstances and timing of injury, should be documented and should accompany the patient to the next echelon of care.

Aggressive cardiovascular support is often necessary in patients wounded in combat. Pre-injury hydration status can be difficult to assess. Patients often appear hypovolemic out of proportion to the degree of injury due to insensible fluid loss from physical exertion of combat combined with constant stress and lack of rest.[24] Patients should be hydrated to provide adequate hemodynamic support and maintain cerebral perfusion pressure, yet not precipitate cerebral and pulmonary edema. If there is clinical evidence of shock, other sources of ongoing blood loss should be vigorously sought.

Entrance and exit wounds are covered with sterile bulky dressings using mild compression for hemostasis. If uncontrollable hemorrhage persists, additional bandages are placed in an attempt to tamponade the bleeding source. Inspecting the wound and removing dressings, clot, and bone fragments can initiate re-bleeding from sites already tamponaded and should be avoided unless definitive intervention is available. This bleeding can be severe and difficult to control, especially if a dural sinus is involved.

After initial stabilization, transfer to a definitive care setting depends on local conditions. Whenever possible, the patient should be evacuated to the closest facility with neurosurgical support, even if this means bypassing intermediate echelons. When this is not feasible, the patient is transferred to the most sophisticated echelon of care available for additional stabilization. Until the patient can be managed by a neurosurgeon, supportive care is given. In some instances, operative intervention by a non-neurosurgeon is the only available treatment. While this has been performed with success, the patient ideally should be treated by a trained neurosurgeon.[25]

For penetrating head injuries, it is important to initiate broad-spectrum antibiotic prophylaxis as early as possible. As mentioned earlier, decreased infection rates have led to a decrease in mortality rates. Penicillin, ampicillin, methicillin, cloxacillin, chloramphenicol, and streptomycin have all been used in recent conflicts with good results.[9–11,24,26,27] No specific regimen appears to be better than others, but coverage for Staphylococcus, Acinetobacter, and Streptococcus species must be of principal concern.[9,27] Patients with penetrating craniocerebral injuries should also be treated for seizure prophylaxis. Steroid use in the management of head injuries remains controversial. Standard doses of corticosteroids such as methylprednisolone or dexamethasone have not been shown to be of significant benefit in closed head injury. High-dose steroid protocols and other free radical scavenging compounds are currently being studied for use in head injuries, and their application to military injuries will await the outcome of these clinical trials.

Preoperative Management

On arrival at the definitive care MTF, the patient is again assessed for overall clinical condition including airway and hemodynamic status. The neurological exam is repeated and compared with earlier exams noting any improvement or deterioration in neurological status that may affect the decision process for appropriate type of operative intervention. Major bleeding from thoracic and abdominal vascular injuries takes precedence over head injuries. In most situations, multiple injuries can be cared for simultaneously.

Hemodynamic support is initiated with crystalloid solutions augmented with colloids depending on the extent of blood loss and availability of blood products. Type-specific or O-negative blood can be used until appropriate cross-matching is performed. Baseline laboratory studies for electrolytes, blood counts, and coagulation status are obtained, if laboratory facilities are available.

For patients with altered mental status and evidence of increased intracranial pressure (ICP), early endotracheal intubation is imperative to maintain cerebral oxygenation. Hyperventilation can be used acutely to help control increased ICP, but should be used in moderation since obtaining arterial blood gas analysis can be problematic in the battlefield setting. Osmotic diuretic agents such as mannitol can also be given for ICP control. When using diuretics, hemodynamic status has to be monitored closely to ensure that the patient is adequately hydrated and not in shock. Resulting diuretic fluid losses can lead to hypotension and decreased cerebral perfusion. Again, the pressures of battle and an austere personnel environment may make evaluating the pre-injury volume status difficult. Serial neurological exams are performed so that a worsening exam can be detected early and corrective measures taken, if possible.

When available, radiographic evaluation of craniocerebral injuries is beneficial for proper operative planning. Most MTFs with neurosurgical support will be able to perform routine radiographic studies, while some field hospitals and hospital ships also have CT capabilities. Plain skull radiographs are used to assess fracture patterns and localized metal fragments. Knowing location of fragments and how the skull fractured can be used to determine the projectile path through the skull and which anatomic structures are involved. Bone fragments within the calvarium indicate secondary projectiles. Fractures over dural sinuses can be evaluated and, when significant, appropriate preoperative planning done for a sinus repair.[24,28] Fractures of the orbit and nasal sinuses increase the risk of infection and delayed mortality. This complication was especially prevalent prior to the development of antibiotics.[29]

The use of CT in wartime scenarios has been limited. The Israeli experience in Lebanon saw widespread use of CT in head-injured patients transferred back to permanent MTFs in Israel for treatment.[10,11,30] Benefits of CT over plain films include accurate assessment of the extent of damage to the brain and skull, determination of projectile path and neurological structures traversed, and the ability to detect mass lesions local and distant to the entrance wound that may not otherwise be found using standard radiographs or during local debridement.[11,14,30] This information is important not only in operative planning, but when combined with the clinical status of the patient; it can be used effectively to triage patients and allocate surgical resources.

Field hospitals and hospital ships with CT equipment were first deployed by the United States during the Persian Gulf War and could be beneficial for patient management in future conflicts. Currently, a great deal of effort and money is being expended to allow wide use of teleradiology in battlefield settings and on ships at sea to provide consultative support by radiologists and other specialists with greater expertise than may be available in the field.

The role of angiography in evaluating penetrating craniocerebral injuries is unclear. With the advent of CT, angiography is rarely indicated preoperatively, especially in the military population. The incidence of traumatic intracranial aneurysms in penetrating injuries is small, 0 to 3.6 percent.[13,31–33] Even with CT evidence of subarachnoid blood, the incidence of traumatic aneurysms is only 3.2 percent. Unless there are significant clinical findings to suggest a ruptured aneurysm, angiography should be reserved for the postoperative period.

SURGICAL MANAGEMENT

Patient Selection

One of the most important aspects of managing penetrating craniocerebral war injuries is determining which patients will benefit from surgery. Multiple casualties arriving simultaneously at the MTF is a real possibility in wartime. However, this has not been the case in several recent conflicts such as Vietnam and Croatia, where head injuries could be treated on an individual basis.[7,34] Limited resources may also place restrictions on patient selection. Faced with the need to select patients for surgery appropriately, it is important to triage patients effectively.

Assuming adequate manpower and equipment resources exist to provide surgery for all potential patients, selection criteria for surgery is based on the mechanism of injury, clinical presentation, and radiographic/laboratory evaluation. Most survivable craniocerebral combat injuries are from low-velocity projectiles, usually in the form of munitions fragments.[10,11,21,34–36] Patients with overwhelming head injuries will die prior to arrival at the MTF if there is any delay in transfer. Patients alive on admission after delayed transfer have a higher chance of survival.[36] When rapid transport is available, many patients will arrive "alive" who might otherwise have succumbed to their injuries in the field. The dilemma then is to determine which of these patients will benefit from surgery.

When deciding which clinical criteria are of prognostic significance for combat craniocerebral injuries, experience can be drawn from the civilian sector and previous military experience. The factors listed in Table 61-5 have been found to be important adjuncts in categorizing patients into groups for prognostic and therapeutic purposes. The most important factor in determining prognosis is admission to the Glasgow Coma Scale (GCS).[8,10,11,18,22,35,37] Most patients presenting with a GCS of 3 and altered brain stem function will not benefit from aggressive surgical intervention. However, GCS alone cannot be used as criteria as 13 to 35 percent of patients with a GCS of 3 to 5 may survive their injuries.[8,11,22,37] Other clinical factors such as pupillary changes, systemic shock, evidence of ongoing infection, and abnormal coagulation status at time of admission have also been associated with increased mortality rates and should be used to help triage patients for operative intervention.[8,11,22,37]

As shown in Table 61-5, radiographic factors can be used in conjunction with clinical status to evaluate severely injured patients for surgical intervention. Plain radiographs can show evidence of ventricular perforation and bihemispheric injuries that contraindicate surgery in moribund patients. Ventricular penetration by the primary projectile indicates a grave prognosis based on the inherent injuries to periventricular, diencephalic structures.

When available, CT criteria are of great benefit in triaging patients with severe penetrating wounds and have been used as the principal justification for CT scanning in battlefield settings. Computerized tomography criteria of injuries crossing the midsagittal or axial midventricular plane, intraparenchymal hemorrhage (possibly indicating disruption of a major vascular structure), and greater than 20 percent contused or damaged brain have been shown to be reliable predictive factors of mortality in penetrating head injuries in the civilian sector.[22,37]

The factors listed in Table 61-5 should be used to help decide which patients have the best chance of survival. Regardless of the criterion used, the selection process must be individualized to each patient and the unique conditions surrounding their admission.

Operative Treatment

The primary goal of surgery in patients with craniocerebral injuries is decompression of accessible mass lesions, debridement of devitalized tissue, and thorough wound closure to prevent infection. After obtaining all necessary radiographic and laboratory testing, the patient is brought to the operating room. If not already done, endotracheal intubation is obtained with care taken to avoid neck injury. Although the incidence of cervical spine injuries in combat-related head injuries is low, clearing the cervical spine of injuries preoperatively can be difficult when resources are limited.

The scalp is widely shaved and prepped around entrance and exit points. This not only makes skin available for rotational flaps, but ensures that no other penetrating wounds are present. When draping the patient, consideration is made for a donor source of fascia (such as facia lata in the thigh) should a duraplasty be needed. Antibiotics and seizure prophylaxis are administered. Depending on the clinical condition, hyperventilation and mannitol can be used for control of increased intracranial pressure and to facilitate wound closure. If a dural sinus injury is expected, ample amounts of crystalloid and colloid solutions should be available and the surgeon should be prepared to repair the sinus.[9]

Surgical Technique

Scalp wounds

Management of the scalp wound is the same in all patients, regardless of type of craniocerebral injury. Adequate skin closure is critical in preventing CSF leaks and infection, complications that significantly affect long-term outcome. The opening of the wound is copiously irrigated and skin edges debrided. Nonviable tissue should be removed rather than risk subsequent necrosis and wound breakdown. After the skin has been debrided, a meticulous closure is performed. The scalp is closed in two layers and should be water-tight and free of significant tension. This may be difficult given the amount of devitalized tissue removed in some cases. Galeal relaxing incisions often allow primary closure to be obtained. If the wound cannot be approximated directly, rotational skin flaps or vascularized skin grafts are used to cover the cranial defect with healthy, vascularized skin tissue. Defects in the scalp resulting from rotational flaps can be covered with skin grafts. The assistance of a plastic surgeon is invaluable in these cases, but neurosurgeons should be familiar with these techniques since plastic surgery support frequently is not available under battlefield conditions.

Tangential (gutter-type) wounds

These injuries, often made by high-velocity missiles glancing off the skull, often have long, elliptical scalp wounds. At surgical exploration, skin edges are first retracted to expose the underlying cranial defect. The scalp wound is lengthened appropriately to expose the entire cranial defect. If the dura is intact, soft, and pulsatile, and if preoperative imaging studies indicate no significant underlying pathology, subdural exploration is not necessary. Loose bone fragments are removed and the edges of the defect are smoothed.

If CT imaging reveals a hematoma or if the dura is discolored and tense at the time of surgery, a craniectomy is performed and the dura opened for exploration of underlying brain. Accessible blood clot is removed with suction and irrigation. Unless otherwise indicated, manipulation of brain should be minimized to avoid injuring viable neural tissue. Dura is closed primarily in a water-tight fashion and the scalp closed appropriately.

If dural penetration is found at exploration, a craniectomy is performed around the skull defect until normal dura is present circumferentially. Superficial fragments of bone and metal are gently removed by forceps and irrigation. Obvious necrotic brain and blood clots are irrigated out of the wound, but vigorous suctioning and debridement of neural tissue should be avoided.

While there is usually not a closed tract from the primary missile in these injuries, fragments of bone or metal may break off and form secondary missiles. Tracts from secondary missiles should be copiously irrigated to remove any additional clot, fragments, or necrotic brain. However, extensive exploration of the tract for fragments not easily visualized should not be performed, especially in eloquent parts of the brain.

In most tangential wounds, the dura is so torn that primary closure is not possible or to do so would place the repair under tension. In these cases, some form of duraplasty is indicated, with donor material coming from autologous sources such as periosteum, temporalis fascia, or facia lata; or from allograft such as Lyodura.[7,24] Dural closure should be in a water-tight fashion to help prevent CSF leaks. This has been shown to be a useful maneuver in recent conflicts.[7,9,10,27]

Penetrating wounds

Several different surgical techniques are used in managing penetrating craniocerebral injuries. The techniques vary depending on the amount of exposure needed and the size of the entrance wound. For cases in which wide exposure is needed but the entrance wound is small, a standard craniotomy flap can be used with the wound being centered on the flap.[38] After retraction of the skin flap, a craniotome is used to create the bone plate, using either the defect in the skull or a separate burr hole for a start site. Exposed dura is opened to allow inspection of the underlying brain and removal of any mass lesions. The missile tract should be irrigated to remove any necrotic tissue and bone or missile fragments, but normal-looking brain should not be extensively explored. Dural closure, primary or by graft, is easily performed with this technique. The entrance site in the bone plate is debrided and the plate fixed by nonabsorbable suture or wire. Likewise, the entrance wound in the scalp is debrided and closed in two layers. The advantage of using a standard craniotomy is increased exposure gained while minimizing the site of craniectomy needed to obtain a similar exposure.[38] This also limits the need for a subsequent cranioplasty.

For larger entrance wounds and skull defects, adequate exposure is often obtained with extension of wound margins. As discussed above with gutter-type wounds, skin edges are retracted to expose the entire cranial defect. The wound is elongated as needed to accomplish this with consideration given for skin flaps to close the wound. Loose bone fragments are removed and a craniectomy performed until normal dura is present circumferentially around the cranial defect. Irrigation is used to remove necrotic brain and fragments from the surface of brain and from along the missile tracts. After closing dura, usually with a duraplasty, the scalp is debrided and repaired as needed.

There has been recent interest in limiting major cranial surgery in patients with penetrating head injuries. Brandvold et al. found that patients with small punctate entrance wounds and no evidence of mass lesions on CT did just as well with debridement and closure of the entrance wound as did patients undergoing a formal cranial procedure in terms of overall mortality and infection.[10] They also reported a decreased incidence in seizures in these patients with less aggressive debridement. Taha et al. had similar results in patients with GCS >10, entry wound < 2 cm, no extra-axial hematoma or intracerebral hemorrhage > 4 cm on CT scan, no exit wound, and who were treated within 6 hours of injury.[26] Patients were treated with wound closure only and 14 days of methicillin. Of 32 conservatively treated patients, only 1 patient (who had a CSF leak) developed an infection. Patients with delayed transfer would not be eligible for this type of management because of the possibility of wound contamination.

Based on these series and others, conservative operative treatment is indicated in patients who are doing relatively well neurologically (GCS > 10), have small entrance wounds, and are seen in the first few hours after injury. Patients with delayed transfer, large wounds, and obvious mass lesions should be treated with standard cranial techniques for debridement, neural decompression, and wound closure. Moribund patients being treated expectantly can also be treated with simple wound closure and observed. If the patient improves neurologically, they are reassessed and treated appropriately.

Until recently, one of the goals of surgery for patients with penetrating head injuries was debridement of the missile tract and removal of all bone and metal fragments.[13,24,39,40] The reasoning behind this aggressive approach was prevention of abscess formation from residual debris. Pursuing this objective often included craniotomy on the opposite side of the entrance wound to remove fragments from the contralateral hemisphere, and reoperation for retained fragments detected on postoperative imaging studies.[24,40]

Current recommendations call for less aggressive debridement of missile and fragment tracts. Deep fragments are removed only if they can be safely removed from the depths of the wound; otherwise they are left in place. Recent studies reveal no increased incidence of infection from retained bone fragments if other risk factors (such as CSF leak, air sinus injury, wound breakdown and large amounts of necrotic tissue) are not present.[10,11,26,27] The primary goal for surgery is decompression of mass lesions, removal of grossly contaminated or necrotic material, and water-tight dural and skin closure to prevent CSF leak and wound breakdown.

Perforating wounds

For both military and civilian populations, perforating injuries to the head generally do poorly because of the high amount of KE needed to penetrate two skull tables. Perforating injuries are treated like penetrating injuries except that two separate wounds must be dealt with. Small entrance wounds can be treated with simple wound closure or craniotomy depending on the neurological condition of the patient, radiographic findings, and time from injury. Exit wounds usually are larger than entrance wounds because of the effects of cavitation. Craniectomy, dural repair, and scalp debridement and repair usually are needed for these wounds.

Dural sinus injuries

Dural sinus involvement has been reported in 10 percent of combat head injuries.[28] Projectile injuries to dural sinuses can lead to massive hemorrhage, especially if unrecognized prior to surgical intervention.[28] Techniques available to manage injuries of the sinus include compression of the defect with collagen sponge, cottonoids, or digit; and use of Fogarty catheters to occlude the proximal and distal segments of the sinus; and temporary shunting.[24,28] Repair of the defect may be performed primarily or with grafting techniques. These repairs should also be bolstered with some type of other material, such as a piece of flattened muscle.[24] Being aware of possible sinus injury before surgery is critical in preoperative planning to allow for appropriate hemodynamic support and to have equipment ready to handle bleeding before it becomes uncontrollable.

Nasal sinus/skull base injuries

Nasal sinus injuries are frequently encountered in combat, occurring in approximately 15 percent of penetrating injuries.[29] These injuries have also been frequently associated with infections.[19,20] Management includes craniotomy or craniectomy, depending on the size of the entrance wound, exenteration of the involved sinus, and a water-tight dural closure.[29] For wounds affecting the skull base, a craniotomy is performed for inspection and repair using intradural grafts.[29,40,41]

PERIOPERATIVE CARE

Monitoring

Types of monitoring equipment available for postoperative management will depend on the sophistication of the field unit. While some MTFs will have capacity for advanced hemodynamic and intracranial pressure monitoring, others will be fortunate to have adequate nursing care. If the patient is able to follow commands and has a neurological exam that can be followed, invasive monitoring is considered unnecessary and will be reserved for patients with a neurological exam that is difficult to follow.

Fluid Management

It is important to get an accurate estimate of the patient's volume status immediately after surgery. As noted earlier, many patients will be hypovolemic before injury. Care must be taken when correcting volume status to avoid decreasing serum osmolarity and overhydrating the patient, which may cause cerebral edema and shock lung in patients with multi-system injury. Judicious use of crystalloid and colloid fluid replacement will allow for maintenance of hemodynamic status and prevent fluid overload. Accurate documentation of parenteral fluid administration, hemodynamic parameters, urinary output, and electrolyte laboratory studies will aid in assessment of volume status.

Infection

One of the most important factors influencing overall mortality in patients with craniocerebral injuries is development of postoperative infection. During World War II, the incidence of cerebral abscess formation went from 27 percent in the early years of the conflict, to 3 percent by war's end.[1] This improvement has been attributed to the introduction and widespread use of penicillin as well as to plastic surgical techniques that improve wound closure. Accordingly, broad spectrum antibiotic coverage should be continued for 10 to 14 days. Recent reports have shown an increasing number of gram-negative infections compared with previous military campaigns, therefore coverage for these organisms must be considered.[27] While antibiotics will not replace good surgical technique, they seem to be valuable in preventing infections.

When infections do occur, they will usually present in the first month. Any evidence of wound breakdown or CSF leak must be treated aggressively, including re-exploration of the wound, when appropriate. If rhinorrhea or otorrhea develop and do not resolve spontaneously or with a lumbar drain, craniotomy for dural repair must be considered early in the management of this problem.[41]

If cerebritis or abscess develops, open debridement is indicated for removal of infected material and necrotic brain. Fragments of bone and metal are also removed, if accessible. In most cases, the nidus of infection will be centered around some type of retained fragment, usually bone.[13,27,39]

Angiography

As noted earlier, the incidence of traumatic aneurysm is low. Hammond found only two cases in his series of 2187 patients from Vietnam. However, the incidence was somewhat higher in the Iran-Iraq and Lebanon conflicts with rates between 1 and 3 percent.[31–33] Levy et al. also found an incidence of 3.2 percent in their civilian population of penetrating gunshot wounds. In recent studies, aggressive debridement of the wound tract was not performed, as opposed to the Hammond series. This may have permitted some arterial injuries to develop into aneurysms. The majority of these lesions resulted from fragment injuries as opposed to gunshot wounds. Clinical presentation of the aneurysm can be from hours to years after the initial injury.[31] Levy et al. recommended angiography for those patients who develop delayed subarachnoid or intracerebral hemorrhages, late deterioration in neurological status (especially if unexpected), or the development of a cranial nerve palsy.[32]

Transfer

When the patient is medically stable, evacuation is arranged to treatment facilities in the rear. Most forward field hospitals have limited bed space. Patients with neurological deficits should be transferred to rehabilitation centers as soon as feasible.

OUTCOME

Mortality

Mortality rates for several military series are presented in Table 61-6. Overall, there has been a general decrease in mortality. This phenomenon is due primarily to widespread use of antibiotics and forward stationing of neurosurgical support allowing definitive treatment to be initiated soon after injury.

Mortality rates from some recent series have not differed from earlier studies. One reason for this apparent lack of improvement, despite improved medical technology, is that severely injured patients are now arriving "alive" at treatment facilities. While these patients are included in admission statistics, their moribund condition precludes effective treatment.[11] If transfer of the patient was delayed, many of these patients would have died prior to arrival at the MTF. Hammon categorized

TABLE 61-6 Combat Craniocerebral Injuries: Mortality Rates in Recent Conflicts

Conflict	Mortality (%)
World War I[19]	29
World War II[20]	14
Korea[24,29]	8–10
Vietnam[13,14,24,34,40]	5–12
Iran-Iraq[8,36]	14–16
Israel-Jordan[10,11,30]	19–24
Croatia[7]	49

these patients as "un-operated expectant" in his review of Vietnam war experience; when these were excluded from other patients who were treated, hospital mortality was reduced from 32 to 11 percent.[13] Aarabi reported a mortality of 8.8 percent in his series of 125 patients in the Iran-Iraq War, but the interval between injury and surgical exploration averaged between 67 to 87 hours.[8] The Brandvold et al. review of the Israeli-Lebanon conflict reported an overall mortality rate of 26 percent, but average time from injury to hospital admission was 2 hours.[10]

The major factor predicting mortality in patients with penetrating craniocerebral head injuries is admission GCS. This is true both for injuries suffered in the civilian[22] or combat setting.[8,10,11,18,35] Other factors predicting mortality in combat head injuries are shown in Table 61-5. Infection is the second most common predictor of mortality and is a leading cause of delayed mortality after initial surgical intervention.[38]

Another important factor in determining mortality is the type of projectile. Bullet wounds produce the majority of fatal penetrating head wounds and shrapnel the majority of survivable wounds.[21] In Vietnam, Hammon found gunshot wounds to have a higher mortality rate (22.7 percent) compared to fragment wounds (7.6 percent).[13] Obviously, high-velocity projectiles produce more significant injuries.

For patients surviving the initial injury and postoperative period, there is a steady decrease in mortality rate with time. Rish et al. studied 1127 patients who survived their initial injuries in the Vietnam War and were alive 1 week after injury.[38] Over a 15-year follow-up period, 8 percent of these patients died, 18 percent of the deaths occurred within the first month of injury, 36 percent within 3 months, and 51 percent within the first year.[38] The causes of death during the first month were related to cerebral injury, infection, extracranial injuries, and pulmonary embolus. At 2 months post-injury, infection, especially in the form of cerebral abscess, became a more common cause of death.[38] During the rest of the first year, post-injury death was usually related to complications arising from prolonged coma.

After the first 2 years, causes of death were similar to those found in noninjured patients. One exception to this trend involved additional patients dying as a result of coma. Another cause of death in five patients between the second and tenth year post-injury was post-traumatic epilepsy. Studies from WWII have also shown post-traumatic epilepsy to be a poor prognostic sign for longevity.[42] Educational level was also found to be a variable in longevity; the higher the pre- and post-injury educational status, the greater the longevity. This finding is probably based more on socioeconomic rather than medical factors.[42]

Functional Status

Despite the extent of their injuries, many patients with penetrating craniocerebral injuries have reasonably good long-term outcomes. Schwab et al., analyzing data from the Vietnam Head Injury Study, found 56 percent of head-injured patients working 15 years after injury compared with 82 percent in a matched control group.[43] It should be noted that most patients examined in this study were victims of low-velocity fragment wounds and 85 percent of patients had no or brief loss of consciousness after injury.[43] Post-traumatic epilepsy, paresis, visual field loss, verbal and visual memory loss, psychological problems, and violent behavior correlated with the inability to work.

How the patient is cared for initially also affects functional outcome. Grosswasser and Cohen compared penetrating head injury patients from the Yom Kippur War (1973) with the Lebanon War (1982).[44] Patients in both conflicts were comparable in age and pre-injury educational level. In the earlier conflict, there were longer delays in transferring patients to definitive care centers. The authors suggested that the shorter transfer times seen in the Lebanon War led to earlier intervention, which produced shorter hospital stays and earlier transfer to rehabilitation centers. While neurological outcome was similar in both groups, there was a significant improvement in work status. This study emphasizes the need for the early transfer of head-injured patients to rehabilitation centers to improve long-term functional outcome.

Cranioplasty

One difficulty encountered with large craniectomy defects from debridement is the need for subsequent cranioplasty. This is especially true in frontal bone defects, which can have significant cosmetic deformities. Timing of this procedure is dependent on the practitioner. If any infectious complications arise in the postsurgical period, corrective surgery is often delayed until one year post-injury, when the risk of infectious complications has presumably decreased.

CONCLUSIONS

Penetrating craniocerebral injuries incurred during military operations remain a devastating problem. While advances in neurosurgical care and antibiotic treatment combined with the ability to rapidly evacuate patients to sophisticated MTFs has improved outcome in many patients, mortality of these injuries remains high. Advances have been made in materials and design for protective equipment for the head, but munitions are designed to defeat protective equipment.[18,21] Penetrating injuries from high-velocity assault weapons at close ranges continue to be lethal.

It is hoped that newer medical therapies now being developed for the care of closed and penetrating head injuries in the civilian population will reduce the morbidity and mortality of craniocerebral injuries encountered on the battlefield.

REFERENCES

1. West CGH: A short history of the management of penetrating missile injuries of the head. *Surg Neurol* 1981; 16:145.
2. Gurdjian ES: The treatment of penetrating wounds of the brain sustained in warfare: A historical review. *J Neurosurg* 1974; 39:157.
3. Zellem RT: Wounded by bayonet, ball, and bacteria: Medicine and neurosurgery in the American Civil War. *Neurosurgery* 1985; 17:850.
4. Kaufman HH: Historical vignette: Treatment of head injuries in the American Civil War. *J Neurosurg* 1993; 78:838.
5. Bellamy RF, Maningas PA, Vayer JS: Epidemiology of trauma: Military experience. *Ann Emerg Med* 1986; 15:1384.
6. Tilney NL: The marrow of tragedy. *Surg Gynecol Obstet* 1983; 157:380.
7. Vrankovic D, Hecimovic I, Splavski B, et al: Management of missile wounds of the cerebral dura mater: Experience with 69 cases. *Neurochirurgia* 1992; 35:150.
8. Aarabi B: Surgical outcome in 435 patients who sustained missile head wounds during the Iran-Iraq War. *Neurosurgery* 1990; 27:692.
9. Aarabi B: Comparative study of bacteriological contamination between primary and secondary exploration of missile head wounds. *Neurosurgery* 1987; 20:610.
10. Brandvold B, Levi L, Feinsod M, et al: Penetrating craniocerebral injuries in the Israeli involvement in the Lebanese conflict, 1982–1985. *J Neurosurg* 1990; 72:15.
11. Levi L, Borovich B, Guilburd JN, et al: Wartime neurosurgical experience in Lebanon, 1982–85. I: Penetrating craniocerebral injuries. *Isr J Med Sci* 1990; 26:548.
12. Jacob E, Setterstrom JA: Infection in war wounds: Experience in recent military conflicts and future considerations. *Milit Med* 1989; 154(6):311.
13. Hammon WM: Analysis of 2187 consecutive penetrating wounds of the brain from Vietnam. *J Neurosurg* 1971; 34:127.
14. Carey ME, Tutton RH, Strub RL, et al: The correlation between surgical and CT estimates of brain damage following missile wounds. *J Neurosurg* 1984; 60:947.
15. Kirkpatrick JB, DiMaio V: Civilian gunshot wounds of the brain. *J Neurosurg* 1978; 49:185.
16. Harvey EN: Studies on wound ballistics, in Andrus EC, Bronk DW, Carden GA Jr, et al (eds): *Advances in Military Medicine.* Boston: Atlantic-Little, Brown, 1948: 191–205.
17. Scott R: Pathology of injuries caused by high-velocity missiles. *Clin Lab Med* 1983; 3:273.
18. Bellamy RF: Ambush. *Milit Med* 1988; 153:378.
19. Cushing H: A study of a series of wounds involving the brain and its enveloping structures. *Br J Surg* 1918; 6:558.
20. Matson DD: *The Treatment of Acute Craniocerebral Injuries Due to Missiles*, Springfield IL: Charles C Thomas, 1948.
21. Carey ME, Sacco W, Merkler J: An analysis of fatal and non-fatal head wounds incurred during combat in Vietnam by U.S. forces. *Acta Chir Scand* 1982; Suppl 508:351.
22. Shaffrey ME, Polin RS, Phillips CD, et al: Classification of civilian craniocerebral gunshot wounds: A multivariate analysis predictive of mortality. *J Neurotrauma* 1992; 9 (Suppl 1):S279.
23. Arishita GI, Vayer JS, Bellamy RF: Cervical spine immobilization of penetrating neck wounds in a hostile environment. *J Trauma* 1989; 29:332.
24. Mathews WE: The early treatment of craniocerebral missile injuries: Experience with 92 cases. *J Trauma* 1972; 12:939.
25. Coupland RM, Pesonen PE: Craniocerebral war wounds: Non-specialist management. *Injury* 1992; 23(1):21.
26. Taha JM, Saba MI, Brown JA: Missile injuries to the brain treated by simple wound closure: Results of a protocol during the Lebanese conflict. *Neurosurgery* 1991; 29:380.
27. Taha JM, Haddad FS, Brown JA: Intracranial infection after missile injuries to the brain: Report of 30 cases from the Lebanon conflict. *Neurosurgery* 1991; 29:864.
28. Kapp JP, Gielchinsky I: Management of combat wounds of the dural venous sinuses. *Surgery* 1972; 71:913.
29. Arendall REH, Meirowsky AM: Air sinus wounds: An analysis of 163 consecutive cases incurred in the Korean War, 1950–1952. *Neurosurgery* 1983; 13:377.
30. Rappaport ZH, Sahar A, Shaked I, et al: Computerized tomography in combat-related craniocerebral penetrating missile injuries. *Isr J Med Sci* 1984; 20:668.
31. Rahimizadeh A, Abtahi H, Daylami MS, et al: Traumatic

cerebral aneurysms caused by shell fragments: Report of four cases and review of the literature. *Acta Neurochir (Wien)* 1987; 84:93.

32. Levy ML, Rezai A, Masri LS, et al: The significance of subarachnoid hemorrhage after penetrating craniocerebral injury: Correlations with angiography and outcome in a civilian population. *Neurosurgery* 1993; 32:532.
33. Achram M, Rizk G, Haddad FS: Angiographic aspects of traumatic intracranial aneurysms following war injuries. *Br J Rad* 1980; 53:1144.
34. Plaut M: War wounds of the central nervous system: Surgical results. *J Trauma* 1972; 12:613.
35. Rish BL, Dillon JD, Weiss GH: Mortality following penetrating craniocerebral injuries: An analysis of the deaths in the Vietnam Head Injury Registry population. *J Neurosurg* 1983; 59:775.
36. Ameen AA: The management of acute craniocerebral injuries caused by missiles: Analysis of 110 consecutive penetrating wounds of the brain from Basrah. *Injury* 1984; 16:88.
37. Levy ML, Masri LS, Lavine S, et al: Outcome prediction after penetrating craniocerebral injury in a civilian population: Aggressive surgical management in patients with admission Glasgow Coma Scale scores of 3, 4, or 5. *Neurosurgery* 1994; 35:77.
38. Rish BL, Dillon JD, Caveness WF, et al: Evolution of craniotomy as a debridement technique for penetrating craniocerebral injuries. *J Neurosurg* 1980; 53:772.
39. Meirowsky AM: The retention of bone fragments in brain wounds. *Milit Med* 1968; 133(11):887.
40. Meirowsky AM, Rish BL, Mohr JP, et al: Definitive care of cerebral missile injuries crossing the midline. *Milit Med* 1980; 145:246.
41. Meirowsky AM, Caveness WF, Dillon JD, et al: Cerebrospinal fluid fistulas complicating missile wounds of the brain. *J Neurosurg* 1981; 54:44.
42. Corkin S, Sullivan EV, Carr FA: Prognostic factors favoring life expectancy after penetrating head injury. *Arch Neurol* 1984; 41:975.
43. Schwab K, Grafman J, Salazar AM, et al: Residual impairments and work status 15 years after penetrating head injury: Report from the Vietnam Head Injury Study. *Neurology* 1993; 43:95.
44. Grosswasser Z, Cohen M: Rehabilitation outcome of combat head injuries: Comparison of the October 1973 War and Lebanon War, 1982. *Isr J Med Sci* 1985; 21:957.

CHAPTER 62

HEAD INJURY IN DEVELOPING COUNTRIES

Wen-Ta Chiu
Ronald E. LaPorte
G. Gururaj
Iftikhar A. Raja
Thomas J. Pentel'enyi
K. A. Bouyoucef
Arnoldo Levy
Ching-Chang Hung

SYNOPSIS

During the past fifty years, most developed and developing countries have followed a pattern of declining infectious diseases and a simultaneously increasing severity of noncommunicable diseases. This pattern has led to a large increase in injury morbidity and mortality rates in a very short period of time. Industrialization and economic growth in developing countries have led to a rapid increase in the number of motor vehicles and motor vehicle-related accidents. As a consequence, with the exception of some countries such as Colombia in which assaults are the leading cause of head injury, in most developing countries traffic accidents are the major cause of head injury.

Head injuries present a variety of problems to developing countries, mainly because of difficulties arising in the treatment of these injuries. Developing countries tend to lag behind in advances of medical technology and do not have adequate medical facilities and equipment to deal with head injuries and their complications. In addition, owing to ongoing industrialization, some of these countries still lack the appropriate transportation and communication facilities to carry out efficient emergency medical services. Developing countries also tend to have an insufficient number of neurosurgeons and trained practitioners. In these countries, trauma care systems are not well developed, and many head injuries are treated by physicians not qualified because of improper training. There are also specific epidemiological factors affecting particular geographic regions. The role of geographic variation is reflected in the higher incidence and mortality rates in rural than in urban areas. Incidence and mortality rates also can be correlated to a country's degree of development, including its quality of transportation, infrastructure, and education.

In order to initiate prevention efforts, it is necessary to establish head injury registries to monitor the frequency and outcomes of head injury, and to use standardized definitions and methodologies to carry out collaborative studies. Programs such as the Multinational Spine and Head Injury Project (SHIP) and "Think First" can aid in the prevention of head injury in developing countries.

INTRODUCTION

Head injury presents difficult and complex problems in developing countries. Treatment is very costly and usually necessitates extensive care. Developing countries often lack sufficient labor power and facilities for such treatment. Currently, there is little knowledge concerning the frequency of head injuries in these countries.

Reviews of the epidemiology of head injury in 1990 by Kraus, and by Jennett and Frankowski, showed that the incidence rates of head injury ranged from 132 to 430/100,000 per year; the mortality rate ranged from 9 to 32 per 100,000 per year.[1–19] However, most of these studies were based on data from westernized countries[3–10,12–19]; studies from developing countries were not included. After 1990, several developing countries, such as Taiwan, Pakistan, India, Burkino Faso, Colombia, and Algeria, began to report population-based studies,[10–23] but the definition and methods differed in each study. Thus, the scope of head injury in these countries is still difficult to map because of problems in establishing standardized approaches. Nevertheless, there is little question that head injuries constitute a major problem in developing countries, potentially more so than in Europe or America, although the patterns may be different.

An epidemiological transition is occurring across the world, with a rapid decline of infectious diseases and an increase in the importance of noncommunicable diseases. This change increases the need for reliable statistics, since epidemiological data form the basis of health-care planning.

INCIDENCE AND MORTALITY RATES OF HEAD INJURY IN DEVELOPING COUNTRIES

It is commonly agreed that the incidence of head injury increases as countries become more industrialized; however, the existing medical systems in most developing countries are grossly inadequate to deal with these problems. A less developed country, such as India or Pakistan, would be expected to have a low incidence rate and a high mortality rate, owing to problems with transport of patients and inadequate treatment facilities. In contrast, a country such as Taiwan that has recently undergone rapid industrialization would be expected to have a higher incidence rate but potentially a lower case fatality rate than less developed countries because of improved care. Furthermore, there is considerable variability in the etiology, incidence, and outcome from injury, even within a particular country, as, for example, between an urban and a rural setting. Note the difference between the statistics for Taipei (urban) and Hualien (rural) in Taiwan (Table 62-2). Some countries may

TABLE 62-1 Incidence and Mortality Rates of Head Injuries in Developing and Developed Countries

	Incidence (/100,000)	Mortality (/100,000)	Year	Case fatality rate (%)
	Developing Countries			
Algeria, Blida	80	5	1989	—
Colombia, Cali	676	120	1990	—
India, Bangalore	150	—	1990	9.6
Pakistan, Multan	81	11	1990	—
Taiwan,				
Taipei	182	19	1988–1992	10.6
Hualien	304	87	1988–1992	28.7
	Developed Countries			
Norway				
Trodelag	200	5.5	1984	2.8
Italy				
San Marino	468	—	1981–1982	—
U.S.A.				
San Diego	180	30	1984	6
Britain				
England	270	9	1981	—
Scotland	313	9	1981	—

have special features, like Colombia which exhibits an extraordinarily high incidence and mortality rate due to social factors. From our limited data of five developing countries (Table 62-1), it can be seen that the data are comparable with what might be expected with development and that they differ from those of westernized countries. It should be emphasized that the definition and methodology are different in each study; therefore, strong conclusions cannot be drawn from these comparisons. Furthermore, great care should be exercised when extrapolating data from a particular region to an entire country. A collaborative study with identical definition and methodology is needed in order to be able to improve the reliability of the data.

CAUSES OF HEAD INJURY IN DEVELOPING COUNTRIES

The major causes of head injury in developing and developed countries are listed in Table 62-2. Traffic accidents account for the largest proportion of head injury (50–75 percent),[10,11] an incidence slightly higher than that of westernized countries (45–60 percent). These include an exceedingly high motorcycle accident rate (80 percent) in Taiwan, and a high pedestrian injury rate (43 percent) and falls-from-moving-vehicles rate (7 percent) in Pakistan. Head injury caused by falls ranges from 15 to 23 percent, which appears to be lower than that in westernized countries. Head injury caused by assaults ranges from 6.5 to 22 percent in developing countries. This feature is similar to that of westernized countries (8 to 11 percent). Pakistan and Colombia have an unusually high percentage of head injuries due to assaults. Agricultural, work, home, and sport injuries also were found in these series.

TREATMENT

Several factors appear to affect the treatment and outcome of head injuries in developing countries: isolation; medical facilities; labor power and training; and specific epidemiological factors.

Isolation

Large areas in many developing countries often tend to be isolated from modern technology and advances in medicine; thus, they may lack adequate knowledge for

TABLE 62-2 Causes of Head Injury in Developing and Developed Countries

	Traffic accidents (%)	Falls (%)	Assaults (%)	Others (%)
	Developing Countries			
Algeria				
Blida (adult)	55.6	—	15.7	18.6
(child)	40.1	—	5.4	49.1
Colombia				
Cali	50	—	22	—
India				
Bangalore (city)	61.6	22.5	10.6	3.6
Pakistan				
Multan (city)	57.6	16	22	—
Taiwan				
Taipei (urban)	64.6	22.9	6.5	6
Hualien (rural)	75.3	15.4	6.5	2.8
	Developed Countries			
Norway				
Trodelag	45	—	8	—
Italy				
San Marino	60	33	—	—
United States				
San Diego	53	31	11	—

TABLE 62-3 Comparison of CT Scanners and Neurosurgeons in Developing Countries and U.S.A.

	Pakistan	State of* Karnataka (India)	City of* Bangalore (India)	Algeria	Colombia	Taiwan	United States
Population (million)	110	45	4	25	33	21	248
Neurosurgeons	43	32	21	69	250	132	3000
Neurosurgeons per million	0.4	0.07	0.5	2.8	7.6	6.3	15
CT scans	27	12	7	8	25	150	over 4000
Incidence rate (per 100,000)	81	150	150	80	676	243	180

* Bangalore is a major metropolitan area within the State of Karnataka in South India.

the optimal treatment of head injury. Furthermore, transportation and communication are relatively insufficient, which leads to inefficient emergency medical service and delay in patient transfer.

Medical Facilities

Medical facilities in developing countries are limited when compared to those in developed countries. Developing countries often lack the medical equipment necessary for routine treatment of head injuries, such as CT scan and intensive care units. The shortage of CT scanners for diagnosis of intracranial hematomas is a very significant problem in developing countries (Table 62-3).

Labor Power and Treatment

Table 62-4 shows that developing countries have fewer neurosurgeons and trained practitioners than do developed countries. As compared to the United States, the ratio of head injuries per neurosurgeon is 13 in Pakistan and 2 to 3 in Taiwan. However, since most of the developing countries do not have a sufficient number of adequate neurosurgeons, and since trauma systems are not well developed, a large proportion of head injuries are treated by general surgeons or other physicians who may lack the training and experience necessary to deal properly with these patients. This situation must change if significant progress is to be made. Furthermore, trauma care is not considered a high-priority issue and head injury is not a professionally "sexy" subject among many physicians. Hence, there is a silent epidemic that receives much less attention than other high-profile elective, and sometimes high-tech, disease entities.

Specific Epidemiological Factors

Taiwan

The pattern of declining infectious diseases and an increasing burden of noncommunicable diseases is characteristic of most countries in the developed and developing world over the last 50 years. Taiwan is an example of this, as there has been an enormous increase in injury morbidity and mortality in a very short period of time.

The problem of head injury in Taiwan is significant because of the very rapid increase in the number of motor vehicles (over 10 million motorcycles and 3 million other vehicles) during the past 20 years owing to rapid industrial and economic growth. This increase has led to a sharp rise in the number of deaths from acci-

TABLE 62-4 Comparison of the Estimates of Head Injury Treated by Each Neurosurgeon per Year in 3 Countries

	Pakistan	Taiwan	United States
Total population	110 million	21 million	248 million
Average incidence rate of head injury	81/100,000	243/100,000	180/100,000
Estimated head injury per year	891,000	52,000	496,000
Neurosurgeons	43	132	3000
Estimated number of head injury treated by each neurosurgeon per year	2070	394	165
Ratio*	12.6	2.4	1

* These ratios assume that all head injury patients are seen by neurosurgeons, which is not the case. The severity of the head injury is not specified. This probably accounts for some of the variability in statistics from different studies.

TABLE 62-5 Head Injuries in Urban (Taipei City) and Rural (Hualien County) Counties in Taiwan, 1988–1991

	1988	1989	1990	1991
Head injury				
Taipei	4692	4724	5062	4955
Hualien	1183	1145	1338	1069

dents, now the third leading cause of death in Taiwan. Of these deaths, over half are related to motor vehicle accidents.

In an effort to clarify the trends of these injuries in Taiwan, five years ago the largest head and spinal cord injury registry in the world was established. This project is being conducted by Head and Spinal Cord Injury Research Group, Neurological Society, R.O.C. (Taiwan). A population-based urban (Taipei City) and rural (Hualien County) comparative study of head and spinal cord injury is in its fifth year of research. Approximately 5000 cases of head injury in Taipei and 1200 cases in Hualien are collected annually, and a total of 30,000 cases of head injury have been registered (Tables 62-5, 62-6). Mild head injuries accounted for 77.7 percent of these cases; moderate and severe head injuries accounted for 9.6 and 12.8 percent, respectively.

Considerable geographic variation was seen in these two areas. The incidence rate and mortality rate were two and four times higher, respectively, in the rural areas. The causes of head injury also were different from those in studies of westernized countries, with a higher traffic accident rate, especially in rural areas. Motorcycles accounted for about 80 percent of the traffic accidents in the rural areas.

Since 1990, this registry has been extended to three other rural counties with a higher motorcycle use rate: Taitong; I-Lan; and Penghu Counties. A result similar to the Hualien study was obtained (Table 62-7). Starting in 1994, this will be the first countrywide program in the world to begin monitoring head injuries. Realizing that it is difficult to compare across registries and countries at this time, we plan to use the work in Taiwan as

TABLE 62-6 Incidence and Mortality Rates of Head Injury in Taiwan Area, 1988–1991

	1988	1989	1990	1991
Incidence (/100,000)				
Taipei	180	177	187	183
Hualien	333	325	332	301
Mortality (/100,000)				
Taipei	23	20	22	20
Hualien	89	75	77	86

TABLE 62-7 Incidence and Mortality Rates of Head Injury in Eastern Taiwan and Penghu County, 1990

	Incidence	Mortality
Hualien	332/100,000	77/100,000
Taitong	273/100,000	84/100,000
I-Lan	357/100,000	57/100,000
Penghu	281/100,000	45/100,000

Total = 3855 cases
Male to female ratio = 2:3
Average incidence rate = 344/100,000
Average mortality rate = 71/100,000

a model and then to make our data comparable with studies in other countries.

Pakistan

Road traffic accidents are responsible for the majority of head injuries in Pakistan (58 percent). Pedestrians hit by vehicles in traffic form the largest subgroup (43 percent), followed by falls from moving vehicles, including trains (7 percent). The rates of vehicle-to-vehicle and all motorcycle-related accidents are only 3.2 and 4.3 percent, respectively. The higher percentage of pedestrian injuries indicates unsatisfactory road conditions and poor education of pedestrians and drivers. Owing to a shortage of private transport, falls from overcrowded vehicles and trains are common.

India

In Bangalore, a major metropolitan city in South India, road traffic accidents (62 percent) and falls (23 percent) are the major causes of head injury. In addition, mortality statistics among two-wheeler drivers are high. Rapid urbanization and motorization without corresponding improvement in road traffic control have been primarily responsible for the high rate of head injuries. India has improved its primary health system, leading to a major reduction of communicable diseases, but head injuries are ever-increasing. With increasing motorization, another problem is lack of specialized trauma centers and physicians to treat head injuries. The magnitude of head injuries is not clearly known at this time. Disappointingly, there is only one area (Bangalore) in India from which incidence data are available.

In addition to Taiwan, Pakistan, and India, a few countries are developing population-based studies of head injury, but have not yet published their data. These include Algeria, Burkina Faso, China, Colombia, Malaysia, and Nigeria. However, there is a great paucity of head injury data from developing countries. Data from most countries of South America, Africa, the Middle East, and Southeast Asia are not available.

SUGGESTIONS AND FUTURE DIRECTIONS

It is important to begin to establish cost-effective systems for monitoring the frequency of these injuries and their outcomes. Moreover, it is essential to be able to forecast the incidence of injuries expected in the future; this is needed for prevention of future head injuries. To accomplish these goals, it is critical to establish head injury monitoring registries in developing countries. In addition, more neurosurgeons and diagnostic and therapeutic facilities are needed to provide better care to head-injured patients.

Epidemiological studies of head injury are needed especially in developing countries because these data: (1) are very important for establishing and shaping policies for the prevention of head injury; (2) help to monitor the outcomes of head injuries; and (3) are generally lacking in most countries. The definitions for monitoring head injury need to be standardized so that data from different countries can be compared and the actual differences identified.

Two specific programs are recommended for head injury prevention in developing countries. One is the Global Spine and Head Injury Prevention Project (SHIP), which is an international collaborative study to monitor head and spinal cord injuries worldwide.[24–28] The purpose of this project is to establish standardized population-based registries across the world in order to evaluate the distribution and determinants of these injuries. There are currently 31 participating centers in 21 countries. These countries include Algeria, Burkina Faso, China, Colombia, France, Hong Kong, Hungary, India, Italy, Japan, Malaysia, Nigeria, Norway, Pakistan, Saudi Arabia, Singapore, South Africa, Spain, Sweden, Taiwan, and the United States. The other program for head injury prevention is the "Think First" project in the United States.[29] "Think First" is a prevention project that has been applied successfully in the United States and can also be applied in developing countries. Financial support from each country's government is required for the implementation of "Think First."

As many developing countries do not currently have the finance and labor power needed to conduct registries or other surveillance of head injury, valuable data are not being collected, making prevention policies difficult to implement. An alternative method for evaluating the incidence rate of head injury in developing countries is by the capture-recapture method, which has been used as a tool for counting birds in forests and fishes in lakes.[30–32] This method could be utilized in counting the incidence of head injuries; however, its potential remains to be evaluated.

A different prevention project should be established in each developing country according to specific causes and situations of head injury, and a priority for each prevention project should be implemented. For example, in Taiwan, head injury due to motorcycle accidents is unusually high; therefore, a priority should be made to prevent motorcycle accidents and to enforce helmet laws. In Pakistan, the prevention of pedestrian injuries and falls from moving vehicles could be set as the highest priority.

CONCLUSION

With the rapid global industrialization effort in developing countries, there has been a corresponding increase in the incidence of head injury. However, we still know little about the frequency with which they occur or their outcomes. It is important to begin to monitor the incidence of these head injuries in order to understand them and to initiate prevention efforts.

ACKNOWLEDGEMENTS

We would like to acknowledge Drs. M. Iqbal Ahmad, Mukhter Ahmad, B. S. Das, Chandramouli, Maria Isabel Gutierrez, Anjum Habib, Tanvir Ul Hassan, Dinesh Mohan, K. V. R. Sastry, D. K. Subbakrishna, and Miguel Velasquez for their contribution.

Special thanks to Drs. Mark Mawe Attah, Ahmed Bou-Salah, Ralph F. Frankowski, Jess Kraus, and Thomas J. Songer for their invaluable assistance. The members of the Global SHIP Project (SHIP Crew) also provided great help on this paper. SHIP Crew: K. A. Bouyoucef; Burkina Faso: A. BouSalah: Yun-Jin Lu, Shu-Yuan Yang: Arnoldo Levy: Jean Luc Truelle: Kwan-Hon Chan: Thomas J. Pentel'enyi: G. Gururaj, Dinesh Mohan: Franco Servadei: Norio Nakamura, Akihiro Takatsu: Rajam Krishnan: Mark Mawe Attah: Tom-Harald Edna: Iftikhar A. Raja: Ahmed M. Alkhani: Sadasivan Balaji: Robert A. Butchart: Santiago Sanchez-Alarcos Ramiro: Ake Nygren: Po-Ya Chang, Wen-Ta Chiu, Shen-Long Howng, Ching-Chang Hung, Chun-Jen Shih, Yeou-Chih Wang: Paul J. Amoroso, Ralph F. Frankowski, Jess F. Kraus, Ronald E. LaPorte, Thomas M. Scott.

This chapter was made possible by the support of the Department of Health, Executive Yuan, R. O. C., the Neurological Society, R. O. C., and the Head and Spinal Cord Injury Research Group; Drs. C. J. Shih, L. S. Lee, Y. H. Shih, L. S. Lin, C. M. Wu, Y. C. Wang, and J. S. Huang.

References

1. Kraus JF: Epidemiology of head injury, in Cooper PR (ed): *Head Injury* (3d ed). Baltimore: Williams & Wilkins, 1993: 1–26.
2. Jennett B, Frankowski RF: The epidemiology of head injury, in Braakman R (ed): *Handbook of Clinical Neurology,* vol 13 (57), New York: Elsevier Science, 1990.
3. Annegars JF, Grabow JD, Kurland LT, et al: The incidence, causes, and secular trends of head trauma in Olmsted County, Minnesota. *Neurology* 1980; 30:912.
4. Kalabeck WD, McLaurin RL, Harris BSH, et al: The national head and spinal cord injury survey: Major findings. *J Neurosurg* 1980; 53 (suppl):S19.
5. Klauber M, Barrett-Conner E, Marshall L, et al: The epidemiology of head injury: A prospective study of an entire community—San Diego, California. *Am J Epidemiol* 1981; 113:500.
6. Kraus JF, Black MA, Hessol N, et al: The incidence of acute brain injury and serious impairment in a defined population. *Am J Epidemiol* 1984; 119:186.
7. Fife D, Faich G, Hollinshed W, et al: Incidence and outcome of hospital-treated head injury in Rhode Island. *Am J Public Health* 1986; 76:773.
8. Cooper KD, Tabbador K, Houser WA, et al: The epidemiology of head injury in the Bronx. *Neuroepidemiology* 1983; 2:70.
9. Jagger J, Levine JI, Jane JA, et al: Epidemiologic features of head injury in a predominantly rural population. *J Trauma* 1984; 24:40.
10. Whitman S, Coonley-Hoganson R, Desai BT: Comparative head trauma experience in two socio-economically different Chicago area communities: A population study. *Am J Epidemiol* 1984; 119:570.
11. Hung CC, Chiu WT, Tsai SC, et al: The epidemiology of head injury in Hualien County, Taiwan. *J Formosan Med Assoc* 1991; 90:1227.
12. Lee LH, Shih YH, Chiu WT, et al: Epidemiologic study of head injuries in Taipei City, Taiwan. *Chin Med J* (Taipei) 1992; 50:219.
13. Tiret L, Hausherr E, Thicoipe M, et al: The epidemiology of head trauma in Aquitaine (France), 1986: A community based study of hospital admission and deaths. *Int J Epidemiol* 1990; 19:133.
14. Edna TH, Cappelan J: Hospital-admitted head injury: A prospective study in Trodelag, Norway, 1979–1980. *Scand J Soc Med* 1984; 12:7.
15. Nestvoid K, Lundar T, Blikra G, et al: Head injuries during one year in a central hospital in Norway: A prospective study. *Neuroepidemiology* 1988; 7:134.
16. Jennett B, MacMillian R: The epidemiology of head injury, *BMJ* 1981; 282:101.
17. Parkison D, Stephesen S, Phillips S: Head injury: A prospective computerized study. *Can J Surg* 1985; 28:79.
18. Servadei F, Bastinnelli G, Naccarato G, et al: Epidemiology and sequelae of head injury in San Marino Republic. *J Neurosurg Sci* 1985; 29:297.
19. Knight R, Burnside J, Boyle L, McClure R: Socioeconomic status and injury: Abstracts. *The Second World Conference On Injury Control,* May 20–23, 1993; 384.
20. Gururaj G, Channabasvanna SM, Das BS, Kaliaperumal VG: Epidemiology of head injuries in Bangalore, South India: Abstracts. *The Second World Conference On Injury Control,* May 20–23, 1993; 225.
21. Krishnan R, Nontak S, Arokiasamy J: Injury surveillance needs in a developing country: Abstracts. *The Second World Conference On Injury Control,* May 20–23, 1993; 384.
22. Gutierrez MI, Velasquez M, Levy A: Epidemiology of head injury in Cali, Colombia: Abstracts. *The Second World Conference On Injury Control,* May 20–23, 1993; 394–395.
23. Bouyoucef KA: Epidemiology of head injury in Algeria. *Personal communication,* August, 1993.
24. Chiu WT, LaPorte RE: The global SHIP: Spine and head-injury prevention project: Abstracts. *The Second World Conference On Injury Control,* May 20–23, 1993; 150–151.
25. LaPorte RE, Chiu WT, Dearwater SR: Applications of the global SHIP in developing and developed countries: Abstracts. *The Second World Conference On Injury Control,* May 20–23, 1993; 151.
26. Alexander E: Global spine and head injury prevention project (SHIP): Editorial. *Surg Neurol* 1992; 38:478–479.
27. Chiu WT, LaPorte RE: SHIP notice. *Surg Neurol* 1993; 39:411.
28. Chiu WT, LaPorte RE: Letter to the editor: *J Trauma:* accepted, 1993.
29. Saul TG, Kelker DB, Burton A: Think first—An educational model for the prevention of brain and spinal cord injury: Abstracts. *The Second World Conference on Injury Control.* May 20–23, 1993; 150.
30. LaPorte RE, McCarty DJ, Tull ES, et al: Counting birds, bees, and NCDs. *Lancet* 1992; 339:494.
31. LaPorte RE, Tull ES, McCarty DJ: Monitoring the incidence of myocardial infarctions: Application of capture-mark-recapture technology. *Int J Epidemiol* 1992; 21(2):258–263.
32. Chiu WT, Dearwater SR, McCarty DJ, et al: Establishment of accurate incidence rates for head and spinal cord injuries in developing and developed countries—A capture-recapture approach. *J Trauma* 1993; 35, 2; 1–6.

CHAPTER 63

SPORTS-RELATED HEAD INJURY

Wayne M. Alves
Richard S. Polin

SYNOPSIS

Differences exist between the treatment of head injury in athletes and treatment in the general population. Foremost are the potential for prophylactic protective measures, access to medical care and follow-up, and the ability to carefully observe and assess the athlete's recovery. Certain sports display established patterns of frequent head injury, allowing identification and interpretation of the concerns particular to head injury in athletes.

Catastrophic injury has been reduced in most prominent organized sports. Neurosurgical treatment of these injuries, which generally involve subdural hematoma and underlying brain contusion, is no different from management of nonathletic brain trauma. Therefore, the diagnosis, management, and recovery from mild head injury and the link between mild and severe head injury will be discussed, with emphasis on classification of such injuries and on practical guidelines to prevent future serious injuries in athletes with a history of previous trauma.

Neurosurgeons should play an aggressive role in the prevention, management, and treatment of sports-induced head injuries. Legislation in the form of improved rules and regulations can have significant impact on incidence and possibly severity of injury. A major issue is the repetitiveness of injuries and the ever-present potential for catastrophic injury.[1–6]

Early appropriate neurosurgical intervention with the same standards of care afforded any head injury victim is needed. The neurosurgeon will need to know the mechanism of injury and the sequence of deterioration of the player or participant. It is important for those who manage injured athletes in the field to provide accurate documentation of loss of consciousness and subsequent neurological deficits.

Assessment of the player or participant is typical for any patient presenting with a history of head trauma. Although heavily used in the evaluation of boxers, EEG does not appear to predict clinical impairment.[7] *Neuropsychological testing has produced inconsistent results, and it has also been difficult to find strong predictive factors for clinical impairment, especially early dysfunction.*[8–10] *This does not argue against the potential value of such assessments.*

BOXING–A MODEL OF CHRONIC BRAIN INJURY

Boxing provides the best model of chronic brain injury, involving multiple relatively low-energy blows to the head over time. Since Harrison Martland's[11] original treatise on the "punch drunk" condition, clinicians and neuropathologists have sought to better define the clinical impairment caused by the chronic brain injury of boxing. Martland aptly described early symptoms of this condition as "uncertainty in equilibrium," "very slight flopping of one foot or leg in walking," and "periods of slight mental confusion." Disease progression includes "slowing of muscular movements," "hesitancy of speech," "tremors of the hands," "nodding movements of the head," and an eventual progression to a parkinsonian state coinciding with severe encephalopathy.

Retrospective examinations of former boxers by Roberts[12] and Johnson[13] have shown a significant percentage of traumatic encephalopathy (17 and 50 percent, respectively), with number of fights and patient age contributing in part to the discrepancy. Neuropathological analysis of the brains of former pugilists, largely performed by Corsellis and colleagues,[14] reveals several important changes, including a high prevalence of fenestrated cavum septum pellucidum formation, neurofibrillary tangles, amyloid angiopathy, perhaps neuritic plaques suggestive of Alzheimer's disease, and degenerative changes in the substantia nigra that resemble those seen in postencephalopathic parkinsonism.

The finding of a fenestrated cavum septum pellucidum seems to be a sensitive marker for *dementia pugilistica*. In Corsellis and colleagues'[14] original report, this finding was evident in 12 of 13 former fighters (an additional 2 had a cavum in association with intraventricular hemorrhage). While many normal individuals harbor this anomaly, only 0.6 percent contained fenestrations, and the cavum in boxers averaged three times larger than in the general population. Isherwood and colleagues[15] found similar lesions on computed tomography scans (CT) in 9 of 16 former fighters. Bogdanoff and Natter[16] prospectively evaluated 1914 consecutive adults obtaining CT scans. They found 14 (0.7 percent) cases of fenestrated cavum septum pellucidum, 6 of whom had a history of boxing or repeated head blows.

Martland[11] noticed the clinical similarities between traumatic encephalopathy and Parkinson's disease. This observation has prompted the search for neuropathological similarities between the two conditions. Brandenburg and Hallervorden[17] first described a loss of pigmented neurons and gliosis in the substantia nigra of an ex-boxer. Corsellis et al.[14] described intense pigment loss in four patients who exhibited pronounced signs of parkinsonism. Overall, they found that 11 of 15 subjects displayed some degree of nigral degeneration with an absence of Lewy bodies, resembling postencephalitic parkinsonism more than the primary disease.

Memory loss is often the earliest symptom noted by the family of the victim of traumatic encephalopathy. The pathological basis for memory disturbance may include mesial temporal neurofibrillary tangle formation, atrophy of the mamillary bodies, disruption of the fornix by septal cavum formation, or generalized cerebral atrophy. Corsellis et al.[14] related the degree of temporal lobe neurofibrillary tangle formation to the degree of memory loss. Studying former amateur fighters, Thomassen et al.[7] found no increased evidence of clinical memory disturbance or dementia, although the ex-fighters performed worse than controls on a test of logical memory.

Former and current boxers have been subjected to a neuropsychological battery to attempt to decipher early clues to future impairment. Testing current pugilists revealed deficits of memory, attention, or reaction time in 15 of 20 active amateurs. Levin and colleagues[10] found statistically significant impairment on a verbal learning test compared with normal controls. Casson et al.[8] examined 15 former and current professional fighters and reported that most subjects displayed abnormalities on at least half the tests in an extensive battery. Thomassen et al.[7] and Haglund and Persson[9] found less pervasive deficits among former boxing amateurs.

Other sports involving possible repeated low-impact blows may also predispose participants to chronic encephalopathy. Electroencephalographic (EEG) changes have been identified in soccer players who frequently head the ball[18] and true traumatic encephalopathy has been witnessed among former national hunt club jockeys.[19]

No single method of analysis conclusively predicts the development of *dementia pugilistica*. Changes develop over time on the neurological, neuroradiographic, neuropsychological, and EEG examinations. As long as boxing remains a sanctioned sport, standard testing of participants should be focused on potential early changes representative of traumatic encephalopathy. These may include new onset of tremor, gait abnormality, memory or attention deficit, or a change in the appearance of the CT scan. One simple step is to perform CT scans at standard intervals in a boxer's career (every 2 years) and after a knockout. The finding of a new cavum septum pellucidum, the increase in size of an existing one, or the progression of cerebral atrophy would provide cause for cessation of boxing. Neuropsychological parameters could invoke a similar role in preventing chronic brain damage in its earliest stages. Amateur boxing has fostered safety precautions that have clearly reduced the rate of both long- and short-term head injury. Consequently, the rate of these abnormalities among boxers who fought only as amateurs is small.

ACUTE ATHLETIC HEAD INJURY

Most modern sports have undergone rule adjustments to minimize the incidence of catastrophic head injury. Turn of the century football caused so many deaths that President Roosevelt considered banning the sport until the violence was curbed. Further legislation, including the elimination of spearing and adoption of helmet specifications in the 1970s, further reduced the rate of catastrophic head injury[5]; nonetheless, precise reporting documents that severe head injury still causes significant morbidity and mortality in football primarily, but in other organized sports as well. The chief difference between severe nonathletic and sports injuries is the preventable nature of the latter. In particular, some of the most tragic cases of brain trauma in athletes result from relatively minor blows potentiated by brain swelling from prior injury. Recognition of and adherence to protocols for return to competition should help minimize these instances of "second-impact syndrome."[2,6]

Epidemiology

The epidemiology of sports head injury is similar to other injury mechanisms in that young males are the typical victims.[4,20–22] While the extreme case of chronic sports-induced brain injury is *dementia pugilistica*, equally important are the pressing acute injuries that regularly present at emergency departments. We especially should not underemphasize the milder forms of brain injury that may appear to be more nuisance than damage, but nonetheless add to considerable morbidity and societal costs.

Local, regional, and national culture defines the kinds and frequencies of injuries that will present. In some sports violence is central, and injury incidence should be expected to be high. Other sports or activities appear to be low-risk for head injuries, but specific positions may be at relatively greater risk, e.g., soccer goalies. What sports or recreational activities are popular and frequent in a given location will determine the incidence and nature of head injuries seen. Table 63-1 lists high-risk organized sports and recreation activities that yield frequent brain injury.

The epidemiology of athletic head injury also will vary with locale. The frequency of injury will increase in younger populations, and the causes will depend on the individual sports popular in the region. Carlsson[20] reported that athletic head injuries within a large Swedish population clustered between the second and fourth decades, with a peak of 5000 incidents per 100,000 people occurring among teenagers. Highest incidences of sports-related head injury occur in rugby in New Zealand,[23] horseback riding and soccer in southern France,[24] American football in the United States,[4] and golf in Scotland.[3] In this country, the National Center for Catastrophic Sports Injury Research in Chapel Hill, NC has accurately compiled the incidence of severe head injury in organized athletic activity. Between the fall of 1982 and the spring of 1989, football provided 34 fatalities from brain injuries and 18 additional cases of devastating head trauma. Other organized sports such as wrestling, baseball, gymnastics, ice hockey, diving, and soccer each provided isolated instances of catastrophic head injury. While football injuries far exceed those from other sports, catastrophic events in that sport have declined from a maximum of 16 per year (1965 to 1974) to the current level of 5 per year (1982 to 1988). Most football fatalities involve subdural hematoma (87 percent).[5]

Mild head injury is a frequent consequence of football. Gerberich et al.[22] reported that 19 percent of high school athletes had experienced at least one minor head trauma. Approximately 70 percent of players returned to competition the same day they lost consciousness. Buckley[1] reported 2124 concussions in college football players over a cumulative 36,000 athlete seasons. About 10 percent (208) of these injuries were severe enough to prevent participation for more than 7 days. Concussions were evenly divided between practices and games.

Boxing federations have also maintained statistics about deaths resulting directly from damage suffered in the ring. McCunney and Russo[25] calculated the annual fatality rate for boxers, which has remained at about 6 deaths per year, to be 0.13 per 1000 participants, making the risk of dying from the sport somewhat less than for college football. Symptoms of minor head injury are almost invariably present, even when fights do not involve knockouts. Jordan[26] found that 262 cases of head and neck injury occurred in 3100 rounds of boxing in New York State. Sercl and Jaros[27] reported that 79 percent of fighters exhibited at least transient neurological signs; in 21 percent the deficit persisted at least 24 h.

The implications for improvement in the care of the head-injured athlete center on two statistics. First, as previously mentioned, only 30 percent of players suffering a loss of consciousness do not return to action on the same day. Second, as reported by Jørgensen and Schmidt-Olsen[28] in a survey of ice hockey accidents, athletic knee injuries are managed by a physician 72 percent of the time, whereas athletic brain trauma is monitored by a physician only 8 percent of the time.

TABLE 63-1 Sports with High Risk of Brain Injury

Organized Sports
Boxing
Football
Professional Horse Racing
Rugby and Australian Football
Ice Hockey
Soccer
Recreational Sports
Hang Gliding
Scuba Diving
Mountaineering
Equestrian Sports
Winter Skiing

Postconcussive Syndrome

Postconcussive syndrome refers to the constellation of signs and symptoms that characterize the period of recovery from acute brain injury. Headache, dizziness, tinnitus, memory disturbance, and difficulty with concentration are hallmarks described by most victims. While these sequelae invariably follow moderate or severe brain injury, they have also been shown to result from minor athletic head trauma. Wilberger[29] reported that over half of high school football players complained of fatigue, dizziness, poor attention, or memory disturbance after minor head injury.

At the University of Virginia a study was undertaken to examine the consequences of head injury from football over the course of the athlete's recovery.[30] Over a 4-year period, 2300 college football players were entered into the study. Each player received preseason baseline testing consisting of a neurobehavioral test protocol and a psychosocial assessment protocol. This battery consisted of Reitan's trailmaking test, Smith's symbol digit test, Gronwall's paced auditory serial addition task, Ammon's quick test, a psychiatric research epidemiology interview, and a review of the patient's subjective symptomatology. Controls consisted of both age-matched students not involved in contact sports and football players who sustained orthopedic injuries during the season.

Approximately 8 percent (183 of 2300) of athletes suffered mild head injuries identified by the team physician or head trainer over the 4-year testing interval. Twelve subjects received multiple instances of trauma, one three times. Only nine (4.7 percent) of the injuries involved a positive loss of consciousness, none longer than 5 min. Transient disorientation (less than 5 min) occurred in half of these subjects, while confusion persisting for greater than an h occurred in 14 percent. The head-injured players had more complaints of headache and dizziness than their age-matched controls at 1 and 5 days after injury, while complaints of difficulty with memory persisted to 10 days posttrauma (Table 63-2). Performance on the neuropsychiatric battery remained impaired until the patients became free of postconcussive symptomatology, with tests aimed at concentration providing the longest sustained impairment (Table 63-3).[30]

The Second-Impact Syndrome

Multiple injuries have been noted to increase the duration and magnitude of postconcussive symptoms. Carlsson et al.[21] found that headache, dizziness, and memory deficit persisted longer in head trauma victims with a history of previous concussions. Wilberger's[29] study of head-injured high school football players included 62 individuals with multiple injuries within one season. Impairment on tests of memory and concentration in these subjects remained at 1 month in 47 percent and at 3 months in 26 percent. Postconcussive subjective complaints also lingered with multiple injuries.

Many isolated case reports detailing malignant brain swelling following relatively minor blows in the setting

TABLE 63-2 Complaints of Headache After Mild Head Injury in Collegiate Football Players

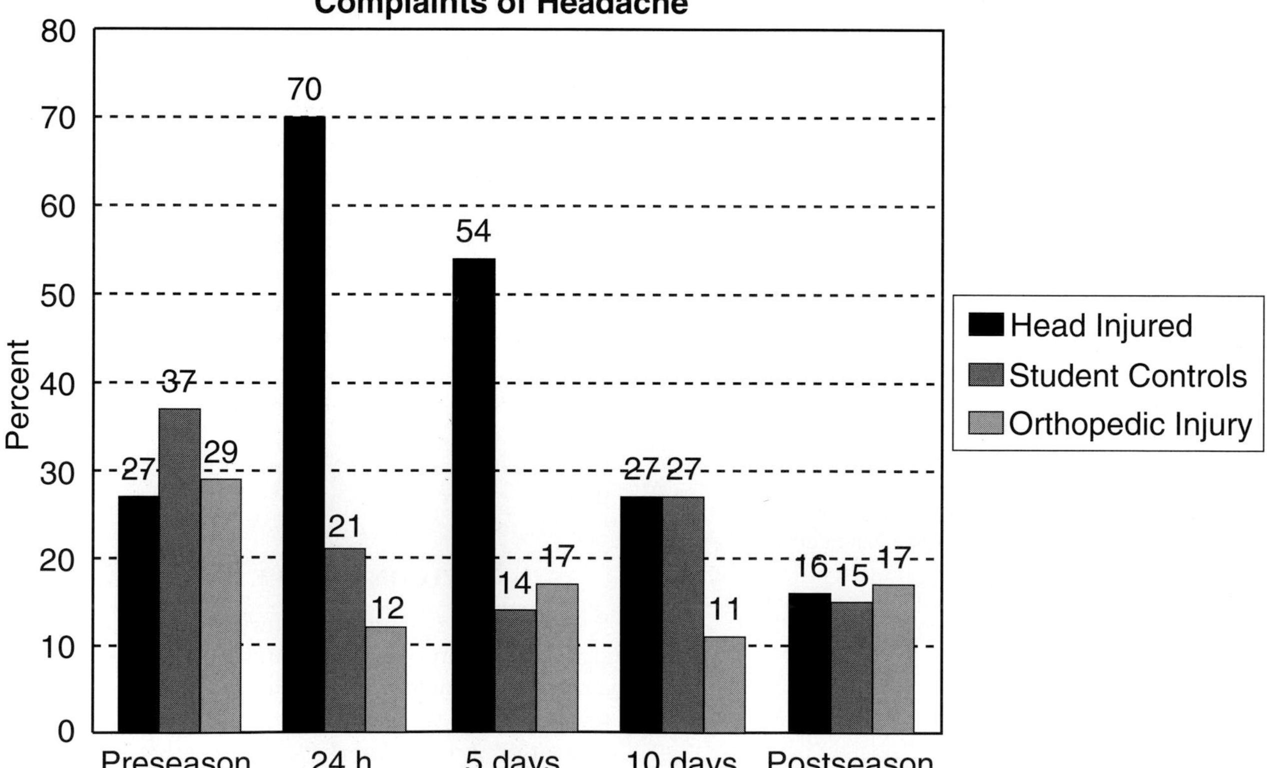

Source: Alves, 1991.[30]

TABLE 63-3 Performance of Football Players Suffering Mild Head Injury on the Paced Serial Addition Test: An Assessment of Attention and Concentration

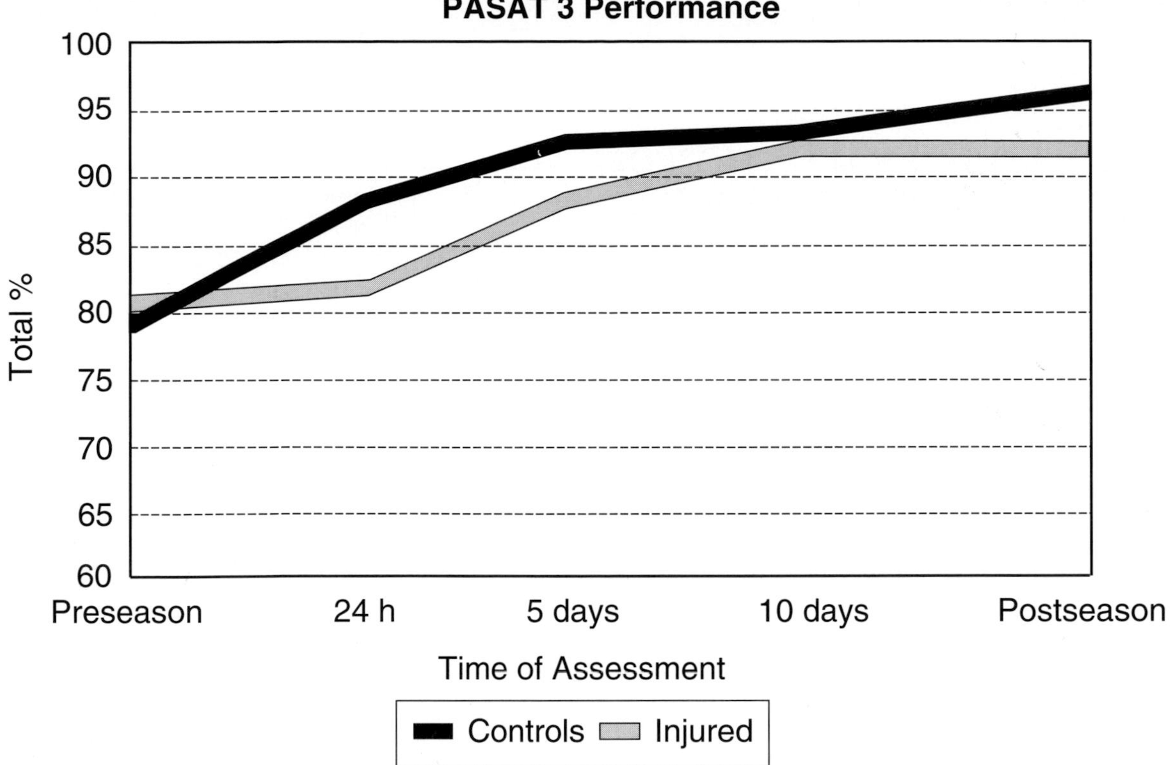

Source: Alves, 1991.[30]

of recent mild head injury have been documented.[6] The National Center for Catastrophic Sports Injury Research found 29 cases of this second-impact syndrome from football alone between 1980 and 1991.[2] The pathophysiology of this entity is believed to involve subclinical brain swelling from a traumatic insult that makes the brain more susceptible to further injury. It is postulated that the first insult disturbs the brain's autoregulatory mechanisms, with consequent vascular congestion and poor brain compliance. This reasoning is difficult to prove in a clinical setting because the first injury, thought to be minor, does not necessitate invasive intracranial pressure monitoring. It is postulated because the presumed poor compliance could lead to rapid deterioration from brain swelling following a relatively minor second impact. Torg and colleagues[31] have described several cases that mimic second-impact syndrome in which the athlete had preexisting encephalitis from mononucleosis. This condition could similarly cause poor compliance due to vasomotor dysfunction. Underscoring the difference between these injuries and the more common presentations of severe athletic brain injuries is the lack of subdural hematoma and the prominence of subacute contusion as the pathological cause of death seen at autopsy.

Treatment of second impact syndrome is particularly problematic in that the patients tend to present with severe intracranial hypertension. Measures to reduce intracranial pressure (ICP) should begin in the field and include rapid intubation and hyperventilation, elevating the head in the reverse Trendelenburg position, and medical reduction of ICP with intravenous mannitol. As these patients tend not to have surgically treatable mass lesions, management of cases refractory to hyperventilation and mannitol includes barbiturates for neuroprotection or, alternatively, bifrontal decompressive craniectomy. Novel pharmaceutical agents, such as the 21-aminosteroid tirilazad mesylate, have shown beneficial effects in experimental models of diffuse head injury and are undergoing clinical trials.

The second-impact syndrome underscores the need to rationally restrict head-injured athletes from return to competition. While it has not been proved in humans, we believe that the postconcussive symptomatology may reflect underlying vasomotor dysfunction and poor brain compliance that can lead to deterioration from a second insult. Even if this is not reliably the case, one should assume underlying alterations in brain compliance among athletes whose headache, dizziness, memory disturbance, and poor attention persist. This assumption leads to our novel criteria for guiding the return to competition among head-injured athletes.

CLASSIFICATION EVALUATION OF SPORTS MILD HEAD INJURY

Before developing strategies to guide return to competition, one must define an appropriate classification of mild neurological head injury. Previous schemes have graded mild athletic brain injury primarily on loss of consciousness and posttraumatic amnesia (PTA) (Table 63-4).[32–34] At the Sports Neurosurgery Center of the Virginia Neurological Institute, we have revised existing analyses to establish the concept that the fundamental nature of the injury should be apparent to the on-site medical supervisor. Therefore, factors such as posttraumatic amnesia, which may persist many hours after otherwise minor head injury, have been deemphasized, while criteria of impairment in the neurological examination have been added. To simplify the latter, the Glasgow Coma Scale (GCS) has been used as an assessment of global neurological functioning.

The majority of injuries in our scheme are termed *Grade I* (Table 63-5). These injuries may involve momentary loss of consciousness; however, the GCS must remain 15 throughout the recovery phase. For purposes of dictating return to activity, Grade 1 injuries with posttraumatic amnesia of greater than 1 h are termed *Grade 1a. Grade 2* injuries may include loss of consciousness or depression of GCS of less than 5 min. Grades 1, 1a, and 2 events may be monitored by the on-site medical personnel (see Fig. 63-1).

Criteria for a *Grade 3* injury include a GCS less than 15 but greater than 12 for up to 1 h, with less than a

TABLE 63-4 Grading Scales for Athletic Mild Head Injury

	Mild: Grade 1	Moderate: Grade 2	Severe: Grade 3
Cantu	No LOC or PTA < 1 h	LOC < 5 min or PTA of 1–24 h	>5 min or PTA > 24 h
Torg[31]	(Grade I–II) No LOC, No amnesia (or PTA only)	(Grade III–IV) LOC < few min. PTA or retrograde amnesia	(Grade V–VI) LOC, (coma) Confusion with amnesia
Colorado Consortium	No LOC Confusion without amnesia	No LOC Confusion with amnesia	LOC

LOC = Loss of Consciousness
PTA = Posttraumatic amnesia

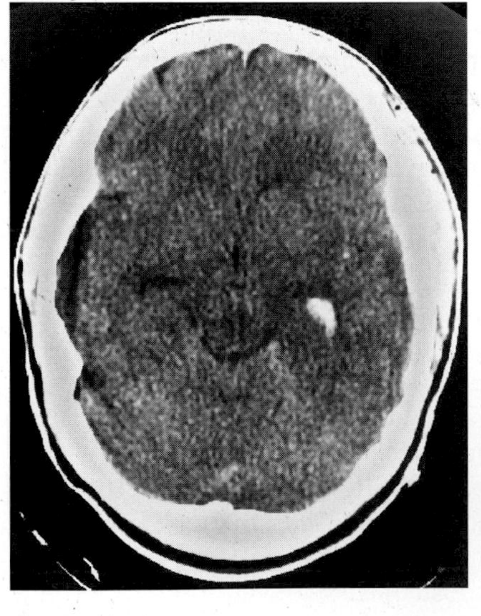
A

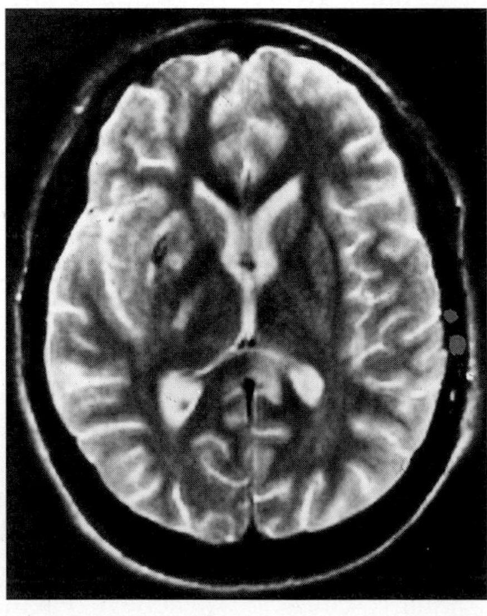
B

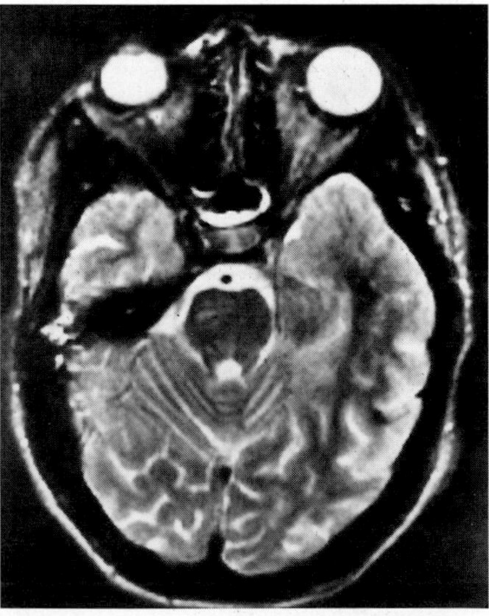
C

Figure 63-1. CT scan taken on a 22-year-old female with GCS 8 after a skiing injury. CT shows intraventricular hemorrhage and diffuse brain swelling (*A*). The patient did not improve substantially despite an absence of elevated ICP. MRI obtained on postinjury day 20 shows evidence of brainstem (*B*), basal ganglia, and corpus callosum (*C*) axonal shear injury on T2-weighted images.

TABLE 63-5 Virginia Neurological Institute Grading Scale for Athletic Mild Head Injury

	LOC	PTA	GCS
Grade 1	momentary	<1 h	GCS 15
Grade 1a	momentary	>1 but <24 h	GCS 15
Grade 2	<5 min	PTA up to 24 h	GCS < 15 for 5 min or less
Grade 3	<5 min	N/A	12 < GCS < 15 for up to 1 h
Grade 4	>5 but <60 min	N/A	GCS <12 for over 5 min or GCS <15 for more than 1 h

5-min loss of consciousness. *Grade 4* injuries may display a GCS of less than 13 for up to 5 min, or a GCS of 13 or 14 that persists past an h. Loss of consciousness may exceed 5 min as well. We advise that individuals with Grade 3 or Grade 4 injuries should not be observed merely at the athletic venue but be transported to a medical facility. Any injury too severe for this scale demands immediate neurosurgical attention (see Fig. 63-2).

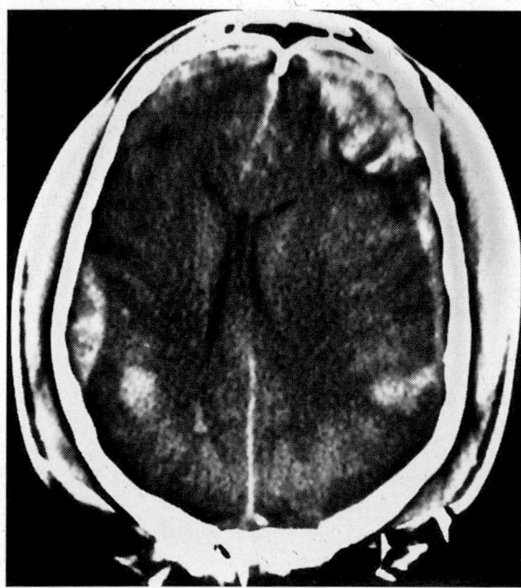

Figure 63-2. Computed tomography scan taken of a 32-year-old male after a skiing accident. The patient was initially GCS 11 but deteriorated rapidly and died two days after injury. CT shows bihemispheric contusions, a right-sided epidural hematoma, and a left-sided subdural hematoma.

Return to Competition

The grounds for allowing athletes to return to competition following head injury have been founded on assessing the severity of the injury and the history of previous trauma. More recently, postconcussive symptomatology has become a factor in allowing participation. Cantu[32–34] established a set of guidelines that factor the patient's history of previous injuries (Table 63-6). Mild concussion dictates return to competition after observation of at least 30 min if the victim is asymptomatic. A second injury sidelines patients for 2 weeks, provided they have been asymptomatic for 1 week. A third mild injury entails termination of the given athletic season. Moderate concussion necessitates an absence of at least 1 week, with a second injury lengthening the interval to 1 month. The athlete with severe concussion defined by persistent loss of consciousness is restricted from participation for 1 month from the time of injury if asymptomatic. The restriction continues indefinitely until the athlete is asymptomatic with mild exertion. A second Grade 3 lesion terminates the athlete's season.

The University of Colorado Consortium[35] requires a minimum of 20 min of asymptomatic observation before return to competition in Grade 1 (confusion without amnesia) head trauma. Athletes suffering confusion with amnesia, but no loss of consciousness (Grade 2) must undergo serial examination over 24 h, with return after 1 week without symptoms. Any patient experiencing loss of consciousness must be asymptomatic for 2 weeks after initial evaluation before being permitted to participate.[35]

The Virginia Neurological Institute guidelines also provide minimum requirements for cessation of participation, but focus on postconcussive symptomatology as the key for physicians to guide the athlete's return (Table 63-7). Grades 1 and 1a injuries necessitate 1 and 2 days absence, respectively. Temporary impairment of consciousness results in longer minimum periods of abstinence. Grade 2 injuries are kept out for 4 days (to cover the interval of maximum brain edema), Grade 3 injuries have a minimum of 1 week without participation, and Grade 4 entails at least 2 weeks free from contact sports. The persistence of postconcussive symptomatology, which in our experience tends to wane between days 5 and 10 after injury, absolutely precludes the athlete from participation. For athletes to be cleared to resume contact sports after mild head injury, they must be both free of subjective complaints and cleared by team medical personnel on 5-min recall of three objects. With all but Grades 1 and 1a injuries, this symptom-free interval must last 48 h prior to reinstatement, and should be tested sequentially under progressively more rigorous practice conditions, i.e., graded return to activity.

TABLE 63-6 Cantu's Return-to-Competition Guidelines Based on Severity of Injury and History of Previous Injury

Concussion Grade	First Concussion	Second Concussion	Third Concussion
Grade 1-Mild	May return when asymptomatic	May return in 2 weeks if asymptomatic for 1 week	Terminate season
Grade 2-Moderate	May return when asympomatic for 1 week	May return in 1 month if asymptomatic for 1 week	Terminate season
Grade 3-Severe	May return in one month if asymptomatic for 1 week	Terminate season	

Cantu, Clinics in Sports Medicine, vol 7, 1988.

Individuals with multiple injuries within the same athletic season are subjected to longer periods of restricted activity. Essentially, each subsequent trauma increases the grade of the injury by 1. Therefore, an athlete suffering a Grade 2 mild head injury after having experienced an uncomplicated Grade 1 injury a few weeks earlier, would be managed as a Grade 3. Any two injuries in which one is termed Grade 4, or any third injury, sidelines the individual for the season (or a minimum of 3 months). Furthermore, multiple injuries would require neurological or neurosurgical clearance prior to return and suggests the need for neuroradiographic evaluation. These steps will certainly sideline some athletes, but is intended if properly administered to minimize the risk of second-impact syndrome.

TABLE 63-7 Virginia Neurological Institute Guidelines for Return to Athletic Competition Providing Minimum Standards with the Caveat that any Postconcussive Symptom Will Prohibit Participation: A Graded Return to Contact Sports is Suggested

Minimum Absence without Postconcussive Symptoms

Grade of Concussion	First Injury	Second Injury	Third Injury
Grade 1	Minimum 1 day	Minimum 4 days	Terminate season
Grade 1a	Minimum 2 days	Minimum 4 days	Terminate season
Grade 2	Minimum 4 days	Minimum 7 days	Terminate season
Grade 3	Minimum 7 days	Minimum 14 days	Terminate season
Grade 4	Minimum 14 days	Terminate season	

Virginia Neurological Institute

PRESCREENING AND EVALUATION

The role of prescreening the prospective participant in organized sports activity is controversial. Traditionally, prescreening of athletes prior to participation in contact sports has analyzed the participant's history and a neurological examination, which is often cursory. A history of headache, ataxia, diplopia, tinnitus, or memory disturbance should prompt investigation prior to participation. The neurological examination should include a fundoscopic examination for signs of papilledema, a detailed cranial nerve examination, evaluation for truncal and extremity ataxia, and a mini mental status examination. Because boxing carries a known risk, we suggest that professional fighters be prescreened with a CT scan. Individuals demonstrating a large cavum septum pellucidum or atrophy inappropriate for age would be excluded from competition. Subsequent scans obtained at regular 2-year intervals or after a knockout could prevent second-impact injuries.

EVALUATION OF HEADACHE

Attention should be given to the evaluation of headache. Athletes are just as prone as other individuals to suffer episodic headache unrelated to trauma; however, given the possibility of chronic subdural hematoma or hydrocephalus in the athlete with only a distant history of head injury, all such participants deserve careful evaluation. The two key points that guide management principles in the athlete with chronic headache are defining the pattern of evolution of the problem and defining any potential traumatic initiating insults. A patient with a stable pattern of headache, not exacerbating in terms of intensity or duration, and not temporally associated with a traumatic blow, may be followed. A change in the pattern of headache demands further investigation.

A CT scan is the first step for patients with a change in the pattern of headache and a distinct traumatic trigger. A CT will demonstrate chronic subdural hematoma, hydrocephalus from previous traumatic subarachnoid hemorrhage, or most cortical contusions. Magnetic resonance imaging (MRI) can better diagnose shear injury and is obtained if the CT is negative and headache does not abate. Any athlete with new unexplained headache or an exacerbation of a baseline headache should be restricted from participation until a source of the headache is determined and addressed or the pain is restored to baseline.[36]

MRI is the first imaging modality for athletes with exacerbation of headache but without a clear history of past head trauma. Of 103 patients with presumed benign headache, Rooke[37] found that 10 harbored intracranial pathology. Retrospectively, 7 of these 10 had lesions that are imaged significantly better on MRI than on CT (Chiari 1 in 3, platybasia in 2, basilar impression in 1, cerebellar hemangioblastoma in 1). As suggested by this list, MRI is clearly superior to CT in detecting pathology in the posterior fossa or skull base and is therefore preferred for initial screening of headache in athletes with no defined traumatic event.

CONCLUSION

The study of athletic head injury provides a unique window for the evaluation, assessment, and ultimately the prevention of brain trauma. Clinicians have improved the evaluation and treatment of injuries, adding neuroradiographic and neuropsychological studies to the routine assessment of mild and moderate head injuries. We have appreciated the clinical situation of traumatic encephalopathy through the sport of boxing. We have realized that the rate of catastrophic brain injury resulting from football, amateur boxing, and ice hockey can be drastically reduced through the use of improved protective headgear, rules that discourage contact with the skull, and adequate on-site supervision. One lingering concern is the need for standardized monitoring of boxers to prevent traumatic encephalopathy. For this task, we postulate that neuropsychological or neuroradiographic abnormalities may predate clinical impairment and identify potential victims before their irreversible decline.

Many sports have retained their inherent risk of head injury but are clearly amenable to preventive intervention. The routine use of appropriate helmets by jockeys has drastically reduced injuries during competition; therefore, the majority of recreational horseback accidents producing head injury that occur in unhelmeted riders are ultimately preventable. Similar measures in other recreational sports like hang gliding, mountaineering, and sledding would prevent some head injuries. These activities are loosely organized, so efforts at safety awareness must be targeted at small groups of participants.

Finally, recognition of the multiplicative nature of repeated mild head trauma has fostered attempts to classify injuries and to regulate more closely both return of athletes to competition and the management of the athlete with headache. The Virginia Neurological Institute classification of head injury seeks to replace existing schemes with criteria that can be employed by on-site team physicians and trainers. We have sought to downplay factors such as posttraumatic amnesia that take hours to days to clear. We do assume a rudimentary knowledge of the GCS for on-site application of this scale. Our criteria for return to participation stress the clearing of postconcussive symptoms as an absolute prerequisite for return to competition. We believe that in some cases these subjective complaints are manifestations of vasomotor dysfunction and poor brain compliance that can precipitate second-impact syndrome. Multiple head injuries receive special attention in terms of mandatory clearance by a neurospecialist before return to competition and stricter time-out limits should be imposed prior to reinstatement. In this field most of the conclusions are not so much derived from hard data as extrapolated from clinical experience. Prospective study of athletic head injury is difficult because most cases never reach medical attention. All efforts, however, to prospectively define risk in athletic head injury are integral to a better definition of the risk of individual insults.

References

1. Buckley WE: Concussions in college football: A multivariate analysis. *Am J Sports Med* 1988; 16:51–56.
2. Cantu RC: Second impact syndrome: Immediate management. *Physician and Sportsmedicine*. 1992; 20:55–66.
3. Lindsay KW, McLatchie G, Jennett B: Serious head injury in sport. *Br Med J* 1980; 281:789–791.
4. Mueller FO: Catastrophic sport injuries, in Mueller FO, Ryan AJ (eds): *Prevention of Athletic Injuries: The Role of the Sports Medicine Team.* Philadelphia: FA Davis, 1991: 26–34.
5. Mueller FO, Blyth CS: Fatalities from head and cervical spine injuries occurring in tackle football: 40 years' experience. *Clin Sports Med* 1987; 6:185–196.
6. Saunders RL, Harbaugh RE: The second impact in catastrophic contact-sports head trauma. *JAMA* 1984; 252:538–539.
7. Thomassen A, Juul-Jensen P, De Fine Olivarius B, et al: Neurological, electroencephalographic and neuropsychological examination of 53 former amateur boxers. *Acta Neurol Scand* 1979; 60:352–362.
8. Casson IR, Sham R, Campbell EA, et al: Neurological and CT evaluation of knocked-out boxers. *J Neurol Neurosurg Psychiatry* 1982; 45:170–174.
9. Haglund Y, Persson HE: Does Swedish amateur boxing lead to chronic brain damage? III. A retrospective clinical neurophysiological study. *Acta Neurol Scand* 1990; 82:353–360.
10. Levin HS, Lippold SC, Goldman A, et al: Neurobehavioral functioning and magnetic resonance imaging findings in young boxers. *J Neurosurg* 1987; 67:657–667.
11. Martland HS: Punch drunk. *JAMA* 1928; 91:1103–1107.
12. Roberts AH: *Brain Damage in Boxers.* London: Pitman, 1969.
13. Johnson J: Organic psychosyndrome due to boxing. *Br J Psychiatry* 1969; 115:45–53.
14. Corsellis JAN, Bruton CJ, Freeman-Browne D: The aftermath of boxing. *Psychol Med* 1973; 3:270–303.
15. Isherwood I, Maudsley C, Ferguson FR: Pneumoencephalographic changes in boxers. *Acta Radiol* 1966; 5:654–661.
16. Bogdanoff B, Natter HM: Incidence of cavum septum pellucidum in adults: A sign of boxer's encephalopathy. *Neurology* 1989; 39:991–992.
17. Brandenburg W, Hallervorden J: Dementia pugilistica mit anatomischem Befund. *Virchows Archiv* 1954; 325:680–709.
18. Tysvaer AT, Storli O: Soccer injuries to the brain. *Am J Sports Med* 1989; 17:573–578.
19. Foster JB, Leiguardia R, Tilley PJB: Brain damage in national hunt jockeys. *Lancet* 1976; 1(7967):981–983.
20. Carlsson GS: Head injuries in a population study. *Acta Neurochir* 1986; (Suppl 36):13–15.
21. Carlsson GS, Svardsodd K, Welm L: Long-term effects of head injury sustained during life in three male populations. *J Neurosurg* 1987; 67:197–205.
22. Gerberich SG, Priest JD, Boen JR, et al: Concussion incidences and severity in secondary school varsity football players. *Am J Publ Health* 1983; 73:1370–1375.
23. Lingard DA, Sharrock NE, Salmond CE: Risk factors of sports injury in winter. *N Z Med J* 1976; 83:69–73.
24. Vigouroux RP, Guillermain P, Verrando R: Neurotraumatology of sportive origin. *Neurochir* 1978; 24:247–250.
25. McCunney RJ, Russo PK: Brain injuries in boxers. *Physician and Sportsmedicine* 1984; 12:53–67.
26. Jordan BD: Neurologic aspects of boxing. *Arch Neurol* 1987; 44:453–459.
27. Sercl M, Jaros O: The mechanisms of cerebral concussion in boxing and their consequences. *World Neurol* 1962; 3:351–357.
28. Jorgensen U, Schmidt-Olsen S: The epidemiology of ice hockey injuries. *Br J Sports Med* 1986; 20:7–9.
29. Wilberger JE: Minor head injuries in American football: Prevention of long term sequelae. *Sports Med* 1993; 15:338–343.
30. Alves WM: Football-induced mild head injury, in Torg JS (ed): *Athletic Injuries to the Head, Neck, and Face.* St. Louis: Mosby Year Book, 1991: 283–304.
31. Torg JS, Beer LA, Vesgo J: Head trauma in football players with infectious mononucleosis. *Physician and Sportsmedicine* 1980; 8:107–110.
32. Cantu RC: Guidelines for return to contact sports after a cerebral concussion. *Physician and Sportsmedicine* 1986; 14:75–83.
33. Cantu RC: Head and neck injuries, in Mueller FO, Ryan AJ (eds): *Prevention of Athletic Injuries: The Role of the Sports Medicine Team.* Philadelphia: FA Davis, 1991: 201–212.
34. Cantu RC: Criteria for return to competition after a closed head injury, in Torg JS (ed): *Athletic Injuries to the Head, Neck, and Face.* St. Louis: Mosby Year Book, 1991: 323–330.
35. Kelly JP, Nichols JS, Filley CM, et al: Concussion in sports: Guidelines for the prevention of catastrophic outcome. *JAMA* 1991; 266:2867–2869.
36. Caccayorin ED, Petro GR, Hochhauser L: Headache in the athlete and radiographic evaluation. *Clin Sports Med* 1987; 6:739–749.
37. Rooke ED: Benign exertional headache. *Med Clin North Am* 1968; 52:801–808.

Clinical Trials in Head Injury

CHAPTER 64

CLINICAL TRIAL DESIGN

Charles F. Contant, Jr.

SYNOPSIS

It is agreed among researchers that the most convincing method for evaluating a new treatment is a prospective randomized clinical trial (PRCT). While useful information can be obtained from controlled observational studies, it is only through a PRCT that a final assessment of the efficacy of a treatment can be made. Although a complete review of clinical trials is beyond the scope of this chapter, the principles of clinical trial design and the tools for designing a simple trial will be presented.

HISTORICAL DEVELOPMENT OF CLINICAL TRIALS

The concept of a clinical trial dates back to biblical times. The Book of Daniel, verses 12 to 15, describes a planned experiment, including observations at enrollment and follow-up. The eleventh-century Arabian Canon of Medicine contains principles for evaluating treatments that include most of the properties of a comparative study. At times, natural experiments provided a comparative study that was reported by insightful observers, such as the one reported by Pare in the early sixteenth century.[1] The first study that is considered to fulfill the criteria for a clinical trial was conducted by Lind in 1747, when he assessed the effect of eating oranges on scurvy among British sailors.[2–4] There was little further development in the conduct of clinical trials until 1923, when R. A. Fisher applied the concept of randomization to experiments conducted in agricultural research.[5,6] In 1930, the Medical Research Council of the United Kingdom appointed a special committee for the conduct of clinical trials.[4,7] In 1931, the first human clinical trial to use random allocation of the treatments was reported by J. B. Amberson, B. T. McMahon, and M. Pinner in a test of sanocrysin in tuberculosis.[8] Further development of multicenter trials, codes of ethics for human experimentation, and the adoption of clinical trials by the U.S. Food and Drug Administration (FDA) occurred during the 1940s to 1960s.[4]

DEFINITION OF TERMS

Friedman and coworkers defined a clinical trial as a prospective study comparing the effect and value of an intervention or interventions with control treatment in human subjects.[9] Meinert added an emphasis on the notion that a trial is a planned experiment and that the study subjects are enrolled and treated and their outcome is assessed over the same period of time.[4] This chapter will use a combination of these definitions as the working definition of a clinical trial: A clinical trial is a planned, prospective study comparing the effect and value of a therapy or another intervention with a control therapy. The trial is conducted with study subjects who are enrolled and treated and whose outcome is assessed over the same period of time. The trial has a defined set of patients to be enrolled, exact specification of the treatments to be used, and a predefined outcome that will be used to compare the effects of the experimental therapy with those of the control therapy. This definition excludes a trial that compares current therapy with historical information, that is, "historical controls." The exclusion of historical controls is somewhat controversial, as some arguments can be made for using such controls.[9,10] The use of historical information is implicit in some of the designs of phase II trials, but the use of these designs should be limited to screening the efficacy of therapies. These definitions do not exclude nonrandomized, unblinded studies, though only trials that are randomized and blinded can provide high-quality information that is considered specifically pure.

The following words will be used with specific connotations. "Treatment" signifies both the experimental therapies and the standard therapy, or control group therapy. Therefore, a comparison of an experimental drug with a standard drug would be a trial with two treatments. "Control group" refers to the patients who are given the standard therapy or a placebo. "Treated group" refers to patients who receive the experimental therapy. While clinical trials are often thought of in the context of drug trials, the term "therapy" will be used to signify a drug or a surgical or medical management intervention. Clinical trials may be conducted at a single site or at many sites simultaneously ("multicenter" trial).

TYPES OF CLINICAL TRIALS

Clinical trials may be characterized as one of four "phases":

Phase I trials: Trials that assess the chemical action and safety of a therapy and are not concerned with treatment efficacy. These trials may include a dose escalation study to determine minimal or maximal safe doses. While of great importance in the development of new therapies, phase I trials will not be dealt with further in this chapter. They are often conducted with normal volunteers by the pharmaceutical industry.

Phase II trials: Trials conducted to provide initial estimates of the efficacy of a therapy and often to refine the dose. Phase II trials are very useful for screening several therapies to determine which treatment should be considered for further development. The proper design of these trials may be rather complicated, though the total sample size requirement is rarely over 200 patients and is often under 100.

Phase III trials: Clinical trials conducted to formally test the hypothesis that the new treatment is better than the standard therapy or control. These trials usually include an assessment of safety and dosing as well. Phase III trials are the last phase in the process of formal approval of drugs by the FDA. Pocock indicated that the treatment should have been shown to be reasonably effective before the conduct of the phase III trial[11] because of the great expense and effort associated with such trials.

Phase IV trials: These trials are generally thought of as postmarketing studies that are performed after the acceptance of a therapy and usually apply to drug treatments. Meinert indicated that the trials should still be randomized and controlled,[4] while Pocock noted that these trials should include monitoring of the adverse events, morbidity, and mortality associated with the treatment.[11] These trials are less clearly defined.

Phase II trials can be used to efficiently determine whether a treatment should be considered a candidate for a large, expensive phase III trial. Phase II trials also can be used to screen several potential therapies to select the most (or least) promising treatment. Phase II trials usually are designed to match the statistical properties inferred from the research question. Therefore, there are no general rules that can be used to design phase II trials. (As with any clinical trial, phase II trials should be designed after consultation with a statistician.[12,13]) The rest of this chapter will focus on issues inherent in designing, conducting, and analyzing a phase III clinical trial. The specific problems associated with neurotrauma patients will be highlighted.

RANDOMIZATION

The introduction of randomization in clinical trials has allowed researchers to use statistical methods to test differences between or among treatment groups. Technically, all statistical tests of hypotheses rely on the selection of a random sample from a larger population. Randomization, in the context of a clinical trial, is done to provide balancing of the known and unknown factors that might be related to the outcome under question. For example, it is well established that the Glasgow Coma Scale (GCS) score is related to outcome from traumatic brain injury.[14] If a treatment were tested in such a way that only GCS 3 through 5 patients were in the treated group and only GCS 6 through 8 patients were in the control group, the effect of the treatment would be masked by the fact that only the very sick patients were treated. While this total imbalance rarely occurs, more subtle imbalances can modify the conclusion of a trial significantly. Tables 64-1 through 64-3 illustrate the problem.

In both groups, there is a clear 20 percent difference in the outcomes favoring the treated group. However, the imbalance in the allocation of patients to the GCS categories reduces the difference to 6.3 percent, with a resulting p value that is unlikely to lead to further interest in the treatment.

One solution to this problem would be for the investigator to balance the allocation to the two GCS categories. That is, each of the categories, or "strata," would have the same number of treated patients. This approach would work and is often done in trial design, as discussed below. If the investigator had perfect knowledge, this approach would allow for a balancing of all the possible factors that might affect outcome. However, it is impossible for an investigator to have such perfect knowledge (if he or she did, why conduct the trial in the first place?). By allocating each subject to the treatments so that there is an equal chance of being placed into any treatment, randomization tends to solve this problem. If there are only two treatments, as above, each patient has an equal, or 50 percent, chance of being allocated to the treated group. On average, then, about half the patients will be in the treated group and the other half will be in the control group. Important factors that could influence outcome will have an equal chance of being assigned to the treated group or the control group. The proportion of patients with a specific risk factor in one treatment group will be about the same as the proportion in the other treatment group. This holds for all known and unknown factors.

A second reason for randomization is control of investigator bias. When there is a random allocation of patients to the treatment arms, the investigator does not have an opportunity to allow known or hidden biases to influence the treatment a particular patient receives. Often, a clinical trial is conducted by investigators who are biased in regard to which therapy is superior. Allowing the investigator to assign subjects to treatments may result in the assignment only of patients who will do well to the treated group, with patients expected to have a poor outcome assigned to the control group. Even with the most objective investigators, unconscious bias may lead to unbalancing the trial. It is very important that all investigator decisions regarding the selection of a patient for a trial be made before the assignment to a particular treatment to avoid even subtle bias.

It is worth noting that randomization does not guarantee perfect balance between the treatment groups. In fact, at the 0.05 significance level, 1 in 20 factors will be significantly unbalanced among the treatment groups. The alpha level (significant p value) used for the trial includes the possibility of this imbalance. However, monitoring the randomization and analysis of the data, incorporating factors that are related to outcome, is important in the conduct of a trial.

Somewhat related to randomization is the issue of intention to treat, which implies that once a study subject

TABLE 64-1 Hypothetical Trial: GCS 3–5

GCS 3–5	Favorable Outcome	Poor Outcome	Total
Treated group	80	120	200 (40% favorable outcome)
Control group	10	40	50 (20% favorable outcome)

$p = 0.0084$.

TABLE 64-2 Hypothetical Trial: GCS 6–8

GCS 3–5	Favorable Outcome	Poor Outcome	Total
Treated group	12	8	20 (60% favorable outcome)
Control group	68	102	170 (40% favorable outcome)

$p = .0866$.

TABLE 64-3 Hypothetical Trial: Combined GCS

Total (GCS 3–8)	Favorable Outcome	Poor Outcome	Total
Treated group	92	128	220 (41.8% favorable outcome)
Control group	78	142	220 (35.5% favorable outcome)

$p = .2030$.

is randomized to a treatment, he or she always stays in that treatment group. In most trials, after randomization, there are problems in a few study subjects which may result in violations of the study protocol. The study subject may die, the wrong drug may be given, or the patient may require therapy that violates the protocol. In these cases, it is tempting to remove the study subject from the trial. The concept of intention to treat would require that the patient be analyzed as he or she was initially randomized. In this way, it is not possible for an unconscious preference for the experiment therapy or the control therapy to affect decisions regarding which patients are deemed to have experienced protocol violations.

Methods of Randomization

Randomization methods generally fall into two classes: fixed allocation and adaptive randomization. The fixed allocation method assigns the treatments to study subjects with a predetermined probability that is constant. A treatment is allocated for all the possible study subjects in the trial. Adaptive allocation allows the probability for a treatment to vary as the trial progresses. To illustrate the two approaches, assume that a trial of a total of 200 patients is to be undertaken and that an experimental therapy is to be compared to a control. Using fixed randomization, each patient is assigned to the treated group or the control group with a probability of 1 in 2. In practice, 200 study identification numbers are generated, and a random number is assigned to each identification number, using a computer program or random number table. Each study subject has the same chance of being assigned to either the control or the experimental therapy. Adaptive randomization changes the allocation of patients to treatment according either to imbalances in the types of patients randomized or to the results of a trial. Using the above example, add the requirement that the 200 patients must be balanced according to the number of males and females in each treatment group. After a short period in which fixed allocation is performed, the number of males and females in each treatment group is determined. Then, if there is an imbalance, the allocation is adjusted so that the imbalance is corrected. If 60 percent of the control subjects are male, the probability of assignment to the control is set slightly higher for females until the percentage of males approaches 50 percent. Adaptive procedures generally are very difficult to carry out and require extensive planning and monitoring. However, they should be considered if the statistical resources are available.

Fixed allocation procedures may be subclassified as simple, blocked, or stratified. Simple randomization was described in the fixed allocation example described above. Random number tables are available in most statistical texts and in the standard statistical tables,[4,15] which include instructions for their use. Computers are commonly used to generate the random numbers. A random number generator produces a number between 0 and 1 (actually, the highest number is not exactly 1 but a number as close as the computer can approach to 1). The range between 0 and 1 is subdivided into ranges according to the number of treatment groups. For two groups, the categories are 0 to 0.49999 and 0.500 to 0.99999. These ranges then are assigned to each treatment group, such as control for 0 to 0.499999 and experimental therapy for 0.5 to 0.99999. With this scheme, the patient identification numbers are associated with a treatment.

Blocked allocation procedures are performed so that the treatment groups will be approximately balanced at any time during the trial. Simple randomization could, by chance, assign 15 controls to the first 20 study identification numbers. While in itself this is not a problem, if there are external factors that may change over time during the trial, this imbalance will produce problems in the analysis. For example, if the residents are assigned to a hospital so that they rotate every 6 months, one will try to block in such a way that each group of residents sees about the same number of control and experimental therapy patients. Another advantage of blocking is that if the trial is terminated early, treatment allocation will be roughly equal at any time point. The size of the block is often in the range of 4 to 20. The randomization is set up to make the number of patients in each treatment group equal at the end of each block. A potential problem with blocked randomization occurs when the block length is known by the investigators and the trial is not double-blinded. In this case, it is possible to infer what the next few treatments will be from the previous few treatments. Therefore, it is essential that the blocking factor not be revealed to the investigators. In unblinded studies, it is possible to infer the block size from the allocation of treatments. In these cases, several different block sizes may be used and may be assigned at random. The actual formation of blocked randomization lists usually is performed using specialized computer programs, such as SAS and S-Plus. Statistical consultation is essential.

The most complex form of fixed allocation randomization is stratified randomization. The purpose of the stratification is to ensure that the treatment groups are balanced with respect to one or more factors that may be related to the patient's outcome. The levels of these factors form the strata. The example shown in Tables 64-1 through 64-3 indicates a situation in which stratified randomization would be useful. The probability of a favorable outcome in the control group is different in the two categories of GCS (20 percent versus 40 percent), although the absolute difference between the treatment and control groups is the same in each category (20 percent). If each GCS stratum had the same number of control and treated patients, the final table would be very different (Tables 64-4 through Tables 64-6).

In this example, the overall results of the trial support the results found in each category of the GCS.

Stratified randomization is essentially simple or block randomization within different "categories" of patients. Two separate lists of treatment assignments are created, one for GCS 3 through 5 and another for GCS 6 through 8. Blocked allocation usually is used. The total number of treatment assignments may reflect the expected proportion of patients in each group, or a larger number of assignments are made than expected in each stratum and the excess not used. In either case, the treatment allocations for each stratum are kept separate so that the assignment of treatment to a particular patient may be made from the GCS category appropriate for that patient. The total number of strata that are practical usually depends on the sample size required, though it is rare for more than two or three risk factors to be used to create strata.

In application to surgical trials, it may be possible to stratify by surgeon when the number of surgeons is small. This approach would help solve one of the persistent problems with trials of surgical techniques, that is, the variation in outcome among different surgeons.

Once the randomization procedure is produced, the individual study identification numbers and their assigned treatments should be packaged in a way that keeps the treatment assignment confidential until a patient is actually randomized. This is usually performed using opaque envelopes with the study identification number and other bookkeeping information on the outside and the treatment to be used written on a card inside the envelope. In multicenter trials, the randomization is often performed centrally, using a computer. Scrupulous accounting of the envelopes should be performed to make certain that the randomization is being performed correctly. Additionally, it is wise to monitor the accrual of patients during the course of the trial and to examine the data in a blinded fashion for imbalances in characteristics of the patients in the treatment arms.

Monitoring the rate of patient accrual can help determine whether there is a reasonable chance that the number of patients required to complete the trial will be available in a reasonable amount of time. A plot of the expected and observed accrual of patients is a helpful method of displaying these data. The plot in Fig. 64-1 illustrates a hypothetical trial with a sample size of 200 at the sixteenth week of accrual in which it was thought that 10 patients per week would be enrolled. During weeks 6 through 10 of the trial, patient accrual was better than expected, but in subsequent weeks, accrual fell behind somewhat. Such data indicate that it may be necessary to increase the duration of the trial slightly.

TABLE 64-4 Stratified Trial: GCS 3–5

GCS 3–5	Favorable Outcome	Poor Outcome	Total
Treated group	44	66	110 (40% favorable outcome)
Control group	22	88	110 (20% favorable outcome)

$p = .0012$.

TABLE 64-5 Stratified Trial: GCS 6–8

GCS 6–8	Favorable Outcome	Poor Outcome	Total
Treated group	66	44	110 (60% favorable outcome)
Control group	44	66	110 (40% favorable outcome)

$p = .0030$.

TABLE 64-6 Stratified Trial: Combined GCS

Total (GCS 3–8)	Favorable Outcome	Poor Outcome	Total
Treated group	110	110	220 (50% favorable outcome)
Control group	66	154	220 (30% favorable outcome)

$p = .0000$.

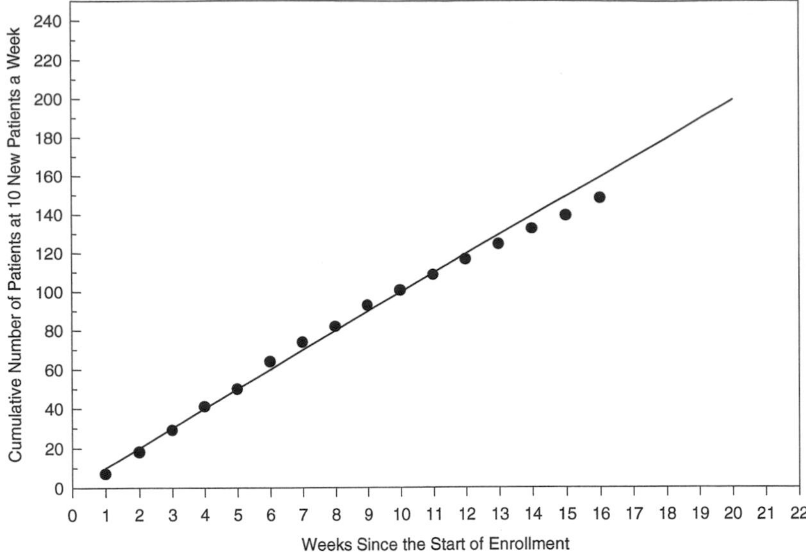

Figure 64-1. Patient accrual plot. Graph of the total number of patients in the trial by the number of weeks since the trial began. The dots indicate the number of patients actually enrolled, and the line indicates the expected number based on the duration of the trial and the number of patients needed. Where the dot is above the line, accrual is better than expected; where it is below the line, the accrual is worse. This is a useful administrative plot.

Blinding

Blinding is another procedure that is used to reduce bias in a trial. These biases may be produced by investigators, patients, or both. Investigators may watch a patient receiving an experimental therapy more closely than a patient receiving the control therapy and therefore see good results earlier or overemphasize minor changes. Conversely, adverse events that would be unimpressive in control patients may be seen as reactions to therapy in the treated group. Results of performance tests, interviews, and assessment of the patient's functioning may be unconsciously influenced by knowledge of the treatment provided. When the patient is aware of the treatment given, he or she may imagine improvements in outcome that are not real or detect side effects of the therapy that do not exist. Thus, both investigator and patient bias may invalidate the results of the study.

Four levels of blinding are recognized. In unblinded, or open label, trials, there is obviously no blinding. Single-blind trials are those in which the investigator is aware of the treatment group but the patient is not. Double-blind trials occur when both the investigator and the patient are unaware of the treatment being given. Triple-blind studies are conducted in such a way that the treatment assignment is not revealed at any time during the course of the study to investigators, patients, or the individuals managing the data. Triple-blind studies are rarely applied outside the multicenter trial setting. Double- and triple-blinded studies are considered the most scientifically valid designs.

Double-blind trials add complexity to the conduct of a study. Both the experimental therapy and the control therapy must be administered so that an observer cannot distinguish between the two. This may require the creation of a placebo which is identical to the experimental therapy in color and mode of administration. Alternatively, the drugs may be packaged so that neither is visible to the investigator. If the drugs are not delivered in a ready-to-administer form, a pharmacist will have to be recruited to prepare the drugs in a manner that maintains the correct treatment assignment while ensuring that blinding is preserved. It will be necessary to have an emergency source of information which can break the blinding if a medical condition arises that requires knowledge of the treatment given. Although double-blinding may increase the problems in the management of the study, the increased scientific validity of the results of the trial justifies the extra time and expense. The standard clinical trial texts contain suggestions for solving some of these administrative problems.[4,9] Occasionally, double-blinding may increase the risk to the patient so significantly that it will be unsafe to perform the trial in such a manner.

Clinical trials of pharmaceutical agents are conducted in neurotrauma patients using double- and triple-blinded designs with little problem. However, comparison of surgical techniques and, to some extent, medical management protocols, cannot be performed in a double-blinded fashion. It is impossible for a surgeon not to know which procedure he or she just performed or for an intensivist not to know which treatment protocol is being followed for a patient. If the patient is comatose and the therapy used does not otherwise have to be revealed to the patient on awakening, the trial may be called single-blinded. In these cases, it is vital that the outcome assessment be made by an investigator who is blinded to the treatment the patient received. If possible, information should be obtained using testing instruments which can be graded by a blinded individual. The determination of the Glasgow Outcome Scale (GOS)[16] score or the Disability Rating Scale (DRS)[17] score must be made by a blinded individual who does not inquire about the therapy the patient received. With these precautions, the information from a single-blinded study will have more scientific credibility.

ETHICAL ISSUES

Human experimentation is an ethically delicate area. The Declaration of Helsinki was issued in 1960 and revised in 1975 and provides general guidelines for ethical medical research. Meinert summarized these guidelines by saying that *"it is unethical to conduct research which is badly planned or poorly executed"* (his italics).[4] He defined three major problems a clinical trial should avoid: bias, inadequate sample size, and failure to publish the findings. Of equal importance is the safeguarding of the rights and privileges of patients. These principles involve the use of informed consent.

Randomization and blinding are mechanisms used to reduce bias in the performance of clinical trials and thus should be used for ethical as well as scientific reasons. Correct calculation of sample size can ensure that an adequate number of patients are seen, and strong leadership by the principal investigators will ensure expeditious completion of the study and publication of the results.

One of the mechanisms used in the United States to evaluate the ethics of a trial are the Institutional Review Boards (IRBs). The committees are formed by all institutions which perform human trials. It is the responsibility of the IRB to review all protocols for human studies and to determine whether a study is ethically and scientifically sound. All proposals for clinical trials must be reviewed by the appropriate IRB before they are begun.

Informed consent should be provided to all patients or patient representatives in a manner that is clear, describes the risks and benefits of the trial, and delineates the rights and responsibilities of the investigators, any pharmaceutical sponsors, and the patient. One of the issues which creates problems for clinical trials in neurotrauma patients is the requirement for informed consent. If the therapy being tested has a short therapeutic window (which is commonly the case), the patient may not be competent to give consent and the appropriate family members may not yet have been found. Unless the IRB will allow consent to be obtained at a later time, the patient cannot be enrolled in the trial. Unfortunately, the remaining patients constitute a small proportion of the total available, and they are likely to be unrepresentative of the entire population of trauma patients. In the second half of 1995 this issue was under review by the appropriate federal agencies.

Clinical trials rarely are conducted in an atmosphere in which the investigators do not hold strong opinions about the efficacy and safety of the treatment being performed. Some proponents of the new therapy may be so convinced of its efficacy that they would consider it unethical to use any other treatment. At times investigators will be convinced that the experimental therapy is completely worthless or worse and so will not choose to participate. In most cases, the investigators tend to hold opinions that are between these extremes and allow them to comfortably conduct the trial.

Many moral and ethical issues may arise during a clinical trial. In all cases, the guidance of the IRB is invaluable in resolving those problems.

DESIGN OF A CLINICAL TRIAL

There are many issues in the design of a clinical trial, some of which are specific to the particular therapy under investigation. The major issues that all clinical trials face are stating the research question, choosing the eligible patients for the trial, selecting the statistical design, selecting and defining the data to be collected, monitoring for adverse events, and administering and managing the trial. Clinical trials which use statistical expertise from the very beginning of the design benefit by avoiding problems before they arise.

FORMULATION OF THE RESEARCH QUESTION

Exact formulation of the research questions the trial is to address is the most important issue in designing a trial. Only with clearly defined research questions can the statistical and managerial issues be evaluated and the appropriate design be created for the trial. The research questions can be divided into three kinds: the primary question, secondary questions, and all other supplementary questions.[9] The primary research question is the question that is most important to the investigators and can be answered. The primary research question provides the basis for the statistical design of the study, selection of an appropriate outcome measure, and the determination of sample size.

In stating the primary research question, as much specificity as possible is needed. Usually the research question begins as a rather vague statement: "Therapy A is better than therapy B in patients with head injury." To refine this statement, the investigators need to consider what they mean by "better" and how much "better" therapy A will be. "Better" is usually indicated by some outcome measure, such as death, or the number of individuals who fall into one or more levels of the GOS. "Better" may mean some other form of outcome, such as that used in the trial of barbituate therapy for increased intracranial pressure. In this study, outcome was defined in terms of the proportion of patients who would not fail intracranial pressure (ICP) control. Failure was defined as exceeding one of three levels of ICP for a specific duration.[18] As recovery from neurotrauma is a prolonged process, the time after injury at which the outcome is assessed must be specified. It is vital that the outcome variables be clearly defined and be evaluated in a reliable manner.

Once the outcome is determined, the amount of improvement that is expected in this outcome must be specified. In designing phase II trials, the difference is defined with two bounds. The first bound describes the amount of benefit that would warrant further study of the therapy, and the second defines the gain that would be too small to be of interest. For example, the phase II trial may be designed so that if the therapy reduces the number of episodes of cerebral perfusion pressure below 60 mmHg by 30 percent or more, the therapy will be considered for future trials. However, if the number of episodes is reduced by 15 percent or less, the benefit will be considered too small to warrant further interest.

Phase III trials require a statement of the minimum benefit expected from the therapy. When the outcome variable is continuous, this improvement usually is defined in terms of an absolute difference in the means of the two populations. Thus, the outcome may be defined as follows: "Patients receiving the experimental therapy will have a mean ICP 10 mmHg less than that of patients receiving the control therapy, measured at 24 h after injury." When one is expressing benefits in terms of dichotomous categorical variables, two forms may be used. The form used most in neurotrauma trials can be expressed as an absolute difference in the proportion of patients experiencing a favorable outcome between the two treatments. For example, "Favorable outcomes (good recovery and moderate disability on the GOS) will occur in 30 percent of the experimental therapy group and in only 20 percent of the control therapy." The difference of 10 percent in the rates of favorable outcome is the expected benefit of the trial. The alternative expression of benefit involves stating the relative rates of occurrence. That is, a trial may be designed using the statement "The probability of a favorable outcome in the experimental group is 1.5 times that seen in the control therapy patients." Both of these examples describe the same type of expected outcome in the trial. However, expressing the treatment effect as 10 percent indicates that the experimental therapy will have 40 percent favorable outcomes if the control therapy results in 30 percent favorable outcomes. If the treatment effect is expressed in terms of the relative proportions of favorable outcome, 30 percent in the control therapy group indicates 45 percent favorable outcomes in the experimental therapy patients. Generally, the relative difference is used when the baseline, or control therapy, proportion is small, while the absolute difference is used for larger baseline rates. In most neurotrauma trials, the absolute difference is used. When the outcome and the expected effect of the experimental therapy are specified, a testable hypothesis is formed from a vague statement.

Once the primary research question is formulated, it is used to determine the overall trial design and sample size. Secondary research questions then should be formulated. These questions may involve collecting observations related to the mechanisms of action of the therapy or may involve secondary endpoints. Often, blood levels of a drug will be determined to relate the patient's outcome to the delivered dose of the drug. An investigator may be interested in determining whether the patients receiving therapy A have a faster recovery or a higher incidence of a side effect of the control therapy. Ancillary questions that are unrelated to the therapy may be addressed as well. For example, the evolution of cerebral contusions in the control group may be studied. Both types of questions should be formulated in the same manner as the primary question, with specification of what will be measured and what is expected from the measurements. When comparison between the therapies is to be performed, the difference should be specified. The difference between the secondary questions and the ancillary questions lies in the importance each has to the overall trial design. The overall trial design should rest on the primary question, and other questions should have a relatively minor impact. While a small increase in the sample size may be considered to ensure an answer to a secondary question, no such increase is likely to answer an ancillary question.

Study Population

The population to be studied must be specified nearly as exactly as the research question is. All clinical trials are conducted on a sample drawn from a larger population. If this were not the case, the results of a trial would apply only to those individuals who were in that trial. Therefore, it is important to decide to whom the results of trial are to be generalized and how the sample included in the trial will be related to this population. If pilot studies indicate that the therapy is efficacious only in a subpopulation, the trial should focus on that type of patient. For example, if the therapy is thought to work only in patients with diffuse injuries, the study should be performed only in patients with such injuries. From these considerations, an inclusion list and an exclusion list are derived. Age, gender, pregnancy, and medical complications may be parts of the eligibility criteria. The trial may be designed to focus only on patients who have a high probability of recovery, and certain concomitant injuries or injury severities will be excluded. The methods for screening and recruiting the patients into the trial should be clearly defined and should reflect the trial's eligibility criteria. At no time should a decision to include or exclude a patient from the trial be performed in violation of the eligibility criteria. When individual judgment is required, these decisions should be well documented. To that end, a log of all patients who present to the center and are not randomized should be maintained. Such a log was maintained by the Barbituate Coma Trial,[18] which found that only 12 percent of 925 patients screened were eligible for the trial. A clear definition of who may be in the trial and who is not in the trial allows readers of the final report of the trial results to decide which patients may benefit from the therapy.

The accessibility of patients needs to be considered. All efforts to guarantee that patients can be followed for the entire course of the study should be considered. A large number of patients in whom the outcome cannot be determined will seriously undermine the utility of the study. If necessary, the eligibility criteria should be modified to focus only on a more stable population. While this change may result in less generalization of the results of the trial, the ability to complete the trial is well worth the difference. If the eligibility criteria result in very slow recruitment of patients into the study, enthusiasm for the study may dwindle, and the long intervals between entering consecutive patients into the study may result in errors. Under these circumstances, it may be necessary to consider relaxing the eligibility criteria or recruiting other centers into a multicenter trial.

Statistical Design

There are a myriad of possible designs for a clinical trial. These designs generally are formulated to reflect the specific research question and start with one of several basic trial designs. The research question and the reference population determine the types of statistical designs that may be used in performing the trial. Almost all the statistical designs used in clinical trials are based on the general experimental designs found in statistics texts. The most basic design for a phase III study is the simple comparison of one treatment with another. In this design, patients are randomly and equally allocated to one of two treatments and are followed, after which their outcome is assessed. The trial is perspective and concurrent. To protect against bias, the trial should be single- or double-blinded. This trial has shown structure in Table 64-7.

TABLE 64-7 Simple Comparison

Therapy A	Therapy B
n1	n2

The number of patients in therapy A, n1, is equal to the number in therapy B, n2. Randomization usually is conducted in a block manner, and the final comparison is extremely simple. This trial may be expanded to include more than one therapy, as in Table 64-8.

The number of therapies in such a trial is often limited to three, though in theory the number is unlimited. When the trial is designed to compare each therapy with a control, the sample sizes are not necessarily equal, as proposed by Dunnett in 1964.[19] When the comparisons of interest are among all the possible therapies, the analysis becomes more difficult. These designs constitute only 38 percent of the trials described by Meinert and associates in 1984.[20]

The most common modification to the single treatment trial is to introduce stratification. In this design, one or more risk factors are used to create strata into which patients are randomized. When more than one stratum is defined, the patients should be randomized into all the combinations of the strata. For example, consider two stratifying variables: GCS and age. GCS will be defined in two categories—3 through 5 and 6 through 8—and age will be formed into three categories—16 through 25, 26 through 35, and 36 through 64. The trial will then have six strata, as in Table 64-9.

The primary comparison is still between the two therapies, but the patients are randomized so that the number of patients in therapy A in a stratum is the same as the number of patients in therapy B in that stratum. The data are analyzed by using special techniques that account for stratification. It is not required that the number of patients in each stratum be the same. Randomization may be established so that there are enough patient identification numbers to take all the expected patients in each stratum, or the number of patients in each stratum may be held to a fixed number per stratum. When stratification is to be performed only to remove the effects of imbalances on the final assessment, the

TABLE 64-8 Multiple Treatment Trial

Therapy A	Therapy B	. . .	Therapy E
n1	n2	. . .	n10

TABLE 64-9 Stratified Design

Stratum	Therapy A	Therapy B
GCS 3–5, age 16–25	n11	n12
GCS 3–5, age 26–35	n21	n22
GCS 3–5, age 36–64	n31	n32
GCS 6–8, age 16–25	n41	n42
GCS 6–8, age 26–35	n51	n52
GCS 6–8, age 36–64	n61	n62

effect on the final sample size is usually small. However, if the trial is designed to look at treatment differences within each stratum, the sample size will be considerably larger. The number of strata that are practical is usually limited to the range of 8 to 12.

One form of stratification that may greatly affect the trial design occurs when the efficacy of the treatment varies across the strata. Such an effect is called a treatment interaction. Using the example data from above, consider the following possibility (Tables 64-10 through 64-12).

The effect of the therapy is large (20 percent improvement in favorable outcomes) in the GCS 6 through 8 stratum but is deleterious in the GCS 3 through 5 stratum (9.9 percent reduction in favorable outcomes). If the trial is designed to treat stratification as only a "covariate," only the results of Table 64-12 will be used to determine the effect of the therapy. The beneficial effect in the GCS 6 through 8 stratum will be lost. The correct analysis of results such as these involves examining each stratum separately. If the trial had been designed to do this, the results would indicate no significant difference in the GCS 3 through 5 group and a strong difference in the GCS 6 through 8 stratum. For this reason, it is extremely important to determine whether the therapy will have roughly the same impact on outcome across strata. Phase II trials should be designed to examine this question if there is a good reason to suspect such an effect.

Stratification is a form of factorial design in which two or more treatments or factors are examined simultaneously in the trial. Stratified trials rarely are designed to examine for differences among the strata and are even less likely to determine whether differences in response exist among strata. A complete factorial design will include provisions for these differences. A factorial design enables the researchers to determine how beneficial each treatment is and provide a comparison of the two treatments. A factorial design can be represented as shown in Tables 64-13 and 64-14.

Table 64-14 is an alternative representation of Table 64-13 and illustrates the similarity of the factorial and stratified designs. The number of patients in each treatment combination (n11, n12, n21, n22) will be the same.

It may be very important in determining the efficacy of a treatment to see whether a common ancillary treat-

TABLE 64-10 Stratified Design with Interaction: GCS 3–5

GCS 3–5	Favorable Outcome	Poor Outcome	Total
Treated group	16	94	110 (14.6% favorable outcome)
Control group	28	82	110 (25.5% favorable outcome)

p = .0431.

TABLE 64-11 Stratified Design with Interaction: GCS 6–8

GCS 6–8	Favorable Outcome	Poor Outcome	Total
Treated group	66	44	110 (60% favorable outcome)
Control group	44	66	110 (40% favorable outcome)

p = .0030.

TABLE 64-12 Stratified Design with Interaction: Combined GCS

Total	Favorable Outcome	Poor Outcome	Total
Treated group	82	138	220 (37% favorable outcome)
Control group	66	154	220 (30% favorable outcome)

p = .1064.

TABLE 64-13 Factorial Design

	Therapy A	
Therapy B	**Absent**	**Present**
Absent	n11	n12
Present	n21	n22

ment modifies the results of the experimental therapy. Two treatments that have been established as effective may be much more effective in combination or may counteract each other. When these situations arise, it may be advisable to design a factorial trial. Two major problems exist when fully factorial designs are applied to clinical trials. First, the sample size is likely to be rather large, more than that required by a simple two-treatment comparison. Second, it may be difficult to persuade two sponsors to support a trial that may show that only one therapy is effective or that the two therapies cancel each other out. However, in specific circumstances, there may be excellent reasons to perform a factorial trial.

The designs discussed above are considered "parallel group" designs, since two or more groups of patients are followed simultaneously. A design in which a patient is treated with both the control and the experimental therapy at two different times is called a "crossover" study. Crossover studies are attractive, since each patient serves as his or her own control. However, the design and proper analysis of crossover trials are difficult, and the application of crossover designs to neurotrauma is very difficult. For such a design to be acceptable, there cannot be a large spontaneous change in the patient's status over time. There must be a time interval between treatments for the effect of the first treatment to dissipate before the second treatment is started. In the context of neurotrauma, where the patient is recovering from the injury and where the outcomes are measured long after the injury, crossover designs are impractical. However, in specific cases, such studies may be feasible. For example, if the therapy is designed to produce an immediate response and the effects of the therapy are very short-lived, a crossover design may be possible.

Another design that occasionally may be useful in neurotrauma is a longitudinal study. In this design, patients are randomized to the treatments and their response is measured repeatedly over time. Such studies provide more information about the patient's status. The repeated measures allow the variation in response "within" the patient to be removed from the comparison of the treatments, allowing for greater power in the trial. When the treatment changes the rate at which a patient recovers, a longitudinal study is very efficient in determining that effect. The major problem with the longitudinal design is that the therapy must have an effect that can be measured fairly early in the course of the patient's recovery. Long-term effects are not easy to demonstrate with this design. There is added expense in the collection of the same information over time, and the analysis of these data is not simple. An example would be to examine the score on some neuropsychological or functional tests as the patient recovers from a head injury. Longitudinal designs probably are underutilized in neurotrauma.

TABLE 64-14 Alternative Representation of a Factorial Trial

Treatment Combination	Number of Patients
No therapy A, no therapy B	n11
Therapy A, no therapy B	n12
Therapy B, no therapy A	n21
Therapy A, therapy B	n22

Sequential trials are designed to examine the results of a trial almost continuously during the conduct of that trial. When a certain excess in the number of patients responding positively to the experimental therapy is reached, the trial is terminated with the conclusion that the therapy is effective. Conversely, when the experimental therapy does not show a clear benefit after a certain number of patients have been randomized, the trial is terminated. The implication is that there is not a meaningful difference between the two treatments. Sequential trials often are used to reduce the sample size and time required to evaluate a treatment and are highly useful in that regard. The outcome must be ascertained shortly after the therapy is given for this design to be effective, and there is a chance that the total sample size required will exceed the number required for a simple trial. However, the use of these trials under applicable circumstances in neurotrauma research probably should be encouraged. An excellent source of information about sequential trials is Whitehead's *The Design and Analysis of Sequential Clinical Trials*.[21]

Data to Collect

Once the basic design of the trial has been determined, the data to be collected must be determined. There are four broad classes of data: outcome data, confounder data, ancillary study data, and administrative data. All four should be included.

The selection of the outcome variable has a major impact on the trial. The research question has defined the outcome that is considered important, and the variables used to assess this outcome must be well defined and reliably measured. Clifton and colleagues[22] have recommended that functional outcome be assessed using the GOS and DRS for severely and moderately head injured patients. Severe patients (GCS 3 through 8) should be assessed using either scale at 6 months after the injury, and moderately injured patients (GCS 9 through 12) should be assessed at 3 months after injury using the DRS. In this paper, behavioral changes were measured using the Neurobehavioral Rating Scale supplemented with measures of attention, memory, language, mental processing, and motor function.

Outcome variables generally are classified in regard to type. Continuous variables are those in which the number of possible values is large. Often, continuous variables are interval, so that the meaning of the difference between any two values is the same regardless of the values. For example, the difference between 30 mmHg and 35 mmHg is the same as the difference between 63 mmHg and 68 mmHg. This does not mean that the impact of the variable on other measures is the same across all values of a continuous variable. A 5-mmHg difference in ICP at 15 mmHg is likely to have less of an effect on the patient's health than will a 5-mmHg difference at 25 mmHg. Measuring the outcome of a trial in terms of a continuous variable often results in a much smaller sample size.

There are some variables that are almost continuous. They measure a large number of possible levels of outcome, but not on a strictly continuous scale. One example is the DRS, which has 31 categories of outcome. The DRS is neither interval nor continuous. However, the large number of possible values may allow the *assumption* of a continuous variable to be used. Careful examination of data from preliminary studies will aid in this determination.

Categorical variables are those which take one of a limited number of values. Mortality is such a variable, as is the GOS. Ethnicity and gender are considered nominal categorical variables, as there is no implied ordering among the categories. GCS and GOS, however, have an implied ordering and are considered ordered categorical variables. When there are only two ordered categories, such as with vital status, ordering provides no information. Where there are multiple ordered categories, analytic techniques exist to take advantage of these properties, resulting in more meaningful and powerful analyses.

Time is a continuous variable that must be defined in terms of a starting time and an endpoint. In most clinical trials, the starting point is defined as the moment the patient was enrolled into the trial. The endpoint is defined by some event, such as death or recovery of a neuropsychological score to a predetermined value. Of course, the choice of endpoint event is determined by the research question. Trials in which the major outcome is defined in this manner are often termed survival trials. The outcome is defined with a "time-to-event" variable.

Care must be taken to collect data that may be required to determine how the treatments were administered. Adequate documentation of when and how the therapy was administered is important in understanding any problems in the therapy unrelated to the direct physiological effect of the therapy. When the experimental therapy is a drug, samples should be taken to document the delivered dose. Of course, these data should be collected for both the experimental and control therapies in a blinded manner if at all possible.

In addition to measuring the variables related to the desired outcome of the trial, it is important to monitor the patients for the occurrence of complications that may be related to the treatments. A list of adverse events may be defined at the beginning of the trial, and the incidence of those events may be monitored. When the therapy is a drug, these events may be related to expected side effects of the compound. If the drug has no specific side effects or if a nondrug therapy is being tested, the adverse events list may be difficult to create. Some form of adverse monitoring is likely to be required by the FDA and most IRBs.

"Confounders" are variables that may have an impact on the effectiveness of the treatment and/or may change the probability that the outcome will be observed. The most obvious covariates often are used as stratification variables, such as the GCS. However, the number of factors that may influence outcome is usually much larger than can be reasonably used for stratification. When these variables are documented, adjustment can be made in the analysis phase of the study to account for their effects on outcome. Such confounders may include evidence of hypoxia or hypotension, some form of classification of the computed tomography (CT) scan,[23] and pupillary reactivity or another brainstem reflex. Events during the course of the treatment that could influence outcome may be important both as covariates and as indicators of an effect of the treatment. The number of times ICP exceeds a specific value and occurrences of jugular venous oxygen desaturations are variables that are likely to be included. Generally, any factor that is important in explaining the results of a trial should be collected.

In addition to confounders that are related to treatment and outcome, a set of variables may be included which are designed to answer ancillary questions. These secondary issues are defined in the process of stating the research questions for the trial, and care must be taken to assure that the data to answer these questions are collected. Often, data collected during a clinical trial are of much higher quality than are those collected during routine clinical observation. If the cost is relatively low, adding a few variables to answer ancillary questions will result in a large return of excellent data.

Though not strictly important for answering the scientific questions posed by a trial, administrative data are extremely important in documenting the individual treatments and the overall quality of the trial. These data may include the lot numbers of treatments, the date and time for each clinical assessment, and information concerning the management of the data. It is always important to include the documents related to informed consent. When the trial is being conducted as part of a submission to the FDA, the administrative data may be defined by the requirements of the regulatory agency. Even in small, locally funded trials, some concern should be given to these data.

Regardless of which items are collected, it is extremely important that the data have the highest quality possible. To ensure such quality, data forms should be clear and easy to use. The data should be edited soon after the form is completed so that any problems can be addressed while the information is fresh. Internal and external validity checks should be incorporated into the data management system. Crucial data related to treatment and outcome may require auditing by reabstraction and verification. It is equally important that the data that will be collected be defined at the start of the study. Performing a retrospective search for the information is usually costly and incomplete and may lead to bias. A balance has to be struck between collecting all possible information and the effort required to collect the information. At some point, the weight of the data collection forms becomes a burden that can detract from the conduct of the trial.

Determination of Adequate Sample Size

An adequate sample size is one of the biggest problems in clinical trials. Unfortunately, too many studies are performed without consideration of whether enough patients will be studied to provide a statistically sound answer to the research question. Good therapies may be discarded needlessly.

To calculate a sample size, several pieces of information are required.

1. Trial design: The kind of trial may have an impact on the sample size, especially if a factorial or survival study is to be performed.
2. Type of outcome variable: Is the outcome variable continuous, ordered categorical, or dichotomous?
3. Minimum treatment effect: In terms of the outcome variable, what is the minimum change that the treatment is likely to produce which is meaningful clinically? For example, this may be expressed as a difference in means, the difference in the percentage of patients having a favorable outcome, or a difference in survival times. Specification of the treatment effect should be based on the results of earlier studies, such as phase II trials. When the outcome involves collapsing the GCS into two categories, the conventional wisdom has been that the trial should be able to detect a 10 percent difference in the outcome proportions in the two groups. It is important to define the difference in outcome probabilities and the baseline probability from which the difference is measured. The standard deviation of dichotomous variables is a function of the baseline probability.
4. Standard deviation of the outcome variable: An estimate of the outcome variable's variation is required. For trials involving proportions, the standard deviation is defined by the proportions. For continuous variables, the standard deviation must be estimated somehow.

Power and Alpha Level

Power is technically defined as the probability of rejecting the null hypothesis when an alternative hypothesis is actually true. The alpha level, or size, is defined as the probability of rejecting the null hypothesis when it is actually true. Both concepts are related to a "truth table" (Table 64-15).

The alpha level is defined as the probability of making a type I error and should be kept fairly low. Power is defined as 1 minus the probability of a type II error. Another way of conceptualizing power is that it expresses the chance that the trial will be a success, given

TABLE 64-15 Truth Table

	Truth	
Trial Results	**Experimental Treatment Effective**	**Experimental Treatment Is Not Effective**
Trial indicates the experimental treatment is effective		Type I error
Trial indicates the experimental treatment is not effective	Type II error	

the treatment differences the investigator expects. Clearly, the investigator would like to have a good chance of conducting a conclusive trial. Usually alpha levels and power are chosen as a matter of custom. An alpha level of 0.05 is almost sacrosanct, and common choices for power are 80 and 90 percent.

One minor point concerning the alpha level should be mentioned. Unless it is absolutely impossible that the difference in outcome could go in the opposite direction from the one specified, a two-sided alpha should be used. If the outcome is expressed as a difference in the amount of height gained by teenagers, a one-sided test may be employed, as loss of height is not likely. As much as such situations are undesirable, the experimental therapy may actually result in *fewer* favorable outcomes than the control therapy, and the trial should be designed to reflect the fact.

The analytic method may have an impact on the sample size requirements. The choice of method usually is implied by the research question, the outcome variable, and the way in which confounders and other covariates are to be incorporated into the analysis. If all these pieces are available, determination of the sample size is a straightforward procedure. Consultation with a statistician is clearly indicated.

To illustrate some of the effects of power, alpha level, and baseline probability on the sample size, several figures are included in this chapter. In all these figures, the sample sizes are expressed in terms of the sample size required per group for a comparison of two treatments, with equal numbers of patients in each group. In Fig. 64-2, a graph of the sample size versus power is shown for a difference in favorable outcomes of 25 to 35 percent and 25 to 45 percent. Figure 64-3 illustrates the sample size versus alpha level for 80 percent power and a difference of 25 to 35 percent. The effect of changes in the baseline probability of a favorable outcome is shown in Fig. 64-4 for 80 percent and 90 percent power. In this graph, the sample size required to detect a 10 percent difference in favorable outcome is graphed against the probability of a favorable outcome in the control group. The experimental therapy is assumed to provide a favorable outcome probability of the baseline rate plus 10 percent.

Figure 64-5 is a three-dimensional plot of the probability of a favorable outcome in an experimental group and a control group and the required sample size to have 80 percent power and an alpha level of 0.05. The sample size is shown on the vertical axis, and values greater than 800 have been truncated to 800. The steep ridge in the center of the graph indicates the rather large increase in sample size needed when the two probabilities are close. Figure 64-6 is a contour plot of the same data. This figure can be used to estimate the approximate sample size needed to detect a difference between two proportions. The sample size needed to have 80 percent power and an alpha of 0.05 to detect the difference between 20 percent and 60 percent falls between 20 and 50 contours. The exact sample size is 28 subjects per group. This plot cannot be used to determine the exact sample size required for the trial, but it can provide a rough estimate of the number of patients needed to detect the difference specified on the vertical and horizontal axes. For a more exact estimate of the sample sizes, Tables 64-16 and 64-17 provide the required sample sizes for the probabilities between 0.05

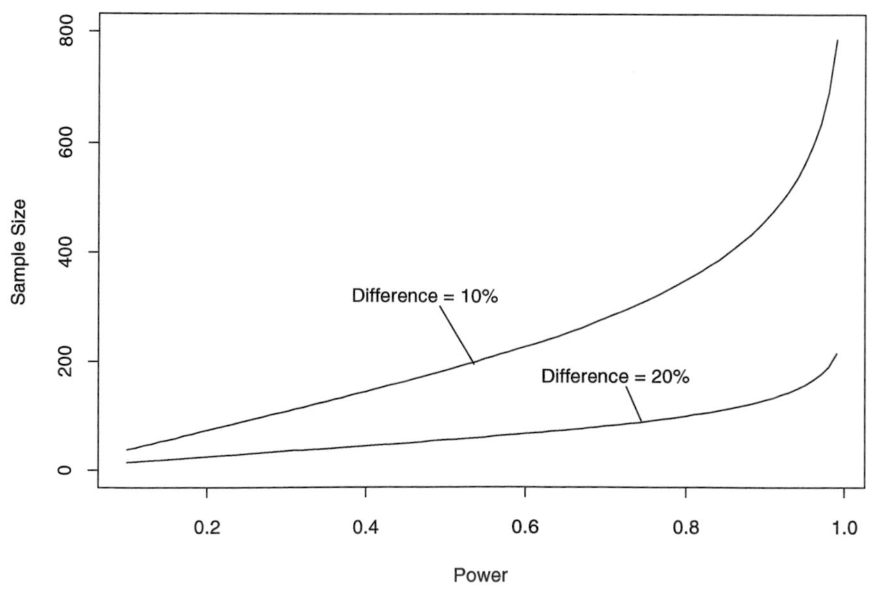

Figure 64-2. Sample size versus power. Two plots of the sample size against the power of the trial where the outcome is two categories (dichotomous) are shown. The change in sample size as power increases is rather small until powers over 90 percent are reached, at which point the sample size increases rapidly. The sample size for a 10 percent difference (25 percent versus 35 percent is larger for all powers compared with the sample size for a 20 percent difference (25 percent versus 45 percent), and the 10 percent difference sample size rises much faster as the power increases. The alpha level for this plot is 0.05.

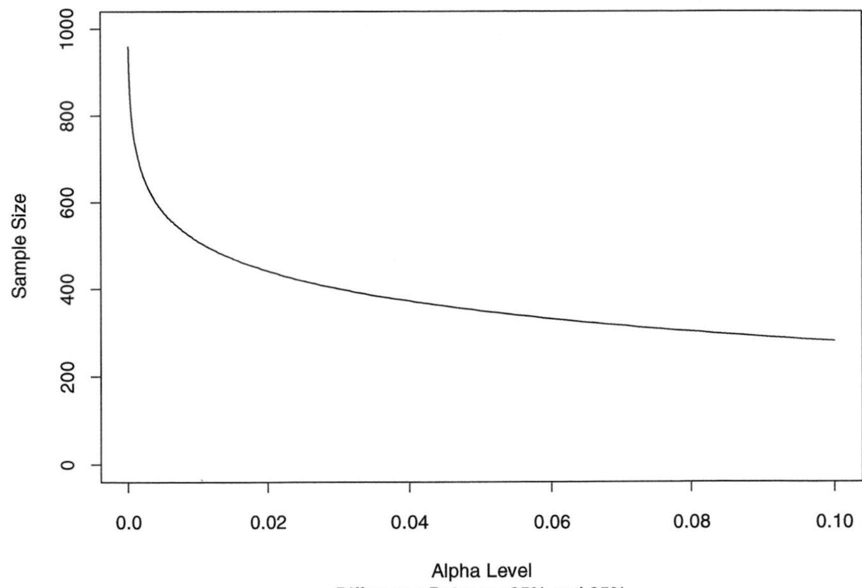

Figure 64-3. Sample size versus alpha level. A plot of the sample size versus the alpha level for a trial which is designed to detect the difference between 25 percent favorable outcomes and 35 percent favorable outcomes is shown. As the alpha level drops below 0.02, the sample size rises rapidly. The power assumed for this graph was 80 percent.

and 0.95 in steps of 0.05. Table 64-16 is based on a power of 80 percent, and Table 64-17 uses a power of 90 percent. To find the required sample size for two probabilities, find the first probability in the columns of the table and the second in the rows. The intersection of the row and column contains the sample size. As an example, using the 80 percent power table, the sample size for a comparison of 0.20 to 0.30 is 313 patients per group. For convenience, the entire table is presented, though it may be seen that the table is symmetrical.

Sample sizes for continuous variables are dependent only on the difference in means, not on the values of the means. The difference between the means usually is converted to standard deviation units by division:

$$\text{Difference in standard deviations} = \frac{\text{mean in experimental therapy} - \text{mean in control therapy}}{\text{standard deviation of the measurement}}$$

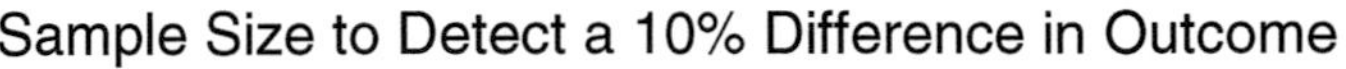

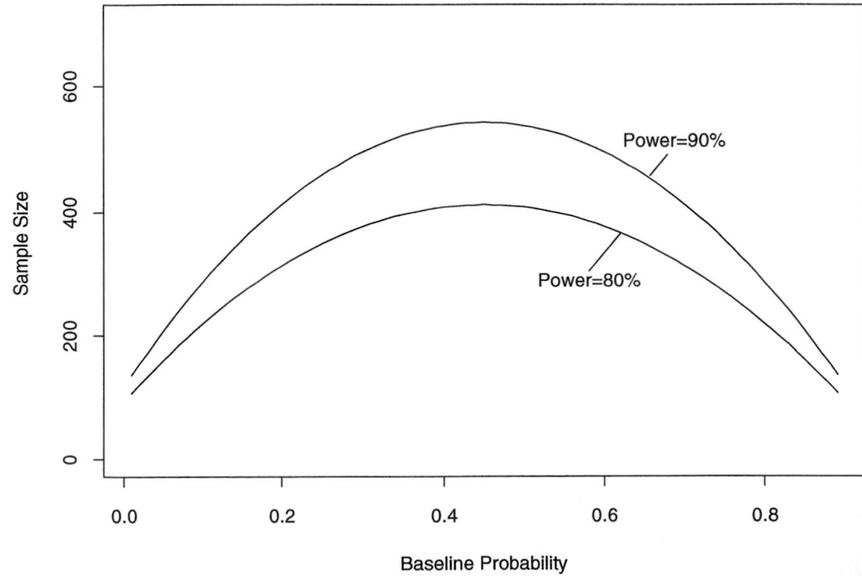

Figure 64-4. Sample size to detect a 10 percent difference in outcome. Two plots of the sample size required to detect a 10 percent difference in a dichotomous outcome—one for 80 percent power and one for 90 percent power—are shown. The baseline probability is that found in the control therapy, and the experimental therapy outcome rate is assumed to be 10 percent above that. This graph indicates the dependence of the sample size on the baseline rate, even for a fixed difference between baseline and experimental outcome rates. The sample size is maximal around the 0.50 baseline probability rate. The alpha level is 0.05.

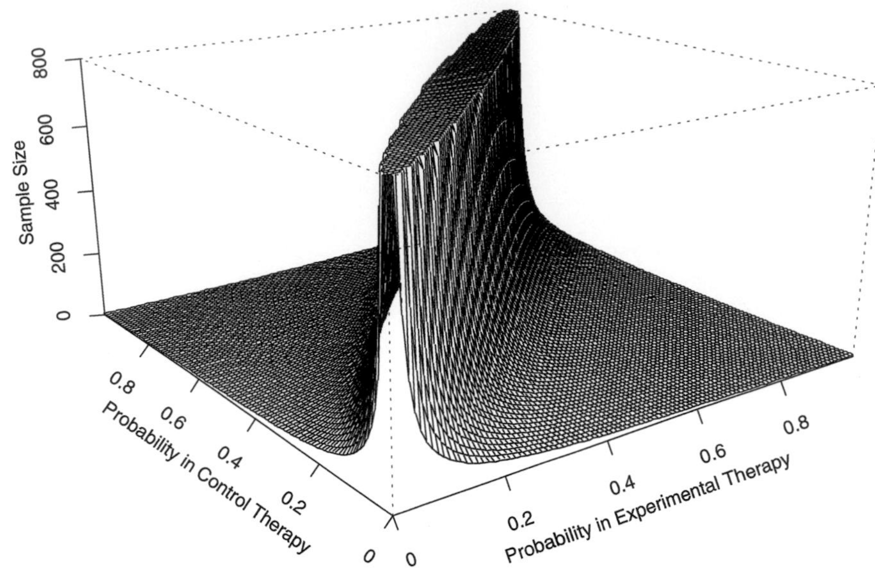

Figure 64-5. Perspective plot of sample size at 80 percent power. A three-dimensional graph of the sample size as a function of the outcome rates in the control therapy and the experimental therapy is shown. When the control and experimental therapy outcome rates are very different, the sample size is small. As the two probabilities approach each other, the sample size climbs rapidly. The alpha level is 0.05.

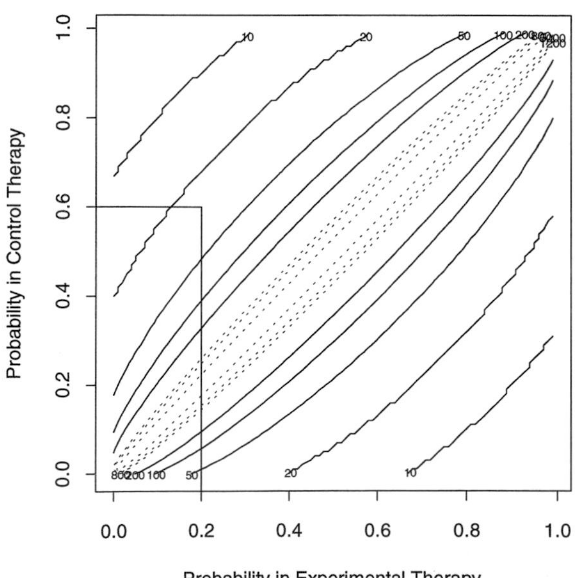

Figure 64-6. Contour plot of sample size at 80 percent power. This is a contour plot of Fig. 64-5. The contour lines indicate the small sample size needed for very different outcome rates and the extremely large sample sizes required for outcome rates that are close to each other. An example using 0.60 and 0.20 is drawn on the graph.

For example, the trial may be designed to detect a 12-mmHg average decrease in cerebral perfusion pressure (CPP) as a result of the experimental therapy. Assuming that the standard deviation of the CPP is 18 mmHg, the difference to be detected is 0.667 standard deviation. Figure 64-7 graphs the sample size versus the difference in terms of standard deviations required for 80% power and an alpha of 0.05. Relatively small sample sizes are required to detect differences that are often of interest. For the 0.67 difference calculated above, the sample size is 37 per group. A graph of sample size versus power for a fixed difference of 0.67 standard deviation is shown in Fig. 64-8. The stairstep nature of the graph reflects the fact that sample sizes are always whole numbers.

Table 64-18 provides a guide to the sample size needed to detect a difference at 80 and 90% power. The difference in standard deviations is shown in the first column, and the sample sizes in the second and third columns.

When the outcome is specified as an ordered categorical variable or if a survival trial is being performed, the same size calculations are more complex. A very good reference for determining sample sizes for a variety of trial designs is Machin and Campbell's *Statistical Tables for the Design of Clinical Trials.*[15] While it is always preferable to consult with a statistician, this book provides a more precise estimation of the required sample size than can be given here.

Administrative Design

In parallel to the statistical design of the trial, the administrative structure of the study should be developed. This

TABLE 64-16 Sample Size for 80 Percent Power

	0.05	0.10	0.15	0.20	0.25	0.30	0.35	0.40	0.45	0.50	0.55	0.60	0.65	0.70	0.75	0.80	0.85	0.90	0.95
0.05		474	160	88	59	43	34	27	22	19	16	14	12	11	9	8	7	7	6
0.10	474		726	219	113	72	51	38	30	25	20	17	15	13	11	10	9	8	7
0.15	160	726		945	270	134	83	57	42	33	26	22	18	15	13	11	10	9	7
0.20	88	219	945		1134	313	151	91	62	45	35	28	22	19	16	13	11	10	8
0.25	59	113	270	1134		1291	349	165	98	66	48	36	28	23	19	16	13	11	9
0.30	43	72	134	313	1291		1417	376	176	103	68	49	37	29	23	19	15	13	11
0.35	34	51	83	151	349	1417		1511	396	183	106	70	49	37	28	22	18	15	12
0.40	27	38	57	91	165	376	1511		1574	408	186	107	70	49	36	28	22	17	14
0.45	22	30	42	62	98	176	396	1574		1605	412	186	106	68	48	35	26	20	16
0.50	19	25	33	45	66	103	183	408	1605		1605	408	183	103	66	45	33	25	19
0.55	16	20	26	35	48	68	106	186	412	1605		1574	396	176	98	62	42	30	22
0.60	14	17	22	28	36	49	70	107	186	408	1574		1511	376	165	91	57	38	27
0.65	12	15	18	22	28	37	49	70	106	183	396	1511		1417	349	151	83	51	34
0.70	11	13	15	19	23	29	37	49	68	103	176	376	1417		1291	313	134	72	43
0.75	9	11	13	16	19	23	28	36	48	66	98	165	349	1291		1134	270	113	59
0.80	8	10	11	13	16	19	22	28	35	45	62	91	151	313	1134		945	219	88
0.85	7	9	10	11	13	15	18	22	26	33	42	57	83	134	270	945		726	160
0.90	7	8	9	10	11	13	15	17	20	25	30	38	51	72	113	219	726		474
0.95	6	7	7	8	9	11	12	14	16	19	22	27	34	43	59	88	160	474	

information is set forth in the protocol. The protocol includes details of the treatment protocol, the methods of data collection, a management scheme for the distribution and administration of the treatments, and methods for monitoring adverse events.

The treatment protocol should specify all aspects of the clinical care of patients in the trial, especially procedures that are related to the experimental and control therapies. This document includes the research question, the inclusion and exclusion criteria, how the patients are to be screened for entry, and how the patients are to be randomized. The methods for administering the treatments are set out in detail, and the steps required to maintain blinding are described. The methods for preparing the treatments for administration and the doses are detailed. Often, the protocol includes the background information used to generate the trial's research questions.

The protocol should describe the timing of data collection and list the variables to be collected at each time point. The method of data collection is specified. Generally, paper forms are created and the data are abstracted onto these forms from the patient record. Special procedures may be documented directly on the

TABLE 64-17 Sample Size for 90 Percent Power

	0.05	0.10	0.15	0.20	0.25	0.30	0.35	0.40	0.45	0.50	0.55	0.60	0.65	0.70	0.75	0.80	0.85	0.90	0.95
0.05		621	207	114	75	55	42	34	28	23	20	17	15	13	11	10	9	7	6
0.10	621		957	286	146	92	65	49	38	31	25	21	18	15	13	11	10	9	7
0.15	207	957		1252	354	174	107	73	54	42	33	27	22	19	16	14	12	10	9
0.20	114	286	1252		1504	412	198	119	80	58	44	35	28	23	19	16	14	11	10
0.25	75	146	354	1504		1714	460	216	128	85	61	46	36	28	23	19	16	13	11
0.30	55	92	174	412	1714		1882	496	230	134	88	63	47	36	28	23	19	15	13
0.35	42	65	107	198	460	1882		2008	523	240	138	90	63	47	36	28	22	18	15
0.40	34	49	73	119	216	496	2008		2092	538	244	140	90	63	46	35	27	21	17
0.45	28	38	54	80	128	230	523	2092		2134	544	244	138	88	61	44	33	25	20
0.50	23	31	42	58	85	134	240	538	2134		2134	538	240	134	85	58	42	31	23
0.55	20	25	33	44	61	88	138	244	544	2134		2092	523	230	128	80	54	38	28
0.60	17	21	27	35	46	63	90	140	244	538	2092		2008	496	216	119	73	49	34
0.65	15	18	22	28	36	47	63	90	138	240	523	2008		1882	460	198	107	65	42
0.70	13	15	19	23	28	36	47	63	88	134	230	496	1882		1714	412	174	92	55
0.75	11	13	16	19	23	28	36	46	61	85	128	216	460	1714		1504	354	146	75
0.80	10	11	14	16	19	23	28	35	44	58	80	119	198	412	1504		1252	286	114
0.85	9	10	12	14	16	19	22	27	33	42	54	73	107	174	354	1252		957	207
0.90	7	9	10	11	13	15	18	21	25	31	38	49	65	92	146	286	957		621
0.95	6	7	9	10	11	13	15	17	20	23	28	34	42	55	75	114	207	621	

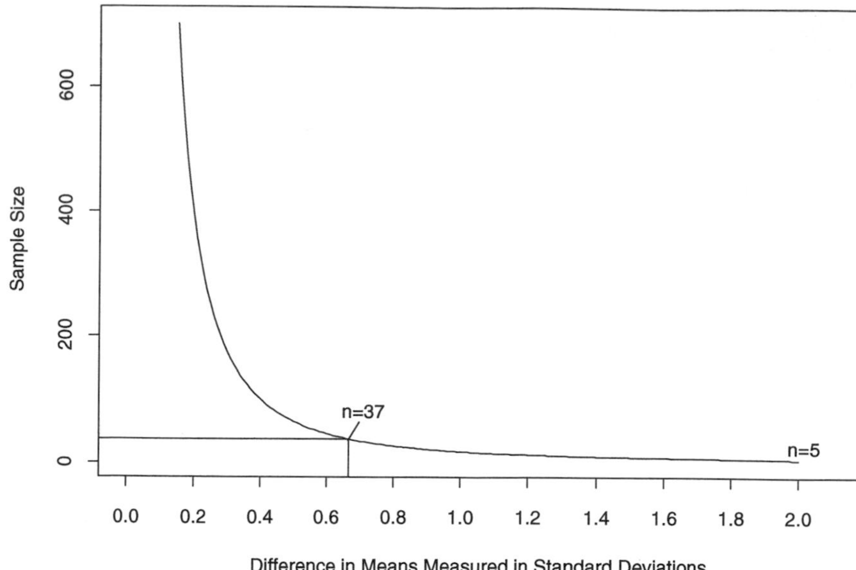

Figure 64-7. Sample size and difference in means—80 percent power. A plot of the sample size versus the difference in means for continuous, normally distributed outcomes is shown. The difference in means is expressed in terms of standard deviations. A difference of 0.67 standard deviation requires a sample size of 37 patients per treatment, while for a difference of 2.0 standard deviations the sample size is only five. The sample size does depend on the baseline value of the means. An alpha of 0.05 and a power of 0.80 were used.

forms. Electronic data collection methods are available but are expensive. The data collection methods should be tested with real data to find possible problems. The protocol should have clear definitions of the outcome variable and should include instructions for ascertaining the outcome. A plan for accounting for any drugs must be specified. A procedure for recording and reporting adverse events is described. Generally, a list of likely adverse events is generated, and the presence of those events is determined on a regular basis. Serious events, including death, are documented more fully, possibly including notification of the IRB, the sponsor, and the FDA. The individual who is to be notified when a serious event occurs and the one who is responsible for making the notification report should be specified. Provisions must be made to break the blind for an individual patient if a medical or other emergency arises. The conditions under which blinding is to be broken should be described, along with the method for breaking the blinding. The protocol should include samples of the in-

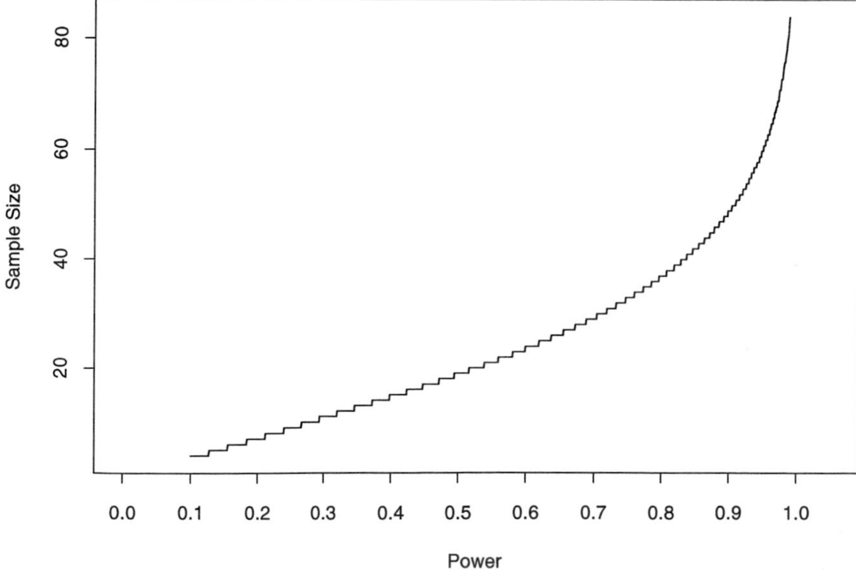

Figure 64-8. Sample size versus power: difference = 0.67 standard deviation. The sample size is plotted against the power for a fixed difference of 0.67 standard deviation. As with the categorical outcomes, the sample size rises steeply as the power increases.

TABLE 64-18 Sample Size for Continuous Outcomes

Difference in Means Expressed in Standard Deviations	Sample Size for 80% Power	Sample Size for 90% Power
0.05	6281	8407
0.15	699	935
0.25	253	338
0.35	130	173
0.45	79	105
0.55	53	71
0.65	39	51
0.75	29	39
0.85	23	31
0.95	19	25
1.05	16	21
1.15	13	17
1.25	12	15
1.35	10	13
1.45	9	11
1.55	8	10
1.65	7	9
1.75	7	8
1.85	6	8
1.95	6	7
2.05	5	6
2.15	5	6
2.25	5	6
2.35	4	5
2.45	4	5

formed consent forms and names of individuals who can answer questions regarding the trial.

Multicenter Trials

Multicenter trials should be conducted only after enough phase II trials have been performed to clarify dose levels and the likely efficacy of the therapy. Often, multicenter phase III trials are conducted after one or more single-center Phase III trials have shown promising results. All the trial designs discussed above can be used in a multicenter trial. Multicenter trials are conducted to provide rapid accrual of patients and allow a timely assessment of the therapies under study. Often, randomization is blocked within the centers, which are treated as stratification factors in the analysis. Multicenter trials require meticulous detail in defining the research questions and standardizing the data definitions. Administratively, a multicenter trial requires an order of magnitude more effort than a single-center trial. However, if the question is pressing and a multicenter trial is the most efficient way to conduct the study, the results may justify the effort.

ANALYSIS OF THE DATA

Data collection should be ongoing during the trial. The data from new patients should be entered into the computerized database when they become available. Checking the data for logical inconsistencies and errors is important. Errors can then be corrected shortly after the patient is last seen, reducing the chance of missing information. Administrative analysis, such as accrual rates, should be performed. If required, interim analyses should be conducted.

All the methods commonly used to analyze data from clinical trials test whether the null hypothesis is to be rejected. Though most hypotheses are formed in what is called the alternative form, statistical tests deal with the null form. For example, the alternative hypothesis may be that therapy A results in 10 percent less mortality than does therapy B. The null form of this hypothesis is that there is no difference in mortality among patients treated with therapy A or therapy B. Statistical tests of this hypothesis can only provide a measure of whether to reject the null hypothesis. The p value that is reported from the statistic is an assessment of the probability that the results actually observed in the trial could have occurred by random chance *if the null hypothesis were actually true.* Therefore, the smaller the p value, the less likely it is that the null hypothesis holds.

A complete description of the analysis of the data from a clinical trial is beyond the scope of this chapter. However, a brief introduction to the various methods that may be used is in order.

Continuous Outcome Measures

For continuous outcome measures, the simplest analysis is the two-group, or unpaired, t test. This method is also the most abused. To be valid, this test must be performed on data that are continuous, are distributed approximately normally, and have nearly the same standard deviation in the two groups. Alternative forms of this procedure to allow for unequal standard deviations are easily applied by computer. When the data are clearly not normally distributed, an alternative is to use a nonparametric method such as the Mann-Whitney test. A mathematical transformation, such as the log function, may result in data that are more normal.

Analysis of variance involves an extension of the t test to more than two treatments or is employed when stratification is used. The errors associated with the data are assumed to be normally distributed, as with the t test. A one-way analysis of variance allows comparison of multiple treatments. A significant difference among the treatments indicates that the means are not all the same and does not imply that any two means are different. A two-way analysis of variance can be used to perform a stratified analysis. Even when stratified randomization is used in the trial, it is always wise to do a stratified analysis, as residual effects of the stratification variable may be present. Analysis of variance can be used to adjust the comparison for the effects of a categorical covariate. Multiway analyses of variance always should be performed with extreme care in regard to the assumptions.

Analysis of covariance is closely related to analysis of variance. In addition to the effects of categorical covariates, analysis of covariance includes the effects of continuous covariates. Analysis of covariance is much like a combination of analysis of variance and regression. Analyses of variance, t-tests and analyses of covariance are all examples of the general linear model.

Categorical Outcome Variables

The most common form of clinical trial in head injury is one in which the outcome is categorical and often dichotomous. The methods used to analyze these outcomes will be given in some detail below. The analysis of categorical variables usually begins with the 2-by-2 table and the chi-square statistic. The chi-square statistic associated with Table 64-3 is 1.620 with Yates continuity correction, yielding a p value of .2030. The hypothesis being tested is that there is no association between the two variables that define the rows and columns of the table. The basic assumption of the test is that the sample size in each cell is large enough for the normality assumptions in the test to be valid. This number is usually 5. When there are fewer than five observations in one or more cells, Fisher's exact test should be employed. The chi-square test can be extended to the case of more than one row and more than one column. Again, the number of observations in each cell should be above five, and if it is not, specialized extensions of Fisher's exact test should be used. For multiple-row and multiple-column tables, the null hypothesis is still that there is no association between the rows and columns.

Stratified analysis of categorical variables is performed by using the Mantel-Haenszel procedure,[24] which is an extension of the ideas proposed by Cochran.[25] This method is based on combining the information across each stratum into a final set of summary values. The details of this method can be found in Fleiss.[26] The differences in proportions of favorable outcome in each stratum are combined, weighted by the inverse of the variance of the difference, so that strata with stronger evidence will receive more weight in the summary.

Application of the procedure to Tables 64-16 and 64-17 reveals a striking result. Instead of p value of .2030, the Mantel-Haenszel adjusted p value is .0025! The adjustment procedure yields a result much closer to the results found in Tables 64-4 through 64-6.

When there are multiple stratification variables, the Mantel-Haenszel procedure will not allow assessment of the effects of each variable. Therefore, the logistic regression model should be used. This model allows for adjustment for stratification variables and confounders. Both categorical and continuous variables may be included as independent variables. The basic model is

$$\Pr(\text{good outcome}) = \frac{e^{\text{sum of effects of treatment, effects of stratification, and effects of covariates}}}{1 + e^{\text{sum of effects of treatment, effects of stratification, and effects of covariates}}}$$

where the effects of treatment, stratification, and covariates are estimated by using a computer program. This formulation of the model is that used by Hosmer and Lemeshow,[27] there are other mathematically equivalent representations of the model. This model is extremely useful in the analysis of clinical trials. The effect of treatment can be adjusted for the effects of the stratification variables and any important covariates. The result is often a more precise measure of the treatment effect. Hosmer and Lemeshow[27] provide an excellent introduction to the intricacies of logistic regression. The logistic regression model can be extended to the case where there are multiple outcomes, such as the five levels of the GOS. When these outcomes are ordered, a form of the model will incorporate that information into the analysis.

Time-To-Event, or Survival Outcome, Variables

The methods of analysis commonly employed with survival data are the Kaplan-Meier estimate of the survival curve[28]; one of several methods of comparing two groups, such as the log-rank statistic[29]; and proportional hazards regression.[30] Kaplan-Meier methods can be used to estimate the survival curve and allow a visual way of exploring the results of the trial. Several methods are available to perform a formal test of the difference in survival between two treatments. One of the most commonly used is the log-rank test, which is analogous to combining a large number of 2-by-2 tables. Proportional hazards regression allows the incorporation of many covariates in the same manner as does logistic regression. Even though survival trials are very common in the cancer and cardiovascular fields, they have had little application to head trauma.

Repeated Measures Analysis

When the outcome variable is assessed repeatedly in the same patient, the measures are often correlated from measurement to measurement. An analysis that does not account for this correlation may provide an incorrect result. The simplest method of analysis of these data is the repeated measures analysis of variance. The data must be continuous with errors that are normally distributed. The data should have been collected at predetermined times during the study, and the number of measurements for each person should be the same. Finally, the within-person correlation should be of a certain pattern. When any of these assumptions are violated, an alternative must be used. These alternatives are difficult to apply and should be performed with great care. The most common longitudinal methods are the random-effects model for longitudinal data[31] and the general estimating equation method.[32]

General Analysis Considerations

If the time and effort have been expended to perform a good clinical trial, the analysis should be of equal quality. Collaboration with a statistician can provide valuable insights into the data that would be missed if the simplest methods available were used. The analysis should rely heavily on graphic displays of the data and displays of the results of the statistical analysis. Interaction between the neurosurgeon and the statistician can lead to high-quality results.

INTERIM ANALYSES

An issue that deserves special mention in the analysis of trial data is whether to perform an interim analysis and the type of analysis to perform. Interim analyses are performed during the course of a trial to determine whether enough evidence exists at that point to declare one treatment superior to the other. The rates of adverse events and complications should be examined simultaneously to assure that the treatments are safe. Interim analyses often are included in a trial for ethical reasons. If, during the course of the trial, there is evidence that the experimental treatment is clearly superior to the control therapy, it may be unethical to continue treating patients with the control therapy. Alternatively, if the rate of adverse events is unacceptably high in the experimental therapy, it may be necessary to stop the trial to avoid putting further patients at risk. When one is considering whether to perform interim analyses, the length of time between randomization and determination of the patient's outcome should be short relative to the time between accruals of new patients. If the interim analysis has to wait for a 6-month outcome to be determined and patients are randomized at the rate of 20 per month, nearly 120 patients will be randomized during the time when the subjects eligible for the interim analysis are being followed. The benefit of performing the analysis is then lost for these 120 patients.

These analyses are often performed blinded to the treatment, and the blind is broken only if the evidence warrants. The O'Brien-Fleming procedure[33] allows for one or more interim examinations of the data. A standard analytic method is applied to the data, and the *p* value for the test is calculated. This value is compared to a value that has been set high enough to preserve the integrity of the overall alpha level of the trial. A recently introduced method is based on "spending" the alpha level over the course of trial so that the number of interim analyses is not necessarily fixed at the outset.[34] One objection to the O'Brien-Fleming procedure is that there is no method for stopping the trial if the evidence indicates that there is no difference between the treatments. Stochastic curtailment is a recently developed technique for dealing with this problem.[35] Regardless of the analyses performed, it is always a good idea to form a committee that will evaluate the results of the analyses. These individuals should not be directly affiliated with the trial or investigators and should be able to provide a detached look at the trial and its progress. For small trials, these committees can be informal, while in larger trials, separation between the committee and the managers of the trial must be maintained.

REPORTING RESULTS

As was suggested earlier, it is unethical not to report the results of a clinical trial. While negative trials are more difficult to publish, some form for disseminating the findings of a negative trial should be found. Positive results are often easily published. To avoid problems when the time comes to prepare manuscripts, the investigators in the trial should agree on a method to assign and share credit. This problem is especially difficult in larger, multicenter trials, which may form publications committees to deal with such matters.

CONCLUSIONS AND RECOMMENDATIONS

This chapter cannot include the large amount of information available to help in the design of a trial. Several general books are excellent sources of information. Those listed here have proved valuable in a neurotrauma setting, but others are likely to be equally valuable. *Fundamentals of Clinical Trials*[9] is a excellent overview of the design and conduct of a trial without being excessively technical. *Clinical Trials; Design, Conduct and Analysis*[4] is a detailed examination of clinical trials, and includes many practical suggestions for use in trial design. From a statistical point of view, the work of Machin and Campbell[15] is valuable. *The Design and Analysis of Clinical Experiments*[26] provides a detailed examination of many of the statistical issues arising from trials. *Recent Advances in Clinical Trial Design and Analysis*[36] describes current development in clinical trials. Also, the journal of the Society for Clinical Trials, *Controlled Clinical Trials*, can be consulted.

The design, conduct, analysis, and reporting of a clinical trial is not a simple task. Medical, ethical, managerial, and statistical issues must be addressed and solved. Simple trials run in a single institution should adopt the same rigorous standards for trial design and data quality used in large multicenter trials funded by the National Institutes of Health (NIH). Even the simplest designs can be destroyed by lack of planning. While a simple trial could be designed using the information in this chapter, the wise investigator will always seek the collaboration of a statistician, especially if the statistician has some knowledge of the field. Neurotrauma trials pose their own set of problems. Obtaining consent for a patient who is comatose and needs early treatment is difficult. Surgical trials are almost impossible to blind, and randomization may be difficult. The sample size required to see outcome differences in the GOS are often very large. However, these are all problems that have solutions, and enlightened and motivated investigators can conduct phase II and phase III trials of high quality. In the field of neurotrauma, where the number of currently available efficacious treatments is low, such trials are extremely important in developing new therapies.

REFERENCES

1. Packard FR: *Life and Times of Ambroise Pare, 1510–1590.* New York: Paul B. Hoeber; 1921.
2. Bull JP: The historical development of clinical therapeutic trials. *J Chronic Dis* 10:218–248, 1959.
3. Lilienfeld AM: Ceteris paribus: The evolution of the clinical trial. *Bull Hist Med* 56:1–18, 1982.
4. Meinert CL, Tonascia S: Clinical trials: Design, conduct, and analysis (abstract). 1986.
5. Fisher RA, MacKenzeie WA: Studies in crop variations: II. The manurial response of different potato varieties. *J Agric Sci* 13:311–320, 1923.
6. Box JF: R. A. Fisher and the design of experiments, 1922–1926. *Am Stat* 34:1–7, 1980.
7. Medical Research Council: Clinical trials of new remedies (annotations). *Lancet* 304, 1931.
8. Amberson JB Jr, McMahon BT, Pinner M: A clinical trial of sanocrysin in pulmonary tuberculosis. *Am Rev Tuberc* 24:401–435, 1931.
9. Friedman LM, Furberg CD, DeMets DL: *Fundamentals of Clinical Trials.* Littleon, Mass: PSG, 1985.
10. Gehan EA, Freireich EJ: Non-randomized controls in cancer clinical trials. *N Engl J Med* 290:198–203, 1974.
11. Pocock SJ: *Clinical Trials: A Practical Approach.* Chichester, UK: Wiley, 1983.
12. Herson J: Statistical aspects in the design and analysis of phase II clinical trials. in Buyse ME, Staquet MJ, Sylvestor RJ (eds): *Cancer Clinical Trials: Methods and Practice.* Oxford, UK: Oxford Medical Publications, 1984.
13. Thall PF, Simon RM: Recent developments in the design of phase II clinical trials, in Thall PF (ed): *Recent Advances in Clinical Trial Design and Analysis.* Boston: Kluwer, 1995:49–72.
14. Teasdale G, Jennett B: Assessment of coma and impaired consciousness: A practical scale. *Lancet* ii:81–84, 1974.

15. Machin D, Campbell MJ: *Statistical Tables for the Design of Clinical Trials*. Oxford, UK: Blackwell, 1987.
16. Jennett B, Bond M: Assessment of outcome after severe brain damage. *Lancet* i:480, 1975.
17. Rappaport M, Hall KM, Hopkins K, et al: Disability rating scale for severe head trauma: Coma to community. *Arch Phys Med Rehabil* 63:118–123, 1982.
18. Eisenberg HM, Frankowski RF, Contant CF, et al: High-dose barbituate control of elevated intracranial pressure in patients with severe head injury. *J Neurosurg* 69:15–23, 1988.
19. Dunnett CW: New tables for multiple comparison with a control. *Biometrics* 20:482–491, 1964.
20. Meinert CL, Tonascia S, Higgins KH: Content of reports on clinical trials: A critical review. *Controlled Clin Trials* 5:328–347, 1984.
21. Whitehead J: *The Design and Analysis of Sequential Clinical Trials*. New York: Ellis Horwood, 1992.
22. Clifton GL, Hayes RL, Levin HS, et al: Outcome measures for clinical trials involving traumatically brain-injured patients: Report of a conference. *Neurosurgery* 31:975–978, 1992.
23. Marshall LF, Marshall SB, Klauber MR, et al: The diagnosis of head injury requires a classification based on computed axial tomography. *J Neurotrauma* 9 (suppl 1):S287–S292, 1992.
24. Mantel N, Haenszel W: Statistical aspects of the analysis of data from retrospective studies of disease. *JNCI* 22:719–748, 1959.
25. Cochran WG: Some methods of strengthening the common chi-squared tests. *Biometrics* 10:417–451, 1954.
26. Fleiss JL: *The Design and Analysis of Clinical Experiments*. New York: Wiley, 1986.
27. Hosmer DW, Lemeshow S: *Applied Logistic Regression*. New York: Wiley, 1989.
28. Kaplan EL, Meier P: Nonparametric estimation from incomplete observations. Journal of the American Statistical Association 53:457–481, 1958.
29. Cox DR, Oakes D: *Analysis of Survival Data*. London: Chapman and Hall, 1984.
30. Cox DR: Regression models and life-tables (with discussion). *JR Statist Soc B* 34:187–220, 1972.
31. Laird NM, Ware JH: Random-effects models for longitudinal data. *Biometrics* 38:963–974, 1982.
32. Zeger SL, Liang KY, Albert PS: Models for longitudinal data: A generalized estimating equation approach. *Biometrics* 44:1049–1060, 1988.
33. O'Brien PC, Fleming TR: A multiple testing procedure for clinical trials. *Biometrics* 35:549–556, 1979.
34. DeMets DL, Lan G: The alpha spending function approach to interim data analysis, in Thall PF (ed): *Recent Advances in Clinical Trial Design and Analysis*. Boston: Kluwer, 1995:1–28.
35. Davis BR, Hardy RJ: Data monitoring in clinical trials: The case for stochastic curtailment. *J Clin Epidemiol* 47:1033–1042, 1994.
36. Thall PF: *Recent Advances in Clinical Trial Design and Analysis*. Boston: Kluwer, 1995.

CHAPTER 65

HEAD INJURY TRIALS–PAST AND PRESENT

Wayne M. Alves
Howard M. Eisenberg

SYNOPSIS

In the 1980s the mortality rate from severe head injury declined from the 50 percent predicted in 1974 to 35 percent.[1,2] Although there is reason to feel encouraged, ensuring survival may not be enough. The impairments and disabilities that result from the damage wrought by a head injury are not always the preferred outcomes. For example, a severely disabled or vegetative survival may not make a clinician feel that this or her efforts on behalf of the patient and the patient's family were worthwhile. Fortunately, the value of early aggressive neurosurgical intervention is reasonably well documented, and one need not take a nihilistic point of view.[3]

A new sense of encouragement has come in the 1990s, the "decade of the brain," as promising novel compounds for preventing or ameliorating the destructive consequences of acute head injury have become available for human testing. Until now there have been few large multicenter efficacy trials in head injury, and the state of the art can still be viewed as being in its infancy. Several compounds are being tested, and it is anticipated that as these and future novel compounds are tested, physicians will acquire knowledge and experience in how best to design, conduct, and analyze data from multicenter randomized clinical trials. As new and even more promising compounds become available for the acute and chronic treatment of head injury and its consequences, clinicians may offer survivors a better than even chance for a reasonable quality of life.

This chapter reviews the major issues in the design of modern clinical trials as they apply to traumatic brain injury. It examines head injury populations in terms of inputs and outcomes relevant for head injury clinical trials. Some of the issues or problems are germane to acute neurological disorders in general, while others are specific to head injury. The chapter briefly mentions areas of potential controversy involving the design, conduct, and analysis of data from current multicenter head injury trials. Finally, previous and current experience with safety and efficacy trials in head injury are discussed. Throughout the following sections, it is assumed that the principle of a closely monitored trial to ensure adequate safety evaluation which meets scientific, clinical, and regulatory standards of excellence has been met. Therefore, safety monitoring in head injury trials will not be discussed in detail.

DESIGN OF HEAD INJURY CLINICAL TRIALS

UNDERLYING LOGIC

The underlying rationale or hypotheses of head injury clinical trials can be phrased as follows. The overlapping pathological processes which are initiated at the time of the traumatic brain injury take several days to cause irreversible cellular damage or death. Early treatment aimed at interrupting or stopping these processes should be able to minimize or prevent their delayed consequences. If these processes are prevented from achieving their full course, one can expect an improvement in brain metabolic or physiological functioning that will result in improved clinical outcomes. The most reasonable way to pursue these hypotheses is to test them with drugs with demonstrated mechanisms of action that can interrupt deleterious processes.

The biomechanical aspects of traumatic brain injury have been well described,[4,5] and head injury clinical trials in the 1980s focused on the control of intracranial pressure. More recently, emphasis has been placed on the secondary mechanisms of brain injury, with special interest in agents that afford global brain protection from ischemia and hypoxic injury. In practice, most head injury trials have focused only on the conventional drug-testing paradigm, which is to give the treatment, assure that it is safe (i.e., it is not detrimental, and complications are manageable), and determine whether the outcome from head injury is better than that of patients who did not receive the drug. In the case of head injury, this paradigm is straightforward and acceptable so long as the treatment is clearly effective. However, if it is not, the reasons for the apparent lack of efficacy may not be easily determined.

Several logical steps in the drug development process lead to a determination of the effectiveness of a novel compound.* These comments are necessarily brief and illustrative, and more detailed discussions are readily available.[6,7] First, the screening and identification of an agent worthy of clinical testing in humans are usually accomplished by using the drug in experimental models of the disease for which it is to be used clinically. Since animal models cannot replicate the entire spectrum and the numerous types of clinical head injury, this initial step is problematic in the case of traumatic brain injury. The fact that preclinical head injury models may be relevant only to a limited number of situations is an obvious limitation which is easily compensated for by the discovery of promising new compounds. It is easy for a new treatment to be extended to clinical conditions for which it was not tested. In that case, the drug's mechanism of action can only be considered putative rather than proven. If an experimentally useful drug fails in clinical trials, one explanation may be that the fidelity of the animal models in reproducing clinically relevant head injury was low and that it therefore was tested in the wrong patient population. Head injury is an instance in which the paradigm of serial animal-then-human testing can seriously limit progress.

Determining that a novel drug treatment in humans is effective for its original purpose ideally requires that several steps be fulfilled.[8] The safety of the compound must be demonstrated at least to the level of effective management of the side effects of the drug. The drug should be delivered to its intended site of action with the anticipated neuropharmacologic effect, and an expected neurophysiological response should be observed. Our ability to identify the neurophysiological response to a drug depends in part on the fidelity of the animal model to the clinical situation. Despite the extensive preclinical testing that precedes the human testing of many new compounds, this ideal often is not realized in practice. A drug may be deemed efficacious even though its mechanism of action remains putative. In practice, demonstration of efficacy requires the observation of a measurable improvement in the outcome of the disease process (i.e., a more favorable outcome in the drug treatment group).

* This section benefited from numerous discussions between one of the authors (WMA) and Thomas A. Gennarelli, M.D., Chairman, Department of Neurosurgery, Hahnemann Medical College, Philadelphia. Any flaws are this author's.

DESIGN CONSIDERATIONS

REQUIREMENTS OF MODERN RANDOMIZED CLINICAL TRIALS

The principles of modern clinical trial design are well established. The current standard is a well-controlled and closely monitored study that involves concurrent control subjects, adequate blinding of treatment, and the random assignment of patients to treatment groups.[9] In modern head injury clinical trials, concurrent controls may consist of subjects who receive a placebo or vehicle treatment, standard management, or both. Preserving the study blind in head injury trials is essential because of the attendant problems of bias, at times admittedly theoretical and subtle, that can creep into the evaluation of clinical outcomes. The current standard is to use double-blind procedures to ensure that the subject and the investigator are unaware of which treatment was received. Management trials such as hypothermia therapy may not permit this. However, one can and should use blinded evaluators for outcome assessment.

Randomization procedures often help preserve the blind in a well-designed and well-executed trial. The current standard of randomizing patients is specifically intended to avoid or minimize bias by ensuring that prognostic factors and unknown or extraneous sources of variation are controlled or balanced across the different treatment groups. In addition, random assignment allows the valid use of statistical tests or procedures for comparison of treatment groups. Equal randomization is the most theoretically attractive procedure for the random assignment of subjects to a trial. All things being equal, this approach minimizes statistical error and maximizes power.[10] The value of equal randomization for achieving the desired statistical balance and for analyzing data should not be underestimated. Anecdotal experience with current head injury trials indicates, however, that the desired statistical balance between treatment groups may be difficult to achieve even with a fairly large number of subjects.

Essential design features of head injury trials

Designing effective evaluations of novel head injury treatments depends on the careful development of methodology for comparing interventions that make use of design features to increase sensitivity (i.e., statistical power) within the constraints imposed by realistic sample size considerations and the naturally occurring heterogeneity of head injury severity and outcome.[11,12] The major issues involve prestratification and other randomization strategies, testing of multiple treatments, and the use of between- and within-subject design features in the presence of the known heterogeneity of head injury. In head injury clinical trials to date, the elemental features of good design have often been present, although not necessarily with the desired frequency.[13]

The *randomized controlled trial* is the essential tool for assessing therapeutic efficacy. The demands of modern clinical trials, coupled with the relative imprecision of the clinical endpoints currently used to evaluate outcome, put limits on the possibility of assessing all the drugs purported to be of benefit in head injury. Before the 1990s, controlled clinical studies to evaluate new head injury treatments seemed to require that an allowance be made for smaller numbers of patients than are typically desired or required for statistical sensitivity.[11,12] In addition, investigators seldom explicitly took into consideration the heterogeneity and complexity of head injury damage and outcome. When one considers the evolution of a therapeutic hypothesis, study designs in which smaller numbers of patients receive a new treatment and all improve might be a helpful first result, but it is more likely that the treatment success-failure ratio will split nearer to 50-50. In the extreme case, no patients improve and researchers are unable to differentiate between an ineffective treatment and those which are effective in specific patient subgroups. Patient selection factors, possibly quite subtle and *despite* random assignment to treatment, typically are the reason why these results are observed.[14]

CURRENT HEAD INJURY TRIALS AND TRIBULATIONS

Current head injury clinical trials are complex, are difficult to manage, and require considerable time to assess endpoints properly. This section considers some of the current issues involved in testing new compounds for head injury that have emerged in the context of past and current head injury trials.

Which Drug of Many?

Many head injury trials could be performed to assess off-the-shelf drugs with presumed therapeutic value in clinical head injury. In addition, there are numerous novel compounds available for testing which provide new hope of finding an efficacious and approvable drug. When there are so many competing compounds or when a new family of compounds is developed and many companies are competing for scarce patients, the question of which drug of the many available should be tested becomes paramount. It has become apparent in the early 1990s that this is not an atypical situation in head injury. Consider, for example, the case of magnesium, which is believed to act by blocking calcium channels associated with the *N*-methyl-D-aspartate (NMDA) receptor and has been shown to be beneficial in animal models.[15,16] Presumably, lower posttraumatic magnesium levels would hamper the normal blocking of the NMDA channel, allowing more calcium entry into the cell. Therefore, reestablishing the magnesium block may prevent cellular injury and improve brain function. Numerous compounds for head injury are in various stages of testing. They are briefly described in Table 65-1 and discussed later in this chapter.

Clinical Testing Of New Compounds

Novel therapies are exciting, and the urgency to find new therapies often leads to attempts to shorten or circumvent the laborious process of testing a new drug for approval. In part, the problem lies in the lack of adequate supportive preclinical data showing that a particular drug has the activity and efficacy implied by those who advocate its use. As competition for scarce patients increases, one can expect to see even greater pressure to skip over critical steps in the drug development process. Conducting necessary studies in parallel is the minimum requirement.

Careful consideration, and control to the extent possible, of the background therapy underlying a head injury clinical trial is essential. This has *not* been an explicit feature of past head injury clinical trials. Dearden and associates[17] long ago recognized the lack of a standardized management regimen as a factor contributing to the limitations of head injury trials. The trade-off is between simplicity and adequate and standardized management reflecting the best possible care available for the patient. In addition, issues such as duration of dosing, adequacy of dosing, and concomitant medications allowed in the trial are all important.

Adequate analysis of safety parameters to ensure adequate documentation of possible drug-related adverse events is a necessary feature of modern head injury clinical trials. In a recently completed phase III head

TABLE 65-1 Drugs Being Tested in Head Injury

Compound Group	Examples*	Expected Mechanism of Action
Barbiturates	Pentobarbital Thiopental	Normalize unresponsive intracranial pressure (ICP)
Corticosteroids	Dexamethasone	ICP control
Lactate buffers	CPC-211 (Cypros) Tromethamine (THAM)	Inhibit accumulation of lactate, reducing cerebral acidosis, and controlling ICP
NMDA antagonists	CGS-19755 (Selfotel, Ciba-Geigy) Cerestat (Cambridge Neuroscience) Dextromethorphan Felbamate Ketamine MK-801 (Fidia) Phencyclidine (PCP) SDZ EAA-494 (Sandoz) SNX-11 (Neurex)	Block or inhibit excitatory amino acids at NMDA receptor site, preventing neuronal death
Calcium antagonists	Nimodipine (Nimotop, Miles)	Prevent hypoxic/ischemic injury by preventing toxic calcium accumulation
Free radical inhibitors	Superoxide dismutase (Dismutec, Stirling) Tirilazad mesylate (Freedox, Upjohn)	Inhibit oxygen-derived free radicals to prevent ischemic injury and reduce threat to structural integrity and function of cell membrane
Phospholipid metabolism	Cytidine diphosphocholine (CDP-choline)	Prevent decrease in cell membrane phospholipids, inhibiting cytotoxic edema pathway
Others	Adenosine agonists (Gensia) Bradykinin antagonist (Bradycor, Cortech) Opiate receptor antagonists (naloxone) Antiadhesion compounds	

* Selected proprietary names and/or companies developing drugs are indicated in parentheses.

injury trial of the novel 21-aminosteroid tirilazad mesylate (Freedox, Upjohn Company), the author's examined over 230 categories of adverse medical events in 13 body systems. In addition to coding the seriousness of the event to comply with regulatory requirements for the reporting of the serious or drug-related adverse medical events associated with a clinical trial, the authors also coded the severity of the event (i.e., an event might be considered severe without being serious, as in the case of severe vomiting). Sorting out the complications associated with the natural history of head injury from the potential complications of a new drug remains a problem.[18] It is also important to keep in mind that if the drug being tested has already been approved for other indications, that does not obviate the need for evaluating toxicity and may well lead to the detection of previously unseen side effects.

Dosing Timing and Regimen

Dosing regimens have seldom been discussed in reports of clinical trials in head injury. Some investigators have acknowledged considerations such as the timing of the administration of the study drug, especially varying time intervals after the injury.[17,19] The dosing regimen is critical and depends on numerous factors, including the half-life of the agent, its bioavailability, and its pharmacokinetics and pharmacodynamics.[20] To a lesser extent, the route of administration may also be relevant, but probably for other reasons relating to dosing. For example, venous irritation at an intravenous (IV) infusion site is not an important problem since head injury patients have central lines through which the study drug may be administered.

The duration of dosing may also be critical in light of the evolution of the diseases of head injury and the time from onset in which physicians need to ensure that a therapeutic level of the "protective agent" is available. Careful definition of the onset and termination of treatment and treatment latency (i.e., the interval from treatment to observable response) is important in the design of effective head injury trials.[21]

Treatment Latency

Time to diagnosis and neurosurgical treatment is no longer controversial in head injury.[3] Of great importance for current head injury clinical trials, however, is an understanding of the time to treatment in which one can expect a drug to have a chance to be effective. In head injury, as in other acute neurological emergencies, it is presumed that the earlier, the better. Four-hour postinjury dosing windows are now common. In addition, the dosing regimen is likely to be a reason given for situations in which data from clinical trials show that a drug does not appear to be efficacious. On a practical level, the average time to dosing of a study drug typically pushes the upper end of the dosing window. This, combined with the potential imprecision of the time when the head injury occurred, calls into question whether drugs are delivered as quickly as they need to be to have the desired effect.

DESIGN ISSUES IN CURRENT HEAD INJURY TRIALS

This section will consider several issues in the design of current head injury trials. It also raises several practical center-related issues in conducting clinical trials that deserve attention. Most current concerns focus on achieving an adequate description of head injury populations that has considerable importance for the clear definition of prognostic and other input variables that serve to define inclusion and exclusion criteria (i.e., pretreatment) and data analysis plans. In addition, there are implications for subsetting head injury populations for post hoc analyses of clinical trials data.

Current head injury trials, like those for other acute neuroemergencies, require multiple endpoints to represent the complete story of damage and outcome. The use of surrogate measures, including brain imaging endpoints, and the possibility of study treatment–induced pathological outcomes create complexity in describing the safety and efficacy of novel compounds. The problem of multiple endpoints also creates statistical problems in that multiple comparisons require an adjustment of the statistical significance.

Fairly simple standards existed for data analysis in past head injury clinical trials. While physicians may have a clear idea of which patients they are interested in testing the drug in, for a variety of reasons, including practicality and measurement error, noise is introduced into the data. In addition, the potential for selection bias is always present. Thus, the basic analysis population of a modern clinical trial is the *intent-to-treat* population, that is, the patients randomized to the arms of the trial whether or not there are errors of classification, randomization, or treatment. In addition, there are compelling reasons to require no missing data in the efficacy analysis; that is, one must have complete outcome data on all randomized patients. Since this is especially difficult to achieve in head injury, imputation rules exist, for example, the "last observation carried forward" procedure. However, these are at best limited practical solutions to a difficult and inescapable problem in head injury trials. Complicating the issue is the possibility that it may be the subjects with better outcomes who are lost to follow-up.

DESCRIBING HEAD INJURY POPULATIONS

HETEROGENEITY OF HEAD INJURY PATHOLOGY

The potentially devastating consequences of head injury are well known.[22,23] Head injury patients are among the sickest patients modern medical practice must deal with. The design of current head injury trials is complicated by interactions of pathological events that are difficult to define and in some cases are poorly understood.[11]

Brain injury is simultaneously heterogeneous and complex. Primary and secondary brain injuries, well-known complicating factors (e.g., hemorrhage and extracranial injuries), and competing risk factors (comorbidities) all influence outcome.[30,32] Current head injury clinical trials are designed against this multifactorial backdrop. A further complication is that factors of lifestyle and the life cycle also play important roles in the incidence of head injury and outcomes. Since there is no singular and easily describable recovery pattern, measurements of recovery have largely been limited to global clinical rating scales such as the Glasgow Outcome Score.[24] In part, these global measures have also been chosen in order to maintain acceptable levels of validity and reliability. However, the multifactorial nature of head injury outcome may require more sophisticated and extensive quality-of-life measures.[25]

INJURY SEVERITY

The Glasgow Coma Scale[26] (GCS) grades coma severity without depending on specific anatomic-clinical correlations and allows physicians to describe the outcomes of head injury in terms of initial inputs.[1] It is now well understood that injury severity is a continuum, although practical classifications into mild, moderate, and severe injury are useful. For example, in the case of GCS 3 through 5, mortality is high and success is generally low. For GCS 6 through 8, aggressive neurosurgical management may be the most important determinant of outcome. The situation is less clear in the case of moderate head injury (GCS 9 through 12), and in the case of GCS 13 through 15, the sequelae may be best handled by disciplines other than neurosurgery. In the current head injury trials, GCS 4 through 12 or some subset of this range typically defines the severity range of the eligible study population.

The value of the GCS in grading coma severity is undeniable, yet the GCS is not the entire story. Aspects of the patient's neurological status, especially pupil reactivity and seizures, are important indicators of injury severity. Gennarelli and colleagues[27] noted that an unstated hypothesis appears to be that injury severity, as determined by the GCS, is the sole determinant of outcome. Data from their seven-center study indicate that pathology or anatomic injury severity may account for as much as 50 percent of the outcome from traumatic brain injury as defined by the Glasgow Outcome Score or mortality. This has profound implications for head injury clinical trials, since it is imperative that balance in pathology be achieved through randomization. Even small, apparently insignificant differences between treatment groups can tamper with the ability to detect or measure treatment effects.

Pathology

Although each case of human head injury may be heterogeneous and complex (i.e., multiplicity of damage), the mechanisms of brain injury are fairly limited. They include diffuse axonal injury, hemorrhage, brain ischemia and brain swelling, brain edema (as a specific cause of swelling), neurotransmitter failure, and "toxic" substances which cross a defective blood-brain barrier.[3,5] The essential questions to answer are, What kind of injuries have occurred? and What single system or whole-body impairments follow those injuries?

Classifying patients into injury severity groups is not an exact science. Nonetheless, it is necessary to be able to identify the natural pathological groups of traumatic brain injury so that designs for head injury clinical trials are more sensitive to drug safety and efficacy evaluations. The key problem in doing this is that the terms that describe head injury are not mutually exclusive and that it is not always clear which should take precedence. How does one factor both anatomic and physiological severity descriptors into a single classification that is clinically meaningful and useful in clinical trials to subset patients for inclusion in trials for stratifying before randomization and for planned and post hoc analyses of data from subpopulations? Current head injury clinical trials require a fairly simple way of describing the pathology in the population of patients enrolled as subjects. The most useful clinical classification based on computed tomography has been provided by the National Traumatic Coma Data Bank investigation team.[28] The intracranial diagnoses based on CT scans recommended by this group are defined in Table 65-2.

Prognostic Factors

Factors which have prognostic value for head injury outcomes are hypotension (shock), hypoxia, age, and, to a lesser extent, gender.[23,29] In addition, isolated severe head injury is less common than multiple trauma and extracranial injuries may interact in synergy with brain injuries in producing unfavorable outcomes.[30] Therefore, several descriptors are essential and form the minimal input into every modern head injury clinical trials design. These descriptors are listed in Table 65-3. How to factor these inputs into preplanned analyses in a straightforward way is uncertain at this time and is likely to remain controversial, although useful information is becoming available in the head injury literature.[28,29,31]

Choice of Trial Endpoints

Endpoints of traumatic brain injury outcome used in current head injury trials include mortality and various

TABLE 65-2 Computed Tomography Classification of Head Injury Pathology

Category	CT Scan Definition
Diffuse injury I	No visible CT pathology
Diffuse injury II	No compression of shift (≤5 mm) and/or no high- or mixed-density lesions greater than 25 ml
Diffuse injury III (swelling)	Compression, no shift, and/or no lesions > 25 ml
Diffuse injury IV (shift)	Shift (> 5 mm), no lesions > 25 ml
Evacuated mass lesion	Any lesion surgically removed
Nonevacuated mass lesion	High- or mixed-density lesion >25 ml not surgically removed

SOURCE: Adapted from Marshall LF, Marshall SB, Klauber MR, et al: The diagnosis of head injury requires a classification based on computed axial tomography. *J Neurotrauma* 9:S287–S292, 1992.

TABLE 65-3 Prognostic Factors That Are Minimal Requisites for Modern Head Injury Clinical Trials

Category	Variables
Demographics	Age
	Sex*
	Race*
Admission status	Hypoxia
	Hypotension (shock, systolic blood pressure (SBP) < 90)
	Seizures
	Temperature†
Injury severity	Glasgow Coma Scale
	Pupillary responses
	Hemiparesis
	Brainstem reflexes
Pathology	Lesion size (hemorrhage or contusion)
	Shift (>5 mm)
	Swelling (status of mesencephalic cisterns)
	Presence of subarachnoid blood

* Gender differences in injury severity, pathology, and outcomes have not been established. Gender and racial/ethnic classifications are included here to indicate their importance for subgroup analyses and regulatory reporting requirements.

† Temperature is added to indicate the potential importance of hypothermia as a brain protectant.

descriptors of mobility and morbidity. What counts as a relevant outcome measure? A stepladder of expected brain injury outcomes might be as follows:

Death
Severe or moderate neurophysical impairments
Personality changes and/or neurobehavioral impairments
Social and behavioral problems
Lack of employability
Reduction in quality of life.

Since lifestyle and life cycle factors are important in recovery, it is difficult to separate the outcomes of head injury from the premorbid characteristics of subjects. Life domains overlap, and we can expect spillover effects as problems in one of life's arenas create problems in others. In addition, some outcomes swamp others. For example, if a patient never returns to work, the economic impact is felt in all life domains. It is questionable whether one ever needs to measure so much. This standard imposes a considerable obligation to determine the probable measurable effects of a new compound and to determine whether the endpoints selected (surrogate physiological measures or long-term clinical endpoints) have the requisite level of precision and sensitivity.

Choice of Clinical Endpoints

A clear definition of relevant clinical outcomes is an essential ingredient of good clinical trial design. This is important since surrogate endpoints may not be acceptable to regulatory agencies, and so one should focus on longer-term clinical endpoints. In past and present head injury trials, the 6-month Glasgow Outcome Score (GOS) has been generally accepted as the primary study endpoint. It is important to consider time to recovery in determining when to best assess efficacy, since selection of the time of assessment can dramatically alter the conclusions of a clinical trial.[11,12,21] Choi and coworkers[32] recently considered the transition of outcome states based on the GOS from 3 to 6 months after injury. They concluded that the 3-month outcome endpoint could satisfactorily serve as the primary endpoint for clinical trials.

Definition Issues and Surrogate Clinical Endpoints

Often the putative mechanism of action is an important secondary endpoint. It is now typical to include mechanistic endpoints as secondary endpoints in clinical trials. For example, if posttraumatic subarachnoid blood reflects a pathology that can be expected to lead to ischemic deficits in a head-injured patient and subsequently a poor outcome, it may be necessary to be able to document the fact that clinical ischemic deficits actually occur and that the drug actually prevents or reduces their incidence. Previously, very few head injury clinical trials used such endpoints. Pitts and Kaktis[33] are a notable exception in using control of intracranial pressure as a primary efficacy endpoint in a trial of high-dose corticosteroids. Dearden and associates[17] later criticized other high-dose steroid studies for not measuring the presumed mechanism of action.

Potential for Pathological Outcomes

In evaluating new drugs or the off-label use of approved drugs, there must always be concern for potential drug-related pathological outcomes. For example, one can imagine "saving" patients who might have died without the drug only to find that they remain in a persistent vegetative state. Even more problematic is the risk of shifting some patients who would have had a "good recovery" or "moderate disability" to an unfavorable outcome category. The practical consequence of this problem for current head injury trials is the imposition of both a "win" and a "no-win" rule. To successfully demonstrate efficacy, one has to observe an increase in the favorable outcome category. In addition, one cannot have a positive study unless one can also show that there is no difference in unfavorable outcomes between the treatment groups. Demonstrating strict equivalence is not required. Rather, it is necessary only to show that one does not exceed a clinically accepted threshold for the observed difference. For example, the "dead" and "vegetative" GOS categories in the study drug group should not exceed those in the placebo group by more than 10 percent.

Time to Recovery and Outcomes Assessment

Current approaches to the management of traumatic brain injury typically assume that patients who sustain a brain injury can expect a better prognosis if treatment is immediate and aggressive.[3] Also assumed is that the outcomes that are expected from a particular type of brain injury are predictable and can therefore serve as an index of drug efficacy. Unfortunately, the shape of head injury outcome distributions is largely unknown. The authors do expect the distribution of the GOS to be U- or J-shaped, but this is far from clear in the case of other outcome measures, especially quality of life. Ideally, one wants a measure that fully ranks all head injury outcomes from best to worst.

Not knowing the nature or shape of head injury outcome distributions also applies to the case of *when* to measure outcome, that is, the time-oriented shape of the outcome distribution. One can imagine a distribution ranging from the subacute phase (at which point surrogate measures may be appropriate) through rehabilitation and then recovery. Depending on lost-to-follow-up patterns and the mix of patients (i.e., inputs), this distribution remains unknown, and even apparently subtle differences in pathology between head injury treatment groups can be reflected in substantial differences in outcome rates.[27,28]

Considerations of Statistical Power

Several issues involving statistical design must be weighed in defining a good head injury clinical trial. A sufficient number of patients is necessary to detect whether an efficacious drug has the desired effect in the treatment population (statistical power). Whether one should stratify patients to improve sensitivity is a difficult decision. For example, one may at a minimum want to stratify randomization to ensure balance in important subsets (e.g., injury severity defined as "moderate" versus "severe" using the GCS). However, there are compelling reasons to suggest that a patient population that includes both severe and moderate head injuries is a group with a significant risk for mortality and morbidity.

It is very difficult to determine whether the head injury trials performed to date were adequately powered for their primary hypotheses. This may in part be a reporting problem best dealt with by journal editors and reviewers but in part may be a potential flaw in the original design of a trial. The current standard for head injury trials is for considerations of statistical power to be given great weight in the planning phase.

Data Analysis Requirements

Data analysis requirements of head injury clinical trials must weigh which analysis populations are relevant. In defining data analysis populations, both scientific and regulatory concerns are at issue. The intent-to-treat population is generally the *randomized* population; that is, subjects are analyzed in the groups into which they were randomized regardless of whether they received the treatment intended. In current head injury trials, this typically serves as the primary analysis population even if there are errors in screening, randomization, or study drug dosing. Screening occurs, a judgment is made to enroll, and dosing begins. Generally, the authors have used the time of mixing of the study drugs as the time of randomization, although this can pose practical problems (e.g., a pharmacy mixing error based on the knowledge that a *possible* subject is being screened). Sometimes the intent-to-treat population is defined as "randomized and receives one dose of study drug" (the *dosed* population) or "randomized plus one dose of study drug plus one outcome evaluation" (the *evaluable* population).

The data analysis window is also a very important consideration in an analysis of data from head injury trials. A "full window" is all data received regardless of whether the data fall within the desired time window for assessment, or "medical window," for example, 3 months plus or minus 2 weeks. A full window would include an outcome received at 4 months after the injury, while the medical window analysis would include only cases within 2 weeks of the 3-month follow-up date.

Regulatory guidelines require a "no missing data" (NMD) analysis, which typically involves imputing a score for patients with missing observations, such as the "last observation carried forward" procedure. In current head injury trials, it may be more sensible to substitute later observations for earlier missing observations. For example, the 12-month GOS, if available, may be a better surrogate for a missing 6-month score than is the 3-month GOS. Regulatory guidelines also require an analysis of center (or investigator) effects, either qualitative or a formal quantitative test for the homogeneity of treatment effects. For example, one might want to examine treatment outcomes stratified by admission severity classes defined as "severe" and "moderate" across centers by using the Mantel-Haenszel procedure or other procedures.[34]

Data Analysis Issues

Current statistical issues in head injury trials relating to data analysis include precision of outcome measures, multiplicity of endpoints, selection biases, and the effects of adjustments to data and subsequent interpretations.

Precision of outcome measures

A difficult problem in head injury clinical trials is that current outcome measures are imprecise and were not designed to assess either physiological responses or functional changes caused by drug treatment effects. Consequently, in determining the effectiveness of a drug, the outcome is evaluated long after the treatment is given, and so large numbers of patients are required. It may be possible to decrease the numbers of patients needed if the outcome measures have been improved or if the drug can be assessed closer to its time of action. Solely measuring functional changes, however, does not remove this difficulty because of the multifactorial functional impairments that follow traumatic brain injury. The issue is whether determining a more direct effect of a drug will truly allow a conclusion about the drug's eventual effectiveness in improving outcome. For example, measurements of infarct volume in stroke patients may not correlate with final patient outcome even if these are not noisy data. If a measurable physiological effect is not present, will the new compound be likely to prove efficacious? The key to this reasoning is choosing an appropriate measure of the drug's physiological effect. However, one may still demonstrate long-term clinical improvement in the drug treatment group without a measurable physiological effect. The cost of not using physiological surrogate endpoints is an increase in sample size requirements. If an incorrect measure is chosen for evaluating a drug, by that measure the drug may prove ineffective when in actuality it has a benefit when measured against another endpoint. It is reasonable to try to determine whether sufficient evidence can be obtained to suggest that it is worth proceeding with more detailed, lengthy, and hence more expensive testing of the drug.

Multiplicity of endpoints

The multifactorial nature of head injury and the need for multiple outcome measures lead to the problem of multiple comparisons. This is especially true since physicians often do not clearly specify or even anticipate all a priori hypotheses. Some correction must be made for the many post hoc comparisons that are inevitably made as data are analyzed. Several practical options for evaluating multiple endpoints are listed below. Although they cannot be discussed in detail here, the reader can consult the references provided. The most frequent adjustment is a Bonferroni procedure, although in certain circumstances a compelling argument can be made for using Hotelling's T^2 procedure,[35] the sum of normalized scores described by O'Brien,[36] stepwise procedures,[37] or some form of combined test. With few exceptions, past and current (completed and published) head injury trials data were analyzed without consideration of this issue or the use of these procedures.

Selection bias

Selection biases which can cloud analysis in head injury trials arise from several sources. Recruitment of patients is largely dependent on postinjury time of arrival in emergency departments and the availability of informed consent. If the treatment window is narrow, say, 4 h, there may be no time to find the appropriate representative to provide informed consent. Ideally, one wants every eligible patient at the site enrolled in the trial. If the site is not properly organized, many eligible patients will be excluded. It will then be difficult to know whether the patients included at that site were truly representative of that site and of the head injury population in general. Patient characteristics and treatments are other potential sources of selection bias. The current regulatory requirement of two independent positive trials to demonstrate efficacy provides investigators with a test data set as long as the blind on the second trial remains intact.

Variation in prognostic factors

Variation in prognostic factors is a major cause of inconclusive findings when one tries to draw conclusions from a clinical trial. Interpretation of the results from a given "sample" of head injury patients can be subtly influenced by shifts in these prognostic factors.[11,12] The major factors are age, injury severity as defined by the GCS and selected features of the neurological exam, hypotension, hypoxia, the incidence of significant extracranial injuries, and the nature of the injuries themselves, that is, pathology.[28,29] The need to categorize and possibly prestratify subjects according to pathology was recognized by several investigators as a limitation of the trials of high-dose steroids conducted during the 1980s that are described later in this chapter. Randomization is no guarantee of balance across treatment groups, especially in diseases as complex and multifactorial as head injury. This has been the experience in critical care medicine clinical trials as well.[38]

The main option in regard to design is to prestratify patients before randomization, generally according to injury severity and other significant variables. These considerations should be developed in the formal statistical plan of the trial before the blind is broken for analysis. How prognostic factors contribute to the observed findings of a specific head injury clinical trial is uncertain but nonetheless is necessary to consider and evaluate. For example, one intuitively knows that small changes in the average age or the proportion of males in a head injury population can alter the observed mortality rate. Similar arguments can be made regarding the distribution and balance of pathology between treatment groups. What one needs to understand is how subtle multivariable imbalances can contribute to the findings of head injury clinical trials. Of course, this is in part the rationale for randomization of a large number of subjects. What to do about this issue is not clear. While a variety of statistical adjustment procedures exist, they have not been used in head injury trials to the extent that they should. In part, this occurs because it is often difficult to draw clear clinical information relevant to drug safety and efficacy from the results of the adjusted models, but many studies also are inadequately powered to allow such analysis (i.e., too few subjects were enrolled in the trials).

UNRESOLVED BIOSTATISTICAL ISSUES

Stopping a clinical trial can occur because of safety reasons, early detection of efficacy, or the futility of continuing the trial because of the low likelihood of a positive result if the trial is completed as planned; that is, the primary endpoint cannot possibly pass the statistical criteria for a positive study. Methods and procedures are available for stopping a trial for any of these reasons.[39]

Scientific interest and the daunting but exciting challenge of demonstrating the efficacy and safety of novel therapeutic compounds create considerable interest in participation in head injury clinical trials. Investigators are often desirous of participating in all the trials currently under way. However, the requirements of multiple-project organization, logistic problems such as overlapping eligibility and background management protocols, potential conflicts of interest, and possible ethical dilemmas indicate that researchers should exercise prudence in allowing concurrent enrollment in multiple trials at the same site.[40]

There are several reasons for defining subsets for subsequent analyses once the primary efficacy analysis has been performed. First, modest but important treatment effects in clinically relevant subpopulations may be hidden. Generally, this problem is considered under the heading of covariate adjustment or stratification. In the case of head injury, subclasses may not have been well defined or may be overidentified (i.e., too many categories).[28] In addition, mechanistic and prognostic classifications may or may not correspond. Current head injury trials should define these subsets in advance of analysis (i.e., before breaking the study blind). The availability of a prior independent trial can be helpful as a test set for defining potentially relevant subpopulations.

OUTCOME ASSESSMENT FOR HEAD INJURY TRIALS

BASIC OUTCOMES PARADIGMS

Several basic paradigms exist for outcomes assessment. Each has a rich tradition in the literature,[25] and the authors can only briefly touch on them in this section. One can concentrate on clinical outcomes such as mortality or measurements of *impairment* of motor function, sensory function, cognition, and behavior. Currently, there is no single validated and reliable scale for doing so, as exists for stroke (the NIH Stroke Scale). A second approach is to measure the *functional status* of the subject, generally by assessing the subject's ability to perform the basic activities of daily living. In addition, this includes measuring depression and anxiety. Reasonably good measures exist, but further validation in head injury populations may be necessary. Several reliable and useful functional status measures are available for the head injury population. The participants of the Houston Conference recommended the Rappaport Disability Rating Score as the most suitable for the head injury population, although the Barthel Index may also be useful as an adjunct measure to the GOS.[41]

A third approach is to assess overall *quality of life*, which may be viewed as the subject's perceived life status relative to his or her functional status. Finally, one can measure traditional economic endpoints such as return to work or days lost from work as well as the preference for or the value placed on alternative health states (i.e., *health utilities*).

CLINICAL OUTCOMES

While there is little to argue about in using mortality as a concrete endpoint for head injury clinical trials, one has to wonder whether much can be done about patients destined to die early from the direct effect of their injuries. Many current head injury clinical trials exclude patients with a GCS of 3 on admission. The most frequently used clinical outcome measure in head injury clinical trials is the 6-month GOS. The GOS provides a simple clinical measure of whole-body impairment, although sometimes there is an attempt to measure the "brain component" of the GOS.

There is less agreement on how to measure various impairments in different neurological systems. Successful and useful measures for clinical trials have been developed in other acute neurological diseases, such as the NIH Stroke Scale for ischemic stroke. An alternative would be the development of an impairment scoring system which provides a consistent and reliable way to "add up" the motor, sensory, cognitive, and behavioral impairments that characterize a head injury survivor. No such measure has been developed to date.

Neurobehavioral Outcomes

It has been typical to use a battery of tests to assess the cognitive status of a patient after a head injury. The participants in the Houston Conference made recommendations for a fairly straightforward and simple approach.[41] Also, the Traumatic Coma Data Bank investigators have provided a very reduced set of measures known to correlate with head injury outcome.[42] However, one should remember that two head injury patients can appear to have the same amount of gross disability, yet in one case it is largely due to neurophysical or cognitive impairments while in the other personality or emotional factors are largely responsible. The measures recommended by the Houston Conference attendees (Table 65-4) include a brief battery of neuropsychological tests and the Neurobehavioral Rating Scale.

Quality-of-Life Outcomes

Quality-of-life (QOL) outcomes are relevant efficacy measures in clinical studies of neurological disease. These measures assume a broader importance in light of current issues in health economics and managed health care. They also offer a way of comparing medical and surgical treatments. Also, such measures may help in differentiating between therapies with marginal differences in clinical outcome. In the future, these may be useful adjuncts to the regulatory approval process if not the primary criteria for approval.

The interest in QOL measurement in neuroscience populations is clearly growing. Until now much of this has been implicit rather than explicit measurement; that is, if one prevents bad outcomes, one ensures a good quality of life. This naive view ignores the fact that, emotionally and socially, some lives may not be worth returning to. Still unresolved is whether researchers should use a generic QOL measure or one adapted for the specific disease of interest. Regardless, at present there are few compelling data regarding the reliability and validity of various QOL measures in head injury populations. Physicians do not even know the nature of the outcome distributions of QOL measures in head injury groups. Thus, the response over time to therapeutic interventions is difficult to gauge with QOL measures. Furthermore, when to ascertain these measures is even more difficult to decide. Not knowing the time course, researchers do not know whether they are using the right point to demonstrate efficacy. Finally, how do numerical differences in QOL measures translate into clinically meaningful terms? This is an important issue in head injury clinical trials, since the victims are largely young, healthy individuals. Survivors may live for a long time, and the natural history of aging after a traumatic brain injury is not described. Usually investigators want to use a comprehensive battery of tests, but this can be difficult in head injury trials in which crisp and relevant assessment protocols are desired.

TABLE 65-4 Recommended Outcome Measures in Head Injury Patients

Domain	Measure Recommended	Appropriate Population
Clinical outcome	Glasgow Outcome Score	Severe and moderate
	Rappaport Disability Rating Score	Severe and moderate
Social adjustment and personality	Neurobehavioral Rating Scale	Severe and moderate
Attention	Digit Symbol	Severe and moderate
	Paced Auditory Serial Addition Task	Moderate only
Memory	Rey Complex Figure	Severe and moderate
	Selective Reminding	Severe and moderate
Language	Controlled Word Association	Severe and moderate
Mental process	Trail Making	Severe and moderate
	Wisconsin Card Sorting	Moderate only
Motor	Grooved Pegboard	Severe and moderate

SOURCE: Adapted from Clifton GL, Hayes RL, Levin HS, et al: Outcome measures for clinical trials involving traumatically brain-injured patients: Report of a conference. *Neurosurgery* 31:975–978, 1992.

Economic Outcomes

Productivity losses (e.g., days lost from work) by the subject constitute a typical socioeconomic endpoint.[43,44] Usually these data are obtained through a questionnaire or interview in which preinjury and posttreatment employment status is documented and compared. Economists have also proposed utility assessment, in which a preference for a given health state versus death or complete health is measured. These measures have a decided advantage in that questionnaire responses in which the patient or caregiver gives his or her own rating scale score for the patient's health state are scored to provide a *population-based* reference for the health state. Less direct measures include visual analogue scales in which the patient or family member indicates the patient's current health status on a scale from poorest to perfect health or responds to QOL questions.

Cost-utility analysis is another important method of evaluating the net social benefit of therapeutic interventions. This approach requires a reasonable measure of utility. The Health Utilities Index (HUI) is a six-question instrument that also asks about different aspects of the patient's health state. Developed by Drummond and coworkers,[45] this instrument is accompanied by scores that can be used to translate the responses into utility values. However, at present the HUI does not contain its own rating scale. It may be necessary to add a generic rating scale or validate the utilities for a brain injury population.

HEAD INJURY TRIALS PAST AND PRESENT

This section reviews the published reports of head injury clinical trials conducted during the 1980s and 1990s (Tables 65-5 and 65-6). Table 65-7 describes the incidence of "favorable outcomes" (defined by the GOS categories "good recovery" and "moderate disability") and the incidence of unfavorable outcome (GOS "dead" and "persistent vegetative state"). Many trials are currently under way and will be briefly mentioned in this section,

TABLE 65-5 Randomized Clinical Trials of High-Dose Corticosteroids in Head Injury

Study	Inclusion Criteria	Exclusion Criteria	Subjects per Arm	Primary Endpoint
Dearden et al, 1986[17]	Severe injury GCS ≤ 8 or GCS > 8 and deterioration	Brain-dead Prior steroid treatment Incorrect administration of study treatment	68 high dose 62 placebo	6-month GOS
Giannotta et al, 1984[19]	GCS ≤ 8	History of peptic ulcer Prior steroid treatment Penetrating injury "Serious" noncerebral injury likely to cause death Undiagnosed/untreated medical condition Pregnancy	38 high dose 34 low dose 16 placebo	6-month GOS
Braakman et al, 1983[50]	Coma (GCS ≤ 8*) Severe nonmissile injury Dosing within 6 h of injury	Brain-dead or expected in 1 h Conscious at initial emergency room exam Prior steroid treatment "Selected dosed patients"	81 high dose 80 placebo	1-month survival
Saul et al, 1981[51]	GCS ≤ 7 Isolated head injury Dosing within 6 h of injury	Injuries causing death within 72 h	50 high dose 50 placebo	6-month GOS
Pitts and Kaktis 1980[33]	Coma on admission or lapse into coma for at least 6 h after admission	ICP monitored < 12 h	36 high dose 22 low dose 18 placebo	ICP up to 72 h
Cooper et al, 1979[52]	Severe injury	Not included in publication	24 high dose† 25 low dose 27 placebo	6-month GOS

* GCS inferred from authors' discussion.

† An additional 21 subjects were available for subsequent analysis, but the detail was insufficient to report in this table.

TABLE 65-6 Randomized Trials of Selected Neurotherapeutic Compounds in Head Injury

Study	Drug	Inclusion Criteria	Exclusion Criteria	Subjects per Arm	Primary Endpoint
Braakman, 1991[56]	Nimodipine	Not obeying commands at entry Dosing within 24 h after injury *and* 12 h not obeying commands 16–70 years old CT scan	Prior treatment confounds evaluation (e.g., paralysis) Systemically unstable Gunshot wound (GSW) Pregnancy Wide nonreacting pupils and motor absent after 2 h Likelihood of death within 24 h due to multiple trauma Unlikely availability for 6-month follow-up	405 drug 411 placebo	6-month GOS*
Muizelaar et al, 1993[59]	Superoxide dismutase	GCS ≤ 8 Age ≥ 15 Unable to follow commands Dosing within 12 h of injury	Brain-dead after resuscitation Penetrating injury Pregnancy	27 high dose 25 middle dose 26 low dose 26 placebo	3-month GOS 6-month GOS (primary not specified)
Wolf et al, 1993[54]	Tromethamine	GCS ≤ 8 Age 16–75	Chronic renal failure Admission creatinine clearance ≤ 30 ml/min Massive blood transfusions for multiple trauma Major visceral injury GSW GCS 3 for whom only supportive care Pregnancy	73 drug 76 control	3-month GOS 6-month GOS 12-month GOS (primary not specified)
Muizelaar et al, 1991[53]	Tromethamine	GCS ≤ 8 after resuscitation and treatment of mass lesions Age ≥ 3	Not stated	36 HV† + drug 36 HV alone 41 NV‡	12-month GOS 3- and 6-month GOS
Maldonado et al, 1991[60]	CDP-choline	GCS 5–10	Open trauma Severe systemic disease	115 drug 101 control	3-month GOS
Teasdale et al, 1990[55]	Nimodipine	Not obeying simple commands within first 24 h after injury	Hemodynamic instability Brain-dead Systemic decompensation (renal, hepatic, pulmonary, or cardiac) Pregnancy	176 drug 175 placebo	6-month GOS

* GOS = Glasgow Outcome Score; GCS = Glasgow Coma Scale.
† HV = hyperventilation.
‡ NV = normal ventilation.

since only a few have been very recently completed and have not generated published reports. The main purpose of this section is to gain an appreciation of the evolution of clinical trials in head injury during the past 15 years. These pioneering efforts set the stage for the current large and complex phase III trials of novel compounds for head injury (Table 65-1).

BARBITURATES (PENTOBARBITAL)

Evidence from nonrandomized clinical studies has indicated a potential benefit of high-dose barbiturates for the control of unresponsive intracranial pressure (ICP).[46–49] In a subsequent multicenter trial, pentobarbital was administered to 80 randomized patients se-

TABLE 65-7 Incidence of Favorable and Unfavorable Outcomes in Head Injury Trials*

A. High-Dose Corticosteroids Trials

Study	*Favorable Outcome, %* Drug	*Favorable Outcome, %* Control	Difference	*Dead and Vegetative, %* Drug	*Dead and Vegetative, %* Control	Difference
Deardon et al, 1986[17]	44.0 (68)	56.5 (62)	−12.5	48.5 (68)	35.5 (62)	+13.0
Giannotta et al, 1984[19]	26.3 (38)	31.2 (16)	−4.9	47.4 (38)	62.5 (16)	−15.1
Braakman et al, 1983[50]	29.6 (81)	32.5 (80)	−1.9	56.8 (81)	61.2 (80)	−4.4
Saul et al, 1981[51]	52.0† (50)	62.0† (50)	−10.0	48.0 (50)	38.0 (50)	+10.0
Pitts and Kaktis, 1980[33]	38.8‡ (58)	32.2‡ (18)	+6.6	60.7 (58)	49.3 (18)	+11.4
Cooper et al, 1979[52]	29.2 (29)	37.0 (37)	−7.8	66.6 (29)	48.1 (37)	+18.5

B. Selected Neurotherapeutic Head Injury Trials

Study	*Favorable Outcome, %* Drug	*Favorable Outcome, %* Control	Difference	*Dead and Vegetative, %* Drug	*Dead and Vegetative, %* Control	Difference
Braakman, 1991[56]	60.5 (405)	59.4 (414)	+1.1	25.4 (405)	28.3 (414)	−2.9
Muizelaar et al, 1993[59]	62.5§ (24)	56.0§ (25)	+6.5	20.8 (24)	36.0 (25)	15.2
Wolf et al, 1993[54]	49.3 (73)	55.3 (76)	−6.0	31.5 (73)	34.2 (76)	2.7
Muizelaar et al, 1991[53]	36.1# (29)	36.6 (37)	−0.5	nr¶	nr	nr
Maldonado et al, 1991[60]	83.4 (115)	81.2 (101)	+2.2	15.7 (115)	9.9 (101)	+5.8
Teasdale et al, 1990[55]	52.0 (176)	49.0 (175)	+3.0	nr	nr	nr

* Favorable outcomes defined as Glasgow Outcome Score categories "good recovery" and "moderate disability." Unfavorable outcome defined as GOS categories "dead" and "persistent vegetative state."

† Favorable outcome includes severe disability category.

‡ High- and low-dose drug groups combined.

§ High-dose drug group.

Drug group = THAM plus hyperventilation. Hyperventilation alone also reported.

¶ nr = not reported; i.e., detail in publication was insufficient to report in this table.

lected from 117 who met final eligibility criteria; the final set of eligible patients represented a reduction from 925 patients initially eligible from preliminary screening.[47] Although pentobarbital was clearly effective in lowering ICP, the results were inconclusive regarding outcome because of the crossover study design. Thus, no definitive statement could be made regarding the efficacy of high-dose barbiturates in improving outcome from head injury.[47] A lengthier discussion of this study by one of the authors of this chapter is available.[11]

High-Dose Corticosteroids (Dexamethasone)

Based on the well-known anti-inflammatory, immunosuppressive, and membrane-stabilizing properties of glucocorticoids, single-center randomized clinical trials of high-dose corticosteroids were conducted from the late 1970s through the mid-1980s. These studies constitute the largest set of modern clinical trials that test a single clinical hypothesis in head injury. The authors examined six published reports that represent the best studies available and are illustrative of the state of the art during this epoch.[17,19,33,50–52] They are described in Table 65-5. The studies were largely double-blind, placebo-controlled trials on patients seen at single neurosurgical centers. Only one study involved two sites, while another used a standard-care control group rather than a placebo.[50,51] These high-dose steroids trials were pioneering in bringing modern clinical trials methodology to head injury even though they involved only one or two centers. These studies also illustrate the refinement of the inputs that define inclusion and exclusion criteria for current head injury trials. However, it is easy to be critical of these studies from the point of view of design or data analysis. For example, the importance of intent-to-treat analysis was not recognized or fully appreciated during this epoch.

The 6-month GOS was the primary efficacy endpoint in four of the six high-dose steroids trials examined, with 1-month survival being used in one study. Pitts and Kaktis[33] were the only investigators to conduct a study with a mechanistic endpoint (increased ICP up to 72 h after injury) as the primary efficacy outcome measure. Although the use of this endpoint makes it impossible to achieve a double-blind study, there are fairly good reasons to consider this a valid and useful surrogate endpoint.

Reporting of the details of past randomized head injury clinical trials has not been consistent or uniform, and so it is difficult to determine whether subject selection (i.e. inclusion and exclusion) was truly consistent across the studies. At a minimum, it is difficult to discern with accuracy how the reported differences in inclusion and exclusion criteria might have influenced the findings or conclusions reached regarding the safety and efficacy of high-dose corticosteroids. Unequal randomization procedures were used in two studies to allocate subjects to the high-dose steroids, low-dose steroids, or placebo arms of the trial. For example, Pitts and Kaktis[33] employed an unequal randomization procedure to enroll 18 (placebo), 22 (low-dose), and 36 (high-dose) subjects in the treatment arms of their trial.

The trials of high-dose steroids were limited to subjects with severe head injury on admission as defined by the admission GCS or subsequent changes in the GCS indicating early neurological deterioration (i.e., before treatment). Exclusion of essentially brain-dead patients or those likely to die early from other injuries was attempted by most investigators, but differences in definition apply, and it is not entirely clear how consistently these exclusion criteria were applied across the studies reviewed. Most investigators excluded penetrating injuries, and later studies in the series excluded patients with prior steroid treatment; this, in addition to issues of safety, could cloud an evaluation of efficacy. Pitts and Kaktis[33] included patients comatose on admission or within 6 h of injury and excluded patients whose ICP was monitored for less than 12 h, children, and patients with impending brain death, open head injuries, or impression fractures. They further acknowledged that there were "posttreatment exclusions." Saul and colleagues[51] also included patients within 6 h of injury with GCS < 8 but excluded all patients with extracranial injuries. In addition, these investigators excluded subjects whose injuries caused death within 72 h after injury, and this might have had an impact on the primary endpoint (the GOS). Braakman and coworkers[50] included subjects with severe nonmissile injury who were in coma on admission when treatment was initiated within 6 h of injury. They restricted admission GCS to 8 or less and excluded patients who were brain-dead on arrival or were expected to die within 1 h, patients who were conscious during the emergency room exam, and patients who had received prior steroid therapy at a treating hospital. They also acknowledged excluding "some dosed patients" from data analysis; that is, they did not use an intent-to-treat analysis. Giannotta and colleagues[19] continued to refine inclusion and exclusion criteria on the basis of safety and efficacy considerations. They excluded patients with a history of peptic ulcer, patients with an undiagnosed or untreated medical condition, patients who had been treated with steroids within 2 weeks of injury, patients with penetrating wounds, and patients with "serious noncerebral injuries" that were likely to cause death. Finally, Dearden and associates[17] excluded patients with prior steroid treatment and those who were brain-dead on admission as well as subjects in whom the study drug was "improperly administered"; that is, they also did not use an intent-to-treat analysis.

Seldom did study reports describe the dosing regimen in terms of the timing or duration of treatment. Dearden and associates[17] dosed subjects for 5 days after injury, with the initial dose typically given within 6 to 8 h after injury. Other investigators did not report the dosing regimen, but when it could be reasonably inferred from the report, 6 h after injury was the preferred time for the initial dose.

There is insufficient information in the published reports to determine whether the studies were adequately powered to detect a clinically relevant difference between the treated and placebo groups. In retrospect, most of the studies might have stopped early anyway. Yet a definitive answer regarding the efficacy of high-dose steroids may not be drawn from the studies reported to date if the apparent safety issue is manageable or is limited to specific patient subpopulations. Several provocative findings were reported that pointed toward the future of clinical trials for acute head injury. Dearden and associates[17] reported that steroid therapy in patients with increased ICP was associated with worse outcomes. This early concern over the possibility of pathological outcomes is manifested today in similar concerns that new compounds might "save" marginal patients (i.e., saved only to remain in a vegetative state) or "push" better outcomes into worse outcome categories. Braakman and colleagues[50] terminated their trial on the grounds of futility when it was determined through sequential analysis procedures that the likelihood of a positive study for the 1-month survival endpoint could not be achieved after 161 subjects were enrolled and matured to the outcome assessment time. Giannotta and coworkers[19] reported a positive mortality effect but acknowledged the possibility of poor outcomes for survivors in the area of speech recovery. Finally, Pitts and Kaktis[33] reported a positive mortality effect but also reported a considerably higher rate of "unconscious, but stable" patients in the treated group in an activity analysis (i.e., by pooling both the low- and high-dose groups and comparing them with placebo). What subsequently happened to those subjects would have been of help in determining the efficacy of the high-dose steroids. It is interesting to note that in the Pitts and Kaktis[33] trial, the "fully recovered" rate in the combined steroid group was higher than it was with placebo.

Lactate Buffer (Tromethamine)

CO_2-induced cerebral vasoconstriction leading to decreased ICP has been the underlying rationale for the use of sustained hyperventilation therapy in the management of head injury patients.[53,54] Of the utmost concern in patients undergoing prolonged severe hyperventilation is managing the risk of diminished cerebral CO_2 leading to an increase in pH and thus initiating a destructive acidosis.[3] The buffer tromethamine (THAM) was proposed to counteract the depletion of bicarbonate buffer in CSF as a result of the short-lived deleterious effect of hyperventilation on CSF pH and subsequent arteriolar diameter. This hypothesis was tested by Muizelaar and coworkers,[53] who conducted a three-arm management trial comparing normal ventilation with sustained hyperventilation alone and with THAM. Table 65-6 summarizes the design of this trial. This single-site trial was randomized, but the nature of the treatment prevented blinding or the use of a placebo control. Patients 3 years and older with a GCS of 8 or less after resuscitation and neurosurgical treatment for mass lesions were eligible for inclusion. Block randomization procedures within strata defined by GCS motor score (GCS_{motor} 1 through 3 and GCS_{motor} 4 through 5) were used to ensure that a balance of key prognostic factors would be achieved. The sample sizes were small (36 to 41 patients per group), and there were insufficient data reported to determine whether the study was adequately powered. Balance appeared to be reasonably achieved for average GCS and other indicators of injury severity.

The THAM study was terminated for safety considerations based on a sequential analysis of the data.[53] Although the primary efficacy endpoint was the 12-month GOS, at 3 months the "hyperventilation alone" group showed a decreased favorable outcome rate compared with the "normal ventilation" group. Age and admission motor score were used as covariates and treatment by covariate interaction terms indicated that the effect was pronounced in the GCS_{motor} 4 through 5 group, and so the study was terminated. When the subjects matured to the final analysis endpoint and the data were later analyzed, the decrease in favorable outcome was no longer evident at 12 months after injury. It is not clear whether survival analysis procedures would have proved useful in this decision making, since it is not clear that the subjects included in the analysis at 3 months were all fully mature. This could subtly bias the observations, since subjects who die are more likely to be included in the samples for comparison. The investigators noted that the THAM group subjects might have been less severely injured. Of course, hindsight and experience are excellent teachers.

Continuing the hope for an effective reversal of the potential adverse effects of prophylactic hyperventilation on early recovery, Wolf and coworkers[54] reported a further study of THAM to reduce cerebral acidosis (and thus ICP) in a 149-patient trial. Four hundred thirty-eight patients were screened to identify the 149 subjects subsequently enrolled in the trial. Patients who were 16 to 75 years old with a GCS of 8 or less were eligible. Patients with chronic renal failure, those admitted with creatinine clearance of 30 ml/min or less, those requiring massive blood transfusions, those with gunshot wounds, and those with a GCS of 3 for whom only supportive measures were given were excluded. Not enough data were provided on the 289 excluded patients to allow an evaluation of the potential selection biases imposed by the screening criteria. For subjects included in the trial, the balance across the treatment groups for age, sex, surgical mass lesions, GCS, and initial recorded ICP was reasonably good.

No significant findings were reported regarding the efficacy endpoints, but the investigators did replicate the finding of a decrease in the percentage of time when ICP was greater than 20 mmHg in the first 48 h after injury. In addition, fewer subjects in the THAM group required barbiturate coma therapy (5.48 percent versus 18.4 percent, $p < .05$), a marker of the treatment intensity level. The authors reported that the THAM-treated subjects were worse at 3 months after injury but that there were no differences between the THAM and control groups at 6 or 12 months after injury.[54]

Calcium Antagonists (Nimodipine)

The largest published phase III multicenter clinical trials in head injury to date have been the studies of the calcium channel blocker nimodipine (Table 65-6). Teasdale and the British/Finnish Group[55] reported a study involving 351 patients treated for 7 days after injury, initially at 1 mg/h and then at 2 mg/h if the patient's blood pressure tolerated it. Braakman and the European Nimodipine Group[56] analyzed data on 819 evaluable patients. Both studies were randomized, double-blind, placebo-controlled trials and used the 6-month GOS as the primary efficacy endpoint. The European group used a block randomized design, assigning subjects to treatment groups within each center to ensure a balance of prognostic factors in the treatment and placebo arms. In both studies a balance of important prognostic factors appeared to be achieved.

Cerebral ischemia is an important mechanism of traumatic brain injury. The British/Finnish group implicated "traumatic vasospasm," while the European group implicated the hypoxic/ischemic damage caused by decreased cerebral blood flow. The major inclusion criterion in the British/Finnish study was "not obeying commands within 24 hours after injury."[55]

The larger European group trial included patients 16 to 70 years old who had a CT scan, were in a stable systemic condition, and were treated within 24 h of injury but within 12 h of not following commands. This design twist would allow for the inclusion of many of the "talk and die" patients while allowing the exclusion of patients who were essentially brain-dead on admission. Both investigator groups were concerned about the use of nimodipine in patients who were systematically or hemodynamically unstable because of a potential complication of drug-induced hypotension and therefore were excluded. The British/Finnish group also excluded patients with pretreatment renal, hepatic, pulmonary, or cardiac complications, which might have led to systemic decompensation. The European group also excluded multiple-trauma patients who were not likely to survive 24 h after injury, and in addition, for the first time, reported an exclusion based on the likely availability for follow-up at 6 months.

In the British/Finnish study, 83 percent of subjects were admitted to the hospital (neurosurgical services) within 6 h after injury and 68 percent entered the study within 12 h after injury. This important fact was seldom reported in past head injury clinical trials. "Favorable outcome" as defined by the GOS ("good recovery" or "moderate disability") was nearly identical in the two treatment groups; 52 percent (nimodipine) versus 49 percent (placebo). The number of dead subjects in the two groups was very close, with most deaths attributed directly to the head injuries.

The European group rejected the hypothesis that nimodipine would increase favorable outcome from 50 percent to 60 percent at 6 months after injury, a 20 percent relative difference. In fact, the 6-month favorable outcome rates were 60.5 percent versus 59.4 percent and the GOS distributions in the two treatment groups were remarkably similar.[56] There was a trend in favorable outcome in the subjects with subarachnoid hemorrhage (SAH) on the baseline CT scan, but this is a post hoc comparison which is being assessed in a follow-up study. The investigators also performed a secondary analysis on all "valid patients," defined as subjects who received at least 80 percent of study doses, but this did not provide further information.

Free Radical Inhibitors (PEG-SOD)

The oxygen radical superoxide anion has been implicated in the pathophysiology of traumatic brain injury.[57,58] The most common presumed pathway is ischemic injury and/or ischemic-reperfusion injury. Control of sustained high ICP and amelioration of vicious secondary insults (i.e., hypoxia, hypotension, and intracranial hypertension) caused by the destructive effects of oxygen free radicals was the rationale for testing polyethylene glycol–conjugated superoxide dismutase (PEG-SOD) in a double-blind, placebo-controlled phase II trial that involved 104 subjects and was conducted at two sites[59] (Table 65-6). The study was a four-arm dose-ranging trial in which high (10,000 units/kg), medium (5,000 units/kg), and low (2,000 units/kg) doses of PEG-SOD were compared with placebo. Patients 15 years or older who were admitted with a GCS of 8 or less and were unable to follow commands after resuscitation were eligible for the study. Initial dosing with the study drug was required within 12 h of injury. Patients likely to be brain-dead after resuscitation and patients with penetrating injuries were excluded. A block randomization strategy was employed to balance prognostic factors within the two participating centers, and this appeared to be reasonably successful with the exception of age in the high-dose (10,000 units/kg) PEG-SOD group (mean, 34 years old) compared with the placebo group (mean, 25 years old). Both the 3-month and 6-month GOS were reported, but the investigators did not report which was considered the primary study endpoint.[59]

There were promising results with respect to ICP control. The percentage of time when ICP exceeded 20 mmHg was less in the 5,000- and 10,000-unit dose groups. The effect size was modest. Further, the 10,000-

unit dose group required less mannitol for the management of ICP on day 2 and day 3 after injury. There was no significant difference in either the 3- or the 6-month GOS outcome endpoints, although there were promising trends.[59] At 3 months, 44 percent of the placebo group were dead or vegetative, versus 20 percent in the 10,000-unit dose group. At 6 months, the dead and vegetative rates were 36 percent and 21 percent in the high-dose and placebo groups, respectively. However, results using a logistic regression model adjusting for age, GCS, and center indicated significantly higher favorable outcome rates in the high-dose group at both 3 months ($p < .03$) and 6 months ($p \leq .04$) after injury. A potential weakness of this analysis, however, was that "severe disability" was included in the definition of "favorable outcome," which represents a departure from past and current usage.[59] If only the "good recovery" and "moderate disability" categories were used to define "favorable outcome," there was no significance ($p = .18$ at 3 months, $p = .71$ at 6 months). Based on these findings, phase III studies were planned and have recently been completed. We are awaiting the final published results.

Phospholipid Metabolism (CDP-Choline)

Decreases in cell membrane phospholipids leading to failure of the sodium-potassium pump and eventually causing cytotoxic edema were the underlying mechanism of cellular damage used to justify the use of citicoline (CDP-choline), a precursor in the synthesis of glycerophospholipids. CDP-choline was tested at a single center in Spain in a group of 216 patients with a history of head injury and a GCS of 5 to 10 on admission[60] (Table 65-6). The study was a single-blind, standard-care controlled trial, and patients with open trauma and severe systemic disease were excluded from eligibility. The 3-month GOS was the primary efficacy endpoint, and other endpoints were posttraumatic symptoms (headaches, dizziness, memory problems), motor dysfunction, IQ, personality changes, and total days in the intensive care unit.

More deaths were observed in the CDP-choline group (18, or 15.7 percent) than in the conventional care control group (10, or 9.9 percent). Only survivors were compared in the final efficacy analysis, and while the CDP-choline group did not appear to differ in terms of favorable outcome (83.5 percent versus 81.2 percent of the controls), 66.9 percent were good recovery compared with 50.5 percent of the controls.[60] While the CDP-choline group was consistently better than the controls in the other endpoints, most of the differences were not statistically significant.

Head Injury Trials in Progress

Head injury clinical trials have become large and complex, with more sophisticated design and logistics: For example, the use of futility analysis, which resulted in the termination of one of the high-dose steroids trials,[50] or the increasing appreciation of pathological outcomes recognized by investigators testing high-dose corticosteroids set the stage for current head injury clinical trials. Contributing to the increasing complexity of current head injury trials is the availability of novel compounds for human testing (Table 65-1).

The past 10 years have been very exciting, as the development of possible treatments for traumatic brain injury has intensified. Clarification of the role of acidosis in the pathogenesis of neuronal damage, the implication of overstimulation of excitatory amino acids (EAA, principally glutamate) in neuronal damage after head injury,[61–64] recognition of the horribly destructive consequences of free radical species,[65–67] and finally the growing recognition that excessive calcium influx is a final common pathway drove many potential solutions[64,68–72] in the form of novel compounds to inhibit EAA, prevent ischemic injury, and eliminate oxygen free radical–induced lipid peroxidation.

Many head injury clinical trials are under way for evaluating these truly novel compounds. As researchers have matured in our trials experience, they have recognized that the demands of testing these compounds are much different from those involved in testing an already approved drug.

Until recently, improvement in clinical trial design and methodology has been incremental. Frustrating our efforts is the growing recognition that increasingly sophisticated critical care serving as the background for testing a new drug may have greater than anticipated efficacy. This was discovered by investigators evaluating high-dose barbiturates for treating intractable ICP. Experienced trial clinicians know that patients seem to do better when they are on a clinical trial. A large number of patients may be screened, but a much smaller number are actually enrolled in a trial. This points to the potential need for adjudication and assessment of reliability in the possible presence of selection bias. While this potential problem may not create difficulty in the assessment of efficacy, investigators may be very limited in their ability to assess the likely effectiveness of a drug for the intended patient population.

There is a need for sharper inclusion and exclusion criteria. The trade-off is between the simplicity of enrollment criteria to ensure an adequate accrual and ease of enrollment in the trial. Reporting of head injury trials has not been adequate, particularly with respect to the background treatment and dosing regimen. Multiple endpoints are required, but investigators have sometimes been reluctant to specify the primary endpoint, that is, the one measure that will determine efficacy, rather than a lengthy list of potential endpoints. Finally, it is understood that ethical concerns must weigh heavily in the conduct of head injury clinical trials and in fact may overwhelm all other issues.

The most aggressive head injury drug development program in the 1990s has been Upjohn's studies of tirilazad mesylate, a novel 21-aminosteroid that is also currently being tested in SAH and stroke. The North American and international phase III tirilazad head injury trials have been completed, and the results are expected soon. We are also eagerly awaiting the results of the phase III PEG-SOD trial. Currently, the phase III Ciba-Geigy CGS-19755 (Selfotel) trial is in the accrual period. A phase II trial of Bradycor, Cortech's bradykinin antagonist, was halted because of safety concerns in another trial for a non-CNS indication. Several other head injury compounds are nearing phase III testing, such as Sandoz's EAA-494 and Cambridge Neuroscience's Cerestat. In addition, Neurex's SNX-11 and an adenosine antagonist are, or may soon be, in early human testing.

What can be expected from the current head injury trials? Table 65-7 summarizes the incidence of favorable outcomes (good recovery and moderate disability) in the published studies reviewed for this chapter. The effect sizes are small to modest. In the case of the high-dose steroid trials, absolute differences were 12 percent or less and generally were unfavorable to the drug group. The relatively small numbers of patients in these trials indicate that it is prudent to interpret the size of these differences with caution. More disturbing are the sizes of differences in the poor outcomes (dead and vegetative), which are unfavorable to the drug group. In two of the steroid trials, the incidence of poor outcomes was lower in the drug groups.[19,50] Yet in the same studies the incidence of favorable outcomes was slightly lower in the drug group. The relatively small numbers of patients make this difficult to interpret. With the exception of the phase II PEG-SOD trial,[59] very small to virtually no differences in favorable outcome were observed (Table 65-7). The modest increase in favorable outcomes (6.5 percent) was complemented by a 15 percent reduction in poor outcomes in favor of the drug group. A fair proportion of these "saves" survived with "severe disability" (as defined by the GOS), and it would be worth knowing more about the quality of their survival. It should be noted that the group sizes were small and that these findings, while encouraging, are not sufficient to establish definitive efficacy. The phase III PEG-SOD trial has recently been completed, and the results should be published soon.

It is likely that the current head injury trials will demonstrate small beneficial effects. For many of the reasons described earlier in this chapter, one should expect a complex pattern of findings in large phase III head injury trials. Simple treatment effects may be difficult to detect against the background noise of the natural history of head injury. Further complicating investigators' ability to detect efficacy is variability in management from patient to patient and center to center. The term "head injury" refers to a complex, multifactorial group of diseases. This complexity must somehow be captured in a simple enough fashion to be of practical use in a clinical trial and yet be faithful to the primary disease. This is a daunting challenge. However, the increasing availability of new compounds to test and the evolution of head injury clinical trials methodology in the past 15 years indicate that there is reason to be optimistic.

References

1. Langfitt TW, Gennarelli TA: Can the outcome from head injury be improved? *J Neurosurg* 56:19–25, 1982.
2. Marshall LF, Eisenberg HM, Jane JA, et al: The outcome of severe closed head injury. *J Neurosurg* 75:S28–S36, 1991.
3. Becker DP: Common themes in head injury, in Becker DP, Gudeman SK (eds): *Textbook of Head Injury.* Philadelphia: Saunders, 1989, pp 1–22.
4. Gennarelli TA, Thibault LE: Biological models of head injury, in Becker DP, Povlishock JT (eds): *Central Nervous System Trauma Status Report.* Bethesda: National Institute of Neurological and Communicative Disorders and Stroke, National Institutes of Health, 1985, pp 391–404.
5. Graham DI, Adams JH, Gennarelli TA: Pathology of brain damage in head injury, in Cooper PR (ed): *Head Injury*, 3d ed. Baltimore: Williams & Wilkins, 1993, pp 91–113.
6. Mathieu M: *New Drug Development: A Regulatory Overview,* rev. 3d ed. Waltham, MA: PAREXEL International, 1994.
7. O'Grady J, Linet OI (eds): *Early Phase Drug Development in Man.* Boca Raton, FL: CRC Press, 1990.
8. Peace KE (ed): *Biopharmaceutical Statistics for Drug Development.* New York: Marcel Dekker, 1988.
9. Meinert CL: *Clinical Trials: Design, Conduct, and Analysis.* New York: Oxford University Press, 1986.
10. Winer BJ: *Statistical Principles in Experimental Design*, 2d ed. New York: McGraw-Hill, 1971.
11. Eisenberg HM: Head and spinal cord injury, in Porter RJ, Schoenberg BS (eds): *Controlled Clinical Trials in Neurological Disease.* Boston: Kluwer, 1990, pp 171–183.
12. Miller JD, Teasdale GM: Clinical trials for assessing treatment for severe head injury, in Becker DP, Povlishock JT (eds): *Central Nervous System Trauma Status Report.* Bethesda: National Institute of Neurological and Communicative Disorders and Stroke, National Institutes of Health, 1985, pp 17–32.

13. Haines SJ: Randomized clinical trials in neurosurgery. *Neurosurgery* 12:259–264, 1983.
14. Fleiss JL: *The Design and Analysis of Clinical Experiments*. New York: Wiley, 1986.
15. McIntosh TK, Vink R, Yamakami I, Faden AI: Magnesium protects against neurological deficit after brain injury. *Brain Res* 482:252–260, 1989.
16. McIntosh TK, Faden AI, Tamakami I, Vink R: Magnesium deficiency exacerbates and pretreatment improves outcome from traumatic brain injury in rats. *J Neurotrauma* 5:17–31, 1988.
17. Dearden NM, Gibson JS, Chir B, et al: Effect of high-dose dexamethasone on outcome from severe head injury. *J Neurosurg* 64:81–88, 1986.
18. Chestnut RM: Medical complications of the head injured patient, in Cooper PR (ed): *Head Injury*, 3d ed. Baltimore: Williams & Wilkins, 1993, pp 459–502.
19. Giannotta SL, Weiss MH, Apuzzo MLJ, Martin E: High dose glucocorticoids in the management of severe head injury. *Neurosurgery* 15:497–501, 1984.
20. Irwin RP, Nutt JG: Principles of neuropharmacology: I. Pharmacokinetics and pharmacodynamics, in Klawans HL, Goetz CG, Tanner CM (eds): *Textbook of Clinical Neuropharmacology and Therapeutics,* 2nd ed. New York: Raven Press, 1992, pp 1–14.
21. Dambrosia JM: Statistical and epidemiological consideration, in Porter RJ, Schoenberg BS (eds): *Controlled Clinical Trials in Neurological Disease.* Boston: Kluwer, 1990, pp 29–51.
22. Kraus JF: Epidemiology of head injury, in Cooper PR (ed): *Head Injury*, 3d ed. Baltimore: Williams & Wilkins, 1993, pp 1–25.
23. Vollmer DG: Prognosis and outcome of severe head injury, in Cooper PR (ed): *Head Injury*, 3d ed. Baltimore: Williams & Wilkins, 1993, pp 553–581.
24. Jennett B, Bond MR: Assessment of outcome after severe brain damage. *Lancet* 1:480–484, 1975.
25. Spilker B (ed): *Quality of Life Assessments in Clinical Trials.* New York: Raven Press, 1990.
26. Teasdale G, Jennett B: Assessment of coma and impaired consciousness: A practical scale. *Lancet* 2:81–84, 1974.
27. Gennarelli TA, Spielman GM, Langfitt TW, et al: Influence of the type of intracranial lesion on outcome from severe head injury: A multicenter study using a new classification system. *J Neurosurg* 56:26–32, 1982.
28. Marshall LF, Marshall SB, Klauber MR, et al: The diagnosis of head injury requires a classification based on computed axial tomography. *J Neurotrauma* 9:S287–S292, 1992.
29. Chesnut RM, Marshall LF, Klauber MR, et al: The role of secondary brain injury in determining outcome from severe head injury. *J Trauma* 34:216–222, 1993.
30. Gennarelli TA, Champion HR, Copes WS, Sacco WJ: Comparison of mortality, morbidity, and severity of 59,713 head injured patients with 114,447 patients with extracranial injuries. *J Trauma* 37:962–968, 1994.
31. Choi SC, Muizelaar JP, Barnes TY: Prediction tree for severely injured patients. *J Neurosurg* 75:251–255, 1991.
32. Choi SC, Barnes TY, Bullock R, et al: Temporal profile of outcomes in severe head injury. *J Neurosurg* 81:169–173, 1994.
33. Pitts LH, Kaktis JV: Effect of megadose steroids on ICP in traumatic coma, in Shulman K, Marmarou A, Miller JD, et al (eds): *Intracranial Pressure IV.* Berlin/Heidelberg/New York: Springer-Verlag, 1980, pp 638–642.
34. Koch GG, Edwards S: Clinical efficacy trials with categorical data, in Peace KE (ed): *Biopharmaceutical Statistics for Drug Development.* New York: Marcel Dekker, 1988, pp 403–457.
35. Morrison DF: *Multivariate Statistical Methods*, 3d ed. New York: McGraw-Hill, 1990.
36. O'Brien PC, Shampo MA: Statistical considerations for performing multiple tests in a single experiment: I. Introduction. *Mayo Clinic Proceedings* 63(8):816–820, 1988.
37. Dunnett CW, Goldsmith CH: When and how to do multiple comparisons, in Buncher CR, Tsay J-Y. (eds): *Statistics in the Pharmaceutical Industry*, 2d ed. New York/Basel/Hong Kong: Marcel Dekker, 1994, pp 481–511.
38. Bowden MI, Bion JF: Drug assessment in critical illness, in Gilbert GS (ed): *Drug Safety Assessment in Clinical Trials.* New York/Basel/Hong Kong: Marcel Dekker, 1993, pp 93–110.
39. Geller NL, Pocock SJ: Design and analysis of clinical trials with group sequential stopping rules, in Peace KE (ed): *Biopharmaceutical Statistics for Drug Development.* New York/Basel/Hong Kong: Marcel Dekker, 1988, pp 489–508.
40. Torner JC: Multiple studies in a single site: Logistical and ethical considerations. Poster presented at the Annual Meeting of the Society for Clinical Trials, Dallas, May 1994.
41. Clifton GL, Hayes RL, Levin HS, et al: Outcome measures for clinical trials involving traumatically brain-injured patients: Report of a conference. *Neurosurgery* 31:975–978, 1992.
42. Levin HS, Gary HE Jr, Eisenberg HM, et al: Traumatic Coma Data Bank Research Group: Neurobehavioral outcome one year after severe head injury: Experience of the Traumatic Coma Data Bank. *J Neurosurg* 73:699–709, 1990.
43. Grabowski HG, Hansen RW: Economic scales and tests, in Spilker B (ed): *Quality of Life Assessment in Clinical Trials.* New York: Raven Press, 1990, pp 61–69.
44. Feeny D, Labelle R, Torrance GW: Integrating economic evaluations and quality of life assessments, in Spilker B (ed): *Quality of Life Assessment in Clinical Trials.* New York: Raven Press, 1990, pp 71–83.
45. Drummond MF, Stoddart GL, Torrance GW: *Methods for the Economic Evaluation of Health Care Programmes.* Oxford, UK: Oxford University Press, 1987.
46. Nordby HK, Nesbakken R: The effect of high dose barbiturate decompression after severe head injury: A controlled study. *Acta Neurochir (Wien)* 72:157–166, 1984.
47. The Comprehensive Central Nervous System Trauma Centers: Eisenberg HM, Frankowski RF, Contant CF, et al: High dose barbiturates control elevated ICP in

patients with severe head injury. *J Neurosurg* 69:15–23, 1988.

48. Schwartz ML, Tator CH, Rowed DW: The University of Toronto head injury treatment study: A prospective randomized comparison of pentobarbital and mannitol. *Can J Neurol Sci* 11:434–440, 1984.
49. Ward JD, Becker DP, Miller JD, et al: Failure of prophylactic barbiturate coma in the treatment of severe head injury. *J Neurosurg* 62:383–388, 1985.
50. Braakman R, Schouten HJA, Blaauw-van Dishoeck M, Minderhoud JM: Megadose steroids in severe head injury: Results of a prospective double-blind clinical trial. *J Neurosurg* 58:326–330, 1983.
51. Saul TG, Ducker TB, Salcman M, Carro E: Steroids in severe head injury: A prospective randomized clinical trial. *J Neurosurg* 54:596–600, 1981.
52. Cooper PR, Moody S, Clark WK, et al: Dexamethasone and severe head injury: A prospective double-blind study. *J Neurosurg* 51:307–316, 1979.
53. Muizelaar JP, Marmarou A, Ward JD, et al: Adverse effects of prolonged hyperventilation in patients with severe head injury: A randomized clinical trial. *J Neurosurg* 75:731–739, 1991.
54. Wolf AL, Levi L, Marmarou A, et al: Effect of THAM upon outcome in severe head injury: A randomized prospective clinical trial. *J Neurosurg* 78:54–59, 1993.
55. The British/Finnish Co-operative Head Injury Trial Group: Teasdale G, Bailey I, Bell A, et al: The effect of nimodipine on outcome after head injury: A prospective randomised control trial. *Acta Neurochir, Suppl (Wien)* 51:315–316, 1990.
56. The European Study Group on Nimodipine in Severe Head Injury: A multicenter trial of the efficacy of nimodipine on outcome after severe head injury. *J Neurosurg* 80:797–804, 1991.
57. McCord JM: Oxygen-derived free radicals in postischemic tissue injury. *N Engl J Med* 312:159–163, 1985.
58. Chan PH, Fishman RA: Transient formation of superoxide radicals in polyunsaturated fatty acid induced brain swelling. *J Neurochem* 35:1004–1007, 1980.
59. Muizelaar JP, Marmarou A, Young HF, et al: Improving the outcome of severe head injury with the oxygen radical scavenger polyethylene glycol-conjugated superoxide dismutase: A Phase II trial. *J Neurosurg* 78:375–382, 1993.
60. Maldonado VC, Perez JBC, Escario JA: Effects of CDP-choline on the recovery of patients with head injury. *J Neurol Sci* 103:S15–S18, 1991.
61. Albers GW, Goldberg MP, Choi DW: *N*-methyl-D-aspartate antagonists: Ready for clinical trial in brain ischemia? *Ann Neurol* 25:398–403, 1989.
62. Faden AI, Demediuk P, Panter SS, Vink R: The role of excitatory amino acids and NMDA receptors in traumatic brain injury. *Science* 244:789–800, 1989.
63. Faden AI, Lemke M, Simon RP, Noble LJ: *N*-methyl-D-aspartate antagonist MK-801 improves outcome following traumatic spinal cord injury in rats: Behavioral, anatomic, and neurochemical studies. *J Neurotrauma* 5:33–45, 1988.
64. Lipton SA, Rosenberg PA: Excitatory amino acids as a final common pathway for neurologic disorders. *N Engl J Med* 330:613–622, 1994.
65. Braughler JM, Hall ED: Central nervous system trauma and stroke: I. Biochemical considerations for oxygen radical formation and lipid peroxidation. *Free Radic Biol Med* 6:289–301, 1989.
66. Hall ED: The neuroprotective pharmacology of methylprednisolone. *J Neurosurg* 76:13–22, 1992.
67. Hall ED, Yonkers PA, Andrus PK, et al: Biochemistry and pharmacology of lipid antioxidants in acute brain and spinal cord injury. *J Neurotrauma* 9(suppl 2):137–142, 1992.
68. Gennarelli TA: Cerebral concussion and diffuse brain injury, in Cooper PR (ed): *Head Injury,* 3d ed. Baltimore: Williams & Wilkins, 1993, pp 137–158.
69. Hubschman OR, Nathanson DC: The role of calcium and cellular membrane dysfunction in experimental trauma and subarachnoid hemorrhage. *J Neurosurg* 62:698–703, 1985.
70. Meldrum B: Possible therapeutic applications of antagonists of excitatory amino acid neurotransmitters. *Clin Sci* 68:113–122, 1985.
71. Helfaer MA, Kirsch JR, Traystman RJ, Rogers MC: Lazaroids: The potential role of 21-aminosteroids in treating critically injured patients, in Chernow B (ed): *The Pharmacologic Approach to the Critically Ill Patient.* Baltimore: Williams & Wilkins, 1994, pp 378–387.
72. Simon RP, Swan JH, Griffiths T, Meldrum BS: Blockade of *N*-methyl-D-aspartate receptors may protect against ischemic damage in the brain. *Science* 226:850–852, 1984.

CHAPTER 66

ECONOMICS OF HEAD INJURY TRIALS

Mary Ellen Cheung Michel

INTRODUCTION

"The most effective argument in favour of randomized clinical trials is that the alternative, practicing in complacent uncertainty, is worse."[1]

The effort needed and resources necessary to mount a trial to demonstrate the efficacy of an intervention are formidable for any disorder, and traumatic brain injury (TBI) certainly presents its own special problems that influence the cost of trials. The need for highly trained personnel, the length of a study to properly assess outcome, and the identification of reliable and sensitive outcome measures are some issues that make clinical trials of TBI extremely costly. But first, of course, is the basic research that leads to the intervention which is to be put to the test. While the cost of drug development is shared by government, industry, and academia, the National Institute of Neurological Disorders and Stroke (NINDS) has been a major contributor to all facets of research on traumatic brain injury. The primary goal has been to provide funding for basic and clinical research aimed at elucidating the underlying mechanisms of injury with a view to preserving or restoring neurological function. It is fortunate that basic research has identified several processes of secondary damage that can hopefully be intercepted. Likewise, clinical investigators have documented the fundamental information on demographics, pathology, routine care, and expected outcome(s) that are necessary to design and carry out randomized trials of treatment in acute head injury. Indeed, several clinical trials of various sizes are now underway in TBI.

One way to estimate cost of head injury trials is to look at what NINDS spends on clinical trials in this field. While one tends to think primarily in terms of direct costs on relevant grants, this is only part of the story. The true costs, over and above the direct costs, include salaries for NINDS employees, indirect grant costs charged by universities, and intramural research devoted to related topics.

A clinical trial is defined as: "a scientific research activity undertaken to define prospectively the effect and value of prophylactic/diagnostic/therapeutic agents, devices, regimens, procedures, etc., applied to human subjects. It is essential that the study be prospective, and that intervention of some sort occur. The choice of number of cases or patients will depend on the hypothesis being tested, but must be sufficient to permit a definite conclusion. Excluded are: Phase I, feasibility, pilot studies, screening phase, or other preparations for the trial itself which must involve intervention related to disease, disorder or abnormal condition. . . ."

At this time, the NINDS supports a multicentered clinical trial of moderate hypothermia to treat severe TBI, and a single-center trial on posttraumatic epilepsy. Both studies with all related costs should be included in an estimate of research outlay. However, a comprehensive cost estimate probably should also include the early phase trials of safety, or pilot studies obtained in support of the larger trials. Indeed, most of the NINDS-supported head injury clinical research centers (P50s) are conducting head injury treatment or monitoring protocols, and use a common database. These costs could be included since they may lead to larger clinical trials. In addition, other clinical studies, deemed *related* to head injury (such as experimental protocols for brain imaging), may also be included. It is easy to see that the actual cost of trials is much greater than just the direct costs of TBI-related studies.

NINDS Budget Overview

NINDS supports clinical research both at NIH and at universities throughout the world. The NINDS Financial Management Branch publishes figures for the major,

TABLE 66-1 NINDS Research Budget FY 1992

	Number	$(Thousands)
Research Projects Grants:*		
Noncompeting	1357	296,200
Administrative Supplement**	54	1332
Competing	443	100,513
Subtotal	1800	398,045
Other Research:		
Careers	173	13,455
Other Rel. Res.	69	3844
Support of NIH Programs		2027
Subtotal	242	19,300
Research Centers (P50):***	42	31,455
Total Research Grants	*2084*	*448,800*
Research Training:		
Individual	164	4175
Institutional	352†	9171
Total, Training	516	13,345
R&D Contracts	50	17,050
Intramural Research	—	75,754
Res. Man. & Supp.	—	25,841
Total, NINDS	—	*580,790*

* See Table 66-2 for details.

** Administrative supplements are funds provided to individual, ongoing grants to offset unforeseen expenses, i.e. equipment failure, increased animal costs. Minority/handicap supplements are also awarded from this category. It does not represent additional numbers of grants, and therefore is not included in the total (1800).

*** Biomedical Research Support program, Minority Biomedical Research Support program.

† Represents number of individual fellows supported on all institutional training grants (T32).

legislated budget categories. An overview of institute funding for clinical trials, along with other types of research, can be obtained. The most recent fiscal year for which figures are complete is 1992 (Table 66-1). For that year, the total budget expended by NINDS was approximately $580 million. NINDS is a midsized institute, and is the sixth largest out of a total of 18*.[2] The Institute is divided into intramural and extramural components. The intramural line item comprises funds expended ($75,754,000) for all the intramural research programs at the Bethesda campus, including clinical protocols, equipment, supplies, and employees. Everything else is extramural and contains expenditures to fund research outside NIH. The extramural budget includes the salaries for NINDS extramural administrative staff, supplies, and overhead costs related to the management of these extramural grants and contracts. ($25,841,000)

* Total appropriation in thousands: NCI $1,951,541; NHLBI $1,191,500; NIAID $960,914; NIGMS $815,134; NIDDK $662,678. *NIH Databook 1992*, page 8.

NINDS Grants

Approximately 80 percent of the NINDS budget is devoted to the extramural programs. The line items that constitute the bulk of the expenditures are: Research Projects Grants; Research Centers; Other Research; Research Training; and Research and Development Contracts. All of these funding mechanisms provide monies to investigators through the direct costs of research, and provide research support to institutions through indirect costs. Clinical trials, as defined, most often occur in the extramural program.

As extramural awards, clinical trials can be funded under several mechanisms, such as grants, contracts, cooperative agreements, or program projects. Costs for the institute vary by mechanism, i.e., contracts are very labor-intensive to review and to manage compared with grants. In addition, contracts are usually funded in specific, predetermined amounts, and are subject to price negotiation as part of the competition. Planning at the institute level involves selecting a mechanism that will consume appropriate amounts of staff time and resources, in addition to the funding that must be provided to investigators. Although the funding of large clinical trials as grants puts most of the administrative burden on the grantee, it does not relieve the institute of oversight responsibility. Regular monitoring visits or committee meetings must be a part of the institute's cost of performing the trial, no matter what mechanism of funding is chosen.

The grant portfolio (1800 awards for $396,713,000) represents approximately 68 percent of the total NINDS budget. So, in 1992, NINDS spent 68 percent of its appropriation on Research Project grants, both basic and clinical science (Table 66-2). Several different grant mechanisms that exist within the category of Research Projects and clinical trials, or the clinical studies that lead up to a large trial, are funded under all of them. Individual investigator awards (R01), FIRST awards for new investigators (R29), Phase I and II small business grants (R43 and R44), and program projects (P01) all support clinical research. The bulk of the institute's outlay in numbers and dollars was (and is) for R01s. There are no concrete funding ceilings on individual research grants (R01s), and some of the large clinical trials funded by NINDS have been funded through this mechanism.

Support for Head Injury Research

The Institute's 1992 outlay for extramural projects on head injury research, summarized in Table 66-3, totaled approximately $29 million. As for the total NINDS, the largest commitment category was to research projects (69 percent). We may note also that the head injury

TABLE 66-2 NINDS Research Project Grants Total FY 1992

	Noncompeting		*Competing*		*Total*	
	No.	**\$(Thousands)**	**No.**	**\$(Thousands)**	**No.**	**\$(Thousands)**
Activity						
P01	75	67,748	19	13,109	94	80,857
R01	1101	210,426	352	80,108	1453	290,534
R29	172	16,070	39	4124	211	20,194
R43	00	00	25	1247	25	1247
R44	9	1956	8	1925	17	3881
Total	1357	296,200	443	100,513	1800	396,713

program has a relatively heavy commitment to large, multidisciplinary grants, with 45 percent of the expended funds devoted to program projects and centers. This structure is due in part to outside influence. In 1991, in response to Congressional language and following recommendations of the 1989 Interagency Head Injury Task Force, NINDS issued a Request for Applications to create new centers in head and spinal cord injury. Three new centers (P50) and six new feasibility centers for head injury (P20) resulted. Most of the head injury centers and program projects include clinical investigations, Phase I treatment trials, or epidemiological studies. These centers devoted anywhere from 5 to 50 percent of their total direct costs to clinical research.

Clinical Trials

Although other funding strategies (e.g., cooperative agreements) are widely used by other institutes at NIH,[2] NINDS funds most extramural clinical trials by either the R01 or contract mechanism (Table 66-4). Programmatically, the total portfolio of clinical trials concentrates on epilepsy and stroke, and the funding mechanisms vary between grants and contracts. The two largest trials on central nervous system injury are both funded as R01s.

The Institute's total costs for extramural trials also involves administrative support. For instance, the reporting and oversight requirements for clinical trials involve interim reviews by a safety monitoring committee, set up and run by NINDS. The costs of these committee meetings are an institute expense, but do not appear in the clinical trials category; rather they are included within Division managerial support. For NIH, in addition to in-house expenses, the cost of clinical trials must include large indirect costs paid to universities. For multisite projects these indirect costs will be charged as direct costs to the parent grant, and will be part of the budget submitted for peer review. Indirect costs vary among universities and medical centers; for six of the NINDS program projects and centers in head injury (University of Pennsylvania, Baylor College of Medicine, Medical College of Virginia, Richmond, University of Miami, UCLA, and University of Washington, Seattle) the rates currently range from 47.5 to 62.5 percent. The rates are negotiated between the federal government and the university, and are subject to further negotiation for particular studies or locations at the site. Over the course of a long trial, these rates can increase,

TABLE 66-3 NINDS Head Injury and Research FY 1992

	Number	**\$(Thousands)**
Research Projects Grants (P01, R01, R23, R29, R43, R44)	39	10,117,839
Centers (P50 & P20)	8	4,282,514
Other Research		
R55 (Shannon)	2	110,000
NRSA		
Individual	0	
Institutional	1	123,990
Intramural Research	1	153,545
Extramural & Intramural Subtotal	51	14,787,888
Program Mgmt Costs		14,948,000*
Total	51	29,735,888

* Includes NINDS overhead costs, extramural research programs (e.g., PET, pain) that support research in head injury.

TABLE 66-4 National Institute of Neurological Disorders and Stroke Clinical Trials FY 1992

	Number	**\$(Thousands)**
Research grants	23	25,732
Research centers	1	528
R&D contracts	10	3822
Intramural research	7	2522
(Total)	41	32,604

and create problems in funding in future years. Interestingly, NIH does not pay indirect costs to foreign institutions, which provides an economical alternative venue in some cases.

In 1992, the "average" R01 clinical trial funded in NINDS cost over $1 million for the first year. This level of expenditure for a single project would certainly affect any program trying to balance clinical, basic, and applied research in head injury. Taken in the broadest perspective, however, the dollars currently spent by NINDS for extramural clinical trials amount to only approximately 5 percent of the total budget; 6 percent of the extramural budget; and 9 percent of the R01 expenditure. This level of support for clinical trials has remained fairly constant for the last several years.

Preparing Budgets for NIH Grants

Several publications have been written by NIH staff to guide investigators preparing applications for grants, including clinical trials.[3] The most common problems identified by reviewers have been distilled into guidelines for investigators (Table 66-5). All mainly emphasize the scientific merit of the project. However, make no mistake that the cost directly reflects on the feasibility of the undertaking, and is a critical part of these applications. Budgets should be sufficient to ensure that the hypothesis proposed will be tested. Unrealistic, "bargain-basement" prices will not be judged favorably, either by the reviewers or the Institute staff. Padded budgets designed to hedge against possible reductions or to support other related research are easily recognized, and will jeopardize the entire enterprise.

TABLE 66-5 Common Deficiencies in Clinical Grant Applications

A. Research Goals
- Lack of new or original ideas
- Diffuse, superficial, or unfocused research plan
- Unimportant or uncertain potential impact

B. Experimental Design
- Uncritical approach
- Unrealistically large amount of work
- Study group or control inappropriate or insufficient
- Technical methodology questionable, unsuited, inappropriate
- Data collection or analysis procedures vague, unsophisticated

C. Investigator
- Inadequate expertise, experience
- Lack of knowledge of published, relevant work
- Insufficient time devoted to project

D. Resources
- Insufficient staff for patient follow-up, clinical assessment, data handling
- Inadequate institutional setting or facilities
- Budgets too large or too small for proposed work

Designing an NIH budget can help to identify study shortcomings, especially regarding personnel and data handling. Appropriate expertise, as well as appropriate levels of time and effort for personnel on the project, are critical for success. In general, including fewer people, with higher levels of commitment, is preferable to rounding up many individuals with small (less than 10 percent time and effort) commitments. The involvement of the heads of several departments for 2 percent of their time inflates the budget and does not necessarily contribute to the goals of the study. Conversely, a dedicated, full-time study nurse will ensure that patients are entered, useful data are collected, and follow-up is completed. The influence of a biostatistician must be very evident throughout the application to ensure good study design, quality control, and data analysis. For large, multicentered trials, the data center is often separate in both location and budget from the clinical centers, and may even be reviewed as a separate application.

COST CONSIDERATIONS IN HEAD INJURY CLINICAL TRIALS

The following budget-busters are faced by all investigators who conduct clinical trials, no matter how the trials are funded. Because of the complexity of head injury and the subsequent complexity of evaluating outcome, the costs for a multicentered efficacy trial are potentially very high. Funding agencies are already concerned about these costs, and conducting economical trials is essential if this type of research is to continue. The following areas are ones in which investigators must tread a fine line between essential costs and unnecessary expense.

Planning to Reduce Costs

An undertaking of the magnitude of a Phase III clinical trial (hundreds of patients, multicentered, randomized, placebo-controlled) requires long and careful planning (see Chap. 64). Development of the trial involves many steps and costs tens of thousands of dollars; but such groundwork will save much more money if the experience gained prevents delays or anticipates obstacles during the larger trial. Of course, the trial will then be based on sound scientific information, and will propose reasonable and achievable goals. Starting a large trial with an ill-conceived research plan, incomplete procedures manual, untested data collection forms, and no experience entering patients wastes money and time. Training is essential for all study personnel on all procedures that will translate into data elements; uniformity of data must be assured across all participating centers for the duration of the trial. A videotape of a "proper" Glasgow Outcome Score or Glasgow Coma Scale could be necessary for residents participating in the trial; the costs of producing the tape could be justified by fewer investigator meetings later in the study. Training is particularly important for neuropsychological endpoints, and special personnel or consultant costs may be justified. "Preliminary data" are essential for all grant applications to NIH, and should be carefully obtained and evaluated by any investigator contemplating a large clinical trial.

Planning for a trial will be a cooperative effort between investigators and sponsor(s), and may include industry, government, or private foundations. All of these groups can provide start-up funding for protocol development, case report forms, data management, or preparation of a manual of operations. Pharmaceutical companies may supply test compounds free of charge; such arrangements should be agreed upon in the early planning stages. Feasibility and logistics should be ironed out by the collection of preliminary data, and plans for mailing specimens, retrieving data, or analyzing vast quantities of safety information well established before a Phase III effort is launched. The goals of trials sponsored by NIH are not necessarily equivalent to those of trials sponsored by industry, and costs will differ. For example, company-sponsored trials often require collection of extensive data on drug safety that would be unnecessary in a purely research driven trial.

Study Design

Principles of cost management for clinical trials have been put forward in many articles[4] and texts,[5] and these tenets certainly should be applied to clinical trials in head injury. Head injury treatment takes place in a very expensive setting—the neurosurgical intensive care unit. Literally hundreds of data elements are collected on each subject as part of routine monitoring. Inclusion of all of these is practically impossible and counterproductive; inclusion of many of them could easily drive costs very high. The message must be to determine the data points that are critical and collect only those data points. In general, use of high-tech measurements greatly inflates costs. Although valuable research information relevant to the treatment of head injury can be gained from PET or MRI scanning, blood flow measurement, or extensive monitoring of numerous ICU parameters, inclusion of such evaluations in a large trial warrants close scrutiny. The temptation to include numerous secondary outcomes, or ancillary studies, should be avoided; a broad, unfocused work scope wastes resources. Of course, layers of complexity will not only inflate costs, but also will jeopardize the integrity of the trial. Investigators should thoroughly consider and justify all data to be collected. If data are collected, then, naturally, they should be analyzed; and all results will affect the conclusions drawn from the trial.

Outcome Measures

The costs of head injury clinical trials are greatly influenced by the complexity of outcome measures and the duration of the postinjury periods chosen for assessment. Selection of outcome measures for TBI trials is still controversial, although the Glasgow Outcome Scale is widely used clinically and in research. The Food and Drug Administration (FDA) regulates applications for new drugs, and thereby sets standards for the trials that assess drug efficacy. For use in a trial that would be submitted to the FDA, outcome measures must be validated and clinically relevant; preservation of life without quality of life is not acceptable. For use in Phase III trials of TBI, the FDA strongly recommends the use of a practical measure of the activities of daily living, and the research community is struggling with the selection of such endpoints. Assessment scales and test batteries exist; however, because of the complexity and variety of deficits that can result from the injury, evaluations are often numerous, lengthy, difficult for patients, and require special expertise to administer. At this time, it may be wise to plan and execute smaller clinical studies aimed at evaluating putative endpoints, before embarking on a large, expensive, and possibly futile trial.

In 1991, NINDS convened a workshop of TBI clinical investigators, including neuropsychologists, neurosurgeons, rehabilitation specialists, as well as representatives of the pharmaceutical industry and government to assess various outcome measures for clinical trials.[6] The participants debated such issues as stratification, acute stage measurements, study duration, as well as selection of functional outcome measures. A test battery to assess outcome was suggested and has been published. The selected tests cover the major domains of activity known to be affected in head injury, and the evaluation can be performed within one and one-half hours. Each element is standardized within its domain and can be administered by a study nurse or technician. Unfortunately, this battery of tests has yet to be validated in a TBI study. It must be noted that this battery consists of several individual elements, and differences could be found among the various parameters tested. At this time, there is no evidence for selection of any one measure over another (e.g., attention versus memory) as a primary outcome measure. Again, smaller clinical studies may be required to define specific parameters for assessment as primary outcome measures in large trials.

Outcome in head injury trials is often measured at monthly, or even yearly, time points, and expense is tied closely to the length of the trial. Trials always become more costly the longer they run, and cost overrun can easily force cancellation or early close-out of a trial. In addition, changes in clinical practice may jeopardize a lengthy effort and render preliminary findings obsolete.

Staffing Costs

Attempts to cut costs by relying on individuals paid primarily from other sources will jeopardize a trial. A technician who is already on a grant, or nurses heavily committed to routine clinical duties are not reasonable choices for major roles in a clinical trial. Full-time (or as close as possible) study nurses and/or clinical coordinators are very important. These people are responsible for patients from informed consent through the final follow-up visit, and long-term follow-up is unrealistic without experienced, dedicated staff.

Principal investigators (PIs) are usually senior people and, therefore, are expensive. Paid time and effort for such a person can run between 20 and 30 percent of their professional time. As the focal point for the study within their institutions, the PI will coordinate efforts among the study personnel and other departments, services, or offices. The PI must attend investigator meetings, monitoring visits, and any other function where changes to the study protocol or other major decisions affecting either budget or science would be made. It is the PI's responsibility to provide staff and resources that will ensure patient recruitment and follow-up. For a large study, the demands on a busy person are great. It is often useful for the PI to have a full-time second-in-command: a coinvestigator who directly assesses patients, responds to study needs after hours, and generally insures that the trial proceeds when the PI is unavailable. At present, federal policy imposes a ceiling of $125,000 on investigator salaries, so for NIH grant applications the costs for these critical personnel may appear unrealistically low.

One cannot compensate for overstaffing on the data collection (clinical) side of a trial by reductions on the data analysis side. Skimping on personnel responsible for data entry, quality control, and statistical analysis may prove disastrous, and may do so after considerable resources have already been expended. To safeguard against the worst case, it is essential to include a senior biostatistician or methodologist, familiar with the design and conduct of clinical trials, as a paid investigator in the trial from its earliest planning stages through the publication of final results. The effort devoted to the trial should reflect actual time and effort, and salaries can certainly run into the range of the NIH ceiling. Here, too, a more junior coinvestigator or study coordinator, with a substantial time commitment, is necessary for large, multicentered trials.

Travel Costs

Proposed follow-up visits for patients are often scheduled at 3, 6, and 12 months postinjury, and these are the occasions where the critical outcome data are obtained. When designing the trial, the necessity and duration of each visit needs to be carefully considered in light of primary and secondary outcomes, and visits eliminated that are unlikely to answer the research question(s).

Once follow-up visits are determined, virtually no effort should be spared to obtain usable data. Compensation for patient travel must certainly be sufficient to meet expenses and provide some incentive, but lavish offers cannot appear to coerce patient consent to participate. Getting patients back to the clinic (or getting staff out to patients) may involve elaborate schemes, from sending birthday cards and making phone calls to dispatching vans with computer hookups. These are necessary, justifiable expenses. Patients lost to follow-up are extremely costly, and often inclusion criteria are crafted so that persons unlikely to be available a year after injury (e.g., homeless, illegal aliens) are not entered.

Regular monitoring or investigator meetings serve to identify problems, and provide an opportunity to handle them quickly. The costs for yearly meetings can be budgeted by investigators, but sponsors may require and fund others. Costs for meetings are burdensome; so, naturally, only essential personnel attend, and only at essential times. The purpose of all meetings should be clear and driven by the progress of the trial, not necessarily scheduled strictly by calendar. Monitoring committee meetings can be useful to identify centers that are not meeting recruitment goals. Funding for nonproductive centers within multicentered trials should be discontinued quickly, and funds either transferred to new centers or to existing centers where patient entry, follow-up, and data handling are satisfactory. Travel for investigators is expensive, but changes to an ongoing study are very expensive—new case report forms, new data collection methods, more staff training, more meeting time, more randomization.

BITING THE BULLET

Total outlay for a trial includes many factors that never appear in budgets submitted by investigators. Those who sponsor trials, whether private industry or public organizations, must also devote huge resources to pursue a single indication. Compensation for time and effort, data management, travel, and overhead are doubly burdensome. Therefore, resources for large clinical trials cannot be made available for every possible receptor antagonist, every inhibitor of secondary damage, every putative mechanism proposed as a factor after head injury. Large clinical trials for head injury are the final step in the total research scheme to bring effective treatments to bear and to eliminate ineffective ones. How much do trials in head injury cost? Is $10,000 per patient too expensive? For a trial using 500 patients that would be $5,000,000 direct costs, plus 50 percent indirect costs, plus 10 percent management costs for 1 year. Should a public funding agency such as NIH devote this large a commitment to a single project? How many patients will be helped? What is the cost/benefit ratio for severe head injury? If there is to be a future for clinical trials in head injury, investigators, regulators, industry, and funding agencies cannot allow these projects to become prohibitively expensive. While much progress has been made, much remains to be done in this field.

ACKNOWLEDGMENTS

Budget information was supplied by Mr. Andrew Baldus, NINDS.

References

1. Bracken MB: Clinical trials and the acceptance of uncertainty. *Br Med J* 1987; 294:1111.
2. *NIH Data Book 1992.* Public Health Service, Department of Health and Human Services, 1992.
3. *Preparing a Research Grant Application to the National Institutes of Health.* NIH Division of Research Grants, Office of Grants Inquiries, 1989.
4. Drummond MF, Davies L: Economic analysis alongside clinical trials. *Int J Tech Assess Health Care* 1991; 7:561.
5. Meinert CL: *Clinical Trials: Design, Conduct, and Analysis.* New York: Oxford University Press, 1986.
6. Clifton GL, Hayes RL, Levin HS, et al: Outcome measures for clinical trials involving traumatically brain-injured patients: Report of a conference. *Neurosurgery* 1992; 31:975.

Organizational Aspects of Neurotrauma

CHAPTER 67

SURVEY OF TRAUMA SYSTEMS

A. Brent Eastman
Jon C. Walsh

SYNOPSIS

Care of the injured patient is man's earliest recorded surgical endeavor, and neurosurgical intervention with trephining of skull is one of the earliest documented surgical procedures. Care of the injured patient has evolved over the centuries with accelerated punctuations of improved care derived from the experience of military conflicts. The concept of trauma centers dates back to the Napoleonic Wars; however, the concept of trauma care systems is a recent innovation. Despite the proven efficacy of such organized care for the severely injured, there are only isolated trauma systems around the world. In the United States, it is estimated that less than 25 percent of the population has access to systematized trauma care.

The components of a trauma care system are well-established, as outlined in the Model Trauma Care System Plan, 1992.[16] *The recent Trauma Care Systems Development Act (1991) has given great impetus to the development of trauma care systems in this country.*

Since neurotrauma is a major component in any population of severely injured patients, it is critical that neurosurgeons be involved in the planning, development, implementation, and maintenance of a trauma care system.

As more states develop trauma care systems, it will be possible to establish a national database and to define standards of care. The ACS/COT is committed to the establishment of a national database through the National Trauma Registry of the American College of Surgeons (TRACS).

The ultimate goal of any trauma care system should be to ensure optimal care to all injured patients, given the available resources.

INTRODUCTION

Injury is the number one public health problem in the United States. It is the fourth leading cause of death for all ages and accounts for more years of productive life lost than cancer and heart disease combined.[1] It is well established that survival from severe injuries is directly related to the time from injury to definitive care. Definitive care is best provided in a qualified trauma center that is part of an organized trauma system. The concept of a trauma care system insures that injured patients are taken expeditiously to the most appropriate facility. The American College of Surgeons' Committee on Trauma has published, *Resources for Optimal Care of the Injured Patient: 1993,* which establishes guidelines for optimal care. This includes specific reference to neurotrauma care and the role of the neurosurgeon in a trauma care system.[2]

Although the trauma center is a key component of acute care for the severely injured, the trauma care system encompasses all phases of care from pre-hospital through acute care and rehabilitation.

It is critical that, within a geographic area committed to a trauma system, the *entire* population of injured patients be considered. Because only 10 to 15 percent of all hospitalized injured patients will require the resources of a designated trauma center, the remaining patients necessarily will be treated in other acute care facilities in the region. An *inclusive system* guarantees that all injured patients will receive optimal care, given available resources, even if they do not require the resources of a designated trauma center.

Trauma care systems may be a paradigm for health care delivery in the United States since several key issues are addressed:

1. Universal access:
   All injured patients are provided optimal care, given available resources, in an inclusive trauma care system.
2. Quality of care:
   Trauma care systems demand careful quality improvement programs, including a trauma registry.
3. Cost-effective care:
   Cost effectiveness is gained by regionalizing care and triaging the most critically injured patients to trauma centers. This provides for optimal utilization of limited resources.

An important contribution to the trauma systems literature is the *1993 Inventory of Trauma Systems.*[3] This document was developed specifically as a tool to assist in the design or refinement of trauma care systems. The inventory provides extensive data on the structural characteristics of trauma systems that were operational in 1993, including information on:

- Trauma system administrative structure and legal authorities
- Trauma center standards, verification and designation
- Pre-hospital care personnel
- Emergency transportation
- Emergency communications
- Medical direction and control
- Field categorization and triage
- Inter-hospital transfer agreements
- System evaluation activities

This chapter will review the historical development of trauma care systems and will detail systems components and operations.

The reader should understand the evolution of trauma care systems as a background to essential concepts of a functional trauma care system. The role of the neurosurgeon will be discussed.

DEVELOPMENT OF TRAUMA CARE SYSTEMS IN THE UNITED STATES

The evolution of trauma systems has paralleled the history of armed conflict. The development of the 'flying ambulance' by Larrey in the Napoleonic Wars was one of the early demonstrations of systematized rapid transport from the site of injury to definitive care. In the American Civil War, injured troops were carried by ambulance transports to battlefield aid stations and to field hospitals.[4]

The lessons of military conflicts continued to advance the care of the injured soldier; yet little was transferred to the civilian sector until the middle of the 20th century. The American College of Surgeons formed the Committee for the Treatment of Fractures in 1922, but had limited influence outside the military until World War II, when quicker transport to definitive care clearly improved outcomes. Further improvements in rapid transport in both Korea and Vietnam added support to the concept of an ideal system of caring for the injured, whether soldier or civilian.[5]

In peacetime, the lessons of the military experience were put to civilian use. Historically, trauma centers were primarily inner city hospitals with de facto trauma center status in that they served high-risk populations. However, in the 1970s an evolution occurred with the development of trauma care systems. A key observation was that too many injured patients were dying unnecessarily after having arrived at a hospital. Several so-called "preventable deaths studies" were performed around the country, and each confirmed that standard emergency room care was unreliable. The National Science Foundation produced the now classic White Paper document in 1966, *Accidental Death and Disability: The Neglected Disease of Modern Society* (National Academy of Science/National Research Council, 1964) identifying trauma as a major national problem and challenging organized medicine to produce a solution. Emergency care providers in many areas took up the challenge by evaluating their own performance and identifying suboptimal care.[5–8] These studies gradually led to the development and implementation of regionalized trauma care systems. It became clear that the ideal was more than rapid transport from the scene of injury to the hospital; optimal care entailed a much deeper commitment of resources from the hospital, including surgeons and the entire support staff. With time it also became clear that systems of trauma care would not survive without the support of all hospitals in the community, as well as the governmental agencies responsible for emergency medical systems planning and organization.

Several systems have matured to such a point that we now have post-system assessment data demonstrating the effectiveness of organized trauma care in reducing morbidity and mortality for the multiply injured patient.[9–12] The new challenges of sustaining effective trauma care systems during times of economic pressures and health care reform are great. The goal must be to make these regionalized programs both clinically successful and economically viable.

NATIONAL STRATEGIES

Although the efficacy of trauma care systems is now well established, it is estimated that less than 25 percent of the geographical area of the United States is served by such systems. The number of hospitals claiming trauma center status is approximately 420, but many of these are functioning in isolation, whether because of political factors (such as the inability to reach consensus as to which hospital in an area should be a trauma center), lack of financial support, or simply lack of an organized trauma care system.[13]

In addition to regional efforts of states, counties, and cities, there has been an increasing national focus on the development of trauma care systems. In 1988, the U.S. Department of Transportation recognized the need for a model curriculum on trauma system development. This curriculum, *The Development of Trauma Systems: A State and Community Guide* (DOTS), marked the first time that the essential components of trauma system development, including system design, planning, and implementation, were fully expressed.[14] The goal of the curriculum was to provide a basic framework for trauma system development in the form of a guide for states and communities that could be taught in an eight-hour course. In 1990, the Centers for Disease Control (CDC) in Atlanta, GA, convened for the second World Conference on Injury Control. Part of that effort was the development of a series of position papers on injury control, one of which was on trauma care systems. This paper was prepared by a panel of experts from across the United States, including physicians, nurses, EMS administrators, epidemiologists, and representatives from governmental agencies.

The basic format of this position paper was:

Where we are
Where we want to be
How we get there[15]

In this paper the concept of an inclusive trauma care system was described. Previous system design had tended to exclude non-trauma center hospitals. However, as only the most severely injured 15 percent of patients require the expanded resources of a designated trauma center, it is critical that the remaining 85 percent receive optimal care as well. The trauma care system was then expanded to include all facilities providing care to persons injured in a geographic region. The goal of the inclusive trauma care system is to match each hospital's trauma care resources with the needs of injured persons.[15] A graphic display (Fig. 67-1) of the inclusive system concept was developed in the CDC paper and was subsequently refined in the *Model Trauma Care System Plan.*[16]

The establishment of trauma systems and the designation of trauma centers is the function of the local Emergency Medical Services (EMS) authority. The development of trauma centers in the United States received great impetus in November, 1990, with the Trauma Care System Planning and Development Act (PL 101-590). This legislation, designed to encourage the establishment of trauma systems in the United States, called for a model trauma care system plan.[16] Much of the trauma systems component of the model trauma care plan was based on the DOTS curriculum and the position paper developed by the CDC at the third National Trauma Control conference held in 1991.[14,15]

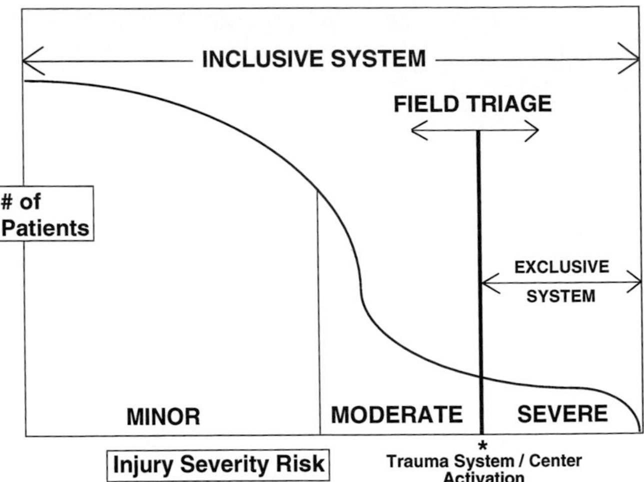

Figure 67-1. Graphic display of the inclusive system. (Reprinted with permission of Health Resources and Services Administration, Public Health Service.)

In the first allocation of grants from the Trauma System Planning and Development Act, 23 states received support to develop trauma care systems. Based on the initial work of the Department of Transportation in developing the DOTS curriculum, the CDC position paper and the subsequent model trauma care plan, a framework has been created on which a trauma care system can be developed.

COMPONENTS OF AN INCLUSIVE TRAUMA CARE SYSTEM

The components of an inclusive trauma care system are described in Fig. 67-2.[2]

This model was based on a concept initially described in the Regional Trauma System Design: Critical concepts 1987[17] and expanded in the CDC position paper; the final version was graphically displayed in the model trauma care system plan and the *Resources for Optimal Care of the Injured Patient: 1993.*

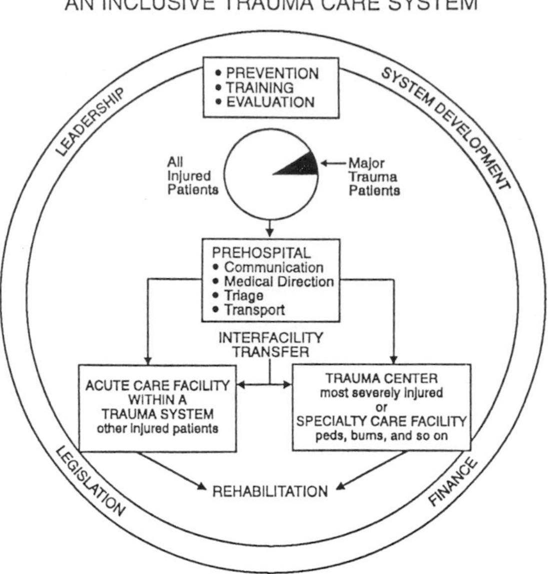

Figure 67-2. Components of inclusive trauma care system. (Reprinted with permission of Health Resources and Services Administration, Public Health Service.)

In evaluating this model from the outer circle through the inner circle to the central core, all essential components of an inclusive trauma care system will be discussed. This discussion is based on the Model Trauma Care System Plan published by the U.S. Department of Health and Human Services, and portions of this chapter are taken directly from that document.[16]

The outer ring falls under the classification of administrative components.

Leadership[16]

The successful development of any system requires a lead agency. The authority of such an agency must be established, since it is responsible for coordinating system design as well as establishing the minimum standards for system performance.

In addition to the lead agency, the successful development of a trauma system requires health care leaders. It is particularly important that there be surgical leadership, since the ultimate success of any system depends on the commitment of trauma surgeons. This includes general surgeons, as well as such subspecialists as neurosurgeons and orthopedic surgeons. In fact, neurosurgical coverage has been a critical factor in the viability of many trauma centers in the United States.[13]

System Development[16]

The planning process for trauma system development is the key to the ultimate success of the system. Many areas will require a comprehensive needs assessment study to determine the magnitude of the injury problem within that geographic area. It will also be necessary to document and quantify the resources available in the area. These resources will vary greatly from area to area, and it is critical that a trauma system be designed based on the unique needs and resources of that particular area. A common error has been to transpose a successful urban trauma system model to a rural area. In fact, the rural situation is very different and the urban model generally does not pertain.

In the spirit of an inclusive trauma care system, it is very important to get all providers involved in the planning process. Equally important is to educate the community about injury and the reason for a trauma care system. An informed public will be a valuable ally in developing and maintaining a trauma care system.

All trauma centers should be carefully integrated with their local EMS system.

Legislation[16]

The development and maintenance of a trauma care system is greatly enhanced by having comprehensive enabling legislation. This legislation should be designed to establish a public lead agency with the authority to plan, develop, implement, and maintain the trauma care system. This will necessarily include the authority to organize data collection in a trauma registry. In the inclusive system, it is imperative that data be obtained from all acute care hospitals who care for injured patients, so that we may better understand the epidemiology of trauma in the region.

Legislation should be designed to provide fiscal support for the trauma care system. Trauma care systems might best be likened to a public utility that must be maintained for the public good.

Finance

The greatest barrier to implementation and the greatest cause of failure of trauma care systems are economic factors. A recent national survey of trauma centers revealed that 80 percent felt that they had major financial problems. Several studies have confirmed that the principal reason for trauma care closure is financial loss.[13]

A study of 25 trauma centers indicated that underfunding results from a combination of the following:[18]

1. Adverse selection—attracting patients who incur above-average costs. It is estimated that the cost of admission of the average patient with traumatic injury is two to three times greater than other hospital admissions of patients with acute illness. A recent study of

95 trauma centers showed the mean cost per patient to be approximately $10,000 in urban areas and $8000 per patient in rural areas.[13]

2. Disproportionate share—attracting a higher proportion of indigent (underinsured and uninsured) patients.[18]

A reimbursement profile of the aggregate data on 95 trauma centers reveals a net margin of −8 percent, shown in Fig. 67-3.[13]

The x axis displays the proportionate distribution of costs by payer class. The y axis reflects the cost recovery ratio (collection/cost).

It is a paradox that the very object of trauma care systems, namely, concentrating the most critically injured patients in a limited number of designated trauma centers, has proved to be the primary cause of center closures and system failure.

The hospital reimbursement crisis is paralleled by inadequate payment of physicians. This has led to a shortage of trauma surgeons—particularly neurosurgeons, who are few in number but whose skills are in high demand. A national survey revealed that 36 percent of trauma centers reported the need to subsidize physicians to maintain trauma center support. Physician support in the form of a guarantee on trauma billing charges has proved successful in some hospitals.[13]

Moving from the outer ring of administrative components to the inner ring of operational and clinical components, there are three key issues:

1. Prevention
2. Training
3. Evaluation[16]

Prevention and Public Education[16]

Inherent to the success of any trauma system is public education. Our failure to educate the public adequately has contributed to the problem of developing trauma care systems. As noted earlier, injury is the number one public health problem in the United States, and it is incumbent on those establishing trauma care systems to convey this to the public they serve to obtain the required support. Many of the other problems, such as inadequate funding, will be more easily solved when the public supports the trauma system.

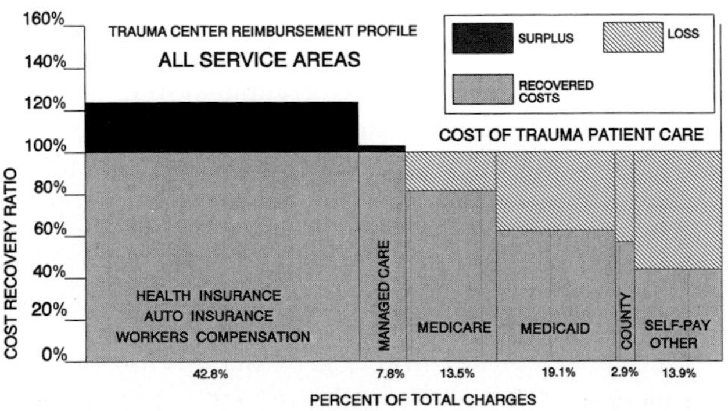

Figure 67-3. The x axis displays the proportionate distribution of costs by payer class. The y axis reflects the cost recovery ration (collection/cost).

Prevention is a critical aspect of a trauma system. It is generally accepted that injury is a potentially preventable problem, and a well-planned community and public information/education and prevention program is an integral part of an effective trauma system. One of the goals of an organized trauma system is to prevent injuries.

Without question, the most cost-effective approach to injury is prevention, and injury is potentially one of the most preventable diseases we encounter. An aggressive system-wide prevention program would reduce the costs of trauma care. In Australia, because of aggressive drunk driving laws, economic savings to the National Auto Insurance Company has resulted in funds for construction of a world-class trauma center. There is currently a surge of interest in the United States regarding the epidemic of violent crime. Because of the injuries resulting from violence, trauma care systems should be at the forefront of developing and implementing violence prevention programs.

Injury prevention programs require a database that can be analyzed to provide information necessary to develop prevention programs based on local needs. Injury surveillance data systems should include systematic reporting of E codes (international classification of diseases, external cause of injury). This will allow for identification of high-risk groups in the injury database. Once identified, specific prevention programs can be devised and implemented.[19]

Three general strategies are commonly used in injury prevention:

1. Persuasion programs designed to alter behavior or guide decision making for increased self-protection (e.g., drunk driving campaigns, seatbelt education, and gun safety).

2. Legislation or enforcement of policies that require individuals to follow protective guidelines (e.g., motorcycle helmet law, seatbelt policy, gun registration).

3. Automatic protection by altering products or the environment (e.g., air bags, smoke alarms, fire-resistant clothing).

Ultimately, a trauma care system can monitor the epidemiology of injury within that system and evaluate the effectiveness of the implemented prevention and public education programs. The data obtained from these epidemiological studies can then provide the support needed for legislative measures, such as gun control and drunk driving laws.

Training[16]

It is incumbent upon any trauma care system to ensure adequately trained personnel to provide trauma care services. This training will include pre-hospital and hospital personnel. Examples of some specialized programs that might be offered:

1. ATLS (Advance Trauma Life Support)
2. Pre-hospital TLS (Pre-hospital Trauma Life Support)
3. Basic Trauma Life Support
4. Trauma Nursing Core Course
5. Pediatric Advanced Life Support and Advanced Pediatric Life Support

Evaluation[16]

Quality improvement (QI) programs are essential to ensure that the standard of care is met in a trauma care system. Fundamental to such a QI program is the acquisition of data on all injured patients transported to acute care facilities. This data retrieval is best accomplished with a system-wide trauma registry that has data points covering all phases of care. It is important that for each phase of care issues of resource utilization, cost effectiveness, and outcome data be considered.

Evaluation of care must be done both in the individual centers and system-wide. An effective model has been a system medical audit process whereby major clinical and system problems are reviewed on a regular basis.[10] The judgments of such a medical audit process can then be given back to the individual facilities so that appropriate quality improvement action may be taken. The most important component of the quality improvement process is translating identified problems into plans of correction. This requires committed and concerted efforts by the trauma leadership to ensure that trauma care-givers are kept informed about improvements in care and corrective action plans. Trauma care systems that have utilized such a quality improvement process have shown that standards of care continue to evolve and improve as a result of the process. Actual meetings with representatives from trauma centers, other acute care facilities, the medical examiner, EMS agency personnel, critical subspecialists, trauma surgeons, and subspecialists such as neurosurgeons have provided a certain cohesiveness to the trauma care system.

Each trauma center must also have a rigorous quality improvement program. This requires regular multidisciplinary meetings of trauma surgeons, orthopaedic surgeons, anesthesiologists, neurosurgeons, and others to discuss critically and take action on quality of care issues within the institution.

The neurosurgeon's participation in both the trauma center and the trauma system quality improvement and evaluation process is critical.

Pre-Hospital Care[16]

Any trauma care system is dependent on efficient and well-organized pre-hospital trauma care. The key components of pre-hospital care are:

1. Public accesss
2. Response by qualified pre-hospital personnel
3. Triage of trauma patients
4. Transport to the nearest appropriate trauma care facility.

Communication

Communication begins with a public access system. The most common telephone access in the United States is via 9-1-1. This service can be significantly improved with enhanced 9-1-1, which permits automatic caller locations. Highway call boxes also should be considered for areas distant from population centers.

The communication network must be integrated to include linkages between:

1. Dispatch to ambulance
2. Ambulance to ambulance
3. Ambulance to hospital
4. Hospital to hospital

In areas with aeromedical transport capabilities, the same linkage must be established as with ground transport ambulances.

A centralized dispatching capability is the best way to ensure provision of resources appropriate to current needs within the trauma care system. This dispatch system should be physician-directed.

The communication component of a trauma care system must have a careful quality improvement program.

Medical direction

The pre-hospital component of trauma system care requires medical direction. In the United States, this generally will be the role of the EMS Medical Director.

Medical direction can be broken down into two basic components:

1. Off-line medical direction protocols. Prospective and retrospective medical functions.
2. On-line medical direction. Concurrent medical functions. On-line medical direction is provided by direct communication with an on-line physician adviser or designee either on-scene or by direct voice communication.

Medical direction of pre-hospital providers is particularly important for patients with severe head injuries. Often decisions must be made rapidly about intubation and administration of medications. It is critical that the neurosurgeons involved in providing neurotrauma care in the trauma centers also have input regarding pre-hospital management of neurotrauma.

Triage

Triage comes from the French word "trier," which referred to the sorting of wool by the early traders.[20]

The same concept of sorting pertains in trauma care systems. Triage is the process by which injured patients are categorized by actual or perceived degree of risk of injury and directed to the most appropriate trauma system facility. Therefore, in a trauma system, the process of triage not only sorts patients by severity of injury but also determines patient distribution to hospitals. This process has major political and economic impact on trauma care providers. It is, therefore, very important that objective triage criteria be established in any trauma care system. The ACS/COT has created an algorithm (Fig. 67-4) that is generally accepted as a basic guideline for triage decision making.[20,21]

The inclusive trauma system model allows a trauma system to establish triage criteria as broad or narrow as the system requires. These criteria will determine the field categorization of the "major trauma patient" who requires trauma center resources and transport to the most appropriate center. The vertical (field triage) line will move right or left depending on the individual trauma system (see Fig. 67-1).

In any trauma care system, there will be some moderately injured patients who will not be identified or appropriately triaged in the field. These patients will not be transported to trauma centers, but later will be found to have injuries that require the resources of a trauma center (undertriage). There must be transfer protocols and written agreements to ensure the prompt transfer of such patients to the nearest appropriate center. Similarly, there will be patients transferred to designated trauma centers who do not require such resources and can be transferred back to their community hospital when appropriate (overtriage).

These transfer protocols become particularly important with health care reform in the United States. With the managed care model predominant, there must be an excellent working relationship between payors and the trauma care providers to allow for regionalized trauma care within the framework of a managed care system.

When combined with a trauma registry and a good system quality improvement program, triage criteria can be adjusted to achieve the optimal balance of sensitivity and specificity in a given trauma care system. The goal of triage is to match patient needs with available resources in order to provide optimal care in the most effective way.

Transportation

A basic precept of trauma care is that survival after major injury is directly related to the interval between injury and definitive care. This is particularly true of the head-injured patient. Therefore, it is critical that patient transport be carefully considered in a trauma care system. This will require coordinated utilization of ground and air transport resources. Decisions about mode of transport for trauma patients should be based solely on the medical needs of the patient.

The system QI program should continuously evaluate the transportation component of the pre-hospital system.

Definitive Care Facilities[2]

The central core of any trauma care system will be the definitive care facilities. In the Inclusive System Model, this will include both trauma centers and other centers, since many less severely injured patients will receive their care at less specialized centers.

The trauma care system should either establish trauma facility standards or adopt those currently available. The guidelines established by the ACS/COT are the most frequently utilized. These guidelines have recently been revised and published in the new *Resources for Optimal Care of the Injured Patient,* 1993.[2] The facilities defined in that document are described below.

Level I

The Level I facility is a regional resource that is a tertiary center central to the trauma care system. Ultimately, all patients who require the resources of the Level I center should have access to it.

In addition to acute care responsibilities, Level I trauma centers have the major responsibility of providing leadership in education, research, and system planning.

Neurosurgical capabilities are essential in Level I.

Level II

The Level II trauma center is a hospital that is also expected to provide initial definitive trauma care regardless of severity of injury. However, depending on geographic location, patient volume, personnel, and re-

TRIAGE DECISION SCHEME

Measure vital signs and level of consciousness

Step 1

Glasgow Coma Scale	<14 or
Systolic blood pressure	<90 or
Respiratory rate	<10 or >29 or
Revised Trauma Score	<11
Pediatric Trauma Score	<9

YES — Take to trauma center; alert trauma team

NO — Assess anatomy of injury

Step 2

- All penetrating injuries to head, neck, torso, and extremities proximal to elbow and knee
- Flail chest
- Combination trauma with burns
- Two or more proximal long-bone fractures
- Pelvic fractures
- Limb paralysis
- Amputation proximal to wrist and ankle

YES — Take to trauma center; alert trauma team

NO — Evaluate for evidence of mechanism of injury and high-energy impact

Step 3

- Ejection from automobile
- Death in same passenger compartment
- Extrication time >20 minutes
- Falls >20 feet
- Rollover
- High-speed auto crash: Initial speed >40 mph; Major auto deformity >20 inches; Intrusion into passenger compartment >12 inches
- Auto-pedestrian/auto-bicycle injury with significant (>5 mph) impact
- Pedestrian thrown or run over
- Motorcycle crash >20 mph or with separation of rider from bike

YES — Contact medical control and consider transport to a trauma center. Consider trauma team alert

NO

Step 4

- Age <5 or >55
- Cardiac disease, respiratory disease
- Insulin-dependent diabetes, cirrhosis, or morbid obesity
- Pregnancy
- Immunosuppressed patients
- Patient with bleeding disorder or patient on anticoagulants

YES — Contact medical control and consider transport to trauma center. Consider trauma team alert

NO — Reevaluate with medical control

WHEN IN DOUBT TAKE TO A TRAUMA CENTER

Figure 67-4. ACS Triage Algorithm (With permission of the Committee on Trauma, American College of Surgeons.[21]) See notes to figure on following page.

sources, the Level II trauma center may not be able to provide the same comprehensive care as Level I centers. Therefore, patients with more complex injuries may have to be transferred to a Level I center (e.g., patients requiring advanced and extended critical care).

Neurosurgical capabilities are essential in Level II.

Level III

The Level III center serves communities that do not have immediate access to Level I or II institutions. Level III trauma centers can provide prompt assessment, resuscitation, emergency operations, and stabilization,

Notes to Figure 67-4

It is the general intention of these triage guidelines to select severely injured patients for trauma center care. When there is doubt, the patient is best evaluated in a trauma center.

Step 1 Physiologic status thresholds are values of the Glasgow Coma Scale, blood pressure, and respiratory rate from which further deviations from normal are associated with less than a 90 percent probability of survival. Used in this manner, prehospital values can be included in the admission trauma score and the quality assessment process.

A variety of physiologic severity scores have been used for prehospital triage and have been found to be accurate. Those scores contained in the triage guidelines are believed to be the simplest to perform and provide an accurate basis for field triage based on physiologic abnormality.

Deterioration of vital signs would necessitate transport to a trauma center.

Step 2 A patient who has normal vital signs at the scene of the accident may still have a serious or lethal injury.

*Step 3** It is essential to look for indications that significant forces were applied to the body.

Evidence of damage to the automobile can be a helpful guide to the change in velocity. Intrusion into the passenger compartment from any direction should prompt consideration of the potential for major injury.

*Step 4** Certain other factors that might lower the threshold at which patients should be treated in trauma centers must be considered in field triage. These include the following:

A. Age Patients over age 55 have an increasing risk of death from even moderately severe injuries. Those younger than age 5 have certain characteristics that may merit treatment in a trauma center with special resources for children.

B. Comorbid Factors The presence of significant cardiac, respiratory, or metabolic diseases are additional factors that may merit the triage of patients to trauma centers.

**Each trauma system and its hospitals should use QI programs to determine use of mechanism of injury and comorbid factors as activators for bypass and trauma team activation.*

Figure 67-4. *Continued.*

and can also arrange for possible transfer to a facility offering definitive care. Prompt availability of general surgeons is essential in a Level III facility. Neurosurgical capabilities are not required.

Level IV

Level IV trauma facilities provide advanced trauma life support prior to patient transfer in remote areas where no higher level of care is available. Such a facility may be a clinic, rather than a hospital, and may or may not have a physician available. The Level IV trauma facility should be an integral part of the inclusive trauma care system.

An inclusive system should leave no facility without direct linkage to a Level I or II trauma center. This insures neurosurgical care for all patients with neurotrauma wherever they are injured.

In addition to the designated Trauma Centers, there may be special care facilities, such as specialized burn centers or comprehensive pediatric centers. The ACS *Resources for Optimal Care of the Injured Patient,* 1993, provides specific criteria for such centers.

Designation[16]

Essential to the development of a trauma care system is the designation of definitive care facilities. The lead agency in the system must have the authority to determine the appropriate number of trauma centers for a given area. The number and location of trauma centers should be determined by geography, population density, available hospital resources, and transportation capabilities. The designation process should limit the number of centers to insure the optimal utilization of resources. The concentration of the most seriously injured patients will enable designated centers to maintain their expertise and to have the volume of patients necessary to support quality of care research and postgraduate education for physicians, nurses, and other health care professionals.

The proper designation of trauma centers is particularly critical with regard to neurotrauma care. Because of the limited number of neurosurgeons compared with most other surgical specialties, it is important to concentrate the patients with head and spine injuries in designated trauma centers that have the resources to provide optimal care.

The phases of the designation process usually include:

1. Creation of a request for proposal (RFP) by the designating agency.
2. Submission of proposals by applicant hospitals.
3. Proposal review.
4. Independent expert site survey to validate the system.
5. Public hearings.
6. Recommendation of designated facilities.
7. Formal designation.

The process of designation should focus on three major areas. Does the facility have the resources to provide optimal trauma care to injured patients? Are the physicians currently practicing at this facility committed to providing a level of trauma care consistent with accepted standards? Can the facility evaluate itself against a set of standards to ensure that the quality of the service delivered meets or exceeds acceptable levels, problems of care are identified and corrected, and care is improved? In addition to the process of initially selecting trauma care facilities based on their ability to meet certain standards, there should be a process for redesignation and "de"-designation. Continual, ongoing monitoring of trauma care performance over time assures a consistent approach to the care of the trauma victim and makes improvements in trauma care an integral part of the trauma system. This process requires trauma patient data from all facilities that care for injured patients. This data retrieval is best accomplished by a trauma registry.

Interfacility Transfer[16]

The system model (Fig. 67-2) indicates that all injured patients within a trauma care system will be triaged, either to a designated trauma center or to other acute care facilities. However, because the triage process is not precise, there will be fewer injured patients transferred inappropriately to trauma centers (overtriage), and, more problematically, seriously injured patients who require the resources of a trauma center transported to nondesignated trauma centers (undertriage). In either case, it is important to have clearly established interfacility transfer agreements.

These transfer agreements are fundamental to the linkage between rural Level III and IV areas and the region's Level I and II trauma centers.

The inclusive trauma care system should ensure that any seriously injured patient will have access to the highest level of care necessary for their injuries.

In any given system, it will frequently be neurotrauma that necessitates transfer of an injured patient to a higher level of care. Therefore, the neurosurgeons should be involved in the establishment of interfacility transfer policies.

Rehabilitation[16]

A critical component of any trauma care system is rehabilitation. This aspect of patient care unfortunately has been underemphasized and delayed until the patient is ultimately referred to a "rehab facility." Optimal care of the injured patient requires that rehabilitation should begin promptly after admission to an acute care facility and should continue through that patient's ultimate recovery. Rehabilitation should include not only the patient's physical condition but also reintegration into society. The results of effective rehabilitation areas are productive members of society.

Neurosurgeons have a particularly important role in establishing an effective rehabilitation component to the trauma system, since most patients requiring rehabilitation will have suffered neurotrauma. Neurosurgical leadership at both the hospital and system level is necessary.

References

1. Rice DP, MacKenzie EJ: *Cost of Injury in the United States: A Report to Congress.* Atlanta: Centers For Disease Control, 1989.
2. Committee on Trauma, American College of Surgeons: *Resources for Optimal Care of the Injured Patient: 1993.* American College of Surgeons, 1993.
3. Bazzoli G, Madura K: *1993 Inventory of Trauma Systems.* The Hospital Research and Educational Trust, 1993.
4. Trunkey DD: Predicting the community's needs: Local solutions to local problems, in West, JG (ed): *Trauma care systems: Clinical, financial and political considerations.* New York: Praeger, 1983:5–10.
5. Cales RH: Concepts in trauma care systems, in Cales RH, Heilig RW Jr (eds): *Trauma care systems: A guide to planning, implementation, operation and evaluation.* Maryland: Aspen, 1986:3–18.
6. Cales RH: Trauma mortality in Orange County: The effect of implementation of a regional trauma system. *Ann Emerg Med* 1984; 13:15–23.
7. Cales RH, Trunkey DD: Preventable trauma deaths: A review of trauma care systems development. *JAMA* 1985; 254:1059–1063.
8. Lowe DK, Gaely HL, Goss F, et al: Patterns of death, complication and error in the management of motor vehicle accident victims: Implications for a regional system of trauma care. *J Trauma* 1983; 23(6):503–509.
9. Ornato JP, Craren EJ, Nelson NM, et al: Impact of improved emergency medical services and emergency trauma care on the reduction in mortality from trauma. *J Trauma* 1985; 25(7):575–579.
10. Shackford SR, Hollingworth-Fridlund P, Cooper GF, et al: The effect of regionalization upon the quality of trauma care as assessed by concurrent audit before and after institution of a trauma system: A preliminary report. *J Trauma* 1986; 26(9):812–820.
11. Shackford SR, Mackersie RC, Hoyt DB, et al: Impact of a trauma system on outcome of severely injured patients. *Arch Surg* 1987; 122:523–527.
12. Eastman AB: Blood in our streets: The status and evolution of trauma care systems. *Arch Surg* 1992; 127:677–681.
13. Eastman AB, Bishop GS, Walsh JC, et al: The economic status of trauma centers on the eye of health care reform. *J Trauma* 1994; in press.
14. National Highway Traffic Safety Administration: *Development of trauma systems: A state and community guide.*

Washington: National Highway Traffic Safety Administration, 1988.

15. *Trauma Care Systems.* Position paper, Third National Injury Control Conference, "Setting the National Agenda for Injury Control in the 1990's." Atlanta, GA, U.S. Department of Health and Human Services, Centers for Disease Control, 1991.
16. U.S. Department of Health and Human Services, Public Health Service: *Model Trauma Care System Plan, Health Resources and Services Administration.* Rockville, MD, September 30, 1992.
17. Eastman AB, Lewis RE, Champion HR, Mattox KL: Regional trauma care systems design: Critical concepts. *Am J Surg.* 1987; 154:79–87.
18. Eastman AB, Rice CL, Bishop GS, et al: An analysis of the critical problem of trauma center reimbursement. *J Trauma* 1991; 31:920–926.
19. Committee on Trauma, American College of Surgeons: *Injury Prevention and Control, in Resources for Optimal Care of the Injured Patient: 1993.* ACS 1993:13–15.
20. Eastman AB, West JG: Trauma: Field triage, in Moore EE, Mattox KL, Feliciano DV (eds): *Trauma* (2d ed). Connecticut, Appleton and Lange, 1991:67–79.
21. Committee on Trauma, American College of Surgeons: Triage decision scheme, in *Resources for Optimal Care of the Injured Patient: 1993,* ACS 1993; 20.

ACKNOWLEDGMENTS

We would like to thank Gail F. Cooper, San Diego Department of Emergency Services, for her insightful comments on this chapter.

A special thanks to our secretary, Mary Jansky, for her efforts in preparing the manuscript.

CHAPTER 68

ROLE OF THE TRAUMA SURGEON IN NEUROTRAUMA

Michael Rhodes

SYNOPSIS

Neurotrauma is the major cause of traumatic death and serious injury in the United States. The sheer volume of neurotrauma has the potential to overwhelm available neurosurgical resources in many areas of the country. The contemporary trauma surgeon is a general surgeon with a genuine interest in and substantial knowledge of care of victims with neurotrauma. General surgeons can work with their neurosurgical colleagues throughout the pre-hospital, resuscitative, surgical, critical care, and rehabilitation phases of neurotrauma care. Jointly developed protocols and clinical conferences can greatly facilitate a better defined role for the general trauma surgeon in neurotrauma.

INTRODUCTION

The term traumatologist, which was popularized in Europe, was used to describe a surgeon capable of operating on the entire spectrum of injury, including head and skeletal trauma. Owing to emerging technological advances and recognition of trauma as a disease, it is current practice in the United States for an injured patient to be cared for by a team of specialists. In reality, all surgical specialists caring for the injured patient are "trauma surgeons;" but, generically, the term has come to refer to a general or thoracic surgeon charged with coordinating the overall care of trauma patients, including those with neurotrauma.

In a study of more than 16,000 head-injured patients admitted to trauma centers, Gennarelli and co-workers found that one-sixth of the patients with head injuries died, one-fourth of patients with isolated head injuries died, and that mortality from head injury was three times greater than for patients without head injury.[1] They concluded that head injury is now the most important cause of traumatic death and remains the greatest challenge facing trauma centers. Therefore, it is clear that neurosurgical availability is a cornerstone to effective trauma care. However, a recent study revealed that half of the hospitals claiming to have neurosurgical services in their emergency departments had difficulty ensuring coverage.[2] Fewer than one-fourth of identified trauma centers in the United States have a neurosurgical residency.[3,4] Inadequate neurosurgical coverage is a common deficiency cited for hospitals attempting to gain verification as trauma centers.[5]

For every neurosurgeon in the United States there are six orthopedic surgeons and ten general surgeons.[6] Given the magnitude of neurotrauma and the limited availability of neurosurgical manpower, a more efficient use of this resource is indicated. The trauma surgeon generally has the responsibility of working with his/her neurosurgical colleagues to provide quality neurotrauma care throughout all phases of management.

PREHOSPITAL CARE

Prehospital care triage guidelines, such as those published by the American College of Surgeons Committee on Trauma, direct most neurotrauma to trauma centers.[7]

Prehospital care airway management, especially with endotracheal intubation, has had a positive effect on head injury treatment results.[8] Prehospital treatment of shock also has had a positive effect.[9] Although this is much more difficult to demonstrate in clinical studies, it is likely that strong emphasis on spine protection has prevented exacerbation of many spinal injuries.

The trauma surgeon frequently is in a position to influence the prehospital care of the patient with neurotrauma. Participation in the training of emergency medical technicians, paramedics, and flight nurses can be done through courses such as Prehospital Trauma Life Support[10] (PHTLS) and Basic Trauma Life Support[11] (BTLS). Active involvement in the Advanced Trauma Life Support (ATLS) course sponsored by the American College of Surgeons Committee on Trauma can influence the management of neurotrauma in referring hospitals.[12] Ongoing involvement by the trauma surgeon in regional Emergency Medical Services (EMS) organizations also can have a very favorable impact on emergency airway management, spine immobilization, and other prehospital efforts toward care of neurotrauma. Although the neurosurgeon is more than welcome to participate in the aforementioned efforts, it is usually more practical for trauma surgeons to interact with the pre-hospital world by working with their emergency medicine colleagues. It is imperative that the trauma surgeon, emergency medicine physician, and neurosurgeon communicate frequently about pre-hospital issues.

EMERGENCY ROOM

Although many patients may have an isolated anatomical injury to the head or spine, the physiological injury is frequently manifest in many organs. In patients with multiple injuries, including the head or spine, the same cerebrospinal protective, diagnostic, and therapeutic techniques apply as in the "isolated" head injury, although the priorities may differ.

In many trauma centers, the trauma surgeon or his designee is the neurosurgical surrogate responsible for initial assessment and treatment of neurotrauma. It is incumbent on the trauma surgeon to be trained to perform an appropriate neurologic assessment. Since the early management of the head-injured patient frequently requires intubation and chemical paralysis, the neurosurgeon may have to depend on the assessment of the trauma surgeon. The trauma surgeon may have to also become skilled at evaluation of spinal x-rays and head CT scans. Recognition of most intracranial hematomas and depressed skull fractures is not difficult. Recognition of compressed cisterns, cerebral edema, and small contusions can be learned with experience and communication. Understanding these lesions and the clinical approach of their neurosurgeon colleagues can allow trauma surgeons to anticipate and facilitate the resuscitation of the patient with neurotrauma. Frequent combined clinical conferences are necessary to provide adequate communication between the trauma surgeon and the neurosurgeon.

The Joint Section on Neurotrauma and Critical Care of the American Association of Neurologic Surgeons and the Congress of Neurologic Surgeons have published minimal standards for neurotrauma care (Table 68-1).[6] In addition, the American College of Surgeons Committee on Trauma has recommended that the neurosurgeon be "promptly available"; that is, upon patient arrival, a neurosurgeon or physician who has been specially trained by the neurosurgeon must be present to begin neurologic diagnosis and therapy. In some institutions this is a neurosurgical resident. However, in many institutions this may be an attending trauma surgeon or general surgical resident at the PGY-4 or PGY-5 level.

Rhodes and co-workers reported a study measuring the impact of selective neurosurgical consultation on neurotrauma care.[13] Utilizing factors of high, moderate, and low risk for significant head injury promoted by the ATLS course[12] (Table 68-2), they developed criteria for urgent, non-urgent, and no neurosurgical consultation (Table 68-3). Urgent consultation required immediate (within four hours) response by the neurosurgeon; non-urgent consultation required patient evaluation within 12 to 24 hours. The remainder of the patients required no consultation and were managed entirely by the trauma service. All patients with head and spine injury, either isolated or with multiple trauma, were admitted to the trauma service and were managed by predetermined clinical protocols under the guidance of the attending trauma surgeon, with neurosurgical telephone

TABLE 68-1 Minimal Standards for Neurotrauma Care

1. Neurosurgeons and trauma surgeon on-call, promptly available, all times
2. 24-hour ED staff—ATLS-trained
3. Operating room—"rapid acceptance"—all times
4. CT scan → "constantly available"
5. MRI—"readily available"
6. Appropriate ICU
7. Bypass plan

SOURCE: Published by the Joint Section of Neurotrauma & Critical Care; AANS-CNS.

Adapted from data.[6]

TABLE 68-2 Risk Factors for Significant Head Injury

Risk		
High	**Moderate**	**Low**
▪ Depressed consciousness ▪ Focal signs ▪ Decreasing consciousness ▪ Penetrating injury ▪ Palpable, depressed fracture	▪ Change of consciousness ▪ Post-traumatic amnesia ▪ Progressive headache ▪ Multiple trauma ▪ Alcohol or drug intoxication ▪ Serious facial injury ▪ Unreliable history ▪ Signs of basilar fracture ▪ Age > 2 years ▪ Possible skull penetration ▪ Post-traumatic seizure ▪ Possible depressed fracture ▪ Vomiting ▪ Suspected child abuse	▪ Asymptomatic ▪ Headache ▪ Dizziness ▪ Scalp hematoma ▪ Scalp laceration ▪ Scalp contusion ▪ Scalp abrasion ▪ Absence of moderate or high-risk criteria

SOURCE: From ACS.[12]

consultation at his/her discretion. The impact on the neurosurgeon's time as measured by frequency and urgency of consultation was then recorded prior to the onset of these protocols and at a four-year interval after the establishment of the protocols. Three standard neurotrauma quality assurance filters were evaluated throughout these two periods (Table 68-4). Table 68-5 shows the results on over 800 patients with head and spine with Abbreviated Injury Score (AIS) ≥1 in each of the periods. The percentage of patients admitted to the Neurosurgical Service was significantly reduced from 16 to 3 percent. Those patients requiring urgent consultation were reduced from 26 to 12 percent, whereas those requiring non-urgent consultation increased slightly from 30 to 33 percent. The most dramatic change was in patients receiving no consultation,

TABLE 68-3 Criteria for Urgent, Non-Urgent, and No Neurosurgical Consultation

Consultation		
Urgent	**Non-Urgent**	**None**
▪ Lateralizing signs[1] ▪ GCS and age < 13 ▪ Open depressed skull Fx ▪ CT with —Mass effect[2] —Compressed cisterns —Massive edema ▪ Unstable C-spine Fx[3] ▪ Incomplete spinal cord[4]	▪ Concussion with mod risk[5] ▪ Skull Fx—nondepressed ▪ Age > 12 ▪ GCS < 13 w/o "urgent" CT —Contusion w/o mass —Minimal edema —Diffuse axonal injury ▪ Complete cord lesion[4] ▪ Stable C-spine Fx	▪ Concussion with low risk ▪ Headache < 24 hrs → Neg CT ▪ Vomiting < 12 hrs → Neg CT ▪ Intoxicated—Neg CT ▪ Fx T/L spine, w/o deficit, non-op

[1] Lateralizing signs—include pupillary asymmetry or nonreactivity, and hemiparesis.

[2] Mass effect—any shift of the septum pellucidum or pineal from the midline is considered significant. However, a shift of 5 mm or more suggests the need for decompressive surgery.

[3] Unstable cervical spine fracture—all C-spine fractures except spinous process fractures should be initially considered unstable until otherwise proven by CT and/or dynamic studies. This is particularly so in the presence of associated neurological deficits.

[4] Incomplete spinal cord injury—the role of surgery and its timing in patients with spinal cord injury have not been established conclusively. With the increasing use of MRI in the early evaluation of these patients, persistent spinal cord compression may be detected. The value of early surgical decompression in patients with complete deficits needs to be re-examined. If there is any role for early surgery, all patients with spinal cord injury—i.e., whether they are complete or incomplete—would qualify for "urgent" neurosurgical consultation.

[5] Concussion with moderate risk (see Table 68-2.)

TABLE 68-4 Neuro QA Filters

- Craniotomy > 4 h for clot
- CT scan > 2 h if GCS < 13
- Delay Dx C-spine Fx

which almost doubled from 28 to 52 percent. The numbers of trauma craniotomies and significant quality concerns as measured by the quality assurance audit filters were not significantly different. This study suggests a more defined role for the trauma surgeon in recognition of the practical limitations of neurosurgical resources, particularly in trauma centers without neurosurgical residents.

OPERATING ROOM

The trauma surgeon is in a position to facilitate the rapid evacuation of epidural, subdural, and intracerebral hematomas. In patients who are hemodynamically stable, rapid resuscitation, CT scan diagnosis, and transport to the operating room can be directed by the resuscitating trauma surgeon. This presents the opportunity to eliminate unnecessary delays by allowing the neurosurgeon to meet the patient in the CT scan suite or, in many instances, in the operating room. In the operating room, ongoing resuscitation and evaluation by the trauma service, including performance of a diagnostic peritoneal lavage, when indicated, can be carried out while preparing the patient for craniotomy. This requires a mature working relationship and sense of trust between the trauma surgeon and neurosurgeon.

Hemodynamically unstable patients with multiple trauma, including neurotrauma, present a special challenge to the trauma team. Thomason and co-workers have shown that the hypotensive multiple trauma patient is eight times more likely to require a laparotomy or thoracotomy than a craniotomy.[14] Fulton and associates, in a retrospective review of 462 consecutive patients with blunt trauma, found that fewer than 5 percent of the patients required neurosurgical intervention and that non-neurosurgical procedures to provide hemodynamic stability should be instituted before attempting a CT scan of the head.[15] Gutman and colleagues prospectively reviewed 646 consecutive trauma patients to evaluate the relative incidence of intracranial mass lesions and severe torso injury after accidental injury.[16] They suggested that victims of motor vehicular crashes who are less than 30 years of age and hypotensive with tachycardia should have diagnostic tests and emergent treatment of severe torso injury prior to detection and treatment of intracranial mass lesions. They further suggested that elderly victims of a fall, particularly those with focal neurologic signs, should prompt a more urgent neurologic diagnosis after initial resuscitation. Wisner and co-workers, in a similar study designed to identify independent predictors of surgical intracranial lesions, found that field intubation and lateralizing signs were significant predictors of such lesions.[17] However, they also found that field intubation was a predictor for laparotomy, leaving the presence of lateralizing signs as the most significant independent predictor of a surgical mass lesion in the multiple trauma patient. They suggested that a patient with a positive diagnostic peritoneal lavage and lateralizing neurologic signs who could be stabilized with ED resuscitation should undergo a CT scan of the head prior to the laparotomy. However, a patient with gross blood on the peritoneal tap or with continued hemodynamic instability should proceed directly to the operating room for laparotomy, prior to CT scan of the head.

The conclusion of the above studies suggests that for most patients presenting with multiple injuries, excluding elderly victims of falls, the likelihood of a significant abdominal or thoracic injury is substantially greater than the presence of a surgical intracranial lesion. If the patient is very unstable hemodynamically, everything possible should be done to restore normal blood pressure and ventilation promptly, including surgery when indicated. However, if the blood pressure can be normalized, a CT scan of the head should be obtained before going to the OR, provided this can be accomplished expeditiously (hence, the need for in-house, 24-hour CT scan capability in Level I trauma centers). Under optimal circumstances, a CT scan of the head generally can be obtained within a few minutes without causing any substantial delay in getting the patient to the OR.

TABLE 68-5 Results[13]

	1986	1990	p
*Head AIS ≥ 1	842	882	ns
m Age	33.2	34.9	ns
m ISS	11.2	10.9	ns
Mortality	10.3%	9.9%	ns
Neuro service	132 (16%)	24 (3%)	<.05
Urgent consult	220 (26%)	106 (12%)	<.05
Non-urgent consult	254 (30%)	290 (33%)	ns
No consult	236 (28%)	462 (52%)	<.05
Craniotomies	62	54	ns
Quality concerns	7	5	ns

* Approximately 12% of each group had associated spine injuries.
SOURCE: From Rhodes.[13]

CRITICAL CARE

Intensive care management of the patient with neurotrauma can be extremely challenging. The multiple trauma victim with associated neurotrauma requires a delicate balance of the competing priorities for managing the various organ systems. Even the anatomically "isolated" head and spine injury patient is prone to develop multiple organ abnormalities, including sinusitis, pulmonary edema, pulmonary barotrauma, atelectasis, pneumonia, diabetes insipidus, and ileus.

Most trauma surgical intensivists are continuing to gain experience with neurotrauma care. This is extending into a joint effort in many neuro-intensive care units. The contemporary trauma surgeon has an obligation to maintain a profound interest in the pathophysiology of head and spine injury. Intracranial pressure, cerebral perfusion pressure, jugular venous bulb oxygen saturation, cerebral blood flow, and cerebral metabolic rate can be effectively assessed only when taken in the context of hemodynamic, ventilatory, and metabolic management of the patient. The trauma surgeon can promote early removal of tubes and devices from the oro- and nasopharynx in these patients; this has been shown to reduce such complications as sinusitis and pneumonia.[18] Early tracheostomies in severely head-injured patients also have the potential to reduce ventilatory days and ICU length of stay.[19,20] Gastrostomy is also useful for providing decontamination of the oropharynx, as well as a route for long-term feeding. Both tracheostomy and gastrostomy can be done safely at the bedside utilizing the percutaneous technique.[21]

REHABILITATION

Aggressive rehabilitation of victims of neurotrauma may be the single most effective phase of trauma care. Traditionally, the trauma surgeon has left that aspect of the patient's care to the rehabilitation team, which usually is led by a physiatrist. It would seem prudent, however, for the trauma surgeon to maintain a very active role in that process. It is not unusual for the trauma surgeon to have been the first point of contact for the patient and the patient's family. This provides the trauma surgeon with the unique privilege of developing a special bond and rapport with the patient and family. Understanding and participating in the rehabilitation of the patient can facilitate an early and coordinated effort. It also allows the trauma surgeon to contribute to long-term outcome studies that will be essential to the ultimate survival of organized trauma care in the United States.

SUMMARY

Neurotrauma is the most significant aspect of trauma care in today's society. The neurosurgical community is making a considerable effort to deal with head and spinal cord injury. However, the sheer magnitude of the problem can be overwhelming to available neurosurgical resources. It is the responsibility of trauma surgeons to support their neurosurgeon colleagues throughout all phases of trauma care. Jointly developed protocols offer a unique opportunity for effective collaborative management. It has been suggested that neurosurgeons may be abdicating their leadership role in head injury management.[22] On the contrary, a defined role of the general surgeon in neurotrauma can allow the neurosurgeon to provide leadership in a more efficient manner.

REFERENCES

1. Gennarelli TA, Champion HR, Sacco WJ, et al: Mortality of patients with head injury and extracranial injury treated in trauma centers. *J Trauma* 1989; 29:1193–1202.
2. *Specialty Coverage in Hospital Emergency Departments.* Office of the Inspector General, U.S. Department of Health and Human Services, August 1992.
3. *Directory of Graduate Medical Educations Programs: 1992–1993.* Chicago: American Medical Association, 1992.
4. Eastman AB, Bishop GS, Walsh JC, et al: The economic status of trauma centers on the eve of health care reform. (Abstract) *J Trauma* 1993; 35:162.
5. Mitchell FL, Thal ER: Trauma center peer review verification program analysis of hospital failures. (Abstract) *J Trauma* 1993; 35:166.
6. Narayan RK, Saul TG, Eisenberg HM, Pitts LH: Neurotrauma care, in *Resources for optimal care of the injured patient: 1993.* Chicago: American College of Surgeons, Committee on Trauma, 1993:41.
7. Krantz BE: Field triage, in *Resources for optimal care of the injured patient: 1993.* Chicago: American College of Surgeons, Committee on Trauma, 1993:20.
8. Baxt WG, Moody P: The impact of advanced prehospital emergency care on the mortality of severely brain-injured patients. *J Trauma* 1987; 27:365–369.
9. Wald S, Fenwick J, Shackford SR: The effect of secondary insults on mortality and longterm disability of severe

head injury in a rural region without a trauma system. (Abstract) *J Trauma* 1993; 34:377–382.

10. The National Association of Emergency Medical Technicians: *Pre-hospital trauma life support* (3d ed). St. Louis: Mosby Lifeline, 1994.
11. Alabama ACEP Staff, Campbell JE: *Basic trauma life support.* Englewood Cliffs NJ: Prentice-Hall, 1985.
12. Advanced Trauma Life Support Program for Physicians: Instructor Manual (5th ed). Chicago: American College of Surgeons, 1993.
13. Rhodes M, Morrow R, Lester M: Selective neurosurgical consultation for trauma. (Abstract) *J Trauma* 1993; 35:979.
14. Thomason M, Messick J, Rutledge R, et al: Head CT scanning versus urgent exploration in the hypotensive blunt trauma patient. *J Trauma* 1993; 34:40–45.
15. Fulton RL, Everman D, Mancino M, Raque G: Ritual head computed tomography may unnecessarily delay lifesaving trauma care. *Surg Gynecol Obstet* 1993; 176:327–332.
16. Gutman MB, Moulton RJ, Sullivan I, et al: Relative incidence of intracranial mass lesions and severe torso injury after accidental injury: Implications for triage and management. *J Trauma* 1991; 31:974–977.
17. Wisner DH, Victor NS, Holcroft JW: Priorities in the management of multiple trauma: Intracranial versus intra-abdominal injury. *J Trauma* 1993; 35:271–278.
18. Seiden AM: Sinusitis in the critical care patient. New Horizons: *The Science and Practice of Acute Medicine* 1993; 1:261–270.
19. Dunham CM, LaMonica C: Prolonged tracheal intubation in the trauma patient. *J Trauma* 1984; 24:120–124.
20. Rodriguez JI, Steinberg SM, Luchetti FA, et al: Early tracheostomy for primary air management in the surgical critical care setting. *Surgery* 1990; 108:655–659.
21. Moore FA, Haenel JB, Moore EE, Read RA: Percutaneous tracheostomy/gastrostomy in brain-injured patients—a minimally invasive alternative. *J Trauma* 1992; 33:435–439.
22. Andrews BT, Narayan RK: Have neurosurgeons abdicated their leadership role in the management of head injury? *Surg Neurol* 1993; 40:1–2.

CHAPTER 69

NEUROTRAUMA CARE–PROBLEMS AND SOLUTIONS

John A. Kusske

SYNOPSIS

The significant scientific and technological strides that have been made in the care of patients with head and spine injuries are apparent in this book. As a result, there appears to have been a major reduction in morbidity and mortality of patients with neurological injuries over the past two decades. At least part of the reason for this improvement in outcomes is the development of prehospital care systems for the initial emergency treatment and rapid transport of patients with injuries. Simultaneously, technological advances in imaging and in the management of intracranial hypertension and spinal cord injury have contributed to this trend. The proliferation of dedicated intensive care units that are equipped to deal with neurological injuries has been another factor that has led to better outcomes. Neurosurgeons in general have also become more aggressive and prompt in their treatment of traumatically induced intracranial hematomas. Most of these advances relate to a well-designed trauma care system with rapid access to enlightened neurosurgical care. The active participation of neurosurgeons is paramount in assuring the smooth functioning of a neurotrauma system. Furthermore, adequate funding of trauma care is critical to the survival of the system. Paradoxically, as the ability to provide improved neurotrauma care has evolved, the entire trauma care system has been put at risk and in some areas is floundering or has never been established.

The specific problems of delivering neurotrauma care will be reviewed as they relate to the success of the trauma system as a whole. Solutions to many of these vexing issues depend to a great extent on health care reform and political will. Other answers depend on the willingness of the neurosurgical community to become more involved in the planning and operation of trauma systems. Although neurosurgeons have been instrumental in the tremendous advances made in neurotrauma care, in certain communities they have also been identified as a weak link in the trauma care chain. The survival of the discipline of neurosurgery may in part depend on the willingness of neurosurgeons to identify themselves as being the responsible primary physicians for the care of CNS and spinal trauma.

TRAUMA CARE SYSTEMS

TRAUMA CARE SYSTEM DESIGN

Trauma care systems are designed to provide care to an injured patient from the time of injury through definitive therapy in an acute care hospital and subsequently during rehabilitation. Ideally, the care is regionalized to match the seriousness of the injury with the available resources in a designated area. The system ideally provides a continuum of care and ensures means of measuring outcomes.[1,2] A variety of providers are needed in a comprehensive trauma system,[3] and a series of steps must be taken to develop such a system.[4] A step-by-step process for the development, management, and analysis of a trauma care system has been described by West and associates.[5] An instructive document for states and counties has been prepared by the National Highway Traffic Safety Administration.[6] Neurosurgeons have initiated and actively participated in trauma care planning in various communities. The principles for neurosurgical participation have been enunciated in various ways over the last several years.[7–9] The American Association of Neurological Surgeons (AANS) and the Congress of Neurological Surgeons (CNS) support the concept of organized neurosurgical trauma care consisting of the appropriate combination of prepared communities and institutions and adequate numbers of committed neurosurgeons.[8]

A 1979 study comparing preventable deaths in a trauma center with those in hospitals without trauma centers was a starting point for the development of trauma care systems in the United States.[10] In 1991, a total of 457 operational state-designated or American College of Surgeons–verified trauma centers were identified in this country, and approximately 20 other hospitals were functioning as trauma centers even though they were not designated.[11] Maryland, Virginia, Pennsylvania, Washington, Oregon, and a few other states have established statewide trauma care systems.[2] Progress toward trauma care systems has been aided by the enactment of the Federal Trauma Care Systems Planning and Development Act (PL101-590) in 1990. This act provides assistance to states for the planning, implementation, and monitoring of trauma systems.

Trauma System Dysfunction

Lack of Systems Nationwide

The efficacy of trauma systems has been verified by multiple studies that show as much as a 50 percent reduction in preventable deaths subsequent to the organization of regional trauma systems.[11–15] Nevertheless, the trauma care system is floundering.

Less than 25 percent of the United States is served by such systems. Many states have not developed systems, and in a number of areas systems that were started subsequently failed.[16] In a 1991 study, the General Accounting Office (GAO) reported that closures occurred primarily because of financial losses sustained from treating uninsured patients and patients covered by Medicaid and other government-assisted programs.[17] In a study of 25 trauma centers, Eastman and colleagues found that underfunding resulted from a combination of adverse factors—including above-average costs and a disproportionate number of indigent patients.[18] These authors pointed out that the object of a trauma care system is to concentrate the most critically injured patients in a limited number of designated trauma centers and that design is the primary cause of system failure. At least 60 trauma centers closed in the 5 years preceding the GAO report.[17]

Closures

The following description of trauma center failures in a major urban area highlights the problems that must be overcome.[19] In 1984, the Los Angeles County Emergency Medical Services Agency (EMS) verified 23 trauma centers, including 10 Level I centers, 10 Level II centers, and 3 rural centers, utilizing criteria enunciated by the American College of Surgeons Committee on Trauma.[4] Two years later seven hospitals had withdrawn from the system, including the third and fourth busiest hospitals, which provided 20 percent of the system's care. The loss left large areas of central and western Los Angeles, including the Los Angeles Airport, the intersections of the Santa Monica and Harbor freeways, and some of the most heavily traveled sections of the San Diego and Hollywood freeways, without an adjacent trauma center. Two major hospitals in the eastern portion of the county also withdrew, leaving large areas to the east of Los Angeles without a nearby facility, including the areas which had been the site of a severe earthquake several months earlier.[19]

There were four reported reasons why these private hospitals that had been designated as trauma centers dropped out of the system.

The first was the very high volume of uninsured patients. The second was the inability to transfer uninsured patients promptly to a county hospital because these hospitals were already operating at or beyond capacity. The third was the steadily growing numbers of trauma cases, which far exceeded the anticipated volume. The fourth was the fact that the volume of uninsured patients interfered with physicians' ability to manage their private practice patients for elective scheduled surgeries and the lack of space in the intensive care units.[19] A hospital that remained in the system was significantly affected by the closures of the other hospitals and saw its trauma caseload more than double, the number of uninsured patients climb from 25 to 55 percent, and the percentage of intensive care unit (ICU) resources devoted to trauma patients soar from 14 to 40 percent. The hospital had to initiate compensatory payments to its neurosurgeons, orthopedic surgeons, and cardiovascular surgeons because of the high volume of uninsured patients they had to treat. Eventually, the county had to redraw the hospital's catchment area to reduce the volume of uninsured trauma patients in order to keep the center in the system.[19] By 1992, 10 of the 23 trauma centers in Los Angeles County had left the system, and in southern California 14 of 32 centers had terminated their contracts with the various EMS agencies.[20] The result of this is that many southern California communities no longer have reliable networks of EMS hospitals, and many institutions have been forced to formally or informally abandon full-service emergency programs. Meanwhile, the demand for emergency services, particularly among the poor, continues to grow at a time when capacity is shrinking.[21] The Los Angeles experience may be reenacted in the future in other large urban areas.

Inadequate Financial Resources

Trauma center closures should be a concern at the national, state, and local levels. Lack of reimbursement for the costs associated with the delivery of emergency and trauma care has been the primary focus of many studies.[22] Several factors seem to be related to the difficulties encountered by trauma centers. These include hospital overcrowding, the perceptions and biases of hospital personnel, lack of revenue-producing activities, and inadequate governmental and private reimbursement.[22] Many hospitals and EMS systems do not have adequate statistical data specific to neurotrauma and emergency care. This became apparent during a study of the delivery of neurotrauma care in Los Angeles County, California.[23] It was determined, for example, that in 1990, of over 11,400 paramedic runs through the 911 system that were classified as neurosurgical, 10,200 (90 percent) did not require the services of a neurosurgeon.[23] This significant overestimation of the volume of neurosurgery emergency patients created a situation that led to a demand by the Los Angeles County EMS office to stop the transport of neurosurgical patients to the designated hospital and instead to take these patients to the nearest hospital. Later, after revision and refinement of the triage criteria, the situation was clarified and the paramedics reverted to taking neurosurgical patients to hospitals designated to receive them.[23]

A survey of neurotrauma delivery models in various other cities in the United States was completed by the task force. The cities included were Dallas, Detroit, Chicago, Baltimore, San Diego, and Sacramento. It was found that most were still in the process of refining their systems and had not specifically addressed their neurosurgical service problems.[23] Furthermore, no cost estimates could be given for neurotrauma care, and data indicating the volume of surgical procedures were not available. To ameliorate this situation, a study was undertaken in Orange County, California, to determine the costs associated with neurotrauma care and ascertain workloads.[24] Neuroregistry data acquired by the Orange County Emergency Services Agency were summarized for the years 1985–1991 and analyzed for the year 1990. Data were obtained on every patient admitted through the EMS system from the four paramedic neurosurgical receiving centers and the three trauma centers. These data included the total hospital charges and estimated charges for neurosurgeons generated by each neurotrauma patient and defined the neurotrauma activity in an urban-suburban county of 2.3 million people. This study showed that in 1990, 241 emergency neurosurgical procedures were performed in Orange County EMS hospitals. The total estimated charges for all 1476 patients entered into the system were $33,016,884. It was clear that the workload related to emergency neurosurgery was not overwhelming. Such efforts will guide other regions in providing efficient, cost-effective emergency neurosurgical care.

Lack of a Reliable Database

The lack of a reliable database for neurotrauma patients has had a major impact on the ability to differentiate between types of patients and document costs. This hinders billing, collecting, and reimbursement negotiations and makes accurate demographic analyses impossible. Without adequate data, decisions related to the delivery of neurotrauma care will be based on perceptions and can lead to inappropriate actions on significant issues. Neurosurgeons and those interested in the efficient delivery of neurotrauma care need to establish systems which track patients from the point of entry through discharge. As Moorhead has demonstrated, perceptions may be a primary determinant in the decisions made about trauma care. Many decisions to alter the patterns of care are based on negative anecdotal information about events, not on factual data.[22]

Many facilities have not documented the costs related specifically to neurotrauma or even to trauma in general. Policies and procedures associated with registration, charges, and billing specific to trauma have not been developed by many institutions. Training for billing and collection personnel is inadequate in many hospitals, and charges in many instances do not reflect all the treatment given. Efficiency in billing and collections could partially ameliorate the financial difficulties faced by trauma centers as they attempt to deal with present and future demands.[22]

Reimbursement by government must more fairly reflect the government's mandate that all persons must receive emergency care without regard to their ability to pay. Governmental payment at both the state and federal levels does not approximate the costs involved, and even these funds have been decreasing as a result of various cost-control strategies. It has been estimated that the cost of unsponsored trauma care totaled $1 billion in 1988 and represented approximately 10 to 12 percent of the $8.3 billion in unsponsored health care provided by U.S. acute care hospitals in that year.[16] One of the major issues has been that of Diagnostic Related Groups (DRGs). In California it has been estimated that up to 9 percent of trauma patients are affected adversely by inappropriate DRG policy.[21] The conclusion of most authors is that there needs to be a differentiation made within the DRG scheme for trauma and emergency care. The Medicaid program in most states seems to utilize similar methods. A trauma/emergency differential which recognizes patient acuity and prolonged treatment times must be incorporated into both programs.

Perceptions and Misconceptions

A perception among neurosurgeons is that trauma patients, particularly if they are indigent, are more likely to sue for malpractice than are other patients.[25] The available evidence suggests that this is not true. Contrary to physicians' perceptions, a representative from a large association of insurance companies has stated that participation in emergency services does not affect the price or availability of malpractice insurance.[25] In Maryland, it has been determined that claims filed by persons enrolled in Medicaid were lower than expected based on population statistics.[26] The GAO found that Medicare and Medicaid patients are less likely than are other patients to file malpractice claims.[17] Another study revealed that indigent and uninsured patients are significantly less likely to initiate malpractice actions.[27] The American College of Obstetricians and Gynecologists completed a review of Medicaid obstetric patients and found no statistically significant difference between the percentages of obstetrics-related malpractice suits filed by women whose care is funded by the Medicaid program and those filed by other patients.[28] This question needs to be addressed in a study directed specifically at claims arising from the emergency room activities of specialists such as neurosurgeons. State initiatives to give physicians some protection from liability in emergency care require further study. The current informational void about malpractice risks in emergency departments clearly has to be corrected.

Health Care Reform

Health care reform will have to address issues of trauma care. Large, vertically integrated health care plans such as Kaiser-Permanente, which has about 5 million covered lives in California, have not participated in any significant way in the trauma system. The planners of health care initiatives in general have not made significant statements about the financing of trauma care, and this issue will have to be addressed. The financial problems faced by trauma centers mirror the economic uncertainty facing the rest of the nation's health care system. The opportunity may exist to establish equitable payment programs for hospitals and physicians who provide sophisticated neurotrauma care. There may be additional opportunities to generate supplemental support for neurotrauma care in the context of the trauma system. Options, as outlined by Champion and Mabee, include the following:

1. Cigarette and alcohol tax
2. Surcharges on driver's license fees, traffic violation penalties, 911 telephone numbers, and motor vehicle registration fees
3. Trauma financing pool—a federal–state–private sector financing pool developed to reimburse qualified centers for documented uncompensated trauma care
4. Adjustment of DRG-based reimbursement
5. Increased reimbursement in return for regional trauma care.[16]

The California experience with these options has not been encouraging. Californians enacted Proposition 99 (tobacco tax) in 1988 to initiate the California Healthcare for Indigents Program. The funds were routinely used by hospitals to cover bad debt resulting from EMS operations, and physicians were attracted to the call panels because of the funding provided by this measure. The tobacco tax was effective in stabilizing the EMS system in southern California. However, the funds were subsequently diverted to other programs, with a 53.5 percent loss to the physician's account and a 26 percent loss to the hospital account. The state, through its passage of SB 612 (1988), gave counties the ability to establish an Emergency Medical Services Fund through an increased penalty assessment on traffic violations. Initially, these funds provided increased reimbursement for EMS providers, but the funds have also been partly directed to other uses by various governments.[20] Furthermore, recent budget reductions for both Medicare and Medicaid make it unlikely that there will be any adjustments for DRG differentials in trauma care.

The development of neurotrauma care in rural areas is also a problem that must be dealt with as attempts are made to refine rural trauma systems in general. These areas face unique problems in providing neurotrauma care. They are generally large land areas with small numbers of people. This creates logistical problems, including prolonged travel times, difficult access, and small hospitals with limited financial and human resources. Mortality rates associated with motor vehicle accidents have been shown to be highest in counties with a low population density.[29] This is thought to be partially related to inadequate access to trauma care in rural areas.

In the current era of managed care, neurotrauma care must be provided in a cost-effective manner in conjunction with fully organized trauma systems. Many of the managed care plans, including large staff model health maintenance organizations (HMOs), do not address the issue of trauma care. Most plans have out-of-network contingencies that provide payment for such services in emergency situations. It is important that neurosurgeons support efforts to continue funding for trauma systems. President Clinton's defunct proposal presented to Congress in early 1994 did not contain any provisions specifically related to trauma systems in its entire 1342 pages.[30]

At present, the establishment of trauma systems and the designation of trauma centers are functions of the local emergency medical services (EMS) authority. The Trauma Care Systems Planning and Development Act (PL 101-590) of 1990 called for a Model Trauma Care System Plan, and this was written in 1992.[31] Recommendations in the model trauma plan are compatible with the criteria established by the American College of Surgeons (ACS) in its most recent iteration of Resources for Optimal Care of the Injured Patient.[32] However, as experience has shown in major urban centers such as Los Angeles, unless adequate funding is available, the well-conceived plans of the ACS will not necessarily lead to the establishment of a viable system.

COBRA AND OTHER DANGERS

A federal statute governing the transfer of patients participating in the Medicare program was enacted in 1986.[33] This legislation was part of the Consolidated Budget Reconciliation Act of 1985 (COBRA), formally known as the Emergency Medical Treatment and Active Labor Law (EMTALL). These laws were amended in 1989 and 1991. Parallel legislation has been promulgated in several states, some of which is more restrictive than the federal statutes.[34] Extensive reviews have been published elsewhere.[35] The state and federal laws were designed to eliminate patient "dumping," that is, the transfer of unstable patients because they are uninsured or otherwise unable to pay for services. This law significantly affects emergency rooms as well as physicians who serve on call. It has been stated that "the country is now embarking on a permanent course in medical care delivery under a federal law that defines the standard of care according to law and not according to medical practice."[36] The process that led to these statutes will be reviewed briefly below, and the many unintended effects will be discussed.

Hospital profitability depends on having a low proportion of patients who are indigent and have no insurance.[37] In an effort to reduce the admissions of indigent patients, hospitals may be motivated to transfer them to publicly supported hospitals.[38,39] During the 1980s, the number of patients transferred increased as support from government funding sources decreased, and it was estimated that as many as 250,000 Americans were dumped in 1987.[40] It became apparent that such transfers delayed definitive medical care for a substantial number of patients who were transferred without regard to their medical stability.[41–43] Studies from public teaching hospitals provided data showing that financial dumping was widespread. The results of a study done at Parkland Hospital in Dallas provided the impetus for Texas to prohibit dumping.[37,44] This legislation was the model for federal action in the 1985 COBRA bill. Interhospital transfers to Cook County Hospital in Chicago rose more than 400 percent between 1980 and 1983.[41] Insurance status was cited by transferring institutions in 87 percent of the instances when these data became known. Of the patients transferred to Cook County, 81 percent were unemployed, minorities predominated, and the average age was 36 years. At Parkland in the first year of their study, 28 percent of interhospital transfers were unannounced, the patients were generally indigent and uninsured, and at least 30 individuals were unstable.[37] Similar data were developed at Highland General Hospital in Oakland, California,[43] and the Regional Medical Center at Memphis.[42] Twenty-seven percent of the economic transfers were judged to be unstable at the time of arrival. Among the vignettes presented in these reports is one describing an uninsured man who became comatose at a private hospital while two neurosurgeons allegedly refused to see him. Subsequent to transfer, a diagnosis of a cerebral contusion was made; the patient did not survive.[43]

These studies demonstrate that patient dumping usually occurs in one direction, that is, toward public hospitals. However, dumping may take other forms as well. For example, physicians in rural areas regularly refer patients to tertiary urban centers when they require services that smaller hospitals lack. Related to this issue, however, was a report of a practitioner in rural North Carolina who attempted to transfer a 35-year-old uninsured woman who had a head injury and was deteriorating to a tertiary facility where the physician had trained. A neurosurgeon at the hospital was contacted and, on hearing that the patient had no insurance, denied the transfer.[45]

In the past it was recognized that the transfer of patients for financial reasons was not sanctioned by the medical community. Many believed that the primary reason for transfer was to offer services to a patient that were not available at the original hospital or to move a patient who had requested a transfer to another institution. Fiscal constraints on medical care were generally thought to have been abolished after the passage of the Medicare and Medicaid acts in 1965. However, the principal reason why dumping has persisted is the continued lack of any health insurance among certain patients.[46] It has been stated that one of the first inquiries made at most hospitals is in regard to a patient's insurance status, which is then clearly marked on the emergency department record. As articulated by Judith Waxman, "We often hear of patients who must disclose their insurance status and ability to pay before they are physically screened to determine the extent of their physical condition." Of course, in this era of shrinking resources, health care providers are not entirely to blame. "Cost shifting," or charging more to those who could afford to pay to provide care for those who could not, was used in the past to support indigent care.[47] With substantial tightening of reimbursement by managed care companies, there is no longer any money to "shift," and hospitals have to carefully assess their reimbursement on every patient group to remain viable.

The federal government is the largest health care consumer through the Medicare and Medicaid programs. During the early 1980s, major changes in the eligibility requirements for Medicaid were enacted. In 1977, Medicaid insured 92 percent of Americans who were defined as poverty-stricken; in 1989, it covered about 40 percent.[47] Along with decreasing rates of reimbursement, many urban areas have seen a larger share of their population fall below the poverty line. In Los Angeles County, California, for example, there was an 18.5 percent increase in the population from 1980 to 1990. At the same time, there was a 42.9 percent increase in the poor population.[48] The unprecedented increase in the transfer rate noted in the Chicago and Oakland studies was ascribed to reductions in Medicaid reimbursement.[41,42] In 1988, hospitals in the United States underwrote $10 billion of indigent health care.[49] Public hospitals, which represent 5 percent of all hospital beds, provided 40 percent of all charity care.[50] From two-thirds to three-fourths of uncompensated care is for uninsured patients. Private hospitals provided for almost one-fourth of uncompensated care in 1982,[50] and it is unlikely that they will be able to significantly accept a larger fraction of these patients in the future.

Physicians and hospitals that violate COBRA laws are subject to severe penalties, including fines, investigation, disciplinary action, increased liability exposure, and criminal prosecution. COBRA also created a private right of action for the alleged violation of the statutes and allows the individual to obtain "those damages available for personal injury under [state] law" and "such equitable relief as is appropriate." The rules apply to all hospitals which are enrolled in the Medicare program and all patients who come to the emergency departments of these hospitals, not just Medicare recipients.[35] Further, in a result apparently not contemplated by Congress, COBRA may be used by malpractice attorneys to pursue a federal cause of action along with or instead of traditional state law claims.[51] In June of 1994 long-awaited federal interim final regulations were promulgated by the U.S. Department of Health and Human Services, Health Care Financing Administration.[52]

Hospitals that maintain an emergency department also must comply with the following other requirements:

Obligation to screen: Each person who presents at an emergency department must be provided with an "appropriate medical screening examination" by a physician for the purpose of determining whether that person has an "emergency medical condition" or is in "active labor."[53] The definition of "emergency medical condition" under federal law is "a medical condition manifested by acute symptoms of sufficient severity (including severe pain), such that the absence of immediate medical attention could reasonably be expected to result in placing the patient's health in severe jeopardy, serious impairment to bodily functions, or serious dysfunction of any bodily organ or part."[54]

Obligation to treat until stabilized: Generally speaking, each person presenting at an emergency department who is determined to have an emergency medical condition must receive, within the capability of the facility, the care, treatment, and/or surgery by a physician necessary to relieve or eliminate the emergency medical condition such that the discharge or transfer of the patient will not cause material deterioration in or jeopardy to the individual's medical condition or expected chances for recovery.[55] This includes the obligation to provide specialty consultation as medically appropriate, such as consultation over the telephone, and personal examination and treatment by a specialist "when determined to be medically necessary jointly by the emergency and specialty physician." The emergency care and treatment must be provided *before* one asks about the patient's ability to pay.[55]

Restrictions on transfer: Federal law does not restrict the transfer of stable patients, except in that it requires certain facilities to accept such transfers (see below).[56] With respect to unstable patients, federal law allows the transfer of these patients only if (1) a patient requests the transfer or (2) a physician certifies that the benefits expected from the transfer outweigh its risk. With respect to the physician's certification that an unstable patient may be transferred, there must be a summary of the risks and benefits on which the certification is based, and this must be signed by the physician.[57] The medical record requirement also includes "the name and address of any on-call physician who has refused or failed to appear within a reasonable time to provide necessary stabilization treatment."[58]

Exceptions to transfer requirements: There are two narrow exceptions to the transfer requirements for unstable patients. There can be a transfer for medical reasons if the patient makes a written request for a transfer after informed discussion about the benefits and risks or if the physician states that "the medical benefits reasonably expected from the provision of appropriate medical treatment at another medical facility outweigh the increased risks to the individual. . . ."[59]

Hospitals' obligations to accept transfers: Hospitals participating in the Medicare program that have "specialized capabilities or facilities" (such as burn units, shock-trauma units, and neonatal intensive care units) or are identified as federal regional referral centers must accept an appropriate transfer of an individual who requires such specialized capabilities or facilities whether or not the patient has been stabilized.[60] The wording "such as burn units, etc." is not meant to be all-inclusive. For example, a hospital that is not officially designated as a trauma center but has a neurosurgeon on call would still be considered to have specialized capabilities and therefore might be expected to serve as a referral hospital for an emergency department without neurosurgical backup. Confusion exists about this portion of the statute.[35] What if a patient requires nonsurgical care but the on-call specialist refuses to accept the transfer? What is the hospital that wants to transfer the patient supposed to do? If the patient needs a transfer because no neurosurgical coverage is available at hospital A, the emergency physician at that hospital documents the refusal and the efforts to stabilize the patient and find an accepting hospital. If there is a neurosurgical unit at hospital B with facilities available, it can be in violation of COBRA if it refuses to accept the patient. The refusing specialist is also at risk if the violation is reported by hospital A. Hospitals have been cited under this relative standard.[35]

Obligations of physicians: The duty to screen and treat patients presenting at the emergency department and certify patients for transfer rests with the emergency department physician. On-call physicians have duties under the law as well. Although the law does not require physicians to serve on call, it does require that if a physician serves on call, he or she cannot refuse the patient on the basis of the patient's race, ethnicity, religion, national origin, citizenship, age, sex, preexisting medical condition, physical or mental handicap, insurance status, economic status, ability to pay, or any other nonmedical reason. Federal law implicitly requires on-call physicians to come to the hospital when medically necessary within a "reasonable period of time" and establishes a mandatory reporting obligation on transferring hospitals when an on-call physician refuses or fails to appear within a reasonable time to provide necessary stabilizing treatment.[61] The name and address of the physician who failed to respond must be submitted to the receiving hospital at the time of transfer, along with the patient's medical records.[61]

Physician penalties: Under federal law, all physicians, including those on call, face a potential fine up to $50,000 for each violation they have committed or for which they are responsible. Under certain circumstances, a physician may be excluded from the Medicare program.[61]

Expanded liability: Any person who is potentially harmed by a violation may bring an action against the responsible hospital or administrative or medical personnel to enjoin the violation. Court decisions have affirmed that the act does not allow a federal cause of action against physicians.[62] Actions against physicians, however, can be joined with COBRA suits against the hospital in federal court, with an adverse affect on physician liability. Hospitals may cross-claim for indemnity against physicians.

Although the statutes apply to individuals who present to a hospital, a recent case before the U.S. Court of Appeals for the Seventh Circuit held that a plaintiff could sue a hospital for violation of the federal emergency transfer law when the hospital by radio directed an ambulance to another hospital, claiming it was on diversion status. In a highly unusual action, the Seventh Court vacated its earlier opinion and issued a new opinion that reached the opposite result.[63] The new and final opinion holds that while the plaintiff could bring suit against the hospital for negligence arising from breach of its common law duty to the patient, the patient could not bring an action under the federal emergency transfer laws. The court stated that the law applied only to an individual who actually comes to the hospital's emergency department. However, hospitals and physicians who serve as base station facilities and directors for local EMS agencies should take care to ensure that any diversion of ambulances based on the hospital's perception of inadequate resources be carefully determined.

Many questions will continue to plague physicians and hospitals in regard to these statutes. There is an urgent need for legislative amendments or interpretive regulations that address certain practical considerations. Specific ambiguities include (1) the definition of "facility capability," (2) what constitutes a transfer, (3) the conditions of the medical screening examination, and (4) the nature of an emergency medical condition.

Federal law requires that treatment be provided as necessary to stabilize the patient "within the staff and facilities available at the hospital."[55] This is not defined in the law, but at least one federal appellate court has held that the provision of a medical screening examination within an emergency room's "capabilities" constitutes good-faith application of the hospital's resources.[64] In states such as California, the definition of "facility capability" is complicated by state law, and basically any service that a hospital reports to the state that it provides must be available for emergency cases at all times.[65]

The definition of "transfer" needs clarification. At present, COBRA defines a transfer to include any movement involving the discharge of an individual outside a hospital's facilities. There are many reasons for a noneconomic transfer, including an error in diagnosis. In such an instance, the hospital may be inadvertently *denying* therapy to a patient and negligently failing to recognize the need for treatment. This suggests that COBRA has transcended its antidumping origins and is taking a step closer to becoming a federal malpractice law.[51]

The term "emergency medical condition" gives rise to numerous questions in regard to what a court may consider "serious" and what "immediate" means in terms of minutes, hours, or days. "Emergency medical condition" is a broad concept that may include conditions that many physicians would not consider true emergencies. Therefore, physicians must be aware that the legal definition of "emergency medical condition" for the purposes of compliance with the transfer laws is not necessarily the same as the clinical definition.

Because of numerous uncertainties in interpreting and implementing emergency transfer laws, physicians are well advised to work with their medical staffs in developing policies that attempt to reduce the burdens imposed by emergency room coverage. All such policies should be incorporated into the medical staff bylaws. Physicians who need legal advice should contact their professional liability carriers or attorneys.

Hospitals are legally responsible for providing on-call coverage in emergency departments. If a hospital is unable to obtain adequate coverage, it may eliminate a particular service or in extreme cases close the emergency department. Although neurosurgeons are not legally bound to be involved in arranging for the provision of on-call coverage, a lack of such involvement invariably leads to conflicts involving emergency department coverage. If the agreement to provide emergency neurosurgery services is a joint decision of the hospital administration and the medical staff, the two parties have an obligation to work together to provide on-call coverage. Neurosurgeons can influence this process by making recommendations to the hospital administration. It is also advisable for medical staffs to draft comprehensive policies regarding reasonable expectations of the neurosurgeons who serve on on-call panels. It is in the best interests of the medical staff to develop policies that are appropriate to the facility, guided by the number and distribution of neurosurgeons available as well as the patient care demands of the hospital and the community. Thus, policies regarding on-call neurosurgeons need to be addressed in a systematic way. On-call activities should be date- and time-specific. There is an inherent conflict between the interest of hospitals in providing an on-call panel of neurosurgeons to serve in the emergency department and the generally voluntary nature of those panels in most hospitals. It is important to remember that while serving on the on-call panel may be voluntary, once a neurosurgeon is designated as the person on call for a facility, there is nothing voluntary about responding to emergency room needs.

The question is often asked whether an on-call neurosurgeon is exposed to COBRA liability when he or she fails to respond for reasons beyond his or her control, as occurs when he or she is tied up in surgery or when there is a breakdown in communication such as a beeper failure. No exceptions to duty are expressly recognized under the law. Moreover, because of the potential for abuse, the authorities are likely to take a dim view of cases in which a physician fails to respond because of reasons allegedly beyond his or her control. Also, the law does not provide an express exception for situations in which the physician is treating another patient. Special questions arise with respect to physicians who have traditionally provided simultaneous on-call coverage to more than one facility. The law does not address this issue, and it is conceivable that the state or federal authorities could attempt to impose liability.

It seems that the best solution to these problems is a working arrangement among the facilities, neurosurgeons, and local EMS in a geographic area. Certain hospitals would be designated to receive neurosurgical trauma patients, and neurosurgeons would be on call only at those facilities. This would avoid the possibility of multiple exposures to liability if trauma patients requiring the attention of a neurosurgeon are dispatched to two or three hospitals where the same neurosurgeon is on call.

NEUROSURGERY PARTICIPATION IN TRAUMA CARE

The participation of neurosurgeons in neurotrauma care has come under scrutiny in both the news media and various government studies. A study completed in 1990 demonstrated that there was a considerable EMS on-call problem in Los Angeles County, California.[66] The problem affected a number of specialties, but particularly neurosurgery, in that 47 percent of the respondents ranked neurosurgery as their biggest problem. From the hospital executives' perspective, physicians' reluctance to accept calls stemmed primarily from inadequate payment levels, followed closely by malpractice liability issues. Also noted prominently were the risks imposed by COBRA legislation and disruption of the physician's practice routines. The EMS on-call problem was so pervasive that a majority of the survey respondents considered closure of their EMS services.

In the print media, examples of criticism of neurosurgeons appeared prominently during the summer of 1991. Headlines such as "Local Emergency Rooms Bar Neurosurgical Patients"[67] and "Neurosurgery Crisis Hits City"[68] were seen. The *Los Angeles Times* story included phrases such as "Head Injuries? No Admittance" and "Neurosurgeons Refuse Patients."[67]

The Office of the Inspector General (OIG) of the Department of Health and Human Services (HHS) also noted that the problem of on-call coverage for emergency rooms throughout the United States was most acute for neurosurgery.[25] Forty-nine percent of hospitals that offered neurosurgery in their emergency departments encountered difficulty ensuring coverage. Sixty-six percent of the specialty physicians surveyed stated that fear of increased malpractice liability had persuaded them not to participate in on-call activities. Forty-seven percent of the physicians considered that the COBRA laws were a serious drawback to participation in emergency care, and 44 percent stated that reimbursement for emergency services was inadequate. Hospital administrators responding to the survey cited a shortage of specialty physicians as the leading factor in their inability to meet this demand. The OIG indicated that many specialists did not want to participate in trauma care because they were engaged in more lucrative activities such as private practice with elective surgery only. More than 90 percent of hospitals in Massachusetts reported specialty coverage problems in 1990.[69]

The OIG report did not consider the support that was needed to provide neurosurgical coverage. Many hospitals that do not have neurosurgical emergency coverage may not be suitable places to provide this service, since they are not properly equipped. The regionalization of emergency neurotrauma care as suggested in the ACS plan is the most appropriate way to link available neurosurgeons with hospitals that have the logistical resources to provide efficient and safe care for these complex problems. Thus, in Los Angeles County, 33 of 103 hospitals met the criteria for neurosurgical receiving centers.[23]

For the system to be sensibly organized and efficiently run, there should be an adequate number of neurosurgeons to provide coverage. It has even been suggested that there may be excessive numbers of neurosurgeons in the United States.[70] However, neurosurgeons must take part in providing emergency care for neurotrauma patients. This is clearly in the best interest of the patients and indeed of neurosurgery. If neurosurgeons abdicate their leadership role in this field, an important aspect of neurosurgery will be gradually taken over by nonneurosurgeons, probably to the detriment of our patients and our specialty.[71]

References

1. Eastman AB, Lewis FR, Champion HR, Mattox KL: Regional trauma care systems design: Critical concepts. *Am J Surg* 154:79, 1987.
2. Eastman AB: Blood in our streets: The status and evolution of trauma care systems. *Arch Surg* 127:677, 1992.
3. American College of Emergency Physicians: Guidelines for trauma care systems. *Ann Emerg Med* 16:459, 1987.
4. American College of Surgeons Committee on Trauma: Resources for the optimally injured patient. Chicago: American College of Surgeons, 1990.
5. West JG, Williams MJ, Trunkey DO, Wolferth CC: Trauma systems current status: Future challenges. *JAMA* 259:3597, 1988.
6. U.S. Dept of Transportation, National Highway Traffic Safety Administration: *Development of Trauma Systems: A State and Community Guide.* Washington, DC: Office of Enforcement and Emergency Medicine, 1991.
7. Guidelines for establishment of trauma centers. *J Neurosurg* 65:569, 1986.
8. Neurotrauma care and the neurosurgeon: A statement from The Joint Section on Trauma of the AANS and CNS. *J Neurosurg* 67:783–785, 1987.
9. Narayan RK, Saul TG, Eisenberg HM, Pitts LH: Neurotrauma care, in (eds) *Resources for the Optimal Care of the Injured Patient.* Chicago: American College of Surgeons Committee on Trauma, 1993: 41–46.
10. West JG, Trunkey DO, Lim RC: Systems of trauma care: A study of two counties. *Arch Surg* 114:455, 1979.
11. Eastern Association for the Surgery of Trauma: *Preliminary survey of US Trauma Centers and State-by-State Analysis of Trauma System Development.* Reston, VA: Timothy Bell and Co., 1991.
12. Cales RH: Trauma mortality in Orange County: The effect of implementation of a regional trauma system. *Ann Emerg Med* 13:1, 1984.
13. U.S. Dept of Transportation, National Highway Safety Administration: *Medical Services Program and Its Relationship to Highway Safety.* Washington, DC: Office of Enforcement and Emergency Medical Services, 1985. Technical Report DOT HS 806832.
14. Champion HR, Teter H: Trauma care systems: The federal role. *J Trauma* 18:877, 1988.
15. Shacksford SR, Hollingsworth-Fridlund P, Cooper GF, Eastman AB: The effect of regionalization upon quality of trauma care as assessed before and after the institution of a trauma system: A preliminary report. *J Trauma* 26:812, 1986.
16. Champion HR, Mabee MS: *An American Crisis in Trauma Care Reimbursement.* Washington, DC: Washington Hospital Surgical Critical Care Services, 1990.
17. United States General Accounting Office: *Trauma Care: Life Saving System Threatened by Unreimbursed Costs and Other Factors.* Washington, DC: General Accounting Office, 1991.
18. Eastman AB, Rice CL, Bishop GS: An analysis of the critical problem of trauma center reimbursement. *J Trauma* 31:920, 1991.

19. Oversight hearing on the financial problems of trauma centers in Los Angeles County, California Legislative Special Committee on Medi-Cal Oversight. Los Angeles, October 22, 1987.
20. Abbate A: *Report to Governor Pete Wilson on Trauma Hospital Reimbursement in Southern California.* Los Angeles: Hospital Council of Southern California, May 1992.
21. *View of the Future.* Los Angeles: Hospital Council of Southern California, 1992.
22. Moorhead GV: *Report on Factors Affecting the Closure of Trauma Centers and Emergency Departments.* Emergency Medical Services Authority, San Joaquin County EMS Agency, August 1990.
23. *Report on Phase II of the On-Call Task Force Analysis.* A Joint Project of the Hospital Council of Southern California, Los Angeles County Medical Association, County of Los Angeles, Department of Health Services and California Association of Neurological Surgeons, September 1991.
24. Kusske JA, Shaver TE, O'Rourke B, Stalcup C: Neurotrauma care: Orange County California. Poster Presentation. American Association of Neurological Surgeons, Boston, April 25, 1993.
25. *Evaluation of Hospital Emergency Room Specialty Services.* OIG Report No. OEI-01-91-00771, August 1992. Subject: "Specialty Coverage in Hospital Emergency Departments."
26. Musman MG: Medical malpractice claims filed by Medicaid and Non-Medicaid recipients in Maryland. *JAMA* 265:2992, 1991.
27. McNulty M: Are poor patients likely to sue for malpractice? *JAMA* 262:1391, 1989.
28. *Hospital Survey on Obstetric Claim Frequency by Patient Payor Category.* Baltimore: American College of Obstetrics and Gynecology, February 1988.
29. Baker SP, Whitfield MA, O'Neill B: Geographic variation in mortality from motor vehicle crashes. *N Engl J Med* 316:1384, 1987.
30. Health Security Act H.R./S.105, 1994.
31. U.S. Public Health Service: *Model Trauma Care System Plan,* September 30, 1992. Rockville, MD: U.S. Department of Health and Human Services, United States Public Health Service, Health Resources and Services Administration, 1992.
32. Eastman AB: Resources for optimal care of the injured patient, 1993. *ACS Bulletin.* 78:21, 1994.
33. 42 U.S.C. §§ 1395cc, 1395dd.
34. California Health and Safety Code §§ 1317 *et seq.*
35. *Emergency Transfer Laws: California Physician's Legal Handbook.* California Medical Association, Chap. 10, 1994.
36. Frew SA: *Patient Transfers: How to Comply with the Law.* Dallas: American College of Emergency Physicians, 1991.
37. Reed WG, Cawley KA, Anderson RJ: Special report: The effect of a public hospital's transfer policy on patient care. *N Engl J Med* 315:1428, 1986.
38. Friedman E: Problems plaguing public hospitals: Uninsured patient transfers, tight funds, mismanagement, and misperception. *JAMA* 257:1850, 1987.
39. Relman A: What are hospitals for? *N Engl J Med* 312:372, 1985.
40. Ansell DA, Schiff RL: Patient dumping: Status implications and policy recommendations. *JAMA* 257:1500, 1987.
41. Schiff RL, Ansell DA, Schlosser JE, et al: Transfers to a public hospital: A prospective study of 467 patients. *N Engl J Med* 314:552, 1987.
42. Kellerman AL, Hackman BS: Emergency department "dumping": An analysis of interhospital transfer to the regional center at Memphis, Tennessee. *Am J Public Health* 78:1287, 1988.
43. Himmelstein DU, Woolhandler S, Harnly M, et al: Patient transfers: Medical practice as social triage. *Am J Public Health* 74:494, 1984.
44. Breitsch LM: Economic patient dumping: Whose life is it anyway? *J Leg Med (Chicago)* 10:433, 1989.
45. Wrenn K: No insurance, no admission. *N Engl J Med* 312:373, 1985.
46. *Equal Access to Health Care: Patient Dumping.* Hearing before the Human Resources and Intergovernmental Relations Subcommittee of the House Committee on Government Operations. 100th Congress, 1st Session, 1987. (Statement of Judith G. Waxman, Oct. 21, 1987.)
47. McClung AL: Your money or your life: Interpreting the federal act against patient dumping. *Wake Forest Law Rev* 24:173, 1989.
48. U.S. Census Report, 1990.
49. Reinhardt U: Economics, ethics and the American health care system. *New Physician* 20:22, 1985.
50. Gage JH, Andrulis CA: Our nation's great public health hospitals. *JAMA* 257:1942, 1985.
51. Metropoulos DG: Son of Cobra: The evolution of a federal malpractice law. *Stanford Law Rev* 45:263, 1992.
52. 42 C.F.R. Part 489, §§ 489.20, 489.24.
53. 42 C.F.R. Part 489, § 489.24(a).
54. 42 C.F.R. Part 489, § 489.24(b).
55. 42 U.S.C. § 1395dd(b).
56. 42 U.S.C. § 1395dd(d).
57. 42 U.S.C. §§ 1395dd(d).
58. 42 U.S.C. §§ 1395dd(c)(2)(C).
59. 42 U.S.C. §§ 1395dd.
60. 42 U.S.C. §§ 1395dd(g).
61. 42 U.S.C. § 1395dd(d).
62. Delancy v. Cade et al. 986 F.2d 387 (10 Cir. 1993).
63. 982 F.2d 230 (7th Cir. 1992).
64. Cleland v. Bronson Health Care Group Inc. 917 F.2d (6th Cir. 1990).
65. California Health and Safety Code §§ 1317.1(h).
66. Study of medical specialist emergency on-call practices of hospitals in Los Angeles County: A joint study of the Hospital Council of Southern California, Los Angeles County Medical Association and the County of Los Angeles, Department of Health Services, 1990.
67. *Local Emergency Rooms Bar Neurosurgical Patients:* Los Angeles Times. Metro Edition, p. 1. August 7, 1991.

68. *Neurosurgery Crisis Hits City:* Glendale Daily News Press, p. 1. August 8, 1991.
69. The state of hospital emergency departments in Massachusetts: Massachusetts Medical Society and Massachusetts Chapter, American College of Emergency Physicians, in cooperation with Massachusetts Hospital Association. January 1991, p. 61.
70. Wennberg JE, Goodman DC, Nease RF, Keller RB: Finding equilibrium in U.S. physician supply. *Health Affairs* 12:89, 1993.
71. Andrews BT, Narayan RK: Have neurosurgeons abdicated their leadership role in the management of head injury? *Surg Neurol* 40:1–2, 1993.

CHAPTER 70

VARIABILITY OF NEUROTRAUMA CARE IN HOSPITALS

Jam B. Ghajar

SYNOPSIS

Over the past two decades, considerable advances have been made in the care of patients with severe head injury, resulting in a steady decline in the mortality rates associated with this condition in centers with a demonstrated interest in neurotrauma. Much of this improvement can be ascribed to a better understanding of the pathophysiology of severe head injury and the resulting improvement in neurocritical care. Unfortunately, only a relatively small proportion of patients with a severe head injury fully benefit from these advances because of the considerable variability in the accepted management of this condition. This chapter outlines the rationale for an intensive care approach to these patients, summarizes the results of a U.S. survey of management practices, and discusses the newly developed practice guidelines for severe head injury.

INTRODUCTION

Intensive care for patients with severe neurological problems has been termed "neurocritical care" and in head-injured patients focuses on reducing secondary injuries such as cerebral hypoperfusion and intracranial hypertension. Overall, there is little published information on neurocritical management in the United States and other industrialized countries. This may be due to the paucity of scientific data supporting one form of treatment compared with another. Consequently, a variety of monitoring and treatment protocols have been developed that are based on clinicians' preferences rather than on scientific evidence. This chapter gives the results of our survey of U.S. neurotrauma centers and reviews practices in other countries.

Intracranial pressure (ICP) is elevated in 50 to 75 percent of patients with severe head trauma,[1] and the duration of elevated ICP above 20 mmHg has been found to be strongly correlated, as an independent prognostic factor, with increased morbidity and mortality in traumatically brain injured (TBI) patients.[2] This is true for patients with mass lesions as well as for those with diffuse brain injury in which intractable intracranial hypertension (ICH) results in mortality rates ranging from 16 to 56 percent.[3–5] Furthermore, primary brain damage suffered at the time of a head injury may be exacerbated by a secondary injury such as cerebral hypoxia or hypoperfusion.[6] These secondary events usually occur immediately after an injury or in the first week and are generally preventable through early cardiopulmonary support and appropriate treatment of ICH in conjunction with ICP monitoring.[5,7] Therapeutic lowering of ICH is based on the finding that persistent ICH is associated with a poor prognosis and that treatment initiated at a lower ICP improves patient outcome.[2,5,8]

OVERVIEW OF PUBLISHED TREATMENT PROTOCOLS

In 1977, Jennett and colleagues[9] reported on the management of severe head injury in three countries by collecting epidemiological data from hospital centers in Glasgow, Scotland; Rotterdam and Groningen, Netherlands; and Los Angeles, California. The city university hospitals in Rotterdam and Groningen served a population of 1 million people. Almost 90 percent of patients with severe head injuries arrived at the hospital within 2 h of injury. In both cities, most of the patients were treated in the neurology department. Rotterdam received a greater percentage of more seriously injured patients, and the care of these patients was not standardized. The Dutch centers reported variations in the proportion of patients receiving osmotic agents, steroids, and controlled respiration and suggested that different treatment regimens did not have a great effect on patient mortality or morbidity, since the patients in the three countries had very similar outcomes.[9] However, in 1983 the centers in Rotterdam and Groningen reported on the outcome of their severe head injury patients treated from 1974 to 1977 and showed a mortality rate of 45 percent in Rotterdam and 63 percent in Groningen. The investigators claimed that Rotterdam's less aggressive treatment accounted for 7.5 percent of the 18 percent difference in the survival rate, while the other 10.5 percent difference in mortality was due to discrepancies in the severity of injury at the two hospitals.[10] This study appeared to support the use of less aggressive therapy to improve outcome; however, the differences in admission criteria and treatment protocols even within the same center made comparison between hospitals difficult.

In Sweden, a study compared the outcome of patients admitted to Uppsala University Hospital before (1980 and 1981) and after (1987 and 1988) the development of a neurosurgical intensive care unit. After the establishment of this unit, the number of favorable patient outcomes increased significantly. Although there were no established guidelines for the treatment of patients in this neurosurgical intensive care unit, the intensive care management for patients in both time periods was described. From 1980 to 1981, conventional neurosurgical operations were performed, but compared with 1987 and 1988 fewer computed tomography (CT) scans were taken and no ICP monitoring was done. Ninety-six percent of the patients received steroids, mannitol was given to 65 percent, and 4 percent received high-dose thiopentone infusion. After the neurosurgical intensive care unit was established, there was intensive critical care and ICP monitoring. Treatment of raised ICP was accomplished by means of controlled hyperventilation, osmotherapy, deep barbiturate coma, and occasionally CSF drainage. During the 1987 to 1988 period, more CT scans were taken, 46 percent of the patients had their ICP monitored, and the patients were kept normovolemic. Steroids, although not part of their treatment, had been administered to 25 percent of the patients before they were admitted to the unit. Mannitol was given to 76 percent of the patients and 14 percent received thiopentone. This study found that outcome improved with the more aggressive mode of treatment during the 1987 to 1988 period, presumably because of continuous neurological monitoring, repeat CT scans for neurologically deteriorating patients, and monitoring and treatment of ICP.[11]

At the University of Edinburgh in Scotland, neurosurgeons advocate targeting specific therapies that depend on the CT scans of severe TBI patients. These clinicians have established a protocol for treating severely head injured patients, and this protocol might have contributed to the observed decreased mortality rate from 50 to 35 percent witnessed over the last 15 years.[12–14] Their concept of management, referred to as targeted therapy for controlling ICH, matches treatment of raised ICP to its cause. The basis of this treatment stems from the concept that an ICP greater than 20 mmHg is seen in a large percentage of head trauma patients and is associated with a poor outcome. In their 1993 study, these researchers reported that of their 215 study patients, 53 percent had an increased ICP > 20 mmHg for 5 or more min.[15] When a patient's ICP rises, a search for the causative factor is initiated, and then that factor is appropriately treated. The Edinburgh group outlined three specific causes of raised ICP and the appropriate targeted treatments: (1) An increase in cerebral blood volume is most appropriately managed with hyperventilation and hypnotic drugs, (2) the therapy of choice for an increase in brain water content is osmotherapy, and (3) an increase in CSF outflow resistance can best be treated with CSF drainage.[16] Other causes of raised ICP, such as head position, hyperthermia, seizures, and an intracranial hematoma, are also diagnosed and treated accordingly.

One of the few severe head injury management protocols that has been published and tested was established by investigators at the Medical College of Virginia. In 1977, these investigators instituted standardized therapy for treating patients with severe head injury. This protocol called for an early diagnosis and surgical evacuation of intracranial mass lesions, followed by treatment of the secondary cerebral injuries caused by hypoxia and brain swelling, using artificial ventilation and continuous monitoring of ICP. ICH (ICP > 40 mmHg) was controlled by increasing ventilation (maintaining Pa_{CO_2} at 25 to 35 mmHg), CSF drainage, and intravenous mannitol bolus doses at 0.5 to 1.0 g/kg. At this time, all patients received dexamethasone and prophylactic anticonvulsant therapy. These investigators concluded that their protocol improved the outcome of severe head injury patients compared with prior studies. In their investigation, 36 percent of their patients made a good recovery, 24 percent were moderately disabled, 8 percent were severely disabled, 2 percent were vegetative, and 30 percent died. Also, it was noted that this therapy did not increase the number of severely disabled or vegetative patients, as some opponents of aggressive treatment would have predicted.[4,8,17]

At the University of San Diego Medical Center, standardized aggressive therapy for the treatment of ICH has also been reported.[3] This group advocated immediate treatment of small rises in ICP to prevent uncontrolled ICH in severely head injured patients. In one study, 100 head trauma patients were managed with this algorithm, which included immediate endotracheal intubation, hyperventilation, and mannitol administration. A CT scan was then used to evaluate these patients. If the scan demonstrated an intracranial lesion, the patient was taken to the operating room for its removal and the insertion of an ICP monitor and then was cared for in the intensive care unit (ICU). If no intracranial lesion was found, the patient went immediately to the ICU, where ICP was monitored. In the ICU, patients were kept sedated, normovolemic, and normothermic, with the head of the bed elevated and with a Pa_{CO_2} of 100 mmHg and a Pa_{O_2} of 27 to 30 mmHg.[3,18,19]

The San Diego management protocol for severe head injury stipulated ICP monitoring in all comatose patients. If ICP rose above 20 mmHg, ventricular drainage was instituted. If the ICP still remained above 20 mmHg, mannitol was administered and a repeat CT scan was performed. Refractory ICPs above 20 mmHg were treated with high-dose barbiturate therapy to prevent additional ICH.[18,19] In this patient study, significant ICH ($ICP > 15$ mmHg) was detected in 53 percent of patients without a surgical lesion and 60 percent of patients who had craniotomies for the evacuation of a hematoma despite treatment with hyperventilation and dexamethasone. The results of the treatment protocol showed that 45 percent of patients had minor or no disability, 15 percent were moderately disabled, 4 percent were severely disabled, 8 percent were in a persistent vegetative state, and 28 percent died. Compared with previous reports, it appeared that severely head injured patients who were treated with this management protocol had a better outcome.[3,18,19]

The protocols described so far have shown improvement in patient outcome when compared retrospectively to the time before a protocol was instituted or in comparison with other centers' data. However, in these studies the effect of ICP monitoring and treatment cannot be separated from other parameters, such as improvements in critical care or brain imaging. Consequently, in 1989 a prospective clinical trial was initiated at Cornell University Medical Center to study the effect of ICP monitoring and treatment versus no monitoring and treatment in severe TBI patients.[20] Forty-nine consecutive patients between ages 16 and 70 who sustained blunt head injury, had a Glasgow Coma Scale (GCS) ≤ 7 for at least 24 h, and did not meet brain death criteria within that time period were studied. One group received ventricular ICP monitoring and was managed according to our staircase ICP protocol (Fig. 70-1), while the other group did not get ICP monitoring or treatment. Patients were assigned to the "ICP-monitored" group or the "nonmonitored" group based on the neurosurgeon on call when a patient was admitted. Other than in terms of ICP monitoring, all patients were managed similarly by a neurotrauma protocol that included intubation and ventilation to a Pa_{O_2} of 100 mmHg and a Pa_{CO_2} of 35 mmHg, CT scans, and prompt evacuation of significant subdural hematomas. Fluid resuscitation in the emergency room was performed according to Advanced Trauma Life Support Program (ATLS) guidelines. Patients were maintained normovolemic and were monitored for blood pressure and arterial Pa_{O_2}, Pa_{CO_2}, and pH with an indwelling arterial line and, if they were hypotensive on admission, with Swan-Ganz monitoring.

Both groups had a similar entry GCS and percentage of evacuated subdural hematomas. The Glasgow Outcome Score for both groups was evaluated at 6 months to 3 years after discharge. Mortality in patients who had ICP monitoring and treatment was approximately four times lower than it was in patients who were not monitored or treated, and the percentage of patients living independently was three times greater in the monitored group. The percentage of patients who were vegetative or dependent was not significantly different between the two groups. Since this was a small pilot study and was not truly randomized, the results should be interpreted with caution. However, the results suggested that outcomes could be improved with the use of ventricular ICP monitoring and treatment, utilizing CSF drainage as the primary modality. These results are encouraging, and past publications were researched to see if any advantage was afforded by CSF drainage in reducing mortality in patients with severe TBI. Fourteen publications, including the above study, were compared and are listed in Table 70-1. When these studies are grouped into no CSF drainage (ICP bolts), sometimes CSF drainage (a mix of bolts and ventriculostomies were used to monitor ICP), and always CSF drainage, a 51 percent improvement in mortality was noted with increased use of ventricular CSF drainage (Table 70-2).[20]

SURVEY OF CURRENT PRACTICES IN SEVERE HEAD INJURY MANAGEMENT IN U.S. TRAUMA CENTERS

Despite the abundance of clinical publications[4,5,7,8,17,21,22] and textbooks[23–26] on the management of severely head injured patients, no previous study had examined practices in head injury care on a nationwide basis. Therefore, a study was undertaken by the Brain Trauma Foun-

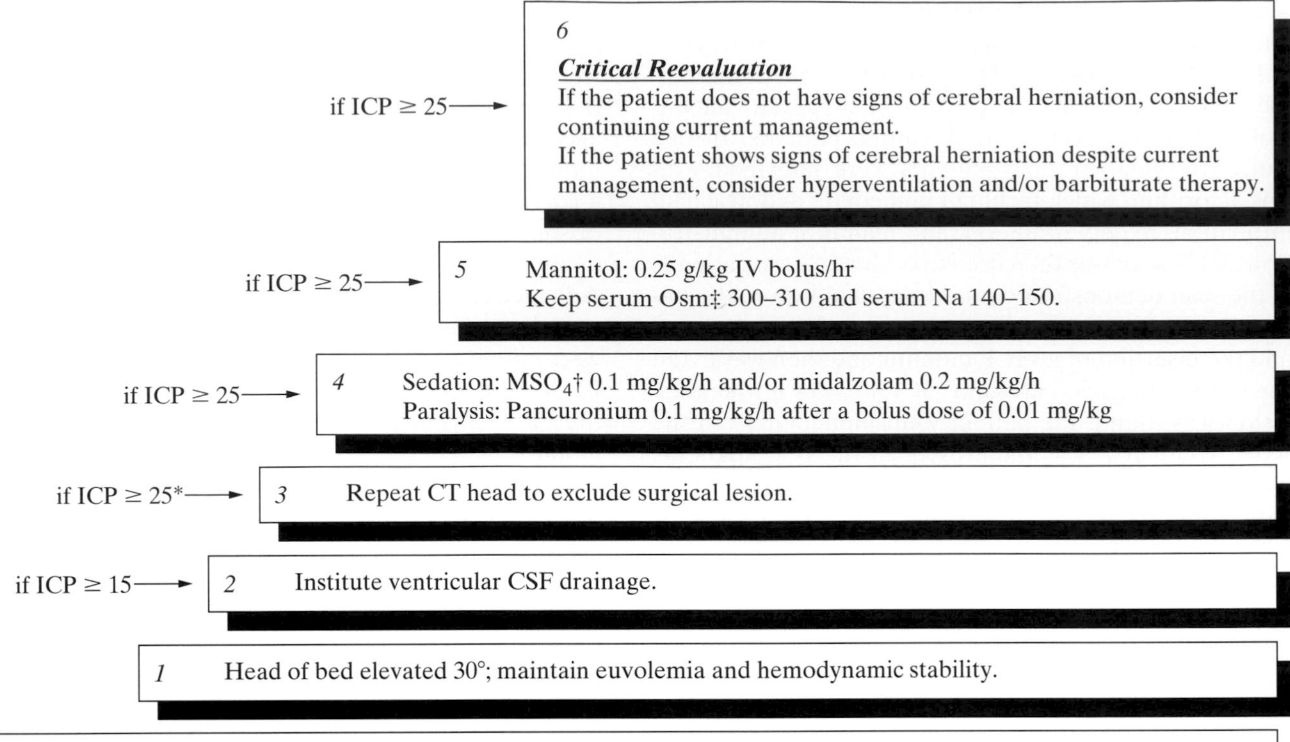

6
Critical Reevaluation
If the patient does not have signs of cerebral herniation, consider continuing current management.
If the patient shows signs of cerebral herniation despite current management, consider hyperventilation and/or barbiturate therapy.
if ICP ≥ 25
5 Mannitol: 0.25 g/kg IV bolus/hr
Keep serum Osm‡ 300–310 and serum Na 140–150.
if ICP ≥ 25
4 Sedation: MSO_4† 0.1 mg/kg/h and/or midalzolam 0.2 mg/kg/h
Paralysis: Pancuronium 0.1 mg/kg/h after a bolus dose of 0.01 mg/kg
if ICP ≥ 25
3 Repeat CT head to exclude surgical lesion.
if ICP ≥ 25*
2 Institute ventricular CSF drainage.
if ICP ≥ 15
1 Head of bed elevated 30°; maintain euvolemia and hemodynamic stability.
The staircase begins with a comatose patient following cardiopulmonary resuscitation, emergent surgical procedures, and with a functioning ventriculostomy in place.

* ICP is measured in mmHg. ICP ≥ 25 is defined as the average ICP over an 8-h period.
‡ Osm = osmolarity.
† MSO_4 = morphine sulfate.

Figure 70-1. The ICP management climb.

TABLE 70-1 Comparison of Outcome: Fourteen U.S. Studies

Study	No. Patients	GCS	ICP Monitor*	CSF Drain	Rx at ICP, mmHg	Outcome G/MD, %	Outcome Dead, %
Jaggi[51]	64	≤9	Bolt	0	>20	47	53
Colohan[52]	122	≤8	Bolt	0	>20	—	41
Smith	37	≤8	Bolt	0	>25	54	35
Wald	170	≤8	Epidural	0	>20	48	41
Saul I	127	≤7	Ventric, bolt	+/0	>25	—	46
Saul II	106	≤7	Ventric, bolt	+/0	>15	54	28
Bowers	200	≤7	Ventric, bolt†	+/0	>20/25	52	36
Becker	160	≤9	Ventric, bolt	+/0	>25/40	60	30
Miller[4]	225	≤9	Ventric, bolt	+/0	>25	56	34
Muizelaar	113	≤8	Ventric, bolt	+/0	>25	39	34
Marion	68	≤8	Ventric	+	‡	51	18
Narayan	207	≤9	Ventric	+	>25	57	34
Rosner	34	≤7	Ventric	+	‡	68	21
Ghajar	34	≤7	Ventric	+	15	59	12

* ICP monitor deemed ventric if ventriculostomy was used in more than 90 percent of patients.
† Only 41 percent of patients were monitored.
‡ Cerebral perfusion pressure maintained at 70–80 mmHg.
GCS = Glasgow Coma Scale; ICP = intracranial pressure; CSF = cerebrospinal fluid; G = good recovery; MD = moderate disability.
0 = not used; + = used.
— = data unavailable.

TABLE 70-2 Average Outcome from Studies Based on CSF Drainage Category

CSF Drainage Category	G/MD, %	Dead, %
Never (0)	49.7	43.0
Sometimes (+/0)	52.2	34.7
Routinely (+)	58.8	21.3

dation and the Aitken Neurosurgery Laboratory at Cornell University Medical College to ascertain current practices in severe head injury management in U.S. hospitals designated as "trauma centers" by the American Hospital Association.

Methods

The trauma centers in this study were selected from the 1991 directory of the American Hospital Association (AHA) hospitals. A trauma center, as defined by the AHA guide, is a state-certified facility that provides emergency care and specialized intensive care to critically ill and injured patients.[27] Six hundred twenty-four trauma centers were listed in the directory. The trauma centers surveyed were randomly selected from that list to provide a representative sample from each state. The survey included trauma centers from rural, suburban, and large metropolitan areas. Bed capacity varied from 100 to 1300, with the larger centers being located in more densely populated urban areas. It was noted that the larger trauma centers were often university- or medical college–affiliated hospitals with an average bed strength of 1000. The rural and suburban trauma centers characteristically were of smaller size, were not usually university-affiliated, and accounted for approximately two-thirds of all the centers surveyed.

The survey of critical care units specifically caring for severely head injured patients was conducted by telephone. Nurse managers, clinical nurse specialists, and staff nurses responsible for neurotrauma care were interviewed because they were the individuals most likely to complete census data and be involved in the daily care of these patients. The survey consisted of 22 questions: 16 multiple choice and 6 requiring subjective responses. The majority of the questions were designed to elicit verifiable information, such as patient census, type of unit, monitoring and treatment techniques, and trauma center level designation.

The collected data represented answers to telephone interviews from 277 trauma centers. Overall, 261 centers (94 percent) participated in the survey. Of the participating centers, 219 (84 percent) acknowledged that they were providers of care for severely head injured patients, while 42 centers (16 percent) stated that they did not provide such care. According to the 1991 AHA directory, there are five states without any formal trauma center designation process. Therefore, the 219 trauma centers in this survey came from the remaining 45 states. Severely head injured patients were defined as patients with postresuscitation GCS scores ≤ 8.[28] To assess reliability and account for differences among respondents, 40 centers (15 percent) were resurveyed 6 months later. This follow-up survey was completed by a nursing professional from a different shift, although the questions were the same.

Trauma Center Designation

Trauma center level designation criteria were only broadly based on the American College of Surgeons (ACS) guidelines published in 1990.[29] The ACS document provides a detailed description of the components necessary for a hospital to be adequately set up to provide a certain level of trauma care. These guidelines are frequently used by state departments of health and emergency medical service (EMS) agencies as a template for developing their own licensing guidelines for trauma centers. The vast majority of "trauma centers" in the United States are either formally designated by their respective states or identify themselves as having a certain level of commitment to trauma care. However, caution should be taken in the use of the term "trauma center." Currently, this term is loosely used. Only about 61 centers nationwide have actually undergone review by the ACS and have successfully completed the designation process (Level I–41, Level II–17, Level III–3). However, the list of ACS-designated trauma centers is not released to the public; thus, no distinction was made in our study between state-designated trauma centers and those designated by the ACS. As shown in Table 70-3, the largest group of respondents came from centers that identified themselves as Level I centers (49 percent), followed by Level II (32 percent) and Level III (2 percent). Interestingly, only 17 percent of the responding hospitals stated that they held no formal trauma center designation. However, the majority of states lack an organized trauma system. Individual hospitals may voluntarily choose to be reviewed by the ACS and receive formal recognition as a trauma center. The vast majority have not done so.

ICU Description and Patient Numbers

The results in Table 70-3 reflect responses to questions regarding patient census, trauma center level designation, the presence of specialty ICUs for neurotrauma patients, and ICU directorship. Table 70-4 summarizes information derived from questions regarding ICP monitoring and modalities used for the treatment of ICH.

TABLE 70-3 Trauma Center Characteristics

Survey Question	Respondents, %
Do you currently take care of patients in acute coma from head injury?	
Yes	84
No	16
What is your trauma center level designation (of those who answered yes to previous question)	
Level I	49
Level II	32
Level III	02
No level	17
Do you have a designated neurological/neurosurgical ICU?	
Yes	34
No	66
How many cases of severe head injury do you receive per month?	
>30	01
15–30	14
8–14	24
4–7	22
1–3	31
<1	08
Who is the director of your ICU?	
Critical care physician	27
Neurosurgeon	21
General surgeon	17
Neurologist	03
Other	30
Do not know	02

ICU = intensive care unit.

Thirty-four percent of the surveyed hospitals had a designated neurological/neurosurgical ICU, and only 24 percent of all units surveyed were under the direction of a neurosurgeon or neurologist (Table 70-3). Specialization of the ICUs was more common in larger hospitals. The smallest hospitals, those with less than 300 beds, relied on one general critical care unit. Hospitals with a larger bed capacity responded more frequently that severely head injured patients were cared for in surgical/trauma or neurological specialty units.

Table 70-3 shows the monthly census data for the trauma centers surveyed. Relatively few centers (15 percent) received more than 15 patients with a severe head injury per month, and 31 percent received only 1 to 3 patients per month. The majority of centers received 4 to 14 head-injured patients per month (46 percent).

ICP Monitoring

ICP monitoring was employed with 75 to 100 percent frequency in the treatment of severely head injured patients in only 77 of the 219 centers surveyed; 16 centers reported never using ICP monitoring. The technique most often used by the units that reported monitoring ICP were ventriculostomy (72 percent) and intraparenchymal fiber-optic catheters (48 percent), followed by subarachnoid bolts (25 percent), epidural devices (15 percent), and subdural catheters (5 percent) (Table 70-4).

Table 70-5 summarizes the differences in frequency of ICP monitoring at Level I, II, and III trauma centers. Level I trauma centers were found to monitor ICP in severely head injured patients more frequently than did Level II and Level III centers. There was also a statistically significant direct correlation between the number of severely head injured patients treated per month and the use of ICP monitoring (Table 70-6, Fig. 70-2).

ICP Treatment Modalities

Eighty-three percent of critical care units reported utilizing hyperventilation and osmotic diuretics as a means of reducing elevated ICP (Table 70-4). The degree of hyperventilation varied considerably, with 57 percent of the units hyperventilating patients with severe head

TABLE 70-4 ICP Monitoring and Treatment of Intracranial Hypertension

Survey Question	Respondents, %
What percentage of severely head injured patients receive ICP monitoring?	
90–100	28
75–90	12
50–75	17
25–50	24
01–25	12
0	07
What types of ICP monitors are used?	
Ventriculostomy	72
Intraparenchymal	48
Subarachnoid	24
Epidural	15
Subdural	05
Which of the following treatments do you use for ICH in >50% of severely head injured patients?	
Osmotic diuretics	83
Hyperventilation	83
Steroids	64
CSF drainage	44
Barbiturates	33
To what extent are patients hyperventilated?	
Pa_{CO_2} >30 mmHg	14
Pa_{CO_2} = 25–30 mmHg	57
Pa_{CO_2} <25 mmHg	29

ICP = intracranial pressure; ICH = intracranial hypertension; CSF = cerebrospinal fluid.

TABLE 70-5 Frequency of ICP Monitoring Correlated with Trauma Center Level*

ICP Monitoring Frequency, %	Level I, %	Level II, %	Level III, %
75–100	51	37	20
50–75	17	13	40
25–50	21	24	20
0–25	11	25	20

* Differences between Level I, Level II, and Level III are statistically significant ($p < .0001$) by contingency table (chi-square) analysis.

injuries to achieve a Pa_{CO_2} between 25 and 30 mmHg and 29 percent of the centers hyperventilating patients to maintain a Pa_{CO_2} less than 25 mmHg.

The use of ventriculostomy catheters for ICP monitoring was employed in 72 percent of the centers, but CSF drainage using ventriculostomy catheters was utilized by only 44 percent of the hospitals. The administration of barbiturates was reported in 33 percent of the units as a treatment for ICH. Steroids were reportedly used more than half the time in 64 percent of the trauma centers (Table 70-4).

Follow-Up Survey

To determine the reliability of the responses from the initial survey, 40 centers (15 percent) were reinterviewed 6 months after the original survey. These responses were compared with those obtained from the same 40 trauma centers in the original survey (Table 70-7). Trauma center level designation, patient census, and presence of specialty units were unchanged between the two surveys. Interestingly, the frequency of ICP monitoring changed significantly; this might have been due to variation in the impressions of the persons surveyed or sensitization to these issues resulting from reports in the press.[30]

No significant changes were noted in the resurveyed group regarding therapies for ICH and the degree of hyperventilation compared with the original survey results. However, a statistically significant difference was noted between the two groups regarding the types of monitoring devices used. This may reflect the greater availability of intraparenchymal monitoring devices.

Discussion

The findings of this survey confirm the impression that practice patterns vary widely and that a patient with a

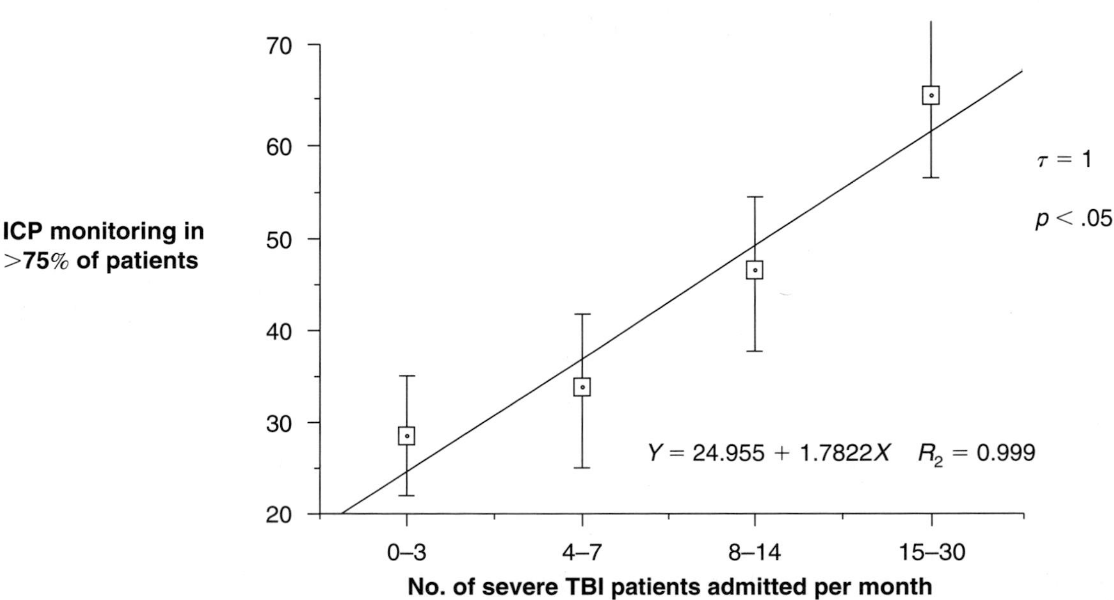

Figure 70-2. Frequency of ICP monitoring versus number of patients admitted per month.

TABLE 70-6 Frequency of ICP Monitoring and Number of Severely Head Injured Patients Admitted per Month*

ICP Monitoring Frequency, %	*Number of Patients per Month*			
	15–30	8–14	4–7	0–3
75–100	65	45	34	28
50–75	06	23	28	13
25–50	10	22	26	35
0–25	19	10	12	24

* Differences between groups are statistically significant ($p < .0001$) by contingency table (chi-square) analysis. Regression analysis reveals a significant linear correlation with $R = 0.999$ and equation of regression $Y = 24.95 + 1.78X$.

TABLE 70-7 Comparison of ICP Monitoring and Treatment of Intracranial Hypertension from Trauma Centers between 1991 and 1992

Survey Question	*Respondents, %*	
	1991	1992
What percentage of severely head injured patients receive ICP monitoring?		
90–100	28	27
75–90	12	43*
50–75	17	17
25–50	24	05†
01–25	12	08
0	7	0*
What types of ICP monitors are used?		
Ventriculostomy	72	65
Intraparenchymal	48	65‡
Subarachnoid	24	0*
Epidural	15	10
Subdural	5	5
Which of the following treatments do you use for ICH in >50% of severely head injured patients?		
Osmotic diuretics	83	73
Hyperventilation	83	80
Steroids	64	43
CSF drainage	44	33
Barbiturates	33	20
To what extent are patients hyperventilated?		
Pa_{CO_2} >30 mmHg	14	10
Pa_{CO_2} = 25–30 mmHg	57	65
Pa_{CO_2} <25 mmHg	29	25

* $p < .001$.
† $p < .01$.
‡ Statistically significant ($p < .05$) differences by *t*-test.
ICP = intracranial pressure; ICH = intracranial hypertension; CSF = cerebrospinal fluid.

severe head injury is likely to be managed quite differently depending on where and by whom that patient receives treatment. The key findings include the fact that ICP monitoring is not used routinely in comatose head injury patients in a significant proportion of hospitals. By contrast, hyperventilation is being empirically and sometimes overaggressively used, a practice that may result in more harm than good.[21,31,38] Finally, steroids are being widely administered despite the lack of evidence of their efficacy in severe head injury.[40–43]

No standardized management guidelines have been developed for severe head injury on a national basis. However, most authorities in the field agree that mortality and morbidity from this condition can be reduced significantly by means of a protocol that includes early intubation (in the field if necessary), rapid transportation to an appropriate trauma center, early CT scanning, and immediate evacuation of an intracranial mass lesion, followed by intensive care in the appropriate unit. The main objectives in the ICU are to maintain adequate cerebral perfusion and avoid medical complications while the brain recovers.

In the late 1970s and thereafter, several researchers reported a significant reduction in mortality in patients with severe brain injury using the intensive management principles outlined above.[3,17] More recent data have helped us better understand why those somewhat empirical protocols worked and resulted in a drop in mortality from around 50 percent[9] to somewhere between 30 and 40 percent.[4] While there has clearly been a fairly dramatic improvement in outcome at severe head injury centers, there remains a great deal of variability in the care of these patients around the country.[32,33]

MAJOR AREAS OF CONCERN

As ascertained by this survey, the typical management of a severely head injured patient in the majority of centers surveyed consisted of hyperventilating the patient to a Pa_{CO_2} of 25 to 35 mmHg, administering osmotic diuretics and steroids, and not monitoring ICP. As was expected, Level I trauma centers, because of their specialized staff and technology, monitored ICP more frequently than did Level II and Level III centers. Also, the frequency of ICP monitoring correlated significantly with the number of severely head injured patients admitted per month (Table 70-6). These survey results draw attention to several aspects of head injury care that merit closer scrutiny.

ICP Management

ICP elevation is a very common and potentially lethal consequence of head injury. Indeed, most of the treatment rendered to these patients, including mannitol, hyperventilation, and barbiturates, exerts its effect either wholly or partially by reducing ICP. Furthermore, it is widely accepted that there are no reliable clinical signs of increasing ICP in a comatose patient until a dilated pupil heralds cerebral herniation. Therefore, it is surprising that ICP monitoring has not become more widely used; this survey indicated that only 28 percent of hospitals monitored ICP in over 90 percent of comatose head-injured patients. Hence, in the majority of hospitals, ICP is being treated empirically with therapies that may be under- or overutilized.

Several factors may contribute to the low utilization of ICP monitoring. This is a somewhat labor-intensive undertaking, requiring trained nurses and physicians to record accurately the data and promptly treat the problem. These resources may be limited, albeit for different reasons, both in smaller hospitals and in already overburdened trauma centers. Whether neurosurgeons are in short supply is subject to debate, but it seems unlikely that there will ever be enough of them to adequately cover all hospitals that wish to receive major trauma patients.[33] ICP monitoring itself is not without risk, with an infection rate of about 6 percent (reported range, 0 to 20 percent) and a major hemorrhage rate of 1 to 2 percent.[7]

Finally, there is the issue of proof of efficacy. While no reasonable physician would ask for proof of the value of blood pressure monitoring during cardiac surgery or the need for serial blood pressure measurements in a patient being treated for hypertension, a controlled trial that demonstrates improved outcomes as a result of ICP monitoring per se is demanded by some before they will accept the additional effort and risk associated with such monitoring. The correlation between high ICP and a poor outcome after a head injury has been amply demonstrated by various groups.[2,3,7,8,17] An extensive body of clinical experience indicates that reducing elevated ICP reduces the risk of herniation and facilitates recovery.[3,5,7,8] There is increasing evidence that a low cerebral perfusion pressure (mean systemic blood pressure minus ICP) is associated with a poor outcome.[2,6,34–37] Measuring ICP directly is the only known way of monitoring cerebral perfusion pressure (CPP). Given these facts, it is difficult to design a clinical trial of the value of ICP monitoring without encountering serious ethical concerns with regard to the nonmonitored group.

Hyperventilation

Hyperventilation has been used for several years as a rapid, effective, and easy method of reducing ICP. However, some evidence convincingly demonstrates that it can be a double-edged sword.[38] The first indication that hyperventilation can be harmful if used aggressively came from a randomized trial in which patients with severe head injury were treated with hyperventilation alone, hyperventilation plus the buffer THAM, or neither.[21] In this trial, the patients who were hyperventilated alone had a retarded recovery compared with the other two groups. Subsequently, it has been shown that hyperventilating patients down to Pa_{CO_2} levels of less than 25 mmHg can result in a higher incidence of transient cerebral hypoxia as evidenced by jugular venous oxygen saturation less than 50 percent.[39] Furthermore, recent data indicate that even these brief periods of cerebral hypoxia, which would go undetected without jugular oxygen saturation monitoring, are associated with markedly worse outcomes in head injury patients.[31] Hence, in adults, hyperventilation should be used only when ICH cannot be controlled by other means, such as ventricular CSF drainage.

In this survey, we found that 83 percent of hospitals reported using hyperventilation in over 50 percent of severely head injured patients. About 29 percent of the respondents used Pa_{CO_2} levels less than 25 mmHg, a level that we now know can be harmful in certain cases.[21,31] Furthermore, since many hospitals were not monitoring ICP, hyperventilation is usually used empirically. In the absence of any objective indicator of when and how much hyperventilation is required, there is considerable potential for overuse of this treatment modality.

Steroids

While steroids are clearly useful in reducing the edema associated with brain tumors, their value in head injury is not clear. In fact, studies to date have been unable to demonstrate any benefit associated with the use of steroids in terms of ICP control or improved outcome from a severe head injury.[40–43] Furthermore, there is some evidence that steroid use may have a deleterious effect on metabolism in these patients.[44,45] It is possible that very high doses of certain steroids may have a beneficial effect in a certain subset of these patients, as was demonstrated with methylprednisolone in spinal cord injury.[46] The new steroid analogue Tirilazad is undergoing clinical trials and may eventually prove to be useful. However, to date, currently available steroids in standard dosage regimens have not been valuable. Nevertheless, 64 percent of respondents are using these agents in over 50 percent of their patients. While this practice is probably not harmful, the potential side effects and the cost of these drugs need to be considered.

MANAGEMENT GUIDELINES

The survey data, which were recently published, indicate that there is considerable variation in the management of severe head injury in the United States.[47] This is due partly to a lack of hard data on which to base practice and partly to the personal prejudices of treating physicians. While the data are by no means conclusive, there is now much more information on which to base practice than there was even 5 years ago. There is no doubt that any suggested practice guidelines will change as our knowledge evolves. However, this seems to be an appropriate time to make a move toward documenting the current state of knowledge in an easily accessible manner.

Guidelines for clinical practice have been developed for various other conditions, including trauma,[29] myocardial infarction,[47] and anesthesia care.[48] While such guidelines could be used against physicians medicolegally, it is more likely that they will be employed to defend physicians against a lawsuit in appropriately managed cases with a less than satisfactory outcome. In fact, the monitoring standards set by the American Board of Anesthesiology[49] have lowered intraoperative patient morbidity and mortality. As a consequence, the number of lawsuits against anesthesiologists has declined, as has the premium for their insurance.[50]

However, great caution needs to be exercised to avoid dogma in the development of practice guidelines. Furthermore, labor-intensive practices such as ICP monitoring may not be practical in all hospitals or in areas where neurosurgical coverage is limited. A triage system for the care of severely injured patients may be helpful in these circumstances so that such patients may be treated at the most appropriate hospital rather than at the closest facility.

In the final analysis, evidence-based practice guidelines are desirable because they can improve the standard of care rendered to patients. If developed with care and sensitivity and updated on a regular basis, such guidelines can help standardize the care of these patients and reduce the mortality and morbidity associated with head injury. Such a document is currently under preparation.

ACKNOWLEDGMENT

The author would like to thank Erica D. Goldberger for her manuscript assistance. This survey was supported by a grant from the Brain Trauma Foundation and the Annie Laurie Aitken Charitable Trust as part of their commitment to the advancement of brain injury research.

REFERENCES

1. Miller JD, Deardon NM, Piper IR, Chan KH: Control of ICP in patients with severe head injury. *J Neurotrauma* 9:S317–S321, 1992.
2. Marmarou A, Anderson RL, Ward JD, et al: Impact of ICP instability and hypotension on outcome in patients with severe head trauma. *J Neurosurg* 75(Suppl):S59–S66, 1991.
3. Marshall LF, Smith RW, Shapiro HM: The outcome with aggressive treatment in severe head injuries. *J Neurosurg* 50:20–25, 1979.
4. Miller JD, Butterworth JF, Gudeman SK, et al: Further experience in the management of severe head injury. *J Neurosurg* 54:289–299, 1981.
5. Saul TG, Ducker TB: Effect of intracranial pressure monitoring and aggressive treatment on mortality in severe head injury. *J Neurosurg* 56:498–503, 1982.
6. Chestnut RM, Gautille T, Blunt BA, et al: Neurogenic shock in the Traumatic Coma Bank (abstract). San Francisco: American Association of Neurological Surgeons Scientific Meeting No. 357, April 1992.
7. Narayan RK, Kishore PRS, Becker DP, et al: Intracranial pressure: To monitor or not to monitor? *J Neurosurg* 56:650–659, 1982.
8. Miller JD, Becker DP, Ward JD, et al: Significance of intracranial hypertension in severe head injury. *J Neurosurg* 47:503–516, 1977.
9. Jennett B, Teasdale G, Galbraith S, et al: Severe head injury in three countries. *J Neurol Neurosurg Psychiatry* 40:291–298, 1977.
10. Gelpke GJ, Braakman R, Habbema JDF, Hilden J: Comparison of outcomes in two series of patients with severe head injuries. *J Neurosurg* 59:745–750, 1983.
11. Warme PE, Bergstrom R, Persson L: Neurosurgical intensive care improves outcome after severe head injury. *Acta Neurochir* (*Wien*) 110:57–64, 1991.
12. Miller JD: Changing patterns in acute management of head injury. *J Neurol Sci* 103:S33–S37, 1991.
13. Miller JD, Dearden NM, Tocher JL: Progress in the management of head injury. *Br J Surg* 79:60–64, 1992.
14. Fowkes FGR, Ennis WP, Evans RC, Williams LA: Admission guidelines for head injuries: Variance with clini-

cal practice in accident and emergency units in the UK. *Br J Surg* 73:891–893, 1986.
15. Miller JD, Piper IR, Dearden NM: Management of intracranial hypertension in head injury: Matching treatment with cause. *Acta Neurochir (Wien)* 57(Suppl):152–159, 1993.
16. Miller JD, Jones PA: The work of a regional head injury service. *Lancet* 1141–1144, 1985.
17. Becker DP, Miller JD, Ward JD, et al: Outcome from severe head injury with early diagnosis and intense management. *J Neurosurg* 47:491–502, 1977.
18. Chestnut RM, Marshall LF: Management of severe head injury, in Ropper AH (ed): *Neurological and Neurosurgical Intensive Care,* 3d ed. New York: Raven Press, 1993: 203–246.
19. Chestnut RM, Marshall LF: Treatment of abnormal intracranial pressure. *Neurosurg Clin North Am* 2(2):267–284, 1991.
20. Ghajar JBG, Hariri RJ, Patterson RH: Improved outcome from traumatic coma using only ventricular cerebrospinal fluid drainage for intracranial pressure control. *Adv Neurosurg* 21:173–177, 1993.
21. Muizelaar JP, Marmarou A, Ward JD, et al: Adverse effects of prolonged hyperventilation in patients with severe head injury: A randomized clinical trial. *J Neurosurg* 75:731–739, 1991.
22. Bowers SA, Marshall LF: Outcome in 200 cases of severe head injury treated in San Diego County: A prospective analysis. *Neurosurgery* 6:237–242, 1980.
23. Becker DP, Gudeman SK: *Textbook of Head Injury.* Philadelphia: Saunders, 1987.
24. Cooper PR: *Head Injury,* 2d ed. Baltimore: Williams & Wilkins, 1987.
25. Marshall LF, Bowers SA: *Neuroscience Critical Care: Pathophysiology and Patient Management.* Philadelphia: Saunders, 1990.
26. Narayan RK: Head Injury, in Grossman RG, Hamilton WJ (eds): *Principles of Neurosurgery.* New York: Raven Press, 1991: 235–292.
27. American Hospital Association: *Guide to the Health Care Field.* Chicago: 1991.
28. Teasdale G, Jennett B: Assessment of coma and impaired consciousness: A practical scale. *Lancet* 2:81–84, 1974.
29. American College of Surgeons Committee on Trauma: *Resources for Optimal Care of the Injured Patient.* Chicago: 1990.
30. Kolata G: Flawed Treatment of Head Injuries Found. *NY Times,* Oct. 16, 1991: C14.
31. Gopinath SP, Robertson CS, Contant CF, et al: Transient jugular venous oxygen desaturation and outcome after head injury. *J Neurol Neurosurg Psychiatry* 57:717–723, 1994.
32. Marshall LF, Eisenberg HM, Jane JA, et al: The outcome of severe head injury. *J Neurosurg* 75:528–536, 1991.
33. Office of the Inspector General, Department of Health and Human Services: *Specialty Coverage in Hospital Emergency Departments.* Washington, D.C.: 1992.
34. Changaris DG, McGraw CF, Richardson JD, et al: Correlation of cerebral perfusion pressure and Glasgow coma scale to outcome. *J Trauma* 27:1007–1013, 1987.
35. Piek J, Chestnut RM, Marshall LF, et al: Extracranial complications of severe head injury. *J Neurosurg* 77:901–907, 1992.
36. Robertson CS, Constant CF, Gokaslan ZL, et al: Cerebral blood flow, arteriovenous difference, and outcome in head injured patients. *J Neurol Neurosurg Psychiatry* 55:594–603, 1992.
37. Rosner MJ, Daughton S: Cerebral perfusion pressure management in head injury. *J Trauma* 30:933–940, 1990.
38. Cold GE: Does acute hyperventilation provoke cerebral oligaemia in comatose patients after acute injury? *Acta Neurochir (Wien)* 96:100–106, 1989.
39. Sheinberg M, Kanter MJ, Robertson CS, et al: Continuous monitoring of jugular venous oxygen saturation in head-injured patients. *J Neurosurg* 76:212–217, 1992.
40. Braakman R, Schouten HJA, Dishoek MB, Minderhound JM: Megadose steroids in severe head injury: Results of a prospective double-blinded clinical trial. *J Neurosurg* 58:326–330, 1983.
41. Cooper PR, Moody S, Clark WK, et al: Dexamethasone and severe head injury: A prospective double blind study. *J Neurosurg* 51:307–316, 1979.
42. Gudeman SK, Miller JD, Becker DP: Failure of high-dose steroid therapy to influence intracranial pressure in patients with severe head injury. *J Neurosurg* 51:301–306, 1979.
43. Saul TG, Ducker TB, Saleman M, et al: Steroids in severe head injury: A prospective randomized clinical trial. *J Neurosurg* 54:596–600, 1981.
44. Robertson CS, Clifton GL, Goodman JC: Steroid administration and nitrogen excretion in the head injured patient. *J Neurosurg* 63:714–718, 1985.
45. Young B, Ott L, Phillips R, et al: Metabolic management of the patient with head injury. *Neurosurg Clin North Am* 2:303–328, 1991.
46. Bracken MB, Shepard MJ, Collins WF, et al: A randomized controlled trial of methylprednisolone or nalonone in the treatment of acute spinal cord injury: Results of the Second National Acute Spinal Cord Injury Study. *N Engl J Med* 322:1405–1411, 1990.
47. Ghajar J, Hariri RJ, Narayan RK, et al: Survey of critical care management of comatose, head-injured patients in the United States. *Crit Care Med* 23:560–567, 1995.
48. American College of Cardiology/American Heart Association Task Force Report: Guidelines for the early management of patients with acute myocardial infarction. *Circulation* 82:664–707, 1990.
49. American Society of Anesthesiologists: *Standards for Basic Intraoperative Monitoring.* Park Ridge, IL: 1986.
50. Eichhorn JH, Cooper JB, Cullen DJ, et al: Standards for patient monitoring during anesthesia at Harvard Medical School. *JAMA* 256:1017–1020, 1986.
51. Jaggi JL, Obrist WD, Gennarelli TA, et al: Relationship of early cerebral blood flow and metabolism to outcome in acute head injury. *J Neurosurg* 72:176–182, 1990.
52. Colohan Austin RT, Alves WM, Gross CR, et al: Head injury mortality in two centers with different emergency medical services and intensive care. *J Neurosurg* 71:202–207, 1989.

CHAPTER 71

MEDICOLEGAL ASPECTS OF HEAD AND SPINAL INJURY

Joseph L. Romano

SYNOPSIS

Medicolegal issues are an integral and important aspect of the care of patients with head and spinal cord injury. Some clinicians have a limited understanding of these matters and may feel intimidated by, and uncomfortable with, this reality of patient care. This chapter succinctly describes these issues. A clear understanding of the legal aspects of such cases can substantially lower clinicians' anxieties and facilitate more effective interactions with the patient, the family, and the various social and legal agencies that deal with the neurotrauma victim.

The chapter is divided into three major sections. The first, "Patient Focus," deals with issues of guardianship, informed consent, self-determination, confidentiality, quality of life, and the right-to-die. The second section, "Resource Focus," describes the nuances of insurance policies and how best to deal with them. The final section, "Legal Focus," discusses the role of the physician in establishing factual evidence—both as the primary caregiver and as an expert witness.

Health care professionals today find themselves in the difficult position of having to deal with the added responsibilities of medicolegal issues during treatment. The rising cost of health care and the legal burdens placed on the health care provider compel them to view the care they provide with a patient focus, a resource focus, and a legal focus. These are all necessary aspects of insuring that the patient receives maximum rehabilitation and utilizes all available resources.

PATIENT FOCUS

According to the American Trauma Society, each year an estimated 500,000 Americans are admitted to hospitals following traumatic brain injuries. An estimated 75,000 to 90,000 of these die annually. Of those who survive, about 70,000 to 90,000 will endure life-long debilitating loss of function; an additional 2000 will exist in a persistent vegetative state. More than one million children sustain head injuries annually.[1]

The medicolegal issues on which health care professionals need to focus to insure the protection of a patient's rights are guardianship, the patient's right of self-determination and informed consent, and the patient's right-to-life/right-to-death decisions.

GUARDIANSHIP

Guardianship is a legal relationship between one individual (the guardian) and an incapacitated individual (the ward). It gives the guardian the duty and the right to act on behalf of the incapacitated party in making decisions that affect the incapacitated person's life. The words "incompetent person" or "incapacitated person" is a "legal term of art," which means that the court has determined that the individual can no longer manage his or her own affairs and needs a guardian.

Faced with the dilemma of a patient with a traumatic brain injury who is obviously incapable of making informed decisions, the health care professional should urge family members to have a guardian appointed to insure proper legal authority to treat. If the patient has had the foresight to prepare a durable power of attorney (also known as a health care proxy) that names an individual to manage his or her medical affairs and money in the event he or she becomes incapacitated, then the appointment of a guardian by the court is unnecessary.

If the medical professional determines that a guardian is required, a petition must be filed in the Orphans' Court in the county where the disabled individual resides or is being treated. The petition essentially requires information concerning the relationship of the proposed guardian to the incapacitated individual, financial information of the incapacitated individual, facts and circumstances that led to the particular injury or illness, and medical documentation. Attorneys should consult with the attending physician, family physician, and all interested family members to determine who should be appointed as guardian. Unless the guardianship is limited by the court in some way, the guardian will manage all of the incapacitated party's personal, medical, legal, and financial affairs.

Upon receipt of a petition for the appointment of a guardian, the court will hold a hearing to determine if there is sufficient medical documentation to appoint a guardian. Although most courts require that the treating doctor testify in person concerning medical aspects of the case, some courts will not require this if the doctor files a notarized medical report or deposition with the court. It is not necessary that the medical report or testimony be from a psychiatrist; any doctor involved in the treatment of the individual can provide the medical documentation or testimony necessary to support the appointment of a guardian. If the treating doctor states that it would be against the best interest of the incapacitated individual to appear in court, the court will usually not require the patient's appearance. However, sometimes the judge will want to visit the incapacitated individual to discuss the appointment of the guardian, especially if the individual is able to communicate his or her wishes. Courts are reluctant to declare a person incapacitated or incompetent unless it is both absolutely necessary and based on proper medical documentation. It is often very difficult for a family member to think about guardianship, but it is crucial that the doctor and the health care team discuss this issue as soon as possible with the family in order to protect the medical and legal interests of the incapacitated individual.

Informed Consent

As early as the 18th century, a physician was legally obligated to obtain a patient's consent. If a physician did not obtain a patient's consent, the patient had a remedy which was compensable under a "battery theory." A "battery" is harmful or offensive bodily contact with a patient without his or her consent. Traditionally, the key element to prove a battery was not the intent of the physician but the absence of patient consent. It is a well established legal principle that health care professionals are responsible for making adequate disclosures of information to the patient and obtaining the patient's informed consent. The basis of the doctrine of informed consent is that the patient has a right to determine what shall be done with his or her own body.

In order for a patient to give "*informed consent*," the health care professional should discuss the following with the patient:

- Diagnosis
- Nature and purpose of treatment
- The desired outcome
- The hazards or risk of the medication, treatment, or proposed health care
- Chances of success or failure
- Alternative procedures that could achieve the desired medical result
- Likely medical consequences without any treatment at all.

"*Actual consent*" occurs when a health care professional has explained the risks, alternative procedures, and expected consequences to a competent adult, to the parent of a minor child, or to the court-appointed guardian.

"*Implied consent*" is a legal theory that evolved because ill or injured individuals were unable to grant a health care professional "actual consent." The most common situation where the court will use the doctrine of implied consent is in a medical emergency. Health care professionals, paramedics, and emergency medical technicians can transport an individual to a facility and treat any individual, adult or minor, in an emergency without anyone's consent, since in an emergency a patient's consent is implied. An emergency exists when a patient is suffering from a life-threatening disease or injury that requires immediate treatment. There is no clear-cut rule as to how long an emergency lasts. It could last from a few days to a week; during this time, medical personnel are permitted to give necessary treatment to the patient at an acute care facility. If it becomes evident that an adult individual will remain in a coma or be otherwise incapacitated for a long period, then family members should be advised that it will be necessary to have a guardian appointed.

Patient Self-Determination Act

Beginning December 1, 1991, the new Patient Self-Determination Act[2] requires that nearly every health care facility advise newly admitted patients of their right to accept or refuse treatment should they become gravely ill. This act applies to hospitals, skilled nursing facilities, home health agencies, hospices, and prepaid organizations that accept Medicaid or Medicare. Patients are entitled by law to state their wishes in documents known as "advance directives." The most common of these are living wills and health care proxies (also known as a "durable power of attorney"). According to a 1991 study by the Gallup Organization, only about 20 percent of adults have living wills or durable powers of attorney. A living will outlines the life-prolonging treatment a patient would choose should he or she become unable to make medical decisions. With health care proxies, patients designate someone to make health care decisions for them. The Patient Self-Determination Act does not require a competency determination, but a health care provider would be prudent to determine the issue of competency before discussing authority to treat, informed consent, living wills, and health care directives. The act requires health care providers to provide adult patients with written notice of: (a) their state law regarding a patient's right to consent to or refuse care and to formulate advance directives regarding health care; and (b) the relevant policies of the particular institution. The provider must inquire whether the patient has executed an advance directive and document the response in the medical record. The provider's staff must be educated on these issues. Compliance with any state law applicable to any advance directives (such as durable power of attorney, living will, etc.) must be insured, and written policies and procedures implementing the above requirements must be maintained. In many hospitals, admissions personnel will make the initial inquiry as to whether a patient has advance directives. However, a facility or health care provider may not require that patients execute advance directives as a condition of admission or treatment.

Confidentiality and Medical Records

Although it is generally conceded that the hospital or physician are the owners of a patient's medical records, both common law and most state laws have recognized a patient's right of access to his or her own medical records. Laws governing access by third parties to a patient's medical records vary from state to state. Some states prohibit certain government agencies and law enforcement officials from obtaining medical information without patient authorization, a subpoena, or a court order. Unfortunately, some hospitals or facilities will release information to insurance companies and other third parties without a proper, specific authorization from the patient. Improper release of medical information to insurance companies, medical assistance, and Social Security can lead to the denial of medical benefits and the limiting of resources for long-term rehabilitation.

Unless the patient or his or her representative specifically denies the medical institution permission to release this information, certain biographical and chronological information provided to a hospital by a patient may be considered "not confidential" and could be released to police, government agencies, or the press. Other information, such as dangerous communicable diseases, poisonings, child abuse, and gunshot wounds, may be available to police or government agencies whether or not the patient consents.

The lack of control over what insurance companies and others do with medical records is the single largest weakness in medical privacy law today.[3] While physicians still swear an oath not to reveal patient information, old-fashioned medical confidentiality has become a notion as quaint as the house call—gradually eroded by court decisions and by the industrialization of medicine.[4] The introduction of computer networks and facsimile machines into health care record keeping and transmission also further complicates efforts to maintain the confidentiality of patient information.[5]

Numerous studies have indicated the wisdom of permitting a patient free and complete access to medical records. According to a study conducted by the Medical Center Hospital of Vermont, when patients are permitted free and complete access to their medical records, cooperation between physician and patient was markedly increased, and patient anxiety was reduced. Eighty percent of patients who had access to their records were more careful about following recommendations for medication after seeing them in writing, and 97 percent worried less about their health care.

A patient, parent, or court-appointed guardian has the right to copy all of his or her medical records. The medical facility should provide these medical records to the patient or patient representative in a prompt manner, since an inordinate delay in providing medical records to a patient or the patient's representative can cause difficulty for the patient in obtaining a second opinion or for discharge planning. It can also give the patient or his or her representative the "wrong idea" that they are not receiving all of the medical records. The hospital or treating medical practitioner is entitled to be reimbursed the cost of copying medical records. An individual can designate a medical copying service as his or her representative to actually copy the medical records, and this often can expedite the procedure.

Right-to-Life/Right-to-Die—Quality of Life Issues

This year, nearly 10,000 people will be neurologically impaired by spinal cord injuries (SCI) resulting from accidents. More than 49 percent of all SCI occur between May and September; weekends account for more than 38 percent of all SCI; if injuries occurring on Fridays were included, this total would jump to 53.1 percent. The overwhelming majority of SCI (about 80 percent) are incurred by males who are, in general, between the ages of 16 and 25 when injured.[6] Statistics vary, but there are approximately 200,000 to 500,000 persons already disabled by SCI from years past.

The rehabilitation and quality of life issues faced by

the spinal cord-injured individual are markedly different from those of the individual with a traumatic brain injury. As previously discussed, the spinal cord-injured individual usually is competent to make his or her own medical decisions, whereas a traumatically brain injured individual often requires a guardian. With modern medical advances, persons with SCI now find themselves confronted with decisions that previously they never had to make. For example, a patient who is a ventilator-dependent quadriplegic must decide whether or not to continue medical treatment and whether or not to remain on a ventilator. Spinal cord-injured patients must deal with these quality of life issues in a climate made much more difficult owing to the dwindling financial resources available to keep pace with modern medical progress.

The advice and guidance of the health care professional for the traumatically brain injured or spinal cord-injured patient who faces quality of life or right-to-life/right-to-die decisions is critically important. Many health care professionals are misinformed or ill-informed concerning the guidelines set forth by the United States Supreme Court on right-to-life/right-to-die issues. As a consequence, many of them adopt an "ostrich" approach. Unlike the right-to-die area, there are no reported United States Supreme Court cases confronting the issue of quality of life/right to refuse treatment by the catastrophically ill or injured individual. It appears that the trend is to permit a competent individual to determine his or her own quality of life and to refuse life-sustaining medical treatment.

The Right to Die is a common law or Old English right based on the right of self-determination; i.e., patients have the right to control what happens to their bodies. The right to die or to decline medical treatment has been codified in the United States Constitution and is embodied in the XIVth Amendment Due Process clause. Therefore, the right to die arises from three places: the common law right of self-determination; the United States Constitution; and the doctrine of informed consent.

In *Karen Quinlan,*[7] her parents requested the New Jersey Court to authorize the discontinuance of a mechanical respirator to sustain the vital processes of their daughter, who was in a persistent vegetative state. The court authorized the removal of the respirator, since Ms. Quinlan had expressly evidenced during her life that she not be sustained by artificial means. In *Quinlan,* the court stated that an individual must have expressed his or her wishes with regard to medical treatment, e.g., hydration and nutrition, while he or she is living. It is not sufficient that a patient wishes to die, or that he or she agrees with the termination of life, if the patient did not expressly indicate his or her wishes before death. The court also indicated that before it would authorize the removal of a respirator or life-sustaining medical treatment, the patient must be in an irreversible, persistent, vegetative state. Usually, the court will require a neurologist or other qualified doctor to testify in court that the person is in a persistent vegetative state. Most times, more than two medical opinions are obtained.

In *Nancy Cruzan,*[8] the United States Supreme Court upheld a state's authority to stop the removal of food, water, or other life-prolonging treatment from permanently unconscious patients whose wishes are unknown or unclear. The Court upheld Missouri's authority to keep Nancy B. Cruzan, a 32-year-old comatose woman, alive despite her parents' desire to withdraw a surgically implanted feeding tube. The woman suffered severe head injuries when she was thrown from her car in a crash and never regained consciousness. The only treatment provided was a gastrostomy tube through which she received food and water. The Court ruled that the United States Constitution does not forbid any state from preserving the life of an incapacitated person unless a surrogate produces "clear and convincing" proof (either by a living will or by testimony in court) that the patient would have wanted to die rather than live in a persistent vegetative state. While the Court did not state that there is a constitutional right to die, it suggested such a right may exist for those individuals who have made a clear declaration of their intention in a document such as a living will.

The *Quinlan* and *Cruzan* decisions underscore the need for a living will, durable power of attorney, and court-appointed guardian. Because of the increasing use and sophistication of medical technology, the legal and medical communities face the issues of *Code vs. No Code* situations, custodial care vs. rehabilitation, quality of life decisions concerning future care, and when to remove life-support systems. The United States Supreme Court's decisions in *Quinlan* and *Cruzan* are a first step toward promulgating standards for the medical/legal community in the right-to-life/right-to-die quality of life area.

RESOURCE FOCUS

Finding adequate health coverage for a brain-injured, spinal cord-injured, or ventilator-dependent patient is a monumental task. Governmental and private insurance have enacted legal, contractual, and practical obstacles that make it very difficult, if not next-to-impossible, to find adequate health benefits for the timely transfer of an individual from a hospital into a rehabilitation facility or skilled nursing facility. To overcome these problems and other obstacles requires knowledge of the myriad regulations concerning reimbursement for catastrophically injured individuals. It is often necessary to marshal a team of doctors, other health care professionals, attorneys, hospital administrators, insurance representatives, and legislators.

The Gallup Organization conducted a survey[9] to document the number of chronic ventilator patients, the cost of keeping them in the hospital, the discharge setting for those patients, and the cost burden absorbed by our health care system. The chronic ventilator patient was defined as one needing mechanical ventilation for at least 6 h a day for 30 days or more. Among the most important findings from this survey are:

1. There are 11,119 chronic ventilator-dependent patients being treated in our hospitals at any time.
2. The daily cost of caring for those patients is $9,012,332.
3. Hospitals must absorb 46 percent of the cost of care for those patients.
4. After it is determined that a chronic ventilator patient can be sent to a postacute care location, the patient must wait approximately 35 days before a bed opens at a qualified facility.
5. While waiting, one patient incurs an additional $27,615 of cost.

It has been estimated that head injuries cost the nation $25 billion a year, and the combined medical costs for spinal cord-injured patients will surpass $2 billion.[10]

The trend in the medical community is toward aggressive treatment of ventilator patients and persons with head and spinal cord injury. To fund this aggressive approach toward treatment and the need for long-term rehabilitation, the legal and medical communities must take a creative approach.

INSURANCE COMPANIES: LIMITATION OF BENEFITS BY CONTRACT

EXCLUSIONS: INSURANCE COMPANY EXCLUDES PAYMENT FOR REQUESTED MEDICAL SERVICES

An "*exclusion*" is when an insurance company relies on a clause in its contract to exclude payment for requested medical services. Examples of commonly used exclusions are: *We will not pay for . . . alcohol-related accidents; drug-related accidents; family exclusion—refusal of payment when a family member is involved in causing the accident; accidents occurring on a recreational vehicle, such as motorcycles, all-terrain vehicles (ATVs), dune buggies, snowmobiles, bicycles, skateboards; AIDS-related illness; and accident or injury occurring outside the United States or its territories.* The use of exclusionary language is an insidious attempt by insurance companies to deny benefits after they have received a premium from the insured. Sadly, what generally occurs is that a patient or family member first learns about an exclusion when they call the insurance company for a claim number and are informed that the insurance company is denying coverage based on the exclusion. For instance, the insurance company will, for the first time, raise the issue that the person was drinking when the automobile accident occurred so they have excluded the requested medical benefit. Family members of catastrophically injured persons should be encouraged to challenge an exclusion. Many times exclusions placed in the insurance policy are void as against public policy, and the needed medical benefit can be recovered. With the advent of managed care, insurance companies will insert more exclusionary clauses into all types of insurance policies in an attempt to deny needed short-term and long-term rehabilitation coverages.

LIMITATIONS

Unlike exclusions, limitations are generally valid and rarely can be successfully challenged in court. Limitations are a contractual matter between the insured and the insurance company, and ideally the insured is informed of the limitations at the time the policy is purchased. Examples of limitations are: *In the event of a catastrophic injury the patient will only receive 30 days of acute or subacute inpatient rehabilitation; the patient is limited to 30 days or 60 days of outpatient treatment; the insurance company will provide a non-motorized but not a motorized wheelchair; the insurance policy will not allow second opinions or certain diagnostic tests without precertification.* Most patients are unaware of the limitations included in their insurance contract or policy until after a serious or catastrophic injury occurs.

DEFINITIONAL EXCLUSIONS

Two issues that consistently arise in connection with the medical treatment of catastrophically injured persons are: (1) whether or not they can continue to make rehabilitative gains; and (2) whether or not the care they are receiving is "custodial care." Most insurance policies either will not pay for custodial care or will pay very limited benefits. Insurance companies argue that they are not responsible for medical services that do not substantially contribute to the improvement of the injured person's condition. With the present health care crisis, insurance companies increasingly press the issue of whether or not medical services contribute substantially to the improvement of the injured person's medical condition.

There are myriad definitions relied upon by insurance companies to deny medical benefits. Most denials based on definitions in the insurance contract fall within three areas:

1. Denial of surgery—payment approved for reconstructive surgery but not for plastic surgery.
2. Denial of rehabilitation services—refusal to pay for continuing rehabilitation unless specific rehabilitative gains are proven by the rehabilitation facility or medical doctor.
3. Limits to long-term care—refusal to pay if care is "custodial" in nature.

MANAGED CARE

The third-party payer system in this country was expressly structured to avoid interference with the doctor/patient relationship. Only a patient's treating doctor or health care professional could determine an individual's course of treatment. Today, with managed care, cost constraints are beginning to change the traditional relationship between patients, third-party payers, and health care providers.[11] Managed care organizations are aggressively using utilization review companies, precertification procedures, auditing, case managers and rehabilitation nurses, and peer review, to limit their exposure. Managed care entities are requiring health care providers to sign preferred provider agreements or other contractual obligations, which place health care professionals in a conflict position, i.e., a health care professional is in the unenviable position of having a contractual obligation to the managed care company to limit costs, while also having a moral and ethical obligation to treat the patient regardless of cost. The challenge for the medical and legal community in a managed care setting will be to deliver appropriate care for the patient in a cost-effective manner.

MEDICAL BENEFITS CAN BE REDUCED BY A SELF-INSURED EMPLOYER

In *Greenburg vs. H & H Music,*[12] John McGann, who had worked at H & H Music Company since 1982, learned in 1987 that he had AIDS and submitted his first claim for reimbursement under the company's group health plan, which provided for lifetime medical benefits of 1 million dollars. After his employer learned that he had AIDS, they immediately reduced his medical benefits from 1 million dollars to a lifetime maximum of $5000. McGann quickly reached the $5000 limit. In 1991, at age 47, McGann died of an AIDS-related illness. Appalling, but perfectly legal, according to two lower federal courts and the United States Supreme Court, which allowed the self-insured employer to change the provisions of the insurance policy in midstream. The Employee Retirement Income Security Act of 1987 (ERISA) does govern self-insurance plans to the extent that employers must provide every benefit they have promised, but ERISA doesn't stop employers from changing their benefit plans, even after a worker has received some benefits; it merely requires employers to keep employees informed of any changes. According to business surveys, an estimated 60 percent of employers now fund their own medical benefits.

The outcome of *Greenburg* could have catastrophic implications for employees, consumers, and the health care community. Self-insured companies may not only refuse to provide coverage for certain costly illnesses and injuries, such as AIDS, ventilator patients, paraplegia, quadriplegia, and traumatic brain injury; they may also drop the coverage after the employee discloses the illness or injury.

Health care providers should educate their staff regarding exclusions and definitions in an insurance policy, managed care limitations, custodial care language, and the court's decision in *Greenburg.* Health care professionals who treat patients suffering from catastrophic injuries should instruct their precertification departments, billing departments, accounting offices, and social work departments to acquire and review the entire health insurance policy and to obtain written confirmation of the maximum medical benefits available under the policy.

LEVERAGE–PAYMENT OF MEDICAL BILLS: INADEQUATE INSURANCE

Subrogation rights are the right of an insurance company, a self-insured employer, or state or federal government agency that pays a patient's medical bills to be repaid for the cost of the medical care they provided from any money received by the patient from a lawsuit or any settlement from a third party. Subrogation rights are provided either by contract or by statute. A private insurance company or governmental agency will issue an insurance booklet that has, by contract, language that gives the insurance company the right to be repaid the amount of their benefits. An illustration of subrogation language is as follows: *When a covered person incurs medical expenses which are payable under contract, workers' compensation or any other similar statute, or payable because legal action is brought against any third party to recover damages for an injury or illness . . . ; The Company is entitled to reimbursement for any payment which a covered person or covered dependent may receive from a third party . . .*

When a benefit payer has subrogation rights, the concept of leverage often can be used to obtain extracontractual benefits. The best way to explain the concept of leverage is to use an example. Johnny is catastrophically injured in a hotel swimming pool accident and there was no lifeguard present. Johnny and his family have no insurance to pay for his medical bills and, though there is a facility that believes it could successfully rehabilitate Johnny from his head and spinal cord injuries, it is unwilling to accept him without insurance. An attorney representing Johnny files a lawsuit against the hotel, claiming that Johnny's injury was in part the result of a defective swimming pool and a lack of a lifeguard at the pool. In the usual leverage situation, the medical facility agrees to treat Johnny with the understanding that it would get paid back the cost of its medical services from the money Johnny receives in his lawsuit, rather than accept a nominal payment from governmental benefits. Leverage can be most useful when the following three factors exist: (1) catastrophically injured person; (2) facility equipped to meet the individual's needs; and (3) no insurance or inadequate insurance.

Extracontractual benefits

In the above scenario involving Johnny injured in the pool accident, let us assume that he had his father's insurance benefits with ABC Insurance Company to pay his medical bills. His father's medical plan was limited to $250,000 in lifetime medical benefits. The cost of Johnny's acute care and acute rehabilitation exceeded the $250,000 limit, and he now needs subacute treatment, as well as life-long nursing care for his head and spinal cord injuries. Extracontractual benefits will often be paid by ABC Insurance Company if an attorney will agree to repay ABC Insurance Company from the proceeds of any third-party litigation. There is an incentive for an insurance company to pay extracontractual benefits for a catastrophically injured individual, since, as in the above example, ABC Insurance Company has already paid $250,000 out of its pocket, and it is in their interest to "pay a little more" if it leads to recovery of the initial $250,000 payment.

Special education benefits: the underutilized benefit

Special education benefits for children are an underutilized method to obtain much-needed medical benefits for the short-term and long-term rehabilitation of catastrophically injured patients. *The Education For All Handicapped Children Act*[13] (EHA), mandates that all states make available to handicapped children a "free appropriate public education" and extensive "due process" procedures. This federal act and the regulations of the United States Department of Education establish procedures by which handicapped children are evaluated, their classifications are determined, and an appropriate program of special education and "related services" is developed and implemented. The program developed for each individual handicapped child is known as an *Individualized Education Program* (IEP), and must be developed jointly by school officials and parents. The special education student's yearly IEP must determine whether that student requires one or more related services, which must be provided at no expense to the parents. The listed examples of related services include: transportation; speech; pathology; audiology; psychological services; physical therapy; occupational therapy; social work services; school health services; early identification/assessment; medical services for diagnosis or evaluation; parent counseling/education; recreation; counseling services; developmental services; corrective services; and other support services. While the list of potential related services is extensive, it must be remembered that a special education student is entitled only to such related services as are documented as necessary by the treating health care professional to allow the student to receive an "appropriate education," i.e., a special education program that provides "educational benefit" to the student. The child's deficits may be further documented by health care providers through the use of computer tomography (CT) scans, electroencephalographs (EEG), magnetic resonance imaging (MRI), evoked potential tests, and neuropsychological tests, whenever appropriate, in order to enable a parent to apply for needed special education benefits. It is incumbent upon the health care community to advise the family of the broad range of "related services" available for payment by the school district so that their child can benefit from the rehabilitation services offered by the health care community. A health care professional's obligation is not solely to provide medical treatment for a patient, but is also to be acquainted with the resources available to implement the needed treatment. Patients and their families faced with a traumatic brain or spinal cord injury assume that the health care professional is aware of the maximum health insurance benefits for which they are eligible to meet rehabilitation needs. It is detrimental to the patient's interests to neglect an available funding resource. Many have argued that identifying available health insurance benefits places an unfair burden on the health care community. Sharing this burden among the health care community, the patient, the patient's family, patient advocates, the school district, a representative of the health insurance company, and the patient's attorney will ensure coordination of all the available health insurance benefits and enable the patient to receive necessary treatment in a consistent and cost-effective manner.

LEGAL FOCUS: AN ISSUE OF PROOF

Brain injury can be present in a person who has never lost consciousness.[14] The alteration of consciousness caused by the blow to the head may instead have taken the form of a period of feeling dazed, confused, or agitated.[15] Persons with mild to moderate brain injury, unlike persons with SCI, are beset by residual problems that usually escape detection in ordinary medical examinations. Because these problems are unidentified or improperly defined, they become more frightening and debilitating to the victim.[16] The doctor has the unenviable position of determining the information necessary to arrive at the correct preliminary diagnosis. The facts are often absent or incorrectly presented, and the medical history may be incomplete. Determination may not have been made as to whether the accident is a new head injury or has aggravated a preexisting psychological or psychiatric disorder. If the doctor knows how the accident or injury occurred and has obtained a complete medical history, the chances of a nondiagnosis or misdiagnosis are lessened. To avoid investigation pitfalls, a medical investigation should be prompt, factually accurate, and thorough.

Health care professionals are called upon to describe or explain the nature of the traumatic brain injury and spinal cord injury to families, insurance companies, and the court. The family's initial concern is usually how long the injured person will be disabled, whether the difficulties will improve, what the long-term limitations will be, and how long medical care will be needed. However, the court and the insurance companies are more realistic in evaluating a person's injury and will request from the medical professional objective or subjective evidence of injury. For an expert witness to be adequately prepared for court testimony, and to insure that the expert provides the most persuasive guidance to the fact finder, a basic understanding of the legal rules and practices that govern expert testimony is essential.

The expert's level of certainty is particularly important where medical testimony is necessary to establish legal "causation," i.e., that a particular injury resulted from the negligent act of the defendant. For example, Jane was being treated for depression; then she was in an auto accident and suffered a head injury. The issue for the court and the jury to determine is whether or not the auto accident "caused" or "aggravated" Jane's preexisting psychological condition. In such cases, it generally is necessary for the plaintiff to produce an expert's opinion that a defendant's negligent act or omission increased the risk of harm to the plaintiff, and that this increased risk was a substantial factor in producing the harm. This opinion must be rendered by the expert to a reasonable degree of medical certainty in order to be admitted by the court.

When someone has suffered a traumatic brain injury in a motor vehicle accident, it is good practice for the emergency room physician to question the other occupants of the car. If there are no passengers to question, or if the others are themselves injured, the physician can speak with the witnesses to the accident, other drivers, paramedics, and police officers. They can describe to the doctor whether the damage to the vehicles involved was minor, moderate, or severe. Questions such as: Was the person ejected from the vehicle, and if so, how far was the person thrown? Was there bleeding from the ears? Was there a period of unconsciousness? Was there evidence of drug or alcohol use? Was the victim wearing a seat belt or a combined seat belt and shoulder harness? Was the air bag inflated? can all be determined at this time. Any details that can be obtained from witnesses to the accident, other occupants of the motor vehicle, investigating police officers, emergency medical technicians, first responders, and paramedics will provide crucial information in the earliest stages of treatment and diagnosis for a traumatic brain injury.

Unlike the spinal cord-injured patient, a head-injured patient often is unable to respond to questions about his or her medical background, or the information obtained is unreliable. A spouse, parent, family member, or next of kin can provide necessary medical history, including family medical history. A complete medical history for a person with a suspected traumatic brain injury should include: Has there been a prior head, neck, or back injury? Is the individual currently undergoing treatment for any medical condition? Is the individual currently taking medication?

Obtaining a complete family medical history and determining whether or not there has been prior psychological or psychiatric treatment or a prior injury to the back or spine is essential to document whether or not the current injury has aggravated a preexisting condition. Too often, the medical practitioner does not learn that the individual he or she is treating was being treated previously for depression or a back injury until many weeks after the first contact with the patient. This causes difficulties for the doctor in documenting that the injury aggravated the preexisting depression or injury.

It is good practice in determining whether or not there is a significant medical problem in an individual's history to contact the family doctor and any other professional treating an individual for a preexisting psychological or psychiatric disorder to determine the medical diagnosis, treatment program, medications ordered, and prognosis. A physician should not rely on his or her staff to make this contact, but should speak personally to the doctors in order to aid the diagnosis.

Medical Providers as Expert Witnesses

One of the most fundamental tenets of American litigation is its insistence upon the most reliable sources of information at trial. "One of the earliest and most pervasive manifestations of this attitude is the rule requiring that a witness who testifies to a fact . . . must have actually observed the fact."[17] However, the law also has long recognized that many human undertakings involve complex disciplines which the average layperson cannot hope to comprehend without additional guidance from those who are learned in the field. Therefore, the law acknowledges that where a controversy involves a science, profession, or occupation "beyond the ken of the average layman"[18] expert testimony is admissible to assist the fact finder in resolving the dispute.

In order for the court to permit such expert testimony, the witness must have sufficient skill, knowledge, or experience in his or her field to make it probable that his opinion will aid the fact finder in its decision. While the court may rule that a certain subject area will require that a member of a given profession, such as a physician, be utilized as the expert witness, a specialist in that particular field is not always legally required, although such expertise is frequently desirable. Finally, the courts generally will not allow the introduction of expert testimony in areas of science that are only experimental, but rather will require that the subject matter of the expert's testimony "be sufficiently established to have gained general acceptance in the particular field to which it belongs."[19] Therefore, opinion evidence will not be admitted if the state of scientific knowledge in a field is not so advanced as to permit a reasonable opinion to be asserted, even by an expert.

Opinion evidence of a traumatic brain injury will be admitted based on computer tomography (CT) scans, x-rays, electroencephalograph (EEG), and magnetic resonance imaging (MRI). Some courts have allowed expert testimony based upon positron emission tomography (PET) scans, evoked potentials, and brain electrical activity mapping (BEAM) tests.

Neuropsychological testing often will demonstrate cognitive deficits of a patient where more traditional testing, such as routine neurological examination, CT scans, x-rays, and MRIs, did not document objective findings of organic impairment. Indeed, one study found that 424 of the 538 patients suffering minor head injuries who were seen for a follow-up 3 months postaccident were entirely normal with regard to neurological evaluations (including EEGs and the 6 percent of those who were given CT scans), even though 8 percent had some minor neurological abnormality on admission to the hospital. However, on neuropsychological examination, the vast majority demonstrated mild impairment (Halstead-Reitan Impairment Index = .5, Category test = 54.7, Tactual Performance Test Location − 4.2, Trails Making Test − 116.0), even though IQ and academic test results were not significantly different from established norms. One-third of the patients who had been gainfully employed before their accident were still unemployed 3 months later, disabled with headaches and memory deficits.[20]

"Objective" neuropsychological testing is in fact little more objective than the psychologist running the tests and is subject to the same contextual bias as the other forensic examinations. Just as one neurologist can find clear evidence of brain damage in a patient whom a second neurologist finds entirely free of impairment, very often "objective" neuropsychological testing will reveal precisely what the examiner hoped to find.[21] Nevertheless, opinion evidence based on "objective testing" will be viewed more favorably by the courts and gives the trial attorney more ammunition in trying to prove or disprove the residual effects of the traumatic brain injury.

As previously mentioned, to the layperson as well as the court, the damages of a spinal cord-injured individual are more obvious than those of an individual who has suffered traumatic brain injury. Just as it is generally difficult to obtain insurance reimbursement for services for the traumatically brain injured, such as group homes, computer programs, and transitional living programs, insurance companies are also reluctant to pay for programs and services for the spinal cord-injured, such as computerized adaptive living devices for the home, motorized wheelchairs, state-of-the-art vans, and other durable medical equipment. Insurance companies will reimburse for, and courts will usually allow testimony concerning, any medical testing or advance if the state of scientific knowledge in the field is so advanced as to permit a reasonable opinion to be asserted by an expert.

When an attorney has determined that the use of a medical expert is strategically valuable and legally admissible, counsel frequently will prepare the case with substantial emphasis upon the anticipated testimony of the expert. A medical expert should expect to be required to answer questions within a particular legal framework in accordance with rules of admissibility and evidence. Since the witness's expertise must first be accepted by the court in order to allow the witness to offer an expert opinion, the witness initially will be asked to testify as to academic and employment credentials, including educational background, relevant work experience, publications authored, and ongoing professional training. Opposing counsel will then be permitted to cross-examine the expert regarding these credentials, and counsel may object to an acceptance of the witness as an expert by the court. Since the standard for acceptance of the qualifications of an expert is generally quite modest, it is relatively rare for a proffered expert to be rejected by the court. However, as the leading scholar on the law of evidence has noted, "The witness must have sufficient skill, knowledge or experience in that field or calling as to make it appear that his opinion or inference will probably aid the trier in his search for truth."[22] If a witness has any reasonable pretension to specialized knowledge on the subject under investigation, he/she may testify, and the weight to be given to this evidence is for the jury to determine.[23]

After a witness in a traumatic brain injury or spinal cord injury case has been accepted as an expert by the court, counsel generally will then provide a factual basis for the witness's opinion. For example, counsel will inquire into the witness's familiarity with the patient and his/her medical condition, the witness's involvement in the treatment of the patient, and the records/documentary materials that the witness reviewed and relied upon in preparing the opinion. After establishing the factual foundation for the expert witness's opinion, counsel will either: (1) ask the witness a direct question to obtain an opinion in the relevant area; or (2) fashion a "hypothetical question" that asks the witness to assume certain facts already presented at trial, and to state an opinion based upon those facts. The former method generally is utilized where the expert witness has firsthand knowledge of the material facts (e.g., the witness was the victim's treating physician), so that the witness may describe his or her own observations and provide an expert opinion therefrom. A hypothetical question is typically used in circumstances where the expert witness does not possess firsthand knowledge of the facts of the case, but rather is presenting an opinion based on the observations and evaluations of other individuals. Finally, after the witness has stated his or her expert opinion, the witness may be asked to relate those facts that support the conclusion reached.

An issue that frequently arises when substantial reliance is placed on expert testimony is the extent to which the expert may rely on reports or statements of others who have not testified in court. This situation occurs when a treating physician is unavailable to provide an expert opinion at trial. In such circumstances, the court must determine whether another physician qualified in the field of inquiry may provide an opinion with regard to the medical condition of the patient that is based only on reports of others, without ever having examined that patient. The clear trend of the law is to permit such an expert opinion to be presented.[24] The Pennsylvania Supreme Court permitted "medical witnesses to express opinion testimony on medical matters based, in part, upon reports of others which are not in evidence, but which the expert customarily relies upon in the practice of his profession."[25] The court also held that expert medical witnesses may rely on reports of laypersons, provided such reports are customarily relied on by experts in the medical field. Consequently, an expert may generally render an opinion based on the reports of others, so long as the expert is prepared to testify that the reports are of the type customarily relied on by colleagues in the field.[26]

When the testifying witness is someone other than the initial treating physician, the witness will have a better foundation on which to base his or her final conclusion of traumatic brain injury if the initial treating physician made a prompt, factually correct, thorough investigation of the circumstances of the accident and the patient's prior medical history and has clearly documented these in his/her notes.

In preparing to testify, an expert must also be aware that he or she will be expected to state that the opinion rendered is held to a reasonable degree of medical certainty.[27] Consequently, the expert witness must carefully avoid the use of such conditional words as "probably" or "maybe." The expert is required to express his or her opinion to a higher degree of certainty. In one case, a doctor was asked whether the plaintiff's condition was caused by the automobile accident that gave rise to the lawsuit. The doctor testified that the accident was "consistent with the injury," and that "there is probably a cause and effect relationship." The court held this testimony to be inadmissible:

> "The issue is not merely one of semantics. There is a logical reason for the rule. The opinion of a medical expert is evidence. If the fact finder chooses to believe it, he can find as fact what the expert gave as an opinion. For the fact finder to award damages for a particular condition to a plaintiff, it must find as a fact that the condition was legally caused by the defendant's conduct. Here, the only evidence offered was that it was 'probably' caused, and that is not enough. Perhaps in the world of medicine nothing is absolutely certain. Nevertheless doctors must make decisions in their own profession every day based on their expert opinions. Physicians must understand that it is the intent of our law that if the plaintiff's medical expert cannot form an opinion with sufficient certainty so as to make a medical judgment, there is nothing on the record with which a jury can make a judgment with sufficient certainty so as to make a legal judgment. Because Mrs. McMahon's testimony was not made with sufficient certainty, it was not legally competent evidence. . . ."[28]

This "certainty requirement" has evolved into a key phrase where counsel will ask an expert to express his or her opinion "to a reasonable degree of medical certainty." It is not required that the expert express an opinion with absolute certainty.

Attorneys are increasingly relying on rehabilitation nurses, case managers, and lifetime planning experts to prepare reports setting forth the lifetime needs of persons with catastrophic head or spinal cord injury. These future cost assessment reports should include: the purpose of the report; the facts of the case; biographical information; diagnosis of the medical problem; school background; work history; family support system; home evaluation; list of all hospitals and treating physicians; list of medical records reviewed; prior health history; itemized cost of all durable medical equipment; medications; therapies; annual doctor visits; nursing care; home modifications; future medical care; recommendations; and prognosis.

Increasingly, insurance companies are reviewing medical charts and submitting cases for peer review before paying medical benefits. If the treating professional has underestimated the traumatic brain injury or spinal cord injury, the difficulties increase in receiving medical reimbursement from an insurance company for future care and in proving the injury at trial.

CONCLUSION

The focus of the health care professional in treating traumatically brain injured and spinal cord-injured patients must necessarily evolve with the current changes in the nation's health care system. Health care professionals should have a patient focus, resource focus, and legal focus. Learning to work within the constraints of new managed care guidelines, speaking "insurance company language," and providing skilled and knowledgeable in-court testimony will maximize a patient's benefits and provide reimbursement to the health care provider for services rendered.

REFERENCES

1. *Trauma Facts 1992.* American Trauma Society, Upper Marlboro, MD.
2. *Patient Self-Determination Act.* Federal Omnibus Budget Reconciliation Act of 1990.
3. Norton C: Absolutely not Confidential, HIPPOCRATES (March–April 1989), quoting Robert Ellis Smith, *The Privacy Journal,* Washington, D.C.
4. Id.
5. Shaw D: "Growing Use of Fax Machines Raises Concern about Corporate Security," *Philadelphia Inquirer,* May 5 1991.
6. Odum MX: *Attention to Prevention.* Woburn MA, National Spinal Cord Injury Association.
7. *In re Quinlan,* 355 A. 2d 647 (NJ 1976).
8. *Cruzan v. Director, Missouri Dept. of Health,* 110 S.CT. 2841 (1990).
9. Milligan S: AARC and Gallup, *AARC Times,* 1991.
10. *Trauma Facts 1992.* American Trauma Society, Upper Marlboro, MD.
11. Griner D: Paying the piper: A third-party payor liability for medical treatment decisions. *Georgia Law Review* (Spring 1991).
12. *Greenburg vs. H & H Music Company, et al,* 113 S.CT. 482 (1992).
13. *The Education For All Handicapped Children Act.* U.S. Public Law 94-142.
14. Davidoff Mark: Neuro-behavioral sequelae of minor head injury—A consideration of post concussive syndrome vs. post traumatic stress disorder. *Cognitive Rehabilitation,* Mar.–Apr. 1988; 52.
15. Levin G., High, Mattis, et al: Minor head injury and the post-concussional syndrome: Methodological issues and outcome studies, in *Neuro-Behavioral Recovery from Head Injury.* 263 1987.
16. Bender: Persisting symptoms after mild head injury—A review of the post-concussive syndrome. *J Clin Exper Neurophysiol* 1986; 323.
17. *McCormick on Evidence,* 2d, Section 10, at 20.
18. *McCormick on Evidence,* 2d, Section 13, at 29.
19. *Frye v. United States,* 293 F. 1013, 1014 (1923) (The first case to consider—and reject—the admissibility of the results of a lie detector examination). *McCormick on Evidence* at 29-31, 489.
20. Rimel et al: Disability caused by minor head injury. Neurosurgery (1981) 9-221-228; *Psychiatry in the Everyday Practice of Law.* Blinder (2d ed), 1982.
21. *Psychiatry in the Everyday Practice of Law.* (2d ed) Blinder, 1982:40.
22. *United States v. Viglia,* 549 F.2d 335 (5th Cir. 1977) (Physician with no experience in treating obesity could render an opinion regarding the use of a controlled substance allegedly used for controlling obesity).
23. *McCormick on Evidence,* 2d, Section 15, at 34-36; Federal Rules of Evidence, Rule 703.
24. *Commonwealth v. Thomas,* 444 Pa. 436, 445, 282 A. 2d 693, 698 (1971).
25. *Commonwealth v. Daniels,* 480 Pa. 340, 390 A. 2d 172 (1978); See also *McCormick on Evidence,* at 34-36.
26. *"Admissibility of Expert Medical Testimony as to Future Consequences of Injury as Affected by Expression in Terms of Probability or Possibility."* 75 A.L.R., 3d 9.
27. *McMahon v. Young,* 442 Pa. 484, 486, 276 A. 2d 534, 535 (1971).
28. *Hamil v. Bashline,* 481 Pa. 256, 392 A. 2d 1280 (1978); *Restatement of Torts,* Section 323.

CHAPTER 72

THE THINK FIRST PROGRAM

Thomas G. Saul
Diana Kelker

SYNOPSIS

The think first program was developed in 1986 by the American Association of Neurological Surgeons and the Congress of Neurological Surgeons with the goal of preventing head and spinal cord injury through education, public awareness, and legislation. This chapter outlines the growth and successes of this program. For methodological reasons, it is difficult to demonstrate the effectiveness of such a program in reducing the incidence of these injuries. However, pilot studies have clearly demonstrated an increased awareness of the problem and an intention to change risky behavior among schoolchildren who have been exposed to the program.

INTRODUCTION

If rehabilitation is the logical and moral extension of trauma care outside the "back door" of the trauma center, it follows that prevention is the logical and moral extension of trauma care outside the "front door." This is the perspective of American neurosurgeons.

Severe head and spinal cord injuries are among the most serious and devastating traumas. It is hard to imagine the impact that such an injury has on the victim, the victim's family, the trauma center, the victim's workplace, the victim's friends and loved ones, the health care system, and society as a whole. Multiply that by the hundreds of thousands of individuals who are injured each year, and one sees a major health care problem. As with traumatic injuries in general, many head and spinal cord injuries are preventable. In most trauma centers, neurosurgeons are responsible for the care of patients with these injuries. It is from this experience that neurosurgeons in the United States have committed themselves to the prevention—not just the treatment—of these injuries. In spite of all the state-of-the-art treatments and innovations discussed in this book, there is no cure for severe head injury and spinal cord injury. Even when we are successful in treating these patients, their lives are altered forever.

The THINK FIRST Program was jointly founded in 1986 by the American Association of Neurological Surgeons and the Congress of Neurological Surgeons. It combines the experiences of two educational programs in Florida and Missouri. THINK FIRST has been built on efforts that were carefully designed and implemented over a multiyear period and that demonstrated the potential to reduce injuries. The primary objective of THINK FIRST is to decrease head and spinal cord injuries, particularly among young persons, through educational, public awareness, and legislative approaches.

DOCUMENTATION OF THE PROBLEM AND NEED FOR PREVENTION

The magnitude of the neurotrauma problem is finally receiving recognition. Traumatic injuries constitute a major public health problem, imposing a greater burden on modern society than do other diseases. Moreover, neural injuries are also the most preventable. For individuals under age 45, injuries remain the leading cause of death, claiming more than 142,000 American lives each year.[1] The total health care bill for traumatic injuries in 1988 was approximately $170 billion.[2] Prevention and control efforts must be developed that are commensurate with the negative impact of this health problem.

Head and spinal cord injuries are the leading causes of morbidity and mortality among American youth. These injuries result in numerous human and economic costs. Approximately 2 million Americans suffer a traumatic brain injury each year.[3] This means that an injury occurs every 15 seconds. Among all patients with brain injuries, 75,000 to 100,000 die within hours of the injury, 500,000 require hospitalization, and 70,000 to 90,000 develop irreversible loss of function. Additionally, 10,000 to 12,000 spinal cord injuries occur each year.[4,5] More than half the individuals suffering a spinal cord injury are less than 24 years old. Lifetime costs for a spinal cord injury and a head injury can exceed $600,000 and $4 million, respectively.[2] These figures do not include the loss of potential income. In addition, there is no way to place a monetary value on the pain and suffering that patients and families endure. The total national bill for traumatic brain injury is approximately $25 billion per year. This includes rehabilitation, support services, and lost income on the part of injured patients.[3,6]

Motor vehicle crashes are the most common cause of spinal cord injuries, accounting for about 50 percent of cases.[7] The majority of these injuries are associated with alcohol intake. Falls are the second leading cause of spinal cord injuries, followed by diving injuries.[8] Sports and recreation injuries account for 10 percent of brain injuries and 7 percent of spinal cord injuries.[9] Approximately 1000 diving-related injuries occur each year,[10] accounting for 10 percent of all spinal cord injuries.[8,11] Ninety-five percent of diving-related spinal cord injuries result in quadriplegia.[11] More than 25 percent of spinal cord injuries and 12 percent of brain injuries result from violent assaults.[3,6] These figures vary among geographic areas and populations.[2]

Society cannot afford the loss of young lives, the high cost of medical treatment of head and spinal cord injuries, and the cost of supporting those who are permanently disabled by these injuries. Unlike some other major health problems, a variety of effective preventive measures are available for trauma. Unfortunately, they are not applied often.[12] Therefore, neurosurgeons must take an active role in trying to prevent these injuries.[13]

THE THINK FIRST PROGRAM

The THINK FIRST Prevention Program is an attempt on the part of the American Association of Neurological Surgeons and the Congress of Neurological Surgeons to fulfill this role. In accordance with U.S. strategic objectives for health promotion and disease prevention, the THINK FIRST message has been synchronized with the 1992 national document *Healthy People 2000.* Two objectives of *Healthy People 2000* are to reduce nonfatal head injuries so that hospitalizations are required for no more than 106 of 100,000 persons and to reduce nonfatal spinal cord injuries so that hospitalizations are limited to no more than 5 per 100,000 persons. The current rates are 124 and 5.9 per 100,000, respectively.[2]

Originally called the National Head and Spinal Cord Injury Prevention Program, THINK FIRST was created by combining the experiences of a model educational program in Florida directed by E. Fletcher Eyster, M.D., and one in Missouri directed by Clark Watts, M.D.[13] THINK FIRST was founded on the principle that by educating individuals who are most at risk for injuries about the consequences of such injuries, one can promote changes in behavior and attitudes that may decrease the incidence of spinal cord and head injuries in this population (Fig. 72-1). Injury prevention can occur effectively by three methods. The first and most effective method is to empirically provide protection devices through product and environmental design. Examples of this are air bags, antilock brakes, and restraint systems in cars. The second method is to mandate through legislation safety behavior, such as laws requiring the use of safety belts and helmets. One of the major public health successes of the decade has been that all 50 states now require safety restraints for young children. This contributed to a 36 percent decline in motor vehicle fatalities for those age 1 through 14 between 1980 and 1984.[14] The effectiveness of safety belts in preventing injury and death in motor vehicle crashes is well documented. Safety belts reduce motor vehicle fatalities by an estimated 40 to 50 percent and serious injuries by 45 to 55 percent.[15] One study found that safety belt use reduced hospital bills by 67 percent.[16] Conversely, repeal of the mandatory use of helmets for motocyclists resulted in a 40 percent increase in the number of fatalities after motorcycle crashes.[17,18] The third and perhaps most challenging method is to persuade individuals who are at risk to alter their behavior. It is to this educational method that THINK FIRST is dedicated. The Centers for Disease Control stated that from 1984 to 1988, "universal use of helmets by all bicyclists could have pre-

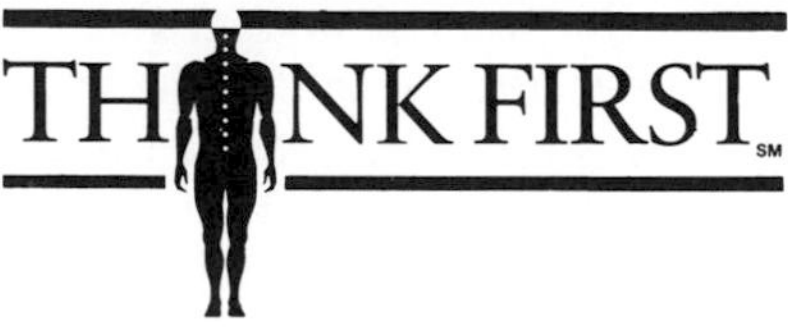

Figure 72-1. THINK FIRST logo.

vented as many as 2500 deaths and 757,000 head injuries."[19] Currently, fewer than 10 percent of all cyclists and 2 percent of cyclists under age 15 wear helmets.[20] Cyclists who wear helmets reduce their risk of brain injury by 85 percent.[21] It is apparent from these statistics that children and parents do not have adequate knowledge regarding the benefit of helmet use while bicycling or simply choose to ignore the facts.

The national THINK FIRST Program has four components: (1) a basic education program, (2) reinforcement activities, (3) general public education efforts, and (4) public policy initiatives.

The primary component of THINK FIRST is an education curriculum directed at the teenage population. The program informs young adults about their vulnerability and the consequences of their risk-taking behavior. Teenagers, who are at the greatest risk for brain and spinal cord injuries, are unaware of the potential consequences of these injuries and often view themselves as invincible. Teens are easily influenced by their peers to engage in risky behaviors and wear safety belts less often than do adults.[22] The THINK FIRST educational curriculum is based on the Health Belief Model of Rosenstock.[23] This model proposes that teenagers must be made aware of the problem and its consequences. They must also believe that there are actions they can take to avoid the risks. Finally, teenagers must realize that the barriers to safe action do not outweigh the benefits of such action. With respect to the THINK FIRST message, the major barrier to success is negative peer pressure.

The THINK FIRST Education Program is delivered primarily through school systems to students in large assemblies or in a classroom format. The presentation consists of four segments. The first part is the showing of a 15-min film, *On the Edge.* This film depicts, through interviews with young people who have survived head and spinal cord injuries, the risk-taking behaviors that led to their injuries and the consequences of those injuries. The second part involves a presentation by a health care professional to inform the students about brain and spinal cord anatomy, the types of injuries, and the epidemiology of these injuries. Types and causes of injuries are discussed, including those involving motor vehicle crashes, drinking, diving, all-terrain vehicles, action sports, and violence. The third part of the program introduces the students to a young person who has sustained a spinal cord or brain injury. This person candidly discusses his or her injury: the cause as well as the physical, emotional, and social consequences. This is followed by questions from the student audience to the injured speaker, who answers the questions openly and honestly. This interaction is perhaps the most effective method for communicating the realities of injury and disability. Paramedics or emergency medical technicians may be included in the presentations to emphasize prevention methods. An optional fourth feature is a wheelchair obstacle course: Volunteer abled-bodied students are put in wheelchairs and asked to negotiate an obstacle course that resembles real-life barriers to the disabled. This is designed to provide additional awareness of the problems confronted in everyday life by people in wheelchairs.

The second primary component of the THINK FIRST Program involves reinforcement activities. No matter how effective the presentation is, it is unlikely that adolescents' behavior can be changed after a 1-h presentation. A continued prevention message helps reinforce the education program in the school. Reinforcement activities include essay and poster contests, repeated exposure to the program, skills training for bystander response, school and community bulletin boards, school health fairs, bike rodeos, alcohol-free prom and graduation events, and the creation of safety clubs. Reinforcement activities in locations associated with high-risk activities also can increase the effectiveness of the program. Swimming pools, ponds, creeks, and beaches can be provided with appropriate preventive signs in collaboration with local civic groups.

The third and fourth components of the THINK FIRST Program pertain to general public awareness initiatives and support of state and federal public policy efforts. Injury prevention programs such as THINK FIRST face a number of challenges. They must increase awareness among key decision makers and the general public, who often are unaware of the magnitude of the injury problem in comparison with other public health issues. THINK FIRST enhances its education efforts with the general public through public service announcements, television talk shows, newspaper feature articles, position papers, and other media events. In addition, the glorification of risk taking and unsafe behaviors by the media and society must be combatted.[24] Public policy initiatives help ensure that injury prevention issues are addressed at the appropriate community and state levels. The THINK FIRST national office in Chicago and the local chapters keep abreast of and support policy issues that can lead to laws that enhance the prevention effort. One of the most pressing goals of the national THINK FIRST Program is the establishment of CNS injury registries in every state. Such registries can provide better data from which meaningful prevention, therapeutic, and rehabilitation programs can be developed. Legislative efforts are being made to increase funding for the prevention, treatment, and rehabilitation of brain and spinal cord injuries. Additionally, a major provision in pending bills is the establishment of a national traumatic brain injury registry.[6] THINK FIRST encourages government research and programs geared toward reducing injuries to the brain and spinal cord. More than one-fourth (28 percent) of the direct costs arising from treatment of these injuries are borne by federal, state, and local governments. In marked contrast to this heavy societal financial burden, the total amount in federal research expenditures for injury is quite low. Research expenditures for injury were estimated at $160 million, compared with National Cancer Institute obligations of $1.4 billion and National Heart, Lung, and Blood Institute obligations of $930 million.[22]

During the first 6 years of its existence, the THINK FIRST Program was completely supported by funds provided by the two national neurosurgical organizations which founded the program. It was soon recognized that because of the magnitude of the problem, it would be difficult for neurosurgeons alone to achieve the long-term goals of the program. Therefore, in October 1990, the THINK FIRST Foundation was created. This enabled other interested people to participate in a tax-free foundation dedicated to prevention. The foundation has facilitated the involvement of both laypeople and professionals outside neurosurgery to influence public policy, collaborate with other prevention organizations, and assure that funding levels are maintained. Building and maintaining strong links with other agencies and organizations with a common mission are essential.[24]

The local THINK FIRST chapters across the country are actively collaborating with Safe Kids, the National Head Injury Foundation, the National Spinal Cord Injury Association, the National Safety Council, MADD, the National Highway and Safety Administration, the U.S. Consumer Products Safety Commission, and the Centers for Disease Control. Additionally, in the fall of 1992, the American Medical Association (AMA) medical student section passed a resolution to increase medical students' involvement in spinal cord and head injury prevention.

EFFICACY

The THINK FIRST Program is strongly committed to measuring and evaluating the program's efficacy. However, objective demonstration of efficacy is not an easy task. Nevertheless, efficacy evaluation is essential for any prevention program. Efficacy is measured in three ways. First, the message is transferred and the knowledge gained can be measured. Second, the effect of knowledge on behavior is measured. For example, participants can be tested to determine whether they used the newly gained knowledge to change their behaviors. Third, the incidence of the disease or injury itself is monitored to show the result, preferably a decrease in that injury.

Socially oriented programs have many intangible variables, making them difficult to standardize and study in a controlled fashion.[13] Several local chapters have conducted studies to critically evaluate the impact of their programs on the behavior and knowledge of young people. The Missouri Head's Up Program, a THINK FIRST local chapter under the direction of Dr. Clark Watts, conducted several studies that showed a positive influence on behavior as well as increased awareness. That group also reported that even several years after exposure, the risk-taking attitudes of 445 students were favorably modified compared with a control group of 379 students who were not exposed to the program.[13] In 1992, the THINK FIRST chapter directed by Dr. Ed Neuwelt in Portland, Oregon, examined the program's impact on the knowledge, attitude, and behavior of high school students. After the program, students were more likely to believe that there were actions they could take to keep from getting injured.[26] In a 1984 Florida study, a decrease in the incidence of spinal cord injuries was reported for counties implementing the Florida THINK FIRST Program compared with nonparticipating counties.[11]

As a national program, THINK FIRST is committed to conducting a multicenter efficacy study of the educational program. Because of all the uncontrollable variables in any geographic location, proving an absolute reduction in the incidence of head and spinal cord injury solely as a result of THINK FIRST may be impossible. Therefore, a study is planned that will measure the effectiveness of the program's ability to transfer information and increase knowledge about injury and its consequences, change students' attitudes toward risk-taking behavior, and increase students' intention to change their risk-taking behavior in favor of safer behavior.

The evaluation tool utilized in this multicenter study will be a self-reporting questionnaire that was created through the collaborative efforts of the THINK FIRST Foundation, the Rehabilitation Institute of Chicago, the Florida Department of Health and Rehabilitative Services, the Baylor College of Medicine, and the Institute of Rehabilitation and Research (TIRR) in Houston. This questionnaire assesses demographic data about the students, including their personal experience with trauma, their knowledge about injury and the consequences of injury, and their attitudes and behaviors with respect to risk-taking activities. In addition, the posttest questionnaire includes five questions that assess their "intent to change their behavior."

This evaluation questionnaire has been pilot tested in two locations in the United States. Pilot tests were conducted in Houston through the Baylor College of

Medicine and TIRR and St. Elizabeth's Hospital in Beaumont, Texas. It also was tested in Chicago through the Rehabilitation Institute of Chicago. The purpose of these pilot tests was to evaluate the validity of the evaluation questionnaire and the ease of implementation of the experimental design. The study was conducted in a two-wave quasi-experimental design. The Chicago pilot test focused on assessing the validity of the questionnaire and the ease of implementation of the design. That study confirmed the validity of the questionnaire. It demonstrated that the students had no difficulty with the questionnaire and that it was completed within a short time frame. The two-wave quasi-experimental design was also easily implemented. It demonstrated that the knowledge questions may not be difficult enough to be able to demonstrate an increase in knowledge as a result of the program. Therefore, we will evaluate the quality of the knowledge questions in our questionnaire. The Chicago study also demonstrated that it is necessary to conduct this multicenter study in sites where there is a THINK FIRST chapter that has been operational for some time to successfully implement the logistics of this study.[27]

The Houston pilot test examined the pretest and posttest results of this study to determine any initial statistical trends. The test was administered to tenth-graders in four schools in Houston and four schools in Beaumont, Texas. There were one experimental group and two control groups in each city. Group I, the experimental group, took the pretest questionnaire; the students were exposed to the THINK FIRST educational assembly and then were given the posttest questionnaire after a 2-week interval. Group II, the first control group, was administered the pretest; the students were not exposed to the educational assembly, and after a 2-week interval they also received the posttest questionnaire. The posttest questionnaire in both groups contained five "intent to change behavior" questions that were not in the pretest. The third group (group III) took the pretest questionnaire, did not receive the educational assembly, and then at 2 weeks took the posttest without the five "intent to change behavior" questions. This therefore was actually a simple repeat of the pretest. The reason for this is that the third group was then exposed to the educational assembly and after 2 weeks was given the complete posttest containing the "intent to change behavior" questions. Thus, in this second wave of the design, the third group actually became another experimental group that increased our numbers. Over 700 individuals took the pretest. There was a 51 percent match rate among the students; that is, the pretest of a particular student was matched perfectly with his or her posttest. This resulted in 368 matched pretests and posttests on which to do an analysis.

The Houston pilot test demonstrated the following: The experimental group—those who attended the THINK FIRST educational assembly—performed statistically significantly higher on the posttest for the questions pertaining to their attitudes and behaviors regarding risk-taking activities than did the control groups. More important, however, those in the experimental group scored higher on the "intent to change behavior" questions. In addition, the third group, which became the experimental group in the second wave, had results similar to those of the original experimental group, indicating that these results are reproducible. The most important thing the Houston test uncovered was a trend to affect the intent to change behavior. There were five questions on the posttests to assess this. Three of five questions reached a statistically significant difference when the control groups were compared with the experimental group. What this means is that students who have attended the THINK FIRST assembly are much more inclined after that assembly to wear helmets, check water depth before they dive, and stop a friend from engaging in risk-taking behavior.[27]

Having performed this pilot testing, the THINK FIRST Foundation is in the process of designing a multicenter efficacy study using a questionnaire that has subsequently been refined. This multicenter study will be conducted at 5 to 10 different geographic locations throughout the United States during the academic year 1994–1995. Through this national study, we hope to document that the THINK FIRST Program can result in an increase of self-reported safety behaviors. It is also possible that through the answers to these questions we will be able to evaluate the rationale of young people's unsafe behaviors and as a result direct our intervention at combatting those thought processes. Furthermore, as the efficacy of our prevention program is documented, we hope that this will increase our chances for further funding for the foundation and its future projects. It is also hoped that in the future, because we have documented efficacy, the current junior high and high school program, as well as the newly developed elementary education curriculum, will have a higher probability of being adopted by school systems throughout the country.

PROGRAM GROWTH

Since its inauguration in 1986, the THINK FIRST Program has grown from the original two chapters to over 200 active local chapters throughout the United States. There are seven "model" chapters that are responsible for training new groups and conducting a THINK

FIRST Program. This training, which is free of charge, includes the THINK FIRST curriculum guide, a slide set, recommendations for acquiring local funding, and guidance in establishing a program. Each group requesting training must have a neurosurgeon as a sponsoring director, who, along with the local coordinator, oversees the program. If a specific group has not been able to find a local neurosurgeon to act as a director, the THINK FIRST national office staff will help locate such a person. Since 1986, the expansion of this program has brought the THINK FIRST message to over 2.7 million students throughout the United States.

THINK FIRST is also active in Canada. In 1991, with the help of the U.S. THINK FIRST Foundation, THINK FIRST Canada was founded and is now operational. In addition, THINK FIRST is currently collaborating with individuals from Chile and Mexico.

FUTURE DIRECTIONS

During these initial years, THINK FIRST has concentrated its educational efforts on the most at-risk group, those age 16 through 24. The program may be more effective if we take our prevention message to a younger age group. The group with the second highest risk consists of those age 6 through 14. Currently, one-third of THINK FIRST presentations in this country are presented in elementary schools. It has become overwhelmingly evident that there is a need to move into that younger age group with the program's message. In other words, it may be easier to "form" behavior than to "change" behavior. To meet this need, the THINK FIRST Foundation is developing an elementary education curriculum. This curriculum, called "THINK FIRST FOR KIDS," targets young people in the 6- to 8-year age group. This age group is the most impressionable and malleable. It is probable that in the future, the current junior high and high school program will become a reinforcement tool within the overall THINK FIRST Program, which will begin in the elementary age group. THINK FIRST FOR KIDS will be a multimodality learning experience for second-graders and third-graders. This program will have an introductory 10-min animated cartoon video starring "Street Smart," a safety superhero with whom the students can identify (Fig. 72-2). This individual will take the students on a journey through five safety modules: vehicular safety, bicycle safety, water safety, playground and sports safety, and weapons safety. A progressive student comic strip will be presented within each module. The teachers will be given an instruction guide that will recommend behavioral and reinforcement activities that can be done in the classroom. This curriculum will also contain classroom poster sets for each module, emphasizing the specific safety principles. In addition, there will be an interactive computer video game for the students. This will be for reinforcement purposes throughout the next several years. It will also have a built-in capacity to test our efficacy through a scoring process.

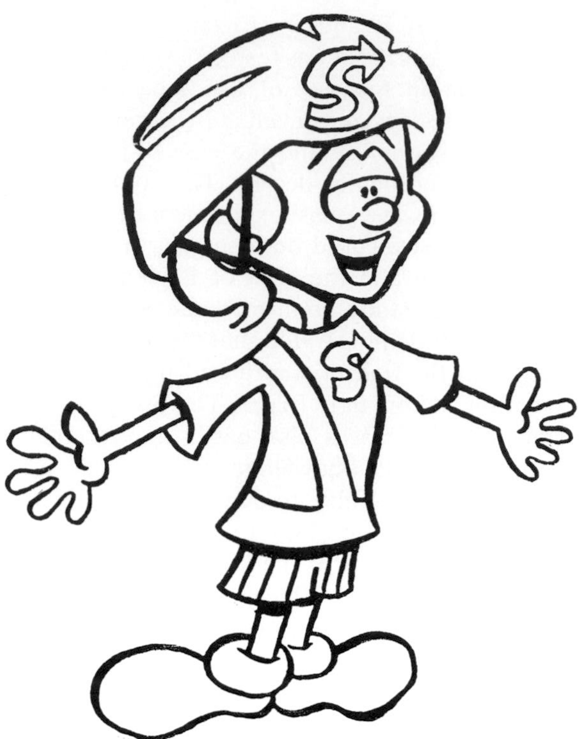

Figure 72-2. Superhero with whom students can identify.

CONCLUSION

The THINK FIRST Foundation has a national office near Chicago in Park Ridge, Illinois. The staff is responsible for curriculum development and implementation, coordination of the training, program expansion, and interfacing with other injury control agencies. A quarterly newsletter, *Prevention Pages,* is available and is distributed to over 8000 people. There is a separate development department within the foundation for the purposes of fund-raising for the Foundation Endowment as well as for special projects such as the elementary education curriculum. Individuals interested in THINK FIRST can contact the national office by calling 708-692-2740 or writing the THINK FIRST Foundation, 22 South Washington Street, Park Ridge, IL 60068.

Many years ago, Dr. Louis Pasteur said, "When meditating over a disease, I never think of finding a remedy for it, but instead a means of preventing it." More recently, one of our contemporary medical statesmen, Dr. C. Evertt Koop, former U.S. surgeon general, stated, "If diseases were killing our children in the proportions that accidents are, people would be outraged and demand that this killer be stopped." Prevention must become an integral part of trauma care, and all individuals who are actively involved in the treatment of trauma patients must extend their commitment to prevention efforts locally, regionally, and nationally.

References

1. National Center of Health Statistics: *Advance Report of Final Mortality Statistics, 1985.* Washington, D.C.: U.S. Government Printing Office, 1987.
2. Public Health Service: *Healthy People 2000: National Health Promotion and Disease Prevention Objectives—Full Report with Commentary.* Washington, D.C.: U.S. Department of Health and Human Services, Public Health Service No. PHS 91-50212, 1991.
3. Interagency Head Injury Task Force Reports. National Institute of Neurological Disorders and Stroke, National Institutes of Health, Bethesda, MD, 1989.
4. Kalsbeek WP, McLaurin RL, Harris BSH III, et al: The national head and spinal cord injury survey: Major findings. *J Neurosurg* 53(suppl):S19–S31, 1980.
5. Kraus JF, Franti RS, Riggins RS, et al: Incidence of traumatic spinal cord lesions. *J Chronic Dis* 28:471–492, 1975.
6. Jones L: Bill Aims to Curb Brain Injury. *American Medical News,* Oct. 19, 1992, pp 3, 9.
7. Carter RE Jr: Traumatic spinal cord injury due to automobile accidents. *South Med J* 70:709–710, 1977.
8. Stover SC, Fine PR (eds): *Spinal Cord Injury: The Facts and Figures.* National Spinal Cord Injury Statistical Center. University of Alabama at Birmingham, 1986.
9. Kraus JF, Conroy C: Mortality and morbidity from injuries in sports and recreation. *Annu Rev Public Health* 5:163–192, 1984.
10. Maiman D, Kunelius D, Weiss H, et al: Diving-associated spinal cord injuries during drought conditions: Wisconsin, 1988. *MMWR* 37:453–464, 1988.
11. Shaw LR, McMahon BT, Bruce JH: The Florida approach to spinal cord injury prevention. *Rehabil Lit* 45:85–89, 1984.
12. Rice, MacKenzie, et al: *1989 Cost of Injury in the U.S.: A Report to Congress.* San Francisco: Institute for Health and Aging, University of California, and Injury Prevention Center, Johns Hopkins University.
13. Eyster EF, Watts C: An update of the National Head and Spinal Cord Injury Prevention Program of the American Association of Neurological Surgeons and the Congress of Neurological Surgeons. *Clin Neurosurg* 38:252–260, 1992.
14. National Highway Traffic Safety Administration: *Fatal Accident Reporting Systems, 1987.* Washington, D.C.: U.S. Department of Transportation, 1988.
15. National Highway Traffic Safety Administration: Final Rule, FMVSS208: Occupant Crash Protection, 49 CPR, Part 571. Washington, D.C.: U.S. Department of Transportation, 1984.
16. Chorba TL, Reinturt D, Hulka BS: Efficacy of mandatory seat-belt use legislation. *JAMA* 260:3593–3597, 1988.
17. National Highway Traffic Safety Administration: *A Report to the Congress on the Effect of Motorcycle Helmet Use Law Repeal: A Case for Helmet Use.* Washington, D.C.: U.S. Department of Transportation, 1980.
18. Watson GS, Zador PL, Wilks A: The repeal of helmet use laws and increased mortality in the United States 1975–1978. *Am J Public Health* 70:529–585, 1980.
19. Sacks JJ, Holmgreen P, Smith SM, et al: Bicycle-associated head injuries and deaths in the United States from 1984 through 1988: How many are preventable? *JAMA* 266:3016–3018, 1991.
20. Goldsmith MF: Campaigns focus on helmets as safety exerts warn bicycle riders to use—and preserve heads. *JAMA* 268:308–310, 1992.
21. Thompson RS, Rivara FP, Thompson DC: A case-control study of the effectiveness of bicycle helmets. *N Engl J Med* 320:1361–1367, 1989.
22. Baker S, O'Neill B, Ginsburg M: *Injury Fact Book,* 2d ed. New York: Oxford University Press, 1989.
23. Rosenstock IM: Historical origin of the health belief model, in Becker MH (ed): *The Health Belief Model and Personal Health Behavior.* Thorofare, N.J.: CB Slack, 1974.
24. National Committee for Injury Prevention and Control: Injury prevention: Meeting the challenge. *Am J Prevent Med* 5(suppl 3):106–108, 1989.
25. Frank RG, Bouman DE, Cain K, et al: A preliminary study of a traumatic injury prevention program. *Psychol Health* 6:129–140, 1992.
26. Avolio AEC, Ramsey FL, Neuwelt EA: Evaluation of a program to prevent head and spinal cord injuries: A comparison between middle and high schools. *Neurosurgery* 31(3):557–562, 1992.
27. Heineman AW, Lemkuhl D, Garvin L, et al: *Prediction of Adolescent Injury Risk Awareness.* Paper presented at Am. Cong. Rehab. Med. Minn., MN, 1994.

PART II

SPINAL CORD INJURY

Overview

CHAPTER 73

HISTORICAL PERSPECTIVES ON SPINAL CORD INJURY

William F. Collins

INTRODUCTION

The most ancient written historical perspective of spinal cord injury is in the Edwin Smith Papyrus, copied about 1700 BC from an earlier Egyptian manuscript written between 2000 and 3000 BC. The writer's conclusion was that spinal cord injury is, "an ailment not to be treated".[10] One can find a description of a decompressive laminectomy in the 7th century by Paulus of Aegina and a description of an instrument for traction reduction of a spinal column dislocation by Aulus Cornelius Celsus in the 16th century.[31] There are sporadic optimistic reports throughout the centuries, such as one in the 18th century by Antrine Louis describing removal of a bullet from a spine or of a laminectomy for spinal cord injury by Henry Cline in the 19th century that was said to improve the condition of the patient even though the latter died some nine days later.

When these reports are considered critically, it is not difficult to reject them as not supporting any definitive therapy. It was not until near the end of the 19th century that experimental studies of spinal cord injury began to elucidate the pathogenesis and the pathology of the response of the spinal cord to injury, and it was not until almost the end of the second decade of the 20th century that improvements in mortality from spinal cord injury occurred. The mortality encountered in treating spinal cord injury had been a continuing reason why the commonest form of treatment for some 5000 years was essentially no active treatment—just as recommended by the writer of the Edwin Smith Papyrus.

Although improvement in survival and functional rehabilitation of the victims of spinal cord injury in the past 60 years has been a significant accomplishment, a treatment to aid recovery of spinal cord function following an injury to the spinal cord was not clinically demonstrated until the 1980s, indicating how early we are in the saga of spinal cord injury and its treatment. Experimental studies of spinal cord injury were well under way by the end of the 19th century, but it was not until the first decade of the 20th century, when Alfred Reginald Allen, a Philadelphia neurologist, devised an impact injury model of spinal cord injury that produced reproducible spinal cord injuries, that experimental evaluation of treatment for spinal cord injury became possible. Allen's development of a drop-weight impact spinal cord injury model that was accurate enough to predict a complete or incomplete injury allowed him to test the effect of proposed treatments in the post-injury period. His paper in the *Journal of the American Medical Association* in 1911 described the impact apparatus and the positive effect, both functionally and histologically, of a longitudinal myelotomy over the area of spinal cord injury in dogs.[2] The improvement he demonstrated supported his two hypotheses: that active treatment of spinal cord injury could have a positive effect on functional outcome; and that the response of the spinal cord to injury caused a portion of the resulting deficit. Allen convinced Dr. Charles Frazier, a prominent Philadelphia neurosurgeon, to perform decompressive laminectomies and myelotomies on three patients with spinal cord injury; then, in a paper in the *Journal of Nervous and Mental Diseases* in 1914 entitled "Histological Changes in the Spinal Cord Due to Impact," he reported the results.[3] Although two of the patients died (reportedly not as a direct result of the operation), all were said to have shown marked neurological improvement following the procedure. A quote from Allen's 1911 paper summarizes his concepts.

"Given as the hypothesis that there is a twofold factor after impact: 1. the direct injury to axon cylinders from the impact; 2. the outpouring of serum and blood into the substance of the cord; given the condition of the closely investing pia-arachnoid and the inability of drainage; given the comparative absence of symptoms after median longitudinal incision into the spinal cord—the corollary which presented itself was: What effect would a median longitudinal incision into the spinal cord have on subjects submitted to hyperimpact?

"The factors suggesting this course were, the need for spinal cord drainage, thereby accomplishing a spinal cord decompression, and the fact the heteromeric neurons in the dog and in man are not of vital importance. In five dogs I have used a hyperimpact of 540 gram-centimeters and then made a medial longitudinal incision from 1 to 1.5 cm in length directly through the impact level and passing altogether through the spinal cord. These dogs made uneventful recoveries showing only slight spasticity and awkwardness in the hind limbs but not enough to prevent running and jumping. This impact would have led to dire consequences had not the median incision been made. The first important step to determine is: How long after injury to the dog's spinal cord can one wait and still obtain the good effect of the drainage from a median longitudinal incision?"

The answer to that question was not completed before Allen enlisted in the United States Army as an infantry officer during World War I and was killed in France near Verdun. His work and his hypothesis that a secondary injury from the response of the nervous system contributes to the resulting neurological deficit has withstood more than 80 years of studies by other investigators. Unfortunately, there was a considerable hiatus before other investigators undertook the experimental study of spinal cord injury.

Although a few investigators experimented with various models of spinal cord injury in the 1920s, it was not until the late 1940s and early 1950s that Freeman and Wright, using a modification of Allen's drop-weight model, reactivated in an organized manner experimental spinal cord injury studies. They obtained evidence that supported Allen's work, demonstrating in the dog that myelotomy done promptly after a contusion of the spinal cord improved the functional outcome.[25] Tarlov, using an epidural compressing balloon, showed in the 1950s that the tracts of the spinal cord could withstand compression for over 12 hours and still recover function, suggesting that decompression of a compressing force within a 12- to 24-hour period, might have therapeutic value.[48] All the studies showed the same pathological lesion following injury—gray matter hemorrhage, necrosis of the central portion of the cord, progressive edema in and destruction of the white matter, and, developing with time, cavitation in the area of injury. This progressive pathological lesion was considered to be further evidence that the response of the nervous system to injury was responsible for a portion of the resulting deficit, and it was called "progressive central hemorrhagic necrosis." It more likely demonstrates the time necessary for the pathological changes to be seen by light microscopy. However, the hypothesis that the response of the nervous system was responsible for a portion of the resulting neurological deficit was a major impetus to a search for some treatment that could alter the response and therefore the outcome after injury.

In the 1960s, Albin and coworkers[1] showed in primates and dogs that hypothermic liquid perfusion of the surface of a traumatized spinal cord had a protective effect, suggesting a possible metabolic cause of the secondary loss of function following injury. Also in the 1960s, Ducker and Hamit[19] demonstrated the protective effect of corticosteroids, with the initial concept being that the steroid decreased the inflammatory response and stabilized neuronal membranes.

In the 1970s, Osterholm and Mathews proposed the hypothesis that norepinephrine accumulation at the site of injury caused a decrease in vascular perfusion and damage to cell membranes.[40,41] Although there was considerable evidence of an increase in biogenic amines at the site of injury, the hypothesis that the amine responsible for the effects at the site of injury was norepinephrine could not be supported by other laboratories. The expanded hypothesis that local accumulation of biogenic amines may be a major cause of damage was, however, an impetus for the National Institute of Neurological Communicative Diseases and Stroke of the NIH to increase its support of research in spinal cord injury.

Within a few years, experimental studies delineated a number of possible mechanisms that could cause a secondary loss of neurological function following spinal cord injury. Griffiths demonstrated early loss of vascular perfusion in the area of injury[30]; Stewart and Wagner[46] demonstrated alteration in vascular permeability with trauma causing edema and, as elsewhere in the central nervous system, the progressive course of edema along white matter tracts following injury. Senter and Venes[44,45] confirmed the decrease of local perfusion in the injured area and demonstrated loss of autoregulation in the spinal cord, beginning some 30 to 40 minutes after injury. With the demonstration of a change in expected outcome with treatment paradigms in an experimental model of spinal cord injury, a number of agents were shown to have positive or negative effects. Most important, this information firmly supported the concepts that the response of the nervous system contributed in part to the neurological deficit in the experimental situation and that the mechanisms were multiple.

The next experimental direction was to identify more specifically and to define the response mechanisms.

It became apparent in the experimental spinal cord injury studies that although the amount and extent of edema related directly to the amount of force applied to produce the injury, considerable edema, both in amount and extent, could accumulate with little effect on local function.[46] Studies of posttraumatic blood vessel morphology demonstrated endothelial damage, intravascular clot, and other evidence of vascular damage as possible causes of the compromised blood flow,[18] but blocking opioid receptors with naloxone or TRH decreased vascular resistance, increasing local perfusion at the site of the injury with a positive effect on the outcome. This suggested that the anatomic changes were not the only cause of the circulatory problem.[20,21]

Correction of the systemic hypotension that often accompanied spinal injury to hypertension was done in experimental spinal cord injury studies in an attempt to increase local perfusion and decrease the neurological loss. The lack of autoregulation that occurred allowed hypertension to cause an increase in hemorrhage and local damage; since hypotension decreased the hemorrhage but also increased the neurological deficit,[36] there was no support for the concept that an increase or decrease in systemic blood pressure would be of therapeutic value. This conclusion supported keeping systemic blood pressure within acceptable perfusion levels for the body as a whole. The rapidity with which gray matter changes occurred made it apparent that cell damage at the site of injury could not be altered by any postinjury treatment, but that blocking the cause of the loss of the white matter tracts might have considerable therapeutic value. The studies also demonstrated a posttraumatic decrease in local O_2, with production of acidosis,[4] a decrease in extracellular calcium with a rapid intracellular influx of calcium,[4,47] and an increase in free iron with lipid peroxidation, hydrolysis, and formation of eicosinoids and free radicals.[15,16,38] With the rapid lipid degradation, the instability of the cell membranes, and the intracellular influx of calcium, there is activation of membrane phospholipids; with depletion of energy stores, there is an impairment in the ability of the membranes to recycle the phospholipids, leading to an increase in fatty acids, especially arachidonic acid, and the production of thrombogens and prostaglandins.[15,16,47] They and the free radicals are capable of further disruption of cellular membranes and microvasculature, leading to the cascade of white matter destruction.[8,16,33,53–55]

This hypothetical basis for a destructive neural process has had considerable experimental support. Since the process appears to feed upon itself until its fuel, the cellular matrix of the nervous system, is consumed, it also suggests directions for possible therapeutic intervention. Some of the putative therapeutic approaches include: free radical scavengers; lipoxygenase inhibitors; phospholipase inhibitors; leukotriene receptor blockers; and calcium channel blockers. Of the many experimental drugs tried, two seemed to have the most effect of controlling axonal degeneration, probably by a combination of stabilizing membranes, decreasing the arachidonic cascade and peroxidation, and increasing vascular perfusion. The drugs were large doses of steroids and the blocking of opioid receptors with naloxone.[8,20,25,33,34,53–55] These findings in experimental animals were the basis for the National Acute Spinal Cord Injury Study (NASCIS) trials, which will be discussed later.

To return to the clinical area. At the turn of the century, mortality following severe spinal cord injury was approximately 90 percent. This allowed the concept that, to be considered, some treatment should not be worse than no treatment. In the United States, Mixter and Chase of Boston suggested operative intervention. They reported two patients who improved with decompressive laminectomies after spinal cord injury.[39] However, a series of some 133 patients treated at the Massachusetts General Hospital, almost half of whom had received surgical intervention that (including Mixter and Chase's patients), was published in 1913 by Hartwell.[35] He did not think that surgery significantly improved the treatment of spinal cord injury. The high mortality of both operated and nonoperated patients in that series supported his opinion. At about this time Allen published the series of three myelotomies done by Frazier.[3] Although he suggested neurological improvement with the operation, the 67 percent mortality also was not very encouraging. It was not until Head and Riddoch in Great Britain, toward the end of World War I, showed that, with special care of the urinary tract, the respiratory system, and the skin, as well as careful attention to the general nutrition of the patients, survival of a majority of patients with severe spinal cord injury was possible. Riddoch also was able to show in that group of patients that the spinal reflexes described by Sherrington existed in humans—thus, the isolated human spinal cord functioned.[43] This meant that supraspinal control of the isolated spinal cord might be possible if techniques for regeneration could be developed.

Unfortunately, most of the spinal cord-injured survivors who had benefited from this intensified acute treatment in Great Britain were not able to function in society and often became nursing home residents, their lives shortened because of skin breakdown and kidney failure.[17] Thus, the acute posttraumatic improvement in mortality seen in the British centers did not significantly change the long-term outcome of spinal cord injury. This supported the concept that there was little reason to prolong the agony of these patients by active treatment, a not uncommon opinion among the doctors caring for them. Hartwell's report on 133 cases of spinal cord injury,[35] almost half of which had surgical therapy, and Allen's report of his experimental findings and Frazier's results on three patients with decompression and myelotomy,[3] however, had, in the United States, sown the seed for invasive treatment of spinal cord injury.

The concept of rapid reduction and, if possible, surgical decompression became the standard for spinal cord injury care. During the 1920s and 30s there were a number of attempts to improve the treatment of the paralyzed patient, Munro's work in Boston on care of the bladder being outstanding. Despite all the efforts, ranging from changing cystostomies to closed and tidal drainage for bladder care, and plaster casts and turning beds for skin protection, the lives of the paralyzed spinal cord patients were short. The patients essentially were nonfunctional.

As the Second World War progressed, the number of soldiers with nervous system wounds, including spinal cord injuries, became almost overwhelming in Great Britain. Riddoch, at that time a brigadier consultant to the Emergency Medical Services for the British Armed Forces, put together plans to develop specialized units for spinal cord injuries. He knew of the concepts of Ludwig Guttmann, who had emigrated from Germany to Great Britain just before the war, and he asked him to set up a spinal cord injury unit at Stoke Mandeville. Thus began the development of the most successful treatment of spinal cord injury up to that time—and, in many respects, up to the present.[24] Guttmann's concept[31] was that spinal cord-injured patients can have, with special care and training, the ability to reenter society as productive members and, if trained correctly, should be able to take care of themselves and minimize the medical problems caused by the cord injury.

This concept evolved into the belief that, after the initial trauma, any additional trauma to the spinal cord from interventional treatment caused loss of spinal cord function and weakened the ability of the patient to overcome the handicaps of the neurological loss.[24,31] A comment from a paper, presented in 1963 by Dr. Guttmann at an Edinburgh conference on spinal cord injury, summarizes his concepts: "The guiding principles in the initial management of the fractured spine resulting in immediate damage to the spinal cord or cauda equina are great gentleness and avoidance of hasty immediate operative procedures such as laminectomy or open reduction as well as forceful conservative procedures by manipulation."

The success of the rehabilitation program supported the acceptance of the concept of noninterventional treatment of spinal cord injuries by a majority of the world's surgeons. The exception was the United States, where rapid, often forceful reduction, frequently with decompression and fusion, not only continued but was the accepted practice. Over the past decade the differences between these extremes of interventional and noninterventional therapy have decreased. It became apparent through study of the outcomes of the different treatment programs for spinal cord-injured patients that, if the program prevented a second injury, protected the skin, respiratory system and renal system, the outcomes essentially were related only to the severity of the injury. If surgery was done only to decompress the cord, with no indication that a progressive neurological deficit from compression of the spinal cord was taking place, surgical morbidity and mortality were added, making the outcome less favorable.[13,14,32,37,42,49,51] If the surgery was done to protect against a second injury, with the reason for needing protection (including, for example, transport), problems with skilled nursing, or an uncooperative or elderly patient, and if it was done with modern anesthesia and surgical techniques, the resulting protection from second injury improved the outcome, compared with patients who might suffer a second injury during their care.

As mentioned above, by the 1970s the experimental work in a number of laboratories had demonstrated that, following injury of the spinal cord, the response of the nervous system to trauma contributed to the resulting neurological deficit.[49] Although a number of agents had been shown experimentally to alter that effect, the consensus was that steroids given in large doses within a few hours of injury were most effective in favorably altering the response. In 1977, under the auspices of the National Institutes of Health, the National Acute Spinal Cord Injury Study Group (NASCIS) was organized. After completing a pilot study, a trial of the use of steroids was begun in February 1979, supported by the National Institute of Neurological Diseases and Stroke.

The first trial (NASCIS I) tested the difference between a low dose and a high dose of methylprednisolone given within 48 h of injury. Both doses were given intravenously in divided amounts for 7 days, with the low dose being 100 mg/d and the high dose 1000 mg/d. The findings indicated no difference between the 2 arms of the study.[6] During the time this study was being done, further experimental findings indicated that the most effective dose was considerably higher than the high dose of methylprednisolone being used.[8,33,34] In addition, Faden's work, which had demonstrated during the same period that the opioid antagonist naloxone improved blood flow and outcome, was confirmed in other laboratories.[20,23,54] After a successful phase I clinical trial of the large dose of naloxone suggested by the studies,[22] naloxone was proposed to be added to the study. At the time the first NASCIS trial was organized, few of the spinal cord injury service directors would agree to treat an injury without steroids; however, by the time of the second NASCIS trial, clinical studies showing lack of effect of steroids on head trauma and the findings in the first NASCIS study changed the opinion of most of these directors, and a placebo arm was added.

The second trial (NASCIS II) had 3 arms: a placebo; methylprednisolone; and naloxone. The drugs were given within 12 h of injury as follows. Methylprednisolone: an intravenous bolus of 30 mg/kg, given within 15 min, followed by 23 h of 5.4 mg/kg. Naloxone: an intravenous bolus of 5.4 mg/kg given within 15 min, followed by 4.0 mg/kg for 23 h. The findings demonstrated that methylprednisolone had a significant positive effect on the outcome if given within 8 h of injury.[7] This finding not only indicated that steroids had an effect, but also that the hypothesis that the response of the nervous system contributed to the resulting neurological deficit following trauma was supported. Since surgery of the nervous system is planned trauma, the effect of methylprednisolone in protecting adjacent nervous tissue during surgery had to be included.

It is important to realize what clinical studies like the NASCIS trials demonstrate. The NASCIS study did not determine what was the best drug, the best dose of that drug, or whether more than one drug would have an added effect. It did not determine that naloxone has no effect, but rather that, within the limitations of its use in that particular trial, an effect on those patients could not be demonstrated. The effect of methylprednisolone shown in the trial was small and suggested that more work was needed to try to increase the effect. The positive effect also makes other trials more difficult to plan,[52] since ethically they must compare their effect with the effect seen with methylprednisolone.

Another clinical trial using G_{M1} ganglioside recently was reported to show enhanced recovery of motor function.[27] The effect was present even when the ganglioside was given as late as 3 d after injury. Although the action of the neuronal gangliosides is not known, experimental evidence suggests that they enhance neuronal sprouting.[11,28,29] Both the timing of when the ganglioside was given and the suggested actions make it unlikely that the effect seen has any relation to the effects of the steroids. As mentioned earlier in this report, there are a number of possible approaches to protect the injured spinal cord and to improve functional outcome. There are also other ways to enhance return of function, as suggested in the ganglioside study, where consideration must include understanding and controlling regeneration in the central nervous system if one is to regain cephalad control of the isolated spinal cord. CNS regenerative ability is not as improbable as once considered. It has been well demonstrated that adult CNS neurons have the ability to regenerate. Aguayo and his colleagues have shown that, with the correct receptive milieu, CNS neurons will regenerate.[5,9] A number of investigators have looked at grafts of fetal tissue as possible bridges and growth factors and at molecular directional molecules as possible means to initiate and control regeneration.[12,26,28]

Although such molecular approaches are exciting, they should not allow one to forget some of the most effective means of altering the effects of spinal cord injury. Because a majority of injuries result from motor vehicle accidents, improvements in motor vehicle design to protect the spinal cords of passengers should be pursued and, along with enforcement of traffic laws, remain a priority. Education in prevention of sport accidents, as proposed in the Think First program initiated by the American Association of Neurological Surgeons, is another important concept. While considerable effort has been spent to control secondary injury from the response of the nervous system, a major problem that remains is second injury from inadequate first aid and emergency transportation. We must improve medical care from first aid through transport and initial hospital care. This, plus trained units for acute hospital care and continuing to improve both the continuing care and rehabilitation of these patients, can have a significant effect on the outcomes. From a historical perspective, the accomplishments of the past few decades suggest that further improvements will occur, with a brighter future for this difficult problem that now, at least, "is a disease to be treated."

References

1. Albin MS, White RJ, Acousta-rua G, Yashon D: Study of functional recovery produced by delayed localized cooling after spinal cord injury in primates. *J Neurosurg* 1968; 29:113–120.
2. Allen AR: Surgery of experimental lesion of spinal cord equivalent to crush injury of fracture dislocation of spinal column: A preliminary report. *JAMA* 1911; 57:878–880.
3. Allen AR: Remarks on the histopathological changes in the spinal cord due to impact. An experimental study. *J Nerv Ment Dis* 1914; 41:141–147.
4. Anderson DK, Means ED, Waters TR, Spears CJ: Spinal cord metabolism following compression trauma to the feline spinal cord. *J Neurosurg* 1980; 53:375–380.
5. Aguayo AJ: Axonal regeneration from injured neurons in the adult mammalian central nervous system, in Cotman CW (ed): *Synaptic Plasticity.* New York: Guilford Press, 1985: 457–484.
6. Bracken MB, Collins WF, Freeman DF, et al: Efficacy of methylprednisolone in acute spinal cord injury. *JAMA* 1984; 251:45–52.
7. Bracken MB, Shepard MJ, Collins WF, et al: A randomized controlled trial of methylprednisolone or naloxone

in the treatment of acute spinal cord injury. *N Engl J Med,* 1990; 322:1405–1411.

8. Braughler JM, Hall ED: Correlation of methylprednisolone pharmacokinetics in cat spinal cord with its effect on [Na+/K+]−ATPase, lipid peroxidation and motor neuron function. *J Neurosurg* 1982; 56:838–844.
9. Bray GM, Aguayo AJ: Exploring the capacity of CNS neurons to survive injury, regrow axons and form new synapses in adult mammals, in Seil FJ (ed): *Neural Regeneration and Transplantation Frontiers of Clinical Neuroscience.* New York: Alan R Liss, 1989: 67–78.
10. Breasted JH: *The Edwin Smith Surgical Papyrus.* Chicago: University of Chicago Press, 1930.
11. Ceccarelli B, Aporti F, Finesso M: Effects of brain gangliosides in functional recovery in experimental regeneration: In, Porcellati G, Ceccerelli B, Tettamanti G (eds) *Ganglioside Function: Biochemical and Pharmacological Implications. Advances in Experimental Medicine and Biology,* New York: Plenum, 1976: 275–293.
12. Commissiong JW, Toffano G: The effect of GM-1 ganglioside on coerulospinal, noradrenergic, adult neurons and on fetal monoaminergic neurons transplanted into the transected spinal cord of the rat. *Brain Res* 1986; 380:205–215.
13. Collins WF: A review and update of experimental and clinical studies of spinal cord injury. *Paraplegia* 1983; 21:204–219.
14. Collins WF, Piepmeier J, Ogle E: The spinal cord injury problem: A review. *Central Nervous Trauma.* 1986, 3, No. 4:317–331.
15. Demediuk P, Saunders RO, Anderson DK, et al: Membrane lipid changes in laminectomized and traumatized cat spinal cord. *Proc Natl Acad Sci* 1985; 82[20]:7071–7075.
16. Demopoulos HB, Flamm ES, Pietrenegro DD, Seligman ML: The free radical pathology and the microcirculation in the major central nervous system disorders. *Acta Physiol Scand* 1980; 492(Suppl):91–119.
17. Dick TBS: Traumatic paraplegia pre-Guttmann. *Paraplegia* 1969; 7:173–178.
18. Dohrmann GJ, Wagner FC Jr, Bucy P: The microvasculature in transitory traumatic paraplegia: An electron microscopic study in the monkey. *J Neurosurg* 1971; 35:263–271.
19. Ducker TB, Hamit HI: Experimental treatments of acute spinal cord injury. *J Neurosurg* 1969; 30:693–697.
20. Faden AI, Jacobs TP, Holaday JW: Opiate antagonist improves neurological recovery after spinal injury. *Science* 1980; 211:493–494.
21. Faden AI, Jacobs TP, Smith MT, Holaday JW: Comparison of thyrotropin-releasing hormone (TRH) and dexamethasone treatments in experimental spinal injury. *Neurology* 1983; 33(6):673–678.
22. Flamm ES, Young W, Collins WF, et al: A phase 1 trial of naloxone treatment in acute spinal cord injury. *J Neurosurg* 1985; 63:390–397.
23. Flamm ES, Young W, Demopoulus HB, et al: Experimental spinal cord injury: Treatment with naloxone. *Neurosurgery* 1982; 10:227–231.
24. Frankel HL, Hancock DO, Hyslop G, et al: The value of postural reduction in the initial management of closed injuries of the spine with paraplegia and tetraplegia. *Paraplegia* 1967; 7:179–192.
25. Freeman LW, Wright TW: Experimental observation of concussion and contusion of the spinal cord. *Ann Surg* 1953; 137:433–443.
26. Gage FH, Buzsaki G: CNS grafting: Potential mechanism of action, in Seil FJ (ed): *Neural Regeneration and Transplantation. Frontiers of Clinical Neuroscience.* New York: Alan R Liss, 1983: 211–226.
27. Geisler FH, Dorsey FC, Coleman WP: Recovery of motor function after spinal cord injury: A randomized, placebo controlled trial with GM-1 gangliosides. *N Engl J Med* 1991; 324(26):1829–1838.
28. Gorio A: Gangliosides as a possible treatment affecting neuronal repair processes, in Waxman SG (ed) *Functional Recovery in Neurological Disease.* New York: Raven Press, 1988: 523–530.
29. Gorio A, DiGuillo AM, Young W, et al: GM-1 effects on chemical, traumatic and peripheral nerve induced lesions of the spinal cord, in Goldberger ME, Gorio A, Murray M (eds) *Development and Plasticity of the Mammalian Spinal Cord* vol 3. Padua, Italy: Liviana Press, 1986: 227–242.
30. Griffiths IR: Spinal cord blood flow after acute spinal cord injury in dogs. *J Neurol Sci* 1976; 27:247–259.
31. Guttmann L: *Spinal Cord Injuries: Comprehensive Management and Research,* 2d ed. London: Blackwell Scientific, 1976.
32. Harris P, Karmi MZ, McClemont E, et al: The prognosis of patients sustaining severe cervical spine injury (C2–C7 inclusive). *Paraplegia* 1980; 18:324–330.
33. Hall ED, Braughler JM: Acute effect of intravenous glucocorticoid pre-treatment on the in vitro peroxidation of cat spinal cord tissue. *Experiment Neurol* 1981; 72:321–324.
34. Hall ED, Braughler JM: Effects of methylprednisolone on spinal cord lipid peroxidation and [Na+/K+]-ATPase activity: Dose response analysis during the first hour after contusion injury in the cat. *J Neurosurg* 1982; 57:247–253.
35. Hartwell JB: An analysis of 133 fractures of the spine treated at the Massachusetts General Hospital. *Boston Med Surg J* 1917; 177:31–41.
36. Lohse DC, Senter HJ, Kauer JS, et al: Spinal cord blood flow in experimental transient paraplegia. *J Neurosurg* 1980; 49:844–853.
37. Maynard FM, Reynolds GG, Fountain S, et al: Neurological prognosis after traumatic quadriplegia. *J Neurosurg* 1979; 50:611–616.
38. McCord JM: Oxygen-derived free radicals in postischemic tissue injury. *N Engl J Med* 1985; 312(3):159–163.
39. Mixter SJ, Chase HM: Operation in spinal cord injuries. *Ann Surg* 1904; 39:495–511.
40. Osterholm JL, Mathews GJ: Altered norepinephrine metabolism following experimental spinal cord injury: I. Relationships to hemorrhagic necrosis and post wound neurological defects. *J Neurosurg* 1972; 36:386–394.
41. Osterholm JL, Mathews GJ: Altered norepinephrine me-

tabolism following experimental spinal cord injury: II. Protection against traumatic spinal cord hemorrhagic necrosis by norepinephrine synthesis blockade with alpha methyl tyrosine. *J Neurosurg* 1972; 36:395–401.

42. Phillipi R, Kuhn W, Zach GA, et al: Survey of the evolution of 300 spinal cord injuries seen within 24 hours after injury. *Paraplegia* 1980; 18:337–346.
43. Riddoch G: The reflex function of the completely divided spinal cord in man compared with those associated with less severe lesions. *Brain* 1917; 40.
44. Senter HJ, Venes JL: Altered blood flow and secondary injury in experimental spinal cord injury. *J Neurosurg* 1978; 49:569–578.
45. Senter HJ, Venes JL: Loss of autoregulation and posttraumatic ischemia following experimental spinal cord trauma. *J Neurosurg* 1979; 50:198–206.
46. Stewart WB, Wagner FC: Vascular permeability changes in contused spinal cord. *Brain Res* 1979; 169:163–167.
47. Stokes BT, Fox P, Hollinden G: Extracellular calcium activity in the injured spinal cord. *Exp Neurol* 1983; 80:561–572.
48. Tarlov IM: *Spinal Cord Compression Mechanisms, Paralysis and Treatment.* Chicago: Thomas, 1957.
49. Tator CH: Acute spinal cord injury: A review of recent studies of treatment and pathophysiology. *Can Med Assoc J* 1972; 107:143–150.
50. Toffano S, Savoini G, Moroni F, et al: GM-1 ganglioside stimulates the regeneration of dopaminergeric neurons in the central nervous system. *Brain Res* 1983; 261:163–266.
51. Young JS, Dexter WR: Neurological recovery distal to the zone of injury in 172 cases of closed traumatic spinal cord injury. *Paraplegia* 1978; 16:39–49.
52. Young W: Strategies for the development of new and better pharmacological treatments for acute spinal cord injury, in Seil FJ (ed): *Neural Injury and Regeneration.* New York: Raven Press 1993: 249–256.
53. Young W, Flamm ES, Demopoulus H, et al: The effect of high dose corticosteroid therapy on blood flow, evoked potentials and extracellular calcium in experimental spinal injury. *J Neurosurg* 1982; 57:667–673.
54. Young W, Flamm ES, Demopoulus H, et al: The effect of naloxone on posttraumatic ischemia in experimental spinal contusion. *J Neurosurg* 1981; 55:209–219.
55. Young W, Yen V, Blight A: Extracellular calcium ionic activity in experimental spinal cord contusion. *Brain Res* 1982; 253:105–113.

CHAPTER 74

THE EPIDEMIOLOGY OF SPINAL CORD INJURY

Jeffrey M. Lobosky

INTRODUCTION

Few, if any, injuries result in the physical and psychological devastation visited upon the victim of spinal cord trauma. Although a serious head injury often will result in lifelong disability, frequently the effects may be subtle, or the individual's perception of those disabilities and their consequences may be altered by the very process that created them. A spinal cord injury, unless accompanied by significant head trauma, leaves the patient fully cognizant of the severity and implications of this unfortunate event. Such a realization can only compound the already tragic circumstances. Severe trauma to one's spinal cord has a profound effect upon a wide array of physiological functions, the loss of which plays an equally crucial role in the patient's psychological well being.

It is both sad and ironic to recognize that spinal cord injuries are truly a product of our advancing societies. Although reported for over two millennia, the dramatic rise in occurrence of these injuries has paralleled the development of industrialized nations and their associated tools. The emergence of automobiles and firearms, in particular, brought a new opportunity for the occurrence of these catastrophes, and in many areas of the United States these two implements compete as leading causes of spinal cord trauma.

Epidemiological studies of spinal cord injuries are invaluable in attempting to identify important medical and sociological factors, such as populations at risk and etiologies. Furthermore, they can be instrumental in the development of prevention strategies that might reduce these events and diminish their cost to society. Incidence and prevalence data allow an estimation of the economic burden associated with spinal cord injury and permit more realistic planning for the utilization of health care dollars. Yet, despite the importance and benefit of this information, valid epidemiological studies are scarce, and much of the literature is weakened by a variety of complicated factors. Fortunately a trend toward regionalized management of the spinal cord-injured patient is emerging that may not only provide improved outcomes but also enhance the ability to amass and interpret epidemiological data.

HISTORICAL PERSPECTIVES

It may be somewhat comforting to modern neurosurgeons that the futility they often experience in treating acute spinal cord injury has been reflected in the medical communications of their predecessors for almost 4000 years. The Egyptian physician Imhotep, serving Pharaoh Zoser III, has been credited with providing the first descriptions of spinal cord injury victims around 1700 BC.[1] The writings were contained in a papyrus purchased in 1862 by Edwin Smith and translated in 1930 by JH Breasted.[2]

In this classic manuscript the author describes 48 case reports, 6 of which pertain directly to spinal cord injury. The physician prescribes specific treatment modalities for those conditions that are expected to result in recovery. More important, he also chronicles patients whose injuries are so devastating that hope for recovery is impossible. Pointedly, these victims are judged by Imhotep as harboring an "ailment not to be treated."[2,3] Thus it appears that even in ancient times the concept of health care rationing was at work.

Galen experimented with laminectomized models to define specific cord levels of injury,[1] but it was not until the 7th century AD that the pessimistic outlook regarding these victims softened. Paulus of Aegina was the first to advocate surgical decompression as a treatment option in acute cord trauma.[3] An omen of the type of problems that would plague future neurosurgeons was described by Louis Antrin in 1762, when he became the first to treat surgically a gunshot wound to the spine. His exercise was indeed a rare one, as opposed to 20th century surgeons, and most spinal cord injury victims of assault or violence either succumbed to the initial insult or to the many complications outlined by Dana in 1876.[4] Unfortunately, in today's society these ancient tragedies are now commonplace.

It is interesting to note that the medicolegal issues now often intertwined in the management of acute spinal cord injuries were prevalent as long ago as the late 1800s. In Ohry's informative monograph on the history of spinal cord injuries, a report is uncovered in *JAMA* by Burry and Andrews that documented relatively enormous cash awards as a result of cord injuries and brought attention to a developing phenomenon of malingering for secondary gain.[3,5]

INCIDENCE OF SPINAL CORD INJURY

Incidence, defined as the number of occurrences in a given population in a discrete geographical region and within a specific time frame, provides us with a tangible understanding of the scope of the problem of spinal cord injury. The available literature concerning the incidence of spinal cord trauma makes obvious that validity and applicability often suffer for a variety of causes. Ergas[6] in 1985 published an insightful review of the various reports of incidence and prevalence of spinal trauma and documented many of the difficulties that can alter the data and thus affect adversely the reliability of the published figures.

Many incidence studies rely heavily on material extracted from the National Hospital Discharge Survey (NHDS), which employs ICD-9-CM codes to classify patients. Errors may arise on the basis of initial miscoding of patients or from the fact that patients admitted on multiple occasions will inflate the number of reported codes, since a single individual may be responsible for several "acute spinal cord injury" admissions. Conversely, at the time of discharge only the primary diagnosis code may be entered, and thus a patient who has suffered multisystem trauma may have the code for spinal cord injury listed as an associated rather than primary condition. This might result in an underreporting of the true incidence.

On occasion, patients rendered quadriplegic or paraplegic from infection, neoplasm, or degenerative disease may be erroneously coded as a spinal cord injury, once again increasing the reported incidence. Finally, many reports list only patients admitted to the hospital, excluding victims who expired at the scene or in the emergency room. Furthermore, it is inevitable that victims of multiple trauma who die immediately will be assumed to have succumbed to their most obvious injury, and an associated spinal cord lesion could easily go unrecognized. This reporting practice may seriously underestimate the true incidence.

Regionalized epidemiological studies can be fraught with their own set of unique problems, which may invalidate their extrapolation to larger geographical entities. For example, a population-based survey of spinal cord injury incidence and prevalence carried out in such temperate climates as Florida or California may show an unusually high number of survivors but not necessarily reflect local occurrence rates. Many victims may have chosen to relocate to these areas *after* their injuries because of more favorable weather conditions, proximity to family, access to services, a more generous welfare system, or other factors. These issues would inflate the incidence of spinal cord injury.

Certain characteristics of a given locale may predispose to cord injury and not be applicable to other geographic regions. Increased rates of motorcycle use, the absence of an enforced mandatory seatbelt law, the prevalence of firearm injuries, or the opportunity for year-long water sport participation may be reflected in higher incidence figures locally, and thus would not be a valid representation of a larger and more diverse population.

Table 74-1 is a compilation of several major reports on the incidence of acute spinal cord injury. One of the classical epidemiological studies in this arena is the highly regarded, carefully designed project by Kraus and coworkers in 1975.[7] Their exhaustive survey of 18 northern California counties remains the gold standard by which others are measured. Kraus reported an annual incidence of 53.4 acute cord injuries per million of the population, but that number included patients who expired at the scene or in emergency departments. When considering only those victims who survived the initial insult and were admitted to the hospital, the number decreased to 32.2 per million.

Although relying on NHDS data, Bracken, Freeman,

TABLE 74-1 Outline of the Major Reports on the Incidence of Spinal Cord Injury in the United States

Authors	Year of Publication	Population	Incidence per Million
Kraus et al.[7]	1975	Northern California	32/53*
Bracken et al.[8]	1981	United States	40
Kalsbeek et al.[16]	1982	United States	50
Fine et al.[10]	1979	Southeastern U.S.	29
Albin et al.[11]	1978	Pennsylvania	50

The report by Kraus cites a figure of 53/million when patients who expired at the scene or in the emergency room were included, but only 32/million if the population was limited to patients admitted to the hospital.

and Hallebrand published an incidence figure for the United States of 40.1 per million in the years 1970–77.[8] This number reflected those patients *admitted* to the hospital alive and correlated well with other epidemiological surveys. Its validity has been sustained by other studies and the study is valuable because of its more national scope. These investigators reported a peak incidence in 1974 and a gradual decline through 1977.

Another national study of spinal cord injury incidence was undertaken by the National Head and Spinal Cord Injury Survey (NHSCIS) sponsored by the NINDS in 1980.[9] Ergas justifiably criticizes this report because of the relatively low numbers (only 31 patients), the failure to address the problem of multiple admissions, and the incongruent finding of a female preponderance of 60 percent in their population pool.[6] Despite these inconsistencies they found an incidence of acute cord injury in the United States to be approximately 50 per million in 1974. This number is not dissimilar to Bracken's finding of 47.6 per million for the same year.[8]

Other regional studies reveal surprisingly similar findings. In 1979, Fine and coworkers reported an incidence of 29.4 per million for a population in the southeastern United States based on admissions to a regional model spinal cord injury treatment center.[10] A 1978 report from Pennsylvania by Albin and colleagues, based on a hospital questionnaire, concluded that in the years 1973–74 there was an incidence of 50 per million spinal cord injuries in the state.[11] Thus, despite dissimilar methods and populations, an annual incidence of approximately 40 cases of acute spinal cord injury per 1 million of population appears to be a reasonable representation in the United States.

Reports from countries outside the United States vary widely in both reported incidence and in the methodology utilized in arriving at the figures. In 1975, Botterell and coworkers published an incidence of 14.7 per million for the Canadian population.[12] Two separate Australian studies found markedly different rates for their population. One, based only on admissions referred to spinal cord injury centers, revealed an incidence of 14.4 per million, whereas the other report included all hospital admissions and found an incidence rate almost double that.[13,14]

These studies, regardless of their shortcomings, provide invaluable information about the impact of acute spinal cord injury on a given population. With an increasing tendency toward regionalization of the care of these victims, more thorough and valid studies on the incidence of spinal cord injury are inevitable and will prove invaluable when planning future health care strategies.

PREVALENCE OF SPINAL CORD INJURY

The term "prevalence" defines the number of spinal cord injury victims within a specific population base who are alive at any given time. As recently as 1975, Kurtzke bemoaned the fact that there existed no good data on the prevalence of spinal cord injury in the United States.[15] This is unfortunate because valid prevalence information may be the single most important clue to the social and economic impact of traumatic cord injury. Reliable figures on the volume of paralyzed patients living in the community provide health care planners with an estimate of the dollars that will be required to support these victims and allow a more rational approach to the development of regional services required.

Just as incidence studies are hampered by methodology, prevalence data suffer from similar shortcomings. Results often are based on calculations derived from incidence data of dubious validity. Some studies extract their figures from household surveys and exclude institutionalized patients; others focus only on individuals hospitalized and fail to take into account those who are cared for at home. Surveying only those patients with complete or near-complete lesions ignores a sizable population of patients whose deficits may have resolved or whose injury has left them with less severe disability.

Kurtzke concluded that in 1971 the prevalence of spinal cord injury approached 41,000, a figure that most agree is a significant underestimation.[15] Ergas cited a report from the California Disability Survey that estimated 32,500 spinal cord injured patients in that state alone.[6] As he points out this figure may be misleading since only two-thirds of the respondents suffered paralysis as a result of trauma, and thus the number would be lower than reported. However, the study also excluded individuals not of working age, so the pool was absent individuals under 18 and over 65 and could lead to an underestimation. Accounting for these criticisms, Ergas estimated a national prevalence of 211,000 for 1978 and 238,000 for 1984.

A 1982 National Head and Spinal Cord Injury Survey (NHSCIS) study published in the *Journal of Neurosurgery* estimated that in 1974 28,000 people were alive with spinal cord injury. This figure calculates a rate of 13 per 100,000 and is far exceeded by all other reported prevalence rates. The inaccuracy is a reflection of the small number of patients studied and the fact that only institutionalized patients were included.[16] A United States Center for Health Statistics report looked instead at all patients with either complete or partial spinal cord injury who resided at home, excluding the institutionalized patients. Their rate of 90 per 100,000 or 191,000 persons in 1977 appears to be a more accurate representation.[17] This figure is almost identical to that arrived at by DeVivo and coworkers, who calculated a prevalence rate of 91 per 100,000 based on an incidence rate of 6600 new occurrences per year and an average life expectancy of 30 years postinjury.[18]

A recent 1990 estimation of 177,000 patients included both institutionalized and non-institutionalized patients residing in the United States in 1988.[19] Utilizing the 1988 population base and extrapolating from prevalence rates in other reports, Harvey and coworkers derived a rate of 72 per 100,000, which fell between the extremes of 13 per 100,000 from the NHSCIS and 112 per 100,000 found by Collins in 1987.[16,20] When considering the inherent difficulties in the published literature it appears reasonable to accept a prevalence figure of 200,000 to 250,000 as the most accurate estimation of the total number of patients with spinal cord injury residing in the United States today. This view is reflected by the National Institute of Neurological Disorders and Stroke (NINDS), which cited a figure of 250,000 in a September 1992 Fact Sheet.[21]

DEMOGRAPHICS OF ACUTE SPINAL CORD INJURY

Every major study reviewed by the author discloses a preponderance of males in the population of spinal cord-injured patients. Although the figures vary somewhat, it appears that at least 75 percent of these victims are male.[7,8,10,15,20,22] The single exception to this trend was reported by Kalsbeek and coworkers in the National Head and Spinal Cord Injury Survey showing a 60 percent *female* majority in their study group.[16] This unusual finding, coupled with the relatively small number of patients, seriously questions the validity of their data.

The reasons for the overwhelming numbers of males suffering cord injury have not been well elucidated, but parallel their higher involvement in other traumatic injuries as well. A plausible explanation is that men tend to engage in more risk-taking activities, both recreationally and in their occupations. Furthermore, they have a higher rate of alcohol and substance abuse than do females, and these injuries frequently are associated with intoxication.

Similar among the reports of injury demographics is the finding of varying rates of occurrence throughout differing age groups. In general, the highest risk group is between the ages of 16 and 30, not unlike head injuries. Spinal cord injury is rare in the pediatric population but can be associated with severe neurological injury without demonstrable radiographic abnormalities (SCIWORA).[23–25] Although the incidence after the age of 30 declines steadily, there exists a second peak in the most elderly population and reflects progressive spondolytic disease and an increased incidence of falls in this group.

The National Spinal Cord Injury Association compiled demographic information on acute spinal cord-injured patients. They reported that 53 percent of these patients were married at the time of their injuries and among those in the working population of 16 to 60, 64 percent were employed when injured.[26]

Spinal cord injury is most likely to occur among whites because of their significant majority among the population; however, the incidence of these injuries is disproportionately represented in the nonwhite races, which are more likely to suffer their injuries as a result of assaults and gunshot wounds.[7,10] The majority of the traumatic events leading to spinal cord injury occur late at night or in the early hours of the morning; as noted above, they are highly correlated with alcohol or drug intoxication.[27]

A seasonal variation has long been appreciated, with a significantly increased rate of occurrence during the summer months.[28] The more frequent use of the motorcycle, higher incidence of assaults, and increased participation in water sports during these months accounts for the almost twofold rise observed in the summer.

A slight preponderance of quadriplegia over paraplegia pervades most of the older literature and remains true today; however, Gibson noted an interesting reversal of the ratio of complete and incomplete lesions, with the latter being reported more frequently in recent studies.[29] This finding may be the result of early intervention and minimization of secondary injury, improved overall treatment strategies, or the regionalization of care, with more sophisticated examination by experienced practitioners who might be more apt to discover subtle remnants of neurological function.

More often than not, the victim of a spinal cord injury suffers trauma to other systems as well. Between 45 and 55 percent of these patients will be discovered to have associated injuries that can seriously affect their ultimate prognosis.[26,28] This fact emphasizes the importance of a thorough initial evaluation to minimize morbidity and enhance recovery.

ETIOLOGY OF ACUTE SPINAL CORD INJURY

Trauma in the United States has reached epidemic proportions in terms of both personal suffering and economic impact on the health care system. In regard to spinal cord injury, the causes are varied yet have been relatively consistent over the last decades, although several interesting observations have emerged in recent years. Most dramatic is the exponential rise in gunshot wounds as a significant etiologic factor; in several large urban areas handguns are responsible for more traumatic paralysis than are automobiles.[30] On a more positive note, rational dialogue has led to rule changes in organized sports that resulted in a drastic reduction in cord injuries suffered by athletes, especially football players.[31,32] If continued incidence reduction is to occur, similar efforts will be necessary in other arenas of trauma prevention. The major causes of spinal cord injury are presented in Table 74-2 and discussed below.

TABLE 74-2 Causes of Acute Spinal Cord Injury and the Estimated Percentage of each Category as Compared to all Causes

Etiology	Estimated Percentage of all Spinal Cord Injuries
Vehicular Trauma	50
Automobiles	
Motorcycles	
Bicycles	
Falls	15–20
Interpersonal Violence	15–20
Gunshot Wounds	
Other Assaults	
Sports and Recreation	10–15
Diving (2/3 of cases in this category)	
Football and Rugby	
Hockey	
Gymnastics	
Wrestling	

Vehicular Accidents

Despite the above remarks, motor vehicle accidents remain the leading cause of spinal cord injury throughout the United States. Most estimates of the causes of cord injury attribute about 50 percent to vehicular accidents, including motorcycles and bicycles. Over one-half of these accidents are single-vehicle collisions; as reported by Kraus,[22] truck drivers and operators of other large vehicles have more than double the rate of cord injuries suffered by occupants in passenger vehicles.[15,22,26,29] Since a significant number of patients injured in motor vehicle accidents suffer multisystem trauma and many die at the scene, the number of cord injuries resulting from this type of accident is no doubt underestimated.

Falls

Whether accidental or an attempted suicide, falls continue to play a prominent role in the etiology of spinal cord injuries, accounting for about 20 percent of the cases in most reports.[7,15,22,26,29,33] In Kurtzke's review of etiologies, the remarkable exception was the study of Tusji out of Fukuoka, where falls were responsible for 44.3 percent of cord injuries—more than twice the number suffered in motor vehicle accidents.[15] This reversal most likely reflects the lower speed limits on Japanese roadways and the generally decreased incidence of drinking and driving in far eastern cultures. As age increases, vehicular accidents become less responsible for traumatic paralysis, and falls assume the lead.[26] As mentioned earlier in this chapter, falls in general are more frequent in the aged population; because of the associated increase in cervical spondolytic stenosis in this group, their risk of cord damage from an even trivial fall is dramatic.

VIOLENT ASSAULT

It is a sad commentary on contemporary American society that although the incidence of spinal cord injury from most causes appears to be diminishing, the overall rate remains steady because of a drastic increase in the number of young people rendered quadriplegic or paraplegic as a result of gunshot wounds. Indeed, information from the National Spinal Cord Injury Association reveals that between 15 and 20 percent of cord injuries result from interpersonal violence,[26] a figure similarly reported by Gibson in his overview of cord injuries.[29] Although the terms "violence" or "assault" may include injuries from penetrating knife wounds or beatings, the vast majority involve the handgun. In a 1989 report, Graham and Weingarden revealed that in the Detroit area over 40 percent of all cord injuries were the result of handgun assaults, surpassing all other causes of acute traumatic spinal cord injury.[30] In the last 5 years, gunshot wounds have equaled motor vehicle accidents as an etiologic factor in the pediatric population at Rancho Los Amigos Rehabilitation Hospital in the greater Los Angeles area.[24]

The typical victim is a young, teen-aged, black male, often assaulted by an individual known to him. The assault frequently occurs in a social setting where alcohol or other intoxicants are being used. There is also frequent association of these injuries with drug activity or gang violence. Although not exclusively, the majority of these incidents occur in urban ghettos; this would explain the almost fourfold higher rate of expected incidence in the nonwhite population reported in several studies.[7,15,24,30] It is interesting to contrast the occurrence of assault-related cord injury in the United States to that in Japan, where strict gun control laws are operable and violence induced cord injury is almost nonexistent.

SPORTS AND RECREATION

Spinal cord injury is the result of activities related to sports and recreation in approximately 10 to 15 percent of affected patients. Within this general category, however, diving accidents account for over two-thirds of these injuries, a figure that is repeated outside the United States as well.[7,15,22,26,29,33–35] As would be expected, these tragedies occur mainly in the summer months and have an overwhelming representation in the male population. Unlike other sports-related injuries that tend to produce incomplete lesions, diving accidents most often result in a complete motor and sensory loss, with the vast majority occurring at the C5-C6 level. Only a minority of the events occur in a swimming pool; most patients are injured in rivers or oceans. Several innovative preventive programs have taken measures to alert the at-risk population to the dangers of river and stream diving in an attempt to reduce the incidence of these potentially preventable tragedies.

Despite the prominence of diving injuries in the etiology of spinal cord trauma, no area has been more carefully researched and reported than American football. Paralysis from football injuries is only one-tenth as common as diving accidents, yet Schneider's classic monograph on the subject awakened the sporting community to the epidemic number of young men whose lives were forever changed as a result of their participation in one of America's favorite pastimes.[29,36] Estimates on the number of individuals suffering a cord injury while engaged in football vary from a low of 1/58,000 participants reported by Mueller and Blyth to a high of 1/7000 found in Maroon's study in Pennsylvania.[32,37] Such data fortunately have led to a widespread appreciation of the size of the problem, resulting in a cooperative effort by organized football and the medical community. As a consequence, rule changes were initiated, and the incidence of football-related quadriplegia declined dramatically (Fig. 74-1).

Outside the United States, different types of contact sports result in cord injuries. The worldwide popularity of rugby, especially in Great Britain and its cultural allies, makes it a significant contributor to the number of sports-related quadriplegics. As in American football, the number of injuries in such countries as England,

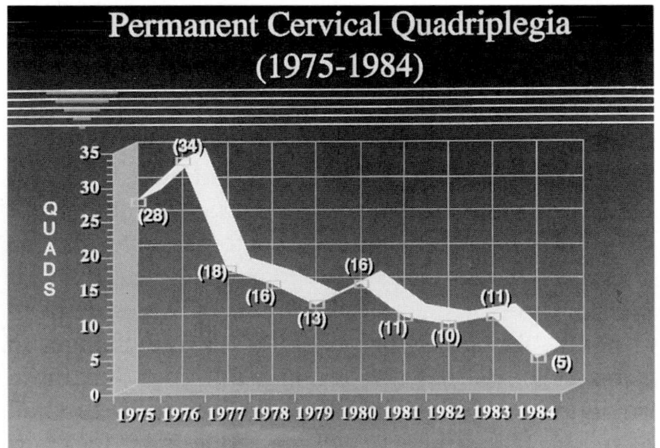

Figure 74-1. Yearly incidence of permanent cervical quadriplegia suffered in all levels of participation in football in the United States from 1975–1984. This figure dramatically demonstrates the effect of rule changes which were instituted after the 1976 season. From Torg et al.[31]

Australia, and New Zealand appears to be declining, but a recent report from South Africa suggests a disturbing reversal of that trend in Cape Province.[38,39]

Significant risks for spinal cord injury have been reported in other team sports as well. Several studies have chronicled the incidence of cord injury in hockey players, and the increasing number reflects the growing violence associated with the sport and society's tolerance and encouragement of such behavior.[40] Other sports with relatively high risk for spinal cord injury include wrestling, gymnastics, hang gliding, and motorcycle and automobile racing.

ECONOMIC IMPACT OF SPINAL CORD INJURY

The catastrophe of acute spinal cord injury has an undeniable impact on both the physical and psychological well-being of the patient and family. Beyond that, however, is the tremendous financial burden visited upon these victims and, often times, society as a whole. A number of studies have attempted to analyze these costs and allowed us to measure the true financial consequences of these injuries. Most reports do an admirable job of reviewing direct costs, such as hospitalization, rehabilitation, residence modification, and long-term care. More difficult is the approximation of indirect costs like lost wages and wasted potential.

Direct costs reflect a variety of factors and can be drastically affected by length of stay, hospital and physician charges, and subsequent rehospitalization rates. As our treatment of acute spinal cord injury has progressed, we have been able to provide survivors with a much better quality of life, shorten their hospital stays, and reduce the necessity for rehospitalization. Surprisingly, despite these advances, adjusted costs for their care continue to rise.

DeVivo and coworkers followed the trends in spinal cord injury demographics from 1973 through 1986 and discovered that during this period the length of stay for both acute hospitalization and rehabilitation declined significantly.[33] For patients treated in regional spinal cord injury care systems, acute hospitalization was reduced from a high of 44.6 days to a low in 1986 of 37.1 days, and rehabilitation confinement was reduced from 97.9 days to 76.6 days. Furthermore, the percentage of patients requiring readmission to the hospital in the subsequent year declined in the study period from 54.9 to 37.5 percent. Despite these significant reductions, the direct costs (adjusted for 1989 dollars) continued a precipitous rise. Mean acute hospital charges increased from $27,194 to $40,789, with rehabilitation charges rising less dramatically from $50,412 to $55,464.

According to the National Spinal Cord Injury Association, the direct costs in 1990 dollars for initial hospitalization and rehabilitation for a quadriplegic are $118,900 and for a paraplegic $85,100.[26] Gibson, on the other hand, broke those costs down for incomplete and complete lesions and found the charges to range from $71,980 (1989 dollars) for an incomplete paraplegic to $153,312 for a complete quadriplegic. He went on to report estimated lifetime costs of $210,379 and $571,854 for the same two categories, respectively.[29]

A thorough and careful analysis of the estimate of direct costs of spinal cord injury was published in 1992 by Harvey and associates and detailed the specifics of out-of-hospital expenses for home modifications and continued care.[41] Using 1988 dollars, they estimated acute costs for an incomplete paraplegic to be about $65,955, and $136,029 for a complete quadriplegic—figures similar to those reported above by Gibson. However, once the patient rematriculates into the community a significant amount of money is required for modifying their environment to accommodate the newly acquired disability. Harvey found that for home modifications alone the new quadriplegic could expect to incur expenses averaging $17,473 and the incomplete paraplegic $8140. A summary of the direct costs published by Harvey is reprinted in Table 74-3.

Of course these tremendous burdens cannot be borne solely by patients and their families. A review of the sources of payment for the care of a spinal cord injury victim reveals that slightly over half of the expenses are covered by private insurers. DeVivo and coworkers found that in 1973 State Departments of Vocational Rehabilitation were responsible for 30.7 percent of payments, but in 1986 that the figure dropped to only 8.9 percent. Workers' compensation contributions during the same period remained constant at about 15 percent, but Medicare as a source of payment doubled from 2.7 to 5.6 percent, reflecting the general increase in population age.[33] In the National Spinal Cord Injury Association Factsheet, the authors report a major difference between sources of payment for acute care and for chronic expenses. In their audit private insurance companies were responsible for 53 percent of expenses for acute care and only 43 percent of the costs for chronic, long-term care. On the other hand, Medicaid covered 25 percent of acute spinal cord-injured patients and 31 percent of those requiring postacute care, while Medicare was responsible for only 5 percent of the acute patients but 25 percent of patients after their initial hospitalization.[26]

Reviewing these figures highlights the tremendous costs associated with a spinal cord injury and the dramatic impact these tragedies have on our entire health

TABLE 74-3 Summary of the Average Direct Costs for the Care of an Acute Spinal Cord Injury Patient in 1988 Dollars. Cost Calculated in 1992 Dollars is Listed in Parentheses

	Total	Complete QUAD	Incomplete QUAD	Complete PARA	Incomplete PARA
Initial Costs					
Hospitalization	95,203	136,029	115,028	101,537	65,955
	(113,291)	(161,874)	(136,883)	(120,829)	(78,486)
Home Modifications	8208	17,473	5969	9344	8140
	(9767)	(20,792)	(7103)	(11,119)	(9686)
Total Costs	103,411	153,502	120,997	110,881	74,095
	(123,059)	(182,667)	(143,986)	(131,948)	(88,173)
Recurring Annual Expenses					
Hospitalization	2958	3484	5169	1975	1384
	(3520)	(4145)	(6151)	(2350)	(1646)
Practitioner	2248	3783	3300	1975	1310
	(2675)	(4501)	(3927)	(2350)	(1558)
Personal Assistance and	6269	14,243	8090	3783	3934
Institutional Care	(7460)	(16,949)	(9627)	(4501)	(4681)
Prescription Drugs	113	304	61	52	138
	(134)	(361)	(72)	(61)	(164)
Nonprescription Items	1686	2468	2043	1712	1328
	(2006)	(2936)	(2431)	(2037)	(1580)
Adaptive Equipment	861	1874	1292	800	449
	(1024)	(2230)	(1537)	(952)	(534)
Total Costs	14,135	26,156	19,955	10,297	8543
	(16,820)	(31,125)	(23,746)	(12,253)	(10,166)

SOURCE: From Harvey et al.[41]

care system. This, and the fact that many of these injuries were avoidable, underscores the importance of prevention in the discussion of future directions in spinal cord injury research.

PREVENTION STRATEGIES

The preceding sections in this chapter serve as a sobering reminder of the enormous physical, psychological, and financial ramifications attendant to a traumatic insult to the spinal cord. Other chapters in this textbook emphasize the relative fragility of the nervous system and underscore the limited ability of the neurosurgeon to reverse the devastating effects of such catastrophes. Probably nowhere else in medicine is the adage "an ounce of prevention is worth a pound of cure" more relevant than in neurological trauma. Yet, despite the epidemic proportions of these events, research funds to develop successful prevention programs remain disappointingly meager. When almost one out of every seven health care dollars are expended on the treatment of the traumatized patient, the importance of these programs cannot be overemphasized.

Prevention goals can be accomplished through a variety of distinctly different strategies. One can attempt to change the behavior of an at-risk population by education, mandate behavioral change through legislative efforts, or, finally, reduce risk by design innovations that add to the inherent safety of the product.

Several programs currently exist across the United States that target the at-risk population for injury and attempt to effect a behavioral change through educational assemblies, the raising of public awareness, and the reversal of peer pressure to engage in activities associated with a disturbingly high incidence of spinal cord injury. Safe Kids Coalition, Students Against Driving Drunk (SADD), and Friday Night Live represent just a few of the many attempts to reach young people with the message of risk reduction. Perhaps the most innovative and comprehensive program to address the issue of injury prevention is the Think First Program pioneered by Drs. Fletcher Eyster and Clark Watts in the early 1980s and adopted by organized neurosurgery soon thereafter. With over 200 active centers across the United States, this ambitious project targets high school students and presents a multifaceted assembly accompa-

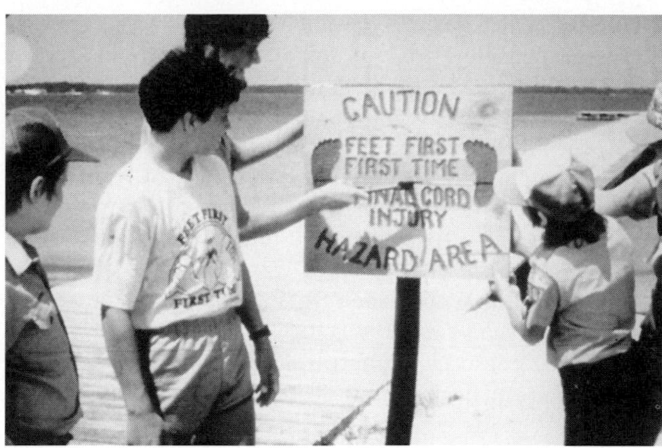

Figure 74-2. Programs such as *THINK FIRST* provide educational assemblies and reinforcement projects such as the one above to alert at risk populations to the importance of preventing a spinal cord injury. (Photograph courtesy of *THINK FIRST*, Park Ridge, Illinois. All rights reserved.)

nied by unique reinforcement strategies in an attempt to influence a positive change in their audience[42] (Fig. 74-2). Recent experience has suggested that presentation at an earlier age may enhance the desired outcome of behavior change; thus, Think First currently is developing a curriculum for younger audiences as well.

Legislative mandates as a manner of enforcing safety practices often are the least popular yet most effective tools in altering risky behavior. As a good example, for two decades significant effort was expended to increase the public's awareness of the important injury reduction benefit of seat belt use. Yet, in spite of these campaigns, only 15 to 20 percent of Americans routinely "buckled up" until the middle of the 1980s, when federal highway funds were contingent upon state laws mandating their use. In the short time since this practice began, seat belt use has increased to over 75 percent in states where these statutes are in place and automobile deaths are on the decline.

Similar legislation requiring the use of motorcycle helmets and bicycle helmets is becoming commonplace, much to the delight of the health care providers who see the positive effect of such laws. However, powerful lobbying groups continue to oppose such enactments, citing freedom of choice as the overriding principle. When, as reported by the National Spinal Cord Injury Association, more than one-half of all spinal cord injury patients require financial support from Medicaid or Medicare, the issue of free choice to act irresponsibly appears moot. Finally, more stringent drunk driving initiatives are playing a major role in the reduction of vehicular trauma as a cause of cord injury.

In the arena of product safety, automobile air bags, automatic restraint systems, and the like contribute to the overall reduction of spinal cord injury incidence. Unfortunately, recent reports document that the gains effected by such measures may be offset by the rise in personal violence and handgun injuries previously discussed in this chapter.[24,30]

As discussed in a preceding section on etiology, major advancements have been made in organized athletics to reduce the risk of spinal cord trauma, especially in American football. Through these concerted efforts of rule changes, altered techniques, and improved conditioning of the cervical musculature, dramatic declines in the incidence of football-related paralysis have been achieved.[31,32]

This success must be carried into other areas with comparable enthusiasm, dedication, and innovation. The catastrophe of spinal cord injury, especially a preventable one, cannot be tolerated nor its economic devastation borne if American society is to continue to advance.

References

1. Ducker TB, Lucas JT, Wallace CA: Recovery from spinal cord injury, in Weiss MH et al (eds): *Clinical Neurosurgery,* vol 30, chap 27. Baltimore: Williams and Wilkins, 1982: 495–513.
2. Breasted JH: *The Edwin Smith Papyrus,* vol 1. Chicago: University of Chicago, 1930: 316–342, 425–428.
3. Ohry A, Ohry-Kossoy K: *Spinal Cord Injuries in the 19th Century: Background, Research and Treatment.* Edinburgh: Churchill Livingstone, 1989.
4. Dana HT: Case of gunshot wound of the spinal cord. Am J Med Sci 1876; 72:120.
5. Burry J, Andrews EW: Medico-legal aspects of some injuries of the spinal cord. *JAMA* 1888; 11:841–844.
6. Ergas Z: Spinal cord injury in the United States: A statistical update. *Central Nervous System Trauma* (vol 2, No 1) Mary Ann Liebert, 1985: 119–32.
7. Kraus JF, Franti CE, Riggins RS, et al: Incidence of traumatic spinal cord lesions. *J Chron Dis* 1975; 28:471–492.
8. Bracken MB, Freeman DH, Hallebrand K: Incidence of acute traumatic hospitalized spinal cord injuries in the United States, 1970–77. *A J Epidemiol* 1981; 113: 615–622.
9. Anderson D, McLaurin R (eds): Report of the national head and spinal cord injury survey. *J Neurosurgery* 1980; 53:524–534.
10. Fine PR, Kuhlemeier KV, DeVivo MJ, Stover SL: Spinal cord injury: An epidemiologic perspective. *Paraplegia* 1979; 17:237–250.
11. Albin MS, Aronica MJ, Black WA, et al: Report, spinal cord injury task force, health advisory council, Dept. of Health, Commonwealth of Pennsylvania. *Pennsylvania Med* 1978; 81:29–54.

12. Botterell EH, Jousse AT, Kraus AS, et al: A model for the future care of acute spinal cord injuries. *Ann Roy Coll of Phys Surg Can* 1975; 8:193–218.
13. Sutton NE: Injuries of the spinal cord: *The Management of Paraplegia and Tetraplegia.* London: Butterworth 1973.
14. Burke DC: Spinal cord injuries. *Austral NZ J Surg* 1977; 47:166–170.
15. Kurtzke JF: Epidemiology of spinal cord injury. *Exper Neurol* 1975: No 3, 48: 163–236.
16. Kalsbeek WD, McLaurin RL, Harris BSH, Miller JD: The national head and spinal cord injury survey: Major findings. *J Neurosurg* 1982; 53, S19–S43.
17. Feller BA: Prevalence of selected impairments in the United States—1977. Vital and Health Statistics, Feb 1981; Series 10, No 134, DHHS Publication (PHS) 81–1562.
18. DeVivo MJ, Fine PR, Maetz HM, Stover SL: Prevalence of spinal cord injury: A reestimation employing life table techniques. *Arch Neurol* 1980; 37:707–708.
19. Harvey C, Rothschild BB, Asmann AJ, Stripling T: New estimates of traumatic spinal cord injury prevalence: A survey based approach. *Paraplegia* 1990; 28:537–544.
20. Collins JG: Types of injuries and impairments due to injuries, in *Vital and Health Statistics.* Series 10, No 159. DHHS Publication (PHS) 87–1587.
21. Oliver NJ: Annual estimates: Stroke and central nervous system trauma. Office of Scientific and Health Reports. Bethesda MD: NINDS, 1992.
22. Kraus JF: Epidemiological apsects of acute spinal cord injury: A review of incidence, prevalence, causes and outcome, in Becker DD, Povlishock JT (eds): *Central Nervous System Trauma Status Report, 1985.* NINCDS 1985: 313–322.
23. Birney TJ, Hanley EN: Traumatic cervical spine injuries in childhood and adolescence. *Spine* 1989; 14:1277–1282.
24. Haffner DL, Hoffer MM, Wiedbusch R: Etiology of children's spinal injuries at Rancho Los Amigos. *Spine,* 1993; 18:679–684.
25. Osenbach RK, Menezes AH: Pediatric spinal cord and vertebral column injury. *Neurosurgery* 1992; 30:385–390.
26. Factsheet No. 2: Spinal cord injury statistical information. Woburn MA: National Spinal Cord Injury Association, 1992.
27. Green BA, Klose KJ, Goldberg ML: Clinical and research considerations in spinal cord injury, in Becker DD, Povlishock JT (eds): *Central Nervous System Trauma Status Report,* 1985. NINCDS, 1985: 341–368.
28. Stover SL, Fine PR (eds): *Spinal Cord Injury: The Facts and Figures.* Birmingham AL: University of Alabama at Birmingham, 1986.
29. Gibson CJ: An overview of Spinal Cord Injury. *Phys Med Rehab Clin North Am* 1992; 3:699–709.
30. Graham PM, Weingarden SI: Victims of gun shootings. *J Adol. Health Care* 1989; 10:534–536.
31. Torg JS, Vegso JJ, Sennett B, Das M: The national football head and neck injury registry. *JAMA* 1985; 254:3439–3443.
32. Maroon JC, Steele PB, Berlin R: Football head and neck injuries—An update, in Carmel PW et al (eds): *Clin Neurosurg* 1979; 27, 414–429.
33. DeVivo MJ, Rutt RD, Black KJ, et al: Trends in spinal cord injury demographics and treatment outcomes between 1973 and 1986. *Arch Phys Med Rehab* 1992; 73:424–430.
34. Tator CH, Edmonds VE, New ML: Diving: A frequent and potentially preventable cause of spinal cord injury. *Can Med Assoc J* 1981; 124:1323–1324.
35. Kewalramani LS, Taylor RG: Injuries to the cervical spine from diving accidents. *J Trauma* 1975; 15:130–142.
36. Schneider RC: Serious and fatal neurosurgical football injuries. *Clin Neurosurg* 1966; 12:226.
37. Mueller FO, Blyth CS: Catastrophic head and neck injuries. *Phys Sportsmed* 1979; 7:71–77.
38. Burry HC, Gowland H: Cervical injury in rugby football—A New Zealand survey. *Br J Sports Med* 1981; 15:56–59.
39. Kew T, Noakes TD, Kettles AN, et al: A retrospective study of spinal cord injuries in Cape Province rugby players, 1963–1989. *S Afr Med* 1991; 80:127–133.
40. Tator CH, Ekong CEU, Rowed DW, et al: Spinal injuries due to hockey. *Can J Neurol Sci* 1984; 11:34–41.
41. Harvey C, Wilson SE, Green CG, et al: New estimates of direct costs of traumatic spinal cord injuries: Results of a nationwide survey. *Paraplegia* 1992; 30:834–850.
42. Watts C, Eyster F: National head and spinal cord injury prevention program of the American association of neurological surgeons and the congress of neurological surgeons. *J Neurotrauma* 1992; 9:S307–S312.

CHAPTER 75

CLASSIFICATION OF SPINAL CORD INJURY BASED ON NEUROLOGICAL PRESENTATION

Charles H. Tator

INTRODUCTION

The most important requirements for the effective management of patients with acute spinal cord injury are accurate clinical assessment of the neurological injury and detailed radiological evaluation of the spinal cord and vertebral column injuries. The most useful assessment of the spinal cord injury is based on the clinical neurological examination,[1] although information from other modalities including pathology, electrophysiology, and imaging also help to define the nature, severity, and mechanism of cord injury. In addition, the clinical neurological examination provides the most useful information for determining the prognosis. The combined clinical and neurological assessment and the radiological and imaging findings allow the clinician to classify the type of spinal cord injury and to develop a rational treatment plan.

The neurological assessment and classification of spinal cord injury must be sufficiently robust and reliable to ensure that serial observations by the same or different observers provide reliable sequential comparisons to assess deterioration or improvement of neurological function. Accurate assessment and classification of neurological function is essential for the management of individual patients, for longitudinal studies at one institution, and for comparison with other institutions, as might occur in research projects.

In 1990 and 1991, the American Spinal Injury Association (ASIA) convened consensus meetings with international representation involving the many disciplines that participate in the management of patients with acute spinal cord injury. The mandate was to develop a new system of classification and evaluation of clinical neurological function in spinal cord injury. In 1992, ASIA, along with the International Medical Society of Paraplegia (IMSOP), published the *International Standards for Neurological and Functional Classification of Spinal Cord Injury.*[2] This new classification is based on the Frankel classification of 1969,[3] with modifications suggested by Tator and coworkers[4] and Waters and associates[5] as described below, and will be referred to here as the ASIA/IMSOP classification. This new method is now the international standard and is strongly recommended for use by all physicians and surgeons managing patients with acute spinal cord injury.

ASIA/IMSOP IMPAIRMENT SCALE

The new ASIA/IMSOP impairment scale shown in Table 75-1 contains five grades of impairment, with Grade A denoting a complete injury; Grades B, C, and D varying levels of incomplete injury; and Grade E a patient with normal motor and sensory spinal cord function. Completeness in Grade A is now defined as absence of sensory and motor function in the lowest sacral segments, S4 and S5, as originally described by Waters and coworkers.[5] Grade B is a patient who has only sensory preservation below the level of injury. Frankel and colleagues[3] originally described Grades C and D on the basis of preserved motor function classified as "useless" in Grade C and "useful" in Grade D, but these were imprecise terms. The new scale defines function more precisely on the basis of the MRC muscle grading system[6]: in Grade C, the majority of key muscles

TABLE 75-1 Classification of Spinal Cord Injury Based on the International Standards for Neurological and Functional Classification of Spinal Cord Injury by the American Spinal Injury Association (ASIA) and the International Medical Society of Paraplegia (IMSOP)

ASIA/IMSOP Impairment Scale		
Grade A	Complete	No motor or sensory function is preserved in the sacral segments S4–S5.
Grade B	Incomplete	Sensory but not motor function is preserved below the neurological level and extends through the sacral segments S4–S5.
Grade C	Incomplete	Motor function is preserved below the neurological level, and the majority of key muscles below the neurological level have a muscle grade less than 3.
Grade D	Incomplete	Motor function is preserved below the neurological level, and the majority of key muscles below the neurological level have a muscle grade greater than or equal to 3.
Grade E	Normal	Motor and sensory function are normal.

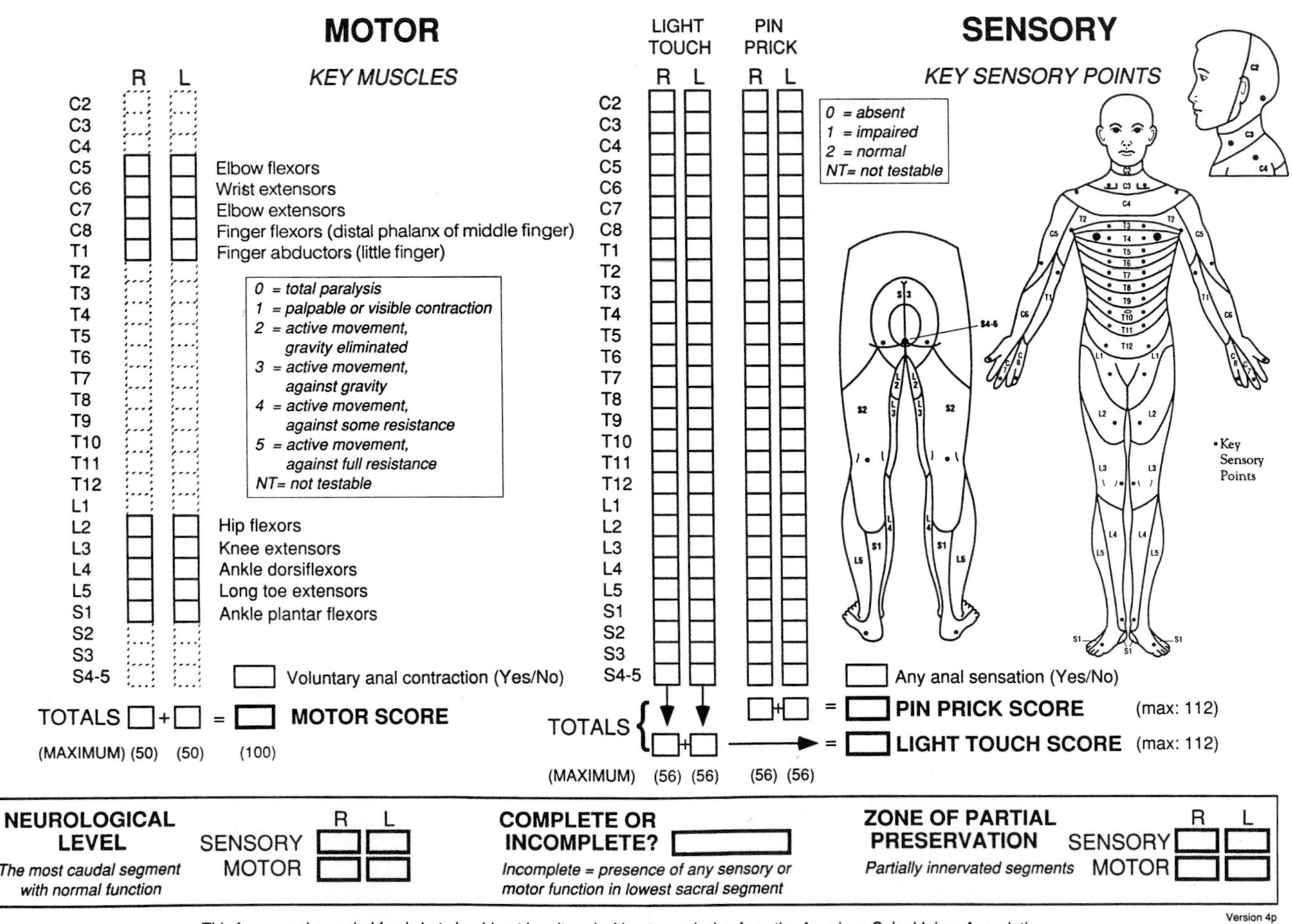

STANDARD NEUROLOGICAL CLASSIFICATION OF SPINAL CORD INJURY

MOTOR

KEY MUSCLES

	R	L	
C2			
C3			
C4			
C5			Elbow flexors
C6			Wrist extensors
C7			Elbow extensors
C8			Finger flexors (distal phalanx of middle finger)
T1			Finger abductors (little finger)
T2			
T3			
T4			
T5			
T6			
T7			
T8			
T9			
T10			
T11			
T12			
L1			
L2			Hip flexors
L3			Knee extensors
L4			Ankle dorsiflexors
L5			Long toe extensors
S1			Ankle plantar flexors
S2			
S3			
S4-5			

0 = total paralysis
1 = palpable or visible contraction
2 = active movement, gravity eliminated
3 = active movement, against gravity
4 = active movement, against some resistance
5 = active movement, against full resistance
NT= not testable

Voluntary anal contraction (Yes/No)

TOTALS ☐+☐ = ☐ MOTOR SCORE
(MAXIMUM) (50) (50) (100)

SENSORY

KEY SENSORY POINTS

	LIGHT TOUCH R	LIGHT TOUCH L	PIN PRICK R	PIN PRICK L
C2				
C3				
C4				
C5				
C6				
C7				
C8				
T1				
T2				
T3				
T4				
T5				
T6				
T7				
T8				
T9				
T10				
T11				
T12				
L1				
L2				
L3				
L4				
L5				
S1				
S2				
S3				
S4-5				

0 = absent
1 = impaired
2 = normal
NT= not testable

Any anal sensation (Yes/No)

TOTALS ☐+☐ = ☐ PIN PRICK SCORE (max: 112)
☐+☐ = ☐ LIGHT TOUCH SCORE (max: 112)
(MAXIMUM) (56) (56) (56) (56)

•Key Sensory Points

NEUROLOGICAL LEVEL — The most caudal segment with normal function — SENSORY R ☐ L ☐; MOTOR R ☐ L ☐

COMPLETE OR INCOMPLETE? ☐ — Incomplete = presence of any sensory or motor function in lowest sacral segment

ZONE OF PARTIAL PRESERVATION — Partially innervated segments — SENSORY R ☐ L ☐; MOTOR R ☐ L ☐

This form may be copied freely but should not be altered without permission from the American Spinal Injury Association

Version 4p GHC 1992

Figure 75-1. Neurological classification of spinal cord injury (ASIA/IMSOP). This diagram contains the principal information about motor, sensory, and sphincter function necessary for accurate classification and scoring of acute spinal cord injuries. The 10 key muscles to be tested for the motor examination are shown on the left, along with the MRC grading system, and the 28 dermatomes to be tested on each side for the sensory examination are shown on the right. The system for recording the neurological level(s), the completeness, and the zone of partial preservation (in complete injuries) are shown at the bottom.

below the neurological level have a muscle grade less than 3; in Grade D, the majority of key muscles below the neurological level have a muscle grade greater than or equal to 3. These modifications are based on the classification of Tator and associates.[4] The new system requires the examination of 10 key muscle groups from ten left and ten right myotomes, and the testing of sensation in 28 left and 28 right dermatomes (Fig. 75-1). Scores are generated on the basis of these examinations. Each of the 10 key muscle groups on each side of the body is scored on the basis of the traditional MRC scale of 0–5, with a total possible score of 100. Scoring of the 28 dermatomes on each side of the body is based on a scale of 0–2 for pinprick, with a total possible score of 112.

COMPLETE VERSUS INCOMPLETE INJURY

The new ASIA/IMSOP grading scale has improved the precision of differentiating between a complete and an incomplete spinal cord injury. To differentiate between the two it is absolutely essential for the clinician to test touch and pinprick sensation in the lowest sacral dermatomes, S4 and S5, perianally at the mucocutaneous junction, as well as deep anal sensation. Also, voluntary motor contraction of the external anal sphincter must be tested by digital examination. The important distinction between complete and incomplete is crucial for planning treatment and for predicting outcome.

Until about 1970, approximately two-thirds of acute spinal cord injuries were complete neurological injuries on admission to tertiary care facilities. Since then, there has been a remarkable change. In the 1990s, approximately two-thirds of spinal cord injuries are incomplete neurological injuries on admission.[7] The reasons for this significant epidemiological change are uncertain, but likely are related to earlier referral to an acute spinal cord injury center, better prehospital first-aid care, including better management of systemic and neurogenic shock, less mishandling by untrained lay people, and other prevention measures such as seat belt usage.

For cervical, thoracic and thoracolumbar cord injuries, the prognosis for neurological recovery is much better for incomplete than complete injuries.[8] Indeed, in the past, it was generally believed that there was no possibility of distal cord recovery in patients with complete spinal cord injury. However, it should be noted that almost all series of large numbers of patients with acute spinal cord injury have included a small percentage of initially complete cases who then showed significant recovery of distal cord function. This fact is well documented in Hansebout's comprehensive review of several large published series of complete cases, in which he found that 1 to 2 percent of complete injuries became ambulatory.[9] It is readily acknowledged that some complete cases with distal cord recovery can be explained on the basis of difficulties encountered in performing the initial neurological assessment of certain patients, including those who are inebriated, under the influence of sedatives or other drugs, in spinal shock, suffering head injury, or who may be uncooperative for other reasons. The present author believes that, after excluding all these difficulties, approximately 1 to 2 percent of complete cord injuries recover some distal cord function, and that early appropriate treatment can increase this number. Support for the concept that some complete cases can recover comes from the work of Dimitrijevic,[10] who identified by means of electrophysiological tests in the subacute or chronic stage some physiologically intact fibers in certain patients considered initially complete (the so-called "discomplete syndrome"). Also, autopsy studies have shown that the cord in most complete cases is still anatomically intact in some areas.[11,12] For example, Bunge and coworkers found pathological evidence for the continuity of neural tissue at the injury site in more than 60 percent of patients with clinically complete injuries.

THE LEVEL OF A SPINAL CORD INJURY

Until recently, there has been inconsistency in the methodology used by clinicians to define the level of a spinal cord injury.[1] Fortunately, the new ASIA/IMSOP classification provides precise methodology for defining the neurological motor and sensory levels, the skeletal level, and the zone of partial preservation (Fig. 75-1). Since normal segments may differ on the two sides, and may differ in terms of motor and sensory function, there may be up to four different segments identified in determining the neurological level, i.e., right sensory, left sensory, right motor, and left motor. The terms "sensory level" or "motor level" are defined as the most caudal segment of the cord with normal sensory or motor function, respectively, on both sides of the body. These levels are determined by neurological examination of a key sensory point in each of the 28 right and 28 left dermatomes and a key muscle in each of the 10 right and 10 left myotomes. The zone of partial preservation is defined as encompassing those dermatomes and myotomes caudal to the neurological level that remain partially inner-

TABLE 75-2 Classification of Acute Spinal Cord or Cauda Equina Injury Syndromes in Trauma Patients

Complete Spinal Cord Injury: ASIA/IMSOP Grade A
- Unilevel—no zone of partial preservation
- Multiple level—with zone of partial preservation

Incomplete Spinal Cord Injury: ASIA/IMSOP Grades B, C, and D
- Cervico-Medullary Syndrome
- Central Cord Syndrome
- Anterior Cord Syndrome
- Posterior Cord Syndrome
- Brown-Séquard Syndrome
- Conus Medullaris Syndrome

Complete Cauda Equina Injury: ASIA/IMSOP Grade A

Incomplete Cauda Equina Injury: ASIA/IMSOP Grades B, C, and D

vated in complete injuries (Table 75-2 and Fig. 75-1). The concept of the zone of partial preservation is very helpful for documenting complete injuries that extend for more than one segment, and these are especially common in the cervical region. The pathological substrate for injuries with a long rostral-caudal extent may be spreading edema, remote hemorrhages, or ischemia.[8]

The skeletal level of an injury is defined as the level of greatest vertebral damage on radiological examination. The skeletal level and the neurological levels may be similar or may differ by one or more segments.

RELATIONSHIPS BETWEEN NEUROLOGICAL LEVEL, SEVERITY OF SPINAL CORD INJURY, AND TYPE OF SPINAL COLUMN INJURY

In the author's analysis of 358 patients with spinal cord injury,[8] the 71 thoracic injuries showed a significantly higher incidence of complete injuries (77.5 percent complete) than did the 202 cervical injuries (60.4 percent complete) or the 85 thoracolumbar cord injuries from T11–T12 to L1–L2 (64.7 percent complete). Anterior dislocations and fracture-dislocations showed a higher percentage of complete cord injuries than did compression fractures or burst fractures. In patients with complete injuries, neurological recovery at one year was greater for cervical injuries, second for thoracic injuries, and lowest for thoracolumbar (T11–T12 to L1–L2) injuries. In incomplete cases, the likelihood of neurological recovery was approximately the same in cervical and thoracic cases and considerably less in thoracolumbar injuries.[8] In all three regions, the incidence and extent of recovery in incomplete injuries was related to the severity of the injury as determined by the initial neurological examination: the less severe the neurological injury at admission, the greater the neurological recovery.

SPINAL SHOCK

Spinal shock occurs in major spinal cord injury and can be a source of considerable confusion to the examiner. Spinal shock is a form of neurogenic shock, and differs in etiology and manifestations from systemic shock, which also can occur in spinal cord-injured patients (for example, a thoracic cord injury with a concomitant aortic injury). Spinal shock consists of the loss of somatic motor, sensory, and sympathetic autonomic function due to spinal cord injury.[13] The more severe the cord injury, and the higher the level of injury, the greater the severity and duration of spinal shock. Thus, spinal shock is most severe in complete upper cervical cord injuries, is less severe in incomplete thoracic injuries, and is minimal in all lumbar cord injuries.

In severe cases, the somatic motor component of spinal shock may consist of paralysis, flaccidity, and areflexia with respect to deep tendon and cutaneous reflexes. The sensory component may consist of anesthesia to all modalities, and the autonomic component may include systemic hypotension and bradycardia and skin hyperemia and warmth. The bradycardia is due to the loss of sympathetic function in the presence of persisting parasympathetic function (unopposed vagotonia). The exact mechanism of spinal shock is unknown, but may be related to a reversible neuronal and axonal membrane dysfunction that results in temporary electrolyte or neurotransmitter imbalance and ensuing deficits in impulse conduction. For example, leakage of intracellular potassium from neuronal cell bodies and axons into the extracellular space may be the principal cause of the conduction defect in spinal shock.

The major difficulty caused by spinal shock with respect to the clinical examination occurs in the first few hours or days after spinal cord injury, when there is an admixture of the physiological, temporary effects of spinal shock and the pathological, more permanent effects of the cord injury itself. Another difficulty is the variable duration of spinal shock. To avoid confusion, it is recommended that the clinician use the following guidelines: (1) assume that the somatic motor and sensory deficits due to spinal shock last only one hour or less and have terminated by the time most patients are examined in the first hospital reached (which in most countries is now within one to four hours of injury); (2) assume that the reflex and autonomic components of spinal shock persist for days to months, depending on the level and severity of the cord injury: (3) conclude that the motor and sensory deficits persisting more than one hour after spinal cord injury are due to pathological changes in the cord rather than the physiological effects of spinal shock. These guidelines reduce the chance of missing a serious spinal cord injury because the examiner mistakenly attributed the observed neurological deficits to spinal shock.

CLASSIFICATION OF INCOMPLETE ACUTE SPINAL CORD INJURY SYNDROMES

Table 75-2 shows the large variety of incomplete acute neurological syndromes that can occur in patients with spinal cord injury. These incomplete syndromes are classified as Grades B, C, or D on the ASIA/IMSOP scale (Table 75-1), provided there is at least some preservation of sensation in the lowest sacral dermatomes, S4 and S5. It is the preservation of sacral sensation that distinguishes these incomplete syndromes from complete syndromes (the latter may have some preserved distal cord sensory function in the zone of partial preservation, but not in the lowest sacral segments). In general, the incomplete syndromes are classified according to the presumed anatomic location of the injury in the transverse plane of the spinal cord (Figs. 75-2 to 75-9). For two reasons, it is useful to categorize the incomplete injuries according to the location of the injury in the cord: first, anatomic characterization of the type of incomplete syndrome provides information about the mechanism of injury, which in turn is useful for the selection of treatment; second, defining the category of incomplete injury helps to determine the prognosis for recovery, because the prognosis varies among the syndromes.

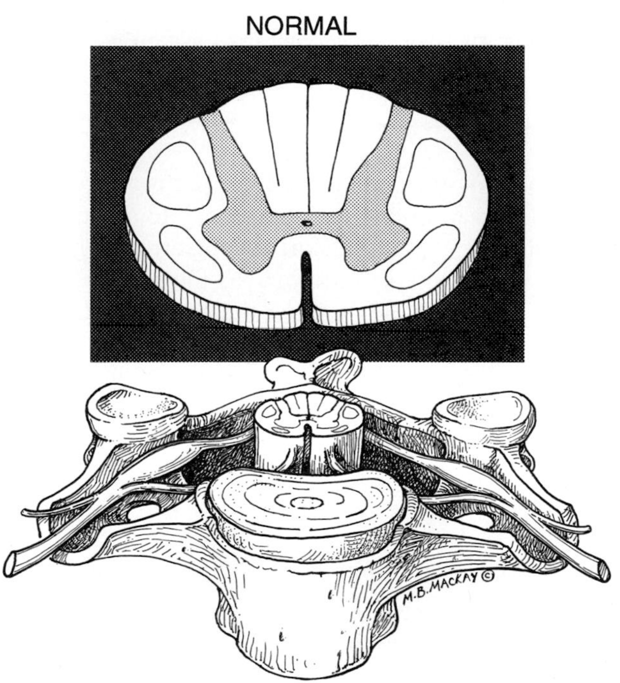

Figure 75-2. The normal spinal cord and spinal column. The normal relationships between the spinal cord, spinal column, and nerve roots are depicted in the midcervical region. For clarity, the dura has been omitted. In the upper diagram, the gray matter is finely stippled, and the corticospinal and spinothalamic tracts are outlined. The intervertebral disk is shown.

CERVICO-MEDULLARY SYNDROME (UPPER CERVICAL CORD TO MEDULLA SYNDROME)

In a high proportion of injuries to the upper cervical cord, there also will be damage to the medulla, due either to direct injury or an accompanying injury to the vertebral arteries. "Cervico-medullary syndrome" is a useful term to describe these cases that involve the upper cervical cord and brainstem, although several other terms have been used, as described below. These injuries may extend caudally to C4 or even lower in the cord, and may extend rostrally to involve the pons.

Schneider was the first to pay special attention to the lesions affecting the upper cervical cord, and he noted that they can occur with or without involvement of the lower medulla. He used a variety of terms to describe them such as the "bulbar-cervical dissociation pattern."[14,15] In its severe form the cervico-medullary syndrome includes respiratory arrest, hypotension, tetraplegia, and anesthesia that can extend from C1–C4. One of the interesting and distinguishing features is the sensory loss over the face conforming to the onion skin or Déjerine pattern. In general, the more cephalad lesions such as occipito-atlantal dislocation have more severe manifestations of brainstem and cranial nerve involvement. The mechanisms of cord or brainstem injury may include traction or compression due to severe dislocation and anteroposterior compression from burst fracture or ruptured disk. Improved first-aid including management of the airway, respiration, and shock accounts for the relatively higher current incidence of these injuries due to the greater number of survivors arriving at neurosurgical centers.

Knowledge of the neuroanatomy of the upper cervical cord and brainstem improves our understanding of the clinical manifestations of this syndrome. The examiner should carefully examine facial sensation in all cervical spinal injuries to detect damage to the fibers of the descending spinal tract of the trigeminal nerve or to the cell bodies in the nucleus of the spinal tract of the trigeminal nerve, which begin in the pons and medulla and extend caudally to at least the C4 cervical segment. Owing to the onion skin or Déjerine pattern of topographic representation, a perioral distribution of sensory loss denotes a lesion in the medulla and upper cervical cord, while a more peripheral facial distribution of sensory loss involving the forehead, ear, and chin denotes a lesion in the cord at C3–C4.

Another important distinguishing characteristic of cervico-medullary injuries is that they may mimic the central cord syndrome, the hallmark of which is greater arm than leg weakness. This clinical pattern is based on the anatomic arrangement of the crossing fibers in the pyramidal tract at the cervico-medullary junction (Fig. 75-4) and has been termed the syndrome of cruciate paralysis of Bell.[16] Schneider[14] found that the pyramidal decussation in the ventrolateral aspect of the cervico-medullary junction is susceptible to compression by either the odontoid process or the anterior rim of the foramen magnum. The motor fibers to the upper extremities decussate rostral and ventral to those of the lower extremities, and then assume a medial position in the lateral corticospinal tract between the medulla and C1 (Fig. 75-4). Conversely, the lower extremity fibers that lie lateral to the arm fibers in the medulla continue caudally in this position to decussate between C1 and C2. By the time these fiber pathways reach the C2 level they have crossed completely to assume a lateral position in the lateral corticospinal tract (Fig. 75-3). Thus, a centrally located injury at the junction of the medulla and the C1 segment of the cord would damage the crossing upper limb fibers and spare the uncrossed lower limb fibers of the corticospinal tract and produce selective bilateral arm paralysis. The syndrome of cruciate paralysis of Bell can result from a variety of injuries involving displacement of the odontoid, which is anatomically adjacent to the rostral decussating arm fibers, including such injuries as fractures of the odontoid, atlanto-axial dislocation, and atlanto-occipital dislocation.[16]

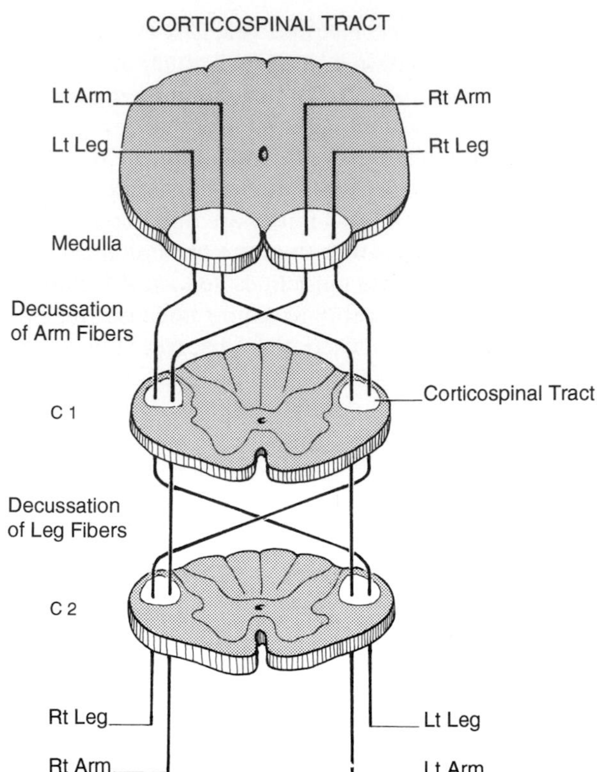

Figure 75-4. The crossing of the axons in the corticospinal tracts. The upper, middle, and lower cross sections show the medulla, the spinal cord at C1, and the spinal cord at C2, respectively. The axons subserving arm function cross the midline between the medulla and C1; those subserving leg function cross between C1 and C2.

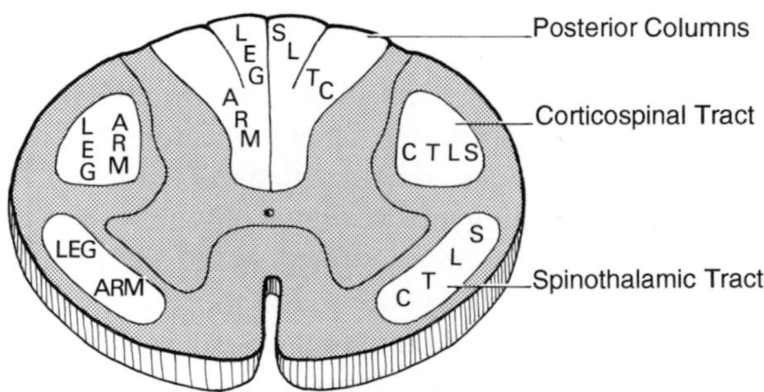

Figure 75-3. Topographical distribution in the posterior columns, corticospinal, and spinothalamic tracts. The location of the axons subserving arm and leg function are shown in the three tracts. Similarly, the locations of the axons subserving sacral (S), lumbar (L), thoracic (T), and cervical function (C) in the three tracts are indicated.

CENTRAL CORD SYNDROME

Schneider described the acute central cervical cord injury syndrome characterized by a disproportionally greater loss of motor power in the upper extremities than in the lower extremities with varying degrees of sensory loss.[14,17] He reported that many cases would recover spontaneously without surgical treatment, even though he thought that acute compression was an etiological factor in many cases. He theorized that many of the cases in older people with cervical spondylosis were due to central hematomyelia and surrounding "edematomyelia" resulting from anteroposterior compression of the cord during hyperextension injury. The cord was compressed between bony bars or spurs anteriorly and infolded ligamenta flava posteriorly (Fig. 75-5), a mechanism suggested earlier by Taylor.[18,19] To explain the pattern of arms showing a worse deficit than the legs, Schneider invoked the presumed lamination of the corticospinal tract with the leg fibers lateral and the arm fibers medial in the cord (Fig. 75-3). The central necrotic areas in pathological specimens appeared to involve principally the presumed location of the medial arm fibers of the corticospinal tracts bilaterally, with relative sparing of the lateral leg fibers. Schneider and coworkers also attributed the upper limb predilection to the involvement of the anterior horn cells in the necrotic center of the cord.[22] It should be noted that the concept of the lamination of corticospinal fibers originally postulated by Foerster in 1936[20] has been challenged by Nathan and Smith,[21] who found that the motor fibers subserving the upper and lower limb movements were intermingled.

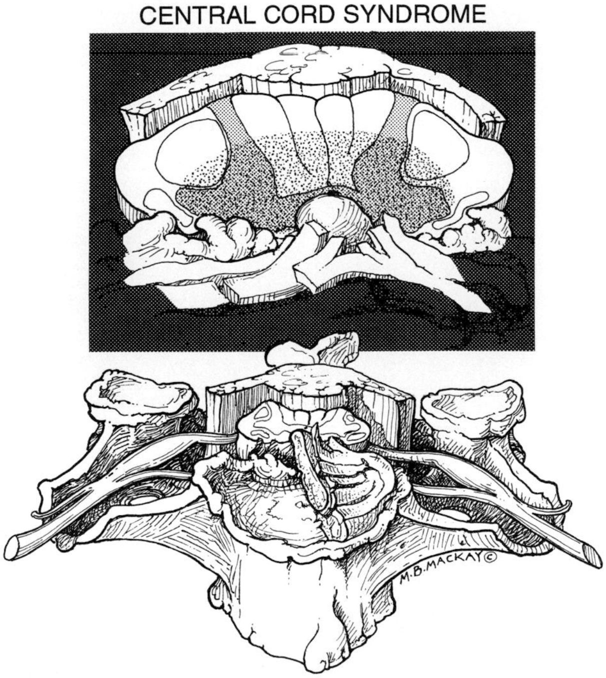

Figure 75-5. Central cord syndrome. The drawing depicts a case of cervical spondylosis with osteoarthritis of the cervical spine including anterior and posterior osteophytes and hypertrophy of the ligamentum flavum. Superimposed is an acute hyperextension injury that has caused rupture of the intervertebral disk and infolding of the ligamentum flavum. The spinal cord is compressed anteriorly and posteriorly. The central portion of the cord shown in rough stippling sustained the greatest damage. The damaged area includes the medial segments of the corticospinal tracts subserving arm function.

In cases of central cord syndrome without cervical spondylosis, stenosis, or other direct bony compression, Schneider postulated a vascular etiology and implicated a number of possible ischemic mechanisms to account for central infarction. The pathophysiological explanations for the central cord syndrome included "watershed" infarcts between zones of spinal medullary artery perfusion, vertebral artery interruption or stretching, anterior spinal artery spasm or vascular occlusion at the site of maximal hyperextension, and venous infarction.[14] Any of these vascular mechanisms might account for the central infarction of the medially located upper limb fibers of the corticospinal tract supplied by the anterior sulcal arteries, which are branches of the anterior spinal artery. Conversely, it is postulated that the laterally located leg fibers of the corticospinal tract might survive these ischemic mechanisms of injury because they are supplied by the arteriae coronae or the pial mesh, which derives its feeders from branches of *both* the anterior and posterior spinal arteries. Schneider and coworkers also implicated selective damage to the microcirculation in the center of the cord with anterior horn cell ischemia as a mechanism for producing the central cord syndrome; they thought that "the higher perfusion demands of the grey matter" might account for "the selective vulnerability of the central grey matter to ischemia."[14]

Recently, Quencer and colleagues[23] analyzed the correlations between the clinical, MR, and pathological findings in 11 patients with central cord syndrome. Most of their cases were elderly patients with cervical spondylosis and/or stenosis, although some of the younger patients had disk herniations or subluxation. All 11 cases had MR imaging, from 18 hours to 2 days after spinal cord injury in 7 patients and from 3 to 10 days after injury in the remaining 4. Autopsy studies of patients with central cord syndrome were available in 3 cases, 2 of whom had MR. Surprisingly, they did not find any evidence of hematomyelia, either on T1- or T2-weighted MR studies or in the pathological specimens. All patients showed hyperintense signals within the cord on gradient echo MR, which the authors attributed to edema. The histological specimens did not show central necrosis, but, rather, the "central grey matter was intact." In the more acute stages, the histological changes were primarily edema and separation of the axon myelin units; at the later stages, there was demyelination and myelin breakdown and breakdown of mainly large axons, especially in the corticospinal tracts but also affecting other areas of the white matter. These investigators concluded that the central cord syndrome is due primarily to "direct mechanical compression of the cord, maximal along its posterolateral aspect" which causes damage to the white matter consisting of edema, myelin breakdown, and axonal disintegration, especially in the corticospinal tracts but also elsewhere in the white matter. Furthermore, since the damage to the corticospinal tracts was diffuse and not concentrated medially in the presumed location of the arm fibers as postulated by Foerster,[20] Quencer and coworkers[23] favored the evidence of Nathan and Smith[21] that the arm and leg fibers are intermingled in the corticospinal tract. To explain the "arms more than legs" deficit of the central cord syndrome, they cited the findings of Phillips and Porter[24] and Eidelberg[25] that in primates the corticospinal tract is critical for hand function, but not for locomotor function of the legs.

Thus, the central cord syndrome appears to have a spectrum of pathological changes ranging from milder, nonhemorrhagic lesions to those with major central hemorrhagic necrosis. It is of interest that Schneider initially admonished against operating on individuals with central cord syndrome because of their good prognosis for spontaneous recovery. Indeed, some of his cases showed very rapid spontaneous clinical recovery. Furthermore, he was particularly distressed to see some patients treated by laminectomy who deteriorated dramatically postoperatively, especially those without demonstrable, persisting compression at the time of surgery. While it is true that many patients with central cord syndrome do make a substantial recovery without surgery, nevertheless many remain with significant deficits,[26] especially with severe impairment of the hands due to a combination of severe weakness and severe proprioceptive loss. Because of these facts, the present author strongly recommends that patients with central cord syndrome who have persisting compression, instability, or neurological deterioration should be considered surgical candidates for decompression, stabilization, or both, similar to patients with other incomplete syndromes. Indeed, with persisting compression it is preferable to decompress the lesion early, but even late decompression has been helpful in patients with central cord syndrome.[27]

ANTERIOR CORD SYNDROME

This syndrome was originally described in the setting of acute cervical trauma by Schneider,[28] who presented two cases of "immediate complete paralysis with hyperesthesia at the level of the lesion and an associated sparing of touch and some vibration sense" in distal dermatomes. These two cases, one of which was a young football player, had ruptured disks (although the football player also had bone fragments in the canal). Both made a substantial recovery following operative removal of the intracanalicular space-occupying lesions. This syndrome in Schneider's view was "a syndrome for which early operative intervention is indicated." It is of interest that Schneider's mentor, E. A. Kahn, had published earlier a report of chronic compressive myelopathy in which he hypothesized that the cord deficits of spasticity, disturbance of gait, and modified sensory changes were due to "mechanical stress factors" in the cord related to the attachment of the dentate ligaments.[29] Kahn wrote that "in anterior spinal cord compression, I believe that with pressure over a period of time, the pyramidal tracts because of the greater stress on them and the large size of the fibres, have more disturbance of conductivity than the pain fibres of the spinothalamic tracts, even though the latter are closer to the compressing mass, be it midline herniated nucleus pulposus or tumor." Kahn also stated that "secondary stress is directly on pyramidal tracts" due to the attachment of the dentate ligaments and that "the leg area is most lateral in the pyramidal tracts, while the hand area is most medial, explaining the usual sparing of the hands." Thus, Kahn's theories of lines of stress and mechanical stress factors in chronic myelopathy were applied by Schneider to explain the clinical findings in acute cord injury. This theory seemed more plausible than the theory previously held in these cases that the

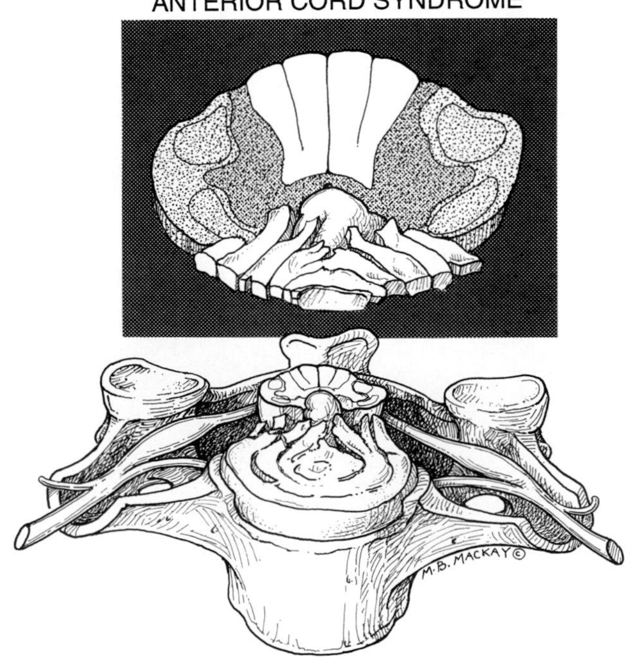

Figure 75-6. Anterior cord syndrome. A large disk herniation is shown compressing the anterior aspect of the cord, resulting in damage (rough stippling) to the anterior and lateral white matter tracts and to the gray matter. The posterior columns remain intact.

deficit was due to compression of the anterior spinal artery, for which there was no direct proof at that time or subsequently.

Most cases of the anterior cord syndrome would be Grade B patients on the ASIA/IMSOP scale with relative sparing of the posterior columns and complete motor paralysis (Fig. 75-6). The prognosis for recovery of other sensory modalities or motor function varies greatly from minimal recovery to excellent recovery of both motor and sensory function.

POSTERIOR CORD SYNDROME

This is an extremely rare type of incomplete syndrome; indeed, many, including the author, have doubted its existence. By definition, it consists of major damage to the posterior aspect of the cord but with some residual functioning of spinal cord tissue anteriorly (Fig. 75-7). Clinically, the patient would have retained spinothalamic function but would have lost movement and proprioception due to damage to the posterior half of the cord, including the corticospinal tracts and posterior columns.

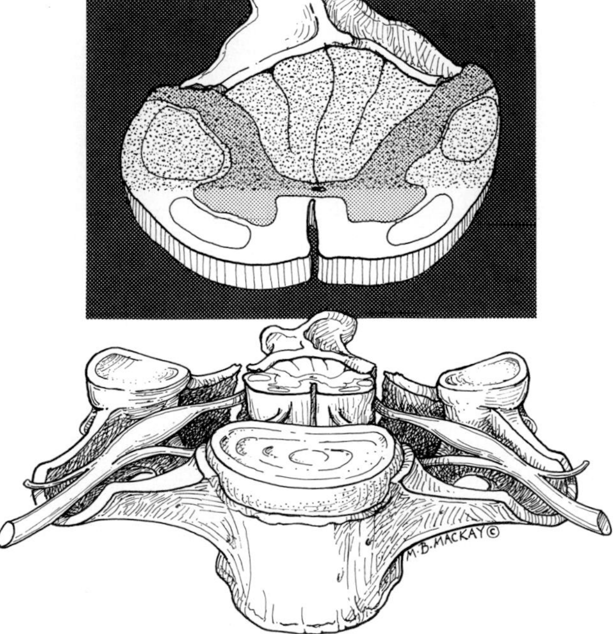

Figure 75-7. Posterior cord syndrome. A laminar fracture is depicted with anterior displacement of the fractured bone and compression of the posterior aspect of the spinal cord. The damaged area of the cord (roughly stippled in the upper diagram) includes the posterior columns and the posterior half of the lateral columns including the corticospinal tracts.

BROWN-SÉQUARD SYNDROME

The Brown-Séquard syndrome[30] results from damage to the lateral half of the spinal cord and is characterized by loss of ipsilateral motor and proprioceptive function and loss of contralateral pain and temperature sensation (Fig. 75-8). The syndrome can be associated with a variety of mechanisms of injury, but in the series of Braakman and Penning[31] was most often observed with hyperextension injuries, although they also had many cases with flexion injuries, locked facets, and compression fractures. Lazorthes and coworkers[32] concluded that the syndrome often signified spinal cord compression from lesions such as a herniated disk.

The Brown-Séquard syndrome may be present immediately after an acute injury, or may become apparent only within days after injury as a gradual evolution from a bilateral incomplete injury. Hybrid combinations of Brown-Séquard and other incomplete syndromes may occur. For example, the author has seen frequent examples of central cord injuries that are quite asymmetric, with the more severely damaged side of the cord showing features of a Brown-Séquard syndrome. The Brown-Séquard syndrome occurs most often after cervical injuries, with less frequent examples occurring in the thoracic cord and conus medullaris. In milder cases, there may be no sphincter deficit. The prognosis for recovery

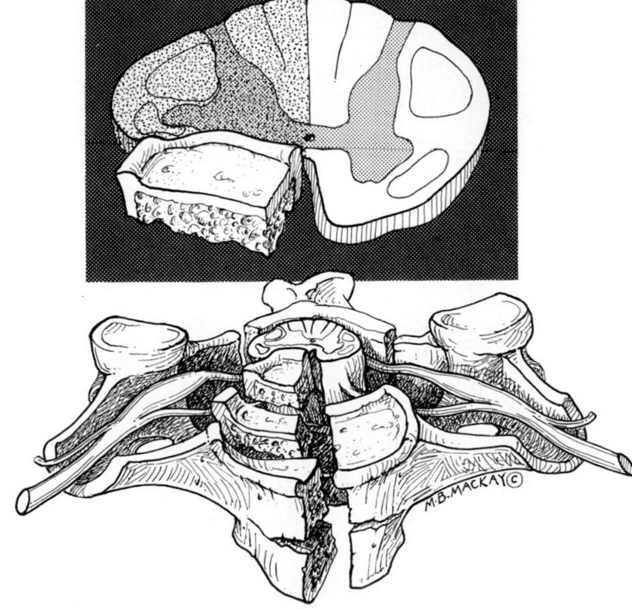

Figure 75-8. Brown-Séquard syndrome. A burst fracture is depicted with posterior displacement of bone fragments and disk, resulting in unilateral compression and damage (rough stippling) to one-half of the spinal cord.

varies widely, but there are many examples of excellent recovery.

CONUS MEDULLARIS SYNDROME

Anatomically, in most patients, almost all of the lumbar cord segments are opposite the T12 vertebral body, and almost all of the sacral cord segments are opposite the L1 vertebral body, with the cord ending opposite the L1–L2 disk space. Since injuries at T11–T12 and T12–L1 are relatively common, because of the mobility of these segments compared with the relatively immobile thoracic segments above, injuries to the conus medullaris are frequent (Fig. 75-9). Indeed, in the author's experience conus medullaris injuries comprised approximately 24 percent of cases of acute spinal cord injury.[8] These injuries usually produce a combinaton of lower motor neuron deficits with initial flaccid paralysis of the legs and anal sphincter, followed in the chronic phase by a combination of some degree of muscle atrophy and spasticity or reflex hyperactivity with possibly extensor plantar responses. The sensory picture may be variable, and in some cases the only evidence of incompleteness is retention of some perianal sensation, an example of sacral sparing. In the more severe conus lesions, the bowel and bladder deficits may be profound, with the ultimate development of a low-pressure, high-capacity neurogenic bladder. This type of lower motor neuron syndrome does not have a very good prognosis for recovery,[8] perhaps because the cell bodies are injured rather than the axons alone as in cauda equina injuries.

CAUDA EQUINA INJURIES

With the cord terminating normally opposite the L1–L2 disk space (Fig. 75-9), injuries at this level or below will involve the roots of the cauda equina, although injuries one or two levels above will also involve

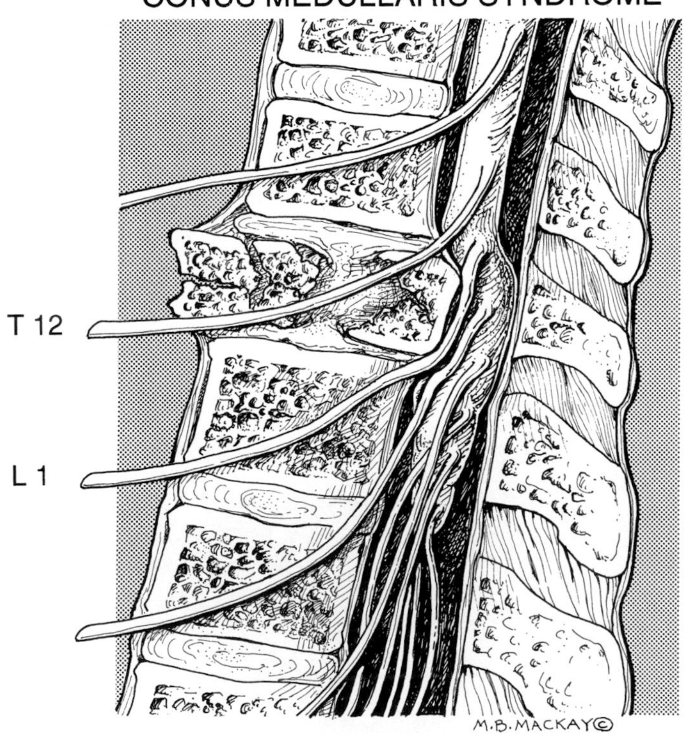

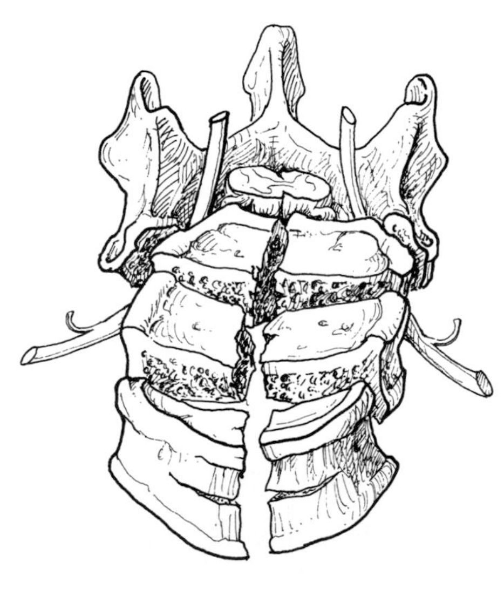

Figure 75-9. Conus medullaris syndrome. A burst fracture of T12 is depicted with posterior dislocation of bone fragments from the vertebral body into the spinal canal resulting in compression of the conus medullaris. Almost all the lumbar cord segments are opposite the T12 vertebral body, so that a severe compression injury at this level could affect all the lumbar and sacral segments of the cord.

the origins of some of the roots comprising the cauda equina. Clinically, these injuries may be either complete in which they would be grade A on the new ASIA/IMSOP scale, while incomplete injuries are of varying severity, ranging from grades B to D. Similar to cord injuries, the motor fibers tend to be more susceptible to trauma, so that incomplete cases always have sensory preservation with or without some motor preservation. Cases with only motor preservation without sensory preservation are extremely rare. The degree of bowel and bladder deficits parallel those found with cord injury. It is said that cauda equina injuries have a much better prognosis for neurological recovery as compared with spinal cord injury because the lower motor neuron inherently has more resilience to trauma, with fewer secondary injury mechanisms and greater regenerative capacity than the upper motor neuron and its tracts.

One of the most interesting and dangerous cauda equina syndromes is associated with acute central disk herniation at L4–L5 or L5–S1, which causes major damage to the sacral roots lying centrally within the dural sac (Fig. 75-10). There may be partial or complete sparing of the lumbar roots, and often sparing of the S1 roots as well, in which case patients may have normal strength in the legs but complete bowel and bladder paralysis and perineal anesthesia. The sacral roots are very delicate and sometimes never recover, even if decompressed expeditiously.

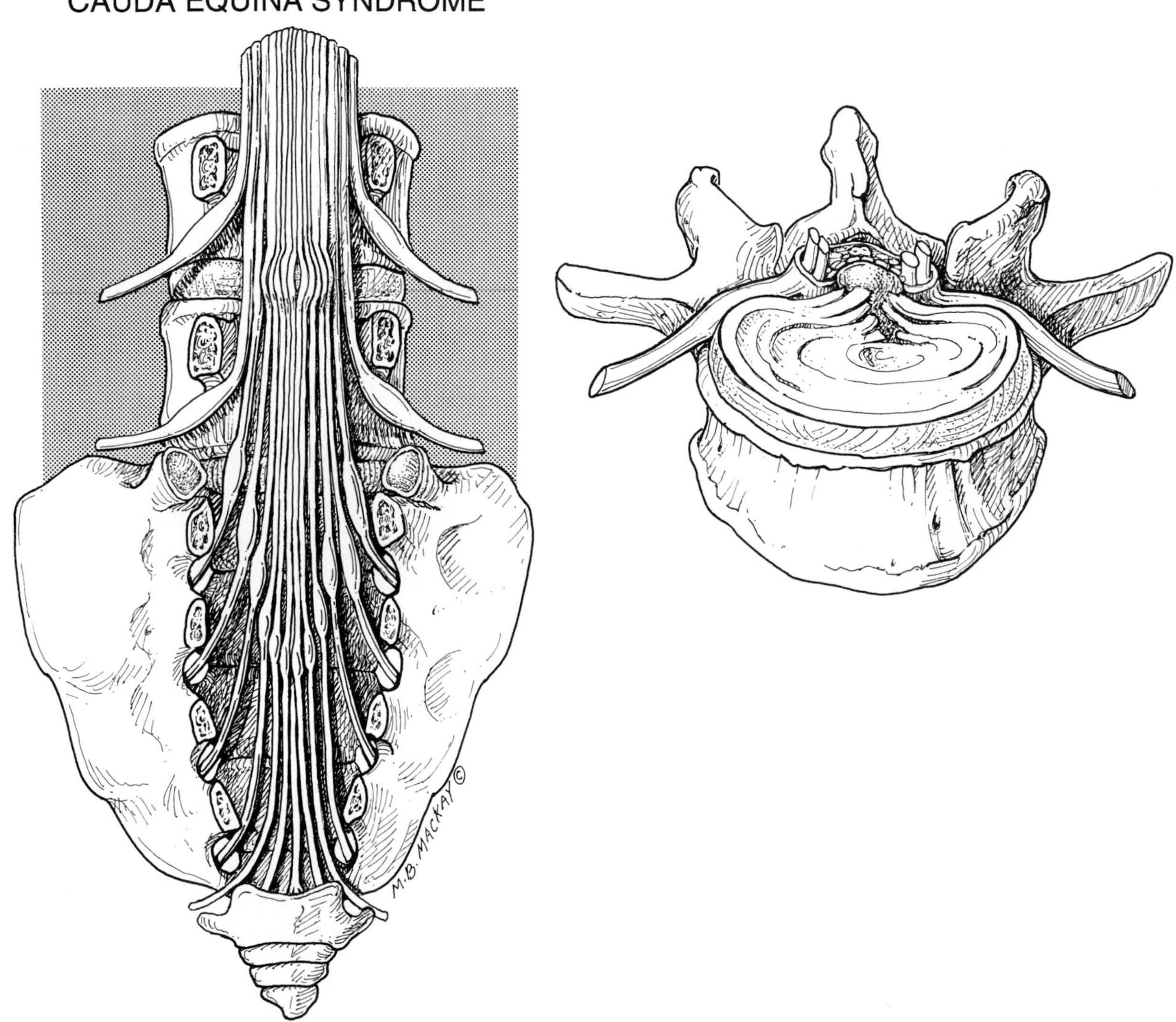

Figure 75-10. Cauda equina syndrome. The drawing shows an acute central disk herniation of L4–L5 with major compression of the central aspect of the cauda equina. The medially placed sacral roots from S2 downward sustain the maximal compression, whereas the more laterally located L5 and S1 roots are completely or partially spared.

REVERSIBLE, TRANSIENT SYNDROMES

A number of complete or incomplete spinal cord injury syndromes (Table 75-3) are reversible or transient, one of the most interesting of which is the "burning hands syndrome" frequently seen in athletes.[33–35] This syndrome is characterized by transient paresthesias and dysesthesias in the upper limbs, especially in the hands, and may exist with or without long tract signs, which if present are usually evanescent.[36] Biemond[37] found pathological changes in the posterior horn of one case with reversible findings and termed the condition contusio cervicalis posterior. Braakman and Penning[36] found that hyperextension was the most frequent mechanism of injury of the transient syndromes. Intramedullary lesions may be demonstrable by MR.[34]

Torg and coworkers[38] described a transient incomplete spinal cord syndrome with sensory and motor deficits lasting up to 48 hours in football players and used the inappropriate term "neurapraxia," which by definition refers to peripheral nerve injuries. They found that all of the patients had radiological spinal abnormalities such as ligamentous instability, disk disease, or spinal stenosis. These transient cord syndromes in athletes are usually bilateral, which distinguishes them from the other syndrome of "stingers" or "burners" in athletes due to unilateral nerve root or brachial plexus lesions (especially traction injury), most of which also are transient.[34,39]

Spinal cord concussion is a transient loss of motor or sensory function of the spinal cord that usually recovers within minutes, but always within hours. In almost all instances, the initial clinical examiner obtains the history that the symptoms are rapidly diminishing and finds no abnormalities on the neurological examination. The exact pathophysiology of spinal cord concussion is unknown, but most likely involves biochemical abnormalities such as leakage of potassium from the intracellular to the extracellular space due either to direct mechanical injury of neuronal cell membranes or secondary to a vascular mechanism, the latter possibility having been implicated by Schneider and associates.[14]

TABLE 75-3 Classification of Reversible, Transient Syndromes of Traumatic Spinal Cord Injury

Burning Hands Syndrome
Contusio Cervicalis
Cord Concussion
Hysteria

ACUTE SPINAL CORD SYNDROME WITHOUT RADIOLOGICAL EVIDENCE OF TRAUMA

In the pediatric population, the syndrome of spinal cord injury without radiological abnormality (SCIWORA) is more common than in adults, representing a significant percentage of spinal cord injuries in children.[40] In general, children with SCIWORA tend to be less severely injured than those with definite evidence of bony injury, but even complete injuries have been described. By definition, the negative radiological examination includes only plain films and tomography, either conventional or CT. If a negative MR was included in the definition, the number of cases would diminish dramatically because of the extreme sensitivity of MR for detecting mild cord injuries and spinal column injuries such as ligamentous injuries and hematomas not usually seen on plain films or CT. Children are more susceptible to these injuries, presumably because of their lax spinal ligaments and the weakness of their paraspinal muscles.

True SCIWORA also can occur in adults (Table 75-4), but is much less frequent than the syndrome of acute spinal cord injury without radiological evidence of trauma (SCIWORET). Patients with SCIWORET have abnormal radiological exams, but the radiographs and CT do not show any evidence of trauma. Prior to the use of CT in spinal trauma, the incidence of SCIWORET in adults with spinal cord injury was approximately 14 percent.[8] The addition of CT has reduced the incidence of SCIWORET to about 5 percent. MR appears to be highly sensitive in detecting spinal cord injury, even mild cases, and has high sensitivity for non-bony spinal column lesions such as ligamentous injuries. Thus, MR would reduce further the incidence of SCIWORET. In adults, cervical spondylosis is the most common underlying associated condition in patients with SCIWORET, but other arthropathies may be

TABLE 75-4 Classification of Acute Traumatic Spinal Cord Injury Syndromes without Radiological Abnormality (SCIWORA) or without Radiological Evidence of Trauma (SCIWORET)

SCIWORA—in children (less commonly in adults)
SCIWORET—in adults (less commonly in children)
Occurs in: Cervical Spondylosis
Spinal Stenosis
Ankylosing Spondylitis
Other Arthropathies
Disk Herniation
Nucleus Pulposus Embolism

associated with a spinal cord injury without radiological evidence of bony trauma. An example would be a minor, radiologically undetectable fracture in a patient with ankylosing spondylitis who develops an epidural hematoma. Acute traumatic disk herniations frequently are not detected by older generation CT scanners, but can easily be diagnosed by MR. Some patients with spinal stenosis, especially in the cervical region may sustain a major spinal cord injury without traumatic changes on plain films or CT. Patients with nucleus pulposus embolism may have profound spinal cord deficits without any radiological evidence of trauma, even when trauma was an antecedent factor.[41] However, MR in these cases would be expected to show evidence of spinal cord infarction. Indeed, the incidence of SCIWORET would likely be 1 to 2 percent of spinal cord injury if high-resolution MR was used to examine the spinal cord and spinal column in all cases.

TRAUMA PATIENTS WITH AN ACUTE SPINAL CORD SYNDROME BUT WITHOUT DIRECT TRAUMA TO THE SPINE

This relatively rare syndrome differs from SCIWORET and SCIWORA in that these patients sustain a lesion of the spinal cord that manifests as an acute spinal cord syndrome, and is associated with trauma, but the trauma is not to the spine (Table 75-5). The syndrome can occur in both children and adults. Keith[42] described four cases in children with major abdominal or thoracic trauma, and concluded that many of them had sustained a vascular injury that caused aortic injury or occlusion of intercostal or lumbar arteries with subsequent occlusion of medullary arteries and spinal cord infarction. Rarely, penetrating injuries such as gunshot wounds can interrupt major arterial feeders to the cord without direct trauma to the spine. Severe hypotension and systemic shock in trauma patients also can result in spinal cord ischemia and infarction, even without causing concomitant cerebral ischemia.

TABLE 75-5 Trauma Patients with an Acute Spinal Cord Syndrome but without Direct Trauma to the Spine

1. With hypotension and systemic shock
2. With vascular injury to feeding artery
   - aorta
   - vertebral artery
3. Anterior spinal artery syndrome

ANTERIOR SPINAL ARTERY SYNDROME

The anterior spinal artery syndrome results from ischemia and infarction of the cord in the distribution of supply of the anterior spinal artery, which includes the anterior two-thirds of the spinal cord. It is generally held that this syndrome is due to obstruction of the anterior spinal artery, the cause of which in most cases is unknown.[43] The syndrome has been associated with a spinal cord angioma, postinfection or vaccination, systemic hypotension, aortic disease, or surgical procedures on the aorta. Clinically, it is characterized by varying degrees of motor weakness and with a dissociated sensory loss involving loss of pain and temperature sense with relative or complete preservation of proprioception. Recently, angiographic evidence of obstruction of the anterior spinal artery has been presented, along with the MRI appearance of the infarcted cord.[44] Although somewhat similar in anatomical distribution to the central cord syndrome, this syndrome is not due to acute spinal cord injury, but may occur in rare instances in trauma patients.

CLASSIFICATION OF CHRONIC POSTTRAUMATIC SPINAL CORD SYNDROMES

A number of important clinical syndromes develop in the subacute and chronic stages after acute spinal cord injury (Table 75-6). Cystic degeneration at the epicenter of the cord injury, mainly in the central region of the cord, but also spreading rostral and caudal, is a frequent sequela of the hemorrhagic necrosis and ischemia of the cord in the acute stage. The greater the acute injury, the greater the tendency to subsequent cyst formation at the injury site and in the rostral-caudal direction. The exact pathophysiology of progressive posttraumatic syringomyelia is unknown,[45] but central cord disruption and arachnoiditis are common antecedents. This clinical syndrome becomes progressive in about 3 percent of cord injuries, and begins months to years later, usually

TABLE 75-6 Classification of Chronic Posttraumatic Spinal Cord Syndromes

1. Posttraumatic syringomyelia
2. Posttraumatic microcystic myelomalacia "Marshy Cord Syndrome"
3. Arachnoiditis
4. Deafferentation Pain Syndromes
   - Neurogenic
   - Myelogenic
   - Cephalogenic
5. Discomplete Syndrome

with the onset of a causalgic type of deafferentation pain. Subsequently, there is further loss of sensory or motor function or both. The motor deficit is usually of the lower motor neuron type at the level of the injury or rostrally, an upper motor neuron type caudal to the level of the injury (if the injury was incomplete), and further loss of bowel or bladder function. The sensory loss tends to be of the spinothalamic type because the cyst formation usually begins centrally, which damages the crossing sensory afferents in the anterior white commissure coursing toward the spinothalamic tract.

The syndrome of posttraumatic microcystic myelomalacia is similar to posttraumatic syringomyelia in that it can cause late deterioration of spinal cord function months to years after spinal cord injury, owing to a progressive lesion in the cord. The new clinical deficits can be identical to posttraumatic syringomyelia. Based on radiology, MRI, and surgical data (since there is no comprehensive pathological study of this condition), the cord shows microcystic degeneration best described as the "marshy cord syndrome."[46] Arachnoiditis is a constant accompaniment and may play a causative role.

Arachnoiditis occurs after spinal cord injuries of all types and severity, even minor injuries. However, some major cord injuries may cause little. The propensity to spread rostrocaudally from the site of injury also varies widely: in some cases it is confined to the epicenter of the lesion; in others there is extensive involvement in the rostrocaudal direction. Connective tissue bridging from the dura to the arachnoid, and from the arachnoid into the injured cord itself, tends to be greater in cases with pial disruption or dural laceration.[47] Otherwise, the etiology of this rare, late posttraumatic syndrome is unknown. Posttraumatic arachnoiditis can cause neurological deterioration in a progressive fashion, either slowly or steplike, the latter suggesting a vascular component due to fibrotic strangulation of subarachnoid arteries or veins supplying or draining the spinal cord.

Various pain syndromes can be present immediately after spinal cord injury, but, fortunately, the majority ultimately abate. However, approximately 25 percent of spinal cord injuries continue to have significant pain syndromes, the most important of which are the neuropathic types of deafferentation pain classified as neurogenic, myelogenic, or cephalogenic, depending on whether the abnormal painful impulses are generated from the damaged nerve roots, spinal cord, or brain.[48]

Dimitrijevic has defined a clinical syndrome termed the "discomplete syndrome" in which clinically complete cases have some evidence of impulse conduction across the lesion site shown by evoked potential testing or some other neurophysiological means.[10] The relevance of this syndrome to clinical management or prognosis is uncertain.

References

1. Michaelis LS, Braakman R: Current terminology and classification of injuries of spine and spinal cord, in Vinken PJ, Bruyn GW (eds): *Handbook of Clinical Neurology,* Amsterdam: North-Holland, 1976: 145–153.
2. *International Standards for Neurological and Functional Classification of Spinal Cord Injury.* American Spinal Injury Association, International Medical Society of Paraplegia—ASIA/IMSOP, Revised, 1992.
3. Frankel HL, Hancock DO, Hyslop G, et al: The value of postural reduction in the initial management of closed injuries of the spine with paraplegia and tetraplegia. *Paraplegia* 1969; 7:179–192.
4. Tator CH, Rowed DW, Schwartz ML: Sunnybrook Cord Injury Scales for assessing neurological injury and neurological recovery, in Tator CH (ed): *Early Management of Acute Spinal Cord Injury.* New York: Raven Press, 1982: 17–24.
5. Waters RL, Adkins RH, Yakura JS: Definition of complete spinal cord injury. *Paraplegia* 1991; 9:573–581.
6. *Aids to Investigation of Peripheral Nerve Injuries.* Medical Research Council War Memorandum, 2d ed. London: HMSO, Revised, 1943.
7. Tator CH, Duncan EG, Edmonds VE, et al: Changes in epidemiology of acute spinal cord injury from 1947 to 1981. Surg Neurol 1993; (40):207–215.
8. Tator CH: Spine-spinal cord relationships in spinal cord trauma. *Clin Neurosurg* 1983; 30:479–494.
9. Hansebout RR: A comprehensive review of methods of improving cord recovery after acute spinal cord injury, in Tator CH (ed): *Early Management of Acute Spinal Cord Injury.* New York: Raven Press, 1982: 181–196.
10. Dimitrijevic MR: Residual motor function in spinal cord injury, in Waxman SG (ed): *Functional Recovery in Neurological Disease.* New York: Raven Press, 1988: 139–155.
11. Kakulas BA: Pathology of spinal injuries. *Cent Nerv Syst Trauma* 1984; 1:117–129.
12. Bunge RP, Puckett WR, Becerra JL, et al: Observations on the pathology of human spinal cord injury. A review and classification of 22 new cases with details from a case of chronic cord compression with extensive focal demyelination. *Adv Neurol* 1993; 59.

13. Kiss ZHT, Tator CH: Neurogenic shock, in Geller ER (ed): *Shock and Resuscitation.* New York: McGraw-Hill, 1993; 421–440.
14. Schneider RC: Traumatic spinal cord syndromes and their management. *Clin Neurosurg* 1973; 20:424–492.
15. Schneider RC: Concomitant craniocerebral and spinal trauma, with special reference to the cervico-medullary regions. *Clin Neurosurg* 1970; 17:266–309.
16. Bell HS: Paralysis of both arms from injury to the pyramidal decussation: "Cruciate paralysis." *J Neurosurg* 1970; 33:376–380.
17. Schneider RC, Cherry GL, Pantek HF: The syndrome of acute central cervical spinal cord injury. *J Neurosurg* 1954; 11:546–577.
18. Taylor AR, Blackwood W: Paraplegia in hyperextension cervical injuries with normal radiographic appearance. *J Bone Joint Surg* 1948; 30B:245–248.
19. Taylor AR: The mechanism of injury to the spinal cord in the neck without damage to the vertebral column. *J Bone Joint Surg* 1951; 33B:543–547.
20. Foerster O: Symptomatologie der erkrankungen des ruckenmarks undseiner wurzeln. *Handb Neurol* 1936; 5:1–403.
21. Nathan PW, Smith MC: Long descending tracts in man: I. Review of present knowledge. *Brain* 1956; 78:248–304.
22. Schneider RC, Thompson JM, Bebin J: The syndrome of the acute central cervical spinal cord injury. *J Neurol Neurosurg Psychiatr* 1958; 21:216–227.
23. Quencer RM, Bunge RP, Egnor M, et al: Acute traumatic central cord syndrome: MRI-pathological correlations. *Neuroradiology* 1992; 34:85–94.
24. Phillips CG, Porter R: Corticospinal neurones: Their role in movement. *Monographs of the Physiological Society,* No. 34. London: Academic Press, 1977.
25. Eidelberg E: Consequences of spinal cord lesions upon motor function, with special reference to locomotor activity. *Prog Neurobiol* 1981; 17:185–202.
26. Bosch A, Stauffer S, Nickel V: Incomplete traumatic quadriplegia: A ten year review. *JAMA* 1971; 216:(3) 473–478.
27. Brodkey JS, Miller CF Jr, Harmody RM: The syndrome of acute central cervical spinal cord injury revisited. *Surg Neurol* 1980; 14:251–257.
28. Schneider RC: A syndrome in acute cervical injuries for which early operation is indicated. *J Neurosurg* 1951; 8:360–367.
29. Kahn EA: The role of the dentate ligaments in spinal cord compression and the syndrome of lateral sclerosis. *J Neurosurg* 1947; 4:191–199.
30. Brown-Séquard CE: *Course of Lectures on the Physiology and Pathology of the Central Nervous System.* Philadelphia: Collins, 1860.
31. Braakman R, Penning L: Injuries of the cervical spine, in Vinken PJ, Bruyn GW (eds): *Handbook of Clinical Neurology.* Amsterdam: North-Holland 1976: 227–380.
32. Lazorthes G, Géraud J, Espagno J, et al: Syndrome de Brown-Séquard et hernie discale cervicale. *Neurochirurgie* 1961; 7:288.
33. Wilberger JE, Maroon JC: Burning hands syndrome revisited. *Neurosurgery* 1987; 20:599–605.
34. Wilberger JE, Maroon JC: Cervical spine injuries in athletes. *Physician Sports Med* 1990; 18:57–70.
35. Maroon JC: Burning hands and football spinal cord injury. *JAMA* 1977; 238:2049–2051.
36. Braakman R, Penning L: *Injuries of the Cervical Spine.* Amsterdam: Excerpta Medica, 1971.
37. Biemond A: Contusio cervicalis posterior. *Med T Geneesk* 1964; 108:1333.
38. Torg JS, Pavlov H, Genuario SE, et al: Neurapraxia of the cervical spinal cord with transient quadriplegia. *J Bone Joint Surg* 1986; 68A:1354–1370.
39. Sallis RE, Jones K, Knopp W: Burners: Offensive strategy for an underreported injury. *Physician Sports Med* 1992; 20:47–55.
40. Pang D, Wilberger JE Jr: Spinal cord injury without radiographic abnormalities in children. *J Neurosurg* 1982; 57:114–129.
41. Kestle JRW, Resch L, Tator CH, Kucharczyk W: Intervertebral disc embolization resulting in spinal cord infarction: Case report. *J Neurosurg* 1989; 71:938–941.
42. Keith WS: Traumatic infarction of the spinal cord. *Can J Neurol Sci* 1974; 1:124–126.
43. Foo D, Rossier AB: Anterior spinal artery syndrome and its natural history. *Paraplegia* 1983; 21:1–10.
44. Takahashi S, Yamada T, Ishii K, et al: MRI of anterior spinal artery syndrome of the cervical spine cord. *Neuroradiology* 1992; 35:25–29.
45. Barnett HJM, Jousse AT: Posttraumatic syringomyelia (cystic myelopathy), in Vinken PJ, Bruyn CH (eds): *Injuries of the Spine and Spinal Cord, vol. 26, Handbook of Clinical Neurology.* Amsterdam: North-Holland, 1976: 113–157.
46. MacDonald RL, Findlay JM, Tator CH: Microcystic spinal cord degeneration causing posttraumatic myelopathy: Report of two cases. *J Neurosurg* 1988; 68:466–471.
47. Tator CH: Pathophysiology and pathology of spinal cord injury, in Wilkins RH, Rengachary SS (eds): *Neurosurgery* (2d ed). New York: McGraw-Hill, 1994: 269–282.
48. Tator CH: Pain following spinal cord injury, in Wilkins RH, Rengachary SS (eds): *Neurosurgery* (2d ed). New York: McGraw-Hill, 1994: 301–307.

CHAPTER 76

SPINAL CORD INJURY PATHOPHYSIOLOGY AND THERAPY

Wise Young

INTRODUCTION

Over 200,000 people in the United States and several million people worldwide have been chronically paralyzed by traumatic spinal cord injury (SCI). About 11,500 people suffer new traumatic SCIs in the United States each year. Most are injured by falls, motor vehicle and bicycle accidents, sports- and work-related accidents, or gunshot or knife wounds. A large majority of the victims are young at the time of injury: 60 percent are injured before age 30, and 70 percent before age 40.[1] More than 90 percent of SCI victims survive and live a nearly normal life span.

Millions of people suffer from nontraumatic injuries of the spinal cord that result from severe vertebral disk disease, spinal curvatures such as scoliosis and kyphoscoliosis, demyelinating disorders such as multiple sclerosis, viral infections, inflammatory disorders, reduced spinal cord blood flow caused by arteriovenous malformations and dissecting aortic aneurysms, tumors outside or within the spinal cord, and the complications of spinal surgery. These causes of spinal cord damage are more prevalent than is trauma.

SCI imprisons its victims with a lifelong sentence of sensory loss, paralysis, and dependence. As a result of the young age, high survival rate, and long life span of its victims, SCI is among the most costly neurological disorders, causing more years of disability than other diseases that have a higher mortality and affect primarily elderly people. For the first time in history, a large number of SCI victims are surviving their injuries; this population is growing and aging.

Current therapy is largely palliative, aimed at preventing injury progression, reducing the complications of sensory loss and paralysis, and teaching patients to cope with their disabilities. Pessimism pervades clinical SCI care from the emergency room through rehabilitation. On the basis of long-established dogma that CNS neurons do not regenerate[2–4] and despite sporadic observations of CNS regeneration in the mammalian central nervous system,[5–13] most clinicians continue to be deeply skeptical that any therapy for chronic SCI can be effective.

This work is supported by grants from the NIH: NS10164, NS15590, and NS32000.

A SCIENTIFIC BASIS FOR HOPE

In 1990, the Second National Acute Spinal Cord Injury Study (NASCIS 2) reported that very high doses of methylprednisolone (MP) significantly improve neurological recovery in human SCI when given shortly after an injury.[14] This study was the first to demonstrate the neuroprotective effect of any treatment for human SCI and gave credence to the hypothesis that progressive tissue damage in an acute spinal cord can be ameliorated with early therapy. Because of the high dose of MP required for beneficial effects, far exceeding the levels required for its action as glucocorticoid hormone, the neuroprotective effects of MP have been attributed to inhibition of lipid peroxidation.[15,16] Many other treatments are neuroprotective in animal spinal cord injury models.[17–28]

Aguayo and coworkers[29–32] demonstrated convincingly that central neurons grow alacritously in peripheral nerves. This finding stimulated an intense search for factors that facilitate or inhibit regeneration in the CNS. The first major breakthrough was the discovery of brain-derived neurotrophic factor (BDNF),[33–35] followed by the identification of the genes for BDNF and other neurotrophins[36,37] that regulate not only the growth but the death of neurons.[38–44] A second breakthrough came with the discovery of CNS proteins that inhibit regeneration.[45–51] Blockade of these proteins promotes functional regeneration in mammalian spinal cords.[52,53]

SCI studies have shown that a small proportion (probably less than 10 percent) of spinal axons can support substantial functional recovery[54–56] and that myelin loss contributes to neurological deficits in SCI.[54,56–62,63,171] Thus, therapies do not need to preserve, restore, or regenerate many axons to allow a patient to achieve functional recovery after SCI.

Studies of acute CNS injury have progressed remarkably during the past 5 years. Much evidence indicates that CNS neurons have complex and robust autodestructive mechanisms that induce neuronal suicide through ubiquitous excitotoxic neurotransmitters[64–77] and "programmed cell death."[39,43,78–83] Cell death and growth share intracellular messengers.[1A] Recent data suggest that glucocorticoids may affect similar intracellular messenger systems,[84–89] including key phosphatases.[90–95] Well-defined pharmaceutical agents are available to manipulate these mechanisms.

The mechanisms responsible for neuronal growth and death in SCI are becoming clear and accessible to manipulation. Most scientists now believe that effective neuroprotective and regenerative therapies are not only possible but likely in the near future, in contrast to the deep pessimism in the clinical arena.

TECHNOLOGICAL ADVANCES

Two major technological obstacles have held back the development of SCI therapies. First, although many SCI models have been used over the years, few have been standardized. Disparate outcome measures are used to evaluate the consequences of injury and therapy. As a result of differences in SCI models and in outcome measures among laboratories, data replication has been inordinately difficult and time-consuming, delaying proposals of treatments to be used in clinical trials. Clinical trials and epidemiological databases have utilized several independent and often incompatible clinical assessment scales to classify and evaluate SCI outcome in clinical trials. Second, many of the most promising and interesting treatments involve organic molecules that must be delivered to the injury site and maintained for long periods. Until recently, there have been few methods available for manipulating the long-term environment of the injury site.

Standardized, reproducible, and predictive animal SCI models are now available for testing therapies. The first multicenter preclinical SCI study began in 1994, based on an SCI model developed at NYU Medical Center.[96,97] Eight leading SCI laboratories have agreed to use the same model and the same outcome measures to test treatments systematically. In addition, the field has agreed on well-defined and validated standards for classifying and documenting neurological recovery in human[98,99] and animal SCI.[100] Since 1991, all clinical trials of SCI therapies worldwide have collected a standardized set of neurological data that allows sharing and comparisons of trial results.

A wealth of new technologies have emerged for manipulating the molecular and cellular environment of the spinal cord. These include transplantation of fetal[101,102] and genetically engineered cells[103–107] that can produce growth factors and guidance molecules, monoclonal antibodies to block growth-inhibiting molecules, and cell surface molecules that stimulate and guide growing axons.[108–114] Viral and other vectors are available for direct delivery and incorporation of genetic materials into cells in an injured spinal cord.

Combined with the scientific advances of the past decade, these technological and organizational developments provide an unprecedented and favorable environment for developing and establishing the efficacy of SCI therapies. For the first time, scientists are optimistic that treatments can be developed, several promising therapies are available for investigation, clinicians are enthusiastic about carrying out clinical trials, major technological obstacles to therapy delivery and evaluation have been overcome, and efficient clinical trial mechanisms are in place. With sufficient resources and effort, we should be able to develop more effective therapies for SCI before the end of the decade.

SPINAL CORD INJURY

The spinal cord links the brain with the body. The human spinal cord contains about 20 million nerve fibers[115] that carry information from the brain to all parts of the body and from the body to the brain. Injury disrupts communication between the body and the brain, leading to loss of motor function and sensory perception below the lesion site. This simple notion has unfortunately led to several common misconceptions about SCI and its consequences.

Common Misconceptions about Spinal Cord Injury

SCI is often viewed as an all-or-none event that is irreversible from the moment of injury. Clinicians have long segregated SCI patients into two distinct categories: those with "complete" loss of neurological function below the injury site and those with partial or "incomplete" loss. The dichotomy between complete and incomplete loss, however, is not absolute. Some functional recovery typically occurs even after severe SCI. For example, NASCIS 2 revealed that patients admitted with so-called complete loss of neurological function recovered on average about 8% of what they had lost, compared with 59 percent in "incomplete" patients.[116] More important, NASCIS 2 revealed that MP significantly improves neurological recovery of "complete" as well as "incomplete" patients. Thus, complete injury does not necessarily indicate complete loss of all connection, and treatments delivered shortly after an injury can preserve some connections that are lost in the aftermath of the injury.

Complete neurological loss is frequently equated to physical disruption of all the axons at the injury site. Complete SCI is sometimes referred to as "transections," although actual spinal cord transections are relatively rare.[117–120] Several studies have shown that many so-called complete patients have evidence of residual connections.[121–124] A more likely and reasonable explanation of the difference between complete and incomplete SCI is that presence of a certain threshold of connections is necessary for functional recovery. The determinants of this threshold are complex and, as described below, probably involve not only the loss of spinal axons but dysfunction of the surviving axons and plasticity of the spinal cord.

While paralysis is the most frequently cited consequence of SCI, paralysis is often the least of the problems that beset SCI victims. Urinary tract dysfunction is the major cause of mortality and morbidity in patients with SCI. Loss of pain sensation leads to decubitus or pressure sores. Many SCI victims suffer from pain and dysesthesias caused by partially disconnected sensory centers in the spinal cord. Residual connections to spinal circuits contribute to spasticity or abnormal muscle activity.[125–128] Pain and spasticity can be so disruptive that many people consent to drugs or surgery to suppress or eliminate the remaining function in the spinal cord in order to escape the agony.

Restoration of walking is the most avidly sought goal of SCI therapy. However, the return of other motor and sensory functions is eminently worthwhile. For example, in patients with cervical injuries that affect hand and arm function, the return of one segmental level may allow a patient to feed himself or herself, transfer from bed to wheelchair without help, drive, or operate a computer keyboard more efficiently. These small but critical capabilities may mean independence, gainful employment, and an active social life as opposed to dependence, poverty, and isolation. Even small therapeutic effects can have major benefits. For example, a more rapid return of automatic bladder emptying will markedly improve an SCI patient's long-term health and reduce hospitalization. Treatments that effectively suppress abnormal spinal cord activity can allow many patients to resume lives otherwise incapacitated by pain and spasticity. Partial restoration of sensation allows patients to protect and feel ownership of their bodies. Better control of blood pressure reduces fatigue and dizziness. Improving diaphragm strength reduces the need for ventilatory assistance and lowers the risk of contracting pneumonia.

Finally, the corticospinal tract is widely assumed to mediate voluntary movements. Corticospinal tract regeneration is consequently a goal of many regeneration experiments.[49,52,53,129] However, the corticospinal tract is neither necessary nor sufficient for complex voluntary forelimb movements in cats.[130–134] Multiple descending pathways, including the rubro-, cortico-, tecto-, and bulbospinal pathways, excite C3 to C5 propriospinal neurons that distribute motor and sensory signals in the cervical spinal cord[135–137] and can mediate complex motor activities in cat forelimbs.[138] Lesions of individual long spinal tracts do not irreversibly eliminate motor control or activity.[139–146] Cutting the corticospinal tract in the spinal cord has relatively little effect on visually guided forelimb movements, whereas higher brainstem pyramidal sections profoundly disturb voluntary movements.[147] Curiously, cutting the dorsal columns several weeks before high pyramidal sections paradoxically increases the rate and extent of motor recovery.[148] These results suggest that multiple ascending and descending pathways[149] influence motor recovery and that regenerating the corticospinal tract may be neither necessary nor sufficient for motor recovery after an SCI.

Recovery from Spinal Cord Injury

Recovery is the rule rather than the exception in SCI patients. Most people recover somewhat from SCI, although slowly over many weeks or even years. NASCIS 2 showed that SCI patients often recover significant motor and sensory function.[14,150] Patients admitted to the hospital with no sensory or motor function below the injury level typically recovered 8 percent of what they had lost. Patients with some neurological function below the lesion recovered 59 percent of what they had lost. MP improved this recovery to 22 percent in severely injured patients to 75 percent in partially injured patients. The difficulty of performing clinical and animal

SCI studies stems in part from a high incidence of recovery even after severe injuries. As a result of the tendency of animals to recover from nearly total losses of spinal tracts, a long-standing criterion for regeneration studies is complete transection of the spinal cord.[4,151]

Animal studies have shown that very few spinal axons can support functional recovery. Many investigators[54,55,139–142,144,152–154] have reported that animals can recover evoked potentials and the ability to walk with as little as 10 percent of their spinal axons. In fact, animals with transected spinal cords can be trained to walk.[155–160] These findings indicate that spinal cords have innate mechanisms for locomotory behavior and give hope that preservation, restoration, or regeneration of relatively few spinal axons can result in substantial motor and sensory recovery.[161]

Spinal cords have remarkable plasticity. Many investigators have reported rapid sprouting of surviving fibers to innervate disconnected spinal cells.[162–167] Sprouting and other mechanisms of plasticity allow a few nerve fibers to carry out the functions of many. Plasticity accounts for the tendency of people with the slightest degree of functional preservation to recover substantial motor and sensory function over the long term.

Axon loss is also not the only reason for neurological deficits in SCI. More than a decade ago, Blight and associates[56,152,168] found that many axons that survive traumatic injury are dysfunctional. Many of these axons have lost part or all of their myelin, a sheath of membranes that insulates axons and improves both the reliability and the speed of signal conduction. In particular, the drug 4-aminopyridine (4-AP), which excites axons by closing potassium (K^+) channels and has been used to treat multiple sclerosis,[169,170] significantly improves conduction in spinal-injured animals[54,59,60] and humans.[61,62,171] This drug improves conduction only while it is being given and has undesirable side effects such as seizures, tachycardia, and hyperthermia. As a result of these side effects, 4-AP may not represent a suitable long-term therapy for chronic SCI. However, it may be useful as a diagnostic tool to detect patients who might benefit from biological remyelination therapy.

Acute, Recovery, and Chronic Phases

The adjectives "acute" and "chronic" are often applied to SCI, and so it is useful to define these terms. SCI can be logically divided into three phases: acute, recovery, and chronic. The acute injury phase refers to a period of progressive damage that starts with the injury and may continue for hours or even days, depending on injury severity. The recovery phase refers to a period during which function returns, starting within hours and extending for months or even years after an injury. The chronic phase refers to a time when functional recovery has reached a plateau. Acute therapies include neuroprotective drugs. Recovery therapies include treatments that increase the rate and extent of functional return. Chronic therapies are aimed at restoring function through remyelination or regeneration or even through elimination of unbalanced or abnormal spinal connections.

Acute phase

Therapeutic studies have contributed substantially to our understanding of acute SCI. Four classes of drugs may be neuroprotective in SCI: antioxidants, neurotransmitter receptor blockers, phosphokinase stimulators, and phosphatase inhibitors. Antioxidants neutralize free radicals or reactive molecules generated by injured cells; free radicals damage cell membranes and proteins.[15,172,173] Spinal axons and cells possess neurotransmitter receptors,[174–179] and some neurotransmitter receptor blockers have been reported to have beneficial effects on SCI models.[180–182] Several glutamate receptor blockers have been reported to be neuroprotective in SCI models.[67,183–186] Phosphokinase modulation by growth factors, neurotransmitters, and hormones may influence endogenous neuroprotective mechanisms.[87,92,187–190] Finally, phosphatases such as calcineurin activate nitric oxide synthetase,[191] receptor channels,[192–195] and voltage-sensitive ionic channels. These factors may contribute to secondary injury.

Recovery phase

Most SCI victims recover to some extent, although slowly over months or even years. Remyelination of axons and plasticity of denervated tissues contribute to recovery. Therapy may increase the rate and extent of remyelination as well as the growth and plasticity of the spinal cord. Examples of therapies include inflammatory factors, since inflammation plays a key role in cell repair and growth. Combinations of inflammatory and anti-inflammatory drugs may selectively enhance the beneficial effects and inhibit the deleterious effects of inflammation.

Chronic phase

Restorative therapies fall into three categories: growth and blockers of growth-inhibiting factors, intracellular messenger modulators, and transplantable cells or materials. The first category includes neurotrophins and other factors that stimulate regeneration and antibodies that bind growth-inhibiting proteins. The second category includes drugs that influence protein kinase and phosphatases that modulate cell growth and differentiation. The third category includes transplantable cells or materials, such as genetically modified fibroblasts, astrocytes, and oligodendrolgia, that express or release factors that are believed to stimulate or guide axonal growth.

THERAPY FOR SPINAL CORD INJURY

NEUROPROTECTIVE THERAPIES

Injury initiates complex responses in the body and the spinal cord. These responses include a cascade of inflammatory mechanisms to clean up cellular debris and repair tissues. However, these mechanisms also release toxic substances that cause further tissue damage, a process called secondary injury. The discovery in 1990 that high-dose MP can improve neurological recovery when given within 8 h after an SCI gave credence to the hypothesis that secondary injury mechanisms occur in the human spinal cord. Secondary injury mechanisms fall into four general categories:

- *Free radicals.* Free radicals are highly reactive molecules that have an extra electron in an outer orbital. Being intermediate products of normal chemical reactions, free radicals accumulate when an injury interrupts chemical reactions. In particular, damaged mitochondria release oxygen free radicals or superoxide. Two ubiquitous enzymes—superoxide dismutase (SOD) and catalase—normally neutralize oxygen free radicals.[196–199] SOD converts superoxide to hydrogen peroxide (H_2O_2), and catalase converts H_2O_2 to oxygen and water. In addition, the brain and spinal cord contain high levels of antioxidants, such as ascorbic acid,[200–207] glutathione,[201,208–210] and vitamin E,[16,202,211–215] which scavenges free radicals. In injured tissues, as a result of increased free radical production, depletion of endogenous antioxidants, and damage to SOD, excess free radicals accumulate and damage lipids and proteins, producing additional free radicals.
- *Excessive calcium influx and excitotoxicity.* Normally, calcium ionic (Ca^{2+}) activity exceeds 1 mM in extracellular fluids and is less than 10^{-7} *M*. Thus, a steep gradient drives Ca^{2+} ions into injured cells through membrane holes, voltage-sensitive Ca^{2+} channels, neurotransmitter receptor-gated channels, and sodium-calcium exchangers.[216,217] Ca^{2+} ions activate enzymes that break down lipids and proteins, such as phospholipases and proteases. Glutamate, an excitatory neurotransmitter, kills neurons by allowing Ca^{2+} and Na^{2+} entry through *N*-methyl-D-aspartate (NMDA) receptor channels. Glutamate and other excitatory amino acids are released into extracellular space in an injured spinal cord.[218] Glutamate receptor blockers are neuroprotective in experimental SCI models.[67,183,219] Recent data suggests that opiates modulate extracellular glutamate release,[186,220–225] perhaps explaining the beneficial effects of opiate receptor blockers in acute SCI.[222,226–233] Incidentally, MP prevents glutamate-induced toxicity in cultured spinal neurons.[234]
- *Eicosanoids and cytokines.* Membrane breakdown in injured cells releases free fatty acids, particularly arachidonic acid. Two enzymes—cyclooxygenase and lipoxygenase—convert arachidonate to prostaglandins and leukotrienes.[235] These inflammatory substances are released in injured spinal cords[213,236–241] and are among the most potent factors known in biology, causing cell swelling.[242–246] and blood flow changes.[239,247–247B] Anti-inflammatory agents such as indomethacin and glucocorticoids significantly reduce eicosanoid release in injured cords.[248,249]
- *Programmed cell death.* Many neurons die during development when they do not reach their intended targets.[42,250] Believed to occur when neurons are deprived of neurotrophins,[43,78,83,251,252] such cell death also results from exposure to low potassium,[187] cytokines,[40] human immunodeficiency viruses,[253–256] and certain hormones.[257] Because this type of cell death requires new protein synthesis,[80,258–261] it is frequently called "programmed" cell death. The dead cell have a distinctive pathological signature, manifesting as shrunken cells with condensed nuclear chromatin, a state called apoptosis,[262] as distinguished from necrosis. Apoptosis is believed to involve excessive Ca^{2+} entry and Ca^{2+}-activated phosphatase.[263] Phosphatase inhibitors such as cyclosporin A[264,265] and FK 506[90,264,266–270] prevent apoptosis. Glucocorticoids also prevent some forms of programmed cell death.[271,272] Programmed cell death is believed to play a role in amyotrophic lateral sclerosis[273] and experimental allergic encephalomyelitis.[274] Injury may well induce apoptotic mechanisms in the spinal cord.

Many drugs interfere with these secondary injury mechanisms.[20,22,23,275] For example, several antioxidants have been reported to be neuroprotective in SCI models.[15,16,172,212,214,236,247,276–279] MP is believed to act in part by scavenging free radicals.[15,17,173,211,248,280–285] Glutamate receptor blockers have been reported to be beneficial in experimental SCI models.[183,184,286A] Likewise, several cyclooxygenase inhibitors are neuroprotective.[238,247–249,286,287] Recent data suggest that the immunosuppressant cyclosporin A, a drug that blocks the phosphatase calcineurin in neurons and lymphocytes, is neuroprotective in SCI.

Thus, there is no lack of potential neuroprotective therapies for acute SCI. The challenge is to identify the most effective treatment or combination of treatments with the least severe side effects for human clinical trials. This is not a trivial undertaking. For example, to assess three treatment doses, three initiation times, and three durations at three injury severity levels, plus vehicle and MP control groups, a preclinical study may have to examine 159 treatment-injury groups. If 10 to 20 experiments are required per group to detect treatment effects, thousands of experiments must be carried out per treatment. Few laboratories have the ability or resources to carry out such tour de force studies.

Recovery-Enhancing Therapies

Recovery from SCI is generally slow, requiring months or even years. Increasing the recovery rate should have a large impact on the medical and rehabilitation costs of SCI. Little attention has been devoted to developing therapies to increase the recovery rate. Since part of the deficit in SCI may be due to atrophy and lack of use of denervated structures, increasing the recovery rate may also improve the extent of recovery. The slow recovery rate in SCI may be due to remyelination and reorganization of spinal circuity. Three categories of drugs may accelerate recovery after SCI:

- *Potassium channel blockers.* Loss of myelin depresses axonal excitability and therefore the reliability and speed of axonal conduction.[288] Several drugs are known to increase the excitability of demyelinated axons. The best known of these is 4-AP, which blocks voltage-sensitive K^+ channels on axons and increases both the duration and the amplitude of signals in axons.[60,63,289–293] As was pointed out above, 4-AP itself is not suitable for long-term use in SCI because of its side effects. However, for short-term therapy lasting several weeks or even months, these side effects are well tolerated by SCI patients[61–63,171] and are justified, especially if the drug improves the rate or extent of recovery.
- *Neurotransmitter receptor agonists.* Spinal axons have receptors to the neurotransmitters GABA,[174,177,178,180,294,295] norepinephrine,[175,176]and serotonin (5-HT).[179] Numerous synthetic agonists are available for each of these neurotransmitters. In addition, several drugs increase endogenous levels of these neurotransmitters by blocking uptake. The 5-HT_2 receptor agonist quipazine,[179] several adrenergic agonists,[175,176] and GABA antagonists[174,177,295–298] have strong excitatory effects on spinal axons, similar to the effects of 4-AP. Antagonists of these receptors have been reported to be neuroprotective in experimental SCI models, particularly GABA,[180] 5-HT,[181,182] and adrenergic[299] antagonists. 5-HT and adrenergic neurotransmitters initiate and modulate locomotory function in animals with transected cords.[155,156,179,223–224E] Finally, 5-HT agonists increase the excitability of spinal cord somatosensory[300,301] and pain systems.[302–304] A recent study showed that the 5-HT antagonist mianserin can depress locomotory recovery in rats after hemisection.[179] Much evidence suggests that neurotransmitters play an important role in the plasticity of injured CNS.[305]
- *Inflammatory factors.* The brain[71,306,307] and spinal cord[158,162–167] have remarkable abilities to reorganize and adapt to injuries. Inflammation is a major stimulus for such reorganization.[308,309] Inflammatory factors therefore may stimulate and accelerate reorganization of the spinal cord. For example, nearly three decades ago, the potent inflammatory stimulant piromen was reported to improve neurological recovery after SCI.[9] Another study[96] recently revealed unexpected antagonism of MP effects by the monosialic ganglioside G_{M1} in acute SCI. The authors consequently suggested that the beneficial effects of G_{M1}[310,311] may be related to the proinflammatory effects of G_{M1}. Inflammatory agents, however, may damage neurons and therefore should be administered carefully and in combination with anti-inflammatory agents. A recent study[312] reported that the potent inflammatory endotoxin lipopolysaccharide (LPS) combined with indomethacin remarkably improves neurological recovery in rats subjected to spinal cord crushes. Indomethacin is a nonsteroidal anti-inflammatory cyclooxygenase inhibitor. Other potentially interesting therapeutic agents for spinal cord injury include interferon, a potent proinflammatory agent[313–315] that has been reported to have beneficial effects on neurological recovery in multiple sclerosis.[316,317]

Anti-inflammatory treatments that are neuroprotective in acute SCI patients may be deleterious to recovery. Glucocorticoids plus nonsteroidal anti-inflammatory agents have been reported to be neuroprotective in animal SCI models.[248,249] However, glucocorticoids also inhibit axonal sprouting.[318–322] Likewise, the serotonin receptor inhibitor mianserin has been reported to be neuroprotective in acute SCI,[181,182] and serotonin is a key neurotransmitter in peripheral inflammatory reactions.[323–328] Prolonged suppression of inflammatory mechanisms may inhibit plasticity and recovery, perhaps explaining the curious finding that MP started more than 8 h after injury tended to reduce recovery.[14,116,150,329]

Several laboratories are beginning to investigate combinations of therapies to deal with the complex cascade of responses to injury. If anti-inflammatory acute SCI treatments are deleterious for recovery and if treatments that enhance recovery may promote secondary injury, a different therapeutic strategy may be necessary. Instead of combination therapy, sequential therapy may be needed. In sequential therapy, different drugs would be given for different phases after SCI, targeting specific needs for neuroprotection, recovery, and ultimately regeneration and restoration.

Regenerative and Restorative Therapies

Spinal regenerative therapy has been a holy grail for neuroscientists since Cajal[2,3] first described the abortive attempts of spinal axons to regenerate. Spinal axons can regenerate in the peripheral nerve environment.[29,31,32,330–337] Inhibition of myelin-associated proteins allows axons to regenerate in adult mammalian spinal cords,[50,52,53,129] especially when combined with the neurotrophin NT3.[129] Electromagnetic fields[338–342] and the inflammatory piromen combined with adrenocorticotropin[9] have also been reported to facilitate regeneration in mammalian spinal cords. Young animals are known to regenerate spinal pathways,[343,344] especially after fetal cell transplants.[345–349] Several molecules on astrocytic[350] and Schwann cell[108,110,113,351–353] surfaces permit central axonal regeneration. Finally, inflammation[308,309] appears to promote axon sprouting.

Thus, much evidence suggests that spinal cord regeneration occurs in young animals in the presence of Schwann cells, young or fetal astroglia, and inflammation and when myelin-associated inhibitory factors are inhibited. The regeneration appears to be facilitated by selected growth factors and electromagnetic fields, although the latter mechanism is controversial and is not well understood.[354] The field is poised for rapid advances. In particular, the development and availability of new technologies for transplantation of fetal[101,102,355–358] and genetically modified cells will allow scientists to modify the environment and deliver growth factors[38] selectively at injury sites.[103–107,359]

Transplanted cells can also be directed at remyelination. Fetal cell transplants include precursor oligodendroglia cells that normally cover central axons with myelin. Several investigators have successfully remyelinated rat spinal cord with transplanted oligodendroglial cells.[360–362] Schwann cells should encourage axonal remyelination and regeneration, since they myelinate peripheral nerve fibers,[363] secrete nerve growth factor,[364] express permissive cellular adhesion molecules,[111] and avidly remyelinate spinal axons.[54,360,365–374] However, Schwann cells do not seem to get along with astrocytes[375,376] and appear to invade only spinal cord areas that have lost astrocytes.[54] Nevertheless, Scwhann cell remyelination improves conduction in chronically injured spinal cords.[54]

SUMMARY

A host of promising neuroprotective, recovery-accelerating, regenerative, and restorative therapies have been reported in animal studies. Remarkable progress has been achieved in understanding the molecular and cellular bases of neural autodestructive mechanisms, mechanisms of axonal dysfunction, factors that inhibit and stimulate axonal regeneration, and remyelination in the spinal cord. Many drugs have been reported to improve behavioral recovery in animal SCI models. Much, however, remains to be done before these treatments can be brought to clinical application.

Only one therapy (MP) has been shown to be neuroprotective in human acute SCI. One treatment (G_{M1}) has been reported to be beneficial in the recovery phase when started 48 h after an SCI and continued for several weeks. One treatment (4-AP) has been shown to improve spinal cord conduction in chronic SCI. Although several therapies have been reported to permit and stimulate spinal cord regeneration, none have been tested in a clinical trial.

Recent scientific advances allow the development of SCI therapies on a rational basis. For example, the hypothesis that inflammatory mechanisms play a role in spinal cord growth and reorganization links SCI research to a vast field of therapeutic candidates. The concept that CNS tissues have proteins that inhibit axonal growth has focused research on agents that block these proteins. The discovery of neurotrophins has led to an intense and productive search for receptors and intracellular messengers that mediate neurotrophic effects. Finally, several classes of drugs have been reported to be neuroprotective in SCI.

A major challenge lies in selecting the best therapies for systematic investigation and clinical trials. Technological advances in SCI models and outcome measures now allow rigorous empirical testing and verification of theories. For the first time, therapies can be assessed systematically and quantitatively in preclinical trials to determine the best dose, timing, duration, combination, and sequential application. Such preclinical testing will reduce the risk of time-consuming and expensive clinical trials.

References

1. National SCI Statistical Center: *Spinal Cord Injury Facts and Figures at a Glance.* Birmingham, AL: National SCI Statistical Center, 1993.

1A. Gould E, McEwen BS: Neuronal birth and death. *Curr Opin Neurobiol* 3:676–682, 1993.

2. Cajal RS: *Degeneration and Regeneration of the Nervous System.* New York: Hoffner, 1928.
3. Cajal RS: Notas preventivas sobre la degeneración y regeneración de las vías nerviosas centrales. *Trab Lab Invest Biol, Univ Madrid* 4:295–301, 1906.
4. Guth L, Brewer CR, Collins WF, et al: Criteria for evaluating spinal cord regeneration experiments. *Exp Neurol* 69:1–3, 1980.
5. Björklund A, Nobin A, Stenevi U: Regeneration of central serotonin neurons after axonal degeneration induced by 5,6-dihydroxytryptamine. *Brain Res* 50:214–220,1973.
6. Foerster AP: Spontaneous regeneration of cut axons in adult rat brain. *J Comp Neurol* 210:335–356, 1982.
7. Harston CT, Morrow A, Kostrzewa RM: Enhancement of sprouting and putative regeneration of central noradrenergic fibers by morphine. *Brain Res Bull* 5:421–424, 1980.
8. Lampert P, Cressman M: Axonal regeneration in the dorsal columns of the spinal cord of adult rats: An electron microscopic study. *Lab Invest* 13:825–839, 1964.
9. McMasters RE: Regeneration of the spinal cord in the rat: Effects of piromen and ACTH upon the regenerative capacity. *J Comp Neurol* 119:113–125, 1962.
10. Piatt J: Regeneration in the central nervous system of amphibia, in Windle WF (ed): *Regeneration in the Central Nervous System.* Springfield, IL: Thomas, 1955: 20–46.
11. Wilson DH, Jagadeesh P: Experimental regeneration in peripheral nerves and the spinal cord in laboratory animals exposed to a pulsed electromagnetic field. *Paraplegia* 14:12–20, 1976.
12. Windle WF: *Regeneration in the Central Nervous System.* Springfield, IL: Thomas, 1955.
13. Wolman L: Axon regeneration after spinal cord injury. *Paraplegia* 4:175–184, 1966.
14. Bracken MB, Shepard MJ, Collins WF, et al: A randomized controlled trial of methylprednisolone or naloxone in the treatment of acute spinal-cord injury: Results of the Second National Acute Spinal Cord Injury Study. *N Engl J Med* 322:1405–1411, 1990.
15. Hall ED: The neuroprotective pharmacology of methylprednisolone. *J Neurosurg* 76:13–22, 1992.
16. Hall ED, Braughler JM, McCall JM: Antioxidant effects in brain and spinal cord injury. *J Neurotrauma* 9:S165–S172, 1992.
17. Nockels R, Young W: Pharmacologic strategies in the treatment of experimental spinal cord injury. *J Neurotrauma* 9:S211–217, 1992.
18. Young W: Acute, restorative, and regenerative therapy of spinal cord injury, in Piepmeier JM (ed): *The Outcome Following Traumatic Spinal Cord Injury.* Mount Kisco, NY: Futura, 1992: 173–197.
19. Young W: Clinical trials and experimental therapies of acute spinal cord injury, in Frankel HL (ed): *Handbook of Clinical Neurology: Spinal Trauma.* Amsterdam: Elsevier 1992: 399–419.
20. Young W: Medical treatments of acute spinal cord injury. *J Neurol Neurosurg Psychiatry* 55:635–639, 1992.
21. Young W: Nonregenerative approaches to spinal cord injury, in Glorio A (ed): *Neuroregeneration.* New York: Raven Press, 1993: 169–184.
22. Young W: Secondary injury mechanisms in acute spinal cord injury. *J Emerg Med* 11:13–22, 1993.
23. Young W: Strategies for the development of new and better pharmacological treatments for acute spinal cord injury. *Adv Neurol* 59:249–256, 1993.
24. Young W: The therapeutic window for methylprednisolone treatment of acute spinal cord injury: Implications for cell injury mechanisms, in Waxman SG (ed): *Molecular and Cellular Approaches to the Treatment of Neurological Disease.* New York: Raven Press, 1993: 191–206.
25. Young W: Neuroprotective therapy for brain and spinal cord injury, in Chernow B (eds): *The Pharmacologic Approach to the Critically Ill Patient,* Third Edition. Baltimore, Williams & Wilkins, 1994: 863–874.
26. Young W: Neurorehabilitation of spinal cord injury. *J Neurol Rehab* 8:3–9, 1994.
27. Young W, Huang P, Kume-Kick J: Cellular, ionic and biomolecular mechanisms of the injury process. *Neurosurg Topics* 21:1995.
28. Young W, Kume-Kick J, Constantini S: Glucocorticoid therapy of spinal cord injury. *Ann NY Acad Sci* 743:241–265, 1994.
29. Aguayo AJ, Benfey M, David S: A potential for axonal regeneration in neurons of the adult mammalian nervous system. *Birth Defects* 19:327–340, 1983.
30. Benfey M, Bunger UR, Vidal SM, et al: Axonal regeneration from GABAergic neurons in the adult rat thalamus. *J Neurocytol* 14:279–296, 1985.
31. David S, Aguayo AJ: Axonal regeneration after crush injury of rat central nervous system fibres innervating peripheral nerve grafts. *J Neurocytol* 14:1–12, 1985.
32. Richardson PM, Issa VM, Aguayo AJ: Regeneration of long spinal axons in the rat. *J Neurocytol* 13:165–182, 1984.
33. Barde YA, Edgar D, Thoenen H: Purification of a new neurotrophic factor from mammalian brain. *Eur Molec Biol Org J* 1:549–553, 1982.
34. Barde YA, Edgar D, Thoenen H: New neurotrophic factors. *Annu Rev Physiol* 45:601–612, 1983.
35. Thoenen H, Korsching S, Barde YA, Edgar D: Quantitation and purification of neurotrophic molecules. *Cold Spring Harb Symp Quant Biol* 2:679–684, 1983.
36. Hohn A, Leibrock J, Bailey K, Barde YA: Identification

and characterization of a novel member of the nerve growth factor/brain-derived neurotrophic factor family. *Nature* 344:339–341, 1990.

37. Leibrock J, Lottspeich F, Hohn A, et al: Molecular cloning and expression of brain-derived neurotrophic factor. *Nature* 341:149–152, 1989.
38. Gage FH, Björklund A: Trophic and growth-regulating mechanisms in the central nervous system monitored by intracerebral neural transplants. *Ciba Found Symp* 126:143–159, 1987.
39. Garcia I, Martinou I, Tsujimoto Y, Martinou JC: Prevention of programmed cell death of sympathetic neurons by the bcl-2 proto-oncogene. *Science* 258:302–304, 1992.
40. Kessler JA, Ludlam WH, Freidin MM, et al: Cytokine-induced programmed death of cultured sympathetic neurons. *Neuron* 11:1123–1132, 1993.
41. Lindsay RM, Barde YA, Davies AM, Rohrer H: Differences and similarities in the neutrotrophic growth factor requirements of sensory neurons derived from neural crest and neural placode. *J Cell Sci [Suppl]* 3:115–129, 1985.
42. Raff MC, Barres BA, Burne JF, et al: Programmed cell death and the control of cell survival: Lessons from the nervous system. *Science* 262:695–700, 1993.
43. Rich KM: Neuronal death after trophic factor deprivation. *J Neurotrauma* 9:S61–69, 1992.
44. Thoenen H, Barde YA, Davies AM, Johnson JE: Neurotrophic factors and neuronal death. *Ciba Found Symp* 126:82–95, 1987.
45. Caroni P, Savio T, Schwab ME: Central nervous system regeneration: Oligodendrocytes and myelin as non-permissive substrates for neurite growth. *Prog Brain Res* 78:363–370, 1988.
46. Caroni P, Schwab ME: Antibody against myelin-associated inhibitor of neurite growth neutralizes nonpermissive substrate properties of CNS white matter. *Neuron* 1:85–96, 1988.
47. Caroni P, Schwab ME: Two membrane protein fractions from rat central myelin with inhibitory properties for neurite growth and fibroblast spreading. *J Cell Biol* 106:1281–1288, 1988.
48. Caroni P, Schwab ME: Codistribution of neurite growth inhibitors and oligodendrocytes in rat CNS: Appearance follows nerve fiber growth and precedes myelination. *Dev Biol* 136:287–295, 1989.
49. Savio T, Schwab ME: Lesioned corticospinal tract axons regenerate in myelin-free rat spinal cord. *Proc. Natl Acad Sci USA* 87:4130–4133, 1990.
50. Schwab ME: Myelin-associated inhibitors of neurite growth. *Exp Neurol* 109:2–5, 1990.
51. Schwab ME, Caroni P: Oligodendrocytes and CNS myelin are nonpermissive substrates for neurite growth and fibroblast spreading in vitro. *J Neurosci* 8:2381–2393, 1988.
52. Schnell L, Schwab ME: Axonal regeneration in the rat spinal cord produced by an antibody against myelin-associated neurite growth inhibitors. *Nature* 343:269–272, 1990.
53. Schwab ME: Regeneration of lesioned CNS axons by neutralization of neurite growth inhibitors: A short review. *J Neurotrauma* 9:S219–221, 1992.
54. Blight A, Young W: Central axons in injured cat spinal cord recover electrophysiological function following remyelination by Schwann cells. *J Neurol Sci* 91:15–34, 1989.
55. Blight A, Young W: Axonal morphometric correlates of evoked potentials in experimental spinal cord injury, in Salzman S (ed): *Neural Monitoring.* New York: Humana Press, 1990: 87–113.
56. Blight AR, DeCrescito V: Morphometric analysis of experimental spinal cord injury in the cat: The relation of injury intensity to survival of myelinated axons. *Neuroscience* 19:321–341, 1986.
57. Blight AR: Delayed demyelination and macrophage invasion: A candidate for secondary cell damage in spinal cord injury. *Cent Nerv Syst Trauma* 2:299–315, 1985.
58. Blight AR: Remyelination, revascularization, and recovery of function in experimental spinal cord injury. *Adv Neurol* 59:91–104, 1993.
59. Blight AR, Gruner JA: Augmentation by 4-aminopyridine of vestibulospinal free fall responses in chronic spinal-injured cats. *J Neurol Sci* 82:155–159, 1987.
60. Blight AR, Toombs JP, Bauer MS, Widmer WR: The effects of 4-aminopyridine on neurological deficits in chronic cases of traumatic spinal cord injury in dogs: A phase I clinical trial. *J Neurotrauma* 8:103–119, 1991.
61. Hansebout RR, Blight AR, Fawcett S, Reddy K: 4-aminopyridine in chronic spinal cord injury: A controlled double-blind, crossover study in eight patients. *J Neurotrauma* 10:1–18, 1993.
62. Hayes KC, Blight AR, Potter PJ, et al: Preclinical trial of 4-aminopyridine in patients with chronic spinal cord injury. *Paraplegia* 31:216–224, 1993.
63. Hayes KC, Potter PJ, Wolfe DL, Hsieh JT, Delaney GA, Blight AR: 4-Aminopyridine-sensitive neurologic deficits in patients with spinal cord injury. *J. Neurotrauma* 11:433–46, 1994.
64. Choi DW: Glutamate neurotoxicity in cortical cell culture is calcium-dependent. *Neurosci Lett* 58:293–297, 1985.
65. Choi DW: Calcium-mediated neurotoxicity: Relationship to specific channel types and role in ischemic damage. *Trends Neurosci* 11:465–469, 1988.
66. Duverger D, Benavides J, Cudennec A, MacKenzie ET: A glutamate antagonist reduces infarction size following focal cerebral ischaemia independently of vascular and metabolic changes. *J Cereb Blood Flow Metab* 7: S144, 1987.
67. Faden AI, Simon RP: A potential role for excitotoxins in the pathophysiology of spinal cord injury. *Ann Neurol* 23:623–626, 1988.
68. Germano IM, Pitts LH, Meldrum BS, et al: Kynurenate inhibition of cell excitation decreases stroke size and deficits. *Ann Neurol* 22:730–734, 1987.
69. Gill R, Foster AC, Woodruff GN: Systemic administration of MK-801 protects against ischemia-induced hip-

pocampal neurodegeneration in the gerbil. *J Neurosci* 7:3343–3349, 1987.

70. Goldberg MP, Viseskul V, Choi DW: N-Methyl-D-aspartate receptors mediate hypoxic neuronal injury in cortical culture. *J Pharmacol Exp Ther* 245:1081–1087, 1987.
71. Isacson O, Sofroniew MV: Neuronal loss or replacement in the injured adult cerebral neocortex induces extensive remodeling of intrinsic and afferent neural systems. *Exp Neurol* 117:151–175, 1992.
72. Koh JY, Choi DW: Vulnerability of cultured cortical neurons to damage by excitotoxins: Differential susceptibility of neurons containing NADPH-diaphorase. *J Neurosci* 8:2153–2163, 1988.
73. McDonald JW, Silverstein FS, Johnston MV: MK-801 protects the neonatal brain from hypoxic-ischemic damage. *Eur J Pharmacol* 140:359–361, 1987.
74. Rothman SM, Olney JW: Excitotoxicity and the NMDA receptor. *Trends Neurosci* 10:299–302, 1987.
75. Rothman SM, Thurston JH, Hauhart RE, et al: Ketamine protects hippocampal neurons from anoxia in vitro. *Neuroscience* 21:673–678, 1987.
76. Stewart GR, Olney JW, Pattikonda M, Snider WD: Excitotoxicity in the embryonic chick spinal cord. *Ann Neurol* 30:750–766, 1991.
77. Tecoma ES, Monyer H, Goldberg MP, Choi DW: Traumatic neuronal injury in vitro is attenuated by NMDA antagonists. *Neuron* 2:1541–1545, 1989.
78. Deckwerth TL, Johnson EM Jr: Temporal analysis of events associated with programmed cell death (apoptosis) of sympathetic neurons deprived of nerve growth factor. *J Cell Biol* 123:1207–1222, 1993.
79. Edwards SN, Tolkovsky AM: Characterization of apoptosis in cultured rat sympathetic neurons after nerve growth factor withdrawal. *J Cell Biol* 124:537–546, 1994.
80. Freeman RS, Estus S, Johnson EM Jr: Analysis of cell cycle-related gene expression in postmitotic neurons: Selective induction of Cyclin D1 during programmed cell death. *Neuron* 12:343–355, 1994.
81. Howard MK, Burke LC, Mailhos C, et al: Cell cycle arrest of proliferating neuronal cells by serum deprivation can result in either apoptosis or differentiation. *J Neurochem* 60:1783–1791, 1993.
82. Martin DP, Ito A, Horigome K, et al: Biochemical characterization of programmed cell death in NGF-deprived sympathetic neurons. *J Neurobiol* 23:1205–1220, 1992.
83. Mesner PW, Winters TR, Green SH: Nerve growth factor withdrawal-induced cell death in neuronal PC12 cells resembles that in sympathetic neurons. *J Cell Biol* 119:1669–1680, 1992.
84. Bailey JM: New mechanisms for effects of anti-inflammatory glucocorticoids. *Biofactors* 3:97–102, 1991.
85. Bollen M, Stalmans W: The structure, role, and regulation of type 1 protein phosphatases. *Crit Rev Biochem Mol Biol* 27:227–281, 1992.
86. Her E, Reiss N, Braquet P, Zor U: Characterization of glucocorticoid inhibition of antigen-induced inositolphosphate formation by rat basophilic leukemia cells: Possible involvement of phosphatases. *Biochim Biophys Acta* 1133:63–72, 1991.
87. Nordeen SK, Moyer ML, Bona BJ: The coupling of multiple signal transduction pathways with steroid response mechanisms. *Endocrinology* 134:1723–1732, 1994.
88. Subramaniam M, Colvard D, Keeting PE, et al: Glucocorticoid regulation of alkaline phosphatase, osteocalcin, and proto-oncogenes in normal human osteoblast-like cells. *J Cell Biochem* 50:411–424, 1992.
89. Zor U, Her E, Braquet P, et al: A novel mechanism of glucocorticosteroid (GC) action in suppression of phospholipase A2 (PLA2) activity stimulated by Ca^{2+} ionophore A23187: Induction of protein phosphatases. *Adv Prostaglandin Thromboxane Leukotriene Res* 21A: 265–271, 1991.
90. Bonnefoy-Berard N, Genestier L, Flacher M, Revillard JP: The phosphoprotein phosphatase calcineurin controls calcium-dependent apoptosis in B cell lines. *Eur J Immunol* 24:325–329, 1994.
91. Liu J: FK506 and cyclosporin, molecular probes for studying intracellular signal transduction. *Immunol Today* 14:290–295, 1993.
92. Moyer ML, Borror KC, Bona BJ, et al: Modulation of cell signaling pathways can enhance or impair glucocorticoid-induced gene expression without altering the state of receptor phosphorylation. *J Biol Chem* 268:22933–22940, 1993.
93. Ohoka Y, Nakai Y, Mukai M, Iwata M: Okadaic acid inhibits glucocorticoid-induced apoptosis in T cell hybridomas at its late stage. *Biochem Biophys Res Commun* 197:916–921, 1994.
94. Schwaninger M, Blume R, Oetjen E, et al: Inhibition of cAMP-responsive element-mediated gene transcription by cyclosporin A and FK506 after membrane depolarization. *J Biol Chem* 268:23111–23115, 1993.
95. Solter PF, Hoffmann WE, Hungerford LL, et al: Assessment of corticosteroid-induced alkaline phosphatase isoenzyme as a screening test for hyperadrenocorticism in dogs. *J Am Vet Med Assoc* 203:534–538, 1993.
96. Constantini S, Young W: The effects of methylprednisolone and the ganglioside GM1 on acute spinal cord injury in rats. *J Neurosurg* 80:97–111, 1994.
97. Huang P, Young W: Relationship of arterial blood gases to spinal cord lesion volumes after graded contusion injury. *J Neurotrauma* 11:547–562, 1994.
98. Ditunno J Jr, Young W, Donovan WH, Creasey G: The international standards booklet for neurological and functional classification of spinal cord injury. American Spinal Injury Association. *Paraplegia* 32:70–80, 1994.
99. Ditunno JFJ, Young W, Donovan WH, et al: *Standards for Neurological Classification of Spinal Cord Injury.* Chicago: American Spinal Injury Association, 1992.
100. Basso M, Beattie M, Bresnahan J, et al: Multicenter analysis of open field test locomotory scores: Role of experience, teamwork, and field conditions on reliability. *J Neurotrauma* (submitted for publication).
101. Reier PJ, Anderson DK, Thompson FJ, Stokes BT: Neural tissue transplantation and CNS trauma: Ana-

tomical and functional repair of the injured spinal cord. *J Neurotrauma* 9:S223–248, 1992.

102. Reier PJ, Stokes BT, Thompson FJ, Anderson DK: Fetal cell grafts into resection and contusion/compression injuries of the rat and cat spinal cord. *Exp Neurol* 115:177–188, 1992.
103. Fisher LJ, Gage FH: Grafting in the mammalian central nervous system. *Physiol Rev* 73:583–616, 1993.
104. Fischer LJ, Raymon HK, Gage FH: Cells engineered to produce acetylcholine: Therapeutic potential for Alzheimer's disease. *Ann NY Acad Sci* 695:278–284, 1993.
105. Kang UJ, Fisher LJ, Joh TH, et al: Regulation of dopamine production by genetically modified primary fibroblasts. *J Neurosci* 13:5203–5211, 1993.
106. Shimohama S, Fisher LJ, Gage FH: Intracerebral grafting of genetically modified cells: Applications to a rat model of Parkinson's disease. *Adv Neurol* 60:744–748, 1993.
107. Suhr ST, Gage FH: Gene therapy for neurologic disease. *Arch Neurol* 50:1252–1268, 1993.
108. Ard MD, Schachner M, Rapp JT, Faissner A: Growth and degeneration of axons on astrocyte surfaces: Effects of extracellular matrix and on later axonal growth. *Glia* 9:248–259, 1993.
109. Horstkorte, R, Schachner M, Magyar JP, et al: The fourth immunoglobulin-like domain of NCAM contains a carbohydrate recognition domain for oligomannosidic glycans implicated in association with L1 and neurite outgrowth. *J Cell Biol* 121:1409–1421, 1993.
110. Lochter A, Schachner M: Tenascin and extracellular matrix glycoproteins: From promotion to polarization of neurite growth in vitro. *J Neurosci* 13:3986–4000, 1993.
111. Martini R, Xin Y, Schachner M: Restricted localization of L1 and N-CAM at sites of contact between Schwann cells and neurites in culture. *Glia* 10:70–74, 1994.
112. Probstmeier R, Fahrig T, Spiess E, Schachner M: Interactions of the neural cell adhesion molecule and the myelin-associated glycoprotein with collagen type I: Involvement in fibrillogenesis. *J Cell Biol* 116:1063–1070, 1992.
113. Schachner M: Cell surface recognition and neuron-glia interactions. *Ann NY Acad Sci* 633:105–112, 1991.
114. Schachner M: The analysis of neural recognition molecules: Benefits and vicissitudes of functional knock-outs using antibodies and gene ablation. *Curr Opinion Cell Biol* 5:786–790, 1993.
115. Blinkov SM, Gletze II: *The Human Brain in Figures and Tables.* New York: Plenum Press, 1968.
116. Young W, Bracken MB: The second national acute spinal cord injury study. *J Neurotrauma* 9:S429–451, 1992.
117. Kakulas BA: Pathology of spinal injuries. *Cent Nerv Syst Trauma* 1:117–129, 1984.
118. Kakulas BA: Pathomorphological evidence for residual spinal cord functions, in Eccles JC, Dimitrijevic MR (eds): *Upper Motor Neuron Function and Dysfunction.* Basel: Karger, 1985: 163–169.
119. Kakulas BA: The clinical neuropathology of spinal cord injury: A guide to the future. *Paraplegia* 25:212–216, 1987.
120. Kakulas BA, Bedbrook GM: A correlative clinicopathological study of spinal cord injury. *Proc Aust Assoc Neurol* 6:123–132, 1969.
121. Cioni B, Dimitrijevic MR., McKay WB, Sherwood AM: Voluntary supraspinal suppression of spinal reflex activity in paralyzed muscles of spinal cord injury patients. *Exp Neurol* 93:574–583, 1986.
122. Dimitrijevic MR: Residual motor functions in spinal cord injury, in Waxman SG (ed): *Functional Recovery in Neurological Disease.* New York: Raven Press, 1988: 139–155.
123. Dimitrijevic, MR, Dimitrijevic M, Faganel J, Sherwood AM: Suprasegmentally induced motor unit activity in paralyzed muscles of patients with established spinal cord injury. *Ann Neurol* 16:216–221, 1984.
124. Dimitrijevic MR, Hsu CY, McKay WB: Neurophysiological assessment of spinal cord and head injury. *J Neurotrauma* 9:S293–300, 1992.
125. Dimitrijevic, MR, Faganel J, Lehmkuhl D, Sherwood AM: Motor control in man after partial or complete spinal cord injury, in Desmedt JE (ed): *Motor Control Mechanisms in Health and Disease.* New York: Raven Press, 1983: 915–926.
126. Dimitrijevic MR, Nathan PW: Studies of spasticity in man: I. Some features of spasticity. *Brain* 90:1–42, 1967.
127. Dimitrijevic MR, Nathan PW, Sherwood AM: Clonus: The role of central mechanisms. *J Neurol Neurosurg Psychiatry* 43:321–332, 1980.
128. Dimitrijevic MR, Sherwood AM: Spasticity: Medical and surgical treatment. *Neurology* 30:19–27, 1980.
129. Schnell L, Schneider R, Kolbeck R, et al: Neurotrophin-3 enhances sprouting of corticospinal tract during development and after adult spinal cord lesion. *Nature* 367:170–173, 1994.
130. Alstermark B, Eide E, Gorska T, et al: Visually guided switching of forelimb target reaching in cats. *Acta Physiol Scand* 120:151–153, 1984.
131. Alstermark B, Lundberg A: Electrophysiological evidence against the hypothesis that corticospinal fibres send collaterals to the lateral reticular nucleus. *Exp Brain Res* 47:148–150, 1982.
132. Alstermark B, Lundberg A, Sasaki S: Integration in descending motor pathways controlling the forelimb in the cat: 10. Inhibitory pathways to forelimb motoneurones via C3-C4 propriospinal neurones. *Exp Brain Res* 56:279–292, 1984.
133. Alstermark B, Lundberg A, Sasaki S: Integration in descending motor pathways controlling the forelimb in the cat: 11. Inhibitory pathways from higher motor centres and forelimb afferents to C3-C4 propriospinal neurones. *Exp Brain Res* 56:293–307, 1984.
134. Alstermark B, Lundberg A, Sasaki S: Integration in descending motor pathways controlling the forelimb in the cat: 12. Interneurones which may mediate descending feed-forward inhibition and feed-back inhibition from the forelimb to C3-C4 propriospinal neurones. *Exp Brain Res* 56:308–322, 1984.

135. Alstermark B, Gorska T, Lundberg A, Pettersson LG: Integration in descending motor pathways controlling the forelimb in the cat: 16. Visually guided switching of target-reaching. *Exp Brain Res* 80:1–11, 1990.
136. Alstermark B, Isa T, Kummel H, Tantisira B: Projection from excitatory C3-C4 propriospinal neurones to lamina VII and VIII neurones in the C6-Th1 segments of the cat. *Neurosci. Res* 8:131–137, 1990.
137. Alstermark B, Isa T, Tantisira B: Projection from excitatory C3-C4 propriospinal neurones to spinocerebellar and spinoreticular neurones in the C6-Th1 segments of the cat. *Neurosci Res* 8:124–130, 1990.
138. Alstermark B, Isa T, Tantisira B: Pyramidal excitation in long propriospinal neurones in the cervical segments of the cat. *Exp Brain Res* 84:569–582, 1991.
139. Eidelberg E: Consequences of spinal cord lesions upon motor function, with special reference to locomotor activity. *Prog Neurobiol* 17:185–202, 1981.
140. Eidelberg E, Nguyen L, Deza L: Recovery of locomotor function after hemisection of the spinal cord in cats. *Brain Res Bull* 16:507–515, 1986.
141. Eidelberg E, Story JL, Walden JG, Meyer BL: Anatomical correlates of return of locomotor function after partial spinal cord lesions in cats. *Exp Brain Res* 42:81–88, 1981.
142. Eidelberg, E, Straehley D, Erspamer R: Relationship between residual hindlimb assisted locomotion and surviving axons after incomplete spinal cord injuries. *Exp Neurol* 56:312–322, 1977.
143. Eidelberg E, Walden JG, Nguyen LH: Locomotor control in macaque monkeys. *Brain* 104:647–663, 1981.
144. Eidelberg E, Yu J: Effects of corticospinal lesions upon treadmill locomotion in cats. *Exp Brain Res* 43:101–103, 1981.
145. Eidelberg E, Yu J: Effects of vestibulospinal lesions upon locomotor function in cats. *Brain Res* 22:179–183, 1981.
146. Yu J, Eidelberg E: Effects of vestibulospinal lesions upon locomotor function in cats. *Brain Res* 22:179–183, 1981.
147. Alstermark B, Isa T, Lundberg A, et al: The effect of low pyramidal lesions on forelimb movements in the cat. *Neurosci Res* 7:71–75, 1989.
148. Alstermark B, Isa T, Lundberg A, et al: The effect of a low pyramidal transection following previous transection of the dorsal column in cats. *Neurosci Res* 11:215–220, 1991.
149. Alstermark B, Lundberg A, Pettersson LG: The pathway from Ia forelimb afferents to the motor cortex: A new hypothesis. *Neurosci Res* 11:221–225, 1991.
150. Bracken MB, Shepard MJ, Collins WF, et al: Methylprednisolone or naloxone treatment after acute spinal cord injury: 1-year follow-up data: Results of the second National Acute Spinal Cord Injury Study. *J Neurosurg* 76:23–31, 1992.
151. Guth L, Albuquerque EX, Deshpande SS, et al: Ineffectiveness of enzyme therapy on regeneration in the transected spinal cord of the rat. *J Neurosurg* 52:73–86, 1980.
152. Blight AR: Cellular morphology of chronic spinal cord injury in the cat: Analysis of myelinated axons by line sampling. *Neuroscience* 10:521–543, 1983.
153. Little JW, Harris RM, Sohlberg RC: Locomotor recovery following subtotal spinal cord lesions in a rat model. *Neurosci Lett* 87:189–194, 1988.
154. Windle WF, Smart JO, Beers JJ: Residual function after subtotal spinal cord transection in adult cats. *Neurology* 8:518–521, 1958.
155. Barbeau H, Rossignol S: Recovery of locomotion after chronic spinalization in the adult cat. *Brain Res* 412:84–95, 1987.
156. Barbeau H, Rossignol S: Initiation and modulation of the locomotor pattern in the adult chronic spinal cat by noradrenergic, serotonergic and dopaminergic drugs. *Brain Res* 546:250–260, 1991.
157. Belanger M, Drew T, Rossignol S: Spinal locomotion: A comparison of the kinematics and the electromyographic activity in the same animal before and after spinalization. *Acta Biol Hung* 39:151–154, 1988.
158. Edgerton VR, Roy RR, Hodgson JA, et al: Potential of adult mammalian lumbosacral spinal cord to execute and acquire improved locomotion in the absence of supraspinal input. *J Neurotrauma* 9:S119–128, 1992.
159. Pearson KG, Rossignol S: Fictive motor patterns in chronic spinal cats. *J Neurophysiol* 66:1874–1887, 1991.
160. Rossignol S: Locomotion of the adult chronic spinal cat and its modification by monoaminergic agonists and antagonists, in Golgberger M (ed): *Development and Plasticity of the Mammalian Spinal Cord.* Padova: Liviana Press, 1986: 323–345.
161. Young W: Recovery mechanisms in spinal cord injury: Implications for regenerative therapy, in Seil FJ (ed): *Neural Regeneration and Transplantation.* New York: Liss, 1988: 157–169.
162. Björklund A, Katzman R, Stenevi U, West KA: Development and growth of axonal sprouts from noradrenaline and 5-hydroxytryptamine neurones in the rat spinal cord. *Brain Res* 31:21–33, 1971.
163. Goldberger ME, Murray M: Restitution of function and collateral sprouting in the cat spinal cord: The deafferented animal. *J Comp Neurol* 158:37–54, 1974.
164. Goldberger ME, Murray M: Patterns of sprouting and implications for recovery of function. *Adv Neurol* 47:361–385, 1988.
165. Murray M, Goldberger ME: Restitution of function and collateral sprouting in the cat spinal cord: The partially hemisected animal. *J Comp Neurol* 158:19–36, 1974.
166. Polistina DC, Murray M, Goldberger ME: Plasticity of dorsal root and descending serotoninergic projections after partial deafferentation of the adult rat spinal cord. *J Comp Neurol* 299:349–363, 1990.
167. Prendergast J, Murray M, Goldberger ME: Sprouting and reflex recovery after spinal nerve lesions in cats. *Exp Neurol* 73: 732–749, 1981.
168. Blight AR: Axonal physiology of chronic spinal cord injury in the cat: Intracellular recording in vitro. *Neuroscience* 10:1471–1486, 1983.
169. Jones RE, Heron JR, Foster DH, et al: Effects of 4-aminopyridine in patients with multiple sclerosis. *J Neurol Sci* 60:353–362, 1983.

170. Stefoski D, Davis FA, Faut M, Schauf CL: 4-Aminopyridine improves clinical signs in multiple sclerosis. *Ann Neurol* 21:71–77, 1987.
171. Hayes KC, Blight AR, Potter PJ, et al: Effects of intravenous 4-aminopyridine on neurological function in chronic spinal cord injured patients: Preliminary observations. *Third IBRO World Conf Neurosci* 1991.
172. Braughler JM, Hall ED: Involvement of lipid peroxidation in CNS injury. *J Neurotrauma* 9:S1–7, 1992.
173. Demopoulos HB, Flamm ES, Seligman MC, et al: Further studies on free radical pathology in the major central nervous system disorders: Effect of very high doses of methylprednisolone on the functional outcome, morphology and chemistry of experimental spinal cord impact injury. *Can J Physiol Pharmacol* 60:1415–1424, 1981.
174. Honmou O, Sakatani K, Young W: GABA and potassium effects on corticospinal and primary afferent tracts of neonatal rat spinal cord dorsal columns. *Neuroscience* 54:93–104, 1993.
175. Honmou O, Young W: Intracellular messengers regulating axonal excitability. *Neuroscience* (in press).
176. Honmou O, Young W: Norepinephrine modulates excitability of neonatal rat optic nerves through calcium-mediated mechanisms. *Neuroscience* (in press).
177. Sakatani K, Chesler M, Hassan AZ: GABA-A receptors modulate axonal conduction in dorsal columns of neonatal rat spinal cord. *Brain Res* 542:273–279, 1991.
178. Sakatani K, Chesler M, Hassan AZ: GABA-sensitivity of dorsal column axons: An in vitro comparison between adult and neonatal rat spinal cords. *Brain Res Dev Brain Res* 61:139–142, 1992.
179. Saruhashi Y, Young W: Opposing effects of serotonergic 5-HT1A and 5-HT2 receptor agonists and antagonists on spinal axon excitability. *Neuroscience* 61:645–653, 1994.
180. Lee M, Sakatani K, Young W: A role of GABA-A receptors in hypoxia induced conduction failure of neonatal rat spinal dorsal column axons. *Brain Res* 601:14–19, 1993.
181. Puniak MA, Freeman GM, Agresta CA, et al: Comparison of a serotonin antagonist, opioid antagonist, and TRH analog for the acute treatment of experimental spinal trauma. *J Neurotrauma* 8:193–203, 1991.
182. Salzman SK, Puniak MA, Liu ZJ, et al: The serotonin antagonist mianserin improves functional recovery following experimental spinal trauma. *Ann Neurol* 30:533–541, 1991.
183. Faden AI, Lemke M, Simon RP, Noble LJ: N-methyl-D-aspartate antagonist MK801 improves outcome following traumatic spinal cord injury in rats: Behavioral, anatomic, and neurochemical studies. *J Neurotrauma* 5:33–45, 1988.
184. Wrathall JR, Bouzoukis J, Choiniere D: Effect of kynurenate on functional deficits resulting from traumatic spinal cord injury. *Eur J Pharmacol* 14:1–4, 1992.
185. Wrathall JR, Teng YD, Choiniere D, Mundt DJ: Evidence that local non-NMDA receptors contribute to functional deficits in contusive spinal cord injury. *Brain Res* 586:140–143, 1992.
186. Yum SW, Faden AI: Comparison of the neuroprotective effects of the N-methyl-D-aspartate antagonist MK-801 and the opiate-receptor antagonist nalmefene in experimental spinal cord ischemia. *Arch Neurol* 47:277–281, 1990.
187. D'Mello SR, Galli C, Ciotti T, Calissano P: Induction of apoptosis in cerebellar granule neurons by low potassium: Inhibition of death by insulin-like growth factor I and cAMP. *Proc Natl Acad Sci USA* 90:10989–10993, 1993.
188. Paliogianni F, Kincaid RL, Boumpas DT: Prostaglandin E2 and other cyclic AMP elevating agents inhibit interleukin 2 gene transcription by counteracting calcineurin-dependent pathways. *J Exp Med* 178:1813–1817, 1993.
189. Puri J, Pierce JH, Hoffman T: Transduction of a signal for arachidonic acid metabolism by untriggered CSF-1 receptor induces an opposite effect to that induced by CSF-1 receptor and its ligand: Separate regulation of phospholipase A2 and cyclooxygenase by CSF-1 receptor/CSF-1. *Prostaglandins Leukotrienes Essent Fatty Acids* 45:43–48, 1992.
190. Zhang H, Li YC, Young AP: Protein kinase A activation of glucocorticoid-mediated signaling in the developing retina. *Proc Natl Acad Sci USA* 90:3880–3884, 1993.
191. Dawson TM, Steiner JP, Dawson VL, et al: Immunosuppressant FK506 enhances phosphorylation of nitric oxide synthase and protects against glutamate neurotoxicity. *Proc Natl Acad Sci USA* 90:9808–9812, 1993.
192. Antoni FA, Shipston MJ, Smith SM: Inhibitory role for calcineurin in stimulus-secretion coupling revealed by FK506 and cyclosporin A in pituitary corticotrope tumor cells. *Biochem Biophys Res Commun* 194:226–233, 1993.
193. Armstrong DL: Calcium channel regulation by calcineurin, a Ca^{2+}-activated phosphatase in mammalian brain. *Trends Neurosci* 12:117–122, 1989.
194. Kameyama M, Hescheler J, Mieskes G, Trautwein W: The protein-specific phosphatase 1 antagonizes the beta-adrenergic increase of the cardiac Ca current. *Pflugers Arch* 407:461–463, 1986.
195. Kostyuk, PG, Lukyanetz EA: Mechanisms of antagonistic action of internal Ca^{2+} on serotonin-induced potentiation of Ca^{2+} currents in helix neurones. *Pflugers Arch* 424:73–83, 1993.
196. Cuevas P, Carceller-Benito F, Reimers D: Administration of bovine superoxide dismutase prevents sequelae of spinal cord ischemia in the rabbit. *Anat Embryol* (*Berl*)179:251–255, 1989.
197. Grabitz K, Freye E, Prior R, et al: The role of superoxide dismutase (SOD) in preventing postischemic spinal cord injury. *Ad Exp Med Biol.* 264:13–16, 1990.
198. Grabitz K, Freye E, Prior R, et al: Does prostaglandin E1 and superoxide dismutase prevent ischaemic spinal cord injury after thoracic aortic cross-clamping? *Eur J Vasc Surg* 4:19–24, 1990.
199. Qayumi AK, Janusz MT, Jamieson WR, Lyster DM: Pharmacologic interventions for prevention of spinal cord injury caused by aortic crossclamping. *J Thorac Cardiovasc Surg* 104:256–261, 1992.

200. Faden AI, Shirane R, Chang LH, et al: Opiate-receptor antagonist improves metabolic recovery and limits neurochemical alterations associated with reperfusion after global brain ischemia in rats. *J Pharmacol Exp Ther* 255:451–458, 1990.
201. Ferris DC, Kume-Kick J, Rice ME: Gender differences in cerebral ascorbate and glutathione. *Soc Neurosci* (in press).
202. Lemke M, Frei B, Ames BN, Faden AI: Decreases in tissue levels of ubiquinol-9 and -10, ascorbate and alpha-tocopherol following spinal cord impact trauma in rats. *Neurosci Lett* 108:201–206, 1990.
203. Pietronegro DD, DeCrescito V, Tomasula JJ, et al: Ascorbic acid: A putative biochemical marker of irreversible neurologic functional loss following spinal cord injury. *Cent Nerv Syst Trauma* 2:85–92, 1985.
204. Rice ME, Cammack J: Anoxia-resistant turtle brain maintains ascorbic acid content in vitro. *Neuroscience Lett* 132:141–145, 1991.
205. Rice ME, Nicholson C: Interstitial ascorbate in turtle brain is modulated by release and extracellular volume change. *J Neurochem* 49:1096–1104, 1987.
206. Rice ME, Pérez-Pinzón MA, Choy Y, Lee E: Ascorbate as an endogenous neuroprotective agent: High levels in turtle brain and protection against oxidative damage in mammalian hippocampal slices (in preparation).
207. Takagi K, Kanemitsu H, Tomukai N, et al: Changes of superoxide dismutase activity and ascorbic acid in focal cerebral ischaemia in rats. *Neurol Res* 14:26–30, 1992.
208. Chan AC: Partners in defense, vitamin E and vitamin C. *Can J Physiol Pharm* 71:725–731, 1994.
209. Mizui T, Kinouchi H, Chan PH: Depletion of brain glutathione by buthionine sulfoximine enhances cerebral ischemic injury in rats. *Am J Physiol* 1992.
210. Ratan RR, Murphy TH, Baraban JM: Oxidative stress induces apoptosis in embryonic cortical neurons. *J Neurochem* 62:376–379, 1994.
211. Anderson DK, Means ED: Alpha-tocopherol, mannitol, and methylprednisolone prevention of $FeCl_2$ initiated free radical induced lipid peroxidation in spinal cord, in Novelli U (ed): *Oxygen Free Radicals in Shock.* Karger: Basel, 1986: 224–230.
212. Anderson DK, Waters TR, Means ED: Pretreatment with alpha tocopherol enhances neurologic recovery after experimental spinal cord compression injury. *J Neurotrauma* 5:61–67, 1988.
213. Hall ED, Braughler JM: Role of lipid peroxidation in post-traumatic spinal cord degeneration: A review. *Cent Nerv Syst Trauma* 3:281–294, 1986.
214. Hall ED, Yonkers PA, Andrus PK, et al: Biochemistry and pharmacology of lipid antioxidants in acute brain and spinal cord injury. *J Neurotrauma* 9:S425–442, 1992.
215. Saunders RD, Dugan LL, Demediuk P, et al: Effects of methylprednisolone and the combination of alpha-tocopherol and selenium on arachidonic acid metabolism and lipid peroxidation in traumatized spinal cord tissue. *J Neurochem* 49:24–31,1987.
216. Young W: Role of calcium in spinal cord injury. *Cent Nerv Syst Trauma* 2:109–114, 1985.
217. Young W: Role of calcium in central nervous system injuries. *J Neurotrauma* 9:S9–25, 1992.
218. Panter SS, Yum SW, Faden AI: Alteration in extracellular amino acids after traumatic spinal cord injury. *Ann Neurol* 27:96–99, 1990.
219. Faden AI, Ellison JA, Nobel LJ: Effects of competitive and noncompetitive NMDA receptor antagonists in spinal cord injury. *Eur J Pharmacol* 175:165–174, 1990.
220. Bakshi R, Faden AI: Competitive and non-competitive NMDA antagonists limit dynorphin A-induced rat hindlimb paralysis. *Brain Res* 507:1–5, 1990.
221. Bakshi R, Newman AH, Faden AI: Dynorphin A-(1-17) induces alterations in free fatty acids, excitatory amino acids, and motor function through an opiate-receptor-mediated mechanism. *J Neurosci* 10:3793–3800, 1990.
222. Faden AI: Dynorphin increases extracellular levels of excitatory amino acids in the brain through a non-opioid mechanism. *J Neurosci* 12:425–429, 1992.
223. Jackson DA, White SR: Thyrotropin releasing hormone (TRH) modified excitability of spinal cord dorsal horn cells. *Neurosci Lett* 92:171–176, 1988.
224. White SR: A comparison of the effects of serotonin, substance P and thyrotropin-releasing hormone on excitability of rat spinal motoneurons in vivo. *Brain Res* 335:63–70, 1985.
224A. Harris-Warrick RM, Cohen AH: Serotonin modulates the central pattern generator for locomotion in the isolated lamprey spinal cord. *J Exp Biol* 116:1–20, 1985.
224B. Hashimoto T, Fukuda N: Contribution of serotonin neurons to the functional recovery after spinal cord injury in rats. *Brain Res* 539:263–270, 1991.
224C. Wallen P, Christenson J, Brodin L, et al: Mechanisms underlying the serotonergic modulation of the spinal circuitry for locomotion in lamprey. *Prog Brain Res* 80:321–327, 1989.
224D. White SR, Neuman RS: Facilitation of spinal motoneurone excitability by 5-hydroxytryptamine and noradrenaline. *Brain Res* 188:119–127, 1980.
224E. Yamazaki J, Ono H, Nagao T: Stimulatory and inhibitory effects of serotonergic hallucinogens on spinal mono- and polysynaptic reflex pathways in the rat. *Neuropharmacol* 31:635–642, 1992.
225. White SR: Serotonin and co-localized peptides: Effects on spinal motoneuron excitability. *Peptides* 2:123–127, 1985.
226. Faden AI: TRH analog YM-14673 improves outcome following traumatic brain and spinal cord injury in rats: Dose-response studies. *Brain Res* 486:228–235, 1989.
227. Faden AI: Opioid and nonopioid mechanisms may contribute to dynorphin's pathophysiological actions in spinal cord injury. *Ann Neurol* 27:67–74, 1990.
228. Faden AI, Holaday JW: A role for endorphins in the pathophysiology of spinal cord injury, in Martin JB, Reichlin S, Bick KL (eds): *Neurosecretion and Brain Peptides.* New York: Raven Press, 1981: 435–446.
229. Faden AI, Jacobs TP: Opiate antagonist WIN 44,441-3 stereospecifically improves neurologic recovery after ischemic spinal injury. *Neurology* 35:1311–1315, 1985.

230. Faden AI, Jacobs TP, Holaday JW: Opiate antagonist improves neurologic recovery after spinal injury. *Science* 211:493–494, 1980.
231. Faden AI, Jacobs TP, Holaday JW: Thyrotropin releasing hormone improves neurologic recovery after spinal trauma in cats. *N Eng J Med* 305:1063–1067, 1981.
232. Faden AI, Jacobs TP, Smith MT: Thyrotropin-releasing hormone in experimental spinal injury: Dose response and late treatment. *Neurology* 34:1280–1284, 1984.
233. Faden AI, Sacksen I, Noble LJ: Opiate-receptor antagonist nalmefene improves neurologic recovery after traumatic spinal cord injury in rats through a central mechanism. *J Pharmacol Exp Ther* 245:742–748, 1988.
234. Ogata T, Nakamura Y, Tsuji K, et al: Steroid hormones protect spinal cord neurons from glutamate toxicity. *Neuroscience* 55:445–449, 1993.
235. Horrocks LA, Demediuk P, Saunders RD, et al: The degradation of phospholipids, formation of metabolites of arachidonic acid, and demyelination following experimental spinal cord injury. *Cent Nerv Syst Trauma* 2:115–120, 1985.
236. Anderson DK, Saunders RD, Demediuk P, et al: Lipid hydrolysis and peroxidation in injured spinal cord: Partial protection with methylprednisolone or vitamin E and selenium. *Cent Nerv Syst Trauma* 2:257–267, 1985.
237. Demediuk P, Daly MP, Faden AI: Changes in free fatty acids, phospholipids, and cholesterol following impact injury to the rat spinal cord. *J Neurosci Res* 23:95–106, 1989.
238. Demediuk P, Faden AI: Traumatic spinal cord injury in rats causes increases in tissue thromboxane but not peptidoleukotrienes. *J Neurosci Res* 20:115–121, 1988.
239. Jacobs TP, Shohami E, Baze W, et al: Thromboxane and 5-HETE increase after experimental spinal cord injury in rabbits. *Cent Nerv Syst Trauma* 4:95–118, 1987.
240. Moreland DB, Soloniuk DS, Feldman MJ: Leukotrienes in experimental spinal cord injury. *Surg Neurol* 31:277–280, 1989.
241. Xu JA, Hsu CY, Liu TH, et al: Leukotriene B4 release and polymorphonuclear cell infiltration in spinal cord injury. *J Neurochem* 55:907–912, 1990.
242. Asano T, Koide T, Gotoh O, et al: The role of free radicals and eicosanoids in the pathogenetic mechanism underlying ischemic brain edema. *Mol Chem Neuropathol* 10:101–133, 1989.
243. Asano T, Shigeno T, Johshita H, et al: A novel concept on the pathogenetic mechanism underlying ischaemic brain oedema: Relevance of free radicals and eicosanoids. *Acta Neurochir [Suppl] (Wein)* 41:85–96, 1987.
244. Bazan NG, Rodriguez de Turco EB: Membrane lipids in the pathogenesis of brain edema: Phospholipids and arachidonic acid, the earliest membrane components changed at the onset of ischemia. *Adv Neurol* 28:197–204, 1980.
245. Chan PH, Fishman RA, Caronna J, et al: Induction of brain edema following intracerebral injection of arachidonic acid. *Ann Neurol* 13:625–632, 1983.
246. Chan PH, Fishman RA, Lee JL: Arachidonic acid induced swelling in incubated rat brain cortical slices: Effect of bovine free serum albumin. *Neurochem Res* 5:629–640, 1984.
247. Hall ED, Wolf DL: A pharmacological analysis of the pathophysiological mechanisms of posttraumatic spinal cord ischemia. *J Neurosurg* 64:951–961, 1986.
247A. Lauritzen M, Hansen AJ, Kronberg D, Wieloch T: Cortical spreading depression is associated with arachidonic acid accumulation and preservation of energy charge. *J Cereb Blood Flow Metab* 10:115–122, 1990.
247B. Pickard JD: Role of prostaglandins and arachidonic acid derivatives in the coupling of cerebral blood flow to cerebral metabolism. *J Cereb Blood Flow Metab* 1:361–384, 1981.
248. Siegal T, Siegal T, Lossos F: Experimental neoplastic spinal cord compression: Effect of anti-inflammatory agents and glutamate receptor antagonists on vascular permeability. *Neurosurgery* 26:967–970, 1990.
249. Siegal T, Siegal T, Shohami E, Shapira Y: Comparison of soluble dexamethasone sodium phosphate with free dexamethasone and indomethacin in treatment of experimental neoplastic spinal cord compression. *Spine* 13:1171–1176, 1988.
250. Truman JW, Thorn RS, Robinow S: Programmed neuronal death in insect development. *J Neurobiol* 23:1295–1311, 1992.
251. Galli G, Fratelli M: Activation of apoptosis by serum deprivation in a teratocarcinoma cell line: Inhibition by L-acetylcarnitine. *Exp Cell Res* 204:54–60, 1993.
252. Linnik MD, Hatfield MD, Swope MD, Ahmed NK: Induction of programmed cell death in a dorsal root ganglia X neuroblastoma cell line. *J Neurobiol* 24:433–446, 1993.
253. Gougeon ML, Garcia S, Heeney J, et al: Programmed cell death in AIDS-related HIV and SIV infections. *Aids Res Hum Retroviruses* 9:553–563, 1993.
254. Groux H, Torpier G, Monte D, et al: Activation-induced death by apoptosis in CD4+ T cells from human immunodeficiency virus-infected asymptomatic individuals. *J Exp Med* 175:331–340, 1992.
255. Muller WE, Schroder HC, Ushijima HD, et al: gp120 of HIV-1 induces apoptosis in rat cortical cell cultures: Prevention by memantine. *Eur J Pharmacol* 226:209–214, 1992.
256. Zauli G, Gibellini D, Milani D, et al: Human immunodeficiency virus type 1 Tat protein protects lymphoid, epithelial, and neuronal cell lines from death by apoptosis. *Cancer Res* 53:4481–4485, 1993.
257. Robinow S, Talbot WS, Hogness DS, Truman JW: Programmed cell death in the Drosophila CNS is ecdysone-regulated and coupled with a specific ecdysone receptor isoform. *Development* 119:1251–1259, 1993.
258. Edwards SN, Buckmaster AE, Tolkovsky AM: The death programme in cultured sympathetic neurones can be suppressed at the posttranslational level by nerve growth factor, cyclic AMP, and depolarization. *J Neurochem* 57:2140–2143, 1991.
259. Gagliardini V, Fernandez PA, Lee RK, et al: Prevention of vertebrate neuronal death by the crmA gene. *Science* 263:826–828, 1994.

260. Hockenbery DM, Zutter M, Hickey W, et al: BCL2 protein is topographically restricted in tissues characterized by apoptotic cell death. *Proc Natl Acad Sci USA* 88:6961–6965, 1991.
261. Villa P, Miehe M, Sensenbrenner M, Pettmann B: Synthesis of specific proteins in trophic factor-deprived neurons undergoing apoptosis. *J Neurochem* 62:1468–1475, 1994.
262. Pittman RN, Wang S, DiBenedetto AJ, Mills JC: A system for characterizing cellular and molecular events in programmed neuronal cell death. *J Neurosci* 13:3669–3680, 1993.
263. Branconnier RJ, Branconnier ME, Walshe TM, et al: Blocking the Ca(2+)-activated cytotoxic mechanisms of cholinergic neuronal death: A novel treatment strategy for Alzheimer's disease. *Psychopharmacol Bull* 28:175–181, 1992.
264. Fruman DA, Mather PE, Burakoff SJ, Bierer BE: Correlation of calcineurin phosphatase activity and programmed cell death in murine T cell hybridomas. *Eur J Immunol* 22:2513–2517, 1992.
265. Little GH, Flores A: Inhibition of programmed cell death by cyclosporin. *Comp Biochem Physiol [C]* 103:463–467, 1992.
266. Bierer BE, Schreiber SL, Burakoff SJ: The effect of the immunosuppressant FK-506 on alternate pathways of T cell activation. *Eur J Immunol* 21:439–445, 1991.
267. Couez D, Pages F, Ragueneau M, et al: Functional expression of human CD28 in murine T cell hybridomas. *Mol Immunol* 31:47–57, 1994.
268. McCarthy SA, Cacchione RN, Mainwaring MS, Cairns JS: The effects of immunosuppressive drugs on the regulation of activation-induced apoptotic cell death in thymocytes. *Transplantation* 54:543–547, 1992.
269. McCarthy SA, Mainwaring MS, Cairns JS: Effects of FK 506 and cyclosporine on T-cell tolerance: Inhibition of a "protective" mechanism that regulates activation-induced apoptosis in developing thymocytes. *Transplant Proc* 23:2925–2927, 1991.
270. Shi YF, Sahai BM, Green DR: Cyclosporin A inhibits activation-induced cell death in T-cell hybridomas and thymocytes. *Nature* 339:625–626, 1989.
271. Holder MJ, Knox K, Gordon J: Factors modifying survival pathways of germinal center B cells: Glucocorticoids and transforming growth factor-beta, but not cyclosporin A or anti-CD19, block surface immunoglobulin-mediated rescue from apoptosis. *Eur J Immunol* 22:2725–2728, 1992.
272. Mailhos C, Howard MK, Latchman DS: Heat shock protects neuronal cells from programmed cell death by apoptosis. *Neuroscience* 55:621–627, 1993.
273. Eisen A, Krieger C: Pathogenic mechanisms in sporadic amyotrophic lateral sclerosis. *Can J Neurol Sci* 20:286–296, 1993.
274. Pender MP, Nguyen KB, McCombe PA, Kerr JF: Apoptosis in the nervous system in experimental allergic encephalomyelitis. *J Neurol Sci* 104:81–87, 1991.
275. Young W: Neuroprotective therapy for brain and spinal cord injury, in Chernow B (ed): *The Pharmacologic Approach to the Critically Ill Patient, Third Edition* Baltimore: Williams & Wilkins, 1994: 863–874.
276. Anderson DK, Means ED: Free radical-induced lipid peroxidation in spinal cord: $FeCl_2$ induction and protection with antioxidants. *Neurochem Pathol* 1:249–264, 1983.
277. Hall ED, Braughler JM, Yonkers PA, et al: U-78517F: A potent inhibitor of lipid peroxidation with activity in experimental brain injury and ischemia. *J Pharmacol Exp Ther* 258:688–694, 1991.
278. Hall ED, Yonkers PA, Horan KL, Braughler JM: Correlation between attenuation of posttraumatic spinal cord ischemia and preservation of tissue vitamin E by the 21-aminosteroid U74006F: Evidence for an in vivo antioxidant mechanism. *J Neurotrauma* 6:169–176, 1989.
279. Jacobsen EJ, McCall JM, Ayer DE, et al: Novel 21-aminosteroids that inhibit iron-dependent lipid peroxidation and protect against central nervous system trauma. *J Med Chem* 33:1145–1151, 1990.
280. Anderson DK, Means ED: Iron-induced lipid peroxidation in spinal cord: Protection with mannitol and methylprednisolone. *J Free Radic Biol Med* 1:59–64, 1985.
281. Bracken MB, Collins WF, Freeman DF, et al: Efficacy of methylprednisolone in acute spinal cord injury. *JAMA* 251:45–52, 1984.
282. Bracken MB, Shepard MJ, Hellenbrand KG, et al: Methylprednisolone and neurological function 1 year after spinal cord injury: Results of the National Acute Spinal Cord Injury Study. *J Neurosurg* 63:704–713, 1985.
283. Hall ED, Braughler JM: Glucocorticoid mechanisms in acute spinal cord injury: A review and therapeutic rationale. *Surg Neurol* 18:320–327, 1982.
284. Hall ED, Braughler JM, McCall JM: New pharmacological treatment of acute spinal cord trauma. *J Neurotrauma* 5:81–89, 1988.
285. Kalayci O, Cataltepe S, Cataltepe O: The effect of bolus methylprednisolone in prevention of brain edema in hypoxic ischemic brain injury: An experimental study in 7-day-old rat pups. *Brain Res* 569:112–116, 1992.
286. Faden AI, Lemke M, Demediuk P: Effects of BW755C, a mixed cyclo-oxygenase-lipoxygenase inhibitor, following traumatic spinal cord injury in rats. *Brain Res* 463:63–68, 1988.
286A. Lucas JH, Wang GF, Gross GW: NMDA antagonists prevent hypothermic injury and death of mammalian spinal neurons. *J Neurotrauma* 7:229–236, 1990.
287. Fujita Y, Shingu T, Kurihara M, et al: Evaluation of a low dose administration of aspirin, dipyridamol and steroid: Therapeutic effects on motor function and protective effects on Na^+-K^+-activated ATPase activity against lipid peroxidation in an experimental model of spinal cord injury. *Paraplegia* 23:56–57, 1985.
288. Waxman SG: Demyelination in spinal cord injury. *J Neurol Sci* 91:1–14, 1989.
289. Birch BD, Kocsis JD, Di-Gregorio F, et al: A voltage- and time-dependent rectification in rat dorsal spinal root axons. *J Neurophysiol* 66:719–728, 1991.
290. Blight AR: Effect of 4-aminopyridine on axonal conduction-block in chronic spinal cord injury. *Brain Res Bull* 22:47–52, 1989.

291. Dubuc R, Rossignol S: The effects of 4-aminopyridine on the cat spinal cord: Rhythmic antidromic discharges recorded from the dorsal roots. *Brain Res* 491:335–348, 1989.
292. Dubuc R, Rossignol S: Unitary discharges in dorsal and ventral roots after the administration of 4-aminopyridine in the cat. *Brain Res* 491:349–355, 1989.
293. Young W, Rosenbluth J, Wojak JC, et al: Extracellular potassium activity and axonal conduction in spinal cord of the myelin-deficient mutant rat. *Exp Neurol* 106:41–51, 1989.
294. Lee MR, Sakatani K, Young W: Interaction of hypoxia and hypothermia on dorsal column conduction in adult rat spinal cord in vitro. *Exp Neurol* 119:140–145, 1993.
295. Sakatani K, Hassan A, Lee M, et al: Nonsynaptic modulation of dorsal column conduction by endogenous GABA in neonatal rat spinal cord. *Brain Res* 662:43–50, 1993.
296. Sakatani K, Black JA, Kocsis JD: Transient presence and functional interaction of endogenous GABA and GABA-A receptors in developing rat optic nerve. *Proc R Soc Lond [Biol]* 247:155–161, 1992.
297. Sakatani K, Hassan AZ, Chesler M: Effects of GABA on axonal conduction and extracellular potassium activity in the neonatal rat optic nerve.*Exp Neurol* 127:291–297, 1994.
298. Sakatani K, Hassan AZ, Ching W: Age-dependent extrasynaptic modulation of axonal conduction by exogenous and endogenous GABA in the rat optic nerve. *Exp Neurol* 114:307–314, 1991.
299. White SR, Black PC, Samathanam GK, Paros KC: Prazosin suppresses development of axonal damage in rats inoculated for experimental allergic encephalomyelitis. *J Neuroimmunol* 39:211–218, 1992.
300. Carstens E, Gilly H, Schreiber H, Zimmermann M: Effects of midbrain stimulation and iontophoretic application of serotonin, noradrenaline, morphine and GABA on electrical thresholds of afferent C- and A-fibre terminals in cat spinal cord. *Neuroscience* 21:395–406, 1987.
301. Saito Y, Collins JG, Iwasaki H: Tonic 5-HT modulation of spinal dorsal horn neuron activity evoked by both noxious and non-noxious stimuli: A source of neuronal plasticity. *Pain* 40:205–219, 1990.
302. Alhaider AA, Lei SZ, Wilcox GL: Spinal 5-HT3 receptor-mediated antinociception: Possible release of GABA. *J Neurosci* 11:1881–1888, 1991.
303. Kiefel JM, Paul D, Bodnar RJ: Reduction in opioid and non-opioid forms of swim analgesia by 5-HT2 receptor antagonists. *Brain Res* 500:231–240, 1989.
304. Zhuo M, Gebhart GF: Spinal serotonin receptors mediate descending facilitation of a nociceptive reflex from the nuclei reticularis gigantocellularis and gigantocellularis pars alpha in the rat. *Brain Res* 550:35–48, 1991.
305. Lipton SA, Kater SB: Neurotransmitter regulation of neuronal outgrowth, plasticity, and survival. *Trends Neurosci* 12:265–270, 1989.
306. Cohen LG, Roth BJ, Wassermann EM, et al: Magnetic stimulation of the human cerebral cortex, an indicator of reorganization in motor pathways in certain pathological conditions. *J Clin Neurophysiol* 8:56–65, 1991.
307. Yamamoto T, Lyeth BG, Dixon CE, et al: Changes in regional brain acetylcholine content in rats following unilateral and bilateral brainstem lesions. *J Neurotrauma* 5:69–79, 1988.
308. Lu X, Richardson PM: Inflammation near the nerve cell body enhances axonal regeneration. *J Neurosci* 11:972–978, 1991.
309. Siegal JD, Kliot M, Smith GM, Silver J: A comparison of the regeneration potential of dorsal root fibers into gray or white matter of the adult rat spinal cord. *Exp Neurol* 109:90–97, 1990.
310. Geisler FH, Dorsey FC, Coleman WP: Recovery of motor function after spinal-cord injury—a randomized, placebo-controlled trial with GM-1 ganglioside. *N Engl J Med* 324:1829–1838, 1991.
311. Geisler FH, Dorsey FC, Coleman WP: GM-1 ganglioside in human spinal cord injury. *J Neurotrauma* 9:S517–S530, 1992.
312. Guth L, Zhang Z, DiProspero NA, et al: Spinal cord injury in the rat: Treatment with bacterial lipopolysaccharide and indomethacin enhances cellular repair and locomotor function. *Exp Neurol* 126:76–87, 1994.
313. Cooley MA, McLachlan K, Atkinson K: Cytokine activity after human bone marrow transplantation: III. Defect in IL2 production by peripheral blood mononuclear cells is not corrected by stimulation with Ca++ ionophore plus phorbol ester. *Br J Haematol* 73:341–347, 1989.
314. Dunn DE, Herold KC, Otten GR, et al: Interleukin 2 and concanavalin A stimulate interferon-gamma production in a murine cytolytic T cell clone by different pathways. *J Immunol* 139:3942–3948, 1987.
315. Rosenbach TO, Zor U, Moshonov S, et al: Induction of acute synovitis in the rat by human interferon. *Clin Exp Rheumatol* 5:35–40, 1987.
316. Durelli L, Bergamini L: Multiple sclerosis: II. A critical assessment of immunotherapy. *Riv Neurol* 59:191–201, 1989.
317. Lin CY: Improvement in steroid and immunosuppressive drug resistant lupus nephritis by intravenous prostaglandin E1 therapy. *Nephron* 55:258–264, 1990.
318. Morse JK, Scheff SW, Dekosky ST: Gonadal steroids influence axon sprouting in the hippocampal dentate gyrus: A sexually dimorphic response. *Exp Neurol* 94:649–658, 1986.
319. Scheff SW, Benardo LS, Cotman CW: Hydrocortisone administration retards axon sprouting in the rat dentate gyrus. *Exp Neurol* 68:195–201, 1980.
320. Scheff SW, Cotman CW: Chronic glucocorticoid therapy alters axon sprouting in the hippocampal dentate gyrus. *Exp. Neurol* 76:644–654, 1982.
321. Scheff SW, Dekosky ST: Steroid suppression of axon sprouting in the hippocampal dentate gyrus of the adult rat: Dose-response relationship. *Exp Neurol* 82:183–191, 1983.
322. Scheff SW, Hoff S, Anderson KJ: Altered regulation of lesion-induced synaptogenesis by adrenalectomy and

corticosterone in young adult rats. *Exp Neurol* 93:456–470, 1986.

323. Cirino G, Peers SH, Flower RJ, et al: Human recombinant lipocortin 1 has acute local anti-inflammatory properties in the rat paw edema test. *Proc Natl Acad Sci USA* 86:3428–3432, 1989.
324. Fedoseev GB, Zhikharev, SS, Goncharova VA, et al: The role of serotonin, histamine and the kallikrein-kinin system in the pathogenesis of asphyxic attacks in bronchial asthma. *Ter Arkh* 64:47–53, 1992.
325. Lindsberg PJ, Yue TL, Frerichs KU, et al: Evidence for platelet-activating factor as a novel mediator in experimental stroke in rabbits. *Stroke* 21:1452–1457, 1990.
326. Morita H: Histamine/serotonin ratio (H/S ratio): A new scale for determining the degree of inflammation in ulcerative colitis (letter). *J Clin Gastroenterol* 15:159–160, 1992.
327. Ngassapa D, Narhi M, Hirvonen T: Effect of serotonin (5-HT) and calcitonin gene-related peptide (CGRP) on the function of intradental nerves in the dog. *Proc Finn Dent Soc* 1:143–148, 1992.
328. Ramos BF, Zhang Y, Angkachatchai V, Jakschik BA: Mast cell mediators regulate vascular permeability changes in Arthus reaction. *J Pharmacol Exp Ther* 262:559–565, 1992.
329. Bracken MB, Holford TR: Effects of timing of methylprednisolone or naloxone administration on recovery of segmental and long-tract neurological function in NASCIS 2. *J Neurosurg* 79:500–507, 1993.
330. Aguayo AJ, Bray GM, Rasminsky M, et al: Synaptic connections made by axons regenerating in the central nervous system of adult mammals. *J Exp Biol* 153:199–224, 1990.
331. Aguayo AJ, David S, Bray GM: Influences of the glial environment on the elongation of axons after injury: Transplantation studies in adult rodents. *J Exp Biol* 95:231–240, 1981.
332. Benfey M, Aguayo AJ: Extensive elongation of axons from rat brain into peripheral nerve grafts. *Nature* 296:150–152, 1982.
333. Bray GM, Vidal SM, Aguayo AJ: Regeneration of axons from the central nervous system of adult rats. *Prog Brain Res* 71:373–379, 1987.
334. Bray GM, Villegas-Perez MP, Vidal-Sanz M, Aguayo AJ: The use of peripheral nerve grafts to enhance neuronal survival, promote growth and permit terminal reconnections in the central nervous system of adult rats. *J Exp Biol* 132:5–19, 1987.
335. David S, Aguayo AJ: Axonal elongation into peripheral nervous system "bridges" after central nervous system injury in adult rats. *Science* 214:931–933, 1981.
336. Munz M, Rasminsky M, Aguayo AJ, et al: Functional activity of rat brainstem neurons regenerating axons along peripheral nerve grafts. *Brain Res* 340:115–125, 1985.
337. So KF, Aguayo AJ: Lengthy regrowth of cut axons from ganglion cells after peripheral nerve transplantation into the retina of adult rats. *Brain Res* 328:349–354, 1985.
338. Borgens RB, Blight AR, McGinnis ME: Behavioral recovery induced by applied electric fields after spinal cord hemisection in guinea pig. *Science* 238:367–369, 1987.
339. Borgens RB, Blight AR, McGinnis ME: Functional recovery after spinal cord hemisection in guinea pigs: The effects of applied electric fields. *J Comp Neurol* 296:634–653, 1990.
340. Borgens RB, Blight AR, Murphy DJ: Axonal regeneration in spinal cord injury: A perspective and new technique. *J Comp Neurol* 250:157–167, 1986.
341. Borgens RB, Blight AR, Murphy DJ, Stewart L: Transected dorsal column axons within the guinea pig spinal cord regenerate in the presence of an applied electric field. *J Comp Neurol* 250:168–180, 1986.
342. Wallace MC, Tator CH, Lewis AJ: Chronic regenerative changes in the spinal cord after cord compression injury in rats. *Surg Neurol* 27:209–219, 1987.
343. Bates CA, Stelzner DJ: Extension and regeneration of corticospinal axons after early spinal injury and maintenance of corticospinal topography. *Exp Neurol* 123:106–117, 1993.
344. Iwashita Y, Kawaguchi S, Murata M: Restoration of function by replacement of spinal cord segments in the rat. *Nature* 367:167–170, 1994.
345. Bregman BS: Spinal cord transplants permit the growth of serotonergic axons across the site of neonatal spinal cord transection. *Brain Res* 431:265–279, 1987.
346. Bregman BS, Goldberger ME: Anatomical plasticity and sparing of function after spinal cord damage in neonatal cats. *Science* 217:553–555, 1982.
347. Commissiong JW, Toffano G: The effect of GM1 ganglioside on coerulospinal, noradrenergic, adult neurons and fetal monoaminergic neurons transplanted into the transected spinal cord of the adult rat. *Brain Res* 380:205–215, 1986.
348. Kunkel BE, Bregman BS: Spinal cord transplants enhance the recovery of locomotor function after spinal cord injury at birth. *Exp Brain Res* 81:25–34, 1990.
349. Kunkel BE, Dai HN, Bregman BS: Recovery of function after spinal cord hemisection in newborn and adult rats: Differential effects on reflex and locomotor function. *Exp Neurol* 116:40–51, 1992.
350. Kliot M, Smith GM, Siegal JD, Silver J: Astrocyte-polymer implants promote regeneration of dorsal root fibers into the adult mammalian spinal cord. *Exp Neurol* 109:57–69, 1990.
351. Appel F, Holm J, Conscience JF, Schachner M: Several extracellular domains of the neural cell adhesion molecule L1 are involved in neurite outgrowth and cell body adhesion. *J Neurosci* 13:4764–4775, 1993.
352. Griffith LS, Schmitz B, Schachner M: L2/HNK-1 carbohydrate and protein-protein interactions mediate the homophilic binding of the neural adhesion molecule P0. *J Neurosci Res* 33:639–648, 1992.
353. Hall H, Liu L, Schachner M, Schmitz B: The L2/HNK-1 carbohydrate mediates adhesion of neural cells to laminin. *Eur J Neurosci* 5:34–42, 1993.
354. Young W: Electrical field effects on neuronal growth

and regeneration, in Carpenter DO, Ayrapetyan S (eds): *Biological Effects of Electric and Magnetic Fields: Beneficial and Harmful Effects.* New York: Academic Press, 1994: 3–11.

355. Grabowski M, Brundin P, Johansson BB: Fetal neocortical grafts implanted in adult hypertensive rats with cortical infarcts following a middle cerebral artery occlusion: Ingrowth of afferent fibers from the host brain. *Exp Neurol* 116:105–121, 1992.
356. Jakeman LB, Reier PJ: Axonal projections between fetal spinal cord transplants and the adult rat spinal cord: A neuroanatomical tracing study of local interactions. *J Comp Neurol* 307:311–334, 1991.
357. Slavin MD, Held JM, Basso DM, et al: Fetal brain tissue transplants and recovery of locomotion following damage to sensorimotor cortex in rats. *Prog Brain Res* 78:33–38, 1988.
358. Soares H, McIntosh TK: Fetal cortical transplants in adult rats subjected to experimental brain injury. *J Neural Transplant Plast* 2:207–220, 1991.
359. Lucidi-Phillipi CA, Gage FH: The neurotrophic hypothesis and the cholinergic basal forebrain projection. *Prog Brain Res* 98:241–249, 1993.
360. Harrison B: Schwann cell and oligodendrocyte remyelination in lysolecithin-induced lesions in irradiated rat spinal cord. *J Neurol Sci* 67:143–159, 1985.
361. Hasegawa M, Rosenbluth J: Transplantation of labeled fetal spinal cord fragments into juvenile myelin-deficient rat spinal cord. *Anat Rec* 229:138–143, 1991.
362. Rosenbluth J, Hasegawa M, Shirasaki N, et al: Myelin formation following transplantation of normal fetal glia into myelin-deficient rat spinal cord. *J Neurocytol* 19:718–730, 1990.
363. Feigin I, Ogata J: Schwann cells and peripheral myelin within human central nervous tissues: The mesenchymal character of Schwann cells. *J Neuropathol Exp Neurol* 30:603–612, 1971.
364. Lindholm D, Heumann R, Meyer M, Thoenen H: Interleukin-1 regulates synthesis of nerve growth factor in non-neuronal cells of rat sciatic nerve. *Nature* 330:658–659, 1987.
365. Blakemore WF: Remyelination by Schwann cells of axons demyelinated by intraspinal injection of 6-aminonicotinamide in the rat. *J Neurocytol* 4:745–757, 1975.
366. Blakemore WF: Observations on remyelination in the rabbit spinal cord following demyelination induced by lysolecithin. *Neuropathol Appl Neurobiol* 4:47–59, 1978.
367. Blakemore WF: Remyelination of CNS axons by Schwann cells transplanted from the sciatic nerve. *Nature* 266:68–69, 1981.
368. Blakemore WF, Crang AJ: The use of cultured autologous Schwann cells to remyelinate areas of persistent demyelination in the central nervous system. *J Neurol Sci* 70:207–223, 1985.
369. Blakemore WF, Crang AJ, Evans RJ, Patterson RC: Rat Schwann cell remyelination of demyelinated cat CNS axons: Evidence that injection of cell suspensions of CNS tissue results in Schwann cell remyelination. *Neurosci Lett* 77:15–19, 1987.
370. Blakemore WF, Crang AJ, Patterson RC: Schwann cell remyelination of CNS axons following injection of cultures of CNS cells into areas of persistent demyelination. *Neurosci Lett* 77:20–24, 1987.
371. Blakemore WF, Welsh CJ, Tonks P, Nash AA: Observations on demyelinating lesions induced by Theiler's virus in CBA mice. *Acta Neuropathol* (*Berl*) 76:581–589, 1988.
372. Graca DL, Blakemore WF: Delayed remyelination in rat spinal cord following ethidium bromide injection. *Neuropathol Appl Neurobiol* 12:593–605, 1986.
373. Harrison BM, Pollard JD: Pattern of Schwann cell remyelination in a spinal cord lesion. *Neurosci Lett* 52:275–280, 1984.
374. Itoyama Y, Webster HD, Richardson EPJ, Trapp BD: Schwann cell remyelination of demyelinated axons in spinal cord multiple sclerosis lesions. *Ann Neurol* 14:339–346, 1983.
375. Blakemore WF: Limited remyelination of CNS axons by Schwann cells transplanted into the sub-arachnoid space. *J Neurol Sci* 64:265–276, 1984.
376. Blakemore WF, Patterson RC: Observations on the interactions of Schwann cells and astrocytes following X-irradiation of neonatal rat spinal cord. *J Neurocytol* 4:573–585, 1975.

Biomechanics

CHAPTER 77

BIOMECHANICS OF CERVICAL SPINE TRAUMA

Ryan S. Glasser
Richard G. Fessler

SYNOPSIS

With the great number of spinal implants presently available, understanding the biomechanical aspects of the injury process and its treatment has never been more important. In most traumatic injuries, the mechanism of injury and the consequences of forces imposed on the cervical spine can be deduced from the clinical history and the radiographs. However, basic scientific study of the biomechanics of the injury continues to provide the necessary background. Some cervical spine injuries remain poorly understood and require further laboratory investigation. In addition, many of the newer spinal implants have not been applied to injury models and then subjected to biomechanical evaluation. Biomechanical understanding of cervical spine traumatic injuries is, and will continue to be, essential knowledge for the surgeon treating these disorders.

INTRODUCTION

Trauma of the cervical spine involves a complex set of events that may result in severe neurological dysfunction. Using biomechanical principles, the traumatic event and its impact on the cervical spine can be broken down into component parts. The direction and magnitude of the force, the impulse (force over time), the posture of the head and neck, and the anatomic location of load impact can combine to produce an injury. A direct relationship exists between the characteristics of the applied loads and the resultant cervical spine injury. This relationship should be reproducible in the laboratory and applicable in the clinical setting.

This chapter focuses on practical applications of biomechanical principles. By understanding normal and abnormal motion and pertinent anatomy, a framework for studying specific traumatic injuries to the cervical spine can be established. This framework, in turn, helps the surgeon formulate treatment options.

APPLIED ANATOMY OF THE CERVICAL SPINE

Upper Cervical Spine

The anatomic characteristics of the upper cervical spine (occiput–C1–C2) are quite different from those of the lower cervical region (C3–T1). The absence of a true C1 vertebral body, the unique ligamentous structures encompassing the dens, and the relative increased spinal canal size all help to explain both normal motion and the consequences of trauma to this region.

The bony ring of the atlas provides a "bridge" between the occiput and the axis (Fig. 77-1). The atlas is thinnest just medial to the lateral mass in the region of the posterior arch where the vertebral artery runs, making this region susceptible to fractures. The occipital condyles, which rest on the lateral masses of C1, permit much more anteroposterior than lateral movement at the occipital-atlantal articulation. This is due primarily to the shallowness of the atlanto-occipital joint in the anteroposterior plane, while the cephalad sloping of the

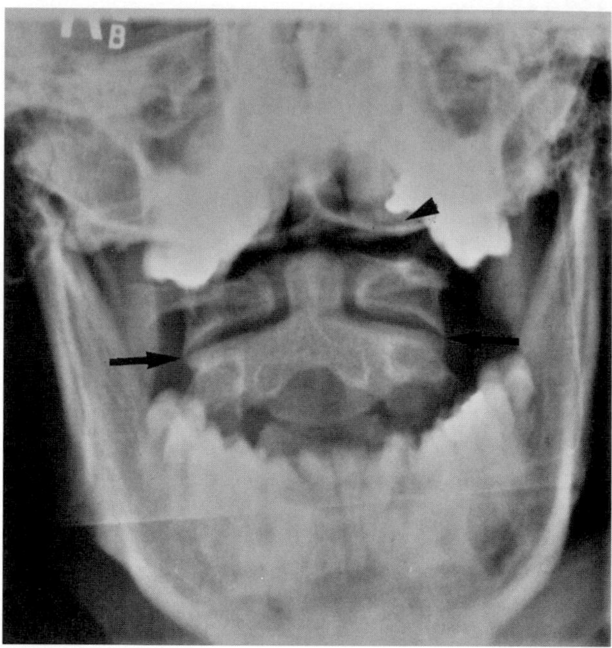

Figure 77-1. The relationship of the atlas with the occipital condyles and the axis can be appreciated in this normal anteroposterior radiograph, open-mouth view. Note the central location of the dens. Also, the lateral margins of the atlanto-axial articulation demonstrate normal, symmetrical alignment (*arrows*). The occipital condyles (*arrowhead*) are partly obscured by the maxilla in this projection, but can be seen to be located above the C1 lateral mass.

lateral aspect of the lateral mass limits excessive lateral motion (Fig. 77-1). In fact, rotation of the occiput on C1 has been thought not to be possible,[1,2] but probably is present, although minimal.[3,4]

The dens extends cephalad, posterior to the anterior arch of C1, and, together with its ligamentous attachments, forms the caudal portion of the occipito-atlanto-axial complex. The ligamentous structures are shown in Fig. 77-2. The primary stabilizing ligament in this region is the transverse ligament, which is attached to a tubercle on the medial aspect of each lateral mass of the atlas. It is at this bony attachment that the transverse ligament is weakest.[5] Of the secondary ligaments, the alar ligament can limit anterior translation of C1 and C2, but predominantly stabilizes in rotation. The alar ligaments actually are comprised of two portions within each ligament. The occipito-alar portion connects the occipital condyles to the lateral tip of the dens, and the atlanto-alar portion attaches from the dens to the lateral mass of the atlas.[6]

Additional stability in the occipital–C1–C2 region is through the other minor ligaments illustrated in Fig. 77-2, as well as the supporting musculature.[7] An extension of the posterior longitudinal ligament, the tectorial membrane, limits excessive motion in both flexion and extension. The anterior atlanto-occipital membrane, a continuation of the anterior longitudinal ligament, interconnects the anterior rim of the foramen magnum with the anterior arch of C1 and primarily restricts excessive extension. The posterior atlanto-occipital membrane functions to limit flexion and is located between the posterior rim of the foramen magnum and the posterior arch of C1. The apical ligament connects the tip of the dens to the occiput, but is not biomechanically significant. More recently, Dvorak and Panjabi identified an additional ligament, the anterior atlanto-dental ligament, that had not previously been described[6] (Fig. 77-2). This ligament connects the inferior aspect of the anterior arch to the dens, in the midline, and may play a role in C1–C2 stability as well.

Lower Cervical Spine

The subaxial cervical spine interconnects the occipital–C1–C2 complex with the fairly rigid thoracic spine. Generally, the motion segments of C2–C3 through C7–T1

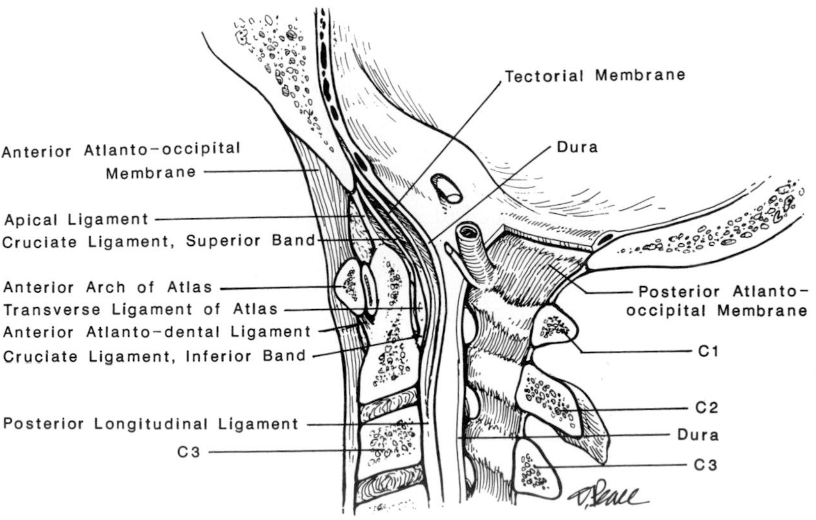

Figure 77-2. Anatomical drawing of the occipital-atlanto-axial region through the midsagittal plane. The relationship of the ligamentous structures to the dens is evident, with two layers of support located posterior to the dens.

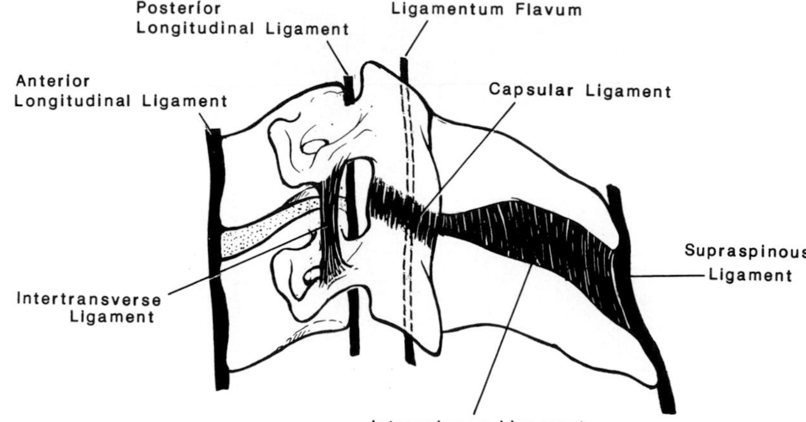

Figure 77-3. Anatomic drawing of the ligamentous structures that support the middle and lower cervical spine. These ligaments, together with the intervertebral discs and muscles, resist the multiaxial forces imposed on the cervical spine.

are included in the discussion of the lower cervical spine. The relatively small vertebral bodies and the transverse foramina from C1 to C6 are among the features that distinguish this region of the spine.

The vertebral bodies gradually enlarge from C3 to L5, which accounts for the increasing capacity to withstand compressive forces as one moves down the spinal column. The bodies are composed of the stronger, inner cancellous bone and are surrounded by cortical bone. At the junction with the intervertebral discs, the endplates appear to be the weakest portion of the body and frequently are the site of fracture when subjected to compressive loads.[8] Extending superiorly from the lateral aspect of the superior endplate are the uncinate processes, which serve primarily to limit posterior translation and lateral displacement.[9] The uncinate processes function to control the anteroposterior translation that occurs during sagittal motion.[10]

The annulus fibrosus attaches to the cartilaginous endplates via elastic fibers known as Sharpey's fibers, although some of the fibers of the annulus attach directly to the anterior and posterior longitudinal ligaments. The annulus is composed of obliquely oriented collagen fibers that resist rotation, tension, and shear forces,[7] but is weakest posterolaterally, the site of most nucleus pulposus herniations.[11,12]

The pedicles project posterolaterally from the bodies, connecting with the lamina, facets, and spinous processes to form the posterior arch. The posterior arch in the cervical region bears a proportionately greater amount of the compressive load than is found elsewhere in the spine. Pal and Sherk found that only 36 percent of the compressive load was borne by the cervical discs and bodies, with the remainder of the load accepted by the posterior elements.[13]

One of the main factors governing the range of motion in the cervical spine is the orientation of the articular surfaces. Facet orientation varies within the cervical spine and is very different than in the thoracic or lumbar spine. At C1–C2, the angle of articulation is horizontal, permitting a large range of axial rotation. From C3–C4 to C7–T1, the angle is 45 degrees, which is conducive to flexion-extension, lateral bending, and, less so, to axial rotation. The orientation of the C2–C3 articular surface is intermediate.[9]

Seven ligaments function to permit normal motion and restrict excessive motion of the cervical spine (Fig. 77-3). In general, the ligaments anterior to the body (intertransverse and anterior longitudinal ligaments) primarily resist extension forces, while those located posteriorly resist flexion forces. This is true because a ligament must be stretched or taut to provide resistance to motion. The ligamentum flavum, located in close proximity to the dura mater, possesses a high content of elastic fibers, which minimizes its length when the ligament is not under stretch.[14,15] When the cervical spine is extended, this property minimizes the likelihood of neural compression by the "buckled" ligamentum flavum.

The capsular ligaments have been shown to be one of the strongest ligaments in the lower cervical spine and to provide stability in flexion.[9,16] Obviously, the motion of the cervical spine is complex, and other structures, such as the intervertebral discs and the supporting musculature, assist the ligaments in resisting multiaxial forces.[17]

GENERAL BIOMECHANICAL PRINCIPLES

KINEMATICS

Kinematics is the study of motion of spinal segments irrespective of the forces that may be applied,[18] and provides a foundation for evaluating cervical spine trauma. A motion segment, or functional spinal unit,

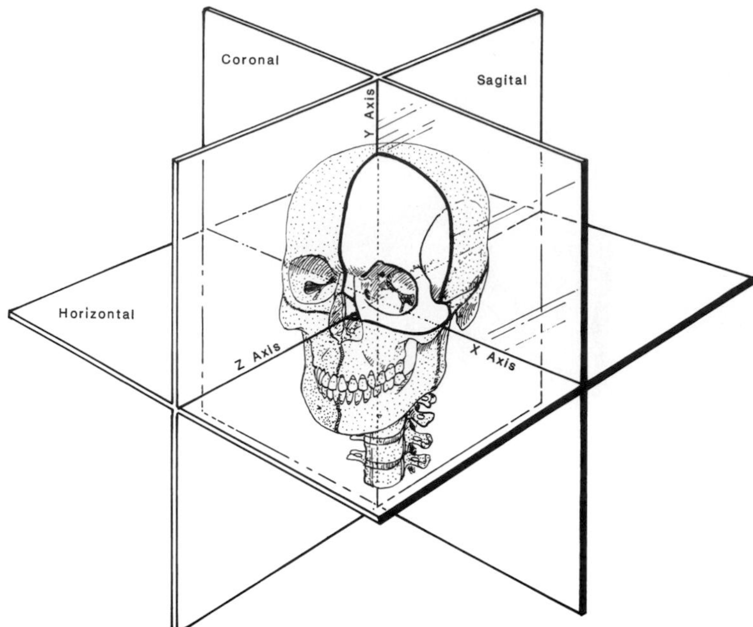

Figure 77-4. Schematic drawing illustrating a three-axes coordinate system. The *x*, *y*, and *z* axes each represent a line in space and provide the foundation for this coordinate system. Movement along the *x* axis describes right and left translation; anterior and posterior translation occurs along the *z* axis; cephalad and caudad motion occurs along the *y* axis. The intersection of two axes forms a plane. The horizontal plane encompasses *x* and *z*; the sagittal plane encompasses *y* and *z*; and the coronal plane involves the *x* and *y* axes.

involves two adjacent vertebrae and the supporting ligaments. This anatomic unit is most often employed during studies of cervical biomechanics.

Coordinate systems have been utilized in an effort to establish a common terminology when discussing the motion of the cervical spine. Panjabi and coworkers recommend a 90-degree angle coordinate system using *x*, *y*, and *z* axes[19] (Fig. 77-4).

When discussing cervical spine motion, the terms "translation" and "rotation" are used to describe the type of motion relative to the three axes. Translation refers to motion along either the *x*, *y*, or *z* axis. For example, forward (or anterior) translation describes movement anterior along the *z* axis, and is a length that can be measured. Rotation refers to angular displacement about one of the axes and can be measured in degrees. Thus, flexion-extension, axial rotation, and lateral bending all describe rotations about the *x*, *y*, and *z* axes, respectively.

As was discussed in the previous section, the anatomic characteristics of the cervical spine determine the range of motion possible at each motion segment. Experimental studies using x-rays[20,21] and CT scans[3] have quantitated the range of motion at each motion segment. Table 77-1 details representative degrees of flexion-extension, lateral bending, and axial rotation at each motion segment of the cervical spine. Over one-half of the axial rotation of the entire cervical spine occurs at C1–C2. The ability to flex and extend, however, is fairly well distributed throughout the cervical spine, but is slightly more at Occ–C1, C1–C2, C4–C5, and the C5–C6 interspace. Lateral bending is greatest from C2–C3 to C4–C5, but becomes sequentially less as one moves down the cervical spine.[9]

The axis upon which cervical spine motion rotates at a given motion segment has come to be known as the "instantaneous" axis of rotation (IAR). The IAR provides a frame of reference when describing movement at a motion segment. This point remains fixed during rotation and is slightly different for each plane of rotation. In reality, motion is almost always multiplanar, but has been broken up into its component parts by convention and because the most commonly used tool to study kinematics, x-ray, images in one plane. The exact location of this point has been debated, but for practical purposes the instantaneous axis of rotation is in the anterior part of the inferior body of the motion segment in question. This location is probably most accurate for flexion-extension and axial rotation,[9,21,22] while lateral bending has not been studied as extensively. The instantaneous axis of rotation for occipital-atlantal motion is somewhat different. As described by

TABLE 77-1 Range of Motion of the Cervical Spine

	Representative Angles (in Degrees)		
	Combined Flexion/Extension	**Lateral Bending**	**Axial Rotation**
Occ-C1	25	5	5
C1-C2	20	5	40
C2-C3	10	10	3
C3-C4	15	11	7
C4-C5	20	11	7
C5-C6	20	8	7
C6-C7	17	7	6
C7-T1	9	4	2

SOURCE: Modified from White and Panjabi[9]

Henke in 1863, it is found just above the tip of the dens for flexion-extension and 2 to 3 cm above the dens for lateral bending.[9,23]

The full range of motion of the cervical spine is not limited to considering each motion separately. Instead, rotational and translational motions frequently are combined to produce complex neck movements.[24] "Coupling" refers to the consistent and simultaneous occurrence of motion about one axis with motion about another axis. In vivo "pure" motion rarely occurs, but rather a main motion predominates, and a coupled motion or motions accompany that motion. Panjabi and coworkers delineated the three-dimensional nature of cervical spine motion by measuring load displacement curves for cadaveric specimens subjected to "pure" loads. They found that with anterior and posterior loading the main motion was translation, and the coupled motions were flexion (with anterior loads) and extension (with posterior loads). After right and left lateral loads, the main motion was lateral translation and the primary coupled motion was axial rotation. Finally, when the spine was rotated about the *y* axis (axial rotation), lateral bending was the coupled motion observed.[25]

Instability

An "unstable" cervical spine is a concept that refers not only to acute posttraumatic instability but also to delayed posttraumatic instability. Clinical instability, as defined by White and Panjabi, is the loss of the ability of the spine to maintain its orientation so that there is no initial or subsequent neurological injury, no deformity, and no incapacitating pain during normal activity.[9] However, the posttraumatic cervical spine may not fall into an obviously "stable" or "unstable" classification, but there may be a continuum where the spine, if subjected to repeated loads, would eventually fail.[26] In vivo, the cervical spine is exposed to multiaxial forces that can be broken down into components in the laboratory. Load-to-failure characteristics of the cervical spine have been defined for the different planes of movement. In general, ligaments tend to fail under tensile or shear forces, but not under compressive forces.[27–29]

Based on the clinical history, the neurological examination and radiographs, a determination of instability often can be made if the biomechanics of the injury are considered. Static and dynamic radiographs have been the mainstay for determining instability in the past. While ligaments are not directly visualized, ligamentous integrity can frequently, but not always, be assessed.

In the upper cervical spine, the integrity of the transverse atlantal ligament (TAL) is the primary determinant of stability, and frequently can be deduced from x-rays. Fielding and associates demonstrated that if the atlanto-dental interval (distance from anterior arch to dens) is > 3 to 4 mm in adults on a lateral radiograph, then the TAL probably is ruptured.[30] Likewise, on an anteroposterior film, if the total overhang of the lateral masses of C1 on C2 is > 7 mm, then the TAL is incompetent.[31] More recently, Dickman and coworkers have also noted the utility of magnetic resonance imaging (MRI) in the assessment of the status of the TAL.[32] Other cogent findings can be gleaned from x-ray when assessing upper cervical spine stability and are listed in Table 77-2.

TABLE 77-2 Radiographic Findings of Occiput-Atlas-Axis Instability

Occiput-C1 axial rotation (one side)	>8°
Occiput-C1 translation	>1 mm movement in flexion/extension
C1-C2 lateral displacement (overhang)	>7 mm total
Atlanto-dental interval	>4 mm
C1-C2 axial rotation	>45°
C1 spine canal diameter	<13 mm

SOURCE: Modified from White and Panjabi[9]

Instability after lower cervical spine trauma has been considered in the context of a three-column[33,34] or a two-column approach.[9,35] In one of the most thorough analyses of ligamentous instability, Panjabi and colleagues employed the two-column theory. They defined the anterior elements as the posterior longitudinal ligament (PLL) and all ligaments anterior to it. The posterior elements were composed of all ligaments posterior to the PLL. From this study, in which they sequentially cut all ligaments, they concluded that if all the posterior elements alone or all the anterior elements alone are incompetent, then instability potentially exists.[35] When applying this two-column approach to clinical situations, one entire column plus one ligamentous structure must be functioning to maintain stability.

Louis describes a three-column theory for assessing stability of the cervical spine. The anterior column is composed of the intervertebral discs, the vertebral bodies, and the ligaments attached to the anterior and posterior aspect of the bodies. A middle column is not a part of this theory, but there are two posterior columns. The posterior columns are mirror images of one another and are comprised of the facet complex on one side, the adjacent lamina, and the ligaments that interconnect the posterior arch on that side. Disruption of any two columns renders the affected motion segment unstable. Louis qualifies instability by differentiating between "permanent ligamentous" and "temporary bony instability." Thus, even if two columns are disrupted, but the injury is predominantly osseous, stability often can be achieved without surgery after a period of immobilization.[33]

Several authors have attempted to assign relative values to abnormal findings of static and dynamic radiographs.[36] This is a useful approach that encourages an overall evaluation of spinal instability by assessing its component parts. The radiographic abnormalities of >11 degrees of sagittal plane translation and >3.5 mm of sagittal plane translation were derived experimentally by White and colleagues and carry a high relative value toward the diagnosis of instability.[16] Other radiographic abnormalities suggestive of instability include interspinous widening, loss of facet parallelism, 50 percent compression of the vertebral body, and loss of the normal cervical lordosis.[33,36] In addition to static x-ray studies, dynamic radiographs indirectly suggest ligamentous injury if excessive translation or angulation is identified.[37] MRI also has been employed in an effort to identify ligamentous injury and may prove useful when the diagnosis of instability is in question.[38]

In addition to radiological criteria, clinical findings such as a neurological deficit must be factored into the diagnostic schema. The presence of a neurological deficit after cervical spine trauma implies that the spinal cord or nerve roots were subjected to either a vascular, mechanical, or chemical insult. Raynor and Koplik propose that the type of neurological injury is directly related to the magnitude of the applied force. For example, milder forces would produce a root syndrome and greater forces would produce a complete physiological transection.[39] Another determinant of the risk of neurological deficit after a traumatic event is the spinal canal diameter. Eismont and colleagues demonstrated that individuals with small sagittal canal diameters were much more likely than those with large canals to suffer neurological dysfunction after cervical fracture dislocations. They found the average sagittal spinal canal diameter of all patients studied to be largest at C1 (23.9 mm) and smallest at C6 (17.7 mm).[40] Clinical instability is not guaranteed in the traumatic case with neurological injury, but in this setting the clinician should certainly be atuned to the radiological clues that might confirm the diagnosis of instability. White and Panjabi suggest that if the trauma is severe enough to result in a neurological deficit, then the integrity of the supporting structures has been altered, possibly permitting reinjury, and represents an unstable spine.[9]

BIOMECHANICAL CONSIDERATIONS IN SPECIFIC INJURIES

Both experimental models and clinical experience have been used in an effort to correlate the mechanism of injury with an expected injury pattern. The biomechanics of some of the more common injuries to the cervical spine have been well characterized, but others have not. Radiographic evaluation often permits identification of the osseous injury, but ligamentous injuries must be deduced indirectly. Understanding the biomechanics of the trauma greatly facilitates recognition of instability associated with cervical spine trauma and allows proper treatment.

Traumatic cervical spine injuries are best divided into upper and lower cervical lesions, since the anatomy and kinematics of these regions differ so much. The mechanism of the injury may, however, be similar in some upper and lower cervical spine traumatic injuries. Factors that dictate where the injury lies are not always clear, but may be related to variations in the strength of the dens or other osseous elements, the supporting musculature, or the spinal canal size.[40]

Most of our understanding of specific injuries comes from retrospective reviews of patients who incurred similar injuries, emphasizing the radiographic findings. While this is very useful information, experimental data on several injuries have greatly enhanced our understanding of the mechanism of injury, the likelihood of stability of the injury, and the usual outcome. Both of these sources are referred to in this discussion of specific injury patterns.

Upper Cervical Spine

Atlanto-occipital Dislocations

Dislocations in this region are usually associated with high energy trauma and often are fatal. They are being diagnosed with increased frequency, however, probably because of improved emergency medical services.[41] Atlanto-occipital dislocations are more common in children than in adults. In children, the occipital condyles are poorly developed, and therefore are not well seated in the lateral mass of the atlas. This makes the atlanto-occipital articulation less stable and more susceptible to dislocation.[9,41] These dislocations represent a group of injuries classified as anterior, posterior, or longitudinal separation by Treynalis and coworkers.[42] Owing to this injury's frequent association with immediate death, its biomechanics are poorly understood.

Anterior dislocation, the most common type in this group, is felt to be caused predominantly by anterior translation, although there may be a component of hyperflexion as well. Conversely, a posterior dislocation occurs as a result of posterior translation, but has been described in association with a fracture of the posterior arch of the atlas, implying a hyperextension element as well.[43] The longitudinal separation or distraction type most likely has a major injury vector in the y axis, but has not been studied in the laboratory.

Fractures of the Atlas

The Jefferson fracture is the best known of the atlantal fractures, involving fractures in two, three, or four places in the ring of the atlas.[44] Two- or three-part fractures are most common and may be located anterior and posterior or, if the force is directed more posteriorly, may be confined to the posterior arch.

The major injury vector in most atlantal fractures is in the *y* axis (axial compression), typically secondary to a direct blow to the vertex of the head (Fig. 77-5). With rotation about the *x* axis in a negative direction (hyperextension), the posterior arch becomes compressed between the occiput and the posterior arch of the axis, often resulting in a fracture of the posterior ring of the atlas.[1]

Fractures of the atlas are typically stable, treated successfully in a Philadelphia collar alone. However, if greater than 7 mm of combined lateral displacement exists radiographically, then the transverse ligament is torn,[45] and the injury is unstable. Despite the incompetent transverse ligament, these injuries typically heal in a halo brace.[46]

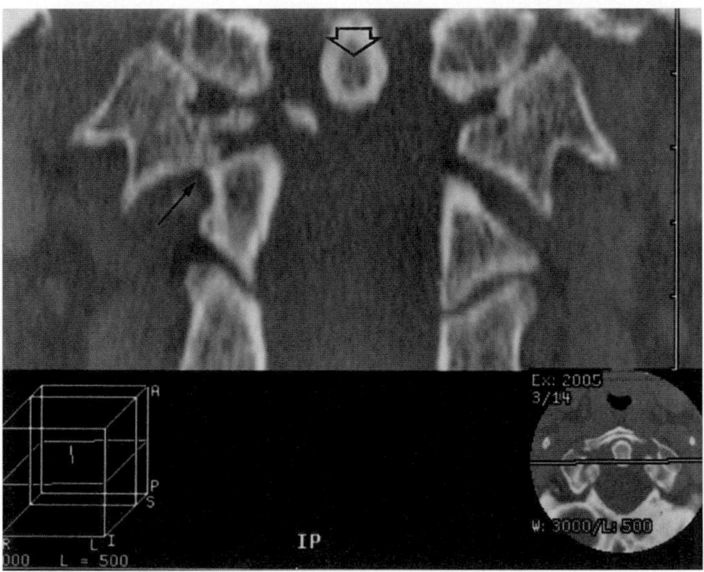

A

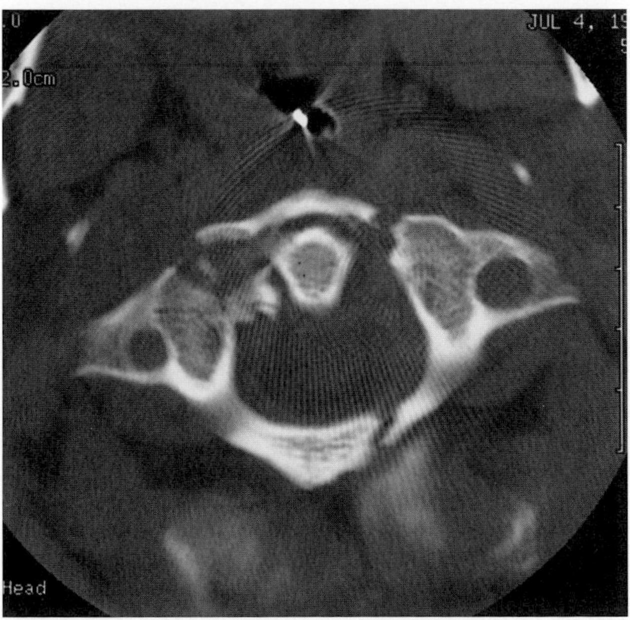

B

Figure 77-5. Radiographs of a 52-year-old man who was involved in a motor vehicle accident. *A*. Reformatted CT scan demonstrates a Jefferson fracture in the coronal plane. Note the malalignment of the lateral margin of the atlantoaxial joint on the right (*small arrow*). The presumed axial compression vector is illustrated by the large arrow. *B*. CT scan, axial cut, shows two fractures of the anterior arch (comminuted on the right) and one fracture of the posterior arch.

Atlanto-axial dislocations and subluxations

Displacements of C1 in relation to C2 secondary to trauma may be either anterior, posterior, or rotatory. They may be associated with fractures, and have different mechanisms.

The major injury vector required to produce an anterior dislocation is one of flexion and anterior translation. This is similar to the mechanism thought to be operative in producing an odontoid fracture with anterior subluxation. When C1–C2 anterior subluxation occurs without a dens fracture, the diameter of the spinal canal is compromised. While traumatic C1–C2 dislocations may be seen without an associated fracture, they are more likely to be associated with a dens fracture.[30,47]

Rotary subluxation is also rare and, as its name implies, due to rotational forces. Dvorak and coworkers implicated an alar ligament injury as a possible cause of C1–C2 rotary instability.[3] They suggested that the alar ligament might fail in a hyperflexion injury with the head also rotated opposite the ruptured ligament.

Traumatic atlanto-axial dislocations frequently are fatal, and therefore are seldom encountered in clinical practice. All the patients with C1–C2 dislocations (without fractures) studied by Fielding and colleagues had severe head injuries as well.[47] Owing to the severe ligamentous injury, these lesions are unstable.

Odontoid fractures

Fractures of the dens have been categorized into three groups by Anderson and D'Alonzo.[48] Since these three fracture types have different mechanisms of injury and different treatments and prognoses, this schema has proved clinically useful.

Type I odontoid fractures are very rare and consist of those fractures that extend obliquely through the tip of the dens. These fractures are stable at the C1–C2 level, but have been described in conjunction with a posterior atlanto-occipital dislocation.[43] The mechanism of injury of the Type I fracture has not been widely studied, but is believed to be due to a combination of translation and compression.[49] However, Althoff demonstrated that the direction of the force vector was the critical determinant of which type of odontoid fracture could be produced experimentally. He found that a fracture similar to Type I fractures would result if this force was applied from a lateral direction, 90 degrees to the midsagittal plane.[49] It has been suggested that Type I odontoid fractures be considered a radiographic sign of atlanto-occiput dislocation and, therefore, potentially unstable.[50]

Type II, the most common odontoid fracture, represents those fractures through the junction of the dens with the body of C2 or slightly higher. This injury may be associated with anterior displacement (most commonly) or with posterior displacement. In an experiment using the isolated axis, Doherty and colleagues recently studied the forces required to produce Type II fractures.[51] They found that a force applied on an oblique plane (45 degrees) between extension and lateral bending reliably produced Type II fractures.[51] Previous studies also implicated an obliquely-directed vector.[9,49,52] If an element of flexion coexisted, anterior subluxation was likely; if extension was combined with translation and directed obliquely, then posterior subluxation was likely. Treatment of Type II fractures is somewhat controversial and is discussed in another chapter.

Type III fractures have been produced experimentally after an anteroposteriorly applied force.[9,49,51,52] The fracture line in this injury runs through the body of C2, below the dens (Fig. 77-6). The Type III dens fracture is rarely unstable; successful fusion usually is possible by nonoperative means (halo bracing).

Traumatic spondylolisthesis of the axis

Traumatic spondylolisthesis of the axis has been well described, since it was the consistent result of judicial hanging. The "hangman's fracture," therefore, is an injury pattern that is fairly well understood. Today, this injury most commonly is due to motor vehicle accidents.

The hangman's fracture actually is a spectrum of injuries, all of which include a fracture bilaterally through the pars interarticularis or the pedicles. Depending on the extent of the injury, the anterior longitudinal ligament is typically torn at C2–C3, with resultant widening of the C2–C3 disc space. There may be C2–C3 subluxation and occasionally bilateral locked facets.[53] Because of the pars fracture, there is a separation of anterior bony elements from the posterior elements and, therefore, a low incidence of neural injury.

The mechanism of injury is thought principally to be one of extension and distraction[9,18] (Fig. 77-7). With these forces, the posterior elements are compressed, and the anterior elements are distracted. However, Saternus and Paul were able experimentally to produce hangman's fractures with a severe hyperflexion injury in isolated atlanto-axial segments.[54] This hyperflexion component may be responsible for the C2–C3 bilateral interfacetal dislocation occasionally seen in hangman's fracture.

Lower Cervical Spine

Injuries involving the subaxial cervical spine are probably best categorized according to the mechanism of injury believed to be involved. Obviously, combined

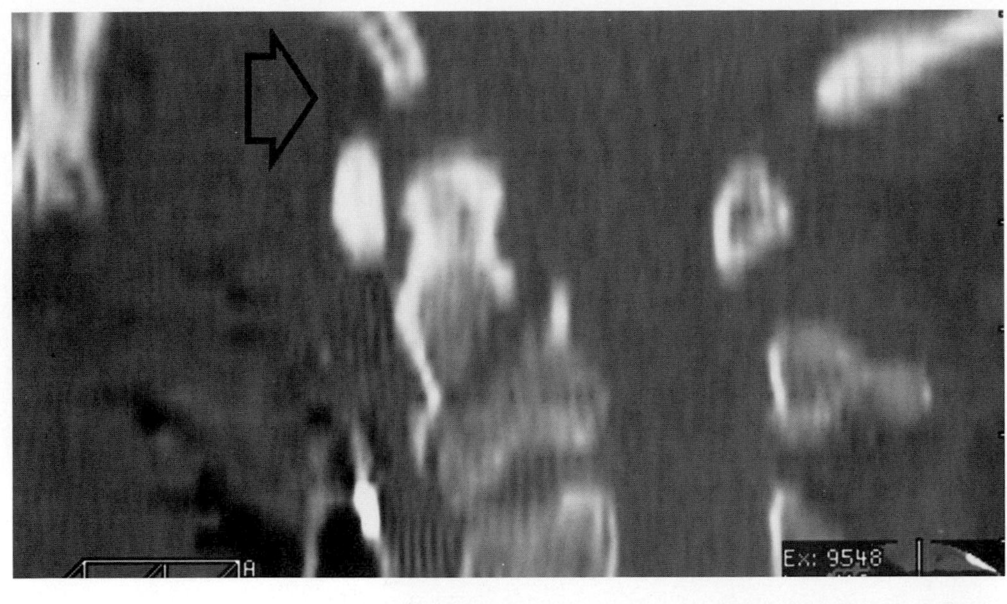

A

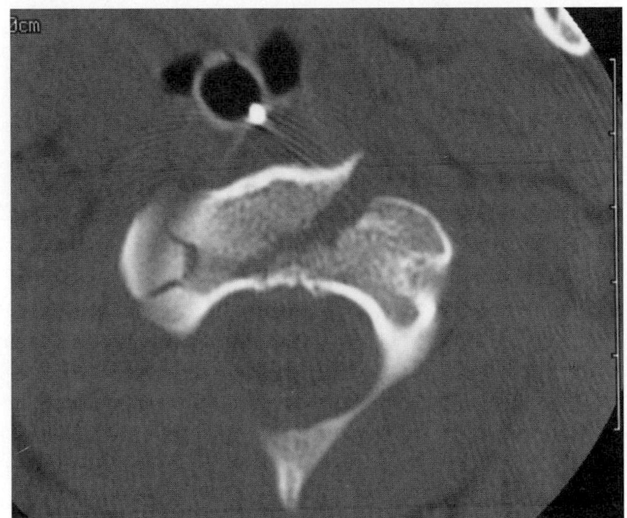

B

Figure 77-6. Radiographs of a young woman who was involved in a motor vehicle accident, striking her forehead on the windshield. *A*. Reformatted CT scan, midsagittal plane, shows a Type III odontoid fracture. The large arrow illustrates the major injury vector directed in an anteroposterior direction, which causes both translation and hyperextension. The injury vector is directed in the sagittal plane in Type III fractures, while the vector in Type II fractures is directed in an oblique plane. *B*. CT scan, axial image, reveals a fracture through the body of C2.

forces may be operative in a given injury pattern, but usually a major injury vector can be identified. Our discussion of the biomechanical considerations of injuries to this region will use a classification similar to that proposed by Allen and colleagues.[27] The mechanism of injury is the primary factor in this schema, while neck posture is considered only indirectly.

Vertical compression

This group of injuries has in common the major injury vector in the *y* axis (axial compression). Torg and coworkers showed that, owing to the normal lordosis of the cervical spine, a slightly flexed posture is required to align the spine vertically.[55] The resulting forces, therefore, impact the spine vertically along the instantaneous axis of rotation with little or no distractive or flexion forces being applied posteriorly or anteriorly. Compression or "burst" fractures are the most common result of an axially applied force, the vertebral body "exploding," possibly with retropulsion into the spinal canal. Alternatively, a simple wedge compression fracture may be produced, characterized by decreased anterior body height and possibly disruption of the superior or inferior endplate.[56] In cadaveric preparations, Selecki and Williams found that after an axial force the discs failed first, causing vertebral body fractures and often subsequent disruptions of the anterior and posterior longitudinal

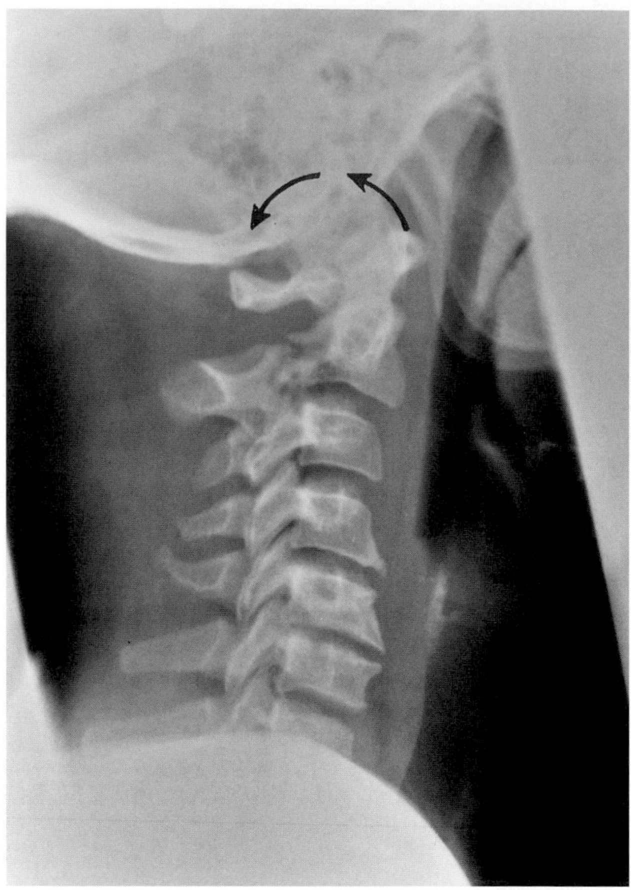

A

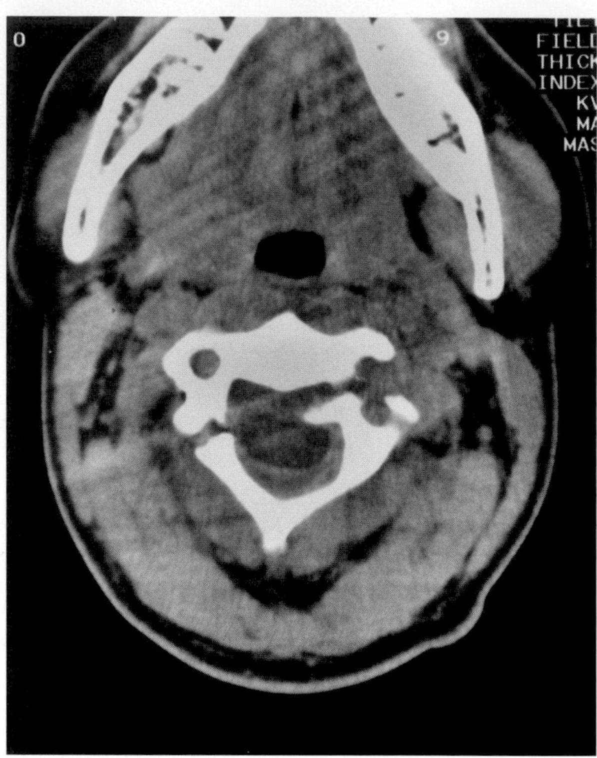

B

Figure 77-7. Radiographs of a 32-year-old woman who sustained a hyperextension injury. *A*. Lateral view shows the pedicle fracture. The presumed injury vector is depicted by the curved arrows, illustrating rotation about the *x* axis. *B*. CT scan, axial image, demonstrates the bilateral fractures.

ligaments.[57] Maiman and colleagues also studied compression injuries in cadavers. They demonstrated that higher forces were required to produce a true axial compression injury compared with flexion-compression or extension-compression injuries.[58] In addition, Panjabi and coworkers found it difficult to create "pure" vertical compression injuries in a porcine model. They did, however, find that vertical compression injuries are rarely unstable.[59] The vertebral body was typically fractured, but the ligaments were intact—the result being a stable injury.

Compression flexion

This group of injuries is common and includes the popularly-used category known as flexion "teardrop" fractures. According to Allen, this injury mechanism was the most likely to produce serious neurological deficit.[27,60] There is, however, a spectrum of severity, as is true of all cervical spine traumatic injuries.

The major injury vector is one of rotation about the *x* axis (flexion), but also an element of compression. The typical diving injury exemplifies this group of injuries. In this situation, the head is hyperflexed when it strikes the floor, and the cervical spine is subjected to a compressive force as well as accentuation of the hyperflexion (Fig. 77-8).

Mild compression flexion injuries primarily affect the anterior vertebral body and may be difficult to distinguish from a "pure" vertical compression injury. With more dramatic forces, the teardrop-shaped fracture of the anterior-inferior segment of the vertebral body may be seen involving the superior vertebra of the involved motion segment. Unfortunately, the posterior aspect of the vertebral body not uncommonly impinges on the spinal cord, causing complete paralysis or an anterior

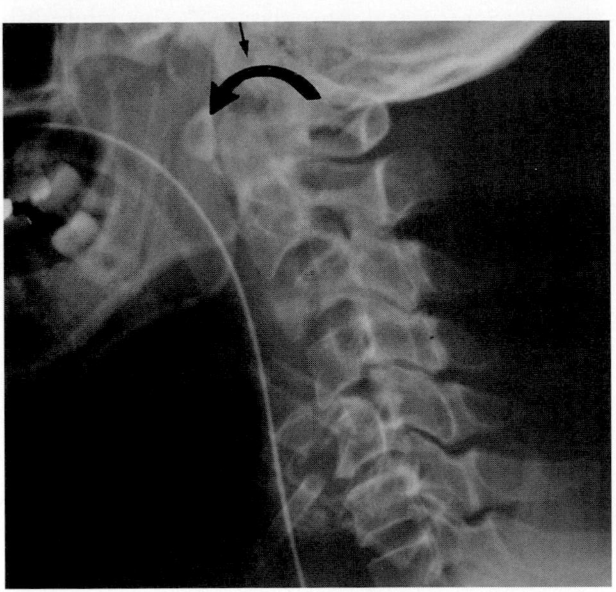

A

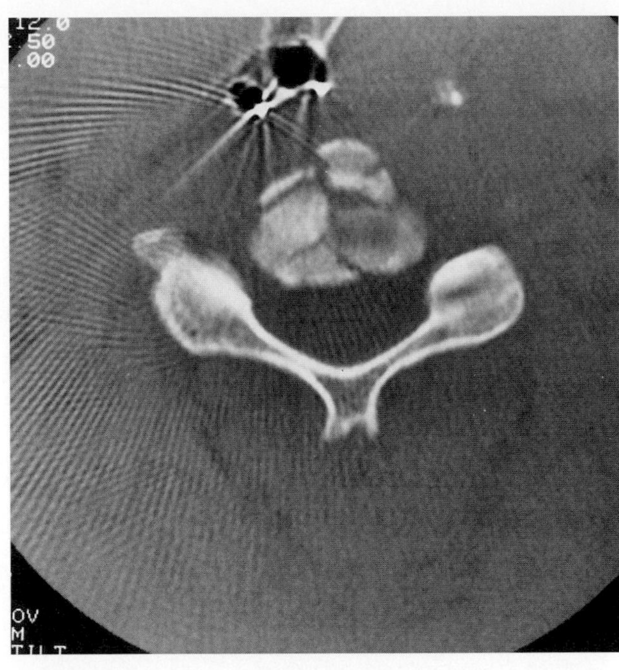

B

Figure 77-8. Radiographs of a 19-year-old man who suffered a compression flexion injury after a diving accident. *A*. Lateral view reveals a fracture of the anterior body of C3, with angulation and subluxation of C2–C3. The curved arrow depicts the flexion nature of the injury; the small arrow illustrates a compressive force acting on the hyperflexed neck. *B*. CT scan, axial image, shows the comminuted fracture of the C3 body.

spinal artery syndrome.[61,62] Posterior arch fractures occur in up to 50 percent of compression flexion injuries.[62]

While it is true that when flexion forces are imposed on the cervical spine an element of distraction occurs posteriorly, this usually does not produce posterior ligamentous injury in compression flexion lesions, as is typically the case in distractive flexion injuries. The compression flexion injuries typically heal in a halo brace, with bony ankylosis occurring in up to 90 percent.[60]

Distractive Flexion

Injuries categorized in this group are seen frequently clinically and range from the "hyperflexion sprain" to bilateral interfacetal dislocation (BID). In contrast to the compressive flexion injuries, there is a predominant rotation about the x axis (torque) with very little compression in this injury pattern. The injury has been described in the past as involving both anterior translation (shear) and flexion forces[63] (Fig. 77-9).

Pathologically, the posterior ligaments are injured early and may be evident radiographically as a widened interspinous distance.[56] Depending on the extent of the trauma, the facet capsules and anterior ligaments may fail as well, resulting in a three-column injury. If there is also an axial rotation or lateral bending component, then unilateral locked facets are likely. While vertebral body fractures are uncommon with distractive flexion injuries, laminar fractures do occur, and were reported in 40 percent of cases of BID.[27]

Since distractive flexion forces principally injure ligamentous structures, often in all three columns, this group of injuries usually is unstable. The hyperflexion sprain is a milder injury of the posterior ligaments or musculature that often heals with conservative management.

Compressive Extension

Hyperextension injuries represent a spectrum of lesions that commonly occur after cervical spine trauma. The mechanism of injury most frequently operative is one of vertical compression with the head in an extended posture.[64]

In Allen's original description, a unilateral vertebral arch fracture was one of the most common injuries and is due to compressive extension forces.[27] With more severe trauma secondary to this major injury vector, anterior ligamentous injury or a fracture-dislocation may be seen. In this situation, the compressive

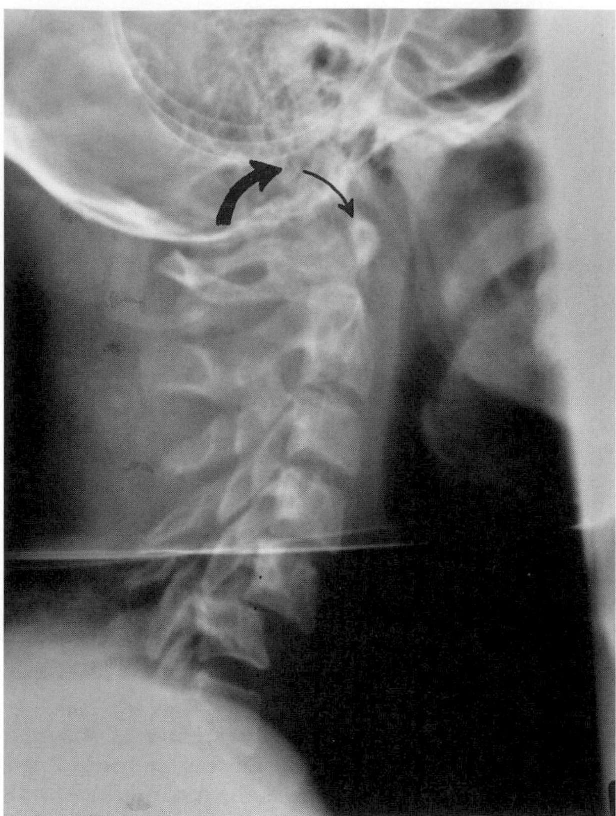

Figure 77-9. Radiographs of a 28-year-old woman who was unrestrained in the back of a pick-up involved in a rear-end collision. This resulted in a C5–C6 bilateral facet dislocation. The large arrow illustrates the hyperflexion load, resulting in some distraction, but little or no compression. As was true in this patient, this injury often causes severe neurological deficit.

forces account for the fractures of the lateral masses, pedicles and lamina, but the extension component causes an avulsion of the superior aspect of the body of the inferior vertebra. Maiman and Yoganandan have shown experimentally that the anterior longitudinal ligament may be injured prior to fractures of the posterior elements.[7] Instability, if present, usually is anterior in compressive extension lesions. However, the milder forms of isolated vertebral arch fractures often are unaccompanied by anterior ligamentous injury and are stable.

Distractive extension

Hyperextension injuries without a compressive element are due to angular displacement about the x axis in the sagittal plane. Several defined injury patterns are best classified in this group. One such injury, whiplash, a commonly used term, is due primarily to hyperextension and may or may not be preceded by hyperflexion.[65] In an experimentally produced whiplash model, Macnab found injuries to the anterior longitudinal ligament (ALL) most commonly, but often found minor tears in the anterior cervical musculature.[66] This injury usually is stable, although this varies with the extent of the ligamentous injury.

Another common scenario for this injury pattern is the elderly patient who falls, strikes the forehead, and suffers an acute cervical spinal cord injury, often with normal radiographs. Marar and Orth studied this injury pattern and suggested that a transient subluxation occurs with a "pinching" of the spinal cord between the vertebral body and the infolded ligamentum flavum.[67] Radiographic evidence of this injury pattern may be subtle; often only widening of the anterior disc space is identified. Since the anterior elements are subjected to distractive forces, the ALL is commonly ruptured, although occasionally facet dislocation also is seen.[67,68] Distractive extension injuries are stable in flexion, but, with disruption of the ALL, are unstable in extension.

Lateral flexion

This group of injuries typically results from an asymmetrically applied compressive force. The cervical spine is bent laterally; because of physiological coupling, it also is rotated axially. This injury may be seen after a blow to the side of the head during football or in a motor vehicle accident.

On the side where the head and neck are bent, the lateral aspect of the body, the lateral mass, and ipsilateral lamina are subjected to compressive forces; the opposite side is under distractive forces. Common sequelae include lateral mass fractures (often sagittally oriented),[69] asymmetric vertebral body fractures, laminar fractures, and possibly unilateral interfacetal dislocation on the side sustaining the distractive forces.[70]

Lee and Woodring reviewed the radiographs of patients with lateral mass fractures and noted a relatively high incidence of neurological deficit (45 percent), and instability (59 percent). Owing to the proximity of the vertebral artery, they also recognized vertebral artery injuries in association with some lateral mass fractures.[69] Lateral flexion injuries were thought to be uncommon,[27] but increasingly are being recognized as likely due to the increased use of CT scanning in the assessment of cervical spinal trauma.[69]

BIOMECHANICAL CONCERNS IN STABILIZATION

Stabilization can be achieved to varying degrees in the cervical spine using external orthoses and internal fixation. Internal fixation has the advantage of providing immediate stabilization, with the rigidity of the stabilization varying among the different techniques. We will review some of the biomechanical characteristics of external orthoses and surgical fixation of the upper and lower cervical spine. This discussion will include data concerning some of the newer spinal implants and comparisons of the various techniques.

External Orthoses

External orthotic devices have been utilized as the sole treatment of cervical spine traumatic injuries or as an adjunct to surgical stabilization. The ability of the various external orthoses to immobilize the cervical spine varies greatly in the three planes of rotation, but also varies within regions of the cervical spine. The more common cervical orthoses, listed in order of least to greatest immobilization afforded, are: soft collar; Philadelphia collar; SOMI (Sternal-Occipital-Mandibular-Immobilizer) brace; four-poster brace; rigid cervicothoracic brace; halo vest; and Minerva body jacket.[71–74]

Johnson and coworkers evaluated the ability to control cervical motion of most of these external orthoses and found immobilization properties similar to those just listed. Using both photographic techniques and x-ray, they were able to quantitate the amount of restricted motion in flexion-extension, lateral bending, and axial rotation. In patients wearing the halo vest, motion was limited to 4 percent of normal in flexion-extension and lateral bending, and to 1 percent of normal in axial rotation. The halo was most effective in the upper cervical spine. The SOMI brace limited flexion in the upper cervical spine, albeit less than the halo, but was relatively less rigid in extension. In the lower cervical region, the cervicothoracic brace was the most effective of the non-halo devices in controlling motion. None of the orthoses, except the halo vest, proved very effective in limiting lateral bending.[71] The Minerva body jacket was not studied by Johnson and colleagues, but probably is as effective at immobilizing as the halo.[72,73]

The halo has been shown to be effective in limiting overall cervical motion by other investigators, but, when movements at each intervertebral level are added, even the halo permits substantial movement.[73,75,76] The phenomenon of "snaking" or serpentine movement is thought to account for the ability of the rigidly immobilized cervical spine to flex at some levels and extend at others while overall movement is minimal. Benzel and coworkers compared "snaking" in patients immobilized with the halo brace and those in a Minerva body jacket. They found 5.2 degrees of overall movement in flexion-extension for both groups, but 23.4 degrees for the halo compared to 14.8 degrees for the Minerva body jacket when the sum of each intervertebral level was evaluated. Motion in the upper cervical spine is poorly controlled by most of the non-halo orthoses. In fact, the only orthosis that effectively controls occiput-C1 motion is the halo vest.[77] Lower cervical spine motion can be more effectively controlled with several of the external orthoses; however, the halo and Minerva body jacket provide the most resistance to motion in this region of the cervical spine as well.

General Biomechanical Principles of Internal Fixation

The goal when applying internal fixation is to achieve an osseous union, thereby stabilizing the motion segment in question. The strength of spinal fusions has been shown to be improved relative to the rigidity of the implant.[78–81] However, all implants ultimately will fail if bony fusion does not occur.[82]

Whether to place the fusion anteriorly or posteriorly is dictated by the location of the instability. Posterior fusions have been performed with good results in the lower cervical spine and with variable results in the upper cervical spine.[83] Typically the fusion mass is secured with wire or laid over the area to be fused, but may be put under compression if placed between adjacent posterior arches. Posterior fusions rely heavily on the method of internal fixation for immediate stability. Anterior intervertebral bone grafts act as spacers and can act to resist compressive forces, but do not resist tensile forces. Internal stabilization of the cervical spine with wire has been used since it was first described by Hadra in 1891,[84] and continues to be an effective method of fixation. Larger wires typically are stronger, and twisting the wire improves the strength of the wire construct.[85] In fact, using double-stranded twisted wire permits the use of smaller wire with superior tensile strength.[86] Newer multistranded cables appear to be stronger than wire and also are more malleable, which makes passage technically easier.[87]

Since internal fixation using screws alone or with some type of plate is being employed increasingly, some general biomechanical principles of screw fixation should be considered. The strength of the screw and, therefore, the construct, depends on several factors. Ideally, the screw will not bend, break, or pull out, and will provide rigid internal fixation, which in turn increases the likelihood of an osseous union. The pull-out strength is determined primarily by the length of the screw, with long, wide screws being best in this regard.[78,80,88] Bicortical screw purchase has been suggested to improve resistance to pull-out.[89,90] Although probably true in the lateral mass,[91] this has been questioned in relation to the anterior cervical spine.[92] The bending strength of the screw is determined primarily by the minor, or inner, diameter.[78,80,88] Finally, the weakest location of an implant secured with screws is the bone-screw interface.[78]

Upper Cervical Spine

The internal fixation of traumatic instability in the upper cervical spine has consisted primarily of posterior constructs. However, odontoid or atlanto-axial screw fixation can be performed from an anterior approach. In addition, an onlay occipital-atlantal fusion can be performed anteriorly, but rarely is required and achieves no immediate stability. The exposure for bilateral anterior C1–C2 screw fixation is difficult; thus, this procedure is infrequently employed. This technique would appear to be very rigid; however, no biomechanical studies have evaluated this procedure. With recent advances in biplanar fluoroscopy, anterior odontoid screw fixation is being used with increased frequency. Doherty and coworkers have performed the only biomechanical analysis of this technique to date.[51] Using isolated C2 vertebrae, they created Type II and Type III fractures and placed a single screw across the fracture site, achieving bicortical purchase. They tested for multidirectional stability and load-to-failure and found stiffness and load-to-failure approximately one-half that of the intact specimens. The load-to-failure of an isolated screw was found to be about one-fourth that of an intact odontoid. Most surgeons, however, attempt to place two screws if the size of the odontoid permits, which probably constitutes a stiffer constant.[93] The primary biomechanical advantage of the anterior odontoid screw fixation over posterior C1–C2 arthrodesis is the preservation of C1–C2 motion (very important in rotation).

Posterior fixation techniques frequently are utilized to treat occipitocervical and atlantoaxial instability. Occipitocervical fusion is rarely required after trauma and should be avoided unless occipital-atlantal instability is present. A fusion from occiput to C2 greatly limits cervical flexion-extension and axial rotation. Upper cervical spinal instability after trauma is much more common at C1–C2 than at the occiput-C1; therefore, internal fixation usually does not require inclusion of the occiput.

Posterior atlantoaxial arthrodesis has been performed using a variety of techniques. Some of these techniques have been subjected to biomechanical tests in the laboratory.[81,94,95] Grob and coworkers compared the multidirectional stability of a Gallie-type fusion, a Brooks-type fusion, posterior C1–C2 transarticular screws, and interlaminar clamps. They found the stability in flexion-extension to be equal in all constructs except the Gallie fusion, which was significantly weaker. Also, when analyzing axial rotation and lateral bending the posterior C1–C2 screws allowed the least motion of all the constructs tested.[96] Montesano and associates support this contention, finding the posterior C1–C2 screws to be stiffer in rotation compared with the Gallie technique. They also demonstrated anteroposterior translation after the Gallie fusion, but no translation in the specimens treated with transarticular screws.[81] The clinical correlate of these biomechanical findings is that the C1–C2 transarticular screws probably are the stiffest of the posterior C1–C2 fusions, implying a higher likelihood of fusion; but the patient's axial rotation is limited more than in the other procedures.[83] The Gallie fusion, which is the most commonly used technique,[97] provides the least amount of immediate stability; if employed, it probably should be supplemented with a halo brace.[98]

Lower Cervical Spine

A vast array of surgical constructs are presently available for stabilizing the lower cervical spine. Anterior constructs consist of plating systems, interbody grafts, and polymethylmethacrylate (PMMA). An extensive list of posterior techniques includes wiring procedures, plates (lateral mass and hook plates), clamps, and PMMA. The biomechanical properties of some of these procedures have been studied and are an important foundation for the selection of the appropriate technique for a given patient. In lower cervical spine trauma, decompression of a spinal cord or root-compromising mass takes precedence over immediate stabilization and dictates whether an anterior or posterior procedure needs to be undertaken initially. More commonly, closed reduction can be achieved without a decompression procedure. Since a flexion injury is the most common mechanism,[27] resultant posterior ligamentous incompetence often must be addressed surgically. We will review some of the pertinent biomechanics of the posterior techniques.

Using isolated vertebrae with ligaments removed, Roy-Camille and colleagues evaluated several posterior fixation techniques under flexion and extension loads. Their findings suggested that interspinous wiring techniques are not effective under extension forces and vary in effectiveness in resisting flexion stresses. Interspinous wiring without a bone graft increases stability in flexion to 33 percent of normal, but is 88 percent of normal if wired through the facets. Lateral mass plates increased stability in flexion to 97 percent of normal, but also provided some resistance in extension, increasing stability by 60 percent.[99]

Gill and coworkers evaluated Rogers interspinous wiring, Halifax interlaminar clamps, and lateral mass plates using cadaveric specimens. They showed that lateral mass plates with bicortical purchase were the stiffest construct, but this did not prove to be statistically significant.[91] Similar findings were obtained by Coe and associates, who also tested Bohlman's triple wiring technique, sublaminar wires, and hook plates, but did not evaluate interlaminar clamps. They concluded that the hook plate and lateral mass plate offered improved control of rotational forces, but overall found all the posterior constructs to be equally effective in resisting flexion, extension, and axial loading.[100] Their group appropriately advises against sublaminar wiring since it provides no biomechanical advantage and has the highest risk of the posterior fixation techniques.[100,101]

Anterior cervical instrumentation has been utilized to treat unstable compression flexion and distractive flexion injuries,[102–104] often in conjunction with a decompressive corpectomy.[103] Cabenela and Ebersol reported successful fusions using anterior cervical plate stabilization for compression flexion injuries. They did, however, use the halo vest as an adjuvant postoperatively, which may have contributed to their success.[103]

Several authors have questioned the use of anterior plate stabilization for flexion injuries,[81,100,105] basing their arguments on biomechanical data. Sutterlin and co-workers tested anterior cervical plates applied to intact motion segments and to motion segments after a simulated distractive flexion injury. They subjected these specimens to both static and cyclical loads. The authors concluded that anterior cervical plates were stiff in extension, but were inadequate in resisting axial and flexion loads, often noting resubluxation of the specimen.[105] Montesano and colleagues results were similar, demonstrating that posterior wiring techniques are superior to anterior plates in resisting flexion.[81] Based on these biomechanical studies, anterior cervical plating alone may not be the ideal method to treat cervical flexion injuries. Conversely, in three-column cervical spine injuries treated with posterior fixation alone, the posterior stabilization may be ineffective, and both a posterior and an anterior fixation on occasion may be required.[106]

References

1. Shapiro R, Youngberg AS, Rothman SLG: The differential diagnosis of traumatic lesions of the occipito-atlanto-axial segment. *Radiol Clin North Am* 1973; 11:505–526.
2. Fielding JW: Cineroentgenography of the normal cervical spine. *J Bone Joint Surg* 1957; 39A:1280–1288.
3. Dvorak J, Panjabi M, Gerber M, Wichmann W: CT-functional diagnosis of rotatory instability of the upper cervical spine. An experimental study on cadavers. *Spine* 1987; 12(3):197–205.
4. Panjabi MM, Dvorak J, Duranceau J, et al: Three-dimensional movements of the upper cervical spine. *Spine* 1988; 13(7):726–730.
5. Dvorak J, Schneider E, Saldinger P, Rahn B: Biomechanics of the craniocervical region: the alar and transverse ligaments. *J Orthop Res* 1988; 6:452–461.
6. Dvorak J, Panjabi MM: Functional anatomy of the alar ligaments. *Spine* 1987; 12:183–189.
7. Maiman DJ, Yoganandan N: Biomechanics of cervical spine trauma. *Clin Neurosurg* 1991; 37:543–570.
8. Rolander SD, Blair WE: Deformation and fracture of the lumbar vertebral end-plate. *Orthop Clin North Am* 1975; 6:75–81.
9. White AA III, Panjabi M: *Clinical Biomechanics of the Spine* (2d ed). Philadelphia: JB Lippincott, 1990.
10. Milne N: The role of zygapophyseal joint orientation and uncinate processes in controlling motion in the cervical spine. *J Anat* 1991; 178:189–201.
11. Delashaw JB, Knego RS, Jane JA: Lumbar disc disease. *Perspect Neurol Surg* 1992; 3(2):1–37.
12. Humzah MD, Soames RW: Human intervertebral disc: Structure and function. *Anat Rec* 1988; 220:337–356.
13. Pal GP, Sherk HH: The vertical stability of the cervical spine. *Spine* 1987; 13(5):447–449.
14. Buckwalter JA, Cooper RR, Maynard JA: Elastic fibers in human intervertebral discs. *J Bone Joint Surg* 1976; 58A:73–76.
15. Nachemson A, Evans J: Some mechanical properties of the third lumbar inter-laminar ligament (ligamentum flavum). *J Biomech* 1968; 1:211–220.
16. White AA III, Johnson RM, Panjabi MM, Southwick WO: Biomechanical analysis of clinical stability in the cervical spine. *Clin Orthop* 1975; 109:85–96.
17. Yoganandan N, Sances A, Maiman DJ, et al: Experimental spinal injuries with vertical impact. *Spine* 1986; 11:855–860.
18. Miz G: Cervical spine instability and biomechanics of treatment, in Errico TJ, Bauer RD, Waugh T (eds): *Spinal Trauma*. Philadelphia: JB Lippincott, 1991: 123–143.
19. Panjabi MM, White AA III, Brand RA: A note on defining body parts configurations. *J Biomech* 1974; 7:385–394.
20. Werne S: Studies in spontaneous atlas dislocation. *Acta Orthop Scand* 1957; 23(suppl):1–150.
21. Lysell E: Motion in the cervical spine. *Acta Orthop Scand* 1969; 123(Suppl):1–61.
22. Dimnet J, Pasquet A, Krag MH, Panjabi MM: Cervical spine motion in the sagittal plane: Kinematics and geometric parameters. *J Biomech* 1982; 15:959–969.
23. Henke W: *Handbuch der Anatomie and Mechanic der Gelenke mit Rucksicht auf Luxationen und Contracturen*. Leipzig, Heidelberg: CF Winter, 1863.
24. Alund M, Larsson SE: Three dimensional analysis of neck motion: A clinical method. *Spine* 1990; 15:87–91.
25. Panjabi MM, Summer DJ, Pelker RR, et al: Three-dimensional load-displacement curves due to forces on the cervical spine. *J Orthop Res* 1986; 4:152–161.
26. Yoganandan N, Maiman DJ, Pintar F, et al: Microtrauma in the lumbar spine: A cause of low back pain. *Neurosurgery* 1988; 23:162–168.
27. Allen BL, Ferguson RL, Lehmann TR, O'Brien RP: A mechanistic classification of closed, indirect fractures and dislocations of the lower cervical spine. *Spine* 1982; 7(1):1–27.

28. King AI, Vulcan AP: Elastic deformation characteristics of the spine. *J Biomech* 1971; 4:413–429.
29. Noyes FR, Delucas JL, Torvik PJ: Biomechanics of anterior cruciate ligament failure: An analysis of strain rate sensitivity and mechanisms of failure in primates. *J Bone Joint Surg* 1974; 56A:236–253.
30. Fielding JW, Cochran GVB, Lawsing JF III, Hohl M: Tears of the transverse ligament of the atlas: A clinical and biomechanical study. *J Bone Joint Surg (Am)* 1974; 56:1683–1691.
31. Spence KF, Decker S, Sell KW: Bursting atlantal fracture associated with rupture of the transverse ligament. *J Bone Joint Surg (Am)* 1970; 52:543–549.
32. Dickman CA, Mamourian A, Sonntag VKH, Drayer BP: Magnetic resonance imaging of the transverse atlantal ligament for the evaluation of atlantoaxial instability. *J Neurosurg* 1991; 75:221–227.
33. Louis R: Stability and instability of the cervical spine, in Kehr P, Weidner A (eds): *Cervical Spine I.* New York: Springer-Verlag, 1987: 21–27.
34. Denis F: Spinal instability as defined by the three-column spine concept in acute spinal trauma. *Clin Orthop Rel Res* 1984; 189:65–76.
35. Panjabi MM, White AA III, Johnson RM: Cervical spine biomechanics as a function of transection of components. *J Biomech* 1975; 8:327–336.
36. Webb JK, Broughton RBK, McSweeny T, Park WM: Hidden flexion injury of the cervical spine. *J Bone Joint Surg* 1976; 58B:322–326.
37. Dvorak J, Froehlich D, Penning L, et al: Functional radiographic diagnosis of the cervical spine: Flexion/extension. *Spine* 1988; 13(7):748–755.
38. Ignelzi RJ: The potential role of low field MR with open design in assessing ligamentous injury in acute cervical trauma. *Surg Neurol* 1993; 39:519–529.
39. Raynor RB, Koplik B: Cervical cord trauma. The relationship between clinical syndromes and force of injury. *Spine* 1985; 10(3):193–197.
40. Eismont FJ, Clifford S, Goldberg M, Green B: Cervical sagittal spinal canal size in spine injury. *Spine* 1984; 9(7):663–666.
41. Reisner A, O'Brien MS: Atlanto-occipital dislocation. *Contemp Neurosurg* 1992; 14(8):1–8.
42. Treynalis VC, Mararo GD, Dunker RO, et al: Traumatic atlanto-occipital dislocation: Case report. *J Neurosurg* 1986; 65:863–870.
43. Eismont FJ, Bohlman HH: Posterior atlanto-occipital dislocations with fractures of the atlas and odontoid process. *J Bone Joint Surg* 1978; 60A(3):397–399.
44. Alker GJ, Oh YS, Leslie EV, et al: Postmortem radiology of head and neck injuries in fatal traffic accidents. *Radiology* 1975; 114:611–616.
45. Spence KF, Decker S, Sell KW: Bursting atlantal fracture associated with rupture of the transverse ligament. *J Bone Joint Surg (Am)* 1970; 52:543–549.
46. Sonntag VKH, Douglas RA: Management of spinal cord trauma. *Neurosurg Clin North Am* 1990; 1(3):729–750.
47. Fielding JW, Hawkins RJ, Ratzan SA: Spine fusion for atlanto-axial instability. *J Bone Joint Surg* 1976; 58A:400–407.
48. Anderson LD, D'Alonzo RT: Fractures of the odontoid process of the axis. *J Bone Joint Surg* 1974; 56A:1163–1174.
49. Althoff B: Fracture of the odontoid process. *Acta Orthop Scand* 1979; 177(suppl):1–95.
50. Scott EW, Haid RW Jr, Peace D: Type I fractures of the odontoid process: Implications for atlanto-occipital instability. *J Neurosurg* 1990; 72:488–492.
51. Doherty BJ, Heggeness MH, Esses SI: A biomechanical study of odontoid fractures and fracture fixation. *Spine* 1993; 18(2):178–184.
52. Mouradian WH, Fietti VG, Cochran GVB, et al: Fracture of the odontoid: A laboratory and clinical study of mechanisms. *Orthop Clin North Am* 1978; 9:985–1001.
53. Effendi B, Roy D, Cornish B, et al: Fractures of the ring of the axis: A classification based on the analysis of 131 cases. *J Bone Joint Surg* 1981; 63B:319–327.
54. Saternus KS, Paul E: Forms of fracture of the dens axis in the applications of ventral flexion force. *Aktuel Traumatol* 1986; 1(1):28–33.
55. Torg JS, Vegso JJ, Sennett B, Das M: The national football head and neck injury registry: 14-year report on cervical quadriplegia, 1971 through 1974. *JAMA* 1985; 254(24):3439–3443.
56. Harris JH Jr, Edeiken-Monroe B: *The Radiology of Acute Cervical Spine Trauma* (2d ed). Baltimore: Williams & Wilkins, 1987.
57. Selecki BR, Williams HBL: Injuries to the cervical spine and cord in man. Australia Medical Association Mervyn Archadall Medical Monograph No. 7. South Wales, Australia: Australian Publishing Co, 1970.
58. Maiman DJ, Sances A Jr, Myklebust JB, et al: Compression injuries of the cervical spine: A biomechanical analyses. *Neurosurgery* 1983; 13(3):254–260.
59. Panjabi MM, Duranceau JS, Oxland TR, Bowen CE: Multi-directional instabilities of traumatic cervical spine injuries in a porcine model. *Spine* 1989; 14:1111–1115.
60. Allen BL Jr: Recognition of injuries to the lower cervical spine, in Cervical Spine Research Society (eds): *The Cervical Spine* (2d ed). Philadelphia: Lippincott, 1993: 283–298.
61. Schneider RC: The syndrome of acute anterior spinal cord injury. *J Neurosurg* 1955; 12:95–122.
62. Fuentes JM, Blancourt J, Vlahovitch, Castan P: Tear drop fractures: Contribution to the study of its mechanics and osteodisco-ligamentous lesions. *Neurochirurgie* 1983; 29:129–134.
63. Bause RJ, Ardran GM: Experimental production of forward dislocation in the human cervical spine. *J Bone Joint Surg* 1978; 60B:239–245.
64. Krag MH: Biomechanics of the cervical spine including bracing, surgical constructs, and orthoses, in Frymoyer JW (ed): *The Adult Spine: Principles and Practice.* New York: Raven Press, 1991: 929–965.
65. McKenzie JA, Williams JF: The dynamic behavior of the head and cervical spine during "whiplash". *J Biomech* 1971; 4:477–490.

66. Macnab I: Acceleration injuries of the cervical spine. *J Bone Joint Surg* 1964; 46A:1797–1799.
67. Marar BC, Orth MC: Hyperextension injuries of the cervical spine: The pathogenesis of damage to the spinal cord. *J Bone Joint Surg* 1974; 56A:1655–1662.
68. Forsyth HF: Extension injuries of the cervical spine. *J Bone Joint Surg* 1964; 46A:1792–1797.
69. Lee C, Woodring JH: Sagittally oriented fractures of the lateral masses of the cervical vertebrae. *J Trauma* 1991; 31:1638–1643.
70. Woodring JH, Goldstein SJ: Fractures of the articular processes of the cervical spine. *AJNR* 1982; 3:239–243.
71. Johnson RM, Hart DL, Simmons EF, et al: Cervical orthoses: A study comparing their effectiveness in restricting cervical motion in normal subjects. *J Bone Joint Surg* 1977; 59A:332–339.
72. Millington PJ, Ellingsen JM, Hauswirth BE, Fabian PJ: Thermoplastic Minerva body jacket—A practical alternative to current methods of cervical spine stabilizations: A clinical report. *Phys Ther* 1987; 67:223–225.
73. Benzel EC, Hadden TA, Saulsberry CM: A comparison of the Minerva and halo jackets for stabilization of the cervical spine. *J Neurosurg* 1989; 70:411–414.
74. Fisher SV, Bowar JF, Awad EA, Gullickson G Jr: Cervical orthoses effect on cervical spine motion: Roentgenographic and goniometric method of study. *Arch Phys Med Rehab* 1977; 58:109–115.
75. Lind B, Sihlbom H, Nordwall A: Forces and motions across the neck in patients treated with halo vest. *Spine* 1988; 13:162–167.
76. Johnson RM, Owen JR, Hart DL, Callahan RA: Cervical orthoses: A guide to their selection and use. *Clin Orthop* 1981; 154:34–45.
77. Wolf JW Jr, Johnson RM: Cervical orthoses, in Cervical Spine Research Society (eds): *The Cervical Spine* (2d ed). Philadelphia: JB Lippincott, 1989: 97–105.
78. Dickman CA, Sonntag VKH, Marcotte PJ: Techniques of screw fixation of the cervical spine. *BNI Q* 1992; 8(2):9–26.
79. Kostuik JP, Smith TJ: Pitfalls of biomechanical testing. *Spine* 1991; 16:1233–1235.
80. Krag MH: Biomechanics of thoracolumbar spinal fixation: A review. *Spine* 1991; 16:584–599.
81. Montesano PX, Juach EC, Anderson PA, et al: Biomechanics of cervical spine internal fixation. *JBJS* 1991; 16(3):510–516.
82. Kaufman HH, Jones E: The principles of bony spinal fusion. *Neurosurgery* 1989; 24:264–270.
83. Glasser RS, Fessler RG: Posterior cervical spine fixation. *Contemp Neurosurg* 1993; 15(12):1–8.
84. Bick EM: An essay on the history of spine fusion operations. *Clin Orthop* 1964; 35:9–15.
85. Schultz RS, Boger JW, Dunn HK: Stainless steel surgical wire in various fixation modes. *Clin Orthop Rel Res* 1985; 198:304–307.
86. Taitsman JP, Saha S: Tensile strength of wire-reinforced bone cement and twisted stainless steel wire. *J Bone Joint Surg* 1977; 59A:419–425.
87. Huhn SL, Wolf AL, Ecklund J: Posterior spinal osteosynthesis for cervical fracture/dislocation using a flexible multistrand cable system: Technical note. *Neurosurgery* 1991; 29:943–946.
88. Krag MH, Frederickson BE, Yuan HA: Spinal instrumentation, in Wiesel SW (ed): *The Lumbar Spine.* Philadelphia: WB Saunders, 1990: 916–940.
89. Caspar W, Barbier DD, Klara PM: Anterior cervical fusion and Caspar plate stabilization for cervical trauma. *Neurosurgery* 1989; 25:491–501.
90. Gofffin J, Plets C, Van den Bergh R: Anterior cervical fusion and osteosynthetic stabilization according to Caspar: A prospective study of 41 patients with fractures and/or dislocations of the cervical spine. *Neurosurgery* 1989; 25:865–871.
91. Gill K, Paschal S, Corin J, et al: Posterior plating of the cervical spine: A biomechanical comparison of different posterior fusion techniques. *Spine* 1988; 13(7):813–816.
92. Maiman DJ, Pintar FA, Yoganandan N, et al: Pull-out strength of Caspar cervical screws. *Neurosurgery* 1992; 31:1097–1101.
93. Montesano PX, Anderson PA, Schlehr F, et al: Odontoid fractures treated by anterior odontoid screw fixation. *Spine* 1991; 16(3):533–537.
94. Hanson PB, Montesano PX, Sharkey NA, Rauschning W: Anatomic and biomechanical assessment of transarticular screw fixation for atlantoaxial instability. *Spine* 1991; 16:1141–1145.
95. Hajeck PO, Lipka J, Hartline P, et al: Biomechanical study of C1–C2 posterior arthrodesis techniques. *Spine* 1993; 18:173–177.
96. Grob D, Dvorak J, Panjabi MM, Hayek J: Dorsal atlanto-axial screw fixation. A stability test in vitro and in vivo. *Orthopade* 1991; 20(2):154–162.
97. Fielding JW: Current concepts review: The status of arthrodesis of the cervical spine. *J Bone Joint Surg* 1988; 70A:1571–1574.
98. White AA III, Panjabi MM: The role of stabilization in the treatment of cervical spine injuries. *Spine* 1984; 9:512–522.
99. Roy-Camille R, Saillant G, Mazel C: Internal fixation of the unstable cervical spine by a posterior osteosynthesis with plates and screws, in Cervical Spine Research Society (eds): *The Cervical Spine* (2d ed). Philadelphia: JB Lippincott, 1987: 390–403.
100. Coe JD, Warden KE, Sutterlin CE III, McAfee PC: Biomechanical evaluation of cervical spinal stabilization methods in a human cadaver model. *Spine* 1989; 14:1122–1131.
101. Geremia GK, Kim KS, Cerullo L, Calenoff L: Complications of sublaminar wiring. *Surg Neurol* 1985; 23:629–634.
102. Bohler J, Gaudernak T: Anterior plate stabilization for fracture-dislocations of the lower cervical spine. *J Trauma* 1980; 20:203–205.
103. Cabenela ME, Ebersol MJ: Anterior plate stabilization

for bursting teardrop fractures of the cervical spine. *Spine* 1988; 13:888–891.

104. de Oliveria J: Anterior plate fixation of traumatic lesions of the lower cervical spine. *Spine* 1987; 12:324–329.

105. Sutterlin CE, McAfee PC, Warden KE, et al: A biomechanical evaluation of cervical spinal stabilization methods in a bovine model. Static and cyclical loading. *Spine* 1988; 13:795–802.

106. Cybulski GR, Douglas RA, Meyer PK, Rovin RA: Complications in three-column cervical spine injuries requiring anterior-posterior stabilization. *Spine* 1992; 17:253–256.

Early Care

CHAPTER 78

PREHOSPITAL MANAGEMENT OF THE SPINALLY INJURED PATIENT

Edward C. Benzel
David Doezema

SYNOPSIS

The treatment of acute spinal cord injury (SCI) has three primary goals: maximized neurological recovery; spinal stabilization; mobilization and rehabilitation. Achieving these goals requires a logical management scheme that begins in the prehospital phase and continues through radiographic diagnoses, acute management, and surgical treatment. Thus, management in the prehospital phase may impact significantly on outcome from the SCI. It has been asserted that 10 to 25 percent of neurological deficits occur as a result of improper prehospital handling; however, available studies offer either minimal data or otherwise unconvincing evidence for such statements.[17,18] *Nevertheless, the chance for deterioration in the early postinjury period is reason for concern.*[10] *The specialized management initiated at the accident scene is vital. Patient stabilization for associated injuries and the systemic effects of the SCI must be accomplished simultaneously with spinal stabilization to minimize secondary insults to the injured cord.*

ACUTE TREATMENT STRATEGIES

The Handling of the Patient

Spinal alignment

The physical handling of the patient is very important during the initial management in the field. Patients need to be extricated from vehicles or rescued from the scene of an accident with great care to minimize the possibility of further spine or spinal cord injury. Although the chance of cervical spine injury is less than 10 percent, the gravity of the potential disability mandates that all multiple trauma victims be treated presumptively as having a spine injury.

Manual stabilization can be used effectively to immobilize the cervical spine. The head should be maintained in a neutral or slightly extended position, with slight distraction. Flexion should be avoided. Most spine injuries that may be iatrogenically worsened following trauma result from a combination of flexion and axial loading. Therefore, management schemes that minimize the reenactment of the forces that caused the injury are theoretically beneficial.

Slight distraction helps maintain spinal alignment and prevents further flexion and spinal compression. It is emphasized that if resistance to the positioning of the head in a neutral position is met, head position should be unaltered. Further injury to an injured spine otherwise may result. Traction should be used minimally, since too much traction may exacerbate the injury or result in subluxation.[19] Furthermore, it is probably inadvisable to recommend traction in the field, since the skill level of prehospital personnel is variable, and excessive traction frequently would be applied. Movements such as the log-rolling maneuver actually can cause considerable spine movement,[20] so that optimal methods of moving spine-injured patients have yet to be proven.

Confining movement by taping

The maintenance of a neutral cervical posture often is accomplished by the manual application of resistance to movement, cervical stabilization, lateral calvarial application of sandbags or towel rolls, and the taping of the calvarium to a transportation board. Taping to control lateral head movement is nearly as effective as when it is combined with a semirigid collar.[21,22] Most patients on a flat backboard are in relative cervical extension, so occipital padding is necessary to attain a more neutral position as well as greater comfort.[23] Confining movement of the head and/or the chest to a spine board by maneuvers such as taping provides sound stability. The agitated patient, however, may apply significant stresses to intermediate segmental levels of the cervical spine. This, indeed, may result in a phenomenon termed "snaking" of the spine.[24] Spinal snaking may result in unexpected and untoward segmental movements in such a manner that excessive segmental distraction/compression or flexion/extension occurs (Fig. 78-1). The restriction of chest excursion by techniques that confine movement, such as taping the chest to a spine board, can aggravate acute or chronic pulmonary processes by exaggerating the restrictive component of pulmonary pathology, and can even produce an important restrictive effect in patients with normal lung function.[25,26] Furthermore, confinement to the supine position places the patient at an increased risk for bronchopulmonary aspiration, owing to an inability to protect the airway by body position alteration during and following emesis. Finally, confining movement may result in increased agitation. This, in turn, may augment movements that stress the spine and spine injury sites, e.g., via snaking, etc.

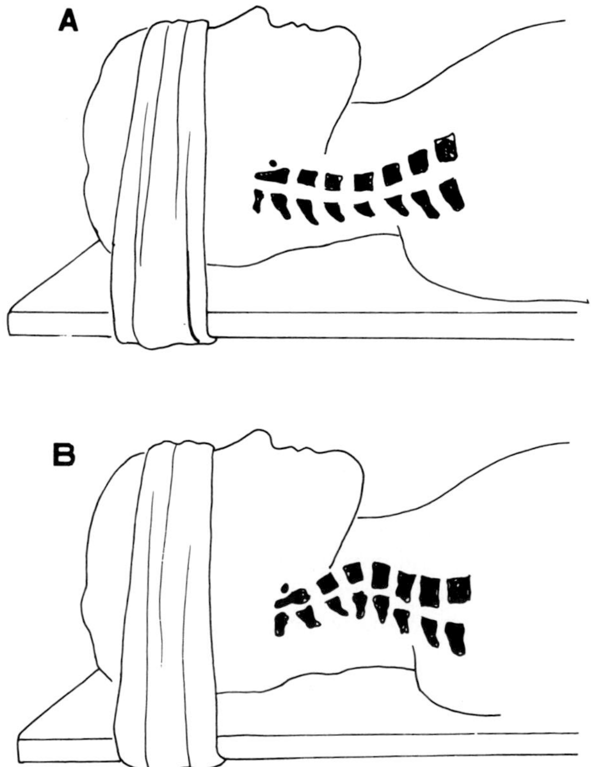

Figure 78-1. The snaking phenomenon occurs when the head and chest are rigidly confined, as observed with the taping of the head to a spine board. Attempted flexion (*A*) and extension (*B*) movements result in unexpected segmental serpentine movements of the cervical spine.

Sand bags

Sand bags may be placed strategically and secured in a manner that does not affect airway protection maneuvers while simultaneously minimizing unwanted snaking movements of the spine. Some physicians, however, are concerned about infection transmission via contamination from inadequately cleaned sand bags.[27] In the field, sand bags may be less practical because they are difficult to secure during transport. Towel rolls taped to the sides of the head may limit lateral movement as efficiently as sand bags. Sand bags or towel rolls are most effectively used in combination with taping and rigid collars.

Collar immobilization

Collar immobilization of the acutely injured patient is associated with two concerns: (1) the risk associated with donning the collar; and (2) the relative ineffectiveness of collar immobilization. There is some risk with collar application. Although some collars require less neck manipulation than others, neck flexion is never completely eliminated. Since neck flexion often may be dangerous, collars should be applied with great care. Furthermore, cervical collars are relatively ineffective in minimizing neck motion.[27] When combined with taping, semirigid collars help to limit flexion and extension, but are not adequate when used alone.[20,21] Newer devices, such as the Vacuum Splint Cervical Collar may restrict movement more effectively than do shorter collars.[27] Cervical collars are most effective in alert ambulatory patients in whom the brace functions as a reminder of the potential for injury. However, in the cerebrally impaired or agitated patient, excessive muscular activity directed at neck motion is relatively unimpeded by collar immobilization.

Manual movement restriction

Perhaps the most effective technique to restrict cervical spine movement appropriately and safely in the combative patient is via manual movement restriction by a knowledgeable care giver. With this technique, a care giver applies movement restrictive forces (continuously monitored via feedback). The arm-chest/hand-mandible technique, with continuous nonthreatening conversation with the patient, is most effective (Fig. 78-2). Manual spine control is limited in the prehospital setting by the difficulty in its employment during transport,

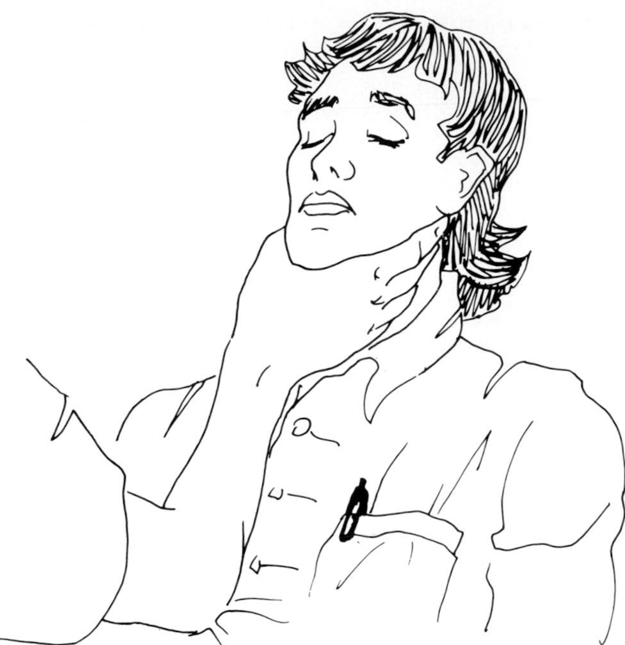

Figure 78-2. The arm/chest-hand/mandible technique of manual movement restriction. Note the arm placed firmly on the chest without breathing restriction. The hand is placed on the mandible in such a manner as to maintain slight extension and to limit movement. Continuous nonthreatening conversation assists in this process in the agitated patient.

when unpredictable stops and turns occur and limited personnel are available to manage the immobilization.

Spine boards

Spine boards are devices to immobilize and transport patients with existing or potential spine injuries. Although spine boards facilitate transportation of injured patients, they also cause excessive restriction of pulmonary function, as discussed above. Furthermore, patients placed on spine boards are less likely to be examined for dorsal injuries. Finally, spine boards may cause excessive pressure to sacral, scapular, calcaneal, and occipital regions. This early postinjury integument injury may lead to subsequent decubiti formation, with the potential for significant morbidity. Therefore, the utility of the spine board must be continuously assessed and reassessed on an individual, patient-specific basis and the patient moved off the board as soon as safe and clinically feasible. New inflatable immobilization devices may improve comfort and reduce the risk of decubiti.

The helmeted patient

Helmeted patients are often best managed initially by leaving the helmet in place. Although the helmet causes the patient's neck to be slightly flexed (an undesirable posture, as discussed above) and may be concealing life-threatening hemorrhage, its removal is not required in the field unless airway problems exist. Removal can risk

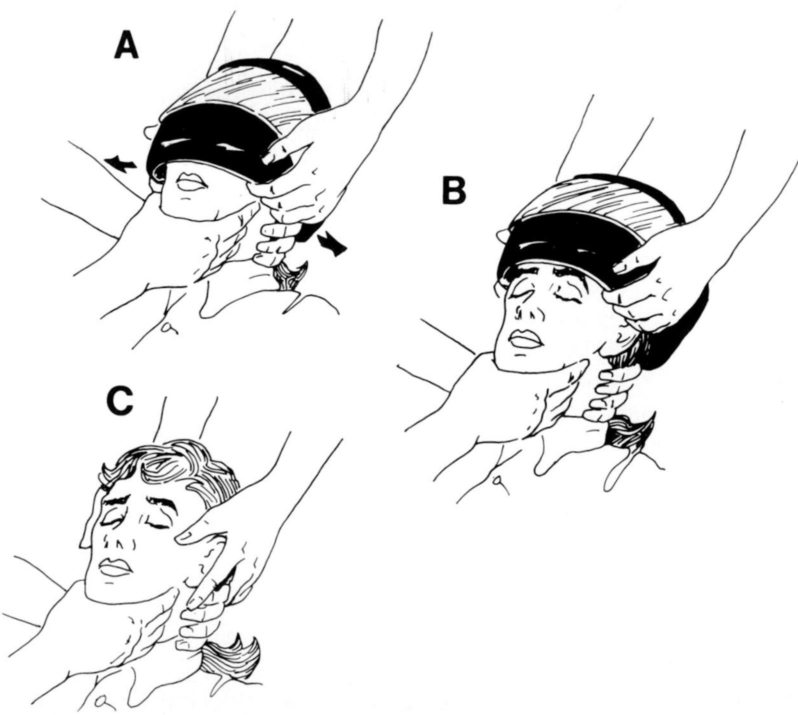

Figure 78-3. Two-person technique of helmet removal.[28]

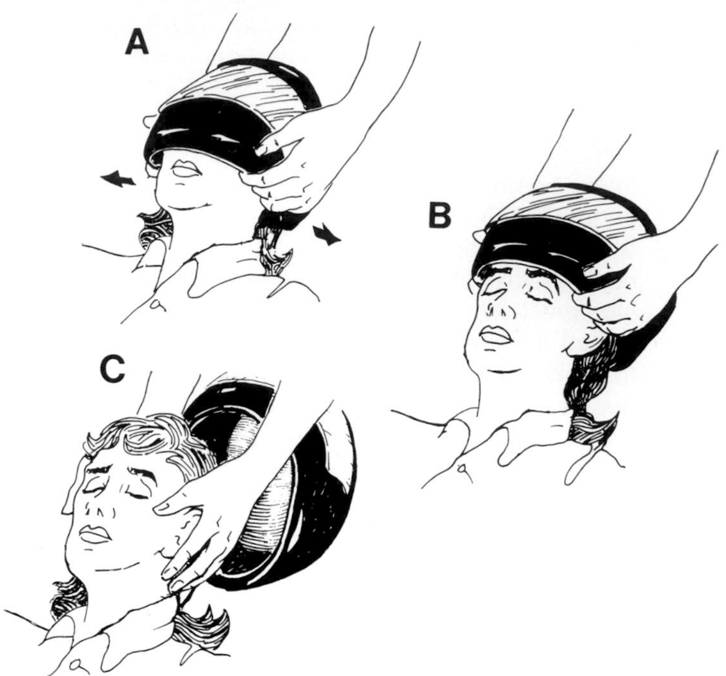

Figure 78-4. One-person technique of helmet removal.[28]

further injury to the cervical spine. The helmet also may be used as an attachment site for the application of traction.

Helmets can be removed safely using the two-person technique recommended by the American College of Surgeons or a one-person technique (Fig. 78-3, 78-4).[28,29] Helmet removal in patients with a documented or potential spine injury is facilitated in some cases by using a cast-saw to cut the helmet in half.

Resuscitation

In general, the American College of Surgeons' protocol for trauma resuscitation applies to patients with spinal cord injury.[30] Life-threatening injuries must be dealt with first, followed by assessment and treatment of spine pathology and other less life-threatening injuries. The spine must be immobilized, and motion of the spine limited as much as possible during resuscitation. In the past this often meant that assessment of life-threatening injuries was delayed while the cervical spine was radiographed. It is now appreciated that the spine can be adequately stabilized during the resuscitation and assessment period.[30]

Medical Management

Airway Management

The inadequately ventilated nonintubated patient requires establishment and maintenance of a patent posterior pharyngeal airway. In a patient with a suspected cervical spine injury, the jaw thrust maneuver should be performed while minimizing manipulation of the neck (Fig. 78-5). A nasopharyngeal or oropharyngeal airway may be used if respirations are adequate; however, usually these are useful only temporarily, and may cause increased movement of the spine in a confused patient by constantly stimulating the gag reflex.

Chin lift, jaw thrust, mask ventilation, and all routes of tracheal intubation may cause movement of the cervical spine.[31,32] Physicians should choose the intubation technique with which they have the greatest experience

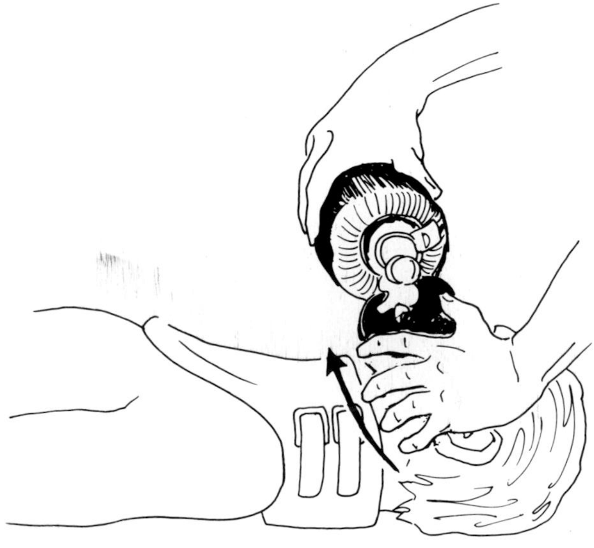

Figure 78-5. The jaw thrust maneuver for the maintenance of a posterior pharyngeal airway.

and skill. If the neck is manually immobilized, endotracheal intubation is safe, provided appropriate precautions are taken.[33–36] Cervical traction may worsen preexisting injuries,[31,37] therefore, manual immobilization without traction should be utilized during endotracheal intubation.[27,30,38]

If the patient cannot be intubated, a surgical cricothyrotomy is the procedure of choice. The attainment of a surgical airway is associated with significant complications.[35,39–42] Emergency cricothyrotomy has a complication rate of 10 to 40 percent, compared with a 45 percent complication rate for tracheotomy.[43–45] This favorable complication rate compared with tracheotomy, and its ease of performance, make cricothyrotomy the procedure of choice for surgical airway in the prehospital and hospital setting.[32,41,46] Some have recommended cricothyrotomy if cervical spine injury is present or highly suspected; however, the low incidence of spine damage with the more rapidly performed tracheal intubation make cricothyrotomy the procedure of last resort for airway access. Furthermore, if a spine injury is, indeed, present, an anterior cervical spine operation may be delayed or complicated by the transtracheal airway procedure.

Ventilation

Once intubation is accomplished, adequate ventilation must be achieved. Multiple factors may be related to pathological ventilation in the spinal cord injury patient. These range from traumatic brain or spinal cord injury (indirect effect on pulmonary function) to direct pulmonary injury (direct effect on pulmonary function). Although nervous system injury does not directly affect pulmonary function, it impacts negatively on ventilation. Ventilation is depressed and ventilation-perfusion defects often are present. These often may be minimized by high tidal volume ventilation.

Direct negative effects on pulmonary function are caused by non-nervous-system trauma such as rib fracture, flail chest, tension pneumothorax, aspiration pneumonitis, etc. Each is best managed by proven treatment regimens, and their management is, in general, not influenced by nervous system trauma.

Respiratory failure in the SCI patient may be present from the moment of impact or may occur insidiously at any time during the acute or chronic phase of the patient's postinjury course. The earlier the presentation of respiratory failure, the more likely it is to be associated with neurogenic dysfunction, e.g., paralysis of primary or accessory respiratory muscles. Later deterioration often is related to direct and indirect components, as well as to fatigue. Parameters for intubation in this situation include arterial oxygenation and carbon dioxide level. An elevated respiratory rate, however, must not be overlooked as an indication of respiratory failure and, thus, for intubation and ventilatory support.

Two factors are unique to the respiratory failure associated with cervical SCI: (1) paradoxical chest wall movement; and (2) the postural dependence of vital capacity.[47] Acute quadriplegia results in paradoxical movements of the chest and abdomen if diaphragm function is present. In this situation, diaphragm movement results in a passive chest wall movement that is opposite (and paradoxical) to movements that occur in the face of normal innervation of the intercostal muscles. This may significantly impair ventilation in the acute phases of injury.

Vital capacity is diminished during the assumption of the upright or Trendelenburg position of the quadriplegic patient. The mass of the abdominal contents pulls the diaphragm caudally (or pushes it rostrally), thus decreasing vital capacity. Therefore, nonsupine positioning should be avoided during the early phases of quadriplegia unless the patient is intubated and ventilated or extenuating circumstances prevail.

Intravascular Volume Status Management

Hypotension and tachycardia are often manifestations of hypovolemia. These classic manifestations of shock, however, may be misleading or absent in patients with spinal cord injury. Because of the sympathectomy effect associated with cervical or high thoracic spinal cord injury, both bradycardia and hypotension are manifestations. This complicates the vascular volume management of the spinal cord injury patient. On the one hand, the presence of hypotension indicates intuitively that volume replacement is indicated; however, hypotension often may exist in the presence of normovolemia. Indeed, the determination of volume replacement in the prehospital and early hospital time frame often is difficult. Without knowing the central venous or left atrial pressure (pulmonary wedge pressure), the determining the etiology of hypotension is difficult. Hypotension may be caused by either a combination of hypovolemia or the sympathectomy effect related to cervical or upper thoracic spinal cord injury. The sympathectomy effect results in hypotension and bradycardia.

The management of hypotension differs, depending on its etiology. If hypotension is caused by hypovolemia, volume replacement is indicated. Central venous and pulmonary artery wedge pressures are low. If a spinal cord neurogenic etiology is present, the central venous or pulmonary artery wedge pressures may be normal, even in the presence of hypotension. In these patients, excessive volume replacement is not indicated—and, in fact, is contraindicated. Overhydration may result in pulmonary edema and respiratory distress syndrome.

Volume replacement, titrated to a central pressure in the range of 6 to 12 mmHg, is clinically appropriate. Since central pressures are not attainable in the field, indirect assessments are necessary. In this vein, clinical assessment often provides indicators of the etiology of hypotension. Cool diaphoretic skin is a manifestation of hypovolemic shock; warm skin is a manifestation of spinal cord neurogenic shock. The former is associated with a low urine output and tachycardia, and the latter with a normal urine output and bradycardia. Assessment of hypovolemia may be difficult for prehospital providers. They usually are encouraged to treat with rapid crystalloid infusion if hypotension is present. Infusing large volumes of fluid should be discouraged if hypotension and tachycardia are not present. For longer transports from primary centers to trauma centers, air transport may offer the advantages of improved transport time and higher skill level of providers.[48] Once the cause of hypotension is determined at the hospital or trauma center to be the nervous system, the blood pressure may be managed with vasopressors or volume expansion, as dictated by direct central pressure measurement.

In cases of extreme shock, type-specific blood is the optimal volume expansion medium. If unavailable or if emergency situations dictate otherwise, type O negative packed cells may be used. Otherwise, normal saline, lactated Ringer's, plasmanate, albumin, or synthetic volume expanders may be employed.

Spinal shock is a manifestation of an acute injury to the spinal cord. In the early postinjury period, an upper motor neuron injury manifests itself clinically as a lower motor neuron injury (hyporeflexia). This phase persists for a variable length of time—usually from several days to several months. Its presence or absence appears to affect outcome minimally and, therefore, has little effect on the acute postinjury management scheme.

Spinal cord perfusion augmentation

As is obvious, the volume status management of the spinal cord injury patient is fraught with the hazard of both under- or overhydration. The optimization of spinal cord blood flow, or, more important, the spinal cord perfusion pressure, offers a theoretical advantage in outcome.[49–52] Therefore, it appears prudent to aggressively manage the intravascular volume status and blood pressure of the spinal cord injury patient. The management scheme should essentially be that of standard protocols for hypovolemic shock.

Lost intravascular volume should rapidly be replaced while intravascular volume status is monitored clinically or via central pressure measurement. Following rapid establishing of euvolemia, normotension should be achieved with pressors (in the range of 110 to 140 mmHg systolic). This scheme should optimize perfusion of the spinal cord. It is emphasized that, in spite of an adequate urine output and an alert patient, relative hypotension (systolic blood pressure less than 100) may adversely affect neurological outcome. It appears prudent to maintain a normotensive state via vasopressors, if necessary, during the acute phase of injury (i.e., from the moment of impact until the end of the first postinjury week).

Methylprednisolone

Although controversial, the second National Acute Spinal Cord Injury Study (NASCIS-II) has played a seminal role in establishing: (1) that there is clinical significance to the secondary injury phenomenon noted in the laboratory; and (2) that the timing of intervention is critical.[53]

The methylprednisolone treatment of spinal cord injury is most likely optimized by initiating treatment as soon following injury as possible. Prehospital treatment may, indeed, optimize therapeutic efficacy. This issue, however, is complicated by such factors as the definition of appropriate patients for such treatment and the known negative side effects of treatment. Nevertheless, patients should be treated, if possible, before transfer from a community hospital to a trauma center.

Gangliosides

Other pharmacological regimens also may be clinically effective. However, only G_{M1} ganglioside has been shown clinically to be so to date.[54] In this study, G_{M1} ganglioside enhanced the recovery of neurological function at the one-year follow-up. Further investigations regarding the efficacy of G_{M1} ganglioside and lazaroids (21-aminosteroids) are currently proceeding.

CONCLUSION

The early postinjury management of the spinal cord injury patient is complicated. Many of the factors involved with management scheme determination are poorly understood and inadequately studied. Nevertheless, by following some of the guidelines presented here and by liberal use of common sense, the care of the spinally injured patient can be optimized.

References

1. Benzel EC, Larson SJ: Functional recovery after decompressive operation for thoracic and lumbar spine fractures. *Neurosurgery* 1986; 19:772–778.

2. Benzel EC, Larson SJ: Functional recovery after decompressive operation for cervical spine fractures. *Neurosurgery* 1987; 20:742–746.
3. Burke DC, Murray DD: The management of thoracic and thoracolumbar injuries of the spine with neurologic involvement. *J Bone Joint Surg* 1976; 58B:72–78.
4. Dickson JH, Harrington PR, Erwin WE: Results of reduction and stabilization of the severely fractured thoracic and lumbar spine. *J Bone Joint Surg* 1978; 60A:799–805.
5. Frankel HL, Hancock DO, Hyslop G, et al: The value of postural reduction in the initial management of closed injuries of the spine with paraplegia and tetraplegia—Part I. *Paraplegia* 1969; 7:179–192.
6. Larson SJ, Holst RA, Hemmy DC, et al: Lateral extracavitary approach to traumatic lesions of the thoracic and lumbar spine. *J Neurosurg* 1976; 45:628–637.
7. Mason RL, Gunst RF: Prediction of mobility gains in patients with cervical spinal cord injuries. *J Neurosurg* 1976; 45:677–682.
8. Schmidek HH, Gomes FB, Seligson D, et al: Management of acute unstable thoracolumbar (T11–L1) fractures with and without neurological deficit. *Neurosurgery* 1980; 7:30–35.
9. Suwanwela C, Alexander E Jr, Davis CH: Prognosis in spinal cord injury, with special reference to patients with motor paralysis and sensory preservation. *J Neurosurg* 1962; 19:220–227.
10. Marshall LF, Knowlton S, Gardin SR, et al: Deterioration following spinal cord injury. *J Neurosurg* 1987; 66:400–404.
11. Tominaga S: Periodical neurological-functional assessment for cervical cord injury. *Paraplegia* 1989; 27:227–236.
12. Piepmeier JM, Jenkins NR: Late neurological changes following traumatic spinal cord injury. *J Neurosurg* 1988; 69:399–402.
13. Chehrazi B, Wagner FC, Collins WF, et al: A scale for evaluation of spinal cord injury. *J Neurosurg* 1981; 54:310–315.
14. Lucas JT, Ducker TB: Motor classification of spinal cord injuries with mobility, morbidity and recovery indices. *Am Surg* 1979; 45:151–158.
15. Maynard FM, Reynolds GG, Fountain S, et al: Neurological prognosis after traumatic quadriplegia: Three year experiment of California regional spinal cord injury care system. *J Neurosurg* 1979; 50:611–616.
16. Tator CH, Rowed DW, Schwartz ML: Sunnybrook Cord Injury Scales for assessing neurological injury and neurological recovery, in Tator CH (ed): *Early Management of Acute Spinal Cord Injury.* New York: Raven Press, 1982: 7–24.
17. Cloward RB: Acute cervical spine injuries. Ciba Monograph, 1980.
18. Toscano J: Prevention of neurological deterioration before admission to a spinal cord injury unit. *Paraplegia* 1988; 26:143.
19. Bivens HG, Ford S, Bezamalinovic Z, et al: The effect of axial traction during orotracheal intubation of the trauma victim with an unstable cervical spine. *Ann Emerg Med* 1988; 17:25–29.
20. McGuire RA, Neville S, Green BA, Watts C: Spinal instability and the log-rolling maneuver. *J Trauma* 1987; 27:525–531.
21. Graziano AF, Scheidel EA, Cline JR, et al: A radiographic comparison of prehospital cervical immobilization methods. *Ann Emerg Med* 1987; 16:1127–1131.
22. Podolsky S, Baraff LJ, Simon RR, et al: Efficacy of cervical spine immobilization methods. *J Trauma* 1983; 23:461–465.
23. Schreger DL, Larmon B, LeGassick T, Blinman T: Spinal immobilization on a flat backboard: Does it result in neutral position of the cervical spine? *Ann Emerg Med* 1991; 20:878–881.
24. Benzel EC, Hadden TA, Saulsbery CM: A comparison of the Minerva and halo jackets for the stabilization of the cervical spine. *J Neurosurg* 1989; 70:411–414.
25. Bauer D, Kowalski R: Effect of spinal immobilization devices on pulmonary function in the healthy nonsmoking man. *Ann Emerg Med* 1988; 17:915–918.
26. Schafermeyer RW, Ribbeck RM, Gaskins J, et al: Respiratory effects of spinal immobilization in children. *Ann Emerg Med* 1991; 20:1017–1019.
27. Rosen PB, McSwain NE, Arata M, et al: Comparison of two new immobilization collars. *Ann Emerg Med* 1992; 21:1189–1195.
28. Meyer RD, Daniel WW; The biomechanics of helmets and helmet removal. *J Trauma* 1985; 25:325–332.
29. Aprahamian C, Thompson BM, Darin JC: Recommended helmet removal techniques in a cervical spine injured patient. *J Trauma* 1984; 24:841–842.
30. American College of Surgeons. *Advanced Trauma Life Support Course Manual.* Chicago: American College of Surgeons, 1989.
31. Aprahamian C, Thompson BM, Finger WA, et al: Experimental cervical spine injury model: Evaluation of airway management and splinting techniques. *Ann Emerg Med* 1984; 13:584–587.
32. Hauswald M, Sklar DP, Tandberg D, Garcia JF: Cervical spine movement during airway management: Cinefluoroscopic appraisal in human cadavers. *Am J Emerg Med* 1991; 9:535–538.
33. Majernick TG, Bieniek R, Houston JB, Hughes HG: Cervical spine movement during orotracheal intubation. *Ann Emerg Med* 1986; 15:417–420.
34. Holley J, Jorden R: Airway management in patients with unstable cervical spine fractures. *Ann Emerg Med* 1989; 18:1237–1239.
35. McGill J, Clinton JE, Ruiz E: Cricothyrotomy in the emergency department. *Ann Emerg Med* 1982; 11:361–364.
36. Rhee KJ, Green W, Holcroft JW, et al: Oral intubation in the multiply injured patient: The risk of exacerbating spinal cord damage. *Ann Emerg Med* 1990; 19:511–514.
37. Bivins HG, Ford S, Bezmalinovic Z, et al: Cervical spine movement during orotracheal intubation. *Ann Emerg Med* 1988; 17:25–29.
38. Walls RM: Airway management. *Emerg Med Clin North Am* 1993; 2:53–60.

39. Bjoraker DG, Neelam BK, Allan CD: Evaluation of an emergency cricothyrotomy instrument. *Crit Care Med* 1987; 15:157–160.
40. Erlandson MJ, Clinton JE, Ruiz E, et al: Cricothyrotomy in the emergency department revisited. *J Emerg Med* 1989; 7:115–118.
41. Miklus RM, Elliott C, Snow N: Surgical cricothyrotomy in the field: Experience of a helicopter transport team. *J Trauma* 1989; 29:506–508.
42. Walls RM: Cricothyrotomy. *Emerg Med Clin North Am* 1988; 6:725–736.
43. Mace SE: Cricothyrotomy, in Roberts JR, Hedges JR (eds): *Clinical Procedures in Emergency Medicine.* Philadelphia: WB Saunders, 1991.
44. Brantigan CO, Grow JB: Cricothyrotomy: Elective use in respiratory problems requiring tracheotomy. *J Thorac Cardiovasc Surg* 1976; 71:72.
45. Kress TD, Balasubramaniam S: Cricothyrotomy. *Ann Emerg Med* 1982; 11:197–201.
46. Spaite DW, Joseph M: Prehospital cricothyrotomy: An investigation of indications, technique, complications, and patient outcome. *Ann Emerg Med* 1990; 19:279–285.
47. Chicoine RE, Ball PA, Gettinger A: Anesthesia and critical care management of spinal cord injury, in Benzel EC, Tator CH (eds): *Contemporary Management of Spinal Cord Injury*. American Association of Neurological Surgeons, 1994.
48. Burney RE, Waggoner R, Maynard FM: Stabilization of spinal injury for early transfer. *J Trauma* 1989; 29:1497–1499.
49. Dolan EJ, Tator CH: The effect of blood transfusion, dopamine, and gamma hydroxybutyrate on posttraumatic ischemia of the spinal cord. *J Neurosurg* 1982; 56:350–358.
50. Dolan EJ, Tator CH: The treatment of hypotension due to acute experimental spinal cord compression injury. *Surg Neurol* 1980; 13:380–384.
51. Frankel HL, Mathias CJ: The cardiovascular system in tetraplegia and paraplegia, in "Injuries of the Spine and Spinal Cord," Part II. *Handbook of Clinical Neurology* 1976; 26:313–333.
52. Haghighi SS, Chehrazi BB, Wagner FC: Effect of Nimodipine-associated hypotension on recovery from acute spinal cord injury in cats. *Surg Neurol* 1988; 29:293–297.
53. Bracken MB, Shepard MJ, Collins WF, et al: A randomized, controlled trial of methylprednisolone or naloxone in the treatment of acute spinal cord injury. *N Engl J Med* 1990; 322:1405–1411.
54. Geisler FH, Dorsey FC, Coleman WP: Recovery of motor function after spinal cord injury: A randomized, placebo-controlled trial with GM-1 ganglioside. *N Engl J Med* 1991; 324:1829–1838.

CHAPTER 79

EMERGENCY MANAGEMENT OF SPINAL CORD INJURY

Randall M. Chesnut

INTRODUCTION

Despite recent advances in our understanding of neuronal injury, repair, and plasticity, the ability of present-day medicine to actively promote neuronal recovery remains limited. As a result, the greatest impact we can make at present on spinal cord injury remains the optimization of the neuronal healing environment and prevention of secondary insults. It is, therefore, critical that vigilant and meticulous care of the spinal cord injury patient be initiated at the time of initial contact and maintained throughout that patient's course. It is the purpose of this chapter to discuss those issues pertinent to the optimal care of the spine trauma patient during the acute-care period directly following the injury.

FUNDAMENTAL CONCEPTS

Several fundamental concepts underlie all aspects of care of the spinal injury patient and must be considered throughout all phases of treatment. One of these is the absolute primacy of the ABCs. As with all types of neurological insult, the maintenance of adequate oxygenation and perfusion of injured tissues is necessary, and not only for optimization of recovery: it appears that even brief periods of hypoperfusion can significantly increase mortality and decrease recovery of function from spinal cord insult.[1] There is an increasing body of evidence that the injured nervous system will not tolerate periods of hypoperfusion that, in most cases, would be considered mild and inconsequential. It is, therefore, critical to monitor the patient's vital signs extremely closely and avoid scrupulously hypotension and hypoxia at all stages of patient care—most specifically during the first several days following the initial trauma.

The other universal concept in spinal cord injury is the assumption that all trauma victims have spinal column/cord injuries until proven otherwise. A corollary to this rule is that no spinal segment can be mobilized until it has been specifically cleared. As we are unable to repair injured neurons, it is critical to avoid repeating or exacerbating the trauma that caused the injury. Therefore, early and strict immobilization of the entire spine from initial contact is a fundamental component of proper treatment. The institution of such practices into trauma resuscitation and triage is felt to be largely responsible for the progressive decrease in the ratio of quadriparesis to paraparesis in multiple trauma patients.[2]

Analysis of the above principles leads to the conclusion that all trauma victims should be treated as proven or potential spinal cord injury patients until specifically cleared. Indeed, the resuscitative measures discussed in this chapter should be applied, to some extent, in the resuscitation of all trauma patients. Therefore, although the fundamental focus here is the emergency treatment of spinal cord injury patients, the spinal column and cord-specific treatment of all trauma victims will be covered.

RESUSCITATION

Initial Evaluation and Treatment

Upon initial presentation at the receiving institution, the spinal injury patient must be afforded the same resuscitation as any multiple trauma patient. Prehospital resuscitation and stabilization issues have been discussed elsewhere in this volume and will not be considered specifically here. In instances where the prehospital resuscitation has been limited, however, the initial management at the receiving institution must incorporate procedures such as immobilization that are otherwise handled in the field. The approach discussed here will encompass maneuvers applicable to a patient presented to the resuscitation team who has not had the benefit of prior medical care. When there has been prehospital stabilization and resuscitation, some of the steps discussed may be skipped or modified, after making certain that they have been adequately managed in the field.

It is important to avoid focusing exclusively on the spinal cord/column injury until a full initial assessment has been carried out. In all instances, the adequacy of the airway and gas exchange as well as hemodynamic stability and the checking of major hemorrhage must be handled straightforwardly. Thus, by establishing and maintaining strict immobilization during the primary and secondary surveys, the axial skeleton and spinal cord can be "placed on hold" while the primary survey and resuscitation are performed (Fig. 79-1).

Initial Immobilization

Cervical immobilization characteristically involves placing sandbags firmly alongside the head and then strapping a 3-inch piece of tape from the edge of the backboard, across the patient's brow, to the other edge of the backboard.[3] This method allows free motion of the jaw and lower face for airway control while maintaining stability as good as any rigid, external orthosis,[4] although a hard cervical collar may be added as a supplement. Soft collars do not provide sufficient immobilization and should not be used.[5,6]

The patient's axial skeleton must be immobilized on a rigid backboard throughout the course of the initial evaluation and resuscitation. If this has not been accomplished in the field, the patient should be placed on a backboard according to the principles discussed elsewhere in this volume. Either cloth tape or nylon seatbelt webbing should be used to secure the patient to

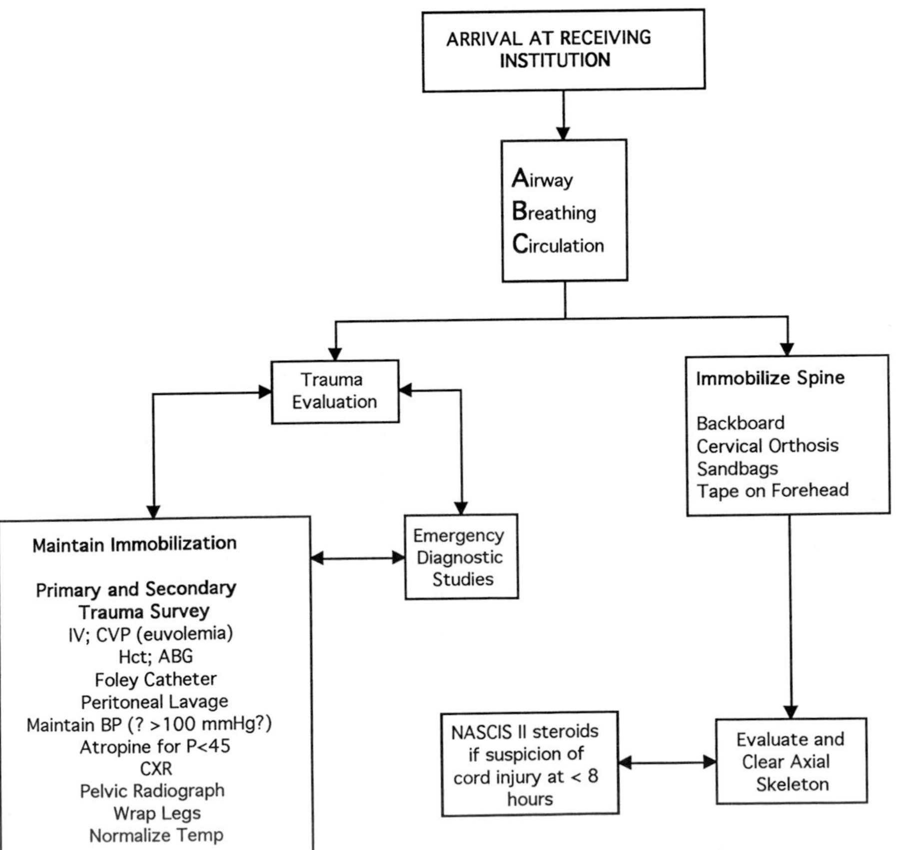

Figure 79-1. Initial trauma evaluation of a patient with a suspected spinal injury. Note the primacy of the ABCs and the use of immobilization to put the spine "on hold" during the resuscitation.

the backboard to prevent loosening during early in-hospital transport or if the patient is combative.

The ABCs and Initial Evaluation

Given the profound disruptions in the autonomic systems responsible for homeostasis that can be associated with spinal cord injury, in addition to the ramifications of a patient with real or potential alterations in sensorimotor function, the inital evaluation must be particularly thorough. Importantly, a period of stable vital signs prior to arrival does not imply absence of serious injury.

Aspiration and shock are the primary causes of death in spinal cord injury victims during the early postinjury period. This underscores the necessity of attending to the ABCs as the first order of treatment in the spinal cord/column injury patient, as in all trauma victims. Owing to the real or potential instability of the axial skeleton in such patients, however, there are important guidelines for management techniques (Fig. 79-2). If the airway is adequate on initial assessment, patients should be stabilized "as they lie" and supplemental oxygen administered via nasal prongs or face mask. If the airway is obstructed, the routine technique of the jaw thrust/neck extension maneuver should be avoided in any patient with an uncleared cervical spine, and the chin-lift substituted. If this does not adequately clear the airway, the cervical spine should be stabilized and the patient intubated. Despite the difficulty and potential hazards of intubation maneuvers, the morbidity of an inadequate airway and the extreme hazard of "crash" intubation under emergency conditions mandate early airway control in any patient where there is a question of a compromised airway.

Intubation must be performed carefully in any patient with an uncleared cervical spine. Intubation may be required because of airway compromise, inadequate ventilation from intercostal or diaphragmatic muscular

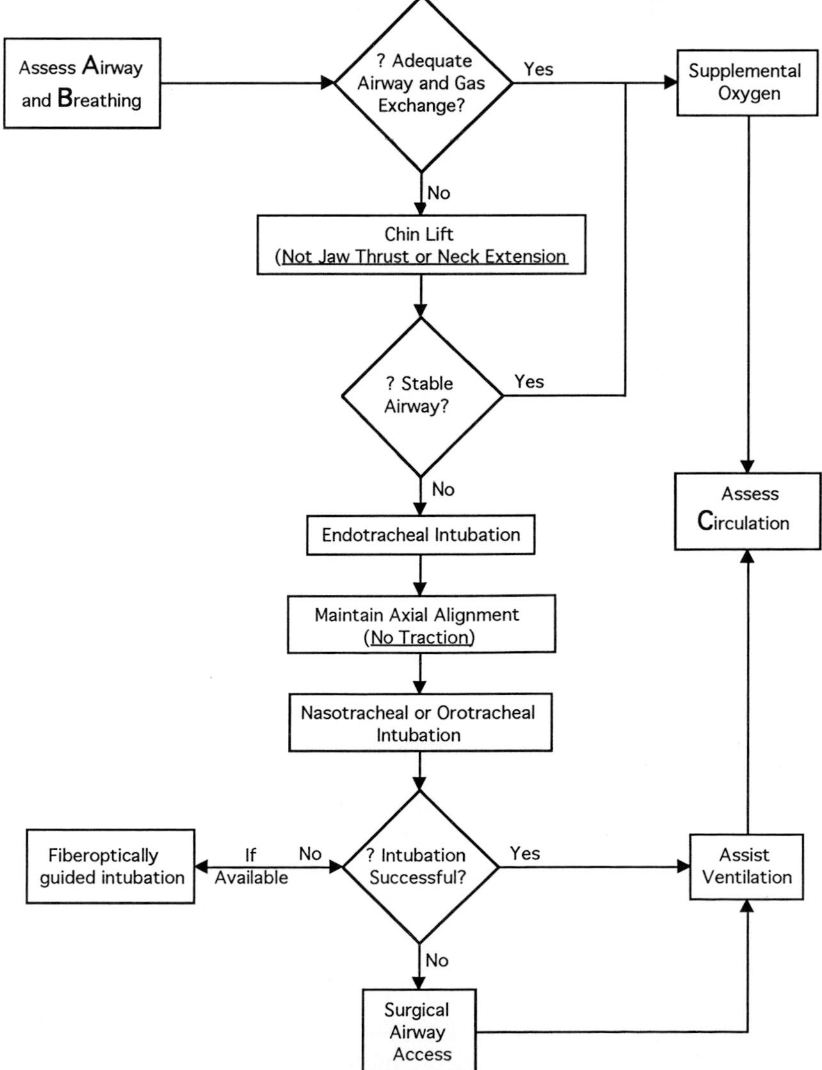

Figure 79-2. Evaluation and treatment of the *A*irway and *B*reathing components of the ABCs during the initial evaluation of the spinal injury patient.

paralysis, or a depressed level of consciousness. During intubation, the head must be maintained in a neutral position. Axial traction should be avoided and certainly must not be overly vigorous, as serious vertebral distraction can result from even moderate traction on an unstable spine during intubation.[7]

Nasotracheal intubation is easier than oral intubation, does not require neck hyperextension, and diminishes the likelihood of aspiration,[8] but the patient must have spontaneous respirations, and the maneuver is much easier if the patient is cooperative. If nasotracheal intubation is not an option, orotracheal intubation will be required, either laryngoscopically-guided or over a flexible fiberoptic bronchoscope. This should be performed gently, with the head and neck immobilized by an assistant. Surgical airway access, such as emergency tracheostomy or cricothyroidotomy, should be avoided if possible, as the wound can compromise later anterior surgical approaches to the cervical spine.

Occasionally, an awake patient with a spinal column/cord injury will maintain the head in a position other than neutral. Such patients should be treated and immobilized "as they lie," and no attempt should be made to correct the abnormal posture. Such a position, whether maintained voluntarily or due to muscle spasm, often represents a conscious or unconscious effort to maintain the cervical spine in a meta-stable position and to avoid further injury.

It is crucial to maintain adequate perfusion pressures (Fig. 79-3).[9] Hypotension not only increases the early morbidity and mortality of spinal cord injury but also appears to decrease the likelihood of an optimal recovery.[1] It is therefore critical to monitor blood pressure closely in any patient with a real or suspected spinal cord injury and to strictly avoid even mild episodes of hypotension (systolic blood pressure < 90 mmHg).

The etiology of hypotension in the spinal cord injury patient is often multifactorial. As in any trauma patient, hypotension due to blood loss must be suspected and volume resuscitation initiated immediately. Intravenous access should be accomplished rapidly and isotonic fluids administered. The Trendelenburg position will increase central venous return, thereby increasing cardiac preload, and will also diminish the risk of aspiration. Military anti-shock trousers (MAST) will also assist volume redistribution. Although neurological deterioration has been associated with inflation of MAST trousers that include a posterior (thoracolumbar) bladder, newer designs eliminate this compartment, which reduces the probability of mobilizing a potentially unstable spinal region.[10]

Hypovolemic hypotension may occur in a relative sense if there is disruption of the descending sympathetic pathways. The loss of peripheral sympathetic drive with decreased peripheral vascular resistance will result in venous pooling and decreased cardiac afterload.[11] In general, when resuscitating a spinal cord injury patient, the adequacy of fluid resuscitation should be established by the early institution of central venous pressure monitoring in order to ensure adequate rehydration while avoiding volume overload. In instances where blood pressure remains low despite apparently adequate fluid resuscitation, a pulmonary artery catheter should be floated for monitoring of filling pressures, systemic vascular resistance, and cardiac output.

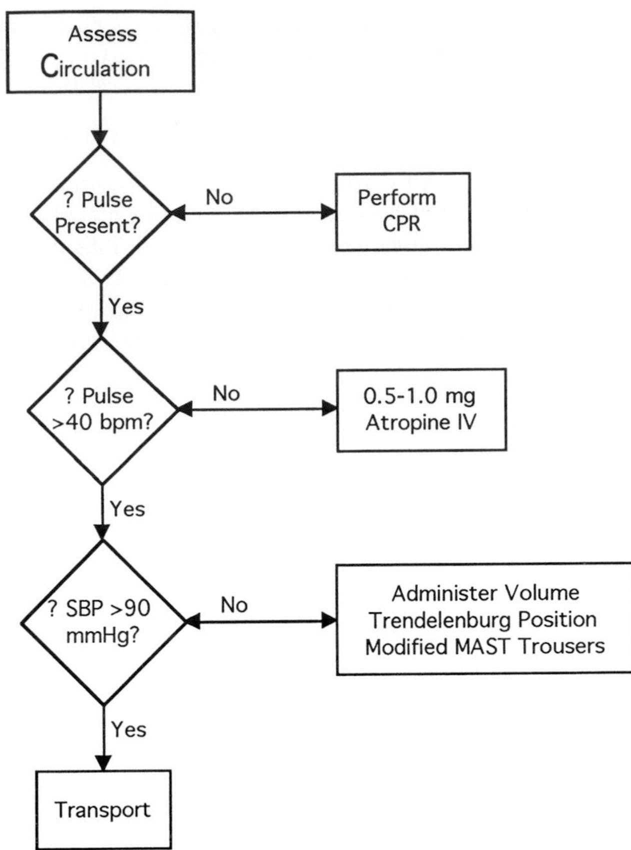

Figure 79-3. Evaluation and treatment of the *C*irculation component of the ABCs during the initial evaluation of the spinal injury patient.

In situations where the blood pressure is refractory to fluid administration and establishment of adequate cardiac preload, volume resuscitation often must be supplemented with such systemic pressors as dopamine or phenylephrine to maintain an adequate perfusion pressure. Although pressors are not substitutes for satisfactory volume resuscitation, the extreme sensitivity of the injured nervous system to even transient hypotension allows them to be used more freely in such a setting, even as a temporizing maneuver while the adequacy of fluid resuscitation is being established or checked.

In instances of complete spinal cord injuries above the cervicothoracic junction, the normal reflex response of tachycardia in response to hypotension will be prevented. Such injuries disrupt the descending sympathetic pathways prior to their exit to the sympathetic chain from which they course to the heart. This not only eliminates the positive inotropic and chronotropic actions of the sympathetic nervous system on the heart, but also leaves the parasympathetic (vagal) pathway uninhibited, with resulting bradycardia. This results in the paradoxical situation of hypotension and bradycardia, which immediately should suggest a severe injury to the cervical spinal cord.

The proper response to such a situation is to increase the cardiac preload by volume loading and redistribution. The bradycardia may be treated by intravenous atropine (0.5–1.0 mg IV) or glycopyrrolate (0.1 mg IV).

An indwelling urinary catheter should be inserted (after checking for urethral disruption in males) to monitor urine outflow and prevent bladder distension in patients with neurogenic urinary retention. In any patient with possible sensory dysfunction, diagnostic peritoneal lavage or abdominal CT imaging should be performed. Altered sensation can blunt or eliminate a patient's ability to complain of abdominal pain, and spinal shock will prevent the development of abdominal muscular rigidity.

Once the ABCs are secure, a rapid head-to-toe secondary survey should be performed. This may provide clues suggesting the possibility and the level of spinal column or cord injury. Scalp or facial injuries suggest possible cervical spine injury. Transabdominal ecchymoses commonly associated with thoracolumbar flexion-distraction injuries related to lap-belt use may be noted. Axial tenderness or deformity also may be present, but immobilization must not be compromised during any such examination. Motor or sensory deficits suggest neurological injury and may indicate the level; these should be noted so that any subsequent neurological changes can be detected.

In addition to the cervical spine x-rays that are part of the initial resuscitation studies, a complete set of spinal radiographs should be obtained. Since 11 percent of fractures associated with a head or spinal cord injury are missed, any patient with a suspected or proven neurological deficit must be cleared with a full set of high quality radiographs.[12]

Disruption of the peripheral sympathetic system can render spinal cord injury patients poikilothermic. Normal body temperature should be restored in such patients by external warming, warmed IV fluids, and heated inspired air if the patient is mechanically ventilated.

The neurological examination included in the second survey should be performed with an eye to determining the presence, severity, and level of neurological dysfunction. If the patient is alert and oriented, a full neurological examination can be carried out and the presence of a spinal cord injury definitively assessed. In the unconscious or uncooperative patient, however, less profound neurological deficits can easily be missed, as the sensorimotor examination often is limited to peripheral extremity withdrawal from noxious stimulation. In such instances, the patient cannot be determined to have an intact CNS when there is no evidence of trauma on a full set of quality axial skeleton radiographs. Even when radiographically cleared, such patients must remain on spinal precautions until more detailed neurological examination is possible after the sensorium clears.

In most instances, strict maintenance of spinal immobilization can be greatly facilitated by obtaining as many of the necessary initial studies as possible while the patient is still immobilized on the initial transport device (e.g., backboard). This minimizes the number of early patient transfers that can compromise immobilization.

An unstable patient who requires emergent, life-saving surgery or other interventional/diagnostic procedures should remain immobilized on the initial transport device throughout all transfers and procedures. Anteroposterior and lateral radiographs of the cervical spine should be obtained as soon as possible, either in the resuscitation unit or the operating theater. The rest of the axial skeletal radiographs can then be obtained when the urgent situation has been stabilized. Although it is incorrect to delay life-saving interventions in order to obtain cervical spine radiographs, and it is rarely possible to clear the cervical spine of an unstable patient during a rocky resuscitation, the early identification of injury types such as cervical dislocations can allow treatment to be initiated in the operating theater or radiology suite at the time of life-saving surgical/radiographic procedures.

EXAMINATION OF THE SPINE AND NEUROLOGICAL SYSTEM

Although the physical examination performed during any secondary survey must be complete and thorough, the examination of the axial skeleton and neurological system bear separate mention in the context of this chapter. The cervical spine can be examined while the patient is supine and always can be done during the secondary survey. Examination of the thoracolumbar spine also should be included in all trauma physical examinations, but requires turning the patient and generally should be done when the patient is log-rolled for removing the backboard. If there is neither a spinal cord injury nor suspicion of instability, the examination can be performed during the secondary survey. If either of these conditions exists, the removal of the backboard will be delayed until the patient is transferred to the nursing bed, and the spine exam should be performed at that time.

Examination of the cervical spine involves carefully palpating the midline and para-median elements from the occiput to as far down the upper thoracic region as possible without compromising immobilization. Because of the large paraspinous muscles, the spinous processes above C7 are difficult to feel, but the presence of point tenderness is suspicious for soft-tissue injury and obviates clearing the spine on a clinical basis in an otherwise asymptomatic patient. The presence of crepitus or widening of an interspinous space should also be noted.

Examination of the thoracolumbar spine should include serial palpation of all interspinous spaces. Point tenderness requires investigation. Widening of an interspinous space is very suggestive of a posterior column ligamentous injury, signs of which should be sought on radiographs of the region. Occasionally, posterior interspinous widening will be the only obvious finding in a patient with a soft tissue Chance fracture. The back should also be quickly inspected visually for spinal deformity as well as for skin lesions that could compromise any needed surgical procedure.

Although a very detailed and sensitive neurological examination is generally difficult to perform during the secondary survey, it is important to determine the patient's degree and level of deficit as early as possible in order to provide a baseline to which all subsequent examinations can be compared. The neurological examination must encompass both spinothalamic and dorsal column sensory functions as well as motor power and reflex activity. Pinprick sensation is the most easily tested sensation, particularly if a Wartenburg pinwheel is available. All dermatomes should be investigated in a serial fashion in order to determine the spinal level of injury and extent of dysfunction. The exam also must be compared side-to-side. When a region of hypesthesia is discovered, the level should be determined from above (intact to impaired) as well as from below (impaired to intact) in order to determine more precisely the actual boundaries as well as to detect the possible existence of a zone of hypesthesia between intact and completely anesthetic zones. All boundaries should be marked on the skin for further examiners.

Fine touch is difficult to examine during the secondary survey because it requires significant concentration by the patient, but an effort should nonetheless be made. A cotton-tipped applicator is useful for performing this exam. Again, the level of any sensory change as well as any side-to-side differences should be noted. Fine touch boundaries should be marked on the patient if different from pinprick.

Optimally, the neurological recording chart should contain a dermatome diagram (Fig. 79-4) on which the

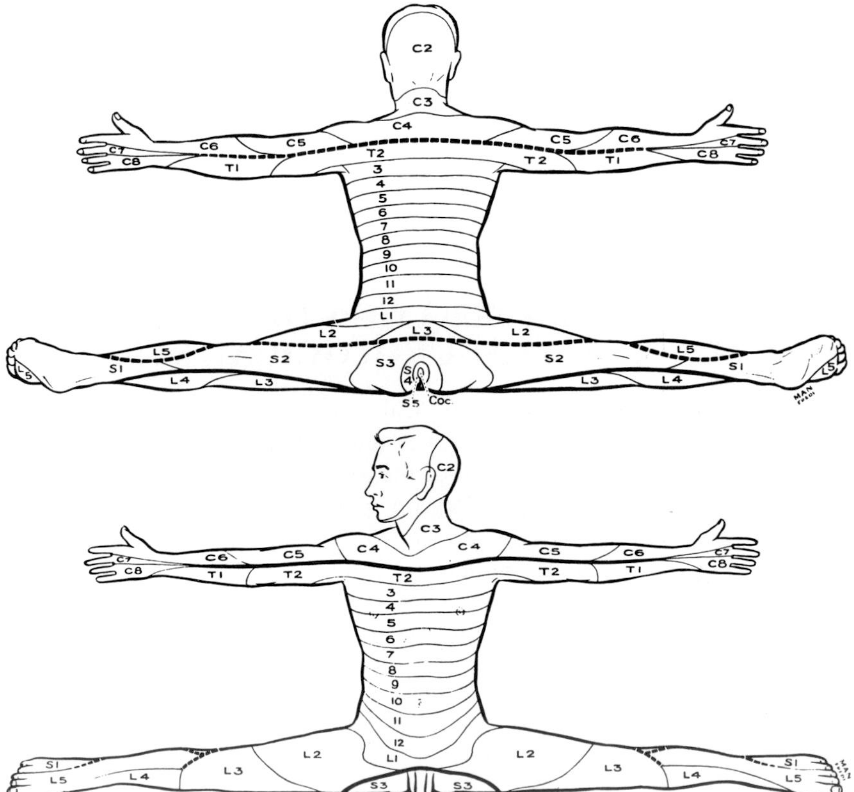

Figure 79-4. Cutaneous innervation dermatomes representing individual spinal segments (after Foerster). Note the "C4 cape" on the anterior and posterior chest (see text). (From Haymaker W, Woodhall B (eds): *Peripheral Nerve Injuries*, 2d ed. Philadelphia, WB Saunders, 1962, with permission.)

details of the sensory examination can be illustrated. One important aspect of the normal dermatomal pattern that is illustrated in Fig. 79-4 is the "C4 Cape." This is where the C4 dermatome directly abuts the T2 dermatome on the upper chest while the intervening C5 through T1 dermatomes are distributed exclusively on the upper extremities. If a distinct hypesthesia is noted at this level, it is important not to interpret this as a C4 sensory level, but, rather, to then perform a careful sensory examination on the adjoining upper extremity in order to clarify the actual neurological level. These levels should then be marked on both the chest and the extremity.

Vibration/joint position sense should also be determined for all extremities using a 128-Hz tuning fork or passive movement of joints. Losses in absolute sensitivity as well as side-to-side variations should be recorded. This is the most likely part of the initial examination to be confounded by preexisting medical conditions, such as diabetic or alcohol-related neuropathic changes.

The motor examination is a critically important part of the initial evaluation because it is objective, unlike the subjective sensory examinations. Motor power should be tested in all groups in all four extremities so that every cervical and lumbar level is tested at least twice (e.g., deltoid and supraspinatus for C5; brachioradialis and pronator for C6, etc.). Power should be recorded using the Royal Medical Council Scale (Table 79-1) for each muscle group. It is important to include the status of voluntary contraction of the anal sphincter as part of the motor examination.

Given the conditions under which it is being performed it is important not to compromise immobilization of the axial skeleton during the motor examination. Therefore, testing motor power in the flexors or extensors of the hip should be avoided until an unstable lumbar fracture has been ruled out. Additionally, the hip should be passively flexed only to a minimal extent during examination of knee flexion and extension power in order to avoid rotating the pelvis and thus mobilizing the lumbar spine.

TABLE 79-1 The Medical Research Council of Great Britain Grading Scale is the most commonly used scale for grading motor function in individual muscle groups. Grade 4 is sometimes subdivided into 4−, 4, and 4+ to reflect varying degrees of weakness against resistance.

Medical Research Council Muscle Grading Scale	
Grade 0	No motor activity.
Grade 1	Palpable muscle contraction. No joint motion.
Grade 2	Complete range of motion with gravity eliminated.
Grade 3	Complete range of motion against gravity.
Grade 4	Complete range of motion against gravity with some resistance.
Grade 5	Complete range of motion against gravity with full resistance.

Deep tendon reflexes (DTRs) should be examined in all extremities for presence and briskness as well as for side-to-side symmetry. DTRs should be graded from zero (absent) through four-plus (hyperactive with generalization or clonus). The presence of clonus should be noted separately. A single absent DTR suggests a root impingement, whereas symmetrical loss of DTRs in the lower extremities (or, rarely, all four extremities) often implies spinal shock. Hyperactive reflexes are consistent with an upper motor neuron lesion but do not limit the lesion to the spinal cord.

Testing for release reflexes, such as Babinski's or Hoffman's, is rarely useful in the acute situation where the subtle differentiation between true- and false-positives is difficult. Additionally, positive findings in isolation are of questionable value. Nevertheless, results should be recorded for the sake of completeness.

Reflexes, such as the anal wink and bulbocavernosus, as well as subconscious, tonic muscle activity, such as anal sphincter tone, should be tested. The anal wink is elicited by applying a mild, noxious (pinprick) stimulus to the perianal region and looking for a puckering of the anus. This is the normal response and should be present in "sacral sparing." The normal bulbocavernosus reflex is contraction of the anal sphincter in response to traction on the penis. It is best felt by inserting a finger into the rectum, during which the presence or absence of normal anal sphincter tone also can be checked. Reflex contraction of the anal sphincter muscles (normal "positive" bulbocavernosus reflex) must be differentiated from the sensation of movement of the Foley balloon when traction is applied to the penis after a Foley catheter has been inserted ("false-positive"). Absence of rectal sphincter tone and the bulbocavernosus reflex in the setting of an acute spinal cord injury suggests spinal shock.

Reflex penile erection ("priapism") may be present initially in males suffering complete spinal cord injuries. It is a release reflex and, if present, is a poor prognostic indicator with respect to recovery of function.

During the sensorimotor examination, it is particularly important to note the degree of patient attention and cooperation (including degree of iatrogenic or recreational intoxication) as well as the presence of confounding injuries such as fractures, abrasions, or lacerations of examined extremities. If there is reason to doubt the accuracy or veracity of the initial examination, the same examiner should repeat the exam as soon as conditions improve (e.g., under quieter circumstances).

Since a deteriorating neurological status mandates urgent intervention, it is particularly important to provide this information to all care-givers. All examinations should be carefully recorded on the same exam document. Additionally, a neurological examination should be performed jointly by both parties during any changes in nursing or physician personnel.

An important aspect of interpretation of results from the neurological and spine examination is integration with historical information. It often is difficult to determine if all or part of the abnormalities found on physical or radiographic examinations are new or manifestations of prior pathology. Neurological deficits, fractures, or physical deformities may be old, and their acuity may not be clear even with a good history. This is particularly true in the instance of the intoxicated or head-injured patient. Therefore, in addition to attending to the initial report by the transport team, it generally is profitable to obtain as much reliable historical information as possible from the patient, relatives, or old medical records. Previous radiographs can be of singular value in assisting in the dating of fractures, even if the films were not performed with bone imaging technique.

A number of neurological syndromes can be seen acutely and should be kept in mind during early examinations. These include spinal shock, the Brown-Seq́uard syndrome, the central cord syndrome, and the anterior cord syndrome. Spinal shock is commonly seen and presents as complete loss of any neurological function below a cord lesion, including segmental and polysynaptic reflex activity and autonomic functions. It appears to result from sudden and profound loss of descending facilitory supraspinal input to the spinal circuitry. Although prognostically ominous, it preempts a quantitative assessment of neurological function distal to the spinal cord injury until it clears. Spinal shock generally resolves within 1 to 2 weeks, although it can persist longer and may be permanent in as many as 15 percent of patients.[13]

The Brown-Seq́uard syndrome results from a lateral, hemicord lesion. Owing to disruption of the descending corticospinal and ascending dorsal column tracts, both of which decussate at the occipitocervical region, paralysis and loss of vibratory and joint-position senses occur ipsilateral to the lesion. Since spinothalamic fibers cross within several segments of their level of cord entry, most pain and temperature sensation loss will be contralateral to the injury. A small patch of ipsilateral hypalgesia often can be found at the level of the cord lesion, however, resulting from damage to fibers within the cord prior to decussation. The Brown-Seq́uard syndrome can result from any type of trauma, although it is more common with penetrating injuries.

The central cord syndrome occurs with injury at the cervical level causing damage to central or paracentral regions of the cord. This syndrome can occur with any injury type but is seen most commonly in patients without a vertebral fracture or instability but, rather, with focal or diffuse narrowing of the cervical canal due to a combination of a small native canal size and spondylotic disease or ossification of the posterior longitudinal ligament. Motor neurons of the upper extremities are injured, many permanently, and descending fibers to the lower extremities also are commonly involved, albeit to varying degrees. Since the motor fibers in the lateral corticospinal tract are laminated, such that those serving the lower extremities are more lateral, motor function is preferentially lost in the upper extremities. Upper extremity weakness is of the lower motor neuron type, whereas an upper motor neuron pattern is seen in the legs.

Vibration and position senses in the upper extremities generally are retained to a much greater extent than are sensations of pain and temperature. Although the dorsal columns usually are spared, there is characteristically damage to decussating spinothalamic fibers at the injury level as well as to the more medial layers of the spinothalamic tract (which arise from cervical regions).

Many patients with traumatic central cord syndromes present in spinal shock, and the syndrome is not recognized until this resolves. The overall presentation is that of three "mores": motor more than sensory; upper extremities more than lower extremities; distal dysfunction (hands) more than proximal. The *forme fruste* of the central cord syndrome is a patient with spastic hands.

The anterior cord syndrome is rare after trauma unless there is an accompanying cardiac arrest, disruption of the descending aorta, or period of profound hypotension. It is caused by interruption of perfusion in the distribution of the anterior spinal artery and is characterized by loss of the spinothalamic sensory and corticospinal motor functions residing in the anterior aspect of the spinal cord while the dorsal columns are spared.

TREATMENT OF ACUTE SPINE INJURY

Early Steroids

In 1990, the NASCIS-II study documented statistically significant improvement in motor function in patients who were prospectively and randomly treated with high-dose methylprednisolone for 24 h compared with those who received treatment with naloxone or placebo.[14,15] Despite the shortcomings of this study, it has established that early, high-dose methylprednisolone treatment of spinal cord injury patients can statistically increase the degree of their improvement as a group. Recent publication of the 1-year follow-up results from this study confirmed the statistical association between neurological improvement and treatment within 8 h.[15] Interestingly, patients treated between 8 and 12 h after injury actually had statistically less improvement than those given placebo. There were no statistically significant complications, albeit there were trends toward increased infection and gastrointestinal hemorrhage in the methylprednisolone-treated group.

As a result of this study, it has now become standard of practice to administer high-dose methylprednisolone to any patient suffering a spinal cord injury (excluding injuries of peripheral nerves or the cauda equina) if the steroid administration can be initiated within 8 h of the injury. The loading dose is 30 mg of intravenous methylprednisolone succinate, given as a bolus over 15 min, followed by a continuous intravenous infusion of 5.4 mg of methylprednisolone succinate per kg per h, initiated 45 min after the loading dose and continued for 23 h. Although, for statistical reasons, the NASCIS-II study was unable to ascertain that there was any increased benefit if the injury-to-steroid interval could be further shortened from 8 h, there is ample laboratory evidence that shortening the period between injury and drug administration is beneficial. Therefore, as soon as it is decided that the patient is a candidate, attempts should be made to initiate treatment as expeditiously as possible. It is to this end that some centers have initiated the administration of the loading dose by field personnel to patients with definite spinal cord injuries.

Currently, the NASCIS-III study is underway to determine the efficacy of a shorter injury-to-treatment interval, the efficacy of extending treatment to 48 h, and the utility of tirilazad (Lazaroid) versus methylprednisolone succinate as the anti-lipid-peroxidation agent during the second 24-h period.

Timing of Imaging Studies

After resuscitation and stabilization, it is important to make a definitive diagnosis in as expeditious a fashion as possible while maintaining strict patient immobilization, so that definitive therapy can be initiated with a thorough clinical understanding of the underlying anatomic pathology. Plain films are easily obtained with the patient remaining on the backboard. In most cases where CT scanning is readily available, computed tomographic imaging of the injured section, including the adjacent sections necessary for possible surgical stabilization, also can be rapidly obtained on the backboard. Plain tomography as well can be performed on the backboard, as can magnetic resonance imaging (MRI) if the backboard is completely nonferrous. These latter two studies, however, are rarely of importance equal to the CT scan in establishing the diagnosis.

The overall goal is to rapidly accomplish all necessary initial diagnostic studies without compromising the initial spinal immobilization by moving the patient from the backboard. This allows limiting the number of breaks in strict immobilization attendant on transferring the patient to and from the chosen nursing bed. In many instances, the only other such transfer necessary will be from the nursing bed to the operating table for definitive decompression and stabilization.

MRI and CT/Myelography in Acute Spinal Injury

If a proven neurological deficit is unexplained by radiographic findings, further studies should be performed to rule out spinal cord compression from a potentially treatable source, such as disk herniation, extra-axial hematoma, or retropulsed bony/soft tissue. Beyond plain CT scanning, the two diagnostic modalities most useful for this purpose are CT myelography and MRI. CT myelography is generally readily available in all centers and requires no special equipment or other physical constraints. It does, however, require significant patient manipulation, necessitates introduction of contrast material into the subarachnoid space, and does not image the spinal cord itself except as a signal void. Additionally, puncture below a complete block may precipitate neurological deterioration, adding hazard to the lumbar route of contrast instillation. The necessity of multiple transfers between the nursing bed, the myelography table, and the CT scanner also presents some risk. One advantage of this technique is that the CT images that follow the myelographic films is the excellent bone definition afforded by CT is very useful for operative planning.

The precise role of MRI in the early care of the spinal cord-injured patient is, as yet, undetermined. The major advantage of MRI scanning is its ability to visualize the spinal cord and identify precisely intra- and extramedullary soft tissue pathology.[16–19] Although the overall anatomic definition is far superior to that of CT myelography (with the exception of bony anatomy), both imaging modalities appear to be reliable in revealing pathology that is useful in determining the acute care treatment.[18,20] The specific capabilities of MRI to reveal the presence of spinal cord edema, hematomyelia, or various degrees of cord transection, however, appear to have some prognostic significance.[17,19] While clearly inferior to CT scanning with respect to delineation of bony pathology, it appears that traumatic vertebral injuries can be reliably identified with modern MRI techniques.[20] MRI signal changes consistent with hemorrhage within ligamentous structures will also outline soft tissue pathology not evidenced by CT myelography, which may be particularly useful in the head-injured patient with a neurological deficit not explained with other imaging modalities.[18,20,21]

Unfortunately, at most institutions, MRI scanning is not available on a 24-hour basis. In addition, the physical environment of the magnet makes the use of ferromagnetic materials impossible, greatly limiting the image of trauma patients requiring mechanical ventilation or other instrument-intensive treatments. Finally, the physical isolation of the patient within the MRI scanning tube not only impedes nursing care but also makes it difficult to monitor the patient visually during imaging. As a result, at most institutions, MRI scanning of the acute spinal cord/column injury patient should remain an elective study best applied to a stable patient with an unexplained or progressive neurological deficit.

Traction/Reduction of Cervical Spine Fractures/Dislocations

Following the initial resuscitation and radiographic evaluation of the patient with an unstable cervical spine injury, traction should be initiated for the purposes of stabilization and, if necessary, reduction. Although other methods, such as Crutchfield tongs or a halo ring, can be used, the most common method of securing traction to the patient's head is with Gardner-Wells tongs. These are applied under local anesthesia, the pins placed just above the pinnae of the ears on an imaginary plane connecting the mastoid processes and the external auditory canals. Prior to the placement of any traction device, it is important to rule out a skull defect that might complicate the application. In the case of Gardner-Wells tongs, the relevant areas of the skull often can be seen on the lateral cervical spine films. If there is any question of a fracture in the temporal regions, a lateral skull film can be obtained or the bone windows of a head CT scan can be inspected, if available. Once the tongs have been applied, traction should be arranged so that it is coaxial with the cervical spine and the initial lateral cervical spine traction radiograph obtained.

Overdistraction must be avoided.[22,23] This is particularly true in fractures of the upper cervical spine (C1, C2) or fractures associated with significant damage to anterior and posterior structures, such as hyperextension-distraction injuries or fracture-dislocations.[22,23] If the purpose of traction is simply to stabilize an injury, 5 lbs is sufficient weight for injuries of the upper cervical spine and 10 lbs usually is sufficient below.

In cases requiring reduction, the approach is much more controversial. It is generally felt beneficial to reduce cervical injuries associated with dislocation.[22,24–26] The accomplishment of reduction is associated with neurological improvement[24,25] as well as diminished frequency of late complications such as pain and instability.[24,26,27] Although anecdotal reports of a correlation between the rapidity of reduction and the degree of neurological improvement have been used to suggest that the reduction of dislocation should be carried out in an urgent fashion,[24,28] the necessity for very rapid reduction remains controversial and, again, the risk of overdistraction must not be ignored.

Neurological injury following reduction of cervical dislocations has been reported and generally is related to the presence of retropulsed disk material.[29,30] Although neurological improvement generally has followed subsequent anterior decompression, this has not always been the case. An alternative would be that every patient have a contrast-enhanced CT scan or an MRI scan of the cervical region prior to reduction. Unfortunately, in the vast majority of such instances, neither imaging modality is readily available, and a protracted delay in the initiation of reduction procedures is undesirable.

Fortunately, there are some early signs that the possibility of retropulsed disk material exists. It has been our experience that such material is generally visible if the soft-tissue windows of the prereduction cervical CT scan are carefully reviewed. Robertson and Ryan[30] reported that disproportionate narrowing of the disk space on plain radiographs is suggestive and should prompt further imaging prior to reduction. Certainly, any instance wherein neurological deterioration follows reduction should be investigated immediately with either a contrast-enhanced CT scan or a cervical MRI scan. If it is certain that there is only the single-level injury in the cervical spine and the patient deteriorates in a situation where neither of these imaging modalities is available, consideration should be given to exploration of the disk space.

In the situation of a cervical dislocation, there are two general approaches toward reduction: manipulation and traction. Although much more widely practiced in Europe and the United Kingdom than in the United States, manual reduction is an effective means for reducing cervical dislocations.[23,31] This technique has the advantage of combining tactile and radiographic feedback with the ongoing ability to perform a neurological examination on the patient in a dynamic setting that markedly enhances the rapidity with which reduction can be performed. Although it can be performed under anesthesia,[23,31] this eliminates active feedback from the patient and is therefore less desirable than reduction under sedation.

Manual reduction at our institution is performed in the operating theater under fluoroscopic guidance with an anesthetist present to administer sedation and other required medications. The goal of sedation is to relax the patient, particularly with respect to muscle spasm, without obtunding the patient's ability to report subjective changes in neurological function. Short-acting and/or reversible agents such as midazolam, fentanyl, or propofol are useful. A C-arm fluoroscope is placed at the level of the cervical spine, and the hands of the manipulator are protected by leaded gloves. The technique of manual reduction is actually reproduction of the angulation that produced the dislocation. This generally requires axial traction and sagittal angulation, which may be supplemented by minor degrees of lateral angulation or rotation. Liberal use of fluoroscopic imaging allows precise control of the process. In occasional cases, it is possible to gain some further degree of direct control of the cervical spine by direct pressure at the level of the fracture. Once the reduction has been accomplished, the neck is slowly returned to the neutral position and axial traction diminished. The patient is then characteristically left in between 5 to 10 lbs of axial traction for stabilization and the necessity for internal versus prosthetic stabilization addressed.

The more commonly used method in the United States is traction employing the attachment of a cord to the Gardner-Wells tongs, the other end of which is affixed to a platform upon which weights can be placed. This system has the disadvantage of being bulky and awkward, and CT scanning with the patient in this sort of traction is difficult to accomplish without potentially destabilizing manipulations of the weight and, therefore, the actual amount of traction applied. This is one of the reasons why it is very helpful to have obtained a quick CT study of the cervical spine prior to the initiation of traction.

The placement of the Gardner-Wells tongs can be varied according to the type of injury. For instance, flexion-distraction injuries such as unilateral or bilateral locked facets generally require flexion forces, and pin placement slightly behind the usual position may be useful.

Considerable controversy exists regarding the actual mechanics of traction-reduction. The general recommendation is a maximum of 5 lbs per vertebral level above the fracture/dislocation. Some authors recommend against using even this much weight for fear of overdistraction.[22] Others site cadaver studies suggesting that the pull-out strength of correctly applied Gardner-Wells tongs is greater than 100 pounds[32] and present reports of successful reduction using such weights in vivo.[24,32,33] We feel that the use of extremely high weights is heroic, carrying with it the significant chance of over-distraction and injury to ligamentous structures at other levels as well as the anecdotally reported catastrophic occurrence of tong pull-out, with immediate and complete loss of traction. In general, traction should be initiated with light weights and increased at 10- to 15-min intervals with attendant radiographs. The axis of traction should be manipulated in order to optimize reduction in a fashion similar to that used during manual reduction. A useful upper limit in most cases is 50 percent of the patient's body weight. As one approaches this limit, careful attention should be paid toward the vectors of traction, so that the weight is optimally applied. If traction is unsuccessful as the threshold is reached, a stepwise tapering back of weights should be accomplished without a delay longer than several hours, and other approaches should be considered. If reduction is accomplished, a similar stepwise diminution in traction also should be undertaken. Final traction weights should be between 5 and 10 lbs.

The administration of muscle relaxants and sedatives during such procedures can greatly facilitate reduction. Again, the goal is to relax the paraspinous muscles without obtundation. It is particularly important to avoid sudden oversedation during traction, as rapid relaxation of paraspinous musculature could allow significant overdistraction without a change in applied weight.

In general, reduction of unilateral or bilateral facets should be possible in 70 to 80 percent of cases[34] by either traction-reduction or manual reduction. Those cases not reduced should be surgically reduced in order to prevent delayed pain and instability.

Multiple Level Spinal Column Injuries

It is important to image the entire spinal axis in any patient with suspected or proven spinal column/cord injury. Multiple, noncontiguous fractures separated by an area of normal spine have been reported to occur in 4 to 5 percent of cases.[35–38] Calenoff and coworkers reported that, for patients whose neurological level identifies and focuses attention on a select region of the vertebral axis (primary injury), a significant number of secondary injuries are missed during the initial evaluation.[37] One clue to the likelihood of a secondary injury was a primary injury at the T2 to T7 level, which, although comprising less than 5 percent of all spinal column injuries, accounted for almost 50 percent of primary injuries in one series of spinal cord-injured patients with multiple level fractures. It is particularly important to pay careful attention to the distal ends of the vertebral column, as almost half of the secondary injuries occur at C1, C2, L4, or L5.[37]

Combined Head and Spinal Cord Injury

Some degree of head injury occurs in at least 25 percent of patients suffering acute spinal cord injury, particularly when the cervical spine is involved.[39] The combination of spinal cord injury and severe head injury (defined as a Glasgow Coma Scale [GCS] score of 8 or less) is less common, with a frequency of 2 to 3 percent. This is probably in part a reflection of the extremely high prehospital mortality of this combination of injuries. Unfortunately, recovery from one of these injuries is significantly complicated by the presence of the other, and this should be taken into account at the time of initial assessment.

Viewed in reverse, the presence of trauma to the head appears to be associated with a significant increase in the likelihood of concomitant cervical spine injury, so that approximately 4 to 6 percent of patients with head trauma will have a cervical spine fracture, two-thirds of which are unstable.[39–43] An additional 2 percent will have injuries to the thoracolumbar spine.[39] Of note, it has been suggested that it is the level of neurological function rather than the presence of injury to the head per se that is most indicative of the presence of a coincident cervical spine fracture.[43] It appears that depression in the level of consciousness to the extent that the GCS score is less than 14 approximately doubles the chance of a cervical spine fracture and the probability that the fracture is associated with a spinal cord injury.[39] Such data strongly underscore the necessity to immobilize absolutely the axial skeleton of any patient with a depressed level of consciousness until a spinal cord/column injury can be definitively ruled out. As many of these injuries occur at the craniocerebral junction—an area less clearly demonstrated on plain radiographs—and the mid- to lower cervical spine, liberal inclusion of CT cuts through the upper cervical spine at the time of brain imaging has been suggested as very useful in demonstrating occult occipitocervical fractures in head-injured patients.[44]

Patient Transfers

Patient transfers are particularly hazardous for the patient with an unstable axial skeleton. Strict axial alignment without rotation must be maintained at all times. At no point during transfer can the axial skeleton be unsupported. Mechnical devices such as slider-boards maintain a rigid undersurface and can facilitate horizontal patient movements. Sling lifts must not be employed unless the sling can be stabilized or substituted by a rigid frame.

Manual transfers, as from an imaging to a nursing bed, must be carefully planned and performed. A particularly useful technique is to place one person at the head of the bed to manage the cervical spine and four sturdy people on one side of the patient who all work their hands completely under the patient and then lift in unison from that side. This allows a sixth person to roll the gurney or other device from beneath the suspended patient and replace it with the receiving bed without requiring the group holding the patient to move.

Despite the best of intentions, such transfers are potentially hazardous, and this added risk must be taken into account when calculating the risk-benefit ratio of any planned maneuver.

TREATMENT ALGORITHMS FOR PATIENTS WITH SUSPECTED SPINAL COLUMN INJURY WITH OR WITHOUT SPINAL CORD INJURY

Figures 79-5 through 79-9 show suggested approaches toward evaluating patients with real or suspected spinal column injury with or without evidence of spinal cord dysfunction. They are intended only as an organizing framework to facilitate emergency evaluation of the spinal injury patient. Most of the injury-specific issues are dealt with in greater detail elsewhere in this text.

For both anatomic and biomechanical reasons, the C-spine is covered separately from the thoracolumbar spine. If more than one insult is suspected, two or more algorithms may be combined.

Clearing the Cervical Spine in Asymptomatic Patients Without Evidence of Neck Injury

Controversy exists over the mechanisms required to clear the cervical spine in the awake, alert, nonintoxicated patient with neither complaints nor physical signs of cervical spine injury. Although the most conservative method would be to obtain a full series of cervical spine radiographs in all patients, such a practice significantly increases the cost and duration of the initial evaluation and may expose the patient to unnecessary radiation. There is now significant evidence that patients who are awake, alert, and not intoxicated, who are neurologically intact (in a satisfactory examination performed with the full attention and cooperation of the patient), and who do not complain of cervical spine pain and are without tenderness or other physical findings suggestive of such injury, may be cleared clinically.[45–48] Notably, all these criteria must be strictly met before clinical clearance is valid (Fig. 79-5).

Of particular note is the necessity for the patient's mental status and attention to be completely unimpeded. Any patient who is intoxicated, who has an abnormal Glasgow Coma Scale score, or is unable to cooperate fully with the examination cannot be cleared clinically. It has also been suggested that the inability of a patient to give full attention to the examiner because

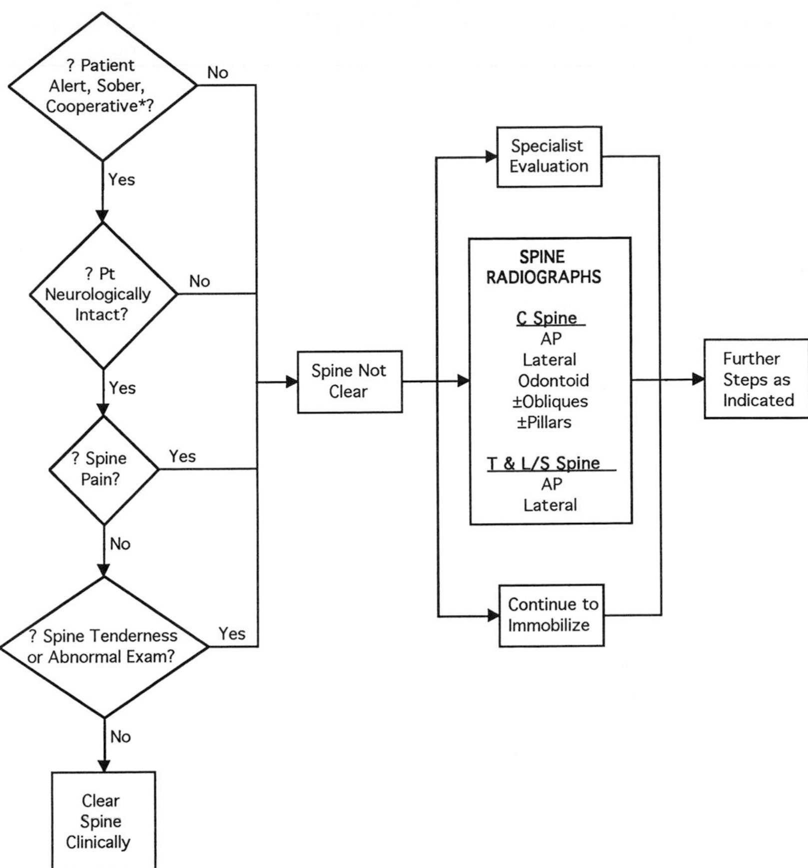

Figure 79-5. The initial spine evaluation when there is a low suspicion of a spine injury. Patients meeting all the criteria in the left column of the decision tree may be cleared clinically if flexion and extension are painless (see text).

of a severely painful injury unrelated to the cervical spine may increase the likelihood of missing a cervical spine injury, and this should be kept in mind when considering clearing the neck.[46]

In a patient who meets all the above criteria, observed flexion-extension should be performed. If this proves asymptomatic, the cervical spine can be cleared clinically. If there is any violation of the above criteria, the cervical spine must be considered unclear and radiographs obtained. Anteroposterior, lateral, and odontoid views are required in any patient whose cervical spine cannot be clinically cleared.[49,50] The cervical spine must continue to be immobilized until radiographically cleared.

Suspected Cervical Spine Injury Without Evidence of Spinal Cord Injury

The approach to the neurologically intact patient with symptoms or signs related to the neck is to expeditiously eliminate or confirm the presence of an injury while maintaining immobilization sufficient to protect against a delayed insult to the cervical cord (Fig. 79-6). The cervical spine should remain mechanically immobilized, and plain anteroposterior, lateral, and odontoid radiographs obtained. If these are normal, oblique ± pillars views should be obtained. If no fracture is revealed, the patient should be maintained in a rigid cervical orthosis.

If the patient is not in a great deal of initial discomfort, flexion-extension films can be performed straightaway. If pain is particularly severe, the patient should remain under observation until the pain abates enough for flexion-extension views to be obtained. Almost universally, these flexion-extension views will be limited in excursion and reliability by splinting of the paraspinous muscles because of pain. Although it has been argued that these early flexion-extension views can be eliminated and done only after the pain has resolved, occasionally evidence of a ligamentous instability can be visualized with early studies. Despite the paraspinous splinting, this will greatly facilitate diagnosis and treatment. Therefore, early flexion-extension views should be performed, even in a patient with mild to moderate discomfort.

Rigid cervical orthosis should not be discontinued on the basis of early flexion-extension views, however, even if there is no motion. Instead, it should be worn until pain has abated, at which point the flexion-extension

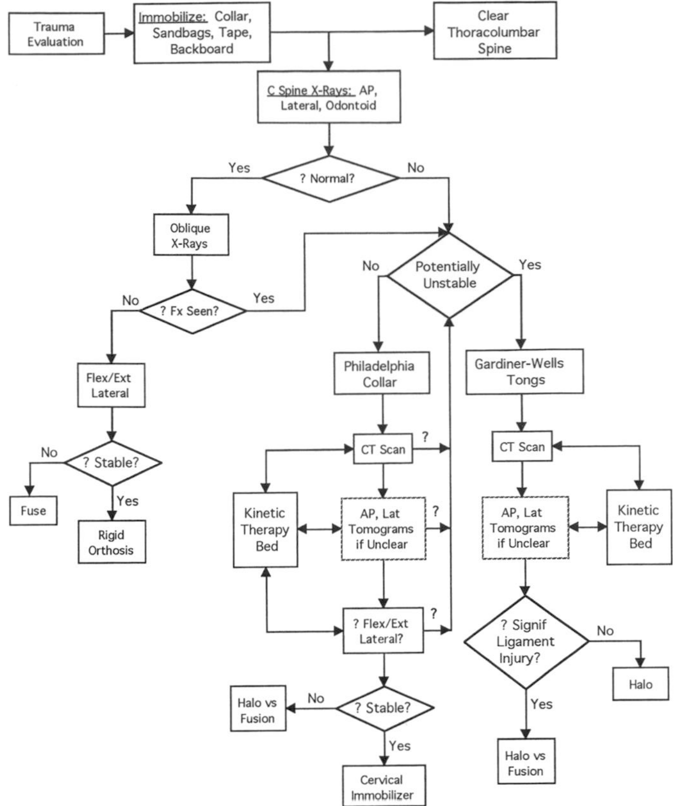

Figure 79-6. The acute management of a patient with a suspected cervical spine injury without neurological deficit.

views can be repeated on an inpatient or outpatient basis as dictated by other injuries. The patient must not be taken out of the rigid cervical orthosis until full and unencumbered flexion-extension views are revealed to be normal.

Occasionally a patient will present with unremarkable cervical spine films but profound neck pain. This is highly suspicious for "internal splinting" of an unstable cervical spine injury. Patients with severe neck pain should not be discharged until the pain has abated enough to allow a reasonable first set of flexion-extension views. If a very high level of suspicion remains despite adequate, negative flexion-extension views, a White-Panjabi stretch test may be performed.[5] This is rarely indicated in the presence of fully satisfactory flexion-extension views. In most cases, if instability is revealed despite the absence of a bony injury, the injury is ligamentous and usually will require fusion.

If a fracture is seen on oblique films, this level should undergo CT scanning for full delineation of the anatomy of the injury. This may be supplemented with AP and lateral tomograms if the injury is unclear. Tomography is particularly useful when the fracture is in the same plane as the CT imaging. This is particularly true with odontoid fractures, which are much better delineated by tomography than by CT imaging, even with reconstructions.

If there is a significant cervical spine fracture, the immediate question is potential instability. Even if it appears to be a stable fracture, the patient should remain immobilized until full imaging is accomplished. This may or may not require lateral flexion-extension views to determine stability. Mobilization must not be allowed until the stability has been determined and the proper mode of stabilization established.

For potentially unstable cervical spine fractures, the patient should be placed in Gardner-Wells tongs after the initial diagnostic CT scan, with traction as applied for stabilization and/or reduction as indicated. Further imaging may be required, but generally should be delayed until the patient has been well stabilized and any necessary reduction has been accomplished. Again, the degree of instability and the component of ligamentous damage will dictate the subsequent definitive treatment.

In most cases, bony injuries will heal, and the goal becomes adequate alignment with anatomic restoration and protection of the cervical cord. Depending on the location and seriousness of the fracture, treatment in a cervical immobilizer or a halo is the most common practice if normal anatomy can be restored and maintained.

Suspected Thoracolumbar Spine Injury Without Evidence of Spinal Cord Injury

Maintaining the thoracolumbar spine in a state of rigid immobilization, AP and lateral radiographs should be obtained (Fig. 79-7). If no fracture or dislocation is disclosed, oblique views may be useful, particularly in the lumbosacral region. If plain film radiographs do not reveal pathology and an area is particularly suspect, CT imaging or AP and lateral tomography may reveal unsuspected fractures or suggest ligamentous disruption. Use of either of these imaging modalities, however, requires some confidence in localizing the region of suspicion. In some cases, the ability of MRI to demonstrate hemorrhage associated with ligamentous disruption may be of use. In general, however, a patient with no evidence of fracture should be nursed with spine precautions until the muscular spasm abates and flexion-extension lateral radiographs may be obtained.

If a fracture is seen, the patient should remain immobilized on the backboard, and CT imaging obtained. In most cases, this will permit both a definitive diagnosis and treatment planning. The patient may then either be placed on the appropriate immobilization bed or taken directly for definitive therapy. In some cases, such as Chance fractures, AP and lateral tomograms may reveal pathology missed by the CT scan and should be

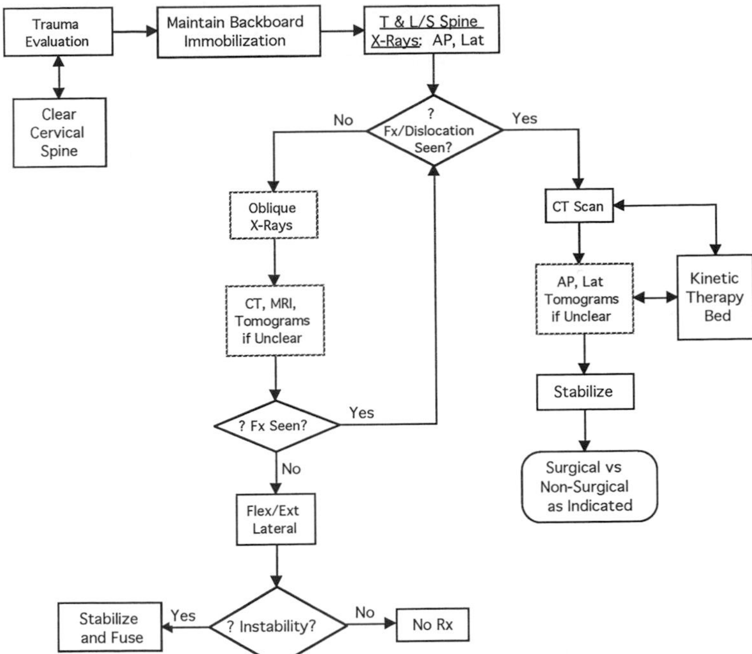

Figure 79-7. The acute management of a patient with a suspected thoracolumbar spine injury without neurological deficit.

considered when there is a possibility that the axis of fracture or dislocation is coplanar with the CT imaging sequence.

Cervical Spinal Cord Injury

In the patient with a neurological deficit, the emphasis changes from determining the presence of a bony lesion and preventing possible injury to defining the skeletal damage and minimizing or reversing the neurological deficit (Fig. 79-8). As soon as the neurological deficit is recognized, the NASCIS-II steroid protocol should be initiated. For the patient with a cervical spinal cord insult, the entire axial skeleton must be immobilized throughout the diagnostic and prestabilization period, utilizing a backboard as well as sandbags or a hard cervical collar, forehead tape during evaluation, and a kinetic treatment bed or Stryker frame with Gardner-Wells tongs and traction for nursing. The initial resuscitation must be carried out, assuming that the patient is unable to subjectively identify any potential pathology below the level of the cervical spine. A full set of skeletal radiographs should be obtained in order not to miss secondary fractures in the thoracolumbar area.

A full series of plain cervical radiographs should be taken in order to define the fracture. If no fracture or dislocation is seen, the patient should remain immobilized and a CT scan obtained, focused at the level indicated by the neurological examination and including at least one motion segment above and below that level. If a definitive injury is demonstrated by CT scan, subsequent treatment will be dictated by these findings. If there is no radiographic evidence of a cervical spine fracture, the likelihood of a significant ligamentous injury should be entertained, and the patient should remain immobilized on a spinal nursing bed. The placement of Gardner-Wells tongs to moderate (10 to 20 lbs) traction may be of use at this point to assist in stabilizing the cervical spine and, perhaps indirectly, decompressing the spinal canal to some extent by unfolding the ligamentum flavum. Further studies, possibly including tomography, CT/myelography, or MRI, can then be planned and obtained when possible. If the injury is well defined by these studies, definitive treatment can be undertaken. If not, flexion-extension views should be obtained, possibly supplemented by a White-Panjabi stretch test to evaluate further ligamentous stability and to allow final planning of treatment.

If a fracture or dislocation is seen, the immediate goals are diagnosis and the institution of appropriate therapy. If there is no need for reduction, a CT scan should be obtained with the patient completely immobilized. A definitive treatment plan can then be formulated and initiated if a firm diagnosis results from the CT scan data. If not, the patient generally should be transferred to the spinal nursing bed until further studies can be obtained as indicated. Depending on the type of injury, its degree of instability, and the amount of ligamentous damage, operative or nonoperative treatment can be planned.

If reduction is necessary, a CT scan should be obtained if one is immediately available; otherwise, reduction should be initiated and CT imaging deferred. Prereduction CT scanning allows refinement in the ap-

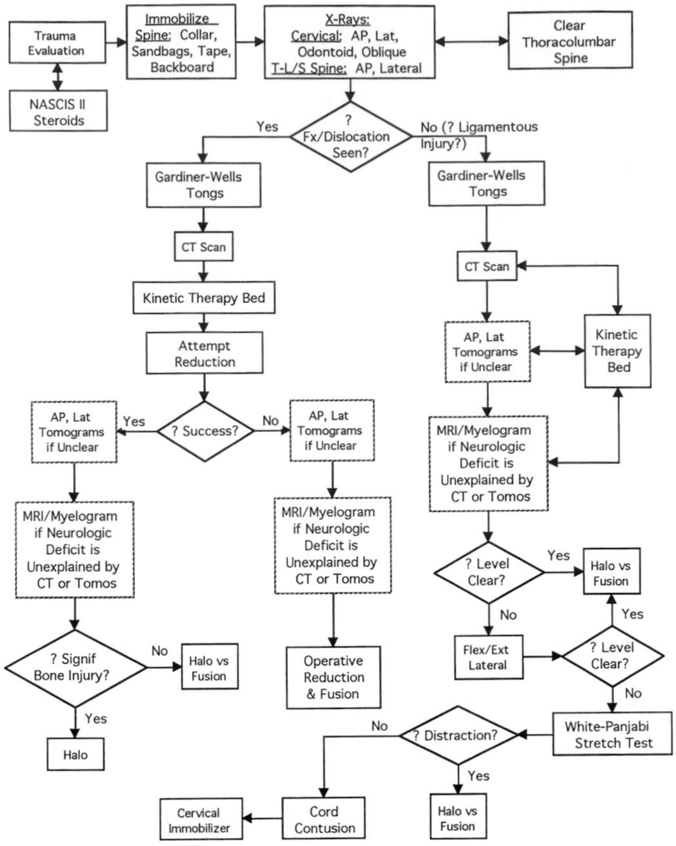

Figure 79-8. The acute management of a patient with a suspected cervical spine injury with a neurological deficit suggesting a cord injury.

proach to reduction based on the degree of dislocation, the presence of associated fractures (particularly joint fractures), and the possibility of unsuspected fracture planes. In addition, careful examination of the soft tissue images often will suggest a large retropulsed disk fragment if such is present. Herniated disk material can present a significant risk to the cervical cord during reduction, suggesting that a prereduction CT/myelogram or MRI should be obtained and that an anterior decompression might be needed as an initial therapeutic step.

If reduction is successful, the need for further imaging can be assessed. If it is not successful, operative reduction will be required, and further imaging should be considered, knowing that intraoperative reduction is performed in the absence of patient feedback outside of electrophysiological recording.

Thoracolumbar Spinal Cord Injury

As with a cervical spine injury, the goal here is to allow full and expeditious diagnosis without placing the patient at risk for further injury (Fig. 79-9). As soon as the neurological deficit is recognized, the NASCIS-II steroid protocol should be initiated. Concomitant with obtaining a full set of thoracolumbar spine radiographs, the cervical spine should be evaluated and cleared, if possible. If the thoracolumbar spine series reveals a fracture or dislocation, the patient usually should be taken immediately to the CT scanner while still on the initial backboard and the definitive pathological anatomy demonstrated. Unless immediate surgery is planned, the patient should then be immobilized in a spinal nursing bed. The necessity for and planning of further diagnostic imaging may then be accomplished and the proper treatment and its time course planned.

If no fracture or dislocation is found on the initial evaluation of a patient with a thoracolumbar cord injury, further imaging is indicated. Oblique films may be useful in the lumbar area and may be obtained at this point. The most definitive evaluation will be the CT scan, which should be straightforwardly obtained without mobilizing the patient from the backboard unless there is a significant delay before the scanner becomes available. If the CT scan reveals the pathology to a satisfactory degree, definitive therapy can be planned. If not, the patient usually should be placed on the spinal nursing bed and further studies planned and obtained under stable, prearranged conditions. Since the absence of an expeditious diagnosis generally means a delayed surgical procedure, subsequent evaluation should be done under planned, stable, and controlled conditions.

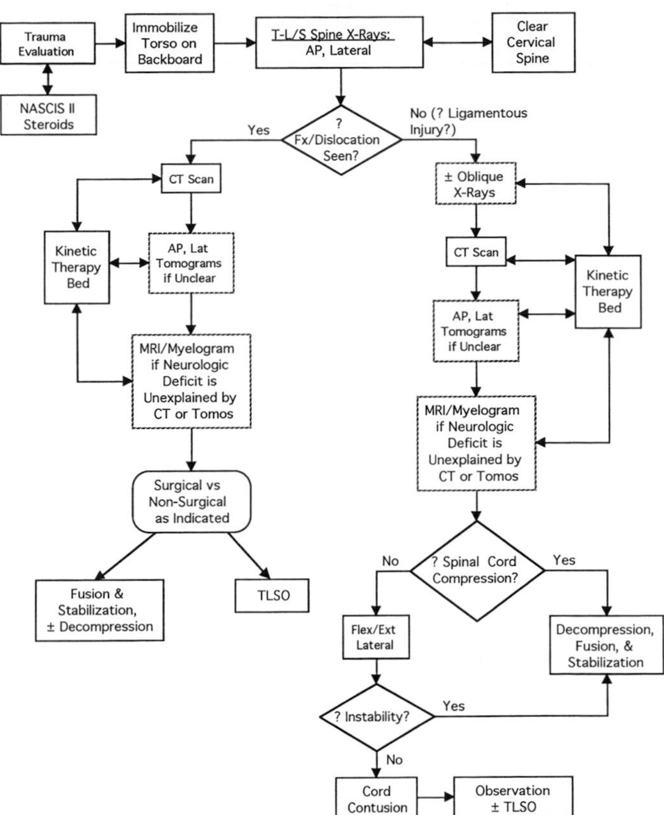

Figure 79-9. The acute management of a patient with a suspected thoracolumbar spine injury with a neurological deficit suggesting a cord injury.

The presence of a fracture or evidence of significant ligamentous injury, with or without concomitant spinal cord compression, generally guides definitive treatment. If no evidence of precise pathology is obtained on static imaging, the patient should be immobilized until paraspinous muscle spasm has resolved and satisfactory flexion-extension views obtained. If no instability is evidenced on these studies, the patient may be very carefully mobilized, generally wearing a TLSO.

References

1. Meguro K, Tator CH: Effect of multiple trauma on mortality and neurological recovery after spinal cord or cauda equina injury. *Neurol Med Chir* 1988; 28:34–41.
2. Gunby P: New focus on spinal cord injury. *JAMA* 1981; 245:1201–1206.
3. Dunford JV: Spinal column trauma, in Baxt W (ed): *Trauma: The First Hour.* Norwalk, CT: Appleton-Century-Crofts, 1984: 171–219.
4. Podolsky SM, Baraff LJ, Simon RR, et al: Efficacy of cervical spine immobilization methods. *J Trauma* 1983; 23:687–690.
5. White AA, Panjabi MM: *Clinical Biomechanics of the Spine.* Philadelphia: JB Lippincott, 1978.
6. Johnson RM, Hart DL, Simmons EF, et al: Cervical orthoses: A study comparing their effectiveness in restricting cervical motion in normal subjects. *J Bone Joint Surg* 1977; 59A:332–339.
7. Bivins HG, Ford S, Bezmalinovic Z, et al: The effect of axial traction during orotracheal intubation of the trauma victim with an unstable cervical spine. *Ann Emerg Med* 1988; 17:25–29.
8. Sellick BA: Cricoid pressure to control regurgitation of stomach contents during induction of anaesthesia. *Lancet* 1961; 2:404–406.
9. Bohlman HH, Ducker TB, Lucas JT: Spine and spinal cord injuries, in Rothman RH, Simeone FA (eds): *The Spine*. Philadelphia: WB Saunders, 1982: 362–371.
10. Rockwell DD, Butler AB, Keats TE, Edlich RF: An improved design of the pneumatic counterpressure trousers. *Am J Surg* 1982; 143:377–379.
11. Troll GF, Dohrmann GJ: Anaesthesia of the spinal cord-injured patient: Cardiovascular problems and their management. *Paraplegia* 1975; 13:162–171.
12. Garland DE, Rhoades ME: Orthopedic management of brain-injured adults: Part II. *Clin Orthop* 1978: 52–56.
13. Kuhn RA: Functional capacity of the isolated human spinal cord. *Brain* 1950; 73:1–51.
14. Bracken MB, Shepard MJ, Collins WF, et al: A randomized, controlled trial of methylprednisolone or naloxone in the treatment of acute spinal-cord injury: Results of the Second National Acute Spinal Cord Injury Study. *N Engl J Med* 1990; 322:1405–1411.

15. Bracken MB, Shepard MJ, Collins WFJ, et al: Methylprednisolone or naloxone treatment after acute spinal cord injury: 1-year follow-up data. Results of the second National Acute Spinal Cord Injury Study. *J Neurosurg* 1992; 76:23–31.
16. Kalfas I, Wilberger J, Goldberg A, Prostko ER: Magnetic resonance imaging in acute spinal cord trauma. *Neurosurgery* 1988; 23:295–299.
17. OBeirne J, Cassidy N, Raza K, et al: Role of magnetic resonance imaging in the assessment of spinal injuries. *Injury* 1993; 24:149–154.
18. Wittenberg RH, Boetel U, Beyer HK: Magnetic resonance imaging and computer tomography of acute spinal cord trauma. *Clin Orthop* 1990: 95–101.
19. Schaefer DM, Flanders A, Northrup BE, et al: Magnetic resonance imaging of acute cervical spine trauma: Correlation with severity of neurologic injury. *Spine* 1989; 14:1090–1095.
20. Silberstein M, Tress BM, Hennessy O: A comparison between M.R.I. and C.T. in acute spinal trauma. *Australas Radiol* 1992; 36:192–197.
21. Emery SE, Pathria MN, Wilber RG, et al: Magnetic resonance imaging of posttraumatic spinal ligament injury. *J Spinal Disord* 1989; 2:229–233.
22. Jeanneret B, Magerl F, Ward JC: Overdistraction: A hazard of skull traction in the management of acute injuries of the cervical spine. *Arch Orthop Trauma Surg* 1991; 110:242–245.
23. Sonntag VK: Management of bilateral locked facets of the cervical spine. Neurosurgery 1981; 8:150–152.
24. Cotler HB, Miller LS, DeLucia FA, et al: Closed reduction of cervical spine dislocations. *Clin Orthop* 1987: 88–93.
25. Shrosbree RD: Neurological sequelae of reduction of fracture dislocations of the cervical spine. *Paraplegia* 1979; 17:212–221.
26. Beyer CA, Cabanela ME: Unilateral facet dislocations and fracture-dislocations of the cervical spine: A review [published erratum appears in *Orthopedics* 1992 May;15(5):545]. *Orthopedics* 1992; 15:311–315.
27. Rorabeck CH, Rock MG, Hawkins RJ, Bourne RB: Unilateral facet dislocation of the cervical spine: An analysis of the results of treatment in 26 patients. *Spine* 1987; 12:23–27.
28. Brunette DD, Rockswold GL: Neurologic recovery following rapid spinal realignment for complete cervical spinal cord injury. *J Trauma* 1987; 27:445–447.
29. Olerud C, Jonsson HJ: Compression of the cervical spine cord after reduction of fracture dislocations: Report of 2 cases. *Acta Orthop Scand* 1991; 62:599–601.
30. Robertson PA, Ryan MD: Neurological deterioration after reduction of cervical subluxation: Mechanical compression by disc tissue. *J Bone Joint Surg [Br]* 1992; 74:224–227.
31. Kleyn PJ: Dislocations of the cervical spine: Closed reduction under anaesthesia. *Paraplegia* 1984; 22:271–281.
32. Star AM, Jones AA, Cotler JM, et al: Immediate closed reduction of cervical spine dislocations using traction. *Spine* 1990; 15:1068–1072.
33. Sabiston CP, Wing PC, Schweigel JF, et al: Closed reduction of dislocations of the lower cervical spine. *J Trauma* 1988; 28:832–835.
34. Bucholz RD, Cheung KC: Halo vest versus spinal fusion for cervical injury: Evidence from an outcome study. *J Neurosurg* 1989; 70:884–892.
35. Bentley G, McSweeney T: Multiple spinal injuries. *Br J Surg* 1968; 55:565–570.
36. Blahd WH, Iserson KV, Bjelland JC: Efficacy of the posttraumatic cross-table lateral view of the cervical spine. *J Emerg Med* 1985; 2:243–249.
37. Calenoff L, Chessare JW, Rogers LF, et al: Multiple level spinal injuries: Importance of early recognition. *Am J Roentgenol* 1978; 130:665–669.
38. Kewalramani L, Taylor RG: Multiple noncontiguous injuries to the spine. *Acta Orthop Scand* 1976; 47:52–58.
39. Michael DB, Guyot DR, Darmody WR: Coincidence of head and cervical spine injury. *J Neurotrauma* 1989; 6:177–189.
40. Hills MW, Deane SA: Head injury and facial injury: Is there an increased risk of cervical spine injury? *J Trauma* 1993; 34:549–553.
41. Kach K, Friedl HP, Imhof HG, Trentz O: [Unstable spinal injuries in cranio-cerebral injuries]. *Schweiz Med Wochenschr* 1993; 123:582–586.
42. Moskopp D, Boker DK, Kurthen M, et al: [Concomitant vertebral trauma in patients with craniocerebral injuries: 34 consecutive patients over 3 years]. *Unfallchirurg* 1990; 93:120–126.
43. Williams J, Jehle D, Cottington E, Shufflebarger C: Head, facial, and clavicular trauma as a predictor of cervical-spine injury. *Ann Emerg Med* 1992; 21:719–722.
44. Kirshenbaum KJ, Nadimpalli SR, Fantus R, Cavallino RP: Unsuspected upper cervical spine fractures associated with significant head trauma: role of CT. *J Emerg Med* 1990; 8:183–198.
45. McNamara RM, Heine E, Esposito B: Cervical spine injury and radiography in alert, high-risk patients. *J Emerg Med* 1990; 8:177–182.
46. Hoffman JR, Schriger DL, Mower W, et al: Low-risk criteria for cervical-spine radiography in blunt trauma: A prospective study. *Ann Emerg Med* 1992; 21:1454–1460.
47. Kreipke DL, Gillespie KR, McCarthy MC, et al: Reliability of indications for cervical spine films in trauma patients. *J Trauma* 1989; 29:1438–1439.
48. Mirvis SE, Diaconis JN, Chirico PA, et al: Protocol-driven radiologic evaluation of suspected cervical spine injury: Efficacy study. *Radiology* 1989; 170:831–834.
49. MacDonald RL, Schwartz ML, Mirich D, et al: Diagnosis of cervical spine injury in motor vehicle crash victims: How many X-rays are enough? *J Trauma* 1990; 30:392–397.
50. Bachulis BL, Long WB, Hynes GD, Johnson MC: Clinical indications for cervical spine radiographs in the traumatized patient. *Am J Surg* 1987; 153:473–478.

CHAPTER 80

CERVICAL, THORACIC, AND LUMBAR ORTHOSES

Curtis A. Dickman
William R. Zerick

INTRODUCTION

Spinal orthotic devices were used as early as the fifth Egyptian dynasty.[1] Today's wide variety of orthotic devices can be used as the sole treatment or as an adjunct to surgery. This chapter reviews the fundamental principles and clinical characteristics of spinal orthoses. Commonly used spinal orthoses are examined, along with their applications and potential complications. The scientific principles and biomechanical efficacy of different spinal orthoses need to be considered to plan rational treatment strategies.

The goal of a spinal orthosis is to limit spinal motion over specific segments. After trauma, an orthosis can be used to reduce load on the vertebral column while fractures heal or while a fusion forms across internally fixated motion segments. Spinal orthoses also may be required as a diagnostic trial, to provide mechanical support, to immobilize the spine, to correct spinal deformity, and to protect the spinal cord and nerve roots. Selection of the proper orthosis is based on the condition being addressed, the general medical condition of the patient, and expectations for compliance. Treatment should be individualized by patient and the extent of spinal injury. One person may be a candidate for a halo external device, but a more compliant patient with an identical injury could be treated with a cervical collar or poster-type orthoses.

PRINCIPLES OF SPINAL IMMOBILIZATION WITH ORTHOSES

The basic tenets of spinal orthoses for traumatic spinal injuries have evolved from principles developed in treating scoliosis.[2,3] The simplest functions of an orthosis are to limit gross motions of the trunk, head, or neck and to reduce segmental spinal motion.[2,3]

Orthoses act by several mechanisms to control spinal motions.[3–6] First, orthoses usually apply forces indirectly to the spine, not by directly fixating the spine. Second, skeletal fixation can be provided by directly fixating the skeleton (e.g., the halo brace). Third, soft tissue structures adjacent to the vertebral column can be compressed, distracted, and immobilized. Finally, restraining devices can provide an irritative reminder for the patient to restrict spinal motion.

Orthotic devices are intended to protect the neural structures, to allow healing of spinal fractures or a spinal fusion, to decrease spinal motion, to maintain spinal alignment, and to correct spinal deformity. Spinal stability can be achieved using an orthosis while the bone and/or ligaments of the spine heal, until the spine can bear full physiological loads.

The effectiveness of immobilization of an orthosis depends on the location and extent of the spinal injury; the design, configuration, and fitting of the orthotic device; and the patient's motion and body habitus. For example, an orthosis will immobilize a thin or inactive patient better than an obese or active patient.

Orthoses also are used postoperatively. The strength of a spinal internal fixation device depends on the patient's bone density, the implant characteristics, and the subsequent stresses acting on the spine. Postoperative orthoses are used as an adjunct to "load share" or to reduce the forces acting to cause failure of the fixation device until the bone fuses solidly. The mechanical requirements of a postoperative orthosis are not usually as stringent as a nonoperative orthosis.

Early orthoses made from plaster casts, metal and/or leather were heavy, bulky, and often uncomfortable. Current orthoses are made from lightweight composite materials and can be custom-molded to make them comfortable, lightweight, and more effective. Brace components commonly are made from thermoplastic materials (e.g., low-density polyethylene or polypropylene). Metal alloys also have been introduced to facilitate spine imaging and to improve the strength-to-weight ratio of the braces.

The effectiveness of the orthosis ultimately depends on proper fit and patient compliance. A halo vest, thoracic brace, or thoracolumbar orthosis should harness the trunk and fit like a saddle on a horse. The orthosis should fit snugly against the soft tissues. Three-point fixation or circumferential fixation can be provided. Contact with bone prominences (e.g., iliac crest, ribs, mandible, etc.) is needed, but the braces must be molded and padded to avoid eroding the skin. Braces that are custom-fitted and reinforced with pads apply the best corrective forces and achieve the best immobilization.

The normal biomechanical characteristics of each spinal segment also determine the effectiveness of an orthosis. The cervical and lumbar motion segments are more difficult to immobilize because they are very flexible and have a much wider range of motion than the thoracic vertebrae. In comparison, the thoracic motion segments are usually fixated more effectively with an orthoses because they are relatively rigid and stiff and because the ribs attach to the thoracic vertebrae.

The vertebrae are rigid structures connected by elastic soft tissue structures (ligaments and discs) and surrounded by viscoelastic soft tissues. The multiple joints and the segmental viscoelastic character of the spine make it difficult to immobilize the spine with an orthosis. Even when corrective forces are applied by an orthosis, "paradoxical motion"—snaking movements of the spine—can still occur. This motion is analogous to the undulations of a snake's body when it is held at both its head and tail.

CERVICAL SPINE ORTHOTIC DEVICES

There are four types of cervical spine orthoses: collars; poster-type orthoses; cervicothoracic orthoses; and halo orthoses (Figs. 80-1, 80-2). Motion control is best achieved through rigid skeletal fixation, which is provided with the halo brace. Orthoses that employ mechanical compression or three-point fixation, such as the

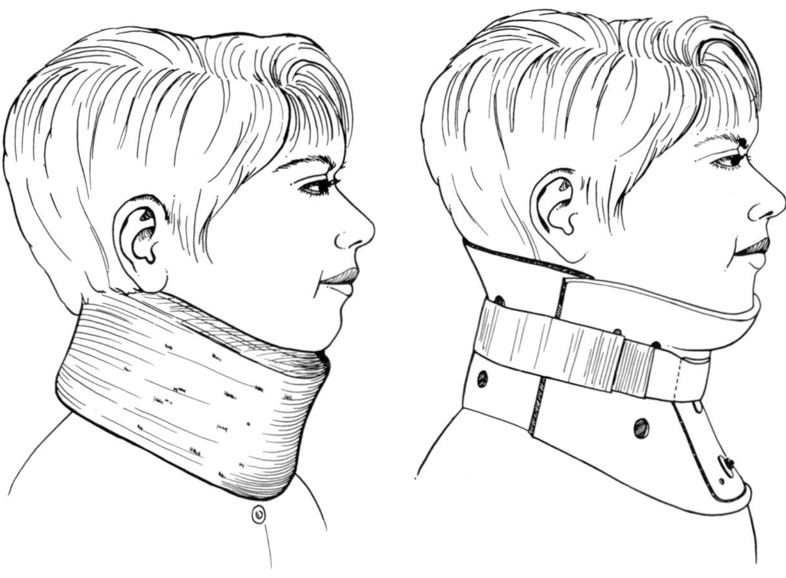

Figure 80-1. *A*. The soft cervical collar is constructed of foam and cloth. *B*. The Philadelphia-type reinforced cervical collar has a mandibular and occipital extension to restrain cervical movements. *C*. Sterno-occipital-mandibular immobilizer (SOMI). This is a three-poster brace that attaches to a sternal plate. *D*. The four-poster brace. *E*. The Yale cervicothoracic collar.

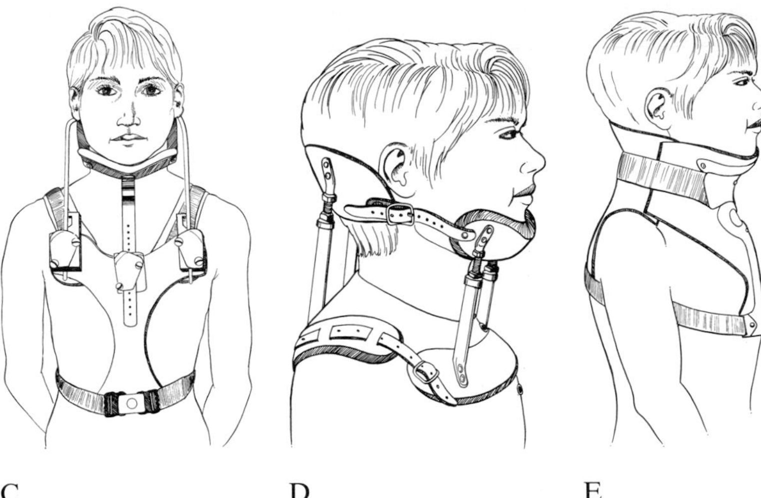

Figure 80-1. *Continued.* C D E

poster-type, provide less motion control. Each type of orthosis will be considered individually. The mechanical immobilization provided by the different cervical orthoses is compared in Fig. 80-3.

Cervical Collars

Cervical collars are the most popular type of cervical orthosis (Fig. 80-1*A*, *B*). They are affordable, comfortable, and require little expertise to apply. Cervical collars provide gentle muscular support, but minimally restrict cervical motion. Cervical collars are relatively ineffective as spinal immobilization devices and act by applying pressure against the soft tissues of the neck and mandible to resist neck movement. There are two types—the soft collar and the reinforced (Philadelphia-type) collar.

Soft collars minimally restrict neck motion.[7–10] A soft cervical collar should be used only when the spine is stable, as with cervical muscle spasm or sprains. Hard collars shaped like the soft collar have been constructed of polyethylene to provide additional support; however, these collars also only minimally restrict cervical motion.

The Philadelphia collar is the most commonly used cervical orthosis for minor injuries and degenerative conditions (Fig. 80-1*B*). The Philadelphia collar provides substantially more restriction of cervical motion than the soft collar (Fig. 80-3). It limits motion best in the sagittal plane (i.e., flexion and extension), but it is less effective for restricting lateral bending and axial rotation. Its mandibular and occipital supports moderately restrict cervical motion. The Philadelphia collar restricts motion better at the upper cervical spine than in the middle or lower cervical segments.

The Malibu collar and Miami collar are reinforced, molded cervical collars similar to the Philadelphia collar. Their height and circumference may be adjusted to permit a more contoured fit and to restrict cervical motion more than the Philadelphia collar.

The use of the "Philadelphia" type collar should be limited to clinical situations where cervical stability is known, e.g., after cervical fusions, with minor fractures, or for muscular injuries. This collar may be used to treat nondisplaced or minimally displaced cervical fractures. In the prehospital setting after an accident, the collar is valuable because it partially restricts movement and is easy to apply. When used with sandbags and tape to restrict head motion on a backboard, satisfactory temporary immobilization of the spine can be achieved.

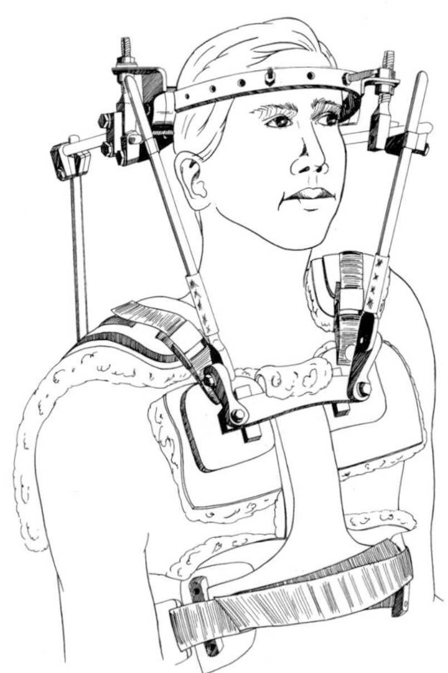

Figure 80-2. The halo brace.

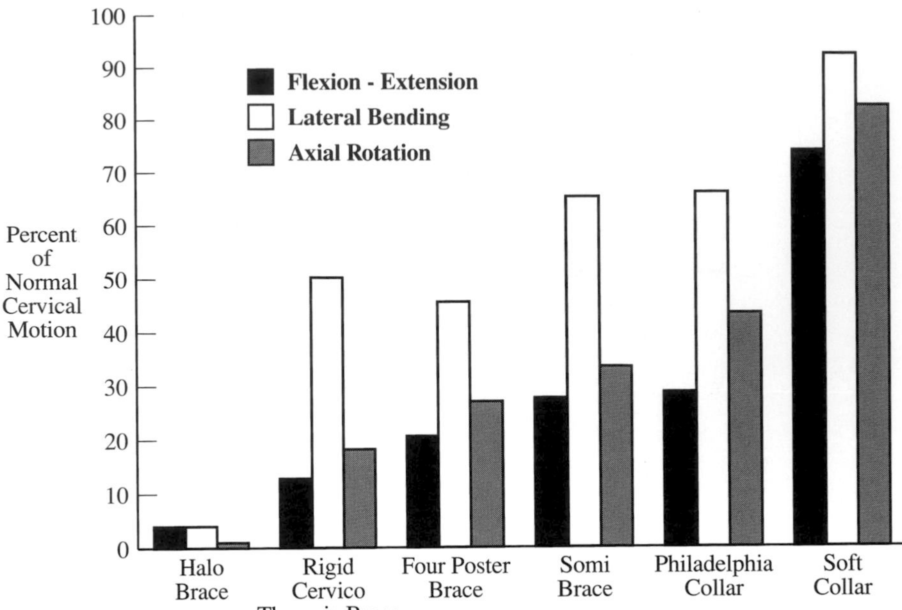

Figure 80-3. Cervical motions allowed by different orthosis in normal subjects. (Based on data from Johnson RM, et al.[14])

Poster Orthoses

Poster orthoses provide more rigid support and can restrict cervical motion slightly better than the Philadelphia collar (Fig. 80-1*C*, *D*, Fig. 80-3). Poster-type orthoses constrain neck motion by fixating the mandible, the occiput, and the thorax. Examples of the poster orthoses are the sterno-occipito-mandibular immobilizer brace (SOMI), a three-poster brace, and the four-poster brace. The prefabricated SOMI brace has mandibular and occipital supports attached to a sternal vest by three adjustable posts (Fig. 80-1*C*). This brace can be applied relatively easily with the patient in a supine position. The four-poster brace is similar to the SOMI brace, but it has four adjustable metal supports that attach to an adjustable chest brace (Fig. 80-1*D*). Compared to the Philadelphia collar, the SOMI brace provides significantly more control of rotation, but it is equally effective for restricting lateral bending and flexion-extension. The four-poster brace restricts more flexion, extension, lateral bending, and axial rotation than the SOMI brace (Fig. 80-3).

Cervicothoracic Orthoses

The Philadelphia collar, four-poster, and SOMI braces control gross cervical motion fairly well, but their principal effect is to restrict motion between C1 and C3. These braces provide little motion control below the C4 level. The Yale collar, a rigid cervicothoracic orthosis, provides better immobilization distal to the C4 level. It has a sternal and chest plate that attaches to a molded, reinforced Philadelphia-type collar (Fig. 80-1*E*). It is easy to apply and usually is well tolerated. The Yale cervicothoracic collar is the most rigid of the nonhalo orthoses (Fig. 80-3).

The cervicothoracic junction, the lower cervical spine, and the upper thoracic spine are difficult to immobilize with an orthosis because the vertebrae are distant from the external sites of fixation and because this is a transition area from a mobile, flexible region to a fixed, rigid region. Four types of orthoses can be used for the cervicothoracic junction: (1) a cervicothoracic orthosis; (2) a halo orthosis; (3) a thoracolumbar sacral orthosis (TLSO) brace with a SOMI extension (i.e., a Milwaukee brace); or (4) a Minerva body jacket.[11] The halo brace and the Minerva jacket provide the most effective fixation of this region.[11]

Halo Brace

The halo brace was designed by Nickel after modification of a device designed to treat facial fractures in pilots.[12,13] The halo brace provides the most rigid immobilization available for the cervical spine (Fig. 80-2). It is the best device to control motion between the occiput and C3. The halo brace achieves skeletal fixation, restricting cervical motion better than any other orthosis. It has become the standard by which the effectiveness of other cervical orthoses are compared.

The first halo braces were attached to a body cast. Blount[2] modified the halo by replacing the cast with a thoracic vest attached to the halo ring by posts. Many modifications have since added to the ease of use, comfort, and efficacy of the halo fixator. Lightweight composite brace materials allow magnetic resonance (MR) imaging compatibility and have made the halo more useful after concurrent brain and spine injuries. The use of partially open, incomplete rings facilitates application. Attachments between the halo ring and posts allow the surgeon to vary the head and neck position to permit fine multiplanar control of cervical alignment. The vests are lightweight; when custom fitted, they minimally restrict respiratory function.

The halo brace is clearly the most effective cervical orthosis for restricting cervical motion; however, it does not completely eliminate all cervical motion.[8,14–16] In normal subjects, the halo brace permits 4 percent of the cervical motion during flexion-extension, 1 percent of axial rotation, and 4 percent of lateral bending (Fig. 80-3). These data were collected on subjects without cervical instability; therefore, the findings should be applied with caution in patients with spinal instability. More spinal motion may occur in the injured spine immobilized with the halo brace.

Wang and coworkers[15] compared the ability of halo vests of different lengths to restrict cervical motion. They wanted to determine whether shortening the vest length to provide more comfort compromised mechanical immobilization. Twenty normal subjects each wore three different vest lengths: (1) a full vest extending to the iliac crests; (2) a short vest extending to the costal margins; and (3) a half vest extending to the level of the nipples. Regardless of the length of the vest, no cervical motion occurred during axial rotation or lateral bending. When flexion-extension was evaluated, no significant differences occurred in motion cephalad to the fifth cervical vertebra. Caudal to C5, the vest that extended to the level of the costal margins provided better immobilization than the half vest, but extending the vest to the level of the iliac crest provided no additional benefit.[15]

The halo brace must be applied properly and fitted correctly to provide effective fixation and to minimize complications. An experienced orthotist is an invaluable asset for the application and ongoing management of a halo device. Since the halo brace is frequently used in clinical practice, we will review the basic techniques for application.

During application of the halo brace, mild sedatives can be administered, but respiratory compromise must be avoided and neurological signs must be monitored closely. The patient remains supine while one person immobilizes the head, applies traction, and maintains cervical alignment. Pin-sites are selected and prepared by shaving the hair and cleansing the skin by sterile techniques. Local anesthesia is achieved by injecting 1% lidocaine solution into the scalp.

Anterolateral pin-sites are positioned approximately 1 cm superior to the orbital rim, cephalad to the lateral two-thirds of the orbit. Medial pin-sites are avoided to avoid penetrating the frontal sinuses. Care also is taken to avoid the anterior aspect of the temporalis muscle. The thin bone over the frontal sinuses, and the thin temporal squamosa are avoided to prevent the pins from penetrating the skull. The posterior pin-sites are selected diagonal to the anterior pins. If the occiput is at the six o'clock position, the posterior pins are at the four and eight o'clock position. Posterior pin-sites are selected to allow 1 cm of clearance between the superior aspect of the ear and the halo ring.

Certain patients may require different pin-sites to allow for differences in head shape. Additional pins may be needed if the forehead is sloped or the skull is thin. A halo ring is selected to allow clearance of 1 cm around the head. The ring is carefully sized to ensure that it does not contact the scalp or is not too large. The halo ring is then positioned with temporary pins. The sterile permanent pins are advanced to the skin, making sure that the pins are perpendicular to the skull.[17] A stab wound at the pin-site does not provide any clinical or mechanical advantage and may cause unnecessary scalp bleeding.[18] After the patient's eyes are closed, the pins are advanced sequentially by 2-in/lb increments with a torque screwdriver. The pins are advanced, alternating the tightening between diagonally opposed pins until a 6- or 8-in/lb (0.90 N/m) torque is reached.[18]

After the halo ring is secured, the posterior halo vest is positioned after carefully lifting the patient's trunk 30° from the bed while maintaining neutral cervical alignment. The patient is then returned to the supine position, the anterior portion of the vest is placed, and the anterior and posterior vest segments are attached to each other. The posts are attached to the vest and to the halo ring. Final pin torque and vest fit are reassessed. A supine lateral cervical spine radiograph is obtained to check the cervical alignment; subsequently, sitting and upright radiographs are obtained. The pins are retightened one day after placement and then as needed. Pin-site care is performed twice daily with half-strength hydrogen peroxide and Betadine ointment.

Several complications associated with the halo brace have been reported.[12,19–25] Complications of the halo brace can be minimized by proper placement of pins, attention to pin-site care, and proper vest and halo ring fitting.[26] The most common complication is a local scalp pin-site infection, which usually can be prevented with meticulous pin-site care. Pin-site infections generally respond to oral antibiotics, local pin-site care, and changing the pin to a new location. When cellulitis or a scalp abscess develops, cultures should be obtained, the patient placed on intravenous antibiotics, and the pin-site changed. Early detection and prevention of pin-site infections are needed to avoid skull osteomyelitis, epidural abscess, or brain abscesses. Fortunately, these complications are uncommon. Other complications of the halo brace include loss of spinal alignment, bone graft migration, decubitus ulcers under the vest, restriction of respiratory function, and others. Serial cervical spine films are warranted during the course of immobilization to evaluate for changes in spinal alignment. Custom-fitted vests may be necessary in patients with kyphotic deformities who are susceptible to skin breakdown or in patients who require special vest sizes (children or obese patients).

THORACIC AND LUMBAR ORTHOSES

The Milwaukee brace or cervicothoracic lumbosacral orthosis, the original standard care of orthotic treatment, was developed for the treatment of scoliosis. Introduced by Blount,[2,3] this brace consists of a body jacket (TLSO) with a SOMI extension. It is used to treat kyphotic deformities or scoliotic deformities with apices above the T8 level.

Thoracic and lumbar spinal orthoses can be divided into four types: corsets, braces, jackets, and spicas (Figs. 80-4–80-6). All are used for the lumbar spine; only braces and jackets are used for the thoracic spine.

Thoracolumbar orthoses act by immobilizing the chest, abdomen, and trunk, secondarily restraining the spine by immobilizing the tissue surrounding it. The thoracolumbar junction, like the cervicothoracic junction, is difficult to immobilize with an orthosis because of the transition from a very rigid to a very mobile region of the spine.

Many braces and jackets have been used for thoracolumbar fixation, such as the Boston Brace, the Wilmington jacket, the Miami TLSO, the Rosenberger orthosis, the Jewett hyperextension brace, the Milwaukee brace, the Taylor brace, the Williams brace, and the chairback brace, among others. These braces act by providing mul-

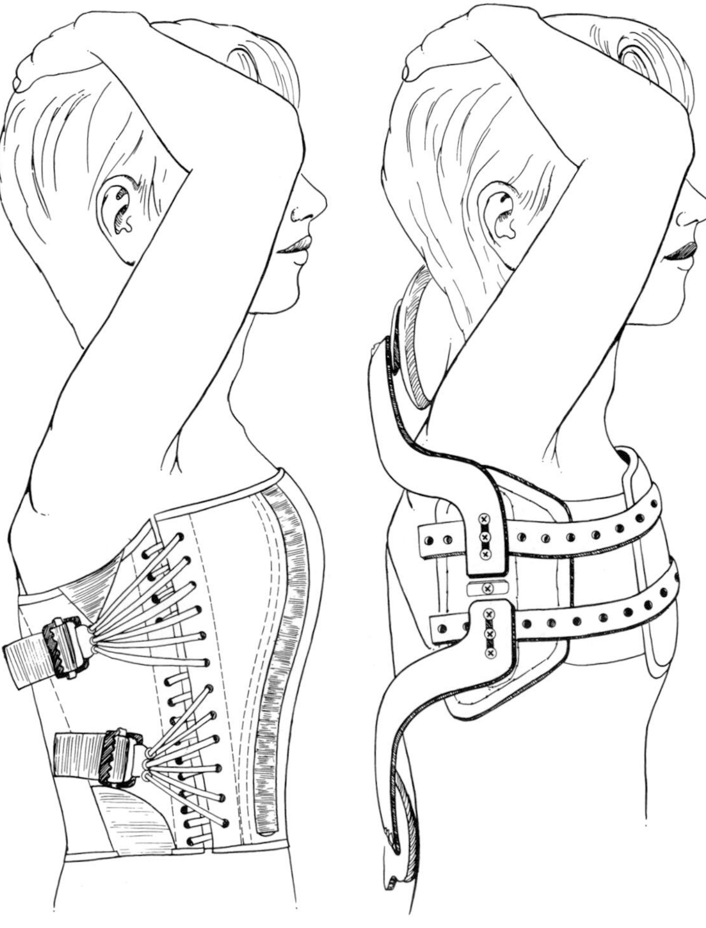

Figure 80-4. (*A*) Lumbar corset brace. (*B*) Jewett hyperextension brace.

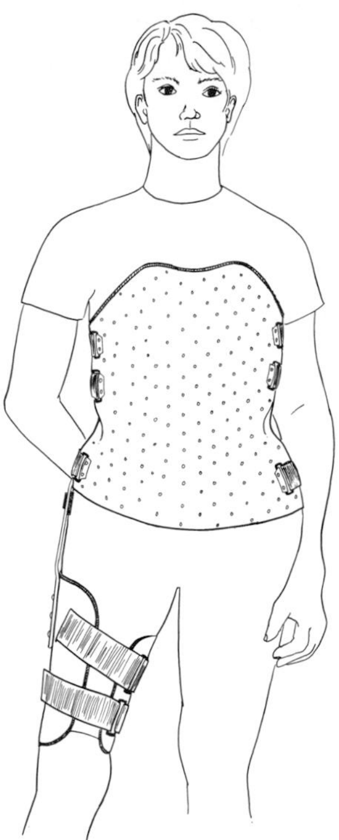

Figure 80-5. Thoracolumbosacral orthosis (TLSO) with a thigh extension.

tiple points of fixation of the torso and by increasing intraabdominal pressure, acting to unload the spine.[27]

The TLSO is a generic term that describes an orthosis that extends from the axillae or mid-chest, across the thoracolumbar junction, to the level of the iliac crests (Figs. 80-5, 80-6). The TLSO usually is a custom-molded jacket made of thermoplastic materials. The TLSO immobilizes the spine from the T8 to the L4 levels and is reasonably effective for treating fractures of the thoracolumbar junction. The brace primarily restricts flexion and extension, with less restriction of lateral bending and axial rotation. Biomechanically, the TLSO provides significantly more rigid immobilization than the corset brace or chairback brace. This type of brace is ineffective for deformities or injuries above the T8 level. Similarly, the TLSO brace poorly restricts motion across the lumbosacral joint. To immobilize the L5 and sacral segments, a thigh extension (i.e., spica extension) is added to the TLSO to reduce motion across the pelvis.

Because the lumbar spine is normally mobile and because of the inability to achieve skeletal fixation, little motion control is achieved with lumbar orthoses. A large amount of soft tissue must transmit the forces applied from the orthotic device to the spine. Trunk support is used with lumbar and thoracolumbar orthoses, causing an increase in intraabdominal pressure that allows transmission of loads from the spinal column to the trunk.

The simplest, least restrictive lumbar orthosis is the corset (Fig. 80-4*A*). Corsets are constructed of canvas with reinforced metal struts. They provide little support or motion restriction, and are used most often in the management of chronic low back pain, acting primarily as an irritative restraint.[5]

Lumbosacral spica orthoses or TLSO jackets with a thigh extension are used to restrict lumbosacral motion. The spica uses three-point fixation and the sleeve principle to limit pelvic and lumbosacral motion. Like the TLSO, spicas are custom-fitted but have a thigh extension that limits pelvic movement.[4,28,29] Patients requiring restriction of movement between L4 and S1 require secure pelvic fixation, generally with a spica or thigh extension.

The mechanical effects of lumbar and lumbosacral orthoses were compared in normal volunteers[28] to evaluate from L1 to L5. The corset reduced midlumbar movements by 33 percent, while the TLSO and spica reduced movement to two-thirds of normal. A jacket with a spica attachment was the most effective combination in reducing low lumbar and lumbosacral motion. It allowed only 12 percent of normal movement at

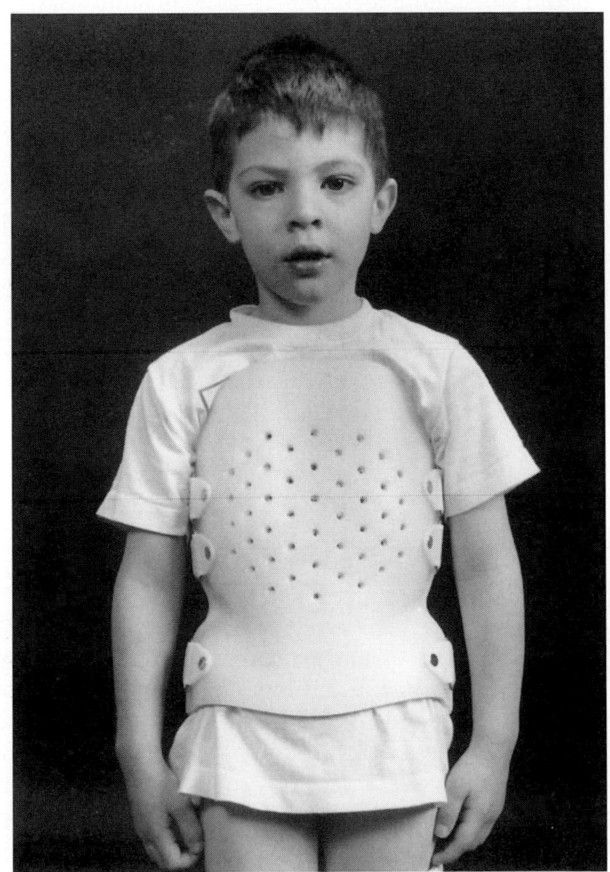

Figure 80-6. A custom-fitted TLSO brace used in a two-year-old boy with a lumbar spine fracture.

L4–L5 and only 8 percent of normal movement at the L5–S1 segment. The effect of the spica, compared with the jacket without the thigh extension, was statistically significant for limiting lumbosacral movement.

ORTHOSES FOR CHILDREN

The mechanisms of action of orthoses are the same in children as in adults. However, special considerations are needed for pediatric orthoses.[3,30,31] The small body sizes and unique individual body habitus require lightweight, custom-fitted orthoses in most children (Fig. 80-6). If orthoses are used for a prolonged period, they will need to be refitted as the child grows. Children's bones heal much more quickly than adults' bones; therefore, prolonged bracing usually is unnecessary.

The risk of noncompliance is high in children. Children tend to disregard their orthoses and resume normal activity if unsupervised. This noncompliance has been implicated in recurrent spinal cord injuries in children.[31] To avoid noncompliance, the child and family should be extensively counseled. Attachments can be added to the orthosis to prevent removal by the unsupervised child.

Cervical collars and poster braces should be used carefully in children because mandibular distraction can cause dental deformities and malocclusion.[3,30]

If the halo brace is needed for a small child, the skull thickness should be assessed with a head CT. Multiple pins are placed (8 to 10 pins) with low pin torques (1- to 2-in-lb), and a custom halo ring and vest are also needed.[30] The halo brace can be used in children as young as two years old.[30]

CONCLUSION

A variety of orthoses are available for immobilization of the cervical, thoracic, and lumbar spine. The type of orthosis used depends primarily on the location of the spine injury, its severity, and the patient's cooperation. Minimally restrictive orthoses are used for muscular injuries. Moderately restrictive orthoses are used for linear, nondisplaced, or minimally displaced fractures. Rigid orthoses are used for comminuted or widely displaced fractures.

A team approach is essential to ensure a successful result from orthotic treatment. The patient, orthotist, nurses, respiratory therapists, and physicians must work together to educate the patient and to minimize complications. Close follow-up and serial spine radiographs are needed to detect complications and failures of treatment, such as loss of alignment, progressive spinal kyphosis, and nonunion. Fractures that fail to heal properly with an orthosis require internal fixation to prevent progressive spinal deformity and neurological injury. Orthoses also can provide an invaluable postoperative adjunct to reduce loads on the fixated spine while the fusion is healing.

REFERENCES

1. Smith GE: The most ancient splints. *Br Med J* 1908; 1:732.
2. Blount WP: Early recognition and prompt evaluation of spinal deformity. *Wis Med J* 1969; 68:245–249.
3. Gavin TM, Shurr DG, Patwardhan AG: Orthotic treatment for spinal disorders, in Weinstein SL (ed): *The Pediatric Spine: Principles and Practice.* New York: Raven Press, 1994: 1795–1827.
4. Sypert GW: Spinal orthotics, in Sundaresan N (ed): *Tumors of the Spine, Diagnosis and Clinical Management.* Philadelphia: Saunders, 1990: 494–503.
5. Sypert GW: External spinal orthotics. *Neurosurgery* 1987; 20:642–649.
6. White AA, Panjabi MM: *Clinical Biomechanics of the Spine.* Toronto: Lippincott, 1978.
7. Colachis SC, Strohm BR: Cervical spine motion in normal women: Radiographic study of effect of cervical collars. *Arch Phys Med Rehabil* 1973; 54:161–169.
8. Hartman JT, Palumbo F, Hill BJ: Cineradiography of the braced normal cervical spine: A comparative study of five commonly used cervical orthoses. *Clin Orthop* 1975; 109:97–102.
9. Johnson RM, Owen JR, Hart DL: Cervical orthoses: A guide to their selection and use. *Clin Orthop* 1981; 154:34–45.
10. Kaufman WA, Lunsford TR, Lunsford BR, Lance LL: Comparison of three prefabricated cervical collars. *Orthot Prosthet* 1986; 39:21–28.
11. Benzel EC, Larson SJ, Kerk JJ, et al: The thermoplastic Minerva body jacket: A clinical comparison with other cervical spine splinting techniques. *J Spin Dis* 1992; 5(3):311–319.
12. Perry J: The halo in spinal abnormalities: Practical factors and avoidance of complications. *Orthop Clin North Am* 1972; 3:69.
13. Perry J, Nickel VL: Total cervical spine fusion for neck paralysis. *J Bone Joint Surg (Am)* 1959; 41A:37.
14. Johnson RM, Hart DL, Simmons EF, et al: Cervical orthoses: A study comparing their effectiveness in restricting cervical motion in normal subjects. *J Bone Joint Surg (Am)* 1977; 59A:332–339.
15. Wang GJ, Moskal JT, Albert T, et al: The effect of halo-vest length on stability of the cervical spine: A study in

normal subjects. *J Bone Joint Surg* (*Am*) 1988; 70A:357–360.

16. Wolf JW, Jones HB: Comparison of cervical immobilization of the cervical spine by halo casts versus halo plastic jackets. *Orthop Trans* 1981; 5:118.
17. Triggs KJ, Ballock RT, Lee TQ, et al: The effect of angled insertion on halo pin fixation. *Spine* 1989; 14:781.
18. Botte MJ, Byrne TP, Garfin SR: Use of skin incisions in the application of halo skeletal fixator pins. *Clin Orthop* 1989; 246:100.
19. Garfin SR, Botte MJ, Byrne TP, Woo SLY: Application and maintenance of the halo skeletal fixator. *Update Spin Dis* 1987; 2:1.
20. Garfin SR, Botte MJ, Nickel VL, Waters RL: Complication in the use of the halo fixation device. *J Bone Joint Surg* (*Am*) 1986; 68A:320–325.
21. Garfin SR, Botte MJ, Triggs KJ, Nickel VL: Subdural abscess associated with halo-pin traction. *J Bone Joint Surg* (*Am*) 1988; 70A:1338.
22. Glaser JA, Whitehill R, Stamp WG, Jane JA: Complications associated with halo-vest: A review of 245 cases. *J Neurosurg* 1986; 65:762–769.
23. Goodman ML, Nelson PB: Brain abscess complicating the use of a halo orthosis. *Neurosurgery* 1987; 20:27–30.
24. Victor DI, Bresnan MJ, Keller RB: Brain abscess complicating the use of halo traction. *J Bone Joint Surg* (*Am*) 1973; 55A:635–639.
25. Whitehill R, Richman JA, Glaser JA: Failure of immobilization of the cervical spine by the halo vest: A report of five cases. *J Bone Joint Surg* (*Am*) 1986; 68A:326–332.
26. Browner CM, Hadley MN, Sonntag VKH, Mattingly LG: Halo immobilization brace care: An innovative approach. *J Neurosci Nurs* 1987; 19:24–29.
27. Nachemson AL, Morris J: In vivo measurements of intradiscal pressure. *J Bone Joint Surg* (*Am*) 1964; 46A:1077–1092.
28. Fidler MW, Plasmans CMT: The effect of four types of support on the segmental mobility of the lumbosacral spine. *J Bone Joint Surg* (*Am*) 1983; 65A:943–947.
29. Norton PL, Brown T: The immobilizing efficiency of back braces. *J Bone Joint Surg* (*Am*) 1957; 39A:111.
30. Dickman CA, Rekate HL, Sonntag VKH, Zabramski JM: Pediatric spinal trauma: Vertebral column and spinal cord injuries in children. Review article. *Pediatr Neurosci* 1989; 15:237–256.
31. Dickman CA, Zabramski JM, Hadley MN, et al: Pediatric spinal cord injury without radiographic abnormalities: Report of 26 cases and review of the literature. *J Spin Dis* 1991; 3(4):296–305.

Imaging Techniques

CHAPTER 81

IMAGING AFTER SPINAL INJURY

Bruce J. Andersen
Warren A. Stringer

INTRODUCTION

Recent advances in neuroradiological techniques to image the bony and soft tissues of the spinal cord have left the clinician with a variety of options when radiographic examinations are needed to diagnose and define the sequelae of trauma to the spinal cord and its surrounding structures. This chapter attempts to show which techniques are most useful for defining the bony anatomy of the spine, its articulations and ligamentous structures, and the spinal cord in the acute care of a trauma patient. Particular attention will be paid to the strengths and weaknesses of each modality, in terms of both anatomic definition and efficacy of use in spine trauma. We will discuss the indications for each imaging modality and the information expected from each. Our overall purpose will be to aid in the selection of imaging techniques used to establish both bony and ligamentous stability and extrinsic compression of the cord following trauma. Although the figures used here to illustrate points made in the text show cervical spine pathology, the same principles apply to imaging at all spinal levels.

HISTORY

Following Roentgen's discovery in 1885, x-rays were immediately applied to skeletal trauma, but their first use in spine trauma did not occur until almost a year later. On November 6, 1886, Cushing took AP and lateral roentgenograms of the cervical spine on a patient with a Brown-Séquard syndrome following a gunshot injury, showing a bullet adjacent to the spinal canal at C5–C6. The use of roentgen rays for spine injury remained limited for many years, partly because of technical limitations, lack of hospital support, and general controversy surrounding the application of radiology to any aspect of skeletal trauma. In 1900 the American Surgical Association concluded that "the routine employment of the x-ray in cases of fracture is not at present of sufficient definite advantage to justify the teaching that it should be used in every case."[1] This conclusion apparently was influenced by the fact that x-rays had led to malpractice suits filed against several of the committee members. The American Surgical Association did not officially reverse this position until 1913.

The next major step in spine imaging was the development of myelography. Dandy introduced air ventriculography in 1918 after numerous attempts to introduce positive contrast agents into the ventricles of dogs proved fatal. The same year he described the concepts of air myelography and spinal canal block. He described a patient in whom a cord tumor was suspected but no block was present, but at surgery was found to have chronic transverse myelitis. Dandy did not actually obtain spinal radiographs in this patient, and the first deliberate air myelogram was done the next year by Jacobaeus. However, he and others concluded that the images obtained by air myelography were too diffuse and too difficult to read for general use. Positive contrast myelography was discovered accidentally in 1921, when Sicard and Forestier inadvertently injected Lipiodol into the lumbar subarachnoid space while attempting an epidural injection. Subsequent introduction of Pantopaque in 1944, metrizamide in the 1970s, and second-generation, water-soluble nonionic agents in the 1980s resulted in progressively improved safety and efficacy of myelography, while the development of C1–C2 puncture techniques and CT "mini-myelograms" greatly increased the applicability of myelography to acute spinal trauma.

Plain film radiography, occasionally supplemented by myelography, remained the only means by which to evaluate the spine until the development of tomography by a number of investigators working independently in the 1930s. This process, with or without intrathecal contrast, became the definitive technique for spine imaging about 1940 and remained so until the development and widespread availability of third-generation CT scanners in the early 1980s.

Computed tomography was introduced by Hounsfield in 1972. Early scanners were quite slow and had poor spatial resolution, resulting in limited usefulness in the spine. The development of faster, higher resolution scanners and software techniques for multiplanar reconstruction around 1978 led to rapid application of CT to spine imaging, including spinal trauma. CT is now the most commonly used form of imaging after plain films.

Magnetic resonance imaging (MRI) has been applied to spine injury since the mid-1980s. Initial studies concentrated on subacute and chronic sequelae of spine trauma. Imaging of acutely injured patients was difficult, owing to relatively slow scanning speeds, low spatial resolution, and the inability to stabilize and monitor patients adequately within the magnetic environment of the scanner. More recently, advanced scanning techniques have decreased the time required and increased the information yield from MRI. Monitoring equipment compatible with high magnetic fields is now available in many centers. MRI is now being used more frequently to evaluate spine trauma and may surpass CT as the secondary test of choice owing to its higher informational yield.

SCREENING EXAMS AND TRIAGE PRIORITIES

When considering the integrity of the bony and ligamentous structures associated with the spinal column of a trauma victim, the radiographic examination should be tailored to demonstrate that the anatomy is normal—or, if not, the extent of alteration of normal structure and articulation. Since many factors control the quality of radiographic procedures, an inability to demonstrate structural or functional pathology does not rule out its presence. In trauma, the primary goal is resuscitation without exacerbation of underlying injuries. If spine pathology cannot be defined in the acute resuscitation phase, immobilization should be maintained until definitive imaging is feasible; the complications associated with prolonged immobilization are minuscule in comparison with the risks of injudicious movement of an undefined spine injury. Immobilization of the cervical spine can be adequately maintained in an appropriate collar. Immobilization of the thoracic and lumbar spine does not require that the patient remain on a backboard. In fact, this may be contraindicated if the patient is anesthetic, comatose, or sedated because these patients have significant risk of developing early pressure ulcers.

Once initial stabilization of airway, breathing, and circulation has occurred, definition of the spinal injury can be addressed. Plain films of the cervical spine, consisting of at least AP, lateral, and odontoid views are required, as is visualization from the basiocciput to the top of T1 on the lateral film. The decision to obtain additional imaging studies depends on whether the patient's pain or neurological deficit is explained by existing studies.

To be considered an adequate evaluation of the traumatized spine, all pain and neurological dysfunction must be explained. Since plain radiographs define only bony pathology, ligamentous injury, disk protrusion, and cord compression or contusions may go undetected and may represent the etiology of neurological dysfunction not readily explained by the normal bony anatomy seen radiographically. Many trauma patients are pharmacologically paralyzed or comatose, so a neurological examination of spinal function may not be obtainable. In these circumstances, a more exhaustive radiological examination is indicated because localizing neurological dysfunction cannot focus our attention on specific areas of potential pathology.

INDICATIONS

The modern radiological armamentarium can easily be overused in the diagnosis of traumatic spinal injury. After screening films have been obtained, the physician must keep in mind that the goal of imaging techniques is to explain specific pain and/or neurological deficits, not to embark on a "fishing expedition." Anatomic abnormalities that are asymptomatic certainly can be found in trauma patients, but defining the symptomatic abnormalities is the goal of imaging of acute spinal trauma. The trauma imaging paradigm should begin with screening examinations that are quick and inexpensive, and then progress to more sophisticated modalities if the etiology of pain or neurological dysfunction remains unexplained. Asymptomatic or incidental findings can be definitively imaged once the patient has been stabilized.

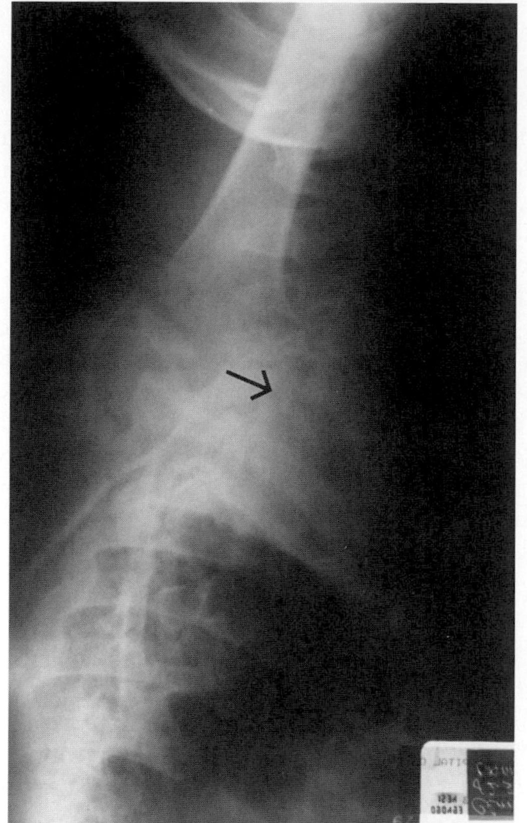

A

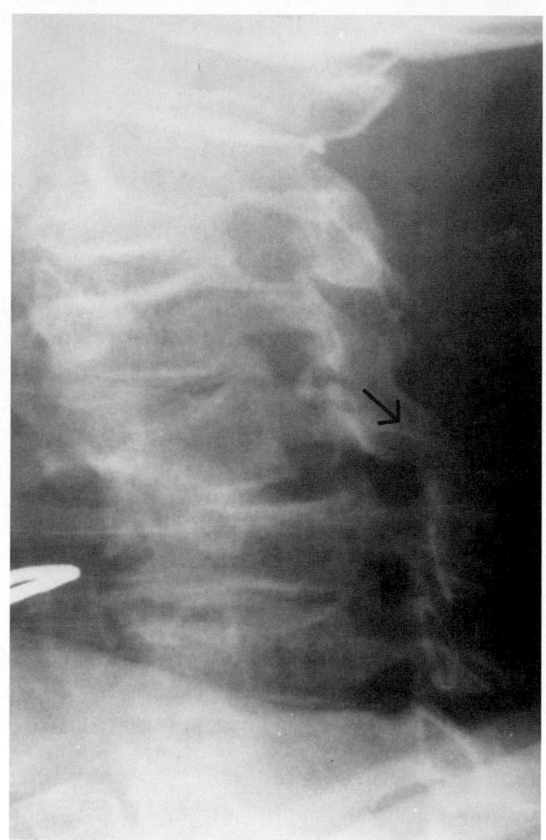

B

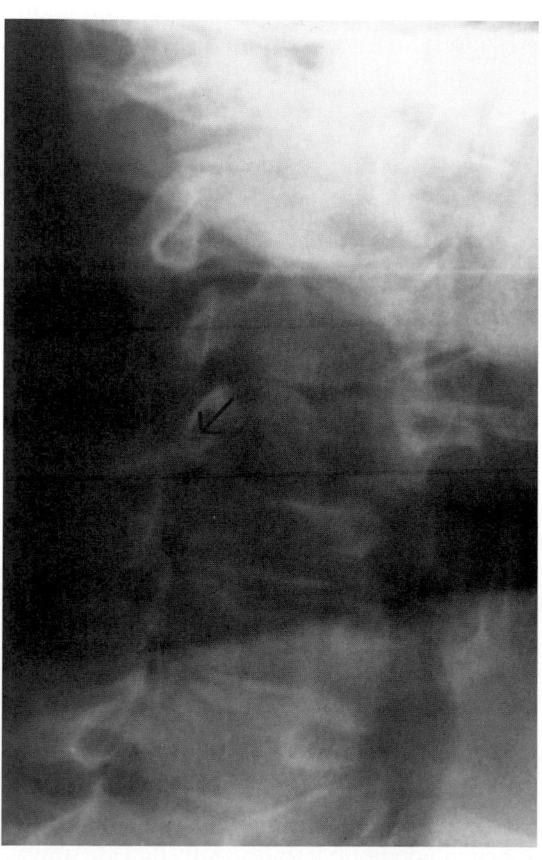

C

Figure 81-1. Swimmer's view (*A*) compared with Supine Oblique (*B*, *C*) views of subluxation. Note the dimensional distortion on the obliques but the ease at which malalignment of vertebral bodies and facets (arrows indicate bilateral facet dislocations) at C7–T1 can be visualized, both without moving the patient's arms.

Plain Films

In all trauma and ATLS protocols, minimal plain films of the cervical spine are requisite (lateral, odontoid, AP), as they define bony anatomy, alignment, soft tissue swelling, and spatial interrelationships between individual bones and are the basis of all other evaluations and treatments. They should be obtained in all polytrauma or neurologically impaired patients, as well as in any neurologically normal patient complaining of neck pain. This basic series of plain films can be obtained without moving the patient; by exposing the film during exhalation with careful traction on the arms, the series usually will show the superior endplate of T1 on the lateral view, thus assuring adequacy of the lateral film. Swimmer's or supine oblique films may be useful in situations where T1 cannot be visualized on lateral views, but supine obliques frequently offer the same information concerning the C7–T1 region, as do swimmer's views, without requiring patient movement (Fig. 81-1). Some authors recommend supine obliques in addition to the above three views in all situations.[2] Supplemental views such as upright obliques or flexion-extension films can be obtained as necessary in conscious, neurologically intact patients.

The lateral view alone will diagnose significant spinal injury in 70 to 90 percent of cases,[3] and addition of the AP and odontoid views increases the rate of diagnosis to about 93 percent.[4]

Computerized Tomography

CT scanning is unmatched in its ability to evaluate subtle fractures and equivocal areas seen on plain films, particularly when reformatted images are considered (Fig. 81-2). The addition of CT scanning of questionable areas seen on plain films or areas of the spine associated with the patient's neurological dysfunction increases the diagnosis rate up to 98 percent.[5] CT is also the best study available for defining the anatomy of the spinal canal and identifying and characterizing displaced bony fragments in the canal or foramina, and can be used to differentiate new from old fractures, fracture from developmental anomaly, and to identify degenerative change. Associated airway and paraspinal soft tissue injury also can be defined. By obtaining sagittal reformatted images, alignment that may have been in question on plain films also can be evaluated, although to be accurate this requires thin, contiguous or overlapping cuts that may take quite a bit of time and require the patient to remain motionless throughout the examination. The nonbony contents of the spinal canal are not seen adequately unless intrathecal contrast is given (Fig. 81-3).

Magnetic Resonance Imaging

MRI has become the gold standard for imaging intramedullary pathology and other intraspinal and paraspinal soft tissues. It also can evaluate ligamentous injury (Fig. 81-4), disk anatomy, intra- and extradural hemorrhages, cord edema (Fig. 81-5), and other fluid collections.[6–12] Root avulsions, dural tears, and pseudomeningoceles, and (with the addition of GRE sequences) direct assessment of vascular flow can be imaged using MR. Major bony fractures and alignment abnormalities are also seen adequately (Fig. 81-6). MRI also is important as an early prognostic indicator of recovery from spinal cord injury.[12–14]

Magnetic Resonance Angiography

With proper technique, direct assessment of vascular flow and anatomy can be achieved without intravenous or intra-arterial contrast agents, but should be considered a screening examination only. Fine detail falls short of that obtained using conventional angiography. Often, adequate evaluation of vascular patency can be obtained from routine transaxial and sagittal MR imaging without special MRA sequences.

Radionuclide Bone Scans

Bone scanning is useful to differentiate new from old fractures and other disruptive injuries. It highlights areas of inflammation and repair, but gives no information concerning anatomy or stability. It has no place in the acute evaluation of traumatic spinal injuries.

Conventional Polytomography

This method of evaluating fractures and alignment has generally been replaced by CT, which has greater speed, near-equal sensitivity, and decreased dependence on patient cooperation and operator skills.[3,4,15] The technique is still of value for very subtle, transaxially oriented fractures, facet injuries, and laminar and spinous process fractures.[3]

Myelography

This technique, when combined with CT scanning, gives accurate anatomic information concerning the relationship between neural and bony structures. In patients unable to undergo MR imaging, it is the only modality available to evaluate accurately the presence of root avulsions, herniated disk, or protruding ligamentous structures impinging on the cord or its roots.

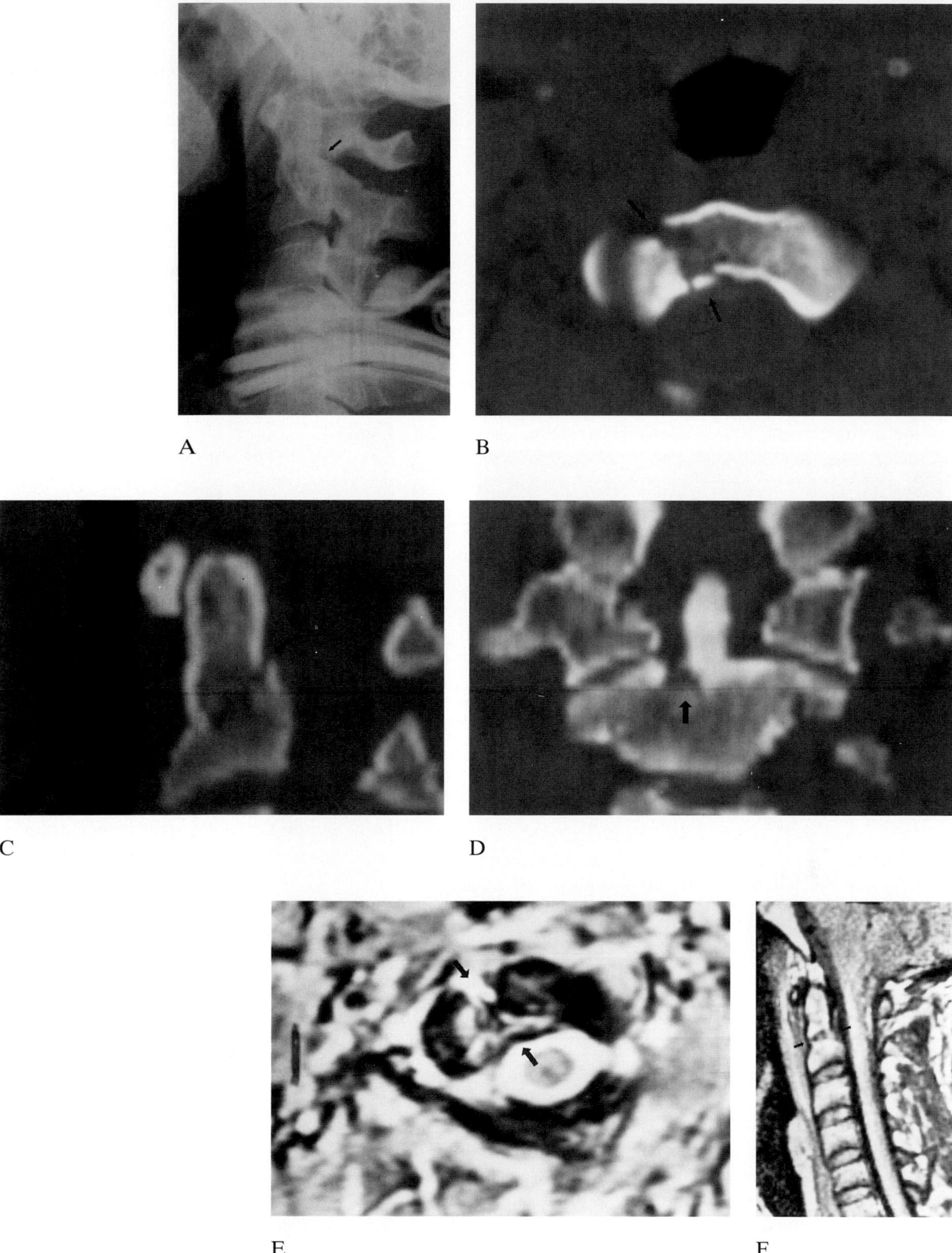

Figure 81-2. Comparison of imaging techniques using a single case of odontoid fracture with arrows indicating the fracture line: *A*. Plain film. *B*. CT axial. *C*. CT sagittal reformatted image. *D*. CT coronal reformatted image. *E*. MR axial image using a gradient echo sequence. Note altered cortical contour and signal characteristics of the marrow discontinuity, hemorrhage, and edema at the fracture site (arrows). *F*. MR sagittal image using a T_1 weighted sequence. Again, the fracture is characterized by cortical discontinuity and altered marrow signal.

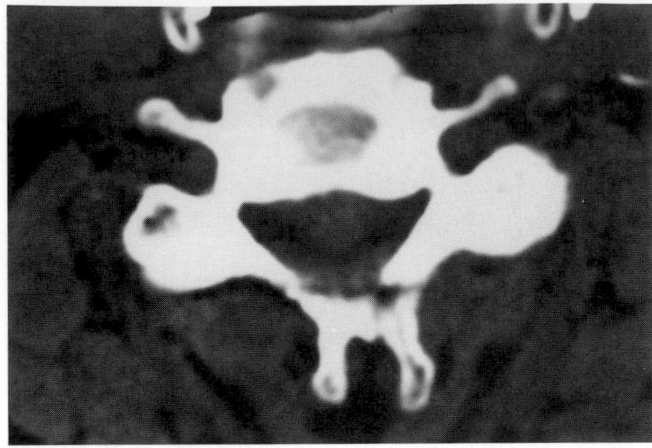

A

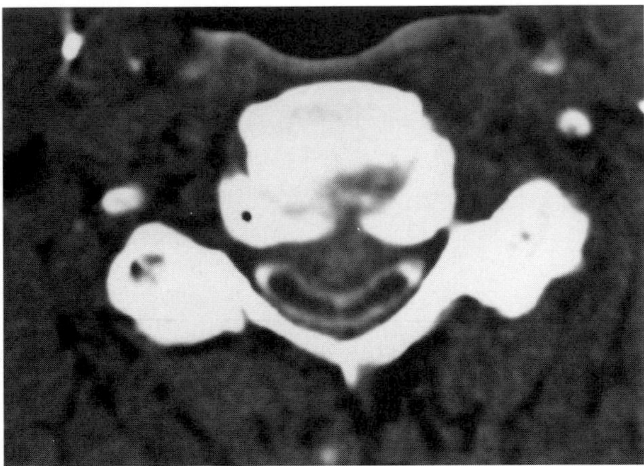

B

Figure 81-3. Plain CT scan of an acute disk herniation (*A*), showing how the addition of intrathecal contrast (*B*) defines lesions (this case illustrates a traumatic disk herniation) compressing the cord.

SPECIFIC PROBLEM AREAS

The goal of imaging spinal trauma is finding and defining acute injuries that cause pain or neurological dysfunction. Within this context, two major problem areas arise: (1) how much definition of anatomy is adequate? and (2) how best to rule out significant pathology in a patient whose neurological examination is either unreliable or unobtainable?

Clinical judgment, risk/benefit ratios, and treatment plans should guide the decision whether to proceed with films available or to spend more time to further define the anatomy. If spinal surgery is the optimal treatment, accurate knowledge of the anatomy is desirable. The extra time required to define that anatomy could bring more benefit to the patient, outweighing the extra risk of further time spent imaging, particularly if instrumentation is contemplated. However, for example, if the plain films show significant subluxation, rapid reduction of the malalignment is probably more in the patient's best interest than prolonged CT scanning to further define the bony anatomy.

When evaluating an immobile, nonresponsive (including those pharmacologically paralyzed) patient, a

Figure 81-4. MR image of ligamentous damage. The anterior longitudinal ligament is lifted off the vertebral body (open arrow points to ALL), and the posterior longitudinal ligament is ruptured (arrow head at PLL rupture).

clinical decision concerning the likelihood of spinal vs. head trauma as the etiology of the patient's lack of extremity movement must be made. If the mechanism of injury or associated soft tissue damage suggests that significant force was delivered to the spinal column during the course of trauma, the possibility that the patient's immobility could be due to a high spinal injury rather than nonresponsiveness from a head injury exists, and appropriate steps should be taken to evaluate the cervical spine if possible.

SPECIFICS OF INTERPRETATION

Plain Films

This series of films, consisting of lateral, AP, odontoid, and occasionally supine obliques will identify most major fractures and malalignments, and will suggest areas of instability that then can either be treated or investigated further.

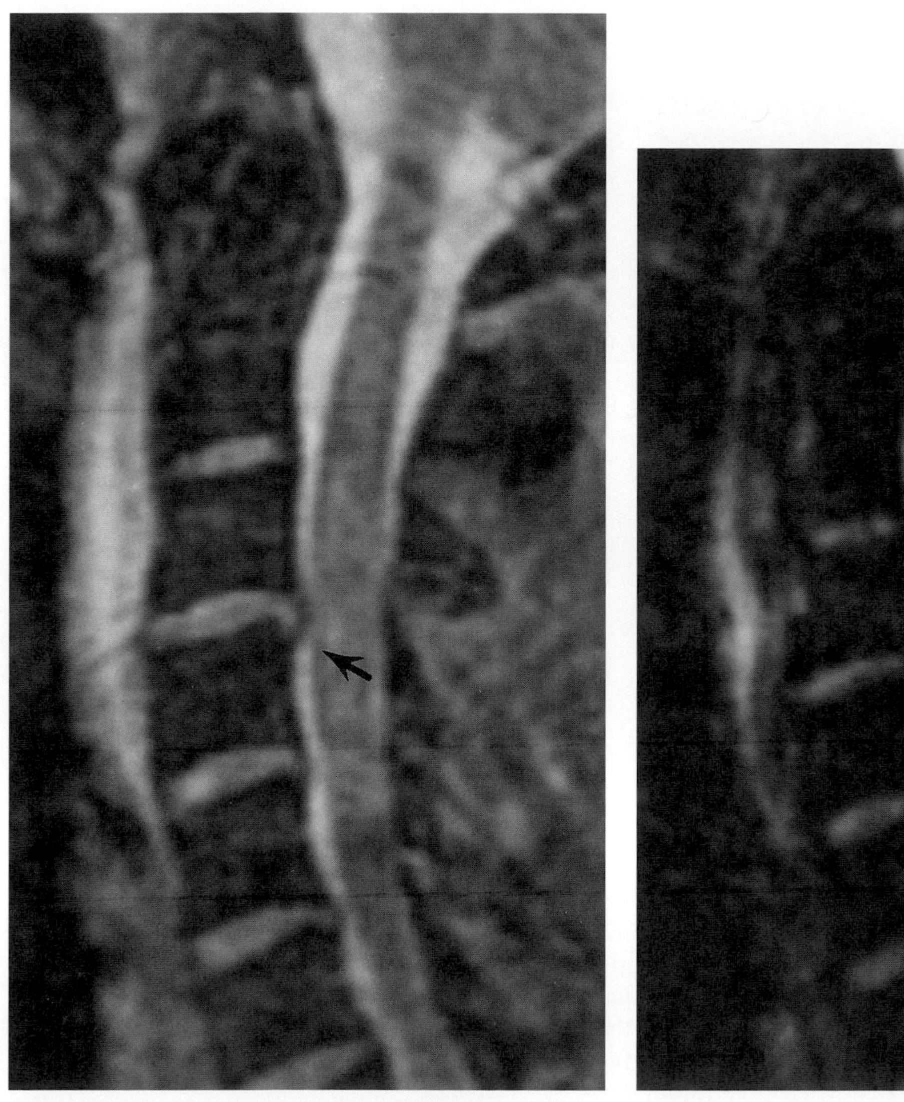

A

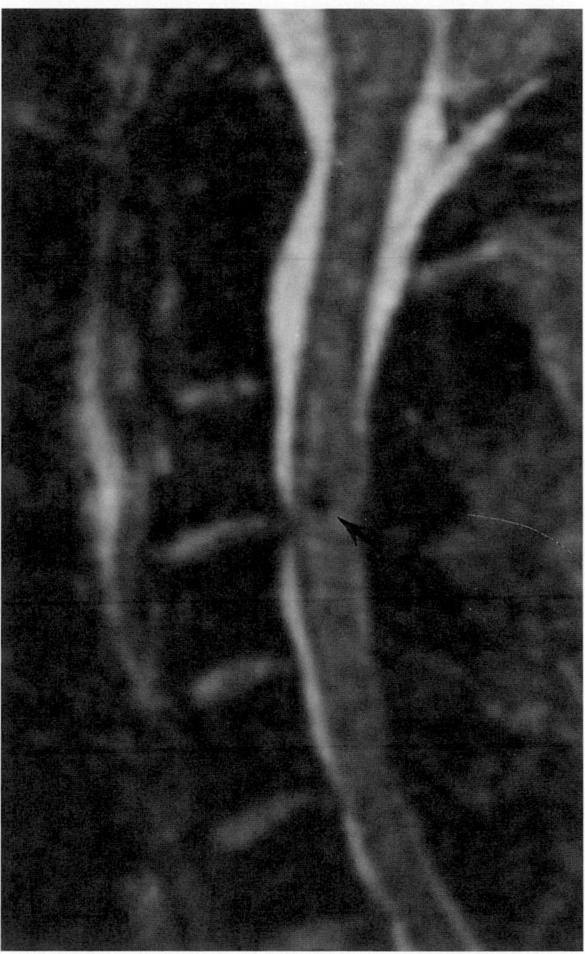

B

Figure 81-5. Series of MR images illustrating the advantages of specific sequences in a single case: *A.* Cord indented by herniated disk best seen on the first echo of a double echo gradient sequence at arrow. *B.* Cord contusion best seen on the second echo of the same double echo gradient sequence at arrow. *C.* Cord edema best seen on the fast spin echo T_2 sequence at arrow.

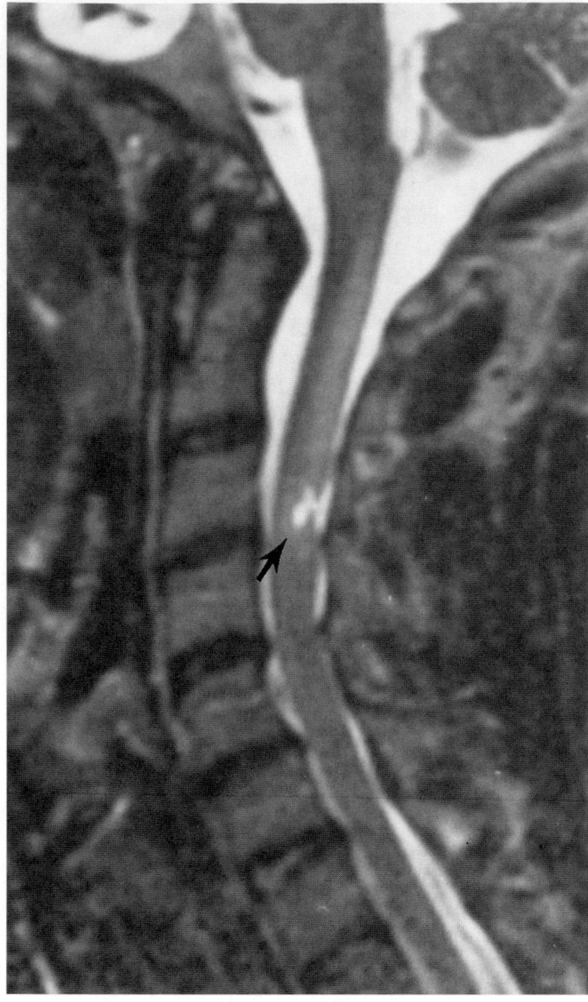

C

Figure 81-5. *Continued.*

LATERAL VIEW (INCLUDING SWIMMER'S VIEW)

These must include the basiocciput to the superior endplate of T1 to be considered adequate. Swimmer's views should be obtained only after good attempts at obtaining standard lateral views (e.g., exposure during exhalation with arm traction) have failed; their frequent poor quality prevents adequate evaluation of anything other than gross malalignment or fracture. Alternatively, supine obliques can adequately image down to T1 without moving the patient (Fig. 81-1). Specific anatomic points to look for include:

- Discontinuity of anterior and posterior vertebral lines, which may indicate anterior or posterior longitudinal ligament damage. Normal variability is up to 2 to 3 mm when anterior osteophytes are ignored.[16–18]
- Discontinuity of spinolaminar line, which may indicate ligamentum flavum damage. Normal AP translational variability is 2 mm.[3,16,18]
- Craniovertebral junction articulations. Normally the occipital condyles rest on the C1 articulating facets and have a maximum sagittal translation of 1 mm.[19] The tip of the clivus should be in apposition with the tip of the dens, regardless of the degree of flexion or extension.[20]
- Preodontoid space which may indicate atlanto-axial instability. Normal translational distance between the ring of C1 and the dens is 3 mm in adults and 4 to 5 mm in children.[3,21,22]
- Interspinous space and angulation may indicate interspinous ligament instability. Normal angulation is

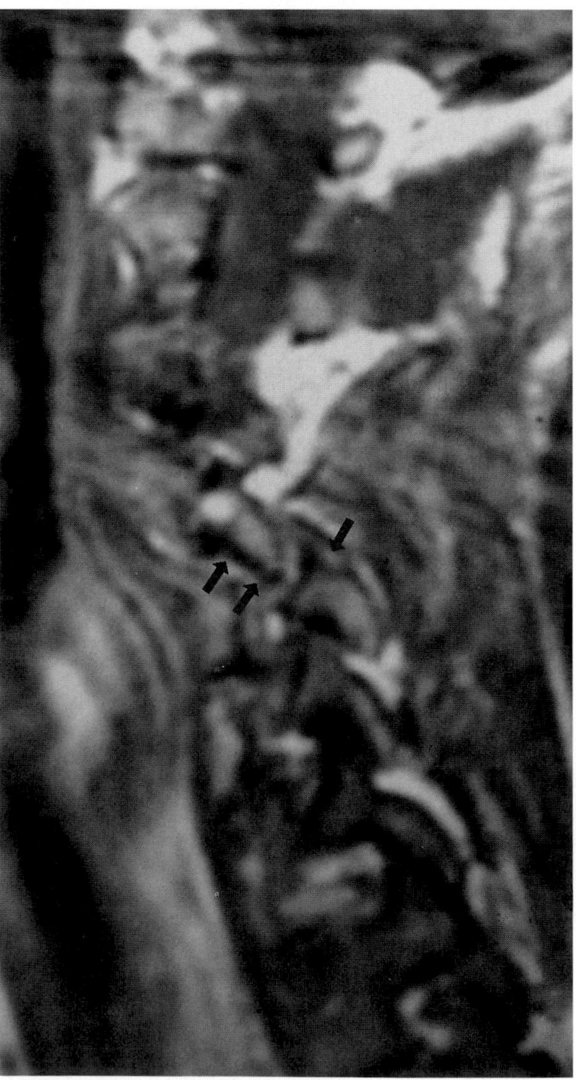

Figure 81-6. MR image of locked facets with arrows pointing to the normally opposed joint surfaces of the subluxed facets.

no more than a 2 mm difference between any three adjacent levels.[3,16]

- Kyphosis or scoliosis may indicate facet damage, compression fracture, or ligamentous instability. Normally, the spinolaminar line and the posterior aspects of the vertebral bodies describe a smooth curve. Acute angulation or discontinuity in the curve of either line is abnormal.
- Disk height or interbody distance may indicate disk rupture or anterior or posterior longitudinal ligament damage. Normal interspace height should be approximately the average of the interspace measurements from the adjacent two levels.
- Prevertebral soft tissue swelling can indicate severity of injury and increase index of suspicion for occult damage. Normal prevertebral soft tissue distance between the anterior vertebral body and the pharyngeal air shadow at C3 is 4 mm at 72 inches (tube-film distance) or 7 mm at 40 inches and at C6 is 22 mm in adults and 14 mm in children at 40 inches.[3,20] These measurements can depend on whether the film was taken during swallowing.[23] Repeat films may be indicated.
- Bony integrity of the ring of C1 and C2 and the connections between the body of C2 and the dens.

AP view

- Lateral alignment, judged by the degree to which the pedicles fall onto a line drawn through those above and below the suspected lesion.
- Interpedicular distance should remain the same or gradually increase by similar increments while descending the spine. Normal variability is 2 mm from the average of the interpedicular distances above and below the level in question.[3]
- Joints of Luschka should have similar-sized joint spaces on either side of the same level and with levels above and below the area in question.
- Lateral displacement or rotation of spinous processes (not to be confused with a bifid spinous process).

Odontoid or open-mouth view

This view should give a clear outline of the dens and the facets of C1–C2. Occasionally, dental structures overlie this anatomy, projecting vertical shadows that may be confused with fractures. Mach lines represent x-ray beam artifacts caused by superimposition of the ring of C1 and the occiput over and behind the dens, resulting in dark horizontal lines that also should not be mistaken for fractures.[23] If in doubt, a repeat film at a slightly different angle should move dental and Mach lines but not fracture lines. Specific anatomy to evaluate includes:

- Bony integrity of entire dens and its junction with the body of C2.
- Articulations between the occipital condyles and the superior facets of C1 should remain intact in all degrees of flexion and extension.
- Articulations between the facets of C1 and C2. The sum of the total overhang (both sides) of the C1 lateral masses when compared with the lateral margins of the superior facets of C2 normally is less than 7 mm.[17]

Oblique views

True obliques are exposed with the film perpendicular to the incident x-ray beam while the patient's neck is rotated 45°. Trauma (supine) obliques are somewhat modified in that the x-ray beam is oriented at the same 45° incident angle to the anatomy, but the film is simply placed on the stretcher lateral to the patient's neck. This avoids patient movement but exaggerates the dimensions of the pedicles and vertebral bodies. These views allow good visualization of the vertebral body and facet alignment and reliably show C7–T1 junctions as an alternative to swimmer's views when lateral films do not show the entire C-spine (Fig. 81-1). Specific anatomy to examine includes:

- Alignment of facets and vertebral bodies
- Integrity of pedicles and neural foramina

Flexion-extension views

These are intended to assess the integrity of ligamentous structures and the function of the facets joints and should be performed in alert, conscious patients to their limits of comfort only. No external force or assistance should be applied. In certain cases in comatose patients, this examination may be performed by neurosurgical personnel actively under fluoroscopy. Specific points to examine include:

- Abnormal motion segments, listheses, or subluxations indicate ligamentous damage. Normal subluxation is 2 to 3 mm in both flexion and extension.[3,18]
- Asymmetrical widening of the interspinous distance indicates interspinal ligament incompetence. Normal motion is within 2 mm of the average distance of the adjacent interspinous distances.[3,18]

Conventional Polytomography

This was the precursor of CT scanning in its ability to define the bony anatomy of a specific slice of bone at

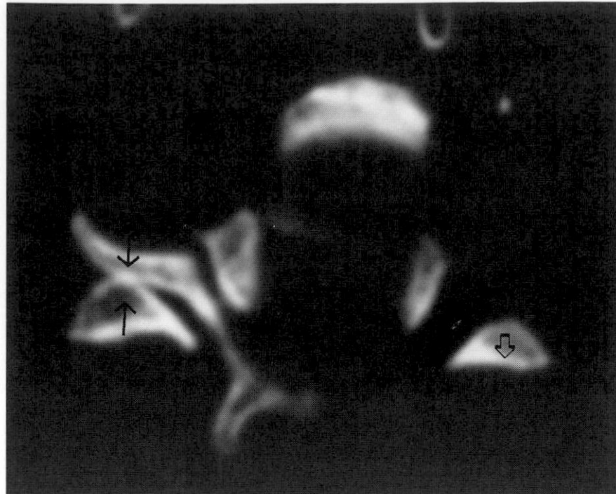

A

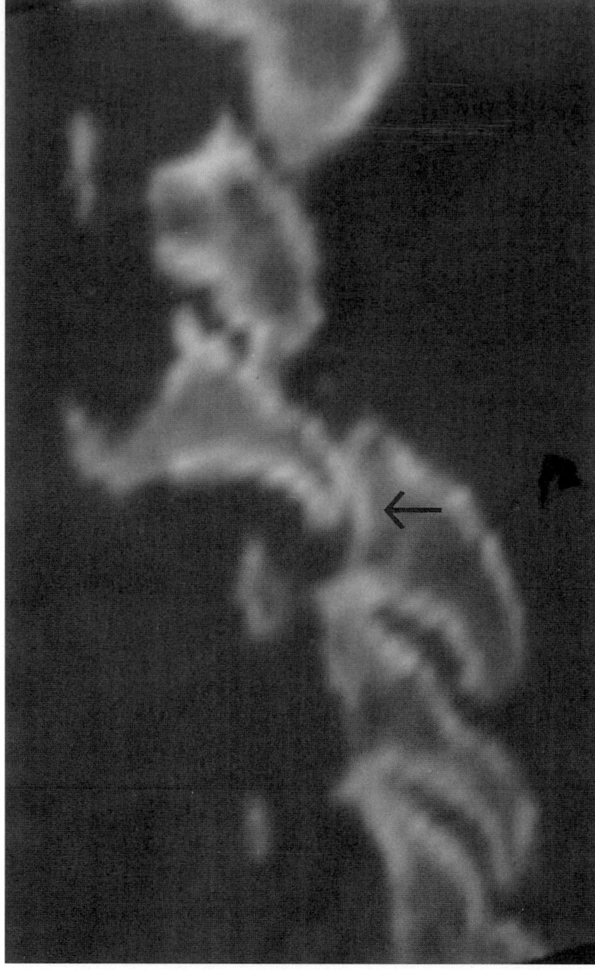

B

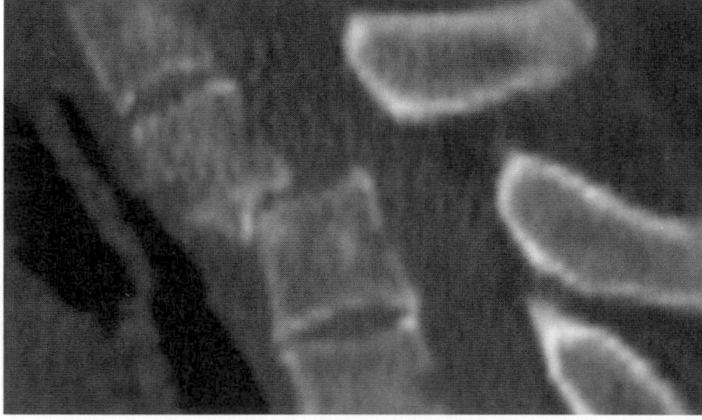

C

Figure 81-7. CT axial (*A*) and sagittal (*B*, *C*) reformatted images of facet disruption with subluxation, facet lock (arrows on *A* and *B*), "empty" facet (open arrow on *A*), and splaying of spinous processes (*C*). Note degree of detail seen when the transaxial scans are obtained using thin, contiguous cuts.

a predetermined depth from the skin surface by rotating the beam of a conventional x-ray head in multiple planes sharing a fixed point of focus within the area in question. Because of its complicated operation, high radiation exposure, and limited informational yield (when compared with CT), polytomography has become of more limited use when imaging spinal trauma and is rarely indicated unless both plain films and CT are inadequate.

Computerized Tomography (CT)

Scans typically are performed with 1.5- to 3-mm transaxial slices in the cervical spine and 3- to 5-mm slices in the thoracic and lumbar spine. This slice thickness will adequately image most fractures and will accumulate enough information to allow sagittal and coronal reformatted images to demonstrate most bony pathology. To evaluate fractures in the plane of the scanner (horizontal or transaxial fractures), thinner cuts (1.5- to 2-mm) and overlapping slices provide the most information on reformatted images. Thin overlapping transaxial cuts reformatted into coronal and sagittal images will adequately show fractures and malalignments in all but the most subtle nondisplaced fractures (Fig. 81-7). Patient motion while obtaining transaxial images for reconstructions can mimic malalignments on the reconstructions, but also will displace any adjacent air columns or soft tissue structures to the same degree within the plane in which the apparent bony step-off is seen.

3-D reconstructions sometimes are helpful, particularly when MR imaging is not possible and plain films are inadequate, although they are not routinely necessary.[24] They can provide a more visually coherent picture of the bony pathology, and, when combined with intrathecal contrast enhancement, its relationship to the cord and thecal sac. Unless thin, overlapping cuts are used to obtain the data for reconstruction, spatial resolution and the ability to discern subtle fractures and malalignments can be lost.

Transaxial and reconstructed scans should be filmed both in "soft-tissue" (width ≈ 300–400, level ≈ 50) and "bone" (width ≈ 2000–4000, level ≈ 400) windows. Soft-tissue windows are necessary to search for epidural hematomata, paraspinal soft-tissue injuries, and disk protrusion, but they obscure bony detail. The best bony detail is obtained by processing the data in a "bone" or "detail" algorithm designed to maximize spatial resolution at the expense of soft-tissue contrast and smoothing.

Intravenous contrast is indicated infrequently in head or spine trauma, and never before the first scan, as areas of enhancement can obscure hemorrhage. Following the initial scan, contrast can be given for other studies as indicated. Once spiral scanners become more widely available, IV contrast may be used in conjunction with scans of the neck to screen for carotid and vertebral artery injury, but this application is experimental at the present time.

Administration of intrathecal contrast prior to CT scanning remains the best alternative for evaluation of extrinsic compression of the thecal sac or roots if MR scanning is not an option (Fig. 81-3). It remains the test of choice for diagnosis of root avulsions, dural tears, and meningocele.

Details of interpretation:

- New cortical breaks have sharp, usually irregular edges that contrast with lower density cancellous bone in the fracture gap, as opposed to older nonunions that tend to smooth out the edges of the fracture. Nutrient foramina may mimic fractures, but are different in that they are typically seen on only one or two slices and have smooth margins (Fig. 81-8).
- Facets should always be seen in pairs. Unpaired, "empty," or "naked" facets indicate fracture or displacement of one or both articular processes (Fig. 81-7).
- Displacement of bone fragments into spinal canal.
- Alignment on reformatted images (Fig. 81-7).
- Disk displacements and other space-occupying lesions impinging upon the thecal sac (seen after administration of intrathecal contrast) (Fig. 81-3).
- Degenerative changes in facets or Luschka joints, and the presence of osteophytes.

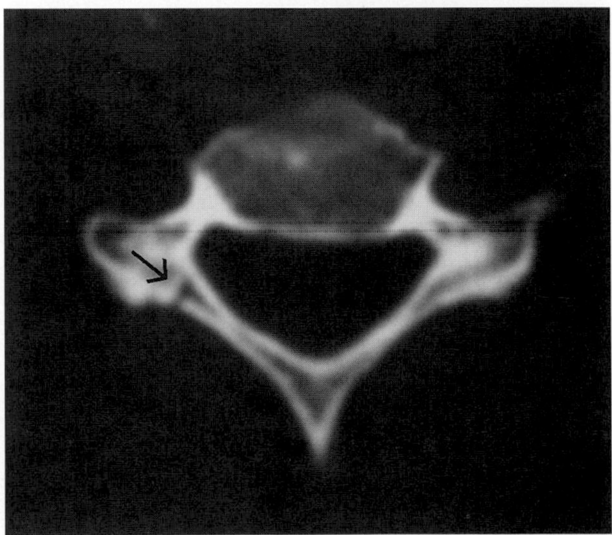

A

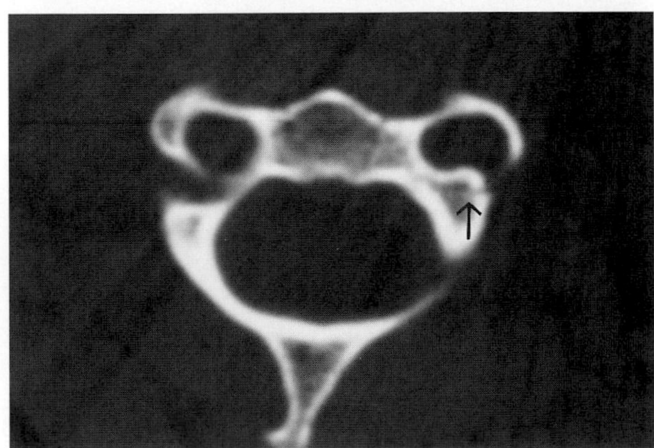

B

Figure 81-8. Comparison of nutrient foramen (*A*) vs. fracture (*B*). Note sharp cortical discontinuity of fracture and the smooth cortical margin of the nutrient foramen, both shown by arrows.

- Old versus acute fractures, old nonunions, congenital malformations.
- Soft tissue swelling, hematomata, or air.

Magnetic Resonance Imaging (MRI)

A bewildering array of imaging sequences is available on most MR scanners, accompanied by initials and acronyms that are cryptic at best. However, the majority of spinal imaging is done with only three main types of sequences, namely spin echo (SE), gradient echo (GRE), and fast spin echo (FSE).

Spin echo images may be T_1, T_2, or "proton density" weighted, depending on the repetition time (TR) and echo time (TE) chosen. T_1 weighted images are characterized by short TR (300–1000 msec) and short TE (15–30 msec) and are recognized by dark CSF. Fat, subacute hemorrhage (older than about 3 days), and gadolinium enhancement are all bright on T_1 weighted images. T_2 weighted images have long TR (1500–3000 msec), long TE (60–120 msec), and have bright CSF signal. Most types of intramedullary pathology are bright on T_2 weighted images, but acute hemorrhage (roughly 6 h to 3 days old) is very dark. Proton density images attempt to balance T_1 and T_2 effects, and some-

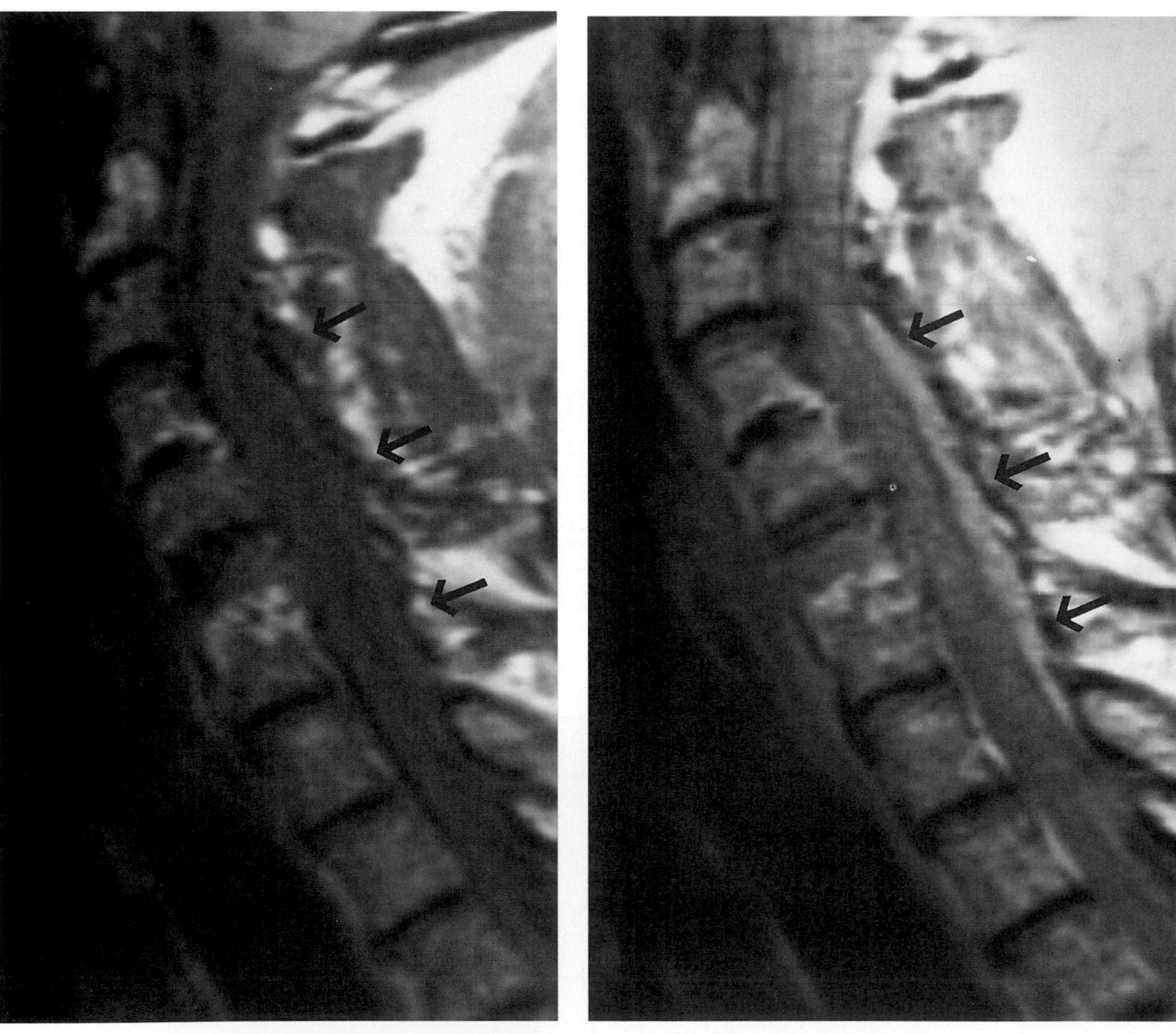

Figure 81-9. Epidural hematoma (arrows) without fracture or subluxation ≈10 hours after injury. Oxygenated hemoglobin is nearly isointense when compared with the spinal cord on T_1 weighted SE sequence (*A*), and hyperintense on double echo FSE proton density weighted (*B*) and T_2 weighted (*C*) images. Also note enlargement and subtle edema of the cord, best seen on the T_2 weighted image (open arrow on *C*), and marked degenerative disease.

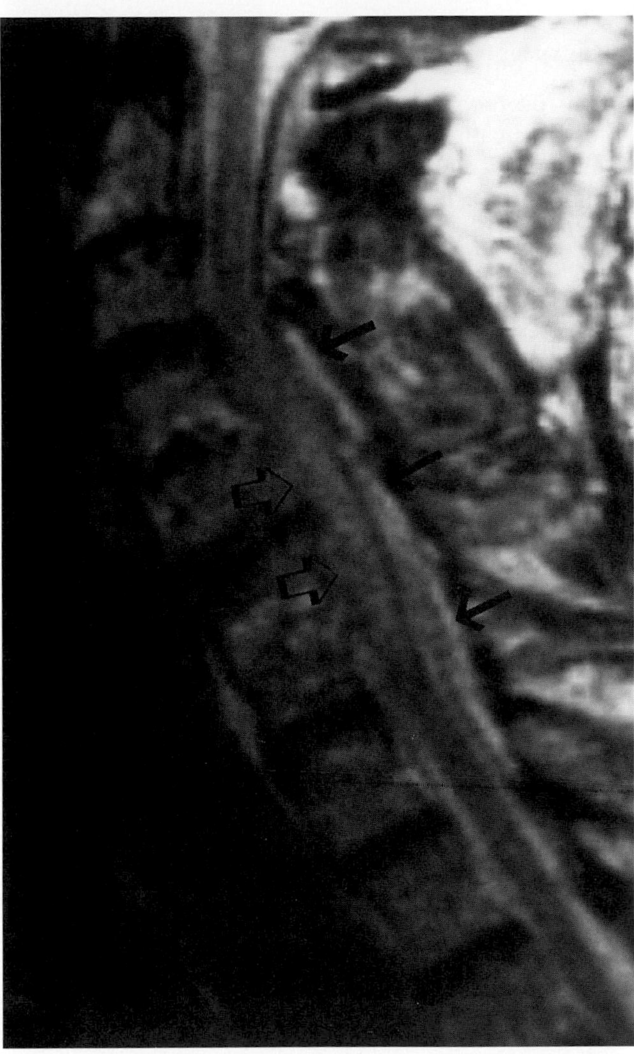

C

Figure 81-9. *Continued.*

times are called "intermediate" or "balanced" images. They have long TR (1500–3000 msec) but short TE (30–60 msec). CSF signal is approximately isointense compared with the spinal cord, but the relationships of vertebral cortex, disk nucleus and annulus, posterior longitudinal ligament, and CSF are often best seen with these images. Most intramedullary pathology is bright on these images, but acute hemorrhage is usually approximately isointense when compared with normal cord (Fig. 81-9).

Gradient echo images typically use a narrow proton "flip angle" to suppress T_1 effects and generate images similar to T_2 weighted SE images in much less time. TR and TE are very short, typically 15–35 msec and 5–15 msec, respectively, with flip angles of 5–20 degrees. These images are usually called T_2* (T_2 star) to differentiate them from the true T_2 images generated by spin echo sequences. A double gradient echo sequence with both proton density and T_2* weighting are available on some scanners with no time penalty and are especially useful in trauma because more information is gathered using the same amount of time as a single echo sequence (Fig. 81-5). T_2* images are more sensitive to acute hemorrhage than true T_2 SE images, but are also more sensitive to artifacts from nearby metal implants. GRE images also may be obtained with T_1 weighting, but these are most often used in MR angiography and have limited utility in routine imaging of the spine.

Fast spin echo is a recently developed imaging process that allows several points within an imaging "slice" to be scanned at once, resulting in an image being obtained in a fraction of the time required for traditional spin echo techniques. TR is long (2000–6000 msec), and single or double echo proton density and T_2 weighted images are obtained using TE of 20–50 msec and 80–120 msec, respectively. Compared to traditional SE T_2 and GRE T_2* images, FSE T_2 weighted images are less sensitive to acute hemorrhage and thus should not be used alone in cases of spine injury. However, they are also less sensitive to metal artifact, and sometimes may be successful in the presence of spinal stabilization hardware or metallic fragments when other sequences are not. Fat suppression may be required to use FSE sequences to best advantage.

Inversion recovery sequences (STIR) are sometimes used to define pathology within bone marrow. They typically have less spatial resolution than other imaging sequences, take longer to acquire, and usually are not done in the setting of trauma.

The choice of imaging sequences will be determined by both the hardware and software of the specific MR scanner available, as well as by the nature and age of the patient's injury. Epidural and intramedullary hemorrhage, in particular, evolves quickly over the first hours to days after the injury, and the specific imaging sequences that will best define it change over this period of time. Other patient factors, such as the level of injury, ability to cooperate with the examination, and presence of metal near the region of interest also play a role. The MR examination should therefore be tailored to each patient individually, but certain general principles apply.

Sagittal and axial orientations are the most useful and should be obtained from normal anatomy above the lesion through normal anatomy below the lesion. Typically, an entire spinal segment (cervical, thoracic, or lumbar) will be examined at once. Coronal orientation is useful for imaging odontoid lesions. Technical points to consider include:

- Rapid sequences are most applicable to trauma: i.e., avoid true T_2 if possible.
- T_2 or T_2* information is needed to diagnose cord edema and intraparenchymal hematomata and liga-

mentous tears, especially in the anterior and posterior longitudinal ligaments and the interspinous ligaments. Information pertaining to ligamentous integrity is best obtained in the sagittal plane.

- Gradient echo sequences are a faster alternative to T_2 spin echo images and show most pathology as well or better. Double gradient echo sequences are available on some scanners and carry with them no additional time penalty. Differing aspects of pathology often show up on one or the other of these scan sequences; which sequences work best for a particular type of pathology often depends on the hardware and software configuration of the MR system. Experience with individual systems will dictate which sequences are most appropriate for specific pathology, particularly in reference to the T_2, FSE, and GRE sequences.
- T_1 sequences are helpful for localization and characterization of the age of hemorrhages.
- Either T_1 or T_2 sequences are useful for evaluation of bony alignment, including facet relationships, marrow changes (e.g., tumor invasion or fracture), and cortical disruptions. Both should be obtained to maximize available information and increase the ease with which it is interpreted. It is difficult to predict which of these standard sequences will be of most value.
- Fast spin echo images should not be used alone as they are insensitive to recent hemorrhages, but they often define the extent of cord edema better than GRE sequences.
- Contrast enhancement has no role in the acute evaluation of spine trauma. It may be useful in follow-up scans to distinguish areas of cord damage from edema, although it probably is not necessary.
- Axial T_2* weighted GRE images often give a "free look" at adjacent vascular structures.

Suggested Screening Protocol (not a rigid algorithm but points 1 through 3 should be obtained in most cases):

1. Sagittal T_1 weighted images, through the facets on each side.
2. Sagittal double echo T_2* gradient echo sequence (single or double echo) through the same anatomy.
3. Axial gradient echo (single or double echo) T_2* sequence through areas of the cord, epidural, or disk abnormality localized on the sagittal sequences.
4. Axial and/or sagittal fast spin echo sequence with both proton density and T_2 weighting if extent of cord edema, compression, epidural fluid collection, or disk herniation remains unclear.
5. Use 3- to 5-mm slice thickness with $\leq$1-mm gap between slices for all sequences.
6. Use a dedicated cervical or surface coil for all sequences.

This protocol should prove adequate for evaluation of bony, ligamentous, dural, and cord pathology in trauma, particularly when "fine tuned" with information obtained from the plain films and neurologic examination (Figs. 81-4–81-6).

MRI AND PROGNOSIS

Recently there have been attempts to correlate MRI findings with the pathophysiological events underlying spinal cord injury and subsequent neurological outcome. Schaeffer in 1988 studied 53 patients with MRI and found the presence of hematomyelia to be associated with a complete spinal cord injury in 92 percent of patients, while contusion/edema was associated with incomplete injury in 81 percent.[25] Kulkarni reported similar findings and indicated that long-term prognosis was poor for neurological improvement when hematomyelia was present on the initial MRI.[15] Mirvis and associates attempted to correlate sequential MRI findings with outcome and suggested that a worsening of an initial MRI abnormality was associated with a poor prognosis.[9] In 1990 Flanders and coworkers reported on 78 patients who were studied with MRI acutely after spinal cord injury. It was noted that all patients with a neurological deficit had intrinsic abnormalities evident in the spinal cord. They also found hematomyelia to be highly predictive of complete spinal cord injury.[12] Yamashita and associates found that the most important prognostic finding on MRI scanning after spinal cord injury was the degree and extent of cord compression. The importance that these varieties of findings may ultimately play in spinal cord injury management remains to be determined.[29]

3-D MRI RECONSTRUCTIONS

These are of doubtful utility in trauma in that they add no new detail to the images already obtained and are labor-intensive to produce. They also result in loss of spatial and/or contrast resolution.

FIELD STRENGTH CONSIDERATIONS

If a choice is available, use high field strength to more accurately define cord anatomy. The presence of cord hemorrhage is a major prognostic factor and is more readily seen using higher field strength machines.[25]

If the patient has been stabilized with metallic implants, a low field strength magnet may allow better visualization of recurrent epidural fluid collections. However, acceptable images also can be obtained using high field strength magnets as long as the metallic implant consists of nonferrous materials. T_1 weighted and FSE T_2 weighted sequences are relatively less sensitive to magnetic artifacts and will be most helpful in imaging patients with implants or metallic fragments.

Magnetic Resonance Angiography (MRA)

This technique may be useful for screening suspected vascular injuries, but is time consuming and often not definitive enough to base surgical treatment upon.

Myelography

Using a water based nonionic contrast material inserted either in the lumbar area or, if the patient cannot be placed in a prone or lateral position, into the C1–C2 interspace, blockages to the flow of contrast can be seen if fluoroscopy is used to follow the progression of contrast up and down the spinal column. Often in trauma this is too time consuming and time can be saved by concentrating on the region of interest with CT scans through those particular areas. The advantages of this combination are that it minimizes movement of a damaged spine, requires considerably less contrast (2–3 ml vs. 5–10 ml), and provides information concerning both the bony anatomy, root sleeve integrity, extrinsic compression, and the relationship between fracture fragments and the spinal cord. Since all that is required is that the intrathecal contrast be administered a few minutes prior to the CT scan (to allow for adequate mixing), contrast can be injected in the emergency department before bringing the patient to the CT scanner (Fig. 81-3). A variant of this technique is known as the "mini-myelogram." With the use of modern contrast agents seizures are extremely rare. The most significant, but distinctly uncommon, morbidity associated with this technique is cord or vertebral artery damage during C1–C2 puncture.[26] Specific anatomic points to examine include:

- Relationships between the thecal sac and bony anatomy.
- Integrity of the dural sleeves surrounding nerve roots.
- Extravasation of contrast into soft tissues, indicating a dural tear or root avulsion.
- Blockage of contrast flow past a fracture segment.
- Extrinsic deformation of the contrast column, suggesting an epidural mass or hematoma.

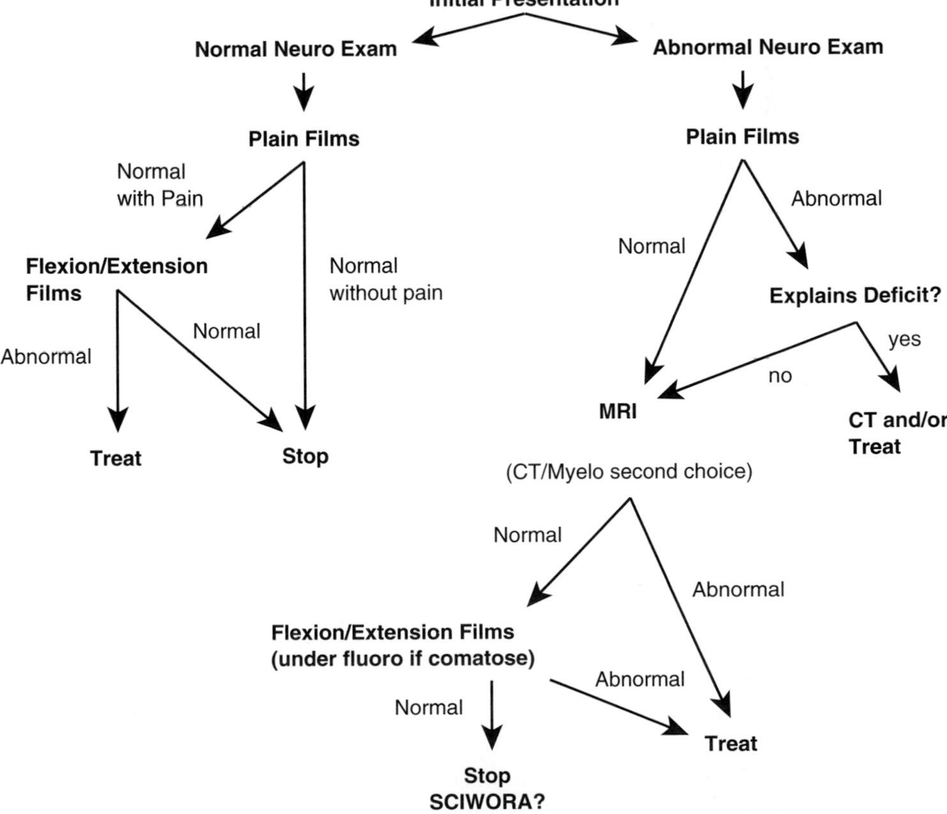

Figure 81-10. Decision tree to guide selection of neuroradiologic techniques when imaging spinal trauma.

Bone Scans

These studies are not indicated in acute trauma. Nevertheless, they can be useful once the patient is stable to determine the age of fractures and perhaps the presence of infection or inflammation. Points to note include:

- Increased activity in the area of anatomic abnormality suggests inflammation and repair processes associated with healing, but can be positive for many months following the initial damage.
- Soft tissue injury will show increased activity, and may give a false-positive reading if trying to determine whether or not an adjacent bony abnormality is in fact a new versus an old fracture or anatomic variant.

CONCLUSION

The imaging of acute spinal trauma is a goal-directed activity designed to diagnose and define anatomic abnormalities that result in pain, instability, or neurological dysfunction. In order to achieve this goal efficiently, the clinician needs to decide whether or not the pain, instability, or neurological dysfunction is explained by the radiological studies in hand. If not, further imaging techniques or imaging of other spinal regions is necessary. Once the etiology of pain, instability, or dysfunction is diagnosed radiographically, treatment paradigms come into play. The nature of some surgical stabilization techniques may require additional studies to allow placement of hardware, etc.

The evaluation of the spine of a comatose, immobile patient requires clinical judgment concerning the likelihood that the patient's immobility may be due to a high spinal injury versus a severe head injury.

Asymptomatic lesions certainly cannot be ignored, but owing to their asymptomatic nature, can be identified, stabilized, and further defined at a more leisurely pace following the stabilization of the trauma patient.

The following is a suggested decision tree to guide the selection of imaging modalities based upon whether or not the radiographs explain the clinically observed abnormality (Fig. 81-10). Specifics concerning treatment are discussed in other chapters.

References

1. Eisenberg RL: *Radiology: An Illustrated History.* St Louis: Mosby, 1992.
2. Goldberg AL, Daffner RH, Schapiro RL: Imaging of acute spinal trauma: An evolving multi-modality approach. *Clin Imaging* 1990; 14:11–16.
3. Murphy MD, Batnitzky S, Bramble JM: Diagnostic imaging of spinal trauma. *Radiol Clin North Am* 1989; 27(5):855–872.
4. Pathria MN, Petersilge CA: Spinal trauma. *Radiol Clin North Am* 1991; 29(4):847–865.
5. Gerrelts BD, Petersen EU, Mabry J: Delayed diagnosis of cervical spine injuries. *J Trauma* 1991; 31:1622–1626.
6. Kerslake RW, Jaspan T, Worthington BS: Magnetic resonance imaging of spinal trauma. *Br J Radiol* 1991; 64:386–402.
7. Davis SJ, Terisi LM, Bradley WC Jr, et al: Cervical spine hyperextension injuries: MR finding. *Radiology* 1991; 180:245–251.
8. Beers GJ, Raque GH, Wagner GG, et al: MR imaging in acute cervical spine trauma. *J Comp Assist Tomog* 1988; 12(5):755–761.
9. Mirvis SE, Geisler FH, Jelenik JJ: Acute cervical spine trauma: Evaluation with 1.5T MR imaging. *Radiology* 1988; 166:807–816.
10. Tarr RW, Drolshagen LF, Kerner TC, et al: MR imaging of recent spinal trauma. *J Comp Assist Tomog* 1987; 11(3):412–417.
11. Goldberg AL, Rothfus WE, Deeb ZL, et al: Hyperextension injuries of the cervical spine: Magnetic resonance findings. *Skeletal Radiol* 1989; 18:238–288.
12. Flanders AE, Schaeffer DM, Doan HT, et al: Acute cervical spine trauma: Correlation of MR imaging findings with degree of neurological deficit. *Radiology* 1990; 177:25–33.
13. Kulkarni MV, McArdle CB, Kopanicky D, et al: Acute spinal cord injury: MR imaging at 1.5T. *Radiology* 1987; 164:837–843.
14. Kulkarni MV, Bondurant FJ, Rose SL, Narayana PA: 1.5 Tesla magnetic resonance imaging of acute spinal trauma. *Radiographics* 1988; 8(6):1059–1082.
15. Acheson MB, Livingston RR, Richardson ML: High resolution CT scanning in the evaluation of cervical spine fractures: Comparison with plain film examination. *AJR* 1987; 148:1179–1185.
16. Daffner RH, Deeb ZL, Goldberg AL, et al: The radiologic assessment of post-traumatic vertebral stability. *Skeletal Radiol* 1990; 19:103–108.
17. White AA III, Panjabi MM: *Clinical Biomechanics of the Spine.* Philadelphia: JB Lippincott, 1978: 283–294.
18. Fielding JW: Normal and selected abnormal motions of the cervical spine from the second cervical vertebra to the seventh cervical vertebra based on cineroentgenography. *J Bone Joint Surg* 1964; 46-A:1779–1781.
19. Wiesel SW, Rothman RH: Occipitoatlantal hypermobility. *Spine* 1979; 4:187–191.
20. Weir DC: Roentgenographic signs of cervical injury. *Clin Orthop* 1975; 109(9):9–17.
21. Fielding JW, Cochran GVB, Lawsing JF III, Hohl M: Tears of the transverse ligament of the atlas. *J Bone Joint Surg* 1974; 56-A:1683–1691.
22. Penning L: Normal movements of the cervical spine. *AJR* 1978; 130:317–326.

23. Harris JH Jr: Acute injuries of the spine. *Semin Roentgenol* 1978; 13:53–68.
24. Hadley MN, Sonntag VKH, Amos MR: Three dimensional computed tomography in the diagnosis of vertebral column pathological conditions. *Neurosurgery* 1987; 21:186–192.
25. Schaeffer DM, Flanders A, Northrup BE: Magnetic resonance imaging of acute cervical spine trauma: Correlation with severity of neurologic injury. *Spine* 1989; 14:1090–1095.
26. Robertson HJ, Smith RD: Cervical myelography: Survey of modes of practice and major complications. *Radiology* 1990; 174:79–83.
27. Pang D, Wilberger JE Jr: Spinal cord injury without radiographic abnormalities in children. *J Neurosurg* 1982; 57:114–129.
28. Pollack IF, Pang D, Sclabassi R: Recurrent spinal cord injury without radiographic abnormalities in children. *J Neurosurg* 1988; 69:177–182.
29. Yamashita Y, Takahashi M, Matsuno Y, et al: Acute spinal cord injury: MRI correlated with myelopathy. *Br J Radiol* 1991; 64:201–209.

Operating Room Management

CHAPTER 82

ANESTHESIA MANAGEMENT OF SPINAL TRAUMA

Edward Teeple, Jr.
Edward K. Heres

INTRODUCTION

Spinal cord trauma, especially involving the cervical spine, although not a frequent occurrence, is assumed to be a common circumstance during the initial management of multiple trauma patients. The "assumption of risk" is an important concept for the care of all trauma patients, since failure to recognize and/or protect against unstable spinal injuries can have grave long-term consequences for these patients. There are approximately 13,000 new cases of traumatic spinal cord injury in the United States each year.[1] Up to 20 percent of these patients may die acutely from associated injuries or from high spinal cord injuries with loss of respiratory function.[2] This chapter will explore the role of the anesthesiologist in the management of acute spinal cord injury, especially cervical spine injury. Each stage of trauma resuscitation will be discussed, including the evaluation of the patient's airway, the adequacy of breathing and circulation, and the issues surrounding the management of tracheal intubation.

As the anesthesiologist approaches a trauma patient, an immediate assessment of spinal injury must be made. If the patient is unconscious or unable to communicate (because of intoxication, immaturity, etc.), an assumption of an unstable injury to the spine is assumed until proved otherwise. Frequently, Advanced Trauma Life Support (ATLS) protocols mandate that cervical collars and rigid backboards be in place.[3] Often the method of securing the head directly conflicts with the ease of airway management, and compromises must be made to achieve both neck stabilization and oxygenation and ventilation. The lack of complaints of pain or positive neurological findings in an intoxicated or confused multiple trauma patient do not negate potential spinal instability or cord injury. The anesthesiologist must be aware of the level of spinal cord injury. As the level of a spinal cord injury rises, the patient will lose increasing degrees of autonomic, sensory, motor, and reflex activity. The higher the level, the greater the physiological impact on the patient. Table 82-1 describes the functional levels of the spine. In the second and third columns, physiological compromises are shown for each spinal level.[4] Initial anesthesia assessment and treatment should follow the ABCs of trauma management.

A IS FOR AIRWAY

A patient with an acute cervical spinal cord injury requires intense respiratory monitoring and care because pulmonary complications are a major cause of initial morbidity and mortality. During the initial management, ensuring a patent airway is critical. In an unconscious patient, airway obstruction usually is relieved by chin lift, jaw thrust, and continuous positive airway pressure or nasal or oral airway insertion. However, chin lift and jaw thrust should be done with caution, since it has been reported that both maneuvers can cause a greater than 5-mm widening of the disk space in a cadaver model with C5 to C6 instability.[5] Placement of an oral or nasal pharyngeal catheter may relieve the obstruction with minimal movement of the cervical spine. If the nasal passage has been traumatized or a suspected basilar skull fracture is present, an oral airway may be used, but this frequently is not tolerated by an

TABLE 82-1 Level of Spinal Injury and Implications for Physiological Stability

Level of Injury	Cardiac	Pulmonary	Other
C1 to C4		Loss of accessory muscles of respiration	Hangman fracture risk with extension; older patients extension with intubation
C3 to C4		Diaphragmatic innervation; loss of respirations	
C5 to C6		If increased, spinal edema can rise to C3 to C4 with loss of respiration	
C4 to C6			Unstable with cervical flexion with intubation
T1 to T4	Cardioaccelerator fibers; bradycardia and sinus arrest can occur, esp. with attempt at intubation Poor fluid tolerance may cause congestive heart failure; higher cardiac output can decrease in short term; may require beta-adrenergic support		
T1 to T12	As level increases, there is more loss of peripheral sympathetic tone, leading to lowered blood pressure, poor tolerance of fluid load, and poikilothermia		
L1 to L2		Loss of control of thoracic and abdominal muscles to maximize breathing and coughing	
S1 to S3			Loss of bladder (urinary retention) and rectal sphincter control (incontinence)

awake patient. In the field, a cricothyroidotomy may be necessary in an unconscious patient to provide emergency access to the airway if more conventional modalities are unsuccessful.

Ventilation should always be assessed while keeping the head in a neutral position. Cervical collars are placed on most of these patients during transport to prevent anterior flexion of the neck. Anterior flexion tends to cause the most severe injury at the C4 through C6 level if it is unstable. These levels are the most common sites of cervical cord injury.[6]

When one is attempting mask ventilation, the mandible is usually extended to achieve an unobstructed airway. Unstable C1-2 fractures, however, tend to worsen the injury if the neck is extended. The odontoid process can compress the cord during extension. A discussion of emergency intubation with a cervical spine injury appears at the end of this chapter.

Oxygen saturation should be maintained at nearly 100% to minimize any potential secondary injury to the spinal cord. Simply giving supplemental oxygen via a rebreathing mask at 6 to 8 liters per minute of oxygen may correct decreases in oxygen saturation without any other airway manipulation.

B IS FOR BREATHING

Once the airway is patent, respiratory depth and rate and oxygen saturation must be assessed. A decision to mask ventilate or intubate and ventilate will be necessary if (1) the respiratory rate is less than 10/min, (2) the vital capacity is less than 15 ml/kg, (3) oxygen saturation is less than 90% (with supplemental oxygen), (4) arterial blood gas Pa_{O_2} is below 60 mmHg and Pa_{CO_2} is above 45 mmHg, (5) pulmonary function tests show a maximum expiratory force of 20 cmH_2O or less or a maximum inspiratory force of 20 cmH_2O or less.

Greater compromise of respiratory function will occur as the level of spinal injury ascends. Intubation may not be required for spinal lesions lower than C6, since diaphragmatic breathing remains intact. However, other compromises of respiratory function may coexist, such as upper airway obstruction, flail chest, pneumothorax, and lung contusion. These complications may require intervention and respiratory support even if the spinal injury is lower.

Injuries at the C5 to C6 level may require prophylactic intubation and ventilation for the first 48 to 72 h after injury. Respiratory support is provided because the loss of function may rise to the C3 to C4 level from secondary spinal edema. The origin of the diaphragmatic fibers is at C3 to C4; hence, diaphragmatic breathing may stop and imperil the patient. The diaphragm, the principal muscle of inspiration, accounts for two-thirds of the air that enters the lungs during quiet breathing.

Just as closed head injuries cause a risk of secondary injury from edema formation, the spinal canal should also be considered a closed space. Arterial carbon dioxide levels greater than 40 mmHg and/or arterial oxygen levels below 60 mmHg may cause increased blood flow and tissue swelling of the injured spinal tissue. Secondary injury to the spine can lead to a worsening downward spiral of injury. Spinal cord compromise can impair normal physiological control processes. Changes in heart rate, blood pressure, respiration, and hormonal function can further increase spinal cord damage and amplify the physiological abnormalities. Optimization of the long-term outcome for these patients requires early aggressive intervention to break this downward spiral. All vital sign parameters must be maintained at levels as normal as possible. If necessary, the decision to intubate and support ventilation should not be delayed until the emergency room if breathing is compromised. The most common cause of immediate preventable death in high spinal injuries is failure to provide an unobstructed airway and ventilation.[6]

Rescuers at the scene and during transport must constantly evaluate the respiratory function and intervene if respirations are compromised. If possible, delaying the attempted intubation until the emergency room may be advantageous. In patients who cannot move their hands, arms, or legs (no innervation below C4), alveolar ventilation is grossly impaired, and these patients always require assisted ventilation or intubation in the acute phase. Patients with intact C5 innervation (can shrug their shoulders) have partial diaphragmatic denervation but usually can breathe adequately if they are not overly anxious and there are no associated thoracic or abdominal injuries. With the neurological deficit at C6 and below, diaphragmatic ventilation is intact, but ventilation is reduced by total intercostal muscle paralysis.[7]

C IS FOR CIRCULATION

Along with the assessment of the airway and respirations, the anesthesiologist may play a role in managing the cardiovascular status of a spinal injury patient. Again, the higher the level of the spinal injury, the worse the physiological derangements.

The sympathetic nervous system exits from the spinal cord at the thoracic level (T1 through T12).[8] The higher the level of the injury, the stronger the tendency toward hypotension and hypothermia. As the injury ascends, more and more of the body's peripheral vasoconstrictor activity is lost. Loss of vasoconstriction impairs blood pressure control, blood volume control, and heat conservation. If the injury is at T7 or higher, the normal adrenal response to stress will be inhibited. In the short term this may cause hypotension. In the longer term and if the spinal injury is above T7, problems with hypertension, myocardial infarction, and stroke can occur. This is due to the loss of higher neuronal inhibitory activity on the reflex adrenal response to lower-level noxious stimuli. This is known as mass reflex or autonomic hyperreflexia.[9,10]

If the level of the spinal injury involves T1 through T4 or higher, this can affect the function of the heart. These segments provide the cardioaccelerator fibers for the heart, controlling the sympathetic tone of the heart. Loss of these segments can cause slowing of the heart rate, decreased response to changes in fluid volume, and decreased cardiac contractility.

The clinical changes seen with the loss of the cardioaccelerator fibers include bradycardia and occasionally full cardiac arrest. The risk of cardiac arrest is high during attempted intubations (vagal stimulus from stimulation of pharynx and trachea can cause bradycardia). The bradycardia can be treated with infusions of dopamine or epinephrine to control hypotension and heart rate and/or atropine boluses to control bradycardia. Isoproterenol may not be ideal because it may further lower blood pressure. Atropine up to 1.2 mg may be required to inhibit the bradycardia that can occur with attempted intubation. Some authors even suggest aggressive pretreatment with atropine before atttempted intubation to avoid the risk of bradycardia.[11] Twenty-two of 83 patients admitted with traumatic quadriplegia had significant bradycardia. Bradycardia does not usually require a pacemaker in spinal cord injury patients, since the heart rate and cardiac output tend to increase and stabilize after 2 to 4 weeks.[12]

Hypotension is also a problem in these patients. Increased venous capacitance, decreased cardiac contractility, and decreased cardiac output can combine to cause hypotension. Problems may arise during trauma resuscitation or subsequent surgery in regard to differentiating the effects of the spinal injury from hypotension caused by blood loss, third spacing of fluids, or anesthesia. Central venous pressure monitoring is necessary to differentiate hypotension and low cardiac output from real hypovolemia and to avoid fluid overload. High-spinal-cord-level patients will not have raised blood pressure or a slow heart rate in response to fluid overload. If fluid overload occurs, this may increase the risk of spinal or cerebral edema.[13]

Central monitoring may also prevent misdiagnosis of the etiology of sudden-onset hypotension in the first 24 to 48 h after an injury. Late-onset sudden hypotension with no apparent etiology may be a result of late-onset spinal shock. Evaluation of the electrocardiogram (ECG) at this time is also important to rule out cardiac contusion or myocardial ischemia. Subendocardial ischemia has been demonstrated in clinical and experimental cord transection at C5 to C6.[14] Other ECG changes noted include sinus pauses, shifting sinus pacemaker, atrial fibrillation, multifocal preventricular contractions, ventricular tachycardia, and ST wave changes.[15]

Hypothermia can also occur as a result of a loss of sympathetic tone. Spinal injury patients are poikilothermic and have no ability to sweat. Hypothermia shifts the oxyhemoglobin dissociation curve to the left, decreasing oxygen delivery. Hypothermia also induces an increased sensitivity of the myocardium to altered calcium and potassium concentrations, increasing the risk of arythmias.[16]

D IS FOR DISABILITY

A brief neurological exam by the anesthesiologist is appropriate as a part of overall management. In confused, pediatric, or intoxicated patients it may not be possible to clinically discern all areas of injury. Twenty percent of spinal injuries can occur at multiple levels, 10 percent of head injuries are associated with cervical spine injuries, and 90 percent of cervical injuries are associated with head injuries.[17] Spinal cord trauma is associated with other injuries 25 to 65 percent of the time.[16]

E IS FOR EXPOSURE/ ENVIRONMENT

Normal patients can become hypothermic after trauma. As was discussed above, high spinal cord lesions can further inhibit temperature regulation and cause quicker onset and more severe temperature loss. Spinal cord injury patients must be monitored for temperature, and if hypothermia occurs, they should be treated aggressively.

INTUBATING A POTENTIAL CERVICAL SPINE INJURY PATIENT

Intubation of a multiple trauma patient is a complicated real-time problem. The difficulty lies in the choice of intubating technique to treat the ventilatory problem. Reasons for intubation can include respiratory failure, closed head injury, known high spinal cord injury, and difficult to control patients.[18] Sometimes the most neurologically damaged patients are the easiest to intubate, since they offer no resistance. An awake, pediatric, or combative patient may offer no options but to proceed with an anesthetic induction even if the airway is abnormal. Attempts to intubate combative patients awake may cause more injury, since the patient may move his or her neck to resist the intubation. The goal of this section is to review various components of the process of intubation and the anesthesiologist's method of assessment and planning for an emergency intubation.[19–27]

Assessment

Assessment may be the most important contribution of the anesthesiologist in the management of a trauma patient. Knowing which patient will be easy is just as important as knowing which patient will be difficult. Difficult airway patients may require more refined intubation techniques.

Normal Airway

The normal airway often may not present a problem for intubation with an intravenous anesthetic and a neuromuscular blocking drug. However, tracheal intubation of a trauma patient with a suspected cervical spine injury can be very challenging to even the most experienced anesthesiologist. In addition to the mandatory cervical spine immobilization, which can make airway management and intubation difficult, multiple trauma patients can present with facial and oropharyngeal bleeding and be in an intoxicated and combative state. These patients are considered to have full stomachs and are at increased risk of aspiration. Cervical spine fractures can cause posterior pharyngeal hematoma and edema formation around the larynx, and this can distort the laryngeal anatomy.[28]

There are a number of articles in the literature from trauma centers reporting low morbidity and mortality rates in trauma patients with potential cervical injuries who were intubated while anesthetized and paralyzed.[29,30] Other articles, while describing a number of complications associated with this approach (multiple intubations, aspirations, and esophageal intubations), still indicated that intubations using anesthetics and neuromuscular blockers were appropriate.[31–34] Most authors report high success rates with intubation, including second and third attempts at intubation. However, it is during these repeated attempts that the potential complications often occur.

Abnormal Airway

If an airway is diagnosed as abnormal before intubation, will attempted intubation under general anesthesia and paralysis have the same low morbidity and mortality rate? Abnormal airways not only are difficult to intubate but can create difficulties in mask ventilating and/or performing a tracheotomy.[35] Successful ventilation and/or tracheotomy may be achieved only at the cost of hyperextension of the neck. Maintenance of a neutral position of the neck is a primary goal in the care of these patients. However, failure to provide adequate ventilation for even short periods can cause swelling and ischemia of the spinal cord or brain if prior tissue injury exists.

The list below contains the most common abnormal airway presentations.[36,37] If these conditions are diagnosed before attempted intubation, an awake intubation should be considered:

Full stomach
Obesity, pregnant
Short mandible
Large tongue
Short neck
Small mouth or decreased range of motion
Limited neck movement
Bleeding in airway
Regurgitation, active vomiting, aspiration
Documented or suspected neck fracture

The presence of these conditions does not contraindicate the use of general anesthesia and paralysis (GA&P) to achieve intubation. There can be modifiers that encourage the use of anesthesia and paralysis even if these increased airway risks are present. For instance, if the patient is combative, confused, uncooperative, or a child, GA&P may be the best alternative. Risks inherent to the patient include the following:

Pediatric
Combative
Disoriented
Uncooperative
Stat vs. semielective intubation

The skill level of the intubator and that of the person performing the potential tracheotomy are important. One anesthesiologist may perform a quick and smooth nasal intubation using topical anesthesia, whereas this same technique could be a disaster with another anesthesiologist or someone with lesser skills in airway management. Skill in the method of intubation is integral to the success of any airway technique.[38] Only the most skilled individuals using techniques they have practiced and are comfortable with should attempt airway control measures in a potential spinal cord injury patient.

METHODS OF INTUBATION

It is important to have some familiarity with the drugs used to establish unconsciousness and paralysis during intubation. The following sedatives are the ones most commonly used:

Fentanyl 0.7 to 2 μg/kg
Midazolam 0.025 to 0.1 mg/kg
Diazepam 0.025 to 0.1 mg/kg

Light sedation can be useful in some cases of awake intubation. The drugs used for this are usually midazolam, diazepam, and/or fentanyl.[39,40] These drugs should be given intravenously and titrated slowly to achieve sedation but avoid respiratory depression or apnea. For maximum effect, waiting 2 min after giving an intravenous (IV) injection is best. Sedation should be avoided in cases were oxygenation or ventilation is at a critical level. Oxygen supplementation before and during the intubation is recommended.

When anesthetic induction with paralysis is planned, the following anesthetics should be used. It is important that in-line traction and preoxygenation precede the drug injections. Suction should be available to remove foreign bodies, blood, and secretions from the oropharynx. This will also aid in visualizing the vocal cords. All three of these agents produce quick unconsciousness. If the patient has had blood loss or is hypovolemic, thiopental sodium and propofol may cause significant drops in blood pressure. Smaller doses of these drugs should be used, or etomidate should be given. Etomidate tends to maintain the pressure at its initial level.

If blood pressure is very low and the patient is unconscious, the drugs listed below should be avoided:

Thiopental 3 to 5 mg/kg
Propofol 2 to 2.5 mg/kg
Etomidate 0.1 to 0.4 mg/kg

There are a number of drugs available that cause neuromuscular block. Certain aspects of each drug and method of use deserve mention here.[32,33,38,41,42]

Succinylcholine is a good agent, since it has a fast onset and wears off quickly (45 s and 6 to 10 min, respectively). It sometimes can increase intracranial pressure as a result of fasciculations; therefore, pretreatment with a small dose of curare (3 mg in an adult) is recommended. Succinylcholine can also precipitate malignant hyperthermia in patients with such a tendency. Succinylcholine can cause bradycardia in children. High spinal injury patients may be more prone to bradycardia. Atropine pretreatment before intubation will minimize this risk. Finally, succinylcholine may cause rises in serum potassium levels in patients with burns or large crush injuries. In these cases, the use of a nondepolarizer may be safer. Succinylcholine can cause dangerous rises in serum potassium levels in parapligic and quadriplegic patients. This results from hypersensitization of the denervated muscle tissue below the level of the lesion. This reaction usually will not occur before 48 h. Thus, succinylcholine is not contraindicated in spinal injury patients at the time of the initial injury.[43] The following drugs may be used to achieve a neuromuscular block:

Depolarizers
Succinylcholine 1 to 2 mg/kg
Nondepolarizers
Vecuronium 0.08 to 0.1 mg/kg
Atracurium 0.3 to 0.5 mg/kg
Rocuronium 0.1 mg/kg

Nondepolarizers can prevent problems that are associated with the use of succinylcholine. However, the nondepolarizing neuromuscular blockers have characteristics that can also create problems.[44–46] Nondepolarizers tend to have a slower onset of neuromuscular block. The increased interval from unconsciousness to intubation increases the risk of oxygen desaturation. The longer the period of unconsciousness and nonintubation, the greater the risk of aspiration. To overcome this, pretreatment of the patient with a small dose of the nondepolarizer is suggested to decrease the onset time of the block. Also, if the dose of the nondepolarizer is increased, the onset time of the block is also shortened. Both of these methods are recommended. However, increasing the dose of the drug can increase the duration of action. If the intubation is unsuccessful, the patient's ventilation will have to be supported until the drug wears off (8 mg vecuronium can last 40 min or longer). As was discussed previously, ventilating a suspected unstable neck fracture is risky. Hence, if an abnormal airway is suspected, awake intubation, using a depolarizing neuromuscular blocker or a smaller dose of the nondepolarizer, is recommended. Rocuronium, a newer neuromuscular blocker, was designed to have the shortest half-life of the nondepolarizers listed above. It may be the agent of choice for emergency intubation using a nondepolarizing drug.[47,48]

Many articles suggest that anesthesia, neuromuscular block, and oral intubation using direct laryngoscopy with in-line cervical traction constitute the most appropriate method for managing a suspected cervical spine injury patient. As was discussed above, there may be times when other methods of achieving airway control are more appropriate. The final decision may depend on the patient's overall condition, the extent of the spinal injury, and the preferences and experience of the anesthesiologist. Various methods of intubation are listed below; they are not listed in order of application:

Awake, no topicalization
Awake, topicalization
Oral visualized
Retrograde wire
Blind nasal[49–52]
Fiber-optic[53]
Lighted stylet[54,55]
Emergency cricothyroidotomy[56–59]
Elective tracheostomy
Slash nonelective tracheostomy
Esophageal obturator[38,60,61]
Laryngeal mask[62,63]

DIRECT LARYNGOSCOPY

The surest and fastest method of intubating the trachea is direct laryngoscopy. Patients can be anesthetized and paralyzed for this procedure. In patients with suspected cervical spine injury, the head and neck are stabilized in the neutral position to minimize spine motion. However, to bring the larynx into view, exposing the vocal cords, atlanto-occipital extension is required. Some authors worry that this neck movement during direct laryngoscopy may injure an unstable spine. Horton and associates[64] showed that during direct laryngoscopy there was significant atlanto-axial extension but minimal movement in the lower cervical spine.[65,66] Therefore, direct laryngoscopy may be more dangerous for those with known or suspected C1 or C2 injuries than for those with lower cervical spine injuries.

Does cervical spine stabilization during laryngoscopy prevent further spinal cord injury? Studies in cadavers and anesthetized volunteers have shown that neck movement was reduced but not prevented by stabilization attempts during direct laryngoscopy.[5] While neck movement has been implicated in neurological injury in acute trauma patients who have not had cervical immobilization, neck movement caused by direct laryngoscopy in patients with in-line cervical traction has not been shown to cause neurological injury.[67,68]

Awake Intubation

Many authors recommend awake tracheal intubation for patients with potential C-spine injuries, believing that this will avoid moving or endangering the spine. This technique is not appropriate if the airway must be secured rapidly. Although the awake technique does not employ atlanto-occipital extension as frequently as does direct laryngoscopy, there is often some neck movement required. Meschino and coworkers[69] have reported a minimal risk of neurological injury in a series of awake intubations.

Awake intubation using blind nasal intubation, fiberoptic intubation, or the lighted stylet method is greatly facilitated by topically anesthetizing the nasal, oropharyngeal, and tracheal passages before the attempted intubation. For the oropharynx and nasal passages, this is accomplished with acetocaine spray or lidocaine gel 2% applied to the tongue. This requires a cooperative patient. For the nasal passage, 2% lidocaine gel is applied to a small nasal trumpet, and the trumpet is carefully slipped into the nasal passage. This is repeated four or five times to minimize the risk of hemorrhage in the nasal passage. For tracheal topical anesthesia (the trachea and the vocal cords), 4% lidocaine 4 ml is injected into the trachea, using a 21-gauge needle. The entry point can be either the cricothyroid membrane or via the trachea (only done by experienced personnel).[70] Proof of the intratracheal position is shown by clear aspiration of bubbles in the syringe before injection of the fluid into the trachea. The lidocaine is injected quickly to create a mist in the trachea. This will anesthetize the cords and trachea in approximately 30 s. In-line cervical traction should be maintained during the tracheal injection. An alternative method for anesthetizing the larynx is a superior laryngeal nerve block.[71,72]

Airway intubation is also facilitated by explaining the process to the patient. When they understand the gravity of the situation, many patients cooperate fully and facilitate the intubation. A full explanation decreases the patient's fear and makes the experience more tolerable.

Once the airway is anesthetized, the method chosen depends on the patient and the anesthesiologist. Blind nasal intubation can be used in patients without suspected basilar skull fractures or nasal trauma. It also may be indicated in anatomically difficult airways where there is bleeding or copious secretion, since secretions or blood can inhibit successful fiber-optic intubation. Hemorrhage often can be prevented by good lubrication of the nasal passage and the choice of a reasonable tube size. In adult males a 7 to 8 internal diameter tube is best. In adult females a 6.5 to 7 internal diameter tube is best. Endotrol (Rtm) endotracheal tubes are preferred because they allow the intubator to adjust the anterior-posterior angle of the tube as it exits the posterior naris. Right and left adjustments are produced by axial rotation of the tube.

In patients with cervical injuries, minimal head and neck motion are allowed. Therefore, the nasal tube has to be rotated and moved anteriorly or posteriorly with the endotrol tube control. It is important to have the patient stick out the tongue during the attempt. This elevates the base of the tongue and epiglottis, exposing the vocal cords to the tip of the endotracheal tube. If needed, gauze can be used to grasp the tongue and pull it forward. The tube should be advanced slowly and only during inspiration, when the cords are open. Tube placement should be adjusted to maximize the audible breath sounds as the cords are approached. Blind nasal intubation is criticized because of a success rate of approximately 67 to 90 percent.[73] However, in patients with obviously abnormal airways and cervical injuries, it may provide a safe alternative method of intubation.

Fiber-optic intubation has the advantage of allowing either nasal or oral awake intubation. It can be more difficult in patients with airway bleeding or excessive secretions. It has a high success rate in experienced hands.[74] Oral intubation may be a preferred method, since sinusitis has been reported as a complication of prolonged nasal intubation.[75,76]

A recent technique for awake intubation is the lighted stylet. In this method, the endotracheal tube is placed over the stylet. The stylet has a light filament with a high-intensity beam. In a topicalized airway, with the room darkened, the stylet is passed blindly under the tongue. As it passes through the cords, it lights the anterior surface of the trachea. When the light can be seen as a small dot pattern on the anterior neck, the stylet has entered the trachea. The stylet is then withdrawn, and the endotracheal tube remains within the trachea.[54,55]

Cricothyroidotomy is a rapid but more invasive technique for securing the airway. It can be difficult to perform and has a high complication rate.[77] Cricothyroidotomy or tracheostomy may be indicated in patients with known anatomic features that predict difficult direct laryngoscopy under normal circumstances, since direct laryngoscopy may be even more difficult in a trauma setting with neck and head stabilization.

Esophageal obturator use is not considered safe as a method for intubation, since the distal portion of the tube may pass into the trachea and prevent ventilation of the lungs. One author felt that if the esophageal obturator is to be used, much time should be spent teaching the users to identify and remove a tracheal occlusion, a potentially lethal complication of this device.[38]

The laryngeal mask has also been suggested for the management of difficult airways. These authors have not had experience with its use in the emergency room. However, some difficulty in placement may occur because of inability to move the head and neck. There is a risk of aspiration using this device. Also, when this technique is used, the anesthesia personnel must stay in attendance, and this is a decided disadvantage.

ANTICIPATION—PART OF THE DECISION PROCESS

One must always assume that a multiple trauma patient has a spinal injury until proved otherwise. When airway control is necessary, using intravenous anesthesia and a neuromuscular block with in-line cervical traction for intubation is considered safe. Intubation of an easy airway is usually uneventful, and fortunately, normal airways constitute the majority of cases. However, if the airway appears abnormal, alternative awake and topicalized methods of intubation or tracheostomy should be considered. Sometimes, even an abnormal airway patient's condition or combativeness may prevent awake intubation attempts. In this case, proceeding to anesthesia with neuromuscular blocking drugs while preparing for immediate emergency tracheostomy by a skilled surgeon is necessary.

Finally, the anesthesiologist's role in the management of a potential cervical spine injury is to help with the intubation. That is not the only skill the anesthesiologist can contribute. Anesthesiologists are also vitally important in providing a risk assessment of the airway. Anticipation of risk is a cornerstone of anesthetic practice and the best means of avoiding potentially bad outcomes. Knowledge of the drugs used for intubation and of safe algorithms for intubation is part of anesthesia practice. The anesthesiologist should strive to communicate with and educate the emergency and surgical staff about how to best use anesthetic drugs and most safely intubate a multiple trauma patient with a potential spinal cord injury. A diagram of a flowchart for intubation is provided (Fig. 82-1).

ANESTHESIA FOR THE TRAUMA PATIENT

Anesthesia management for trauma patients follows the guidelines discussed above. A few additional points can be addressed.

Anesthesia often must occur on an emergency basis. The patient may have been intubated and ventilated in the emergency room or in the field. When the patient

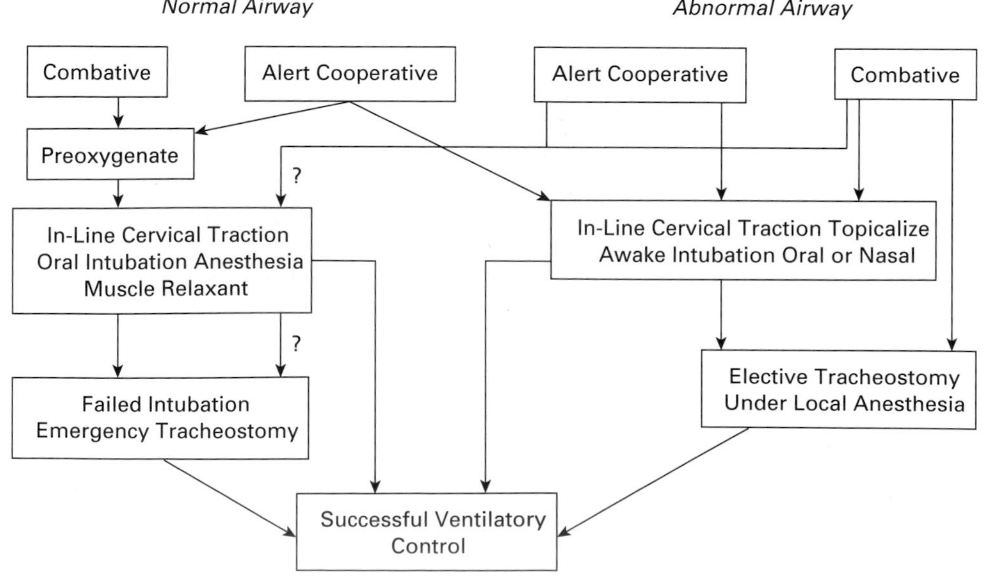

Figure 82-1. Algorithm for intubation of cervical injury.

is brought to the operating room, diligent placement of the patient on the operating room table is imperative. Careful log-rolling must be done. The patient's neural axis must be maintained in a straight neutral position during the move and the final positioning for surgery. The same neutral position must be maintained when the patient is taken off the table.

If the surgery is not required immediately and the patient is cooperative, greater consideration can be given to awake intubation techniques. If an awake intubation is performed, this can also allow for awake positioning. Awake positioning allows the patient to help determine the most comfortable and nonpainful position before the induction of anesthesia.[78,79] The patient can be tested for intact neurological function before going to sleep. Some anesthesiologists feel that this is one more check that can be used to protect the patient from any nerve damage caused by positioning.

Heat loss during anesthesia is often a problem.[80] In spinal injury patients with high lesions, this is a common problem. Careful attention to keeping the patient warm during surgery is important.

Blood loss and volume replacement often occur during surgery.[81] Again, high-level paraplegics and quadriplegics tend to have lower normal blood pressures, a worse ability to tolerate fluid overload, and larger venous capacity than normal patients. Fluid management in these patients is made easier by using a central venous pressure monitor during lengthy surgical procedures or wherein large losses of blood are anticipated.

These patients have a decreased ability to clear secretions as a result of the loss of abdominal and intercostal muscle function. Frequently, when these patients are placed in the prone position for surgery, mucus plugs occlude the endotracheal tube and completely obstruct ventilation. This problem may be minimized by placing a sterile 0.9% sodium chloride solution down the endotracheal tube after intubation and performing multiple suctions to clear the thick secretions from the airway. This should be performed while the patient is still in the prone position. If increased difficulty ventilating occurs during surgery in the prone position in patients with high spinal injuries, a mucus plug causing the obstruction should be considered.

The final important consideration during anesthesia is the patient's compromised ability to ventilate. If possible, measurements of the patient's preanesthesia pulmonary function and arterial blood gases can help in determining the appropriate time to extubate the patient after anesthesia and surgery. Normal values for these patients can be very different from those of patients without spinal cord lesions. Conservative weaning protocols should be used to extubate these patients gradually. There are several good review articles on this topic.[82,83]

References

1. Kraus JF, Franti CE, Borhani NO, et al: Incidence of traumatic spinal cord lesions. *J Chronic Dis* 28:471–492, 1975.
2. Kraus JF, Franti CE, Borhani NO, et al: Survival with acute spinal cord injury. *J Chronic Dis* 32:269–283, 1979.
3. Alexander RH, Proctor HJ: *Advanced Trauma Life Support Course for Physicians*, 5th ed. Chicago: American College of Surgeons, 1993: chap 2.
4. Netter FH, *The CIBA Collection of Medical Illustrations.* Volume I: *Nervous System Anatomy and Physiology*. West Caldwell, N.J.: Ciba Geigy, 1984: 70, 128.
5. Majernick TG, Bieniek R, Houston JB, et al: Cervical spine movement during orotracheal intubation. *Ann Emerg Med* 15:417–420, 1986.
6. Aprahamian C, Thompson B, Fingen W, Darm J: Experimental cervical spine injury model: Examination of airway splinting techniques. *Ann Emerg Med* 13:584–587, 1984.
7. Gatz AJ: *Manter's Essentials of Clinical Neuroanatomy and Neurophysiology*, 4th ed. Philadelphia: Davis, 1972: 23.
8. Miller RD (ed): *Anesthesia,* 2d ed. New York: Churchill Livingstone, 1986: 948.
9. Newfield P, Cottrell JE: *Handbook of Neuroanesthesia: Clinical and Physiologic Essentials*. Boston: Little, Brown, 1983: 341–342.
10. Desmond J: Paraplegia: Problems confronting the anaesthesiologist. *Can Anaes Soc J.* 17(5):435–451, 1970.
11. Doolan LA, O'Brien JF: Safe intubation in cervical spine injury. *Anaesth Intensive Care* 13:319–324, 1985.
12. Winslow EB, Lesch M, Talano JV, et al: Spinal cord injuries associated with cardiopulmonary complications. *Spine* 1:809–812, 1986.
13. Wilson RH, Whiteside MC, Moorehead RJ: Problems in diagnosis and management of hypovolaemia in spinal injury. *Br J Clin Pract* 47(4):224–225, 1993.
14. Altose MD. Pulmonary mechanics, in Fishman AP (ed): *Pulmonary Diseases and Disorders.* New York: McGraw-Hill, 1980: 359.
15. Greenholt JH, Reichenbach D: Cardiac injury and subarachnoid hemorrhage: Clinical pathologic correlation. *J Neurosurg* 30:521–531, 1969.
16. Kopaniky DR, Frost EAM: Management of spinal cord trauma, in Frost EAM (ed): *Clinical Anesthesia in Neurosurgery.* Boston: Butterworth, 1984: 375.
17. Schreibman DL, MacKenzie CF: The trauma victim with an acute spinal cord injury, in Matjesko MJ (ed): *Problems in Anesthesia: Anesthesia and Trauma*. Philadelphia: Lippincott, 1990: 459–460.
18. Schwartz DE, Matthay MA, Cohen NH: Death and other complications of emergency airway management in critically ill adults: A prospective investigation of 297 tracheal intubations. *Anesthesiology* 82(2):367–376, 1995.
19. Deem S, Bishop MJ: Evaluation and management of the difficult airway (review). *Crit Care Clin* 11(1):1–27, 1995.
20. Stauffer JL: Medical management of the airway (review). *Clin Chest Med* 12(3):449–482, 1991.

21. Williamson R: Tracheal intubation and cervical injury (letter). *Can J Anaesth* 40(8):797–798, 1993.
22. Palmer AR: Tracheal intubation and cervical injury (letter, comment). *Can J Anaesth* 40:470–471, 1993.
23. Drummond JC: Tracheal intubation and cervical injury (letter, comment). *Can J Anaesth* 39(9):1000–1001, 1992.
24. Cohn SM, Lyle WG, Linden CH, Lancey RA: Exclusion of cervical spine injury: A prospective study. *J Trauma* 31(4):570–574, 1991.
25. Smale JR, Kutty K, Ohlert J, Cotter T: Endotracheal intubation by paramedics during in-hospital CPR. *Chest* 107(6):1655–1661, 1995.
26. Vilke GM, Hoyt DB, Epperson M, et al: Intubation techniques in the helicopter. *J Emerg Med* 12(2):217–224, 1994.
27. Holley J, Jorden R: Airway management in patients with unstable cervical spine fractures. *Ann Emerg Med* 18(11):1237–1239, 1989.
28. Biby L, Santora AH: Prevertebral hematoma secondary to whiplash injury necessitating emergency intubation. *Anesth Analg* 70:112–114, 1990.
29. Murphy-Macabobby M, Marshall WJ, Schneider C, Dries D: Neuromuscular blockade in aeromedical airway management. *Ann Emerg Med* 21(6):664–668, 1992. *Klin Monatsbl Augenheilk* 200(1):43–47, 1992.
30. Ligier B, Buchman TG, Breslow MJ, Deutschman CS: The role of anesthetic induction agents and neuromuscular blockade in the endotracheal intubation of trauma victims. *Surg Gynecol Obstet* 173(6):477–481, 1991.
31. Holley J, Jorden R: Airway management in patients with unstable cervical spine fractures. *Ann Emerg Med* 18(11):1237–1239, 1989.
32. Nakayama DK, Waggoner T, Venkataraman ST, et al: The use of drugs in emergency airway management in pediatric trauma. *Ann Surg* 216(2):205–211, 1992.
33. Rotondo MF, McGonigal MD, Schwab CW, et al: Urgent paralysis and intubation of trauma patients: Is it safe? *J Trauma* 34(2):242–246, 1993.
34. Rhee KJ, Green W, Holcroft JW, Mangili JA: Oral intubation in the multiply injured patient: The risk of exacerbating spinal cord damage. *Ann Emerg Med* 19(5):511–514, 1990.
35. Rhee KJ, O'Malley RJ, Turner JE, Ward RE: Field airway management of the trauma patient: The efficacy of bag mask ventilation. *Am J Emerg Med* 6(4):333–336, 1988.
36. Jambor CR, Steedman DJ: Acute gastric dilation after trauma. *J R Coll Surg Edinb* 36(1):29–31, 1991.
37. Davies JM, Weeks S, Crone LA, Pavlin E: Difficult intubation in the parturient (review). *Can J Anaesth* 36(6):668–674, 1989.
38. Pepe PE, Zachariah BS, Chandra NC: Invasive airway techniques in resuscitation (review). *Ann Emerg Med* 22:393–403, 1993.
39. Omoigui S: *The Anesthesia Drug Handbook.* Chicago: Mosby, 1992.
40. Barash PG, Cullen BF, Stoelting RK (eds): *Clinical Anesthesia.* New York: Lippincott, 1989.
41. Roberts DJ, Clinton JE, Ruiz E: Neuromuscular blockade for critical patients in the emergency department. *Ann Emerg Med* 15(2):152–156, 1986.
42. Redan JA, Livingston DH, Tortella BJ, Rush BF Jr: The value of intubating and paralyzing patients with suspected head injury in the emergency department. *J Trauma* 31(3):371–375, 1991.
43. Frost EAM (ed): *Clinical Anesthesia In Neurosurgery.* Boston: Butterworth, 1984: 210.
44. Taboada JA, Rupp SM, Miller RD: Refining the priming principle for vecuronium during rapid-sequence induction of anesthesia. *Anesthesiology* 64(2):243–247, 1986.
45. Deepika K, Bikhazi GB, Mikati HM, et al: Facilitation of rapid-sequence intubation with large-dose vecuronium with or without priming. *J Clin Anesth* 4(2):106–110, 1992.
46. Brandom BW, Meretoja OA, Taivainen T, Wirtavuori K: Accelerated onset and delayed recovery of neuromuscular block induced by mivacurium preceded by pancuronium in children. *Anesth Analg* 76(5):998–1003, 1993.
47. Wright PM, Caldwell JE, Miller RD: Onset and duration of rocuronium and succinylcholine at the adductor pollicis and laryngeal adductor muscles in anesthetized humans. *Anesthesiology* 81(5):1110–1115, 1994.
48. Magorian T, Flannery KB, Miller RD: Comparison of rocuronium, succinylcholine, and vecuronium for rapid-sequence induction of anesthesia in adult patients. *Anesthesiology* 79(5):913–918, 1993.
49. Nakajima M, Lee YE, Nakazawa T, et al: Pneumothorax, subcutaneous emphysema and mediastinal emphysema in transnasally intubated patients (Japanese). *Nippon Geka Hokan* 58(6):522–526, 1989.
50. Wilkinson JA, Mathis RD, Dire DJ: Turbinate destruction—a rare complication of nasotracheal intubation. *J Emerg Med* 4(3):209–212, 1986.
51. Danzl DF, Thomas DM: Nasotracheal intubations in the emergency department. *Crit Care Med* 8(11):677–682, 1980.
52. Hartung HJ, Osswald PM, Vossmann H: Experiences with nasotracheal intubation in the primary management of severe facial burns of face and neck (author's transl) (German). *Anasthesiol Intensivther Notfallmed* 15(1):7–11, 1980.
53. Dellinger RP: Fiberoptic bronchoscopy in adult airway management. *Crit Care Med* 18(8)882–887, 1990.
54. Debo RF, Colonna D, Dewerd G, et al: Cricoarytenoid subluxation: Complication of blind intubation with a lighted stylet. *Ear Nose Throat J* 68(7):517–520, 1989.
55. Vollmer TP, Stewart RD, Paris PM, et al: Use of a lighted stylet for guided orotracheal intubation in the prehospital setting. *Ann Emerg Med* 14(4):324–328, 1985.
56. Boyd SW, Benzel EC: The role of early tracheotomy in the management of the neurosurgical patient. *Laryngoscope* 102(5):559–562, 1992.
57. Lewis RJ: Tracheostomies: Indications, timing, and complications (review). *Clin Chest Med* 13(1):137–149, 1992.
58. DeLaurier GA, Hawkins ML, Treat RC, Mansberger

AR Jr: Acute airway management: Role of cricothyroidotomy. *Am Surg* 56(1):12–15, 1990.
59. Dayal VS, el Masri W: Tracheostomy in intensive care setting. *Laryngoscope* 96(1):58–60, 1986.
60. Smith JP, Bodai BI, Seifkin A, et al: The esophageal obturator airway: A review [review]. *JAMA* 250(8): 1081–1084, 1983.
61. Don Michael TA: Esophageal obturator airway. *Med Instr* 11(6):331–333, 1977.
62. Asai T, Morris S: The laryngeal mask airway: Its features, effects and role (review). *Can J Anaesth* 41(10):930–960, 1994.
63. Pothmann W, Eckert S, Fullekrug B: Use of the laryngeal mask in difficult intubation (German). *Anaesthetist* 42(9):644–647, 1993.
64. Horton WA, Fahy L, Charters P: Disposition of cervical vertebral, atlanto-axial joint, thyroid and mandible during x-ray laryngoscopy. *Br J Anaesth* 63:435–438, 1989.
65. Vander Krol L, Wolfe R: The emergency department management of near-hanging victims. *J Emerg Med* 12(3):285–292, 1994.
66. Fox MW, Onofrio BM, Kilgore JE: Neurological complications of ankylosing spondylitis. *J Neurosurg* 78(6):871–878, 1993.
67. Riggins R, Kraus J: The risk of neurologic damage with fractures of the vertebrae. *J Trauma* 17:126–133, 1977.
68. Hastings RH, Marks JD: Airway management for trauma patients with potential cervical spine injuries. *Anesth Analg* 73:471–482, 1991.
69. Meschino A, Devitt JH, Schwartz ML, Koch JP: The safety of awake tracheal intubation in cervical spine injury. *Can J Anaesth* 35:131–132, 1988.
70. Ovassapian A, Krejcie TC, Yelich SJ, Dykes MH: Awake fibreoptic intubation in the patient at high risk of aspiration. *Br J Anaesth* 62(1):13–16, 1989.
71. Reasoner DK, Warner DS, Todd MM, et al: A comparison of anesthetic techniques for awake intubation in neurosurgical patients. *J Neurosurg Anesth* 7(2):94–99, 1995.
72. Gotta AW, Sullivan CA: Anaesthesia of the upper airway using topical anaesthetic and superior laryngeal nerve block. *Br J Anaesth* 53(10):1055–1058, 1981.
73. Ovassapian A, Yelich S, Dykes M, Brenner E: Failed nasotracheal intubation: Incidence and causes of a failure. *Anesth Analg* 62:692–695, 1983.
74. Ovassapian A, Dykes M: The role of fiberoptic endoscopy in airway management. *Semin Anesth* 6:93–104, 1987.
75. Hansen M, Poulsen MR, Bendixen DK, Hartmann-Anedersen F: Incidence of sinusitis in patients with nasotracheal intubations. *Br J Anaesth* 61:231–232, 1988.
76. Kronberg FG, Goodwin WJ Jr: Sinusitis in intensive care unit patients. *Laryngoscope* 95(8):936–938, 1985.
77. McGill J, Clinton J, Ruiz E: Cricothyroidotomy in the emergency department. *Ann Emerg Med* 11:361–364, 1982.
78. Frost EAM (ed): *Clinical Anesthesia in Neurosurgery.* Boston: Butterworths, 1984: 211.
79. Lee C, Barnes A, Nagel EL: Neuroleptanalgesia for awake pronation of surgical patients. *Anesth Analg* 56:276, 1977.
80. Attia M, Engel P: Thermoregulatory set point in patients with spinal cord injuries (spinal man). *Paraplegia* 21(4):233–248, 1983.
81. Wilson RH, Whiteside MC, Moorehead RJ: Problems in diagnosis and management of hypovolaemia in spinal injury. *Br J Clin Pract* 47(4):224–225, 1993.
82. Moeschler O, Ravussin P: Anesthesia of patients with injury to the cervical spine (French). *Ann Fr Anesth Reanim* 11(6):657–665, 1992.
83. Cucchiara RF, Michenfelder JD: *Clinical Neuroanesthesia.* New York: Churchill Livingstone, 1990: 328–341.

CHAPTER 83

CERVICAL SPINE STABILIZATION: SURGICAL TECHNIQUES

Iain H. Kalfas

INTRODUCTION

Techniques for stabilizing the cervical spine have advanced significantly over the past decade. An improved understanding of spinal biomechanics has led to the development of a variety of internal fixation devices designed to supplement or replace standard arthrodesis techniques. Although initially developed to manage posttraumatic cervical instability, these stabilization devices and techniques are now broadly used to treat degenerative, neoplastic, and iatrogenic cervical instability as well. The broad spectrum of cervical spine instability necessitates both a thorough understanding of spine biomechanics and the stabilization options available to assure that a specific technique is appropriately selected for each individual problem.

The modern surgical management of cervical spine injuries began in 1891, when Hadra reported wiring the spinous processes of the sixth and seventh cervical vertebrae to reduce a fracture of the seventh cervical vertebra.[44] In 1910, Pilcher reported an unsuccessful attempt to reduce an atlanto-axial dislocation. Although arthrodesis had not been his intention, a dense mass of callus fortuitously developed between the occiput and the axis, resulting in the first reported fusion of the cervical spine.[62]

Since that time, a variety of techniques for arthrodesis of the cervical spine have been developed and modified. Although the selection of a surgical approach is limited primarily to an anterior, a posterior, or a combined anterior-posterior approach, the variety of instrumentation and bony arthrodesis techniques available can be confusing. There is no single, optimal stabilization procedure for all cases of cervical spine instability. Each technique has its own advantages and disadvantages. Furthermore, several options may be suitable for a specific instability problem. Although the nonoperative management of cervical spine instability is still appropriate in isolated instances, surgical treatment is indicated in most cases. The purpose of this chapter is to review the specific surgical options.

INDICATIONS AND ADVANTAGES OF SURGICAL STABILIZATION

Spinal instability, as defined by White and Panjabi, is the inability of the spine under physiological loads to prevent initial or additional damage to the spinal cord or nerve roots, incapacitating deformities, or pain from structural changes.[80] The indications for spinal stabilization vary and include unstable conditions arising from traumatic, degenerative, infectious, and neoplastic disorders, as well as iatrogenic instability caused by a wide laminectomy. The specific stabilizing technique chosen depends on the nature of the injury or destabilizing disorder, the presence of persistent spinal cord compression, the degree of neurological injury, and the skills and preferences of the surgeon.

The primary goal in managing cervical spine instability is to minimize further neurological injury and painful spinal deformity and to promote the recovery of the spinal cord and nerve roots. This goal requires a stable, healed osseomusculoligamentous complex that will prevent further injury of the neural elements and offer the best opportunity for pain-free function.

Prolonged immobilization by cervical traction was previously the method most frequently used to stabilize the cervical spine. Although often successful, this method is infrequently used today because of poor patient tolerance and the potential for systemic complications associated with the required lengthy period of bed rest. Furthermore, the complications associated with prolonged immobilization can occur at a higher rate and be more devastating than will complications associated with operative intervention.

Using halo immobilization alone eliminates the need for prolonged bed rest because the cervical spine is satisfactorily stabilized externally while healing takes place. Although this method avoids the hazards of prolonged bed rest, it often does not stabilize certain complex fractures and severe ligamentous injuries, resulting in delayed instability and the need for open stabilization.[25]

Surgical management of the unstable cervical spine has the advantage of producing immediate stability without the need for prolonged bed rest or, in most cases, halo immobilization. Morbidity and mortality from these procedures are relatively low, and often are related more to the injury than to the operative treatment. However, the timing of surgery after injury and, in some instances, the indications for surgery are still controversial. These topics are beyond the scope of this chapter, but their consideration is as important as the technical aspects of each stabilization procedure. The surgeon must have a thorough working knowledge of the mechanisms of spinal injury and spinal biomechanics before attempting to manage cervical instability.

The surgical approaches for the cervical spine include an anterior, a posterior, and a combined approach. The choice of approach should be based on the integrity of the bony elements, the location of neural compression, and the mechanism of injury.

Anterior cervical stabilization is indicated for significant ventral cord compression resulting from involvement of the vertebrae or intervertebral disk.[26,50] Frequently, an anterior decompression of the neural elements may itself destabilize the cervical spine, necessitating a stabilization procedure. This is most common after the removal of one or more vertebrae.

Posterior stabilization is indicated for significant disruption of the posterior bony or ligamentous structures of the cervical spine with minimal or no involvement of the vertebrae itself. It is the preferred approach in most cases of spinal instability caused by a flexion injury, including posterior ligamentous injury, anterior dislocation, bilateral facet dislocation, and simple wedge compression fractures. Flexion rotation injuries causing unilateral facet dislocation may require posterior cervical stabilization if closed reduction is unsuccessful.[26,66,69]

A combined approach is indicated when both the anterior and posterior bony and/or ligamentous structures are significantly injured. In this case, sufficient decompression or stabilization cannot be achieved by either an anterior or posterior approach alone. The combined approach is indicated in more extensive cervical injuries, such as flexion teardrop fractures, vertical compression burst fractures with significant posterior ligamentous injury, and bilateral facet dislocation with an associated herniated disk compressing the ventral cord.

STABILIZATION USING AN ANTERIOR APPROACH

The anterior approach for decompression and stabilization of the cervical spine was introduced in the 1950s. Although initially devised to manage cervical degenerative disc disease, this approach is now also used for more complex decompression and stabilization procedures involving the removal of one or more vertebrae.[22,50,81]

Most anterior cervical decompression procedures are coupled with the insertion of a bone graft to provide long-term spinal stability. A number of clinical series have demonstrated that the success rates for anterior cervical fusion range from 74 to 98 percent, with graft dislodgement occurring at a rate of 2 to 5 percent.[41,65,70,79] In multilevel fusions, pseudoarthrosis can occur at a rate as high as 33 percent.[79] In cases of cervical trauma, graft extrusion rates range from 10 to 29 percent, and persistent postoperative deformity rates range from 38 to 64 percent.[8,18,77] These rates of fusion failure, graft dislodgement, and postoperative cervical deformity recently stimulated the development of anterior plate fixation devices for the cervical spine.

For several decades, orthopedic surgeons have used metal plates and screws to hold two bone fragments in approximate alignment.[53] Studies of fracture healing using plate osteosynthesis have shown that optimal results are achieved by absolute immobilization and compression of the fracture fragments. The rigid plate, coupled with screws that insert into the vertebral bodies adjacent to the bone graft, creates a construct that resists a variety of potential distortional forces, including flexion, extension, and rotational and lateral forces. Additionally, when a bone graft beneath the plate is held in contact under load, the plate becomes part of the load-bearing, cross-sectional area, further stabilizing the construct.[23]

In 1975, Herrmann first described the application of a metal plate to the anterior cervical spine.[47] Although others reported variations of this approach, the technique met with limited acceptance because of the difficulty of plate application, the risk of neurological injury, and the potential for screw loosening and subsequent fixation failure.[11,14,40]

Anterior cervical plate fixation advanced when Caspar introduced a new plating system (Fig. 83-1).[19] This system consists of a standardized and universal set of instruments, retractors, distractors, and osteosynthetic plates and fixation screws of various lengths. The Caspar system, when coupled with intervertebral body bone grafting, stabilizes the cervical spine immediately without the need for postoperative halo immobilization. It meets all the criteria for optimal fracture healing or graft incorporation—specifically, anatomic realignment, absolute immobilization, bone-to-bone contact, and compression of the fracture fragments or the bone graft. The disadvantage is that the system requires that the screws used for plate fixation ideally engage both the anterior and posterior vertebral body cortex. This specification introduces the potential for direct neurological injury if a drill bit or screw passes beyond the posterior vertebral body cortex into the spinal canal. The incidence of this complication is low, but the necessary precautions do add to the difficulty and length of the procedure.

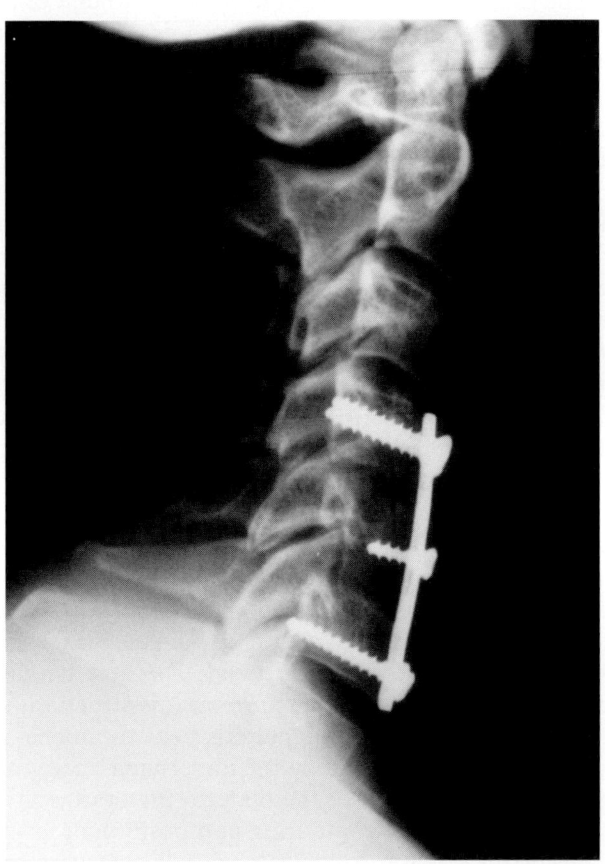

Figure 83-1. Lateral cervical radiograph demonstrating Caspar plate instrumentation following a C5 corpectomy and strut graft reconstruction.

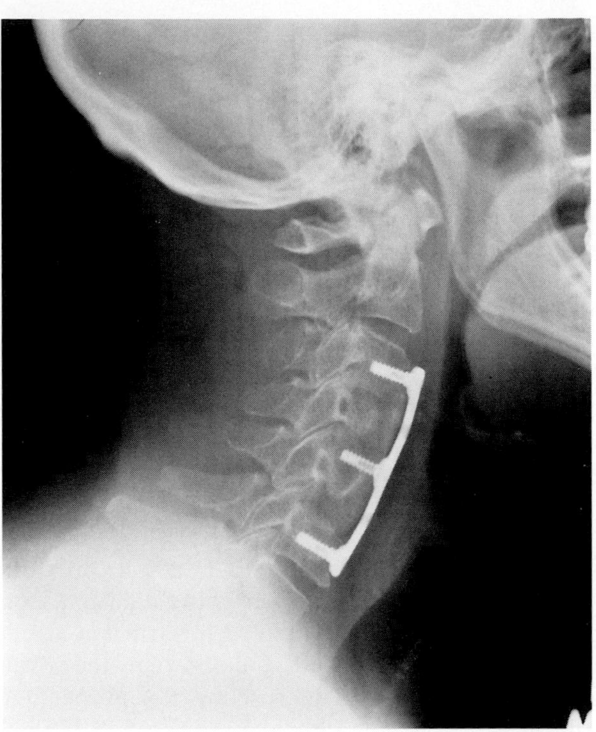

Figure 83-2. Lateral cervical radiograph demonstrating the cervical spine locking plate following a C4 and C5 corpectomy and strut graft reconstruction.

Morscher recently developed an anterior plate system that provides the mechanical advantage of internal fixation but reduces the risk of neurological injury associated with screw fixation of the posterior vertebral body cortex[59] (Fig. 84-2). The Cervical Spine Locking Plate (CSLP) system uses an anchor screw that has a hollow, expandable head. After the anchor screw is inserted, a second, smaller locking screw is placed in the head of the anchor screw. This screw expands the head of the anchor screw, compressing it against the inner walls of the plate hole. This enhanced screw-plate fixation eliminates the need for screw fixation in the posterior cortex of the vertebrae and minimizes the need for intraoperative fluoroscopy required by the Caspar system. The risk of neurological injury, the degree of technical difficulty, and the length of the procedure are all reduced.

Caspar Plate Fixation

The procedure for Caspar plate fixation has been described in detail.[19,76] Exposure is made through the standard anterior approach using either a transverse or oblique incision along the medial border of the sternocleidomastoid muscle. The appropriate diskectomy, corpectomy, or both, is performed, and a bone graft is positioned. The optimal source for an anterior cervical graft is either the fibula or the iliac crest. Although autogenous bone is preferred, an allograft also may be used.

After graft insertion, an osteosynthetic plate of appropriate length is selected. Plates short enough to bridge a single disk space or long enough to span three or four vertebrae are available. The plate is properly positioned when the screws can be placed into the midvertebral body at each end of the plate. The plate should not overlap an intact disk space, as this overlap will contribute to screw loosening and eventual fixation failure.

Under lateral fluoroscopic guidance, holes are drilled in the superior and inferior vertebrae adjacent to the bone graft. The depth of the advancing drill is controlled by both adjusting a drill guide and observing the advancing drill under real-time fluoroscopy. For proper screw fixation, the drill hole should pass through both the anterior and posterior cortex of each vertebra. The depth of each hole is measured, the hole is tapped, and the appropriate length fixation screw is tightened in place so that both vertebral cortices are engaged. Additional screws also may be passed through the plate into the graft to minimize the risk of graft dislodgement. Postoperatively, a cervical collar is worn for 8 to 12 weeks. Halo immobilization rarely is required.

Caspar and others have reported that, in their experience, the osteosynthetic plate technique is associated with a minimal incidence of neurological morbidity, pseudoarthrosis, or fixation failure. Screw loosening can occur and may require reoperation to remove the system. However, the Caspar plate system is generally a safe and effective means of stabilizing the cervical spine.[20,39,76]

Cervical Spine Locking Plate System Fixation

The Cervical Spine Locking Plate (CSLP) system improves on the Caspar system in that the screws placed into the vertebrae are required to engage only the anterior cortex. This system includes two different screws. The anchor screw is 4.0 mm in diameter and 14 mm long; it is placed through the plate holes into the vertebral body or bone graft. The anchor screw has a hollow head surrounded by a segmented, expandable collar. A shorter locking screw 1.8 mm in diameter is then inserted into the head of the anchor screw, forcing the collar of the anchor screw against the inner walls of that plate hole. This design effectively locks the screw to the plate, minimizing the possibility that the anchor screw will back out. This locking screw feature also eliminates the need for screw fixation in the posterior cortex of the vertebral body and significantly reduces the potential for neural injury secondary to screw insertion.

A second stabilizing feature of the CSLP system involves the angulation of the anchor screws when passed through the plate. The rostral end of each plate is indicated by an arrow at that end. The two rostral screw holes are specifically designed so that screws passed through these holes are inclined superiorly and medially. The two caudal screw holes are angled medially in a plane perpendicular to the plate. This configuration reduces the potential for failure at the screw-bone interface, thus limiting the potential for screw and plate backout and eliminating the need for bicortical screw placement.

The titanium composition of the CSLP system is an additional advantage. Titanium is highly biocompatible, with minimal risk for metal sensitivity. Furthermore, the titanium composition allows better postoperative radiographic imaging with minimal distortion, particularly in magnetic resonance imaging.

The CSLP system application is similar to that of the Caspar plate. Because the screws of this system do not engage the posterior vertebral body cortex, fluoroscopy is not required. After the standard exposure, and localization and decompression of the affected levels, the bone graft is positioned. The appropriate length cervical spine locking plate is selected and placed over the bone graft and the two adjacent vertebrae. The plate length is correct if the two pairs of holes on either end of the plate are positioned just beyond the ends of the bone graft and over the ajacent vertebrae. The plate should not overlap an intact disk space, as this overlap will increase the risk of screw loosening and fixation failure.

If necessary, the plate may be bent to conform better to the curvature of the anterior cervical spine. In this case, a slightly longer plate should be selected, because any bending will reduce the plate length. The underlying bone surface should be inspected for elevated bony ridges that prevent the plate from sitting flush on the graft and adjacent vertebral bodies. If present, these ridges are removed with a drill or rongeur. Excessive bending of the plate should be avoided because bending can fatigue the metal and compromise its structural integrity. Furthermore, if the plate is bent too much, its center may ride too high over the underlying bone graft, compromising fixation of the plate to the graft.

After satisfactory contouring and positioning of the plate, two holes are drilled in each adjacent vertebral body. The holes are tapped, and the anchor screws are inserted. Additionally, one or two holes can be drilled in the bone graft itself and a screw placed through each hole to fix the plate to the graft. Locking screws are then placed in the head of each anchor screw and tightened firmly. The patient is placed in a hard cervical collar postoperatively for approximately 8 to 12 weeks.

Preliminary reports of anterior cervical plate fixation using the CSLP system have indicated favorable results.[72] No occurrences of pseudoarthrosis or iatrogenic injury resulting from screw insertion have been reported, and the incidence of postoperative screw migration has been minimal.

Both the Caspar and CSLP systems have been used following single- or multilevel corpectomies in managing cervical spondylosis, trauma, vertebral body neoplasms, and posttraumatic or postlaminectomy kyphosis. Their use is not advocated following a single-level anterior diskectomy and interbody fusion. However, these systems may be beneficial following a multilevel anterior interbody fusion or following a single-level anterior interbody fusion when that level previously has been decompressed posteriorly (a laminectomy or foraminotomy).

Contraindications to the use of both the Caspar and CSLP system in the cervical spine include unsatisfactory bone for screw fixation (i.e., osteoporosis) or an infectious process (i.e., wound infection or vertebral osteomyelitis). The use of anterior plate fixation in cases of cervical trauma, particularly flexion injuries, is limited. Although the plating technique can be used to manage a vertebral body fracture or traumatic disk herniation, it must be coupled to a posterior stabilization procedure when significant posterior bony or ligamentous disruption is evident. Furthermore, anterior cervical plating does not effectively stabilize a flexion-dislocation injury. Biomechanical studies have shown anterior cervical plate fixation to be inferior to conventional posterior stabilization techniques in the management of this injury.[74]

Upper Cervical Screw Fixation

The surgical management of atlanto-axial instability traditionally has involved a posterior approach using one of several wire fixation and bone graft techniques. The posterior stabilization procedures advocated by Gallie, Brooks, and others have been used primarily for managing odontoid fractures, os odontoideum, or atlanto-axial instability associated with rheumatoid arthritis.[13,37,52,56] All these techniques effectively achieve stability at the atlanto-axial level, but occasionally may fail and result in a pseudoarthrosis at the fracture site or in the fusion construct. Additionally, a standard posterior atlanto-axial fusion may at times be technically unfeasible (i.e., absence or fracture of the posterior arch of C1).

For these reasons, atlanto-axial fusion using an anterior approach has been suggested. Fang and Ong introduced the anterior transoral interbody method in 1962 to stabilize the upper cervical spine.[32] This method, however, carries the added risk of exposing a nonvascularized bone graft to a contaminated operative field. It has never been widely accepted as a means of stabilizing the atlanto-axial junction.

Bohler and others reported the anterior placement of a single screw passed superiorly through the C2 body into the base of the odontoid to stabilize displaced odontoid fractures.[10,12,54] This technique provides an alternative to the standard posterior C1–C2 stabilization procedure.

Barbour, in 1971, described an anterior technique of atlanto-axial fusion using two vitallium screws to transfix the atlanto-axial joints in cases of odontoid fractures. He reported this technique was satisfactory, providing rigid internal fixation that allows early mobilization. Odontoid fractures usually heal well when this technique is used.[7]

Bohler's technique for anterior transodontoid screw fixation has been described in detail.[10,38] The procedure is performed with the patient supine. One or two C-arm fluoroscopes are positioned for intraoperative visualization of the upper cervical spine in both an anteroposterior and a lateral plane.

A transverse incision is made at the C5 level, and dissection is carried down to the level of the anterior cervical vertebrae. The dissection is extended rostrally along the anterior longitudinal ligament to expose the inferior aspect of the C2 vertebra. Under direct fluoroscopic guidance, a 2-mm drill is positioned along the inferior margin of the C2 vertebra and directed parallel to the midline sagittal plane. The drill is angled posteriorly to enter the odontoid. The odontoid is fixed with one or two 3.5-mm diameter screws. A single screw can reduce and fix an odontoid fracture satisfactorily. Two screws provide better rotational control, but the dens must be large enough to accommodate both screws. No bone grafting is performed. Postoperatively, a cervicothoracic orthosis is worn for 8 to 12 weeks (Fig. 83-3).

The advantage of odontoid screw fixation is that normal atlanto-axial rotation is preserved. This technique can be used for odontoid fractures only when the transverse ligament is intact. If the transverse ligament is disrupted, fixation of the odontoid will not immobilize C1. The integrity of the transverse ligament can be directly assessed by magnetic resonance imaging.[29]

Barbour's[7] C1–C2 transfacetal screw fixation involves the same operative exposure. The C1–C2 facet joints are identified laterally and decorticated with an angled curette to promote fusion. The entry point for screw insertion is the groove between the vertebral body and the superior C1 facet. The screws are directed rostrally and slightly laterally into the lateral masses of C1. Single, 3.5-mm diameter screws are placed in each facet

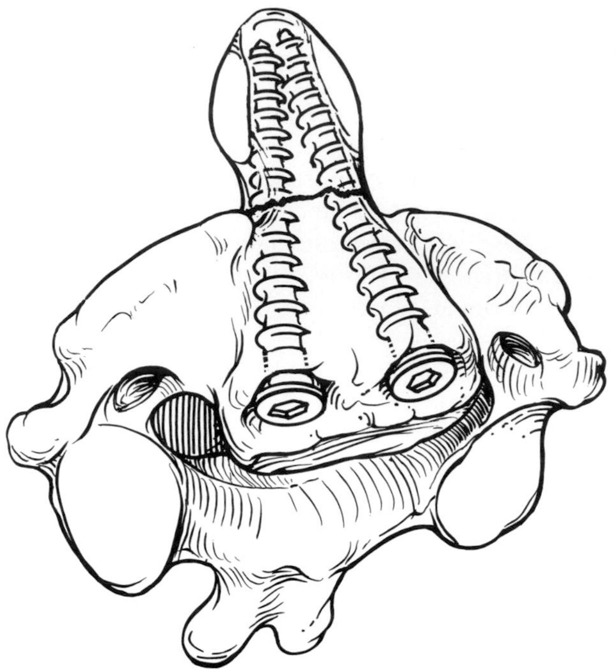

Figure 83-3. Anterior transodontoid screw fixation. One screw is satisfactory. Two screws provide better rotational control.

under fluoroscopic guidance. This technique rigidly stabilizes C1–C2, but sacrifices all motion at this level (Fig. 83-4).

Although these two fixation techniques do not represent the procedures of choice for atlanto-axial instability, they do offer alternatives to the standard posterior stabilization procedures if a posterior approach is not feasible or persistent pseudoarthrosis develops. Furthermore, if the posterior arch of C1 is absent, the anterior screw-fixation technique is preferable to an occiput-C2 fusion because it preserves motion at the occipital-C1 level.[38]

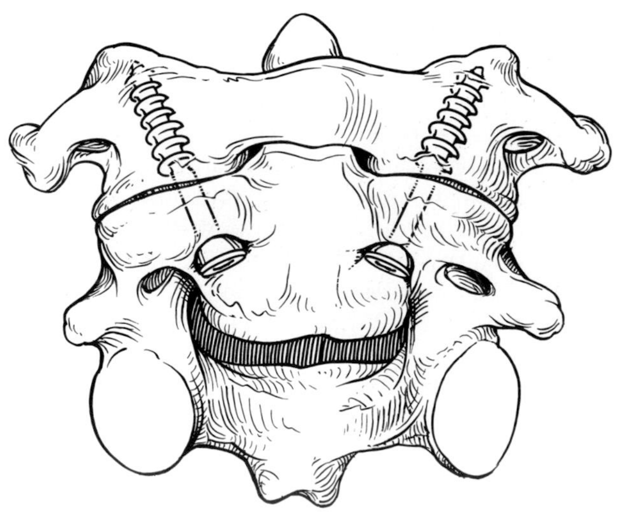

Figure 83-4. Anterior atlanto-axial facet screw fixation.

STABILIZATION USING A POSTERIOR APPROACH

Posterior stabilization of the cervical spine is indicated when the stabilizing integrity of posterior bony or ligamentous structures is disrupted.[3,26,69] Several posterior stabilization techniques are available, and most are reasonably effective in achieving spinal stability. In the past, most of these techniques involved a combination of wire and bone fixation. However, the recent introduction of instrumentation devices has greatly expanded the options for posterior stabilization.

Occipito-Atlantal Arthrodesis

The indication for occipital-cervical fusion is instability of the occipito-atlantal joint or atlanto-axial instability with a structurally deficient posterior atlantal arch. Occipital-cervical fusion is also indicated in cases of basilar impression with upward migration of the odontoid process into the foramen magnum.[24,63,78] However, it is not indicated for the management of atlanto-axial instability when the C1 arch is intact. This problem is best managed with an atlanto-axial stabilization procedure, because it allows greater cervical motion and has a lower rate of pseudoarthrosis than an occipital-cervical fusion.[34,56]

Occipito-atlantal instability is most commonly associated with trauma[2] but also may be seen with rheumatoid arthritis,[24] congenital anomalies,[46] and neoplasms[45] involving the upper cervical spine. Treatment is initially directed toward reduction and stabilization with external fixation, followed by occipito-atlantal arthrodesis. Halo immobilization permits adjustments in reduction and aids in maintaining the correct position during and after surgery. Anterior arthrodesis is technically impractical at this level, although it has been performed.[32]

A posterior approach is technically more feasible. Two methods have been used in the past. The first involves onlay bone grafting using corticocancellous bone from the iliac crest placed between the occiput and C2. The second, more commonly used, method involves wiring cancellous bone to the posterior arch of the atlas and to the adjacent occiput. If the posterior atlantal arch is absent or deficient, however, the graft is extended to include the second cervical vertebra.[33,84]

Several recent technical innovations have been applied to these two traditional techniques of occipital-cervical fusion. Ransford and coworkers in 1986 described the application of a contoured metal loop that is wired in place and supplemented with iliac cancellous bone graft. Following posterior exposure of the craniocervical junction, two small holes are drilled in the lower occipital bone on either side of the midline, approximately 1 cm from the margin of the foramen magnum. A wire is passed through these holes. Sublaminar wires are passed at three vertebral levels immediately caudal to the craniocervical junction. The occipital and sublaminar wires are then secured to a Wisconsin or Luque rod that conforms to the craniocervical region. Cancellous bone grafts are placed in the lateral gutters of the upper cervical spine to augment a bony fusion.[64]

Sonntag and associates describe using a large, threaded Steinmann pin contoured to the appropriate shape and wired in place with occipital and sublaminar wires. Cancellous bone chips are then placed in the lateral gutters. When the C1 posterior arch is absent, a unicortical plate of iliac crest graft is wired to each arm of the Steinmann pin, thus suspending it over the defect. This construct is believed to facilitate osteocyte migration and incorporation of the bone graft into the overall construct.[28]

Occipital-cervical fusion using a Y-shaped screw plate also has been described.[42] Screws are placed through the Y plate into the occiput and C1–C2 facet joints. The screw plate is supplemented with cancellous bone grafts. Screw plates secured to the cervical vertebrae rigidly fix the spine. However, screws placed in the occipital bone at the midline may be biomechanically suboptimal. The occipital bone is relatively thin; therefore, short screws must be used in the occiput to minimize the risk of cerebellar injury. Such screws increase the rate of screw pull-out and fixation failure.

Atlanto-Axial Stabilization

Atlanto-axial instability has many causes, varied presentations, and potential complications. Four types of atlanto-axial instability have been described: (1) traumatic (odontoid fracture); (2) inflammatory (rheumatoid arthritis, retropharyngeal infection); (3) congenital (os odontoideum); and (4) neoplastic. The indications for atlanto-axial fusion vary depending on the cause, type, and degree of instability and the activity of the patient. Although a number of techniques have been described, it is imperative that the procedure selected provides immediate stability through wire fixation, screw fixation, or both, and long-term stability with a bone graft. Although fusions using acrylic (instead of bone) have been described, acrylic is a foreign substance and loses, rather than gains, strength with age, unlike bone.[31,82,84]

In 1910, Mixter and Osgood described a patient with atlanto-axial instability successfully treated by fixing the posterior arch of the atlas to the spinous process of the axis with a silk thread.[58] Gallie popularized posterior atlanto-axial arthrodesis in 1939 by discussing a principle of "fastening the two vertebrae together by fine steel wire passed around the lamina or spines . . . and . . . bone grafts laid in the spines or on the lamina and articular facets."[37] He provided no description, however, of a specific technique employing these principles.

McGraw and Rusch[56] and Fielding[35] elaborated on Gallie's method. After posterior exposure of the atlanto-axial complex, a looped wire is passed under the posterior atlantal arch and through or behind the C2 spinous process. A unicortical iliac crest graft is notched to conform to the C2 spinous process and is laid on the lamina of C1 and C2. The two free ends of the wire are then brought over the top of the graft to secure it. Cancellous grafts are placed in the lateral gutters. The disadvantage of laying the bone graft on the lamina of C1 and C2 instead of between the laminae is the potential for further displacing an odontoid fracture into the spinal canal as the wire is tightened and the lamina of C1 and C2 are drawn together. This possibility is a greater problem when the initial displacement of the odontoid fracture is posterior.

Brooks and Jenkins, in 1978, described a wedge compression method of atlanto-axial arthrodesis that improves on Gallie's midline wiring method. Instead of passing the midline wire underneath the arch of the atlas and through or behind the C2 spinous process, two separate looped wires are passed under the lamina of both C1 and C2. These wires can then be moved laterally from the midline. Two tricortical iliac crest grafts are beveled and placed in the C1–C2 interlaminar space on each side of the midline. The sublaminar wires are tightened to secure them. This method gives a much more rigid construct that resists rotation.[13] It also prevents further displacement of an odontoid fracture when the wires are tightened. The disadvantage of this method is that two sublaminar wires are passed across two levels, increasing the potential for iatrogenic neural injury.

A recent innovation in the atlanto-axial fixation techniques of Gallie and Brooks has been described.[61] After exposure of the atlanto-axial complex, the inferior margin of the posterior atlantal arch and the superior margin of the C2 lamina and spinous processes are decorticated. A twisted 24-gauge looped wire (three twists/cm) is passed under the C1 arch and behind the C2 spinous process. Tensile tests have determined that braided 24-gauge looped wire has the same strength as a single strand 18-gauge wire but is more malleable and easier to use.[75] Alternatively, a steel or titanium cable specifically designed for use with spinal instrumentation can be used.[71]

Following passage of the wire or cable, a 2-cm section of tricortical iliac crest graft is obtained. The superior cortical surface of the graft is removed, producing a rectangular graft with two opposing cortical surfaces and two cancellous surfaces. The graft is positioned in the C1–C2 interlaminar space so that the two cancellous surfaces contact the decorticated C1 and C2 laminae. The placement of cancellous bone against cancellous bone facilitates graft incorporation, while the two cortical surfaces provide the graft with its inherent strength. The two free strands of wire or cable are then brought around the spinous process of C2 and tightened to secure the graft. Cancellous bone chips are placed laterally. The patient is placed in a halo brace for approximately 8 to 12 weeks postoperatively (Fig. 83-5).

The advantage of this interspinous fusion procedure is that it prevents further displacement of a posteriorly displaced odontoid fracture. Additionally, it has the same degree of resistance to rotational forces as the Brooks technique but has less risk during wire or cable passage. A review of this technique showed a 97 percent fusion rate in 36 patients.[30]

Posterior C1–C2 Screw Fixation

In 1987, Magerl and Seemann reported a technique of atlanto-axial stabilization using transarticular screw fixation.[55] This technique has an advantage over more conventional atlanto-axial stabilization procedures in that it more immediately stabilizes the C1–C2 complex, eliminating the need for a halo brace postoperatively. It is not intended to be used alone, but instead is combined with one of the standard wire and bone fixation procedures previously described.

The patient is placed in the prone position and a C-arm fluoroscope is positioned to give a lateral view of the upper cervical spine. Proper alignment of the C1–C2 level is then confirmed. A standard posterior exposure of the C1–C2 complex is performed and initial stabilization is achieved using any of the standard wire and bone fixation techniques.

Because a relatively flat angle of approach is needed to place screws across the C1–C2 facet joint, Magerl's original technique required exposure of the entire cervical spine. However, such exposure is unnecessary if two separate, smaller incisions are made on either side of the midline at the cervicothoracic junction (C7–T1). A guide tube is then passed through the cervicothoracic incisions and brought out into the operative field at the C1–C2 level. Instruments designed specifically to place the C1–C2 screws are passed through the guide tube, and the screws are placed. This approach limits the surgical exposure to the C1–C2 level.

Before placing the screws, the C1–C2 facet joints are exposed bilaterally. The C2 nerve root and the associated venous plexus immediately posterior to the facet joint are identified and dissected from the underlying facet joints. A curette can be inserted into the facet joints to strip the synovial surface to facilitate joint fusion.

The appropriate drill and screw trajectory is determined using lateral C-arm fluoroscopy. The drill and screw should be directed toward the anterior C1 arch on the lateral view. The entry point for screw insertion

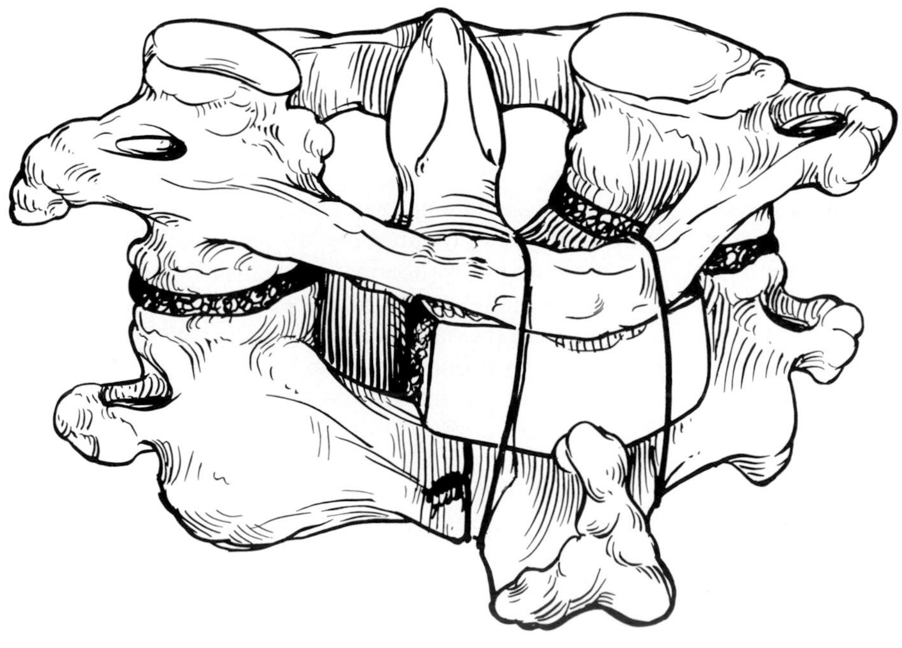

Figure 83-5. Posterior C1–C2 interspinous wire and graft fixation.

is the caudal aspect of the C2 lamina, approximately 1 to 2 mm lateral to the lateral edge of the spinal canal. A nerve hook can be inserted under the caudal edge of the C2 lamina to identify the medial wall of the C2 pars articularis, which is the lateral margin of the spinal canal. The guide tube is positioned through the two small stab incisions made at the C7–T1 level. The central obturator is removed and an inner drill guide placed. Under fluoroscopic guidance, a pilot hole is drilled through the C2 lateral mass into the C1 lateral mass. The drill and inner drill guide are removed. The hole is tapped, and the appropriate length 4.0-mm diameter titanium screw is positioned. The screw length usually varies from 36 to 40 mm in length. The procedure is then repeated on the other side. Proper positioning of the screw can be determined by inspection of the facet joint. The screw should be visible or palpable in the facet joint. The patient is then immobilized in a cervical collar for 6 to 8 weeks postoperatively[5] (Fig. 83-6).

To avoid injury to neural or vascular structures in this area, a thorough preoperative anatomic assessment is imperative. A CT scan through the C1–C2 area will indicate aberrant positioning of the vertebral artery foramina. If the foramina position is too medial, a screw should not be placed on that side.

Grob and associates reported a preliminary experience with this technique in 1991. A stable fusion was obtained in all but one of 161 patients. Screw malpositions were noted in 15 percent but did not result in cord or vertebral artery injury.[43]

Mid- and Lower Cervical Spine Arthrodesis

As in the upper cervical spine, a variety of surgical options are available to stabilize the mid- to lower cervical spine.[16,17,31,36,48,60,83] The interspinous process wiring and bone grafting approach described by Rogers in 1942 is most commonly used for posterior stabilization.[67] However, several variations of the Rogers method have been described, including a technique introduced by Benzel and Kesterson.[9] As in the Rogers method, wire is passed through a hole made in the base of the upper spinous process and then around the base of the lower spinous process. The wire is tightened, drawing the two spinous processes together. However, in addition to placing onlay cancellous bone over the laminae and facets as Rogers described, a split-thickness, tricortical iliac crest graft is compressed bilaterally against the involved medial laminae and spinous processes. These grafts are held in place with a wire running between the spinous process and encircling the grafts, thus compressing the spinous processes between them.

Despite adequately stabilizing against translational forces, interspinous wiring alone is less effective in stabilizing against rotational forces. For this reason, bilateral facet-spinous process wiring was introduced to maximize the rotational stability of the cervical spine.[15] After realignment of the cervical spine and exposure of the posterior elements, the facet joint capsules and articular cartilage are removed with a curette. A hole

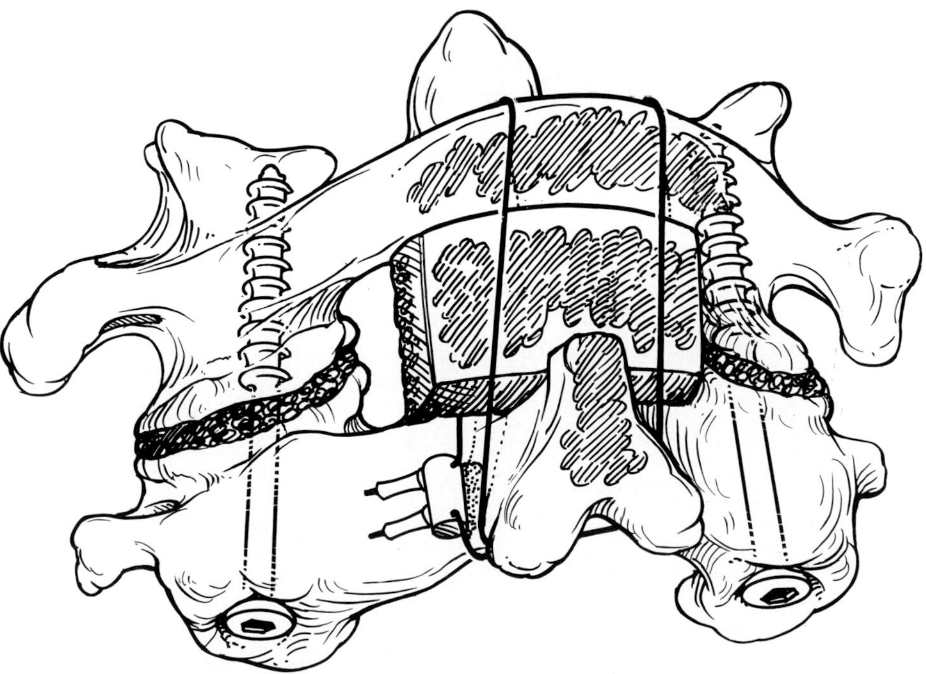

Figure 83-6. Posterior C1–C2 screw fixation combined with interspinous wire and graft fixation.

is drilled through the inferior facets of the upper vertebrae, perpendicular to the articular surface. Double-braided, 24-gauge, stainless steel wires are passed through the holes, brought out through the facet joint, and tightened around the lower spinous process. Corticocancellous bone is then placed over the decorticated posterior elements. Although this technique effectively stabilizes the cervical spine, the integrity of the fusion depends on an intact facet. In addition to traumatic disruption, one or both facets may be disrupted as the wires are tightened, further compromising stabilization.

Stabilization of the cervical spine may, on occasion, be required in the case of disrupted or absent posterior elements (i.e., following cervical laminectomy). Robinson first advocated posterior lateral facet fusion in 1960.[66] Callahan and coworkers, in 1977, popularized a technique in which corticocancellous struts of the iliac crest are positioned over denuded facets on each side of a laminectomy defect and then secured by the bilateral facet wiring technique previously described. In the original series, solid fusion was achieved in 50 of 51 patients with this method.[16]

Other techniques of posterior cervical stabilization include variations using methylmethacrylate and wire or sublaminar wiring with bone grafting. Methylmethacrylate has the advantage of immediately immobilizing the cervical spine and may be used when bone grafting is not feasible. Wire, Kirschner pins, and wire mesh have all been used in conjunction with methylmethacrylate, serving as stabilizing templates for the acrylic.[1,21,52] The disadvantage of acrylic, however, is that it does not bind to bone, weakens with time, and remains a permanent foreign body.[31,83]

Sublaminar wiring gives the most stabilization when immobilizing the cervical spine after a flexion injury, but there are inherent risks when passing these wires under the lamina.[57] Because the neural canal above C2 is wide (2.0 cm), sublaminar wires can be used safely at these levels. Below C2, however, the relatively small size of the canal in relation to the spinal cord can make the blind passage of sublaminar wires hazardous. In addition, when passed under three laminae, the wire tends to bow anteriorly, thereby narrowing the neural canal and compressing the spinal cord. Sublaminar wiring should therefore be avoided in the mid- and lower cervical spine.

Interlaminar (Halifax) Clamp Fixation

Holness and coworkers described the use of interlaminar clamps for cervical spine fixation in 1984.[48] The indication for this technique is posterior ligamentous injury with minimal or no posterior bony element fracture. The system also has been used in the case of atlanto-axial instability, although this approach is not as widely accepted as are other stabilization procedures. It is not indicated if a significant vertebral body injury exists, unless combined with an anterior stabilization procedure.

To apply interlaminar clamps, the patient is placed in the prone position. To expose the cervical spine, a standard posterior approach is performed. An appropriately shaped, stainless steel clamp consisting of two pairs of free arms joined by an adjustable screw is selected and applied to the adjoining laminae of the involved levels. The clamps fit over the rostral laminar edge of the superior vertebrae and the caudal laminar edge of the inferior vertebrae. Up to three vertebral levels can be fixed with the clamp. The clamps are applied bilaterally, and each should span the same number of vertebral levels. Any required decompressive procedure is performed before the clamp is applied. If posterior element fractures are present, the clamp may be applied unilaterally to the opposite nonfractured side.

After application of the clamp, the screw connecting the two halves of the clamp is tightened. A bone graft is not required, but can be used. Postoperatively, the patient is immobilized in a cervical collar for 8 to 12 weeks. Holness reported satisfactory results in 51 patients, with only two requiring reoperation for dislodged clamps (Fig. 83-7).

When used to stabilize the atlanto-axial complex, the two ends of the clamp are placed around the superior margin of the C1 arch and the inferior margin of the C3 lamina. The C3 lamina is used because the shape and obliqueness of the inferior C2 lamina does not permit the lower clamp to be positioned satisfactorily. This technique is best suited for anteriorly displaced odontoid fractures as opposed to posteriorly displaced odontoid fractures. Tightening the clamp may produce a traction effect on the posteriorly displaced odontoid fracture, drawing it further into the neural canal.

Posterior Cervical Plate Fixation

Posterior stabilization of the cervical spine using plates and screws was introduced by Roy-Camille and associates.[68] This technique has been used in Europe for many years, but has only recently gained acceptance in North America.

Biomechanical testing of posterior cervical plate fixation has shown it to be superior to posterior wiring, especially in extension and torsion.[27] Clinical reports to date are also encouraging, indicating a high rate of fusion; alignment is satisfactorily maintained.[4,27] Although neurological or vascular complications related to plate and screw insertion have not been reported, injury to the vertebral artery or cervical nerve roots can occur if the proper insertion technique is not followed.

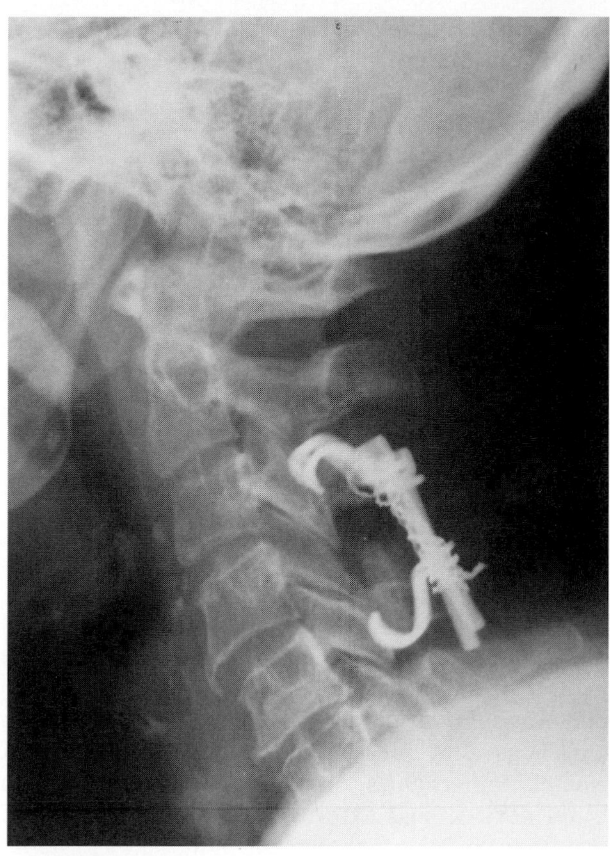

Figure 83-7. Lateral cervical radiograph demonstrating C3–C6 interlaminar clamp fixation.

The indications for posterior cervical plating include cervical subluxation without significant vertebral body fracture, postlaminectomy instability, bilaminar or spinous process fractures that preclude operative stabilization with interspinous wires, and recurrence of subluxation or angulation despite halo immobilization. This technique is contraindicated when the bone of the cervical spine is severely osteoporotic.

The posterior cervical plate is applied after adequate realignment and exposure of the posterior elements.[27] An awl is used to pierce the cortical bone of the involved articular pillars. Holes are drilled with a 2-mm drill bit in the center of the articular pillars. The drill is angled slightly rostrally (10 to 20°) and laterally (20 to 30°) to avoid the vertebral artery and exiting nerve root. The rostral angulation places the drill approximately parallel to the adjacent facet joints. The lateral angulation positions the drill in a plane nearly parallel to the exiting nerve root and away from the vertebral artery.

When one motion segment is to be stabilized, holes are drilled bilaterally in the articular pillars of the two adjacent vertebrae. When two motion segments are to be stabilized, holes are drilled bilaterally in the articular pillars of each of the three adjacent vertebrae. The plates are positioned over the drill holes and secured with self-tapping cancellous bone screws.

Several posterior cervical plating systems are available. Most of these systems incorporate titanium plates and screws for postoperative radiographic compatibility.

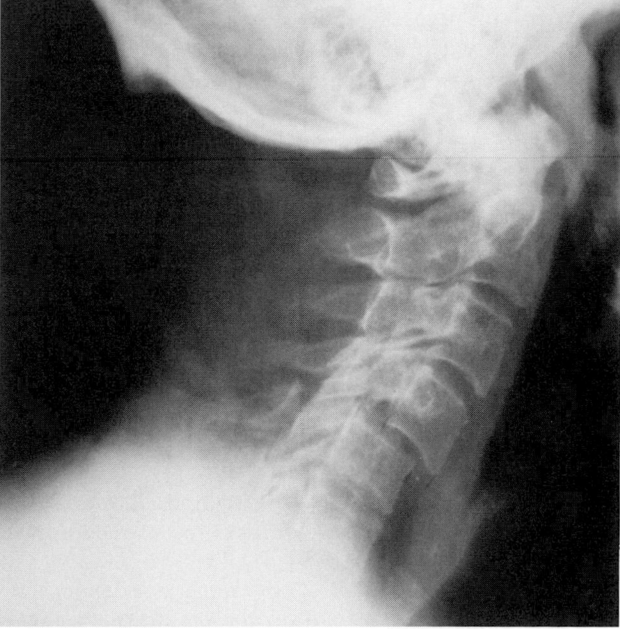

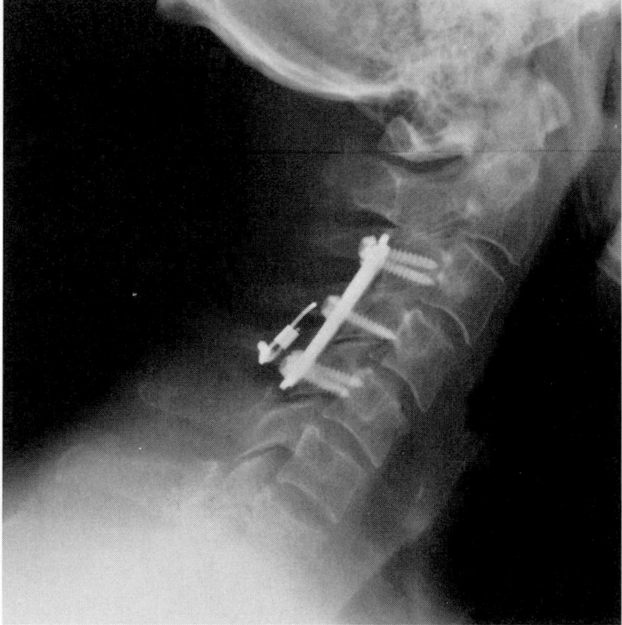

Figure 83-8. Preoperative (left) and postoperative lateral cervical radiograph (right) demonstrating a traumatic C4–C5 subluxation stabilized by posterior lateral mass plates extending from C3 to C5. C3 was included in the construct because of a fractured lateral mass on the right side at C4.

The plates vary in length and generally have two to four screw holes each. Two-hole plates are used when there is instability at one level, as occurs with ligamentous disruption at the facet joints. Three-hole plates are used to stabilize two motion segments when there is instability at two levels, injury to two disk spaces, comminution of a vertebral body, or injury to a lateral mass or pedicle that precludes using that vertebral element to achieve stability. Plates with more than four holes are rarely required, but are available when three or more motion segments need to be immobilized. Bone grafting is not routinely performed, although small fragments of bone from the spinous processes may be removed and impacted into the facet joint(s) spanned by each plate. Postoperatively, the patient is immobilized in a cervical collar for 8 to 12 weeks. Halo immobilization is not required (Fig. 83-8).

PRINCIPLES OF CERVICAL SPINE STABILIZATION

Despite the wide selection of stabilization techniques for the cervical spine, several general principles apply to all methods. When surgically stabilizing the cervical spine, immobilizing as few levels as possible is critical. The fusion of additional levels not only decreases the chance that the fusion will mature into a solid construct, but also causes excessive immobility when the fusion matures appropriately. This immobility may then produce discomfort as well as accelerate the degenerative changes at the spinal levels above and below the fusion.[6,49]

Regardless of the stabilizing technique used, bony fusion is critical to the long-term maintenance of the surgically stabilized spine. External splints provide only partial immobility. Metallic internal fixation devices and methylmethacrylate serve only as temporary immobilizing constructs and will ultimately fatigue and fail over time. A solid bony fusion, however, will last indefinitely.[51]

The ultimate goal of spinal fusion is to create a fusion mass of the appropriate size and structure in the shortest period of time. This goal can be achieved by attending to three well-recognized principles in bone graft surgery: (1) adequate preparation of the graft bed; (2) selection of the appropriate graft (i.e., autograft vs. allograft, corticocancellous bone vs. cancellous bone); and (3) an adequate period of postoperative immobilization of the fusion site. When these principles are adhered to, solid fusion will usually occur in three months.[51]

Systemic problems such as malnutrition, severe systemic illness, antimetabolic drugs, or myelosuppressive drugs can impede bone graft incorporation. Local problems such as infection, foreign bodies, radiation necrosis, malignancy, and sclerotic or osteopenic bone may also compromise the success of a graft. With insufficient postoperative immobilization, vascularization of the graft will be insufficient, and, consequently, fibrocartilage development will predominate.[73] Although the nonunion rate in cervical spine arthrodesis procedures is small, it usually is the result of inadequate postoperative immobilization time.[57]

SUMMARY

In summary, because of the virtually unlimited combination of injuries and disorders that can affect the cervical spine, no single stabilizing procedure can be advocated for all situations. As our understanding in the areas of spinal biomechanics, bone graft properties, internal fixation devices, and external immobilization has improved, advances have been made in the surgical stabilization of the cervical spine. These innovations are not necessarily intended to replace proven methods that traditionally have been employed, but rather add to the armamentarium of available stabilizing techniques. With this broader selection of techniques, managing patients with an unstable cervical spine can be even more appropriately individualized.

REFERENCES

1. Alexander E: Posterior fusions of the cervical spine. *Clin Neurosurg* 1981; 28:273–296.
2. Alker GJ Jr, Oh YS, Leslie EV: High cervical spine and craniocervical junction injuries in fatal traffic accidents: A radiological study. *Orthop Clin North Am* 1978; 9:1003–1010.
3. An HS: Internal fixation of the posterior cervical spine. *Semin Spine Surg* 1992; 4:142–151.
4. Anderson PA, Henley MB, Grady MS, et al: Posterior cervical arthrodesis with AO reconstruction plates and bone graft. *Spine* 1991; 16:S72–S79.
5. Apfelbaum RI: C1–2 posterior transarticular screw fixation (abstract). *Joint Section on Disorders of the Spine and Peripheral Nerves*, 1993; 40.
6. Baker WC, Thomas TG, Kirkaldy-Willis WH: Changes in the cartilage of the posterior intervertebral joints after anterior fusion. *J Bone Joint Surg Br* 1969; 51B:736–746.

7. Barbour JR: Screw fixation and fractures of the odontoid process. *S Austral Clin* 1971; 5:20–24.
8. Bell GD, Bailey SI: Anterior cervical fusion for trauma. *Clin Orthop* 1977; 128:155–158.
9. Benzel EC, Kesterson L: Posterior cervical interspinous compression wiring and fusion for mid to low cervical spine injuries. *J Neurosurg* 1989; 70:893–899.
10. Bohler J: Anterior stabilization for acute fractures in non-unions of the dens. *J Bone Joint Surg Am* 1982; 64A:18–27.
11. Bohler J, Gaudermak T: Anterior plate stabilization for fracture dislocations of the lower cervical spine. *J Trauma* 1980; 20:203–205.
12. Borne GM, Bedou GL, Pinaudeau M, et al: Odontoid process fracture osteosynthesis with a direct screw fixation technique in nine consecutive cases. *J Neurosurg* 1988; 68:223–226.
13. Brooks AL, Jenkins EB: Atlanto-axial arthrodesis by the wedge compression method. *J Bone Joint Surg Am* 1978; 60A:279–284.
14. Brown JA, Havel P, Ebraheim N, et al: Cervical stabilization by plate and bone fusion. *Spine* 1988; 13:236–240.
15. Cahill DW, Bellegarrigue R, Ducker TB: Bilateral facet to spinous process fusion: A new technique for posterior spinal fusion after trauma. *Neurosurgery* 1983; 13:1–4.
16. Callahan RA, Johnson RM, Margolis RN, et al: Cervical facet fusion for control of instability following laminectomy. *J Bone Joint Surg Am* 1977; 59A:991–1002.
17. Capen DA, Nelson RW, Zigler J, et al: Surgical stabilization of the cervical spine: A comparative analysis of anterior and posterior spine fusions. *Paraplegia* 1987; 25:111–119.
18. Capen DA, Garland DE, Waters RL: Surgical stabilization of the cervical spine. *Clin Orthop* 1985; 196:229–237.
19. Caspar W: Anterior cervical fusion and interbody stabilization with the trapezial osteosynthetic plate technique. *Aesculap Scientific Information Leaflet* S-039. Burlingame, CA: Aesculap Instruments Corp, 1986.
20. Caspar W: Anterior stabilization with trapezoid osteosynthetic technique in cervical spine injuries, in Kehr B, Weidner A (eds) *Cervical Spine*. New York: Springer-Verlag, 1987: 198–204.
21. Clark CR, Keggi KJ, Panjabi MM: Methylmethacrylate stabilization of the cervical spine. *J Bone Joint Surg* 1984; 66A:40–46.
22. Cloward RB: The anterior approach for removal of ruptured cervical disks. *J Neurosurg* 1958; 15:602–614.
23. Cochran G: *A Primer of Orthopaedic Biomechanics*. New York: Churchill Livingstone, 1982: 180–198.
24. Conaty JP, Mongan ES: Cervical fusion in rheumatoid arthritis. *J Bone Joint Surg Am* 1981; 63A:1218–1227.
25. Cooper PR: Operative management of cervical spine injuries. *Clin Neurosurg* 1988; 34:650–674.
26. Cooper PR: Stabilization of fractures and subluxations of the middle and lower cervical spine. *Contemp Neurosurg* 1988; 10:1–6.
27. Cooper PR, Cohen A, Rosiello A, Koslow M: Posterior stabilization of cervical spine fractures and subluxations using plates and screws. *Neurosurgery* 1988; 23:300–306.
28. Dickman CA, Douglas RA, Sonntag VKH: Occipitocervical fusion: Posterior stabilization of the craniovertebral junction and upper cervical spine. *BNI Quarterly* 1990; 6(2):2–14.
29. Dickman CA, Mamourian A, Sonntag VKH: Magnetic resonance imaging of the transverse atlantal ligament for the evaluation of atlanto-axial instability. *J Neurosurg* 1991; 75:221–227.
30. Dickman CA, Sonntag VKH, Papadopoulos SM, Hadley MN: The interspinous method of posterior atlanto-axial arthrodesis. *J Neurosurg* 1991; 74:190–198.
31. Eismont FJ, Bohlman HH: Posterior methylmethacrylate fixation for cervical trauma. *Spine* 1981; 6:347–353.
32. Fang HSY, Ong GB: Direct anterior approach to the upper cervical spine. *J Bone Joint Surg Am* 1962; 44A:1588–1604.
33. Fielding JW: The status of arthrodesis of the cervical spine. *J Bone Joint Surg Am* 1988; 70A:1571–1574.
34. Fielding JW: Normal and selected abnormal motion of the cervical spine from the second cervical vertebrae to the seventh cervical vertebrae based on cineroentgenography. *J Bone Joint Surg Am* 1964; 46A:1779–1791.
35. Fielding JW, Hawkins RJ, Ratzan SA: Spine fusion for atlanto-axial instability. *J Bone Joint Surg Am* 1976; 58A:400–407.
36. Fuji T, Yonenobu K, Fujiwara K, et al: Interspinous wiring without bone grafting for non-union or delayed union following anterior spinal fusion of the cervical spine. *Spine* 1986; 11:982–987.
37. Gallie WE: Fractures and dislocations of the cervical spine. *Am J Surg* 1939; 46:495–499.
38. Geisler FH, Cheng C, Poka A, et al: Anterior screw fixation of posteriorly displaced type II odontoid fractures. *Neurosurgery* 1989; 25:30–38.
39. Goffin J, Plets C, Van den Bergh: Anterior cervical fusion and osteosynthetic stabilization according to Caspar: A prospective study of 41 patients with fractures and/or dislocations of the cervical spine. *Neurosurgery* 1989; 25:865–871.
40. Goodman J, Seligson D: The anterior cervical plate. *Spine* 1983; 8:700–706.
41. Gore DR, Sepic SB: Anterior cervical fusion for degenerated or protruded discs. *Spine* 1986; 9:667–671.
42. Grob D, Dvorak J, Panjabi M, et al: Posterior occipitocervical fusion: A preliminary report of a new technique. *Spine* 1990; 16:S17–S24.
43. Grob D, Jeanneret B, Aebi M, Markwalder T: Atlanto-axial fusion with transarticular screw fixation. *J Bone Joint Surg Br* 1991; 73B:972–976.
44. Hadra BE: Wiring of the spinous process in Pott's disease. *Trans Am Orthop Assoc* 1891; 4:206–211.
45. Hastings DE, MacNab I, Lawson V: Neoplasms of the atlas and axis. *Can J Surg* 1968; 11:290–296.
46. Hensinger RN, Lang JE, MacEwen GD: Klippel-Feil syndrome: A constellation of associated anomalies. *J Bone Joint Surg Am* 1974; 56A:1246–1253.
47. Herrmann HD: Metal plate fixation after anterior fusion of unstable fracture dislocation of the cervical spine. *Acta Neurochir* (*Wien*) 1975; 32:101–111.

48. Holness RO, Huestis WS, Howes WJ, et al: Posterior stabilization with an interlaminar clamp in cervical injuries: Technical note and review of the long-term experience with the method. *Neurosurgery* 1984; 14:318–322.
49. Hunter LY, Braunstein EM, Bailey RW: Radiographic changes following anterior cervical fusion. *Spine* 1980; 5:399–401.
50. Jacobs B: Anterior cervical spine fusion. *Surg Ann* 1976; 8:413–446.
51. Kaufman HH, Jones E: The principles of bony spinal fusion. *Neurosurgery* 1989; 24:264–270.
52. Kelly DL Jr, Alexander E Jr, Davis CH Jr, et al: Acrylic fixation of atlanto-axial dislocations. *J Neurosurg* 1972; 36:366–367.
53. Lane AW: *The Operative Treatment of Fractures*. London: Medical Publishing, 1914.
54. Lesoin F, Autricque A, Franz K, et al: Transcervical approach and screw fixation for upper cervical spine pathology. *Surg Neurol* 1987; 27:459–465.
55. Magerl F, Seemann PS: Stable posterior fusion of the atlas and axis by transarticular screw fixation, in Kehr P, Weidner A (eds): *Cervical Spine*. New York: Springer-Verlag, 1987: 322–327.
56. McGraw RW, Rusch RM: Atlanto-axial arthrodesis. *J Bone Joint Surg Br* 1973; 55B:482–489.
57. Meyer PR Jr: *Surgery of Spine Trauma*. New York: Churchill Livingstone, 1989.
58. Mixter SJ, Osgood RB: Traumatic lesions of the atlas and axis. *Ann Surg* 1910; 51:193–207.
59. Morscher E, Sutter F, Jennis M, Olerud S: Die Vordere Verplattung der Halswirbelsaule mit dem Hohlschrauben-plattensystem. *Der Chirurg* 1986; 57:702–707.
60. Murphy MJ, Daniaux H, Southwick WO: Posterior cervical fusion with rigid internal fixation. *Orthop Clin North Am* 1986; 17:55–65.
61. Papadopoulos SM, Dickman CA, Sonntag VKH: Atlanto-axial stabilization in rheumatoid arthritis (abstract). *Joint Section on Disorders of the Spine and Peripheral Nerves*, 1990: 80.
62. Pilcher LS: Atlanto-axial fracture-dislocation. *Ann Surg* 1910; 51:208–211.
63. Rana NA, Hancock DO, Taylor AR, et al: Upward translocation of the dens in rheumatoid arthritis. *J Bone Jont Surg Br* 1973; 55B:471–477.
64. Ransford AO, Crockard HA, Pozo JL, et al: Craniocervical instability treated by contoured loop fixation. *J Bone Joint Surg Br* 1986; 68B:173–177.
65. Riley LH, Robinson RA, Johnson KA, Walker AE: The results of anterior interbody fusion of the cervical spine. *J Neurosurg* 1969; 30:127–133.
66. Robinson RA: Anterior and posterior cervical spine fusions. *Clin Orthop* 1964; 35:34–62.
67. Rogers WA: Treatment of fracture-dislocation of the cervical spine. *J Bone Joint Surg* 1942; 24:245–258.
68. Roy-Camille R, Mazel C, Saillant G: Treatment of cervical spine injuries by a posterior osteosynthesis with plates and screws, in Kehr P, Weidner A (eds): *Cervical Spine*. New York: Springer-Verlag, 1987: 163.
69. Sherk HH, Snyder B: Posterior fusions of the upper cervical spine: Indications, techniques and prognosis. *Orthop Clin North Am* 1978; 9:1091–1099.
70. Simmons EH, Bhalla SK: Anterior cervical discectomy and fusion. *J Bone Joint Surg Br* 1969; 51B:225–236.
71. Songer M, Spencer D, Meyer P: The use of sublaminar cables to replace luque wires. *Spine* 1991; 16:418–421.
72. Suh PB, Kostuik JP, Esses SI: Anterior cervical plate fixation with the titanium hollow screw plate system: A preliminary report. *Spine* 1990; 15:1079–1081.
73. Sumner-Smith G: *Bone in Clinical Orthopedics. A Study in Comparative Osteology*. Philadelphia: WB Saunders, 1982.
74. Sutterlin CE, McAfee PC, Warden KE, et al: A biomechanical evaluation of cervical spinal stabilization methods in a bovine model. *Spine* 1988; 13:795–802.
75. Taitsman JP, Saha S: Tensile strength of wire-reinforced bone cement and twisted stainless wire. *J Bone Joint Surg Am* 1977; 59A:419–425.
76. Tippets RH, Apfelbaum RI: Anterior cervical fusion with the Caspar instrumentation system. *Neurosurgery* 1988; 22:1008–1013.
77. Van Peteghem PK, Schweigel JF: The fractured cervical spine rendered unstable by anterior cervical fusion. *J Trauma* 1979; 19:110–114.
78. Wertheim SB, Bohlman HH: Occipitocervical fusion: Indications, technique and long-term results in thirteen patients. *J Bone Joint Surg Am* 1987; 69A:833–842.
79. White AA, Southwick WO, DePonte RJ, et al: Relief of pain by cervical spine fusion for spondylosis. *J Bone Joint Surg Am* 1973; 55A:525–534.
80. White A, Panjabi MM: Clinical instability of the spine, in Evarts CM (ed): *Surgery of the Musculoskeletal System*. New York: Churchill-Livingstone, 1983: 97–106.
81. Whitecloud TS, LaRocca SH: Fibular strut graft in reconstructive surgery of the cervical spine. *Spine* 1976; 1:33–43.
82. Whitehill R, Reger SI, Kett RL, et al: Reconstruction of the cervical spine following anterior vertebral body resection: A mechanical analysis of a canine experimental model. *Spine* 1984; 9:240–245.
83. Whitehill R, Stowers SF, Fechner RE, et al: Posterior cervical fusions using cerclage wires, methylmethacrylate cement and autogenous bone graft. An experimental study of a canine model. *Spine* 1987; 12:12–22.
84. Wiesel SW, Rothman RH: Occipito-atlantal hypermobility. *Spine* 1979; 4:187–191.

CHAPTER 84

TIMING OF SURGICAL INTERVENTION AFTER SPINAL CORD INJURY

Azik Wolf
Jack E. Wilberger, Jr.

INTRODUCTION

The appropriate timing of surgical intervention in the cervical spinal cord-injured (SCI) patient is controversial. The single, widely accepted indication for early surgical intervention is documented neurological deterioration in association with ongoing spinal canal compromise from disc or bone fragments, hematoma, or unreduced subluxation. In general, there is much less urgency about surgery, primarily for spinal stabilization, as traction or devices such as roto-beds, almost always provide excellent immobilization until the patient is in optimal condition for operation. The traditional neurosurgical approach has thus been to stabilize the SCI medically over periods sometimes extending weeks before intervention. This has been felt necessary to reduce both neurological and systemic complications from the surgery. Recently, however, renewed concerns over the high incidence of the complications of prolonged immobilization in SCI patients before and after delayed surgical intervention have led some to reconsider the appropriateness of early operative intervention. Additionally, there are currently several strong advocates of early surgical spinal decompression, especially in an incomplete spinal cord injury in an attempt to ameliorate neurological dysfunction and/or facilitate neurological recovery.

The goals of early definitive surgical therapy are to provide a maximal environment for neurological recovery, to facilitate early mobilization and thus avoid adverse systemic and psychological effects related to prolonged bedrest, to create the opportunity for an earlier start of the rehabilitation process, to reduce the difficulties of nursing care, and to decrease overall expenses. Arguments against early intervention have included the following: (1) initial trials of early surgery promoted by the medical community's growing understanding of a patient's adverse physiological response to prolonged immobilization showed no improvement in overall outcome; (2) early intervention may be precluded by the admitting medical facility's lack of intensive care capability, specific equipment, and experienced personnel required to perform such surgery, necessitating patient transfer to a specialty referral center and thus delaying surgery; (3) acute systemic trauma, need for life-saving interventions, and hemodynamic/respiratory instability may further compromise the patient's recovery; (4) surgery to insure alignment and stabilization may be implemented only after the failure of other primary treatment modalities; and (5) the risk of neurological deterioration after spinal cord trauma may be increased with early surgery.

HISTORICAL PERSPECTIVE

Traditionally, neurosurgeons have been cautioned against early surgical intervention for spinal stabilization after cervical SCI. The two primary reasons for this caution have been concerns over the high risk of systemic—especially pulmonary—complications and over contributing to neurological deterioration with early surgery.

Many authors have addressed the complications attendant on the management of acute cord injury.[1–3] Heiden and coworkers in 1975 carefully documented their experience with systemic complications in 356 complete and incomplete injuries after anterior cervical fusions, laminectomy, and nonsurgical management.[3] In the 157 patients with incomplete SCI, there was a 29 percent systemic complication rate after anterior cervical fusion or laminectomy versus a 20 percent rate from nonsurgical management. In the 199 patients with complete SCI, no significant neurological recovery was seen regardless of the type or timing of surgical intervention. Thirty-seven percent of the nonsurgical group had one or more systemic (severe pulmonary, thrombophlebitis, pulmonary embolism, gastrointestinal hemorrhage, infection) complications, while complications developed in 50 percent of those undergoing anterior cervical fusion. In addition, the pulmonary complications rate was 46 percent if anterior fusion was performed within the first week of injury, compared with 27 percent if the surgery was delayed one to four weeks after spinal cord injury. Such information led these authors to conclude that early operative intervention (<1 week post-SCI) is associated with "unacceptable morbidity."

Marshall and coworkers in 1987 comprehensively addressed the issue of neurological deterioration after spinal cord injury.[4] One-third of all cases of neurological deterioration were directly attributed to surgical intervention. Out of 134 patients undergoing surgery, four patients (2.9 percent) suffered a significant neurological deterioration. A direct correlation was established between timing of operative intervention and risk of neurological deterioration. Four of 26 patients (15.3 percent) undergoing spinal surgery within five days of spinal cord injury deteriorated, while none of 44 undergoing surgery from five to ten days after SCI had any neurological sequelae. Marshall thus strongly advocated that "early surgical intervention on the cervical spine should be performed under only one circumstance: to avoid further deterioration in neurological function."

In spite of such concerns, however, there have been at various times proponents of "early" surgical intervention, primarily for the purposes of earlier patient mobilization. Raynor in 1967 advocated early anterior fusion after SCI, indicating that "anterior fusion usually allows earlier mobilization of the patient and can help the morale factor in addition to simplifying nursing care."[5] Raynor reported his experience with early anterior fusion in 14 patients. The time from SCI to surgery ranged from four to 56 days. No comments were made about postoperative systemic complications; however, no neurological deterioration related to surgical intervention occurred. In spite of supporting such early intervention, Raynor did caution that "unless neurological deterioration develops, the patient with moderate to severe injury to the cervical spine should be allowed several days to a week for the spine to stabilize."

Norrell in 1970, citing concerns over prolonged immobilization of SCI patients, advocated a "radical departure" in the management of spinal injury. Early anterior fusion was felt to offer the advantages of providing mechanical stability, protecting the nervous tissue, and decreasing pain as well as allowing early mobilization. Results of early surgery in 31 patients were presented to support such an approach. The time from SCI to surgery ranged from one to 19 days, with a mean of four days. There were two deaths and four cases of "marked respiratory instability" in the series. Norrell concluded that surgery could be safely undertaken "during the first week following injury."[6] However, Norrell reversed his position somewhat in 1980 regarding surgery after quadriplegia—"it should be delayed for 12–21 days with the understanding that surgery carries a significant risk and the only indication is to reduce the time of recumbency."[7]

EARLY SURGICAL INTERVENTION AND SYSTEMIC COMPLICATIONS

In general, it is known that spinal cord-injured patients are susceptible to many systemic and neurological complications regardless of the treatment undertaken. The techniques of immobilization and prolonged immobilization itself may further increase the complication rate. Even though surgery was associated with neurological complications in one-third of Marshall's patients, as noted previously, the remaining two-thirds were directly attributable to the techniques of immobilization—halo application, Stryker frame or roto-bed rotation, skeletal traction application. In addition, the complications of prolonged immobilization and the susceptibility of the spinal cord-injured patient to these complications is well known. The best available current information about the risks of such complications comes from the National Acute Spinal Cord Injury Study. Of 478 patients treated at spinal cord injury centers from 1986 to 1988, there was a 30 percent incidence of pneumonia, 18.6 percent decubiti, 4.6 percent thrombophlebitis, and 2.8 percent pulmonary embolism.[8,9]

Noting these concerns, more contemporary studies do not support significant inherent risks in rapid surgical intervention after spinal cord injury. Wilberger in 1991 reported on a comparative study of early versus late spinal stabilization after cervical spinal cord injury. Of 100 patients with cervical injuries, 88 underwent surgical intervention—39 within 24 hours of injury and 49 from 24 hours to three weeks after injury.[10] The incidence of systemic, medical complications (pneumonia, thrombophlebitis, pulmonary embolism, decubiti) were reduced by over 50 percent when comparing early versus late stabilization groups. In addition, the incidence of postsurgical neurological deterioration was 0 percent in the early and 2.5 percent in the late stabilization group. Levi and associates reviewed the records of 103 consecutive patients with mid- to lower cervical spine trauma admitted to the Shock Trauma Center in Baltimore between 1985 and 1990.[11] Of the 103 patients, 45 underwent early surgery (mean 11.7 hours), 35 of whom had complete neurological deficits. The complications rate was similar between the early and delayed surgical groups (Table 84-1). With regard to pulmonary status, skin care, and deep vein thrombosis prophylaxis, there was unmeasured but obvious ease in management of the patients who had no need for prolonged traction. The mean number of chest physiotherapy and suction procedures during the first week differed significantly between the early and delayed groups: 6.0 versus 9.86 procedures/24 hours, respectively, $p = 0.04$. The patients' mean classification scores in terms of hours of care during each day of the first postinjury week were similar: 23.1 and 21.8 in the early and delayed groups, respectively. The length of stay until discharge to rehabilitation program was shorter by a mean of 6.5 days in the early subgroup of these patients. One patient (1.9 percent) in the early subgroup died of Adult Respiratory Distress Syndrome (Table 84-1).

A recent reanalysis of data from the National Acute Spinal Cord Injury Study demonstrated that the complications rate was somewhat decreased (10.3 vs. 8.4 percent, $p > 0.05$) in those patients who underwent surgical intervention in the overall treatment of their spinal cord injury. Additionally, no neurological deterioration was attributable to the type or timing of surgery.[12]

Several authors recently have shown a trend toward shorter hospital stays and earlier rehabilitation in patients treated with aggressive surgical intervention.[10,11]

Thus, if operative intervention is felt necessary after spinal cord injury, assuming the patient is otherwise medically stable, there do not appear at present to be significant increased risks attendant on early aggressive intervention. On the contrary, the period of immobilization and the associated medical complications may be lessened considerably by early intervention.

EARLY SURGICAL INTERVENTION AND NEUROLOGICAL RECOVERY

The question of enhancing or promoting neurological recovery by surgical intervention is for the most part presently unresolved. Intuitively and anecdotally it appears reasonable to consider early spinal canal and spinal cord decompression in an effort to improve neurological recovery. Consider the recently reported MRI study of Yamashita and coworkers indicating that the most important predictive factor for neurological recovery was the degree and extent of extrinsic cord compression.[13] Hadley and colleagues, in a recent study of cervical facet fracture dislocation, found a correlation between the time to realignment/decompression of the

TABLE 84-1 Hospitalization Data

	Incomplete Deficit			*Complete Deficit*		
Parameter	**Early (n = 10)**	**Delayed (n = 40)**	**T/A[a] (n = 50)**	**Early (n = 35)**	**Delayed (n = 18)**	**T/A (n = 35)**
Time to surgery						
Range (days)	1	2–77	1–77	1	2–45	1–45
Mean	1	13	10.6[b]	1	13	5.1[b]
Stabilization method						
Caspar plate	7	25	32	33	16	49
Iliac crest bone graft alone	3	15	18	2	2	4
Mean number of chest physiotherapy interventions/day				6	9.86	7.30[b]
Complications						
Per patient	0.60	0.45	0.48	1.31	1.89	1.51
Number of patients	5	13	18	28	18	46
Length of stay	19.9	22.0	21.6	38.7	45.2	40.9

[a] T/A, total or average

[b] Statistically significant ($p < 0.05$).

spinal canal and the potential for neurological recovery—all cases of significant neurological recovery that occurred in patients reduced within eight hours of injury.[14] For the most part, however, it has been impossible to determine whether in relationship to surgical treatments the extent of neurological recovery is due to the treatment itself or to the degree and extent of the primary injury to the spinal cord.

It is well known that there is a rate of spontaneous neurological recovery even in complete injury irrespective of treatment approaches. Frankel, in developing his classic spinal cord injury grading system three decades ago, noted that approximately 8 percent of patients with initially complete injuries had recovery of useful lower extremity motor function.[15] A contemporary report of thoracolumbar injuries with complete spinal cord injury found that 25 percent of all patients regained two or more Frankel grades without surgical intervention. The NASCIS II data likewise support a not insignificant degree of spontaneous neurological recovery.[8,9]

A few would argue that early, aggressive surgical intervention is warranted even in the face of an initially complete spinal cord injury. Such proponents point to the belief that persistent compression of the spinal cord may exacerbate the secondary injury cascade that normally occurs after spinal cord injury. Indeed, there is some experimental evidence that rapid decompression within the first 24 hours of injury may improve outcome. In addition, there have been a number of anecdotal experiences in which significant, unexpected neurological recovery occurred after some form of surgical intervention. Nevertheless, available data would not appear to support such contentions (Table 84-2). Of 199 patients with complete spinal cord injury, Heiden and coworkers found no evidence of significant neurological recovery regardless of the type or timing of surgical intervention. In a comparative study of early (<24 hours) versus late anterior decompressive surgery in 53 patients with complete cervical spinal cord injury, Levi and associates could not document any significant differences between the groups when comparing motor and functional outcome (Table 84-3). Similarly, in evaluation of 34 patients with complete SCI secondary to bilateral facet dislocation, 7 (20.6 percent) of the 34 improved their grades; one gained ambulation. The rates of improvement were not statistically significant between those undergoing acute (26.7 percent) or delayed (18.8 percent) reduction and/or surgery ($p = 0.46$). In a recent Scoliosis Research Society study of over 1000 thoracolumbar injuries, similarly no advantages could be seen in regard to Frankel grade improvement or functional outcome in surgically versus nonoperatively treated patients.

Even in the presence of an initially incomplete spinal cord injury there is no clear compelling evidence of neurological benefits from surgical intervention. In the

TABLE 84-2 Results in Different Series of Patients with Complete Cord Deficits[a]

Series (Ref. no.)	Number	Died (%) DC	Died (%) FU	Improved (%) DC	Improved (%) FU	Ambulatory FU
Frankel et al., 1969 (15)[b]	123			34.1		8.9
Heiden et al., 1975 (3)[c]	199					1.0
Tator et al., 1982 (16)	232	17.0	26.0	9.5	12	2.6
Horsey et al., 1977–1978 (17)	27	3.7	3.7	11.1	11.1	
Lucas & Ducker, 1979 (18)[d]	56	13.0	13.0			
Young & Dexter, 1978–1979 (19)[e]	49				16.3	2.0
Maynard et al., 1979 (20)[f]	68			8.8	19.4	1.6
Marshall et al., 1987 (4)	69					1.3
Benzel & Larson, 1987 (21)[g]	35		8.6		0.0	
Weinshel et al., 1990 (22)[h]	81			4.4	12.3	2.5
Levi et al., 1991 (11)	53	1.9	1.9	9.4	34.0	3.8
Total (no.)	992	52/403	83/526	80/519	79/461	26/874
(%)		12.9	15.8	15.4	17.1	3.0

[a] DC, discharge; FU, follow-up
[b] No surgery
[c] 5.5% underwent anterior decompressive surgery within 2 days
[d] All underwent anterior decompression and/or fusion
[e] 26% underwent surgery via an anterior approach
[f] 41% underwent decompressive surgery within the first month
[g] All underwent surgery within a mean of 21.5 days
[h] All underwent surgery (anterior or posterior) within a mean of 13 days

TABLE 84-3 Follow-up Data[a]

	Incomplete Deficit			*Complete Deficit*		
Parameter	**Early (n = 10)**	**Delayed (n = 40)**	**T/A (n = 50)**	**Early (n = 35)**	**Delayed (n = 18)**	**T/A (n = 35)**
Mean Yale motor score						
Admission	2.76	3.85	3.63	0.38	0.30	0.35
Discharge	3.40	4.27	4.10	0.55	0.50	0.53
6 weeks	4.40	4.78	4.69	0.70	0.77	0.74
6 months	4.70	4.70	4.70	0.98	0.80	0.94
12 months	4.90	4.90	4.90	1.03	1.42	1.20
Mean improvement rate (admission-discharge)	37.20	45.00	43.50	3.90	4.40	4.10
Mean neurological grade						
Admission	4.10	5.45	5.18	1.00	1.00	1.00
Complications						
Discharge	4.80	5.74	5.53	1.12	1.06	1.10
12 months	6.00	6.59	6.47	2.01	1.93	2.03
Number of patients improved						
Discharge	5	9[b]	14	4	1	5
12 months	7	17[b]	24	16	7	23

[a] T/A, total or average

[b] Eight patients who were intact at admission were excluded.

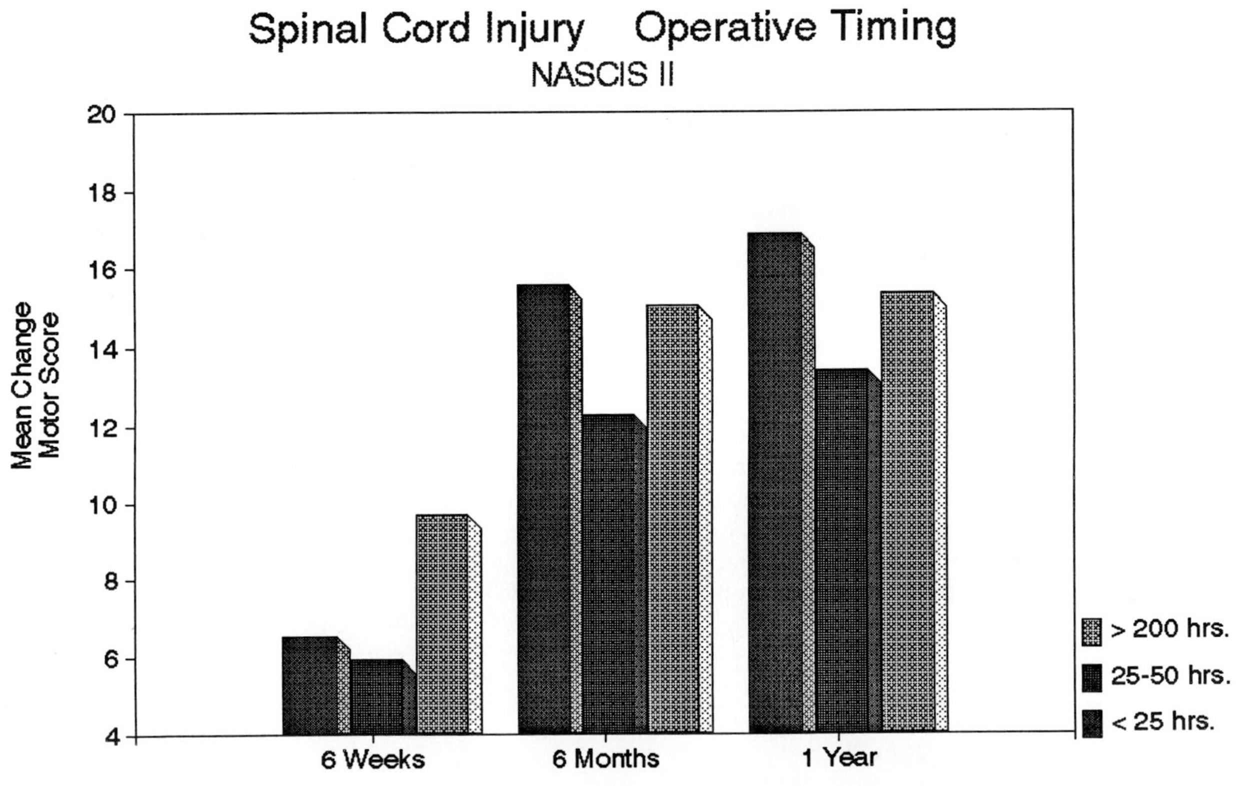

Figure 84-1. NASCIS II—Effects of surgical timing on long-term neurological outcome.

Levi study, 53 patients with incomplete cervical spinal cord injury were also studied in regard to early versus late anterior decompression. While some trends were noted toward improved neurological recovery in the early group, no statistically significant difference could be documented when comparing motor and functional outcome (Table 84-3).

In a recent reanalysis of surgical treatment data on the 487 patients treated in the NASCIS II study, no statistically significant benefits could be documented in neurological recovery related to the type or timing of surgical intervention in both complete and incomplete spinal cord injury. Sixty percent of these patients underwent surgical treatment for decompression and/or spinal realignment. Ultimately, neither the surgical intervention itself nor its absolute timing showed any enhanced neurological improvement over those treated nonoperatively. There was, however, a trend of improved neurological recovery in patients undergoing surgery within 24 hours of injury and in those whose surgery was delayed more than 200 hours after injury. Patients operated upon at 26 to 50 hours after injury, tended to have the least neurological recovery. However, none of these differences were statistically significant (Fig. 84-1).

It must be borne in mind that all the studies reporting to show an advantage or disadvantage to a given surgical procedure and its timing in regards to neurological recovery are retrospective in nature and have not been randomized with respect to the many important variables that may affect neurological recovery. In addition, recent data from animal studies as well as clinical trials suggest that any therapeutic interventions aimed at enhancing neurological recovery may have a narrow time "window of opportunity"—as early as eight hours after injury. Until it becomes feasible to undertake a large scale prospective randomized clinical trial, the surgical treatment of spinal cord injury to enhance neurological recovery will remain problematic. The decision whether or not to pursue early surgery must include a careful analysis of a variety of factors including but not necessarily limited to: (1) the presence of an irreducible, anatomic, compressive lesion; (2) the relative systemic risks; (3) the need for multiple procedures; (4) associated multiple trauma; (5) the presence of a neurological deficit attributable to a compressive lesion; and (6) neurological deterioration following attempts at reduction.

CONCLUSION

Contemporary studies have shown that early surgery after SCI does not increase the complication rate or induce any other adverse effects compared with delayed surgery. It is thus not unreasonable to consider prompt spinal reduction and decompression (either nonoperative or surgical) and early internal stabilization so that patients have the maximum advantage affordable by early mobilization and rehabilitation.

Anecdotal and intuitive impressions that neurological recovery can be positively influenced by aggressive, early surgical intervention are strong and pervasive, but have yet to be borne out by randomized studies.

Ultimately, the decision of whether and when to intervene surgically after SCI will depend on a number of institutional and patient-related variables that cannot be prescribed by rigid protocol.

References

1. Wagner FC, Chehrazi B: Early decompression and neurological outcome in acute cervical spinal cord injuries. *J Neurosurg* 1982; 56:699–705.
2. Bohlman HH: Indications for late anterior decompression and fusion for cervical spinal cord injuries, in Tator CH (ed): *Early Management of Acute Spinal Cord Injury*. New York: Raven Press, 1982: 315–333.
3. Heiden JS, Weiss MH, Rosenberg AW, et al: Management of cervical spinal cord trauma in Southern California. *J Neurosurg* 1975; 43:732–736.
4. Marshall LF, Knowlton S, Garfin SR, et al: Deterioration following spinal cord injury: A multicenter study. *J Neurosurg* 1987; 66:400–404.
5. Raynor RB: Severe injuries of the cervical spine treated by early anterior interbody fusion and ambulation. *J Neurosurg* 1968; 28:311–316.
6. Norrell H, Wilson CB: Early anterior fusion for injuries of the cervical portion of the spine. *JAMA* 1970; 214:525–530.
7. Norrell H: The early management of spinal injuries. *Clin Neurosurg* 1980; 27:385–400.
8. Bracken MB, Shepherd MJ, Collins WF, et al: A randomized control trial of methylprednisolone or naloxone in the treatment of acute spinal cord injury. *N Engl J Med* 1990; 322:1405–1411.
9. Bracken MB, Shepherd MJ, Collins WF, et al: Methylprednisolone or naloxone treatment after acute spinal cord injury: One year follow-up data. Results of the second National Acute Spinal Cord Injury Study. *J Neurosurg* 1992; 76:23–31.
10. Wilberger JE: Diagnosis and management of spinal cord trauma. *Curr Adv Manag Major Trauma* 1990; 1:83–84.
11. Levi L, Wolf A, Regheb J, et al: Anterior decompression in cervical spine trauma: Does the timing of surgery affect the outcome? *Neurosurgery* 1991; 29:216–222.
12. Wilberger JE, Duh MS, Bracken MB: Surgical treatment of spinal cord injury—the NASCIS II Experience. AANS Annual Meeting, Boston, MA, April 1993, abstract book:75.
13. Yamashita Y, Takashi M, Masuno Y, et al: Acute spinal cord injury: MRI correlated with myelopathy. *Br J Radiol* 1991; 64:201–209.

14. Hadley MN, Fitzpatrick B, Sonntag VK, Brown CM: Facet fracture—dislocation injuries of the cervical spine. *Neurosurgery* 1992; 30:661–666.
15. Frankel HL, Hancock DO, Hyslop G, et al: The value of postural reduction in the initial management of closed injuries of the spine with paraplegia and tetraplegia. *Paraplegia* 1969; 7:179–192.
16. Tator CH, Rowed DW, Schwartz ML: Sunnybrook Cord Injury Scales for assessing neurological injury and neurological recovery, in Tator CH (ed): *Early Management of Acute Spinal Cord Injury*. New York: Raven Press, 1982: 7–24.
17. Horsey WJ, Hudson AR, Tucker WS: Indications, technique and results of anterior cervical fusion after cervical spine injury, in Tator CH (ed): *Early Management of Acute Spinal Cord Injury*. New York: Raven Press, 1982: 305–313.
18. Lucas JL, Ducker TB: Morbidity, mortality and recovery rates of patients with spinal cord injuries undergoing anterior decompressive procedures of fusion or both. *Surg Forum* 1979; 28:451–453.
19. Young JS, Dexter WR: Neurological recovery distal to the zone of injury in 172 cases of closed, traumatic spinal cord injury. *Paraplegia* 1979; 16:39–49.
20. Maynard FM, Reynolds GC, Fountain S, et al: Neurological prognosis after traumatic quadriplegia. Three years' experience of California Regional Spinal Cord Injury Care System. *J Neurosurg* 1979; 50:611.
21. Benzel EC, Larson SJ: Functional recovery after decompressive spine operation for cervical spine fractures. *Neurosurgery* 1987; 10:742–746.
22. Weinshel SS, Maiman DJ, Beok P, Scales L: Neurologic recovery in quadriplegia following operative treatment. *J Spin Dis* 1990; 3:244–249.

CHAPTER 85

INTENSIVE CARE MANAGEMENT OF SPINAL CORD INJURY

Gerald E. Rodts, Jr.
Regis W. Haid, Jr.

Intensive care management of the patient suffering an acute spinal cord injury requires careful immobilization of the spine and thoughtful attention to the multitude of neurological and medical problems that result from neurological compromise and immobility. The highest incidence of morbidity and mortality occur within the first two weeks following injury. This chapter will discuss the recommended methods of initial cervical traction, spinal reduction, and orthotic immobilization. Equally as important is the intensive care management of the cardiopulmonary, gastrointestinal, urological, dermatological, and emotional problems that develop. Diligent medical therapy beginning on admission to the intensive care unit (ICU) may maximize neurological recovery and shorten the time necessary to mobilize the patient and initiate physical and occupational therapy.

ADMISSION

In most medical centers, the patient with a spinal cord injury will arrive in the intensive care unit in a rigid cervical collar taped to a backboard. Transfer to the ICU bed may be further complicated by arm or leg splints and traction. Multitrauma patients also may have undergone emergency external pelvic fixation, thoracotomy, laparotomy, and/or craniotomy. The physician should immediately confirm respiratory and hemodynamic stability and perform a detailed neurological examination.[1] The severity of spinal cord injury can be quantified by measurement with the Frankel scale and/or the American Spinal Injury Association (ASIA) motor score (see Chapter 75). The Frankel scoring system divides neurological disability into five grades, which measure function below the level of injury ranging from normal function (E) to complete loss of motor and sensory function (A). The main limitation of the Frankel scoring system is its categorization of injury into five discrete groups, whereas the injury and recovery are actually on a continuum.[2] The ASIA clinical scale measures function in five key muscles in each extremity. Motor function ranges from 0 (no movement) to 5 (full strength); therefore, the total score ranges from 0 (quadriplegia) to 100 (normal motor function). Although this system overcomes the strict categorization of the Frankel scale, it fails to identify a unique anatomic site for any improvement that may occur.[3] Together, these two scales (though imperfect) provide a useful monitoring system for current status and prognosis.

Any patient with neurological deficit and/or any evidence of cervical spine instability on plain radiograph should be immobilized. It is important to remove the paralyzed patient from the backboard as soon as possible to prevent skin breakdown. Prior selection of an appropriate bed support is critical because preservation of skin integrity is essential to the optimal care of the spinal cord-injured patient. Mattresses are available in four basic varieties: foam; gel; air-filled; and water-filled. These four types of support offer variable degrees of ability to minimize shear forces and pressure gradients present at the skin surface by deforming to accommodate prominent deep areas yet conform with concave areas of the body as well. Other ideal qualities of a bed support include temperature control, adequate air-moisture exchange, stability for transfers and weight shifting, automated continuous position change, and affordability.[4] Air- and water-filled beds provide excellent protection from skin maceration, but do not maintain adequate spinal immobilization in concert with a traction system and tend to compromise respiratory function. Gel mattresses adjust to movement and mimic adipose tissue in providing greater cushion for the body frame, but are expensive. Polymer foams provide good protection from skin maceration and are lightweight. They can be cut and modified as desired. Most foam mattresses, however, are affected by temperature changes and are irreversibly damaged by sunlight. In addition, they wear out easily and are not readily cleanable.

For patients with spinal cord injury and paralysis, the Rotorest bed represents a superior bed support system. This device rotates continuously 24 hours per day and affords excellent support and stabilization of the spine while providing physiological movement of the patient. An assortment of flaps and hatches allow access to important body areas to enhance nursing care without compromising spinal stability. It is designed to accommodate in-line cervical traction and can even be used as an operating table if necessary. The foam mattress is lined with gortex, which allows excellent air-moisture exchange. Similar models, like the Stryker frame and the circoelectric bed (like the air- and water-filled beds) are less able to maintain spinal stability and are more apt to compromise respiratory function.[5] The Stoke-Eggerton bed provides good stability, but the patient remains in one position for two hours, increasing the risk of skin maceration compared with the Rotorest bed.

CERVICAL SPINE IMMOBILIZATION

Cervical traction has two purposes: spinal immobilization and fracture reduction. The authors propose that 5 to 10 pounds of traction is safe with most injuries (except atlanto-occipital dislocation or severe atlanto-axial injuries) and can augment immobilization provided by a rigid orthosis. Although it is somewhat controversial, we believe that reduction of a fractured, dislocated spine should not be attempted in patients with neurological deficit and/or evidence of spinal instability until a radiographic imaging study such as MRI or myelography with CT scanning has been performed. Thin-section axial CT scans alone may be revealing if these other modalities are not immediately available. Prompt imaging can rule out the presence of a ventral mass lesion such as hematoma, ruptured intervertebral disc, or bone fragment in the canal. Extension and traction force in the presence of a ventral mass lesion can result in secondary neurological injury.[6] This initial radiographic screening can identify patients who should undergo surgical decompression prior to intraoperative or external reduction. The University of Michigan protocol for acute spinal cord injury requires that an imaging study be performed within the first two hours of admission and application of cervical traction (personal correspondence, Steve Papadopoulos, University of Michigan).

The reduction and temporary stabilization of cervical spine fracture/dislocations using increasing increments of traction force applied through skull tongs was first introduced by Crutchfield in 1933.[7] The older models of tongs (still used in many countries today) were placed well above the largest diameter of the skull (near the superior temporal ridge) and were easy to pull out; therefore, the maximum weight that could be applied was limited (18 pounds). Gardner introduced in 1973 a simple two-pin, spring-loaded tong.[8] This model has been improved, and the current tongs (Gardner-Wells, Zimmer Corp., and Trippi tongs) can be placed below the equator (largest diameter) of the skull. This provides excellent purchase of the skull bone and allows for substantial traction forces to be applied with far less risk of pin displacement. There is low risk of tong-skull interface failure, even at loads of 65 pounds or greater.[9]

The application of Gardner-Wells tongs is simple and can be done with local anesthesia and the patient in the recumbent position (on the backboard). Some authors have demonstrated that 98 percent of patients on a backboard are in a relatively extended position.[10] It is best to place a towel or pad approximately 1.5 inches wide underneath the occipital area to establish a more neutral position of the spine. Tape and sandbags are carefully removed. The hair above the pinnae is shaved and prepared with betadine scrub. Local anesthetic with 1% lidocaine usually is sufficient, though short-acting intravenous agents such as midazolam or lorazepam also may be used with caution. The usual site for skeletal traction in the neutral position is two finger-breadths directly above the peak of the pinna on each side. This technique may be altered, however, to treat specific injuries. For instance, placement of the pins slightly posterior to the aforementioned position will create a traction vector resulting in slight flexion, which may be useful in reducing locked facets.[11] Hyperextension injuries with disruption of the anterior longitudinal ligaments also may require more posterior pin placement to achieve neutral alignment.[12] In situations where application of a halo vest device for prolonged immobilization is anticipated or if more manipulation for realignment is required, it is more efficient to directly apply an open halo head ring with a removable bale attachment. The bale attachment allows for application of in-line traction (Fig. 85-1) This avoids the step of removing the Gardner-Wells tongs for secondary placement of the halo ring following successful reduction and thereby eliminates the patient discomfort of two separate pin applications. Many open ring devices are available (PMT, Bremer, ACE) and are composed of alloys that are MRI-compatible and provide tensile strength equivalent to the traditional closed (complete) ring models.[13] The open back makes placement relatively easy with the patient in the supine position and requires no repositioning. It also improves MRI imaging by avoiding a circular configuration that may distort high-field imaging. The ring should be placed two finger-breadths above the ears posteriorly and one finger-breadth above the lateral one-third of the eyebrows anteriorly. Common errors to avoid include failure to place the two anterior pins posterolateral enough in the frontal bone to avoid supraorbital nerve injury. Placement of the ring higher than two finger-breadths above the eyebrows or pinnae incurs greater risk of pin movement owing to the decreasing diameter of the skull in the cephalad direction (Fig. 85-2). The distance between the ring and scalp should be symmetrical throughout to avoid an imbalance in applied pin forces. The torque force applied to the skull pins should not exceed 6 to 8 inch-lbs to avoid skull fracture.[14] In children with immature skulls, a greater number of pins should be placed to distribute the torque applied to each pin. Four to eight pins are used and tightened to a torque that is safe relative to the patient's skull bone maturity. For example, 5 ft-lbs of torque is recommended for children over the age of four years. Below that age, one pound per year of age is suggested.[15] Intracranial hemorrhage or even brain abscess is a potential albeit rare complication of inner table fracture.[16] The site of attachment of the bale can be altered as with Gardner-Wells pins so that different traction strategies can be executed.

A simple guideline suggested by Crutchfield uses five pounds for each level below the occiput down to the level of the lesion. For example, up to 30 pounds of weight can be safely applied for an injury at the C6 level. Most practitioners begin with 5 to 10 pounds of weight regardless of the level of injury and add weight in increments of 10 pounds. The total amount of weight that can be used to achieve closed cervical reduction is controversial. Most authors agree that up to 65 pounds or more can be used safely, and cadaver studies have demonstrated mechanical tolerance of 100 pounds in the adult.[10] These latter studies, however, do not provide data on cord function and should be interpreted with extreme caution. The total weight eventually achieved is not as important as the amount of weight added in each increment. Greater incremental weight increases can result in neurological deterioration thought to be due to vascular compromise and distraction of the neural elements. For these reasons, great caution should be exercised with elderly patients, injuries of the upper cervical spine, coexistent spondylosis, or significant soft tissue disruption. Careful serial neurological examinations are mandatory after every change in traction weight and should be accompanied with a portable lateral cervical spine radiograph for confirmation of satisfactory alignment and distraction. Portable traction devices are available for safe, efficient transport from the ICU to the radiology suite for CT scanning, tomograms, and other necessary studies.[17]

The amount of time that should be allotted for closed spinal reduction is determined by the patient's neurolog-

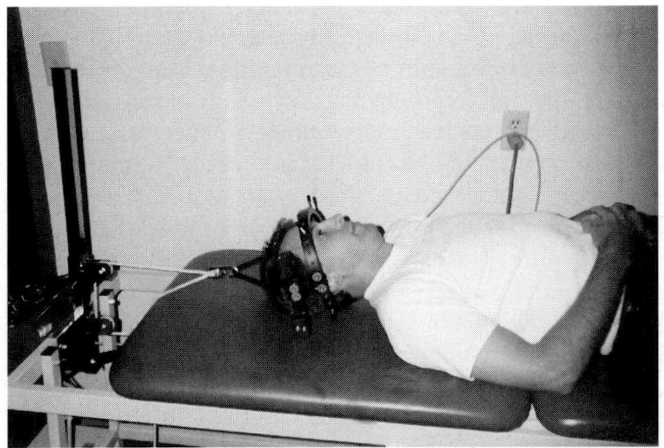

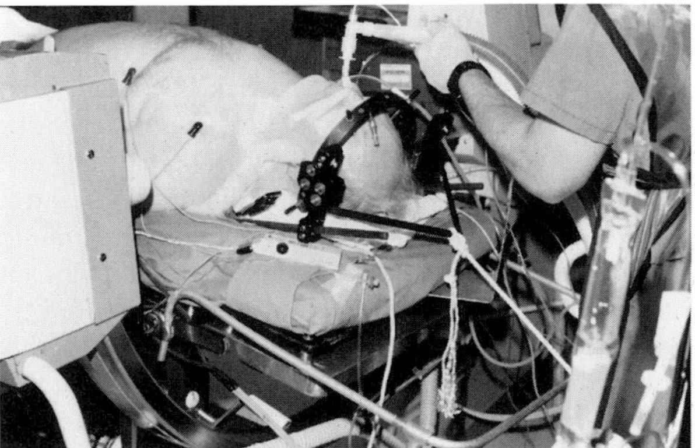

Figure 85-1. Photographs of patients with a halo ring and bale device for cervical traction that is easily converted to a vest device following reduction.

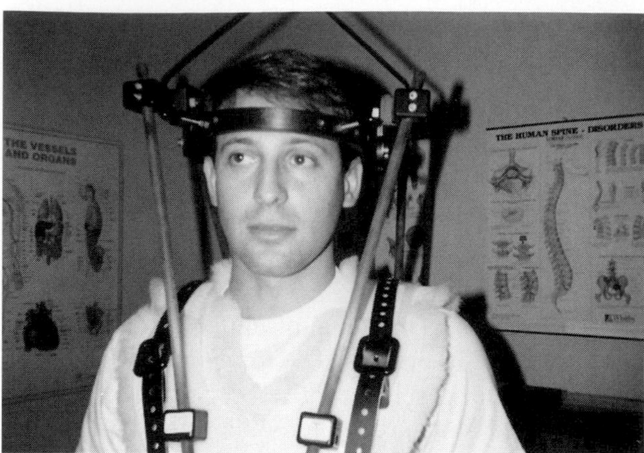

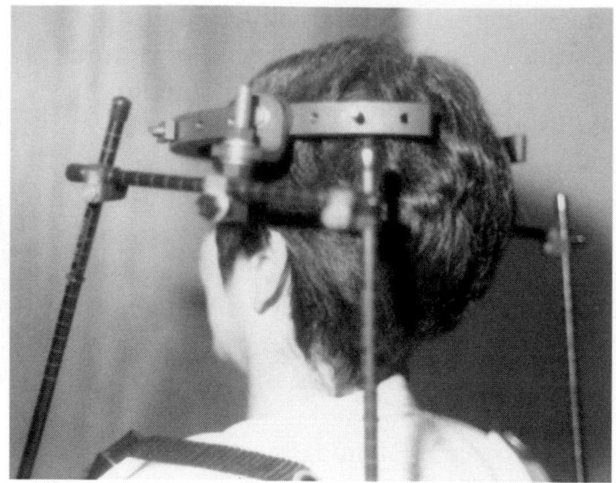

Figure 85-2. Incorrect (left) placement of halo ring above the largest equator of the skull (note distance between pinna of ear and ring) and correct location of ring (right).

ical condition and the philosophy of the treating physician.[18] In a patient with a partial spinal cord injury, failure to achieve reduction over several hours (with the maximal weight judged for the level of injury) will require consideration of open (surgical) reduction and fusion. Though there is a paucity of literature to confirm that early reduction alters the outcome of spinal cord function,[19] it is generally accepted that the most optimal milieu for neurological recovery in the incomplete patient includes prompt bony realignment. For patients with a complete spinal cord level, rapid reduction usually is not practiced and greater time can be allowed to achieve closed realignment.

A significant deterrent to successful cervical reduction is paraspinal muscle spasm and rigidity. Intravenous narcotics (morphine sulfate, 1–5 mg via IV push per hour for adults) and oral or parenteral benzodiazepines (diazepam, 5–10 mg orally or IV every six to eight hours for adults) are very useful in relieving pain and spasm, but should be used very cautiously in combination. Any sedative agent can compromise cardiopulmonary function and will diminish the consciousness of the patient during examination when feedback is critical. Furthermore, excessive sedation may allow overdistraction with or without a change in traction weight, causing secondary cord injury. The use of general anesthesia and pharmacological paralytic agents for aggressive manipulation of the spine is used in a few centers in this country, but most physicians prefer manipulation to be performed in an awake patient and defer to open reduction in those patients who fail traction.[20,21]

If spinal reduction is achieved with traction, the weight is lowered incrementally to one-half or one-third the maximal weight for placement of the halo vest.[22,23] Most patients can be safely rotated continuously in the Rotorest bed or log-rolled at frequent intervals by an experienced neurosurgical nursing staff for skin care, cleaning, and general mobilization.

Cardiopulmonary Considerations

Many organ systems are affected by spinal cord injury, none as potentially lethal in the acute phase as hemodynamic and respiratory compromise.[24,25] Interruption of descending sympathetic fibers diminishes normal vasoconstrictor tone, resulting in hypotension, venous pooling, and decreased preload on the heart. Vagal predominance causes bradycardia, and this may be an important sign distinguishing hypotension due to functional sympathectomy from that due to hemorrhagic, septic, or hypovolemic shock. In any cord-injured patient with hypotension, placement of a pulmonary artery catheter (Swan-Ganz), is optimal for monitoring central venous pressure, pulmonary capillary wedge pressure, cardiac output, and systemic vascular resistance. Administration of bolus volumes of crystalloid fluid to treat hypovolemia and hypotension may result in pulmonary edema and congestive heart failure in the paralyzed patient and probably should be avoided. Crystalloid may be contraindicated if there is an associated head injury. Colloid solutions of albumin and hetastarch (Plasmanate, Hespan) are effective volume expanders and often are necessary in conjunction with intravenous cardiovascular stimulants such as phenylephrine (Neo-Synephrine, 10 mg in 500 ml dextrose, to run at 40–60 μg/min or 40–60 drops/min [20 drops/ml]) and dopamine: 400 mg in 250 ml D_5W, 4-50 μg/min). These agents increase peripheral vascular resistance (e.g., neosynephrine, via alpha receptor stimulation) and increase cardiac output (e.g. dopamine, via myocardial beta$_1$ receptor interaction), respectively. Continuous ECG and arterial blood pressure monitoring is mandatory, with frequent electrolyte testing for the first seven to ten days following injury.[26] In the subacute phase, fludrocortisone and ergotamine maybe helpful in maintaining intravascular volume and blood pressure.[27] A baseline 12-lead ECG should be performed on admission. Any patient suspected of an associated cardiac contusion (chest contusion, pneuomothorax, etc.) should have serial ECG examinations and CPK/MB enzyme fraction determination. One should anticipate possible arrhythmias or diminished pump function from any cardiac muscular injury. Bradycardia can be symptomatic, requiring atropine sulfate administration (0.5–1.0 mg IV) or even transvenous electrical pacing. Atropine should be kept at the bedside during the first few days following spinal cord injury. All patients with any evidence of cord injury should be monitored very closely for development of respiratory difficulty, even if they arrive on admission to the ICU breathing spontaneously without prior endo- or nasotracheal intubation in the emergency department. Normal respiration involves abdominal, intercostal, diaphragmatic, and (in certain circumstances) accessory muscles of respiration (sternocleidomastoid, scalenes, and trapezius). High cervical injuries (at C4 and above) result in loss of all muscular components of breathing and will have required immediate intubation at the scene of the accident or in the ER. Prevertebral soft tissue swelling can compromise the airway during initiation of cervical traction and should be considered during halo placement.[28] Patients with lower levels of quadriplegia who seem to be respiring adequately in the immediate post-injury period may be relying solely on the accessory muscles of respiration. Moreover, the neurological deficit can rise one to two spinal levels in the acute period. These patients can appear stable at first and then rapidly or insidiously fatigue over the following hours or days. With paralysis of the diaphragm (phrenic nerves, C3–5), intercostal and abdominal muscles, the hemidiaphragms are pushed passively upward during expansion of the upper rib cage by accessory muscles, resulting in inward movement of the abdomen during inspiration.[29] The reverse occurs during expiration, and this phenomenon is collectively referred to as paradoxical abdominal breathing. Functional residual capacity (FRC), tidal volume and inspiratory and expiratory reserve volumes (IRV and ERV) are significantly diminished and residual volume (RV) is markedly increased. When combined with inevitable atelectasis and poorly cleared secretions, a ventilation-perfusion (V/Q) mismatch is created, resulting in hypoxemia. In these patients, the sitting position or elevation of the thorax will lower the paralyzed diaphragm and improve respiratory function. On the contrary, if the patient has a lower injury with partial diaphragm function, assuming the Trendelenberg position (and shifting the diaphragm cephalad) lengthens innervated muscle fibers and creates a mechanical advantage that increases excursion on inspiration. Furthermore, functional vital capacity (FVC) is reduced in sitting patients with some diaphragm function as the paralyzed abdominal muscles allow gravity to pull the viscera and diaphragm further caudad in the abdominal cavity. Elastic abdominal binders may be useful in counteracting this effect.

A baseline arterial blood gas should be obtained with serial tests at least every six hours during the first two to three days. A pulse oximeter should be used continuously to monitor oxygen saturation. Charting the p_{CO_2} in graph form is helpful in detecting a dangerous trend toward hypercapnia. Hypoxia, hypercapnia, and acidosis are not only deleterious to cardiac and pulmonary function, but also may cause significant secondary insult to the existing spinal cord injury. With the patient in traction or manual immobilization in the neutral position, prompt fiberoptic nasotracheal, endotracheal, or even digital (under life-threatening instances) intubation should be carried out in a patient who is clearly fatiguing on clinical examination and/or in whom blood gas analysis indicates inadequate oxygenation and CO_2 exchange. The endotracheal route can be used even if the patient is fixed in the neutral position with the aid of manual cricoid pressure; this reduces the risk of nasal mucosal injury, pain, bleeding, bacteremia, chronic paranasal sinusitis, and sepsis.[30] If the initial intubation is via the nasotracheal route, the tube should be exchanged for an endotracheal tube after five days.[31]

Continuous positive pressure can reduce atelectasis and improve FRC. The assist-control (AC) mode of ventilation will be necessary for patients with high cervical level who are unable to initiate any degree of inspiration. Synchronized intermittent ventilation (SIMV) is appropriate in patients with some respiratory function and can continuously train the muscles that have remained innervated. Positive end-expiratory pressure (PEEP) may be necessary in severely hypoxic patients with atelectasis and airway collapse, but this modality also may diminish venous return from the cord and may be contraindicated in patients with an associated brain injury.

Patients who do retain innervation of respiratory muscles should be aggressively weaned from ventilatory support once they are medically stable. Problems such as hospital-acquired pneumonia, tracheomalacia, oxygen toxicity, oral/nasal mucosal ulceration with sinusitis, and hemodynamic compromise and other complications of prolonged intubation can be avoided. Depending on the degree of weakness and length of intubation, patients may require many days or more in the IMV mode, with progressively shorter rest periods at night. Ultimately, long periods of weaning with a T-tube or continuous positive airway pressure (CPAP) will prepare the patient for a successful extubation. Useful parameters predictive of successful weaning include a vital capacity of >1 liter, maximal inspiratory pressure of <-30 cm H_2O, minute ventilation of <10 liters, alveolar-arterial oxygen tension difference (AAD02) of <350 mmHg, and p_{CO_2} of <50 mmHg.[32] Failure to maintain adequate respiration is common in SCI patients intubated from more than one week and/or with significant diaphragm or accessory muscle weakness. Again, the caretaker is urged to recognize the slow, quiet deterioration of the paralyzed patient before significant hypoxia, hypercapnia, and acidosis are present.

Tracheostomy may facilitate optimal pulmonary toilet and respiratory training. This procedure, however, should not be performed if there is any potential need for an anterior surgical approach for spinal cord decompression and spinal stabilization. Postural chest percussion and drainage, inhalant therapy with bronchodilators and expectorants (Mucomist, Alupent, Bronkosol, normal saline), and bronchoscopic therapy (in cases of severe lung collapse) can result in a 33 percent decrease in the time complete ventilator dependence is needed.[33] Despite these aggressive efforts, however, some patients will require long-term ventilator support. For patients with complete paralysis at or above C3, implantable radiofrequency phrenic nerve stimulators currently offer an alternative to prolonged ventilator dependence.

Deep Vein Thrombosis

Deep vein thrombosis has been reported to occur in 81 to 100 percent of spinal cord patients with complete spinal lesions and in 8 to 9.3 percent of those with partial spinal cord injury.[34,35] Venous pooling secondary to paralysis and lack of muscular contraction in the lower extremities and abdominal viscera is the major factor in this increased risk.[36] In some trauma patients, hypercoagulability and vessel damage play an important role. The combination of stasis of flow, vessel wall damage, and hypercoagulable state is referred to as Virchow's triad. Surgical intervention, delay in transfers and increased age also increase risk.[37] The incidence of PE was 4.6 percent in the acute phase of injury (4.3 percent for paraplegia and 4.8 percent for quadriplegia), and is the cause of death in approximately 4 percent of patients during the initial hospitalization.[36] The actual peak incidence is at one month post-injury, and pulmonary embolism occurs in 45 percent of all patients, though rarely within the first week of injury.[40] Venous thrombosis is best treated with prevention, and aggressive measures should be instituted as part of the initial intensive care management of the paralyzed patient.

External sequential pneumatic compression stockings can lower the incidence of DVT, but have not been clearly shown to lower the rate of PE.[38] However, since the stockings are simple to use and involve little to no risk to the patient, they are recommended for use. As the condition of the patient permits, vigorous passive and (if not completely paralyzed) active ranging of all four extremities should be performed. Subcutaneous aqueous heparin in not recommended during the acute phase of injury, as it may extend areas of parenchymal cord hemorrhage and may be contraindicated in settings of multiorgan trauma. After several days or one week, subcutaneous heparin (5000 units every 8 hours) can be started in most cases without incident.[39,40] Even with subcutaneous heparin, Green reported a 33 percent DVT rate.[41] Intravenous catheter placement should be avoided below the level of the subclavian vein; femoral and lower extremity catheters are associated with higher risk of venous thrombosis in the paralyzed patient.[42]

Clinical detection of deep venous thrombosis in the paralyzed patient can be difficult, as there usually are few physical signs and symptoms. Sensory loss obfuscates the classic triad of tenderness, edema, and a positive Homan's sign. One should have an extremely high index of suspicion in the debilitated patient and a low threshold for noninvasive Doppler monitoring—a technique with 90 percent accuracy in detecting complete occlusion of the deep venous systems. False-negative results, however, can be be found in incomplete venous occlusion. Impedence plethysmography, a technique that correlates changes in venous blood flow with changes in resistance to an electrical signal passing through the affected extremity, can be useful more distally in the lower extremity, but the technique is only 50 percent accurate.[43] Radiolabeled fibrinogen screening is expensive, carries a high false-positive rate (7.7 percent) and has associated (albeit low) risks of liver damage and radiation injury.[44] Venography remains the gold standard for detection of venous thrombosis, but may be logistically difficult.

Signs and symptoms of pulmonary embolism also may be absent or misleading. The typical findings of tachypnea, pleuritic chest pain, dyspnea, and tachycardia may not be present owing to disruption of sensory and autonomic pathways. The patient may merely appear diaphoretic and/or febrile. Other sources of fever (especially urinary tract infection or pneumonia) are extremely common, but one should remain alert to the possibility of pulmonary embolism. Blood gas analysis will reveal decreased oxygen saturation and p_{O_2} (usually below 80 mmHg) and decreased p_{CO_2}. If the patient is physically able to mount a tachypneic response, a respiratory alkalosis will be present. A pleural effusion may be present on chest x-ray, but commonly the film appears unchanged from previous studies. Ventilation-perfusion scans are accurate in most patients in detecting a V/Q mismatch consistent with pulmonary embolism, but often this test will be interpreted as equivocal and a pulmonary angiogram will be necessary. Angiography has the benefit of allowing for simultaneous placement of a vena cava filter (Greenfield filter). This is useful in cases where anticoagulation with intravenous heparin is judged to be contraindicated owing to proximity in time to the spinal cord injury or the presence of head or other injuries. Wilson and co-workers recently presented data that arguably supported the use of prophylactic vena cava insertion in patients with spinal cord injury. Their one-year patency rate as measured by duplex scan was 81.8 percent. There were no complications associated with filter insertion, and no patients developed PE after the procedure.[45]

Gastrointestinal Considerations

In the first few days of spinal cord injury, decompression of distended viscera and prophylaxis against stress ulceration of the stomach and duodenum constitute two important early steps in intensive care management. Disorders of the gastrointestinal (GI) tract can be caused by direct trauma to abdominal organs, neuroendocrine response to GI stress, and abrupt loss of nervous control.[46] After initial stabilization, nutrition and bowel function are primary concerns. The goal is to deliver maximal caloric support while maintaining daily bowel evacuation.

Acute abdominal distension in the paralyzed patient presents many preventable risks. Gastric dilatation is seen most commonly with cervical and high thoracic lesions, and leads to third spacing of fluids and hypovolemia. Diaphragmatic excursion and respiration are severely compromised and aspiration of gastric contents leads to pneumonia and further deterioration. A nasogastric or (in the presence of facial or skull-base fractures) orogastric tube should be placed immediately for decompression and removal of stomach contents. Intravenous fluid replacement should be maintained with ml for ml replacement of NG tube outputs. A plain anteroposterior radiograph of the chest is taken to confirm proper placement of the tube in the stomach.

The reported incidence of acute ulceration in patients with SCI is approximately 5 percent, but is likely to be higher owing to failure of recognition in many cases.[47,48] Endogenous steroid release, iatrogenic steroid administration, and increased acetylcholine due to unopposed vagal stimulation contribute to the increased risk. The risk rises substantially if the clinical condition includes respiratory compromise, multiple injuries, early surgical procedures, or pre-existing stomach pathology. When the airway is adequately protected and a gastric or duodenal tube is in place, antacids such as Mylanta (30 ml) should be administered every six hours. Intravenous H_2-(histamine)-receptor blockers (cimetidine, ranitidine, pepsid) are continuously administered. These agents can cause CNS depression (though ranitidine has fewer CNS effects) and should be used cautiously in the presence of associated head injury. Most H_2-blockers interfere with hepatic microsomal metabolism and can alter the pharmakokinetics of warfarin sodium, benzodiazepines, and anticonvulsants.[49] Exacerbation of coexistent renal or hepatic dysfunction is another recognized side-effect. All patients should be monitored closely with continuous BP and heart rate monitoring. Serum hematocrit should be checked twice daily and guaiac test are performed on all stools, Gastric pH is monitored every two to four hours and antacid doses are adjusted to keep $pH > 4.5$. Paralyzed, insensate patients rarely complain of localized pain, so anorexia of unknown cause, tachycardia, shoulder-tip pain, or vague, nonlocalized abdominal discomfort should be earnestly investigated. For stable patients, low-pressure continuous suction, iced saline lavage, antacids (IV and enteral), and prompt, judicious use of blood transfusion constitute the preliminary treatment of gastroduodenal hemorrhage. Bedside endoscopy performed by a gastroenterologist or general surgeon has low morbidity and can be done in the ICU. Endoscopy has an 85 percent accuracy in diagnosing the site of bleeding and can be used in therapy.[50] Patients in need of laparotomy can be rapidly identified.

In addition to gastric decompression and ulcer prevention in the acute post-injury phase, attention should be directed toward meeting the nutritional requirements of the traumatized, paralyzed patient.[51] Clinical factors such as the presence of multi-organ trauma, young age of the typical SCI victim, cord level of injury, degree of respiratory support, infection or fever, and healing requirements must be identified.[52] Immediately following injury, there is typically a gain in weight due to fluid sequestration, and lower body temperature and basal metabolic rate. Within 24 hours, there is a shift to catabolism enhanced by the endogenous release and iatrogenic administration of glucocorticoids. There is weight loss due to mobilization of retained fluids, decreased body fat, and decreased lean body mass due to breakdown of protein in muscle. Metabolism of protein yields amino acids, which provide nitrogen substrates for caloric energy via gluconeogenesis. Maximal nitrogen loss occurs between the fourth and fifth days. Glycogen and fat are metabolized to yield glucose and fatty acids. Glucose is utilized by the central nervous system, immune system, and in wound healing. Fatty acids are used for cardiac and skeletal muscle and respiratory energy needs.

Overshooting energy requirements, on the other hand, can worsen hypermetabolism, hyperglycemia, and increased CO_2 production, and can compromise respiratory function and cause hepatic steatosis. It is wrong to use nitrogen balance calculations to assess nutritional effectiveness in SCI patients since denervation of large muscle masses below the level of the cord lesion leads to a negative nitrogen balance in the acute period. Measurement with bedside charts or monitoring of energy expenditure offers a more reliable estimation. Once the patient is beyond the acute phase, the clinician must be aware of decreasing caloric requirements. After one to two weeks, the SCI patient's basal metabolic rate (BMR) will decrease. Body fat content rises as lean body mass (especially muscle) decreases. In fact, in the stable, post-acute quadriplegic patient, actual mean energy expenditure is 67 to 80 percent of expected.[53,54] Whereas most acute, critically ill patients require 30 to 40 kcal/kg/day, subacute or chronic quadriplegic patients require approximately 22.7 kcal/kg/day, and paraplegic patients approximately 27.9 kcal/kg/day.[55]

Because of ileus, associated head or abdominal injuries, aspiration pneumonia, cervical traction, or other complicating factors, oral or enteral feeding may be delayed for days or even weeks.[56] Though few data are available for SCI patients, parenteral nutrition has been shown to decrease morbidity and mortality in brain injury.[57] Peripheral total parenteral nutrition (PPN), in the form of 1000 ml of 8.5 percent amino acids, 1000 ml of 10 percent dextrose, and trace elements, can be mixed to deliver 2 liters of 5 percent dextrose per 24 hours. This solution is hypocaloric for most acutely ill patients, however, and most intensivists add 500 ml of 20 percent Intralipid. The efficaciousness of PPN, however, is limited, owing to the sensitivity of small- and medium-sized veins to hyperosmolar solutions. Central total parenteral nutrition (TPN) is the method of choice (via subclavian or internal jugular catheter) to deliver maximal energy needs, and many authors advocate starting the patient on TPN within the first 24 to 48 hours of injury.[58] When starting, graded increases in glucose concentration are recommended to avoid complications of hyperglycemia (>250 mg/dl) and glucosuria. In general, patients are susceptible to fluid overload owing to diminished vascular resistance and low salt tolerance. Other complications include prolonged hyperinsulinemia, hyperphosphatemia, hypermagnesemia, and increased urinary excretion of bone minerals in the early phase of cord injury.[59]

Physiological feeding via the alimentary tract is preferred and should be instituted as soon as clinically appropriate. For patients unable to swallow or protect their airway, a nasogastric or (preferably) a nasoduodenal tube can be placed easily. Nasogastric tubes allow for bolus feedings, which are more physiological although they carry the risk of aspiration. Gastric aspirates should be checked every hour and feedings started if they are less than 50 ml. Initial concentrations of full strength Osmolite or Isocal at a rate of 30 ml/hour can be increased slowly until nutritional requirements are met. Residual volumes are aspirated hourly, and feedings are held for 30 minutes if volumes exceed 75 ml.

In cases of delayed gastric emptying, small-bore, distally-weighted nasoduodenal (ND) tubes are useful. They are more difficult to place, however, and the small intestine is less tolerant of large or rapid infusions, which can cause fluid and electrolyte shifts and diarrhea. It usually is not possible to aspirate residual volume, owing to the extended length and narrow caliber of ND tubing. Advantages include lower risk of aspiration and consistent delivery of nutrients to the small intestine. Invasive modes, such as gastrostomy or jejunostomy, should be deferred for several weeks to allow for possible recovery of eating ability.

A critically important yet often overlooked or underestimated component of GI management is evacuation of the bowels. Following SCI there is usually immediate fecal incontinence, followed by constipation and lack of bowel movements for three to seven days. Normally, when the rectum is distended by fecal matter, there is a reflex relaxation of the internal anal sphincter and an increase in external anal sphincter tone (the anorectal reflex). In an upper motor neuron bowel (lesion above the conus medullaris), the internal anal sphincter is stimulated by the enteric nervous system to maintain resting tone. With SCI, there usually is little or no control of the external sphincter, and it rapidly relaxes, allowing for automatic defecation. Since the internal anal sphincter is relexively relaxed, defecation can be initiated by digital stimulation or suppositories to maintain a regular bowel schedule.[46] Presence of a bulbocavernosus or anal reflex indicates that rectal stimulation will likely result in bowel evacuation. This is not the case with lower motor neuron injury of the spine. With lesions below the conus, there is loss of the anorectal reflex, and digital stimulation is not helpful.

The most physiological way to maintain regular bowel habits is dietary fiber. The addition of 10 to 20 grams of fiber per day is recommended. If the patient is not able to take oral bran fiber, other bulk fibers can be given by NG or ND tube, such as psyllium hydrophobic mucilloid (Metamucil, Prodiem). Stool softeners like dioctyl sodium sulfosuccinate (Colace) are effective, but should be administered with caution in the SCI patient. Sulfosuccinate has a detergent-like action in increasing the water content of stool, but also can disrupt rectal mucous membranes and cause increased absorption of medications.[26] Harsh laxatives are not intended for prolonged use; they can result in rectal mucosal irritation, bleeding, cramping, or autonomic dysreflexia. Osmotic laxatives such as synthetic dissacharides (Lactulose) which are not split by intestinal enzymes are useful. They are broken down into organic acids by gut bacteria, resulting in acidification of the stool and reduced ammonia absorption. The result is increased water in the stool.

The recommended dose is 2 to 7.5 grams once or twice per day. Glycerine suppositories are gentle and also useful in stimulating defecation.

Enemas are potentially harmful procedures in the SCI patient. In particular, soapsuds enemas should be avoided; they cause mucosal damage, Na^+/K^+ imbalance, and hypovolemia (by drawing excess water into the colon). Saline and oil retention enemas can be used to assist in passage of stools, but large volumes should be avoided as they can initiate an autonomic crisis.

Urological Considerations

The primary urological goal in the intensive care management of acute spinal cord injury is maintenance of satisfactory renal function and an efficient means of bladder emptying. The initial evaluation must rule out an anatomic lesion in the genitourinary (GU) tract, as this organ system is commonly associated with spinal cord injury. Second, one must assess the level of neurological function (upper versus lower motor neuron bladder). This determination is crucial to deciding upon the best method of bladder emptying. The overall goal is maintenance of renal blood flow and sufficient glomerular filtration, control of acid-base balance, elimination of urine, and prevention of urinary tract infection.

Initial assessment of the multitrauma patient will reveal a high incidence of GU tract injury. Regardless of whether hematuria is present, a complete evaluation including CT scan of the abdomen and pelvis and/or intravenous pyelogram is indicated for the immediate work-up in patients with visceral trauma.[60] If the bladder or urethra is suspected to have been injured, cystography or retrograde urethrography are performed. After several days to two weeks, spinal cord shock may result in loss of all reflex activity below the level of injury. Internal urinary sphincter closure is maintained, however, thus blocking micturition and necessitating placement of a urethral catheter.[61] If no blood is seen at the urethral meatus, a small-bore catheter (12, 14 French) is placed for the first 24 to 48 hours to monitor urine output closely. To avoid urethral injury catheters should not be placed in patients with frank hematuria or in males with priapism.[62] In these cases, a suprapubic tube is placed by the urologist.

The initial neurological examination can reveal important information for the continued urological management of the SCI patient. The bulbocavernosus reflex is elicited by pinching the glans penis or clitoris or by applying a gentle tug on the urethral catheter. The response is contraction of the perianal musculature. If intact, this reflex indicates integrity of the conus micturition (parasympathetic) center and lower sacral elements.[63,64] If spinal cord shock is present, the striated muscles of the pelvic floor are the first to regain relex activity, followed by the detrusor muscle fibers. In an upper motor neuron bladder (with the lesion above the conus), reflex bladder contractions recur but initially are weak and not enough to open the bladder neck and proximal urethra. These contractions gradually increase in power to provide spontaneous voiding. Prompt placement of the urethral or suprapubic catheter is critical; even two to three hours of bladder dilatation can cause a delay in the return of reflex activity and prolong the time invasive techniques are needed for bladder emptying. Once the patient is stable, the indwelling catheter is removed and intermittent catheterization is performed every six hours. The timing is then adjusted so that 300 to 350 ml of urine are removed with each catheterization. Clean, intermittent catheterization reduces weeks, patients with upper motor neuron bladders can be tested for spontaneous voiding ability. Prophylactic antibiotics have not been shown to decrease the incidence of clinically significant urinary tract infections and should not be used. Treatment is justifiable if the patient is ill or febrile and no other source of infection is identified. Bacteriuria is practically unavoidable in SCI, and usually is tolerated by the patient. Routine surveillance cultures are recommended every few days in the first few weeks to identify potential pathogens and to assess the degree of pyuria.

In quadriplegic patients with suprasacral lesion, spontaneous voiding is acceptable if intravesical pressure in urodynamic studies is not significant ($<$60–70 cm H_2O) and residuals are small ($<$75 ml) and uninfected. Male patients can use a condom catheter. Though no satisfactory external collection device is available for females, high-absorbance pads can be used. With upper motor neuron bladders, detrusor contractions and bladder emptying can be elicited by suprapubic tapping. Problems arise when spastic contraction of the external striated sphincter obstructs bladder emptying when reflex detrusor contraction occurs in response to regular bladder distension. This pathological condition is referred to as detrusor-sphincter dyssynergia and occurs when normal signals from the pontine-mesencephalic reticular formation do not cross the level of cord injury to coordinate afferent signals of bladder distension with efferent impulses to inhibit external sphincter contraction. In fact, the higher the cord level of injury, the greater the incidence of detrusor-sphincter dyssynergia. Alpha sympatholytics (phentolamine, phenoxybenzamine, prazosin) and skeletal muscle relaxants (dantrolene, baclofen) can be used to depress the external sphincter.[65] If bladder hyperreflexia is present, causing too-frequent detrusor contraction, bladder musculature can be relaxed with anticholinergics (propantheline, atropine) or smooth muscle relaxants (oxybutinin).[66] Along with decreasing detrusor pressure, bladder capacity is increased, thereby increasing the time interval between voiding. Surgical therapy for external sphincter spasticity such as transurethral sphincterotomy should be postponed for several months to a year to allow for potential recovery of coordinated bladder contraction and external sphincter relaxation. The ultimate goal is to achieve a "balanced bladder" state in which voiding is not more frequent than every two hours and residual urine is <100 ml in a low-pressure system.

In paraplegic patients with suprasacral (upper motor neuron) lesions, spontaneous voiding into an external device is possible if vesical voiding pressures are low. If intravesical pressures are high and/or there is detrusor hyperreflexia, the first line of management is to paralyze the bladder pharmacologically to create a low pressure system. Oxybutinin (Ditropan), propantheline, and flavoxate are the medications of choice. Ditropan can be started at 5 mg bid and increased to 5 mg qid if needed. Manual depression of the bladder (Crede maneuver) can create very high vesical pressures and should be avoided.

In paraplegic patients with a lower motor neuron (arreflexic) bladder, a different approach is necessary. For many patients, abdominal straining or manual compression of the bladder (Crede maneuver) will result in satisfactory emptying. Intermittent catheterization is reserved for patients with high residual volumes (>100 ml). In-dwelling catheters increase the risk of urethrocutaneous fistulae, urethritis, bladder calculi, contractures, and urosepsis and should be avoided. The urine should be acidified with daily oral ascorbic acid or cranberry juice intake.

In addition to these complications, inadequate bladder emptying can result in very harmful autonomic crises. This response, referred to as autonomic dysreflexia, is found in patients with lesions above most of the sympathetic outflow from the cord (T6). Afferent signals from a distended bladder enter the cord below the lesion, ascend in the lateral funiculi to the level of the lesion, and activate sympathetic reflexes along the way. The lack of descending inhibitory control results in a massive outflow of sympathetic discharge, resulting in hypertension, diaphoresis above the level of the lesion, piloerection, restlessness, anxiety, pounding headache, flushing of the face, and paroxysmal bradycardia. Other less common cause of autonomic dysreflexia include visceral distension (fecal impaction), cold air stimulation of the skin (especially after cleaning), catheterization, testicular torsion, or excessive anal stimulation (digital disimpaction).[67] Treatment consists of removing the stimulus promptly. For severe hypertension, hydralazine or IV nitroprusside (100 mg/ml in 5 percent dextrose starting at rate of 1 mg/kg/min) can be instituted. Ganglionic blocking agents such as phentolamine, trimethophan, pentolamine, and amyl nitrate have been used with variable success. Phenoxybenzene, an alpha-receptor blocker, is another alternative medication. Though autonomic crises can be severe in the early phases of SCI, they are usually less severe six to 12 months later.

OPTIMAL MEDICAL MANAGEMENT

The best current initial medical and pharmacological therapy of spinal cord injury must be based on the potentially reversible pathophysiological changes that occur related to reduction in spinal cord blood flow and oxygenation and the beneficial effects that have been demonstrated with high-dose methylprednisolone treatment.

Because of the known tendency of spinal cord perfusion to fall abruptly acutely after spinal cord injury, systemic blood pressure should be vigorously supported, and, on occasion, mild hypertension induced to assure adequate spinal cord blood flow for at least the first 12 to 24 hours following injury. Tator's group in Toronto have consistently shown that re-establishing normotension alone does not necessarily ensure restoration of adequate blood flow in the injured spinal cord.[9,10] Fluid resuscitation is a keystone to the initial therapy. Even in the absence of associated systemic injury, however, it may be very difficult to maintain an adequate perfusion pressure in the presence of vasogenic spinal shock. Vasogenic spinal shock occurs frequently with mid- to upper level cervical injuries as a result of sympathetic vascular denervation and peripheral vasodilatation. Fluid resuscitation should consist of an appropriate combination of crystalloid and colloid solutions or blood replacement, depending on the presence of associated injury. In most instances, lactated Ringer's or normal saline is the best initial fluid to employ. If, despite adequate fluid replacement, the blood pressure cannot be normalized or elevated slightly, pressors such as dopamine or Neo-Synephrine may be instituted. An additional temporary measure in improving peripheral vascular resistance after spinal cord injury may be the use of the pneumatic antishock garment.

As spinal cord blood flow depends not only on perfusion pressure, but on blood rheology as well, it is important to consider measures to reduce blood viscosity, thereby increasing perfusion. Decreased viscosity can be achieved maximally with blood hematocrits in the range of 33 to 37 percent. The use of Plasmanate, Albuminsol, Dextran or other similar volume-expanding agents can be helpful.

Maintenance of adequate tissue oxygenation is also important in the first hours following spinal cord injury.

Inadequate oxygenation of the injured region of the cord will only hasten the pathophysiological cascade that occurs. Careful attention must be paid to airway maintenance, intubation, and assisted ventilation when necessary to maintain satisfactory blood P_{O_2} levels.

If treatment can be initiated within eight hours of injury, methylprednisolone should be given as a bolus of 30 mg/kg intravenously, followed by continuous infusion of 5.4 mg/kg/h for 23 hours. Methylprednisolone should not be given if more than eight hours have elapsed since the spinal cord injury.

References

1. Chestnut RM, Marshall LF: Early assessment, transport, and management of patients with posttraumatic spinal instability, in Cooper PR (ed): *Management of posttraumatic spinal instability*. AANS Publications Committee, Neurosurgical Topics, Park Ridge, IL, 1990.
2. Tominaga S: Periodical, neurological-functional assessment for cervical cord injury. *Paraplegia* 1989; 27:227–236.
3. Geisler F, Dorsey F, Coleman W: Recovery of motor function after spinal-cord injury—a randomized, placebo-controlled trial with GM-1 ganglioside. *N Engl J Med* 1991; 324:26:1829–1838.
4. Krouskop TA: The role of mattresses and beds in preventing pressure sores, in Lee By, Ostrander LE, Cochran GVB, Shaw WW (eds): *Spinal cord injured patient: Comprehensive management*. Philadelphia: WB Saunders, 1991.
5. Green BA, et al: The acute management of spinal cord injury, in Lee BY, Ostrander LE, Cochran GVB, Shaw WW (eds.): *The spinal cord injured patient: Comprehensive management*. Philadelphia: WB Saunders, 1991.
6. Doran SE, Papadopoulos SM, Ducker TB, Lillehei KO: Magnetic resonance imaging documentation of coexistent traumatic locked facets of the cervical spine and disc herniation. *J Neurosurg* 1993; 79:341–345.
7. Crutchfield NG: Skeletal traction for dislocation of the cervical spine. Report of a case. *South Surgeon* 1933; 2:156–159.
8. Gardner WJ: Principle of spring loaded points for cervical traction. Technical note. *J Neurosurg* 1973; 39:543–544.
9. Star A, Jones A, Cotler J, et al: Immediate closed reduction of cervical spine dislocations using traction. *Spine* 1990; 10:1068–1072.
10. Schriger DL, Baxter L, LeGassick T, Blinman T: Spinal immobilization on a flat backboard: Does it result in neutral position of the cervical spine? *Ann Emerg Med* 1991; 8:878–881.
11. Wong AMK, Leong CP, Chen CM: The traction angle and cervical intervertebral separation. *Spine* 1992; 17(2):136–138.
12. Chestnut RM, Marshall LF: Early assessment, transport, and management of patients with posttraumatic spinal instability, in Cooper PR (ed): *Management of posttraumatic spinal instability*. AANS Publications Committee, Neurosurgical Topics, Park Ridge, IL, 1990.
13. Hadley MN: Spinal orthoses, in Cooper PR (ed): *Management of Posttraumatic Spinal Instability*. AANS Publications Committee, Neurosurgical Topics, Park Ridge, IL, 1990.
14. Rizzolo SJ, Piazza MR, Cotler JM, et al: The effect of torque pressure on halo pin complication rates. *Spine* 1993; 18(15):2163–2166.
15. Mandabach M, Ruge JR, Yoon SH, McLone DG: Pediatric axis fractures: Early halo immobilization, management and outcome. *Pediatr Neurosurg* 1993; 19:225–232.
16. Williams FH, Nelms DK, McGaharan KM: Brain abscess: A rare complication of halo usage. *Arch Phys Med Rehab* 1992; 73(5):490–492.
17. Kinnaird R, Jelsma R: A portable traction device for cervical fractures. *J Neurosurg* 1992; 76:544–545.
18. Wagner FC: Injuries to the cervical spine and spinal cord, in Youmans JR (ed): *Neurological surgery*, (3d ed) Philadelphia: WB Saunders, 1990.
19. Weiss MH: Mid- and lower cervical spine injuries, in Wilkens RH, Rengachary SS (eds): *Neurosurgery*, New York: McGraw-Hill, 1985:1708–1716.
20. Green BA: Response to "Management of locked facets of the cervical spine," by Maiman D, Barolat G, Larson S. *Neurosurgery* 1986; 18(5):546–547.
21. Sonntag V: Management of bilateral locked facets of the cervical spine. *Neurosurgery*, 1981; 8(2):150–152.
22. Maiman D, Barolat G, Larson S: Management of bilateral locked facets of the cervical spine. *Neurosurgery*, 1986; 18(5):542–547.
23. Rockswold GL, Bergman TA, Ford SE: Halo immobilization and surgical fusion: Relative indications and effectiveness in treatment of 140 cervical spine injuries. *J Trauma* 1990; 30(7):893–898.
24. Martinez JA: Spinal cord syndromes and spinal shock, in McSwain NE, Martinez JA (eds): *Cervical spine trauma*, New York, 1989.
25. Zejdlik CP: *Management of spinal cord injury*, 2d ed. Boston: Jones and Bartlett, 1992.
26. Hanak M, Scott A: *Spinal cord injury: An illustrated guide for health care professionals*. New York: Springer, 1983.
27. Groomes TE, Huang CT: Orthostatic hypotension after spinalcord injury: treatment with fludrocortisone and ergotamine. *Arch Phys Med Rehabil* 1991; 72:56–58.
28. Meakem TD, Meakem TJ, Rappaport W: Airway compromise from prevertebral soft tissue swelling during placement of halo-traction for cervical spine injury. *Anesthesiology* 1990; 73:775–776.
29. Giffin JP, Grush K: Spinal cord injury treatment and the anesthesiologist, in Lee BY, Ostrander LE, Cochran GVB, Shaw WW (eds): *The spinal cord injured patient: Comprehensive management*. Philadelphia: WB Saunders, 1991.
30. Weber RK: Respiratory management of acute cervical cord injuries, in Tator CH (ed): *Early management of acute spinal injury*. New York: Raven Press, 1982.
31. Bindsher L: Respiratory care. *Curr Opinion Anesthesiol* 1989; 2:173–177.

32. LaSala PA, Frost EAM: Intensive care management of spinal cord injury, in Alderson JD, Frost EA (eds): London: Butterworths, 1990.
33. McMichan JC, Westbrook PR: Pulmonary dysfunction following traumatic quadriplegia. *JAMA* 1980; 243:528.
34. Watson W: Venous thrombosis and pulmonary embolism in spinal cord injury patients. *Paraplegia* 1978; 16:113–121.
35. Waring WP, Karunas RS: Acute spinal cord injuries and the incidence of clinically occurring thromboembolic disease. *Paraplegia* 1991; 29(1):8–16.
36. Lee BY: Management of peripheral vascular disease in the spinal cord injured patient, in Lee BY, Ostrander LE, Cochran GVB, Shaw WW: *The spinal cord injured patient: Comprehensive management*. Philadelphia: Saunders, 1991.
37. Kulkarni JR, Burt AA, Tromans AT, Constable PD: Prophylactic low dose heparin anticoagulant therapy in patients with spinal cord injuries: A retrospective study. *Paraplegia* 1992; 30(3):169–172.
38. Black PM, Baker MF, Snook CP: Experience with external calf compression in neurology and neurosurgery. *Neurosurgery* 1986; 18(4):440–444.
39. Caprini JA, Araelus JI, Traverso JI, et al: Low molecular weight heparins and external pneumatic compression as options for venous thromboembolism prophylaxis: A surgeon's perspective. *Semin Thromb Hemostas* 1991; 17:356–366.
40. Merli GJ: Management of deep vein thrombosis in spinal cord injury. *Chest* 1992; 102(Suppl 6):652S–657S.
41. Green D, Hull RD, Mammen EF, et al: Deep vein thrombosis in spinal cord injury. Summary and recommendations. *Chest* 1992; 102(6 Suppl):633S–635S.
42. Meredith JW, Young JS, O'Neil EA, et al: Femoral catheters and deep venous thrombosis: A prospective evaluation with venous duplex sonography. *J Trauma* 1993; 35(2):187–191.
43. Watts C, Gaede S, Pulliam MW: Problems associated with multiple trauma, in Youmans JR (ed): *Neurological Surgery*. Philadelphia: Saunders, 1990:2554–2561.
44. Sautter RO, Larson DE, Bhattacharyya SK, et al: The limited utility of fibrinogen K-125 leg scanning. *Arch Intern Med* 1983; 139:148–153.
45. Wilson TI, Rogers FB, Wald SL, et al: Prophylactic vena cava filter insertion in patients with traumatic spinal cord injury: Preliminary results. *Neurosurgery* 1994; 35(2):234–239.
46. Seaton T, Hollingworth R: GI complications in spinal cord injuries, in Block RF, Basbaum M (eds): *Management of spinal cord injury*. Baltimore: Williams & Wilkins, 1986.
47. Kraft C: Bladder and bowel management in spinal cord injury, in Buchanan LE, Nawoczenski DA (eds): *Spinal cord injury: Concepts and management approaches*. Baltimore, Williams & Wilkins, 1987.
48. Kewalramani S: Neurogenic gastroduodenal ulceration and bleeding associated with spinal cord injuries. *J Trauma* 1979; 19(4):259–265.
49. Segal JF, Brunnemann SR: Clinical pharmacokinetics in patients with spinal cord injuries. *Clin Pharmacokinet* 1989; 17(2):109–129.
50. Tanaka M, Uchiyama M, Kitano M: Gastroduodenal disease in chronic spinal cord injuries: An endoscopic study. *Arch Surg* 1979; 114:185–187.
51. Kuric J, Lucas CE, Ledgerwood AM, et al: Nutritional support: A prophylaxis against stress bleeding after spinal cord injury. *Paraplegia* 1989; 27(2):140–145.
52. Nikas DL: Pathophysiology and nursing interventions in acute spinal cord injury. *Trauma Q* 1988; 4(3):23–44.
53. Kearns PJ, Pipp TL, Qurik M, et al: Nutritional requirements in quadriplegics. Meeting of the American Society of Parenteral and Enteral Nutrition, Washington, DC, Jan. 23–26, 1983.
54. Kolpeck J, Oh G, Record K, et al: Comparison of urinary urea nitrogen excretion and measured energy expenditure in spinal cord injury and nonsteroid-treated severe head trauma patients. *J Parent Ent Nutr* 1989; 13(3):277–80.
55. Cox S, Weiss S, Posunick E, et al: Energy expenditure after spinal cord injury: An evaluation of stable rehabilitating patients. *J Trauma* 1985; 25(5):419–423.
56. Norton JA, Oh LG, McClain C, et al: Intolerance to enteral feeding in the brain injured patient. *J Neurosurg* 1988; 68:62–6.
57. Young B, Oh L, Twyman D: The effect of nutritional support outcome from severe head injury. *J Neurosurg* 1987; 67:668–676.
58. Green BA, Eismont FJ: Acute spinal cord injury: A systems approach. *CNS Trauma* 1984; 1:173–195.
59. Kirveli O, Askanazi J: Anaesthetic care for spinal injuries: parenteral nutrition, in Alderson JD, Frost EA (eds): *Spinal cord injuries: Anaesthetic and associated care*. London: Butterworths, 1990.
60. Owens GF, Addonizio JC: Urologic evaluation and management of the spinal cord injured patient, in Lee BY, Cochran GVB, Shaw WW (eds): *The spinal cord injured patient: Comprehensive management*. Philadelphia: Saunders, 1991.
61. McGuire EJ: Immediate management of the inability to void, in Parsons KF, Fitzpatrick JM (eds): *Practical urology in spinal cord injury*. London: Springer-Verlag, 1991.
62. Graham SD: Present urological treatment of spinal cord injury patients. *J Urol* 1981; 26:1.
63. Krishnan KR: General considerations in the management of the urinary tract, in Parsons KF, Fitzpatrick JM (eds): *Practical urology in spinal cord injury*. London: Springer-Verlag, 1991.
64. Perlow DL, Dionko AC: Predicting lower urinary tract dysfunctions in patients with spinal cord injury. *Urology* 1981; 18:531.
65. Heerschorn S, Gerridzen RG: The management of the neurogenic bladder, in Bloch RF, Basbaum M (eds): *Management of spinal cord injuries*. Baltimore: Williams & Wilkins, 1986.
66. Staskin DR, Krone RJ: A practical approach to urodynamic evaluation, in Parsons KF, Fitzpatrick JM (ed): *Practical urology in spinal cord injury*. London: Springer-Verlag, 1991.
67. Pearman JW, England EJ: *The urologic management of the patient following spinal cord injury*. Springfield, IL: Charles C Thomas, 1973.

CHAPTER 86

APPLICATION OF EVOKED POTENTIAL MONITORING IN SPINAL CORD INJURY

Gary Shurman
Paul Lobaugh
Jack E. Wilberger, Jr.

INTRODUCTION

Historically, somatosensory evoked potentials (SSEPs) were first applied to the study of spinal cord injury (SCI) over 50 years ago.[1] Since that time, researchers and clinicians have disagreed over the utility of evoked potentials (EPs) as diagnostic and prognostic tools after SCI. More recently, the controversy has focused on the role of intraoperative EPs during spinal surgery. Additionally, the current, although limited, clinical application of motor evoked potentials (MEPs) has renewed interest in defining the application and interpretation of neurophysiological data relative to the diagnosis, treatment, and prognosis of the spinal cord-injured patient.

EVOKED POTENTIAL GENERATION AND ACQUISITION

SSEPs have been extensively investigated and analyzed for generator sources, effects of stimulus variables, effects of subject variables, and effects of disease, lesions, and injury on receptor transmission pathways and cortical generators.[2,3]

Stimulation of a mixed or sensory nerve as well as dermatomal fields begins the chain of electrical events culminating in the SSEP wave form. For lower extremity SSEPs, the neural volley is initiated at a distal site such as the posterior tibial nerve at the ankle and propagated along the nerve to the spinal cord. This propagated volley may be detected at any point along the nerve by using surface electrode recording techniques that are routinely done with nerve conduction velocity studies. The incoming volley is synapsed at the dorsal horn cells of the dorsal root ganglion and propagated through the ascending dorsal columns of the spinal cord. Some investigators have described a stationary, far-field potential that is optimally recorded at the L1 vertebral level and is believed to represent this synchronized synaptic discharge activity. This response, however, is technically quite difficult to acquire. The next order synapse that can be recorded reliably is the potential generated in brainstem structures, most likely the lateral meniscus, and referred to as the foramen magnum response. From this point, the signal is relayed via third-order neurons to both the thalamus and primary sensory cortex.

The upper extremity SSEP is best acquired by stimulation of median or ulnar nerve at the wrist. A large amplitude wave is generated by propagation of the impulse through the brachial plexus. This is typically referred to as the Erb's point potential and can be visualized optimally by electrode recording over the supraclavicular fossa. Subsequent transmission to the spinal cord and brainstem to the sensory cortex is identical to that from lower extremity stimulation sites.

The primary clinical criticism of SSEPs is the fact that their conduction primarily to the dorsal columns of the spinal cord limits their usefulness and applicability except in situations where the dorsal columns are either preferentially affected or the spinal cord is globally "injured." The importance of the dorsal column in this process has been emphasized by a number of investigators. One of the most widely reported studies is that of Cusick et al. who demonstrated in monkeys that selective segmental lesions of the dorsal columns resulted in almost complete attenuation of associated cortical evoked responses. Conversely, isolated segmental dorsal column preservation allowed for intact transmission.[4] Other investigators, however, have found evidence of conduction of SSEPs to pathways other than the dorsal column. Ziganow, in a clinical study, found that intact spinothalamic tract functioning was necessary for optimization of certain components of the SSEP wave form.[5] Nevertheless, most clinicians would agree that at best SSEPs provide only inferential information concerning ascending tracts other than those in the dorsal columns. These anatomic considerations obviously must be borne in mind in clinical applications of SSEPs to SCI.

The importance of technique for acquisition of reliable EP wave form data must be emphasized. The SSEP is easily contaminated by patient artifact or by environmental sources, such as 60-cycle electrical artifact or other radiofrequency sources. The anatomic location of stimulation and stimulus parameters of rate, duration, current type, and direction, as well as intensity, must be uniform across patients in order to assure that clinical data are not influenced by environmental variables. Normative data for latency and amplitude of the primary EP response peaks have been established; however, each institution clinically applying EPs to SCIs should develop their own normative data to confirm that it compares favorably with that reported in the literature.

The MEP was first described in 1980 by Mertan and Morton and has been investigated with increasing vigor over the subsequent years.[2,6,7] Motor evoked potentials are produced by synchronized, excitatory volleys in corticospinal pathways. MEPs can be initiated by either cortical or direct spinal cord stimulation. Both magnetic and electrical forms of stimulation have been studied. With cortical stimulation at each anterior horn cell synapse, an excitatory postsynaptic potential is generated. If there is sufficient temporal and spatial summation of potentials, the anterior horn cell will fire and trigger a motor unit/muscle response. Thus, responses can be monitored in both peripheral nerve (neurogenic) or muscle (myogenic). With direct spinal cord stimulation, electrodes can be placed either epidurally or in adjacent spinous processes. Subsequent neurogenic or myogenic responses can be recorded.

The pros and cons of magnetic versus electrical stimulation and the specific issues of MEP acquisition and interpretation are dealt with in several recent reviews. Presently, however, MEP techniques are considered investigational, and clinical applications have not been approved by governmental regulatory agencies in North America.

REVIEW OF EP STUDIES IN SPINAL CORD INJURY

Application of EP studies to the laboratory investigation of spinal cord injury in animal models has been notable over the past 15 years. Various species (rat, dog, cat, hog, rabbit, and monkey) and injury methods (static compression, dynamic compression, vascular disruption, spinal cord transection, and spinal cord distraction) have been studied with EPs.

The research to date on animal models of SCI would support several observations. First, SSEPs change after SCI and appear reversible in proportion to the magnitude of trauma. This generalization applies across species and injury methods and is applicable to both SSEPs and MEPs. Several studies have noted that direct spine recordings are more sensitive and/or specific to injury changes and patterns than are surface-recorded cortical SSEPs. Conflicting data exist as to the relative merits of SSEP versus MEP. Some studies report MEP as being more sensitive to traumatic injury changes in spinal cord conduction; others note that SSEPs are more sensitive to changes in conduction due to compressive or distractive forces. Second, SSEP is absent when the stimulation site is distal to a complete spinal cord injury/transection. Third, SSEP varies in proportion to the magnitude of injury. However, normal SSEPs may be present with significant spinal cord injury.

Clinical research on SSEPs in spinal cord injury began appearing over 20 years ago. Early reports by McGarry and others described significant alterations in SSEPs as studied in small groups of SCI patients.[8] The general postulate from these studies was that SCI would result in an overall reduction in SSEP amplitude and increase in latency and a general loss of wave form integrity.[9–12]

DIAGNOSTIC AND PROGNOSTIC UTILITY

The past 20 years have seen over 60 reported studies that deal with the diagnostic and prognostic significance of SSEP monitoring after SCI.

A number of clinicians and investigators have attempted to correlate changes in EP amplitude, latency, and wave form with both the diagnosis and prognosis of SCI. However, in spite of their regular application for over two decades, there remains little consensus over the place of EPs in this regard.[12–15]

In 1978, Rowed and Tator[16] reported that while a variety of SSEP abnormalities are seen with incomplete SCI, wave forms are invariably absent with complete SCI. They also suggested that the more normal the SSEP after SCI, the greater the likelihood and magnitude of neurological recovery, with clinical improvement paralleling improvements in the SSEP tracings. In the intervening years, these findings have both been confirmed and challenged. Emphasizing the limitations of SSEPs, York et al.[15] reported on 71 patients with complete SCI, finding over 20 percent with retained tibial or peroneal EPs even though no motor or sensory function was regained during 1 year of follow-up. In 43 incomplete SCI patients, these authors were not able to predict clinical recovery with wave form or latency analysis. They did, however, suggest that the combination of absent SSEPs and a clinically incomplete SCI portended little if any neurological recovery.[16]

Ziganow[5] studying 25 incomplete SCI patients concluded that certain attributes of the SSEP wave form were encountered with statistically significant greater frequency in patients who ultimately had marked neurological recovery: large amplitudes within the initial 80 milliseconds; shorter latency and greater amplitude of the first major positive wave; increased wave form complexity. Similar findings were reported by Li et al.[12] utilizing quantitative SSEP analysis. Interpeak latency across the SCI site and the amplitude of the early cortical responses were the most powerful predictors of neurological recovery at 6 months.[5]

Thus, based on these as well as a number of other studies, it appears reasonable to conclude that SCI patients with absent SSEPs acutely postinjury have little likelihood of useful neurological recovery regardless of whether their injury is clinically complete or incomplete. Any other prognostic implications for SSEPs remain unclear.

There have been very few published reports on MEPs after SCI. MacDonell and Donnan recently concluded that MEPs provide little if any useful information after acute SCI. In 25 SCI patients, magnetic MEPs could not be elicited either at rest or during attempts at voluntary contraction in patients who had no clinical evidence of volitional movement. This was true even for initially paralyzed muscles which subsequently recovered. Compared to normal controls, MEP thresholds were elevated even for muscles innervated above the level of injury. Repeat testing at 6 weeks after injury continued to show abnormalities which did not improve in parallel with neurological recovery.[17]

INTRAOPERATIVE EVOKED POTENTIALS

Although EP monitoring is increasingly advocated as an operative adjunct to spine/spinal cord surgery, a number of factors must be considered in its application. The neural pathways at risk must be amenable to monitoring and the opportunity for corrective intervention must exist if the EPs change significantly. Unfortunately, the operating room is often a hostile environment for EP acquisition and interpretation. One of the major considerations in this regard is the effect of general anesthetic agents on cortical EPs. All general anesthetic agents produce latency increases and changes in amplitude. The effects of most agents are additive, and the dose-related effects of inhaled anesthetics have been well documented. For example, nitrous oxide alone will slightly depress amplitude, but has little effect on latency. Since changes in the EP relative to preoperative baseline may appear similar whether the cause is surgical or anesthetic, one needs to be able to differentiate between sources of alteration.

All cortically generated waves of SSEP are affected by volatile inhalation anesthetics. A number of studies have documented EP changes due to various minimal alveolar concentrations (MAC) of halothane, enflurane, and isoflurane. Although there is considerable individual patient variation to various end-tidal MAC, general patterns and subsequent guidelines are apparent. More than one-half of patients demonstrate SSEP cortical wave from decrement at 1.0% MAC of isoflurane with 60% nitrous oxide, while all patients demonstrate severe alterations and/or complete abolishment of cortical EPs at 2% MAC with 60% nitrous oxide. Inhalation anesthetics have little if any effect on the brainstem components of SSEPs.

Intravenous anesthetics affect cortical SSEPs significantly less than do inhalation anesthetics. Narcotics such as fentanyl or sufentanil alter cortical SSEPs only in high doses, but responses still can be visualized. Interestingly, bolus administration of fentanyl has a much greater effect on cortical EPs than does a steady-state infusion. Barbiturates such as thiopental or pentobarbital have little effect on cortical and no effect upon subcortical SSEP. Reports indicate that SSEPs can be adequately monitored even under barbiturate-induced coma. Initial reports suggest that propofol has minimal latency shift/amplitude reduction effects on the SSEP and offers promise as an effective adjunct in neuroanesthesia.

Optimal anesthetic protocol in conjunction with EP monitoring is the "balanced" technique of narcotic with nitrous oxide. Jellinek and others have proposed a total intravenous anesthesia to provide large amplitude median nerve cortical SSEP, which may be extremely helpful in cervical surgery.[18] At the least, shared communication between the individual performing the monitoring and the anesthetist together with a coordinated plan stressing safe and effective anesthesia with adequate EP signals will lead to the optimal protocol. While no single technique will perfectly satisfy each member of the neurosurgical team, compromise through common goals usually will provide for an effective neuromonitoring environment.

Similar anesthetic problems can be encountered with MEP monitoring as well. Jellinek et al. studied the effects of nitrous oxide anesthesia on motor evoked responses utilizing N_2O concentrations of 20 to 70 percent.[18] They observed that a progressive increase in N_2O concentration clearly correlated with a progressive increase in latency and a decrease in amplitude of the MEPs. These authors recommended avoidance of N_2O concentrations of greater than 50 percent when attempting MEP monitoring. In a related article studying propofol, a reduction in response amplitude to 7 percent of baseline was seen utilizing this anesthetic technique.[19] Concerns arise even when utilizing a "balanced" technique of neuroanesthesia; Calancie described dramatic attenuation and/or elimination of myogenic responses to motor cortical stimulation with the addition of as little as 0.4% isoflurane.[20]

In spite of the above considerations, SSEPs have been commonly applied to cervical and thoracolumbar spine and spinal cord surgery. Presently, monitoring of the lumbosacral spine with SSEP for surgery caudal to the lumbar plexus is not usually performed owing to the relative insensitivity of mixed nerve SSEP to disruption. Utilizing SSEPs, C8 to T1 spinal cord levels can be studied via median or ulnar nerve stimulation in combination with the lower extremity mixed nerve. Bipolar surface electrodes are placed in a cathode proximal orientation above the course of the nerve at the wrist, ankle, popliteal fossa, fibular head, or, alternatively, along the ulnar groove at the elbow. The palmar wrist surface and medial ankle surface are most often utilized for stimulation sites, although the previously mentioned choices provide alternative access to the patient with limb anomalies or obstruction of primary stimulation sites by intravenous catheters, wounds, etc. Disposable pregelled adhesive stimulating electrodes are available commercially and are preferred because they maintain adhesiveness and uniform electrical impedance over periods of up to 20 h. Subdermal needle electrodes are a viable alternative to surface electrodes in cases where perfuse perspiration, sclerotic or edematous skin tissue, or obesity are obstacles to effective transdermal electrical excitation.

Intensity required for stimulation can be calculated based on a number of factors. One commonly accepted approach is to determine the amount of current (expressed in milliamperes) required to evoke a visibly detectable thenar or plantar twitch. Current intensity is then increased to twice this threshold value and maintained at this level throughout the case. A second approach is to set the level at a predetermined number for all patients. With either approach a maximum level of 50 milliamperes should be established; this is universally sufficient to evoke the SSEP supramaximally but not high enough to cause dermal damage. The stimulus duration should optimally be between 200 to 300 μsec. Increasing duration will result in greater delivery of energy to the nerve, and this may be used as higher intensity is required—but maximal available current is limited to 30 to 40 milliamperes.

Stimulus rates should include a delivery scheme that allows for rapid collection of data for averaging yet provides a sufficient time window to visualize the relevant bioelectric activity and excludes rhythmic extraneous nonbiological electrical signals (noise). A rate approximating 5 stimuli per second is usually sufficient for this purpose.

Baseline studies should be conducted immediately following induction of anesthesia. It is important to acquire preincision data prior to positioning the patient. SSEPs are collected immediately following positioning to ensure that tracings have not been altered.

Baseline traces are stored in computer memory and displayed online for analysis of peak latency and peak to trough amplitude of primary peripheral brainstem and cortical components. These components are first measured for the most distal latency (brachial plexus at the supraclavicular fossa or tibial nerve at the popliteal fossa). Normal latencies for these peaks are approximately 10 msec ($\pm$ 2 msec) depending on limb length, temperature, predisposing factors such as peripheral neuropathy, etc. Amplitudes are not compared to normal value tables as the variants associated with amplitude and far field evoked potentials is 10 times greater than latency variants. Thus, each patient becomes their own control at baseline and for the duration of the surgical case.

Brainstem components from stimulation of each extremity are then measured for peak N14 (wrist) and peak N31 (ankle). The difference between brainstem and peripheral latency is calculated to assess conduction time across the spinal segment. Typical ranges of conduction time are 3.8 to 5 msec for upper extremity and 20.5 to 26 msec for lower extremity stimulation respectively.

Cortical SSEPs that serve a dual purpose are collected simultaneously with a more caudal response. First, they represent redundant information regarding conduction via dorsal column spinal tract and are useful should the brainstem signal be lost due to technical/equipment malfunction or excessive electrical interference. Second, cortical SSEP data may be useful as a rudimentary index of brain neuroelectric activity. Instances of spinal monitoring have been reported in which surgical and/or anesthetic misadventures, excessive and unanticipated blood loss, or embolism were detected by disturbances in the cortical SSEPs.

Many schemes for defining stability versus change of response have been described. Nash et al. first applied SSEP monitoring in a large series of spine surgical cases.[21] They established criteria of 50 percent or more reduction in peak-to-peak amplitude of the cortical response as a marker of significant change related to surgical intervention. Loder et al.[22] defined significant change as greater than 10 percent latency increase or 50 percent amplitude reduction in a series of patients undergoing spinal surgery for deformity. Jones et al. concluded that 30 to 50 percent reduction in overall amplitude of SSEP was not associated with clinical sequelae, whereas loss of more than 50 percent of overall amplitude and/or loss of one or more components of the multiphasic response collected from the epidural space correlated with postoperative neurological deficits.[23] Most centers that have adopted the 50 percent amplitude, 10 percent latency criteria, a significant change from baseline during clinical spinal cord monitoring, found this to provide adequate sensitivity and specificity.

Given the anatomic limitations of SSEPs, a method of monitoring ventral spinal cord tracts has been actively sought. In this regard, various authors have reported good correlation between MEPs and postoperative motor function. Three methods of intraoperative monitoring of MEPs are currently in use. Transcranial electrical stimulation may be applied and responses recorded from the spinal cord and peripheral nerves. Another method involves directly stimulating the spinal cord electrically and recording from peripheral nerve sites. Finally, transcranial magnetic stimulation may be applied with subsequent recording from either muscle or peripheral nerve.

In one of the earlier studies, Levy et al. found no new motor deficits in patients who had MEP amplitudes that did not attenuate to less than 33 percent of baseline values. However, complete loss of the MEP was always associated with a postoperative motor deficit.[7,24]

In a more comprehensive study, Zenter found that MEP amplitudes spontaneously vary by more than 50 percent before intervention of any type. The author established a lower limit of 25 to 43 percent of baseline as being clinically important and recommended warning the surgeon when amplitudes attenuated to less than one-third of baseline. Changes in latency were much more difficult to evaluate and provided no useful monitoring information. The author, however, did report two patients who had normal postoperative neurological function in spite of loss of all intraoperative MEP waveforms.[25]

References

1. Pool JE: Electrospinogram, spinal cord action potentials recorded from a paraplegic patient. *J Neurosurg* 1945; 3:192–198.
2. Amassian VE, Stewart M, Quirk J, Rosenthal JL: Physiologic basis of motor effects of a transient stimulus to the cerebral cortex. *Neurosurgery* 1987; 20:74–93.
3. Powers SK, Bolger CA, Edwards MSB: Spinal cord pathways mediating somatosensory evoked potentials. *J Neurosurg* 1982; 57:472–482.
4. Cusick JE, Mykehust JB, Larson SJ, Sances A: Spinal cord evaluation by cortical evoked response. *Arch Neurol* 1979; 36:140–143.
5. Ziganow S: Neurometric evaluation of the cortical somatosensory evoked potential in acute and complete spinal cord injuries. *Electroenceph Clin Neurophysiol* 1986; 65:86–93.
6. Day BL, Rothwell JC, Thompson PD, et al: Motor cortex stimulation in intact man. *Brain* 1987; 110:1191–1209.
7. Levy WJ, McCaffrey M, Haghighi S: Clinical experience with motor and cerebellar evoked potential monitoring. *Neurosurgery* 1987; 20:169–182.
8. McGarry J, Friedgood DL, Woolsey R, et al: Somatosensory evoked potentials in spinal cord injury. *Surg Neurol* 1984; 22:341–343.
9. Beric A: Cortical somatosensory evoked potentials in spinal cord injury patients. *J Neurol Sci* 1992; 107:50–59.
10. Dimitrijevic MR, Shu CY, McCay B: Neurophysiological assessment of spinal cord and head injury. *J Neurotrauma* 1992; 9:5293–5300.
11. Kovindha A, Miahachal R: Short latency SSEPs of the tibial nerves and spinal cord injuries. *Paraplegia* 1992; 30:502–506.
12. Li C, Houlden DA, Rowed DW: Somatosensory evoked potentials and neurological grades as predictors of outcome in acute spinal cord injury. *J Neurosurg* 1990; 72:600–609.

13. Perot PL, Vera CL: Scalp recorded SSEPs to stimulation of nerves in the lower extremities and evaluation of patients with spinal cord trauma. *Ann NY Acad Sci* 1982; 388:359–386.
14. Sedgwick EM, El-Negary E, Frankel H: Spinal cord potentials in traumatic paraplegia and quadriplegia. *J Neurol Neurosurg Psychiatry* 1980; 43:823–830.
15. York DH, Watts C, Raffensberger M, et al: Utilization of SSEP's in spinal cord injury: Prognostic limitations. *Spine* 1983; 8:832–839.
16. Rowed DW, McLean JAG, Tator CH: Somatosensory evoked potentials in acute spinal cord injury: Prognostic value. *Surg Neurol* 1978; 9:203–210.
17. MacDonell RAL, Donnan GA: Magnetic cortical stimulation in acute spinal cord injury. *Neurology* 1995; 45:303–305.
18. Jellinek D, Platt M, Jewkes D, Symon L: Effects of nitrous oxide on motor evoked potentials recorded from skeletal muscle in patients under total anesthesia with intravenously administered prophofol. *Neurosurgery* 1991; 29:558–562.
19. Jellinek D, Jewkes D, Symon L: Noninvasive intraoperative monitoring of motor evoked potentials under prophofol anesthesia: Effects of spinal surgery on the amplitude and latency motor evoked potentials. *Neurosurgery* 1991; 29:551–557.
20. Calancie B, Klose J, Baier S, Green BA: Isoflurane-induced attenuation of motor evoked potentials caused by electrical motor cortex stimulation during surgery. *J Neurosurg* 1991; 74:897–904.
21. Nash CL, Lorig RA, Schatzinger LA, Brown RH: Spinal cord monitoring during operative treatment of the spine. *Clin Orthop* 1977; 126:100–105.
22. Loder R, Thomson G, LaMont R: Spinal cord monitoring in patients with nonidiopathic spinal deformities using somatosensory evoked potentials. *Spine* 1990; 15:286–292.
23. Jones SJ, Edgar MA, Ransford AO, Thomas NP: A system for the electrophysiological monitoring of spinal cord during operations for scoliosis. *J Bone Joint Surg* (*Br*) 1983; 65:134–139.
24. Levy WJ, McCaffrey M, Haghighi S: Motor evoked potential as a predictor of recovery in chronic spinal cord injury. *Neurosurgery* 1989; 20:138–142.
25. Zenter J: Noninvasive motor evoked potential monitoring during neurosurgical operations on the spinal cord. *Neurosurgery* 1989; 24:709–712.

Therapeutic Agents

CHAPTER 87

PHARMACOLOGICAL RESUSCITATION FOR SPINAL CORD INJURY

Jack E. Wilberger, Jr.

INTRODUCTION

The potential for pharmacologically improving neurological outcome after spinal cord injury has for decades been the goal of both basic neuroscientists and clinicians. Since most paralyzing spinal cord injuries are the result of incomplete anatomic damage to the spinal cord, typically a not insignificant amount of viable neural tissue—neurons, axons, and tracts—is left to support potential neurological recovery. Indeed, it has been shown that an increase in neural tissue survival from 3 to 6 percent at the injury site may be sufficient to allow for significant return of neurological function.[50] Unfortunately, however, the unique pathophysiological response of the spinal cord to injury results in progressive secondary or delayed damage, rendering potential recoverable tissue nonviable and the neurological destruction permanent. Pharmacological inhibition of this pathophysiological process thus might hold promise for preserving neurological function and/or enhancing recovery. Abundant basic research supports the use of a number of pharmacological agents to attenuate various components of the pathophysiological cascade with promising neurological benefits. However, until recently, transfer of such benefits to the clinical setting has been contradictory and disappointing. Results from the National Acute Spinal Cord Injury Study and the GM-1 ganglioside trial have given new impetus to clinical trials of pharmacotherapy for spinal cord injury.

PATHOPHYSIOLOGICAL RESPONSE TO SPINAL CORD INJURY

For several minutes following severe impact injury to the spinal cord, the cord may look grossly and histologically normal. Detailed animal studies of impact spinal cord injury, however, have delineated the sequence of pathological events that transform this normal appearance into one of total focal necrosis and inflammation within 24 to 48 hours of injury. The mechanical disruption of axons and neurons at the time of impact injury has been termed primary neural injury, while the progressive pathological and physiological changes occurring subsequently are known as secondary neural injury.

From a pathological standpoint, light microscopy shows petechial hemorrhages in the central cord gray matter within 30 minutes of injury. Initially confined to the areas in the anterior horns and about the central canal, these hemorrhages coalesce over several hours and extend into the posterior gray matter and white matter. Each hemorrhage, for the most part, appears to circumscribe a single vessel and may result from tears in the vessel walls.[47] Two hours after injury, an invasion of inflammatory cells begins—microglia and polymorphonuclear leukocytes. Nearly half of the cord's cross-sectional area becomes necrotic by the fourth hour after injury. Edema fluid, thought to be primarily vasogenic, begins to appear within six hours of injury. If the initial impact is severe, the entire cross-sectional area of the cord will be edematous and necrotic within 48 hours of impact injury. Occasionally, a small rim of white matter may remain. Weeks after injury, only a contracted scar consisting of astrocytes, fibroblasts, and collagen will remain.

Significant physiological derangements accompany the pathological changes. Within two hours of injury there is a significant reduction in spinal cord blood flow—from 40 to 50 ml per 100 g of tissue per minute to less than 20 ml per 100 g of tissue per minute in the gray matter, while initial white matter blood flow may rise slightly.[41,51] Severe vascular congestion develops and leads to extravasation of red cells and protein-rich edema fluid, causing cord swelling, a rise in interstitial pressure, and further reduction of cord perfusion. Oxygen tensions fall and carbon dioxide tensions rise. Vascular autoreactivity is lost, and hypoxia, ischemia, and infarction ensue.[40]

Many biochemical mechanisms have been implicated in the evolution of the pathological changes and physiological derangements that occur after spinal cord injury. One of the first and still most controversial biochemical events studied in traumatized spinal cord tissue is postinjury elevations of norepinephrine. In 1972, Osterholm and Mathews reported a doubling of norepinephrine levels in the spinal cord of injured cats within 30 minutes of injury; at one hour, the levels were increased fourfold. It was thus proposed that the decrease in spinal cord blood flow after impact injury was directly related to the elevated norepinephrine levels.[39] Since that time, attention has been focused on a number of other biochemical events: ionic shifts of sodium and potassium and calcium[53,54]; lysosomal and phospholipase activation[9,13]; release of vasoactive and neurotoxic substances such as prostaglandins, thromboxanes, and excitatory neurotransmitters[33]; activation of opiate receptors[23,24]; and lipid peroxidation secondary to generation of oxygen free radicals (Fig. 87-1).[15,16]

The complexity of the known and postulated biochemical reactions and interactions is thus readily appreciated, leading to an understanding of the enormous difficulty in choosing a specific area for pharmacological intervention. It is primarily for this reason that, over the years, most pharmacological treatment has been

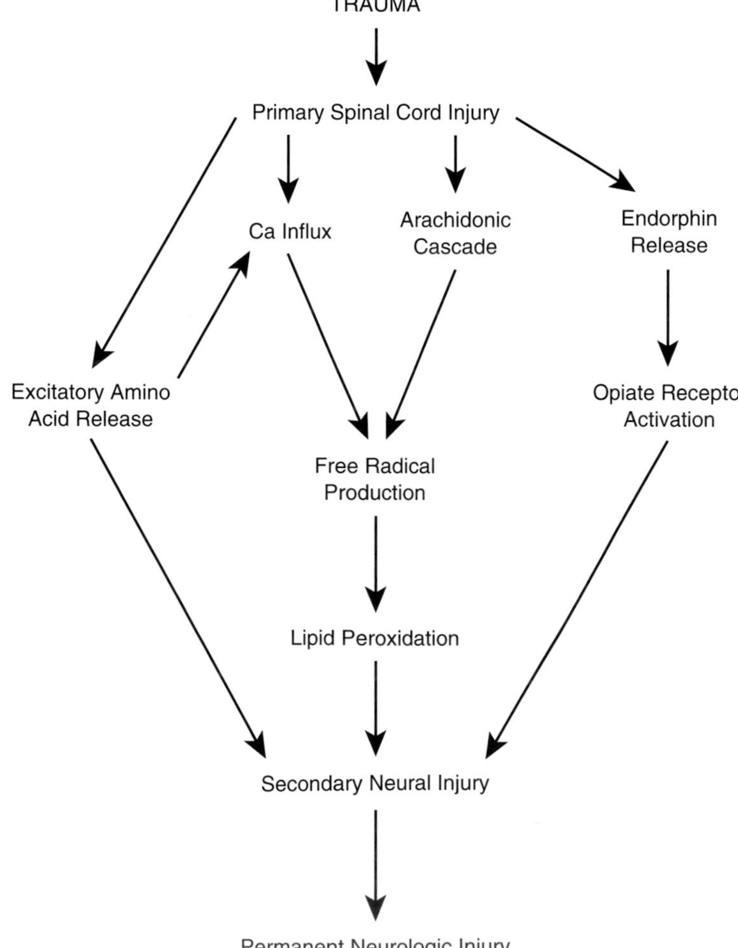

Figure 87-1. Potential biochemical pathways of secondary injury and opportunities for pharmacological interventions.

aimed at the hemodynamic rather than the biochemical changes that occur in the injured cord. Ducker studied a variety of volume expanders and vasoactive agents—dextran, methyldopa, phenoxybenzamine—and found few, if any, benefits in experimental cord injury.[18,19] Dimethylsulfoxide (DMSO) diminishes platelet aggregation as well as thrombus formation in blood vessels; however, it has shown only limited efficacy in animal spinal cord injury models.[34] Calcium channel blockers have been shown to increase spinal cord blood flow in animals after experimental cord trauma. However, associated systemic and subsequent spinal cord hypotension limits their usefulness.[30] Dolan and Tator studied the effects of blood transfusion, dopamine, and gamma hydroxybutyrate on posttraumatic ischemia of the spinal cord. They found in a lab model that this treatment regimen significantly improved blood flow in both the gray and white matter and also held advantages for ultimate neurological recovery in the treated animal.[17] In a similar vein, Kobrine and associates found that intravenous lidocaine will produce elevations in cord blood flow after injury.[36] Basic studies such as these have led to the hypothesis that elevation of systemic blood pressure may improve neurological recovery after acute spinal cord injury. However, clinically, such hypotheses have yet to be definitively proven.

In recent years, experimental interest in pharmacological agents has refocused on biochemical events, with two receiving considerable attention—lipid peroxidation and opiate receptor activation. Additionally, promotion of neural regeneration after injury by pharmacological intervention has generated considerable interest.

OPIATE RECEPTORS

In the early 1980s, Faden and coworkers found that spinal cord injury in cats causes release of endorphin-like substances into the bloodstream. They reasoned that these substances, which have marked peripheral vascular effects, may be responsible for the reduced perfusion to the spinal cord after spinal cord injury.[22–24] Endorphins are endogenous opiate compounds that act via opiate receptors in the brain and spinal cord. Thus, opiate receptor blockers such as naloxone and thyrotropin releasing hormone (TRH) theoretically should prevent significant reductions in spinal cord blood flow due to posttraumatic endorphin release. Several independent laboratories reported that naloxone, given in doses (2–10 mg/kg) far exceeding levels at which the drug normally antagonizes opiate receptors, improved spinal cord blood flow and functional neurological recovery in animals. Faden and associates reported significant neurological recovery in both rat and cat models.[23,24] Young and colleagues and Flamm and coworkers reported improved spinal cord blood flow and somatosensory evoked potentials as well as a greater ability to walk in a cat model of spinal cord injury after treatment with naloxone.[26,52]

The exact mechanism of the naloxone effect in spinal cord injury has not been clearly elucidated. It has been theorized that endogenous opiates play a role in the posttraumatic ischemia that develops following such injuries and that naloxone, by blocking the influence of these opiates, ameliorates the associated ischemia. Another theory is that naloxone acts by increasing cardiac output to the spinal cord without significant associated rise in mean systemic arterial pressure.

TRH is also a potent antiopiate substance. Several investigators have found TRH to be as effective as naloxone in preventing the drop in spinal cord blood flow following injury and also equally effective in improving neurological recovery.[25] There is some additional evidence that TRH-mediated stimulation of thyroid hormone production may have some direct beneficial effect on the injured spinal cord.[45]

LIPID PEROXIDATION

Oxygen-derived free radical species are important mediators of several forms of tissue damage: ischemic and traumatic. Free radicals are very reactive species produced in the normal course of cellular reactions but controlled by such endogenous systems as superoxide dismutase, catalase, and peroxidase, and by naturally occurring antioxidants such as vitamin E and ascorbic acid. With superimposed trauma, ischemia, and disruption of mitochondrial electron transport systems, free radical production rapidly exceeds the cell's ability to neutralize them. One important target of the free radicals is the cell membrane. Lipid peroxidation at the cellular membrane level is a chain reaction that alters or destroys the polyunsaturated tails of membrane phospholipids. The structural integrity and functions of cell membranes are irreversibly changed during membrane lipid peroxidation. Extracellular calcium can enter the cell, resulting in the activation of calcium-dependent phospholipases and protein kinases. Phospholipases, once activated, will cleave fatty acids from phospholipids and cause additional changes in the chemical composition and physiological state of the cell membrane. Demopoulous and co-workers were the first to propose that free radical-mediated lipid peroxidation catalyzed by iron and copper from extravasated blood is involved in the microcirculatory damage and subsequent autodestruction that occurs after cord injury.[15,16] Subsequent studies have shown that more than 50 percent of tissue phospholipids may be broken down within a few hours of spinal cord injury.[14]

Given such mechanisms, lipid peroxidation inhibitors, free radical scavengers, and antioxidants theoretically should provide powerful pharmacological advantages in treating spinal cord injury.

Steroids are potent inhibitors of lipid peroxidation and indeed have been studied extensively in experimental spinal cord injury. The first in vitro study to demonstrate the effectiveness of steroids in reducing lipid peroxidation was reported by Hall and Braughler.[31] Spinal cord tissue from animals pretreated with a 30 or 60 mg/kg dose of methylprednisolone showed significantly less lipid peroxidation than untreated animals. As early as 1969, Ducker and Hamit showed improved motor recovery in beagle dogs when dexamethasone was given after a severe contusion model.[18–20] In rapid succession 11 other steroid studies appeared in the literature. Eight found significantly enhanced motor recovery in treated animals, two found that steroids improved the histological appearance of the injured cord, and one found no benefits from steroid therapy.[19] Such results led to the optimistic and widespread clinical use of steroids, but yielded no evidence of significant clinical benefits. Subsequent investigations have shown that steroid dose and timing of treatment are highly important in affecting lipid peroxidation. Means and Anderson demonstrated that very high doses of methylprednisolone are required to improve the histological outcome and microvascular perfusion as well as to reduce lipid peroxidation in compressed feline spinal cords.[3,10] Hall and Braughler studied the dose-response relationship between methylprednisolone and reduction in lipid peroxidation, protein degradation, and metabolic dysfunction in injured cat spinal cords. They found a narrow, bell-shaped curve where the positive effects peak at 30 mg/kg, are barely significant at 15 mg/kg, and become deleterious at 60 mg/kg. They also demonstrated an eight-hour window for treatment after spinal cord injury.[10,11] Hall has recently theorized that the optimal duration of treatment with methylprednisolone may be for at least several days after spinal cord injury. During this time, intracord hemorrhage is being resorbed and the hemoglobin present may continue to drive the lipid peroxidation process. Such information set the stage for further and more rational clinical trials of steroids in spinal cord injury.

Steroids have been shown to have a number of other effects in spinal cord injury models: prevention of posttraumatic ischemia, reversal of intracellular calcium accumulation, prevention of neurofilament degradation, and inhibition of prostaglandin formation.

The newly developed 21-aminosteroid, tirilazad, performs multiple functions in inhibiting lipid peroxidation—it scavenges reactive oxygen species and lipid radicals, protects membranes by decreasing membrane fluidity, and inhibits radical-mediated proteolysis. Tirilazad has shown impressive activity in models of acute spinal cord injury in cats.[2,38] When given within 30 minutes and four hours of a moderately severe compression injury, four-week neurological recovery is significantly improved. A recently completed study initiated treatments 30 minutes, and two, four, and eight hours after injury. Animals whose treatment was delayed for up to four hours after trauma had a significant improvement after four weeks, recovering nearly 70 percent of normal neurological function by that time. In contrast, delaying treatment until eight hours resulted in a very poor recovery indistinguishable from vehicle-treated animals with 14 percent of normal neurological recovery. Several studies have also shown the ability of tirilazad to prevent or reverse the typically seen posttraumatic spinal ischemia.

In spite of being a steroid derivative, addition of the amino group has eliminated all steroid side effects such as immunosuppression and hyperglycemia, thus potentially allaying concerns over high-dose clinical usage. Tirilazad has successfully passed through preclinical safety and Phase I clinical trials and is currently being evaluated in a Phase III clinical spinal cord injury trial.

NEURAL REGENERATION

An alternative pharmacological approach to promoting neurological recovery after spinal cord injury has been in the area of regeneration research. Several strategies—axonal bridges, neuronotropic factors, blockade of neurite outgrowth inhibitors—have been explored with positive but generally modest results.[1,32,43]

Recently, interest has refocused on the gangliosides as potential mediators of neuronal regeneration. Most of the lipids constituting the neuronal plasma membrane are gangliosides. By inserting into normal or damaged neuronal membranes, gangliosides may modify membrane protein activity. In vitro, they have been shown to promote sprouting and neurite outgrowth from motor neurons.[4] In vivo, gangliosides potentiate neuronotropic factor effects.

Early studies with mechanical lesions have demonstrated improved neurological outcomes with GM-1 treatment in nigrostriatal pathway injuries.[46] GM-1 has also been shown to enhance recovery after spinal cord injury in cats.[29]

GM-1 has gone through a limited Phase II/III clinical trial and is currently being studied extensively in Europe and the United States.

CLINICAL STUDIES

In spite of promising laboratory results for the variety of pharmacological agents, demonstration of any reproducible clinical effectiveness has been slow in coming. One reason for this is the difficulty in conducting rigorously controlled randomized clinical trials in spinal cord injury with large enough patient populations to draw clear and statistically significant conclusions. Another reason is the general complexity of spinal cord injury and the variety of treatment approaches. Such considerations must be borne in mind when evaluating clinical results indicating efficacy or lack thereof for a given pharmacological agent in spinal cord injury.

Steroid and Naloxone Trials

Excluding anecdotal reports and nonrandomized trials of various steroids in spinal cord injury, the first randomized controlled trial of steroids was undertaken by the National Acute Spinal Cord Injury Study (NASCIS I), a consortium of ten major United States spinal cord injury centers. Begun in 1977, this trial took five years to complete, with results being published by Bracken and coworkers in 1984.[7] In a double-blinded fashion, patients with complete and incomplete spinal cord injury randomized to high-dose methylprednisolone (1000-mg bolus, 250 mg every six hours for 10 days) versus conventional-dose methylprednisolone (100-mg bolus, 250 mg every six hours for 10 days). No patient was denied what was considered to be therapeutic steroids, and treatment was continued for ten days after injury. Data from 330 patients were collected and subjected to rigorous statistical analysis. Ultimately, there was no statistical difference ($p < 0.05$) in the sensory or motor recovery of the high-dose steroid group versus the conventional-dose group, while such complications as mortality and postoperative wound infections were much more common in the high-dose treatment group. Even though there were no control patients in the study, the overall results strongly suggested that steroids given in this dose and manner—up to 24 hours after spinal cord injury—were of no benefit in improving neurological recovery. Although considered an epidemiological success for its ability to collect and follow such a large group of spinal cord injured patients, the results of NASCIS I were called into question on several fronts: there was no placebo group in the trial; the dose of methylprednisolone was too low, based on the 30 mg/kg dose-response relationship established by Hall and Braughler; the time to treatment was too long for any possible beneficial therapeutic effect to be seen.

Considering these concerns and taking into account available laboratory information on spinal cord injury, a second clinical trial was initiated in 1985—NASCIS II. Three treatment groups were delineated—methylprednisolone, 30 mg/kg-bolus, followed by 5.4 mg/kg/hour for 23 hours; naloxone 5.4 mg/kg-bolus, followed by 4.0 mg/kg/hour for 23 hours; and a placebo. Only patients in whom treatment could be initiated within 12 hours of spinal cord injury were randomized. NASCIS II took five years to complete, and its results were published in 1990.[8]

A total of 487 patients were randomized for treatment and followed for at least one year after spinal cord injury—162 received methylprednisolone, 154 naloxone, and 171 placebo. The average time from spinal cord injury to treatment was 8.7 hours. Spinal cord injury was complete in 60 percent and incomplete in 40 percent. Detailed neurological examination documenting motor and sensory function were performed on admission, at six weeks, at six months, and one year after injury.

Patients treated within eight hours of injury with the methylprednisolone regimen evidenced statistically significant improvements in both motor and sensory compared to naloxone and placebo, regardless of whether the spinal cord injury was initially complete or incomplete. Patients treated after eight hours, regardless of regimen, did not show similar gains (Fig. 87-2). The odds of a methylprednisolone-treated patient improving motor function were greater than two to one compared with other therapies; the odds of improving sensory function were three to one. Patients receiving naloxone within eight hours of spinal cord injury also showed neurological gains compared with placebo patients, but the gains were one-half to two-thirds of those seen in the methylprednisolone-treated patients. The advantage of having received methylprednisolone was still evident at one-year follow-up. However, a disturbing trend became apparent at one year—in those patients treated after eight hours, placebo patients were neurologically better than those who had received methylprednisolone or naloxone. However, this difference was not statistically significant.

A recent reanalysis of the NASCIS II data indicated that the most significant recovery of neurological func-

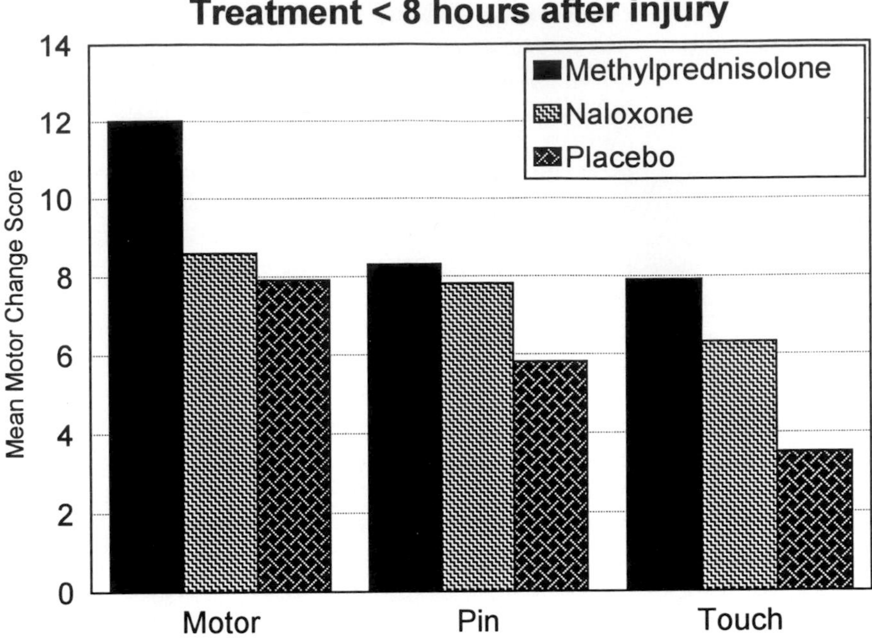

A

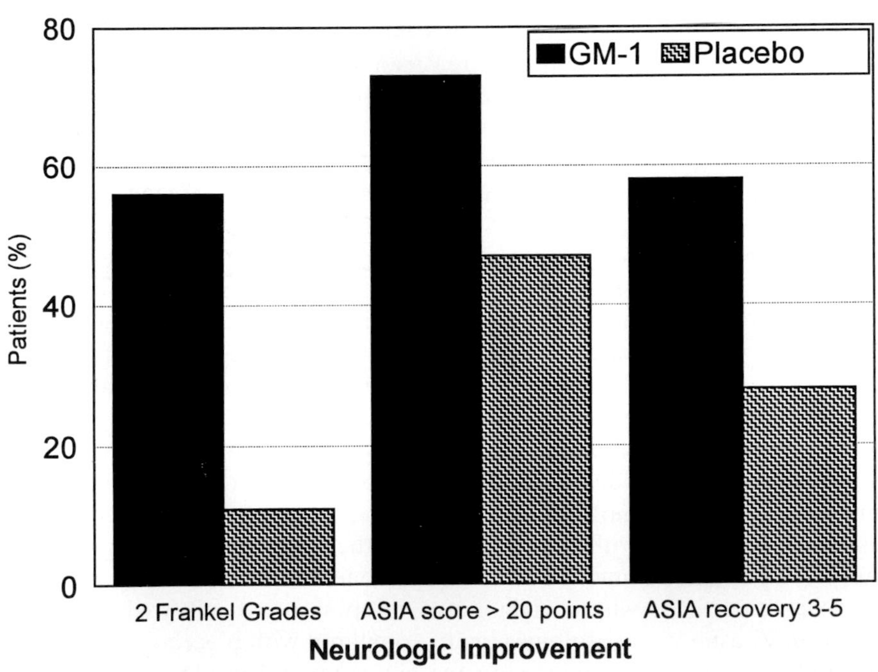

B

Figure 87-2. *A*. Improvement in motor scores at 1 year following spinal cord injury (NASCIS II). *B*. GM-1 Ganglioside Study. Neurological and Functional Improvements.

tion occurs below the level of the lesion in the spinal cord. This means that methylprednisolone is most likely preserving, stabilizing, and allowing recovery of the long white matter tracts rather than having a significantly beneficial effect on the motor neurons at the level of the injury.[6]

The NASCIS II trial has been hailed as a major breakthrough in the treatment of spinal cord injury. While neurological improvement was definitely demonstrated, the gains were small and the functional significance of these gains has been called into question. Nevertheless, NASCIS II has provided the most encouraging clinical evidence yet found that pharmacological intervention may be able to ameliorate the secondary neurological injury after spinal cord injury. Given the effectiveness of naloxone, NASCIS II also provided the first clear clinical evidence that multiple processes contribute to the secondary injury and that more than one pharmacological agent may be necessary to enhance neurological recovery.

A NASCIS III trial was initiated in late 1991. This randomized trial is comparing the NASCIS II treatment regimen with 48 hours of methylprednisolone and the new lipid peroxidation inhibitor, tirilazad. All patients are being treated within eight hours of injury. As of early 1995, approximately 400 patients have been entered in the trial, which should be completed by mid-1995.

TRH Trial

A limited clinical trial of TRH was undertaken in 20 patients from 1986 to 1988 by Pitts and coworkers at the San Francisco General Hospital. Treatment was begun within 12 hours of injury in a randomized blinded fashion with either placebo or TRH—0.2 mg/kg IV bolus, followed by 0.2 mg/kg/hour for six hours. Outcome at 12 months after spinal cord injury was assessed based on the NASCIS sensorimotor recovery score. Patients were divided into four groups for the purposes of analysis: group 1—placebo/complete spinal cord injury; group 2—TRH/complete spinal cord injury; group 3—placebo/incomplete spinal cord injury; group 4—TRH/incomplete spinal cord injury. The median change in sensorimotor score from admission to the end of the study for group 1 was 13 ($n = 3$); group 2, 6.5 ($n = 4$); group 3, 7.5 ($n = 6$); and group 4, 24 ($n = 7$).

The physiological and subjective changes associated with TRH infusion were tachycardia, headache, urinary urgency, and a flushed sensation. In two patients, development of significant hypertension required temporary cessation of drug infusion.

Given the small sample size, statistical analysis for patients with complete spinal cord injury was not feasible. For incomplete spinal cord injury patients, there was no significant difference between placebo- or TRH-treated groups. However, once again, the samples were small and there was a clear trend of improved scores in the TRH-treated patients.

These results have led investigators to propose a broader clinical trial of TRH in spinal cord injury.

GM-1 Trial

In 1991, Geisler and coworkers reported the results of a prospective, randomized, placebo-controlled, double blind study of GM-1 ganglioside in acute spinal cord injury. Thirty-four patients (16 GM-1, 18 placebo) were followed for one year, with neurological recovery determined by both Frankel grades and ASIA motor scores. All patients were treated with steroids prior to receiving the GM-1 drug (the NASCIS II regimen was not used as these results were not known at the time of the study) and received daily intravenous doses of GM-1, beginning within 72 hours of the spinal cord injury and extending for 18 to 32 days.[27,28]

GM-1-treated patients overall demonstrated significant improvements in ultimate neurological outcome when compared with patients receiving placebo. Of those patients who could potentially improve two or more Frankel grades, 50 percent of GM-1 patients did so, while only 7.1 percent of placebo patients achieved this degree of recovery ($p = 0.033$). There was significantly greater mean neurological improvement at one-year follow-up in GM-1 patients as compared to placebo ($p = 0.047$). Sixty-eight percent of GM-1 patients had motor recoveries of more than 20 points on the ASIA scale compared with 38.9 percent of the placebo group. In the GM-1 group, 30.9 percent of the paralyzed motor groups remained paralyzed and 51.7 percent recovered to 3-5 muscle strength; in the placebo group, 65.5 percent remained paralyzed, with 25.3 percent recovering to this degree.

The small sample size in this study precluded detailed analysis of other aspects of spinal cord injury or its treatment that may impact on outcome. It should be noted that in spite of the neurological improvements demonstrated, both groups of patients were "functionally equivalent" at one year's follow-up.

Analysis of the degree and extent of recovery has led Geisler to conclude that GM-1 is effective by virtue of its ability to increase the proportion of surviving or effective axons through the injury site—similar to the findings of the recent NASCIS study. As noted previously, the exact mechanisms by which this effect is exerted remain to be determined.

Currently, a large scale multicenter clinical trial of GM-1 is ongoing, with a targeted completion date of 1995–1996. All patients in this trial are receiving the NASCIS II methylprednisolone protocol before being treated with GM-1.

FUTURE OF SPINAL CORD INJURY CLINICAL RESEARCH

Ultimately, the primary measure of the success or failure of any current or future pharmacological treatment of spinal cord injury is the enhancement of functional neurological recovery. In addition to demonstrating the beneficial effect of methylprednisolone and establishing a therapeutic window of eight hours, NASCIS II clearly showed that there is a not insubstantial spontaneous recovery of neurological function, even in patients with initially complete cord injuries. A 12 to 15 point improvement was noted in the motor and sensory scores in placebo-treated patients. In addition, the GM-1 study results are strongly suggestive of enhanced neurological recovery based on pharmacological intervention. It has been shown in animal studies that return of neurological function may depend on a very small number of surviving spinal tracts or axons—up to 90 percent of tracts may be destroyed without the loss of locomotion.[5,21,44] Blight and Decrescito have recently shown that some spinal cord-injured cats walk normally with as few as 10 percent of their original axon population after spinal cord injury.[5] Such information suggests that few, if any, spinal cord injuries are truly complete and nonrecoverable. The problem has been determining the true extent of the injury in any given spinal cord injury patient in the clinical setting. Recent studies done with magnetic resonance imaging suggest that this modality ultimately may provide useful information about in vivo pathophysiological changes after spinal cord injury. MRI not only provides good anatomic definitions of spinal injury, but is the only available imaging modality capable of delineating intrinsic spinal cord abnormalities—cord transection, hematomyelia, swelling, contusions, ischemia—after spinal cord injury.[35] Shaefer in 1988 was one of the first to attempt to correlate the intrinsic cord abnormalities with clinical neurological findings. His group studied 53 patients with MRI and found that the presence of hematomyelia was associated with a complete spinal cord injury in 92 percent of patients, while contusion and edema were associated with incomplete spinal cord injury in 81 percent.[42] Kulkarni and associates reported similar findings and indicated that long-term prognosis was poor for neurological recovery when hematomyelia was present on the initial MRI.[37] Recently, Wilberger and coworkers reported on sequential MRI changes after spinal cord injury and found a correlation between the evolutionary changes in the intrinsic cord abnormalities and the subsequent neurological recovery or lack thereof.[48] Further refinement of such information may provide a clinical basis for determining the true extent of spinal cord injury and to follow the effects of pharmacological interventions based on direct MRI imaging of the pathophysiological cord changes after spinal cord injury.

Renewed interest in neural regeneration and spinal cord transplantation and the possibility of pharmacologically modulating these responses are currently generating considerable research activity. The identification of "early response" genes involved in CNS regeneration and their activation by intranuclear chemicals suggests that they may be amenable to therapeutic modulation.[44]

The confluence of decades of animal and laboratory research and clinical treatment of spinal cord injury have led to the beginnings of a potentially effective pharmacological approach to the treatment of spinal cord injury. New clinical trials are on the horizon for methylprednisolone, tirilazad, TRH, and GM-1 ganglioside; other compounds are being intensively studied for their potential application in the clinical setting. The results of NASCIS II and the GM-1 trial have led to renewed hope and interest in this area. The ability to further enhance neurological recovery to a level of functional significance is the current goal of all clinical and basic spinal cord injury research in the area of pharmacological resuscitation.

References

1. Aguayo AJ, Benfey M, David S: A potential for axonal regeneration in neurons of the adult mammalian nervous system. *Birth Defects* 1983; 19:327–340.
2. Anderson DK, Braughler JM, Hall ED, et al: Effects of treatment with U-74006F on neurological outcome following experimental spinal cord injury. *J Neurosurg* 1988; 69:562–567.
3. Anderson DK, Saunders RD, Demediuk P, et al: Lipid hydrolysis and peroxidation in injured spinal cord: Partial protection with methylprednisolone or vitamin E and selenium. *CNS Trauma* 1985; 2:257–267.
4. Barletta E, Bremer EG, Culp LA: Neurite outgrowth in dorsal root neonatal hybrid clones modulated by ganglioside GM-1 and disintegrins, *Exp Cell Res* 1991; 193:101–111.
5. Blight AR, Decrescito V: Morphometric analysis of experimental spinal cord injury in the cat: The relation of injury intensity to survival of myelinated axons. *Neuroscience* 1986; 19:321–341.
6. Bracken MD, Holford TR: Effects of timing of methylprednisolone or naloxone administration on recovery of segmental and long-tract neurological function in NASCIS II. *J Neurosurg* 1993; 79:500–507.
7. Bracken MD, Collins WF, Freeman DF, et al: Efficacy of methylprednisolone in acute spinal cord injury. *JAMA* 1984; 251:45–52.
8. Bracken MD, Shepherd JJ, et al: A randomized controlled trial of methylprednisolone or naloxone in the treatment of acute spinal cord injury: The results of the National Acute Spinal Cord Injury Study. *N Engl J Med* 1990; 322:1405–1411.
9. Braughler JM, Duncan LA, Chase RL: Interaction of lipid peroxidation and calcium in the pathogenesis of neuronal injury. *CNS Trauma* 1985; 2:269–283.
10. Braughler JM, Hall ED: Correlation of methylprednisolone pharmacokinetics in cat spinal cord with its effects on (Na+K) ATP-ase, lipid peroxidation and motor neuron function. *J Neurosurg* 1983; 56:838–844.
11. Braughler JM, Hall ED, Means ED, et al: Evaluation of an intensive methylprednisolone sodium succinate dosing regimen in experimental spinal cord injury. *J Neurosurg* 1987; 67:102–105.
12. Campbell JV, Decrescito V, Tomasula JJ, et al: Effect

of antifibrinolytic and steroid therapy on the contused spinal cord of cats. *J Neurosurg* 1974; 40:726–733.

13. Clendenon NR, Allen N, Ito T, et al: Response of lysosomal hydrolase of adult spinal cord and cerebral spinal cord fluid to experimental trauma. *Neurology* 1978; 28:78–84.
14. Demediuk P, Saunders RD, Anderson DK, et al: Membrane lipid changes in laminectomized and traumatized cat spinal cord. *Proc Natl Acad Sci USA* 1985; 82:7071–7075.
15. Demopoulos HB, Flamm ES, Pietronigro DD, et al: Free radical pathology and the microcirculation in the major central nervous system disorders. *Acta Physiol Scand* 1980; 492:91–119.
16. Demopoulos HB, Flamm ES, Seligman M: Membrane perturbations in central nervous system injury: Theoretical basis for free radical damage and a review of the experimental data, in Popp AJ (ed): *Neurotrauma.* New York: Raven Press, 1979: 63–78.
17. Dolan EJ, Tator CH: The effect of blood transfusion, dopamine and gamma hydroxybutyrate on post traumatic ischemia of the spinal cord. *J Neurosurg* 1982; 56:350–358.
18. Ducker TB: Experimental injury of the spinal cord, in Vinkin PJ, Bruyn GW (eds): *Handbook of Clinical Neurology,* vol 25. Amsterdam: North Holland, 1976: 9–26.
19. Ducker TB, Hamit HF: Experimental treatments of acute spinal cord injury. *J Neurosurg* 1969; 30:693–697.
20. Ducker TB, Salcman M, Daniell HB: Experimental cord trauma: III. Therapeutic effect of immobilization and pharmacologic agents. *Surg Neurol* 1978; 10:71–78.
21. Eidelberg E, Walden J, Nguyen L: Locomotor control in Macaque monkeys. *Brain* 1981; 104:647–663.
22. Faden AI, Jacobs TP, Holaday JW: Comparison of early and late naloxone treatment in experimental spinal injury. *Neurology* 1982; 32:677–681.
23. Faden AI, Jacobs TP, Holaday JW: Opiate antagonist improves neurologic recovery after spinal injury. *Science* 1981; 211:493–494.
24. Faden AI, Jacobs TP, Mougey E, et al: Endorphins and experimental spinal injury: Therapeutic effects of naloxone. *Ann Neurol* 1981; 10:326–332.
25. Faden AI, Jacobs TP, Holaday JW: Thyrotropin releasing hormone improves neurologic recovery after spinal trauma in cats. *N Engl J Med* 1981; 305:1063–1067.
26. Flamm ES, Young W, Demopoulos HB, et al: Experimental spinal cord injury: Treatment with naloxone. *Neurosurgery* 1982; 10:227–231.
27. Geisler FH, Dorsey FC, Coleman WP: GM-1 ganglioside in human spinal cord injury. *J Neurotrauma* 1992; 9(2):5517–5530.
28. Geisler FH, Dorsey FC, Coleman SP: Recovery of motor function after spinal cord injury—A randomized, placebo controlled trial with GM-1 ganglioside. *N Engl J Med* 1991; 326:1829–1838.
29. Gorio A, DiGiulio AM, Young W, et al: GM-1 effects on chemical, traumatic and peripheral nerve induced lesions to the spinal cord, in Goldberger ME (ed): *Development and Plasticity of the Mammalian Spinal Cord.* Padova: Liviana Press, 1986: 227–242.
30. Guha A, Tator CH, Piper I: Effect of calcium channel blocker on post traumatic spinal cord blood flow. *J Neurosurg* 1987; 66:423–430.
31. Hall ED, Braughler JM: Acute effects of intravenous glucocorticoid pretreatment on the in vitro peroxidation of cat spinal cord tissue. *Exp Neurol* 1981; 73:321–324.
32. Hohn A, Liebrock J, Bailey K, Barde YA: Identification and characterization of a novel member of the nerve growth factor/brain-derived neurotropic factor family. *Nature* 1990; 344:338–341.
33. Hsu CY, Halushka PV, Hogan EL, et al: Alterations of thromboxane and prostacyclin levels in experimental spinal cord injury. *Neurology* 1985; 35:1003–1009.
34. Jacob SW, Herschler R: Biologic actions of dimethylsulfoxide, in: *Conference of the Biological Action of Dimethylsulfoxide.* New York Academy of Science, New York, 1974.
35. Kalfas I, Wilberger J, Goldberg A, Prostko ER: Magnetic resonance imaging in acute spinal cord trauma. *Neurosurgery* 1988; 23:295–299.
36. Kobrine AI, Evans DE, LeGrys DC, et al: Effect of intravenous lidocaine on experimental spinal cord injury. *J Neurosurg* 1984; 60:595–601.
37. Kulkarni MV, McArdle CB, Kopanicky D, et al: Acute spinal cord injury: MR imaging at 1.5 T. *Radiology* 1987; 164:837–843.
38. McCall JM, Braughler JM, Hall ED: A new class of compounds for stroke and trauma: Effects of 21-amino steroids on lipid peroxidation. *Acta Anaesthesiol Belg* 1927; 38:417–420.
39. Osterholm JL, Mathews GJ: Altered norepinephrine metabolism following experimental spinal cord injury: Part I. Relationship to hemorrhagic necrosis and post wounding neurological deficits. *J Neurosurg* 1972; 36:386–394.
40. Osterholm JL: The pathophysiological response to spinal cord injury: The current status of related research. *J Neurosurg* 1974; 40:5–33.
41. Sandler AN, Tator CH. Review of the effects of spinal cord trauma on vessels and blood flow in the spinal cord. *J Neurosurg* 1972; 45:638–646.
42. Schaefer DM, Flanders A, Northrup BE, et al: Magnetic resonance imaging of acute cervical spine trauma: Correlation with severity of neurologic injury. *AJNR* 1989; 14(3):1090–1095.
43. Schwab ME: Regeneration of lesioned CNS axons by neutralization of neurite growth inhibitors: A short review. *J Neurotrauma* 1992; 9(1):S219–221.
44. Skaper SD, Leon A: Monosialogangliosides, neuroprotection and neuronal repair processes. *J Neurotrauma* 1992; 9(2):5507–5516.
45. Tator CH, Van der Jagt EHC: Effect of exogenous thyroid hormones on functional recovery of the rat after acute spinal cord compression injury. *J Neurosurg* 1980; 53:381–394.
46. Toffano G, Savioni G, Moroni F, et al: GM-1 ganglioside stimulates the regeneration of dopaminergic neurons in the central nervous system. *Brain Res* 1983; 261:163–166.

47. Wagner FC, Dohrmann GJ, Bucy PC: Histopathology of transitory traumatic paraplegia in the monkey. *J Neurosurg* 1981; 35:272–276.
48. Wilberger JE: Sequential MRI after spinal cord injury. *AANS Abstracts Book,* April 1991.
49. Windle WF: Concussion, contusion and severance of the spinal cord, in Windle WF (ed): *The Spinal Cord and Its Reactions to Traumatic Injury.* New York: Marcel Dekker, 1980: 205–217.
50. Young W: Recovery mechanism in spinal cord injury: Implications for regenerative therapy, in Seil FT (ed): *Neural Regeneration and Transplantation.* New York: Liss, 1989: 157–169.
51. Young W: Blood flow metabolic and neurophysiologic mechanisms in spinal cord injury, in Becker D, Poblishok JT (eds): *Central Nervous System Trauma Status Report.* Bethesda: NIH, NINCDS, 1985: 463–473.
52. Young W, Flamm ES, Demopoulos HB, et al: The effect of naloxone on post traumatic ischemia in experimental spinal contusion. *J Neurosurg* 1981; 55:209–219.
53. Young W, Koreh I: Potassium and calcium changes in injured spinal cords. *Brain Res* 1986; 365:42–53.
54. Young W, Flamm ES, Demopoulos HB, et al: Tissue Na, K and Ca changes in regional cerebral ischemia: Their measure and interpretation. *CNS Trauma* 1986; 3:215–234.

Complications and Sequelae

CHAPTER 88

THE ACUTE COMPLICATIONS OF SPINAL CORD INJURY

David W. Cahill
G. R. Rechtine

INTRODUCTION

All spinal cord injuries produce immediate and usually obvious neurological deficits. The physical and psychological trauma attendant upon these losses, both in the victim and the family, is an illness as dramatic as any encountered in clinical medicine. Yet, with the exception of high cervical cord injuries associated with complete respiratory failure, it is rarely the spinal cord injury itself that proves fatal. The great majority of deaths attributable to acute spinal cord injury actually result from the complications of the initial injury and its associated neurological deficit.

Prior to the advent of modern respiratory care techniques, the majority of quadriplegic cervical cord-injured patients died of secondary pulmonary difficulties. Quadriplegics and many paraplegics who survived in the initial postinjury phase succumbed months or years later of urologic problems, such as sepsis or renal failure. Before World War I, no more than one-third of quadriplegics survived beyond a few months postinjury.[1] Today, a quadriplegic who survives the first year may expect a virtually normal life expectancy.[2]

Though many spinal cord injuries produce truly devastating changes in the victim's physical capacities and psychological well-being, modern spinal cord injury teams can minimize secondary insults and save lives in the acute and chronic postinjury periods, thus restoring the injured patient's fundamental right to choose to return to a functional existence within the confines of his or her disability.

HYPERACUTE COMPLICATIONS

Hypotension

A complete or near complete injury to the cervical or upper thoracic cord often is associated with functionally total sympathectomy (Table 88-1). The loss of vasoconstrictor tone in trunk and lower extremities, as well as beta-adrenergic cardiostimulatory effect, often produces a clinical picture of hypotension with paradoxical bradycardia as the patient is evaluated in the field or in the emergency room. This condition is best treated with sympathomimetic agents, such as dopamine or dobutamine, rather than with massive volume expansion, if it can be clearly established that there is no associated visceral or extremity injury causing occult hemorrhage and blood loss. However, in the acutely cord-injured patient, massive hemorrhage into the chest, abdomen, or even thigh may produce no physical symptoms. In the face of life-threatening hypotension, volume resuscitation is often the best part of valor until it is clearly established that there is no associated injury with occult bleeding. No amount of vasoconstrictor drug will save the life of someone who has lost three or four liters of blood into the chest or abdomen. It is especially urgent to perform appropriate CT scans or diagnostic lavage in the cord-injured elderly patient, who may quickly progress to congestive heart failure and pulmonary edema from overvigorous fluid resuscitation.

As with any trauma victim in shock, appropriate mon-

TABLE 88-1 Hyperacute Complications

Hypotension/Shock
- Sympathectomy effect
- R/O Blood Loss

Bradycardia
- With or without hypovolemia

Hypothermia
- With or without infection

Hypoventilation/Respiratory Failure
- Occiput–C2: all respiratory function lost; lower cranial nerve palsies
- C3–C4: diaphragm and intercostals out; pharynx/larynx function preserved
- C5–T1: intercostals out; diaphragm preserved
- T2–T12: variable intercostal loss (Beware associated ARDS secondary to aspiration or drowning at time of injury)

Iatrogenic Complications
- Dislocation with secondary spinal cord injury
- Decubiti secondary to prolonged spine board maintenance

Gastrointestinal bleeding
- With or without steroids
- With or without mini-dose heparin

Ileus
- Abdominal distension/vomiting
- Aspiration

itoring of central venous or pulmonary artery pressures is mandatory to reestablish physiological parameters.

Acute Pulmonary Complications

The act of respiration in the normal individual requires the functional integrity of the pontomedullary brainstem and cranial nerves supplying the pharynx and larynx, the cervical cord segments innervating the diaphragm (C3, C4, C5), and the thoracic cord segments innervating the intercostal musculature (T2–T12).

With spinal column injuries involving the bony segments above C4, none of these neural elements may be functional. With fractures involving the occiput, C1, or C2, brainstem injury may impair glottic function or even the transmission of respiratory drive impulses from the brainstem to the cervical cord. Fractures at C3 or C4 and occasionally lower may eliminate both diaphragm and intercostal function. These lesions often are associated with complete respiratory arrest at the time of injury. Resuscitation at the scene may be life-saving, but secondary hypoxic brain injury often impedes rehabilitation. Incomplete injuries at these levels often result in permanent respiratory insufficiency, necessitating chronic ventilatory support and/or diaphragmatic pacing.

With bony injuries at C5–T2, upper airway and diaphragm function usually is preserved, though intercostal function is lost. This common clinical picture usually results in the loss of about half of total preinjury respiratory capacity. Paradoxical chest constriction with diaphragmatic contraction is often seen. These individuals usually are independent of external support in the absence of secondary pulmonary insults, but may quickly become ventilator-dependent if there is associated COPD, pneumonia, ARDS secondary to drowning, pulmonary embolism, or even intraabdominal pathology leading to decreased diaphragmatic excursion.

With bony injuries at T8 or below, there is usually little if any respiratory muscle compromise, yet the inability to stand and hence decompress the diaphragm, may lead to basal segment atelectasis with secondary pneumonia and sometimes life-threatening respiratory insufficiency. This is especially likely in obese patients and smokers.

Though the "Feet First" program appears to be successfully decreasing the number of shallow-water diving accidents, this mechanism of injury still accounts for a significant proportion of cervical cord injuries among young men, especially in coastal areas. The pulmonary complications of drowning are often not apparent on initial radiographs. In this subset of patients, initially adequate respiratory function may quickly deteriorate in the subsequent 24 to 48 hours. The treating physician must be prepared for a rapid neutral neck position intubation if oxygen saturation declines.

As is often apparent on MRI, edema of the cord may extend several segments above and below the visualized spine fracture. In cases of lower cervical fractures, ascending cord edema may impair diaphragmatic function in the several days after injury, necessitating ventilator support temporarily. In most cases, diaphragm function returns as the edema resolves and the patient is able to reestablish respiratory independence.

Harris and Reines noted that the risks of death and significant postinjury complications among the spinal cord injured were directly correlated with age and the results of pulmonary function parameters.[3] In their series, survivors averaged 28 years of age; those who succumbed averaged 53. Of survivors who developed significant pulmonary complications, initial postinjury, forced vital capacity (FVC) averaged 1100ml and Pa_{O_2} 76 mmHg. Of those free of such problems, FVC averaged 1850ml and Pa_{O_2} 90 mmHg.

Almost 40 years ago, Cameron and associates found that, unlike intact individuals whose respiratory capacities are maximal in the upright position, quadriplegics reached their best function when supine.[4] Since quadriplegics have no extensor tone in the major muscle groups of the dorsal spine, the sitting posture leads to collapse of the thorax on the abdomen, telescoping the abdominal contents onto the undersurface of the diaphragm and impairing diaphragmatic excursion.

Over the past 15 years, Green and colleagues and workers at many other spinal cord injury centers have clearly established the benefits of kinetic beds in maximizing respiratory function and minimizing pulmonary complications among quadriplegic patients.[5] Rosner and coworkers documented a significantly decreased pulmonary arteriovenous shunt fraction when patients were nursed on a kinetic bed as opposed to a standard hospital bed.[6] Though RotoBed therapy adds significantly to hospital costs in the short term and to the difficulty of patient transfer for diagnostic or therapeutic procedures, it is reasonably well established that overall improvements in pulmonary management decrease short-term morbidity and hence acute care hospitalization time, and thus are clearly worth the trouble.

The pulmonary compromise secondary to cord injury may lead to life-threatening complications not simply related to hypoventilation. The lack of intercostal function may render cough ineffective or impossible. Without a functional cough, the patient may find it impossible to clear bronchial mucus plugs or even oropharyngeal secretions. Recurrent mucus plugging is a common cause of acute respiratory insufficiency and even death in the early period after cord injury. Frequent tracheal bronchial suctioning and careful pulmonary toilet and physiotherapy are mandatory. This is particularly true in the elderly, smokers, and the homeless or malnourished, many of whom are often relatively dehydrated at the time of injury.

Aspiration of stomach or oropharyngeal contents is very common at the time of initial spinal cord injury and not uncommon after the patient is in the hospital in the first several days after injury. Obviously aspiration is more common in patients who are not intubated than in those who are. Ileus is very common after thoracic or cervical spine injury and may further contribute to the risk of aspiration. Nasogastric suctioning is usually advisable for the first two or three days after cord injury and sometimes for much longer. It should also be remembered that the clinical and radiographic sequelae of aspiration may take days to evolve fully. Initially adequate blood gas analysis and negative chest x-ray may provide a false sense of security.

Hypoexpansion of the chest produces chronic atelectasis, which predisposes to pneumonia. Hospital-acquired organisms in the period following initial stabilization may produce a vehement pneumonitis often resistant to many or most antibiotics. Inadequate cough predisposes to suboptimal bronchial clearance of infectious debris, mandating vigorous respiratory therapy and aggressive medical care. The pneumonia usually is treatable. It nonetheless remains the most common cause of death among quadriplegics in the first year after injury. Most of these deaths occur during the initial hospitalization.[2]

Aggressive preemptive pulmonary care is therefore critical for any immobilized patient—most particularly the patient with a cervical spinal cord injury whose breathing is entirely diaphragmatic. Promotion of full lung expansion and avoidance of ventilation perfusion mismatching must be facilitated by patient positioning without compromising immobilization. Constant vigilance for early evidence of ventilatory compromise, atelectasis, or pneumonia is important. Oxygen saturation should be monitored continuously during the early course via pulse oximetry. Bedside spirometry, including peak expiratory flow rate and vital capacity done on a daily basis, can provide early warning of impending ventilatory compromise. Besides impeding gas exchange, decreased tidal volume will promote pneumonia and atelectasis. When pneumonia or atelectasis occurs, it should be treated aggressively at its earliest appearance with respiratory therapy and increased incentive spirometry, supplemented with flexible bronchoscopy as indicated. Any significant deterioration in oxygenation, ventilation, or spirometry values should be investigated immediately. A number of complications besides pulmonary disease can interfere with pulmonary function, including fatigue, inadequate nutrition, embarrassment of the diaphragm by abdominal distension, pain, etc. Other less common but nonetheless important causes of deterioration in respiratory function include cardiac disease, pulmonary embolism, oversedation, and ascension of the spinal cord injury. Such etiologies should be investigated when the cause of respiratory compromise is not readily apparent.

Immobilization Beds

An integral component of the acute care of spinal cord injury is the management of the patient in an appropriate bed. One must be able to rely on the bed to maintain spinal stability and alignment while at the same time allowing easy nursing access and an ability to reposition the patient frequently in an attempt to lessen the complications of immobilization. As noted previously, the two most commonly utilized special beds are the wedge turning frame (Stryker frame) and the kinetic treatment table (RotoBed).

The importance of "mobilizing" the patient in spinal traction cannot be overemphasized. In general, it is well known that spinal cord-injured patients are susceptible to many systemic complications, regardless of the treatment undertaken. The techniques of immobilization and prolonged immobilization itself may further increase the complications rate. The best current available information about risks of such complications comes from the National Acute Spinal Cord Injury Study.[7] In 478 patients treated at spinal cord injury centers from 1986 through 1988, there was a 30 percent incidence of pneumonia, 18.6 percent decubiti, 4.6 percent thrombophlebitis, and 2.8 percent pulmonary embolism.

The Stryker frame has been in widespread use for many decades; however, its potential inadequacies in immobilizing the cervical spine were first pointed out by Slabaugh and Nickel in 1978.[8] The frame is a narrow canvas-covered structure that is lightweight and simple to use. It is recommended that patients be turned from the supine to the prone position every two hours while on this frame. During turning, the patient is wedged between the two pieces of the frame to protect against loss of spinal immobilization.

Slabaugh pointed out three specific concerns with the Stryker frame: loss of immobilization with turning; diminished pulmonary vital capacity; development of decubiti in unusual locations. One case was presented of loss of alignment of a C5–C6 subluxation on turning from the supine to the prone position. They also found 13 to 16 percent decrements in vital capacity going from the prone to the supine positions on the frame. Finally, a number of occipital decubitus ulcers were encountered.[8]

The kinetic treatment table is a bulky apparatus. However, it automatically and continually rotates the patient in a cradlelike fashion through an arc of 125 degrees. Added supports are used to maintain arms, legs, and trunk in proper position and can be easily removed for nursing or other therapeutic interventions. In addition, there are supports for the side of the head to prevent any rotation when the bed is in motion.

The benefits of kinetic therapy have been described in a number of reports. Green and coworkers reported a series of 105 acute spinal cord injuries treated on a kinetic bed, with only a 1.9 percent incidence of significant pulmonary complications.[9] Brackett and Condon compared complications in patients treated on both Stryker frames and kinetic beds.[10] Of the 14 complete spinal cord injuries immobilized on Stryker frames, 46 percent had severe pulmonary problems; of these, almost one-third went on to respiratory failure and death. However, none of the 17 patients managed on kinetic beds had any severe pulmonary problems, and no deaths were reported. The total days spent in the intensive care unit was 45 percent greater for those on the Stryker frame compared with those treated on a kinetic bed.

Recently, McGuire and associates examined the efficacy of immobilization of the spine, comparing the two beds.[11] Using a cadaver model, unstable injuries were produced in both cervical and lumbar spine. The spines were then rotated on the beds, as is typically done in clinical management. With the unstable lumbar injuries on the Stryker frame, significant anteroposterior displacement, angular movement, and distraction were seen at the injury site on turning the model from the supine to the prone position; no similar movements were identifiable with the spine on a kinetic bed. Similarly, with an unstable cervical spine injury, turning from the supine to the prone position on the Stryker frame resulted in considerable change in the degree of distraction and angular movement. No such changes were seen with the spine on the kinetic bed.

Based on the above information, it does not appear that the Stryker frame is suitable for patients with severely unstable complicated spine injuries or for those with preexisting pulmonary problems. There should be additional concerns about its use in obese patients or in patients with marked agitation or restlessness. When the frame is used, the patient should be carefully checked after each turn for any new complaints or neurological findings. Arterial blood gases or pulse oximetry should be monitored continually to watch for arterial desaturation when going from one position to another. Finally, a lateral spine x-ray should be made in both the supine and prone positions on at least one occasion to ensure that clinically unexpected significant spine movement is not occurring.

The kinetic bed will rotate the patient automatically in a 125-degree arc every 4 to 5 minutes and can be stopped in any position to facilitate nursing care. The patient's back can be assessed through one of the several hatches on the underside of the bed so as to minimize patient movement. The side supports are easily removed to provide for ranging of the extremities. The kinetic bed, however, is not without potential problems. In a previous study, Marshall and colleagues reported one patient neurologically deteriorating in the course of rotation on the RotoBed.[12] Additionally, spine surgery generally is not possible while the patient remains on a kinetic bed. Nevertheless, for complex spine injuries, especially those associated with spinal cord injury, the kinetic bed offers significant advantages in patient management.

Fever or Hypothermia

The sympathectomy effect of spinal cord injury leads to vasodilatation and hypothermia. The inability to shiver eliminates this mechanism for generating heat. Hence, in addition to being relatively hypotensive and bradycardic, the acutely cord-injured patient often is hypothermic, irrespective of whether he or she is septic or well. Acute sepsis may have few associated vital sign alterations among the quadriplegic. Absence of fever should never dissuade the treating physician from pursuing the appropriate workup if there is any reason to suspect infection.

Temperature homeostasis tends to recover in most patients over time, but most nonetheless remain partially poikilothermic when exposed unprotected to higher or lower ambient temperatures. In the subacute or chronic phase after cord injury, spasticity and/or autonomic dysreflexia may produce falsely elevated body temperature in the absence of infection. This is rarely the case in the acute postinjury period.

Associated Injuries

The usual symptoms or even signs of somatic injuries often are inapparent with concomitant cord injury. It is critically important to evaluate thoracic, abdominal, extremity, and lower spinal contents, assuming that they are injured until proved otherwise. Acute cord injury with deficit does not mean that lower spinal or lower extremity fractures should not be treated. Initial therapy must always assume that the patient may recover some or all of his or her deficit.

In treating associated injuries, however, the risks of pressure ulceration and respiratory compromise must constantly be borne in mind. The development of pressure sores secondary to casts, inadvertent phrenic nerve injury during surgery, pneumothorax secondary to central line placement, etc., can prove life-threatening.

Perhaps the most devastating complication is a worsened neurological deficit secondary to an iatrogenic spinal dislocation acquired while moving a patient with a spinal fracture for a diagnostic or therapeutic procedure. However, though immobilization is critical until stability is reestablished, this policy must never be so rigid as to preclude adequate diagnostic testing or therapy.

Gastrointestinal Bleeding

There is an increased risk of gastric bleeding with any type of physical or psychological trauma. This risk is exacerbated further by chronic steroid administration and may be made even worse by hyperacute megadose steroid administration. The NASCIS II Trial found a 4.5 percent incidence of gastric hemorrhage in a 24-hour megadose methylprednisolone group versus a 3 percent incidence in the placebo group.[7] Epstein and coworkers found no increase in the incidence of GI bleeding, however, with the use of "minidose" heparin for deep venous thrombosis prophylaxis in spinal cord-injured patients.[13] There is clearly, however, increased incidence of gastric hemorrhage with full therapeutic anticoagulation. Thus, spinal cord-injured patients are naturally at risk for GI hemorrhage and may be at increased risk secondary to necessary therapeutic interventions.

Prophylaxis against GI hemorrhage clearly results in decreased risk of this complication. There appears to be no significant difference in results for the various methods of prophylaxis. Routine oral antacids are quite effective if given frequently in high doses and titrated against the gastric pH. H2-blockers and mucosal protective agents (Sucralfate) are equally effective if given in appropriate dosages. Cost, ease of administration, and side effects are the factors to be considered in deciding which form of prophylaxis is most appropriate in a given case. Combinations of two or more prophylactic agents often are appropriate in patients with known ulcer histories.

SUBACUTE COMPLICATIONS

Deep Venous Thrombosis and Pulmonary Embolism

The protean nature of deep venous thrombosis (DVT) and pulmonary embolism (PE) mandates particular attention to these disease entities in the spinal injury patient. DVT occurs in approximately 15 percent of paralyzed patients, accompanied by pulmonary embolism in about half that number (Table 88-2).[14] DVT prophylaxis should be initiated as soon as possible. Intermittent compression stockings should be utilized if there are no contraindications. Low-dose heparin should be started as soon as the patient has stabilized from the multiple trauma and any needed operative procedure. Early mobilization also will be of use in preventing DVT. In any patient in whom low-dose heparin administration is contraindicated and who must remain immobilized, strong consideration should be given to placement of an inferior vena cava filter.

The possibility of pulmonary embolism also should be kept in mind whenever there is respiratory compromise that is not straightforwardly explained. Arterial blood gas values characteristically are not helpful in the absence of a very large embolus, and the chest radiograph will not be diagnostic unless there has been frank pulmonary infarction. If the clinical suspicion arises, a ventilation perfusion study often is the first diagnostic approach; however, based on the results of the PIOPED study, the only absolutely diagnostic VQ scan results are "normal" or "high probability."[15] The significant occurrence of both false-positive and false-negative results relegates intermediate VQ scan results as nonabsolute. Since many spinal cord injury patients have some element of pulmonary dysfunction, which almost eliminates the possibility of a normal ventilation scan, and since complete anticoagulation is rather undesirable during the acute course in such patients, pulmonary

TABLE 88-2 Subacute Complications

Secondary Respiratory Failure
- Mucus plugging
- Atelectasis
- Pneumonia
- Pulmonary embolism

Deep Vein Thrombosis
- Almost universal
- PE prophylaxis mandatory

Bladder/Bowel dysfunction
- Priapism
- Urinary retention with bladder overdistension
- Bladder may be spastic or flaccid
- Sphincters may be spastic or flaccid
- Vesicosphincteric dyssynergia
- Fecal impaction
- Rectal overdistension ± tear
- Hemorrhoids

Skin Breakdown/Decubiti
- Beware prolonged spine board use for diagnostic or therapeutic procedures
- RotoBeds turned off don't help!

Inadequate Nutrition

Autonomic Dysreflexia
- Usually secondary to overdistension of bowel or bladder

Age and chronic disease increase all risks of spinal cord injury
- –COPD → Pulmonary Cx
- –ASCVD → Coronary + Cerebral Cx
- –Degenerative spinal stenosis → Neurological Cx
- –Prostate hypertrophy → Urological Cx
- –Osteoporosis → Orthopedic Cx

angiography often is required following an intermediate VQ scan report and indeed is the initial study of choice in many instances. Although an inferior vena cava filter is a viable alternative to systemic anticoagulation, it is not without serious short- and long-term complications, including recurrent pulmonary embolism.

Bowel and Bladder Dysfunction

The complex autonomic and voluntary innervation of the bladder and the sphincter may be disordered in various ways in the face of spinal cord injury. Unfortunately, the classic teaching that an upper motor neuron injury produces a spastic bladder whereas a lower motor neuron injury produces a hypotonic bladder is very simplistic and often incorrect. In any case, the autonomic (sympathetic) innervation of the vesical sphincter and voluntary innervation of the pelvic diaphragm ("external sphincter") are at least as important for function as the contractile state of the parasympathetically innervated detrusor muscle.

Upon admission after spinal cord injury, two common genitourinary complications must be dealt with immediately. In males with cervical injuries, priapism is common and makes catheterization difficult. Though usually self-limited, local urologic measures sometimes are necessary for control. The more important acute issue is urinary retention and overdistension of the bladder.

Urinary retention is present in almost every spinal cord injury acutely. Whether retention is secondary to detrusor flaccidity, autonomic or voluntary sphincter hyperactivity, or some form of vesicosphincteric dyssynergia, the acute therapy is the same—bladder catheterization.

It is recommended that an indwelling bladder catheter be used until resuscitation and stabilization have been accomplished, associated injuries are treated, and fluid intake can be safely restricted, after which intermittent catheterization may be safely instituted. Institution of an intermittent catheterization regimen while the patient is hemodynamically unstable or still requires large amounts of fluid is contraindicated. The incidences of urosepsis and secondary hypotonic bladder due to overdistention have been dramatically decreased by using these techniques. Controversy exists over whether or not to use prophylactic antibiotics routinely in all cord-injured patients with indwelling or intermittent catheters.

In the subacute and chronic period after cord injury, the management of the bladder depends on the results of complete urodynamic evaluation and may range from spontaneous voiding into a condom catheter or diaper to complex urological surgical procedures. The majority of cervical cord-injured patients void spontaneously once the period of spinal shock and cord edema has passed.

Bowel management in the acute phase after injury must consider both ends of the gastrointestinal tract. As noted above, ileus is very common in the first few days after cord injury. Abdominal distension impairs diaphragmatic excursion and further increases the likelihood of vomiting, risking aspiration. In either case, respiratory status may be acutely compromised. Nasogastric decompression is very important. This is rarely needed for more than a few days in the absence of associated abdominal injury.

At the opposite end of the bowel, autonomic denervation of the colon and rectum and voluntary denervation of the abdominal wall and pelvic diaphragm make voluntary defecation impossible. Fecal impaction can become quite severe in only a few days. Untreated abdominal distension, hemorrhoids, and even a rectal tear may occur. It is generally recommended that stool softeners be used on a twice-a-day basis and every-other-day rectal suppositories begun immediately after admission. Oral laxatives and enemas are used as necessary until a regular bowel routine is established. Digital evacuation of the rectum is often necessary two or three times weekly in the acute period. Early attention to the bowel regimen is especially important in elderly patients or chronic laxative abusers.

Skin Complications and Decubiti

Though decubiti are more likely to develop in the subacute or chronic period after cord injury, it is likely that mismanagement in the acute phase may predispose to this complication.[17] All cord-injured patients will develop pressure sores if not managed appropriately and if allowed to sit or lie in a fixed position for prolonged periods. This includes lying on a hospital bed or on a kinetic bed that is not moving.

A recent study found that any patient kept on a spine board for as long as eight hours after mobilization in the field was predisposed to the development of decubiti.[18] Keeping the patient on the spine board makes it very easy for EMT personnel, emergency room personnel, and various consultants to resuscitate, stabilize, obtain diagnostic studies, and operate on associated injuries—but is nonetheless inappropriate. Presacral, trochanteric, calcaneal, occipital, and scapular pressure sores are far easier to prevent than to treat. Extensive plastic surgical procedures often are needed for closure.

Curry and Casady found that the risk of decubiti was linearly related to the length of time a patient was kept on the spine board, although the actual sore may develop only days or weeks later.[18] There is little valid reason to keep a cord-injured patient on a spine board once he or she has arrived at the receiving center and has been initially evaluated.

Nutrition

As with all forms of major trauma, calorie and nitrogen requirements are very high in the initial few days after injury. Post-cord-injury ileus or associated abdominal injuries may preclude external alimentation acutely. Currently it is recommended that oral or enteral alimentation be begun as soon as possible after the injury. If enteral alimentation cannot be started within three days of admission, parenteral alimentation should be considered and maintained until the bowel is functional. However, no amount of alimentation will prevent the often dramatic weight loss that follows cord injury.

Autonomic Dysreflexia

The phenomena of hypertension, bradycardia, and piloerection, along with profuse sweating of the head and upper extremities, compose a form of autonomic crisis occasionally seen in the acute phase after spinal cord injury.[19] Even in a chronic phase, autonomic crises are becoming progressively less common with better education of patients and families on the necessity of good bowel and bladder management. Nonetheless, the hypertension seen in this syndrome can be dramatic and life-threatening. Though any form of stimulation may trigger the storm, visceral stimulation is usual; most commonly overdistension of bladder or rectum. Visceral stimulation during barium enema, colonoscopy, cystoscopy, etc., also may initiate the crisis.[20] Therapy must always first eliminate the source of stimulation (stop the procedure, empty the bowel, disimpact the rectum, etc.) and then control the hypertension if it persists. Repeated episodes of autonomic dysreflexia occasionally may warrant prophylactic sympatholytic therapy.

Age and the Risk of Complications

In Florida, there has been a large experience with the management of spinal cord injuries in the elderly. While the typical central cord syndrome secondary to hyperextension of the stenotic spondylitic cervical spine is most common, any form of cervical or thoracolumbar cord injury may occur. Diffuse degenerative spine disease, chronic pulmonary disease, arteriosclerotic vascular disease, hypertension, and benign and malignant prostate disease are all very common in the elderly and increase the risks of all the complications discussed previously. Hypotension in the face of stenotic coronary or cerebral arteries predisposes to myocardial infarction or stroke. Chronic obstructive lung disease related to smoking may make an otherwise independent patient ventilator-dependent. Prostate disease adds another complicating dimension to bladder management. Osteopenia makes recurrent or multiple spine or long bone fractures likely.

The care of elderly cord-injured patients requires anticipation of likely complications in order that they may be treated expeditiously or prevented. In treating the infirm elderly, however, one must never lose sight of the likely long-term outcome. Therapeutic decisions must be tempered with judgment.

CONCLUSION

Five thousand years ago, the author of the Egyptian document now called The Edwin Smith Papyrus warned of the hopelessness of treating patients with quadriplegia.[21] In the subsequent centuries, little progress has been made in reversing the deficits that attend upon the initial cord trauma. We have therefore concerned ourselves here with the more measurable accomplishments in the prevention and management of secondary complications. Dramatic improvements have been made in saving lives after cord injury and in the surgical repair of the broken spine.

Our function as spinal cord injury physicians is not unlike our function in most other areas of medicine. It is to help patients and their families deal with serious illnesses by maximizing residual function and preventing secondary insults. In the acute management of spinal cord injury, a lot has been accomplished.

References

1. Hartwell JB: An analysis of 133 fractures of the spine treated at the Massachusetts General Hospital. *Boston Med Surg J* 1917; 177:31–41.
2. Ducker TB, Lucas JT, Wallis CA: Recovery from spinal cord injury. *Clin Neurosurgery* 1983; 30:495–513.
3. Harris R, Reines HD: Prevention of pulmonary complications in spinal cord injury with the roto rest bed, in Green BA, Summer WR (eds): *Continuous Oscillation Therapy: Research and Practical Applications.* Miami: University of Miami Press, 1986:56–62.
4. Cameron GS, Scott JW, Jousse AT, Botterell EG: Diaphragmatic respiration in the quadriplegic patient and the effect of position on his vital capacity. *Ann Surg* 1955; 141:451–456.
5. Green BA, Summer WR (eds): *Continuous Oscillation Therapy: Research and Practical Applications.* Miami: University of Miami Press, 1986.
6. Rosner MJ, Coley I, Elias Z: Oscillating therapy and pulmonary shunt fraction after severe spinal cord injury, in Green BA, Summer WR (eds): *Continuous Oscillation Therapy: Research and Practical Applications.* Miami: University of Miami Press, 1986:79–83.
7. Bracken MB, Shepard MJ, Collins WF, et al: A randomized controlled trial of methylprednisolone or naloxone in the treatment of acute spinal cord injury. *N Engl J Med* 1990; 322:1405–1411.
8. Slabaugh PB, Nickel VL: Complications with use of the Stryker frame. *J Bone Joint Surg* 1978; 60A:2222–2223.
9. Green BA, Green KL, Klose KJ: Kinetic therapy for spinal cord injury. *Spine* 1983; 8:722–728.
10. Brackett TO, Condon N: Comparison of the wedge turning frame and kinetic treatment table in the acute care of spinal cord injury patients. *Surg Neurol* 1984; 22:53–56.
11. McGuire RA, Green BA, Eismont FJ, Watt C: Comparison of stability provided to the unstable spine by the kinetic therapy table and the Stryker frame. *Neurosurg* 1988; 22:842–845.
12. Marshall LF, Knowlton S, Garfin SR, et al: Deterioration following spinal cord injury: A multicenter study. *J Neurosurg* 1987; 66:400–404.
13. Epstein N, Hood DC, Ransohoff J: Gastrointestinal bleeding in patients with spinal cord trauma. *J Neurosurg* 1981; 54:16–20.
14. Casas ER, Sanchez MP, Arais CR, et al: Prophylaxis of venous thrombosis and pulmonary embolism in patients with acute traumatic spinal cord lesions. *Paraplegia* 1976; 14:178–183.
15. PIOPED: Value of the ventilation perfusion scan in acute pulmonary embolism: Results of the prospective investigational pulmonary embolism diagnosis. Pioped Investigators. *JAMA* 1990; 263:2753–2759.
16. Krane RJ, Siroky MB (eds): *Clinical Neurourology.* Boston: Little, Brown, 1991.
17. Linares HA, Mawson AR, Suarez E, Biundo JJ: Association between pressure sores and immobilization in the immediate post injury period. *Clin Ortho* 1987; 10:517–573.
18. Curry K, Casady L: The relationship between extended periods of immobility and decubitus ulcer formation in the acutely spinal cord injured individual. *J Neurosci Nurs* 1992; 24:185–189.
19. Appenzeller O: *The Autonomic Nervous System* (3d ed). Amsterdam: North Holland, 1982.
20. Fleischman S, Shah P: Autonomic dysreflexia: An unusual radiologic complication. *Diag Radiol* 1977; 124:695–697.
21. Breasted JH: *The Edwin Smith Surgical Papyrus,* vol 1. Chicago: University of Chicago Press, 1930.

CHAPTER 89

LATE SEQUELAE OF SPINAL CORD INJURY

Joseph M. Piepmeier

INTRODUCTION

Clinical studies from spinal cord injury treatment centers have provided the majority of useful reports concerning the neurological outcome and long-term sequelae following traumatic spinal cord injury. Most studies of spinal cord-injured patients demonstrate remarkable similarities in patient epidemiology, the location and mechanism of injury, severity of initial neurological deficits, and recovery statistics. Only the treatment methods and conclusions regarding the effectiveness of therapy are different.

It is clear that a patient's neurological outcome and ultimate functional capabilities relate directly to the severity and location of their initial neurological impairment. As a practical guide to evaluating outcome, patients can be divided into two groups: those with total loss of motor and sensory function (complete injury) at the time of injury and those with some retained neurological function (partial injury) distal to the cord lesion.[1,3,20] Regardless of the type of treatment, patients with complete injuries not only have a significantly less favorable prognosis for recovery, but also have more complications and longer hospitalizations. Patients with partial lesions have a much more favorable prognosis for significant improvement in neurological function, and many regain sufficient movement and sensation to achieve functional independence.

Even with the recent findings from randomized clinical trials that show improvement in recovery with pharmacological treatment, the severity of the initial injury to the cord remains the most important factor in predicting outcome.[4,5,7] Rehabilitation therapy has been the primary method of optimizing a patient's functional capabilities and preventing complications that have a deleterious effect on recovery.[21] However, spinal cord-injured patients are susceptible to a variety of neurological and systemic problems that occur at a time remote from the injury, and these patients frequently require neurosurgical intervention to halt or reverse these problems. This chapter will review some of the most significant issues as they relate to the neurological outcome and sequelae of traumatic cord injury.

NEUROLOGICAL VS. FUNCTIONAL OUTCOME

The interpretation of outcome results following traumatic cord injury depends on the method of measuring the patient's impairments.[6,7,11,17,19,22] The most sensitive clinical method of measurement is a careful neurological examination. This type of evaluation typically grades motor function according to force of movement in representative muscle groups and sensory perception by the ability to detect different stimuli in the dermatomes caudad to the lesion.[3,5,7,10,11,17] This information then is used to quantify neurological function according to a numerical scale. Changes in the neurological examination are evaluated by changes in a numerical score. While a graded neurological examination can detect even small changes in motor and sensory function, it is vulnerable to variations in grading by different examiners, and it provides little direct information regarding the functional significance of these numerical changes. This type of evaluation most commonly has been applied in clinical studies where the ability to detect even small changes in the neurological examination relate to statistical considerations on outcome.

Functional scales typically do not quantify the relative differences in motor power and sensory perception.[3,6,7,10,16,19] They interpret outcome by evaluating how changes influence the patient's ability to perform daily activities. Functional scales are less susceptible to variations in measurement by examiners. However, because they are less sensitive to fluctuations in the neurological examination, the impact of therapy on neurological recovery may not be detected as readily. The major advantage is that changes in functional status are more highly correlated with changes in the patient's abilities and life-style. The optimal method for evaluating recovery should include the ability to quantify changes in the neurological examination as well as a functional scale that determines whether these neurological changes result in a life-style change for the individual.

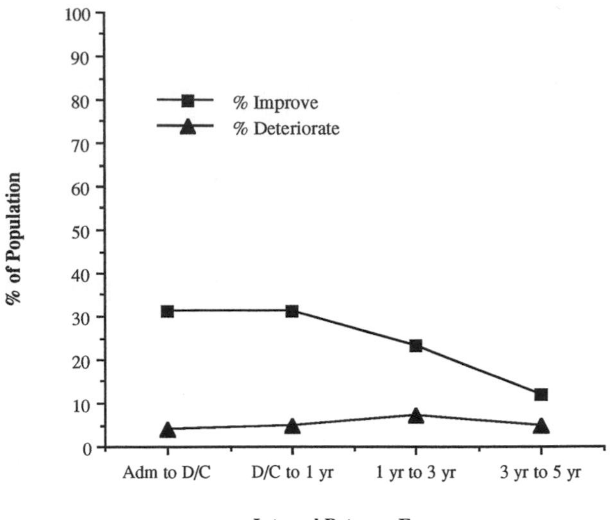

Figure 89-1. Graph demonstrating the incidence of delayed improvement and deterioration in spinal cord injured patients over five years after injury. The percentages indicate the number of patients who lost or gained one or more Frankel grades in the indicated time interval.

NEUROLOGICAL SEQUELAE

Virtually all clinical studies demonstrate that the more severe the spinal cord injury, as determined by the initial neurological examination, the less likely significant recovery will occur.[3,6,22,23] Patients with complete loss of motor and sensory function below the level of injury clearly have a worse prognosis than those with some retained motor power or sensory perception. In other words, the amount of recovery is inversely proportional to the severity of the initial trauma, and the more neurological function that is retained, the greater the patient's chances of improving. Neurological improvement has been demonstrated in 14 to 30 percent of patients with complete lesions by one year.[1,6,9–12] However, fewer than 5 percent of these patients will regain the ability to walk. In contrast, patients with retained function following injury have a significantly better prognosis for ambulating within one year. For example, patients with motorplegia but preserved sensation (primarily posterior column function) have a 34 to 72 percent chance of walking.[1,6,9–12] Patients with preserved movement, even if it is very weak, have a 50 to 93 percent incidence of recovering the ability to walk.[1,6,9–12] These numbers reflect an assessment of functional capabilities within the first year after injury. Data concerning late changes in neurological and functional abilities are more difficult to find. A discussion of delayed improvement and deterioration (after the first year) is presented below (Fig. 89-1).

DELAYED IMPROVEMENT

Most reports on recovery and neurological outcome compare a patient's status at the time of initial evaluation with the status at discharge from the hospital or at one year. This method of reporting clinical results implies that significant changes in the patient's status does not occur after this time. While it has generally been reported that the maximal recovery of neurological function as measured by quantifying the neurological examination or by functional scales occurs within the first few months after injury, significant changes in the patient's status may continue for several years. However, even these late changes follow a pattern similar to the one-year results. Late improvements occur less frequently in patients with more severe injuries.

Although an accurate assessment of the incidence of delayed (after the first year) recovery has not been established, continued improvements can be detected in nearly 25 percent of spinal cord-injured patients by three years and in an additional 12 percent by five years.[10] Because the numbers of patients studied for this extended period are small, these findings raise the potential for overestimating the frequency of delayed changes. Within these limitations it has been found that although useful motor function returned in 3 percent of patients with initial complete injuries, no patients who remained plegic for one year regained motor power after this time period.[10] However, around 10 percent of the patients who maintain complete injuries for one year will regain some sensory perception at three years, and an additional 10 percent will be found to perceive crude sensation below the level of injury at five years. It should be noted that none of the delayed improvements noted were associated with changes in the patient's functional capabilities.[10] These findings may not impact the lifestyle of the patient, but they present the basis for speculation regarding the ability of the spinal cord to recover, even at this late time.

For patients with incomplete injuries the chances for recovery and the frequency of delayed improvement are greater. Of the patients with even modest retained motor power in the lower extremities who subsequently recover the ability to walk, approximately 50 percent will achieve this status after the first year. Nearly one-third of patients with motorplegia but retained sensation achieve the ability to ambulate after one year.[10]

Physiotherapy may be an important reason why patients with retained movement regain functional use of their legs. However, rehabilitation provides a reasonable explanation for only half of the patients who experience delayed improvement. Although the reasons for delayed changes in functional status for the remainder have not been determined precisely, these data support the importance of continued neurological evaluation and physiotherapy for many years following injury.

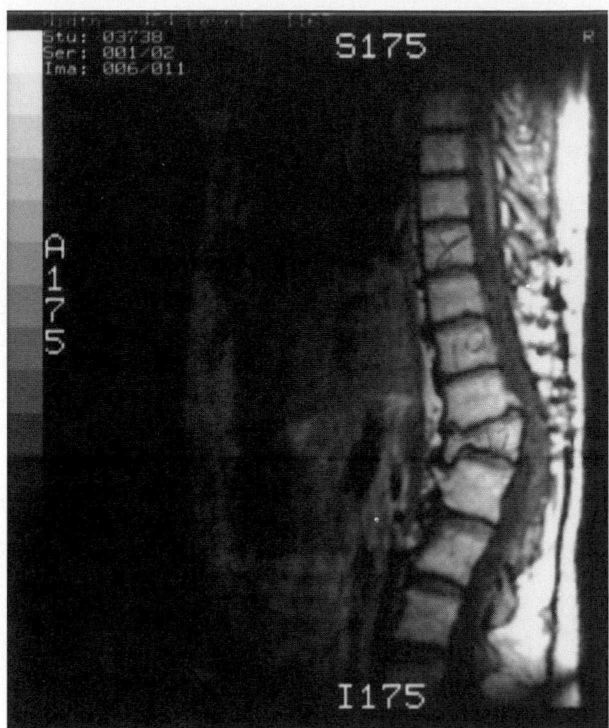

Figure 89-2. Sagittal MRI of the thoracic cord with ascending sensory loss seven years following a complete spinal cord injury at T12. The study demonstrates loss of cord as high as T8.

Delayed Deterioration

An accurate assessment of the incidence of late deterioration in neurological function remains unknown. Most reported series indicate that the incidence of deterioration is low, likely reflecting the expertise of specialized spinal cord injury treatment centers.[6,8–12,24] However, several factors have been identified that are associated with loss of function. In general, it has been found that the frequency of late deterioration appears to be stable over several years following injury. That is to say, between 1 and 2 percent of patients will lose function each year during the first five years.[10] The incidence of loss of function also correlates with the severity of the injury; the more profound the initial impairment, the greater the risk of delayed functional loss.

The majority of causes of late deterioration in neurological function result from systemic complications from the spinal injury or to delayed changes within the cord at the injury site. Deterioration in the patient's status is an indication for investigation, and high-resolution imaging techniques can provide detailed information concerning the region of interest (Fig. 89-2). Several pathological changes have been identified and associated with late deterioration, including posttraumatic cysts, tethering, atrophy, delayed spinal deformity, fibrosis, residual cord compression, and subarachnoid cysts.[24–26] These problems may become clinically relevant by causing motor and/or sensory loss, pain, change in posture, increased spasticity, or autonomic dysfunction. Since many of these problems have similar clinical presentations, imaging is important in determining a cause.

The results of medical and surgical correction of spinal deformities and intrinsic cord lesions associated with late deterioration need more critical evaluation. However, in appropriately selected patients, it has been found that deterioration can be stopped; in some cases treated early, reversal of new deficits may be possible.[24–26]

RADIOLOGICAL EVALUATION

The evaluation of the spinal cord injured patient has been facilitated by noninvasive high-resolution imaging. While recent studies suggest that magnetic resonance imaging (MRI) findings within a few days of injury correlate with outcome,[28] high-resolution imaging studies also can provide critical information concerning the likely causes of late deterioration in status. It is generally held that computed tomography (CT) offers detailed images of the spine and can be very useful for evaluating late bone deformity and poor healing of fractures.[25] MRI provides high-resolution images of the cord and intrinsic cord pathology.[25] However, both of these imaging techniques are limited by imaging artifacts that arise from metallic instrumentation typically overlying the area of maximal interest. When necessary, contrast myelography with tomography may be needed to investigate the spinal cord in regions obscured by metallic artifact. On occasion, metallic implants have been removed to permit a better examination of the spinal cord.

Indications for Evaluation

The new onset of neurological deterioration, change in posture, or deterioration in functional status are indications for radiological evaluation. When imaging studies reveal a likely cause for the new findings, treatment options should be carefully considered. The widespread use of high-resolution imaging also has caused problems in management by identifying altered anatomy and intrinsic cord lesions that commonly occur and are not necessarily reasons for deterioration nor indications for intervention. Consequently, imaging findings must be considered carefully, since correction of altered anatomy on imaging may not achieve the desired result (Fig. 89-3). In selected cases, late intervention can enhance recovery; however, under most circumstances, correction of an intrinsic cord lesion will halt the progression of a new deficit (Fig. 89-4).

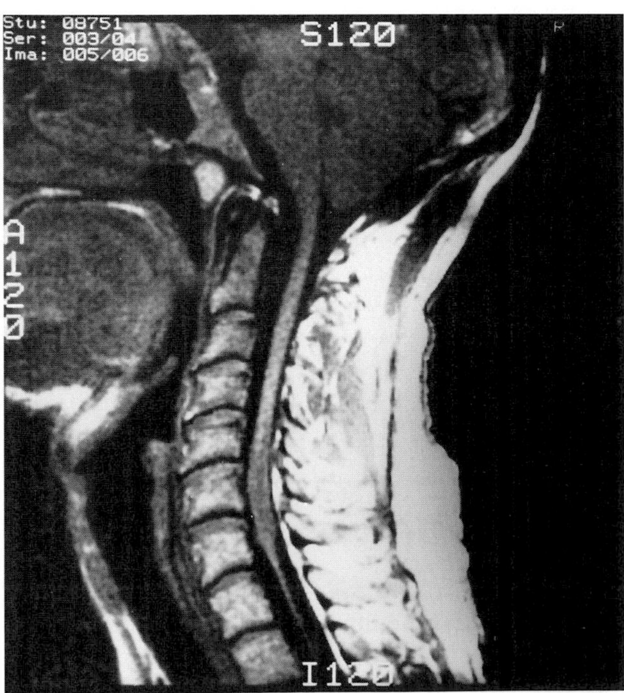

Figure 89-3. Sagittal MRI of the cervical spine in a patient with progressive loss of sensory function four years following trauma thought to be caused by spondylosis. The imaging study clearly demonstrates atrophy of the distal cord as the cause of progressive deterioration.

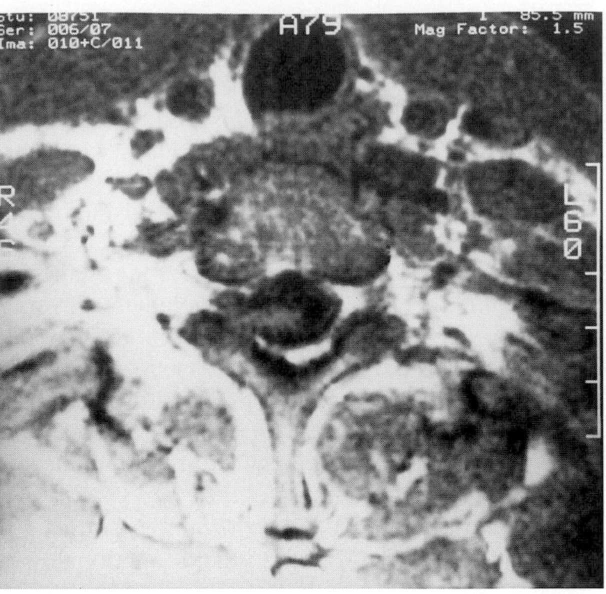

Figure 89-4. Axial MRI of the cervical spine in a patient with progressive myelopathy eight years following cervical root avulsion. Tethering of the cord at the site of avulsion was corrected surgically, resulting in neurological improvement.

Interpretation of Imaging Findings

Since the region of injury will not have normal anatomy, one must determine whether MRI and CT findings represent a new lesion or merely the persistence of a stable lesion. The decision to correct an intrinsic cord lesion is facilitated by obtaining a baseline study that can be used for comparison with later imaging studies. This is particularly true for the treatment of posttraumatic cystic cavitation. Cavitation at the site of trauma is common in patients with severe cord injuries.[25] However, there is little compelling evidence to indicate that surgical drainage offers any advantage to the patient unless the cysts are considered to be the cause of an ascending lesion or deterioration in patients with retained cord function (Fig. 89-5). Similarly, cord compression from residual canal compromise may have little relationship to the patient's current problems. There have been isolated reports of significant improvement following surgical correction of compressive lesions, even late after injury.[25,26] This appears to be most often reported with lesions in the cauda equina or at the thoracolumbar junction.[29] However, surgery for late cord compression often results in loss of spinal stability and the need for fusion and prolonged immobilization. While these problems do not preclude the importance of preserving cord and root function, they must be con-

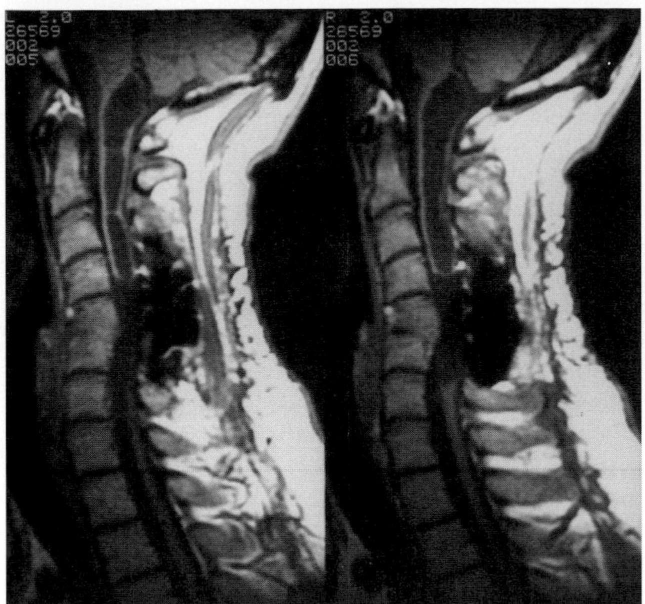

Figure 89-5. Sagittal MRI of the cervical spine in a patient with ascending neurological deficits five years following a complete spinal injury at C5. The posttraumatic cyst was treated surgically, resulting in neurological improvement.

sidered prior to offering the patient a surgical procedure.

DELAYED SPINAL INSTABILITY

A major concern in the management of spinal cord injury is reestablishing stability in the injured spinal elements. For the purposes of this chapter, spinal instability is defined as the mechanical failure of the spine to support the axial skeleton and protect the spinal cord.

Disruption caused by fracture and dislocation of vertebral segments is relatively easy to demonstrate, whereas ligamentous injury may not become apparent until time and weight-loading reveal delayed instability. Consequently, deformity resulting from mechanical failure may not become apparent until late, and may reach medical attention because of neurological loss, pain, or functional impairment from changes in posture and gait.[26] Paralysis can result in further deterioration of the axial and extremity skeleton associated with osteomalacia, heterotopic bone formation, fractures, and flexion deformity.

Kyphosis

Spinal cord injury is associated with paralysis of paraspinous muscles and loss of this important element in maintaining stability.[26] The natural history of instability leads to kyphosis. These deformities can bring functional impairment (chin on chest) in the cervical region or altered cardiopulmonary function in the thoracic region. Once this problem is identified, it may progress to the point of impairment in nearly 50 percent of patients, and surgical correction is often the only reliable method of correction. Anterior surgical approaches frequently are required to release the deformity and to decompress the cord. When the deformity is treated early, prior to autofusion, reduction of the deformity and posterior stabilization may be sufficient to prevent further progression. Posttraumatic kyphosis is commonly associated with postlaminectomy patients when the potential long-term consequences of posterior decompression are not adequately considered. Because the posterior elements have been altered by surgery and have failed to secure stability, both an anterior and posterior approach often are required to correct the deformity.[26]

Scoliosis

Although scoliosis is not as common as kyphosis following traumatic cord injury, this deformity may occur, particularly in the pediatric population.[26,27] Altered muscle tone and restriction of mobility to a wheelchair contribute to this problem. Once identified, scoliosis tends to be progressive. Progressive scoliosis causes a change in functional status that results from altered posture. External immobilization and bracing can, at times, halt the progression; however, since the mechanisms that led to this deformity are permanent, surgical correction and stabilization frequently are required.

Pseudarthrosis

Pseudarthrosis is the failure of a fracture to heal sufficiently to regain mechanical stability. While the incidence of this problem varies according to different authors, it is clear that the risk is increased when a dislocation has not been reduced.[26] Pseudarthrosis is commonly associated with pain that increases with mechanical stress and progressive deformity associated with weight-bearing. Since by definition a pseudarthrosis is not fixed, it usually can be reduced and fused by a posterior approach. When the anterior pseudarthrosis is stabilized (usually by compression rods) spontaneous fusion commonly occurs.[26]

Prevention of Delayed Instability

Posttraumatic spinal deformity cannot always be prevented, but the incidence of this problem can be reduced by adequate immobilization and/or spinal fixation and fusion following injury. It is important to monitor these patients closely, particularly in the pediatric population, where the growing spine is susceptible to more rapid changes and these problems may be magnified. Progressive spinal deformity can contribute to delayed cord compression.[25,26] This typically results from inadequate immobilization or premature removal of a spinal orthosis, an inability to recognize the severity of soft tissue injury to ligaments, or missed second spinal injuries that become clinically significant following the addition of weight-bearing from mobilization. The incidence of delayed deformity is increased in surgical patients treated with posterior decompression without fusion or in children who develop deformity as they grow. Radiographic monitoring of spinal alignment is important for identifying early signs of spinal deformity. Because these problems tend to be progressive, intervention to prevent progression may reduce the frequency of late spinal cord compression. Flexion and extension views are helpful in identifying patients with excessive mobility and provide a warning that a patient is at risk for delayed spinal deformity.

REHABILITATION

General Concepts

Functional capabilities following cord injury are the most significant concerns for the patient. It is clear that improvement in a single cervical cord level may dramatically change a patient's independence and significantly influence his/her life-style. Patients with retained function at the C7 level or below potentially can gain a large measure of independence, whereas patients with lesions at C5 or above will need assistance for almost all activities of daily living.[21] The application of assistive devices and appropriate surgical procedures (tendon transfers) may increase the patient's use of the upper extremities for many daily activities.

Spinal cord injury and paralysis influence the patient's functional capabilities in a systemic way. Skin integrity, bowel and bladder function, respiratory sufficiency, infection, autonomic dysreflexia, cardiovascular instability, deep venous thrombosis, flexion deformity and spasticity, pain, psychological adjustment, and temperature regulation all are important issues for the chronically paralyzed patient.[30,31] Improvements in rehabilitation management have had an impact on the complications of paralysis. For example, long-term follow-up data indicate that as many as 50 percent of cord-injured patients will experience skin breakdown, but life-threatening sepsis from infected skin ulcers is becoming less common.[21] During the 1960s, urinary sepsis was the most common cause (60 percent) of late fatality in this population.[21] This number has been reduced to less than 4 percent with appropriate management. Spasticity and pain continue to be major long-term complications. Some success in treatment of these problems has been achieved with intrathecal medication and functional electrical stimulation. New devices are under development to use as implantable systems for continuous use.

The significance of these chronic complications has become more apparent because careful patient management has resulted in longer life expectancy for the paralyzed patient. The long-term needs of the spinal cord-injured patient require the expertise of clinicians from a variety of disciplines. Coordination of the management of complications and health problems for the paralyzed patient is best handled through a multidisciplinary clinic, typically under the direction of a rehabilitation specialist. Early intervention to prevent complications from becoming life-threatening problems, the use of adaptive equipment, and the support services provided by these clinics can increase the patient's chances of regaining some measure of functional independence.[2]

Mortality

The highest mortality risk occurs within the first post-injury year. For those who survive the first year, 10 percent will die within the next six years. Mortality statistics indicate that the patient's age at the time of injury and the severity and level of trauma directly influence survival.[33] More than 90 percent of patients with incomplete lesions under the age of 25 are alive after 12 years, whereas, nearly 80 percent of quadriplegic patients over 50 will not survive 12 years following injury.[33] The major causes of late mortality in this patient population (renal failure, sepsis, respiratory failure, suicide) are a direct result of complications from paralysis.

CONCLUSION

There have been significant improvements in the rehabilitation of the cord-injured patient, but identifying a management technique that significantly improves neurological recovery has been more problematic. This difficulty results in part because, although most clinical studies have presented very similar findings regarding the incidence of neurological recovery, these studies often make different recommendations for intervention and treatment. Consequently, while some consider early surgical intervention to be beneficial, others have found nonsurgical treatment as effective, and neither treatment method has significantly improved neurological recovery for the past 30 years.[32] Furthermore, many studies include a small number of patients whose recovery is significantly better than would be predicted but cannot identify a cause for these favorable results.

The recent findings from the National Acute Spinal Cord Injury Study and the Maryland Institute for Emergency Medical Services Institute suggest that pharmacological intervention will have an important future role in influencing neurological and functional recovery.[4,5,7] These studies indicate that pharmacological intervention can halt or reverse the progression of cord damage from secondary injury and that there is a window of time following trauma when therapy is most effective. It is anticipated that this research will provide the basis for more effective methods to increase the chances of neurological recovery and change the management of these patients. It is too early to evaluate the long-term consequences of pharmacological therapy. However, the final analysis of any proposed treatment should include an assessment of the long-term consequences for the spinal cord-injured patient.

Traumatic spinal cord injury occurs in an instant but has life-long effects. While most research and clinical study in this patient population has focused on the early management following trauma, it is clear that these patients need continuous medical observation for the rest of their lives. Spinal cord injury treatment centers have produced significant improvements in patient management; however, vigilant care cannot eliminate the risk of serious complications nor can it offer these patients a normal life expectancy. Until medical research can identify an effective method of reversing paralysis, society will have an obligation to consider environmental adaptations that will increase the paralyzed patient's chances of returning to a productive life-style.

References

1. Collins W, Piepmeier J, Ogle E: The spinal cord injury problem—A review. *CNS Trauma* 1987; 4:317–332.
2. Piepmeier J: *The Outcome Following Traumatic Spinal Cord Injury.* New York: Futura, 1992.
3. Piepmeier J, Collins W: Recovery of function following spinal cord injury, in Vinken P, Bruyn G, Klawans H, Frankel H (eds): *Handbook of Clinical Neurology,* vol 61. Amsterdam: Elsevier, 1993:269–277.
4. Bracken M, Shephard M, Collins W, et al: Methylprednisolone or naloxone treatment after acute spinal cord injury: 1-year follow-up data. Results of the second National Acute Spinal Cord Injury Study. *J Neurosurg* 1991; 76:23–31.
5. Bracken M, Shephard M, Collins W, et al: A randomized clinical trial of methylprednisolone and naloxone used in the initial treatment of acute spinal cord injury. *N Engl J Med* 1990; 322:1405–1411.
6. Frankel H, Hancock D, Melzak J, et al: The value of postural reduction in the initial management of closed injuries of the spine with paraplegia and tetraplegia. *Paraplegia* 1969; 7:179–192.
7. Geisler F, Dorsey F, Coleman W: Recovery of motor function after spinal cord injury: A randomized placebo-controlled trial with GM-1 ganglioside. *N Engl J Med* 1991; 324:1829–1838.
8. Marshall L, Knowlton S, Garfin S, et al: Deterioration following spinal cord injury: A multicenter study. *J Neurosurg* 1987; 66:400–404.
9. Maynard F, Reynolds G, Fountain S, et al: Neurological prognosis after traumatic quadriplegia: Three-year experience of California regional spinal cord injury care system. *J Neurosurg* 1979; 50:611–616.
10. Piepmeier J, Jenkins N: Late changes in neurological examinations following traumatic spinal cord injury. *J Neurosurg* 1988; 69:399–402.
11. Tator C, Rowed D, Schwartz M: Sunnybrook Cord Injury Scales for assessing neurological injury and neurological recovery, in Tator CH (ed): *Early Management of Acute Spinal Cord Injury.* New York: Raven Press, 1982: 7–24.
12. Young J, Dexter W: Neurological recovery distal to the zone of injury in 172 cases of closed traumatic spinal cord injury. *Paraplegia* 1978; 16:39–49.
13. Ducker T, Russo L, Bellegarrique R, Lucas J: Complete sensorimotor paralysis after cord injury: Mortality, recovery and therapeutic implications. *J Trauma* 1979; 19:837–840.
14. Tator C, Duncan E, Edmonds V, et al: Comparison of surgical and conservative management in 208 patients with acute spinal cord injury. *Can J Neurol Sci* 1987; 14:60–69.
15. Lucas J, Ducker T: Morbidity, mortality and recovery rates of patients with spinal cord injuries undergoing anterior decompression procedures or fusion or both. *Surg Forum* 1977; 28:451–452.
16. Wilcox E, Stauffer S: Follow-up of 423 consecutive patients admitted to the spinal cord center, Rancho Los Amigos hospital, 1 January to 31 December 1967. *Paraplegia* 1972; 10:115–122.
17. Cherazi B, Wagner F, Collins W, Freeman D: A scale for evaluation of spinal cord injury. *J Neurosurg* 1981; 54:310–315.
18. Bosch A, Stauffer S, Nickle V: Incomplete traumatic quadriplegia: A ten-year review. *JAMA* 1971; 216: 473–478.
19. Bernard E, Minaire P, Girard R, Bourret J: Results of rehabilitation in central cord syndromes. *Paraplegia* 1977; 14:259–261.
20. Piepmeier J: The management of the cervical fracture, in Long D (ed): *Current Therapy in Neurological Surgery.* Philadelphia: BC Decker, 1985:171–201.
21. Arnold P: Rehabilitation of patients with spinal cord injury, in Piepmeier J (ed): *The Outcome Following Traumatic Spinal Cord Injury.* New York: Futura, 1992: 89–118.
22. Wagner F, Zusman E: Neurological recovery following traumatic spinal cord injury, in Piepmeier J (ed): *The Outcome Following Traumatic Spinal Cord Injury.* New York: Futura, 1992: 1–12.

23. Piepmeier J: Acute cervical spinal cord injury. *Neurosurg Consult* 1990; 1:2.
24. Marshall L, Garfin S: Incidence and causes of neurological deterioration following spinal cord injury, in Piepmeier J (ed): *The Outcome Following Traumatic Spinal Cord Injury.* New York: Futura, 1992: 13–30.
25. Wilberger J, Maroon J, Whiting D: Radiographic investigation of the post-spinal cord injury patient, in Piepmeier J (ed): *The Outcome Following Traumatic Spinal Cord Injury.* New York: Futura, 1992: 31–56.
26. Murphy M, Lieponis J: Long-term orthopedic considerations of spinal cord injury, in Piepmeier J (ed): *The Outcome Following Traumatic Spinal Cord Injury.* New York: Futura, 1992: 57–88.
27. Sonntag V, Dickman C: Pediatric spinal cord injury, in Piepmeier J (ed): *The Outcome Following Traumatic Spinal Cord Injury.* New York: Futura, 1992: 139–172.
28. Bondurant F, Colter H, Kulkarni M, et al: Acute spinal cord injury: A study using physical examination and magnetic resonance imaging. *Spine* 1990; 15:161–168.
29. Maiman D, Larson S, Benzel E: Neurological improvement associated with late decompression of the thoracolumbar spinal cord. *Neurosurg* 1984; 14:302–307.
30. Baskin D, Azordegan P: Non-neurological complications of spinal cord injury, in Piepmeier J (ed): *The Outcome Following Traumatic Spinal Cord Injury.* New York: Futura, 1992: 119–138.
31. Piepmeier J, Lehmann K, Lane J: Cardiovascular instability following acute cervical spinal cord trauma. *CNS Trauma* 1985; 2:153–160.
32. Piepmeier J, Thibodeau L: Spinal cord injury research. Pathways for the future, in Mall K (ed): *Advances in Trauma* Chicago: Yearbook, 1986: 267–289.
33. Geisler W, Jousse A: Life expectancy following traumatic spinal cord injury, in Vinken P, Bruyn G, Klawans H, Frankel H (eds): *Handbook of Clinical Neurology,* vol. 61. Amsterdam: Elsevier, 1993:250–253.

CHAPTER 90

SPASTICITY ASSOCIATED WITH SPINAL CORD INJURY

Paul G. Loubser

INTRODUCTION

Spasticity may be regarded as a clinical syndrome characterized by a persistent increase in involuntary muscle tone following stretch. This response to stretch is typically velocity-dependent, i.e., increasing the rate of muscle stretch increases tone. The other characteristics of spasticity include four phenomena: hypertonia; hyperactive tendon reflexes; clonus; and spread of reflex responses beyond the stimulated muscle.[1]

Rigidity is a term reserved for hypertonia that is uniform throughout the range of muscle movement and not velocity-dependent. Extrapyramidal rigidity occurs in Parkinson's disease; decerebrate (extensors) and decorticate (flexors and extensors) rigidity occurs secondary to head injury. Dystonia is also associated with hypertonia, but refers to a syndrome of hyperkinetic, repetitive, patterned movements, characterized by twisting, that may occur spontaneously or following voluntary movements. It occurs secondary to a variety of CNS disorders.

Injury or lesions of the CNS that are upper motor neuron in type characteristically produce spasticity. In contrast, lower motor neuron lesions occur secondary to disease or injury to the anterior horn cell, peripheral motor nerve, or myoneural junction, and are associated with hypotonia, hyporeflexia, weakness, and muscle atrophy.

The exact prevalence and severity of spasticity in spinal cord injury (SCI) is not known at present. This is due to differences in classification systems, clinical neurophysiological testing methodologies, and paucity of controlled studies comparing drug effect with placebo and correlating change in spasticity with functional status. Spasticity can cause skin breakdown from recurrent friction or trauma secondary to uncontrolled movements. Personal hygiene may be compromised when access to certain anatomic regions (groin, axilla) is obstructed by stiff joints. Chronic untreated spasticity may lead to contractures, heterotopic ossification, and joint dislocation.[2] From a functional standpoint, spasticity interferes with activities of daily living and such functional abilities as movements and wheelchair transfers.[3] Sleep interruption occurs, driving a vehicle is impossible, and muscle hypertonia may be extremely painful. Using the World Health Organization model of disability, spinal spasticity creates additional handicaps and compounds the disability produced by SCI.[4]

PATHOPHYSIOLOGY OF SPASTICITY

Neurophysiology of Motor Function

An understanding of the basic neuroanatomy and physiology of motor function is needed to comprehend the pathophysiology of spinal spasticity. A motor unit consists of an alpha motor neuron and the motor fibers that innervate extrafusal muscle fibers. Small alpha motor neurons innervate small "red" slowly fatiguing muscle fibers; large nerve fibers innervate large "white" rapidly fatiguing fibers. Furthermore, small alpha motor neurons are largely responsible for motor tone, while large alpha motor neurons act when power and speed are needed.

Muscle spindles are specialized encapsulated sensory receptors within skeletal muscle that consist of several "intrafusal" muscle fibers attached to connective tissue within the muscle belly. Afferents from muscle spindles include rapidly-conducting, large-diameter Group Ia fibers (changes in muscle length) and smaller Group II afferents (static length). These spindles are passively shortened when extrafusal muscle fibers contract, thereby providing the CNS with muscle length activity information. Gamma motor fibers innervate these small intrafusal muscle fibers and produce spindle contraction when extrafusal fibers are stretched, termed the "gamma fusimotor system." Therefore, activation of gamma motor neurons is closely linked to alpha motor activity.[5]

When an agonist muscle is stretched, reciprocal inhibition of the antagonist muscle occurs via Group Ia interneurons, acting to prevent motor discord.[6] Further control is provided by Renshaw cells, which are connected by axons to alpha motor neurons, providing recurrent feedback and modulating motor activity. Simultaneously, Renshaw cells send inhibitory signals to Ia interneurons associated with alpha motor neurons of antagonist muscle groups, so that, as the agonist contracts, the antagonist relaxes. This arrangement is referred to as the "Renshaw circuit" (Fig. 90-1).[7]

Profound supraspinal influences also may affect spinal motor circuits. The lateral vestibulospinal tract of the pontine reticular activating system facilitates extensor alpha and gamma motor neurons.[8] The lateral reticulospinal system of the medullary reticular activating system innervates extensor motor neurons and Ia interneurons. The corticorubrospinal system excites contralateral flexor alpha and gamma motor neurons, while the pyramidal corticospinal tracts exert potent flexor-facilitory and extensor-inhibitory effects via large spinal tracts.

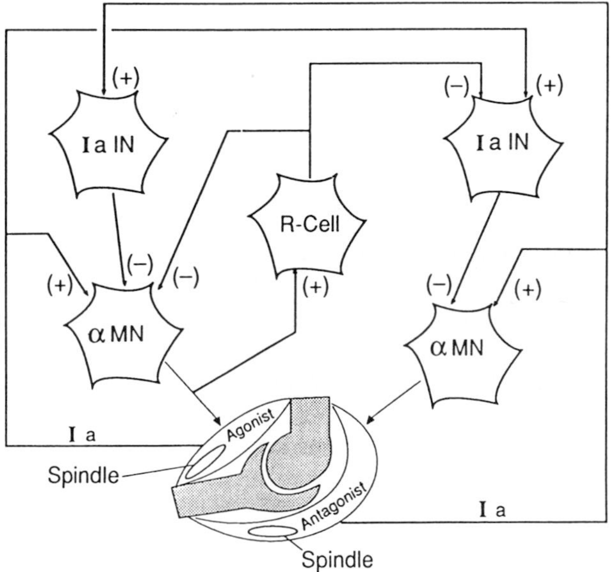

Figure 90-1. Renshaw circuit. (From Whitlock JA[7]).

Neurophysiology of Spinal Spasticity

The neurophysiology of spasticity is indeed complex and has undergone considerable speculation and theoretical refinement over the last 30 years. One of the earliest theories on the mechanism of spinal spasticity is the "gamma release hypothesis," which postulates that descending inhibitory influences on gamma motor neurons are interrupted. In turn, gamma motor neurons become extremely sensitive to local and supraspinal facilitatory influences. However, Delwaide has advanced this theory by suggesting that Ia interneurons are the prime source of inhibition, and that spasticity is produced by removing facilitation of Ia interneurons, termed the "presynaptic inhibition hypothesis."[9] "Axonal sprouting" is also thought to be an important element underlying temporal changes in muscle tone following injuries to the CNS. Ashby and Verrier suggest that hypertonia is produced as new dorsal roots sprout, which fill synaptic vacancies left by degenerating supraspinal fibers and are devoid of presynaptic inhibition.[10] Lance suggests that increased central motor neuron excitability accounts for spread of hyperreflexia through muscles following propagation of vibration waves through a limb.[11] Dimitrijevic and coworkers suggested that clonus is produced by a central oscillatory mechanism that develops secondary to functional reorganization within the spinal cord,[12] while Rack and colleagues suggest that clonus occurs secondary to selfsustaining oscillation of the stretch reflex arc.[13]

Intrinsic muscle stiffness is a dynamic variable influenced by muscle length, degree of length change, and speed of movement. Nichols and Houk postulate that spindle-mediated autogenic reflexes compensate for variations in intrinsic muscular responses to changes in length.[14] However, animal research has demonstrated that chronic imposed shortening of muscle length combined with active contractility produce reduction in the number of sarcomeres and increased stiffness.[15] These changes possibly account for Herman's observations that early spasticity without contracture reflects primarily reflex effect.[16] Once contracture develops, reflex activity declines, and rate-independent stretch resistance occurs in muscle as a viscoelastic force.

Exteroceptive hyperreflexia refers to the response to afferents in skin and subcutaneous tissue subserving touch, pressure, and temperature. This response is commonly referred to as "spasms" and is characterized by exaggerated reactions to cutaneous stimuli, such as lightly stroking the foot. Profound bilateral flexor responses ensue that may or may not be admixed with extensor responses. This response subserves no useful purpose and may actually move a limb toward a noxious stimulus. Little is known about the physiology of this response, which is complex, polysynaptic, and influenced by multiple descending systems.[7]

TREATMENT

The goals of any treatment modality for spasticity should be not only reduction of spasticity, but, if possible, optimization of function. Therefore, voluntary function and strength should be preserved. Pain may also occur secondary to spasticity, requiring specific treatment above and beyond the reduction of muscle tone.

Physical Modalities

Several noninvasive physical modalities may be used effectively to decrease spasticity. These agents decrease tone in the spastic muscle or facilitate antagonist muscle tone producing "reciprocal inhibition."[17]

Sustained local cold directly inhibits a spastic muscle. Skin receptors are inhibited by cold, spindle sensitivity is decreased, and nerve conduction velocity delayed.[18] Monosynaptic reflexes may decrease 34 percent in amplitude following cold application to the legs.[19] Local cold may be applied by using a cold pack, ice pack, or a towel with crushed ice. Twenty minutes of application will provide approximately 30 min of relaxation, at which time range of motion and other exercises may be attempted. Quick icing of antagonist muscles may relax spastic muscles by reciprocal inhibition, although results may be unpredictable.[19,20] An evaporative coolant spray such as ethyl chloride may decrease skin temperature below 10°C, in turn reducing spasticity.

The use of topical local anesthetics (benzocaine) sprayed across the surface of a spastic muscle produces three to four hours of spasticity reduction.[21] However, in a controlled placebo study, benzocaine ointment failed to produce objective reduction of lower extremity spasticity.[17]

Heat also reduces muscle tone, increases muscle blood flow and tendon extensibility, and decreases fusimotor efferent activity.[22] Neutral warmth may be applied by wrapping an extremity in a blanket for 10 to 20 min, producing short-duration reduction of spasticity. A hydrocollator pack applied directly to the muscle raises not only skin temperature but also muscle temperature. Firing rate of muscle spindles decreases at 42°C,[23] although the mechanism of spasticity reduction is probably that of "counterirritation." Short-term reduction of spasticity is produced so that range of motion and stretching may be accomplished. A paraffin dip of 52 to 54°C also provides temporary reduction of tone and should be followed by stretching and splinting. Fluidotherapy or the dry whirlpool combines the effects of light stroking massage with those of superficial heat.[24] The Hubbard tank or large whirlpool also combines heat, massage, and some sedation to decrease muscle spindle excitability. In addition, heating the hypothalamus decreases fusimotor activity, which may reduce spasticity from 30 min to 12 h.[25] Ultrasound may be applied to a spastic agonist muscle, producing heat. A dose of at least 1.5 watts/cm^2 increases thigh muscle temperature 4.5°C when applied in a light stroking manner across the muscle for 10 to 20 min.[26] Tendon extensibility also increases in response to ultrasound.[27]

Electrical stimulation may be used in several ways to decrease spasticity. Most often, stimulation is provided to the antagonist to produce reciprocal inhibition, but may also be performed on the spastic muscle itself to reduce tone.[28] Various devices are available, each with specific waveforms and parameters of electrical stimulation. Stimulation of an antagonist muscle for 10 min may produce up to 3 h of spasticity reduction, although, in most patients, as much as 8 h per day for at least 2 to 3 weeks may be required before significant decreases in spasticity occur. Thirty-five to 50 pps is the recommended starting frequency of stimulation. "Russian" or high-frequency stimulation at 2500 pps may produce direct relaxation of a spastic muscle.[29] Proposed mechanisms include relaxation secondary to muscle fatigue and decreased muscle fiber excitability.[30] This form of stimulation may be painful and associated with strengthening of the spastic muscle over time. Transcutaneous electrical nerve stimulation (TENS), a form of electrical stimulation used mainly for pain control, also may reduce spasticity. TENS is associated with lower intensity of stimulation; however, Bajd and coworkers demonstrated reduction of quadriceps spasticity following 20 min of TENS applied over the L3–L4 dermatome in 6 SCI patients.[31] Acupuncture-like TENS is characterized by a much lower frequency of stimulation ($<$50 pps), producing rhythmic muscle contraction, which increases muscle blood flow.[32] Dimitrijevic and associates demonstrated reduction of the flexor reflex in paraplegic patients following acupuncture-like TENS.[33]

Electromyographic biofeedback provides immediate feedback of muscle activity to patients, and, from a theoretical standpoint, has significant potential for reducing spasticity. Patients should be motivated and should understand the complexities of this modality. Training is first directed toward relaxing the spastic muscle, followed by strengthening the antagonist.[34] Dual channel feedback of agonist-antagonist groups optimizes this form of therapy. Biofeedback-assisted relaxation training also may reduce spasticity secondary to generalized relaxation.[34,35] Advanced biofeedback techniques incorporate training of individual muscles with devices that monitor joint position. An electrogoniometer provides feedback of joint range of motion, and can be used as a monitor of severity of spasticity.[36] Newer biofeedback devices also incorporate electrical stimulation, so that stimulation-induced relaxation may be complemented with antagonist training and strengthening. However, a study by Winchester and colleagues found no change in spasticity following 4 weeks of EMG feedback and electrical stimulation.[36]

High-frequency (>70 Hz) vibration of antagonist muscles may produce reciprocal inhibition,[37] whereas low-frequency vibration produces generalized relaxation.[38] Application of high-frequency vibration to a muscle or tendon produces reflex contraction termed the tonic vibration reflex.[39] Ideally, the muscle should be stretched to maximize reciprocal inhibition, which may last 20 to 30 min.

Studies by Foley[40] and Odeen[41] have demonstrated that repeated maintained stretch reduces spasticity significantly, increasing passive range of motion an average of 48 percent. This can be maintained by use of prone standers, Buck's traction, or casting. Manual pressure on tendons reduces the amplitude of the H-reflex and eases range of motion of spastic muscles.[42] Other forms of manual pressure include air splints and elastic bandages. Occupational and physical therapists have developed a sophisticated approach to spasticity management using elaborate splints and casts, particularly for the upper extremities.[43] Spasticity is reduced and contractures may be prevented by aggressive use of these modalities. Unfortunately, splinting also may cause muscle atrophy, which has led to the development of dynamic splints that allow for some movement about joints.[44] Inhibitory casting of a spastic extremity also may be associated with tone reduction. Possible mechanisms include neutral warmth, pressure, and decreased cutaneous input with subsequent reduction of alpha and gamma motor neuron excitability and sensitivity of spindle response to stretch.[43] Plastic materials generally are used for splints, such as Orthoplast or Orthoform, although plexiglass may be applied. Casts are usually made of plaster or fiberglass, and initially are solid. Eventually, solid casts are bivalved to be worn at night or during certain times of day. Ankle-foot orthoses may be fabricated based on the results of casts to accommodate patterns of spasticity such as equinovarus.[44] Serial casting describes the repetitive application of casts, following gradual stretch of muscles and increases in range of motion of a joint. Casts and splints are also of benefit when applied in conjunction with regional anesthetic procedures. With all these techniques, much care must be taken to ensure adequate circulation and to minimize skin pressure and pain.

Several other physical modalities are available, each providing short-term reduction of spasticity. Slow rocking, weight-bearing, joint mobilization, and massage all reduce spasticity, either via generalized relaxation or by reducing spindle sensitivity.[17] Low-power laser treatments and acupuncture are used by some therapists to reduce spasticity, although no objective evidence exists that they produce prolonged reduction of spasticity.

Pharmacological Management

An impressive array of pharmacological agents that reduce spasticity are currently available. Oral pharmacological agents form the mainstay of spasticity management; most often, in conjunction with physical modalities, spasticity is reduced to manageable levels or to a point where the risk of contractures is minimized.

Oral Agents

Dantrolene sodium acts peripherally on the muscle fiber, uncoupling excitation/contraction by inhibition of calcium release.[45] Deep tendon reflexes, resistance to passive motion, spasms, and clonus are all reduced. In some patients, activities of daily living also are improved.[46] Dosage ranges from 50 to 800 mg/day, although optimal dosage is 100 to 200 mg/day. Rarely are dosages greater than 400 mg/day needed. Adverse effects include weakness, drowsiness, lethargy, dizziness, paresthesias, nausea, vomiting, and diarrhea. Liver damage, demonstrated by abnormal liver function tests, also may occur in approximately 1.8 percent of patients receiving high doses for more than 60 days.[47] Dantrolene should be used for patients who have spasticity and retention of good voluntary strength or for patients with complete paralysis and spasticity in whom weakness is not a concern.[48]

Diazepam is one of the oldest benzodiazepines and the most widely used antispasticity medication. Diazepam potentiates the presynaptic inhibitory action of gamma aminobutyric acid (GABA), an inhibitory neurotransmitter.[49] The active metabolite is desmethyldiazepam. When compared to placebo, diazepam has been demonstrated to increase spasticity in SCI patients in several studies.[50,51] Diazepam is effective in reducing resistance to passive movement, deep tendon reflexes, and muscle spasms. However, muscle rigidity is not reduced by diazepam, and anecdotal evidence suggests that diazepam is more effective in incomplete SCI lesions than in complete lesions.[48] Dosage ranges from 4 to 30 mg/day, although dosages as high as 60 to 80 mg/day may be necessary. Side effects include sedation, weakness, depression, ataxia, memory loss, and dependence. Patients on high dosages of diazepam may experience withdrawal symptoms—in particular, convulsions—if the drug is rapidly withdrawn, or if the benzodiazepine antagonist flumazenil is administered.

Baclofen is one of the most effective oral antispasticity medications used for spasticity control. Although baclofen is an analogue of GABA (Fig. 90-2), an inhibitory neurotransmitter, potentiation of GABA or a GABAergic effect may not be its sole mechanism of action.[52] Instead, glutamate, an excitatory neurotransmitter, may be inhibited by baclofen.[53] Baclofen reduces resistance to stretch, spasms, and clonus and decreases muscle EMG activity. Improved passive and active movements may be observed, although Pederson and coworkers reported decreased strength and ambulation with baclofen.[54] Dosage ranges from 30 to 100 mg/day, and increases must be made incrementally. Common side effects include drowsiness, fatigue, muscle weakness, dizziness, and paresthesias. Abrupt withdrawal may lead to symptoms similar to an organic brain syndrome, with hallucinations, convulsions, and coma.[55] Unfortunately, comparative studies of diazepam, dantrolene, and baclofen are completely lacking in SCI patients, although several studies have been conducted in patients with multiple sclerosis. These studies suggest that of the three agents, oral baclofen is the most efficacious.[48]

Other oral agents have also been used to control spasticity. Clonidine, an alpha$_2$-agonist appears to act at multiple levels within the spinal cord and brainstem, decreasing sympathetic outflow and reducing afferent reflex arc input.[56] Two studies have evaluated oral clonidine, each reporting drug efficacy in reducing spasms and resistance to passive stretch.[56,57] In both studies, side effects were prominent, including postural hypotension and depression. A 62 percent success rate was noted in one study in which 0.4 mg/day was administered, although clonidine was judged less effective than baclofen.[57] Tizanidine, another alpha$_2$-agonist, acts similarly

CL
H2N—CH2—CH
CH2
COOH
BACLOFEN

H2N—CH2—CH2
CH2
COOH
GABA

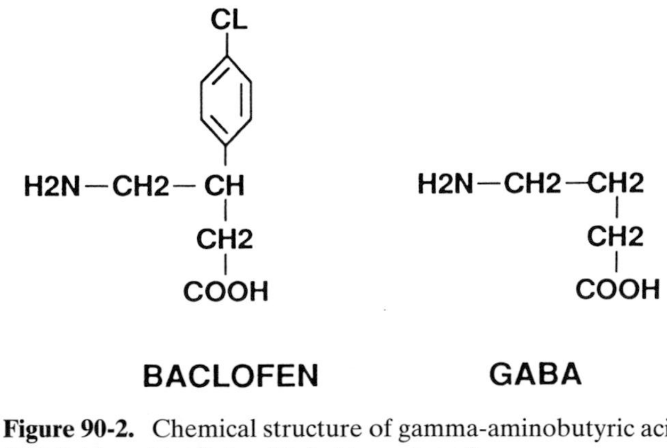

Figure 90-2. Chemical structure of gamma-aminobutyric acid (GABA) and baclofen (β-4-chlorophenyl).

to clonidine,[58] but has fewer hemodynamic side effects. No experience is available in SCI patients, although studies in patients with MS and cerebral spasticity suggest that it may be as effective as baclofen and diazepam and is associated with less weakness.[59,60] Sedation remains a prominent side effect at a dosage of 6 to 36 mg/day. Various other agents have been tried without beneficial results, including cyclobenzaprine, glycine, and chlorpromazine. Patients often report that inhaled tetrahydrocannibinol reduces spasticity, although these effects may be secondary to its general relaxant properties.[48]

Intrathecal Pharmacotherapy

The availability of implanted infusion pumps has presented a new avenue of therapy for spasticity. In 1983, the observations of Struppler and coworkers that epidural morphine reduced flexor spasms secondary to MS led to further investigation of the use of intrathecal morphine for spasticity control.[61] Two groups of researchers have demonstrated that adequate control of spasticity may be achieved with a continuous infusion of intrathecal morphine.[62,63] When intrathecal morphine is used for pain control, significant tolerance may occur, requiring massive dosage escalation. However, similar tolerance phenomena have not been observed when intrathecal morphine is used for spinal spasticity control.[63] The action of intrathecal morphine in spinal spasticity is thought to occur secondary to inhibition of polysynaptic pathways.[62]

The awareness of the intrathecal space as a novel route of drug delivery led to further studies of continuous intrathecal baclofen pharmacotherapy by Penn and Kroin.[64] As indicated above, the molecular structure of baclofen resembles GABA (Fig. 90-2). Passage across the blood-brain barrier is limited; dosage increases to achieve effective concentrations of drug within the spinal cord following oral administration often are associated with cerebral side effects. Administration intrathecally bypasses the blood-brain barrier, delivering larger concentrations of drug to active sites within the spinal cord.[65] In turn, intrathecal dosages are much smaller, e.g., 25 to 1200 μg/day. The actual mechanism of action is complex but may involve presynaptic inhibition of spinal reflexes, via GABA (β) receptors,[52] or even a postsynaptic action.[66] Many studies worldwide have confirmed the effectiveness of this drug in controlling spasticity and improving functional abilities and activities of daily living.[65,67–75] Intrathecal baclofen decreases spasms, deep tendon reflexes, passive resistance to stretch, and truncal tone in a dose-dependent and predictable manner (Fig. 90-3). Intrathecal baclofen also is being studied in other forms of spasticity following head injury, in cerebral palsy,[76] and in pediatric patients.[77]

A. Control

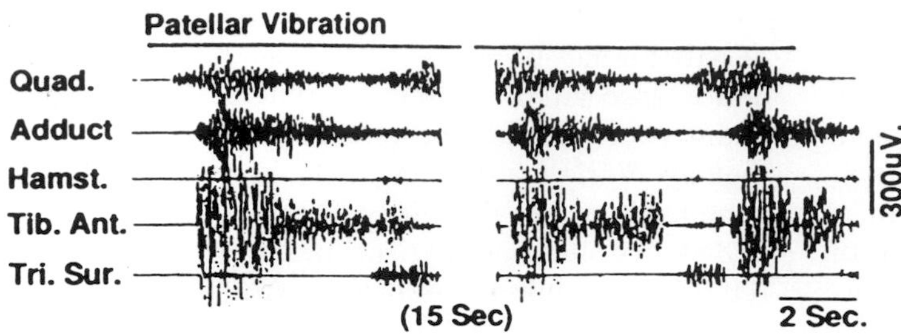

B. During Intrathecal Baclofen

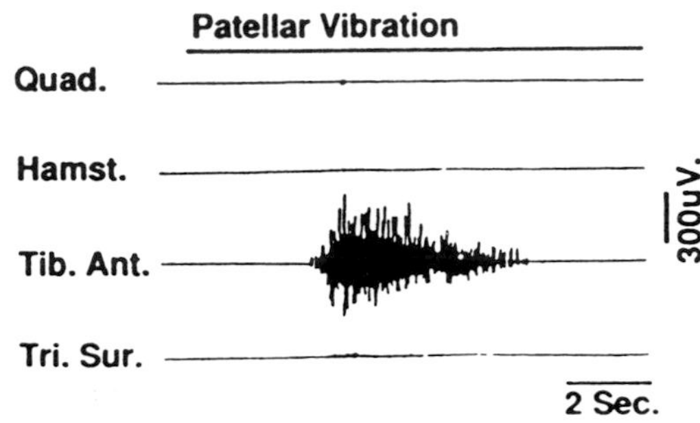

Figure 90-3. Change in polyelectromyography during intrathecal baclofen infusion. (From Loubser PG et al.[65])

However, the effectiveness of intrathecal baclofen in SCI patients who ambulate is uncertain. If patients depend on their spasticity for strength during ambulation, for example, quadriceps tone, intrathecal baclofen will weaken lower extremities and worsen ambulation.[65] Upper extremity spasticity also is difficult to control with intrathecal baclofen, because the drug is delivered in the lumbar spinal canal, and local cerebrospinal fluid (CSF) concentrations of baclofen in the cervical region are significantly lower compared with the lumbar intrathecal space. Although baclofen flows rostrally within the intrathecal space,[78] increasing drug delivery to

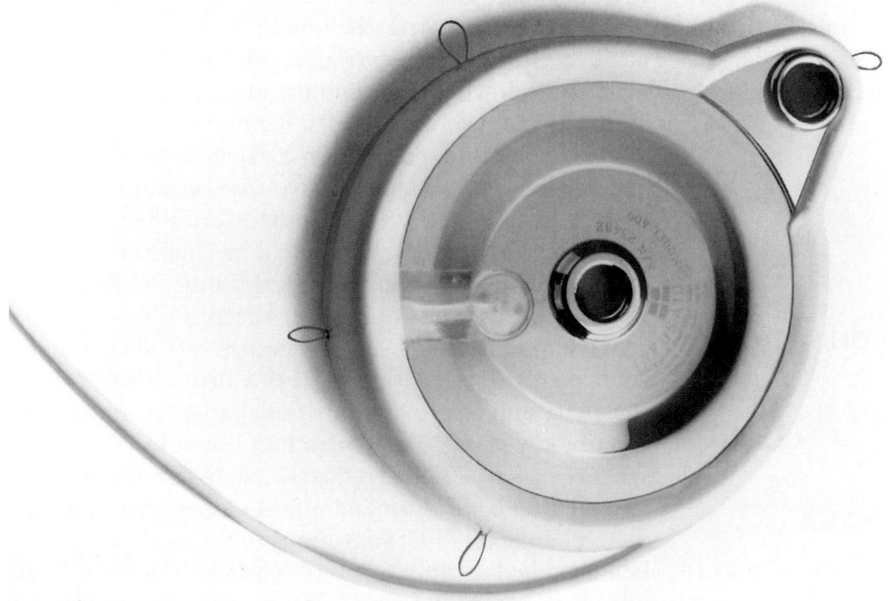

Figure 90-4. Infusaid 400 constant flow infusion pump. (From Infusaid, Inc., Norwood, MA.)

achieve higher cervical concentrations also increases the risk of drug toxicity. Dangers of intrathecal baclofen mainly involve overdosage phenomena when the drug reaches brainstem regions, producing sedation and eventual coma.[52,78] Typical tolerance phenomena are not seen with intrathecal baclofen, although dosage increases occur during the initial 12 months of therapy, eventually reaching a plateau.[79] Intrathecal baclofen decreases musculoskeletal pain associated with spasticity, although neurological pain symptoms such as dysesthesias and paresthesias usually are unaffected. However, a recent study reported alleviation of dysesthetic pain following intrathecal baclofen, implicating the involvement of GABA (β) receptors in deafferentation pain.[80]

An implanted infusion pump and intrathecal catheter are required for intrathecal pharmacotherapy. Two forms of implanted infusion pumps are available. Constant infusion pumps deliver a fixed daily volume; variable flow devices are adjustable. The Infusaid 400 is an example of a constant flow infusion pump (Fig. 90-4), although at present not specifically approved for intrathecal baclofen therapy. The Medtronic Synchromed is a microprocessor-based pump approved for intrathecal baclofen therapy (Fig. 90-5) in which solution flow rates may be varied by computerized telemetry. This flow rate may be lowered to enable pump reservoir refills (18 ml) every 3 months. Pumps are implanted in the lower quadrant of the abdomen and connected to a catheter placed in the lumbar intrathecal space with the tip at T12–L1. Loubser and Narayan reported that placing the catheter at higher levels is associated with less spasticity reduction in the lower extremities,[81] i.e., the catheter should be placed in spinal cord regions associated with spasticity.[82] Drug gradually flows rostrally and is absorbed into the spinal cord. The Synchromed has a limited battery life of 3 to 5 years, requiring surgical replacement. Other problems related to these pumps include catheter breakage, migration, plugging with fibrotic material, pump pocket infections, and meningitis. If pump or catheter malfunction is suspected, Indium DPTA isotope may be injected into the pump, and passage through the catheter and intrathecal space observed.

The efficacy of intrathecal baclofen has been compared to intrathecal morphine, midazolam, and tizanidine in SCI patients with spasticity. Intrathecal morphine and midazolam produce less reduction of spasticity compared to intrathecal baclofen, while intrathecal tizanidine is virtually ineffective.[83] Unfortunately, the safety of applying various agents intrathecally in the absence of animal studies that exclude the possibility of neurotoxicity should be questioned. Administration of midazolam epidurally has been studied in conjunction with neurophysiological testing; these studies revealed dramatic reductions in spasticity.[84] However, systemic drug absorption from the epidural space is significant, and side effects are prominent.

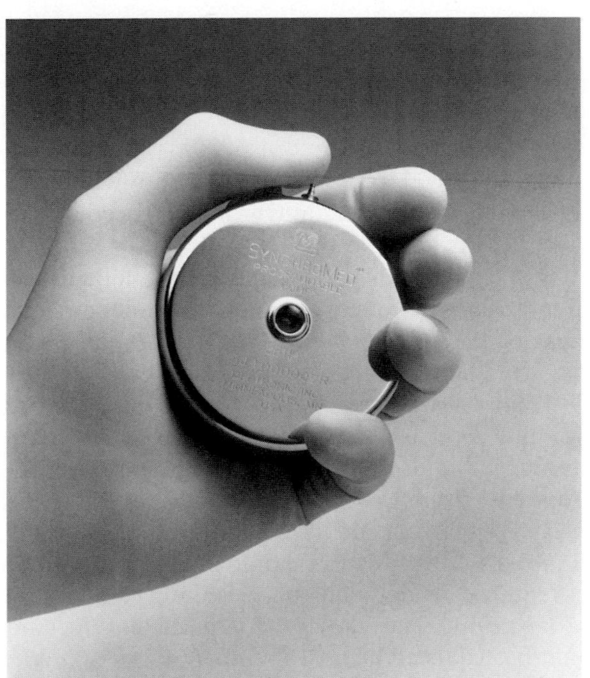

Figure 90-5. Synchromed variable flow programmable infusion pump. (From Medtronic, Inc., Minneapolis, MN.)

Regional anesthetic interventions

Several studies have demonstrated that regional anesthetic interventions or nerve blocks have a prominent role in the management of spasticity. In general, two types of procedures exist—diagnostic (short-term) and therapeutic (long-term) interventions. Diagnostic procedures may be used to assess joint range of motion, ambulation potential, or presence of contractures. Therefore, they attempt to increase understanding of how severe spasticity of a particular muscle or group of muscles may be, whether joint contracture contributes to joint deformity, or whether any improvements in functional activities/abilities occur secondary to reduction of spasticity. Therapeutic injections are aimed at long-term spasticity control by increasing joint range of motion, decreasing passive resistance to stretch and intensity of deep tendon reflexes, or facilitating placement of casts and splints. These interventions are based on the principle that injection of an anesthetic substance adjacent to a nerve produces conduction blockade.

A variety of local anesthetic formulations are currently available for use with diagnostic nerve blocks, such as lidocaine, bupivacaine, etidocaine, and chloroprocaine. Each agent manifests varying pharmacodynamic properties depending on the concentration of agent used.[85] For example, 0.5% lidocaine or 0.25% bupivacaine produces mainly sensory blockade, whereas 1.5% lidocaine or 0.75% bupivacaine includes motor blockade.[85] Etidocaine is a unique local anesthetic in that it preferentially blocks motor fibers.[85] Use of a low concentration of local anesthetic for a nerve block produces interruption of only the sensory arc of the reflex, whereas a higher concentration also will affect the motor component, producing additional muscle relaxation. Volume of local anesthetic injection is also important, since larger nerves such as the sciatic nerve will require 20 to 30 ml for blockade compared with the ulnar nerve, which may require only 5 ml. Local anesthetics also have an expected or known duration of effect. For example, nerve blocks with lidocaine and bupivacaine last approximately 60 to 90 and 90 to 120 min, respectively.[85] The duration of effect is important, since testing and joint measurements should be performed while the block is active. In general, local anesthetic blockade does not produce long-term reduction of spasticity. However, if aggressive range of motion is performed while the block is in effect, "carry-over" effects will last for several days. The use of repeated local anesthetic nerve blocks via an implanted catheter in conjunction with aggressive range of motion has been advocated by some researchers,[86] although long-term use of local anesthetics may be associated with neurotoxic side effects (nerve damage) and bone marrow suppression.[87]

In order to produce long-term reduction of spasticity, neurolytic agents are needed. Neurolytic agents continue to create some controversy among clinicians because they are neurodestructive in nature, and their use from a therapeutic standpoint in SCI appears to be contradictory. Phenol or carbolic acid is the most popular neurolytic agent currently in use (Fig. 90-6). Considerable information is available describing its pharmacological and therapeutic effects. Phenol is soluble at room temperature and is prepared by pharmacists to produce an aqueous mixture of 5 to 10 percent. Concentrations above 8 percent start to precipitate at room temperature, requiring constant agitation of the suspension prior to injection; concentrations below 5 percent do not possess significant neurolytic action.[88] Phenol denatures protein and produces neurolysis.[88] Although researchers initially thought that phenol produced selective neurolysis of gamma motor fibers, phenol produces nonselective destruction of all nerve fiber types.[89] The neurolytic effect is marked by disruption of the myelin sheath, either segmentally or completely, and eventual Wallerian degeneration with surrounding inflammation.[90,91] The destructive effect peaks at 7 to 10 days, whereafter some regrowth of the nerve fiber commences.[92] This process of regrowth occurs over the next 30 to 90 days, although scarring and fibrosis are prominent.[92]

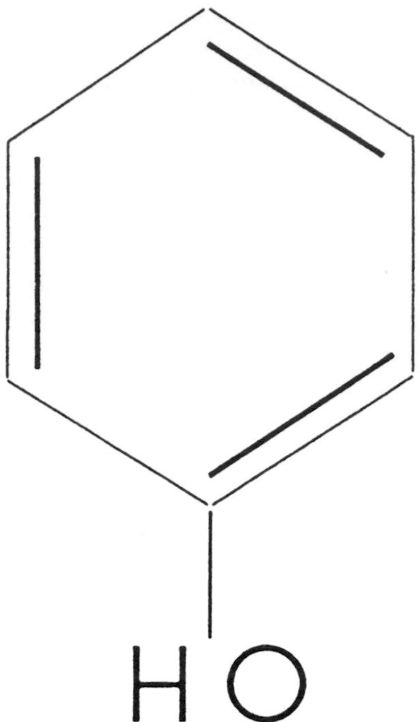

Figure 90-6. Chemical structure of phenol.

The pharmacology of phenol is important since this influences decision-making and therapeutic choices. Phenol initially produces an immediate local anesthetic action that lasts from 3 to 8 h.[88] Thereafter, some spasticity returns, but gradually fades over the next seven days as neurolysis continues. Recovery from neurolysis may be associated with return of spasticity, and interventions may need to be repeated. The duration of spasticity reduction following a neurolytic procedure is the subject of considerable debate, with most reports suggesting 2 to 6 months.[93–95] Many factors influence this response, such as volume of phenol injected, technical success of the block, adjunctive antispasticity medications or modalities such as splints, and severity of spasticity. With large fibers, phenol injected adjacent to the nerve may produce eccentric neurolysis of only part of the nerve,[91] requiring repeated injections to produce a therapeutic response. However, with repeated injections, nerve scarring and fibrosis occur, so that the duration of spasticity reduction should increase. Use of phenol requires a detailed understanding of regional neuroanatomy. The choice of a particular technique should be balanced against therapeutic goals.[96] Where possible, motor nerves should be identified and injected as opposed to mixed nerves with both motor and sensory components. Sensory blockade will be associated with numbness and with time, a 2 to 32 percent incidence of dysesthesias may develop in the distribution of that nerve.[96]

Other available neurolytic agents include ammonium sulfate and glycerol, which are weak and unsuited to spasticity management. Ethyl alcohol is a potent agent producing neurolytic actions similar to phenol in concentrations from 50 to 100 percent.[97] Its main disadvantage is the high incidence of dysesthesias, hyperesthesias, and skin irritation should any agent leak into surrounding tissues.

Specific nerve blocks have selected indications. In the lower extremities, obturator blocks are used to decrease hip adductor tone. Femoral nerve blocks are aimed at decreasing quadriceps tone, so that spasticity-producing hip flexion and knee extension may be reduced. Sciatic blocks are aimed at hamstring hypertonicity; tibial blocks will reduce clonus and equinovarus deformities. More invasive procedures include paravertebral neurolysis, in which phenol is deposited at the intervertebral foramina of L2–L5 in order to decrease the innervation of the psoas major, a potent hip flexor.[94] Phenol also may be administered epidurally via a catheter in the L2 region.[98] Termed epidural phenol radiculolysis,[99] three daily injections are needed to produce complete neurolysis of roots. In the epidural space, the dura mater appears to limit the neurolytic effect of phenol.[100] Phenol also may be injected intrathecally at L1–L2 in order to reach intradural rootlets. This procedure has a long historical basis, termed "anterior chemical rhizotomy" by Nathan in 1959.[101] A small volume of high-concentration phenol (20%) is used, and careful positioning required because spread of intrathecal phenol occurs by gravity. Phenol is mixed in glycerine, which retards the delivery of phenol to nerve sites, thus maximizing neurolytic effect. In the upper extremities, neurolytic blocks are used less frequently. Motor branches of the brachial plexus may be injected or peripheral nerves at the elbow and wrist are selected. However, in the upper extremity, motor point blocks (MPB) are more suitable.

The motor point on a muscle is identified by finding that area of muscle that contracts in response to minimal amounts of electrical current. It represents the point where motor fibers actually enter the muscle tissue itself, or where motor endplates cluster.[102] Therefore, injection of agent at this point selectively reduces muscle tone, while preserving some voluntary function.[96] MPBs may be performed on any muscle,[103–105] although a large muscle (for example, quadriceps) may require as many as 20 motor point injections. The technique is time-consuming and requires an electrical stimulator and insulated needle (Fig. 90-7). Use of a local anesthetic agent implies a diagnostic MPB, while injection of phenol has been termed "intramuscular neurolysis" by Halpern.[89] Volume of agent injected at each point depends on the size of the muscle treated, but ranges from 0.5 to 2 ml per point. MPBs are particularly suited to the upper extremity, where elbow flexion deformities may be corrected with MPBs of biceps and brachioradialis. In the lower extremity, a gastrocnemius MPB will control clonus while preserving some ankle plantarflexion. MPB may produce some muscle and tissue swelling, requiring ice application, elevation, removal of casts and splints, and oral anti-inflammatory agents.

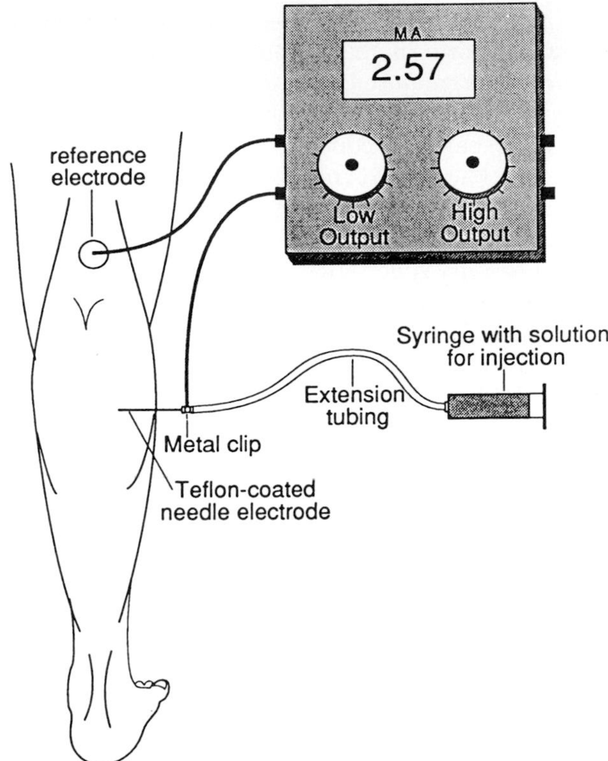

Figure 90-7. Motor point blockade—equipment/technique. (From Glenn MB.[96])

Surgical Management

The use of intrathecal pharmacology in conjunction with implanted pumps and the application of neurolytic agents and regional anesthetics for spasticity control have been described above. Destructive surgical procedures for spasticity control have a long history, but are used infrequently at present. Foerster's rhizotomy of posterior roots was for many decades the only partially effective surgical modality for spasticity.[106] However, spasticity recurred, and the procedure was associated with loss of sensation. Rhizotomy of anterior roots was associated with a more prolonged response, although the procedure required an extensive laminectomy.[107] Refinement of the posterior rhizotomy by performing selective or partial section of rootlets was thought to avoid complete loss of muscle tone and spare some useful spasticity.[108] Sindou and coworkers modified this approach further by performing a lesion through the dorsal root entry zone (DREZ), again aiming at preservation of some sensation and useful tone and voluntary muscle function.[109]

Another destructive procedure is the dorsal longitudinal or "T" myelotomy first described by Bischof.[110] This procedure interrupts the reflex arcs that connect the posterior and anterior horns of the spinal cord and is reported to be highly effective.[111–112] Disadvantages include an extensive laminectomy, voiding difficulties, and sensory disturbances. The recent interest in spinal cord neural regeneration techniques (cellular implants, nerve growth factors) has led many researchers and clinicians to shy away from major destructive surgical procedures that are irreversible. Similar concerns surround the subject of surgical neurectomy, although selective motor neurectomies or open surgical motor neurolysis may be indicated for certain clinical problems.[113] The latter procedure is performed by surgically exposing a nerve and motor branches (for example, musculocutaneous, tibial) and selectively applying phenol to these branches.[114] Trainer and colleagues described the successful performance of intrapelvic obturator neurectomies for severe hip adductor spasticity refractory to nerve blocks.[115]

Percutaneous radiofrequency rhizotomy is performed by placing a thermistor electrode at the intervertebral foramen paraspinally from T12–L5. Nerve localization is obtained with a fluoroscope and electrical stimulator similar to the technique used for paravertebral phenol neurolysis. 120°C of heat applied for 120 s at each level effectively electrocoagulates the nerve. Kenmore,[116] Kasdon and Lathi,[117] and Herz and coworkers[118] have all reported high rates of success for this procedure, including minimal loss of sensory and voluntary function and a low recurrence of spasticity.

Dorsal column stimulation (DCS) or epidural spinal cord stimulation is performed by placing a stimulating electrode in the cervical, thoracic, or lumbar epidural space of the spinal cord. The electrode is implanted surgically and connected to a subcutaneous pulse generator. Various parameters of electrical stimulation may be delivered via four to eight electrode sites on the epidural lead. DCS has become quite popular for chronic low-back pain control, although its use for spasticity management is not firmly established. In 1973, Cook and Weinstein first described reduction of spasticity in a patient with MS receiving DCS.[119] Subsequently, various clinical research groups have attempted to establish objectively a clear role for this modality in spasticity management. DCS usually does not produce an immediate effect on spasticity, and comparisons with placebo are difficult to conduct. A recent review of the value of DCS in spasticity management concluded that, of the approximately 20 clinical reports in the literature, DCS still remains experimental, should be restricted to a few centers with the necessary expertise, and still requires extensive study to confirm its efficacy.[120] However, DCS may be preferable to intrathecal baclofen in SCI patients with upper extremity spasticity or in SCI patients with spasticity who ambulate.

The development of contractures or heterotopic ossification secondary to uncontrolled spasticity requires the consultation of an orthopedic surgeon and is beyond the scope of this discussion.

CONCLUSION

A wide array of therapeutic interventions are available to reduce spasticity. Spasticity is a multidisciplinary problem that requires the expertise of several different specialists. In most modern rehabilitation centers, the primary management of spasticity falls within the realm of physical medicine and rehabilitation. However, in more severe injuries, other specialists, including anesthesiologists, neurologists, neurosurgeons, and orthopedists are needed to deliver more complex and invasive modalities.

REFERENCES

1. Bishop B: Spasticity: Its physiology and management: Part III. Identifying and assessing the mechanisms underlying spasticity. *Phys Ther* 1977; 57:385.
2. Dralle D, Muller H, Zierski J: A short historical review of spasticity, in Muller H, Zierski J, Penn RD (eds): *Local-spinal Therapy of Spasticity.* New York: Springer-Verlag, 1988: 3–16.
3. Gans BM, Glenn MB: Introduction, in Glenn MB, Whyte J (eds): *Practical Management of Spasticity in Children and Adults.* Philadelphia: Lea & Febiger, 1990: 1–7.
4. World Health Organization: *International Classification of Impairments, Disabilities and Handicaps: A Manual of Classification Relating to the Consequences of Disease.* Geneva: 1980.
5. Valbo AB, Hagbarth KE, Torebjork HE, Wallin BG: Activity in human peripheral nerves. *Physiol Rev* 1979; 59:919.

6. Hultborn H, Illert M, Santini M: Convergence of interneurons mediating the reciprocal Ia inhibition of motor neurons. *Acta Physiol Scand* 1976; 96:193.
7. Whitlock JA: Neurophysiology of spasticity, in Glenn MB, Whyte J (eds): *Practical Management of Spasticity in Children and Adults.* Philadelphia: Lea & Febiger, 1990: 8–33.
8. Rhines R, Magoun HW: Brain stem facilitation of cortical motor responses. *J Neurophysiol* 1946; 9:219.
9. Delwaide PI: Human monosynaptic reflexes and presynaptic inhibition, in Desmedt JE (ed): *New Developments in Electromyography and Clinical Neurophysiology.* Basel: Karger, 1973: 508–522.
10. Ashby P, Verrier M: Neurophysiologic changes in hemiplegia. *Neurology* 1976; 26:1145.
11. Lance JW: Pathophysiology of spasticity and clinical experience with baclofen, in Feldman RG, Young RR, Koeller WP (eds): *Spasticity: Disordered Motor Control.* Chicago: Yearbook, 1980: 185–203.
12. Dimitrijevic MR, Nathan PW, Sherwood AM: Clonus: The role of central mechanisms. *J Neurol Neurosurg Psychiatry* 1980; 43:321.
13. Rack PMH, Ross HF, Thilman AF: The ankle stretch reflexes in normal and spastic subjects. *Brain* 1984; 107:637.
14. Nichols TR, Houk JC: Reflex compensation for variations in the mechanical properties of muscle. *Science* 1973; 131:182.
15. Gallego R, Kuno M, Nunez R: Dependence of motor neuron properties on the length of immobilized muscle. *J Physiol (Lond)* 1979; 291:179.
16. Herman R: The myotatic reflex: Clinicophysiologic aspects of spasticity and contracture. *Brain* 1970; 93:273.
17. Giebler KB: Physical modalities, in Glenn MB, Whyte J (eds): *Practical Management of Spasticity in Children and Adults.* Philadelphia: Lea & Febiger, 1980: 118–148.
18. Kunesch E, Freund HJ: Peripheral neural correlates of cutaneous anesthesia induced by skin cooling in man. *Acta Physiol Scand* 1987; 129:247.
19. Knutsson E, Mattson E: Effects of local cooling on monosynaptic reflexes in man. *Scand J Rehabil Med* 1969; 1:126.
20. Umphred DA, McCormack GL: Classification of common facilitatory and inhibitory treatment techniques, in Umphred DA (ed): *Neurological Rehabilitation.* St. Louis: CV Mosby, 1985: 72–117.
21. Sabbahi MA, DeLuca CJ, Powers WR: Topical anesthesia: A possible treatment method for spasticity. *Arch Phys Med Rehabil* 1981; 62:310.
22. Lehmann JF, deLateur BJ: Diathermy and superficial heat and cold therapy, in Kottke FJ, Stillwell GK, Lehmann JF (eds): *Krusen's Handbook of Physical Medicine and Rehabilitation,* (3d ed). Philadelphia: WB Saunders, 1982: 275–350.
23. Valenza J, Rossi C, Parker R, Henley EJ: A clinical study of a new heat modality. *J Am Podiatr Assoc* 1979; 69:440.
24. Borrell RM, Parker R, Henley EJ, et al: Comparison of in vivo temperatures produced by hydrotherapy, paraffin wax treatment, and fluidotherapy. *Phys Ther* 1980; 60:1273.
25. Von Euler C, Soderberg MK: The influence of hypothalamic thermoceptive structures on the EEG and gamma motor activity. *EEG Clin Neurophysiol* 1957; 9:391.
26. Lehmann JF, Stonebridge JB, deLateur BJ, et al: Temperatures in human thighs after hot pack treatment followed by ultrasound. *Arch Phys Med Rehabil* 1978; 59:472.
27. Lehmann JF, deLateur BJ: Therapeutic heat, in Lehman JF (ed): *Therapeutic Heat and Cold,* (3d ed). Baltimore: Williams & Wilkins, 1982: 404–562.
28. Lee WJ, McGovern JP, Duvall EN: Continuous tetanizing (low voltage) currents for relief of spasm. *Arch Phys Med* 1950; 31:766.
29. Greathouse DG, Nitz AJ, Matulionis DH, Currier DP: Effects of short-term electrical stimulation on the ultrasound of rat skeletal muscles. *Phys Ther* 1986; 66:946.
30. Nitz AJ, Dobner JJ: High intensity electrical stimulation effect on thigh musculature during immobilization for knee sprain. *Phys Ther* 1987; 67:219.
31. Bajd T, Gregoric M, Vodovnik L, Benko H: Electrical stimulation in treating spasticity resulting from spinal cord injury. *Arch Phys Med Rehabil* 1985; 66:515.
32. Mohr T, Akers TK, Wessman HC: Effect of high voltage stimulation on blood flow in the rat hind limb. *Phys Ther* 1987; 67:526.
33. Dimitrijevic MR, Faganel J, Gregoric M, et al: Habituation: Effects of regular and stochastic stimulation. *J Neurol Neurosurg Psychiatry* 1972; 35:234.
34. Basmajian JV: Biofeedback in rehabilitation: A review of principles and practices. *Arch Phys Med Rehabil* 1981; 62:469.
35. Wolf SL, Binder-Maclead SA: Electromyographic biofeedback applications to the hemiplegic patient. *Phys Ther* 1983; 63:1404.
36. Winchester P, Montgomery J, Bowman B, Hislop H: Effects of feedback stimulation training and cyclical electrical stimulation on knee extension in hemiparetic patients. *Phys Ther* 1983; 63:1096.
37. Eklund G: Some physical properties of muscle vibrators used to elicit tonic propioceptive reflexes in man. *Acta Soc Med Upsal* 1971; 76:271.
38. Johnson MD, Hensel CL, Matheson DW: Vibration effects on 3 measures of relaxation. *Percept Mot Skill* 1982; 54:1071.
39. Bishop B: Spasticity: Its physiology and management: Part IV. *Phys Ther* 1977; 57:396.
40. Foley J: The stiffness of spastic muscle. *J Neurol Neurosurg Psychiatry* 1961; 24:125.
41. Odeen I: Reduction of muscular hypertonus by long-term muscle stretch. *Scand J Rehabil Med* 1981; 13:93.
42. Goad RA, Ricks NR: Pressure modalities in the treatment of the hypertonic limb. *Neurology Rep* 1984; 8(3):63.
43. Feldman PA: Upper extremity casting and splinting, in Glenn MB, Whyte J (eds): *The Practical Management of Spasticity in Children and Adults.* Philadelphia: Lea & Febiger, 1990: 149–166.

44. Hylton N: Dynamic casting and orthotics, in Glenn MB, Whyte J (eds): *The Practical Management of Spasticity in Children and Adults.* Philadelphia: Lea & Febiger, 1990: 167–200.
45. Pinder RM, Grogden RN, Speight TM: Dantrolene sodium: A review of its pharmacological properties and therapeutic efficacy in spasticity. *Drugs* 1977; 13:3.
46. Monster AW: Spasticity and the effects of dantrolene sodium. *Arch Phys Med Rehabil* 1974; 55:373.
47. Utili R, Boitnott JK, Zimmerman HJ: Dantrolene-associated hepatic injury: Incidence and character. *Gastroenterology* 1977; 72:610.
48. Whyte J, Robinson KM: Pharmacologic management, in Glenn MB, Whyte J (eds): *The Practical Management of Spasticity in Children and Adults.* Philadelphia: Lea & Febiger, 1990: 201–226.
49. Davidoff RA: Antispasticity drugs: Mechanism of action. *Ann Neurol* 1985; 17:107.
50. Corbett M, Frankel HL, Michaelis L: A double blind cross-over trial of Valium in the treatment of spasticity. *Paraplegia* 1972; 10:19.
51. Wilson LA, McKechnie AA: Oral diazepam in the treatment of spasticity in paraplegia: A double blind trial and subsequent impressions. *Scott Med J* 1966; 11:46.
52. Zieglbansberger W, Howe JR, Sutor B: The neuropharmacology of baclofen, in Muller H, Zierski J, Penn RD (eds): *Local-spinal Therapy of Spasticity.* New York: Springer-Verlag, 1988: 37–49.
53. Puil E: Actions and interactions of S-glutamate in the spinal cord, in Davidoff RA (ed): *Handbook of the Spinal Cord,* vol 1. New York: Marcel Dekker, 1983: 105–169.
54. Pederson E, Arlien-Soborg P, Grynderup V, Henriksen O: GABA derivative in spasticity. *Acta Neurol Scand* 1970; 46:257.
55. Roy CW, Wakefield IR: Baclofen psychosis: Case report. *Paraplegia* 1986; 24:318.
56. Nance PW, Shears AH, Nance DM: Clonidine in spinal cord injury. *Can Med Assoc J* 1985; 133:41.
57. Donovan WH, Carter RE, Rossi CD, Wilderson MA: Clonidine effect on spasticity: A clinical trial. *Arch Phys Med Rehabil* 1988; 69:193.
58. Lopierre Y, Bouchard S, Tansey C, et al: Treatment of spasticity with tizanidine in multiple sclerosis. *Can J Neurol Sci* 1987; 14:513.
59. Bass B, Weinshenker B, Rice GPA, et al: Tizanidine versus baclofen in the treatment of spasticity in patients with multiple sclerosis. *Can J Neurol Sci* 1988; 15(1):15.
60. Bes A, Eysette M, Pierrot-Deseilligny E, et al: A multicenter, double-blind trial of tizanidine, a new antispasticity agent, in spasticity associated with hemiplegia. *Curr Med Res Opin* 1988; 10:(10):709.
61. Struppler A, Burgmayer B, Ochs GB, Pfeiffer HG: The effect of epidural application of opioids on spasticity of spinal origin. *Life Sci* 1983; 33:607.
62. Erickson DL, Blacklock JB, Michaelson MA, et al: Control of spasticity by implantable continuous flow morphine pump. *Neurosurg* 1985; 16:215.
63. Loubser PG, Sharkey P, Dimitrijevic M: Control of chronic spasticity following spinal cord injury with intrathecal morphine. *Anesth Analg* 1988; 67:S135.
64. Penn RD, Kroin JS: Long-term intrathecal baclofen infusion for treatment of spasticity, *J Neurosurg* 1987; 66:181.
65. Loubser PG, Narayan RK, Sandin KJ, et al: Continuous infusion of intrathecal baclofen: Long-term effects on spasticity in spinal cord injury. *Paraplegia* 1991; 29:48.
66. Azouvi P, Roby-Brami A, Biraben A, et al: Effect of intrathecal baclofen on the monosynaptic reflex in humans: Evidence for a postsynaptic action. *J Neurol Neurosurg Psychiatry* 1993; 56:515.
67. Broseta J, Garcia-March G, Sanchez-Ledesma MJ, et al: Chronic intrathecal baclofen administration in severe spasticity. *Stereotact Funct Neurosurg* 1990; 54:147.
68. Penn RD, Savoy SM, Corcos D, et al: Intrathecal baclofen for severe spinal spasticity. *N Engl J Med* 1989; 320:1517.
69. Lazorthes Y, Sallerin-Caute B, Verdie JC, et al: Chronic intrathecal baclofen administration for control of severe spasticity. *J Neurosurg* 1990; 72:393.
70. Ochs G, Struppler A, Meyerson BA, et al: Intrathecal baclofen for long-term treatment of spasticity: A multicentre study. *J Neurol Neurosurg Psychiatry* 1989; 52:933.
71. Sahuquillo J, Muxi T, Noguer M, et al: Intraspinal baclofen in the treatment of severe spasticity and spasms. *Acta Neurochir (Wien)* 1991; 110:166.
72. Siegfried J, Rea GL: Intrathecal application of baclofen in the treatment of spasticity. *Acta Neurochir Suppl* 1987; 39:121 (Suppl).
73. Hugenholtz H, Nelson RF, Dehoux E, Bickerton R: Intrathecal baclofen for intractable spinal spasticity—a double-blind cross-over comparison with placebo in 6 patients. *Can J Neurol Sci* 1992; 19:188.
74. Muller H, Zierski J, Dralle, et al: Intrathecal baclofen in spasticity, in Muller H, Zierski J, Penn RD (eds): *Local-spinal Therapy of Spasticity.* New York: Springer-Verlag, 1988: 156–214.
75. Penn RD: Intrathecal baclofen for spasticity of spinal origin: 7 years of experience. *J Neurosurg* 1992; 77:236.
76. Albright AL, Cervi A, Singletary J: Intrathecal baclofen for spasticity in cerebral palsy. *JAMA* 1991; 265:1418.
77. Armstrong RW, Steinbok P, Farrell K, et al: Continuous intrathecal baclofen treatment of severe spasms in 2 children with spinal cord injury. *Dev Med Child Neurol* 1992; 34:731.
78. Muller H, Zierski J, Dralle D, et al: Pharmacokinetics of intrathecal baclofen, in Muller H, Zierski J, Penn RD (eds): *Local-spinal Therapy of Spasticity.* New York: Springer-Verlag, 1988: 223–226.
79. Akman NM, Loubser PG, Donovan WH, et al: Intrathecal baclofen: Does tolerance occur? *Paraplegia* 1993; 31:516.
80. Herman RM, Dluzansky SC, Ippolito R: Intrathecal baclofen suppresses central pain in patients with spinal lesions: A pilot study. *Clin J Pain* 1992; 8:338.
81. Loubser PG, Narayan RK: Effect of subarachnoid cath-

eter position on the efficacy of intrathecal baclofen for spinal spasticity. *Anesthesiology* 1993; 79:611.

82. Hugenholtz H, Nelson RF, Dehouz E: Intrathecal baclofen—the importance of catheter position. *Can J Neurol Sci* 1993; 20:165.
83. Muller H, Zierski J: Clinical experience with spinal morphine, midazolam and tizanidine in spasticity, in Muller H, Zierski J, Penn RD (eds): *Local-spinal Therapy of Spasticity*. New York: Springer-Verlag, 1988: 143–150.
84. Dahm LS, Beric A, Dimitrijevic MR, Wall PW: Direct spinal effect of a benzodiazepine (Midazolam) on spasticity in man. *Stereotact Funct Neurosurg* 1989; 53:85.
85. Tucker GT, Mather LE: Properties, absorption and disposition of local anesthetic drugs, in Cousins MJ, Bridenbaugh PO (eds): *Neural Blockade in Clinical Anesthesia and Management of Pain,* (2d ed). Philadelphia: JB Lippincott, 1988: 45–85.
86. Keenan ME: The orthopedic management of spasticity. *J Head Trauma Rehabil* 1987; 2:62.
87. Scott DB, Cousins MJ: Clinical pharmacology of local anesthetic agents, in Cousins MJ, Bridenbaugh PO (eds): *Neural Blockade in Clinical Anesthesia and Management of Pain,* (2d ed). Philadelphia: JB Lippincott, 1988: 86–121.
88. Wood KM: The use of phenol as a neurolytic agent: A review. *Pain* 1978; 5:205.
89. Halpern D: Histologic studies in animals after intramuscular neurolysis with phenol. *Arch Phys Med Rehabil* 1977; 58:438.
90. Schaumberg HN, Byck R, Weller RO: The effect of phenol on peripheral nerves: A histological and electrophysiological study. *J Neuropathol Exp Neurol* 1970; 29:615.
91. Burkel WE, McPhee M: Effect of phenol injection into peripheral nerve of rat: Electron microscope studies. *Arch Phys Med Rehabil* 1950; 51:391.
92. Mooney V, Frykman G, McLamb J: Current status of intraneural phenol injections. *Clin Orthop* 1969; 63:122.
93. Khalili AA: Physiatric management of spasticity by phenol nerve and motor point block, in Ruskin AP (ed): *Current Therapy in Physiatry*. Philadelphia: WB Saunders, 1984: 464–474.
94. Meelhuysen FE, Halpern D, Quast J: Treatment of flexor spasticity of hip by paravertebral lumbar spinal nerve block. *Arch Phys Med Rehabil* 1964; 49:36.
95. Halpern D, Meelhuysen FE: Duration of relaxation after intramuscular neurolysis with phenol. *JAMA* 1967; 200:1152.
96. Glenn MB: Nerve blocks, in Glenn MB, Whyte J (eds): *The Practical Management of Spasticity in Children and Adults*. Philadelphia: Lea & Febiger, 1990: 227–258.
97. May O: The functional and histological effects of intraneural and intraganglionic injections of alcohol. *Br Med J* 1912; 1:465.
98. Tardieu G, Tardieu C, Hariga J, Gagnard L: Treatment of spasticity by injection of dilute alcohol at the motor point or by epidural route. *Dev Med Child Neurol* 1968; 10:555.
99. Loubser PG: Intrathecal alcohol injection guided by electrical localization of spinal routes. *Anesth Analg* 1990; 70:115.
100. Racz GB, Heavner J, Haynsworth R: Repeat epidural phenol injections in chronic pain and spasticity, in Lipton S, Miles J (eds): *Persistent Pain*. Orlando: Grune & Stratton, 1985: 157–179.
101. Nathan PW: Intrathecal phenol to relieve spasticity in paraplegia. *Lancet* 1959; 2:1099.
102. Walthard KM, Tchicaloff M: Motor points, in Licht S (ed): *Electrodiagnosis and Electromyography,* (3d ed). New Haven: Elizabeth Licht, 1971: 153–170.
103. Garland DE, Lilling M, Keenan ME: Percutaneous phenol blocks to motor points of spastic forearm muscles in head-injured adults. *Arch Phys Med Rehabil* 1984; 65:243.
104. Easton JKM, Ozel T, Halpern D: Intramuscular neurolysis for spasticity in children. *Arch Phys Med Rehabil* 1979; 60:155.
105. Halpern D, Meelhuysen FE: Phenol motor point block in the management of muscular hypertonia. *Arch Phys Med Rehabil* 1966; 47:659.
106. Foerster O: On the indications of the excision of posterior spinal nerve roots in men. *Surg Gynecol Obstet* 1913; 16:463.
107. Munro D: The rehabilitation of patients totally paralysed below the waist: With special reference to making them ambulatory and capable of earning a living: I. Anterior rhizotomy for spastic paraplegia. *N Engl J Med* 1945; 223:453.
108. Fraioli B, Guidetti B: Posterior partial rootlet section in the treatment of spasticity. *J Neurosurg* 1977; 46:618.
109. Sindou M, Millet MF, Mortamais J, Eysette M: Results of selective posterior rhizotomy in the treatment of painful and spastic paraplegia secondary to multiple sclerosis. *Appl Neurophysiol* 1982; 45:335.
110. Bischof W: Die longitudinale myelotomie. *Zentralbl Neurochir* 1951; 11:79.
111. Toennis W, Bischof W: Ergebnisse der lumbalen myelotomie nach Bischof. *Zentralbl Neurochir* 1962; 23:120.
112. Putty TK, Shapiro SA: Efficacy of dorsal longitudinal myelotomy in treating spinal spasticity: A review of 20 cases. *J Neurosurg* 1991; 75:397.
113. Benzel EC, Barolat-Romano G, Larson SJ: Femoral obturator and sciatic neurectomy with iliacus and psoas muscle section for spasticity following spinal cord injury. *Spine* 1988; 13:905.
114. Garland DE, Lucie RS, Waters RL: Current uses of open phenol nerve block for adult acquired spasticity. *Clin Orthop Rel Res* 1982; 165:217.
115. Trainer N, Bowser BL, Dahm LS: Obturator nerve block for painful hip in adult cerebral palsy. *Arch Phys Med Rehabil* 1986; 67:829.
116. Kenmore D: Radiofrequency neurotomy for peripheral pain and spasticity syndromes. *Contemp Neurosurg* 1983; 58:895.
117. Kasdon DL, Lathi ES: A prospective study of radiofrequency rhizotomy in the treatment of posttraumatic spasticity. *Neurosurgery* 1984; 15:526.

118. Herz DA, Parsons KC, Pearl L: Percutaneous radiofrequency foraminal rhizotomies. *Spine* 1983; 8:729.

119. Cook AW, Weinstein SP: Chronic dorsal column stimulation in multiple sclerosis. *NY State J Med* 1973; 73:2868.

120. Krainick JU, Waisbrod H, Gerbershagen HU: The value of spinal cord stimulation in treatment of disorders of the motor system, in Muller H, Zierski J, Penn RD (eds): *Local-spinal Therapy of Spasticity*. New York: Springer-Verlag, 1988: 245–252.

Rehabilitation

CHAPTER 91

REHABILITATION ASSESSMENT AND MANAGEMENT IN THE ACUTE SPINAL CORD INJURY (SCI) PATIENT

John F. Ditunno, Jr.

INTRODUCTION

Acute SCI care requires the cooperation of the surgical team and the rehabilitation team. The surgical team is highly skilled, oriented to reduce worsening of the neurological deficit by stabilization with drugs, traction, and the surgical correction of structural abnormalities of the spine and associated injuries. The rehabilitation team is highly skilled and oriented to the assessment and maintenance of multiple body systems affected by the neurological deficit in order to restore, substitute, or modify function and ultimately return the patient to the community. Neither is limited to these primary approaches alone; both utilize other interventions and may rely on additional consultations to restore the individual to the highest level of independent function. This chapter will deal with the rehabilitation teams' approach to acute SCI assessment, making a prognosis, and setting goals of early management. The acute SCI phase will be defined as the first one to three weeks postinjury or until the patient is transferred to the acute rehabilitation unit.

SYSTEMS ASSESSMENT

The systems involved include the neuromusculoskeletal and skin, genitourinary and gastrointestinal, and often the cardiovascular and pulmonary systems. Disruption of the individuals' personal and societal relationships require assessment of psychosocial and vocational domains. The systems are discussed in the following order: neurological; immobilization (musculoskeletal); bladder; bowel; lungs (heart); extremities (vascular); and skin. The first two systems should always be assessed as the first priority.

NEUROLOGICAL

Accurate and precise examination on admission and daily thereafter provides the basis for determining deterioration, improvement, and prognosis of neurological impairments. The standard assessment and prognosis based on the neurological examination will be covered below. Fluctuation in the neurological findings is common in the initial 72 hours, either because of progression of the lesion or rapid improvement, and caution is advised in making a definitive prognosis.[1] Associated head injury,[2,3] endotracheal tubes, and various drugs may present complications, but most often determination of neurological level, completeness of the lesion, motor and sensory scores, and the ASIA impairment scale is possible. A change in motor score provides a rapid and reliable method for clinicians to communicate change. Patients and families should be informed of the positive potential for recovery, self-care, and ambulation as early as possible, and future goals should be outlined.

IMMOBILIZATION

Instability of the spine prior to surgical stabilization with or without a halo brace or body jacket requires definition and communication to the nursing staff and therapists. Vigorous strengthening exercises to the upper extremities in a cervical lesion and even range of motion exercise to the hips with a thoracolumbar fracture may be contraindicated. Postoperative mobilization out of bed with or without braces and mobilization of associated fractures of the extremities requires consistent guidelines agreed to by protocol between the surgical and rehabilitation teams. A decrease in motor score needs immediate attention and may require reassessment of spine stability or alignment. Associated fractures of the upper or lower extremities occur in 9.5 percent of cases,[4] and the extent of weight-bearing and time lines should be defined for upper extremities required for transfers and for lower extremities for ambulation. This process may delay the rehabilitation program and may require temporary placement until a patient is able to participate in more intensive therapy. The staging of this plan because of associated fractures should be defined within the first week in order to identify the alternative disposition and to maximize days spent in the appropriate unit.

Bladder

Bladder training begins when fluids are restricted to 1800 ml and intermittent catheterization is implemented, usually within the initial days or weeks postinjury. Often fluids are not restricted during the perioperative period or because of pulmonary complications; if so, an indwelling Foley catheter should be taped to the abdomen to prevent penile uretheral angle erosion and fluids in excess of 3000 ml per 24-hour period. The goal is to keep the urine sterile or to achieve a sterile urine prior to discharge; this condition has been shown to have significantly fewer upper tract complications long-term.[5] Premature removal of the catheter without attention to urine analysis, urine culture, and postvoiding residuals predisposes to upper tract infection. Some physicians will prescribe antibiotics several days before and after removal of the indwelling catheter; others will use antibiotics only in the presence of significant bacteriuria. Daily inspection on rounds of the color and clarity of the urine will alert the clinician to blood, bile, or underhydration.

Bowel

The initiation of bowel training may not be possible in the first week because of ileus, which occurs in 8 percent of cases,[6] abdominal surgery, or other reasons for withholding food. However, a bowel routine of stool softeners, suppositories, and timed evacuation should begin as soon as possible. Use of narcotic analgesics and the neurological impairment itself contribute to constipation, obstipation, and fecal impaction. This presents additional problems in quadriplegia, because abdominal distension can compromise diaphragmatic excursion, contributing to atelectasis or pneumonia. If hyperalimentation is provided by vein or the gastrointestinal route, attention to evacuation and prevention of obstipation is still necessary.

Lungs/Heart

Care of the lungs in the acute phase is determined by the risk of complications. Atelectasis of three days' duration and/or pneumonia developed in 80 percent of C4–C5 complete tetraplegic patients admitted to a regional center,[7] while less than 20 percent developed these complications with a lower lesion. Four out of five patients had left lower lobe involvement, which is most likely because of the difficulty in placing a suction catheter into the left mainstem bronchus. Respiratory complications remain the leading cause of morbidity and mortality acutely. Respiratory tract infection in the first two weeks carries a high incidence of recurrence after discharge, and respiratory complications continue to be the leading cause of death long-term in quadriplegia.[8] Aggressive treatment and surveillance of vital capacity is indicated during rehabilitation and follow-up. Vital capacity can increase approximately 1000 ml over the subsequent four- to five-month period, and breathing exercises with pulmonary toilet are essential.[9] Adult respiratory distress syndrome, an occasional complication, may result in reduced lung compliance and may require extended periods of weaning[10] if the patient is ventilator-dependent. The vital capacity is the manual muscle test of the diaphragm[11] and should be monitored daily in the acute phase. Hemopneumothorax is common in thoracic lesions but seldom leads to long-term complications. With stabilization of medical complications and associated injuries, training to increase vital capacity and clear secretions is begun in this phase and continued throughout the rehabilitation period.

Bradycardia secondary to unopposed vagal stimulation in the high tetraplegic patient may require short-term cardiac pacing, but rarely is a problem in the subacute phase.[12,13] As this risk declines after four to six weeks, however, the emergence of autonomic hyperreflexia with hypertension and bradycardia due to a distended bladder or bowel can occur. This is rarely seen in a new injury in the acute phase.

Extremities

During the initial four to six weeks following injury, attention to prevention of deep vein thrombosis (DVT) in the paralyzed lower extremities and subsequent pulmonary embolism takes priority, and discontinuation of external pneumatic compression (EPC) is not warranted because the patient is being mobilized. In the past decade a number of studies[14,15] have shown that a 70 percent or greater incidence of DVT can be reduced to less than 10 percent by preventive measures. The use of prophylactic heparin and EPC must be defined in the acute injury and perioperative period by the surgical team, preferably by protocol. Mobilization of fractures has been covered above, but with casts and external fixation compression may not be possible and other prophylactic alternatives may be indicated. Although prevention has dramatically reduced the incidence of DVT and pulmonary emboli, it still occurs, requiring therapeutic levels of anticoagulation. Precaution in stretching hamstrings is necessary in such patients because significant hemorrhage does occur in the hamstring muscle,[16] and therapists should be advised to avoid vigorous stretching. Heterotopic ossification(HO) may occur in 30 to 50 percent of patients, but less than 5 percent will have contracture of the joint significant enough to result in disability in sitting and transfers.[17] At times DVT is associated with HO, and either condition may result in swelling with pitting edema of the lower extremity.

Skin

Skin care requires attention to the prevention of pressure and shear forces at all phases of care. The sacrum area accounts for 55 percent of all severe pressure sores.[4] Patients are at risk in the acute phase during transportation and in the emergency room while immobilized on the hard spinal board owing to instability of the spine. In cases where reduction is difficult or risks to instability persist, as in patients with ankylosing spondylitis with fracture and deformity, pressure relief must be defined for the nursing staff by the physician in the initial admission orders. While nurses and therapists provide important monitoring of these problems, physicians need to establish the priorities for mobilization or restrictions based on daily assessment. If the patient is mobilized out of bed in the sitting position, pressure relief is indicated every 20 to 30 minutes, or more often depending on the tolerance of the skin based on inspection.

The organization of the above discussion permits an approach that may be utilized on daily rounds. The systems can be outlined for the physician in the acronym NIBBLES. Contrary to what it suggests, it is a huge bite and a lot for the physician to digest who manages patients in the acute phase and sees them on a daily basis following the acute injury. It does organize the approach by body systems and the related functional goals for restoration of mobility, continence of feces and urine, and cardiovascular and pulmonary endurance to support self-care and ambulation activities. Clearly it should include, in addition, attention to vital signs, laboratory values, and input from other clinicians.

Assessment of the impact on the patient and family runs concurrently with the management of the body systems. Attention to the emotional support of the patient and family involves the entire team of physicians, nurses, and therapists, but speech therapists, social workers, and psychologists are able to provide special interventions. The respirator-dependent patient or any patient on temporary ventilatory support may have difficulty communicating with nurses (although many nurses are skilled in lip reading), physicians, therapists, or family members in the first few weeks post-SCI. A speech therapist may facilitate communication by providing special equipment. A physician and social worker who meets with the family at some length during the first week to discuss anticipated complications, neurological and functional recovery, strategy and timing for return to home, and disposition alternatives is key to alleviating anxieties and enlisting patient and family as members of the team. While depression is common in the acute phase, it is less of a problem long-term.[18] Patients and families often request and appear to benefit from support from psychologists, social workers, and, in certain settings, from other families. In the first few weeks vocational potential and early goals should be positively presented as correlations of independence in self-care and ambulation. Sexual function and capacity for having children and parenting are frequently concerns and should be discussed in the acute phase, especially if raised by the patient or family.

For these reasons, the rehabilitation physician should be involved from the day of injury to direct the care by the team of physical, occupational, and speech therapists, social workers, and psychologists. The rehabilitation physician also must assist the surgical team in facilitating appropriate care by nurses and other therapists toward mobilization, care of bladder, bowel, lung, and skin. The plan developed in the acute phase by the surgical and rehabilitation team continues under the supervision of the rehabilitation physician upon patient transfer to the acute rehabilitation unit, usually within days or weeks of injury.

The goals for self-care and ambulation are defined for the ongoing rehabilitation phase based in large part on the initial neurological assessment in the acute phase. Therefore, newly agreed upon international standards[19] are important to SCI surgeons and rehabilitation clinicians for proper categorization of injuries, prognosis, and determination of good rehabilitation outcomes.[20,21] The following material is included and made available with the permission of Aspen Publishers, Inc. This supplements and expands on the previous neurological discussion.

NEUROLOGICAL EXAMINATION

The neurological examination involves motor and sensory testing and must be performed accurately and periodically to assess patients properly. The key muscles to test and the specific points of the sensory examination are as discussed and illustrated in Chapter 75. There are five muscles listed for each extremity; these are the same for the right and left sides. The modalities of light touch and pinprick (pain) are examined separately and recorded for 23 vertebral segments, also on the right and left sides. From these examinations, the neurological level or the motor and sensory level for the right and left sides is derived, and the lesion is categorized as complete or incomplete. Most clinicians describe the severity and extent of injury on the basis of the neurological level of the injury and its degree of completeness. The neurological examination also will reveal the extent of partially innervated segments or the zone of partial preservation (ZPP), which is important in determining the degree of completeness of the injury. Other scales and indices utilized in the standards, such as motor scores, sensory scores, and impairment scales (formerly Frankel grades), also are derived from this baseline examination. These scales and indices are used by clinicians and investigators to describe the extent of the impairment to monitor neurological recovery or deterioration.

Functional assessment measures are usually not employed until the patient is stabilized and mobilized because they relate to activities of daily living (ADLs) such as self-care and mobility functions. The term tetraplegia (quadriplegia) refers to paralysis of the lower extremities plus any involvement of the upper extremities above T2, whereas paraplegia refers to normal upper extremity function and any paralysis of the lower extremities due to a lesion of the spinal cord or cauda equina.

Muscle testing is based on strength grading of the key muscles on a scale of 0 to 5. Each key muscle represents a motor segment. In the upper extremity, elbow flexors represent C5, elbow extensors C7, wrist extensors C6, finger flexors C8, and finger abductors T1. In the lower extremity, hip flexors represent L2, knee extensors L3, ankle dorsiflexors L4, ankle plantar flexors S1, and toe extensors L5. The grading system scores no movement of the muscle on voluntary effort as 0, trace contraction as 1, movement through the joint range of motion with gravity eliminated as 2, range of motion against gravity as 3, range of motion with moderate resistance as 4, and range of motion against full resistance as 5. This system of muscle grading is quite reliable, although errors are not uncommon clinically, and even trained personnel will require periodic evaluation in carrying out the test. For example, function of the elbow extensor (C7) may be graded erroneously as present because the patient can voluntarily flex the forearm (C5) against gravity and the forearm is observed to extend passively upon relaxation. This can be misleading in management decisions and upon review of the medical record.

By convention, the motor neurological level is considered normal when the grade for the key muscle of the specific motor segment is 3 or higher, provided that the next key muscle cephalad is graded as 4 or 5. Therefore, accuracy in determining motor levels is based on the accuracy of grading the key muscles. Because the motor score is a summation of the individual motor grades of all 20 key muscles in the upper, lower, right, and left extremities, skill in manual muscle testing is essential.

The sensory neurological level is determined by identifying the most caudal segment with normal response to both pinprick and light touch for each side. The sensory score is the summation of the results of testing of the 23 dermatomes for the right and left sides and has a maximum value of 112 for each modality. Partially innervated segments are determined by findings on examination of impaired strength and/or impaired perception of pinprick and light touch; these findings help define the ZPP. They also contribute to the distinction between a complete and an incomplete lesion, but here again caution is advised to avoid errors in either examination or interpretation. The recent revision of the definition of a complete lesion requires absence[22] of all voluntary movement and any sensation in the lowest sacral segment (S4–S5), irrespective of the number of partially innervated segments in the ZPP. If, however, there is voluntary contraction of the anal sphincter or any sensation in S4–S5, then the injury is considered incomplete.

This distinction frequently requires careful examination in a less than ideal environment (emergency department) and in patients who are not always able to cooperate fully because of anxiety or impaired cognition. Because of these conditions as well as evidence from large trials[23] that a small but significant number of complete lesions convert to incomplete ones, clinicians should avoid making an absolute statement regarding poor prognosis for the first few days after injury. Spinal shock, or the absence of all reflexes, is a period during which one cannot prognosticate accurately. Because there is no clear understanding of spinal shock,[24] its presence adds little to the need for caution in prognostication already stated.

The baseline examination not only aids in defining a complete lesion, but also permits the derivation of the ASIA Impairment Scale (formerly the Frankel grades; see Fig. 91-1) and determination of the presence of incomplete clinical syndromes. This system of measuring neurological function and impairment allows one to link neurological recovery to gains in human performance. The daily human performance of necessary activities, or ADLs, usually is expressed in terms of self-care and mobility functions. The new ASIA standards recommend the Functional Independence Measure (FIM) as the definitive functional assessment measure; it is the most widely utilized measure in the United

ASIA IMPAIRMENT SCALE

☐ **A = Complete:** No motor or sensory function is preserved in the sacral segments S4-S5.

☐ **B = Incomplete:** Sensory but not motor function is preserved below the neurological level and extends through the sacral segments S4-S5.

☐ **C = Incomplete:** Motor function is preserved below the neurological level, and the majority of key muscles below the neurological level have a muscle grade less than 3.

☐ **D = Incomplete:** Motor function is preserved below the neurological level, and the majority of key muscles below the neurological level have a muscle grade greater than or equal to 3.

☐ **E = Normal:** Motor and sensory function is normal.

CLINICAL SYNDROMES

☐ Central Cord
☐ Brown-Séquard
☐ Anterior Cord
☐ Conus Medullaris
☐ Cauda Equina

Figure 91-1. The ASIA Impairment Scale. The new ASIA standards recommend the Functional Independence Measure (FIM).

States today. The FIM includes, under self-care, eating, grooming, bathing, dressing the upper body, dressing the lower body, and toileting. In addition to self-care, the FIM evaluates another 12 activities grouped under sphincter control, mobility, locomotion, communication, and social cognition. These functions are graded on seven levels from requiring no help to requiring total assistance. The assessments are usually performed by rehabilitation clinicians and staff after the patient has been mobilized in the days or weeks after SCI. The need for future modification of the FIM is discussed below.

The second National Acute Spinal Cord Injury Study (NASCIS II) has reported small but significant improvement in neurological recovery when large doses of methylprednisolone are given in the first eight hours after injury[23,25] (e.g., 30 mg/kg IV over 15 minutes, with a subsequent maintenance infusion of 5 mg/kg/h over the next 24 hours). Administration of a ganglioside (GM-1) was recently reported to be of benefit in an initial study,[26] and a large multicenter trial has been initiated.

In 1991, NASCIS III began evaluation of tirilazad in combination with methylprednisolone. These drugs, their proposed mechanism of action, and their place in the medical treatment of acute SCI have been well described.[27] Various assessments such as motor and sensory scores were used in the NASCIS II trials, but these scores differ sufficiently from other databases that utilize the ASIA standards so that the results could not be compared (NASCIS II used seven muscles per extremity to calculate the motor score rather than the five muscles per extremity recommended by the ASIA standards, and some of the muscles were different). Although the GM-1 study utilized the ASIA standards, neither study used a measure of ADLs. The NASCIS III trials have adopted essentially the revised ASIA standards, and the multicenter trial of GM-1 utilizes the ASIA neurological classification and an alternative assessment for ambulation. The Model SCI programs have utilized the ASIA standards and their revisions for almost 10 years, so that more than 40 centers conducting trials in SCI management have adopted the revised ASIA standards, and most of these use both the neurological and the functional classifications. In addition, these standards have received initial endorsement by the International Medical Society of Paraplegia. The revised ASIA standards thus should provide a powerful tool to clinicians and clinical investigators throughout the world for the evaluation not only of neuropharmacological agents but of surgical and rehabilitation interventions as well.[27]

RECOVERY OF NEUROLOGICAL FUNCTION IN SCI

The recovery of neurological function after SCI is divided into recovery at the zone of injury and recovery distal to the zone of injury. This distinction is necessary because recovery at the zone of injury in a complete lesion is most frequently confined to several segments and occurs predominantly in the area of lower motor neuron injury, whereas recovery distal to the zone of injury primarily represents recovery of upper motor neurons or long tracts. In cauda equina lesions, which are injuries to the spinal roots within the spinal column, the recovery is more typical of root level recovery. Therefore, the mechanisms are somewhat different. Recovery at the zone of injury recently has been demonstrated to involve peripheral sprouting of motor terminals[28] in addition to resolution of conduction (neuropraxia) and muscle strength. Long tract recovery is probably due to remyelinization and possible central sprouting. Improvement in neurological function always occurs after SCI, even in complete lesions, at the zone of injury. Recovery at the zone of injury has been almost exclusively studied in cervical lesions in terms of recovery of upper extremity muscle strength. A multicenter study of motor levels in 150 complete C4, C5, and C6 injuries reported recovery of strength in elbow flexors, wrist extensors, and elbow extensors continuing for up to two years.[29] Of patients with some muscle strength from the spinal segment below the intact level, 80 to 90 percent recovered strength to grade 4 or 5 within the initial hospital stay of four to six months. Of those patients with no muscle strength from the segment below the intact level, however, only 25 to 35 percent showed recovery to grade 3 to 5 by four to six months, but this percentage more than doubled after discharge (Fig. 91-2). Certain areas of the United States now require earlier discharge of tetraplegic patients, long before their maximum recovery of function.[30]

Incomplete cervical lesions tend to recover sooner than complete lesions at the site of injury and distal to the site. It remains unclear whether this recovery is actually greater, however. Studies of recovery below the zone of injury have been based on Frankel grades modified by the ASIA standards. Patients with injuries that remain complete (A) for longer than one week usually will not recover useful neurological function below the ZPP (D) even though function may improve one to two segments at the ZPP (#12 and 13 of the article). Several studies[31,32] that initially showed 5 to 10 percent of injuries classified as A converting to D were called into question by Maynard in 1979, who objected that most patients with injuries so classified had had associated head injury, which made accurate initial examination improbable.

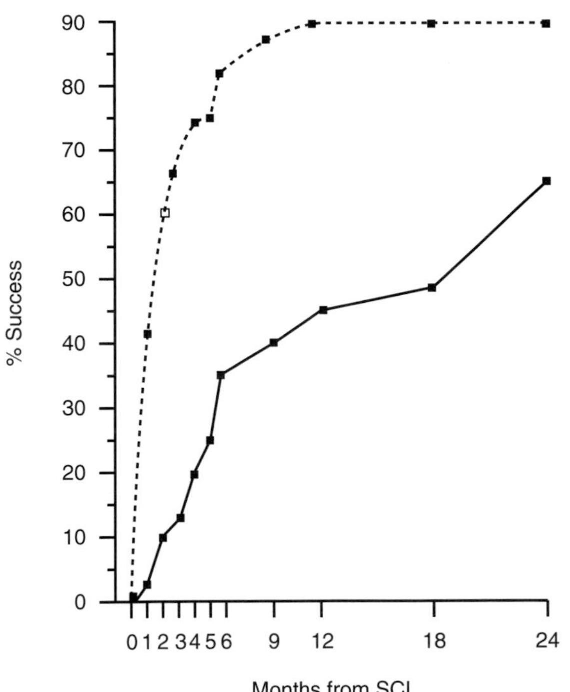

Figure 91-2. Percentage of success recovery vs. discharge.[29]

In light of recent reports of pharmacological agents used in the acute phase of SCI[23,25,26] it is unclear how many complete lesions convert to incomplete ones. Of patients who have any voluntary movement in their lower extremities distal to the injury site, more than 80 percent will show useful motor function recovery (D or better).[33] Although most studies[34] have been retrospective, a recent prospective study[35] from our center showed that eventual walking could be predicted on the basis of initial and follow-up tests of motor strength in the quadriceps. Patients with some initial quadriceps strength whose muscle tests improved to grade 3 or higher by two months had an excellent prognosis for becoming household or community walkers by one year; those whose tests improved after two months did not do as well ($P = 0.002$).

In central cord syndromes in which lower extremity strength is greater than upper extremity strength, it has been reported[36] that more than 50 percent of patients will become ambulatory. A recent report[37] from our center compared the outcome of central cord syndromes in young adults to that in patients older than 50 years (central cord syndromes are frequently associated with less severe trauma and spinal stenosis in younger patients). More than 90 percent of young patients who presented with, or evolved to, a central cord injury were ambulating at the time of discharge. Only about 40 percent of patients older than 50 years were able to walk at discharge ($P < 0.002$).

Brown-Séquard syndrome, or hemisection of the cord, carries as good a prognosis for ambulation as central cord injuries in young patients.[36] Prognosis in anterior cord syndrome varies according to the type of sensation that is spared. Crozier and colleagues[38] reported that 90 percent of patients with complete paralysis but with preservation of pinprick sensation in the sacral segments were ambulating by discharge. Only 20 percent of patients with touch sensation alone became ambulatory. These investigators suggested proximity of the lateral spinal thalamic tracts, which carry pinprick sensation to the corticospinal tracts (which in turn carry the long axons for ambulation) as the reason for this recovery.

The FIM, originally developed for the rehabilitation industry to demonstrate burden of care socially and economically, is also used as a monitor of quality of care. Hamilton and DeVivo[39] compared FIM data and showed significant changes or improvements in self-care or mobility among patients with SCI during a rehabilitation stay, but it was unclear how much of the improvement was due to spontaneous recovery and how much was due to training. The FIM has been demonstrated to be a reliable and valid instrument in patients with mixed disabilities and has shown good reliability in SCI patients.[40] Its reliability for social cognition and communication activities, however, is less than for other types of activities. Also, it has not been demonstrated to be valid for precisely measuring recovery in subpopulations such as tetraplegics.[19] Zafonte and associates,[41] in a recent report, showed that patients with C7 motor levels on one side were capable of independence in most feeding activities measured by the Quadriplegia Index of Function (QIF),[42] but the FIM would have scored most of these patients as requiring supervision. The QIF is also more discriminating for upper extremity motor scores than the FIM.[43] It is conceivable that the FIM will require further modification to fit SCI subpopulations.[21] Tables have been developed for various textbooks[13] that describe function in terms of neurological levels of injury. Although they serve a useful purpose for students, these guidelines are only crude estimates of self-care ability and will require refinement as standards for neurological and functional assessment evolve.

The rehabilitation approach to SCI assessment in the acute phase by the clinicians has been outlined in terms of body systems. Neurological, immobilization (musculoskeletal), bladder, bowel, lung, extremities, and skin status should be evaluated on a daily basis in order to formulate short- and long-term functional goals. Self-care and ambulation outcome is based on the initial neurological assessment. The new international standards should provide clinicians the opportunity for uniformity in the categorization of the severity of the injury and determining the potential for recovery and improvement of function.

References

1. Brown PJ, Marion RJ, Herbison GJ, Ditunno JF: The 72-hour exam in a predictor of recovery in motor complete quadriplegia. *Arch Phys Med Rehabil* 1991; 72:546–548.
2. Davidoff G, Thomas P, Johnson MB, et al: Closed head injury in acute traumatic spinal cord injury—incidence and risk factors. *Arch Phys Med Rehabil* 1988; 69(10):869–872.
3. Maynard FM, Reynolds GG, Fountain S, et al: Neurological prognosis after traumatic quadriplegia. *J Neurosurg* 1979; 50:611–616.
4. Stover SL, Fine PR: *Spinal Cord Injury: The Facts and Figures.* Birmingham: University of Alabama, 1986.
5. Stover SL: Management of bacteriuria and infection in neurogenic bladder. *Med Rehabil Clin North Am* 1993; 4(2):343–362.
6. Gore RM, Mintzer RA, Calenoff L: Gastrointestinal complications of spinal cord injury. *Spine* 1981; 6(6):538–544.
7. Fishburn MJ, Marino RJ, Ditunno JF: Atelectasis and pneumonia in acute spinal cord injury. *Arch Phys Med Rehabil* 1990; 71:197–200.
8. DeVivo MJ, Black KJ, Stover SL: Causes of death during the first 12 years after spinal cord injury. *Arch Phys Med Rehabil* 1993; 74(3):248–254.
9. Carter RE: Intermittent catheterization: A small warning. *Emerg Med* 1974; 6(4):274–275.
10. Peterson JR, Ditunno JF: Failure of initial weaning parameters to predict ultimate ventilator dependence: The case of a patient with traumatic C4 quadriplegia complicated by the adult respiratory distress syndrome and hemidiaphragmatic paralysis. *J Am Paraplegia Soc* 1992; 15:114.
11. Macklem PT: Muscular weakness and respiratory function. *N Engl J Med* 1986; 314(12):775–776.
12. Naso F: Cardiovascular problems in patients with spinal cord injury. *Phys Med Rehabil Clin North Am* 1992; 3(4):741–750.
13. Staas WE et al: Rehabilitation of the spinal cord injured patient, in DeLisa JA (ed): *Rehabilitation Medicine: Principles and Practice,* (2d ed). Philadelphia: JB Lippincott, 1993: 886–915.
14. Merli GJ, Crabbe SJ, Doyle L, et al: Mechanical plus pharmacological prophylaxis for deep vein thrombosis in acute spinal cord injury. *Paraplegia* 1992; 30(8):558–562.
15. Green D, Lee MY, Ito V, et al: Fixed vs adjusted dose heparin in the prophylaxis of thromboembolism in spinal cord injury. *JAMA* 1988; 260(9):1255–1258.
16. Chen YT, Gershkoff AM: Lower extremity hemorrhage in spinal cord injured patients receiving therapeutic anticoagulation. *Arch Phys Med Rehabil* 1984; 65(5):263–266.
17. Venier L, Ditunno JF: Heterotopic ossification in the paraplegic patient. *Arch Phys Med Rehabil* 1971; 52:475–479.
18. Richards JS: Psychological adjustment to SCI during the first post-discharge year. *Arch Phys Med Rehabil* 1986; 67(6):362–365.
19. American Spinal Injury Association (ASIA): *Standards for Neurological and Functional Classification of Spinal Cord Injury.* Chicago, 1992.
20. Ditunno JF: Functional assessment measures in CNS trauma. *J Neurotrauma* 1992; 9:5301–5305.
21. Ditunno JF: New spinal cord injury standards—1992. *Paraplegia* 1992; 30:90–91.
22. Waters RL, Adkins RH, Yakura JS: Definition of complete spinal cord injury. *Paraplegia* 1991; 9:573–581.
23. Bracken MB, Shepard MJ, Collins WF, et al: A randomized controlled trial of methylprednisolone or naloxone in the treatment of acute spinal cord injury. *N Engl J Med* 1990; 322:1405–1411.
24. Illis LS: Clinical evaluation and pathophysiology of the spinal cord in the chronic stages, in, Willis J. (ed); *Spinal Cord Dysfunction Assessment.* Oxford: Oxford University Press, 1988: 260–290.
25. Bracken MB, Shepard MJ, Collins WF, et al: Methylprednisolone or naloxone treatment after acute spinal cord

injury: 1-year follow-up data. Results of the second National Acute Spinal Cord Injury Study. *J Neurosurg* 1992; 76:23–31.

26. Geisler FH, Dorsey FC, Coleman WP: Recovery of motor function after spinal cord injury—A randomized placebo controlled trial with GM1 ganglioside. *N Engl J Med* 1991; 324:1829–1838.
27. Young W: Medical treatment of acute spinal cord injury. *J Neurol Neurosurg Psychiatry* 1992; 55:635–639.
28. Marino RJ, Herbison GJ, Ditunno JF: Peripheral sprouting in the zone of partial preservation in motor complete spinal cord injury. *J Am Paraplegia Soc* 1992; 15:122.
29. Ditunno JF, Stover SL, Freed MM, Ahn JH: Motor recovery of the upper-extremities in traumatic quadriplegia: A multicenter study. *Arch Phys Med Rehabil* 1992; 73:431–436.
30. Madorsky J: Personal communication, 1992.
31. Frankel HL, Hancock DO, Hyslop G, et al: The value of postural reduction in the initial management of closed injuries of the spine with paraplegia and tetraplegia. *Paraplegia* 1969; 7:179–192.
32. Young JS, Dexter WR: Neurological recovery distal to zone of injury in 172 cases of closed, traumatic spinal cord injury. *Paraplegia* 1979; 16:39–49.
33. Folman Y, Masri WE: Spinal cord injury: Prognostic indicators. *Injury* 1989; 20:92–93.
34. Hussey RW, Stauffer ES: Spinal cord injury: Requirements for ambulation. *Arch Phys Med Rehabil* 1973; 54:544–547.
35. Zorn GW, Crozier KS, Cheng LL, et al: Quadriceps recovery in Frankel C spinal cord injury. *J Am Paraplegia Soc* 1991; 14:90.
36. Bosch A, Stauffer ES, Nickel VL: Incomplete traumatic quadriplegia: A ten-year review. *JAMA* 1979; 216:473.
37. Penrod LE, Hegde SK, Ditunno JF: Age effect on prognosis for functional recovery in acute, traumatic central cord syndrome. *Arch Phys Med Rehabil* 1990; 71:963–968.
38. Crozier KS, Graziani V, Ditunno JF, Herbison GJ: Prognosis for ambulation based on sensory examination in patients who are initially motor complete. *Arch Phys Med Rehabil* 1991; 72:119–121.
39. Hamilton BB, DeVivo MJ: Functional enhancement, in *Spinal Cord Injury: The Model.* Proceedings of a National Consensus Conference on Catastrophic Illness and Injury, Atlanta, GA. Georgia Regional Spinal Cord Injury Care System, Shepherd Center for Treatment of Spinal Injuries, 1990.
40. Hamilton BB, Laughlin JA, Granger CV, Kayton RM: Interrater agreement of the seven level Functional Independence Measure (FIM). *Arch Phys Med Rehabil* 1991; 72:790.
41. Zafonte RD, Demangone DA, Herbison GJ, Ditunno JF: Daily self-care in quadriplegic subjects. *Neurorehabilitation* 1991; 1:17–24.
42. Gresham GE, Labi ML, Dittmar SS, et al: The quadriplegia index of function (QIF): Sensitivity and reliability demonstrated in a study of thirty quadriplegic patients. *Paraplegia* 1986; 24:38–44.
43. Knight P, Huang M, Marino RJ, et al: Evaluating self-care in quadriplegia: Superiority of the Quadriplegia Index of Function over the Functional Index Measure. *J Am Paraplegia Soc* 1992; 15:144.

Special Groups

CHAPTER 92

PEDIATRIC SPINAL CORD INJURY

John G. Piper
Arnold H. Menezes

SYNOPSIS

Traumatic spinal cord injury is a significant cause of morbidity and mortality that carries tremendous costs to our society. While spine injuries are uncommon in the pediatric population, the young age of these patients magnifies the impact of these devastating problems. The pattern of pediatric spinal column and spinal cord injury differs significantly from adults and requires distinct approaches to diagnosis and treatment. The pediatric spine is in a dynamic state of development, differing anatomically as well as biomechanically from the adult spine. This chapter will focus on the distinct nature of pediatric spinal column and spinal cord injury. Specific differences in epidemiology, pattern of injury, diagnosis, treatment, and outcome will be highlighted.

EPIDEMIOLOGY

Spinal column and spinal cord injuries are uncommon in the pediatric population. Pediatric spine injury accounts for only 2.7 to 9.4 percent of all spinal injuries.[22,27,28,32,33,35,56,69] Eighteen to 21 injuries per million population per year occur in the pediatric age group, compared with adults who have from 53 to 68 injuries per million per year.[10,32] Approximately one-half of pediatric patients with spinal column injury also have associated spinal cord injury.[27,28] Also, spinal injuries in the pediatric population have a higher mortality, with death occurring 2.5 times more often than in adults.[27,28] However, it is important to note that many of these reviews may underestimate the true incidence of spinal column and spinal cord injury in the pediatric population. This is mainly related to referral patterns, but also is influenced by the fact that patients at either extreme of neurological deficit—who either die at the scene or have very mild injuries not requiring hospitalization—may not be included.[2,15]

DEVELOPMENTAL ANATOMY AND BIOMECHANICS

Configurations of the vertebrae change dramatically from infancy through early childhood, reaching an adult form by the age of 8 years.[30,51,52,56] Several intrinsic and extrinsic factors of the pediatric spine alter its biomechanics, producing a pattern of spinal column injury that differs from that of adults. On one hand, these may predispose the child to spinal cord and ligamentous injury at certain levels because of immaturity; however, at the same time they act to decrease the overall incidence of spinal column fracture compared with adolescents and adults.[26,30,32,33,52,53,65]

Intrinsic factors that predispose to injury include the wedge shape of vertebral bodies in the infant and childhood spine which are not fully ossified. While this lack of ossification protects against fractures through the vertebral body, the wedge shape allows excessive motion in flexion and extension. When fractures do occur in the pediatric spine, they tend to affect the cartilaginous endplate, especially in areas of active growth.[4] Furthermore, the uncinate processes in childhood are small, and the facets, particularly in the cervical spine, have a more horizontal orientation. Therefore, the facet joints and uncovertebral joints provide less stability. The stabilizing ligaments of the pediatric spine have more laxity compared with the adult spine, and the paraspinous muscles do not reach full maturity until puberty. Extrinsic factors that affect stability of the pediatric spine are largely related to differences of body habitus in the child compared with the adult. The child's head is proportionally larger compared to the body, which increases the forces exerted on the spine and shifts the fulcrum of flexion and extension from the low cervical level to the C2–C3 level.

DISTRIBUTION OF FRACTURES

Changes in these intrinsic and extrinsic factors help explain the varying distribution of fractures which occur in the pediatric population under the age of 8 years compared with older children.[22,28,44,49,50,56] Several series have found that patients under the age of 8 to 10 years tend to have fractures at the craniovertebral junction and subaxial levels down to C5.[26,30,32,33,52,53,65] There is a relative sparing of the lower cervical spine. Thoracolumbar spine fractures also occur, with a peak incidence at T10.[56] After approximately 10 years of age, the spine has reached a mature state, and patients begin to engage in activities similar to the adult population, predisposing them to a similar pattern of fractures. In adults the craniovertebral junction can be affected; however, fractures of the cervical spine more commonly involve the cervicothoracic junction.[26,50,56] Thoracolumbar spine fractures are also common in this group.

ETIOLOGY OF SPINAL COLUMN AND SPINAL CORD INJURY

Motor vehicle accidents are by far the most common cause of spinal cord and spinal column injuries in the pediatric population, representing 20 to 65 percent.[26,30,56,58] Motorcycle accidents are also common in adolescents. However, in the infant and young pediatric age group, pedestrian/auto accidents are particularly common.[32,33] Hadley and coworkers found that children under 9 years of age had an incidence of pedestrian/auto related injuries 10 times greater than children 15 years or older.[26] Another important cause of injuries are falls, representing 15 to 20 percent of the total injuries.[26,30] Some series focusing on early childhood report this as the most the common etiology.[56] Analogous to pedestrian/auto injuries, these are also more common in younger children, being seen two to four times more often than in adolescent and teenage patients. Various sport activities are also common causes of pediatric spinal injury. These account for 10 to 15 percent of spinal column injuries in most series, with some reports approaching 32 percent of cases.[25,32,33,49,50,56] Much less frequent are traumatic birth injuries, accounting for 10 to 15 percent of cases, and penetrating injuries such as gunshot and stab wounds.[32,33,50]

MECHANISMS OF SPINAL COLUMN AND SPINAL CORD INJURY

The basic mechanisms of spinal cord injury are analogous to those in the adult population. These include flexion, compression, distraction, hyperextension, rotation, penetrating injuries, and vascular/ischemic insults.[5,18,43–45,50,52,59,62] Mechanical forces can be exerted in an isolated form; however, they occur more often in combination (i.e., flexion/compression, flexion/dislocation, etc.). Some generalizations can be made about location of spinal column injury and neurological deficits based on the type of forces involved in the injury. Flexion/dislocation injuries often produce devastating neurological deficits related to severe ligamentous disruption and facet dislocations (Fig. 92-1). Flexion/compression injuries produce vertebral body compression fractures, subluxation, and posterior ligamentous disruption. Axial loading forces are associated with burst fractures of the vertebral body, which may produce retropulsion of bone fragments and severe neurological injury. In the pediatric population this most frequently involves the superior endplate adjacent to the intervertebral disk. The neural arches are splayed laterally; however, the ligamentous structures may be relatively spared. Hyperextension forces produce fractures of the facets and the posterior elements. In addition, extension places traction on the anterior longitudinal ligament, producing avulsion fractures of the vertebral body. Flexion, extension, distraction, and rotatory forces are all important at the occipito-atlantal and atlanto-axial articulations. Birth injuries are often caused by excessive traction in hyperextension. Penetrating trauma to the pediatric spine is quite uncommon; however, with the increasing violence in our society, this can be expected to increase. Finally, vascular and ischemic mechanisms have been implicated as the cause of spinal cord injury in patients without radiographic abnormalities.

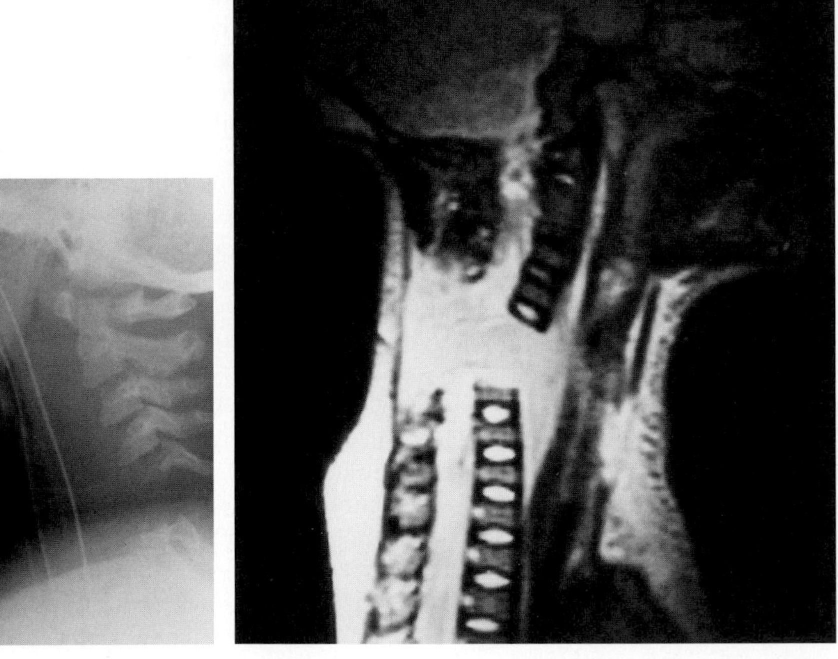

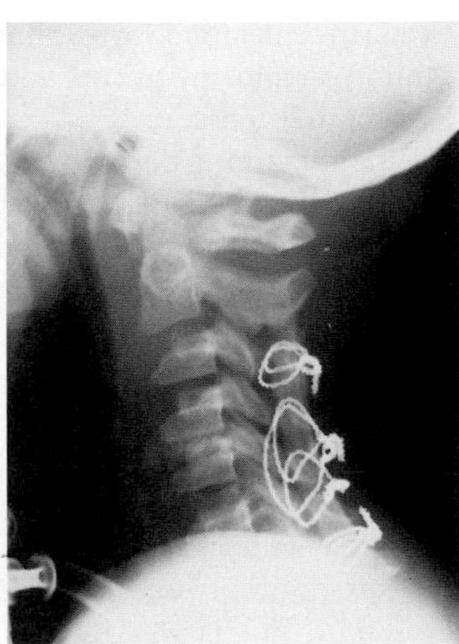

A B C

Figure 92-1. *A*. Lateral cervical radiograph of an eight-year-old child involved in a motor vehicle accident. Severe flexion-distraction injury at C5–C6 is demonstrated, with avulsion of the spine. Note the massive prevertebral space. *B*. Parasagittal T2 weighted MRI of the cervical spine demonstrates the distraction between the proximal and distal segments and a large pseudomeningocele. The avulsion fracture occurred at the vertebral endplate. *C*. Lateral cervical radiograph obtained after reapproximation of the spine and dorsal fusion with rib grafts and sublaminar wire.

CLASSIFICATION OF PEDIATRIC SPINE INJURIES

A convenient classification system for pediatric spine injuries has been developed.[25,26,50] Four specific groups can be identified: those with isolated fractures; those with fractures combined with subluxation; those with subluxation without evidence of fracture; and spinal cord injury without radiographic abnormality (SCIWORA).[50,52] Overall, the most common injuries in pediatric patients are isolated fractures, which occur in 40 to 45 percent of cases. However, these are common only in patients with spinal maturity above the age of 9 years.[25,50] The paucity of fractures before this age is related to the lack of ossification of the vertebral column, which makes it resistant to fracture. The next most common injury is the fracture combined with subluxation, which likewise occurs in adolescent and teenage patients, being rare before spinal maturity. Isolated subluxations are more common in younger children and result from severe ligamentous injury without bony disruption.[50] Finally, spinal cord injury without radiographic abnormalities follows a similar age pattern of isolated subluxation, being two to three times more common before eight years of age.[25,26,50,56] Some generalizations can be made regarding the risk of spinal cord injury with various types of spinal column injury. Osenbach and Hadley have both reviewed large institutional series and demonstrated a two- to threefold higher risk of neurological deficit in patients with subluxation, whether isolated or combined with a fracture.[25,50]

NEUROLOGICAL DEFICITS IN PEDIATRIC SPINAL INJURY

The incidence of neurological deficits from spinal column injury in the pediatric age group varies widely, exceeding 50 percent in some series.[25,50,56] These neurological deficits can be complete or incomplete, with incomplete injuries presenting as several varying syndromes. Complete injury indicates total loss of motor and sensory function below the level of the injury. Kewalramani and coworkers and Burke found a strong association between pediatric spine injury and complete neurological deficits with 69 to 95 percent of their patients having complete deficits, respectively.[16,32,33] However, the incidence of complete injuries reported by Anderson and coworkers and Ruge and associates were less than 20 percent.[3,56]

The remaining patients in all of these series had varying types of incomplete injuries. The anterior cord syndrome describes injury to the anterior and lateral funiculi, with loss of motor function as well as pain and temperature sensation. Posterior column functions are preserved. Common causes of anterior cord syndrome include traumatic disk herniation, retropulsed bone fragments, and such vascular injuries as anterior spinal artery infarction. The central cord syndrome is very common with all types of spinal column injury, given the susceptibility of the central gray matter to injury. However, this is an especially common pattern in spinal cord injury without radiographic abnormality (SCIWORA).[49,50,56] Central cord syndrome is easily recognized in cervical spine injuries, where injury to the central gray matter produces weakness of the upper extremities with relative sparing of white matter destined for the lower extremities. Often these patients will show improvement in neurological function with follow-up. Finally, the Brown-Séquard syndrome may be seen in spinal column injury; however, it rarely appears in a pure form. This syndrome describes hemisection or hemi-injury to the spinal cord, affecting motor and dorsal column function ipsilateral to the lesion and pain and temperature sensation contralateral to the lesion. Penetrating injuries such as stab wounds or gunshot wounds are more strongly associated with this neurological pattern.

RADIOGRAPHIC AND OTHER IMAGING TECHNIQUES

The evaluation of a potential pediatric spine injury presents numerous problems, ranging from difficulty obtaining adequate imaging studies to poor detection of ligamentous injuries with static radiographs. Therefore, a multimodality imaging approach has been adopted to minimize the risk of an overlooked injury. The evaluation begins with cervical, thoracic, and lumbar spine radiographs in the frontal and lateral planes. Cervical spine evaluation also includes oblique x-rays, an open-mouth odontoid view, as well as swimmer's views when needed. A complete spine evaluation is required, since 16 percent of patients with spine injury will have multiple levels of involvement.[25,26] Of obvious importance is the open-mouth view for evaluation of the craniovertebral junction, where injuries commonly occur in this age group. While lower cervical spine injuries are less common, they still occur, and thorough evaluation of the cervicothoracic junction is required, with visualization down to the upper thoracic vertebrae. Given the high incidence of ligamentous injury, flexion/extension films should be considered with suspected spinal injury. Areas of suspicion can be further evaluated by computed tomography (CT) to define the presence of fractures, which often are difficult to visualize on plain films, particularly when they involve the facets or posterior elements. Tomograms or CT reconstructions are also helpful for detecting fractures, assessing facet joint integrity, and determining alignment.[61] However, alignment can be difficult to assess on CT reconstructions if movement has occurred between images. For evaluation of the spinal cord, myelogram with follow-up CT scan has been used extensively in the past. However, with the advent of MRI, clear delineation of the spinal cord and subarachnoid space is possible. Traumatic epidural hematomas, traumatic disk herniation, and ligamentous injury are also easily documented.[49,50,56] Therefore, MRI has replaced myelographic techniques at our institution unless otherwise contraindicated. MRI has proved particularly valuable in evaluating the craniovertebral junction in occipito-atlantal (O-A) dislocation, which will be discussed later.

MANAGEMENT OF PEDIATRIC SPINE INJURY

In many respects the acute management of pediatric patients with spinal injuries parallels that in adult patients. Preservation of blood pressure within the normal range as well as administration of oxygen may help limit ischemic injury.[59] If blood pressure cannot be maintained with fluid administration, dopamine or Neo-Synephrine may facilitate maintenance of a normal blood pressure. However, there are several differences between the management of adult and pediatric spine injuries that warrant discussion. Immediate immobilization in a collar and backboard with universal spine precautions should be followed in both groups.[25,26,50] However, selecting the right type of immobilization is important in the pediatric age group. Herzenberg and coworkers reported that the combination of adult backboards and the relatively large size of the child's head places the cervical spine in flexion, which can be undesirable when there is a possible injury.[29] Therefore, they recommend either the use of specialized pediatric backboard equipment for transportation or modification of adult boards to accommodate the pediatric patient.

Pharmacological intervention in spinal cord injury is being explored. Earlier reports of the use of steroid intervention were equivocal[10,11]; however, a recent national prospective randomized trial of methylprednisolone has demonstrated benefit, when given within 8 hours of injury, and therefore should be considered in all patients with spinal cord injury.[12,13] A loading dose of methylprednisolone of 30 mg/kg is given in the first h, followed by infusion of 5.4 mg/kg/h for 23 h. Evaluation of the treatment in experimental models of spinal cord injury using calcium channel blockers, iron chelators, free radical scavengers, and antagonists of excitatory amino acids is progressing. While these interventions hold promise, they have not yet been shown to be of clinical value.

REDUCTION OF SPINAL COLUMN INJURY

Once the patient sustaining a spine injury has been stabilized and baseline diagnostic tests performed, options for reduction of fractures or subluxations can be entertained. However, given the relative small size of pediatric patients and the high incidence of ligamentous injury, extreme caution must be used if traction is undertaken.[43,44,51,60] The inappropriate use of traction may produce overdistraction and progressive neurological dysfunction. This has been clearly shown in longitudinal occipito-atlantal dislocations (Type II).[44,60] When a severe cervical ligamentous injury is suspected, consideration can be given to manual positioning under fluoroscopic guidance with the patient in a halo ring.[44,51] This will frequently succeed in reducing injuries in the very young, minimizing the risk of overdistraction (e.g., occipito-atlantal dislocations). In older pediatric patients or in patients who fail to reduce with manual positioning under radiographic guidance, cervical traction can be considered. After approximately the age of 1 year, halo rings or crowns can be applied with caution. MRI-compatible devices can facilitate further spine evaluations. Crown halo rings applied in children from 1 to 4 years of age should utilize at least 6 to 8 pins, with each pin not exceeding 2 in/lbs. of torque; however, caution is needed because skull perforation can occur.[51] Traction is then implemented, but should not initially exceed 1 to 2 lb in patients under 2 years. Frequent films should be obtained to exclude overdistraction, and extreme care must be exercised when adding further weight. Fractures of the thoracic and lumbar spine are treated much as in adults.

EXTERNAL STABILIZATION

The majority of pediatric patients sustaining a spinal column injury with or without associated spinal cord injury can be managed by some kind of external stabilization.[16,25,26,48,50] Only 16 to 27 percent of the pediatric spine injuries ultimately require surgical intervention.[25,56] The simplest cervical orthosis used is the Philadelphia cervical collar or similar hard collars. These can be used safely in mild ligamentous injuries or stable fractures for added support; however, they are insufficient to treat unstable injuries because they limit cervical spine mobility by only 29 to 66 percent.[67] Yale braces, SOMI braces, four-poster braces, or other similar orthoses offer an intermediate level of immobilization of the craniovertebral junction and may offer superior immobilization of the lower cervical spine.[67] These are difficult to fit in the young children and also may lead to skin breakdown and dental malocclusion with long-term use. Halo vests offer the greatest immobilization of the craniovertebral junction, and thus are important devices in the conservative management of pediatric spinal column injuries.[67] This is particularly true since the craniovertebral junction and upper cervical spine are a common site of injury in patients under the age of 10. These can also be used effectively in lower cervical spine injuries. As previously mentioned, halo devices for children aged 4 years or younger utilize 6 to 8 pins, each with less than 2 in./lb of torque. This evenly distributes the pressure throughout the circumference of the skull. Care should be taken to avoid sutures in infants. If any question exists about adequate calvarial thickness, CT scans can clearly define skull thickness prior to application of this device. In patients who are not candidates for halo vests, custom thermoplastic vests combined with collars have been shown to immobilize the cervical spine and craniovertebral junction nearly as efficiently as the halo apparatus. Thoracolumbosacral orthoses can be used in thoracolumbar spine fractures in children after an initial period of recumbency of 6 weeks' duration. These orthoses may help minimize the risk and slow progression of spinal deformities, which unfortunately are quite common in pediatric patients with neurological dysfunction. One final caution: no matter what level of the child's spine is affected or what orthosis is implemented, numerous radiographs should be obtained while slowly mobilizing the patient from recumbency to assure that adequate immobilization is being provided and that slumping into the orthosis has not occurred. If the orthosis fails to maintain alignment, operative intervention should be considered.

SURGICAL TREATMENT

Most pediatric spinal injuries are successfully managed by reduction followed by external stabilization; however, in specific instances surgical intervention is either preferable or required[26,50] (Fig. 95-1). Traditional indications for acute surgical intervention for adult patients also apply in the pediatric age group. Patients with a progressive neurological deficit resulting from an unstable fracture or dislocation will benefit from surgical intervention. Furthermore, surgery should be considered in instances where adequate reduction of a fracture is not possible with traction, or if external stabilization proves to be insufficient. Further indications include spinal epidural hematomas and traumatic disk herniations. Patients who have significant compression of the neural elements by bony fragments but otherwise have a partial but stable neurological deficit could be considered for surgical decompression.[44,51,63] While some may disagree with this approach, it is felt that removal of persistent compressive pathology may foster neurological improvement. There is no clear evidence to suggest that acute surgical intervention will benefit those with complete spinal cord lesions.[26,33] In the authors' own experience of 93 traumatic spinal cord injuries in pediatric patients, acute surgical intervention did not alter the degree or rate of neurological recovery compared with conservative management.[50] Gunshot wounds or other open injuries may require debridement and closure of cerebrospinal fluid leaks, but, as with closed injuries, surgery will not improve neurological outcome in those with complete deficits. Finally, posttraumatic spinal deformity or persistent instability despite an adequate period of external immobilization are delayed indications for operative intervention.

Surgical intervention may involve decompression of the neural elements as well as stabilization and fusion. The operative approach undertaken is dictated by the location of compression, degree of instability, and the integrity of various bony and ligamentous structures.[24,25,44,50,65] Most cervical spine injuries can be approached posteriorly, allowing for both decompression and fusion; however, certain instances require an anterior approach, such as traumatic cervical disk herniations or ventral compression from a severely comminuted vertebral body fracture with retropulsed bone. Fusion procedures performed in children should be modified to preserve the greatest mobility and growth potential. Therefore, the fusion should be limited to the vertebrae immediately around the unstable segments whenever possible. Fusion constructs used in adults, such as rib and iliac crest, may not always be appropriate in children. In neonates, ribs are often insubstantial, precluding their use. In older children, fractured posterior elements or developmental deficiency may preclude certain types of posterior fusion procedures. Given the small spinal canal in toddlers and young children, passage of sublaminar wires may be contraindicated. In such cases, an onlay bone graft may be adequate to achieve bony fusion when combined with postoperative immobilization in a halo vest. A final note: wires should never be used alone. They do not provide adequate stability in the absence of bony fusion.

While cervical spine injuries represent the largest group of pediatric spinal injuries, thoracolumbar spine fractures do occur. Most often these fractures occur at the thoracolumbar junction. The forces involved are severe flexion and compression, which produce extreme instability commonly associated with neurological deficits. Given the constraints that exist for conservative management, early operative intervention with internal reduction and stabilization combined with fusion often is preferred. Early mobilization and rehabilitation are also facilitated by this approach. A variety of internal fixation systems are marketed for spinal stabilization. Selection of a system depends on a variety of factors, such as the level of injury, the need for distraction, and location of neural element compression.

SPECIFIC INJURIES

Occipito-Atlantal Dislocations

Occipito-atlantal dislocations were once considered rare and nearly always fatal.[15,54,60] Reports of occasional survivors have recommended dorsal occipito-cervical fusions to overcome the tremendous instability associated with these injuries.[60] However, since the advent of MRI, previously overlooked cases of occipito-atlantal dislocation with mild-to-moderate neurological deficits have been identified, prompting us to reevaluate their management.

On plain radiographs occipito-atlantal dislocations

can be identified by various techniques[54,60]; however, the most widely accepted technique is the Powers' ratio.[54] This is calculated by taking the distance between the basion to the posterior arch of C1 and dividing it by the distance between the opisthion and the anterior arch of C1. Under normal circumstances this ratio averages 0.77, with ratios greater than 1 being pathological. However, in our personal series this was diagnostic in only 39 percent of cases. Inaccurate results occur with posterior dislocations as well as with associated injuries of the craniovertebral junction. Furthermore, longitudinal dislocations may also yield false-negatives. We have therefore relied on MRI as the diagnostic gold standard of occipito-atlantal dislocations. MRI can demonstrate clival epidural hematomas, ligamentous injury and soft tissue swelling, and cervicomedullary junction compression and injury.

Most patients with occipito-atlantal dislocation have severe ligamentous injury and require occipito-cervical fusion.[60] This is particularly true of patients with longitudinal dislocations, posterior dislocations, or if the injury is initially unrecognized with progression to chronic instability. However, select patients have been treated with halo vests following reduction. Selection criteria include the acute presentation of an anterior dislocation (without *any* longitudinal component) occurring in a pediatric or young adult patient with only a mild-to-moderate deficit. In this select group, a trial of halo immobilization is warranted, with fusion reserved for those who fail external immobilization or if the halo is adequate to maintain alignment.

Atlanto-axial Instability

Instability of the atlanto-axial complex can present in many forms. Anterior or posterior subluxations are frequently associated with odontoid fractures; however, instability can develop from injury to the transverse and other associated ligaments[43,45] (Fig. 92-2). Unlike adult patients, where the predental space should not exceed 3 mm, pediatric patients may have predental spaces up to 5 mm under normal circumstances. If this dimension exceeds 5 mm, injury to the transverse ligament is suspected.[43,66] The integrity of the transverse ligament is important in treating anterior and posterior atlanto-axial instability, since patients with injury to the transverse ligament often require dorsal cervical fusion, whereas those with an intact transverse ligament are treated successfully with halo immobilization.[45]

A second group of atlanto-axial injuries are the rotatory luxations where the skull and C1 are rotated on C2 with the dens serving as the axis of rotation (Fig. 92-3). This region is difficult to visualize on plain radiographs, and CT of the craniovertebral junction with reconstructions often will be required to clearly define rotation of the atlas on the axis.[45] Fielding and colleagues classified atlanto-axial rotatory luxations depending on the integrity of the transverse ligament and other supporting ligamentous structures.[21] With an intact transverse ligament, rotation will not exceed 35°, and these injuries are easily realigned with traction followed by halo immobilization. However, when the transverse ligament is disrupted, rotation can exceed 40°, resulting in facet interlock, which requires dorsal cervical fusion.[43,45]

Odontoid Fractures of Childhood

Spine fractures are uncommon in young children, but when they occur they often affect the odontoid process.[20,24,57,61] Odontoid fractures of infancy and early childhood differ from adult odontoid injuries in that the "fracture" typically occurs through the neurocentral synchondrosis and is an avulsion (Fig. 92-4). Both flexion and extension injury can produce odontoid fractures. Since open-mouth odontoid views are difficult to obtain in children, CT can be quite helpful.[61] Untreated or inadequately treated injuries also may lead to os odontoideum formation with chronic instability. There is great controversy over operative and nonoperative treatment of adult odontoid fractures, particularly Type II fractures. However, pediatric odontoid fractures are easily treated with halo vests, achieving good rates of union.[45,61]

Hangman's Fractures of Childhood

Hangman's fracture describes a bipedicular fracture of the axis vertebra that is uncommon in childhood.[45,64] This injury typically is produced by hyperextension in which further movement of the C2 body is prevented by the inferior facets, resulting in a fracture in the weakest area, the pars interarticularis. After the injury, the body of C2 and C1 often will sublux anteriorly. Plain radiographs and CT are both useful for diagnosis, and treatment consists of halo immobilization after alignment is reestablished.[45,64]

SPINAL CORD INJURY WITHOUT RADIOGRAPHIC ABNORMALITY

Reports of spinal cord injury without visible fracture or dislocation appeared in the literature as early as 1907.[1,38] Pang and Wilberger first coined the term "spinal

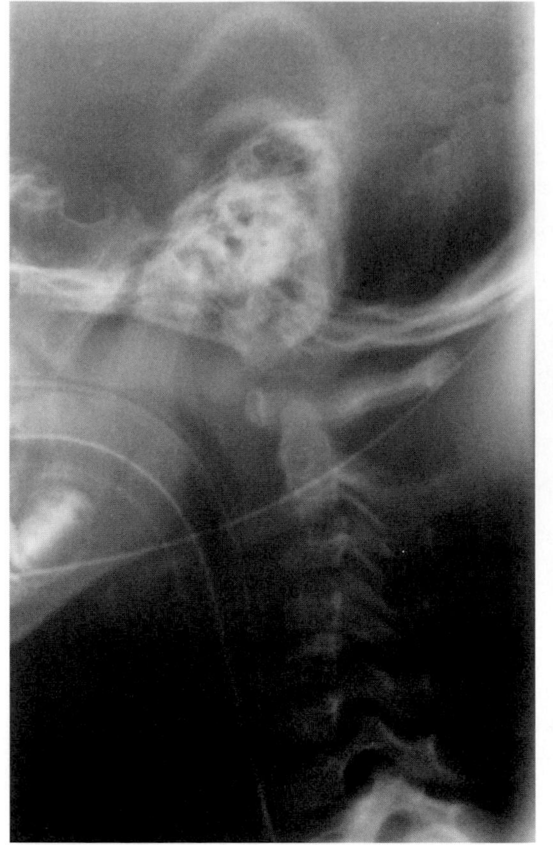

A

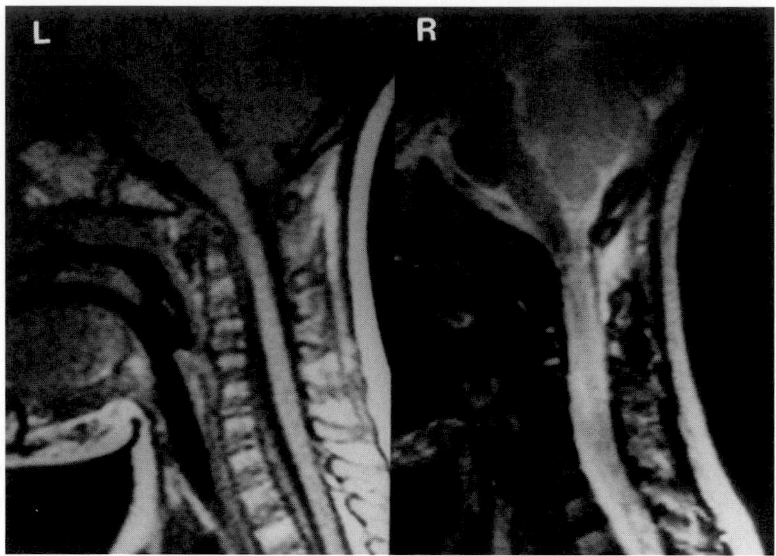

B

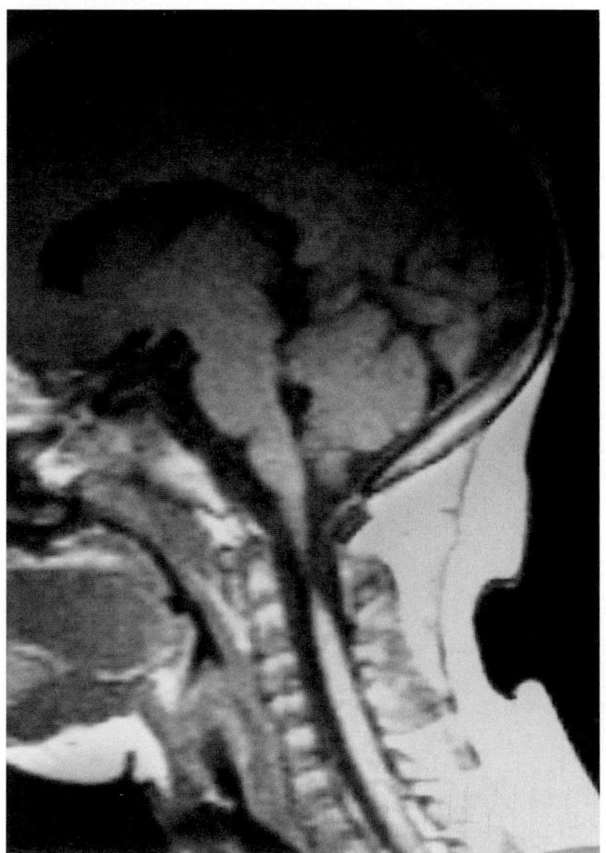

C

Figure 92-2. *A.* Lateral cervical radiograph obtained in a four-year-old motor vehicle accident victim showing a markedly enlarged prevertebral space. The occipital condyles are bare and there is widening of the dorsal atlanto-axial space. *B.* Composite of midsagittal craniovertebral junction MRI in the T1 (left) and T2 (right) weighted modes performed within one day of injury. Note the dorsal location of the odontoid tip, edema in the dorsal atlanto-axial region, and high signal intensity in the cervicomedullary junction. *C.* Midsagittal T1 weighted MRI of the head and neck made one year after injury. Note the atrophy of the spinal cord at the cervicomedullary junction.

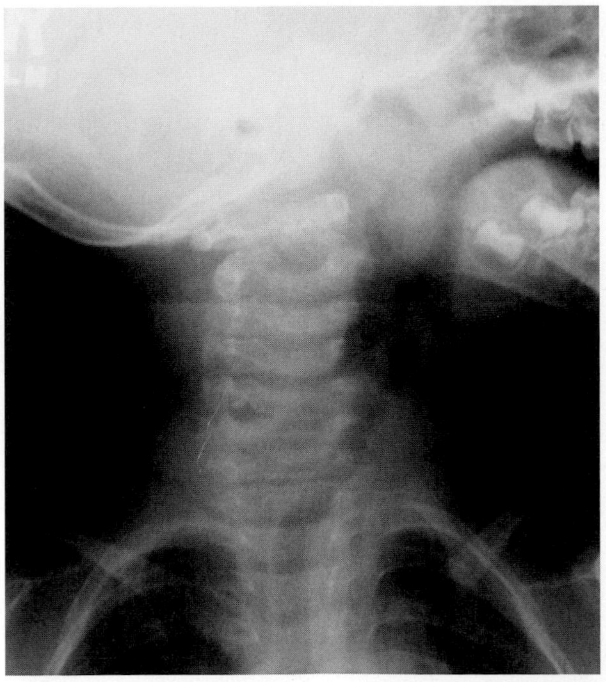

A

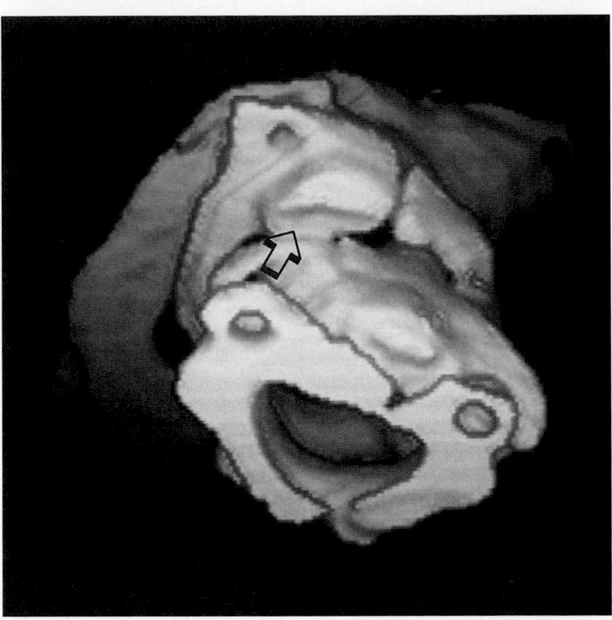

B

Figure 92-3. *A.* Plain radiograph (AP) of a child who sustained an atlanto-axial rotatory luxation. Note the total rotation of the head to a lateral position. *B.* Follow-up CT of the cervical spine with 3-D reconstruction reveals facet interlocking (arrow) from rotation in excess of 40°.

cord injury without radiographic abnormality" or SCIWORA to describe these injuries.[52] Compared with adults, SCIWORA is quite common in pediatric age groups. Hadley and coworkers reported that 33 percent of pediatric spine injuries with deficit were attributable to SCIWORA.[25,26] However, other reports vary widely, ranging from 5 to 70 percent of pediatric spinal injuries, depending on the series.[25,26,49,50,56] The neurological deficit can come on rapidly, or as late as 54 hours.[1,49,50,52,62] Often the neurological pictures resemble a central cervical cord syndrome.[16,18,62]

Multiple etiological factors have been implicated in SCIWORA. Early theories implicated laxity of the ligaments, which allowed transient subluxation and subsequently recoil to establish normal alignment. This transient subluxation was felt to produce the neurological deficit seen in this disorder (flexion recoil theory).[38,44] Hyperextension also has been implicated as a cause of neurological deficit by producing buckling of the ligamentum flavum. Both of these factors can produce up to 50 percent canal narrowing.[52] SCIWORA also may represent an ischemic injury or infarction of the spinal cord.[1,18,49,52] Typically SCIWORA will produce a pattern consistent with central cord syndrome, and preferentially affects the cervical spine.[5,9] Flexion injuries have been correlated with upper cervical spine deficits whereas extension injuries tend to affect the lower cervical spine.[49,52] Finally, cases of pediatric SCIWORA appear to be associated with more severe deficit than in adults.[50,53] The incidence of SCIWORA appears to be decreasing concurrent with the advent of MRI, which can detect occult fractures, ligamentous injury, traumatic disk herniations, and epidural hematomas that previously may have been overlooked.

COMPLICATIONS FROM PEDIATRIC SPINAL INJURY

Aggressive surgical and medical management of spinal column and spinal cord injury combined with aggressive rehabilitation has led to an increased number of children surviving these devastating injuries. Many common problems seen in pediatric patients with paraplegia or

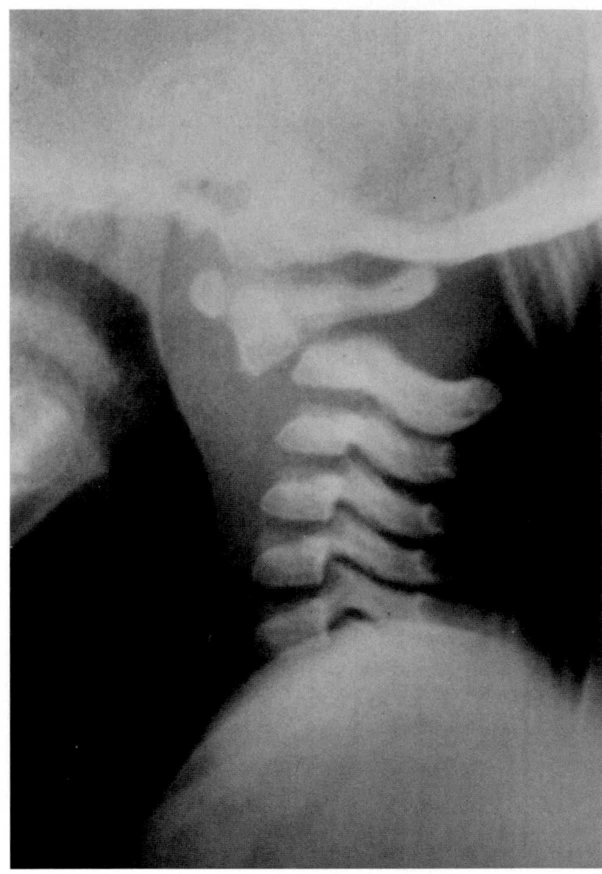

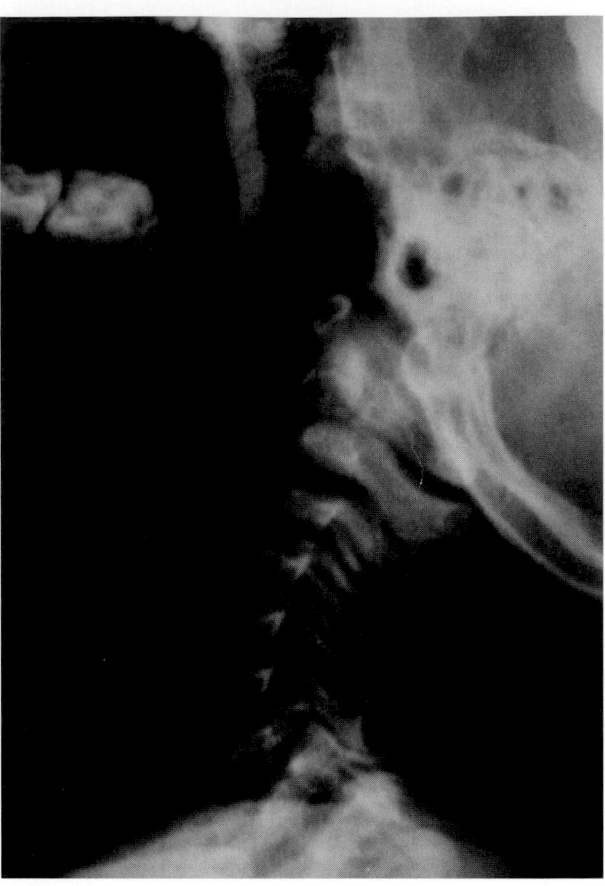

A B

Figure 92-4. *A.* Lateral cervical spine radiograph in a three-year-old following a motor vehicle accident. Note the avulsion odontoid fracture with severe anterior atlanto-axial dislocation. *B.* Lateral cervical radiograph made three months after halo immobilization. There is satisfactory realignment with fracture healing.

quadriplegia parallel those seen in adults, including genitourinary tract infections, pneumonia, decubitus ulcers, and myositis ossificans.

Posttraumatic spinal deformity can occur at any age; however, it appears to develop much more frequently in early childhood than in adolescents or adults. Several factors can be implicated to account for this high frequency. With any age group, postural muscles supporting the trunk may be paralyzed, resulting in asymmetric forces being exerted on the developing spinal column, particularly with respect to muscles of rotation.[5,55] More specific to early childhood are injuries to the growth plates of the spine. Analogous to long bone injuries, epiphyseal damage interferes with growth, and this effect frequently is asymmetrical.[4,55] Together these factors contribute to the high rate of scoliosis, kyphosis, and lordosis following spinal cord injuries in children, being of greatest importance during phases of rapid growth.[4,55]

Severe deformities may predispose to the development of further medical complications. Decubitus ulcers may form from abnormal weight-bearing on the ischial tuberosities. Also if the curve exceeds 60°, cardiopulmonary function may be compromised. Progressive neurological deficit is also possible.

The incidence of progressive spinal deformity has been identified in 84 to 100 percent in children sustaining spinal cord injury.[6,17,36,40] Factors that predispose to the development of posttraumatic spinal deformity include young age at the time of injury, severity of neurological deficit, level of injury, and the presence of spasticity.[6,9,14,34,36,39,46,68] Laminectomy appears to predispose to development of spinal deformity.[39] Because of the high rate of spinal deformity in pediatric spinal cord injuries, several authors have recommended operative intervention with fusion. A more prudent method of treatment involves bracing of the thoracolumbar spine when curves exceed 20° to 30°. Surgical intervention and fusion should await spinal maturity whenever possible. Laminectomies should be avoided in the preadolescent group, if possible.[40,44]

PROGNOSIS

Reports of outcome following spinal cord injury in pediatric patients are mixed. Many children with spinal cord injuries die at the scene or soon after presentation for medical care.[2,15,32,33] Frequently these patients have high cervical injuries. However, children who survive spinal cord injury and are discharged have a longer five-year survival than seen in other age groups.[7,32,33,37,41,47] The prognosis for recovery of neurological function also varies substantially. Some authors feel that children have an improved prognosis, perhaps from greater "plasticity" of the CNS; however, others feel that their outcome is relatively poor.[16,33,50] What seems clear from all studies, though, is that the best predictor of good outcome is the initial neurological status of the patient. Those with complete injuries have a dismal outlook for useful neurological recovery.[19,25,26,41,50]

CONCLUSION

Because the pediatric spine is in a process of rapid development below the age of 8 to 9 years, there are distinct differences in the patterns of spinal cord and spinal column injuries seen in infancy and early childhood compared with older children and adults. Young children tend to have injuries affecting the craniovertebral junction and upper cervical spine. Adolescent and teenage patients have patterns of injury that resemble adults, affecting the cervicothoracic and thoracolumbar junctions. Some features of the spine in early childhood offer protection, such as resistance to fractures; however, ligamentous laxity and incomplete development of bony structures lead to greater risk of subluxation.

Although many pediatric patients succumb to their injuries at the scene, improvements in emergency medical services and treatment, combined with the recognition of important differences between pediatric and adult spinal columns and cord injuries has improved survival. Most injuries can be managed nonoperatively with halo immobilization or other orthoses. Furthermore, pharmacological agents such as methylprednisolone have shown promise in improving neurological outcome. Finally, care of these children does not end with their discharge from the hospital. Aggressive follow-up is required to diagnose early any possible complicating factors such as progressive spinal deformity.

REFERENCES

1. Ahmann PA, Smith SA, Schwartz JF, Clark DB: Spinal cord infarction due to minor trauma in children. *Neurology* 1975; 25:301–307.
2. Alker GJ, Oh YS, Leslie EV: High cervical spine and craniocervical junction injuries in fatal traffic accidents: A radiological study. *Ortho Clin North Am* 1978; 9:1003–1010.
3. Anderson JM, Schutt AH: Spinal injury in children: A review of 156 cases seen from 1956 through 1978. *Mayo Clin Proc* 1980; 55:499–504.
4. Aufdermaur M: Spinal injuries in juveniles: Necropsy findings in twleve cases. *J Bone Joint Surg* 1974; 56B:513–519.
5. Babcock JL: Spinal injuries in children. *Pediatr Clin North Am* 1975; 22:487–500.
6. Banniza VB, Paeslack UK: Scoliotic growth in children with acquired paraplegia. *Paraplegia* 1974; 11:277–284.
7. Banta JV: Rehabilitation of pediatric spinal cord injury: The Newington Children's Hospital experience: *Conn Med* 1984; 48:14–18.
8. Barnett HJM, Bottrell EH, Jouse AT, et al: Progressive myelopathy as a sequel to traumatic paraplegia. *Brain* 1966; 89:159–174.
9. Bedbrook GM: Correction of scoliosis due to paraplegia sustained in pediatric age group. *Paraplegia* 1977–78; 15:90–96.
10. Bracken MG, Freeman DH Jr, Hellenbrand K: Incidence of acute traumatic hospitalized spinal cord injury in the United States, 1970–1977. *Am J Epidemiol* 1981; 113:615–622.
11. Bracken MG, Shepard MJ, Hellenbrand KA, et al: Methylprednisolone and neurological function 1 year after spinal cord injury: Results of the National Acute Spinal Cord Injury Study. *J Neurosurg* 1985; 63:704–713.
12. Bracken MB, Shepard MJ, Collins WF, et al: A randomized, controlled trial of methylprednisolone or naloxone in the treatment of acute spinal-cord injury: Results of the second National Acute Spinal Cord Injury Study. *N Engl J Med* 1990; 322:1405–1411.
13. Bracken MB, Shepard MJ, Collins WF, et al: Methylprednisolone or naloxone treatment after acute spinal cord injury: 1-year follow-up data. *J Neurosurg* 1992; 76:23–31.
14. Bradford DS: Deformities of the thoracic and lumbar spine secondary to spinal injury, in Bradford DS, Lonstein JE, Moe JH, et al (eds): *Moe's Textbook of Scoliosis and Other Spinal Deformities,* (2d ed). Philadelphia: Saunders, 1987: 435–463.
15. Bucholz RW, Burkhead WF: The pathological anatomy of fatal atlanto-occipital dislocations. *J Bone Joint Surg* 1979; 61A:248.
16. Burke DC: Traumatic spinal paralysis in children. *Paraplegia* 1974; 11:268–276.

17. Campbell J, Bonnett C: Spinal cord injury in children. *Clin Orthop* 1975; 112:114–123.
18. Choi JU, Hoffman HJ, Hendrick EB, et al: Traumatic infarction of the spinal cord in children. *J Neurosurg* 1986; 65:608–610.
19. Ducker TB, Lucas J, Wallace CA: Recovery from spinal cord injury. *Clin Neurosurg* 1983; 30:495–513.
20. Ewald FC: Fracture of the odontoid process in a seventeen-month-old infant treated with a Halo. *J Bone Joint Surg* 1971; 53A:1636–1640.
21. Fielding JW, Hawkins RJ, Hensinger RN, Francis WR: Atlantoaxial rotary deformities. *Orthop Clin North Am* 1978; 9:955–967.
22. Fielding JW: Cervical spine injuries in children, in Sherk HH, Dunn EJ, Eismont FJ, et al (eds): *The Cervical Spine.* Philadelphia: JB Lippincott, 1983: 268–281.
23. Gabriel KR, Crawford AH: Identification of acute posttraumatic spinal cord cyst by magnetic resonance imaging: A case report and review of the literature. *J Pediatr Orthop* 1988; 8:710–714.
24. Gaufin LM, Goodman SJ: Cervical spine injuries in infants: Problems in management. *J Neurosurg* 1975; 42:179–184.
25. Hadley MN: Pediatric spine injuries, in Camins MD and O'Leary PF (eds): *Disorders of the Cervical Spine.* Baltimore: Williams & Wilkins, 1992: 311–316.
26. Hadley MN, Zabramski JM, Browner CM, et al: Pediatric spinal trauma: Review of 122 cases of spinal cord and vertebral column injuries. *J Neurosurg* 1988; 68:18–24.
27. Hamilton MG, Myles ST: Pediatric spinal injury: Review of 174 hospital admissions. *J Neurosurg* 1992; 77:700–704.
28. Hamilton MG, Myles ST: Pediatric spinal injury: Review of 61 deaths. *J Neurosurg* 1992; 77:705–708.
29. Herzenberg JE, Hensinger RN, Dedrick DK, Phillips WA: Emergency transport and positioning of young children with cervical spine injuries: The standard backboard may be hazardous (abstract). *J Bone Joint Surg* 1989; 71B:347.
30. Hill SA, Miller CA, Kosnik EJ, Hunt WE: Pediatric neck injuries. A clinical study. *J Neurosurg* 1984; 60:700–706.
31. Kao CC, Chang LW, Bloodworth JR: The mechanism of spinal cord cavitation following spinal cord transection. *J Neurosurg* 1977; 46:745–755.
32. Kewalramani LS, Kraus JF, Sterling HM: Acute spinal-cord lesions in a pediatric population: Epidemiological and clinical features. *Paraplegia* 1980; 18:206–219.
33. Kewalramani LS, Tori JA: Spinal cord trauma in children: Neurological patterns, radiologic features, and pathomechanics of injury. *Spine* 1980; 5:11–18.
34. Kilfoyle RM, Foley JJ, Norton PL: Spine and pelvic deformity in childhood and adolescent paraplegia: A study of 104 cases. *J Bone Joint Surg* 1965; 47A:659–682.
35. Kraus JF: Epidemiological aspects of acute spinal cord injury: A review of incidence, prevalence, causes, and outcomes, in Becker DP, Povlishock JT (eds): *Central Nervous System Trauma Status Report.* Bethesda MD: National Institute of Neurological and Communicative Disorders and Stroke, National Institutes of Health, 1985: 313–322.
36. Lancourt JE, Dickson JH, Carter RE: Paralytic spinal deformity following traumatic spinal-cord injury in children and adolescents. *J Bone Joint Surg* 1981; 63A:47–53.
37. Letts M, Kaylor D, Gouw G: A biomechanical analysis of halo fixation in children. *J Bone Joint Surg* 1988; 70B:277–279.
38. Lloyd S: Fracture dislocation of the spine. *Med Rec* 1907; 71:465–470.
39. Lonstein JE: Post-laminectomy spine deformity, in Bradford DDS, Lonstein JE, Moe JH, et al (eds): *Moe's Textbook of Scoliosis and Other Spinal Deformities,* (2d ed). Philadelphia: WB Saunders, 1987: 271–305.
40. Mayfield JK, Erkkila JC, Winter RB: Spine deformity subsequent to acquired childhood spinal cord injury. *Am Acad Orthop Surgeons* 1979; 3:281–282.
41. Maynard FM, Reynolds GG, Fountain S, et al: Neurological prognosis after traumatic quadriplegia: Three-year experience of California regional Spinal Cord Injury Care System. *J Neurosurg* 1979; 50:611–616.
42. McComas DF, Frost JL, Schochet SS: Posttraumatic syringomyelia with paroxysmal episodes of unconsciousness. *Arch Neurol* 1983; 40:322–324.
43. Menezes AH: Traumatic lesions of the craniovertebral junction, in VanGilder JC, Menezes AH, Dolan K (eds): *Textbook of Craniovertebral Junction Abnormalities.* Mt. Kisco NY: Futura, 1987.
44. Menezes AH, Godersky JC, Smoker WRK: Spinal cord injury, in McLaurin RL, Schutt L, Venes JL, Epstein F (eds): *Pediatric Neurosurgery: Surgery of the Developing Nervous System,* (2d ed). Philadelphia: WB Saunders, 1989: 298–317.
45. Menezes AH, Muhonen MG: Management of occipitocervical instability, in Cooper PR (ed): *Management of Post-traumatic Spine Instability.* Park Ridge IL: AANS, 1990: 65–76.
46. Menezes AH, Smoker WRK, Dyste GH: Syringomyelia, Chiari malformations, and hydromyelia, in Youmans JR (ed): *Neurological Surgery,* (3d ed). Philadelphia: WB Saunders, 1990: 1454–1455.
47. Mesard L, Carmody A, Mannarino E, Ruge D: Survival after spinal cord trauma. A life table analysis. *Arch Neurol* 1978; 35:78–83.
48. Mubarak SJ, Camp JF, Vuletich W, et al: Halo application in the infant. *J Pediatr Orthop* 1989; 9:612–614.
49. Osenbach RK, Menezes AH: Spinal cord injury without radiographic abnormality (SCIWORA) in children. *Pediatr Neurosci* 1989; 15:168–175.
50. Osenbach RK, Menezes AH: Pediatric spinal cord and vertebral column injury. *Neurosurgery* 1992; 30:385–390.
51. Pang D, Hanley EN: Special problems of spinal stabilization in children, in Cooper PR (ed): *Management of Post-traumatic Spinal Instability.* Park Ridge IL: AANS, 1990: 181–206.
52. Pang D, Wilberger JE Jr: Spinal cord injury without radiographic abnormality in children. *J Neurosurg* 1982; 57:114–129.
53. Papavasiliou V: Traumatic subluxation of the cervical spine during childhood. *Orthop Clin North Am* 1978; 9:945–954.
54. Powers B, Miller MD, Kramer RS, et al: Traumatic ante-

rior atlanto-occipital dislocation. *Neurosurgery* 1979; 4:12–17.
55. Roaf R: Scoliosis secondary to paraplegia. *Paraplegia* 1970; 8:42–47.
56. Ruge JR, Sinson GP, McLone DG, Cerullo LJ: Pediatric spinal injury: The very young. *J Neurosurg* 1988; 68:25–30.
57. Savader SJ, Martinez C, Murtaugh F: Odontoid fracture in a nine-month-old infant. *Surg Neurol* 1985; 24:529–532.
58. Shannon N, Symon L, Logue A, et al: Clinical features, investigation and treatment of post-traumatic syringomyelia. *J Neurol Neurosurg Psychiatry* 1981; 44:35–42.
59. Tator CH, Fehlings MG: Review of the secondary injury theory of acute spinal cord trauma with emphasis on vascular mechanisms. *J Neurosurg* 1991; 75:15–26.
60. Traynelis VC, Marano GD, Dunker RO, Kaufman HH: Traumatic atlanto-occipital dislocation. *J Neurosurg* 1986; 65:863–870.
61. Vining DJ, Benzel EC, Orrison W: Childhood odontoid fractures evaluated with computerized tomography. *J Neurosurg* 1992; 77:795–798.
62. Walsh JW, Stevens DB, Young AB: Traumatic paraplegia in children without contiguous spinal fracture or dislocation. *Neurosurgery* 1983; 12:439–445.
63. Weinshel SS, Maiman DJ, Baek P, Scales L: Neurologic recovery in quadriplegia following operative treatment. *J Spinal Disord* 1990; 3:244–249.
64. Weiss MH, Kaufman B: Hangman's fracture in an infant. *Am J Dis Child* 1973; 126:268–269.
65. Wickboldt J, Sorensen N: Anterior cervical fusion after traumatic dislocation of the cervical spine in childhood and adolescence. *Childs Brain* 1978; 4:120–128.
66. Wilberger JE Jr.: *Spinal Cord Injuries in Children.* Mount Kisco NY: Futura, 1986.
67. Wolf JW Jr., Johnson RM: Cervical orthoses, in Sherk HH, Dunn EJ, Eismont FJ, et al (eds): *The Cervical Spine.* Philadelphia: Lippincott, 1989: 97–105.
68. Yasuoka S, Peterson HA, Maccarty CS: Incidence of spinal column deformity after multilevel laminectomy in children and adults. *J Neurosurg* 1982; 57:441–445.
69. Zambramski JM, Browner CM, Rekate H, Sonntag VKH: Pediatric spinal cord and vertebral column injuries. *BMI Quarterly* 1986; 2:11–17.

CHAPTER 93

SPINAL CORD INJURY OCCURRING IN OLDER INDIVIDUALS*

R. Edward Carter
Daniel E. Graves

SYNOPSIS

Spinal cord injury in the elderly has a higher incidence than any other age group. This older age group tends to be predominantly male. The trauma, usually secondary to a fall, may occur without a cervical fracture. The most common neurological finding is a central cord syndrome of spinal cord injury secondary to a hyperextension injury. It is characterized by more motor impairment of the upper extremities than of the lower extremities, bladder dysfunction, and varying degrees of sensory loss. The older patients show less return of motor recovery and less return of voluntary bowel and bladder function following a traumatic central cord syndrome. Complications are more frequent in the older age group, and length of survival is decreased, with cardiovascular and respiratory problems being the major causes of death.

INTRODUCTION

Although most spinal cord injuries in the United States occur in persons between 15 and 45 years of age, approximately 7 percent of all such injuries are sustained by persons 60 or older. The incidence of spinal cord injury among the elderly is 11 in 100,000, a rate higher than that for any other age group.[1] Uniquely, among this older age group the injuries have different etiologies than in younger groups. In addition, survival decreases with increasing age at injury; there is a greater percentage of spinal cord trauma occurring without skeletal fractures, cervical spondylosis usually with stenosis, and more incomplete than complete neural injuries.

Many of the statistics cited in this report are taken from data collected by the National Spinal Cord Injury Statistical Center (NSCISC). This collection includes all patients treated within 1 year of injury at any one of the 13 current Regional Model Spinal Cord Injury Systems (referred to hereafter as model systems) sponsored by the National Institute on Disability and Rehabilitation Research (NIDRR).

DEMOGRAPHICS

Analysis of over 15,000 cases in the national database reveals that almost half were in the group 25 years of age and under, while only slightly over 1000 cases were 60 years and above. In the group of 25 years of age or under, males predominated over females by 83 to 17 percent; in the group over 60, males predominated by only 74 to 26 percent. The causes of spinal cord injury in the older age group are considerably different from those of the younger group. In this latter group, the leading cause remains motor vehicle crashes, with gunshot wounds and sporting injuries close behind. The group 60 years and older, as seen in Table 93-1, shows a slightly decreased incidence of motor vehicle crash injuries and certainly many fewer by gunshot wounds and sporting activities. However, atraumatic causes are much increased over the younger group, and perhaps the most significant change in etiology is a fourfold

* Preparation of this manuscript was supported in part by grant #H133N00016 from the National Institute on Disability and Rehabilitation Research (NIDRR), Department of Education, Washington, DC, USA.

TABLE 93-1 Distribution of Injury Etiology by Age Group

Etiology	25 or younger (%)	60 or older (%)
Motor vehicle crash	12	54
Motorcycle crash	38	30
Other vehicle crash	<1	8
Gunshot wound	4	4
Falls	18	3
Water sports	14	1
Sports	6	<1
Atraumatic	8	<1
Other	<1	<1
Number of patients	7384	1032

increase in the number of injuries created by falls. In a review by Hardy in 1977, of 141 patients with cervical injury without skeletal damage, 70 percent were over the age of 50, with falls stated as the most common cause.[2] Weingarden and Graham in 1989 reported on a series of spinal cord injury patients over the age of 50 admitted to the Southeastern Michigan Spinal Cord Injury System between 1983 and 1988. Seventy-five patients over 58 years were admitted during this period, and 58 (77 percent) of these were injured secondary to a fall.[3] The mean age for the total group was 65.3 years, with 31 patients (53 percent) being over 60. The circumstances of the fall were classified into: (1) falling downstairs (23 cases); (2) falling from a height, such as a porch or balcony (19 cases); and (3) falling on a level surface (16 cases). In 10 of the latter cases, the fall was preceded by loss of consciousness. Interestingly enough, 31 of the 58 patients (53 percent) were noted to have consumed some alcohol prior to their fall. Nurick noted that the average rate of alcohol use prior to injury was about 30 to 40 percent in paraplegics and quadriplegics, while this rate increased to approximately 68 percent in central cord syndrome.[4]

NEUROLOGICAL

Analysis of neurological classification upon discharge from the initial rehabilitation center reveals that complete injuries are less common in the group of patients above 60 years of age, consisting of 32 percent. In patients 25 or younger, 53 percent were complete injuries. The Frankel B classification, consisting of preserved sensation only, was essentially the same incidence in both younger and older age groups. Motor preservation,

TABLE 93-2 Distribution of Frankel Grade by Age Group

Frankel Rating	25 or younger (%)	60 or older (%)
A	53	32
B	11	9
C	9	19
D	27	40
Number of patients	7384	1032

both nonfunctional and functional, tended to be considerably higher in the older age group. In summary, it appears that slightly over 50 percent of the spinal cord injuries in patients over 60 result in incomplete quadriplegia. Complete quadriplegia, paraplegia, and incomplete paraplegia occur in 16 to 17 percent in this older age group, as seen in Table 93-2.

Schneider and coworkers reported in 1954 on a syndrome of acute central cervical spinal cord injury that occurred most frequently in severe hyperextension injuries.[5] This syndrome was characterized by disproportionately more motor impairment of the upper than of the lower extremities, bladder dysfunction (usually urinary retention), and varying degrees of sensory loss below the level of the lesion. The pattern seen most frequently in older individuals sustaining a fall resulting in spinal cord injury is that of central cord syndrome. It occurs almost exclusively in the cervical area, involving the central gray matter and the more medial white matter, producing greater weakness in the upper limbs than in the lower limbs and sacral sensory sparing.[6] This type of injury is caused most commonly by cervical hyperextension. Neurological recovery usually occurs earliest and to the greatest extent in the lower extremities, and is followed in sequence by the bladder, upper extremities, and finally the hands.

NEUROPATHOLOGY

Taylor in 1951 demonstrated that there may be extensive impingement of structures into the cervical canal without damage to the vertebral column.[7] He believed that the injury was caused by hyperextension of the cervical spine without temporary dislocation, and that the agent that impinges on the cord is the forward-bulging ligamentum flavum. In a later study by Quencer and coworkers in 1992, magnetic resonance images of 11 consecutive cases of acute traumatic central cord syndrome secondary to closed injury to the spine were analyzed.[8] These cases were then correlated with gross pathological and histological features of three cervical spinal cord injuries obtained postmortem from patients with this syndrome, including two patients studied by MRI. Ten of the 11 patients had preexisting cervical spondylosis and/or spinal canal stenosis. In this study, the MRIs indicated that the damage was predominantly to the white matter and that intramedullary hemorrhage is not a necessary feature of the syndrome—and is, in all probability, an uncommon event. It was suggested that the most common mechanism of injury in the acute traumatic central cord syndrome may be direct compression of the cervical spinal cord by buckling of the ligamenta flava into an already narrowed cervical spinal canal. This would explain the predominance of axonal injury in the white matter of the lateral columns. Indeed, in the original article by Schneider and associates, it was pointed out that central cord syndrome also may be associated with cervical arthritis, certain cervical compression fractures, and special types of hyperextension or flexion fracture-dislocations of the cervical spine.[5] They also felt that surgical decompression of the spinal cord was contraindicated in this syndrome.

GENDER

Spinal cord injury is basically male-predominant. Satomi and Herabayaski and Roth and Lawler found a four-to-one male-to-female ratio in patients of all ages with central cord syndrome.[9,10] Others have found that the male/female ratio is essentially two-to-one in reviewing cases of cervical spondylosis. Friedenberg and Miller found that 60 percent of patients with degenerative disk disease of the cervical spine were male.[11] Nurick, in a review of patients with cervical spondylitic myelopathy, found a two-to-one male preponderance.[4]

AGE AND PROGNOSIS

From a standpoint of prognosis, the study by Penrod and coworkers in 1990 found a definite age effect correlating with prognosis.[12] Fifty-one subjects were studied, with 30 being younger than 42 years of age and 21 over 50 years. The younger group was much more successful in becoming independent in ambulation and ability to perform independently the activities of daily living. The younger group also had a much higher percentage for independent control of bowel and bladder. These authors concluded that younger patients showed significantly greater recovery after traumatic central cord syndrome injuries than did older patients in all aspects of function. More of the older patients had consumed alcohol immediately prior to their injury. In addition, 57 percent of the older subjects did not have cervical fractures; of those without fractures, 10 of the 12 were noted as having degenerative disk disease or stenosis.

SKELETAL

A review of 4565 cases in the National Spinal Cord Injury database reveals that only 1 percent of patients 25 years of age or younger had spinal stenosis; in the group over 60, the incidence of spinal stenosis was 18 percent. Similarly, there was a history of cervical spondylosis in only 0.2 percent of the younger group, compared with 23 percent in those over 60. Ankylosing spondylitis was present as a contributing etiology in 0.3 percent of cases in the younger group and in 13 percent in the group 60 years and over.

COMPLICATIONS

Complications are interesting to compare between the younger age group (below 25 years) and the older age group (above 60), as seen in Table 93-3. For example, deep venous thrombosis has essentially the same incidence in both groups, while pulmonary embolism is reported at 2 percent in the younger group and 6 percent in the older group.

A significant difference in methods of bladder drainage is noted in the older age group, which has almost three times the frequency of indwelling catheters to manage their bladder drainage compared with the younger patients. Also, only half of the older group are catheter-free or use an external catheter. During care in the model system, the incidence of bacteriuria over 100,000 colonies per ml is the same in both groups and approximates 87 to 84 percent. Kidney stones in a report of over 15,000 cases are apparent in 2 percent of the older age group, compared with 0.1 percent of the younger group. Contractures appear to be the same in both age groups (3 to 5 percent). Conversely, heterotopic ossification appears to be three times more common in the younger age group. As one might anticipate,

TABLE 93-3 Prevalence of Medical Complications and Preexisting Conditions of Age Groups Expressed in Percentages

Complication/Condition	Number of Cases (n = 4600)*	Percentage of Age Group Presenting Complication	
		25 or younger	*60 or over*
Urinary tract infection	3649	87	84
Hypertension	386	<1	38
Pneumonia	641	11	24
Atelectasis	831	17	23
Heart disease**	401	<1	19
Diabetes mellitus	135	<1	15
Deep vein thrombosis	573	11	11
Aspiration	154	2	10
Obstructive pulmonary disease	131	1	9
Pulmonary embolism	158	2	6
GI hemorrhage	124	3	5
Heterotopic ossification	224	6	2
Kidney stones**	57	<1	2
Scoliosis	46	1	<1

* Because of changes in the data collected, some variables were collected for only a portion of the patients.
** Based on 15,130 patients.

scoliosis in the younger age group occurs in approximately 1 percent and is quite a bit higher than the 0.5 percent reported for the older age group. GI hemorrhage is almost twice as frequent in those over 60. Aspiration is approximately five times more common in the older age group, and atelectasis occurs in 23 percent of the older patients compared with 17 percent of the younger group. Diabetes mellitus is more common in the older group by 15 to 0.3 percent. Hypertension, as expected, is more common by 38 to 1 percent, and heart disease by 19 to 1 percent in the older group. Pneumonia appears twice as often, and COPD is eight times more common in the older age group.

SPECIAL CONSIDERATIONS—ACUTE MANAGEMENT

Several important systems deserve special attention in the acute posttraumatic stage of spinal cord injury in older individuals; namely, respiratory, urological, nutritional, and functional. From a respiratory standpoint, the patient with cervical or high thoracic injury should be treated as having respiratory insufficiency until proven otherwise.

The work of breathing is considerably increased in quadriplegics. In addition, the major difficulty of respiration is the severe weakness of forced expiration—coughing.[13] Intermittent positive pressure breathing should be initiated as early as possible posttrauma to evacuate mucus and prevent pooling of the normal endobronchial secretions, recognizing that these may be increased in patients with a history of smoking and/or previous respiratory disease. The intermittent positive pressure breathing (IPPB) should have nebulization with mucolytics and bronchodilators. Each treatment must be followed first by chest clapping or percussion to mobilize mucus and then by assistive coughing to evacuate the mucus, preventing its pooling, reinfection, and/or atelectasis. Incentive respirometry can be used subsequently to continue strengthening of the respiratory musculature. Also the assistive muscles of respiration, namely those in the neck, should not be forgotten. Isometrics and later resistive exercises for the neck musculature should be initiated as soon as spine stability permits.

It is not infrequent for spinal cord patients immediately posttrauma to develop acute gastric dilatation and/or ileus. If this is prolonged for several days, intravenous hyperalimentation must be initiated. When tolerated, the patient should be started gradually on a progressively increasing diet regimen supplemented by high protein and high caloric intake between meals and at bedtime. Hypercatabolism is increased in spinal cord injury in older individuals, due mostly to protein loss from denervated musculature as well as bed rest. Protein replacement prevents severe hypoproteinemia, thus helping to prevent pressure ulcers on anesthetized surfaces.

Turning the patient and bed positioning also should have high priority. Turning from side to back to side should be done at least every 2 h to preserve skin integrity, but mostly from the standpoint of preventing pooling of mucus in the endobronchial tree, which can lead to atelectasis/infection. It should be remembered that, along with oral hyperalimentation, a daily bowel program should be instituted with adequate bulk intake, stool softener and/or laxative, and a daily suppository for evacuation. From a functional standpoint, the older patient with spinal injury should be mobilized as rapidly as possible. Surgical procedures for stabilization should be done as soon as possible so that the patient can begin mobilization and enter an active program of physical and occupational therapy. This will further assist the return of a normal appetite and return of the patient's blood chemistries to normal. In addition, because of age, immobility, and paralysis, it would be highly recommended that the patient start on a low-molecular weight heparin, such as enoxaparin, for prevention of deep venous thrombosis and, more specifically, pulmonary embolism.

The urinary tract may be involved with complications, both early and late. This is due in part to the lack of normal voluntary neural control of voiding, decreased local blood circulation, and the stress of injury and possible surgery. Exogenous corticosteroids can result in lowered host resistance and a decreased immune response. Major complications usually involve three systems: the respiratory system; the skin; and the urinary system. The first two usually are manifested by a complication that is either visible or that results in obvious localized symptoms. The urinary tract, on the other hand, may present with a symptom only of fever, although associated ileus or acute gastric dilatation are not uncommon. As soon as they are admitted to a trauma center, patients should be placed on a closed system indwelling catheter that is taped either to the lower abdominal midline or the medial thigh, and given prophylactic antibacterial coverage. This system can be kept sterile for several weeks. As soon as the patient can tolerate a restriction of fluids to approximately 400 ml every 4 h, this closed system catheter can be removed and the patient placed on intermittent catheterization every 4 h. Oral intake must be adjusted so that the catheterized volumes do not exceed bladder capacity. This method, particularly in males, obviates having an indwelling catheter continually in the urethra, which can result in acute urethritis, periurethral abscess, epididymitis, testicular abscess, etc. With intermittent catheterization, the urine should be kept sterile, avoiding this excessive trauma. This method can be continued until the patient's immune system, host resistance, and general health have returned to normal.

In the rehabilitation phase, after the patient has been in an acute trauma center, the preceding areas still need to be addressed. The patient will continue to need strengthening of the respiratory muscles that contribute to inspiration and expiration. This is particularly important in quadriplegics and in high paraplegics, and can be accomplished through continued use of an incentive respirometer two to three times daily, breathing exercises, and IPPB. Nutritional requirements should continue to be monitored so that hypoproteinemia and electrolyte imbalance do not occur. Intermittent catheterization is continued as long as feasible, but could be converted to a closed system Foley catheter if a higher intake of liquids is required.

Functionally, the patient should be kept out of bed to his or her tolerance in a progressive wheelchair sitting program. This sitting program is limited by the patient's fatigue, skin tolerance to pressure over the seated surface, and postural hypotension. Postural hypotension may be ameliorated by an abdominal binder, thigh-length elastic hose, and progressive increases in sitting angles and duration as tolerated. If further assistance is needed, sodium chloride, 1 g 4 times daily, may be employed. In addition, 25 mg of ephedrine, 30 to 45 min prior to wheelchair sitting twice a day, may be utilized. As a last resort, Florinef, 0.5 mg to 0.1 mg daily, may be given to assist in sodium retention, expansion of blood volume, and control of postural hypotension. At the current time, it is recommended that low-molecular weight heparin be given subcutaneously twice daily for a period of 3 to 4 weeks and then once daily for a total of 3 to 4 months from onset of trauma. This is done to prevent deep venous thrombosis and pulmonary embolism.

Penrod and coworkers reported that younger patients showed significantly greater recovery after traumatic central cord syndrome than older patients in all aspects of function.[12] They felt that the older age group had a greater percentage of medical complications both before and after their spinal cord injuries, and were uncertain of the extent to which this increase of medical complications contributed to the poorer outcome of older patients. It is possible that there are other factors, such as the effect of blood supply to the spinal cord and the effect of spondylosis and cervical stenosis. With advancing age, arteriosclerosis of the vertebral arteries and fibrosis of the smaller arterial vessels may compromise the blood supply to the spinal cord. Breig and associates, using fresh cadavers, found that cervical spondylosis causes deformity of the anterior horn cells of the gray matter as well as of the lateral columns.[14]

They also believed that this direct mechanical injury, combined with a decreased vascular supply, caused even greater damage to the spinal cord. The younger and older age groups had roughly equivalent recovery of lower extremity motor scores following central cord injury. However, the upper extremity motor scores showed better recovery in the younger age group.

SURVIVAL

Mesard and coworkers found a higher proportion of paraplegic than quadriplegic patients surviving in every age category.[15] The likelihood for survival after injury was influenced by age and by level of injury for both paraplegics and quadriplegics. In a study by DeVivo, the cumulative 12-year survival rate percentages for persons injured between 1973 to 1984 and treated at model spinal cord injury systems were calculated in the 50 years-plus age group.[16] Survival percentage was 18 percent for complete quadriplegia and 53 percent for incomplete quadriplegia with onset of injury at 50 years and over. This compares with 87 percent of complete quadriplegia and 95 percent of incomplete quadriplegia surviving 12 years postinjury in the 25 years and under group.

CAUSES OF DEATH

Analysis of 1422 cases in the National Spinal Cord Injury database shows that in the 60 years of age and over group, heart disease and respiratory disease account for 58 percent of deaths. In the group below 25 years of age, these diagnoses comprised only 35 percent of deaths. Whiteneck and coworkers, in the publication *Aging with Spinal Cord Injury,* demonstrated that 45 percent of all spinal cord injury survivors were over 45 years, with 20 percent being over 60 years of age.[17] Percentage of spinal cord injuries occurring in people over 60 was 5 percent in 1981 and 6 percent in 1991.

Whiteneck and coworkers, studied spinal cord injured patients in the 1940s, 1950s, and 1960s in Britain who within 1 year were known to have survived the first year of injury.[17] A total of 834 patients were studied. Of these, 362 (43 percent) are known to have died, and 7 percent were lost to follow-up. Of the 412 known survivors, only 19 could not be successfully contacted. The surviving percentage at 10 years posttrauma was 85 percent, and at 40 years posttrauma was 35 percent. The most dramatic differences resulted from analysis by age at injury. The median survival for those injured before 30 years of age was 43 years, while the median survival for those injured at 50 years of age and over was 11 years. It appeared that cardiovascular and respiratory deaths became relatively more frequent with aging. This suggests that as time passes the causes of death among individuals with spinal cord injuries move away from such classics as renal failure and begin to approximate the causes of death of the nondisabled population. In their *Spinal Cord Injury—The Facts and Figures,* Stover and colleagues reported on 10-year survivals with traumatic spinal cord injury by age and injury.[18] This indicated a survival of 93 percent at 10 years in the 10- to 19-years-of-age group at onset of injury. By comparison, the survival was 52 percent at 10 years in the 60- to 69-years-of-age group, and 32 percent in the 70-years-of-age and above group. It is well known that the greatest mortality risk lies in the first year posttrauma; once past this, mortality rates tend to diminish significantly.

ACKNOWLEDGMENTS

The Model Regional Spinal Cord Injury Case Systems funded by the National Institute on Disability and Rehabilitation Research contributed data to the National Spinal Cord Injury Statistical Center data set, which was used in this study. Preparation of this manuscript was supported in part by Grant #H133N0016 from the NIDRR, Department of Education, Washington, DC, USA.

References

1. Kalsbeek WD, McLaurin RL, Harris BSH, Miller JD: The national head and spinal cord injury survey: Major findings. 1980; *J Neurosurg* 53:S19–S31.
2. Hardy A: Cervical spinal cord injury without bony injury. *Paraplegia* 1977; 14:296–305.
3. Weingarden SI, Graham PM: Falls resulting in spinal cord injury: Patterns and outcomes in an older population. *Paraplegia* 1989; 27:423–427.
4. Nurick S: The pathogenesis of the spinal cord disorder associated with cervical spondylosis. *Brain* 1972; 95:87–100.
5. Schneider RC, Cherry G, Pantek H: The syndrome of acute central cervical spinal cord injury, with special reference to the mechanics involved in hyperextension injuries of cervical spine. *J Neurosurg* 1954; 11:546–577.
6. American Spinal Injury Association: *Standards for Neurological Classification of Spinal Injury Patients.* Chicago: American Spinal Injury Association, 1987.

7. Taylor AR: The mechanism of injury to the spinal cord in the neck without damage to the vertebral column. *J Bone Joint Surg* 1951; 33-B:543–547.
8. Quencer RM, Bunge RP, Egnor M, et al: Acute traumatic central cord syndrome: MRI-pathological correlations. *Neuroradiology* 1992; 34:85–94.
9. Satomi K, Herabayaski K: Clinical analysis of central cervical cord injury. Proceedings American Spinal Injury Association, 14th meeting, abstracts, 1988.
10. Roth J, Lawler M: Functional outcome of central cord syndrome. Proceedings American Spinal Injury Association, 14th meeting, abstracts, 1988.
11. Friedenberg Z, Miller W: Degenerative disc disease of the cervical spine. *J Bone Joint Surg* 1983; 45:1171–1177.
12. Penrod LE, Hedge SK, Ditunno JF Jr.: Age effect on prognosis for functional recovery in acute, traumatic central cord syndrome. *Arch Phys Med Rehabil* 1990; 71:963–967.
13. Carter RE: Respiratory management, including ventilator care in tetraplegia and diaphragmatic pacing, in Frankel HL (ed): *Handbook of Clinical Neurology,* vol. 17(61): *Spinal Cord Trauma.* Amsterdam: Elsevier 1992: 261–273.
14. Breig A, Turnbull I, Hassler O: Effects of mechanical stresses on the spinal cord in cervical spondylosis: A study on fresh cadaver material. *J Neurosurg* 1966; 25:45–56.
15. Mesard L, Carmody A, Mannarino E, Ruge D: Survival after spinal cord trauma. *Arch Neurol* 1978; 35:78–83.
16. DeVivo MJ: Prognostic factors for long-term survival after spinal cord injury. *Am J Epidemiol* 1989; 130:847–848.
17. Whiteneck GG, Charlifue SW, Gerhart KA, et al: *Aging with Spinal Cord Injury.* New York: Demos, 1993.
18. Stover SL, Fine PR, Go BK, et al: *Spinal Cord Injury: The Facts and Figures.* Birmingham: University of Alabama, 1986.

CHAPTER 94

PENETRATING SPINAL CORD INJURY

Richard K. Simpson, Jr.
Daniel P. Robertson
Raj K. Narayan

INTRODUCTION

The first description of penetrating spinal injury (PSI) is credited to Ambroise Paré in 1567. However, the most famous incident occurred at the Battle of Trafalgar on October 21, 1805.[1,2] Toward the end of the struggle against the Spanish and French fleets, at approximately 1:15 PM, Admiral Horatio Nelson suddenly fell to his knees. "They have done for me at last, Hardy," Nelson exclaimed to his able flag captain. Hardy replied, "I hope not." Nelson then said, "Yes, my backbone is shot through." The ship's surgeon, Dr. Beatty, rushed to his assistance and said, "My Lord, unhappily for our Country, nothing can be done for you." Shortly thereafter, when victory was at hand, Nelson died. Although this pessimistic attitude toward PSI has persisted over the centuries, the prognosis following such an injury is not uniformly dismal, especially if associated injuries are properly managed. Issues related to management of PSI remain controversial, for example, surgical versus nonsurgical therapy, timing of surgery, and the use of steroids.

Civilian PSI was reported infrequently prior to the Vietnam war; in general, treatment of civilian injuries paralleled the military philosophy current at the time. The earliest series of battlefield-incurred PSI can be found in records from the American Civil War. There were 642 cases of PSI documented in the *Medical and Surgical History of the War of the Rebellion,* which represented a very small proportion of the total number of casualties.[3] Most injuries occurred to the thoracolumbar region, although wound location often was not reported. Operative intervention was not discussed, presumably reflecting the nonavailability of adequate surgical facilities at that time. The overall mortality was reportedly 55 percent.

WORLD WAR I

Battlefield PSI was treated with greater frequency, often by surgeons specializing in neurological injuries, after the introduction of antiseptic surgical techniques. A report by Harvey Cushing discussing the outcome of 32 cases of PSI during World War I suggested that mortality rates had increased whether or not operation was performed.[4] The mortality rates were similar to a series of 175 cases reviewed by Frazier.[5] The higher mortality, if not an artifact of data collection, was felt to be the result of more powerful and accurate missiles. Perhaps Hanson represented the opinion of that era when he stated, "War wounds of the spine were particularly distressing . . . one scarcely knew where to begin, if to begin at all."[6] Indications for surgery were not well defined, and treatment often consisted of debridement of the wound with little to no manipulation of the dura or cord.

WORLD WAR II

Prior to the onset of World War II, there was no standard of care for PSI. The discovery of antibiotics and the surgical techniques developed during World War I influenced military philosophy. A policy was formulated to encourage prompt operative intervention if there was a reasonable chance that the spinal cord was not completely destroyed. Treatment consisted of laminectomy, debridement, foreign body removal, and limited exploration of intradural injuries, followed by dural grafts, if necessary. According to Matson, PSI, in some form, was reported in nearly 12 percent of battlefield injuries.[7] Approximately half of these sustained severe associated chest or abdominal wounds. Results from 1260 cases reported by Spurling illustrate a remarkable decrease in operative mortality, compared with the preantibiotic era, and 15 percent of patients were reported to have improved neurologically—usually those with incomplete deficits.[8] The routine placement of indwelling urethral catheters, better care of paralyzed patients, and use of blood products certainly influenced clinical outcome.

THE KOREAN WAR

Surgical lessons learned in World War II and logistical advances in casualty evacuation and transportation to organized forward and base hospitals were decisive in the formulation of a new treatment policy during the Korean War, as discussed by Meirowsky.[9] Operative intervention during the acute phase of neurological injury was thought to reduce delayed morbidity and mortality. When the patient's general condition permitted, wound debridement, laminectomy, and intradural exploration were performed in all cases of PSI. The dura was opened, even if it had not been penetrated. Postponement, but not omission, of surgery was acceptable. Mierowsky discussed several cases of neurological improvement following prolonged, delayed surgery for PSI. Of the 359 cases discussed, nearly half of the patients with complete paraplegia or quadriplegia and the vast majority with incomplete deficits improved postoperatively.

THE VIETNAM WAR

The philosophy of operating on all cases of PSI continued into the Vietnam War and was largely based on the reported success of spinal surgery during the Korean War. There has been no compilation of all cases of PSI from this relatively recent military experience, although, several smaller series have been reported.[10–12] A representative series by Jacobson and Bors revealed that, although operative mortality was slightly less than that seen during the Korean War, no neurological improvement was observed in patients with complete neurological injuries.[11] Approximately 25 percent of patients with incomplete deficits improved postoperatively. The discrepancy between results in the Korean and Vietnam Wars is unclear and may reflect sampling error in the latter report or differences in the definitions and documentation of deficits in the two series. Results from a more recent series of battlefield injuries from Lebanon and Israel indicate that the prognosis for postoperative neurological recovery remains poor. Ohry and Rozin concluded that the role of operative intervention is not certain.[13] However, in their series of 31 patients, neurological improvement was seen in 50 percent of the surgically treated patients and in only 38 percent of those treated conservatively, although this may represent sampling bias.

CIVILIAN STUDIES

Epidemiological studies reveal that the vast majority of civilian patients sustaining PSI are young males. In a recent series by Six and associates, nearly 80 percent were male, generally between 21 and 30 years of age.[14] The same age and sex distribution has been reported from very large series of gunshot wounds (GSW) by Stauffer and coworkers and stab wounds (SW) by Peacock and associates.[15,16] Race has been discussed only occasionally. In a recent report by Simpson and coworkers, 53 percent of cases were black, 28 percent were Latin American, 18 percent were white, and 1 percent were Asian.[17] The racial distribution described by Six and associates is similar and probably reflects multiple social factors inherent in urban populations.[14]

WEAPON TYPE

In general, the offending caliber or type of weapon is often unknown. However, gunshot wounds (GSW) seen in civilian practice usually are caused by small caliber bullets from handguns. As discussed by Miller, and Six and associates, 0.22-, 0.25-, 0.32-, and 0.38-caliber weapons are commonly used.[14,18] Injuries from large-caliber and more powerful weapons resembling those seen in military combat, such as 0.357-, 0.44-, 0.45-caliber handguns as well as bullets from rifles and shotgun pellets are not seen as frequently.[19,20] The composition of bullets also can vary, although most are made of lead.

Although delayed response to injury has often been attributed to copper-jacketed fragments, which have been reported to cause an exaggerated granulomatous response, an inflammatory tissue reaction also can occur in response to steel and glass.[21–23] Lacerating injuries usually are the result of knives; however, a wide variety of weapons can be used, including scissors, bicycle spokes, and sharpened broomsticks.[24]

WOUND LOCATION

Most PSI wounds are to the thoracic spine; lumbosacral and cervical injuries occur with somewhat less frequency.[15,18,20,24,25] This probably reflects the relative proportion of these cord segments. Spinal injuries at more than one site are highly unusual in civilian PSI. A study of 114 patients by Jacobson and Bors showed that 13 percent of patients had cervical, 54 percent had thoracic, and 33 percent had lumbosacral spine injuries, and other large series are in general agreement.[11] Lacerating injuries (non-GSW PSI), as reported by Peacock and coworkers, were seen most frequently in the thoracic region as well (64 percent).[15] The cervical spine and lumbosacral spine were involved in 29 percent and 7 percent of cases, respectively.

NEUROLOGICAL INJURY

Neurological deficits as a result of PSI may be broadly classified as: (1) complete neurological deficit, including sensory, motor, and sphincter function, below the level of injury; (2) incomplete neurological deficit, whereby some function remains at all cord segments; and (3) cauda equina injuries. Benzel and associates, and Coleman and coworkers found that most (57 percent) patients had complete neurological deficits.[26,27] Only 26 percent had incomplete and 17 percent had cauda equina injuries. Stauffer and colleagues, in 185 cases, also found 57 percent to be complete and 43 percent to be incomplete injuries.[16] Yashon and coworkers found that 52 percent of cases involved complete neurological deficits, 13 percent were incomplete deficits, and 35 percent were cauda equina or conus medullaris injuries.[28] Lacerating PSI often results in incomplete neurological deficit. Peacock and colleagues reported that 58 percent of SW had a variant of the Brown-Séquard type lesion.[15] Only 22 percent of cases had classic hemisection of the cord; the remainder had complete paraplegia or quadriplegia.

MECHANISM OF INJURY

The differences between military and civilian PSI in terms of clinical outcome, percentage of patients with complete neurological deficits, and appearance of the cord have been attributed to the mechanism of tissue damage. Blast or concussive forces causing temporary neurological impairment are thought to occur more frequently in PSI sustained by projectiles with high velocities.[18] Although most studies regard the kinetic energy ($\frac{1}{2}\ mv^2$) released by a missile as being responsible for tissue damage, Yashon has proposed that velocity is the most important factor in determining the injury potential of a projectile, expressed as a function of power (mv^3).[20] In general, weapons used in cases of civilian PSI have muzzle velocities of 600 to 1100 ft/s, whereas military weapons range from 2000 to 4000 ft/s.[18,20] Shrapnel, for brief distances, also travel at high velocities and have been reported to be responsible for nearly a third of wartime PSI.[11]

Supporting the concept of concussive injury in the military setting are many reported cases of normal-appearing spinal cords at laminectomy by Frazier, Haynes, Meirowsky, and Six and associates.[5,9,14,29] "Shock wave" or indirect cord injury was thought to be responsible for neurological impairment. The transient nature of deficits was also proposed, in part, to be the result of resolving edema. Such concussive forces are less likely to occur from weapons usually responsible for civilian PSI. Neurological impairment in civilian PSI, therefore, is more likely to be the result of direct spinal cord or root damage. A patient with direct injury to nervous tissue, such as that caused by a knife, small caliber handgun, or buckshot, is less likely to show neurological improvement. The pathological features of spinal cords that had sustained an indirect blast injury or a direct penetrating injury have been studied in detail by Wolman and Frazier, respectively.[5,30]

MANAGEMENT PHILOSOPHY

For the past 30 years the need for laminectomy, intradural exploration, and wound debridement in cases of civilian PSI has been debated. Treatment of civilian PSI has paralleled management of battlefield PSI. Since the Korean war, many surgeons have maintained that all cases of civilian PSI require exploration.[9] This philosophy is reflected by Scarff, who stated that, "All compound injuries of the spine should be explored at the earliest possible moment...."[31] Recent studies have suggested that civilian PSI differs in some respects from battlefield PSI.[17] These studies conclude that the indications for neurosurgical intervention may differ from the military guidelines. Although considerable ambiguity exists, the relatively few civilian studies reported to date have concluded that neurological deterioration or an incomplete neurological deficit is an indication for surgery.[26,28] Wound debridement and exploration for purposes of infection prophylaxis and prevention of CSF leakage are frequently stated surgical indications.[16,32] Decompression and fragment removal are also commonly regarded indications for operation.[18,25] However, the reports concerning the actual benefits of decompressive laminectomy and intradural exploration in civilian PSI are conflicting.

WOUND DEBRIDEMENT

Stauffer and coworkers, in a large series, reported that the overall complication rate was higher in patients subjected to surgery.[16] Approximately 16 percent of patients had postoperative wound infections, CSF leakage, or spinal instability. None of the conservatively managed patients had such complications. Heiden and associates, in their series, reported that 18 percent of patients had meningitis, wound infections, spinal abscesses, or vertebral instability if an operation was performed, and that no conservatively treated case had such a complication.[32] Likewise, Maier and colleagues found a much higher rate of delayed infection in patients who had undergone aggressive wound debridement.[33] However, Bricker and coworkers failed to see such complications in patients sustaining major associated injuries to the chest or abdomen.[34] Romanick and associates, in a study of 20 patients, urged early operative intervention for infection prophylaxis, particularly if the abdomen was penetrated.[35] Infection was encountered in 88 percent of patients sustaining an associated colon injury. No patients had infections if the gastrointestinal tract was not entered or if penetration was limited to the stomach or small bowel. A high rate of complications due to infections was seen in associated neck wounds by Jones and colleagues.[36] If the trachea or esophagus was penetrated, patients were considered to be at high risk for infection if wound exploration, thorough debridement of bone and soft tissue, and drainage were not implemented.

FRAGMENT REMOVAL

Fragment removal has been described as an indication for operation, although there is considerable debate. In recent reviews by Carey and by Miller, surgical intervention was suggested if bone, clot, or metallic fragments could be visualized radiographically within the spinal canal.[18,25] However, Yashon and coworkers hold a contradictory viewpoint.[28] In their large series, no neurological improvement was seen in patients subjected to surgery for fragment removal. No infections occurred in patients where fragments remained if high-dose antibiotic coverage was administered. These observations were supported by Stauffer and associates in their series of 185 patients.[16] There are, however, several case reports showing delayed neurological deterioration or radicular pain secondary to retained or migrating missile fragments.[23,37] Osteomyelitis as a delayed complication from PSI has been observed by Guttmann, Jones and coworkers, and Malik and colleagues.[19,36,38] Radicular symptoms secondary to a herniated nucleus pulposus has occurred as a rare, yet delayed complication from GSW.[39] Several cases of delayed, acute lead intoxication from retained bullet fragments have been reported by Grogan and coworkers and Linden and associates.[40,41] Retained copper-jacketed bullets also have been associated with neurotoxicity, as reported by Dell and Baum, and Messer and Cerza.[42,43]

NEUROLOGICAL DETERIORATION

A worsening neurological examination is an uncommon feature in the clinical evaluation of civilian PSI. Yashon and associates, in their series of 65 patients, had 2 patients with progressing deficits.[28] Both patients underwent laminectomy, neither improved, and both died of complications from their injuries. Heiden and coworkers had a similar experience in their series of 38 patients.[32] Only 1 patient had surgery for deteriorating neurological function, with no postoperative improvement. However, Wilson has concluded, from his single case, that progressing neurological injury remains an absolute indication for neurosurgical intervention.[44] Recent reports of battle-inflicted PSI continue to support the philosophy that neurological deterioration is a certain indication for neurosurgical intervention.[13] Guttmann's review of an extensive civilian and wartime experience also concluded that worsening neurological deficit was extremely uncommon and proposed that neural damage was likely the result of the immediate injury rather than delayed secondary effects.[19]

INCOMPLETE DEFICITS

When incomplete injury was an indication for surgical intervention, Stauffer and coworkers found that 71 percent of patients improved neurologically following surgery.[16] However, 76.5 percent of patients with incomplete deficits treated conservatively improved. Yashon and colleagues discussed five cases of incomplete spinal cord injury.[28] Two patients had undergone laminectomy; neither patient improved. In contrast, a recent study by Benzel and associates, and Coleman and coworkers state that 100 percent of surgically-treated patients with incomplete injuries showed improvement in spinal cord and/or radicular function.[26,27] However, 75 percent of the nonsurgically-treated patients also improved. Six and colleagues, in a study of 59 patients, reported that no difference in the ultimate outcome was attained by surgically treating PSI, regardless of preoperative neurological function.[14]

CAUDA EQUINA LESIONS

Benzel and coworkers reported that radicular improvement occurred in 100 percent of cauda equina-injured patients.[26] However, this rate of improvement occurred in both operative and nonoperative groups. Little and DeLisa reported that functional recovery from PSI can occur over a 13- to 16-year period if treated only with aggressive physical therapy.[45] Yashon and associates reported the results of operation in 16 of 23 cauda equina-injured patients and found no major neurological improvement.[28] Although preservation of sphincter function is often a goal of surgery, in this series, of the patients suffering sphincter dysfunction, all had persistent bowel and bladder incontinence postoperatively.

Miller, however, has suggested that aggressive treatment of cauda equina injuries by decompression and dural repair is warranted because of the likelihood of functional recovery.[18] Chronic pain from root compression also may be prevented by operation. Results from Comarr and Kaufman, and Cybulski and coworkers also support neurosurgical intervention for cauda equina injuries.[46,47] The latter series showed improvement in 56 to 100 percent of the surgically-treated patients. This contention is supported by Carey in a recent review.[25] Fragments of bone or metal and hematomas were said to deserve special surgical attention if present within the cauda equina, particularly if incomplete neurological deficits were present.

LACERATING INJURIES

Lacerating injuries of the spinal cord or cauda equina are not common in the United States. However, SW occur with relatively high frequency in South Africa. Peacock and coworkers, studying 450 cases, suggested that the only indications for surgery were a retained knife blade, persistent CSF leakage, or abscess formation.[15] Only 4 percent of patients in their series had surgery for lacerating PSI. A study of 314 cases of SW to the spine by Lipschitz was basically in agreement.[24] No patient with complete cord or cauda equina transection improved. Of the patients with incomplete neurological deficits, 14 percent recovered completely, and the remainder showed some improvement. Delayed myelopathy secondary to small retained fragments of a knife blade or glass has been reported to occur up to 8 years after the initial injury. A recent study by De Villers and Grant, and a comment by Schmidek, however, suggested that early surgical intervention in the case of SW to the upper cervical cord region, including debridement, foreign body removal, and repair of dural or vascular rents is advisable.[48,49] Injuries to this region often include lacerations to the vertebral artery and veins with concomitant risk of false aneurysm formation, arteriovenous fistulas, and vascular occlusion. Delayed neurological impairment from vascular compromise also has been reported to occur following GSW to the craniocervical junction.[50]

SHOTGUN WOUNDS

Shotgun wounds, in general, are more serious surgical injuries because considerable soft tissue loss usually occurs. Four cases of shotgun wounds of the spine reported by Sights, were complicated by concurrent severe abdominal or chest injury.[51] The deficits ranged from normal neurological exam to complete paraplegia. No generalizations regarding treatment were suggested. A preliminary report by Simpson and coworkers included five patients who had sustained PSI from shotgun blasts.[17] Deficits ranged from radicular symptoms from spinal root avulsion to complete paraplegia secondary to transection of the cord. Associated injuries were extensive and complex resulting in very long hospitalizations (up to 18 months) and multiple nonneurosurgical operations.

Because these patients often have a complicated hospital course and such PSI wounds occur infrequently, no generalizations regarding treatment have been offered. However, a recent autopsy study of a paraplegic patient who sustained a shotgun wound to the thoracic spine 14 years prior to his death revealed numerous intradural epidermoids and lipomata thought to be the result of traumatic implantation.[52] Delayed neurological symptoms from buckshot have been reported by Daniel and Smith in a patient who sustained shotgun PSI seven years earlier.[53]

ASSOCIATED INJURIES

Several recent reviews have concluded that associated injuries occur in only 25 percent of patients sustaining civilian PSI, but in 67 percent or more of patients sustaining wartime PSI.[11] However, the current surgical management of civilian PSI has been greatly influenced by the presence of coexistent visceral, bronchial, or esophageal penetration.[25] Bricker and associates, studying 15 cases of PSI, including SW and shotgun injuries, recommended that exploration of the spinal canal be performed through the neck, chest, or abdomen during nonneurosurgical procedures.[34] This would take advantage of exposed vertebrae and missile tracts and not subject the patient to a second operation.

Jones and coworkers, in reviewing GSW to the neck, found that broad-spectrum antibiotics, debridement of devitalized tissue, immobilization of the cervical spine, and wound drainage were essential in order to prevent complications from tracheal or esophageal penetration.[36] Romanick and colleagues found that in GSW patients with colon injuries, abdominal exploration and debridement was indicated.[35] Infections such as meningitis, diskitis, and osteomyelitis were often delayed up to 11 weeks after injury, if treated conservatively. No infections were seen in PSI patients with coexistent small bowel and/or stomach penetration. Fatal meningitis was reported by Wilson as a delayed consequence of colon injury and PSI.[44] However, Maier and coworkers found that delayed abscess formation and osteomyelitis were seen more frequently in patients undergoing aggressive debridement than in conservative care.[33] Approximately 29 percent of patients treated surgically and 4 percent of conservatively managed patients had delayed complications.

Injuries to other organs associated with SW are uncommon. Peacock and associates found only 30 cases in their review of 450 patients.[15] Pneumothorax or hemothorax was the most common, accounting for 80 percent of associated injuries. Gentleman and Harrington have suggested that although complications occur more frequently if bowel or bronchus was entered, the role of neurosurgical intervention was small.[54] Prophylactic antibiotic administration for prevention of meningitis was recommended.

BAYLOR CASE REVIEW

In an attempt to validate the relatively arbitrary criteria suggested by the limited literature on the subject of civilian PSI, an extensive review of such cases treated at Ben Taub General Hospital was made. This review, like all others of civilian or military PSI, was retrospective and nonrandomized. A concise summary of the cases at Baylor College of Medicine has been reported previously.[55]

Patient Population

One hundred and sixty patients with PSI were treated between 1980 and 1986.[55] This series included 142 GSW, including 5 shotgun injuries, and 18 SW to the spinal cord or cauda equina. Twenty-seven percent of the injuries were cervical, 54 percent thoracic, and 19 percent lumbosacral cord or cauda equina injuries. The average age was 29 years and ranged from 7 to 75 years. Males accounted for 94 percent and females 6 percent. Associated injuries of the esophagus, trachea, bronchi, or bowel occurred in 107 (67 percent) of patients. The most frequent associated injury was pneumothorax, followed by injury to a hollow viscus. Virtually all patients received antibiotics regardless of whether surgery was performed. Antibiotic type, dosage, interval, and length of treatment varied. On admission, 94 (66 percent) of the 142 GSW and 4 (22 percent) of the 18 SW patients had complete paraplegia or quadriplegia. Approximately 48 (34 percent) of GSW and 14 (78 percent) of SW patients had incomplete neurological deficits. Plain x-rays were obtained in all cases. Other methods of evaluation were infrequently used.

It should be stated that statistical comparisons have been made between groups of patients treated in certain different ways. While such comparisons are interesting and do yield certain insights into the problem, they are not technically accurate, because the groups being compared are not necessarily comparable (being non-randomized). This limitation is, however, true of any retrospective study.

Surgical Intervention

Neurosurgical operations were undertaken in 31 (22 percent) GSW patients and 6 (33 percent) SW patients. The stated indications for surgery were varied, and often multiple. In general, the operation consisted of a laminectomy with intradural exploration and fragment removal. Thirty-four operative patients had laminectomies, 1 patient had only a soft tissue exploration, and in 2 patients the operative details were not clearly reported. Of the 35 patients with sufficient documentation, 20 had intradural explorations. Of these patients, 12 had primary repair of the dura, and 8 had a dural graft. Along with a laminectomy and/or intradural exploration, 20 patients had removal of a foreign body, 9 had only wound debridement, and 6 had only bony decompression.

Gunshot Wounds

Of the surgically treated patients with gunshot wounds and complete paraplegia or quadriplegia, 2 (13 percent) improved, 13 (81 percent) were unchanged, and 1 (6 percent) worsened postoperatively. Without surgery, 12 (15 percent) improved, 64 (82 percent) remained unchanged, and 2 (3 percent) worsened. This was not a statistically significant difference between the groups. Of the surgically-treated GSW patients with incomplete neurological deficits, 6 (40 percent) improved, 6 (40 percent) remained unchanged, and 3 (20 percent) worsened postoperatively. If treated conservatively, 19 (58 percent) improved, 8 (24 percent) showed no change, and 6 (18 percent) deteriorated. No statistical difference existed between these two groups.

Stab Wounds

There were only 4 stab wound patients with complete deficits in our series. Of the 2 treated surgically, one improved and one showed no change. Of the 2 treated conservatively, both remained unchanged. There were 14 SW patients with incomplete deficits. Four of these patients had neurosurgical intervention. Postoperatively, 2 improved, 1 worsened, and 1 was unchanged. Among the 10 patients managed conservatively, 7 improved and 3 showed no change. No statistical difference between these groups was identified.

Shotgun Wounds

There were 5 patients in our series who suffered shotgun wounds to the spine. All 5 patients survived despite extensive associated soft tissue injuries. Four of these patients had complete neurological deficits, and 1 had an incomplete injury. Neurological function remained unchanged in each case. All patients had neurosurgical as well as general surgical treatment of their injuries. None of the patients had neurosurgical complications, although 4 had protracted hospital stays secondary to complications arising from their associated injuries. These types of penetrating spinal injuries are often thought to be "distinct entities" and are discussed in detail in an earlier study.[56]

Cauda Equina Study

Our original study of PSI was expanded to include 1987–1989 for the study of penetrating injuries restricted to the cauda equina. During this period, 33 patients with penetrating injuries to the cauda equina were admitted. Thirty were gunshot injuries, and 3 were stab wounds. Twenty-nine patients (88 percent) had incomplete neurological deficits. Of these, 15 (52 percent) had surgery, and of this patient group, 7 (47 percent) improved, 7 (47 percent) showed no change, and 1 (6 percent) worsened. Fourteen patients (48 percent) with incomplete deficits were treated conservatively, 10 (71 percent) improved, and 4 (29 percent) had no change. Four patients (12 percent) had complete deficits, 3 of whom had surgery, and all improved. One patient with a complete deficit was treated conservatively and did not improve. Ten patients (34 percent) had bowel or bladder dysfunction, and none improved regardless of the type of treatment. Complications occurred in 5 (28 percent) of operative patients and 1 (7 percent) conservatively treated patient. These results indicate that early neurosurgical intervention for penetrating injury of the cauda equina may be beneficial, particularly if the neurological injury is complete, but carries an increased risk of complication. Curiously, 2 patients with incomplete lesions that improved postoperatively had significant posterolateral disk herniations as a direct result of the bullet traversing the disk space.[57] These observations have recently been reported as a detailed comparison between penetrating injuries involving either the cauda equina or the spinal cord.[58]

Associated Injuries

One hundred and seven patients in our series had associated injuries. These were defined as injuries not involving the spine, cord, or cauda equina and requiring nonneurosurgical intervention. These injuries occurred to the neck in 25 (23 percent), chest in 23 (21 percent), abdomen in 33 (31 percent), and multiple sites in 26 (25 percent) of cases. Of these 107 patients, 67 (63 percent) had complete neurological injuries and 40 (37 percent) had incomplete deficits. All 107 patients underwent surgical exploration and repair of their visceral injuries. Neurosurgical procedures were also performed for decompression of the neural elements and wound debridement in 19 of these patients. No statistically significant difference in neurological outcome was found in patients with or without neurosurgical intervention, regardless of the presence of associated injuries, the mechanism of injury, or the extent of the neurological deficit. This controversial topic has been the focus of a separate study.[59] Of interest are cases described by Fischer and coworkers that indicate cervical spinal cord injuries may be avoided if penetration involves facial structures. These structures are thought to act as a biological shield.[60]

Dexamethasone Therapy

Forty-two percent of all patients received steroid therapy. Improvement was observed in 32 percent of these patients, no change was noted in 55 percent, and 5 percent deteriorated neurologically. Although the dosage and interval varied, patients in general received 4 to 6 mg dexamethasone every 4 to 6 h intravenously. Of patients not receiving steroids, 30 percent improved, 66 percent remained unchanged, and 4 percent worsened. These differences were not statistically significant.

Operative Indications

Nearly half (41 percent) of the operative patients in our large series underwent a neurosurgical operation for wound debridement and exploration. Although neurosurgical intervention did not appear to influence outcome, the complication rate was higher in surgically-treated patients than in those managed conservatively. Approximately 24 percent (9) of the surgically treated patients in our series were operated upon for removal of retained fragments, debridement, and decompression. Postoperatively, 2 improved and 7 remained unchanged, results that are similar to the overall series. Only 7 patients were operated upon in our series in response to neurological deterioration. Postoperatively, 3 improved, 3 showed no change, and 1 worsened—results that are, again, not clearly different from our overall series.

Complications

Only 7 percent ($8/123$) of the conservatively managed group had neurological complications including meningitis, CSF leakage, pseudomeningocele, wound infection, and spinal instability. On the other hand, 22 percent ($8/37$) of the surgically-managed patients had these complications postoperatively. Complications occurred in 9 percent ($9/107$) of patients with associated injuries and in 13 percent ($7/53$) of patients without associated injuries. While the difference in complication rate between the surgical patients and conservatively treated groups was statistically significant, the influence of associated injuries on complication rates was not. The mortality rate was 4 percent ($7/160$), with all deaths the result of severe associated injuries.

Patient Evaluation

An accurate neurological examination is of the utmost importance in evaluating a patient with PSI. In our series, each patient was subjected to many examinations by several different physicians at admission, and in follow-up. Minor discrepancies in findings were often seen in the records, resulting in some difficulty in interpreting data. Our results suggest that the short-term goals of neurosurgical intervention, e.g., neurological improvement and the prevention of complications, are difficult to achieve. In fact, neurological complications occurred with greater frequency in patients who had a neurosurgical procedure other than local wound care. However, as in other series, most of our patients were followed for a relatively short period. The average follow-up by Stauffer and coworkers was 3 years, Romanick and associates 31 months, and Yashon and colleagues less than 2 years.[16,28,35] The long-term effects of surgery, however, have yet to be clarified.

Delayed neurological deterioration has been found to occur as a result of retained fragment including bullets, knives, glass, or buckshot.[21,23,53] Neurological sequelae from PSI after extended periods have been attributed to migration of fragments, granulomatous reaction, persistent local trauma, delayed osteomyelitis, spinal instability, epidermoid and lipomata formation, and acute lead toxicity.[19,21,23,36,37,39–41,52,53] Such delayed consequences of PSI warrant reconsideration of operative intervention in cases of civilian PSI.

Although the need for urgent operative intervention as a definitive treatment of civilian PSI remains debatable, each case should be individualized, particularly because of systemic complications from coexistent injuries to other parts of the body. In patients who are to undergo surgical intervention, precise localization of the bony and neural injury is paramount. Examination alone, using dermatomal patterns and motor function loss, or missile entrance, exit, and trajectory, have proved to be an inaccurate method of wound localization. Kislow has shown that the suspected site of cord or cauda equina injury, based on cutaneous or neurological examination, can differ from the level of bony injury by several segments in over 40 percent of patients.[61]

RADIOLOGICAL EVALUATION

The diagnostic benefit of plain films of the spine, both anteroposterior and lateral views, has been advocated since the beginning of the century.[5,6] However, there are several reports of bony injuries discovered at operation that were not seen on x-ray.[62] Likewise, dependence on the location of metallic fragments has been criticized because of the tendency of bullets to ricochet within the body.[19] Computed tomography has been reported to be a more precise method of localizing small fractures. A large series by Post and coworkers concluded that CT of the spine was an adequate method of localizing PSI and obviated the need for myelography.[62] Recently, Yashon and associates questioned the need for myelography in PSI.[28] In fact, Post and coworkers and Yashon and associates have admonished against myelography, using either oil-based or water-based contrast, owing to the possibility of arachnoiditis and neurological disturbances associated with their use.[28,62] However, Benzel and colleagues found that CT of the spine was of limited value because of: (1) the degree of artifact caused by metallic fragments; and (2) precise soft tissue definition was lacking.[26] A recent study by Vogt and Narayan demonstrated that U.S. ammunition, except for steel shotgun pellets, is nonmagnetic in nature.[63] MRI scanning may therefore eventually play a useful role in evaluating these cases.

ELECTROPHYSIOLOGICAL TESTS

Standard electrophysiological diagnostic procedures, such as an electromyogram and/or nerve conduction velocity, have limited utility in the evaluation of acute PSI.[64] Sophisticated techniques are currently available that may be of considerable use regarding initial assessment, intraoperative monitoring, and long-term evaluation of PSI cases. Somatosensory evoked potentials (SSEPs) and, recently, corticomotor evoked potentials (CMEPs), have been suggested by Simpson and coworkers and Baskin and associates to offer some degree of objective, quantitative, and reproducible form of neurological evaluation.[65,67]

SUMMARY OF CURRENT GUIDELINES

Immediate broad spectrum antibiotic administration and antitetanus prophylaxis are recommended in current studies of civilian PSI.[18,25] Operation is performed when the patient's general medical condition permits. Often, associated injuries require immediate attention in order to preserve life. Bricker and colleagues recommend that neurosurgical procedures should be performed while the patient is explored for associated chest or abdominal injuries.[34] Severe neurological deficits require special attention because of the potential for various acute and chronic complications. Recommendations for the general management of acute spinal cord trauma patients have been described in detail elsewhere by Green and Klose.[68]

Pharmacological Treatment

Pharmacological therapy in spinal cord injury has been recently and extensively reviewed by Yashon.[69] Many agents have been used in an attempt to reverse or limit the neurological deficits caused by damage to the spinal cord or cauda equina.[69] Several agents have been shown to favorably influence neurological recovery in experimental animals.[70] Steroid treatment of spinal cord injury had been widely used for many years, and currently is recommended in blunt acute spinal cord injury.[70] Unfortunately, high-dose steroid administration may not alter neurological recovery following PSI. Results from our limited study show no clear beneficial effects.

Surgical Approach

If operation is to be performed, a standard posterior approach via laminectomy is the most common. Although there are many variations on performing a laminectomy, several operative hazards can be encountered because of the penetrating force exerted by the missiles and consequent bone and soft tissue destruction. However, certain details not of concern in routine laminectomy require special attention in cases of PSI.[9]

In general, current recommendations are that a longitudinal incision be centered over the involved lamina and extended to include one intact lamina both above and below the wound. Although a subperiosteal resection of the paraspinous muscles from the lamina should be performed, sharp dissection of the muscles is recommended in the immediate area of comminution and depression. The bony damage is carefully surveyed, and the interspinous ligaments are also sharply divided. Spinous processes of the involved site and the immediate cephalad and caudad processes are removed with bone-cutting instruments, taking great care not to disturb loose bony or metallic fragments. At this point, devitalized soft tissue can be identified and debrided, and the wound thoroughly irrigated with warmed saline. Beginning with normal tissue cephalad to the wound, small rongeurs are used to carefully remove the lamina bilaterally, and the ligamentum flavum is removed to expose intact dura. Removal of adjacent depressed and comminuted bony fragments or pieces of metal can be done more easily and safely with this technique. All fragments are removed, and lateral exposure is gained. Facets are spared if possible. The caudad lamina is then removed to allow visualization of the entire wounded segment.

Several surgeons advocate intradural inspection of the cord regardless of whether the dura has been violated to determine if an occult hematoma exists.[9] However, others recommend that if there is no evidence of CSF leakage and the dura appears intact, no intradural exploration is necessary. It is useful at this point to utilize intraoperative ultrasonography to determine if a cryptic intradural hematoma or fragment is present. If not, the wound could be closed after thoroughly irrigating the intraspinal compartment. If the dura obviously has been violated, it can be opened along the axis of the cord until normal tissue is visualized, and secured laterally with stay sutures. The cord is carefully inspected and hematoma or fragments removed. Blood should be prevented from entering the subarachnoid space. The damaged dura is debrided, as are the proximal and distal ends of the damaged cord. After thoroughly irrigating the intrathecal compartment, the dura is either closed primarily or a dural graft is used. Roots are decompressed if necessary, and the wound is tightly closed to prevent CSF leakage. Spinal instability is an occasional concern, but as a general rule instrumentation for stabilization is not performed at the time of acute operation.

Postoperative Care

All patients with PSI need to be followed carefully to prevent, detect, and treat complications as they arise. All patients are put on a standard care protocol used for spinal cord injury. Particular care is given to pulmonary, urinary, and skin care in those patients with neurological impairment. Rehabilitation efforts should be initiated as soon as possible.

CONCLUSIONS

The results from our large series indicate that neurosurgical operations did not clearly influence neurological recovery from PSI. The influence of surgical treatment on outcome did not appear to be dependent on the type of neurological injury or its location. Although the sample size was small, an exception may be complete cauda equina lesions. In addition, the administration of dexamethasone did not appear to influence overall neurological outcome. Coexistent visceral injuries also did not appear to affect recovery. However, the incidence of neurological complication was higher in the surgically managed patients compared with those managed conservatively. While, as pointed out earlier, this analysis is limited by the retrospective, nonrandomized nature of the data, it certainly casts doubts on some traditionally held beliefs regarding PSI.

References

1. Keynes G: *The Apologie and Treatise of Ambroise Paré.* New York: Dover, 1968: 175, 205, 218–219.
2. Walker D: *Nelson, A Biography.* Trafalgar, New York: Dial Press/James Wade, 1978: vol 2, 499–501.
3. Medical and surgical history of the war of the rebellion, in Frazier CH (ed): *Surgery of the Spine and Spinal Cord.* New York: Appleton, 1918: 464.
4. Cushing H: Organization and activities of the neurological service, American expeditionary forces, in Hanson AM (ed): *The Medical Department of the United States Army in the World War, Surgery.* Washington: US Government Printing Office, 1927: 749–758.
5. Frazier CH: Stab and gunshot wounds to the spine, in Frazier CH (ed): *Surgery of the Spine and Spinal Cord.* New York: Appleton, 1918: 457–497.
6. Hanson AM: Management of gunshot wounds of the head and spine in forward hospitals, AEF, in Hanson AM (ed): *The Medical Department of the United States Army in the World War, Surgery.* Washington: US Government Printing Office, 1927: 776–794.
7. Matson DD: The management of acute compound battle-incurred injuries of the spinal cord, in Woodhall B (ed): *The Medical Department of the United States Army. Surgery in World War II, Neurosurgery.* Washington: US Government Printing Office, 1959: 31–65.

8. Spurling RG: The European theater of operations, in Woodhall B (ed): *The Medical Department of the United States Army. Surgery in World War II, Neurosurgery,* Washington: US Government Printing Office, 1959: 25–30.
9. Meirowsky AM: Penetrating spinal cord injuries, in Coates JB, Meirowsky AM (eds): *Neurological Surgery of Trauma.* Washington: US Government Printing Office, 1965: 257–344.
10. Jacobs GB, Berg RA: The treatment of acute spinal cord injuries in a war zone. *J Neurosurg* 1971; 34:164–167.
11. Jacobson SA, Bors E: Spinal cord injury in Vietnamese combat. *Paraplegia* 1970; 7:263–281.
12. Plaut M: War wounds of the central nervous system: Surgical results. *J Trauma* 1972; 12:613–619.
13. Ohry A, Rozin R: Acute spinal cord injuries in the Lebanon War, 1982. *Israel J Med Sci* 1984; 20:345–349.
14. Six E, Alexander E, Kelly DL, et al: Gunshot wounds to the spinal cord. *South Med J* 1979; 72:699–702.
15. Peacock WJ, Shrosbree RD, Key AG: A review of 450 stabwounds of the spinal cord. *South Afr Med J* 1977; 51:961–964.
16. Stauffer ES, Wood RW, Kelly EG: Gunshot wounds of the spine: Effects of laminectomy. *J Bone Joint Surg* 1979; 61:389–392.
17. Simpson RK, Venger BH, Narayan RK: Penetrating spinal cord injury in a civilian population: A retrospective analysis (1980–1985). *Surg Forum* 1986; 37:494–496.
18. Miller CA: Penetrating wounds of the spine, in Wilkins RH, Rengachary SS (eds): *Neurosurgery.* San Francisco: McGraw-Hill, 1985: vol 2, 1746–1748.
19. Guttmann L: Gunshot injuries of the spinal cord, in Guttmann L (ed): *Spinal Cord injuries. Comprehensive Management and Research.* Oxford: Blackwell, 1976: 177–187.
20. Yashon D: Missile injuries of the spinal cord and cauda equina, in Yashon D (ed): *Spinal Injury.* New York: Appleton-Century-Crofts, 1986: 285–305.
21. Jones FD, Woolsey RE: Delayed myelopathy secondary to retained intraspinal metallic fragment. *J Neurosurg* 1981; 55:979–982.
22. Ott K, Tarlov E, Crowell R, Papadakis N: Retained intracranial metallic foreign bodies: Report of two cases. *J Neurosurg* 1976; 44:80–83.
23. Wu WQ: Delayed effects from retained foreign bodies in the spine and spinal cord. *Surg Neurol* 1986; 25:214–218.
24. Lipschitz R: Stab wounds of the spinal cord, in Vinken PJ, Bruyn GW (eds): *Handbook of Clinical Neurology.* New York: American Elsevier, 1976: vol 25, 197–207.
25. Carey ME: Brain and spinal wounds caused by missiles, in Long DM (ed): *Current Therapy in Neurological Surgery 1985–1986.* Toronto: BC Decker, 1985: 114–117.
26. Benzel EC, Hadden TA, Coleman JE: Civilian gunshot wounds to the spinal cord and cauda equina. *Neurosurgery* 1987; 20:281–285.
27. Coleman JE, Benzel EC, Hadden T: Gunshot wounds to the spinal cord and cauda equina in civilians. *Surg Forum* 1986; 37:496–498.
28. Yashon D, Jane JA, White RJ: Prognosis and management of spinal cord and cauda equina bullet injuries in sixty-five civilians. *J Neurosurg* 1970; 32:163–170.
29. Haynes WG: Acute war wounds of the spinal cord. *Am J Surg* 1946; 72:424–433.
30. Wolman L: Blast injury of the spinal cord, in Vinken PJ, Bruyn GW (eds): *Injuries of the Spine and Spinal Cord. Handbook of Clinical Neurology.* New York: American Elsevier, 1976: vol 25, 221–225.
31. Scarff JE: Injuries to the vertebral column and spinal cord, in Brock S (ed): *Injuries of the Brain and Spinal Cord and their Coverings.* New York: Springer, 1960: 568.
32. Heiden JS, Weiss MH, Rosenberg AW, et al: Penetrating gunshot wounds of the cervical spine in civilians: Review of 38 cases. *J Neurosurg* 1975; 42:575–579.
33. Maier RV, Carrico CJ, Heimbach DM: Pyogenic osteomyelitis of axial bones following civilian gunshot wounds. *Am J Surg* 1979; 137:378–380.
34. Bricker DL, Waltz TA, Telford RJ, Beall AC Jr: Major abdominal and thoracic trauma associated with spinal cord injury. *J Trauma* 1971; 11:63–75.
35. Romanick PC, Smith TK, Kopaniky DR, Oldfield D: Infection about the spine associated with low-velocity-missile injury to the abdomen. *J Bone Joint Surg* 1985; 67:1195–1201.
36. Jones RE, Bucholz RW, Schaefer SD, et al: Cervical osteomyelitis complicating transpharyngeal gunshot wounds to the neck. *J Trauma* 1979; 19:630–634.
37. Karim NO, Nabors MW, Golocovsky M, Cooney FD: Spontaneous migration of a bullet in the spinal subarachnoid space causing delayed radicular symptoms. *Neurosurgery* 1986; 18:97–100.
38. Malik GM, Sapico FL, Montgomerie JZ: Severe vertebral osteomyelitis in patients with spinal cord injury. *Arch Int Med* 1982; 142:807–808.
39. Mariottini A, Delfini R, Ciappetta P, Paolella G: Lumbar disc hernia secondary to gunshot injury. *Neurosurgery* 1984; 15:73–75.
40. Grogan DP, Bucholz RW: Acute lead intoxication from a bullet in an intervertebral disc space. *J Bone Joint Surg* 1982; 63:1180–1182.
41. Linden MA, Manton WI, Stewart RM, et al: Lead poisoning from retained bullets: Pathogenesis, diagnosis, and management. *Ann Surg* 1982; 195:305–313.
42. Dell M, Baum H: Retained intraspinal bullet—an illustrative case report. *Neurosurg Rev* 1989; 12:67–70.
43. Messer H, Cerza P: Copper jacketed bullets in the central nervous system. *Neuroradiology* 1976; 12:121–129.
44. Wilson, TH: Penetrating trauma of colon, cava, and cord. *J Trauma* 1976; 16:411–413.
45. Little JW, DeLisa JA: Cauda equina injury: Late motor recovery. *Arch Phys Med Rehab* 1986; 67:4547.
46. Comarr A, Kaufman A: A survey of the neurological results of 858 spinal cord injuries: A comparison of patients treated with and without laminectomy. *J Neurosurg* 1956; 13:95–106.
47. Cybulski G, Stone J, Kant R: Outcome of laminectomy for civilian gunshot injuries of the terminal spinal cord and cauda equina: Review of 88 cases. *Neurosurgery* 1989; 24:392–397.
48. De Villiers JC, Grant AR: Stab Wounds at the craniocervical junction. *Neurosurgery* 1985; 17:930–936.
49. Schmidek HH: Comments. "De Villiers JC, Grant AR:

Stab wounds of the craniocervical junction." *Neurosurgery,* 1985; 17:936.

50. Grant JMF, Yeo JD, Sears WR, Copeman MC: Arterial Brown-Séquard's syndrome after a penetrating injury of the spinal cord at the cervicomedullary junction. *Med J Aust* 1985; 142:84–85.
51. Sights WP: Ballistic analysis of shotgun injuries to the central nervous system. *J Neurosurg* 1969; 31:25–33.
52. Smith CML, Timperley WR: Multiple intraspinal and intracranial epidermoids and lipomata following gunshot injury. *Neuropath Appl Neurobiol* 1984; 10:235–239.
53. Daniel EF, Smith GW: Foreign-body granuloma of intervertebral disc and spinal canal. *J Neurosurg* 1960; 17:480–482.
54. Gentleman D, Harrington M: Penetrating injury of the spinal cord. *Injury* 1984; 16:7–8.
55. Simpson RK Jr, Venger BH, Narayan RK: Treatment of acute penetrating injuries of the spine: A retrospective analysis. *J Trauma,* 1989; 29:42–46.
56. Simpson RK Jr, Venger BH, Fischer DK, et al: Shotgun injuries of the spine: Neurosurgical management of five cases. *Br J Neurosurg* 1988; 2:321–326.
57. Robertson DP, Simpson RK Jr, Narayan RK: Lumbar disc herniation from a gunshot wound to the spine: A report of two cases. *Spine* 1991; 16:994–995.
58. Robertson DP, Simpson RK Jr: Penetrating injuries restricted to the cauda equina: A retrospective analysis. *Neurosurgery* 1992; 31:265–270.
59. Venger BH, Simpson RK Jr, Narayan RK: Neurosurgical intervention in penetrating spinal trauma associated with visceral injuries. *J Neurosurg* 1989; 70:514–518.
60. Fischer DK, Simpson RK Jr, Narayan RK, Mattox KL: Shielding of the spinal cord by cervical and facial structures in penetrating trauma. *Neurochirurgia* 1991; 34:37–41.
61. Kislow VA: Clinical peculiarities of war wounds of the spinal cord. *Bull War Med* 1944; 4:705.
62. Post MJ, Green BA, Quencer RM, et al: The value of computed tomography in spinal trauma. *Spine* 1982; 7:417–431.
63. Vogt MW, Narayan RK: The magnetic properties of bullets and other metallic objects as they relate to MRI. *Proceedings of the Annual Meeting of the Congress of Neurological Surgeons.* Baltimore MD, October, 1987.
64. Lieberman JS: Neuromuscular electrodiagnosis, in Youmans JR (ed): *Neurological Surgery.* Philadelphia: WB Saunders, 1982: 617–635.
65. Baskin DS, Simpson RK Jr: Corticomotor and somatosensory evoked potential evaluation of acute spinal cord injury in the rat. *Neurosurgery* 1987; 20:871–877.
66. Simpson RK, Baskin DS: Corticomotor evoked potentials in acute and chronic blunt spinal cord injury in the rat: Correlation with neurological outcome and histological damage. *Neurosurgery* 1987; 20:131–137.
67. Simpson RK, Blackburn JG, Martin HF, Katz S: Peripheral nerve fiber and spinal cord pathway contributions to the somatosensory evoked potential. *Exp Neurol* 1981; 73:700–715.
68. Green BA, Klose KJ: Acute spinal cord injury: Emergency room care and diagnosis, medical and surgical management, in Green BA, Marshall LF, Gallager TJ (eds): *Intensive Care for Neurological Trauma and Disease.* New York: Academic Press, 1982: 249–271.
69. Yashon D: Pharmacological treatment, in Yashon D (ed): *Spinal Injury.* New York: Appleton-Century-Crofts, 1986: 319–332.
70. Simpson RK, Hsu CY, Dimitrijevic MR: The experimental basis for early pharmacological intervention in spinal cord injury. *Paraplegia* 1991; 29:364–372.

CHAPTER 95

SPORTS-RELATED SPINAL CORD INJURY

Robert Cantu
Robert C. Cantu
Jack E. Wilberger, Jr.

SYNOPSIS

"Pro football is a violent, dangerous sport. To play it other than violently would be imbecilic," according to the late Vince Lombardi.[19] *Many sports hold the potential for serious permanent spine and spinal cord injury. Fortunately, the incidence of catastrophic spine and spinal cord injuries has dramatically declined in the past 10 to 15 years. This decline is in part attributable to the development of sports-related spine injuries registries, the elucidation of the pathomechanics of these injuries, and the implementation of appropriate preventive measures. This chapter focuses on sports-related spinal cord and nerve injuries, ranging from the mild "stinger" syndrome to complete quadriplegia. Epidemiology, etiology, and treatment of these injuries will be reviewed, concluding with recommendations on return to competition and prevention.*

EPIDEMIOLOGY

The list of athletic pursuits with the potential for catastrophic injury is extensive.[8,12,13,15,27,29,32] Sports bearing the highest risk of spinal cord injury include: auto racing; motorcycle racing; diving; hang gliding; football; and gymnastics. Sports considered "high-risk" include: horseback riding; ice hockey; mountain climbing; parachuting; ski jumping; sky gliding; snowmobiling; trampolining; and wrestling.[4]

In 1977, the National Collegiate Athletic Association (NCAA) initiated funding for a national survey of catastrophic football injuries, which was conducted at the University of North Carolina at Chapel Hill. In 1982, research was expanded to include all sports for both men and women, and a National Center of Catastrophic Sports Injury Research was established.

Of the school sports, football is associated with the greatest number of catastrophic injuries, but the incidence for injury per 100,000 participants is higher in a number of other sports (Table 95-1). Paralyzing injuries in football have been dramatically reduced when recent data are compared with data from the late 1960s and early 1970s.[23] From 1971 to 1975 there were 259 cervical spine injuries (4.1 per 100,000 players), and 99 cases of permanent quadriplegia (1.58 per 100,000 players). A careful evaluation of the data collected during that time led to the conclusion that one of the main contributing factors was inadequate head protection, and the problem was corrected with helmet redesign. As a result, the head became a primary contact point in blocking and tackling. Identifying this resultant problem provided the primary impetus for 1976 NCAA football rule changes, which were intended to abolish the use of the head as an offensive weapon. After 1978, the incidence of spine injuries (1.3 per 100,000) and quadriplegia (0.4 per 100,000) declined dramatically and have remained relatively stable.[28] There were 12 serious injuries in football in 1991—10 in high school and two in college football. All of the serious cases involved head or neck injuries. Most of the catastrophic injuries in football involve the cervical spine. In a recent review of 34 spinal cord injuries, the most common level involved was C6. Only four of these 34 made a complete recovery.

In gymnastics, the trampoline has been the source of most spine injuries. Zimmerman first called attention to this problem in 1956.[37] However, it was not until 1960 when Ellis and coworkers presented five cases of

TABLE 95-1 High School/College Sports Direct Injuries per 100,000 Participants

	Male		
Sport	**Fatalities**	**Nonfatal***	**Serious****
Baseball	0.07/0.98	0.17/0.00	0.15/0.49
Football	0.25/0.40	0.75/2.00	0.81/6.00
Gymnastics	1.75/0.00	1.75/11.25	0.00/11.15
Ice Hockey	0.43/0.00	1.73/2.48	0.86/7.45
Track	0.17/0.30	0.13/0.60	0.13/0.60
Wrestling	0.08/0.00	0.66/1.31	0.37/0.00

* Nonfatal permanent neurological impairment

** Serious initial neurological impairment with complete recovery

quadriplegia associated with the trampoline and called for the institution of specific regulations for this sport that the magnitude of the problem was recognized.[8] From 1955 through 1978, 114 cases of quadriplegia from trampoline use were reported.[1] Several authors observed that most injuries occurred in experienced, expert, and elite trampolinists. In 1976, the American Academy of Pediatrics issued a policy statement recommending that trampolines be banned from use as part of the physical education program in grammar schools, high schools, and colleges and also be abolished as a competitive sport. In 1978, the NCAA took a less strong position and issued a series of guidelines that recommended optional and voluntary use of the trampoline with increased attention to the risks involved and acquisition of appropriate skills on the equipment. Almost simultaneously, in 1978 the National Gymnastic Catastrophic Injury Registry was established at the University of Illinois to collect data on gymnastics-related spine and spinal cord injuries. Since increased attention has been focused on the problem, only 20 severe injuries have been reported, with 14 occurring on the trampoline. Based on such data, in 1981 the American Academy of Pediatrics softened its stand on banning the trampoline and instead called for a trial period of limited and controlled use.[2]

In the mid-1970s a perceived significant increase in hockey-related spine injuries led to the formation of the Canadian Committee on the Prevention of Spine and Head Injuries Due to Hockey. Tator and Edmonds reported that from 1948 to 1973 there were no spinal cord injuries among hockey players, whereas from 1977 through 1981 hockey became the second most common cause of spinal cord injury resulting from sports or recreational activities.[27] From 1977 through 1983 the Committee documented 42 spine injuries with 28 cases of spinal cord injury. Careful analysis indicated that most resulted from a vertex blow to the head as a result of pushing or checking into uncushioned boards. As a result, in 1983 the Committee issued guidelines aimed at decreasing the incidence of spine injuries in hockey: better enforcement of rules against boarding and cross-checking; institution of rules against pushing or checking from behind; development of neck muscle conditioning programs; better player education regarding neck injuries; and helmet redesign to improve shape and shock absorbency. Primarily as a result of these efforts, spine injuries have decreased by more than 50 percent since 1984.

ETIOLOGY

The propensity of the cervical spine to sports-related injury is borne out by the fact that, in football, all documented spinal cord injuries have occurred in the cervical spine. The pathomechanics of spine injuries in athletes appears to be similar regardless of the sport involved. Until the mid-1970s, hyperflexion of the cervical spine was thought to be the primary mechanism of spine injuries in athletes. However, careful analysis of these injuries by Torg and coworkers clearly established axial loading as the most common important pathophysiological factor.[31] Under normal circumstances, forces transmitted to the cervical spine are primarily dissipated by the cervical muscles, which allow for lateral bending, flexion, and extension. This injury dissipation is most effective with the neck in an anatomic position—slightly extended because of normal cervical lordosis. However, when the neck is slightly flexed (approximately 30°) and the normal lordosis is eliminated, the cervical spine becomes a single, straight, segmented column: thus any forces are transmitted directly to the bones, ligaments, and discs rather than to the muscles. When an athlete's head strikes another player, the ground, or the bottom of a pool, the cervical spine is compressed between the decelerated head and the force of the trunk. When sufficient force is applied, the bones, ligaments, and/or discs fail, resulting in various injuries (Fig. 95-1).[3,29,30]

The validity of this pathophysiology of athletic spine injuries has been underscored by many authors. For example, Scher studied spine injuries in rugby and stated: "When the neck is slightly flexed, the spine is straight. If significant force is applied to the vertex, the force is transmitted down the long axis of the spine. When the force exceeds the energy-absorbing capacity of the structures involved, cervical spine flexion and dislocation will result."[22] Similarly, the most common mechanism of 28 severe hockey-related spinal cord injuries studied by Tator and Edmonds occurred from vertex impacts with the neck slightly flexed.[26] The importance of these pathomechanics is also well established in diving injuries.[26]

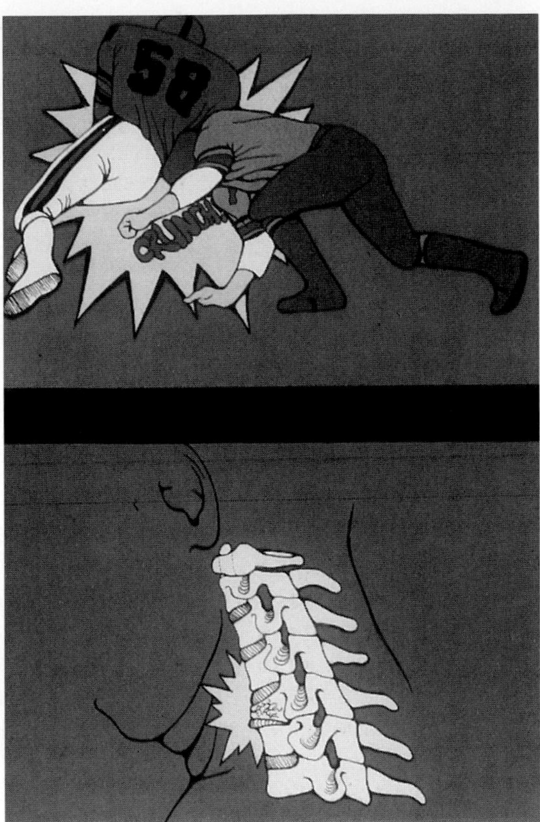

Figure 95-1. Pathomechanics of athletic-related spine and spinal cord injury.

When this mechanism is understood, it becomes clear that athletes occasionally use techniques and maneuvers that may place the cervical spine at risk of injury. Thus, more effective training, conditioning, and preventive measures can be instituted to decrease further the incidence of the more serious injuries.

INJURY CLASSIFICATION AND TREATMENT

There are generally few questions over the management of serious spine or spinal cord injuries in athletes. If the patient is fully conscious, cervical fracture or cervical cord injury usually is accompanied by rigid cervical muscle spasm and pain, which immediately alerts the athlete and the physician to the presence of such an injury. It is the unconscious athlete who is unable to say his neck hurts with lax cervical musculature who is most susceptible to cord injury if one does not think of the possibility of an unstable cervical spine fracture. With an unconscious or obviously neck-injured athlete, it is important that no neck manipulation occur on the field.

The athlete should be carefully questioned about the presence of any neck pain, weakness, numbness, or burning paresthesias. The burning hands syndrome has been classically described in association with athletic spine injury. First elucidated by Maroon in 1977 and refined by Wilberger in 1987, the syndrome is now recognized as a variant of the central cord syndrome.[18,34] The characteristic complaint is of burning paresthesias and dysesthesias in both arms or hands and occasionally in the legs; weakness does not occur. Burning hands syndrome has been associated with a bony or ligamentous spine abnormality in approximately 50 percent of affected individuals. Thus, any athlete with this syndrome should be treated as having a significant spinal cord injury until proven otherwise.

The initial on-field examination is crucial to subsequent evaluation and treatment, and should be limited to assessment for airway patency, adequate circulation, and generalized neurological function. If neurological complaints or findings are short-lived or improve over minutes, then transportation to a medical facility and diagnostic evaluation can proceed in a routine manner. If, however, the athlete is unconscious, complaining of significant ongoing neurological symptoms, or is manifesting any abnormal neurological findings, transportation and treatment must be immediate. In either case, whenever there is a suspicion of spine injury, the athlete should be transported on a fracture board. The head should be secured in a neutral position with the helmet taped to the board. Alternatively, sandbags can be used to stabilize the neck laterally. If available, a rigid cervical collar can be applied. Unless there are significant problems with the athlete's airway and breathing, the helmet should be left in place until it can be carefully removed in a more controlled setting.

STINGERS

"Stingers" or "burners" are colloquial terms used by athletes and trainers to describe a set of symptoms that involve pain, burning, and/or tingling down an arm, occasionally accompanied by localized weakness. The symptoms typically abate within seconds or minutes, rarely persisting for days or longer. It has been estimated that a stinger will occur at least once during the career of over 50 percent of athletes.[6]

There are two typical mechanisms by which stingers may occur—traction on the brachial plexus or nerve root impingement within the cervical neural foramen. The majority of high-school level injuries are of the brachial plexus type, while most at the college level and virtually all in the professional ranks result from a pinch phenomenon within the neural foramen.

The brachial plexus stinger commonly involves a forceful blow to the head from the side, but also can result from head extension or shoulder depression while the head and neck are fixed. Nerve root impingement usually occurs when the athlete's head is driven toward his shoulder pad. The dorsal spinal nerve root ganglion lies close to the posterior intervertebral facet joints, and is pinched when the neural foramen is compressed.

With either type of stinger the athlete experiences a shocklike sensation of pain and numbness radiating into the arm and hand. The symptoms typically are purely sensory in nature, and most commonly involve the C5 and C6 dermatomes. On occasion, weakness also may be present. The most common muscles involved include the deltoid, biceps, supraspinatus, and infraspinatus.

Stingers are always unilateral and almost never involve the lower extremities. Thus, if symptoms are bilateral and/or involve the legs, then the burning hands syndrome with all its implications must be considered.

When not associated with any neck pain or limitation of neck movement, if all motor and sensory symptoms clear within seconds to minutes, the athlete may safely return to competition. This is especially true if the athlete has experienced similar symptoms. If there are any residual symptoms or complaints of neck pain, return should be deferred pending further workup.

On rare occasions a stinger may result in prolonged sensory complaints or weakness. In such a situation an MRI of the cervical spine should be considered to look for a herniated disc or other compressive pathology. If symptoms persist for more than two weeks, then electromyography should allow for an accurate assessment of the degree and extent of injury.

Some athletes seem predisposed to a series of recurrent stingers. It has been suggested that repeated stinger injuries over many years may lead to proximal arm weakness and constant pain. Thus, if an athlete suffers two or more stingers, particularly in rapid succession, consideration can be given to the use of high shoulder pads supplemented by a soft cervical roll, which should limit lateral neck flexion and extension. Examining and/or changing the athlete's blocking and tackling techniques or changing the player's position also may be helpful in preventing recurrences. If, despite these interventions, stingers repeatedly recur, cessation of the causative athletic activity may be necessary.

SERIOUS SPINE INJURY

Case report: a 14-year-old boy sustained a C3–C4 fracture dislocation during competitive diving. No neurological injury occurred. Posterior cervical wiring and fusion were performed, and recovery was uneventful. The patient was not allowed to return to diving but was allowed to participate in other competitive sports. He developed an interest in gymnastics and went on to become a state high school champion by age 18. During one competition while performing on uneven horizontal bars, he fell. Immediate quadriplegia secondary to an odontoid fracture resulted (Fig. 95-2). The patient remained ventilator-dependent.

For athletes who have suffered an unstable fracture or fracture dislocation of the cervical spine and who have undergone spinal fusion, a return to any sport involving risk of further spine injury raises strong concerns. Even in the presence of an apparently stable spine as seen on flexion and extension radiographs, continued participation may not be advisable. While the above case may have been a chance occurrence—an accidental fall from the apparatus is the most common cause of

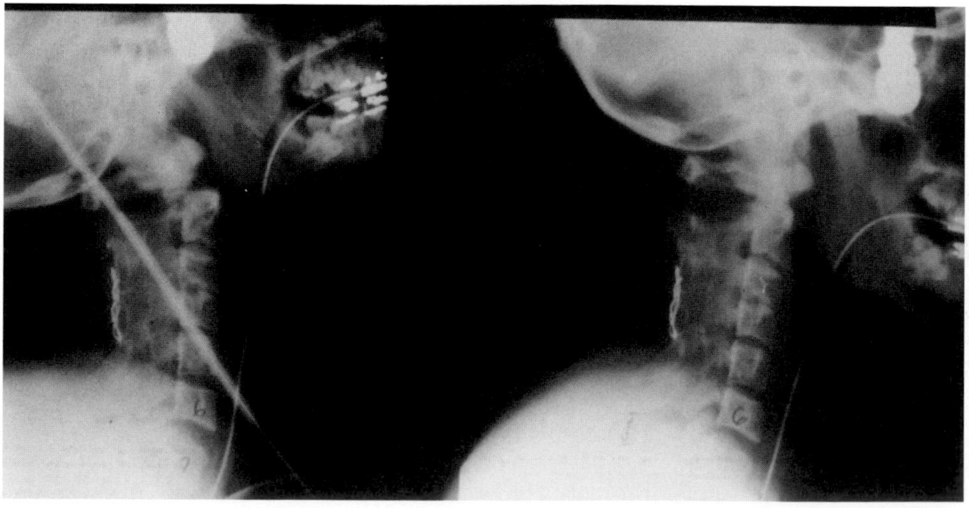

Figure 95-2. Odontoid fracture in an 18-year-old gymnast with prior posterior cervical fusion.

quadriplegia in gymnastics—there are no experimental or clinical data to help physicians predict the stability of healed spinal fractures or fusions when they are placed under extreme degrees of mechanical stress.[33] There is increased mechanical stress above and below fused spinal segments, and repetitive microtrauma to a "stiff" spine exacerbates this stress.[10] Torg and coworkers estimated that the forces involved in a football tackle may approach 18 Gs.[29] Some attempt has been made to assess spinal strength following spinal injury with a Cybex dynamometer.[21] The Cybex has been particularly useful in assessing muscle strength, power, and endurance, but its applicability to the spine has yet to be determined. In fact, there is no evidence that the injured cervical spine is made stronger than normal by fusion. Thus, in the absence of any objective ability to measure the degree of dynamic stress stability of the spine, any healed fracture (with the exception of chip fractures, minor wedge/compression, isolated laminar, or spinous process fractures) and any injury that has required internal stabilization is highly suspect in its ability to withstand further challenges from contact sports.

This raises the question of what competitive sports, if any, a spine-injured athlete could safely resume without significant risk to neurological or spinal integrity. Once again there is little information to guide us. It has been reported that spine surgeons do not feel that fusion of the cervical spine is a contraindication to participation in contact sports unless at C1 or C2. However, laminectomy, disc surgery, and spinal instrumentation have been considered contraindications to continued participation.[13,18] There are a number of college and professional athletes who have had disc surgery or fusions for various nontraumatic reasons (cervical disc disease, spondylosis, spondylolisthesis) and participate without difficulty or apparent increased risk of injury. The American Academy of Pediatrics has classified sports according to degree of contact, impact, and exertion involved in order to help physicians determine the appropriateness of allowing children with serious spine trauma to participate in these endeavors (Table 95-2). Given the lack of any more objective data, these guidelines may be reasonable for adult athletes as well.

TABLE 95-2 American Academy of Pediatrics Sports Classification

Contact/Collision	*Limited Contact/Impact*
Football	Baseball
Boxing	Basketball
Soccer	Diving
Ice Hockey	Gymnastics
Wrestling	Skiing
Strenuous/Noncontact	***Moderate Strenuous/Noncontact***
Aerobics	Badminton
Running	Cycling
Swimming	Table Tennis
Tennis	
Track	
Nonstrenuous/Noncontact	
Archery	
Golf	
Riflery	

MINOR SPINE INJURY

Case report: a 19-year-old linebacker developed neck pain after a hard tackle during a college game. The neurological examination was normal. Cervical x-rays obtained several days later because of persistent neck pain showed a C5 anterior wedge fracture. The athlete was treated with a cervical collar for three months and was advised not to play football for the season. He returned to play the next season. He played for several National Football League and U.S. Football League teams for the next six to seven years without incident until, at age 27, he experienced neck pain and right arm tingling after a tackle on a kickoff play. Results of the neurological examination were normal. Cervical spine films in flexion and extension as well as MRI in flexion and extension showed the old C5 wedge fracture but no new trauma, spinal canal compromise, or evidence of instability. He was allowed to return to football after his symptoms resolved.

As noted previously, there are no definite data that fully assess spinal stress tolerance after injury. The wedge fracture in this patient withstood repeated stress without evidence of long-term instability. Thus, isolated wedge fractures and chip fractures of the vertebral body in the absence of subluxation, laminar fracture, and spinous process fracture would seem to pose no long-term problem once adequate healing has occurred. However, there may be an exception to this general rule if there is greater than 11° of angular deformity of the endplate of the vertebral body fracture compared with the adjoining normal vertebra. White and coworkers suggested that such a degree of deformity may predispose one to chronic instability.[33] When such an injury occurs, the athlete should discontinue all contact and competitive sports for at least six months. If the athlete is asymptomatic and if dynamic films show fracture healing without evidence of instability, then return to competition is unlikely to be associated with a significant risk of further injury.

SPRAIN/STRAIN—LIGAMENTOUS INJURY

Most cervical injuries will involve a ligament sprain, muscle strain, or contusion. With such injuries there is no neurological or osseous injury, and return to competition can occur when the athlete is free of neck pain with and without axial compression, range of motion is full, and the strength of the neck is normal. Cervical x-rays should show no subluxation or abnormal curvatures. If the athlete has a neck profile of maximal weight, they can pull with the neck in flexion, extension, and to each side. It is preferable that they not return to competition until they are asymptomatic and can perform to the level of their preinjury profile.

> *Case report:* a 22-year-old ice hockey forward complained of severe localized neck pain after being cross-checked into the boards during a game. His neurological exam was normal. His cervical spine films in flexion and extension showed 5 mm of active movement at the C2–C3 level. He wore a hard cervical collar for four weeks, by which time his symptoms had resolved. Repeated cervical spine flexion-extension films showed no evidence of ongoing abnormalities. He was allowed to return to hockey after another four weeks. Additional films showed no abnormality.

It is well known that ligament damage may accompany a cervical spine injury and can occur in the absence of bony injury. Generally, this is minor and self-limited, but on occasion it may result in progressive instability, cervical spine deformity, and spinal cord injury. There are guidelines to assist in determining ligament stability. Under normal circumstances, conditions permit very little motion between the cervical vertebrae. In cadaver studies with all ligaments intact, horizontal movement of one vertebral body on the next does not exceed 3.5 mm, and the angular displacement of one vertebral body on the next is always 11° or less. Only when most of the restraining ligaments are injured or destroyed do motions in excess of this occur.[33] In the clinical setting, measurements of the horizontal or angular displacement can be made on neutral or flexion-extension radiographs.

Incipient severe ligamentous injury in the acutely injured athlete may not be recognized because a normal degree of spinal ligamentous laxity in younger patients is generally accepted, and cervical muscle spasm, which may compensate for ligamentous instability, may be present. For these reasons, when any subluxation is seen after a sports-related injury, the patient should wear a hard cervical collar and flexion-extension films of the cervical spine should be repeated two to four weeks after injury. If the films show no evidence of progression or if there is a return to normal, it is unlikely that any significant injury has occurred, and the athlete can most likely return safely to his or her competitive sport.

TRANSIENT NEUROLOGICAL DEFICITS

The development of transient neurological deficit may occur in association with sports. A 1984 survey of over 500 NCAA football programs (with a total of over 39,000 players) found that the incidence of transitory paresis and paresthesias was 1.3 per 10,000 participants and the incidence of numbness and tingling was 6.0 per 10,000 participants.[32]

> *Case report:* a 27-year-old NFL linebacker experienced transient upper and lower extremity paralysis and numbness after tackling a 255-pound opponent. The patient made contact sufficient to dent the forehead portion of his helmet and appeared to sustain an axial load injury with some hyperextension. Paralysis lasted four minutes. Then, over the next 10 to 20 minutes, motor and sensory function returned, beginning in the lower extremities. On arrival at the hospital, the patient was complaining of a burning sensation across his neck and shoulders. He denied any loss of consciousness, and there was no loss of bowel or bladder control. On physical examination, higher cortical functions were intact. Motor exam was 5/5 throughout and reflexes were 2+ and symmetrical, except the ankles, which were 1+ and symmetric. Plantar response was downgoing bilaterally. Sensory exam was intact to light touch and pin prick. Cerebellar exam was intact. Plain films of the cervical spine showed no evidence of fracture, dislocation, subluxation, or degenerative disc disease. The canal

height measured within normal limits: 15 mm at C3–C4; 17 mm at C5; and 20 mm at C6. MRI showed no evidence of fracture, canal compromise, or contusion. Flexion and extension views of the cervical spine showed no instability. Cervical CT and MRI showed a functional reserve of cerebrospinal fluid around the spinal cord (Fig. 95-3).

To determine the relevant risk of future neurological consequences to athletes, Ladd and Scranton conducted a retrospective analysis on 117 quadriplegic athletes studied in the National Football Head and Neck Registry. None reported any episodes of transient motor weakness prior to their permanent cord injury. Only one reported prior transient sensory symptoms.[16]

When faced with an athlete who has suffered a transient neurological deficit, the physician must do a thorough workup to rule out bony or ligamentous injury to the spine. Plain cervical spine films with flexion and extension views are essential. A computed tomography scan and/or polytomography may be necessary to evaluate subtle bony injuries. If no bony or ligamentous abnormalities are identified in a patient with transient neurological deficit, the physician must rule out ongoing extrinsic cord or nerve root compression or intrinsic cord abnormalities. This is most readily accomplished by MRI. Somatosensory evoked potentials also may prove useful in documenting physiological cord dysfunction. Special concerns should be raised if any intrinsic abnormalities are seen on MRI or are documented by somatosensory evoked potentials as this provides direct evidence of an overt, though mild, spinal cord injury and should preclude a return to sports. If no evidence of spinal cord injury is found and no bony or ligamentous problems are identified, then return to competition probably is safe. A second episode of transient neurological deficit should initiate another complete workup. If all the studies remain normal, a return to competition need not be precluded; however, concerns should be raised about the recurrent nature of the problem and consideration given to limiting further athletic activity.

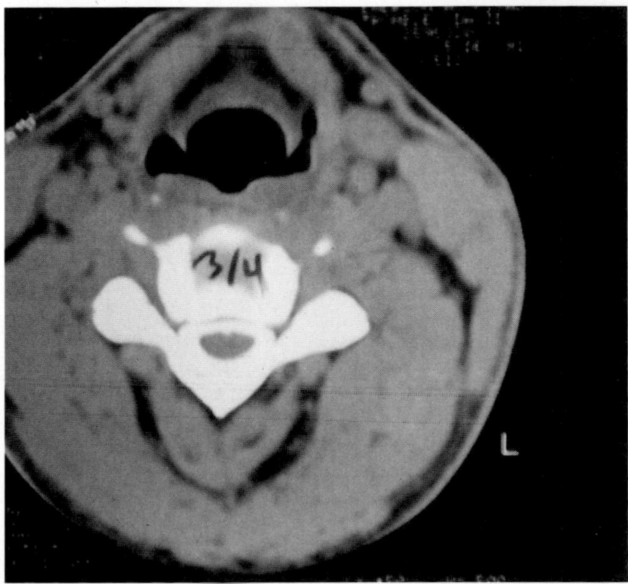

Figure 95-3. Contrast CT showing functional reserve of CSF around the cord at C3–C4.

CERVICAL STENOSIS

Case report: a young male first injured his neck as a high school football player in 1987. Upon making what he remembers to be a head-up tackle, he fell to his side, unable to get up or roll onto his back. Sensation and motor movement were absent from the neck down. Gradually, motor function and sensation returned, first in the feet and then his hands. He could not move his head because of cervical spasm, and any attempt produced jabs of pain running from his neck to his head. After several minutes he was able to stand and walk off the field unassisted, though his legs felt very weak. His neck was rigid on the sidelines and he did not return to play. No x-rays were taken at that time and no medical attention was sought. The patient played the following week with a neck collar. He reported his neck was rigid, and he performed poorly. He did not play the next two weeks owing to continued rigidity and severe neck pain. Three weeks after the injury, because of persistent neck pain and stiffness, he sought medical attention at a sports medicine facility. There, cervical spine x-rays were taken. Though canal heights were not measured, subsequent review of these films revealed canal heights of 12 mm, consistent with spinal stenosis. Two weeks later, the patient returned to competition, his neck pain and stiffness relieved. He played his senior season without further cervical symptoms.

The following fall as a college freshman on a full athletic scholarship, the patient squatted to make a tackle, hitting face-to-face and chest-to-chest. With head tilted up, his face mask made first contact. He fell backward on the ground, unable to move, and had no sensation from the neck down. Over the next few minutes, movement began to return to his right side and he felt patchy sensation to his left side. He was transported to the hospital, where physical examination showed the presence of a Brown-Séquard syndrome with right-sided sensory loss and a nearly flaccid left side. X-rays, CTs, and MRIs were taken. The films revealed cervical stenosis and posterior disc herniation at the C3–C4 level with displacement of the cord and thecal sac to the right. Edema was found within the spinal cord from C2 to C5 (Fig. 95-4). After surgery and extensive rehabilitation, the patient recovered to a spastic quadriparetic state.

Cervical spinal canal stenosis in the athlete may be a developmental or congenital condition or may be caused by acquired degenerative changes in the spine. It is well known that long-term sports participation predisposes the athlete to degenerative changes. When the minimum anteroposterior diameter of the cervical spine in the general population is compared with that of patients with cervical spondylitic myelopathy, it is clear that a substantial number of individuals have a constitutionally narrow spinal canal. The central question, however, is whether a narrow canal alone predisposes to the development of myelopathy. In sports, most attention is focused on developmental spinal stenosis as a result of dramatic cases of spinal cord injury associated with a congenitally small spinal canal in several football players. In spite of this, however, there is little information concerning the risk of an asymptomatic narrow canal in an athlete. Schneider has been quoted as collecting "large series of cases of athletes who sustained an injury to the neck and who were later discovered to have stenosis of the cervical spine." Permanent neurological deficit, quadriplegia, or death occurred in a high percentage of these athletes. However, no details are available from these series.[10,23,24]

In a study at the University of Iowa, all football recruits underwent routine cervical spine films. While multiple preexisting neck injuries were found—disc compression, vertebral body compression fractures, posterior element fractures—no comment was made on the incidence of cervical stenosis.[9] Similarly, while the

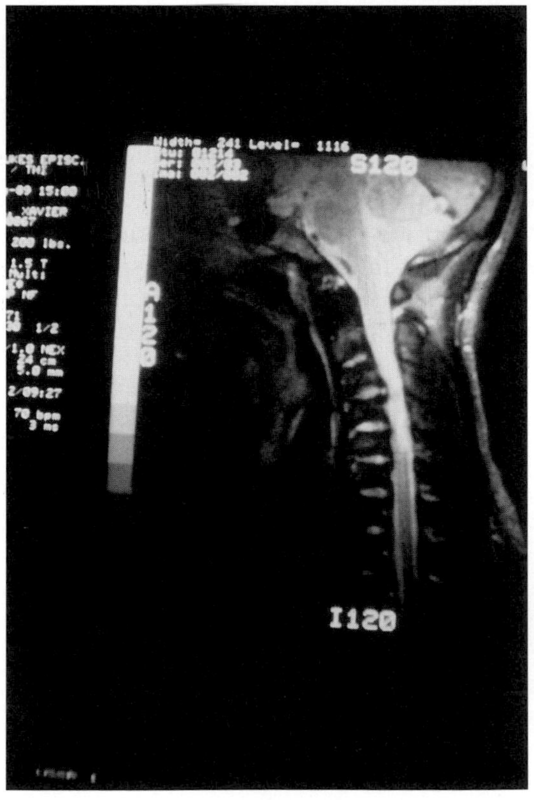

A

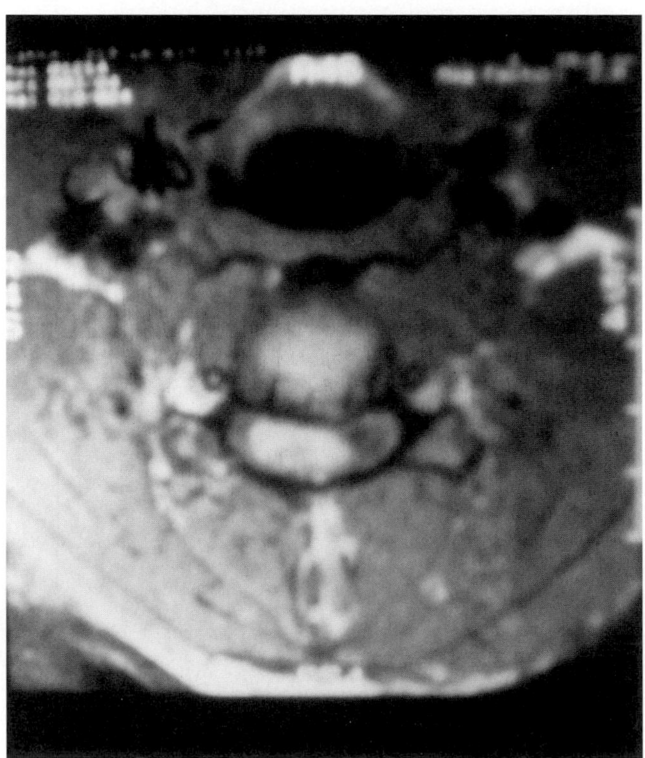

B

Figure 95-4. Sagittal (*A*) and axial (*B*) T2-weighted MRI images demonstrating disc herniation at C3–C4, displacement of spinal cord, poor functional reserve of CSF, and spinal cord ischemia/contusion extending from C2 to C5.

National Football Head and Neck Registry maintains excellent statistics, no specific information is available on the rate of cervical stenosis associated with such injuries.

Some debate exists, however, over the definition of spinal stenosis. In the past, the AP diameter of the spinal canal measured from the posterior aspect of the vertebral body to the most anterior point on the spinal laminar line was used to determine the presence of stenosis. General consensus has been that between C3 and C7, canal heights are normal above 15 mm and spinal stenosis is present below 13 mm. Resnick feels that CT and myelography are the most sensitive diagnostic modalities in determining spinal stenosis.[20] He points out that plain x-rays failed to appraise the width of the spinal cord and thus are not useful when stenosis results from ligamentous hypertrophy or disc protrusion. Ladd and Scranton state that the AP diameter of the spinal canal is "unimportant" if there is total impedance of the contrast medium.[16] They argue that an enhanced myelogram is needed in the injured athlete since CT alone fails to reveal dural compression adequately. Thus, spinal stenosis cannot be defined by bony measurements alone.[14] "Functional" spinal stenosis, defined as loss of the CSF around the cord or in more extreme cases deformation of the spinal cord whether documented by contrast, CT, myelography, or MRI, is a more accurate measure of stenosis. The term "functional" is taken from the radiographic term "functional reserve" as applied to the protective cushion of CSF around the spinal cord in a nonstenotic canal. In a recent study where MRI was used to document the presence or absence of spinal stenosis in 11 athletes rendered quadriplegic, six had functional stenosis.[5]

Anyone with developmental or spondylitic narrowing of the spinal canal is especially at risk for neurological injury during hyperextension.[7] Generally an anteroposterior diameter of less than 15.5 mm and a cross-sectional area of less than 55 mm^2 puts an individual at high risk.[36] When the neck is hyperextended, the sagittal diameter of the spinal canal is further compromised by as much as 30 percent by infolding of the interlaminar ligaments. Thus, it is understood how hyperextension is the mechanism most likely to compromise further an already narrow spinal canal and lead to neurological symptoms. However, as previously noted, axial loading combined with flexion rather than hyperextension is the most important factor in sports-related spinal cord injury. Thus, the athlete might be at less risk than expected.

Whether cervical stenosis in an athlete increases the risk of spinal cord injury has yet to be resolved. Increased attention soon may be focused on this question, and several professional football teams now require detailed investigations of the cervical and lumbar spine (some including MRIs) as a prerequisite to the draft process. Presently there are no good guidelines to help the physician manage an athlete with a narrow asymptomatic cervical spinal canal. When such an abnormality is encountered, management must be individualized according to the patient's symptoms, the degree of canal stenosis, and the perceived risk of permanent neurological injury.

CONCLUSION

Careful study of the pathomechanics and epidemiology of sports-related spine injuries brings to light many common features. The incidence increases as the sport becomes increasingly violent and aggressive. Improperly conditioned neck muscles and lack of knowledge of the proper techniques of the sport put the athlete who sustains a blow to the head at significant risk for a spine injury. Improper helmet fit and the use of the head as an offensive weapon are also common features. While recognition of these features has resulted in a dramatic reduction in catastrophic athletic spine injury, the athlete remains at risk for less severe spine injury.

General guidelines can be formulated for the management of athletes with stably healed major or minor spine fractures, transient neurological deficits, and asymptomatic cervical stenosis. However, the decision to allow a return to competitive sports must be individualized. Thus, when such injuries occur, the physician must consider spine and spinal cord integrity as well as the athlete's expectations of future sports participation.

References

1. American Academy of Pediatrics Committee on Accident and Poison Prevention: *Trampolines.* Evanston IL: American Academy of Pediatrics, 1976.
2. American Academy of Pediatrics Committee on Accident and Poison Prevention and Committee on Pediatric Aspects of Physical Fitness, Recreation and Sports: *Trampoline II. Pediatrics* 1981; 67:438–439.
3. Burstein AW, Otis JC, Torg JS: Mechanisms and pathogenics of athletic injuries to the cervical spine, in Torg JS (ed): *Athletic Injuries to the Head, Neck and Face.* Philadelphia: Lea & Fibiger, 1982: 119–149.
4. Cantu RC: Head and spine injuries in the young athlete, in Micheli LJ (ed): *Injuries in the Young Athlete.* Philadelphia: WB Saunders, 1988: 459–472.
5. Cantu RC: Functional cervical spinal stenosis: A contraindication to participation in contact sports. *Med Sci Sports Exerc* 1993; 25(3).

6. Clark KS: Prevention: an epidemiologic view, in Torg JS (ed): *Athletic Injuries to the Head, Neck and Face.* Philadelphia: Lea & Fibiger, 1982: 15–26.
7. Eismont FJ, Clifford S, Goldberg M, et al: Cervical sagittal spinal canal size in spinal injury. *Spine* 1984; 9:663–666.
8. Ellis WB, Green D, Holzatfel NR, et al: The trampoline in serious neurological injuries: A report of five cases. *JAMA* 1960; 174:1673–1676.
9. Feldick HG, Albright JP: Football survey reveals "missed" neck injuries. *Physician Sports Med* 1976; 4:77–81.
10. Firooznia H, Ahn J, Rafii M, et al: Sudden quadriplegia after a minor trauma: The role of pre-existing spinal stenosis. *Surg Neurol* 1985; 23:165–168.
11. Friedman RJ, Micheli LJ: Acquired spondylolisthesis following scoliosis surgery. *Clin Orthop* 1981; 190:132–135.
12. Frykman G, Hilding S, Hopp PA: Studs matta kan orsaka allvarlig. *Skador Lakartidingen* 1970; 67:5862–5864.
13. Funk FJ, Wells RE: Injuries of the cervical spine in football. *Clin Orthop* 1975; 109:50–58.
14. Herzog RJ, Weins JJ, Dillingham MF, Sontag MJ: Normal cervical spine morphometry and cervical spinal stenosis in asymptomatic professional football players. *Spine* 1991; 16:178–186.
15. Kewalramani LS, Taylor RG: Injuries to the cervical spine from diving accidents. *J Trauma* 1975; 15:130–142.
16. Ladd AL, Scranton PE: Congenital cervical stenosis presenting as transient quadriplegia in athletes. *J Bone Joint Surg* 1986; 68:1371–1374.
17. Maroon JC: Burning hands and football spinal cord injury. *JAMA* 1977; 238:2049–2051.
18. Micheli LJ: Sports following spinal surgery in the young athlete. *Clin Orthop Rel Res* 1985; 198:152–157.
19. O'Brien M: *Vince—a Personal Biography of Vince Lombardi.* New York: Morrow, 1987: 16.
20. Resnick D: Degenerative disease of the spine, in *Diagnosis of Bone and Joint Disorders.* Philadelphia: WB Saunders, 1981: 1408–1415.
21. Rolander SD: Motion of the lumbar spine with special reference to the stabilizing effect of a posterior fusion. *Acta Orthop Scand* 1966; (suppl) 9E:1–6.
22. Scher AT: Vertex impact in cervical dislocation in rugby players. *South African Med J* 1981; 59:227–228.
23. Schneider RS, Reifel E, Grisler H, et al: Serious and fatal football injuries involving the head and spinal cord. *JAMA* 1961; 177:362–367.
24. Schneider RC: Serious and fatal neurosurgical football injuries. *Clin Neurosurg* 1966; 12:226–236.
25. Tator CH, Edmonds VE, Duncan EG: Catastrophic sports and recreational injuries in Ontario: Causes and prevention. American Association of Neurological Surgeons Annual Meeting, Washington, 1989.
26. Tator CH, Edmonds VE, New ML: Diving: A frequent and preventable cause of spinal cord injury. *Can Med Assoc J* 1981; 124:1323–1324.
27. Tator CH, Edmonds VE: National survey of spinal injuries in hockey players. *Can Med Assoc J* 1984; 130:875–880.
28. Torg JS, Vegso JJ, Sennett B, et al: The National Football Head and Neck Injury Registry: Fourteen-year report of cervical quadriplegia, 1971–1984. *JAMA* 1985; 254:3439–3443.
29. Torg JS, Yu A, Pavlov H, et al: Cervical quadriplegia resulting from axial loading injuries. Cinematographic, radiographic, kinematic and pathologic analysis. *Orthop Trans* (to be published).
30. Torg JS: Epidemiology, pathomechanics and prevention of athletic injuries to the cervical spine. *Med Sci Sports Exerc* 1985; 17:295–303.
31. Torg JS, Pavlov H, Genuano SE, et al: Neuropraxia of the cervical spinal cord with transient quadriplegia. *J Bone Joint Surg* 1986; 68A:1354–1370.
32. Torg JS, Das M: Trampoline-related quadriplegia: Review of the literature and reflections on the American Academy of Pediatrics position statement. *Pediatrics* 1984; 74:804–812.
33. White AA, Johnson RM, Panjabi MM, et al: Biomechanical analysis of clinical stability in the cervical spine. *Clin Orthop Rel Res* 1975; 109:85–96.
34. Wilberger JE, Maroon JC: Burning hands syndrome revisited. *Neurosurgery* 1987; 20:599–605.
35. Wilberger JE, Maroon JC: Cervical spine injuries in athletes. *Physician Sports Med* 1990; 18:27–47.
36. Yu YL, Stevens JM, Kendal B, et al: Cord shape and measurements in cervical spondylitic myelopathy and radiculopathy. *Am J Neuroradiol* 1983; 4:839–842.
37. Zimmerman HM: Accident experience with trampolines. *Res Q* 1956; 27:452–455.

CHAPTER 96

CHRONIC PAIN ASSOCIATED WITH SPINAL CORD INJURY

Paul G. Loubser
William H. Donovan

SYNOPSIS

Chronic pain is a significant problem among patients with spinal cord injury (SCI). The reported prevalence varies widely, although clinical studies using accepted pain measurement tools and adequate controls are generally lacking. Two major categories of chronic SCI pain are identified—neurological and nonneurological. Segmental, central, and visceral pain comprise the neurological group, while musculoskeletal and psychogenic pain fall within the nonneurological category. Mechanisms of nociception underlying chronic SCI pain are not generally agreed upon, although magnetic resonance imaging, clinical neurophysiological testing, and diagnostic regional anesthesia may elucidate the source of pain. Treatment involves maximizing rehabilitative function with physical modalities and oral pharmacological agents, including nonnarcotic analgesics, antidepressants, and anticonvulsants. Dorsal root entry zone (DREZ) lesioning of affected segments is an accepted surgical treatment modality for chronic SCI pain. The use of epidural spinal cord stimulation has been associated with mixed results; intrathecal pharmacotherapy represents a promising new avenue for future research.

HISTORICAL PERSPECTIVES

The care of patients with spinal cord injury (SCI) has undergone dramatic improvements in the last 20 years. However, chronic pain management in SCI patients continues to be a difficult clinical problem for primary care physicians who, while seeking to alleviate pain and suffering, also must attempt to preserve all remaining neurological function and as much capability for independent daily living as possible. Experienced practitioners specializing in pain management uniformly regard chronic pain following SCI as being one of the most complex pain problems, often proving refractory to medical and surgical treatment. Many references describe various clinical syndromes, the prevalence of these syndromes in particular patient populations, and different hypotheses of nociception. However, it is clear that placebo-controlled studies that compare various treatments and use accepted pain measurement tools and double-blind based protocols are few and far between.

Undoubtedly, one factor responsible for the paucity of objective data on chronic SCI pain has been the medical practitioner's difficulty in recognizing that pain may occur in areas insensate to cutaneous stimulation. The early references to SCI pain having a "phantom" quality indicated that some manner of imagination was active or that these symptoms were sinister. More recently, these sensations have been collectively regarded as "altered sensations" or "discomfort," but standardized terminology and nosologies acceptable to the disciplines involved in chronic SCI pain are lacking. Furthermore, few multidisciplinary pain treatment programs focus exclusively on chronic SCI pain. However, recent research advances in the field of pain of spinal cord origin are providing important leads and new foundations for clinical strategies. These have been augmented by the recent surge of interest in neuraxial stimulation and spinal pharmacological treatments using implanted devices. We attempt to elucidate further what is currently known about chronic SCI pain, what treatments are currently available, and what future directions exist.

Scope of the Problem

Prevalence

The prevalence of chronic pain following SCI has been the subject of several studies, although large variations in the reported incidence appear to be related to the pain assessment methodology, i.e., the subjective techniques that use verbal reports to estimate pain severity. Botterell reported that 94 percent of 125 SCI patients experienced pain; 30 percent of these reported that the pain was disabling.[10] Woolsey reported that 67 percent of SCI patients experienced pain, which was severe in 18 percent.[68] In the largest published clinical series, Davis reported that 126 out of 471 patients reported pain so severe as to require active steps, including anterolateral cordotomy, paravertebral alcohol injection, and systemic ammonium chloride infusion.[18] In all three studies, a lower incidence of pain was noted in cervical injuries compared with injuries to the thoracic spine and cauda equina. In contrast, Holmes found a higher incidence of pain in cervical SCI.[34] Richards reported a 77 percent incidence of pain in 75 SCI patients, with greater severity associated with greater age, intelligence, anxiety, and a more negative psychosocial situation.[57] Nepomuceno surveyed 200 SCI patients: while only 25 percent reported the intensity of pain as severe, 44 percent of the respondents indicated that pain did interfere with their daily activities.[53] Burke's classic study comparing pain in SCI patients in Australia and the United States, reported incidences of 14 and 45 percent, respectively.[11] This study further showed a higher incidence of pain in association with laminectomy and delayed hospital admission. Frisbie found 55 incidents of pain in 66 patients surveyed (83 percent) with chronic pain, 58 percent of whom regarded it as severe.[26] Lamid compared two groups of SCI patients, one inpatient and one outpatient, using self-rating pain measurements, an activity check list, and a drug-use rating scale.[39] They found an almost fourfold higher incidence of pain in inpatients. In a carefully conducted pain assessment, Beric evaluated 178 SCI patients and found that 88 patients (49 percent) complained of pain and altered sensations.[3] Pain also occurred less frequently in cervical SCI patients in this series. Rintala as part of a large study examining community-based services for SCI patients completed a telephone survey of 640 patients with SCI in which 350 patients were asked to report on their pain.[60] One hundred and eight (31 percent) of the respondents (31 male, 78 female) reported the presence of severe pain. More pain was observed in paraplegics than quadriplegics in this study also. A postal survey of 615 patients by Rose produced some sobering data—16 percent reported that it was their pain, not their paralysis, that prevented them from working.[62] Eighty-three percent of those working reported that pain interfered with work, and 59 percent reported that pain produced sleep disturbance. Richards studied 56 SCI patients and found a higher incidence of pain in patients with bullet injuries.[58] This finding agrees with those reported by Rintala, who similarly found a higher incidence of pain in patients with SCI as a result of violence. Davidoff as well, comparing 19 SCI patients with function-limiting dysesthetic pain to a cohort of 147 SCI patients, discovered a higher incidence of pain among those injured by gunshot and among those with incomplete injuries.[16] A study by Cohen on 49 SCI patients indicated that pain following SCI was regarded as less of a threat to general well-being, compared with a group of patients with chronic pain secondary to other disorders.[13] This study further suggested that the Minnesota Multiphasic Personality Inventory was not a valid measure of the impact of pain in patients with SCI. Eighty-five SCI males were studied by Dew to evaluate the contribution of physical versus psychological variables to individual's long-term perceptions of themselves.[20] A higher level of education and a longer duration of hospitalization were associated with higher levels of perceived pain. Summers evaluated psychosocial factors in 54 SCI patients using a variety of questionnaires and psychological assessment tools,[64] demonstrating that anger and negative cognitions were associated with greater pain severity.

Studies that rely on self-reporting techniques include many variables and subjective factors that influence the accuracy of the results. Furthermore, new definitions of pain have recently emerged so that what one author termed "phantom pain," may now be regarded as "central pain." This may account for the wide range (5 to 94 percent) of reported incidences of chronic SCI pain in several studies.[12] In addition, grading the severity of pain is very difficult because no objective pain scales are widely available. Therefore, other yardsticks must be used, such as the amount of medication ingested or the effect on functional status. Nonetheless, the bulk of the evidence extant suggests that between 30 and 40 percent of people with SCI experience severe, disabling pain.

Aggravation of Disability

The World Health Organization's (WHO) recent classification of impairment, disability, and handicap places in perspective the potential effect that chronic pain has on the SCI patient.[69] In the WHO model, impairment is defined as "any loss or abnormality of psychological, physiological or anatomical structure or function." Disability is defined as "any restriction or lack of ability (resulting from an impairment) to perform an activity in the manner or within the range considered normal for a human being." Handicap is defined as "a disadvantage, for a given individual, resulting from an impairment or a disability, that limits or prevents the fulfillment of a role that is normal." Applying this model to

SCI, paralysis and sensory loss produced by SCI is the primary impairment, in turn producing disabilities in such areas as personal care, mobility, and dexterity. In SCI, handicap in the following areas bears special relevance to chronic pain: occupation; social integration; and economic self-sufficiency. Building on the WHO model and applying this to the SCI rehabilitation model, one may conclude that chronic pain imposes an additional handicap for a given degree of disability. Rehabilitation on the one hand, aims at minimizing disability for a given degree of impairment, while on the other hand it concentrates on minimizing handicap for a given degree of disability. Within this context, the significance of chronic SCI pain on the overall function of the patient is multidimensional, since it impedes not only restoration of maximal function for a given degree of disability, but also affects quality of life, including emotional stability, ability to work, and social reintegration.

Clinical Presentation

As stated previously, several clinical syndromes have been described, each with several subtypes. There is as yet no uniformly agreed upon classification system available to practitioners providing medical care to patients with SCI. The terms "neuropathic," "neurogenic," and "deafferentation" abound in the literature, although not often used by those involved in SCI medicine. From a practical standpoint, chronic SCI pain can be divided into discrete entities using either phenomenological or etiological approaches. It must be remembered, however, that not all pain experienced in SCI people is neuropathic.

Syndromes

One of the best-known syndromes of SCI pain involves the wide distribution of burning, dysesthetic pain below the level of SCI. These dysesthesias may occur in conjunction with such altered sensations as allodynia and hyperpathia. Several different terms have been used to describe this type of pain, including phantom pain syndrome, function-limiting dysesthetic pain syndrome, and central dysesthesia (deafferentation) syndrome.

Cauda equina or *conus-cauda equina syndrome* refers to a collection of pain symptomatologies resulting from injuries to the distal portion of the spinal cord. Pain occurs typically in the buttocks, perineum, and/or lower extremities, often with combinations of dysesthesias and neuralgic pain in the thighs, calves, or feet.

A further variant has been termed "double lesion syndrome" by neurophysiologists to describe the presence of an occult lumbosacral lesion in conjunction with an incomplete cervical SCI.[4]

Transitional zone pain refers to pain that occurs at or just caudad to the sensory level of anesthesia. Within the area that pain is perceived, sensation may be absent or altered. It is frequently described as being tight, burning, cramping, and bilateral. This has also been termed "junctional" pain by some practitioners. A variation of this, termed "end-zone" pain, refers to pain that is segmental in nature, follows a sclerotomal or musculoskeletal distribution, but is unilateral and asymmetrical.

Classification

Chronic SCI pain may be divided into several major categories. The syndromes described above fall into each of these categories. Burke originally described three categories of SCI pain: root pain; visceral pain; and dysesthesia.[11] Donovan labeled five discrete categories as follows: segmental; central; visceral; musculoskeletal; and psychogenic.[21] Essentially, chronic SCI pain may be divided into two major categories—neurological and nonneurological. Neurological pain, also termed neuropathic, neurogenic, or deafferentation pain, comprises the segmental, central, and visceral categories. Nonneurological pain comprises the musculoskeletal and psychogenic categories.

Musculoskeletal

Also referred to as "orthopedic" pain or "nociceptive" pain by some practitioners, this form of pain occurs secondary to stimulation or irritation of nociceptors within bone, muscle, and soft tissues. A myriad of etiological factors can cause this pain in SCI patients, including muscle atrophy, muscle weakness, muscle and joint contractures, arthritic changes (particularly in the facet joints), and sequelae of surgery (spinal instrumentation and fusion, laminectomy, etc.). Also included in this category are myofascial pain syndromes, fibromyalgias, and other arthritic conditions associated primarily with immobility secondary to SCI. When present, they may confuse examiners because the pain may be felt below the neurological level of injury. The neurological level however, is determined from examination of sensation in the skin. Innervation of deeper structures does not necessarily conform to innervation of the skin. Thus, pain arising from strain of the latissimus dorsi may be felt in the back or side of the trunk in a C7 "complete" quadriplegic. Spasticity may also produce discomfort and cramping sensations in the lower extremities and abdominal muscles for those retaining innervation of parts of those structures.

Segmental

Also termed "radicular" or "peripheral," this pain follows a segmental or dermatomal distribution, and is secondary to involvement of particular nerve root radicles. As described above, this includes transitional zone pain, cauda equina syndrome, etc. The dermatomal distribution of pain suggests mechanical nerve root impingement, traction, entrapment, or distortion by either bone or meningeal scarring. It is not clearly known whether involvement of nerve roots is associated with aberrant conduction/processing of sensory input within the dorsal horn cell or substantia gelatinosa.

Central Pain

The delineation of central pain following SCI and other forms of neurological injury is an area that is now generating considerable interest and research. The term "central" is used to denote that the origin of nociception occurs within the spinal cord, i.e., proximal to nerve roots (which are part of the peripheral nervous system). It may involve the dorsal horn cells, including the substantia gelatinosa, diffusely and/or any level of ascending somatosensory tracts at more than one location, including the lower brainstem or thalamus. Central pain is typically described as burning or stinging in quality and can be extremely disabling. It is diffuse and therefore does not follow a dermatomal distribution; it has no definite symmetry or radiation pattern, and may fluctuate in response to weather, diurnal rhythms, emotional status, and may be worsened by the slightest movements.

Visceral Pain

Abdominal pain may occur in high-thoracic and cervical SCI patients despite varying degrees of sensory anesthesia and/or paralysis. Despite interruption of spinal sensory pathways, autonomic connections to the viscera and mesentery may remain intact, e.g., via the vagus nerve or via the sympathetic chain. In most cases, a comprehensive diagnostic workup will point to the source of pain, i.e., gallbladder, bowel, bladder, kidney, etc., and appropriate treatment will alleviate pain. However, a study by Juler of 36 SCI patients with visceral disease suggests that the diagnosis may be delayed in spinal injuries above the splanchnic outflow.[35] Sometimes no apparent etiology or source of pain may be identified. This form of chronic visceral pain is "idiopathic" and poorly understood. Little is known about its exact prevalence and its significance to patients with SCI. However, it may represent a form of central pain.

Psychogenic

This pain is associated with obvious psychsomatic or psychiatric disturbances. True psychogenic pain syndromes such as somatization disorder, conversion disorder, hypochondriasis, and factitious disorder are not specifically unique to patients with SCI. Factors such as depression, anxiety, attention-seeking behavior, secondary-gain, and addiction clearly will influence the severity of pain symptomatologies, and are probably present to some degree in many patients with chronic SCI pain. Depression and substance addiction can lower one's pain threshold and interfere with coping mechanisms. Therefore, it is important for the clinician to determine early on, if the pain is perceived as "worse," whether this represents an intensification of noxious stimuli or a decreased ability to cope with the usual intensity. Our experience using diagnostic spinal anesthesia to assess SCI pain has been helpful in this regard and has yielded surprisingly low incidence of placebo responses, suggesting that psychological factors alone are not as significant as previously thought.[45]

Other

Several other pain disorders may occur quite frequently but are not included in standard classifications. Sympathetically maintained pain (SMP), also known as reflex sympathetic dystrophy and causalgia, is divided into three distinct stages based on chronicity and autonomic disturbances.[1,14] The Roberts hypothesis, which suggests that SMP occurs secondary to hyperresponsiveness of dorsal horn cells innervated by unmyelinated C fibers over A-delta afferents from mechanoreceptors, is widely accepted.[61] However, the exact role that SMP plays in chronic SCI pain is unclear. Sympathetic blocks and/or surgical sympathectomy have achieved variable success.[12] However, there are several similarities between SMP and neuropathic SCI pain, and recent evidence suggests that it may be an important cause of upper extremity pain and swelling in quadriplegics.[28,67]

THEORIES OF ORIGIN

Central pain following SCI remains an area of ongoing research and speculation. Thus far, most research has focused on the subject of deafferentation pain, the results of which may be applied to chronic SCI pain. Two broad approaches are identifiable from the literature, one being neurophysiological and the other neuropharmacological.[56,66]

Neurophysiological Mechanisms

Several hypotheses have been forwarded to explain central pain, including irritation of spinothalamic and lemniscal systems, irritation of the sympathetic system, diversion of pain impulses to the hypothalamus, loss of inhibitory thalamic pain mechanisms, and activation of secondary pathways.[56] Levitt and Pagni further differentiate central and peripheral deafferentation pain states.[40,56] However, one of the most plausible theories is one put forward by Melzack and Loeser, who suggested that central pain occurred secondary to "pattern-generating mechanisms" emanating from dorsal horn cells and the somatosensory projection systems.[49] These mechanisms are thought to occur at multiple levels above the level of spinal injury.[43] A more recent hypothesis, proposed by Beric, suggests that in patients with incomplete SCI lesions disproportionate transmission of spinothalamic and dorsal column information to the thalamus and lower brainstem results in widespread dysesthesias.[5]

Neuropharmacology

Ascending and descending spinal cord function derives from a composite myriad of nerve fibers, receptors, neurotransmitters, and ligands. Different classes of receptors including opioid, adrenergic, serotonergic, glycinergic, and GABAergic modulate activity of the dorsal horn.[47] Animal research has focused on determining whether agonists and antagonists applied intrathecally have any effect on sensory processing.[15] However, the complexity of applying this information to SCI pain makes the securing of a good animal model very difficult. Allodynia evoked by the local intrathecal action of strychnine in animals is similar to pain associated with spinal cord injury.[70] Yaksh's studies with various spinal agonists and antagonists suggest that trophic changes in glycine receptor function is predominantly implicated in this form of pain.[70] GABA is also thought to play an important role, although our clinical experiences with its intrathecal application for spasticity control suggest that it is not an effective antinociceptive agent for dysesthesias associated with SCI.[46] The use of opiates, encephalins, or endorphins in neuropathic SCI pain is controversial. Most research has shown that opiates are uniformly inefficient in relieving neuropathic pain,[2] although recent animal evidence suggests that larger doses may be needed to compensate for the loss of presynaptic mu receptors.[7] Very little information exists with regard to the neuraxial application of opioids or other agents. Glynn et al. reported their experiences with epidural morphine, a mu agonist; buprenorphine, a kappa agonist; and clonidine, an alpha-adrenergic agonist, in 15 patients with chronic deafferentation pain secondary to SCI.[32] Five patients reported pain relief following epidural morphine, while an additional two patients reported pain relief following epidural buprenorphine.[32] However, the use of neuraxial opioids for chronic SCI pain is an unresearched area where factors such as patient selection, health care costs, and drug tolerance are important issues. Stevens recently demonstrated in rats using a chronic intrathecal infusion model, that sufentanil was associated with less receptor down-regulation and "tolerance" compared to other narcotic agents.[63] An additional neurotransmitter involved in both central and peripheral nociceptive transmission is substance P. Capsaicin, available as a cream, has been demonstrated to deplete unmyelinated C fibers of substance P, in turn producing analgesia in various neuropathic pain conditions such as a diabetic neuropathy, herpetic neuralgia, and rheumatoid arthritis.[6] Its efficacy in SCI pain is still unknown.

Factors Intensifying Pain

Several clinical studies and our own experience demonstrate that the severity of pain perception is influenced by many factors including those associated with increased nociceptive spinal input, just as is found in the able bodied, e.g., bladder infection, paronychia, and urolithiasis. Other factors such as spasticity, the weather, and one's psychological status, i.e., anxiety and depression also influence the perception of pain, the latter perhaps by lowering the pain threshold. Exercise, work, and other distractions can affect pain perception by competing for attention from cognitive centers.

DIAGNOSIS

Clinical Assessment

The patient's initial perception of discomfort and/or altered sensations in relation to the actual SCI will assist the practitioner in characterizing the pain. Burke divided SCI pain into "early" and "late" forms, the early form reflecting the tissues' responses to acute injury. As in other forms of injury this generally passes quickly and should no longer be present after several weeks. Pain may be considered chronic when it has been present for over 6 months, whether its duration is based on the patient's reports or a physician's observations. As with any chronic pain condition, a thorough clinical assessment should provide information about the character, frequency, and distribution of pain. Descriptive words should be noted such as aching, burning, stinging, stabbing, etc., in order to determine whether pain is dysesthetic or neuralgic in quality. A pain diary, in which the patient keeps daily records of pain symptomatology may shed light on special factors such as sleep disturbance and interference with activity patterns. The relationship between pain and activity, rest, and posture should be clearly identified, as well as medication ingestion patterns. Factors decreasing or aggravating pain should be recorded. While the physician should be aware of the distinct pain entities discussed above, frequently one may see a combination of pain symptomatologies. Patients may complain of episodic lightning pains down a particular lower extremity, while superimposed on this, he/she feels a continuous background of burning pain. Physical examination should identify typical clinical signs that may point to a particular pain category, such as joint pain, trigger points, allodynia, hyperpathia, or vasomotor and sudomotor changes. Several pain measurement tools are available to the clinician, such as the traditional 10-cm visual analogue scale, pain distribution diagram, the McGill Pain Questionnaire, the Sternbach Pain and Intensity Profile, the Zung Pain and Distress Scale, etc. Their use often assists the practitioner in following patients over extended intervals, so that serial comparisons of pain severity and response to treatment can be performed.

In addition, it is imperative that an appraisal of the patient's psychological condition be performed, so that obvious psychological conditions can be identified and treated. In particular, it must be recognized that factors such as secondary gain or drug-seeking behavior will significantly affect the severity and chronicity of the pain. Depression, anxiety, and addiction will require a psychiatrist's consultation, since successful treatment of chronic SCI pain can be difficult to impossible in the presence of these conditions.

Once the clinical nature of pain has been determined, the practitioner may be able to decide if the pain is neurological or nonneurological. However, if not initially discernible on clinical grounds, additional testing may be indicated.

Diagnostic Procedures

Magnetic resonance imaging (MRI)

Syrinx formation in the spinal cord (posttraumatic syringomyelia) rostral to the spinal cord lesion, may present with ascending sensory loss and motor weakness. Frisbie reviewed 55 occurrences of chronic SCI pain, and demonstrated 11 of these to be associated with syringomyelia.[26] Using clinical criteria, pain due to syringomyelia may begin below the level of SCI in incomplete lesions. However, when this pain ascends above the level of paralysis a syrinx should strongly be suspected. MRI is then indicated to confirm the presence of a syrinx. Pain associated with syringomyelia is usually effectively alleviated by surgical drainage of the cyst.

Clinical neurophysiology

Several clinical neurophysiological tests may also assist in the diagnosis of SCI pain syndromes. According to Beric, central dysesthesia syndrome may be diagnosed by correlating clinical signs with evidence of disproportionate spinothalamic and posterior column function.[5] This may be determined by performing discrete sensory quantification studies in the areas of pain. Using a Marstock stimulator, the response to heat and cold pain and to vibration is assessed and measured. This provides information about the balance of ascending spinal cord transmission of impulses.[27] The demonstration of abnormal lumbar somatosensory evoked potentials in an incomplete quadriplegic or high paraplegic may provide clues as to the presence of an occult lumbosacral lesion (double-lesion syndrome), in those who present with lower extremity or perineal segmental pain.[4] Some of the patients will also have areflexic bladders. The use of various electrical parameters of percutaneous electrical stimulation in painful areas may also shed light on whether increasing sensory input from a certain area improves or aggravates pain. This information may be helpful in subsequent treatment with transcutaneous electrical nerve stimulation (TENS).

Regional anesthetics

The use of local anesthetic agents in the assessment and management of chronic SCI pain is quite commonplace.[8] A diagnostic regional anesthetic is performed by injecting the agent at a particular anatomic site, usually in close proximity to a particular nerve or nerve plexus. The use of an electrical stimulator and stimulating needle assists the practitioner in precise localization of the nerve. Confirmation of adequate conduction blockade is obtained by demonstration of sensory anesthesia, motor paralysis, or temperature change. Several factors may be manipulated in order to vary the regional anesthetic including the type of local anesthetic, its concentration, the volume, or the addition of vasoconstrictor agents. Duration of conduction blockade may vary according to these parameters.

Regional anesthetics shed light on mechanisms of nociception. The cessation of pain following conduction blockade suggests that the source of nociception emanates from the area included within the distribution of the regional anesthetic.[36] In contrast, a negative response suggests that the origin of nociception occurs proximal to the area of conduction blockade, possibly even "centrally." However, the response to a particular procedure should not be considered completely indicative of a certain pain mechanism. Confirmation of adequate conduction blockade may be more difficult in patients with varying degrees of sensory anesthesia following SCI, particularly in complete SCI patients. Several subjective factors may confound the response to conduction blockade. It is important to compare a positive response following a particular local anesthetic to a placebo agent (saline) to exclude false-positive responses. Similarly, a negative response to a local anesthetic may be repeated at a different time to exclude false-negative responses. Systemic effects of local anesthetics may also influence the perception of pain, so that total dosage of local anesthetic should be kept to a minimum. It should also be borne in mind that a positive response to a placebo should not be used to "label" a pain as being psychogenic. Mount demonstrated that 35 percent of patients exhibit placebo responses when tested with a variety of agents.[50] The duration of response to a local anesthetic may also outlast the predicted or expected duration of action for that local anesthetic, termed "carry-over" effect. Even a physiologically "correct" response to a regional anesthetic is rarely used as the basis for a destructive procedure. Although pain may be temporarily relieved by chemical or surgical nerve destruction, it soon returns, often in greater intensity or with more disabling characteristics.[65]

While individual nerve trunk blocks (e.g., femoral, tibial, ulnar, etc.) as described above may be useful in pain localized to discrete areas, diagnostic spinal or subarachnoid anesthesia represents a useful modality in assessing more diffuse chronic SCI pain. Based on the original "differential" method described, use of this modality has been previously reported.[45] In this technique, the source of the "neural pain generator" may be localized by varying the height of the spinal anesthetic to affect neuraxial regions that are caudad, at, or rostral to the actual SCI level. However, this procedure may be influenced by certain anatomic and pharmacological factors. Spinal canal obstruction should be excluded in lumbar and thoracic SCI since cephalad spread of local anesthetic would be impeded. In turn, this might produce false-negative responses. Cisternography, which is performed by injecting the radioisotope indium DPTA intrathecally via lumbar puncture, objectively identifies spinal canal obstruction. In lieu of cisternography, an MRI, CT scan, or myelogram also may verify spinal canal patency. Furthermore, since increased CSF protein concentration invariably accompanies spinal canal obstruction, the effect of protein binding on local anesthetic action also requires consideration. Local scarring and fibrosis, such as occurs following arachnoiditis, also may interfere with spread of local anesthetic intrathecally. In patients with obvious spinal canal obstruction, other regional anesthetic techniques may be considered, such as extradural anesthesia or paravertebral somatic anesthesia.

The role of diagnostic sympathetic blocks in the assessment of chronic SCI pain is not clearly established. Several reports describe the response to sympathetic blockade in chronic SCI pain as unpredictable.[24,38] However, sympathetic blockade of the stellate ganglion in the neck or lumbar paravertebral chain with local anesthetic may provide evidence of sympathetic involvement or a sympathetically maintained pain syndrome. In contrast, the absence of a positive response to a sympathetic block, suggests that pain is independent of a sympathetic mechanism (sympathetically independent pain, SIP).

Scintigraphy

If patients present with strong clinical evidence of SMP, a technetium triple-phase bone scan may provide further confirmatory evidence. Kozin reported that scintigraphy was more specific than routine roentgenography in detecting reflex sympathetic dystrophy.[37] Gellman further reported that scintigraphy will be positive earlier than would conventional bone roentgenograms.[28] However, disuse atrophy of bone secondary to paralysis may mimic the patchy demineralization seen in SMP conditions.

TREATMENT

Rehabilitative Care

The initial treatment of chronic SCI pain requires a broad comprehensive approach and application of simple physical modalities. Any factors that work to the detriment of the SCI patient's health will often worsen or contribute to the severity of pain. In nonneurological forms of pain, factors such as posture, lumbar support, appropriate activity levels, exercise, spasticity control, and correct wheelchair prescription will help prevent fatigue and aggravation of pain. As mentioned previously, stress, depression, and psychological factors must be addressed separately. In neurological pain conditions, any form of stimulation below the level of injury may aggravate pain. Frequently, intensification of pain may herald the onset of a urinary tract infection, bladder stones, decubitus ulceration, or paronychia. By correcting these medical problems, pain may return to a more manageable intensity, where other modalities may be effective.

Simple physical modalities may modulate pain intensity, including local heat or cold, massage, acupressure, and physical therapy. Based on the Melzack and Wall's Gate Control theory, surface electrical stimulation (TENS, FES, NMS) can be extremely effective in reducing nonneurological pain, although its efficacy in neurological pain is unpredictable. Davis demonstrated that only one-third of 31 SCI patients treated with TENS obtained significant relief of pain.[18] Acupuncture, which involves the placement of needles at certain points along meridians, has an uncertain place in neurological SCI pain. In chronic musculoskeletal SCI pain, in combination with electrical stimulation, termed "electroacupuncture," it may be as efficacious as TENS, although controlled studies addressing its use in chronic SCI pain have never been performed.

Pharmacological Approaches

Oral

Oral pharmacological agents form the mainstay of chronic pain control in SCI pain. Simple analgesics such as salicylates, acetaminophen, nonsteroidal anti-inflammatory agents, and related agents including methocarbamol, cyclobenzaprine, and carisoprodol will ameliorate musculoskeletal discomfort, but will have little effect on neurological pain. Other agents such as antidepressants and anticonvulsants have been found to be far more effective. Although a large body of literature exists on the use of these agents in neuropathic and deafferentation pain, few controlled studies have been performed specifically in SCI patients. Therefore, the use of these agents in SCI patients is based mainly on anecdotal or empirical grounds.[23]

Tricyclic antidepressant drugs are thought to modulate pain by inhibiting uptake of norepinephrine and serotonin, thereby potentiating the inhibitory action of the brainstem on dorsal horn cells. A variety of agents have been used for neuropathic pain, including amitriptyline, desipramine, clomipramine, and imipramine; however, the choice of agent is guided by the efficacy and incidence of side effects. In the authors' experience, amitriptyline works best, and the anticholinergic side effects usually are tolerable. Two studies have assessed the use of antidepressants in SCI patients. Heilporn used combinations of melitracin and TENS in 11 SCI patients with dysesthetic pain, reporting relief of pain in 8 patients.[33] Davidoff assessed the action of the antidepressant trazodone in 19 SCI patients with chronic dysesthetic pain, using a double-blind placebo-controlled methodology.[17] Trazodone selectively inhibits serotonin and norepinephrine uptake in a ratio of 25:1, and is thought to produce greater analgesia and fewer anticholinergic side effects compared with nonselective agents such as amitriptyline. However, trazodone failed to produce significant analgesia compared with placebo, suggesting that its use in chronic dysesthetic SCI pain may be limited.

Another class of agents commonly used are anticonvulsants, including phenytoin, carbamazepine, sodium valproate, and clonazepam. Anticonvulsants exert "membrane-stabilizing" effects by preventing excessive discharge from damaged neurons, although each agent has a specific site of action. For example, phenytoin acts on axonal membranes and on synaptic transmission, while sodium valproate increases brain GABA (and, presumably, presynaptic inhibition). Controlled studies describing the use of these agents in SCI patients are lacking, although Gibson reports two cases of "denervation hyperpathia" associated with paraplegia responding to carbamazepine.[29]

A miscellaneous group of oral pharmacological agents may also be considered on empirical grounds, including baclofen, mexilitene, clonidine, and opioids. When pain is caused by severe spasticity, baclofen may produce relief by controlling spasticity. The use of opioids in chronic SCI pain is controversial. In nonneurological or nociceptive pain states, short-term use of opioids clearly is efficacious. However, the tolerance phenomena and physical dependence that accompany long-term ingestion detract significantly from its clinical usage. Furthermore, as previously discussed, the analgesic action of narcotics in neurological pain is unpredictable. Notwithstanding the recommendations by Farkash et al. that narcotics be used after all reasonable methods of pain control have failed,[23] suggesting that dependence and toxicity with chronic opioid usage are overstated, the authors believe they have no place in the treatment of chronic pain in nonterminal conditions.

Regional anesthetics

Trigger-point injections may be used in patients with characteristic myofascial syndromes. Sympatholysis (either sympathetic blocks or intravenous regional anesthesia) may be applied in patients who have SMP. The use of diagnostic blocks, discussed previously, also may have therapeutic potential. In certain patients, the duration of pain relief may outlast the expected duration of local anesthetic action, termed "carryover" effect. As demonstrated by Kibler in selected patients,[36] this effect may be prolonged for as long as 60 hours or may even be permanent. Patients demonstrating prolonged analgesia following diagnostic regional anesthetics may therefore benefit from repeated or even continuous regional anesthetic procedures in an attempt to maximize this "carryover" effect. The exact mechanism underlying this type of response is not clearly known. The use of oral and intravenous local anesthetic agents (systemic) in the management of chronic neuropathic pain has also been described.[9] Intravenously administered local anesthetics (procaine, lidocaine, chloroprocaine) at a dosage sufficient to produce a measurable blood concentration is associated with significant analgesia in patients with a variety of neuropathic pain disorders. In turn, the response to an intravenous local anesthetic agent may be used to guide subsequent treatment with oral agents. Two oral agents are currently available, tocainide and mexilitene. Unfortunately, tocainide is associated with severe side effects, and mexilitene is currently regarded as the preferred agent.[30] Local anesthetics are thought to produce analgesia by a concentration-dependent blockade of axoplasmic sodium channels on peripheral nerves.

In contrast to their demonstrated efficacy in the treatment of spasticity, especially for complete lesions, neurolytic agents such as phenol and alcohol, in the authors' opinion, do not have a major role in chronic SCI pain management. The effects of denervation associated with these agents include sensory anesthesia, loss of voluntary movement, muscle atrophy, loss of sacral functions (e.g., bladder), and such complications as anesthesia dolorosa, neuritis, scar formation (arachnoiditis), and dysesthesias. However, pain related to spasticity may respond to reduction of muscle tone per se, and in this setting hypertonicity may be controlled with selective nerve trunk, intrathecal, or intramuscular neurolyses.

There are few clinical experiential data on the use of neuraxial pharmacological delivery systems in the treatment of chronic SCI pain. Glynn et al. reported their experiences in 15 SCI patients with chronic pain.[32] Five responded to epidural morphine, while seven responded to epidural clonidine but not to morphine. Glynn further recommends epidural testing/treatment with a variety of agents, including local anesthetics, midazolam, and ketamine.[31] Our experience in patients with SCI pain receiving intrathecal baclofen or spasticity control suggests that while it produces reduction of nonneurological pain (related to spasticity), the effects on neurological pain are not impressive.[46] However, the technological advances associated with implanted neuraxial pharmacological delivery systems has opened an important therapeutic avenue. As such, using an implanted system, with or without an infusion pump, a pharmacological agent can be administered epidurally or intrathecally, effecting drug delivery directly to the presumed site of the neural pain generator. While considerable information exists on the use of neuraxial narcotics in acute postsurgical and chronic cancer pain, the use of various agents and delivery systems in chronic SCI pain must still be regarded as experimental, requiring carefully controlled studies and patient safeguards. The authors regard this as an exciting area for future research.

Surgical Procedures

Certain presentations of musculoskeletal SCI pain may benefit from surgical intervention. For example, pain produced by Harrington or other stabilizing metallic rods may be abruptly relieved by surgical removal. Pain produced by a posttraumatic syrinx will respond to immediate drainage. However, several destructive surgical procedures have been described for chronic SCI pain and all except one (dorsal root entry zone lesioning, DREZ), are currently regarded as either ineffective, crude, unpredictable, or irreversible. Although pain relief may be observed for a short interval following these procedures, invariably pain returns, often in conjunction with secondary neuropathic pain symptoms produced by the surgical lesion itself. A brief review of these procedures is provided here for historical interest only, since all have been abandoned.

Dorsal rhizotomy describes a procedure in which the sensory roots are divided, either intradurally or extradurally. In cordotomy, either open or percutaneous, the anterior spinothalamic tracts subserving pain and temperature function are divided, often requiring a bilateral approach. Commissural myelotomy describes the surgical interruption of the decussating pain and temperature fibers in the midline commissures of the spinal cord. Cordectomy describes the surgical excision of a segment of spinal cord tissue; transverse myelotomy describes the division of the spinal cord, usually one to two segments rostral to the area of SCI.

In contrast, DREZ lesioning of the spinal cord has an established role in chronic SCI pain management. The technique of DREZ coagulation was originally described by Nashold.[52] The DREZ is made up of part of the dorsal nerve roots, superficial layers of the dorsal horn (Rexed Zones I through V and Lissauer's tract). A lesion in this area produced either by radiofrequency or laser coagulation will interrupt transmission of nociceptive information via the spinothalamic tracts. Although originally described for pain secondary to brachial plexus avulsion, several reports confirm its utility in chronic neurological SCI pain. Nashold performed DREZ in 13 patients with chronic SCI pain, achieving 50 percent or more relief of pain in 11 patients.[51] Unfortunately, three patients developed major surgical complications, including loss of voluntary movement in certain muscles and loss of reflex bladder control. Five years later, Friedman reviewed results in 56 patients with chronic SCI pain followed for 6 months—6 years following DREZ. Twenty-eight patients (50 percent) demonstrated good pain relief, while 23 patients (41 percent) reported poor pain relief.[25] They further suggested certain prognostic indicators, in that patients with segmental types of pain, extending caudally below the SCI level for several dermatomes or unilaterally, demonstrated the best response to the procedure. Only 32 percent of patients with diffuse pain responded favorably. Almost all patients in this series noted a postoperative rise in sensory level. Recently, Young reviewed the effects of DREZ in 78 patients, of whom 26 presented with chronic SCI pain.[71] In particular, radiofrequency lesioning was compared to the CO_2 laser technique. His findings generally were more favorable than those of Nashold, in that 16 (>50 percent) of the SCI patients demonstrated pain relief. Significantly, 83 percent of patients with cauda equina injuries responded to the procedure. Young further concluded that human DREZ lesions were reliably produced using the radiofrequency lesioning technique.

A nondestructive surgical modality useful in SCI pain management is spinal stimulation. In this technique, also termed epidural or dorsal column stimulation (DCS), a stimulating electrode is placed within the dorsal epidural space and connected to an implantable stimulator. Various commercial devices are now approved for use in patients, the latest models having versatile programmable features in which frequency, polarity, choice of electrode combination, pulse width, and amplitude of stimulation may be varied. Unfortunately, two reports in 1980 and 1981 by Richardson and Long, respectively, suggested that there was very little reason to pursue its development or application in SCI pain.[44,59] This was corroborated in a recent study demonstrating a poor success rate in 16 patients with SCI pain.[48] However, recently, North and colleagues updated their results in 62 patients with chronic pain of various etiologies using the more advanced DCS electrode systems.[54] They concluded that a majority of patients reported greater than 50 percent pain relief, and that multichannel programmable devices were associated with greater efficacy. Their goal of treatment in DCS was to cover the painful area with electrical stimulation sensations termed "superposition of paresthesias." Unfortunately, only five patients in North's series had chronic SCI pain, with two demonstrating adequate pain relief; however, their study design and results suggest that DCS may have a greater role in chronic SCI pain management.

An extension of the implantable stimulator concept is applied in deep brain stimulation (DBS). Although first used 30 years ago, stimulation of selected thalamic areas may produce analgesia in certain central pain conditions.[41] However, a recent review of advances in this field suggested that of the 42 clinical studies of thalamic stimulation in humans, only 2 were well-controlled.[22] Furthermore, considerable disagreement exists among various neurosurgeons, and the results of this modality are unpredictable. The future of this modality in SCI pain is not clear at this time.

FUTURE DIRECTIONS

The following areas represent promising avenues for further clinical research in chronic SCI pain. Controlled clinical studies addressing oral pharmacological management of chronic SCI pain are sorely needed to formulate clinical and empirical guidelines. However, these studies must include placebos and control variables to ensure a homogeneous patient population. Attention should be focused on central pain syndromes, since these by far are the most severe and disabling of all SCI pain categories. The use of DCS should be reexamined specifically in patients with SCI pain, using the more advanced multichannel, programmable devices. The administration of neuraxial pharmacological agents also needs further exploration to find agonists or antagonists of the various receptor-neurotransmitter classes that may modulate nociceptive input to the dorsal horn cells without undue toxicity or tolerance.

ACKNOWLEDGMENTS

Supported in part by a grant from The National Institute on Disability and Rehabilitation Research, U.S. Department of Education, Grant Number H133N00016-91. The authors thank Dr. Marcus J. Fuhrer for providing a scholarly review of the manuscript.

REFERENCES

1. Andrews LG, Armitage KJ: Sudeck's atrophy in traumatic quadriplegia. *Paraplegia* 1971; 9:159–165.
2. Arner S, Myerson BA: Lack of analgesic effect of opioids on neuropathic and idiopathic forms of pain. *Pain* 1988; 33:11–23.
3. Beric A: Altered sensation and pain in spinal cord injury, in Dimitrijevic MR, Wall PD, Lindblom U (eds): *Recent Achievements in Restorative Neurology.* London: Karger, 1990: 27–36.
4. Beric A, Dimitrijevic MR, Light JK: A clinical syndrome of rostral and caudal spinal injury: Neurological, neurophysiological and urodynamic evidence for occult sacral lesion. *J Neurol Neurosurg Psychiatry* 1987; 50:600–606.
5. Beric A, Dimitrijevic MR, Lindblom U: Central dysesthesia syndrome in spinal cord injury patients. *Pain* 1988; 34:109–116.
6. Bernstein JE, Bickers DR, Dahl MV, Roshal JY: Treatment of chronic postoperative neuralgia with topical capsaicin. *J Am Acad Dermatol* 1987; 17:93–96.
7. Besson JM, Lombard MC, Zajac JM, et al: Deafferentation, nociceptive dorsal horn neurons and opioids, in Dimitrijevic MR, Wall PD, Lindblom U (eds): *Recent Achievements in Restorative Neurology.* London: Karger, 1990: 143–151.
8. Boas RA: Diagnostic and therapeutic nerve blocks in

altered sensation and pain, in Dimitrijevic MR, Wall PD, Lindblom U (eds): *Recent Achievements in Restorative Neurology.* London: Karger, 1990: 17–26.
9. Boas RA, Covino BG, Shahnarian A: Analgesic responses to IV lignocaine. *Br J Anaesth* 1982; 54:501–505.
10. Botterell EH, Callaghan JC, Jousse AT: Pain in paraplegia: Clinical management and surgical treatment. *Proc R Soc Med* 1953; 47:281–288.
11. Burke DC: Pain in paraplegia. *Paraplegia* 1973; 10:297–313.
12. Burke DC, Woodward JM: Pain and phantom sensation in spinal paralysis, in Vinken PJ, Bruyn GW (eds): *Handbook of Clinical Neurology,* Amsterdam: North Holland, 1976; 26:489–499.
13. Cohen MJ, McArthur DL, Vulpe M, et al: Comparison of chronic pain from spinal cord injury to chronic pain of other origins. *Pain* 1988; 35:57–63.
14. Cremer SA, Maynard F, Davidoff G: The reflex sympathetic dystrophy syndrome associated with traumatic myelopathy: Report of 5 cases. *Pain* 1989; 37:187–192.
15. Davidoff RA, Hackman JC: Drugs, chemicals, and toxins: Their effects on the spinal cord, in Davidoff RA (ed): *Handbook of the Spinal Cord.* New York: Marcel Dekker, 1983; 10:409–476.
16. Davidoff RA, Guarracini M, Roth E, et al: Trazodone hydrochloride in the treatment of dysesthetic pain in traumatic myelopathy: A randomized, double-blind, placebo-controlled study. *Pain* 1987; 29:151–161.
17. Davidoff RA, Roth E, Guarracini M, et al: Function-limiting dysesthetic pain syndrome among traumatic spinal cord injury patients: A cross-sectional study. *Pain* 1987; 29:39–48.
18. Davis R, Lentini R: Transcutaneous nerve stimulation for treatment of pain in patients with spinal cord injury. *Surg Neurol* 1975; 4:100–101.
19. Davis L, Martin J: Studies upon spinal cord injuries. *J Neurosurg* 1947; 4:483–491.
20. Dew MA, Lynch KA, Ernst J, et al: A causal analysis of factors affecting adjustment to spinal cord injury. *Rehab Psychol* 1985; 30:39–46.
21. Donovan WH, Dimitrijevic MR, Dahm L, Dimitrijevic M: Neurophysiological approaches to chronic pain following spinal cord injury. *Paraplegia* 1982; 20:135–146.
22. Duncan GH, Bushnell MC, Marchand S: Deep brain stimulation: A review of basic research and clinical studies. *Pain* 1991; 45:49–59.
23. Farkash AE, Portenoy RK: The pharmacological management of chronic pain in the paraplegic patient. *J Am Paraplegia Soc* 1986; 9:41–50.
24. Freeman LW, Heimburger RF: Surgical relief of pain in paraplegic patients. *Arch Surg* 1947; 55:433–440.
25. Friedman AH, Nashold BS: DREZ lesions for relief of pain related to spinal cord injury. *J Neurosurg* 1986; 65:465–469.
26. Frisbie JH, Aguilera EJ: Chronic pain after spinal cord injury: An expedient diagnostic approach. *Paraplegia* 1990; 28:460–465.
27. Fruhstorfer H, Lindblom U, Schmidt WG: Method for quantitative estimation of thermal thresholds in patients. *J Neurol Neurosurg Psychiatry* 1976; 39:1071–1075.
28. Gellman H, Eckert RR, Botte MJ, et al: Reflex sympathetic dystrophy in cervical spinal cord injury patients. *Clin Orthop* 1988; 233:126–131.
29. Gibson JC, White LE: Denervation hyperpathia: A convulsive syndrome of the spinal cord responsive to carbamazepine therapy. *J Neurosurg* 1971; 35:287–290.
30. Glazer S, Portenoy RK: Systemic local anesthetics in pain control. *J Pain Symptom Mgmt* 1991; 6:30–39.
31. Glynn C, Teddy PJ: Assessment and management of the patient with spinal cord injury and pain, in Alderson JD, Frost EAM (eds): *Spinal Cord Injuries, Anaesthetic and Associated Care.* London: Butterworths, 1990: 139–166.
32. Glynn C, Teddy PJ, Jamous MA, et al: Role of spinal noradrenergic system in transmission of pain in patients with spinal cord injury. *Lancet* 1986; ii:1249–1250.
33. Heilporn A: Two therapeutic experiments on stubborn pain in spinal cord lesions: Coupling melitracen-flepenthixol and transcutaneous nerve stimulation. *Paraplegia* 1977; 25:368–372.
34. Holmes G: Pain of central origin, in Hoebe PB (ed): *Contributions to Medical and Biological Research.* New York: Raven, 1919; 1:235–246.
35. Juler GL, Eltorai IM: The acute abdomen in spinal cord injury patients. *Paraplegia* 1985; 23:118–123.
36. Kibler RF, Nathan PW: Relief of pain and paraesthesiae by nerve block distal to a lesion. *J Neurol Neurosurg Psychiatry* 1960; 23:91–98.
37. Kozin F, Ryan LM, Carerra GF, Soin JS: The reflex sympathetic dystrophy syndrome (RSDS). *Am J Med* 1981; 70:23–30.
38. Krueger EG: Management of painful states in injuries of the spinal cord and cauda equina. *Am J Phys Med* 1960; 39:103–110.
39. Lamid S, Chia LS, Kohli A, Cid E: Chronic pain in spinal cord injury: Comparison between inpatients and outpatients. *Arch Phys Med Rehabil* 1985; 66:777–778.
40. Levitt M, Levitt JH: The deafferentation syndrome in monkeys: Dysesthesias of spinal origin. *Pain* 1981; 10:129–147.
41. Levy RM, Lamb S, Adams JE: Treatment of chronic pain by deep brain stimulation: Long term follow-up and review of the literature. *Neurosurgery* 1987; 21:885–893.
42. Lindblom U: Classification and assessment of altered sensation and pain, in Dimitrijevic MR, Wall PD, Lindblom U (eds): *Recent Achievements in Restorative Neurology.* London: Karger, 1990: 7–16.
43. Loeser JD, Ward AA, White LE: Chronic deafferentation of human spinal cord neurons. *J Neurosurg* 1968; 29:48–50.
44. Long ML, Erickson D, Campbell J, North R: Electrical stimulation of the spinal cord and peripheral nerves for pain control. *Appl Neurophysiol* 1981; 44:207–217.
45. Loubser PG, Donovan WH: Diagnostic spinal anaesthesia in chronic spinal cord injury pain. *Paraplegia* 1991; 29:25–36.
46. Loubser PG, Narayan RK, Sandin KJ, et al: Continuous infusion of intrathecal baclofen: Long-term effects on spasticity in spinal cord injury. *Paraplegia* 1991; 29:48–64.
47. MacDonald RL: Neuropharmacology of spinal cord and dorsal root ganglion neurons in primary dissociated cell

culture, in Davidoff RA (ed): *Handbook of the Spinal Cord*. New York: Marcel Dekker, 1993; 9:381–407.

48. Meglio M, Cioni B, Prezioso A, Talamonti G: Spinal cord stimulation (SCS) in deafferentation pain. *PACE* 1989; 12:709–712.
49. Melzack R, Loeser JD: Phantom body pain in paraplegics: Evidence for a central "pattern generating mechanism" for pain. *Pain* 1978; 4:195–210.
50. Mount BM: Psychological and social aspects of cancer pain, in Wall PD, Melzack R (eds): *Textbook of Pain,* (2d ed). London: Churchill Livingstone, 1989: 610–623.
51. Nashold BS, Bullit E: Dorsal root entry zone lesions to control pain in paraplegics. *J Neurosurg* 1981; 55:414–419.
52. Nashold BS, Ostdahl RH: Dorsal root entry zone lesions for pain relief. *J Neurosurg* 1979; 51:59–69.
53. Nepomuceno C, Fine PR, Richards JS, et al: Pain in patients with spinal cord injury. *Arch Phys Med Rehabil* 1979; 60:595–608.
54. North RB, Ewend MG, Lawton MT, Piantadosi S: Spinal cord stimulation for chronic, intractable pain: Superiority of "multichannel" devices. *Pain* 1991; 44:119–130.
55. Pagni CA: Pathophysiology of central pain, in Dimitrijevic MR, Wall PD, Lindblom U (eds): *Recent Achievements in Restorative Neurology*. London: Karger, 1990: 56–61.
56. Pagni CA: Central pain due to spinal cord and brain stem damage, in Wall PD, Melzack R (eds): *Textbook of Pain,* (2d ed). London: Churchill Livingstone, 1989: 634–655.
57. Richards JS, Meredith RL, Nepomuceno C, et al: Psychosocial aspects of chronic pain in spinal cord injury. *Pain* 1980; 8:355–366.
58. Richards JS, Stover SL, Jaworski T: Effect of bullet removal on subsequent pain in persons with spinal cord injury secondary to gunshot wound. *J Neurosurg* 1990; 73:401–404.
59. Richardson RR, Meyer PR, Cerullo LJ: Neurostimulation in the modulation of intractable paraplegic and traumatic neuroma pains. *Pain* 1980; 8:75–84.
60. Rintala DH, Hart KA, Fuhrer MJ: Self-reported pain in persons with chronic spinal cord injury. *Am Paraplegia Soc* 1991; 14:83.
61. Roberts WJ: A hypothesis on the physiological basis for causalgia and related pains. *Pain* 1986; 24:297–311.
62. Rose M, Robinson JE, Ells P, Cole JD: Pain following spinal cord surgery: Results from a postal survey. (Letter) *Pain* 1988; 34:101–102.
63. Stevens CW, Yaksh TL: Potency of infused antinociceptive agents is inversely related to magnitude of tolerance after continuous infusion. *J Pharmacol Exp Therap* 1989; 250:1–8.
64. Summers JD, Rapoff MA, Varghese G, et al: Psychosocial factors in chronic spinal cord injury pain. *Pain* 1991; 47:183–189.
65. Sweet WH: Deafferentation pain after posterior rhizotomy, trauma to a limb and herpes zoster. *Neurosurgery* 1984; 15:928–932.
66. Tasker RR: Pain resulting from central nervous system pathology: Central pain, in Bonica JJ (ed): *Management of Pain*. Philadelphia: Lea & Febiger, 1990: 264–283.
67. Wainapel SF: Reflex sympathetic dystrophy following traumatic myelopathy. *Pain* 1984; 18:345–349.
68. Woolsey RM: Chronic pain following spinal cord injury. *J Am Paraplegia Soc* 1986; 9:39–40.
69. World Health Organization: *International Classification of Impairments, Disabilities, and Handicaps: A Manual of Classification Relating to the Consequences of Disease*. Geneva, 1980.
70. Yaksh TL: Pharmacological studies suggesting the role of spinal receptor systems in the anomalous encoding of high and low threshold cutaneous stimuli, in Dimitrijevic MR, Wall PD, Lindblom U (eds): *Recent Achievements in Restorative Neurology*. London: Karger, 1990: 132–142.
71. Young RF: Clinical experience with radiofrequency and laser DREZ lesions. *J Neurosurg* 1990; 72:715–720.

PART III

BASIC RESEARCH

CHAPTER 97

AN OVERVIEW OF BRAIN INJURY MODELS

John T. Povlishock

INTRODUCTION

This chapter and the next review some of the commonly used animal models of traumatic brain injury that attempt to replicate, with varying degrees of fidelity, features seen in humans who sustain a nonmissile injury. As will be noted, few animal models faithfully replicate the full spectrum of human traumatic brain injury; thus, to some degree, each animal model must be seen as a compromise between fully replicating the human situation and generating data that have relevance to at least one of the factors associated with human head injury. The central problem associated with the modeling of human traumatic brain injury lies in the nature of human injury. In the case of nonmissile injury, it is clear that in humans, the cause and biomechanical forces associated with each injury are not necessarily the same. Clearly, falling from a ladder or being thrown from a horse are quite different from sustaining a motor vehicle or auto-pedestrian accident. Because of this diversity, it is apparent that no single animal model can faithfully reproduce all the potentially diverse conditions associated with human traumatic brain injury. In fact, if all animal modeling were driven to fully replicate the full spectrum of human injury, this would most likely prove an unattainable task.

In view of these considerations, what follows is an attempt to provide an overview of many of the currently employed animal models of traumatic brain injury. In this overview, the type of the animal models employed will be described, along with the features of human traumatic brain injury that they are presumed to model. This overview will focus on animal models of nonmissile or closed head injury, with no consideration given to injuries of the missile type.

HISTORICAL PERSPECTIVE ON ANIMAL MODELING

In the context of nonmissile injury, the historical basis for animal modeling goes back well over a hundred years, with the primary focus being on unraveling the phenomenon of traumatically induced concussion. In the early studies of Witkowski,[1] frogs were subjected to blows to the head to observe their behavioral response to that injury. Interestingly, to determine whether concussion had its basis in a brain parenchymal versus a microvascular response, Witkowski removed the hearts of frogs before injury, a procedure compatible with viability for at least several minutes. When injured, the frogs demonstrated an immediate loss of consciousness or stunning, thus demonstrating that the brain was responsible for this behavioral response independent of any vascular mechanism. These rather straightforward early studies regarding the role of the brain versus that of its microvasculature in the genesis of concussion have long been overlooked, and today, many of the same themes are being revisited.

By the turn of the century, limited experimentation on animal modeling resumed. Again, primarily to understand the phenomenon of concussion, various investigators subjected animals to blows to the head and subsequently studied their behavioral, physiological, and histological responses.

The modern era of traumatic brain injury modeling began in the early 1940s with the pioneering work of Denny-Brown and Russell,[2,3] who focused on two models of injury, one involving acceleration concussion and the other involving percussion concussion. For acceleration concussion, Denny-Brown and Russell subjected the unrestrained heads of animals to various forms of impact that resulted in acceleration of the head and neck as well as the brain. Using these approaches, Denny-Brown and Russell showed that the unrestrained head was more prone to injury after mechanical loading than was the restrained head, demonstrating that acceleration of the brain is an important component in the pathobiology of injury and concussion. In the percussion concussion models, Denny-Brown used a piston-driven device to elicit mechanical loading of the brain and subsequent pathobiological responses. Using then-current anatomic, physiological, and functional studies, Denny-Brown and Russell provided a wealth of information on the brain's response to injury under these loading conditions.

CONTEMPORARY PERSPECTIVES

The pioneering work of Denny-Brown and Russell has set the stage for further model development that continues to fall into the categories originally classified by those investigators. Within the past 20 years, Denny-Brown's acceleration concussion models have led to the development of the inertial acceleration and impact acceleration models. In this context, inertial acceleration is defined as involving acceleration of the head without impact. To date, as reviewed by Gennarelli,[4] such inertial models have been used in primates,[5–10] cats,[11] and swine.[12,13] Unlike the inertial acceleration models, impact acceleration models involve direct impacts that elicit both focal loading and diffuse strains throughout the brain. Typically, such models provide impact through an impactor, a piston or weight dropped directly onto the skull, or a steel plate affixed to the skull to minimize local skull loading and fracture.

To date, impact acceleration models have been used in primates,[14–18] cats,[19,20] mice,[21] and rats.[22–27] In relation to the inertial injury models, their highest development is seen in the subhuman primate models first developed and described by Ommaya and Gennarelli,[8] with subsequent refinement by Gennarelli and coworkers. These models utilized subhuman primates subjected to impulsive nonimpact loading conditions in which the head was constrained to move only in certain directions. Further, the impact was regulated so that the head could move only a certain distance in a specific path, assuring that the response of the head was exactly the same in each experiment. In this fashion, either angular accelerations or translational accelerations could be produced, with the resulting pathobiology and neurological sequelae carefully characterized. In the early experience with these models, it was recognized that concussion could be produced only with angular acceleration despite the fact that pathological change reflected in contusions and subdural and subarachnoid hemorrhage could be seen with injuries involving either translational or angular acceleration.[5,8,28–32]

To further explore the genesis of concussion and determine whether more prolonged traumatic unconsciousness or coma could be generated in the same model, Gennarelli and colleagues initiated further change in the system, using a thermoplastic helmet attached to a lifter pivoted 60 degrees by a driven thrust column in 2 to 4 ms.[33–39] Using this approach, these investigators were consistently able to reproduce concussion, and they began to appreciate that such concussion was associated with axonal damage scattered throughout the brain.[40,41] With further modification, which involved angular accelerations with longer pulse durations (5 to 10 ms), the duration of traumatic unconsciousness was prolonged, and with the prolonged unconsciousness, axonal damage was readily recognized.[7,42] These experiments gave rise to the seminal observation that the direction of head movement was important in the process by demonstrating that movement of the head in the coronal plane, instead of the sagittal plane, produced prolonged unconsciousness and generated the same type of decebrate and decorticate responses seen in severely head-injured humans.[43,44]

At present, inertial injury models have provided some of the most complete insight into the pathobiology of the events that occur in traumatically brain-injured humans. Through the exploration of translational and angular acceleration in these models, Gennarelli and colleagues have been able to reproduce the full spectrum of human head injury, ranging from subconcussive responses to immediate death. Importantly, in addition to mimicking the spectrum of human traumatic brain injury, these models have been able to replicate the full pathobiology of human traumatic brain injury, ranging from contusional change and mass lesion formation to diffuse axonal injury.

Despite the relative elegance of these models and their implications for understanding human traumatic brain injury, subhuman primate studies utilizing inertial injury have not been conducted routinely for multiple reasons, including but not limited to the cost of the studies and the size of the animals involved in assessment. More recently, because of these issues, Gennarelli and colleagues have modified this model to adapt it for use in miniature swine. While this model of acceleration injury has not been fully characterized, preliminary studies suggest that it has promise as a model of human traumatic brain injury.[12,13]

Paralleling the development of these inertial injury models, significant development and refinement of percussion concussion models have occurred. Such models, which include both fluid and rigid percussion varities, employ a rather fluid pulse or a mechanically driven piston to rapidly compress the brain and thus elicit its elastic deformation in a fashion purportedly consistent with that which occurs in traumatic brain injury (see Chap. 100). To date, these fluid percussion and rigid percussion models have been used in a host of experimental animals, including rats,[45–76] cats,[77–94] ferrets,[95] and pigs.[96]

In general, in the fluid percussion models, a craniectomy is made midway between the bregma and the vertex, and within this craniotomy site a central injury shaft is inserted. The shaft is connected to a fluid-filled reservoir which is closed by a piston (plunger) surrounded by rings. When the fluid-filled reservoir is impacted by the pendulum, a pressure pulse is generated, which in turn travels through the cylinder and the central injury shaft to strike the intact dura of the experimental animal. In most cases, the injuries are measured in terms of atmospheric pressure and generally are allowed to range from 15 to 30 ms in duration. Biomechanical characterization of this model shows maximal strain development in the brainstem, with more modest involvement of the cortical and subcortical regions; this is consistent with the known pathophysiology of the model.[97] Typically, midline fluid percussion models reveal histopathologic change in the foci anatomically related to the site of percussion injury in addition to more widespread change throughout the brainstem. When the pressure pulse is centrally placed, modest bilateral cortical and dorsal hippocampal changes are found, while in the brainstem, the central midbrain tegmentum, the lateral pons, and the midventral medulla also are commonly involved.

While all fluid percussion insults originally were directed at the midline,[48,93] with time, placement of the fluid pressure pulse in more lateral positions also was used.[65] Such injuries tended to cause unilateral focal neocortical and hippocampal change, with a more modest involvement of the brainstem. Recently, these lateral cortical injury models have been modified to include contralateral cranial opening to allow for more widespread axonal injury. Additionally, the model has been modified to utilize a parasagittal placement of the fluid pressure pulse, which again triggers its own subset of histopathologic change.[47,98]

Similar to the fluid percussion models that employ a fluid pulse injected into the neuraxis to elicit movement of the brain, other related models use a rigid piston or indentor placed within the craniotomy site.[48,99,100] The piston then is allowed to strike the intact dura, allowing for the rapid loading of the underlying cortical tissue. Unlike the inertial injury devices employed in primates and swine, the underlying goal of both the fluid percussion and rigid interior models of injury is not to faithfully replicate the full spectrum of human traumatic brain injury. Rather, it is thought that when the brain is injured, general injury processes can be dissected out, evaluated, and subjected to various therapeutic interventions. In this regard, the fluid percussion injury and rigid indention have gained widespread use in rodents, as a large number of animals can be employed and thus large scale preclinical drug trials can be conducted.

In the preceding passages, the author has attempted to characterize some of the more common models used for the study of the pathobiology of traumatic brain injury. The remainder of this chapter will attempt to characterize the structural and functional changes that are known to occur in these animal models. While it is beyond the scope of this chapter to review every animal model and its specific structural and functional sequelae, the author will attempt to present in general terms known structural and functional changes and relate them where possible to specific model systems. To assist the reader in linking observed structural and functional

TABLE 97-1 Utility of Animal Models in Replicating Human Traumatic Brain Injury

Model	Contusion	Subarachnoid Hemorrhage	Acute Subdural Hematoma	Intra-parenchymal Hemorrhage	Neuronal Loss	Axonal Injury	Blood-Brain Barrier Disruption	Altered Brain Metabolism	Altered Blood Flow	Altered Vascular Responses
Central fluid percussion	+	++	−	+	+	+	++	++	++	+
Lateral fluid percussion	+	++	−	+	++	+	++	++	++	+
Rigid indentation	++	++	+	+	+	+	++	?	?	?
Inertial injury	+++	+++	+++	+++	+++	+++	?	?	?	?
Impact acceleration	±	++	−	+	++	++	++	++	++	?

Note: ± = inconstant; ? = no data exist; + = duplicates to some degree; ++ = duplicates with greater fidelity; +++ = duplicates with the greatest fidelity.

SOURCE: Modified from Gennarelli TA: Animate Models of Human Head Injury. *J Neurotrauma* 11:363, 1994.

changes with specific animal models, Table 97-1 is provided to supplement the text.

STRUCTURAL CHANGES

Similar to the situation described for the pathology of nonmissile brain injury in humans (see Chap. 4), the structural changes associated with experimental traumatic brain injury have been organized in the framework of focal versus diffuse change. In the context of focal injury, contusion, hematoma formation, and neuronal cell loss have received considerable attention, while in relation to diffuse traumatically induced change, the focus has been on diffuse axonal injury and diffuse microvascular damage reflected in either overt vascular damage or disruption of the blood-brain barrier.

Focal Changes

Contusion

Much as in the human condition, contusions have been described in virtually all animal models of traumatic brain injury. They have been described in relation to fluid percussion and rigid percussion insults as well as inertial and impact acceleration injuries. In terms of percussion injuries, contusion is seen to develop incidentally to the sight of mechanical loading, and as such, its genesis is directly dependent on the severity and duration of the percussion insult. While investigators in the field of animal experimentation have assumed that there is only one type of contusion, most have lost sight of the fact that in traumatically brain-injured humans, contusion may take multiple forms. The contusion seen with fluid percussion injuries and some rigid percussion insults involves hemorrhagic damage at the gray-white interface with relative initial sparing of the overlying cortical gray matter.[45,47,50,65] Such contusional change appears to be reminiscent of a gliding contusion seen in traumatically brain-injured humans rather than bearing similarities to the more overt contusional changes associated with cortical movement against the overlying bony surface (surface contusion) (see Chap. 4). Some models of rigid indention, however, cause extensive hemorrhage scattered throughout the cortical gray matter,[95] and in this situation, they are more reminiscent of the surface contusions described in traumatically brain-injured humans. In virtually all animal models of traumatic brain injury, both gliding-like and surface-like contusions go on over time to show necrosis, ultimately resulting in the formation of a cystic cavity walled off by gliotic tissue.

Hematoma formation

Unlike the human situation, epidural hematoma formation is not a feature of most experimental traumatic brain injuries. This is easy to appreciate, however, when one understands that in humans, the presence of an epidural hematoma is associated with skull fracture, which is not a major feature of most animal models. Despite the fact that epidural hematoma is not routinely modeled in experimental models of traumatic brain injury, subdural hematomas can be studied. They have been reproduced in inertial injury models, particularly the subhuman primate model as refined and characterized by Gennarelli and coworkers.[7] While subdural hematoma formation also has been reported to occur with the use of rigid indention,[95] it has not been well characterized, and thus its overall significance remains to be determined.

Intraparenchymal hematoma formation has been described in various animal models of traumatic brain injury. In general, this hematoma formation is reserved for the most severe forms of injury. In the percussion models, hematoma formation appears to be confined to the brain stem, with occasional subcortical involvement.[45,47,50,65,66,93] In the inertial injury models, hematoma formation can occur scattered throughout the central white matter as well as the basal ganglia, again being most conspicuous in the most severe forms of traumatic brain injury.

Neuronal loss

The issue of neuronal loss has been addressed only recently in the field of traumatic brain injury. While historically many researchers have focused on posttraumatic chromatolytic change within the brainstem as a measure of traumatically induced unconsciousness, more contemporary studies have not attended to this issue. Recently, however, more attention has been focused on the potential for traumatically induced neuronal loss in order to better understand some of the functional and behavioral changes associated with experimental traumatic brain injury. Typically, most information regarding neuronal cell loss has evolved in relation to fluid percussion injury models, particularly those utilizing lateral injuries. In these models, neuronal cell loss has been described in mild to moderate traumatic brain injuries that generally are not associated with the induction of overt contusional change. Such neuronal loss has been described in the parieto-occipital cortex, the CA3 subsector of the dorsal hippocampus, and the hilus of the dentate gyrus.[57,72]

Using a midline fluid percussion insult, comparable cell loss has not been described[59]; however, this was most likely a function of the severity of the injury used as well as the specific biomechanical features of the central injury model. Interestingly, using a parasagittal fluid percussion injury, Dietrich and colleagues described irreversible neuronal damage in the neocortex, the C3 and C4 subsectors of the hippocampus, and the lateral thalamus.[47] In addition to the neuronal loss described in the fluid percussion models in rodents, neuronal loss has been described in the inertial injury model utilized at the University of Pennsylvania.[101] In those studies, hippocampal neuronal loss has been described, with the suggestion that it occurred independent of any hypoxic or ischemic insult. Instead, it has been speculated that this loss was a direct result of the excitatory amino acid storm triggered by the traumatic injury. Although to date the issue of cell loss in traumatically brain-injured humans has not received much attention, some recent reports have addressed this issue. After traumatic injury in humans, Ross and colleagues[102] have shown the loss of thalamic reticular neurons, which they also have linked to a neuroexcitatory-mediated event. Similarly, in the human hippocampus, neuronal cell loss has been described and correlated with the neurotransmitter storm associated with a traumatic brain event.[103]

Diffuse Changes

Diffuse axonal injury

While virtually every model of traumatic brain injury has been reported to demonstrate diffuse axonal injury reminiscent of that seen in traumatically brain-injured humans, these assertions do not appear to be fully justified. On the one hand, it is clear that most models of traumatic brain injury result in the occurrence of axonal damage; on the other hand, it is clear that in most cases, this axonal damage is rather limited and generally is confined to discrete anatomic loci rather than being diffusely scattered throughout the neuraxis. In both central and lateral fluid percussion injuries, damage and/or reactive axons can be found scattered primarily throughout brainstem, with some subcortical involvement.[50,79,80,89,104–106] In the lateral rigid percussion model as modified by opening the contralateral cranium, an increased number of subcortically distributed damaged axons are found,[105] yet again, these axons appear to be confined to the contralateral opening site. Thus, while most animal models show varying distributions of axonal damage, they do not replicate the full distribution of reactive axonal change seen in traumatically brain-injured humans, where they are found scattered throughout the subcortical white matter, corpus callosum, and brainstem (see Chap. 4). The animal model most reminiscent of humans in terms of axonal injury is the inertial injury model developed by Gennarelli and colleagues.[7] In their work, subhuman primates subjected to angular acceleration elicit a full array of reactive axonal change throughout the subcortical white matter, the corpus callosum, the internal capsule, the dorsal lateral quadrant of the brainstem, and the pontomedullary junctions that is reminiscent of humans.[7]

Diffuse deafferentation

In both the human and the animal modeling literature, the concept of traumatically induced target deafferentation has received little consideration. Obviously, if any injury to an animal or human results in scattered axonal injury, scattered or diffuse deafferentation of the axons' target sites will occur. Such scattered deafferentation has been best described in the cat model of fluid percussion brain injury, and the neuroplastic responses triggered by such target deafferentation have been considered in the same model.[80] While target deafferentation in traumatically brain-injured humans is an obvious consequence of diffuse axonal injury, its characterization in terms of deafferentation and potential neuroplastic change has been addressed in only the most simplistic fashion[92]; obviously, much work is required in this area.

Diffuse Microvascular Change

Disruption of the blood-brain barrier

Virtually all animal models of traumatic brain injury demonstrate perturbation of the blood-brain barrier.[45,47,74,75,91,98] This disruption has been detected primarily through the passage of serum proteins, which normally are confined to the vascular compartment by the intact barrier. With traumatic brain injury, disruption of the barrier properties allows for the exudation of these substances from the blood to the brain front. To date, the passage of endogenous albumin and immunoglobulins has been followed in addition to the passage of exogenously administered tracers such as horseradish peroxidase and radiolabeled serum albumin. While it is not possible in this chapter to describe the distribution of traumatically induced barrier change in the various models of traumatic brain injury, it should be noted that most of these models involve local barrier changes related to the site of mechanical leading as well as diffuse changes that most likely are related to strains generated by the traumatic event. Disruption of the blood-brain barrier has been noted in the fluid percussion and rigid percussion models as well in various acceleration models in which the sites of barrier change again are consistent with the sites of mechanical loading and diffuse tissue strains. For example, in fluid percussion models, the midline bilateral permeability change is seen in the neocortex, dorsal hippocampus, and subcortical white matter as well as throughout the brainstem.[45,98] In contrast, the lateral fluid percussion model appears to evoke more unilateral change involving the same anatomic sites.[98]

Mechanistically, little effort has been made to better understand the cellular substrates that underlie the observed traumatically induced disruption of the blood-brain barrier. While in many cases overt damage to the microvasculature is responsible for the movement of tracers from the blood to the tissue front, in other cases the endothelium remains intact, and alternative mechanisms must be proposed. To date, cleaving of the endothelial tight junctions and increased vesicular activity in addition to direct membrane perturbation have been proposed as potential substrates for the passage of various substances through the blood-brain barrier.[91] In general, this traumatically induced barrier perturbation appears to be rather transient, resolving within the first day after injury.[91] Interestingly, this profile of traumatically induced permeability change is quite reminiscent of that described in traumatically brain-injured humans, using gadolinium contrast studies.

FUNCTIONAL CHANGE

Neuroexcitation

Traumatically brain-injured animals, particularly those subjected to fluid percussion insults, have been shown to undergo a net phase of traumatically induced neuroexcitation. This phase has been documented through various approaches, including the use of microdialysis as well as receptor antagonism. Specifically, in fluid percussion injury models, microdialysis has confirmed a rise in the excitatory amino acid levels in the first minutes after an injury.[107,108] The overall rise of these excitatory amino acids appears to be dependent on the severity of the injury in addition to technical aspects regarding whether the probe was positioned before or after the traumatic insult. The fact that these neurotransmitters are responsible for traumatically induced morbidity has been shown by multiple laboratories using the same animal model systems. Specifically, through the use of multiple receptor antagonists targeting the glutamate/N-methyl-D-aspartate as well as the cholinergic/muscarinic receptor populations, it has been shown that these strategies provide considerable protection if they are initiated either before or immediately after the induction of the traumatic insult.[55,56,60–62,108–115] To date, using the fluid percussion brain-injury model, these strategies have been shown to afford behavioral protection and prevent the loss of neuronal elements after the induction of a secondary posttraumatic insult.

Whether comparable changes are ongoing in brain-injured humans has remained a matter of debate, as these patients cannot be routinely monitored within minutes of the traumatic event. Recent microdialysis studies from Scandinavia[116] and the United States, however, suggest that the traumatic episode can trigger sustained rises in excitatory amino acids which can be detected in the brain parenchyma several hours after the injury.

Cerebral Metabolism

The issue of cerebral metabolic change after traumatic brain injury also has been investigated in various animal models of traumatic brain injury (see Chap. 110). In early descriptive studies using the midline fluid percussion model in the cat, the use of ^{14}C 2-deoxyglucose demonstrated a relative reduction in brain glucose metabolism, with only scattered foci demonstrating enhanced glucose metabolic activity.[81,82]

In a more recent work utilizing the fluid percussion model in rodents, a somewhat different profile of glucose metabolism was described. Specifically, through the efforts of Hovda and coworkers, fluid percussion injury was recognized to result in an immediate hypermetabolism, which in turn was followed by a period of generalized hypometabolism.[117–118] Again, these studies utilized ^{14}C 2-deoxyglucose to assess relative changes in glucose metabolism. In rodent models of fluid percussion brain injury, these periods of hypermetabolism have been equated with the period of neuroexcitation, with the suggestion that the hypermetabolism was a direct result of the brain's attempt to maintain ionic homeostasis after traumatically induced neuroexcitation (see Chap. 110). While the correlation of these metabolic events seen in animals with head-injured humans is tenuous, it is not unreasonable to speculate that comparable metabolic changes occur in humans and may be contributors to traumatically related morbidity. Obviously, further research in this area is required.

Brain Electrical Activity

Information regarding electrical activity after a traumatic injury is relatively modest. With EEG analyses, most researchers concur that concussion is associated with a suppression of EEG activity.[93,119] In general, all contemporary reports suggest that concussion evokes varying responses, ranging from high-amplitude slow-wave activity that appears to approximate the duration of unconsciousness to frank EEG suppression that parallels the concussive episode. Similar to the changes reported in EEG activity with traumatic brain injury, somatosensory evoked potential studies also have revealed abnormalities. The early work of Ommaya and Gennarelli[8] demonstrated that the somatosensory evoked response, or at least the P_2 component of that response, was abolished with the onset of concussion. In addition to these analyses of EEG and somatosensory evoked responses, more recent studies have unmasked other examples of traumatically induced electrophysiological change. Specifically, literature is just emerging that shows that traumatic brain injury suppresses the induction of long-term potentiation (LTP), which is presumed to be the physiological substrate of learning and memory in the hippocampus.[70,120] The same studies also have suggested that with this suppression of LTP induction, the traumatic injury causes local changes in neuronal excitability.[70]

Alterations in Blood Flow

In addition to the functional changes that occur in relation to the brain parenchyma, experimental traumatic brain injury evokes a host of functional changes in the brain's intrinsic vasculature. In both traumatically brain-injured animals and humans, data suggest that traumatic brain injury elicits changes in cerebral blood flow. Again, primarily using the fluid percussion brain injury models in both the cat and the rat, there have been attempts to fully characterize the blood flow changes seen in both the early and late posttraumatic periods. Through the use of laser Doppler[69] as well as radioactive microspheres[121] and iodoantipyrine tracers,[122] a picture of the flow changes associated with traumatic brain injury is beginning to emerge. Specifically, using the lateral fluid percussion model in rodents,[121] McIntosh and coworkers described the early period of posttraumatic hypoperfusion, which is followed in turn by normalization of blood flow. Interestingly, the same flow pattern has been shown to occur in the midline fluid percussion model in rodents, where early hypoperfusion has been observed.[69] The key question in these studies is whether such hypoperfusion reaches ischemic levels. While the actual flows reported to date are not within the ischemic range, some represent an overall reduction of blood flow in the range of 50 percent. Interestingly, despite these rather consistent changes described in rodent models of fluid percussion brain injury, the cat fluid percussion model has not yielded comparable results. In fact, the use of radioactive microspheres in cats has shown a period of posttraumatic hyperemia followed by a normalization of flows rather than the profile of hypoperfusion followed by normalization described in brain-injured rodents.[123]

Impaired Vascular Reactivity

Accompanying the flow abnormalities described above, impaired vascular responses have been described in many of the currently used animal models of traumatic brain injury. In these models, and in particular in the fluid percussion model in cats, impaired autoregulation has been described after traumatic brain injuries of varying severity.[124,125] In addition to impaired autoregulation, these models have demonstrated an inability of the pial arterioles to respond to normal changes in blood gas P_{CO_2} and P_{O_2}.[126,127] Further, the same pial vessels demonstrate abnormal endothelial dependent responses after a traumatic brain injury.[128,129] Normally, agents such as acetylcholine induce vasodilation through the release of endothelial-derived relaxing factors (EDRF), which in turn act on the vascular smooth muscle. In traumatic brain injury, however, the normal vasodilatory endothelial-dependent response is converted to vasoconstriction. In fact, in the early posttraumatic period, the topical application of acetylcholine constricts pial arterioles and abolishes the responses of larger vessels. Interestingly, similar abnormalities also are observed in response to the vasoconstrictor influences of serotonin, which also leads to an impaired response in the early period after an injury.[129] While it is beyond the scope of this chapter to consider these issues fully, many of the changes in vascular reactivity described above have been directly related to the traumatically induced production of oxygen radicals generated as a by-product of the increased metabolism of arachidonate.[130–134] In this pathway, the production of the superoxide anion and the hydroxyl radical appears to be involved in the generation of these vascular abnormalities. In the case of both experimental and human traumatic brain injury, the vascular abnormalities described above all suggest that the injured brain is not prepared to deal on the vascular front with a systemic challenge that it would otherwise tolerate well. In this context, one could easily envision how relatively modest hypotensive or hypoxic insults could translate into devastating injury for an already compromised brain.

SUMMARY AND CONCLUSIONS

This chapter has provided an overview of some of the major models of traumatic brain injury currently in use. The author has attempted to provide insight into precisely how these models injure the brain and what morphopathological responses they evoke. While it is clear that no single animal model can fully replicate the spectrum of human traumatic brain injury, it is equally obvious that most can reproduce multiple features of human traumatic brain injury which subsequently can be analyzed and evaluated. With the exception of the inertial injury models used in subhuman primates, no other animal model fully replicates the spectrum of human traumatic brain injury. However, there is no doubt that most animals models replicate important features of the human condition and thus allow for the continued study and analysis of processes similar to those ongoing in traumatically brain-injured man.

References

1. Witokowski L: Ueber Gehirnerschutterung. *Virchows Arch A Pathol Anat Histopathol* 69:498, 1877
2. Denny-Brown D: Cerebral concussion. *Physiol Rev* 25:296, 1945.
3. Denny-Brown D, Russell WR: Experimental cerebral concussion. *Brain* 64:93, 1945.
4. Gennarelli TA: Animate models of human head injury. *J Neurotrauma* 11:357, 1993.
5. Ommaya AK, Hirsch AE, Flamm ES, Mahone RH: Cerebral concussion in the monkey: An experimental model. *Science* 153:211, 1966.
6. Higgins LS, Schmall RA: A device for the investigation of head injury effected by non-deforming head accelerations, in *11th Stapp Car Crash Conference Proceedings*. New York: Society of Automotive Engineers, 1967; 35–46.
7. Gennarelli TA, Thibault LE, Adams JH, et al: Diffuse axonal injury and traumatic coma in the primate. *Ann Neurol* 12:564, 1982.
8. Ommaya AK, Gennarelli TA: Cerebral concussion and traumatic unconsciousness: Correlation of experimental and clinical observations on blunt head injury. *Brain* 97:633, 1974.
9. Ono K, Kiruchi A, Nakamura M, et al: Human head tolerance to sagittal impact: Reliable estimation deduced from experimental head injury using subhuman primates and human cadaver skulls, in *24th Staff Car Crash Conference Proceedings.* New York: SAE, 1980:101.
10. Tsubokawa T, Yamamoto T, Miyazaki S, et al: Pathogenic mechanism of cerebral concussion due to rotational angular acceleration impact. *Neurol Med Chir (Tokyo)* 21:657, 1981.
11. Nelson LR, Auen EL, Bourke RS, Barron KD: A new head injury model for evaluation of treatment modalities (abstract). Proceedings of the Society for Neuroscience 5:516, 1979.
12. Ross DT, Meaney DF, Sabol M, et al: Distribution of diffuse axonal injury following inertial closed head injury in miniature swine. *Exp Neurol* 126:1, 1994.
13. Ross DT, Meaney DF, Thibault LE, Gennarelli TA: Distribution of diffuse axonal injury following inertial closed head injury in miniature swine (abstract). Proceedings of the Society for Neuroscience 19:1486, 1993.
14. Folz EL, Schmidt RP: The role of the reticular formation in the coma of head injury. *J Neurosurg* 13:145, 1956.
15. Gosh HH, Gooding E, Schneider RC: The lexan calvarium for the study of cerebral responses to acute trauma. *J Trauma* 10:370, 1970.
16. Kobrine AI, Kempe LG: Studies in head injury: I. An experimental model of closed head injury. *Surg Neurol* 1:34, 1973.
17. Shatsky SA: Flash x-ray cinematography during impact injury, in *17th Stapp Car Crash Conference Proceedings.* New York: SAE, 1973:361.
18. Sekino H, Nakamura N, Kiruchi A, et al: Experimental head injury in monkeys using rotational acceleration impact. *Neurol Med-Chir (Tokyo)* 20:27, 1979.
19. Langfitt TW, Tannanbaum HM, Kassell NF: The etiology of acute brain swelling following experimental head injury. *J Neurosurg* 24:47, 1966.
20. Torhneim PA, Linwinicz BH, Hirsch CS, et al: Acute responses to blunt head trauma: Experimental model and gross pathology. *J Neurosurg* 59:431, 1983.
21. Hall ED, Yonkers PA, McCall JM, Braughler JM: Effects of the 21-aminosteroid U74006F on experimental head injury in mice. *J Neurosurg* 68:456, 1988.
22. Bean JW, Beckman DL: Centrogenic pulmonary pathology in mechanical head injury. *J Appl Physiol* 27:807, 1969.
23. Bakay L, Lee JC, Lee GC, Peng J-R: Experimental cerebral concussion: I. An electron microscopic study. *J Neurosurg* 47:525, 1977.
24. Huger F, Patrick G: Effect of concussive head injury on central catecholamine levels and synthesis rates in rat brain regions. *J Neurochem* 33:89, 1979.
25. Goldman H, Hodgson V, Morehead M, Murphy S: Cerebrovascular changes in a rat model of moderate closed-head injury. *J Neurotrauma* 8:129, 1991.
26. Marmarou A, Foda MAA-E, Van Den Brink W, et al: A new model of diffuse brain injury in rats. *J Neurosurg* 80:291, 1990.
27. Shapira Y, Shohami E, Sidi A, et al: Experimental closed head injury in rats: Mechanical pathophysiologic, and neurologic properties. *Crit Care Med* 16:258, 1988.
28. Gennarelli TA, Thibault LE: Biological models of head injury, in Povlishock J, Becker BP (eds): *Central Nervous System Trauma Status Report.* William Byrd Press, Richmond, Va., 1985:392.
29. Gennarelli TA, Ommaya AK, Thibault LE: Comparison of linear and rotational acceleration in experimental cerebral concussion, in *15th Stapp Car Crash Conference Proceedings.* New York: SAE, 1971:797–803.
30. Gennarelli TA, Thibault IE, Ommaya AK: Pathophysiologic responses to rotational and translational acceleration of the head, in *16th Stapp Car Crash Conference Proceedings.* New York: SAE, 1972:296–308.
31. Ommaya AK, Gennarelli TA: Correlations between the biomechanics and pathophysiology of head injury, in Sano K, Ischii S (eds): *Neural Trauma.* New York: American Elsevier, 1974:275–289.
32. Ommaya AK, Thibault L: Head and spinal injury toler-

ance with no direct head impact. *Proceedings of the International Conference on the Biokinetics of Impacts.* Lyon: IRCOBI, 1973:311–319.

33. Abel JM, Gennarelli TA, Segawa H: Incidence and severity of cerebral concussion in the rhesus monkey following sagittal plane angular acceleration, in *22nd Stapp Car Crash Conference Proceedings.* New York: SAE, 1978:33–53.
34. Gennarelli TA, Adams JH, Graham DI: Acceleration induced head injury in the monkey: I. The model, its mechanical and physiological correlates. *Acta Neuropathol (Berl)* VII (suppl):23, 1981.
35. Gennarelli TA, Abel JM, Adams H, Graham DI: Differential tolerance of frontral and temporal lobes to contusion induced by angular acceleration, in *23rd Stapp Car Crash Conference Proceedings.* New York: SAE, 1979:563–586.
36. Adams JH, Graham DI, Gennarelli TA: Neuropathology of acceleration induced head injury in the subhuman primate, in Grossman RG, Glidenberg PL (eds): *Head Injury: Basic and Clinical Aspects.* New York: Raven Press, 1982:141–150.
37. Gennarelli TA, Thibault LE: Biomechanics of acute subdural hematoma. *J Trauma* 22:680, 1982.
38. Graham DI, Adams JH, Gennarelli TA: Head injury neuropathology, in Ommaya AK (ed): *Consensus of Head and Neck Injury Criteria.* National Highway Traffic Safety Administration, Washington, DC 1983:235–246.
39. Gennarelli TA, Jane J, Thibault LE, Stewart O: Axonal damage in mild head injury demonstrated by the nauta method, in Villiani R (ed): *Advances in Neurotraumatology.* Amsterdam: Excerpta Medica, 1983:37–40.
40. Jane JA, Steward O, Gennarelli T: Axonal degeneration induced by experimental noninvasive minor head injury. *J Neurosurg* 62:96, 1985.
41. Jane J, Rimel RW, Pobereskyn LH, et al: Outcome and pathology of minor head injury, in Grossman RG (ed): *Seminars in Neurological Surgery.* New York: Raven Press, 1982:229–238.
42. Adams JH, Graham DI, Gennarelli TA: Acceleration induced head injury in the monkey: II. Neuropathology. *Acta Neuropathol (Berl)* VII (suppl):26, 1981.
43. Gennarelli TA, Thibault LE: Experimental production of prolonged traumatic coma in the primate, In Villiani R (ed): *Advances in Neurotraumatology.* Amsterdam: Excerpta Medica, 1982:31–33.
44. Adams JH, Gennarelli TA, Graham DI, et al: Diffuse axonal head injury in non-missile head injury, in Villiani R et al (eds): *Advances in Neurotraumatology.* Amsterdam: Excerpta Medica, 1983:53–58.
45. Cortez SC, McIntosh TK, Noble LJ: Experimental fluid-percussion brain injury: Vascular disruption and neuronal and glial alterations. *Brain Res* 482:271, 1989.
46. DeWitt DS, Kong DL, Lyeth BR, et al: Experimental traumatic brain injury elevates brain prostaglandin E2 and thromboxane B2 levels in rats. *J Neurotrauma* 5:303, 1988.
47. Dietrich WD, Alonso O, Halley M: Early microvascular and neuronal consequences of traumatic brain injury: A light and electron microscopic study in rats. *J Neurotrauma* 11:289, 1994b.
48. Dixon CE, Clifton GL, Lighthall JW, et al: A controlled cortical impact model of traumatic brain injury in the rat. *J Neurosci* 39:253, 1991.
49. Dixon CE, Lighthall JW, Anderson TE: Physiologic, histopathologic, and cineradiographic characterization of a new fluid-percussion model of experimental brain injury in the rat. *J Neurotrauma* 5:99, 1988.
50. Dixon CE, Lyeth BG, Povlishock JT, et al: A fluid-percussion model of experimental brain injury in the rat. *J Neurosurg* 67:110, 1987.
51. Enters EK, Pascua JR, McDowell KP, et al: Blockade of acute hypertensive response does not prevent changes in behavior or in CSF acetylcholine (TBI). *Brain Res* 476:271, 1992.
52. Hamm RJ, Dixon CD, Gbadebo DM, et al: Cognitive deficits following traumatic brain injury produced by controlled cortical impact. *J Neurotrauma* 9:11, 1992.
53. Hicks RR, Smith DH, Lowenstein DH, et al: Mild experimental brain injury in the rat induces cognitive deficits associated with regional neuronal loss in the hippocampus. *J Neurotrauma* 10:405, 1993.
54. Hovda DA, Yoshino A, Kawamata T, et al: Diffuse prolonged depression of cerebral oxidative metabolism following concussive brain injury in the rat: A cytochrome oxidase histochemistry study. *Brain Res* 567:1, 1991.
55. Jenkins LW, Lyeth BG, Lewelt W, et al: Combined pretrauma scopolamine and phencyclidine attenuate posttraumatic increased sensitivity to delayed secondary ischemia. *J Neurotrauma* 5:275, 1988.
56. Kawamata T, Katayama Y, Hovda DA, et al: Administration of excitatory amino acid antagonists via microdialysis attenuates the increase in glucose utilization seen following concussive brain injury. *J Cereb Blood Flow Metab* 12:12, 1992.
57. Lowenstein DH, Thomas MJ, Smith DH, McIntosh TK: Selective vulnerability of dentate hilar neurons following traumatic brain injury: A potential mechanistic link between head trauma and disorders of the hippocampus. *J Neurosci* 12:4846, 1990.
58. Lyeth BG, Hayes RL: Cholinergic and opioid mediation of traumatic brain injury. *J Neurotrauma* 9:S463, 1992.
59. Lyeth BG, Jenkins LW, Hamm RJ, et al: Prolonged memory impairment in the absence of hippocampal cell death following traumatic brain injury in the rat. *Brain Res* 526:249, 1990.
60. Lyeth BG, Ray M, Hamm RJ, et al: Postinjury scopolamine administration in experimental traumatic brain injury. *Brain Res* 569:281, 1992.
61. McIntosh TK, Vink R, Soares H, et al: Effects of the N-methyl-D-aspartate receptor blocker MK-801 on neurologic function after experimental brain injury. *J Neurotrauma* 6:247, 1989.
62. McIntosh TK, Vink R, Soares H, et al: Effect of non-competitive blockade of N-methylD-aspartate receptors on the neurochemical sequelae of experimental brain injury. *J Neurochem* 55:1170, 1990.

63. McIntosh TK, Vink R, Yamakami I, Faden AI: Magnesium protects against neurological deficit after brain injury. *Brain Res* 482:252, 1989.
64. McIntosh TK, Faden AI, Bendall MR, et al: Traumatic brain injury in the rat: Alterations in brain lactate and pH as characterized by ^{1}H and ^{31}P nuclear magnetic resonance. *J Neurochem* 49:1530.
65. McIntosh TK, Vink R, Noble L, et al: Traumatic brain injury in the rat: Characterization of a lateral fluid percussion model. *Neuroscience* 28:233, 1989.
66. McIntosh TK, Noble L, Andrews B, Faden AI: Traumatic brain injury in the rat, characterization of a midline fluid-percussion model. *Cent Nerv Syst Trauma* 4:119, 1987.
67. Miazaki S, Newlon P, Goldberg S, et al: Cerebral concussion suppresses hippocampal long-term potentiation (LTP) in rats, in Marmarou A, Hoff J (eds): *Intracranial Pressure*. New York: Springer, vol 7, 1991:651–653.
68. Miyazaki S, Katayama Y, Lyeth BG, et al: Enduring suppression of hippocampal long-term potentiation following traumatic brain injury in rat. *Brain Res* 585:335, 1992.
69. Muir JK, Boerschel M, Ellis EF: Continuous monitoring of posttraumatic cerebral blood flow using laser-doppler flowmetry. *J Neurotrauma* 9:355, 1992.
70. Reeves TM, Lyeth BG, Povlishock JT: Long-term potentiation deficits and excitability changes following traumatic brain injury. *Exp Brain Res* 106:248–256, 1995.
71. Smith DH, Okiyama K, Thoms MJ, et al: Evaluation of memory dysfunction following experimental brain injury using the Morris Water Maze. *J Neurotrauma* 8:259, 1991.
72. Soares HD, McIntosh TK: Subcortical neuronal degeneration following experimental rat brain injury (abstract). Proceedings of the Society for Neuroscience 17, 1992.
73. Sutton RL, Lescaudron L, Stein DG: Unilateral cortical contusion injury in the rat: Vascular disruption and temporal development of cortical necrosis. *J Neurotrauma* 10:135, 1993.
74. Tanno H, Nockels RP, Pitts LH, Noble LJ: Breakdown of the blood-brain barrier after fluid percussive brain injury in the rat: I. Distribution and time course of protein extravasation. *J Neurotrauma* 9:21, 1992.
75. Tanno H, Nockels RP, Pitts LH, Noble LJ: Immunolocalization of heat shock protein after fluid percussion brain injury and relationship to breakdown of the blood-brain barrier. *J Cereb Blood Flow Metab* 13:116, 1993.
76. Vink R, Head VA, Rogers PJ, et al: Mitochondrial metabolism following traumatic brain injury in rats. *J Neurotrauma* 7:21, 1990.
77. Cheng CLY, Povlishock JT: The effect of head injury on the visual system: A morphological characterization of reactive axonal change. *J Neurotrauma* 5:47, 1988.
78. Ellison MD, Erb DE, Kontos HA, Povlishock JT: Recovery of impaired endothelium-dependent relaxation after fluid-percussion brain injury. *Stroke* 20:911, 1989.
79. Erb DE, Povlishock JT: Axonal change with severe head injury. *Acta Neuropathol (Berl)* 76:347, 1988.
80. Erb DE, Povlishock JT: Neuroplasticity following traumatic brain injury: A study of GABAergic terminal loss and recovery in the cat dodral lateral vestibular nucleus. *Exp Brain Res* 83:253, 1991.
81. Hayes RL, Katayama Y, Jenkins LW, et al: Regional rates in glucose utilization in the cat following concussive head injury. *J Neurotrauma* 5:121, 1988.
82. Hayes RL, Pecura CM, Katayama Y, et al: Activation of midbrain cholinergic sites implicated in unconsciousness following cerebral concussion in the cat. *Science* 223:301, 1984.
83. Hayes RL, Stalhammar D, Povlishock JT, et al: A new model of concussive brain injury in the cat produced by extradural fluid volume loading: II. Physiological and neuropathological observations. *Brain Inj* 1:93, 1987.
84. Kontos HA, Povlishock JT: Oxygen radicals in brain injury. *Cent Nerv Syst Trauma* 3:257, 1986.
85. Kontos HA, Wei EP: Endothelium-dependent responses after experimental brain injury. *J Neurotrauma* 9:349, 1992.
86. Marmarou A, Shima K: Comparative studies of edema produced by fluid percussion injury with lateral and central modes of injury in cats. *Adv Neurol* 52:233, 1994.
87. Povlishock JT: Traumatically induced reactive axonal change without concomitant change in focal related neuronal somata and dendrites. *Act Neuropathol (Berl)* 70:53, 1986.
88. Povlishock JT, Becker DP: The fate of reactive axonal swellings induced by head injury. *Lab Invest* 52:540, 1985.
89. Povlishock JT, Becker DP, Cheng CLY, Vaughan GW: Axonal change in minor head injury. *J Neuropathol Exp Neurol* 42:225, 1983.
90. Povlishock JT, Becker DP, Miller JD, Dietrich WD: The morphologic substrates of concussion? *Acta Neuropathol (Berl)* 47:1, 1979.
91. Povlishock JT, Becker DP, Sullivan HG, Miller JD: Vascular permeability alterations to horseradish peroxidase in experimental brain injury. *Brain Res* 153:223, 1978.
92. Povlishock JT, Erb DE, Astruc J: Axonal response to traumatic brain injury. Reactive axonal change, deafferentation, and neuroplasticity. *J Neurotrauma* 9:S189, 1992.
93. Sullivan HG, Martinez J, Becker DP, et al: Fluid-percussion model of mechanical brain injury in the cat. *J Neurosurg* 45:520, 1976.
94. Wei EP, Dietrich WD, Povlishock JT, Kontos HA: Functional, morphologic, metabolic abnormalities of the cerebral microcirculation after concussive brain injury in cats. *Circ Res* 46:37, 1980.
95. Lighthall JW: Controlled cortical impact: A new experimental brain injury model. *J Neurotrauma* 5:1, 1988.
96. Valadka AB, Marqueen TJ, Shah J, Povlishock JT: Diffuse axonal injury in the micropig: Evidence for progressive axonal change demonstrating temporal heterogeneity. *J Neurotrauma* (in review).

97. Thibault LE, Meaney DF, Anderson BJ, Marmarou A: Biomechanical aspects of a fluid percussion model of brain injury. *J Neurotrauma* 9:311, 1992.
98. Schmidt RH, Grady MS: Regional patterns of blood-brain barrier breakdown following central and lateral fluid percussion injury in rodents. *J Neurotrauma* 10:415, 1993.
99. Gennerelli TA, Thibault LE, Goldstein D, et al: Axonal injury in the rat cerebral cortex in a modified rigid indenter cortical impact model. *J Neurotrauma* 9:60, 1992.
100. Lighthall JW, Goshgarian HG, Pinderski CR: Characterization of axonal injury produced by controlled cortical impact. *J Neurotrauma* 7:65, 1990.
101. Kotapka MJ, Gennarelli TA, Graham DI, et al: Selective vulnerability of hippocampal neurons in acceleration-induced experimental head injury. *J Neurotrauma* 8:247, 1991.
102. Ross TD, Graham DI, Adams JH: Selective loss of neurons from the thalamic reticular nucleus following severe human head injury. *J Neurotrauma* 10:151, 1993.
103. Koptapka MJ, Graham DI, Adams JH, Gennarelli TA: Hippocampal pathology in fatal human head injury without high intracranial pressure. *J Neurotrauma* 11:317, 1994.
104. Schweitzer JB, Park MR, Einhaus SL, Robertson JT: Ubiquitin marks the reactive swellings of diffuse axonal injury. *Acta Neuropathol* (*Berl*) 85:503, 1993.
105. Gennarelli TA, Thibault LE, Ross DT, Meaney D: Enhancement of axonal damage in the forebrain during contralateral craniectomy during controlled cortical impact injury in the rat (abstract). Proceedings of the Society for Neuroscience 15, 1990.
106. Yaghami A, Povlishock JT: Traumatically induced reactive change as visualized through the use of monoclonal antibodies targeted to the neurofilament subunits. *J Neuropathol Exp Neurol* 51:158, 1992.
107. Faden AI, Demediuk P, Panter SS, Vink R: The role of excitatory amino acids and NMDA receptors in traumatic brain injury. *Science* 244:798, 1989.
108. Katayama Y, Becker DP, Tamura T, Hovda DA: Massive increases in extracellular potassium and the indiscriminate release of glutamate following concussive brain injury. *J Neurosurg* 73:889, 1990.
109. Hayes RL, Chapouris R, Lyeth BG, et al: Pretreatment with phencyclidine (PCP) attenuates long-term behavioral deficits following concussive brain injury in the rat. *Soc Neurosci Abstr* 13:1254, 1987.
110. Hayes RL, Jenkins LW, Lyeth GB: Neurotransmitter-mediated mechanisms of traumatic brain injury: Acetylcholine and excitatory amino acids. *J Neurotrauma* 9:S173, 1992.
111. Hayes RL, Jenkins LW, Lyeth BG, et al: Pretreatment with phencyclidine, an N-methyl-D-aspartate-receptor antagonist, attenuates long-term behavioral deficits in the rat produced by traumatic brain injury. *J Neurotrauma* 5:529, 1988a.
112. Jenkins LW, Lyeth BG, Lewelt W, et al: Muscarinic and NMDA receptor blockade attenuates increased post-traumatic vulnerability to cerebral ischemia. *J Cereb Blood Flow Metab* 9:S750, 1989.
113. Lyeth BG, Dixon CE, Hamm RJ, et al: Effects of anticholinergic treatment on transient behavioral suppression and physiological responses following concussive brain injury to the cat. *Brain Res* 448:88, 1988.
114. Lyeth BG, Dixon CE, Jenkins LW, et al: Effects of scopolamine treatment on long-term behavioral deficits following concussive brain injury to the rat. *Brain Res* 452:39, 1988b.
115. Lyeth BG, Jenkins LW, Hamm RJ, et al: Pretreatment with MK-801 reduces behavioral deficits following traumatic brain injury (TBI) in rats. *Soc Neurosci Abstr* 15:1113, 1989.
116. Persson L, Hillered L: Chemical monitoring of neurosurgical intensive care patients using intracerebral microdialysis. *J Neurosurg* 76:72, 1992.
117. Yoshino A, Hovda DA, Kawamata T, et al: Dynamic changes in local cerebral glucose utilization following cerebral concussion in rats: Evidence of a hyper- and subsequent hypometabolic state. *Brain Res* 561:106, 1991.
118. Yoshino A, Hovda DA, Katayama Y, et al: Hippocampal CA3 lesions prevents postconcussive metabolic dysfunction in CA1. *J Cereb Blood Flow Metab* 12:996, 1992.
119. Ommaya AK, Rockoff SD, Baldwin M: Experimental concussion: A first report. *J Neurosurg* 21:249, 1964.
120. Miyazaki S, Katayama Y, Lyeth BG, et al: Enduring suppression of hippocampal long-term potentiation following traumatic brain injury in rat. *Brain Res* 585:335, 1992.
121. Yamakami I, McIntosh TK: Effects of traumatic brain injury on regional cerebral blood flow in rats as measured with radiolabeled microspheres. *J Cereb Blood Flow Metab* 9:117, 1989.
122. DeWitt DS, Prough DS, Taylor CL, Whitley JM: Reduced cerebral blood flow, oxygen delivery, and electroencephalographic activity after traumatic brain injury and mild hemorrhage in cats. *J Neurosurg* 76:812, 1992a.
123. Jenkins LW, Marmarou A, Lewelt W, Becker DP: Increased vulnerability of the traumatized brain to early ischemia, in Baethmann A, Go KG, Unterberg A (eds): *Mechanisms of Secondary Brain Damage.* New York: Plenum. 1986:173–281.
124. Lewelt WL, Jenkins LW, Miller JD: Autoregulation of cerebral blood flow after experimental fluid percussion injury of the brain. *J Neurotrauma* 53:500, 1980.
125. DeWitt DS, Prough DS, Taylor CL, et al: Regional cerebrovascular responses to progressive hypotension after traumatic brain injury in cats. *Am J Physiol* 263:H1276, 1992.
126. Wei EP, Dietrich WD, Povlishock JT, et al: Functional morphological and metabolic abnormalities of the cerebral microcirculation after concussive brain injury in cats. *Circ Res* 46:37, 1980.
127. Kontos HA, Wei EP, Povlishock JT: Pathophysiology of vascular consequences of experimental concussive brain injury. *Trans Am Clin Climatol Assoc* 30:111, 1981.

128. Ellison MD, Erb DE, Kontos HA, Povlishock JT: Recovery of impaired endothelium-dependent relaxation after fluid-percussion brain injury in cats. *Stroke* 20, 911, 1989.
129. Kontos HA, Wei EP: Endothelium-dependent responses after experimental brain injury. *J Neurotrauma* 9:349, 1992.
130. Kontos HA, Wei EP, Christman CW, et al: Free oxygen radicals in cerebral vascular response. *Physiologist* 26:265, 1983.
131. Kontos HA, Wei EP, Povlishock JT, Christman CW: Oxygen radicals mediate the cerebral arteriolar dilation from arachidonate and bradykinin in cats. *Circ Res* 55:295, 1984.
132. Wei EP, Christman CW, Kontos HA, Povlishock JT: Effects of oxygen radicals on cerebral arterioles. *Am J Physiol* 248:157, 1985.
133. Wei EP, Kontos HA, Ellison MD, Povlishock JT: Oxygen radicals in arachidonate-induced increased blood-brain barrier permeability to proteins. *Am J Physiol* 251:H693, 1986.
134. Kontos HA, Povlishock JT: Oxygen radicals in brain injury. *Cent Nerv Syst Trauma* 3:257, 1986.

CHAPTER 98

FLUID PERCUSSION AND CORTICAL IMPACT MODELS OF TRAUMATIC BRAIN INJURY

C. Edward Dixon
Ronald L. Hayes

BRIEF HISTORY OF TBI MODELS

INTRODUCTION

Several investigators have developed animal models of mechanical brain injury in an attempt to reproduce various aspects of the biomechanical responses, neurological syndromes, and pathology observed in human closed-head injury. Such models are necessary in order to determine brain injury mechanisms and to develop and test potential modes of therapy. A variety of experimental techniques have been developed, including closed-head impact models,[14,49,70,79] open-head impact models,[10,13,27,44,56,75] and acceleration injury.[59]

Two of the most widely employed TBI models are open-head impact techniques and fluid percussion and controlled cortical impact. As detailed below, fluid percussion produces brain injury by rapid injection of fluid into the closed cranial cavity. Cortical impact models utilize a pneumatic piston to deform a controllable volume of exposed cortex over a range of impact velocities. As Figs. 98-1 and 98-2 illustrate, in recent years rodent fluid percussion models have become the most commonly used models. Also, investigators increasingly are using cortical impact models. In this chapter, we will briefly review and compare the two models and their primary outcome measures. We will also review current controversies regarding the use of these models. Finally, we will discuss the future challenges, such as model standardization and development of preclinical criteria for therapy assessment.

INTRODUCTION TO RODENT MODELS

ADVANTAGES

The use of the laboratory rat provides a number of advantages in studying experimental TBI. These advantages include: (1) precise knowledge of age and genetic background of the animals; (2) existence of normative data for a wide range of physiological and behavioral variables; (3) compatibility with a number of neurochemical and molecular techniques not readily employed in larger species; (4) low purchase price and animal care costs; (5) high resistance to infection; and (6) economical use of expensive radioisotopes and drugs owing to low animal body weight.

DISADVANTAGES

The primary disadvantages include: (1) differences in brain structure and mass complicate biomechanical studies; (2) potential for seizures; (3) no prolonged unconsciousness; (4) less axonal injury; and (5) inability to test for more complex and/or subtle behavioral deficits.

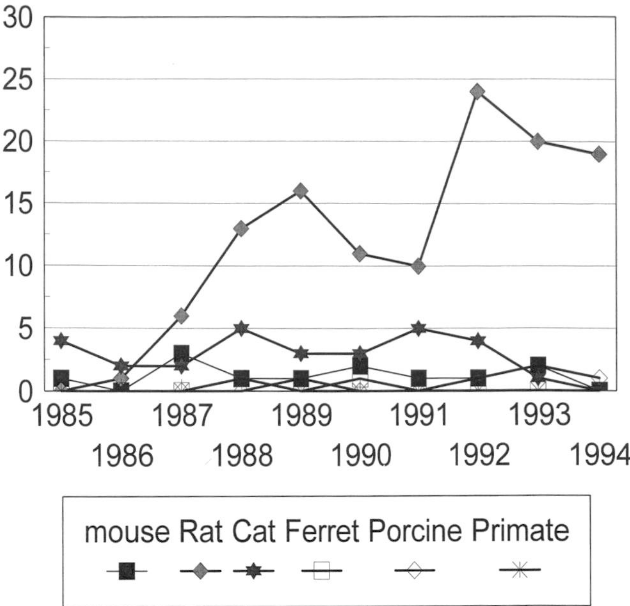

Figure 98-1. Approximate yearly number of peer-reviewed publications using experimental traumatic brain injury models divided by species. Data was gathered by searching Medline from 1985 to Sep. 1994 and by surveying back issues of the *Journal of Neurotrauma.* The graph indicates a substantial increase in the use of rats in experimental brain injury research during the last decade.

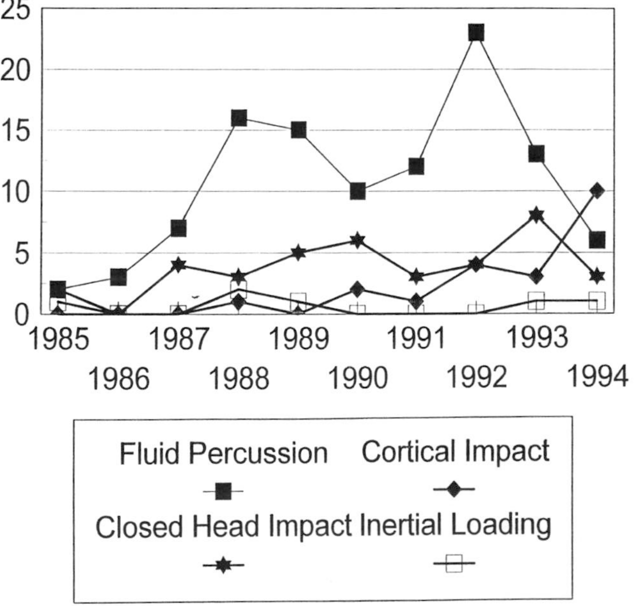

Figure 98-2. Approximate yearly number of peer-reviewed publications using experimental traumatic brain injury models divided by model. Data were gathered by searching Medline from 1985 to Sep. 1994 and by surveying back issues of the *Journal of Neurotrauma.* The graph suggests that fluid percussion has been the most frequently used experimental model over the last decade. Data from 1994 indicate an increase in the use of cortical impact models.

BRIEF HISTORY OF CURRENT MODELS

Fluid Percussion

Fluid percussion models produce graded levels of brain injury associated with rapid injection of small volumes of saline into the closed cranial cavity. The classic technique uses a pendulum hammer to hit the end of a plunger within a fluid-filled tube.[13,51,75] The pressure pulse is delivered through a craniotomy to induce a brief intracranial pressure increase and associated deformation of neural tissue. The technique does not attempt to reproduce precisely the array of events following closed-head injury in humans, in which injury results from rapid acceleration-deceleration of the head, usually with impact to intact skull. Rather, fluid percussion brain injury successfully produces graded levels of injury associated with predictable neurological, physiological, and histological changes comparable to those observed in human brain injury.[3,5,13,20,30,40,81] As others have pointed out, efforts to reproduce directly the mechanisms of human brain injury usually resulted in models that do not reliably reproduce the neurological deficits or pathologies seen clinically.[39] Furthermore, when other techniques are used, such as extracranial impact to the intact skull or nonimpact acceleration of the head, it is more difficult to quantify directly and control the forces producing brain deformation, and measurements of brain displacement have not been precise.[26,39] Fluid percussion injury in the rat reproduces many of the features of head injury observed in other models and species. Thus, this animal model represents a useful experimental approach to studies of pathological changes similar to those seen in human head injury.

Controlled Cortical Impact

The controlled cortical impact technique was developed so that the biomechanical events contributing to injury could be analyzed by establishing a quantifiable relationship between measurable engineering parameters, such as force, velocity, or deformation, and the magnitude of tissue damage and/or functional impairment. The application of a constrained stroke pneumatic impactor allows accurate, reliable, and independent control of the deformation parameters over a wide range of contact velocities, and has been demonstrated in spinal cord injury models to produce contusion and to allow a reproducible gradation of injury outcome severity.[1,38]

Experimental TBI, employing a pneumatic impactor, has been well characterized in the laboratory ferret[42,43] and rat.[16] In general, the injury responses resembled aspects of severe closed-head injury in humans. In contrast to fluid percussion models of traumatic brain injury,[13,15,28,44] the cortical impact model of experimental brain injury uses a known impact interface and a measurable, controllable impact velocity and cortical deformation. These controlled mechanical variables enable the amount of deformation and the change in deformation over time to be accurately determined.

PRIMARY OUTCOME MEASURES

Behavior

Motor

If a specific protocol employs short-acting anesthetics, then acute neurological suppression can be assessed by using a battery of tests that have been shown to be sensitive to varying magnitudes of both fluid percussion[13,46] and controlled cortical impact models of TBI.[8,16] This battery, which includes tests analogous to motor components of the Glasgow Coma Scale,[78] allows quantification of various features of the suppression of the animal's responsiveness to external stimuli and relationships between durations of behavioral suppression and magnitudes of injury.

Vestibulomotor function has been assessed using beam balance and beam walking tasks. The beam balance task consists of measuring the animal's latency to balance on a beam up to 60 seconds. The beam walking task, originally devised by Feeney et al.,[19] allows the assessment of more refined locomotor activity in the context of a learned avoidance task. Prior to injury, rats are trained to escape a bright light and loud white noise by traversing a narrow wooden beam to enter a darkened goal box at the opposite end of the beam.

Composite neurological scores, in which the scores of several neurological tests are summed up to a single numerical value, have been frequently used to assess the extent of global neurological deficit following lateral fluid percussion brain injury.[18,51] Finally, when assessing cognitive deficits, measurement of task-specific motor functioning is necessary to control for nonspecific—and thus possibly confounding—motor deficits. For example, performance in the Morris water maze task should be independent of the animal's ability to swim.

Cognitive

Memory deficits are one of the most persistent sequelae of non-missile head injury in humans.[41] These memory disturbances include a period of transient post-traumatic amnesia characterized by gross confusion and inability to commit new information to memory. After the resolution of post-traumatic amnesia, many patients exhibit persistent memory disturbances. Recently, animal models of TBI have been used to examine cognitive deficits following injury. Lyeth et al.[47] evaluated memory deficits following fluid percussion brain injury with the radial-arm maze. They found that working memory was impaired for up to 15 days after injury. In the reference memory aspect of the task, no differences were observed between the injured and uninjured animals. Working memory has also been assessed for 7 days after fluid percussion TBI with a delayed-matching-to-sample procedure. In this study working memory deficits were observed at the longer delay intervals (>20 sec) for 4 days following TBI. These data suggest that animals exhibit transitory deficits in working memory following fluid percussion TBI. Smith et al.[72] demonstrated significant memory dysfunction in the Morris water maze test 42 hours after lateral fluid percussion injury. Hamm et al.[27] showed spatial memory performance deficits in the Morris water maze task on days 11 to 15 and 30 to 34 following cortical impact in rats. Morris water maze performance is also impaired following bilateral frontal cortical impact injury.[33] Thus, many laboratories have consistently reported that traumatic brain injury can produce spatial memory deficits in rats. Importantly, spatial memory may represent a rodent analogue for declarative memory studied in humans and thought to be importantly mediated by temporal lobe function.[88] However, the neural substrates serving spatial memory in rats are not entirely clear. While hippocampal function seems to be important for spatial memory, other data in rats suggest that the cortex may also be critical for spatial memory performance.[4]

Morphology

Histopathological studies in TBI models is an important outcome measure because it can be clinically validated by direct comparison with human diagnostic images or postmortem specimens. Historically, studies of traumatic brain injury have focused on the production of overt structural alterations such as hemorrhages, contusion, and diffuse axonal injury. There is little doubt that structural damage can occur in both animals and humans following TBI.[64]

Diffuse axonal injury

Clinical studies suggest that diffuse axonal injury may be a factor in mild to moderate TBI in humans.[60] These neuropathological studies suggest a continuum of diffuse axonal injury severity in which the lesions are mechanical in origin and are caused by stretching and tearing of nerve fibers and small blood vessels. This postulated continuum of severity is also supported by neuropathological studies in animals following experimental mild head injury.[34,64] In general, axonal injury appears to occur less in rats than in larger species in both fluid percussion and controlled cortical impact models. There seems little doubt that diffuse axonal injury is a reliable consequence of mechanical trauma in humans and animals. Recent advances in our understanding of the pathobiology of trauma suggest that mechanical injury may not be restricted to axons but may also more generally include neuronal processes including dendrites.[63] Thus, diffuse axonal injury may be viewed as one subset of diffuse injury to neuronal processes. Whether or not similar or different mechanisms underlie damage to axons and dendrites remains to be determined.

Contusion

Apart from subarachnoid hemorrhage, cortical contusions are probably the most common clinical macroscopic findings.[74] Cortical contusion is generally not a prominent feature of central fluid percussion injury.[47] This probably reflects the distributed nature of cortical loading in the technique.[15] In contrast, lateral fluid percussion can result in contusions either at the site of injury[51] or lateral to and remote from the site of injury.[12] Cortical contusions are primary features of cortical impact models.[16,42] Cortical impact studies[76] indicate that contusions produce slowly progressing cystic cavities at mild-to-moderate magnitudes of injury, with larger cavities and almost total loss of contused tissue and underlying white matter occurring at late periods after more severe impact.

Cell death

For many years a major misconception has clouded the study of neural injury mechanisms—namely, that behavioral deficits are necessarily caused by structural injury. Unlike the study of most other forms of excitotoxic brain insults, such as ischemia or epilepsy, TBI studies have not commonly employed magnitudes of injury that produce overt cell death.[35,47] This research strategy has recently provided compelling evidence that mild and moderate traumatic brain injury can produce enduring pathological alterations in neural function not accompanied by light or electron microscopic tissue damage.[48]

As discussed above, mild and moderate TBI without contusion can produce prolonged spatial memory deficits in rats that persist for as long as 15 days after injury.[47] In that study no qualitative or quantitative evidence of neuronal death was observed in rats showing persistent memory deficits. Additionally, no overt evidence of axonal injury was observed in any forebrain structure, including major intrinsic and extrinsic connecting hippocampal pathways. In contrast to midline fluid percussion injury, lateral fluid percussion can produce cell loss in the CA3 region of the hippocampus[7,72] as well as cell loss in the hilar regions.[31,45] However, lateral fluid percussion does not always produce detectable hippocampal cell loss.[67,80] Qualitative light microscopic examinations following central controlled cortical impact have not been reported to produce hippocampal cell loss.[14,27]

While fluid percussion injury produces axonal injury and intraparenchymal hemorrhages,[64] it also produces histopathological changes different from those seen in severe human head injury. Fluid percussion at high injury magnitudes is primarily a model of brain stem injury.[71] Localized brain stem injury is not a primary feature of severe human traumatic brain injury.[54]

Neurotransmitters

Acute release

Studies with microdialysis sampling have confirmed EAA neurotransmitter release from hippocampal regions immediately after both fluid percussion and cortical impact TBI in the rat. Katayama et al.[37] reported a 90 percent increase in glutamate within 2 minutes after moderate fluid percussion TBI which returned to baseline within 4 minutes. A much larger magnitude of EAA release was reported by Faden et al.[17] In their study, moderate fluid percussion TBI associated with contusions produced 282 and 273 percent increases in glutamate and aspartate, respectively, while severe injury produced increases of 940 and 1849 percent in glutamate and aspartate, respectively. Peak concentrations occurred within 10 minutes and remained elevated for more than 1 hour. More recently, controlled cortical impact in rats has been reported to produce transient increases in dialysate concentrations of aspartate and glutamate.[61] Fold increases in aspartate and glutamate normalized within 20 to 30 minutes following moderate cortical impact and took >60 minutes to normalize following severe cortical impact.

Acetylcholine (ACh) levels also have been reported to change in brain and CSF following TBI. In a preliminary report by Gorman et al.,[24] hippocampal ACh levels (measured by microdialysis) increased 74 percent above control within 5 to 10 minutes after fluid percussion TBI. Saija et al.[68,69] found that ACh turnover rate (measured by a phosphoryl [$^2H_9$]choline method) increased in the brainstem 73 and 50 percent at 12 minutes and 4 hours, respectively, after moderate fluid percussion TBI in the rat. TBI did not produce increased ACh turnover in every region. Thus, moderate TBI appears to produce a transient release of ACh and increased cholinergic neuronal activity in some brain regions for several hours after injury.

Receptor changes

Measurements of changes in receptor binding following TBI have identified specific receptor populations affected by the injury process. Our laboratories have demonstrated decreased binding to both cholinergic and glutamatergic receptor binding following TBI. Moderate fluid percussion TBI without contusion produced significant changes in NMDA but not in quisqualate or kainate glutamate receptor subtypes in the rat.[53] Binding of [^{3}H]glutamate to NMDA receptors was reduced by 15 to 30 percent from control values in cerebral cortex at 5 minutes, 3 hours, and 24 hours after injury. NMDA binding in hippocampal CA1 and dentate gyrus was significantly lower (12 to 15 percent) only at 3 hours after injury. We have not yet determined whether these reductions in binding represent changes in receptor number (B_{max}) or affinity (K_d). The predominant changes seen only in the NMDA receptor suggest that the EAA agonist-receptor interactions produced by moderate TBI occur predominantly at this receptor subtype. The pathological role of this receptor subtype in TBI is further supported by the protection afforded by administration of NMDA antagonists.

Moderate fluid percussion TBI without contusion produced significant changes in receptor binding following TBI, and thus identified specific receptor populations affected by the injury process. TBI can significantly alter the binding sites of muscarinic receptors in hippocampus and neocortex for as long as 15 days after TBI.[20] A recent examination of the binding responses of M1 and M2 muscarinic receptor subtypes found decreased [^{3}H]-AFDX384 binding in the M2 receptor subtype at 24 hours in hippocampal CA2–3 region and dorsal blade of the dentate gyrus.[4] These reductions in receptor binding may persist for even longer periods and contribute to enhanced sensitivity to cholinergic antagonists after TBI.

Ion Shifts and Second Messengers

The earliest measurable neurochemical change following experimental TBI are ionic shifts. Several studies have provided evidence that experimental traumatic brain injury produces widespread neuronal depolarization[32,37,77] as measured by large increases in extracellular potassium (K_e^+). Increases in K_e^+ can result from mechanical deformation of voltage-gated K^+ channels[36] or from the opening of ligand-gated ion channels by neurotransmitters. In more severe magnitudes of injury involving hemorrhage and contusion, nonspecific breakdown of the plasma membrane may result in a massive outward shift of K^+.

A series of experiments using microdialysis techniques[37] found a short lasting two-fold increase in K_e^+ within 2 minutes after mild fluid percussion TBI. Administration of tetrodotoxin (TTX), which potently depresses neural firing, reduced the increase in K_e^+, while cobalt, which blocks Ca^{++} channels necessary for excitotoxic release of neurotransmitters, did not, thereby suggesting that the increased K_e^+ resulted from neuronal discharges and not from neurotransmitter release. Moderate TBI produced a larger (five-fold) and longer lasting increase in K_e^+ which was not blocked by TTX but was partially blocked by cobalt, suggesting that neurotransmitter release was recruited to increase depolarization as injury severity increased. Furthermore, kynurenic acid, an EAA antagonist, significantly reduced, but did not eliminate, the K_e^+ increase following moderate TBI, indicating that release of EAA transmitters (see below) significantly contributes to the increase in K_e^+ following TBI. Thus, following moderate TBI, tissue deformation is likely to open ion channels, resulting in an efflux of K^+ of sufficient magnitude to induce indiscriminate neurotransmitter release and further depolarization.

TBI can produce long-term increases in calcium ion levels. Increased total tissue calcium ion levels has been reported 48 hours following lateral fluid percussion TBI.[72] Increased calcium accumulation has been reported in the hippocampus for several days after injury.[21]

Molecular Changes

TBI can produce membrane depolarization and excessive excitatory neurotransmitter release, which may lead to increases of intracellular free calcium levels.[29] These processes activate calcium-dependent enzymes, including protein kinase C (PKC), which is known to play an important role in signal transduction. Changes in PKC activity have been implicated in a variety of neuronal functions associated with normal and pathological events.[50,57,58,82] Using the midline fluid percussion model, significant increases in PKC activity have been observed at 1 hour and 3 hours post-injury. Additionally, there was a significant increase in PKC levels in membrane fraction 3 hours, but not 1 hour, after injury.

Stimulation of protein kinases, such as PKC, can modulate the activity of transcription factors via protein phosphorylation.[9,22,85] Activation of these transcription factors alters the expression of downstream genes, some of which encode other transcription factors. This cascade of events ultimately may lead to the alteration of expression of later-effector genes, which may change the functional properties of nerve cells.[23,55] An oncoprotein mediator of gene expression, c-fos, was evaluated in the central fluid percussion model of traumatic brain injury.[62] An increase in c-fos-positive neurons was found in CA1 pyramidal neurons at 15 minutes following mild and moderate fluid percussion TBI. At 1 hour, significant increases were found only following mild TBI. By 24 hours, the number of c-fos-positive at both injury levels was not different from sham controls. The time course of c-fos expression also has been examined following lateral cortical impact injury.[8,86] C-fos protein was induced 1 hour after cortical impact and persists up to 3 hours. Immunohistochemical studies showed more extensive c-fos immunoreactivity following lateral cortical impact than following mild and moderate central fluid percussion TBI.[62] Therefore, it is possible that the functional deficits observed following TBI may be, in part, attributable to the pathophysiological expression of specific neuronal late-effector genes.

COMPARISON OF FLUID PERCUSSION TO CONTROLLED CORTICAL IMPACT MODELS

Advantages and Disadvantages

Fluid percussion in cortical impact models is best understood as a complementary approach to modeling a continuum of varying magnitudes of traumatic brain injury. Central fluid percussion injury is a useful model of mild-to-moderate diffuse brain injury without significant mass lesion effects. In contrast, cortical impact injury and lateral fluid percussion injury more closely approximate the severe levels of supratentorial involvement associated with lesions and contusions. Thus, the advantages of fluid percussion models reside primarily in their simplicity and their ability to produce significant disturbances in brain physiology in the absence of overt pathology at the light microscopic level. However, fluid percussion injury allows relatively little control over, or measurement of, biomechanical events accompanying injury. In addition, central fluid percussion injury produces significant brain stem involvement, even at relatively low injury magnitudes; at higher injury magnitudes it can produce brain stem collapse and death. Although cortical impact devices produce significant cortical damage even at lower injury magnitudes, cortical impact devices provide accurate measurement and control of a number of biomechanical parameters. In addition, since there is little brain stem involvement at most injury magnitudes commonly employed, mortality is relatively less than observed in central fluid percussion injury. Typically, investigators interested in neuropharmacological and signal transduction cascades unconfounded by changes in morphopathology or cerebral blood flow have employed central fluid percussion injury. In contrast, investigators interested in more severe levels of injury associated with focal ischemia contusion and evolving cell death and necrosis have employed cortical impact or lateral fluid percussion injury.

Neuropathology

While the fluid percussion technique reproduces a number of clinically relevant pathophysiological responses, it has two important limitations. First, fluid percussion brain injury is difficult to analyze biomechanically. Studies of fluid percussion biomechanics have been confined to analyzing fluid pulse parameters as indirect indices of the mechanical loading of the brain.[73] Furthermore, the fluid pulse enters the calvarium and disperses diffusely within the epidural space, as demonstrated by high-speed cineradiography,[15] making the tissue displacement difficult to quantify. The second limitation is that, while fluid percussion injury produces axonal injury and intraparenchymal hemorrhages,[64] it also produces histopathological changes different from those seen in severe human head injury. Fluid percussion at high injury magnitudes is primarily a model of brain stem injury.[71] Localized brain stem injury is not a primary feature of severe human traumatic brain injury.[54] Apart from subarachnoid hemorrhage, cortical contusions are probably the most common clinical macroscopic findings.[74] With some exceptions,[51] cortical contusion is generally not a prominent feature of fluid percussion injury.

Histopathological similarities and differences exist between the rat-controlled cortical impact model and the rat fluid percussion model. At moderate- and high-injury magnitudes, both models produced a similar distribution of intraparenchymal hemorrhages and axonal injury in the brain. Also, similar to the ferret cortical impact model,[43] the rat model produced profound axonal injury at the cerebellar peduncles. Histopathology in the cerebellar peduncles has been reported to be a common feature following blunt head injury in humans.[54] Unlike fluid percussion models, cortical contusion and cavitation are common features of the cortical impact model.

Cerebral Blood Flow

Studies of cerebral blood flow employing both microspheres[84,87] and iodoantipyrine[11] have been conducted in central and lateral rat fluid percussion models of TBI.

These studies examined flow times ranging from 5 minutes to 6 hours after injury. Although investigators have consistently reported flow reductions in some brain regions, no studies have reported flows approaching ischemic values. However, greater flow reductions were observed in contusional TBI models, suggesting a greater possibility for focal ischemia to occur in those models. In addition, Yamakami and McIntosh[84] reported in a rat lateral fluid percussion TBI model that prolonged focal oligemia at the site of fluid percussion injury was associated with the development of cystic necrosis at 4 weeks post-injury, implying that disturbances in cerebral blood flow contributed to tissue necrosis. Thus, possible post-traumatic ischemic episodes in that model may have also contributed to neurotransmitter-mediated excitotoxic injury. While significantly less is known about CBF responses to cortical impact injury, recent preliminary data demonstrated focal complete ischemia confined primarily to the cortical region surrounding the site of injury.[6]

CURRENT CONTROVERSIES

As with most animal models of clinical pathology, controversies surround the relevance of individual models to specific pathological features of human head injury and their usefulness as predictors of therapeutic efficacy in humans. A recent conference sponsored by the National Institutes of Health attempted to develop a framework for addressing these issues.[66] However, to date there is no formal consensus on either of them. This absence of consensus is largely attributable to our incomplete understanding of the most relevant pathobiological mechanisms in varying magnitudes of human brain injury. In addition, since there are to date no demonstrably effective therapies for human head injury, it is difficult to assess the predictive validity of varying models for assessing therapies useful in humans.

FUTURE CHALLENGES

Model Standardization

In recent years, a number of variations have been made to both rat fluid percussion and cortical impact models. Variations to the rat fluid percussion model include: (1) site of injury (e.g., central vs. lateral); (2) anesthetic regimen, including ventilatory support; (3) method of affixing the injury tube over the craniotomy; (4) interval from injury tube implantment and injury; (5) length and material of the connecting tube; and (6) the aperture of the injury tube. Different combinations of these variations can result in profoundly different injury profiles. For example, relocating the site of injury from the vertex to a more lateral orientation can change the model from one that produces a diffuse moderate brain injury with little detectable histopathology[47] to one that produces a more focal contusion and cell loss.[52]

Variations to the basic rat controlled cortical impact model include the: (1) site of injury (central vs. lateral); (2) size and shape of the impact tip; (3) amount of clearance between the impact tip and the edge of the craniotomy; (4) amount of deformation; (5) impact velocity; (6) use of secondary craniotomies to direct the movement of tissue; (7) angle of impact; and (8) anesthetic regimen, including ventilatory support.

While all of the above variations illustrate the ingenuity of investigators in adapting the models to their specific needs, they also illustrate an increasing lack of standardization. As indicated above, our current knowledge of the pathobiology of human head injury suggests that efforts of widespread standardization may be premature. However, it would seem reasonable to identify specific components of the pathobiology of trauma (i.e., excitotoxic cascades, diffuse injury to axons and dendrites) which may be optimally modeled by specific models.

Future Directions

Considerable progress has been made in understanding spinal cord injury with regard to developing a standardized model for preclinical assessments of drugs potentially useful for treating the acute phase of spinal cord injury. In the near future, similar efforts should be attempted for traumatic brain injury. These efforts will not only require the acceptance of one and/or a limited number of preclinical models. They also will require the establishment of rigorous criteria for determining whether or not preclinical assessments of an agent warrant clinical testing. These criteria should include, minimally, a determination of whether or not the putative therapeutic agent improves outcome. Thus, end-point assessments will become a critical feature of model standardization efforts, since investigators must agree upon the most relevant outcome measures, including behavioral assessments, assessments of cerebral blood flow, neurochemical changes, and/or histopathological alterations. Other preclinical criteria include assessments of whether or not the agents will ultimately be suitable for human use. Recent experience with NMDA receptor antagonists and alleged neuronal vacuolization should sensitize investigators to the careful selection of agents with minimal toxic potential. Ideally, preclinical assessments should also provide data on the pathophysiological processes being treated. While this is not a strong prerequisite for preclinical assessments, data suggesting a mechanism of action that is operative in humans would further support the clinical utility of the therapy.

In conclusion, rodent models of traumatic brain injury have had considerable influence on the progress of investigations in our field since their introduction in 1987. While rodent models of fluid percussion injury in traumatic brain injury are probably not sufficient to reproduce the entire spectrum of human head injury, their utility has made possible rapid advances in our understanding of a number of pathobiological mechanisms of trauma, including receptor-coupled cascades, changes in cerebral blood flow, and, more recently, molecular alterations. Future refinements in rodent models and the development of new models such as the porcine fluid percussion model[83] should further facilitate increased understanding of the mechanisms of trauma and lead to improved treatment of the traumatically brain-injured patient.

References

1. Anderson TE: A controlled pneumatic technique for experimental spinal cord contusion. *J Neurosci Meth* 1982; 6:327–333.
2. Becker DP, Miller JD, Sweet RC, et al: Head injury management, in Popp AJ, et al (eds): *Neural trauma.* New York: Raven Press, 1979:313–328.
3. Becker DP: The temporal genesis of primary and secondary brain damage in experimental and clinical head injury. *NATO Advanced Workshop on Mechanisms of Secondary Brain Damage.* Mauls: Sterzing, Italy, 1984.
4. Berger-Sweeney T, Heckers S, Mesulam MM, et al: Differential effects of spatial navigation on immuntoxin-induced cholinergic lesions of the medial septal area and nucleus basalis magnocellularis. *J Neurosci* 1994; 14(7):4507–4519.
5. Bruce DA, Langfitt TW, Miller JD, et al: Regional cerebral blood flow, intracranial pressure, and brain metabolism in comatose patients. *J Neurosurg* 1973; 38:131–144.
6. Bryan RM, Cerian L, Roberson C: Regional cerebral blood flow after controlled cortical impact injury in rats. *Proceedings of Eleventh Annual Neurotrauma Symposium,* 1993.
7. Cortex SC, McIntosh TK, Noble LJ: Experimental fluid percussion brain injury: Vascular disruption and neuronal and glial alterations. *Brain Res* 1989; 482:271–282.
8. Dash PK, Moore AN, Ginty D, Dixon CE: Spatial memory deficits, increased phosphorylation of the transcription factor CREB and induction of the AP-1 complex following lateral cortical impact. (In Press) 1994.
9. Dash PK, Karl KA, Colicos MA, et al: cAMP response element-binding protein is activated by Ca2 + /calmodulin—as well as cAMP-dependent protein kinase. *Proc Natl Acad Sci USA* 1991; 88:5061–5065.
10. Denny-Brown D, Russell WR: Experimental cerebral concussion. *Brain* 1941; 64:93–164.
11. DeWitt DS, Hayes RL, Lyeth BG, et al: Effects of traumatic brain injury on cerebral blood flow and metabolism: Autoradiographic studies. *Anesth Rev* 1988; 15:31–32.
12. Dietrich WD, Alonso O, Busto R, et al: Post-traumatic brain hypothermia reduces histopathological damage following concussive brain injury in the rat. *Acta Neuropathol* 1994; 87:250–258.
13. Dixon CE, Lyeth GB, Povlishock JT, et al: A fluid percussion model of experimental brain injury in the rat. *J Neurosurg* 1987; 67:110–119.
14. Dixon CE, Hamm RJ, Taft WC, Hayes RL: Increased anticholinergic sensitivity following closed skull impact and controlled cortical impact traumatic brain injury in the rat. *J Neurotrauma* 1994; 11(3):275–287.
15. Dixon CE, Lighthall JW, Anderson TE: A physiologic, histopathologic, and cineradiographic characterization of a new fluid percussion model of experimental brain injury in the rat. *J Neurotrauma* 1988; 5(2):91–104.
16. Dixon CE, Clifton GL, Lighthall JW, et al: A controlled cortical impact model of traumatic brain injury in the rat. *J Neurosci Meth* 1991; 39:253–262.
17. Faden AI, Demediuk P, Panter SS, Vink R: The role of excitatory amino acids and NMDA receptors in traumatic brain injury. *Science* 1989; 244:798–800.
18. Faden AI: Comparison of a single and combination drug treatment strategies in experimental brain trauma. *J Neurotrauma* 1993; 10(2):91–100.
19. Feeney DM, Boyeson MG, Linn RT, et al: Responses to cortical injury. I. Methodology and local effects of contusion in the rat. *Brain Res* 1981; 211:67–77.
20. Fieschi C, Sakurada O, Sokoloff L: Local cerebral glucose utilization during resolution of embolic experimental ischemia. *Adv Neurol* 1978; 20:223–229.
21. Fineman I, Hovda D, Smith M, et al: Concussive brain injury is associated with a prolonged accumulation of calcium: A ^{45}Ca autoradiographic study. *Brain Res* 1993; 624:94–102.
22. Ginty DD, Kornhauser JM, Thompson MA, et al: Regulation of CREB phosphorylation in the suprachiasmatic light and a circadian clock. *Science* 1993; 260:238–241.
23. Goelet P, Castellucci VF, Schacher S, Kandel ER: The long and short of long-term memory: A molecular approach. *Nature* 1986; 322:519–522.
24. Gorman LK, Fu K, Hovda DA, et al: Analysis of acetylcholine release following concussive brain injury in the rat. *J Neurotrauma* 1989; 6:203.
25. Gorman LK, Shook BL, Becker DP: Traumatic brain injury produces impairments in long-term and recent memory. *Brain Res* 1993; 614:29–36.
26. Gurdijan ES, Lissner HR, Webster JE, et al: Studies on experimental concussion: Relation of physiologic effect to time duration of intracranial pressure increase at impact. *Neurology* 1954; 4:674–681.

27. Hamm RJ, Dixon CE, Gbadebo DM, et al: Cognitive deficits following traumatic brain injury produced by controlled cortical impact. *J Neurotrauma* 1992; 9:11–20.
28. Hayes RL, Stalhammer DA, Galinat BJ, et al: A new model of concussive brain injury in the cat produced by extradural fluid volume loading. II. Physiological and neuropathological observations. *Brain Injury* 1987; 1:93–112.
29. Hayes RL, Jenkins LW, Lyeth BG: Neuropharmacological mechanisms of traumatic brain injury: Acetylcholine and excitatory amino acids. *J Neurotrauma* 1992; 9(suppl 1):S173–S187.
30. Hayes RL, Pechura CM, Katayama Y, et al: Activation of pontine cholinergic sites implicated in unconsciousness following cerebral concussion in the cat. *Science* 1984; 223:301–303.
31. Hicks RR, Smith DH, Lowenstein DH, et al: Mild experimental brain injury in the rat induces cognitive deficits associated with regional neuronal loss in the hippocampus. *J Neurotrauma* 1993; 10(4):405–414.
32. Hubschmann OR, Kornhauser D: Effects of intraparenchymal hemorrhage on extracellular cortical potassium in experimental head trauma. *J Neurosurg* 1983; 59:289–293.
33. Hoffman SW, Fulop Z, Stein DG: Bilateral frontal cortical contusion in rats: Behavioral and anatomic consequences. *J Neurotrauma* 1994; 11(4):417–431.
34. Jane JA, Steward O, Gennarelli T: Axonal degeneration induced by experimental noninvasive minor head injury. *J Neurosurg* 1985; 62:96–100.
35. Jenkins LW, Lyeth BG, Hayes RL: The role of agonist-receptor interactions in the pathophysiology of mild and moderate head injury, in Hoff JT, Anderson TE, Cole T (eds): *Contemporary Issues in Neurological Surgery: 1. Mild to Moderate Brain Injury.* Boston: Blackwell Scientific, 1989:47–61.
36. Julian FJ, Goldman DE: The effects of mechanical stimulation on some electrical properties of axons. *J Gen Physiol* 1962; 46:297–313.
37. Katayama Y, Becker DP, Tamura T, Hovda DA: Massive increases in extracellular potassium and the indiscriminate release of glutamate following concussive brain injury. *J Neurosurg* 1990; 73:889–900.
38. Kearney PA, Ridella SA, Viano DC, Anderson TW: Interaction of contact velocity and cord compression in determining the severity of spinal cord injury. *J Neurotrauma* 1988; 5(3):187–208.
39. Langfitt TW, Obrist WD: Cerebral blood flow and metabolism after intracranial trauma, in Krayenbuhl H (ed): *Progress in Neurological Surgery.* Basel: Karger, 1981:14–48.
40. Lewelt W, Jenkins LW, Miller JD: Autoregulation of cerebral blood flow after experimental fluid percussion injury of the brain. *J Neurosurg* 1980; 53:500–511.
41. Levin HS: Outcome after head injury: General considerations and neurobehavioral recovery. Part II. Neurobehavioral recovery, in Becker DP, Povlishock JT (eds): *Central Nervous System Status Report.* Washington: NINCDS and NIH, 1985:281–299.
42. Lighthall JW: Controlled cortical impact: A new experimental brain injury model. *J Neurotrauma* 1988; 5(1):1–15.
43. Lighthall JW, Goshgarian HG, Pindeerski CR: Characterization of axonal injury produced by controlled cortical impact. *J Neurotrauma* 1990; 7(2):65–76.
44. Lindgren S, Rinder L: Experimental studies in head injury. I. Pressure propagation in "percussion concussion." *Biophysik* 1966; 3:174–180.
45. Lowenstein, et al: Selective vulnerability of dentate. *J Neurosci* 1992; 12(12):4846.
46. Lyeth BG, Dixon CE, Hamm RJ, et al: Effects of scopolamine treatment on long-term behavioral deficits following concussive brain injury to the rat. *Brain Res* 1988; 452:39–48.
47. Lyeth BG, Jenkins LW, Hamm RJ, et al: Prolonged memory impairment in the absence of hippocampal cell death following traumatic brain injury in the rat. *Brain Res* 1990; 526:249–258.
48. Makiyama Y, Jenkins LW, Lyeth BG, et al: An ultrastructural analysis of the CA1 sector of the excitotoxic rodent hippocampus following mild and moderate traumatic brain injury. *Acta Neuropathol* (IN REVIEW???) 1991.
49. Marmarou A, Abd-Elfattah MA, VanDenBrink W, et al: A new model of diffuse brain injury in rats: Part 1. Pathophysiology and biomechanics. *J Neurosurg* 1994; 80:291–300.
50. Masliah E, Cole GM, Hansen LA, et al: Protein kinase C alteration is an early biochemical marker in Alzheimer's disease. *J Neurosci* 1991; 11(9):2759–2767.
51. McIntosh TK, Nobel L, Andrews B, Faden AI: Traumatic brain injury in the rat: Characterization of a midline fluid-percussion model. *CNS Trauma* 1987; 4(2):119–134.
52. McIntosh TK, Vink R, Yamakami I, et al: Traumatic brain injury in the rat: Characterization of a midline fluid percussion model. *J Neurosci* 1989; 28(1):233–244.
53. Miller LP, Lyeth BG, Jenkins LW, et al: Excitatory amino acid receptor subtype binding following traumatic brain injury. *Brain Res* 1990; 526(1):103–107.
54. Mitchell DE, Adams JH: Primary focal impact damage to the brain stem in blunt head injuries: Does it exist? *Lancet* 1973; ii:215–218.
55. Morgan JI, Curran T: Stimulus-transcription coupling in the nervous system: The inducible proto-oncogenes fos and jun. *Ann Rev Neurosci* 1991; 14:421–451.
56. Nillson B, Ponten U, Voigt G: Experimental head injury in the rat. Part I. Mechanics, pathophysiology and morphology in an impact acceleration trauma model. *J Neurosurg* 1977; 47:241–251.
57. Nishizuka Y: The molecular heterogeneity of protein kinase C and its implications for cellular regulation. *Nature* 1988; 334:661–665.
58. Nishizuka Y: Intracellular signaling by hydrolysis of phospholipids and activation of protein kinase C. *Science* 1992; 358:607–614.
59. Ommaya AK, Gennarelli TA: Cerebral concussion and traumatic consciousness: Correlation of experimental and clinical observations on blunt head injuries. *Brain* 1974; 97:633–654.
60. Oppenheimer DR: Microscopic lesions of the brain fol-

lowing head injury. *J Neurol Neurosurg Psychiatry* 1968; 31:299–306.
61. Palmer AM, Marion DW, Botscheller ML, et al: Traumatic brain injury-induced excitotoxicity assessed in a controlled cortical impact model. *J Neurochem* 1993; 61:2015–2024.
62. Phillips LL, Belardo ET: Expression of c-fos in the hippocampus following mild and moderate fluid percussion brain injury. *J Neurotrauma* 1992; 9:323–333.
63. Postmantur R, Hayes RL, Dixon CE, Taft WC: Neurofilament 68 and neurofilament 200 protein levels decrease after traumatic brain injury. *J Neurotrauma* (In Press).
64. Povlishock JT, Becker DP, Cheng CLY, Vaughan GW: Axonal change in minor head injury. *J Neuropathol Exp Neurol* 1983; 42:225.
65. Povlishock JT, Becker DP: Fate of reactive axonal swelling induced by head injury. *Lab Invest* 1985; 52:540–552.
66. Povlishock JT, Hayes RL, Michel ME: Workshop on animal models of traumatic brain injury. *J Neurotrauma* (In Press).
67. Prasad MR, Tagaret CM, Smith D, et al: Decreased alpha 1-adrenergic receptors after experimental brain injury. *J Neurotrauma* 1992; 9:269–279.
68. Saija A, Hayes RL, Lyeth BG, et al: Effect of concussive head injury on central cholinergic neurons. *Brain Res* 1988; 452:303–311.
69. Saija A, Robinson SE, Lyeth BG, et al: Effect of scopolamine and traumatic brain injury on central cholinergic neurons. *J Neurotrauma* 1988; 5:161–169.
70. Shapira Y, Shohami E, Side A: Experimental closed head injury in rats: Mechanical, pathophysiologic, and neurologic properties. *Crit Care Med* 1988; 16(3):255–265.
71. Shima K, Marmarou A: Evaluation of brain stem dysfunction following severe fluid percussion head injury to the cat. *J Neurosurg* 1991; 72:270–277.
72. Smith DH, Okiyama K, McIntosh TK: Ketamine and magnesium attenuate memory loss after experimental brain injury. *Soc Neurosci Abstr* 1991; 17:66.
73. Stalhammer D, Galinat BJ, Allen AM, et al: A new model of concussive brain injury in the cat produced by extradural fluid volume loading: II. Physiological and neuropathological observation. *Brain Injury* 1987; 1:93–112.
74. Strich SJ: Lesions in the cerebral hemispheres after blunt head injury. *J Clin Pathol* 1970; 23(suppl 4):166–171.
75. Sullivan HG, Martinez J, Becker DP, et al: Fluid percussion model of mechanical brain injury in the cat. *J Neurosurg* 1976; 45(5):520–534.
76. Sutton RL, Lescaudron L, Stein DG: Unilateral cortical contusion injury in the rat: Vascular disruption and temporal development of cortical necrosis. *J Neurotrauma* 1993; 10(2):135–149.
77. Takahashi H, Manaka S, Sano K: Changes in extracellular potassium concentration in cortex and brain stem during the acute phase of experimental closed head injury. *J Neurosurg* 1981; 55:708–717.
78. Teasdale G, Jennett B: Assessment of coma and impaired consciousness: A practical scale. *Lancet* 1974; 2:81–84.
79. Tornheim PA, Linwicz BH, Hirsch CS, et al: Acute responses to blunt head trauma: Experimental model and gross pathology. *J Neurosurg* 1983; 59:431–438.
80. Yoshino XO, Hovda DA, Katayama Y, et al: Hippocampal CA3 lesion prevents postconcussive metabolic dysfunction in CA1. *J Cerebr Blood Flow Metab* 1992; 12:996–1006.
81. Wei EP, Dietrich WD, Povlishock JT, et al: Functional, morphological, and metabolic abnormalities of the central microcirculation after concussive brain injury in cats. *Circ Res* 1980; 46:37–47.
82. Wieloch T, Cardell M, Bingren H, et al: Changes in the activity of protein kinase C and the differential subcellular redistribution of its isozymes in the rat striatum during and following transient forebrain ischemia. *J Neurochem* 1991; 56:1227–1235.
83. Valadka AB, Povlishock JD, Shah J, Walker S: Reactive axonal change in a micropig model of brain injury: Evidence for a human-like progression of axonal change. *Neurosci Abstr* 1993; 19:1485.
84. Yamakami I, McIntosh TK: Effects of traumatic brain injury on regional cerebral blood flow in rats as measured with radiolabeled microspheres. *J Cerebr Blood Flow Metab* 1989; 9:117–124.
85. Yamamoto KK, Gonzales GA, Biggs WH, Montminy MR: Phosphorylation-induced binding and transcriptional efficacy of nuclear factor CREB. *Nature* 1988; 334:494–498.
86. Yang K, Mu XS, Xue JJ, et al: Increased expression of c-fos mRNA and AP-1 transcription factors after cortical impact injury in rats. *Molec Brain Res* (In Press), 1994.
87. Yuan XQ, Prough DS, Smith TL, Dewitt DS: The effects of traumatic brain injury on regional cerebral blood flow in rats. *J Neurotrauma* 1988; 5(4):289–301.
88. Zola-Morgan S, Squire LR: Medical temporal lesions in monkeys impairs memory of a variety of tasks sensitive to human amnesia. *Behav Neurosci* 1985; 99:22–34.

CHAPTER 99

EXPERIMENTAL MISSILE WOUNDING OF THE BRAIN

Michael E. Carey

THE PROBLEM

Gunshot wounds to the brain account for more than 30,000 civilian deaths yearly in the United States.[1] For soldiers engaged in ground combat, head wounds (largely of the brain) have accounted for almost half of all deaths since World War II.[2] My interest in the problem of brain wounding developed after serving as a neurosurgeon in Vietnam. Upon returning to the United States and reviewing war wound literature, it became apparent that very little was known about brain wounding from missiles in modern biological terms.[3–25] Amazingly, fewer than 25 laboratory papers had ever been published where a brain wound from a missile had been replicated in an anesthetized animal and the effects on the brain studied.

PHYSICAL CORRELATES OF MISSILE WOUNDING

Missile wounding can only be understood in terms of the physical interactions between the missile and the tissue(s) through which it passes. The primary destructive effect of a missile interacting with tissue is caused by the crushing action of the missile itself.[26–30] Besides this direct action, however, a missile moving in a water or tissue medium generates three distinct types of pressures within the medium it transits.[27,28,31]

Juxta-Missile Pressure

Extremely high pressures (thousands of atmospheres) are generated just in front of and at right angles to a moving missile owing to flow of the surrounding medium around the missile. The pressure is confined to the missile's immediate vicinity.

Longitudinal "Strong" Shock Wave Pressure

When a missile strikes an object, a high-pressure compression front or shock wave is formed that moves spherically away from the missile strike-point. A blunt missile may cause a "strong" shock wave if it impacts with a strike velocity as low as 60 percent of the velocity of sound in the medium. The velocity of the shock wave in tissue approximates the velocity of sound in water (1460 m/sec) (Fig. 99-1). The longitudinal, "strong" shock pressure wave initially has a very steep front, but its shape and duration may be changed with propagation through a medium, particularly one that is not homogeneous, such as tissue. As it travels, therefore, the steep front of a "strong" shock wave will become less steep and, finally, will assume the characteristics of an "ordinary" pressure wave (see below). In water, the peak pressure of a "strong" shock wave may exceed 80 atmospheres (atm), but the entire "strong" shock wave event lasts only about 10 microseconds. In the absence of a fluid-to-air interface, "strong" pressure waves are thought not to cause tissue damage because their brief duration prevents transfer of sufficient energy to surrounding tissues to distort and tear them.[29]

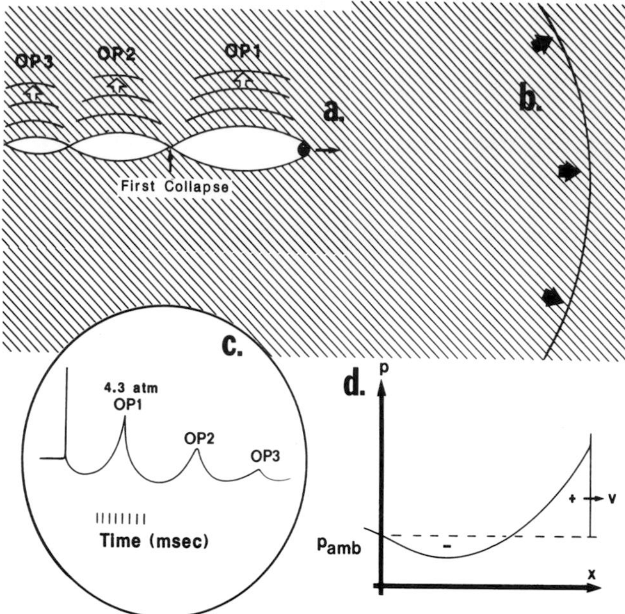

Figure 99-1. Missile (*black circle*) (*A*) traveling through medium (*hatched*). The "strong" shock wave (*B*) moves with the speed of sound in the medium. The shape of the strong shock wave is depicted in *d*. It has an extremely sharp front, represented by the vertical line. Its velocity through the medium is indicated by *v*. The extremely high over pressure, *p*, lasts but microseconds. Owing to kinetic energy transfer, tissue molecules are thrust radially away from the missile's path, creating an over-pressure laterally, *OP1*, and a near-vacuum (*white area*) directly behind the missile. Once thrust aside, the molecules of the medium tend to fall back to their original position (*first collapse*), but then move laterally again to set up another over-pressure in the medium, *OP2*. This cycle is repeated, *OP3*, until the kinetic energy is expended. Overpressures caused by radial displacement of tissue molecules are depicted in *c*. These "ordinary" pressure waves last milliseconds and cause tissue damage about the wound track. We hypothesize that they also cause damage at a distance in the brain.

Pressure Waves from Kinetic Energy Transfer ("Ordinary" Pressure Waves)

When a missile passes through tissue, kinetic energy is transferred to nearby tissue elements that are propelled radially from the missile track, thereby increasing pressure in this tissue. A large subatmospheric temporary cavity forms directly behind the missile as a consequence of the radial movement of tissue away from the missile path. When the elastic limit of the outwardly displaced tissue is reached, the tissue falls inward from whence it was displaced. This cycle may be repeated several times before the deranged tissue comes to rest around the permanent track created by the missile. The oscillating, outward and inward rush of tissue creates long-lasting (milliseconds) lower amplitude (20- to 30-atm) pressure waves that propagate widely throughout the medium and may distort and damage tissues at a distance from the site of actual missile injury[27,28,31] (Fig. 99-1).

THE ENERGY OF WOUNDING

The kinetic energy (KE) of any missile equals 0.5 × missile mass × (missile velocity).[2] The amount of tissue damage caused by a missile may be correlated with the amount of missile KE deposited within the tissue by the missile.[29,30] The missile kinetic energy of deposit (KE_d) = $KE_{en} - KE_{ex}$, where KE_{en} = missile kinetic energy of entry, and KE_{ex} = missile kinetic energy of exit. If a missile is retained within the tissue, $E_{ex} = 0$, and all missile energy will be deposited within the tissue. If a missile exists, only *part* of its kinetic energy will be deposited. The same amount of energy may be deposited by a small-mass missile with a large velocity or a greater-mass missile with smaller velocity. Kinetic energy deposited by a missile is partitioned between that which directly crushes tissues in its path and that which displaces tissues adjacent to the missile track.[26] The latter is less destructive than the former owing to the elastic properties of the displaced tissue which may be deformed without being irrevocably destroyed (L Sturdivan, Edgewood Arsenal, Edgewood, MD, personal communication, 1988).

MISSILE-CAUSING BRAIN WOUNDS

Most wounds in modern combat are caused by small fragments, not by bullets.[32] Eighty percent of all wounds sustained at Dunkirk were caused by "splinters" 5 mm or less in diameter,[33] and missile fragments weighing 110 to 220 mg inflicted most fatal brain wounds in American soldiers in Vietnam (Carey ME: Unpublished data from analysis of casualties surveyed by the Wound Data and Munitions Effectiveness Team, WDMET, in Vietnam).

A bullet has a streamlined shape that allows it to maintain a high velocity over many hundreds of yards. Bullet velocity decreases linearally with distance. Because of their high velocities, military bullets possess enormous energies that can create very destructive "ordinary" pressure waves that may widely disrupt the brain. WDMET data provided an instance of fatal brain wound by an AK47 round fired from 400 yards.

Owing to their irregular, nonaerodynamic shape, fragments lose velocities and kinetic energies exponentially over distance. Lighter fragments lose velocity and energy with particular rapidity. Yards from the site of an ordnance explosion the typical shell fragment has lost much of its initial kinetic energy. While such a fragment may penetrate the skull, the amount of tissue destruction caused directly by its crushing effect may be small. The "ordinary" pressure waves that it sets up may not widely disrupt brain tissue because the fragment does not deposit much energy within the brain. If its trajectory does not cross vital brain structures, such a missile, producing relatively little brain destruction, may be quite compatible with life, although it may cause a discrete neurological injury.

This fundamental difference between bullets and fragments accounts for the fact that approximately 90 percent of all brain wounds operated on by neurosurgeons in Vietnam were caused by fragments. Brain wounds caused by bullets and seen by neurosurgeons undoubtedly were caused by tangential wounds, where only *part* of the bullet's energy was deposited within the brain, or by spent rounds (as by ricochet), where the bullet's kinetic energy was greatly reduced and the energy deposited within the brain also reduced.

In the past among American civilians it was not uncommon to see nonfatal .22-caliber bullet wounds to the brain because the kinetic energy associated with such bullets is low (in the KE range of some shell fragments). Currently, bullet wounds to the brain in American civilians are highly lethal because higher velocity (and energy) bullets are being used. Forty-four magnum bullets have velocities and energies in the range of military bullets.

PRIOR EXPERIMENTS ON BRAIN WOUNDS IN ANESTHETIZED ANIMALS

During the 19th century clinicians and physiologists had an intense interest in physiological, anatomic, and clinical events associated with brain trauma. They recognized that blunt trauma to the head caused respiratory and circulatory changes in addition to coma.[34] Using anesthetized dogs, Horsley in 1893 concluded that a bullet wound to the brain could be fatal by causing apnea. Such a brain wounded individual might conceivably recover provided respiratory support were given.[3] He hypothesized that the respiratory arrest was produced by brain stem anemia consequent to missile-induced increased intracranial pressure. In 1943, Webster and Gurdjian, wounding anesthetized dogs, essentially confirmed these observations on apnea.[4] When animals were wounded through a closed cranial vault, respiratory effects became more profound with increasing missile energy. Like Horsley, these investigators hypothesized that the increased intracranial pressure produced by the bullet affected medullary respiratory centers. This respiratory effect could be prevented by craniectomy prior to wounding.

Gerber and Moody in 1972 developed a brain missile wound model wherein an anesthetized Rhesus monkey was wounded through a 7-mm diameter trephine by a pellet gun.[6] They concluded that the most important single variable correlating with death was decreased carotid blood flow (and, by inference, cerebral blood flow). Respiratory effects were not prominent.

Djordevic et al. in 1976 used anesthetized dogs to study the intracranial pressure effects of brain wounding by 870-mg spheres.[8] Missile velocities ranged from 122 to 785 m/s. Increased postwounding ICP was attributed to intracranial bleeding and an increase in CSF outflow resistance. Vasodilatation was not felt to be a factor in ICP elevation.

Crockard et al. expanded Gerber's model, again using anesthetized Rhesus monkeys.[9–13,15,16] The brain wound was caused by a 310-mg missile fired through a 7-mm occipital trephine. Missile energies from 0.49 to 5.02 Joules (J) were created by using missile velocities from 56 to 180 m/s. Wounds of 5 J were highly lethal, primarily by their respiratory effects, while those of 0.49 J produced few physiological changes. Wounds of 1.26 J (missile velocity = 90 m/s) produced transient bradycardia, respiratory slowing, and increased tidal volume. Arterial blood gases, however, were unchanged. In subsequent experiments, the prominent effects of missile wounding on brain stem function were noted, but apnea was not notable in these investigators' "standard" 1.26-J wound. A highly accurate prediction of animal survival following a brain wound of this energy could be made from cerebral blood flow (radioactive xenon clearance), the cerebral metabolic rate of lactate, and MABP from 30 to 60 minutes after brain wounding. Follow-up experiments indicated that brain wounding in spontaneously breathing Rhesus monkeys was associated with decreased cardiac output (CO) and that this, in turn, might be the underlying cause of diminished CBF associated with brain wounding.[21] Opposed to the earlier works of Horsley, Webster, and Gurdjian, these experiments focused on cerebral blood flow rather than respiration as the critical factor in a fatal missile wound to the brain.

Maynard et al. modified the Gerber-Crockard model, wounding anesthetized baboons with a 4.8-mm, 411-mg steel sphere through a trephine placed posterior to the left coronal suture.[23] This resulted in a bifrontal wound track. Intracranial pressure was monitored by bilateral piezoelectric transducers. In various experiments missile impact energies ranged from 7.2 to 29.2 J. With missile passage, brief (0.5 msec), energy-dependent intracranial overpressure developed that ranged from 68 to 330 psi (470–2270 kPa) in the left-sided pressure transducer and 105 to 570 psi (720–3900 kPa) on the right.

Ten of 11 wounded animals failed to maintain spontaneous respirations after wounding. Respiratory complications were common with missile energies above 7 J; as higher missile energies were used, postwounding apnea was the rule, either immediately after wounding or within an hour. All apneic animals were placed on a respirator. It could not be determined whether the respiratory changes were a function of missile energy deposit or whether they occurred in an all-or-none way above some threshold energy deposit.

All wounded animals also exhibited hypotension, bradycardia, ECG changes, and CO reductions. The postwounding CO decrements were related to a so-called "scaled energy" term (missile impact energy/animal mass) which provided a linear relationship between "scaled energy" and CO reduction. A simpler analysis made by this author from Maynard's data also shows a linear trend between missile impact energy and CO reduction in nine animals where missile velocity was measured: impact energy 7 J, CO reduction 12 percent (N = 2); missile impact energy 17 J, CO reduction 32 percent (N = 5); missile impact energy 28 J, CO reduction 59 percent (N = 2). Neural reflexes both sympathetic and parasympathetic, were thought to underlie the cardiovascular changes because they occurred within seconds of missile impact. These investigators noted that both sympathetic and parasympathetic outflows are modulated by hypothalamic and brain stem areas, and histological examination of the wounded brains revealed that both the hypothalamus and brain stem exhibited perivascular ring hemorrhages from the indirect effects of missile energy.

DEVELOPMENT OF A CONTEMPORARY BRAIN WOUND MODEL

When considering the conduct of further experiments on brain missile wounds, there appeared little point in studying massively destructive, nonsurvivable brain wounds like those caused by a high energy-of-deposit missile such as a military bullet. Rather, it was thought that the most efficacious laboratory model should replicate survivable brain wounds such as those caused by a lower energy-of-deposit missile, i.e., a small shell fragment or possibly a *low* energy bullet, e.g., a 0.22-caliber. The excellent experiments of Gerber, Crockard, Brown, Levett, and Maynard[6,9–21,23] provided many valuable insights concerning brain wounding, and the use of a subhuman primate with a human brain configuration (brain stem more or less at right angles to the midaxial plane of the cerebral hemispheres) was appealing. Wounding through a trephine with a large-mass, slow-moving, heavy projectile did not, however, accord with the usual fragment wound of the brain encountered in combat, where most survivable brain wounds are caused by small, higher-velocity fragments that enter through the frontal or parietal bone. Thus, the criteria for more realistic and useful models would include: (1) wounding through an intact skull; (2) a small, high velocity missile; (3) frontal entry; and (4) a cerebral hemisphere missile trajectory.

In our model development a laboratory gun was made by Mr. Robert Carpenter of the Edgewood Arsenal, Edgewood, MD, recognizing that the smallest feasible missile that could readily be fired would be a 2-mm diameter sphere, weighing 31.7 mg. While most missiles causing brain wounds are not spherical, spheres are often utilized in wound simulation experiments to simplify mathematical analysis of missile-media interactions.[35] Furthermore, one could envision little difference in the brain injury variables that would result from an injury caused by a round, smooth missile versus an irregularly shaped one.

In our chosen model (Fig. 99-2), a solenoid release valve activated by direct current was placed between

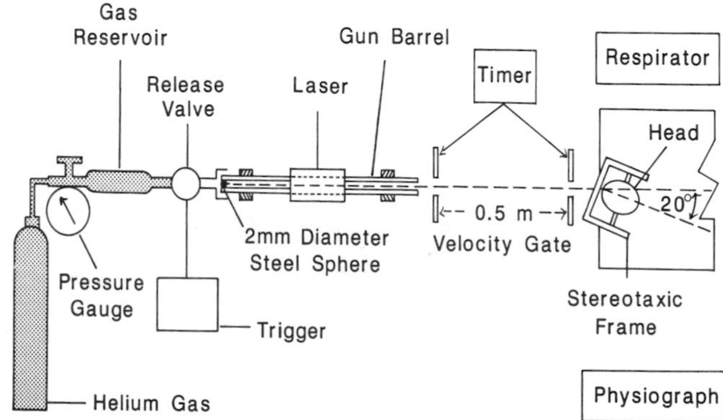

Figure 99-2. Experimental set up: Helium is used as the propellant because of its great coefficient of expansion. Direct current is used to trigger the solenoid release valve because alternating current gave inconstant missile speed, presumably because of different valve opening rates. A laser beam allowed very precise aiming. Missile velocity was measured by the velocity gate from which missile KE was calculated. The stereotaxic frame is about 0.5 m from the velocity gate.

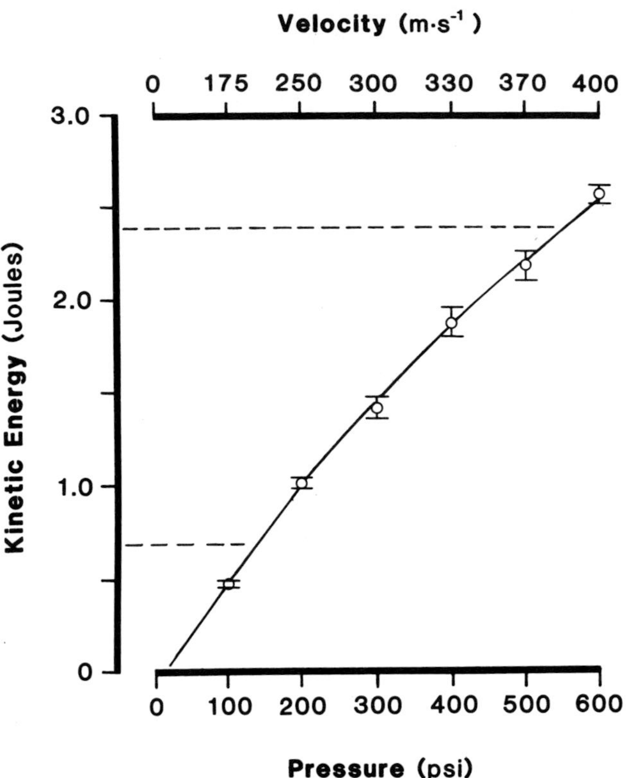

Figure 99-3. Gas reservoir pressure, sphere velocity, and calculated sphere KE, five shots each point. Note the restricted possible wound energies (*dotted lines*); we wished to study a nonfatal missile wound. Skull penetration required 0.7 J; 67 percent of cats died from apnea at 2.4 J.

the gas storage tank and the gun. This provided missile velocities very closely related to the helium charge (Fig. 99-3). Missile accuracy was within 1 to 2 mm over the short range.

The Choice of an Experimental Animal

Several considerations determined the choice of experimental animal: (1) appropriateness relative to physiological variables to be studied; (2) mass of the missile relative to the mass of the brain; and (3) cost, not only of the animal but also of radioactive isotopes and microspheres to be utilized in characterizing the animal model. This latter factor, in particular, mandated that a small animal be used. While the rat would seem most desirable in studies of this nature, the use of a 31.7-mg missile to injure a 1.0-gm brain would generate a missile mass 374 times larger than the mass of a missile documented to cause fragment wounds to the brain in humans. Thus, an animal with a larger brain was required. The cat was deemed a more appropriate choice because of its brain size—approximately 25 gm—and because it has been widely used and characterized in a wide range of neurological investigations.[36–39] Further, unlike dogs, cats have a more uniform cranial shape; after fixation in a sterotaxic frame, one has a high expectation of producing a consistent brain wound.

Arguments against the use of cats can be found in the facts that (1) the missile-to-brain ratio was still 7 to 15 times too large; (2) the cat has a bony tentorium not present in humans; and (3) the cat's neuraxis is not aligned as in humans. Nevertheless, it was thought that the positive scientific aspects of using the cat far outweighed the negatives.

Pentobarbital anesthesia was selected for use in cats because it has been widely used in brain edema and cerebral blood flow studies.[36–39] With pentobarbital, both brain blood flow and metabolism are simultaneously reduced; flow and metabolism thus remain coupled. (Personal communication, John Michenfelder MD, Professor of Anesthesia Research, Mayo Medical School, November 1989.)

Animal Preparation

In this model cats were deeply sedated with IP pentobarbital and then infiltrated in the groin with 1 percent local xylocaine. The femoral vein was cannulated for further IV pentobarbital as needed. Other required vascular lines were then placed and an endotracheal tube inserted. A 5-cm midline scalp incision was made and the skin reflected laterally. The outer wall of the right frontal sinus was removed because preliminary experiments showed that the small, lightweight missile merely glanced off the sloping outer wall of the right frontal sinus without bony penetration. Removal of the outer wall allowed the sphere to strike the nearly vertical, intact posterior bony sinus wall, perforate the skull, and penetrate the brain. When appropriate, intracranial pressure was monitored by a Camino ICP monitor placed through a small left parietal trephine. The EEG was monitored via small steel skull screws. For studies evaluating the effect of missile wounding on respiration, the animals were allowed to breathe spontaneously prior to wounding. After wounding these cats were given respiratory support via ventilator as needed. For cerebral blood flow studies where control of Pa_{CO_2} was critical, the animals were paralyzed with Gallamine and artificially ventilated. After surgical preparation the cats were placed in a stereotaxic frame facing the barrel of the pellet gun.

Because we wished to generate a nonfatal brain wound, the missile trajectory was placed in a cerebral hemisphere, away from midline and brain stem structures. The initial trajectory was parasagittal, 2 to 3 mm from the falx cerebri. Missile impact on the bony tentorium almost directly over the brain stem, however, resulted in prominent cardiovascular changes in many animals, not analagous to the human condition. To minimize this effect, the missile trajectory was altered to slant 20 degrees laterally away from the midline. Serial coronal sections showed that after penetrating the right frontal tip, the 2-mm missile track was usually in cerebral hemisphere white matter between the outer corner of the lateral ventrical and the cortical gray. In order to relate all observed physiological effects to missile energy deposited within the brain, it was a requisite that the missile not exit the skull ($KE_{ex} = 0$). It was determined that a threshold missile energy 0.5 J to .07 J was needed to produce frequent skull perforation through the posterior wall of the right frontal sinus. Missile energy of 0.9 J assured bone perforation and brain penetration. Missiles with energies as high as 2.4 J rarely exited the skull but caused severe respiratory problems in a high percentage of cats. As had been noted by prior investigators, significant intracranial bleeding was not a common problem.[6,11] In this respect, the experimental paradigm also mirrored the clinical situation.[40]

Findings in this Model of Brain Wounding

It quickly became apparent that wounding through the intact skull produced prominent respiratory effects even at low missile energies, even though the missile track was at least 2 cm from the brain stem.[41] To conserve animals, if a cat became apneic after wounding, it was placed on a respirator, which was removed at 1-minute intervals to see whether spontaneous respiration had returned. If respiration had not returned, ventilatory support was continued until spontaneous respiration had recovered or for 2 hours, when the experiment was terminated. Six minutes of apnea is fatal for a cat; therefore, in a retrospective analysis relating missile energy to apnea, we considered cessation of respiration for longer than 6 minutes to be a "fatal apnea." These experiments showed that missile-induced fatal apnea is a direct function of missile energy deposit. A 0.9-J missile caused fatal apnea in 14 percent of cases, a 1.4-J missile produced fatal apnea 40 percent of the time, while a 2.4-J missile caused 67 percent of the cats to become fatally apneic (Fig. 99-4). Surprisingly, but in accord with Horsley's original observations,[3] following respiratory support of up to 2 hours many apneic cats recovered spontaneous respiration, and when recovered appeared neurologically intact (Fig. 102-4). These respiratory effects of brain wounding were also accorded with those of Webster and Gurdjian, who wounded anesthetized animals through an intact skull.[4] It appears that the significant effects of low-energy deposit missiles upon respiration were masked in Gerber's[6] and Crockard's[11,12] Rhesus monkey and Maynard's baboon experiments[23] in which their use of skull trephination attenuated the missile's effect on respiration. Thus, Crockard et al.[11,12] noted no significant respiratory effects with a 1.3-J missile, while almost 40 percent of our animals sustained a fatal apnea with a 1.4-J wound. Wounding through a trephine required missile energies of 5 to 7 J to cause a prominent respiratory effect.[11,12,23] Our data suggest that in a cerebral hemispheral missile wounding not involving midline or brain stem structures, the crucial physiological effect determining life or death is the missile's effect on medullary respiratory centers. Provision of timely respiratory support therefore may allow recovery of spontaneous respiration and prevent death. Missile wounding also may reduce cardiac output but significant cardiac output reductions occur at missile energies significantly greater than that required to cause

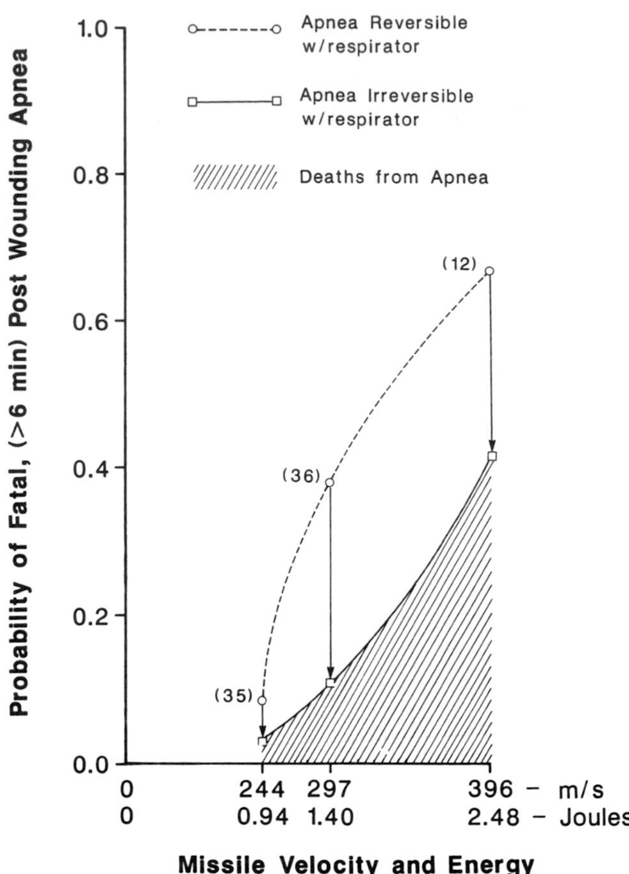

Figure 99-4. Missile energy and the probability of causing fatal apnea. Fatal apnea, *dotted line*, was highly dependent on missile energy of deposit. With timely artificial ventilation many cats resumed breathing. Immediate respiratory support lowers the probability of permanent apnea, *solid line*. The likelihood of permanent apnea, *shaded area,* theoretically could be decreased by measures (i.e., drugs) enhancing recovery of respiratory mechanisms.

apnea. Clinically, unless timely respiratory resuscitation occurs, the overriding effect of apnea would make any possible effects of CO reduction moot.

Our experiments also suggest that after bone penetration a rather narrow limit of allowable missile energies exists (in our model 0.7 J to 2.4 J) before the effects of increased missile energy deposit gravely affects respiratory function and produces death in a very high percentage of animals. By inference, humans sustaining a missile wound to a cerebral hemisphere also have a relatively narrow window of missile energies compatible with life before the indirect effects of the propagated "ordinary" pressure waves irreversibly affect medullary respiratory centers. Pearce et al.[35] in a series of parietal impact wounds showed that a 900-gm sphere required about 15 J to penetrate the parietal bone of a prepared human skull. A 90-J sphere penetrated the skull and transited both cerebral hemispheres, while a 250-J sphere severely disrupted the entire calvarium and produced a large cone-shaped temporary cavity in the gelatin filling the skull. This latter wound clearly would be fatal. Since missiles that have the energy to transit two cerebral hemispheres are known to produce severe brain wounds, clinically, one may estimate the range of survivable hemispheral missile energy deposits in humans to be approximately 15 to 90 J or less. If the permissible range of missile energies in our model (0.7 to 2.4 J) is relevant, the range of survivable missile energies for humans sustaining a cerebral hemisphere wound would be between 15 and 51 J (maximum $KE_d = 3.4 \times$ penetration energy).

In subsequent experiments we demonstrated that, following a brain wound producing a brief transient apnea, some cats rapidly regained a normal respiratory rate and survived; others resumed spontaneous breathing, but at a reduced rate.[42] These latter cats eventually developed permanent apnea 10 to 20 minutes after their injury. Reductions in cardiac output were not a prominent feature in these fatally wounded cats. Mean brain stem rCBF (microspheres) in cats with respiratory depression fell from a control of 33 $\pm$ 5 ml/100 g/min to 25 $\pm$ 4 ml/100 g/min. This mild rCBF reduction after wounding resulted in a brain stem blood flow well above ischemic levels (15 ml/100/min).[43] Thus, contrary to Horsley's hypothesis, it does not appear that brain stem ischemia is responsible for that apnea seen following a hemispherical missile wound. Biological factors that distinguish animals that succumb to apnea following brain wounding from those that don't remain to be elucidated. Treatments for such impaired respiration can be devised.

In this animal model, brain stem nuclear and hypothalamic catecholamines were also evaluated following a 2.4-J brain wound associated with death from apnea in greater than 50 percent of the animals.[44] Despite the severe brain stem effects associated with such a wound, and although epinephrine was significantly reduced in the raphe nuclei as well as in several hypothalamic and brain stem sites, brain stem or hypothalamic biogenic amines were never totally depleted. The monaminergic systems in these structures appeared to reflect a generalized stress response pattern seen not only with missile wounding but also with elevated intracranial pressure. This suggests that a severe brain wound likely to cause early death does not do so by totally disrupting the hypothalamic and brain stem biogenic amine system. Whether the response of and relative maintenance of the catecholamine system after brain wounding is indicative of other chemical mediator systems in the brain stem is unknown.

At present we hypothesize, as did Horsley, Webster, and Gurdjian, that the fatal effect of a hemispherical missile wound that does not severely disrupt the brain or directly damage vital, midline structures stems from the propagated "ordinary" pressure waves of missile energy deposit. The propagated "ordinary" pressure waves most notably affect respiratory nuclei that lie just under the floor of the fourth ventricle in close proximity to the CSF compartment. Whether this location makes them particularly susceptible to mechanical or chemical insults transmitted through or by the CSF remains to be determined. Possibly the superficial location of respiratory neurons or the long, complex respiratory circuits cause the respiratory system to be preferentially impaired following even low energy missile wounds and/or other forms of head injury. Cardiovascular function, although disturbed by head injury, is not usually destroyed. The location of cardiovascular control nuclei deeper in the core of the medulla, away from the floor of the fourth ventricle may explain why increased missile energy is required to cause cardiac output decreases. If a brain-wounded individual survives a bout of transient apnea, specific treatments may then be required to prevent concomitant or delayed cardiac output reduction.

Brain edema occurs following traumatic brain injury, and we sought to measure its significance in brain wounding from missiles.[45] Brain edema (wet weight–dry weight method) following missile wounding appeared confined to the region surrounding the missile track. It was not severe, and had the characteristics of vasogenic edema (VBE). Following missile wounding (as in cold injury) VBE edema peaked in 48 to 72 hours and then receded to baseline values within a week (Fig. 99-5).

With our sampling techniques we could not ascertain any differences in the amount of VBE or its time course between a 0.9-J or a 1.4-J missile injured groups. This lack of a distinct graded response in the production of VBE in the cerebral hemisphere was most likely related to the fact that the missile energies allowable for a nonfatal wound were too restricted and that the variance

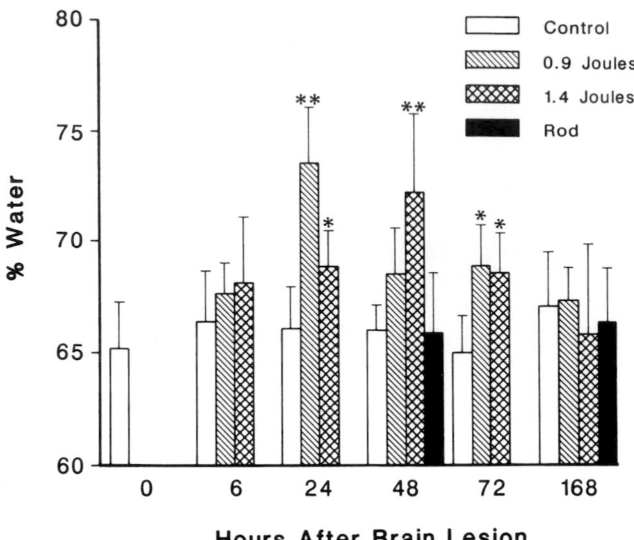

Figure 99-5. Percentage of brain water in white matter about the missile track. Tissue sodium also rose while tissue potassium remained constant characteristic of vasogenic brain edema. Note that at 48 hours a 2-mm rod injury (a lowering energy cutting injury) was not associated with any increase in water. (Means ± S.D. $**p < 0.01$; $*P < 0.05$ of control.)

in the amount of VBE produced by a missile of either energy was too great to allow for the dissemination of those edematous changes seen with missiles of such close energies. The lack of a distinct, graded response in this hemispherical pathobiological event is in great contradistinction to missile effect on medullary respiratory function, where a distinct, graded physiological effect occurred with missiles of very close energies, 0.9 and 1.4 J.

Coagulopathy has been well described following head injury.[46] We showed that 2 hours following missile wounding total platelets are significantly decreased, but by 6 hours they had returned to normal. Fibrinogen levels decreased 4 hours after injury and were depressed at 6 hours.[47]

Drug Studies

The experimental missile wound model has been used to test agents that might improve physiological or overall brain function after injury. Using Gerber's and Crockard's missile wound model, it was demonstrated that mannitol given shortly after wounding markedly improved CPP, CBF, and $CMRO_2$ out of proportion to any observed ICP reduction, possibly through direct effects on blood flow and metabolism.[14,16,18] DMSO also improved postwounding MABP, CPP, CBF, and $CMRO_2$ through poorly understood mechanisms.[19,20]

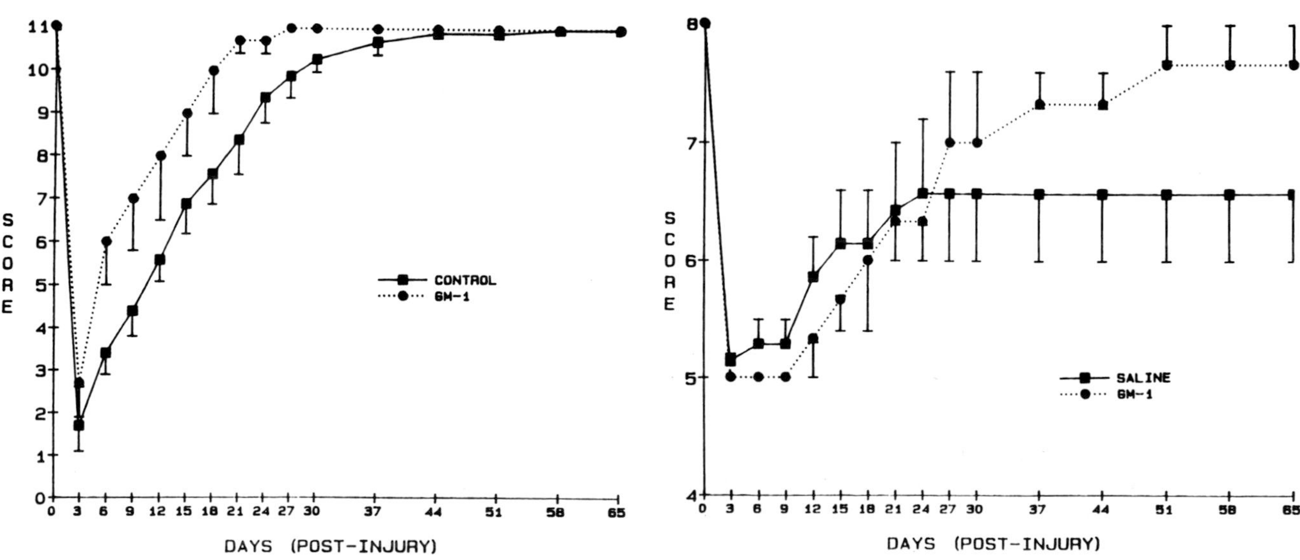

Figure 99-6. (*Left*) Before wounding, cats were trained to traverse an elevated beam to achieve a tunafish reward. Ability was scored on an 11-point scale before and after wounding and treatment with GM1 ganglioside. Balance beam performance appeared to return more quickly following treatment.

(*Right*) A normal cat will withdraw its forelimb when a front paw guard hair touches a surface, even though the cat cannot see the surface. This nonvisual placing test was evaluated by a four-point score before and after wounding and treatment with GM1 ganglioside, which seemed to enhance placement performance.

In our laboratory Soblosky and Sarna developed a detailed cat behavioral paradigm that allowed accurate behavioral assessment of wounded cats allowed to awaken from anesthesia. Although their behavior was depressed for a few days following anesthesia and injury, no cat manifested any evidence of pain. We evaluated the neuroprotective effect of GM1 ganglioside given IP at 20 mg/kg 10 minutes after wounding and continued daily for 10 days. Unfortunately, these experiments were terminated before statistical significance could be achieved. The missile wound-GM1 ganglioside data are presented, however, because they suggest that the GM1 ganglioside is neuroprotective after missile wound injury, accelerating and enhancing recovery of neural function (Fig. 99-6).

ACKNOWLEDGEMENTS

Experiments cited from the LSU Brain Trauma Laboratory were performed by Drs. George Sarna, Dan Torbati, Joseph Soblosky, and Deepak Awasthi under U.S. Army Contracts DAMD17-83-C-3145 and DAMD17-86-C-6098. Opinions expressed are those of the author and are not to be construed as an official Department of the Army position.

REFERENCES

1. Kaufman HH: Civilian gunshot wounds to the head. *Neurosurgery* 1993; 32:962.
2. Carey ME: Learning from traditional combat mortality and morbidity data used in the evaluation of combat medical care. *Milit Med* 1987; 152:6.
3. Horsley V: The destructive effects of small projectiles. *Nature* 1894; 50:104.
4. Webster JE, Gurdjian ES: Acute physiological effects of gunshot and other penetrating wounds of the brain. *J Neurophysiol* 1943; 6:255.
5. Aleksandrov LN, Dyskin EA, Ozeretskovskii LB, et al: Mechanisms of gunshot wound of the cranium and brain (experimental study). *Vestn Khir (USSR)* 1970; 104:81.
6. Gerber AM, Moody RA: Craniocerebral missile injury in the monkey: An experimental physiological model. *J Neurosurg* 1972; 36:43.
7. Clemedson CJ, Falconer B, Frankenberg L, et al: Head injury caused by small-caliber, high velocity bullets. An experimental study. *Z Rechtsmed* 1973; 73:103.
8. Djordevic M, Lofgren J, Steiner H, et al: Intracranial pressure effects of missiles, in Beks JWF, Bosch DA, Brock M (eds): *Intracranial Pressure III.* New York: Springer-Verlag, 1976:79.
9. Crockard HA, Brown FD, Calica AB, et al: ICP CVR and cerebral metabolism following experimental missile injury, in Beks JWF, Bosch DA, Brock M (eds): *Intracranial Pressure III.* New York: Springer-Verlag, 1976:73.
10. Calica AB, Crockard HA, Mullan JF: Predicting injury to the brain—the death equation. *Surg Forum* 1976; 27:470.
11. Crockard HA, Brown FD, Johns LM, et al: An experimental cerebral missile injury model in primates. *J Neurosurg* 1977:776.
12. Crockard HA, Brown FD, Calica AB, et al: Physiological consequences of experimental cerebral missile injury and use of data analysis to predict survival. *J Neurosurg* 1977; 46:784.
13. Crockard HA, Brown FD, Trimble J, et al: Evoked potentials, cerebral blood flow and metabolism following cerebral missile trauma in monkeys. *Surg Neurol* 1977; 7:281.
14. Brown FD, Johns LM, Jafar JJ, et al: Systemic and cerebral hemodynamic response to mannitol after cerebral missile injury. *Surg Forum* 1978; 29:525.
15. Crockard HA, Johns L, Levett J, et al: "Brainstem" effects of experimental cerebral trauma, in Popp AJ, et al (eds): *Neural Trauma.* New York: Raven Press, 1979:19.
16. Brown FD, Johns LM, Crockard HA, et al: Response to mannitol following experimental cerebral missile injury, in Popp AJ, et al (eds): *Neural Trauma.* New York: Raven Press, 1979:281.
17. Brown FD, Johns LM, Mullan JF: DMSO treatment in an experimental missile injury. *Surg Forum* 1979; 30:444.
18. Brown FD, Johns L, Jafar JJ, et al: Detailed monitoring of the effects of mannitol following experimental head injury. *J Neurosurg* 1979; 50:423.
19. Brown FD, Johns LM, Mullan S: Dimethylsulfoxide in experimental brain injury, with comparison to mannitol. *J Neurosurg* 1980; 53:58.
20. Brown FD, Johns L, Mullan S: Dimethylsulfoxide therapy following penetrating brain injury. *Ann N Y Acad Sci* 1983:245.
21. Levett JM, Johns LM, Replogle RL, et al: Cardiovascular effects of experimental cerebral missile injury in primates. *Surg Neurol* 1980; 13:59.
22. Allen IV, Scott R, Tanner JA: Experimental high-velocity missile head injury. *Injury* 1982; 14:183.
23. Maynard RL, Cooper GJ, Evans VA, et al: Pathophysiological effects of experimental medium velocity penetrating head injury. CDE Technical Note No: 567, CDE, Porton Down, Salisbury, Wilts, England.
24. Allen IV, Kirk J, Maynard RL, et al: An ultrastructural study of experimental high velocity penetrating head injury. *Acta Neuropathol (Berl)* 1983; 59:277.
25. Allen IV, Crockard HA, Maynard RL, et al: Pathological changes following experimental medium velocity penetrating head injury. New York: Raven Press, 1982.
26. Fackler ML: What's wrong with the wound ballistics literature and why. San Francisco: Letterman Army Institute of Research, 1987.
27. Harvey EN, Korr IM, Oster G, et al: Secondary damage in wounding due to pressure changes accompanying the passage of high velocity missiles. *Surgery* 1947; 21:218.

28. Harvey EN, McMillen JH, Butler EH, et al: Mechanisms of wounding, in Coats JB Jr (ed): *Wound Ballistics.* Washington: Office of the Surgeon General, 1962:Chap 2.
29. Janzon B: *High Energy Missile Trauma.* Goteborg: Minab/Gotab, 1983.
30. Owen-Smith MS: *High Velocity Missile Wounds.* London: Edward Arnold, 1981.
31. Harvey EN, McMillen JH: An experimental study of shock waves resulting from the impact of high velocity missiles on animal tissues. *J Exp Med* 1947; 85:321.
32. Beyer JC, Arisma JK, Johnson DW: Enemy ordnance material, in Coats JB Jr (ed): *Wound Ballistics.* Washington: Office of the Surgeon General, 1962:Chap 1.
33. Burns BD, Zuckerman S: The wounding power of small bomb and shell fragments. British Ministry of Supply Advisory Council on Scientific Research and Technical Development, RC 350 (7 Oct 1942).
34. Polis A: Récherches experimentales sur la commotion cérebral. *Rev Chir* 1884; 273:645.
35. Pearce BP, Stauber MC, Watkins FP: Physical effects of the penetration of head simulants by steel spheres. NATO: Defence Research Study Group II, 1983. Ref: Ptn/IL2801/801/83.
36. Pappius HM, McCann WP: Effects of steroids on cerebral edema in cats. *Arch Neurol* 1969; 20:207.
37. Long DM, Maxwell RE, Choi KS, et al: Multiple therapeutic approaches in the treatment of brain edema induced by a standard cold lesion, in Reulen HJ, Schurmann K (eds): *Steroids and Brain Edema.* New York: Springer-Verlag, 1972:87.
38. Ginsberg MD, Budd WW, Welsh FA: Diffuse cerebral ischemia in the cat: I. Local blood flow during severe ischemia and recirculation. *Ann Neurol* 1978; 3:482.
39. Shalit MN, Cotev S: Interrelationship between blood pressure and regional cerebral blood flow in experimental intracranial hypertension. *J Neurosurg* 1974; 40:594.
40. Carey ME, Young HF, Mathis JL: The neurosurgical treatment of craniocerebral missile wounds in Vietnam. *Surg Gynecol Obstet* 1972; 135:386.
41. Carey ME, Sarna GS, Farrell JB, et al: Experimental missile wound to the brain. *J Neurosurg* 1989; 71:754.
42. Torbati D, Jacks AF, Carey ME, et al: Cerebral cardiovascular and respiratory variables after an experimental brain missile wound. *J Neurotrauma* 1922; 9:Suppl 1:5143.
43. Hossman KA, Hossman V, Tayagi S: Microsphere analysis of local cerebral and extracerebral blood flow after complete ischemia of the cat brain for one hour. *J Neurol* 1978; 218:275.
44. Soblosky JS, Rogers NL, Adams JA, et al: Central and peripheral biogenic amine effects of brain missile wounding (BMW) and increased intracranial pressure. *J Neurosurg* 1992; 76:119.
45. Carey ME, Sarna GS, Farell JB: Brain edema following an experimental missile wound to the brain. *J Neurotrauma* 1990; 7:1, 13.
46. Kaufman HH, Moake JL, Olson JD, et al: Delayed and recurrent intracranial hematomas related to disseminated intravascular clotting and fibrinolysis in head injury. *Neurosurgery* 1980; 7:445.
47. Awasthi D, Rock WA, Carey ME, et al: Coagulation changes after an experimental missile wound to the brain in the cat. *Surg Neurol* 1991; 36:441.

CHAPTER 100

THE NEED FOR CONTINUED DEVELOPMENT OF EXPERIMENTAL MODELS OF BRAIN INJURY

Thomas E. Anderson
James W. Lighthall

INTRODUCTION

The development of an experimental model for brain injury is shaped by the investigator's objectives. Differing scientific objectives and goals may result in different yet equally valid models, each appropriate to specific questions. The most appropriate model for studying axonal injury may not be as useful in studies of cortical contusions or diffuse brain swelling, for instance. And a focus on injury biomechanics places different constraints on the design of the model and the experimental measurements than does evaluation of pharmacological efficacy for a specific component of brain tissue pathophysiology or functional outcome. Despite potentially different objectives, however, certain experimental criteria are shared by every useful brain injury model. The injury response, specified in physiological, behavioral, or anatomic terms, must be reproducible and quantifiable over a continuum of injury severities which are clinically relevant. Often, the most valuable data are found in transition or threshold regions of the experimental injury severity.

Clinically, brain injuries include both diffuse and focal injuries. Diffuse injuries consist of brain swelling, concussion, and diffuse axonal injury. Focal injuries include epidural hematoma, subdural hematoma, intracerebral hematoma, and brain contusions. The development of various experimental brain injury models continues to be driven by a desire to reproduce these pathologies individually and in combination and to do so in a reproducible and predictable manner. If the injury technique is designed to be relevant to hypothesized biomechanics and the pathophysiology of clinical injury, the critical factor becomes the production of functional and anatomic sequelae comparable to those seen clinically in a human closed head injury.

Ideally, the mechanical input to the brain will mimic, at least in part, the biomechanics of human brain injury. A reproducible well-defined mechanical input can simplify the interpretation of the pathophysiological, biomechanical, and biochemical mechanisms of the resultant injury. Indeed, early attempts to replicate the biomechanics of human head injury were only partially successful in reproducing the pathology that was observed clinically. In large part, this reflected differences in both the size and the geometry of the experimental animal brain in comparison with the human brain. Even primate experimental models differ significantly in brain size and somewhat in geometry from the human. This creates a challenge in terms of creating sufficient brain accelerations to cause an injury relevant to human closed head injury without also causing skull fracture.

By contrast, models which directly deform the brain can create local tissue deformation which is controllable and potentially analyzable. The argument can be made that if the local tissue pathology is comparable to clinical observations, the local tissue biomechanical deformation which initiates the response may be comparable to the local deformation that occurs in clinical brain injury, regardless of the gross brain injury which initiates the local response. One can further argue on the same basis that in vitro models can provide valuable information and insights regarding thresholds for axonal or vascular injury.

The various classes of models ranging from closed head impact to in vitro studies, will be discussed with exemplars. The strengths and limitations of each approach are indicated as well. This review is intended to provide examples and general considerations for model development rather than to be an exhaustive review of all the models which have been used.

HEAD IMPACT MODELS

Primate Studies

Head unrestrained

Controlled impact to the unrestrained head of nonhuman primates was pioneered by Denny-Brown and Russell.[1,2] These experiments established impact to the unrestrained head as a common experimental technique, since it was observed that when the head was held fixed, concussion was less likely to result from impact. The evaluation of neurological and physiological indicators of injury severity was carried out in fully anesthetized animals, and this limited analysis of the injury outcome to brainstem reflexes and systemic physiological changes.

Gurdjian and associates used an impact piston with a 1-kg mass to strike the head of an anesthetized primate in a predetermined location on the skull. Physiological parameters, impact force, and head acceleration were monitored in an effort to determine thresholds for concussion and coma, coup and contrecoup contusions, and relative brain motions.[3,4] In later experiments, a molded protective skullcap was used to prevent fracture. Ommaya and others also used this technique with slight variations to evaluate changes in intracranial pressure, behavior, systemic physiology, cerebral metabolism, and histopathology after an impact injury to the primate skull.[5,6]

Constraint of head motion in these impact studies was provided only by the neck, and this resulted in complex and ill-characterized three-dimensional head movement. Severity was determined through selection of impactor velocity, impactor mass, material used as an interface, and impactor contact area. Although a range of injury severities could be produced, injury mechanisms remained complex, including local skull deformation, development of pressure gradients or shear strains in the brain tissue, and relative motion between the brain and the skull. Technically, it is not feasible to separate these biomechanical components of the injury event to allow more detailed analysis of mechanisms.

Head restrained

A number of studies have therefore constrained, at least partially, head motion during and after impact, typically to a single plane, in an effort to increase the reproducibility of the injury outcome.[7,8] An analysis of the pathophysiology and the relation of impact biomechanics to outcome in these studies indicates that partial control of head motion does not represent a significant improvement in the gradation and reproducibility of impact parameters and outcome severity compared with an unconstrained head.

Nonprimate Studies

Direct impact of the head also has been applied to nonprimate species, with a variety of studies using the rat as an experimental model.[9–12] The relatively small size and moderate cost of rodents make their use attractive for studies requiring large numbers of subjects for analysis of histopathologic and behavioral responses. In general, the biomechanical analysis of head and brain dynamics after head impact in rodents was hampered by an unspecified degree of head restraint or support. Typically, moderate impact to a rat head resulted in either no identifiable injury or immediate convulsions associated with apnea. Serious injuries resulted in either fatality or a brief period of unconsciousness, usually indicated by absence of the righting reflex.[13,14]

Convulsive activity produced in this model may affect the outcome and must be considered in interpreting the cerebral metabolic, neurophysiological, and EEG changes which follow injury. The histopathologic evidence of neural injury is typically restricted to the lower brainstem, in contrast to clinical observations. The injury tolerance curve is extremely steep, changing from no injury to fatality over a narrow range of injury parameters, perhaps as a result of the small size and mass of the rodent brain and the necessarily high levels of head acceleration which must therefore be induced to cause injury, raising the likelihood of skull fracture. In addition, the lissencephalic nature of the cortex does not allow complete modeling of all the changes occurring in the human brain, which has a complex structure of gyri and sulci, and the physiological responses of rodents to traumatic brain injury differ in some respects from those of humans.

Head impact studies performed in cats, using a captive-bolt pistol to deliver the impact, have been most extensively developed by Tornheim and colleagues.[15,16] Impacts delivered to the coronal suture cause a reproducible contusion with associated edema and skull fracture. The captive-bolt head impact model has been used successfully to test the efficacy of antiedema drugs. Subsequent experiments have used an oblique lateral impact, with the head resting on a collapsible hex-cell support.[16] This model is useful for studies of cerebral contusion and resultant edema, though reliable gradation of impact severity is still needed.

The various direct head impact methods for nonprimates all suffer from a high degree of variability in the response. This variability may result from a lack of control over the precise conditions of the impact, an absence of control of head dynamic response, inconsistent impactor-skull interface parameters, variability in skull thickness, and a relatively steep injury outcome curve, in which a slight variation in impact energy may cause a large variation in injury outcome. As a result, the expected variability resulting from biological differences is confounded by the mechanical variability of the injury event, necessitating a large number of experiments to obtain a representative sample of pathophysiological response. In addition, the uncontrolled injury biomechanics make analysis of brain injury biomechanics difficult at best.

HEAD ACCELERATION MODELS

Free Head Motion

As in head impact models, various head acceleration models have been developed, some of which tightly control the motions of the head while others allow free head motion. Free head acceleration is attained through an abrupt deceleration of a moving frame to which the rest of the body is firmly affixed. This produces a whiplash head motion and can result in concussion.[17,18] These studies have been performed in nonhuman primates, since the anatomic relationships between brain, brainstem, and spinal cord are most similar to those of humans, as is the ratio of brain mass to head mass. In any whole head acceleration model, the geometry and mass distribution significantly affect brain impact dynamics and the resultant injury. A major difference between head impact and head acceleration models is the relative absence of skull fracture in the acceleration models; however, in human head injury, the range of induced accelerations which produce injury experimentally is attained only when head impact occurs.

Constrained Head Motion

Since unconstrained head dynamics make the analysis of injury biomechanics difficult, the majority of studies using head acceleration techniques have employed some type of helmet and linkage to control head motions.[19–21] Such a system controls the path direction, path length, and duration of acceleration, so that the head motion is comparable for experiments with a comparable input. In addition, controlled head acceleration reduces the incidence of skull fracture and local skull deformation, which are common occurrences when impact techniques are used.

Primate studies

The most extensive series of experiments using constrained head motion to study brain injury was initiated by Ommaya and Gennarelli and continued by Gennarelli and Thibault. These investigators were able to produce graded anatomic and functional injury severities, including prolonged (>30 min) traumatic unconsciousness, in nonhuman primates.[19] This series of experiments was based on the findings of an earlier head acceleration study which had indicated that loss of consciousness was more readily produced by high levels of angular acceleration than by high levels of translational acceleration.[20–22]

The device and control linkage were designed to allow high levels of angular acceleration to be delivered to the primate head without skull fracture.[19] The acceleration pulse was biphasic, with a relatively long, ramp-like acceleration phase that was followed by an abrupt deceleration phase. Injury was presumed to occur as a result of the deceleration phase. Diffuse axonal injury was observed in the subcortical white matter, comparable to the pathophysiology observed in clinical brain injury.[19,23–25] The spectrum of injury ranged from mild, subconcussive brain injury with only sparse histological evidence of axonal damage, through prolonged (hours to days) traumatic coma with extensive axonal injury throughout the white matter and brainstem, to immediately fatal injury. Histopathologic evaluation shows a high degree of comparability to clinical brain injury pathology, substantiating the relevance of the technique. However, the injury device is complex and costly to duplicate and requires the collaboration of medical scientists and biomechanical engineers for implementation and meaningful data interpretation.

Nonprimate studies

Nelson and colleagues developed a controlled nonimpact head acceleration model in the cat, using repetitive head accelerations.[26,27] Oscillations delivered at 1200 to 1400 per minute were combined with induced posttraumatic hypoxia or ischemia. Injury severities were categorized into three outcomes: immediate fatality, delayed mortality, and extended coma. Although clinical brain injury typically involves a period of hypoxia or relative cerebral ischemia, the relevance of rapid, repetitive accelerations of the head to human brain injury biomechanics is unclear. This technique induces a consistent range of injury with a reproducible percentage distribution in each of the three outcome categories but did not allow prediction of the injury severity which is likely to result from a specific exposure. Hence, testing for pharmacological efficacy is based on changes in the percentage distribution of outcomes among the three functional categories, leading to increased sample sizes and impairing the interpretation of biomechanical and pathophysiological mechanisms.

DIRECT BRAIN DEFORMATION MODELS

Nonpenetrating focal deformation of cortical tissue has been employed as an alternative to head impact and induced acceleration models of brain injury and has some potential advantages for biomechanical analysis of the injury event and the relation of brain tissue deformation to injury outcome.

Distributed functional and histopathologic changes are consistently observed using the fluid percussion brain injury technique initially developed by Lindgren and colleagues in the rabbit.[28,29] In this technique, a brief fluid pressure pulse is applied to the dural surface at the vertex of the brain through a craniotomy. The procedure has been modified frequently to employ different pulse parameters and locations of the applied pressure pulse, including lateral techniques, and has been applied to cats and rats to generate a range of brain injury, from mild to severe.[30–40]

The pressure pulse is delivered via a fluid column to the intact dura and results in functional changes accompanied by subcortical axonal damage and brainstem pathology. A graded, reproducible range of injury severities can be produced. Cortical contusion at the site of pressure application typically occurs only in lateral fluid percussion injury. Global changes in cerebral blood flow, reactivity to CO_2, and autoregulation also are observed. The mechanics of the fluid percussion injury model are poorly understood and probably differ from closed head injury in humans.[33,39] However, the pathophysiological changes offer a reasonable model for studying mechanisms for brainstem injury, contusion, and secondary CNS-metabolic abnormalities. The ability to produce contusion, graded brainstem injury, and subcortical axonal injury makes the fluid percussion technique useful for those aspects of clinical brain injury, and the lateral fluid percussion technique provides a useful model for cortical contusion.[41] Also, in cats, fluid percussion injury can produce concussion with flaccidity resembling coma which persists up to 4 h.[34,42]

From a theoretical point of view, since brain tissue injury is initiated by induced stresses and pressures in the cerebrum and brainstem, direct cortical deformation may be used to study closed head injury if it results in a comparable pattern of intracerebral forces in the brain and a comparable anatomic and functional injury outcome. Since the functional changes and histopathology are in many aspects comparable to clinical brain injury, these models are widely used for studies of pharmacological intervention and chronic treatment approaches.

Direct focal cortical compression has been produced by using weight drop devices.[43] Both localized cortical contusions and distributed cerebral metabolic effects were observed, though pathological changes in neural and vascular elements were observed predominantly in the impact region.[44] In particular, functional consequences of importance to clinical brain injury were not produced using this technique. Local damping of input force by dural and cortical tissue might have effectively prevented propagation throughout the remainder of the brain; the absence of biomechanical data on brain deformations in these injury models prevents any further conclusions.

Dynamic mechanical compression of the brain surface also has been shown to produce pathological and functional outcomes similar to human brain injury.[45,46] This technique elicits a range of pathological responses similar to those described for other brain injury models and allows independent control over contact velocity and amount of brain compression to permit biomechanical studies. The technique has been applied successfully in rats as well, and this will facilitate behavioral studies of learning and memory loss and testing of the efficacy of pharmacological intervention.[31,47] Axonal injury is observed at 3 and 5 days after injury for moderate to severe injury parameters. Axonal injury was observed in subcortical white matter, including the corpus collosum, stria medullaris, and internal capsule; thalamic relay nuclei, including the lateral geniculate and pulvinar; and the midbrain, pons, and medulla. Axonal injury also was evident in the white matter of the cerebellar folia and the region of the deep cerebellar nuclei.

When lateral cortical impact is used in combination with a contralateral craniotomy, the pattern of axonal injury is concentrated in the corpus callosum in the plane across the midline established by the craniotomy sites. Behavioral assessment also showed functional coma consisting of decorticate and decerebrate rigidity, followed by muscle flaccidity and inability to maintain sternal recumbence lasting up to 36 h after 8.0 m/s impacts and concluding with impaired movement and control of the extremities. It is clear that a wide spectrum of responses can be produced by manipulating the velocity and depth of the cortical impact.

Another model which falls under the heading of direct deformation, although of CNS axons rather than brain tissue, is the optic nerve stretch lesion model described by Gennarelli and coworkers.[48] In this model, the optic nerve is subjected to brief dynamic tensile loading. The resultant stretch causes axonal lesions which are reminiscent of the diffuse axonal injury seen in humans with moderate to severe head injury. Approximately 17 percent of the axons demonstrated injury in this model in the absence of vascular injury. This model not only simplifies the geometric and size issues but allows the investigator to test directly for the axonal injury threshold. Knowledge of the tensile load magnitude which will lead to axonal injury is needed in mathematical modeling of brain injury and aids in the interpretation of in vivo experimental studies.

IN VITRO MODELS

In vitro models of brain injury differ fundamentally from in vivo models in that the goal is not the reproduction of gross or even tissue-level injury but rather the reproduction of cellular injury and investigation of the mechanism at the cellular and subcellular levels.[49,50] Thus, it is not required, though it may be preferred, to reproduce the mechanical forces which are believed to act at the cellular level in the initiation of injury. Indeed, the experimental approaches used with in vitro models have included direct neurite transection by cutting; injury by laser irradiation to generate photobiological or pressure wave insults, depending on energy density; and mechanical injury using various methodologies. In all cases, the resultant pathology in the nerve cell body and processes is directly accessible to analysis. As a further benefit, the local physiological environment is under experimental control and no anesthetic is required in the culture. At the same time, the investigator must remember that the secondary pathophysiological response which occurs in vivo and which undoubtedly contributes to the final functional and pathological result does not occur in vitro. Therefore, it is necessary to evaluate in vitro data continually in the context of in vivo responses to ensure proper interpretation and consideration of factors, such as ischemia and hypoxia, which may not be included in a particular in vitro model.

While the in vitro models represent highly simplified systems and in fact have been developed and used successfully precisely because they are simplified and remove many interacting influences, it is possible to introduce additional complexity to the model in a stepwise manner. This allows direct study or pathophysiological mechanisms and separation of mechanical versus physiological factors.

PHYSICAL MODELS

Physical models provide a useful tool for evaluating the severity of brain deformation which probably is produced by a particular injury model and determining the reproducibility of brain dynamics after the injury event. This is important from the standpoint of validation for mathematical models and the development of local injury threshold criteria. Thibault and associates probably have conducted the most extensive program of the physical modeling of brain injury, using a variety of plastic cylinders and brain cavity simulators filled with gel material to emulate the brain's mechanical properties.[51] The physical model provides a unique opportunity to directly measure deformations deep in the brain tissue when a transparent simulant is used. Typically, a partial thickness of the simulant is poured, a grid is inked on the surface, and the balance of the brain simulant is poured. When accelerations are then applied to the model, deformations at the depth of the grid can be quantified, representing the deformation expected in the brain tissue. These studies have been used to identify deformation occurring in brain tissue during closed head acceleration or direct brain loading, such as fluid percussion, and to define injury threshold levels on the basis of the calculated strain. They also have been used to partially validate mathematical model predictions of deformations during experimental injury and thus further refine the models' accuracy.

CONCLUSIONS

Experimental brain injury can be created by using a variety of techniques, ranging from head impact to direct brain deformation Fig. 100-1. In addition, cellular pathophysiology and local biomechanical injury initiation can be addressed directly, using in vitro and physical models, respectively. Each approach has advantages and limitations, and no single model reproduces the full pathophysiological and functional injury features and the range of injury severity observed in human head injury. Finally, all in vivo models have the complicating factor of anesthetic protocol, just as in vitro models are affected by factors such as the extracellular medium, fluid exchange rates if applicable, and temperature, all of which are under the experimenter's control. To facilitate interlaboratory comparisons, attention should be paid to the age and sex of the animals. Also, physiological parameters, including blood gases, blood glucose, blood

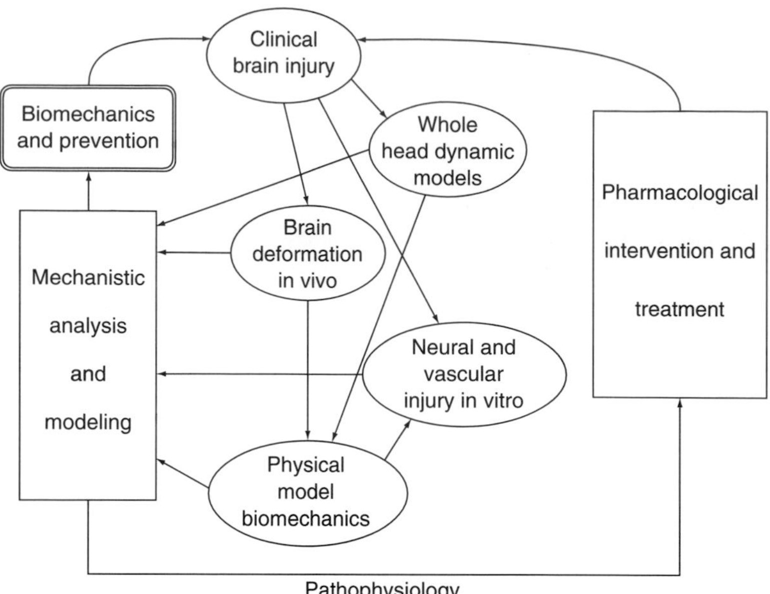

Figure 100-1. Schematic representation of injury model types and postulated interactions. The goal of analysis is prevention and/or treatment of clinical brain injury. Each model category represents a simplification of the complex biomechanics and pathophysiology of clinical brain injury. Arguably, the clinical realism is greatest at the top of the chart and decreases toward the bottom, although control of injury mechanics and physiology increases from top toward the bottom. Through model simplification and consequent recombination and analysis of the data, necessary information for improved understanding of both injury biomechanics and injury physiological response can be obtained. These advances will facilitate a reduced incidence of and improved treatments for clinical brain injury.

pressure, and body temperature, should be monitored routinely.

Differing scientific objectives and goals may result in different yet equally valid models, each appropriate to specific questions. This is consistent with the conclusion of a recent National Institute of Neurological Disorders and Strokes-sponsored workshop on experimental models for brain injury, which found that no single model of brain injury could be embraced as the "gold standard" (Table 100-1).[52] However, for all experimental models, the injury response, specified in physiological, behavioral, or anatomic terms, must be reproducible and quantifiable over a continuum of injury severities which are clinically relevant. The development of the various experimental brain injury models has been driven by an intent to reproduce clinically observed features of

TABLE 100-1

Injury or model	Clinical relevance	Experimental control	Other factors	Treatment	Prevention
Clinical injury	++++	−−	Variable	Validate	Utilize
Whole head dynamic models	+++	++ (potentially)	Present and controllable	Preclinical trials	Validate
Direct brain deformation in vivo	++	+++	Present and controllable	Develop and test	Develop and validate
Neural and vascular in vitro	−− (cellular mechanism)	++++	Tissue culture issues	Prescreen	Cell-level injury criteria
Physical models	−−−	++++ (mechanics)	Not relevant	Not relevant	Measure gross deformation

Advantages and limitations of the various experimental injury models by category. "Other factors" includes considerations such as anesthesia for the experimental models, life support for both the models and clinical injury, and physiological influences, including blood alcohol, blood sugar levels, loss of blood, and other associated injuries, for clinical brain injury. Degree of clinical relevance and control of injury parameters are represented from ++++ (highly relevant or controlled) to −−− (little direct relevance or control).

brain injury pathology and behavioral dysfunction either individually or in combination.

Head impact models have been developed in both primate and nonprimate animal models, and although a range of injury severities are produced, injury mechanisms remain complex and partially understood. These mechanisms include local skull deformation, development of pressure gradients or shear strains in the brain tissue, and relative motion between the brain and the skull. Although some studies have attempted to evaluate the effects of rotational and translational head acceleration separately, careful biomechanical analysis of the experiments clearly shows that skull impact produces both rotational and translational acceleration components in all cases.

This makes analysis difficult in regard to definition of injury criteria and complicates the analysis of therapeutic interventions. Impact techniques have been only partially successful at producing a spectrum of clinically relevant injury in the rat. Skull fracture commonly occurs at impact severity levels insufficient to produce prolonged coma. Moreover, the occurrence of skull fracture in the rat is not well correlated with injury severity, and postinjury convulsive activity may affect outcome and must be considered in the interpretation of the cerebral metabolic, neurophysiological, and EEG changes which follow injury.

Head acceleration models, by contrast, do not always involve skull fracture and the resultant complications of injury mechanisms. Avoidance of skull fracture requires careful attention to experimental design but can be achieved readily, particularly in larger animal models. These techniques have been most successful in large animal models, since the acceleration levels necessary to cause brain injury increase substantially as the size of the brain decreases. Even for larger brains, the acceleration levels required are high, and for humans they typically occur only with head impact. As a result, the mechanism required to produce injury is complex and costly to duplicate and requires a team of medical scientists and biomechanical engineers to implement and maintain.

Brain injury produced by the fluid percussion technique includes pathophysiological changes which offer a reasonable model for studying mechanisms for brainstem injury, contusion, and secondary CNS metabolic abnormalities. The ability to produce contusion, graded brainstem injury, and subcortical axonal injury continues to make the fluid percussion technique a useful model for those aspects of clinical brain injury, and the lateral fluid percussion technique provides a useful model for cortical contusion. Also, fluid percussion injury can produce concussion in cats with flaccidity resembling coma, which persists up to 4 h.

From a theoretical point of view, since brain tissue injury is initiated by induced stresses and pressures in the cerebrum and brainstem, direct cortical deformation may be used to study closed head injury if it results in a comparable pattern of intracerebral forces in the brain and a comparable anatomic and functional injury outcome. Dynamic mechanical compression of the brain surface also has been shown to produce pathological and functional outcomes similar to human brain injury. In addition to eliciting a range of pathological responses similar to those described for other brain injury models, direct cortical contusion allows independent control over contact velocity and amount of brain compression, which is needed in biomechanical studies to determine a tissue-level criterion for brain injury. This technique has been applied successfully in rats, and this will facilitate behavioral studies of learning and memory loss and testing of the efficacy of pharmacological intervention.

There are several advantages to using a single, controlled mechanical input to produce a brain injury. If the mechanical input is designed to be quantifiable and graded, correlations can be made between the brain deformation parameters, including applied force, the amount of deformation and its time history, and the resultant pathology and functional changes. Such analysis will ultimately lead to enhanced understanding of the interaction between the physical input, the severity of the physiological injury response, and the functional outcome. The restriction to one quantifiable mechanical input variable facilitates the biomechanical analysis of an experimental brain injury. Parallel analysis utilizing physical and analytic modeling of tissue deformation will then allow correlation to the more complex dynamics of human brain injury through derivation of brain tissue biomechanical parameters which produce transient neurological changes, coma, or fatality.

In vitro models provide a means of directly addressing postulated pathophysiological mechanisms at the cellular level and bring much of the sequence of injury response under the active control of the experimenter. They also provide a means to separate immediate, biomechanically induced injury to axonal processes and other neural tissue elements from secondary pathology resulting from the injury response and local metabolic changes. And through consideration of potential mechanisms, it becomes possible to experimentally simulate the proposed (or measured) injury physiological response and address the interaction of mechanically initiated and physiologically embellished pathologies. Finally, physical models enable the experimentalist and modeler to simulate brain motions and derive information about the internal deformations which are likely to occur. This provides information as input into the in vitro studies, setting appropriate deformation levels for experimental study, and assists in the validation of computational models of brain injury.

Despite the many successful models for various aspects of human brain injury, to date there is no single model which is entirely satisfactory in producing the complete clinical picture using a well-defined and controlled biomechanical input. As a result, continued development of experimental models for specific aspects of clinical brain injury is needed to further our understanding of brain injury mechanisms and facilitate the evaluation of specific interventions. Indeed, a multiplicity of models, each simulating one or more aspects of clinical brain injury, provides a more robust test of potential therapeutic interventions which may warrant clinical trials. Since no single model is ideal in providing the complete pathophysiological response and since all involve anesthetics and some degree of experimenter control of physiology (baseline, injury response, or both) to increase reproducibility, this mutiplicity of models increases the likelihood that a successful intervention approach which has been validated in several laboratories may prove to be successful clinically.

References

1. Denny-Brown D, Russel WR: Experimental cerebral concussion. *Brain* 64:93–164, 1941.
2. Denny-Brown D: Cerebral concussion. *Physiol Rev* 25:296–325, 1945.
3. Gurdjian ES, Lissner HP, Webster HP, et al: Studies on experimental concussion: relation of physiologic effect to time duration of intracranial pressure increase at impact. *Neurology* 4:674–681, 1954.
4. Gurdjian ES, Roberts VL, Thomas LM: Tolerance curves of acceleration and intracranial pressure and protective index in experimental head injury. *J Trauma* 6:600–604, 1966.
5. Ommaya AK, Hirsch AE, Flamm ES, Mahone RH: Cerebral concussion in the monkey: An experimental model. *Science* 153:211–212, 1966.
6. McCullough D, Nelson KM, Ommaya AK: The acute effects of experimental head injury on the vertebrobasilar circulation: Angiographic observations. *J Trauma* 11:422–428, 1971.
7. Langfitt TW, Tannanbaum HM, Kassel NF: The etiology of acute brain swelling following experimental head injury. *J Neurosurg* 24:47–56, 1966.
8. Shatsky SA, Evans DE, Miller F, Martins AN: High-speed angiography of experimental head injury. *J Neurosurg* 41:523–530, 1974.
9. Goldman H, Hodgson V, Morehead M, et al: Cerebrovascular changes in a rat model of moderate closed head injury. *J Neurotrauma* 8:129–144, 1991.
10. Hall E: High-dose glucocorticoid treatment impairs neurologic recovery in head-injured mice. *J Neurosurg* 62:882–887, 1985.
11. Shapira Y, Shohami E, Sidi A, et al: Experimental closed head injury in rats: Mechanical, pathophysiologic and neurologic properties. *Crit Care Med* 16:258–265, 1988.
12. Shaw NA: A simple device for experimentally concussing the rat. *Physiol Behav* 35:637–639, 1985.
13. Govons SR, Govons RB, Van Huss WD, Heusner WW: Brain concussion in the rat. *Exp Neurol* 34:121–128, 1972.
14. Nilsson B, Ponten U, Voigt G: Experimental head injury in the rat: I. Mechanics, pathophysiology, and morphology in an impact acceleration trauma. *J Neurosurg* 47:241–251, 1978.
15. Tornheim PA, McLaurin RL, Thorpe JF: The edema of cerebral contusion. *Surg Neurol* 5:171–175, 1976.
16. Tornheim PA, Linwicz BH, Hirsch AE, et al: Acute responses to blunt head trauma; Experimental model and gross pathology. *J Neurosurg* 59:431–438, 1983.
17. Ommaya AK, Hirsch AE: Tolerances for cerebral concussion from head impact and whiplash in primates. *J Biomech* 4:13–31, 1971.
18. Ommaya AK, Corrao P, Letcher FS: Head injury in the chimpanzee: Biodynamics of traumatic unconsciousness. *J Neurosurg* 39:167–177, 1973.
19. Gennarelli TA, Thibault LE, Adams JH, et al: Diffuse axonal injury and traumatic coma in the primate. *Ann Neurol* 12:564–574, 1982.
20. Ommaya AK, Gennarelli TA: Cerebral concussion and traumatic unconsciousness: Correlation of experimental and clinical observations on blunt head injuries. *Brain* 97:633–654, 1974.
21. Unterharnscheidt FJ: Pathomorphology of experimental head injury due to rotational acceleration. *Acta Neuropathol (Berl)* 12:200–204, 1969.
22. Gennarelli TA, Thibault LE: Experimental production of prolonged traumatic coma in the primate, in Villiani R (ed): *Advances in Neurotraumatology*. Amsterdam, Excerpta Medica, 1983:31–33.
23. Adams JH, Doyle DI: Diffuse brain damage in non-missile head injury, in Anthony PP, MacSween RNM (eds): *Recent Advances in Histopathology*. Edinburgh: Churchill Livingstone, 1984; 241–257.
24. Adams JH, Graham DI, Gennarelli TA: Contemporary neuropathological considerations regarding brain damage in head injury, in Becker DP, Povlishock JT (eds): *Central Nervous System Trauma Status Report*. NINCDS Publication, 1985.
25. Jane JA, Steward O, Gennarelli T: Axonal degeneration induced by experimental noninvasive minor head injury. *J Neurosurg* 62:96–100, 1985.
26. Nelson LR, Auen EL, Bourke RS, Barron KD: A new head injury model for evaluation of treatment modalities. *Neurosci Abstr* 5:516, 1979.
27. Nelson LR, Auen EL, Bourke RS, et al: A comparison of animal head injury models developed for treatment modality evaluation, in Grossman RG, Gildenberg PL (eds): *Head Injury: Basic and Clinical Aspects*. New York: Raven Press, 1982:117–128.
28. Lindgren S, Rinder L: Experimental studies of head injury: I. Some factors influencing results of model experiments. *Biophysik* 2:320–329, 1965.
29. Rinder L: Concussive response and intracranial pressure changes at sudden extradural fluid volume input in rabbits. *Acta Physiol Scand* 76:352–360, 1969.
30. Dixon CE, Clifton GL, Lighthall JL, et al: A controlled

cortical impact model of traumatic brain injury in the rat, *J Neurosci Methods* 39:253–262, 1991.
31. Dixon CE, Lyeth GB, Povlishock JT, et al: A fluid percussion model of experimental brain injury in the rat: Neurological, physiological, and histopathological characterizations. *J Neurosurg* 67:110–119, 1987.
32. Hayes RL, Stalhammar D, Povlishock JT, et al: A new model of concussive brain injury in the cat produced by extradural fluid volume loading: II. Physiological and neurophysiological observations. *Brain Inj* 1:93–112, 1987.
33. Hayes RL, Katayama Y, Young HF, Dunbar JG: Coma associated with flaccidity produced by fluid-percussion concussion in the cat: I. Is it due to depression of activity within the brainstem reticular formation? *Brain Inj* 2:31–49, 1988.
34. McIntosh TK, Noble L, Andrews B, Faden AI: Traumatic brain injury in the rat: Characterization of a midline fluid-percussion model. *CNS Trauma* 4:119–134, 1987.
35. McIntosh TK, Vink R, Noble L, et al: Traumatic brain injury in the rat: Characterization of a lateral fluid-percussion model, *Neuroscience* 28:233–244, 1989.
36. Marmarou A, Shima K: Comparative studies of edema produced by fluid percussion injury with lateral and central modes of injury in cats. *Adv Neurol* 52:233–300, 1990.
37. Povlishock JT, Becker DP, Sullivan HG, Miller JD: Vascular permeability alterations to horseradish peroxidase in experimental brain injury. *Brain Res* 153:223–239, 1978.
38. Povlishock JT, Becker DP, Cheng CLY, Vaughan GW: Axonal change in minor head injury. *J Neuropathol Exp Neurol* 42:225–242, 1983.
39. Stalhammar D, Galinat BJ, Allen AM, et al: A new model of concussive brain injury in the cat produced by extradural fluid volume loading: I. Biomechanical properties. *Brain Inj* 1:79–91, 1987.
40. Sullivan HG, Martinez J, Becker DP, et al: Fluid percussion model of mechanical brain injury in the cat. *J Neurosurg* 45:520–534, 1976.
41. Povlishock JT, Erb DE, Astrue J: Axonal response to traumatic brain injury: Reactive axonal change, deafferentiation and neuroplasticity. *J Neurotrauma* 9:S189–200, 1992.
42. Katayama Y, Young HF, Dunbar JG, Hayes RL: Coma associated with flaccidity produced by fluid-percussion concussion in the cat: II. Contribution with activity in the pontine inhibitory system. *Brain Inj* 2:51–66, 1988.
43. Feeney DM, Boyson MG, Linn RT et al: Responses to cortical injury: I. Methodology and local effects of contusions in the rat. *Brain Res* 211:67–77, 1981.
44. Dail WG, Feeney DM, Murray HM, et al: Responses to cortical injury: II. Widespread depression of the activity of an enzyme in cortex remote from a focal injury. *Brain Res* 211:79–89, 1981.
45. Lightall JW: Controlled cortical impact: A new experimental brain injury model. *J Neurotrauma* 5:1–15, 1988.
46. Lightall JW, Goshgarian HG, Pinderski CR: Characterization of axonal injury produced by controlled cortical impact, *J Neurotrauma* 7:65–76, 1990.
47. Hamm RJ, Dixon CE, Gradebo DM, et al: Cognitive deficits following traumatic brain injury produced by a controlled cortical impact, *J Neurotrauma* 9:11–19, 1992.
48. Gennarelli TA, Thibault LE, Tipperman R, et al: Axonal injury in the optic nerve: A model simulating diffuse axonal injuries in the brain. *J Neurosurg* 71:244–253, 1989.
49. Kim-Lee MH, Stokes BT, Anderson DK: Intracellular calcium dynamics and cerebral injury, modeling various insults in vitro. *Brain Res* 613:156–159, 1993.
50. Lucas JH: In vitro models of mechanical injury. *J Neurotrauma* 9:117–120, 1992.
51. Thibault LE, Meaney DF, Anderson BJ, et al: Biomechanical aspects of a fluid percussion model of brain injury. *J Neurotrauma* 9:311–322, 1992.
52. Povlishock JT, Hayes RL, Michel ME, McIntosh TK: Workshop on animal models of traumatic brain injury. *J Neurotrauma* 11:723–32, 1994.

Experimental Spinal Cord Injury Models

CHAPTER 101

AN OVERVIEW OF SPINAL CORD INJURY MODELS

Andrew R. Blight

INTRODUCTION—THE USES OF ANIMAL MODELS

The value of relevant animal models is clear to anyone seriously engaged in biomedical research. The issues involved in establishing and validating such models are perhaps less obvious. Genetic or infectious diseases may be difficult to reproduce, even in closely related species, but tissue mechanics and basic cell biological properties in response to injury are more readily generalized, and mechanical trauma can be produced in many ways, some of them quite simple. Validation of injury models, on the other hand, is hindered by the complex, arbitrary and ill-defined nature of mechanical trauma in the clinical setting. The capacity for proliferation of models against a background of uncertain validity has led to persistent misgivings about methodology in this field. As a result, attention has tended to be distracted from more important questions of biology and medicine.

Animal models of acute spinal cord injury have been used for two principal purposes: investigation of injury mechanisms and testing potential therapies. At times, these two goals are shared within a given study, but they are distinct in the requirements they place on the model. Evaluation of experimental therapy has tended to dominate over any concerted attempt to understand the underlying pathological processes. The developers of injury models consequently have stressed properties that benefit testing of therapy rather than investigation of mechanism. At the same time, the effort to validate these models by parallel investigation of human injuries has been minimal, and continues to be fraught with difficulty.

The chief requirements for experimental testing are convergent. The model should be as restricted and repeatable as possible, so that differences between experimental and control populations can be detected with the smallest practical numbers of cases. The injury should be convenient to perform and be readily reproducible in different laboratories. These restrictions require several decisions to be made on the basis of incomplete information, including the selection of species, position of the injury, class of anesthesia, and the type of mechanical damage, including determination of speed, direction, displacement, force, and the area and nature of the interface.

Studies of biological mechanism, on the other hand, benefit from a divergent approach that examines the significance of differences between species, anesthetics, types of injury, and even between individual animals subjected to similar procedures. While the proliferation of models increases the logistic problem of testing potential treatments, it may help the investigation of injury mechanisms, provided the studies are well designed and properly interpreted. There is a case for both divergent and convergent approaches, but some danger of confusion exists unless the object of the research is clearly borne in mind. Also, it should be recognized that an arbitrary convergence on a particular model of convenience is essentially a gamble. It may emerge later that the particular properties of the chosen model are not broadly relevant to the clinical problem or may be specifically insensitive for testing a particular experimental therapy.

Differences exist also in the suitability of various measures of outcome in the two cases. For testing therapy, there is a natural tendency to concentrate on global functional deficits by analogy with the clinical interest in improved neurological outcome in human subjects. Indeed, in order for an experimental treatment to attract sufficient support to initiate a clinical trial it must show evidence of affecting functional outcome. Attention has concentrated on grading overall recovery of locomotion, since this is the most accessible behavior in most animals and appears directly relevant to clinical goals. To some extent, however, efficacy at this level in animal models is illusory, since there is only a tenuous relation between the neural basis of locomotory behavior in laboratory animals (especially rodents) and that of man. Also, it is difficult or impossible to evaluate many of the clinically important aspects of quality of life in animals, particularly with regard to chronic pain and spasticity and bowel and bladder function. Eventually, assessment of effects on quality of life must be carried out in human clinical trials.

Perhaps more important, there is only an indirect relation between focal damage to the thoracic spinal cord and recovery of locomotory function in animals. To understand more about the mechanisms of damage and recovery, as well as the mechanisms of putative treatments, it is necessary to gather information more directly about the actual tissue damage, both through direct examination with quantitative histopathology and through more directly related measures of physiological function in damaged nerve fiber tracts.

A BRIEF HISTORY

Animal experiments on spinal cord injury began in the nineteenth century, with interests in both axonal regeneration and the nature of contusion injury. The animal models developed at that time were quite varied but usually grimly simple in approach. Some of these early studies are summarized by Spiller,[1] who was concerned by the questionable existence of spinal "concussion" without vertebral fracture, and what the pathological basis of such a phenomenon might be. Kirchgaesser[2] had previously drawn attention to the role of damage to nerve fibers as an underlying cause of post-traumatic paralysis. A more complete chronology of early experimentation is given by Yeo,[3] including reference to some of the less quantitative models that continued to appear far into the twentieth century.

The first well-controlled animal model of spinal cord injury was described by Allen in 1911.[4,5] The technique of weight-drop contusion he established has been refined and adapted over the years, but the central principle of using gravity to standardize the mechanical impact on the cord was powerful, and has persisted in brain and spinal cord injury research, despite the introduction of numerous alternatives. Many improvements have been made regarding the control and monitoring of the impact, and much has been achieved in understanding the physical variables and their biological significance.[6] In recent years, artificial means of acceleration have been used to produce spinal cord injury devices that are capable of generating and recording a wider range of impact parameters.[7–11] Although these are more difficult to reproduce from place to place, they have the potential for making an important contribution by freeing the investigator from the restraints of gravitationally derived impact velocities.[12]

A separate line of injury modeling was initiated by Tarlov in a remarkably detailed series of studies to define the gradation of neurological deficits with increasing compression of the spinal cord.[13–16] He used a balloon catheter or a pneumatically driven mechanical plunger to compress the spinal cord in awake or anesthetized dogs. Subsequent investigators have employed a variety of different techniques to produce controlled compression of the spinal cord, including the use of balloon catheters,[17–20] inflatable cuffs,[21] static weights,[22–26] or screws.[27,28] The clinical relevance of slow and maintained compression models is somewhat limited and is distinct from that of the rapid contusion techniques.

A number of independent models of injury have been developed using clips[29,30] or forceps[31–33] to produce relatively brief compression of the spinal cord. These methods share some of the properties of both contusive and compressive models. It is possible to assemble a continuum of techniques, varying in their "impact" velocity and their duration of compression over a wide range. Each of these may be relevant to some proportion of clinical injuries, although the degree to which the pathological processes differ between them has been addressed only rarely. At a gross level, the long-term outcome from all these various insults seems remarkably similar, but there are no data regarding the quantitative clinical relevance of any given method.

Most modern animal models have used injury to the exposed spinal cord under direct visualization for the advantages this gives in standardizing the degree of damage. A closed impact model in dogs has been described,[34] but has not been used for neurological studies, and apparently does not produce histopathology similar to that seen in direct contusion or in clinical studies. An alternative closed-injury model is provided by naturally occurring vertebral disc herniation injuries in dogs, which can be used to examine either chronic[35] or more acute[36] treatments. The natural variability of these injuries can be reduced by rigorous criteria for selection of subjects, and they provide a unique opportunity to examine closed injuries to unanesthetized animals.

Several other laboratory models of injury have been used to examine particular aspects of spinal cord pathology, including distraction injuries,[37–41] ischemic lesions,[42–45] and a wide variety of cutting[46–48] and aspiration lesions.[49,50] These issues and models lie outside the scope of a short review directed primarily at the issue of modeling acute blunt trauma to the spinal cord.

CURRENT TECHNIQUES

Chapters 102 and 103 will deal specifically with two current models designed for improved testing of pharmacological therapies. They derive essentially from the contusion technique of Allen. Some common features of these two models should be noted. They both use the rat as experimental animal. They employ open (post-laminectomy) dorsal contusion injuries of a single segment of the lower thoracic spinal cord under general anesthesia. The measured mechanical parameters of the injury are primarily displacement of the dorsal surface of the cord and/or applied force.[10,51] The consequences of injury are monitored through behavioral deficits—locomotion, posture, balance, righting. These same characteristics are shared by a third recent model of injury,[52–54] which is planned to form the basis of a series of multi-center studies of experimental therapy. It seems almost certain that the bulk of pre-clinical pharmacological testing in the near future will be carried out with these particular model characteristics, which makes it timely to examine the rationale for some of these choices.

THE CHOICE OF INJURY PARAMETERS

Biomechanical Issues

The biomechanical nature of spinal cord contusion or compression can be understood in outline, even though we lack the quantitative details needed for an accurate mathematical model of the process. A large proportion of clinical injuries and almost all laboratory models of acute trauma involve localized displacement of tissue. The spinal cord consists of a complex, readily compressible gel-like parenchyma in the form of an irregular cylinder contained within a closely fitting, flexible, fluid-filled dural tube that is resistant to stretch. This tube, in turn, is contained within a rigid, segmented, and more loosely fitting vertebral canal. The parenchymal gel is interwoven with a meshwork of vasculature, the larger elements of which are accompanied by collagenous reinforcement that provides localized variations in tensile strength. Injuries to this system typically are produced by local compression of the dural tube, which causes its cross-section to flatten into a form that contains a

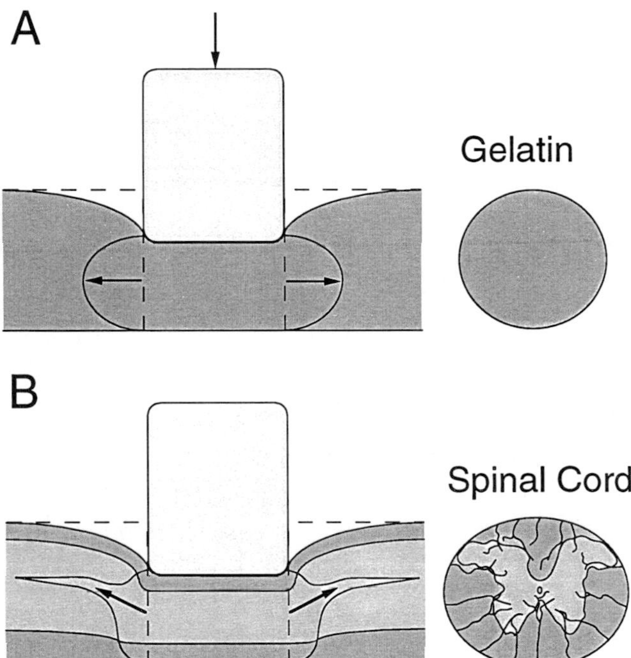

Figure 101-1. *A*. Data derived from a gelatin model of the spinal cord, showing that the parenchymal contents of the dural tube are pushed out from under the site of compression. The bowing out of the gel was made visible by running ink through the vertical midline of the tube before compression[56] (*vertical dashed lines*). *B*. The spinal cord itself presents more complex properties. The outer part of the tissue is partly reinforced by the collagenous ensheathment of blood vessels and by the higher membrane content of the white matter. The paucity of bridging between dorsal columns and central gray matter by vascular or neural processes may be responsible for a weakness in this area that allows extrusive forces to separate the tissue elements,[55] leading to a spindle-shaped area of hemorrhage and necrosis. Distortion of more superficial tissue is reduced by this "breaking out" of the extrusion in the central part of the cord, and this may account for the rapid decrease in displacement with distance from the center of the lesion seen radiographically.[39]

smaller volume per unit length. The parenchymal contents of that length are then distorted and extruded in both longitudinal directions from the center of the compression, causing shearing and stretch of tissue elements (Fig. 101-1). The degree of damage to cells of the parenchyma will depend on several extrinsic variables: the degree of compression; the length of compressed cord; and the speed of compression and its ultimate duration. The damage will also depend on variables intrinsic to the cord: the cross-sectional area at the site of impact and rostral and caudal to it; the local vascular morphology; the tissue pressure; and the resilience of the spinal meninges (Fig. 101-2).

Various injury models have approached this mechanical sequence of injury at different points, as summarized in Fig. 104-2. The weight-drop contusion technique specifies the energy delivered to the system in terms of the weight/height combination. This energy is transferred to the spinal cord and any supporting tissues when the dropped weight and cord collide, either directly or through a resting interface. The force applied to the cord varies with the weight, height, and the resistance offered by the cord and supporting structures, which will affect the rate of deceleration. In particular, the peak force may vary considerably even if the integrated force (impulse of force) remains more stable from one impact to another. This variability in the force applied to the cord can be overcome in several ways, as for example by use of larger weights placed directly on the cord without impact, or by using force-calibrated aneurysm clips.

The displacement of the surface of the cord produced by a given force, however, itself depends on several factors. The area of the impinging interface will affect the degree of compression, as will the resistance offered by the tissue as a result of its viscoelastic and hydrodynamic properties, and the rigidity of its support. Techniques of controlled surface displacement using pneumatic, electrical, or mechanical drives can circumvent this variability in surface displacement by using whatever force is necessary to produce a given displacement in a set time. The degree of extrusion of tissue produced by a displacement of the surface of the cord will depend again on the interface area, but also on the cross-sectional area of the spinal cord. It may also depend, in some cases, on the cross-sectional area of the vertebral canal, since the ability of the cord to distort laterally can be restricted. The technique of compressing the cord to a set thickness between two surfaces allows the residual volume of tissue at the site of compression to be specified. This brings the technique closer to the damaging element of the injury, although the actual

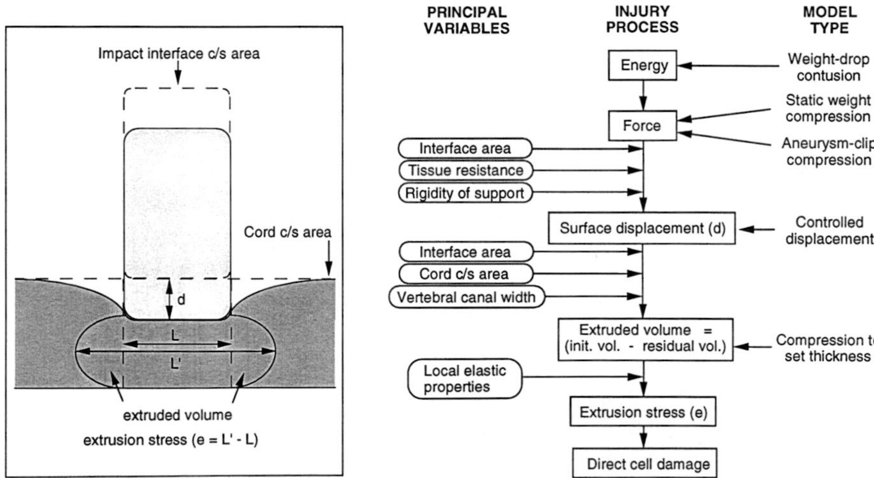

Figure 101-2. A diagram of the process of injury (*inset*), derived as in Fig. 104-1, and a summary of the different approaches to controlled injury. The extruded volume of tissue is a function of the degree of depression (d), the area of the interface between compression and cord, and the cross-sectional area of the cord itself. The extrusion stress on individual elements of the cord will depend on the extruded volume and its distribution. Various injury models have addressed this injury process in different ways. Weight-drop contusion specifies the energy of the impact through the weight and the height above the cord from which it is dropped. Both static weight compression and clip-compression determine the force that is applied to the surface of the cord for a set time. Electrically or pneumatically controlled displacements can specify independently the speed and overall displacement of the cord surface. Compression to a set thickness controls the residual volume of tissue at the peak of compression; subtraction of this residual volume from the initial volume of tissue under the compression device gives the extruded volume.

pattern of extrusion will still be affected by the local elastic properties of the spinal cord, which may be particularly dependent on the individual form of the vasculature.

The mechanical consequences of compression are similar, no matter how the chosen length of spinal cord is compressed. Concern has been expressed at times about the form of the interface between imposed force and the spinal cord, with different designs producing a saddle-shape, a rounded end, circular or square cross-section, dorsal, ventral, or lateral compression. These issues are mostly of little consequence by comparison with the overall length of the cord compressed or the degree and speed of compression. In most models of injury there is little sign of direct shearing damage from the edges of the interface between cord and applied force. The pattern of destruction of nerve fibers is from the inside out, which reflects the central extrusion of the cord contents.[6,55,56] As in any material, the damaging effect of deformation will depend on the rate at which it occurs as well as on the total extent of deformation. This is particularly true at high rates of displacement, such as are involved in weight-drop contusion techniques or their electromechanically or pneumatically produced counterparts.

Most injury models have made an arbitrary or convenient selection of all injury variables except the degree and/or speed of compression, which is initially explored to determine the requirement for a suitable level of neurological outcome. Another variable that might receive more attention is the length of cord compressed. Since the amount of cellular damage relates more to the volume of displaced tissue than to the absolute displacement of any given point on the surface, a relatively small compression of a greater length of cord will produce as much disruption as a profound compression of a shorter length. However, the type of damage will differ under these circumstances. In particular, compression over a short length of cord may require so much focal distortion that shearing damage may be added to the compressive and extrusive components.[57] Local shearing will result in more variable outcome in terms of histopathology and function, since shearing is even more dependent on the local characteristics of the tissue and the form of the interface. These considerations also raise the problem of scale in animal models of trauma. The human spinal cord is severalfold larger than that of the typical rodent subject, although the dimensions of nerve cells and nerve fibers are much more similar. This means that a typical human spinal cord injury involves greater distances on the cellular scale, which may lead to distinct pathological problems not well reproduced by focal contusion in small animals. Among the most important of these are the diffusion distance from the pial vasculature and the subarachnoid space, and the number of consecutive internodes of each nerve fiber that may be affected by parenchymal disruption.

The Principles of Different Mechanical Approaches

The weight-drop technique arose from the concept that it was necessary to standardize the energy delivered to the spinal cord. This was a reasonable extrapolation from simple materials science, but is not necessarily valid in the case of a complex structure like the spinal cord. In one particular regard it was clearly ill-founded. The idea that the severity of the injury would be related to the product of weight and height of the drop, the so-called "gm-cm," seems to have been based on the idea that the potential energy of the suspended weight was the determining element in the injury produced. The demonstration that this was not the case required several decades of empirical research, and the misconstructed "gm-cm" unit is still not entirely eradicated from the fringes of the literature. Beyond this simple error, however, is the fact that the energy delivered to the spinal cord as a mechanical *system* is not simply related to the amount of cellular damage that this will produce.

The cellular elements of the spinal cord experience a certain distortion at a certain rate, which depend on both the impulse of the force of impact and the mechanical properties of the system, including most importantly the elasticity of the dura and the tissue fluid pressure (including the momentary blood pressure). The distortion also depends on the mechanical support given to the spinal cord itself (see below). In the case of clip-compression of the spinal cord,[29] the same consideration of system biomechanics is required, although in this case there is not the additional problem of cord stabilization.

The use of forceps to produce compression of the spinal cord to a set thickness[33] has the dual advantages of making tissue volume displacement independent of the overall biomechanics and of avoiding the problem of stabilized support.

An advantage of pneumatic or electromechanical production of cord compression is that the rate and amount of displacement of the surface of the tissue can be controlled independently of the properties of the spinal cord as a mechanical system.[10] The final displacement of the dorsal surface of the dura is predetermined by the injury device and does not depend on interaction between a decelerating weight and the biomechanical variables. There is still a problem of biological variability, however, in that the properties of tissue displacement may still be altered for a given compression of the dorsal surface of the spinal cord by variations in cord size and interstitial fluid pressure. In practice, this does not seem to result in an unacceptable level of variability in outcome when combined with careful selection of animal subjects.[58]

Stabilization and Monitoring

The problem of stabilization has been reviewed elsewhere,[6] but has not been entirely resolved within the field. The amount of damage done to the tissue by a given collision depends on the rigidity of the support. The reliability of the model also depends on the consistency of that support. As a simple example, a weight of 10 gm dropped 20 cm onto the cat spinal cord, rigidly supported by a fixed vertebral body, creates a lesion similar in extent to that produced by a 20-gm weight from the same height on the unsupported cord.[56] Without separate stabilization, the thorax absorbs much of the impact.[59] A number of means of support have been devised. The currently most popular technique is to clamp surrounding dorsal vertebral spines.[10,51,52,58] Although this does not produce a completely rigid support,[52] it does reduce the variability and increase the speed and severity of the impact from that seen with an otherwise unsupported vertebral column. The problem is avoided in those models where the cord is compressed between two surfaces[29,33,60] rather than subjected to unidirectional impact against the floor of the vertebral canal.

Vertebral Level

Most experimental studies have concentrated on thoracic spinal cord injury for a number of practical reasons. The associated neurological deficits are largely the result of axonal damage at the site of injury as opposed to direct damage to gray matter. The deficits produced are less debilitating to the animal than those experienced with severe cervical injuries, and this facilitates post-injury care and maintenance. The thoracic spinal cord is relatively regular in cross-section compared with cervical and thoracic enlargements. Despite these benefits, there are several drawbacks to thoracic injuries. The first is that cervical injuries are more common and present a more profound clinical problem. The second is that small changes in the segmental distribution of deficits would be difficult to detect in the thoracic injury by comparison with a lesion that involved limb innervation directly. A cervical model of injury has been developed,[61] and is likely to be particularly useful for certain types of experimental therapeutic studies, although there is no reason to expect that the *axonal* pathophysiology of cervical and thoracic injuries is significantly different. At the other extreme, it has been suggested that sacrocaudal injuries offer the advantage of definable behavioral effects with minimal behavioral deficits and systemic complications.[62] Other laboratories have used a lumbar site of injury,[24] which offers the advantage of a larger cord cross-section without the debilitating effects on the experimental animal of a severe cervical injury.

Anesthesia and Physiological Variables

All current animal models of spinal cord injury are prepared with general anesthesia, and all forms of general anesthesia interact to some extent with pathophysiological mechanisms of neural injury. The degree to which this interaction affects the observations made is difficult to determine because testing without anesthesia is not ethically possible. There is no compelling evidence from comparison of different anesthetics to indicate that this represents a profound problem, as long as it is recognized that the anesthetic is part of the injury model. A recent study showed a clear difference between the outcome from injury in rats anesthetized with halothane, nitrous oxide, or sodium pentobarbital.[63] This study indicated that halothane anesthesia allows more axonal survival during or immediately after a similar physical insult, either by altering the response of the tissue to deformation or interfering with secondary pathological processes. Such effects of anesthesia on injury may be particularly important in evaluating the effects of pharmacological therapies, where the likelihood of interaction between different neurologically active drugs is quite high.[64]

Linked to the question of anesthesia is the issue of maintenance of physiological variables. The most important of these is core temperature, since anesthesia generally disrupts temperature control. Cooling can be extremely rapid in small animals, and the temperature can greatly affect the response of the nervous system to injury.[65–70] Adequate thermostatic control of core temperature should be a prerequisite for any animal model. The possibility of controlling respiration and blood pressure is more problematic, since this represents an interference with the results of trauma as much as, if not more than, that of anesthesia. While it may be important to monitor effects of particular treatment regimens on respiration and blood pressure, there does not seem to be a compelling argument for the introduction of artificial respiration or pharmacological stabilization of blood pressure in thoracic injury models.

Species Differences

A range of species has been used for studies of blunt spinal cord injury. The majority in the past used dogs, cats, and primates. Most current studies use rats, and this species is likely to dominate even more in the future. Few researchers have examined species outside this small group, although injury models have been used in sheep,[20,71] pigs,[40] ferrets,[7] rabbits,[72,73] and guinea pigs.[33] There has been little direct comparative study, but the broad elements of pathophysiology appear to be similar in the different animal models. One clear difference has emerged in recent studies of the guinea pig, which shows a remarkable delay in the onset of functional deficits after a moderately severe injury to the spinal cord.[33,74,75] Although there is some evidence of delayed changes in other models of injury, the guinea pig is qualitatively different in its early response, and these secondary changes are more easily detectable. Recent studies comparing rat and guinea pig, using essentially identical methodology, confirm that the two species respond quite differently to the same insult (Gruner and Blight, unpublished observations). The pronounced difference in behavioral response may be based on significant differences in pathophysiology. While no prescription can be made for choice of species at this time, it seems important to continue to explore such differences as may exist, both because of the insights they are likely to provide on mechanism and because we do not yet know which responses may be clinically significant.

Severity

The issue of injury severity is central to the potential of animal studies to study secondary injury mechanisms and their treatment. If injuries are extremely severe, the spinal cord is essentially transected immediately, and there is no treatment of subsequent pathology that is likely to restore function unless extensive regeneration of axons can be achieved. If injuries are too moderate, then spontaneous recovery will be so fast and effective as to mask potential therapeutic benefits. Most injury models for acute trauma have therefore concentrated on moderately severe trauma that allows limited amounts of spontaneous recovery in a proportion of the subjects. Testing of therapy, and particularly comparison of efficacy, must eventually be carried out in a range of injury intensities, since any given treatment may have different effects against a different background of severity.[76]

MEASURES OF OUTCOME

The principal techniques used to define long-term outcome in spinal cord injury are behavioral and histopathological. Evoked potentials and other electrophysiological techniques have been used mainly for acute monitoring of the effects of injury or as confirmatory evidence of changes seen behaviorally. A greater variety of outcome measures have been used in studies of acute pathophysiology.

Histopathological studies have shown a consistent pattern of tissue damage in all forms of injury to the spinal cord, with central necrosis leading to cystic cavitation and gliosis, usually with rostrocaudal extensions, particularly in to the region around the central canal and the ventral aspect of the dorsal column.[77,78] The basis of this spindle-shaped lesion form appears to be biomechanical,[6,56,57] although necrosis and cystic cavitation may also extend longitudinally under the action of delayed pathophysiological mechanisms. Quantitative examination of axonal survival at the center of chronic experimental injuries has shown a smoothly graded loss of axons with depth from the pial surface.[33,56,79] Despite this, it has proved possible in a number of laboratories to define subjectively a "rim" of surviving white matter,[58,61,80–83] the size of which correlates with the severity of injury and recovery of behavioral function. A correlation has also been seen between the severity of motor deficits following injury and the loss of serotonin immunoreactivity in the ventral gray matter of the lumbar cord.[84] Subjectively defined areas of white matter survival are adequate for analysis of treatment effects, and are much more efficient than quantitative morphometry, although they tell us little about potential mechanisms of action or about the mechanisms of secondary cell damage that may be affected by any given treatment. Mechanistically relevant information can be gained from techniques that allow definition of specific and quantitative cellular effects. This requires electron microscopy, high-resolution light microscopy, or careful evaluation of physiological or biochemical changes.

Most studies of chronic outcome in animal models of spinal cord injury have used some measure of recovery of locomotory function. Grading systems have evolved from the basic classification derived by Tarlov and collaborators from studies on the effects of compression injury in dogs,[14,16] to more recent detailed schemes for evaluating open-field movements in rats.[81,83,85–88] Other measures of function, such as various limb reflexes, the "inclined plane test,"[89] grid-walking,[10,81] and footprint analysis,[90,91] have been added to incorporate a wider range of more quantitative comparisons. As in the case of open-field locomotion, however, these tests evaluate a complex and poorly understood mix of sensory, motor, and integrative activity, none of which relates directly and exclusively to the injury under study. Such global measures of neurological outcome add little to our understanding of the original deficits or the mechanisms of recovery of function. Using such measures as open-field locomotion to evaluate the efficacy of acute treatments is analogous to the histological determination of areas of white matter "survival." They give useful, semiquantitative comparisons but do not illuminate cellular pathology or mode of therapeutic action. Questions of cell biology and pathology are better addressed by more specific measures more directly related to the actual injury produced, by using microscopic anatomy, electrophysiology, reflex physiology, or biochemical techniques.

Important acute measures of injury outcome include blood flow,[92–96] tissue ion concentrations, and extracellular activities,[95,97,98] as well as changes in extracellular or tissue levels of a range of other substances, including metabolites[99–102] and potentially toxic neurotransmitters.[103–105] While such measures give important insights into pathological and experimental therapeutic mechanisms, the links between these changes and the long-term neurological outcome are not yet sufficiently established to use these as sufficient determinants of efficacy for evaluation of experimental therapy.

However, given the difficulty and prohibitive cost of performing multiple long-term studies on drug efficacy in animal models of central nervous system trauma, it has been proposed that ionic measurements, in particular, may be used as a valuable screening method for determining the quantity of tissue disruption at 24 hours after injury.[98] This appears to be a valuable technique, and is soundly based in an understanding of cellular pathophysiology, although it is restricted to treatments that affect cell damage occurring within the first day after injury, and it has not been established that this is the only or even the principal time at which secondary damage takes place following central nervous system injury.[74] Magnetic resonance imaging studies have been introduced recently, particularly in relation to acute changes in hemorrhage and edema,[106–108] and considerable improvements in the utility of these techniques is likely,[109] but they have not (at the time of writing) been able to add significantly to our knowledge of laboratory injuries or the evaluation of treatments. Similarly, magnetic resonance spectroscopy is likely to add much to our understanding of acute metabolic and blood flow changes as the technology advances.[73,110]

ACHIEVEMENTS OF ANIMAL MODELS

Perhaps the principal contribution of animal studies has been the concept of central hemorrhagic necrosis, based on histopathological observations over time from injury. From the earliest studies of Allen,[4] the idea of delayed secondary damage to the spinal cord spreading from a region of central disruption has raised the hope of finding ways to intervene in the process and improve long-term outcome. Numerous studies, reviewed elsewhere in this text, have added cell biological and biochemical details to the initial histopathological picture, showing a complex sequence of events in the injured tissue, beginning with an immediate disruption of ionic distribution between intra- and extracellular spaces, and release of a variety of neuroactive substances, progressing through energy depletion and lactic acidosis, to delayed hypoperfusion, vascular occlusion, intense inflammatory responses, and demyelination. Free radical damage to membranes has been identified as an important common biochemical mechanism in this succession of pathological events.[111,112]

With changing fashions in the mainstream of biomedical sciences, a wide range of possible therapeutic approaches have been taken to experimental spinal cord injury, and a surprising number of such approaches have appeared to produce beneficial effects. This is probably as much a reflection of the complexity of the pathological events involved as it is of our optimism and resourcefulness as investigators. Initially, there was a concentration on physical methods, including myelotomy, cooling, superfusion, and tissue oxygenation. Over the last 20 years, a large number of experimental pharmacological treatments have been examined in animal models, more than a dozen in considerable detail.[113,114] Currently, there is much interest in a complexly nested set of biochemical events involving the toxicity of excitatory amino acids, the involvement in this toxicity of free radical mechanisms, including the endogenous production of nitric oxide, and the delayed contribution of inflammatory cells to excitotoxic and free radical damage.

Determining the optimal form of any single therapy requires extensive testing. Application of corticosteroids to reduce swelling of the injured cord was one of the first pharmacological approaches examined.[115] Many years of research in animal models was then required to identify the need for a readily soluble form of the drug and extremely high doses, maintained for some hours.[116,117] Even then, when applied to clinical trials, it was not initially possible to deliver the drug with optimally short latency.[118,119] Given the large number of patients required to evaluate the effects of an acute treatment, clinical testing will continue to lag far behind detection of promising approaches in animal models. This highlights the importance of being able to perform comparative studies of different regimens and combinational approaches in a variety of animal models.[53,76,120] The relative efficacy of different compounds must be explored in animals since clinical evaluation is prohibitively slow and ethically complex, and relative efficacy is likely to vary between species and injury types and severities.

MODEL VALIDATION

Final validation of injury models can come only from confirmation by clinical studies, particularly controlled clinical trials of experimental therapies that have shown efficacy in animals. Few such experimental approaches have been tested clinically.[121–123] Even for those few, quantitative comparison of outcome with animal studies is practically impossible, particularly because of difficulties in the rapid delivery of experimental drugs.

Results of animal experiments, combined with those of the recent National Acute Spinal Cord Injury Study (NASCIS) trial of high-dose methylprednisolone[119,121,122] indicate that post-injury treatments can produce a reduction in functional deficits and perhaps tissue damage, but that both effects appear small relative to overall functional loss and tissue destruction in spinal cord contusion. These modest changes may reflect the actual significance of secondary damage, but this has yet to be proved. There are almost certain to be multiple pathological mechanisms, their relative roles different in individual types of injury. Nonetheless, these modest beginnings have partially validated the use of animal models for identification of therapeutic benefits.

OUTSTANDING QUESTIONS

Given the current narrow focus of animal models for preclinical testing, it is important to continue to explore the mechanisms of injury on a broader front. Researchers in this field have struggled for the best part of the century with the phenomenon of "secondary injury." They have tried to treat it by disparate means and at times seem to have succeeded, if only modestly. Surprisingly little has been discovered in the process about the actual properties of "secondary injury." We do not know what is damaged, when it is damaged, by what agents it is damaged, or how it is damaged—although there has been no shortage of ideas on the last two points. Above all, we do not know how much of the chronic damage that we see is secondary, rather than a direct consequence of acute mechanical trauma. We do not know whether it is reasonable to assume that secondary mechanisms are consistent from one injury or one injury model to another. This dilemma was expressed in a succinct review by Collins and Kauer in 1979.[124] It should not be surprising that we have made little progress in resolving the dilemma in the intervening 15 years, since so little attention has been devoted to the effort.[74]

Looking back over the history of any branch of science, we are struck by the fact that the practitioners were able to think, to communicate, and to experiment constructively without knowing the key phenomena with which they were dealing, but simply having names to apply to them, even if those names in retrospect corresponded to no identifiable objects or phenomena in the real world as we know it. Progress has much to do with the recognition of a lack of correspondence between the words we use and the reality about which we try to speak. The nature of everyday scientific inquiry is such that there is great resistance to questioning that correspondence until the mismatch is painfully obvious. The study of acute spinal cord injury would benefit greatly from a critical examination of the concept of secondary injury. There is remarkably little physiological or behavioral evidence of secondary loss, either in man or animal models. Morphological evidence, which has fueled the concept since the beginning, is extremely ambiguous. Like a number of metabolic measures, the slow deterioration of the histopathology may be a reflection of the rate of degenerative processes rather than a reflection of loss of viability. Determining the primary mechanical damage in a contusive injury model is technically challenging; and without a measure of primary injury it is very difficult to deduce what is secondary.

The past and current unsettled and diversified state of injury models results from the uncoordinated activity of a succession of investigators and small research groups following their own particular lines of investigation. This is a natural and healthy stage in the evolution of research and should not be regarded as a shortcoming that cries out for an imposed standard. The mechanics of an eventual solution are central to the scientific method—the successive testing of key hypotheses by critical experiment—and only need to be exercised to be effective.

SUMMARY AND CONCLUSIONS

Animal models of acute spinal cord trauma have been produced by many variations on a few simple themes for more than 80 years. These models have provided the best and sometimes the only practical way to examine mechanisms of injury and to test potential treatments. Simplified and well-defined systems for testing therapy are possible in animal models, although this requires several arbitrary choices to be made, and the clinical relevance of any finding is guaranteed to be limited. Much has been learned about the biomechanics and cell biology of injury, although no overall synthesis is yet possible. Laboratory studies of animal models will not simplify the problem of spinal cord injury, but they provide the only practical access to its solution. There is a particular need to grapple with the hypothesis of secondary cell damage in spinal cord trauma and to attempt to identify, define, and quantify the phenomenon, even if it appears to lose some of its motivational potency in the process.

References

1. Spiller WG: A critical summary of recent literature on concussion of the spinal cord, with some original observations. *Am J Med Sci* 1899; 118:190–198.
2. Kirchgaesser G: Weitere experimentelle Untersuchungen über Rückenmarkserschütterung. *Z Nervenheilk* 1898; 13:422–431.
3. Yeo JD: A review of experimental research in spinal cord injury. *Paraplegia* 1976; 14:1–11.
4. Allen AR: Surgery of experimental lesion of spinal cord equivalent to crush injury of fracture dislocation of spinal column: A preliminary report. *JAMA* 1911; 57:878–880.
5. Allen AR: Remarks on the histopathological changes in the spinal cord due to impact: An experimental study. *J Nerv Ment Dis* 1914; 41:141–147.
6. Blight A: Mechanical factors in experimental spinal cord injury. *J Am Paraplegia Soc* 1988; 11:26–34.
7. Anderson TE: A controlled pneumatic technique for experimental spinal cord contusion. *J Neurosci Meth* 1982; 6:327–333.
8. Nacimiento AC, Bartels M, Herrmann H-D, Loew F: Reflex activity and axonal conduction in the L-7 spinal cord segment following experimental compression trauma. *J Neurosurg* 1985; 62:898–905.
9. Noyes D: An electromechanical impactor for producing experimental spinal cord injury in animals. *Med Biol Eng Comp* 1987; 25:335–340.
10. Somerson SK, Stokes BT: Functional analysis of an electromechanical spinal cord injury device. *Exp Neurol* 1987; 96:82–96.
11. Stokes BT, Noyes DH, Behrmann DL: An electromechanical spinal injury technique with dynamic sensitivity. *J Neurotrauma* 1992; 9:187–196.
12. Kearney PA, Ridella SA, Viano DC, Anderson TE: Interaction of contact velocity and cord compression in determining the severity of spinal cord injury. *J Neurotrauma* 1988; 5:187–208.
13. Tarlov IM, Klinger M, Vitale S: Spinal cord compression studies: I. Experimental techniques to produce acute and gradual compression. *Arch Neurol Psychiatry* 1953; 70:813–819.
14. Tarlov IM: Spinal cord compression studies: III. Time limits for recovery after gradual compression in dogs. *Arch Neurol Psychiatry* 1954; 71:588–597.
15. Tarlov IM, Klinger H: Spinal cord compression studies: II. Time limits for recovery after acute compression in dogs. *Arch Neurol Psychiatry* 1954; 71:271–290.
16. Tarlov IM: *Spinal Cord Compression: Mechanisms of Paralysis and Treatment.* Springfield, IL: Charles C Thomas, 1957.
17. Martin SH, Bloedel JR: Evaluation of experimental spinal cord injury using cortical evoked potentials. *J Neurosurg* 1973; 39:75–81.
18. Griffiths IR: Vasogenic edema following acute and chronic spinal cord compression in the dog. *J Neurosurg* 1975; 42:155–165.
19. Hansebout RR, Van der Jagt RHC, Sohal SS, Little JR: Oxygenated fluorocarbon perfusion as treatment of acute spinal cord compression injury in dogs. *J Neurosurg* 1981; 55:725–732.
20. Hitchon PW, McKay TC, Wilkinson TT, et al: Methylprednisolone in spinal cord compression. *Spine* 1989; 14:16–22.
21. Tator CH, Deecke L: Value of normothermic perfusion, hypothermic perfusion, and durotomy in the treatment of experimental spinal cord trauma. *J Neurosurg* 1973; 39:52–64.
22. Wakefield CL, Eidelberg E: Electron microscopic observations of the delayed effects of spinal cord compression. *Exp Neurol* 1975; 48:637–646.
23. Anderson DK, Prockop LD, Means ED, Hartley LE: Cerebrospinal fluid lactate and electrolyte levels following experimental spinal cord injury. *J Neurosurg* 1976; 44:715–722.
24. Anderson DK, Means ED, Waters TR, Spears CJ: Spinal cord energy metabolism following compression trauma to the feline spinal cord. *J Neurosurg* 1980; 53:375–380.
25. Anderson DK, Braughler JM, Hall ED, et al: Effects of treatment with U-74006F on neurological outcome following experimental spinal cord injury. *J Neurosurg* 1988; 69:562–567.
26. Black P, Markowitz RS, Cooper V, et al: Models of spinal cord injury: Part 1. Static load technique. *Neurosurgery* 1986; 19:752–761.
27. Gooding MR, Wilson CB, Hoff JT: Experimental cervical myelopathy. Effects of ischemia and compression of the canine cervical spinal cord. *J Neurosurg* 1975; 43:9–17.
28. al-Mefty O, Harkey HL, Marawi I, et al: Experimental chronic compressive cervical myelopathy. *J Neurosurg* 1993; 79:550–561.
29. Rivlin AS, Tator CH: Effect of duration of acute spinal cord compression in a new acute cord injury model in the rat. *Surg Neurol* 1978; 10:39–43.
30. Rivlin AS, Tator CH: Regional spinal cord blood flow in rats after severe cord trauma. *J Neurosurg* 1978; 49:844–853.
31. Naka Y, Nakai K, Itakura I, et al: Alteration of nerve fibers in minor spinal cord injury of guinea pig. *Soc Neurosci Abstr* 1985; 11:591.
32. Guth L, Barrett CP, Donati EJ, et al: Essentiality of a specific cellular terrain for growth of axons into a spinal cord lesion. *Exp Neurol* 1985; 88:1–12.
33. Blight AR: Morphometric analysis of a model of spinal

cord injury in guinea pigs, with behavioral evidence of delayed secondary pathology. *J Neurol Sci* 1991; 103:156–171.
34. Wennerstrand J, Jönsson A, Arvebo E: Mechanical and histological effects of transverse impact on the canine spinal cord. *J Biomech* 1978; 11:315–331.
35. Blight AR, Toombs JP, Bauer MS, Widmer WR: The effects of 4-aminopyridine on neurological deficits in chronic cases of traumatic spinal cord injury in dogs: A phase I clinical trial. *J Neurotrauma* 1991; 8:103–119.
36. Borgens RB, Toombs JP, Blight AR, et al: Effects of applied electric fields on clinical cases of complete paraplegia in dogs. *Restor Neurol Neurosci* 1993; 5:305–322.
37. Myklebust JB, Maiman DJ, Cusick JF: Axial tension model of spinal cord injury. *J Am Paraplegia Soc* 1988; 11:50–55.
38. Maiman DJ, Myklebust JB, Ho KC, Coats J: Experimental spinal cord injury produced by axial tension. *J Spinal Dis* 1989; 2:6–13.
39. Maiman DJ, Coats J, Myklebust JB: Cord/spine motion in experimental spinal cord injury. *J Spinal Dis* 1989; 2:14–19.
40. Owen JH, Naito M, Bridwell KH, Oakley DM: Relationship between duration of spinal cord ischemia and postoperative neurologic deficits in animals. *Spine* 1990; 15:618–622.
41. Salzman SK, Mendez AA, Dabney KW, et al: Serotonergic response to spinal distraction trauma in experimental scoliosis. *J Neurotrauma* 1991; 8:45–54.
42. van Harreveld A, Marmont G: The course of recovery of the spinal cord from asphyxia. *J Neurophysiol* 1939; 2:101–111.
43. Zivin JA, Venditto JA: Experimental CNS ischemia: Serotonin antagonists reduce or prevent damage. *Neurology* 1984; 34:469–474.
44. Watson BD, Prado R, Dietrich WD, et al: Photochemically induced spinal cord injury in the rat. *Brain Res* 1986; 367:296–300.
45. Prado R, Dietrich WD, Watson BD, et al: Photochemically induced graded spinal cord infarction: Behavioral, electrophysiological, and morphological correlates. *J Neurosurg* 1987; 67:745–753.
46. Bregman BS, Kunkel-Bagden E, Reier PJ, et al: Recovery of function after spinal cord injury: Mechanisms underlying transplant-mediated recovery of function differ after spinal cord injury in newborn and adult rats. *Exp Neurol* 1993; 123:3–16.
47. Reier PJ, Stokes BT, Thompson FJ, Anderson DK: Fetal cell grafts into resection and contusion/compression injuries of the rat and cat spinal cord. *Exp Neurol* 1992; 115:177–188.
48. Borgens RB, Blight AR, Murphy DJ: Axonal regeneration in spinal cord injury: A perspective and new technique. *J Comp Neurol* 1986; 250:157–167.
49. Reier PJ, Bregman BS, Wujek JR: Intraspinal transplantation of embryonic spinal cord tissue in neonatal and adult rats. *J Comp Neurol* 1986; 247:275–296.
50. Blight AR, McGinnis ME, Borgens RB: Cutaneous trunci muscle reflex of the guinea pig. *J Comp Neurol* 1990; 296:614–633.
51. Panjabi MM, Wrathall JR: Biomechanical analysis of experimental spinal cord injury and functional loss. *Spine* 1988; 13:1365–1370.
52. Gruner JA: A monitored contusion model of spinal cord injury in the rat. *J Neurotrauma* 1992; 9:123–126.
53. Young W: Secondary injury mechanisms in acute spinal cord injury. *J Emerg Med* 1993; 11:13–22.
54. Constantini S, Young W: The ganglioside GM1 antagonizes neuroprotective effect of methylprednisolone in rat spinal cord injury. *J Neurosurg* 1994; 80:97–111.
55. McVeigh JF: Experimental cord crushes with especial reference to the mechanical factors involved and subsequent changes in the areas of the cord affected. *Arch Surg* 1923; 7:573–600.
56. Blight AR, DeCrescito V: Morphometric analysis of experimental spinal cord injury in the cat: The relation of injury intensity to survival of myelinated axons. *Neuroscience* 1986; 19:321–341.
57. Breig A, Renard M: Healing of spinal cord injuries by biomechanical activation of growth of ruptured medullary tissue, in Ghista DN, Frankel HL: *Spinal Cord Injury Medical Engineering.* Springfield, IL: Charles C Thomas, 1986:59–99.
58. Behrmann DL, Bresnahan JC, Beattie MS, Shah BR: Spinal cord injury produced by consistent mechanical displacement of the cord in rats: Behavioral and histologic analysis. *J Neurotrauma* 1992; 9:197–217.
59. Dohrmann GJ, Panjabi MM, Banks D: Biomechanics of experimental spinal cord trauma. *J Neurosurg* 1978; 48:993–1001.
60. Ford RWJ: A reproducible spinal cord injury model in the cat. *J Neurosurg* 1983; 59:268–275.
61. Schrimscher GW, Reier PJ: Forelimb motor performance following cervical spinal cord contusion injury in the rat. *Exp Neurol* 1992; 117:287–298.
62. Ritz LA, Friedman RM, Rhoton EL, et al: Lesions of cat sacrocaudal spinal cord: A minimally disruptive model of injury. *J Neurotrauma* 1992; 9:219–230.
63. Salzman SK, Mendez AA, Sabato S, et al: Anesthesia influences the outcome from experimental spinal cord injury. *Brain Res* 1990; 521:33–39.
64. Faden AI: Comment: Need for standardization of animal models of spinal cord injury. *J Neurotrauma* 1992; 9:169–170.
65. Albin MS, White RJ, Acosta-Rua G, Yashon D: Study of functional recovery produced by delayed localized cooling after spinal cord injury in primates. *J Neurosurg* 1968; 29:113–120.
66. Hansebout RR, Tanner JA, Romero-Sierra C: Current status of spinal cord cooling in the treatment of acute spinal cord injury. *Spine* 1984; 9:508–511.
67. Morikawa E, Ginsberg MD, Dietrich WD, et al: The significance of brain temperature in focal cerebral ischemia: Histopathological consequences of middle cerebral artery occlusion in the rat. *J Cerebr Blood Flow Metab* 1992; 12:380–389.
68. Green EJ, Dietrich WD, van-Dijk F, et al: Protective effects of brain hypothermia on behavior and histopathology following global ischemia in rats. *Brain Res* 1992; 580:197–204.

69. Ginsberg MD, Globus MY, Dietrich WD, Busto R: Temperature modulation of ischemic brain injury—a synthesis of recent advances. *Prog Brain Res* 1993; 96:13–22.
70. Stys PK, Waxman SG, Ransom BR: Effects of temperature on evoked electrical activity and anoxic injury in CNS white matter. *J Cerebr Blood Flow Metab* 1992; 12:977–986.
71. Yeo JD, Stabback S, McKenzie B: Central necrosis following contusion to the sheep's spinal cord. *Paraplegia* 1977; 14:276–285.
72. Salzman SK, Hirofuji E, Llados EC, et al: Monoaminergic responses to spinal trauma: Participation of serotonin in the posttraumatic progression of neural damage. *J Neurosurg* 1987; 66:431–439.
73. Vink R, Noble LJ, Knoblach SM, et al: Metabolic changes in rabbit spinal cord after trauma: Magnetic resonance spectroscopy studies. *Ann Neurol* 1989; 25:26–31.
74. Blight AR: Remyelination, revascularization and recovery of function in experimental spinal cord injury, in Seil FJ: *Advances in Neurology, Vol. 59: Neural Injury and Regeneration.* New York: Raven Press, 1993:91–104.
75. Blight AR: Effects of silica on the outcome from experimental spinal cord injury: Implication of macrophages in secondary tissue damage. *Neuroscience* 1994;60: 263–273.
76. Young W: Strategies for the development of new and better pharmacological treatments for acute spinal cord injury, in Seil FJ: *Advances in Neurology, Vol. 59: Neural Injury and Regeneration.* New York: Raven Press, 1993:249–256.
77. Bresnahan JC, King JS, Martin GF, Yashon D: A neuroanatomical analysis of spinal cord injury in the rhesus monkey (Macaca mulatta). *J Neurol Sci* 1976; 28: 521–542.
78. Bresnahan JC, Beattie MS, Stokes BT, Conway KM: Three-dimensional computer-assisted analysis of graded contusion lesions in the spinal cord of the rat. *J Neurotrauma* 1991; 8:91–101.
79. Blight AR: Cellular morphology of chronic spinal cord injury in the cat: Analysis of myelinated axons by line-sampling. *Neuroscience* 1983; 10:521–543.
80. Noble L, Wrathall J: Spinal cord contusion in the rat: Morphometric analyses of alterations in the spinal cord. *Exp Neurol* 1985; 88:135–149.
81. Bresnahan JC, Beattie MS, Todd F, Noyes DH: A behavioral and anatomical analysis of spinal cord injury produced by a feedback-controlled impaction device. *Exp Neurol* 1987; 95:548–570.
82. Noble LJ, Wrathall JR: Correlative analyses of lesion development and functional status after graded spinal cord contusive injuries in the rat. *Exp Neurol* 1989; 103:34–40.
83. Behrmann DL, Bresnahan JC, Beattie MS: A comparison of YM-14673, U-50488H, and nalmefene after spinal cord injury in the rat. *Exp Neurol* 1993; 119:258–267.
84. Faden AI, Gannon A, Basbaum AI: Use of serotonin immunocytochemistry as a marker of injury severity after experimental spinal trauma in rats. *Brain Res* 1988; 450:94–100.
85. Gale K, Kerasidis H, Wrathall J: Spinal cord contusion in the rat: Behavioral analysis of functional neurologic impairment. *Exp Neurol* 1985; 88:123–134.
86. Wrathall JR, Pettigrew RK, Harvey F: Spinal cord contusion in the rat: Production of graded, reproducible injury groups. *Exp Neurol* 1985; 88:108–122.
87. Kerasidis H, Wrathall J, Gale K: Behavioral assessment of functional deficits in rats with contusive spinal cord injury. *J Neurosci Meth* 1987; 20:167–189.
88. Bresnahan JC, Beattie MS, Shah BR: Spinal cord injury produced by consistent mechanical displacement of the cord in rats: Behavioral and histologic analysis. *J Neurotrauma* 1992; 9:197–218.
89. Rivlin A, Tator C: Objective clinical assessment of motor function after experimental spinal cord injury in the rat. *J Neurosurg* 1977; 1977:577–581.
90. De Medinacelli L, Freed WJ, Wyatt RJ: An index of functional condition of rat sciatic nerve based on measurement from walking tracks. *Exp Neurol* 1982; 77:634–643.
91. Kunkel-Bagden E, Dai HN, Bregman BS: Methods to assess the development and recovery of locomotor function after spinal cord injury in rats. *Exp Neurol* 1993; 119:153–164.
92. Senter HJ, Venes JL: Altered blood flow and secondary injury in experimental spinal cord trauma. *J Neurosurg* 1978; 49:569–578.
93. Ducker TB, Salcman M, Lucas JT, et al: Experimental spinal cord trauma. II. Blood flow, tissue oxygen, evoked potentials in both paretic and plegic monkeys. *Surg Neurol* 1978; 10:64–70.
94. Fehlings MG, Tator CH, Linden RD: The relationships among the severity of spinal cord injury, motor and somatosensory evoked potentials and spinal cord blood flow. *Electroenceph Clin Neurophysiol* 1989; 74: 241–259.
95. Young W: Blood flow, metabolic and neurophysiological mechanisms in spinal cord injury, in Becker DP, Povlishock JT: *Central Nervous System Trauma Status Report.* Bethesda, MD: NIH, NINCDS, 1985:463–473.
96. Sandler AN, Tator CH: Review of the effect of spinal cord trauma on the vessels and blood flow in the spinal cord. *J Neurosurg* 1976; 45:638–646.
97. Young W, Koreh I: Potassium and calcium changes in injured spinal cords. *Brain Res* 1986; 365:42–53.
98. Young W: Rapid quantification of tissue damage for assessing acute spinal cord injury therapy. *J Neurotrauma* 1992; 9:151–153.
99. Braughler JM, Hall ED: Lactate and pyruvate metabolism in injured cat spinal cord before and after a single large intravenous dose of methylprednisolone. *J Neurosurg* 1983; 59:256–261.
100. Anderson DK, Means ED: The effect of laminectomy on spinal cord blood flow, energy metabolism and ATPase activity. *Paraplegia* 1985; 23:58.
101. Faden AI, Yum SW, Lemke M, Vink R: Effects of TRH-analog treatment on tissue cations, phospholipids

and energy metabolism after spinal cord injury. *J Pharm Exp Ther* 1990; 255:608–614.
102. Halt PS, Swanson RA, Faden AI: Alcohol exacerbates behavioral and neurochemical effects of rat spinal cord trauma. *Arch Neurol* 1992; 49:1178–1184.
103. Liu D, Valadez V, Sorkin LS, McAdoo DJ: Norepinephrine and serotonin release upon impact injury to rat spinal cord. *J Neurotrauma* 1990; 7:219–227.
104. Liu D, Thangnipon W, McAdoo DJ: Excitatory amino acids rise to toxic levels upon impact injury to the rat spinal cord. *Brain Res* 1991; 547:344–348.
105. Panter SS, Yum SW, Faden AI: Alteration in extracellular amino acids after traumatic spinal cord injury. *Ann Neurol* 1990; 27:96–99.
106. Hackney DB, Asato R, Joseph PM, et al: Hemorrhage and edema in acute spinal cord compression: Demonstration by MR imaging. *Radiology* 1986; 161:387–390.
107. Weirich SD, Cotler HB, Narayana PA, et al: Histopathologic correlation of magnetic resonance imaging signal patterns in a spinal cord injury model. *Spine* 1990; 15:630–638.
108. Duncan EG, Lemaire C, Armstrong RL, et al: High-resolution magnetic resonance imaging of experimental spinal cord injury in the rat. *Neurosurgery* 1992; 31:510–517.
109. Ford JC, Hackney DB, Joseph PM, et al: A method for in vivo high resolution MRI of rat spinal cord injury. *Magn Reson Med* 1994; 31:218–223.
110. Vink R, Knoblach SM, Faden AI: ^{31}P magnetic resonance spectroscopy of traumatic spinal cord injury. *Magn Reson Med* 1987; 5:390–394.
111. Braughler JM, Hall ED: Central nervous system trauma and stroke. I. Biochemical considerations for oxygen radical formation and lipid peroxidation. *Free Rad Biol Med* 1989; 6:289–301.
112. Hall ED, Braughler JM: Central nervous system trauma and stroke. II. Physiological and pharmacological evidence for involvement of oxygen radicals and lipid peroxidation. *Free Rad Biol Med* 1989; 6:303–313.
113. Young W: Medical treatments of acute spinal cord injury [editorial]. *J Neurol Neurosurg Psychiatry* 1992; 55:635–639.
114. Faden AI: Experimental neurobiology of central nervous system trauma. *Crit Rev Neurobiol* 1993; 7:175–186.
115. Ducker TB, Hamit HF: Experimental treatments of acute spinal cord injury. *J Neurosurg* 1969; 30:393–397.
116. Hall ED, Braughler JM: Glucocorticoid mechanisms in acute spinal cord injury: A review and therapeutic rationale. *Surg Neurol* 1982; 18:320–327.
117. Braughler JM, Hall ED: Current application of "high dose" steroid therapy for CNS injury. *J Neurosurg* 1985; 62:806–810.
118. Young W, Bracken MB: The second national acute spinal cord injury study. *J Neurotrauma* 1992; 9:S397–405.
119. Bracken MB, Holford TR: Effects of timing of methylprednisolone or naloxone administration on recovery of segmental and long-tract neurological function in NASCIS 2. *J Neurosurg* 1993; 79:500–507.
120. Faden AI: Comparison of single and combination drug treatment strategies in experimental brain trauma. *J Neurotrauma* 1993; 10:91–100.
121. Bracken MB, Shepard MJ, Collins WF, et al: A randomized, controlled trial of methylprednisolone or naloxone in the treatment of acute spinal-cord injury. *N Engl J Med* 1990; 322:1405–1461.
122. Bracken MB, Shepard MJ, Collins WF, et al: Methylprednisolone or naloxone treatment after acute spinal cord injury: 1-year follow-up data. *J Neurosurg* 1992; 76:23–31.
123. Geisler FH, Dorsey FC, Coleman WP: Recovery of motor function after spinal cord injury—a randomized, placebo-controlled trial with GM-1 ganglioside. *N Engl J Med* 1991; 324:1829–1838.
124. Collins WF, Kauer JS: The past and future of animal models used for spinal cord trauma, in Popp AJ, Bourke RS, Nelson LR, Kimelberg HK: *Neural Trauma.* New York: Raven Press, 1979:273–279.

CHAPTER 102

WEIGHT-DROP MODELS OF EXPERIMENTAL SPINAL CORD INJURY

Jean R. Wrathall

INTRODUCTION

Among the animal models devised to mimic human traumatic spinal cord injury (SCI), models based on impact produced by dropping a weight onto the exposed dura have been most frequently chosen for studies on basic pathophysiology and for preclinical testing of potential therapeutic interventions. The weight-drop models of SCI offer the advantages of clinical relevance and both conceptual and mechanical simplicity. Most of our basic understanding of the consequences of SCI originated from weight-drop models. In this chapter, the development and characterization of weight-drop models will be reviewed with special attention to current models that use the laboratory rat.

A SCI model involves production of an experimental injury and evaluation of the outcome. Thus, biomechanical, histopathological, behavioral, and electrophysiological consequences of weight-drop injury must be reviewed. Emphasis will be on the relationship between injury and outcome parameters and on methods presently used by investigators seeking to understand basic mechanisms of injury.

Sources of variability and ways to enhance consistency will be discussed, both within a single laboratory and among different laboratories studying SCI. The advantages and disadvantages of weight-drop models compared to other types of models will be considered. Finally, a brief prospectus will discuss how improved models for SCI research can be developed and suggest desirable attributes for future models.

HISTORICAL BACKGROUND

The deleterious effects of spinal cord injury were noted by the Egyptians nearly 5000 years ago.[1] The earliest recorded experimental studies were conducted by Galen in 177 AD.[2] He performed spinal cord transections of dogs, pigs, and goats, and recognized that resulting functional loss differed with the segmental level of the injury. Later, the histological consequences of surgical lesions were extensively studied by Ramon y Cajal.[3] He described the degeneration of axons in the rostral and caudal ends of a lesioned cord and a resulting widening of the gap at the site of the lesion.

Attempts to model the spinal cord contusion that characterizes most human SCI began late in the nineteenth century. These early experimental studies, reviewed by Dohrman[4] and Yeo,[5] used a variety of approaches to produce an impact injury in an intact animal. Investigators attempted striking the animal's back, dropping it from a height, and also used vibrating, centrifugation, and explosive forces. Although injury could be produced, the results were variable.

Allen's Introduction of the Weight-Drop Technique

Allen's approach was somewhat different.[6] Instead of creating an impact in the intact animal (closed impact injury), he performed a laminectomy to expose the dura so that a controlled force could be applied directly to the spinal cord (open impact injury). Location of the injury site became easier to standardize, and estimation of the force applied to the spinal cord became possible.

Allen devised a weight-drop apparatus[6] with which "a given weight could be dropped from a known height thereby producing a known impact." Allen dropped a weight through a guide tube oriented vertically and perpendicular to the spinal cord. The impact was expressed as the product of the weight in grams and the height in centimeters. An impact of about 300 gm-cm applied to the lower thoracic cord of a dog resulted in complete spastic paraplegia that was transient and from which the animals largely recovered by 7 to 10 days after injury. Dogs subjected to an impact of 400 gm-cm or more usually suffered permanent paraplegia. Histological studies of tissue in acute periods after SCI showed intramedullary hemorrhage and edema that appeared maximal at 4 hours after trauma.[7]

Although many other techniques to produce contusion injury have been described in the past 80 years, modifications of Allen's technique have proved to be suitable for a variety of studies on pathophysiological mechanisms and for preclinical testing of potential therapeutic interventions. Further, Allen's technique has been successfully modified for a variety of mammalian species.

Use of the Weight-Drop Technique in Larger Experimental Animals

Using a canine model, Amako in 1936[8] demonstrated that early gray matter hemorrhage was followed later by cavity formation. In the 1950s Freeman and Wright reported beneficial functional effects of myelotomy after experimental contusive injury.[9] Their hypothesis was that hemorrhage and edema formation increased pressure within the tissue and led to secondary damage. Myelotomy could relieve some of this pressure. Later, intravenous infusion of the osmotic agent urea to reduce edema after injury also was reported to lead to improved functional outcome.[10]

In the late 1960s interest in experimental studies of spinal cord contusion surged. Investigators examined therapeutic potential of treatments that might reduce secondary damage after SCI due to tissue swelling. By extending and modifying Allen's canine techniques for use on both dogs and monkeys, Albin and co-workers[11–13] demonstrated that local hypothermia applied within 4 hours of injury could mitigate the functional deficits produced by weight-drop injury. Later application proved ineffective. Ducker and Hamit,[14] using a canine weight-drop model, reported that local hypothermia and steroids reduced cord swelling and functional impairment. Shortly thereafter, a beneficial effect of steroids after weight-drop injury in monkeys was reported.[15] The therapeutic potential of corticosteroids subsequently was examined in dozens of experimental studies in the 1970s and 80s, many based on the weight-drop injury model. Although results from some studies were negative, or at best equivocal, sufficient data were obtained to support large-scale clinical trials that eventually provided evidence of the therapeutic benefit of methylprednisolone.[16]

A second deleterious consequence of SCI that began to be studied in detail was the injury-induced fall in tissue blood flow and oxygenation. Kelly and colleagues,[17] using a dog model, found reduced spinal cord oxygen pressure, and Ducker and Perot[18] demonstrated that this was associated with reduced blood flow in the injured segment. Beginning in the 1970s a series of studies using various experimental techniques of increasing sophistication demonstrated effects of contusion in reducing tissue blood flow, oxygen tension, and energy sources.[19] This led to testing new agents that might improve blood flow. In addition, agents originally used to reduce edema were re-examined for effects on blood flow. Thus, steroids, originally used to combat tissue edema, were later found to enhance blood flow after SCI.[20,21]

Hyperbaric oxygen treatment was another approach to compensate for reduced tissue oxygenation. Using weight-drop models in primates and dogs, respectively, Hertzog[22] and Kelly[17] reported improved outcome with hyperbaric oxygen treatment. Unfortunately, clinical trials have not been adequate to establish clearly whether there is value in such treatment. The current status of this approach to mitigating effects of SCI is reviewed in Chap. 110.

Another approach to the problem of blood flow reduction was based on inhibiting endogenous factors that lead to tissue hypoperfusion after SCI. Initially, Osterholm and co-workers believed that norepinephrine (NE) was a major factor.[23,24] Subsequent studies failed to confirm NE accumulation at the injury site, but the potential involvement of other vasoactive neurotransmitters, such as dopamine or endogenous opioids, provided the initial rationale for examining the therapeutic potential of opioid antagonists. In the early 1980s, using a feline weight-drop model, Faden and co-workers first demonstrated improved neurological outcome by treatment with naloxone.[25] Beneficial functional effects were confirmed and improved spinal cord blood flow and somatosensory evoked potentials documented by Young et al.[26] and Flamm et al.[27] Such data were the basis for including naloxone in a large-scale clinical trial.[16] However, at the dosage used, less clinical improvement was detected than with methylprednisolone.

Through the 1970s and 1980s many other studies of pathophysiological mechanisms and tests of potentially therapeutic agents were undertaken using weight-drop models of SCI, primarily in dogs and cats, but also in monkeys, sheep, and rabbits. However, by the 1990s most investigators had switched to rat models of SCI. Several factors contributed to the switch, including societal pressures for reduced use of larger mammals in research, financial pressures coupled with the need for large-scale screening of potential therapeutic agents, and the essential demonstration that reproducible spinal cord contusions could be produced in the rat.

Use of the Weight-Drop Technique in the Laboratory Rat

For some time it was thought that the weight-drop technique would not produce consistent SCI in the rat. Instead, other procedures, such as rapidly compressing the cord with an aneurysm clip,[28] were used to model contusion injuries in this species. As late as 1983, in a direct comparison of three methods, the aneurysm clip, compression due to inflation of an extradural balloon, and the weight-drop technique, the latter was found "unreliable for experimental spinal cord injury in the rat." [29] However, within a few years, modifications of the weight-drop technique were reported that allowed the production of graded and reproducible injury groups in the rat.[30] This and similar models have now been adopted in a number of other laboratories.[31–38] Much of the experimental work on spinal cord injury of the past 10 years has utilized such models.

It was quickly established that the pathophysiology after weight-drop injury in the rat[39–42] was, as expected, similar to that previously reported in larger species, including primates.[43] Further, quantitative measures of histopathology significantly correlated to functional deficits as measured by behavioral tests.[41,42] With respect to pathophysiological mechanisms, studies with rat weight-drop models revealed the importance of Ca^{++} accumulation in axonal degeneration.[40] Later, with the establishment of a relationship between ischemic brain injury and excitatory amino acid (EAA) receptors, leading to Ca^{++}-mediated neurotoxicity, rat weight-drop models were used to examine the role of EAA receptors in SCI.[44] Several laboratories have now independently found that antagonists of these receptors can reduce functional deficits, and in some cases, histopathology, after standardized SCI in a rat.[34,35,44–46] Most recently, a rat weight-drop model of injury has been chosen for use by the multicenter group now performing preclinical testing of a series of agents of potential benefit to patients with SCI (Young, personal communication).

BIOMECHANICS

The weight-drop technique uses the force of gravity to produce a consistent impact on the exposed spinal cord. In versions used in larger mammals a vented guide tube is positioned over the dura at the site of a laminectomy. A weight is allowed to fall from a given height directly onto the dura, or by hitting an "impounder" pre-positioned on the spinal cord.

The Problem of the GM-CM Descriptor

Although Allen expressed impact in terms of gm-cm force, this appealingly simple descriptor is not a valid measure of the actual impact force. Biomechanical studies in the 1970s using feline weight-drop models demonstrated that varying the weight and height used to create a specific "gm-cm impact" yields very different impact forces and histopathological lesions. Dohrman and Panjabi[47] analyzed cord deformation and resulting lesion volume in cats subjected to a "400 gm-cm" trauma using the following combinations: 5 g × 80 cm, 10 g × 40 cm, 10 g × 20 cm, 40 g × 10 cm, and 80 g × 5 cm. The volume of the lesions varied almost tenfold among the different groups. Heavier weights falling a shorter distance imparted a higher impulse (force over time) and produced a larger lesion. With only three cats used in each group, the reproducibility of the lesions within the group was not evaluated. However, it was clear from this study that, rather than "gm-cm of impact," both height and weight must be specified to produce a known injury with the weight-drop technique.

With further biomechanical analyses[48] using a larger group of cats (n = 40), it was possible to distinguish force acting on the spinal cord from total force acting on cord and thorax. Using a weight-drop device with a piezoelectric force transducer and a displacement transducer, the investigators recorded both force and displacement (deformation) before and after removing the spinal cord. By subtracting the data in the latter case from those obtained with the spinal cord in place, the force acting on the cord per se was estimated. A hyperbolic relationship was observed between the distance traveled by the weight and the force of impact on the spinal cord, with the greater weights (falling a shorter distance) producing the greatest force.

Taking Advantage of Gravity

Hung et al.[49,50] used high-speed cinematography in concert with a displacement transducer to further evaluate biomechanical aspects of weight-drop injury in cats. They identified the effects on cord displacement of static load by using a heavy "impounder" resting on the spinal cord and recording the cross-sectional area of the "impounder" tip. For a feline model they recommended using a 20-g weight, a 5-mm diameter impounder weighing 0.1 to 0.5 g, and varying the height from which the weight is dropped to produce consistent contusion injury of differing severity. However, data on the reproducibility of the force of impact and cord deformation in animals injured under the same conditions were not reported. Thus, the biomechanical studies of the 1970s identified sources of previously unexplained interlaboratory variability, such as the use of different weight-height combinations and impounder designs, indicated the importance of determining force and impulse, and suggested design principles for weight-drop devices to take advantage of the inherent constancy of gravity.

A Weight-Drop Device for the Rat

In order to develop a weight-drop model in the rat, a device was designed that allowed incorporation of a force transducer (strain gauge) to allow routine measurement of impact force and impulse.[30,51] Figure 102-1 shows this weight-drop device. The strain gauge is mounted on a brass "C-ring" that is attached to a Teflon impounder fitted loosely on a vertical metal rod. For use, the impounder (tip diameter 2.4 mm) is slowly lowered onto the dura until the top of the C-ring reaches a line scribed on the metal rod. The "preload" on the cord, because of the weight of the impounder and C-ring, is 0.06 newtons. The vertical metal rod passes through a 10-g cylindrical weight that is positioned at one of several specified distances from the scribed line by means of a pin passed through holes at different heights from which the weight can be dropped. When the pin is withdrawn the weight falls on the C-ring, deforming it so as to stimulate the strain gauge, and, at the same time, causing the impounder to rapidly impact the dura. The response of the strain gauge, calibrated against a dynamic load cell, is used to calculate the maximum force (newtons) and impulse (newton/sec) when the weight is dropped from different heights.[51] Table 102-1 shows the average maximum force and impulse recorded from groups of rats in which the 10-g weight was dropped 2.5, 5.0, or 17.5 cm. In Table 102-2, the results of linear regression analyses are shown. There is an extremely high correlation between the height from which the weight is dropped and both maximum force ($r = .96$, $p < 0.0001$) and impulse ($r = 0.97$, $p < 0.0001$) on the spinal cord. The consistency of the impact on the spinal cord at a given height is very good: the standard error is less than 2.5 percent of the mean force or impulse. There is also significant correlation between these biomechanical descriptors of the initial impact and the chronic functional deficits,[51,52] somatosensory evoked potentials,[53] and histopathology seen at one month after SCI.[41,42] However, these outcomes show greater variability than the initial mechanical impact, suggesting the importance of biological as well as biomechanical factors on the long-term consequence of contusion injury. Nevertheless, with this rela-

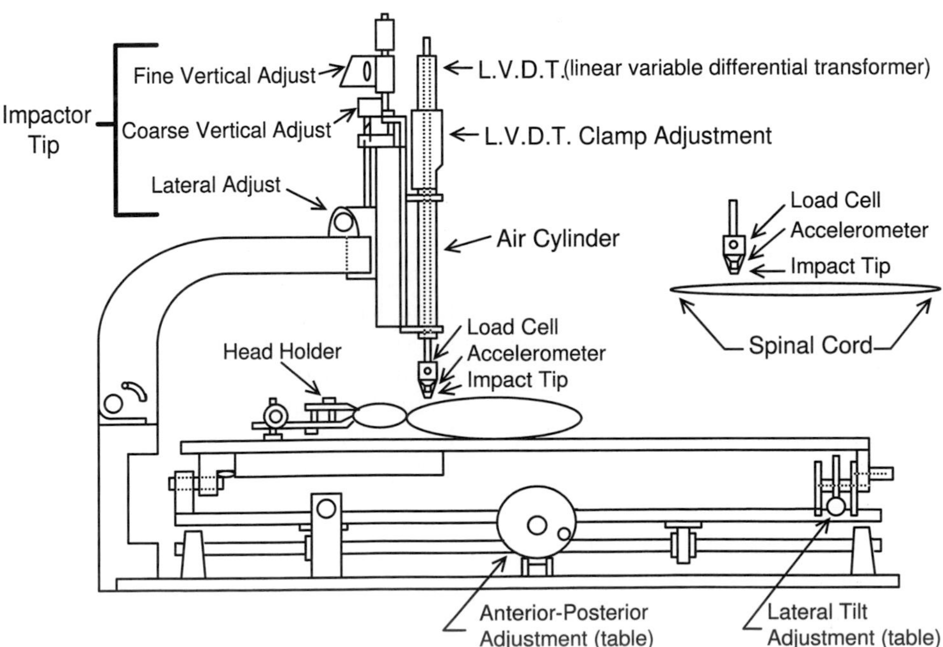

Figure 102-1. Weight-drop device for producing graded contusive spinal cord injury in the rat.[30] *Left:* The device consists of a Teflon impounder (i) attached to a brass C-ring on which a strain gauge (sg) may be mounted. The impounder/C-ring assembly is loose-fitted onto a rod passing through a 10-g weight (w) held at specified heights by means of a pin that can be withdrawn to allow the weight to drop. *Right:* Prior to lowering the impounder of the device onto the dura at T8, the spinal cord is stabilized by means of angled Allis clamps applied to the spinous processes of T7 and T9. The rat is suspended by these clamps to isolate the cord from movements of, and cushioning by, the thorax.

TABLE 102-1 Graded Contusive Injury in the Rat Produced with a Weight-Drop Technique*

Injury Description	Mild	Moderate	Severe
I. Biomechanics			
Height of drop (cm)—10-g weight	2.5	5.0	17.5
Maximum impact force (newtons)	18.4 ± 0.5	28.0 ± 0.5	55.9 ± 1.3
Impulse (newton-sec)	4.16 ± 0.1	6.32 ± 0.1	13.0 ± 0.3
II. Chronic Histopathology			
Lesion volume (mm^2)	1.87 ± 0.64	2.51 ± 0.24	7.35 ± 1.4
Lesion length (mm)	5.75 ± 1.25	9.21 ± 1.25	13.32 ± 1.91
Residual white matter at epicenter (percent)	38.6 ± 5.7	11.3 ± 2.7	2.8 ± 1.5
III. Chronic Hindlimb Functional Deficit			
Motor score (mode)	4	2	1
Inclined plane (angle)	47.0 ± 1.8	36.7 ± 2.7	26.5 ± 0.7
Combined behavioral score	27.1 ± 3.3	58.3 ± 4.1	81.8 ± 3.4
IV. Chronic Sematosensory Evoked Potentials			
Area (mm^2)	103.0 ± 17.6	29.9 ± 13.5	16.3 ± 7.9
Peak (μV)	126.5 ± 11.5	40.6 ± 15	26.9 ± 13.3
SEP detected	100%	54.5%	36.4%

* Data from published papers[30,41,42,51–53] with contusion injury produced with the weight-drop device shown in Fig. 102-1.

TABLE 102-2 Correlation Between Injury and Outcome Measures in a Rat Weight-Drop Model*

	N	Correlation Coefficient	P
I. Relationship between WD Height and Initial Impact			
Maximum force	64	0.96	<.0001
Impulse	34	0.97	<.0001
Chronic Histopathology			
Lesion volume	33	0.71	<.0005
Lesion length	29	0.60	<.0005
Residual white matter	26	−0.68	<.0005
Chronic Hindlimb Deficits			
Inclined plane angle	30	−0.74	<.0001
Combined behavioral score	30	0.80	<.0001
Chronic SEP			
Area	44	0.55	<.0001
Amplitude	44	0.65	<.0001
II. Initial impact and chronic functional deficit (CBS)			
Force (newtons)	64	0.68	<.0001
Impulse (newton-sec)	34	0.79	<.0001
III. Histopathology and chronic functional deficit (CBS)			
Lesion volume (mm^3)	33	0.68	<.0001
Lesion length (mm)	29	0.68	<.0001
Residual white matter (mm^2)	26	−0.91	<.0001
IV. SEP and chronic functional deficit (CBS)			
Area	44	0.60	<.0001
Amplitude	44	0.78	<.0005

* Data from published papers[41,51,53] with contusion injury produced with the weight-drop device shown in Fig. 102-1.

tively simple and inexpensive device, groups of rats with graded lesions and neurological impairment are produced, and these, or similar rat weight-drop models have been used extensively in the past decade to study basic pathophysiological mechanisms and to evaluate potential therapeutic strategies.[31–38,41,42,44–46,54]

A new weight-drop device for the rat has recently been described.[55] To alleviate any effect of impounder preload on the spinal cord, the impounder was eliminated. Instead the whole impactor is positioned directly on the dura with an electrical circuit used to monitor contact with the dura. Both impact velocity and cord compression are measured. With routine measurement of both these parameters, injury standards can be set, and any cases falling outside of the chosen specifications eliminated to reduce the variability of injury group.

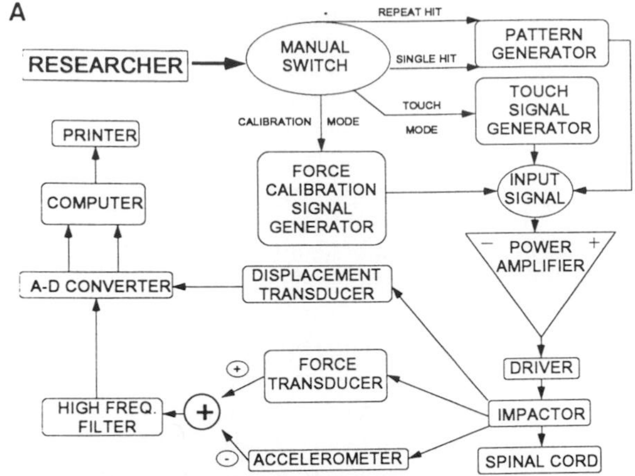

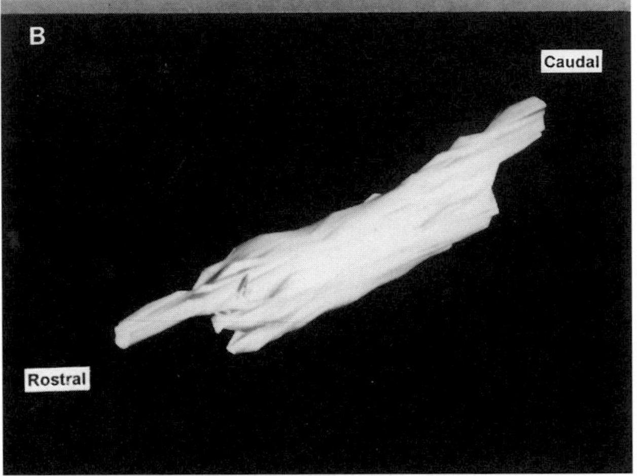

Figure 102-2. Development of histopathological lesions after graded contusive injury in the rat.[42] *A, C, E.* Lesions produced when the 10-g weight is dropped 2.5 cm. *B, D, F.* Lesion from a 17.5-cm weight drop. *A, B.* At 24 hours after injury, the epicenters are characterized by hemorrhage and the appearance of tears and cavities within the tissue. *C, D.* At 1 week after injury large central cavities are present; in the more severe injury, most of the spinal cord tissue has been lost. *E, F.* At 4 weeks after injury the less severe injury site (*E*) is characterized by a central cavity surrounded by a rim of residual white matter. With severe injury (*F*) spinal cord tissue is completely lost and replaced with a loose network of non-neuronal cells.

HISTOPATHOLOGY

One of the major reasons that weight-drop models of injury have been so much used is because, since the time of Allen,[7] it has appeared that the observed histopathology was similar to that of patients with SCI. A basic feature is the observation of initial hemorrhage, particularly associated with the central gray matter, followed at later time periods by the loss of spinal cord tissue and the appearance of cavities. Thus, the pathology of spinal cord contusion is often described as central hemorrhagic necrosis. Anatomic methods used to study the histopathological consequence of SCI, and the results of such studies, have been the subject of a recent review.[56]

Central Hemorrhagic Necrosis

Based on studies over decades using a variety of species,[39–43,57–64] major features of this histopathology may be summarized, with examples shown from our own studies in the rat (Fig. 102-2). (1) The gray matter of the cord is more sensitive to injury than the white matter. Central hemorrhage and necrosis appears in the gray matter with lower impact force and appears earlier in time than in the white matter. (2) With mild and moderate impact, the white matter tracts appear intact immediately after injury although they may be nonfunctional (spinal shock). (3) Spreading tissue necrosis begins to be evident several hours after injury. This is associated with hemorrhage and edema. The lesion spreads centrifugally to involve first the pericentral and later (depending on the severity of the original contusion) the more superficial white matter. It also extends rostrally and caudally from the initial site of injury. Three-dimensional reconstructions of the fully developed lesions indicate a football-like area of necrosis.[60] Areas of vacuolation and finally cavitation develop within the necrotic zone that subsequently may be partially filled with a glial scar.

Quantitative Analyses

Quantitative time-course studies have shown that the development of the chronic lesion is a slow process.[42]

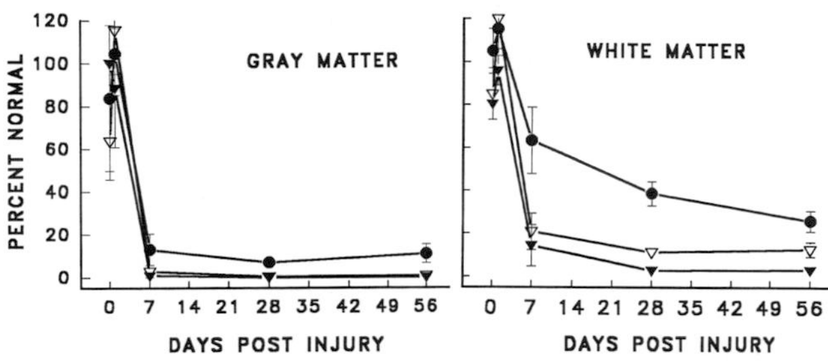

Figure 102-3. Time course of tissue loss in a rat weight-drop model.[42] Spinal cord injury produced with a 10-g weight dropped 2.5 (●), 5.0 (▽), or 17.5 (▼) cm. Data from morphometric analyses of lesion epicenters[42] showing transient swelling of the cord at 1 day with extensive tissue loss by 1 week after injury. Gray matter loss is virtually complete by 1 week after 5.0- and 17.5-cm weight drop. In the 2.5-cm group, a small amount of residual gray matter remains. White matter loss occurs more slowly and continues to occur between 1 and 4 weeks after injury. The rate of loss appears slowest with the 2.5-cm weight drop injury. In the chronic injury site, the amount of residual white matter depends on the height of the initial weight drop.

Although the major necrosis occurs in the first week after injury, tissue loss continues during the second and third week. A comparison of the time course after different degrees of initial impact (10-g weight-dropped 2.5, 5.0, or 17.5 cm), as shown in Fig. 102-3, also indicates that more severe impact leads to more rapid loss of tissue and an approximation of the chronic lesion parameters at an earlier time post-injury. This suggests that secondary factors leading to delayed necrosis may play a significant role in overall tissue loss and consequent functional deficits, especially after less severe impact injury. Support for this hypothesis has come from recent studies with an antagonist of a class of EAA receptors thought to be involved in delayed neurotoxicity. Local application of the antagonist, NBQX, to the injury site 15 minutes after weight-drop injury (10 g × 2.5 cm) leads to a dose-dependent reduction in the loss of gray and white matter and a correlated reduction in chronic hindlimb deficits.[46]

One of the hallmarks of SCI is the partial or complete loss of sensation and voluntary motor function below the level of the injury due to the interruption of long ascending sensory and descending motor tracts. Thus, the relationship between impact severity and loss of white matter tracts is of some interest. In weight-drop models a significant relationship between impact severity and loss of white matter has been shown[41,42] (Tables 102-1, 102-2). Further, there is also a significant correlation between impact and axonal loss, as measured by a line sampling procedure,[65] and an injury dose-response relationship for at least one specific descending motor control pathway, the serotonergic fibers from the brain stem.[66]

Comparison with Histopathology of SCI Patients

Recently the question has been raised whether the central hemorrhage necrosis characteristic of experimental contusion injury models is, in fact, typical of SCI patients. In a report of 23 new human cases, Bunge and colleagues[67] found that one-quarter of the spinal cords (6/23) showed the typical contusion/cyst pathology modeled so well by impact injury devices. Others demonstrated laceration due to gunshot wounds, massive compression, or a newly described pathology, termed "solid cord syndrome," characterized by white matter demyelination. However, the sample of patients is small, and may not be representative of the majority of SCI patients. For example, the average age was 51 compared with 20.5 for the 450 patients in a recent clinical trial.[16] Other recent studies of human histopathology (Kakulas, personal communication) continue to indicate the importance of central hemorrhagic necrosis in most patients with SCI. Thus, those attempting to model human SCI will be most interested in additional data from MRI and histopathological studies of tissue from patients.

FUNCTIONAL DEFICITS

The most important consequence of SCI is the resulting sensory and motor deficits, especially those due to loss of axons in long tracts to and from higher centers. Thus, any SCI model must include an outcome measure to assess these functional deficits. In weight-drop models, two major approaches have been used, behavioral tests of functional deficits and electrophysiological measurements of axonal conduction through the injury site.

Behavioral Testing

Methods for behavioral testing of functional impairment after experimental spinal cord trauma have recently been reviewed.[68] The most commonly used behavioral tests in weight-drop models were initially developed by investigators using other models of injury. Thus, Tarlov and Klinger[69] developed a neurological scale to rate open field locomotion in dogs subjected to SCI through the inflation of a balloon catheter inserted into the vertebral canal. Variations of this Tarlov scale have been widely used ever since. For example, in our rat weight-drop model we use a motor score in which rats are graded in open field locomotion: 0, if no hindlimb movement is seen; 1, for barely perceptible movement; 2, frequent movement without weight-bearing; 3, weight support with a few steps; 4, walking with only mild deficits; 5, normal use of hindlimbs on locomotion.[30]

In larger experimental mammals versions of the Tarlov score have generally been the only behavioral evaluation used. However, in these species the scale is now often expanded.[70] An expanded version for the laboratory rat is currently being tested with rats injured by both weight-drop and controlled impact devices (Bresnahan and Beattie, personal communication).

Although the clinical significance of rating locomotion cannot be doubted, there has been concern about the highly subjective nature of such assessment. Consequently attempts were made to introduce more objective behavioral tests. This movement has been associated with the switch to rat models of SCI.

The inclined plane test was introduced by Riulin and Tator[71] for use in a rat model of injury based on compression of the spinal cord with an aneurysm clip. In this test the maximum angle at which the rat can maintain its position is measured (Fig. 102-4*J*). The use of hindlimb reflex tests in the rat was suggested by De La Torre[72] and first incorporated into a protocol for evaluating weight-drop injury by Gale et al.[52] Reflexes such as toespread, righting, placing, and hindlimb withdrawal in response to extension, pressure, and brief pain, as well as the reflex to lick the feet in response to moderate heat are evaluated (Fig. 102-4*A–H*). Initially, at one day after SCI, rats are areflexic (grade 0). Later, at weekly evaluations, reflex responses may return, but may be hypoactive (grade 1), normal (grade 2), or hyperactive (grade 3). Recovery in various reflex tests, the inclined plan, and a test of ability to swim (Fig. 102-4*I*) are differently sensitive to severity of contusive injury,[73] and can therefore be used to supplement evaluation of locomotion per se to calculate a combined behavioral score (CBS).

The CBS[52] is an overall estimate of hindlimb functional deficit that ranges from 0 in normal rats to 100 in rats that are abnormal in all tests. It was developed on the basis of initial injury dose-response studies. The CBS is calculated based on evaluation of the motor score, inclined plane performance, swimming, and responses in 7 hindlimb reflex tests.[52,73] The CBS exhibits a normal distribution and is suitable for parametric statistical anslysis, in contrast to neurological rating scales that require the use of nonparametric statistics. Although CBS correlates with major component tests such as the motor score and inclined plane test, it has greater statistical power than the individual tests, making it particularly useful in evaluating potential therapeutic agents for SCI.[45,46] The chronic CBS at 1 month after SCI is significantly correlated to the degree of initial injury, functional impairment as measured by somatosensory evoked potentials, and histopathology (Table 102-2). In particular there is a very high correlation ($r = -0.91$) between CBS and residual white matter at the lesion epicenter.[42,43]

With weight-drop and other models of contusive SCI, functional deficits typically are maximal shortly after injury and then demonstrate some decrease, i.e., recovery of function, over time after injury. The degree of recovery varies with severity of injury, as seen in Fig. 102-5, where results from a rat weight-drop model are shown with CBS used as a measure of overall functional deficits. Groups of rats with different degrees of initial impact severity cannot be distinguished at 1 day after SCI due to "spinal shock." However, by 1 week the injury groups begin to be apparent, and by 3 weeks the chronic functional deficit pattern is established. The

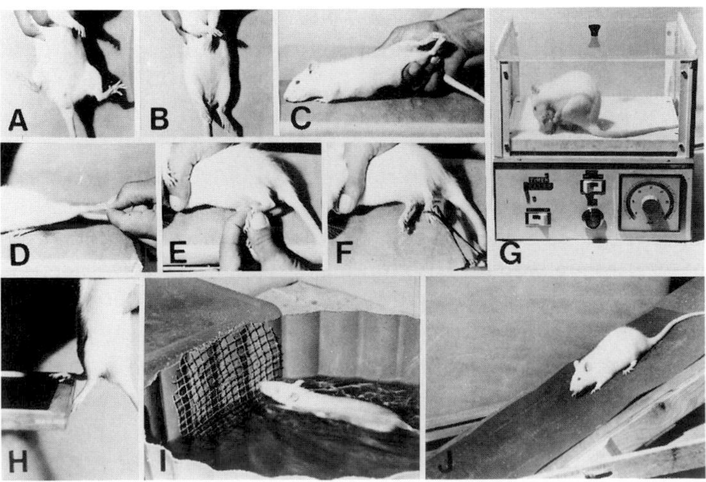

Figure 102-4. Behavioral tests used in a rat weight drop injury.[73] *A*. Normal toespread reflex. *B*. Absence of toespread reflex in a rat after spinal cord injury. *C*. The righting reflex. *D*. The extension withdrawal reflex *E*. Testing hindlimb withdrawal in response to pressure. *F*. Withdrawal in response to brief pain. *G*. Licking the foot, in response to moderate heat. *H*. Placing reflex. *I*. Testing use of the hindlimbs in swimming. *J*. The inclined plane test to determine the maximum angle at which the rat can maintain position.

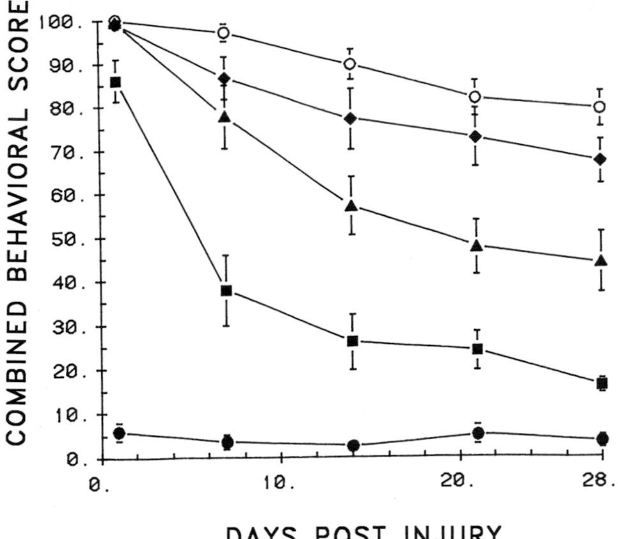

Figure 102-5. Changes in functional deficits over time in a rat weight drop model. Individual test results are used to calculate a Combined Behavioral Score[52] that estimates overall impairment. The score can range from 0 in a normal rat to 100 in a rat with no detected hindlimb function. Results from an initial injury dose-response experiment[52] in which groups of rats (n = 9–10 each group) were injured with the 10-g weight dropped 17.5 (○), 10 (◆), 5 (▲), 2.5 (■), or 0 (●) cm. All of the injured rats demonstrate nearly complete functional loss at 1 day, but show partial recovery thereafter. The extent of recovery depends on the height of the initial weight drop, but, by 3 weeks, functional deficits have stabilized, and the chronic deficits are apparent.

chronic deficit remains stable between 3 and 8 weeks after SCI,[42] and even in the least severe group (10 g × 2.5 cm weight-drop), the deficit is retained through at least 6 months after injury (Wrathall, unpublished).

In recent years there has been a move to further refine behavioral testing of rats with contusive SCI. One change has been to evaluate locomotion more extensively by challenging rats to walk across a grid that requires precise placement of the paws to avoid errors ("footfalls"). This type of evaluation was first introduced for a controlled impact model,[74] but has also been used in the "mild" weight-drop model.[75] With more severe injury, the error rate is too high for this to be a useful test. Other measures of locomotion, such as footprint analysis, also have been used.[76] In the course of development of a new controlled impact model,[77] the sensitivity of different measures of locomotor function were compared.[78] Power analyses indicate that evaluation of open field locomotion, inclined plane performance, and grid walking were more useful measures (i.e., had greater statistical power) than were stride length, base of support, and other measures based on footprint analyses.

Electrophysiological Evaluations

Somatosensory and more recently, motor evoked potentials (SEP, MEP) have been the most commonly used methods for electrophysiological assessment because of the ease of the techniques involved and their relative lack of invasiveness. In a recent critical review Blight has discussed the use of these and other electrophysiological methods in SCI research.[79] Thus, recordings of evoked potentials have been used (1) acutely, to monitor the effect of impact[80–83] and (2) to assess conduction on the chronically injured spinal cord.[53,84,85]

Acute recordings have confirmed an immediate conduction block after weight-drop injuries and have sometimes been continued long enough to demonstrate a partial recovery followed by a secondary loss.[84,86] The initial block is believed to result from an ionic disequilibrium that prevents conduction immediately after injury.[79] The recovery of ionic homeostasis a few hours after injury allows the reappearance of partial conduction through axons that survive the initial mechanical trauma. Then secondary injury processes result in loss of additional axons, and conduction fails again for this reason.

Electrophysiological evaluation of the chronically injured spinal cord has been used in an attempt to obtain an objective measure of the integrity of long axonal tracts, and sometimes to assess any enhancing effect of therapeutic interventions. Unfortunately, the relationship between the electrophysiological measures most commonly used and axonal integrity is not as straightforward as it might appear.[79] For example, although a significant injury dose response relationship for SEP amplitude at 1 month post-injury was found in a rat model of weight-drop injury,[53] this was due primarily to increasing numbers of rats with no detectable SEP as impact intensity increased (Table 102-1). Regression analyses of SEP parameters and either initial injury intensity or quantitative measures of tissue pathology indicated lower correlation than did those obtained with behavioral measures of functional integrity (Table 102-2).

Results from detailed studies on chronic SEP using a feline weight-drop model explain some of the difficulties in attempting to use SEPs to assess the chronically injured spinal cord.[79,84] Numbers of surviving axons in the dorsolateral quadrants of the spinal cord 6 weeks after SCI were compared with quantitative evaluations of the SEP in the animal. Significant recovery of SEP was noted with only 2 to 4 percent of surviving axons at the injury site, but spinal cords with similar numbers of axons also exhibited no SEP. This might be explained by the different relative contribution of axons of different diameter to the SEP, as SCI is known to result preferentially in loss of larger diameter axons.[87] However, a detailed analysis of axon diameters leads to the generation of a theoretical conduction potential much different (and less) from that seen in the actual SEP.[79]

It is this sort of experience—as well as the somewhat invasive and often terminal nature of the electrophysiological assessment protocols that have typically been used—that argues against the routine use of SEPs for evaluating the functional integrity of the chronically injured spinal cord in experimental animals. However, other electrophysiology approaches may be very useful to answer questions of how organization of the spinal cord is altered by injury and interventions after injury. Evaluation of vestibular and auditory startle responses[88] as well as motor evoked potentials[89] are other approaches that have been examined in animals with weight-drop injury. More recently, Thompson et al.[90] re-examined the effects of SCI on the H-reflex and used evaluation of these effects to study the consequence of spinal cord transplants on descending control of reflex activity after contusive injury.

SOURCES OF VARIABILITY

When discussing the variability of experimental SCI produced with weight-drop techniques, it is important to distinguish between inter- and intralaboratory variability. Historically, a great deal of the former is accounted for by lack of appreciation of the biomechanical principles involved. For example, as discussed earlier in this review, "400 gm-cm impacts" in laboratories using different height-weight combinations are unlikely to produce similar lesions, because the impact forces will be different. Other biomechanical factors, discussed below, can contribute to both inter- and intralaboratory variability. Surgical procedures and even choice of anesthetic[36] also can affect the degree of injury. In addition, even with great attention to control of all possible experimental parameters, there appears to be inherent biological variability, even using relatively inbred strains of laboratory rats. As in any biological research, the answer to unavoidable variability lies in appropriate experimental design and statistical analyses. Thus, any group doing research with weight-drop (or other) models of SCI should assess the variability in relevant outcome measures that they experience and should use power analyses to determine the appropriate sample sizes for their experiments. But first, known sources of variability should be eliminated.

Mechanical

Weight-drop devices can appear deceptively simple. However, apparently minor alterations in a design can affect the force of impact and resulting lesion. For example, some years ago a second laboratory sought to duplicate the weight-drop device we had described for rats. However, although their machinist worked from drawings we supplied, he did not use brass for the "C-ring" but a somewhat different alloy with different elastic properties. Less force was transmitted to the spinal cord and the rats had consistently less severe injuries than we had produced with the original device. Comparison of both force and impulse was used to detect the source of this difference. Thus, while it may be unnecessary routinely to measure impact parameters once a model has been established, it is critical to do so initially to determine whether a new device produces impacts similar to those whose outcomes have been well characterized. Other potential sources of interlaboratory variation may stem from the size, shape, and weight of the "impounder," as well as the degree of "bounce" leading to secondary and tertiary impacts, with a specific device.

Both inter- and intralaboratory variability is introduced if the spinal cord is not sufficiently stabilized prior to weight-drop. Any slight movement of the spinal cord with breathing and the cushioning effect of the thorax affects the force and consistency of impact on the spinal cord. One approach to this problem taken in a cat weight-drop model was to use a curved metal "anvil" that was slipped under the spinal cord.[91] In the rat model that we developed we stabilized the cord by clamping the vertebral spines (T7 and T9) immediately adjacent to the laminectomy site (T8) with custom-angled Allis clamps (standard rat spinal clamps were too large for the delicate thoracic vertebra) and held the rat suspended by these vertebra during the weight-drop procedure.[30]

Lack of vertical alignment leads to asymmetrical lesions. If the lesion is to be consistent, the impact—and thus the weight-drop device—must be carefully aligned at a right angle with respect to the spinal cord, both in the rostral-caudal and right-left coordinates, and positioned mid-sagittally. Further, the spinal cord must be truly horizontal if the experimenter wants to take advantage of the constancy of gravitational force. Over the course of 10 years' experience with the rat weight-drop model, increased variability has most often been traced to asymmetrical lesions (seen in histopathogical examination) and typically associated with a new surgeon (see below).

Surgical

Experiments by Salzman and colleagues have demonstrated that the anesthetic agent chosen for surgery can result in altered outcome in a rat weight-drop injury model.[36] Other likely sources of variability associated with surgery include differences in the size of the laminectomy, and how much surrounding tissue that contributes to the overall stability of the vertebral column is removed. The surgery should be standardized if consistent lesions are to be produced. Physiological factors such as blood loss and body temperature are also important and need to be controlled. Finally, as experienced surgeons tend to produce more consistent SCI, the importance of training and practice should not be underestimated.

BIOLOGICAL

Even with very constant impact produced by weight-drop[30] or controlled impact devices,[74,78] the chronic morphological and functional outcome of SCI displays variability. Much of this may be due to biological factors difficult or impossible to control. However, biological variability can be decreased by using genetically similar animals of the same size, specified sex, etc. This is one of the advantages of the rat models of injury as compared to the use of mongrel dogs and cats of different sizes, ages, etc. The chosen spinal cord level may also affect variability. In an early study we compared the behavioral outcome of injury at the T8 and T12 levels (Wrathall and Pettegrew, unpublished). One group of rats ($n = 10$ per) was injured at T8 with the weight-drop device shown in Fig. 102-1, and the second at T12 with the same device using an impounder with a 3.0-mm tip, because of the greater diameter of the cord at T12. The same surgeon did both series and then repeated the study a second time. The results showed that the standard deviations were more than twice as great when the contusions were produced at T12 as compared to T8.

ADVANTAGES AND DISADVANTAGES OF USING WEIGHT-DROP MODELS

A primary advantage of weight-drop and other impact models of SCI lies in their clinical relevance. Most spinal cord injuries are believed to be due to rapid flexion-extension of the vertebral column, resulting in a contusion of the cord when the vertebral bone hits the spinal cord (see Chapters 76 and 77). The result is immediate mechanical trauma as well as the initiation of secondary events (e.g., ischemia, release of excitotoxins, etc.) that can lead to further injury. Nonimpact models such as surgical lesions (transection, hemisections), ischemic lesions, and compression models, cannot model all of the relevant clinical events after SCI as well as impact models can. Evidence to support the contention that impact models adequately model human SCI include the similarity in histopathology to that reported in patients and the success of weight-drop models in predicting therapeutic potential for agents later tested in clinical trials.[16] However, certain caveats must be acknowledged. Only a few agents have so far progressed from testing in animal models to large-scale randomized clinical trials. We do not currently have enough information about the ability of various animal models to predict successful therapeutic agents for humans with SCI or to say whether distinctions between various animal models are significant. In addition, a recent histological evaluation of a series of human spinal cords after injury indicates a significant number of cases where the histopathology is not similar to impact injury models. In this study[67] more than 25 percent of patients (7/23) demonstrated a massive (and permanent) compression of the spinal cord not modeled by any current animal model. Others (6/23), injured by gunfire, demonstrated laceration of the spinal cord—and probably could be modeled only by a combination of contusion and surgical lesion.

Within the context of impact models that produce spinal cord contusion, weight-drop devices are attractive because they are simple to construct and maintain, thus inexpensive and readily exportable. The primary disadvantage is the difficulty in obtaining information on biomechanical parameters of the injury and the design compromises that result. Thus, in a rat model we used a design with a brass C-ring imposed between the weight and the impounder (Fig. 102-1). However, the weight of this assembly resting on the spinal cord and its rebound (bounce) after the weight-drop undoubtedly affect the resulting contusion injury. Further, with this design we do not get information on actual cord deformation. In a recently described new rat weight-drop device,[55] these two problems have been solved, but the device is larger so that the immediately adjacent vertebra cannot be clamped for maximal spinal column stabilization. The controlled impact devices discussed in Chapter 103 generally obviate these difficulties, because the electronic circuitry controlling the impact can generally be used to obtain biomechanical information as well as potentially producing more consistent impacts. However, such devices are complicated and expensive, and their use has not been widespread.

PROSPECTUS

There are several reasons to believe that models of the future will improve. Increasing availability and decreasing cost of computerized control units may allow widespread use of much more sophisticated injury devices, whether gravity or electromechanical force is used. Models undoubtedly also will be improved by the use of more sophisticated outcome measures. However, the greatest potential improvements depend on our knowledge of human injury. MRI and other noninvasive imaging techniques should allow us to accumulate data about the development and chronic appearance of the injury sites we are trying to model. Even more important is feedback from human clinical trials. Experimental models of SCI are used to investigate mechanisms of injury that serve as a basis for developing therapeutic approaches to SCI. As more data from human clinical trials are obtained, the types of animal models and outcome measures that predict those results can be determined. Based on this feedback, improved models and outcome measures can be developed that are more predictive, less expensive, and easier to use. These, in turn, will facilitate the large-scale preclinical screening efforts that will be needed to develop the most effective therapeutic strategies to reduce the consequences of SCI.

References

1. Breasted JH: *The Edwin Smith Surgical Papyrus*. Chicago: University of Chicago Press, 1930; I:337–342.
2. Galen, in Duckworth, WLH (transl), Lyons MC, Towers B (eds): *On Anatomical Procedures*. Cambridge: Cambridge University Press, 1962:22–26.
3. Ramon y Cajal S, in May RM (transl), *Degeneration and Regeneration of the Nervous System*. London: Oxford University Press, 1928.
4. Dohrmann GJ: Experimental spinal cord trauma. A historical review. *Arch Neurol* 1972; 27:468–474.
5. Yeo JD: A review of experimental research in spinal cord injury. *Paraplegia* 1976; 14:1–11.
6. Allen AR: Surgery of the experimental lesion of spinal cord equivalent to crush injury of fracture dislocation of spinal column. *JAMA* 1911; 57:878–890.
7. Allen AR: Remarks on histopathological changes in the spinal cord due to impact. An experimental study. *J Nerv Ment Dis* 1914; 41:141–147.
8. Amaka T: Surgical treatment of spinal cord injury by blunt forces: Experimental study. *J Japn Surg Soc* 1936; 37:1843–1874.
9. Freeman LW, Wright TW: Experimental observations of concussion and contusion of the spinal cord. *Ann Surg* 1953; 137:433–443.
10. Joyner J, Freeman LW: Urea and spinal cord trauma. *Neurology* 1961; 13:69–72.
11. Albin MS, White RJ, Locke GE, Kretchmer HE: Spinal cord hypothermia by localized perfusion cooling. *Nature* 1967; 210:1059.
12. Albin MS, White RJ, Yashon D, et al: Functional and electrophysiologic limitations of delayed spinal cord cooling after impact trauma. *Surg Forum* 1968; 19:423–424.
13. Albin MS, White RJ, Acosta-Rua G, et al: Study of functional recovery produced by delayed localized cooling after spinal cord injury in primates. *J Neurosurg* 1968; 29:113–120.
14. Ducker TB, Hamit HF: Experimental treatments of acute spinal cord injury. *J Neurosurg* 1969; 30:393–397.
15. Black P, Moskowitz RS: Experimental spinal cord injury in monkeys: Comparison of steroids and local hypothermia. *Surg Forum* 1971; 22:409–411.
16. Bracken MB, Shepherd MJ, Collins WF, et al: A randomized, controlled trial of methylprednisolone or naloxone in the treatment of acute spinal cord injury. Results of the second national acute spinal cord injury study. *N Engl J Med* 1990; 322:1405–1411.
17. Kelly DL Jr., Lassiter KRL, Calogero JA, et al: Effects of local hypothermia and tissue oxygen studies in experimental paraplegia. *J Neurosurg* 1970; 33:554–563.
18. Ducker TB, Perot PL Jr.: Spinal cord oxygen and blood flow in trauma. *Surg Forum* 1971; 22:412–445.
19. Tator CH: Ischemia as a secondary neural injury, in Salzman SK, Faden AI (eds): *The Neurobiology of Central Nervous System Trauma*. New York: Oxford University Press, 1994:209–215.
20. Anderson DK, Means ED, Waters TR, Green ES: Microvascular perfusion and metabolism in injured spinal cord after methylprednisolone treatment. *J Neurosurg* 1982; 56:106–113.
21. Young W, Flamm ES: Effect of high dose corticosteroid therapy on blood flow evoked potentials and extracellular calcium in experimental spinal cord injury. *J Neurosurg* 1982; 57:667–673.
22. Hartzog JT, Fisher RG, Snow C: Spinal cord trauma: Effect of hyperbaric oxygen therapy. *Proc Annu Clin Spinal Cord Inj Conf* 1969; 17:70–71.
23. Osterholm JL, Matthews GJ: Altered norepinephrine metabolism following experimental spinal cord injury. I. Relationship to hemorrhagic necrosis and post-wounding neurological deficits. *J Neurosurg* 1972; 36:386–394.
24. Osterholm JL, Matthews GJ: Altered norepinephrine metabolism following experimental spinal cord injury. II. Protection against traumatic spinal cord hemorrhagic necrosis by norepinephrine synthesis blockade with alpha methyl tyrosine. *J Neurosurg* 1972; 36:395–401.
25. Faden AI, Jacobs TP, Holaday JW: Opiate antagonist improves neurologic recovery after spinal cord injury. *Science* 1981; 211:493–494.
26. Young W, Flamm ES, Demopoulos HB, et al: Naloxone ameliorates posttraumatic ischemia in experimental spinal contusion. *J Neurosurg* 1981; 55:205–219.
27. Flamm ES, Young W, Demopoulos HB, et al: Experimental spinal cord injury: Treatment with naloxone. *Neurosurgery* 1982; 10:227–231.
28. Rivlin AS, Tator CH: Effect of duration of acute spinal cord compression in a new acute cord injury model in the rat. *Surg Neurol* 1978; 10:39–43.
29. Khan M, Griebel R: Acute spinal cord injury in the rat: Comparison of three experimental techniques. *J Can Sci Neurol* 1983; 10:161–165.
30. Wrathall JR, Pettegrew RK, Harvey F: Spinal cord contusion in the rat: Production of graded, reproducible injury groups. *Exp Neurol* 1985; 88:108–122.

31. Black P, Markowitz RS, Molt JT, et al: Models of spinal cord injury: Part 3. Dyanmic-load technique. *Neurosurgery* 1988; 22:51–60.
32. Sadanaga KK, Ohnishi T: Chlorpromazine protects rat spinal cord against contusion injury. *J Neurotrauma* 1989; 6:153–161.
33. Kwo S, Young W, DeCrescito V: Spinal cord sodium, potassium, calcium and water concentration changes in rats after graded contusion injury. *J Neurotrauma* 1989; 6:13–24.
34. Faden AI, Ellison JA, Noble LJ: Effects of competitive and non-competitive NMDA receptor antagonists in spinal cord injury. *Eur J Pharmacol* 1990; 175:165–174.
35. Gomez-Pinella F, Tram H, Cotman CW, Nieto-Sampedro M: Neuroprotective effect of MK-801 and U-50488H after contusive spinal cord injury. *Exp Neurol* 104: 118–124.
36. Salzman SK, Mendez AA, Sabato S, et al: Anesthesia influences the outcome from experimental spinal cord injury. *Brain Res* 1990; 521:33–39.
37. Xu J, Hsu CY, Junker H, et al: Kininogen and kinin in experimental spinal cord contusion. *J Neurochem* 1991; 57:975–680.
38. Thompson FJ, Reier PJ, Lucas CC, Parmer R: Altered patterns of reflex excitability subsequent to contusion injury of the rat spinal cord. *J Neurophysiol* 1992; 68:1473–1486.
39. Ballentine JD: Pathology of experimental spinal cord trauma. I. The necrotic lesion as a function of vascular injury. *Lab Invest* 1978; 39:236–253.
40. Ballentine JD: Pathology of experimental spinal cord trauma. II. Ultrastructure of axons and myelin. *Lab Invest* 1978; 39:254–266.
41. Noble LJ, Wrathall JR: Spinal cord contusion in the rat: Morphometric analyses of alteration in the spinal cord. *Exp Neurol* 1985; 88:135–149.
42. Noble LJ, Wrathall JR: Correlative analyses of lesion development and functional status after graded spinal cord contusive injuries in the rat. *Exp Neurol* 1989; 103:34–40.
43. Bresnahan J, King J, Martin G, Yashon D: A neuroanatomical analysis of spinal cord injury in the rhesus monkey (*Macaca mulatta*). *J Neurol Sci* 1976; 28:521–542.
44. Faden AL, Simon RP: A potential role for excitotoxins in the pathophysiology of spinal cord injury. *Ann Neurol* 1988; 23:623–626.
45. Wrathall JR: Effect of kynurenate on functional deficits from traumatic spinal cord injury. *Eur J Pharmacy* 1992; 218:273–281.
46. Wrathall JR, Choiniere D, Ten YD: Dose-dependent reduction of tissue loss and functional impairment after spinal cord trauma with the AMPA/kainate antagonist NBQX. *J Neuroscience* 1994; 14:6598–6607.
47. Dohrmann GJ, Panjabi MM: Standardized spinal cord trauma: Biomechanical parameters and lesion volume. *Surg Neurol* 1976; 6:263–267.
48. Dohrmann GJ, Panjabi MM, Banks D: Biomechanics of experimental spinal cord trauma. *J Neurosurg* 1978; 48:993–1001.
49. Hung TK, Albin MS, Brown TD, et al: Biomechanical responses to open experimental spinal cord injury. *Surg Neurol* 1975; 4:271–276.
50. Hung TK, Lin HS, Albin MS, et al: The standardization of experimental impact injury to the spinal cord. *Surg Neurol* 1979; 11:470–477.
51. Panjabi MM, Wrathall JR: Biomechanical analysis of experimental spinal cord injury and functional loss. *Spine* 1988; 13:1365–1370.
52. Gale K, Kerasidis H, Wrathall JR: Spinal cord contusion in the rat: Behavioral analysis of functional neurological impairment. *Exp Neurol* 1985; 88:123–134.
53. Raines A, Dretchen KL, Marx K, Wrathall JR: Spinal cord contusion in the rat: Somatosensory evoked potentials as a function of graded injury. *J Neurotrauma* 1988; 5:151–160.
54. Noble LJ, Wrathall JR: Distribution and time course of protein extravasation in the rat spinal cord after contusive injury. *Brain Res* 1989; 482:57–66.
55. Gruner JA: A monitored contusion model of spinal cord injury in the rat. *J Neurotrauma* 1992; 9:123–128.
56. Noble LJ: Anatomical assessment of spinal cord injury, in Salzman SK, Faden AI (eds): *The Neurobiology of Central Nervous System Trauma.* New York: Oxford University Press, 1994:99–108.
57. Assenmacher DR, Ducker TB: Experimental traumatic paraplegia: The vascular and pathological changes seen in reversible and irreversible spinal cord lesions. *J Bone Joint Surg* (*Am*) 1971; 53:671–680.
58. Ducker TB, Kindt GW, Kempe LG: Pathological findings of acute spinal cord injury. *J Neurosurg* 1971; 35:700–708.
59. Green BA, Wagner FC Jr.: Evolution of edema in the acutely injured spinal cord: A fluorescence microscopic study. *Surg Neurol* 1973; 1:98–101.
60. Osterholm JL: *The Pathophysiology of Spinal Cord Trauma.* Springfield, IL: Charles C Thomas, 1978.
61. Rawe SE, Lee WA, Perot PL: The histopathology of experimental spinal cord trauma. The effect of systemic blood flow. *J Neurosurg* 1978; 48:1002–1007.
62. Wagner FC, Dohrmann GJ, Bucy PC: Histopathology of transitory traumatic paraplegia in the monkey. *J Neurosurg* 1971; 35:272–276.
63. Wagner FC, Dohrmann GJ: Alterations in nerve cells and myelinated fibers in spinal cord injury. *Surg Neurol* 1975; 3:125–133.
64. Yeo JD, Payne W, Hinwood B, Kidman AD: The sequential pathological changes in experimental contusion injury of the spinal cord. *J Bone Joint Surg* (*Br*) 1975; 58:253–259.
65. Blight AR, DeCrescito V: Morphometric analysis of experimental spinal cord injury in the cat: The relation of injury intensity to survival of myelinated axons. *Neuroscience* 1986; 19:321–341.
66. Faden AI, Gannon A, Basbaum AI: Use of serotonin immunoreactivity as a marker of injury severity after experimental spinal cord trauma in rats. *Brain Res* 1988; 450:94–100.
67. Bunge RP, Puckett WR, Becarra JL, et al: Observation on the pathology of human spinal cord injury. *Adv Neurol* 1993; 59:75–89.

68. Wrathall JR: Behavioral analyses in experimental spinal cord trauma, in Salzman SK, Faden AI (eds): *The Neurobiology of Central Nervous System Trauma.* New York: Oxford University Press, 1994:79–85.
69. Tarlov IM, Klinger H: Spinal cord compression studies II. Time limits for recovery after gradual compression dogs. *Arch Neurol Psychiatry* 1954; 71:272–290.
70. Anderson DK, Braughler JM, Hall ED, et al: Effects of treatment with U-74006F on neurological outcome following experimental spinal cord injury. *J Neurosurg* 1988; 69:562–567.
71. Rivlin AS, Tator CH: Objective clinical assessment of motor function after experimental spinal cord injury in the rat. *J Neurosurg* 1977; 47:577–581.
72. De La Torre JV: Spinal cord injury models. *Prog Neurobiol* 1984; 22:289–344.
73. Kerasidis H, Wrathall J, Gale K: Behavioral assessment of functional deficit in rats with contusive spinal cord injury. *J Neurosci Methods* 1987; 20:167–189.
74. Bresnahan JC, Beattie MS, Todd FD, Noyes DH: A behavioral and anatomical analysis of spinal cord injury produced by a feedback-controlled impactation device. *Exp Neurol* 1987; 95:548–570.
75. Wrathall JR, Teng YD, Choiniere D, Mundt D: Evidence that local non-NMDA receptors contribute to functional deficits in contusive spinal cord injury. *Brain Res* 1992; 586:140–143.
76. Stokes BT, Reier PJ: Fetal grafts alter chronic behavioral outcome after contusion damage to the adult rat spinal cord. *Exp Neurol* 1992; 116:1–12.
77. Stokes BT, Noyes DH, Behrmann DL: An electromechanical spinal injury technique with dynamic sensitivity. *J Neurotrauma* 1992; 9:187–195.
78. Behrmann DL, Bresnahan JC, Beattie MS, Shah BR: Spinal cord injury produced by consistent mechanical displacement of the cord in rats: Behavioral and histologic analysis. *J Neurotrauma* 1992; 9:197–217.
79. Blight AR: Electrophysiological approaches to mechanisms of central nervous system trauma, in Salzman SK, Faden AI (eds): *The Neurobiology of Central Nervous System Trauma.* New York: Oxford University Press, 1994:41–56.
80. Donaghy RMP, Numoto M: Prognostic significance of sensory evoked potential in spinal cord injury. *Proc Annu Clin Spinal Cord Inj Conf* 1969; 17:251–257.
81. Ducker TR, Salcman M, Lucas JT, et al: Experimental spinal cord trauma. II. Blood flow, tissue oxygen, evoked potentials in both paretic and plegic monkeys. *Surg Neurol* 1978; 10:64–70.
82. Baskin DS, Simpson RK: Corticomotor and somatosensory evoked potential evaluation of acute spinal cord injury in the rat. *Neurosurgery* 1987; 20:871–877.
83. Zileli M, Schramm J: Motor versus somatosensory evoked potential changes after acute experimental spinal cord injury in the rat. *Acta Neurochir* (*Wien*) 1991; 108:140–147.
84. Blight AR, Young W: Axonal morphometric correlates of evoked potential in experimental spinal cord injury, in Salzman S (ed): *Neural Monitoring in the Prevention of Intraoperative Injury.* Clifton, NJ: Humana Press, 1990:87–113.
85. Simpson RK, Baskin DS: Corticomotor evoked potential in acute and chronic blunt spinal cord injury in the rat: Correlation with neurological outcome and histological damage. *Neurosurgery* 1987; 20:131–137.
86. D'Angelo CM: The H-reflex in experimental spinal cord trauma. *J Neurosurg* 1973; 2:791–805.
87. Blight AR: Cellular morphology of chronic spinal cord injury in the cat: Analysis of myelinated axons by line sampling. *Neuroscience* 1983; 10:521–542.
88. Gruner JA: Comparison of vestibular and auditory startle responses in the rat and cat. *J Neurosci Meths* 1989; 27:13–23.
89. Gruner JA, Kersun JM: Assessment of functional recovery after spinal cord injury in rats by reticulospinal-mediated motor evoked responses. *Electroencephalogr Clin Neurophysiol* 1991; 43(suppl):297–311.
90. Thompson FJ, Reier PJ, Parmer R, Lucas CC: Inhibitory control of reflex excitability following contusion injury and neural tissue transplantation. *Adv Neurol* 1993; 59:1473–1486.
91. Ford RWJ: A reproducible spinal cord injury model in the cat. *J Neurosurg* 1983; 59:268–275.

CHAPTER 103

SPINAL CORD INJURY MODELING AND OUTCOME ASSESSMENT

Bradford T. Stokes
Philip J. Horner

INTRODUCTION

Improvements in the design of devices that produce experimental spinal cord injury have vastly reduced the variability in outcome measures assessed after injury. While some controversy still exists about the best method to achieve such aims, all workers agree that monitoring of biomechanical variables during the injury process is necessary to insure reliable outcomes. The precision of such monitoring is also critical to insure that a clear distinction can be made between the contributions during the injury process of spinal tissue characteristics on the one hand and of device reliability (e.g., accurate and reproducible mechanical operation) on the other. Certain physiological factors (e.g., blood pressure, tissue stiffness, size of the subdural space, etc.) that could represent intrinsic variability in a particular model must also be assessed to make certain that their contributions to the injury process can be determined. This chapter will emphasize those modeling systems that allow control and monitoring of the relevant injury variables during rapid contusion of the spinal cord. Since one assumes that such paradigms mimic events occurring during human injury, models presented here are relevant to issues of therapeutic intervention, biomechanics, and pharmacological treatments discussed elsewhere in this text. Readers are also referred to a more detailed discussion of these modeling issues in the following reviews.[1–5]

MODELS

Extensive progress has been made in the area of spinal cord injury modeling with devices that attempt to minimize the injury-induced variability. An example of such progress using the weight-drop principle is found in Chap. 102. A careful control of vertebral column stability, monitoring of the relevant variables such as spinal cord displacement during the injury sequence, and avoidance of impounder devices that complicate assessment of injury biomechanics all characterize such advances. Here, however, we will discuss two newer generation devices that control injury biomechanics during the injury itself and therefore allow greater precision or actual determination of injury outcomes. With such control, variables of interest such as contact velocity, displacement, spinal preloading, etc. can be preset to allow a single independent variable. Other monitored variables (e.g., force) also can be used to assess tissue stiffness, preinjury meningeal stiffness, or a variety of other important injury determinants.

The first of these devices, the constrained stroke pneumatic impactor (Fig. 103-1), was pioneered by the research group in the General Motors Research Laboratories.[2,6,7] It has generally been used to injure the cervical spinal region (generally C6 or C7) with the vertebral column intact. By maintaining the normal structure of the spinal column, certain artifacts associated with a laminectomy procedure (e.g., size of laminectomy site,

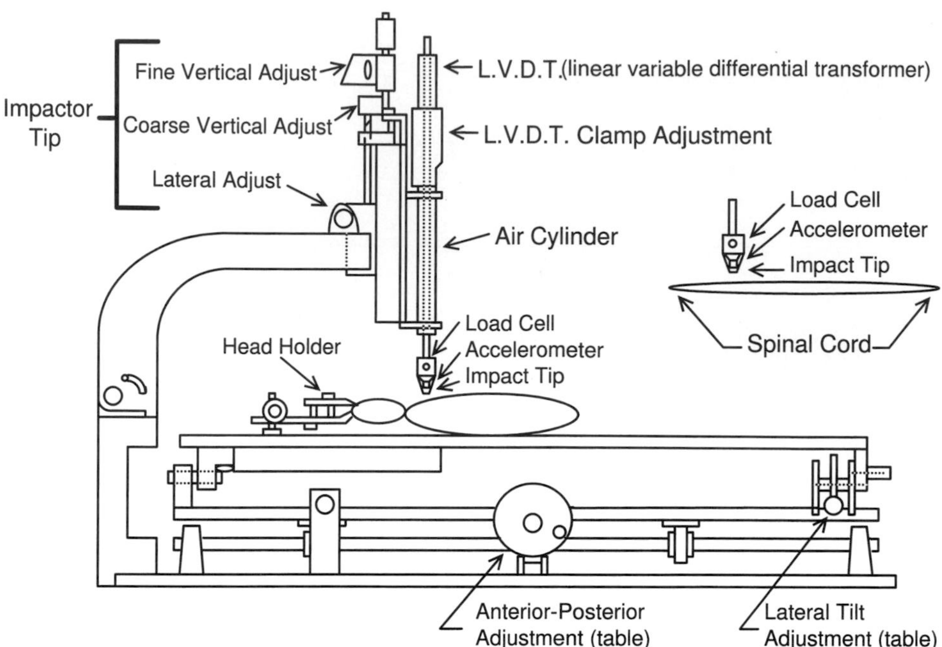

Figure 103-1. Impactor schematic shows key components of the controlled cortical impact device and head holder. Note that the table is adjustable in the horizontal plane for centering of the impactor tip; also it tilts about the rostral-caudal axis to enable lateral as well as side impacts. The impactor itself is driven by a pneumatic cylinder (the air-valving electronics are not shown), which provides control of compression velocity and duration, while the vertical adjustment provides control of amount of compression. The impactor tip incorporates an accelerometer and load cell, which enables calculation of "compensated load," that is, the actual load generated after inertial effects of the impactor mass are subtracted. The LVDT provides accurate tracking of the deformation of the tissue itself.

etc.) are thus avoided, and close approximation of the human injury process is achieved. The technique allows independent control of either rate or magnitude of vertebral displacement. Alternative methodologies to this pneumatic device are limited but include a system developed at the Ohio State University that allows a range of independent variables to be predetermined (i.e., probe velocity, displacement, preload duration and magnitude, starting point biomechanics, etc.). The device has been used for a wide variety of studies over the last decade that collectively support the hypothesis that quantifiable and reproducible injuries are possible in rodents.[2,4,8,9] Furthermore, by using sensitive monitoring devices in the current open-loop device configuration, it has been possible to monitor essential elements of the biomechanical tissue response during the injury process.[4,5,10] Inadequate biomechanical information provided by weight drop devices during this period of time is thus largely avoided.[1,2,11–13] The definition of the inherent biomechanical characteristics of the tissues being compressed or injured by the advancing probe under these circumstances is therefore possible and should provide an understanding of how various tissue compartments might be differentially affected by the injury process.

DEVICE DESIGN

Each of the injury devices are designed to meet specific experimental requirements. In the case of the General Motors device, the instrument was constructed to mimic head and spinal injuries produced by high-speed motor vehicle accidents. When used to produce such spinal injuries, the pneumatically controlled shaft of an impounder arm is adjusted by a crosshead frame to control the amount of vertebral dislocation (see Fig. 103-1). Solenoid devices independently control the rate (0.5 to 7 m/sec) and degree (10 to 75 percent compression) of displacement of the impactor with a reasonable degree of reproducibility (+/− 5 percent). Duration of compression can also be preselected from 10 msec to several seconds. Testing has revealed that the rate of compression is constant even after tissue impact, and thus a constant velocity of impactor movement after vertebral contact can be achieved. Outcome measures also have been assessed to insure that adjustments in injury severity result in the predicted variety of injury deficits as discussed below.

In practice, use of the Ohio State device is simplified

by recent design innovations. Figure 103-2*A* presents a schematic of the new injury device and a rat spinal cord lesion reconstructed at 3 months post-injury. The entire design was based on previous successes with earlier versions of the device. The present configuration has been simplified to allow for more general use of the instrument. In this latest version, displacement is precisely controlled and the open-loop feedback from the force transducer is used to assess the variability of stiffness in the spinal compartment. Depending on the nature of the injury paradigm, the researcher selects one of four modes of impactor operation. The repeat-hit is used for probe adjustment with no animal present and the single-hit mode is used for actually making the injuries. Alternatively, the touch mode provides dural surface sensing, and the force calibration setting is used as its name indicates.

During injury production (hit mode), the power amplifier (Ling shaker) produces a rapid movement of transducer elements, detectors, and the impactor probe to a position approximately 1.0 mm from the start point in approximately 8 to 10 msec. The assembly then contacts a mechanical stop. An adjustable stop nut on the threaded shaft of the driver provides necessary adjustment of the positive stop to allow various displacement ranges (0.6 to 1.2 mm) and, thus, injury magnitudes. Sensing devices include a number of transducer elements used to measure the force and displacement variables accurately during the injury sequence. The impedance head attached to the impactor probe contains two transducers: (1) a rugged piezoelectric force transducer and (2) an accelerometer. As is evident from Fig. 103-2*A*, the signal from the accelerometer is subtracted from the total force signal to correct for the component of force used to accelerate the mass of the impactor shaft (i.e., mass ahead of the force gauge). The removal of this small amount of force therefore allows a true measure of the force transmitted to the spinal compartment. The third transducer is a no-contacting type displacement transducer that is mounted above the stop-nut assembly and that uses a separate aluminum disk as its target. Charge amplifiers collect all the signals from the transducers and distribute them to an A/D converter for appropriate storage in computer files. Impulse, velocity, power, and energy are calculated off-line from the displacement or force data and stored in disk memory. The pattern generator has been considerably simplified from the original design.[12] It now works in open-loop configuration and is the source of the impact signal for the power amplifier. It allows for electronic centering of the probe via the driver and controls the amplitude, slope, and timing of the impact pattern or probe removal. Normally, such adjustments of the pattern generator are not made unless one wishes to vary signal waveforms to test hypotheses about contributions of probe velocity,

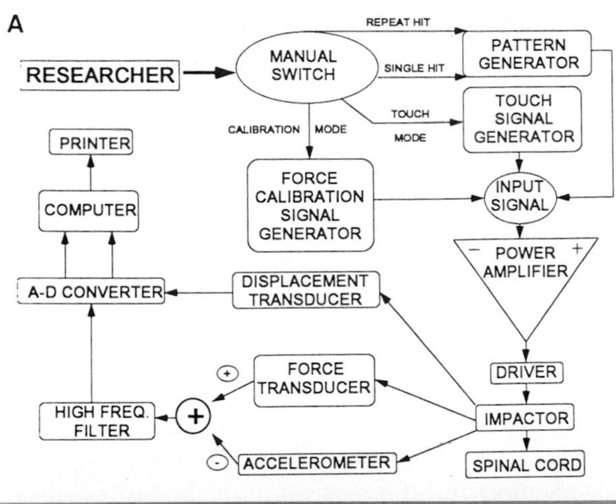

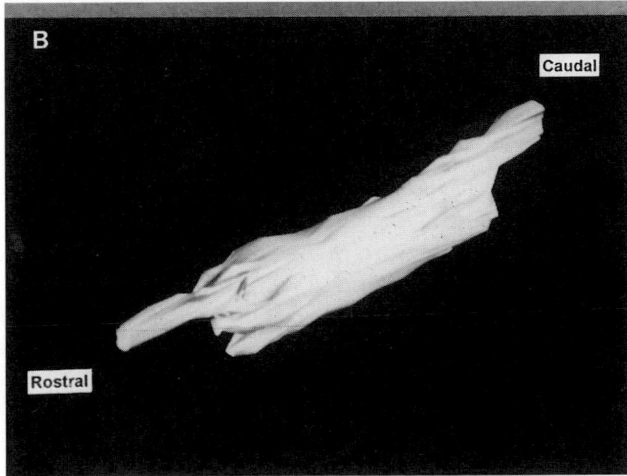

Figure 103-2. Device schematic and lesion characteristics using the Ohio State injury device. The top (*A*) illustration provides a simplified representation of the flow of information or operator decision points during its operation. Thus, by choosing the various modes of operation (repeat, single, touch, or calibration), a researcher can effect a signal output that controls the numerous phases of instrument use. The output signal from the generators is provided via a power amplifier to a powerful electromagnet (Ling shaker) that moves the impactor probe itself. Each phase of calibration, touch, or actual impact is actively sensed by the appropriate transducers that in turn allow storage of all information. *B.* A three-dimensional computer reconstruction of a contused spinal cord from an injured animal. The injury epicenter is approximately one-half the distance between the rostral and caudal poles in this 8-cm reconstruction of a spinal lesion 3 months post-injury. Injury epicenter was at T9; white and gray matter regions of individual spinal sections were traced each 500μ from counterstained paraffin sections using a microscope interface to a SUN 3260 graphics work station (CARP Software).[28]

duration of impact, or speed of probe retraction to the injury process. Calibration of the device is easily achieved with mechanical gauges whose accuracy can be checked in a number of ways.[5]

In summary, the injury device is therefore designed

for simplicity of operation. It relies on the stability and accuracy of the transducer systems and the dial gauge for overall calibration. The transducers attached to the impactor probe provide independent electrical signals proportional to the displacement and/or acceleration of the probe and force transmitted by the probe during impact. Appropriate mechanical variables are therefore independently sensed and subsequently used to judge the success of an individual impact paradigm. In practice, such a design results in surprisingly similar lesions that take on predictable three-dimensional shapes when totally reconstructed from histological sections (Fig. 103-2*B*). Note the greater amounts of destruction of tissue at the lesion epicenter in this 3-month post-lesion reconstruction and the dissection of the lesion into the base of the respective dorsal funiculi rostral and caudal to the lesion site.

Reproducibility of displacement and force profiles that produce these spinal lesions are illustrated in Fig. 103-3. Data (*A*) obtained on a single day from five spinal cords reveal the variability of these measures during a given experiment. Note the consistency of the displacement profiles, which are predetermined by the positive mechanical stop. Variance in the force profiles monitored during the same five trials demonstrates the variability of spinal cord stiffness between individual animals. In addition, results from a similar analysis performed on a different day (*B*) indicates that similar biomechanical outcomes are achieved between animal groups. Peak displacement (mm) in these groups that

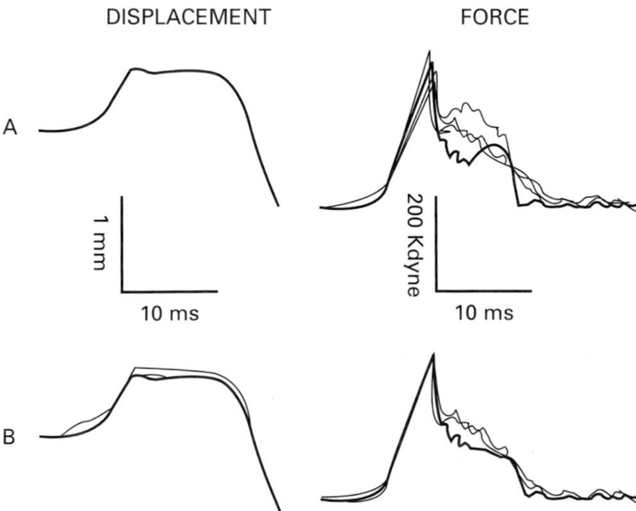

Figure 103-3. Reproducibility of displacement and force profiles using the Ohio State injury device. Data from individual animals were superimposed, using a digital oscilloscope and X–Y plotter to see how well animal data from one experiment (*A*) were reflected in those from another day 2 weeks later (*B*). Traces are in real time and magnitude.

was selected to be at 0.9 mm was actually .912 +/− .001 (SEM) in *A* and .913 +/− .001 in *B*. Peak force (Kdyne), however, was more variable because of intrinsic biomechanical differences in the spinal compartment [*A* = 269 +/− 8.2; *B* = 260 +/− 7.8). Since calibration of the device is checked daily during use, these comparisons represent fair estimates of the control of impact parameters with this particular instrument design.

INJURY BIOMECHANICS AND SOURCES OF ERROR

It has now become clear that direct shear forces probably contribute little to the axonal disruption that results from brief compression injuries. Rather, it is the brief viscoelastic distortion of tissue parenchyma away from the injury site within the meningeal compartment that results in much of the immediate damage. Thus, the control of velocity[2] is an important characteristic of devices that hope to mimic the process of human injury. A variety of biological variables (i.e., basal tension on the meninges, blood pressure, tissue hydrostatic pressure, relative size of the spinal cord or its vertebral envelope, and the placement of spinal rootlets) influence the flexibility or stiffness of the spinal compartment at rest and during the active injury process. They undoubtedly play a role in the mechanical to biological transfer function that occurs at the tip of the impactor probe. Each of these factors also could be considered sources of error in a given injury paradigm, and therefore directly affect the predictability of outcome measures.

The Ohio State device was engineered to measure some of these characteristics during the injury process by predetermining an injury variable instead of passively monitoring outcome variables, as is done during weight drop procedures. After experimenting with a closed-loop analogue computer device that allowed an assessment of these biomechanical contributors, displacement was chosen as the independent variable. As mentioned above, a mechanical stop was also added to the present device to insure the accuracy of probe movements.[5] Force feedback from transducer elements under these displacement-controlled conditions thus allows an accurate measurement of tissue characteristics before, during, and after the injury sequence.

Considerations were given in the new design to the control of each phase of the injury cycle. First, a reproducible biomechanical starting point was determined because the initial experiments revealed up to 50 percent variability in the stiffness of the meningeal envelope in different animals. It was also known that small variations (<0.1 mm) in displacement of the spinal compartment could result in large errors in outcome assessments (up to 2 points on the open-field chronic behavioral scale described below), and the small size of the laminectomy site made surface determination difficult; therefore, simply determining probe contact with the dural surface was not considered to be sufficient. Instead, the dural surface is actively sensed during minimal probe vibration ($+/- 15\mu$) and an initial start point (3000 dynes peak-to-peak) is selected by slowly advancing the probe to this position before the injury sequence is begun. The small dimpling that this produces on the dural surface does not produce detectable injury to the underlying spinal cord. Because the surface of the spinal compartment can be monitored in this way, there is no need for making a large laminectomy site, a major contributor to spinal instability during the injury process itself.

With a measured opening at a single laminectomy site and rigid fixation of the rostral and caudal vertebral processes with Allis clamps, this procedure also eliminates large movements of the vertebral column during injury. We verified this assumption using an older version of the Ohio State injury device.[14] In this configuration (closed-loop, analogue computer-controlled), a large magnitude spinal displacement paradigm (1.50 mm) was used to produce injuries. Force feedback recorded the peak force necessary to produce this displacement. The spinal cord was then removed and hemostasis achieved. The injury device was then programmed for the same peak force that was monitored during the displacement program, i.e., a force profile was predetermined for the next injury sequence. The empty, rigidly fixed spinal column was then impacted in the same way as before with the new predetermined force profile and displacement monitored. The combination of vertebral fixation and small laminectomy site in these trials limited vertebral movement to only 10 percent of its original peak displacement (<.1 mm). The latest version of the injury device utilizes displacements from 0.7 to 1.1 mm. It is estimated that vertebral column movement is a good deal less with this lower displacement range.

The Ohio State device has therefore allowed direct estimates of the contribution of some of these biomechanical factors to the injury process. Furthermore, a variety of device characteristics eliminate other sources of measurement or biological errors that determine the injury sequence. True force measurements are obtained as above by elimination of the force error introduced by the acceleration of the injury probe. Such force profiles are used to detect errors in probe displacement that might occur when the probe inadvertently strikes tissue other than spinal cord (e.g., bone or muscle) during the injury sequence. In addition, the rapid removal of the probe from the spinal surface is effected by fast reversal of the power driver. This eliminates the possibility of any secondary bounces or probe contact with the recoiling spinal compartment, a known source of error in spinal injury.[15,16] All these factors combine to allow a control of injury parameters not previously possible; the resultant determination of behavioral or neuropathological outcome measures has very small coefficients of variation. In a practical sense, this results in the ability to use small groups of animals to test various therapeutic stratagems after spinal cord injury.[9]

OUTCOME VARIABLES

A variety of outcome measures have been used to characterize the degree of spinal injury using the General Motors and Ohio State injury devices. Each device in its own way allows a unique selection of certain impact parameters to achieve experimental aims. For instance, one of the critical measures evaluated with the General Motors pneumatic device has been the somatosensory evoked response. It has been possible on the basis of such evoked potential analysis to separate axonal conduction block from the degree of hemorrhagic necrosis by selecting appropriate injury parameters.[17] The wide range of possible compression rates and the possibility of combining sustained compression with more dynamic injuries make this an instrument of choice for those who wish to model combinations of these factors in the acute and chronic injury process. Such an approach may be appropriate for those whose models require that vertebral displacement be followed by static compression, a process directly relevant to the clinical situation.

The Ohio State device has also been evaluated using a variety of outcome measures. These have included a range of histopathological assessments and behavioral evaluations. To a large degree, one assumes that control of the biomechanical properties described above results in a decrease in the variance of these outcomes. Such reasoning, however, might be flawed if the initial impact parameters were predictive only of acute injury outcomes and not those associated with delayed autolysis that might be produced by a separate set of mechanisms such as autoimmune phenomena.[18,19] This may be of particular importance when one attempts to estimate lesion volumes from biomechanical predictors.[8,9] While lesion shape is nearly biconical, as predicted from force distributions, terminal regions of the lesion distribute into the base of the dorsal funiculi rostral and caudal to the lesion site. This late-developing white matter destruction may be determined by factors other than the original injury biomechanics. It does appear, however, that although lesion shape might be modified from such changes, impact parameters as measured above are very predictive of the percentage of cross-sectional area spared at the lesion epicenter, lesion volume, and lesion length.[9]

Experience with the Ohio State device has also allowed the creation of animal groups that show both acute and chronic behavioral outcomes that are consistently predicted by the measured impact parameters and the consistency of the lesion cytopathology. This is in concert with the need for an increasing variety of methods to assess recovery of function, as has been previously described.[20,21] In this context, it is important to remember that maintaining a separation of scoring in different trials may be necessary (as opposed to an overall combination neuroscoring system), since any particular behavioral trial may correlate best with other pathophysiological changes only at a specific post-injury time.[13] We have attempted to follow such behavioral alterations in both the acute and chronic post-injury stages to allow greater precision in mechanistic approaches to therapeutic interventions. These most often are described as generalized tests of motor (or sensory-motor) function that are sometimes supplemented with other trials in specific experiments.

At Ohio State, behavioral testing after spinal injury usually begins on the first postoperative day with several different assessments: (1) a modified Tarlov scale to indicate general locomotor abilities; (2) an inclined plane test sensitive to postural abilities; and (3) a grid-walking test designed to assess tactile and proprioceptive abilities. Variations on these general schemes include the videotaping of animals crossing a static beam (gait analysis) or reaching with forelimbs for food rewards after cervical cord lesions.[22,23] The first three of these are emphasized here since they have become somewhat standardized in most laboratories and are relatively simple to perform.

The open-field scoring assessment has become the most reliable, albeit somewhat subjective, way to characterize general motor behavior after spinal injury. It is currently being made even more quantifiable for use in the MASCIS pharmacological trials in experimental spinal cord injury. Generally animals are adapted to the test equipment, and on two separate days prior to surgery and behavioral pretests are conducted and scored. Open-field walking is graded on a modified Tarlov scale from 0 to 5—0 representing flaccid paralysis and 5 a normal gait and base of support without toe drags.[24–26] As indicated in Table 103-1, an updated variation of this general theme has allowed more discriminative assessment of hindlimb motor capacities.

Two examiners, blind to the various groups to be tested, score all animals every 2 to 4 days post-injury for the first week post-injury and weekly thereafter. A second test, inclined plane analysis, tests the animals' ability to compensate posturally for displacement in space. The animal is placed in three positions (head up, right side up, and left side up) and scored as an average for the three positions. The third examination, designated as grid walking (GW) analysis, tests the animals' ability to properly place the hindlimbs on grid bars during locomotion. This test requires fore- and hindlimb coordination, and therefore hindlimb support is necessary before this behavioral test can be used. The animal is placed on a wire mesh (4 × 4 cm grid spaces) for 3-minute periods, and the number of hindfoot falls through the mesh is recorded. The quotient of footfalls per second of ambulation is used as the final measure of this task. If the animals accumulate less than 30 s of locomotion time, the test is repeated. Animals are evaluated on postoperative days 3, 8, 14, and 21 for this and for the inclined plane test. If injury parameters are carefully selected (see discussion of Ohio State device above), it is possible to create distinct populations of experimental animals that show a titering of behavioral responses according to injury severity (Fig. 103-4).

Nonparametric statistics (e.g., Kruskall-Wallis ANOVA) are used to analyze open-field scores. Standard repeated-measures ANOVA and post hoc comparisons are used for other measures as necessary. In this way, a highly reproducible analysis of motor capacities may be conducted in partially injured subjects and the outcome measures evaluated for positive or negative effects after therapeutic interventions. These behavioral

TABLE 103-1 Open Field Walking Scale

Score	Description
0	No spontaneous movement
	0.7 Slight movement
1	Movement in the hip and/or knee, none at ankle
	1.3 Active movement at hip or knee, none at ankle
	1.7 Questionable synergy at ankle
2	Movement of limb in all three major joints
	2.3 Attempts at support
	2.7 Support in stance only
3	Active support, uncoordinated gait
	3.3 Intermittent bouts of coordinated gait
	3.7 Lack of control of ankle or foot, walks on knuckles or on medial surface of foot
4	Coordination of forelimbs and hindlimbs in gait
	4.3 Improved hindlimb postural support, abdomen not low to ground, few toe drags
	4.7 One or two toe drags, slight unsteadiness turning at full speed
5	Normal gait and base of support, no loss of balance on fast turns, no toe drags

SOURCE: *Experimental Neurology,* 1993; 119:258–267.

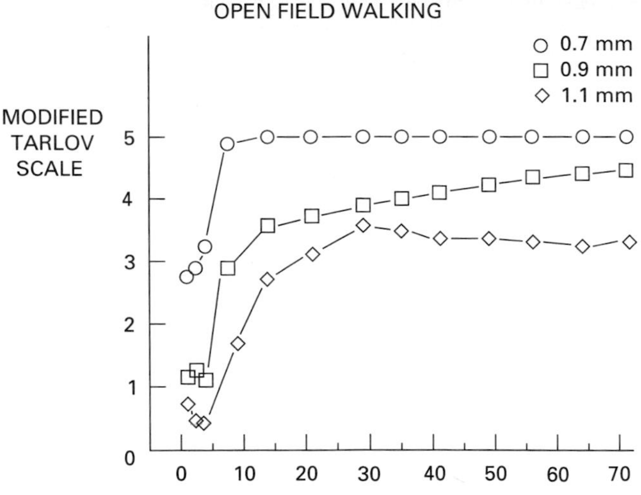

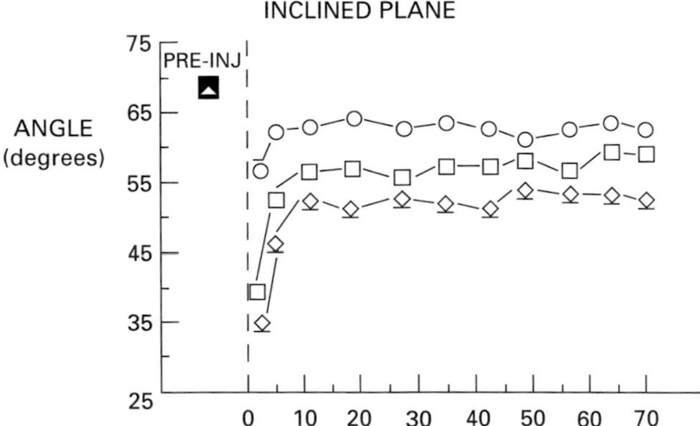

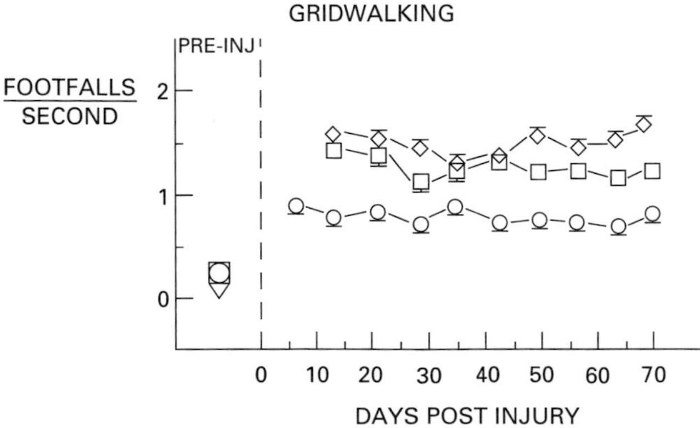

Figure 103-4. Behavioral outcomes of three groups of different injury severity. Peak displacement of the impact probe was varied (0.7, 0.9, and 1.1 mm) in an attempt to create a number of experimental populations that showed variable outcomes dependent on injury intensity. Initial outcomes were markedly different as were chronic recovery profiles for each of the behavioral characteristics assessed (open-field analysis, inclined plane stability, and grid walking footfalls). Control over small variations in peak displacement thus creates large, but predictable, changes in biological outcome measures.

approaches, however, are limited in that they fail to predict specific anatomic losses[27] and may permit masking of behavioral capacities that require the use of motivational stressors in order to be seen.

Other attempts have also been made to enhance the discrimination of behavioral trials involving spinal injured animals. Recent trials using video analysis of beam walking[22] or attempts to obtain food rewards[23] are examples of such approaches. Others have attempted a combination of food rewards and gait analysis[28] in situations that evoke a more goal-directed behavior. Such attempts, while valuable, may also be specific for only certain ranges of injury severity and may require larger numbers of animals for appropriate power analysis.[9]

The recent use of electromyography to assess the specific roles of certain muscles in hindlimb responses after spinal injury has allowed the description of even more definitive deficits.[27] The transition from such individual assessment of evoked muscle responses to behavioral tasks of longer duration has also begun with the assessment and/or conditioning of H-reflexes in the chronically injured animal.[29] The potential of long duration monitoring (24 hours or longer) is particularly promising in that the appearance of spastic limb behaviors could be characterized and potentially modified with reflex training. Finally, additional stimulus-response paradigms in awake animals that involve known descending pathways (e.g., acoustic startle) are being used to characterize loss of conductivity in these dysfunctional fiber systems.[30] Our ability to find new ways to elicit reflex responses in muscles affected by these injuries and to adopt new methods of noninvasively stimulating motor responses (e.g., magnetic stimulators) undoubtedly will contribute to mechanistic explanations of a variety of present interventional strategies (e.g., transplants, pharmaceuticals, etc.) being used to modify the injury process.

SUMMARY

It is now clear that, with the devices described above, a wide and predictable range of spinal cord injuries and behavioral outcomes can be produced.[5,9,12,13,24,25,31] Force, displacement, or velocity can be chosen as the independent variable during the injury sequence, but simplicity of design favors displacement paradigms. It is also of importance to verify the contact velocity in a given model, however, since Kearney et al.[2] have shown that at higher velocities shear forces can play an appreciable role in the injury process.

Much work has therefore been directed at reducing, if

not eliminating, many of the major design disadvantages found in earlier methods of spinal injury. One can avoid the use of weight drop height as a predictor of subsequent outcomes and eliminate the adverse effects documented by others due to post-impact bounce and tube friction.[15,16] The addition of touch circuitry in the Ohio State device has also allowed a determination of a known starting point for subsequent impact paradigms, a factor that contributes greatly to injury consistency and reliability. Furthermore, monitoring of two mechanical parameters (displacement and force) is necessary to insure a reliable hit paradigm and to give information about the variability in stiffness of the individual spinal compartments.[32]

In this review, a number of relatively simple impact devices have been described; these are constructed from readily available components and produce controllable injuries in a realistic time frame. Such devices provide the needed degree of precision and impact strength to apply such techniques to a range of species and impact parameters to mimic injuries that might occur in the human population. They also provide the flexibility to predetermine temporal characteristics of injury paradigms in a more precise way than previously possible. Each in its own way is therefore preferred for the study of the changes in spinal biomechanics that occur during contusion injury in experimental populations.

REFERENCES

1. Panjabi MM, Wrathall JR: Biomechanical analysis of experimental spinal cord injury and functional loss. *Spine* 1988; 13:1365.
2. Kearney PA, Ridella SA, Viano DC, Anderson TE: Interaction of contact velocity and cord compression in determining the severity of spinal cord injury. *J Neurotrauma* 1988; 5:187.
3. Blight A: Mechanical factors in experimental spinal cord injury. *J Am Paraplegia Soc* 1988; 11:26.
4. Stokes BT: Experimental spinal cord injury: A dynamic and verifiable injury device. *J Neurotrauma* 1992; 9(2):129.
5. Stokes BT, Noyes DH, Behrmann DL: An electromechanical spinal injury device with dynamic sensitivity. *J Neurotrauma* 1992; 9:187.
6. Anderson TE: A controlled pneumatic technique for experimental spinal cord contusion. *J Neurosci Methods* 1982; 6:327.
7. Anderson TE: Effects of acute alcohol intoxication on spinal cord vascular injury. *CNS Trauma* 1986; 3:183.
8. Bresnahan JC, Beattie MS, Stokes BT, Conway KM: Three-dimensional computer-assisted analysis of graded contusion lesions in the spinal cord of the rat. *J Neurotrauma* 1991; 8(2):91.
9. Behrmann DL, Bresnahan JC, Beattie MS, Shah BR: Spinal cord injury produced by consistent displacement of the cord in rats: Behavioral and histological analysis. *J Neurotrauma* 1992; 9(3):197.
10. Anderson TE, Stokes BT: Experimental models for spinal cord injury research: Physical and physiological considerations. *J Neurotrauma* 1992; 9(suppl 1):S135.
11. Molt JT, Nelson LR, Poulos DA, Bourke RS: Analysis and measurement of some sources of variability in experimental spinal cord trauma. *J Neurosurg* 1979; 50:784.
12. Noyes DH: An electromechanical impactor for producing experimental spinal cord injury in animals. *Med Biol Eng Comp* 1987; 25:335.
13. Beattie MS, Stokes BT, Bresnahan JC: Experimental spinal cord injury: Strategies for acute and chronic intervention based on anatomic, physiologic and behavioral studies, in Stein DG, Sabel BA (eds): *Pharmacologic Approaches to the Treatment of Brain and Spinal: Cord Injury.* New York: Plenum Publishing, 1988:43.
14. Somerson SK: *Analysis of an Electro-mechanical Spinal Cord Injury Device.* Columbus: The Ohio State University, Thesis, 1986.
15. Koozekanani SH, Vise WM, Hashemi RM, McGhee RB: Possible mechanisms for observed pathophysiological variability in experimental spinal cord injury by the method of Allen. *J Neurosurg* 1976; 44:429.
16. Ford RW: A reproducible spinal cord injury model in the cat. *J Neurosurg* 1983; 59:268.
17. Anderson TE: Spinal cord injury: Experimental dissociation of hemorrhagic necrosis and subacute loss of axonal conduction. *J Neurosurg* 1985; 62:115.
18. Popovich PG, Streit WJ, Stokes BT: Differential expression of MHC Class II antigen in the contused rat spinal cord. *J Neurotrauma* 1993; 10:37.
19. Popovich PG, Reinhard JF, Jr., Flanagan EM, Stokes BT: Elevation of the neurotoxin quinolinic acid occurs following spinal cord trauma. *Brain Res* 1994; 633:348.
20. Goldberger ME, Bregman BS, Vierck CJ, Jr., Brown M: Criteria for assessing recovery of function after spinal cord injury: Behavioral methods. *Exp Neurol* 1990; 107:113.
21. Goldberger ME: The use of behavioral methods to predict spinal cord plasticity. *Res Neurol Neurosci* 1991; 2:339.
22. Kunkel-Bagden E, Bregman BS: Spinal cord transplants enhance the recovery of locomotor function after spinal cord injury at birth. *Exp Brain Res* 1990; 81:25.
23. Schrimsher GW, Reier PJ: Forelimb motor preformance following cervical spinal cord contusion injury in the rat. *Exp Neurol* 1992; 117:287.
24. Bresnahan JC, Beattie MS, Todd FD, 3d., Noyes DH: A behavioral and anatomical analysis of spinal cord injury produced by a feedback-controlled impaction device. *Exp Neurol* 1987; 95:548.
25. Somerson SK, Stokes BT: Functional analysis of an electromechanical spinal cord injury device. *Exp Neurol* 1987; 96:82.
26. Behrmann DL, Bresnahan JC, Beattie MS: A comparison of YM-14673, U-50488H, and Nalmefene after spinal cord injury in the rat. *Exp Neurol* 1993; 119:258.

27. Gruner JA, Wade CK, Menna G, Stokes BT: Myoelectric evoked responses versus locomotor recovery in chronic spinal cord injured rats. *J Neurotrauma* 1993; 10:327.
28. Stokes BT, Reier PJ: Fetal grafts alter chronic behavioral outcome after contusion damage to the adult rat spinal cord. *Exp Neurol* 1992; 116:1.
29. Wolpaw JR, Carp JS: Adaptive plasticity in spinal cord. *Adv Neurol* 1993; 59:163.
30. Akino M, Stokes BT: Acoustic startle responses (ASR) as an index of recovery after spinal cord injury in the rat. *J Neurotrauma* 1994; (abstract) 11:1:101.
31. Noyes DH: Correlation between parameters of spinal cord impact and resultant injury. *Exp Neurol* 1987; 95:535.
32. Noyes DH, Bresnahan JC: Spinal cord lesion volume and impact parameters. *Biophys J* 1981; 33:93a.

Injury Mechanisms and Therapies

CHAPTER 104

FREE RADICALS AND LIPID PEROXIDATION

Edward D. Hall

INTRODUCTION

After CNS trauma, neural degeneration occurs through a combination of primary and secondary mechanisms. While primary mechanical disruption of CNS parenchyma and blood vessels is obviously important, much of the neural injury that follows blunt injury to the brain or spinal cord is due to a cascade of neurochemical and pathophysiological events set in motion by the primary mechanical insult. Clinical support for this concept has been provided by the results of the second National Acute Spinal Cord Injury Study (NASCIS II) which showed that treatment of spinal cord-injured patients beginning within the first 8 hours post-injury with a 24-hour dosing regimen of the glucocorticoid steroid methylprednisolone produces a significant improvement in neurological recovery over a 6- or 12-month follow-up.[1,2] Thus, the fact that an acute pharmacological treatment can modify the neurological course implies that there is indeed a modifiable secondary neurodegenerative process that is triggered by the initial injury. This secondary injury process involves a complex interplay of multiple mechanisms. Available evidence suggests that the principal players are excessive release of the excitatory amino acid neurotransmitter glutamate (Chap. 106), intracellular calcium overload (Chap. 107), activation of the arachidonic acid cascade, and the induction of oxygen free radical-induced lipid peroxidation. It is important to note that these processes are interwoven with positive feedback loops serving to amplify the preceding events.

There is now extensive experimental support for the early occurrence and pathophysiological importance of oxygen radical formation and cell membrane lipid peroxidation in the injured nervous system.[3–7] The radical-initiated peroxidation of neuronal, glial, and vascular cell membranes and myelin is catalyzed by free iron released from hemoglobin, transferrin, and ferritin by either lowered tissue pH or oxygen radicals. Lipid peroxidation is a geometrically progressing process that spreads over the surface of the cell membrane, causing impairment to phospholipid-dependent enzymes, increased membrane permeability, disruption of ionic gradients, and, if severe enough, membrane lysis.

The purpose of this chapter is to review the evidence for the involvement of free radicals in acute CNS injury and their relationship to other secondary degenerative mechanisms and specific pathophysiological events. Much of this information has been obtained from investigations demonstrating the protective efficacy of oxygen radical scavengers and lipid antioxidant agents in experimental models of acute spinal cord or head injury. However, it is important first to provide a mechanistic understanding of the basics of free radical biochemistry, the sources of oxygen radicals in the injured nervous system, and the initiation and propagation phases of membrane lipid peroxidation.

CHEMISTRY OF FREE RADICAL PRODUCTION AND LIPID PEROXIDATION

Superoxide Radical

The chemistry of oxygen free radical production and the process of lipid peroxidation have been extensively reviewed.[3,5,8,9] Only those aspects of oxygen radical production and lipid peroxidation that are key to a discussion of their involvement in CNS trauma will be considered here.

The primary radical for initial consideration is superoxide ion (O_2^-). Within the injured nervous system, a number of possible sources of superoxide radical may be operative within the first minutes and hours after injury, including: the arachidonic acid cascade (i.e., prostaglandin synthase and 5-lipoxygenase activity); enzymatic of autoxidation of biogenic amine neurotransmitters (e.g., dopamine, norepinephrine, 5-hydroxytryptamine); mitochondrial leak; xanthine oxidase activity; and the oxidation of extravasated hemoglobin. Perhaps over the first few post-injury hours and days, activated microglia and infiltrating neutrophils and macrophages provide additional sources of superoxide.

Superoxide, which is formed by the single electron reduction of oxygen, may act as either an oxidant or reductant. While superoxide itself is reactive and can, for example, reduce Fe^{III} to Fe^{II} [8] or cause the release of Fe^{II} from ferritin,[10] its direct reactivity toward biological substrates in aqueous environments is questioned.[9] Moreover, once formed, superoxide undergoes spontaneous dismutation to form H_2O_2 in a reaction that is markedly accelerated by the enzyme superoxide dismutase (SOD).[11]

$$\begin{array}{c}\text{SOD} \rightarrow \\ O_2^- + O_2^- + 2H^+ \rightarrow H_2O_2 + O_2\end{array}$$

In solution, superoxide actually exists in equilibrium with the hydroperoxyl radical ($HO_2^{\cdot}$).

$$O_2^- + H^+ \rightarrow HO_2^{\cdot}$$

The pKa of this reaction is 4.8 and the relative concentrations of O_2^- and $HO_2^{\cdot}$ depends on the H^+ concentration. Therefore, at a pH around 6.8, the ratio of $O_2^-/HO_2^{\cdot}$ is 100/1, whereas at a pH of 5.8, the ratio is only 10/1. Thus, under conditions of tissue acidosis of a magnitude known to occur within the severely injured nervous system, a significant amount of the superoxide formed will exist as hydroperoxyl radical.

Compared with superoxide, $HO_2^{\cdot}$ is considerably more lipid soluble and is a far more powerful oxidizing or reducing agent.[9] Therefore, as the pH of a solution falls and the equilibrium between O_2^- and $HO_2^{\cdot}$ shifts in favor of $HO_2^{\cdot}$, superoxide becomes more reactive, particularly toward lipids. In addition, while the dismutation of O_2^- to H_2O_2 is exceedingly slow at or near neutral pH in the absence of SOD, $HO_2^{\cdot}$ will dismutate to H_2O_2 far more readily at acidic pH values, since the rate constant for $HO_2^{\cdot}$ dismutation is on the order of 10^8 times greater than for O_2^-. Thus, in an acidic environment, O_2^- is: (1) converted to the more reactive, more lipid soluble $HO_2^{\cdot}$ and (2) its rate of dismutation to H_2O_2 is greatly increased.

Iron and Formation of Hydroxyl Radical

The CNS is an extremely rich source of iron and its regional distribution varies in parallel with the sensitivity of various regions to in vitro lipid peroxidation.[12] Under normal circumstances, low molecular weight forms of redox active iron in the brain are maintained, as in other tissues, at extremely low levels. Extracellularly in plasma, the iron transport protein transferrin tightly binds iron in the Fe^{III} form. Intracellularly, Fe^{III} is sequestered by the iron storage protein ferritin. While both ferritin and transferrin have very high affinity for iron at neutral pH and effectively maintain iron in a noncatalytic state,[10] both proteins readily give up their iron at pH values of 6.0 or less. In the case of ferritin, its iron can also be released by reductive mobilization by O_2^-.[13,14] Once iron is released from ferritin or transferrin it can actively catalyze oxygen radical reactions.[14] Therefore, within the traumatized CNS environment, where pH is typically lowered, conditions are favorable for the potential release of iron from storage proteins.

A second source of catalytically active iron is hemoglobin. Hemorrhage resulting from mechanical trauma is an obvious source of hemoglobin. While hemoglobin itself has been reported to stimulate oxygen radical reactions,[15] it is more likely that iron released from hemoglobin is responsible for hemoglobin-mediated lipid peroxidation. Iron is released from hemoglobin by H_2O_2 or by lipid hydroperoxides (LOOH),[16] and this release is further enhanced as the pH falls to 6.5 or below. Therefore, hemoglobin may catalyze oxygen radical formation and lipid peroxidation either directly or through the release of iron by H_2O_2, LOOH, and/or acidic pH.

Free iron or iron chelates participate in free radical reactions at two levels. First of all, the autoxidation of Fe^{II} results in the formation of O_2^-:

$$Fe^{II} + O_2 \rightarrow Fe^{III} + O_2^-$$

The reverse reaction or reduction of Fe^{III} to Fe^{II} by O_2^- also occurs and competes with the dismutation of O_2^- for available O_2^-. In theory, Fe^{II} autoxidation could result in the redox cycling of iron due to the reaction of O_2^- produced with Fe^{III}. Secondly, Fe^{II} is also oxidized in the presence of H_2O_2 (Fenton's reaction) to form hydroxyl radical ($^{\cdot}OH$) or perhaps a ferryl ion (Fe^{III}-OH).

$$Fe^{II} + H_2O_2 \rightarrow Fe^{III} + {}^{\cdot}OH + OH^-$$
$$Fe^{II} + H_2O_2 \rightarrow Fe^{III}OH + OH^-$$

Either $^{\cdot}OH$ or $Fe^{III}OH$ are extraordinarily potent initiators of lipid peroxidation.

Peroxynitrite-Mediated Hydroxyl Radical Formation

Another mechanism of hydroxyl radical formation has recently been identified.[17,18] It is known that endothelial cells, neutrophils, macrophages, and microglia can produce two radicals, superoxide and nitric oxide ($^{\cdot}NO$), from nitric oxide synthetase. The two species can combine to form peroxynitrite anion ($OONO^-$). The peroxynitrite will then undergo protonation (pKa = 6.8), thus becoming peroxynitrous acid (ONOOH). However, ONOOH is an unstable acid that can readily decompose to give hydroxyl radical and nitrogen dioxide ($^{\cdot}NO_2$).

$$O_2^{\bar{\cdot}} + {}^{\cdot}NO \rightarrow ONOO^- + H^+ \rightarrow ONOOH \rightarrow {}^{\cdot}NO_2 + {}^{\cdot}OH$$

Via this mechanism, another source of the highly reactive $^{\cdot}OH$ may be operative within the injured CNS. Moreover, $^{\cdot}NO_2$ may similarly initiate lipid peroxidation or nitrate and inactivate cellular proteins. A particularly attractive aspect of this scenario is that peroxynitrite has a relatively long half-life and thus is potentially more diffusible compared with either superoxide or $^{\cdot}OH$. Therefore, it may offer a mechanism by which free radical damage may occur at a site remote from the actual location of oxygen radical formation. Figure 104-1 summarizes the likely sources of $O_2^{\bar{\cdot}}$ and ultimately $^{\cdot}OH$ in the injured nervous system.

Lipid Peroxidation

In addition to its role in the formation of $^{\cdot}OH$, ferryl ion ($Fe^{III}OH$) and other iron-oxygen complexes, iron also profoundly promotes the process of lipid peroxidation. Indeed, the role of iron in the initiation of lipid peroxidation has been a subject of considerable interest.[19,20] There is no question that iron catalyzes the formation of various radicals as described above. Recent studies have in fact demonstrated the early occurrence of increased $^{\cdot}OH$ levels in the injured brain.[21,22] Initiation of lipid peroxidation occurs when a radical species attacks and removes an allylic hydrogen from an unsaturated fatty acid (LH), resulting in a radical chain reaction:

$$LH + R^{\cdot} \rightarrow L^{\cdot} + RH$$

$$L^{\cdot} + O_2 \rightarrow LOO^{\cdot}$$

$$LOO^{\cdot} + LH \rightarrow LOOH + L^{\cdot}$$

Once lipid peroxidation begins, iron may participate in driving the process as lipid hydroperoxides (LOOH) formed through initiation are decomposed by reactions with either Fe^{II}, Fe^{III}, or their chelates:

$$LOOH + Fe^{II} \rightarrow LO^{\cdot} + OH^- + Fe^{III}$$

$$LOOH + Fe^{III} \rightarrow LOO^{\cdot} + Fe^{II}$$

Both of the reactions of LOOH with iron have acidic pH optima.[23] During in vitro lipid peroxidation, the major pathway for oxidation of Fe^{II} appears to be decomposition of LOOH. Either alkoxyl ($LO^{\cdot}$) or peroxyl ($LOO^{\cdot}$) radicals arising from LOOH decomposition by iron can initiate so-called lipid hydroperoxide-dependent lipid peroxidation resulting in chain branching reactions:

$$LOO^{\cdot} + LH \rightarrow LOOH + L^{\cdot}$$

or

$$LO^{\cdot} + LH \rightarrow LOH + L^{\cdot}$$

Thus, in a membrane, lipid peroxidation need not be initiated by a primordial inorganic oxygen radical,

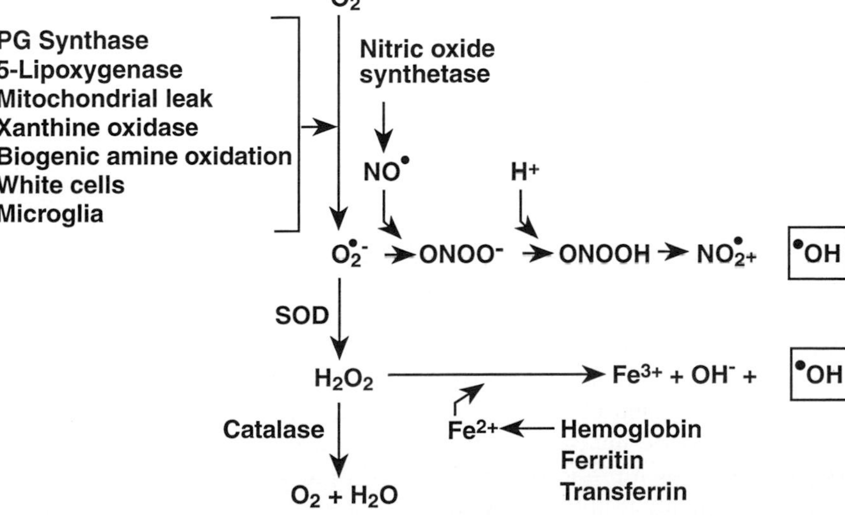

Figure 104-1. Sources of superoxide ($O_2^{\bar{\cdot}}$) and hydroxyl ($^{\cdot}OH$) radicals in the injured central nervous system.

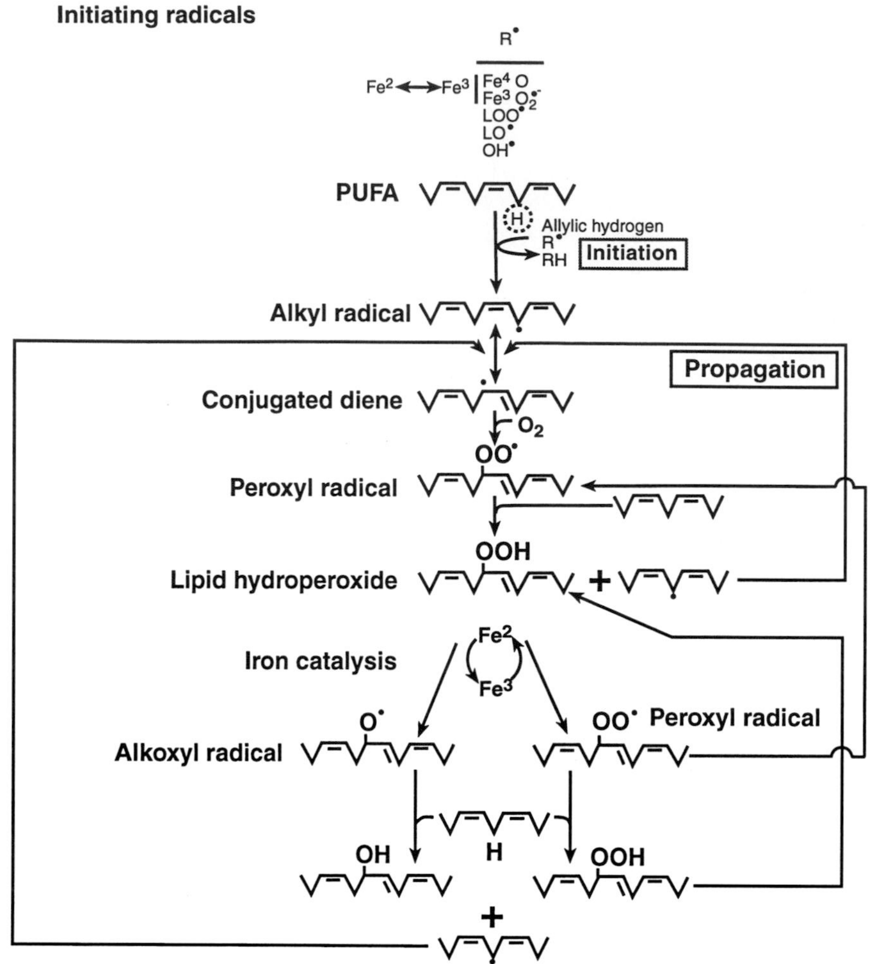

Figure 104-2. Chemistry of the initiation and propagation phases of cell membrane lipid peroxidation.

provided that LOOH and a source of iron are available. In that regard, the presence of pre-existing LOOH within normal healthy cell membranes is a subject for consideration. One would suspect that cells would not have evolved defense mechanisms against radical damage and lipid peroxidation (e.g., superoxide dismutase, catalase, glutathione reductase) unless a need existed. During normal cellular energy metabolism, oxygen radicals and H_2O_2 are produced, and estimated steady state concentrations are on the order of 10^{-9} M or higher, depending on the tissue and radical in question.[9] Thus, unless cellular defenses against radical production and damage are 100 percent efficient, a certain fraction of radicals would be expected to escape cellular scavenging processes and result in lipid peroxidation. Indeed, it has been proposed that oxidation of fatty acids within membranes and their hydrolysis by phospholipases is involved in the normal turnover of membrane lipid.[24,25] From the standpoint of lipid peroxidation during CNS trauma, it may be unnecessary to distinguish between true initiation by a primordial radical and lipid hydroperoxide-dependent lipid peroxidation, since sufficient LOOH may pre-exist in normal membranes to allow for the latter to occur.[26] Figure 104-2 displays in graphic form the initiation and propagation phases of membrane lipid peroxidation.

A final point concerning free radicals and lipid peroxidation should be noted before considering their specific role in CNS injury. Central nervous tissue appears to provide an especially avid environment for the occurrence of oxygen radical generation and uncontrolled lipid peroxidative reactions. Reasons for this include a high content of iron in many brain regions[12] and a high proportion of membrane phospholipids containing such polyunsaturated fatty acids as linoleic acid (18:2) and arachidonic acid (20:4) that are sensitive to peroxidation.

OXYGEN RADICAL MECHANISMS IN SPINAL CORD INJURY

Perhaps the most convincing body of information concerning the occurrence of oxygen radical-induced lipid

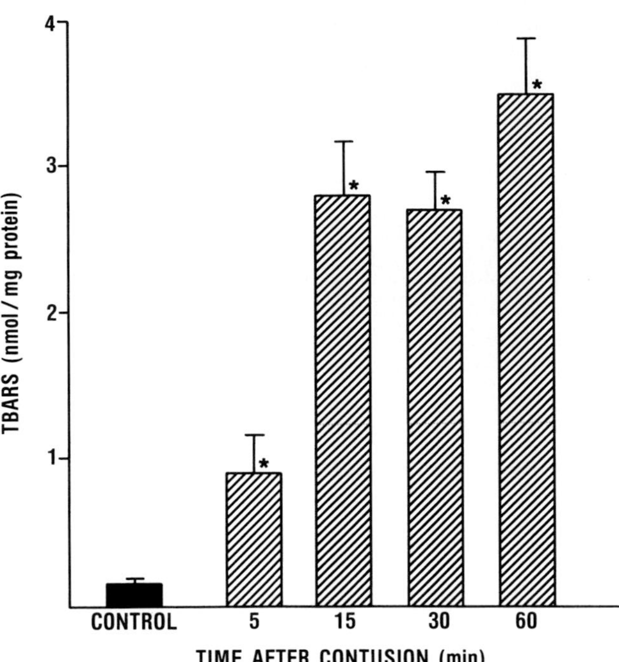

Figure 104-3. Time course of lipid peroxidation in segments of whole cat spinal cord subjected to a moderately severe (400 g-cm) contusion injury. TBARS = thiobarbituric acid reactive substances, mainly malonyldialdehyde. Values = means ± standard error. Asterisks indicate $p < 0.05$ vs. control uninjured spinal cord. Spinal cord tissue was removed from separate groups of animals at the indicated times after injury, homogenized, incubated at 37°C for 60 minutes and lipid peroxidation products measured. (From Hall[6] with permission.)

peroxidation has been gleaned from studies on experimental acute spinal cord injury. As discussed above, the injured CNS provides a fertile environment for the generation of oxygen radical and lipid peroxidation reactions. Biochemical indices of early oxygen radical reactions in the injured spinal cord (contusion or compression injuries) include: an increase in polyunsaturated fatty acid oxidation products such as malonyldialdehyde,[27–29] a decrease in tissue cholesterol and the appearance of cholesterol oxidation products[30,31]; the radical and lipid hydroperoxide-sensitive activation of guanylate cyclase and consequent increase in cGMP[27,28]; a decrease in spinal tissue antioxidant levels (e.g., alpha tocopherol, ascorbate)[32,33]; and the early inhibition of lipid peroxidation-sensitive membrane-bound enzymes such as $Na^+ + K^+$-ATPase.[34,35] Figure 104-3 shows the time course of early post-traumatic lipid peroxidation in the contused cat spinal cord. As early as 5 minutes after moderately severe contusion injury, a significant increase in lipid peroxidation products is apparent within the injured spinal cord segment.

Role in Post-Traumatic Ischemia

Strong support for a pathophysiological role of lipid peroxidative reactions has been provided by investigations showing that the pharmacological inhibition of lipid peroxidation can attenuate the development of post-traumatic spinal cord ischemia. Post-traumatic ischemia is believed to contribute to secondary spinal cord tissue degeneration.[36,37] It is caused by progressive microvascular damage and consequent impairment of microvascular autoregulation, induction of arteriolar spasm, and microthrombosis.[5,34]

The first of these investigations concerns the finding of a close correlation between the ability of a single large IV dose of the glucocorticoid steroid methylprednisolone to inhibit spinal cord lipid peroxidation[27,28] and its coincident action to retard post-traumatic hypoperfusion after severe blunt trauma.[39,40] In both cases, a 30 mg/kg IV dose was required, with lower and higher steroid doses being less effective or ineffective. Moreover, the methylprednisolone dose-response curves describing the inhibition of post-traumatic spinal lipid peroxidation and attenuation of secondary hypoperfusion are essentially identical to that describing the concomitant prevention of early post-injury lactic acid accumulation,[41] a biochemical index of post-traumatic hypoperfusion and ischemic metabolism.

Based on the atypical pharmacological characteristics of methylprednisolone's effects on the injured spinal cord (e.g., requirement for high doses), it was postulated that the steroid's antioxidant and neuroprotective actions (i.e., inhibition of lipid peroxidation and related pathophysiological events) were not dependent on glucocorticoid receptors. This led to the discovery of a novel series of 21-aminosteroids that are potent lipid peroxidation inhibitors but devoid of glucocorticoid receptor-mediated activities.[42] One of these, tirilazad mesylate (U-74006F), has been extensively examined on the development of post-traumatic spinal cord ischemia in cat models of compression and contusion-induced spinal injury.[43,44] In one of these experiments,[43] pentobarbital-anesthetized cats received a compression spinal cord injury to the exposed L3 segment followed by a single bolus injection of vehicle of U-74006F (0.3, 1, 3, or 10 mg/kg) at 30 minutes post-injury plus a second dose half the size of the first at 2.5 hrs. In vehicle-treated cats, there was the typical progressive decline in spinal white matter blood flow. By 4 hours post-injury, SCBF had decreased by 42 percent. In contrast, the 4-hour spinal blood flow in cats treated with any of the three highest dose levels of U-74006F was significantly maintained in comparison with the vehicle-treated cats. U-74006F has also been shown to retard post-traumatic ischemia development in a severe contusion injury model.[44] The mechanism of action of U-74006F in antagonizing post-traumatic ischemia development is clearly linked to an inhibition of oxygen radical-mediated microvascular lipid peroxidation based on the concomitant action of U-74006F to attenuate an injury-induced decline in spinal tissue vitamin E at the same doses that reduce post-traumatic ischemia.[43]

Additional pharmacological evidence for a role of lipid peroxidation in the development of post-traumatic spinal cord hypoperfusion comes from demonstrations that pretreatment with large doses of bona fide antioxidants can also inhibit post-traumatic hypoperfusion. For instance, pre-injury treatment for several days with large oral doses of alpha tocopherol (i.e., vitamin E)[36] or acute pretreatment with a single IV dose of ascorbic acid (i.e., vitamin C)[45] significantly limits the secondary decline in spinal blood flow after contusion injury.

Role in Post-Traumatic Axonal Degeneration

In addition to microvascular damage and consequent development of hypoperfusion in the injured spinal cord, oxygen radical-mediated lipid peroxidation also may be directly involved in the degeneration of spinal axons after injury. Studies have examined this possibility within the context of the anterograde (i.e., Wallerian) degeneration of surgically sectioned cat motor nerve fibers. Specifically, the surgical transection of cat soleus motor axons at the greater sciatic foramen, followed 48 hours later by an assessment of neuromuscular function in the in vivo soleus nerve-muscle preparation, has been shown to provide a reproducible model for the study of the early consequences of neuronal degeneration.[46] In this model, the 48-hour degenerating motor axons and nerve terminals display subtle, but important, defects in neuromuscular transmission and excitability that can be quantified by a number of functional tests. Studies with this system have shown that intensive pretreatment with methylprednisolone,[46] which possesses antioxidant activity,[38] can significantly retard the degenerative process, as evidenced by a significant neuromuscular functional preservation at 48 hours after axon section. Relative to neuronal degeneration in the injured spinal cord, the early and repeated administration of antioxidant doses of methylprednisolone has indeed been shown to result in significantly greater long-term structural preservation following blunt cord injury in cats.[47]

In subsequent experiments, an attempt was made to investigate further the possible role of lipid peroxidation in the anterograde degeneration process via pretreatment with compounds that are specific antioxidants. In one series of experiments, cats were intensively pretreated for 5 days with daily oral doses of d-alpha tocopherol (200 IU) and selenium (50 μg) prior to nerve section.This treatment was also found to significantly retard the anterograde degeneration process. A preservation of neuromuscular function was observed in terms of (1) a greater soleus muscle contractile response to low frequency nerve stimulation; (2) a better maintenance of tetanic contractile tension during high frequency nerve stimulation; and (3) a more rapid recovery from curare-induced neuromuscular block.[48]

The 21-aminosteroid U-74006F has similarly been demonstrated to slow the rate of anterograde degeneration of motor axons and nerve terminals after experimental injury in the cat soleus nerve degeneration model.[49] These results strongly suggest a fundamental mechanistic role of oxygen radical-mediated lipid peroxidation in the anterograde axonal degenerative process.

Effects of Antioxidants on Post-Traumatic Neurological Recovery

In addition to demonstrating the occurrence of acute post-traumatic oxygen radical reactions and their association with pathophysiological events, the establishment of their importance relative to other factors depends on a demonstration that with their interruption chronic neurological recovery can be enhanced. Thus, attempts have been made to show that early treatment of spinal cord-injured animals with bona fide antioxidants or agents with antioxidant properties can beneficially affect sensory and motor recovery.

In this vein, a series of experiments was conducted to examine the ability of intensive dosing with methylprednisolone begun early (30 minutes) after moderately severe spinal cord compression injury to improve chronic functional recovery and spinal tissue preservation in cats. As cited earlier, the early administration of methylprednisolone has been shown to reduce post-traumatic spinal cord lipid peroxidation.[27,30,31] Based on the dose-response and time-action characteristics of methylprednisolone, an intensive methylprednisolone dosing regimen has been tested involving an initial 30 mg/kg IV dose at 30 minutes post-injury, followed by a 48-hour maintenance dosing regimen calculated to maintain effective antioxidant spinal tissue concentrations of the steroid over that time period. The cats were then evaluated (blind) on a weekly basis for 4 weeks for walking, running, and stair climbing ability, after which histological analysis of the spinal injury site was performed. In comparison to vehicle-treated animals, the methylprednisolone-treated cats showed a significantly better recovery by 2 weeks post-injury. A reduction in 4-week post-traumatic spinal tissue loss also was observed, and its degree correlated inversely

($r = -0.88$) with the neurological recovery score.[47] These results show that a dosing regimen centered on the inhibition of post-traumatic lipid peroxidation and related processes (e.g., post-traumatic ischemia) is associated with both enhanced structural preservation and functional recovery.

The results of the second National Acute Spinal Cord Injury Study (NASCIS II) constitutes a major milestone in the search for therapeutic interventions that will interfere significantly with secondary post-traumatic spinal cord degeneration and thereby ameliorate the devastating neurological consequences of spinal cord injury,[1,2] as noted above. In that study, methylprednisolone was demonstrated to improve the 6- and 12-month recovery after spinal cord injury, compared with placebo-treated patients, when administered in an intensive 24-hour intravenous antioxidant dosing regimen that began within 8 hours after injury. The dose level and dosing regimen (30 mg/kg IV bolus plus 5.4 mg/kg/h 23-hr infusion) were derived from pharmacological investigations that focused on inhibition of post-traumatic lipid peroxidation as the therapeutic target.

The 21-aminosteroid U-74006F has also been investigated for its ability to promote neurological recovery of cats[50,51] following a moderately severe compression injury to the lumbar spinal cord. Beginning at 30 minutes after injury, the animals received a 48-hour intravenous regimen of vehicle (sterile water) or U-74006F in a random and blinded protocol similar to that employed in earlier studies with methylprednisolone.[16] Initial U-74006F doses ranged from 0.01 to 30 mg/kg. Two additional maintenance doses, half the size of the initial dose, were given at 2.5 and 6 hours after injury, followed by a 42-hour constant IV infusion. Total 48-hour doses ranged from 0.16 to 160 mg/kg. The animals were neurologically evaluated on a weekly basis for 4 weeks using an 11-point scale that graded their post-traumatic walking, running, and stair-climbing ability. At 4 weeks after injury, vehicle-treated animals uniformly remained paraplegic, with a mean recovery score of 2.2 (i.e., 20 percent of normal). In contrast, cats that received 48-hour doses of U-74006F ranging from 1.6 to 160.0 mg/kg showed significantly better recovery, regaining approximately 75 percent of normal neurological function. The 4-week recovery scores varied from 5.5 to 8.0. Additional studies in a rat model of compressive spinal injury have confirmed the beneficial effects of U-74006F on post-traumatic neurological recovery.[52,53]

Moreover, high-dose pretreatment with vitamin E (1000 IU orally once daily for 5 days) has also been shown to promote the chronic recovery of spinal cord-injured cats.[54] This is consistent with its ability to prevent post-traumatic spinal cord ischemia[36] and lipid peroxidation[30] and with the hypothesis that oxygen radical generation and lipid peroxidation are important mediators of post-traumatic spinal cord pathophysiology and degeneration.

Therapeutic Window for Inhibition of Lipid Peroxidation

Further studies suggest that the 21-aminosteroid U74006F retains its efficacy in promoting post-traumatic recovery after experimental spinal cord injury even when initiation of treatment is delayed to 4 hours post-injury.[51] However, while there is still some residual efficacy apparent when administration is withheld until 8 hours post-injury, it is much less than when treatment is begun within the first 4 hours. Thus, the opportunity for limiting the impact of post-traumatic lipid peroxidation appears to be 8 hours.

Similarity of Peroxidative and Mechanical Spinal Injuries

Additional evidence for a role of oxygen radical formation and lipid peroxidation in post-traumatic spinal cord degeneration has come from studies comparing the neuropathology of mechanical injuries with those produced by microinjection of ferrous chloride into the spinal cord.[55] While circumstantial, the similarities between the neurochemical and neuroanatomic pathology of iron and trauma-induced spinal injury in cats are striking. In both cases, the degenerative changes begin within the central gray matter and spread in a centrifugal fashion to include the surrounding white matter. Furthermore, as with studies of mechanical trauma, pretreatment with a 30 mg/kg IV dose of methylprednisolone has been shown to significantly protect against the iron-induced myelopathy.[56] Likewise, coinjection of the hydroxyl radical scavenger mannitol along with the ferrous chloride exerts a protective effect.[56]

OXYGEN RADICAL MECHANISMS IN HEAD INJURY

Time Course and Location of Oxygen Radical Formation

Multiple studies in cats subjected to fluid percussion injury have demonstrated the early generation of superoxide radicals in injured brain in terms of the colorimetrically measured reduction of nitroblue tetrazolium applied to the brain surface via a cranial window.[7,57–59] Moreover, it has been further disclosed in those studies that the generation of oxygen radicals occurs in parallel with secondary injury to the brain microvasculature and interference with cerebral blood flow autoregulation.[7,57,58] In recent work, the time course and intensity of brain ˙OH generation have been examined in male CF-1 mice during the first hour after moderate or severe concussive head injury.[21] Hydroxyl radical production has been measured using the salicylate trapping method in which the production of 2,3 and/or 2,5 dihydroxybenzoic acid (DHBA) is used as an index of brain ˙OH formation. In mice injured with a concussion of moderate severity, a 60 percent increase in ˙OH formation is observed by 1 min post-injury compared to that observed in uninjured mice. The peak in ˙OH formation occurs at 15 min post-injury (+67.5 percent). At 30 min, the increase in ˙OH loses significance, indicating that the post-traumatic rise in brain ˙OH formation is a transient phenomenon. Saline perfusion of the injured mice to remove the intravascular blood eliminates the injury-induced increase in ˙OH, but does not affect the baseline levels seen in uninjured mice. This suggests that the source of the increased ˙OH in the injured mice is the microvasculature, probably the endothelium. The administration of the 21-aminosteroid lipid antioxidant U-74006F, which possesses ˙OH scavenging properties and localizes in brain microvascular endothelium,[42,60] also attenuates the post-traumatic rise in ˙OH, further supporting the fact that the increase in ˙OH radical formation is at least initially microvascular in origin.[21] A similar, transient rise in ˙OH has also been demonstrated in the rat controlled cortical impact injury model[22] (Fig. 104-4).

Evidence for the early post-traumatic occurrence of lipid peroxidation in injured brain has recently been provided in rat head injury models. Using the lipid peroxyl radical trap phenyl-N-butyl nitrone (PBN) and electron spin resonance detection to measure peroxidation, an increase in PBN spin adducts has been seen in fluid percussion-injured brain by 5 min post-injury.[61] More recently, the highly sensitive HPLC-chemiluminescence method for measuring lipid hydroperoxides (phosphatidylcholine hydroperoxide) has been employed in the rat controlled cortical impact model to show that there is indeed a significant increase in brain lipid peroxidation as early as 5 min post-injury.[22] However, in contrast to the transient rise in ˙OH levels, the increase in lipid peroxidation continues to increase with time (Fig. 107-4).

Role in Post-Traumatic Microvascular Damage

Following moderately severe injury, there is a secondary cerebral (pial) arteriolar dilation together with a loss of normal reactivity to vasoactive agents or to maneuvers including elevations in arterial p_{CO_2} and a decline in blood pressure.[7] This occurs concomitantly with the appearance of focal endothelial lesions and a reduction in oxygen utilization by the pial vascular wall.

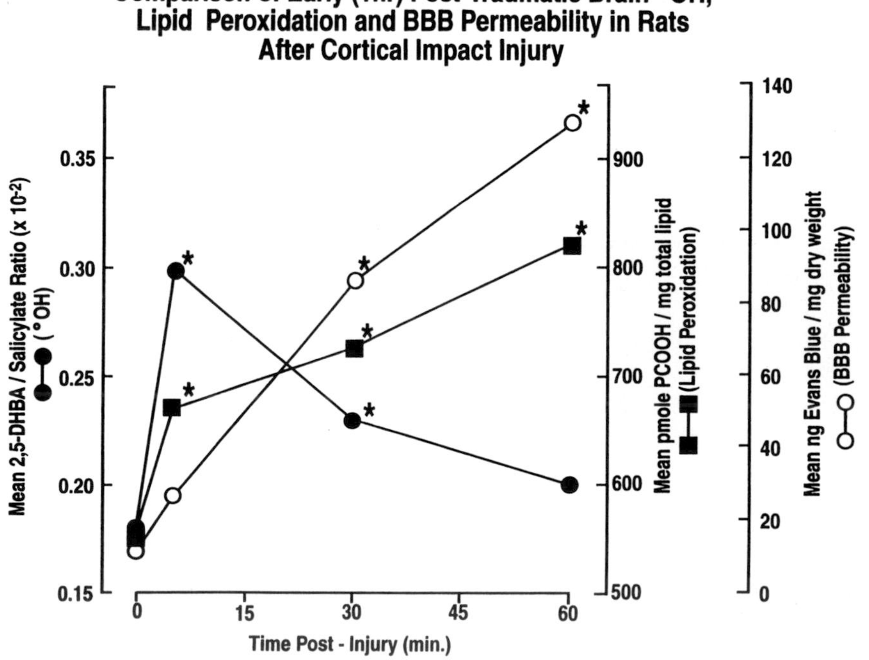

Figure 104-4. Time courses of hydroxyl radical (˙OH) formation, lipid peroxidation (phosphatidylcholine, PCOOH) and blood-brain barrier (BBB) disruption, Evan's blue extravasation following unilateral controlled cortical impact injury in rats. Values = means at each time point. Asterisks indicate $p < 0.05$ vs. sham uninjured animals. (From Smith et al.[22] with permission.)

At a biochemical level, one of the earliest effects of neural injury is activation of brain phospholipase C (PLC)[62] and a consequent rise in tissue levels of cyclooxygenase products (prostanoids) of arachidonic acid.[63] A connection between this and the post-traumatic cerebral microvascular damage is based on the observation that arachidonate or prostaglandin endoperoxide (PGG_2) application to the brain surface causes arteriolar damage similar to that following fluid percussion brain injury.[7,57] However, it is believed that the principal mediators of the microvascular damage are oxygen radicals generated as by-products of the prostaglandin synthase reaction during the conversion of arachidonate to the prostaglandins.[64] Thus, a mechanistic cascade of: (1) injury-induced PLC (and probably PLA_2) liberation of membrane arachidonate; (2) prostaglandin synthase activation and superoxide generation; and (3) oxygen radical-mediated endothelial damage has been proposed. Pharmacological support for this cascade of events has been provided by studies showing that either cyclooxygenase inhibitors (e.g., indomethacin), which would inhibit arachidonate metabolism and the associated free radical generation, or free radical scavengers (e.g., superoxide dismutase, mannitol) attenuate post-traumatic brain microvascular damage.[7,57–59]

Similarly, prostanoid levels also increase dramatically in the injured spinal cord during the first post-traumatic hour.[30,65,66] Consistent with the concept that this increase plays an important pathophysiological role is the observation that pretreatment with cyclooxygenase inhibitors such as ibuprofen and meclofenamate attenuate post-traumatic spinal cord ischemia.[36] It is conceivable that the liberated eicosanoids such as prostaglandin $F_{2\alpha}$, which is a potent vasoconstrictor, or thromboxane A_2, which is a potent vasoconstrictor and platelet aggregation promoter, play a role in the blood flow compromise. However, as in the case of head injury,[7] it is perhaps the oxygen radical burst, associated with prostanoid production,[64] that is mainly responsible for microvascular damage and blood flow compromise. In line with this is the finding that intensive antioxidant dosing[36,39,43–45] consistently limits secondary post-traumatic spinal cord ischemia.

Role in Post-Traumatic Edema

Related to the post-traumatic microvascular damage is the pathophysiological process of vasogenic brain edema that represents a disruption of blood-brain barrier integrity, resulting in brain parenchymal sodium and protein accumulation and osmotic fluid expansion of the brain extracellular space. Clinically, this is reflected by an increase in intracranial pressure, which can cause secondary compressive injury to vital brain structures.

Extensive investigations have provided data suggesting an important role for an arachidonic acid-derived oxygen radical-mediated process.[67] In vitro experiments have shown that when rat brain cortical slices are incubated with arachidonic acid, there is a transient burst of superoxide and lipid hydroperoxide formation that correlates with fluid accumulation (i.e., swelling) in the slices. Further, in vivo studies have shown that arachidonic acid injection into brain can produce vasogenic edema as measured by extravasation of the protein tracking dye Evans' blue.[67,68] In line with a role of free radical-mediated lipid peroxidation, the 21-aminosteroid lipid antioxidant U-74006F has been demonstrated to attenuate arachidonic acid-induced blood-brain barrier disruption.[68,69]

Microinjection of ferrous iron (i.e., ferrous chloride) has also been shown to produce focal vasogenic edema in rat brain, the degree of which is correlated with tissue levels of the lipid peroxidation product malonyldialdehyde. Pretreatment with vitamin E (600 mg/kg intramuscularly once daily for 5 days) together with selenium (5 ppm in the drinking water) reduced the iron-induced edema and lipid peroxidation.[70] Similarly, U74006F can also reduce iron-induced blood-brain barrier opening.[69]

Recent work clearly shows a relationship between post-traumatic free radical formation and induction of vasogenic brain edema. For example, data have been obtained from the mouse head injury model showing that severe concussive injury results in an increase in brain $^{\cdot}OH$ levels coincident with an increase in blood-brain barrier permeability.[71] Similarly, Fig. 104-4 illustrates that there is a progressive opening of the blood-brain barrier (i.e., Evans' blue extravasation) in the rat controlled cortical impact model that follows slightly behind the time course of $^{\cdot}OH$-induced lipid peroxidation. Further support for the mechanistic connection between oxygen radical formation, lipid peroxidation, and post-traumatic opening of the blood-brain barrier comes from studies with the lipid antioxidant 21-aminosteroid U-74006F. U-74006F acts to reduce post-traumatic opening of the blood-brain barrier in the mouse concussive head injury[71] and rat controlled cortical impact models.[22] Consistent with this reduction in post-traumatic blood-brain barrier opening, which would lead to vasogenic brain edema, U-74006F has been shown to attenuate post-traumatic brain edema in the rat model of fluid percussion head injury.[72]

Role in Post-Traumatic Subarachnoid Hemorrhage-Induced Vasospasm

Subarachnoid hemorrhage (SAH) is a common sequela of severe head injury that may contribute to post-traumatic ischemic neurological injury via the gradual induction of delayed vasospasm. The time course of delayed SAH-induced vasospasm correlates well with the gradual oxidation of hemoglobin within the subarachnoid blood clot which is associated with the production of oxygen radicals.[73,74] Indeed, while the pathogenesis of delayed vasospasm is likely to be multifactorial, vascular lipid peroxidation and the consequent loss of endothelium-dependent relaxation is believed to play a key role.[73] Consistent with this concept, intrathecal administration of the radical scavenger superoxide dismutase[75] or repeated systemic injection of the 21-aminosteroid lipid peroxidation inhibitor U-74006F[76–80] have been shown to decrease the magnitude of SAH-induced delayed vasospasm in experimental models. The reduction in angiographic vasospasm is correlated with a reduction in lipid peroxidation products within the subarachnoid clot.[80]

In addition to an effect of U-74006F to retard delayed spasm of the major vessels, the compound has also been shown to attenuate SAH-induced microvascular hypoperfusion during the first few hours after experimental SAH.[81] A portion of this acute maintenance of brain blood flow is attributable to a blunting of the progressive post-SAH rise in intracranial pressure.[81] This latter action is in turn paralleled by a limitation of an SAH-triggered damage to the blood-brain barrier (and associated vasogenic edema) by the 21-aminosteroid.[69] Therefore, based on extensive pharmacological evidence, it is apparent that vascular lipid peroxidation, triggered by oxygen radicals generated in the subarachnoid blood, plays an important role in three aspects of post-traumatic SAH: delayed vasospasm; acute hypoperfusion (i.e., acute vasospasm); and an increase in blood-brain barrier permeability.

Clinical support for a role of lipid peroxidation in SAH pathophysiology has also been provided. In recent Phase II[42] and Phase III[83] trials in aneurysmal SAH, an intensive dosing protocol with U-74006F (tirilazad mesylate) plus the calcium channel blocker nimodipine, beginning within the first 48 hours, has been shown to significantly decrease clinical vasospasm and mortality, and to improve the incidence of "good recovery" (Glasgow Outcome Scale) at 3 months in comparison to treatment with nimodipine alone.

Effects of Antioxidants on Post-Traumatic Neurological Recovery and Survival

As in the case of spinal cord injury discussed earlier in this chapter, the most convincing evidence of the significance of oxygen radical processes in acute head injury is obtained from published reports of the ability of early administration with free radical scavengers or antioxidants to improve post-traumatic neurological recovery and survival. In this regard, there is also evidence that the neuroprotective properties of methylprednisolone, extensively studied in spinal cord injury, are applicable to brain injury. For instance, the steroid has been shown to enhance the early recovery of mice subjected to a moderately severe concussive head injury when administered 5 min post-injury.[84] The dose-response curve for this effect is remarkably similar to that discussed above for spinal cord injury. A 30 mg/kg IV dose was observed to be optimal, while lower (15 mg/kg) and higher (60 and 120 mg/kg) doses were ineffective. However, in more severe injuries, the dose-response curve is shifted to the right such that a 60 mg/kg IV dose is required to improve early recovery.[85] This suggests that the intensity of post-traumatic lipid peroxidation, and thus the dose of an antioxidant required to block the process, is proportional to the severity of the injury.

Consistent with the beneficial effect of antioxidant doses of methylprednisolone in experimental head injury, one controlled clinical trial has shown that a high-dose regimen begun within 6 h after severe injury (Glasgow Coma Scale = 3-8) with a 30 mg/kg IV bolus can significantly increase survival and the recovery of speech.[75] However, while these data are suggestive, flaws in the study prevent it from being definitive. For instance, there were three groups of patients, a placebo group, a low-dose methylprednisolone group (100 mg IV bolus plus 8 days of tapered maintenance dosing), and the high-dose group (30 mg/kg IV bolus plus tapered dosing). There was clearly no difference between the placebo and low-dose groups, but only when these two groups were combined post-hoc and statistically compared to the high-dose group could the significant effect on survival and speech recovery be demonstrated. Furthermore, the effect was only demonstrable if those patients over 40 years of age were excluded, also post-hoc. Thus, an additional trial would be required in order to determine the efficacy of methylprednisolone in brain injury. However, one must consider that glucocorticoid dosing in head injury may be a two-edged sword. The positive edge is the inhibition of post-traumatic lipid peroxidation; the negative side is the fact that glucocorticoid dosing can produce neurotoxicity in certain neuronal populations[87] and has been documented to exacerbate ischemic neuronal injury.[88]

In that regard, experiments have demonstrated the efficacy of the nonglucocorticoid 21-aminosteroid U-74006F in acute head injury in terms of an improvement in the early neurological recovery and survival of head-injured mice.[89] This potent lipid peroxidation inhibitor has been further reported to improve post-traumatic survival[72] and neurological recovery[90] in rats subjected to moderately severe fluid percussion head injury.

Additional experiments in a cat model of severe cortical contusion injury have shown that U-74006F significantly reduces post-traumatic lactic acid accumulation in cerebral cortex and subcortical white matter.[91] This biochemical effect suggests an improved maintenance of cerebral blood flow in the injured brain. As noted above, U-74006F reduces progressive post-traumatic ischemia development in experimental cat spinal cord injury.[43,44] A similar action may provide the explanation for the reduction of post-traumatic lactate levels in the injured brain. Currently, U-74006F (tirilazad mesylate) is being examined in multi-center Phase III clinical trials to ascertain its ability to improve neurological recovery in moderate and severe head injury.

More recently, the cerebral antioxidant activity of the 21-aminosteroid U-74006F has been enhanced by replacing the steroid functionality—which possesses only weak antioxidant activity without the complex amino substitution—with a more potent and effective antioxidant. A series of compounds have been synthesized in which the steroid of U-74006F has been replaced by the antioxidant ring structure (i.e., chromanol) of alpha tocopherol (vitamin E). One of these compounds, U-78517F, has been demonstrated to have predictably more potent effects in regard to inhibition of lipid peroxidation and enhancement of early neurological recovery of head-injured mice.[92] Furthermore, an iron-chelating dextran-desferrioxamine conjugate is also protective in the mouse head injury model, underscoring the importance of iron in post-traumatic lipid peroxidative pathophysiology.[93]

Further clinical evidence of the role of free radicals in head injury has been preliminarily provided by a Phase II trial of polyethylene glycol (PEG)-conjugated SOD in severe head injury (Glasgow Coma Scale = 3-8). In the PEG-SOD-treated patients, there was a decrease in the incidence of death and persistent vegetative state at 3 or 6 months post-injury.[94] Phase III trials are in progress to assess more completely the cerebroprotective efficacy of PEG-SOD administered as a single IV dose within the first 8 post-injury hours.

SUMMARY

This chapter has reviewed the current state of knowledge regarding the occurrence and possible role of oxygen radical generation and lipid peroxidation in acute neurotrauma. Four criteria required to establish the pathophysiological importance of oxygen radical reactions have been met, at least in part. First of all, oxygen radical generation and lipid peroxidation are early biochemical events subsequent to either brain or spinal cord injury. Second, they are linked to pathophysiological processes including loss of microvascular autoregulation and hypoperfusion, SAH-induced vasospasm, vasogenic edema, failure of energy metabolism, and anterograde axonal degeneration. Third, there is a striking similarity between the pathology of blunt mechanical injury to CNS tissue and that produced by chemical induction of peroxidative injury. Fourth, and most convincing, is the repeated observation that compounds that inhibit lipid peroxidation or scavenge oxygen radicals can block post-traumatic pathophysiological processes and promote functional recovery and survival in experimental studies.

It should be kept in mind that the generation of oxygen radicals and lipid peroxidative damage to microvascular, neuronal, and glial membranes is intimately linked to excitotoxic and calcium overload mechanisms. In relation to excitotoxicity, oxygen radicals have been shown to promote glutamate release,[95] while glutamate infusion into brain has been documented to stimulate OH production.[96] Thus, excitatory amino acid release and oxygen radical formation are reciprocal post-traumatic processes. Concerning the issue of intracellular calcium accumulation (i.e., overload), several mechanisms of post-traumatic oxygen radical formation including arachidonic acid release and enzymatic oxidation and xanthine oxidase activation are triggered by increased intracellular calcium. Indeed, increased intracellular calcium produces an enhancement of oxygen radical-induced lipid peroxidation.[3] Moreover, membrane lipid peroxidation exacerbates calcium overload by enhancing calcium permeability and intracellular release[3] and by impairing the function of the membrane calcium pumping mechanisms.[97]

Figure 104-5 displays an attempt to partially integrate these and related mechanisms in the process of secondary post-traumatic tissue injury. The relative importance of oxygen radicals and lipid peroxidation in this scheme ultimately depends on whether it can be demonstrated convincingly that early application of effective anti-free radical or antiperoxidative agents can promote survival and neurological recovery after CNS injury in humans. The results of the NASCIS II clinical trial, which have shown that an antioxidant dosing regimen with methylprednisolone begun within 8 hours after spinal cord injury, can enhance chronic neurological recovery[1,2] strongly support the significance of lipid peroxidation as a post-traumatic degenerative mechanism. However, ongoing Phase III trials with the more selective and effective antioxidant U-74006F (tirilazad mesylate) and the radical scavenger PEG-SOD will give a more clear-cut answer as to the therapeutic importance of inhibition post-traumatic free radical reactions in the injured central nervous system.

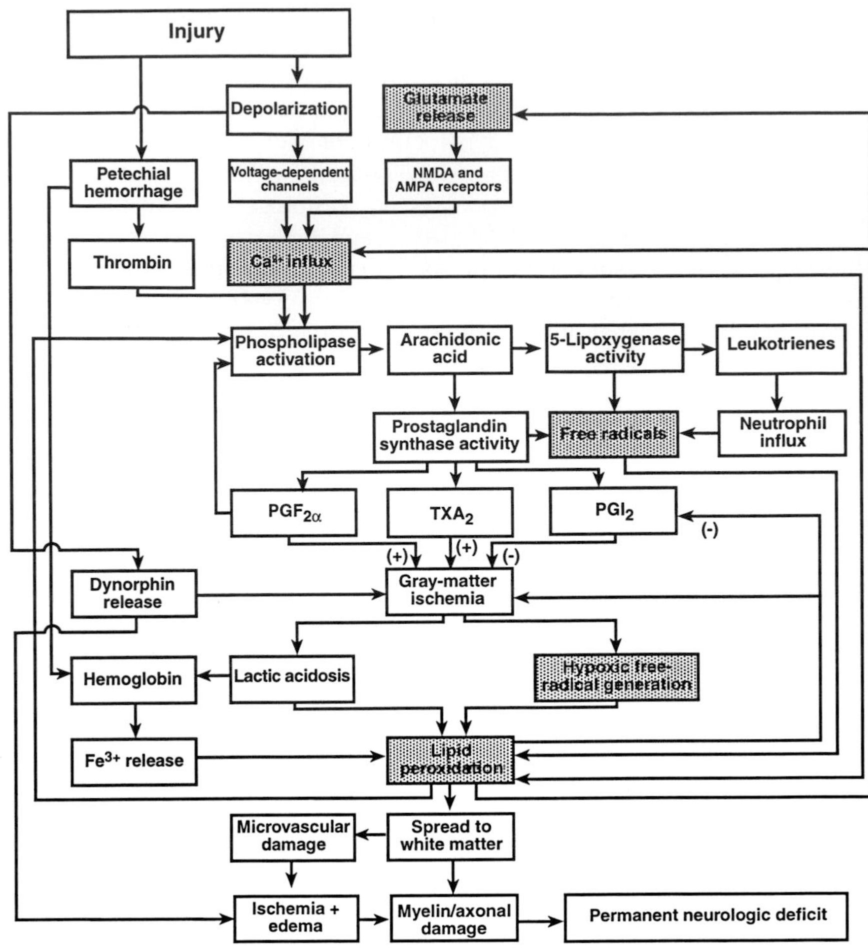

Figure 104-5. Interplay of free radical-lipid peroxidative, excitotoxic, and calcium overload mechanisms involved in secondary injury to the brain or spinal cord.

REFERENCES

1. Bracken MB, Shepard MJ, Collins WF, et al: A randomized controlled trial of methylprednisolone or naloxone in the treatment of acute spinal cord injury. *N Engl J Med* 1990; 322:1405–1411.
2. Bracken MB, Shepard MJ, Collins WF, et al: Methylprednisolone or naloxone treatment after acute spinal cord injury: 1 year follow-up data. *J Neurosurg* 1992; 76:23–31.
3. Braughler JM, Hall ED: Central nervous system trauma and stroke: I. Biochemical considerations for oxygen radical formation and lipid peroxidation. *Free Rad Biol Med* 1989; 6:289–301.
4. Hall ED, Braughler JM: Central nervous system trauma and stroke: II. Physiological and pharmacological evidence for the involvement of oxygen radicals and lipid peroxidation. *Free Rad Biol Med* 1989; 6:303–313.
5. Demopoulos HB, Flamm ES, Pietronigro DD, Seligman ML: The free radical pathology and the microcirculation in the major central nervous system disorders. *Acta Physiol Scand* 1980; 492(suppl):91–119.
6. Hall ED, Brauglher JM: Free radicals in CNS injury, in Waxman SG (ed): *Molecular and Cellular Approaches to the Treatment of Neurological Disease*. New York: Raven Press, 1993:81–105.
7. Kontos HA, Povlishock JT: Oxygen radicals in brain injury. *CNS Trauma* 1986; 3:257–263.
8. Aust SD, Morehouse LA, Thomas CE: Role of metals in oxygen radical reactions. *J Free Rad Biol Med* 1985; 1:3–25.
9. Halliwell B, Gutteridge JMC: *Free Radicals in Biology and Medicine.* Oxford: Claredon Press, 1985.
10. Gutteridge JMC: Antioxidant properties or proteins ceruloplasmin, albumin and transferrin: A study of their activity in serum and synovial fluid from patients with rheumatoid arthritis. *Biochim Biophys Acta* 1986; 869:119–127.
11. Fee JA: On the question of superoxide toxicity and the biological function of superoxide dismutases, in King TE, Mason HS, Morrison M (eds): *Oxidases and Related Redox Systems*. New York: Pergamon Press, 1982:101–149.
12. Zaleska MM, Floyd RA: Regional lipid peroxidation in rat brain *in vitro:* Possible role of endogenous iron. *Neurochem Res* 1985; 10:397–410.
13. Koster JF, Slee RG: Ferritin, a physiological iron donor for microsomal lipid peroxidation. *FEBS Lett* 1986; 199:85–88.
14. Thomas CE, Morehouse LA, Aust SD: Ferritin and superoxide-dependent lipid peroxidation. *J Biol Chem* 1985; 260:3275–3280.

15. Sadrzadeh SM, Graf E, Panter SS, et al: Hemoglobin, a biological Fenton reagent. *J Biol Chem* 1984; 259:14354–14356.
16. Gutteridge JMC: Iron promoters of the Fenton reaction and lipid peroxidation can be released from hemoglobin by peroxides. *FEBS Lett* 1986; 201:291–295.
17. Beckman JS, Beckman TW, Chen J, et al: Apparent hydroxyl radical production by peroxynitrite: Implications for endothelial injury from nitric oxide and superoxide. *Proc Natl Acad Sci USA* 1990; 87:1620–1624.
18. Radi R, Beckman JS, Bush KM, Freeman BA: Peroxynitrite-induced membrane lipid peroxidation: The cytotoxic potential of superoxide and nitric oxide. *Arch Biochem Biophys* 1991; 288:481–487.
19. Braughler JM, Duncan LA, Chase RL: The involvement of iron in lipid peroxidation: Importance of ferric to ferrous ratios in irritation. *J Biol Chem* 1986; 261:10282–10289.
20. Minotti G, Aust SD: The requirement for ferric in initiation of lipid peroxidation by ferrous hydrogen peroxide. *J Biol Chem* 1987; 262:1098–1104.
21. Hall ED, Andrus PK, Yonkers PA: Brain hydroxyl radical generation in acute experimental head injury. *J Neurochem* 1993; 60:588–594.
22. Smith SL, Andrus PK, Zhang JR, Hall ED: Direct measurement hydroxyl radicals, lipid peroxidation and blood-brain barrier disruption following unilateral cortical impact injury in the rat. *J Neurotrauma* 1994; 11:393–404.
23. O'Brien PJ: Intracellular mechanisms for the decomposition of a lipid peroxide. I. Decomposition of a lipid peroxide by metal ions, nerve compounds and nucleophiles. *Can J Biochem* 1969; 47:485–492.
24. Sevanian A, Kim E: Phospholipase A_2 dependent release of fatty acids from peroxidized membranes. *J Free Rad Biol Med* 1985; 1:263–271.
25. van Kuijk FJGM, Sevanian A, Handelman GJ, Dratz EA: A new role for phospholipase A_2: Protection of membranes from lipid peroxidation damage. *TIBS* 1987; 12:31–34.
26. Zhang JR, Andrus PK, Hall ED: Age-related phospholipid hydroperoxides measured by HPLC-chemiluminescence and their relation to hydroxyl radical stress. *Brain Res* 1994; 639:275–282.
27. Hall ED, Braughler JM: Effects of intravenous methylprednisolone on spinal cord lipid peroxidation and $Na^+ + K^+$-ATPase activity: Dose-response analysis during 1st hour after contusion injury in the cat. *J Neurosurg* 1982; 57:247–253.
28. Kurihara M: Role of monoamines in experimental spinal cord injury. Relationship between $Na^+ + K^+$-ATPase and lipid peroxidation. *J Neurosurg* 1985; 62:743–749.
29. Milvy P, Kari S, Campbell JB, Demopoulos HB: Paramagnetic species and radical products in cat spinal cord. *Ann NY Acad Sci* 1973; 222:1102–1111.
30. Anderson DK, Saunders RD, Demediuk P, et al: Lipid hydrolysis and peroxidation in injured spinal cord: Partial protection with methylprednisolone or vitamin E and selenium. *CNS Trauma* 1985; 2:257–267.
31. Demopoulos HB, Flamm ES, Seligman ML, et al: Further studies on free radical pathology in the major central nervous system disorders: Effects of very high doses of methylprednisolone on the functional outcome, morphology and chemistry of experimental spinal cord impact injury. *Can J Physiol* 1982; 60:1415–1424.
32. Pietronigro DD, Hovsepian M, Demopoulos HB, Flamm ES: Loss of ascorbic acid from injured feline spinal cord. *J Neurochem* 1983; 41:1072–1076.
33. Saunders RD, Dugan LL, Demediuk P, et al: Effects of methylprednisolone and the combination of alpha tocopherol and selenium on arachidonic acid metabolism and lipid peroxidation in traumatized spinal cord tissue. *J Neurochem* 1987; 49:24–31.
34. Anderson DK, Means ED: Pathophysiological mechanisms in acute spinal cord trauma: Effects of decompartmentalized iron on cellular membranes, in Dacey RG, Winn HR, Rimel RW, Jane JA (eds): *Trauma of the Central Nervous System.* New York: Raven Press, 1985:297–308.
35. Clendenon NR, Allen H, Gordon WA, Bingham WG: Inhibition of $Na^+ + K^+$-activated ATPase activity following experimental spinal cord trauma. *J Neurosurg* 1978; 49:563–568.
36. Hall ED, Wolf DL: A pharmacological analysis of the pathophysiological mechanism of post-traumatic spinal cord ischemia. *J Neurosurg* 1986; 64:951–961.
37. Young W: Blood flow, metabolic and neurophysiological mechanisms in spinal cord injury, in Becker DB, Povlishock JT (eds): *Central Nervous System Trauma Status Report.* Bethesda: NIH, 1985:463–474.
38. Hall ED, Braughler JM: Acute effects of intravenous glucocorticoid pretreatment on the *in vitro* peroxidation of cat spinal cord tissue. *Exp Neurol* 1981; 73:321–324.
39. Hall ED, Wolf DL, Braughler JM: Effects of a single large dose of methylprednisolone sodium succinate on experimental posttraumatic spinal cord ischemia: Dose-response and time-action analysis. *J Neurosurg* 1984; 61:124–130.
40. Young W, Flamm ES: Effect of high-dose corticosteroid therapy on blood flow, evoked potentials, and extracellular calcium in experimental spinal injury. *J Neurosurg* 1982; 57:667–673.
41. Braughler JM, Hall ED: Lactate and pyruvate metabolism in injured cat spinal cord before and after a single large intravenous dose of methylprednisolone. *J Neurosurg* 1983; 59:256–261.
42. Hall ED, McCall JM, Means ED: Therapeutic potential of the lazaroids (21-aminosteroids) in CNS trauma, ischemia and subarachnoid hemorrhage. *Adv Pharmacol* 1994; 28:221–268.
43. Hall ED, Yonkers PA, Horan KL, Braughler JM: Correlation between attenuation of posttraumatic spinal cord ischemia and preservation of vitamin E by the 21-aminosteroid U-74006F: Evidence for an in vivo antioxidant action. *J Neurotrauma* 1989; 6:169–176.
44. Hall ED: Effect of the 21-aminosteroid U74006F on posttraumatic spinal cord ischemia. *J Neurosurg* 1988; 68:462–465.
45. Hall ED, Braughler JM: Role of lipid peroxidation in post-traumatic spinal cord degeneration: A review. *CNS Trauma* 1986; 3:281–293.
46. Hall ED, Wolf DL: Methylprednisolone preservation of

motor nerve function during early degeneration. *Exp Neurol* 1984; 84:715–720.

47. Braughler JM, Hall ED, Means ED, et al: Evaluation of an intensive methylprednisolone sodium succinate dosing regimen in experimental spinal cord injury. *J Neurosurg* 1987; 67:102–105.
48. Hall ED: Intensive anti-oxidant pretreatment retards motor nerve degeneration. *Brain Res* 1987; 413:175–178.
49. Hall ED, Yonkers PA: Preservation of motor nerve function during early degeneration by the 21-aminosteroid antioxidant U74006F. *Brain Res* 1990; 513:244–247.
50. Anderson DK, Braughler JM, Hall ED, et al: Effects of treatment with U-74006F on neurological recovery following experimental spinal cord injury. *J Neurosurg* 1988; 69:562–567.
51. Anderson DK, Hall ED, Braughler JM, et al: Effect of delayed administration of U74006F (tirilazad mesylate) on recovery of locomotor function following experimental spinal cord injury. *J Neurotrauma* 1991; 8:187–192.
52. Holtz A, Gerdin B: Blocking weight-induced spinal cord injury in rats: Therapeutic effect of the 21-aminosteroid U-74006F. *J Neurotrauma* 1991; 8:239–245.
53. Holtz A, Gerdin B: Efficacy of the 21-aminosteroid U-74006F in improving neurological recovery after spinal cord injury in rats. *Neurol Res* 1992; 14:49–52.
54. Anderson DK, Waters TR, Means ED: Pretreatment with alpha tocopherol enhances neurologic recovery after spinal cord compression injury. *J Neurotrauma* 1988; 6:61–68.
55. Anderson DK, Means ED: Lipid peroxidation in spinal cord. FeCl2 induction and protection with antioxidants. *Neurochem Path* 1983; 1:249–264.
56. Anderson DK, Means ED: Iron-induced lipid peroxidation in spinal cord: Protection with mannitol and methylprednisolone. *J Free Rad Biol Med* 1985; 1:59–64.
57. Kontos HA, Wei EP, Povlishock JT, et al: Cerebral arteriolar damage by arachidonic acid and prostaglandin G_2. *Science* 1980; 209:1242–1245.
58. Wei EP, Kontos HA, Dietrich WD, et al: Inhibition by free radical scavengers and by cyclooxygenase inhibitors of pial arteriolar abnormalities from concussive brain injury in cats. *Circ Res* 1981; 48:95–103.
59. Kontos HA, Wei EP: Superoxide production in experimental brain injury. *J Neurosurg* 1986; 64:803–807.
60. Audus KL, Guillot FL, Braughler JM: Evidence for 21-aminosteroid association with the hydrophobic domains of brain microvessel endothelial cells. *Free Rad Biol Med* 1991; 11:361–371.
61. Torbati D, Church DF, Carey ME, Pryor WA: Generation of free radicals immediately after closed head injury in rat brain. *FASEB J* 1991; 5:A891.
62. Wei EP, Lamb RG, Kontos HA: Increased phospholipase C activity after experimental brain injury. *J Neurosurg* 1982; 56:695–698.
63. Ellis EF, Wright KF, Wei EP, Kontos HA: Cyclooxygenase products of arachidonic acid metabolism in cat cerebral cortex after experimental concussive brain injury. *J Neurochem* 1991; 37:892–896.
64. Kukreja RC, Kontos HA, Hess ML, Ellis EF: PGH synthase and lipoxygenase generate superoxide in the presence of NADH and NADPH. *Circ Res* 1986; 59:612–619.
65. Hsu CY, Halushka PV, Hogan EL, et al: Alteration of thromboxane and prostacyclin levels in experimental spinal cord injury. *Neurology* 1985; 35:1003–1009.
66. Jonsson HT, Daniell HB: Altered levels of PGF in cat spinal cord tissue following traumatic injury. *Prostaglandins* 1976; 11:51–61.
67. Chan PH, Longar S, Fishman RA: Oxygen-free radicals: Potential edema mediators in brain injury, in Inaba Y, Klatzo I, Spatz M (eds): *Brain Edema.* Tokyo: Springer-Verlag, 1985:317–323.
68. Hall ED, Travis MA: Inhibition of arachidonic acid-induced vasogenic brain edema by the non-glucocorticoid 21-aminosteroid U74006F. *Brain Res* 1988; 451:350–352.
69. Zuccarello M, Anderson DK: Protective effect of a 21-aminosteroid on the blood-brain barrier following subarachnoid hemorrhage in rats. *Stroke* 1989; 20:367–371.
70. Willmore LJ, Rubin JJ: Effects of antiperoxidants on FeCl2-induced lipid peroxidation and focal edema in rat brain. *Exp Neurol* 1984; 83:62–70.
71. Hall ED, Yonkers PA, Andrus PK, et al: Biochemistry and pharmacology of lipid antioxidants in acute brain and spinal cord injury. *J Neurotrauma* 1992; 9(suppl): 425–442.
72. McIntosh T, Banbury M, Smith D: The novel 21-aminosteroid U74006F attenuates cerebral oedema and improves survival after brain injury in the rat. *Acta Neurochir* 1992; 51(suppl):329–330.
73. Asano T, Matsui T, Takuwa Y: Lipid peroxidation, protein kinase C and cerebral vasospasm. *Crit Rev Neurosurg* 1991; 1:361–379.
74. Sano K, Asano T, Tanishima T, Sasaki T: Lipid peroxidation as a cause of cerebral vasospasm. *Neurol Res* 1980; 2:253–272.
75. Macdonald RL, Weir BKA, Runzer TD, et al: Effect of intrathecal superoxide dismutase and catalase on oxyhemoglobin-induced vasospasm in monkeys. *Neurosurgery* 1992; 30:529–539.
76. Vollmer DG, Kassell NF, Hongo K, et al: Effect of the nonglucocorticoid 21-aminosteroid U-74006F on experimental cerebral vasospasm. *Surg Neurol* 1989; 31:190–194.
77. Steinke DE, Weir BKA, Findlay JM, et al: A trial of the 21-aminosteroid U-74006F in a primate model of chronic cerebral vasospasm. *Neurosurgery* 1989; 24:179–186.
78. Zuccarello M, Marsch JT, Schmitt G, et al: Effect of the 21-aminosteroid U-74006F on cerebral vasospasm following subarachnoid hemorrhage. *J Neurosurg* 1989; 71:98–104.
79. Kanamaru K, Weir BKA, Findlay JM, et al: A dosage study of the effect of the 21-aminosteroid U-74006F on chronic cerebral vasospasm in a primate model. *Neurosurgery* 1989; 27:29–38.
80. Kanamaru K, Weir BKA, Simpson I, et al: Effect of 21-aminosteroid U-74006F on lipid peroxidation in subarachnoid clot. *J Neurosurg* 1991; 74:454–459.
81. Hall ED, Travis MA: Effects of the non-glucocorticoid 21-aminosteroid U-74006F on acute cerebral hypoperfusion following experimental subarachnoid hemorrhage. *Exp Neurol* 1989; 102:244–248.
82. Zuccarello M, Anderson DK: Protective effect of a 21-

aminosteroid on the blood-brain barrier following subarachnoid hemorrhage in rats. *Stroke* 1989; 20:367–371.

83. Kassell NF, Haley EC, Alves W, Hansen CA: Phase III trial of tirilazad in aneurysmal subarachnoid hemorrhage. *J Neurosurg* 1994; 80:383A.

84. Hall ED: High-dose glucocorticoid treatment improves neurological recovery in head-injured mice. *J Neurosurg* 1985; 62:882–887.

85. Hall ED, McCall JM, Chase RL, et al: A non-glucocorticoid steroid analog of methylprednisolone duplicates its high-dose pharmacology in models of central nervous system trauma and neuronal membrane damage. *J Pharmacol Exp* 1987; 242:137–142.

86. Giannotta SL, Weiss MH, Apuzzo MLJ, Martin E: High dose glucocorticoids in the management of severe head injury. *Neurosurgery* 1984; 15:497–501.

87. Sapolsky RM: A mechanism for glucocorticoid toxicity in the hippocampus: Increased vulnerability to metabolic insults. *J Neuroscience* 1985; 5:1228–1232.

88. Sapolsky RM, Pulsinelli W: Glucocorticoids potentiate ischemic injury to neurons: Therapeutic implications. *Science* 1985; 229:1397–1399.

89. Hall ED, Yonkers PA, McCall JM, Braughler JM: Effect of the 21-aminosteroid U74006F on experimental head injury in mice. *J Neurosurg* 1988; 68:456–461.

90. Sanada T, Nakamura T, Nishmura MC, et al: Effect of U-74006F on neurological function and brain edema after fluid percussion injury in rats. *J Neurotrauma* 1993; 10:65–71.

91. Dimlich RVW, Tornheim PA, Kindel RM, et al: Effects of a 21-aminosteroid (U-74006F) on cerebral metabolites and edema after severe experimental head trauma, in Long D, et al (eds): *Advances in Neurology*. New York: Raven Press, 1990; 52:365–375.

92. Hall ED, Braughler JM, Yonkers PA, et al: U78517F, a potent inhibitor of lipid peroxidation with activity in experimental brain injury and ischemia. *J Pharmacol Exp Ther* 1991; 258:688–694.

93. Panter SS, Braughler JM, Hall ED: Dextran-coupled deferoxamine improves outcome in a murine model of head injury. *J Neurotrauma* 1992; 9:47–53.

94. Muizelaar JP, Marmarou A, Young HF, et al: Improving the outcome of severe head injury with the oxygen radical scavenger polyethylene glycol-conjugated superoxide dismutase: A phase II trial. *J Neurosurg* 1993; 78:375–382.

95. Pellegrini-Giampetro DE, Cherici G, Alesiani M, et al: Excitatory amino acid release and free radical formation may cooperate in the genesis of ischemia-induced neuronal damage. *J Neuroscience* 1990; 10:1035–1041.

96. Boisvert DPJ, Schreiber C: Interrelationship of excitotoxic and free radical mechanisms, in Krieglstein J, Oberpichler H (eds): *Pharmacology of Cerebral Ischemia.* Stuttgart: Wissenshaftliche Verlaggesellschaft, 1992:1–10.

97. Rohn TT, Hinds TR, Vincenzi FF: Ion transport ATPases as targets for free radical damage: Protection by an aminosteroid of the Ca^{2+} pump ATPase and Na^{+}/K^{+} pump ATPase of human red blood cell membranes. *Biochem Pharmacol* 1993; 46:525–534.

CHAPTER 105

DEATH BY CALCIUM: A WAY OF LIFE

Wise Young

INTRODUCTION

Calcium (Ca^{2+}) ions are widely acknowledged to be essential messengers of life. Ca^{2+} ions initiate and regulate mitosis, motility, growth, secretion, and many other crucial cell functions. A surfeit of Ca^{2+}, however, is deadly to cells, particularly neurons. Small elevations of intracellular Ca^{2+} activity ($[Ca^{2+}]_i$) above 1 μM will activate entire families of phospholipases, proteases, and nucleases which attack and rapidly digest cellular proteins, lipids, and DNA. Since extracellular Ca^{2+} ionic activity ($[Ca^{2+}]_e$) normally exceeds 1.0 mM and intracellular Ca^{2+} ionic activity ($[Ca^{2+}]_i$) is typically five orders of magnitude lower, a huge gradient of Ca^{2+} is poised to flood injured cells.

First recognized in spinal cord injury,[1,2] the tendency for progressive tissue damage appears to be a general property of central nervous tissues, perhaps accounting for the exquisite vulnerability of the brain and spinal cord to trauma, ischemia, and anoxia. The existence of autodestructive mechanisms in neurons is a central paradox in biology. Why should neurons, undoubtedly crucial to survival and unable to regenerate or repair themselves, possess hair-trigger autodestructive mechanisms. For example, why have vertebrates evolved an elaborate bony structure to protect the spinal cord and then endow the spinal cord with suicidal tendencies?

Ca^{2+}-activated autodestructive mechanisms may be neuroprotective. Profound and prolonged depressions of extracellular Ca^{2+} activity ($[Ca^{2+}]_e$) occur in contused spinal cords.[3,4] Total tissue calcium concentrations ($[Ca]_t$) increase.[5,6,7] We propose that Ca^{2+}-induced autodigestion releases large amounts of phosphates and phosphatides that buffer and lower $[Ca^{2+}]_e$.[8,9]

Lowering $[Ca^{2+}]_e$ is an efficient and effective means of reducing Ca^{2+} entry into surrounding cells.[10] The mechanism is robust, does not require nor consume energy, and is selectively triggered only in severely injured cells. The process eliminates moribund cells that would otherwise consume precious metabolic resources and protect neighboring cells. The presence of an endogenous neuroprotective mechanism that staves off tissue damage may be one reason why some neuroprotective drugs can be given several hours after injury and still be effective.[11]

Students of CNS trauma have long grappled with Ca^{2+}-mediated autodestructive mechanisms in isolation. Viewing it as "pathology," most neuroscientists ignored the phenomenon until recent evidence accumulated to show that Ca^{2+}-mediated autodestructive mechanisms play a major role in development. Many neurons die during development, due to Ca^{2+}-mediated excitotoxicity,[12,13] apoptosis, or programmed cell death mechanisms.[14–16]

In this chapter, we shall review some of the mechanisms by which Ca^{2+} ions kill neurons, how CNS tissues protect neurons against Ca^{2+} floods but at the same time use Ca^{2+} to initiate programmed cell death.

Ca^{2+}-MEDIATED AUTODESTRUCTIVE MECHANISMS

Calcium has been aptly called the "final common path of cell death."[17] Because Ca^{2+} is an essential messenger in many cellular processes, excessive rises of $[Ca^{2+}]_i$ will shut down virtually all anabolic and metabolic cell functions, with the exception of mechanisms that seem designed to destroy the cells. Ca^{2+} ions will bind to mitochondria and disrupt electron transport.[18] Incomplete oxidation and other sources of free radicals combine with other Ca^{2+}-activated mechanisms to contribute to lipid peroxidation.[19] In addition, Ca^{2+} ions activate several families of intracellular enzymes that attack and digest proteins, lipids, and even nucleic acid, as well as induce release of inflammatory mediators that complete the destruction of the cells.

Ca^{2+}-activated proteases attack both structural and functional proteins in cells. Examples of the former include neurofilament[20–22] and myelin basic protein.[23–25] The latter includes ATPases,[26–29] superoxide dismutase,[30–33] and probably other enzymes. Damage to enzymes is likely contribute to prolonged dysfunction and eventual demise of injured cells. However, loss of enzyme activities is also a general manifestation of cell death, and Ca^{2+}-activated proteases may simply be disabling these enzymes in already moribund cells.

Ca^{2+} ions also activate several classes of phospholipases in neurons. The best known include phospholipases.[34,35] Phospholipases cleave membrane phospholipids to release arachidonic acid,[36] a primary substrate from which prostaglandins and leukotrienes are formed.[37,38] These eicosanoids are potent vasoactive and inflammatory mediators that contribute to the sequelae of tissue damage, including the delayed loss of blood flow.[39,10]

Finally, Ca^{2+} ions stimulate nucleases that break down DNA.[15,40–43] Nuclease-induced DNA breakdown is involved in and characteristic of a form of programmed cell death called "apoptosis,"[44–48] although the mechanisms of such programmed cell death are still not clearly understood.

There is clearly no dearth of mechanisms by which excessive Ca^{2+} can initiate a cascade of autodestructive responses to kill cells. Nature seems to have left no stone unturned when installing autodestructive mechanisms in neurons. Given the presence of such mechanisms, the more difficult question is, How do neurons survive a lifetime of exposure to a high Ca^{2+} environment and repeated episodes of ischemia and trauma that all neurons sooner or later experience? On heuristic grounds alone, neurons must have evolved robust and fool-proof mechanisms to protect themselves against the dangers of being flooded with Ca^{2+} at the slightest injury.

INTRACELLULAR Ca^{2+} BUFFERING

Ca^{2+} ionic activity is tightly regulated inside cells. Besides regulating Ca^{2+} entry and egress through transmembrane channels and Ca^{2+} transport mechanisms, such as Ca^{2+} ATPase[49,50] and Na : Ca exchange,[51–59] neurons also possess specialized mechanisms for binding or buffering $[Ca^{2+}]_i$.

Intracellular organelles such as sarcoplasmic or endoplasmic reticulum not only bind Ca^{2+} but have specialized mechanisms such as the ryanodine receptor[60–62] to control intracellular Ca^{2+} release. In myocytes, both Ca^{2+}-activated and Na^+-activated[62] Ca^{2+} release inside cells comes in part from sarcoplasmic reticulum.[64] At certain $[Ca^{2+}]_i$ levels, sarcoplasmic reticulum engages in rhythmic or phasic release of Ca^{2+}.[65] Finally, L-type calcium channels are present in sarcoplasmic reticulum, serving as sensors for voltage dependent Ca^{2+} release inside cells.[36] Endoplasmic reticulum likewise appears to regulate $[Ca^{2+}]_i$ in neurons.

Mitochondria are storehouses of intracellular Ca^{2+}.[18,66–69] Cytoplasmic pH and Ca^{2+} binding of mitochondria are inversely related.[18,70] Large amounts of Ca^{2+} accumulate in mitochondria in ischemic nervous tissues.[71] Mitochondria possess specialized pores that allow Ca^{2+} entry and exit.[72–76] Oxidative stress and toxins such as doxorubicin and cis-platinum open these mitochondrial pores.[76–83] Mitochondria thus cannot take up and store large amounts of Ca^{2+} but possess specialized mechanisms for releasing these stores under some circumstances.

Neurons possess remarkable Ca^{2+} binding capacity. More than 20 years ago, Baker et al.[51,84–86] showed that Ca^{2+} ions are rapidly bound by axoplasmic substances and do not diffuse when injected into squid axons, in contrast to Na^+ or K^+ ions, which diffuse long distances. Other data suggest that CNS tissues have a huge excess of Ca^{2+} buffering capacity. For example, in injured cat spinal cords, extracellular Ca^{2+} falls from >1.0 mM to

<100 μM within minutes and remains depressed for hours.[3,41] Since even complete equilibration between intra- and extracellular compartments should lower $[Ca^{2+}]_e$ to only 200 μM, injury must be releasing large amounts of Ca^{2+} binding substances, capable of reducing and maintaining $[Ca^{2+}]_e$ at low levels for many hours despite Ca^{2+} pouring in from surrounding tissues and vascular compartments.

Ca^{2+} BUFFERING AS AN ENDOGENOUS NEUROPROTECTIVE MECHANISM

The ability of cells to buffer Ca^{2+} must be the first line of defense against excessive rises in $[Ca^{2+}]_i$ in injured cells. No other mechanism can adequately defend against the onslaught of Ca^{2+} that rushes into cells after trauma or ischemia. Transmembrane pumps and Na : Ca exchangers are ineffective when confronted with membrane holes. Likewise, shutting down voltage-gated or receptor-gated Ca^{2+} channels is not enough. One effective approach is to endow neurons with enough Ca^{2+} binding capacity to neutralize large amounts of Ca^{2+} entering cells.

Central nervous tissues possess a large excess of Ca^{2+} binding capacity, sufficient to bind many times the total amount of free Ca^{2+} present at the tissue. For example, in spinal cord injury, total calcium ($[Ca]_t$) increases at the injury site.[7,8] Within 3 hours after injury, $[Ca]_t$ rises from 2.1 to 3.6 μmol/g. Since $[Ca^{2+}]_e$ is normally 1.2 mM or 1.2 μmol/g, extracellular volume is 0.80-0.90, and $[Ca^{2+}]_i$ is negligible low (<0.001 μmol/g), the amount of free Ca^{2+} is normally less than 0.24 μmol/g. An increase of 1.5 μmol/g represents more than six times the amount of free Ca^{2+} in the tissue before injury. In ischemic cerebral cortices, $[Ca]_t$ may exceed 6 μmol/g.[6,87] In unpublished studies of ischemic cerebral tissues at 7 days, we have observed Ca concentrations as high as 25 μmol/g.

The Ca^{2+} binding substances must be able to buffer $[Ca^{2+}]_e$ to <10 μM and to bind as much as 20 to 30 μmol Ca^{2+} per g of tissue. While nervous tissues possess many proteins that bind Ca^{2+} avidly, such as calmodulin, these proteins do not exceed 3 to 5 μmol/g. Phosphates and phosphatides are likely to be the Ca^{2+} binding substances. Both products of phospholipid breakdown and bind Ca^{2+}. Brain and spinal cord have very high concentrations of phosphate,[88] exceeding 100 μmol/g. Injury may release as much as 60 percent of total tissue phosphates over several hours.

Ca^{2+}-activated neuronal autodestructive mechanisms have major advantages for the tissue. First, these mechanisms would rapidly, selectively, and unerringly eliminate severely injured cells that have been flooded by Ca^{2+} beyond their initial cytoplasmic Ca^{2+} buffering capacity. Rapid elimination of these cells would prevent consumption of precious metabolic resources by cells that probably would not survive. Second, rapid autodigestion of the cells would rapidly release large amounts of phosphates and phosphatides to reduce and maintain $[Ca^{2+}]_e$ at low levels, protecting neighboring cells. Third, the process is robust. It neither requires nor consumes ATP.

Eventually, $[Ca^{2+}]_e$ must return to normal levels. However, by this time, many partially injured cells may have recovered. Thus, by altruistically sacrificing themselves, severely injured neurons may save some of their neighbors. The delay in tissue damage due to $[Ca^{2+}]_e$ may be partially responsible for the therapeutic time window that allow neuroprotective drugs to be given many minutes or hours after injury[11,89] and still be effective. It may also explain why very rapid restoration of blood flow may be deleterious to injured brains and spinal cords.

NEUROTRANSMITTER RECEPTOR-GATED CALCIUM CHANNELS

A major role of glutamate in neuronal death is now firmly established in developmental neurobiology and is becoming accepted as a major mechanism of secondary tissue damage in cerebral ischemia, traumatic brain and spinal cord injury.[41,90–107] Much evidence suggests that the N-methyl-D-aspartate (NMDA) receptor contributes to "excitoxic" death by allowing Ca^{2+} to enter neurons.[12,13,108–110]

Some details of how glutamate receptors contribute to traumatic brain and spinal cord injury in vivo, however, are still unclear. First, the sites of glutamate action have not been clearly established in some cases. For example, in spinal cord injury, glutamate receptors have not yet been reported on spinal axons, although they are clearly present on spinal neurons.[111] Since the neurological consequences of spinal cord injury are largely due to white matter damage, the beneficial effects of glutamate receptor blockers in injured spinal cords may be indirectly mediated by other neurotransmitters or toxins. Second, the timing of glutamate release is a problem. Microdialysis studies have shown rapid and transient rises of extracellular glutamate levels associated with cerebral ischema,[112–114] and brain trauma.[91,102,107,115–119] The Ca^{2+} inrush from NMDA receptors should occur too fast to be blocked by receptor antagonists given hours or even minutes after injury. Third, a phenomenon called spreading depression repeatedly releases glutamate in brain[120–123] and is not always associated with tissue damage.[124] Finally, neuronal glutamate receptors inactive rapidly after exposure to glutamate and are effectively shut down by acidosis,[125] thus limiting the amount of Ca^{2+} that would enter neurons. If neurons can buffer large amounts of Ca^{2+}, why should the relatively small amounts of Ca^{2+} entering through glutamate receptors kill neurons?

Glutamate may indirectly contribute to neuronal death by means other than Ca^{2+} entry through NMDA channels. For example, astrocytes contain glutamate receptors.[126–129] In addition, several other neurotransmitter receptors control Ca^{2+} channels: acetylcholine,[130–135] serotonin,[136,137] and histamine. In addition, we have recently discovered that spinal axons possess GABA,[138–140] norepinephrine,[141] and serotonin receptors. Finally, recent evidence suggest that neurons possess highly specific mechanisms to initiate programmed cell death without requiring high or prolonged elevations of $[Ca^{2+}]i$.

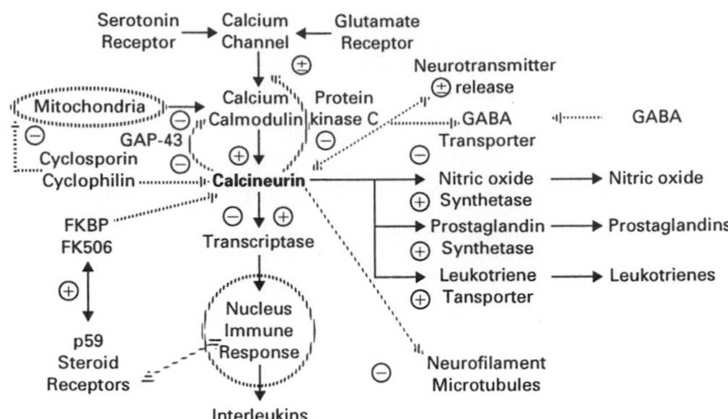

Figure 105-1. Reported actions of calcineurin and related intracellular messengers. Solid arrows indicate positive or stimulatory effects while the shaded arrows indicate modulatory effects. Calcium ions entering the cells through voltage-sensitive and neurotransmitter gated channels combine with calmodulin to activate calcineurin. Calcineurin dephosphorylates the serine-threonine sites of many proteins and enzymes, including neurofilaments, microtubules, neuromodulin (GAP-43), transcriptases that induce immune and inflammatory responses, protein kinase C, nitric oxide synthase, prostaglandin synthase, and leukotriene transporters. The immunosuppressant agents cyclosporin and FK506 inhibit calcineurin by binding respectively to cyclophilin and FK binding protein (FKBP). Cyclosporin also blocks Ca^{2+} pores on mitochondrial membranes while FK506 interacts with cytoplasmic steroid receptors and the heat-shock protein.

Ca^{2+}-ACTIVATED PHOSPHATASES AND APOPTOSIS

Much recent evidence suggests that Ca^{2+} initiates programmed death of neurons. Specifically, Ca^{2+} ions activate several families of phosphatases that dephosphorylate a wide variety of intracellular enzymes. These phosphatases include the Type 1, Type 2A, and Type 2B phosphatases. Type 1 phosphatases are modulated by insulin and other hormonal receptors and regulate many crucial cellular processes including glycogen metabolism, calcium transport, muscle contraction, intracellular transport, protein synthesis, and cell division.[142] Type 2B phosphatases include calcineurin,[143,144] a phosphatase that induces immune and inflammatory responses[145,146] in lymphocytes and neurons.

Calcineurin is present in neurons[147] and lymphocytes,[148–150] but apparently not astrocytes.[151,152] In the presence of Ca^{2+} and calmodulin, calcineurin dephosphorylates enzymes at serine-threonine sites. For example, calcineurin turns on transcriptases[153–159] that induce expression and synthesis of interleukins,[155,157] prostaglandin,[160] and nitric oxide.[161–164] In addition, calcineurin modulates voltage-sensitive and receptor-gated Ca^{2+} channels,[165–168] neurotransmitter release,[168–170] and transmembrane ionic[171] and leukotriene transport.[172–175] Figure 105-1 summarizes some reported actions of calcineurin.

Much evidence suggests that calcineurin contributes to apoptosis and secondary injury in a variety of tissues. During development, T-lymphocytes exposed to and activated by native antigens are programmed to die. Cyclosporin, a specific inhibitor of calcineurin,[176–179] prevents this form of apoptosis. Likewise, both cyclosporin and FK506 (a macrolide antibiotic that also inhibits cyclosporin) prevents antigen-induced apoptosis of B-lymphocytes.[148,180] In a study of thyroxin-induced regression of bull-frog tadpole tails,[181] cyclosporin blocked the tail resorption. Recent studies reported that calcineurin inhibitors are neuroprotective in endothelin-induced cerebral ischemia,[182] ischemia-reperfusion injury of brain,[183] and heart,[74] toxic and anoxic injury to hepatocytes.[184–188] Type 1 and 2a phosphatases also may be involved in apoptosis. For example, calyculin A inhibits Type 1 and Type 2a phosphatases and prevents apoptosis in Burkitt's lymphoma.[189] On the other hand, okadaic acid, another Type 1 and 2a phosphatase inhibitor, apparently can cause apoptosis in a variety of mammalian cells, including primary hepatocyte cultures, a human mammary carcinoma cell line, human neuroblastoma cell line, rat pituitary adenoma, and rat promyelocytic cells.[190]

SUMMARY AND CONCLUSIONS

Neurons live in a sea of Ca^{2+} that threatens to flood them as a consequence of the slightest injury. Neurons also possess Ca^{2+}-activated enzymes that will rapidly and completely digest protein, membrane, and even DNA of the cells. The presence of such Ca^{2+}-activated autodestructive mechanisms in the longest-lived cells of our body is puzzling. Neurons must possess robust and fool-proof mechanisms for defending themselves against Ca^{2+} floods.

Central nervous tissues have evolved a remarkable capacity to bind and buffer Ca^{2+} ions. Nervous tissues contain high concentrations of phosphates. Autodigestion of severely injured neurons releases large amounts of phosphates and phosphatides that bind Ca^{2+}. Ion-selective recordings have shown that $[Ca^{2+}]_e$ falls and remains depressed for hours after injury, despite continued Ca^{2+} diffusion from surrounding tissues and vascular compartments. At the same time, total tissue $[Ca]_t$ increases by 40 to 60 percent, representing several times the amount of free Ca^{2+} available in the tissue before injury. Thus, neurons possess excessive Ca^{2+} binding capacity, sufficient to bind not only all the free Ca^{2+} in the tissue but also Ca^{2+} diffusing from surrounding tissues and vascular compartments. Eventually, however, $[Ca^{2+}]_e$ must return, and secondary injury occurs. The post-traumatic depression of $[Ca^{2+}]_e$ may explain why some neuroprotective treatments can be given hours after injury and still be effective.

Ca^{2+}-activated autodestructive mechanisms are advantageous to the organism for several reasons. First, such mechanisms rapidly eliminate moribund cells, preventing wasteful consumption of precious metabolic resources by cells that are likely to die. Second, owing to the high concentrations of phosphates in neural tissues, complete digestion of the cells will release sufficient phosphates and phosphatides to buffer and maintain $[Ca^{2+}]_e$ at low levels for many minutes or even hours. Third, the mechanism is robust and does not require or utilize ATP or oxygen, both of which may be scarce at the injury site. Fourth, lowering $[Ca^{2+}]_e$ is the most efficient and effective means of reducing transmembrane Ca^{2+} gradients and slowing Ca^{2+} entry into surrounding cells. Thus, by sacrificing severely injured cells that will probably die anyway, the organism reduces risk to neighboring cells and the energy burden of restoring Ca^{2+} homeostasis in these cells.

Central nervous tissues, however, seem to have evolved ways to circumvent their own protective mechanisms when initiating programmed cell death or apoptosis. During development, large numbers of neurons die if they do not reach or connect the appropriate target. Glutamate receptors contribute to such programmed cell death, by allowing Ca^{2+} entry through glutamate receptor-gated Ca^{2+} channels. However, these receptors generally inactivate rapidly and also are effectively shut down by acidosis, limiting the amount of Ca^{2+} entry. It is unclear how and why a limited amount of Ca^{2+} entering cells through neurotransmitter receptor-gated channels would be so toxic.

Finally, small amounts of Ca^{2+} can initiate programmed cell death by activating calcineurin, a Type 2B phosphatase that triggers immune and inflammatory responses leading to apoptosis. Calcineurin inhibitors such as cyclosporin have been reported to prevent lymphocytic and neuronal apoptosis, as well as secondary injury in cerebral and myocardial ischemia.

REFERENCES

1. Allen AR: Surgery of experimental lesion of spinal cord equivalent to crush injury of fracture dislocation of spinal column. A preliminary report. *JAMA* 1911; 57:878–880.
2. Allen AR: Remarks on histopathological changes in spinal cord due to impact: an experimental study. *J Nerv Ment Dis* 1914; 41:141–147.
3. Young W, Flamm ES: Effect of high dose corticosteroid therapy on blood flow, evoked potentials, and extracellular calcium in experimental spinal injury. *J Neurosurg* 1982; 57:667–673.
4. Young W, Yen V, Blight A: Extracellular calcium activity in experimental spinal cord contusion. *Brain Res* 1982; 253:115–123.
5. Kwo S, Young W, DeCrescito V: Spinal cord sodium, potassium, calcium, and water concentration changes in rats after graded contusion injury. *J Neurotrauma* 1989; 6:13–24.
6. Young W, Hadani M, Rappaport ZH, et al: Tissue Na, K, and Ca changes in regional cerebral ischemia: Their measurement and interpretation. *CNS Trauma* 1986; 3:215–234.
7. Young W, Koreh I: Potassium and calcium changes in injured spinal cords. *Brain Res* 1986; 365:42–53.
8. Young W: Role of calcium in spinal cord injury. *CNS Trauma* 1985; 2:109–114.
9. Young W: Ca paradox in neural injury: A hypothesis. *CNS Trauma* 1986; 3:235–251.
10. Young W: Role of calcium in central nervous system injuries. *J Neurotrauma* 1992; 9:S9–25.
11. Young W: The therapeutic window for methylprednisolone treatment of acute spinal cord injury: Implications

for cell injury mechanisms, Waxman SG (ed): in *Molecular and Cellular Approaches to the Treatment of Neurological Disease.* New York: Raven Press, 1993:191–206.

12. Olney JW: Excitotoxin-mediated neuron death in young and old age. *Prog Brain Res* 1990; 86:37–51.
13. Rothman SM, Olney JW: Excitotoxicity and the NMDA receptor. *Trends Neurosci* 1987; 10:299–302.
14. Deckwerth TL, Johnson EM Jr: Temporal analysis of events associated with programmed cell death (apoptosis) of sympathetic neurons deprived of nerve growth factor. *J Cell Biol* 1993; 123:1207–1222.
15. Joseph R, Li W, Han E: Neuronal death, cytoplasmic calcium and internucleosomal DNA fragmentation: Evidence for DNA fragments being released from cells. *Brain Res Mol Brain Res* 1993; 17:70–76.
16. Truman JW, Thorn RS, Robinow S: Programmed neuronal death in insect development. *J Neurobiol* 1992; 23:1295–1311.
17. Schanne FAX, Kane AB, Young EE, Farber JL: Calcium dependence of toxic cell death: A final common pathway. *Science* 1979; 206:700–702.
18. Chance B: The energy-linked reaction of calcium with mitochondria. *J Biol Chem* 1965; 240:2729–2748.
19. Braughler JM, Duncan LA, Goodman T: Calcium enhances in vitro free radical-induced damage to brain synaptosomes, mitochondria, and cultured spinal cord neurons. *J Neurochem* 1985; 45:1288–1293.
20. Iwasaki Y, Yamamoto H, Iizuka H, et al: Suppression of neurofilament degradation by protease inhibitors in experimental spinal cord injury. *Brain Res* 1987; 406:99–104.
21. Kamakura K, Ishiura S, Suzuki K, et al: Calcium-activated neutral protease in the peripheral nerve which requires μM order Ca^{2+}, and its effect on the neurofilament triplet. *J Neurosci Res* 1985; 13:391–403.
22. Pant NC, Gainer H: Properties of a calcium-activated protease in squid axoplasm which selectively degrades neurofilament proteins. *J Neurobiol* 1980; 11:1–12.
23. Banik NL, Hogan EL, Power JM, Whetstine LJ: Degradation of cytoskeletal proteins in experimental spinal injury. *Neurochem Res* 1982; 7:1465–1475.
24. Banik NL, Hogan EL, Whetstine LJ, Balentine JD: Changes in myelin and axonal proteins in $CaCl_2$-induced myelopathy in rat spinal cord. *CNS Trauma* 1984; 1:131–138.
25. Banik NL, McAlhaney WW, Hogan EL: Calcium-stimulated proteolysis in myelin: Evidence for a Ca^{2+}-activated neutral proteinase associated with purified myelin of rat CNS. *J Neurochem* 1985; 45:581–588.
26. Faden AI, Chan PH, Longar S: Alterations in lipid metabolism, Na^+,K^+-ATPase activity, and tissue water content of spinal cord following experimental traumatic injury. *J Neurochem* 1987; 48:1809–1816.
27. Hall ED, Braughler JM: Effects of methylprednisolone on spinal cord lipid peroxidation and (Na^+-K^+)-ATPase activity: dose response analysis during the first hour after contusion injury in the cat. *J Neurosurg* 1982; 57:247–253.
28. Seddik Z, Habib YA, el, SE: The prognostic value of the brain sodium-potassium ATPase enzyme concentration in head injury. *Childs Nerv Syst* 1991; 7:135–138.
29. Vink R, Faden AI, McIntosh TK: Changes in cellular bioenergetic state following graded traumatic brain injury in rats: Determination by phosphorus 31 magnetic resonance spectroscopy. *J Neurotrauma* 1988; 5:315–330.
30. Grabitz K, Freye E, Prior R, et al: The role of superoxide dismutase (SOD) in preventing postischemic spinal cord injury. *Adv Exper Med Biol* 1990; 264:13–16.
31. Kontos HS, Wei EP: Superoxide production in experimental brain injury. *J Neurosurg* 1986; 64:803–807.
32. Shohami E, Shapira Y, Rosenthal J, Reches A: Superoxide dismutase activity is not affected by closed head injury in rats. *J Basic Clin Physiol Pharmacol* 1991; 2:103–109.
33. Tokuda Y, Uozumi T, Kawasaki T: The superoxide dismutase activities of cerebral tissues, assayed by the chemiluminescence method, in the gerbil focal ischemia/reperfusion and global ischemia models. *Neurochem Internat* 1993; 23:107–114.
34. Hirata F, Notsu Y, Iwata M, et al: Identification of several species of phospholipase proteins by radioimmunoassay for lipomodulin. *Biochem Res Comm* 1982; 109:223–230.
35. Wei EP, Lamb RG, Kontos HA: Increased phospholipase C activity after experimental brain injury. *J Neurosurg* 1982; 56:695–700.
36. Flower RJ, Blackwell GJ: The importance of phospholipase A2 in prostaglandin biosynthesis. *Biochem Pharmacol* 1976; 25:285–291.
37. Kontos HA, Wei EP, Povlishock JT, et al: Cerebral arteriolar damage by arachidonic acid and prostaglandin G2. *Science* 1980; 209:1242–1245.
38. Pickard JD: Role of prostaglandins and arachidonic acid derivatives in the coupling of cerebral blood flow to cerebral metabolism. *J Cereb Blood Flow Metab* 1981; 1:361–384.
39. D'Avella D, Germano A, Santoro G, et al: Effect of experimental subarachnoid hemorrhage on CSF eicosanoids in the rat. *J Neurotrauma* 1990; 7:121–129.
40. Batistatou A, Greene LA: Internucleosomal DNA cleavage and neuronal cell survival/death. *J Cell Biol* 1993; 122:523–532.
41. Dessi F, Charriaut-Marlangue C, Khrestchatisky M, Ben-Ari Y: Glutamate-induced neuronal death is not a programmed cell death in cerebellar culture. *J Neurochem* 1993; 60:1953–1955.
42. Okamoto M, Matsumoto M, Ohtsuki T, et al: Internucleosomal DNA cleavage involved in ischemia-induced neuronal death. *Biochem Biophys Res Commun* 1993; 196:1356–1362.
43. Pittman RN, Wang S, DiBenedetto AJ, Mills JC: A system for characterizing cellular and molecular events in programmed neuronal cell death. *J Neurosci* 1993; 13:3669–3680.
44. Diana A, Setzu M, Sirigu S, Diaz G: Nuclear patterns of apoptotic and developing neurons of superior cervical ganglion of newborn rat. *Int J Dev Neurosci* 1993; 11:773–780.

45. Loo DT, Copani A, Pike CJ, et al: Apoptosis is induced by beta-amyloid in cultured central nervous system neurons. *Proc Natl Acad Sci USA* 1993; 90:7951–7955.
46. Mesner PW, Winters TR, Green SH: Nerve growth factor withdrawal-induced cell death in neuronal PC12 cells resembles that in sympathetic neurons. *J Cell Biol* 1992; 119:1669–1680.
47. Pender MP, Nguyen KB, McCombe PA, Kerr F: Apoptosis in the nervous system in experimental allergic encephalomyelitis. *J Neurol Sci* 1991; 104:81–87.
48. Shi YF, Szalay MG, Paskar L, et al: Activation-induced cell death in T cell hybridomas is due to apoptosis. Morphologic aspects and DNA fragmentation [published erratum appears in *J Immunol* 1990; Dec 1;145(11):3945]. *J Immunol* 1990; 144:3326–3333.
49. Futawatari K, Kowada M, Nishino K: Ultracytochemical study of Ca^{2+}-ATPase activity in isolated, superoxide-treated rat brains. *Neurol Med Chir* 1989; 29:369–376.
50. Nishie I, Anzai K, Yamamoto T, Kirino Y: Measurement of steady-state Ca^{2+} pump current caused by purified Ca^{2+}-ATPase of sarcoplasmic reticulum incorporated into a planar bilayer lipid membrane. *J Biol Chem* 1990; 265:2488–2491.
51. Baker PF, Blaustein MP, Hodgkin AL, Steinhardt RA: The influence of calcium on sodium efflux in squid axons. *J Physiol* (*Lond*) 1969; 200:431–458.
52. Barzilai A, Rahamimoff H: Stoichiometry of the sodium-calcium exchanger in nerve terminals. *Biochemistry* 1987; 26:6113–6118.
53. Blaustein MP: Sodium/calcium exchange and the control of contractility in cardiac muscle and vascular smooth muscle. *J Cardiovasc Pharmacol* 1988; 12:S56–68.
54. Blaustein MP, Ratzlaff RW, Kendrik NK: The regulation of intracellular calcium in preynaptic nerve terminals. *Ann NY Acad Sci* 1978; 307:195–212.
55. Gill DL, Chueh SH, Whitlow CL: Functional importance of the synaptic plasma membrane calcium pump and sodium-calcium exchanger. *J Biol Chem* 1984; 259:10807–10813.
56. Hilgemann DW: Numerical approximations of sodium-calcium exchange. *Prog Biophys Mol Biol* 1988; 51:1–45.
57. Kaczorowski GJ, Slaughter RS, Garcia ML, King VF: The role of sodium-calcium exchange in excitable cells. *Biochem Soc Trans* 1988; 16:529–532.
58. Kaczorowski GJ, Slaughter RS, King VF, Garcia ML: Inhibitors of sodium-calcium exchange: identification and development of probes of transport activity. *Biochim Biophys Acta* 1989; 988:287–302.
59. Korn SJ, Horn R: Influence of sodium-calcium exchange on calcium current rundown and the duration of calcium-dependent chloride currents in pituitary cells, studied with whole cell and perforated patch recording. *J Gen Physiol* 1989; 94:789–812.
60. Brillantes AB, Ondrias K, Scott A, et al: Stabilization of calcium release channel (ryanodine receptor) function by FK506-binding protein. *Cell* 1994; 77:513–523.
61. Priori SG, Corr PB: Mechanisms underlying early and delayed afterdepolarizations induced by catecholamines. *Am J Physiol* 1990; 258:H1796–1805.
62. Timerman AP, Ogunbumni E, Freund E, et al: The calcium release channel of sarcoplasmic reticulum is modulated by FK-506-binding protein. Dissociation and reconstitution of FKBP-12 to the calcium release channel of skeletal muscle sarcoplasmic reticulum. *J Biol Chem* 1993; 268:22992–22999.
63. Leblanc N, Hume JR: Sodium current-induced release of calcium from cardiac sarcoplasmic reticulum [see comments]. *Science* 1990; 248:372–376.
64. Kirino Y, Shimizu H: Ca^{2+}-induced Ca^{2+} release from fragmented sarcoplasmic reticulum: a comparison with skinned muscle fiber studies. *J Biochem* (*Tokyo*) 1982; 92:1287–1296.
65. Briggs GM, Morgan JP, Gwathmey JK: Inhibition of aftercontractions and phasic calcium release by yohimbine in ferret papillary muscle. *Eur J Pharmacol* 1989; 170:281–284.
66. Brinley FJJ, Tiffert T, Scarpa A: Mitochondria and other calcium buffers of squid axon studied in situ. *J Gen Physiol* 1978; 72:101–127.
67. Carafoli E, Crompton M: The regulation of intracellular calcium by mitochondria. *Ann NY Acad Sci* 1978; 307:269–284.
68. Carafoli E, Lehninger AL: A survey of the interaction of calcium ions with mitochondria from different tissues and species. *Biochem J* 1971; 122:681–690.
69. Lehninger AL, Reynafarje B, Vercesi A, Tew WP: Transport and accumulation of calcium in mitochondria. *Ann NY Acad Sci* 1978; 307:160–176.
70. Poole ?, Wilson P, A? Regulation of intracellular pH in the myocardium; relevance to pathology. *Mol Cell Biochem* 1989; 89:151–155.
71. Kumar K, Goosmann M, Krause GS, et al: Ultrastructural and ionic studies in global ischemic dog brain. *Acta Neuropathol* (*Berl*) 1987; 73:393–399.
72. Crompton M, Ellinger H, Costi A: Inhibition by cyclosporin A of a Ca^{2+}-dependent pore in heart mitochondria activated by inorganic phosphate and oxidative stress. *Biochem J* 1988; 255:357–360.
73. Griffiths EJ, Halestrap AP: Further evidence that cyclosporin A protects mitochondria from calcium overload by inhibiting a matrix peptidyl-prolyl cis-trans isomerase. Implications for the immunosuppressive and toxic effects of cyclosporin. *Biochem J* 1991; 274:611–614.
74. Griffiths EJ, Halestrap AP: Protection by cyclosporin A of ischemia/reperfusion-induced damage in isolated rat hearts. *J Mol Cell Cardiol* 1993; 25:1461–1469.
75. Savage MK, Jones DP, Reed DJ: Calcium- and phosphate-dependent release and loading of glutathione by liver mitochondria. *Arch Biochem Biophys* 1991; 290:51–56.
76. Solem LE, Wallace KB: Selective activation of the sodium-independent, cyclosporin A-sensitive calcium pore of cardiac mitochondria by doxorubicin. *Toxicol Appl Pharmacol* 1990; 121:50–57.
77. Chen G, Jaffrezou JP, Fleming WH, et al: Prevalence of multidrug resistance related to activation of the mdr1

gene in human sarcoma mutants derived by single-step doxorubicin selection. *Cancer Res* 1994; 54:4980–4987.
78. Fardel O, Ratanasavanh D, Loyer P, et al: Overexpression of the multidrug resistance gene product in adult rat hepatocytes during primary culture. *Eur J Biochem* 1992; 205:847–852.
79. Jiang XR, Macey MG, Collins PW, Newland AC: Characterization and modulation of drug transport kinetics in K562 c1.6 daunorubicin-resistant cell line. *Br J Haematol* 1994; 86:547–554.
80. Larsson R, Bergh J, Nygren P: Combination of cyclosporin A and buthionine sulfoximine (BSO) as a pharmacological strategy for circumvention of multidrug resistance in small cell lung cancer cell lines selected for resistance to doxorubicin. *Anticancer Res* 1991; 11:455–459.
81. Mutch DG, Herzog TJ, Chen CA, Collins JL: The effects of cyclosporin A on the lysis of ovarian cancer cells by cisplatin or adriamycin. *Gynecol Oncol* 1992; 47:28–33.
82. Petrini M, Mattii L, Sabbatini AR, et al: Activity of different revertant agents on multidrug resistance: in vitro evaluation of their combination. *Int J Tissue React* 1994; 15:17–23.
83. Speeg KV, Maldonado AL: Effect of the nonimmunosuppressive cyclosporin analog SDZ PSC-833 on colchicine and doxorubicin biliary secretion by the rat in vivo. *Cancer Chemother Pharmacol* 1994; 34:133–136.
84. Baker PF: The regulation of intracellular calcium. *Symp Soc Exp Biol* 1972; 30:67–88.
85. Baker PF: Transport and metabolism of calcium ions in nerve. *Prog Biophys Mol Biol* 1972; 24:177–223.
86. Baker PF, Hodgkin AL, Ridgeway EB: Depolarization and calcium entry into squid giant axons. *J Physiol (London)* 1971; 218:709–755.
87. Rappaport ZH, Young W, Flamm ES: Regional brain calcium changes in the rat middle cerebral artery occlusion model of ischemia. *Stroke* 1987; 18:760–764.
88. Auerbach S, Young W: A method for regional determination of total phosphate in rat brain. *CNS* 1987; 4:53–61.
89. Young W: Secondary injury mechanisms in acute spinal cord injury. [Review]. *J Emerg Med* 1993; 1:13–22.
90. Allen BT, Davis CG, Osborne D, Karl I: Spinal cord ischemia and reperfusion metabolism: the effect of hypothermia. *J Vasc Surg* 1994; 19:332–339.
91. Bakshi R, Faden AI: Competitive and non-competitive NMDA antagonists limit dynorphin A-induced rat hindlimb paralysis. *Brain Res* 1990; 507:1–5.
92. Danielisova V, Chavko M: Amelioration of ischemic spinal cord damage by postischemic treatment with propentofylline (HWA 285). *Brain Res* 1992; 590:321–324.
93. Demediuk P, Daly MP, Faden AI: Effect of impact trauma on neurotransmitter and nonneurotransmitter amino acids in rat spinal cord [published erratum appears in *J Neurochem* 1990 Feb;54(2):724]. *J Neurochem* 1989; 52:1529–1536.
94. Faden AI, Ellison JA, Noble LJ: Effects of competitive and noncompetitive NMDA receptor antagonists in spinal cord injury. *Eur J Pharmacol* 1990; 175:165–174.
95. Faden AI, Lemke M, Simon RP, Noble LJ: N-methyl-D-aspartate antagonist MK801 improves outcome following traumatic spinal cord injury in rats: Behavioral, anatomic, and neurochemical studies. *J Neurotrauma* 1988; 5:33–45.
96. Faden AI, Simon RP: A potential role for excitotoxins in the pathophysiology of spinal cord injury. *Ann Neurol* 1988; 23:623–626.
97. Long JB, Rigamonti DD, Oleshansky MA, et al: Dynorphin A-induced rat spinal cord injury: evidence for excitatory amino acid involvement in a pharmacological model of ischemic spinal cord injury. *J Pharmacol Exp Ther* 1994; 269:358–366.
98. Madden KP, Clark WM, Kochhar A, Zivin JA: Efficacy of LY233053, a competitive glutamate antagonist, in experimental central nervous system ischemia. *J Neurosurg* 1992; 76:106–110.
99. Marsala M, Sorkin LS, Yaksh TL: Transient spinal ischemia in rat: Characterization of spinal cord blood flow, extracellular amino acid release, and concurrent histopathological damage. *J Cereb Blood Flow Metab* 1994; 14:604–614.
100. McBurney RN, Daly D, Fischer JB, et al: New CNS-specific calcium antagonists. *J Neurotrauma* 1992; 2:S531–S543.
101. Meldrum BS, Swan JH, Leach MJ, et al: Reduction of glutamate release and protection against ischemic brain damage by BW 1003C87. *Brain Res* 1992; 593:1–6.
102. Panter SS, Faden AI: Pretreatment with NMDA antagonists limits release of excitatory amino acids following traumatic brain injury. *Neurosci Lett* 1992; 136:165–168.
103. Rokkas CK, Helfrich L, Jr, Lobner DC, et al: Dextrorphan inhibits the release of excitatory amino acids during spinal cord ischemia. *Ann Thorac Surgery* 1994; 58:312–319.
104. Steinberg GK, Kunis D, Saleh J, DeLaPaz R: Protection after transient focal cerebral ischemia by the N-methyl-D-aspartate antagonist dextrorphan is dependent upon plasma and brain levels. *J Cereb Blood Flow Metab* 1991; 11:1015–1024.
105. Tymianski M, Wallace MC, Spigelman I, et al: Cell-permeant Ca^{2+} chelators reduce early excitotoxic and ischemic neuronal injury in vitro and in vivo. *Neuron* 1993; 11:221–235.
106. von Euler M, Seiger A, Holmberg L, Sundstrom E: NBQX, a competitive non-NMDA receptor antagonist, reduces degeneration due to focal spinal cord ischemia. *Exper Neurol* 1994; 129:163–168.
107. Yum SW, Faden AI: Comparison of the neuroprotective effects of the N-methyl-D-aspartate antagonist MK-801 and the opiate-receptor antagonist nalmefene in experimental spinal cord ischemia. *Arch Neurol* 1990; 47:277–281.
108. Choi DW: Excitotoxic cell death [Review]. *J Neurobiol* 1992; 23:1261–1276.
109. Rothman S, Olney JW: Glutamate and the pathophysiology of hypoxic ischemic brain damage. *Ann Neurol* 1986; 19:105–111.
110. Stewart GR, Olney JW, Pattikonda M, Snider WD:

Excitotoxicity in the embryonic chick spinal cord. *Ann Neurol* 1991; 30:750–766.

111. Regan RF, Choi DW: Glutamate neurotoxicity in spinal cord cell culture. *Neuroscience* 1991; 43:585–591.
112. Benveniste H, Drejer J, Schousboe A, Diemer NH: Elevation of the extracellular concentrations of glutamate and aspartate in rat hippocampus during transient cerebral ischemia monitored by intracerebral dialysis. *J Neuorchem* 1984; 43:1369–1374.
113. Benveniste H, Jorgensen MB, Sandberg M, et al: Ischemic damage in hippocampal CA1 is dependent on glutamate release and intact innervation from CA3. *J Cereb Blood Flow Metab* 1989; 9:629–639.
114. Drejer J, Benveniste H, Diemer NH, Schousboe A: Cellular origin of ischemia-induced glutamate release from brain tissue in vivo and in vitro. *J Neurochem* 1985; 45:145–151.
115. Faden AI: Dynorphin increases extracellular levels of excitatory amino acids in the brain through a non-opioid mechanism. *J Neurosci* 1992; 12:425–429.
116. Faden AI, Demediuk P, Panter SS, Vink R: The role of excitatory amino acids and NMDA receptors in traumatic brain injury. *Science* 1989; 244:798–800.
117. Katayama Y, Becker DP, Tamura T, Hovda DA: Massive increases in extracellular potassium and the indiscriminate release of glutamate following concussive brain injury. *J Neurosurg* 1990; 73:889–900.
118. Katayama Y, Becker DP, Tamura T, Ikezaki K: Early cellular swelling in experimental traumatic brain injury: A phenomenon mediated by excitatory amino acids. *Acta Neurochir* 1990; 51(suppl):271–273.
119. Kawamata T, Katayama Y, Hovda DA, et al: Administration of excitatory amino acid antagonists via microdialysis attenuates the increase in glucose utilization seen following concussive brain injury. *J Cereb Blood Flow Metab* 1992; 12:12–24.
120. Aitken PG, Jing J, Young J, Somjen GG: Ion channel involvement in hypoxia-induced spreading depression in hippocampal slices. *Brain Res* 1991; 541:7–11.
121. Evans D, Smith JC: Seizure activity and cortical spreading depression monitored by an extrinsic potential-sensitive molecular probe. *Brain Res* 1987; 409:350–357.
122. Moghaddam B, Gruen RJ, Roth RH, et al: Effect of L-glutamate on the release of striatal dopamine: in vivo dialysis and electrochemical studies. *Brain Res* 1990; 518:55–60.
123. Szerb JC: Glutamate release and spreading depression in the fascia dentata in response to microdialysis with high K^+: role of glia. *Brain Res* 1991; 542:259–265.
124. Nedergaard M, Hansen AJ: Spreading depression is not associated with neuronal injury in the normal brain. *Brain Res* 1988; 449:395–398.
125. Giffard RG, Monyer H, Christine CW, Choi DW: Acidosis reduces NMDA receptor activation, glutamate neurotoxicity, and oxygen-glucose deprivation neuronal injury in cortical cultures. *Brain Res* 1990; 506:339–342.
126. Ahmed Z, Lewis CA, Faber DS: Glutamate stimulates release of Ca^{2+} from internal stores in astroglia. *Brain Res* 1990; 516:165–169.
127. Chan PH, Chu I: Mechanisms underlying glutamate-induced swelling of astrocytes in primary culture. *Acta Neurochir* 1990; 51(suppl):7–10.
128. Kimelberg HK, Rose JW, Barron KD, et al: Astrocytic swelling in traumatic-hypoxic brain injury. Beneficial effects of an inhibitor of anion exchange transport and glutamate uptake in glial cells. *Mol Chem Neuropathol* 1989; 11:1–31.
129. Noble LJ, Hall JJ, Chen S, Chan PH: Morphologic changes in cultured astrocytes after exposure to glutamate. *J Neurotrauma* 1992; 9:255–267.
130. Hayes RL, Jenkins LW, Lyeth BG: Neurotransmitter-mediated mechanisms of traumatic brain injury: acetylcholine and excitatory amino acids. *J Neurotrauma* 1992; 9:S173–187.
131. Lyeth BG, Hayes RL: Cholinergic and opioid mediation of traumatic brain injury. *J Neurotrauma* 1992; 2:S463–S474.
132. Robinson SE, Foxx SD, Posner MG, et al: The effect of M1 muscarinic blockade on behavior and physiological responses following traumatic brain injury in the rat. *Brain Res* 1990; 511:141–148.
133. Saija A, Hayes RL, Lyeth BG, et al: The effect of concussive head injury on central cholinergic neurons. *Brain Res* 1988; 452:303–311.
134. Saija A, Robinson SE, Lyeth BG, et al: The effects of scopolamine and traumatic brain injury on central cholinergic neurons. *J Neurotrauma* 1988; 5:161–170.
135. Yamamoto T, Lyeth BG, Dixon CE, et al: Changes in regional brain acetylcholine content in rats following unilateral and bilateral brainstem lesions. *J Neurotrauma* 1988; 5:69–79.
136. Osterholm JL, Bell J, Meyer R: Experimental effects of free serotonin on the brain and its relation to brain injury: Part 1: The neurological consequences of intracerebral serotonin injections. Part 2: Trauma induced alterations in spinal fluid and brain. Part 3. Serotonin-induced cerebral edema. *J Neurosurg* 1969; 31:408–421.
137. Salzman SK, Puniak MA, Liu ZJ, et al: The serotonin antagonist mianserin improves functional recovery following experimental spinal trauma. *Ann Neurol* 1991; 30:533–541.
138. Honmou O, Sakatani K, Young W: GABA and potassium effects on corticospinal and primary afferent tracts of neonatal rat spinal cord dorsal columns. *Neuroscience* 1993; 54:93–104.
139. Lee M, Sakatani K, Young W: A role of GABA-A receptors in hypoxia induced conduction failure of neonatal rat spinal dorsal column axons. *Brain Res* 1993; 601:14–19.
140. Sakatani K, Hassan A, Lee M, et al: Non-synaptic modulation of dorsal column conduction by endogenous GABA in neonatal rat spinal cord. *Brain Res* 1993; 662:43–50.
141. Honmou O, Young W: Norepinephrine modulates excitability of neonatal rat optic nerves through calcium-mediated mechanisms. *Neuroscience* 1995;?
142. Bollen M, Stalmans W: The structure, role, and regulation of type 1 protein phosphatases. *Crit Rev Biochem Mol Biol* 1992; 27:227–281.
143. Klee CB, Crouch TH, Krinks MH: Calcineurin: A calci-

um- and calmodulin-binding protein of the nervous system. *Proc Natl Acad Sci* 1979; 76:6270–6273.
144. Klee CB, Draetta GF, Hubbard MJ: Calcineurin. *Adv Enzymol Relat Areas Mol Biol* 1988; 61:149–200.
145. Schreiber S: Chemistry and biology of the immunophilins and their immunosuppressive ligands. *Science* 1991; 251:283–287.
146. Schreiber SL: Immunophilin-sensitive protein phosphatase action in cell signalling pathways. *Cell* 1992; 70:365–368.
147. Guerini D, Hubbard MJ, Krinks MH, Klee CB: Multiple forms of calcineurin, a brain isozyme of the calmodulin-stimulated protein phosphatase. *Adv Second Messenger Phosphoprotein Res* 1990; 24:242–247.
148. Bonnefoy-Berard N, Genestier L, Flacher M, Revillard JP: The phosphoprotein phosphatase calcineurin controls calcium-dependent apoptosis in B cell lines. *Eur J Immunol* 1994; 24:325–329.
149. Clipstone NA, Crabtree GR: Identification of calcineurin as a key signalling enzyme in T-lymphocyte activation. *Nature* 1992; 357:695–697.
150. Fruman DA, Klee CB, Beirer BE, Burakoff SJ: Calcineurin phosphatase activity in T lymphocytes is inhibited by FK-506 and cyclosporin A. *Proc Natl Acad Sci USA* 1992; 89:3686–3690.
151. Chung E, Dvorozniak MT, Van-Woert MH, Li HC: Regional distribution of calcium/calmodulin-dependent phosphatase activity of calcineurin in rat brain. *Res Commun Chem Pathol Pharmacol* 1989; 64:357–371.
152. Goto S, Nagahiro S, Korematsu K, Ushio Y: Striatonigral involvement following transient focal cerebral ischemia in the rats: an immunohistochemical study on a reversible ischemia model. *Acta Neuropathol* 1993; 85:515–520.
153. Chang CD, Mukai H, Kuno T, Tanaka C: cDNA cloning of an alternatively spliced isoform of the regulatory subunit of Ca^{2+}/calmodulin-dependent protein phosphatase (calcineurin B alpha 2). *Biochim Biophys Acta* 1994; 1217:174–180.
154. Jain J, McCaffrey PG, Miner Z, et al: The T-cell transcription factor NFATp is a substrate for calcineurin and interacts with Fos and Jun. *Nature* 1993; 365:352–355.
155. Kubo M, Kincaid RL, Ransom JT: Activation of the interleukin-4 gene is controlled by the unique calcineurin-dependent transcriptional factor NF(P). *J Biol Chem* 1994; 269:19441–19446.
156. McCaffrey PG, Perrino BA, Soderling TR, Rao A: NF-ATp, a T lymphocyte DNA-binding protein that is a target for calcineurin and immunosuppressive drugs. *J Biol Chem* 1993; 268:3747–3752.
157. Nghiem P, Ollick T, Gardner P, Schulman H: Interleukin-2 transcriptional block by multifunctional Ca^{2+}/calmodulin kinase. *Nature* 1994; 371:347–350.
158. Rao A: NF-ATp: a transcription factor required for the co-ordinate induction of several cytokine genes. [Review]. *Immunology Today* 1994; 15:274–281.
159. Schreiber SL, Crabtree GR: The mechanism of action of cyclosporin A and FK506. *Immunol Today* 1992; 13:136–142.
160. Stroebel M, Goppelt-Struebe M: Signal transduction pathways responsible for serotonin-mediated prostaglandin G/H synthase expression in rat mesangial cells. *J Biol Chem* 1994; 269:22952–22957.
161. Busse R, Luckhoff A, Mulsch A: Cellular mechanisms controlling EDRF/NO formation in endothelial cells. *Basic Res Cardiol* 1991; 2:7–16.
162. Dawson TM, Steiner JP, Dawson VL, et al: Immunosuppressant FK506 enhances phosphorylation of nitric oxide synthase and protects against glutamate neurotoxicity [see comments]. *Proc Natl Acad Sci USA* 1993; 90:9808–9812.
163. Fast DJ, Lynch RC, Leu RW: Cyclosporin A inhibits nitric oxide production by L929 cells in response to tumor necrosis factor and interferon-gamma. *J Interferon Res* 1993; 13:235–240.
164. Mittal CK, Jadhav AL: Calcium-dependent inhibition of constitutive nitric oxide synthase. *Biochem Biophys Res Comm* 1994; 203:8–15.
165. Armstrong DL: Calcium channel regulation by calcineurin, a Ca^{2+}-activated phosphatase in mammalian brain. *Trends Neurosci* 1989; 12:117–122.
166. Kostyuk PG, Lukyanetz EA: Mechanisms of antagonistic action of internal Ca^{2+} on serotonin-induced potentiation of Ca^{2+} currents in Helix neurones. *Pflugers Arch* 1993; 424:73–83.
167. Lieberman DN, Mody I: Regulation of NMDA channel function by endogenous $Ca^{(2+)}$-dependent phosphatase. *Nature* 1994; 369:235–239.
168. Nichols RA, Suplick GR, Brown JM: Calcineurin-mediated protein dephosphorylation in brain nerve terminals regulates the release of glutamate. *J Biol Chem* 1994; 269:23817–23823.
169. Halpain S, Girault JA, Greengard P: Activation of NMDA receptors induces dephosphorylation of DARPP-32 in rat striatal slices. *Nature* 1990; 343:369–372.
170. Halpain S, Greengard P: Activation of NMDA receptors induces rapid dephosphorylation of the cytoskeletal protein MAP2. *Neuron* 1990; 5:237–246.
171. Mendoza I, Rubio F, Rodriguez-Navarro A, Pardo JM: The protein phosphatase calcineurin is essential for NaCl tolerance of Saccharomyces cerevisiae. *J Biol Chem* 1994; 269:8792–8796.
172. Bohme M, Buchler M, Muller M, Keppler D: Differential inhibition by cyclosporins of primary-active ATP-dependent transporters in the hepatocyte canalicular membrane. *FEBS Lett* 1993; 333:193–196.
173. Bohme M, Muller M, Leier I, et al: Cholestasis caused by inhibition of the adenosine triphosphate-dependent bile salt transport in rat liver. *Gastroenterology* 1994; 107:255–265.
174. Kadmon M, Klunemann C, Bohme M, et al: Inhibition by cyclosporin A of adenosine triphosphate-dependent transport from the hepatocyte into bile [see comments]. *Gastroenterology* 1993; 104:1507–1514.
175. Leier I, Jedlitschky G, Buchholz U, Keppler D: Characterization of the ATP-dependent leukotriene C4 export carrier in mastocytoma cells. *Eur J Biochem* 1994; 220:599–606.

176. Fruman DA, Mather PE, Burakoff SJ, Bierer BE: Correlation of calcineurin phosphatase activity and programmed cell death in murine T cell hybridomas. *Eur J Immunol* 1992; 22:2513–2517.
177. McCarthy SA, Cacchione RN, Mainwaring MS, Cairns JS: The effects of immunosuppressive drugs on the regulation of activation-induced apoptotic cell death in thymocytes. *Transplantation* 1992; 54:543–547.
178. McCarthy SA, Mainwaring MS, Cairns JS: Effects of FK506 and cyclosporine on T-cell tolerance: inhibition of a "protective" mechanism that regulates activation-induced apoptosis in developing thymocytes. *Transplant Proc* 1991; 23:2925–2927.
179. Shi YF, Sahai BM, Green DR: Cyclosporin A inhibits activation-induced cell death in T-cell hybridomas and thymocytes. *Nature* 1989; 339:625–626.
180. Genestier L, Dearden-Badet MT, Bonnefoy-Berard N, et al: Cyclosporin A and FK506 inhibit activation-induced cell death in the murine WEHI-231 B cell line. *Cell Immunol* 1994; 155:283–291.
181. Little GH, Flores A: Inhibition of programmed cell death by cyclosporin. *Comp Biochem Physiol* [*c*] 1992; 103:463–467.
182. Sharkey J, Butcher SP: Immunophilins mediate the neuroprotective effects of FK506 in focal cerebral ischemia. *Nature* 1994; 371:336–339.
183. Shiga Y, Onodera H, Matsuo Y, Kogure K: Cyclosporin A protects against ischemia-reperfusion injury in the brain. *Brain Res* 1992; 595:145–148.
184. Broekemeier KM, Carpenter-Deyo L, Reed DJ, Pfeiffer DR: Cyclosporin A protects hepatocytes subjected to high Ca^{2+} and oxidative stress. *FEBS Lett* 1992; 304:192–194.
185. Carini R, Parola M, Dianzani MU, Albano E: Mitochondrial damage and its role in causing hepatocyte injury during stimulation of lipid peroxidation by iron nitriloacetate. *Arch Biochem Biophys* 1992; 297:110–118.
186. Imberti R, Nieminen AL, Herman B, Lemasters JJ: Synergism of cyclosporin A and phospholipase inhibitors in protection against lethal injury to rat hepatocytes from oxidant chemicals. *Res Commun Chem Pathol Pharmacol* 1992; 78:27–38.
187. Pastorino JG, Snyder JW, Serroni A, et al: Cyclosporin and carnitine prevent the anoxic death of cultured hepatocytes by inhibiting the mitochondrial permeability transition. *J Biol Chem* 1993; 268:13791–13798.
188. Snyder JW, Pastorino JG, Attie AM, Farber JL: Protection by cyclosporin A of cultured hepatocytes from the toxic consequences of the loss of mitochondrial energization produced by 1-methyl-4-phenylpyridinium. *Biochem Pharmacol* 1992; 44:833–835.
189. Song Q, Lavin MF: Calyculin A, a potent inhibitor of phosphatases-1 and -2A, prevents apoptosis. *Biochem Biophys Res Commun* 1993; 190:47–55.
190. Boe R, Gjertsen BT, Vintermyr OK, et al: The protein phosphatase inhibitor okadaic acid induces morphological changes typical of apoptosis in mammalian cells. *Exp Cell Res* 1991; 195:237–246.

CHAPTER 106

CELL-MEDIATED INJURY

Chung Y. Hsu
Zhong Y. Hu
S. Kathleen Doster

SYNOPSIS

Trauma to the brain and spinal cord resulting in an immediate physical injury is frequently followed by further tissue damage that may progress over a period of hours or days after the initial insult. This phenomenon has been called secondary injury.[177,81] *Among a number of pathophysiological processes that may contribute to secondary injury, cell-mediated processes caused by post-traumatic inflammation have been increasingly recognized. Acute inflammation is associated with inflammatory mediator production, polymorphonuclear neutrophil (PMN) infiltration, platelet deposition, endothelial cell (EC) injury and activation, increased vascular permeability, and edema formation.*[51] *In addition, activation and proliferation of monocytic cells, both microglial and blood-borne, may occur. Inflammatory responses after CNS injury may have substantial pathophysiological implications*[86] *and may be an important determinant of the ultimate outcome.*[85] *In this chapter, we discuss cell-mediated secondary injury after brain and spinal cord trauma in the context of a post-traumatic inflammatory reaction.*

INFLAMMATORY REACTION: CONCEPT AND CONSEQUENCE

The hallmark of acute inflammation is the infiltration of PMNs, which are the primary effector cells. This is triggered by expression of cell adhesive molecules (CAMs), endothelial cell injury with resultant impairment of surface anticoagulant mechanism, and generation of inflammatory mediators. Tissue destruction in acute inflammation has been largely ascribed to the actions of PMNs, which generate free radicals and release proteases.[3,11,167] Both free radicals and proteases may cause vascular injury to sustain the PMN-EC interaction.[106] Normal ECs are essential for maintaining the integrity of vasculature and preventing intravascular clotting. ECs, once injured, become active participants in inflammation and cause their own destruction.[27] PMN activation by inflammatory mediators is enhanced by ECs.[75] Injured ECs can stimulate PMNs, platelets, and activate coagulation pathways. Interaction of platelets and ECs through lipid inflammatory mediators has been extensively studied in both normal and pathological conditions.[121] Platelets are also inflammatory cells[27,51] and, like PMNs, release inflammatory mediators (TXA2, 12-HETE, PAF, and serotonin) and proteolytic enzymes.[51] The actions of platelets and PMNs are mediated by common factors such as thromboxane, prostaglandins, leukotrienes, PAF, CAMs, and cytokines. The synergistic interaction of platelets and PMNs has been recognized only recently.[43,112] Platelet-dependent PMN-mediated tissue injury in nephritis[91] exemplifies the interaction of platelets and PMNs in inflammation. The interaction among PMNs, platelets, and ECs in acute inflammation and that engaging macrophage or microglia, ECs, and injured neural tissue in the subacute phase of post-traumatic inflammatory reaction are very complex and involve redundant activating mechanisms making pharmacological intervention a difficult task.

CELLULAR MECHANISM OF INFLAMMATION

An evolving concept of inflammation has emerged from recent cell and molecular biology studies of animal models of inflammation.[146] At the cellular level, EC injury leading to CAM expression may be a primary mechanism to attract leukocytes and platelets with resultant production of inflammatory mediators and extravasation of inflammatory cells. Cellular elements of inflammatory reaction have been extensively described after traumatic and ischemic CNS injury.

Post-Traumatic EC Injury

Spinal cord injury

Vascular injury probably plays an important role in the progressive injury of the spinal cord after traumatic insult. Endothelial damage[6,38,68,69,92,128] and vasogenic edema[82,83] proceed or develop in parallel with neuronal damage.[6,7] Damage to vascular endothelium has been noted immediately following spinal cord injury as a consequence of primary mechanical injury.[6,82,128,68,69,92,38,67,148,66,160] However, the vascular injury has been shown to progress[6,82,128,68,69] and extend beyond the level of initial mechanical injury,[92,160] suggesting involvement of secondary factors.

Brain injury

EC injury and blood-brain barrier dysfunction reflected by increased vascular permeability and vasogenic brain edema have been extensively described in animal models of traumatic brain injury.[138] While some of these models were associated with hemorrhagic lesions,[32,156] others, especially the more recent studies, have clearly illustrated that EC injury after brain injury can be dissociated from hemorrhage.[138,62,150,151]

Post-Traumatic PMN Infiltration

Infiltration of acute inflammatory cells, notably PMNs, into the injured spinal cord has been shown in morphological and enzymatic studies.[6,7,117,174] Recently, PMN infiltration into the traumatized brain[144,13,122] also has been noted.

Post-Traumatic Platelet Deposition

Platelet deposition is seen early after impact injury to the spinal cord.[6,63] Platelet deposition has also been well documented in ischemic brain.[40] Platelet accumulation has not yet been morphologically characterized in traumatized brain. Endothelial injury exposes platelets to basement membranes, resulting in adhesion, then aggregation, shape change, degranulation, and the liberation of arachidonic acid.[43] Degranulation releases inflammatory mediators (TXA2, 12-HETE, PAF, and serotonin) and proteolytic enzymes.[27] These, in turn, cause disruption of endothelium and activation of PMNs. PMNs are also potent inducers of platelet activation, which may be mediated by PMN-derived proteases.[43]

Mononuclear Cell Response

Response to CNS injury may be characterized, under certain pathological conditions, by a predominantly mononuclear infiltrate. To what extent this reaction is derived from the microglia in the CNS or from the recruitment of monocytic cells from the peripheral blood cannot be easily determined. There is ample evidence to support the contention that the microglia are indeed the resident macrophages of the CNS.[135,155] Microglia possess antigenic markers of the mononuclear phagocyte lineage and generate inflammatory mediators shared by monocytic inflammatory cells. This repertoire includes proteases, major histocompatibility antigens, and cytokines.[39]

Experimental evidence suggests that microglia activation after CNS injury may be detrimental. Microglia have been implicated in the pathogenesis of neuronal degeneration in a number of conditions including acquired immune deficiency syndrome (AIDS), Alzheimer's disease, Parkinson's disease, and others[155] where excitotoxins may play an important role.[24] In excitotoxin-induced CNS injury, axonal injury and demyelination were correlated with the extent of monocytic cell infiltration.[29,136] Irradiation reduces both the inflammatory response and the damage of the myelinated axons.[28] These findings are in agreement with a "bystander effect" of CNS inflammatory reaction noted for nearly two decades.[171]

Spinal cord injury

An association of axonal damage and macrophage infiltration has been noted in a number of animal models of spinal cord injury.[162,71,15] In a spinal cord ischemia-reperfusion model, Giulian and Robertson[60] noted that reduction of mononuclear phagocytes by chloroquine or colchicine was accompanied by improved neurological function and neuronal survival. Blight[16] has extensively and elegantly reviewed the role of macrophage in traumatic spinal cord injury, using the framework of a post-traumatic inflammatory reaction.

Brain injury

Microglia may cause neuronal degeneration by releasing soluble neurotoxic factors that may be blocked by NMDA antagonists.[59,61] Interleukin-1 level[55] was increased in brain after stabbing injury and was shown to be generated by ameboid microglia.[56,57] Microglia may also contribute to wound healing after traumatic brain injury by promoting astrogliosis and angiogenesis.[58] The exact roles of microglia in the injured CNS remain to be fully characterized. The neurotoxic and neurotrophic effects of microglia may be exerted at different stages after injury involving different mechanisms.[21,54,61,62]

INFLAMMATORY MEDIATORS

Cellular reaction in inflammation is mediated by a variety of mediators. The recruitment of circulating leukocytes into inflammatory foci involves the expression of surface molecules on ECs and leukocytes. Interaction among inflammatory cells including PMNs, macrophages, platelets and ECs is facilitated by cytokines and inflammatory mediators. In a brief review below, the mediators of inflammation will be arbitrarily divided into four broad categories: (1) adhesive molecules; (2) cytokines; (3) lipid inflammatory mediators; and (4) nitric oxide.

Cell Adhesion Molecules (CAMS)

Expression of CAMs is a dynamic process requiring de novo gene expression in response to a variety of proinflammatory stimuli particularly the generation of cytokines (see below). CAMs can be divided into those expressed by the circulating leukocytes and those expressed by ECs.

Leukocyte-derived CAMS

There are two important types of leukocyte-derived CAMs: leukocyte integrins and L-selectin. Leukocyte integrin family consists of at least 13 alpha/beta heterodimers with the ligand specificity of each integrin determined by both the alpha and beta chains. Integrins mediate both cell adhesion to extracellular matrix and cell-cell adhesion. The most familiar integrins in inflammation and immune function are LFA-1 (CD11a/CD18), Mac-1 (CD11b/CD18), and gp 150/95 (CD11c/CD18). The classification, structure, and function of integrins have been recently reviewed[148] and are beyond the scope of this chapter. L-selectin is constitutively expressed on circulating leukocytes and is probably involved in transient and reversible binding of leukocytes to the endothelium.

EC-derived CAMS

CAMs derived from ECs can be categorized into endothelial selectins and CAMs that belong to a immunoglobulin superfamily. Endothelial selectins are represented by E-selectin and P-selectin that are similar to L- also found, in addition to ECs, in platelets. P-selectin can be rapidly translocated to the cell surface upon activation. Both E-selectin and P-selectin are CAMs for PMNs, macrophages, and subpopulation of T-lymphocytes. ECs express three CAMs that share similar sequence domains of immunoglobulins: ICAM-1, ICAM-2, and VCAM-1. ICAM and VCAM stand respectively for intercellular and vascular CAMs. ICAM-1 is a single glycoprotein with five Ig-like domains which is expressed by ECs and a variety of other cells including leukocytes. ICAM-1 is constitutively expressed by ECs at low levels but can be drastically increased in response to inflammation. ICAM-2 is similar to ICAM-2 but contains only two Ig-like domains. It is constitutively expressed by ECs and but is not increased by cytokine activation. Both ICAM-1 and ICAM-2 are counter-receptors of LFA-1. VCAM-1 is a cytokine-responsive endothelial CAM with Ig-like domains that are counter-receptors of CAMs expressed by monocytes and lymphocytes. EC-derived CAMs have also been extensively reviewed.[12] CAM expression after brain or spinal cord injury remains to be explored. Post-traumatic inflammation is likely to engage CAMs in the EC interaction with inflammatory cells.

Cytokines

Cytokines are soluble proteins released by activated inflammatory cells. Cytokines mediate the bidirectional communication between cells to facilitate and perpetuate the inflammatory processes. The diversity of cytokines and their complex actions make a detailed description of each individual cytokine beyond the scope of this chapter. The brief summary below is intended only to introduce the general properties and common actions of cytokines. Readers interested in more detailed review of this topic are referred to a number of excellent reviews published recently.[88,110,111,118]

Cytokines are polypeptides or glycoproteins of low molecular weight (with monomeric forms of 25 to 30 kd) which exert their actions by binding to specific receptors. These receptors may be present on the secreting cell, nearby cells, or distant targets. Most cytokine actions entail new mRNA transcription, leading to cell proliferation, differentiation, or expression of new proteins (e.g., CAMs). Most cytokines have potent effects on hematopoietic cells and vascular endothelium. Overall effects of cytokine expression and release by inflammatory cells are pro-thrombotic and pro-inflammatory. Systemic effects of selected cytokines include induction of fever (tumor necrosis factor [TNF], interleukin-1 [IL-1], interleukin-2 [IL-2], interferons [INFs]), stimulation of the production of acute phase proteins (TNF, IL-1, IL-6, and INF-gamma), and cachexia (TNF, IL-1, and

INF-gamma). Increased IL-1, IL-2, IL-6, and TNF levels have been reported after brain or spinal cord injury.[54,115,129,130,116,173,107,109,176,154,63,152]

Lipid Inflammatory Mediators

Like cytokines, lipid inflammatory mediators also play crucial roles in cellular interaction in acute inflammation. Activation of AA metabolism is a key event in inflammation.[169,86,49] Inflammatory mediators derived from AA include prostaglandins (PGs), thromboxane (TX) A2, and leukotrienes (LTs), which are collectively called eicosanoids. PGs and TXA2 are generated via cyclooxygenase pathway.[172] PGs, particularly PGE2 and PGI2, enhance vascular permeability induced by other inflammatory mediators such as BK, histamine, complement fragment (Cr5a), and platelet activating factor (PAF).[27] TXA2 is the major eicosanoid released by platelets. It causes aggregation and endothelial adhesion of platelets and PMNs.[27] Aspirin and most of the newly available nonsteroidal anti-inflammatory drugs are cyclooxygenase inhibitors.[84,22] Glucocorticoids are among the most potent anti-inflammatory agents. The beneficial effects of methylprednisolone in spinal cord injury in animal models[2] and humans[17] has been ascribed to its antioxidant effect.[18] It is plausible that anti-inflammatory effect of methylprednisolone also contributes, at least in part, to its neuroprotective effect.[85] Recent development of new anti-inflammatory drugs has been directed toward the lipoxygenase pathway of AA, namely lipoxygenase. Lipoxygenases catalyze the formation of LTs, hydroxyeicosatetraenoic acids (HETEs), hydroperoxyeicosatetraenoic acids (HPETEs), and others. The roles of LTs in inflammation have been well established. LTB4 is one of the most potent chemoattractants.[46] LTC4 and LTD4 promote vascular permeability and act synergistically with LTB4 and other mediators in the inflammatory process.[143,105] The exact roles of HETEs, HPETEs and other lipoxygenase metabolites in the inflammatory process remain to be fully defined.[127,121] They may serve as chemoattractants and mediate the interaction of PMNs, platelets, and ECs.[169] AA metabolites derived from a third (cytochrome P-450) pathway also have to be fully investigated for their roles in inflammation.[1]

Another new avenue for modulating inflammation concerns platelet-activating factor (PAF). PAF belongs to the lipid class 1-O-alkyl-2-acetyl-sn-glycero-3-phosphocholine. Its release from cell membrane is closely coupled to activation of AA metabolism. PAF enhances platelet aggregation and PMN adhesion to ECs and increases vascular permeability. PAF also stimulates AA metabolism. The roles of PAF as a key inflammatory mediator has also been established.[72] Activation of arachidonate metabolism leading to the increased formation of lipid inflammatory mediators has been well documented in the literature.[41,42,166,37,82,174]

Activation of arachidonate metabolism may be partly caused by the activation of kininogen-kinin cascade. Kininogens are acute phase reactants and precursors of kinins. Synthesis and release of kininogens into plasma are increased in inflammation or following tissue injury.[140] Kinins including bradykinin (BK), Lys-BK, and T-kinin are peptide inflammatory mediators. They are released from kininogens by proteolytic enzymes, including kallikreins, calpains, PMN-derived proteases, and others. Activation of several other proteolytic cascades (coagulation, fibrinolysis, and complement) after tissue injury also triggers kinin release from kininogens.[105] At least part of the pro-inflammatory action of kinins is mediated by AA metabolites. BK activates AA metabolism by stimulating phospholipases.[30] BK may also increase vascular permeability and protein extravasation independent of, but enhanced by, AA metabolites.[51] Recent studies in a rat SCI model indicate that there is increased accumulation of kininogen and its conversion to pro-inflammatory kinins in the injured spinal cord.[175,87] In addition to their primary role as inflammatory mediators, kinins also may sustain the activation of phospholipases leading to a progressive accumulation of eicosanoids.[97,98] Kininogen-kinin system has also been associated with the secondary vascular changes in experimental traumatic head injury.[42]

Nitric Oxide

Nitric oxide (NO) is the first example of a completely new signaling molecule, a departure from the classic concept of the conventional inflammatory mediators such as cytokines (proteins), kinins (peptides), and arachidonic acid (AA) and its derivatives (fatty acids). NO is in contrast to cytokines, kinins, or eicosanoids, which possess complex structures and depend for their action on a complementary fit to specific receptors. The conventional agonist-receptor interaction triggers cell signal processes through second messengers and protein kinases. NO is a simple radical gas and soluble in both water and lipid. It is freely diffusible in the cellular environment. The reactivity of NO is related to its redox state, as is oxygen's, both forming redox couples. NO and O_2 react with each other, yielding strongly oxidizing molecules such as nitrogen dioxide and peroxynitrite. These oxidants are potentially more toxic than NO itself. When small amounts of NO are formed (i.e., in the physiological state from the constitutively expressed NOS or cNOS),[44] they preferentially bind to heme (e.g., heme-containing enzyme, guanyl cyclase). When large amounts of NO are released (i.e., under pathological conditions from the inducible NOS or iNOS),[44] they may bind to thiols or through nitrosylation or nitration reactions with cellular proteins, lipids, or DNA to cause oxidative injury. Peroxynitrite, a highly reactive and toxic free radical species generated from NO reaction with superoxide, may be an example of NO autotoxicity in pathological conditions.[9]

NO SYNTHASE (NOS)

NO is derived from L-arginine (L-arg) by hydroxylation of the nitrogen in the guanidino group. L-citrulline is the byproduct. This reaction is catalyzed by NO synthase (NOS). It requires reduced pyridine nucleotides, reduced biopteridine, and calmodulin as cofactors. NOS can be divided into constitutive (cNOS) and inducible NOS (iNOS). Three NOS isozymes (I: neuronal cNOS; II: iNOS in activated cells, including PMNs, ECs, and glial cells; and III: endothelial cNOS) have been isolated, representing three distinct gene products.[124,48] Endothelial cNOS undergoes post-transitional modification following stimulation by agonists such as acetylcholine or BK. This is a calcium-dependent process. Endothelial cNOS is active only in the presence of calcium and calmodulin.[19] Activation of cNOS (which usually occurs in physiological conditions) leads to a transient release of a small quantity of NO. iNOS is different from cNOS in that it is functionally calcium-independent. iNOS contains calmodulin tightly bound to each subunit of the enzyme.[23] It is presumed that calmodulin is incorporated into iNOS during synthesis, resulting in a permanent activation of the enzyme throughout its life. Expression of iNOS in certain pathological conditions is usually accompanied by a sustained release of large amounts of NO a thousand times higher than that catalyzed by cNOS.[4] Massive NO release by iNOS is only limited by the extent of its expression, availability of substrate (L-arg), and cofactors including NADPH, tetrahydrobiopertin (BH_4), and reduced thiol. In the absence of L-arg, NOS can generate superoxide and hydrogen peroxide.[44,78,96,139] iNOS can be induced in virtually every nucleated somatic cell. Endotoxin and selected cytokines, especially in combination, are known to be the major stimuli to induce glial, PMN, and EC iNOS expression in inflammation.[104] iNOS has also been called cytokine-inducible NOS or immune/inflammatory NOS.[8] iNOS induction by cytokine stimuli are at the transcriptional level requiring mRNA synthesis and are under the control of signaling processes (e.g., protein kinase C or tyrosine kinases) that regulate gene expression.[52,133,45] In many cases, changes in NO production are correlated with similar changes in iNOS regulation, which occurs at a pre-translational step such as transcription or mRNA stability.[124] iNOS mRNA levels thus correlate well with iNOS activity under most circumstances. The organization of bovine endothelial iNOS gene has recently been elucidated. The gene was noted to contain several putative transcription factor binding sites including AP-1, TNF responsive element, and an NF-kB site. Others have also reported DNA regulatory sequences within the promotor-regulatory region of NF-IL-6, interferon response elements.[124] The identification of these regulatory elements is consistent with the observation that inflammatory signals including cytokines (ILs, TNF, INFs) induce iNOS expression at the transcriptional level.[142,159]

NOS INHIBITORS

The synthesis of NO from L-arg can be inhibited by analogues of L-arg. Examples of these are N^6-monomethyl-L-arginine (L-NMMA), N^G-nitro-L-arginine (L-NNA), and N^G-nitro-L-arginine methyl ester (L-NAME). These NOS inhibitors act by competing with L-arg at the active site of NOS. They may also compete with L-arg for the arginine transporter system that regulates cellular L-arg levels, thereby reducing NO synthesis.[124] The competitive inhibition of NO synthesis by L-NMMA or L-NAME can be reversed by adding higher concentration of L-arg. Other inhibitors of NOS are such guanidino derivatives as aminoguanidine, which was thought to be mainly an inhibitor of iNOS.[33] Ebselen (2-phenyl-1,2-benzisoselemazol-3-(2H)one) is a selenium-containing antioxidant that inhibits both cNOS and iNOS. 7-nitro idazole (7-NI) is thought to be a specific inhibitor of neuronal NOS. Besides NOS inhibition, NO action also can be blocked by oxyhemoglobin. At least part of the action of NO (especially in physiological conditions) is through the activation of soluble guanyl cyclase, which can be blocked by methylene blue.[4,44] These inhibitors are useful pharmacological tools for assessing the role of NO in a wide variety of pathological conditions. Studies based on NOS inhibition or blocking NO actions have revealed that the involvement of NO in inflammation may be more complicated than previously thought. In endotoxin-induced sepsis or a number of experimental inflammation models,[157,149,74,124] NOS inhibition has been noted to be either beneficial or detrimental.[124,77,153,33,120,99,132] NO has been called the "Jekyll and Hyde" of inflammation.[119] Neuronal cNOS was thought to mediate NMDA-induced neuronal death under hypoxic/ischemic condition.[35,36] The literature on effects of NOS inhibitors on ischemic brain injury was equally confused.[103,44] NO can be a friend or foe, depending on experimental ischemic condition.[25] The application of a neuronal cNOS knockout transgenic mouse model,[89] however, has firmly confirmed the hypothesis pioneered by Dawson and colleagues[35,36] that activation of neuronal cNOS contributes to ischemic brain injury. NOS inhibitors have profound CBF effects[90,44] that may compound their pharmacological actions. It is likely that variable amounts of NO and its redox state may play different roles at different stages of disease processes.[25,108,44] The presence of different cellular and humoral mediators may also contribute to the variable effects caused by pharmacological modulation of NO synthesis or action.[124] The roles of nitric oxide cascade in traumatic brain and spinal cord injury remain to be delineated.

NO INTERACTION WITH OTHER INFLAMMATORY MEDIATORS

NO has emerged as a central figure in inflammatory reaction. NO may mediate the pro-inflammatory actions of such pro-inflammatory mediators as cytokines and bradykinin (BK) and may act synergistically with AA and its derivatives, eicosanoids.

Cytokines and Cell Adhesive Molecules (CAMs)

Certain cytokine actions are thought to be mediated by NO.[94,31,158] NOS is induced by pro-inflammatory cytokines such as TNF, IL1, IL2, and INF[163,95,125,168,157,34,64,102,141,100,164,170] in several types of cells and is suppressed by anti-inflammatory cytokines such as TGF or IL4, IL-8, and IL10.[76,114,134] NOS expression may depend on relative dominance of either pro- or anti-inflammatory cytokines at various stages of the inflammatory process.[76,26] Cytokines may interact synergistically in the induction of iNOS.[124,14,170] NO also may mediate cytokine-induced cell death, including apoptosis.[5] In a number of experimental paradigms, the roles of cytokines and NO could not be clearly distinguished.[93,31] Interaction of NO and cytokines may also create another positive feedback loop, as has been shown in a lung inflammation model.[170]

The accumulation of leukocytes in the inflammation sites results from their increased adhesiveness to ECs. In addition to the inflammatory mediators, CAMs play pivotal roles in this interaction. Expression of CAMs is a dynamic process requiring de novo gene expression in response to a variety of pro-inflammatory stimuli, particularly the generation of cytokines. NOS inhibitors have been shown to increase platelet and leukocyte adhesion to the normal endothelium.[101,137,131] These observations suggest that, under physiological conditions, NO may reduce endothelial adhesiveness. However, in pathological conditions, NO may mediate cytokine enhancement of CAM expression.[10,47]

Kinin-eicosanoid cascade

BK-induced increase in vascular permeability in skin inflammation is suppressed by NOS inhibitor, L-NAME, suggesting that BK may also contribute to endothelial NO production under pathological conditions.[133] NO interaction with eicosanoids has also been noted in a renal inflammation model in which NO also enhance PG release.[65] Together, these findings suggest that a positive feedback system engaging kinin-eicosanoid and NO cascades may be triggered under experimental inflammation.

Glial NO

In normal brain, the major source of NO synthesis is probably neuronal cNOS.[19] iNOS is expressed in glial cells in culture following incubation with lipopolysac-

TABLE 106-1 Cellular Elements and Key Mediators of Secondary CNS Injury

Cell Types	CAMs	Cytokines	Lipid Mediators	Type of Injury
PMN	L-selectin Mac-1	IL-1, IL-2, IL-6, TNF	LTB4, PGE2, PAF	Traumatic brain and spinal cord injury
Platelet	P-selectin		TXB2, PAF	Traumatic spinal cord injury, ischemic brain injury
Endothelial Cell	E-selectin ICAM	IL-1, IL-2, TNF	PGI2, PAF	Traumatic brain and spinal cord injury, ischemic brain injury
Macrophage or Microglia	L-selectin Mac-1	IL-1, IL-2, IL-6	TXB2, PAF	Traumatic brain and spinal cord injury

(Nitric oxide is synthesized and released by all the inflammatory cells listed in this table. Adapted with modification from Morganti-Kossmann et al, 1992[123]).

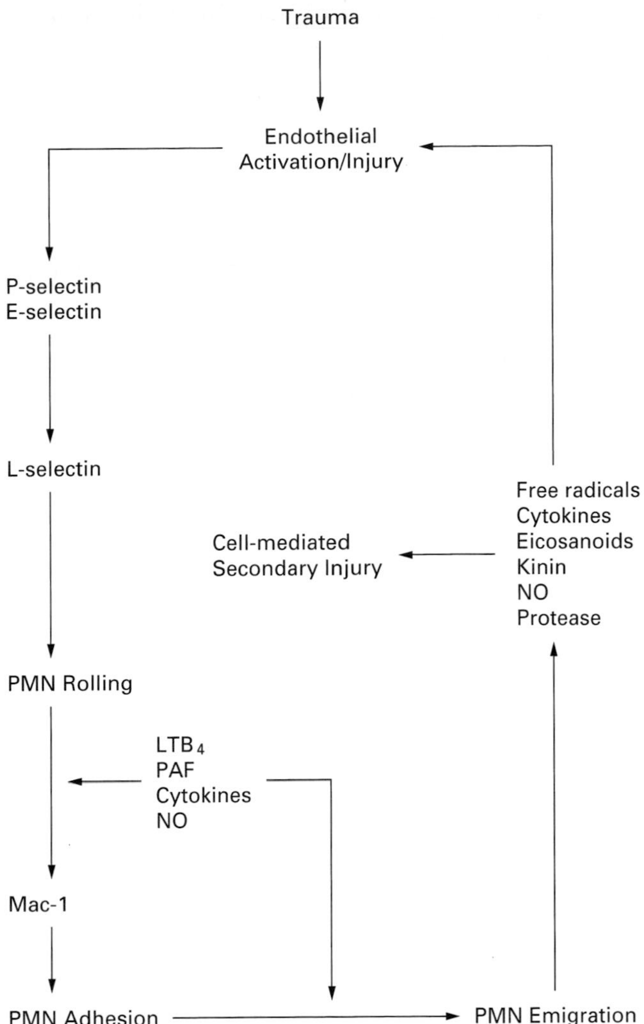

Figure 106-1. A simplified scheme of cell-mediated secondary injury after CNS trauma. Effects of selected inflammatory mediators on PMNs interacting with injured or activated ECs are depicted, based on a framework of post-traumatic inflammatory reaction.

charide (LPS) and/or cytokines.[50,145,79] A similar if not identical iNOS can also be expressed in C6 glioma cell line.[126] NADPH diaphorase is a marker enzyme of neurons expressing cNOS. After global or focal cerebral ischemia, reactive astrocytes showed intense expression of NADPH-diaphorase and iNOS in a double-labeling study.[162] Brain inflammation caused by mycoplasma led to glial synthesis of cytokines, eicosanoids, and induction of NOS.[20] As noted above, NO produced by neuronal cNOS has been implicated in mediating excitotoxic or hypoxic/ischemic neuronal death. Hewett and colleagues[79] noted glial iNOS expression after exposure to cytokines and endotoxin. Expression of glial iNOS accentuated NMDA-mediated neuronal death.[80] Endothelial injury was noted to be a trigger of the expression of iNOS in the vascular smooth muscle.[73] Glial swelling is a major factor in certain types of brain edema (e.g., hepatic encephalopathy and Reye's disease). Microglia also plays a key role in cell-mediated brain injury after ischemic or traumatic insult. Microglia express iNOS in response to brain injury.[80,162] The role of glial NOS in postischemic and post-traumatic inflammatory reaction and cell-mediated injury is not known.

CONCLUSION

Extensive studies in animal models of brain and spinal cord injury have yielded results supporting the hypothesis of cell-mediated second injury in the setting of a post-traumatic inflammatory reaction. Table 106-1 shows the cellular elements and the mediators that may be involved in these processes.[123] Figure 106-1 depicts a simplified scheme of cell-mediated injury involving inflammatory mediators. Understanding the cellular and molecular mechanism of second injury will facilitate future development of novel therapeutic interventions directed at the post-traumatic inflammatory process to reduce cell-mediated injury.

ACKNOWLEDGMENT

Works from the authors' lab cited in this review were supported in part by NIH grants NS25545, NS28995, NS32000, NS32636, and by Vivian L. Smith Foundation for Restorative Neurology. We thank Ms. Vickie Reckamp for the preparation of this manuscript.

REFERENCES

1. Amruthesh SC, Falck JR, Ellis EF: Brain synthesis and cerebrovascular action of epoxygenase metabolites of arachidonic acid. *J Neurochem* 1992; 58:503–510.
2. Anderson DK, Braughler JM, Hall ED, et al: Effect of treatment with U74006F on neurological recovery following experimental spinal cord injury. *J Neurosurg* 1988; 69:562–567.
3. Anderson BO, Brown JM, Harken AH: Current research review: Mechanisms of neutrophil-mediated tissue injury. *J Surg Res* 1991; 51:170–179.
4. Anggard E: Nitric oxide: Mediator, murderer, and medicine. *Lancet* 1994; 343:1199–1206.
5. Ankarcrona M, Dypbukt JM, Brune B, Nicotera P: Interleukin1 beta.

6. Balentine JD: Pathology of experimental spinal cord trauma. I. The necrotic lesion as a function of vascular injury. *Lab Invest* 1978; 39:236–253.
7. Balentine JD: Pathology of experimental spinal cord trauma. II. Ultrastructure of axons and myelin. *Lab Invest* 1978; 39:254–266.
8. Bastian NR, Hibbs JB Jr: Assembly and regulation of NADPH oxidase and nitric oxide synthase. *Curr Opin Immunol* 1994; 6:131–139.
9. Beckman JS, Beckman TW, Chen J, et al: Apparent hydroxyl radical production by peroxynitrite: Implications for endothelial injury from nitric oxide and superoxide. *Proc Natl Acad Sci USA* 1990; 87:1620–1624.
10. Bereta M, Bereta J, Georgoff I, et al: Methylxanthines and calcium-mobilizing agents inhibit the expression of cytokine-inducible nitric oxide synthase and vascular cell adhesion molecule-1 in murine microvascular endothelial cells. *Exp Cell Res* 1994; 212:230–242.
11. Bernofsky C: Nucleotide chloramines and neutrophil-mediated cytotoxicity. *FASEB* 1991; 5:295–300.
12. Bevilacqua MP: Endothelial-leukocyte adhesion molecules. *Annu Res Immunol* 1993; 11:767–804.
13. Biagas KV, Uhl MW, Schiding JK, et al: Assessment of posttraumatic polymorphonuclear leukocyte accumulation in rat brain using tissue myeloperoxidase assay and vinblastine treatment. *J Neurotrauma* 1992; 9(4):363–371.
14. Blazka ME, Harry GJ, Luster MI: Effect of lead acetate on nitrite production by murine brain endothelial cell cultures. *Toxicol Appl Pharmacol* 1994; 126:191–194.
15. Blight AR: Delayed demyelination and macrophage invasion: A candidate for secondary cell damage in spinal cord injury. *Cent Nerv Syst Trauma* 1985; 2:299–315.
16. Blight AR: Macrophages and inflammatory damage in spinal cord injury. *J Neurotrauma* 1992; 9[suppl I]:S83–S91.
17. Bracken MB, Shepard MJ, Collins WF, et al: A randomized, controlled trial of methylprednisolone or naloxone in the treatment of acute spinal-cord injury. *N Engl J Med* 1990; 322:1405–1411.
18. Braughler JM, Pregenzer, Chase RL, et al: Novel 21-amino substituted steroids as potent inhibitors of iron-dependent lipid peroxidation. *J Biol Chem* 1987; 262:10438–10440.
19. Bredt DS, Snyder SH: Isolation of nitric oxide synthetase, a calmodulin-requiring enzyme. *Proc Natl Acad Sci USA* 1990; 87:682–685.
20. Brenner T, Yamin A, Gallily R: Mycoplasma triggering of nitric oxide production by central system glial cells and its inhibition by glucocorticoids. *Brain Res* 1994; 641:51–56.
21. Brown MC, Perry VH, Lunn ER, et al: Macrophage dependence of peripheral sensory nerve regeneration: Possible involvement of nerve growth factor. *Neuron* 1991; 6:359–370.
22. Chen ST, Lin TN, Lee TK, Hsu CY: Non-steroidal anti-inflammatory drugs in stroke, in Lewis AJ, Furst D (eds): *Non-Steroidal Anti-Inflammatory Drugs: Mechanism and Clinical Use.* 2d ed. New York: Marcel Dekker, 1994:55–70.
23. Cho HJ, Xie Q, Calaycay J, et al: Calmodulin is a subunit of nitric oxide synthase from macrophages. *J Exp Med* 1992; 176:599–604.
24. Choi DW: Glutamate neurotoxicity and diseases of the nervous system. [Review] *Neuron* 1988; 1(8):623–634.
25. Choi DW: Nitric oxide: Friend or foe to the injured brain? *Proc Natl Acad Sci USA* 1993; 90:9741–9743.
26. Cifone MG, Festuccia C, Cironi L, et al: Induction of the nitric oxide-synthesizing pathway in fresh and interleukin 2-cultured rat natural killer cells. *Cell Immunol* 1994; 157(1):181–194.
27. Clark RAF, Henson PM: *The Molecular and Cellular Biology of Wound Repair. New Joints.* Boston, MTP Press, 1988.
28. Coffey PJ, Perry VH, Allen Y, et al: Ibotenic acid induced demyelination in the central nervous system: A consequence of a local inflammatory response. *Neurosci Lett* 1988; 84:178–184.
29. Coffey PJ, Perry V, Rawlins JN: An investigation into the early stages of the inflammatory response following ibotenic acid-induced neuronal degeneration. *Neurosci* 1990; 35:121–135.
30. Conklin BR, Burch RM, Steranka LR, et al: Distinct bradykinin receptors mediate stimulation of prostaglandin synthesis by endothelial cells and fibroblasts. *J Pharmacol Exp Ther* 1988; 244:646–649.
31. Corbett JA, McDaniel ML: Reversibility of interleukin-1 beta-induced islet destruction and dysfunction by the inhibition of nitric oxide synthase. *Biochem J* 1994; 299:719–724.
32. Crockard A, Kang J, Ladds G: A model of focal cortical contusion in gerbils. *J Neurosurg* 1982; 57:203–209.
33. Cross AH, Misko TP, Lin RF, et al: Aminoguanidine, an inhibitor of inducible nitric oxide synthase, ameliorates experimental autoimmune encephalomyelitis in SJL mice. *J Clin Invest* 1994; 93:268–290.
34. Damoulis PD, Halushka PV: Cytokines induce nitric oxide production in mouse osteoblasts. *Biochem Biophys Res Commun* 1994; 201:924–931.
35. Dawson VL, Dawson TM, London ED, et al: Nitric oxide mediates glutamate neurotoxicity in primary cortical cultures. *Proc Natl Acad Sci USA* 1991; 88:6368–6371.
36. Dawson VL, Dawson TM, Bartley DA, et al: Mechanisms of nitric oxide-mediated neurotoxicity in primary brain cultures. *J Neurosci* 1993; 13:2651–2661.
37. Demediuk P, Saunders RD, Anderson DK, et al: Membrane lipid changes in laminectomized and traumatized cat spinal cord. *Proc Natl Acad Sci USA* 1985; 82:7071–7075.
38. Demopoulos HB, Yoder M, Gutman EG, et al: The fine structure of endothelial surfaces in the microcirculation of experimentally injured feline spinal cords. *Scanning Electron Microsc* 1978; 11:677–682.
39. Dickson DW, Lee SC, Mattiace LA, et al: Microglia and cytokines in neurological disease, with special reference to AIDS and Alzheimer's disease. *Glia* 1993; 7:75–83.
40. Dietrich WD, Dewanjee S, Prado R, et al: Transient platelet accumulation in the rat brain after common

carotid artery thrombosis. An ^{111}In-labeled platelet study. *Stroke* 1993; 24:1534–1540.

41. Ellis EF, Wright KF, Wei EP, Kontos HA: Cyclooxygenase products of arachidonic acid metabolism in cerebral cortex after experimental concussive brain injury. *J Neurochem* 1981; 37:892–896.
42. Ellis EF, Chao J, Heizer ML: Brain kininogen following experimental brain injury: Evidence for a secondary event. *J Neurosurg* 1989; 71:437–442.
43. Faint RW: Platelet-neutrophil interactions: Their significance. *Blood Reviews* 1992; 6:83–91.
44. Faraci FM, Brian JE: Nitric oxide and the cerebral circulation. *Stroke* 1994; 25:692–703.
45. Feinstein DL, Galea E, Reis D: Norepinephrine suppresses inducible nitric oxide synthase activity in rat astroglial culture. *J Neurochem* 1993; 60:1945–1948.
46. Ford-Hutchinson A, Brag M, Doig M: Leukotrienes B_4, a potent chemokinetic and aggregating substance released from polymorphonuclear leukocytes. *Nature* 1980; 286:264.
47. Forstermann U, Nakane M, Tracey WR, Pollock JS: Isoforms of nitric oxide synthase: Functions in the cardiovascular system. *Eur Heart J* 1993; 14 Suppl I: 15.
48. Forstermann U, Closs EI, Pollock JS, et al: Nitric oxide synthase isozymes. Characterization, purification, molecular cloning, and functions. *Hypertension* 1994; 23:1121–1131.
49. Fletcher JR: Eicosanoids: Critical agents in the physiological process and cellular injury. *Arch Surg* 1993; 128:1192–1196.
50. Galea E, Reis DJ, Feinstein DL: Cloning and expression of inducible nitric oxide synthase from rat astrocytes. *J Neurosci Res* 1994; 37:406–414.
51. Gallin JI, Goldstein IM, Snyderman R: *Inflammation: Basic Principles and Clinical Correlates.* New York: Raven Press, 1992.
52. Geng YJ, Wu Q, Hansson GK: Protein kinase C activation inhibits cytokine-induced nitric oxide synthesis in vascular smooth muscle cells. *Biochim Biophys Acta* 1994; 1223:125–132.
53. Giulian D, Tomozawa Y, Hindman H, Allen RL: Peptides from regenerating central nervous system promote specific populations of macroglia. *Proc Natl Acad Sci USA* 1985; 82:4287–4290.
54. Giulian D, Lachman LB: Interleukin-1 stimulation of astroglial proliferation after brain injury. *Science* 1985; 228:497–499.
55. Giulian D, Baker TJ, Shih LC, Lachman LB: Interleukin 1 of the central nervous system is produced by ameboid microglia. *J Exp Med* 1986; 164:594–604.
56. Giulian D: Ameboid microglia as effectors of inflammation in the central nervous system. *J Neurosci Res* 1987; 18:132–133, 155–171.
57. Giulian D, Chen J, Ingeman JE, et al: The role of mononuclear phagocytes in wound healing after traumatic injury to adult mammalian brain. *J Neurosci* 1989; 9(12):4416–4429.
58. Giulian D, Vaca K, Noonan CA: Secretion of neurotoxins by mononuclear phagocytes infected with HIV-1. *Science* 1990; 250:1593–1596.
59. Giulian D, Robertson C: Inhibition of mononuclear phagocytes reduces ischemic injury in the spinal cord. *Ann Neurol* 1990; 27:33–42.
60. Giulian D, Vaca K, Corpuz M: Brain glia release factors with opposing actions upon neuronal survival. *J Neurosci* 1993; 13:29–37.
61. Giulian D: Reactive glia as rivals in regulating neuronal survival. *Glia* 1993; 7:102–110.
62. Goldman H, Hodgson V, Morehead M, et al: Cerebrovascular changes in a rat model of moderate closed-head injury. *J Neurotrauma* 1991; 8:129–144.
63. Goodman JC, Robertson CS, Grossman RG, Narayan RK: Elevation of tumor necrosis factor in head injury. *J Neuroimmunol* 1990; 30:213–217.
64. Goureau O, Hicks D, Courtois Y, De Kozak Y: Induction and regulation of nitric oxide synthase in retinal Muller glial cells. *J Neurochem* 1994; 63:310–317.
65. Granger DN, Kubes P: The microcirculation and inflammation: Modulation of leukocyte endothelial cell adhesion. *J Leukoc Biol* 1994; 5:662–675.
66. Green BA, Wagner FC: Evolution of edema in the acutely injured spinal cord: A fluorescence microscopic study. *Surg Neurol* 1973; 1:98–101.
67. Griffiths IR, Miller R: Vascular permeability to protein and vasogenic oedema in experimental concussive injuries to the canine spinal cord. *J Neurol Sci* 1974; 22:291–304.
68. Griffiths IR, McCulloch M, Crawford RA: Ultrastructural appearances of the spinal microvasculature between twelve hours and five days after impact injury. *Acta Neuropathol* 1978; 43:205–211.
69. Griffiths IR, Burns N, Crawford AR: Early vascular changes in the spinal gray matter following impact injury. *Acta Neuropathol* 1978; 41:33–39.
70. Griffiths IR, McCulloch MC: Nerve fibers in spinal cord impact injuries. *J Neurol Sci* 1983; 58:335–349.
71. Haberl RL, Anneser F, Kodel U, Pfister HW: Is nitric oxide involved as a mediator of cerebrovascular changes in the early phase of experimental pneumococcal meningitis? *Neurol Res* 1994; 16:108–112.
72. Hanahan DJ: Platelet activating factor: A biologically active phosphoglyceride. *Ann Rev Biochem* 1986; 55:483–509.
73. Hansson GK, Geng YJ, Holm J, et al: Arterial smooth muscle cells express nitric oxide synthase in response to endothelial injury. *J Exp Med* 1994; 180:733–738.
74. Harbrecht BG, Stadler J, Demetrics AJ, et al: Nitric oxide and prostaglandins interact to prevent hepatic damage during murine endotoxemia. *Am J Physiol* 1994; 266:G1004–1010.
75. Harlan JM: Leukocyte-endothelial interactions. *Blood* 1985; 65:513–525.
76. Hausmann EH, Hao SY, Pace JL, Pamely MJ: Transforming growth factor beta 1 and gamma interferon provide opposing signals to lipopolysaccharide-activated mouse mouse macrophages. *Infect Immunol* 1994; 62:3625–3632.
77. Hecker M, Sessa WC, Harris HJ, et al: The metabolism of L-arginine and its significance for the biosynthesis of endothelium-derived relaxing factor: Cultured endothe-

lial cells recycle L-citrulline to L-arginine. *Proc Natl Acad Sci USA* 1990; 87:8612–8616.

78. Heinzel B, John M, Klatt P: Ca^{2+}/calmodulin-dependent formation of hydrogen peroxide by nitric oxide synthase. *Biochem J* 1992; 281:627–630.
79. Hewett SJ, Corbett JA, McDaniel ML, Choi DW: Interferons gamma and interleukin beta induce nitric oxide formation from primary mouse astrocytes. *Neurosci Lett* 1993; 164:229–232.
80. Hewett SJ, Csernansky CA, Choi DW: Selective potentiation of NMDA induced neuronal injury following induction of astrocytic iNOS. *Neuron* 1994; 13:487–494.
81. Hovda DA, Becker DP, Katayama Y: Secondary injury and acidosis. *J Neurotrauma* 1992; 9[Suppl I]: S47–S60.
82. Hsu CY, Halushka PV, Hogan EL, et al: Alteration of thromboxane and prostacyclin levels in experimental spinal cord injury. *Neurology* 1985; 35:1003–1008.
83. Hsu CY, Norris JW, Hogan EL, et al: Pentoxifylline in acute nonhemorrhagic stroke—a randomized, placebo-controlled double blind trial. *Stroke* 1988; 19:716–723.
84. Hsu CY and Hogan EL (1989): Antiplatelet agents in acute cerebral ischemia: In: Fisher M, ed., *Medical Therapy of Acute Stroke*, Marcel Dekker, New York, pp 73–95.
85. Hsu CY, Dimitrijevic MR (1990): Methylprednisolone in spinal cord injury: Possible mechanism of action. *J Neurotrauma* 7:115–119.
86. Hsu CY, Liu TH, Xu J, Hogan EL and Chao J (1990): Lipid inflammatory mediators in ischemic brain edema and injury. In: Bazan NG, eds. *Lipid Mediators in Ischemic Brain Damage and Experimental Epilepsy.* New Trends Lipid Mediators Res. Basel, Karger, vol 4, pp. 85–112.
87. Hsu CY, Lin TN, Xu J, Hogan EL and Chao J (1994): Kinins and related inflammatory mediators in CNS injury. In: Salzman SK and Faden AI, eds. *Neurobiology of CNS Trauma. FASEB Series*, in press.
88. Hsu CY, Doster K, Hu ZY (1995): Cell-mediated injury. In: Narayan K, Wilberger JE Jr, Povlishock JT (eds). *Neurotrauma: A Comprehensive Textbook of Head and Spinal Injury.* McGraw Hill Companies, New York.
89. Huang Z, Huang PL, Panahian N, Dalkara T, Fishman MC, Moskowitz MA (1994): Effects of cerebral ischemia in mice deficient in neuronal nitric oxide synthase. *Science* 265:1883–5.
90. Iadecola C, Pelligrino DA, Moskowitz MA, Lassen NA: Nitric oxide synthase inhibition and cerebrovascular regulation. *J Cereb Blood Flow Metab.* 14:175–92.
91. Johnson RJ, Alpers CE, Pritzc P, et al. (1988): Platelets mediate neutrophil-dependent immune complex nephritis in the rat. *J Clin Invest* 82:1225–1235.
92. Kapadia SE (1984): Ultrastructural alteration in blood vessels of the white matter after experimental spinal cord trauma. *J Neurosurg* 61:539–544.
93. Ketteler M, Border WA, Noble NA (1994): Cytokines and arginine in renal injury and repair [editorial]. *Am J Physiol* 267:F197–207.
94. Kilbourn RG, Owen Schaub LB, Cromeens DM, Gross SS, Flaherty MJ, Santee SM, Alak AM, Griffith OW (1994): N^G-methyl-arginine, an inhibitor of nitric oxide formation, reverses mediated hypotension in dogs. *J Appl Physiol* 76:1130–7.
95. Kinugawa K, Takahashi T, Kohmoto O, Yao A, Aoyagi T, Momomura S, Hirata Y, Serizawa T (1994): Nitric oxide mediated effects of interleukin-6 on $[Ca^{2+}]$ and cell contraction in cultured chick ventricular myocytes. *Circ Res* 75(2):285–95.
96. Klatt P, Schmidt K, Uray G, Mater B (1993): Multiple catalytic functions of brain nitric oxide synthase. *J Biol Chem* 268:14781–14787.
97. Kontos HA, Wei EP, Povlishock JT, Christman CW: Oxygen radicals mediate the cerebral arteriolar dilatation from arachidonate and bradykinin. *Circ Res* 1984; 55:295–303.
98. Kontos HA, Wei EP, Ellis EF, et al: Appearance of superoxide anion radical in cerebral extracellular space during increased prostaglandin synthesis in cats. *Circ Res* 1985; 57:142–151.
99. Konturek SJ, Szlachcic A, Dembinski A, et al: Nitric oxide in pancreatic secretion and hormone induced pancreatitis in rats. *Int J Pancreatol* 1994; 15(1):19–28.
100. Kosaka H, Sakaguchi H, Sawai Y, et al: Effect of interferongamma on nitric oxide hemoglobin production in endotoxin treated rats and its synergism with interleukin 1 or tumor necrosis factor. *Life Sci* 1994; 54:1523–1529.
101. Kubes P, Kurose I, Granger DN: NO donors prevent integrin-induced leukocyte adhesion but P-selectin-dependent rolling in postischemic venules. *Am J Physiol* 1994; 267:H931–937.
102. Kunz D, Muhl H, Walker G, Pfeilschifter J: Two distinct signaling pathways trigger the expression of inducible nitric oxide synthase in rat renal mesangial cells. *Proc Natl Acad Sci USA* 1994; 91:5387–5391.
103. Kuo PC, Slivka A: Nitric oxide decreases oxidant mediated hepatocyte injury. *J Surg Res* 1994; 56:594–600.
104. Leibovich SJ, Polverini PJ, Fong TW, et al: Production of angiogenic activity by human monocytes requires an arginine/nitric oxide synthase dependent effector mechanism. *Proc Natl Acad Sci USA* 1994; 91:4190–4194.
105. Lewis GP: *Mediators of Inflammation.* Bristol: Wright, 1986.
106. Lewis RE, Granger HJ: Neutrophil-dependent mediation of microvascular permeability. *Fed Proc* 1986; 45:109–113.
107. Lindholm D, Castren E, Kiefer R, et al: Transforming growth factor-beta 1 in the rat brain: Increase after injury and inhibition of astrocyte proliferation. *J Cell Biol* 1992; 117:395–400.
108. Lipton SA, Choi YB, Pan ZH, et al: A redox based mechanism for the neuroprotective and neurodestructive effects of nitric oxide and related nitroso compounds [see comments]. *Nature* 1993; 364:626–632.
109. Logan A, Frautschy SA, Gonzalez AM, et al: Enhanced expression of transforming growth factor beta 1 in the rat brain after a localized cerebral injury. *Brain Res* 1992; 587:216–225.
110. Lowry SF: Cytokine mediators of immunity and inflammation. *Arch Surg* 1993; 128:1235–1241.
111. Mantovani A, Bussolino F, Dejana E: Cytokine regula-

tion of endothelial cell function. *FASEB* 1992; 246:2591–2599.

112. Marcus AJ, Safier LB, Ullman HL, et al: Inhibition of platelet function in thrombosis. *Circulation* 1985; 72:698–701.
113. Maxwell WL, Whitfield PC, Suzen B, et al: The cerebrovascular response to experimental lateral head acceleration. *Acta Neuropathol (Berl)* 1992; 84:289–296.
114. McCall TB, Palmer RM, Moncada S: Interleukin-8 inhibits the induction of nitric oxide synthase in rat peritoneal neutrophils. *Biochem Biophys Res Commun* 1992; 186:680–685.
115. McClain CJ, Cohen D, Ott L, et al: Ventricular fluid interleukin-1 activity in patients with head injury. *J Lab Clin Med* 1987; 110:48–54.
116. McClain C, Cohen D, Phillips R, et al: Increased plasma and ventricular fluid interleukin-6 levels in patients with head injury [see comments]. *J Lab Clin Med* 1991; 118:225–231.
117. Means ED, Anderson DK: Neuronophagia by leukocytes in experimental spinal cord injury. *J Neuropathol Exp Neurol* 1983; 42:707–719.
118. Merrill JE: Tumor necrosis factor alpha, interleukin 1 and related cytokines in brain development: Normal and pathological. *Dev Neurosci* 1992; 14:1–10.
119. Miller MJ, Chotinaruemol S, Sadowska-Krowicka H, et al: Nitric oxide: The Jekyll and Hyde of gut inflammation. *Agents Actions* 1993; 39 Spec No: C180–182.
120. Miller MJ, Munshi UK, Sadowska Krowicka H, et al: Inhibition of calcium dependent nitric oxide synthase causes ileitis and leukocytosis in guinea pigs. *Dig Dis Sci* 1994; 39:1185–1192.
121. Moncada S, Higgs EA: Metabolism of arachidonic acid. *Ann NY Acad Sci* 1988; 522:445–463.
122. Moreno-Flores MT, Bovolenta P, Nieto-Sampedro M: Polymorphonuclear leukocytes in brain parenchyma after injury and their interaction with purified astrocytes in culture. *Glia* 1993; 7(2):146–157.
123. Morganti-Kossmann MC, Kossmann T, Wahl SM: Cytokines and neuropathology. *Trends Pharmacol Sci* 1992; 13:286–291.
124. Morris SM Jr, Billiar TR: New insights into the regulation of inducible nitric oxide synthesis. *Am J Physiol* 1994; 266:E829–839.
125. Muhl H, Kunz D, Pfeilschifter J: Expression of nitric oxide synthase in rat glomerular mesangial cells mediated by cyclic AMP. *Br J Pharmacol* 1994; 112:1–8.
126. Murphy S, Simmons ML, Agullo L, et al: Synthesis of nitric oxide in CNS glial cells [see comments]. *Trends Neurosci* 1993; 16:323–328.
127. Needleman P, Turk J, Jakschik BA, et al: Arachidonic acid metabolism. *Ann Rev Biochem* 1986; 55:69–102.
128. Nemecek S, Petr R, Suba P, et al: Longitudinal extension of oedema in experimental spinal cord injury: Evidence for two types of post-traumatic oedema. *Acta Neurochir* 1977; 37:7–12.
129. Nieto-Sampedro M, Chandy KG: Interleukin-2-like activity in injured rat brain. *Neurochem Res* 1987; 12:723–727.
130. Nieto-Sampedro M, Berman MA: Interleukin-1-like activity in rat brain: Sources, targets, and effect of injury. *J Neurosci Res* 1987; 17:214–219.
131. Niu XF, Smith CW, Kubes P: Intercellular oxidative stress induced by nitric oxide synthesis inhibition increases endothelial cell adhesion to neutrophils. *Circ Res* 1994; 74:1133–1140.
132. Novogrodsky A, Vanichkin A, Patya M, et al: Prevention of lipopolysaccharide induced lethal toxicity by tyrosine kinase inhibitors. *Science* 1994; 264:1319–1322.
133. Paul W, Douglas GJ, Lawrence L, et al: Cutaneous permeability responses to bradykinin and histamine in the guinea pig: Possible differences in their mechanism of action. *Br J Pharmacol* 1994; 111:159–164.
134. Perrella MA, Yoshizumi M, Fen Z, et al: Transforming growth factor-beta 1, but not dexamethasone, downregulates nitric-oxide synthase mRNA after its induction by interleukin-1 beta in rat smooth muscle cells. *J Biol Chem* 1994; 269:14595–14600.
135. Perry VH, Gordon S: Macrophages in the nervous system. *Int Rev Cytol* 1991; 125:203–244.
136. Perry VH, Andersson P-B: Glial symposium: The inflammatory response in the CNS. *Neuropathol Appl Neurobiol* 1992; 18:454–459.
137. Pietersma A, De Jong N, Koster JF, Sluiter W: Effect of hypoxia on adherence of granulocytes to endothelial cells in vitro. *Am J Physiol* 1994; 267:H874–879.
138. Povlishock JT: The morphopathologic responses to experimental head injuries of varying severity, in Becker DP, Povlishock JT (eds): *Central Nervous System Trauma Status Report.* NIH, NINCDS, 1985:443–452.
139. Pou S, Pou WS, Brebt DS, et al: Generation of superoxide by purified brain nitric oxide synthase. *J Biol Chem* 1992; 267:24173–24176.
140. Proud D, Kaplan AP: Kinin formation: Mechanisms and role in inflammatory disorders. *Ann Rev Immunol* 1988; 6:49–83.
141. Punjabi CJ, Laskin JD, Hwang SM, et al: Enhanced production of nitric oxide by bone marrow cells and increased sensitivity to macrophage colony-stimulating factor (CSF) and granulocyte-macrophage CSF after benzene treatment of mice. *Blood* 1994; 83(11):3255–3263.
142. Robinson LJ, Weremowicz S, Morton CC, Michel T: Isolation and chromosomal localization of the human endothelial nitric oxide synthase (NOS3) gene. *Genomics* 1994; 19:350–357.
143. Samuelsson B: Leukotrienes: Mediators of immediate hypersensitivity reaction and inflammation. *Science* 1983; 220:568–575.
144. Schoettle RJ, Kochanek PM, Magargee MJ, et al: Early polymorphonuclear leukocyte accumulation correlates with the development of posttraumatic cerebral edema in rats. *J Neurotrauma* 1990; 7:207–217.
145. Simmons ML, Murphy S: Induction of nitric oxide synthase in glial cells. *J Neurochem* 1992; 59:897–905.
146. Slogan DJ, Wood MJ, Charlton HM: Leucocyte recruitment and inflammation in the CNS. *Trends Neurosci* 1992; 15:276–278.
147. Smyth SS, Joneckis CC, Parise LV: Regulation of vascular integrins. *Blood* 1993; 81:2827–2843.

148. Stewart WB, Wagner FC: Vascular permeability changes in the contused feline spinal cord. *Brain Res* 1979; 169:163–167.
149. Stefanovic-Racic M, Stadler J, Georgescu HI, Evans CH: Nitric oxide and energy production in articular chondrocytes. *J Cell Physiol* 1994; 159:274–280.
150. Tanno H, Nockels RP, Pitts LH, Noble LJ: Breakdown of the blood-brain barrier after fluid percussive in the rat. Part 1: Distribution and time course of protein extravasation. *J Neurotrauma* 1992; 9:21–32.
151. Tanno H, Nockels RP, Pitts LH, Noble LJ: Breakdown of the blood-brain barrier after fluid percussive in the rat. Part 2: Effect of hypoxia on permeability to plasma proteins. *J Neurotrauma* 1992; 9:335–347.
152. Taupin V, Toulmond S, Serrano A, et al: Increase in IL-6, IL-1 and TNF levels in rat brain following traumatic lesion. Influence of pre- and post-traumatic treatment with Ro5 4864, a peripheral-type (p site) benzodiazepine ligand. *J Neuroimmunol* 1993; 42:177–185.
153. Tiao G, Rafferty J, Ogle C, et al: Detrimental effect of nitric oxide synthase inhibition during endotoxemia may be caused by high levels of tumor necrosis factor and interleukin-6. *Surgery* 1994; 116:332–337; discussion 337–338.
154. Tchelingerian JL, Quinonero J, Booss J, and Jacque C: Localization of TNF alpha and IL-1 alpha immunoreactivities in striatal neurons after surgical injury to the hippocampus. *Neuron* 1993; 10:213–224.
155. Thomas WE: Brain macrophages: Evaluation of microglia and their functions. *Brain Res Rev* 1992; 17:61–74.
156. Tornheim PA: Traumatic edema in head injury, in Becker DP, Povlishock JT (eds): *Central Nervous System Trauma, Status Report.* NIH, NINCDS, 1985:431–442.
157. Tsujino M, Hirata Y, Imai T, et al: Induction of nitric oxide synthase gene by interleukin-1 beta in cultured rat cardiocytes. *Circulation* 1994; 90:375–383.
158. Turco J, Winkler HH: Relationship of tumor necrosis factor alpha, the nitric oxide synthase pathway, and lipopolysaccharide to the killing of gamma interferon-treated macrophage-like RAW264.7 cells by *Rickettsia prowazekii. Infect Immunol* 1994; 62:2568–2574.
159. Venema RC, Nishida K, Alexander RW, et al: Organization of the bovine gene encoding the endothelial nitric oxide synthase. *Biochim Biophys Acta* 1994; 1218:413–420.
160. Wagner FC Jr, Stewart WB: Effect of trauma dose on spinal cord edema. *J Neurosurg* 1981; 54:802–806.
161. Wakefield CL, Eidelberg E: Electron microscopic observations of the delayed effects of spinal cord compression. *Exp Neurol* 1975; 48:637–646.
162. Wallace MN, Bisland SK: NADPH-diaphorase activity in activated astrocytes represents inducible nitric oxide synthase. *Neuroscience* 1994; 59:905–919.
163. Walter R, Schaffner A, Schoedon G: Differential regulation of constitutive and inducible nitric oxide production by inflammatory stimuli in murine endothelial cells. *Biochem Biophys Res Commun* 1994; 202:450–455.
164. Wang MH, Cox GW, Yoshimura T, et al: Macrophage-stimulating protein inhibits induction of nitric oxide production by endotoxin- or cytokine-stimulated mouse macrophages. *J Biol Chem* 1994; 269:14027–14031.
165. Wang SC, Rossignol DP, Christ WJ, et al: Suppression of lipopolysaccharide-induced macrophage nitric oxide and cytokine production in vitro by a novel lipopolysaccharide antagonist. *Surgery* 1994; 116:339–346; discussion 446–447.
166. Wei EP, Kontos HA, Dietrich WD, et al: Inhibition by free radical scavengers and by cyclooxygenase inhibitors of pial arteriolar abnormalities from concussive brain injury in cats. *Circ Res* 1981; 48:95–103.
167. Weiss SJ: Tissue destruction by neutrophils. *N Engl J Med* 1989; 320:365–376.
168. Welsh N: A role for tyrosine kinase activation in interleukin-1 beta induced nitric oxide production in the insulin producing cell line RINm-5F. *Biosci Rep* 1994; 14(1):43–50.
169. Williams KI, Higgs GA: Eicosanoids and inflammation. *J Pathol* 1988; 156:101–110.
170. Willis RA, Nussler AK, Fries KM, et al: Induction of nitric oxide synthase in subsets of murine pulmonary fibroblasts: Interleukin-6 production. *Clin Immunol Immunopathol* 1994; 71:231–239.
171. Wisniewski HM, Bloom BR: Primary demyelination as a non-specific consequence of a cell-mediated immune reaction. *J Exp Med* 1975; 141:346–359.
172. Wolfe LS: Eicosanoids: Prostaglandins, thromboxane, leukotrienes and other derivatives of carbon-20 unsaturated fatty acids. *J Neurochem* 1982; 38:1–14.
173. Woodroofe MN, Sarna GS, Wadhwa M, et al: Detection of interleukin-1 and interleukin-6 in adult rat brain, following mechanical injury, by in vivo microdialysis: Evidence of a role for microglia in cytokine production. *J Neuroimmunol* 1991; 33:227–236.
174. Xu J, Hsu CY, Liu TH, et al: Leukotriene B4 release and polymorphonuclear cell infiltration in spinal cord injury. *J Neurochem* 1990; 55:907–912.
175. Xu J, Hsu CY, Junker H, et al: Kininogen and kinin in experimental spinal cord injury. *J Neurochem* 1991; 57:975–980.
176. Yan HQ, Banos MA, Herregodts P, et al: Expression of interleukin (IL)-1 beta, IL-6 and their respective receptors in the normal rat brain and after injury. *Eur J Immunol* 1992; 22:2963–2971.
177. Young W: Blood flow, metabolic and neurophysiological mechanisms in spinal cord injury, in Becker D, Povlishock JT (eds): *Central Nervous System Trauma, Status Report.* Bethesda: NINCDS 1985:463.
178. Zhuang J, Shackford SR, Schmoker JD, Anderson ML: The association of leukocytes with secondary brain injury. *J Trauma* 1993; 35(3):415–422.

CHAPTER 107

TRAUMATIC BRAIN INJURY AND EXCITATORY AMINO ACIDS

Douglas H. Smith
Tracy K. McIntosh

INTRODUCTION

A common misconception concerning traumatic brain injury (TBI) is that the outcome depends on the extent of physical neuronal damage occurring immediately at the moment of trauma. However, recent evidence exists suggesting that delayed or secondary neurochemical events may contribute substantially to neuronal cell loss and dysfunction. These secondary events are thought to include the acute and marked release of excitatory amino acid (EAA) neurotransmitters and the subsequent overexcitation of EAA receptors, with resultant neuronal death and neurological dysfunction. This hypothesis has become testable since the recent availability of novel EAA receptor antagonists that may be used to potentially reverse the secondary injury cascade. We will review the current literature, which implicates EAAs as pathological factors in TBI, and examine the differential effects between the various classes of novel EAA receptor antagonists, which have recently been evaluated for their potential therapeutic efficacy in the treatment of TBI.

EXCITATORY AMINO ACID RECEPTORS

EAA neurotransmitters such as glutamate (glu) and aspartate (asp) have long been known to be involved in excitatory neurotransmission function of CNS neurons.[11,41,111] In addition, glu has more recently been found to be one of the most prevalent neurotransmitters in the CNS.[62,78] While glu binds all EAA receptors, selective EAA ligands have been used to characterize at least three major classes of EAA receptor subtypes, each with distinct properties. The EAA receptor subtype selectively bound by the ligand *N*-methyl-D-aspartate (NMDA), is a receptor complex that includes a receptor-mediated voltage-dependent divalent and monovalent cation channel. When bound by NMDA or glu, the ion channel is opened. However, a voltage dependent block by Mg^{2+}, which binds within the opened ionophore, must then be overcome, typically by depolarization of the neuron, in order to allow an influx of Ca^{2+} and Na^{+} and an efflux of K^{+}.[19,33,84] In addition to EAA binding, activation of the NMDA receptor also requires binding of glycine to a distinct strychnine-insensitive binding site on the NMDA receptor.[34,40] Additional modulation of the NMDA receptor has been demonstrated by Zn^{2+}, which also binds via a distinct site and is thought to inhibit glycine binding,[114] and by polyamines, which may either enhance or inhibit NMDA receptor activation by binding at yet another distinct site.[83] In addition to the NMDA receptor, another class of EAA ionotropic receptors selectively binds either kainate (KA) or α-amino-3-hydroxy-5-methyl-4-isoxazole propionate (AMPA), which are associated with EAA receptor-mediated monovalent cation channels. These receptors are collectively referred to as "non-NMDA" receptors. Activation of these receptors results in the opening of their associated ion channel in a non-voltage-dependent manner, allowing the exchange of monovalent cations (influx of Na^{+}, efflux of K^{+}).[21,84,114] Recent studies, however, have demonstrated that unique subtypes of these AMPA/KA receptors may also be permeable to Ca^{2+}.[32] Although AMPA receptors have previously been referred to as quisqualate (QA) receptors, QA (now recognized as nonselective), was found to bind to a third class of EAA receptor subtype, the metabotropic EAA receptor.[91] Unlike the ionotropic EAA receptors, this metabotropic EAA receptor acts through a second messenger system. The binding of glutamate or QA to this receptor will activate phospholipase C resulting in the generation of inositol triphosphate (IP_3), leading to the release of bound intracellular Ca^{2+},[87,102] thus increasing the concentration of intracellular free calcium ($[Ca^{2+}]_i$) through a different mechanism than NMDA receptor-mediated Ca^{2+} influx.

Exogenous Modulation of Excitatory Amino Acid Receptor Activation

Identifications of multiple modulatory sites on EAA receptors, particularly on the NMDA receptor, have enabled investigators to develop several classes of compounds, acting through different mechanisms, which may antagonize or inhibit EAA receptor activity. Owing to the sheer number of compounds that have been synthesized, we will limit the discussion here to agents evaluated in brain trauma research.

Competitive NMDA Receptor Antagonists

3-(2-carboxypiperizin-4yl)-propyl-1-phosphonic acid (CPP) and 2-amino-5-phosphovaleric acid (APV), which bind directly to the NMDA/glu site, have been shown to inhibit NMDA activity in vitro.[70] However, CPP and APV are lipophobic compounds, with poor blood-brain barrier permeability, necessitating intracerebral administration for biological activity in vivo. More recently developed compounds, including cis-4-(phosphomethyl)-2-piperidine carboxylic acid (CGS19755) and (+/−)-(25R,4R5)-4-(1H-tetrazol-5yl-methyl)piperidine-2-carboxylic acid (LY233053), appear to have a greater blood-brain barrier permeability and may be administered parenterally.[71,102A]

NMDA Receptor Channel Blockade

NMDA receptor activation may also be noncompetitively (allosterically) antagonized by compounds that bind within the opened receptor-associated ionophore in a distinct location from magnesium. Although several synthetic compounds have been shown to bind at this site within the ion channel, no endogenous ligands have as yet been identified. Phencyclidine (PCP) and ketamine, previously identified as dissociative anesthetics, have been shown to bind within the NMDA receptor channel.[37] In addition, the antitussive compound, dextromethorphan and its derivative, dextrorphan, also antagonize the NMDA receptor through channel blockade. All of these compounds have also been shown to bind to the σ opiate receptor.[37] A related compound, dizocilopine (MK801), has more recently been synthesized, demonstrating excellent CNS penetration and high potency at the NMDA receptor with weak σ opiate receptor affinity.[112] However, MK801 as well as ketamine and PCP have been shown to produce pathological changes in neurons, including vacuolization of neurons in the cingulate gyrus,[77] and induce expression of the stress protein, heat shock protein (HSP),[89] causing debate concerning the potential therapeutic utility versus the possible inherent neurotoxicity of these compounds. Recently, a nonpsychotropic cannabinoid, HU-211 (7-hydroxy-tetrahydrocannabinol-1,1-dimethylheptyl), has also been shown to selectively antagonize the NMDA receptor by binding within the ionophore.

Modulation of the NMDA Receptor by Magnesium

The component of the excitatory postsynaptic current mediated by NMDA receptors in vitro has a slow onset and very long decay phase relative to AMPA/KA receptors, which is thought to result from the voltage-sensitive block within the NMDA receptor-associated ionophore by Mg^{2+}, strongest between membrane potentials of −80 and −40 mV.[48,73] Loss of magnesium homeostasis may disrupt NMDA-mediated neurotransmission, and has been suggested to play a major role in the pathogenesis of brain injury as described below. Correction of hypomagnesemic states may be accomplished by exogenous administration of magnesium salts (i.e., $MgCl_2$ and $MgSO_4$),[51] thus restoring the potentially compromised voltage-dependent block of the NMDA receptor.

NMDA Receptor-Associated Glycine Site Modulation

In addition to the absolute requirement of glycine binding for NMDA receptor activation, modulation of the NMDA receptor-associated glycine site has been shown to affect binding properties at other domains within the NMDA receptor. Uniquely, activation of the glycine site not only potentiates NMDA receptor binding, but also enhances binding of channel blocking compounds.[39,84] Conversely, antagonism of the glycine site inhibits binding of NMDA receptor ligands, thus indirectly inhibiting the binding of ligands with affinity sites within the ionophore.[50] In addition, agonists acting at the glycine site have been shown to have substantial enhancing effects on learning and memory, presumably by enhancing potentiation of the NMDA receptor.[24,26,64] What is perplexing about this regulatory site, especially with regard to potential enhancement, is that under normal conditions there appears to be sufficient extracellular glycine available to maximally saturate all sites.[34] A possible explanation for this paradox may be related to the identification of an endogenous NMDA receptor-associated glycine site antagonist, kynurenate (KYNA), which may function as an endogenous modulator of neuronal excitability. The concentration of endogenous KYNA, which also acts as a competitive antagonist of AMPA/KA receptors, has been shown to increase with aging and neurodegenerative disorders.[9,65] These data suggest that *endogenous* antagonism of EAA receptors by endogenous neurochemicals such as KYNA may play an important role both in the modulation of normal EAA neurotransmission and in mediating pathological circumstances.

In addition to KYNA, other compounds have been synthesized that demonstrate varying selectivity and affinities for the NMDA receptor-associated glycine site. These compounds include indole-2-carboxylic acid (I2CA), which has been shown to selectively antagonize the glycine site,[30] and 6-cyano-7-nitroquinoxaline-2,3-dine (CNQX), a quinoxalinedione derivative initially developed to selectively antagonize AMPA/KA receptors, but has since been shown to also antagonize the NMDA receptor-associated glycine site.[29,39] Compounds such as CNQX and KYNA, shown to antagonize both NMDA and AMPA/KA receptors, frequently are referred to as *broad spectrum EAA receptor antagonists.*

Modulation of the NMDA receptor-associated polyamine binding site

It has been demonstrated that the endogenous polyamine compounds, spermidine and spermine, enhance NMDA receptor activation, while putrescine inhibits NMDA receptor activation. These polyamines bind to the NMDA receptor via a site distinct from glutamate and glycine.[83] Although activation of the polyamine site is not a requirement for NMDA receptor activation, the potential endogenous enhancement or inhibition of NMDA function mediated through this binding site may be analogous to endogenous modulation of the glycine binding site. This additional modulatory site further demonstrates the complexity of regulatory mechanisms involved in NMDA receptor function. Similar to antagonism of the glycine site, competitive antagonism of the polyamine site has been shown to inhibit the binding of ligands to the NMDA receptor and to the binding site within the receptor-associated ionophore.[85] In addition to putrescine, synthetic competitive antagonists of the polyamine binding site, including ifenprodil and its derivative, eliprodil (SL82.0715), also have been shown to antagonize NMDA receptor activation.[4]

AMPA/KA receptor antagonism

To date, selective competitive AMPA/KA antagonists, such as NBQX (2,3-dihydroxy-6-nitro-7-sulfamoyl-benzo(F)quinoxaline),[90] have not been evaluated in brain trauma models. However, the broad spectrum EAA antagonists, KYNA and CNQX, which demonstrate antagonism of the AMPA/KA and NMDA receptors, have been utilized in models of experimental brain injury (see below). It has recently been observed that AMPA/KA receptors may also be *noncompetitively* antagonized by the 2,3-benzodiazepine muscle relaxant, GYKI 52466 (1-(4-aminophenyl)-4-methyl-7,8-methylenedioxy-5H-2,3-benzodiazepine HCl), which has been shown to be both highly selective and potent. Antagonism of AMPA/KA receptors may indirectly affect NMDA receptor function by inhibiting depolarization of the neuron, thus maintaining the voltage-dependent block by magnesium of the NMDA receptor.

Metabotropic receptor modulation

Selective activation of this most recently identified EAA receptor subtype, leading to phosphoinositide hydrolysis, has been demonstated by 1S,3R-amino-1,3-cyclopentanedicarboxylic acid (ACPD), while nonselective activation has been demonstrated by QA, which also stimulates AMPA receptors. Noncompetitive antagonism of the EAA metabotropic receptor has been demonstrated by D,L-2-amino-3-phosphonopropionate (AP3). However, the role of the metabotropic receptor in the pathogenesis of traumatic brain injury has yet to be elucidated, and, to date, no studies have demonstrated pharmacological efficacy with either antagonists or antagonists of this receptor. Nonetheless, studies in various laboratories are currently underway to evaluate modulation of this receptor for brain trauma therapy.

EAA release inhibition

In addition to direct antagonism or blockade of EAA receptor function, modulation of EAA receptor activity also may be accomplished by inhibition of EAA release. Lamotrigine (3,5-diamino-6-[2,3-dichlorophenyl]-1,2,4-triazine) and its more potent derivatives, BW 1003C87 (5-[2,3,5-trichlorophenyl]pyrimidine-2,4-diamine ethane sulfonate) and 619C89 (4-amino-2-(4-methyl-1-piperazinyl)-5-(2,3,5-trichlorophenyl) pyrimidine mesylate monohydrate have been shown to inhibit veratrine- but not K^+-stimulated glutamate release, potentially by reducing ion flux through voltage-gated Na^+ channels.[58,59,102A] (Schematic representation of the pharmacological modulation of EAA receptors is shown in Fig. 107-1.)

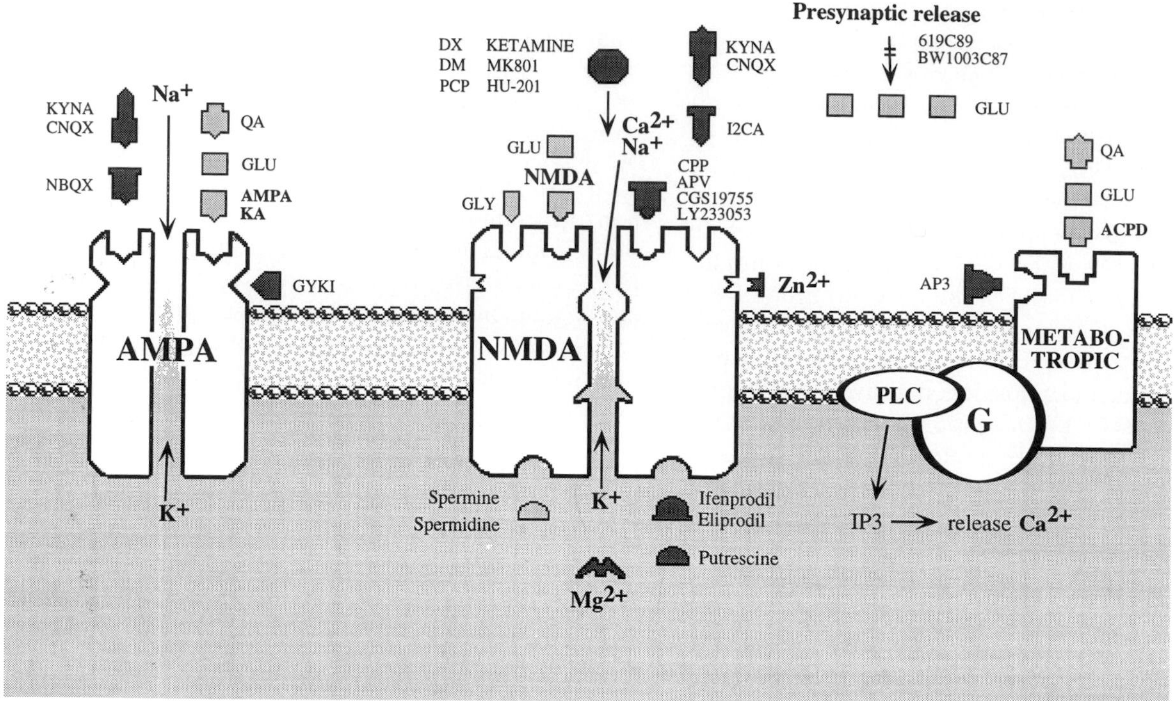

Figure 107-1. Schematic representation of excitatory amino acid receptors and their effectors, relevant to current brain trauma research. Light-filled ligands—agonists; dark-filled ligands—antagonists. Code: ACPD—1S,3R-amino-1,3-cyclopentanedicarboxylic acid; AMPA—α-amino-3-hydroxy-5-methyl-4-isoxazole propionate; AP3—D,L-2-amino-3-phosphonopropionate; HU211, LY233053, 619C89 with their chemical names as now found on the new revised table; APV—2-amino-5-phosphovaleric acid; BW1003C87—5-[2,3,5-trichlorophenyl]pyrimidine-2,4-diamine ethane sulfonate; CGS19755—*cis*-4-(phosphomethyl)-2-piperidine carboxylic acid; CNQX—6-cyano-7-nitroquinoxaline-2,3-dine; CPP—3-(2-carboxypiperizin-4yl)-propy-1-phosphonic acid; DM—dextromethorphan; DX—dextrorphan; G—G protein; glu—glutamate; gly—glycine; GYKI—GYKI 52466 (1-(4-aminophenyl)-4-methyl-7,8-methylenedioxy-5H-2,3-benzodiazepine HCl I2CA—indole-2-carboxylic acid; IP3—inositol triphosphate; KYNA—kynurenate; MK801—dizocilopine; NBQX—2,3-dihydroxy-6-nitro-7sulfamoyl-benzo(F)quinoxaline; PCP—phencyclidine; PLC—phospholipase C; QA—quisqualate.

EXCITATORY AMINO ACID NEUROTOXICITY

Early in vitro experiments by Olney and colleagues demonstrated that EAA neurotransmitters applied directly to neurons produced cell swelling, vacuolization, and eventual cell death.[74,75] EAA neurotransmitters also produce seizures and general CNS neuronal death when administered in vivo.[42,57,76] These observations led to the concept of "excitotoxicity," by which EAA neurotransmitters become neurotoxic in pathological circumstances and contribute to the tissue damage within the CNS in a variety of disorders, including neurodegenerative disorders (e.g., Alzheimer's disease, Parkinson's disease, Huntington's disease, amyotrophic lateral sclerosis, epilepsy, cerebral hypoxia, ischemia, and trauma).[3,5,17,20,22,25,82,86] This excitotoxic sequela is thought to arise from an overactivation of the various EAA receptor subtypes, causing a massive influx of Na^+ and efflux of K^+ through KA and AMPA receptor-associated channels, depolarizing the neurons and subsequently overcoming the voltage-dependent block by Mg^{2+} of the NMDA receptor ionophore and allowing a large influx of Ca^{2+} into the neuron.[8,48,86] Young and others have proposed that an increase in $[Ca^{++}]_i$ is the final common pathway for neuronal death following spinal cord injury.[116] Although the exact mechanisms underlying EAA-mediated cell death are not well understood, Choi has postulated that following the sustained release of glutamate with prolonged postsynaptic excitation: (1) early accumulation of intracellular Na^+ (through AMPA and KA receptor gated ionophores) leads to acute neuronal swelling; and (2) delayed Ca^{2+} influx (through the NMDA receptor ionophore) causes a cascade of metabolic disturbances within the neuron.[5] More recently, the increase in $[Ca^{2+}]_i$ following an excitotoxic event has also been linked to both the influx of Ca^{2+} through non-NMDA receptors (KA and AMPA receptors)[31,32] and to the IP_3-mediated release of Ca^{2+} from intracellular stores following EAA stimulation of the metabotropic receptor.[87,102]

EAA NEUROTOXICITY AND TRAUMATIC BRAIN INJURY

The suggestion that EAA excitotoxicity plays a role in the pathophysiological sequelae of CNS trauma has been substantiated, in part, by studies employing both experimental models of brain injury and in vivo intracerebral microdialysis techniques, which have demonstrated an acute and marked increase in extracellular EAAs following trauma. However, major differences in the magnitude and duration of post-traumatic EAA release have been reported. While Katayama and colleagues[35] observed a four- to fivefold increase in extracellular EAA release following lateral fluid percussion (LFP) brain injury in the rat, Palmer et al.[79] observed an 81- to 144-fold increase following controlled cortical impact of mild and moderate severity, and Faden et al.[18] reported a 280-fold increase in extracellular EAAs following LFP injury. Further evidence substantiating post-traumatic EAA neurotoxicity has been observed by characterizing changes in cation homeostasis following experimental brain injury. Using atomic absorption spectrophotometry, total tissue concentrations of Na^+ and Ca^{2+} appear to be increased following lateral fluid percussion (LFP) brain injury in the rat, while the total tissue concentrations of K^+, Mg^{2+}, and Zn^{2+} appear to decrease.[100,101,106,107] In addition, extracellular K^+ concentration has been observed to increase substantially following LFP brain injury,[35] which may play a role in the further release of EAAs. Intracellular free magnesium concentrations ($[Mg^{2+}]_i$), measured by ^{31}P MRS, have been shown to decrease dramatically following LFP injury[110] and following a new rotational acceleration model of diffuse axonal injury in miniature swine.[96] This decrease in $[Mg^{2+}]_i$ following LFP injury was found to correlate with the severity of neurological motor dysfunction.[53] The decrease in $[Mg^{2+}]_i$ may be an important initial step in the excitotoxic process, since Mg^{2+} not only provides a voltage-dependent block of the NMDA receptor, but also plays a global role in cellular physiology and bioenergetics.[15]

Another series of studies linking EAA neurotoxicity with the pathophysiological sequelae of brain injury concerns the effects of trauma on cognition. EAA neurotransmission has been shown to play a major role in normal cognitive process. Long-term potentiation (LTP), demonstrated as the long-term enhancement of monosynaptic connections following short neuronal tetanization, has been shown to be mediated, in part, by the influx of calcium through NMDA receptors.[2,6,7] LTP is considered the synaptic analogue of memory,[69] since studies have demonstrated that antagonists acting at the NMDA receptor induce both blockade of LTP and a cognitive impairment.[6,12,67,68] LTP also may be blocked following antagonism of the EAA metabotropic receptor,[1] suggesting that LTP is related to an increase of $[Ca^{2+}]_i$ from both intracellular (IP_3 activation) and extracellular (NMDA- or KA/AMPA-mediated) sources. Through excitotoxic processes, damage to and/or dysfunction of the EAA receptor network might therefore impede production of normal LTP and thus disrupt normal cognitive processes. Indeed, in the clinical setting, the most common and most persistent sequela of brain trauma is cognitive dysfunction.[43]

Bilateral damage to the hippocampus and other limbic structures has been shown to play a major role in the development of memory disorders.[43,81] The hippocampus, which specifically appears to be involved with spatial learning and memory,[16] has a high density of EAA receptors.[63,72] Following experimental midline fluid percussion (MFP) brain injury in the rat, decreases in NMDA receptor binding have been observed in the hippocampus following injury,[60] and LTP has been found to be suppressed in this model.[61] Moreover, a learning deficit has been observed following MFP brain injury, using an eight-arm radial maze technique.[46] More recently, several groups have characterized both learning and memory deficits following experimental brain injury, using neurobehavioral tests such as the Morris water maze,[66] and have performed detailed histopathological analyses in search of potential anatomic substrates responsible for these deficits. In the LFP model of brain injury in the rat, profound retrograde amnesia (loss of memory of events that occurred prior to injury) of the spatial water maze task has been observed following brain injury.[91] The magnitude of selective hippocampal neuronal cell loss in the CA3 region ipsilateral to the area of cortical damage and bilaterally in the hilus of the dentate gyrus observed following LFP brain injury has been found to correlate with the severity of this post-traumatic memory loss.[93] This correlation has even been observed following *mild* experimental brain injury.[27] In addition, the presence of abnormal hyperexcitability of dentate granule cells has been observed to correlate with the loss of dentate hilar neurons following LFP injury.[44] A mouse model, CCI, has also been shown to produce memory dysfunction and hippocampal cell loss in a distribution similar to that seen in the rat LFP model of brain injury.[94] Moreover, in a model of unilateral neocortical contusion in the rat, a consistent post-traumatic loss of neurons has been observed in the ipsilateral CA3 and dentate hilar regions of the hippocampus, which is associated with a deficit in LTP production and a dysfunction of spatial learning in the Morris water maze.[103] In contrast to the above observations, in experimental brain injury models of MFP and CCI in the rat, severe learning dysfunction has been demonstrated in the absence of overt cell loss in the hippocampus.[13,23,46] However, in both the MFP and CCI rat models of brain injury, a decrease of microtubule-associated protein (MAP)2 has been observed in the hippocampus, using Western blotting and immunohistochemical techniques,[104,105] suggesting that cytoskeletal damage has occurred in this brain region in the absence of overt cell loss. Moreover, following LFP injury, immunohistochemical techniques have revealed bilateral expression of the stress protein, heat shock protein (HSP)72,[52] and loss of MAP2[95] in the hippocampus in regions not associated with cell loss. More recently, alterations in mRNA expression of HSP, the proto-oncogene c-fos, and the glucose-regulated proteins (GRP), GRP-78, and GRP-92, have been documented following LFP injury in regions without overt cell loss.[45] These findings have led several investigators to postulate that post-traumatic cognitive deficits may result, in part, from excitotoxic events specifically targeting the hippocampus, inducing either overt neuronal cell loss, cellular stress, and/or dysfunction, thereby disrupting normal synaptic transmission. Further evidence of a potential mechanistic link between post-traumatic EAA neurotoxicity, cognitive deficits, and hippocampal dysfunction has recently been proposed by studies demonstrating that EAA receptor antagonists may attenuate post-traumatic spatial memory dysfunction and protect neurons in the hippocampus (see below).

PHARMACOLOGICAL INTERVENTION OF EAA TOXICITY FOLLOWING TRAUMATIC BRAIN INJURY

Several pharmacological compounds affecting EAA neurotransmission systems have been assessed to date in at least four models of experimental brain injury. Unlike CNS hypoxia/ischemia research, in which pharmacological efficacy is determined primarily by histological evaluation of neuroprotective effects, investigations in the field of brain trauma have relied more on neurochemical, metabolic, and behavioral outcome measures, owing to difficulty in histopathological characterization and interpretation. However, several recent studies have begun to identify EAA receptor antagonists that can limit histopathological damage following experimental brain injury. The following is a compendium of studies utilizing EAA receptor antagonists and effectors, grouped according to outcome parameters, which have demonstrated efficacy in the treatment of traumatic brain injury.

Effects on Cerebral Edema Formation

Significant, regional cerebral edema formation has been demonstrated in a variety of experimental brain injury models using both the wet weight/dry weight and microgravimetric density gradient techniques.[47,88,101] This edema formation has been postulated to originate from both cytotoxic and vasogenic sources. Cytotoxic edema may arise, in part, from an excitotoxic event, in which astrocytic and neuronal swelling may occur subsequent to increased intracellular Na^+ concentrations producing an osmotic gradient. Vasogenic edema may result from an opening of the blood-brain barrier following trauma, which has been observed following LFP brain injury.[10] Owing to the potential role of EAA in mediating post-traumatic cerebral edema formation, several compounds that block EAA receptor activation have been evaluated for their effects in attenuating cerebral edema. The NMDA receptor channel blocker, MK801, has been shown to reduce regional cerebral edema formation in the LFP model of injury (1 mg/kg, IV, 15 min post-injury)[55] and in the weight-drop model of brain injury (3 mg/kg, intraperitoneally, 1 h post-injury).[88] Post-traumatic cerebral edema has also been shown to be attenuated with post-injury administration of the NMDA receptor channel blockers, dextromethorphan (10 mg/kg, IV, 15 min post-injury)[56] and $MgCl_2$ (300 μmol, IV infusion, 15 min post-injury).[99,90B] Recently, the nonpsychotropic cannabinoid, HU211 (7-hydroxy-tetrahydrocannabinol 1,1-dimethylheptyl) (25 mg/kg, IV) improved cerebral edema formation even if treatment was delayed two hours following weight-drop brain injury.[90B] The NMDA receptor-associated glycine site antagonist I2CA (20 mg/kg, IV, 15 min post-injury) and the broad spectrum EAA antagonist KYNA (300 mg/kg, IV, 15 min post-injury), which antagonizes both the glycine site and the AMPA/KA binding site, have been found to be effective in reversing regional post-traumatic edema in the cortex, hippocampus, and thalamus.[100] BW1003C87 (10 mg/kg, IV, 15 min post-injury), acting as a presynaptic glutamate release inhibitor, has also been shown to decrease regional cerebral edema.[99] However, the competitive NMDA receptor antagonists, CGS19755 (10 and 30 mg/kg, IV, 15 min post-injury) and CPP (10 and 100 μg, intracerebroventricular [ICV], 15 min post-injury) have demonstrated no effect on post-traumatic cerebral edema formation,[56,92] suggesting that noncompetitive NMDA receptor antagonists may be superior to competitive antagonists in reducing post-traumatic regional cerebral edema. It is important to note that, in most brain injury models, even the most efficacious compounds do not reduce edema in the maximal injury sites, which demonstrate the most profound swelling, possibly because of the predominance of vasogenic edema in these regions. Efficacy is typically demonstrated in cortical regions adjacent to the maximal injury site and in the hippocampus, in which cytotoxic mechanisms may play a greater role in edema formation, and may therefore be more responsive to EAA receptor antagonism.

Total Tissue Cation Concentration Effects

Disturbances in cation homeostasis may play an important role in the pathogenesis of the secondary injury cascade (see above). Using the LFP model of brain injury, changes in the regional concentrations of Na^+, K^+, Ca^{2+}, Mg^{2+}, and Zn^{2+}, characterized using atomic absorption spectroscopic techniques,[101,106,107] have been shown to be attenuated with several EAA receptor antagonists. MK801 (1 mg/kg, IV, 15 min post-injury), was shown to decrease local post-traumatic increase in tissue [Na^+].[55] KYNA (300 mg/kg, IV, 15 min post-injury) was found to reduce the post-traumatic regional increase in [Ca^{2+}], while I2CA (20 mg/kg, IV, 15 min post-injury) prevented regional decreases in [K^+], [Zn^{2+}], and [Mg^{2+}] and increases in [Na^+].[100] In a weight-drop model of brain injury, ketamine (180 mg/kg, i.p.), administered up to 2 hours following injury, attenuated increases in tissue Ca^{2+} and decreases in tissue Mg^{2+}.[90A] These results suggest that post-traumatic administration of EAA receptor antagonists, acting at different binding sites of the EAA receptors, may help to maintain post-traumatic cation homeostasis, potentially attenuating secondary neurotoxic events.

Intracellular Free [Mg^{2+}] and Bioenergetics

In addition to the effects of inhibition of EAA receptor activity on the maintenance of *total tissue* Mg^{2+} concentrations following LFP brain injury, ^{31}P MRS studies have demonstrated that pharmacological intervention with EAA receptor antagonists may also maintain post-traumatic *intracellular free* Mg^{2+} homeostasis. A decrease in tissue bioenergetic status, reflected by a decline in the PCr/Pi ratio of brain tissue, was shown to be improved following treatment designed to inhibit EAA receptor activity. Compounds demonstrating efficacy by maintaining both [Mg^{2+}]$_i$ levels and the PCr/Pi ratio include MK801 (1 mg/kg, IV, 15 min post-injury)[55] and dextrorphan (10 mg/kg, IV, 30 min post-injury).[18] In addition, $MgSO_4$ (15 mEq/liter blood) administered IV 5 min prior to LFP injury prevented the post-traumatic decline in [Mg^{2+}]$_i$.[110]

Extracellular [K^+], Metabolism, and Glutamate Release

Katayama and colleagues[35] have used intracerebral microdialysis techniques in an LFP model of brain injury to demonstrate that a massive, post-traumatic increase in extracellular [K^+] could be attenuated by *in situ* administration of 1 to 25 mM KYNA, in a dose-dependent fashion. Subsequently, Panter and Faden,[80] also utilizing intracerebral microdialysis techniques, demonstrated that NMDA receptor antagonists may attenuate the post-traumatic release of EAAs following LFP brain injury. In this study, glutamate release in animals treated 15 min prior to LFP brain injury with dextrorphan (10 mg/kg, IV) or CGS19755 (30 mg/kg, IV) was shown to be reduced compared to nontreated brain-injured animals. The results from these studies may suggest that by blocking post-traumatic K^+ efflux following treatment with EAA receptor antagonists, subsequent K^+-mediated release of EAAs may be attenuated.

Kawamata and colleagues[36] also noted that the marked increase observed in cortical glucose utilization (using ^{14}C-2-deoxyglucose autoradiography techniques) following LFP injury could be reduced in areas infused, via microdialysis, with the broad spectrum EAA antagonists KYNA (10 mM) or CNQX (300 μM and 1 mM), or following intraparenchymal infusion of the competitive NMDA receptor antagonist APV (100 μM, 1 mM and 10 mM). These data suggest that post-traumatic metabolic changes are due, in part, to EAA toxicity and may be attenuated by EAA receptor antagonism.

Histological Neuroprotective Effects

Recently, three compounds, KYNA, Eliprodil, and 619C89 have been shown to attenuate histological damage in experimental models of brain injury. These are the first reported cases of histological neuroprotection following experimental brain injury. However, a previous study by Jenkins and colleagues (1988),[33A] which combined MFP brain injury with subsequent cerebral ischemia, demonstrated that PCP (4 mg/kg), administered intraperitoneally in combination with the muscarinic receptor blocker, scopolamine (1 mg/kg), 15 min prior to MFP brain injury, attenuated neuronal cell death associated with the post-traumatic delayed secondary ischemia.

In LFP brain injury, KYNA (300 mg/kg, IV, 15 min post-injury), was found to prevent selective hippocampal neuronal cell loss in the CA3 region, but not in the dentate hilar region.[28] This effect may reflect differential windows of therapeutic opportunity between these two regions, as evidenced by studies demonstrating that post-traumatic cell loss in the dentate hilar region appears to occur more rapidly than that in the CA3 region. More recently, sparing of hippocampal neurons following LFP brain injury has also been observed with treatment using 619C89 (30 mg/kg, IV) when administered 15 min prior to injury.[102A]

In a new model of LFP brain injury, utilizing high performance liquid chromatography (HPLC) equipment to induce the fluid pressure pulse, a relatively defined lesion is produced unilaterally in the parietal cortex.[108] The volume of this lesion has been shown to be reduced dramatically following treatment with Eliprodil, which antagonizes the NMDA receptor by binding to the polyamine modulatory site. Dosing regimens of Eliprodil (10 mg/kg, ip) given 15 min, 6 h, and 24 h after injury and then bid for the following 6 days, and delayed treatments with the initial dose at 12 h and 18 h all demonstrated neuroprotective efficacy.[109] These results were compared to treatment with MK801 (0.6 mg/kg, ip) administered 6 h, 24 h, then bid for the following 6 days, which did not demonstrate a significant effect on lesion volume. The encouraging results from this study are the first to suggest that, for cortical neurons, a large post-traumatic window may exist for therapeutic intervention.

Neurological Motor Effects

Hayes and colleagues,[25] in the first study evaluating the efficacy of an EAA receptor antagonist in a model of brain injury, demonstrated that treatment with PCP 15 min prior to MFP brain injury, at doses of 1, 2, and 4 mg/kg, ip, significantly attenuated long-term neurological deficits in a dose-dependent fashion. Subsequent studies with other NMDA receptor channel blockers demonstrated that both dextrorphan (10 mg/kg, IV, 30 min post-trauma)[18] and dextromethorphan (10 mg/kg, IV, 15 min post-injury)[92] significantly improved neurological motor deficits following LFP injury. In addition, MK801 (1 mg/kg, IV) administered 15 min prior to LFP injury also improved post-LFP injury motor outcome, while animals treated 15 min post-injury with MK801 failed to demonstrate any neurological improvement.[53] In contrast, in a weight-drop model of brain injury, MK801 (3 mg/kg, ip) administered 1 hour post-injury improved neurological motor outcome.[88] In the same weight-drop model of brain injury, HU-211 (25 mg/kg, i.p.) improved neurologic motor outcome even with treatment delayed up to 2 h following injury.[90B] Treatment with $MgSO_4$ (15 mEq/liter blood) 5 min prior to LFP injury and with $MgCl_2$ (12.5 and 125 μmol IV infusion) and 30 min following LFP injury have also been shown to attenuate post-traumatic motor dysfunction.[51,54] Although the competitive antagonist, CPP (100 μg, ICV) administered 5 min pre-LFP injury improved motor outcome,[18] CPP at the same dose and route administered 15 min following injury showed no beneficial effect.[56] Post-LFP injury treatment with another competitive antagonist, CGS19755 (10, 20, and 30 mg/kg, IV, 15 min post-injury) also did not demonstrate beneficial effects on motor outcome.[92] Other compounds demonstrating efficacy in their ability to improve neurological motor outcome following LFP brain injury include the broad spectrum EAA receptor antagonist, KYNA (300 mg/kg, IV, 15 min post-injury), the selective NMDA receptor-associated glycine site antagonist, I2CA (20 and 50 mg/kg, IV, 15 min post-injury) and with inhibition of glutamate release using 619C89 (30 mg/kg, IV, 15 min prior to injury).[100,102A] These results suggest that noncompetitive NMDA receptor antagonists may be superior to competitive antagonists in the treatment of post-traumatic neurological motor deficits.

Effects on Cognition

Since cognitive deficits are the most significant clinical aspects of post-traumatic sequelae, several compounds that modulate EAA receptor activity have been evaluated in the experimental LFP model of brain injury. Compounds acting at EAA receptors shown to significantly improve post-traumatic memory function include the broad spectrum EAA antagonist KYNA (300 mg/kg, IV, 15 min post-injury), the selective glycine site antagonist, I2CA (20 and 50 mg/kg, IV, 15 min post-injury),[100] the NMDA receptor channel blocker, ketamine (4 mg/kg, IV, 15 min post-injury), and $MgCl_2$ (125 μmol, IV infusion, 15 min post-injury).[98] Combination treatment with both ketamine and $MgCl_2$ at the same doses also improved post-traumatic memory function without any additive effect.[98] We have recently observed that the AMPA/KA noncompetitive receptor antagonist, GYKI (2 mg/kg) administered following injury at 15 min (IV) and 60 min (ip) and that the competitive NMDA receptor antagonist, LY233053 (100 mg/kg, IV) given 15 min following injury,[21A,31A] also improve cognitive outcome. Moreover, we have recently found that the use-dependent sodium channel antagonist, 619C89

TABLE 107-1 Pharmacological Modulation of EAA Neurotoxicity in Models of Experimental Brain Injury

	Compound	Model	Effects
Competitive NMDA Receptor Antagonists	CPP	LFP	Improves motor outcome[1]
	CGS 19755	LFP	Decreases glutamate release[2]
	APV	LFP	Decreases hypermetabolism[3]
	LY233053	LFP	Improves cognitive outcome[4]
NMDA receptor channel blockers	PCP	MFP	Improves motor outcome[5]
	MK801	LFP	Improves motor outcome[6]; decreases cerebral edema, maintains cation homeostasis, maintains $[Mg^{2+}]_i$ and bioenergetic status[7]
		Weight drop	Improves motor outcome, decreases cerebral edema[8]
	Ketamine	LFP	Improves cognitive outcome[9]
		Weight drop	Maintains cation homeostasis[10]
	Dextromethorphan	LFP	Improves motor outcome[11]; decreases cerebral edema[12]
	Dextrorphan	LFP	Improves motor outcome, maintains $[Mg^{2+}]_i$, improves bioenergetic status[1]; decreases glutamate release[2]
	HU-211	Weight drop	Improves motor outcome; decreases cerebral edema[13]
NMDA voltage-sensitive block	$MgCl_2$	LFP	Improves cognitive outcome[9]; improves motor outcome[14]; decreases cerebral edema[15]
	$MgSO_4$	LFP	Improves motor outcome, maintains $[Mg^{2+}]_i$[16]
Selective-NMDA receptor glycine antagonists	12CA	LFP	Improves cognitive and motor outcome, decreases cerebral edema, maintains cation homeostasis[17]
Ifenprodil-like NMDA receptor antagonists	Eliprodil	HPLC-LFP	Neuroprotection of cortical neurons[18]
Broad spectrum EAA receptor antagonists	KYNA	LFP	Improves cognitive and motor outcome, decreases cerebral edema, maintains cation homeostasis[17]; decreases release of K^+[19]; decreases hypermetabolism[3]; neuroprotection of hippocampal neurons[20]
	CNQX	LFP	Decreases hypermetabolism[3]
Selective AMPA/KA non-competitive-receptor antagonists	GYKI 52466	LFP	Improves cognitive outcome[21]
EAA release inhibitors	619C89	LFP	Improves cognitive outcome[22]; neuroprotection of hippocampal neurons; improves motor outcome[23]
	BW1003C87	LFP	Decreases cerebral edema[15]

Compounds demonstrating efficacy in models of experimental brain injury. Abbreviations: **Compounds:** *APV*—2-amino-5-phosphovaleric acid; *BW1003C87*—5-[2,3,5-trichlorophenyl] pyrimidine-2,4-diamine ethane sulfonate; *CGS19755*—*cis*-4-(phosphomethyl)-2-piperidine carboxylic acid; *CNQX*—6-cyano-7-nitroquinoxaline-2,3-dine; *CPP*—3-(2-carboxypiperizin-4yl)-propy-1-phosphonic acid; *GYKI 52466*—1-(4-aminophenyl)-4-methyl-7,8-methylenedioxy-5H-2,3-benzodiazepine; *HU-211*—7-hydroxy-tetrahydrocannabinol 1, 1-dimethylheptyl; *12CA*—indole-2-carboxylic acid; *KYNA*—kyurenate; *LY233053*—(+/−)-(2SR,4RS)-4-(1H-tetrazol-5ylmethyl)pipieridine-2-carboxylic acid; *MK801*—dizocilopine; *PCP*—Phencyclidine; *619C89*—4-Amino-2-(4-methyl-1-piperazinyl)-5-(2,3,5-trichorophenyl) pyrimidine mesylate monohydrate. **Brain injury models:** *HPLC*—high performance liquid chromatography pump LFP; *LFP*—lateral fluid-percussion; *MFP*—midline fluid-percussion

References:

1 Faden AI et al *Science* **244,** 789–800, 1989
2 Panter SS et al *Neurosci Lett* **136,** 165–168, 1992
3 Kawamata T et al *J Cereb Blood Flow Metab* **12,** 12–24, 1992
4 Glatt BS et al *J Neurotrauma* **12,** 118, 1995 (Abstract)
5 Hayes RL et al *J Neurotrauma* **5,** 259–274, 1988
6 McIntosh TK et al *J Neurotrauma* **6,** 247–259, 1989
7 McIntosh TK et al *J Neurochem* **55,** 1170–1179, 1990
8 Shapira Y et al *J Neurotrauma* **7,** 131–139, 1990
9 Smith DH et al *Neurosci Lett* **157,** 211–214, 1993
10 Shapira Y et al *J Cereb Blood Flow Metab* **13,** 962–968, 1993
11 Smith DH et al *FASEB Journal* **4(3),** 773, 1990 (Abstract)
12 McIntosh TK et al *Excitatory Amino Acids,* 247–253, 1992
13 Shohami E et al *J Neurotrauma* **10,** 109–119, 1993
14 McIntosh TK et al *Brain Res* **482,** 252–260, 1989
15 Okiyama K et al *J Neurochem* **64(2),** 802–809, 1995
16 McIntosh TK et al *J Neurotrauma* **5,** 17–31, 1988
17 Smith DH et al *J Neurosci* **13,** 5383–5392, 1993
18 Toulmond S et al *Brain Res* **620,** 32–41, 1993
19 Katayama Y et al *J Neurosurg* **73,** 889–900, 1990
20 Hicks RR et al *Brain Res* **655,** 91–96, 1994
21 Hylton C et al *J Neurotrauma* **12,** 124, 1995 (Abstr)
22 Voddi MD et al *J Neurotrauma* **12,** 146, 1995 (Abstr)
23 Sun F-Y and Faden AI *Brain Res* **673,** 133–140, 1995

(20 mg/kg, IV) administered 15 min following injury also attenuates post-LFP injury cognitive dysfunction.[110A] The positive effects of these compounds on post-traumatic memory function help to confirm the hypothesis of the role of EAAs in the selective delayed damage to cognitive systems. In particular, the post-traumatic effects of KYNA on memory, hippocampal neuronal sparing, maintenance of Ca^{2+} homeostasis in the hippocampus, and attenuation of edema formation in the hippocampus supports the concept of a mechanistic link between post-traumatic EAA neurotoxicity, cognitive dysfunction, and hippocampal damage.

In contrast to attenuation of cognitive dysfunction following brain injury, cognitive enhancement of persistent post-traumatic learning deficits also has been demonstrated following LFP injury. In a Morris water maze learning paradigm, it was observed that the notropic piracetam-like cognitive enhancer, BMY-21502, (10 mg/kg) administered subcutaneously 30 min prior to the learning paradigm significantly improved learning performance. Although no direct link to EAA neurotransmission systems by BMY-21502 has been identified, it has been shown to enhance LTP in slice preparations.[37] Table 107-1 summarizes the efforts, to date, of EAA receptor modulation in the treatment of traumatic brain injury.

CONCLUSIONS

These data support the role of EAA neurotransmitters in the delayed pathophysiological sequelae of traumatic brain injury. It appears that an acute and marked release of EAA neurotransmitters occurs following trauma, targeting regions in the brain rich in EAA receptors, including the hippocampus, and initiating a cascade of metabolic disturbances that lead to secondary neuronal cell destruction or damage. Because of the delayed nature of this damage, several methods of therapeutic intervention appear to be efficacious, including inhibition of EAA release, competitive and noncompetitive antagonism of EAA receptors, and voltage-dependent blockade of the NMDA receptor. Although Toulmond and colleagues[109] have elegantly demonstrated a neuroprotective effect of the EAA receptor antagonist, Eliprodil, with the initial dose delayed as late as 18 hours post-injury, a well-defined critical window of therapeutic opportunity in brain trauma has yet to be discerned, and much work needs to be performed to identify the most promising compound or combination of compounds in the treatment of traumatic brain injury. Nevertheless, owing to the promising potential efficacy of EAA receptor inhibition following brain trauma, clinical studies have been initiated evaluating the effects of the competitive NMDA receptor antagonist, CGS 19755, and the magnesium salt, $MgSO_4$, in the treatment of human head injury.

References

1. Aronica E, Frey U, Wagner M, et al: Enhanced sensitivity of "metabotropic" glutamate receptors after induction of long-term potentiation in rat hippocampus. *J Neurochem* 1991; 57:376–383.
2. Bliss TVP, Lomo T: Long-lasting potentiation of synaptic transmission in the dentate area of the anaesthetized rabbit following stimulation of the perforant path. *J Physiol (Lond)* 1973; 232:331–356.
3. Bosley TM, Woodhams PL, Gordon RD, Balazs R: Effect of anoxia on the stimulated release of amino acid neurotransmitters in the cerebellum in vitro. *J Neurochem* 1983; 40:189–201.
4. Carter C, Rivy JP, Scatton B: Ifenprodil and SL 82.0715 are antagonists at the polyamine site of the N-methyl-D-aspartate (NMDA) receptor. *Eur J Pharmacol* 1989; 164:611–612.
5. Choi DW: Glutamate neurotoxicity in cortical cell culture is calcium dependent. *Neurosci Lett* 1985; 58: 293–297.
6. Collingridge GL, Bliss TVP: NMDA receptors—their role in long-term potentiation. *Trends Neurosci* 1987; 10:288–293.
7. Collingridge GL, Davies SN: NMDA receptors and long-term potentiation in the hippocampus, in Watkins JC, *The NMDA Receptor.* Collingridge GL (eds): Oxford IRL Press, 1989: 123–135.
8. Collingridge GL, Lester RAJ: Excitatory amino acid receptors in the vertebrate central nervous system. *Pharmacol Rev* 1989; 41:143–210.
9. Connick JH, Carla V, Moroni F, Stone TW: Increase in kynurenic acid in Huntington's disease motor cortex. *J Neurochem* 1989; 52:985–987.
10. Cortez SC, McIntosh TK, Noble L: Experimental fluid percussion brain injury: Vascular disruption and neuronal and glial alterations. *Brain Res* 1989; 482:271–282.
11. Curtis DR, Watkins JC: The pharmacology of amino acids related to gamma-aminobutric acid. *Pharmacol Rev* 1965; 17:347–392.
12. Davis S, Butcher SP, Morris RGM: The NMDA receptor antagonist D-2-amino-5-phosphonopentanoate (DAP5) impairs spatial learning and LTP in vivo at intracerebral concentrations comparable to those that block LTP in vitro. *J Neurosci* 1992; 12:21–34.
13. Dixon CE, Clifton GL, Lighthall JW, et al: A controlled cortical impact model of traumatic brain injury in the rat. *J Neurosci Methods* 1991; 39:253–262.
14. Dovevan SD, Rogawski MA: GYKI 52466, a 2,3-benzodiazepine, is a highly selective, noncompetitive antagonist of AMPA/kainate receptor responses. *Neuron* 1993; 10:51–59.

15. Ebel H, Gunther T: Magnesium metabolism: A review. *J Clin Chem Clin Biochem* 1980; 8:257–270.
16. Eichenbaum H, Stewart C, Morris RGM: Hippocampal representation in place learning. *J Neurosci* 1990; 10(11):3531–3542.
17. Evenly S, Tecoma ES, Monyer H, et al: Traumatic neuronal injury in vitro is attenuated by NMDA antagonists. *Neuron* 1989; 2:1541–1545.
18. Faden AI, Demediuk P, Panter SS, Vink R: The role of excitatory amino acids and NMDA receptors in traumatic brain injury. *Science* 1989; 244:789–800.
19. Fields RD, Yu C, Nelson PG: Calcium, network activity, and the role of NMDA channels in synaptic plasticity in vitro. *J Neurosci* 1991; 11(1):134–146.
20. Ford LM, Sanberg PR, Norman AB, Fogelson MH: MK-801 prevents hippocampal neurodegeneration in neonatal hypoxic-ischemic rats. *Arch Neurol* 1989; 46:1090–1096.
21. Foster A, Fagg G: Neurobiology. Taking apart NMDA receptors. *Nature* 1987; 329:395–396.
21A. Glatt BS, Raghupathi R, Gennarelli TA, McIntosh TK: Effect of simultaneous blockade of opiate and glutamate receptors on neurobehavioral outcome following experimental brain injury. *J Neurotrauma* 1995; 12:118.
22. Gupta RK, Gupta P, Moore KD: NMR studies of intracellular metal ions in intact cells and tissues. *Ann Rev Biophys Bioeng* 1984; 13:221–246.
23. Hamm RJ, Dixon CE, Gbadebo DM, et al: Cognitive deficits following traumatic brain injury by controlled cortical impact. *J Neurotrauma* 1992; 9:11–20.
24. Handelmann GE, Nevins ME, Mueller LL, et al: Milacemide, a glycine prodrug, enhances performance of learning tasks in normal and amnestic rodents. *Pharmacol Biochem Behav* 1989; 34:823–828.
25. Hayes RL, Jenkins LW, Lyeth BG, et al: Pretreatment with phencyclidine, an N-methyl-D-aspartate antagonist, attenuates long-term behavioral deficits in the rat produced by traumatic brain injury. *J Neurotrauma* 1988; 5:259–274.
26. Herberg LJ, Rose IC: Effects of D-Cycloserine and Cycloleucine, ligands for the NMDA-associated strychnine-insensitive glycine site, on brain-stimulation reward and spontaneous locomotion. *Pharmacol Biochem Behav* 1990; 36:735–738.
27. Hicks RR, Smith DH, Lowenstein DH, et al: Mild experimental brain injury in the rat induces cognitive deficits correlate with regional neuronal loss in the hippocampus. *J Neurotrauma* 1993; 10(4):405–414.
28. Hicks RR, Smith DH, McIntosh TK: Kynurenate is neuroprotective following experimental brain injury in the rat. *Brain Res* 1994; 655:91–96.
29. Honore T, Davies SN, Drejer J, et al: Potent and competitive antagonist at non-NMDA receptors by FG-9041 and FG-9065. *Soc Neurosci Abstr* 1987; 17:383.
30. Huettner JE: Indole-2-carboxylic acid: A competitive antagonist of potentiation by glycine at the NMDA receptor. *Science* 1989; 243:1611–1613.
31. Hume RI, Dingledine R, Heinemann S: Identification of a site in glutamate receptor subunits that controls calcium permeability. *Science* 1991; 253:1028–1031.
31A. Hylton C, Perri B, Voddi M, Smith D, Raghupathi R, Tarnawa L et al. Non-NMDA antagonist GYKI 52466 enhances spatial memory after experimental brain injury. *J Neurotrauma* 1995; 12(1):124.
32. Iino M, Ozawa S, Tsuki K: Permeation of calcium through excitatory amino acid receptor channels in cultured rat hippocampal neurons. *J Physiol (Lond)* 1990; 424:151–165.
33. Jahr CE, Stevens CF: A quantitative description of NMDA receptor-channel kinetic behavior. *J Neurosci* 1990; 10(6):1830–1837.
33A. Jenkins LW, Lyeth BG, Lewelt W, Moszynski K, DeWitt DS, Balster RL et al: Combined pretrauma scopolamine and phencyclidine attenuate posttraumatic increased sensitivity to delayed ischemia. *J Neurotrauma* 1988; 5(4):275–287.
34. Johnson JW, Ascher P: Glycine potentiates the NMDA response in cultered mouse brain neurons. *Nature* 1987; 325:529–531.
35. Katayama Y, Becker D, Tamura T, Hovda DA: Massive increases in extracellular potassium and the indiscriminate release of glutamate following concussive brain injury. *J Neurosurg* 1990; 73:889–900.
36. Kawamata T, Katayama Y, Hovda DA, et al: Administration of excitatory amino acid antagonists via microdialysis attenuates the increase in glucose utilization seen following concussive brain injury. *J Cereb Blood Flow Metab* 1992; 12:12–24.
37. Kemp JA, Foster AC, Wong EHF: Non-competitive antagonists of excitatory amino acid receptors. *Trends Neurosci* 1987; 10:294–298.
38. Kessler M, Baudry M, Lynch G: Quinoxaline derivatives are high-affinity antagonists of the NMDA receptor-associated glycine sites. *Brain Res* 1989; 489:377–382.
39. Kessler M, Terramani T, Lynch G, Baudry M: A glycine site associated with N-methyl-D-aspartic acid receptors: Characterization and identification of a new class of antagonists. *J Neurochem* 1989; 52:1319–1328.
40. Kleckner NW, Dingledine R: Requirement for glycine in activation of NMDA receptors expressed in Xenopus oocytes. *Science* 1988; 241:835–837.
41. Krnjevic K: Chemical nature of synaptic transmission in vertebrates. *Physiol Rev* 1974; 54:418–540.
42. Lapin IP: Convulsant action of intracerebroventricularly administered l-kynurenine sulphate, quinolinic acid and other derivatives of succinic acid, and effects of amino acids: Structure-activity relationships. *Neuropharmacology* 1982; 21:1227–1233.
43. Levin HS: Outcome after head injury. Part II. Neurobehavioral recovery, in: *Status Report on Central Nervous System Trauma Research.* Bethesda: National Institute of Neurological and Communicative Disease and Stroke, 1985: 281–299.
44. Lowenstein DH, Thomas M, Smith DH, McIntosh TK: Selective vulnerability of dentate hilar neurons following traumatic brain injury: A potential mechanistic link between head trauma and disorders of the hippocampus. *J Neurosci* 1992; 12:4846–4853.
45. Lowenstein DH, Gwinn RP, Seren MS, et al: Increased expression of mRNA encoding Calbindin-D28k, the

glucose-regulated proteins, or the F2kDA heat-shock protein in three models of acute CNS injury. *Mol Brain Res* 1994; 22(1–4):299–308.

46. Lyeth BG, Jenkins LW, Hamm RJ, et al: Prolonged memory impairment in the absence of hippocampal cell death following traumatic brain injury in the rat. *Brain Res* 1990; 526:249–258.
47. Marmarou A, Poll W, Shulman K, Bhagavan H: A simple gravimetric technique for measurement of cerebral edema. *J Neurosurg* 1978; 49:530–537.
48. Mayer M, Westbrook G: The physiology of excitatory amino acids in the vertebrate central nervous system. *Prog Neurobiol (Oxford)* 1987; 28:197–276.
49. Mayer ML, Westbrook GL: The action of N-methyl-D-aspartic acid on mouse spinal neurones in culture. *J Physiol (Lond)* 1985; 361:65–90.
50. McDonald JW, Penney JB, Johnston MV, Young AB: Characterization and regional distribution of strychnine-insensitive <3H> glycine binding sites in rat brain by quantitative receptor autoradiography. *Neuroscience* 1990; 35:653–668.
51. McIntosh TK, Vink R, Yamakami I, Faden AI: Magnesium deficiency exacerbates and pretreatment improves outcome following traumatic brain injury in rats. 31P Magnetic resonance spectroscopy and behavioral studies. *J Neurotrauma* 1988; 5:17–31.
52. McIntosh TK, Soares H, Gonzalez M, Sharp F: Heat shock protein expression in rat brain after experimental brain injury. *Neurosci Abstr* 1989; 15:132.
53. McIntosh TK, Vink R, Soares H, et al: Effects of N-methyl-D-aspartate receptor blocker MK-801 on neurological function after experimental brain injury. *J Neurotrauma* 1989; 6:247–259.
54. McIntosh TK, Vink R, Yamakami I, Faden AI: Magnesium protects against neurological deficit after brain injury. *Brain Res* 1989; 482:252–260.
55. McIntosh TK, Vink R, Soares H, et al: Effects of noncompetitive blockade of N-methyl-D-aspartate receptors on the neurochemical sequelae of experimental brain injury. *J Neurochem* 1990; 55:1170–1179.
56. McIntosh TK, Smith DH, Hayes R, et al: Role of excitatory amino acid neurotransmitters in the pathogenesis of traumatic brain injury, in Simon RP (ed): *Excitatory Amino Acids* New York: Thieme 1992: 247–253.
57. McLennan H, Huffman RD, Marshall KC: Patterns of excitation of thalamic neurones by amino-acids and by acetylcholine. *Nature* 1968; 219:387–388.
58. Meldrum BS, Swan JH, Leach MJ, et al: Reduction of glutamate release and protection against ischemic brain damage by BW 1003C87. *Brain Res* 1992; 593:1–6.
59. Miller AA, Sawyer DA, Roth B, et al: Lamotrigine, in: Meldrum BS, Porter RI (eds): *New Anticonvulsant Drugs*. London: John Libbey, 1986: 165–177.
60. Miller LP, Lyeth B, Jenkins L, et al: Excitatory amino acid receptor subtype binding following traumatic brain injury. *Brain Res* 1990; 526:103–107.
61. Miyazaki S, Katayama Y, Lyeth BG, et al: Enduring suppression of hippocampal long-term potentiation following traumatic brain injury in rat. *Brain Res* 1992; 585:335–339.
62. Monaghan DT, Bridges RJ, Cotman C: The excitatory amino acid receptors: Their classes, pharmacology, and distinct properties in the function of the central nervous system. *Annu Rev Pharmacol Toxicol* 1989; 29:365–402.
63. Monaghan DT, Cotman C: Identification and properties of N-methyl-D-aspartate receptors in rat brain plasma membranes. *Proc Natl Acad Sci* 1986; 83:7532–7536.
64. Monahan JB, Handelmann GE, Hood WF, Cordi AA: D-Cycloserine, a positive modulator of the N-methyl-D-aspartate receptor, enhances performance of learning tasks in rats. *Pharmacol Biochem Behav* 1989; 34:649–653.
65. Moroni F, Russi P, Carla V, Lombardi G: Kynurenic acid is present in the rat brain and its content increases during development and aging processes. *Neurosci Lett* 1988; 94:145–150.
66. Morris RGM: Developments of a water maze procedure for studying spatial learning in the rat. *J Neurosci Methods* 1984; 11:47–60.
67. Morris RGM, Anderson E, Lynch GS, Baudry M: Selective impairment of learning and blockade of long-term potentiation by an N-methyl-D-aspartate receptor antagonist. *Nature* 1986; 319:774–776.
68. Morris RGM: Synaptic plasticity and learning: Selective impairment of learning in rats and blockade of long-term potentiation in vivo by the N-methyl-D-aspartate receptor antagonist AP5. *J Neurosci* 1989; 9:3040–3057.
69. Morris RGM, Baker M: in Squires L, Butters N (eds): *The Neuropsychology of Memory*. New York: Guilford, 1983: 521–535.
70. Murphy DE, Schneider J, Boehm C, et al: Binding of $[^3H]$3-(2-carboxypiperazin-4-yl)propyl-1-phosphonic acid to rat brain membranes: A selective, high affinity ligand for N-methyl-D-aspartate receptors. *J Pharmacol Exp Ther* 1987; 240:778–784.
71. Murphy DE, Hutchinson AJ, Hurt SD, et al: Characterization of the binding of $[^3H]$-CGS 19755: A novel N-methyl-D-aspartate antagonist with nanomolar affinity in rat brain. *Br J Pharmacol* 1988; 95:932–938.
72. Nakanish S: Molecular characterization of the family of metabotropic glutamate receptors, in Simon R (ed): *Excitatory Amino Acids*. New York: Time Medical Publishers, 1992: 21–22.
73. Nowak L, Bregestovski P, Ascher P, et al: Magnesium gates glutamate-activated channels in mouse central neurons. *Nature* 1984; 307:462–465.
74. Olney JW: Glutamate induced retinal degeneration in neonatal mice: Electron microscopy of the actively evolving lesion. *Science* 1969; 134:719–721.
75. Olney JW: Inciting excitotoxic cytocide among central neurons. *Adv Exp Biol Med* 1986; 203:631–645.
76. Olney JW, Price M, Salles K, et al: MK-801 powerfully protects against N-methyl aspartate neurotoxicity. *Eur J Pharmacol* 1987; 141:357–361.
77. Olney JW, Labruyere J, Price M: Pathological changes induced in cerebrocortical neurons by phencyclidine and related drugs. *Science* 1989; 244:1360–1362.
78. Olverman HF, Jones AW, Watkins JC: <3H> D-2-

amino-5-phosphonopentanoate as a ligand for N-methyl-D-aspartate receptors in the mammalian central nervous system. *Neuroscience* 1988; 26:1–15.

79. Palmer AM, Marion DW, Botscheller ML, et al: Traumatic brain injury-induced excitotoxicity assessed in a controlled cortical impact model. *J Neurochemistry* 1993; 61:2015–2024.
80. Panter SS, Faden AI: Pretreatment with the NMDA antagonists limits release of excitatory amino acids following traumatic brain injury. *Neurosci Lett* 1992; 136:165–168.
81. Parkin AJ: Amnesic syndrome: A lesion-specific disorder? *Cortex* 1984; 20:479–508.
82. Patel SC, Papachristou DN, Patel YC: Quinolinic acid stimulates somatostatin gene expression in cultured rat cortical neurons. *J Neurochem* 1991; 56:1286–1291.
83. Ransom RW, Stec NL: Cooperative modulation of [^{3}H]MK-801 binding to the N-methyl-D-aspartate receptor-ion channel complex by L-glutamate, glycine and polyamines. *J Neurochem* 1988; 51:830–836.
84. Reynolds IJ, Miller RJ: Multiple sites for the regulation of the N-methyl-D-aspartate receptor. *Mol Pharmacol* 1988; 33:581–584.
85. Robinson TN, Robertson C, Cross AJ, Green AR: Modulation of [^{3}H]-dizocilpine ([^{3}H]-MK-801) binding to rat cortical N-methyl-D-aspartate receptors by polyamines. *Mol Neuropharmacol* 1990; 1:31–35.
86. Rothman S, Olney JW: Glutamate and the pathophysiology of hypoxic ischemic brain damage. *Ann Neurol* 1986; 19:105–111.
87. Schoepp D, Bockaert J, Sladeczek F: Pharmacological and functional characteristics of metabotropic excitatory amino acid receptors. *Trends Pharmacol Sci* 1990; 11:508–515.
88. Shapira Y, Yadid G, Cotev S, et al: Protective effect of MK-801 in experimental brain injury. *J Neurotrauma* 1990; 7:131–139.
89. Sharp F, Jasper P, Hall J, et al: MK-801 and ketamine induce heat shock protein HSP72 in injured neurons in posterior cingulate and retrosplenial cortex. *Ann Neurol* 1991; 30:801–809.
90. Sheardown MJ, Nielsen EO, Hansen AJ, et al: 2-3-Dihydroxy-6-nitro-7-sulfamoyl-benzo(F)quinoxaline: A neuroprotectant for cerebral ischemia. *Science* 1990; 247:571–574.

90A. Shapiro Y, Lam AM, Artro AA, Eng C, Soltow L: Ketamine alters calcium and magnesium in brain tissue following experimental brain injury in rats. J. Cereb. Blood. Flow Metab 1993; 13(6):962–968.

90B. Shohami E, Novikov M, Mechoulam R: A nonpsychotropic cannabinoid, HU211, has cerebroprotective effects after closed head injury in the rat. *J Neurotrauma* 1993; 10(2):109–119.

91. Sladeczek F, Pin JP, Recasens M, et al: Glutamate stimulates inositol phosphate formation in striatal neurones. *Nature* 1985; 317:717–719.
92. Smith DH, Thomas M, Soares H, McIntosh TK: Differential effects of competitive and non-competitive N-methyl-D-aspartate (NMDA) receptor antagonists in experimental brain injury. *FASEB J* 1990; 4(3):773.
93. Smith DH, Okiyama K, Thomas M, et al: Evaluation of memory dysfunction following experimental brain injury using the Morris water maze. *J Neurotrauma* 1991; 8:259–269.
94. Smith DH, Soares H, Perlman K, et al: Characterization of a mouse model of cortical contusion: cognitive and histopathologic effects. *J Neurotrauma* 1995; 12(2):169–178.
95. Hicks RR, Smith DH, McIntosh TK: Temporal response of microtubule associated protein 2 immunoreactivity following experimental brain injury in rats. *Brain Res* 168(1–2):151–160, 1995.
96. Smith DH, Lenkinski RE, Meaney DF, et al: Experimental diffuse axonal injury in minature swine: Metabolic consequences. *J Neurotrauma* 1994; 11(1):128.
97. Smith DH, Lowenstein DH, Hicks RR, et al: Experimental brain injury induces long-term memory dysfunction associated with bilateral hilar neuronal cell loss. *Neurosci Abstr* 1993; 18(1):170.
98. Smith DH, Okiyama K, Gennarelli TA, McIntosh TK: Magnesium and ketamine attenuate cognitive dysfunction following experimental brain injury. *Neurosci Lett* 1993; 157:211–214.
99. Smith DH, Okiyama K, Simon R, McIntosh TK: Pre- and post-synaptic inhibition of glutamate attenuates cerebral edema following experimental brain injury. *Neurosci Abstr* 1993; 19:1877.
100. Smith DH, Okiyama K, Thomas M, McIntosh TK: Effects of the excitatory amino acid receptor antagonists kynurenate and indole-2-carboxylic acid on behavioral and neurochemical outcome following experimental brain injury. *J Neurosci* 1993; 13:5383–5392.
101. Soares H, Thomas M, Cloherty K, McIntosh TK: Development of prolonged cerebral edema following experimental brain injury in the rat. *J Neurochem* 1992; 58:1845–1852.
102. Sugiyama H, Ito I, Hirono C: A new type of glutamate receptor linked to inositol phospholipid metabolism. *Nature* 1987; 325:531–533.

102A. Sun F-Y, Faden AI: Neuroprotein effects of 619C89, a use-dependent sodium channel blocker, in rat traumatic brain injury. *Brain Res* 1995; 673:133–140.

103. Sutherland RJ, Sutton RL, Feeney DM: Traumatic brain injury in the rat produces anterograde but not retrograde amnesia and impairment of hippocampal LTP. *J Neurotrauma* 1993; 10:65–68.
104. Taft WC, Yang K, Dixon EC, Hayes RL: Microtubule-associated protein 2 levels decrease in hippocampus following traumatic brain injury. *J Neurotrauma* 1992; 9:281–290.
105. Taft WC, Varahrami P, Bao J, et al: Diminished MAP2 immunoreactivity following cortical impact brain injury. *Soc Neurosci Abstr* 1993; 19:1880.
106. Thomas M, Breault D, Nolan B, et al: The effects of experimental brain injury on regional cation concentrations. *Neurosci Abstr* 1990; 16:777.
107. Thomas MJ, Breault D, Nolan B, et al: Regional brain concentration of sodium and potassium after experimental brain injury. *Neurosci Abstr* 1991; 17:168.
108. Toulmond S, Duval D, Serrano A, et al: Biochemical

and histological alterations induced by fluid percussion brain injury in the rat. *Brain Res* 1993; 620:24–31.

109. Toulmond S, Serrano A, Benavides J, Scatton B: Prevention by eliprodil (SL 82.0715) of traumatic brain damage in the rat. Existence of a large (18 h) therapeutic window. *Brain Res* 1993; 620:32–41.

110. Vink R, McIntosh TK, Demediuk P, et al: Decline in intracellular free Mg^{2+} is associated with irreversible tissue injury following brain trauma. *J Biol Chem* 1988; 263:757–761.

110A. Voddi M, Perri B, Smith DH, Leach M, McIntosh TK: The use-dependent sodium channel antagonist 619C89 attenuates memory dysfunction following experimental brain injury. *J. Neurotrauma* 1995; 12(1):146.

111. Watkins JC, Evans RH: Excitatory amino acid transmitters. *Annu Rev Pharmacol Toxicol* 1981; 21:165–204.

112. Wong EHF, Knight AR, Woodruff GN: <3H> MK-801 labels a site on the N-methyl-D-aspartate receptor channel complex in rat brain membranes. *J Neurochem* 1988; 50:274–281.

113. Yeh, G-C, Bonhaus DW, McNamara JO: Evidence that zinc inhibits N-methyl-D-aspartate receptor-gated ion channel activation by noncompetitive antagonism of glycine binding. *Mol Pharmacol* 1990; 38:14–19.

114. Young AB, Fagg G: Excitatory amino acid receptors in the brain: Membrane binding and receptor autoradiographic approaches. *Trends Pharmacol Sci* 1990; 2:126–133.

115. Young W: The post-injury response in trauma and ischemia. Secondary injury or protective mechanisms? *CNS Trauma* 1987; 4:27–51.

CHAPTER 108

METABOLIC DYSFUNCTION

David A. Hovda

Cerebral metabolism has been measured and analyzed in many pathophysiological states of CNS injury. In studies of cerebral ischemia,[1–15] cerebral metabolism has been used to demonstrate the effects of a severe reduction in cerebral blood flow, dramatically revealing the consequences of energy failure. In addition to ischemia studies, metabolic experiments conducted after cortical ablations[16–21] or freeze lesion[22–26] have revealed a marked reduction in metabolism in regions of the brain remote from the site of injury. Finally, in traumatic brain injury, metabolic studies have been conducted in order to demonstrate the pathophysiological sequelae of metabolic changes not necessarily linked to cell death.

The study of cerebral metabolism has classically been used to determine the degree and extent of fuel consumption and/or delivery. Under this broad heading, studies related to oxygen or glucose consumption, rate of lactate or CO_2 production, and changes in pH or alteration in cerebral blood flow all can be characterized as measurements of cerebral metabolism in the normal central nervous system (CNS). However, although these measures may be intricately related to one another, there is now a growing body of evidence that, in both the normal intact and the damaged CNS, the results of one measurement do not necessarily imply a corresponding result in another. For example, in the normal brain, cells appear to have a preference for glucose over oxidative metabolism when membranes are exposed to ionic fluxes.[27] As first described in the heart,[28] this energy compartmentalization has been demonstrated to occur within the CNS. This "preference" appears to be due to the fact that oxidative phosphorylation continuously runs at near peak capacity. Consequently, any dynamic increase in the demand for energy is satisfied through the production of ATP via glycolysis. Such dynamic demands for energy occur at any time there is an ionic imbalance across the cell membrane.

Although this principle has been put forth by several investigators,[27,29,30] it has probably been most convincingly shown by the work of Ackermann and Lear (1989).[27] In developing a double-label autoradiographic technique for measuring the rate of glycolysis and oxidative phosphorylation, Ackermann and Lear[27] were able to determine which metabolic substrate would be used to support a dynamic change in ionic disturbance. Although different converging experiments were conducted, the most striking experiment occurred when animals were exposed to a flashing light stimulus. The superior colliculus exhibited a marked increase in glucose utilization, but no increase in oxidative metabolism. This principle of selective activation of glycolysis in the presence of ionic perturbation has been confirmed by others,[31] and appears to be well accepted within the neuroscience literature for the intact brain in a normal "steady state."

In the injured CNS,[32,33] the close physiological relationships associated with a "steady state" (e.g., between cerebral blood flow and metabolism) can become markedly altered for various periods of time. Consequently, measurements of one metabolic substrate or by-product cannot be used to infer information about another. In addition to the uncoupling phenomenon, anatomic changes, including the loss of cells or innervation, further complicate the interpretation of metabolic measurements. With such a complex array of factors influencing the way cerebral metabolism is measured and interpreted, even in the normal brain, an important question arises as to the validity of metabolic measurements made in the injured brain where the physiological "steady state" may be dramatically altered. Consequently, the interpretation of metabolic changes following CNS injury must be conducted with close scrutiny to neurochemistry, cerebral perfusion, and injury-induced anatomic changes.

Given these restrictions and possible complications, the study of cerebral metabolism following traumatic injury to the CNS provides at least three general investigative attributes that can and should be exploited. First, measurements of metabolism, when combined with other techniques, can provide important information regarding cellular pathophysiology. Second, measurements of metabolism offer the opportunity to delineate regions of the brain affected by different types of trauma. In most experimental studies of CNS injury, morphological analysis of cell death is used to determine the extent of damage. Although this morphological analysis is a critical dependent variable needing to be addressed in all studies of experimental traumatic brain injury, it is well known that morphological damage may be insufficient to predict functional impairment. Finally, although more work is needed in order to understand how specific mechanistic relationships are altered following brain injury, cerebral metabolism does reflect cellular function. Consequently, metabolic measurements may be used in predicting neurological outcome.

A review of all the metabolic work in different CNS injury models would exceed the scope of this chapter. Therefore, emphasis will be placed on traumatic brain injuries that incorporate a biomechanical component. This does not imply that other injury models are invalid or inherently uninteresting. However, those models typically address a different set of issues with regard to injury than what will be discussed in the following pages.

TRAUMA-INDUCED IONIC FLUX—A TRIGGER FOR METABOLIC DYSFUNCTION

The ionic fluxes similar to those seen following traumatic brain injury have been proposed to result in the selective activation of glycolysis.[29,30,34,35] It is thought that this activation of glycolysis represents a dynamic increase in energy demand used to drive membrane pumps in order to re-establish cellular ionic homeostasis. Consequently, in order to understand the degree and extent of this acute metabolic change following brain injury, a clear understanding of the ionic flux must be achieved.

The assessment of ionic perturbation has been conducted after many different types of injury to the brain, with the greatest number of experiments conducted in models of ischemia-hypoxia. Measurement of ionic fluxes related to cerebral metabolism following traumatic brain injury are not as numerous, however; potassium,[34,36–38] calcium,[39–41] and magnesium[41–44] have been studied using multiple techniques, including total tissue dissection,[38] NMR spectroscopy,[42,44,45] ion-specific microelectrodes,[37] and cerebral microdialysis.[34] The results from these studies indicate that each ion has its own post-traumatic profile in both extent and duration of change.

Potassium

Several earlier studies have indicated that a massive increase in extracellular potassium concentration $[K^+]_e$ occurs in response to experimental traumatic brain or spinal cord injury.[36,46,47] Nonspecific breakdown of the plasma membrane may explain an increase in $[K^+]_e$, particularly in regions of the brain subjected to localized contusions[36,47] or intracerebral hemorrhages.[46] However, an increase in $[K^+]_e$ has also been reported following concussive brain injury[34,36] which, although it transmits a mechanical stress to wide areas of the brain, does not result in overt morphological damage. This increase in $[K^+]_e$, following concussive brain injury, could be explained in terms of a K^+ flux through voltage-gated K^+ channels associated with neuronal discharges, since deformation of neural tissue alone can produce sufficient depolarization resulting in neuronal firing.[48] Furthermore, several lines of evidence suggest that intense neuronal discharges occur at the initial moment following concussive brain injury,[49,50] and recently it has been shown that at least some of the K^+ flux associated with mild (but not severe) concussion can be blocked with tetrodotoxin administered via microdialysis.[34]

Another possible explanation for the increase in $[K^+]_e$ is due to an opening of ligand-gated ion channels as a result of an indiscriminate release of neurotransmitters. Among the various neurotransmitters, the excitatory amino acids (EEAs), especially glutamate, appear to be the most likely candidates to produce such a large ionic flux.[51–53] EAAs activate kainate and AMPA receptors opening channels permeable to both sodium and potassium as well as N-methyl-D-aspartate (NMDA) receptors permeable to calcium as well as sodium and K^+.[51–53] In a recent work,[34] the level of the EAA glutamate was seen to increase in conjunction with the increase in K^+ following fluid percussion brain injury. Furthermore, by administering (in situ) the EAA blocker kynurenic acid, the injury-induced increase in $[K^+]_e$ is greatly reduced.[34]

Regulation of Extracellular Potassium

The brain normally possesses a powerful mechanism for the uptake of elevated $[K^+]_e$[54–56] including the uptake of $[K^+]_e$ by glial cells.[57–59] These mechanisms are effective enough to rapidly balance any $[K^+]_e$ increase resulting from neuronal discharges and to maintain $[K^+]_e$ below a limit ranging from 6 to 10 mM.[54,60–62] This limit cannot be surpassed, even with seizure activity.[61,62] The small increase in $[K^+]_e$, expressed as the difference between pre- and postconcussion concentrations ($[K^+]_d$) and seen following a very minor concussion,[34] is likely to have stayed below the physiological ceiling of $[K^+]_e$, since this increase appears to reflect intense neuronal discharges.

In contrast, a larger increase in $[K^+]_d$, seen following more severe concussive injury,[34] appears to penetrate the physiological ceiling level. It has been shown that the recovery rate of a dialysis system for K^+ (in vivo) decreases during ischemia, presumably due to shrinkage of the extracellular space,[63] which may result in a decrease of effective surface area of the dialysis system. In addition, shrinkage of the extracellular space has been demonstrated following concussive brain injury.[64] Therefore, it is likely that a relationship between observed changes in $[K^+]_d$ and actual level of $[K^+]_e$ following the injury is not linear. Comparison with the increase in $[K^+]_d$, induced by ischemia, suggests that the actual level of $[K^+]_e$ following severe concussive injury may have increased to approximately 70 percent of the maximum level attained by ischemia. Since $[K^+]_e$ reaches 80 mM during ischemia,[65–67] it appears reasonable to conclude that $[K^+]_e$ can increase far beyond that physiological ceiling level following concussive brain injury. This conclusion is in agreement with the results of earlier studies using ion-sensitive electrodes (in vivo).[36,68,69]

Potassium in Other Pathological States

Potassium changes have also been shown in a variety of pathological conditions in which $[K^+]_e$ is elevated due either to excessive release[61,70–74] or to impaired uptake.[65–67,74] In ischemia or anoxia, an initial slow increase in $[K^+]_e$, presumably due to impaired uptake to a level ranging from 6 to 10 mM, is followed by a steep increase to a level ranging from 50 to 60 mM.[65–67,74] Also, an abrupt $[K^+]_e$ increase has also been shown with electrical stimulation resulting in an excessive release of $[K^+]_e$ due to neuronal dischargers. When the $[K^+]_e$ in the cortex exceeds this level during electrical stimulation or K^+ application, further massive $[K^+]_e$ increase (termed "spreading depression") is abruptly elicited.[70–75]

There are, in fact, a number of similarities between the large $[K^+]_e$ observed following severe concussive brain injury[34] and spreading depression.[70,74] For example, spreading depression propagates, even in the presence of TTX,[72,76] much faster than simple diffusion of K^+ and is dependent on the presence of Ca^{2+}.[70,73] Although the $[K^+]_e$ increase following concussive brain injury occurs simultaneously in wide areas of the brain,[36,64,69,77] in contrast to a true "spreading" depression, the underlying mechanism(s) may be similar. From the work of Katayama et al. (1990),[34] it appears, in concussive brain injury, that $[K^+]_e$ initially increases due to sudden intense neuronal discharges. Then, when the level of $[K^+]_e$ surpasses the physiological ceiling, neurotransmitters are rapidly released, resulting in much greater K^+ fluxes. If this is the case, the large $[K^+]_e$ increase following concussive brain injury resistant to (in situ) administration of tetrodotoxin[34] can be explained as a result of the propagation of these processes from the release of neurotransmitters from adjacent brain areas employing mechanisms similar to the propagation of spreading depression.

Calcium

In addition to the increase of $[K^+]_e$, calcium (Ca^{2+}) accumulation has been studied following brain injury as induced by both cerebral ischemia[78–83] and spinal cord contusion.[84–87] Following a contusion to the spinal cord, measurements of extracellular ionic and total Ca^{2+} changes indicate a shift from the blood and extracellular space into injured cells,[84–87] with extracellular Ca^{2+} decreasing primarily at the site of trauma and remaining low for several hours.[85,86] Furthermore, the affected cells appear to have the capacity of managing an enormous increase of intracellular Ca^{2+} through proposed buffering mechanisms.[86] When these cells are actually damaged, these mechanisms would be directly exposed to the extracellular space, forming a "calcium sink" attracting Ca^{2+} away from nearby tissue.[85,86,88] Measurements of total Ca^{2+} (both extra- and intracellular) revealed a dramatic increase, following injury, far above presurgical levels.

Few studies have addressed Ca^{2+} accumulation following cerebral traumatic brain injury. This neglect is surprising given the important role Ca^{2+} plays in secondary cell death,[89,90] which would subsequently alter cerebral metabolism. One report[39] has shown some evidence of increased Ca^{2+} in a few cells of the dorsal hippocampus following cerebral contusion. However, there was no attempt to quantify this effect nor to delineate its extent or duration. The importance of measuring Ca^{2+} following traumatic brain injury is underscored by work showing a close relationship between Ca^{2+} and the increase in $[K^+]_e$.[34] By utilizing the microdialysis technique, the administration of cobalt (a Ca^{2+} channel blocker) significantly reduces the amount of $[K^+]_e$ typically seen following severe traumatic brain injury.[34] Given the important role Ca^{2+} plays on secondary cell death,[89,90] this ion deserves more attention in studies of experimental brain injury.

In more recent work,[40] the extent and duration of Ca^{2+} flux following a lateral fluid percussion brain injury in the rat was assessed using ^{45}Ca autoradiography. Animals were studied in the following time periods after the insult: immediately, 6; 24; and 96 hours. In addition, cell suspension studies were conducted to determine the extent of cellular flux of ^{45}Ca. The results from this work indicated that in animals who exhibited no gross morphological damage, ^{45}Ca accumulation following injury was exhibited primarily within the ipsilateral cerebral cortex, dorsal hippocampus, and striatum. This accumulation continued for several days, returning to control levels by the fourth day after injury, and could be substantially reduced with administration of an N-type Ca^{2+} channel blocker.[91,92] In animals that sustained morphological damage, the contusion site exhibited a marked accumulation of ^{45}Ca which did not resolve spontaneously over the course of four days.

Magnesium

A review of the important role magnesium plays in CNS physiology is beyond the scope of this chapter. Furthermore, an excellent review on magnesium and how it relates to traumatic brain injury already exists.[93] However, given that magnesium is important for both glycolysis and oxidative phosphorylation,[94–96] magnesium must be at least briefly discussed when addressing the concept of an injury-induced metabolic dysfunction.

Utilizing magnetic resonance spectroscopy, several studies reported a marked decrease in intracellular magnesium following experimental traumatic brain injury.[44,97–101] When total tissue analysis was conducted, the injury-induced decrease in magnesium was present for as long as 24 hours following injury. Given the abovementioned importance of magnesium in metabolic processes, its reduction following traumatic brain injury could have implications for cerebral metabolic recovery. However, direct measurements of magnesium flux and its relationship to post-traumatic cerebral metabolism have yet to be conducted.

ACUTE METABOLIC CHANGES FOLLOWING TRAUMATIC BRAIN INJURY

Response of Glucose Metabolism

Several studies[10–12] addressing the cerebral metabolic rate of glucose (lCMRglc: μM/100g/min) have been conducted during the acute period following cerebral ischemia. These studies describe an intermediate zone of increase in lCMRglc between normal and infarcted regions of the brain. However, few reports exist using this same [^{14}C]2-deoxy-D-glucose (2DG) autoradiographic technique during the acute period following experimental traumatic brain injury.

Shah and West (1983),[102] in what appears to be the first study using the 2DG methodology very early after experimental traumatic brain injury, reported that at 10 minutes after a concussive insult the relative uptake of [^{3}H] deoxy-D-glucose was significantly higher (111 percent of control). The rest of the brain regions studied, including the hypothalamus, hippocampus, and striatum, exhibited no significant change. Interestingly, when animals were studied 20 minutes after injury, there was no evidence of change in 2DG uptake in any of the regions measured. These authors speculated that, although they were unable to calculate rates of glucose utilization, the changes in uptake may be related to a trauma-induced spreading depression.

In another autoradiographic study,[103] lCMRglc was measured in rats 1, 2, 4, and 24 hours after a fluid percussion injury severe enough to result in cortical contusions. In addition, electrophysiological studies were conducted evaluating the presence of a DC potential along with EEG monitoring. The results from this work indicated that in all animals, across all time points, the core of the contusion exhibited a marked reduction in lCMRglc. When animals were studied 2 hours after injury ($N = 6$), evaluation of lCMRglc within the cerebral cortex indicated that most animals ($N = 4$) exhibited normal or a slight increase in glucose metabolism with two animals showing a marked increase. These authors concluded that the pattern of changes in lCMRglc resembled that of cortical spreading depression since a negative DC potential, concomitant with EEG suppression in the injured cerebral cortex, was observed frequently during the first 2 hours.

A similar 2DG study was conducted 1 hour following a fluid percussion injury in the cat.[104,105] However, unlike the above studies conducted in the rodent, the only evidence of an injury-induced increase in lCMRglc was restricted to the dorsomedial pontine tegmentum. The remaining cortical and subcortical regions revealed a marked depression in metabolism. In this particular study, the increase of metabolism seen within the brain stem was thought to be related to unconsciousness and not due to an ionic disturbance.

In more recent work, quantitative glucose utilization has been studied systematically following experimental traumatic brain injury in rats. Both lateral[106–108] and midline[109] fluid percussion models of traumatic brain injury have been studied with 2DG experiments being conducted at preselected intervals after the insult. Immediately following a lateral insult, the entire cerebral cortex, primarily ipsilateral to the side of the injury cap, exhibited an 81 percent increase in lCMRglc compared to controls, with rates reaching above 120μmol/100g/min[108] (Fig. 108-1). If a midline-oriented fluid percussion was conducted, the acute increase in glucose metabolism was seen bilaterally[109] (Fig. 108-2). The injury-induced

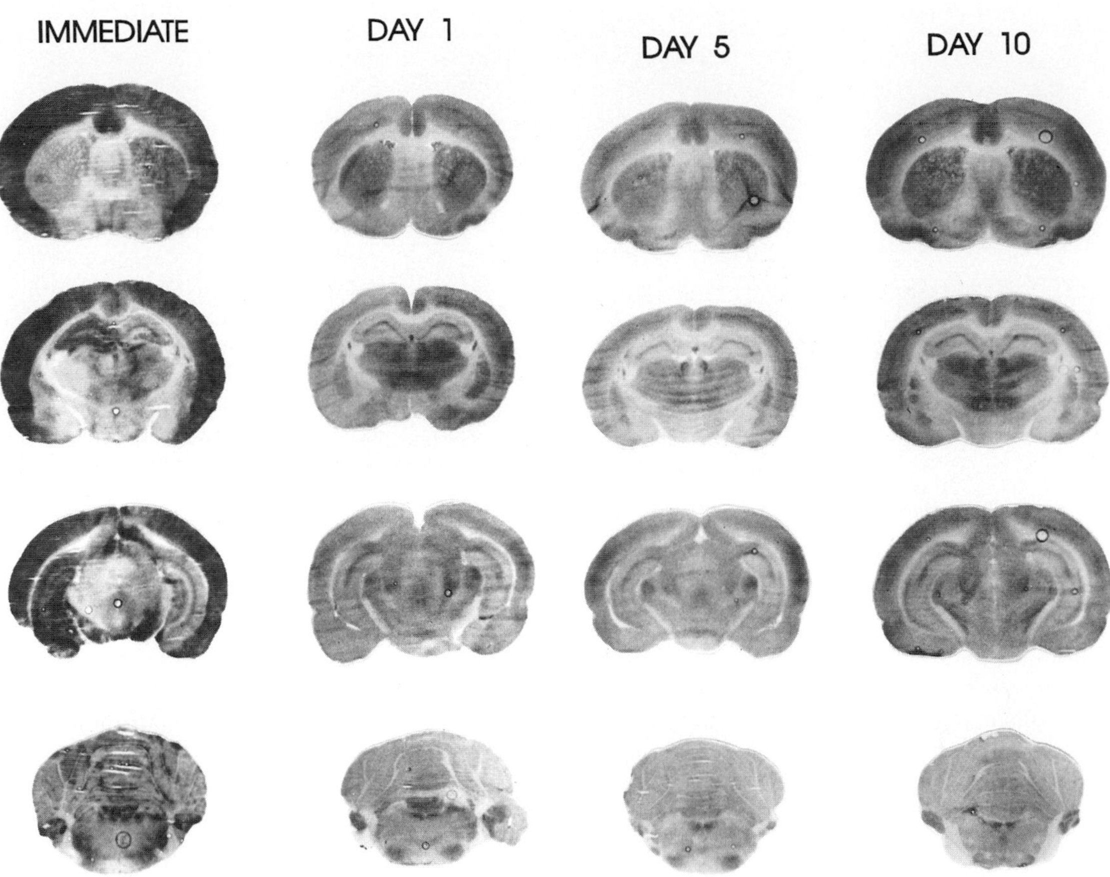

Figure 108-1. Coronal 2DG autoradiographs through the caudate/putamen, dorsal hippocampus, brain stem and cerebellum processed immediately, 1, 5, and 10 days following a lateral fluid percussion brain injury. Note the increase in glycolysis evident immediately following injury, primarily in the side (*left*) ipsilateral to the introduction of the fluid percussion. This increase in metabolism gave way to a metabolic depression by 6 hours and was maintained for as long as 5 days. (From Yoshino et al.[109] with permission.)

increase in ICMRglc was also pronounced within the hippocampus[106] and was still present when animals were studied 30 minutes after the insult.

As discussed previously, this injury-induced increase in glucose metabolism is thought to be the result of cellular ionic fluxes that dramatically change the extracellular milieu. Given that the time frame of the increase in glycolysis is most closely matched to the time frame of the massive release of K^+ following fluid percussion injury,[34] this ion appears to be a likely candidate.

It is now well accepted that a major factor contributing to the release of K^+ is the stimulation of EAA receptors by the injury-induced release of glutamate.[34] One of the more convincing experiments leading to this conclusion involved the preinjury (in situ) administration (via microdialysis) of the broad spectrum EAA antagonist, kynurenic acid. The dialysis of this compound markedly attenuated the increase in K^+ flux typically seen following fluid percussion.[34] In order to determine if the injury-induced release of K^+ plays a significant role in the metabolic changes seen after injury, a similar experimental design was employed. However, instead of measuring K^+, glucose utilization was assessed in the cerebral cortex in which EAA antagonists were administered prior to a fluid percussion insult.[109] The EAA antagonists consisted of kynurenic acid, 2-amino-5-phosphonovaleric acid (APV), a selective N-methyl-D-aspartate (NMDA) receptor antagonist, and 6-cyano-7-nitrogen oxaline-2,3-dine (CNQX), a non-NMDA receptor antagonist. In another related study utilizing the same design,[110] cobalt, a calcium channel blocker, was also infused through the microdialysis probe. The results from these studies indicated that the EAA antagonists were effective (in a dose response fashion) in reducing the demand for glucose metabolism following experimental traumatic brain injury. The calcium channel blocker, cobalt, had very little effect (Fig. 108-2). This fact, coupled with the different results be-

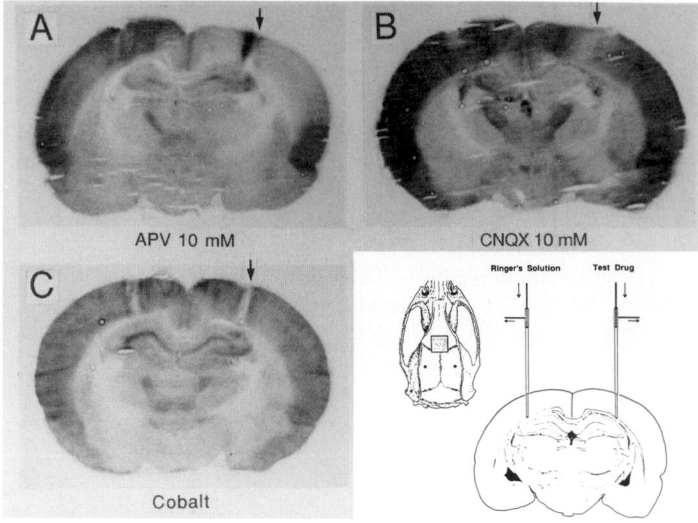

Figure 108-2. The effect of excitatory amino acid antagonists (*A*) 2-amino-5-phosphonovaleric acid (APV), a selective N-methyl-D-aspartate (NMDA) receptor antagonist and (*B*) 6-cyano-7-nitrogen oxaline-2,3-dine (CNQX), a non-NMDA receptor antagonist along with (*C*) cobalt, a calcium channel blocker on their ability to reduce the hyperglycolysis typically seen following a central fluid percussion injury. The diagram depicts the positioning of the injury cap (*shaded area*) and the positioning of the two microdialysis probes through which these compounds where infused prior to insult. Note the effect of the NMDA antagonist APV (see *A*) on the increase in glycolysis.

tween APV and CNQX, leads to the conclusion that, although all subtypes of the glutamate receptor appear to be involved in the injury-induced increase in glucose metabolism, the NMDA receptor may play a major role.

The acute increase in glucose metabolism following traumatic brain injury has also been well documented in an experimental model of subdural hematoma.[111] Two hours after inducing the hematoma, a severe reduction in glucose metabolism (using 2DG) was seen within the cortex beneath the hematoma (ICMRglc <5). This region was verified histologically as a zone of infarction. A band of markedly increased ICMRglc was seen in the peri-ischemic zone surrounding the infarcted tissue and throughout the hippocampus bilaterally. The increase in ICMRglc within both the cortex and hippocampus was markedly reduced in rats pretreated with the NMDA antagonist (E)-4-(3-phosphonoprop-2 enyl) piperazine-2-carboxylic acid (CPP). This study complements the previously mentioned work and again points to the important role the ligand-gated receptor NMDA may play in the metabolic dysfunction seen following traumatic brain injury.

The hypothesis that the increase in glucose utilization seen immediately following experimental traumatic brain injury is due to the increase of the extracellular concentration of K^+ appears quite supportable. However, many other mechanisms activated by traumatic brain injury could result in an increase in the concentration of the ^{14}C isotope in a particular region of the brain, thereby providing misleading information in 2DG experiments.

THE USE OF 2DG AUTORADIOGRAPHY SOON FOLLOWING BRAIN INJURY

With the use of the 2DG method[112] soon following an insult to the brain, some of the basic "steady state" assumptions, including the lump constant, may be violated. In studies of cerebral ischemia where cerebral blood flow is purposefully restricted, adjustments have been proposed in calculations of ICMRglc due to alterations in the lump constant and the K values.[113,114] Others have limited their description to the ICMRglc results in terms of ratios.[12] However, in a model of concussion using the fluid percussion device, a number of observations indicate that many of the methodological requirements for the 2DG method are met. First, there is no histopathology (e.g., hemorrhage or contusion), and, although some authors have reported a breakdown of the blood-brain barrier,[115] ICMRglc calculation, even within the region of blood-brain barrier breakdown, indicated that the mechanisms of glucose transport were not grossly disturbed.[116] Second, the levels of brain glucose are not significantly altered following low levels of fluid percussion brain injury,[117] indicating that the lump constant is not changed. Finally, plasma glucose levels following this type of concussion stay within the acceptable limits for the 2DG method.[116]

There are, however, some concerns regarding cerebral blood flow (CBF) following this type of injury. Some authors have reported, even with severe fluid percussion injury, CBF stays within normal limits 60 minutes after the insult.[118] In addition, when compared to preinjury baseline, radioactive microsphere measurements indicate a decrease in CBF, primarily within the cerebral hemispheres, beginning 30 min following trauma.[119] However, when compared to sham controls, rates for CBF (ml/100g/min) in all regions measured were significantly depressed by up to 50 percent (rates = 65–82).[119] Others have also reported an immediate and marked reduction of CBF in all brain regions following a concussive brain injury.[120] This depression lasted anywhere from 30 minutes to 1 hour. By 2 hours following trauma, the rates for CBF returned to normal

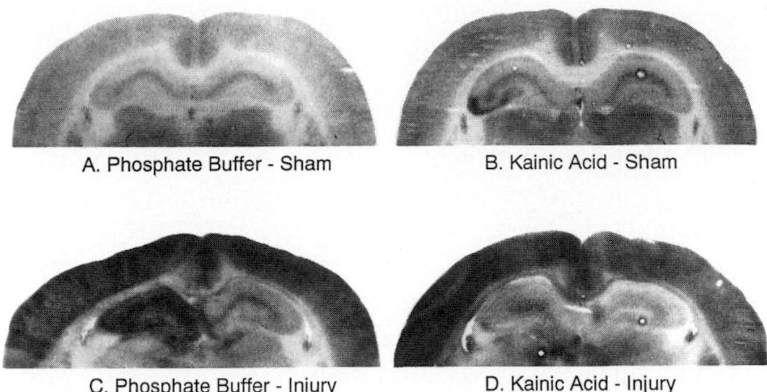

Figure 108-3. Coronal 2DG autoradiographs through the dorsal hippocampus processed immediately following a lateral (*left*) fluid percussion or sham injury from animals that were previously injected intraventricularly with either vehicle or kainic acid. Note that, in the animal receiving the vehicle injection, the fluid percussion injury produced an increase of glucose metabolism within both the cerebral cortex and the ipsilateral hippocampus. In contrast, the animal receiving the kainic acid injection exhibited an increase in glucose metabolism immediately following fluid percussion only within the cerebral cortex with the ipsilateral hippocampus, particularly the CA1 region, being spared from the injury-induced hyperglycolysis. (From Yoshino, et al.[106] with permission.)

values. Finally, following an impact acceleration injury, CBF was shown to be immediately increased (50 percent) above normal values and then quickly decreased to approximately 40 percent of control rates.[121] However, within 40 minutes CBF returned to normal values.

Most of these issues have been addressed in a recent study[106] designed to determine if endogenous glutamate innervation from CA_3 to the CA1 region of the hippocampus can provide an anatomic basis to support the glutamate-ionic-metabolic hypothesis while controlling for the above-mentioned possible confounding variables. In this study, the CA1 glutamatergic innervation from CA3 was removed by intraventricular injection of kainic acid (5 percent) 5 days prior to induction of a lateral fluid percussion brain injury. In these CA_3-lesioned rats, the 2DG experiment, conducted immediately following brain injury, revealed the characteristic increase in ICMRglc within the cerebral cortex but no evidence of any increase in glucose utilization within CA1 compared to controls (Fig. 108-3). These results support the conclusion that the injury-induced increase in glucose metabolism is due to an endogenous process involving the EAA glutamate, and further supports the validity of the ICMRglc measurements during the acute period following fluid percussion brain injury.

Given the above results and the confirmation of an injury-induced hyper-glycolysis utilizing arterial-venous difference measurements,[30] the 2DG method is most likely a valid and reliable technique for measuring glucose uptake following a concussive brain injury. However, care must be taken regarding the interpretation of ICMRglc during the first few minutes following insult if CBF is reduced to levels that could violate the assumptions required for quantification.

Response of Oxidative Metabolism

In baboons, arterial-venous differences for oxygen following mild (40 lb/sq in; duration = 50 ms) concussion delivered via an air gun indicated that the cerebral metabolic rate for oxygen ($CMRO_2$) was increased by 7 percent during the first minute following injury. However, following severe concussion (duration = 150 ms) $CMRO_2$ was reduced significantly during the first 5 minutes following trauma.[122] In measurements of energy metabolism following an impact acceleration injury, adenosine diphosphate (ADP) was increased at 1 and 4 minutes following trauma in the pons and medulla,[123] with oxygen utilization being increased during the first few minutes following trauma.[121] Therefore, apparently, in the traumatic injury model oxidative metabolism may be disrupted for only the first few minutes following injury. This has been thought to be due to an injury-induced disruption of mitochondrial functions. However, in a study[124] measuring the capacity of oxidative phosphorylation in mitochondria following a fluid percussion brain injury, there was no significant alteration in the ADP per oxygen consumption ratio or in state 3 respiratory rate (ADP stimulated). These results indicate that, unlike ischemia, traumatic brain injury does not cause uncoupling of ATP synthesis from respiration, and brain mitochondria are quite resistant to trauma-induced injury. This is supported by results indicating that during the first 10 minutes following a fluid percussion in cats there is a transient increase in the level of oxidized cytochrome a, a_3 as measured by the dual-wavelength reflection spectrophotometry technique via a cranial window.[125]

Lactate Accumulation

The perturbation of ionic gradients across the neuronal cell membrane, like those described above following brain injury, activate energy-dependent ion pumps,[126–130] resulting in an increase in glucose metabolism and substrate supply. Similar results have been reported during the acute period following traumatic brain injury.[68,122,123,131,132] This sudden increase in energy metabolism has been shown to produce a decline in high-energy phosphates which may stimulate anaerobic glycolysis.[30,117,133] One natural consequence of such changes would be the accumulation of lactate and the development of intracellular acidosis.[117,133] Previous observations indicate that lactate definitely increases in cerebral spinal fluid as well as in brain tissue during the initial 60 minutes following diffuse fluid percussion brain injury.[117,134] Severe fluid percussion injury causes progressive, longer-lasting lactate accumulation, presumably because of cell disruption.[134]

Evidence for an ionic flux-induced lactate accumulation is present in studies of spreading depression in which the passage of a single wave is accompanied by an increase of extracellular K^+, a decrease in the level of glucose concentration and tissue pH, and an increase in lactate.[135–140] The metabolic and, consequently, lactate changes persist much longer than the period of transient depolarization,[135,137] and recovery to normal levels is not observed until 10 minutes following repolarization.[137] In other studies, the local application of kainate (5 nmol), an excitatory neurotoxin, can produce an immediate transient increase in lactate concentration in the extracellular space as measured by microdialysis. Again, the changes in lactate concentration are quite enduring, lasting for more than 30 minutes.[141] In a study utilizing electroconvulsive shock (50 Hz for 1 s) as a global neuronal stimulus causing generalized seizures for 30 to 45 s, an immediate increase in extracellular lactate, as demonstrated by microdialysis, with this increase being sustained for more than 20 minutes.[141] As predicted, given the relationship between glucose metabolism and lactate production, the electroconvulsive shock-induced increase in lactate was attenuated when glycolysis was inhibited by 2-deoxyglucose-6-phosphate.[141]

In models of general brain injury, an increase in extracellular K^+ has been reported following fluid percussion injury for 3 to 5 minutes across wide brain regions.[36,63,69,77] Since the metabolic derangements characteristic of a fluid percussion are due to the ionic flux through EAA activated channels, there may be a causal relationship between EAA release and the massive ionic fluxes, and between the massive ionic fluxes and subsequent lactate accumulation. Changes in levels of lactate in the extracellular space are readily evaluated with microdialysis,[141,142] and the increase in extracellular lactate measured by microdialysis quickly responds to local inhibition of glycolysis with 2-deoxyglucose-6-phosphate. These results indicate that changes in lactate detected by this method reflect metabolism occurring in tissue directly adjacent to the probe.[141]

Recently, two important papers have been published that address the changes in extracellular lactate following experimental traumatic brain injury. Using a weight drop model, Nilsson et al. (1993)[142] demonstrated that in the rat there was a four- to fivefold increase in the dialysate concentration, which did not return to normal levels until 80 minutes after the insult. When the severity of the injury was increased, a more pronounced elevation of lactate was exhibited (approximately sevenfold) which did not return to normal levels until after 2 hours. This increase in extracellular lactate concentration was thought to be due to a combination of an increase in energy demand due to the injury-induced neurochemical changes in conjunction with a decrease in cerebral blood flow.

Evidence now indicates that at least some of the increase in extracellular lactate seen after traumatic brain injury is due to the massive ionic flux of K^+.[143] As reported by Kawamata et al. (1994),[143] when cerebral microdialysis was conducted following a fluid percussion brain injury, the increase in lactate concentration was attenuated if the EAA antagonist kynurenic acid was administered (in situ) prior to the insult. As reported previously,[34] this same antagonist markedly reduced the amount of K^+ flux following injury. The relationship was further demonstrated when the non-energy-dependent K^+ uptake mechanism of glial cells was restricted prior to injury via the administration of barium.[143] In these experiments the increase in extracellular lactate following injury was markedly increased and the duration of the increase was prolonged.[143] Consequently, it now appears that the EAA-induced ionic flux is very closely related to both the increase in glycolysis and the increase in extracellular lactate seen following cerebral insult.

Earlier in vitro and in vivo studies had indicated deleterious effects of lactate accumulation on brain tissue.[144–150] It has been reported that when lactate accumulates at high concentrations, cell membranes are damaged, cellular function is altered, a breakdown of the blood brain barrier is seen, and widespread brain edema is induced. Recent studies have established detrimental effects of lactate accumulation in ischemic brain injury on postischemic recovery.[146,147,149] Thus, lactate accumulation appears to represent a subcellular dysfunctional state of traumatized neuronal cells and is likely to be related to their vulnerability to secondary ischemic injury.[151–153] Therefore, investigation of the mechanism of the lactate accumulation will be an important step toward defining mechanism of neuronal dysfunction in traumatic brain injury.

CHRONIC CHANGES IN CEREBRAL METABOLISM—A MAP OF REGIONAL DYSFUNCTION FOLLOWING TRAUMA

The previous work illustrates how studies of cerebral metabolism can be used to test specific hypotheses regarding the cellular pathophysiology of traumatic brain injury. However, assessment of cerebral metabolism can provide important information regarding what regions of the brain have been affected by the insult. Clinically, as well as experimentally, it is difficult to be confident of the extent of neuronal dysfunction following trauma. In most cases, emphasis is placed on the degree and extent of morphological damage and/or cell death. Although the assessment of structural damage is an important factor in determining what areas of the brain have been affected by the injury, these measurements alone do not reveal the entire consequence of trauma.

As described above, during the acute period following a lateral fluid percussion, the entire cerebral cortex and underlying hippocampus ipsilateral to the site of injury exhibit a marked increase in glucose metabolism. This pattern of metabolic dysfunction occurs in the face of very little morphological damage and suggests that this injury is diffuse in nature both in terms of cortical and subcortical effects. Consequently, one would predict that neurological functions that depend on these structures would be disrupted.

This pattern of injury-induced metabolic change is much different in models of CNS trauma in which a local cortical contusion is implemented. In recent work[154] addressing the metabolic changes following a cortical impact injury, glucose utilization was also found to be increased within the cerebral cortex. However, unlike fluid percussion, when the piston was introduced laterally the increase was restricted to the cortex surrounding the contusion. However, changes in glucose utilization were similar to fluid percussion injury in that the underlying hippocampus also exhibited a marked increase in glucose uptake. Since this cortical contusion injury model produces more cellular degeneration than that introduced by fluid percussion, an anatomic interpretation would suggest that cortical contusion was the more severe of these two injuries. In contrast, if the severity of the injury were determined using metabolic markers, abnormal patterns of glucose utilization appear to be much more extensive following fluid percussion and therefore would suggest that the diffuse injury was more severe, at least during the acute period.

These types of comparisons regarding injury severity between two different experimental models of traumatic brain injury are, to some degree, artificial. The severity of an injury is more often determined in terms of behavioral outcome than by metabolic alterations. However, it should be stressed that the determination of the functional characteristics of an injury in metabolic terms will not only facilitate the prediction of the resulting neurological deficits, but will also dictate the types of therapeutic treatments to be attempted.

A case in point is when comparisons are made between suction ablation[21,155] and traumatic injury studies. The brain injury literature contains an enormous number of investigations in which portions of the cerebral cortex are surgically aspirated and animals are studied in terms of recovery of function.[155–157] This work has led to very important discoveries about how the brain responds to perturbation, particularly in terms of understanding neuroplasticity.[158] Although the authors of these investigations are quite correct in stating that this work has implications for future treatment of brain-injured patients, the direct link to trauma may be a bit removed, given the lack of biochemical and neurochemical alteration.

In recent work,[159] the acute period of suction ablation was studied both in terms of neurochemistry and metabolism. In general, it was discovered that, unlike in traumatic injury, suction ablation caused very little change in extracellular ionic concentration and relatively little evidence of an increase in glucose metabolism. Consequently, this injury model, presumably due to its lack of biomechanical characteristics, does not provide many of the ionic and metabolic consequences characteristic of trauma. As with the discussion of the differences between fluid percussion and cortical contusions, statements regarding severity of injury between trauma and suction ablation are most likely irrelevant. They simply represent different types of injury as detected using metabolic studies.

Long-Term Effects on Glucose Metabolism

The alteration of glucose metabolism is not restricted to the first hour following concussive brain injury. Beginning 6 hours after a diffuse fluid percussion, many regions of the brain go into a state of hypometabolism lasting up to 10 days[109] (Fig. 108-1). This metabolic depression appears to have the physiological consequences seen in similarly prepared animals, since neurobehavioral deficits are present during this same period after injury.[160] The phenomenon of a diffuse metabolic depression has also been reported following cerebral ischeemia,[12,161] tumor,[162,163] cortical freezing lesions,[22,25,29,164] and sensorimotor cortex ablations.[21,165] Although this metabolic diaschisis appears to be a relatively common phenomenon, the mechanisms behind its presentation are not understood.

One possibility is that the depression reflects a prolonged metabolic disruption due to the ionic perturbations seen after injury. Many of the ionic and metabolic changes occurring over the first few minutes following a fluid percussion brain injury are also seen following ischemia. The difference is that following diffuse fluid percussion injury secondary cell death does not usually occur, whereas following ischemia secondary cell death, primarily within the CA1 layer of the hippocampus, is well documented.[83,166–169] However, the fluid percussion injury may produce a level of ionic flux and metabolic derangement, which, although sublethal, may disrupt cellular processes for several days, rendering the cells vulnerable.

An example of this state of an injury-induced vulnerability has been reported. If a fluid percussion brain injury is followed in 1 hour by a sublethal level of ischemia (middle cerebral artery occlusion for 5 minutes), cells normally surviving either insult independently, now die.[170] Furthermore, the time of onset of the increase in extracellular K^+ seen following complete cerebral ischemia is shortened if the brain sustains a previous fluid percussion injury.[171] Therefore, from the above-mentioned studies, cells subjected to a fluid percussion become vulnerable and presumably require time (duration as yet unknown) to recover their stability.

Several studies have reported long-term cellular disruptions following concussive injury that could contribute to the resulting metabolic depression. Protein synthesis, as studied autoradiographically,[172,173] is reduced in many regions of the brain following diffuse fluid percussion lasting from minutes to hours. Additionally, as previously described, Ca^{2+} accumulates in many regions of the brain after concussion for at least two days, thereby extending the period of post-traumatic ionic disturbance.[40] Finally, oxidative metabolism appears to be unaffected during the first few minutes following fluid percussion injury. However, beginning as soon as 24 hours after the insult and lasting up to 10 days, oxidative capacity is markedly reduced, indicating that glycolysis is not the only metabolic pathway affected.[174]

Other factors that may contribute to the depression of glucose utilization following fluid percussion include the disturbance of cerebral blood flow[119,120,175] and the accumulation of lactic acid.[117,176,177] Long-term decreases in CBF following trauma has been postulated[69] to be due to the coupling of flow to metabolism, injury-induced cell swelling, acidosis (due to H^+ and/or lactic acid accumulation), and the release of angio-action factors. Consequently, if there is a sustained change in CBF following traumatic brain injury, the depression of glucose utilization may only reflect the alteration in cerebral perfusion.

The formation of lactic acid has been well documented following ischemia[178–181] and has also been reported to occur following fluid percussion injury.[117,176,177] Although many investigators have attributed the increase of lactic acid to impairment of mitochondrial functions,[117,134,182,183] others have reported that mitochondrial functions are not disrupted following fluid percussion brain injury.[124] Therefore, the accumulation of lactate is most likely due to hyperglycolysis. Regardless of the source, increased levels of lactic acid have been associated with cellular acidosis[117,137,176,178–180,182,184–186] and can, thereby, produce long-term intracellular dysfunctions that could be reflected in the depression of glucose utilization.

In other models of brain injury, the long-term metabolic depression has been attributed to remote effects of neurotransmitters.[21,24] In pharmacological work, catecholamine stimulation via amphetamine administration has been shown to alleviate the metabolic depression typically seen following sensorimotor cortex ablation in the rat.[21]

In studies of traumatic lesions, the resulting depression of glucose metabolism has been attributed to the disruption of serotonin[24] and norepinephrine functioning.[21,24,187,188] In general, these studies propose that the remote functional depression of glucose metabolism following brain injury represents a reduction of neuromodulation of specific neurotransmitters. However, whether these changes in neurotransmitter functions are independently responsible for the metabolic depression or whether these disruptions reflect the end result of the ionic and/or neurochemical cascade initiated by the trauma remains to be determined.

Long-Term Effects on Oxidative Metabolism

As reviewed previously, several studies have addressed how oxidative metabolism is altered during the first few minutes following experimental injury. However, few studies exist in which oxidative metabolism has been studied chronically. To address long-term changes in oxidative metabolism following disuse,[189–199] denervation,[196,200,201] cortical ablation,[202,203] cortical contusion,[204,205] or ischemia,[206] cytochrome oxidase (CO) histochemistry has been employed. This histochemical method has been used extensively to obtain a relative measure of oxidative capacity of neural tissue.[196] As described in a review by Wong-Riley (1989),[196] using the osmiophilic reagent 3,3′-diaminobenzidine as an electron donor, it is oxidatively polymerized to a noncoalescing, nondroplet indamine polymer osmiophilic and detectable at both the light and electron microscope levels. Since the reaction requires continued reoxidation of cytochrome c by cytochrome oxidase for adequate accumulation of a visible product, this reaction essentially demonstrates cytochrome oxidase activity localizing cytochrome c on the outer surface of the inner mitochondrial membrane. It has previously been shown within the CNS, contributions from endogenous catalyses and peroxidase are negligible.[207] Finally, the specificity of the reaction to oxidative metabolism was verified by complete inhibition with potassium cyanide.[208]

Typically, the final reaction is qualitatively described; however, others have utilized optical densitometry for quantification.[198,202,203,208] This method of quantification appears to be justified as long as the factors influencing the density of the reaction in vitro are controlled.[209] In fact, the intensity of the reaction product detected with optical density has been shown to be closely correlated (r = .90) with cytochrome oxidase activity measured spectrophotometrically in punch biopsies of the brain.[208]

Utilizing the CO histochemical technique, a few preliminary studies suggest, following concussion brain injury[210] or cortical ablation,[211] oxidative metabolism was reduced for at least several days, particularly within the cerebral cortex and underlying hippocampus. Although these studies provide important insights into the regional differentiation of oxidative metabolic changes following brain injury, the degree or duration of these changes has yet to be defined.

In a recent comprehensive study,[174] rats were studied histochemically measuring the degree of CO activity present within different structures at different times following a lateral fluid percussion in brain injury. By far, the most affected region within the hemisphere ipsilateral to the fluid percussion site was the cerebral cortex. This region exhibited a general depression of oxidative metabolism 1 day following injury. However, by the second day, the depression alleviated and subsequently returned by day 3. This injury-induced decrease in CO activity became even more pronounced, reaching its greatest extent by 5 days and returning to presurgical levels within 10 days. Of the regions within the cortex studied, the temporal cortex was the most affected, reaching levels twice as depressed as any other cortical region measured.

In addition to the cerebral cortex, subcortical structures, including the hippocampus, thalamus, brain stem, and cerebellum, also were studied. Of these other structures, only the hippocampus exhibited a marked depression in CO activity. In brief, the dorsal and ventral hippocampus regions did not exhibit any change in CO activity 24 hours after injury. However, by 3 days, both of these regions exhibited a decrease in CO activity, with this depression being more evident within the ventral hippocampus. Like the cerebral cortex, this injury-induced depression of oxidative metabolism returned to near normal levels within 10 days.

THE IONIC AND METABOLIC CASCADE: IMPLICATIONS FOR RECOVERY OF FUNCTION

It now appears to be well established that following traumatic brain injury a series of events (e.g., ionic fluxes, metabolic disruption) are put in motion that are causally related but different in extent and duration (Fig. 108-4). To understand the time course of these individual post-traumatic, secondary injury events is critical in order not only to determine what kind of

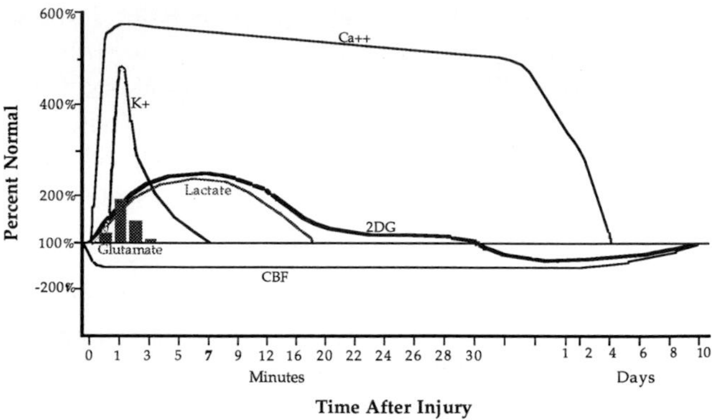

Figure 108-4. A summary of the neurochemical-neurometabolic cascade following an experimental fluid percussion brain injury in the rat. Note that each component has its own time duration and extent of effect. The calcium curve is derived from nonparametric measurements of ^{45}Ca density. (See reference[40].)

treatments should be designed for the head-injured patient, but at what time they would be effective. Of particular importance is the long-term disruption in metabolic processes that may delineate a period of time following injury when the brain is functionally compromised and consequently may be extremely vulnerable to a second insult.

Although major advances have been made in understanding the post-traumatic neurochemical and neurometabolic cascade, questions still remain. For example, the concept of an injury-induced ionic flux is now well established; however, we still do not have a firm understanding of the channel(s) involved. The different contribution of voltage-dependent and ligand-activated channels needs to be clarified in order to determine the appropriate targets for channel and/or receptor blocking agents. In addition, the reasons why the increase in energy demand of cells subjected to altered ionic environments is satisfied by a selective increase in glycolysis, even in the presence of oxygen and adequate CBF, must be understood. Answering these questions regarding the acute effects of trauma may contribute to our understanding of the more chronic metabolic changes related to recovery of function.

The depression of metabolic functioning following injury to the brain has been reported in many different studies.[3,14,16,22,25,161,202,212–217] In addition to the possible mechanisms proposed earlier, the depression could simply reflect changes in cerebral perfusion, neuronal degeneration, anatomic reorganization, or the imbalance of excitation and inhibition. Whatever the mechanism(s), there is ample evidence to suggest that this long-term metabolic depression reflects a depression of neuronal functioning and, thereby, contributes to the neurological deficits exhibited following injury.

The concept of a functional depression being responsible for neurological deficits is not new and is probably best known under the descriptions of diaschisis.[218–220] However, many of the early descriptions were based on neurological deficits that could not be explained given the morphological understanding of the lesion. Attempts have been made at uncovering this depression by electrophysiological means.[221–223] However, it wasn't until metabolic imaging methods were developed, allowing for accurate regional assessment, that the depression was characterized. To review all the animal and human studies in which a metabolic depression remote from the site of the lesion is documented would exceed the aims of this chapter, especially since there are already excellent reviews on this topic.[224–227] What has been lacking is a clear understanding of the functional implications of this depression. Few studies exist where metabolic and behavioral studies are conducted simultaneously over the course of recovery following brain injury.

Early attempts at correlating functional to metabolic recovery were conducted in an ischemia model measuring postischemic cerebral blood flow.[228] However, there was no indication that the neurological recovery was related to cerebral blood flow recovery. Consequently, it was concluded that improved postischemic blood flow could not be used as a criterion for assessing interventions without reference to metabolic demand.

This metabolic demand issue was addressed in a cortical freezing lesion model in the rat.[164] In this study, both metabolic (2DG) and behavioral experiments were conducted 1, 3, and 6 days after a unilateral injury. During the early time points, animals exhibited asymmetries in somatosensory responsiveness, a decrease in running wheel activity, and difficulty in coordinating limb movements. At the completion of behavioral testing on day 3, ICMRglc demonstrated a widespread depression in glucose utilization, primarily within the cerebral cortex ipsilateral to the lesion. The degree and extent of the lesion-induced metabolic depression was significantly correlated to the severity of the behavioral deficits. When animals were studied 6 days after the lesion, only deficits in limb coordination remained. At this time point, ICMRglc measurements indicated that the depression of glucose metabolism had spontaneously alleviated. Consequently, this study provided strong evidence that the behavioral changes following brain injury were a manifestation of a widespread functional depression as determined by the decrease in glucose utilization.

As previously described[35,106,108] (Fig. 108-4) most of the general post-trauma time scale of cerebral metabolic changes have been documented for a lateral fluid percussion brain injury. Consequently, the analysis of the rate of spontaneous recovery of both sensorimotor as well as cognitive functions following the same injury would allow a similar comparison between metabolism and behavior in a model of traumatic brain injury. Our recent behavioral studies indicate that deficits persist as long as the metabolic depression is present (Fig. 108-5). More importantly, the recovery of behavioral function was correlated with the recovery of metabolic function in the appropriate region(s). For example, following a lateral fluid percussion injury, both the cerebral cortex and underlying hippocampus become metabolically depressed beginning 6 hours after the insult. Although both structures recover spontaneously in terms of metabolism, the rate of recovery is much different. The hippocampus returns close to normal levels within 5 days. However, it takes as long as 10 days before the cerebral cortex returns to pre-injury metabolic baseline levels. In the assessment of neurological deficits, cognitive function, as measured on a Morris water maze, returned toward normal levels within 5 days, whereas sensorimotor deficits as measured on a beam-walking task did not completely recover until after 10 days.

If there does exist a behavioral-metabolic relationship, then pharmacological agents shown to increase the rate of behavioral recovery following traumatic brain injury should result in corresponding changes in metabolism. In this vein, catecholamine agonists (e.g. D-amphetamine) have been well documented as having the capacity to increase the rate of functional recovery in both animals[93,229–243] and man.[230,244] Consequently, this agent should have a similar impact in terms of metabolic recovery. To determine if the behavioral-metabolic relationship would still be maintained we extended our work to incorporate the post-traumatic treatment of animals with D-amphetamine. This pharmacological study indicated that animals that received a single injection of D-amphetamine (2 mg/kg, ip) 3 hours after a lateral fluid percussion injury exhibited a marked increase in the rate of recovery of sensorimotor functions. When these same animals were studied metabolically, the rate of recovery of glucose utilization matched the rate of behavioral recovery (Fig. 108-5). Consequently, it now appears that cerebral metabolism may become an important outcome measure to determine the therapeutic effectiveness of treatments for traumatic brain injury.

SUMMARY

Studies of cerebral metabolism have provided important insights into the mechanisms and consequences of the ionic flux initiated by the insult and propagated via

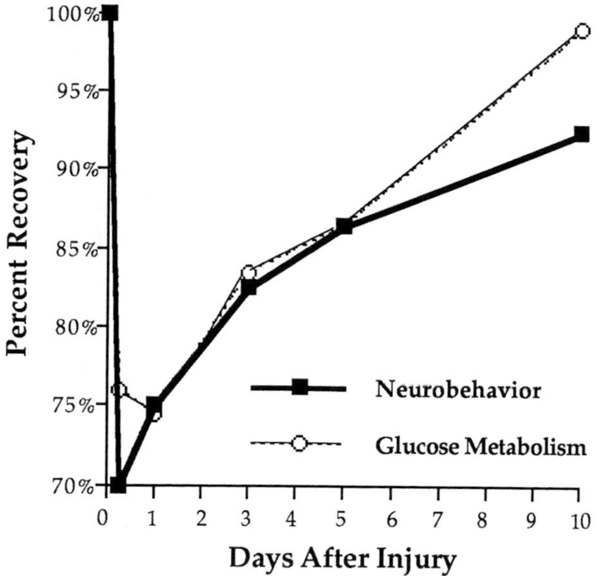

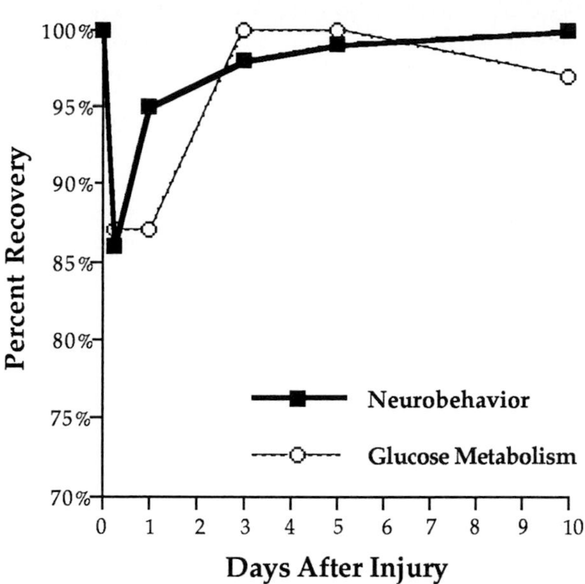

Figure 108-5. General comparisons of behavioral versus metabolic recovery in animals treated with saline (*left*) or D-amphetamine (*right*) following a moderate, lateral fluid percussion injury. Amphetamine was adminstered (2 mg/kg ip) 3 h after the insult and resulted in an enhanced recovery of both metabolism and behavioral function.

ligand-gated ion channels. Furthermore, imaging techniques offer the ability to discriminate regions of the brain that may be functionally, but not yet structurally, affected by traumatic brain injury. Consequently, different types of injury can now be further characterized in terms of functional impairment instead of relying on anatomic and/or neurological findings. In addition, the assessment of metabolic functioning appears to be directly correlated with neuronal functioning, and thus, can provide important information about the state of behavioral deficits as they pertain to recovery of function.

Several years ago, many of the methods and techniques described over the course of this discussion on metabolic dysfunction following injury were restricted to the laboratory. However, with the development of positron emission tomography (PET/SPECT Imaging in Head Injury, Michael Caron, see Chap. 11) and human cerebral microdialysis (Biochemical Monitoring, Clay Goodman and Richard Simpson, see Chap. 40), similar types of investigations and/or measurements can now be made in patients who have endured head injury. Consequently, the achievements of recent years in our understanding of the cellular pathophysiology of brain injury can now begin to be applied to the human condition.

ACKNOWLEDGMENTS

I would like to acknowledge Drs. Katayama, Kawamata, Yoshino, Lee, and Becker for their contribution to much of the above-mentioned work. This work was supported by NS30308 and the Lind Lawrence Foundation.

REFERENCES

1. Ginsberg MD: Local metabolic responses to cerebral ischemia. *Cerebr Brain Metab Rev* 1990; 2:58.
2. Jorgensen MB, Wright DC, Diemer NH: Postischemic glucose metabolism is modified in the hippocampal CA1 region depleted of excitatory input or pyramidal cells. *J Cereb Blood Flow Metab* 1990; 10:243.
3. Beck T, Wree A, Schleicher A: Glucose utilization in rat hippocampus after long-term recovery from ischemia. *J Cereb Blood Flow Metab* 1990; 10:542.
4. Chokl J, Greenberg J, Reivich M: Regional cerebral glucose metabolism during and after bilateral cerebral ischemia in the gerbil. *Stroke* 1983; 14:568.
5. Suzuki R, Yamaguchi T, Kirino T, et al: The effects of 5-minute ischemia in mongolian gerbil: 1. Blood-brain barrier, cerebral blood flow, and local cerebral glucose utilization changes. *Acta Neuropathol* 1983; 60:207.

6. Pulsinelli WA, Levy DE, Duffy TE: Regional cerebral blood flow and glucose metabolism following transient forebrain ischemia. *Ann Neurol* 1982; 11:499.
7. Diemer NH, Siemikowicz E: Increase in 2-deoxyglucose uptake in hippocampus, globus pallidus and substantia nigra after cerebral ischemia. *Acta Neurol Scand* 1980; 61:56.
8. Beck T, Wree A, Schleicher A: Postichemic glucose utilization in rat hippocampal layers. *Brain Res* 1990; 510:74.
9. Nedergaard M, Diemer NH: Experimental cerebral ischemia: barbiturate resistant increase in regional glucose utilization. *J Cereb Blood Flow Metab* 1988; 8:763.
10. Nedergaard M, Jakobsen J, Diemer NH: Autoradiographic determination of cerebral glucose content, blood flow and glucose utilization in focal ischemia of the rat brain: Influence of the plasma glucose concentration. *J Cereb Blood Flow Metab* 1988; 8:100.
11. Nedergaard M, Astrup J: Infarct rim: Effect of hyperglycemia on direct current potential and [^{14}C]2-deoxyglucose phosphorylation. *J Cereb Blood Flow Metab* 1986; 6:607.
12. Shiraishi K, Sharp FR, Simon RP: Sequential metabolic changes in rat brain following middle cerebral artery occlusion: A 2-deoxyglucose study. *J Cereb Blood Flow Metab* 1989; 9:765.
13. Nedergaard M: Mechanisms of brain damage in focal cerebral ischemia. *Acta Neurol Scand* 1988; 77:1.
14. Ginsberg MD, Reivich M, Giandomenico A, Greenberg JH: Local glucose utilization in acute focal cerebral ischemia: Local dysmetabolism and diaschisis. *Neurology* 1977; 27:1042.
15. Braughler JM, Hall ED: Central nervous system trauma and stroke I. Biochemical considerations for oxygen radical formation and lipid peroxidation. *J Free Radic Biol Med* 1989; 6:289.
16. Dauth GW, Gilman S, Frey KA, Penney JB: Basal ganglia glucose utilization after recent precentral ablation in the monkey. *Ann Neurol* 1985; 17:431.
17. Gilman S, Dauth GW, Frey KA, Penney JB: Experimental hemiplegia in the monkey: Basal ganglia glucose activity during recovery. *Ann Neurol* 1987; 22:370.
18. Hosokawa S, Kato M, Aiko Y, Shima F: Altered local cerebral glucose utilization by unilateral frontal cortical ablations in rats. *Brain Res* 1985; 343:8.
19. Sharp F, Evans KL: Bilateral [^{14}C]2-deoxyglucose uptake by motor pathways after unilateral neonatal cortex lesions in the rat. *Dev Brain Res* 1983; 6:1.
20. Cooper RM, Thurlow GA, Rooney BJ: 2-Deoxyglucose uptake and histologic changes in rat thalamus after neocortical ablations. *Exp Neurol* 1984; 83:134.
21. Feeney DM, Sutton RL, Boyeson MG, et al: The locus coeruleus and cerebral metabolism: Recovery of function after cortical injury. *Physiol Psych* 1985; 13:197.
22. Pappius HM, Wolfe LS: Effects of indomethacin and ibuprofen on cerebral metabolism and blood flow in traumatized brain. *J Cereb Blood Flow Metab* 1983; 3:448.
23. Pappius HM: Local cerebral glucose utilization in thermally traumatized rat brain. *Ann Neurol* 1981; 9:484.
24. Pappius HM: Significance of biogenic amines in functional disturbances resulting from brain injury. *Metab Brain Dis* 1988; 3:303.
25. Pappius HM: Dexamethasone and local cerebral glucose utilization in free-traumatized rat brain. *Ann Neurol* 1982; 12:157.
26. Pappius HM: Brain injury: New insights into neurotransmitter and receptor mechanisms. *Neurochem Res* 1991; 16:941.
27. Ackermann RF, Lear JL: Glycolysis-induced discordance between glucose metabolic rates measured with radiolabeled fluorodeoxyglucose and glucose. *J Cereb Blood Flow Metab* 1989; 9:774.
28. Weiss J, Hiltbrand B: Functional compartmentation of glycolytic versus oxidative metabolism in isolated rabbit heart. *J Clin Invest* 1985; 75:436.
29. Andersen BJ, Marmarou A: Energy compartmentalization in neural tissue. *J Cereb Blood Flow Metab* 1989; 9(suppl 1);S386.
30. Andersen BJ, Marmarou A: Isolated stimulation of glycolysis following traumatic brain injury, in Hoff JT Betz AL (eds): *Intracranial Pressure VII.* Berlin: Springer-Verlag, 1989: 575–580.
31. Adachi K, Cruz N, Sokoloff L, Dienel G: CMR_{glc} during cortical spreading depression: Assays with [6-^{14}C]glucose or [^{14}C]deoxyglucose (abstr). *Soc Neurosci* 1993; 19:1223.
32. Lewelt W, Jenkins LW, Miller JD: Autoregulation of cerebral blood flow after experimental fluid percussion injury of the brain. *J Neurosurg* 1980; 53:500.
33. Dirnagl U, Pulsinelli WA: Autoregulation of cerebral blood flow in experimental focal brain ischemia. *J Cereb Blood Flow Metab* 1990; 10:327.
34. Katayama Y, Becker DP, Tamura T, Hovda DA: Massive increases in extracellular potassium and the indiscriminate release of glutamate following concussive brain injury. *J Neurosurg* 1990; 73:889.
35. Hovda DA, Becker DP, Katayama Y: Secondary injury and acidosis. *J Neurotrauma* 1992; 9(suppl 1):S47.
36. Takahashi H, Manaka S, Sano K: Changes in extracellular potassium concentration in cortex and brain stem during the acute phase of experimental closed head injury. *J Neurosurg* 1981; 55:708.
37. Kaminogo M, Mori K: Post-traumatic early fits and $[K^+]$o (abstr). *J Neurotrauma* 1990; 7:108.
38. Soares HD, Thomas M, Cloherty K, McIntosh TK: Development of prolonged focal cerebral edema and regional cation changes following experimental brain injury in the rat. *J Neurochem* 1992; 58:1845.
39. Cortez SC, McIntosh TK, Noble LJ: Experimental fluid percussion brain injury: Vascular disruption and neuronal and glial alterations. *Brain Res* 1989; 482:271.
40. Fineman I, Hovda DA, Smith M, et al: Concussive brain injury is associated with a prolonged accumulation of calcium: A ^{45}calcium autoradiographic study. *Brain Res* 1993; 624:94.
41. Smith DH, Okiyama K, Thomas MJ, McIntosh TK: Effects of the excitatory amino acid receptor antagonists kynurenate and indole-2-carboxylic acid on behavioral and neurochemical outcome following experimental brain injury. *J Neurosci* 1993; 13:5383.

42. McIntosh TK, Faden AI, Yamakami I, Vink R: Magnesium deficiency exacerbates and pretreatment improves outcome following traumatic brain injury in rats: 31P magnetic resonance spectroscopy and behavioral studies. *J Neurotrauma* 1988; 5:17.
43. McIntosh TK, Vink R, Yamakami I, Faden AI: Magnesium protects against neurological deficit after brain injury. *Brain Res* 1989; 482:252.
44. Vink R, McIntosh TK, Demediuk P, et al: Decline in intracellular free Mg^{2+} is associated with irreversible tissue injury after brain trauma. *J Biol Chem* 1988; 263:757.
45. Vink R, Faden AI, McIntosh TK: Changes in cellular bioenergetic state following graded traumatic brain injury in rats: Determination by phosphorus 31 magnetic resonance spectroscopy. *J Neurotrauma* 1988; 5:315.
46. Hubschmann OR, Kornhauser D: Effects of intraparenchymal hemorrhage on extracellular cortical potassium in experimental head trauma. *J Neurosurg* 1983; 59:289.
47. Young W, Koreh I, Yen V: Effects of sympathectomy on extracellular potassium activity and blood flow in experimental spinal cord contusion. *Brain Res* 1982; 253:115.
48. Julian FJ, Goldman DE: The effects of mechanical stimulation on some electrical properties of axons. *J Gen Physiol* 1962; 46:297.
49. Hayes RL, Katayama Y, Young HF, Dunbar JG: Coma associated with flaccidity produced by fluid-percussion concussion in the cat. I: Is it due to depression of activity within the brainstem reticular formation? *Brain Injury* 1988; 2:31.
50. Walker AE, Kolloros JJ, Case TJ: The physiological basis of concussion. *J Neurosurg* 1944; 1:103.
51. Cotman CW, Iverson LL: Excitatory amino acids in the brain—focus on NMDA receptors. *TINS* 1987; 10:263.
52. Habiltz JJ, Langmoen IA: Excitation of hippocampal pyramidal cells by glutamate in the guinea-pig and rat. *J Physiol* 1982; 325:317.
53. Mayer ML, Westbrook GL: Cellular mechanisms underlying excitotoxicity. *TINS* 1987; 10:59.
54. Heinemann U, Lux HD: Ceiling of stimulus induced rises in extracellular potassium concentration in the cerebral cortex of cat. *Brain Res* 1977; 120:231.
55. Katzman R: Maintenance of a constant brain extracellular potassium. *Fed Proc* 1976; 35:1244.
56. Orkand RK: Functional consequences of ionic changes resulting from electrical activity. *Fed Proc* 1980; 39:1515.
57. Ballanyi K, Grafe P, Bruggencate CT: Ion activities and potassium uptake mechanisms of glial cells in guinea-pig olfactory cortex slices. *J Physiol* 1987; 382:159.
58. Kuffler SW: Neuroglial cells: Physiological properties and a potassium mediated effect of neuronal activity on the glial membrane potential. *Proc R Soc Lond* 1967; 168:1.
59. Paulson OB, Newman EA: Does the release of potassium from astrocyte endfeet regulate cerebral blood flow? *Science* 1987; 237:896.
60. Hotson JR, Sypert GW, Ward AA: Extracellular potassium concentration changes during propagated seizures in neocortex. *Exp Neurol* 1973; 34:20.
61. Moody W, Futamachi KJ, Prince DA: Extracellular potassium activity during epileptogenesis. *Exp Neurol* 1974; 42:248.
62. Sypert GW, Ward AA: Changes in extracellular potassium activity during neocortical propagated seizures. *Exp Neurol* 1974; 45:19.
63. Katayama Y, Cheung MK, Alves A, Becker DP: Ion fluxes and cell swelling in experimental traumatic brain injury: The role of excitatory amino acids, in Hoff JT, Betz AL (eds): *Intracranial Pressure VII.* Berlin: Springer-Verlag, 1989: 584–588.
64. Katayama Y, Cheung MK, Gorman L, et al: Increase in extracellular glutamate and associated massive ionic fluxes following concussive brain injury (abstr). *Soc Neurosci* 1988; 14:1154.
65. Astrup J, Rehcrona S, Siesjö BK: The increase in extracellular potassium concentration in the ischemic brain in relation to the preischemic functional activity and cerebral metabolic rate. *Brain Res* 1980; 199:161.
66. Hansen AJ: Extracellular potassium concentration in juvenile and adult rat brain cortex during anoxia. *Acta Physiol Scand* 1977; 99:412.
67. Hansen AJ: The extracellular potassium concentration in brain cortex following ischemia in hypo- and hyperglycemic rats. *Acta Physiol Scand* 1978; 102:324.
68. Dewitt DS, Jenkins LW, Wei EP, et al: The effects of fluid percussion brain injury on regional and total cerebral blood flow and pial vessel diameter. A Combined pial window and microsphere study. *J Neurosurg* 1986; 64:787.
69. Tsubokawa T: Cerebral circulation and metabolism in concussion. *Neurol Surg* 1983; 11:563.
70. Nicholson C, Kraig RP: The behavior of extracellular ions during spreading depression, in Zeuthen T (ed): *The Application of Ion-Selective Electrodes.* New York: Elsevier, North-Holland, 1981: 217–238.
71. Prince DA, Lux HD, Neher E: Measurements of extracellular potassium activity in cat cortex. *Brain Res* 1973; 50:489.
72. Sugaya E, Takato M, Noda Y: Neuronal and glial activity during spreading depression in cerebral cortex of cat. *J Neurophysiol* 1975; 38:822.
73. Van Harreveld A: Two mechanisms for spreading depression in chicken retina. *J Neurobiol* 1978; 9:419.
74. Vyscocil F, Kriz N, Bures J: Potassium selective microelectrodes used for measuring the extracellular brain potassium during spreading depression and anoxic depolarization in rats. *Brain Res* 1973; 39:255.
75. Somjen GG, Giacchino JL: Potassium and calcium concentrations in interstitial fluid of hippocampal formation during paroxysmal responses. *J Neurophysiol* 1985; 53:1098.
76. Tobiasz C, Nicholson C: Tetrodotoxin resistant propagation and extracellular sodium changes during spreading depression in rat cerebellum. *Brain Res* 1982; 241:329.
77. DeSalles AAF, Jenkins LW, Anderson RL, et al: Extracellular potassium activity following concussion. A microelectrode study in the cat (abstr). *Soc Neurosci* 1986; 12:967.
78. Dienel GA: Regional accumulation of calcium in postischemic rat brain. *J Neurochem* 1984; 43:913.

79. Choi DW: Calcium-mediated neurotoxicity: Relationship to specific channel types and role in ischemic damage. *TINS* 1988; 11:465.
80. Kato H, Kogure K, Nakano S: Neuronal damage following repeated brief ischemia in the gerbil. *Brain Res* 1989; 479:366.
81. Sakamoto N, Kogure K, Ohtomo H: Disturbed Ca^{2+} homeostasis in the gerbil hippocampus following brief transient ischemia. *Brain Res* 1986; 264:372.
82. Rappaport ZH, Young W, Flamm ES: Regional brain calcium changes in the rat middle cerebral artery occlusion model of ischemia. *Stroke* 1987; 18:760.
83. Deshpande JK, Siesjö BK, Wieloch T: Calcium accumulation and neuronal damage in the rat hippocampus following cerebral ischemia. *J Cereb Blood Flow Metab* 1987; 7:89.
84. Stokes BT, Fox P, Hollinden G: Extracellular calcium activity in the injured spinal cord. *Exp Neurol* 1983; 80:561.
85. Young W, Yen V, Blight A: Extracellular calcium ionic activity in experimental spinal cord contusion. *Brain Res* 1982; 253:105.
86. Young W, Koreh I: Potassium and calcium changes in injured spinal cords. *Brain Res* 1986; 365:42.
87. Happel RD, Smith KP, Banik NL, et al: Ca^{2+}-accumulation in experimental spinal cord trauma. *Brain Res* 1981; 211:476.
88. Young W, Flamm ES: Effect of high dose corticosteroid therapy on blood flow, evoked potentials, and extracellular calcium in experimental spinal injury. *J Neurosurg* 1982; 57:667.
89. Schanne FAX, Kane AB, Young EE, Farber JL: Calcium dependence of toxic cell death: A final common pathway. *Science* 1979; 206:700.
90. Choi DW: Ionic dependence of glutamate neurotoxicity. *J Neurosci* 1987; 7:369.
91. Badie H, Smith ML, Hovda DA, et al: Omega-conopeptide reduces the extent of calcium accumulation following traumatic brain injury (abstr). *Soc Neurosci* 1993; 19:1485.
92. Hovda DA, Fu K, Badie H, et al: Administration of an omega-conopeptide one hour following traumatic brain injury reduces ^{45}calcium accumulation. *Acta Neurochir* 1994; 60(suppl):521.
93. McIntosh TK: Novel pharmacologic therapies in the treatment of experimental traumatic brain injury: A review. *J Neurotrauma* 1993; 10:215.
94. Ebel H, Gunther T: Magnesium metabolism: A review. *J Clin Chem Biochem* 1980; 8:257.
95. Garfinkel L, Garfinkel D: Magnesium regulation of the glycolytic pathway and the enzymes involved. *Magnesium* 1985; 14:60.
96. Aikawa JK: *Magnesium: Its Biologic Significance.* Boca Raton: CRC Press, 1981.
97. Vink R, McIntosh TK, Demediuk P, Faden AI: Decrease in total and free magnesium concentation following traumatic brain injury in rats. *Biochem Biophys Res Commun* 1987; 149:594.
98. Vink R, McIntosh TK, Weiner MW, Faden AI: Effects of traumatic brain injury on cerebral high-energy phosphates and pH: A 31P magnetic resonance spectroscopy study. *J Cereb Blood Flow Metab* 1987; 7:563.
99. Vink R, McIntosh TK: Pharmacological and physiological effect of magnesium on experimental traumatic brain injury. *Magn Reson* 1990; 3:163.
100. Vink R, McIntosh TK, Yamakami I, Faden AI: ^{31}P NMR characterization of graded traumatic brain injury in rats. *Magn Reson Med* 1988; 6:37.
101. Vink R, McIntosh TK, Romhanyi RS, Faden AI: Opiate antagonist nalmefene improves intracellular free Mg^{2+}, bioenergetic state, and neurologic outcome following traumatic brain injury in rats. *J Neurosci* 1990; 10:3524.
102. Shah KR, West M: The effect of concussion on cerebral uptake of 2-deoxy-D-glucose in rat. *Neurosci Lett* 1983; 40:287.
103. Sunami K, Nakamura T, Ozawa Y, et al: Hypermetabolic state following experimental head injury. *Neurosurg Rev* 1989; 12:400.
104. Wilson JA, Pentland B, Currie CT, Miller JD: The functional effects of head injury in the elderly. *Brain Injury* 1987; 1:183.
105. Hayes RL, Pechura CM, Katayama Y, et al: Activation of pontine cholinergic sites implicated in unconsciousness following cerebral concussion in the cat. *Science* 1984; 223:301.
106. Yoshino A, Hovda DA, Katayama Y, et al: Hippocampal CA3 lesion prevents post-concussive metabolic dysfunction in CA1. *J Cereb Blood Flow Metab* 1992; 12:996.
107. Hovda DA, Katayama Y, Yoshino A, et al: Pre- or postsynaptic blocking of glutamatergic functioning prevents the increase in glucose utilization following concussive brain injury, in Globus M, Dietrich WD (eds): *The Role of Neurotransmitters in Brain Injury.* New York: Plenum Press, 1993: 327–332.
108. Yoshino A, Hovda DA, Kawamata T, et al: Dynamic changes in local cerebral glucose utilization following cerebral concussion in rats: Evidence of a hyper- and subsequent hypometabolic state. *Brain Res* 1991; 561:106.
109. Kawamata T, Katayama Y, Hovda DA, et al: Administration of excitatory amino acid antagonists via microdialysis attenuates the increase in glucose utilization seen following concussive brain injury. *J Cereb Blood Flow Metab* 1992; 12:12.
110. Kawamata T, Hovda DA, Yoshino A, et al: Administration of excitatory amino acid antagonists via microdialysis prevents the increase in glucose utilization seen immediately following concussive brain injury (abstr). *Soc Neurosci* 1990; 16:778.
111. Inglis F, Kuroda Y, Bullock R: Glucose hypermetabolism after acute subdural hematoma is ameliorated by a competitive NMDA antagonist. *J Neurotrauma* 1992; 9:75.
112. Sokoloff L, Reivich M, Kennedy C, et al: The [^{14}C]deoxyglucose method for the measurement of local cerebral glucose utilization: Theory, procedure, and normal values in the conscious and anesthetized albino rat. *J Neurochem* 1977; 28:897.

113. Ginsberg MD, Reivich M: Use of the 2-deoxyglucose method of local cerebral glucose utilization in the abnormal brain: Evaluation of the lumped constant during ischemia. *Acta Neurol Scand* 1979; 60(suppl 72):226.
114. Nakai H, Matsuda H, Takara E, et al: Changes in lumped and rate constants in experimental cerebral ischemia. Intra-animal comparison before and after middle cerebral artery occlusion. *Neurol Med Chir (Tokyo)* 1988; 28:11.
115. McIntosh TK, Vink R, Noble L, et al: Traumatic brain injury in the rat: Characterization of a lateral fluid-percussion model. *Neuroscience* 1989; 28:233.
116. Hayes RL, Katayama Y, Jenkins LW, et al: Regional rates of glucose utilization in the cat following concussive head injury. *J Neurotrauma* 1988; 5:121.
117. Yang MS, Dewitt DS, Becker DP, Hayes RL: Regional brain metabolite levels following mild experimental head injury in the cat. *J Neurosurg* 1985; 63:617.
118. Dewitt DS, Rosner MJ, Becker DP, Hayes RL: Measurement of local blood flow and glucose metabolism within the same tissue samples in the feline CNS (abstr). *Soc Neurosci* 1981; 7:376.
119. Yuan X-Q, Prough DS, Smith TL, Dewitt DS: The effects of traumatic brain injury on regional cerebral blood flow in rats. *J Neurotrauma* 1988; 5:289.
120. Yamakami I, McIntosh TK: Effects of traumatic brain injury on regional cerebral blood flow in rats as measured with radiolabeled microspheres. *J Cereb Blood Flow Metab* 1989; 9:117.
121. Nilsson B, Nordstrom C-H: Experimental head injury in the rat. Part 3: Cerebral blood flow and oxygen consumption after concussive impact acceleration. *J Neurosurg* 1977; 47:262.
122. Meyer JS, Kondo A, Normura F, et al: Cerebral hemodynamics and metabolism following experimental head injury. *J Neurosurg* 1970; 32:304.
123. Nilsson B, Ponten U: Experimental head injury in the rat. Part 2: Regional brain energy metabolism in concussive trauma. *J Neurosurg* 1977; 47:252.
124. Vink R, Head VA, Rogers PJ, et al: Mitochondrial metabolism following traumatic brain injury in rats. *J Neurotrauma* 1990; 7:21.
125. Duckrow RB, LaManna JC, Rosenthal M, et al: Oxidative metabolic activity of cerebral cortex after fluid-percussion head injury in the cat. *J Neurosurg* 1981; 54:607.
126. Bull RJ, Cummins JT: Influence of potassium on the steady-state redox potential of the electron transport chain in slices of rat cerebral cortex and the effect of ouabain. *J Neurochem* 1973; 21:923.
127. Lewis DV, Schuette WH: NADH fluorescence and $[K^+]o$ changes during hippocampal electrical stimulation. *J Neurophysiol* 1975; 38:405.
128. Lothman E, LaManna J, Cordingley G, et al: Responses of electrical potential, potassium levels, and oxidative metabolic activity of the cerebral neocortex of cats. *Brain Res* 1975; 88:15.
129. Mayevsky A, Chance B: Repetitive patterns of metabolic changes during cortical spreading depression of the awake rat. *Brain Res* 1974; 65:529.
130. Rosenthal M, LaManna JC, Yamada S, et al: Oxidative metabolism, extracellular potassium and sustained potential shifts in cat spinal cord in situ. *Brain Res* 1979; 162:113.
131. Nelson SR, Lowry OH, Passonneau JV: Changes in energy reverses in mouse brain associated with compressive head injury, in Caveness WF, Walker AE, (eds): *Head Injury.* Philadelphia: Lippincott, 1966: 444–447.
132. Nilsson B, Nordstrom C-H: Rate of cerebral energy consumption in concussive head injury in the rat. *J Neurosurg* 1977; 47:274.
133. Becker DP: Brain acidosis in head injury: A clinical trial, in Becker DP, Povlishock JT (eds): *Central Nervous System Trauma Status Report—1985.* Richmond: Byrd Press, 1985: 229–242.
134. Inao S, Marmarou A, Clarke GD, et al: Production and clearance of lactate from brain tissue cerebrospinal fluid, and serum following experimental brain injury. *J Neurosurg* 1988; 69:736.
135. Csiba L, Paschen W, Mies G: Regional changes in tissue pH and glucose content during cortical spreading depression in rat brain. *Brain Res* 1985; 336:167.
136. Gjedde A, Hansen AJ, Quistorff B: Blood-brain glucose transfer in spreading depression. *J Neurochem* 1981; 37:807.
137. Krivanek J: Some metabolic changes accompanying Leao's spreading cortical depression in the rat. *J Neurochem* 1961; 6:183
138. Shinohara M, Rapoport S, Sokoloff L: Cerebral glucose utilization: Local changes during and after recovery from spreading cortical depression. *Science* 1979; 203:188.
139. Somjen GG: Acidification of interstitial fluid in hippocampal formation caused by seizures and by spreading depression. *Brain Res* 1984; 311:186.
140. Kocher M: Metabolic and hemodynamic activation of postischemic rat brain by cortical spreading depression. *J Cereb Blood Flow Metab* 1990; 10:564.
141. Kuhr WG, Korf J: Extracellular lactic acid as an indicator of brain metabolism: Continuous on-line measurement in conscious, freely moving rats with intrastriatal dialysis. *J Cereb Blood Flow Metab* 1988; 8:130.
142. Nilsson P, Hillered L, Ponten U, Ungerstedt U: Changes in cortical extracellular levels of energy-related metabolites and amino acids following concussive brain inury in rats. *J Cereb Blood Flow Metab* 1990; 10:631.
143. Kawamata T, Katayama Y, Hovda DA, et al: Lactate accumulation following concussive brain injury: The role of ionic fluxes induced by excitatory amino acids. *Brain Res* 1995; 674:196.
144. Friede RL, Van Houten WH: Relations between post mortem alterations and glycolytic metabolism in the brain. *Exp Neurol* 1961; 4:197.
145. Gardiner M, Smith ML, Kagstrom E, et al: Influence of blood glucose concentration on brain lactate accumulation during severe hypoxia and subsequent recovery of brain energy metabolism. *J Cereb Blood Flow Metab* 1982; 2:429.
146. Kalimo H, Rehncrona S, Soderfelt B, et al: Brain lactic

acidosis and ischemic cell damage. II. Histopathology. *J Cereb Blood Flow Metab* 1981; 1:313.
147. Kalimo H, Rehncrona S, Soderfelt B: The role of lactic acidosis in ischemic nerve cell injury. *Acta Neuropathol* 1981; 7:135.
148. Myers RE: A unitary theory of causation of anoxic and hypoxic brain pathology. *Adv Neurol* 1979; 26:195.
149. Rehncrona S, Rosen I, Siesjö BK: Brain lactic acidosis and ischemic cell damage. I. Biochemistry and neurophysiology. *J Cereb Blood Flow Metab* 1981; 1:297.
150. Siemkowicz E, Hansen AJ: Clinical restitution following cerebral ischemia in hyponormo- and hyperglycemic rats. *Acta Neurol Scand* 1978; 58:1.
151. Becker DP, Jenkins LW, Rabow L: The pathophysiology of head trauma, in Miller TA, Rowlands BJ (eds): *The Physiological Basis of Modern Surgical Care.* St. Louis: Mosby, 1987: 763–788.
152. Jenkins LW, Marmarou A, Lewelt W, Becker DP: Increased vulnerability of the traumatized brain to early ischemia, in Baethmann A, Go GK, Unterberg A (eds): *Mechanisms of Secondary Brain Damage.* New York: Plenum Press, 1986: 273–282.
153. Ishige N, Pitts LH, Berry I, et al: The effects of hypovolemic hypotension on high-energy phosphate metabolism of traumatized brain in rats. *J Neurosurg* 1988; 68:129.
154. Hovda DA, Sutton RL, Adelson PD, et al: Dynamic changes in cerebral glucose metabolism and blood flow following cerebral cortical contusion (abstr). *J Cereb Blood Flow Metab* 1993; 13(suppl 1):S574.
155. Finger S, Stein DG: Brain Damage and Recovery: Research and Clinical Perspectives. New York: Academic Press, 1982.
156. Feeney DM, Sutton RL: Pharmacotherapy for recovery of function after brain injury. *CRC Crit Rev Neurobiol* 1987; 3:135.
157. *Brain Injury and Recovery: Theoretical and Controversial Issues.* New York: Plenum Press, 1988.
158. *Synaptic Plasticity.* New York: Guilford Press, 1985.
159. Adelson PD, Ogawa H, Hovda DA, et al: Acute alterations in cerebral metabolism and glutamate concentrations following suction-ablation injury (abstr). *J Neurotrauma* 1992; 9:56.
160. Tandian D, Romhanyi RS, Hovda DA, et al: Amphetamine enhances both behavioral and metabolic recovery following fluid percussion brain injury. *J Neurotrauma* 1991; (In Press)
161. Kushner M, Alavi A, Reivich M, et al: Contralateral cerebellar hypometabolism following cerebral insult: A positron emission tomographic study. *Ann Neurol* 1984; 15:425.
162. Hossman KA, Niebuhr I, Tamura M: Blood flow and metabolism in the rat brain during experimental tumor development. *Acta Neural Scand* 1979; 72:576.
163. Patronas NJ, Chiro GD, Smith BH, et al: Depressed cerebellar glucose metabolism in supratentorial tumors. *Brain Res* 1984; 291:93.
164. Colle LM, Holmes LJ, Pappius HM: Correlation between behavioral status and cerebral glucose utilization in rats following freezing lesion. *Brain Res* 1986; 397:27.
165. Sutton RL, Hovda DA, Chugani HT: Time course of local cerebral glucose utilization (LCGU) alteration after motor cortex ablation in the rat (abstr). *Soc Neurosci* 1989; 15:128.
166. Benveniste H, Jorgensen MB, Sandberg M, et al: Ischemic damage in hippocampal CA1 is dependent on glutamate release and intact innervation from CA3. *J Cereb Blood Flow Metab* 1989; 9:629.
167. Sheardown MJ, Nielsen EA, Hansen AJ, et al: 2,3-Dihydroxy-6-nitro-7-sulfamoyl - benzo(F)quinoxaline: A neuroprotectant for cerebral ischemia. *Science* 1990; 247:571.
168. Gill R, Kemp JA: Protection of CA1 pyramidal cell function by MK-801 following ischaemia in the gerbil. *Neurosci Lett* 1989; 105:101.
169. Thilmann R, Xie Y, Kleihues P, Kiessling M: Persistent inhibition of protein synthesis precedes delayed neuronal death in postischemic gerbil hippocampus. *Acta Neuropathol* 1986; 71:88.
170. Jenkins LW, Moszynski K, Lyeth BG, et al: Increased vulnerability of the mildly traumatized rat brain to cerebral ischemia: The use of controlled secondary ischemia as a research tool to identify common or different mechanisms contributing to mechanical and ischemic brain injury. *Brain Res* 1989; 477:211.
171. Katayama Y, Tamura T, Becker DP, Kawamata T: Traumatic brain injury facilitates potassium flux during secondary ischemic insult (abstr). *Neurotrauma Soc* 1989; 6:200.
172. Ogawa H, Hovda DA, Badie H, Becker DP: ^{14}C-leucine incorporation following fluid percussion injury: No definitive role for glutamate (abstr). *J Cereb Blood Flow Metab* 1993; 13(suppl 1):S575.
173. Ogawa H, Hovda DA, Becker DP: Cerebral protein synthesis in the rat: Further studies following fluid percussion injury (abstr). *J Neurotrauma* 1992; 9:395.
174. Hovda DA, Becker DP: Concussion produces dynamic changes in metabolism and calcium accumulation resulting in prolonged neurological deficits. *Nimodipine: Pharmacological and Clinical Results in Cerebral Ischemia,* A. Scriabine, G.M. Teasdale, D. Tettenborn, & W. Young (Eds) Proceedings of the Second International Symposium on Nimodipine, Miami Beach, Florida, USA, April 25–28, 1990, pp 235–240.
175. Yamakami I, Yamaura A, Makino H, McIntosh TK: Effects of traumatic brain injury on regional cerebral blood flow and electroencephalogram (abstr). *J Neurotrauma* 1990; 7:101.
176. Inao S, Kuchiwaki H, Sugita K, Marmarou A: Significance of lactate production and clearance in brain tissue, CSF and serum following experimental brain injury (abstr). *J Neurotrauma* 1990; 7:100.
177. Kawamata T, Katayama Y, Hovda DA, et al: Administration of kynurenic acid via microdialysis attenuates lactate accumulation following concussive brain injury in rats. *J Neurotrauma* 1991; (In Press)
178. Kleihues P, Hossmann K-A, Pegg AE, et al: Resuscitation of the monkey brain after one hour complete ischemia. III. Indications of metabolic recovery. *Brain Res* 1975; 95:61.

179. MacMillan V: Cerebral Na^+, K^+-ATPase activity during exposure to and recovery from acute ischemia. *J Cereb Blood Flow Metab* 1982; 2:457.
180. Robertson CS, Goodman JC, Grossman RG, Priessman A: Reduction in spinal cord postischemic lactic acidosis and functional improvement with dichloroacetate. *J Neurotrauma* 1990; 7:1.
181. Hillered L, Hallstrom A, Segersvard S, et al: Dynamics of extracellular metabolites in the striatum after middle cerebral artery occlusion in the rat monitored by intracerebral microdialysis. *J Cereb Blood Flow Metab* 1989; 9:607.
182. Unterberg AW, Andersen BJ, Clarke GD, Marmarou A: Cerebral energy metabolism following fluid-percussion brain injury in cats. *J Neurosurg* 1988; 68:594.
183. Valentino RJ, Curtis AL, Parris DG, Wehby RG: Antidepressant actions on brain noradrenergic neurons. *J Pharmacol Exp Ther* 1990; 253:833.
184. Becker DP, Verity MA, Povlishock JT, Cheung M: Brain cellular injury and recovery—Horizons for improving medical therapies in stroke and trauma. *West J Med* 1988; 148:670.
185. Vink R, Noble LJ, Knoblach SM, et al: Metabolic changes in rabbit spinal cord after trauma: Magnetic resonance spectroscopy studies. *Ann Neurol* 1989; 25:26.
186. Schurr A, Rigor BM: Cerebral ischemia revisited: New insights as revealed using in vitro brain slice preparations. *Experientia* 1989; 45:684.
187. Boyeson MG, Feeney DM: Intraventricular norepinephrine facilitates motor recovery following sensorimotor cortex injury. *Pharmacol Biochem Behav* 1990; 35:497.
188. Boyeson MG, Bach-y-Rita P: Determinants of brain plasticity. *J Neuro Rehab* 1989; 3:35.
189. Hyde GE, Durham D: Cytochrome oxidase response to cochlea removal in chicken auditory brainstem neurons. *J Comp Neurol* 1990; 297:329.
190. Eckenrode TC, Barr GA, Battisti WP, Murray M: Acetylcholine in the interpeduncular nucleus of the rat: Normal distribution and effects of deafferentation. *Brain Res* 1987; 418:273.
191. Land PW, Akhtar ND: Chronic sensory deprivation affects cytochrome oxidase staining and glutamic acid decarboxylase immunoreactivity in adult rat ventrobasal thalamus. *Brain Res* 1987; 425:178.
192. Kageyama GH, Wong-Riley M: Differential effect of visual deprivation on cytochrome oxidase levels in major cell classes of the cat LGN. *J Comp Neurol* 1986; 246:212.
193. Wong-Riley MTT, Merzenich MM, Leake PA: Changes in endogenous reactivity to DAB induced by neuronal inactivity. *Brain Res* 1978; 141:185.
194. Wong-Riley MTT, Welt C: Histochemical changes in cytochrome oxidase of cortical barrels after vibrissal removal in neonatal and adult mice. *Proc Natl Acad Sci USA* 1980; 77:2333.
195. Wong-Riley M: Changes in the visual system of monocularly sutured or enucleated cats demonstrable with cytochrome oxidase histochemistry. *Brain Res* 1979; 171:11.
196. Wong-Riley MTT: Cytochrome oxidase: An endogenous metabolic marker for neuronal activity. *TINS* 1989; 12:94.
197. Jen LS, Zhao LP, Chau RMW: Cytochrome oxidase activity in the rat retina following unilateral thalamic lesion. *Neurosci Lett* 1989; 103:133.
198. Kageyama GH, Meyer RL: Laminar histochemical and cytochemical localization of cytochrome oxidase in the goldfish retina and optic tectum in response to deafferentation and during regeneration. *J Comp Neurol* 1988; 278:521.
199. Warren R, Remblay N, Dykes RW: Quantitative study of glutamic acid decarboxylase-immunoreactive neurons and cytochrome oxidase activity in the normal and partially deafferented rat hindlimb somatosensory cortex. *J Comp Neurol* 1989; 288:583.
200. Barr GA, Eckenrode TC, Murray M: Normal development and effects of early deafferentation on choline acetyltransferase, substance P and serotonin-like immunoreactivity in the interpeduncular nucleus. *Brain Res* 1987; 418:301.
201. Wong-Riley M, Riley DA: The effect of impulse blockage on cytochrome oxidase activity in the cat visual system. *Brain Res* 1983; 261:185.
202. Hovda DA, Sutton RL, Feeney DM: Recovery of tactile placing after visual cortex ablation in cat: A behavioral and metabolic study of diaschisis. *Exp Neurol* 1987; 97:391.
203. Hovda DA, Villablanca JR: Sparing of visual field perception in neonatal but not adult cerebral hemispherectomized cats. Relationship with oxidative metabolism of the superior colliculus. *Behav Brain Res* 1990; 37:119.
204. Sutton RL, Lescaudron L, Stein DG: Unilateral cortical contusion injury in the rat: Vascular disruption and temporal development of cortical necrosis. *J Neurotrauma* 1993; 10:135.
205. Weisend MP, Salazar RA, Feeney DM: Sensorimotor cortex contusion but not ablation increases cytochrome oxidase activity in rat auditory and entorhinal cortex. *J Neurotrauma* 1991; (In Press)
206. Wagner KR, Kleinholz M, Myers RE: Delayed onset of neurologic deterioration following anoxia/ischemia coincides with appearance of impaired brain mitochondrial respiration and decreased cytochrome oxidase activity. *J Cereb Blood Flow Metab* 1990; 10:417.
207. Wong-Riley MTT: Endogenous peroxidatic activity in brainstem neurons as demonstrated by their staining with diaminobenzidine in normal squirrel monkeys. *Brain Res* 1976; 108:257.
208. Darriet D, Der T, Collins RC: Distribution of cytochrome oxidase in rat brain: Studies with diaminobenzidine histochemistry in vitro and [^{14}C]cyanide tissue labeling in vivo. *J Cereb Blood Flow Metab* 1986; 6:8.
209. Silverman MS, Tootell RBH: Modified technique for cytochrome oxidase histochemistry: increased staining intensity and compatibility with 2-deoxyglucose autoradiography. *J Neurosci Methods* 1987; 19:1.
210. Becker DP, Shook BL, Gorman L, Katayama Y: Histochemical and behavioral changes following experimental brain injury in rat (abstr). *Soc Neurosci* 1989; 15:131.

211. Sutton RL, Chen MJ, Hovda DA, Feeney DM: Effects of amphetamine on cerebral metabolism following brain damage as revealed by quantitative cytochrome oxidase histochemistry (abstr). *Soc Neurosci* 1986; 12:1404.
212. Graf R, Kataoka K, Rosner G, Heiss W-D: Cortical deafferentation in cat focal ischemia: Disturbance and recovery of sensory functions in cortical areas with different degrees of cerebral blood flow reduction. *J Cereb Blood Flow Metab* 1986; 6:566.
213. Lagreze HL, Levine RL, Pedula KL, et al: Contralateral flow reduction in unilateral stroke: Evidence for transhemispheric diaschisis. *Stroke* 1987; 18:882.
214. Kiyosawa M, Pappata S, Duverger D, et al: Cortical hypometabolism and its recovery following nucleus basalis lesions in baboons: A PET study. *J Cereb Blood Flow Metab* 1987; 7:812.
215. Dail WG, Feeney DM, Murray HM, et al: Responses to cortical injury: II. Widespread depression of the activity of an enzyme in cortex remote from a focal injury. *Brain Res* 1981; 211:79.
216. Naritomi H: Transtentorial diaschisis: Reduction of cerebellar blood flow caused by supratentorial local cerebral ischemia in the gerbil. *Stroke* 1983; 14:213.
217. Deuel RK, Collins RC: Recovery from unilateral neglect. *Exp Neurol* 1983; 81:733.
218. Riese W: *Principles of Neurology in the Light of History and Their Present Use.* New York: Coolidge Foundation, 1950.
219. von Monakow C: Diaschisis [1914, trans by G. Harris], in Pribram KH (ed): *Brain and Behavior, I: Mood States and Mind.* Baltimore: Penguin, 1969: 27–36.
220. von Monakow C: *Neue Gesichtspunkte in der Frage Nach der Lokalisation im Grosshirm.* Wiesbaden: Bergman, JF, 1910.
221. Glassman RB: Recovery following sensorimotor cortical damage: Evoked potentials, brain stimulation and motor control. *Exp Neurol* 1971; 33:16.
222. West JR, Deadwyler SA, Cotman CW, Lynch GS: An experimental test of diaschisis. *Behav Biol* 1976; 18:419.
223. Glassmann RB, Malamut BL: Recovery from electroechcephalographic slowing and reduced evoked potentials after somatosensory cortical damage in cats. *Behav Biol* 1976; 17:333.
224. Meyer JS, Obara K, Muramatsu K: Diaschisis. *Neurol Res* 1993; 15:362.
225. Meyer JS: Does diaschisis have clinical correlates? *Mayo Clin Proc* 1991; 66:430.
226. Pantano P, Baron JC, Samson Y, et al: Crossed cerebellar diaschisis. *Brain* 1986; 109:677.
227. Fiorelli M, Blin J, Bakchine S, et al: PET studies of cortical diaschisis in patients with motor hemi-neglect. *J Neurol Sci* 1991; 104:135.
228. LaManna JC, Crumrine RC, Jackson DL: No correlation between cerebral blood flow and neurologic recovery after reversible total cerebral ischemia in the dog. *Exp Neurol* 1988; 101:234.
229. Sutton RL, Weaver MS, Feeney DM: Drug-induced modifications of behavioral recovery following cortical trauma. *J Head Trauma Rehabil* 1987; 2:50.
230. Davis JN, Crisostomo EA, Duncan P, et al: Amphetamine and physical therapy facilitate recovery of function from stroke: Correlative animal and human studies, in Raichle ME, Powers WJ (eds): *Cerebrovascular Diseases.* New York: Raven Press, 1987: 297–306.
231. Feeney DM, Hovda DA: Reinstatement of binocular depth perception by amphetamine and visual experience after visual cortex ablation. *Brain Res* 1985; 342:352.
232. Hovda DA, Sutton RL, Feeney DM: Amphetamine-induced recovery of visual cliff performance after bilateral visual cortex ablation in cat: Measurements of depth perception thresholds. *Behav Neurosci* 1989; 103:574.
233. Sutton RL, Hovda DA, Feeney DM: Amphetamine accelerates recovery of sensorimotor function following bilateral frontal cortex ablation in cat. *Behav Neurosci* 1989; 103:837.
234. Hovda DA, Feeney DM: Amphetamine and experience promote recovery of function after motor cortex injury in cat. *Brain Res* 1984; 298:358.
235. Feeney DM, Hovda DA: Amphetamine and apomorphine restore tactile placing after motor cortex injury in cat. *Psychopharmacology* 1983; 79:67.
236. Midgley GC, Tees RC: Reinstatement of orienting behavior by D-amphetamine in rats with superior colliculus lesions. *Behav Neurosci* 1986; 100:246.
237. M'Harzi M, Willig F, Costa JC, Delacour J: D-amphetamine enhances memory performance in rats with damage to the fimbria. *Physiol Behav* 1988; 42:575.
238. Goldstein LB: Amphetamine-facilitated functional recovery after stroke, in Ginsberg MD, Dietrich WD (eds): *Cerebrovascular Diseases.* New York: Raven Press, 1989: 303–308.
239. Hurwitz BE, Dietrich WD, McCabe PM, et al: Amphetamine-accelerated recovery from cortical barrel-field infarction: Pharmacological treatment of stroke, in Ginsberg MD, Dietrich WD (eds): *Cerebrovascular Diseases.* New York: Raven Press, 1989: 309–318.
240. Feeney DM, Gonzales A, Law WA: Amphetamine, haloperidol and experience interact to affect rate of recovery after motor cortex injury. *Science* 1982; 217:855.
241. Goldstein LB, Davis JN: Post-lesion practice and amphetamine-facilitated recovery of beam-walking in the rat. *Restor Neurol Neurosci* 1990; 1:311.
242. Feeney DM, Sutton RL: Catecholamines and recovery of function after brain damage, in Stein DG, Sabel BA (eds): *Pharmacological Approaches to the Treatment of Brain and Spinal Cord Injury.* New York: Plenum Press, 1988: 121–142.
243. Sutton RL, Feeney DM: α-Noradrenergic agonists and antagonists affect recovery and maintenance of beam-walking ability after sensorimotor cortex ablation in the rat. *Restor Neurol Neurosci* 1992; 4:1.
244. Crisostomo EA, Duncan PW, Propst M, et al: Evidence that amphetamine with physical therapy promotes recovery of motor function in stroke patients. *Ann Neurol* 1988; 23:94.

CHAPTER 109

PHARMACOLOGICAL TREATMENT APPROACHES FOR BRAIN AND SPINAL CORD TRAUMA

Alan I. Faden

INTRODUCTION

The theoretical basis for use of pharmacological treatment strategies in CNS trauma derives from the concept of delayed or secondary tissue injury.[1] First proposed near the turn of the century, this concept has been well supported by experimental studies during the past decade as well as by the demonstration that pharmacological treatments following spinal cord injury in humans reduce long-term neurological deficits.[2,3] Because hypotheses regarding delayed injury mechanisms have served as the basis for evaluation of drug therapies, it is important to understand both the nature of the interactive secondary injury cascade and its temporal profile.

SECONDARY TISSUE INJURY AFTER TRAUMA

Mechanical injury to the central nervous system causes rapid breakdown of cell membranes; subsequent phospholipid hydrolysis through the activation of phospholipases results in the release of polyunsaturated free fatty acids, including arachidonic acid, within minutes of trauma.[4–6] It has been shown that polyunsaturated free fatty acids are capable of directly injuring brain tissue and contributing to tissue edema, in part by inhibiting Na^+, K^+-ATPase.[7] Subsequent enzymatic degradation and/or metabolism lead to production of a variety of potentially toxic byproducts, including thromboxanes and leukotrienes,[8–12] as well as free radicals.[13,14] Also within minutes of trauma, there is a release of platelet activating factor (PAF), possibly through the action of phospholipase A_2; PAF can reduce tissue blood flow and disrupt the blood-brain barrier, and is thought to be directly toxic to neurons through the action of a specific ligand-gated calcium channel.[15–17] Release of eicosanoids may also exacerbate tissue damage through effects on cerebral or spinal cord blood flow, and may induce inflammatory responses.[8–12] Free radicals can also contribute to the injury process in a variety of ways, including the peroxidation of lipid membranes and associated effects on lipid-dependent enzymes, including Na^+, K^+-ATPase.[13,14]

Within 10 to 15 minutes of trauma there is a marked release of excitatory amino acids, principally glutamate,[18–20] which causes damage through NMDA receptor and possibly AMPA-kinate receptor mechanisms.[20–21] The injurious effects of NMDA receptor activation involve both Na^+ and Ca^{2+} influx,[21] as well as the induction of nitric oxide synthetase to produce nitric oxide; the latter, in the presence of free radicals, yields the toxic peroxynitrite moiety.[22] Activation of NMDA receptors also appears to play an important role in the induction of certain immediate early response genes, which subsequently may affect the transcription of other potential injury factors.[23]

Additional proinflammatory factors appear in the first hours after trauma, including cytokines [such as tumor necrosis factor alpha (TNFα) and interleukin 1 beta (IL-1β)] as well as kinins, among others.[24–26] Within the first hours after injury, increases are found in potentially pathogenic neurotransmitters or neuromodulators, such as serotonin,[27,28] norepinephrine,[28,29] acetylcholine,[30,31] and endogenous opioids.[32,33] Certain of these factors, particularly IL-1β, appear to play an important role in inducing an astroglial response to injury.[34] Astrocytic reactions may modulate the injury response by affecting various biochemical changes: acidosis,[35] excitotoxicity,[36] the activity of certain oxidative[37] and lysosomal enzymes,[38] and regenerative capabilities.[39]

Although important biochemical alterations continue well beyond the first hours of trauma,[4] such changes have not been well delineated. Information about these more delayed events is clearly needed and may provide the basis for pharmacological treatments that substantially expand the presently recognized therapeutic window.

EVALUATION OF PHARMACOLOGICAL TREATMENTS: IMPORTANT CAVEATS

A large variety of experimental methods and species have been used to study neurotrauma.[1] Although many of the proposed injury factors have been identified across a number of injury models, there may be important pathophysiological differences among them. For example, impact-induced spinal cord injury tends to cause substantial reductions in spinal cord blood flow,[40] whereas fluid percussion-induced traumatic brain injury results in more modest declines of cerebral blood flow.[41] The time frame for release of certain endogenous factors may also vary across different experimental models. For example, following fluid percussion-induced traumatic brain injury in rats, production of cytokines such as IL-1β occurs within the first hours of injury and peaks at about 8 hours[25]; in contrast, following invasive brain injury, peak production of IL-1β occurs at 2 days after trauma.[42] Treatment strategies based on antagonizing cytokine effects clearly must differ in these two types of brain injuries.

Another obvious consideration, but one too often ignored, is the fact that demonstration of effectiveness of pharmacological agents depends on choice of outcome measures that are capable of being modified by the treatment. Generally, ED_{50} models are preferred because too severe or too modest levels of injury may obscure potential treatment effects.

Drugs may also differ markedly with regard to their dose-response profiles. For example, therapeutic effects of naloxone and structurally related opioid receptor antagonists such as nalmefene show relatively narrow, bell-shaped dose-response curves with diminishing effects at doses only slightly higher or lower than optimal levels.[43] In contrast, the benzomorphan opioid receptor antagonist WIN44,441-3 (quadrazocine) has a very broad effective dose-response range.[44] Additionally, optimal therapeutic dose in one injury model or species may not necessarily translate to another model or species, making it imperative that pharmacological studies include adequate dose-response evaluations.

Because virtually all of the in vivo injury model systems that are employed require anesthetized animals, it is important to recognize that a particular anesthetic agent may modify (by either enhancing or antagonizing) the consequences of the drug being studied. For example, we have found that the TRH analogue YM14673 significantly improves motor recovery after impact spinal cord injury in rats anesthetized with pentobarbital alone, but shows no protective effects in animals anesthetized with pentobarbital plus ketamine.[45] Moreover, anesthetic agents themselves may markedly shift injury curves.[46]

Treatment time and knowledge of a drug's pharmacokinetics represent additional important considerations and, once again, may vary considerably across species. For example, the therapeutic efficacy of high-dose methylprednisolone in experimental spinal cord trauma in rats may be limited to the first 2 hours after injury (Wise Young, personal communication), but may extend to as long as 8 hours in humans.[3] Although optimal treatment strategies clearly require an understanding of the metabolism of the drug in the species being studied, this has rarely been possible in preclinical neurotrauma evaluations.

Inadequate design, or failure to use appropriate statistics, may also serve to critically affect the interpretation of drug treatment studies. For example, the use of an insufficient number of animals may contribute to a Type II statistical error, that is, concluding that there is an absence of treatment effect where one is actually present. Rarely have investigators used a power analysis based on expected differences between treated and control animals with reference to a particular outcome measure. Use of incorrect data analyses may serve to yield either false-negative or false-positive conclusions. Specific examples include: (1) failure to perform repeated measures of analysis where the value of a variable followed over time may affect its subsequent level; (2) failure to correct for multiple comparisons; (3) failure to utilize one-tailed evaluations when justified by the hypothesis being tested; (4) failure to utilize nonparametric statistics where data are either noncontinuous, or do not follow a normal distribution (e.g., as often occurs for percentage change comparisons). For all these reasons, one should be particularly cautious in giving equal weight to negative and positive drug treatment studies, unless the negative study attempted to follow precisely the methodology of a previously published positive study, or unless the study has adequately addressed such key issues as dose-response, pharmacokinetics, choice of appropriate outcome variable and model, and use of appropriate statistical methods.

DRUG TREATMENT STRATEGIES

A large number of drugs has been used in experimental models of CNS trauma with some reported success. The scope of this review is limited to classes of treatment that have most experimental support, or that reflect a persuasive underlying hypothesis regarding pathobiology.

Drugs Related to Membrane Alterations or Degradation

Steroids

Corticosteroids, particularly methylprednisolone, have been used for many years in experimental neurotrauma, initially based on their purported ability to stabilize lysosomal membranes or to reduce tissue edema.[45] Whereas many positive experimental studies using corticosteroids have been reported, a number of negative reports also have appeared.[45,47] Reasons for such differences may relate to injury model, but are more likely attributable to the type of steroid and the steroid dose.[47] It has been demonstrated in vitro that only very large doses of methylprednisolone (in the range of 30 to 60 mg/kg) significantly inhibit lipid peroxidation, providing the hypothetical basis for recent studies employing large doses.[48] Such doses of methylprednisolone have indeed been found to improve spinal cord blood flow, to reduce post-traumatic decreases in extracellular Ca^{++}, and to improve behavioral outcome after experimental spinal cord injury.[47,49] Moreover, in a large randomized multicenter clinical study, methylprednisolone—administered as a 30 mg/kg intravenous bolus injection, followed by 5.4 mg/kg/h over the ensuing 23 hours—was found to significantly enhance neurological recovery in human spinal cord injury when the drug was administered within the first 8 hours of trauma.[2,3,50] This study contrasted with the nonpositive results from earlier cooperative studies that used smaller doses of methylprednisolone,[51] as well as negative findings from a number of clinical trials of human head injury in which different steroid preparations or lower doses were utilized.[52–54]

Other compounds that inhibit lipid peroxidation also have protective activity in neural trauma models. Most notably among these have been the 21-aminosteroids (lazaroids).[55] One such compound, U-74006F or tirilazad mesylate, has been shown to improve behavioral recovery following traumatic brain injury in mice,[56] to reduce post-traumatic brain edema in rats,[57] and to limit post-traumatic ischemia[58] and improve neurological outcome[59] following spinal cord injury in cats. Although methylprednisolone and lazaroids have been proposed to work by inhibiting trauma-induced lipid peroxidation, it is likely that all mechanisms of action for these compounds have not been fully characterized.

Free Radical Scavengers and Antioxidants

Traumatic injuries cause release of free radicals by a number of mechanisms,[60–62] along with a decrease in the levels of endogenous antioxidants such as ascorbate (vitamin C), alpha-tocopherol (vitamin E), retinoic acid (vitamin A), and ubiquinones.[63–65] Treatment with vitamin C or vitamin E has been shown to provide protection in various models of CNS injury including trauma, but generally requires pre-injury administration.[14,66–68] Other agents that act as antioxidants or free radical scavengers have also been found to be beneficial; these include, among others, deferroxamine[69,70] and superoxide dismutase.[71–73]

Drugs that Inhibit Arachidonic Acid Metabolism

Potentially toxic products of arachidonic acid metabolism include thromboxanes, peptidyl-leukotrienes, hydroxy-eicosatetraenoic acids, and free radicals. The two major enzymatic pathways by which arachidonic acid is metabolized are cyclooxygenase and lipoxygenase. Both cyclooxygenase inhibitors and mixed cyclooxygenase-lipoxygenase inhibitors have been effective when administered following experimental spinal cord injury. Traumatic spinal cord ischemia in cats was reduced following administration of either cyclooxygenase inhibitors alone (meclofenamic acid or ibuprofen), or a combination of the thromboxane synthetase inhibitor (U63447A) plus a stable PGI_2 analogue (ciprostene).[74] In contrast, a 5-lipoxygenase inhibitor (piriprost) was not effective at the doses studied. A cyclooxygenase inhibitor, combined with other agents, was found to improve neurological recovery following traumatic spinal cord injury in cats.[75] Moreover, the mixed cyclooxygenase-lipoxygenase inhibitor BW7544C was shown to improve recovery following impact spinal cord injury in rats.[76] Interestingly, oligomeric prostaglandins related to PGE_1 may also be protective in rat spinal cord trauma.[77] Studies that utilize specific thromboxane or leukotriene receptor antagonists have not been reported to date, nor have strategies been employed attempting to inhibit 12-lipoxygenase or 15-lipoxygenase pathways.

GANGLIOSIDES

Potential use of gangliosides in CNS trauma has received considerable attention following a report that GM_1 treatment significantly improved neurological recovery in humans following spinal cord injury, even though the drugs were not administered until approximately 72 hours after trauma.[78] Several experimental studies have also reported that administration of gangliosides can facilitate regeneration or neurological recovery in models of CNS injury.[79,80] Potential mechanisms underlying possible effects of gangliosides may include modulation of protein kinase C,[81] release of growth factors,[82] or inhibition of release of excitatory amino acids.[83] More extensive preclinical studies of ganglioside treatment in CNS trauma are needed, as well as further studies directed to possible mechanisms of action.

DRUGS THAT MODIFY ACTIONS OF MONOAMINES

A role for catecholamines in the pathophysiology of CNS trauma remains uncertain. Studies in the 1970s suggested a pathophysiological role for both norepinephrine and dopamine in spinal cord injury.[84,85] However, changes in the levels of these catecholamines, as well as pharmacological manipulation studies, have been controversial.[45] Some studies have suggested that blockade of catecholamine synthesis or catecholamine receptors may be beneficial in spinal cord injury.[84,86] Chlorpromazine has been reported to improve motor recovery following spinal cord injury in rats,[87] and the selective destruction of descending catecholaminergic systems using 6-hydroxy-dopamine injections has been found to enhance motor recovery following spinal cord compression.[88]

There is a well-demonstrated sympatho-adrenal response following traumatic brain injury[89,90] which may be modified by clonidine, an $alpha_2$ agonist.[91] Whether treatment with norepinephrine or norepinephrine agonists is beneficial in traumatic brain injury is unclear. Whereas one study demonstrated that intraventricular administration of norepinephrine improved recovery following unilateral ablation of the sensorimotor cortex in rats,[92] a study by the same group failed to find a potential effect of the alpha agonist methoximine.[29] Clearly, more experimental work is required to clarify the role(s) for catecholamines in brain or spinal cord trauma pathophysiology, and to determine whether modulation of catecholamine production or catecholamine receptor interactions may have a therapeutic role.

There is more support for the role of acetylcholine in the secondary injury response. Experimental studies have shown that post-traumatic behavioral depression after brain injury is mediated in part through activation of cholinergic systems in brain stem.[30,31,93] Moreover, it has been found that cholinergic antagonists such as scopolamine can reduce behavioral deficits following fluid percussion-induced traumatic brain injury in rats.[94,95] Earlier clinical studies, although not well controlled, suggested a potential protective effect for atropine in traumatic brain injury.[96] However, a recently attempted double-blind randomized controlled clinical trial of scopolamine in traumatic brain injury was terminated prematurely because of psychomimetic side effects.[97] It should also be noted that, experimentally, protective effects of scopolamine have been found only when administered within 15 minutes post-injury,[98] suggesting that this approach may be limited as a clinical strategy.

Serotonin levels are increased rapidly following brain or spinal cord injury, and may be associated with post-injury edema formation.[28,99,100] Combined $5\text{-HT}_1/5\text{-HT}_2$ receptor antagonists [mianserin and (S)-emopamil] have been found to improve motor recovery after spinal cord injury, in contrast to 5-HT_2 antagonists which proved less effective.[45,101,102] Inhibition of 5-HT synthesis using P-chlorophenylalanine also was shown to reduce the depression of local cerebral glucose utilization following focal brain injury induced by freezing.[103]

GLUTAMATE RECEPTOR ANTAGONISTS

Traumatic injuries to the brain or spinal cord cause the release of large amounts of glutamate and aspartate into the extracellular space; peak levels occur within the first 15 minutes.[18–20,104] Increased extracellular levels of these excitatory amino acids correlate with injury severity.[18] In vitro studies have shown that glutamate receptors—particularly N-methyl-D-aspartate (NMDA) receptors—mediate delayed cell death caused by excitatory amino acids through influx of calcium.[21] Exogenous NMDA, when administered intrathecally, exacerbates the response to trauma; this action is not duplicated by the stereoisomer N-methyl-L-aspartate, which has a lower affinity for the NMDA receptor.[105] Both competitive and noncompetitive NMDA antagonists have been shown to improve outcome following traumatic spinal cord injury in rats.[105,106] Beneficial effects were found following either central or systemic administration, and protective actions were noted with regard to biochemical and anatomical behavioral outcome measures.[106–108] A number of groups have also demonstrated protective effects of NMDA antagonists following traumatic brain injury.[20,109–111] Again, protective effects were seen with a variety of antagonists, including competitive and noncompetitive antagonists. The latter have included infusion of magnesium salts.[112,113] Treatment with NMDA antagonists was found not only to improve neurological function, but to cause recovery in early metabolic changes, including changes in cellular bioenergetic state and free intracellular Mg levels.[20,114] A preliminary, double-blind, randomized trial of magnesium treatment suggested a protective effect in clinical head injury.[97]

Little work has been published to date using non-NMDA ionotropic glutamate-specific antagonists. However, preliminary results have suggested that blockade of AMPA kinate receptors with NBQX may be highly protective in rat traumatic spinal cord injury.[115] Use of another such antagonist, CNQX, was found to reduce post-traumatic cortical glucose utilization after fluid percussion-induced brain trauma in rats.[116]

Calcium Channel Antagonists

It has been proposed that entry of Ca through voltage dependent channels may contribute to secondary tissue injury.[117] Early results using Ca channel antagonists such as the dihydropyridines in experimental spinal cord injury did not support this hypothesis.[118–120] In part, this may reflect the hypotensive actions of these compounds, as support of blood pressure in combination with nimodipine treatment, has proved effective.[121] (S)-emopamil, which acts both as a 5-HT antagonist and as a Ca channel antagonist, has been found to improve motor recovery and cognitive function, as well as to reduce cerebral edema and the post-traumatic decline of regional cerebral blood flow following fluid percussion-induced traumatic brain injury in rats.[122,123] This drug also improves motor recovery following traumatic spinal cord injury in rats.[124] Whereas earlier clinical studies suggested that nimodipine might improve outcome following clinical head injury,[125] more recent double-blinded, controlled, randomized studies of both nimodipine[126] and nicardepine[127] have failed to show benefits for these agents.

Opiate Receptor Antagonists

Endogenous opioids may contribute to secondary injury following CNS trauma through a variety of mechanisms which include reduction of blood flow and release of excitatory amino acids, or through effects on ionic homeostasis and cellular bioenergetic state.[128] Dynorphin-like immunoreactive compounds accumulate in injured tissue following brain or spinal cord trauma in proportion to injury severity.[32,33] Administered intrathecally, dynorphin produces paralytic injury that simulates spinal cord injury with regard to behavioral, biochemical, and anatomic changes.[129–131] Administration of subinjury doses of dynorphin exacerbates the responses to both traumatic brain and spinal cord injury.[129,132] In addition, treatment with antibodies to dynorphin, but not to other endogenous opioids, reduces motor deficits following traumatic spinal cord injury.[129] Protective effects of opioid receptor antagonists have been found across a number of laboratories and models.[101,133–144] Beneficial actions have been shown for structurally different opioid receptor antagonists and are stereospecific—supporting the concept that certain pathophysiological changes in CNS trauma are mediated by opioid receptors.[128] Most significant effects have occurred utilizing drugs that have enhanced activity at kappa opioid receptors.[101,137–139,141–143] In these various models, opiate receptor antagonists have been shown to improve post-traumatic blood flow changes,[133,134,141] ionic alterations,[142–144] cellular bioenergetic state,[142,143] electrophysiology[134,135,138,140,141] histological changes,[137,138] and behavioral outcome.[133,136–139,141–143] Some laboratories have failed to find protective effects with opioid receptor antagonists[145–148]; differences may relate to methodological issues such as dosage level, experimental model, or outcome measure. Although first reports of the randomized clinical study comparing naloxone and methylprednisolone to placebo in human spinal cord injury indicated that naloxone treatment produced no statistically significant effect,[50] re-analysis of the study data with focus on nonsegmental changes suggests a significant beneficial effect for naloxone treatment.[3] It should be noted that in this clinical study the dose of naloxone used was probably too high, being on the descending portion of the bell-shaped, or inverted U-shaped, response curve.[128]

The suggestion that kappa opioid receptors may mediate pathophysiological responses in CNS trauma has been questioned by the observation that certain kappa agonist compounds may themselves be neuroprotective.[149] This apparent discrepancy may be explained by the demonstration of the existence of kappa isoreceptors.[150–152] Kappa agonists showing protective effects in CNS injury are active at the $kappa_1$ isoreceptor, yet these kappa agonists have little activity at the $kappa_2$ site in contrast to dynorphin.[151] Interestingly, the most potent opioid receptor antagonist in the treatment of CNS trauma—WIN44,441-3 (quadrazocine)[141]—has been shown to have the highest activity at the $kappa_{2\beta}$ isoreceptor.[153]

TRH and TRH Analogues

TRH was initially utilized in the treatment of spinal cord trauma because of its ability to antagonize at a physiological level many of the actions of endogenous opioids.[154] This tripeptide can also antagonize several other factors that have been implicated in secondary tissue injury following trauma, including platelet activating factor,[155] peptidyl-leukotrienes,[156] and excitatory amino acids.[157,158] TRH treatment improves neurological outcome in a variety of experimental models of spinal cord trauma.[159–161] Protective effects are dose-related and are found even when treatment is delayed as long as 24 hours after trauma.[162] Treatment with TRH has also been found to improve outcome after experimental traumatic brain injury.[163,164]

Because of the extremely short half-life of TRH, a variety of more stable TRH analogues has been evaluated in CNS trauma models. In general, analogues that preserve the integrity of the C-terminus have been found to be highly protective in injury models, whereas those that modify the C-terminal peptide have no demonstrated protective actions.[165] Compounds found to be effective include the pyroglutamyl-substituted analogues CG-3509,[166] CG-3703,[165,167,168] and YM-14673,[101,137,169–171] as well as the histidyl (imidazole)-substituted analogues 2,4 di-iodo(Im) TRH and 4(5)NO_2 (Im) TRH.[172] Beneficial effects for these various analogues have been demonstrated in a variety of species and models, including cat spinal cord[166] and brain trauma,[167] rabbit spinal cord injury,[168] and rat spinal cord[101,137,165,168–170,172] and brain trauma.[169,171] In addition to markedly enhancing post-traumatic behavior recovery following either brain or spinal cord trauma, these compounds have been found to attenuate lipid degradation,[168] restore ionic homeostasis,[167,168] and enhance cellular bioenergetic state.[167] Several laboratories have now compared effects of TRH or TRH analogue treatment with other major classes of pharmacotherapies in CNS trauma. Faden and colleagues showed that treatment with TRH or TRH analogues is more effective than treatment with an opioid receptor antagonist.[173] Behrmann et al. reported that treatment with YM14673 is significantly better than that with optimal dose methylprednisolone[170] or the opioid receptor antagonist nalmefene[137] in improving outcome after rat spinal cord trauma. Puniak et al. found that YM14673 provides better protection than either a 5-HT antagonist or nalmefene following rat spinal cord injury.[101] Faden showed that YM14673 treatment was superior to treatment with nalmefene or the NMDA antagonists dextrorphan and magnesium.[174] Thus, in direct testing, TRH analogues appear to be superior to other major classes of treatments that have been studied to date. In a preliminary randomized trial using TRH infusions in human spinal cord injury, there was a suggestive clinical benefit to TRH treatment in patients with incomplete injuries.[174A]

Platelet Activating Factor Antagonists

PAF administered intrathecally causes profound dose-dependent decreases in spinal cord blood flow that are receptor-mediated.[16] Pretreatment with several structurally indifferent PAF receptor antagonists has been found to improve neurological recovery following fluid percussion-induced traumatic brain injury in rats.[17] However, treatment after trauma was not beneficial, suggesting that this class of compounds is likely to have little clinical utility.[17]

OTHER TREATMENT STRATEGIES

Several reports have suggested a potential therapeutic role for anion transport inhibitors.[175,176] Kimelberg et al. have shown that the anion exchange inhibitor L-644,711 reduces mortality, EEG abnormalities, and neurological deficits following traumatic-hypoxic brain injury in cats.[175]

A variety of studies have implicated the cytokines TNFα and IL-1β in traumatic brain injury.[24,25,42] One report has found protection against postischemic brain injury using a recombinant form of the endogenous IL-1 receptor antagonist.[177] Other potential treatment strategies that may antagonize IL-1β effects include the use of monoclonal antibodies, and possibly the endogenous compound lipocortin-1.[178] TNF antibodies are also available and may provide a basis for future experimental treatment strategies.

In traumatic brain injury, few treatments have been evaluated that have sought specifically to attenuate the post-traumatic inflammatory response. This strategy has, however, been examined in a spinal cord ischemia model that showed that the compounds chloroquine and colchicine significantly reduce postischemic inflammatory changes and limit subsequent tissue damage.[179]

It is also important to remember that post-injury reactive responses, including the release of neurotrophic factors, may continue for weeks.[180] Treatment with neurotrophic factors can enhance neuronal survival in various brain lesion models,[180,181] but has not yet been shown to enhance functional recovery in standardized trauma models.

Combination treatment strategies have been utilized with, at most, limited success. In a recent study, Faden found no additive or synergistic effects among a TRH analogue, an opioid receptor antagonist, and NMDA antagonists, when used in combination.[174] Indeed, effects of the TRH analogue and the NMDA antagonist were mutually inhibitory, raising potential concerns about the use of combination treatment strategies. Sequential or serial treatment strategies, based on recognition of the temporal profile of the secondary injury cascade, may provide a promising future approach.

FUTURE DIRECTIONS

Further delineation of the pathophysiological mechanisms involved in secondary tissue damage after CNS trauma are likely to suggest additional novel treatment strategies. Better elucidation of the time course for the appearance of specific injury factors may lead to better treatment. Demonstrated effectiveness of methylprednisolone[2] and, more recently, naloxone[3] in the treatment of human spinal cord injury has provided strong support for the concept of secondary injury, and for the use of animal model systems to evaluate novel experimental treatment strategies. The recent establishment of a consortium of experimental spinal cord injury centers to evaluate new drug treatments, and the proposal to establish a similar consortium for experimental traumatic brain injury, should markedly enhance the evaluation of experimental treatments for potential clinical use.

REFERENCES

1. Faden AI: Experimental neurobiology of central nervous system trauma. *Crit Rev Neurobiol* 1993; 7(3/4): 175–186.
2. Bracken MB, Shepard MJ, Collins WF, et al: A randomized controlled trial of methylprednisolone or naloxone in the treatment of acute spinal cord injury: Results of the second national acute spinal cord injury study. *N Engl J Med* 1990; 322:1405–1411.
3. Bracken MB, Holford TR: Effects of timing of methylprednisolone or naloxone administration on recovery of segmental and long-tract neurological function in NASCIS 2. *J Neurosurg* 1993; 79:500–507.
4. Faden AI, Chan PH, Longar S: Alterations in lipid metabolism, (Na^+, K^+)-ATPase activity, and tissue water content of spinal cord following experimental traumatic injury. *J Neurochem* 1987; 48:1809–1816.
5. Demediuk P, Clendenon NR, Means ED, et al: Changes in lipid metabolism in traumatized spinal cord. *Prog Brain Res* 1985; 63:211–226.
6. Wei EP, Lamb RG, Kontos HW: Increased phospholipase C activity after experimental brain injury. *J Neurosurg* 1982; 56:695–698.
7. Chan PH, Fishman RA: The role of arachidonic acid in vasogenic brain edema. *Fed Proc* 1984; 43:210–213.
8. Hsu CY, Halushka PV, Hogan EL, et al: Alteration of thromboxane and prostacyclin levels in experimental spinal cord injury. *Neurology* 1985; 35:1003–1009.
9. Demediuk P, Faden AI: Traumatic spinal cord injury in rats causes increases in tissue thromboxane but not peptidoleukotrienes. *J Neurosci* 1988; 20(1):115–121.
10. Shohami E, Shapira Y, Sidi A, Cotev S: Head injury induces increased prostaglandin synthesis in rat brain. *J Cereb Blood Flow Metab* 1987; 7:58–63.
11. Kiwak KJ, Moskowitz MA, Levine L: Leukotriene production in gerbil brain after ischemic insult, subarachnoid hemorrhage and concussive injury. *J Neurosurg* 1985; 62:865–869.
12. DeWitt DS, Kong DL, Lyeth BG, et al: Experimental traumatic brain injury elevates brain prostaglandin E_2 and thromboxane B_2 levels in rats. *J Neurotrauma* 1988; 5:303–313.
13. Kontos H, Povlishock J: Oxygen radicals in brain injury. *J Neurotrauma* 1986; 3:257–263.
14. Hall E, Braughler J: Role of lipid peroxidation in posttraumatic spinal cord degeneration—a review. *J Neurotrauma* 1986; 3:281–294.
15. Yue T-L, Feuerstein GZ: Platelet-activating factor—a putative neuromodulator and mediator in the pathophysiology of brain injury. *Crit Rev Neurobiol* 1994; 8(1/2):11–24.
16. Faden AI, Halt P: Platelet-activating factor reduces spinal cord blood flow and causes behavioral deficits after intrathecal administration in rats through a specific receptor mechanism. *J Pharmacol Exp Ther* 1992; 261(3):1064–1070.
17. Faden AI, Tzendalian P: Platelet-activating factor antagonists limit glycine changes and behavioral deficits after brain trauma. *Am J Physiol* 1992; 263:R909–R914.
18. Panter SS, Yum SW, Faden AI: Alteration in extracellular amino acids after traumatic spinal cord injury. *Ann Neurol* 1990; 27:96–99.
19. Nilsson P, Hillered L, Ponten U, Ungerstedt U: Changes in cortical extracellular levels of energy-related metabolites and amino acids following concussive brain injury in rats. *J Cereb Blood Flow Metab* 1990; 10:631–637.
20. Faden AI, Demediuk P, Panter SS, Vink R: The role of excitatory amino acids and NMDA receptors in traumatic brain injury. *Science* 1989; 244:798–800.
21. Choi DW: Ionic dependence of glutamate neurotoxicity. *J Neurosci* 1987; 7:369–379.
22. Lipton SA: Prospects for clinically tolerated NMDA antagonists: Open-channel blockers and alternative redox states of nitric acid. *Trends Neurosci Sci* 1993; 16(12):527–532.
23. Dragunow M, Goulding M, Faull RLM, et al: Induction of c-fos mRNA and protein in neurons and glia after traumatic brain injury: Pharmacological characterization. *Exp Neurol* 1990; 107:236–248.
24. Giulian D, Chen J, Ingeman J, et al: The role of mononuclear phagocytes in wound healing after traumatic injury to adult mammalian brain. *J Neurosci* 1989; 9(12):4416–4429.
25. Taupin V, Toulmond S, Serrano A, et al: Increase in IL-6, IL-1 and TNF levels in rat brain following traumatic lesion. *J Neuroimmunol* 1993; 42:177–186.
26. Xu J, Hsu CY, Chao S, et al: Kininogen and kinin in experimental spinal cord injury. *J Neurochem* 1991; 57:975–980.
27. Salzman S, Mendez AA, Dabney KW, et al: Serotonergic response to spinal distraction trauma in experimental scoliosis. *J Neurotrauma* 1991; 8:45–54.
28. Liu D, Valadez V, Sorkin LS, MacAdoo DJ: Norepinephrine and serotonin release upon impact injury to rat spinal cord. *J Neurotrauma* 1990; 7:219–227.

29. Feeney DM, Westerberg VS: Norepinephrine and brain damage: Alpha noradrenergic pharmacology alters functional recovery after cortical trauma. *Can J Psychol* 1990; 44:233–252.
30. Hayes R, Stonnington H, Lyeth B, et al: Metabolic and neurophysiologic sequelae of brain injury: A cholinergic hypothesis. *J Neurotrauma* 1986; 3:163–173.
31. Saija A, Hayes R, Lyeth B, et al: The effect of concussive head injury on central cholinergic neurons. *Brain Res* 1988; 452:303–311.
32. McIntosh TK, Head VA, Faden AI: Alterations in regional concentrations of endogenous opioids following traumatic brain injury in the cat. *Brain Res* 1987; 425:225–233.
33. Faden AI, Molineaux CJ, Rosenberger JG, et al: Endogenous opioid immunoreactivity in rat spinal cord following traumatic injury. *Ann Neurol* 1985; 17:386–390.
34. Giulian D, Lachman LB: Interleukin-1 stimulation of astroglial proliferation after brain injury. *Science* 1985; 228:497–499.
35. Chelser M: The regulation and modulation of pH in the nervous system. *Prog Neurobiol* 1990; 34:401.
36. Kimelberg HK, Pang S, Treble DH: Excitatory amino acid-stimulated uptake of $^{22}Na^{+}$ in primary astrocyte cultures. *J Neurosci* 1989; 9:1141–1149.
37. Friede RL: The enzymatic response of astrocytes to various ions in vitro. *J Cell Biol* 1964; 20:5–15.
38. Vijakan VK, Cotman CW: Lysosomal enzyme changes in young and aged control and entorrhinal-lesioned rats. *Neurobiol Aging* 1983; 4:13.
39. Boloventa P, Wandosell F, Nieto-Sampedro M: CNS glial scar tissue: A source of molecules which inhibit central neurite outgrowth, in Yu ACH, Hertz L, Norenberg MD, Sykova E, Waxman SG (eds): *Neuronal-Astrocytic Interactions: Implications for Normal and Pathological CNS Function.* Amsterdam: Elsevier, 1992; 94:367–379.
40. Sandler AN, Tator CH: Review of the effect of spinal cord trauma on the vessels and blood flow in the spinal cord. *J Neurosurg* 1967; 5:638–646.
41. Yamakami I, McIntosh TK: Effects of traumatic brain injury on regional blood flow in rats measured with radiolabelled microspheres. *J Cereb Blood Flow Metab* 1989; 9:117–124.
42. Woodroofe MN, Sarna GS, Wadhwa M, et al: Detection of interleukin-1 and interleukin-6 in adult rat brain, following mechanical injury, by in vivo microdialysis: Evidence of a role for microglia in cytokine production. *J Neuroimmunol* 1991; 33:227–236.
43. Faden AI, Sacksen I, Nobel LJ: Opiate receptor antagonist nalmefene improves neurological recovery after traumatic spinal cord injury in rats through a central mechanism. *J Pharmacol Exp Ther* 1988; 245:742–748.
44. McIntosh TK, Hayes RL, DeWitt DS, et al: Endogenous opioids may mediate secondary damage after experimental brain injury. *Am J Physiol* 1987; 253:E565–E574.
45. Faden AI, Salzman SK: Experimental pharmacology, in Salzman S, Faden AI (eds): *The Neurobiology of CNS Trauma.* New York: Oxford University Press, 1994; 22:227–244.
46. Halt PS, Swanson RA, Faden AI: Alcohol exacerbates behavioral and neurochemical effects of rat spinal cord trauma. *Arch Neurol* 1992; 49:1178–1184.
47. Braughler JM, Hall ED: High dose methylprednisolone and CNS injury. *J Neurosurg* 1988; 64:985–986.
48. Braughler JM, Hall ED: Correlation of methylprednisolone levels in cat spinal cord with its effect on $[Na^{++}K^{+}]$-ATPase, lipid peroxidation, and alpha motor neuron function. *J Neurosurg* 1982; 56:838–844.
49. Young W, Flamm ES: Effect of high dose corticosteroid therapy on blood flow, evoked potentials and extracellular calcium in experimental spinal contusion. *J Neurosurg* 1982; 55:209–219.
50. Bracken BM, Shepard MJ, Collins WF Jr, et al: Methylprednisolone or naloxone treatment after acute spinal cord injury: 1-year follow-up data. Results of the second National Acute Spinal Cord Injury Study. *J Neurosurg* 1992; 76:23–31.
51. Bracken MB, Collins WF, Freeman DF, et al: Efficacy of methylprednisolone in acute spinal cord injury. *JAMA* 1984; 251:45–52.
52. Cooper PR, Moody S, Clark WK, et al: Dexamethasone and severe head injury: A prospective double blind study. *J Neurosurg* 1979; 51:307–316.
53. Gudeman SK, Miller JD, Becker DP: Failure of high dose steroid therapy to influence intracranial pressure in patients with severe head injury. *J Neurosurg* 1979; 51:301–306.
54. Braakman R, Schouten HJA, Blaauw-van Dishoeck M, et al: Megadose steroids in severe head injury, results of a prospective double-blind trial. *J Neurosurg* 1983; 58:326–330.
55. Braughler JM, Pregenzer JF, Chase RL: Novel 21-aminosteroids as potent inhibitors of iron-dependent lipid peroxidation. *J Biol Chem* 1987; 262:10438–10440.
56. Hall ED, Yonkers PA, McCall JM, Braughler JM: Effects of the 21-aminosteroid U-74006F on experimental head injury in mice. *J Neurosurg* 1988; 68:456–461.
57. McIntosh TK, Thomas M, Smith DF, Banbury M: The novel 21-aminosteroid U74006F attenuates cerebral edema and improves survival after brain injury in the rat. *J Neurotrauma* 1992; 9:33–46.
58. Hall ED: Effects of the 21-aminosteroid U-74006F on post-traumatic spinal cord ischemia in cats. *J Neurosurg* 1988; 68:462–465.
59. Anderson DK, Braughler JM, Hall ED, et al: Effect of treatment with U-74006F on neurological outcome following experimental spinal cord injury. *J Neurosurg* 1988; 69:562–567.
60. Hall ED, Wolf DL: A pharmacological analysis of the pathophysiological mechanisms of post-traumatic spinal cord ischemia. *J Neurosurg* 1986; 64:951–961.
61. Panter SS, Faden AI: Biochemical changes and secondary injury from stroke and trauma, in Young RR, Delwade PJ (eds): *Principles and Practice of Restorative Neurology,* New York: Butterworths, 1992: Chap 4.
62. Kontos H, Povlishock J: Oxygen radicals in brain injury. *J Neurotrauma* 1986; 3:257–263.
63. Lemke M, Frei B, Ames BN, Faden AI: Decreases in tissue levels of ubiquinol-9 and -10, ascorbate and alpha-

tocopherol following spinal cord impact trauma in rats. *Neurosci Lett* 1990; 108:201–206.

64. Anderson DK, Means ED: Iron-induced lipid peroxidation in spinal cord: Protection with mannitol and methylprednisolone. *J Free Radic Biol Med* 1985; 1:59–64.
65. Pietonegro DD, Hovsepian M, Demopoulos HB, Flamm ES: Loss of ascorbic acid from injured feline spinal cord. *J Neurochem* 1983; 41:1072–1076.
66. Yoshida S, Busto R, Ginsberg MD, et al: Compression-induced brain edema: Modification by prior depletion and supplementation of vitamin E. *Neurology* 1983; 33:166–172.
67. Clifton GL, Lyeth BG, Jenkins LW, et al: Effect of D1 α-tocopherol succinate and polyethylene glycol on performance tests after fluid percussion brain injury. *J Neurotrauma* 1989; 6:71–81.
68. Anderson DK, Waters TR, Means ED: Pretreatment with α-tocopherol enhances neurologic recovery after experimental spinal cord injury. *J Neurotrauma* 1988; 5:61–68.
69. Ikeda Y, Ikeda K, Long DM: Protective effect of the iron chelator deferroxamine on cold-induced brain edema. *J Neurosurg* 1989; 71:233–238.
70. Panter SS, Braughler JM, Hall ED: Dextran-coupled deferroxamine improves outcome in a murine model of head injury. *J Neurotrauma* 1992; 9:47–53.
71. Wei EP, Kontos HA, Dietrich WD, et al: Inhibition by free radical scavengers and by cyclooxygenase inhibitors of pial arteriolar abnormalities from concussive brain injury in cats. *Circ Res* 1981; 48:95–103.
72. Lim KH, Connolly M, Rose D, et al: Prevention of reperfusion injury of the ischemic spinal cord: Use of recombinant superoxide dismutase. *Ann Thorac Surg* 1986; 42:282–286.
73. Chan P, Longar S, Fishman R: Protective effects of liposome-entrapped superoxide dismutase on post-traumatic brain edema. *Ann Neurol* 1987; 21:540–547.
74. Hall ED, Wolf DL, Braughler JM: Pathophysiology, consequences and pharmacological prevention of post-traumatic CNS ischemia, in Gilad GM, Gorio A, Kreutzberg GW (eds): *Processes of Recovery from Neural Trauma.* Berlin: Springer-Verlag, 1986: 63–73.
75. Hallenbeck JM, Jacobs TP, Faden AI: Combined PGI_2, indomethacin, and heparin improve neurological recovery after spinal trauma in cats. *J Neurosurg* 1983; 58:749–754.
76. Faden AI, Lemke M, Demediuk P: Effects of BW755C, a mixed cyclooxygenase lipoxygenase inhibitor following traumatic spinal cord injury in rats. *Brain Res* 1988; 463:63–68.
77. Ohnishi ST, Barr JK, Katagi C, Katsukasa M: Protection of rat spinal cord against contusion injury by new prostaglandin derivatives. *Arnzneim-Forsch/Drug Res* 1989; 39:236–239.
78. Geisler FH, Dorsey FC, Coleman WP: Recovery of motor function after spinal cord injury: Randomized placebo trial with GM_1 ganglioside. *N Engl J Med* 1991; 324:1829–1838.
79. Bose B, Osterholm JL, Kalia M: Ganglioside-induced regeneration and reestablishment of axonal continuity in spinal cord transected rats. *Neurosci Lett* 1986; 63:165–169.
80. Karpiak SE, Li YS, Mahadik SP: Ganglioside treatment: Reduction of CNS injury and facilitation of functional recovery. *Brain Inj* 1987; 1:161–170.
81. Magel E, Louis J-C, Aguilera J, Yavin E: Gangliosides prevent ischemia-induced down regulation of protein kinase C in fetal rat brain. *J Neurochem* 1990; 55:2126–2131.
82. Cuello AC, Garofalo L, Kenigsberg RL, Maysinger D: Gangliosides potentiate in vivo and in vitro effects of nerve growth factor on central cholinergic neurons. *Proc Natl Acad Sci USA* 1989; 86:2056–2060.
83. Nicoletti F, Cavallaro S, Bruno S, et al: Gangliosides attenuate NMDA receptor-mediated excitatory amino acid release in cultured cerebellar neurons. *Neuropharmacology* 1989; 28:1283–1286.
84. Osterholm JL, Matthews GJ: Altered norepinephrine metabolism following experimental spinal cord injury. Part 1: Relationship to hemorrhagic necrosis and post-wounding neurological deficits. *J Neurosurg* 1972; 36:386–394.
85. Naftchi NE, Demeny M, DeCrescito V: Biogenic amino concentrations in traumatized spinal cords of cats. Effect of drug therapy. *J Neurosurg* 1974; 40:52–57.
86. Dow-Edwards D, DeCrescito V, Tomasula JJ, Flamm ES: Effect of aminophylline and isoproterenol on spinal cord blood flow after impact injury. *J Neurosurg* 1980; 53:385–390.
87. Sadanaga K, Ohnishi ST: Chlorpromazine protects rat spinal cord against contusion injury. *J Neurotrauma* 1989; 6:153–161.
88. Yone K: Role of endogenous norepinephrine in microcirculation after experimental acute spinal cord injury. *J Jpn Orthop Assoc* 1988; 62:389–398.
89. Rosner MJ, Newsome HH, Becker DP: Mechanical brain injury: The sympathoadrenal response. *J Neurosurg* 1984; 61:76–86.
90. Hamill RW, Woolf PD, McDonald JV, et al: Catecholamines predict outcome in traumatic brain injury. *Ann Neurol* 1987; 21:438–443.
91. Payen D, Quintin L, Plaisance P, et al: Head injury: Clonidine decreases plasma catecholamines. *Crit Care Med* 1990; 18:392–395.
92. Boyeson MG, Feeney DM: Intraventricular norepinephrine facilitates motor recovery following sensorimotor cortex injury. *Pharmacol Biochem Behav* 1990; 35:497–501.
93. Hayes R, Pechura VM, Katayama Y, et al: Activation of pontine cholinergic sites implicated in unconsciousness following cerebral concussion in the cat. *Science* 1984; 223:301–303.
94. Lyeth BG, Dixon CE, Hamm RJ, et al: Effects of anticholinergic treatment on transient behavioral suppression and physiological responses following concussive brain injury to the rat. *Brain Res* 1988; 448:88–97.
95. Lyeth BG, Dixon CE, Jenkins LW, et al: Effect of scopolamine pretreatment on long term behavioral deficits following concussive brain injury in the rat. *Brain Res* 1988; 452:39–48.

96. Ward A Jr: Atropine and the treatment of closed head injury. *J Neurosurg* 1950; 7:398–401.
97. McIntosh TK: Novel pharmacologic therapies in the treatment of experimental traumatic brain injury: A review. *J Neurotrauma* 1993; 10(3):215–256.
98. Lyeth BG, Ray M, Hamm RJ, et al: Postinjury scopolamine administration in experimental traumatic brain injury. *Brain Res* 1992; 569:281–286.
99. Salzman SK, Mendez AA, Dabney KW, et al: Serotonergic response to spinal distraction trauma in experimental scoliosis. *J Neurotrauma* 1991; 8:45–54.
100. Pappius HM, Dadoun R: Effects of injury on the indoleamines in cerebral cortex. *J Neurochem* 1987; 49:321–325.
101. Puniak MA, Freeman GM, Agresta CA, et al: Comparison of a serotonin antagonist, opioid antagonist and TRH analog for the acute treatment of experimental spinal trauma. *J Neurotrauma* 1991; 8:193–203.
102. Salzman SK, Puniak MA, Liu T-J, et al: The serotonin antagonist mianserin improves the functional recovery following experimental spinal trauma. *Ann Neurol* 1991; 521:33–39.
103. Pappius HM, Dadoun R, McHugh M: The effect of p-chlorophenylalanine on cerebral metabolism and biogenic amine content of traumatic brain. *J Cereb Blood Flow Metab* 1988; 8:324–334.
104. Katayama Y, Cheung MK, Alves A, Becker DP: Ion fluxes and cell swelling in experimental traumatic brain injury: The role of excitatory amino acids, in Hoff JT, Betz AL (eds): *Intracranial Pressure VII.* Berlin: Springer-Verlag, 1989: 584–588.
105. Faden AI, Simon RP: A potential role for excitotoxins in the pathophysiology of spinal cord injury. *Ann Neurol* 1988; 23:623–626.
106. Faden AI, Ellison JA, Noble LJ: Effects of competitive and noncompetitive NMDA receptor antagonists in spinal cord injury. *Eur J Pharmacol* 1990; 175:165–174.
107. Faden AI, Lemke RP, Simon RP, Noble LJ: N-methyl-D-aspartate antagonist MK-801 improves outcome following traumatic spinal cord injury in rats: Behavioral, anatomical and neurochemical studies. *J Neurotrauma* 1988; 5:33–45.
108. Gomez-Pinilla F, Tram H, Cotman CW, Nieto-Sampedro M: Neuroprotective effect of MK-801 and U-50488H after contussive spinal cord injury. *Exp Neurol* 1989; 104:118–124.
109. McIntosh TK, Vink R, Soares H, et al: Effects of N-methyl-D-aspartate receptor blocker MK-801 on neurologic function after experimental brain injury. *J Neurotrauma* 1989; 6:247–259.
110. Hayes RL, Jenkins LW, Lyeth BG, et al: Pretreatment with phencyclidine, an N-methyl-D-aspartate antagonist, attenuates long-term behavioral deficits in the rat produced by traumatic brain injury. *J Neurotrauma* 1988; 5:259–274.
111. Shapira Y, Yadid G, Cotev A, et al: Protective effect of MK-801 in experimental brain injury. *J Neurotrauma* 1990; 7:131–139.
112. Vink R, McIntosh TK, Demediuk P, et al: Decline in intracellular free Mg^{++} is associated with irreversible tissue injury after brain trauma. *J Biol Chem* 1988; 263:757–761.
113. McIntosh TK, Faden AI, Yamakami I, Vink R: Magnesium deficiency exacerbates and pretreatment improves outcome following traumatic brain injury in rats: ^{31}P Magnetic resonance spectroscopy and behavioral studies. *J Neurotrauma* 1988; 5:17–31.
114. McIntosh TK, Vink R, Soares H, et al: Effect of noncompetitive blockade of N-methyl-D-aspartate receptors on the neurochemical sequelae of experimental brain injury. *J Neurochem* 1990; 55:170–179.
115. Wrathall JR, Yang DT, Choiniere D, Mundt DJ: Evidence that local non-NMDA receptors contribute to functional deficits in contusive spinal cord injury. *Brain Res* 1992; 586:140–143.
116. Kawamata T, Katayama T, Hovda DA, et al: Administration of excitatory amino acid antagonists via microdialysis attenuates the increase in glucose utilization seen following concussive brain injury. *J Cereb Blood Flow Metab* 1992; 17:12–24.
117. Young W: The role of calcium in spinal cord injury. *CNS Trauma* 1985; 2:109.
118. Cheng MK, Robertson C, Grossman RG: Neurological outcome correlated with spinal evoked potentials in a spinal cord ischemia model. *J Neurosurg* 1984; 60:786–795.
119. Faden AI, Jacobs TP, Smith MT: Evaluation of the calcium channel antagonist nimodipine in experimental spinal cord ischemia. *J Neurosurg* 1984; 60:796–799.
120. Ford WJ, Malm DN: Failure of nimodipine to reverse acute experimental spinal cord injury. *CNS Trauma* 1985; 2:9–17.
121. Ross IB, Tator CH: Further studies of nimodipine in experimental spinal cord injury in the rat. *J Neurotrauma* 1991; 8:229–239.
122. Okiyama K, Smith DH, Gennarelli TA, McIntosh TK: Evaluation of a novel calcium channel blocker (S)-emopamil on regional cerebral edema and neurobehavioral function after experimental brain injury. *J Neurosurg* 1992; 77:607–615.
123. Okiyama K, Smith DH, Gennarelli TA, McIntosh TK: (S)-emopamil attenuates regional cerebral blood flow reductions following experimental brain injury. *J Neurotrauma* 1994; 11(1):83–95.
124. Salzman SK, Chavin JM, Wang L, et al: S-emopamil improves functional recovery from experimental spinal trauma. *J Neurotrauma* 1993; 9:69.
125. Kostron H, Twerdy K, Stampfl G, et al: Treatment of the traumatic cerebral vasospasm with the calcium channel blocker nimodipine. *Neurol Res* 1984; 6:29–32.
126. Teasdale G: A randomized trial of nimodipine in severe head injury: HIT 1. *J Neurotrauma* 1991; 9:S545–S550.
127. Compton JS, Lee T, Jones NC, et al: A double-blind placebo controlled trial of the calcium entry blocking drug nicardipine in the treatment of vasospasm following severe head injury. *Br J Neurosurg* 1990; 4:9–16.
128. Faden AI: Role of endogenous opioids and opioid receptors in central nervous system injury, in Herz A (ed): *Handbook of Experimental Pharmacology. Vol 104/II*

Opioids II. Berlin: Springer-Verlag, 1993: Chap 43, 325–341.

129. Faden AI: Opioid and non-opioid mechanisms may contribute to dynorphin's pathophysiological actions in spinal cord injury. *Ann Neurol* 1990; 27:67–74.
130. Bakshi R, Newman AH, Faden AI: Dynorphin A-(1-17) induces alterations in free fatty acids of excitatory amino acids, and motor function through an opiate receptor-mediated mechanism. *J Neurosci* 1990; 10:3793–3800.
131. Bakshi R, Ni R, Faden AI: N-methyl-D-aspartate and opioid receptors mediate dynorphin-induced spinal cord injury: Behavioral and histological studies. *Brain Res* 1992; 580:255–264.
132. McIntosh TK, Romhanyi R, Yamakami I, Faden AI: Exacerbation of traumatic brain injury following central administration of kappa-opiate receptor agonists. *Soc Neurosci Abstr* 1988; 14:1152.
133. Faden AI, Jacobs TP, Holaday JW: Endorphins in experimental spinal injury: Therapeutic effect of naloxone. *Ann Neurol* 1981; 10:326–332.
134. Young W, Flamm ES, Demopoulos HB, et al: Naloxone ameliorates post-traumatic ischemia in experimental spinal contusion. *J Neurosurg* 1981; 55:209–219.
135. Inoue Y: Evoked spinal potentials in the Wistar rat: Effect of cord compression and drugs. *Nippon Seikeigeka Gakkai Zasshi* 1986; 60:777–785.
136. Arias MJ: Effect of naloxone on functional recovery after experimental spinal cord injury in the rat. *Surg Neurol* 1985; 23:440–442.
137. Behrmann DL, Bresnahan JC, Beattie MS: A comparison of YM-14673, U-50488H, and nalmefene after spinal cord injury in the rat. *Exp Neurol* 1993; 119:258–267.
138. Faden AI, Sacksen L, Noble LJ: Opiate receptor antagonist nalmefene improves neurologic recovery after traumatic spinal cord injury in rats through a central mechanism. *J Pharmacol Exp Ther* 1988; 245:742–748.
139. Faden AI, Takemori AE, Portoghese TS: κ-selective opiate antagonist norbinaltorphimine improves outcome after traumatic spinal cord injury in rats. *CNS Trauma* 1987; 4:227–237.
140. Hayes R, Galinet BJ, Kulkarne P: Effects of naloxone on systemic cerebral responses to experimental concussive brain injury in cats. *J Neurosurg* 1983; 58:720–728.
141. McIntosh TK, Hayes RL, DeWitt DS, et al: Endogenous opioids may mediate secondary damage after experimental brain injury. *Am J Physiol* 1987; 253:E565–E574.
142. Vink R, McIntosh TK, Rhomhanyi R, Faden AI: Opiate antagonist nalmefene improves intracellular free Mg^{2+}, bioenergetic state, and neurologic outcome following traumatic brain injury in rats. *J Neurosci* 10:3524–3530.
143. Vink R, Portoghese PS, Faden AI: Kappa-opioid antagonist improves cellular bioenergetics and recovery after traumatic brain injury. *Am J Physiol* 1991; 261: R1527–R1532.
144. Stokes BT, Hollinden G, Fox P: Improvement in injury induced hypocalcia by high-dose naloxone intervention. *Brain Res* 1984; 290:187–190.
145. Hoerlein BF, Redding RW, Hoff EJ, McGuire JA: Evaluation of naloxone, crocetin, thyrotropin releasing hormone, methylprednisolone, partial myelotomy and hemilaminectomy in the treatment of acute spinal cord trauma. *J Am Anim Hosp Assoc* 1985; 2:67–77.
146. Wallace MC, Tator CH: Failure of naloxone to improve spinal cord blood flow and cardiac output after spinal cord injury. *Neurosurgery* 1986; 18:428–432.
147. Black P, Markowitz RS, Keller S, et al: Naloxone and experimental spinal cord injury: Part 1. High dose administration in a static load compression model. *Neurosurgery* 1986; 19:905–908.
148. Holtz A, Nystrom B, Gerdin B: Blocking weight-induced spinal cord injury in rats: Effects of TRH or naloxone on motor function recovery and spinal cord blood flow. *Acta Neurol Scand* 1989; 80:215–220.
149. Hall ED, Wolf DL, Althaus JS, Von Voigtlander PF: Beneficial effects of kappa opioid antagonist U50488H in acute CNS trauma models. *Brain Res* 1987; 435:174–180.
150. Gouarderes C, Attali B, Audigier Y, Cros J: Interaction of selective mu and delta ligands with the $kappa_2$ subtype of opiate binding sites. *Life Sci* 1983; 33(suppl 1): 175–178.
151. Zukin RS, Eghbali M, Olive D, et al: Characterization and visualization of rat and guinea pig κ-opiate receptors: Evidence of κ_1 and κ_2 receptors. *Proc Natl Acad Sci USA* 1988; 85:4061–4065.
152. Clark JA, Liu L, Price M, et al: Kappa opiate receptor multiplicity: Evidence of two U50,488-sensitive κ_1 subtypes and a novel κ_3 subtype. *J Pharmacol Exp Ther* 1989; 251(2):461–468.
153. Rothman RB, Bykov V, deCosta BR, et al: Interaction of endogenous opioid peptides and other drugs with four kappa opioid binding sites in guinea pig brain. *Peptides* 1990; 11:311–331.
154. Holaday JW, Tseng LF, Loh HH, Li CH: Thyrotropin releasing hormone antagonizes beta-endorphin hypothermia and catalepsy. *Life Sci* 1978; 22:1537–1543.
155. Feuerstein G, Lux WE Jr, Snyder R, et al: Hypotension produced by platelet-activating factor is reversed by thyrotropin-releasing hormone. *Circ Shock* 1984; 13:255–260.
156. Lux WE Jr., Feuerstein G, Faden AI: Alteration of leukotriene D4 hypotension by thyrotropin releasing hormone. *Nature* 1983; 302:822–824.
157. Renaud LP, Blumne HW, Pittman QJ, et al: Thyrotropin-releasing hormone selectively depresses glutamate excitation of cerebral cortical neurons. *Science* 1979; 205:1275–1276.
158. Yoshida M, Izumi K, Nakashini T: Effects of thyrotropin-releasing hormone (TRH) on glutamate-induced seizures in rats. *Tohoku J Exp Med* 1987; 152:311–317.
159. Faden AI, Jacobs TP, Holaday JW: Thyrotropin-releasing hormone improves neurological recovery after spinal trauma in cats. *N Engl J Med* 1981; 305:1063–1067.
160. Arias MJ: Treatment of experimental spinal cord injury with TRH, naloxone and dexamethasone. *Surg Neurol* 1987; 28:335–338.
161. Hashimoto T, Fukuda N: Ameliorating effect of TRH on neurologic impairment induced by spinal cord compression in rats. *Jpn J Pharmacol* 1989; 49(suppl):312P.

162. Faden AI, Jacobs TP, Smith MT: Thyrotropin-releasing hormone in experimental spinal cord injury: Dose response and late treatment. *Neurology* 1984; 34:1280–1284.
163. Manaka S, Sano K: Thyrotropin-releasing hormone tartrate (TRH-t) shortens concussion effects following head impact in mice. *Neurosci Lett* 1978; 8:255–258.
164. Fukuda N, Yoshiaki S, Nagawa Y: Behavioral and EEG alterations with brain stem compression and effect of thyrotropin-releasing hormone (TRH) in chronic cats. *Folio Pharmacol Japan* 1979; 75:321–331.
165. Faden AI, Sacksen I, Noble LJ: Structure-activity relationships of TRH analogs in experimental spinal injury. *Brain Res* 1987; 448:287–293.
166. Faden AI, Jacobs TP: Effect of TRH analogs on neurologic recovery after experimental spinal trauma. *Neurology* 1985; 35:1331–1334.
167. McIntosh TK, Vink R, Faden AI: An analog of thyrotropin-releasing hormone improves outcome after brain injury: ^{31}P NMR studies. *Am J Physiol* 1988; 254:R785–R792.
168. Faden AI, Yum SW, Lemke M, Vink R: Effects of TRH-analog treatment on tissue cations, phospholipids and energy metabolism after spinal cord injury. *J Pharmacol Exp Ther* 1990; 255(2):608–614.
169. Faden AI: TRH analog YM-14673 improves outcome following traumatic brain and spinal cord injury in rats: Dose-response studies. *Brain Res* 1989; 486:228–235.
170. Behrmann DL, Bresnahan JC, Beattie MS: Modelling of acute spinal cord injury in the rat: Neuroprotection and enhanced recovery with methylprednisolone and YM-14673. *Exp Neurol* 1994; 126:61–75.
171. McIntosh TK, Fernyak S, Hayes RL, Faden AI: Beneficial effect of the nonselective opiate antagonist naloxone hydrochloride and the thyrotropin-releasing hormone (TRH) analog YM-14673 on long-term neurobehavioral outcome following experimental brain injury in the rat. *J Neurotrauma* 1993; 10(4):373–384.
172. Faden AI, Labroo VM, Cohen LA: Imidazole-substituted analogs of TRH limit behavioral deficits after experimental brain trauma. *J Neurotrauma* 1993; 10(2):101–108.
173. Faden AI, Jacobs TP, Smith MT, Holaday JW: Comparison of thyrotropin-releasing hormone, naloxone and dexamethasone treatments in experimental spinal cord injury. *Neurology* 1983; 33:673–678.
174. Faden AI: Comparison of single vs. combination drug strategies in experimental brain trauma. *J Neurotrauma* 1993; 10(2):91–100.
174A. Treatment with thyrotropin releasing hormone (TRH) in patients with traumatic spinal cord injury. *J Neurotrauma* 12(3):235–243, 1995.
175. Kimelberg HK, Cragoe EJ Jr, Nelson LR, et al: Improved recovery from a traumatic-hypoxic brain injury in cats by intracisternal injection of an anion transport inhibitor. *CNS Trauma* 1987; 4:3–14.
176. Baron KD, Dentinger MP, Kimelberg HK, et al: Ultrastructural features of a brain injury in the cat. I. Vascular and neurological changes and the prevention of astroglial swelling by L-644,711. *Acta Neuropathol* 1990; 39:340–350.
177. Relton JK, Rothwell NJ: Interleukin-1 receptor antagonist inhibits ischaemic and excitotoxic neuronal damage in the rat. *Brain Res Bull* 1992; 29:243–246.
178. Black MD, Crossman CF, Relton JK, Rothwell NJ: Lipocortin-1 inhibits NMDA receptor-mediated neuronal damage in the striatum of the rat. *Brain Res* 1992; 585:135–140.
179. Giulian D, Robertson C: Inhibition of mononuclear phagocytes reduces ischemic injury in the spinal cord. *Ann Neurol* 1990; 27:33–42.
180. Hagg T, Louis J-C, Longo F, Varon S: Neurotrophic factors, growth factors and CNS trauma, in Salzman S, Faden AI (eds): *The Neurobiology of CNS Trauma.* New York: Oxford University Press, 1994; 23:245–265.
181. Arenas E, Persson H: Neurotrophin-3 prevents the death of adult central noradrenergic neurons in vivo. *Nature* 1994; 367:368–371.

CHAPTER 110

NONPHARMACOLOGICAL STRATEGIES—MODERATE HYPOTHERMIA

W. Dalton Dietrich

INTRODUCTION

The potential neuroprotective effects of *profound* hypothermia during and following central nervous system injury have long been recognized in the laboratory as well as under various clinical settings.[1–4] For example, in the 1950s, moderate hypothermia (30°C) revolutionized cardiac surgery. Although early clinical studies utilizing whole body hypothermia after brain or spinal cord injury were largely positive, some unconvincing results were also reported. The routine use of hypothermia as a therapeutic approach was largely abandoned in the 1960s because of management problems and unwanted side effects, including shivering, arrhythmias, and increased blood viscosity. Further, the development of alternative pharmacological approaches to brain protection, including the use of barbiturates, was thought to provide comparable protection.

More recently, experimental studies of brain injury have indicated that *profound* (<30°C) reductions in brain or spinal cord temperature are not necessary to demonstrate histopathological or behavioral protection with hypothermia. Investigations using varied animal models of brain injury demonstrated that, in some instances, only a 1- or 2-degree decrease in brain or core temperature can be effective in protecting the CNS from injury. Alternatively, raising brain temperature only a couple of degrees *above* normothermic levels post-injury has been shown to significantly worsen outcome. Based on these data, a resurgence in the potential use of therapeutic hypothermia in various animal models of CNS injury has occurred. This chapter reviews recent experimental data obtained in animal models of brain injury demonstrating the beneficial effects of mild-to-moderate hypothermia and considers potential mechanisms underlying such hypothermic protection.

BRAIN ISCHEMIA

TRANSIENT GLOBAL ISCHEMIA

INTRAISCHEMIC HYPOTHERMIA

Models of global ischemia most closely represent the clinical condition of cardiac arrest where cerebral blood flow is transiently reduced. In early studies of global ischemia, moderate-to-deep hypothermia was shown to increase the tolerance of the brain to ischemic insults.[5–9] For example, in one extreme case, White and associates interrupted brain circulation for 60 min in primates, reducing the brain temperature to 5–8°C.[10] In 1962, Hirsch and Muller suggested that *small* differences in brain temperature could affect behavioral outcome following complete global ischemia.[11] Their results showed that postischemic survival time was linear as a function of brain temperature and suggested that a difference of 1–2°C was enough to alter ischemic outcome. Only recently have experimental studies using reproducible models of brain ischemia been undertaken to determine whether small variations in brain temperature could affect histopathological outcome (Table 110-1).

In 1987, Busto and colleagues first demonstrated that rectal temperature unreliably reflected brain temperature during periods of global forebrain ischemia.[12] Studies in which direct brain temperature measurements

TABLE 110-1 Hypothermia in Experimental Global Cerebral Ischemia

Study	Year	Species	Cooling	°C, Duration	Outcome Measures
Busto et al.[12]	1987	Rat	During	33 and 30°C, 20 min	Pathology, 3 days
Dempsey et al.[13]	1987	Gerbil	During	30–31°C, 40 min	Edema, leukotrienes, 2 h
Busto et al.[14]	1989	Rat	After	30°C, 3 h	Pathology, 3 days
Chopp et al.[15]	1989	Cat	During and after	26.8–34.6°C, 16 min and 1.5–2 h	NMR/pH/Metabolites, 2 h
Clifton et al.[16]	1989	Gerbil	During	32–35°C, 5 min	Pathology, 7 days
Dietrich et al.[17]	1990	Rat	During	30 and 33°C, 20 min	Blood-brain-barrier, 1 h
Minamisawa et al.[18]	1990	Rat	During	35°C, 5, 10, 15 min	Pathology, 7 days
Welsh et al.[19]	1990	Gerbil	During	32.5–35.5°C, 5 min	Pathology, 7 days
Carroll and Beek[20]	1992	Gerbil	During and after	28–32°C, 5 min	Pathology, 4 days
			After	28–32°C, 0.5–6 h	Pathology, 4 days
Chen et al.[21]	1992	Rat	During	30°C, 15 min	pH/Pathology, 7 days
Green et al.[22]	1992	Rat	During	30°C, 12.5 min	Behavior/Pathology, 2 months
Kuluz et al.[23]	1992	Rat	During and after	24–30°C, 90 min	Pathology, 7 days
Coimbra, Wieloch[24]	1994	Rat	After	32.5–33.5°C, 5 h	Pathology, 7 days

were conducted in anesthetized rats demonstrated that during a 20-min ischemic period, brain temperature could drop as much as 3–4°C more than rectal temperature. By manipulating and monitoring brain temperature, the importance of small differences in intraischemic brain temperature on histopathological outcome was quantitatively documented. Thus, decreasing intraischemic brain temperature from 36°C to 34°C significantly protected *selectively vulnerable* brain regions, including the CA1 hippocampus and dorsolateral striatum. These novel data also indicated that small temperature variations might have been responsible for the inconsistent histopathological consequences reported after global ischemia.[25]

In a gerbil model of forebrain ischemia, Clifton and associates also demonstrated that body temperature during the ischemic insult had a dramatic impact on cell damage.[16] In that study, a 2°C drop in body temperature provided 100 percent protection to the CA1 hippocampus. These data confirmed that rigorous attention to temperature measurements was necessary to determine the protective effect of any pharmacological agent. In a rat model of forebrain ischemia, Minamisawa and colleagues studied the influence of brain and body temperature on ischemic damage and confirmed that brain temperature dropped during the global ischemic period, even when body temperature was kept constant.[18] Intentionally lowering temperature to 35°C markedly reduced neuronal necrosis in selective brain regions. These studies stressed that the biochemical events responsible for selective neuronal vulnerability were extremely temperature sensitive.

In a gerbil model of bilateral ischemia, Welsh and colleagues regulated the temperature of the body and head to define the degree of hypothermia required to diminish CA1 hippocampal ischemic injury.[19] Reduction of head temperature to 35.5°C and 32°C diminished histological injury in a dose-dependent manner. These authors also stressed the importance of temperature considerations in pharmacological studies of ischemic protection. Interestingly, under normothermic conditions, nicardipine, a drug that previously had been shown to be neuroprotective, failed to diminish ischemic injury. Selective brain cooling also appears to protect the cerebral cortex from histopathological damage after *prolonged* (30 min) global ischemia.[23]

Although histopathological measures are useful in providing a gross index of neurological state, they cannot reveal more subtle changes capable of significantly compromising brain function. In this regard, the effects of moderate hypothermia on the neurobehavioral and functional consequences of global ischemia have also been explored. Green and colleagues demonstrated that intraischemic hypothermia (30°C) during a 12.5-min ischemic period attenuated the neurobehavioral consequences of global ischemia.[22] In a functional study following global ischemia, accelerated recovery of glucose utilization at 24 h after ischemia was documented with intraischemic hypothermia.[26] In that study, activation studies also indicated that the postischemic brain recovered normal responsiveness to peripheral activation faster when intraischemic brain temperature was decreased to 30°C. The protective effect of hypothermia on reversibility of neuronal function was also investigated using the hippocampal slice.[27,28] Okada and colleagues showed that the period of oxygen and glucose deprivation during which neurons could recover function was extended by hypothermia (21–28°C).[27] Taken together, these studies indicate histopathological, behavioral, and functional protection with intraischemic hypothermia following periods of global forebrain ischemia.

Moderate hypothermic protection has been also demonstrated in models of cardiac arrest and cardiopulmonary bypass. Leonov and colleagues examined the effect of mild (34°C) hypothermia in a reproducible dog cardiac arrest model in which ice-water immersion of the cranium was started at cardiac arrest time 3 min and continued to resuscitation at 60 min post-arrest.[29] Behavioral and histopathological outcome scores at 96 h were improved compared to normothermic animals. In a cat model of cardiac arrest and cardiopulmonary resuscitation, Horn et al. demonstrated that selective hypothermia (25–30°C) protected against early signs of neuronal injury.[30] In a pig model of cardiopulmonary bypass (CPB), moderate hypothermia (27°C) prevented neuronal degeneration and astrocytic swelling after 2 h.[31] Thus, moderate hypothermia initiated during and after cardiac arrest or CPB is neuroprotective in several animal models.

In contrast to hypothermia, mild *hyperthermia* has been shown to aggravate the ischemic damage seen in models of global ischemia.[18,32,33] In one study, the neuropathological consequences of global forebrain ischemia were assessed under normothermic (37°C) versus mild hyperthermic (39°C) conditions.[32] Compared to normothermic rats, rats subjected to intraischemic hyperthermia showed increased mortality rate and severity of histopathological damage. The maturation rate of ischemic cell injury was also accelerated compared to normothermia. In another study, the inhibition of postischemic hyperthermia by halothane was shown to attenuate histopathological injury.[33] The importance of intraischemic and postischemic mild hyperthermia on ischemic outcome is important since stroke or cardiac arrest patients can present with a range of head and body temperatures and may experience fever. Thus, measures that would attenuate even mild hyperthermic episodes could potentially limit injury propagation.

Postischemic Hypothermia

Whether or not postischemic brain hypothermia can protect the brain following a transient ischemic insult is an important question from the clinical perspective, where measures could be initiated, for example, to lower brain temperature following cardiac arrest, transient ischemic attacks (TIAs), or acute stroke. In 1989, Busto and colleagues examined whether moderate brain hypothermia (30°C) during the acute recirculation period could protect the CA1 hippocampus from histopathological injury.[14] Partial protection of the CA1 hippocampal subsector was documented at 3 days when the 3-h hypothermic period was initiated at 5 min but not 30 min into the recirculation period. The question of postischemic hypothermic intervention after variable durations of forebrain ischemia has been addressed by Chopp and colleagues.[35] Although significant protection of the hippocampus was demonstrated after 8 min of normothermic ischemia, no protection was detected after a 12-min ischemic insult.

In 1992, Chen and colleagues failed to demonstrate histopathological protection with postischemic hypothermia after 12 min of forebrain ischemia.[36] However, in a dog model of ventricular fibrillation cardiac arrest (17 min), moderate hypothermia (32°C) initiated during recirculation and continued for 3 h reduced the overall brain histologic damage score at 96 h compared with normothermic animals.[37] Taken together, these findings indicate that the *therapeutic window* for postischemic hypothermia is relatively narrow and that ischemic duration and severity may be important factors in determining whether postischemic hypothermia can protect the brain.

The temporal restraints of neuronal protection by postischemic hypothermia have also been examined by Carroll and Beek by varying the duration of the postischemic hypothermic period (0.5 to 6 h).[20] While 6 h of immediate postischemic hypothermia resulted in significant histopathological protection, no protection was seen when a 1-h hypothermic period was investigated. In another study, a period of hypothermia (32.5–33.5°C) of 5 h, initiated 2 h postischemia, also provided significant protection of the CA1 hippocampus.[24] Thus, the duration of the postischemic hypothermic period appears to be a significant factor in determining the beneficial effects of postischemic hypothermia. This fact may help explain the negative findings reported by Welsh and Harris with postischemic hypothermia of either a 1- or 2-h duration.[38]

While intraischemic hypothermia (30°C) provides histopathological protection up to 2 months following transient global ischemia,[22] the issue of whether *chronic protection* occurs with postischemic hypothermia has only recently been examined. In one study, postischemic hypothermia following 10 min of global forebrain ischemia was initiated 5 min into the recirculation period and extended for 3 h.[39] Although significant protection of the CA1 hippocampus was seen at postischemic days 3 and 7, no protection was documented at 2 months (Fig. 110-1). These data indicate that brain hypothermia of a limited postischemic duration provides only temporary protection from normothermic global ischemia. Chronic indicators of neuronal survival and function appear to be necessary when questions regarding postischemic therapeutic strategies are addressed.

Focal Brain Ischemia

Permanent Occlusion

In contrast to models of transient global ischemia that lead to selective neuronal necrosis, models of focal brain ischemia generally produce brain infarction. Thus, the hypothermic conditions that could potentially protect the brain from these different pathologies may vary. Deep hypothermia—in other words, less than 25°C—

TABLE 110-2 Hypothermia in Permanent and Transient Focal Cerebral Ischemia

Study	Year	Species	Cooling	°C, Duration	Outcome Measures
Rosomoff[41]	1957	Dog	During (P)	25°C, 120 min–4 h	Pathology, 18–22 days
Hagerdal et al.[42]	1978	Rat	During (P)	27°C, 25 min	Metabolites, 25 min
Berntman et al.[43]	1981	Rat	During (P)	34°C, 20 min	Metabolites, 20 min
Onesti et al.[44]	1991	Rat	During (P)	24°C, 1 h	Morphology, 1 day
Chen et al.[45]	1992	Rat	During and after (T)	30°C, 3 h	Pathology, 4 days
Morikawa et al.[46]	1992	Rat	During (P)	30°C, 4 h	Pathology, 3 days
			During (P)	30°C, 2 h	Pathology, 3 days
			During (T)	30°C, 2 h	Pathology, 3 days
Xue et al.[47]	1992	Rat	During (P)	30°C, 6 h	Pathology, 6 h
			During (T)	32°C, 3 h	Pathology, 21 h
			During (T)	32°C, 1.5 h	Pathology, 3 days
			During (T)	32°C, 3 h	Pathology, 3 days
			During and after (T)	32°C, 6 h	Pathology, 3 h
Lo and Steinberg[48]	1992	Rat	During (P)	30–33°C	Evoked potentials
Moyer et al.[49]	1992	Rat	During (P)	33°C	T1 and T2, 4 h
Ridenour et al.[50]	1992	Rat	During (P)	33°C, 2 h	Morphology, 4 days
			During (T)	33°C, 1 h	Morphology, 4 days
Zhang et al.[51]	1993	Rat	After (T)	30°C, 3 h	Pathology, 1 week

P = Permanent MCA occlusion; T = Transient MCA occlusion

unquestionably protects the brain against focal brain ischemia. Classic studies by Rosomoff demonstrated that profound hypothermia protected against permanent middle cerebral artery (MCA) occlusion in dogs and monkeys.[40,41] More recently, the effects of more moderate reductions in brain temperature have been studied in focal ischemia models that result in reproducible patterns of brain infarction (Table 110-2). Morikawa and colleagues compared normothermic (36°C) and hypothermic (30°C) rats with permanent MCA occlusion plus hypotension.[46] Although they demonstrated no significant decrease in infarct volume with hypothermia, an interaction between infarct area and temperature was shown by repeated measures of analysis. Onesti and colleagues demonstrated that the reduction of temporalis muscle temperature to 24°C for 1 h after MCA occlusion significantly decreased cortical infarct volume compared to normothermic controls.[44] In a more recent study by Xue and colleagues, mild hypothermia (rectal temperature 32°C, brain temperature 31°C) was shown to reduce the volume of neocortical infarction following permanent MCA occlusion.[47] In that study, hypothermia was extended throughout the 6-h study period. Thus, it appears that in conditions of permanent focal ischemia, profound hypothermia and/or extended periods of hypothermia may be necessary to protect the brain.

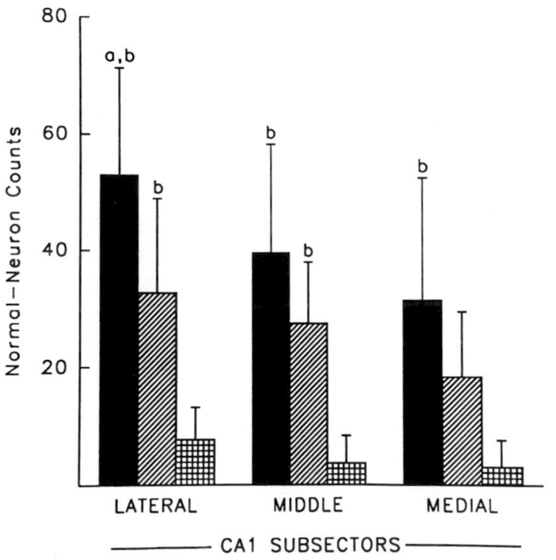

Figure 110-1. Normal-neuron cell counts in hippocampal CA1 subsectors of rats with postischemic hypothermia (means ± SD). *Filled bars*, 3-day survival; *hatched bars*, 7-day survival; *cross-hatched bars*, 2-month survival. [*different from 7-day data; [b]different from 2-month data (repeated-measures analysis of variance followed by Bonferroni test, $p < 0.05$)]. (From[39].)

TRANSIENT FOCAL ISCHEMIA

In contrast to the inconsistent results seen with permanent focal ischemia, moderate hypothermia has been shown to be protective in several models of *transient* MCA occlusion (Table 110-2). Morikawa and colleagues demonstrated that selective brain hypothermia (30°C) during the 2-h period of reversible MCA occlusion significantly reduced infarct volume.[46] Likewise, Chen et al. reported that whole body hypothermia (30°C) in-

TABLE 110-3 Moderate Hypothermia in Experimental Head Trauma

Study	Year	Species	Cooling	°C, Duration	Outcome Measures
Clifton et al.[59]	1991	Rat	Before and after	36–30°C, 1 h	Behavior, 5 days
Jiang et al.[60]	1992	Rat	Before and after	30°C, 1 h	BBB, 1 h
Lyeth et al.[61]	1993	Rat	15-min and 30-min delay	30°C, 1 h	Behavior, 5 days
Taft et al.[62]	1993	Rat	Before and after	30°C, 3 h	Microtubule associated protein 2, 3 h
Palmer et al.[63]	1993	Rat	Before and after	32–33°C	Pathology, 14 days
Dietrich et al.[64]	1994	Rat	5-min delay	30°C, 3 h	Pathology, 3 days

BBB = blood-brain barrier

duced prior to ischemia and maintained for 2 h following MCA occlusion and 1 h reperfusion also decreased histopathological injury.[45] In 1992, Ridenour and colleagues reported that more moderate levels of hypothermia (33°C) during the 1-h ischemic period and first hour of reperfusion reduced infarct volume by 48 percent versus the normothermic group.[50] Finally, Zhang and colleagues have recently reported that both immediate or *delayed* hypothermia (32°C) also leads to infarct reduction.[51] Their results are important in that they imply that hypothermic interventions initiated after a period of cerebrovascular occlusion and subsequent recanalization could potentially aid in reducing structural damage.

BRAIN TRAUMA

Deep hypothermia as a means of cerebral protection in the neurosurgical setting has met with various problems.[52,53] A common problem encountered, for example, during aneurysm surgery has been postoperative bleeding during rewarming after profound hypothermia (10–18°C). The potential clinical utility of moderate hypothermia was, however, demonstrated in severe brain-injured patients as early as 1958.[54] More recently, clinical investigations using systemic hypothermia (32–33°C) have reported evidence of improved neurological outcome in patients with severe nonpenetrating brain injury.[55,56] Therapeutic hypothermia in traumatized patients is also effective in attenuating intracranial hypertension,[57] while not adversely affecting the incidence of delayed intracerebral hemorrhage.[58]

In an early experimental study, Mullan et al. demonstrated in dogs subjected to cerebral trauma that hypothermia (28–33°C) actually *increased* the mortality rate as compared to the normothermic group.[52] In recent experimental studies, the effects of moderate hypothermia were evaluated in well-characterized rodent models of traumatic brain injury (TBI) (Table 110-3). Clifton and colleagues investigated the effect of systemic hypothermia (30–36°C) following fluid percussion brain injury[59] and reported a significant reduction in mortality with 30°C as well as reduced deficits in beam walking, beam balance, and body loss compared with normothermic (38°C) rats. Again using the fluid percussion model, Lyeth and colleagues investigated the effects of a 1-h post-injury hypothermic period (30°C) on behavioral outcome.[61] Although both normothermic and 30-min post-injury hypothermic groups exhibited significant beam balance and beam walking deficits on days 1 and 5 after TBI, the 15-min post-injury hypothermic group exhibited beam walking deficits only on day 1. These data indicated a therapeutic window for moderate hypothermia of less than 30 min after TBI in rats.

Histopathological protection with moderate hypothermia has also recently been reported in models of TBI.[63,64] In one study, the effects of post-traumatic brain hypothermia (30°C) were investigated using a fluid percussion trauma model resulting in hemorrhagic contusion and selective neuronal necrosis.[64] In normothermic animals (37°C), necrotic neurons were observed within ipsilateral cortical regions, hippocampal CA3 and CA4 subsectors and thalamus. Post-traumatic brain hypothermia (30°C for 3 h) initiated at 5 min after injury reduced the overall sum of cortical necrotic neurons as well as contusion volume (Fig. 110-2). These experimental data suggest that histopathological protection may be possible in head-injured patients where early cooling can be initiated.

SPINAL CORD TRAUMA

Although some studies have reported negative results with local spinal cord cooling following traumatic spinal cord injury, most studies have noted beneficial effects (Table 110-4). In early experimental studies by Albin

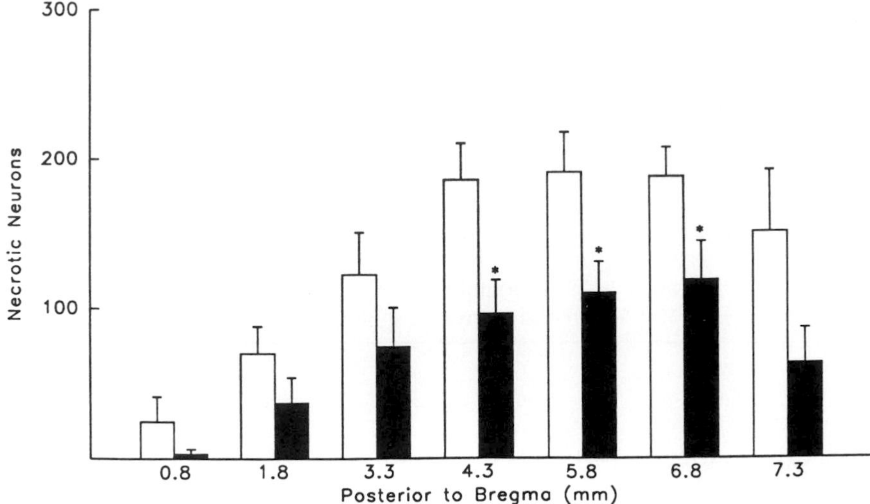

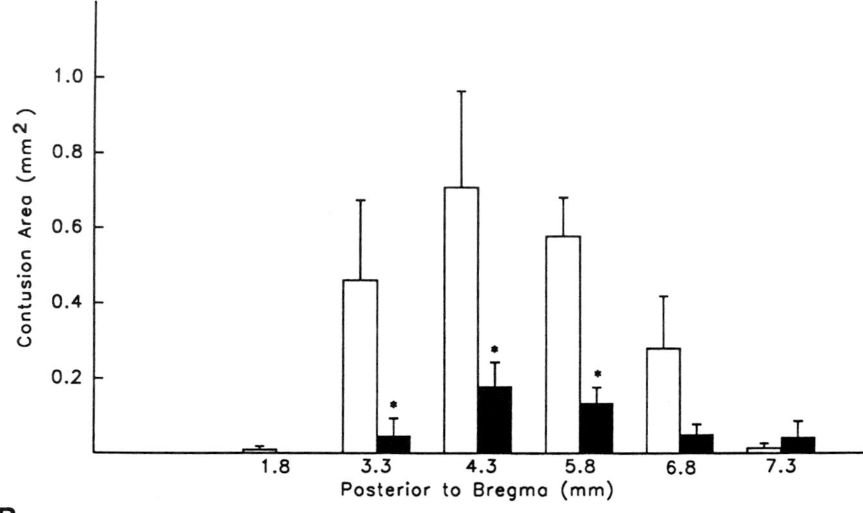

Figure 110-2. Bar graphs of mean ± SEM number of (*A*) cortical necrotic neurons per microscopic field and, (*B*) contusion area at several coronal levels. Data taken from normothermic (*clear bars*) and post-traumatic hypothermic rats (*black bars*). (*significantly different from normothermia by the Kruskal-Wallis one-way analysis by ranks.) (From[64].)

and colleagues, selective spinal cord cooling to about 12°C resulted in marked neurological and functional recovery up to two months after injury.[65,66] The beneficial effects of local hypothermia have also been demonstrated when the hypothermic manipulation is delayed hours after the injury. For example, in a study by Ducker and Hamit, local spinal cord hypothermia (3°C) for a 3-h period was effective in improving recovery of neurological function when begun 3 h after injury.[67]

In a study by Wells and Hansebout, local hypothermia to 6°C was effective in minimizing the functional deficits seen in dogs even when initiated 4 h after compression of the thoracic cord.[76] Interestingly, local cooling for 1 or 18 h was less effective than 4 h, suggesting that a critical duration of hypothermia was most effective and its beneficial effects decreased if that time was exceeded. In a study by Green and colleagues, the effects of regional hypothermia (6–18°C) initiated at 1 and 5 h post-injury were investigated in a cat model of spinal cord contusion.[71] Although both hypothermic manipulations appeared to decrease edema formation and hemorrhage, the degree of protection was greatest when hypothermia was initiated in the earlier post-injury period. Additional studies using reproducible models of spinal cord injury are needed to clarify whether more moderate levels of hypothermia are effective in attenuating injury.

SPINAL CORD ISCHEMIA

Studies designed to test the therapeutic potential of hypothermia on spinal cord ischemia grew out of a need to protect the spinal cord during surgical procedures

TABLE 110-4 Hypothermia in Experimental Spinal Cord Trauma

Study	Year	Species	Cooling	°C, Duration	Outcome Measures
Albin et al.[65]	1965	Dog	Before and after	12°C, 25 h	Behavior, 2 months
Albin, et al.[66]	1968	Monkey	Before and 4-h delay	10°C, 3 h	Behavior, 3 months
Ducker and Hamit[67]	1969	Dog	3-h delay	3°C, 3 h	Behavior, 4–6 months
Kelly et al.[68]	1970	Dog	Before and 4-h delay	12–13°C, 2.5–3 h	Behavior, Pathology, 3 months
Black and Marowitz[69]	1971	Monkey	1-h delay	4–8°C, 5 h	Behavior, 2 weeks
Campbell et al.[70]	1973	Cat	3-h delay	4°C, 3 h	Behavior, 90 days
Green et al.[71]	1973	Cat	1- and 5-h delay	6–18°C, 3 h	Pathology, 3 h
Tator and Deecke[72]	1973	Monkey	3-h delay	5°C, 3 h	Behavior/Pathology, 3 months
Hansebout et al.[73]	1975	Dog	Before and after	4°C, 4 h	Behavior, 7 weeks
Eidelberg et al.[74]	1976	Ferret	1-h delay	10°C, 3 h	Behavior, 4 weeks
Kuchnor and Hansebout[75]	1976	Dog	15-min delay	6°C, 4 h	Behavior, 48 days
Wells and Hansebout[76]	1978	Dog	4-h delay	6°C, 1–8 h	Behavior, 1–56 days
Martinez and Green[77]	1992	Rat	Before and after	31–32°C, h	Pathology, 3 days

requiring aortic clamp cross-clamping (Table 110-5). In an early study by Vacanti and Ames, a temperature reduction of 3°C during temporary occlusion of the abdominal aorta increased the duration of ischemia that could be reversibly sustained.[78] In 1986, Robertson and colleagues showed that moderate hypothermia (30°C) also increased the duration of ischemia required to produce neurological deficits.[79] In that study in rabbits, hypothermia was associated with a higher percentage demonstrating persistent spinal somatosensory evoked potentials (SSEPs) and retaining normal motor function up to 48 hours after ischemia.

In more recent studies, different methods of cooling the spinal cord have been investigated, including spinal cord perfusion as well as epidural cooling techniques. Berguer and colleagues used an extracorporeal perfusion system consisting of a heat exchanger and pump to infuse cooled saline into the subarachnoid space (L6).[80] In that study, spinal cord hypothermia initiated 50 min prior to the cross-clamping of the aorta improved functional recovery graded at 24 h. In another study in rabbits, Vanicky and colleagues used a modified epidural cooling technique to assess hypothermic protection (<15°C).[82] This study indicated that deep spinal cord hypothermia produced by epidural perfusion cooling provided effective protection against spinal cord ischemia. Since regional ischemia can be a consequence of spinal cord trauma, it would be important in future studies to determine whether postischemic hypothermia could also protect the spinal cord from a transient ischemic insult.

MECHANISMS OF HYPOTHERMIC PROTECTION

Temperature is known to affect many normal biological processes. Thus, it would not be too surprising to predict that hypothermic protection from injury would involve not one but multiple pathophysiological processes. Indeed, this feature of brain cooling could explain why hypothermic protection is routinely reported and demonstrated under many different types of brain injury. The following section attempts to summarize current thinking regarding basic mechanisms of hypothermic protection.

TABLE 110-5 Hypothermia in Experimental Spinal Cord Ischemia

Study	Year	Species	Cooling	°C, Duration	Outcome Measures
Vacanti and Ames[78]	1984	Rabbit	During	34.0–36.8°C, 25 min	Behavior/24 h
Robertson et al.[79]	1986	Rabbit	During	30°C, 25–50 min	SSEPs, Behavior, 48 h
Berguer et al.[80]	1992	Dog	During	19–12°C, 45 min	Behavior/Pathology, 24 h
Naslund et al.[81]	1992	Rabbit	During	30°C, 21 min	Behavior/Pathology, 5 days
Vanicky et al.[82]	1993	Rabbit	During	<15°C, 20–60 min	Behavior/Pathology, 2 days
Marsala et al.[83]	1993	Dog	During	28.5°C, 40 min	Behavior/SSEP, Pathology, 2 days

Metabolic Consequences

Hypothermia may protect CNS tissue from injury by reducing metabolism.[84,85] Brain cooling slows O_2 consumption and CO_2 production approximately 7 percent per degree C.[84] In 1978, Nordstrom and Rehncrona documented that, at a body temperature of 23°C, cerebral oxygen consumption was reduced to about 15 percent of normal control values.[86] Using the 2-deoxyglucose technique for determining local rates of glucose utilization in the CNS, McCulloch and colleagues measured glucose utilization in rats under normothermic (37.4°C) and hypothermic (31.8°C) conditions.[87] Importantly, the magnitude of temperature-related alterations in glucose use displayed considerable regional heterogeneity (reduced 35 to 50 percent from normothermics). Using in vivo P-31 nuclear magnetic resonance (NMR) spectroscopy, Chopp and colleagues investigated the metabolic effects of three levels of hypothermia (26.8°C, 32.1°C, 34.6°C) on global cerebral ischemia and recirculation in cats.[15] Although normothermic and hypothermic animals exhibited significant reductions in cerebral intracellular acidosis during ischemia and recirculation, a more rapid return of metabolites was seen during recirculation with hypothermia.

Since hypothermia lowers metabolism and energy demand, hypothermic protection may relate to the preservation of cytoplasmic ATP stores and the sustained maintenance of normal transmembrane ion and neurotransmitter gradients.[9] In this regard, Welsh and colleagues documented that decreasing head temperature to 32.5°C *delayed* but did not prevent the depletion of ATP within the hippocampus during a 5-min ischemic insult (Fig. 110-3).[19] In an earlier study, Busto and colleagues demonstrated that tissue levels of ATP, phosphocreatine, glucose, and glycogen were depleted to similar degrees following 20 min of hypothermic (30°C) or normothermic (36°C) ischemia.[12] Additional data also demonstrated that ischemic protection with intraischemic hypothermia also was not associated with *reduced* lactate accumulation.[12,88] Thus, although cerebral hypothermia may not prevent the eventual depletion of ATP or lactate accumulation during a prolonged ischemic period, hypothermia may delay ATP depletion during the initial ischemic period. Thus, it is conceivable that, during brief ischemic periods, the effects of hypothermia on ATP depletion may play an important role in cerebral protection.

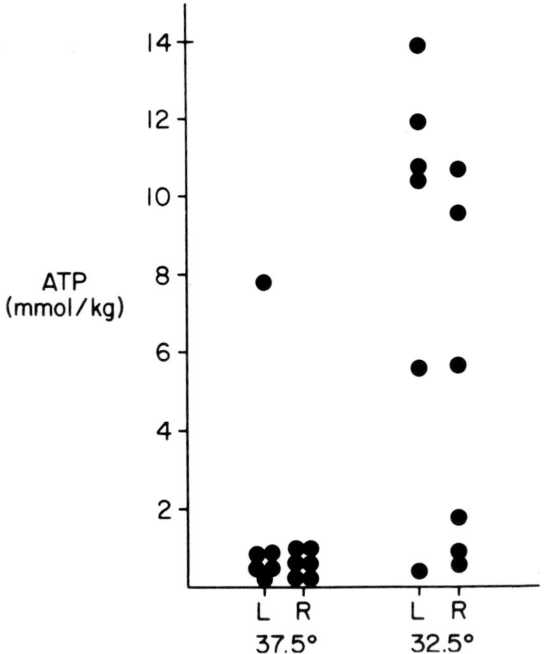

Figure 110-3. Effects of 2-min ischemia on ATP levels in CA1 hippocampus of normothermic and hypothermic gerbils. Head temperature was regulated at 37.5°C or 32.5° in two groups of six animals during ischemia for 2 min. Each point represents the ATP concentration in the CA1 subfield of the left (*L*) or right (*R*) hippocampus of individual animals. ATP levels are given as mmol/kg (dry wt). (From[19].)

Hemodynamic Consequences of Hypothermia

To date, investigations documenting the hemodynamic consequences of hypothermia in the brain and spinal cord have reported conflicting data. In 1954, Rosomoff demonstrated that systemic hypothermia down to 25°C significantly lowered cerebral blood flow (CBF) in dogs.[6] Consistent with this finding, Sakamoto and Monafo showed that systemic hypothermia down to 27.7°C also significantly reduced blood flow.[89] In contrast, however, Kuluz and colleagues recently reported that during selective brain cooling (30.9°C), cortical blood flow as measured by laser Doppler flowmetry increased 215 percent over control values (Fig. 110-4).[90] It should be stressed that, in this study, core temperature was maintained at normal levels. Thus, hypothermic levels (profound versus moderate), as well as methods of cooling (systemic versus selective), may be key factors in determining the local hemodynamic consequences of hypothermia. Hypothermia-induced elevations in CBF would likely attenuate ischemic severity and thereby promote protection.

The consequences of hypothermia on spinal cord blood flow have also resulted in contrasting findings. In 1985, Hansebout and colleagues demonstrated that local cooling in the spinal cord down to 16°C decreased blood flow to 50 percent of normothermic values.[91] Sakamoto and Monafo reported that local hypothermia (25–28°C) also reduced blood flow in the cooled and adjacent cortical segments.[92,93] In contrast, Zielonka and colleagues

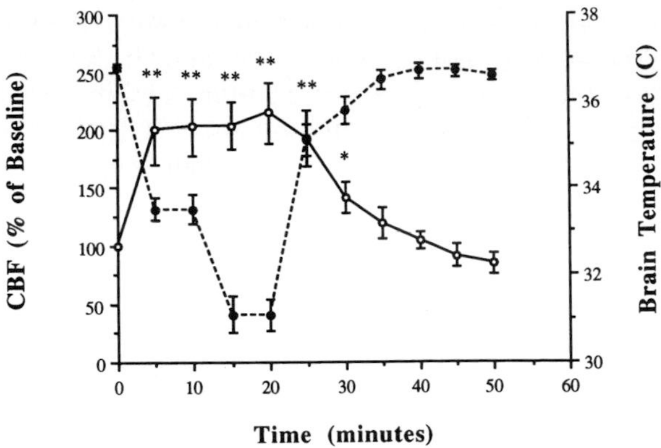

Figure 110-4. Changes in cerebral blood flow (CBF, *open circles*) and brain temperature (*closed circles*) during 20 min of selective brain cooling and 30 min of rewarming. Values are means ± SE. $*p < 0.05$, $**p < 0.01$ for comparisons to baseline. (From[90].)

have reported increases in blood flow within the cooled cord segment (13–16°C).[94] Interestingly, in hypothermic rats with transected spinal cords, spinal cord blood flow is either unchanged or lower in caudal cord segments compared with normothermic cord-transected controls.[95] Thus, prior spinal cord transection or injury may affect the hemodynamic consequences of local spinal cord cooling.

Excitotoxicity

Considerable evidence has implicated excitatory amino acids, particularly glutamate and aspartate in the evolution of ischemic and traumatic brain damage.[96–98] Extracellular levels of excitatory amino acids are increased in response to a variety of insults and glutamate antagonists have been shown to confer protection after CNS injury. In reference to hypothermic protection, moderate levels of hypothermia (33 and 30°C) are known to attenuate the rise in the extracellular levels of striatal glutamate and dopamine after global ischemia (Fig. 110-5).[99] In addition, Baker and colleagues have shown, in hypothermic rabbits (29°C), that ischemia-induced increases in extracellular glutamate, aspartate, and glycine are reduced in the hippocampus.[100] In gerbil hippocampus, levels of extracellular glutamate were also reduced to about half when the intraischemic brain temperature was lowered by 2°.[101] Thus, intraischemic hypothermia is extremely effective in attenuating the acute rise in extracellular levels of neurotransmitters after global ischemia.

In some models of experimental brain injury, moderate hypothermia also has been shown to affect the neurochemical response of injury. For example, Lyeth and colleagues demonstrated that hypothermia (30°C) induced prior to TBI reduced the elevations in cerebrospinal levels of acetylcholine.[102] However, using a controlled cortical impact model of brain injury, Palmer and colleagues demonstrated that hypothermia (32°C) reduced mean lesion volume *without* attenuating injury-induced elevations in interstitial concentrations of glutamate and aspartate.[63] The neurochemical responses to trauma and hypothermic interventions may depend on injury models, the severity of the traumatic insult, as well as regional sampling procedures.

Hypothermia induced at variable periods after injury may also affect *delayed* or secondary excitotoxic processes. Andine and colleagues recently reported a late (at 8 h) rise in extracellular glutamate and aspartate in the hippocampus following 20 min of global ischemia.[103] In a multiple ischemic insult paradigm, Lin and colleagues documented a delayed rise in extracellular glutamate in the striatum at 3 h recirculation.[104] Recently, immediate postischemic hypothermia, combined with delayed MK-801 treatment (postischemic days 3, 5, and 7), led to chronic protection of the CA1 hippocampus.[105] Together, these data indicate a potential for post-injury hypothermia affecting excitotoxic processes.

Primary excitotoxic-mediated brain injury has also been shown to be temperature sensitive. In a recent investigation by McDonald and colleagues, postnatal day 7 rats received intrastriatal injections of the glutamate agonist N-methyl-D-aspartate (NMDA) and then were exposed for 2 h to a range of ambient temperatures.[106] Between 25 and 40°C, a linear relationship between temperature and NMDA-induced histopathological injury was documented. Thus, in addition to

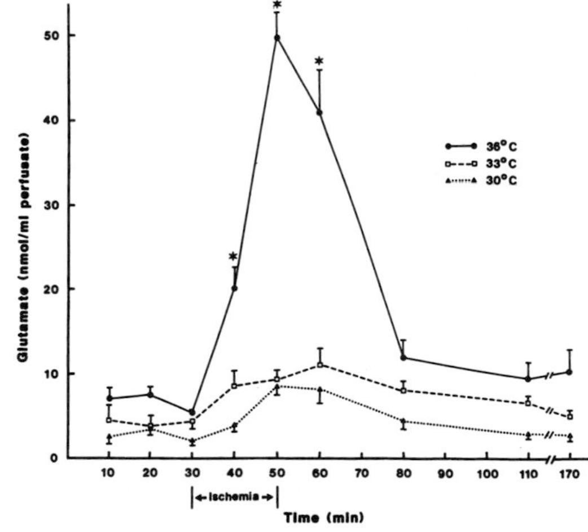

Figure 110-5. Line plot of time-course changes in the perfusate levels of glutamate(nmol/ml) in animals whose intraischemic brain temperature was maintained at 36°C (n = 10), 33°C (n = 4), and 30°C (n = 8). The data presented are means ± SEM. Statistical significance was assessed by two-way ANOVA. (From[99].)

affecting the presynaptic release of neurotransmitters, hypothermia may also influence postsynaptic excitotoxic processes that may occur over extended post-injury periods.

Blood-Brain Barrier

It has been hypothesized that alterations in blood-brain barrier (BBB) permeability following brain injury contribute to injury processes by allowing the passage of water, blood-borne exogenous substances, including ions and neurotransmitters, into the brain parenchyma.[107] Recent studies have investigated the importance of brain and body temperature on the microvascular consequences of brain ischemia and trauma, and my laboratory has explored the importance of intraischemic brain temperature on alterations of the BBB.[17] As is well known, normothermic animals displayed acute BBB permeability to the protein tracer horseradish peroxidase following global ischemia; yet, when hypothermia to 30 or 33°C was employed, consistent BBB changes did not occur. Conversely, when intraischemic brain temperature was elevated to 39°C, BBB damage was exacerbated in comparison to the normothermic series. In normal rats, Krantis demonstrated a hypothermia-induced reduction in the permeation of radiolabeled tracers across the BBB.[108] In addition, Dempsey and colleagues demonstrated, following bilateral carotid artery occlusion in gerbils, that moderate hypothermia of 30 to 31°C reduced postischemic edema formation.[13] Thus, the brain and body temperature appear to be a critical factor in determining the acute BBB consequences of brain ischemia.

The effects of moderate hypothermia on BBB disruption following traumatic brain injury have also been investigated. Jiang and colleagues documented patterns of increased vascular permeability to endogenous serum albumin (IgG) in normothermic and hypothermic (30°C) rats.[60,109] In hypothermic rats, albumin immunoreactivity was greatly reduced compared with normothermic rats. Further, the acute hypertensive response to trauma was significantly depressed in hypothermic animals. Additional studies are needed to determine the effects of hypothermia on other trauma-induced microvascular abnormalities, including secondary ischemia and impaired autoregulation.

Effect of Hypothermia on Protein Induction and Degradation

The 72K-dalton heat shock protein (HSP-72) and other proteins common to the heat shock response are induced in rodent models of brain injury. Importantly, the induction of HSP-72 has been associated with protection in some models of neural injury.[110] Recently, Chopp and colleagues examined the effects of ischemic hypothermia (30°C) on the induction of HSP-72.[111] Although intense HSP-72 immunoreactivity was demonstrated after normothermic forebrain ischemia, intraischemic hypothermia inhibited HSP-72 expression. Thus, HSP induction does not appear to be a potential mechanism by which hypothermia protects against ischemic cell damage.

Taft and colleagues recently investigated the effects of hypothermia (30°C) on hippocampal microtubule-associated protein 2 (MAP-2) following traumatic brain injury.[62] Previously, these investigators reported a loss of hippocampal MAP-2 levels following fluid percussion brain injury.[112] In their recent study, no significant reductions in MAP-2 were seen in the hypothermic-injured group. Using a model of global ischemia, Miyazawa et al. have also reported that mild hypothermia alleviated the decrease in postsynaptic MAP-2 immunostaining at 7 days after ischemia.[113] In terms of structural and behavioral protection with hypothermia, these observations are important since MAP-2 is a principal component of microtubules that participate in many cellular functions, including axoplasmic transport and membrane stabilization. In a model of global ischemia, intraischemic hypothermia (30°C) has recently been shown to attenuate the reduction in protein kinase C activity compared to normothermia.[114] Thus, hypothermic attenuation of injury-induced loss or activation of specific proteins could contribute to the overall neuroprotective effect of brain cooling.

Intracellular Calcium Accumulation

Excessive increases in intracellular calcium are believed to participate in neuronal vulnerability to various brain injuries.[115] Recently, Mitani and colleagues have investigated the temperature dependence of hypoxia-induced calcium accumulation in a hippocampal slice preparation.[116] When hippocampal slices were superinfused with a hypothermic medium (35, 33, or 31°C), calcium accumulation as a consequence of anoxic depolorization was delayed in a temperature-dependent manner. In a recent in vivo study by Araki and colleagues, alterations in cortical cytosolic free calcium were investigated with the intracellular calcium indicator Endo-1 following focal cerebral ischemia.[117] In hypothermic animals where brain temperature was maintained at 31.5 to 32°C, a significantly smaller increase in calcium signal was observed compared with normothermic animals. In addition, EEG recovery in the hypothermic group during the latter phase of recirculation was significantly better than the normothermic group. These data suggest that mild hypothermia may owe part of its protective effect on ischemic neuronal injury to its ability to attenuate increases in cytosolic free calcium.

Reperfusion Injury

Experimental data obtained in the heart, lung, kidney, and brain indicate that reperfusion of ischemic tissue results in irreversible injury.[118] In the myocardium, for example, reperfusion is accompanied by adhesion of neutrophils to the vascular endothelium leading to capillary luminal plugging, permeability alterations, and a no-reflow phenomenon.[119] Indirect evidence for reperfusion injury following brain ischemia also has been demonstrated.[120,121] In reference to hypothermic protection, studies have shown that in addition to affecting the BBB consequences of global ischemia (see above), intraischemic temperature manipulations affect the profile of early postischemic white blood cell accumulation.[122] Interestingly, while intraischemic hyperthermia (39°C) increased the frequency of luminal white blood cells compared with normothermia (37°C), leukocyte accumulation was depressed under hypothermic (30°C) ischemic conditions. Reversible platelet dysfunction has also been reported with varying degrees of hypothermia.[123] Thus, brain temperature may be an important factor in contributing to postischemic white blood cell accumulation or platelet activation and its associated reperfusion injury.

Numerous reports have implicated oxygen radicals in the pathogenesis of reperfusion injury.[124,125] In a recent study by Boisvert, free radical formation was measured by the hydroxylation of salicylic by hydroxyl radicals to produce 2,5-dihydroxybenzoic acid (2,5-DHBA).[126] Interestingly, baseline measurements performed while maintaining head temperature at 34 or 38°C revealed a marked effect of brain temperature on 2,5-DHBA production. More recently, Baiping and colleagues have also provided evidence for moderate hypothermia attenuating lipid peroxidation following global ischemia.[127] These findings indicate that variations in brain temperature, including moderate hypothermia, may significantly affect the generation of free radicals and lipid peroxidation after brain injury.

PHARMACOLOGY AND HYPOTHERMIA

Some agents capable of prolonging survival or protecting the brain from ischemic insults have been found to induce mild hypothermia.[128–131] Based on recent experimental data showing that mild decreases in brain temperature can protect against injury, these degrees of drug-induced hypothermia may be sufficient to explain some of their protective effects. In 1990, Buchan and Pulsinelli demonstrated that 1 mg/kg of MK-801 in gerbils subjected to 5 min of bilateral carotid artery occlusion rendered postischemic animals comatose and hypothermic for several hours compared with saline-treated animals.[128] In subsequent experiments, animals pretreated with MK-801 but maintained normothermic during and after forebrain ischemia demonstrated no protection. In a gerbil model of 5 min bilateral carotid artery occlusion, Corbett and colleagues demonstrated that the protective effect on brain damage of MK-801, 3 mg/kg, was again associated with hypothermia (31.1°C).[129] In a separate group of animals where body temperature was maintained at normothermic levels, MK-801 provided no protection against hippocampal cell loss or spatial memory. Taken together, these data indicate that the protective effects of MK-801 may be largely a consequence of drug-induced hypothermia.

Barbiturates have a long history of neuroprotection in models of ischemia and trauma.[86,131] In a recent study by Sternau and colleagues, the question of whether barbiturate protection in global ischemia involved temperature-dependent mechanisms was investigated.[132] Pretreatment with thiopental (40 mg/kg) protected the ischemic brain when intraischemic brain temperature was allowed to fall spontaneously to 32 to 30°C. However, when intraischemic brain temperature was maintained at normothermic levels (36–37°C), thiopental failed to protect hippocampal neurons. Most recently, the muscarinic cholinergic partial agonist, U-80816E, has also been shown to have hypothermic properties.[130] U-80816E reduced brain temperature 2.2°C lower than saline-treated animals. When treated gerbils were subjected to ischemia but placed in a heated chamber that prevented the hypothermic effects, no cerebral protection was observed with U-80816E. These studies support the concept that various drugs with neuroprotective qualities may protect by temperature-dependent mechanisms. In the clinical arena, pharmacologically induced hypothermia may be an advantageous method of reducing body temperature and promoting CNS protection.

Pharmacotherapy in conjunction with hypothermia may represent a necessary treatment protocol after CNS injury. For example, in several experimental studies, hypothermia in combination with barbiturates has been shown to have an additive effect on CBF and oxygen consumption.[86] In the setting of global forebrain ischemia, recent studies have also assessed the beneficial effects of combining hypothermia with pharmacotherapy. In one study, the beneficial effects of postischemic hypothermia and the NMDA antagonist dextromethorphan were examined.[133] Combined therapy with hypothermia plus dextromethorphan protected the neocortex from injury in excess of the protection conferred by either hypothermia or dextromethorphan alone. More recently, Ikonomidou and colleagues have shown that hypothermia enhances the protective effect of MK-801 against hypoxic-ischemic brain damage in infant rats.[134] Thus, synergistic therapeutic protection in CNS injury may be possible. There is a great need for future studies to examine combination therapies involving mild hypothermia and pharmacological agents directed at specific pathomechanisms.

SUMMARY

Mild-to-moderate hypothermia has now been shown to be neuroprotective in many models of brain injury. In contrast, small elevations in brain temperature over normothermic levels dramatically worsen outcome. Since temperature fluctuations may have profound effects on many pathomechanisms, careful attention to brain or body temperature is necessary in any model of brain injury. Nevertheless, temperature manipulations represent a powerful tool with which to influence outcome and thereby investigate pathomechanisms. It is now known that various drugs that confer neuroprotection induce mild hypothermia. Pharmacological studies aimed at brain or spinal cord protection need to address the potential for drug-induced temperature changes. The use of brain cooling or pharmacological strategies to reduce brain temperature, possibly in combination with selective receptor blockers, may also prove useful in the treatment of the various types of CNS injury. In the clinic, delayed hypothermic treatment may be advantageous in limiting injury-induced damage and by extending the therapeutic window for pharmacological therapy.

ACKNOWLEDGMENTS

This work was supported by USPHS Grants NS-30291, NS-27127, and NS-05820. The author thanks Helen Valkowitz for typing the chapter.

References

1. Dietrich WD: The importance of brain temperature in cerebral injury. *J Neurotrauma* 1992; 9(suppl 2):476–485.
2. Ginsberg MD, Sternau LL, Globus MY-T, et al: Therapeutic modulation of brain temperature: Relevance to ischemic brain injury. *Cerebrovasc Brain Metab Rev* 1992; 4:189–225.
3. Lucas JH, Emery DG, Wang G, et al: In vivo investigations of the effects of nonfreezing low temperatures on lesioned and uninjured mammalian neurons. *J Neurotrauma* 1994; 11:35–61.
4. Safar P: Cerebral resuscitation after cardiac arrest: A review. *Circulation* 1986; 74(suppl IV):138–153.
5. Hirsch HA, Bolte A, Schandig A, Tonnis D: Uber die Wiederbelebung des Gehirns bei Hypothermie. *Pflugers Arch* 1957; 265:328–336.
6. Rosomoff HL, Holaday DA: Cerebral blood flow and cerebral oxygen consumption during hypothermia. *Am J Physiol* 1954; 179:85–88.
7. Rosomoff HL: Experimental brain injury during hypothermia. *J Neurosurg* 1955; 16:177–187.
8. Rosomoff HL: Protective effects of hypothermia against pathological processes of the nervous system. *Ann NY Acad Sci* 1959; 80:475–486.
9. Kramer RS, Sanders AP, Lesage AM, et al: The effect of profound hypothermia on preservation of cerebral ATP content during circulatory arrest. *J Thorac Cardiovasc Surg* 1968; 56:699–709.
10. White RJ, Austin PE, Austin JC, et al: Recovery of the subhuman primate after deep cerebral hypothermia and prolonged ischaemia. *Resuscitation* 1973; 2:117–122.
11. Hirsch H, Muller HA: Funktionelle und histologische Veranderungen des Kaninchengehirns nach kompletter Gehirnischamie. *Pflugers Arch* 1962; 275:277–291.
12. Busto R, Dietrich WD, Globus MY-T, et al: Small differences in intraischemic brain temperature critically determine the extent of ischemic neuronal injury. *J Cereb Blood Flow Metab* 1987; 7:729–738.
13. Dempsey RJ, Combs DJ, Maley ME, et al: Moderate hypothermia reduces postischemic edema development and leukotriene production. *Neurosurgery* 1987; 21: 177–181.
14. Busto R, Dietrich WD, Globus MY-T, Ginsberg MD: Postischemic moderate hypothermia inhibits CA1 hippocampal ischemic neuronal injury. *Neurosci Lett* 1989; 101:299–304.
15. Chopp M, Knight R, Tidwell CD, et al: The metabolic effects of mild hypothermia on global cerebral ischemia and recirculation in the cat: Comparison to normothermia and hyperthermia. *J Cereb Blood Flow Metab* 1989; 9:141–148.
16. Clifton GL, Taft WC, Blair RE, et al: Conditions for pharmacologic evaluation in the gerbil model of forebrain ischemia. *Stroke* 1989; 20:1545–1552.
17. Dietrich WD, Busto R, Halley M, Valdes I: The importance of brain temperature in alterations of the blood-brain barrier following cerebral ischemia. *J Neuropathol Exp Neurol* 1990; 49:486–497.
18. Minamisawa H, Smith M-L, Siesjo BK: The effect of mild hyperthermia (39°C) and hypothermia (35°C) on brain damage following 5, 10 and 15 min of forebrain ischemia. *Ann Neurol* 1990; 28:26–33.

19. Welsh FA, Sims RE, Harris VA: Mild hypothermia prevents ischemic injury in gerbil hippocampus. *J Cereb Blood Flow Metab* 1990; 10:557–563.
20. Carroll M, Beek O: Protection against hippocampal CA1 cell loss by post-ischemic hypothermia is dependent on delay of initiation and duration. *Metab Brain Dis* 1992; 7:45–50.
21. Chen H, Chopp M, Jiang Q, Garcia JH: Neuronal damage, glial response and cerebral metabolism after hypothermic forebrain ischemia in the rat. *Acta Neuropathol* 1992; 84:184–189.
22. Green EJ, Dietrich WD, van Dijk F, et al: Protective effects of neural hypothermia on behavior following global cerebral ischemia. *Brain Res* 1992; 580:197–204.
23. Kuluz JW, Gregory GA, Yu ACH, Chang Y: Selective brain cooling during and after prolonged global ischemia reduces cortical damage in rats. *Stroke* 1992; 23:1792–1797.
24. Coimbra C, Wieloch T: Moderate hypothermia mitigates neuronal damage in the rat brain when initiated several hours following transient cerebral ischemia. *Acta Neuropathol* 1994; 87:325–331.
25. Vibulsresth S, Dietrich WD, Busto R, Ginsberg MD: Failure of nimodipine to prevent ischemic neuronal damage in rat. *Stroke* 1987; 18:210–216.
26. Dietrich WD, Busto R, Alonso O, et al: Intraischemic brain hypothermia promotes postischemic metabolic recovery and somatosensory circuit activation. *J Cereb Blood Flow Metab* 1991; 11(suppl)11:S854.
27. Okada Y, Tanimoto M, Yoneda K: The protective effect of hypothermia on reversibility in the neuronal function of the hippocampal slice during long lasting anoxia. *Neurosci Lett* 1988; 84:277–282.
28. Taylor CP, Weber ML: Effect of temperature on synaptic function after reduced oxygen and glucose in hippocampal slices. *Neuroscience* 1993; 52:555–562.
29. Leonov Y, Sterz F, Safar P, et al: Mild cerebral hypothermia during and after cardiac arrest improves neurologic outcome in dogs. *J Cereb Blood Flow Metab* 1990; 10:57–70.
30. Horn M, Schlote W, Henrich HA: Global cerebral ischemia and subsequent selective hypothermia. *Acta Neuropathol* 1991; 81:443–449.
31. Laursen H, Waaben J, Gefke K, et al: Brain histology, blood-brain barrier and brain water after normothermic and hypothermic cardiopulmonary bypass in pigs. *Eur J Cardio-thorac Surg* 1989; 3:539–543.
32. Dietrich WD, Busto R, Valdes I, Loor Y: Effects of normothermic versus mild hyperthermic forebrain ischemia in rats. *Stroke* 1990; 21:1318–1325.
33. Kuroiwa T, Bonnekoh P, Hossmann K-A: Prevention of postischemic hyperthermia prevents ischemic injury of CA_1 neurons in gerbils. *J Cereb Blood Flow Metab* 1990; 10:550–556.
34. Takino M, Okada Y: Hyperthermia following cardiopulmonary resuscitation. *Intensive Care Med* 1991; 17:419–420.
35. Chopp M, Chen H, Dereski MO, Garcia JH: Mild hypothermic intervention after graded ischemic stress in rats. *Stroke* 1991; 22:37–43.
36. Chen H, Chopp M, Van de Linde AMQ, et al: The effects of post-ischemic hypothermia on the neuronal injury and brain metabolism after forebrain ischemia in the rat. *J Neurol Sci* 1992; 107:191–198.
37. Leonov Y, Sterz F, Safar P, Radovsky A: Moderate hypothermia after cardiac arrest of 17 minutes in dogs. *Stroke* 1990; 21:1600–1606.
38. Welsh FA, Harris VA: Postischemic hypothermia fails to reduce ischemic injury in gerbil hippocampus. *J Cereb Blood Flow Metab* 1991; 11:617–620.
39. Dietrich WD, Busto R, Globus MY-T, Ginsberg MD: Intraischemic but not postischemic brain hypothermia protects chronically following forebrain ischemia in rats. *J Cereb Blood Flow Metab* 1993; 13:541–549.
40. Rosomoff HL: Hypothermia and cerebral vascular lesions. I. Experimental interruption of the middle cerebral artery during hypothermia. *J Neurosurg* 1956; 13:244–255.
41. Rosomoff HL: Hypothermia and cerebral vascular lesions. II. Experimental middle cerebral artery interruption followed by induction of hypothermia. *Arch Neurol* 1957; 78:454–464.
42. Hagerdal M, Welsh FA, Keykhah MM, et al: Protective effects of combinations of hypothermia and barbiturates in cerebral hypoxia in the rat. *Anesthesiology* 1978; 49:165–169.
43. Berntman L, Welsh FA, Harp JR: Cerebral protective effect of low-grade hypothermia. *Anesthesiology* 1981; 55:495–498.
44. Onesti ST, Baker CJ, Sun PP, Solomon RA: Transient hypothermia reduces focal ischemic brain injury in the rat. *Neurosurgery* 1991; 29:369–373.
45. Chen H, Chopp M, Zhang ZG, Garcia JH: The effect of hypothermia on transient middle cerebral artery occlusion in the rat. *J Cereb Blood Flow Metab* 1992; 12:621–628.
46. Morikawa E, Ginsberg MD, Dietrich WD, et al: The significance of brain temperature in focal cerebral ischemia: Histopathological consequences of middle cerebral artery occlusion in the rat. *J Cereb Blood Flow Metab* 1992; 12:380–389.
47. Xue D, Huang Z-G, Smith KE, Buchan AM: Immediate or delayed mild hypothermia prevents focal cerebral infarction. *Brain Res* 1992; 587:66–72.
48. Lo EH, Steinberg GK: Effects of hypothermia on evoked potentials, magnetic resonance imaging, and blood flow in focal ischemia in rabbits. *Stroke* 1992; 23:889–893.
49. Moyer DJ, Welsh FA, Zaber EL: Spontaneous cerebral hypothermia diminishes focal infarction in rat brain. *Stroke* 1992; 23:1812–1816.
50. Ridenour TR, Warner DS, Todd MM, McAllister AC: Mild hypothermia reduces infarct size resulting from temporary but not permanent focal ischemia in rats. *Stroke* 1992; 23:733–738.
51. Zhang R-L, Chopp M, Chen H, et al: Postischemic (1 hour) hypothermia significantly reduces ischemic cell damage in rats subjected to 2 hours of middle cerebral artery occlusion. *Stroke* 1993; 24:1235–1240.
52. Mullan S, Raimondi AJ, Suwanwela C: Effect of hypo-

thermia upon cerebral injuries in dogs. *Arch Neurol* 1961; 5:545–551.

53. Drake CG, Barr WK, Coles JC, Gergely NF: The use of extracorporeal circulation and profound hypothermia in the treatment of ruptured intracranial aneurysm. *J Neurosurg* 1964; 21:575–581.
54. Lazorthes G, Campan L: Hypothermia in the treatment of craniocerebral traumatism. *J Neurosurg* 1958; 15:162–167.
55. Clifton GL, Allen S, Barrodale P, et al: A phase II study of moderate hypothermia in severe brain injury. *J Neurotrauma* 1993; 10:263–273.
56. Marion DW, Obrist WD, Carlier PM, et al: The use of therapeutic moderate hypothermia for patients with severe head injuries: A preliminary report. *J Neurosurg* 1993; 79:354–362.
57. Shiozaki T, Sugimoto H, Taneda M, et al: Effect of mild hypothermia on uncontrollable intracranial hypertension after severe head injury. *J Neurosurg* 1993; 79: 363–368.
58. Resnick DK, Marion DW, Darby JM: The effect of hypothermia on the incidence of delayed traumatic intracerebral hemorrhage. *Neurosurgery* 1994; 34:252–256.
59. Clifton GL, Jiang JY, Lyeth BG, et al: Marked protection by moderate hypothermia after experimental traumatic brain injury. *J Cereb Blood Flow Metab* 1991; 11:114–121.
60. Jiang JY, Lyeth BG, Kapasi MZ, et al: Moderate hypothermia reduces blood-brain barrier disruption following traumatic brain injury in the rat. *Acta Neuropathol* 1992; 84:495–500.
61. Lyeth BG, Jiang JY, Liu S: Behavioral protection by moderate hypothermia initiated after experimental traumatic brain injury. *J Neurotrauma* 1993; 10:57–64.
62. Taft WC, Yang K, Dixon CE, et al: Hypothermia attenuates the loss of hippocampal microtubule-associated protein 2 (MAP2) following traumatic brain injury. *J Cereb Blood Flow Metab* 1993; 13:796–802.
63. Palmer AM, Marion DW, Botscheller ML, Redd EE: Therapeutic hypothermia is cytoprotective without attenuating traumatic brain injury-induced elevations in interstitial concentrations of aspartate and glutamate. *J Neurotrauma* 1994; 10:363–372.
64. Dietrich WD, Alonso O, Busto R, et al: Post-traumatic brain hypothermia reduces histopathological damage following concussive brain injury in the rat. *Acta Neuropathol* 1994; 87:250–258.
65. Albin MS, White RJ, Locke GE: Treatment of spinal cord trauma by selective hypothermic perfusion. *Surg Forum* 1965; 16:423–424.
66. Albin MS, White RJ, Acosta-Rua G, Yashon D: Study of functional recovery produced by delayed localized cooling after spinal cord injury in primates. *J Neurosurg* 1968; 29:113–120.
67. Ducker TB, Hamit HF: Experimental treatments of acute spinal cord injury. *J Neurosurg* 1969; 30:693–697.
68. Kelly DL Jr, Lassieter KRL, Calogero JA, Alexander E Jr: Effects of hypothermia and tissue oxygen studies in experimental paraplegia. *J Neurosurg* 1970; 33:554–563.
69. Black P, Markowitz RS: Experimental spinal cord injury in monkeys: Comparison of steroids and local hypothermia. *Surg Forum* 1971; 22:409–411.
70. Campbell JB, DeCrescito V, Tomasula JJ, et al: Experimental treatment of spinal cord contusion in the cat. *Surg Neurol* 1973; 1:102–106.
71. Green BA, Khan T, Raimondi AJ: Local hypothermia as treatment of experimentally induced spinal cord contusion: Quantitative analysis of beneficent effect. *Surg Forum* 1973; 24:436–438.
72. Tator CH, Deecke L: Value of normothermic perfusion, hypothermic perfusion, and durotomy in the treatment of experimental acute spinal cord trauma. *J Neurosurg* 1973; 39:52–64.
73. Hansebout RR, Kuchner EF, Romero-Sierra C: Effects of local hypothermia and of steroids upon recovery from experimental spinal cord compression injury. *Surg Neurol* 1975; 4:531–536.
74. Eidelberg E, Staten E, Watkins CJ, Smith JS: Treatment of experimental spinal cord injury in ferrets. *Surg Neurol* 1976; 6:243–246.
75. Kuchnor EF, Hansebout RR: Combined steroid and hypothermia treatment of experimental spinal cord injury. *Surg Neurol* 1976; 6:371–376.
76. Wells JD, Hansebout RR: Local hypothermia in experimental spinal cord trauma. *Surg Neurol* 1978; 10:200–204.
77. Martinez-Arizala A, Green BA: Hypothermia in spinal cord injury. *J Neurotrauma* 1992; 9(suppl 2):S497–S505.
78. Vacanti FX, Ames A III: Mild hypothermia and Mg^{++} protect against irreversible damage during CNS ischemia. *Stroke* 1984; 15:695–698.
79. Robertson CS, Foltz R, Grossman RG, Goodman JC: Protection against experimental ischemic spinal cord injury. *J Neurosurg* 1986; 64:633–642.
80. Berguer R, Porto J, Fedoronko B, Dragovic L: Selective deep hypothermia of the spinal cords prevents paraplegia after aortic cross-clamping in the dog model. *J Vasc Surg* 1992; 15:62–72.
81. Naslund TC, Hollier LH, Money SR, et al: Protecting the ischemic spinal cord during aortic clamping. *Ann Surg* 1992; 215:409–416.
82. Vanicky I, Marsala M, Galik J, Marsala J: Epidural perfusion cooling protection against protracted spinal cord ischemia in rabbits. *J Neurosurg* 1993; 79:736–741.
83. Marsala M, Vanicky I, Galik J, et al: Panmyelic epidural cooling protects against ischemic spinal cord damage. *J Surg Res* 1993; 55:21–31.
84. Michenfelder JD, Theye RA: The effects of anesthesia and hypothermia on canine cerebral ATP and lactate during anoxia produced by decapitation. *Anesthesiology* 1970; 33:430–439.
85. Michenfelder JD: The hypothermic brain, in Michenfelder JD (eds): *Anesthesia and the Brain: Clinical, functional, metabolic and vascular correlates.* New York: Churchill, 1988: 23–34.
86. Nordstrom C-H, Rehncrona S: Reduction of cerebral blood flow and oxygen consumption with a combination of barbiturate anesthesia and induced hypothermia in the rat. *Acta Anaesth Scand* 1978; 22:7–12.

87. McCulloch J, Savaki HE, Jehle J, Sokoloff L: Local cerebral glucose utilization in hypothermic and hyperthermic rats. *J Neurochem* 1982; 39:255–258.
88. Natale JE, D'Alecy LG: Protection from cerebral ischemia by brain cooling without reduced lactate accumulation in dogs. *Stroke* 1989; 20:770–777.
89. Sakamoto T, Monafo WW: Regional blood flow in the brain and spinal cord of hypothermic rats. *Am J Physiol* 1989; 247:H785–H790.
90. Kuluz JW, Prado R, Chang J, et al: Selective brain cooling increases cortical cerebral blood flow in rats. *Am J Physiol* 1993; 265:H824–H827.
91. Hansebout RR, Lamont RN, Kamath V: The effects of local cooling on canine spinal cord blood flow. *Can J Neurol Sci* 1985; 12:83–87.
92. Sakamoto T, Monafo WW: The effect of hypothermia on regional spinal cord blood flow in rats. *J Neurosurg* 1989; 70:780–784.
93. Sakamoto T, Monafo WW: Regional spinal cord blood flow during local cooling. *Neurosurgery* 1990; 26:958–962.
94. Zielonka JS, Wagner FC Jr, Dohrmann GJ: Alterations in spinal cord blood flow during local hypothermia. *Surg Forum* 1974; 25:434–435.
95. Sakamoto T, Iwai A, Monafo WW: Regional blood flow in transected rat spinal cord during hypothermia. *Am J Physiol* 1990; 259:H1649–H1654.
96. Benveniste H: The excitotoxic hypothesis in relation to cerebral ischemia. *Cerebrovasc Brain Metab Rev* 1991; 3:213–245.
97. Choi DW, Rothman SM: The role of glutamate neurotoxicity in hypoxic-ischemic neuronal death. *Ann Rev Neurosci* 1990; 13:171–182.
98. Faden AI, Demediuk P, Panter SS, Vink R: The role of excitatory amino acids and NMDA receptors in traumatic brain injury. *Science* 1989; 244:798–800.
99. Busto R, Globus MY-T, Dietrich WD, et al: Effect of mild hypothermia on ischemia-induced release of neurotransmitters and free fatty acids in rat brain. *Stroke* 1989; 20:904–910.
100. Baker AJ, Zornow MH, Grafe MR, et al: Hypothermia prevents ischemia-induced increases in hippocampal glycine concentrations in rabbits. *Stroke* 1991; 22:666–673.
101. Mitani A, Kataoka K: Critical levels of extracellular glutamate mediating gerbil hippocampal delayed neuronal death during hypothermia: Brain microdialysis study. *Neuroscience* 1991; 42:661–670.
102. Lyeth BG, Jiang JY, Robinson SE, et al: Hypothermia blunts acetylcholine increase in CSF in traumatically brain injured rats. *Soc Neurosci Abstr* 1991; 17:165.
103. Andine P, Orwar O, Jacobson I, et al: Changes in extracellular amino acids and spontaneous neuronal activity during ischemia and extended reflow in the CA1 of the rat hippocampus. *J Neurochem* 1991; 57:222–229.
104. Lin B, Globus MY-T, Dietrich WD, et al: Differing neurochemical and morphological sequelae of global ischemia. *J Neurochem* 1992; 59:2213–2223.
105. Lin B, Dietrich WD, Busto R, et al: Postischemic brain hypothermia combined with delayed MK-801 treatment protects chronically after global ischemia in rats. *Stroke* 1994; 25:254.
106. McDonald JW, Chen C-K, Trescher WH, Johnston MV: The severity of excitotoxic brain injury is dependent on brain temperature in immature rat. *Neurosci Lett* 1991; 126:83–86.
107. Povlishock JT, Dietrich WD: The blood-brain barrier in brain injury: An overview, in Globus MY-T, Dietrich WD (eds): *The Role of Neurotransmitters in Brain Injury.* New York: Plenum Publishing, 1992: 265–269.
108. Krantis A: Hypothermia-induced reduction in the permeation of radiolabelled tracer substances across the blood-brain barrier. *Acta Neuropathol* 1983; 60:61–69.
109. Jiang JY, Lyeth BG, Clifton GL, et al: Relationship between body and brain temperature in traumatically brain-injured rodents. *J Neurosurg* 1991; 74:492–496.
110. Barbe MF, Tyell M, Gower DJ, Welch WJ: Hyperthermia protects against light damage in the rat retina. *Science* 1988; 241:1817–1820.
111. Chopp M, Li Y, Dereski MO, et al: Hypothermia reduces 72-kDa heat-shock protein induction in rat brain after transient forebrain ischemia. *Stroke* 1992; 23:104–107.
112. Taft WC, Yang K, Dixon CE, Hayes RL: Microtubule associated protein 2 levels decrease in hippocampus following traumatic brain injury. *J Neurotrauma* 1992; 9:281–290.
113. Miyazawa T, Bonnekoh P, Hossmann K-A: Temperature effect on immunostaining of microtubule-associated protein 2 and synaptophysin after 30 minutes of forebrain ischemia in rat. *Acta Neuropathol* 1993; 85:526–532.
114. Busto R, Globus MY-T, Neary JT, Ginsberg MD: Regional alterations of protein kinase activity following transient cerebral ischemia: Effects of intraischemic brain temperature modulation. *J Neurochem* 1994; 63:1095–1103.
115. Siesjo BD: Cell damage in the brain: A speculative synthesis. *J Cereb Blood Flow Metab* 1981; 1:155–185.
116. Mitani, Kadoya F, Kataoka K: Temperature dependence of hypoxia-induced calcium accumulation in gerbil hippocampal slices. *Brain Res* 1991; 159–163.
117. Araki N, Greenberg JH, Sladky JT, Reivich M: Effects of mild hypothermia on the changes of intracellular calcium in focal ischemia. *J Cereb Blood Flow Metab* 1991; 11(suppl 2):S843.
118. Dietrich WD: Morphological manifestations of reperfusion injury in brain. *Ann NY Acad Sci* 1994; 723:15–24.
119. Schmid-Schonbein GW: Capillary plugging by granulocytes and the no-reflow phenomenon in the microcirculation. *Fed Proc* 1987; 46:2397–2401.
120. Jenkins LW, Povlishock JT, Lewelt W, et al: The role of postischemic recirculation in the development of ischemic neuronal injury following complete cerebral ischemia. *Acta Neuropathol* 1981; 55:205–220.
121. Pulsinelli WA, Brierley JB, Plum F: Temporal profile of neuronal damage in a model of transient forebrain ischemia. *Ann Neurol* 1980; 11:491–498.
122. Dietrich WD, Halley M, Valdes I, Busto R: Interrelationships between increased vascular permeability and

acute neuronal injury damage following temperature controlled brain ischemia in rats. *Acta Neuropathol* 1991; 81:615–625.

123. Valeri CR, Cassidy G, Khuri S, et al: Hypothermia-induced reversible platelet dysfunction. *Ann Surg* 1987; 205:175–181.
124. Kontos HA: Oxygen radicals in CNS injury. *Chem Biol Interactions* 1989; 72:229–255.
125. Chan PH, Schmidley JW, Fishman RA, Longar SM: Brain injury, edema, and vascular permeability changes induced by oxygen-derived free radicals. *Neurology* 1984; 34:315–320.
126. Boisvert DP: In vivo assessment of hydroxyl free radical production in the brain. *J Cereb Blood Flow Metab* 1991; 11(suppl 2):S637.
127. Baiping L, Xiujuan T, Hongwei C, et al: Effect of moderate hypothermia on lipid peroxidation in canine brain tissue after cardiac arrest and resuscitation. *Stroke* 1994; 25:147–152.
128. Buchan A, Pulsinelli WA: Hypothermia but not the N-methyl-D-aspartate antagonist, MK-801, attenuates neuronal damage in gerbils subjected to transient global ischemia. *J Neurosci* 1990; 10:311–316.
129. Corbett D, Evans S, Thomas C, et al: MK-801 reduced cerebral ischemic injury by inducing hypothermia. *Brain Res* 1990; 514:300–304.
130. Hall ED, Andrus PK, Pazara KE: Protective efficacy of a hypothermic pharmacological agent in gerbil forebrain ischemia. *Stroke* 1993; 24:711–715.
131. Hagerdal M, Keykhah M, Perez E, Harp JR: Additive effects of hypothermia and phenobarbital upon cerebral oxygen consumption in the rat. *Acta Anaesth Scand* 1979; 23:89–92.
132. Sternau L, Dietrich WD, Busto R, Kraydieh S: Barbiturates fail to protect the normothermic brain from ischemic injury. *Stroke* 1991; 22:129.
133. Ginsberg MD, Globus MY-T, Busto R, Dietrich WD: The potential of combination pharmacotherapy in cerebral ischemia, in Krieglstein J, Oberpichler H. (eds): *Pharmacology of Cerebral Ischemia.* Stuttgart: Wissenschaftliche Verlagsgesellschaft mbH, 1990: 499–510.
134. Ikonomidou C, Mosinger JL, Olney JW: Hypothermia enhances protective effect of MK-801 against hypoxic/ischemic brain damage in infant rats. *Brain Res* 1989; 487:184–187.

CHAPTER 111

INTRASPINAL TRANSPLANTATION OF FETAL TISSUE: THERAPEUTIC POTENTIAL FOR SPINAL CORD REPAIR

Dena R. Howland
Paul J. Reier
Douglas K. Anderson

Spinal cord injury (SCI) is one of the more physically, psychologically, and socially devastating human afflictions. The sociological and financial burdens associated with SCI are staggering.[1,2] The effects of SCI are pervasive and affect multiple biological systems, including the sensorimotor, respiratory, gastrointestinal, urinary, and reproductive systems.[2,3] As the result of advances in critical care and rehabilitation medicine, many patients now survive their injuries and have life spans that extend as long as 40 years post-injury.[2,3] These individuals, however, live with severe disabilities because there is currently no treatment or therapeutic regimen that can significantly enhance recovery of function. Thus, it is vital to discover ways to reconstruct or repair the injured spinal cord that will restore some degree of function. Effective treatment for SCI would have a dramatic, positive effect on both the quality of life for the spinal cord-injured and their families and on health care costs.[1,2]

The outlook for identifying safe and effective therapies for SCI has improved dramatically in the last decade. Pharmacological treatments in animal models have been shown to protect the injured spinal cord during the acute phases of injury.[4,5] Two of these therapies have been tested in clinical trials, where they improved the neurological function in humans with SCI.[6–8] Although the mechanisms by which function is preserved are not completely understood, these treatments may protect the damaged spinal cord by suppressing secondary injury processes activated by the initial mechanical trauma.[4,9,10] The benefits of these treatments, however, are limited to segments near the lesion site, and no functional improvements have been reported in chronic cases of SCI.

There are several evolving treatment paradigms that may promote greater sparing and recovery of function in both the acute and chronic phases of SCI. One approach is to modify the terrain through which axons elongate. For example, elimination of oligodendrocytes by x-irradiation or the use of antibodies against myelin components enhanced the growth of late-growing corticospinal fibers in the unlesioned newborn rat[11] and promote growth of the transected corticospinal tract in young[12] and adult[13] rat spinal cords.

Another promising strategy currently being evaluated is the transplantation of fetal neural tissue and specific cell types isolated from both the central and peripheral nervous systems. The potential for neural tissue grafts to promote axonal growth was first demonstrated by using peripheral nerve.[14–16] A piece of sciatic nerve inserted at the lesion site and into an appropriate target area formed a conduit for the elongation of a small number of axons in the adult rat. This was the first demonstration that central nervous system (CNS) axons had the intrinsic capacity to regenerate if they were provided a permissive terrain over which to grow. Subsequently, fetal tissue from a variety of CNS sites was shown to promote axonal growth in the spinal cord[17–23] and to enhance locomotor function.[19,24–30] Although our understanding of transplant mechanisms is limited, transplantation strategies are appealing because they have the potential to utilize a variety of specific and nonspecific mechanisms to restore function. Specific mechanisms include the regeneration and/or sprouting of supraspinal and segmental pathways[12,19,26,31] as well as the reinnervation of targets.[28,32,33] Nonspecific mechanisms include the provision of neurotransmitters,[32,34] trophic support,[32,34] and/or an appropriate substrate for growth.[19,26,31,35–37]

The purpose of this chapter is to identify transplantation principles and methods that result in surviving, functional intraspinal grafts and review the anatomical and functional effects of intraspinal grafting in neonatal and adult experimental animals. Finally, the potential role of fetal CNS grafting to repair the injured spinal cord in humans will be discussed.

FACTORS INVOLVED IN SUCCESSFUL NEURAL GRAFTING

Many factors are critical for the survival, development, and function of embryonic transplants in the CNS. Within the past two decades, some of these elements have been identified. These include the age of the donor, revascularization of the transplant, the host immune response and the region of the CNS used as donor tissue. We have shown recently that the time between injury and grafting, and surgical manipulation (debridement) of the injury site may limit transplant-mediated recovery of function.[31] These two factors will be described within the context of the findings from our laboratories that are presented later in this chapter.

Age of the Donor

Tissue from early gestational periods, when neurogenesis is ongoing and the dependence on oxygen is reduced, exhibits the greatest capacity to survive, develop, organize normally and integrate with the host.[38,39] In addition, the proliferative and migratory capacity of the cells from these early developmental stages may increase the transplant area available for attachment. In contrast, adult neuronal tissue usually does not survive transplantation or integrate permanently with the host.[40–42] Any surviving grafts of adult CNS tissue typically are small, necrotic and do not enhance function.

Revascularization of the Transplant

Rapid vascularization of the transplanted tissue by the host's vasculature is required for optimal transplant survival and growth in experimental animal models.[22,43–45] Within 1 day of transplantation, capillaries from the host grow into the transplant.[38,46,47] Inadequate access to, or extensive damage of, host vasculature results in very small transplants or in transplant demise.[22,47] The placement of the transplant close to well-vascularized surfaces of the host, therefore, is critical to transplant survival and growth. It is uncertain whether vascular growth results from the presence of the transplant or is a reactive sprouting phenomenon due to damage sustained by the host capillaries in the lesioning process.

Histocompatibility and the Immunological Response

The immunological reactions to transplants in the CNS are complex and may depend on several parameters including species, age of the host, and the formation of a blood brain barrier (for review see[48]). Central nervous system transplants may be more or less rapidly rejected depending on the genetic disparity between the donor and the host.[49] For example, while allografts can survive for extended periods, xenografts are generally rejected[50,51] (Anderson et al., unpublished observation). Even those xenografts that survive and integrate initially into the host tissue are still ultimately eliminated.[52,53] Survival of both xenografts and allografts can be enhanced, however, by the continued use of immunosuppressive drugs.[24,28,54] In contrast, neuronal grafts with few antigenic immunological differences from those of the host survive permanently (i.e., greater than 6 months).[21,49,55] The formation of a blood brain barrier in transplanted tissue(s) may decrease the likelihood of an immune response but does not provide a barrier to all components of the immune system and may allow at least limited passage of immunocompetent cells.[48] Some transplants never form a blood brain barrier.[47] With respect to transplantation, therefore, the CNS is not an immunologically privileged site.

There is a less intense immunological rejection of xenografts in neonatal hosts, as opposed to those in adult hosts. This difference suggests that host age may have an affect on the immune response.[56] The decreased immunological response in the neonate may result from the immaturity of the immune system. Subsequent grafts or trauma, however, may evoke immune rejection of an apparently permanent xenograft[56] or allograft (Howland et al., unpublished observations) in a neonatal host. Ultimately, the antigenicity affects the survival of the transplant. No particular host-graft combination, therefore, appears to be completely exempt from immunological reaction.[49]

ANATOMIC EVIDENCE FOR SUCCESSFUL GRAFTING

Common to a variety of SCI models, there are a number of anatomic features used to indicate successful intraspinal grafting. These anatomic features include: (1) survival and differentiation of the transplant and (2) integration and axonal connectivity between the transplant and host.

TRANSPLANT SURVIVAL AND DEVELOPMENT

Numerous studies have demonstrated that fetal neural tissue transplants survive in the CNS of both newborn[19,22,26,57] and adult hosts.[19,20,22,24] In addition, embryonic neural tissue will differentiate and show cytoarchitectural organization characteristics of the original tissue origin irrespective of the age of the recipient.[20,22,24,26,39,57,58]

AGE OF THE HOST AND AXONAL CONNECTIVITY

The amount of axon growth that occurs between the host and transplant is affected by characteristics of both the recipient and graft. Axonal connections between the host and grafted tissue are established in both neonatal and adult animals.[19,22,24,26] The age of the host, however, is inversely related to the amount of connectivity established between the host spinal cord and the graft. The growth of long projecting host afferent systems is much greater when the fetal transplant is placed into the partially lesioned neonatal spinal cord[17–19,22,59] than in the spinal cord of adults with similar lesions.[22] In adults, long-distance projections generally terminate a few millimeters beyond the host-transplant interface. In contrast, long-distance projections in neonates can grow extensively throughout the transplants and even cross the caudal transplant-host interface and grow into the denervated caudal spinal cord.[17–19,26,59]

Several factors underlie the more extensive growth of neonatal host systems in the presence of a transplant. One is the greater anatomic plasticity in the developing system compared with that in the mature system. For example, in addition to regenerating axons, late developing axons can also contribute to the more extensive transplanted-mediated growth seen in the neonatal spinal cord.[17,59]

Afferents have also been shown to extend from transplants into the spinal cord of the adult rat.[21,60] It has been hypothesized that these projections from the caudal portion of the graft, combined with descending host projections into the rostral regions of the transplant, could provide the neuronal basis for a functional relay between host and graft. In this case the transplant would not just be a passive substrate for growth but would be an active participant in relaying neuronal information. Evidence that axons from transplant neurons extend into the ventral root and continue at least as far as the midthigh in the rat sciatic nerve[23] may identify another possible relay circuit by the transplant. The extent of transplant-derived afferent growth may be linked to the transplant cell population. Human telencephalic neuroblasts transplanted into the excitotoxically lesioned adult rat striatum extend as far as the cervical spinal cord, a distance of approximately 20 mm.[60] This study suggests that such extensive outgrowth may result from the human neurons' normally protracted development in vivo and indicates that these cells are likely to remain in an actively elongating state for a prolonged period after transplantation. It is also possible that the xenograft neurons do not recognize the growth inhibitory molecules of another species.[61] Although a few other studies have reported elongation of similar distances without human tissue[22] they involved transplantation into a neonatal host.

GLIAL SCARRING AND AXONAL CONNECTIVITY

Glial scarring at the host-graft interface has long been thought to inhibit axonal growth into or out of a transplant (for review see[62]). When there is a dense gliosis at the host-graft interface, the integration between the transplant and host is poor.[22] Host axons appear to travel along graft-host borders until a continuous neurophil without gliosis is reached and then enter the transplant.[21]

It has been proposed that introduction of a fetal transplant into the lesion site may decrease the amount of scarring.[22,38,63] Houle[64] showed that the glial scar was discontinuous following transplantation of fetal spinal cord (FSC) tissue 6 to 8 weeks after a hemisection lesion in the spinal cord of the adult rat. In some instances, as much as 60 percent of the host-graft interface was free of a glial scar. Similarly, we have found that following transplantation of fetal CNS tissue into a chronic compression lesion of the adult cat spinal cord, there is little evidence of a glial scar.[24] Host-graft integration in the chronically injured cat spinal cord appears to be greater than that seen in the chronic spinal cord contusion injury of the adult rat. The slower maturing fetal cat CNS tissue may have a greater capacity than the faster developing fetal rat tissue to remove an existing glial scar and, therefore, to increase host-graft integration.

Source of Fetal Neuraxis as Donor Material and Axonal Connectivity

The source of neural transplant tissue in the spinal cord is critical for mediating connectivity of the host with the transplant. The choice of donor neural tissue can be generally divided into four groups: homotypic, heterotypic, homotopic, and heterotopic. Homotypic transplants share common features (such as transmitters) with the damaged tissue, e.g., FSC or fetal brain stem (FBSt) tissue into spinal cord. Heterotypic transplants are donor tissues that do not share common characteristics with the portion of the neuraxis into which they are transplanted, e.g., fetal neocortex (FNCx) or hippocampus into spinal cord. Homotopic transplants are a subset of homotypic transplants in that these grafts are from the same part of the CNS as the region of the neuraxis into which they are grafted, e.g., FSC into spinal cord. Conversely, heterotopic transplants are from a different part of the CNS, e.g., FBSt into spinal cord.

Homotypic intraspinal transplants promote greater host axonal growth than do heterotypic transplants. This finding may be associated with the capacity of neurons within the homotypic graft to project to the appropriate terminal fields in the host[28,32,33] and for homotypic tissue to provide a better terrain for axonal growth.[20] Moreover, homotypic grafts also form greater numbers of permanent synapses between host axons and grafted neurons than is seen with heterotypic transplants.[20,65] Enhanced growth and behavioral benefits achieved with homotopic transplants versus heterotopic transplants may be due to the presence of system-specific cues for axonal growth and synapse formation and, hence, a greater potential to form polysynaptic relays.

EFFECTS OF TRANSPLANTS ON BEHAVIORAL RECOVERY

The use of transplants to repair circuits, promote survival of axotomized neurons, or supply neurotransmitters to a denervated region is clinically meaningless unless the pathway restoration and neuronal activity improves functional recovery. The survival of a transplant, however, does not automatically confer functional effects on the host.[31,66–68] The choices of transplant origin, host system and behavioral assessment to evaluate functional effect are critical.

There have been a limited number of behavior studies evaluating the affects of transplants in the spinal cord on locomotor development or recovery. Most of these studies used the rat as an animal model. In both neonatal[19,27] and adult rats,[19,25,28–30] FSC transplants have been shown to affect some characteristic(s) of locomotion in animals with partial spinal cord injuries. The mechanisms underlying transplant enhanced recovery have not yet been well defined.

Transplants and Recovery of Motor Function in the Neonatal Rat

Functional recovery following intraspinal transplantation, like anatomic connectivity, is greater overall in the neonate than the adult.[19,27] Fetal spinal cord transplants placed into a thoracic hemisection of the spinal cord in neonatal rats have been shown to affect locomotor function quantitatively.[19,27] Neonatal rats with thoracic overhemisections that received transplants demonstrated a more normal base of support and amount of hindlimb rotation ipsilateral to the lesion than did neonatal rats with a hemisection alone or adult rats with a transplant. Fetal transplants also have been reported to affect locomotor function in neonatal rats with complete spinal cord transections.[69] Using a qualitative evaluation procedure, rats that received transplants appears to have almost normal coordination and foot placement and demonstrated the ability to walk, run and climb. The results of this study are difficult to interpret because the completeness of the initial lesions is difficult to discern. There is a striking similarity in the cytoarchitecture of the grafts and the host spinal cords. Additionally the projections of the corticospinal tract through the apparent edge of the grafts look similar to the rerouting of developing corticospinal axons around a lesion site following partial SCI.[70,71] These projections are dissimilar to the dense plexus of supraspinal fibers previously found throughout fetal transplants in the neonatally lesioned rat spinal cord.[18]

Transplants and Recovery of Motor Function in the Adult Rat

Although the influence of transplants on recovery of function is more robust in the neonate than in the adult, transplants have been shown to promote the recovery of both autonomic[32] and locomotor[19,25,30] function in adult, spinal cord-injured rats. Privat et al[32] demonstrated that raphe transplants placed into the spinal cord below the level of a complete transection restored penile reflexes. Bernstein and Goldberg[25] placed homotypic transplants into the third cervical segment of adult rats whose fasciculus gracilis had been severed bilaterally.

Animals with transplants were able to cross a narrow platform with a significant improvement in foot slips and recoveries in comparison to lesion-only controls. Bregman and colleagues[19] placed FSC into acute over-hemisections in the thoracic spinal cord of adult rats. Animals with transplants improved foot placement accuracy while crossing a grid and a more normal hindlimb stride length during overground locomotion than non-transplanted controls. Stokes and Reier[30] used a reproducible contusion injury of the thoracic spinal cord in the adult rat. Ten days after injury, one group of rats received suspensions of FSC tissue whereas a control group received only glucose-saline injections. Although there was no improvement in the performance of the transplant recipients on generalized motor tasks (i.e., Tarlov open-field, inclined plane, grid walking), the animals with transplants showed a statistical significant improvement in base of support and stride length. This recovery was seen as early as 1 week after grafting. These few studies strongly suggest that intraspinal transplants enhance recovery of function in the adult rat under a variety of lesioning conditions.

Although the rodent has contributed significantly to our understanding of intraspinal transplantation and continues to be an indispensable animal model, we are also evaluating the effects of intraspinal transplantation on recovery of locomotor function in the neonatal[26] and adult cat.[24,31] We have chosen the cat as a model due to the extensive literature on the control of locomotion in this species. Thus, the cat model provides insights to the recovery of locomotor function that are still difficult to appreciate in other experimental models.

The Spinalized Kitten

We used three groups of kittens to study the effects of homotopic embryonic transplants on locomotor function following SCI: normal kittens,[72] spinal kittens,[73] and kittens that received a fetal transplant.[26] Normal kittens were not subjected to any surgical procedures. Spinal kittens had their low thoracic spinal cords completely transected within 48 hours of birth. Kittens with transplants had solid grafts of FSC tissue placed into their lesion cavities during the same surgical procedure in which the spinal cords were transected. The fetal graft tissue was taken from embryonic day 20 to embryonic day 26 (E20–E26).

The locomotor activity of all kittens was initially observed within 24 hours of birth or surgery. Thereafter, kittens were evaluated and trained four to six times per week for 5 months. Three types of locomotion were evaluated: (1) bipedal treadmill locomotion during which the forelimbs stand on a stationary platform and the hindlimbs step in response to a moving treadmill belt; (2) quadrupedal treadmill locomotion during which all four limbs are placed on the moving treadmill belt; and (3) overground locomotion during which the animals cross a 12″-wide runway. These three types of locomotion evaluate different levels of neural control (Fig. 111-1). Coordinated hindlimb walking on a treadmill (bipedal locomotion) can be accomplished using only intraspinal networks that are located in the lumbosacral spinal cord. These intraspinal networks are composed of the hindlimb spinal pattern generators for locomotion (SPGL) and peripheral afferents.[74–77] Coordination of all four limbs while walking on a treadmill belt (quadrupedal treadmill locomotion) requires communication between the SPGL of the hindlimbs and the fore-

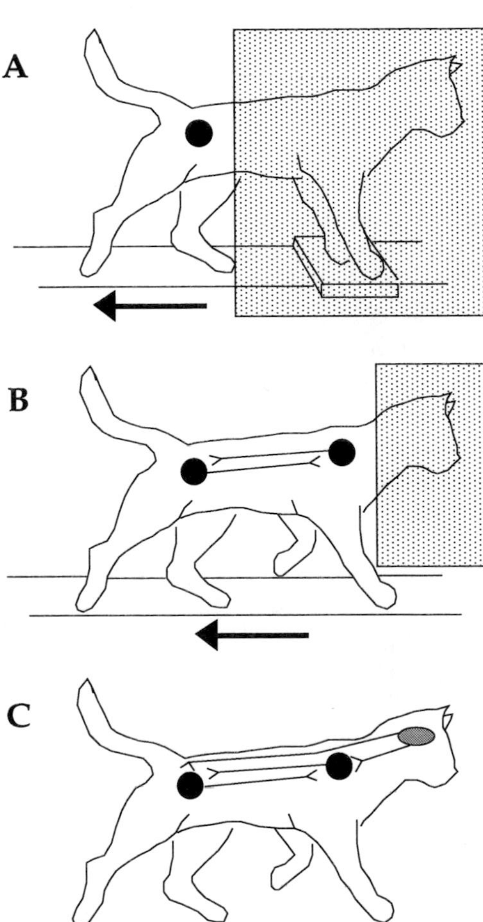

Figure 111-1. Three types of cat locomotion.

A. Bipedal treadmill locomotion requires only intraspinal networks (SPGL) and peripheral afferents located in the lumbosacral spinal cord.

B. Quadrupedal treadmill locomotion is characterized by forelimb-hindlimb coordination. This coordination requires neural connectivity between the forelimb and hindlimb SPGL. Quadrupedal treadmill locomotion can be accomplished without cortical control.

C. During overground locomotion, the spinal circuitry is influenced by descending supraspinal systems.

limbs.[78–81] Both types of treadmill locomotion, therefore, are spinally mediated. During voluntary overground locomotion, the spinal circuitry is influenced by descending supraspinal systems.[82–95] After the kittens were weaned, all forms of locomotion were conditioned to a food reward. Three aspects of quadrupedal locomotion (treadmill and overground) were quantitatively assessed from videotapes of the kittens' performances. Balance was assessed by counting the number of step cycles interrupted by a fall. Weight support was assessed by counting the number of step cycles during which the animal's body was continually supported above the walking surface. Interlimb coordination was assessed in two ways: (1) the E1–F interlimb phase interval, which looks at the timing of these step cycle subphases between ipsilateral limbs, and (2) the interlimb swing phase coordination test, which looks at the pairing of the hindlimb swing phase with the swing phase of another limb.

Normal kittens did not consistently show bipedal treadmill locomotion during the first postnatal month. Kittens with spinal transections, however, consistently stepped on the treadmill within 48 to 72 hours of lesioning. This indicates that the SPGL of the hindlimbs, located in the caudal spinal cord, are capable of functioning at birth. The activity of the SPGL are probably suppressed by descending inhibitory influences in the normal kitten.

Normal kittens developed full weight support, good balance and coordination between the hindlimbs and the forelimbs during overground locomotion by 4 weeks of age. A low thoracic spinal transection severely disrupted the development of overground locomotion. Some spinal animals developed partial hindlimb weight support during overground locomotion around 11 weeks of age. By 15 weeks, the spinal kitten with the best locomotor performance (which was dramatically different from all other spinal kittens) showed full weight support during 42 percent of its step cycles, which decreased to 26 percent by 20 weeks. No spinal kitten ever developed coordination between the hindlimbs and forelimbs. Introduction of an embryonic transplant at the time of transection accelerated and enhanced the development of overground locomotion. By 5 to 6 weeks of age, spinal kittens with transplants showed full hindlimb weight support in an average of 29 percent of their step cycles. This percentage increased to an average of 85 percent by 20 weeks. Balance also improved over the 5-month study period. By 20 weeks, on average, 7 percent of the stepcycles were interrupted by a fall in spinal kittens with transplants. This is in stark contrast to the average of 87 percent of the stepcycles in spinal-only kittens. Statistical analysis showed that both weight support and balance (evaluated by the number of falls) were significantly better in kittens with transplants than spinal-only animals at 15 and 20 weeks of age. Most spinal kittens with transplants coordinated the hindlimbs with the forelimbs at 20 weeks of age. This coordination during quadrupedal treadmill and overground locomotion strongly suggests that neural connections had been formed between the forelimb and hindlimb SPGL. Immunocytochemical analysis of the transection-transplantation sites indicated that the axons of descending supraspinal systems (noradrenergic and serotonergic), as well as segmental systems (sensory afferents), grew extensively into the transplants. Although the mechanisms remain to be clarified, these systems provide a basis for at least part of the superior overground locomotion of spinal kittens with transplants.

Chronic Compression Injuries in Adult Cats

In adult cats we have used a static loading (compression) model to produce spinal cord injury in the upper lumbar segments. Fetal CNS tissue was grafted into the resulting chronic injury cavities 2 to 30 weeks post-injury. Graft tissue was either FSC from embryonic day 21 to embryonic day 24 (E21–E24), FBSt from E21–E38, FNCx from E38, or a mixture of FSC and FBSt. Sham operated controls did not receive a fetal graft. All cats were immunosuppressed with cyclosporine A, starting the day prior to grafting. The injury,[96–101] transplantation methods, and results[24,28,31] have been described in detail previously.

Locomotor function was evaluated on a weekly basis pre-injury, post-injury, and for up to 30 weeks post-grafting. Two methods of locomotor evaluation were used. In initial studies, locomotion was assessed using a categorical assessment scale that rated each cat's ability to walk, change gait, and climb stairs.[96–98,101] A score was assigned for each performance category, the sum of which served as an index of generalized locomotor function. Eleven was the highest score and indicated normal or pre-injury function, while zero was the lowest and indicated complete paraplegia. In more recent studies, conditioned overground locomotion was evaluated. Cats were trained to cross horizontal runways and a ladder for a food reward. The runways varied in width from 2 to 12 inches and the flat 1-inch rungs of the ladder were spaced 6 inches apart. It was first determined whether an animal could cross a runway or ladder using its hindlimbs. If the cat was successful in crossing, the time to cross and the number of errors in hindlimb foot placement were determined from slow motion analysis of videotapes. Hindlimb footfall errors occur when placement of the foot causes it to miss or slip off the runway or ladder surface.

Fetal spinal cord, FBSt, and FNCx tissue, either implanted as solid pieces or as suspensions of dissociated cells, survived transplantation and were well vascularized. Healthy grafts were found 6 to 30 weeks post-grafting in 25 of 29 animals. The basic histological characteristics of the FSC and FBSt grafts into chronic compression lesions of the cat spinal cord have been described previously[24] and were similar to characteristics described for grafts into contusion lesions of the rat spinal cord.[28–30] Both neuronal and glial elements were seen. Tissue from two of the four animals without viable FSC or FBSt grafts showed active rejection of the transplant. These grafts showed significant lymphocytic infiltration and spongiform degeneration. Additionally, the rejection process appeared to be restricted to the grafts. Cyclosporine A had been discontinued in one of these animals 2.5 months prior to sacrifice (4 months post-grafting).

Recovery of locomotor function was seen in some cats that received homotypic grafts (FSC, FBSt, or both) between 2 and 9 weeks post-injury. This recovery appeared to be permanent and was assessed using the categorical rating scale. Approximately 40 percent of lost function was recovered in six of the eight cats receiving homotypic grafts. No functional improvement was seen in the cats that received grafts of FNCx or non-neuronal tissue.[24,31] Thus, while tissue from different regions of the fetal neuraxis survived, only those animals that received homotypic transplants showed an improvement in motor performance based on our categorical rating scale. This enhanced function may be, in part, due to a greater capacity of homotypic transplants to establish polysynaptic relays across the lesion than heterotypic transplants. Theoretically, it has also been suggested that a homotypic graft may serve as a tissue bridge through which axons could regenerate in the adult animal from the rostral and caudal spinal regions.[102,103]

Deterioration of locomotor performance during the last month of survival was seen in two cats that initially had shown an improvement. In both instances, the decline in locomotor function was correlated with graft rejection.

Improvement in locomotor performance suggests that homotypic grafts introduced 2 to 9 weeks post-injury can enhance recovery of hindlimb locomotor function. Moreover, the correlation between deterioration of locomotor performance and graft rejection suggests that permanent graft survival is necessary to maintain motor functions that have been enhanced by the transplant.

Thirteen additional cats that received solid grafts of FSC or FBSt tissue 8 to 31 weeks post-injury were trained and evaluated using the horizontal runways and ladder. After transplantation, the locomotor performance of three cats improved. These cats were able to perform tasks (i.e., cross narrower runways and the ladder) that they were not able to accomplish prior to transplantation. In four animals, function appeared to be unchanged by transplantation (i.e., there was no change in the ability of these cats to cross runways). Immediately after transplantation, six cats showed an immediate, permanent loss of function. They were either unable to support weight without aid or could no longer cross even the widest runway.

In this series of 13 cats, the post-grafting function appeared to be dependent on at least two factors, the time interval between injury and grafting and whether or not the lesion site was debrided at the time of grafting. The three cats that showed improved locomotor function were grafted 8 to 15 weeks following injury with little or no debridement of the lesion cavity. The four animals that showed no change in their post-graft locomotor performance received grafts 11 to 23 weeks after injury with no debridement of the lesion cavities. The six cats that showed an immediate loss of locomotor function post-grafting received grafts 10 to 31 weeks after injury. The lesion cavities of this last group of animals were extensively debrided prior to transplantation. The locomotor performance of a parallel group of four control animals was unchanged. These four animals received sham transplants (Gelfoam or media) with no lesion debridement, 14 to 29 weeks post-injury.

Effect of Delay Periods Between Injury and Grafting

These preliminary findings indicate that cats with some improvement in post-graft locomotor function had, on average, the shortest injury to graft interval. Animals whose function was either unchanged or declined after transplantation had a longer delay between injury and grafting. This suggests that there may be a "therapeutic window" following injury during which homotypic grafts must be introduced in order to enhance locomotion. Following injury the spinal cord shows some plastic features in an attempt to repair itself. Some of these features include sprouting[104–106] and the unmasking of latent functions in existing pathways.[107] If placed during the acute or subchronic post-injury phases, a graft may magnify the ongoing inherent plastic capabilities of the host CNS. It is also possible that grafts implanted during this early phase of recovery may rescue fibers or circuits that would otherwise undergo progressive degeneration.[28] In the established lesions, however, neuron death and fiber degeneration have occurred and remodeling in the spared systems has stabilized. This relative dormant nature of the chronic spinal lesion may contribute to the decreased functional efficacy of homotypic fetal grafts placed in established lesions.

EFFECT OF LESION DEBRIDEMENT ON TRANSPLANT-MEDIATED RECOVERY OF FUNCTION

These initial results suggest that it is likely that graft mechanisms which enhance locomotion may be adversely affected by injury to the host spinal cord at the time of grafting. Immediate and permanent loss of function was seen following transplantation only in those cats whose lesion cavity was debrided prior to grafting. This sudden decline in function suggests that it was the surgical procedure and not the graft that damaged the host spinal cord. Any loss of function due to overgrowth of the grafts would be expected to occur over several weeks, not immediately.

This loss of function suggests that removal of the scar tissue that had formed at the lesion site damaged adjacent, spared host systems. Scar tissue anastomosis tightly with the host neuropil[108] and host fibers are seen within this scar tissue.[109] Thus, removal of the scar would damage host fibers in and immediately adjacent to the lesion. In addition, it is possible that the same secondary pathophysiological events that contributed to the destruction of the spinal cord following the original injury[9,110] may be reactivated by the debridement procedure. Regardless of the mechanism(s), the benefits of removing the scar tissue in order to place the graft in contact with healthy neuropil appears to be negated by the damage that this procedure causes to remodeled systems in the host spinal cord.

It is conceivable, therefore, that debridement of the original lesion in preparation for the grafting of solid pieces of fetal tissue might cause an additional loss of host systems that could mask or minimize any graft-mediated improvement of locomotor performance. This may be particularly true for the more established lesions which appear to be the most susceptible to surgical manipulation. Consequently, a permanent loss of spared function due to debridement plus grafting may argue for the exclusive use of less invasive approaches for placing donor tissue such as injection of dissociated CNS tissue. Injections of cell suspensions cause relatively little damage to the spared host structures they penetrate in contrast to the surgical incisions (frequently with debridement) that must be made when placing a solid graft into a chronic lesion.

Pharmacological treatment of the recipient at the time of transplantation may enhance functional recovery by suppressing the progression of any surgically-induced secondary injury processes. Vitamin E, methylprednisolone sodium succinate (MP), and Trilizad mesylate have all been shown to restrict progression of secondary injury processes.[96–98] In addition, the same pathophysiological processes that damage host tissue could also kill large numbers of the grafted cells. Other work currently ongoing in our laboratories shows that there is a rapid loss of intraspinal fetal graft tissue by 4 days post-grafting.[111,112] Nonetheless, clusters of surviving cells proliferate to produce a graft that fills the lesion cavity by 1 month. If the rats are treated with high doses of MP for the first 4 hours after grafting, the amount of surviving graft tissue appears to be increased at 4 days post-grafting.[112] Rescue of grafted tissue that is destined to die may augment the effects of a transplant. This enhanced early survival of grafted tissue may mean an earlier, more robust, supply of transplant produced neurotrophic and/or neurotropic factors. These factors could increase host-graft neuritic interactions and the number of host fibers and neurons that are rescued. Thus, future studies need to focus on the functional benefits of solid and suspension grafts in combination with the use of pharmacological agents to identify the most effective transplantation procedure(s).

POSSIBLE MECHANISMS OF GRAFT-MEDIATED ACTIVITY

There appear to be at least four potential mechanisms underlying transplant-mediated recovery of function: (1) rescue of host neurons or fibers destined to die; (2) neuronal replacement; (3) reconnectivity across the lesion by formation of polysynaptic relays between host and graft neurons or by axons that use the transplant as a bridge; and (4) supply of neurotransmitters, and neurotrophic and neurotropic factors. These four mechanisms could enhance recovery of function in a variety of SCI models (i.e., resection, suction, or contusion/compression-type lesions). However, an additional mechanism may be operative following the contusion/compression injury. This type of injury is characterized by a central cavity surrounded by a rim of spared white matter. It is likely that the spared tissue contains both functional and dysfunctional fibers. Perhaps grafts can enhance recovery of function in this type of lesion by re-establishing conduction in some of these intact but dysfunctional pathways. The graft tissue could modify the physiological environment of the lesion site,[113,114] block potassium channels in the spared fibers,[115–117] remyelinate demyelinated fibers,[118–120] or provide a glial population capable of transferring sodium channels to the spared axons of the host.[121]

LONG-RANGE IMPLICATIONS OF INTRASPINAL GRAFTING FOR SPINAL CORD INJURED HUMANS

Although fetal tissue transplantation is still experimental, current clinical studies in which mesencephalic tissue from aborted fetuses is placed into individuals with Parkinson's disease[122,123] suggests that this approach may be an effective therapy for certain neurodegenerative diseases. In neurodegenerative processes, as well as in SCI,[124–128] cells and fiber tracts that are essential for normal function are destroyed. Currently, the best option for replacing these cells and lost circuitry is the use of fetal neural tissue. Tissue from the adult CNS is not a viable option for spinal cord repair or the treatment of neurodegenerative diseases because adult neurons are differentiated and lack the ability to proliferate. Adult CNS tissue also dies rapidly upon separation from its blood supply. In addition, the immunogenic characteristics of adult tissue, relative to that of fetal tissue, enhance its chances of rejection by the recipient's immune system.

The potential for fetal tissue transplantation to evolve into a successful treatment for SCI, theoretically, appears to be greater than other current medical treatments. This is because of the multiple mechanisms by which intraspinal fetal transplants may enhance both suprasegmental and segmental function. For example, voluntary motor control could be re-established if fetal neural grafts can restore connectivity, whether through novel connections, rescue of degenerating fibers, or enhancement of intact but dysfunctional pathways in the host. Similar mechanisms might also enhance involuntary autonomic functions.

Fetal tissue transplantation may also be useful to retard deterioration of spared function. Twenty percent of all traumatic SCI cases are complicated by syringomyelia.[129] The spinal shunts that are currently used to drain the expanding syrinx, however, do not permanently halt the progression of syringomyelia.[130] Progression of the syrinx causes pain, increased spasticity, and motor and sensory loss rostral to the original lesion.[131] Since it has been shown that fetal neural tissue grows and can completely fill spinal defects,[24,26] fetal tissue placed into a syrinx may act as a plug. A fetal tissue plug might prevent the accumulation of fluid believed to cause expansion of the syrinx.

In addition to its more immediate clinical implications, fetal neural transplantation is also a vital research tool. Fetal tissue research is providing, and will continue to provide, the clues necessary to identify alternative sources of donor tissue. With current technology, cell lines are being genetically engineered to produce various neurotrophic[132–134] and neurotropic molecules.[135,136] In the future, transplantation of these genetically designed cells may be more therapeutic for select diseases or injury processes than the mixture of cells found in fetal tissue. Alternatively, the benefits of intraspinal fetal transplants may be enhanced by co-transplants of genetically engineered cells. If other sources of donor material prove to be a viable approach to the treatment of SCI as well as other disorders of the nervous system, then the need for fetal tissue may be temporary and the controversy surrounding its use moot.

The evolving literature on the functional benefits of intraspinal transplantation with fetal tissue as well as the availability of usable fetal tissue from voluntary abortions makes it an attractive, although experimental, option for medical treatment. It is difficult to ignore the number of individuals that suffer with SCI who might benefit each year if tissue salvaged from legally aborted fetuses was used for intraspinal transplantation. The medical use of fetal tissue needs to be separated from the controversy surrounding abortion and viewed as donated human tissue that has therapeutic potential[137] in addition to its value as a vital research tool.

ACKNOWLEDGMENTS

The work from our laboratories described in this chapter was supported in part by the Department of Veterans Affairs (D.K.A.), the American Paralysis Association (D.K.A.), the Spinal Cord Research Foundation of the Paralyzed Veterans of America (D.K.A.), the National Institutes of Health (P.J.R., NIH PO1 NS27511), the C.M. and K.E. Overstreet (D.K.A.) and Mark F. Overstreet (P.J.R.) Endowments for Spinal Cord Injury Research at the University of Florida College of Medicine, and the Florida Brain and Spinal Cord Injury Rehabilitation Trust Fund.

References

1. Berkowitz M, Harvey C, Greene CG, et al: *The Economic Consequences of Traumatic Spinal Cord Injury.* New York: Demos Publications, 1992.
2. Tator CA: Epidemiology and general characteristics of the spinal cord injured patient, in: Benzel ED, Tator CH (eds): *Contemporary Management of Spinal Cord Injury.* American Association of Neurological Surgeons, 1995; 9–13.
3. Singh RVP, Suys S, Villanueva PA: Prevention and treatment of medical complications, in: Benzel ED, Ta-

tor CH (eds): *Contemporary Management of Spinal Cord Injury.* American Association of Neurological Surgeons, 1995; 195–215.
4. Anderson DK: Antioxidant therapy in experimental spinal cord injury. *Restor Neurol Neurosci* 1991; 2:169–172.
5. Beattie MS, Stokes BT, Bresnahan JC: Experimental spinal cord injury. Strategies for acute and chronic intervention based on anatomic, physiological, and behavioral studies, in: Stein DG, Sabel BA (eds): *Pharmacological Approaches to the Treatment of Brain and Spinal Cord Injury.* New York: Plenum Press, 1988: 43–47.
6. Bracken MB, Shepard MJ, Collins WF Jr et al: A randomized controlled trial of methylprednisolone or naloxone in the treatment of acute spinal cord injury. *N Engl J Med* 1990; 322:1405–1411.
7. Bracken MB, Shepard MJ, Collins WF Jr et al: Methylprednisolone or naloxone treatment after acute spinal cord injury: 1-year follow-up data. *J Neurosurg* 1992; 76:23–31.
8. Geisler FH, Dorsey FC, Coleman WP: Recovery of motor function following spinal cord injury–a randomized, placebo-controlled trial with GM-1 ganglioside. *N Engl J Med* 1991; 324:1829–1838.
9. Anderson DK, Thomas CE: Mechanisms and role of oxygen free radicals in CNS pathology, in: Recent Advances in the Treatment of Neurodegenerative Disorders and Cognitive Dysfunction *Proceedings of the International Academy for Biomedical and Drug Research CINP President's Workshop.* Basel: Karger, 1994: 119–124.
10. Hall ED, Yonkers PA, Andrus PK, et al: Biochemistry and pharmacology of lipid antioxidants in acute brain and spinal cord injury. *J Neurotrauma* 1992; 9(Suppl 2):S425–S442.
11. Schwab ME, Schnell L: Channeling of developing rat corticospinal tract axons by myelin-associated neurite growth inhibitors. *J Neurosci* 1991; 11:709–721.
12. Schnell L, Schwab ME: Axonal regeneration in the rat spinal cord produced by an antibody against myelin-associated neurite growth inhibitors. *Nature* 1990; 343:269–272.
13. Kunkel-Bagden E, Schnell L, Dai HN, et al: Does the regrowth of injured corticospinal fibers elicited by antibodies to neurite growth inhibitors lead to recovery of motor function? *Soc Neurosci Abstr* 1993; 23:681.
14. Aguayo A, David S, Richardson P, et al: Axonal elongation in peripheral and central nervous system transplants. *Adv Cell Neurobiol* 1982; 3:215–234.
15. David S, Aguayo A: Axonal elongation into peripheral nervous system "bridges" after central nervous system injury in adult rat. *Science* 1981; 214:931–933.
16. Richardson PM, McGuinness UM, Aguayo AJ: Axons from CNS neurones regenerate into PNS grafts. *Nature* 1980; 284:264–265.
17. Bernstein-Goral H, Bregman BS: Spinal cord transplants support the regeneration of axotomized neurons after spinal cord lesions at birth: A quantitative double labelling study. *Exper Neurol* 1993; 23:118–132.
18. Bregman BS: Spinal cord transplants permit growth of serotonergic axons across the site of neonatal spinal cord transections. *Dev Brain Res* 1987; 34:265–279.
19. Bregman BS, Kunkel-Bagden E, Reier PJ, et al: Recovery of function after spinal cord injury: Mechanisms underlying transplant-mediated recovery of function differ after spinal cord injury in newborn and adult rats. *Exper Neurol* 1993; 123:3–16.
20. Itoh Y, Tessler A: Regeneration of adult dorsal root axons into transplants of fetal spinal cord and brain—a comparison of growth and synapse formation in appropriate and inappropriate targets. *J Comp Neurol* 1990; 302:272–293.
21. Jakeman LB, Reier PJ: Axonal projections between fetal spinal cord transplants and the adult rat spinal cord: A neuroanatomical tracing study of local interactions. *J Comp Neurol* 1991; 307:311–334.
22. Reier PJ, Bregman BS, Wujek JR: Intraspinal transplantation of embryonic spinal cord tissue in neonatal and adult rats. *J Comp Neurol* 196; 247:275–296.
23. Tessler A, Himes BT, Houle J, et al: Regeneration of adult dorsal root axons into transplants of embryonic spinal cord. *J Comp Neurol* 1988; 270:537–548.
24. Anderson DK, Reier PJ, Wirth ED III et al: Delayed grafting of fetal CNS tissue into chronic compression lesions of the adult spinal cord. *Restor Neurol Neurosci* 1991; 2:309–325.
25. Bernstein JJ, Goldberg WJ: Fetal spinal cord homografts ameliorate the severity of lesion-induced hindlimb behavioral deficits. *Exper Neurol* 1987; 98:633–644.
26. Howland DR, Bregman BS, Tessler A, et al: Transplants enhance locomotion in neonatal kittens whose spinal cords are transected: A behavioral and anatomical study. *Exper Neurol* 1995; 135:123–145.
27. Kunkel-Bagden E, Bregman BS: Spinal cord transplants enhance the recovery of locomotor function after spinal cord injury at birth. *Exper Brain Res* 1990; 81:25–34.
28. Reier PJ, Anderson DK, Stokes BT: Neural tissue transplantation and CNS trauma: Anatomical and functional repair of the injured spinal cord. *J Neurotrauma* 1992; 9(Suppl 1):S223–S248.
29. Reier PJ, Stokes BT, Thompson FJ, et al: Fetal cell grafts into resection and contusion/compression injuries of the rat and cat spinal cord. *Exper Neurol* 1992; 115:177–188.
30. Stokes BT, Reier PJ: Fetal grafts alter chronic behavioral outcome after contusion damage to the adult rat spinal cord. *Exper Neurol* 1992; 116:1–12.
31. Anderson DK, Howland DR, Reier PJ: Characteristics of intraspinal grafts and locomotor function after spinal cord injury, in: Juurlink B, Kulyk W, Krone P, Verge V, Doucette R (eds): Neural Cell Specification: Molecular Mechanisms and Neurotherapeutic Implication *Proceedings of the Third Altschul Symposium.* New York: Plenum Press, 1995.
32. Privat A, Mansour H, Rajaofetra N, et al: Intraspinal transplants of serotonergic neurons in the adult rat. *Brain Res Bull* 1989; 22:123–129.
33. Reier PJ, Anderson DK, Schrimsher GW, et al: Neural

cell grafting; Anatomical and functional repair of the spinal cord, in: Salzman S, Faden AI (eds): *The Neurobiology of Central Nervous System Trauma.* Oxford: Oxford University Press, 1994: 288–311.

34. Yakovleff A, Roby-Brami A, Guezard B, et al: Locomotion in rats transplanted with noradrenergic neurons. *Brain Res Bull* 1989; 22:115–121.
35. Kliot M, Smith GM, Siegal JD, et al: Astrocyte-polymer implants promote regeneration of dorsal root fibers into the adult mammalian spinal cord. *Exper Neurol* 1990; 109:57–69.
36. Li Y, Raisman G: Schwann cells induce sprouting in motor and sensory axons in the adult rat spinal cord. *J Neurosci* 1994; 14:4050–4063.
37. Xu XM, Guenard V, Kleitman N, et al: Axonal regeneration into Schwann cell-seeded guidance channels grafted into transected adult rat spinal cord. *J Comp Neurol* 1995; 351:145–160.
38. Das GD: Development of neocortical transplants, in: Bjorkland A, Stenevi U (eds): *Neural Grafting in the Mammalian Central Nervous System.* Amsterdam: Elsevier, 1985: 101–123.
39. Kromer LF, Bjorklund A, Stenevi U: Intracephalic embryonic neural implants in the adult rat brain. I. Growth and mature organization of brainstem, cerebellar, and hippocampal implants. *J Comp Neurol* 1983; 218:433–459.
40. Azmitia ECA: Serotonin-hippocampal model indicates adult neurons survive transplantation and aged target may be deficient in a soluble serotenergic growth factor. *Ann NY Acad Sci* 1987; 495:362–376.
41. Ignacio V, Collins VP, Suard IM, et al: Survival of astroglial cell lineage from adult brain transplants. *Devel Neurosci* 1989; 11:174–178.
42. Palaoglu S, Benli K, Pamir N, et al: Examination of autologous and embryonic cortical brain tissue transplantation to adult brain cortex in rats. *Surg Neurol* 1988; 29:183–190.
43. Berry M: Transplantation and regeneration of neural tissue in the central nervous system. *Curr Opin Neurol Neurosurg* 1988; 1:1068–1076.
44. Iversen SD, Dunnett SB: Functional compensation afforded by grafts of foetal neurones. *Prog Neuropsychobiol Psychiatry* 1989; 13:453–467.
45. Nornes H, Bjorklund A, Stenevi U: Reinnervation of the denervated adult spinal cord of rats by intraspinal transplants of embryonic brain stem neurons. *Cell Tissue Res* 1983; 230:15–35.
46. Krum JM, Rosenstein JM: Patterns of angiogenesis in neural transplant models: I. Autonomic tissue transplants. *J Comp Neurol* 1987; 258:420–434.
47. Svendgaard NA, Bjorklund A, Hardebo JE, et al: Axonal degeneration associated with a defective blood-brain barrier in cerebral implants. *Nature* 1975; 255:334–337.
48. Widner K, Brundin P: Immunological aspects of grafting in the mammalian central nervous system. A review and speculative synthesis. *Brain Res Rev* 1988; 13:287–324.
49. Poltorak M, Freed WJ: Immunological reactions induced by intracerebral transplantation: Evidence that host microglia but not astroglia are the antigen-presenting cells. *Exper Neurol* 1989; 103:222–233.
50. Finsen BR, Sorenson B, Castellano B, et al: Leukocyte infiltration and glial reactions in xenografts of mouse brain tissue undergoing rejection in the adult rat brain. A light and electron microscopical immunocytochemical study. *J Neuroimmunol* 1991; 32:159–183.
51. Freed WJ, Dymecki J, Poltorak M, et al: Intraventricular brain allografts and xenografts: Studies of survival and rejection with and without systemic sensitization, in: Gash DM, Sladek JR Jr (eds): *Progress in Brain Research.* Amsterdam: Elsevier, 1988: 233–241.
52. Booss J, Baumann N, Collins P, et al: Host response during successful engraftment of fetal xenogenic astrocytes: Predominance of microglia and macrophages. *J Neurosci Res* 1991; 30:455–462.
53. Suard IM, Collins VP, Ignacio V, et al: Implantation of rabbit embryo brain fragments into newborn mice: Integration and survival of xenogeneic astrocytes. *J Neurosci Res* 1989; 23:172–179.
54. Finsen B, Poulsen PH, Zimmer J: Xenografting of fetal mouse hippocampal tissue to the brain of adult rats: Effects of cyclosporin A treatment. *Exp Brain Res* 1988; 70:117–133.
55. Gonzalez MF, Sharp FR, Loken JE: Fetal frontal cortex transplanted to injured motor/sensory cortex of adult rats. Reciprocal connections with host thalamus demonstrated with WGA-HRP. *Exper Neurol* 1988; 99:154–165.
56. Rao K, Lund RD, Kunz HW, et al: Immunological implications of xenogeneic and allogeneic transplantation to neonatal rats. *Prog Brain Res* 1988; 78:281–286.
57. Himes BT, Goldberger ME, Tessler A: Grafts of fetal central nervous system tissue rescue axotomized Clarke's nucleus neurons in adult and neonatal operates. *J Comp Neurol* 1994; 339:117–131.
58. Jakeman LB, Reier PJ, Bregman BS, et al: Differentiation of substantia gelatinosa-like regions in intraspinal and intracerebral transplants of embryonic spinal cord tissue in the rat. *Exper Neurol* 1989; 103:17–33.
59. Bregman BS, Bernstein-Gora H: Both regenerating and late-developing pathways contribute to transplant-induced anatomical plasticity after spinal lesions at birth. *Exp Neurol* 1991; 112:49–63.
60. Wictorin K, Brundin P, Gustavil B, et al: Reformation of long axon pathways in adult rat central nervous system by human forebrain neuroblasts. *Nature* 1990; 347:556–558.
61. Davies SJA, Field PM, Raisman G: Long interfascicular axon growth from embryonic neurons transplanted into adult myelinated tracts. *J Neurosci* 1994; 14:1596–1612.
62. Reier PJ, Houle JD: The glia scar: Its bearing on axonal elongation and transplantation approaches to CNS repair, in Waxman SG (ed): *Advances in Neurology.* New York: Raven Press, 1988: 87–138.
63. Houle JD, Reier PJ: Transplantation of fetal spinal cord tissue into the chronically injured adult rat spinal cord. *J Comp Neurol* 1988; 269:537–547.

64. Houle J: The structural integrity of glial scar tissue associated with a chronic spinal cord lesion can be altered by transplanted fetal spinal cord tissue. *J Neurosci Res* 1992; 31:120–130.
65. Bregman BS, Kunkel-Bagden E: Effect of target and nontarget transplants on neuronal survival and axonal elongation after injury to the developing spinal cord. *Prog Brain Res* 1988;78:205–212.
66. Lee MH, Rabe A: Neocortical transplants in the microencephalic rat brain. *Morph Behav Brain Res Bull* 1988; 21:813–824.
67. Pallini R, Fernandez E, Gangitano C, et al: Studies on embryonic transplants to the transected spinal cord of adult rats. *J Neurosurg* 1989; 70:454–462.
68. Szeifert GT, Ladocsi T, Zagon A, et al: Transplantation of cultured embryonic spinal cord grafts into the hemisected spinal cord of adult rabbits. *Surg Neurol* 1989; 32:273–280.
69. Iwashita Y, Kawaguchi S, Murata M: Restoration of function by replacement of spinal cord segments in the rat. *Nature* 1994; 367:167–170.
70. Bernstein DR, Stelzner DJ: Plasticity of the corticospinal tract following midthoracic spinal injury in the postnatal rat. *J Comp Neurol* 1983; 221:382–400.
71. Schreyer DJ, Jones EG: Growing corticospinal axons bypass lesions of neonatal rat spinal cord. *Neuroscience* 1983; 9:31–40.
72. Howland DR, Bregman BS, Tessler A, et al: The development of quadrupedal locomotion in the kitten. *Exper Neurol* 1995; 135:93–107.
73. Howland DR, Bregman BS, Tessler A, et al: Development of locomotor behavior in the spinal kitten. *Exper Neurol* 1995; 135:108–122.
74. Grillner S, Zangger P: On the central generation of locomotion in the low spinal cat. *Exper Brain Res* 1979; 34:241–261.
75. Guiliani CA, Smith JL: Stepping behaviors in chronic spinal cats with one hindlimb deafferented. *J Neurosci* 1987; 7:2537–2546.
76. Kato M: Chronically isolated half spinal cord generates locomotor activities in the ipsilateral hindlimb of the cat. *Neurosci Res* 1990; 9:22–34.
77. Kato M: Chronically isolated lumbar half spinal cord, produced by hemisection and longitudinal myelotomy, generates locomotor activities of the ipsilateral hindlimb of the cat. *Neurosci Lett* 1989; 98:149–153.
78. Miller S, Van der Meche FGA: Coordinated stepping of all four limbs in the high spinal cat. *Brain Res* 1976; 109:395–398.
79. Miller S, van der Burg J, Van der Meche FGA: Coordination of movements of the hindlimbs and forelimbs in different forms of locomotion in normal decerebrate cats. *Brain Res* 1975; 91:217–237.
80. Miller S, Reitsma DJ, Van der Meche FGA: Functional organization of long ascending proprio-spinal pathways linking lumbosacral and cervical segments in the cat. *Brain Res* 1973; 62:169–188.
81. Miller S, van der Burg J: The function of long propriospinal pathways in the coordination of quadrupedal stepping in the cat, in: Stein RB, Pearson KG, Smith RS, Redford JB (eds): *Control of Posture and Locomotion.* New York: Plenum Press, 1973: 561–577.
82. Amos A, Armstrong DM, Marple-Horvat DE: Changes in the discharge patterns of motor cortical neurones associated with volitional changes in stepping in the cat. *Neurosci Lett* 1990; 109:107–112.
83. Armstrong DM: Review lecture, the supraspinal control of mammalian locomotion. *J Physiol* 1988; 405:1–37.
84. Armstrong DM: The motor cortex and locomotion in the cat, in: Grillner S, Stein PSG, Stuart DG, Forssberg H, Herman RM (eds): *Neurobiology of Vertebrate Locomotion.* London: Macmillan Press, 1986: 121–137.
85. Barbeau H, Rossignol S: Initiation and modulation of the locomotor pattern in the adult chronic spinal cat by noradrenergic, serotonergic and dopaminergic drugs. *Brain Res* 1991; 546:250–260.
86. Drew T: Motor cortical cell discharge during voluntary gait modification. *Brain Res* 1988; 457:181–187.
87. Garcia-Rill E, Skinner RD: The mesencephalic locomotor region. I. Activation of a medullary projection site. *Brain Res* 1987; 411:1–12.
88. Garcia-Rill E, Skinner RD: The mesencephalic locomotor region. II. Projections to reticulospinal neurons. *Brain Res* 1987; 411:13–20.
89. Martin JH, Ghez C: Red nucleus and motor cortex: Parallel motor systems for the initiation and control of skilled movement. *Behav Brain Res* 1988; 28:217–223.
90. Mori S, Kawahara K, Sakamoto T, et al: Setting and resetting the level of postural muscle tone in decerebrate cats by stimulation of the brainstem. *J Neurophysiol* 1982; 48:737–748.
91. Mori S, Nishimura C, Kurakami C, et al: Controlled locomotion in the mesencephalic cat: Distribution of facility and inhibitory regions within pontine tegmentum. *J Neurophysiol* 1978; 41:1580–1591.
92. Mori S, Shik ML, Yagodnitsyn AS: Role of pontine tegmentum for locomotor control in mesencephalic cat. *J Neurophysiol* 1977; 40:284–295.
93. Orlovsky GN: The effect of different descending systems on flexor and extensor activity during locomotion. *Brain Res* 1972; 40:359–371.
94. Orlovsky GN: Activity of vestibulospinal neurons during locomotion. *Brain Res* 1972; 46:85–98.
95. Shik ML, Severin FB, Orlovsky GN: Control of walking and running by means of electrical stimulation of the midbrain. *Biophysics* 1966; 11:755–765.
96. Anderson DK, Braughler JM, Hall ED, et al: Effects of treatment with U-74006F on neurological outcome following experimental spinal cord compression injury. *J Neurosurg* 1988; 69:562–567.
97. Anderson DK, Waters TR, Means ED: Pretreatment with alpha tocopherol enhances neurological recovery after experimental spinal cord compression injury. *J Neurotrauma* 1988; 5:61–68.
98. Anderson DK, Saunders RD, Demediuk P, et al: Lipid hydrolysis and peroxidation in injured spinal cord. Partial protection with methylprednisolone and vitamin E. *CNS Trauma* 1985; 2:257–267.

99. Anderson DK, Means ED, Waters TR, et al: Spinal cord energy metabolism following compression trauma to the feline spinal cord. *J Neurosurg* 1980; 53:375–380.
100. Anderson DK, Prockop LD, Means ED, et al: Cerebrospinal fluid lactate and electrolyte levels following experimental spinal cord injury. *J Neurosurg* 1976; 44:715–722.
101. Means ED, Anderson DK, Waters TR, et al: Effect of methylprednisolone in compression trauma to the feline spinal cord. *J Neurosurg* 1981; 55:200–208.
102. Nornes H, Bjorklund A, Stenevi U: Transplantation strategies in spinal cord regeneration, in Sladek JR, Jr., Gash DM (eds): *Neural Transplants—Development and Function.* New York: Plenum Press, 1984.
103. Reier PJ: Neural tissue grafts and repair of the injured spinal cord. *Neuropathol Appl Neurobiol* 1985; 11:81–104.
104. Liu CN, Chambers WW: Intraspinal sprouting of dorsal root axons. *Arch Neurol Psychiatry* 1958; 49:46–61.
105. Murray M, Goldberger ME: Replacement of synaptic terminals in lamina II and Clarke's nucleus after unilateral lumbosacral dorsal rhizotomy in adult cats. *J Neurosci* 1986; 6:3205–3217.
106. Zhang B, Goldberger ME, Murray M: Proliferation of SP- and 5HT-containing terminals in lamina II of rat spinal cord following dorsal rhizotomy: quantitative EM-immunocytochemical studies. *Exper Neurol* 1993; 123:51–63.
107. Alstermark B, Lundberg A, Pettersson LG, et al: Motor recovery after serial spinal cord lesions of defined descending pathways in cats. *Neurosci Res* 1987; 5:68–73.
108. Barrett CP, Donati EJ, Guth L: Differences between adult and neonatal rats in their astroglial response to spinal injury. *Exper Neurol* 1984; 84:374–385.
109. Reier PJ, Stensaas LJ, Guth L: The astrocytic scar as an impediment to regeneration in the central nervous system, in Kao CC, Bunge RP, Reier PJ (eds): *Spinal Cord Reconstruction.* New York: Raven Press, 1983: 163–196.
110. Means ED, Anderson DK: The pathophysiology of acute spinal cord injury, in Davidoff RA (ed): *Handbook of the Spinal Cord.* New York: Marcel Dekker, Inc., 1987: 19–61.
111. Theele DP, Reier PJ: Possible pathophysiological and immunological influences on intraspinal fetal graft growth and survival. *Am Soc Neural Transpl* 1995; 2:31.
112. White TE, Schrimsher GW, Anderson DK, et al: Pharmacological neuroprotection (NP) and early viability of intraspinal fetal grafts. *Soc Neurosci Abstr* 1995; 21:821.
113. Barres BA, Loroshetz WJ, Chun LL, et al: Ion channel expression by white matter glia—The type-1 astrocyte. *Neuron* 1990; 5:527–544.
114. Stokes BT, Reier PJ: Oxygen treatment in intraspinal fetal grafts: Graft-host relations. *Exper Neurol* 1991; 111:312–323.
115. Blight AR: Effect of 4-aminopyridine on axonal conduction-block in chronic spinal cord injury. *Brain Res Bull* 1989; 22:47–52.
116. Blight AR, Toombs JP, Bauer MS, et al: The effects of 4-aminopyridine on neurological deficits in chronic cases of traumatic spinal cord injury in dogs: A phase I clinical trial. *J Neurotrauma* 1991; 8:103–118.
117. Hansebout RR, Blight AR, Fawcett S, et al: Aminopyridine in chronic spinal cord injury: A controlled, double-blind, crossover study in eight patients. *J Neurotrauma* 1993; 10:1–18.
118. Blight AR: Cellular morphology of chronic spinal cord injury in the cat: Analysis of myelinated axons by line-sampling. *Neuroscience* 1983; 10:521–543.
119. Blight AR: Axonal physiology of chronic spinal cord injury in the cat: Intracellular recording in vitro. *Neuroscience* 1983; 10:1471–1486.
120. Rosenbluth J, Hasegawa M, Shirasaki N, et al: Myelin formation following transplantation of normal fetal glia into myelin-deficient rat spinal cord. *J Neurocytol* 1990; 19:718–730.
121. Waxman SG: Demyelination in spinal cord injury and multiple sclerosis: What can we do to enhance functional recovery? *J Neurotrauma* 1992; 9(Suppl1):S105–S117.
122. Freed CR, Breeze RE, Rosenberg NL, et al: Therapeutic effects of human fetal dopamine cells transplanted in a patient with Parkinson's disease. *Prog Brain Res* 1990; 82:715–721.
123. Freed CR, Breeze RE, Rosenberg NL, et al: Transplantation of human fetal dopamine cells for Parkinson's disease. Results at 1 year. *Arch Neurol* 1990; 47:505–512.
124. Bunge RP, Puckett WR, Becerra JL, et al: Observations on the pathology of human spinal cord injury. *Adv Neurols* 1993; 59:75–89.
125. Dohrmann GJ: Experimental spinal cord trauma. *Arch Neurol* 1972; 27:468–473.
126. Guth L, Reier PJ, Barrett CP, et al: Repair of the mammalian spinal cord. *Trends Neurosci* 1983; 6:20–24.
127. Guth L, Albuquerque EX, Deshpande SS, et al: Ineffectiveness of enzyme therapy on regeneration in the transected spinal cord of the rat. *J Neurosurg* 1980; 52:73–86.
128. Wagner FC, Jr., VanGilder JC Dohrmann GJ: Pathological changes from acute to chronic in experimental spinal cord trauma. *J Neurosurg* 1978; 48:92–98.
129. Squier M, Lehr RP: Post-traumatic syringomyelia. *J Neurol Neurosurg Psychiatry* 1994; 57:1095–1098.
130. Sgouros S, Williams B: A critical appraisal of drainage in syringomyelia. *J Neurosurg* 1995; 82:1–10.
131. Glasauer FE, Czrny JJ: Hyperhidrosis as the presenting symptom in post-traumatic syringomyelia. *Paraplegia* 1994; 32:423–429.
132. Schinstine M, Kawaja MD, Gage FH: Intracerebral delivery of growth factors: potential application of genetically modified fibroblasts. *Prog Growth Factor Res* 1991; 3:57–66.
133. Sendtner M, Schmalbruch H, Stockli KA, et al: Ciliary neurotrophic factor prevents degeneration of motor neurons in mouse mutant progressive motor neuronopathy. *Nature* 1992; 358:502–504.
134. Suhr ST, Gage FH: Gene therapy for neurologic disease. *Arch Neurol* 1993; 50:1252–1268.

135. Kennedy TE, Serafini T, de la Torre JR, et al: Netrins are diffusible chemotrophic factors for commissural axons in the embryonic spinal cord. *Cell* 1994; 78:425–435.
136. Serafini T, Kennedy TE, Galko MJ, et al: The netrins define a family of axon outgrowth-promoting proteins homologous to C. elegans UNC-6. *Cell* 1994; 78:409–424.
137. Gefland G, Levin TR: Fetal tissue research: Legal regulation of human fetal tissue transplantation. *Washington and Lee Law Review* 1993; 50:647–694.

INDEX

Page numbers followed by an *f* indicate figures. Page numbers followed by a *t* indicate tabular material.

B

C

E

F

G

H

I

J

K

O

P

Q

T

U

V

W

X

Y

Z

ISBN 0-07-045662-3

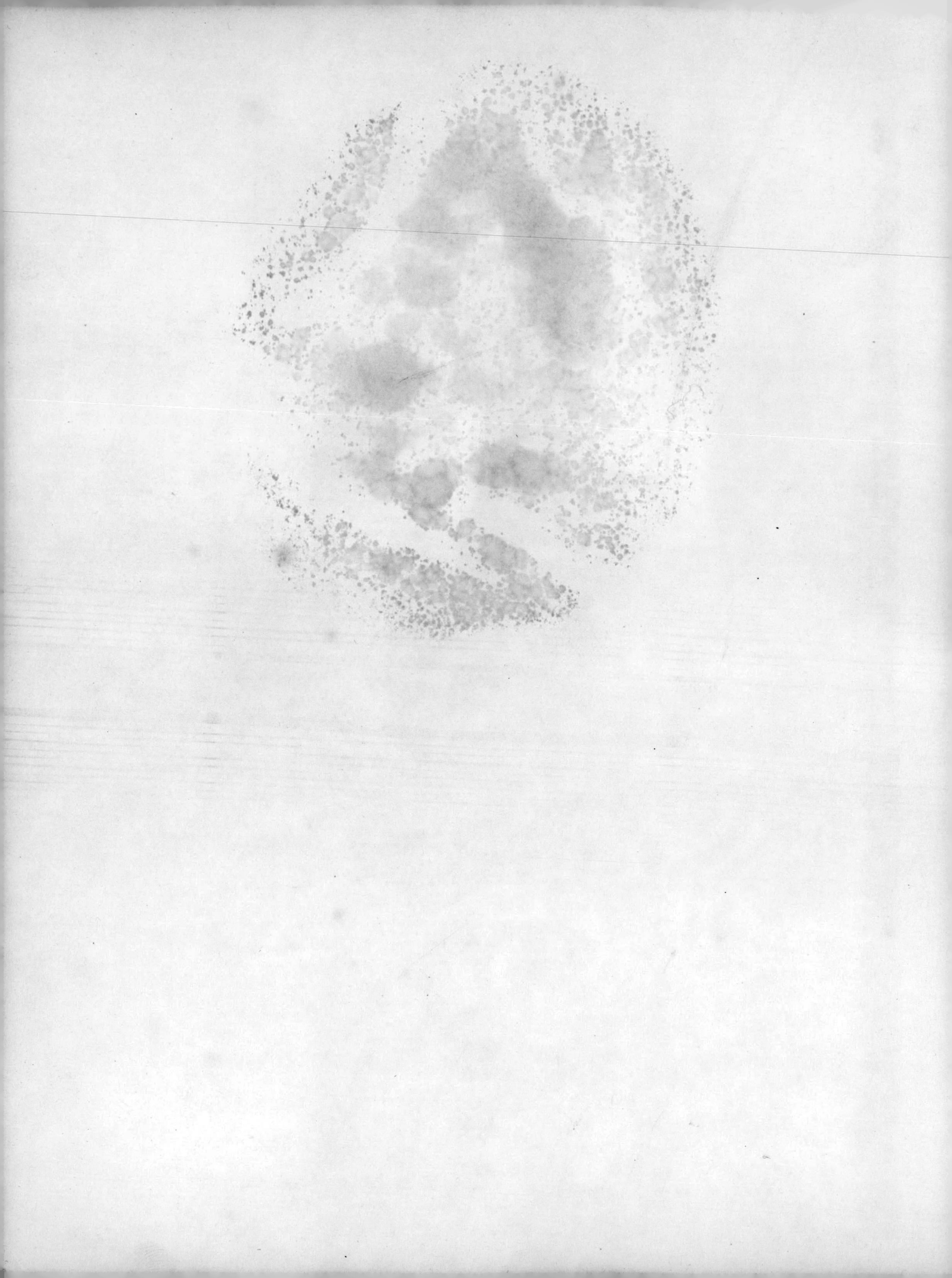